Coté and Lerman's

A Practice *of* Anesthesia
for Infants *and* Children

Coté and Lerman's

A Practice *of* Anesthesia *for* Infants *and* Children

Charles J. Coté, MD, FAAP

Professor of Anaesthesia (Emeritus)
Harvard Medical School
Division of Pediatric Anesthesia
MassGeneral Hospital for Children
Department of Anesthesia, Critical Care and Pain Management
Massachusetts General Hospital
Boston, Massachusetts

Jerrold Lerman, MD, FRCPC, FANZCA

Clinical Professor of Anesthesia
Staff Anesthesiologist
John R. Oishei Children's Hospital,
Jacobs School of Medicine and Biomedical Sciences
Buffalo, New York

Brian J. Anderson, MB, ChB, PhD, FANZCA, FCICM

Professor of Anesthesiology
University of Auckland;
Paediatric Anaesthetist and Intensivist
Paediatic Intensive Care Unit
Auckland Children's Hospital
Auckland, New Zealand

ELSEVIER

ELSEVIER

1600 John F. Kennedy Blvd.
Ste 1800
Philadelphia, PA 19103-2899

A PRACTICE OF ANESTHESIA FOR INFANTS AND CHILDREN, SIXTH EDITION

ISBN: 978-0-323-42974-0

Notices

Previous editions copyrighted 2013, 2009, 2001, 1993, and 1986.

Library of Congress Cataloging-in-Publication Data
Names: Coté, Charles J., editor. | Lerman, Jerrold, editor. | Anderson, Brian J., editor.
Title: A practice of anesthesia for infants and children / [edited by] Charles Coté, Jerrold Lerman, Brian J. Anderson.
Other titles: Coté and Lerman's a practice of anesthesia for infants and children.
Description: Sixth edition. | Philadelphia, PA : Elsevier, [2019] | Preceded by: Coté and Lerman's a practice of anesthesia for infants and children / [edited by] Charles J. Coté, Jerrold Lerman, Brian J. Anderson. 5th ed. c2013. | Includes bibliographical references and index.
Identifiers: LCCN 2017051074 | ISBN 9780323429740 (hardcover : alk. paper)
Subjects: | MESH: Anesthesia | Child | Infant
Classification: LCC RD139 | NLM WO 440 | DDC 617.9/6083–dc23 LC record available at https://lccn.loc.gov/2017051074

Executive Content Strategist: Dolores Meloni
Senior Content Development Specialist: Laura Schmidt
Publishing Services Manager: Catherine Jackson
Project Manager: Tara Delaney
Design Direction: Ryan Cook
Cover Photography: J. Stefaniak, Medical Photographer, Women and Children's Hospital of Buffalo, Buffalo, New York

Printed in China.

Last digit is the print number: 9 8 7 6 5 4 3 2

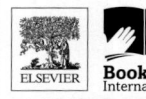

Working together to grow libraries in developing countries

www.elsevier.com • www.bookaid.org

We dedicate the sixth edition of A Practice of Anesthesia for Infants and Children *to physicians around the world who have the pleasure and responsibility of caring for children in the operating room, ICU, and other venues where anesthesia services are vital such as radiology, cardiac catheterization laboratory, and sedation services such as oncology. In particular, we acknowledge those practitioners who take care of children and deliver the best possible care with limited resources and at times with antiquated equipment, limited drugs, electricity, and even the availability of oxygen. Our specialty has grown exponentially in the past 30 years and as a result of new licensing laws, medications are now more thoroughly investigated before they are released for use in children. Ultrasound technology has made regional anesthesia and invasive line insertion far safer than in the past. The quality of airway devices continues to improve. Noninvasive continuous cardiac output devices may provide the next generation of monitors to safeguard the care of our children. Depth of anesthesia monitors also continue to evolve, but still remain unreliable in younger children; we hope that advances will ensure greater reliability in the infant and young child to assess the depth of anesthesia as well as to enable differentiation of moderate from deep sedation and deep sedation from general anesthesia.*

We also dedicate this book to the children to whom we provide anesthesia daily and to their parents/guardians to assure them that their children will receive the highest standard of care and will be as safe as possible from harm. Our specialty continues to investigate the possible adverse effects of anesthetics on the developing brain to determine whether the findings in newborn animals are simply laboratory curiosities or are in fact translatable and potentially harmful to infants and children. Evidence at this time neither confirms nor refutes significant injury to the developing human brain. The challenge we face in our daily work is to reassure parents that anesthesia and the drugs we use are safe (to the best of our current knowledge) and that they do not pose real and substantive risks for their children.

This edition of A Practice of Anesthesia for Infants and Children *highlights key advances and questions in our specialty that we hope will continue to inspire anesthesiologists worldwide through the text, the web-based videos and illustrations, and the pocket shortcut card and phone app (Pedi Anesth).*

Charles J. Coté
Jerrold Lerman
Brian J. Anderson

CONTRIBUTORS

Trevor L. Adams, MD
Assistant Professor
University of Washington
Department of Anesthesiology and Pain Medicine
Seattle Children's Hospital
Seattle, Washington
Essentials of Hematology

Adam C. Adler, MS, MD, FAAP
Assistant Professor
Baylor College of Medicine
Department of Anesthesiology, Perioperative and Pain
    Medicine
Division of Cardiothoracic Anesthesiology
Texas Children's Hospital
Houston, Texas
Mechanical Circulatory Support

Warwick A. Ames, MBBS, FRCA
Associate Professor
Duke University School of Medicine
Pediatric Anesthesiology
Duke University Medical Center
Duke Children's Hospital and Health Center
Durham, North Carolina
Essentials of Nephrology

Brian J. Anderson, MB, ChB, PhD, FANZCA, FCICM
Professor of Anesthesiology
University of Auckland
Paediatric Anaesthetist and Intensivist
Paediatic Intensive Care Unit
Auckland Children's Hospital
Auckland, New Zealand
*Orthopedic and Spine Surgery; Pharmacokinetics and Pharmacology of
    Drugs Used in Children; The Practice of Pediatric Anesthesia; Total
    Intravenous Anesthesia and Target-Controlled Infusion*

Dean B. Andropoulos, MD, MHCM
Professor
Anesthesiology and Pediatrics
Vice Chair for Clinical Affairs
Department of Anesthesiology
Baylor College of Medicine
Anesthesiologist-in-Chief
Department of Anesthesiology, Perioperative and Pain
    Medicine
Texas Children's Hospital
Houston, Texas
Cardiopulmonary Bypass and Management

Martin B. Anixter, MD
Assistant Professor of Anesthesia
University of Pittsburgh School of Medicine
Department of Anesthesiology
Children's Hospital of Pittsburgh at UPMC
Pittsburgh, Pennsylvania
Organ Transplantation

Philip Arnold, BM, FRCA
Honorary Lecturer
University of Liverpool
Consultant Anaesthetist
Jackson Rees Department of Anaesthesia
Alder Hey Children's Hospital
Liverpool, United Kingdom
Medications for Hemostasis

Robert Baker, MD
Pain Management Fellow
University of Cincinnati College of Medicine
Cincinnati Children's Hospital Medical Center
Cincinnati, Ohio
Chronic Pain

M.A. Bender, MD, PhD
Associate Professor
Pediatrics
University of Washington School of Medicine;
Director
Sickle Cell and Hemoglobinopathy Program
Odessa Brown Children's Clinic
Clinical Research Division
Fred Hutchinson Cancer Research Center
Seattle, Washington
Essentials of Hematology

Charles B. Berde, MD, PhD
Professor of Anaesthesia and Pediatrics
Harvard Medical School
Chief, Division of Pain Medicine
Department of Anesthesiology, Perioperative and Pain
    Medicine
Boston Children's Hospital
Boston, Massachusetts
Acute Pain

Laura K. Berenstain, MD
Associate Professor Clinical Anesthesia
University of Cincinnati College of Medicine
Staff Anesthesiologist Division of Pediatric Cardiac Anesthesia
Department of Anesthesiology
Cincinnati Children's Hospital Medical Center
Cincinnati, Ohio
Mechanical Circulatory Support

Brian Blasiole, MD, PhD
Assistant Professor of Anesthesiology
University of Pittsburgh School of Medicine
Department of Anesthesiology
The Children's Hospital of Pittsburgh of UPMC
Medical Director for Sedation Services and Offsite Anesthesia
Pittsburgh, Pennsylvania
Organ Transplantation

Adrian T. Bösenberg, MB ChB, FFA(SA)
Professor
University of Washington School of Medicine
Pediatric Anesthesiologist
Anesthesiology and Pain Management
Seattle Children's Hospital
Seattle, Washington
Pediatric Anesthesia in Developing Countries

Karen A. Brown, MD
Professor
McGill University Medical School
Queen Elizabeth Hospital of Montreal Foundation Chair in Pediatric Anesthesia
Department of Anesthesia
The Montreal Children's Hospital, McGill University Health Center
Montreal, Quebec, Canada
Otorhinolaryngologic Procedures

Roland Brusseau, MD
Instructor in Anaesthesia
Harvard Medical School
Senior Assistant in Perioperative Anesthesia
Department of Anesthesia and Perioperative Medicine
Boston Children's Hospital
Boston, Massachusetts
Fetal Intervention and the EXIT Procedure

James Gordon Cain, MD, MBA, FAAP, DABA
Professor and Vice Chair of Anesthesiology
West Virginia University School of Medicine
Department of Anesthesiology Quality Officer
WVU Medicine Chief of Pediatric Anesthesiology
West Virginia Children's Hospital
Morgantown, West Virginia
Organ Transplantation

Vidya Chidambaran, MD, MS
Associate Professor, Anesthesia and Pediatrics
University of Cincinnati College of Medicine
Director, Perioperative Pain Management
Cincinnati Children's Hospital
University of Cincinnati
Cincinnati, Ohio
Pharmacogenomics

Franklyn P. Cladis, MD, FAAP
Associate Professor of Anesthesiology
The University of Pittsburgh School of Medicine
Department of Anesthesiology
The Children's Hospital of Pittsburgh of UPMC
Program Director, Pediatric Anesthesiology Fellowship
The Children's Hospital of Pittsburgh of UPMC
Pittsburgh, Pennsylvania
Organ Transplantation

Rebecca E. Claure, MD
Clinical Professor
Stanford University School of Medicine
Stanford, California
Department of Anesthesiology, Perioperative and Pain Medicine
Medical Director, Perioperative Services
Packard Children's Hospital Stanford
Palo Alto, California
Essentials of Endocrinology

Jeffrey B. Cooper, PhD
Professor of Anaesthesia
Harvard Medical School
Department of Anesthesia, Critical Care and Pain Medicine
Massachusetts General Hospital
Executive Director Emeritus
Center for Medical Simulation
Boston, Massachusetts
Simulation in Pediatric Anesthesia

Charles J. Coté, MD
Professor of Anaesthesia (Emeritus)
Harvard Medical School
Division of Pediatric Anesthesia
MassGeneral Hospital for Children
Department of Anesthesia, Critical Care and Pain Management
Massachusetts General Hospital
Boston, Massachusetts
Burn Injuries; Pharmacokinetics and Pharmacology of Drugs Used in Children; Preoperative Evaluation, Premedication, and Induction of Anesthesia; Pediatric Equipment; Procedures for Vascular Access; Regional Anesthesia; Sedation for Diagnostic and Therapeutic Procedures Outside the Operating Room; Strategies for Blood Product Management, Reducing Transfusions, and Massive Blood Transfusion; The Pediatric Airway; The Practice of Pediatric Anesthesia

Joseph P. Cravero, MD
Associate Professor of Anaesthesia
Harvard Medical School
Senior Associate
Department of Anesthesiology, Perioperative, and Pain
    Medicine
Boston Children's Hospital
Boston, Massachusetts
*Anesthesia Outside the Operating Room; Sedation for Diagnostic and
    Therapeutic Procedures Outside the Operating Room*

Peter M. Crean, MB BCh, FRCA, FFARCSI
Consultant Paediatric Anaesthetist
Department of Anaesthesia
Royal Belfast Hospital for Sick Children
Belfast, United Kingdom
Essentials of Neurology and Neuromuscular Disorders

Andrew J. Davidson, MBBS, MD, FANZCA
Professor
Department of Paediatrics
University of Melbourne
Staff Anaesthetist
Anaesthesia and Pain Management
Royal Children's Hospital, Melbourne
Director
Melbourne Children's Trials Centre
Murdoch Children's Research Institute
Melbourne, Victoria, Australia
Surgery, Anesthesia, and the Immature Brain

Peter J. Davis, MD
Professor of Anesthesiology and Pediatrics
University of Pittsburgh School of Medicine
Dr. Joseph H. Marcy Endowed Chair in Pediatric Anesthesia
Anesthesiologist-in-Chief
Children's Hospital of Pittsburgh of UPMC
Pittsburgh, Pennsylvania
Essentials of Hepatology; Organ Transplantation

James A. DiNardo, MD, FAAP
Professor of Anaesthesia
Harvard Medical School
Chief, Division of Cardiac Anesthesia
Francis X. McGowan, Jr., M.D. Chair in Cardiac Anesthesia
Boston Children's Hospital
Boston, Massachusetts
Cardiac Physiology and Pharmacology

Michael J. Eisses, MD
Associate Professor of Anesthesia
University of Washington School of Medicine
Department of Anesthesiology and Pain Medicine
Seattle Children's Hospital
Seattle, Washington
Essentials of Hematology

John E. Fiadjoe, MD, FAAP
Associate Professor of Anesthesiology and Critical Care
Perelman School of Medicine at the University of Pennsylvania
Department of Anesthesiology and Critical Care
The Children's Hospital of Philadelphia
Philadelphia, Pennsylvania
Plastic and Reconstructive Surgery; The Pediatric Airway

Paul G. Firth, MBChB, BA
Assistant Professor of Anesthesia
Harvard Medical School
Attending Anesthesiologist
Department of Anesthesia, Critical Care and Pain Medicine
Massachusetts General Hospital
Boston, Massachusetts
Essentials of Pulmonology

John W. Foreman, MD
Professor, Emeritus
Duke University School of Medicine
Department of Pediatrics
Duke Children's Hospital and Health Center
Durham, North Carolina
Essentials of Nephrology

Natalie Forshaw, MBChB (Hons), FRCA
Paediatric Anaesthetist
Department of Paediatric Anaesthesia
Great Ormond Street Hospital
London, Great Britain
Interventional Cardiology

Michelle A. Fortier, PhD
Associate Professor
University of California–Irvine School of Medicine
Department of Anesthesiology and Perioperative Care
Orange, California
Perioperative Behavioral Stress in Children

Sandeep Gangadharan, MD
Assistant Professor of Pediatrics
Hofstra-Northwell School of Medicine
Pediatric Critical Care Medicine
Cohen Children's Medical Center
New Hyde Park, New York
Cardiopulmonary Resuscitation

Ralph Gertler, MD
University Medical Center Hamburg-Eppendorf
Klinik für Anaesthesie
Operative und Allgemeine Intensivmedizin, Notfallmedizin
Klinikum Links der Weser
Bremen, Germany
Cardiopulmonary Bypass and Management; Essentials of Cardiology

Elizabeth A. Ghazal, MD
Associate Professor of Anesthesiology
Loma Linda University School of Medicine
Department of Anesthesiology
Loma Linda, California
Preoperative Evaluation, Premedication, and Induction of Anesthesia

Kenneth Goldschneider, MD
Professor, Clinical Anesthesia and Pediatrics
University of Cincinnati College of Medicine
Department of Anesthesiology
Director, Pain Management Center
Cincinnati Children's Hospital Medical Center
Cincinnati, Ohio
Chronic Pain

Erin A. Gottlieb, MD
Associate Professor of Anesthesiology
Baylor College of Medicine
Department of Anesthesiology, Perioperative and Pain
    Medicine
Texas Children's Hospital
Houston, TX
Cardiopulmonary Bypass and Management

Eric F. Grabowski, MD, ScD
Associate Professor of Pediatrics
Harvard Medical School
Director, Massachusetts General Hospital Comprehensive
    Hemophilia Treatment Center
Co-Director, Pediatric Stroke Services
Director, Cardiovascular Thrombosis Laboratory
Department of Pediatrics
Hematology/Oncology
Massachusetts General Hospital
Boston, Massachusetts
*Strategies for Blood Product Management, Reducing Transfusions, and
    Massive Blood Transfusion*

Kelly L. Grogan, MD
Assistant Professor
University of Pennsylvania, Perelman School of Medicine
Department of Anesthesiology and Critical Care Medicine
The Children's Hospital of Philadelphia
Philadelphia, Pennsylvania
Mechanical Circulatory Support

Padma Gulur, MD
Professor
Duke University School of Medicine
Department of Anesthesiology
Durham, North Carolina
Perioperative Behavioral Stress in Children

Charles M. Haberkern, MD, MPH
Professor
University of Washington School of Medicine
Department of Anesthesiology and Pain Medicine
Professor
Department of Pediatrics (adjunct)
Seattle Children's Hospital
Seattle, Washington
Essentials of Hematology

Gregory B. Hammer, MD
Professor
Department of Anesthesiology, Perioperative and Pain
    Medicine
Department of Pediatrics
Stanford University School of Medicine
Stanford, California
Director of Research
Department of Anesthesiology and Pain Management
Packard Children's Hospital Stanford
Palo Alto, California
Anesthesia for Thoracic Surgery

Raafat S. Hannallah, MD, FAAP, FASA
Professor Emeritus of Anesthesiology and Critical Care
    Medicine and of Pediatrics
The George Washington University School of Medicine and
    Health Sciences
Division of Anesthesiology, Pain and Perioperative Medicine
Children's National Health System
Washington, DC
Otorhinolaryngologic Procedures

Tom G. Hansen, MD, PhD
Associate Research Professor
University of South Denmark
Lead Consultant Pediatric Anesthesiologist
Anesthesiology and Intensive Care—Pediatrics
Odense University Hospital, Odense
Department of Clinical Research—Anesthesiology
Odense, Denmark
General Abdominal and Urologic Surgery

Jeana E. Havidich, MD, MS
Associate Professor
Geisel School of Medicine at Dartmouth
Dartmouth-Hitchcock Medical Center
Department of Anesthesiology and Pediatrics
Children's Hospital at Dartmouth
Lebanon, New Hampshire
The Postanesthesia Care Unit and Beyond

Steen W. Henneberg, MD, PhD
Associate Professor
Uppsala University
Uppsala, Sweden
Consultant
Department of Anesthesiology
Copenhagen University Hospital
Copenhagen, Denmark
General Abdominal and Urologic Surgery

James Houghton, BSC (hons), MBChB, FANZCA
Paediatric Anaesthetist
Department of Paediatric Anaesthesia
Starship Children's Hospital
Auckland, New Zealand
Total Intravenous Anesthesia and Target-Controlled Infusion

Andre L. Jaichenco, MD
Pediatric Anesthesiologist
Director of the Fellowship Program for Pediatric Anesthesia
Chief of the Anesthesia Service of the National Pediatric
    Hospital
Ciudad Autónoma de Buenos Aires
Buenos Aires, Argentina
Infectious Disease Considerations for the Operating Room

Zeev N. Kain, MD, MBA
President
American College of Perioperative Medicine
Chancellor's Professor
Anesthesiology & Pediatrics & Medicine
Executive Director
Center of Stress & Health
University of California School of Medicine, Irvine
Orange, California
Professor (adjunct)
Yale Child Study Center
Yale University School of Medicine
New Haven, Connecticut
Perioperative Behavioral Stress in Children

Richard F. Kaplan, MD
Professor of Anesthesiology
George Washington University
Children's National Medical Center
Washington, DC
*Sedation for Diagnostic and Therapeutic Procedures Outside the
    Operating Room*

Manoj K. Karmakar, MD, FRCA
Professor of Anaesthesia
The Chinese University of Hong Kong
Director of Paediatric Anaesthesia
Department of Anaesthesia and Intensive Care
Prince of Wales Hospital, Shatin
Hong Kong, China
Ultrasound-Guided Regional Anesthesia

T. Bernard Kinane, MD
Associate Professor of Pediatrics
Harvard Medical School
Pediatrics
Massachusetts General Hospital
Boston, Massachusetts
Essentials of Pulmonology

Elliot J. Krane, MD
Professor
Stanford University School of Medicine
Stanford, California
Department of Anesthesiology, Perioperative and Pain
    Medicine
Department of Pediatrics
Director, Pain Management
Packard Children's Hospital Stanford
Palo Alto, California
Essentials of Endocrinology

Wing H. Kwok, MB ChB, FANZCA
Clinical Associate Professor
Consultant Anaesthetist
Anaesthesia and Intensive Care
Prince of Wales Hospital, Shatin
Hong Kong, China
Ultrasound-Guided Regional Anesthesia

Vasco Laginha Rolo, MD
Consultant Paediatric Anaesthetist
Birmingham Children's Hospital
Birmingham, United Kingdom
Anesthesia for Children Undergoing Heart Surgery

Jennifer E. Lam, DO
Associate Professor of Anesthesia and Pediatrics
University of Cincinnati College of Medicine
Director, Cardiac Anesthesia Fellowship
Cincinnati Children's Hospital Medical Center
Cincinnati, Ohio
*The Extremely Premature Infant (Micropremie) and Common
    Neonatal Emergencies*

Mary Landrigan-Ossar, MD, PhD, FAAP
Assistant Professor of Anaesthesia
Harvard Medical School
Senior Associate in Perioperative Anesthesia
Anesthesiology, Perioperative, and Pain Medicine
Boston Children's Hospital
Boston, Massachusetts
*Anesthesia Outside the Operating Room; Sedation for Diagnostic and
    Therapeutic Procedures Outside the Operating Room*

Gregory J. Latham, MD
Associate Professor
University of Washington School of Medicine
Department of Anesthesiology and Pain Medicine
Seattle Children's Hospital
Seattle, Washington
*Perioperative Management of the Oncology Patient; Essentials of
    Hematology*

Jerrold Lerman, MD, FRCPC, FANZCA
Clinical Professor of Anesthesia
Staff Anesthesiologist
John R. Oishei Children's Hospital,
Jacobs School of Medicine and Biomedical Sciences
Buffalo, New York
*General Abdominal and Urologic Surgery; Pharmacokinetics and
    Pharmacology of Drugs Used in Children; Malignant
    Hyperthermia; Pediatric Equipment; Plastic and Reconstructive
    Surgery; The Practice of Pediatric Anesthesia*

Luciana Cavalcanti Lima, PhD
Professor
Medicine
Faculdade Pernambucana de Saúde
Pediatric Anesthesiologist
Instituto de Medicina Integral Prof. Fernando Figueira
Recife, Pernambuco, Brazil
Infectious Disease Considerations for the Operating Room

Ronald S. Litman, DO
Professor of Anesthesiology and Pediatrics
University of Pennsylvania Perelman School of Medicine
Department of Anesthesiology and Critical Care
The Children's Hospital of Philadelphia
Philadelphia, Pennsylvania
The Pediatric Airway

Andreas W. Loepke, MD, PhD, FAAP
Professor of Anesthesiology and Critical Care
University of Pennsylvania Perelman School of Medicine
Associate Chief, Cardiac Anesthesia
Department of Anesthesiology and Critical Care Medicine
Children's Hospital of Philadelphia
Philadelphia, Pennsylvania
Surgery, Anesthesia, and the Immature Brain

Christine L. Mai, MD
Instructor in Anaesthesia
Harvard Medical School
Department of Anesthesia, Critical Care and Pain Medicine
Massachusetts General Hospital
Boston, Massachusetts
Simulation in Pediatric Anesthesia

Bruno Marciniak, MD
Pôle d'Anesthésie Reanimation
Centre Hospitalier Régional et Universitaire
Lille, France
Growth and Development

J. A. Jeevendra Martyn, MD, FRCA, FCCM
Professor of Anaesthesia
Harvard Medical School
Anaesthetist-in-Chief
Shriners Hospital for Children
Director, Clinical and Biochemical Pharmacology Laboratory
Department of Anesthesiology
Massachusetts General Hospital
Boston, Massachusetts
Burn Injuries

Linda J. Mason, MD
Professor of Anesthesiology and Pediatrics
Loma Linda University School of Medicine
Loma Linda, California
Director of Pediatric Anesthesia
Department of Anesthesiology
Loma Linda University Medical Center
Loma Linda, California
Preoperative Evaluation, Premedication, and Induction of Anesthesia

Linda C. Mayes, MD
Arnold Gesell Professor
Yale School of Medicine
Yale Child Study Center
New Haven, Connecticut
Perioperative Behavioral Stress in Children

Craig D. McClain, MD, MPH
Associate Professor of Anaesthesia
Harvard Medical School
Senior Associate in Perioperative Anesthesia
Department of Anesthesiology, Perioperative and Pain
  Medicine
Boston Children's Hospital
Boston, Massachusetts
Fluid Management; Pediatric Neurosurgical Anesthesia

Angus McEwan, MB ChB, FRCA
Consultant Paediatric Anaesthetist
Great Ormond Street Hospital
Great Ormond Street
London, United Kingdom
Anesthesia for Children Undergoing Heart Surgery

Michael L. McManus, MD, MPH
Associate Professor of Anaesthesia (Pediatrics)
Harvard Medical School
Senior Associate
Anesthesia and Critical Care Medicine
Boston Children's Hospital
Boston, Massachusetts
Fluid Management

Julianne Mendoza, MD
Clinical Assistant Professor
Stanford University School of Medicine
Department of Anesthesiology, Perioperative and Pain
  Medicine
Stanford, California
Procedures for Vascular Access

Frederick G. Mihm, MD
Professor of Anesthesia
Stanford University School of Medicine
Division Chief, Critical Care Medicine
Department of Anesthesiology, Perioperative and Pain
  Medicine
Stanford, California
Procedures for Vascular Access

Wanda C. Miller-Hance, MD
Professor
Anesthesiology and Pediatrics
Baylor College of Medicine
Associate Director of Pediatric Cardiovascular Anesthesiology
Director of Intraoperative Echocardiography for Pediatrics
  (Cardiology) and Anesthesiology
Texas Children's Hospital
Houston, Texas
*Anesthesia for Noncardiac Surgery in Children With Congenital
  Heart Disease; Essentials of Cardiology*

Pooja Nawathe, MD, FAAP, CHSE
Assistant Professor of Pediatrics Step IV, David Geffin School
    of Medicine, University of California Los Angeles
Assistant Professor of Pediatrics, Cedars Sinai Medical Center
Associate Director, Congenital Cardiac ICU
Pediatrics and Heart Institute
Cedars Sinai Medical Center
Los Angeles, California
Cardiopulmonary Resuscitation

Jerome Parness, MD, PhD, FAAP
Professor
Anesthesiology
Adjunct Professor
Pharmacology and Chemical Biology
University of Pittsburgh School of Medicine
Children's Hospital of Pittsburgh of UPMC
Pittsburgh, Pennsylvania
Malignant Hyperthermia

David M. Polaner, MD, FAAP
Professor
Departments of Anesthesiology and Pediatrics
University of Colorado School of Medicine;
Attending Pediatric Anesthesiologist
Director of Transplant Anesthesia
Children's Hospital of Colorado
Aurora, Colorado
Chairman, Steering Committee
Pediatric Regional Anesthesia Network
Acute Pain; Regional Anesthesia

Ellen Rawlinson, MA (Hons), MBBChir, MRCP, FRCA, MA
Consultant Paediatric Anaesthetist
Anaesthesia
Great Ormond Street Hospital
London, United Kingdom
Interventional Cardiology

Erinn T. Rhodes, MD, MPH
Assistant Professor
Department of Pediatrics
Harvard Medical School
Director of Endocrinology Healthcare Research and Quality
Boston Children's Hospital
Boston, Massachusetts
Essentials of Endocrinology

Faith J. Ross, MD, MS
Assistant Professor
University of Washington School of Medicine
Department of Anesthesiology and Pain Medicine
Seattle Children's Hospital
Seattle, Washington
Perioperative Management of the Oncology Patient

Patrick A. Ross, MD
Associate Professor of Clinical Anesthesiology and Pediatrics
David Geffin School of Medicine, University of California Los
    Angeles;
Anesthesiology Critical Care Medicine
Children's Hospital Los Angeles
Los Angeles, California
Pediatric Equipment

Echo Rowe, MD
Clinical Assistant Professor
Stanford University School of Medicine
Department of Anesthesiology, Perioperative and Pain
    Medicine
Stanford, California
Packard Children's Hospital Stanford
Palo Alto, California
Essentials of Endocrinology

Senthilkumar Sadhasivam, MD, MPH
Professor of Anesthesia
Indiana University School of Medicine
Riley Children's Hospital
Indianapolis, Indiana
Pharmacogenomics

Charles L. Schleien, MD
Chairman and Professor
Hofstra-Northwell School of Medicine, Cohen Children's
    Medical Center
Department of Pediatrics
New Hyde Park, New York
Cardiopulmonary Resuscitation

Annette Y. Schure, MD, DEAA
Instructor in Anaesthesia
Harvard Medical School
Senior Associate in Cardiac Anesthesia
Department of Anesthesiology, Perioperative and Pain
    Medicine
Boston Children's Hospital
Boston, Massachusetts
Cardiac Physiology and Pharmacology

Julia F. Serber, MD
Aegis Anesthesia
Grapevine, Texas
The Pediatric Airway

Erik S. Shank, MD
Assistant Professor of Anaesthesia
Harvard Medical School
Division Chief
Division of Pediatric Anesthesia, Department of Anesthesia and
    Critical Care
Massachusetts General Hospital
Associate Chief
Department of Anesthesia
Shriners Hospital for Children
Boston, Massachusetts
Burn Injuries

Sulpicio G. Soriano, MD
Professor of Anaesthesia
Harvard Medical School
Department of Anesthesiology, Critical Care and Pain
    Medicine
Endowed Chair in Pediatric Neuroanesthesia
Boston Children's Hospital
Boston, Massachusetts
Pediatric Neurosurgical Anesthesia

James P. Spaeth, MD
Associate Professor of Anesthesia and Pediatrics
University of Cincinnati College of Medicine
Director, Division of Cardiac Anesthesia
Cincinnati Children's Hospital Medical Center
Cincinnati, Ohio
*The Extremely Premature Infant (Micropremie) and Common
    Neonatal Emergencies*

James E. Squires, MD, MS
Assistant Professor
The University of Pittsburgh School of Medicine
Department of Pediatrics
Children's Hospital of Pittsburgh of UPMC
Pittsburgh, Pennsylvania
Essentials of Hepatology

Robert H. Squires, MD
Professor
The University of Pittsburgh School of Medicine
Department of Pediatrics
Medical Director, Liver Transplant
Department of Pediatric Gastroenterology
Children's Hospital of Pittsburgh of UPMC
Pittsburgh, Pennsylvania
Essentials of Hepatology

Christopher P. Stowell, MD, PhD
Associate Professor of Pathology
Harvard Medical School
Director, Blood Transfusion Service
Department of Pathology
Massachusetts General Hospital
Boston, Massachusetts
*Strategies for Blood Product Management, Reducing Transfusions, and
    Massive Blood Transfusion*

Paul A. Stricker, MD
Associate Professor of Anesthesiology and Critical Care
Perelman School of Medicine at the University of Pennsylvania
Department of Anesthesiology and Critical Care Medicine
The Children's Hospital of Philadelphia
Philadelphia, Pennsylvania
Plastic and Reconstructive Surgery; The Pediatric Airway

Santhanam Suresh, MD, FAAP
Professor of Anesthesiology and Pediatrics
Northwestern's Feinberg School of Medicine
Arthur C. King Professor and Chair
Department of Pediatric Anesthesiology
Ann & Robert H Lurie Children's Hospital of Chicago
Chicago, Illinois
Regional Anesthesia

Alexandra Szabova, MD
Associate Professor
University of Cincinnati College of Medicine
Clinical Anesthesia and Pediatrics
Cincinnati Children's Hospital Medical Center
Cincinnati, Ohio
Chronic Pain

Demian Szyld, MD, EdM
Attending Physician
Department of Emergency Medicine
Brigham and Women's Hospital
Senior Director
Institute for Medical Simulation
Center for Medical Simulation
Boston, Massachusetts
Simulation in Pediatric Anesthesia

Andreas H. Taenzer, MS, MD
Associate Professor
Geisel School of Medicine
Hanover, New Hampshire
Department of Anesthesiology, Pediatrics and the Dartmouth
    Institute
Children's Hospital at Dartmouth
Lebanon, New Hampshire
The Postanesthesia Care Unit and Beyond

Sandya Tirupathi, MBBS, DA, MRCPCH
Consultant Paediatric Neurologist
Department of Neurology
Royal Belfast Hospital for Sick Children
Belfast, United Kingdom
Essentials of Neurology and Neuromuscular Disorders

Joseph R. Tobin, MD
Professor Emeritus
Anesthesiology
Wake Forest School of Medicine
Winston-Salem, North Carolina
Ophthalmology

Marissa G. Vadi, MD, MPH
Assistant Professor
Loma Linda University School of Medicine
Department of Anesthesiology
Loma Linda, California
Preoperative Evaluation, Premedication, and Induction of Anesthesia

Susan T. Verghese, MD
Professor of Anesthesiology and Pediatrics
The George Washington University School of Medicine and
    Health Sciences
Division of Anesthesiology, Pain and Perioperative Medicine
Children's National Health System
Washington, DC
Otorhinolaryngologic Procedures

David B. Waisel, MD
Associate Professor of Anaesthesia
Harvard Medical School
Department of Anesthesiology, Perioperative and Pain
    Medicine
Boston Children's Hospital
Boston, Massachusetts
Ethical Issues in Pediatric Anesthesiology

Samuel H. Wald, MD, MBA
Clinical Professor
Stanford University School of Medicine
Department of Anesthesiology, Perioperative and Pain
    Medicine
Stanford, California
Procedures for Vascular Access

Benjamin J. Walker, MD
Associate Professor
University of Wisconsin School of Medicine and Public Health
Department of Anesthesiology
American Family Children's Hospital
Madison, Wisconsin
Acute Pain

R. Grey Weaver, Jr., MD
Professor of Ophthalmology
Wake Forest School of Medicine
Winston-Salem, North Carolina
Ophthalmology

David E. Wesson, MD
Professor of Surgery and Pediatrics
Baylor College of Medicine
Associate Surgeon-in-Chief
Texas Children's Hospital
Houston, Texas
Trauma

Delbert R. Wigfall, MD
Professor of Pediatrics; Associate Dean of Medical Education
Duke University School of Medicine
Pediatric Nephrology
Duke Children's Hospital and Health Center
Durham, North Carolina
Essentials of Nephrology

Niall C. Wilton, MRCP, FRCA
Clinical Director of Anaesthesia and Operating Rooms
Department of Paediatric Anaesthesia
Starship Children's Hospital
Auckland, New Zealand
Orthopedic and Spine Surgery

Joseph I. Wolfsdorf, MB BCh
Professor of Pediatrics
Harvard Medical School
Director, Diabetes Program,
Division of Endocrinology
Boston Children's Hospital
Boston, Massachusetts
Essentials of Endocrinology

David A. Young, MD, MEd, MBA, FAAP
Professor of Anesthesiology
Baylor College of Medicine
Department of Anesthesiology, Perioperative, and Pain
    Medicine
Texas Children's Hospital
Houston, Texas
Trauma

PREFACE

A Practice of Anesthesia for Infants and Children, Sixth Edition, has continued to evolve from its humble beginnings in 1986 with only 304 pages in the 1st edition to more than 1200 pages in the current edition. Founding coeditors of this text Dr. John Ryan and Dr. Nishan Goudsouzian retired, and Dr. I. David Todres succumbed to lymphoma. Dr. Jerrold Lerman joined as a coeditor for the 4th edition, and Dr. Brian J. Anderson joined for the 5th edition; the addition of Dr. Anderson broadened the clarity and insight into basic pharmacology in all chapters.

The current edition includes 109 authors from five continents, 22 of whom are new contributors. The book continues to be a highly respected, evidence-based synopsis of the practice of pediatric anesthesia reflecting a broad perspective from a host of international experts. As was the case in past editions, many of the authors are board-certified in pediatrics and anesthesiology, surgery, and a number of pediatric subspecialties, enhancing the basic understanding of hematology, pulmonology, cardiology, nephrology, hepatology, and neurology. As in the last edition, the book is divided into 10 color-coded sections: Introduction, Drug and Fluid Therapy, The Chest, The Heart, The Brain and Glands, The Abdomen, Other Surgeries, Emergencies, Pain, and Special Topics. This format allows the reader to find chapters and topics of interest easily and quickly. We have shifted all but a few selected references for each chapter to the accompanying Expert Consult website with hypertext links to the original publications in an effort to contain the size of the book. Color illustrations, photographs, and graphics maximize clarity and enhance visual appeal; many new video clips, figures, tables, and appendices are also available online.

In keeping with our mission to create a comprehensive text, we have again sought contributions from a number of pediatric subspecialists who share their perspectives and insights into basic pediatric physiology and the pathophysiologic implications of disease in children. In each case, the specialists have been paired with a pediatric anesthesiologist to ensure that the basic science is intertwined with a practical clinical perspective. These are the "Essentials" chapters.

Maintaining the past tradition, the largest chapter of the book is the pharmacology chapter, which now includes more than 2000 references. The chapter is written by all three editors, reflecting their different perspectives in pediatric pharmacology. We have maintained discussion of older and less frequently used medications to address the wide range of practices globally. The pediatric airway chapter includes an extensive discussion of supraglottic devices as well as emergency airway management strategies and equipment currently available for use in infants and children. There are many online videos illustrating their use.

All chapters on specialized topics, such as thoracic anesthesia, orthopedics, plastic surgery, general and urologic surgery, ophthalmology, otorhinolaryngology, burns, and cardiac topics, including physiology, cardiac surgery, cardiopulmonary bypass, medications for hemostasis, cardiac assist devices, and cardiac catheterization laboratory, have been updated.

The chapter on anesthesia in the developing brain has been substantively redacted to reflect the current state of knowledge on this subject and includes a comprehensive table of all published studies on this topic at the time of publication. Thus, readers are provided with ready access to the most important publications in this area. Chapters concerning anesthesia for extremely premature infants, the ex-utero intrapartum treatment procedure, trauma, and infectious diseases have also undergone significant revision.

Three new chapters focus on pharmacogenomics and the implications regarding drug interactions and drug metabolism, total intravenous anesthesia (TIVA), and on the perioperative management of oncology patients. The pharmacogenomic chapter underscores genetic implications of predicting drug effects and illustrates genetic variants that result in complications that are increasingly important in the day-to-day clinical management of patients. TIVA is becoming an increasingly popular technique as programmable pumps for drug delivery become more accessible.

The last 13 chapters of the book include management of trauma, cardiopulmonary resuscitation, malignant hyperthermia, ultrasound-guided regional anesthesia, management of acute and chronic pain, anesthesia outside the operating room, PACU, sedation for diagnostic and therapeutic procedures, vascular access, infectious disease, medical simulation, and the exceedingly important topic of pediatric anesthesia in developing countries.

It should be noted that our text is accompanied by a website that contains many supplemental pictures, tables, figures, and video clips that will enhance the readers' experiences. The pocket reference card that provides general recommendations for doses of commonly used medications by weight and other useful guides such as LMA sizes, ETT sizes, and other quick references has now been expanded to include a phone-based application for both Android and iPhones that can be found with the search words "Pedi Anesth" that was sponsored by the Starship Children's Hospital in Auckland New Zealand. The phone application provides immediate weight-based dosing of all commonly used medications and other helpful algorithms. Additionally, the expanded version of the phone application contains color illustrations of common congenital heart lesions courtesy of Elsevier, as well as many additional tables and treatment algorithms.

As with all previous editions, this revision involved quite a journey reflecting a microcosm of the world and life in general. Many contributors again experienced various challenges such as loss of loved ones, personal crises, illness, and others during the writing of their chapters. Despite all these obstacles the authors have succeeded in crafting masterful chapters to create what we hope you will agree is an up-to-date, state-of-the-art text in pediatric anesthesia.

Once again, while assembling this new edition, the editors spent many days, evenings, and weekends debating controversial issues and crafting the language of the chapters such that all chapters were edited and reviewed by all three editors and common ground reached. This is an especially useful exercise since it improves the readability of the text and represents a fusion of the USA, Canadian, and New Zealand approaches to and understanding of pediatric anesthesia, which combines our global experience and understanding.

We believe that *A Practice of Anesthesia for Infants and Children*, Sixth Edition, continues to provide the framework for residency and fellowship training in pediatric anesthesia globally and will continue to be a valuable resource for passing the subspecialty boards in pediatric anesthesiology, as well as a resource for practicing pediatric anesthesiologists and other pediatric care providers around the world.

Charles J. Coté
Jerrold Lerman
Brian J. Anderson

ACKNOWLEDGMENTS

We wish to thank our wives, husbands, significant others, children, friends, secretaries, and staff members who lent their support to this wonderful international family of experts that has come together to produce *A Practice of Anesthesia for Infants and Children*, Sixth Edition. In particular, we wish to thank the departments of anesthesiology, pediatrics, surgery, and internal medicine around the world who supported the academic endeavors of their staff and thus made it possible for them to contribute to the sixth edition. We thank Elsevier for their continued support of international education in less medically advanced countries by providing a variety of textbooks, including *A Practice of Anesthesia for Infants and Children*, to Fellows of the World Federation of Societies of Anesthesiologists as well as other fledgling programs, particularly those in sub-Saharan Africa. It is through such international endeavors that we ensure the global availability of the most recent advances in our specialty.

The editors wish to dedicate this edition of the book to honor the passing of Richard J. Kitz, MD, the chairperson who gave Dr. Coté the editorship of this book in 1982. Without his foresight, encouragement, and support, this book may never have been created.

Charles J. Coté
Jerrold Lerman
Brian J. Anderson

CONTENTS

VIDEO CONTENTS

INTRODUCTION

The Practice of Pediatric Anesthesia

CHARLES J. COTÉ, JERROLD LERMAN, AND BRIAN J. ANDERSON

IN THIS CHAPTER, WE outline the basis of our collective practice of pediatric anesthesia. These basic principles of practice can be applied regardless of the circumstances; they provide the foundation for safe anesthesia.

Preoperative Evaluation and Management

PARENTS AND CHILD

Anesthesiologists must assume an active role in the preoperative assessment of children. Ideally, the same anesthesiologist who performs the preoperative evaluation will anesthetize the child. The preoperative evaluation should include a complete review of the birth, medical, surgical and family histories; a review of the medical record; evaluation and review of laboratory, radiologic, and other investigations; and physical examination of every child who is to be anesthetized (see Chapter 4). When appropriate, the child should receive preoperative medical therapy to optimize his or her medical conditions (e.g., a child with reactive airway disease) before receiving anesthesia. In addition, the emotional state of the child and family must be considered and appropriate psychological and, if necessary, pharmacologic support provided. The anesthesia team, working in concert with surgical colleagues, nursing, and child-life specialists (e.g., the use of iPad, movies, play therapy, or games) should find appropriate and creative techniques to prepare the child and family for the surgical experience (e.g., using videotapes, booklets, hospital tours, and/or trained paramedical personnel). The marked increase in the number of outpatient surgical procedures has reduced the time available for the anesthesiologist to interact with the family and the child

preoperatively. Despite the reduced contact time, these support strategies should continue to be included in the preoperative assessment.

Familiarity with a child's clinical and psychological status as well as the parental concerns is essential to delivering quality anesthesia care. To achieve the very best outcome for each child, it is essential to meet with the child and the parents (or caregiver or legal guardian) together and establish rapport preoperatively. If the family speaks a different language than the anesthesiologist, then a medical interpreter should be sought.

Many developmental issues are related to the hospital experience. For example, toddlers fear separation from their parents, younger children fear mutilation from their surgery, and teenagers fear loss of control, awareness, and pain (see Chapter 3). When conducting the preoperative interview, speak directly to the child (who is old enough to understand [usually age 5 years and older]) and explain what anesthesia involves and what will transpire when they enter the operating room in terms that are age appropriate. Children at the age of reason have the same fears as adults but may have greater difficulty articulating them. For example, identify the key elements that distinguish "sleep" from anesthesia medicine from the sleep they experience at home. Explain that even if children undergo anesthesia for hours, they will feel as if they were unconscious for only a few minutes. Children should be reassured that unlike sleep at home, *the anesthetic prevents them from feeling anything during surgery, that they will not wake up during the procedure, and that they will awaken after the surgery.*

How anesthesia will be induced should be explained to the child in terms that are appropriate for the child's developmental level. For young children, one can describe that he/she will breathe "laughing gas" through a flavored mask, with a flavor that he/she chooses. Older children can be given the option to receive anesthesia either intravenously (IV) with nitrous oxide by mask, topical local anesthesia cream (e.g., eutectic mixture of local anesthetics [EMLA]) or vapocoolant such as Pain Ease (Gebauer Chemicals, Cleveland, OH) to establish IV access painlessly; or if they are afraid of needles, they may choose to receive anesthesia by an inhalational induction. Child-life specialists can be particularly helpful in demonstrating the anesthesia mask and circuit, illustrating that an IV is just a plastic tubing and not a needle and even decorating the mask with stickers and picking flavored scents.

If the parents will be present at induction of anesthesia, it is preferable that they attend a preoperative instructional session during which a typical induction is described along with the child's responses, perhaps complemented by a video of an induction. The parents should be instructed on how they might assuage their child's concerns, and questions from the parents should be answered. It is challenging to expect parents to cope with their child's induction without providing any preoperative instruction and teaching. Specific changes that might be observed in their child during anesthetic induction can be addressed as follows:

1. As your child is anesthetized, his or her eyes may roll up: "You might see your child's eyes roll up and this might be disturbing to you, but this is completely normal and expected; it happens to all of us when we fall asleep; it is just that we are not looking for it."

2. "As children fall asleep the structures in the neck relax so they may snore or make other noises from their throat; if your child does this, it is completely normal."

3. "As the anesthetic reaches the brain, the brain sometimes gets excited and causes movements of the arms and legs that are without purpose, or it may cause them to turn their head from side to side. This means the anesthetic is having its effect and even though your child appears to be partly awake, he or she has received enough anesthesia to ensure that he or she does not remember this."

4. "If your child becomes frightened, we will increase the amount of the anesthesia medicine rapidly and calm your child as quickly as possible."

5. If anesthesia is induced intravenously, the parents should be informed that their child might suddenly become limp, stop moving and breathing, and appear pale. These are all normal reactions.

At the same time, parents should not be pressured to be present for induction of anesthesia. If the parents are present at induction, it must be clear that they may be asked to leave the operating room if a new or additional risk to the child surfaces during the induction. Parents should be informed that their presence at induction is for their child's benefit and that their presence is a privilege, not a right. Moreover, in some circumstances it may not be in the child's best interest for parents to be present at induction, such as when the health care team could be distracted when everyone's attention should be focused on the child.

A simple explanation of the monitors to be used during anesthesia can be interesting to children and reassuring to parents. For example, the pulse oximeter can be described as a *"Band-Aid–like device"* that lights up red and measures the oxygen in the bloodstream during anesthesia and recovery. It is very helpful as an early warning indicator of low oxygen levels in the perioperative period. The blood pressure cuff can be characterized as an *"arm*

hugger" or *"muscle tester";* and the electrocardiogram leads can be called *"little sticky things that let us watch your heart beat but don't hurt at all."* Simple descriptions of the measurements may also be soothing. For example, *"We measure the amount of oxygen you (your child) are (is) breathing, we measure the amount of the anesthesia medicines you (your child) are (is) breathing, and we measure the carbon dioxide you (your child) are (is) breathing out to ensure that your (your child's) breathing is just right throughout the anesthesia."* Sometimes asking teenagers if they have studied carbon dioxide in school science class helps them to better understand the monitors and provides reassurance, as well as making it more interesting.

These preemptive discussions are meant to attenuate the parents' anxiety at a time when we need to focus on the child. It is common for parents to decline to be present during induction after hearing these explanations.

To prepare children for recovery from anesthesia, it is useful to describe our strategies to minimize emesis and pain after surgery. In emetogenic surgery and in children who are prone to emesis, prophylactic antiemetic therapy will be administered during anesthesia. If pain is anticipated during recovery, analgesics will be administered during anesthesia either in the form of a regional block and/or parenteral analgesics and supplemented in the recovery room should the child experience further pain. Anesthesiologists can provide valuable assistance in this respect because of their knowledge of the pharmacology of sedative and opioid medications (see Chapter 7), as well as their ability to perform neuraxial and peripheral nerve blocks (see Chapters 42 to 44). If special monitoring is required in the operating room or postoperatively, this should be explained and the child assured that the IV catheters, airway devices, and all invasive monitoring devices will be placed after induction of anesthesia to avoid causing discomfort and will be removed as soon as the child's postoperative condition permits. The possible need for postoperative intensive care, including assisted ventilation, should be anticipated and fully discussed with the parents and child (if the child is of an appropriate age) in circumstances that warrant such discussion.

The anesthesiologist who sits down with the family, who speaks slowly and clearly while answering questions, and who is neither distracted nor in a rush to leave, presents a much more sincere and caring impression to both the child and parents than the anesthesiologist who stands tapping his or her toes while interviewing the family, who speaks quickly, and whose body language points toward the door as if he or she is looking to exit the interview as quickly as possible. The detail with which this information is presented will vary from child to child and family to family, as well as with the anesthesiologist's understanding of the needs of the child and family. The anesthetic prescription should not be recited in a cold and technical manner, but rather with communication that addresses the parents' and the child's questions and concerns. This dialogue is frequently afforded too little time, leaving the parents and child insecure and apprehensive, their questions unanswered. Body language is especially important during this preoperative interview. But by the end of the interview, the child and parents should understand that you will be providing the quality of care that ensures the child's safety during anesthesia, thus reducing the child's and parents' anxiety.

THE ANESTHESIOLOGIST

Anesthesiologists must fully understand the proposed surgical, medical, or investigative procedure to facilitate the planning of an appropriate level of monitoring and selection of anesthetic drugs and technique. They must anticipate the needs of the surgeon or proceduralist in terms of positioning the child, the need for or avoidance of muscle relaxants, considerations regarding specific procedures (e.g., the surgeon's need to monitor motor and sensory evoked potentials may influence choices of anesthetic technique), IV fluids and blood products (see Chapters 9 and 12), as well as the need to alleviate perioperative anxiety and pain. For complex cases, the anesthesiologist and surgeon should formulate a plan and convey it to the parents and child preoperatively. Any important medical issues that require clarification should be investigated during the preoperative evaluation by consulting appropriate medical consultants as indicated. Consultant recommendations must be carefully reviewed and should reflect the consultant's understanding of the anesthesia process and what you require regarding the child's medical condition to assist you in the delivery of anesthesia (see Chapters 11, 13, 16, 24, 27, 28, and 30).

All children should fast preoperatively. Infants must receive special consideration; prolonged abstinence may lead to dehydration or hypoglycemia (see Chapters 4 and 9). Children may surreptitiously circumvent the preoperative fasting orders, especially if the period of fasting is prolonged or other children in the vicinity have food. One must always be prepared for the possibility of a full stomach and its sequelae. For example, the risk of pulmonary aspiration of gastric contents is increased in some children (e.g., those who ate a meal just before a trauma, those who had previous esophageal surgery, or those with a hiatus hernia). In these children, the anesthetic management should be modified to minimize the risk of regurgitation and aspiration. Preoperative consideration must be given to proper psychological support, appropriate premedication, and the timing of the premedication (see Chapters 3 and 4). Psychological support of the child and parents must never be neglected, no matter how calm they might appear. Premedication may be administered on the ward or in the waiting area; however, in children at risk for desaturation or cardiorespiratory compromise, the child may require monitoring and/or close observation. Critically ill children must be accompanied by skilled staff who will ensure continued infusions of vasoactive medications and who are skilled in the management of any emergencies that could arise during transport (see Chapter 39). In some, premedication may be omitted because of the critical nature of a child's illness or because a child is especially cooperative.

Informed Consent

The benefits and risks of the anesthetic procedure must be presented in clear, easily understood terms. At the same time, it is important not to present this information in a manner that unduly frightens the child or parents. The details of such a presentation will depend, in part, on the severity of the underlying medical and surgical conditions and how these affect anesthetic management and the planned procedure. Thus, risk can be presented in general terms, such as the following:

■ "The risks of anesthesia depend on the health of the child. For example, if a child has a heart, lung, or kidney disorder, or so on, then the risk from anesthesia is increased. In your child's case, these are our concerns" (and then elaborate the particular patient's issues, such as reactive airway disease, apnea of prematurity, etc.). "Knowing these problems ahead of time makes it easier for us and reduces the anesthetic risk for your child because we can modify our anesthetic prescription according to your child's specific needs. However, there is

always the possibility of allergic or unusual responses to anesthetic medications that we cannot predict even if your child has had anesthesia before, and that is why we shall carefully observe and monitor your child throughout the anesthetic as I have described."

We are designing the "anesthetic prescription" specifically for the particular needs of their child, and this notion should be described exactly this way to the parents. We are physicians and not technicians, and just as the pediatrician writes a prescription for antibiotics, anesthesiologists write the treatment prescription for anesthesia and administer it.

If a child is critically ill or has a disease process that is an immediate threat to his or her life, then this must be explained to the family. If a parent asks about the mortality risk, then all one can say is that the mortality related to anesthesia in most advanced countries is very small—less risky than crossing a busy thoroughfare on foot. Statistically, the incidence varies from one in several hundred thousand for healthy children undergoing routine procedures to a much greater rate for those who are critically ill. Nonetheless, the mortality for any specific child cannot be predicted with certainty. Recent concerns regarding possible anesthetic agent–induced neurotoxicity in young children (see Chapter 25) have been expressed by parents of young children during the preoperative visit. We should remind parents that the decision to proceed with anesthesia and surgery is a balance of the benefits and risks of both anesthesia and surgery and that the absence of substantive human data that anesthetics cause harm to young children combined with the sensitivity of our monitors to detect untoward events and our experience should allay their concerns.

Operating Room and Monitoring

For the anesthesiologist to successfully carry out a proposed anesthetic plan, the child's medical record must be examined for pertinent information before induction of anesthesia. For children who have already been assessed preoperatively, the record should be reviewed again for new information that may have been added since the initial evaluation. It is most important that the child's identification bracelet is checked, especially if the anesthetizing team is different from the preoperative evaluation team. A "time-out" and checklist for nurses, surgeon, and anesthesiologist to confirm the child's name, the planned surgical procedure, and the site of the surgical procedure (right or left side or bilateral); airway concerns; the need for prophylactic antibiotics; allergies and anaphylaxis; and availability of special equipment and large bore IV access are also reviewed. It is also important to confirm whether antibiotics were administered on the ward or in the ICU to avoid double-dosing of antibiotics. This review constitutes a vital safety net in the operating room (Fig. 1.1). All equipment for induction and maintenance of anesthesia, including suction and all necessary monitoring devices, must be checked by the anesthetic team and operational before induction of anesthesia (see Chapters 4 and 52).

Monitoring should be appropriate for the child's clinical condition and the surgical procedure. In every situation, basic monitoring is essential; to this are added special monitoring devices as they become necessary. The basic monitors are the anesthesiologist's eyes, ears, and hands, which confer the ability to observe a child's color and chest movements, to listen for heart tones and breath sounds, and to palpate the arterial pulse and temperature of the skin. A precordial or esophageal stethoscope is

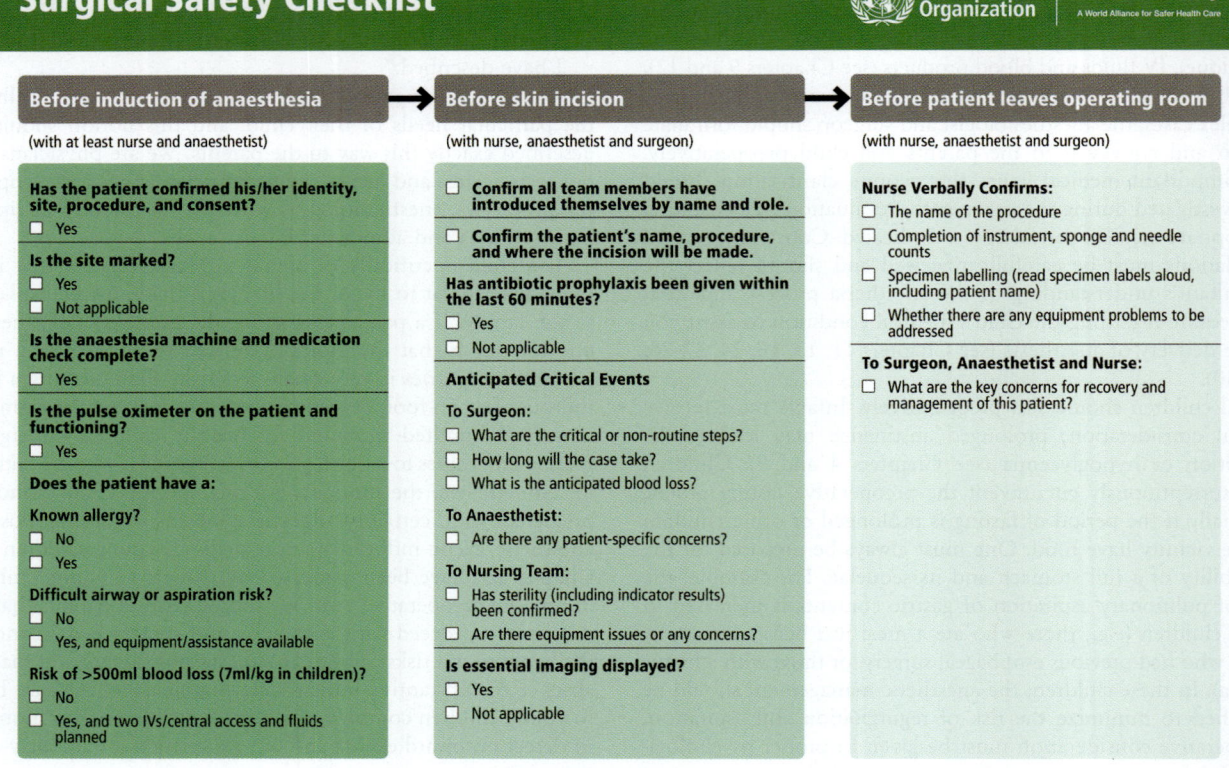

FIGURE 1.1 WHO Surgical Safety Checklist. (From World Health Organization, Geneva, 2009. Available from: http://www.who.int/patientsafety/safesurgery/en/.)

a very useful and simple device to monitor heart sounds and the quality of breath sounds, even when our attention is focused away from physiologic monitors. All children, except those undergoing the briefest noninvasive procedures, should have IV access to allow for fluid administration and to provide a route for rapid and predictable drug administration. If IV access is already in place, its patency should be checked preoperatively. The size of the catheter should be confirmed in case a larger cannula is required to administer large volumes of fluid or blood during surgery. If so, the new catheter should be placed after induction of anesthesia. A balanced salt solution is an appropriate fluid to infuse in most children undergoing elective surgery, although glucose-containing solutions may be preferred in specific circumstances (see Chapter 9). Continuous monitoring of the electrocardiogram, temperature, inspired oxygen concentration, oxygen saturation, expired carbon dioxide, and serial blood pressure determination are considered routine. Expired carbon dioxide monitors (especially those that display the waveform) and pulse oximetry are extremely important in the early detection of potential anesthetic-related events that, if undetected, could result in serious morbidity or mortality. Identifying the anesthetic agent and monitoring its concentration breath by breath is also helpful but not mandatory. The role of wakefulness-monitoring devices in children remains unestablished, especially in children younger than 2 years of age (see Chapters 7 and 52). Near-infrared spectroscopy is being used increasingly during cardiac surgery; it provides a useful monitor of cerebral (i.e., organ) oxygenation. The routine use of noninvasive continuous cardiac output monitors will likely provide the next generation of operating room monitoring (see Chapter 52), providing an early warning of evolving adverse hemodynamic events and the response to corrective measures (e.g., the administration of blood, crystalloid, vasopressor, vagolytic).

Invasive hemodynamic monitoring (e.g., direct arterial blood pressure, central venous pressure) may be required for major surgery if extensive blood loss or major fluid shifts are anticipated, or if a child is medically unstable. Urine output provides indirect data of the intravascular volume and organ perfusion in the presence of normal renal function. Monitoring urinary output is particularly useful for prolonged operations, for procedures involving major blood loss, when there is the potential for rapid or massive blood loss, when wide variations in blood pressure and fluid balance can be anticipated, or during induced hypotensive anesthesia. *In general, if a particular variable would be monitored in an adult, then the same approach should be adopted for a child.*

Invasive monitors are sometimes forsaken in a child because the pediatric anesthesiologist considers that the risk/benefit ratio does not justify their use. However, when the benefits outweigh the risks, these monitors provide an accurate estimate of blood pressure, cardiac output, filling pressures, and cardiac and pulmonary function. In turn, they provide a safe mechanism for assessing the response to pharmacologic interventions, as well as the responses to administration of blood products, fluids, and vasoactive medications (see Chapter 52).

A cautionary note: As monitoring has become more sophisticated, anesthesiologists have become more distanced than ever from their patients. Relying totally on monitoring devices to detect clinical abnormalities is dangerous. *The focus must always be on the child and the surgical field. Electronic monitors may fail, and if the anesthesiologist focuses too much attention on the monitor in an effort to interpret it, rather than attending directly to the child, the child may suffer.* This is the reason a precordial stethoscope is so useful; strong heart sounds in the face of failed monitors provide some degree of assurance that the child is not in severe trouble. The tone of the pulse oximeter should be audible by everyone in the operating room to identify a decreasing oxygen saturation. *Silencing the monitor and its alarms for an extended period of time is a serious breach of safety and practice standards.* One of the editors is aware of a child for whom all monitor alarms and sounds were disabled during anesthesia who was discovered dead at the conclusion of the procedure after an unrecognized, unintended tracheal extubation. All monitors should be functioning and their alarms audible at all times during anesthesia of infants and children.

Induction and Maintenance of Anesthesia

Significant differences in the physiology, pharmacology, and development of a child mandate that the anesthesiologist not consider the child simply a small adult. In an infant, the rate of uptake of inhalation anesthetic agents is more rapid than in an adult. Similarly, protein binding, volume of distribution, and effect-site time constants for some drugs in infants may be less than in adults, resulting in more rapid responses to a given dose. Thus, if changes need to be made, the inspired concentration of an inhalation agent should be adjusted more gradually and the doses of medication diluted and titrated more carefully than in older children and adults (see Chapter 7).

In principle, the approach to an anesthetic procedure in a child is similar to that in an adult. However, in practice it is often advisable to modify the sequence of applying the monitors. In a relatively stable child, induction of anesthesia may proceed with only a pulse oximeter and possibly a precordial stethoscope; the remaining monitors are applied after induction. This sequence often avoids a prolonged preinduction phase during which a child may have more time to become anxious and distressed. In a struggling, upset child, some monitors may display accurate values before induction of anesthesia, whereas others may not. For example, the pulse oximeter may not provide reliable values in a struggling child until the finger or toe is motionless. In critically ill children, however, omitting some monitors to avoid upsetting them is imprudent, especially if it compromises the child's well-being during anesthesia. Thus, the management of the child during induction of anesthesia should be tailored to the child's behavior and illness severity.

Clinical Monitors

In children as in adults, monitoring begins with the basic observations of a child's general condition: the heart rate, blood pressure, respirations, and temperature. The most important aspect of basic monitoring consists of using the senses of sight, hearing, and touch to integrate all the data provided by patient observations and the monitors.

SIGHT

Observing a child's chest excursions (depth and symmetry), the color of the nail beds, oral mucosa, and capillary refill provides vital information regarding the adequacy of ventilation and perfusion. Observation of the surgical field provides an immediate indication of the extent of fluid shifts and blood loss, the color of the blood in the surgical field, evidence of muscle relaxation, depth of anesthesia, and various physiologic problems that may occur during the surgery (e.g., surgical retraction causing venous obstruction).

HEARING

Listening to the pitch of the pulse oximeter as well as the heart tones and breath sounds through a precordial or esophageal stethoscope provides instant and continuous feedback about oxygenation (pulse oximeter), heart rate and rhythm, an impression of the cardiac output (changes in intensity of heart sounds), and the adequacy of ventilation (wheezing, stridor, laryngeal spasm, no air exchange). This information is particularly helpful in diagnosing arrhythmias, hypovolemia, anesthetic overdose, and airway obstruction. It may also be helpful to listen to the sounds of surgery, such as the sudden change in the noise of the suction device with rapid blood loss or the surgeon's comments regarding technical difficulties with the procedure.

TOUCH

Intermittently examining a child—especially palpating peripheral pulses and the skin—provides information that may confirm the auditory input about heart rate, cardiac output, blood pressure, perfusion, and temperature.

Airway and Ventilation

The most important consideration in the safe practice of pediatric anesthesia is to ensure a patent airway. Airway obstruction occurs readily because of the unique characteristics of the infant and child airway (see Chapter 14). Thus, the anesthesiologist must be constantly vigilant of the airway to ensure that it remains patent at all times, particularly during mask anesthesia. In this case, the expired carbon dioxide tension may underestimate the true carbon dioxide tension because of a poor mask fit and/or air leaks combined with an obstructed airway. Airway obstruction may lead to hypoventilation, although the causes of hypoventilation may be central (opioids or inhalation agents) or peripheral (muscle relaxants) in origin. The capnogram is usually very accurate during mask anesthesia with a circle breathing circuit. Failure to detect an appropriate end-tidal carbon dioxide tension suggests inadequate ventilation, a mask leak, or reduced pulmonary blood flow, with the result that the child's condition may deteriorate from lack of an adequate airway or dilution of the anesthetic gas concentrations.

Although it is desirable to optimize ventilation by maintaining an arterial carbon dioxide pressure within the normal range (35 to 45 mm Hg), most healthy infants and children are not harmed by mild to moderate hypoventilation provided arterial oxygenation is maintained; however, severe overventilation has the capacity to reduce cerebral perfusion.

Constant monitoring of the inspired concentration of oxygen, the expired concentration of carbon dioxide, and the oxygen saturation is a valuable adjunct to the senses of sight, hearing, and touch. *Failure to ventilate adequately is probably the most important factor in the morbidity and mortality of children undergoing anesthesia.*

Fluids and Perfusion

Appropriate intraoperative fluid management is especially important in infants and children. Because of the relatively small blood volumes of infants and children, hypovolemia may develop rapidly after what may appear to be a trivial amount of blood loss. Fluid shifts may occur in infants because they fasted for a prolonged period. Replacement of lost blood and basic fluid administration must be carefully titrated (using rate-limiting devices) because overhydration readily occurs. The anesthesiologist should have a clear plan for the type and volume of fluid for perioperative administration. Preoperative calculation of maintenance, deficit, and potential third-space losses helps in formulating this fluid management plan, although for children older than 1 year of age, the fluid replacement strategy has been greatly simplified. A well-planned outline results in a rational and safe approach to both fluid maintenance and correction of fluid deficit and losses (see Chapters 9 and 12). The anesthesiologist should have immediate access to indwelling IV cannulae; line obstructions, loose connections, disconnections, or interstitial cannulae result in children not receiving the intended fluid therapy or medications or infusing them into the subcutaneous space, sometimes with disastrous consequences.

Conduct of the Anesthesia Team

The anesthesiologist must concentrate exclusively on the child and the monitors throughout the procedure. The child's safety is in his or her hands, and any inattention may place the child's life in jeopardy. Should members of the anesthesia team need to replace each other during the anesthetic, it is essential that the "baton of responsibility" be passed by communicating all of the relevant aspects of the child's health, as well as of the anesthetic and surgery that have occurred up to that time. All drugs on the anesthesia machine must be clearly labeled by name and dosage; the use of bar code scanners and automatic labeling devices with color coding are particularly useful. For infants, dilution of drugs or the use of tuberculin syringes may improve the safety of drug administration by limiting the amount of drug in each syringe and allowing more accurate dose administration, although a disproportionate amount of the small volumes of a drug—as in the case of undiluted drugs administered from a tuberculin syringe—may be trapped in the dead space of claves and/or stopcocks, resulting in an underdosing of the drug.

Ongoing communication between the anesthesiologist and surgeon is important if the anesthesiologist is to anticipate potential changes in a child's physiologic status resulting from surgical manipulations and deal with them immediately, appropriately, and effectively.

The conclusion of an anesthetic procedure is fraught with potential problems. The anesthesiologist should not be left alone in the operating room without a nurse or other physician, nor should he or she relax vigilance while a child is awakening and during transport to the recovery room or intensive care unit. It is during this stage that airway obstruction, desaturation, vomiting and aspiration, and emergence delirium are likely to occur.

Records of an anesthetic procedure must be accurate and complete; however, anesthesiologists must avoid the compulsion to complete these during the procedure if a child's condition warrants his or her full attention. The increasing availability of anesthesia information management systems (AIMS) provides an accurate history of physiologic parameters and frees the anesthesiologist to focus on the patient; however, filling in "required" check boxes can be a distraction, particularly at the conclusion of anesthesia.

The Postanesthesia Care Unit

In most jurisdictions, the department of anesthesiology is responsible for the postanesthesia care unit (PACU). Accordingly, the anesthesiologist's responsibility to a child continues into the PACU. Transport to the PACU must be carried out with appropriate monitoring, attention to a clear airway and adequate ventilation, oxygenation, and perfusion. If necessary, battery-powered infusion pumps should be used to maintain accurate infusions of vasoactive drugs. If needed, oxygen should be administered by face mask. Oxygen saturation may be monitored during transport; administering oxygen while monitoring pulse oximetry renders the oximeter a poor reflection of ventilation. Nevertheless, oxygen should be provided during transport to children who have not fully awakened. These children should be transported in the "tonsil position" or "recovery position" (lateral decubitus position) for two major reasons: (1) the dimensions of the upper airway are greater in this position than supine and (2) should vomiting occur, the regurgitant material will flow out of the mouth, away from the larynx and will be identified immediately. This position also allows head extension. The mask should be observed for condensation with each breath to assess the respiratory rate as well as gas movement with respiration.

On arrival in the PACU, a summary of the medical and surgical problems of the child, important intraoperative events—including the timing of antibiotics, analgesics, local anesthetics, or nerve blocks—and details of the anesthetic prescription are given to the PACU personnel. Appropriate social and family histories (marital status) should also be provided to the PACU staff (e.g., nervous parents, history of child abuse or neglect) to help ease social issues that may occur in PACU. The PACU must be equipped with age- and size-appropriate monitoring and resuscitation equipment. Vital signs (oxygen saturation, heart rate, blood pressure, respirations, temperature, and pain score) should be recorded on admission to the PACU and serially during the PACU stay (see Chapter 47). If appropriate, specific instructions should be given relating to oxygen requirements, ongoing fluid management, laboratory tests (e.g., hematocrit, blood gases, electrolytes, and coagulation profile) and radiographs. Once the anesthesiologist confirms that the child's vital signs are stable and has completed the information handover, it is important to take even a brief moment to meet with the parents to confirm that their child is recovering from the anesthetic without (if true) issues or difficulties. They would be interested in knowing how their child tolerated the anesthetic and what they might expect when they visit their child in the recovery room. If the child requires special attention (airway issues, hypotension, possible ongoing blood loss, obstructive sleep apnea, and so on) in the PACU, then the anesthesiologist should reassess the child personally while reassuring the parents before the child is discharged or make appropriate arrangements for postoperative monitoring.

Postoperative Visit

For children who had ambulatory surgery, it is helpful for a member from the anesthesia team to call the family at home on postoperative day one or two to determine their level of satisfaction and identify any complications that may have occurred. Children who were admitted to the hospital overnight should be visited before

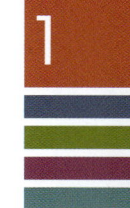

discharge to assess the postanesthetic clinical course and discuss the child's reaction to the anesthetic. A note documenting the visit should also be included in the child's record. These visits help the public understand the role of anesthesiology in the operating room and beyond as a vital medical specialty.

Summary

This introductory chapter presents fundamental aspects for the safe practice of pediatric anesthesia. The chapters that follow elaborate on these principles with our collective experience used to guide the practicing anesthesiologists as well as those in training. Key principles for the safe practice of pediatric anesthesia are repeated throughout the book to emphasize their importance and are supplemented with a range of perspectives on clinical and controversial issues.

Growth and Development

BRUNO MARCINIAK

GROWTH IS A COMPLEX succession of phenomena that starts with the fusion of two cells and matures by 9 months into a complex organism known as a fetus. This phenomenally complex process not only produces a human being, it also traces the history of species with each and every fetus through embryology. Development is more than a simple increase in the number of cells; it includes interactions between the cells and interactions between the fetus and the environment, effects that are modulated by intracellular and intercellular signaling.[1]

It is incumbent upon the physician to understand the developmental changes that occur to the fetus and infant over time, and how these changes affect both responses to diseases and to drug pharmacokinetics and pharmacodynamics.

Normal and Abnormal Growth and Maturation

Growth is the quantitative increase in physical development of the body, whereas maturation is the genetic, biologic, and physical development of the child; both phenomena occur during pregnancy and continue after birth. Prenatal growth is the most important phase in development, comprising organogenesis in the first 8 weeks (embryonic growth), followed by the functional development of organ systems and maturation of the fetus (fetal growth). Rapid growth occurs particularly in the second trimester; a major increase in weight from subcutaneous tissue and muscle mass occurs in the third trimester. The duration of gestation and the weight of an infant are important correlates that vary with ethnicity, maternal environment, and pathology (Table 2.1).

By convention, the term *prematurity* has been applied to neonates who weigh less than 2500 g at birth. However, the designation *preterm neonate* may be more appropriate, defined as an infant born before 37 completed weeks of gestation. A *term or full-term neonate* is an infant born between 37 and 42 completed weeks of gestation. *A postterm neonate* is one born after 42 completed weeks of gestation.

Preterm neonates are further classified according to their actual birth weight. A low–birth-weight (LBW) neonate weighs less than 2500 g regardless of the duration of the pregnancy. A very low–birth-weight (VLBW) neonate weighs less than 1500 g, and an extremely low–birth-weight neonate weighs less than 1000 g. More recently, neonates that weigh less than 750 g at birth are referred to as "*micropremies*"; very limited information has been published regarding the anesthetic management of this vulnerable subpopulation of neonates (see Chapter 37). Common neonatal problems as they relate to age and birth weight are presented in Table 2.2.

After birth, physical growth continues at a rapid pace during the first 6 months of extrauterine life but slows by about 2 years of age. Physical growth accelerates a second time during the pubertal period. A simple way to remember how rapidly infants grow is that birth weight doubles by 6 months of age and triples by 1 year. Length doubles by 4 years of age. This scale, however, does not consistently affect all organs or organ functions. It is important to correctly and precisely assess the stage of development of the

TABLE 2.1	The Relationship of Gestational Age to Weight
Gestation (weeks)	**Mean Weight (g)**
28	1165 ± 109
32	1760 ± 128
36	2621 ± 274
40 (full term)	3351 ± 448

Data from Naeye RL, Dixon JB. Distortions in fetal growth. *Pediatr Res* 1978;12:987–991.

TABLE 2.3	Neurologic and External Physical Criteria to Assess Gestational Age	
Physical Examination	**Preterm (<37 weeks)**	**Term (≥37 weeks)**
Ear	Shapeless, pliable	Firm, well formed
Skin	Edematous, thin skin	Thick skin
Sole of foot	Creases on anterior third	Whole foot creased
Breast tissue	<1-mm diameter	>5-mm diameter
Genitalia		
Male	Scrotum poorly developed	Scrotum rugated
	Testes undescended	Testes descended
Female	Large clitoris, gaping labia majora	Labia majora developed
Limbs	Hypotonic	Tonic (flexed)
Grasp reflex	Weak grasp	Can be lifted by reflex grasp
Moro reflex	Complete but exhaustible (>32 weeks)	Complete
Sucking reflex	Weak	Strong, synchronous with swallowing

child because any substantial deviations warrant an investigation of the cause. For example, height and weight are important metrics of maturity, although other factors may also impact maturity,[2] including those that cause excessive weight gain or prevent normal weight gain (Figs. 2.1 and 2.2).

Gestational Age Assessment

The gestational age of an infant may be assessed in one of three ways. The most accurate means of assessing gestational age is by measuring the crown-rump length of the fetus during a first-trimester ultrasonographic examination. A second method involves calculating gestational age from the first day of the mother's last menstrual period, but this is commonly inaccurate and can result in errors. Alternately, the Dubowitz scoring system is a well-accepted method that combines neurologic and physical criteria of the neonate to provide an accurate assessment of gestational age.[3,4] A summary of the significant neurologic and physical signs of maturity is presented in Table 2.3.

WEIGHT AND LENGTH

Growth is assessed by changes in weight, length, and head circumference. Percentile charts are valuable for monitoring the child's growth and development. Deviations in growth from the past percentile are more significant than any single measurement (Figs. 2.3 and 2.4). Weight is a more sensitive index of well-being,

TABLE 2.2	Common Neonatal Problems With Respect to Weight and Gestation	
Gestation	**Relative Weight**	**Neonatal Problems at Increased Incidence**
Preterm (<37 weeks)	SGA	Respiratory distress syndrome
		Apnea
		Perinatal depression
		Hypoglycemia
		Polycythemia
		Hypocalcemia
		Hypomagnesemia
		Hyperbilirubinemia
		Viral infection
		Thrombocytopenia
		Congenital anomalies
		Maternal drug addiction
		Fetal alcohol syndrome
	AGA	Respiratory distress syndrome
		Apnea
		Hypoglycemia
		Hypocalcemia
		Hypomagnesemia
		Hyperbilirubinemia
	LGA	Respiratory distress syndrome
		Hypoglycemia: infant of a diabetic mother
		Apnea
		Hypocalcemia
		Hypomagnesemia
		Hyperbilirubinemia
Normal (37-42 weeks)	SGA	Congenital anomalies
		Viral infection
		Thrombocytopenia
		Maternal drug addiction
		Perinatal depression
		Hypoglycemia
	AGA	—
	LGA	Birth trauma
		Hyperbilirubinemia
		Hypoglycemia: infant of a diabetic mother
Postmature (>42 weeks)	SGA	Meconium aspiration syndrome
		Congenital anomalies
		Viral infection
		Thrombocytopenia
		Maternal drug addiction
		Perinatal depression
		Aspiration pneumonia
		Hypoglycemia
	AGA	—
	LGA	Birth trauma
		Hyperbilirubinemia
		Hypoglycemia: infant of a diabetic mother

AGA, Appropriate for gestational age; *LGA*, large for gestational age; *SGA*, small for gestational age.

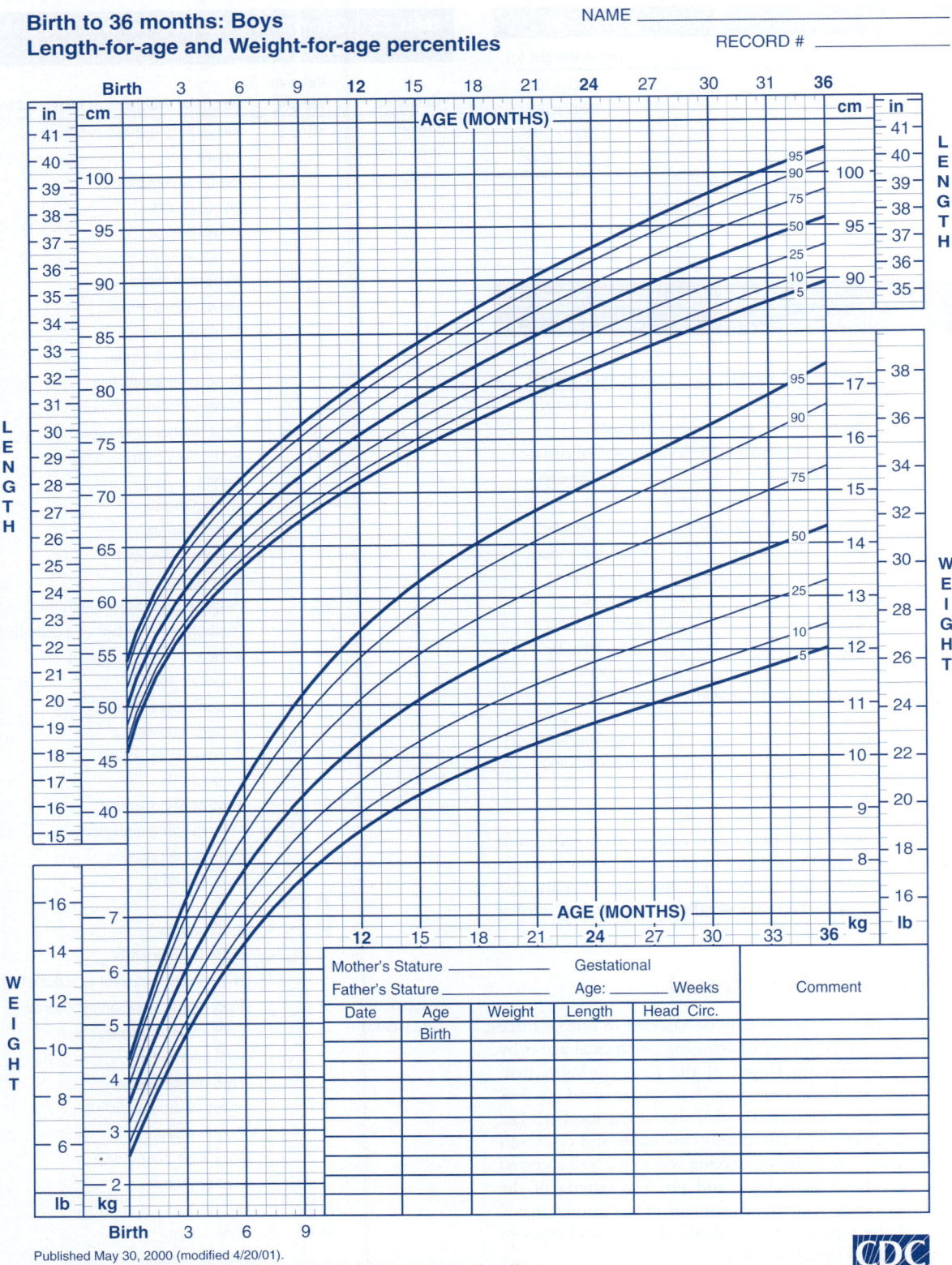

Birth to 36 months: Boys
Length-for-age and Weight-for-age percentiles

NAME _____

RECORD # _____

Published May 30, 2000 (modified 4/20/01).
SOURCE: Developed by the National Center for Health Statistics in collaboration with
the National Center for Chronic Disease Prevention and Health Promotion (2000).
http://www.cdc.gov/growthcharts

FIGURE 2.1 Growth Chart for Boys. (From the National Center for Chronic Disease Prevention and Health Promotion (2000). http://www.cdc.gov/growthcharts Published May 30, 2000 (modified 4/20/01).)

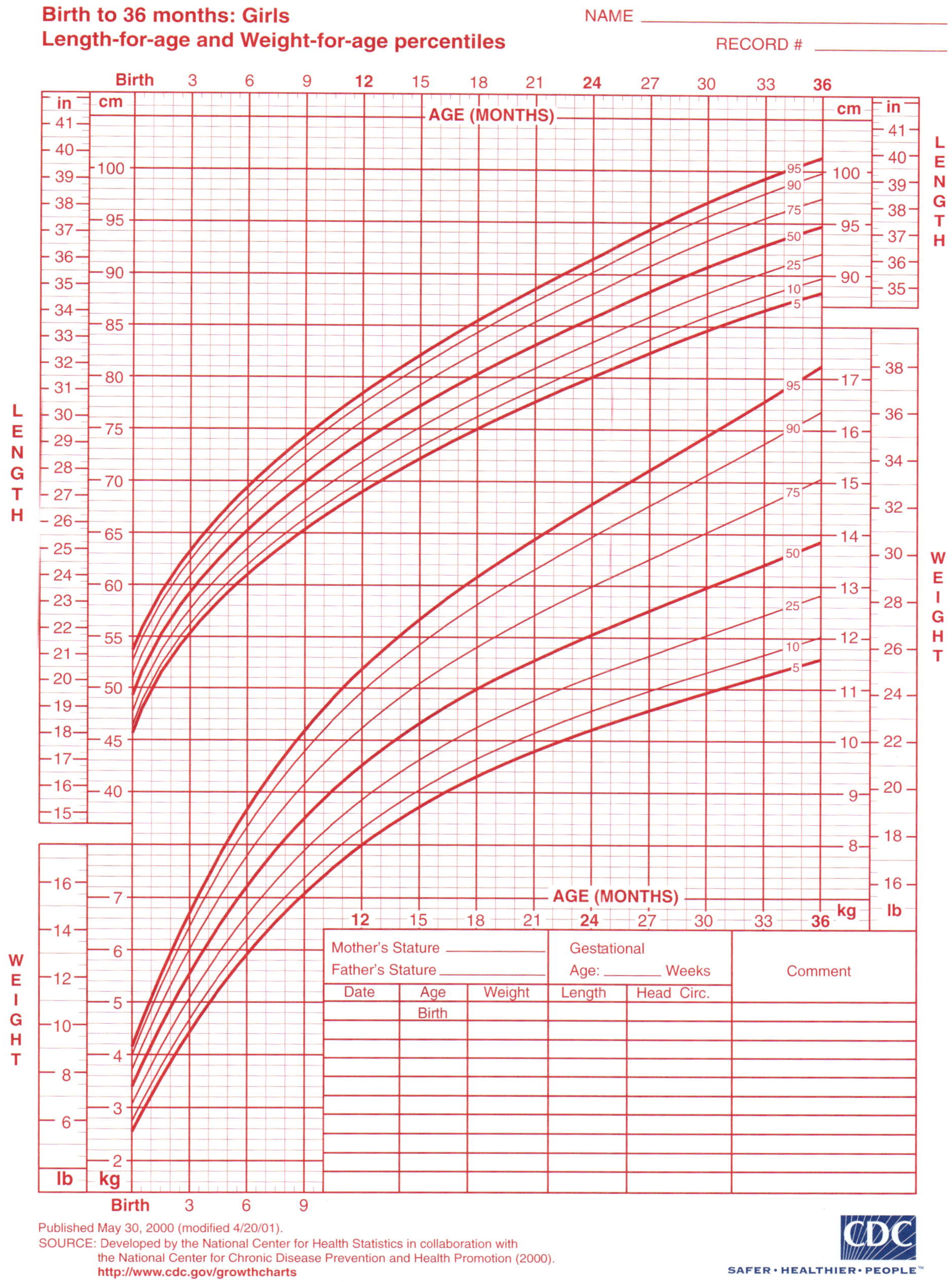

Birth to 36 months: Girls
Length-for-age and Weight-for-age percentiles

NAME _____

RECORD # _____

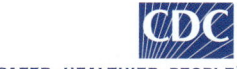

Published May 30, 2000 (modified 4/20/01).
SOURCE: Developed by the National Center for Health Statistics in collaboration with
the National Center for Chronic Disease Prevention and Health Promotion (2000).
http://www.cdc.gov/growthcharts

FIGURE 2.2 Growth Chart for Girls. (From the National Center for Health Statistics in collaboration with the National Center for Chronic Disease Prevention and Health Promotion (2000). http://www.cdc.gov/growthcharts Published May 30, 2000 (modified 4/20/01).)

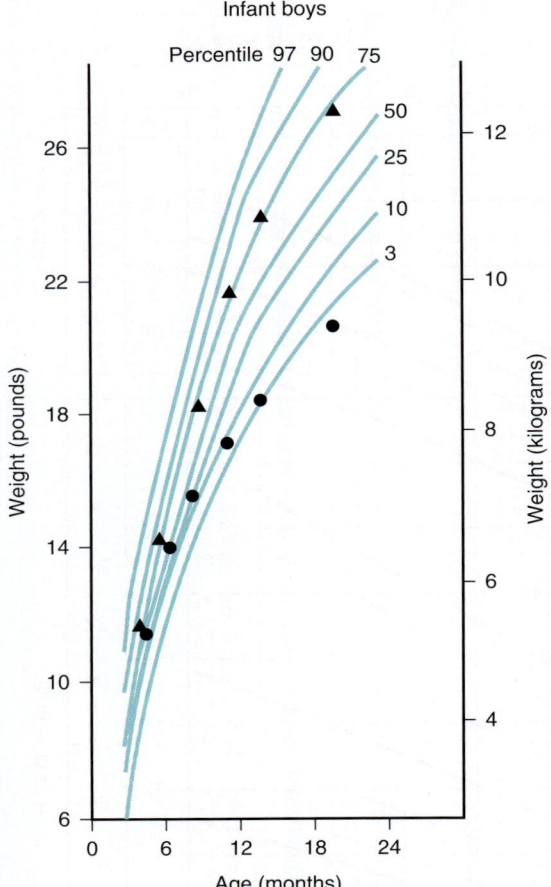

Infant boys

FIGURE 2.3 Postnatal Growth Curve (Weight) for Term Male Infants. This figure represents normal growth curves. *Triangles* indicate a normal child. *Circles* demonstrate failure to thrive in a child with severe renal failure.

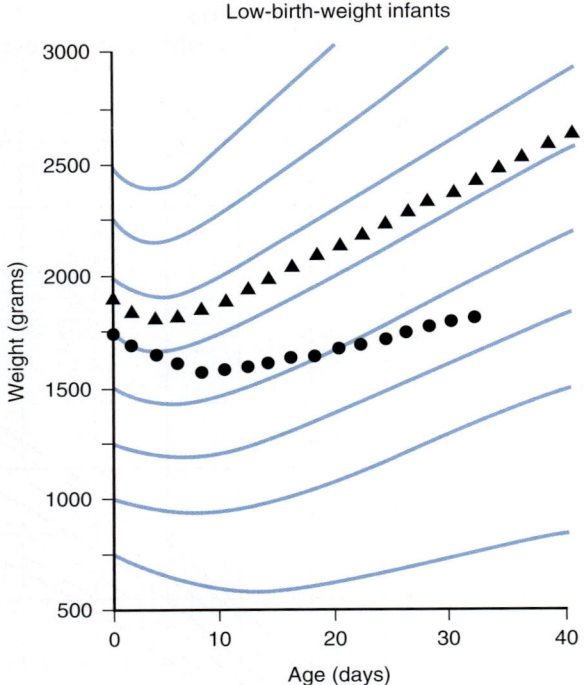

Low-birth-weight infants

FIGURE 2.4 Postnatal Growth Curve (Weight) for Preterm Infants. This figure represents normal growth curves for preterm infants. *Triangles* indicate a normal preterm infant. *Circles* demonstrate failure to thrive in an infant with bronchopulmonary dysplasia.

illness, or poor nutrition than length or head circumference and is the most commonly used measurement of growth. Changes in weight reflect changes in muscle mass, adipose tissue, skeleton, and body water; as a result, weight is a nonspecific metric of growth. Measurement of length provides the best indicator of skeletal growth because it is not affected by changes in adipose tissue or water content.

Term neonates may lose 5% to 10% of their body weight during the first 24 to 72 hours after birth from loss of body water. However, by 7 to 10 postnatal days, they have returned to their birth weight. An average daily increase of 30 g (210 g/week) is expected during the first 3 months after birth, after which an increase of 70 g each week is expected for the subsequent 10 to 12 months (Table 2.4).

When graphing the weight of a preterm neonate on a growth chart, it is common to use the neonate's corrected gestational age (postmenstrual age; postconception age is taken from conception and is approximately 2 weeks less) instead of his or her chronologic age (postnatal age [i.e., from birth]) during the first 2 years of the infant's life to correct for prematurity.

Weight and length are important metrics of growth, although other changes affect the composition of the body itself, especially the total body water, which decreases at the expense of the extracellular compartment during infancy. Adult proportions are

TABLE 2.4 Approximate Relationship of Age to Weight

Age (years)	Weight (kg)
1	10
3	15
5	19
7	23

Corresponding equation for 18 months to 8 years of age is: Wt (kg) = 2 × Age (years) + 9.
For age >8 years: Wt (kg) = 3 × Age (years).

TABLE 2.5 Relationship of Age to Body Water

Age	Body Water (%)	Extracellular	Intracellular
Fetus	90	60	25
Preterm	80	55	30
Full-term	70	50	35
6-12 months	60	30	40

achieved by approximately 1 year of age (see Fig. 7.8).[5,6] These changes in the distribution of water throughout the body have important implications for drug dosing and distribution in the neonate and infant. Males have a greater percentage of water, whereas females have a slightly greater percentage of fat. The percentage decrease in extracellular water is greater than the decrease in total body water because of the simultaneous increase in intracellular water (Table 2.5).[7]

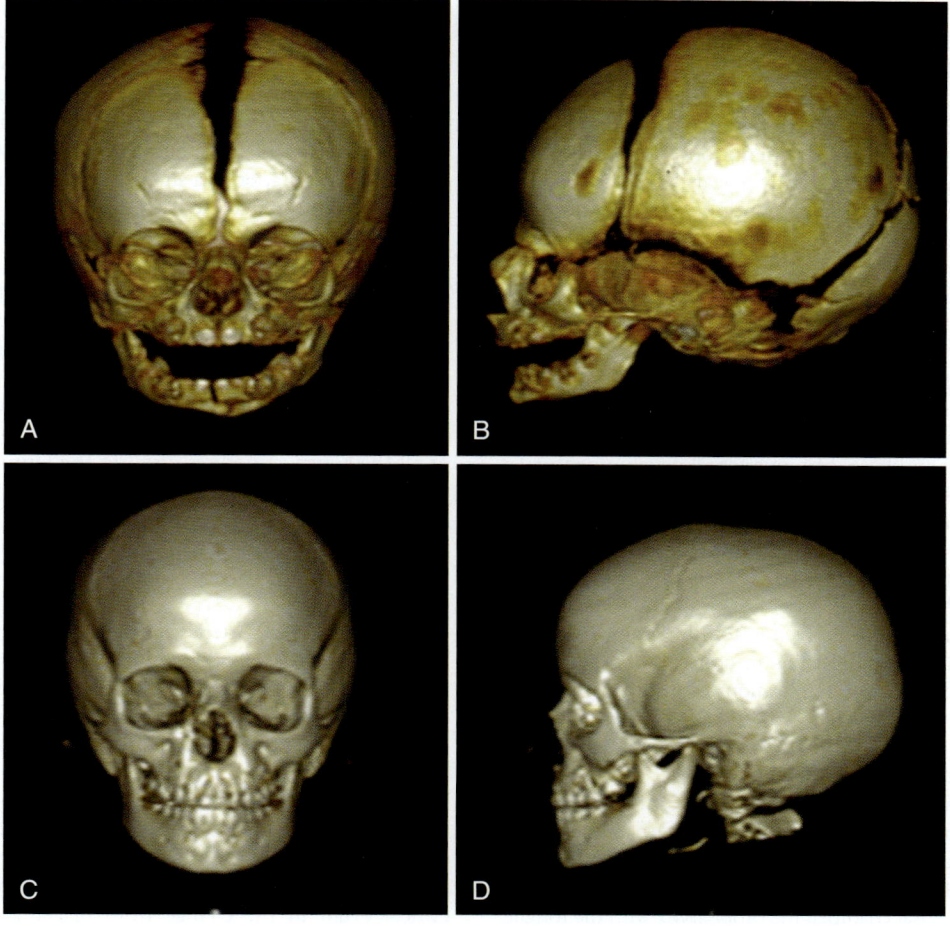

FIGURE 2.5 Cranial Development. **A** and **B** depict the skull of a neonate with wide-open suture. **C** and **D** depict the skull of a 7-year-old boy with fused sutures.

Another, more precise metric to assess development is to calculate the body surface area (BSA).[8] BSA can also be described using an allometric equation with an exponent of ⅔ (see Chapter 7):

$$BSA \propto weight^{2/3}$$

HEAD CIRCUMFERENCE

Head size reflects the growth of the brain and correlates with intracranial volume and brain weight. Changing head circumference reflects head growth and is a part of the total body growth process; it may or may not indicate underlying involvement of the brain. An abnormally large or small head may indicate abnormal brain development, which must alert the anesthesiologist to possible underlying neurologic problems. A large head may indicate a normal variation, familial feature, or pathologic condition (e.g., hydrocephalus or increased intracranial pressure), whereas a small head may indicate a normal variant, familial feature, or pathologic condition such as craniosynostosis or abnormal brain development.

During the first year of life, head circumference normally increases 10 cm, and in the second year increases 2.5 cm. By 9 months of age, head circumference reaches 50% of adult size, and by 2 years it is 75%. Head circumference is closely followed on standard percentile growth curves. As with weight, deviations in the growth of the head from its past percentile are more significant than a single measurement.

The anterior fontanel should be palpated to assess whether it is sunken (dehydration) or bulging abnormally (suggesting increased intracranial pressure as in hydrocephalus, infection, hemorrhage, or increased partial pressure of carbon dioxide in the arterial blood [$PaCO_2$]). If it is bulging, the sutures should be palpated for abnormal separation as a result of increased intracranial pressure. The anterior fontanel closes between 9 and 18 months of age; the posterior fontanel closes by 2 to 4 months of age (Fig. 2.5). Cranial molding occurs particularly in LBW neonates and is usually of no clinical importance.

FACE

Although the cranial vault increases rapidly in size, the face and base of the skull develop at a slower rate. At birth, the mandible is small; but as a child develops, forward growth occurs, reducing the obliquity of the mandibular angle. Failure of prenatal development of the mandible may be associated with severe congenital defects (e.g., Pierre Robin sequence, Treacher Collins, or Goldenhar syndromes). These syndromes often have other associated anomalies. After 2 years of age, the cranial vault increases only marginally in size, whereas the facial configuration undergoes substantive changes. The maxilla grows rapidly to accommodate the developing teeth. In addition, the frontal sinuses develop by 2 to 6 years of age, and the maxillary, ethmoidal, and sphenoidal sinuses appear after 6 years of age.

TEETH

The first tooth, usually a lower incisor, erupts at approximately 6 months after birth (deciduous dentition). Thereafter, one tooth usually erupts each month until all 20 primary deciduous teeth are present by 28 months of age. Preterm infants may show severe enamel hypoplasia in their primary dentition.[9,10]

Permanent teeth begin to appear by 6 years, with the shedding of the deciduous teeth; this process continues over the next 6 to 8 years. Some hereditary disorders such as Down syndrome, as well as others including cerebral palsy, medications (e.g., tetracycline), and nutritional defects can lead to abnormally developed teeth.

Airway and Respiratory System

Airway development includes a large number of structures, including the cranial vault and base, craniovertebral development, face, branchial apparatus, larynx, and oral cavity.

These structures are involved not only in the respiratory function (to provide enough oxygen and to remove carbon dioxide) but also in separating the circulation of air from the swallowing of liquid and food. A variety of processes, including ventilation, perfusion, and diffusion, are involved in fulfilling these functions. Specifically, the anesthesiologist has to consider these developmental changes because of their implications in airway management and ventilation.

UPPER AIRWAY DEVELOPMENT

During development, the upper airway of the infant undergoes major anatomic modifications that include changes in size, shape, and interrelationships; this is particularly prominent during the first few years of life.

The face and the nasal chamber, the oropharynx with the tongue, and the laryngotracheal lumen are the three main components of the upper airway. Development of the neurocranium leads to maturation of the cranial vault and skull base, whereas development of the viscerocranium leads to the skeletal portions of the face. The primordial areas involved in forming the covering of the tongue appear early in the second month of development.

The skull base grows rapidly until age 6 years, with relatively slower growth thereafter. The cranial base flexes postnatally in a rapid growth trajectory that is complete by 2 years of age.

The depth of the nasopharynx increases as a result of remodeling of the palate as well as changes in the angulation of the skull base. During childhood, the soft tissues of the pharyngeal structures surrounding the upper airway increase proportionally to the skeletal structures. After birth, the dimensions of the nasal cavity increase very rapidly. During the first year of life, the total minimal cross-sectional area increases by 67% and the volume of the anterior 4 cm of the nasal airways by 36%.[11,12]

The volume of the oral cavity in the neonate is proportionally less than that in the adult, primarily because of the shorter mandibular ramus. The volume of the oral cavity greatly increases during the first 12 months because of rapid growth in the height of the mandibular ramus.

In the neonate, the tongue contains considerably less fat and soft tissue compared with that in the adult, but it is large relative to the dimensions of the mouth, with relatively larger extrinsic musculature and a less developed superior longitudinal muscle, resulting in a flat dorsal surface with poor lateral mobility (see also Chapter 14).

The larynx is developed embryologically from ectodermal, endodermal, and mesodermal tissues that are derived from the third, fourth, and sixth branchial arch and pouch apparatus. The development of the larynx and airway in the neonate is outlined in detail in Chapter 14. The laryngeal opening (epiglottis and vocal cords) in a neonate and 2-year-old boy are shown in Fig. 2.6. Note the long, omega-shaped epiglottis and the pearly white vocal cords in the neonate.

RESPIRATORY SYSTEM DEVELOPMENT

The development of the respiratory system begins during week 4 of gestation. Three "laws" that describe the temporal development of the airways, alveoli, and pulmonary vessels govern normal lung growth.

Airways: The bronchial tree down to and including the terminal bronchioles forms by week 16 of gestation. The acinus, consisting of all the airway structures distal to the terminal bronchiole and the entire gas-exchanging apparatus, develops throughout the remainder of gestation.

Alveoli: Alveoli develop mainly after birth, increasing in number until approximately 8 years of life and in size until growth of the chest wall ceases.

Pulmonary vessels: Arteries and veins accompanying the bronchial tree form by week 16 of gestation. Those vessels lying within the acinus follow the development of the alveoli. Both the appearance and growth of arterial smooth muscle lag behind the sprouting of new vessels and are not completed until late adolescence.

TRANSITION TO AIR BREATHING

Fetal breathing movements have been detected as early as 11 weeks of gestational age; they are interspersed with long periods of apnea and produce little tidal movement of lung fluid.[13,14] The critical event in the change from placental to pulmonary gas exchange is the first inspiration, which initiates pulmonary ventilation, promotes the clearance of lung fluid, and triggers the change from the fetal to the neonatal pattern of circulation.

The first breath is a gasp that generates a transpulmonary distending pressure of 40 to 80 cm H_2O.[15] This moves the tracheal fluid (100 times more viscous than air), overcomes surface forces that develop as the air–fluid interface reaches the small airways, and overcomes tissue resistance. In some neonates, the removal of lung fluid may be delayed, producing the syndrome called *transient tachypnea of the newborn*.[16,17] Tachypnea lasts for 24 to 72 hours and is associated with a characteristic chest radiographic appearance consisting of increased perihilar markings, fluid in the interlobar fissures, and streaky linear opacities in the parenchyma.

With the onset of pulmonary ventilation, pulmonary blood flow sharply increases. Decreased pulmonary vascular resistance (PVR) and increased peripheral systemic vascular resistance (loss of the umbilical circulation) are the two crucial events involved in the immediate transition from the fetal circulation to the normal postnatal pattern. The increase in systemic afterload causes an immediate closure of the flap valve mechanism of the foramen ovale and reverses the direction of shunt through the ductus arteriosus. Until these fetal shunt pathways close anatomically, the pattern of circulation is unstable. Increased pulmonary vascular reactivity in response to hypoxia and acidosis may precipitate a reversal to right-to-left shunting ("flip-flop" circulation) (see also Chapter 18).

In the first few minutes after birth, a state of "normal" asphyxia exists as a result of the impaired placental blood flow during

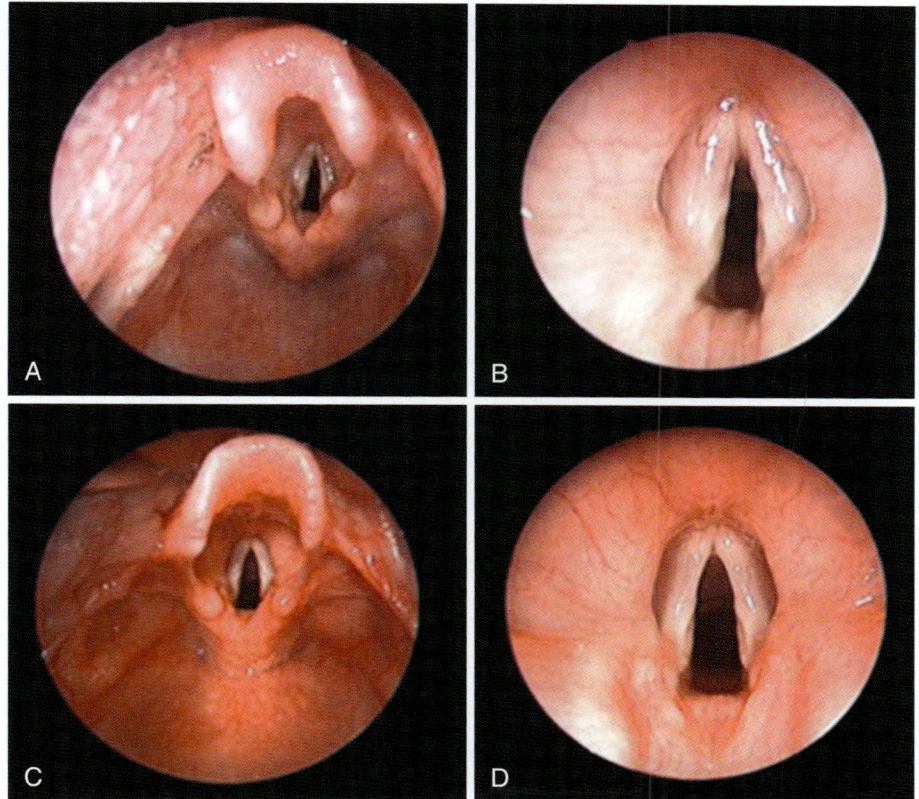

FIGURE 2.6 Larynx Development From Neonate to 2 Years Old. The larynx in the neonate (**A** and **B**), with the long epiglottis (**A**) and the vocal cords (**B**, close-up). The larynx in a 2-year-old (**C** and **D**) with a shorter epiglottis (**C**) and the vocal cords (**D**, close-up).

labor. The partial pressure of oxygen in arterial blood (PaO_2) and pH are reduced, whereas the $PaCO_2$ is increased immediately after birth, but these partial pressures change rapidly in the first hours after birth. Extrapulmonary shunting through fetal channels and intrapulmonary shunting, probably through unexpanded regions of the lung, persist for some time after birth, so that in neonates the physiologic right-to-left shunt is about three times that in adults.[18]

MECHANICS OF BREATHING

Chest Wall and Respiratory Muscles

The accessory muscles of inspiration are relatively ineffective in infants because of an unfavorable configuration of the rib cage. In infancy, the ribs extend horizontally from the vertebral column, moving little with inspiration.[19] Hence, the cross-sectional area of the thoracic cage remains fairly constant throughout the breathing cycle. In fact, inspiration depends almost exclusively on the descent of the diaphragm. These factors increase the workload on the diaphragm, rendering it at risk for fatigue, particularly in the preterm infant.

The chest wall of a neonate is floppy because it consists of noncalcified cartilage, its musculature is poorly developed, and the ribs are incompletely calcified.[20,21] As the work of breathing increases, diaphragmatic displacement must also increase to overcome these deficiencies and maintain the tidal volume. The increased workload may lead to diaphragmatic fatigue and respiratory failure or apnea, especially in preterm infants.[22,23]

Muscle strength depends on the presence of an adequate number of type I (slow twitch, high oxidative capacity) muscle fibers to respond to an increased workload. The diaphragm of the neonate and more critically, the preterm infant, has limited number type I (slow twitch, high oxidative capacity) muscle fibers (see Fig. 14.11). This compounds the risk for respiratory failure in the developing infant.

Elastic Properties of the Lung

Changes in the static pressure–volume relationship of the lungs during growth are caused by increases in volume and changes in the elastic properties of lung tissue. Volume is the principal factor that determines lung compliance, which increases throughout childhood. Specific lung compliance remains relatively constant throughout childhood.[24,25] In contrast, specific compliance of the chest wall declines throughout childhood and adolescence, reflecting the progressive calcification of the ribs and the increasing bulk of the thoracic muscles.

Static Lung Volumes

A detailed description of static lung volumes based on body weight is presented in Table 2.6.

Total Lung Capacity

Adults have a much greater total lung capacity (TLC) than infants (Fig. 2.7). This difference reflects the fact that TLC is an effort-dependent variable, dependent on the strength and efficiency of

TABLE 2.6	Age-Dependent Respiratory Variables						
	Newborn	**6 months**	**12 months**	**3 years**	**5 years**	**12 years**	**Adult**
F (breaths/minute)	50 ± 1	30 ± 5	24 ± 6	24 ± 6	23 ± 5	18 ± 5	12 ± 3
TV (mL)	21	45	78	112	270	480	575
(mL/kg)	6–8						6–7
V_E (mL/minute)	1050	1350	1780	2460	5500	6200	6400
(mL/kg per minute)	200–260						90
V_A (mL/minute)	665		1245	1760	1800	3000	3100
(mL/kg per minute)	100–150						60
V_D/V_T	0.3						0.3
V_{O_2} (mL/kg per minute)	6–8						3–4
VC (mL)	120			870	1160	3100	4000
FRC (mL)	80			490	680	1970	3000
(mL/kg)	30						30
TLC (mL)	160			1100	1500	4000	6000
(mL/kg)	63						82
pH	7.3–7.4		7.35–7.45				7.35–7.45
Pa_{O_2} (mm Hg)	60–90		80–100				80–100
Pa_{CO_2} (mm Hg)	30–35		30–40				37–42

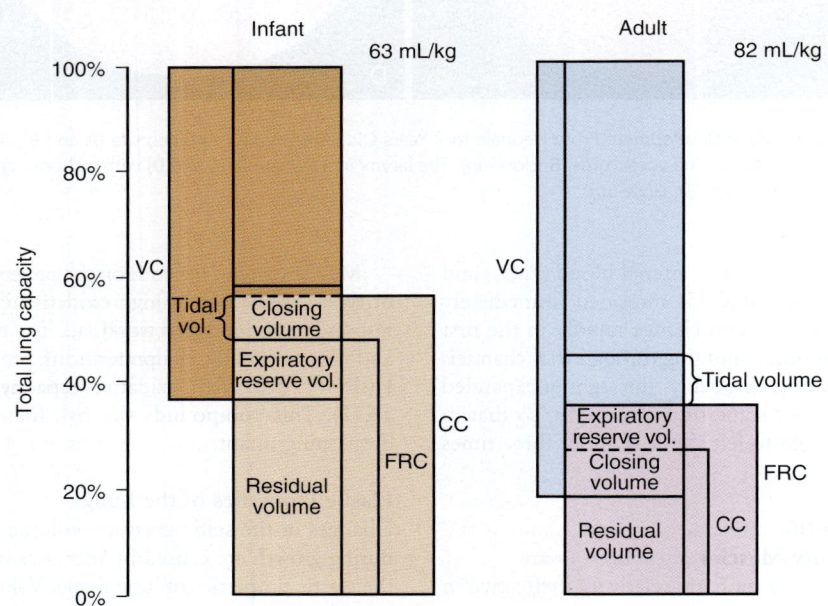

FIGURE 2.7 Lung Volumes in Infants and Adults. Note that in infants, tidal volume breathing occurs at the same volume as closing volume. *CC*, Closing capacity; *FRC*, functional residual capacity; *VC*, vital capacity. (Modified from Nelson NM. Respiration and circulation after birth. In: Smith CA, Nelson NM, eds. *The Physiology of the Newborn Infant*. Springfield, IL: Charles C Thomas; 1976; 207.)

the inspiratory muscles, which can be estimated by the maximum inspiratory pressure at functional residual capacity (FRC). An adult can generate negative pressures in excess of 100 cm H_2O; a neonate can generate pressures as great as 70 cm H_2O, a surprisingly large value considering the weaknesses cited above. This has been attributed to the small radius of curvature of the infant's rib cage, which by the Laplace relationship converts a small tension into a large pressure gradient.[26]

Functional Residual Capacity

FRC normalized to weight (per kilogram) is constant throughout development, although the mechanical factors on which it is based differ in infants and adults.[27] FRC is the volume of gas within the lungs at end of expiration, when the outward forces of the chest wall are balanced against the inward, elastic recoil of the lungs (Fig. 2.8). In the supine neonate, FRC is small, in part because the weak outward forces of the compliant chest wall are

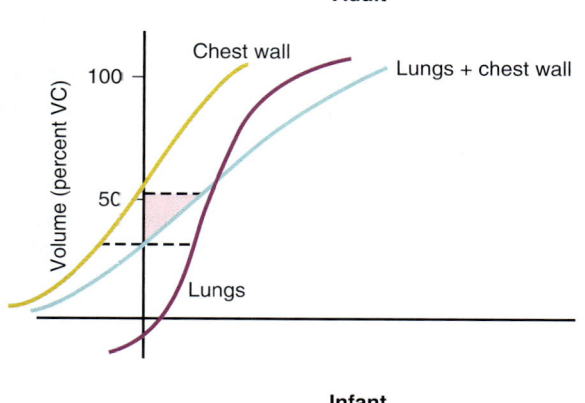

Adult

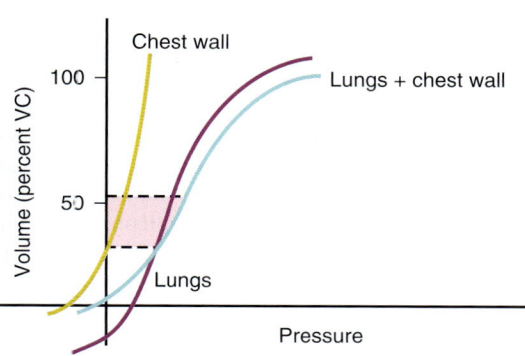

Infant

FIGURE 2.8 Compliance curves for the chest wall (yellow), lungs (purple), and thorax (combination of chest wall and lungs [blue]) in infants and adults. (Modified and reproduced with permission from Pérez Fontán JJ, Haddad GG. Respiratory physiology. In: Behrman RE, Kliegman RM, Jenson HB, eds. *Nelson Textbook of Pediatrics*. 17th ed. Philadelphia: WB Saunders; 2003:1363.)

more than offset by the elastic recoil of the lungs. In addition, the large abdomen pushes the diaphragm upward. The neonate may increase the FRC by exhaling against a closed glottis.

An important clinical implication of the dynamic control of FRC is that an apneic infant has a disproportionately smaller reserve of intrapulmonary oxygen on which to draw than a similarly affected adult. This, combined with their increased metabolic rate, contributes to the rapid development of hypoxemia if the airway becomes compromised in the anesthetized infant.

Closing Capacity

As exhalation proceeds to completion, small airways in dependent regions of the lung close, leading to air trapping in the affected areas. Closing capacity is closely related to age, decreasing throughout childhood and adolescence and increasing thereafter throughout adult life (see Fig. 2.7). This pattern of change has been related to the development and deterioration of lung elastic tissue and its effect on recoil pressure. The latter is the principal determinant of transmural pressure and therefore patency of the smallest airways, which lack intrinsic stability because they contain no cartilage.

Closing volume is within the range of tidal breathing in many older adults and some children younger than 10 years (see Fig. 2.7). It is not possible to measure closing volume in children younger than 5 years, but because the elastic recoil pressure is small in infancy (see Fig. 2.8), some airways likely remain closed throughout tidal breathing. This notion is supported by the finding that infants have a large "trapped gas volume" that is not in free communication with the conducting airways. Age-related changes in PaO_2, which parallel the changes in the difference between FRC and closing volume, may also be related to airway closure.[28]

AIRWAY DYNAMICS
Resistance and Conductance
Airway resistance decreases markedly with growth from 19 to 28 cm H_2O/L per second in neonates to less than 2 cm H_2O/L per second in adults.[27,28] Airway resistance is greater in preterm than in full-term infants. On the other hand, specific airway conductance (reciprocal of resistance) is greater in preterm infants but decreases steadily during the first 5 years of life.[29,30]

Distribution of Resistance
The distribution of airway resistance changes markedly at approximately 5 years of age. Airway resistance per gram of lung tissue is constant at all ages in the "central airways" (trachea to the twelfth to fifteenth bronchial generation), whereas it decreases markedly at approximately 5 years of age in the "peripheral airways" (i.e., distal to the twelfth to fifteenth generation to the alveoli).

Inspiratory and Expiratory Flow Limitation
Tracheal compliance in neonates is twice that of adults; it is even greater in preterm infants and appears to be a consequence of cartilaginous immaturity. The functional importance of this finding is that dynamic collapse of the trachea may occur with inspiration and expiration (see Fig. 14.10).

Regulation of Breathing
In neonates as in adults, PaO_2, $PaCO_2$, and pH control ventilation, with PaO_2 acting mainly through peripheral chemoreceptors in the carotid and aortic bodies and $PaCO_2$ and pH acting on central chemoreceptors in the medulla. In contrast to the adult, an infant's response to hypercapnia is not potentiated by hypoxia, but the latter may actually depress the hypercapnic ventilatory response in term and preterm infants.[31,32]

High concentrations of oxygen depress respiration in the neonate, whereas low concentrations stimulate it. The hypoxic response, however, is not consistent. Initially, hypoxia restores respiration to baseline but thereafter it depresses it. This pattern of response persists in normal term infants throughout the first week of life but may persist longer in preterm neonates. After this initial period, the response to persistent hypoxia gradually transitions to the adult response, which is a sustained increase in ventilation.[33,34]

Periodic breathing commonly occurs in neonates. This should be distinguished from clinical apnea, which occurs in as many as 25% of all preterm infants, especially in the most severely preterm infant. Apnea of prematurity may be a life-threatening condition. In this situation, the apneas may be prolonged and associated with desaturation of arterial oxygen, bradycardia, and loss of muscle tone. The frequency of these apneas increases in the presence of other organ pathology such as intraventricular hemorrhage.

Prematurity is an important risk factor for life-threatening apnea in neonates and infants undergoing general anesthesia.[35] The risk of postanesthetic respiratory depression is inversely related to gestational age and postconception age at the time of anesthesia (Fig. 4.7 and E-Fig. 4.5).[36] There is a general consensus that infants may be at risk for postoperative apnea up to 60 weeks after conception.[36,37]

The reduced PaO_2 of neonates is compensated by a greater oxygen-carrying capacity as a result of increased hemoglobin concentrations, which decline during the first several weeks of life. At birth, the hemoglobin (Hb) content of the blood is 50% fetal hemoglobin. The position of the oxyhemoglobin dissociation curve depends on the ratio of adult to fetal hemoglobin. At birth, the increased fetal hemoglobin content shifts the curve to the left of the adult curve (from a P_{50} of 27 for Hb A to a P_{50} of 19 for Hb F). During the first week after birth, the curve shifts to the right, reflecting the transition from fetal to adult hemoglobin formation.[24] Normal $PaCO_2$ and pH are somewhat reduced in the neonatal period compared with later infancy (see Table 2.6).

Cardiovascular System

An understanding of cardiovascular development is important for anesthesiologists. This section briefly considers developmental changes in heart rate, blood pressure, cardiac output, and the electrocardiogram; more detailed descriptions are found in Chapters 16 and 18.

HEART RATE

Autonomic control of the heart in utero is mediated predominantly through the parasympathetic nervous system. It is only shortly after birth that sympathetic control begins to appear, although the parasympathetic nervous system continues to dominate in childhood, waning only as adolescence is reached. In neonates, the heart rate may have a wide variation that is within normal limits. The mean heart rate in neonates in the first 24 hours of life is 120 beats per minute. It increases to a mean of 160 beats per minute at 1 month, after which it gradually decreases to 75 beats per minute at adolescence (Table 2.7).[38]

In older children, a significant number of arrhythmias and conduction abnormalities are also encountered, with marked fluctuations in heart rate caused by variations in autonomic tone.

BLOOD PRESSURE

Mean systolic blood pressure in neonates and infants increases from 65 mm Hg in the first 12 hours of life to 75 mm Hg at 4 days and 95 mm Hg at 6 weeks. There is little change in mean systolic pressure between 6 weeks and 1 year of age and even between 1 year and 6 years; thereafter, systolic pressure gradually increases with age.[39,40] These measurements apply to infants and children who are awake and calm. The blood pressure in preterm infants in the first 12 hours is less than that in full-term infants; a gradual increase in blood pressure occurs after birth—68/43 mm Hg on day 1 of life compared with 90/55 mm Hg on day 90 of life (Table 2.8).[41,42] Blood pressure measured in the lower extremity is less than in the upper extremity in children.[43] It has also been noted that infants with birth asphyxia and those who require mechanical ventilation have reduced blood pressures.

Blood pressure in adolescents and adults who were born premature is greater than in those who were born full-term. However, with the slower fetal growth in preterm neonates, LBW was not identified as an independent predictor of this greater blood pressure later in life.[44]

CARDIAC OUTPUT

Determination of cardiac output and blood pressure allows calculation of systemic vascular resistance. It provides important information relating to the left ventricular afterload and allows rational application of vasoactive (e.g., vasoconstrictor, vasodilator) and inotropic drugs. Measurement of cardiac output may be carried out by the Fick method (using oxygen extraction) or thermodilution using a pulmonary artery flow-directed catheter. In neonates, the latter technique is rarely used because shunts at the atrial and ductal levels introduce errors when interpreting the results.

Pulsed Doppler determinations of cardiac output provide reasonable noninvasive estimates of cardiac output for clinical application in neonates. Cardiac output, normalized for body weight, in neonates between 780 and 4740 g at birth, remains fairly constant, changing only 10% over this weight range.[45] The range of cardiac output in both full-term and preterm neonates is 220 to 350 mL/kg per minute, two- to threefold greater than in adults.[45,46] Between birth and the end of the first year, mean cardiac output (normalized for body weight or surface area) remains fairly constant at 204 ± 45 mL/kg per minute.[47] The relatively large cardiac output (in milliliters per minute per kilogram) in neonates reflects their greater metabolic rate (on a weight basis) and oxygen consumption compared with adults. Basal metabolic rate has been shown to increase as size decreases in all species[48] (see Chapter 7).

Pulsed Doppler estimation of cardiac output has also been found useful in assessing left ventricular myocardial dysfunction in neonates after perinatal asphyxia and acidosis, as well as its response to therapy.[49,50] In older children, measurements of cardiac

TABLE 2.7	The Relationship Between Age and Heart Rate[a]
Age	**Mean Heart Rate in Beats per Minute (range)**
Premature	120–170
0–3 months	100–150
3–6 months	90–120
6–12 months	80–120
1–3 years	70–110
3–6 years	65–110
6–12 years	60–95
>12 years	55–85

Data from Hartman ME, Cheifetz IM. Pediatric emergencies and resuscitation. In: Kliegman RM, Stanton ST BF, Geme III JW, Schor NF, Behrman RE, eds. *Nelson Textbook of Pediatrics.* 19th ed. Philadelphia: Elsevier; 2011:280.
[a]Note that the heart rate will be lower during sleep or during anesthesia.

TABLE 2.8	The Relationship Between Age and Blood Pressure[a]	
	Normal Blood Pressure (mm Hg)	
Age	*Mean Systolic*	*Mean Diastolic*
Premature	55–75	35–45
0–3 months	65–85	45–55
3–6 months	70–90	50–65
6–12 months	80–100	55–65
1–3 years	90–105	55–70
3–6 years	95–110	60–75
6–12 years	100–120	60–75
>12 years	110–135	65–85

Data from Hartman ME, Cheifetz IM. Pediatric emergencies and resuscitation. In: Kliegman RM, Stanton ST BF, Geme III JW, Schor NF, Behrman RE, eds. *Nelson Textbook of Pediatrics.* 19th ed. Philadelphia: Elsevier; 2011:280.
[a]Note that the blood pressure will be lower during sleep or during anesthesia.

output are necessary in circulatory shock.[51] New noninvasive techniques using changes in impedance hold promise for the future (see Chapter 52; Figs. 52.9 and 52.10).

NORMAL ELECTROCARDIOGRAPHIC FINDINGS

The P wave reflects atrial depolarization and varies little with age. The PR interval increases with age (mean value for the first year is 0.10 sec, increasing to 0.14 sec at 12 to 16 years).[52] The duration of the QRS complex increases with age, but prolongation greater than 0.10 sec is abnormal at any age.

At birth, the QRS axis is right sided, reflecting the predominant right ventricular intrauterine development. It shifts leftward in the first month as left ventricular muscle hypertrophies. Thereafter, the QRS follows a gradual change toward a left-sided axis.

In addition, T waves are upright in all chest leads. Within hours, they become isoelectric or inverted over the left chest; by the seventh day, the T waves are inverted in V_4R (V_4 position under the right clavicle), V_1, and across to V_4. From then on, the T waves remain inverted over the right chest until adolescence, when they become upright over the right side of the chest again. Failure of T waves to become inverted in V_4R and V_1 to V_4 by 7 days may be the earliest electrocardiographic evidence of right ventricular hypertrophy (see also Chapter 16).[53,54]

Renal System

The complex development of the human kidney begins in week 4 of gestation and continues into adulthood. Serious renal malfunction is usually associated with growth retardation.

Urine production begins in utero at 10 to 12 weeks of gestation and is excreted into the amniotic cavity, helping to maintain amniotic fluid volume. The fetus maintains its metabolic homeostasis through the placenta. It is only after birth that the kidney assumes this responsibility. More than 90% of neonates will have voided urine within the first 24 hours after birth. All normal neonates should void by 48 hours after birth; otherwise, they should be investigated for anomalies including posterior urethral valves.[55]

Tubular function begins to develop after 34 weeks of gestation and reaches adult levels by 2 years of age.[56] The number and function of the Na^+/K^+-ATPase transporters are reduced at birth, although their activity increases 5- to 10-fold in the postnatal period. All transporters that rely on the Na^+ gradient are also reduced in function. The renal tubular threshold for resorption of Na^+, glucose, and bicarbonate are decreased in the neonatal period; hence, they are at increased risk for hyponatremia, osmotic polyuria, and metabolic acidosis, respectively.

Nephrogenesis is complete by 36 weeks of gestation. Renal blood flow and glomerular filtration rate (GFR) are reduced and correlate with gestational age. GFR is 20% to 25% of adult rates at term. They increase rapidly in the postnatal period as the result of an increase in cardiac output and a decrease in renal vascular resistance. Adult rates are achieved by approximately 2 years of age[57] (see Fig. 7.12). A reduced GFR significantly affects the ability of the neonate to excrete saline and water loads, as well as drugs. At birth, the serum creatinine concentration reflects the maternal concentration, but this value decreases during the first days after birth. As a result of the rapid growth and increase in muscular mass, normal serum creatinine values increase with age and are greater in males. Creatinine clearance slowly increases in neonates, reaching adult values between 2 and 3 years of age.

In utero, the fetus maintains a mild respiratory acidosis, with a similar plasma bicarbonate concentration, but a greater $PaCO_2$ than its mother. After birth, plasma bicarbonate concentration and $PaCO_2$ are reduced in neonates and infants compared with older children and adults. In addition, the basal acid production in neonates is comparatively greater than in adults and they are less able to respond to an acid load. Endogenous acid production in small children is between 50% and 100% greater per kilogram than adults. This is primarily due to the deposition of Ca^{2+} in bone, a process that produces 0.5 to 1 mEq/ L of acid per day. Bicarbonate absorption from the gastrointestinal tract is an important source of base to neutralize this nonvolatile acid, and in part, explains the tendency of infants to become profoundly acidotic when suffering from gastroenteritis. The neonate or infant is living near its limit of acid compensation and is therefore prone to develop acidosis during the course of an acute illness or starvation.

Neonates and preterm infants are obligate salt losers; they cannot excrete a large salt load or concentrate urine effectively. Immaturity of distal tubular function and relative hypoaldosteronism explain why preterm infants are at increased risk for hyperkalemia.[58]

Digestive and Endocrine System

HEPATIC SYSTEM

Development of the liver and bile ducts begins as an outgrowth of the foregut; by 10 weeks of gestation, the biliary tract has completed its development. The vitelline veins give rise to the portal and hepatic veins. Hepatic sinusoids form the ductus venosus, the bridge between the hepatic vein and the inferior vena cava. Most umbilical venous blood from the placenta passes through the ductus venosus to the inferior vena cava. The remainder passes via the portal vein through the liver to the hepatic veins. The portal venous drainage to the left lobe is less than to the right lobe, leading to a relative underdevelopment of the left lobe. The ductus venosus closes soon after birth.[59]

At 12 weeks of gestation there is evidence of gluconeogenesis and protein synthesis; at 14 weeks, glycogen is found in liver cells. Although by late gestation liver cell morphology is similar to that of adults, the functional development of the liver is immature in neonates and more so in preterm infants. The liver has a major role in metabolism, controlling carbohydrate, protein, and lipid delivery to the tissues. Toward the end of pregnancy, large amounts of glycogen appear in the liver, and, as a result, preterm and small-for-gestational-age (SGA) infants accrue smaller stores of glycogen and are prone to develop hypoglycemia. Bile acid secretion in neonates is reduced, and malabsorption of fat occurs.

The liver is the site for the synthesis of proteins; this process is active in fetal and neonatal life. In fetal life, the main serum protein is alpha-fetoprotein. This protein first appears at 6 weeks of gestation and reaches a peak at 13 weeks. Albumin synthesis starts at 3 to 4 months of gestation and approaches adult values by birth; in preterm infants, the level is reduced. Proteins involved in clotting are also formed in the liver, but their concentrations in preterm and full-term neonates are less than normal for the first few days after birth. Hematopoiesis occurs in the fetal liver, with peak activity at 7 months of gestation. After 6 weeks of age, hematopoiesis is confined to the bone marrow except under pathologic conditions, such as hemolytic anemia (see Chapter 30).

The capacity to enzymatically break down proteins is reduced at birth but matures rapidly throughout the first year, reaching

TABLE 2.9	Causes of Jaundice in Neonates
Excess bilirubin production	
Impaired uptake of bilirubin	
Impaired conjugation of bilirubin	
Defective bilirubin excretion	
Increased enterohepatic circulation of bilirubin	

TABLE 2.10	Pathologic Causes of Jaundice in Neonates
Antibody-induced hemolysis (Rh and ABO)	
Hereditary red blood cell disorders (e.g., glucose-6-phosphate dehydrogenase deficiency, which gives rise to hemolysis from drugs or infection)	
Infections (e.g., neonatal hepatitis, sepsis, severe urinary tract infections)	
Hemorrhage into the body (e.g., intracerebral)	
Biliary atresia	
Metabolic (e.g., hypothyroidism, galactosemia)	

adult levels by adolescence. This is particularly important in preterm infants, in whom the intake of a large protein load can result in dangerously high levels of serum amino acid concentrations and the subsequent development of a metabolic acidosis. In addition to less effective hepatic metabolism, altered drug binding by serum proteins and immature renal function contribute to the disposition of proteins (see also Chapter 7).

Physiologic Jaundice

Hyperbilirubinemia (defined as a total serum bilirubin level >5 mg/dL) is a particularly important problem in neonates. About 60% of term and 80% of preterm neonates develop jaundice in the first week of life, with a total bilirubin concentration exceeding 5 mg/dL.[60] Several mechanisms account for the jaundice (Table 2.9).[61,62] In term neonates, the normal total bilirubin concentration is usually less than 5 mg/dL (86 μmol/L) and is rarely greater than 12 mg/dL without a risk factor, peaking on the third to fourth postnatal day. In preterm infants, the bilirubin concentration peaks at 10 to 12 mg/dL on the fifth to seventh postnatal day. After this period, the concentration gradually decreases, reaching adult values (<2 mg/dL) by 1 to 2 months in both term and preterm infants. The concentration of indirect bilirubin is also increased in the first few days after birth. The cause of nonhemolytic physiologic hyperbilirubinemia is excessive bilirubin production from breakdown of red blood cells and increased enterohepatic circulation of bilirubin with deficient hepatic conjugation as a result of decreased uridine 5-diphospho-glucuronyl transferase activity (UGT1A1, see Chapters 7 and 30). The relationship between breastfeeding and hyperbilirubinemia has been well documented. It is usually delayed in onset (after the third postnatal day), its cause remains unclear, and it occurs in about 1% of breastfeeding infants. An earlier hypothesis ascribing it to inhibition of UGT activity by 3α, 20β-pregnanediol activity has not been substantiated. In addition, genetic variants may affect bilirubin metabolism.[63,64]

Important pathologic causes of jaundice in neonates are presented in Table 2.10. The relative rarity of cholestasis is in sharp contrast with the very common finding of jaundice during the first weeks of life, and therefore, a false diagnosis of physiologic or breast milk jaundice is easily made. Symptoms indicative of cholestasis such as dark urine and pale stools are often unrecognized.[65]

Once the distinction between physiologic and hemolytic hyperbilirubinemia has been made, the underlying cause can then be treated and efforts can be directed at preventing bilirubin induced encephalopathy (kernicterus) by the use of phototherapy and, in selected cases, exchange transfusions. Phototherapy reduces serum bilirubin concentrations by converting bilirubin through structural photoisomerization and photooxidation into excretable products.[66] There are risks and consequences to phototherapy, particularly in VLBW infants.[67] However, phototherapy is not associated with the development of benign or malignant melanocyte lesions.[68]

Sick preterm infants are especially at risk for kernicterus and are more aggressively treated at reduced bilirubin concentrations than full-term infants. Increasingly common is a form of cholestatic jaundice in LBW infants receiving hyperalimentation for prolonged periods. The mechanism of the jaundice is unclear, although it has been attributed to the inhibition of bile flow by amino acids.[69] Promising therapies for hyperbilirubinemia in LBW infants may include the use of tin-mesoporphyrin, which inhibits the production of bilirubin.[70]

GASTROINTESTINAL TRACT

In an embryo, the digestive tract consists of the developing foregut and hindgut. These rapidly elongate so that a loop of gut is forced into the yolk sac. At 5 to 7 weeks, this loop twists around the axis of the superior mesenteric artery and returns to the abdominal cavity. Maturation occurs gradually from the proximal to the distal end. Blood vessels and nerves (Auerbach and Meissner plexuses) are developed by 13 weeks of gestation and peristalsis begins. The pancreas arises from two outgrowths of the foregut; a diverticulum of the foregut gives rise to the liver.

Enzyme levels of enterokinase and lipase increase with gestational age but are reduced at birth compared with older children. Full-term neonates and preterm neonates handle protein loads reasonably well, although preterm neonates may have difficulty with large loads. Fat digestion is limited, particularly in preterm neonates, who absorb only 65% of adult levels. Neonatal duodenal motility undergoes marked maturational changes between 29 and 32 weeks of gestation. This is one factor limiting tolerance of enteral feeding before 29 to 30 weeks of gestation. Central nervous system abnormalities will delay these maturational changes.[71]

Swallowing is a complex process under central and peripheral control. The reflex is initiated in the medulla, through cranial nerves to the muscles that control the passage of food through the pharyngoesophageal sphincter. In the process, the tongue, soft palate, pharynx, and larynx all are smoothly coordinated. Any pathologic condition of these structures can interfere with normal swallowing. Neuromuscular incoordination, however, is more likely to be responsible for any dysfunction. This is particularly evident when the central nervous system has sustained damage either before or during delivery.

Lower esophageal sphincter pressures are reduced at birth but increase steadily, reaching adult values by 3 to 6 weeks postnatal age. Daily vomiting or "spitting up" is reported in half of all infants between 0 and 3 months of age and in up to two-thirds of infants 4 to 6 months of age.[72] Most of these infants suffer no ill effect ("happy spitters") and grow normally.[73] This condition usually begins in the first weeks after birth and resolves spontaneously by 9 to 24 months of age as solid food is introduced and the child assumes the upright position. Between 1:300 and 1:1000 infants have gastroesophageal reflux significant enough to warrant treatment to prevent complications.[74]

Meconium is the material contained in the intestinal tract before birth. It consists of desquamated epithelial cells from the intestinal tract, bile, pancreatic and intestinal secretions, and water (70%). Meconium is usually passed in the first few hours after birth; virtually all term neonates pass their first stool by 48 hours. However, passage of the first stool is usually delayed in LBW neonates, possibly because of immaturity of bowel motility and lack of gut hormones as a result of delayed enteral feeding. Meconium ileus occurs in cystic fibrosis or Hirschsprung disease.

The gastrointestinal transit time in the neonate is less than that in the adult but increases with age. The normal physiologic range of stool frequency varies greatly (from 10 times per day to 1–2 times per week)[75] and more often in breastfed infants. The frequency of bowel movements gradually decreases during the first years of life, reaching adult habits at about 4 years of age.

Necrotizing enterocolitis (NEC) is an acquired gastrointestinal disease associated with significant morbidity and mortality in prematurely born neonates. The disease affects about 10% of preterm neonates weighing less than 1500 g or 1% to 5% of all neonatal intensive care unit admissions (see also Chapter 37).

PANCREAS

The placenta is impermeable to both insulin and glucagon. The islets of Langerhans in the fetal pancreas, however, secrete insulin from week 11 of fetal life; the amount of insulin secretion increases with age. After birth, the insulin response is related to gestational and postnatal ages and is more mature in term infants.

Maternal hyperglycemia, particularly when uncontrolled, results in hypertrophy and hyperplasia of the fetal islets of Langerhans. This leads to increased levels of insulin in the fetus, affecting lipid metabolism and giving rise to a large, overweight neonate characteristic of a mother with diabetes (infant of a diabetic mother, IDM). Hyperglycemia alone is not instrumental in this effect; an IDM may also be the result of an increase in serum amino acids in diabetic mothers. Hyperinsulinemia of the fetus persists after birth and may lead to rapid development of serious hypoglycemia. In addition to severe hypoglycemia, the incidence of congenital anomalies is increased in these neonates.

Neonates who are SGA are frequently hypoglycemic, possibly as a result of malnutrition in utero. In addition, hepatic glycogen stores are inadequate, and deficient gluconeogenesis exists. Preterm neonates may be hypoglycemic without demonstrable symptoms, necessitating close monitoring of blood glucose levels.

Full-term neonates undergo a metabolic adjustment postnatally with regard to glucose. Studies have defined values abnormal glucose concentrations as follows: plasma glucose concentrations less than 35 mg/dL in the first 3 hours after birth; less than 40 mg/dL between 3 and 24 hours; and less than 45 mg/dL after 24 hours.[76] It is important to recognize that neonates may develop serious hypoglycemia that could lead to irreversible central nervous system damage, even though they may demonstrate few or no signs and symptoms. Other neonates may present with seizures, but signs may also be subtle (e.g., lethargy, somnolence, and jitteriness).

Hyperglycemia (plasma glucose ≥150 mg/dL) occurs in stressed neonates, particularly in LBW neonates receiving glucose-containing solutions. Hyperglycemia commonly occurs in neonates and infants during elective surgery under general anesthesia; infusion of glucose-containing solutions may increase the risk of hyperglycemia.

Thus it is advisable that intraoperative glucose concentrations be monitored. A study in infants undergoing surgery under general anesthesia showed that postsurgical plasma glucose values were significantly greater than postinduction values; insulin changes, however, were minimal.[77] The risk of hyperglycemia is considerably greater in infants weighing less than 1000 g compared with infants 2000 g or greater.[78] Hyperglycemia may also lead to osmotic diuresis and dehydration and has been associated with an increased incidence of intraventricular hemorrhage and a neurologic handicap. It is recommended that intraoperative glucose-containing solutions be administered with an infusion pump and only run at basal rates (see also Chapter 9).

Hematopoietic and Immunologic System

The blood volume in a full-term neonate depends on the time of cord clamping, which modifies the volume of placental transfusion. The blood volume is 93 mL/kg when cord clamping is delayed after delivery, compared with 82 mL/kg with immediate cord clamping.[79] Within the first 4 hours after delivery, however, fluid is lost from the blood and the plasma volume contracts by as much as 25%. The larger the placental transfusion, the greater the loss of fluid in the first few hours after birth, resulting in hemoconcentration. The blood volume in preterm infants is greater (90 to 105 mL/kg) than in full-term neonates because of increased plasma volume.

HEMOGLOBIN

The normal range of hemoglobin in the neonate is 14 to 20 g/dL. The site of sampling must be considered when interpreting these values for the diagnosis of neonatal anemia or hyperviscosity syndrome. Capillary sampling (e.g., heel stick) generally overestimates the true hemoglobin concentration because of stasis in peripheral vessels that decreases the volume of plasma and causes hemoconcentration. The net effect may be an increase in hemoglobin concentration by as much as 6 g/dL; venipuncture is preferred over capillary sampling. In 1% of infants, fetal-maternal transfusion before the umbilical cord is cut may explain many of the "lower normal" hemoglobin values reported.

Erythropoietic activity from the bone marrow decreases immediately after birth in both full-term and preterm infants. The cord blood reticulocyte counts of 5% persist for a few days and decline below 1% by 1 week. This is followed by a slight increase to 1% to 2% by the 12th week, where it remains throughout childhood. Preterm infants have greater reticulocyte counts (up to 10%) at birth. Abnormal reticulocyte values generally reflect hemorrhage or hemolysis.

In term neonates, the hemoglobin concentration decreases during the 9th to 12th weeks to reach a nadir of 10 to 11 g/dL (hematocrit 30% to 33%) but increases thereafter. This decrease in hemoglobin concentration is the result of a decrease in erythropoiesis and, to some extent, to a shortened life span of the red blood cells. In preterm infants, the decrease in the hemoglobin concentration is greater and directly related to the degree of prematurity; also, the nadir is reached earlier (4 to 8 weeks).[80] In infants weighing 800 to 1000 g, the decrement may reach a very small concentration, 8 g/dL. This "anemia" (physiologic anemia of the newborn) is a normal physiologic adjustment to extrauterine life. Despite the reduction in hemoglobin, the oxygen delivery to the tissues may not be compromised because of a shift of the oxygen-hemoglobin dissociation curve (to the right), secondary to an increase of 2,3-diphosphoglycerate.[81] In addition, fetal hemoglobin is replaced by adult hemoglobin, which also results in a shift in the same direction. In neonates, especially preterm neonates, reduced hemoglobin concentrations may be associated with apnea and tachycardia.[82] Vitamin E administration does not prevent anemia of prematurity; no significant difference was noted between vitamin E–supplemented and unsupplemented groups in terms of hemoglobin concentration, reticulocyte and platelet counts, or erythrocyte morphology in infants at 6 weeks of age.[83] Infants with anemia of prematurity have an inadequate production of erythropoietin (the primary regulator in erythropoiesis). Some centers now use recombinant human erythropoietin in VLBW infants to stimulate erythropoiesis and decrease the need for transfusions.[44,84]

After the third month, the hemoglobin concentration stabilizes at 11.5 to 12 g/dL until about 2 years of age. The hemoglobin concentration in full-term and preterm infants is comparable after the first year. Thereafter, there is a gradual increase in the hemoglobin concentration to mean values at puberty of 14 g/dL for females and 15.5 g/dL for males (see also Chapter 10).

LEUKOCYTE AND IMMUNOLOGY

The white blood cell count may normally reach 21,000/mm^3 in the first 24 hours of life and 12,000/mm^3 at the end of the first week, with the number of neutrophils equaling the number of lymphocytes. The white blood cell count then decreases gradually, reaching adult values by puberty. At birth, neutrophil granulocytes predominate but rapidly decrease in number so that from the first week of life through 4 years of age, the lymphocyte is the predominant cell. After the fourth year, the values approximate adult values. Neonates have an increased susceptibility to bacterial infection, which is related in part to immaturity of leukocyte function. Sepsis may be associated with a minimal leukocyte response or even with leukopenia. Spurious increases in the white blood cell content may be due to drugs (e.g., epinephrine). The incidence of neonatal sepsis correlates inversely with gestational age and may be as great as 58% in VLBW infants.[85]

PLATELETS

Thrombocytopenia is a common hematologic finding in neonates, occurring in 1% to 2% of healthy term neonates.[86] Mechanical ventilation has been associated with a significant decrease in the platelet count in neonates.[87] There appears to be an inverse correlation between gestational age or birth weight and the severity of platelet reduction. A study of neonatal thrombocytopenia and its impact on hemostatic integrity showed that thrombocytopenic infants are at greater risk for bleeding than equally sick nonthrombocytopenic infants (see Chapters 10, 20, and 37).

COAGULATION

At birth, vitamin K–dependent factors (i.e., II, VII, IX, and X) are 20% to 60% of adult values; in preterm infants, the values are even less. The result is prolonged prothrombin times, normally encountered in full-term and preterm neonates. Synthesis of vitamin K–dependent factors occurs in the liver, which, being immature, produces relatively small concentrations of coagulation factors, even with the administration of vitamin K. It takes several weeks for the levels of coagulation factors to reach adult values; the deficit is even more pronounced in preterm neonates. Vitamin K prophylaxis has been evaluated,[88] and the evidence demonstrates that the majority of cases of neonatal vitamin K deficiency occur in normal neonates. Thus all neonates should receive prophylactic vitamin K soon after birth to prevent hemorrhagic disease of the neonate. Its omission could lead to serious and life-threatening consequences, especially if surgery is undertaken. However, in theory, the increasing risk of bleeding is balanced by the protective effects of physiologic deficiencies of coagulation inhibitors, as well as by the decreased fibrinolytic capacity. Developmental hemostasis should be considered, as well as laboratory variations of coagulation tests that may render any diagnosis of bleeding disorder in infants difficult to establish.[89,90]

Infants of mothers who have received anticonvulsant drugs during pregnancy may develop a serious coagulopathy similar to that encountered with vitamin K deficiency.[91] Administration of Vitamin K$_1$ to neonates usually reverses this bleeding tendency, but deaths have occurred despite therapy. Other risk factors include maternal use of drugs such as warfarin, rifampin, and isoniazid. Breastfeeding may also be associated with severe vitamin K deficiency; exclusively breastfed infants should receive vitamin supplementation.

POLYCYTHEMIA

Neonatal polycythemia (central hematocrit greater than 65%) occurs in 3% to 5% of full-term neonates.[92] Using M-mode echocardiography, a study of neonates demonstrated an increase in PVR with hyperviscosity.[93] Partial exchange transfusion to reduce the hematocrit and decrease the blood viscosity improves systemic and pulmonary blood flow and oxygen transport, although one review questioned the efficacy when the exchange transfusion was conducted after 6 hours of life in asymptomatic infants.[94] The increased organ blood flow should prevent the cardiovascular and neurologic symptoms associated with the hyperviscosity syndrome.

Neurologic Development and Cognitive Development Issues

NEUROLOGIC DEVELOPMENT

Reduction of perinatal mortality during the past decade has not resulted in the expected reduction in the prevalence of cerebral palsy (1/500 live births). The most common etiologies of cerebral palsy are perinatal ischemic stroke, white matter disorder, and intrauterine inflammation.[95] Less than 5% of cases of cerebral palsy result from perinatal asphyxia. The strongest predictors of cerebral palsy appear to be congenital anomaly (congenital heart disease in particular), low birth weight, low placental weight, multiple fetuses, preterm delivery, intrauterine infection, or abnormal fetal position before labor and delivery.[96]

The nervous system is anatomically complete at birth; functionally it remains immature with the continuation of myelination and synaptogenesis. Myelination is usually complete by 7 years of age. An infant's normal mental development depends on the maturation of the central nervous system. This development may be affected by physical illness, inadequate psychosocial support, or poor nutrition. In a randomized trial of diet in preterm babies, a suboptimal diet resulted in reduced intelligence quotients 7 to 8 years later.[97]

The potential adverse effects of many medications used to provide anesthesia on the developing brain of animal models show how delicate this organ is and how its development may be affected by environmental agents (see Chapter 25). Two studies in humans lend support to the notion that a brief exposure to general anesthesia does not harm young children.[98,99]

The rate of brain growth is different from the growth rate of other body systems. The brain has two growth spurts: neuronal cell multiplication between 15 and 20 weeks of gestation and glial cell multiplication commencing at 25 weeks and extending into the second year of life. Myelination continues into the third year. Malnutrition during this phase of neural development may have profound handicapping effects.

Plasma membrane transport selectively promotes the passage of essential substrates such as glucose, organic acids, and amino acids across the blood-brain barrier. Hypoxemia and ischemia may lead to a breakdown in this barrier, with resulting edema and increased intracranial pressure. Injury to the blood-brain barrier may result from abnormal entry of calcium or formation of free radicals. Further studies of the mechanism of this breakdown will lead to rational approaches to therapy. In preterm neonates stressed by hypoxia, the blood-brain barrier may become particularly permeable to the water-soluble unbound bilirubin, with possible damage to the brain.[100]

Full-term neonates show various primitive reflexes including the Moro response and grasp reflex. Milestones of development are useful indicators of mental and physical development guiding expectations for both normal and abnormal development. These milestones represent the *average child*, but there is a range of maturation of different body functions that are within the normal range.[101] The Denver Developmental Screening Test is useful for assessing these milestones. The test focuses on four areas of development: (1) gross motor function, (2) fine motor and adaptive skills, (3) language, and (4) personal and social skills. Developing infants rapidly acquire motor skills beginning with control of posture in a cephalocaudal direction; this begins with head control and rapidly progresses to sitting, standing, walking, and finally running (Table 2.11).

Adaptive skills are performed through well-coordinated fine motor movements (Table 2.12). Abnormal development may be reflected in a delay in appearance of a particular milestone or in its pathologic persistence with maturation in a child. For example, at 5 months, a child reaches and retrieves objects, frequently placing them in his or her mouth. As an infant matures, however, this behavior pattern usually ceases at 12 to 13 months of age; in infants with developmental delay, this oral practice may continue for a longer period of time.

Language development correlates closely with cognitive skills (Table 2.13). Personal and social skills are modified by environmental factors and cultural patterns (Table 2.14). Development of walking, speech, and sphincter control is most important. For appropriate evaluation consider familial patterns, level of intelligence, and physical illness. Deafness may cause delayed speech.

INTERACTIONS WITH THE EXTERNAL WORLD DURING GROWTH AND DEVELOPMENT

The environment with all its potential toxins and pollutants may have a direct influence on growth and development, interfering with both physiologic and pathologic aspects. For the two past decades, we have known that programmed cell death (or apoptosis)

is part of normal development[102] and that triggering factors result from both evolutionary pathways and external influences. This occurs at both anatomic and functional levels and opens the potential for many and varied investigations. Neurogenesis, particularly in specific parts of the brain such as the hippocampus, has long been thought to occur only during development, but recent evidence has shown that it continues throughout human life and both genetics and inflammation may hold the keys to neurodegenerative disorders.[103,104] Implications of an interaction between memory and its influence on degenerative neurologic diseases are now firmly established.[105] Anesthetic drugs have been shown to adversely affect the developing brain in rodents and primates, but with the discovery of neurogenesis in adults, we now know that similar changes occur in adults as well.[106–108] However, recent evidence suggests it is quite unlikely that anesthetics affect the neurobehavioral changes in human infants and toddlers (see also Chapter 25).

Evidence has confirmed that the functional aspect of brain development in the fetus is far more complex than previously thought and is not limited just to the last weeks before birth.[109] A waking-like brain state exists that is present earlier in gestation and inducible with maternal behavioural changes and external stimuli (e.g., music).[110] These factors may have long-term neurodevelopmental effects and the beginning of memorization likely occurs earlier than previously thought.[111] A mother's voice, heartbeat, speech, and language all impact the fetal neural plasticity.[112–115]

In addition, a large number of interactions between the neonate and the external world exist. The child has some direct influences on his or her external environment. The ethnologic concept of

TABLE 2.12	Relationship of Fine Motor/Adaptive Milestones to Age	
Fine Motor/Adaptive Milestones	**Age**
Grasps rattle	3 months
Passes cube hand to hand	6 months
Pincer grip	1 year
Imitates vertical line	2 years
Copies circle	3 years

TABLE 2.13	Relationship of Language Milestones to Age
Language Milestones	**Age**
Squeals	1.5–3 months
Turns to voice	6 months
Combines two words	1.5 years
Composes short sentences	2 years
Gives entire name	3 years

TABLE 2.11	Relationship of Motor Milestones to Age
Motor Milestone	**Age**
Supports head	3 months
Sits alone	6 months
Stands alone	12 months
Balances on one foot	3 years

TABLE 2.14	Relationship of Personal-Social Milestones to Age
Personal-Social Milestones	**Age**
Smiles spontaneously	3 months
Feeds self crackers	6 months
Drinks from cup	1 year
Plays interactive games	2 years

"baby schema" was proposed by Lorenz,[116] who suggested that some type of positive features can result in a positive response in the human.[117,118] Infantile physical features, such as a round face and big eyes, are perceived as cute and motivate caretaking behavior in the human, with the evolutionary function of enhancing offspring survival. This has been observed across animal species.[119] A baby's smile, for example, can increase the speed of the caring response[120,121] and narrow the intentional focus of the mother independently of face recognition.[122,123] Comparisons between neurophysiologic and neuropsychological studies are difficult but may prove an important confounding factor in our search to understand the complexities of human growth and development.

ACKNOWLEDGMENT

The author acknowledges the prior contributions of Ronald Gore, Jonathan H. Cronin, Robert M. Insoft, and I. David Todres to this chapter.

ANNOTATED REFERENCES

Friis-Hansen B. Body water compartments in children: changes during growth and related changes in body composition. *Pediatrics*. 1961;28:169-181.
This classic paper describes body water compartments in children and their changes with age. Results still hold true and are widely used today.

Holliday MA, Segar WE. The maintenance need for water in parenteral fluid therapy. *Pediatrics*. 1957;19:823-832.
Another classic paper outlining fluid requirements in children. The paper served as a reference for many years but has come under recent criticsm and a reanalysis of fluid and electrolyte requirents in children.

Ameisen JC. On the origin, evolution, and nature of programmed cell death: a timeline of four billion years. *Cell Death Differ*. 2002;9:367-393.
This paper discusses how programmed cell death is a genetically regulated process of cell suicide that is central to the development, homeostasis and integrity of multicellular organisms. Dysregulation of mechanisms controlling cell suicide plays a role in the pathogenesis of a wide range of diseases. The author explores these processes that also have relevance to current debate concerning the effects of anaesthesia on neonatal development.

Kotecha S. Lung growth for beginners. *Paediatr Respir Rev*. 2000;1:308-313.
A great primer that can be used as a foundation for further learning.

Nowakowski RS, Hayes NL. CNS development: an overview. *Dev Psychopathol*. 1999;11:395-417.
Another classic paper that serves as a great primer.

Sottas C, Cumin D, Anderson BJ. Blood pressure and heart rates in neonates and preschool children; an analysis from ten years of electronic recording. *Pediatr Anesth*. 2016;26:1064-1070.
Blood pressure in children undergoing anesthesia is generally lower than that observed in healthy awake children. There is concern about what is an acceptable lower limit, particularly in the very young. The authors review observed blood pressure from a single institution involving 54,896 anaesthetics in children younger than 6 years. A mean blood pressure drop of 28.6% was noted in infants 0-10 weeks of age.

A complete reference list can be found online at ExpertConsult.com

Perioperative Behavioral Stress in Children

3

PADMA GULUR, MICHELLE A. FORTIER, LINDA C. MAYES, AND ZEEV N. KAIN

INTEREST IN CHILDREN'S PERIOPERATIVE behavior has increased dramatically over the past 20 years. Specifically, the recognition of the importance of developmental factors in perioperative research has created a dramatic growth of investigation in this area. In this chapter, we discuss developmental considerations that are relevant to the child's perioperative experience (cognitive development, attachment and separation, temperament). We then offer a review and synthesis of recent data on preoperative anxiety and maladaptive behavioral and cognitive outcomes associated with surgery and anesthesia.

Developmental Issues

COGNITIVE DEVELOPMENT AND UNDERSTANDING OF ILLNESS

The perioperative period is stressful for many individuals undergoing surgery, and this is especially true for children. Children's stress during the perioperative period results from multiple sources, one of which is a limited understanding of illness and the need for surgery. Early developmental theorists (e.g., Piaget,[1,2] Werner[3]) suggested that a child's understanding of illness changes qualitatively as cognitive maturation occurs. The most widely cited model for understanding a child's perspective on illness posits that the child's understanding of illness evolves from prelogical explanations, such as phenomenalism (e.g., magical thinking), to concrete-logical explanations, such as contamination (e.g., eating bad food), to formal-logical explanations (e.g., physiologic causes), and differences in understanding occur according to the child's differentiation between the self and others.[4]

Children's understanding of the treatments for illnesses is thought to follow a similar developmental pattern. In terms of surgery, a child's concepts are particularly underdeveloped. Young children have difficulty defining "an operation," suggesting that it is the same as being sick, going for a doctor's checkup, or taking a nap.[5] Given these developmental considerations, it is not surprising that young children are more likely to have misconceptions about hospitalization and surgery than are older children and adults[6] and therefore are at unique and disparate risk for perioperative stress.

ATTACHMENT

Attachment style is another developmental consideration unique to children in the perioperative setting. Although adults also undergo separation from family, the separation of children from their parents is particularly stressful and affected by the parent-child relationship.

Coping with separation is inevitable and necessary for a child's normal, healthy development.[7] Separation experiences, such as saying good-bye at school or sleeping overnight at a friend's house, facilitate normal childhood psychological growth and personality organization by mobilizing opportunities for learning and adaptation. Other separation experiences, especially those occurring in the context of loss, illness, or other stressors, can precipitate states of confusion, anger, and anxiety. Brief separations, such as those associated with surgery, are most stressful for infants, toddlers, and preschool-aged children. Indeed, for school-aged children, responses to separation may reflect, in part, response patterns established early in the preschool years.[7] For children with biologically based vulnerabilities, such as a sensitivity to novelty and changes in routines, even expected separations may impose a greater degree of stress than for less sensitive children.[7] Similarly, for children with developmental delay, separation may be experienced with a degree of anxiety and developmental stress more like that experienced by a younger child.

Attachment affects a child's response to separation and is shaped through early experiences with the primary caregiver. Through these interactions, an infant has the opportunity to develop a sense of trust and security in the reliability and predictability of his or her relationship and the world.[8] The style of attachment exhibited by infants is evident in their responses to brief separations from the primary caregiver and is conceptualized as *secure*, *insecure*, or *anxious*.

Children who are more "securely attached" to their parents deal more adaptively with the stress of brief separation and with the novelty of the hospital experience. Such children are more willing to explore their world and respond positively to their caregivers' return, using the caregivers as a secure, stable base from which to approach strangers and new situations.[9,10] In contrast, children classified as "anxiously attached" to their parents tend to be distressed in unfamiliar situations, like the perioperative environment, even in the presence of their caregivers. When their parents return after brief separations, these children exhibit anger and distress and avoid physical contact. Another form of "insecure attachment" is avoidance. Avoidant children do not explore their surroundings as much as securely attached infants, rarely show distress at separation, and tend to ignore their parents on reuniting. Conversely, "insecurely attached" children are more easily distressed by even brief separations and spend more time trying to stay close to their parents.

TEMPERAMENT

Responses of young children to the stress of the perioperative period also reflect the child's temperament. Temperament refers to stable emotional and behavioral responses (e.g., emotionality, activity, attention, reactivity, sociability) that appear in infancy and are thought to be primarily genetic in nature.[11] Three main dimensions have been proposed to classify infant temperament: emotionality, activity, and sociability.[12] *Emotionality* refers to the ease with which an infant becomes aroused or anxious, especially in situations that might lead to fear, such as perioperative settings. *Activity* refers to the infant's customary level of energy and intensity of behavior. *Sociability* reflects the infant's tendency to approach or avoid others. These behavioral dimensions of temperament are also reflected in physiologic responses related to anxiety.[13,14] In long-term studies, infants who are inhibited in the face of novelty continue to be so through early school age.[15] Thus, temperament as a behavioral descriptor appears to characterize an enduring cluster of traits reflecting reactivity and anxiety regulation in the face of novelty.

In light of these issues, the child's developmental level is an important consideration relating to the child's perioperative behavior. The remainder of this chapter addresses specific behavioral issues related to surgery in children, including anxiety in the preoperative period and postoperative behavioral outcomes, such as emergence delirium, sleep, and other maladaptive behavioral changes.

Preoperative Anxiety

Anxiety in children undergoing anesthesia and surgery is characterized by feelings of tension, apprehension, and nervousness.[16] This response is attributed to separating from parents, loss of control, uncertainty about anesthesia, and uncertainty about the surgery and its outcome.[16] It is estimated that 40% to 60% of children develop significant fear and anxiety before their surgery.[17] Furthermore, separation from parents and induction of anesthesia have been found to be the most stressful times during the surgical and anesthesia experience. Some children verbalize their fears explicitly, whereas others express their anxiety only by behavioral changes. Children may appear scared or agitated, breathe deeply, tremble, stop talking or playing, and start to cry. Some may wet or soil themselves, display increased motor tone, and actively attempt to escape from medical personnel.[18] These behaviors may give children some sense of control in the situation and thereby diminish the damaging effects of a sense of helplessness.[16,18] In addition to the behavioral manifestations detailed here, several studies have documented that anxiety before surgery is associated with neuroendocrine changes, such as increased serum cortisol, epinephrine, growth hormone, and adrenocorticotropic hormone levels, as well as increased natural killer cell activity.[19,20] Significant correlations between heart rate, blood pressure, and behavioral ratings of anxiety have also been reported.[21,22]

RISK FACTORS

Preoperative anxiety is a clinically important phenomenon that should be treated as any other clinical phenomenon or disease. In epidemiologic terms, *all* diseases are characterized operationally by risk factors, interventions, and outcomes; preoperative anxiety is no exception. We review the phenomenon of preoperative anxiety using the classic epidemiologic model of a disease (Fig. 3.1).

Identifying the risk factors for preoperative anxiety is important because the routine use of pharmacologic and behavioral interventions is associated with both advantages and disadvantages. Routine administration of sedative premedication may increase indirect pharmacy costs, the need for nursing staff, and appropriately monitored bed space in the preoperative holding area. Children undergoing extremely brief outpatient procedures (<30 minutes) may also experience delayed discharge. Similarly, behavioral preparation programs administered preoperatively are associated with increased hospital operational costs. Likewise, anxious children can use hospital resources that would be reduced with appropriate pharmacologic preparation. Thus, identifying children who are at a particularly high risk for developing extreme anxiety and distress before surgery would help guide the most effective use of limited resources.

Variation in children's behavioral responses to the perioperative experience has its origin in at least four domains:
- Age and developmental maturity
- Previous experience with medical procedures and illness
- Individual capacity for affect regulation and trait (baseline) anxiety
- Parental state (situational) and trait anxiety

Previous studies that examined the behavioral responses to induction of anesthesia in children did so in terms of these four domains.[23-27] Children between the ages of 1 and 5 years are at greatest risk for developing extreme anxiety and distress. This is not surprising because separation anxiety often does not peak until 1 year of age and children older than 5 years can more easily cope with new situations. A history of previous stressful medical encounters, such as previous hospitalization, affects how a child reacts to new medical encounters; these are important risk factors for preoperative anxiety. Children who are shy and inhibited, as identified by temperament tests, and those who lack good social adaptive abilities are also at increased risk for developing anxiety and distress before surgery.[27]

Parental characteristics also have a strong influence on a child's behavior. Children of parents who are more anxious, children of parents who use avoidance coping mechanisms, and children of separated or divorced parents all appear to be at high risk for developing preoperative anxiety.[28] Because children of anxious parents are more likely to experience high levels of preoperative anxiety, it is important to identify the predictors of increased *parental* preoperative anxiety. Parent gender (mothers are more anxious than fathers[29]), the child's age (<1 year), children with repeated hospital admissions, and the child's temperament are all predictors of increased parental preoperative anxiety.[28,30-32] Identification of children and parents who are at the greatest risk for preoperative anxiety and distress allows for appropriate intervention for this "at-risk" population.

BEHAVIORAL INTERVENTIONS

Pharmacologic (e.g., premedication) and behavioral (e.g., psychological preparation programs) interventions are used to attenuate preoperative anxiety and distress in children and their parents.[17,33]

Behavioral perioperative stress

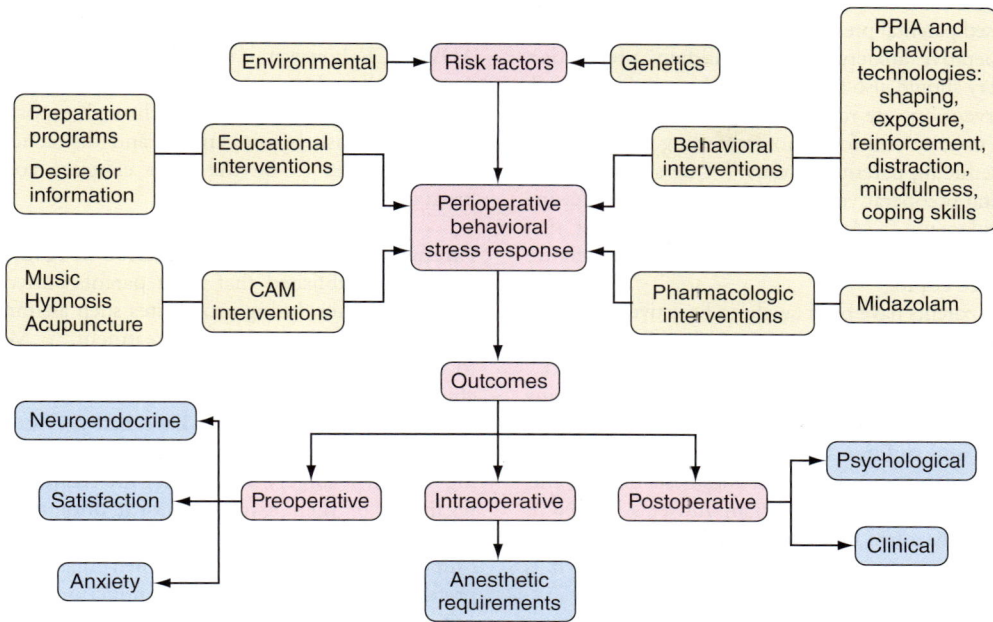

FIGURE 3.1 Operational Overview of Perioperative Anxiety. *CAM,* Complementary alternative medicine; *PPIA,* parental presence during induction of anesthesia.

Preoperative Preparation Programs

Psychological preparation for children undergoing anesthesia and surgery has been widely advocated. These preparation programs may provide narrative information, an orientation tour of the operative facility, role rehearsal using dolls, modeling using videotapes or a puppet show, child-life preparation, or coping education and relaxation skills.[34–36]

Although there is general agreement in the medical community regarding the benefit of preparation programs, recommendations regarding the content of behavioral preoperative preparation differ widely. Early programs were information oriented and often incorporated modeling techniques using videos or a puppet show.[37,38] These techniques were augmented in the late 1980s with child-life preparation and coping skills education.[35] Child-life specialists are trained individuals who facilitate development of coping skills and the adjustment of children and parents to the perioperative environment by providing play experiences, presenting information about events and procedures, and establishing supportive relationships with children and parents.[36] Currently, the development of coping skills is considered the most effective preoperative intervention, followed by modeling, play therapy, operating room (OR) tour, and printed material.[39] Interestingly, coping skills preparation with child life specialists was associated with less anxiety on the day of surgery when compared with lesser rated techniques; however, no differences were found immediately or up to 2 weeks after surgery.[40] Thus, from a cost-effectiveness point of view, one must decide whether the additive cost of child life specialists justifies the reduction in anxiety that occurs *only* during the preoperative period.

It is important that preparation programs are age-appropriate and tailored to the individual child's needs. Several variables influence the responses of children to preparation programs.[28]

For example, children who are 6 years of age or older benefit the most if they participate in a preparation program more than 5 days before the scheduled surgery and benefit the least if they participate in one only 1 day before surgery. In fact, older children prepared a week in advance showed an *increase* in anxiety level during and immediately after the preparation program, but they demonstrated a gradual decrease in anxiety during the 5 days before the day of surgery.[41] To prevent excessive anticipatory anxiety, older children should have sufficient time to process the new information and to rehearse newly acquired coping skills. It is also important to realize that there may be a *negative* effect of a preparation program in children younger than 3 years of age. This may be a result of their inability to distinguish fantasy from reality.[1] A reality-based preparation program may do little to calm young children and may even exacerbate anxiety or sensitize the young child to the surgery. From age 3 to 6 years, children demonstrate an increasing ability to distinguish fantasy from reality and by the age of 6 this distinction is usually accomplished.[1] Therefore, to provide the most benefit, both the age of the child and timing must be factored into delivery of the program.

In addition to age and timing, previous experience in a hospital setting also influences the effectiveness of a preparation program. A child who was previously hospitalized is more likely to develop an exaggerated emotional response to a behavioral preoperative preparation program and the perioperative experience.[28,41–43] Information about what will occur, as demonstrated by sensory expectation and doll play, does *not* provide new information for these children. Furthermore, if the child has had a previous negative medical experience, the routine preparation may increase anxiety by triggering negative memories. In this case, alternative behavioral interventions, such as extensive individualized coping skills training combined with desensitization and actual practice, may be better suited and indicated.[42]

Because increased parental preoperative anxiety has been shown to increase preoperative anxiety in their children, preparation programs for surgery should also be directed at parents.[23] Although a number of interventions are routinely used to reduce a child's anxiety, there is a paucity of information regarding interventions directed toward reducing parental anxiety.[44] One study demonstrated that parental preoperative anxiety decreased after viewing an educational videotape.[45] Most studies to date suggest that preoperative preparation programs for children reduce preoperative anxiety and enhance coping.[35,41,46]

Children whose parents have been taught to be active in distracting their child during stressful medical events may evidence reduced anxiety compared with parents who receive no intervention.[47] Indeed, this was the case in a randomized controlled trial evaluating a family-centered behavioral preparation program (ADVANCE) (Table 3.1). Parents and children who received ADVANCE were less anxious before and during induction of anesthesia than parents and children who did not receive this program. In fact, ADVANCE was as successful as midazolam in managing children's compliance with and anxiety at induction of anesthesia (Table 3.2).[48] It is important to note that ADVANCE also decreased the time spent in the postanesthesia care unit and decreased the analgesic requirements during the postoperative period. A major disadvantage of ADVANCE, however, is its high cost and personnel requirements. Accordingly, efforts to dismantle this multimodal intervention indicate that behavioral shaping through exposing children to the anesthesia mask before surgery and distraction on the day of surgery proved to be the most effective components of the program.[49]

Parental Presence During Induction of Anesthesia

It is well established that most parents and children prefer to remain together during procedures such as immunization, bone marrow aspiration, and dental treatment.[50,51] Most parents prefer to be present during induction of anesthesia regardless of the child's age or previous surgical experience.[52,53] This is the case even for those parents who have had previous experience with pharmacologic interventions. Indeed, parents of children undergoing repeated surgery were likely to request parental presence regardless of their experience with prior parental presence or premedication with midazolam.[54] That is, even if children were calm after midazolam during their first surgery, parents still preferred to be present during induction of anesthesia during subsequent surgeries.

It is important to note, however, that parental presence during induction of anesthesia (PPIA) does not necessarily equate with appropriate choice of interventions. For example, mothers who were most highly motivated to be present at induction of anesthesia also reported high levels of anxiety and their children were more distressed at induction.[55] In fact, more than 90% of parents report some degree of anxiety during the anesthesia induction process.[56] The most upsetting factors include seeing their child become flaccid during induction and separation from their child.[56] This observation was confirmed in a study that examined heart rate, blood pressure, and skin conductance levels in mothers as they observed their child's induction of anesthesia.[57] Mothers who were present during induction of anesthesia showed a moderate increase in heart rate and blood pressure (Fig. 3.2). However, no cardiac arrhythmias or ischemic episodes were noted. Another

TABLE 3.1	The ADVANCE Preoperative Preparation Program

Anxiety reduction

Distraction on the day of surgery

Video modeling and education before surgery

Adding parents to the child's surgical experience and promoting family-centered care

No excessive reassurance—a suggestion made to parents for communication with children about surgery

Coaching of parents by researchers to help them succeed

Exposure/shaping of the child via induction mask practice (the mask placed over the child's nose and mouth to deliver anesthetic drugs)

Reproduced with permission from Kain ZN, Caldwell-Andrews AA, Mayes LC, et al. Family-centered preparation for surgery improves perioperative outcomes in children: a randomized controlled trial. *Anesthesiology* 2007;106:65-74.

TABLE 3.2	Perioperative Outcomes of the ADVANCE Program

| | STUDY GROUP | | | | | |
	Control (n = 99)	Parental Presence (n = 94)	Advance (n = 96)	Midazolam (n = 98)	P VALUE[e]	EFFECT SIZE (95% CI)[f]
Children's Anxiety (mYPAS)						
Holding area	36 ± 16	35 ± 16	31 ± 12[a]	37 ± 17	0.001	0.54 (0.78–0.30)
Introduction of mask at induction	52 ± 26	50 ± 26	43 ± 23[b]	40 ± 24	0.018	0.33 (0.58–0.08)
Postanesthesia Care Unit						
Fentanyl consumption (μg/kg)	1.37 ± 2.00	0.81 ± 1.00	0.41 ± 1.00[c]	1.23 ± 2	0.016	0.54 (0.75–0.24)
Time until discharge (min)	120 ± 48	122 ± 44	108 ± 46[d]	129 ± 44	0.040	0.34 (0.60–0.09)

Reproduced with permission from Kain ZN, Caldwell-Andrews AA, Mayes LC, et al. Family-centered preparation for surgery improves perioperative outcomes in children: a randomized controlled trial. *Anesthesiology* 2007;106:65-74.

CI, Confidence interval; *mYPAS*, modified Yale Preoperative Anxiety Scale.

ADVANCE group anxiety scores:

[a]Significantly less than those in all other groups, $P < 0.01$.

[b]Significantly less than those in the control and parental presence groups, $P < 0.05$.

[c]Significantly less than those in the control and midazolam groups, $P < 0.01$.

[d]Significantly less than those in the midazolam group, $P < 0.01$.

[e]P values for parental presence and control groups = 0.07.

[f]Cohen's *d* effect sizes were calculated for the intervention group vs. other groups combined.

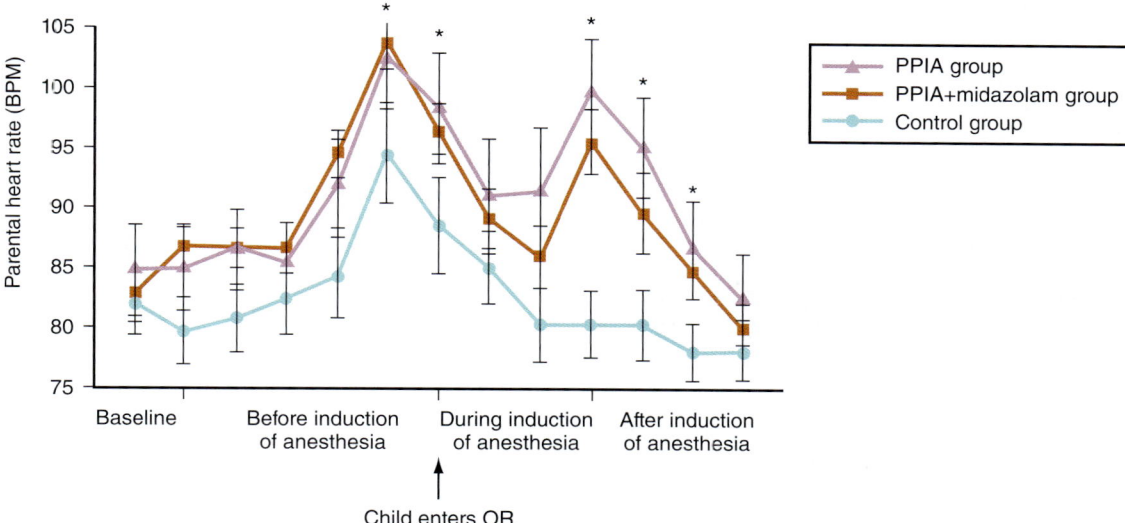

FIGURE 3.2 Changes in Parental Heart Rate From Baseline Measurement Until After Induction of Anesthesia. Data are reported as mean ± SE (standard error). *Asterisks* indicate time points at which differences between groups are statistically significant (*P* < .05). *BPM*, Beats per minute; *OR*, operating room; *PPIA*, parental presence during induction of anesthesia. (From Kain ZN, Caldwell-Andrews AA, Mayes LC, et al. Parental presence during induction of anesthesia: physiological effects on parents. *Anesthesiology* 2003;98:58-64.)

study examined whether parental auricular acupuncture would reduce parental preoperative anxiety and thus allow children to benefit from PPIA.[58] A multivariate model demonstrated that children whose mothers had received the acupuncture intervention were less anxious on entrance to the OR and during placement of the anesthesia mask on their child's face.

Potential benefits from PPIA include minimizing the need for premedication and avoiding the screaming and struggling of the child that may result on separation from the parents. Whether PPIA decreases child anxiety during induction and affects the long-term behavior effects of surgery and anesthesia remains controversial. Common objections to PPIA include concern about disruption of the OR routine, compromising operative sterility, crowded ORs, and possible adverse parental reactions. For some children, their behavioral response to stress may be more negative when a parent is present than when the parent is absent.[59] In several reports, PPIA resulted in disruptive behavior, parents refusing to leave the room when requested, and even removal of a child from the OR by a grandmother during the second stage of anesthesia.[60,61] However, one report has described a 4-year experience with 3086 children in a freestanding ambulatory surgery center in which no parent needed to be escorted from the OR because of undue anxiety and only two parents developed syncope, with prompt recovery.[62] Despite objections, the prevalence of PPIA is becoming more common in the United States. In fact, there was an increase in the overall prevalence in PPIA from 1995 to 2002, and geographic differences in PPIA use decreased during the 7-year period but more recent data are lacking (Fig. 3.3).[63,64]

Evidence to date has been ambivalent regarding the routine use of PPIA.[65–67] Although early studies suggested that PPIA reduced anxiety and increased cooperation,[68,69] more recent investigations indicate that routine PPIA may *not* always be beneficial.[65–67] Characteristics of the parent and child have an impact on the effectiveness of parental presence. For example, older children

(>4 years), children with a "calm" and less active baseline temperament, parents with less situational anxiety, and parents with lower external locus of control, benefit most from PPIA.[30,65] The match between parent and child anxiety level also appears to be important. Calm children with anxious parents do more poorly during induction compared with calm children with calm parents or anxious children with either calm or anxious parents.[30] When interpreting the results of these studies, however, several factors should be considered. First, the design of a randomized controlled study, while considered a gold standard in research, may *not* reflect the practice of *all* anesthesiologists. That is, although a randomized controlled study is applicable to centers that offer PPIA for *all* parents, it may not be applicable to centers in which each request for PPIA is considered individually based on personality characteristics of each child and parent. Such centers may have different results with PPIA than were demonstrated in experimental studies. Second, allowing PPIA without adequate preparation of the parent may be counterproductive. Some parent behaviors, such as criticism, excessive reassurance, and commands, are associated with greater distress.[70]

Given these drawbacks, interest in this area has begun to shift toward an emphasis on what parents actually do during induction of anesthesia. The development of a new tool for assessing child and adult behavior in the perioperative setting (Perioperative Child-Adult Medical Procedure Interaction Scale [P-CAMPIS]) has been developed to facilitate such research (Fig. 3.4).[71] Preliminary validation of this measure indicates that parental behavior affects the child's anxiety during induction, much as it affects a child's distress during immunizations.

The Preoperative Interview

Although not obvious, the preoperative interview is a behavioral intervention that is routinely administered to *all* children undergoing anesthesia and surgery.[72] It is clear that anesthesiologists have an ethical and legal responsibility to disclose to children and

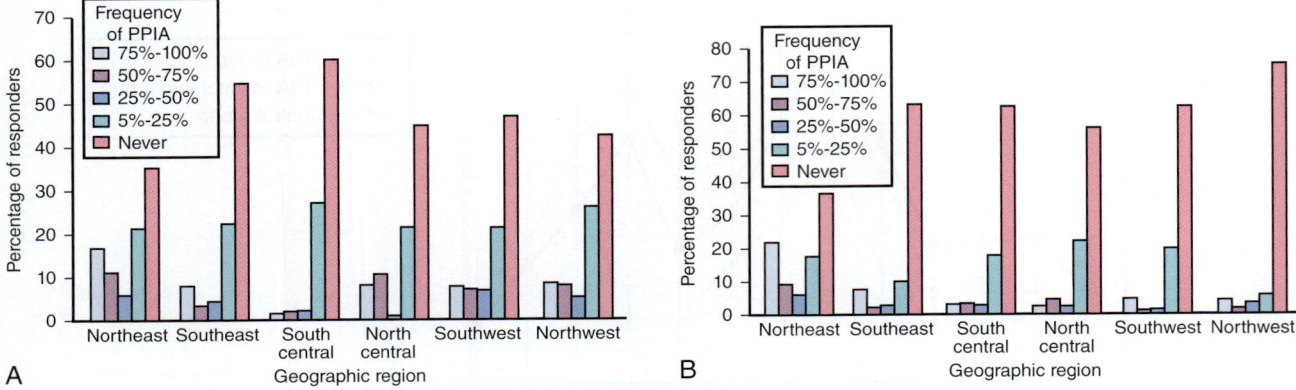

FIGURE 3.3 A, Frequency of parental presence during induction of anesthesia (*PPIA*) practice in the United States as of 2002. **B**, Frequency of PPIA practice in the United States as of 1995/1996. Data reported are medians (range, 0%–100%). (From Kain ZN, Caldwell-Andrews AA, Krivutza DM, et al. Trends in the practice of parental presence during induction of anesthesia and the use of preoperative sedative premedication in the United States, 1995-2002: results of a follow-up national survey. *Anesth Analg.* 2004;98:1252-1259.)

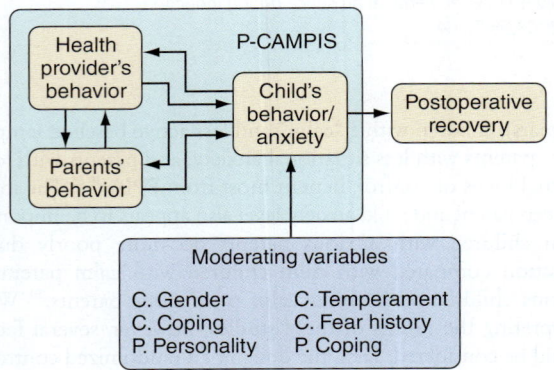

FIGURE 3.4 The conceptual framework that underlies the relation between a child's preoperative anxiety, parental behaviors, health care providers' behaviors, moderating variables, and postoperative recovery. *C*, Child; *P*, parent; *P-CAMPIS*, Perioperative Child-Adult Medical Procedure Interaction Scale. (From Caldwell-Andrews AA, Blount RL, Mayes LC, Kain ZN. Behavioral interactions in the perioperative environment: a new conceptual framework and the development of the perioperative child-adult medical procedure interaction scale. *Anesthesiology* 2005;103:1130-1135.)

parents detailed anesthetic risk information when obtaining informed consent, but how far this disclosure must extend remains controversial. A common reason given for not providing detailed anesthetic risk information is that it may increase the child's or parents' anxiety. Comparative studies investigating anxiety levels in adult patients given a limited amount of information, versus more detailed information concerning procedural and anesthetic risks, report conflicting results. Although early studies provided mixed data regarding whether detailed information delivered preoperatively increased anxiety,[73–75] several studies in the United States and Australia have demonstrated that patients and parents who received detailed information, including numerical estimates of anesthesia-related complications, were no more anxious than those given minimal information regarding risks.[76–78] Furthermore, parents have expressed their desire to have as much perioperative information about their child's surgery as possible,[77] and even

children have expressed a desire for detailed perioperative information, including information about pain, anesthesia, and potential complications.[79] Thus, the presentation of very detailed anesthetic information of what might go wrong should not increase parental or patient anxiety and has the advantage of allowing for fully informed choices. It should be emphasized, however, that anesthesiologists should note the particular coping style of the parents. Parents use different strategies to cope with or handle difficult, unclear, or unpleasant life experiences, such as a child undergoing surgery. Whereas some parents try to avoid information about unpleasant or unclear situations ("avoidance behavior"), others may seek any available information ("monitoring behavior").[80] Although a "monitoring" parent will benefit from a large amount of perioperative information, an "avoiding" parent may react to the information with increased anxiety and distress. Thus, the amount of information provided should be tailored to the needs of the individual parent.

HEALTH CARE PROVIDER INTERVENTIONS

In addition to behavioral interventions targeting children and their parents, a promising new line of research supports the use of behavioral interventions targeting health care providers—both anesthesiologists and nurses. Specifically, an empirically derived intervention titled Provider-Tailored Intervention for Perioperative Stress (P-TIPS) was shown to be successful in changing anesthesiologist and nurse behaviors in the perioperative setting and represents a new clinical avenue for decreasing perioperative anxiety in children.[81] The development of P-TIPS was based on research documenting that adult behaviors (parents and health care providers) affect children's distress during invasive medical procedures, including surgery. Specifically, the use of distraction, nonprocedural talk, and humor are conceptualized as "coping promoting" behaviors and have been shown to decrease children's distress.[82–88] Conversely, adults' use of reassurance, apology, empathy, criticism, or allowing the child too much control over the medical procedure are conceptualized as "distress promoting" behaviors and lead to increased distress in children.[82,87–90] With P-TIPS, a new behavior that affected child distress also emerged: medical reinterpretation (i.e., reconceptualizing medical experiences and equipment as nonthreatening) and was found to increase a child's coping when used with medical experiences that were in the child's immediate environment, but it increased distress when used in reference to objects outside the immediate environment.[87]

Preliminary investigation revealed that P-TIPS was successful at both increasing desired behaviors (coping promoting) and decreasing undesired (distress promoting) behaviors among health care providers.[81] Both resident and attending anesthesiologists were included in this study and evidenced behavior change, as did OR nurses, who were charged with changing their own as well as parent behaviors in the perioperative setting. In fact, nurses demonstrated appropriate behavior change and, in turn, parents demonstrated increases in desired and decreases in undesired behaviors. One important benefit to the type of approach offered by P-TIPS is that it is not necessary to conduct individual training with parents of children undergoing surgery; rather, health care providers who interact with multiple children and parents are targeted, which reduces both logistical and financial constraints of behavioral interventions.

PHARMACOLOGIC INTERVENTIONS

The primary goals of administering a premedication to children are to facilitate an anxiety-free separation from their parents and a smooth, stress-free induction of anesthesia. Other effects that may be achieved by pharmacologic preparation of the child include amnesia, anxiolysis, prevention of physiologic stress (e.g., avoiding tachycardia in patients with cyanotic congenital heart disease), and analgesia (see Chapter 4).

The pattern of use of sedative premedications in the United States has evolved between 1996 and 2002. In 1996, premedication was least often prescribed for children younger than 3 years of age and most often for adults younger than 65 years of age (25% vs. 75%).[63] Premedication prescriptions also varied substantively with the geographic location. In 2002, a follow-up study revealed that the use of premedications in children had increased from 30% to 50%, whereas geographic variability had diminished compared with the results of the 1996 survey (Fig. 3.5).[64] In both surveys, the most commonly used sedative premedicant was midazolam; when data from several surveys were reviewed, it was noted that anesthesiologists in the United States who allowed

PPIA the *least* were those who prescribed sedative premedication the most.[63,91] Thus, most anesthesiologists in the United States use either parental presence or sedative premedication to attenuate preoperative anxiety in children.

PHARMACOLOGIC INTERVENTIONS VERSUS BEHAVIORAL INTERVENTIONS

When pharmacologic interventions are directly compared with behavioral interventions, children receiving a sedative are less anxious and more compliant than those who are accompanied to the OR by a parent.[67] Interestingly, parental anxiety also decreased when the child was premedicated. When sedative premedication and PPIA were compared, the combination of PPIA and sedative premedication was more effective than medication alone for reducing anxiety in the parents and improving parent satisfaction.[92] However, PPIA offered no additional anxiolysis for children who received a premedication preoperatively. Nonetheless, parents who accompanied their sedated children into the ORs were themselves less anxious and more satisfied both with the separation process and with the overall anesthetic, nursing, and surgical care provided. It is important to note that these parents had no preparation for their presence at anesthesia induction. Premedication combined with an advanced behavioral preparation resulted in similar outcomes on child and parent anxiety at induction and child compliance with induction.[48] Furthermore, children who received behavioral preparation evidenced significantly less emergence delirium and required less analgesia in the recovery room compared with those who received only premedication.

In conclusion, although sedative premedications are effective for treatment of preoperative anxiety, they should *not* be used routinely in all children undergoing surgery. Their use should be directed to children who are at a significant risk for developing preoperative anxiety. Variables, such as age, duration of surgery, and potential recovery delays, should also be considered. Nonetheless, it is important that premedication is not withheld if the premedication would likely benefit the child. For example, a child undergoing a very brief procedure who is very anxious would likely benefit from a premedication regardless of the negative effects on recovery and discharge.

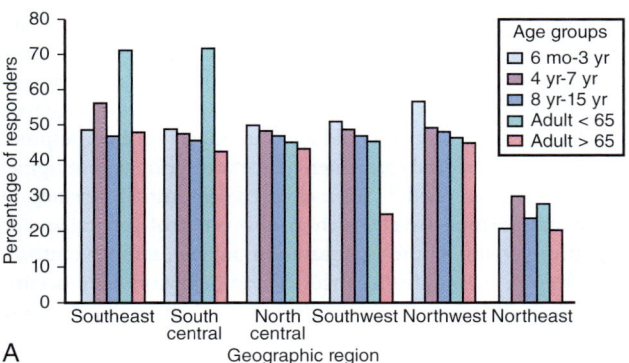
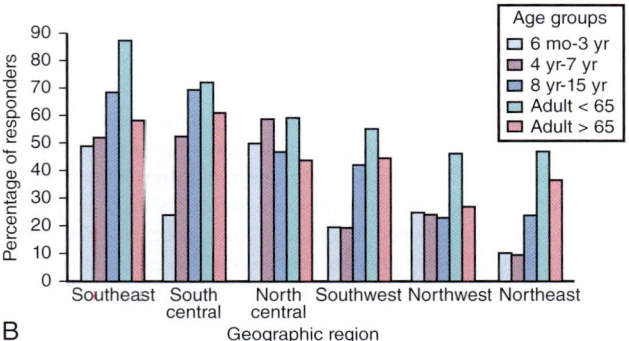

FIGURE 3.5 A, Frequency of sedative premedication practice in the United States as of 2002. **B**, Frequency of sedative premedication practice in the United States as of 1996. Data reported are medians (range, 0%-100%). (From Kain ZN, Caldwell-Andrews AA, Krivutza DM, et al. Trends in the practice of parental presence during induction of anesthesia and the use of preoperative sedative premedication in the United States, 1995-2002: results of a follow-up national survey. *Anesth Analg.* 2004;98:1252-1259.)

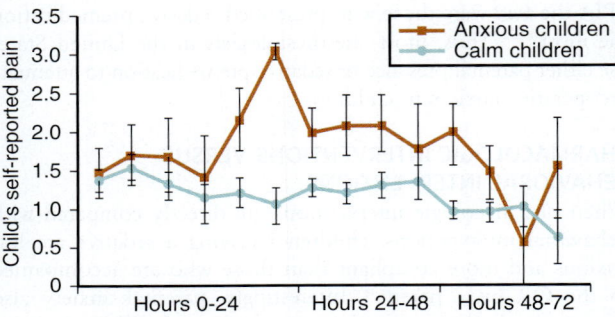

FIGURE 3.6 Children's self-reported postoperative pain as a function of preoperative anxiety. (From Kain ZN, Mayes LC, Caldwell-Andrews AA, et al. Preoperative anxiety, postoperative pain, and behavioral recovery in young children undergoing surgery. *Pediatrics* 2006;118:651-658.)

Postoperative Outcomes

Anxious children experience significantly more pain both during the hospital stay and during the first 3 days at home[93] (Fig. 3.6). During home recovery, anxious children also consume more codeine and acetaminophen compared with nonanxious children. Anxious children also had a greater incidence of emergence delirium (9.7% vs. 1.5%), postoperative anxiety, and sleep problems compared with nonanxious children. Preoperative anxiety in young children undergoing surgery is associated with a more painful postoperative recovery and a greater incidence of disrupted sleep and other problems.[93] Moreover, one study suggests that perioperative anxiety, rather than just preoperative anxiety, is associated with poorer surgical outcomes.[94] Children have traditionally been labeled as anxious or nonanxious after their anxiety was assessed before surgery, such as in the presurgical holding area or at the point of induction in the OR. By contrast, this study examined anxiety in children throughout the perioperative continuum (pre- and postoperatively) and replicated findings of associations between perioperative anxiety and both postoperative pain and new-onset behavioral changes.[94]

The assumption that minimal preoperative anxiety predicts good postoperative outcomes underlies many interventions that attenuate preoperative anxiety. To date, preoperative preparation studies in adult patients have used diverse postoperative outcome measures, including intensity of pain, analgesic requirements, postsurgical complications, length of hospital stay, patient satisfaction, blood cortisol levels, changes in blood pressure and heart rate, and behavioral indexes of recovery.[95–103] Reviews of this research, while critical of the methodology, concluded that psychologically prepared adult patients may have improved postoperative recovery.[96,104–106] As noted previously, children who received the ADVANCE preoperative program were less anxious preoperatively and experienced a reduced incidence of emergence delirium, had a briefer stay in the recovery area, reported less postoperative pain, and required fewer analgesics compared with a control group.[48]

EMERGENCE DELIRIUM

The first maladaptive behavioral change in children that may be evident after surgery is emergence delirium. This phenomenon is characterized by nonpurposeful restlessness and agitation, thrashing, crying or moaning, and disorientation in the recovery room.

Published studies have reported that up to 80% of all children undergoing surgery and anesthesia develop emergence delirium.[107] However, in many of these studies, emergence delirium was not distinguished from pain as the scale to measure emergence delirium had not been validated, pain was present contemporaneously with the delirium, and analgesics were used to treat the delirium. In fact, the range of incidence of delirium using a validated scale in nonpainful surgery is 15% to 50%. Factors that are known to increase the incidence of emergence delirium include young age (2–6 years), preoperative anxiety (although controversial), and the type of anesthetic (sevoflurane, desflurane, and isoflurane ≫ total intravenous anesthesia [TIVA], halothane).[107–109] Other factors such as previous surgery and the type of procedure (painful ≫ nonpainful) may affect the incidence of delirium but more than likely were identified because of poorly designed studies. Rapid emergence and depth of anesthesia do not predict delirium. Furthermore, preoperative anxiety, emergence delirium, and postoperative maladaptive behavior changes have been shown to be closely related phenomena. One study found that the odds of children experiencing marked symptoms of emergence delirium increased in proportion to their preoperative anxiety scores, and that the odds of the onset of new maladaptive behavioral changes also increased with the presence of emergence delirium.[93] Thus the child's preoperative anxiety may help to identify those who are more likely to develop adverse postoperative phenomena, such as emergence delirium and postoperative behavioral changes.

SLEEP CHANGES

Changes in sleep patterns in the postoperative period have been well documented in adults and children. One study reported that 47% of children experienced sleep disturbances after anesthesia[110] and approximately 14% of children showed decreases in percentage of time spent asleep (in both rapid eye movement [REM] and non-REM sleep) after surgery. The most common predictor of sleep difficulties after surgery has been postoperative pain,[111] but psychological variables have also been shown to be important. Specifically, parental personality measures of anxiety and child measures of externalizing behavior have both been found to predict sleep efficiency in children after surgery.

OTHER BEHAVIORAL CHANGES

In addition to sleep, changes in daytime behavior in children after surgery and anesthesia have also been documented. As many as 60% of children undergoing outpatient surgery may develop negative *postoperative* behavioral changes within 2 weeks after surgery.[112–114] These negative behaviors include sleep and eating disturbances, separation anxiety, apathy, withdrawal, and new-onset enuresis.[23,94,114] In fact, some children may develop long-lasting psychological effects that could have an impact on their responses to subsequent medical care. Interference with normal development has also been described.[115] Some children demonstrate new negative behaviors postoperatively, such as new onset of general anxiety, nighttime crying, enuresis, separation anxiety, temper tantrums, and sleep or eating disturbances. These behaviors may occur in up to 44% of children 2 weeks after surgery; about 20% continue to demonstrate negative behaviors up to 6 months postoperatively.[23] The postoperative negative behavioral changes are likely the result of an interaction between the distress the child experiences during the perioperative period and the individual personality characteristics of the child. Previously, variables such as the age and temperament of the child and the state and trait anxiety of the parent have been identified as predictors for the occurrence of negative postoperative behavioral changes.[23] There are a paucity of data, however, regarding a possible association between the distress the child experiences during induction of anesthesia and the occurrence of these negative postoperative behavioral changes. One investigation concluded that extreme anxiety, such as that which occurs with a "stormy induction" of anesthesia, was associated with an increased incidence of postoperative negative behavioral changes.[109] The investigators recommend that anesthesiologists advise parents of children who are anxious during induction of anesthesia of the increased likelihood that their children will develop postoperative negative behavioral changes, such as nightmares, separation anxiety, and aggression toward authority.[109]

Because the anxiety level of the child and parent in the preoperative holding area predicts negative postoperative behavioral problems,[23] it can be hypothesized that if sedative premedications reduce the anxiety of the child and the parents in the preoperative holding area, these agents may also reduce negative postoperative behavioral outcomes.[70] One study found that children who were premedicated exhibited a reduced incidence of negative behavioral changes during week 1 after surgery.[116] These data suggest that reducing preoperative anxiety may improve the child's behavior not only preoperatively, but also immediately postoperatively.[116]

Intraoperative Clinical Outcomes

It is commonly held that increased preoperative anxiety is associated with increased intraoperative anesthetic requirements.[117,118] However, this is based on early studies of questionable scientific validity[119,120]; many of these studies did not use validated scales to measure anxiety or control for potential confounding variables, such as sedative premedication and the surgical procedure.[22] One investigation indicated that an increased baseline (i.e., trait) anxiety is associated with increased intraoperative anesthetic requirements in adults. The investigators in that study controlled for the surgical procedure, used bispectral electroencephalographic analysis (bispectral index) monitoring to ensure the same anesthetic depth in all patients, and used a TIVA technique to ease the calculation of the anesthetics used.[121] As such, it does seem clear that an increased baseline, or trait, anxiety is associated with increased intraoperative anesthetic requirements.

Although several review articles suggest that increased anxiety before surgery and anesthesia is associated with postoperative nausea and vomiting,[122] experimental data suggest that a child's anxiety in the preoperative holding area is not predictive of postoperative nausea and vomiting either in the postanesthesia care unit or at home.[123]

Summary

Approximately 3 million children undergo anesthesia and surgery in the United States every year and 40% to 60% of them are believed to develop behavioral stress before their surgery. Multiple interventions have been proposed to attenuate the preoperative behavioral stress response, however; there is a trend toward a *reduction* in both behavioral and pharmacologic preoperative interventions aimed at children. One possible reason for this trend may be that some physicians believe that reducing parental anxiety during the preoperative period is a surrogate outcome. Rather than evaluating the effects of various preoperative interventions on the transient preoperative behavior, some believe that we should concentrate on research directed at demonstrating that a reduction in preoperative anxiety can dramatically change

postoperative outcomes. It is well established that low levels of preoperative anxiety are associated with good postoperative behavioral recovery, whereas moderate and high levels of preoperative anxiety are associated with poor postoperative behavioral recovery. What is unknown is whether there is an association between preoperative anxiety and postoperative clinical recovery; quality research needs to examine these associations. Furthermore, shifting research focus toward development of economically and clinically feasible interventions that can be delivered to the large numbers of children undergoing surgery each year is vital. Accordingly, incorporating web-based technologies and changes in institutional practice (i.e., changing health care provider behaviors) represent two promising new avenues of intervention.

ANNOTATED REFERENCES

Fortier MA, Bunzli E, Walthall J, et al. Web-based tailored intervention for preparation of parents and children for outpatient surgery (WebTIPS): formative evaluation and randomized controlled trial. *Anesth Analg.* 2015;120:915-922.

WebTIPS is a newly developed, web-based intervention for preparation of parents and children for surgery that can be accessed in the home setting multiple times by families before and after surgery. This paper reported on both formative evaluation and preliminary efficacy using a randomized controlled trial (RCT) of the impact of WebTIPS of children's and parents' preoperative anxiety. A multimethod trial examining both qualitative and quantitative data from 13 families in which a family member had recently undergone surgery or had an upcoming surgery revealed that WebTIPS was well received by parents and children. The RCT demonstrated significant effects with moderate effect sizes (Cohen's d = 0.59 and 0.63) on children's preoperative anxiety at entrance to the operating room and introduction of the anesthesia mask, respectively. Parents in the WebTIPS group were also significantly less anxious compared with parents in the control group in the preoperative holding area (Cohen's d = 0.65).

Kain ZN, Caldwell-Andrews AA, Mayes LC. Parental intervention choices for children undergoing repeated surgeries. *Anesth Analg.* 2003;96:970-975.

Children were assigned to parental presence at induction (PPIA), premedication with midazolam, PPIA + premedication, or no intervention at initial surgery. Children were then followed up at subsequent surgery and parental preference for intervention was assessed. Of parents whose children were assigned to PPIA, 70% would choose PPIA as an intervention again. Of those assigned to premedication, only 23% would choose premedication again. Regardless of prior intervention, parents at subsequent surgery favored PPIA. Children's and parents' anxiety also affected parental preference for intervention.

Kain ZN, Fortier MA, Chorney JM, Mayes L. Web-based tailored intervention for preparation of parents and children for outpatient surgery (WebTIPS): development. *Anesth Analg.* 2015;120:905-914.

This study described the development of a Web-based Tailored Intervention for Preparation of parents and children undergoing surgery (WebTIPS). A multidisciplinary task force was comprised and determined that WebTIPS would consist of the most up-to-date, empirical evidence for preparing children and their parents for the surgical process and would be delivered via the web using an intake, matrix, and output modules covering the four temporal divisions of surgery (home before surgery, waiting area and anesthesia induction, postanesthesia care unit, home after surgery). The child component includes strategies such as information provision, modeling, play, and coping skills training and is fully animated. The parent component includes information provision, coping skills training, and cognitive and behavioral anxiety management skills (e.g., imagery, diaphragmatic breathing) and makes use of various multimedia modes (e.g., text, video, motion graphics).

Kain ZN, Mayes LC, Caldwell-Andrews AA, et al. Preoperative anxiety and postoperative pain and behavioral recovery in young children undergoing surgery. *Pediatrics.* 2006;118:651-658.

This study assessed preoperative anxiety and postoperative pain and behavioral outcomes after surgery in 241 children. Children who displayed more preoperative anxiety were rated as having higher pain after surgery by their parents. Anxious children also consumed more analgesics at home after surgery and were more likely to experience emergence delirium and postoperative sleep disturbances.

Martin SR, Chorney JM, Tan ET, et al. Changing healthcare providers' behavior during pediatric inductions with an empirically based intervention. *Anesthesiology.* 2011;115:18-27.

This study described the development and evaluation of a new intervention (P-TIPS) focused on changing health care provider and parent behaviors in the perioperative setting to reduce children's preoperative anxiety. The intervention consisted of training providers and parents to increase use of behaviors empirically shown to promote children's coping (e.g., nonprocedural talk, humor, medical reinterpretation) and decrease use of behaviors shown to increase children's distress (e.g., reassurance, empathy, apology). The intervention was shown to successfully alter provider and parent behaviors, with meaning increases in rates of desired behaviors at anesthesia induction (average anesthesiologist Cohen's d = 0.97, *average nurse Cohen's* d = 1.59) *and show positive effects on children's preoperative anxiety.*

A complete reference list can be found online at ExpertConsult.com

Preoperative Evaluation, Premedication, and Induction of Anesthesia

4

ELIZABETH A. GHAZAL, MARISSA G. VADI, LINDA J. MASON, AND CHARLES J. COTÉ

Preparation of Children for Anesthesia

FASTING

Infants and children are fasted before sedation and anesthesia to minimize the risk of pulmonary aspiration of gastric contents. In a fasted child, only the basal secretions of gastric juice should be present in the stomach. In 1948, Digby Leigh recommended a 1-hour preoperative fast after clear fluids.[1] Subsequently, Mendelson reported a number of maternal deaths that were attributed to aspiration at induction of anesthesia.[1a,1b] During the intervening 20 years, the fasting interval before elective surgery increased to 8 hours after all solids and fluids. In the late 1980s and early 1990s, an evidence-based approach to the effects of fasting intervals on gastric fluid pH and volume concluded that fasting more than 2 hours after clear fluids neither increased nor decreased the risk of pneumonitis should aspiration occur.[2–10] In the past, the risk for pneumonitis was reported to be based on two parameters: gastric fluid volume greater than 0.4 mL/kg and pH less than 2.5; however, these data were never published in a peer-reviewed journal.[1a,11] In a monkey, 0.4 mL/kg of acid instilled endobronchially, equivalent to 0.8 mL/kg aspirated tracheally, resulted in pneumonitis.[12] Using these corrected criteria for acute pneumonitis (gastric residual fluid volume >0.8 mL/kg and pH <2.5), studies in children demonstrated no additional risk for pneumonitis when children fast for only 2 hours after clear fluids.[2–9]

The incidence of pulmonary aspiration in modern routine elective pediatric or adult cases without known risk factors is small.[13–16] This small risk is the result of a number of factors including the preoperative fasting schedule. The half-life to empty clear fluids from the stomach is approximately 15 minutes (Fig. 4.1); as a result, 98% of clear fluids exit the stomach in children by 1 hour. Clear liquids include water, fruit juices without pulp, carbonated beverages, clear tea, and black coffee. Although fasting for 2 hours after clear fluids ensures nearly complete emptying of the residual volume, extending the fasting interval to 3 hours introduces flexibility in the operative schedule. The potential benefits of a 2-hour fasting interval after clear fluids include a reduced risk of hypoglycemia, which is a real possibility in children who are debilitated, have chronic disease, are poorly nourished, have metabolic dysfunction, or are preterm or formerly preterm infants.[17–20] Additional benefits include decreased thirst, decreased hunger (and thus reduced temptation that the fasting child will "steal" another child's food), decreased risk for hypotension during induction, and improved child cooperation.[2,11,21]

A scheduled operation on a preterm infant or neonate may occasionally be delayed, thus extending the period of fasting to a point that could be potentially dangerous (i.e., from hypoglycemia or hypovolemia). In this circumstance, the infants should be given glucose-containing intravenous (IV) maintenance fluids before induction of anesthesia. Alternatively, if the period may be protracted, the infant should be offered clear fluids orally until 2 hours before induction.

Breast milk, which can cause significant pulmonary injury if aspirated,[22] has a very high and variable fat content (determined by maternal diet), which will delay gastric emptying.[21] *Breast milk should not be considered a clear liquid.*[23] Two studies estimated the gastric emptying times after clear fluids, breast milk, or formula in full-term and preterm neonates.[24,25] The emptying times for

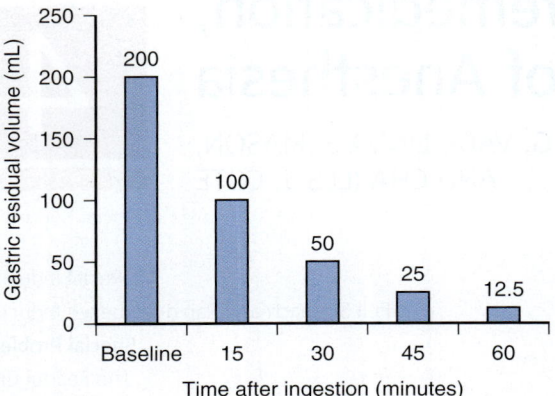

FIGURE 4.1 Clear liquids are rapidly absorbed from the stomach with a half-life of approximately 15 minutes. In this figure, for example, 200 mL of apple juice would be reduced to 12.5 mL after 60 minutes. (Data abstracted from Hunt JN, MacDonald M. The influence of volume on gastric emptying. *J Physiol* 1954;126:459-474.)

TABLE 4.1	Preoperative Fasting Recommendations in Infants and Children
Clear liquids[a]	2 hours
Breast milk	4 hours
Infant formula	6 hours[b]
Solids (fatty or fried foods)	8 hours

From Warner MA, Caplan RA, Epstein B. Practice guidelines for preoperative fasting and the use of pharmacologic agents to reduce the risk of pulmonary aspiration: application to healthy patients undergoing elective procedures. A report by the American Society of Anesthesiologists Task Force on Preoperative Fasting. *Anesthesiology* 1999;90:896–905.
[a]Include only fluids without pulp, clear tea, or coffee without milk products.
[b]Some centers allow plain toast (no dairy products) up to 6 hours prior to induction.

breast milk in both age groups were substantively greater than for clear fluids, and the gastric emptying times for formula were even greater than those for breast milk. With half-life emptying times for breast milk of 50 minutes and for formula of 75 minutes, fasting intervals of at least 3.3 hours for breast milk and 5 hours for formula are required. More importantly, perhaps, was the large (15%) variability in gastric emptying times for breast milk and formula in full-term infants (E-Fig. 4.1). Based in part on these data, the Task Force on Fasting of the American Society of Anesthesiologists (ASA) issued the following guidelines: for breast milk, 4 hours; and for formula, 6 hours (Table 4.1).[26]

Children who have been chewing gum must dispose of the gum by expectorating it, not swallowing it. Hansen and Rune[27] reported a 70% increase in gastric fluid volume in the first 15 minutes after initiating gum chewing, almost all from swallowing saliva. Chewing gum also increases gastric pH in children, leaving no clear evidence that it affects the risk of pneumonitis should aspiration occur.[28] A systemic review and meta-analysis of preoperative gum chewing in both children and adults concluded that chewing gum is unlikely to lead to a meaningful increase in the risk of major morbidity from pulmonary aspiration.[29] Consequently, we recommend that if the gum is discarded, then elective anesthesia can proceed without additional delay. If, however, the child swallows the gum, then surgery should be canceled, because aspirated gum at body temperature may be very difficult to extract from a bronchus or trachea.

Children can never be trusted to fast. Therefore, anesthesiologists must always be suspicious and question children just before induction as to whether they have eaten or drunk anything (although the veracity of the answer may always be questioned as well). It is not unusual to find bubble gum, candy, or other food in a child's mouth. This is another reason to ask children to open their mouth fully and stick out their tongue during the preoperative examination of the airway.

When the anesthesiologist suspects that the child has a full stomach, induction of anesthesia should be adjusted appropriately. The incidence of pulmonary aspiration of gastric contents during elective surgery in children ranges from 1 : 1163 to 1 : 10,000, depending on the study.[13–15,30,31] In contrast, the frequency of pulmonary aspiration in children undergoing emergency procedures

is several times greater, 1 : 373 to 1 : 4544.[30,31] Risk factors for perianesthetic aspiration included neurologic or esophagogastric abnormality, emergency surgery (especially at night), ASA physical status 3 to 5, intestinal obstruction, increased intracranial pressure, increased abdominal pressure, light anesthesia, obesity, and the skill and experience of the anesthesiologist.[14,31]

The majority of aspirations in children occur during induction of anesthesia, with only 13% occurring during emergence and extubation. In contrast, 30% of the aspirations in adults occur during emergence. Bowel obstruction or ileus was present in the majority of infants and children who aspirated during the perioperative period in one study, with the risk increasing in children younger than 3 years of age.[30] A combination of factors predisposes the infant and young child to regurgitation and aspiration, including decreased competence of the lower esophageal sphincter, excessive air swallowing while crying during the preinduction period, strenuous diaphragmatic breathing, and a shorter esophagus. In one study, almost all cases of pulmonary aspiration occurred either when the child gagged or coughed during airway manipulation or during induction of anesthesia when neuromuscular blocking drugs were not provided or before the child was completely paralyzed.[30]

When children do aspirate, the morbidity and mortality are exceedingly small for elective surgical procedures and generally reflect their ASA physical status; most patients with clinical status of ASA 1 or 2 who aspirate clear gastric contents have minimal to no sequelae.[13,30] If clinical signs of sequelae from an aspiration in a child are going to occur, they will be apparent within 2 hours[30]; mortality is exceedingly low and estimated to be between 0 and 1 : 50,000.[13,14,30]

PIERCINGS
Body piercing is common practice in adolescents and young adults. Single or multiple piercings may appear anywhere on the body. To minimize the liability and risk of complications from metal piercings, they should be removed before surgery. Complications that may occur if they are left in situ during anesthesia are listed in E-Table 4.1.[32–34]

PRIMARY AND SECONDARY SMOKING
Primary Smoking
Unfortunately, cigarette smoking is not only limited to adults. Each day, 3800 American adolescents smoke their first cigarette and of these, more than 50% will become regular smokers. The annual burden of smoking-attributable mortality remains high

with 5.6 million youth currently 0 to 17 years of age projected to die prematurely from a smoking-related illness.[35] Even though the rate of new cigarette smokers in North America has declined over the past 2 decades, this has been offset with an increase in use of other nicotine products such as electronic cigarettes (e-cigarettes). Many factors, including lack of regulation at the federal level, "harmless water vapor" messaging, a strong social media presence with celebrity endorsements, and flavors targeting a young audience ("Cupcake," "Alien Blood," "Cherry Crush," "Chocolate Treat," etc.) play a significant role in influencing initiation of e-cigarette use in this age group.[36] A national survey indicated that e-cigarette use was at an all-time high among high school students at 13.4%, which was more prevalent than conventional cigarette use at 9.2%.[37] Youth e-cigarette users are more likely than nonusers to report initiation of conventional cigarettes within a year.[38]

Smoking is known to increase blood carboxyhemoglobin concentrations, decrease ciliary function, decrease functional vital capacity (FVC) and the forced expiratory flow in midphase ($FEF_{25\%-75\%}$), and increase sputum production. There is extensive evidence that smokers undergoing surgery are more likely to develop wound infections and postoperative respiratory complications.[39] Although stopping smoking for 2 days decreases carboxyhemoglobin levels and shifts the oxyhemoglobin dissociation curve to the right, stopping for at least 6 to 8 weeks is necessary to reduce the rate of postoperative pulmonary complications.[40,41]

Current harmful effects of e-cigarette use focus on nicotine exposure, the potential for these products to be a gateway to cigarette use, and the possibility of exposure to harmful flavoring chemicals such as diacetyl (2,3-butanedione).[42] This chemical is used to give foods a buttery or creamy flavor and has been shown to cause acute-onset bronchiolitis obliterans.[43,44] Data are lacking on long-term exposure and health effects of the use of e-cigarettes given the limited time span these products have been in the marketplace.

The perioperative period is the ideal time to abandon the smoking habit permanently, and anesthesiologists can perhaps play a more active role in facilitating this process. Physician communication with adolescents regarding smoking cessation has been shown to positively impact their attitudes, knowledge, intentions to smoke, and quitting behaviors.[45] In summary, during the preoperative visit with adolescents, anesthesiologists should inquire about cigarette smoking and emphasize the need to stop the habit by offering measures to ameliorate the withdrawal (e.g., nicotine patch).

Secondary Smoking

A national survey in the United States revealed the percentage of children 3 to 19 years of age without asthma exposed to environmental tobacco smoke (ETS) decreased from 57.3% to 44.2% from 1999 to 2010 while a higher percentage of children with asthma (54.0%) were exposed to ETS.[46]

Studies have shown that children exposed to ETS are more likely to have asthma, otitis media,[47] atopic eczema, hay fever,[48] and dental caries.[49] There is also an increased rate of lower respiratory tract illness in infants with ETS exposure.[50,51] A recent systemic review and meta-analysis revealed a nearly 2-fold increase in risk of hospitalization for an asthma exacerbation in children with asthma and ETS in westernized countries.[52] This is the first time this risk has been quantified and will enable health care providers to convey the harmful effects of ETS to parents about aggravation of asthma.

Several authors have demonstrated that ETS results in increased perioperative airway complications in children. In one study,[53] urinary cotinine, the major metabolite of nicotine, was used as a surrogate marker of ETS. A strong association was found between passive inhalation of tobacco smoke and airway complications on induction and emergence from anesthesia. A prospective investigation in Australia provided further insight on the effect of the smoking habits of different family members; the risk for perioperative adverse respiratory events was higher when children were exposed to maternal or both parents smoking than when only the father smoked.[54] Respiratory adverse events include laryngospasm, bronchospasm, airway obstruction, oxygen desaturation (<95%), severe or sustained cough, and stridor in the postanesthesia care unit (PACU).

The evidence for adverse perioperative events in children from ETS is clearly overwhelming. During the preoperative visit, the anesthesiologist should ascertain the child's exposure to ETS by asking parents or guardians about smoking within the household. This is an opportune time to educate parents and guardians about the dangers of ETS for their children.

PSYCHOLOGICAL PREPARATION OF CHILDREN FOR SURGERY

The perioperative period is stressful and anxiety-provoking for the child and family; many parents express more concern about the risks of anesthesia than those of the surgery. The factors that influence the ability of the child and family to cope with the stress of surgery include family dynamics, the child's developmental and behavioral status and cultural biases, and our ability to explain away misperceptions and misinformation. Because of logistics and today's practice constraints, there is limited time to evaluate family dynamics and establish rapport. It is therefore vital for the anesthesiologist to interact directly with the child in a manner consistent with the child's level of development. A specific child-oriented approach by the anesthesiologist, surgeon, nurses, and hospital staff is required.

Although the preoperative evaluation and preparation of children are similar to those of adults from a physiologic standpoint, the psychological preparation of infants and children is very different (see also Chapter 3). Many hospitals have an open house or a brochure to describe the preoperative programs available to parents before the day of admission.[55] However, printed material should not replace verbal communication with nursing and medical staff.[56] Anesthesiologists are encouraged to participate in the design of these programs so that they accurately reflect the anesthetic practice of the institution. The preoperative anesthetic experience begins when parents are first informed that the child is to have surgery or a procedure that requires general anesthesia. Parental satisfaction correlates with the comfort of the environment and the trust established between the anesthesiologist, the child, and the parents.[57] If parental presence during induction is deemed to be in the child's best interest, a parental educational program that describes what the parent can expect to happen if he or she accompanies the child to the operating room (OR) can significantly decrease parents' anxiety and increase their satisfaction.[58] The greater the understanding and amount of information the parents have, the less anxious they will be, and this attitude, in turn, will be reflected in the child.[59,60]

Informed consent should include a detailed description of what the family can anticipate and our role to protect the welfare of the child. Before surgery, the anesthetic risks should be discussed in clear terms but in a reassuring manner by describing the measures that will be taken to carefully and closely monitor the safety of the child. Mentioning specific details and the purpose of the various monitoring devices may help diminish the parents' anxiety by demonstrating to them that the child will be anesthetized with the utmost safety and care. A blood pressure cuff will *"check the blood pressure,"* an electrocardiographic monitor will *"watch the heartbeat,"* a stethoscope will help us *"to continuously listen to the heart sounds,"* a pulse oximeter will *"measure the oxygen in the bloodstream,"* a carbon dioxide analyzer will *"monitor the breathing,"* an anesthetic agent monitor will *"accurately measure the level of anesthesia,"* and an IV catheter will be placed *"to administer fluid and medications as needed."* Children who are capable and their parents should be given ample opportunity to ask questions preoperatively. Finally, they should be assured that our "anesthetic prescription" will be designed specifically for their child's needs, taking into account the child's underlying medical conditions and the needs of surgery to ensure optimal conditions for surgery, the safety of the child, and analgesia.

It has been shown that parents desire comprehensive perioperative information, and that discussion of highly detailed anesthetic risk information does not increase parent's anxiety level.[61] Inadequate preparation of children and their families may lead to a traumatic anesthetic induction and difficulty for both the child and the anesthesiologist, with the possibility of postoperative psychological disturbances.[62] Numerous preoperative educational programs for children and adults have evolved to alleviate some of these fears and anxiety. They include preoperative tours of the ORs, educational videos, play therapy, magical distractions, puppet shows, anesthesia consultations, and child-life preparation.[63] The timing of the preoperative preparation has been found to be an important determinant of whether the intervention will be effective. For example, children older than 6 years of age who participated in a preparation program more than 5 to 7 days before surgery were least anxious during separation from their parents, those who participated in no preoperative preparation were moderately anxious, and those who received the information 1 day before surgery were the most anxious. The predictors of anxiety correlated also with the child's baseline temperament and history of previous hospitalizations.[64] Children of different ages vary in their response to the anesthetic experience (see also Chapter 3).[65] Even more important may be the child's trait anxiety when confronted with a stressful medical procedure.[66]

Child Development and Behavior

Understanding age-appropriate behavior in response to external situations is essential. Age-specific perioperative anxieties are outlined in E-Table 4.2 (see also Chapter 3 for further discussion of risk factors for preoperative anxiety). Special aspects of a child's perception of anesthesia should be anticipated; children often have the same fears as adults but are unable to articulate them. The reason and need for a surgical procedure should also be carefully explained to the child. It is important to reassure children that anesthesia is not the same as the usual nightly sleep, but rather a special sleep caused by the medicines we give during which they cannot be awakened and no matter what the surgeon does, they cannot feel pain. Many children fear the possibility that they will wake up in the middle of the anesthetic and during surgery. They should be reassured that they will awaken only after the surgery is completed.

The words the anesthesiologist uses to describe to the child what can be anticipated must be carefully chosen, because children think concretely and tend to interpret the facts literally. Examples of this are presented by the following anecdotes:

Example 1: A 4-year-old child was informed that in the morning she would receive a "shot" that would "put her to sleep." That night, a frantic call was received from the mother, describing a very upset child; the child thought she was going to be "put to sleep" like the veterinarian had permanently "put to sleep" her sick pet.

Example 2: A 5-year-old child admitted for elective inguinal herniorrhaphy received a heavy premedication and was deeply sedated on arrival in the OR. After discharge, the parents frequently discovered him wandering about the house at night. On questioning, the child stated that he was "protecting" his family. He stated: "I don't want anyone sneaking up on you and operating while you are sleeping."

In the first example, the child's concrete thought processes misunderstood the anesthesiologist's choice of words. The second case represents a problem of communication: the child was never told he would have an operation.

The importance of proper psychological preparation for surgery should not be underestimated. Often, little has been explained to both patient and parents before the day of surgery. Anesthesiologists have a key role in defusing fear of the unknown if they understand a child's age-related perception of anesthesia and surgery (see Chapter 3). They can convey their understanding by presenting a calm and friendly face (smiling, looking at the child, and making eye contact), offering a warm introduction, touching the patient in a reassuring manner (holding a child's or parent's hand), and being completely honest. Children respond positively to an honest description of exactly what they can anticipate. This includes informing them of the slight discomfort of starting an IV line or giving an intramuscular premedication, the possible bitter taste of an oral premedication, or breathing our magic laughing gas through the flavored mask.

The postoperative process, from the OR to the recovery room, and the onset of postoperative pain should be described. Encourage the child and family to ask questions. Strategies to maintain analgesia should be discussed, including the use of long-acting local anesthetics; nerve blocks; neuraxial blocks; patient-controlled, nurse-controlled, or parent-controlled analgesia or epidural analgesia; or intermittent opioids (see also Chapters 42, 43, and 44).

As children age, they become more aware of their bodies and may develop a fear of mutilation. Adolescents frequently appear quite independent and self-confident, but as a group, they have unique problems. In a moment their mood can change from an intelligent, mature adult to a very immature child who needs support and reassurance. Coping with a disability or illness is often very difficult for adolescents. Because they are often comparing their physical appearance with that of their peers, they may become especially anxious when they have a physical problem. In general, they want to know exactly what will transpire during the course of anesthesia. Adolescents are usually cooperative, preferring to be in control and unpremedicated preoperatively. The occasional overly anxious or rambunctious adolescent, however, may benefit from preanesthetic medication.

Monitoring the attitude and behavior of a child is very useful. A child who clings to the parents, avoids eye contact, and does not speak is very anxious. A self-assured, cocky child who "knows it all" may also be apprehensive or frightened. This know-it-all behavior may mask the child's true emotions, and he or she may decompensate just when cooperation is most needed. In some cases, nonpharmacologic supportive measures may be effective.

In the extremely anxious child, supportive measures alone may be insufficient to reduce anxiety, and premedication is indicated.

Identifying a difficult parent or child preoperatively is not always easy, especially if the anesthesiologist first meets the child or family on the day of surgery and has limited time to assess the situation. Occasionally, we receive a warning regarding a difficult parent or child from the surgeon or nursing staff, based on their encounters with the family. With experience, some anesthesiologists are able to identify difficult parents and children during the short preoperative assessment and make appropriate adjustments to the anesthetic management plan.

The "veterans" or "frequent flyers" of anesthesia can also be difficult in the perioperative period. They have played the anesthesia and surgical game before and are not interested in participating again, especially if their previous experiences were negative. These children may benefit the most from a relatively heavy premedication; reviewing previous responses to premedication will aid in the adjustment of the current planned premedication (e.g., adding ketamine and atropine to oral midazolam to achieve a greater depth of sedation).

It is important to observe the family dynamics to better understand the child and determine who is in control, the parent or the child. Families many times are in a state of stress, particularly if the child has a chronic illness; these parents are often angry, guilt ridden, or simply exhausted. Ultimately, the manner in which a family copes with an illness largely determines how the child will cope.[67] The well-organized, open, and communicative family tends to be supportive and resourceful, whereas the disorganized, noncommunicative, and dysfunctional family tends to be angry and frustrated. Dealing with a family and child from the latter category can be challenging. There is the occasional parent who is overbearing and demands total control of the situation. It is important to be empathetic and understanding but to set limits and clearly define the parent's role. He or she must be told that the anesthesiologist determines when the parent must leave the OR; this is particularly true if an unexpected development occurs during the induction.

Parental Presence During Induction

One controversial area in pediatric anesthesia is parental presence during induction. Some anesthesiologists encourage parents to be present at induction, whereas others are uncomfortable with the process and do not allow parents to be present. Inviting a parent to accompany the child to the OR has been interpreted by some courts as an implicit contract on the part of the caregiver who invited the parent to participate in the child's care; in one case, the institution was found to have assumed responsibility for a mother who suffered an injury when she fainted.[68] Each child and family must be evaluated individually; what is good for one child and family may not be good for the next.[69–72] (See Chapter 3 for a full discussion of this and other anxiolytic strategies in children.)

If the practice of having parents present at induction is to work well, then the anesthesiologist must be comfortable with such an arrangement. No parent should ever be forced to be present for the induction of anesthesia, nor should any anesthesiologist be forced into a situation that compromises the quality of care he or she affords a child in need.

Parents must be informed about what to anticipate in terms of the OR itself (e.g., equipment, surgical devices), in terms of what they may observe during induction (e.g., eyes rolling back, laryngeal noises, anesthetic monitor alarms, excitation), and when they will be asked to leave. They must also be instructed regarding their ability to assist during the induction process, such as by comforting the child, encouraging the child to trust the anesthesiologist, distracting the child, and consoling the child (Videos 4.1 and 4.2). Personnel should be immediately available to escort parents back to the waiting area at the appropriate time. Someone should also be available to care for a parent who wishes to leave the induction area or who becomes lightheaded or faints. An anesthesiologist's anxiety about parents' presence during induction decreases significantly with experience.[73]

Explaining what parents might see or hear is essential. We generally tell parents the following:

As you see your child fall asleep today, there are several things you might observe that you are not used to seeing. First, when anyone falls asleep, the eyes roll up, but since we are sleeping we do not generally see it. You may see your child do that today, and I do not want you to be frightened by that—it is expected and normal. The second thing is that as children go to sleep from the anesthesia medications, the tone of the structures in the neck decreases, so that some children will begin to snore or make vibrating noises. Again, I do not want you to be frightened or think that something is wrong. We expect this, and it is normal. The third thing you might see is what we call "excitement." As the brain begins to go to sleep, it can actually get excited first. About 30 to 60 seconds after breathing the anesthesia medications, your child might suddenly look around or suddenly move his or her arms and legs. To you it appears that he or she is awakening from anesthesia or that he or she is upset. In reality, this is a good sign, because it indicates to us that your child is falling asleep and that 15 to 30 seconds later he or she will be completely anesthetized. Also, you should know that even though your child appears to be awake to you, in reality he or she will not remember any of that. As soon as your child loses consciousness, we will ask you to give your child a kiss and step out of the operating room.

This kind of careful preparation provides to the parents the confidence that the anesthesiologist really knows what he or she is talking about, and it avoids frightening the parents. In general, the more information provided, the lower the parental anxiety levels. A child-life specialist in surgical services may also prove valuable to the anesthesiologist by calming and preparing both children and parents for the OR experience (see "Inhalation Induction" later in this chapter for further details).

Occasionally, the best efforts to relieve a child's anxiety by parental presence or administration of a sedative premedication (or both) are not successful, and an anticipated smooth induction may not go as planned. There are three options that may be used depending on the age of the child: (1) renegotiating (which is seldom successful), (2) holding the mask farther away from the child's face, or (3) suggesting an IV or intramuscular induction. If an intramuscular shot or IV induction is proposed, the child will usually choose the mask. If the situation is totally out of control, either elective surgery can be rescheduled or intramuscular ketamine can be used if the parents choose to proceed. These situations are particularly difficult for the parents and the caregivers but must be handled on an individual basis.

HISTORY OF PRESENT ILLNESS

The medical history of a child obtained during the preanesthetic visit allows the anesthesiologist to determine whether the child is optimized for the planned surgery, to anticipate potential problems due to coexisting disease, to determine whether appropriate laboratory or other tests are available or needed, to select optimal premedication, to formulate the appropriate anesthetic plan including perioperative monitoring, and to anticipate postoperative concerns

TABLE 4.2 | Review of Systems: Anesthetic Implications

System	Factors to Assess	Possible Anesthetic Implications
Respiratory	Cough, asthma, recent cold	Irritable airway, bronchospasm, medication history, atelectasis, infiltrate
	Croup	Subglottic narrowing
	Apnea/bradycardia	Postoperative apnea/bradycardia
Cardiovascular	Murmur	Septal defect, avoid air bubbles in IV line
	Cyanosis	Right-to-left shunt
	History of squatting	Tetralogy of Fallot
	Hypertension	Coarctation, renal disease
	Rheumatic fever	Valvular heart disease
	Exercise intolerance	Congestive heart failure, cyanosis
Neurologic	Seizures	Medications, metabolic derangement
	Head trauma	Intracranial hypertension
	Swallowing incoordination	Aspiration, esophageal reflux, hiatus hernia
	Neuromuscular disease	Neuromuscular relaxant drug sensitivity, malignant hyperpyrexia
Gastrointestinal/hepatic	Vomiting, diarrhea	Electrolyte imbalance, dehydration, full stomach
	Malabsorption	Anemia
	Black stools	Anemia, hypovolemia
	Reflux	Possible need for full-stomach precautions
	Jaundice	Drug metabolism/hypoglycemia
Genitourinary	Frequency	Urinary tract infection, diabetes, hypercalcemia
	Time of last urination	State of hydration
	Frequent urinary tract infections	Evaluate renal function
Endocrine/metabolic	Abnormal development	Endocrinopathy, hypothyroid, diabetes
	Hypoglycemia, steroid therapy	Hypoglycemia, adrenal insufficiency
Hematologic	Anemia	Need for transfusion
	Bruising, excessive bleeding	Coagulopathy, thrombocytopenia, thrombocytopathy
	Sickle cell disease	Hydration, possible transfusion
Allergies	Medications	Possible drug interaction
Dental	Loose or carious teeth	Aspiration of loose teeth, bacterial endocarditis prophylaxis

including pain management and postoperative ventilatory needs. The history of the present illness is described to the physicians by the parents and verified by the referring or consultant surgeon's notes. If the child is old enough, it is helpful to obtain the child's input. The history should focus on the following aspects:

- A review of all organ systems (Table 4.2) with special emphasis on the organ system involved in the surgery
- A review of patient and parental smoking history
- Medications (over-the-counter and prescribed) related to and taken before the present illness, including herbals and vitamins, and when the last dose was taken
- Medication allergies with specific details of the nature of the allergy and whether immunologic testing was performed
- Previous surgical and hospital experiences, including those related to the current problem
- Timing of the last oral intake, last urination (wet diaper), and vomiting and diarrhea. It is essential to recognize that decreased gastrointestinal motility often occurs with an illness or injury.

In the case of a neonate, problems that may have been present during gestation and birth may still be relevant in the neonatal period and beyond (E-Table 4.3). The maternal medical and pharmacologic history (both therapeutic and drug abuse) may also provide valuable information for the management of a neonate requiring surgery.

PAST/OTHER MEDICAL HISTORY

The past medical history should include a history of all past medical illnesses with a review of organ systems, previous hospitalizations (medical or surgical), childhood syndromes with associated anomalies, medication list, herbal remedies, and any allergies, especially to antibiotics and latex. Whether the child was full-term or preterm at birth should be discerned; if preterm, any associated problems should be noted, including admission to a neonatal intensive care unit, duration of tracheal intubation, history of apnea or bradycardia (including oxygen treatment, home apnea monitor, intraventricular hemorrhage), and congenital defects.

Examination of previous surgical and anesthesia records greatly assists in planning the anesthesia. Particular attention should be paid to any difficulties encountered with airway management, venous access, or emergence. The response to or need for premedication and the route of administration used should be noted.

Herbal Remedies

The use of herbal medicinal products has become increasingly popular, likely driven by the notion that "natural" substances have fewer side effects. A survey in five geographically diverse centers in the United States found that 3.5% of pediatric surgical patients had been given herbal supplements or homeopathic remedies 2 weeks prior to surgery.[74] The findings of the National

Health Interview Survey confirm a similar prevalence rate in which natural product usage among children age 0 to 17 years amounts to 3.9%.[75] Herbal medicine use is more common in adults; 32% of adult surgical patients take one or more herb-related compounds.[76] Nearly 70% of adults failed to disclose their use of herbal remedies when asked about medications during routine perioperative assessment. Herbal medicines are regulated as food supplements under the Dietary Supplement Health and Education Act of 1994 and as such manufacturers are not required to demonstrate safety or efficacy before placing a product on the market.[77] Without the Food and Drug Administration (FDA) regulation, there are no quality assurance requirements for manufacturing and labeling and much variation can occur in each preparation.[78] Anesthesiologists should include specific inquiries regarding the use of these medications because of the potential for adverse effects and drug interactions.

Herbal medicines are associated with cardiovascular instability, coagulation disturbances, potentiation of sedation, and immunosuppression.[79] The most commonly used herbal medications reported are garlic, ginseng, *Ginkgo biloba*, St. John's wort, and *Echinacea*,[80] with *Echinacea* and other herbal medicines for the treatment of coughs and colds taking the lead in the pediatric population.[74,81] The three "g" herbals, together with feverfew *(Tanacetum parthenium)*, potentially increase the risk of bleeding during surgery. The amount of active ingredient in each preparation and the dose taken may vary, thus making detection of a change in platelet function and other subtle coagulation disturbances difficult. St. John's wort is the herb that most commonly interacts with anesthetics and other medications, usually via a change in drug metabolism, because of potent inducing effects on the cytochrome P-450 enzymes (e.g., CYP3A4) and P-glycoprotein. A potentially fatal interaction between cyclosporine and St. John's wort has been well documented.[82–85] Heart, kidney, or liver transplant recipients who were stabilized on a dose of cyclosporine experienced decreased plasma concentrations of cyclosporine and, in some cases, acute rejection episodes after taking St. John's wort. A summary of the most commonly used herbal remedies and their potential perioperative complications is shown in E-Table 4.4.

To avoid potential perioperative complications, the ASA has encouraged the discontinuation of all herbal medicines 2 weeks before surgery,[86] although this recommendation is not evidence based. Recognizing that this is not always feasible, the ASA further recommends that anesthesiologists have knowledge of herbal medications and their potential interactions. Each herb should be carefully evaluated using standard resource texts, and a decision should be made regarding the timing of or need for discontinuation as determined on a case-by-case basis.[87]

Anesthesia and Vaccination

Children may present for surgery after having been recently immunized. The anesthesiologist and surgeon must then consider (1) whether the immunomodulatory effects of anesthesia and surgery might affect the efficacy and safety of the vaccine and (2) whether the inflammatory responses to the vaccine will alter the perioperative course.

What do anesthesiologists think about anesthesia and vaccination? An international survey[88] revealed that only one-third of responding anesthesiologists had the benefit of a hospital policy, ranging from a formal decision to delay surgery to an independent choice by the anesthesiologist. Sixty percent of respondents would anesthetize a child for elective surgery within 1 week of receiving a live attenuated vaccine (such as oral polio vaccine or measles,

mumps, and rubella [MMR] vaccine), whereas 40% would not. The survey also revealed that 28% of anesthesiologists would delay immunization for 2 to 30 days after surgery.

A scientific review of the literature associating anesthesia and vaccination in children resulted in recommendations for the care of children under these circumstances.[89] The review demonstrated a brief and reversible influence of vaccination on lymphoproliferative responses that generally returned to preoperative values within 2 days. Vaccine-driven adverse events (e.g., fever, pain, irritability) might occur but should not be confused with perioperative complications. Adverse events to inactivated vaccines such as diphtheria-tetanus-pertussis (DPT) become apparent from 2 days and to live attenuated vaccines such as MMR from 7 to 21 days after immunization.[89] Therefore appropriate delays between immunization and anesthesia are recommended by type of vaccine to avoid misinterpretation of vaccine-associated adverse events as perioperative complications. Because children remain at risk of contracting vaccine-preventable diseases, the minimum delay seems prudent, especially in the first year of life. Likewise, it seems reasonable to delay vaccination *after* surgery until the child is fully recovered. These recommendations were adopted in a consensus guideline by the Association of Paediatric Anaesthetists of Great Britain and Ireland,* though to date, the US Centers for Disease Control and Prevention does not have a policy regarding the timing of vaccinations and surgery. Other immunocompromised patients, such as human immunodeficiency virus (HIV)-positive children, cancer patients, and transplant recipients, have distinct underlying immune impairments, and the influence of anesthesia on vaccine responses has not been comprehensively investigated.

Allergies to Medications and Latex

The details pertaining to all allergies to medications and materials should be described in the child's record. These include the age of onset, frequency, severity, investigations, and treatments. The vast majority of reported allergies on children's charts are either nonimmunologic reactions or known (or unknown) drug adverse effects. The most common medication- and hospital-related allergies in children are penicillin and latex allergy.

Most cases of reported penicillin allergy consist of a maculopapular rash after oral penicillin. This occurs in 1% to 4% of children receiving penicillin or in 3% to 7% of those taking ampicillin, usually during treatment.[90] Rarely are signs or symptoms that suggest an acute (immunoglobulin E–mediated) allergic reaction present (i.e., angioedema), and even less frequently is skin testing conducted to establish penicillin allergy. Given the frequency of penicillin allergy, most of these unverified allergies in fact are not allergies to penicillin but rather minor allergies to the dye in the liquid vehicle or a consequence of the (viral) infection. If the child has not received penicillin for at least 5 years since the initial exposure and has not been diagnosed with a penicillin allergy by an immunologist or allergist, then a reexposure is warranted. If the child has been tested immunologically for penicillin allergy, then it is best to avoid this class of antibiotics. Although there is a 5% to 10% cross-reactivity between first-generation cephalosporins and penicillin, there is no similar cross-reactivity with second- and third-generation cephalosporins. To date, there have been no fatal anaphylactic reactions in penicillin-allergic children from a cephalosporin.[90]

---

*See http://www.apagbi.org.uk/sites/default/files/images/Final%20Immunisation%20apa.pdf (accessed March 27, 2016).

Latex allergy is an acquired immunologic sensitivity resulting from repeated exposure to latex, usually on mucous membranes (e.g., children with spina bifida or congenital urologic abnormalities who have undergone repeated bladder catheterizations with latex catheters, those with more than four surgeries, those requiring home ventilation). It occurs more frequently in atopic individuals and in those with certain fruit and vegetable allergies (e.g., banana, chestnut, avocado, kiwi, pineapple).[91-97] For a diagnosis of latex anaphylaxis, the child should have personally experienced an anaphylactic reaction to latex, skin-tested positive for anaphylaxis to latex, or experienced swelling of the lips after touching a toy balloon to the lips or a swollen tongue after a dentist inserted a rubber dam into the mouth.[97] The avoidance of latex within the hospital will prevent acute anaphylactic reactions to latex in children who are at risk.[98] Latex gloves and other latex-containing products should be removed from the immediate vicinity of the child. Prophylactic therapy with histamine H_1- and H_2-receptor antagonists and steroids do not prevent latex anaphylaxis.[91,99] Latex anaphylaxis should be treated by removal of the source of latex, administration of 100% oxygen, acute volume loading with balanced salt solution (10 to 20 mL/kg repeated until the systolic blood pressure stabilizes), and administration of IV epinephrine (1 to 10 µg/kg according to the severity of the anaphylaxis). In some severe reactions, a continuous infusion of epinephrine alone (0.01 to 0.2 µg/kg per minute) or combined with other vasoactive medications may be required for several hours.

Family History

It is important to inquire about a family history, particularly focusing on a number of conditions, including malignant hyperthermia, muscular dystrophy, prolonged paralysis associated with anesthesia (pseudocholinesterase deficiency), sickle cell disease, bleeding (and bruising) tendencies, and drug addiction (drug withdrawal, HIV infection). The precise relationship to the proband must be documented.

LABORATORY DATA

The laboratory data obtained preoperatively should be appropriate to the history, illness, and surgical procedure. Routine hemoglobin testing or urinalysis is not indicated for most elective procedures; the value of these tests is questionable when the surgical procedure will not involve clinically important blood loss.[100] There are insufficient data in the literature to make strict hemoglobin testing recommendations in healthy children. A preoperative hemoglobin value is usually determined only for those who will undergo procedures with the potential for blood loss, those with specific risk factors for a hemoglobinopathy, former preterm infants, and those younger than 6 months of age. Coagulation studies (platelet count, international normalized ratio [INR], and partial thromboplastin time [PTT]) may be indicated if major reconstructive surgery is contemplated, especially if warranted by the medical history, and in some centers before tonsillectomy. In addition, collection of a preoperative type-and-screen or type-and-crossmatch sample is indicated in preparation for potential blood transfusions depending on the nature of the planned surgery and the anticipated blood loss.

In general, routine chest radiography is not necessary; studies have confirmed that routine chest radiographs are not cost-effective in children.[101,102] The oxygen saturation of children who are breathing room air is very helpful. Baseline saturations of 95% or less suggest clinically important pulmonary or cardiac compromise and warrant further investigation.

Selective preoperative laboratory tests, such as electrolyte and blood glucose determinations, renal function tests, blood gas analysis, blood concentrations of seizure medication and digoxin, electrocardiography, echocardiography, liver function tests, computed tomography (CT), magnetic resonance imaging (MRI), or pulmonary function tests, should be performed when appropriate. These tests may be ordered after consideration of specific information obtained from sources such as medical records, patient interview, physical examination, and the type and invasiveness of the planned procedure and anesthesia.

PREGNANCY TESTING

Although pregnancy rates among teenagers in the United States are declining,[103] a small percentage of adolescents may still present for elective surgery with an unsuspected pregnancy. Birth rates for teenagers in the United States declined to historic lows in 2014, to 24.2 births/1000 females aged 15–19 compared with 2003 when the birth rate in that age group was 41.6 births/1000.[103,104] The birth rate for girls aged 10 to 14 years also declined from 0.6/1000 in 2003[104] to 0.3/1000 in 2014.[103] However, routine preoperative pregnancy testing in adolescent girls may present ethical and legal dilemmas, including social and confidentiality concerns. This places the anesthesiologist in a predicament when faced with a question of whether to perform routine preoperative pregnancy screening. Each hospital should adopt a policy regarding pregnancy testing to provide a consistent and comprehensive policy for all females who have reached menarche.

A survey of members of the Society for Pediatric Anesthesia practicing in North America revealed that pregnancy testing was routinely required by approximately 45% of the respondents regardless of the practice setting (teaching versus nonteaching facilities).[100] A retrospective review of a 2-year study of mandatory pregnancy testing in 412 adolescent surgical patients[105] revealed that the overall incidence of positive tests was 1.2%. Five of 207 patients aged 15 years and older tested positive, for an incidence of 2.4% in that age group. None of the 205 patients younger than the age of 15 years had a positive pregnancy test. A prospective study of 261 menarcheal patients 10 to 34 years of age revealed 3 pregnancies but none of 107 children <15 years.[106]

The most recent ASA Task Force on Preanesthesia Evaluation recognized that a history and physical examination may not adequately identify early pregnancy and issued the following statement: *"The literature is insufficient to inform patients or physicians on whether anesthesia causes harmful effects on early pregnancy. Pregnancy testing may be offered to female patients of childbearing age and for whom the result would alter the patient's management."*[107] Because of the risk of exposing the fetus to potential teratogens and radiation from anesthesia and surgery, the risk of spontaneous abortion, and the risk of apoptosis reported in the rapidly developing fetal animal brain (see Chapter 25), elective surgery with general anesthesia is not advised during early pregnancy. Therefore, if the situation is unclear, and when indicated by medical history, it is best to perform a preoperative pregnancy test. If the surgery is required in a patient who might be pregnant, then using an opioid-based anesthetic such as remifentanil and the lowest concentration of inhalational agent or propofol that provides adequate anesthesia is preferred.

Premedication and Induction Principles

GENERAL PRINCIPLES

The major objectives of preanesthetic medication are to (1) allay anxiety, (2) block autonomic (vagal) reflexes, (3) reduce airway secretions, (4) produce amnesia, (5) provide prophylaxis against pulmonary aspiration of gastric contents, (6) facilitate the induction of anesthesia, and (7) if necessary, provide analgesia. Premedication may also decrease the stress response to anesthesia and prevent cardiac arrhythmias.[108] The goal of premedication for each child must be individualized. Light sedation, even though it may not eliminate anxiety, may adequately calm a child so that the induction of anesthesia will be smooth and a pleasant experience. In contrast, heavy sedation may be needed for the very anxious child who is unwilling to separate from his or her parents.

Factors to consider when selecting a drug or a combination of drugs for premedication include the child's age, ideal body weight, drug history, and allergic status; underlying medical or surgical conditions and how they might affect the response to premedication or how the premedication might alter anesthetic induction; parent and child expectations; and the child's emotional maturity, personality, anxiety level, cooperation, and physiologic and psychological status. The anesthesiologist should also consider the proposed surgical procedure and the attitudes and wishes of the child and the parents.

The route of administration of premedicant drugs is very important. Premedications have been administered by many routes, including the oral, nasal, rectal, buccal, IV, and intramuscular routes. Although a drug may be more effective and have a more reliable onset when given intranasally or intramuscularly, most pediatric anesthesiologists refrain from administering parenteral medication to children without IV access. Many children who are able to verbalize report that receiving a needle puncture was their worst experience in the hospital.[109,110] In most cases, medication administered without a needle will be more pleasant for children, their parents, and the medical staff. Oral premedications do not increase the risk of aspiration pneumonia unless large volumes of fluids are ingested.[111] In general, the route of delivery of the premedication should depend on the drug, the desired drug effect, and the psychological impact of the route of administration. For example, a small dose of oral medication may be sufficient for a relatively calm child, whereas an intramuscular injection (e.g., ketamine) may be best for an uncooperative, combative, extremely anxious child. Intramuscular administration may be less traumatic for this type of child than forcing him or her to swallow a drug, giving a drug rectally, or forcefully holding an anesthesia mask on the face.[112]

Since Waters'[113] classic work in 1938 on premedication of children, numerous reports have addressed this subject. Despite the wealth of studies, no single drug or combination of drugs has been found to be ideal for all children. Many drugs used for premedication have similar effects, and a specific drug may have various effects in different children or in the same child under different conditions.

MEDICATIONS

Several categories of drugs are available for premedicating children before anesthesia (Table 4.3). Selection of drugs for premedication depends on the goal desired. Drug effects should be weighed against potential side effects, and drug interactions should be considered. Premedicant drugs include tranquilizers, benzodiazepines, barbiturates, nonbarbiturate sedatives, opioids, ketamine, α2 agonists, and drugs that increase gastric motility.

Tranquilizers

The major effect of tranquilizers is to allay anxiety, but they also have the potential to produce sedation. This group of drugs includes the benzodiazepines, phenothiazines, and butyrophenones. Benzodiazepines are widely used in children, whereas phenothiazines and butyrophenones are infrequently used.

TABLE 4.3	Doses of Drugs Commonly Administered for Premedication	
Drug	**Route**	**Dose (mg/kg)**
Barbiturates		
Methohexital	Rectal	(10% solution) 20–40
	Intramuscular	(5% solution) 10
Thiopental	Rectal	(10% solution) 20–40
Benzodiazepines		
Diazepam	Oral	0.1–0.5
	Rectal	1
Midazolam	Oral	0.25–0.75
	Nasal	0.2
	Rectal	0.5–1
	Intramuscular	0.1–0.15
Lorazepam	Oral	0.025–0.05
Phencyclidine		
Ketamine[a]	Oral	3–6
	Nasal	3
	Rectal	6–10
	Intramuscular	2–10
α₂-Adrenergic Agonist		
Clonidine	Oral	0.004
Opioids		
Morphine	Intramuscular	0.1–0.2
Meperidine[b]	Intramuscular	1–2
Fentanyl	Oral	0.010–0.015 (10–15 µg/kg)
	Nasal	0.001–0.002 (1–2 µg/kg)
Sufentanil	Nasal	0.001–0.003 (1–3 µg/kg)

[a]With atropine 0.02 mg/kg.
[b]Only a single dose is recommended due to metabolites that may cause seizures.

Benzodiazepines

Benzodiazepines calm children, allay anxiety, and diminish recall of perianesthetic events. At low doses, minimal drowsiness and cardiovascular or respiratory depression are produced.

Midazolam, a short-acting, water-soluble benzodiazepine with an elimination half-life of approximately 2 hours, is the most widely used premedication for children.[114,115] The major advantage of midazolam over other drugs in its class is its rapid uptake and elimination.[116] It can be administered intravenously, intramuscularly, nasally, orally, and rectally with minimal irritation, although it leaves a bitter taste in the mouth or nasopharynx after oral or nasal administration.[117-123] Most children are adequately sedated after receiving a midazolam dose of 0.025 to 0.1 mg/kg intravenously, 0.1 to 0.2 mg/kg intramuscularly, 0.25 to 0.75 mg/kg orally, 0.2 mg/kg nasally, or 1 mg/kg rectally.

Orally administered midazolam is effective in calming most children and does not increase gastric pH or residual volume.[124,125] Evidence suggests that the required dose of midazolam increases as age decreases in children, similar to that for inhaled agents and IV agents.[126] An increased clearance in younger children contributes to their increased dose requirement.[127] A number of medications that affect the cytochrome oxidase system significantly affect the first-pass metabolism of midazolam, including grapefruit juice, erythromycin, protease inhibitors, and calcium-channel blockers that decrease CYP3A4 activity, which in turn increases the blood concentration of midazolam and prolongs sedation.[128-134] Conversely, anticonvulsants (phenytoin and carbamazepine), rifampin, St. John's wort, glucocorticoids, and barbiturates induce the CYP3A4 isoenzyme, thereby reducing the blood concentration of midazolam and its duration of action. The dose of oral midazolam should be adjusted in children who are taking these medications.

Concerns have been raised about possible delayed discharge after premedication with oral midazolam. Oral midazolam, 0.5 mg/kg, administered to children 1 to 10 years of age, did not affect awakening times, time to extubation, postanesthesia care unit, or hospital discharge times, after sevoflurane anesthesia.[135] Similar results have been reported in children and adolescents after 20 mg of oral midazolam; however, detectable preoperative sedation in this group of children was predictive of delayed emergence.[136] In children aged 1 to 3 years undergoing adenoidectomy as outpatients, premedication with oral midazolam, 0.5 mg/kg, slightly delayed spontaneous eye opening by 4 minutes and discharge by 10 minutes compared with placebo; children who had been premedicated, however, exhibited a more peaceful sleep at home on the night after surgery.[137]

Likely the greatest effect of oral midazolam on recovery occurs with its use in children undergoing myringotomy and tube insertion, a procedure that normally takes 5 to 7 minutes. After oral midazolam premedication (0.5 mg/kg), induction of anesthesia with propofol, and maintenance with sevoflurane, emergence and early recovery were delayed by 6 and 14 minutes, respectively, in children 1 to 3 years of age compared with unpremedicated children, although discharge times did not differ.[138] Increased postoperative sedation may be attributed to synergism between propofol and midazolam on γ-aminobutyric acid (GABA) receptors.[139]

Although anxiolysis and a mild degree of sedation occur in most children after midazolam, a few develop undesirable adverse effects. Some children become agitated after oral midazolam.[140] If this occurs after IV midazolam (0.1 mg/kg), IV ketamine (0.5 mg/kg) may reverse the agitation.[141]

Anxiolysis and sedation usually occur within 10 minutes after intranasal midazolam[142]; nasal administration is not well accepted because it produces irritation, discomfort, and a burning aftertaste.[143-145] Another theoretical concern for the nasal route of administration of midazolam is its potential to cause neurotoxicity via the cribriform plate.[123] There are direct connections between the nasal mucosa and the central nervous system (CNS) (E-Fig. 4.2). Medications administered nasally reach high concentrations in the cerebrospinal fluid very quickly.[146-148] To date, no such sequelae have been reported. Because midazolam with preservative has been shown to cause neurotoxicity in animals, we recommend only preservative-free midazolam for nasal administration.[149,150]

Sublingual midazolam (0.2 mg/kg) has been reported to be as effective as, and better accepted than, intranasal midazolam.[151] Oral transmucosal midazolam given in three to five small allotments (0.2 mg/kg total dose) placed on a child's tongue (8 months to 6 years of age) was found to provide satisfactory acceptance and separation from parents in 95% of children.[152]

Diazepam is used only for premedication of older children. In infants and especially preterm neonates, the elimination half-life of diazepam is markedly prolonged because of immature hepatic function (see Chapter 7). In addition, the active metabolite (desmethyldiazepam) has pharmacologic activity equal to that of the parent compound and a half-life of up to 9 days in adults.[153] The most effective route of administration of diazepam is intra-venous, followed by oral and rectal. The intramuscular route is not recommended because it is painful and absorption is erratic.[154-158] The average oral dose for premedicating healthy children with diazepam ranges from 0.1 to 0.3 mg/kg; however, doses as large as 0.5 mg/kg have been used.[159] The recommended dose of rectal diazepam is 1 mg/kg, and the peak serum concentration is reached after approximately 20 minutes.[160] Compared with rectal midazolam, rectal diazepam is less effective.[161]

Lorazepam (0.05 mg/kg) is reserved primarily for older children. Lorazepam causes less tissue irritation and more reliable amnesia than diazepam. It can be administered orally, intravenously, or intramuscularly and is metabolized in the liver to inactive metabolites. Compared with diazepam, the onset of action of lorazepam is slower and its duration of action is prolonged. The IV formulation of lorazepam is avoided in neonates because it may be neurotoxic.[162,163]

Barbiturates

Barbiturates are infrequently used for premedication as they have been replaced by oral midazolam. The advantages of barbiturates include minimal respiratory or cardiovascular depression, anticonvulsant effects, and a very low incidence of nausea and vomiting.

The relatively short-acting barbiturates *thiopental* and *methohexital* may be given rectally as a 10% solution in the presence of the parents who may hold the toddler until he or she is sedated.[164] The usual dose of rectal thiopental or methohexital is 30 mg/kg via a shortened suction catheter, which produces sleep in about two-thirds of the children within 15 minutes.[165-169] In some cases, the sedation may be profound, resulting in airway obstruction and laryngospasm. Hence, all children should be closely monitored with a source of oxygen, suction, and a means for providing ventilatory support; rectally administered methohexital has been reported to cause apnea in children with meningomyelocele.[170,171] Children chronically treated with phenobarbital or phenytoin are more resistant to the effects of rectally administered methohexital, probably because of enzyme induction.[166,172]

Additional disadvantages of rectal methohexital include unpredictable systemic absorption, defecation after administration, and hiccups. Contraindications to methohexital include hypersensitivity, temporal lobe epilepsy, and latent or overt porphyria.[173-175] Rectal methohexital is also contraindicated in children with rectal mucosal tears or hemorrhoids because large quantities of the drug can be absorbed, resulting in respiratory or cardiac arrest.

Nonbarbiturate Sedatives

Chloral hydrate and *triclofos* are orally administered nonbarbiturate drugs used to sedate children; both have slow onset times and are relatively long acting. Recommended dosing is outlined in Chapters 7 and 48. Chloral hydrate is rarely used by anesthesiologists because it is unreliable, has a prolonged duration of action, is unpleasant to taste, and is irritating to the skin, mucous membranes, and gastrointestinal tract. Use in neonates is not recommended because of impaired metabolism.[176,177] Commercially prepared chloral hydrate is no longer available in the United States but a powdered form can be reconstituted by the hospital pharmacy for oral administration.

Opioids

Opioids may be useful to provide analgesia and sedation in children who have pain preoperatively, but they also confer side effects, including nausea, vomiting, respiratory depression, sedation, and dysphoria. Therefore all children who receive an opioid premedication should be continuously observed and monitored with pulse oximetry.

Morphine sulfate, 0.05 to 0.1 mg/kg intravenously, may be given to children with preoperative pain. It is also effective when given orally; rectal administration is not recommended owing to erratic absorption. Neonates are more sensitive to the respiratory depressant effects of morphine, and it is rarely used to premedicate that age group.[178]

Fentanyl was introduced in a "lollipop" delivery system known as oral transmucosal fentanyl citrate (OTFC) for premedication in children in the United States but is no longer available for that indication, in part due to the high incidence of preoperative nausea and vomiting. Its current use is to treat breakthrough cancer pain. Fentanyl has also been administered nasally (1 to 2 µg/kg) but primarily after induction of anesthesia as a means of providing analgesia in children without IV access.[179]

Sufentanil is 10 times more potent than fentanyl and is administered nasally in a dose of 1.5 to 3 µg/kg. Children are usually calm and cooperative, and most separate from their parents with minimal distress.[142] In a study that compared the adverse effects of nasally administered midazolam and sufentanil, midazolam caused more nasal irritation, whereas sufentanil caused more postoperative nausea and vomiting and reduced chest wall compliance. In addition, children in the sufentanil group were discharged approximately 40 minutes later than those in the midazolam group.[144] The potential adverse effects and prolonged hospital stay after nasal sufentanil make it an unpopular choice for premedication.

Tramadol is a weak µ-opioid receptor agonist whose analgesic effect is mediated via inhibition of norepinephrine reuptake and stimulation of serotonin release. Tramadol is devoid of action on platelets and does not depress respirations in the clinical dose range.[180] Serum concentrations peak by 2 hours after oral dosing with clinical analgesia maintained for 6 to 9 hours. Tramadol is metabolized by CYP2D6 and is subject to variable responses based on polymorphisms of this enzyme.[181] IV tramadol (1.5 mg/kg) given before induction of general anesthesia has been compared with local infiltration of 0.5% bupivacaine (0.25 mL/kg) for ilioinguinal and iliohypogastric nerve blocks. Tramadol was as effective as the regional blocks in terms of pain control, although the incidence of nausea and vomiting was greater in the tramadol group. Time to discharge was similar in both groups.[182]

Butorphanol is a synthetic opioid agonist-antagonist with properties similar to those of morphine that can be administered nasally.[183] The most frequent adverse effect is sedation that resolves approximately 1 hour after administration. A dose of 0.025 mg/kg administered nasally immediately after the induction of anesthesia was shown to provide good analgesia after myringotomy and tube placement at the expense of an increased incidence of emesis at home compared with nonopioid analgesics such as acetaminophen.[184]

When fentanyl or other opioids are combined with midazolam, they produce more respiratory depression than opioids or midazolam alone.[185] If opioids are used in combination with other sedatives such as benzodiazepines, the dose of each drug should be appropriately reduced to avoid serious respiratory depression. For example, if fentanyl is indicated to control pain in a child who has already received midazolam, the fentanyl dose should be titrated in small increments (0.25 to 0.5 µg/kg) to prevent desaturation and hypopnea or apnea.

Codeine is a prodrug that must undergo *O*-demethylation in the liver to produce morphine to provide effective analgesia. The usual oral dose of oral codeine is 0.5 to 1.5 mg/kg with an onset

of action within 20 minutes and a peak effect between 1 and 2 hours. The elimination half-life of codeine is 2.5 to 3 hours. The combination of codeine with acetaminophen is effective in relieving mild to moderate pain. Importantly, between 5% and 10% of children lack the cytochrome isoenzyme (CYP2D6) required for this conversion and therefore do not derive analgesic benefit. On the other hand, a very small percentage of children are ultrarapid metabolizers who rapidly convert this prodrug to morphine (see Chapters 6 and 7 for further discussion). As a result, they will have excessive blood levels of morphine and the potential for severe adverse effects such as respiratory depression and cardiac arrest, particularly if excessive or frequent doses of codeine are prescribed. Children with obstructive sleep apnea have been shown to have altered mu receptors and increased analgesia; thus a normal dose in such children can be a relative overdose.[186–191] As a result of deaths following tonsillectomy, the FDA issued a black box warning regarding the use of codeine in children undergoing tonsillectomy.[192] Most children's hospitals have now removed codeine from their formulary as a result of these concerns.[193]

Ketamine

Ketamine is a phencyclidine derivative that produces dissociation of the cortex from the limbic system, producing reliable sedation and analgesia while preserving upper airway muscular tone and respiratory drive.[194] Ketamine may be administered by IV, intramuscular, oral, nasal transmucosal, and rectal routes. The disadvantages of ketamine include sialorrhea, nystagmus, an increased incidence of postoperative emesis, and possible undesirable psychological reactions such as hallucinations, nightmares, and delirium, although to date no psychological reactions have been reported after oral ketamine. Concomitant administration of midazolam may eliminate or attenuate these emergence reactions.[195,196] The addition of atropine or glycopyrrolate is recommended to decrease the sialorrhea caused by ketamine.[197]

Intramuscular ketamine is an effective means of sedating combative, apprehensive, or developmentally delayed children who are otherwise uncooperative and refuse oral medication. A low dose of 2 mg/kg is sufficient to adequately calm most uncooperative children within 3 to 5 minutes so that they will accept a mask for inhalation induction of anesthesia and does not prolong hospital discharge times even after brief procedures.[112] However, the combination of intramuscular ketamine (2 mg/kg) and midazolam (0.1 to 0.2 mg/kg) significantly prolongs recovery and discharge times, making the ketamine-midazolam combination less suitable for brief ambulatory procedures.[198]

Larger doses of intramuscular ketamine are particularly useful for the induction of anesthesia in children in whom there is a desire to maintain a stable blood pressure and in whom there is no venous access, such as those with congenital heart disease. Larger doses (4 to 5 mg/kg) sedate children within 2 to 4 minutes, and very large doses (10 mg/kg) induce deep sedation that may last from 12 to 25 minutes. Larger doses and repeated doses may be associated with hallucinations, nightmares, vomiting, and unpleasant, as well as prolonged, recovery from anesthesia.[112,199] Concentrations of ketamine of 100 mg/mL are available in the United States and several other countries for intramuscular injection. It is imperative to label these syringes to avoid a syringe swap with syringes containing more dilute concentrations of ketamine.

Oral ketamine alone and in combination with oral midazolam is an effective premedication and has been used to alleviate the distress of invasive procedures (e.g., bone marrow aspiration) in pediatric oncology patients.[200,201] In a dose of 5 to 6 mg/kg, oral ketamine alone sedates most children within 12 minutes and provides sufficient sedation in more than half of the children to permit establishing IV access.[198,202] A larger dose of 8 mg/kg prolongs recovery from anesthesia, although by 2 hours the recovery was no different from that after 4 mg/kg.[203] Oral doses of up to 10 mg/kg have been described as a premedicant for children having procedures for burns; the relative bioavailability was 45%, and absorption was slow with an absorption half-life of 1 hour.[204]

The combination of oral midazolam (0.5 mg/kg) and ketamine (3 mg/kg) provides more effective preoperative sedation than either drug alone. This oral lytic cocktail is a good alternative for children who were not adequately sedated with oral midazolam alone and did not prolong recovery after surgical procedures that lasted more than 30 minutes.[205]

Nasal ketamine in a dose of 6 mg/kg is also an effective premedication for children, with sedation developing by 20 to 40 minutes.[206] In theory, nasally administered ketamine could cause neural tissue damage if it reaches the cribriform plate (see E-Fig. 4.2). Because the preservative in ketamine is neurotoxic, preservative-free ketamine may be safer to administer by the nasal route, although this has not been established.[207] If ketamine is given by this route, we recommend the 100 mg/mL concentration to minimize the volume that must be instilled.

Rectal ketamine (5 mg/kg) produces good anxiolysis and sedation within 30 minutes of administration.[208] However, the rectal route does not provide reliable absorption.

α_2-Agonists

Clonidine, an α_2-agonist, causes dose-related sedation by its effect in the locus coeruleus.[209] It acts both centrally and peripherally to reduce blood pressure, thereby attenuating the hemodynamic response to intubation.[210] Clonidine appears to be devoid of respiratory depressant properties, even when administered in an overdose.[209] The sedative and CNS properties of clonidine reduce the minimum alveolar concentration (MAC) of sevoflurane for tracheal intubation[211] and the concentration of inhaled anesthetic required for the maintenance of anesthesia,[212–214] without prolonging emergence from anesthesia nor leading to airway-related complications.[215]

During the first 12 hours after surgery, oral clonidine (4 µg/kg) reduced the postoperative pain scores and the requirement for supplementary analgesics.[216,217] In children scheduled for tonsillectomy, those who received oral clonidine (4 µg/kg) exhibited more intense anxiety on separation and during induction than those who received oral midazolam (0.5 mg/kg). Even though discharge readiness, postoperative emesis, and 24-hour analgesic requirements were similar in both groups, midazolam was judged to be the better premedicant for children undergoing tonsillectomy.[218] Oral clonidine (4 µg/kg) reduces the incidence of vomiting after strabismus surgery compared with a placebo, clonidine (2 µg/kg), and oral diazepam (0.4 mg/kg).[219]

Although oral clonidine offers several desirable qualities as a premedication, particularly sedation and analgesia, the need to administer it 60 minutes before induction of anesthesia makes its use impractical in busy outpatient settings.[218]

Dexmedetomidine is a sedative with properties that are similar to those of clonidine except that it has an 8-fold greater affinity for the α_2-adenoreceptors than clonidine. Based on bioavailability studies in adults,[220] it is well absorbed through the oral mucosa. In a study of 13 children aged 4 to 14 years, of whom 9 had neurobehavioral disorders, an oral dose of 2 µg/kg of dexmedeto-

midine provided adequate sedation for a mask induction within 20 to 30 minutes of administration. It was postulated that a larger dose of 3 to 4 µg/kg might be more effective.[221]

Intranasal administration of 3 µg/kg dexmedetomidine produced greater success with auditory brainstem response testing than oral chloral hydrate with a more rapid onset of sedation and more rapid return to baseline activity.[222]

In children with burns, both 2 µg/kg intranasal dexmedetomidine and 0.5 mg/kg oral midazolam administered 30 to 45 minutes before induction of anesthesia provided adequate conditions for induction of anesthesia and emergence, although dexmedetomidine produced more sleep preoperatively.[223] Oral midazolam (0.5 µg/kg given 30 minutes before surgery), oral clonidine (4 µg/kg given 90 minutes before surgery), and transmucosal dexmedetomidine (1 µg/kg given 45 minutes before surgery) all produced similar preanesthetic sedation and response to separation from parents in a comparative trial, although children who received dexmedetomidine and clonidine experienced attenuated mean arterial pressure and heart rate preoperatively and reduced pain scores postoperatively compared with midazolam.[224]

Antihistamines

Antihistamines are rarely used for premedication in children, in part because their sedative effects are quite variable. They are very rarely given to infants but may occasionally be indicated for older children, especially those who are hyperkinetic.

Hydroxyzine is mainly administered for its tranquilizing properties[225,226]; it also has antiemetic, antihistaminic, and antispasmodic properties, with minimal respiratory and circulatory effects. It is commonly administered with other classes of drugs as an intramuscular "cocktail" in a dose of 0.5 to 1.0 mg/kg.

Diphenhydramine is an H_1-receptor blocker with mild sedative and antimuscarinic effects. The dose in children is 2.5 to 5 mg/kg per day (maximum 300 mg/d) in four divided doses orally, intravenously, or intramuscularly. Although the duration of action is 4 to 6 hours, it does not appear to interfere with recovery from anesthesia.[227] The combination of oral diphenhydramine (1.25 mg/kg) and oral midazolam (0.5 mg/kg) has been used to provide sedation for healthy children undergoing MRI.[228] The combination was more effective than midazolam alone without a delay in discharge and recovery times.

Anticholinergic Drugs

In the past, anticholinergic agents were used (1) to prevent the undesirable bradycardia associated with some anesthetic agents (halothane and succinylcholine), (2) to minimize the autonomic vagal reflexes manifested during surgical manipulations (e.g., laryngoscopy, strabismus repair), and (3) to reduce secretions. The most commonly used anticholinergic drugs are atropine, scopolamine, and glycopyrrolate. Anticholinergics also provide undesirable effects, including tachycardia, dry mouth, skin erythema, and hyperthermia, as a result of inhibited sweating. Atropine and scopolamine cross the blood-brain barrier and may cause CNS excitation manifested as agitation, confusion, restlessness, ataxia, hallucinations, slurred speech, and memory loss if given in excessive doses.

Because most modern inhalational anesthetics are not associated with bradycardia and succinylcholine is infrequently used in children, the routine use of an anticholinergic drug is not generally warranted. Most anesthesiologists administer these agents only when indicated, such as before IV succinylcholine, combined with ketamine, before laryngoscopy and intubation in neonates, and when surgery stimulates vagal reflexes, such as during strabismus repair. In the majority of cases, anticholinergics need not be given preoperatively but rather should be given after IV access is established.

The recommended doses of anticholinergics are *atropine*, 0.01 to 0.02 mg/kg, and *scopolamine*, 0.005 to 0.010 mg/kg. Atropine is more commonly used and blocks the vagus nerve more effectively than scopolamine, whereas scopolamine is a better sedative, antisialogogue, and amnestic. Infants who are at risk for or show early evidence of a slowing of the heart rate should receive the atropine before the heart rate actually decreases to ensure a prompt onset of effect to maintain cardiac output.[229] *Glycopyrrolate* is a synthetic quaternary ammonium compound that does not cross the blood-brain barrier. It is twice as potent as atropine in decreasing the volume of oral secretions, and its duration of effect is three times greater. The recommended dose of glycopyrrolate (0.01 mg/kg) is half that of atropine. The routine use of an anticholinergic drug for the sole purpose of drying secretions is probably unwarranted, because a dry mouth can be a source of extreme discomfort for a child. Therefore, it is best to reserve the use of glycopyrrolate for specific indications such as to limit sialorrhea associated with ketamine.

Topical Anesthetics

The child's exaggerated fear of the needle makes topical anesthetic creams an attractive alternative to intradermal infiltration and intramuscular injections. There are several needleless methods to minimize procedural pain, each with its own limitations.

EMLA cream (eutectic mixture of local anesthetic; Astra Zeneca, Wilmington, DE) is a mixture of two local anesthetics (2.5% lidocaine and 2.5% prilocaine). One-hour application of EMLA cream to intact skin with an occlusive dressing provides adequate topical anesthesia[230] for a variety of superficial procedures, including IV catheter insertion, lumbar puncture, vaccination, laser treatment of port-wine stains, and neonatal circumcision.[231–236] However, EMLA causes venoconstriction and skin blanching, both of which obscure superficial veins, making IV cannulation more difficult.[237] The prilocaine in EMLA may cause methemoglobinemia,[238] although a 1-hour application at a maximum dose of 1 g did not induce methemoglobinemia when applied to intact skin in full-term neonates and infants younger than 3 months of age.[239] Lidocaine toxicity has been reported when EMLA was applied to mucosal membranes for extended periods.[240]

Ametop gel is a topical local anesthetic (4% tetracaine) available in the United Kingdom, Europe, and Canada (Smith & Nephew, Lachine, Quebec) but not in the United States. Its indications are identical to those of EMLA, but its properties are different. When applied to intact skin under an occlusive dressing, it anesthetizes the skin within 30 to 40 minutes, and it produces no venoconstriction or skin blanching and zero risk of methemoglobinemia.

ELA-Max (4% lidocaine; Ferndale Laboratories, Ferndale, MI) is another topical anesthetic cream that decreases the pain associated with dermatologic procedures[241] and IV catheter insertion after only a 30-minute application.[242] ELA-Max causes some blanching of the skin like EMLA, but to a lesser extent, and dilates the veins better than EMLA.[243]

The *S-Caine Patch* (ZARS, Inc., Salt Lake City, UT) is a eutectic mixture of lidocaine and tetracaine (70 mg of each per patch) that uses a controlled heating system to accelerate delivery and effectiveness of the local anesthetic. After 20 minutes of application, the pain associated with venipuncture is reduced. This patch causes mild and transient local erythema and edema and no blanching of the skin.[244]

Needle-free injection systems for lidocaine are also available for pain-free insertion of IV cannulae or other needle-based procedures such as lumbar puncture.[245,246] One such system is the needleless jet injection system (J tip) (NDC:8164-2001 National Medical Products, Inc., Irvine, CA) that provides local anesthetic at the site of administration in less than 1 minute. The device uses air, instead of a needle, to deliver 0.25 mL of local anesthetic subcutaneously prior to IV insertion. In one study, jet-delivered lidocaine was found to be no more effective than jet-delivered placebo in providing local anesthesia for needle insertion and both may provide superior analgesia compared with no device use; the majority of patients receiving the jet device reported that they would request this for future needle insertions.[247] In a retrospective study, the use of the J tip did not affect first-attempt success for IV line placement in children.[248]

Nonopioid Analgesics

Acetaminophen is the most common nonopioid analgesic used for treatment of postoperative pain in children. It can be administered orally preoperatively, rectally immediately after induction of anesthesia but before the start of surgery, or intravenously (where available) once IV access has been established.

The oral doses of acetaminophen for antipyresis, 10 to 15 mg/kg, are as effective as ketorolac, 1 mg/kg,[249] given 10 or more minutes postoperatively for myringotomies and tube placement.[250] Oral acetaminophen is very rapidly absorbed with a bioavailability of 0.9-1.[250] Neonates may have a lower incidence of hepatotoxicity because the immature hepatic enzyme systems in neonates produce less toxic metabolites than in older children.[251–253] When given preemptively, acetaminophen has opioid-sparing properties that enhance analgesia in children after tonsillectomy.[254,255] Preoperative oral acetaminophen and codeine provided superior analgesia to acetaminophen alone after myringotomy and tube placement.[256] However, in children undergoing tonsillectomy, there was no difference in the level of pain control provided by acetaminophen and acetaminophen with codeine. Postoperative oral intake was significantly higher in children treated with acetaminophen alone.[257] A relationship between concentration and analgesic effect for pain relief after tonsillectomy has been observed in children. An effect compartment concentration of 10 mg/L was associated with a reduction of pain by 2.6 units (using a visual analogue scale ranging from 0 to 10).[258]

The time to the peak blood concentration of acetaminophen after rectal administration of 10, 20, and 30 mg/kg ranges between 60 and 180 minutes after administration. In addition, the equilibration half-time between plasma and effect compartment is approximately 1 hour.[258] This slow absorption and delayed effect-site concentrations require acetaminophen administration immediately after induction of anesthesia to provide sufficient time to achieve therapeutic blood concentrations by the end of surgery (primarily for operations that will take 1 hour or longer).[259] Furthermore, doses of 10 to 30 mg/kg rectal acetaminophen may not achieve peak or sustained blood concentrations that ensure effect (Fig. 4.2). Thus, an initial dose of rectal acetaminophen of 40 mg/kg has been recommended, followed by 20 mg/kg rectally every 6 hours. This dosing regimen was subsequently confirmed.[260] After 45 mg/kg rectal acetaminophen, the mean maximum blood concentration was 13 μg/mL (range 7 to 19 μg/mL), and the mean time to that maximum concentration was approximately 200 minutes.[261] Several other studies of single-dose rectal administration reported similar results.[261,262]

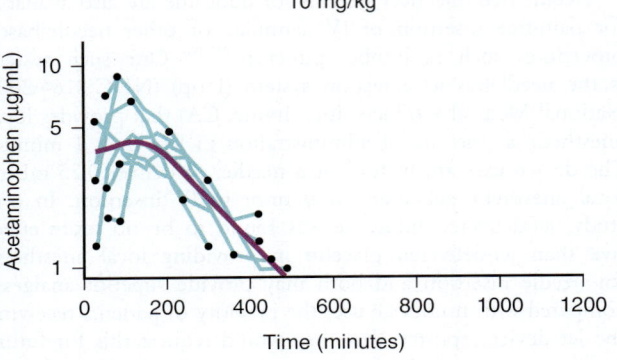

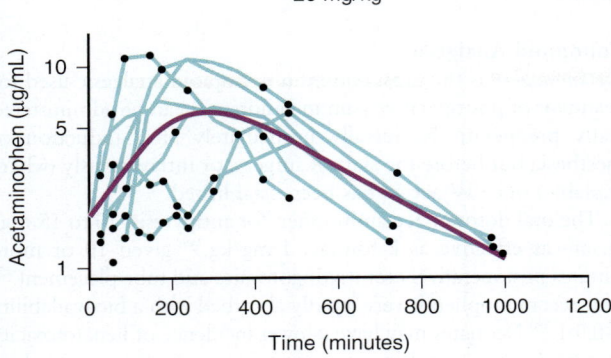

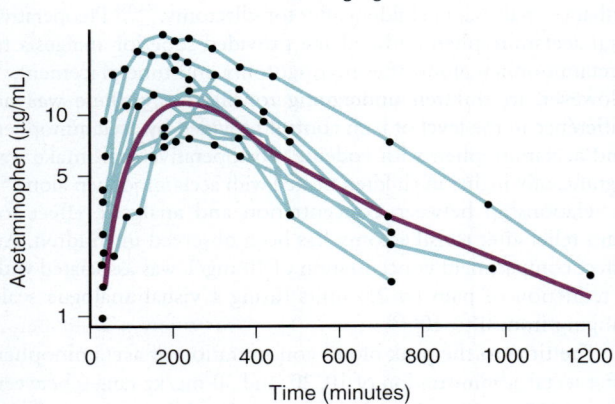

FIGURE 4.2 Acetaminophen concentrations after rectal administration of 10, 20, or 30 mg/kg were recorded. Values for serum concentration of acetaminophen (*solid circles, teal lines*) are plotted against time for each child. Thick (*magenta*) lines indicate "average" values. Note that only children who received 30 mg/kg achieved the antipyretic threshold of 10 to 20 μg/mL, but that even at this dose that range was not sustained. These data suggest the need to use a larger loading dose (approximately 40 mg/kg) followed by subsequent doses of 20 mg/kg every 6 hours; see text for details. (From Birmingham PK, Tobin MJ, Henthorn TK, et al. Twenty-four-hour pharmacokinetics of rectal acetaminophen: an old drug with new recommendations. *Anesthesiology* 1997;87:244-252.)

Until further safety data are developed, the initial dose of rectal acetaminophen should not exceed 40 to 45 mg/kg with a total 24-hour dose of not more than 75–100 mg/kg to avoid hepatic toxicity. Acetaminophen administered rectally in a loading dose of 40 mg/kg and then 20 mg/kg either orally or rectally

every 6 hours after elective craniofacial surgery yielded greater plasma concentrations and lower pain scores than for those who received oral acetaminophen; this was in part related to some children vomiting the oral acetaminophen.[263] Note that these are excessive oral doses that cannot be recommended.

Excessive fasting, a very large loading dose of acetaminophen, and sevoflurane anesthesia may deplete glutathione stores and thus contribute to the development of hepatic failure.[264] The coadministration of antiepileptic drugs has also been implicated in hepatotoxicity from acetaminophen.[265] *Because hepatic toxicity is a real and potentially fatal complication of an acetaminophen overdose, a complete medication history of acetaminophen consumption and concomitant drugs should be completed preoperatively, and the recommended maximum daily dose should not be exceeded.*

Different IV formulations of acetaminophen are available in some countries.[266] One is a prodrug of acetaminophen (*propacetamol*) with a bioavailability of 50%. It may be administered in a dose of 30 mg/kg (15 mg/kg acetaminophen) every 6 hours to children 2 to 15 years of age. In a placebo-controlled trial in febrile children, this dose of propacetamol was superior to placebo.[267] Pharmacokinetic studies indicate that such a dose of propacetamol maintains mean steady-state blood concentrations of acetaminophen of 10 μg/mL.[268] Therapeutic blood concentrations are achieved in neonates 10 days of age or younger with 15 mg/kg of propacetamol 4 times daily, but neonates older than 10 days require twice the dose, or 30 mg/kg, at the same frequency.[269] Hemostatic effects of large (60 mg/kg) doses of propacetamol in adult volunteers showed transient but reversible inhibition of platelet aggregation as well as decreased thromboxane activity. Although these effects were less than those after ketorolac (0.4 mg/kg), the combination of acetaminophen and ketorolac may prolong these effects.[270]

IV acetaminophen, known as *paracetamol* in other countries, became commercially available in the United States in 2011. Paracetamol (15 mg/kg) was compared with propacetamol, 30 mg/kg, for postoperative pain relief after inguinal hernia repair. The outcomes were similar, but IV paracetamol was better tolerated at the injection site.[271]

Several investigations examined IV acetaminophen use in pediatric populations. In a study of 50 children, ages 2 to 5 years, undergoing elective adenoidectomy or adenotonsillectomy, IV acetaminophen 15 mg/kg or rectal acetaminophen 40 mg/kg resulted in equivalent pain scores. The time to the first rescue analgesic in the rectal acetaminophen group (median 10 hours, attributed to its slow absorption) was greater than in the IV acetaminophen group (median 7 hours), although few children in either group required any rescue analgesics during the first 6 hours.[272] IV acetaminophen (15 mg/kg) has been compared with intramuscular meperidine 1 mg/kg in children undergoing tonsillectomy. When compared with meperidine, IV acetaminophen resulted in comparable analgesia but less sedation and earlier readiness for discharge.[273] In children undergoing dental restoration with the same medications and doses, children in the acetaminophen group had greater pain scores but earlier readiness for recovery room discharge.[274] A study of 45 healthy children, ages 5 months to 5 years, presenting for primary cleft palate repair found that IV acetaminophen 12.5 mg/kg (age <2 years) or 15 mg/kg (age 2–5 years) every 6 hours for 24 hours resulted in improved analgesia and decreased postoperative opioid requirements.[275] Administration of IV nonnarcotic analgesics may also result in decreased nausea and vomiting compared with oral medications. Twenty-eight children undergoing craniosynostosis correction were random assigned to receive either oral ibuprofen (10 mg/kg) and acetaminophen (15 mg/kg) versus IV ketorolac (0.5 mg/kg) and acetaminophen (15 mg/kg). There were significantly more vomiting episodes in the group receiving oral medication.[276]

The US FDA has approved IV acetaminophen for use in children 2 years and older. The recommended dose for children 2 to 12 years old weighing less than 50 kg is 15 mg/kg every 6 hours or 12.5 mg/kg every 4 hours with a maximum of 75 mg/kg per day. Use in children younger than 2 years is considered off-label. Practitioners in the United States who choose to use IV acetaminophen off-label should consider reduced dosage for patients younger than 2 years of age. In infants 1 month to 2 years of age, dosing from the pharmacokinetic data suggests a dose reduction of 33%, 10 mg/kg every 4 hours or 12.5 mg/kg every 6 hours, with a maximum dose of 50 to 60 mg/kg per day. In full-term neonates up to 28 days of age, the dose of IV acetaminophen should be reduced by 50% to 7.5 mg/kg every 6 to 8 hours with a maximum daily dose of 30 mg/kg. This dosing regimen produces a similar pharmacokinetic profile as in children older than 2 years of age.[277,278] The major concern in this age group is accidental overdose of acetaminophen and hepatic toxicity. Three near-fatal cases of infants who received 10- and 20-fold overdoses of IV acetaminophen have been reported.[279,280] In many instances, overdose errors resulted for dosages calculated in milligrams, but administered in milliliters.[281] Careful documentation of the dose of IV acetaminophen is warranted in infants.[282]

Antiemetics

Antiemetic administration should be considered in children undergoing high-risk procedures such as tonsillectomy and strabismus repair as well as those who have a history of motion sickness or prior history of postanesthesia nausea and vomiting. The uses of these medications are presented elsewhere in the text (see Chapters 7, 33, and 34).

Corticosteroids

Children who have been taking chronic corticosteroid therapy (e.g., for asthma, Crohn disease, lupus, acute lymphocytic leukemia) and those who have discontinued chronic corticosteroid therapy in the past 6 months may suffer from suppression of the hypothalamic-pituitary-adrenal axis.[283] There is a paucity of evidence to support the need for supplemental corticosteroids in children in the perioperative period who have been receiving long-term corticosteroid therapy. In the past, hypotension was reported in those who were receiving long-term corticosteroid therapy and underwent general anesthesia or another stress. This may be attributed to hypovolemia. Nonetheless, many endocrinologists continue to recommend a dose of supplemental corticosteroids before or shortly after induction of anesthesia for "stress" corticosteroid coverage. The usual recommended dose is 1 to 2 mg/kg of hydrocortisone intramuscularly or intravenously or an equivalent dose of dexamethasone (0.05 to 0.1 mg/kg) approximately 1 hour before the induction of anesthesia or as soon as IV access is established. For more complicated operations, the corticosteroid dose may be repeated every 6 hours for up to 72 hours (see Chapter 27).

Insulin

Optimal management of diabetic children undergoing surgery entails maintaining glucose homeostasis, avoiding hyperglycemia with resultant osmotic diuresis, impaired wound healing, increased infection rate, and avoiding hypoglycemia. Anesthesiologists should work together with the endocrinologist or primary care physician to design a plan for each child's specific diabetes treatment regimen, glycemic control, intended surgery, and anticipated postoperative care. Diabetes mellitus is the most common endocrine problem encountered in children. The preoperative fasting time should be the same as that recommended for nondiabetic children. Every attempt should be made to schedule these children as the first case of the day to minimize the fasting period. Preoperative laboratory tests generally include hematocrit, serum electrolytes, and glucose levels; blood glucose concentrations should be measured at frequent intervals during the perianesthetic period. Several protocols have been crafted to control the blood sugar in children who are diabetic[284]; these are described in more detail in Chapter 27 (see also Figs. 27.1 to 27.9, which describe a variety of management strategies).

Antibiotics

Antibiotics are frequently administered to prevent or reduce infection in surgical patients. Surgical site infection (SSI) accounts for 14% to 16% of nosocomial infections in the United States.[285] A recent retrospective review identified the overall rate of SSI in children undergoing a variety of surgical procedures as approximately 2.4%.[286] SSI increases morbidity and mortality and adds greatly to the cost of hospitalization.[287] The appropriate timing of antibiotics is now a source of performance benchmarking for some insurance carriers, making communication with surgeons essential for the success of this anesthesiology-directed quality assessment measure. Current guidelines define appropriate antibiotic prophylaxis for SSI as administration within 60 minutes prior to incision.[288] Intraoperative redosing is needed if the duration of the procedure exceeds two drug half-lives or there is excessive blood loss. Pediatric doses provided in these guidelines are based on pharmacokinetic data and the extrapolation of adult efficacy data to pediatric patients. *"With a few exceptions (e.g., aminoglycoside dosages), pediatric dosages should not exceed the maximum adult recommended dosages. If dosages are calculated on a milligram-per-kilogram basis for children weighing more than 40 kg, the calculated dosage may exceed the maximum recommended dosage for adults; adult dosages should therefore be used".*[288] Recommended doses and redosing intervals for commonly used antibiotics for surgical prophylaxis are listed in Table 4.4.

For prophylaxis against endocarditis in children with structural heart disease, antibiotics should ideally be administered either intravenously 30 to 60 minutes or orally 1 hour before the induction of anesthesia and surgery. In reality, in children these antibiotics are usually administered after induction of anesthesia and establishment of IV access (see also Tables 16.2 and 16.3).[289]

Antacids, H_2-Receptor Antagonists, and Gastrointestinal Motility Drugs

The risk of aspiration during induction of or emergence from anesthesia may be increased in children who are developmentally delayed, have gastroesophageal reflux, have experienced previous esophageal surgery, had a difficult airway, were obese, or had undergone a traumatic injury. Preanesthetic administration of drugs that reduce gastric fluid volume and acidity may decrease the risk of pulmonary acid aspiration syndrome (Table 4.5).[1,290] Gastric fluid pH may be increased by drinking a nonparticulate antacid such as sodium citrate; particulate antacids should be avoided because they can cause severe pneumonitis if aspirated.

Cimetidine and *ranitidine* are H_2-receptor antagonists that decrease gastric acid secretion, increase gastric fluid pH, and reduce gastric

TABLE 4.4 Current American Society of Hospital Pharmacists Recommendations for Surgical Antibiotic Prophylaxis (Weight-Normalized)

Antibiotic	Recommended Child Dose (mg/kg but not to exceed adult dose)	Recommended Adult Dose	Recommended Repeat Intraoperative Dosing Interval (Hours) or >15% EBV Loss
Ampicillin-sulbactam	50 (Ampicillin component)	3 g	2
Ampicillin	50	2 g	2
Aztreonam	30	2 g	4
Cefazolin	30	2 g; use 3 g if >120 kg	4
Cefuroxime	50	1.5 g	4
Cefotaxime	50	1 g	3
Cefoxitin	40	2 g	2
Cefotetan	40	2 g	6
Ceftriaxone	50–75	2 g	NA
Ciprofloxacin	10	400 mg	NA
Clindamycin	10	900 mg	6
Ertapenem	15	1 g	NA
Fluconazole	6	400 mg	NA
Gentamicin	2.5; based on dosing weight	5 mg/kg; based on dosing weight single dose	Single dose
Levofloxacin	10	500 mg	NA
Metronidazole	15; neonates <1200 g: 7.5 mg/kg (single dose)	500 mg	NA
Moxifloxacin	10	400 mg	NA
Piperacillin-tazobactam	Infants 2–9 months: 80 mg/kg of piperacillin component; Children >9 months and ≤40 kg: 100 mg/kg of piperacillin component	3.375 g	2
Vancomycin	15	15 mg/kg	NA

EBV, estimated blood volume.
Originally published in Bratzler DW, Dellinger EP, Olsen KM, et al. Clinical practice guidelines for antimicrobial prophylaxis in surgery. *Am J Health Syst Pharm.* 2013;70(3):195-283. © [2013], American Society of Health-System Pharmacists, Inc. All rights reserved. Adapted with permission.

TABLE 4.5 Doses of Antacids, H₂-Receptor Antagonists, and Gastrointestinal Motility Drugs

Drug	Dose
Antacids	
Bicitra (oral)	30 mL (0.5–1 mL/kg up to 30 mL)
Prokinetic	
Metoclopramide (IV)	0.1–0.15 mg/kg
H₂-Receptor Antagonists	
Cimetidine (IV)	5–10 mg/kg
Ranitidine (PO/IV)	2–2.5 mg/kg
Famotidine (PO/IV)	0.5 mg/kg (not to exceed 40 mg/day)

residual volume.[291,292] These drugs can be given orally, intravenously, or intramuscularly.

Metoclopramide is often administered with an H₂-receptor antagonist to increase lower esophageal sphincter tone, relax the pyloric sphincter and the duodenal bulb, and promote gastric emptying by increasing peristalsis of the duodenum and jejunum. The drug effect is apparent 30 to 60 minutes after oral administration and 1 to 2 minutes after IV administration.[293] Adverse effects such as extrapyramidal signs relate to the effect of metoclopramide on the CNS through blockade of dopaminergic receptors.

Induction of Anesthesia

PREPARATION FOR INDUCTION

Adequate preparation includes warming the OR and ensuring that warming devices are functioning properly (e.g., heat lamps, warming blanket, forced air warmer) before the child's arrival, especially for young infants. The preinduction checklist should include a variety of sizes of masks, oral airways, laryngoscope blades, tracheal tubes (one-half size larger and one-half size smaller than the anticipated size), an appropriate size laryngeal mask airway (LMA), and functioning wall suction. The anesthesia machine and monitoring equipment should be prepared before the child's arrival in the OR to ensure that all appropriate equipment is on hand and to minimize any last-minute commotion. One of the most essential monitors used during the induction of anesthesia is the precordial stethoscope. The bell from the stethoscope should have a double-stick adhesive attached and ready for application before induction. A chair or stool for the child's parent to sit on helps avoid fainting episodes should the parent be present at induction of anesthesia. Ensuring a quiet, calm OR environment, free of clanging instruments and loud conversations among the staff, allows for a smoother and less upsetting induction.

There are a variety of techniques for inducing general anesthesia. The technique used depends on a number of factors, including the child's developmental age, understanding and ability to cooperate, and previous experiences; the presence of a parent; and the interaction of these factors with the child's underlying medical or surgical conditions.

INHALATION INDUCTION

The most common method of inducing anesthesia in children is inhalation by mask of the nonpungent inhalational anesthetic agent sevoflurane or halothane. The anesthesiologist should be flexible and adapt an approach that suits the child, depending on age, degree of sedation, and cooperation.

If the child is already asleep on arrival in the OR, it is possible to use the "steal induction" technique. The child is not touched or disturbed. After priming of the breathing circuit with N_2O in O_2, the mask is gently placed near the child's face and gradually brought closer and closer until it is gently applied to the face. After the child has been breathing N_2O for 1 to 2 minutes, sevoflurane is administered in a single stepwise increase in concentration to 8% (halothane may be delivered in increasing concentrations as tolerated). Adequate monitoring must be instituted as soon as possible, and the child is then transferred to the operating table. This technique is atraumatic and avoids exposing the child to the strange OR surroundings while awake. However, it is possible that the child may suffer psychological harm when he or she awakens to pain without realizing what has transpired.

If a parent wishes to accompany a young child to the OR, we may allow the child to remain in the parent's lap for the induction. We request that the child be sitting facing forward in the parent's lap so that there is free access to the child's face. It is vital to instruct the parent that he or she must hold the child in a "bear hug"—that is, with the arms tightly wrapped around the child and holding the child's arms in such a way that the child cannot reach up to the face mask—and to warn the parents that as the child loses consciousness, the child will become limp. This approach can be difficult with either an inexperienced anesthesiologist or a very strong child who vigorously rotates his or her neck from left to right, preventing the tight application of a face mask. It is also important to have an experienced individual in front of the child and parent to hold onto the child as induction proceeds and help place the child on the OR table after successful induction. At this point, we invite the parent to kiss their child and then the parent is escorted to the waiting room (E-Fig. 4.3A and B).

The optimal induction sequence in toddlers is to avoid making them feel vulnerable by having the children pick a flavor of lip balm to flavor the mask and having them seated (not lying supine) on the OR bed with the back supported by the anesthesiologist's chest or on the anesthesiologist's or the parent's lap (E-Fig. 4.4A, Video 4.2). They may be distracted by asking them to try to "blow up the balloon" by taking deeper and deeper breaths, where the balloon refers to the reservoir bag. If the child is seated on the parent's or anesthesiologist's lap, it is strongly advised that this be undertaken only with children who are wearing diapers or are sitting on a thick blanket to limit the spread of urine should the bladder empty during induction. The anesthesia machine should be within easy reach during such an induction to allow control of the bag, pop-off valve, and vaporizer without interruption. An assistant should be at hand to help position and hold the child when needed. Other distraction techniques may be used, including allowing them to bring their favorite toy or security blanket into the OR (see E-Fig. 4.4B). Older children may be distracted by allowing them to play electronic handheld games or to watch a movie on a portable electronic device.

Child-life specialists are helpful allies in preparing patients and parents to cope with the stress and uncertainty surrounding anesthesia and surgery. Such specialists are trained to explain procedures and equipment to children in age-appropriate language,

and to introduce coping strategies to reduce anxiety such as therapeutic medical play. For example, children may be less afraid of an anesthesia face mask if allowed to hold the mask in the preoperative holding area, apply a scented flavor of their choosing, and decorate the mask with stickers. One technique often used by child-life specialists is to distract children by allowing them to play electronic handheld games on a portable electronic device. In this scenario, the child-life specialist accompanies the child to the OR, with the child continuing to play his or her preferred game on the portable electronic device during transport. The child-life specialist holds the device for the patient so that the handheld game may be continued as the face mask is applied and the anesthetic induction begins (Video 4.3).

Some children refuse to have the face mask placed anywhere near their face. They may have an unknown fear of masks or may have been traumatized previously with high concentrations of sevoflurane or halothane administered at the outset through the face mask, without premedication or pretreatment with nitrous oxide. One solution to this problem is to remove the mask, place the elbow of the breathing circuit between one's fingers, and then cup your hands below the child's chin. Because nitrous oxide is heavier than air, cupped hands act like a reservoir. The hands are gradually brought closer and closer to the face, while the child is distracted, until they gently cover the mouth. Once the child is becoming sedated, 8% sevoflurane can be introduced and the mask placed on the face. Younger infants who refuse a mask may be soothed by placing one's small finger ("pinky") in the child's mouth to suck on as the face mask is gently advanced to the nose and mouth for an inhalation induction (Fig. 4.3A and B).

Inhalation With Sevoflurane

The traditional mask induction of anesthesia is accomplished by placing the mask lightly on the child's face and administering a mixture of N_2O in O_2 (2:1) for 1 or 2 minutes until the full effect of N_2O is achieved. Offering children the choice of a scented mask or "sleepy air," such as bubble gum or strawberry flavor, applied to the inside of the face mask may disguise the odor of the plastic. Sevoflurane is then introduced and can be rapidly increased to 8% in a single stepwise increase, without significant bradycardia or hypotension in otherwise healthy children. After anesthesia is induced, the sevoflurane concentration should be maintained at the maximum tolerable concentration until IV access is established, but this concentration should be reduced if controlled ventilation is initiated to avoid overdose. The reason for maintaining delivery of a high concentration of sevoflurane is to minimize the risk of awareness during the early period of the induction sequence. Data from unmedicated children (aged ≥3 years) indicate that sevoflurane is associated with small increases in heart rate, although the heart rate does decrease to 80 to 100 beats/minute in some children after breathing sevoflurane for a period of time.[294] In contrast to halothane,[295] sevoflurane does not increase the myocardial sensitivity to epinephrine.[296] In a study of three techniques for delivering sevoflurane for induction of anesthesia, minimal differences were detected among the three: incremental increases in sevoflurane (2%, 4%, 6%, and 7%) in oxygen, a high concentration of sevoflurane (7%) in oxygen, and a high concentration of sevoflurane in a 1:1 mixture of N_2O and O_2.[297] When N_2O was added, there was a decreased time to loss of the eyelash reflex and a decreased incidence of excitement during the induction. Agitation or excitement in early induction (shortly after loss of eyelash reflex) with sevoflurane has been observed; this is discussed in detail in Chapter 7.

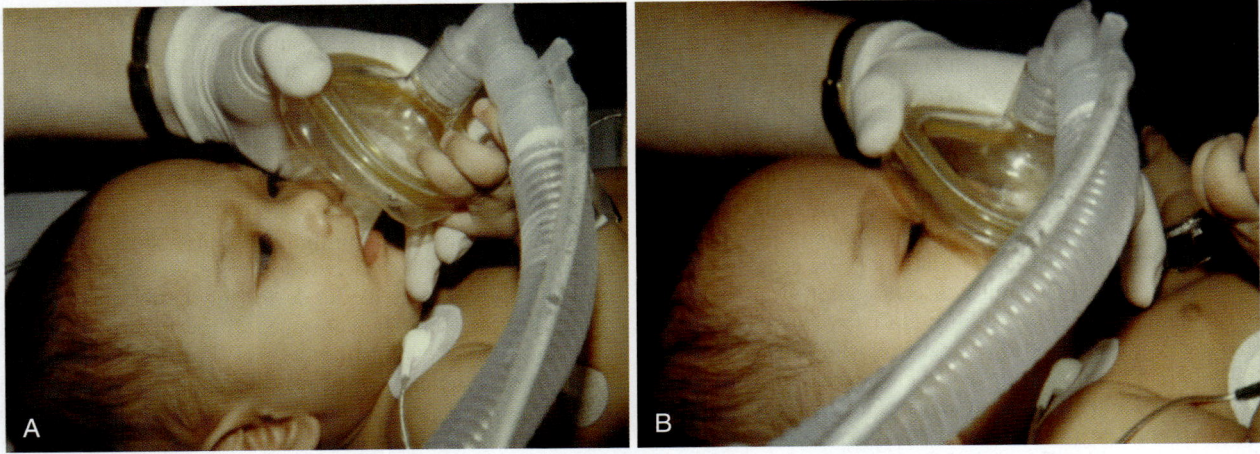

FIGURE 4.3 A, Infants 6 months of age or younger are often consoled during induction by placing the little finger ("pinky finger") of your hand in their mouth while you hold the face mask near their face with the rest of the hand. In general, they are so hungry that they will stop crying and eagerly suckle on your pinky finger. **B,** As the infant loses consciousness, the intensity of the suckling diminishes, the pinky finger is gently removed, and the face mask is fully applied.

Inhalation Induction With Halothane

Halothane has largely been replaced by sevoflurane for inhalation induction of anesthesia because of halothane's slower wash-in and emergence and greater incidence of bradycardia, hypotension, and arrhythmias. When anesthesia is induced with halothane, the inspired concentration is gradually increased by 0.5% every two to three breaths up to 5%. Alternatively, a single-breath induction of anesthesia with 5% halothane can yield a rapid induction of anesthesia without triggering airway reflex responses.[298]

The inspired concentration of halothane should be decreased as soon as anesthesia is established to avoid heart rate slowing and myocardial depression. The child will autoregulate the depth of anesthesia as long as he or she is allowed to breathe spontaneously; however, if respirations are controlled, then anesthetic overdose may easily occur (see Chapter 7).[299,300] Halothane sensitizes the heart to catecholamines, and ventricular arrhythmias may commonly be seen, especially during periods of hypercapnia or light anesthesia.[301]

If vital signs become abnormal during induction, the concentration of halothane should be reduced or discontinued and the circuit flushed with 100% oxygen. If bigeminy or short bursts of ventricular tachycardia occur, then the following strategies should be considered: (1) hyperventilation (to reduce the arterial carbon dioxide tension [$PaCO_2$]), (2) deepening of the halothane anesthesia, or (3) changing to an alternate potent inhalation agent.[301] There is no role for IV lidocaine to treat these arrhythmias.

During inhalation induction with either sevoflurane or halothane, if the oxygen saturation decreases (and there is no mechanical cause for the desaturation such as partial dislodgment of the oximeter probe, patient clenching of fingers or toes, or blood pressure cuff inflating), 100% oxygen should be administered until the oxygen saturation returns to normal while the cause of the desaturation is addressed. If the cause of the desaturation is not related to upper airway obstruction, the most common cause in a healthy child is a ventilation-perfusion mismatch due to segmental atelectasis. Recruitment of alveoli may be achieved by applying a sustained inflation of the lungs to 30 cm H_2O for 30 seconds or as tolerated.[302] This may be difficult to complete before

tracheal intubation because the stomach may inflate. In such a case, recruitment should be abandoned. Alternatively, mild to moderate upper airway obstruction from collapse of the hypopharyngeal structures or the development of mild laryngospasm causes hypoventilation and desaturation. In general, this upper airway obstruction is readily relieved by gently applying a tight mask fit, closing the pop-off valve sufficiently to generate 5 to 10 cm of positive end-expiratory pressure, and allowing the distending pressure of the bag to stent open the airway until the child is adequately anesthetized to tolerate the placement of an oral airway (see Fig. 14.10 and Fig. 33.10). Cephalad pressure should be applied to the superior pole of the condyle of the mandible to sublux the temporomandibular joint because this maneuver opens the mouth and pulls the tongue off the posterior and nasopharyngeal walls, opening the laryngeal inlet.[303] This maneuver may supplant the need for an oral airway. It is very important to avoid applying digital pressure to the soft tissues of the submental triangle because this pushes the tongue and soft tissues into the hypopharynx, occluding the oropharynx and nasopharynx. If the child develops symptomatic bradycardia, then oxygenation and ventilation must first be established, followed by IV atropine (0.02 mg/kg) and, if necessary, chest compressions and IV epinephrine (see Chapter 40).

Inhalation Induction With Desflurane

Desflurane is very pungent, as evidenced by severe laryngospasm (49%), coughing, increased secretions, and hypoxemia during induction.[304] Therefore, *desflurane is not recommended for inhalation induction in children* but may be used safely for maintenance of general anesthesia after the trachea has been intubated.

Hypnotic Induction

Hypnosis can reduce anxiety and pain in children with chronic medical problems and those undergoing painful procedures[305,306] as well as reduce preoperative anxiety. Hypnosis is an altered state of consciousness with highly focused attention, based on the principle of dissociation.[307] Hypnosis results in a state of inner absorption that leads to a reduction in awareness of immediate physical surroundings and experiences. Children are more likely to be absorbed in fantasy, and their natural power of play makes them more hypnotizable than adults.[308] Although an anesthesiologist may not have training in hypnosis, he or she can use hypnotic suggestions to help children even though an actual trance state is not induced. It may be helpful to engage children in age-appropriate scenarios, such as going to the zoo, a fancy tea party, a baseball game, or flying a jet. Words should be spoken slowly and rhythmically with descriptions of sights and sounds that are familiar to the child as well as repeated suggestions of "feeling good." The hypnotic suggestions distract the child so that the smell of the anesthetic agent becomes the scent of the zoo animals, the tea brewing, the aviation fuel, and so on. Any number of stories can be told with the same result as long as one remembers to repeatedly say things that can be identified by the child and that fit with what the child is experiencing at the time of induction.

When hypnosis was administered 30 minutes before surgery, it significantly reduced preoperative anxiety at the time of face mask application and the frequency of behavior disorders postoperatively when compared with oral midazolam (0.5 mg/kg).[309] Hypnosis provided a relaxed state of well-being and enabled children to actively participate in anesthesia, thus leaving them with a pleasant memory. Unlike the anterograde amnesia associated with midazolam, hypnosis offers the benefit of maintaining a pleasant memory to prevent fear during future anesthetics.

Modified Single-Breath Induction

The single-breath induction technique is especially appealing to children who desire to fall asleep "really fast" with a face mask, because loss of consciousness is achieved much more rapidly than with a traditional escalating-dose technique. It works best with older children, although some as young as 3 years of age can be anesthetized with this technique if they are cooperative. Before beginning, the child should be coached through a mock induction by instructing him or her to "breathe in the biggest breath possible" through the mouth (not the nose) and then "breathe all the way out until there is no more air in the lungs." If the child is used to swimming and holding the breath underwater, this makes the exercise much easier. Once this has been practiced a few times, then a practice run is repeated with only the mask (no circuit) on the face.

Before induction, the circuit and reservoir bag are primed with 70% N_2O in O_2 and the maximum concentration of halothane or sevoflurane the vaporizer can deliver. This is achieved by running modest fresh gas flows through the circuit and intermittently emptying the reservoir bag manually into the scavenger system (i.e., with the circuit Y-connector occluded). Once the circuit is primed with the maximum concentration of inhalation agent, the mask is placed on the Y-connector, then the distal end of the circuit is occluded (to avoid contaminating the OR), and the child is instructed to take a deep breath of room air and to exhale all the air and hold expiration. The face mask is then placed securely over the child's mouth and nose while he or she is instructed to take in the "deepest breath ever through the mouth" and "hold it, now just breathe normally." Loss of consciousness, as noted by loss of the eyelash reflex, occurs within 15 to 30 seconds after this vital capacity breath (Fig. 4.4A, B and C, and Video 4.4).[298,310]

INTRAVENOUS INDUCTION

IV induction is usually reserved for older children, those who request an IV induction, those with a previously established

IV catheter, those with potential cardiovascular instability, and those who need a rapid-sequence induction (RSI) because of a full stomach. There are many different options as far as medications that can be used for an IV induction in a child (Table 4.6). Ideally, all children should breathe 100% oxygen before IV induction; if the face mask is met with objections, oxygen may be insufflated without a mask by simply holding the Y-connector of the circuit between your fingers over or near the child's face.

Thiopental

Thiopental (sodium pentothal) has been replaced by propofol as the most commonly used IV induction agent. The recommended induction dose of thiopental in healthy, unpremedicated children is 5 to 6 mg/kg[311]; neonates require a smaller dose (3 to 4 mg/kg).[312] Debilitated or severely ill patients, those who are hypovolemic, and those who have been premedicated may also require a smaller dose for induction of anesthesia. The beta-elimination half-life of thiopental in neonates is twice that in their mothers (15 vs. 7 hours), so a single dose may produce excessively prolonged effect in neonates.[313] This drug is no longer available in the United States.

Methohexital

Methohexital is an ultra-short-acting oxybarbiturate that is infrequently used for IV induction (1.0 to 2.5 mg/kg)[314]; premedicated children require a smaller dose. Recovery after IV administration is more rapid than after thiopental.[315] Larger doses cause skeletal muscle hyperactivity, myoclonic movements, and hiccups.[314] Pain at the injection site is common, necessitating pretreatment with IV lidocaine.

Propofol

Propofol is the most commonly used IV induction agent in children. The induction dose of propofol varies with age: the median effective dose (ED_{50}) for a satisfactory induction in healthy infants 1 to 6 months old is 3.0 ± 0.2 mg/kg, and in healthy children 10 to 16 years old it is 2.4 ± 0.1 mg/kg.[316] The 95% effective dose (ED_{95}) in healthy unpremedicated children 3 to 12 years of age is 2.5 to 3.0 mg/kg.[317] The early distribution half-life is about 2 minutes, and the terminal elimination half-life is about 30 minutes.[318] Clearance is very large (2.3 ± 0.6 L/minute) and exceeds liver blood flow.[318] Advantages to propofol for induction of anesthesia include a reduced incidence of airway-related problems (e.g., laryngospasm, bronchospasm), more rapid emergence,[319,320] and a reduced incidence of nausea and vomiting.[321,322] The major disadvantage of propofol is pain at the site of injection, especially when administered in small veins (e.g., the back of the hand).[316] The administration of lidocaine (0.5 to 1.0 mg/kg) while applying tourniquet pressure proximal to the injection site (mini-Bier block) for 30 to 60 seconds before injecting the propofol effectively eliminates the pain in more than 90% of patients. However, younger children may not tolerate even the discomfort from the Bier block, which is the reason to consider using nitrous oxide as an alternative and equally effective strategy (see Chapter 7). Other techniques reported to attenuate the pain include mixing lidocaine (0.5 to 1 mg/kg) with the propofol (but this should be done within 60 seconds of administration of the propofol), refrigerating the propofol, pretreating with an opioid or ketamine, and diluting propofol to a 0.5% solution.[323–331]

In addition to its use as an induction agent, propofol can be administered by infusion for total IV anesthesia (see

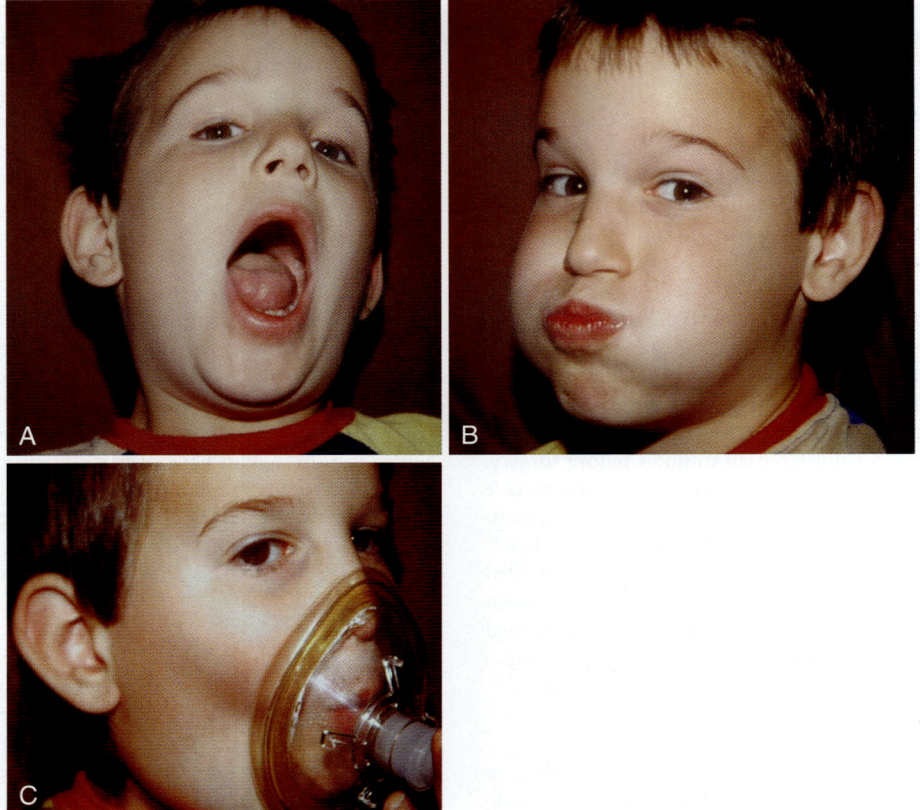

FIGURE 4.4 A single-breath induction is another useful method that is most appropriate for children 5 to 10 years of age. It is important to practice several times without the mask attached to the circuit before the actual induction (see text for details of preparing the circuit). This allows the child to become familiar with the feel of the mask as it is applied to the face and to properly time the sequence of events. **A** and **B,** Typically, we ask the child to take "the biggest breath possible and hold it." Then we ask the child to "breathe all the way out until you have no more air in your lungs and hold it" and place the face mask on the child's face. **C,** We then ask the child to take in "the biggest breath you have ever taken, hold it, then breathe normally." If a full vital capacity breath is taken with a good mask seal around the mouth and nose, most children will lose their lid reflex within 15 to 30 seconds, which is similar to IV induction agents.

TABLE 4.6	Doses of Commonly Used IV Induction Agents
Drug	**Dose (mg/kg)**
Thiopental or thiamylal[a]	5–8
Methohexital	1–2.5
Propofol	2.5–3.5
Etomidate	0.2–0.3
Ketamine	1–2

[a]No longer available in the United States.

Chapters 7 and 8) because of its relatively low context-sensitive half-life. It is especially useful for pediatric patients undergoing non-OR procedures such as CT, MRI, radiotherapy, bone marrow biopsy, upper and lower gastrointestinal endoscopy, and lumbar puncture.

Etomidate

Etomidate is a hypnotic induction agent that provides marked cardiovascular stability. Etomidate is available for use in the United States and several other countries, but it is not available in many others because of concern for adrenal suppression. It is indicated for the induction of anesthesia in children with sepsis, cardiac instability, cardiomyopathy, or hypovolemic shock. The recommended induction dose is 0.2 to 0.3 mg/kg depending on the cardiovascular status of the child. Etomidate causes pain and myoclonic movements when injected intravenously[332] and may suppress adrenal steroid synthesis (see also Chapter 7).[333]

Ketamine

Ketamine is a very useful induction agent for children with cardiovascular instability, especially in hypovolemic states, or for those who cannot tolerate a reduction in systemic vascular resistance, such as those with aortic stenosis or congenital heart disease in whom the balance between pulmonary and systemic blood flow is vital for maintaining cardiovascular homeostasis. In children whose circulation is already maximally compensated by endogenous catecholamines, ketamine is a myocardial depressant that can result in systemic hypotension.[334] The induction dose of ketamine in healthy children is 1 to 2 mg/kg. The dose should be reduced in the presence of severe hypovolemia. Smaller doses of IV ketamine (0.25 to 0.5 mg/kg) have also been used successfully for procedural sedation.

Ketamine causes sialorrhea, psychomimetic side effects (hallucinations, nightmares), and postoperative nausea and vomiting. The administration of an antisialagogue and midazolam is recommended to attenuate these side effects.

INTRAMUSCULAR INDUCTION

Although it is preferable to avoid intramuscular injections in children, there are occasions when this route may be indicated, such as for the uncooperative child or adolescent who refuses all other routes of sedation (oral, intranasal, IV), those susceptible to malignant hyperthermia, those with congenital heart disease, and those who have poor venous access. In infants, but especially in older children, intramuscular ketamine is a very useful medication because it is available in a concentrated solution (100 mg/mL) (see earlier discussion).[112]

RECTAL INDUCTION

Rectal drug administration is ideally suited for an extremely frightened young child who rejects other forms of premedication and for those who are developmentally delayed. It is usually limited to children younger than 5 or 6 years of age or smaller than 20 kg, owing to volume limitations on the fluid injected and concern over emotional consequences. Methohexital, thiopental, ketamine, and midazolam have all been investigated as agents for rectal induction. For unpremedicated children, the induction doses are 30 mg/kg thiopental and methohexital,[335] 1.0 mg/kg midazolam,[336] and approximately 5 mg/kg ketamine.

Disadvantages of rectal drug administration include failure to induce anesthesia because of poor drug bioavailability or defecation and delayed recovery from anesthesia after brief procedures resulting from the variability of rectal drug absorption. Conversely, there can be a very rapid drug uptake, leading to respiratory compromise.

FULL STOMACH AND RAPID-SEQUENCE INDUCTION

A full stomach is one of the most common problems that pediatric anesthesiologists face. The preferred method to secure the airway in the presence of a full stomach is IV rapid sequence induction (RSI). Before this is undertaken, the anesthesiologist must ensure that the proper equipment is at hand (Table 4.7). After IV access is established, the child should breathe 100% oxygen (preoxygenated) if possible. Studies of adult patients demonstrated that oxygen saturation remains greater than 95% for 6 minutes after only four vital capacity breaths of 100% oxygen.[337] Similar studies have not been performed in either cooperative or uncooperative children; however, without preoxygenation, younger infants and children desaturate very rapidly after induction of anesthesia and much

TABLE 4.7	Necessary Equipment for Rapid-Sequence Intubation
Functioning laryngoscope blades and handles (two)	
Suction (two)	
Anesthetic medications	
Checked anesthesia workstation and breathing circuit	
Tracheal tubes of appropriate sizes	
Tracheal tube stylets	
Functioning monitors (including pulse oximeter, blood pressure cuff, and precordial stethoscope)	

more rapidly than older children and adults.[338,339] One study demonstrated a more rapid increase in the inspired oxygen concentration in infants compared with older patients and that preoxygenation to a fractional concentration of O_2 in expired gas (FEO_2) of 0.9 can be achieved in 100 seconds.[340] Even with a crying child, it is possible to increase the arterial oxygen tension (PaO_2) by enriching the immediate environment with high gas flows of oxygen.

Preoxygenation should not be carried out in a manner that upsets a child. Premedication (e.g., IV midazolam, 0.05 to 0.1 mg/kg) in divided doses may alleviate fear and anxiety before induction. It is important to preoxygenate children to avoid positive-pressure ventilation before tracheal intubation because positive-pressure ventilation might distend the already full stomach, leading to regurgitation and aspiration. After preoxygenation (and atropine 0.02 mg/kg), anesthesia is induced with IV thiopental (5 to 6 mg/kg),[311] propofol (3 to 4 mg/kg),[341,342] ketamine (1 to 2 mg/kg), or etomidate (0.2 to 0.3 mg/kg), followed immediately by 2 mg/kg of succinylcholine. Succinylcholine is still the paralytic agent of choice for rapid onset and short duration. However, high-dose rocuronium may be used as an alternative muscle relaxant for RSI if succinylcholine is contraindicated. Intubating conditions 30 seconds after 1.2 mg/kg rocuronium were similar to those after 1.5 mg/kg succinylcholine.[343] The mean time to return 25% of the twitch response was 46 ± 23 minutes (range, 30 to 72 minutes) for rocuronium compared with 5.8 ± 3.3 minutes (range, 1.5 to 8.2 minutes) for succinylcholine. However, if thiopental is used for induction of anesthesia and followed by rocuronium, the thiopental must be cleared from the tubing before the rocuronium is administered to prevent thiopental from precipitating.[344] The availability of the new reversal agent (sugammadex) for rocuronium (and potentially vecuronium) may reduce concern about the risks associated with a prolonged duration of action of rocuronium, particularly in the presence of a difficult airway, and eliminate the need for IV succinylcholine (see Chapter 7). Suggamadex was approved for use by the US FDA in November 2015. The ability to immediately reverse nondepolarizing neuromuscular blocking agents must be weighed against the short duration of action of succinylcholine when selecting a paralytic agent for RSI.

Cricoid pressure (Sellick maneuver) should be applied as anesthesia is induced, and the pressure should be maintained until the tracheal tube has been successfully placed between the vocal cords.[345,346] By obliterating the esophageal lumen, cricoid pressure is intended to prevent regurgitated material from passing from the stomach to the pharynx. Before induction of anesthesia, the cricoid ring is palpated between the thumb and the middle finger and as soon as the child loses consciousness, pressure is steadily increased using the index finger. To prevent passive gastroesophageal reflux, a force of 30 to 40 N (3 to 4 kg of force) must be applied to the upper esophagus (in adults), which creates an intraluminal pressure of approximately 50 cm H_2O in the upper esophagus.[347] However, active vomiting may create esophageal pressures in excess of 60 cm H_2O that could overcome cricoid pressure and result in regurgitation and pulmonary aspiration. Alternatively, if cricoid pressure is not relieved immediately, spontaneous rupture of the esophagus (Boerhaave syndrome) may occur. Hence, the contraindications to cricoid pressure should be carefully reviewed to avoid complications from this maneuver (Table 4.8). Gastric insufflation is prevented in children by cricoid pressure during mask ventilation with peak inspiratory pressures up to 40 cm H_2O.[348] The Sellick maneuver should seal the

TABLE 4.8	Contraindications to Cricoid Pressure
Contraindication	**Potential Complication**
Active vomiting	• Possible rupture of esophagus
Airway issues	• Fractured cricoid cartilage may be made worse. • Sharp foreign body in larynx may result in further laryngeal injury.
Esophageal issues	• Zenker diverticulum • Sharp foreign body in upper esophagus may result in further esophageal injury.
Vertebral/neurologic issues	• Unstable cervical spine may result in spinal cord injury. • Sharp foreign body in the neck may result in injury to other structures in the neck.

From Thiagarajah S, Lear E, Keh M. Anesthetic implications of Zenker's diverticulum. *Anesth Analg* 1990;70:109-111

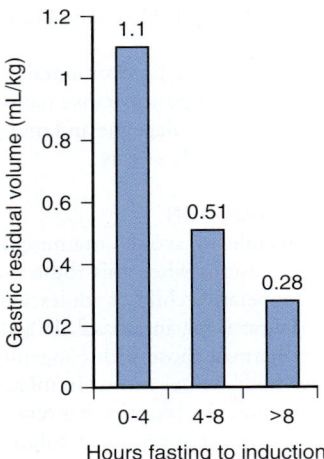

FIGURE 4.5 Mean gastric residual volume is plotted against hours of fasting before anesthetic induction in emergency pediatric cases. These data suggest that a 4-hour fast, if it does not compromise patient safety, may reduce gastric residual volume and therefore reduce (but not eliminate) risk for aspiration. (Data abstracted from Schurizek BA, Rybro L, Boggild-Madsen NB, Juhl B. Gastric volume and pH in children for emergency surgery. *Acta Anaesthesiol Scand.* 1986;30:404-408.)

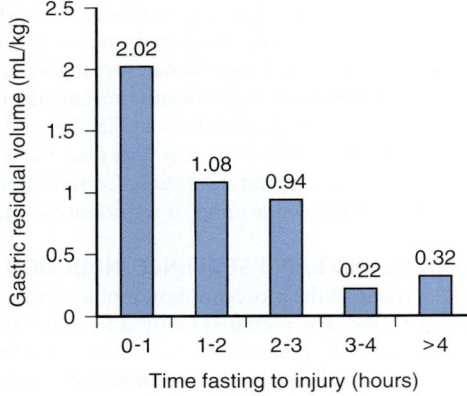

FIGURE 4.6 Mean gastric residual volume is plotted against time from last food ingestion to time of injury. These data suggest that the longer the time from ingestion to injury, the lower the risk for pulmonary aspiration of gastric contents. Also, if more than 4 hours has elapsed between the time of last food ingestion and time of injury, the risk is similar to that for patients with routine fasting. However, even with a 4-hour fasting time period, these patients must still be treated as though they have a full stomach. It should be noted that these volumes also relate to the severity of injury (increased volumes with increased injury severity). (Data abstracted from Bricker SRW, McLuckie A, Nightingale DA. Gastric aspirates after trauma in children. *Anesthesia* 1989;44:721-724.)

esophagus in the presence of a nasogastric tube,[349] but removal of the nasogastric tube before intubation provides a better mask fit on the face and exposure for laryngoscopy and intubation. If the nasogastric tube is left in place, leaving it open to atmospheric pressure will vent liquid and gas present in the stomach.

The results of surveys from the United Kingdom showed that cricoid pressure was used in only 40% to 50% of children in whom it was indicated.[350,351] Reluctance to apply cricoid pressure may be attributed to a number of reasons, including the indications for its use and how often it is applied with the correct position and pressure.[352–354] In adults evaluated with MRI, the esophagus was situated lateral to the cricoid cartilage in more than 50% of patients without cricoid pressure and was laterally displaced more than 90% of the time when cricoid pressure was applied.[355] In addition, cricoid pressure may distort the anatomy of the upper airway, making laryngoscopy more difficult, and it must sometimes be released to facilitate a clear view of the larynx and tracheal intubation, particularly in infants.[356] Cricoid pressure also decreases the tone of the upper and lower esophageal sphincters.[347,357] However, properly applied cricoid pressure can facilitate intubation with RSI and mask ventilation.

Evidence suggests that the gastric residual volume in children undergoing emergency surgery is greater if a child is anesthetized within 4 hours after hospital admission (1.1 mL/kg).[358] If, on the other hand, surgery can be delayed for at least 4 hours, then the mean gastric residual volume is on average much less (0.51 mL/kg)[358]; this gastric residual volume is in fact similar to that observed in children who have fasted for routine surgical procedures (Fig. 4.5).[1] This does not imply that these children should not be regarded as having a full stomach; rather, the risk may be somewhat reduced if surgery can be delayed several hours. In addition, evidence suggests that in emergency cases, the gastric residual volume depends, in part, on the time interval between the last food ingestion and the time of the injury as well as the severity of the injury.[358] Children who last ate more than 4 hours before the injury have a gastric residual volume similar to those who fasted as if it were elective surgery (Fig. 4.6). *There is some comfort in these numbers, but one should never consider such children as not having a full stomach but rather as having a less full stomach.* Additionally, the possible value of H_2-receptor blocking agents, metoclopramide, and clear antacids may be considered, but their use in this regard is not evidence based.

A modified RSI may be preferred in small infants who will likely desaturate during brief periods of apnea and will therefore require assisted ventilation before the trachea is secured. Despite face mask ventilation prior to intubation, there were no cases of pulmonary aspiration in a retrospective cohort analysis of 1001 pediatric patients who underwent modified RSI.[359] Neonates may be intubated while awake if indicated; this may provide a greater margin of safety because it preserves spontaneous ventilation as well as laryngeal reflexes. Skillfully performed awake intubation in neonates is not associated with either significant adverse cardiovascular responses or neurologic sequelae[360] and may be preferred in infants with hemodynamic instability.[361]

Special Problems

THE FEARFUL CHILD

This is a difficult problem without a satisfactory solution. The child's fear is generally based on the child's developmental status, the hospital environment, and the impending surgery. This is why it is so vital that as much information as possible be presented and queries as to why the child is afraid are so important. Frequently, a few well-directed questions and honest answers will resolve most of the child's concerns. Often, allowing a parent to hold the child during induction of anesthesia or allowing the child to hold the anesthetic mask himself or herself will stop the flow of tears and settle the child's emotional upheaval. In other situations, one commonly practiced solution is to use intramuscular ketamine.

AUTISM

Autism spectrum disorder (ASD) is a neurodevelopmental disorder characterized by impairment in social and communication skills, restricted interests, repetitive behavior, and for some, touch, visual, taste, or sound hypersensitivity. Children present early in life but deficits may not become fully manifest until social communication demands exceed capabilities.[362] The diagnosis is based on observation and assessment of behavior and cognition and is aided by validated assessment tools. The fifth edition of *Diagnostic and Statistical Manual of Mental Disorders* (DSM-V) adopted the umbrella term ASD, which includes autism, Asperger syndrome, and pervasive developmental disorder.[363] How prevalence estimates will be affected by the new criteria remains to be assessed.

ASD was diagnosed in 1 in 68 (14.6 per 1000) children aged 8 years residing in US Autism and Developmental Disabilities Monitoring Network sites in 2012,[364] which is an increase over previous estimates of 1 in 88 (11.3 per 1000). The increased prevalence is likely due to broader diagnostic criteria, increased public awareness, and the development of more sensitive screening tools. Autism affects boys more commonly than girls with an overall prevalence ratio of 4.5.[364] Global prevalence of ASD is thought to be approximately 1%.[365] More than 70% of individuals with autism have concurrent medical (gastrointestinal, seizures, insomnia, mitochondrial disease), developmental (intellectual disability), or psychiatric problems (social anxiety disorder, attentive-deficit/hyperactivity disorder [ADHD], oppositional defiant disorder).[362]

Behavior and cognitive training is the most effective therapy for ASD, but it must be initiated at an early age to achieve the best possible neurologic improvement. The existing pharmacologic management for ASD has not been promising in treating core symptoms but has been effective in decreasing the burden of emotional and behavioral problems.[366] Antipsychotic drugs have been shown to effectively reduce repetitive behaviors in children with autism, but associated side effects limit their use to patients with severe impairment.[367] Serotonin reuptake inhibitors may reduce repetitive behaviors, although findings are inconsistent.[367–369] The effect of stimulants on symptoms of ADHD occurring in children with ASD requires more study but shows promise and has been recommended.[370] It is critical for the anesthesiologist to be familiar with these medications and their potential interactions with anesthetic agents (see Table 4.9).[371,372]

TABLE 4.9	Commonly Used Pharmacologic Agents for Children With Autism Spectrum Disorder	
Medication	Target Symptoms	Potential Adverse Effects
Antipsychotics: Haloperidol Risperidone Aripiprazole	Aggression, irritability, self-injury	Weight gain, sedation, extrapyramidal symptoms, hypotension with general anesthesia and proarrhythmic properties (risperidone)
Atypical Antipsychotic: Clozapine	Repetitive behaviors	Agranulocytosis, hyperthermia, cardiac conduction problems, hypotension. Discontinuation can cause dystonia dyskinesia, delirium, and psychosis
Selective Serotonin Reuptake Inhibitors (SSRIs): Fluoxetine Citalopram	Repetitive behaviors	Agitation, gastrointestinal symptoms; reduced platelet aggregation and increased transfusion risk
Stimulants: Methylphenidate Amphetamines	Hyperactivity, inattention	Insomnia, decreased appetite, weight loss, headache, irritability, may increase anesthetic requirement, increase risk of hypertension and arrhythmias, lower seizure threshold and interact with vasopressors
Melatonin	Insomnia	No side effects recorded

The perioperative period can be a stressful time for children with ASD; they do not respond well to changes in routine and may challenge the ingenuity of the anesthesiologist. They are very sensitive to stimuli such as light, sound, touch, and pain and may be unable to articulate concerns they have. The hospital setting is anxiety-provoking and usually upsets most autistic children until they become totally disruptive and uncooperative.

The anesthesiologist's approach to the autistic child depends on the severity of the disorder. Information regarding the child's previous anesthetic experience, assessment of the child's behavior and idiosyncrasies, and bonding with parents or caregivers should be accomplished during the preanesthetic visit. The family should be encouraged to bring favorite toys, electronic devices, and other comforting items. Collecting pertinent information about baseline behavior, triggers of emotional outbursts, and signs of escalating anxiety is invaluable.[373] Sedative premedication can work very well in these children. The decision to administer premedication needs to be made on an individual basis (see "Premedication and Induction Principles"). Oral midazolam (0.5 to 1 mg/kg)[374] is the most commonly used preoperative anxiolytic for children, although other choices include oral ketamine (6 mg/kg)[202] and a combination of oral midazolam (0.5 mg/kg) and ketamine (3 to 6 mg/kg).[205] Oral dexmedetomidine (mean dose 2.6 μg/kg) has also provided adequate sedation prior to induction of anesthesia in children with ASD.[375] Some of these children may have problems with certain textures and tastes; administering oral premedication in a favorite drink should be considered in the context of NPO guidelines. The overly anxious child may be uncooperative with oral medication and may require intramuscular ketamine. Parents can also offer insight into which strategies would make their child's life easier during this difficult time. It is important to take the time to address parental concerns and establish a trusting relationship with the family. In a recent retrospective review, no difference in the perioperative experience was found between children with ASD and healthy children undergoing dental rehabilitation, including no apparent difference in complications, postoperative pain, and time to discharge. The only significant difference was found in the type and the route of administration of the premedication where children with ASD had a higher rate of nonstandard premedication (ketamine intramuscularly with and without midazolam, intranasal ketamine, or an IV line placed preoperatively for IV premedication).[376]

There is great variation in the severity of autism and hospital needs of these children.[377] The focus for optimal management of these children in one institution was on early communication to provide a flexible and individualized admission process and anesthetic plan.[377] A quiet room, scheduling the case as early in the day as possible, minimizing the waiting period, and involving a child-life specialist may offer advantage preoperatively for more severe cases.[373]

Intraoperative goals should include adequate analgesia, prophylaxis of postoperative nausea and vomiting, and optimal intraoperative hydration to allow early removal of the IV cannula, which may prevent negative emotional outbursts in the recovery room. Finally, the appropriate use of parents in the postanesthesia care unit can facilitate the transition from surgery to recovery. Studies have shown that children who are reunited with their parents sooner require less pain medication and are discharged earlier in an ambulatory setting.[378]

ANEMIA

The minimum hematocrit necessary to ensure adequate oxygen transport in children has not been well established. Preoperative hemoglobin testing, however, is of limited value in healthy children undergoing elective surgery when minimal blood loss is expected.[379] Children with chronic anemia, such as those with renal failure, do not require preoperative transfusion because of compensatory mechanisms, such as increased 2,3-diphosphoglycerate, increased oxygen extraction, and increased cardiac output. Elective surgery for children who are anemic should take into consideration their medical history, underlying diseases (e.g., hemoglobinopathies, von Willebrand, sickle cell, other factor deficiency), the nature of the surgery, and its urgency. Most pediatric anesthesiologists would recommend a hematocrit greater than 25% before elective surgery in the absence of chronic disease. If significant blood loss is anticipated and the surgery is elective, then the cause of anemia should be investigated and treated and the surgery postponed until the hematocrit is restored to the normal range. *Healthy children scheduled for elective surgery that is not expected to cause substantive bleeding should not routinely receive a blood transfusion just to bring their hematocrit to an arbitrary limit such as 30%.*

Physiologic anemia of infancy occurs between 2 and 4 months of postnatal age. At this time, there is an increased production of hemoglobin A and an increase in red cell 2,3-diphosphoglycerate, which contribute to a right shift of the oxygen-hemoglobin dissociation curve (see Chapter 10). Therefore, in infants 2 to 4 months of age, a reduced hemoglobin value is acceptable. Anemia, with a hematocrit of less than 30%, in formerly preterm infants represents a special category of patients who may have an increased incidence of postoperative apnea (see later discussion), but transfusion is still not recommended.[380]

TABLE 4.10	Differential Diagnosis of a Child With a Runny Nose
Noninfectious Causes	
Allergic rhinitis: seasonal, perennial, clear nasal discharge; no fever	
Vasomotor rhinitis: emotional (crying); temperature changes	
Infectious Causes	
Viral infections	
Nasopharyngitis (common cold)	
Flu syndrome (upper and lower respiratory tract)	
Laryngotracheal bronchitis (infectious croup)	
Viral exanthems	
Measles	
Chickenpox	
Acute bacterial infections	
Acute epiglottitis	
Meningitis	
Streptococcal tonsillitis	

UPPER RESPIRATORY TRACT INFECTION

The child with a nonpurulent active or recent upper respiratory tract infection (URI; within 4 weeks) often presents a conundrum, even for the most experienced anesthesiologist. Between 20% and 30% of all children have a runny nose during a significant part of the year. A differential diagnosis of a child with a runny nose is presented in Table 4.10. In the preanesthetic evaluation, we must rely on history, physical examination, and, rarely, laboratory data to decide whether to proceed with the anesthesia.

A number of perioperative anesthetic risks have been studied in children with URIs.[381] The risk of postintubation croup was similar in children who had an active URI and those who did not.[382] Bronchospasm occurs more frequently in children whose tracheas are intubated and who have active URIs.[383] The incidence of bronchospasm in children with a URI (41:1000) is 10-fold greater than it is in those without a URI.[384] The incidence of laryngospasm in children with a URI (96:1000) is 5-fold greater than it is in children without a URI (17:1000).[385] The incidence of minor but not major intraoperative hemoglobin desaturation events in children with a URI is greater than in those without a URI.[383] Lastly, the incidence of all respiratory-related adverse events combined in children with a URI was 9-fold greater than in those without a URI and 11-fold greater in children who had a URI and required tracheal intubation.[386]

When a tracheal tube and LMA were compared in children with a URI, the incidence of mild bronchospasm, major desaturation events, and overall respiratory events was reduced in the presence of a LMA, although the incidence of laryngospasm was similar with the two airway devices.[387,388]

Prognostic factors of adverse anesthetic events in children with URIs who were scheduled for elective surgery include the type of airway management (tracheal intubation > LMA); a parent's statement that the child has a "cold"; the presence of nasal congestion, snoring, passive smoking; the induction agent (thiopental > halothane > sevoflurane ~ propofol); sputum production; and whether the neuromuscular agent was antagonized.[389] Reactive airway disease and a history of prematurity have also been associated with adverse outcomes in children with URIs.[390] Age has not been an independent predictor of adverse events in children with URIs in most studies, although one study suggested that the incidence of bronchospasm in infants younger than 6 months with active URIs was greater (20.8% vs. 4.7%, $P = .08$) than in older children.[391] In this study, the greatest incidence of adverse respiratory events occurred in children undergoing airway surgery (e.g., tonsillectomy and adenoidectomy, direct laryngoscopy, bronchoscopy).

Cancellation of cardiac surgery carries special import because of the risk that the child's heart will deteriorate or the disease process will progress (e.g., pulmonary hypertension), as well as the extensive time, materials, and personnel committed to a planned case. In a prospective study of children scheduled for cardiac surgery, the incidences of respiratory adverse events (29.2% vs. 17.3%, $P < .01$), multiple postoperative complications (25% vs. 10.3%, $P < .01$), and bacterial infection (5.2% vs. 1.0%, $P = .01$) were greater in those with a URI than in those without.[392]

A national survey suggested that more experienced anesthesiologists are less likely to cancel surgery because of the presence of a URI.[393] Cancellation may also impose emotional and economic burdens on the parents.[394,395] Factors that should be considered when deciding whether to proceed with elective surgery in a child with a URI are summarized in Table 4.11.

Insofar as which techniques will help to prevent complications from a URI, pretreating healthy children who either had a URI within the preceding 6 weeks or had an active URI with bronchodilators, either inhaled ipratropium or albuterol, before anesthesia provided no benefit.[396] However, in another study, children with a recent URI (≤2 weeks in duration) who received preoperative salbutamol experienced a significantly reduced incidence of laryngospasm, bronchospasm, oxygen desaturation (<95%) and severe coughing with an LMA or tracheal tube.[397] Humidification, IV hydration, and anticholinergics may also decrease perioperative complications,[393] although the results of

at least one study suggested that glycopyrrolate did not reduce the incidence of perioperative adverse respiratory events when it was given after induction of anesthesia to children with URIs.[398] Use of LMAs coated with topical lidocaine in children with URIs was associated with decreased postoperative coughing[399,400] and lower overall perioperative complication rates.[400]

If the decision is made to postpone anesthesia, then how long should one wait before administering general anesthesia to a child? Bronchial hyperreactivity, which is associated with URIs in children, shows spirometric changes in the lungs for as long as 7 weeks after a URI.[401,402] Although studies suggest that surgery should be postponed for at least 7 weeks after resolution of a URI, this plan is impractical because most children will be infected with a new URI by that time. Postponing surgery until 2 weeks after resolution of the URI is a common but as yet unproven strategy. In fact, some data suggest that the incidence of adverse respiratory events is just as great in this population as it is in those who were anesthetized during the acute phase of the URI.[403,404] This 2-week waiting period may be acceptable in a child with uncomplicated nasopharyngitis.[405] Unfortunately, there is no consensus on the optimal time interval before surgery is rescheduled. In a survey of anesthesiologists, most wait 3 to 4 weeks before proceeding with surgery.[393] The rationale for this time period is that the risk of respiratory complications is unchanged for 4 to 6 weeks.[391]

In conclusion, good judgment, common sense, clinical experience, a measured discussion with the surgeon, and informed consent from the parents or guardians must be used when deciding whether to proceed or postpone the surgery. All of these deliberations and discussions including the risks and benefits should be documented in the chart (see Chapter 13 for additional discussion and perspectives).

OBESITY

There are a variety of definitions for childhood obesity. In children and adolescents aged 2 to 19 years, the CDC defines obesity as a body mass index (BMI) at or above the 95th percentile for age, as defined by the 2000 CDC growth charts for normal children.[406] Overweight is defined as a BMI between the 85th and 95th percentiles. The World Health Organization uses standard deviations (BMI z scores) from the mean BMI for age to define childhood overweight and obesity.* A third standard developed by Cole[407] uses pooled international data to provide age-specific and gender-specific BMI cutoff points for childhood obesity.

The prevalence of childhood obesity is rapidly increasing worldwide. Globally, the World Health Organization estimates 42 million children under the age of 5 years were overweight or obese in 2013.† In the United States, approximately 8% of infants and toddlers had high weight for recumbent length, and 17% of children aged 2 to 19 years were obese per CDC standards in 2011-12.[406] The majority of childhood overweight and obesity cases are caused by excessive caloric intake and relative lack of physical activity, with the remaining cases resulting from conditions such as endocrine disorders, neurologic dysfunction, and genetic syndromes (e.g., Prader-Willi).[408]

Obesity is a complex endocrine state and is associated with numerous comorbidities (Table 4.12). The incidences of these

TABLE 4.11	Factors Affecting Decision for Elective Surgery in a Child With Upper Respiratory Tract Infection
Proceed With Caution	**Consider Cancellation**
• Child has "just a runny nose," no other symptoms, "much better"	• Parents confirm symptoms: fever, malaise, cough, poor appetite, just developed symptoms last night
• Active and happy child	• Lethargic, ill-appearing
• Clear rhinorrhea	• Purulent nasal discharge
• Clear lungs and symptoms have leveled off or have improved	• Wheezing, rales that do not clear
• Older child	• Child <1 year, former premie
• Social issues: hardship for parents to be away from work, insurance will run out	• Other factors: history of reactive airway disease, major operation, endotracheal tube required
• No fever	• Fever >38.5°C
• Outpatient procedure that will not expose immunocompromised children to possible infectious agent	• Inpatient procedure that may result in exposure of immunocompromised children to viral/bacterial infection

From Tait AR, Malviya S. Anesthesia for the child with an upper respiratory tract infection: still a dilemma? *Anesth Analg.* 2005;100:59-65.

*See http://www.who.int/dietphysicalactivity/childhood_what/en (accessed April 23, 2016).
†See http://www.who.int/mediacentre/factsheets/fs311/en (accessed April 23, 2016).

TABLE 4.12	Comorbidities Associated With Childhood Obesity
Affected Organ System	**Obesity-Related Comorbidity**
Respiratory system	• Bronchial hyperreactivity • Asthma (present in 30%) • High incidence of upper airway infections • Obstructive sleep apnea (present in 13%–59%)
Cardiovascular	• Hypertension (present in 20%–30%) • Left ventricular hypertrophy (in adolescents)
Endocrine	• Metabolic syndrome (present in 40%–50% of obese adolescents) • Dyslipidemia (hyperlipidemia and hypercholesterolemia) • Polycystic ovarian syndrome
Gastrointestinal	• Gastroesophageal reflux (present in 20% of severely obese children) • Asymptomatic steatosis hepatis (present in 80%). Could progress to hepatic fibrosis, nonalcoholic acute steatohepatitis or rarely cirrhosis.
Neurologic/psychological	• Pseudotumor cerebri • Low self-esteem • Poor school performance
Orthopedic	• Slipped femoral epiphysis

From Mortensen A, Lenz K, Abildstrom H, Lauritsen TLB. Anesthetizing the obese child. *Paediatr Anaesth.* 2011;21:623-629.

TABLE 4.13	Dosage of IV Anesthetics in Obese Children	
Drug	**Induction Dose Based on**	**Maintenance Dose Based on**
Thiopental	LBW	
Propofol	LBW	TBW
Synthetic opioids (fentanyl, alfentanil, and sufentanil)	TBW	LBW
Morphine	IBW	IBW
Remifentanil	LBW	LBW
Nondepolarizing neuromuscular blockers	IBW	IBW
Succinylcholine	TBW	
Sugammadex	TBW	

From Mortensen A, Lenz K, Abildstrom H, Lauritsen TLB. Anesthetizing the obese child. *Paediatr Anaesth.* 2011;21:623-629.
TBW, total body weight; *LBW*, lean body weight; *IBW*, ideal body weight.

comorbidities increase as BMI and the duration of obesity increase.[409] Weight loss may reduce perioperative risk factors.

Obese children have a higher incidence of perioperative adverse respiratory events compared with normal-weight children.[410,411] Functional residual capacity, expiratory reserve volume, forced expiratory volume in 1 second, and diffusion capacity are all reduced. High closing volumes may cause atelectasis and right-to-left intrapulmonary shunting.[412] Bronchial hyperreactivity and asthma are highly prevalent amongst obese children. A review of over 2200 referrals to a pediatric asthma specialist in the United States found that nearly 30% of patients with physician-diagnosed asthma were obese.[413] Asthma incidence and severity rose with increasing BMI. In addition, a cross-sectional study of 1129 preadolescent children found that overweight children with BMI greater than the 90th percentile for age had twice the risk of developing URIs, an independent risk of perioperative respiratory complications, compared with children with lower BMI (please refer to "Upper Respiratory Tract Infections" in this chapter for further discussion of risk).[414]

Obstructive sleep apnea syndrome (OSAS) affects 13% to 59% of obese children (see further).[415–417] Children with OSAS may display increased sensitivity to opioids. Opioids should be carefully titrated to respiratory responses. If apnea is seen after small doses of opioids, further doses of opioids should be reduced and respirations must be closely monitored. Similarly, caution must be used when administering benzodiazepines for premedication in obese children with OSAS given the risk of respiratory depression. If the child is regularly managed with continuous positive airway pressure (CPAP) or biphasic positive airway pressure (BiPAP), this therapy should be maintained postoperatively until the child is awake and can maintain a patent airway.

Obese children have increased blood volume, stroke volume, and cardiac output.[418] Hypertension is present in 20% to 30% of obese children; the incidence of hypertension increases with increasing BMI.[419,420] Blood pressure should be measured preoperatively and exercise tolerance determined to establish whether cardiopulmonary compromise exists.

Significant obesity leads to insulin resistance; nearly half of obese adolescents suffer from the metabolic syndrome and are at high risk of developing type 2 diabetes mellitus.[421] Fasting blood glucose levels should be obtained preoperatively, as type 2 diabetes mellitus may be present but undiagnosed.[422] Adolescents with type 2 diabetes mellitus display adverse measures of cardiac structure and function positively related to BMI and blood pressure.[423] Preoperative electrocardiography and echocardiography should be considered in obese diabetic children with suspected cardiac disease.

Childhood obesity is a risk factor for gastroesophageal reflux. Up to 20% of severely obese children have symptoms of gastroesophageal reflux, compared with 2% of normal-weight children.[424] Despite the increased prevalence of symptomatic reflux, gastric fluid volumes are identical across all BMI categories (when corrected for ideal body weight) and regardless of fasting interval. Overweight and obese children with gastroesophageal reflux may be allowed clear liquids 2 hours before surgery, similar to normal-weight children.[425]

Preoperative height, weight, blood pressure, heart rate, pulse oximetry, and fasting glucose level should be documented for all obese children. A thorough airway examination must be performed. The risk of difficult mask ventilation is higher in obese children than in normal-weight children.[411,426,427] Jaw thrust and CPAP are useful in reducing upper airway collapse during spontaneous ventilation. Equipment for difficult intubation should be readily available prior to the induction of anesthesia. Vascular access may be difficult to establish in obese children.

IV drug dosing is problematic as the pharmacokinetics of most anesthetics are affected by obesity. Unfortunately, there are few pharmacokinetic studies of obese children and data to guide drug dosing are limited. Drug doses for induction of anesthesia may be calculated based on the patient's total body weight, ideal body weight, or lean body weight (Table 4.13). In general, hydrophilic drugs should be dosed according to ideal body weight. One notable exception is succinylcholine, which should be dosed according to total body weight owing to increased pseudocholinesterase activity in obese children (see also Chapters 6 and 7).[428]

OBSTRUCTIVE SLEEP APNEA SYNDROME

Sleep apnea is a sleep-related breathing disorder in children characterized by a periodic cessation of air exchange, with apnea episodes lasting longer than 10 seconds and an apnea-hypopnea index (AHI) indicating that the total number of obstructive episodes per hour of sleep is greater than 1 (AHI 1-5 = mild OSA, 6-10 = moderate OSA, >10 = severe OSA).[429] Sleep apnea may be defined as central (absent gas flow, lack of respiratory effort), obstructive (absent gas flow, upper airway obstruction, and paradoxical movement of rib cage and abdominal muscles), or mixed (due to both CNS defect and obstructive problems). Diagnosis is made by clinical assessment (see later discussion), nocturnal pulse oximetry, or polysomnography studies.

OSAS is manifested by episodes that disturb sleep and ventilation. These episodes occur more frequently during rapid eye movement (REM) sleep and increase in frequency as more time is spent in REM sleep periods as the night progresses. OSAS occurs in children of all ages (about 2% of all children) but is more common in children 3 to 7 years of age. It occurs equally in boys and girls, although the prevalence is greater in African American and Hispanic children compared with Caucasians.[430–433]

Signs of OSAS are sleep disturbances (including daytime sleepiness), irritability, night terrors, nocturnal enuresis, snoring loud enough to be heard through a closed door, pauses and/or gasps during the night, failure to thrive resulting from poor intake due to tonsillar hypertrophy, speech disorders, and decreased size (decreased growth hormone release during disturbed REM sleep). With the worldwide increase in childhood obesity, the presence of obesity in children with OSAS exacerbates the signs and symptoms of OSAS. Parents of obese children should be specifically asked about such signs and symptoms. This syndrome can cause significant cardiac, pulmonary, and CNS impairment caused by chronic oxygen desaturation. Indeed, both OSAS and obesity are systemic inflammatory responses.[434] When they occur together in a child, the severity of the signs and symptoms are greater than if only one had occurred, and resolution of the OSAS after tonsillectomy is less likely. In children with OSAS and morbid obesity, the incidences of hypertension and diabetes are greater than in the absence of these disorders. Therefore, it is important to evaluate the cardiovascular status; although right ventricular dysfunction with pulmonary hypertension is classic, biventricular hypertrophy can develop. It is more likely to occur in children with severe OSAS but has been reported in children with only mild OSAS.[435] Cardiac evaluation is recommended for any child with signs of right ventricular dysfunction, systemic or pulmonary hypertension, or multiple episodes of desaturation below 70% (see also Fig. 33.7). Electrocardiography and chest radiography are insensitive diagnostic tests; rather, echocardiography is recommended.[436] Relief of the tonsillar/adenoidal obstruction can reverse many of these disorders and prevent progression of others (pulmonary hypertension and cor pulmonale) within 6 months after tonsillectomy, although approximately 30% of children with severe OSAS will not have resolution of the OSAS after tonsillectomy.

Children with OSAS may be premedicated with caution with oral midazolam. Despite an incidence of self-limited preoperative desaturation of less than 1.5%, postpremedication monitoring of hemoglobin saturation in these children would seem reasonable.[437]

Avoidance of premedication may, however, be more advantageous postoperatively.

Factors for children who are at increased risk for postoperative upper airway obstruction after tonsillectomy and/or adenoidectomy for OSAS include age younger than 2 years, craniofacial anomalies, failure to thrive, hypotonia, morbid obesity, previous upper airway trauma, cor pulmonale, a polysomnogram with a respiratory distress index greater than 40 or O_2 saturation nadir less than 85%, and a child undergoing an additional uvulopalatopharyngoplasty.[438] *Nocturnal desaturation to less than 85% upregulates the genes responsible for control of opioid receptors, resulting in an increased sensitivity to opioids; opioid requirement is reduced by approximately 50%, making standard doses of opioids a relative overdose in children with severe OSA.* This has been demonstrated in both animals and humans.[439,440] To attenuate the risk of perioperative respiratory complications, opioids should be carefully titrated to the respiratory responses during surgery, and if an increased sensitivity to opioids is detected, all perioperative opioids should be reduced accordingly (see Chapter 33 for further details).[441]

There is increasing evidence of marked ethnic variations in the cytochromes responsible for drug metabolism (see also Chapters 6 and 7). In 8% to 10% of children, a defect in CYP2D6 renders them unable to convert codeine to morphine. Codeine administration results in virtually no analgesia in such children. On the other hand, a small percentage of children (0.5% to 2%) have a duplication of the cytochrome portion responsible for codeine metabolism. Codeine is rapidly converted to morphine, yielding much higher blood levels in these "ultrarapid metabolizers" compared with children with normal cytochromes. This may lead to a relative morphine overdose, and has resulted in fatalities in children with OSA.[187–189] As a result, the FDA has added a boxed warning to codeine-containing products and recommends against the use of codeine, especially with "round-the-clock dosing," in children following tonsillectomy (see also previous discussion).*

If nocturnal upper airway obstruction continues after tonsillectomy, ancillary strategies that have been met with variable success have been used: nasal CPAP or BiPAP, nasal steroids, oxygen therapy, and weight loss, although nasal CPAP/BiPAP is rarely tolerated in children.[438]

The American Academy of Pediatrics (AAP) Clinical Practice Guidelines[442,443] provide recommendations for inpatient monitoring of children at high risk for postoperative complications who have OSAS and are undergoing adenotonsillectomy (Table 4.14). These guidelines advocate that high-risk patients undergo surgery in a facility capable of treating complex pediatric patients and be hospitalized overnight for close monitoring. In addition to the AAP guidelines, the ASA considers this such a growing problem for both adults and children that they also have formulated a Practice Guideline. Tables 4.15 and 4.16 (modified for children) help to clarify the identification and assessment of children potentially at risk for OSAS and offer a proposed (although as yet unvalidated) risk assessment scoring system.[443] This system attempts to characterize those patients who are at significantly increased risk for perioperative complications.

Despite these practice guidelines and risk identification scoring systems, a worrisome number of children with OSA have died or suffered neurologic injury as a result of apnea after tonsillectomy. A survey of Society for Pediatric Anesthesia members and review

---

*See http://www.fda.gov/Safety/MedWatch/SafetyInformation/SafetyAlertsforHumanMedicalProducts/ucm315627.htm (accessed March 29, 2016).

of the ASA Closed Claims Project yielded 111 reports of adverse events between 1990 and 2010 in children undergoing tonsillectomy.[444] Death or neurologic injury occurred in 77% of these cases. Nearly half of the events within 24 hours of the procedure occurred after hospital discharge. Children who fulfilled ASA criteria to be at risk for OSA were more likely to have the adverse event attributed to apnea, whereas all others were more likely to have the event attributed to hemorrhage. Patients at increased perioperative risk secondary to OSA must be closely monitored for apnea and should not be discharged from the recovery area to an unmonitored setting (i.e., home or unmonitored hospital bed) until no longer at risk of postoperative respiratory depression.[443]

Among children 1 to 18 years of age with OSAS, those without complicating medical conditions such as neuromuscular disease, obesity, or craniofacial abnormalities but with mild sleep apnea may have either no or some improvement in their airway obstruction on the night of surgery. Based on current literature, one may consider discharging children 3 to 12 years of age home on the day of surgery after an extended period of observation (4 to 6 hours) if they meet these criteria. However, those with moderate to severe OSA (particularly obese children) may actually experience worse OSA on the night of their surgery.[445,446] These children should receive reduced doses of opioids and be admitted for overnight monitoring with pulse oximetry and an apnea monitor.[447]

ASYMPTOMATIC CARDIAC MURMURS

The presence of a cardiac murmur is a common finding in children[448] and may have significant anesthetic implications. A history should be obtained to delineate the nature of the murmur. In most cases, the parents will report that the murmur was detected previously by the child's pediatrician and determined to be an "innocent flow murmur" without any anatomic or physiologic abnormalities. When a pediatric cardiologist confirms the classic

---

TABLE 4.14	American Academy of Pediatrics Clinical Practice Guidelines: Risk Factors for Postoperative Respiratory Complications in Children With OSAS Undergoing Adenotonsillectomy

Younger than 3 years of age

Severe OSAS on polysomnography

Cardiac complications of OSAS

Failure to thrive

Obesity

Craniofacial anomalies

Neuromuscular disorders

Current respiratory infection

From Clinical practice guideline: diagnosis and management of childhood obstructive sleep apnea syndrome. *Pediatrics* 2012;130:576-584.
OSAS, obstructive sleep apnea syndrome.

TABLE 4.15	Candidate Criteria for Identification and Assessment of OSA[a]

A: Clinical Signs and Symptoms Suggesting Obstructive Sleep Apnea (OSA)

1. Predisposing physical characteristics

a. ≥95th percentile for age and gender
b. Craniofacial abnormalities affecting the airway (e.g., Down syndrome)
c. Anatomic nasal obstruction
d. Tonsils nearly touching or touching in the midline (kissing tonsils)

2. History of apparent airway obstruction during sleep (two or more of the following are present; if patient sleep is not observed by another person, then only one of the following needs to be present)

a. Snoring (loud enough to be heard through a closed door)
b. Frequent snoring
c. Observed pauses in breathing during sleep
d. Awakened from sleep with choking sensation
e. Frequent arousal from sleep
f. Intermittent vocalizations during sleep
g. Parental report of restless sleep, difficulty breathing, or struggling respiratory efforts during sleep
h. Child with night terrors
i. Child sleeps in unusual positions
j. Child with new-onset enuresis

3. Somnolence (one of the following is present)

a. Frequent daytime somnolence or fatigue despite adequate "sleep"
b. Falls asleep easily in a nonstimulating environment (e.g., watching television, reading, riding in, or driving a car) despite adequate "sleep"
c. Parent or teacher comments that the child appears sleepy during the day, is easily distracted, is overly aggressive, or has difficulty concentrating
d. Child is often difficult to arouse at usual awakening time

B: Determination of Severity

a. If a child has signs or symptoms in two or more of the above categories, there is a significant probability that he or she has OSA. The severity of OSA may be determined by sleep study. If a sleep study is not available, such patients should be treated as though they have moderate sleep apnea unless one or more of the signs of symptoms above is severely abnormal (e.g., weight ≥95th percentile for age and gender, respiratory pauses that are frightening to the observer, child regularly falls asleep within minutes after being left unstimulated without another explanation), in which cases patients should be treated as though they have severe sleep apnea.

b. If a sleep study has been done, the result should be used to determine the perioperative anesthetic management of a child. (Review the polysomnogram for evidence of nocturnal desaturations <85%, which increases sensitivity to opioids). However, because sleep laboratories differ in their criteria for detecting episodes of apnea and hypoxemia, the Task Force recommends that the sleep laboratory's assessment (none, mild, moderate, or severe) take precedence over the actual apnea-hypopnea index (AHI, the number of episodes of sleep-disordered breathing per hour). If the overall severity is not indicated, it may be determined by using the following table:

Severity of OSA	Adult AHI	Pediatric AHI
None	0–5	0
Mild OSA	6–20	1–5
Moderate OSA	21–40	6–10
Severe OSA	>40	>10

Modified from Practice guidelines for the perioperative management of patients with obstructive sleep apnea: an updated report by the American Society of Anesthesiologists Task Force on Perioperative Management of Patients with Obstructive Sleep Apnea. *Anesthesiology.* 2014;120:268-286.
[a]Note: This table has been modified for children; the scoring system is intended only as a guide and has not been validated.

TABLE 4.16	OSA Risk Scoring System: Example[a]

A. Severity of Sleep Apnea Based on Sleep Study (or Clinical Indicators if Sleep Study Is Not Available: Point Score 0–3[b,c])
Severity of OSA

None	0
Mild	1
Moderate	2
Severe	3

B. Invasiveness of Surgery and Anesthesia: Point Score 0–3
Type of surgery and anesthesia

Superficial surgery under local or peripheral nerve block anesthesia without sedation	0
Superficial surgery with moderate sedation or general anesthesia	1
Peripheral surgery with spinal or epidural anesthesia (with no more than moderate sedation)	1
Peripheral surgery with general anesthesia	2
Airway surgery with moderate sedation	2
Major surgery with general anesthesia	3
Airway surgery with general anesthesia (e.g., tonsillectomy)	3

C. Requirement for Postoperative Opioids: Point Score 0–3
Opioid requirement

None	0
Low-dose oral opioids (tonsillectomy)	1
High-dose oral opioids, parenteral or neuraxial opioids	3

D. Estimation of Perioperative Risk—Overall Score Equals the Score for "A" Plus the Greater of the Score for "B" or "C": Possible Score 0–6[d]

Modified from Practice guidelines for the perioperative management of patients with obstructive sleep apnea: an updated report by the American Society of Anesthesiologists Task Force on Perioperative Management of Patients with Obstructive Sleep Apnea. *Anesthesiology* 2014;120:268-286.

[a]Note: This table has been modified for children. A scoring system similar to this table may be used to estimate whether a child is at increased perioperative risk of complications from OSA. This example has not been clinically validated, and such a scoring system is simply meant to provide guidance.

[b]One point may be subtracted if a patient has been on continuous positive airway pressure (CPAP) for noninvasive positive-pressure ventilation before surgery and will be using his or her appliance consistently during the postoperative period.

[c]One point should be added if a child with mild or moderate OSA also has a resting arterial carbon dioxide tension greater than 50 mm Hg.

[d]Children with a score of 4 may be at increased perioperative risk from OSA; children with a score of 5 or 6 may be at significantly increased perioperative risk from OSA.

TABLE 4.17	Grading of Heart Murmurs
Grade I	Heard only with intense concentration
Grade II	Faint, but heard immediately
Grade III	Easily heard, of intermediate intensity
Grade IV	Easily heard, palpable thrill/vibration on chest wall
Grade V	Very loud, thrill present, audible with only edge of stethoscope on chest wall
Grade VI	Audible with stethoscope off the chest wall

Modified from Emmanouilides GC, Allen HD, Riemenschneider TA, Gutgesell HP. *Moss and Adams Heart Disease in Infants, Children, and Adolescents Including the Fetus and Young Adult.* 5th ed. Baltimore: Williams & Wilkins; 1995.

TABLE 4.18	Symptoms and Signs of Heart Disease

Feeding difficulties: disinterest, fatigue, diaphoresis, tachypnea, dyspnea
Poor exercise tolerance
Tachypnea, dyspnea, grunting, nasal flaring, and intercostal, suprasternal, or subcostal retractions
Frequent respiratory tract infections (a result of compression of airways by plethoric vessels leading to stasis of secretions and atelectasis)
Central cyanosis (involving warm mucous membranes: tongue and buccal mucosa) or poor capillary refill
Absent or abnormal peripheral pulses

Modified from Pelech AN. Evaluation of the pediatric patient with a cardiac murmur. *Pediatr Clin North Am.* 1999;46:167-188.

clinical features of an innocent murmur, an echocardiogram seldom reveals heart disease, especially if the child is older at presentation.[449] *However, even an experienced cardiologist can occasionally make a misdiagnosis; the only certain means to exclude a structural defect within the heart is with an echocardiogram.*[450] "Appropriate use criteria" for initial transthoracic echocardiography in outpatient pediatric cardiology have been established in a joint project with the American College of Cardiology, the American Society of Echocardiography, and the Society of Pediatric Echocardiography to support the clinical decision as to the appropriateness of care delivered to the pediatric patient.[451] A presumptively innocent murmur with no symptoms, signs, or findings of cardiovascular disease and a benign family history is rated as a "rarely appropriate" indication. In general, nonpathologic murmurs occur during systole and are soft and nonradiating with normal feel to peripheral

pulses; there are normal blood pressures in both upper and lower extremities. However, if the murmur is harsh and difficult to localize, if there are bounding pulses, if the murmur is louder than grade II/VI, or if it is accompanied by other findings (Tables 4.17 and 4.18), then further evaluation is warranted.[452] If the murmur has not been detected previously, referral to a pediatric cardiologist is indicated or an echocardiogram by an experienced pediatric echocardiographer should be obtained before induction of anesthesia.[453]

FEVER

The presence of a low-grade fever before elective surgery poses a dilemma whether to proceed with anesthesia or to delay. In general, if a child has only 0.5°C to 1.0°C of fever and no other symptoms, this degree of fever is not a contraindication to general anesthesia. However, if the fever is associated with a recent onset of rhinitis, pharyngitis, otitis media, dehydration, or any other sign of impending illness, it is prudent to postpone the procedure. If the planned surgery is of an urgent nature, every effort should be made to reduce the fever before induction of anesthesia, primarily to reduce oxygen demands. Reduction of the fever should not include administration of aspirin, because aspirin may interfere with platelet function and is associated with Reye syndrome. Ibuprofen may be associated with an increase in bleeding time[454] and should be avoided before surgery. On the other hand, acetaminophen has no effect on platelet function and is an excellent antipyretic. It is rapidly absorbed when administered orally, producing adequate blood concentrations within several minutes. In contrast, rectal administration requires at least 60 minutes to achieve a significant blood concentration.[259,455] There is no evidence

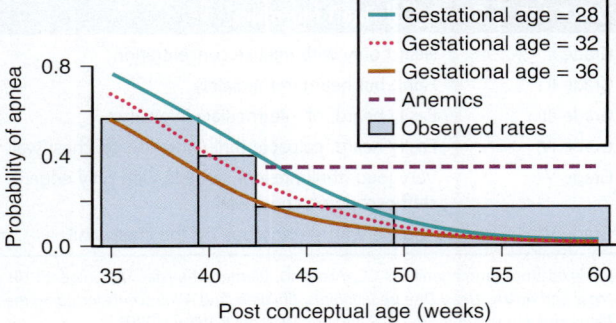

FIGURE 4.7 The predicted probability of apnea for all infants was inversely related to gestational age at the time of birth and postconception age at the time of surgery. The probability of apnea was the same regardless of post-conception age or gestational age for infants with anemia *(dashed magenta line)*. (From Coté CJ, Zaslavsky A, Downes JJ, et al. Postoperative apnea in former preterm infants after inguinal herniorrhaphy: a combined analysis. *Anesthesiology.* 1995;82:807-808.)

that an existing fever predisposes to a malignant hyperthermic reaction.[456]

POSTANESTHESIA APNEA IN FORMER PRETERM INFANTS

Former preterm infants have a multitude of residual problems owing to intensive care therapy, prolonged intubation, and still-maturing organogenesis. The incidence of subglottic stenosis is increased and they are prone to perioperative respiratory complications.[457] At the time of surgery they may or may not have apnea spells, although they often appear normal for their age; a number of prospective studies have defined the population at greatest risk for postoperative apnea.[380,457–466] Former preterm infants <44 weeks postconception age (PCA) are at a greater risk for apnea after general anesthesia than are those older than 44 weeks PCA.[467] In an analysis of eight published prospective papers from four institutions conducted over 6 years, the incidence of apnea varied inversely with both the gestational age and PCA (E-Fig. 4.5).[467] For example, consider two infants who are now 45 weeks PCA: one was born at 28 weeks and the other at 32 weeks of gestation. The risk of apnea in the 28-week gestational age infant is twice that in the 32-week gestational age infant (Fig. 4.7).[467] Similarly, consider two infants of the same gestational age: one anesthetized at 45 weeks PCA and the other at 50 weeks PCA; the younger-PCA infant would be at greater risk for postoperative apnea. The recognition of apnea events depends on the type of device used to monitor the infants (E-Fig. 4.5); simple observation and impedance pneumography are more likely to miss apneic events than continuous recording devices.[467–469] Preterm infants with anemia (hematocrit <30%) are more prone to apnea, and the incidence is unrelated to PCA or gestational age (see Fig. 4.7).[380,467] It appears that the risk for apnea exceeds 1% with statistical certainty until approximately 56 weeks PCA in infants with a gestational age of 32 weeks or 54 weeks PCA in those with a gestational age of 35 weeks, if one excludes anemic infants and those with obvious apnea in the recovery room. This analysis determined that (1) apnea was strongly and inversely related to both gestational age and PCA; (2) ongoing apnea at home is a risk factor; (3) small-for-gestational-age infants are protected from apnea compared with appropriate- and large-for-gestational-age infants; (4) anemia is a significant risk factor, particularly for infants of more than 44 weeks PCA; and (5) a

history of necrotizing enterocolitis, neonatal apnea, respiratory distress syndrome, bronchopulmonary dysplasia, or operative use of opioids or muscle relaxants did not correlate with postoperative apnea.[467] Each clinician must decide how to balance the risk of an unrecognized apnea with the benefit of proceeding with the surgery in terms of cost savings and not hospitalizing the infant for overnight monitoring.[470] The most practical and appropriate plan is to admit and monitor all formerly preterm infants who are less than 60 weeks PCA until they are free of apnea for a minimum of 12 hours.

One study examined the effects of inhalation agents; four anesthetic techniques were compared: sevoflurane induction and maintenance, halothane induction and maintenance, halothane induction/desflurane maintenance, and thiopental induction/desflurane maintenance.[471] No major episodes of apnea occurred in any of the 40 former preterm infants who were <60 weeks PCA and undergoing hernia repair, although there was at least one episode of breath-holding or self-limited apnea in each group. In view of the small sample size in this study, the upper 95% confidence interval that no apnea episodes will occur in all formerly preterm infants is only 92%. *Although the majority of former preterm infants in our microanalysis were anesthetized with halothane,[467] apnea has been reported with all anesthetics, including sevoflurane, desflurane, and regional anesthesia (spinal or caudal epidural, discussed later).*[472–474]

The preoperative evaluation of these infants requires reserving a monitored bed postoperatively and a clear discussion with the family regarding the perioperative risks of anesthesia and apnea. If the child is receiving theophylline or caffeine preoperatively, this therapy should be continued postoperatively.[475] If the child is not receiving theophylline or caffeine, there is no evidence to support the administration of aminophylline postoperatively, but there is weak evidence that caffeine (10 mg/kg) may reduce postoperative apnea spells in high-risk infants.[465,466] The pharmacokinetics of caffeine in preterm and full-term neonates suggest that a single IV dose of caffeine will have a clinical effect that may last for several days. However, the pharmacokinetics of caffeine change dramatically with age: in older infants (e.g., those who are 60 weeks PCA), the half-life of caffeine is reduced to approximately 5 hours (E-Fig. 4.6).[476] A Cochrane review of prophylactic caffeine in formerly preterm infants concluded that although caffeine can be used to prevent postoperative apnea, bradycardia, and episodes of oxygen desaturation, there was insufficient evidence to adopt this as routine anesthetic practice.[477] *If caffeine is administered to a former preterm infant, postoperative admission and overnight respiratory monitoring are still required, because caffeine is not 100% effective in preventing postoperative apnea.*

Apnea may be related to many causes besides prematurity (Fig. 4.8); the most common causes after surgery, however, relate to metabolic derangements, pharmacologic effects, or CNS immaturity. Metabolic causes of apnea such as hypothermia, hypoglycemia, hypocalcemia, acidosis, and hypoxemia should be avoided (see Chapter 37). However, pharmacologic effects on respirations cannot be avoided because most drugs used in anesthesia depress the respiratory system either directly or indirectly.[478] Respiratory depression is probably even more likely to occur in neonates who have an immature respiratory center; residual anesthetic action may contribute to the development of postoperative apnea.[479] In addition, most drugs or inhalation agents decrease muscle tone of the upper airway, thus contributing to the development of upper airway obstruction, more labored breathing, fatigue, and subsequent apnea.[464] Potent inhalation anesthetic agents also decrease intercostal muscle tone, reducing functional residual

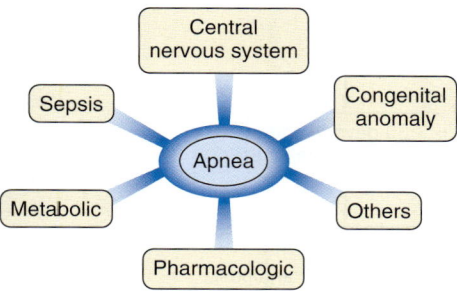

FIGURE 4.8 Apnea, defined as the absence of movement of air at the mouth or nose, may have many causes. Those that anesthesiologists are most often involved with are of metabolic, pharmacologic, or respiratory origins.

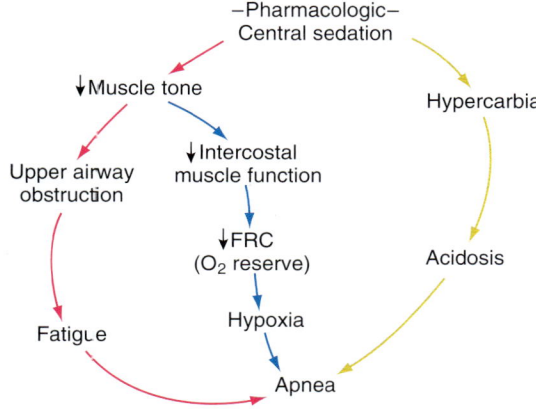

FIGURE 4.9 Pharmacologic interventions may result in several sequences of events leading to apnea. *FRC,* functional residual capacity.

capacity and thereby increasing the propensity to develop hypoxemia (Fig. 4.9).[480]

Regional anesthesia has been used to reduce the risk of postoperative apnea.[459,481–483] A multicenter, multinational study comparing general anesthesia with spinal anesthesia (the GAS study) for former preterm and full-term infants found no difference in the incidence of apnea comparing spinal to general anesthesia (~6% in former preterm infants). However, the severity of the apnea was less and the incidence was lower in the first 30 minutes in the PACU following spinal anesthesia.[474,484] Thus spinal anesthesia may offer potential advantages; however, several infants who had spinal anesthesia experienced life-threatening events many hours after discharge from PACU (similar to our 1995 analysis).[467] Thus although spinal anesthesia offers advantage, it does not eliminate our need for vigilance. In addition, since all of the infants in the general anesthesia group were anesthetized with sevoflurane compared with the 1995 study, in which all were anesthetized with halothane, the use of a more modern anesthetic agent did not seem to have any salutary effects on apnea as some practitioners have suggested.

A Cochrane review found *"no difference in the effect of spinal compared to general anesthesia on the overall incidence of postoperative apnoea, bradycardia, oxygen saturation, need for postoperative analgesics or respiratory support."*[485] Additive drugs used to prolong the duration of a spinal or caudal block, such as clonidine, or sedatives, such as midazolam and dexmedetomidine, have been associated with postoperative or intraoperative apnea.[486–490] Spinal anesthesia is

also associated with a significant failure rate (20% in some studies) and the need for multiple attempts to achieve accurate placement of the needle,[474,491,492] although in experienced hands, the success rate for placing a spinal block was 97.4% and an adequate level of spinal anesthesia was achieved in 95.4% of infants.

Since our microanalysis in 1995,[467] much has changed: new inhalation agents have replaced halothane, artificial surfactant has rescued many infants, and improved respiratory strategies have reduced barotrauma-induced chronic pulmonary disease. Although it would seem logical that these advances should have reduced the incidence of postanesthesia apnea in former preterm infants, little has changed. *Despite these medical advances, former preterm infants should not be anesthetized as outpatients even when a regional technique has been used; they require admission for postoperative monitoring overnight for apnea.*

With respect to full-term neonates, three reports have described infants who developed apnea after apparently uneventful general anesthesias.[493–495] Therefore, if a full-term infant who is younger than 44 weeks PCA demonstrates any abnormality of respiration after anesthesia, we recommend that they be admitted overnight for apnea monitoring. The algorithms in Fig. 4.10 can be used as a decision tree for outpatient surgery in term and former preterm infants.

HYPERALIMENTATION

The anesthesiologist frequently encounters chronically ill infants and children who are unable to tolerate enteral feedings and are therefore maintained on total parenteral nutrition (TPN). It is important to identify the composition and rate of administration of these fluids so that potential intraoperative complications can be avoided. Most of these solutions are hypertonic, have high glucose content, and must be administered through a centrally placed IV route.

The basic principles of care are as follows:

1. Avoid contaminating the line. It is best not to puncture the line for administering medications or changing fluid.
2. Do not discontinue the glucose-containing solution, because the relative hyperinsulinemic state could induce hypoglycemia, the signs of which might be masked by general anesthesia. In contrast, intralipid infusions should be discontinued before surgery, because it is a culture medium if contaminated.
3. An infusion device should be used at all times so that the rate of infusion is constant. Accidental rapid infusion of large amounts of TPN fluid can cause a hypertonic nonketotic coma.[496] There is no consensus on the intraoperative management of TPN solutions. Some clinicians reduce the infusion rate by 33% to 50% to avoid hyperglycemia resulting from a reduced metabolic rate due to the effects of anesthetic agents and a reduced body temperature, whereas others leave the infusion rate unchanged to avoid intraoperative hypoglycemia.
4. Perioperative and intraoperative monitoring of glucose, potassium, sodium, and calcium, as well as acid-base status, is important for long procedures.
5. Preoperative confirmation of correct intravascular line placement (radiography or aspiration of blood) is important to avoid intraoperative complications such as hydrothorax or hemothorax.

DIABETES

Diabetes mellitus is the most common endocrine problem encountered in children. Preoperative assessment should include a thorough knowledge of the child's insulin schedule. The preoperative fasting

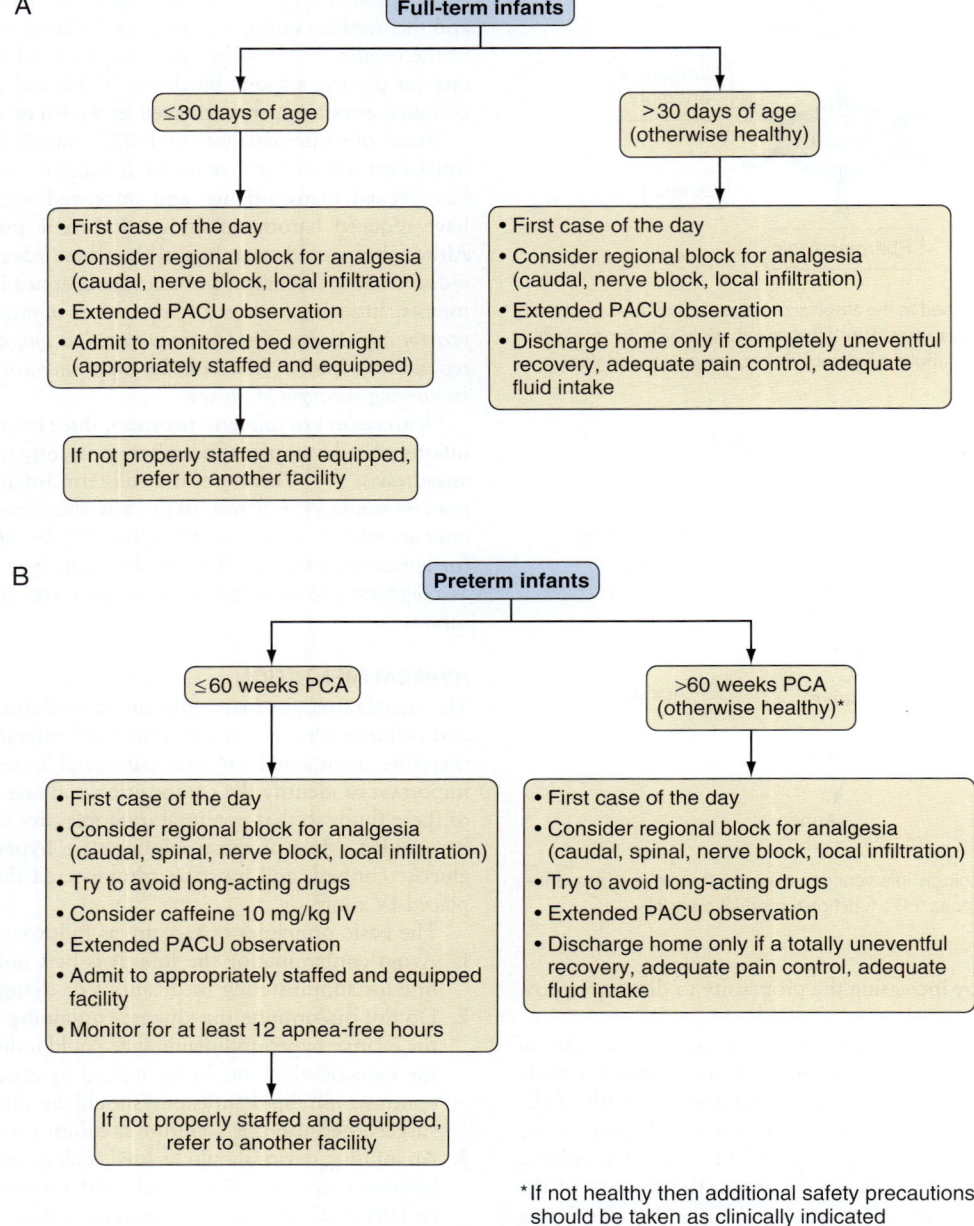

A

Full-term infants

≤30 days of age

- First case of the day
- Consider regional block for analgesia (caudal, nerve block, local infiltration)
- Extended PACU observation
- Admit to monitored bed overnight (appropriately staffed and equipped)

If not properly staffed and equipped, refer to another facility

>30 days of age (otherwise healthy)

- First case of the day
- Consider regional block for analgesia (caudal, nerve block, local infiltration)
- Extended PACU observation
- Discharge home only if completely uneventful recovery, adequate pain control, adequate fluid intake

B

Preterm infants

≤60 weeks PCA

- First case of the day
- Consider regional block for analgesia (caudal, spinal, nerve block, local infiltration)
- Try to avoid long-acting drugs
- Consider caffeine 10 mg/kg IV
- Extended PACU observation
- Admit to appropriately staffed and equipped facility
- Monitor for at least 12 apnea-free hours

If not properly staffed and equipped, refer to another facility

>60 weeks PCA (otherwise healthy)*

- First case of the day
- Consider regional block for analgesia (caudal, spinal, nerve block, local infiltration)
- Try to avoid long-acting drugs
- Extended PACU observation
- Discharge home only if a totally uneventful recovery, adequate pain control, adequate fluid intake

*If not healthy then additional safety precautions should be taken as clinically indicated

FIGURE 4.10 Algorithms used as a decision tree for outpatient surgery in term infants **(A)** and in former preterm infants **(B)**. *PACU*, postanesthesia care unit; *PCA*, postconceptional age.

time should be the same as that recommended for nondiabetics. Every attempt should be made to schedule a diabetic child as the first case of the day to minimize the fasting period. Several protocols have been advocated for glycemic control in diabetics. An IV infusion that contains 5% glucose and electrolytes at a maintenance infusion rate should be started to avoid hypoglycemia. Blood glucose concentrations should be monitored just prior to induction, intraoperatively, and postoperatively until the child is back on a routine schedule. A more detailed discussion of the perioperative management of the child with diabetes is presented in Chapter 27.

BRONCHOPULMONARY DYSPLASIA

Bronchopulmonary dysplasia (BPD) is a form of chronic lung disease associated with prolonged mechanical ventilation and oxygen toxicity in preterm neonates. Antenatal glucocorticoids, surfactant therapy, and gentle ventilation strategies to minimize lung injury have changed the clinical characteristics of BPD.[497] The current definition of BPD has been validated in early infancy and determines three levels of severity (mild, moderate, or severe) using gestational age, oxygen dependence at 36 weeks and post-conceptual age, total duration of oxygen supplementation, and positive pressure requirements.[498,499] The clinical manifestations of BPD include tachypnea, dyspnea, and airway hyperactivity, as well as oxygen dependence. These infants suffer from hypoxemia, hypercarbia, abnormal functional airway growth, tracheomalacia, bronchomalacia, subglottic stenosis, increased pulmonary vascular resistance, and congestive heart failure. Pulmonary function abnormalities, including a reduced functional residual capacity, reduced diffusion capacity, airway obstruction, and reduced exercise tolerance, may persist into the school-age years.[500] Even in the postsurfactant era, retrospective studies estimate a 25% to 35% prevalence of pulmonary hypertension among extremely low–birth-weight infants with BPD requiring prolonged positive pressure ventilation and is an important determinant of mortality.[501] These children are often cared for at home on oxygen therapy with diuretics, digoxin, and β₂-agonists. Preoperative preparation should focus on optimizing oxygenation, reducing airway hyperactivity, and correcting electrolyte abnormalities caused by chronic diuretic therapy. Particular attention should be paid to fluid balance and avoiding excessive hydration. Adequate expiratory time to avoid excessive positive-pressure ventilation is important, and the potential for subglottic stenosis may necessitate using a smaller than expected tracheal tube. The possibility of pulmonary hypertension and right ventricular dysfunction should be considered and, when indicated, evaluated via electrocardiogram and echocardiography. Stress-dose steroid administration is indicated in children with a history of corticosteroid use in the past 6 months.

SEIZURE DISORDER

Management of children with seizure disorders requires a knowledge of the antiseizure medications, medication schedule, and possible interactions between these medications and anesthetic drugs. The stress of surgery and anesthesia may lower the seizure threshold and cause a seizure. Seizure medications should be continued until the time of elective surgery. Characterization of the clinical manifestations of the seizure is useful to be able to diagnose potential seizures postoperatively. If the child is expected to have a significant problem with oral intake postoperatively, then a game plan with the child's neurologist should be developed to build a transition to IV antiseizure medications. Preoperative and postoperative management of anticonvulsant blood concentrations may also ensure proper therapeutic effect (see also Chapter 24).

A ketogenic diet, which is high in fat and low in protein and carbohydrate, has been used to treat some patients with refractory seizures since the 1920s.[502] The classic ketogenic diet uses a 4:1 ratio of fat to carbohydrate and protein. The exact mechanism by which the diet works is unclear. A recent resurgence in interest has resulted in more patients presenting to the OR while consuming ketogenic diets.

A retrospective study examined the perioperative courses of nine children on ketogenic diets who received general anesthesia for surgical procedures lasting between 20 minutes and 11.5 hours.[503] The children continued their ketogenic diets until made NPO for the surgical procedure and resumed the diets postoperatively. All patients were in ketosis, as demonstrated by preoperative serum β-hydroxybutyrate levels. Medications used for general anesthesia varied but included fentanyl, halothane, isoflurane, sevoflurane, nitrous oxide, propofol, thiopental, and ketamine. Only carbohydrate-free solutions were administered intravenously. Glucose levels remained stable intraoperatively, even during the longer procedures. However, there was a tendency for children following ketogenic diets to develop metabolic acidosis during the longer procedures. No other perioperative complications were reported, and children appeared to recover from anesthesia at a usual rate. None of the patients were noted to have increased seizure activity postoperatively. Several additional case reports also describe successful administration of general anesthesia to children following ketogenic diets without adverse events.[504–506]

Unfortunately, there are no consensus guidelines providing clear recommendations for the management of patients undergoing general anesthesia while following a ketogenic diet. Some centers advocate tapering or discontinuing ketogenic diets prior to general anesthesia, while others allow patients to continue ketogenic diets during the perioperative period.[503] The plan for perioperative ketogenic diet management should be discussed with the patient's neurologist or nutritionist preoperatively. For longer procedures, serum pH or bicarbonate levels should be checked preoperatively and at routine intervals intraoperatively (e.g., every 2 to 3 hours) to monitor for acidosis. Serum pH and bicarbonate monitoring should be continued postoperatively until the patient restarts a full ketogenic diet. IV bicarbonate may be required for correction of acidosis. Long-term (>2 hours) propofol infusions, which impair fatty acid oxidation, are not recommended in patients following ketogenic diets as fatal propofol infusion syndrome has been described, but brief infusion should not be problematic (see also Chapter 24).[507,508]

SICKLE CELL DISEASE

Whenever a child presents with either sickle cell disease or sickle cell trait, the anesthetic and postanesthetic management must be modified (see also Chapters 10 and 13). It is important to obtain a detailed family history, and if the child has not been previously tested, a sickle preparation should be obtained. If a sickle test is positive and the surgery is elective, then surgery should be postponed pending hemoglobin electrophoresis to more carefully delineate the nature of the hemoglobinopathy. It must be emphasized that the status of hydration and oxygenation is critical for all children with sickle cell disease or trait. A secure IV route with hydration of at least 1.5 times maintenance is recommended well into the postoperative period, especially after procedures in which ileus may result. Meticulous attention to detail to ensure stable cardiovascular and ventilatory status establishes adequate oxygenation to prevent sickling. Pulse oximetry is of particular value in managing these children by providing an early warning of desaturation. Children with hemoglobin SC are especially at risk because they have a relatively normal hemoglobin level yet are extremely vulnerable to sickling. Further recommendations regarding management of these children, including indications for preoperative transfusion to bring the hemoglobin concentration to 10 g/dL, are discussed in Chapter 10.

ACKNOWLEDGMENT

We wish to thank John F. Ryan, MD; Letty M.P. Liu, MD; I.D. Todres, MD; Nishan G. Goudsouzian, MD; and Leila Mei Pang, MD, for their prior contributions to these topics.

ANNOTATED REFERENCES

Coté CJ, Posner KL, Domino KB. Death or neurologic injury after tonsillectomy in children with a focus on obstructive sleep apnea: Houston, we have a problem! *Anesth Analg.* 2014;118:1276-1283.
Identifies factors leading to deaths or neurologic injury after tonsillectomy caused by apparent apnea in children. Children with severe obstructive sleep apnea may have heightened analgesic and respiratory sensitivity to opioids. Respiratory

monitoring continued throughout first- and second-stage recovery, as well as on the ward during the first postoperative night, reduces adverse events.

Davidson AJ, Morton NS, Arnup SJ, et al. Apnea after awake regional and general anesthesia in infants—do we have an answer? *Anesthesiology.* 2015;123:38-54.

This multicenter, multinational study comparing general anesthesia with spinal anesthesia (the GAS study) for former preterm and full-term infants found no difference in the incidence of apnea in the general anesthesia compared to regional anesthesia group. The incidence and severity of apnea were lower in the first 30 minutes in the PACU following spinal anesthesia compared with general anesthesia.

Gasche Y, Daali Y, Fathi M, et al. Codeine intoxication associated with ultrarapid CYP2D6 metabolism. *N Engl J Med.* 2004;351:2827-2831.

This article first raised awareness of "ultrarapid metabolizers," individuals with duplications in CYP2D6, the cytochrome responsible for codeine metabolism. Affected individuals may experience relative drug overdoses at normal drug doses, especially in the setting of obstructive sleep apnea.

Jones LJ, Craven PD, Lakkundi A, et al. Regional (spinal, epidural, caudal) versus general anaesthesia in preterm infants undergoing inguinal herniorrhaphy in early infancy. *Cochrane Database Syst Rev.* 2015;(6):CD003669.

The review found "no difference in the effect of spinal compared to general anesthesia on the overall incidence of postoperative apnea, bradycardia, oxygen saturation, need for postoperative analgesics or respiratory support."

Kain ZN, Mayes LC, Wang SM, Hofstadter MB. Postoperative behavioral outcomes in children: effects of sedative premedication. *Anesthesiology.* 1999;90:758-765.

Premedication of children with midazolam is not only beneficial in reducing preoperative anxiety but also results in fewer negative behavioural changes during the first postoperative week.

Practice advisory for preanesthesia evaluation: an updated report by the American Society of Anesthesiologists Task Force on Preanesthesia Evaluation. *Anesthesiology.* 2012;116(3):522-538.

An updated practice advisory for preanesthesia evaluation including preoperative testing based on "analysis of expert opinion, clinical feasibility data, open forum commentary and consensus surveys."

Schwengel DA, Sterni LM, Tunkel DE, Heitmiller ES. Perioperative management of children with obstructive sleep apnea. *Anesth Analg.* 2009;109:60-75.

An excellent review article on the diagnosis, treatment, and anesthetic management of children with obstructive sleep apnea syndrome.

Taghizadeh N, Davidson A, Williams K, et al. Autism spectrum disorder (ASD) and its perioperative management. *Paediatr Anaesth.* 2015;25:1076-1084.

An excellent review article surveying the current literature on autism spectrum disorder and its perioperative management.

Tait AR, Malviya S, Voepel-Lewis T, et al. Risk factors for perioperative adverse respiratory events in children with upper respiratory tract infections. *Anesthesiology.* 2001;95:299-306.

Several risk factors for perioperative adverse respiratory events in children were identified: use of an endotracheal tube (<5 years of age), history of prematurity, history of reactive airway disease, paternal smoking, surgery involving the airway, presence of copious secretions, and nasal congestion.

Wang Z, May SM, Charoenlap S, et al. Effects of secondhand smoke exposure on asthma morbidity and health care utilization in children: a systemic review and meta-analysis. *Ann Allergy Asthma Immunol.* 2015;115:396-401.

This review and meta-analysis found that children with asthma and secondhand smoke exposure are "nearly twice as likely to be hospitalized with asthma exacerbation and more likely to have lower pulmonary function test results."

A complete reference list can be found online at ExpertConsult.com.

Ethical Issues in Pediatric Anesthesiology

5

DAVID B. WAISEL

CLINICIANS MUST TAKE SERIOUSLY "the experience, perspective, and power of children."[1] Clinicians should treat every child and family with the grace and consideration with which they would want their own child and family treated. Taking the experience of children seriously means involving interested children in developmentally appropriate decision making. Clinicians should not solicit a child's views without intending to consider them. *Pro forma* solicitations are harmful.

Treating every child like your own means taking time to allow premedication to work, even if it leads to criticism for a delayed anesthesia start time. It means rigorously following sterile practice protocols for central lines. It means patiently explaining anesthetic options to the parents as many times as needed.

Bioethics helps motivated physicians to identify and resolve ethical dilemmas. Solving ethical dilemmas is not solely a matter of being moral. Consider a child with an upper airway respiratory infection. Usually the surgery would be postponed, but suppose the child has missed two previous surgical dates because of an unstable home situation. While the clinician is explaining the risks of proceeding, the mother distractedly requests to proceed with surgery because "we're already here." The clinician has to determine what is in the child's best interest by balancing the risks of proceeding with those of not proceeding, the duty to ensure that the child receives necessary health care, the weight to be given to the mother's consent to proceed, and the duty to "do no harm." Mindful clinicians will seek to identify lurking conflicts of interest in considering whether to proceed.

Informed Consent

The American Academy of Pediatrics (AAP) bases pediatric informed consent on assent, informed permission, and the best interest standard.[1]

THE INFORMED CONSENT PROCESS

Assent: The Role of the Patient

Although most children cannot legally consent to medical care, children should share in decision making to the extent that their development permits (Table 5.1). As children grow older, participa-

tion in decision making should increase, depending on both their maturity and the consequences involved in the decision.

School-age children are developing decision-making capacity, so anesthesiologists should seek both informed permission from the parent and assent and participatory decision making from the child. School-age children are capable of using logic and reason and are able to define and relate multiple aspects of a situation. Such situations may include whether to sedate a 6-year-old before an inhalation induction, whether to use an inhalation or intravenous induction of anesthesia in an 8-year-old, and whether to insert an epidural in a 12-year-old.

Many adolescents older than 14 years of age have the ability to use abstract thought, apply complex reasoning, foresee outcomes, simultaneously evaluate multiple options, and understand concepts such as probability. Although some adolescents have cognitive abilities similar to those of adults, adolescents may be hindered by insufficient psychosocial and emotional development and they may not have developed a reasonably stable set of values.[2] Anesthesiologists should try to fulfill the ethical requirements of consent while obtaining assent. Situations involving these aspects include obtaining consent from a 16-year-old for a sedated thoracic epidural placement for a pectus repair.

Informed Permission, the Best Interest Standard and the Harm Threshold Standard

Parents have traditionally acted as the surrogate decision makers for their children, and legally they give consent. However, surrogate consent does not fulfill the spirit of consent, which is based on obtaining an individualized autonomous decision from the patient receiving the treatment. The AAP has suggested that the proper role for the surrogate decision maker is to provide *informed permission*.[1] Informed permission has the same requirements as informed consent, but it recognizes that the doctrine of informed consent cannot apply.

The *best interest standard* requires decision makers to select the objectively best care. It acknowledges that the cornerstone of informed consent, the right to self-determination, is inapplicable when it is impossible to know or surmise from previous interactions a child's likely preference. Using this standard requires determining

TABLE 5.1	Graduated Involvement of Minors in Medical Decision Making[a]	
Age	**Decision-Making Capacity**	**Techniques**
<6 years	None	Best interests standard
6–12 years	Developing	Informed permission Informed assent
13–18 years	Mostly developed	Informed assent Informed permission
Mature minor	Developed, as legally determined by a judge, for a specific decision. Although particulars vary by state, the mature minor doctrine in general requires adolescents to be at least 14 years old and tends to permit decisions of lesser risk.	Informed consent
Emancipated minor	Developed as determined by statutes defining eligible situations (e.g., being married, in the military, economically independent).	Informed consent

[a]This broad outline should be viewed as a guide. Specific circumstances should be taken into consideration.

(1) who will make the decision and (2) what is the best care. The difficulties arise in assuming that there is always one best choice, because if there is, it should not matter who makes the decision. In our society, acceptable decision making is broadly defined. Parents capable of participating in the decision-making process are the appropriate primary decision makers because of society's respect for the concept of the family and the assumption that parents care greatly for their children. Although a child's preferences cannot be known, it is reasonable to assume that because children will incorporate some of the parents' values as they mature, parental values are a good first approximation for the child's future values. A few have questioned the presumption that parents are the best decision makers.[3] Objections center on the legitimacy of the parents' knowledge of the preferences of the child's future self. Although these concerns are theoretically interesting and help clinicians understand the complexities of the best interest standard, the standard is that parents have extensive leeway in determining what is in their child's best interest.

The best interest of a child can be defined by what choices fall outside the range of acceptable decision making. Criteria to make this determination include the extent of harm to the child from the intervention or its absence, the likelihood of success, and the overall risk-to-benefit ratio.

The best interest standard can guide treatment among acceptable options and determine the limits of parental decision-making authority, but the best interest standard can be indeterminate, particularly for the decision to attempt to limit parental authority. Given the broad reluctance to override parents, limiting parental authority is a high-stakes decision.

Some suggest using a harm threshold standard rather than a best interest standard to determine whether to limit parental authority. The standard for whether a decision exceeds the harm threshold is if a parental decision threatens the health and safety of the child, which is a "lower standard" than whether the decision

is one of the "best" options. This harm threshold is a standard similar to the one in assessing for child maltreatment. Whether this concept of harm threshold is a new cognitive approach or is already used in determining best interest depends in large part about how the borders of acceptable decision making are established; some clinicians may use the harm threshold in determining acceptable decision making and others may not.[4–8]

The harm threshold standard needs further clarification. It may not help clarify the best interest standard and it may not be useful in court, given the inconsistency in how courts assess cases.[9,10] Nonetheless, at the very least, it provides another conceptual way of evaluating whether a treatment is outside acceptable boundaries.

Disclosure

The "reasonable person" standard—the legal standard for most of the United States, Canada, and other countries—requires that the information disclosed be sufficient to satisfy a hypothetical reasonable person. This standard does not define exactly what information should be given, and it does not take into account the patient's desires and needs. The "subjective person" standard suggests that informed consent should be matched to the wants and needs of the decision makers. Although this patient-centered consent better fulfills the spirit of informed consent, its greater ambiguity makes it difficult to use as a legal standard.

Rather than rely on a rote informed consent process, anesthesiologists should seek to satisfy the needs of the decision makers by meeting their information and decision-making needs. Patients and surrogates differ in the extent to which they prefer to receive information and to participate in decision making.[11,12] In general, 10% to 15% of patients may prefer less information than their peers. Overall, most patients want some form of shared decision making.[12]

Anesthesiologists should inform families about matters that the anesthesiologist feels must be communicated and about options that affect the perioperative experience (e.g., regional versus general anesthesia)[13] and then ask whether the decision makers wish to know more. By being attentive to the words and actions of the decision makers, anesthesiologists can tailor the process. It is rare to be found liable for informed consent malpractice issues. The standard for being liable is that there is a duty, a breach of that duty, and a harm directly related to the breach of the duty. Liability in informed consent requires that the information not shared would have affected the patient's choices. Forming a bond with the parents is more effective in reducing malpractice lawsuits.[14]

Performing patient-centered informed consent often requires communication of the anesthesiologist's opinion along with an explanation of the supporting reasons. With this information, the decision makers are better able to determine which anesthetic approach provides the most desired benefits.

Decision makers often overrate the extent of their knowledge about risks and benefits.[15] We can increase the likelihood of the decision makers having sufficient knowledge by modifying practices. For example, informed consent documents often use poorly formatted, dense, incomprehensible text written at too high a reading level for most decision makers.[16] Straightforward language written at an eighth-grade reading level with reader-friendly formatting permits better understanding and thus better decision making about risk, benefits, and options.[17]

Patients may have difficulty understanding quantitative aspects of risk. Risks should be presented as absolute data (e.g., occurs 10% of time) rather than relative data compared with other treatments (e.g., decreases the risk by 50%).[18,19] Some decision

<table>

TABLE 5.2	Recommendations for Risk Communication to Patients[19]

1. Consider presenting only the information that is most critical to the patient's or parents' decision making, even at the expense of completeness.
2. Use language at the eighth-grade level to improve understanding of written and oral communications.
3. Present data using absolute risks and frequencies.
4. Use pictorial recommendations to communicate statistics when appropriate.
5. The order in which risks and benefits are presented may affect risk perceptions. The last topic presented has more weight in decision making.
6. Recognize that comparative risk information (e.g., the average person's risk) is persuasive as well as informative.

makers may understand frequencies better, so it is wise to include both absolute and frequency data. For example, the statement *"If she has regional anesthesia, she has a 20% chance of postoperative vomiting, which means 2 of 10 people will have postoperative vomiting, and if she has general anesthesia, she has a 40% chance of postoperative vomiting, which is 4 of 10 people will have postoperative vomiting. That means that 20 more people of 100 will have postoperative vomiting if we use general anesthesia"* is better than *"She has a 100% more likely chance of postoperative vomiting with general anesthesia as compared with regional anesthesia."* Pictorial representations improve understanding. In the above example, a graphic may be a picture of 10 people, with regional anesthesia having 2 people in one color and general anesthesia having an additional 2 people in a different color, showing the increased risk.

Risk perceptions may be affected by whether risks or benefits are presented last.[19] For example, oncology patients gave more weight to the last topic discussed, even though risks and benefits were presented in the same conversation.[20] Table 5.2 lists recommendations on communications.

Informed Refusal

The requirements to achieve an informed refusal of a procedure are similar to the requirements for informed consent such that decision makers should be substantially well versed about the risks, benefits, and alternatives before declining. When parents refuse what clinicians believe is necessary care for a child who cannot participate in the decision making process, clinicians may invoke the best interest standard or incorporate the harm threshold standard. This situation is more complicated when the child expresses significant decision-making capacity and refuses nonemergent procedures. Anesthesiologists should respect the right of children (typically those over the age of 10 years) not to assent to a procedure, and they should not coerce the child to proceed. In children, particularly adolescents, the distinction between persuasion and coercion is critical. *Persuasion*, the act of using argument and reason to influence a patient's decision, is appropriate. *Coercion*, the outright use of a credible threat, manipulation, or misleading information, is not. Achieving the child's assent may necessitate further discussions with the child, parents, and other providers, and such discussions may best take place away from the operating room.

Consider a 15-year-old who is scheduled for an elective knee arthroscopy. The day before the procedure, she gave assent and her parents gave informed permission for anesthesia and surgery.

She is now crying in the preoperative area and refusing to cooperate. Rather than forcibly or surreptitiously sedating her, the anesthesiologist should discuss her concerns. If she is unable to discuss the issues, the anesthesiologist should consider removing her from the area and giving her time to regain composure before readdressing the situation. Simple actions often allow the situation to be resolved. If the withdrawal of assent was in part related to anxiety, the child may assent to receiving ample premedication before returning to the holding area. Anesthesiologists must obtain her assent before administering the sedation, however, and not simply assume that forceful or surreptitious administration is justified.

"Doctor, If This Were Your Child, What Would You Do?"

Clinicians should respond to requests for advice by using medical facts to explain how different paths support specific values so that decision makers can choose the most concordant path.[21–23] However, the question, *"If this were your child, what would you do?"* can be asked for a number of different reasons, forcing clinicians to put the question into a broader context. Do not duck this question. Not responding to this question may frustrate and confuse decision makers.

For example, parents may be declaring that they are having difficulty comprehending the overwhelming information and need help making a reasonable decision. Perhaps they are actually asking what would give their child the best chance of getting better. In this situation, clinicians should explain the reasons and values underlying their personal choice. Parents may be looking for support that they are making the right choice in an untenable situation. Clinicians should answer with their best judgment if they agree with the family. If they disagree, clinicians should lend support through comments such as *"Other parents in the same situation have made the same choice,"* or by acknowledging that it is normal to feel uncertain.[22] If the family persists in asking what they should do, clinicians may wish to acknowledge that their choice might have been different. Clinicians should emphasize, however, that parental values are more valid than clinician values when choosing for their own child.

Parents may be asking for help in making a life-altering decision. One approach to this question is to offer a process for answering the question (e.g., *"I would talk with the chaplain"*). Clinicians should feel comfortable admitting that they are unable to determine what they would do if in the same situation. Honesty reinforces the difficulty of the decision for the parents.

Disclosure and Apology of Medical Errors

Hiding medical errors is indecent and breaches informed consent.[24] Fear of consequences, inadequate support, limited trust in the institution, and lack of education prevent physicians from disclosing and apologizing appropriately.[25–28] Forthrightly disclosing medical errors, although upsetting, often strengthens the patient–physician relationship.[29,30] Learning about a hidden medical error destroys trust and rapidly triggers legal action.

Physician apologies or sympathetic comments often are prohibited as legal evidence of wrongdoing, but disclosures of errors are permitted as legal evidence.[30–32] Apologizing may influence whether patients pursue legal action and whether such action is successful.[31,33] Sincere (not *pro forma*!) apologies and subsequent redress to prevent future occurrences improves the patient–physician relationship, minimizing the likelihood of legal action.

Physicians without expertise in disclosure and apology often botch the process. Disclosure is a process over time. Initial disclosure should take place as soon as possible after an event and should center on the medical implications. Do not speculate about cause or fault. When disclosing, it is wise to bring along an appropriate colleague who can help with the disclosure by providing psychological support for the patient and family. Soon thereafter, a specific, permanent liaison to the family should be identified. The liaison should be available to arrange meetings, explain the results of the investigation into the cause of the event, and describe plans to prevent future events. The liaison should be trained and experienced in apology and disclosure (e.g., a colleague in risk management).

An apology expresses regret or sorrow. Sincere apologies followed by consistent actions are priceless; insincere apologies are costly. It is always appropriate to apologize for the adverse effects of an event and although the standard teaching is that physicians should not assume responsibility for an event before an investigation is performed, it seems bizarre to dissemble about clear errors. As an example, after reassuring the parents that their child is unharmed, I would readily admit that because I had inadvertently given a muscle relaxant instead of an anticholinesterase, their child will require a brief stay in the intensive care unit until ready for tracheal extubation. To evade responsibility (e.g., "Somehow one drug was given when another was intended") for a clear error mocks the apology.

Different strategies are being tested to improve disclosure and apology. An approach called "disclosure, apology, and offer" shows promise.[34] Open disclosure, prompt and fair compensation, and a vigorous defense of acceptable care leads to a transparency that reduces adversarial relationships, contributes to patient safety, and curtails legal action and costs.[34–36] Success in this program requires aligning of incentives of the clinician and hospital system. Differing incentives, such as in whether to settle or not, lead to distrust and doom the program.

SPECIAL SITUATIONS IN PEDIATRIC INFORMED CONSENT
Confidentially for Adolescents
The obligation to maintain confidentiality requires clinicians to protect patient information from unauthorized and unnecessary disclosure.[37] Confidentiality is necessary for an open flow of information.[38–40] Clinicians enhance trust by interviewing the adolescent in private, acknowledging the adolescent's concerns about confidentiality, and keeping promises. Emancipated and mature minors have a right to complete confidentiality. For other adolescents, if maintaining confidentiality entails minimal harm, clinicians should encourage adolescents to be forthright with parents but respect their decision not to be. If maintaining confidentiality may result in serious harm to the adolescent, clinicians may be ethically justified in notifying the parents. State laws vary in their extent of requirements.

The Pregnant Adolescent
Anesthesiologists face confidentially issues when an adolescent has a positive pregnancy test before anesthesia. Given the principles of confidentiality, it is ethically appropriate to inform only the adolescent.[41,42] Because locales may statutorily prohibit sharing pregnancy information with anyone other than the adolescent, anesthesiologists must share this information with the adolescent without letting the parents know.[43] Anesthesiologists should involve pediatricians, gynecologists, and social workers with expertise in adolescent issues in this discussion.

Matters become more complex if the clinicians and adolescent believe the case should be postponed, and the adolescent chooses not to inform her parents about the pregnancy test.[44] Anesthesiologists must be careful not to inadvertently inform the parents of the pregnancy test while postponing anesthesia and surgery. Nor should anesthesiologists betray the adolescent by saying, "The case is postponed. If you want to know why, ask your daughter." Although such a statement is factually true and within the letter of the law of confidentially, terse obliqueness scorns the spirit of confidentially.

The desire to tell the parents is understandable. But, I would suggest that clinicians who feel that way are too narrowly applying their own experiences and expectations. Not all parents are wise and gentle, and not all homes are safe and healthy. Confidentiality statutes specifically address concerns about child abuse in pregnant adolescents.

The extent to which anesthesiologists should protect the adolescent's confidentiality is debatable. Nonetheless, because the parents have no legal right to that information, I believe that more active deception, although less desirable, is appropriate if necessary. Successful deception avoids initiating diagnostic evaluations or treatment and does not unduly worry parents. For example, do not attribute the delay to "hearing a new murmur." Vague, unremarkable reasons such as "an oncoming cold" are best.

It is rare to condone deception.[45,46] Deception should not be undertaken without serious reservations. But, under certain circumstances, the obligation to the patient may supersede prohibitions on deception. At times, the harms of not deceiving outweigh the harms of deceiving.

The Adolescent and Abortion
Even though pediatric patients who are pregnant may be statutorily or by practice emancipated, many states require some form of parental involvement, such as parental consent or notification, before an elective abortion.[47] If a state requires parental involvement, the ability of the minor to circumvent this regulation by seeking relief from a judge, known as judicial bypass, must be available. Requirements and enforcement of statutes vary from state to state.[47,48] The need for parental involvement in a minor's planned abortion is not always legally straightforward, and it may be best to consult with hospital counsel in determining these issues. Although this is an area in which honorable people disagree, note that both the AAP and the American Medical Association (AMA) have affirmed these rights.[48,49]

Children of Jehovah's Witnesses
Jehovah's Witnesses interpret biblical scripture as prohibiting transfusion therapy because blood holds the "life force" and anyone who takes blood will be "cut off from his people" and not earn eternal salvation.[50–52] For adults, it is a "matter of conscience" whether they accept transfusion products. Adults may refuse potentially life-sustaining transfusion therapy because it is assumed they are making an informed decision about the risks and benefits of transfusion. However, based on the obligations of the state to protect the interests of incompetent patients, courts have uniformly intervened when parents desire to refuse transfusion therapy on behalf of their children. Based on the mature minor doctrine, older adolescents who are able to articulate significant decision-making capacity and maturity have been permitted to refuse potentially life-sustaining transfusion therapy.[53] Most clinicians start considering this option when the patient is 16, but younger children have been permitted to refuse potentially life-sustaining transfusion therapy.[54]

Obtaining informed permission and assent for the care of a ward of a Jehovah's Witness should address transfusion therapy. Anesthesiologists should clarify which therapy is acceptable.

Synthetic colloid solutions, dextran, erythropoietin, desmopressin, and preoperative iron are usually acceptable. Note that erythropoietin is available in two forms: lyophilized, and dissolved in saline with trace concentrations of albumin. Jehovah's Witnesses who accept albumin will accept either formulation, whereas those who refuse albumin should be offered the lyophilized formulation. Some Jehovah's Witnesses accept the removal and return of blood in a continuous loop (e.g., cell saver blood). The family should understand, however, that in a life-threatening situation, the anesthesiologist will seek a court order authorizing the administration of life-sustaining blood. When the likelihood of requiring blood is high or the local judiciary is not very familiar with case law for Jehovah's Witnesses, the anesthesiologist may choose to obtain a court order in advance of the operation.

A common concern is the sudden need for an emergent transfusion in a healthy child undergoing a low-risk procedure. In emergencies, based on the obligation to protect children, anesthesiologists should take the legally correct and ethically appropriate action to protect the child by transfusing blood without a court order. A court order may then be sought if desired.

Clinicians may wonder if they should change their transfusion triggers for a child of a Jehovah's Witness. It may be appropriate for clinicians to delay transfusion as compared with their usual practices in an effort to honor the parents' preferences and in recognition of our inadequate knowledge of when to transfuse. Other clinicians, while acknowledging the difficulty in knowing when to transfuse, believe it is appropriate to use their usual transfusion triggers, in the belief that the requirement is to treat this child of a Jehovah's Witness as you would treat any other child.

Decision makers may consider postponing a procedure that can be delayed until the child is of sufficient age and maturity to decide about transfusion therapy. The complexity is whether the delay may increase the risk or decrease the likelihood of a good outcome. This decision requires the same balancing act as for determining best interest for a child. Relevant factors include the quantitative and qualitative change in risk or benefit. Consider that it may be easier to wait on a procedure that is purely cosmetic than on a procedure for which waiting has a small chance of leading to permanent injury. If individual clinicians choose to honor the wishes of a mature minor, they must ensure the fidelity of the agreement by making certain that postoperative and on-call clinicians will honor the mature minor's wishes.

Emergency Care
Anesthesiologists should provide necessary emergent care for minors who do not have a parent available to give legal consent.[55,56] Emergencies include problems that could cause death, disability, and the increased risk of future complications.

The right of an adolescent to refuse emergency care treatment turns on the adolescent's decision-making capacity and the resulting harm from refusal of care. If the harm is significant and the adolescent's rationale is decidedly short-term or filled with misunderstanding, it becomes necessary to consider whether the adolescent has sufficient decision-making capacity for this decision. In this situation, it may be appropriate to consider what is in the best interest of the adolescent. For example, a 15-year-old football player with a cervical fracture might refuse emergency stabilization, stating that he does not want to live life without football. Most would hold that his conclusion overly values short-term implications, especially in light of the suddenness of the injury, and that he should receive emergency treatment.

THE IMPAIRED PARENT
Parents may be unable to fulfill surrogate responsibilities because of acutely impaired judgment, such as being intoxicated.[57] Clinicians have to weigh the benefits of waiting for appropriate legal consent against what is in the best interest of the child. It may be in the child's best interest to proceed with a routine procedure in the situation of an impaired parent who is unable to give legal consent. Clinicians may wish to consult legal and risk management colleagues for guidance.

End-of-Life Issues

FORGOING POTENTIALLY LIFE-SUSTAINING TREATMENT
Perioperative Limitations on Life-Sustaining Treatment
The concept of limiting potentially life-sustaining medical treatment (LSMT) is the same for children as it is for adults. Decision makers choose to limit LSMT because they do not consider the potential burdens worth the potential benefits.[58,59] The AAP, the American Society of Anesthesiologists (ASA), and the American College of Surgery mandate "required reconsideration" of any limitations on LSMT before proceeding to the operating room.

Although the term "Do Not Resuscitate" (DNR) is commonly used, the term "Life-Sustaining Medical Treatment" is becoming more common. One purpose of this shift is to emphasize that desired limitations on medical treatment are continuous rather than dichotomous. The term "potentially" is often used to modify LSMT to emphasize the uncertainty about whether a therapy will be life-sustaining.

Reevaluation of LSMT preferences for the perioperative period starts with clarifying the patient's goals for the proposed surgery and end-of-life care (Table 5.3). Anesthesiologists should involve the patient, family, and other clinicians such as surgeons, intensivists, and pediatricians in determining what is in the best interest of the child.

Benefits of potentially LSMT include an improved quality of life and prolongation of life under certain circumstances. Burdens

TABLE 5.3	Components of a Pediatric Perioperative Life-Sustaining Medical Treatment Discussion

- Planned procedure and anticipated benefit to child
- Advantages and opportunities of having specific, identified clinicians providing therapy for a defined period
- Likelihood of requiring resuscitation
- Reversibility of likely causes for resuscitation
- Description of potential interventions and their consequences
- Chances of successful resuscitation, including improved outcomes of witnessed arrests compared with unwitnessed arrests
- Ranges of outcomes with and without resuscitation
- Responses to iatrogenic events
- Intended and possible venues and types of postoperative care
- Postoperative timing and mechanisms for reevaluation of the limitations on life-sustaining medical treatment
- Establishment of an agreement (which may include a full resuscitation status) through a goal-directed approach
- Documentation

Adapted from Truog RD, Waisel DB, Burns JP. DNR in the OR: a goal-directed approach. *Anesthesiology* 1999;90:289-295; and Fallat ME, Deshpande JK. Do-not-resuscitate orders for pediatric patients who require anesthesia and surgery. *Pediatrics* 2004;114:1686-1692.

include intractable pain and suffering, disability, and events that cause a decrement in the quality of life, as viewed by the patient.[60,61] These guidelines help in considering short- and long-term goals and putting into appropriate context specific fears such as long-term ventilatory dependency, pain, and suffering.

Legitimate procedures for a child with limitations on LSMT include procedures that decrease pain, provide vascular access, enable the child to be at home, treat an urgent problem unrelated to the primary problem (e.g., appendicitis), or treat a problem that may be related but is not considered a terminal event (e.g., bowel obstruction). However, seeking these interventions does not obviate the desire to avoid potential postresuscitation burdens such as need for extensive ventilator support, cognitive deficits, or physical limitations.

The goal-directed approach for perioperative limitations on LSMT permits decision makers to guide therapy by prioritizing outcomes rather than procedures. After defining desirable outcomes, decision makers ask anesthesiologists to use their clinical judgment to determine how specific interventions will affect achieving the specific goals. Predictions about the success of interventions made at the time of the resuscitation are more accurate than predictions made preoperatively, when the quality and nature of the problems are unknown. Therapy may be guided by goals rather than specific procedures (as is done on the ward), because during the perioperative period children are cared for by dedicated anesthesiologists for brief, defined periods. It is helpful to define a goal-directed approach by discussing the acceptable burdens, the desirable benefits, and the likelihood of distinct outcomes. Most decision makers choose a goal-directed approach of desiring therapy if the interventions and burdens were temporary and reversible (i.e., if they could return to the present state without suffering too much).

Prior determination of acceptable postoperative LSMT is less critical in pediatrics, because usually parents are available in the postoperative period to make decisions regarding therapy. Nonetheless, when a sufficiently mature child participates in discussions about LSMT, anesthesiologists should ensure that the discussion incorporates the child's preferences for postoperative trials of therapy. The willingness to undergo a trial of therapy indicates a belief that the burdens of the trial (e.g., a few days of ventilator support) may be worth the benefits (e.g., extubation of the trachea) initially, but at some point, the increasing burdens may not be worth the decreasing likelihood of the benefits. Flexibly inherent in the goal-directed approach is that it promotes trials of therapy to evaluate whether said therapy achieves its desired goals. This is particularly important given our ever-changing knowledge about the outcomes of resuscitation.[62]

A time-limited trial of therapy is *"an agreement between clinicians and a patient/family to use certain medical therapies over a defined period to see if the patient's condition improves or deteriorates according to the agreed on clinical outcomes."*[63] The results of a time-limited trial can help decision makers determine whether to continue therapy or shift to comfort care measures. Knowing the results of a burdensome therapy makes withdrawing a therapy that does not achieve the identified goals more ethically stout than simply withholding the therapy and not knowing what the effects of the therapy would be.

Iatrogenic problems such as cardiac arrest do not obviate decisions to limit LSMT.[64] To decision makers, the cause of the arrest is irrelevant. Decision makers care about the factors they considered in requesting limited resuscitation, including the likelihood of successful resuscitation and physical and mental status after the arrest. The benefits of continued therapy after certain types of iatrogenic arrests should be addressed as part of the perioperative discussion.[64]

The "temporary and reversible" goal-directed perioperative DNR order can be documented as *"The patient desires resuscitative efforts during surgery and in the postanesthesia care unit (PACU) only if the adverse events are believed to be both temporary and reversible, in the clinical judgment of the attending anesthesiologists and surgeons."* With the patient's permission, anesthesiologists may want to include selected family members in the reevaluation discussion to enable the best communication of the patient's preferences.

Barriers to Honoring Preferences for Resuscitation

Barriers to honoring limitations center on clinician attitudes, time pressures, and inadequate knowledge about policy, law, and ethics.[64–71] Although required reconsideration has been accepted for more than 20 years, and there has been some improvement, anesthesiologists and surgeons still have inadequate knowledge and practices about perioperative LSMT.[72–74] Deficiencies include lack of knowledge about required reconsideration, infrequent preoperative determination of the presence of an advance directive, and inadequate willingness to care for patients with perioperative limitations on LSMT.[75] On the whole, however, it seems that the extent of knowledge and practices is institution-dependent.

Anesthesiologists may falsely believe that law or hospital policy requires full resuscitation during the perioperative period. Clinicians who act in accordance with statutory requirements are often explicitly protected from liability when they honor a child's or family's refusal of resuscitation. Given the well-established right of children and parents to refuse medical treatment and the paucity of cases finding clinicians liable for honoring limitations on LSMT, the risk of liability for honoring an appropriately documented perioperative limitation on LSMT is not high and is likely to be less than the risk of not honoring the limitations.

Physicians Orders for Life-Sustaining Treatment

Physician orders for life-sustaining treatment (POLST) were designed in part to improve honoring resuscitation preferences and are becoming more common in pediatric patients. POLST have two main advantages compared with other forms of advance directives. POLST have the advantages of being a medical order that is valid across different locations, including schools. These features will likely increase compliance with the documented preferences, particularly in terms of emergency medical treatment. The POLST document defines code status and preferences for medical interventions, typically documented as full treatment, trial of treatment, and selective treatment.[76] Although clinicians feel that POLST limited unwanted resuscitation and that the declared preferences were durable, some clinicians report difficulty in using the form or having it honored across locations.[77–81] Research is needed to help optimize POLST practices.[80,82]

Potentially Inappropriate Interventions

It is more helpful to think about potentially inappropriate interventions instead of futile treatments. An intervention is futile only if it cannot accomplish a physiologic goal. A more common and difficult dilemma is how to handle potentially inappropriate interventions. Interventions may be inappropriate when *"there is no reasonable expectation that the patient will improve sufficiently to survive outside the acute care setting, or when there is no reasonable expectation that the patient's neurologic function will improve sufficiently to allow the patient to perceive the benefits of treatment."*[83] This useful concept may be less useful to pediatric decision making given the relatively sparse specific outcome data for the very young.[84,85]

Treatments with small likelihoods of success may be considered inappropriate because of the burden to the child, cost, or uncertain benefit. Discussions about inappropriate treatment should bear in mind the goals of the treatment and the likelihood of achieving a defined result. When offering the likelihood of a result, clinicians should be clear whether the information used to form the estimation is based on intuition, clinical experience, or rigorous scientific studies. Scoring systems that are useful for population predictions in determining potentially inadvisable care should be considered as contributory but not determinative for decision making for individuals.

Parents and clinicians may disagree about therapy for a child near the end of life. Hospitals should have defined processes to help resolve conflict about applying potentially inappropriate interventions (Table 5.4).[86]

IMPROVING COMMUNICATION IN PEDIATRIC INTENSIVE CARE UNITS

Pediatric intensivists should emphasize interdisciplinary communication, tailor the communication style to the parents, and maximize meaningful parental participation in the child's care.[87,88] The goal is to be an empathic professional who establishes compassionate relationships with the child and family by managing emotional, informational, and care needs. In almost all conversations, clinicians should explain the meaning of the conversation in terms of overall care.

Patient-centered characteristics—such as asking questions, using empathic statements, increasing the amount of parental contributions to the conversation, and focusing on psychosocial and lifestyle issues as compared with medical issues—improved parent satisfaction during family conferences.[89] When wanting to convey sympathy to patients and families, wish statements, such as *I wish things were different*, seem effective.[90] Table 5.5 lists characteristics of good communication in the intensive care unit.

TABLE 5.4	Steps for Conflict Resolution of Requests for Potentially Inappropriate Treatment in Intensive Care Units[86]

1. Before initiation of and throughout the formal conflict-resolution procedure, clinicians should enlist expert consultation to aid in achieving a negotiated agreement.

2. Surrogate(s) should be given clear notification in writing regarding the initiation of the formal conflict-resolution procedure and the steps and timeline to be expected in this process.

3. Clinicians should obtain a second medical opinion to verify the prognosis and the judgment that the requested treatment is inappropriate.

4. There should be case review by an interdisciplinary institutional committee.

5. If the committee agrees with the clinicians, then clinicians should offer the option to seek a willing provider at another institution and should facilitate this process.

6. If the committee agrees with the clinicians and no willing provider can be found, surrogate(s) should be informed of their right to seek case review by an independent appeals body.

7. a. If the committee or appellate body agrees with the patient or surrogate's request for life-prolonging treatment clinicians should provide these treatments or transfer the patient to a willing provider.

   b. If the committee agrees with the clinicians' judgment, no willing provider can be found, and the surrogate does not seek independent appeal or the appeal affirms the clinicians' position, clinicians may withhold or withdraw the contested treatments and should provide high-quality palliative care.

From: Bosslet GT, Pope TM, Rubenfeld GD, et al. An official ATS/AACN/ACCP/ESICM/SCCM policy statement: responding to requests for potentially inappropriate treatments in intensive care units. *Am J Respir Crit Care Med.* 2015;191(11):1318-1330. doi:10.1164/rccm.201505-0924ST.

TABLE 5.5	Parents' Desires for Communication in the Intensive Care Units

1. **Honest and complete information** should be tailored to the parents' needs and information-receiving preferences. Comprehension of the child's potential trajectories permits better participation in care and a greater chance of appropriate end-of-life care.

2. **Ready access to staff** should include periodic scheduled informal visits to the bedside and the availability of e-mail interactions. The goal is to provide the parents with easy and frequent opportunities to have their questions answered, with sufficient repetition and clarification of the "big picture."

3. To maximize successful **communication**, clinicians should actively assess the parents' preferences for communication and decision making. This includes considering how to relate information to parents when clinicians have different management opinions. Parents frequently recognize that there are differences between options, and some prefer to hear the range of options, whereas others prefer to hear only the recommended option.

4. **Emotional expression and support by staff** are critical to parents. To do this successfully, clinicians should adapt their style to parents' preferences. Most clinicians should adopt practices that give parents more room to control the conversation, including talking less, listening more, and tolerating silence as parents gather themselves to continue communicating.

5. Parents respond and benefit from the **relational aspects of compassion, mercy, authenticity, and integrity**. More colloquially, the relational aspect is referred to as "being there"—interacting with the parents as a caring person with feelings and emotions. For example, although some clinicians may believe it is inappropriate to show emotion, parents appreciate compassion and some level of distress at the sharing of bad news, rather than cold hard professionalism.[88]

6. **Preservation of the integrity of the parent-child relationship** means enabling parents to continue in their self-identified and prominent role as decision maker and protector. Loss of this role harms parents and may impair their ability to participate in decision making for the child.

7. **Faith and spiritual matters** are highly personal, and parents may feel uncomfortable expressing their faith in an institutional setting. Spiritual matters should be accepted and integrated into the intensive care unit practice to assist those who benefit from spiritual support.

8. **Parents' lifelong views of these events** are profoundly colored by vivid memories and strong feelings about seminal discussions. How difficult discussions are handled and the quality of the communication among clinicians and families often become the basis for the family's lifelong narrative of these events.

Modified from Meyer EC, Ritholz MD, Burns JP, Truog RD. Improving the quality of end-of-life care in the pediatric intensive care unit: parents' priorities and recommendations. *Pediatrics* 2006;117:649-657.

TABLE 5.6	Ethical Issues Surrounding Donation After Cardiac Death (DCD)
Ethical Issue	**Discussion Points**
Should interventions be permitted prior to withdrawal of care?	The burdens from the interventions are not in the best interests of the child. On the other hand, the burdens of the interventions are mostly theoretical and may improve the quality of the transplanted organs.
Should withdrawal of therapy occur in the intensive care unit (ICU) or in the operating room?	Withdrawing therapy in the operating room may increase the quality of the organs transplanted. Withdrawing therapy in the ICU is likely to be less jarring to the family and more consistent with the premise of withdrawing therapy for the child's benefit. In addition, it may remove some of the awkwardness that may occur if the child does not die within the defined interval.
Who should withdraw therapy?	To be consistent with the premises of withdrawal of therapy, it should be the same person who would normally withdraw therapy from the child. Even if the decision is made to withdraw therapy in the operating room, an anesthesiologist who has not been caring for the child should not be asked to withdraw therapy because of the physical location of the event.
How long should cessation of cardiac function exist for a child to be declared dead?	Proposed times may be based on the premises of how long it would take to autoresuscitate compared with how long it would take to be resuscitated through medical intervention.
What are the contents of a good DCD policy?	Acceptable interventions before withdrawing therapy Acceptable locations of withdrawing therapy Amount of time to wait until death before forgoing procurement Which individual should withdraw therapy What to do if the family will not leave after death is declared

ORGAN DONATION AFTER CARDIAC DEATH

In organ procurement after a declaration of death through neurologic criteria (i.e., brain death), the child is declared dead before being brought to the operating room. The organs are then retrieved while total body homeostasis is maintained through mechanical ventilation, pharmacologic therapy, and other standard resuscitative techniques.

Concern about the limited availability of organs for transplantation has resulted in the now widely accepted concept of donation after cardiac death (DCD).[71,91,92] In DCD the child is not declared dead before being brought to the operating room for organ retrieval. Instead, after it is determined that therapy should be withdrawn based on a standard benefits and burdens assessment, the child is brought to the operating room and therapy is withdrawn. If the child dies after life-sustaining therapy is withdrawn, he or she is declared dead by cardiac criteria and the organs are retrieved. Ethical issues regarding DCD protocols center on whether the protocols seriously alter the dying process by shifting decision making away from the best interest of the dying child and by interfering with the family's ability to be with their dying child (Table 5.6).

Clinical and Academic Practice Issues

PEDIATRIC RESEARCH

The anesthesiologist Henry K. Beecher was one of the first to propose that pediatric research had different requirements compared with adult research.[93] Pediatric research is closely examined because children are incapable of consenting to experiments and because the developing child is at greater risk for long-term harm.[94] Federal guidelines give four categories of pediatric research, with each ascending category requiring greater scrutiny of the risk-to-benefit ratio, especially in research without therapeutic benefit for the subject (Table 5.7). Whereas obtaining the assent of the child whenever possible is important for therapeutic medical procedures, it is absolutely essential in the context of research, along with the informed permission of the parents.

Minimal Risk

Minimal risks are defined as those risks that are not greater in and of themselves than those ordinarily encountered in daily life

TABLE 5.7	Federal Classification of Pediatric Research

1. Research not involving greater than minimal risk
   a. IRB determines minimal risk
   b. IRB finds and documents that adequate provisions are made for soliciting assent from children and permission from their parents or guardians
2. Research involving greater than minimal risk but presenting the prospect of direct benefit to the individual subject
   a. IRB justifies the risk by the anticipated benefit to the subjects
   b. The relationship of the anticipated benefit to the risk is at least as favorable as that presented by available alternative approaches
   c. Adequate provisions are made for assent and permission
3. Research that involves greater than minimal risk and no prospect of direct benefit to the individual subject but is likely to yield generalizable knowledge about the subject's disorder or condition
   a. IRB determines that the risk represents a minor increase over minimal risk
   b. The intervention or procedure presents experiences to subjects that are reasonably commensurate with those inherent in their actual or expected medical, dental, psychological, social, or educational situations
   c. The intervention or procedure is likely to yield generalizable knowledge…which is of vital importance for the understanding or amelioration of the subject's disorder or condition
   d. Adequate provisions are made for assent and permission
4. Research not otherwise approvable, which presents an opportunity to understand, prevent, or alleviate a serious problem affecting the health or welfare of children

Where research is covered by numbers 3 and 4 above and permission is to be obtained from parents, both parents must give their permission unless one parent is deceased, unknown, incompetent, or not reasonably available, or when only one parent has legal responsibility for the care and custody of the child.
IRB, institutional review board.
From U.S. Department of Human Services: 45 CFR 46 Subpart D. Additional Protections for Children Involved as Subjects in Research.

or during the performance of routine physical or psychological examinations. Most interpret this to mean the risks encountered in daily life by healthy children, such as running in the backyard, playing sports, or riding in a car.[95-97] A less favored relative interpretation uses as a benchmark those risks encountered in the daily lives of children who will be enrolled in the research. In other words, if a child were living in a manner that exposed the child to risk (e.g., undergoing repeated general anesthesia), then it would be acceptable to expose the child up to that level of risk in a study.

Individuals are poor at estimating the risk levels of activities and often correlate risk to familiarity, control of the activity, and reversibility of the potential harms. Institutional review boards may reject low-risk studies because they involve unfamiliar matters while approving studies that have excessive risks.

Minor Increase Over Minimal Risk

The pediatric research category that involves *"greater than minimal risk and no prospect of direct benefit to the individual subject but is likely to yield generalizable knowledge about the subject's disorder or condition … which is of vital importance"*[98] is based on the idea that it is acceptable to expose a child to a "minor increase over minimal risk" under certain conditions. Parsing the regulation may help clarify this somewhat unhelpful definition. One suggestion has been that "minor increase" means that the pain, discomfort, or stress must be transient, reversible, and not severe.[99] The condition of the subject should be used to mean a set of characteristics *"that an established body of scientific or clinical evidence has shown to negatively affect children's health and well-being or to increase the risk of developing a health problem in the future."* Interpreting "condition" to include "having the potential to have the condition" permits otherwise healthy children to participate in research for diseases that they may develop (e.g., cellulitis). Vital importance implies that the evidence supporting the relevance of the study should require a higher order of proof.

Socioeconomic Concerns and Distribution of Risk

Socioeconomically disadvantaged children living in urban areas may be overrepresented in research studies because urban academic centers in disadvantaged areas perform the majority of clinical research.[100] Children living in socioeconomically disadvantaged areas are often more affected by diseases associated with their environment, such as asthma or nutritional disorders complicated by limited access to stocked grocery stores. One could argue that this unequal burden of risk, primarily manifested by greater participation of socioeconomically disadvantaged children in research studies, is reasonable because these children are more likely to develop these diseases and therefore are more likely to benefit from the research. Most reject that view and believe that in some sense, socioeconomically advantaged patients gratuitously gain the benefits of the research without sharing the risks. The disproportionate risk borne by one segment of society compared with another likely breeches the most accepted interpretation of the core ethical value of justice.

Socioeconomically disadvantaged families may be more likely to be influenced by the small gifts offered to research participants. Aside from compensating for costs (e.g., parking vouchers), gifts should not of themselves encourage participation. The problem is that gifts that represent a small expression of gratitude for some families may provide an incentive for participation for socioeconomically disadvantaged families.[100]

Imperative for Pharmacologic Research

Through the mid-1990s, more than 70% of new molecular entities were without pediatric drug labeling. Inadequate information exposed children to age-specific adverse reactions, ineffective treatment owing to inappropriate dosing, and lack of access to new drugs because physicians tended to prescribe less effective, known medications. Inadequate research into pediatric drugs forced physicians to prescribe drugs in nonstandard ways, such as sprinkled or crushed tablets. Even when there is some pediatric labeling, there is scant labeling for children younger than 2 years of age. In 2009 a survey of a Canadian pediatric tertiary hospital found that even when comparing off-label (see below) use with contemporary pediatric references (an unofficial and very liberal interpretation), 16% of drug administrations during the perioperative period were considered off-label. Based on a more traditional standard of the *Canadian Compendium of Pharmaceutical Specialties*, 55% of drugs administered were used off-label.[101] Neonatology and pediatric intensive care units are particularly at risk for off-label use. In a study of more than 65,000 patients, drugs that were considered to have high-risk status or high priority for study by the Food and Drug Administration [FDA] were used off-label in 85% of patients.[102] Off-label drugs included dexmedetomidine, dopamine, hydromorphone, lorazepam, and milrinone.

The following selective history highlights the overall intent to ensure that (1) children get the same benefits of pharmacologic advances as adults and (2) research is performed in the youngest children. Readers should also learn from this history that persistent advocacy is often required before regulatory change can be successfully obtained. In 1962 the Kefauver-Harris Amendments (passed after the thalidomide disaster) required that drug companies demonstrate safety and efficacy before marketing a drug. Because the vast majority of drugs did not undergo pediatric-specific investigation, this requirement actually led to less pediatric labeling, with the package insert (drug label) often reading, *"Safety and efficacy have not been demonstrated for children <12 years,"* because of the expense of getting this information. In 1994 the U.S. FDA began requiring sponsors to explain why pediatric labeling cannot occur but did not require sponsors to perform pediatric studies (see Chapter 7).

The 1997 FDA Modernization Act and the 1998 Final Rule were legislative initiatives designed to gain more data from drug companies through pediatric studies in exchange for the benefit of an additional 6 months of patent exclusivity. This effort was further codified with the passage of the Best Pharmaceuticals for Children Act (BPCA) in 2002. With these requirements, the FDA now had the legal power to mandate pediatric studies if a new drug might be used in a substantial number of children, if it might provide a meaningful therapeutic benefit, or if inadequate labeling could pose significant risks. The pharmaceutical industry responded with an explosion of pediatric studies. However, the exclusivity provision did not encourage study of generic drugs or drugs with insufficient sales. Further, once exclusivity was credited for older pediatric age groups, there was no incentive to conduct studies in younger groups.

In December 2003 the Pediatric Research Equity Act (PREA) required pediatric studies for all drugs and biologic products with a new indication, new dosage form, new route, new dosing regimen, or new active ingredient. Studies need to evaluate safety, efficacy, dosing and administration for a drug intended use for a specific pediatric subpopulation. Studies could be waived if they were impracticable, if the therapy would be ineffective or unsafe in pediatric patients, or if there would be no meaningful therapeutic benefit over existing therapies and the moiety would not be used in a substantial number of children.

In 2012 the Food and Drug Administration Safety and Innovation Act (FDASIA) made the BPCA and PREA permanent. The FDASIA initiated new requirements such as a Pediatric Study

Plan, which included an outline of the studies including study objectives, design, statistical approach, age of patients, relevant outcomes, and a timeline. An increased focus on the youngest patients included requiring that neonates be included in studies unless the disease did not affect neonates or studies were not feasible or safe. The FDASIA offered priority review for therapies for rare pediatric diseases. Through August 2016 the FDA granted pediatric exclusivity for 217 drugs.[103] In 2014 the FDA put in similar requirements for medical devices intended for use in children. Other nations have adopted similar regulatory requirements and incentives to encourage drug research.[104,105]

MANAGING POTENTIAL CONFLICTS OF INTEREST

A *conflict of interest* is *"a set of conditions in which professional judgment concerning a primary interest (such as a patient's welfare or the validity of research) tends to be unduly influenced by a secondary interest."*[106] Because these conditions in an individual are internal, they are best characterized by describing situations that may create the potential for conflicts of interest. Focusing on potential conflicts of interest moves the concept away from attacking an individual's morals and toward more uniform definitions. Potential conflicts of interest may be induced by financial, personal, and professional benefits such as prestige, promotion, and personal gratification.[107] Anesthesiologists should be mindful of these potential conflicts and attempt to identify them to better understand the likelihood of compromised judgment.

Conducting Research

Perhaps the most powerful conflict in conducting research is the loss of equipoise that can come from originating and developing an idea. Other sources of conflict related to research center on academic promotion and reputation. Research disclosures do not help identify conflicts of interest. In one study, only 80% of physicians disclosed payments related to the research, and only 50% disclosed payments from the same company but unrelated to the product being discussed. Indirect payments were just as likely to influence behavior as direct payment.[108]

In 2009 an anesthesiologist was falsifying data that had encouraged multimodal pain therapy. Concerns of an internal reviewer brought about the internal investigation that found significant irregularities in the research. Major journals retracted articles. The editor of *Anesthesia and Analgesia* was quoted as saying, *"We are left with a large hole in our understanding of this [multimodal pain therapy]."*[109,110] The editor of the journal called the scandal *"a tragedy"* for the profession, for patients, and for the anesthesiologist involved personally. Given that the anesthesiologist's studies were *"robust"* and influential, *"the big chunk of what people have based their [multimodal] protocol on is gone."* It is important to emphasize that the anesthesiologist's coauthors were deceived by him and were not complicit. If fact, they assisted in assessing the legitimacy of articles that were not retracted.[110]

Conflicts of interest also come from industry support of research. To be clear, the academic-anesthesia-industry research complex is necessary to continue the rapid advancement of science. Rigorous oversight minimizes these abuses.[111] Researchers need to be involved in trial development, must have access to raw data, and must be able to publish without the company's authorization. Cozy relationships between powerful members of the local academic community and industry should be examined and brought to light to minimize influence and potential conflicts of interest.[112]

Financial relationships among physicians, researchers, hospitals and industry are publicly available through the Open Payments

TABLE 5.8	Strategies Used by Drug Companies to Influence Physicians

1. Teach sales people subtle verbal and nonverbal techniques to influence physicians.
2. Instruct sales people to misdirect and to dissemble when questioned about possible complications.
3. Cherry-pick which data are distributed to physicians.
4. Prohibit distribution of studies that may criticize the product. (One strategy is to classify concerning studies as background studies and then prohibit distribution of background studies.)
5. Seek "opinion leaders" to speak in favor of the product.
6. Continue the well-established gift-giving strategy to subconsciously curry favor with the physician and to develop a positive association about the product and the company.

program in the Sunshine Act (section 6002) of the Patient Protection and Affordable Care Act.[113,114] This program *"collects information about the payments drug and device companies made to physicians and teaching hospitals for things like travel, research, gifts, speaking fees and meals."*[115,116] From August 2013 through 2015, the Open Payments program reported data from 812,000 physician payments valued at more than 5 billion dollars.[117] The actual benefits from the Open Payments program are unclear.[118–121]

Interaction With Industry

Interaction with industry affects clinicians' prescribing behavior, often through unconscious feelings of gratitude, obligation, or fellowship.[112,122–125] Because clinicians are mostly unaware of the social dynamic industry is creating, clinicians can legitimately assert they do not consciously adjust their clinical practice, but stealthily creating familiarity and good feelings for a product or an individual is a core competency in advertising.

Be cynical about advertisements. Clinicians should independently evaluate information supplied by industry because they commonly overstate benefits and understate risks (Table 5.8).

Risks associated with industry misrepresentation will increase as increasing clinician workload decreases time for study. For these reasons, it is instructive to look more closely at this problem. Evidence published in the 2000 Vioxx Gastrointestinal Outcomes Research (VIGOR) study indicated that rofecoxib (Vioxx) dramatically increased the rate of myocardial infarction in patients. In 2001 the FDA determined that clinicians should be made aware of the cardiovascular effects of rofecoxib, and in 2004 it was withdrawn from the market. Congressman Henry Waxman later wrote the following[126]:

> Merck, the manufacturer of Vioxx, ... has an excellent reputation within the drug industry and supports many products, such as vaccines, that are medically essential but not very profitable. ... Yet as we learned, even a company like Merck can direct its sales force to provide clinicians with a distorted picture of the relevant scientific evidence.

On February 7, 2001 the Arthritis Drugs Advisory Committee of the FDA voted unanimously that physicians should be made aware of VIGOR's cardiovascular results. The next day, Merck sent a bulletin to its rofecoxib sales force [which] ordered, *"DO NOT INITIATE DISCUSSIONS ON THE FDA ARTHRITIS ADVISORY COMMITTEE ... OR THE RESULTS OF THE ... VIGOR STUDY."* It advised that if a physician inquired about VIGOR, the sales representative should indicate that the study showed a gastrointestinal benefit and then say, *"I cannot discuss the study with you."*

Merck further instructed representatives to show those doctors who asked whether rofecoxib caused myocardial infarction a pamphlet called "The Cardiovascular Card." This pamphlet, prepared by Merck's marketing department, indicated that rofecoxib was associated with $\frac{1}{8}$ the mortality from cardiovascular causes of that found with other antiinflammatory drugs.

The Cardiovascular Card did not include any data from the VIGOR study. Instead, it presented a pooled analysis of preapproval studies, in most of which small doses of rofecoxib were used for a short period. None of these studies were designed to assess cardiovascular safety. In fact, FDA experts had publicly expressed *"serious concerns"* about using preapproval studies as evidence of the drug's cardiovascular safety:

> [B]ut it would be a mistake to restrict the lessons learned to a single company. The testimony we heard indicated that Merck's marketing practices may be less aggressive and more ethical than many of its competitors.

Production Pressure

Production pressure is *"the internal or external pressure on the anesthetist to keep the operating room schedule moving along speedily."*[127] Almost half of surveyed anesthesiologists reported seeing what they considered unsafe anesthetic practices in response to this production pressure.[128] As a consequence, anesthesiologists may not want to take the time to allow a child to ask questions about the anesthetic, to adequately premedicate an anxious child, or to engage the parents in a lengthy discussion about postponing the surgery in a child with a cold. Anesthesiologists should be cognizant of their level of skill. For example, the "routine" tonsillectomy may be beyond some anesthesiologists' ability in a child with multiple congenital deficits. Anesthesiologists have an obligation to the patient and themselves to only provide care that is within their skills and to recognize when economic and administrative pressures may induce them to do otherwise.

PHYSICIAN OBLIGATIONS, ADVOCACY, AND GOOD CITIZENSHIP

An implicit social contract obligates physicians to serve society beyond direct patient caring. Society enables medical students, physicians in training, and physicians to train, perform research, and, perhaps most importantly, learn from and with patients. In return, society expects pediatric anesthesiologists to *"manage all things pediatric anesthesia"* (Table 5.9).[129–134] Clinicians should participate in relevant community advocacy, such as reducing variations in pediatric care secondary to issues like race, insurance status, and language barriers.[135–137]

Individual anesthesiologists do not need to fulfill every obligation. "Units" of anesthesiologists, such as private practice groups, academic departments, and state societies, should fulfill these obligations collectively.

Participating in Patient Safety Efforts

Medical errors come from human mistakes and system flaws.[138,139] Parents in particular are interested in medical errors. In one study, 39% of parents felt obligated to be vigilant for medical errors in their child's care.[140] Clinicians have an obligation to work to reduce system flaws, including participating in quality improvement activities and data collection, following policies meant to improve care in high-risk situations (e.g., nosocomial infections), and actively engaging in policies designed to reduce medical errors, such as

TABLE 5.9	Examples of Obligations of Anesthesiologists to Participate and Advocate
Obligations of Pediatric Anesthesiologists[129–131,133,135–137,152,153]	
Treat every child with the grace and consideration you would want for your child and family	
Tailor the perioperative experience to the individual	
Respond to problems that may harm children (e.g., impaired colleagues)	
Practice mindfulness and critical self-reflection	
Actively engage in continuing medical education	
Support advancement of the science	
Participate in quality improvement initiatives such as Wake Up Safe	
Participate in professional organizations such as the Society for Pediatric Anesthesia and the American Academy of Pediatrics Section on Anesthesiology and Pain Medicine	
Prepare future generations through teaching, mentoring, creating opportunities, and developing systems to enable anesthesiologists to fulfill these obligations	
Community Advocacy and Participation	
Raise public awareness about a health or social issue	
Participate in public advocacy and lobbying	
Work toward eliminating racial disparities in care	
Encourage a medical society to act on an issue that concerns the public health	
Serve in a local organization, political interest group, or political organization	
Topics of particular relevance to pediatric anesthesiologists: • Pediatric obesity • Pediatric sedation safety in hospitals and non-hospital facilities • Child abuse • Health care access • Role of subspecialty training in improving care for children	

universal standards of patient identification.[141] Clinicians should also participate in the data collection of national and international databases.

Although clinicians may not see the big picture and therefore resent doing "extra" steps, it is vital for clinicians to accept on faith that participation is good patient care.[129] Surreptitiously circumventing policies may harm patients, does not permit remediation of the policy, and weakens the fidelity of the entire system, encouraging others to *"make their own rules."*

Clinicians also have an obligation to report potential medical errors. Although the "blame-free" approach is well touted, clinicians perceive significant barriers to honestly reporting near-misses, hindering improved patient safety. Institutional barriers center on inadequate procedures and lack of trust in the administration.[142] When clinicians believe that policies are harmful or unnecessary, they are obligated to raise these questions through appropriate channels, particularly to address institutional barriers to reporting patient safety events.

Treating Suffering

Cassel described suffering as an intensely personal feeling that can be defined as *"the state of severe distress associated with events that threaten the intactness of the person."*[143] Suffering should be considered when managing pain, and adequate steps should be taken to find and alleviate sources of suffering. Factors that contribute to a child's suffering include not knowing the origin or meaning of the pain, believing that pain is a punishment, and fearing that the pain will never be relieved. Anesthesiologists minimize suffering by clearly communicating about these issues with parents and children and affording children as much control of their care as possible.

Suspicion of Child Maltreatment

Child maltreatment includes acts of physical abuse, sexual abuse, emotional abuse, and neglect.[144-146] Anesthesiologists should be particularly sensitive to bruises or burns in the shape of objects, injuries to soft tissue areas such as the upper arms, unexplained mouth and dental injuries, fractures in infants, height and weight less than the fifth percentile, and injuries that are not explained by the history (see Fig. 39.2). Children with physical or mental handicaps are particularly prone to abuse.[147] Anesthesiologists, like all physicians, are legally required to report the suspicion of child abuse or neglect to appropriate authorities. Indeed, in most jurisdictions, a physician can be criminally prosecuted if found liable for failing to report suspected child abuse.

THE ETHICS CONSULTATION SERVICE

The ethical dilemmas that occur in the practice of anesthesiology may be difficult for the practitioner to resolve alone. Ethics committees and their consulting services act in an advisory role to help clinicians, patients, and families amicably resolve ethical dilemmas. Anesthesiologists may find ethics consultation helpful with questions about informed consent, decision-making capacity, and resuscitation decisions and in resolving disagreements among patients, families, and clinicians.

Although most ethics consultation services use a small group (typically three people) to perform consultations, some use the entire committee and some use a single individual.[148] Physicians, nurses, social workers, chaplains, administrators, and laypeople serve on ethics committees and perform consultations. Common characteristics of ethics consultation services are that they permit anyone to request an ethics consultation; that they require notification (not permission) of the patient, parents, and attending physician prior to the consultation; and that choosing to follow the recommendations is wholly voluntary. Ethics committees are also available to consult on policy development and to organize continuing educational programs.

For pediatric ethics consultations, the attending physician requested the majority of consults, but consult requests were also commonly received from nurses, social workers, nurse practitioners, and families.[149] Typical ethical concerns were on end-of-life care, goals of care, prognosis, quality of life, parental decision making, pediatric assent, cultural differences, professional obligations, and disagreement among professionals.[149,150] Ethics consultations seems to work efficiently, reaching consensus promptly and consistently.

The opinions of ethicists may differ from the opinions of subsets of physicians. For example, when interpreting the best interest standard for a neonate, ethicists are more likely to consider the infant's interests and the effects on the family. Neonatologists were influenced by parents' wishes, but were more likely to consider only the infant's interests and were less likely to consider the effects on the family.[151] After consultations, clinicians feel greater satisfaction in managing cases with ethical conflicts, not only because of their heightened awareness of the expert consulting services available, but also because of their increased knowledge and comfort in dealing with these issues.

ANNOTATED REFERENCES

Cassel EJ. The nature of suffering and the goals of medicine. *N Engl J Med.* 1982;306:639-646.

Physicians relieve suffering. Cassel's 30-year-old treatise is the unparalleled explanation of suffering.

Committee on Bioethics, American Academy of Pediatrics. Informed consent, parental permission, and assent in pediatric practice. *Pediatrics.* 1995;95:314-317.

This article is the basis of informed consent for children. Pay particular attention to the introduction, in which Dr. William Bartholome (in abstentia) exhorts clinicians to respect "the experience, perspective and power of children".

Gruen RL, Pearson SD, Brennan TA. Physician-citizens: public roles and professional obligations. *JAMA.* 2004;291:94-98.

Gruen et al. provide a thoughtful perspective on the public and professional obligations of physicians. They provide a path on how to fulfill these obligations.

Kon AA, Shepard EK, Sederstrom NO, et al. Defining futile and potentially inappropriate interventions: a policy statement from the Society of Critical Care Medicine Ethics Committee. *Crit Care Med.* 2016;44(9):1769-1774. doi:10.1097/CCM.0000000000001965.

This article elegantly describes the characteristics of potentially inappropriate intervention and provides practical advice about implications.

Lang K, Dupree C, Kon A, Dudinski D. Calling out implicit racial bias as a harm in pediatric care. *Camb Q Healthc Ethics.* 2016;25(3):540-552. doi:10.1017/S0963180116000190.

A thorough, readable and nonjudgmental analysis of one of those problems we prefer not to discuss—differences in care by race.

Quill TE. "I wish things were different": expressing wishes in response to loss, futility, and unrealistic hopes. *Ann Intern Med.* 2001;135(7):551. doi:10.7326/0003-4819-135-7-200110020-00022.

A short paper that changes the way you think about communicating with the patient or family during difficult times. The "wish" statement initiates deeper discussion and conveys empathy and being on the "same side of the fence" with the patient and family.

Shafer SL. Tattered threads. *Anesth Analg.* 2009;108:1361-1363.

Shafer elegantly articulates the harms of false data.

Waxman HA. The lessons of Vioxx: drug safety and sales. *N Engl J Med.* 2005;352:2576-2578.

Waxman's recounting of public testimony eviscerates the reassuring murmurings of industry.

A complete reference list can be found online at ExpertConsult.com.

Pharmacogenomics

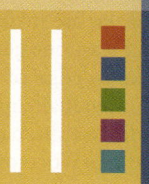

6

VIDYA CHIDAMBARAN AND SENTHILKUMAR SADHASIVAM

U.S. PRESIDENT WILLIAM CLINTON, when announcing the relative completion of the Human Genome Project in July 2000, stated *"With this profound new knowledge, humankind is on the verge of gaining immense new power to heal. Genome science will have a real impact on all of our lives—and even more, on the lives of our children. It will revolutionize the diagnosis, prevention, and treatment of most, if not all, human disease."*[1] This marked the beginning of enhanced interest and vigor in the development of personalized medicine, which simply stated, means "right treatment for the right patient at the right time." This is especially relevant in anesthesia and analgesia as the perioperative period is a state of stress, inflammation, pain, and hemodynamic and metabolic shifts superimposed on chronic disease; all factors have interindividual variability in response.[2] Moreover, use of multiple drugs in a short course of time, as occurs in the perioperative period, introduces variability in metabolism and drug-drug interactions that can be dangerous. This is because genetic factors contribute to an estimated 50% of the variability in drug responses,[3] and it is reported that 59% of drugs are involved in adverse drug reactions and metabolized by at least one gene with variants that affect its metabolism.[4] Hence, knowledge of pharmacogenomics (PG) and its applications for individualizing anesthetic care is critical.[5,6] In this chapter, we discuss the basics and current understanding of PG relevant to the practice of pediatric anesthesia.

Historical Perspectives

The current understanding of personalized medicine is traceable to the writings of Hippocrates, the "father of Western medicine," who lived in the fifth century BCE.[7] Anecdotally, it is said that in 510 BCE, Pythagoras noted that ingestion of fava beans caused a potentially fatal reaction in some, but not all, individuals.[8] The "seeds" of modern genetics were sown by Gregor Mendel, who presented his research on experiments in plant hybridization in 1865. Multiple scientists received Nobel Prizes for ground-breaking discoveries of "nuclein" (Albrecht Kossel in 1910), the double-helical structure of the nucleic acid (Watson, Crick, and Wilkins in 1962), cracking the genetic code (Nirenberg, Khorana, Holley in 1968), and pioneering DNA sequencing methods (Sanger, Gilbert, Berg in 1980). These revolutionized the science of genetic sequencing and in 2003, the Human Genome Project successfully completed the unraveling of the approximately 3 billion DNA base pairs that make up the human genome. Anesthesia is in no way a silent bystander in the history of PG. Some of the initial discoveries of genetic effects on drugs were related to interactions involving barbiturates in patients with porphyria (1937),[9] cholinesterase deficiency leading to succinylcholine-induced prolonged apnea (1957)[10] and malignant hyperthermia (1962).[11]

Basic Concepts and Nomenclature

The term "pharmacogenetics" was coined by Friedrich Vogel of Heidelberg, Germany, in 1959.[12] It refers to the role of genetic variation affecting drug response or adverse reactions to drugs. A broader term, "pharmacogenomics," was introduced in the 1990s with emergence of the Human Genome Project and the development of the genome sciences, encompassing all genes in the genome that may determine drug responses.[13] We now know that the human genome contains about 21,000 genes. The most common type of allelic variation is a single-nucleotide polymorphisms (SNP) when two alternative bases occur at an appreciable frequency in a population (>1%).[14] Other genetic variations are called mutations (incidence <1%), which may be duplications, deletions, insertions, translocation, or inversion of DNA segments. However, since more than one codon (triplet of nucleotides) code for the same amino acid, not all mutations cause structural changes in the protein (called nonsense variant), whereas others do change the protein (called missense variant).

Cells use a two-step process of transcription (DNA to messenger RNA [mRNA]) and translation (mRNA to amino acid) to read each genetic code and produce amino acid sequences that make up proteins. Since proteins function as receptors, enzymes, and transporters for drugs, it was conventionally thought that exonic variants with "functional" roles in genes would affect protein structure and hence be of clinical significance. However, we now understand that the process is not quite as simple as previously thought. Transcription could be affected by alternative splicing and differential gene expression (depending on regulatory variants, microRNA, epigenetic factors), translation by RNA degradation,

or inefficient translation. Moreover, protein formation depends on translation initiation sequences and then posttranslational modifications. Furthermore, protein expression varies in different parts of the body, affected by age, environmental conditions, and disease.[15] This complexity has given rise to various genomic technologies with exciting clinical potential for applications. Consequently, genotype may not always equate with a distinct phenotype in any particular individual.

Transcriptomics is the study of all mRNA molecules in the cell. For example, repeated exposure to high doses of ketamine, an N-methyl-D-aspartate (NMDA) receptor antagonist, can alter expression of apoptotic relevant genes and increase NMDA receptor gene expression in developing neurons (postnatal day 7 rat pup brains).[16]

Proteomics is the large-scale study of proteins, particularly their structures and functions. Tools of proteomic research mainly involve separation and elimination of contaminants with enzymes (e.g., DNAase, RNAase, denaturing agents) followed by protein separation by size (one- or two-dimensional polyacrylamide gel electrophoresis), cleavage into peptides and analysis by mass spectrometry (MS) (commonly matrix-assisted laser desorption time of flight [MALDI-ToF], electrospray ionization, surface-enhanced laser desorption time of flight [SELDI-ToF], and tandem MS/MS).[17] This is based on the property that six or more amino acids define a peptide sequence that can be used to identify the gene that coded for them.[18] Chromatin immunoprecipitation (ChIP) is a type of immunoprecipitation experimental technique used to investigate the interaction between proteins and DNA in the cell. It aims to determine whether specific proteins are associated with specific genomic regions, such as transcription factors on promoters or other DNA binding sites, and is an important investigational tool.

Proteomics has applications in identifying differential expression in the spinal cord after peripheral nerve injury in rat models,[19] including specific dorsal horn proteins involved in transmission and modulation of noxious information, cellular metabolism, plasma membrane receptor trafficking, oxidative stress, apoptosis, and degeneration under neuropathic pain conditions.[20] Proteomics has enabled identification of protein-binding sites of inhalation anesthetics.[21] After desflurane anesthesia, protein expression levels in the rat brain remained altered for at least 72 hours, which lends strength to the notion that the physiologic effects of anesthesia outlast the immediate postoperative period.[22,23] Effects on proteomic expression (proteins broadly classified into groups involved in cytoskeletal/neuronal growth, cellular metabolism, signaling, and cell stress/death responses) on the brain of rats were studied after sevoflurane and propofol anesthesia. The authors showed that proteins concerned with cell death and stress responses were downregulated by both agents, but they had variable effects on proteins in the other groups. Proteins such as ULIP-2 and dihydropyrimidinase-like 2 (DPYSL2; associated with cytoskeletal/neuronal growth) were regulated in opposite directions by propofol and sevoflurane. They also found that sevoflurane had more pronounced effects on a wider range of proteins and over an apparently greater duration than propofol. These findings revealed that sevoflurane could be considered a more disruptive anesthetic agent and suggest that the agents have different underlying mechanisms of protein regulation.[24] It is expected that in the future, proteomics will revolutionize preoperative risk stratification as well as approaches to anesthetic and analgesic drug delivery as they relate to specific protein binding.[15]

Metabolomics is the systematic study of the unique chemical fingerprints that specific cellular processes leave behind. Metabolomics of the live rodent brain differ during isoflurane and propofol anesthesia, with greater concentrations of lactate and glutamate characteristic of isoflurane anesthesia.[25] The use of high-resonance magnetic spectroscopy to measure metabolomics raises exciting avenues for noninvasive recognition of anesthesia-induced brain effects in humans and may be a way of recognizing differential anesthesia-induced apoptosis or neurotoxicity observed in the young, immature brain after exposure to anesthesia (see Chapter 25). Similarly, metabolic profiling of hearts exposed to sevoflurane and propofol in the isolated working rat heart model revealed distinct regulation of fatty acid and glucose oxidation, which could have clinical implications for the responses of a diseased heart under anesthesia.[26]

Another exciting field is of *epigenetics,* which encompasses nonstructural DNA modifications that control gene expression by altering transcription via histone modification and changes of DNA methylation.[27] The concept was initially proposed as a bridge between an organism's heritable genome and environmental influences[28]; such environmental influences are evident from reports of a high frequency of epigenetic differences between aging monozygotic twins.[29]

DNA methylation involves the addition of a methyl group to the 5′ carbon of the cytosine pyrimidine ring in a DNA dinucleotide by DNA methyltransferase enzymes (DNMT1, DNMT3A, DNMT3B), converting it into 5-methylcytosine. Regions in the DNA (60% in gene promoter regions) have been identified where cytosine and guanine appear next to each other in repeating sequence, held together by phosphodiester bonds, and are called CpG islands. Methylation has been found to prevent binding of transcription factors[30] or attracting methylated DNA-binding proteins that repress transcription, leading generally to gene silencing.[31,32] DNA methylation analysis either involves pyrosequencing of bisulfite-treated DNA or use of commercial arrays. There has been immense interest in the role of epigenetics in the transition from acute to chronic pain,[33] the functional regulation of μ-opioid receptors, the main receptor for endogenous as well as exogenous opioids,[34] and neuropathic pain.[35]

Histone deacetylation is modification of nucleosomes (histone octamers and surrounding DNA) that involves acetylation of the exposed *N*-terminal tails of histone by histone acetyl transferases (HATs)[36]; this alters chromatin structure and makes it less compact, thus allowing transcription factors to bind more easily. This results in increased gene expression, especially when located in gene promoter regions. This is analyzed using ChIP, and more recently, combined with sequencing (ChIP-seq).[37] An example of epigenetics as therapeutic targets for pain is provided by the study of the rat brainstem nucleus raphe magnus. This is important for central mechanisms of chronic pain, persistent inflammatory, and neuropathic pain where epigenetic suppression of *GAD2* (the gene that encodes glutamic acid decarboxylase 65 [GAD65], a γ-aminobutyric acid [GABA] synthetic enzyme that regulates pain) transcription through histone deacetylase (HDAC)-mediated histone hypoacetylation, results in impaired GABA synaptic inhibition. Importantly, HDAC inhibitors strongly increased GAD65 activity, restored GABA synaptic function, and relieved sensitized pain behavior, proving to have therapeutic potential.[38]

Epigenetics has been lauded as a possible "epicenter" for future anesthesia research.[39] The 20,000 genes that code for proteins account for only 1.5% of DNA. The National Human Genome Research Institute Encyclopedia of DNA Elements (ENCODE) project was implemented to elucidate the regulatory elements affecting gene expression, with the intention of understanding the role of the unaccounted (98.5%) DNA.[40] Small nucleolar RNAs, long noncoding RNAs, small interfering RNA (siRNA), and microRNA are now included in the list along with known messenger, transport, and ribosomal RNA. *MicroRNAs* are small (19-22 nucleotides) noncoding RNA that bind to mRNA via base pairing with complementary sequences and cause gene silencing or degradation. A short (5-7 nucleotides) sequence in the mature microRNA determines the specificity of binding to mRNAs, so microRNAs can bind multiple mRNAs, and one mRNA can be bound to multiple microRNAs simultaneously. Isoflurane protects mouse hearts from ischemia-reperfusion injury by a microRNA-21–dependent mechanism.[41] Since endogenous microRNAs in tissue can be easily increased or decreased with chemical mimics and inhibitors, this finding may hold clinical relevance for future therapeutic strategies to modulate cardiac gene regulation.

Hepatic Metabolism and Developmental Pharmacogenetics

Metabolism of many drugs involves the *cytochrome P-450 (CYP) enzyme* system. Multiple isoforms of the cytochrome P-450 enzyme system exist with different substrate specificities for different drugs.[42-44] Induction and inhibition of these enzymes by different drugs and chemicals requires a thorough understanding of both the nomenclature of the cytochrome P-450 system as well as the specific isoforms responsible for metabolism of the drugs used in pediatric anesthesia. There are both genetic and ethnic polymorphisms leading to clinically important differences in the capacity to metabolize drugs; these differences can make individual drug responses unpredictable.[45-50] In the future it may be possible to tailor drug doses to the individual's requirements by determining the child's unique metabolic capacity.[50,51]

CYTOCHROMES P-450: PHASE I REACTIONS

Cytochromes P-450 are heme-containing proteins that provide most of the phase I drug metabolism for lipophilic compounds in the body. The generally accepted nomenclature of the cytochrome P-450 isozymes begins with CYP and groups enzymes with more than 36% DNA homology into families designated with an Arabic number followed by alphanumeric letters for the subfamily of closely related proteins (>77% homology) followed by a number for the specific gene—for example, CYP3A4.[52,53] Isozymes that are important in human drug metabolism are found in the *CYP1, CYP2,* and *CYP3* gene families. Table 6.1 outlines the P-450 isozymes and their common substrates, inducers, inhibitors, and polymorphisms.

DEVELOPMENTAL CHANGES OF SPECIFIC CYTOCHROMES

For many drugs, metabolism in neonates is reduced and correlates with fewer cytochrome P-450 enzymes in the hepatic microsomes.[54] Although the concentrations of CYP enzymes increase with gestational age, they may reach only 50% of adult values at term.[54] In neonates, reduced cytochrome P-450 decreases clearance for many drugs, including theophylline, caffeine, diazepam, phenytoin, and phenobarbital.[43,44,55-59] Although many isozymes are immature in the neonate, some P-450 isozymes exhibit near-adult activity, whereas others produce unique metabolic pathways in the neonatal

P450 Enzymes	Selected Substrates	Inducers	Inhibitors	Number of Variants Identified	Examples of Variants	Effect on Enzyme Activity
CYP2B6	Ketamine Methadone Propofol Meperidine	Carbamazepine (S)[a] Phenobarbital Phenytoin Rifampin (S)[a] Efavirenz (W)[c]	Clopidogrel (W)[f] Ticlopidine (W)[f] Prasugrel (W)[f]	>28	*6(516G>T, 785A>G) *16 *5 (172H-262K-487C)	Decreased

CYP2C9	NSAIDs Diclofenac Ibuprofen, Naproxen, Indomethacin
	Others
	  Celecoxib
	  Warfarin
	  Oral hypoglycemic (tolbutamide, glipizide)
	  Phenytoin
		Carbamazepine (M)[b]
		Rifampin (M)[b]
		Phenobarbital (W)[c]
		St. John's wort (W)[c]
			Amiodarone (M)[e]
			Fluconazole (M)[e]
				>30	*2 (430C>T)
					*3 (1075A>G)
						Decreased

CYP2C19	Antiepileptics Diazepam
	Midazolam Phenytoin,
	Phenobarbitone
	Others
	  PPIs
	  TCA
	  SSRI
	  MAOI
	  Clopidogrel
		Rifampin, (M)[b]
		Efavirenz, Ritonavir
		St. John's wort
			Fluconazole (S)[d]
			Fluvoxamine (S)[d]
			Ticlopidine (S)[d]			

CYP2D6	Codeine
	Dextromethorphan
	Oxycodone
	Hydrocodone
	Tramadol
	Ondansetron
	Dolasetron
	Palonosetron
	Tropisetron
	Antidepressants
	  Amitriptyline
	  Imipramine
	  Fluoxetine
	  Duloxetine
	  Paroxetine
		None known	Bupropion (S)[d]
			Fluoxetine (S)[d]
			Paroxetine (S)[d]
			Quinidine (S)[d]
			Duloxetine (M)[e]
			Amiodarone (W)[f]
			Cimetidine (W)[f]
			Celecoxib (W)[f]
			Methadone (W)[f]
				>100	PM: two inactive alleles (*3-*8, *11-*16, *19-*21, *38, *40, *42)
					IM: two decreased-activity alleles (*9,*10, *17, *29, *36, *41) or carrying one active (*1, *2, *33, *35) and one inactive (*3-*8, *11-*16, *19-*21, *38, *40, *42) allele, or carrying one decreased-activity (*9, *10, *17, *29, *36, *41) and one inactive allele (*3-*8, *11-*16, *19-*21, *38, *40, *42)
					UM: a gene duplication in absence of inactive (*3-*8, *11-*16, *19-*21, *38, *40, *42) or decreased-activity (*9, *10, *17, *29, *36, *41) alleles	

CYP2E1	Volatile agents
	  Halothane
	  Isoflurane
	  Enflurane
	  Desflurane
	  Methoxyflurane
	APAP
	Caffeine
		Ethanol
		Isoniazid
			Disulfiram	13	*5 (-1293G>C, 1053C>T)	Increased

CYP3A4.5	Benzodiazepines
	  Diazepam
	  Midazolam
	  Triazolam
	  Alprazolam
	Opioids
	  Morphine
	  Meperidine
	  Fentanyl
	  Sufentanil
	  Remifentanil
	  Alfentanil
	  Methadone
	Granisetron
	Amide group (LA)
		Carbamazepine (S)[a]
		Efavirenz (M)[b]
		Nevirapine (M)[b]
		Phenobarbital
		Phenytoin (S)[a]
		Pioglitazone
		Rifabutin (W)[c]
		Rifampin (S)[a]
		St. John's Wort (S)[a]
		Aprepitant (W)[c]
		Prednisone (W)[c]
			HIV antivirals (S)[d]
			Ketoconazole (S)[d]
			Clarithromycin (S)[d]
			Erythromycin (M)[e]
			Grapefruit juice (M)[e]
			Verapamil (M)[e]
			Diltiazem (M)[e]
			Aprepitant (M)[e]
			Atorvastatin (W)[f]
			Cimetidine (W)[f]
			Isoniazid (W)[f]
			Oral contraceptives (W)[f]
				>50	CYP3A4*1B
					CYP3A5*3
					CYP3A4*1G
						Increased
						Nonfunctional
						Decreased

W: Weak; M: Moderate; S: Strong

(a) Strong Inducers: ≥80% decrease, (b) Moderate Inducers: 50-80% decrease, (c) Weak Inducers: 20-50% decrease in AUC of a substrate

(d) Strong inhibitor: >5-fold increase, (e) Moderate inhibitor: 2-5 fold increase, (f) Weak inhibitor: <2-fold increase in the AUC of a substrate

EM, extensive metabolizer; *IM*, intermediate metabolizer; *LA*, local anesthetics; *MAOI*, monoamine oxidase inhibitor; *PM*, poor metabolizer; *PPIs*, proton pump inhibitors; *SSRI*, selective serotonin reuptake inhibitor; *TCA*, tricyclic antidepressant; *UM*, ultrarapid metabolizer.

From U.S Food and Drug Administration. Drug development and drug interactions: table of substrates, inhibitors and inducers. http://www.fda.gov/Drugs/Development ApprovalProcess/DevelopmentResources/DrugInteractionsLabeling/ucm093664.htm#4; http://medicine.iupui.edu/clinpharm/ddis/clinical-table/.

TABLE 6.2	Developmental Genetics for Important Hepatic Enzymes in the Neonate and Clinical Consequences	
Enzymes	**Developmental Patterns**	**Clinical Consequences**
Uridine diphosphoglucuronyltransferase (UDP-GT) Substrates Morphine Acetaminophen Lorazepam	Ontogeny is isoform specific. In general, adult activity is achieved by 6-18 months of age.	Infants <3 months of age need lower morphine doses due to reduced clearance.[60]
Sulfotransferase Substrates Acetaminophen Dopamine	Ontogeny seems to be more rapid than UDP-GT; however, it is substrate specific. Activity for some isoforms may exceed adult values during infancy and childhood (e.g., that responsible for acetaminophen metabolism).	Higher APAP-sulfate formation in neonates provides "relative protection" from glucuronide formation deficiency.[61]
CYP1A2 Acetaminophen Caffeine	Not present to an appreciable extent in human fetal liver. Adult levels reached by 4 months of age and may be exceeded in children 1-2 years of age.	
CYP2C9	Not apparent in fetal liver. Inferential data using phenytoin disposition as a nonspecific pharmacologic probe suggest low activity during the first week of life, with adult activity reached by 6 months of age and peak activity reached by 3-4 years of age.	Large interpatient variability for ibuprofen effects is due to low levels of CYP2C9 in premature infants.[62]
CYP2C19	CYP2C19 activity can be detected by 8 weeks of gestation and remains unchanged throughout gestation and at birth. Over the first 5 months of postnatal age, CYP2C19 activity increases linearly. Adult activity is reached by 10 years of age.	Allelic variations of CYP2C19 produce PM phenotypes, which increase systemic exposure to PPI in neonates.[63] Diazepam half-life is prolonged in PM phenotype (CYP2C19 *2/*2, *3/*3, *2/*3), causing delayed emergence from anesthesia.[64]
CYP2D6	Low to absent in fetal liver but uniformly present at 1 week of postnatal age. Poor activity (~20% of adult values) at 1 months of postnatal age. Adult competence reached by 3-5 years of age. Metabolism inhibited by cimetidine.	All newborns (<2c weeks) are PM phenotypes, susceptible to drug toxicity, although genetic variability contributes more than ontogeny to variability at all ages.[65]
CYP3A4	CYP3A4 has low activity in the first month of life, with approach toward adult levels by 6-12 months postnatally	Clearance of midazolam affected: adults>full-term neonates>preterm neonates.[66] Cisapride accumulation in neonates due to inadequate metabolism might explain QTc prolongation on ECG due to cisapride.[67]
CYP3A7	CYP3A7 is functionally active in the fetus; ~30%-75% of adult levels of CYP3A4.	

APAP, acetaminophen; ECG, electrocardiogram; PM, poor metabolizer; PPI, proton pump inhibitor.
Adapted from Leeder JS, Kearns GL. Pharmacogenetics in pediatrics: implications for practice. Pediatr Clin North Am. 1997; 44:55–77.[53]

period that invalidate broad generalizations about neonatal drug metabolism. Developmental patterns and clinical consequences of relevant genes are summarized in Table 6.2.

Cytochrome P4501A2 (CYP1A2) accounts for much of the metabolism of caffeine (1,3,7-trimethylxanthine)[69,70] and theophylline (1,3-dimethylxanthine)[71,72]; these methylxanthines are frequently used to treat neonatal apnea and bradycardia. CYP1A2 activity is nearly absent in the fetal liver and remains minimal in the neonate.[73] This limits N-3- and N-7-demethylation of caffeine in the neonate. Renal clearance, the other method of elimination, is also immature[74] and elimination in preterm and term neonates is consequently poor[75,76]; these developmental issues hold important clinical implications for drug dosing and the timing between serial doses for the treatment of apnea of prematurity.[77-79] Adult levels of activity are reached between 4 and 6 months postnatally.[80,81] A similar pharmacokinetic pattern of reduced metabolism at birth occurs with theophylline in which CYP1A2 catalyzes N-3-demethylation and 8-hydroxylation.[71] Theophylline clearance reaches adult rates by 4 to 5 months, which coincides with the changes in CYP1A2 activity as reflected in urine metabolite patterns.[82]

Other P-450 enzymes that are reduced or absent in the fetus include CYP2D6 and CYP2C9.[66,83,84] CYP2D6 has minimal activity (<5% of adult activity) in the last trimester but matures quickly in the first month postnatally to 50% to 75% of adult values, with large interindividual variability. CYP2C9, which is responsible for the metabolism of nonsteroidal antiinflammatory drugs (NSAIDs), warfarin, and phenytoin, has minimal activity antenatally[83] but develops rapidly postnatally[59,85] from 21% of adult values immediately after birth to peak (adult) activity by 3 months, when expressed as milligrams per kilogram per hour.[86] CYP2E1 activity is minimal in utero, increasing by the third trimester, but surges within the first 24 hours postnatally and then increases steadily reaching adult activity levels by 1 year of age.[87] Infants younger than 90 days postnatal age have decreased expression of CYP2E1 activity in vitro and slower metabolism of substrates during this early infant period compared with older infants, children, and adults.[88]

CYP3A is the most important cytochrome involved in drug metabolism. It comprises the majority of adult human liver cytochrome P-450 (see Table 6.1) and metabolizes a broad range of drugs.[89] CYP3A is detectable during embryogenesis as early as

17 weeks, primarily in the form of *CYP3A7*,[73] and reaches 75% of adult activity by 30 weeks gestation.[66] It has been hypothesized that this is due to the potential protective role of *CYP3A7* in preventing retinoic acid–induced human embryotoxicity.[90] In vivo, *CYP3A* activity appears to be mature at birth[91]; however, there is a poorly understood postnatal transition from the fetal *CYP3A7* to the predominant adult isoform *CYP3A4*.[92,93]

CYP2D6 is involved in the metabolism of β-blockers, antiarrhythmics, antidepressants, antipsychotics, and codeine. It is either absent or less than 1% of adult values in the fetus[94] and is eventually expressed postnatally (see Table 6.1).[66,95] O-demethylation begins postnatally with rapid maturation of this enzyme system irrespective of the gestational age at birth, although activity may remain less than 25% of adult values at 5 years of age. Interestingly, CYP2D6 is a noninducible enzyme whose activity, however, may vary with certain disease states, including malignancy, cigarette smoking, and some chronic inflammatory diseases (rheumatoid arthritis).[96]

PHASE II REACTIONS

The other major route of drug metabolism, designated phase II reactions, involves synthetic or conjugation reactions that increase the hydrophilicity of molecules to facilitate renal elimination.[97,98] The phase II enzymes include glucuronosyltransferase, sulfotransferase, N-acetyltransferase, glutathione S-transferase, and methyl transferase. The phase II enzymes also show developmental changes during infancy that influence drug clearance (see Table 6.2).[44,99–101]

Most conjugation reactions have limited activity during fetal development.[102] One of the most familiar synthetic reactions in young infants involves conjugation by uridine diphosphoglucuronosyltransferases (UGTs). This enzyme system includes numerous isoforms and is also responsible for glucuronidation of endogenous compounds, such as bilirubin (*UGT1A1*).[102] As with the maturation of bilirubin conjugation, UGT activity is limited immediately postnatally and the different isoforms mature at different rates postnatally.[103] Dose adjustments are often needed to avoid toxicity in neonates from drugs that require conjugation by UGT for clearance. Experience with chloramphenicol in the 1960s illustrated this lesson when neonates received standard pediatric doses of chloramphenicol without understanding the immaturity of UGT and its role in the elimination of chloramphenicol. Infants accumulated high concentrations of chloramphenicol and developed fatal circulatory collapse, a condition known as the gray baby syndrome.[104,105] Although the clearance of chloramphenicol is low during the neonatal period, appropriate dosage adjustments and monitoring allow safe treatment of preterm and term infants with chloramphenicol.[106]

Morphine, acetaminophen (APAP), dexmedetomidine, and lorazepam are all cleared by glucuronide conjugation. The major steps in the metabolic disposition of morphine in children and adults are glucuronidation in the 3- and 6- positions.[107] The limited ability of neonates to glucuronidate morphine necessitates dosage adjustment.[108–110] Morphine clearance,[109,111] in particular 3- and 6-glucuronide formation, is limited at birth and increases with birth weight,[110] gestational age,[42] and postnatal age.[107,108] Morphine clearance, expressed per kilogram, approaches adult values by 1 month.[108,112] However, size models such as the per kilogram model confound interpretation and clearance does not reach adult values until at least 5 to 6 months when scaled using allometry (see Chapter 7).[109,113] Overall, the maturation of UGT enzymes varies among isoforms, but, in general, adult activity is reached within the first 2 years of life.[53] The time courses of maturation of drug metabolism for morphine,[114,115] APAP,[116] and glomerular filtration rate (GFR)[117] are strikingly similar (see Fig. 7.11) with 50% of size-adjusted adult values reached between 8 and 12 weeks after full-term delivery. Drugs cleared predominantly by UGT that convert the parent compound into a water-soluble metabolite excreted by the kidneys have clearance maturation profiles matching GFR maturation.

In contrast to glucuronosyltransferase, the sulfotransferase enzyme system is well developed in the neonate, and for some compounds it may compensate for limited glucuronidation. Thus, drugs like APAP, which undergoes primarily glucuronidation in the adult, also undergo sulfate conjugation in neonates. Hence, the half-life of APAP is only moderately prolonged in neonates compared with older infants and adults.[61,118,119] This occurs because of the increased volume of distribution of the drug in neonates, and as explained earlier, increased sulfation of the drug, leading to a greater percent of the dose excreted as the APAP-sulfate conjugate.[61,119–122] However, this does not confer safety from hepatotoxicity because the toxic metabolite is created through the oxidative pathway mediated by *CYP2E1*. This is detailed later in this chapter.

ALTERATIONS IN BIOTRANSFORMATION AT BIRTH

Transition from the intrauterine to the extrauterine environment is associated with major changes in blood flow. There may also be an environmental trigger for the expression of some metabolic enzyme activities, resulting in a slight increase in maturation rate above that predicted by postmenstrual age.[123,124] Many biotransformation reactions, especially those involving certain forms of cytochrome P-450, are inducible before birth through maternal drug exposure, cigarette smoke, or other inducing agents. Postnatal biotransformation reactions may also be induced through drug exposure or slowed by hypoxia/asphyxia, organ damage, and/or illness. The reduced thiopental clearance estimated from data when the drug was given to control neonatal seizures caused by hypoxic-ischemic insults may not be applicable to healthy neonates undergoing anesthesia.[125,126]

Genomics of Drug Metabolism, Exposure, and Effects

Genetic variations can have impact on both pharmacokinetics and pharmacodynamics. Single-nucleotide changes or polymorphisms (SNPs) in the DNA sequence in CYP enzymes usually decrease but may also increase metabolic activity for a specific drug or drug substrate.[13] Some of the explanations for variations in drug responses within large populations described as "biologic variation" likely relate to genetic differences in drug metabolism, receptor binding, and intracellular coupling to effector mechanisms. A genetic cause for individuals who were either fast or slow acetylators (N-acetyltransferase, NAT) of isoniazid was identified in the 1950s.[127] Pseudocholinesterase deficiency causing prolonged apnea after succinylcholine deficiency was identified around the same time, although a more obscure variant, the Cynthiana (C5) or Neitlich variant that possesses much more activity that the usual plasma cholinesterase, causes an extremely brief duration of action of succinylcholine.[10,128,129] After recognizing that certain individuals demonstrated exaggerated hypotensive responses to debrisoquine, the enzyme responsible for its metabolism, CYP2D6, was also one of the early drug-metabolizing enzyme deficiencies identified.[130–132]

TABLE 6.3 CYP2D6 Polymorphisms and Recommendations for Codeine Therapy

Likely Phenotype[a]	Activity Score[c]	Examples of Diplotypes	Implications for Codeine Metabolism	Recommendations for Codeine Therapy[b]	Classification of Recommendation for Codeine therapy	Considerations for Alternative Opioids
Ultrarapid metabolizer (~1%–2% of patients)	>2.0	*1/*1xN, *1/*2xN	Increased formation of morphine following codeine administration, leading to higher risk of toxicity	Avoid codeine use due to potential for toxicity.	Strong	Alternatives that are not affected by this CYP2D6 phenotype include morphine and nonopioid analgesics. Tramadol, and to a lesser extent hydrocodone and oxycodone, are not good alternatives because their metabolism is affected by CYP2D6 activity.
Extensive metabolizer (~77%–92% of patients)	1.0–2.0	*1/*1, *1/*2, *2/*2, *1/*41, *1/*4, *2/*5, *10/*10	Normal morphine formation	Use label-recommended age- or weight-specific dosing.	Strong	
Intermediate metabolizer (~2%–11% of patients)	0.5	*4/*10, *5/*41	Reduced morphine formation	Use label-recommended age- or weight-specific dosing. If no response, consider alternative analgesics such as morphine or a nonopioid.	Moderate	Monitor tramadol use for response.
Poor metabolizer (~5%–10% of patients)	0	*4/*4, *4/*5, *5/*5, *4/*6	Greatly reduced morphine formation following codeine administration, leading to insufficient pain relief	Avoid codeine use due to lack of efficacy.	Strong	Alternatives that are not affected by this CYP2D6 phenotype include morphine and nonopioid analgesics. Tramadol, and to a lesser extent hydrocodone and oxycodone, are not good alternatives because their metabolism is affected by CYP2D6 activity; these agents should be avoided

[a]Frequency estimates in Caucasians.
[b]Crews KR, Gaedigk A, Dunnenberger HM, et al. Clinical Pharmacogenetics Implementation Consortium guidelines for cytochrome P450 2D6 genotype and codeine therapy: 2014 update. *Clin Pharmacol Ther* 2014;95(4):376–382.
[c]Some investigators define patients with an activity score of 0.5 and 1.0 as intermediate metabolizers and define patients with an activity score of 1.5 and 2.0 as extensive metabolizers. Classifying patients with an activity score of 1.0 as extensive metabolizers in this guideline is based on data specific for formation of morphine from codeine in these patients. https://www.pharmgkb.org/guideline/PA166104996

Variability in the clinical response to codeine prompted investigations into genetic variants or polymorphisms of *CYP2D6*. This enzyme is mapped to chromosome 22 at 22q13.1. Fifty-five polymorphisms of *CYP2D6* have been described to date with a frequency that exceeds 1% of the population.[133] These include both functional and nonfunctional polymorphisms and gene duplication. The polymorphisms are numbered with *1 denoting the normal or wild allele (the * denotes an allele) (Table 6.3). The mutant alleles, *3, *4, *5, *6, and*9, for example, confer no CYP2D6 activity.[96,133,134] The latter polymorphisms account for more than 90% of the poor metabolizers (PM). Variants *2, *10, and *17 have modestly reduced activity and are referred as intermediate metabolizers (IM).[96] To further complicate the genetic pattern, multiple copies of the same genes[134] may be present in some individuals, resulting in bizarre phenotypes. The wide array of *CYP2D6* polymorphisms of codeine may be summarized into three broad categories: PM (negligible morphine produced [PM]), extensive metabolizers (normals [EM]), and ultra-extensive metabolizers (rapid and large amounts of morphine [UM]). Up to 10% of Caucasians and 30% of Hong Kong Chinese are PM, rendering codeine an ineffective analgesic in these children.[96]

Alternately, 29% of the Ethiopian and 1% of Swedish, German, and Chinese populations are UM, rendering codeine a dangerous analgesic as excessive doses of morphine may be rapidly produced after codeine is administered.[96] The frequency of *CYP2D6* polymorphisms, particularly in children who are PM, may be more common and more varied than previously thought. Earlier studies had shown that individuals might also possess normal or reduced metabolic activity (PM) for debrisoquine and sparteine.[132,135] The frequency of PM varied among ethnic groups, occurring in approximately 7% of Americans in the United States[45] and less than 1% of Chinese and Japanese.[136] The clinical relevance of *CYP2D6* polymorphisms on codeine metabolism are described later in this chapter. Allele frequencies in different races of the various relevant variants related to pharmacokinetics of anesthetic and analgesic drugs are given in Table 6.4.

Pharmacogenomics of Pain and Analgesia

One of the fundamental goals of a pediatric anesthesiologist is to have a comfortable patient in the postoperative period and beyond. Opioids remain the most commonly used medications

TABLE 6.4 Race and Allelic Frequencies of Common Variants Affecting Drug PK/PD

Genetic Variant and Population		EU TSI	North American/CEU	AA/ASW	North African MKK/YRI LWK	Hispanic/ MXL/MEX	ME	JPT	Asian/GIH	CHD CHB	Misc.
CYP2B6*6 516G>T, rs3745274 785A>G, rs2279343		0.284 0.214	0.27	0.298 0.462	0.366 0.421 0.33 0.455	0.284 0.273		0.204	0.421 0.188	0.17 0.19	
OPRM1 A118G		0.162	0.155	0.035	0.032 0 0.009	0.198		0.469	0.416	0.426 0.361	0.210 (Ash. Jews)
COMT Val158Met rs4680 G>A		0.451	0.478	0.272	0.271 0.313 0.294				0.395 0.526		
UGT2B7, 161C/T, 802C/T[a]		C 0.51 T 0.49	C 0.46, T 0.53	C 0.68 T 0.32				C 0.73 T 0.26	C 0.73 T 0.26		
ABCB1 C3435T[b]		0.466	0.534	0.188	0.152 0.117	0.460	0.37 0.38 0.26	0.478	0.597	0.417	
CYP2D6[c,d]	UM	0.08–0.1	0.043	0.049	0.29 (Oceania)	0.017	0.12–0.20			0.009	
	PM	0.01–0.09	0.077	0.019–0.073	0.018–0.19	0.022–0.066	0.032	0	0.018–0.048	<0.001	
CYP2C9*2[e]		0.13	0.015		0.016	0.057–0.07			0.024		
CYP2C19*2[e]		0.128	0.157		0.15	0.083–0.097			0.278		0.355 (AUS)
CYP3A5*3[f]		0.90			0.20				0.75		

Certain studies are region or population specific; the regions or populations are indicated in parentheses. Unless stated by references pertaining to the gene italicized in the left-hand column, the references for the frequencies noted in the table were obtained from www.pharmgkb.org (5/24/2016). Please note that since more than one reference has been used for some genetic variants, a range of frequencies has been reported. Also, the definitions of ethnic groups may not have been strictly the same among different studies.

AA, African Americans; Ash. Jews, Ashkenazi Jews; ASW, African ancestry in Southwest United States; AUS, Australia; CEU, Utah residents with Northern and Western European ancestry from the Centre d'Etude du Polymorphisme Humain (CEPH) collection; CHB, Han Chinese in Beijing, China; CHD, Chinese in Metropolitan Denver, Colorado; EM, extensive metabolizer; EU, European; GIH, Gujarati Indians in Houston, Texas; IM, intermediate metabolizer; JPT, Japanese in Tokyo, Japan; LWK, Luhya in Webuye, Kenya; ME, Middle East; MEX, Mexican; Misc., miscellaneous; MXL, Mexican ancestry in Los Angeles, California; MKK, Maasai in Kinyawa, Kenya; PM, poor metabolizer; UM, ultrarapid metabolizer; TSI, Toscani in Italia; YRI, Yoruba in Ibadan, Nigeria.

[a]Saito K, Moriya H, Sawaguchi T, et al. Haplotype analysis of UDP-glucuronocyltransferase 2B7 gene (UGT2B7) polymorphisms in healthy Japanese subjects. Clin Biochem. 2006;39(3):303–308.

[b]Ameyaw MM, Regateiro F, Li T, et al. MDR1 pharmacogenetics: frequency of the C3435T mutation in exon 26 is significantly influenced by ethnicity. Pharmacogenetics. 2001;11(3):217–221.

[c]Ingelman-Sundberg M, Sim SC, Gomez A, Rodriguez-Antona C. Influence of cytochrome P450 polymorphisms on drug therapies: pharmacogenetic, pharmacoepigenetic and clinical aspects. Pharmacol Ther. 2007;116(3):496–526.

[d]Bernard S, Neville KA, Nguyen AT, Flockhart DA. Interethnic differences in genetic polymorphisms of CYP2D6 in the U.S. population: clinical implications. Oncologist. 2006;11(2):126–135.

[e]Sistonen J, Fuselli S, Palo JU, et al. Pharmacogenetic variation at CYP2C9, CYP2C19, and CYP2D6 at global and microgeographic scales. Pharmacogenet Genomics. 2009;19(2):170–179.

[f]Rodriguez-Antona C, Sayi JG, Gustafsson LL, et al. Phenotype-genotype variability in the human CYP3A locus as assessed by the probe drug quinine and analyses of variant CYP3A4 alleles. Biochem Biophys Res Commun. 2005;338(1):299–305.

to provide analgesia in the perioperative period. However, safe and effective analgesia is still not achievable in about 50% of children[137,138] because of interindividual differences in pain perception and drug responses partly explained by PG.[139]

PAIN PERCEPTION AND GENETICS

Pain is both a subjective experience and a biopsychosocial phenomenon. It is well known that there is tremendous interindividual variability in pain responses, particularly in adolescents experiencing postoperative pain. Animal studies have identified genetic markers in more than 400 genes that affect nociception; these are presented in the Pain Genes Database, an interactive web browser of pain-related transgenic knockout studies.[140]

Neurotransmitters such as catecholamines (epinephrine, norepinephrine, and dopamine) are vital components in the pain perception pathway. Catecholaminergic neurons in the solitary nucleus integrate visceral and somatic sensory information when inflammation is present peripherally.[141,142] One of the genes that affect this pathway is catechol-O-methyltransferase (COMT) that codes for the enzyme COMT involved in degradation of catecholamines. Decreased COMT activity increases catecholamines and leads to increased pain. Four common SNPs (rs6269, rs4633, rs4818, and rs4680) are involved. SNP rs4680 is coded by 472G>A, which causes the substitution of valine by methionine at amino acid position 158 (Val158Met). These four SNPs define low pain sensitivity (LPS: GCCG$_{val}$), average pain sensitivity (APS: ATCA$_{met}$), and high pain sensitivity (HPS: ACCG$_{val}$) haplotypes.[143,144] The presence of these haplotypes was shown to cause differences in mRNA structure, enzymatic activity, and protein levels in cells expressing COMT.[145] The LPS haplotype exhibited the highest enzymatic activity, whereas the HPS haplotype exhibited the lowest enzymatic activity and protein levels in cells expressing COMT. Variations within COMT are associated with experimental pain responses to heat, cold, pressure, and mechanical stimuli. In addition, the COMT genotype is predictive of chronic pain in fibromyalgia, temporomandibular joint disorder,[143] and postsurgical pain.[146] Although there have been conflicting reports of Val/Val genotypes requiring larger doses of morphine in cancer patients[147] compared with Met/Met's larger pain ratings in experimental studies,[148] it is possible that population differences, haplotype differences, and other gene interactions might contribute to these contradictory observations. In a pediatric study involving 149 children undergoing tonsillectomy, associations of COMT SNPs (rs6269, rs4633, rs4818, and rs4680) and haplotypes with maximum pain scores and morphine consumption were studied. In addition to haplotype differences in morphine requirement, the authors found that minor allele carriers of COMT SNPs were approximately three times more likely to require analgesic interventions than homozygotes of major alleles.[68]

The metabolism of phenylalanine and the synthesis of serotonin, dopamine, epinephrine, norepinephrine, and nitric oxide (NO) are reliant on adequate cellular levels of tetrahydrobiopterin (BH4), an essential cofactor of enzymes involved in their synthesis (hydroxylases and NO synthases). GTP cyclohydroxylase 1 (GCH1), the rate-limiting enzyme responsible for the synthesis of BH4, is regulated by gene GCH1. GCH1 transcription is induced in the presence of inflammatory markers and nerve injury, leading to increased BH4 production and increased NO production; NO sensitizes transient receptor potential vanilloid subfamily type 1 (TRPV1) and subfamily ankyrin repeats type 1 (TRPA1), causing increased calcium influx into the neuron and increased pain responses.[149] Concomitantly, loss-of-function haplotype

defined by 3 polymorphisms (rs8007267G<A, rs3783641A<T, and rs10483639C<G) was associated with decreased GCH1 activity in vitro and with pain protection in experimental pain models in volunteers[150] and in patients undergoing diskectomy for persistent radicular low back pain.[151] There have been negative association studies since, but whether the association is spurious or dependent on the effect size is not clear because of multiple confounding variables.

Combinatorial genetics likely contribute to a greater extent than single genes in predicting variability. In 201 Caucasians undergoing abdominal surgery, the authors tested associations among morphine consumption, postoperative pain, and SNPs within opioid receptor μ-1 (OPRM1), COMT, uridine-5′diphosphate glucose-glucuronosyltransferase-2B7 (UGT2B7, and estrogen receptor (ESR1) gene loci to elucidate genetic predictors of opioid consumption. Age and 9 SNPs in ESR1, OPRM1, and COMT explained the greatest proportion of variance of morphine consumption (10.7%; P = 0.001). Three SNPs in ESR1, OPRM1, and COMT explained 5% of the variance (P = 0.007). There was also an interaction between rs4680 in COMT and rs4986936 in ESR1 (P = 0.007) on opioid consumption.[152]

There are also some congenital conditions that lead to insensitivity to pain, caused by pathogenic mutations in genes such as the neurotrophic tyrosine kinase receptor type 1 gene (NTRK1) and nerve growth factor-β (NGFB) with an anhidrosis phenotype.[153] Various mutations of the sodium channel voltage-gated type IX, alpha subunit SCN9A gene leading to nonfunctional alpha subunits of NaV1.7 channels inhibit the generation and transmission of nerve signals, leading to pain insensitivity along with anosmia.[75] For a comprehensive overview of PG and pain, please refer to review articles beyond the scope of this chapter.[139,154]

Genetic Variations Affecting Opioid Pharmacokinetics

Pharmacogenetics affecting enzyme activity have been shown to affect both drug exposure and effect, leading to either decreased effectiveness or increased toxic effects of the drug. The U.S. Food and Drug administration (FDA) has issued warnings and guidelines for pharmacogenetics pertaining to the effects of some drugs used in pediatric anesthesia practice.

CODEINE

Codeine is a weak opioid endorsed by the World Health Organization as the second step on the analgesic ladder for cancer pain and has been used routinely for postoperative and breakthrough pain in chronic sufferers. It is a prodrug with a 200-fold weaker affinity for μ-opioid receptors than morphine. Although 80% of the administered drug is inactivated by glucuronidation to codeine-6-glucuronide by UGT2B7 and N-demethylation to norcodeine by CYP3A4, 5% to 10% of codeine undergoes O-demethylation to morphine, its active form via CYP2D6[155] (Fig. 6.1) Without O-demethylation, codeine confers a small fraction of the analgesic potency of morphine, and much of its analgesic effect is likely contributed by a metabolite, codeine 6-glucuronide.[156]

A small proportion of the population (ranging from 2%-10% in different ethnic groups) are CYP2D6 PM and thus have limited analgesia with codeine.[76,157] Alternative analgesics should be sought in children who are PM.

Recently, the safety and efficacy of codeine in children who are UM have been called into question. The frequency of UM

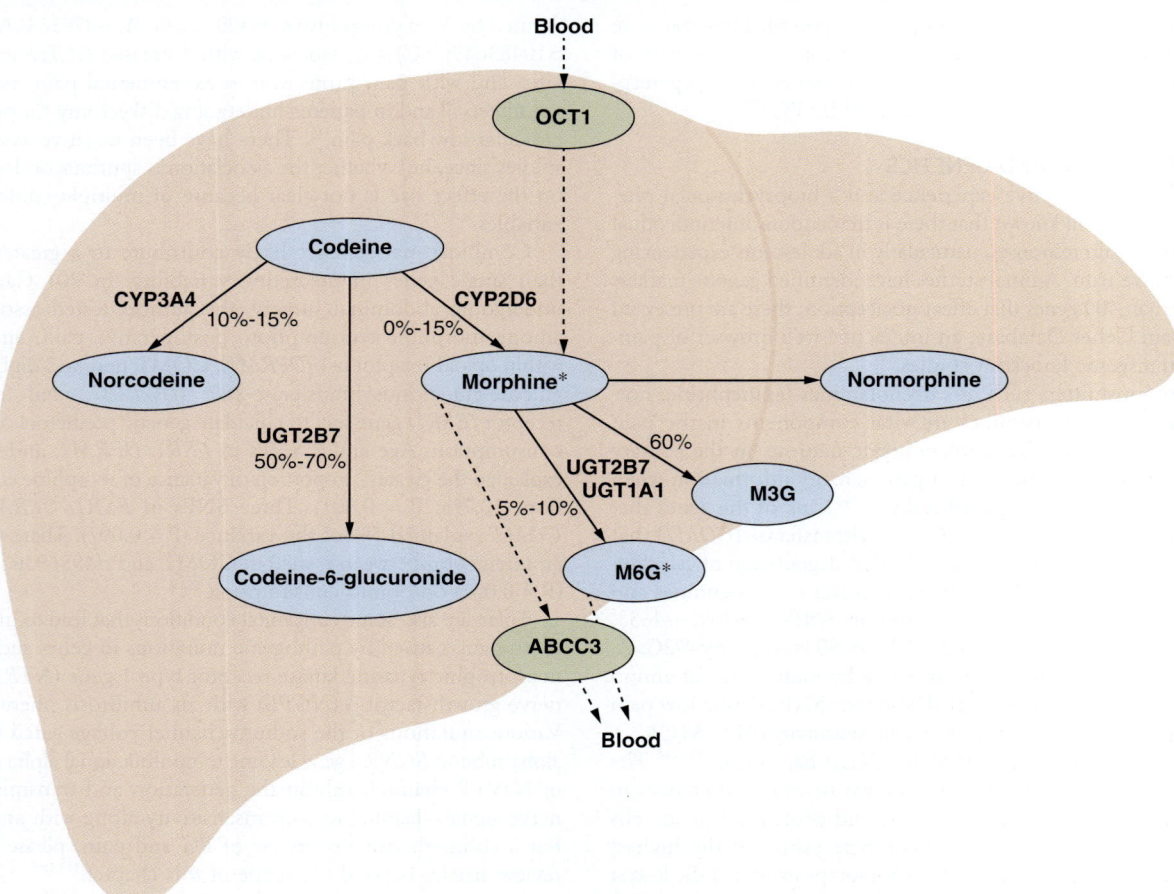

FIGURE 6.1 Diagrammatic presentation of the candidate genes involved in the pharmacokinetic pathway of codeine and morphine in the liver. Codeine, a prodrug is converted to active form* morphine primarily by cytochrome (*CYP2D6*). Approximately 50% to 70% of codeine is converted to codeine-6-glucuronide by uridine glucuronosyl-transferase (*UGT2B7*); 10% to 15% of codeine is *N*-demethylated to norcodeine by cytochrome P450 enzyme (*CYP3A4*). Both these metabolites have a similar affinity to codeine for the μ-opioid receptor. Between 0% and 15% of codeine is *O*-demethylated to morphine by *CYP2D6*, the most active metabolite*, which has 200-fold greater affinity for the μ-opioid receptor compared with codeine. Morphine is mainly (60%) glucuronidated to morphine-3-glucuronide (M3G), while 5% to 10% is glucuronidated to morphine-6-glucuronide (M6G) primarily by *UGT2B7*, and to a lesser extent, *UGT1A1*. M6G is the active metabolite with a higher affinity for the μ-opioid receptor. *OCT1* is a hepatic transporter responsible for transporting morphine from blood into liver cells. *ABCC3* is a hepatic efflux transporter and it transports morphine and morphine glucuronides from liver cells into blood.

genotypes is substantive from 1% in Denmark and Finland, 10% in Greece and Portugal, and 29% in Ethiopia.[158] Children with *CYP2D6* polymorphisms who also have upregulated opioid receptors as a result of chronic intermittent nocturnal hypoxia (obstructive sleep apnea) may be particularly vulnerable to a mishap after regular codeine use.[159] Consequently, the wide clinical response to a standard (or less than standard) dose of codeine necessitates careful monitoring in those with compromised cardiorespiratory status. Several deaths or near-deaths have been reported with "standard" doses of oral codeine in children later found to be UM.[160,161] A fatality after codeine administration was reported in a healthy 2-year-old boy given weight-appropriate codeine doses after adenotonsillectomy; he died on the second postoperative day. Increased blood concentrations of morphine (32 ng/mL) and reduced codeine concentrations (0.70 ng/mL) were found. Genotyping revealed functional duplication of the *CYP2D6* allele.[160] This was followed by further reports[162,163] that ultimately led to new

regulations by the FDA, European Medicines Agency, and the U.K. Medicines and Healthcare Products Regulatory Agency. Restrictions were placed on pediatric use, and some centers have removed codeine from their formularies.[164] The 2012 Clinical Pharmacogenetics Implementation Consortium (CPIC) guidelines for *CYP2D6* genotype and codeine therapy were updated in 2014.[165] This guideline recommends using alternative analgesics to codeine in patients who are *CYP2D6* PM or UM (see Table 6.2). A new *boxed warning*, the FDA's strongest warning, was added to the drug label of codeine-containing products about the risk of codeine in postoperative pain management in children. The warning specifies that *"Health care professionals should prescribe an alternate analgesic for post-operative pain control in children who are undergoing tonsillectomy and/or adenoidectomy. Codeine should not be used for pain in children following these procedures"* (http://www.fda.gov/Drugs/DrugSafety/ucm339112.htm). It should be noted that these same concerns apply to children requiring analgesia for greater than one day

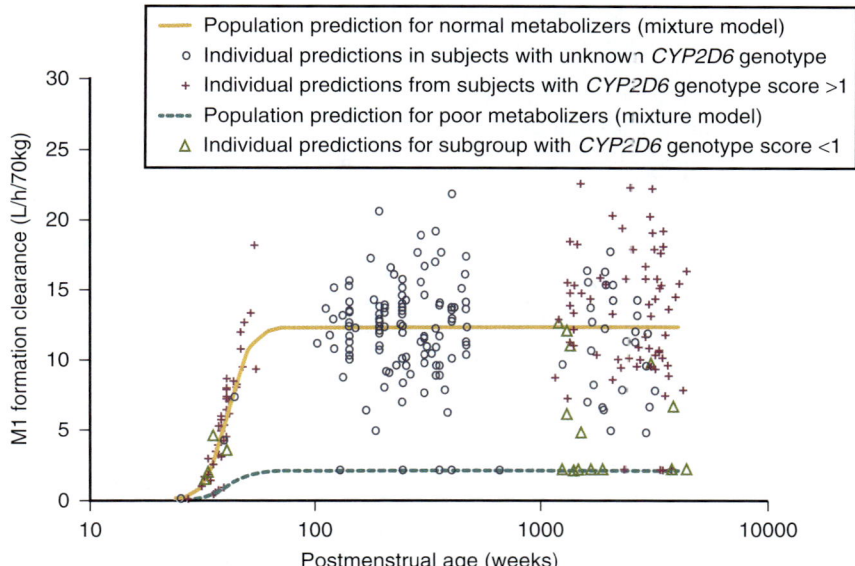

FIGURE 6.2 Maturation of tramadol formation clearance (CLPM) to O-desmethyl tramadol (M1 metabolite) labeled according to the availability of an individual *CYP2D6* genotype activity score. There is a distinct group of patients who are poor metabolizers identified by the phenotype *(dashed line)*. Not all subjects with a low genotype *CYP2D6* activity (n = 20) are included in this poor metabolizer group. (From Allegaert K, Holford NHG, Anderson BJ, et al. Tramadol and o-desmethyl tramadol clearance maturation and disposition in humans: a pooled pharmacokinetic study. *Clin Parmacokinet.* 2015;54(2):167–178. Used with permission from Springer.)

regardless of the surgical procedure, particularly obese children who may have obstructive sleep apnea (see also Chapter 33).

There are also safety concerns for breastfed babies whose mothers take codeine for pain relief. This was highlighted in 2006 with the report of death in a breastfed infant after codeine was administered to the mother; she was an UM of codeine and analysis of her breast milk revealed a very large blood concentration of morphine, 87 ng/mL.[166] Hence, the safest advice is to avoid codeine whenever possible as it is unlikely that the *CYP2D6* activity for any individual will be known; those with high levels of activity may suffer from toxicity, while those with low levels will suffer unnecessary pain. Others have taken a more active posture by identifying the 2D6 isoforms in their patients—in this case, children with sickle cell disease—and determined which patients would benefit from or suffer from codeine administration for chronic pain.[167] Although pharmacokinetic studies show increased conversion of codeine to morphine in *CYP2D6* UM versus EM,[168] it is important to remember that because of hitherto unknown factors, there is substantial variability within patients genotyped as EM, some of whom may have UM phenotypes.[162]

TRAMADOL

Tramadol is a weak opioid agonist metabolized by many pathways, including *CYP2D6*-mediated oxidation to *O*-desmethyltramadol, which has a 200-fold greater affinity for μ-opioid receptors than the parent drug.[169] Tramadol exerts its analgesic activity through complementary mechanisms: activating the μ-opioid receptor mainly by *O*-desmethyltramadol and weak inhibition of norepinephrine and serotonin reuptake (mainly tramadol). For children who are *CYP2D6* PM, both the plasma concentrations for the active metabolite and analgesia are less than with the EM, whereas for those who are 2D6 UM, both the plasma concentrations and analgesia and side effects are greater than in those who are EM.[170-172]

However, as with codeine, genotype may not predict phenotype in all individuals. Not all subjects who are genotype *CYP2D6 PM* (n = 20) have slow clearance of its active metabolite (Fig. 6.2)[173]

HYDROCODONE

Hydrocodone is metabolized by *CYP2D6* to hydromorphone, which has 10- to 33-fold greater affinity for opioid receptors than hydrocodone. While pharmacokinetic studies have shown that the peak concentrations of hydromorphone in PM are less, there is no conclusive clinical evidence of *CYP2D6* genotype on its effects.[174,175]

OXYCODONE

Oxycodone is a semisynthetic opiate agonist; about 11% of the drug is *O*-demethylated by *CYP2D6* to the active metabolite oxymorphone, which has a 40-fold greater affinity and 8-fold greater opioid potency compared with oxycodone itself. The remaining 89% of the drug is *N*-demethylated by *CYP3A* to noroxycodone, a metabolite with weak antinociceptive properties. Both metabolites, oxymorphone and noroxycodone, are further degraded to noroxymorphone by *CYP2D6* and *CYP3A*.[176] The greatest oxymorphone/oxycodone concentration ratios occur in UM and the smallest occur in PM. The noroxycodone/oxycodone ratio and daily oxycodone escalation rate are greater in cancer patients with the *CYP3A5*3/*3* genotype.[177] Although postoperative analgesic requirement is less in UM,[178,179] other studies in postsurgical patients and cancer patients detect clinical differences among the genotypes.[180,181]

MORPHINE

Approximately 60% of morphine is glucuronidated to morphine-3-glucuronide (M3G). Only 5% to 10% is glucuronidated to morphine-6-glucuronide (M6G), principally by *UGT2B7* in the liver, and in part, by *UGT1A1* and *UGT1A8*.[182] M6G is an active metabolite, with slower onset and more prolonged duration of action compared with morphine.[183] It is uncertain whether *UGT2B7* variants affect morphine PKPD. *UGT2B7*-840G allele and the -161 C>T SNP are associated with reduced glucuronidation of morphine,[184,185] although other studies refuted this finding. There was no correlation between 12 SNPs of *UGT2B7* and the morphine glucuronide/morphine serum ratios among 175 patients with normal hepatic and renal function who received long-term oral morphine therapy.[186]

In vitro studies have suggested that morphine has low transporter-independent permeability and 60% of total hepatic uptake is transporter dependent. Hence, there is an interest in the genetics of various hepatic transporters known to play a significant role in the disposition of morphine and its metabolites based on in vitro studies and mice.[182,187–192] *OCT1*, a member of the organic cation transporters (OCT), is predominantly expressed in the sinusoidal membrane of the human liver and mediates cellular uptake of morphine into hepatocytes (see Fig. 6.1). Approximately 10% of Caucasians are compound homozygous carriers of one of the four common coding polymorphisms for *OCT1* (Arg61Cys, Gly401Ser, Gly465Arg, and deletion of Met420) that result in reduced or lost *OCT1* transporter activity and greater plasma concentrations of morphine.[193] *OCT1* genotypes play a significant role in IV morphine clearance in children undergoing tonsillectomy.[194] Morphine clearance in homozygotes of loss-of-function *OCT1* variants (*OCT1*2–*5/*2–*5*) was reduced (20%) compared with the wild type (*OCT1*1/*1*) and heterozygotes (*OCT1*1/*2–*5*).[194] The relatively common allelic frequencies of defective *OCT1* variants among Caucasians may explain their reduced morphine clearance and possibly greater frequencies of adverse events compared with African American children.

Another transporter belonging to the ATP-binding cassette (ABC) subfamily, *ABCC3*, is expressed in the basolateral membranes of hepatocytes and is an efflux transporter of M3G and M6G from the hepatocyte into the bloodstream (see Fig. 6.1). *ABCC3* SNP -211T (rs4793665) is located in the promoter region of the gene and has been reported to alter hepatic mRNA expression[195] and contribute to reduced efflux of morphine glucuronides.[196] In children undergoing tonsillectomy, in addition to the effects of polymorphisms of *OCT1* genotype on morphine pharmacokinetics, the C/C polymorphisms of *ABCC3* -211C>T significantly increased the transformation of morphine-6-glucuronide and morphine-3-glucuronide by ~40% compared with the C/T+T/T genotypes.[197] Similarly, in 316 children undergoing tonsillectomy, *ABCC3* variants rs4148412 (A allele) and rs729923 (allele G) caused a 2.36 (95% confidence interval [CI] = 1.28-4.37, P = 0.0061) and 3.7 (95% CI 1.47-9.09, P = 0.005) times increased odds ratio of morphine-induced respiratory depression, leading to prolonged postoperative care unit stay. These clinical associations were supported by increased formation clearance of morphine glucuronides in children with rs4148412 AA and rs4973665 CC genotypes in this cohort, as well as an independent spine surgical cohort of 67 adolescents.[198] Homozygotes with the 3435C>T variant of another ABC efflux transporter of morphine, *ABCB1*, expressed large cerebrospinal fluid concentrations of morphine. This efflux transporter is responsible for removing unwanted medications and toxins from the central nervous system and gastrointestinal tract. The *ABCB1* 3435 C>T allele is linked to greater analgesia with morphine in cancer-related pain and reduced morphine requirements in mixed chronic pain population.[199,200] Following tonsillectomy, children with GG and GA genotypes of

ABCB1 polymorphism rs9282564 have been shown to have fourfold higher risks of respiratory depression, resulting in prolonged hospital stays.[201]

METHADONE

Methadone is primarily cleared by hepatic *CYP2B6* to its inactive metabolite. Of the many variants of the very polymorphic gene *CYP2B6*, one of the most common and clinically significant variant allele is *CYP2B6*6* (516G>T, Q172H; 785A>G, K262R), which markedly reduces *CYP2B6* expression and activity.[202] Concomitantly, S-methadone concentrations were greater in *CYP2B6*6* homozygotes compared with heterozygotes and noncarriers, and these *CYP2B6*6* patients had reduced dose requirements.[203,204] In fact, genetic influence is found to be greater for oral than IV methadone and S- than R-methadone.[205]

Genetic Variations Affecting Opioid Pharmacodynamics

Genetic modulation of the density of opioid receptors, affinity, or coupling affects the variability in the intersubject responses to opioids. In a study of 121 adult twin pairs who were randomly assigned to receive alfentanil or placebo, there was significant heritability for respiratory depression (30%), nausea (59%), and drug disliking (36%), as well as significant familial effects for sedation (29%), pruritus (38%), dizziness (32%), and drug liking (26%) after alfentanil administration.[206,207]

OPIOID RECEPTOR (*OPRM1*)

This gene, located on chromosome 6q24-q25, is a member of the G protein–coupled receptor family and of major interest as it codes for the μ-opioid receptor, a molecular binding site of all clinically effective opioids and endogenous opioid peptides like β-endorphin.[208] It is widely distributed throughout the nervous system (periaqueductal grey area, in the substantia gelatinosa area in dorsal horn of the spinal cord, in the olfactory bulb, the cerebral cortex, the amygdala) as well as the gastrointestinal tract. This gene mediates opioid-induced analgesia and adverse effects including respiratory depression, and constipation. One of the most commonly studied SNPs of *OPRM1* is A118G (rs1799971), in which guanine (G) is substituted for an adenine (A) at base 118, which in turn causes the amino acid exchange at position 40 of the μ-opioid receptor protein from asparagine to aspartic acid (N40D), that leads to the loss of an *N*-glycosylation site in the extracellular region of the receptor.[209] The allele frequency shows a racial bias; it is greater in the Asian population (50%) than in Caucasians (10.5%–18.8%) and African Americans (5%–15%).[210]

In vitro studies have shown reduced cell-surface receptor binding site availability for morphine in cells expressing the G variant compared with the A variant, less efficient agonist-induced receptor signaling in postmortem human brain tissue in 118G carriers, and 1.5- to 2.5-fold increased mRNA expression in 118A human brain cells compared with the G variant.[211–213] An in vivo study investigating the effects of A118G genotype on μ-opioid receptor binding potential in human brains using carfentanil positron emission tomography, found that smokers homozygous with the wild-type AA genotype exhibited significantly greater levels of receptor binding potential than smokers carrying the G allele in the bilateral amygdala, left thalamus, and left anterior cingulate cortex.[214] In contrast, the variant receptor had a threefold greater binding affinity for endogenous β-endorphins with potentially different connotations for pain sensitivity but not analgesic response to opioids.[215]

In accordance with the mechanistic findings mentioned previously, several studies in adults have shown that the opioid requirements (morphine, M6G, fentanyl, and alfentanil) were greater and the adverse effects such as nausea less in postoperative patients and volunteers with the GG/AG genotypes compared with those with the AA genotypes at the A118G SNP.[216–223] In postsurgical Asian adult patients undergoing knee arthroplasty, hysterectomy, and cesarean section,[216,217,221] carriers of the G allele had greater pain scores and greater morphine requirements than those with the AA genotypes. In a prospective genotype-blinded study of 88 healthy adolescents undergoing spine fusion for idiopathic scoliosis, the risk of morphine-induced respiratory depression in patients with the AA genotype was greater (odds ratio 5.6, 95% CI = 1.4–37.2, P = 0.03) compared with the AG/GG genotypes.[224] Similar results in human volunteers found a two to four times greater dose of alfentanil to produce the same level of analgesia as the wild type, and a 10- to 12-fold greater dose for the same level of respiratory depression in the homozygous 118GG volunteers.[225] However, no association was found for the A118G effects on morphine-6-glucuronide–induced respiratory depression (measured by the isocapnic acute hypoxic ventilatory response) and PONV after fentanyl.[222,226] A meta-analysis of the OPRM1 A118G effects concluded that the evidence that homozygous GG carriers of A118G exhibited slightly greater opioid requirements and slightly less nausea was weak.[227]

In addition to the rs1799971 (A118G) variant, a novel C-T variant (rs563649) has been identified in the 5′ untranslated region of the spliced isoform MOR1K that is preferentially expressed in the medulla oblongata.[228] This variant had the strongest single contribution to measured pain sensitivity responses in 196 pain-free European and American females. The C-T variant is located within a structurally conserved internal ribosome entry site upstream of exon 13 and affects both mRNA levels and translation efficiency of MOR1K isoforms. Strong linkage disequilibrium was identified between rs563649 and rs1799971, and the minor T allele of rs563649 tagged a 6-SNP (AGTCTG) haplotype associated with great pain sensitivity. Haplotype combinations rather than single variants may be a better predictor of OPRM1 effects.

BLOOD-BRAIN BARRIER TRANSPORTER (*ABCB1*)

P-glycoprotein (P-gp), a surface phosphoglycoprotein encoded by *ABCB1* and a member of the superfamily of ABC transporters, is an ATP-dependent drug efflux transporter. P-gp is expressed on the epithelial surface at the intestinal lumen, biliary canaliculi, renal proximal tubule, and in the choroid plexus as the blood-brain barrier (BBB). Morphine, fentanyl, methadone, sufentanil, alfentanil, morphine-6-glucuronide, and loperamide are all confirmed P-gp substrates.[188,229–232] Variations in the *ABCB1* efflux transporter at the BBB can significantly alter cerebral penetration and pharmacokinetics of opioids.[233] The most commonly studied variants in the coding region of *ABCB1* are c.1236C>T (rs1128503), c.2677G>T/A (rs2032582), and c.3435C>T (rs1045642) and these are in strong linkage disequilibrium.[234] *ABCB1* genotypes 1236 TT, 2677TT, and 3435TT, together with the 1236TT genotype alone, were associated with early and profound respiratory suppression in adults given intravenous (IV) fentanyl during spinal anesthesia.[235,236] The homozygous diplotype (GG-CC at c.2677G>T/A and c.3435C>T) were shown to have borderline association with morphine-associated postoperative nausea or vomiting (PONV)[234]; however, in another report of adults treated

with morphine, a combined effect of 3435T of *ABCB1* and 80A of *OPRM1* was associated with increased pain relief but had no influence on the incidence of adverse effects.[199]

Another SNP that has been studied is *rs9282564,* a nonsynonymous polymorphism with a threefold greater maximum velocity for adenosine triphosphatase activity compared with the wild type.[237] Children with GG and GA genotypes of *ABCB1* rs9282564 have a greater risk for respiratory depression after tonsillectomy, resulting in prolonged PACU stays. Each additional copy of the minor allele (G) of the *ABCB1* SNP, rs9282564, increased the odds of respiratory depression that resulted in a 4.7-fold (95% CI: 2.1-10.8) greater duration of stay in PACU. This variant allele had also been reported to have a modest effect in reducing the trough levels of methadone.[238] Haplotypes of SNPs at positions 61, 1199, 1236, 2677, and 3435 influenced methadone requirements in opioid-dependent and nondependent patients, but they did not predict opioid dependence.[239] However, others have reported contradictory results that there was no association between *ABCB1* polymorphisms and the trough plasma concentrations, methadone dose, or methadone response.[240]

OPIOID-CANNABINOID SYSTEM INTERACTIONS

Fatty acid amide hydrolase (*FAAH*), opioid and cannabinoid systems reciprocally and synergistically, modulate functions at multiple levels. *FAAH* codes for an enzyme that hydrolyzes anandamide, the "bliss" molecule. Inhibition of *FAAH* increases the bioavailability of anandamide and thereby augments analgesia; this offers a potential therapeutic target for treating pain.[241,242] Five specific *FAAH* SNPs, including a missense variant (rs324420) that affects *FAAH* stability, were reported to be associated with more than twofold greater risk for refractory PONV in children undergoing tonsillectomy.[243]

Genes of Addiction

There is a genetic component to addiction, and variations of particular genes can predispose to addiction. This is especially relevant in adolescence and early adulthood, which is the prime time when these addictions happen. It is believed that 40% to 60% of the risk is genetic, regardless of the drug of addiction.[244] There were 34.2 million people in the United States (age ≥12 years) in 2011 who had used an opioid for nonmedical use sometime in their lives, and approximately 13% of high school seniors reported using prescription opioids such as oxycodone and hydrocodone.[245,246] A precursor to addiction is opioid exposure, including prescription opioids, and family history suggests genetic vulnerability for opioid use disorder.[247] A meta-analysis of 5-hydroxytryptamine (serotonin) 2A receptor gene (*HTR2A*) genotypes at SNPs rs6313 and rs6311 from available genetic association studies from different populations showed their contribution to genetic susceptibility to substance use disorders, especially alcohol dependence.[248] Certain variants of the glutamate receptor, the NMDA 2A (*GRIN2A*) gene that encodes the 2A subunit of the NMDA receptor, were shown to be involved in the development of heroin addiction.[249] Likewise, the dopamine D1 receptor (*DRD1*), which modulates opioid reinforcement, reward, and opioid-induced neuroadaptation, and the μ-1 opioid receptor gene (*OPRM1*), a target of opioids, also had variants that predicted opioid dependence or protection thereof, in association studies.[250] The A118G SNP of the *OPRM1* gene is the most studied and has been associated with phenotypes including opioid dependence and other substance dependencies.[251,252]

Nonsteroidal Antiinflammatory Drugs and Genetics

NSAIDs act by inhibiting cyclooxygenase enzymes (COX-1 and COX-2) coded for by the prostaglandin endoperoxide synthase genes, *PTGS I* and *II*. Commonly used NSAIDs such as ibuprofen and diclofenac undergo phase 1 detoxification (*CYP2C9* for S(+)-ibuprofen; *CYP2C8* for R(-)-ibuprofen; *CYP2C9* and *CYP3A4* for diclofenac)[253,254] followed by glucuronidation (mainly *UGT2B7*).[255] Multidrug resistance-associated proteins 2 (*MRP2/ABCC2*) and breast cancer resistance protein (*BCRP/ABCG2*) affect biliary excretion of diclofenac glucuronides, and *MRP3/ABCC3* was the main efflux transporter from liver to blood.[256] Dubin-Johnson syndrome is caused by acquired or hereditary deficiency of *ABCC2*, leading to increased concentration of bilirubin glucuronides.[257] As diclofenac shares the same *ABCC2* transporter pathway, it should be prescribed to those individuals with caution to avoid adverse reactions to diclofenac, particularly hepatotoxicity.[258]

There are two frequent allelic variants for *CYP2C9-CYP2C9*2* (430C>T Arg144Cys) and *CYP2C9*3* (1075A>C Ile359Leu) that decrease the activity in a number of in vitro and in vivo studies. *CYP2C9*2*, *3, and *CYP2C8*3* allelic variants reduce ibuprofen metabolism and/or clearance.[259] However, *CYP2C8*3* is in strong linkage disequilibrium with the *CYP2C9*2* variant, making it difficult to distinguish whether the effects are due to *CYP2C8* or *CYP2C9*. Investigations into the association between *CYP2C9* and *CYP2C8* polymorphisms and response to ibuprofen therapy for patent ductus arteriosus closure in extremely preterm neonates showed that greater gestational age and non-Caucasian ethnicity were associated with ibuprofen response, but not the *CYP2C* polymorphism.[260] Gastroduodenal bleeding was strongly associated with *CYP2C9*3* carriers as opposed to noncarriers (adjusted odds ratio 7.3) in adults given NSAIDs, including diclofenac, ibuprofen, celecoxib, and naproxen.[261] These findings were reproduced by some[262] but not by others.[263]

Ketorolac, another nonselective COX inhibitor, is safe for use in neonates.[264] Nonetheless, in children (unlike adults), ketorolac does not significantly penetrate cerebrospinal fluid. The transporter gene, *MDR-1*, has been implicated in drug transport across the BBB.[265] Moreover, animal studies have shown developmental differences in COX-1 expression in the spinal cord, likely explaining the lack of analgesic efficacy of ketorolac in 3 day-old compared with 21-day-old pups[266] and 2-week-old compared with 4-week-old rats.[267] The authors extrapolated that *"should similar deficits occur in humans, COX-1 inhibitors may exhibit reduced efficacy in infants."*[267] However, this lack of effectiveness was not observed in clinical studies of ketorolac in neonates, in whom analgesia was achieved in 94.4%.[264]

Selective COX-2 inhibitors produce less inhibition of COX-1 and are expected to have short-term gastrointestinal safety benefits, although, their long-term benefits are inconclusive.[268] COX-2 mRNA and protein expression are increased in the presence of gastric mucosal lesions, suggesting that they may be involved in the repair process of those lesions.[269] Thus selective COX-2 inhibition might disturb the COX-2 enzyme–mediated protective prostaglandin production.

Celecoxib, a COX-2 inhibitor metabolized by *CYP2C9*, has been investigated for *CYP2C9* variant effects on its pharmacokinetics. In a study in volunteers, those with the *CYP2C9*1/*3* and *CYP2C9*3/*3* variants experienced a greater concentration exposure (2-fold and 7.7-fold, respectively) and maximum concentration (1.5-fold and 1.8-fold, respectively) and a reduced clearance (2.3-fold and 10-fold, respectively) than those with the *CYP2C9*1/*1* variant.[270] A case report described severe drug-induced gastropathy in an IM of the *CYP2C9* gene, presumably resulting from prolonged drug exposure.[271] Children given celecoxib who had the genotype *CYP2C9*3* had less pain and improved functional recovery after tonsillectomy.[272] Celecoxib is currently on the FDA biomarker list, cautioning use in *CYP2C9* PM (dose reduction by 50% or alternate medication).

Acetaminophen and Genetics

APAP is primarily converted to two pharmacologically inactive conjugates: glucuronide (52%–57%) and sulfate (30%–44%), with a minor fraction undergoing oxidation to a reactive metabolite N-acetyl-p-benzoquinoneimine NAPQI (5%–10%).[273] *UGT1A1*, *UGT1A6*, *UGT1A9*, and *UGT2B15* are involved in APAP glucuronidation,[274] whereas a family of cytosolic enzymes, called *sulfotransferases* (*SULT*), are involved in the APAP sulfation (*SULT1A1*, *SULT1A3*).[275] APAP is bioactivated to the reactive intermediate (NAPQI)[276] by three CYP-450 isoforms: *CYP3A4*, *CYP2E1*, and *CYP1A2* of which *CYP2E1* is the most important. The contribution of *CYP3A4* to the production of NAPQI is controversial.[277,278] NAPQI is then conjugated with the sulfhydryl group of glutathione to form a nontoxic conjugate. APAP overdoses initially saturate sulfation, followed by glucuronidation; increased NAPQI production depletes glutathione stores, leading the NAPQI to bind to intracellular hepatic macromolecules to produce cell necrosis and damage.

Infants younger than 90 days postnatal age express less *CYP2E1* activity in vitro compared with older infants, children, and adults,[88] *CYP3A4* appears during the first week after birth, whereas *CYP1A2* appears later.[279] *CYP3A4* and *CYP1A2* activity in 12- to 48-month-old children exceeds that of all other stages of development and could potentially increase NAPQI production in 1- to 4-year-olds,[280] but this is favorably offset by an increased capacity to conjugate the drug with sulfate in this same age group. Nonetheless, two 10-fold overdoses of APAP and two reports of multiple doses from multiple caregivers who were unaware of the other doses[281] have been reported in infants and underscore the need for extreme care when administering and documenting IV acetaminophen.[282] Both infants with the massive APAP overdoses recovered fully.

UGT1A polymorphism c.2042C>G (rs8330) is associated with increased human liver APAP glucuronidation, an increased *UGT1A* exon 5a/5b splice variant/mRNA ratio, and decreased risk of unintentional APAP-induced acute liver failure.[283] Individuals carrying the *CYP3A5* rs776746 A allele were overrepresented among patients with acute liver failure who had intentionally overdosed with APAP with an odds ratio of 2.3 (95% CI = 1.1- 4.9, P = 0.034), although this was not significant after adjusting for multiple comparison testing.[284]

Chronic Pain, Persistent Postoperative Pain, and Genetics

Acute pain thresholds, in contrast to chronic pain levels, are less genetically determined (with estimated heritability scores of 22%–55%).[285] Chronic pain conditions of the neck and back pain in monozygotic versus dizygotic twins showed a heritable component of up to 60%.[286] Imbalances in β₂-adrenergic receptor *(ADRβ2)* function increase the vulnerability to chronic pain conditions.[287] An association between a potassium channel modulatory subunit (KCNS1, also called Kv9.1) polymorphism and pain phenotype was identified in five of six independent chronic pain cohorts (including post–limb amputation and postmastectomy pain). The *KCNS1* allele missense rs734784 is one of the first described prognostic indicators of chronic neuropathic pain risk.[288]

Dramatically altered gene expression is also found in patients who subsequently develop persistent postoperative pain, with at least 10% of the transcriptome being dysregulated in traumatic injury models of neuropathic pain. These mechanisms involve sensitization of peripheral nociceptors (transient receptor potential, *TRPA1/TRPV1*),[289,290] central signaling systems affecting dorsal horn plasticity (for example, brainderived neurotrophic factor, *BDNF*),[291] and neuroimmune mechanisms including proinflammatory mediators (*interleukins, IL-6*, tumor necrosis factor *TNF*).[292] In chronic pain conditions such as inflammatory bowel disease, abdominal pain has been associated with increased capsaicin receptor *TRPV1* expressing sensory fibers in colonic biopsies.[293] The gene *BDNF*, a member of the neurotrophin family, also increased expression in colonic mucosa, along with structural alterations, suggesting contributions to the visceral hyperalgesia seen in these patients.[294] Systems that affect the distribution of δ- and μ-opioid receptors (*OPRM1*) also control heat pain, mechanical pain, opioid effects, and nerve injury–induced mechanical hypersensitivity.[295,296] Voltage-gated calcium channels control trafficking/pain conduction from the dorsal root ganglion to the presynaptic terminals at the dorsal horn[297] (*CACNA1A*), leading to hyperalgesia and allodynia, probably resulting from increased calcium-dependent release of pronociceptive neurotransmitters such as glutamate and substance P. Epigenetic effects on pain are illustrated by an epigenome study in identical twins, which showed the role of the *TRPA1* promoter in pain sensitivity,[298] association of *COMT* methylation with socioeconomic status,[299] and DNA demethylation at specific CpG sites in the *IL1B* promoter in response to inflammation.[300]

Pharmacogenomics Affecting Anesthesia

Genetics influence both the pharmacokinetics and pharmacodynamics of some agents commonly used in pediatric anesthesia, and hence could affect perioperative outcomes.

INTRAVENOUS ANESTHETICS

Propofol

The main enzyme that metabolizes propofol in hepatic as well as renal cortical microsomes is *UGT1A9* (53%), with secondary contribution from hydroxylation (38%), mainly through the *CYP2B6 and CYP2C9* in the liver.[301] Infants younger than 10 months have only 10% and at 1.3 years they have about 50% of adult CYP2B6 activity levels.[302] Very little is known about the developmental changes in *UGT1A9*. However, there is a 100-fold interindividual variability in activity of these enzymes throughout life. Propofol clearance varies more than 300% in the neonatal period with genetics thought to exert a greater influence on its clearance than age.[124,303] SNPs of *UGT1A9* affect glucuronidation: 2152C>T, -440C>T, -331T>C, -275T>A, and 98T>C.[304] In vitro studies of UGT1A9 expression from DNA isolated from Japanese volunteers showed that transversion of 766G>A in the *UGT1A9* gene that results in the substitution of amino acid D256N affected propofol glucuronidation kinetics.[305]

Propofol exerts its hypnotic actions by activation of the central inhibitory neurotransmitter GABA-A controlled by the *GABRE* gene.[306] Adverse effects of propofol have been described, including a rare but life-threatening complication called propofol infusion syndrome,[307] but it is not clear if genetic factors play a role. Although investigators report the time to loss of verbal contact and a bispectral index less than 70 varied 6.6- and 4.3-fold, respectively; after propofol induction in adults, there was 15.5- to 111-fold variability in the time to emergence, and the clearance of propofol varied greatly. However, there were no associations between variations in *CYP2B6* (R487C, K262R, and Q172) variants or *GABRE* variants (mRNA358G/T, 20118C/T, 20326C/T, and 20502A/T) and the observed interindividual variability in response.[308] To date, there is no conclusive evidence of PG variations affecting clinical outcomes with propofol anesthesia.

Dexmedetomidine is metabolized extensively in the liver by glucuronidation (*UGT1A4, UGT2B10*)[309,310] and hydroxylation, mediated by *CYP2A6*.[311] There is high interindividual variability in response to dexmedetomidine,[312] for which the role of CYP2A6 SNPs was evaluated for their effect on clearance. However, the studies concluded that CYP2A6 variants studied did not alter dexmedetomidine pharmacokinetics.[313,314] The sedative and anxiolytic effects of dexmedetomidine are mediated by subtypes of the α₂-adrenergic receptors, mainly by α-2A (*ADRA-2A*). Since receptor sensitivity would be expected to affect dexmetomidine pharmacodynamics, variants affecting *ADRA2A* have been studied. The effects of *ADRA2A* C1291G polymorphism on dexmedetomidine response were studied in 110 patients undergoing coronary artery bypass grafting. It was found that those with the G allele were less sedated than those with the C allele.[315] Similarly, certain SNPs were also found to be associated with statistically significant interindividual differences in blood pressure changes.[316]

INHALATIONAL ANESTHETICS

Inhalational anesthetics act through a different site on the *GABAA* receptor. Preschool-age children with the AA genotype in the *GABAγ2* nucleotide position 3145 in intron A/G exhibited a greater incidence of emergence agitation, compared with the non-AA genotype, after sevoflurane anesthesia.[317] The human melanocortin-1 receptor (*MC1R*) gene is expressed on the surface of melanocytes and affects melanin biosynthesis and pigmentation. Sex specificity in response to κ-opioid agonists has been demonstrated in both mice and humans. Women with two variant *MC1R* alleles displayed significantly greater analgesia from the κ-opioid, pentazocine, than all other groups.[318] Women with three particular mutations of the *MC1R* gene (R151C, R160W, and D294H) had increased desflurane anesthetic requirements.[319] Moreover, those with inactive variants had a particular phenotype of red hair and pale skin, lending credence to the perception of altered anesthetic and analgesic requirements in redheads. They are metabolized primarily by *CYP2E1* in the liver to varying degrees.[320] Although the tendency of halothane hepatitis to cluster in families points to a genetic contribution, the hereditary mechanisms involved have not been defined.[133]

Nitrous Oxide

The effects of genetic variants on nitrous oxide action are related to its inhibitory actions on methionine synthesis whose activated form, S-adenosylmethionine, is the principal substrate involved in the formation of the myelin sheath, neurotransmitters, and DNA synthesis in rapidly proliferating tissues. We know that nitrous oxide irreversibly oxidizes the cobalt atom of vitamin B₁₂, thereby inhibiting the activity of the cobalt-dependent enzyme methionine synthase, which is the catalyst for the formation of methionine. Hence, in a patient who has a deleterious mutation in the 5,10-methylenetetrahydrofolate reductase (MTHFR) gene, exposure to nitrous oxide can lead to neurologic deterioration. This occurred in a male infant whose neurologic status unexpectedly deteriorated; the infant died after two exposures to nitrous oxide for lumbar puncture.[321] Postmortem analysis showed 5,10-methylenetetrahydrofolate reductase deficiency in this infant's fibroblasts and a complex combination of mutations in his MTHFR gene, including C677T and A1298C SNPs associated with a reduction in the enzyme activity. Patients who were homozygote for these variants developed greater plasma concentrations of homocysteine after nitrous oxide anesthesia.[322] Although mitigated by B vitamin infusions, this was not found to be related to an increase in perioperative troponin.[323]

BENZODIAZEPINES

Midazolam exerts its primary effects by reversible interactions with the inhibitor GABA receptor in the central nervous system. It is primarily metabolized by the *CYP3A4/CYP3A5* enzymes in the liver to its hydroxyl derivatives. Hepatic CYP3A4 activity is reduced in neonatal versus adult livers, resulting in reduced midazolam clearance in the former.[324] Midazolam is metabolized mainly by hepatic hydroxylation (*CYP3A4*), followed by glucuronidation of the hydroxymetabolites.[325] *CYP3A7* is the dominant CYP3A enzyme in utero; it is expressed in the fetal liver and appears to have activity from as early as 50 to 60 days after conception. There appears to be a temporal switch in the immediate perinatal period and *CYP3A4* expression increases dramatically after the first postnatal week. Hepatic *CYP3A4* activity begins to dramatically increase at about 1 week of age, reaching 30% to 40% of adult expression by 1 month.[83] Drugs/foods that may interfere with the cytochrome isoforms that metabolize midazolam (*CYP3A4*) include grapefruit juice, erythromycin, calcium channel blockers, and protease inhibitors.[326–329] The net effect is to prolong the duration of action of midazolam.

Diazepam, which is mainly metabolized by the CYP2C19 enzyme[330] to desmethyldiazepam, acts by binding to a specific subunit on the GABAA receptor.[331] CYP2C19 polymorphisms found to affect diazepam clearance and emergence from general anesthesia in Japanese patients were classified as follows: no variants, *1/*1 (EM); one variant, *1/*2 or *1/*3 (intermediate metabolizers [IM]); and two variants, *2/*2, *2/*3 or *3/*3 (PM).[64] The presence of a SNP (G681A) of the CYP2C19 gene was found to be associated with impaired metabolism of diazepam in a gene-dosage effect manner (fourfold greater half-life in homozygotes and twofold greater half-life in heterozygotes carrying the SNP) in Chinese patients.[332] The human GABA-A receptor α-4 subunit is a unique diazepam-insensitive binding site, and it is hypothesized that variations at this site might explain differences in diazepam sensitivity among individuals.[333] A Pro385Ser (1236C>T) amino acid substitution in the human GABA-A α-6 subunit has also been found to play a role in benzodiazepine sensitivity.[334]

NEUROMUSCULAR BLOCKING DRUGS

Pseudocholinesterase deficiency and malignant hyperthermia are pharmacogenetic disorders recognized in the 1960s; the latter is discussed elsewhere (see Chapter 41). Butyrylcholinesterase (BChE) or pseudocholinesterase is the enzyme that hydrolyzes neuromuscular blocking agents such as succinylcholine and mivacurium, as well as ester local anesthetic agents. Deficient activity of the enzyme leads to prolonged apnea from succinylcholine and is caused by several factors, including genetic variants that affect the function of the enzyme.[335] More than 30 variants of the gene (BChE, 3q26.1-q26.3) have been described of which the two most common are the A (atypical) (209A>G, Asp70Gly) and the K (Kalow) variants (1615G>A, Ala539Thr).[336] The homozygosity incidence for the A variant is 3 : 1000 in Caucasians but may be as great as 1 : 175 individuals in some ethnicities in Iraq, Iran, and South India.[337,338] The BChE activity is decreased by 70% in A homozygotes and about 30% in the K homozygotes. Duration of apnea after 1.0 to 1.5 mg/kg of succinylcholine increases from 5 to 10 minutes in homozygous normal to 10 to 20, 20 to 35, and 35 to 60 minutes in heterozygous one abnormal gene, heterozygous two abnormal gene, and homozygous abnormal gene accordingly (see also Chapter 7).[339]

LOCAL ANESTHETICS

The effect of pseudocholinesterases on ester local anesthetics (LA) are less relevant in modern anesthesia. The more commonly used amide LAs, lidocaine and bupivacaine, are metabolized by *CYP3A4*; ropivacaine metabolized by *CYP1A2*. *CYP1A2* is not fully matured before age 3 years, and *CYP3A4* is not mature at birth, with the predominant fetal enzyme being *CYP3A7*. These developmental delays may explain increased risk for toxicity of amide LA in infants younger than 6 months of age.[340] Local anesthetics are sodium channel blockers; hence genetic mutations within the *sodium channel gene* are likely to cause variable binding and efficacy for these drugs. In vitro experiments have shown that the N395K mutation in the *SCN9A* gene attenuates the inhibitory effect of lidocaine on the Nav1.7 channels and produces greater resistance to lidocaine.[341] One case report indicated that bupivacaine induced electrocardiographic and arrhythmic manifestations of the Brugada syndrome in silent carriers of a cardiac sodium channel SCN5A missense mutation, leading to a reduction in sodium current by whole-cell patch-clamping analysis.[342] Lidocaine also acts on vanilloid receptors belonging to the *TRPA1* and *TRPV1* family on sensory neurons, whereby calcitonin gene-related peptide (CGRP), a vasodilatory and nociceptive transmitter, is released.[343,344] A point mutation induced at residue R701 of *TRPV1* led to diminished lidocaine sensitivity in mice.[344] Similar to inhalation anesthesia, *MC1R* variants (phenotypes with red hair) have been found to be more sensitive to thermal pain with reduced subcutaneous lidocaine effectiveness.[345]

Perioperative Outcomes

POSTOPERATIVE NAUSEA AND VOMITING

A genome-wide association study on motion sickness in 80,494 individuals concluded that 35 SNPs involved in balance, glucose homeostasis, and other nervous system roles played an important part in motion sickness and likely, PONV as well.[346] In addition, correlations have been reported between A2A2 alleles at the dopamine D2 receptor (*DRD2*) (Taq1A SNP)[347,348] as well as rs2165870 SNP in the promoter region of the M3 muscarinic acetylcholine receptor (*CHRM3*) gene with PONV.[349] *CYP2D6* is the enzyme that metabolizes commonly used agents for PONV, such as the 5-HT$_3$ receptor antagonists (ondansetron, palonosetron, and dolasetron), which are less effective in *CYP2D6* UM. The incidence of vomiting (and hence ondansetron failure) in women undergoing surgery with three *CYP2D6* copies was significantly greater compared with those with two copies, but not from those with one copy. When analyzed by genotype, the incidence of vomiting in PM, IM, EM, and UM were 8%, 17%, 15%, and 45%, respectively (P < 0.01).[350] Only granisetron is primarily metabolized by *CYP3A4* and may have a better effect in *CYP2D6* UM patients.[351] Although palonosetron is metabolized by 2D6, its duration of action is independent of its clearance because it binds allosterically and exhibits positive cooperativity with the 5-HT₃ receptor, deforming the conformational structure of the receptor, which takes 36 to 48 hours to return to normal.

PERIOPERATIVE BLEEDING

Postoperative bleeding after cardiac surgery has been associated with SNPs of coagulation proteins and platelet glycoproteins (GPIaIIa-52C>T and 807C>T, GPIb alpha 524C>T, tissue factor -603A>G, prothrombin 20210G>A, tissue factor pathway inhibitor-399C>T, and angiotensin-converting enzyme [ACE] deletion/insertion).[352] Plasminogen activator inhibitor 1 (PAI-1) attenuates the conversion of plasminogen to plasmin, and the use of plasminolytic inhibitors may be subject to PAI-1 variants. In a study that evaluated the effectiveness of tranexamic acid (TXA) for reducing postoperative chest tube blood loss in adults undergoing cardiac bypass, patients with plasminogen activator inhibitor-1 5G/5G homozygotes who did not receive TXA showed more postoperative bleeding than those with other *PAI-1* genotypes. Those with 5G/5G homozygotes who received TXA showed the greatest blood-sparing benefit.[353]

HEMODYNAMIC RESPONSE

The β2-adrenergic (β2-ADR) receptor is a member of the 7-transmembrane domain family of receptors which is encoded by a gene located on chromosome 5 (β2-ADR, 5q31-q32). The β2-adrenergic receptor controls vascular and bronchial smooth muscle tone, and hence controls both response to bronchodilators and may contribute to vasopressor responses after laryngoscopy[354,355] and regional anesthesia. While nine β2-ADR variants have been described,[356] the most extensively studied are the Arg16Gly and the Gln27Glu variants, which are in linkage disequilibrium. Mechanistically, it appears that 16Gly variants have enhanced agonist-induced β-ADR downregulation, while the Arg16 genotype shows complete absence of downregulation,[357] which implies that Arg16 and Gln27 homozygotes will be more sensitive to β₂-agonist effects. In accordance, blood pressure variability after neuraxial anesthesia was found to be predicted by variant Arg16Arg (less hypotension)[358] and Glu27 (more hypotension)[359] in two different studies. Similarly, phenylephrine dose was increased by 200 μg in women with the Arg16 homozygous genotype compared with those with the Gly16 homozygous genotype while undergoing cesarean delivery under spinal anesthesia.[360] A detailed review of the *β2-ADR* gene can be found elsewhere.[361]

EFFECT ON OTHER PERIOPERATIVE OUTCOMES

Genetic risk factors have been identified for perioperative cardiac ischemia and arrhythmias,[362] as well as neurologic outcomes such as cognitive dysfunction/stroke,[363] which are beyond the scope of this chapter. Readers are referred to a review on perioperative outcomes for further elaboration.[6] There is a potential mechanistic pathway for perioperative cardiac ischemia and stroke influenced by inflammatory superseded thrombosis-related genes. Associations between specific genetic variants and perioperative

renal compromise,[364] protection against sepsis,[365] inflammatory response, and graft rejection after heart and lung transplants[366] have also been described.

Ancestry/Race and Genetics

The "Out of Africa" theory of human migration advocates for a common origin of human races.[367] The definitions of "race" defined by physical characteristics and "ethnicity" based on sociocultural factors are complicated by genetic admixture and interracial mating.[368] Consequently, genetic studies often use ancestry information markers (AIMs), which are a set of haploid makers (mitochondrial DNA or Y-chromosome haplotypes) or multiple unlinked autosomal markers that are diploid, that exhibit substantially different frequencies between populations from different geographic regions as a basis for race. An ideal AIM should have one allele that is fixed (i.e., allele frequency of 1.0) in one ancestral population and not present in the other,[369] but since the level of genetic variation between human populations is only 5% to 10%, there are challenges with genetic ancestry inference.[370]

The influence of race and ethnicity exists in frequency distribution of polymorphisms of genes encoding drug-metabolizing enzymes, transporters, and receptors.[371] As mentioned earlier, examples are the ethnic differences of pharmacokinetic enzymes such as CYP2D6; UM phenotypes, which are more prevalent among Sub-Saharan populations and low among Caucasians; and in *OPRM1*, where the frequency of the A118G allele is estimated to be much higher in the Asian (46%) compared with European and African American populations (5% to 25%).[210] African American children clear morphine more rapidly than their Caucasian counterparts, which is likely due to differences in allele frequencies for *OCT1* variants.[194,372]

Race has been associated with an unequal burden of perioperative pain and opioid adverse effects in children. Caucasian children had less postoperative pain and more opioid-related adverse effects postoperatively despite reduced opioid doses after tonsillectomy.[372] African American and Hispanic patients also have reduced tolerance for experimentally induced pain compared with Caucasians.[373,374] In another cohort of children who had tonsillectomies, ethnicity affected morphine-induced outcomes; children of Latin ethnicity had more adverse effects from morphine compared with those of non-Latin ethnicity. No genetic variants examined contributed to these differences.[375] While most studies have focused on Caucasian and African American group differences, some studies have reported reduced pain tolerance in Asian Americans compared with non-Hispanic whites.[376] These findings assume importance as race can affect differential treatment of groups, and while this will lead to individualization, it can also lead to overtreatment or undertreatment if it is unclear whether the differences are genetic versus based on race.

Racial disparities are reported in the prescription of opioid analgesics for management of postoperative pain.[377] African Americans and Hispanic Americans were prescribed fewer analgesics than their non-Hispanic white counterparts; these two groups also took their analgesics less frequently than prescribed and experienced limited pain relief from analgesic medications.[378] This has been contradicted by other studies showing decreased opioid requirements and higher sensitivity in African Americans.[379] The effects of race and ethnicity may be medication-specific and affected by numerous contextual factors and should be interpreted with care.[380]

Pharmacogenomics Methods

COMMON GENOTYPING METHODS

There are many options for genotyping. The most commonly used for anesthesia and pain-related pharmacogenetic research and clinical practice are the candidate gene approach and SNPs testing. Other more comprehensive and expensive genotyping include genome-wide association study (GWAS) platforms with 500,000 to 5 million SNPs, whole-exome sequencing (WES), and whole-genome sequencing (WGS) with different depth of coverages. In the past decade, the overall the cost of genotyping has decreased significantly. With the whole-exome and whole-genome sequencing approaches, large amounts of genetic data are typically generated per patient; analyzing and associating any clinical outcome or condition would require a large sample size and complex and robust analytical methods.

COMMON LIMITATIONS OF GENETIC RESEARCH STUDIES AND INTERPRETATION OF GENETIC STUDIES

Interpretation of genetic studies is often limited by study inadequacies (e.g., lack of adequate sample sizes needed to analyze multiple genes or polymorphisms), mostly owing to the expense of genetic testing and population stratification for different racial and ethnic backgrounds. Moreover, publication bias; the winner's curse; statistical and bioinformatics analytical challenges in adjusting for gene and environmental interactions; the lack of reproducibility of results in independent and external cohorts; and the inability to validate genetic associations with mechanistic studies also lead to inadequate proof for clinical implementation of genetic information in clinical care to personalize interventions and care. In addition to genetic risk factors, other factors may influence clinical outcome measures. Thus pharmacogenetic studies also need to be complemented by epigenetic, proteomic, transcriptomic, and metabolomic information to gain additional knowledge and insight to improving personalized care.

CURRENT COSTS OF GENOTYPING AND THIRD-PARTY COVERAGE FOR GENOTYPING

Currently, access to preoperative genotyping, robust evidence to change clinical practice based on underlying genetic risk factors, affordability, and payer coverage for genetic testing are limited. As compelling evidence for personalization of perioperative care based on genetic risk factors (e.g., *CYP2D6* and codeine-related deaths, *RYR1* and malignant hyperthermia) increases, there will be better adaptability of routine preoperative genotyping and coverage of such services by third-party payers. For example, many third party-payers are covering perioperative *CYP2D6* genotyping for prescription of oral opioids in our pediatric institution.

Genetic Counseling

Another ethical fallout of pharmacogenomic research, especially in pediatrics, is the need for genetic counseling. Findings need to be conveyed to children and parents. Assistance with interpretation of incidental findings from secondary analyses may be required. Genetic counselors help patients and their families understand and adapt to the medical, psychological, and familial implications of genetic contributions to clinical outcomes and/or disease, and need to be an integral part of such research efforts. Genetic counseling has been provided traditionally for single-gene conditions (e.g., malignant hyperthermia and *RYR1* gene). As we transition from single-gene testing and genetic counseling to a full genomic medicine approach, clinical implications will get more complex for most of health care professionals.[381] One potential solution would be development of clinical outcome or disease-related multigenic clinical decision support algorithms for more effectively helping patients and health care professionals.

Clinical Translation: Bench to Bedside: Where Are We Now?

As we routinely use the global positioning system to navigate maps and roads, in the future, it is anticipated that we will use a genomic prescribing system (GPS) to proactively identify underlying genetic risks and guide personalized care.[382] Proactive identification of patients at risk of adverse perioperative outcomes is an important first step in guiding personalized interventions, preferably with electronic health record (EHR)-implemented clinical decision support integrating genetic risk factors and their implications for clinical interventions.

To implement pharmacogenomics-based clinical decision support, there is a need for more robust study designs, independent validations, larger study populations, and robust statistical approaches.[383,384] To realize the promise of personalized medicine to perioperative care, we need better evidence in terms of validating clinical association studies engaging physicians, patients, the pharmaceutical industry, health care, payers, and policy makers.

In the field of perioperative pain management and opioid responses, polymorphisms of genes involved in pain pathways (*COMT*[68]), morphine's pharmacokinetics (*OCT1*[194]), ABC B1 and C3 genes (*ABCB1*[201] and *ABCC3*[194,197,198,385]), and pharmacodynamics[139,165,386–390] (*FAAH*[391]), and opioid μ-receptor 1 (*OPRM1*[224]) play a major role in determining postoperative clinical and economic outcomes. These genetic risk factors relevant to opioid pharmacogenetics and surgical pain management have translational promise to improve clinical practice and outcomes. Since genetic association studies do not explain causality, additional research to identify biologic and mechanistic pathways would be needed for better insight to risk stratification and targeted interventions influencing the mechanistic pathways.

Conclusion

Pharmacogenetics pertaining to anesthesia is still an evolving field with exciting prospects in the future, so that anesthesia and analgesia can be individualized using a reactive rather than "trial and approach" strategy. It is important to realize that genetics needs to be combined with other factors to make an individualized approach comprehensive. Completion of the Human Genome Project, as well as rapidly accumulating data in this field from knock-in and knock-out genetic animal models, laboratory-based cell line experiments, and human studies poses a huge challenge in the understanding, education, and interpretation of results and applicability. An average proteomic experiment, for example, might generate 10,000 to 1,000,000 individual data points, with countless potential interactions between data points. Hence, a few web-enabled resources may be worth mentioning, especially given the daily updates that happen with current publications (Table 6.5).

The ultimate goal of pharmacogenetics research is clinical translation. Examples of translational potential include the proposed genomic prescribing system to guide therapy,[382] the genotype-based dosing of opioids based on *OPRM1*, *COMT*, and *MC1R*,[392,393]

TABLE 6.5	Online Resources for Current Pharmacogenomics Information
Online Resource	**Description and Uses**
The Pharmacogenomics Knowledgebase www.pharmgkb.org	A comprehensive resource that curates knowledge about the impact of genetic variation on drug response for clinicians and researchers. This knowledge base can be searched by gene, drug or clinical phenotype, and provides in-depth information about pharmacogenomics, curated publications to clinical implementation guidelines.
Encyclopedia of DNA Elements (ENCODE) Consortium www.encodeproject.org	Provides a comprehensive parts list of functional elements in the human genome, including elements that act at the protein and RNA levels, and regulatory elements that control cells and circumstances in which a gene is active.
Genotype-Tissue Expression (GTEx) project www.gtexportal.org	This project provides the scientific community a resource with which to study human gene expression and regulation and its relationship to genetic variation. This project collects and analyzes multiple human tissues from donors for this purpose. By analyzing global RNA expression within individual tissues and treating the expression levels of genes as quantitative traits, variations in gene expression that are highly correlated with genetic variation can be identified as expression quantitative trait loci (eQTLs).

and genetic risk signatures for opioid-induced respiratory depression.[389] The Electronic Medical Records and Genomics (eMERGE) Network, announced in September 2007, is a National Institutes of Health –organized and –funded consortium of U.S. medical research made up of nine institutions with unique and valuable pioneer experience using a variety of commercial and homegrown EHRs. The challenges and solutions for integrating genomic data into the EHR, creation of integrated genomic decision support, and the human and electronic processes, including standards required for such successful integration, are still a work in progress.[394,395]

In conclusion, the future of precision medicine was aptly described and emphasized by President Barack Obama in his State of the Union address on January 20, 2015: "*I want the country that eliminated polio and mapped the human genome to lead a new era of medicine—one that delivers the right treatment at the right time.*"[396]

ANNOTATED REFERENCES

Andrzejowski P, Carroll W. Codeine in paediatrics: pharmacology, prescribing and controversies. *Arch Dis Child Educ Pract Ed*. 2016;101(3): 148-151.
This article highlights the safety and efficacy aspects of codeine use in children, a very contemporary and important topic. The authors discuss the developmental pharmacology, pharmacokinetics, pharmacodynamics, and pharmacogenetics of codeine in children, how this relates to prescribing, as well as the practical issues and the recent regulatory framework surrounding its use.

Chidambaran V, Mavi J, Esslinger H, et al. Association of OPRM1 A118G variant with risk of morphine-induced respiratory depression following spine fusion in adolescents. *Pharmacogenomics J*. 2015;15(3):255-262.
This article is the first clinical study to show that the opioid receptor polymorphism A118G influences susceptibility to morphine-induced respiratory depression in children.

Chidambaran V, Venkatasubramanian R, Zhang X, et al. ABCC3 genetic variants are associated with postoperative morphine-induced respiratory depression and morphine pharmacokinetics in children. *Pharmacogenomics J*. 2017;17(2):162-169.
This article presents the first study to report association of ABCC3 variants with both morphine pharmacodynamics (opioid-related respiratory depression) and morphine pharmacokinetics (metabolite formation) in two independent surgical cohorts.

Crews KR, Gaedigk A, Dunnenberger HM, et al. Clinical Pharmacogenetics Implementation Consortium guidelines for cytochrome P450 2D6 genotype and codeine therapy: 2014 update. *Clin Pharmacol Ther*. 2014;95(4):376-382.
This article summarizes the evidence from the literature supporting the association of CYP2D6 activity and polymorphisms, provides therapeutic recommendations for codeine based on the CYP2D6 genotype, and includes essential guidelines for prescribing pediatric providers.

Sadhasivam S, Chidambaran V, Zhang X, et al. Opioid-induced respiratory depression: ABCB1 transporter pharmacogenetics. *Pharmacogenomics J*. 2015;15(2):119-126.
This article shows that ABCB1 polymorphisms may affect blood-brain barrier transport of morphine, and therefore individual response to its central analgesic and adverse effects in postsurgical children.

A complete reference list can be found online at ExpertConsult.com.

7 Pharmacokinetics and Pharmacology of Drugs Used in Children

BRIAN J. ANDERSON, JERROLD LERMAN, AND CHARLES J. COTÉ

Hydrocodone	Dexmedetomidine
Methadone	Chloral Hydrate
Fentanyl	**Antihistamines**
Alfentanil	Diphenhydramine
Sufentanil	Cimetidine, Ranitidine, and Famotidine
Remifentanil	**Antiemetics**
Butorphanol and Nalbuphine	Metoclopramide
Codeine	5-Hydroxytryptamine Type 3–Receptor Antagonists
Tramadol	Neurokinin 1 and Other Antiemetics
Tapentadal	**Anticholinergics**
Acetaminophen	Atropine and Scopolamine
Nonsteroidal Antiinflammatory Agents	Glycopyrrolate
Ketorolac	**Antagonists**
Benzodiazepine Sedatives	Naloxone
Midazolam	Naltrexone
Diazepam	Methylnaltrexone
Other Sedatives	Flumazenil
Clonidine	Physostigmine

THE PHARMACOKINETICS AND PHARMACODYNAMICS of most medications in children, especially neonates, differ from those in adults.[1] Children exhibit different pharmacokinetics (PK) and pharmacodynamics (PD) from adults because of their immature renal and hepatic function, different body composition, altered protein binding, distinct disease spectrum, diverse behavior, and dissimilar receptor patterns.[2–8] PK differences necessitate modification of the dose and the interval between doses to achieve the desired concentration associated with a clinical response and to avoid toxicity.[9–12] In addition, some medications may displace bilirubin from its protein binding sites and possibly predispose to kernicterus in premature neonates.[13–18] Drug effect (PD) may be influenced by altered capacity of the end organ, such as the heart or bronchial smooth muscle, to respond to medications in children compared with adults. In this chapter we discuss basic pharmacologic principles as they relate to drugs commonly used by anesthesiologists.

Pharmacokinetic Principles and Calculations

Changes in drug concentrations within the body over time are referred to as *pharmacokinetics*. The principles and equations that describe these changes can be used to adjust drug doses rationally to achieve more effective drug concentrations at the site of action.[19,20] The equations in this section are intended for general and practical use, whereas the more rigorous mathematical intricacies of PK are covered elsewhere.[21,22]

Within the body, a drug may diffuse between several body fluids and tissues at different rates, yet the consistent change in its circulating concentration may be used to characterize its kinetics and to guide dosages. The rate of removal of drug from the circulation is usually described using either first-order or zero-order exponential equations. The difference between these two types of rates has important implications for drug treatment.

FIRST-ORDER KINETICS

Most drugs are cleared from the body with first-order exponential rates in which a constant fraction or constant proportion of drug is removed per unit of time. Because the proportion of drug cleared remains constant, the greater the concentration, the greater the amount of drug removed from the body. Such rates can be described by exponential equations that fit the following form:

$$C = C_0 e^{-kt} \qquad \text{Eq. 7.1,}$$

where C is the concentration at time t, C_0 is the starting concentration (a constant determined by the dose and distribution volume), e is the base of the natural logarithm ($\sim$2.71828), and k is the elimination rate constant with units of time^{-1}. First-order indicates that the exponent is raised to the first power ($-kt$ in Eq. 7.1). Second-order equations are those that are raised to the second power, such as $e^{(z)2}$. First-order exponential equations, such as Eq. 7.1, may be converted to the form of the equation of a straight line ($y = mx + b$, where x and y are variables [e.g., time and concentration], m is the slope parameter, and b is a constant) by taking the natural logarithm of both sides, after which they may be solved by linear regression.

$$\ln C = \ln C_0 + (-kt) \qquad \text{Eq. 7.2}$$

If ln C (i.e., natural logarithm of C) is graphed versus time, the slope is $-k$, and the intercept is ln C_0. If log C (i.e., common logarithm of C) is graphed versus time, the slope is $-k/2.303$, because ln x equals 2.303 log x. When graphed on linear-linear axes, exponential rates are curvilinear and on semilogarithmic axes, they produce a straight line.

HALF-LIFE

Half-life, the time for a drug concentration to decrease by one-half, is a familiar exponential term used to describe the kinetics of many drugs. *Half-life is a first-order kinetic process because the same proportion or fraction of the drug is removed during equal periods of time.* As described earlier, the greater the starting concentration, the greater the amount of drug removed during each half-life.

Half-life can be determined by several methods. If concentration is converted to the natural logarithm of concentration and graphed versus time, as described in Eq. 7.2, the slope of this graph is the elimination rate constant, k. For both accuracy and precision, at least three concentration-time points should be used to determine the slope, and they should be obtained over an interval during which the concentration decreases at least by half. In clinical practice, for infants and small children, however, k is often estimated from just two concentrations obtained during the terminal elimination phase. With multiple data points, the slope of ln C versus time may be calculated easily by least squares linear regression analysis. Half-life ($T_{1/2}$) may be calculated from the elimination rate constant, k (time^{-1}), as follows:

$$T_{1/2} = \frac{Natural\ Logarithm(2)}{k} = \frac{0.693}{k} \qquad \text{Eq. 7.3}$$

Graphic techniques may be used to determine half-life from a series of timed measurements of drug concentration. The concentration-time points should be graphed on semilogarithmic axes and used to determine the best-fitting line either visually or by linear regression analysis. This approach is illustrated in Fig. 7.1, in which the least squares regression line has been fitted to the concentration-time points and crosses a concentration of 20 µg/mL at 100 minutes and a concentration of 10 µg/mL at 200 minutes. The concentration decreased by one-half in 100 minutes, so the half-life is 100 minutes. The elimination rate constant is 0.693/100 per minute or 0.00693 per minute.

Elimination half-life is of no value for characterizing the disposition of many intravenous (IV) anesthetic drugs during dosing periods relevant to anesthesia. A more useful concept is that of the context-sensitive half-time (CSHT) where "context" refers to the duration of the infusion. This is the time required for the plasma drug concentration to decrease by 50% after terminating the infusion.[23] The CSHT is the same as the elimination half-life for a one-compartment model and does not change with the duration of the infusion. However, most drugs in anesthesia conform to multiple compartment models and the CSHTs are markedly different from their respective elimination half-lives.

CSHT may be independent of the duration of the infusion (e.g., remifentanil, 2.5 minutes); be moderately affected (propofol, 12 minutes at 1 hour, 38 minutes at 8 hours); or display marked prolongation (e.g., fentanyl, 1 hour at 24 minutes, 8 hours at 280 minutes). This is a result of the return of drug from peripheral compartments to plasma after stopping the infusion. Peripheral compartment sizes and clearances in children differ from adults and at termination of the infusion, more or less drug remains in the body in children for any given plasma concentration compared with adults. The CSHT for propofol in children, for example, is greater than that in adults.[24] The CSHT gives insight into the PK of a drug, but the parameter may not be clinically relevant; the percentage decrease in concentration required for recovery from the drug effect is not necessarily 50%.

FIRST-ORDER SINGLE-COMPARTMENT KINETICS

The number of exponential equations required to describe the change in concentration determines the number of compartments. Although a drug may diffuse among several tissues and body fluids, its clearance often fits first-order, single-compartment kinetics if it quickly distributes homogeneously within the circulation and is removed rapidly from the circulation through metabolism or excretion. This may be judged visually if a semilogarithmic graph of the change in drug concentration fits a single straight line. Kinetics may appear to be single-compartment, when they are really multiple compartments, if drug concentrations are not measured soon enough after IV administration to detect the initial distribution phase (α phase).

FIRST-ORDER MULTIPLE-COMPARTMENT KINETICS

If drug concentrations are measured several times within the first 15 to 30 minutes after IV administration as well as during a more prolonged period, more than one elimination phase is often present. This can be observed as a marked change in slope of a semilogarithmic graph of concentration versus time (Fig. 7.2). The number and nature of the compartments required to describe the clearance of a drug do not necessarily represent specific body fluids or tissues. When two first-order exponential equations are required to describe the clearance of drug from the circulation, the kinetics are described as first-order, two-compartment (e.g., central and peripheral compartments) that fit the following equation (see Fig. 7.2):

$$C = Ae^{-\alpha t} + Be^{-\beta t}, \qquad \text{Eq. 7.4}$$

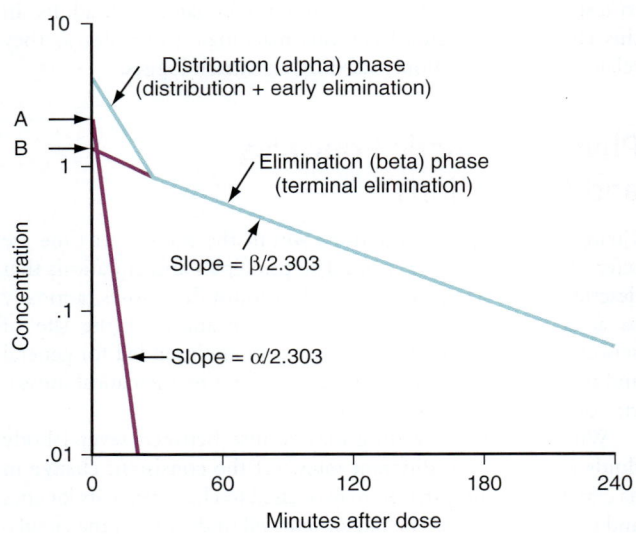

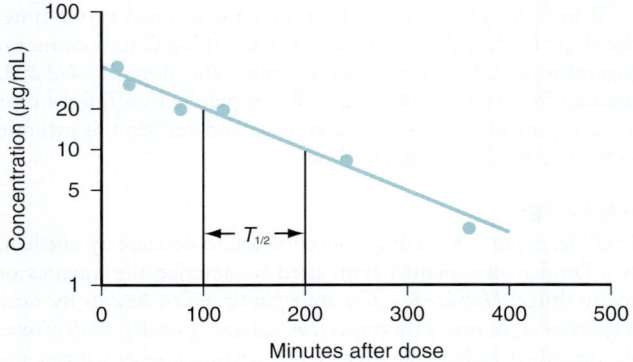

FIGURE 7.1 Graphic determination of half-life. Half-life can be determined from a series of concentration-time points on a semilogarithmic graph if the kinetics are first-order exponential. The concentrations are plotted on semilogarithmic axes; the best-fit line is drawn through the points; convenient concentrations are chosen that decrease in half, such as 20 µg/mL and 10 µg/mL, as illustrated; and the interval between those concentrations is the half-life, which is 100 minutes in the illustration.

FIGURE 7.2 Two compartment kinetics in a semilogarithmic graph. The initial rapid decrease in serum concentration reflects distribution and elimination followed by a slower decrease because of elimination. A is the concentration at time 0 for the distribution rate. Subtraction of the initial decrease in concentration resulting from elimination, using the concentrations from the elimination line extrapolated back to time 0 at B, produces the lower line with a steep slope = α(distribution rate constant)/2.303. The terminal elimination phase has a slope = β(elimination rate constant)/2.303.

where concentration is C, t is time after the dose, A is the concentration at time 0 for the distribution rate represented by the purple line graph with the steepest slope, α is the rate constant for distribution, e is base of natural logarithm, B is the concentration at time 0 for the terminal elimination rate, and β is the rate constant for terminal elimination. Rate constants indicate the rates of change in concentration and each corresponds to the slope of the respective line divided by 2.303 for logarithm concentration versus time.

Such two-compartment or biphasic kinetics are frequently observed after IV administration of drugs that rapidly distribute out of the central compartment of the circulation to a peripheral compartment. In such situations, the initial rapid decrease in concentration is referred to as the α or distribution phase and represents distribution to the peripheral (tissue) compartments in addition to drug elimination. The terminal (β) phase begins after the inflection point in the line when elimination starts to account for most of the change in drug concentration. To determine the initial change in concentration as a result of distribution (see Fig. 7.2), the change in concentration that results from elimination must be subtracted from the total change in concentration. The slope of the line representing the difference between these two rates is the rate constant for distribution.

These parameters (A, B, α, β) have little connection with underlying physiology, and an alternative parameterization is to use a central volume and three rate constants (k_{10}, k_{12}, k_{21}) that describe drug distribution between compartments. Another common method is to use two volumes (central, V1; peripheral, V2) and two clearances (CL, Q). Q is the intercompartment clearance, and the volume of distribution at steady state (Vdss) is the sum of V1 and V2. A more detailed mathematical discussion may be found elsewhere.[19,22]

Although many drugs demonstrate multiple-compartment kinetics, traditional studies of kinetics in neonates did not include enough samples immediately after dosing to identify more than one compartment. For clinical estimates of dose and dosing intervals, it is often not necessary to use multiple-compartment kinetics. To minimize cost, limit blood loss, and simplify PK calculations, dose adjustments are often based on only two plasma concentrations (peak and trough), and linear, single-compartment kinetics (such as that of gentamicin and vancomycin) is assumed. Because the elimination rate constant should be determined from the terminal elimination phase, it is important that peak concentrations of multiple-compartment drugs not be drawn prematurely—that is, during the initial distribution phase. If drawn too early, the concentrations will be greater than those during the terminal elimination phase (see Fig. 7.2), which will overestimate the slope and the terminal elimination rate constant. Population modeling has improved analysis and interpretation of such data.[25,26]

ZERO-ORDER KINETICS

The elimination of some drugs occurs with loss of a *constant amount per time, rather than a constant fraction per time.* Such rates are termed zero-order, and because $e^0 = 1$, the change in the amount of drug in the body fits the following equation[27]:

$$-dA/dt = k_0, \qquad \text{Eq. 7.5}$$

where dA is the change in the amount of drug in the body (in milligrams), dt is the change in time, and k_0 is the elimination rate constant with units of amount per unit time. After solving this equation, it has the following form:

$$A = A_0 - k_0 t, \qquad \text{Eq. 7.6}$$

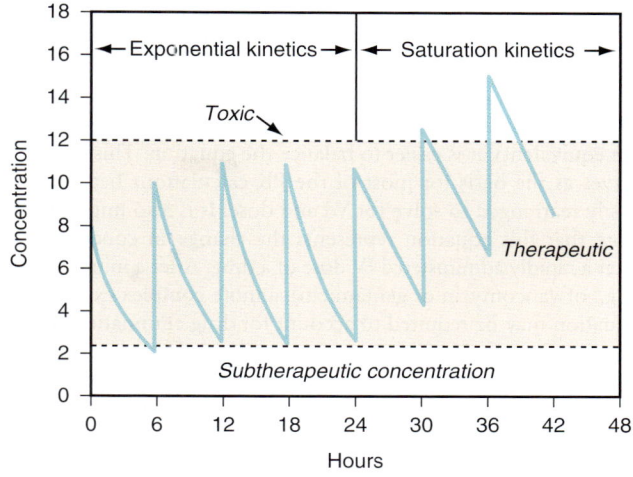

FIGURE 7.3 Transition from exponential to saturation kinetics. During every-6-hour dosing, concentrations during the first 24 hours reflect exponential kinetics with a half-life of 3 hours ($k = 0.231$/hour) followed by a change to saturation kinetics at 24 hours with elimination of 1 mg/hour, leading to drug accumulation to toxic concentrations.

where A_0 is the initial amount of drug in the body and A is the amount of drug in the body (in milligrams) at time t.

Zero-order (also known as Michaelis-Menten) kinetics may be designated saturation kinetics, because such processes occur when excess amounts of drug saturate the capacity of metabolic enzymes or transport systems. In this situation, only a constant amount of drug is metabolized or transported per unit of time. If kinetics are zero order, a graph of serum concentration versus time is linear on linear-linear axes and is curved when graphed on linear-logarithmic (i.e., semilogarithmic) axes. Clinically, first-order elimination may become zero order after administration of excessive doses or prolonged infusions or during dysfunction of the organ of elimination. Certain drugs administered to neonates exhibit zero-order kinetics at therapeutic doses and may accumulate to excessive concentrations, including thiopental, theophylline, caffeine, diazepam, furosemide, and phenytoin. Some drugs (e.g., phenytoin, ethyl alcohol) may exhibit mixed-order kinetics (i.e., first order at low concentrations and zero order after enzymes are saturated at greater concentrations). For these drugs, a small increment in dose may cause disproportionately large increments in serum concentrations (Fig. 7.3).

APPARENT VOLUME OF DISTRIBUTION

The apparent volume of distribution (Vd) is a mathematical term that relates the dose to the circulating concentration observed immediately after administration. It might be viewed as the volume of dilution that can be used to predict the change in concentration after a dose is diluted within the body (i.e., a scaling factor). Vd does not necessarily correspond to a physiologic body fluid or tissue volume, hence the designation "apparent." For drugs that distribute out of the circulation or bind to tissues, such as digoxin, Vd may reach 10 L/kg, a physical impossibility for a fluid compartment in the body. This illustrates the mathematical nature of Vd. The units used to express concentration are amount per unit volume, and dose is expressed as the amount per kilogram and the Vd as volume per kilogram that dilutes the dose to produce the concentration as the ratio:

$$\text{Concentration (mg/L)} = \frac{\text{Dose (mg/kg)}}{\text{Vd (L/kg)}} \qquad \text{Eq. 7.7}$$

If concentration is expressed with the unconventional units of milligrams per liter rather than micrograms per milliliter (which are equivalent), it is easier to balance the equation. This equation serves as the basis for most of the PK calculations because it is easily rearranged to solve for Vd and dose. It is also important to note that this equation represents the change in concentration after a rapidly administered IV dose of a drug. After a mini-infusion (e.g., of vancomycin or gentamicin), a more complex exponential equation may be required to account for drug elimination during the time of infusion. For neonates in whom drug elimination is relatively slow, only a small fraction of drug is eliminated during the time of infusion, and such adjustments can be omitted, whereas more complex equations may be needed in older children.

Knowledge of the apparent Vd is essential for dose adjustments. Vd may be calculated by rearranging Eq. 7.7:

$$\text{Vd (L/kg)} = \frac{\text{Dose (mg/kg)}}{\text{C (postdose)} - \text{C (predose) (mg/L)}} \qquad \text{Eq. 7.8}$$

The concentration after a drug infusion, C (postdose), must be measured after the distribution phase to avoid overestimating the peak concentration that would, in turn, lead to an erroneously low Vd. For the first dose, the predose concentration is 0.

Pharmacokinetic Example

The following example illustrates the application of these PK principles using a four-step approach: (1) calculate Vd; (2) calculate half-life; (3) calculate a new dose and dosing interval based on a desired peak and trough; and (4) check the peak and trough of the new dosage regimen.

For example, vancomycin was administered in a dose of 15 mg/kg IV over 60 minutes every 12 hours. The plasma concentrations were measured on the third day of treatment (presumed steady state). The predose or trough concentration was 12 mg/L; the peak concentration, measured 60 minutes after the *end* of the infusion, was 32 mg/L:

$$\text{Vd (L/kg)} = \frac{15 \text{ mg/kg}}{32 \text{ mg/L} - 12 \text{ mg/L}}$$
$$= 0.75 \text{ L/kg}$$

Step 1: Substituting the data into Eq. 7.8, we calculate Vd.

Step 2: At steady state, peak and trough concentrations reach the same levels after each dose. The time between the peak and trough concentrations is 10 hours—that is, 12 hours minus 1 hour infusion minus 1 hour to peak concentration. Half-life may be solved by rearranging Eq. 7.2 to solve for *k* (elimination rate constant) and substituting the calculated *k* into Eq. 7.3. In this case, the calculated elimination rate constant is 0.098/hour and the corresponding half-life is 7.1 hours. However, a practical and clinically applicable "bedside" approach may be used without need for logarithmic calculations. For example, the plasma concentration decreased from 32 to 16 mg/L in one half-life and then from 16 to 12 mg/L in a fraction of the second half-life. At the end of the second half-life, the concentration would have decreased to 8 mg/L. Because 12 mg/L is the midpoint between the first and second half-lives, 1.5 half-lives have elapsed during the 10 hours between the peak and trough. Thus if one assumes a linear decline, the half-life may be estimated as 6.67 hours

(10 hours ÷ 1.5 half-lives). Note that the error between the actual half-life of 7.1 hours and the estimated half-life (6.67 hours) is a result of the linear assumptions of this calculation between half-lives. In fact, first-order elimination is a nonlinear process and concentration will actually decline from 32 mg/L to 22.6 mg/L during the first 50% of the first half-life rather than from 32 mg/L to 24 mg/L using this linear approach. The same occurs during subsequent half-lives. However, the small error associated with this method is often acceptable for rapid bedside estimates of PK parameters.

Step 3: A new dosage regimen must be calculated if the concentrations are unsatisfactory. Accordingly, one must decide on a desired peak and trough concentration. If, for example, the desired vancomycin peak and trough concentrations were 32 mg/L (20–40 mg/L) and 8 mg/L (5–10 mg/L), respectively, then Eq. 7.8 may be rearranged to solve for the new dose:

$$\begin{aligned} \text{Dose (mg/kg)} &= \text{Vd (L/kg)} \times [\text{C (peak desired)} \\ &\quad - \text{C (trough desired) (mg/L)}] \\ \text{Dose (mg/kg)} &= 0.75 \text{ L/kg} \times (32 \text{ mg/L} - 8 \text{ mg/L}) \\ \text{Dose (mg/kg)} &= 18 \text{ mg/kg} \end{aligned} \qquad \text{Eq. 7.9}$$

The current dose produces a peak of 32 mg/L that is in the recommended therapeutic range, and extending the dosing interval to 2 half-lives (hours) after the peak is reached (2 hours after beginning the dose infusion) will produce a trough concentration of 8 mg/L. The dose interval should be increased to 16 hours and the dose increased to 18 mg/kg.

Step 4: Estimating peak and trough concentrations with the new regimen provides a good double-check against a mathematical error. Sixteen hours after the 15 mg/kg dose is administered (or approximately 2 half-lives after the measured peak), the trough should be approximately 8 mg/L. At this time, administration of 18 mg/kg will increase the concentration by 24 mg/L (assuming a Vd of 0.75 L/kg) to a peak concentration of 32 mg/L.

REPETITIVE DOSING AND DRUG ACCUMULATION

When multiple doses are administered, the dose is usually repeated before complete elimination of the previous one. In this situation, peak and trough concentrations increase until a steady-state concentration (C_{ss}) is reached (see Fig. 7.3). The average C_{ss} (AvgC_{ss}) can be calculated as follows[20]:

$$\begin{aligned} \text{AvgC}_{ss} &= \frac{1}{\text{Clearance}} \times \frac{f \times D}{\tau} \\ &= \frac{1}{k \times \text{Vd}} \times \frac{f \times D}{\tau} \end{aligned} \qquad \text{Eq. 7.10}$$

$$= \frac{1.44 \times T_{1/2}}{\text{Vd}} \times \frac{f \times D}{\tau} \qquad \text{Eq. 7.11}$$

In Eqs. 7.10 and 7.11, f is the fraction of the dose that is absorbed, D is the dose, τ is the dosing interval in the same units of time as the elimination half-life, *k* is the elimination rate constant, and 1.44 equals the reciprocal of 0.693 (see Eq. 7.3). The magnitude of the average C_{ss} is directly proportional to the ratio of $T_{1/2}/\tau$ and D.[20]

STEADY STATE

Steady state occurs when the amount of drug removed from the body between doses equals the amount of the dose.[28,29] Five half-lives are usually required for drug elimination and distribution among tissue and fluid compartments to reach equilibrium. When all tissues are at equilibrium (i.e., steady state), the peak and trough concentrations are identical after each dose. However, before this time, constant peak and trough concentrations after intermittent doses, or constant concentrations during drug infusions, do not prove that a steady state has been achieved because the drug may still be entering and leaving deep tissue compartments. During continuous infusion, the fraction of steady-state concentration that has been reached can be calculated in terms of multiples of the drug's half-life.[20] After 3 half-lives, the concentration is 88% of that at steady state. When changing doses during chronic drug therapy, the concentration should usually not be rechecked until several half-lives have elapsed, unless elimination is impaired or signs of toxicity occur. Drug concentrations may not need to be checked if symptoms improve.

LOADING DOSE

If the time to reach a constant concentration by continuous or intermittent dosing is excessive (e.g., 3–5 half-lives), a loading dose may be used to reach the target concentration or plateau in the concentration more rapidly. Propofol is usually given as a loading dose before establishing an infusion for anesthesia.[24] The same principle is applied to the initial treatment with digoxin, which has a 35- to 69-hour half-life in term neonates and an even greater half-life in preterm infants.[30] Use of a loading dose increases the circulating concentration of drug earlier in the therapeutic course. Loading doses must be used cautiously, because they increase the likelihood of drug toxicity, as has been observed with loading doses of digoxin.[3,5,6,30]

Dose calculations using a one-compartment model (see Eq. 7.9) may not be applicable to many anesthetic drugs that are characterized using multi-compartment models. The use of V1 (central Vd) results in a loading dose that is too large, whereas the use of Vdss (Vd at steady-state) results in a loading dose that is too small. Too large a dose may cause transient toxicity, although slowing the rate of administration may prevent excessive concentrations during the distributive phase.

The time to peak effect (Tpeak) depends on the clearance and effect-site equilibration half-time ($T_{1/2}$keo). At a submaximal dose, Tpeak is independent of dose. At supramaximal doses, maximal effect will occur earlier than Tpeak and persist for a greater duration because of the shape of the response curve (see later discussion). The Tpeak concept has been used to calculate optimal dose for initial boluses,[31] because V1 and Vdss poorly reflect the required scaling factor. A new parameter, the Vd at the time of peak effect-site concentration (*Vpe*) is used and calculated as follows:

$$Vpe = \frac{V1}{\left(Cpeak/C_0\right)},\qquad \text{Eq. 7.12}$$

where C_0 is the theoretical plasma concentration at $t = 0$ after the bolus dose, and *Cpeak* is the predicted effect-site concentration at the time of peak effect-site concentration. Loading dose (*LD*) can then be calculated as

$$LD = Cpeak \times Vpe \qquad \text{Eq. 7.13}$$

Population Modeling

Pediatric anesthesiologists have embraced the population approach for investigating PK and PD. This approach, achieved through nonlinear mixed-effects models, provides a means to study variability in drug responses among individuals representative of those in whom the drug will be used clinically. Traditional approaches to interpretation of time-concentration profiles relied on "rich" data from a small group of subjects. In contrast, mixed effects models can be used to analyze "sparse" data (two to three samples) from each one of a large number of subjects. Sampling times are not crucial for population methods and can be fit around clinical procedures or outpatient appointments. Sampling time bands rather than exact times is equally effective and allows flexibility in children.[31,32] Interpretation of truncated individual sets of data or missing data is also possible with this type of analysis, rendering it particularly useful for pediatric studies. Population modeling also allows pooling of data across studies to provide a single robust PK analysis rather than comparing separate smaller studies that are complicated by different methods and analyses.

Mixed-effects models are "mixed" because they describe the data using a mixture of fixed and random effects. Fixed effects predict the average influence of a covariate, such as weight, as an explanation of some of the variability between subjects in a parameter like clearance. Random effects describe the remaining variability among subjects that are not predictable from the fixed effect average. Explanatory covariates (e.g., age, size, renal function, sex, temperature) can be introduced that explain the predictable part of the between-individual variability. Nonlinear regression is performed by an iterative process to find the curve of best fit.[33,34]

Pediatric Pharmacokinetic Considerations

Growth and development are two major aspects of children not readily apparent in adults. How these factors interact is not necessarily easy to determine from observations because they are quite highly correlated. Drug clearance, for example, may increase with weight, height, age, body surface area (BSA), and creatinine clearance. One approach is to standardize for size before incorporating a factor for maturation.[35]

SIZE

Clearance in children 1 to 2 years of age, expressed as liters per hour per kilogram, is commonly greater than that observed in older children and adolescents. This is a size effect and is not because of bigger livers or increased hepatic blood flow in that subpopulation. This "artifact of size" disappears when allometric scaling is used. *Allometry* is a term used to describe the nonlinear relationship between size and function. This nonlinear relationship is expressed as

$$y = a \cdot Body\ Mass^{PWR}, \qquad \text{Eq. 7.14}$$

where y is the variable of interest (e.g., basal metabolic rate [BMR]), a is a scaling parameter, and *PWR* is the allometric exponent. The value of *PWR* has been the subject of much debate. BMR is the most common variable investigated, and camps advocating for a *PWR* value of ⅔ (i.e., BSA) are at odds with those advocating a value of ¾. Support for a value of ¾ comes from investigations that show the log of BMR plotted against the log of body weight produces a straight line with a slope of ¾ across all species studied, including humans. Clearance is a metabolic process and the log of clearance plotted against the log of body weight also produces a straight line with a slope of ¾ when different species are studied. Fig. 7.4 exemplifies this for tramadol.[36] Fractal geometry

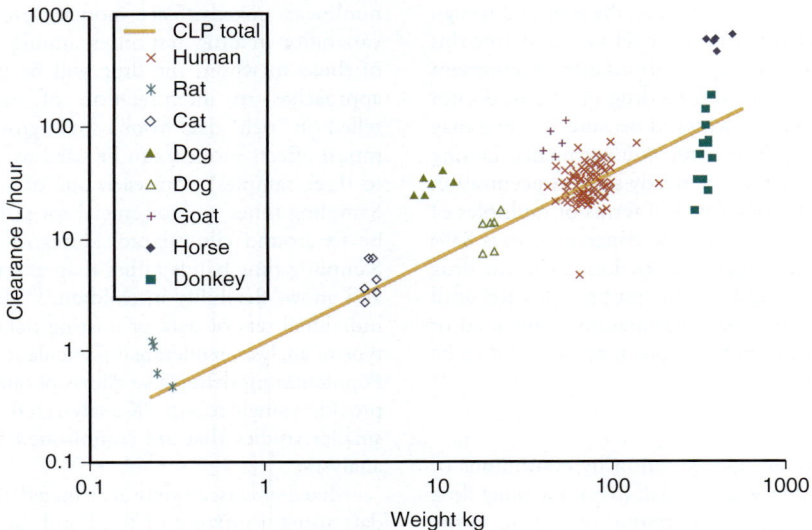

FIGURE 7.4 Weight-predicted tramadol total clearance *(CLP total)* compared with human allometric prediction *(solid line)* using a ¾-power exponent *(solid line)*. (From Holford SD, Allegaert K, Anderson BJ, et al. Parent-metabolite pharmacokinetic models for tramadol—tests of assumptions and predictions. *J Pharmacol Clin Toxicol.* 2014;2[1]:1023–1034, with permission.)

mathematically explains this phenomenon. The ¾-power law for metabolic rates was derived from a general model that describes how essential materials are transported through space-filled fractal networks of branching tubes.[37] A great many physiologic, structural, and time-related variables scale predictably within and between species with weight (*W*) exponents (*PWR*) of ¾, 1, and ¼, respectively.[38]

These exponents have applicability to PK parameters; for example, the exponent for clearance (CL) is ¾, volume (V) is 1, and half-time ($T_{1/2}$) is ¼.[38] The factor for size (*Fsize*) for total drug clearance may be expressed as

$$Fsize = \left(\frac{W}{70}\right)^{3/4} \qquad \text{Eq. 7.15}$$

Remifentanil clearance in children aged 1 month to 9 years is similar to adult rates when scaled using an allometric exponent of ¾.[39] Nonspecific blood esterases that metabolize remifentanil are mature at birth.[40]

MATURATION

Allometry alone is insufficient to predict clearance in neonates and infants from adult estimates for most drugs.[41,42] The addition of a model describing maturation is required. The sigmoid hyperbolic or Hill model[43] has been found useful for describing this maturation process (*MF*):

$$MF = \frac{PMA^{Hill}}{TM_{50}^{Hill} + PMA^{Hill}} \qquad \text{Eq. 7.16}$$

The TM_{50} describes the maturation half-time, while the Hill coefficient relates to the slope of this maturation profile. Maturation of clearance begins before birth, suggesting that postmenstrual age (*PMA*) would be a better predictor of drug elimination than postnatal age (*PNA*).[38] Fig. 7.5 shows the maturation profile for dexmedetomidine, expressed as both the standard per-kilogram model and by using allometry. Clearance is immature in infancy.

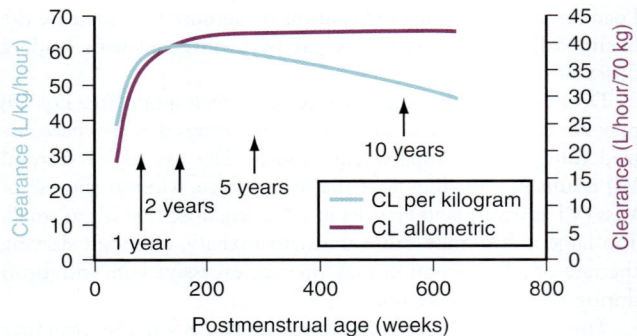

FIGURE 7.5 The clearance (*CL*) maturation profile of dexmedetomidine, expressed using the per-kilogram model and the allometric ¾-power model. This maturation pattern is typical of many drugs cleared by the liver or kidneys. (Data extracted from Potts AL, Anderson BJ, Warman GR, et al. Dexmedetomidine pharmacokinetics in pediatric intensive care—a pooled analysis. *Paediatr Anaesth.* 2009;19(11):1119–1129.)

Clearance, expressed as per kilogram, is greatest at 2 years of age, decreasing subsequently with age. This "artifact of size" disappears with use of the allometric model. Appropriate size scaling shows that the PK in children (>2 years old) is similar to adults. Maturation changes are generally completed within the first 2 years of postnatal life; consequently, infants may be considered as immature children, whereas children are just small adults.[44]

ORGAN FUNCTION

Changes associated with normal growth and development can be distinguished from pathologic changes describing organ function.[35] Morphine clearance is reduced in neonates because of immature glucuronide conjugation, but clearance was lower in critically ill neonates than healthier cohorts,[45–47] possibly attributable to reduced hepatic function. The impact of organ function alteration may be concealed by another covariate. For example, positive-pressure ventilation may be associated with reduced morphine clearance.[48] This effect may be attributable to a consequent reduced hepatic blood flow with a drug that has perfusion limited clearance (e.g., propofol, morphine).

Creatinine clearance is commonly used as a measure of renal function and dictates dose of those drugs cleared by that organ. Renal function in children can be estimated using formulae that allow estimation of glomerular filtration rate (GFR) from clinical characteristics.[49] These formulae use simple markers such as height, plasma creatinine concentration and BSA. Estimation of GFR is acceptable in adults, but prediction is poor in children with a GFR value less than 40 mL/minute.[50] We might expect the maturation of creatinine clearance, a marker for GFR, to reflect the influences of size, maturation, and organ function. Estimation methods such as those of Schwartz incorporate a size factor (body length or height) and a scaling factor (k) that is age dependent (e.g., k = 0.33 for premature neonates; k = 0.45 for term infants 0–1 year; k = 0.55 for 1–12 years; k = 0.7 for 13- to 21-year old adolescent males[51–53]):

$$GFR = \frac{k \cdot height}{Serum\ Creatinine} \qquad \text{Eq. 7.17}$$

Creatinine clearance estimation overpredicts GFR in children, possibly because of tubular secretion. Tubular reabsorption may also create inaccuracies in premature neonates. Dosing of renally cleared drugs in premature neonates should be based on size- and maturation-based predictions of GFR alone, and serum creatinine should not be used as a base until creatinine production rate predictions in this age group are better established. Pharmacokinetic parameters (P) can be described in an individual as the product of size (Fsize), maturation (MF), and organ function (OF) influences, where Pstd is the parameter value in a standard size adult without pathologic changes in organ function[35]:

$$P = Pstd \cdot Fsize \cdot MF \cdot OF \qquad \text{Eq. 7.18}$$

Pharmacodynamic Models

Pharmacokinetics is what the body does to the drug, while *pharmacodynamics* is what the drug does to the body. The precise boundary between these two processes is ill defined and often requires a link describing movement of drug from the plasma to the effect site and its target. Drugs may exert effects at nonspecific membrane sites, by interference with transport mechanisms, by enzyme inhibition or induction, or by activation or inhibition of receptors.

MINIMAL EFFECTIVE CONCENTRATION
The minimal effective analgesic concentration can be established by titration of an analgesic to achieve satisfactory pain at rest or with a painful stimulus. Blood assay for analgesic drug concentration at these times can be used to determine the effective concentration. Further blood assays when pain recurs or when further analgesics are required improve the accuracy of assessment. This technique has been used to determine the minimal effective analgesic concentration of oxycodone.[54]

SIGMOID EMAX MODEL
The relation between drug concentration and effect may be described by the Hill equation or Emax model (see maturation model above)[43]:

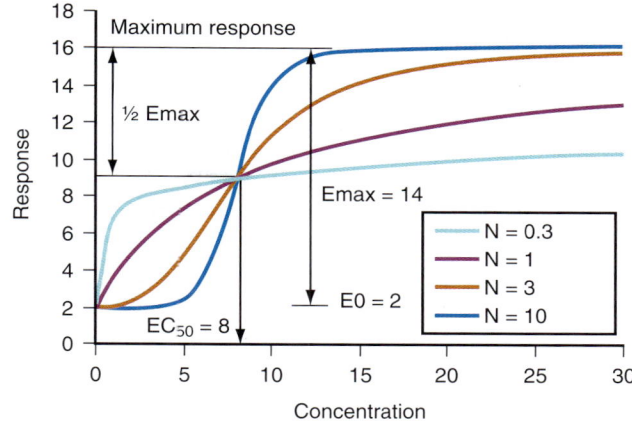

FIGURE 7.6 The sigmoid Emax model is commonly used to describe the relationship between drug response and concentration. Changing the Hill coefficient (*N*) dramatically alters the shape of the curve.

$$Effect = E_0 + \frac{(Emax \cdot Ce^N)}{(EC_{50}^N + Ce^N)}, \qquad \text{Eq. 7.19}$$

where E_0 is the baseline response, *Emax* is the maximum effect change, *Ce* is the concentration in the effect compartment, EC_{50} is the concentration producing 50% Emax, and *N* is the Hill coefficient defining the steepness of the concentration-response curve (Fig. 7.6). Efficacy is the maximum response on a dose or concentration-response curve. EC_{50} can be considered a measure of potency relative to another drug, provided N and Emax for the two drugs are the same.

This model has been used to describe propofol PD in children 1 to 16 years of age using bispectral index as an effect measure. The E_0 was estimated as 93.2, Emax –83.4, EC_{50} 5.2 mg/L, and *N* 1.4.[55] Similar relationships have been described in other groups of children.[56,57] Remifentanil hypotensive effects[58] and acetaminophen analgesic effects[59] in children have also been described using this model.

QUANTAL EFFECT MODEL
The potency of anesthetic vapors may be expressed by minimum alveolar concentration (MAC), and this is the concentration at which 50% of subjects move in response to a standard surgical stimulus. MAC appears, at first sight, to be similar to EC_{50}, but is an expression of quantal response rather than magnitude of effect. There are two methods of estimating MAC. Responses can be recorded over the clinical dose range in a large number of subjects and logistic regression applied to estimate the relationship between dose and quantal effect; the MAC can then be interpolated. Large numbers of subjects may not be available, so an alternative method is often used. The "up-and-down" method described by Dixon[60,61] estimates only the MAC rather than the entire sigmoid curve.[62] It usually involves a study of only one concentration in each subject and, in a sequence of subjects, each receives a concentration depending on the response of the previous subject; the concentration is either decreased if the previous subject did not respond or increased if they did. The MAC is calculated either as the mean concentration of equal numbers of responses and no responses or is the mean concentration of pairs of "response–no response." This technique has also been used to determine the EC_{50} of local anesthetic drugs used in central blockade.[63–65]

LOGISTIC REGRESSION MODEL

When the pharmacologic effect is difficult to grade, then it may be useful to estimate the probability of achieving the effect as a function of plasma concentration. Effect measures, such as movement/no movement or rousable/nonrousable, are dichotomous. Logistic regression is commonly used to analyze such data and the interpolated EC_{50} value refers to the probability of response. For example, an EC_{50} of 0.52 mg/L for arousal after ketamine sedation in children has been estimated using this technique.[66]

Linking Pharmacokinetics With Pharmacodynamics

A simple situation in which drug effect is directly related to concentration does not mean that drug effects parallel the time course of concentration. This occurs only when the concentration is low in relation to EC_{50}. In this situation the half-life of the drug may correlate closely with the half-life of drug effect. Observed effects may not be directly related to serum concentration. Many drugs have a short half-life but a long duration of effect. This may be attributable to induced physiologic changes (e.g., aspirin and platelet function) or may be a result of the shape of the Emax model. If the initial concentration is very high in relation to the EC_{50}, then drug concentrations 5 half-lives later, when we might expect a minimal concentration, may still exert considerable effect.

There may also be a delay as a result of transfer of the drug to the effect site (e.g., neuromuscular blockers [NMBDs]), a lag time (e.g., diuretics), physiologic response (e.g., antipyresis), active metabolite (e.g., valdecoxib), or synthesis of physiologic substances (e.g., warfarin). A plasma concentration-effect plot can form a hysteresis loop because of this delay in effect. Hull and Sheiner introduced the effect compartment concept for NMBDs.[67,68] A single first-order parameter ($T_{1/2}$keo) describes the equilibration half-time. This mathematical trick assumes that the concentration in the central compartment is the same as that in the effect compartment at equilibrium, but that a time delay exists before drug reaches the effect compartment. The concentration in the effect compartment is used to describe the concentration-effect relationship.[69]

Adult $T_{1/2}$keo values are well described (e.g., morphine, 16 minutes; fentanyl, 5 minutes; alfentanil, 1 minute; propofol, 3 minutes). This $T_{1/2}$keo parameter is commonly incorporated into target-controlled infusion pumps to achieve a rapid effect-site concentration. The adult midazolam $T_{1/2}$keo of 5 minutes may be prolonged in the elderly, resulting in overdose if this is not recognized during dose titration.[67]

The $T_{1/2}$keo for propofol in children has been described. As expected, a shorter $T_{1/2}$keo with decreasing age based on size models has been observed.[55,68] Similar results have been demonstrated for sevoflurane and changes in the electroencephalogram (EEG).[70] If the effect site is targeted and Tpeak is anticipated to be later than it actually is because it was determined in a teenager or adult, this will result in excessive dose in a young child.

Drug Distribution

PROTEIN BINDING

Acidic drugs (e.g., diazepam, barbiturates) tend to bind mainly to albumin, whereas basic drugs (e.g., amide local anesthetic agents)

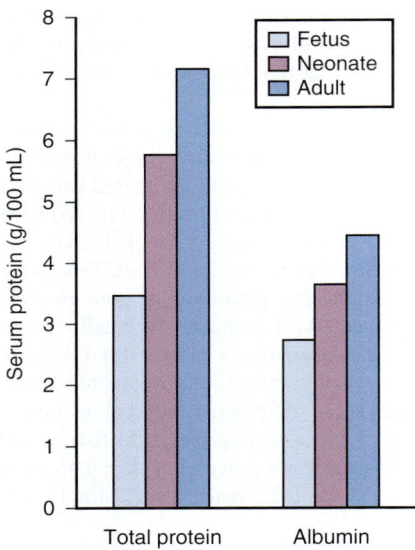

FIGURE 7.7 Changes in total serum protein and albumin values that occur with maturation. Note that total protein and albumin are less in fetuses than in neonates and less in neonates than in adults. The result may be altered pharmacokinetics and pharmacodynamics for drugs with a high degree of protein binding, because less drug is protein bound and more is available for clinical effect in the neonate and fetus. (Data from Ehrnebo M, Agurell S, Jalling B, et al. Age differences in drug binding by plasma proteins: studies on human foetuses, neonates and adults. *Eur J Clin Pharmacol.* 1971;3(4):189–193.)

bind to globulins, lipoproteins, and glycoproteins. In general, plasma protein binding of many drugs is decreased in the neonate relative to the adult in part because of reduced total protein and albumin concentrations (Fig. 7.7).[71] Many drugs that are highly protein bound in adults have less of an affinity for protein in neonates (E-Fig. 7.1).[71–75] Reduced protein binding increases the free fraction of medications, thus providing more free medication and greater pharmacologic effect.[2–4,6,76] This effect is particularly important for medications that are highly protein bound, because the reduced protein binding increases the free fraction of the medication to a greater extent than for low protein-bound drugs. For example, phenytoin is 85% protein bound in healthy infants but only 80% in those who are jaundiced. This equates to a 33% increase in the free fraction of phenytoin when jaundice occurs (E-Fig. 7.2). Differences in protein binding may have considerable influence on the response to medications that are acidic and are therefore highly protein bound (e.g., phenytoin, salicylate, bupivacaine, barbiturates, antibiotics, theophylline, and diazepam). In addition, some medications, such as phenytoin, salicylate, sulfisoxazole, caffeine, ceftriaxone, diatrizoate (Hypaque), and sodium benzoate, compete with bilirubin for binding to albumin (see E-Fig. 7.2). If large amounts of bilirubin are displaced, particularly in the presence of hypoxemia and acidosis, which open the blood-brain barrier (BBB), kernicterus may result.[a] Because these metabolic derangements often occur in sick neonates coming to surgery, special care must be taken when selecting medications for the anesthetic.[78] Medications that are basic (e.g., lidocaine or alfentanil) are generally bound to plasma α_1-acid glycoprotein (AAG); AAG concentrations in preterm and term infants are reduced but are

---

[a]References 14, 15, 72, 75, 77, and 78.

similar to those in adults by 6 months, although between patient variability is high (e.g., AAG 0.32–0.92 g/L).[79] Therefore for a given dose, the free fraction of a drug is greater in preterm and term infants.[79–81] In contrast to drugs bound to plasma proteins, unbound lipophilic drugs passively diffuse across the BBB, equilibrating very quickly. This may contribute to bupivacaine's propensity for producing seizures in neonates. Decreased protein binding, as in the neonate, results in a greater proportion of unbound drug that is available for passive diffusion.

These binding changes in neonates differ from adults in whom protein binding changes are important for the relatively unusual case of a drug that is more than 95% protein bound, with a high extraction ratio and a narrow therapeutic index, that is given parenterally (e.g., IV lidocaine), or a drug with a narrow therapeutic index that is given orally and has a very rapid $T_{1/2}$keo (e.g., antiarrhythmic drugs; propafenone, verapamil).[82]

Maturational changes in tissue binding also affect drug distribution. Myocardial digoxin concentrations in infants are 6-fold greater than those in adults, despite similar serum concentrations. Erythrocyte/plasma concentration ratios of digoxin in infants are one-third smaller during loading digitalization than during maintenance digoxin therapy. These findings are consistent with a greater Vd of digoxin in infants and may explain, in part, the unusually large therapeutic doses needed in infants.[83]

BODY COMPOSITION

Preterm and term infants have a much greater proportion of body weight in the form of water than do older children and adults (Fig. 7.8).[8] The net effect on water-soluble medications is a greater Vd in infants, which in turn increases the initial (loading) dose, based on weight, to achieve the desired target serum concentration and clinical response.[2–4,84,85] Term neonates often require a greater loading dose (milligrams per kilogram) for some medications (e.g., digoxin, succinylcholine, and aminoglycoside antibiotics) than older children.[84–88] However, neonates also tend to be sensitive to the respiratory, neurologic, and circulatory effects of many medications and therefore tend to be more responsive to these effects at reduced blood concentrations than are children and adults. Preterm infants are usually more sensitive than term neonates and in general require even smaller blood concentrations.[2] On the other hand, dopamine may increase blood pressure (BP) and urine output in term neonates only at doses as large as 50 µg/kg per minute. This dose, which would induce intense vasoconstriction in adults, suggests that neonates are less sensitive in their cardiovascular responsiveness.[3,86,89–92] *It is important to carefully titrate the doses of all medications that are administered to preterm and term infants to the desired response.*

Compared with children and adolescents, preterm and term neonates have a smaller proportion of body weight in the form of fat and muscle mass; with growth, the proportion of body weight composed of these tissues increases (Fig. 7.9).[2,3,8,90,93–95] Therefore medications that depend on their redistribution into muscle and fat for termination of their clinical effects likely have a larger initial peak blood concentration. These medications may also have a more sustained blood concentration because neonates have less tissue for redistribution of these medications. An incorrect dose may result in prolonged undesirable clinical effects (e.g., barbiturates and opioids may cause prolonged sedation and respiratory depression). The possible influence of small muscle mass on the response to NMBDs is exemplified by achieving neuromuscular blockade at smaller serum concentrations in infants.[86]

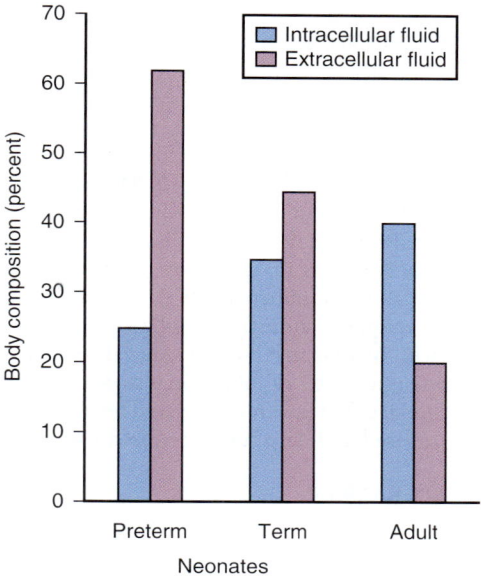

FIGURE 7.8 Changes in the intracellular and extracellular compartments that occur with maturation. Note the large proportion of extracellular water in preterm and term infants. This large water compartment creates an increased volume of distribution for highly water-soluble medications (e.g., succinylcholine, gentamicin) and may account for the large (by weight) loading dose required for some medications to achieve a satisfactory clinical response. (Data from Friis-Hansen B. Body composition during growth. In vivo measurements and biochemical data correlated to differential anatomical growth. *Pediatrics* 1971;47(1 Suppl 2):264+.)

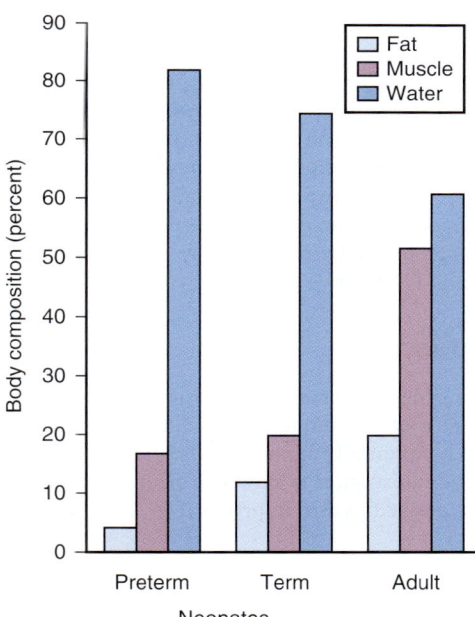

FIGURE 7.9 Changes in body content for fat, muscle, and water that occur with maturation. Note the small percentage of fat and muscle mass in preterm and term infants. These factors may greatly influence the pharmacokinetics and pharmacodynamics of medications that redistribute into fat (e.g., barbiturates) and muscle (e.g., fentanyl) because there is less tissue mass into which the drug may redistribute. (Data from Friis-Hansen B. Body composition during growth. In vivo measurements and biochemical data correlated to differential anatomical growth. *Pediatrics* 1971;47(1 Suppl 2):264+.)

REGIONAL BLOOD FLOWS

There are differences in relative organ mass and regional blood flow that change with growth and development during the first few months of life in addition to physiologic changes at birth. Kidney and brain receive an increasing proportion of the cardiac output, while the proportion to the liver decreases. The proportional mass of the head and liver are much greater in the infant than in the adult.[96] Mean CBF peaks in early childhood (70 mL/minute per 100 g) at about 3–8 years of age[97]; flows in both neonates and adults are less (50 mL/minute per 100 g).[98] The highly lipophilic drugs used for anesthetic induction rapidly achieve concentration equilibrium with brain tissue, but the reduced cerebral perfusion means that onset time after IV induction is slower in neonates that in early childhood. Offset time is also delayed because redistribution to the well-perfused and deep, underperfused tissues is less.

BLOOD-BRAIN BARRIER

The BBB is a network of complex tight junctions between specialized endothelial cells that restricts the paracellular diffusion of hydrophilic molecules from the blood to the brain substance. There are specific transport systems selectively expressed in the barrier endothelial cell membranes that mediate the transport of nutrients into the central nervous system (CNS) and of toxic metabolites out of the CNS. Small molecules can cross into fetal and neonatal brains more readily than they do into adult brains.[99] BBB function improves throughout fetal brain development, reaching maturity at term.[99] This maturation explains why kernicterus is more common in the preterm than the term neonate. BBB breakdown or alterations in transport systems may occur in some diseases. Proinflammatory substances and specific disease-associated proteins often mediate BBB dysfunction.[100] Fentanyl is actively transported across the BBB by a saturable adenosine triphosphate (ATP)-dependent process, while ATP-binding cassette proteins such as P-glycoprotein actively pump out opioids such as fentanyl and morphine.[101] P-glycoprotein modulation significantly influences brain opioid distribution and onset time and magnitude and duration of analgesic response.[102] Modulation may occur during disease processes, increased temperature, or other substances (e.g., verapamil, magnesium).[101] Genetic polymorphisms affecting P-glycoprotein–related genes may explain some individual differences in CNS-active drug sensitivity (see also Chapter 6).[103]

Absorption

Anesthetic drugs are mainly administered through the IV and inhalational routes, although premedication and postoperative pain relief is commonly administered enterally. Drug absorption after oral administration is slower in neonates than in children because of delayed gastric emptying (Fig. 7.10).

ENTERAL

Adult enteral absorption rates may not be reached until 6 to 8 months after birth.[104,105] Congenital malformations (e.g., duodenal atresia), co-administration of drugs (e.g., opioids), or disease characteristics (e.g., necrotizing enterocolitis) may further affect the variability in absorption. Delayed gastric emptying and reduced clearance may dictate reduced doses and frequency of repeated drug administration. For example, a mean steady-state target acetaminophen concentration greater than 10 mg/L at trough can be achieved by an oral dose of 25 mg/kg per day in preterm neonates at 30 weeks, 45 mg/kg per day at 34 weeks, and

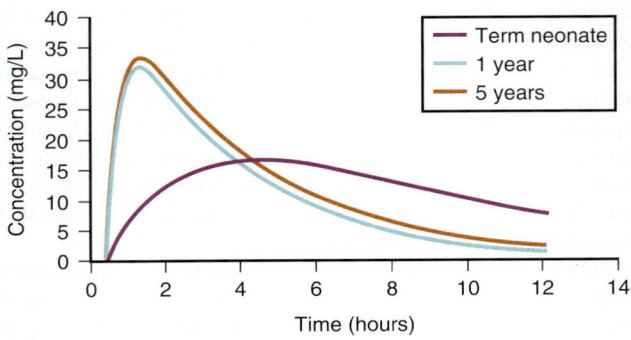

FIGURE 7.10 Simulated mean predicted time-concentration profiles for a term neonate, a 1-year-old infant, and a 5-year-old child given paracetamol elixir. The time to peak concentration is delayed in neonates because of slow gastric emptying and reduced clearance. (Reproduced with permission from Anderson BJ, van Lingen RA, Hansen TG, Lin YC, Holford NH. Acetaminophen developmental pharmacokinetics in premature neonates and infants: a pooled population analysis. *Anesthesiology* 2002;96(6):1336–1345.)

60 mg/kg per day at 40 weeks PMA.[106] Because gastric emptying is slow in preterm neonates, dosing may only be required twice a day.[106] In contrast, the rectal administration of some drugs (e.g., thiopental, methohexital) is more rapid in neonates than adults. However, the interindividual absorption and relative bioavailability (F) variability after rectal administration may be more extensive compared with oral administration, making rectal administration less suitable for repeated administration.[107] The frequent passage of stools in the neonate may render suppository use ineffective. Variable absorption and bioavailability has resulted in respiratory arrest when repeat opioids are administered by the rectal route to children.[108]

CUTANEOUS

The larger relative skin surface area, increased cutaneous perfusion, and thinner stratum corneum in neonates increase systemic exposure of topical drugs (e.g., corticosteroids, local anesthetic creams, antiseptics). Neonates have a greater tendency to form methemoglobin because of reduced methemoglobin reductase activity compared with older children. Furthermore, fetal hemoglobin is more readily oxidized by drugs such as prilocaine compared with adult hemoglobin. Combined with an increased transcutaneous absorption, these have resulted in reluctance to apply repeat or large surface area application of topical local anesthetics, such as EMLA (eutectic mixture of local anesthetics [lidocaine-prilocaine]) cream, in this age group.[109] Similarly, cutaneous application of iodine antiseptics in neonates may result in transient hypothyroidism.

INTRAMUSCULAR

The intramuscular (IM) route is frowned upon in children. Although bioavailability is high and approaches unity for most drugs, absorption is delayed compared to the IV route. Ketamine, however, remains popular, and peak concentrations are reached within 10 minutes after 4 mg/kg.[110]

NASAL

Exploration of alternative delivery routes in young children has centered on the nasal passages.[111] Nasal diamorphine 0.1 mg/kg, used in the United Kingdom for forearm fracture pain in the emergency room, is rapidly absorbed as a nasal spray in 0.2 mL of sterile water, with peak morphine plasma concentrations (Tpeak) occurring at 10 minutes.[112] Nasal S-ketamine (2 mg/kg) results in peak plasma concentrations of 355 ng/mL within 18 minutes.[113] Nasal fentanyl (150 µg/mL) 1.5 µg/kg given to children (3–17 years) for fracture pain resulted in good analgesia; peak concentrations occurred at 13 minutes.[114,115] There remain concerns that intranasal drugs may pass through the posterior nasopharynx or irritate the vocal cords.[116]

Advances in aerosol delivery devices have improved dosing accuracy. Administration of ketorolac (15 mg [weight 30–50 kg] or 30 mg [weight >50 kg]) to adolescents by the intranasal route resulted in a rapid increase in plasma concentration (time to peak concentration was 52 ± 6 minutes) and may be a useful therapeutic alternative to IV injection. A target concentration of 0.37 mg/L in the effect compartment was achieved within 30 minutes and remained above that target for 10 hours.[117] The nasal passages change with age and so it would not be surprising if absorption by that route did not also change with age. Drug combinations may show benefits over single-drug therapy. Formulations containing two drugs may improve analgesia by additivity while decreasing adverse effects.[118]

Buccal and sublingual administration, like the nasal route, offer ease of administration, rapid systemic absorption, and avoidance of hepatic first-pass metabolism.[119] Midazolam administered by the buccal surface is now more popular than rectal administration for the acute management of seizures.[120]

Bioavailability

The oral bioavailability of a drug may be affected by (1) interactions with food when feeding is frequent in the neonate (e.g., phenytoin[121]), (2) use of adult formulations that are divided or altered for pediatric use (nizatidine[122]), and (3) lower cytochrome P450 enzyme activity in the intestine. The last factor may cause an increased bioavailability of midazolam because CYP3A activity is reduced.[123] The use of drug vials designed for adult use may result in dose inaccuracy when proportioned for pediatric use, causing a relative increase or decrease in assumed bioavailability.[124]

Dose accuracy is lost when buccal and sublingual administration is attempted because those routes require prolonged exposure to the mucosal surface. Infants find it difficult to hold the drug in their mouth for the requisite retention time (particularly if taste is unfavorable) and this results in more swallowed drug or drug spat out than in adults.[125] If the drug has a high first-pass effect, then the lower relative bioavailability results in lower plasma concentrations. Although many analgesics are available in an oral liquid formulation, taste is a strong determinant of compliance and unpalatable preparations may be refused.[126] Taste preferences change with age.

First-pass effect impacts bioavailability and contribution of active metabolites to effect. The oral bioavailability of clonidine is low (F = 0.55) in children 3 to 10 years of age. Consequently, larger oral doses of clonidine (per kilogram) are required when this formulation is used to achieve concentrations similar to those reported in adults.[127] Oral absorption is slow (absorption half-time 0.45 hours), and peak concentrations are not reached until 1 hour. Similarly, oral ketamine needs to be given in doses of up to 10 mg/kg to achieve therapeutic effect in children 1 to 8 years of age who have suffered burns.[128] Not only was bioavailability reduced (F = 0.45) but absorption was also slow; absorption half-time was 59 minutes, and between-subject variability in this cohort was substantive.[128] Analgesic effect, however, may be supplemented by the increased concentration of the active metabolite norketamine.

Metabolism and Excretion

The main routes by which drugs and their metabolites leave the body are the hepatobiliary system, the kidney, and the lung. Microsomal enzyme activity can be classified into three groups[129]:

1. Mature at birth but decreasing with age (e.g., CYP3A7 responsible for methadone clearance in neonates)
2. Mature at birth and sustained through to adulthood (e.g., plasma esterases that clear remifentanil)
3. Immature at birth

The last group accounts for the majority of enzymatic activity; the concentrations, and activities of many microsomal enzymes are reduced or absent in the neonate.

HEPATIC METABOLISM

The liver is the most important organ in drug metabolism. Hepatic enzymatic drug metabolism usually converts the medication from a less polar state (lipid-soluble) to a more polar, water-soluble compound (see later discussion). The enzyme activities responsible for drug clearance are reduced in the neonate. However, clearance depends on enzyme activity, organ blood flow, and organ size; these change independently with age. Half-life is often used to describe maturation. The elimination half-lives of diazepam, thiopental, and phenobarbital are markedly increased in neonates compared with adults (i.e., the elimination half-life for thiopental in the neonate [17.9 hours] is almost three times that in children [6.1 hours] and 50% greater than that in adults [12 hours]) (E-Fig. 7.3).[74,76,130,131] In general, the half-lives of medications that are eliminated by the liver are prolonged in neonates, decreased in children 4 to 10 years of age, and reach adult values in adolescents, mirroring clearance changes with age (see Fig. 7.5). Half-life is confounded by clearance (CL) and volume (Vd); both change independently with age.

$$T_{1/2} = \frac{Ln(2) \cdot Vd}{CL} \qquad \text{Eq. 7.20}$$

Consequently, clearance is a better parameter to gauge maturation.

Some medications are extensively metabolized by the liver or other organs (e.g., the intestines or lungs) and are referred to as having high extraction ratios. This extensive metabolism produces a "first-pass" effect in which a large proportion of an enteral dose is inactivated as it passes through the organ before reaching the systemic circulation (e.g., propranolol, morphine, and midazolam). Clearance of these drugs is commonly termed "perfusion limited." In contrast, drugs with low intrinsic clearance (diazepam, phenytoin, aspirin) are termed "capacity limited."

Metabolism via cytochrome P-450 in the intestinal wall may also occur during drug absorption.[132–134] Competition between drugs for these intestinal wall enzymes may increase the bioavailability of one drug over another. The relative bioavailability of phenylephrine was increased when coadministered with acetaminophen owing to competition for gut wall sulfate conjugation.[135,136] Certain foods (e.g., grapefruit juice) may also induce or inhibit intestinal cytochromes, resulting in food–drug interactions.[137] The concentrations of these enzymes in neonates are less than in older children. These enzymes may also be affected by diseases such as cystic fibrosis or celiac disease.[138,139]

The opening or closing of a patent ductus may have profound effects on drug delivery to metabolizing organs in preterm infants.[140,141] The ability to metabolize and conjugate medications improves considerably with age as a result of both increased enzyme activity and increased delivery of drug to the liver. Other factors influence the rate of hepatic maturation and metabolism (e.g., sepsis and malnutrition may slow maturation, whereas previous exposure to anticonvulsants, such as phenytoin or phenobarbital, may hasten maturation).[142–144]

Metabolism through biotransformation to more polar forms is required for many drugs before they can be eliminated. Two types of drug biotransformation can occur: phase I and phase II reactions. Phase I reactions transform the drug via oxidation, reduction, or hydrolysis. Phase II reactions transform the drug via conjugation reactions, such as glucuronidation, sulfation, and acetylation, into more polar forms.[145,146] Hepatic drug metabolism activity appears as early as 9 to 22 weeks gestation, when fetal liver enzyme activity may vary from 2% to 36% of adult activity.[147] It is inaccurate to generalize that the preterm neonate cannot metabolize drugs; rather, the specific pathway(s) of drug metabolism must be considered.

PHASE I REACTIONS: CYTOCHROME P-450

Metabolism of many drugs involves the cytochrome P-450 (CYP) enzyme system. Multiple isoforms of the CYP enzyme system exist with different substrate specificities for different drugs.

Induction and inhibition of these enzymes by different drugs and chemicals requires a thorough understanding of both the nomenclature of the CYP system, as well as the specific isoforms responsible for metabolism of the drugs used in pediatric anesthesia. There are both genetic and ethnic polymorphisms that may lead to clinically important differences in the capacity to metabolize drugs; these differences can make individual drug responses in some cases unpredictable. Epigenetics is a young and new area of research that examines variable but heritable differences in gene expression without modifications to the DNA sequence. This subject is discussed further in Chapter 6.

CYPs are heme-containing proteins that provide most of the phase I drug metabolism for lipophilic compounds in the body.[148] The generally accepted nomenclature of the cytochrome P-450 isozymes begins with CYP, and group enzymes with more than 36% DNA homology subgrouped into families designated with an Arabic number, followed by letters for the subfamily of closely related proteins (>77% homology), followed by a number for the specific enzyme gene, such as CYP3A4.[149,150] Isozymes that are important in human drug metabolism are found in the *CYP1*, *CYP2*, and *CYP3* gene families. Table 7.1 outlines the CYP isozymes and their common substrates.

TABLE 7.1	Developmental Patterns and Activities for Important Cytochrome P-450 Enzymes (Phase I Reactions) in the Neonate			
Enzymes	**Selected Substrates**	**Inducers**	**Inhibitors**	**Developmental Changes**
CYP1A2	Acetaminophen, caffeine, theophylline, warfarin	Cigarette smoke, charcoal-broiled meat, omeprazole, cruciferous vegetables	α-Naphthoflavone	Not present to an appreciable extent in human fetal liver. Adult levels reached by 4 months of age and may be exceeded in children 1–2 years of age. Inhibited by phenobarbital and phenytoin.
CYP2A6	Warfarin, nicotine	Barbiturates	Tranylcypromine	
CYP2C9	Diclofenac, phenytoin, torsemide, *S*-warfarin tolbutamide	Rifampin	Sulfaphenazole, sulfinpyrazone	Not apparent in fetal liver. Inferential data using phenytoin disposition as a nonspecific pharmacologic probe suggests low activity during the first week of life, with adult activity reached by 6 months of age and peak activity reached by 3–4 years of age. Metabolism induced by rifampin and phenobarbital and inhibited by cimetidine.
CYP2C19	Phenytoin, diazepam, omeprazole, propranolol	Rifampin	Tranylcypromine	
CYP2D6	Amitriptyline, captopril, codeine, dextromethorphan, fluoxetine, hydrocodone, ondansetron, propafenone, propranolol, timolol	None known	Fluoxetine, quinidine	Low to absent in fetal liver but uniformly present at 1 week of postnatal age. Poor activity (approximately 20% of adult values) at 1 month of postnatal age. Adult competence reached by 3–5 years of age. Metabolism inhibited by cimetidine.
CYP3A4	Acetaminophen, alfentanil, amiodarone, budesonide, carbamazepine, diazepam, erythromycin, lidocaine, midazolam, nifedipine, omeprazole, cisapride, theophylline, verapamil, *R*-warfarin	Carbamazepine, dexamethasone, phenobarbital, phenytoin, rifampin	Azole antifungals, ethinyl estradiol, naringenin, troleandomycin, erythromycin	CYP3A4 has low activity in the first month of life, which approaches adult levels by 6–12 months postnatally.
CYP3A7	Dehydroepiandrosterone, ethinyl estradiol, various dihydropyrimidines	Carbamazepine, rifampin, phenytoin, dexamethasone, phenobarbital	Azole antifungals, erythromycin, cimetidine	CYP3A7 is functionally active in the fetus; approximately 30% to 75% of adult levels of CYP3A4.

Adapted from Leeder JS, Kearns GL. Pharmacogenetics in pediatrics: implications for practice. *Pediatr Clin North Am.* 1997;44(1):55–77.

For many drugs, the reduced metabolism in neonates relates to reduced total quantities of CYP enzymes in the hepatic microsomes.[151] Although the concentrations of CYP enzymes increase with gestational age, they may reach only 50% of adult values at term. Most isozymes are immature in the neonate, but some CYP isozymes exhibit near-adult activity, whereas others produce unique metabolic pathways in the neonatal period that invalidate broad generalizations about neonatal drug metabolism (see Table 7.1). Developmental changes of specific cytochromes are discussed in Chapter 6.

PHASE II REACTIONS

The other major route of drug metabolism, designated phase II reactions, involves synthetic or conjugation reactions that increase the hydrophilicity of molecules to facilitate renal elimination.[145,146] The phase II enzymes include glucuronosyltransferase, sulfotransferase, N-acetyltransferase, glutathione S-transferase, and methyltransferase. The phase II enzymes also show developmental changes during infancy that influence drug clearance (Table 7.2).[152–155]

Most conjugation reactions have limited activity during fetal development.[156] One of the most familiar synthetic reactions in young infants involves conjugation by uridine diphosphoglucuronosyltransferases (UGTs). This enzyme system includes numerous isoforms and is also responsible for glucuronidation of endogenous compounds, such as bilirubin (by UGT1A1).[156] As with the maturation of bilirubin conjugation, UGT activity is limited immediately postnatally and the different isoforms mature at different rates postnatally.[157] Dosage adjustments are often needed to avoid toxicity in neonates from drugs that require conjugation by UGT for clearance. Experience with chloramphenicol in the 1960s illustrated this lesson when neonates received standard pediatric doses of chloramphenicol without understanding the immaturity of UGT and its role in the elimination of chloramphenicol. Infants accumulated large concentrations of chloramphenicol and developed fatal circulatory collapse, a condition known as the gray baby syndrome.[158–160] Although the clearance of chloramphenicol is poor during the neonatal period, appropriate dosage adjustments and monitoring allow safe treatment of preterm and term infants with chloramphenicol.[161]

Morphine, acetaminophen, dexmedetomidine, and lorazepam also undergo glucuronidation. The major steps in the metabolic disposition of morphine in children and adults is glucuronidation in the 3- and 6-position.[162,163] The limited ability of neonates to metabolize morphine by glucuronidation necessitates dosage adjustment.[46,164,165] Detailed studies have shown that morphine clearance,[164,166] in particular 3- and 6-glucuronide formation, is limited at birth and increases with birth weight,[165] gestational age,[148] and postnatal age.[46,163] In some studies, morphine clearance, expressed as per kilogram, approaches adult values by 1 month,[46,167] although others reported that clearance does not reach adult values until at 5 to 6 months.[164,168] Overall, the maturation of glucuronosyltransferase enzymes varies among isoforms but, in general, adult activity is reached by 6 to 18 months of age.[150] Some of the confusion relating to maturation rates is attributable to the use of the per-kilogram size model. The use of allometry with a maturation model has assisted understanding. The time courses of maturation of drug metabolism for morphine,[45] acetaminophen,[169] dexmedetomidine,[170] and GFR[171] are strikingly similar (Fig. 7.11) with 50% of size-adjusted adult values reached between 8 and 12 weeks (TM_{50}) after full-term delivery. All three drugs are cleared predominantly by UGT that converts the parent compound into a water-soluble metabolite that is excreted by the kidneys; the clearance maturation profiles of these drugs matches that of GFR maturation. Glucuronidation is also the major metabolic pathway of propofol metabolism, although multiple CYP isoenzymes, including CYP2B6, CYP2C9, or CYP2A6, contribute to its metabolism and cause a faster maturation profile than expected from glucuronide conjugation alone.[172] A phase I reaction (CYP3A4) is the major enzyme system for oxidation of levobupivacaine, and clearance through this pathway is faster than those associated with UGT maturation.[45,169,171,173–176]

In contrast to glucuronosyltransferase, the sulfotransferase enzyme system is well developed in the neonate, and for some compounds it may compensate for limited glucuronidation. In adults, the primary pathway for acetaminophen metabolism is glucuronidation, yet its half-life is only moderately prolonged in neonates compared with older infants and adults.[177–179] This occurs partly because of the increased Vd in neonates (Eq. 7.20) and partly because the neonate forms more sulfate than glucuronide conjugate, leading to a greater percent of the dose excreted as the acetaminophen-sulfate conjugate.[106,178–181] Unfortunately, this does not confer safety from hepatotoxicity. The toxic metabolite is created through the oxidative pathway mediated by CYP2E1.

ALTERATIONS IN BIOTRANSFORMATION

Transition from the intrauterine to the extrauterine environment is associated with major changes in blood flow. There may also be an environmental trigger for the expression of some metabolic enzyme activities, resulting in a slight increase in maturation rate above that predicted by PMA.[172,175] Many biotransformation

TABLE 7.2	Developmental Patterns for Important Conjugation (Phase II) Reactions in the Neonate	
Enzymes	**Selected Substrates**	**Developmental Patterns**
Uridine diphosphoglucuronyltransferase (UDP-GT)	Chloramphenicol, morphine, acetaminophen, valproic acid, lorazepam	Ontogeny is isoform specific. In general, adult activity is achieved by 6–18 months of age. May be induced by cigarette smoke and phenobarbital.
Sulfotransferase	Bile acids, acetaminophen, cholesterol, polyethylene, glycols, dopamine, chloramphenicol	Ontogeny seems to be more rapid than UDP-GT; however, it is substrate specific. Activity for some isoforms may exceed adult values during infancy and childhood (e.g., that responsible for acetaminophen metabolism).
N-Acetyltransferase 2	Hydralazine, procainamide, clonazepam, caffeine, sulfamethoxazole	Some fetal activity present by 16 weeks. Virtually 100% of infants between birth and 2 months of age exhibit the slow metabolizer phenotype. Adult activity present by 1–3 years of age.

Adapted from Leeder JS, Kearns GL. Pharmacogenetics in pediatrics: implications for practice. *Pediatr Clin North Am.* 1997;44(1):55–77.

reactions, especially those involving certain forms of CYP, are inducible before birth through maternal exposure to drugs, cigarette smoke, or other inducing agents. Postnatally, biotransformation reactions may be induced through drug exposure (see Tables 7.1 and 7.2) and may be slowed by hypoxia, asphyxia, organ damage, and/or illness. The reduced thiopental clearance estimated from data when the drug was given to control neonatal seizures that resulted from hypoxic-ischemic insults may not be applicable to healthy neonates undergoing anesthesia.[182,183]

EXTRAHEPATIC ROUTES OF METABOLIC CLEARANCE

Many drugs undergo metabolic clearance at extrahepatic sites. Remifentanil and atracurium are degraded by nonspecific esterases in tissues and erythrocytes. Clearance, expressed per kilogram, is increased in younger children,[39,184–187] likely attributable to size, because clearance is similar when scaled to a 70-kg person using allometry.[39] Nonspecific blood esterases that metabolize remifentanil are mature at birth.[40]

Ester local anesthetics are metabolized by plasma butyrylcholinesterase, which is thought to be reduced in neonates. The in vitro plasma half-life of 2-chloroprocaine in umbilical cord blood is twice that in maternal blood,[188] but there are no in vivo studies of the effects of age on its metabolism. Succinylcholine clearance is increased in neonates when expressed as per kilogram, suggesting butyrylcholinesterase activity is mature at birth.[189,190]

RENAL EXCRETION

Renal function in preterm and term infants is less efficient than in adults, even after adjusting for the differences in body weight. This reduced efficiency is related to the combination of incomplete glomerular development, low perfusion pressure, and inadequate osmotic load to produce full countercurrent effects.[191–196] However, glomerular filtration and tubular function both develop rapidly during the first few months of life,[171] and are nearly mature by 20 weeks of age, and fully mature by 2 years of age (Figs. 7.11 and 7.12).[192–196] For these reasons, *drugs that are excreted primarily through glomerular filtration or tubular secretion, such as aminoglycoside and cephalosporin antibiotics, have a prolonged elimination half-life in neonates* (E-Fig. 7.4).[197–199]

In the presence of renal failure, one or two doses of drugs that are excreted via the kidneys often achieve and maintain prolonged therapeutic drug concentrations if there is no alternate pathway of excretion. Whenever administering a medication to a preterm or term infant, one must consider the contribution of renal function in the clearance of both the drug and any active metabolite.

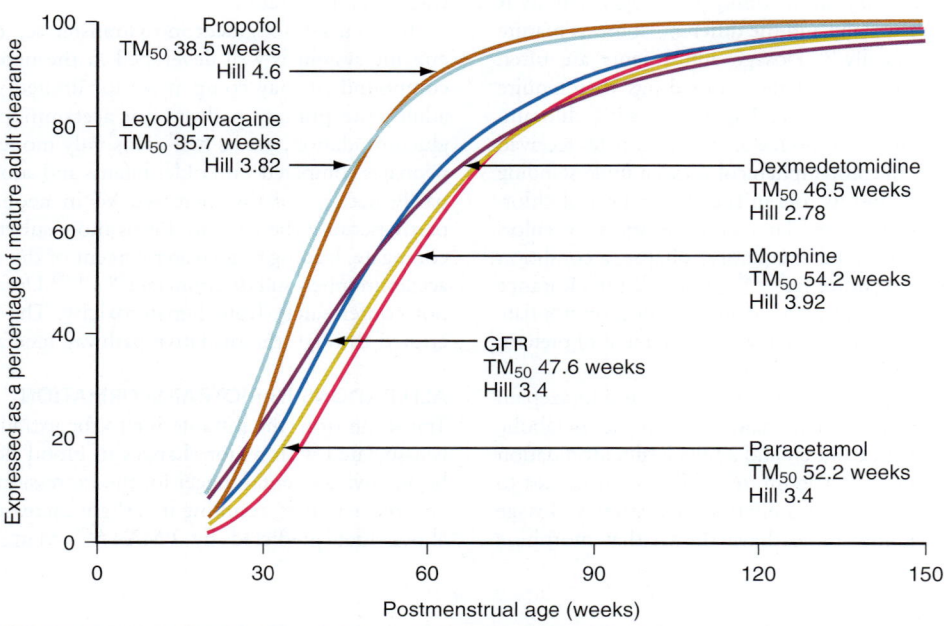

FIGURE 7.11 Clearance maturation, expressed as a percentage of mature clearance, of drugs where glucuronide conjugation (paracetamol, morphine, dexmedetomidine) plays a major role. These profiles are closely aligned with glomerular filtration rate (*GFR*). In contrast, cytochrome P-450 isoenzymes also contribute to propofol and levobupivacaine metabolism and cause a faster maturation profile than expected from glucuronide conjugation alone. *Hill*, Hill coefficient; *TM$_{50}$*, maturation half-time. (Maturation parameter estimates from Anderson BJ, Holford NH. Mechanistic basis of using body size and maturation to predict clearance in humans. *Drug Metab Pharmacokinet.* 2009;24(1):25–36; Anand KJ, Anderson BJ, Holford NH, et al. Morphine pharmacokinetics and pharmacodynamics in preterm and term neonates: secondary results from the NEOPAIN trial. *Br J Anaesth.* 2008;101(5):680–689; Potts AL, Warman GR, Anderson BJ. Dexmedetomidine disposition in children: a population analysis. *Paediatr Anaesth.* 2008;18(8):722–730; Allegaert K, Hoon JD, Verbesselt R, Naulaers G, Murat I. Maturational pharmacokinetics of single intravenous bolus of propofol. *Paediatr Anaesth.* 2007;17(11):1028–1034; Chalkiadis GA, Anderson BJ. Age and size are the major covariates for prediction of levobupivacaine clearance in children. *Paediatr Anaesth.* 2006;16(3):275–282; Rhodin MM, Anderson BJ, Peters AM, et al. Human renal function maturation: a quantitative description using weight and postmenstrual age. *Pediatr Nephrol.* 2009;24(1):67–76; Anderson BJ, Holford NH. Tips and traps analyzing pediatric PK data. *Paediatr Anaesth.* 2011;21(3):222–237.)

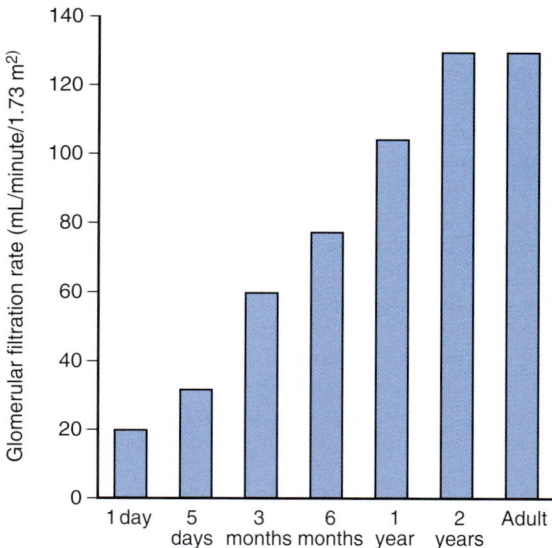

FIGURE 7.12 Changes in glomerular filtration rate versus age. Note the rapid development of glomerular function during the first year of life. Abnormal or immature renal function may delay drug excretion. (Data from Chantler C. *Clinical Pediatric Nephrology*. Philadelphia: JB Lippincott; 1976.)

The PK and PD of the old muscle relaxant, curare, exemplify the complex interaction of increased Vd, smaller muscle mass, and decreased rate of excretion as a result of immaturity of glomerular filtration. The initial dose (per kilogram) of curare needed to achieve neuromuscular blockade is similar in infants and adults.[86] In infants, however, this blockade is achieved at reduced serum concentrations compared with older children or adults, corresponding to differences in muscle mass and receptor immaturity. A larger Vd (total body water) accounts for the equivalent dose for each kilogram of body weight, and the reduced glomerular function in infants compared with older children or adults accounts in part for the longer duration of action.[86] As in the case of drugs excreted by the liver, there is a triphasic developmental response to drugs excreted by the kidneys when expressed as per kilogram (see Fig. 7.5): a prolonged half-life in neonates (immature renal function), a shortened half-life in young children, and a greater elimination half-life in adolescents and adults (size-related).

Reduced protein binding in neonates and preterm infants increases the free fraction of drugs delivered to the kidneys and liver for metabolism; however, reduced clearance results in a greater potential for toxicity.[2,3,5,6] An important example is the immature clearance of bupivacaine, which resulted in large plasma concentrations that increased sufficiently to cause seizures in neonates treated with epidural infusions at rates greater than that at which it was metabolized.[200]

Central Nervous System Effects

Laboratory data have demonstrated that the lethal dose in 50% of neonatal animals (LD_{50}) for many drugs depends on age: the LD_{50} is significantly less in neonatal than in adult animals.[201,202] The sensitivity of human neonates to most of the sedatives, hypnotics, and opioids is clinically well known and may in part be related to increased brain permeability (immature BBB or damage to the BBB) for some medications.[203–209] Laboratory studies

have demonstrated greater brain concentrations of morphine and amobarbital in infant than in adult animals.[210]

However, respiratory depression, measured by CO_2 response curves or arterial oxygen tension, is similar from 2 to 570 days after birth at the same morphine blood concentration.[211] Altered PK may contribute to the increased sensitivity to morphine in neonates. A reduced clearance and a reduced Vd in neonates will result in greater plasma concentrations in this age group compared with older children given similar weight-scaled doses,[212,213] and this greater concentration contributes more to respiratory depression than the increased brain permeability in those who were not premature.

Drugs that are not particularly lipid soluble may enter the brain more easily in neonates with incomplete myelination than in infants where the BBB is intact.[203,204,210,214] When considering the use of any centrally acting medication in children younger than 1 year of age, and particularly those less than 48 weeks PMA, one must balance the potential risks and benefits. The dose must be carefully calculated and titrated to the minimum dose that achieves the desired response. Careful monitoring of vital signs is critical because prolonged effects or adverse clinical responses may occur in children at any age, but particularly in infants in whom CNS maturation may be incomplete.

Pharmacodynamics in Children

Children's responses to drugs have much in common with the responses in adults.[215] The perception that drug effects differ in children may be attributed to the patchy study of drugs in pediatric populations who have size- and maturation-related effects, as well as different diseases. Neonates and infants, however, often have altered PD. For example, the increased sensitivity of the neonate to morphine compared with children may be attributable, in part, to altered PK (reduced clearance, smaller Vd), but it may also be a reflection of the developmental regulation of opioid receptors.[216]

The MAC for most inhalational anesthetics is less in neonates than in infants, which in turn is greater than that observed in children and adults.[217] The MAC of isoflurane in preterm neonates less than 32 weeks gestation is 1.28%, and that in neonates 32 to 37 weeks gestation is 1.41%.[218] This value increases to 1.87% by 6 months of age before decreasing again throughout childhood.[218] The cause of these age-related differences is uncertain and may relate to maturational changes in cerebral blood flow (CBF), γ-aminobutyric acid (GABA) class A receptor numbers, or developmental shifts in the regulation of chloride transporters.[219–221]

Neonates have an increased sensitivity to the effects of NMBDs.[86] The reason for this is unknown, but it is consistent with the observation that there is a 3-fold reduction in the release of acetylcholine from the infant rat phrenic nerve as well as a relatively reduced muscle mass.[222–225] The increased Vd, however, means that a single NMBD dose (calculated as milligrams per kilogram) in the neonate results in blockade at a reduced plasma concentration while the decreased clearance prolongs the duration of effect.

Both the coagulation[226,227] and the fibrinolytic systems[228–231] are immature at birth. Consequently, the target plasma concentration of antifibrinolytic drugs required to achieve similar effects in neonates is less than that in adults. Although the concentration of ε-aminocaproic acid (EACA) required to inhibit fibrinolysis in adult plasma in vitro is 130 mg/L, the concentration required in neonatal plasma is much smaller, 50 mg/L.[232,233] The dose of EACA must be adjusted in neonates because of both the immaturity of their antifibrinolytic clearance pathways and the coagulation cascade.

Cardiac calcium stores in the endoplasmic reticulum are reduced in the neonatal heart because of immaturity. Exogenous calcium has greater impact on contractility in this age group than in older children and adults. Conversely, neonates may suffer cardiac arrest if given the calcium antagonist, verapamil.[234] Immaturity of myocardial potassium channels prolongs the QT interval in neonates; neonates exhibit a greater sensitivity toward QTc (corrected QT) interval prolongation compared with older children. This made them more sensitive to sotalol given for supraventricular tachycardia (SVT).[235]

Amide local anesthetic agents induce blocks of briefer duration and require a larger weight-scaled dose to achieve similar dermatomal levels when given by subarachnoid block to infants. This may be due, in part, to myelination, spacing of the nodes of Ranvier, the length of nerve exposed, increased relative volume of CSF, as well as other size factors. There is an age-dependent expression of intestinal motilin receptors and the modulation of gastric antral contractions in neonates. Prokinetic agents may not be useful in very preterm infants, partially useful in older preterm infants, and useful in full-term infants. Similarly, bronchodilators in infants are less effective because of the paucity of bronchial smooth muscle that can cause bronchospasm.

Drug effects in neonates may not be evident until later in life. Neonates and young children may suffer permanent effects resulting from a stimulus applied at a sensitive point in development. For example, congenital hypothyroidism, if untreated, causes lifelong phenotypic changes. The incidence of vaginal carcinoma in children of mothers treated with stilboestrol during pregnancy is great.[236]

Corticosteroids are associated with growth retardation in children with asthma.[237] There are concerns that neonatal exposure to some anesthetic agents (e.g., ketamine, midazolam) may cause widespread neuronal apoptosis and long-term memory deficits (see Chapter 25).

MEASUREMENT OF PHARMACODYNAMIC ENDPOINTS

Outcome measures are more difficult to assess in neonates and infants than in children or adults. Measurement techniques, disease and pathology differences, inhomogeneous groups, recruitment issues, ethical considerations, and endpoint definitions for establishing efficacy and safety often confuse interpretation of the measures.[238]

Common effects measured in infancy include anesthesia depth, pain responses, depth of sedation, and intensity of neuromuscular blockade. A common effect measure used to assess depth of anesthesia is the EEG or a modification of detected EEG signals (spectral edge frequency, bispectral index [BIS], entropy). Physiologic studies in adults and children indicate that EEG-derived anesthesia depth monitors can provide an imprecise and drug-dependent measure of arousal. Although the outputs from these monitors do not closely represent any true physiologic entity, they can be used as guides for anesthesia, and in so doing, may improve outcomes in adults. In older children the physiology, anatomy, and clinical observations indicate the performance of the monitors may be similar to that in adults. In infants, however, their use cannot be supported in theory or in practice at this time.[239,240] During anesthesia, the EEG in infants is fundamentally different from the EEG in older children; there remains a need

for specific neonate-derived algorithms if EEG-derived anesthesia depth monitors are to be used in neonates.[241,242] Examples of problems with BIS monitoring in infants and young children include the observations that BIS numbers paradoxically increase when sevoflurane concentrations exceed 3% (1.2 × MAC), there is often a difference between the right and left sides of the brain, equivalent MAC values yield different BIS values with each agent, and values in children tend to be greater than those in adults at equivalent MAC values (see also Chapter 52).[243-247]

The Children's Hospital of Wisconsin Sedation Scale has been used to investigate ketamine in the emergency department.[66,248] However, despite the use of such scales in procedural pain or sedation studies, few behavioral scales have been adequately validated in this setting and interobserver variability can be substantial.[249-251] Most scores are validated for the acute, procedural setting and are less robust for subacute or chronic pain or stress.

THE TARGET CONCENTRATION APPROACH

The goal of treatment is the target effect. A PD model is used to predict the target concentration given a target effect. Population estimates for the PD model parameters and covariate information are used to predict typical PD values in a specific patient. Population estimates of PK model parameter estimates and covariate information are then used to predict typical PK values in a typical patient. For example, a dexmedetomidine steady-state target concentration of 0.6 μg/L may be achieved with an infusion of 0.33 μg/kg per hour in a neonate, 0.51 μg/kg per hour in a 1-year-old, and 0.47 μg/kg per hour in an 8-year-old.[176] This target concentration strategy is a powerful tool for determining the clinical dose.[252] Monitoring the drug concentrations in serum and Bayesian forecasting may be used to improve the dose in individual patients.

This target effect approach is intrinsic to pediatric anesthesiologists using target-controlled infusion systems (see also Chapter 8). These devices target a specific plasma or effect-site concentration in a typical individual and this concentration is assumed to have a typical target effect. The target concentration is one that achieves a target therapeutic effect (e.g., anesthesia) without excessive adverse effects (e.g., hypotension). Unfortunately, these devices have still not been approved by the Food and Drug Administration (FDA) for use in the United States.

DEFINING TARGET CONCENTRATION

An effect-site target concentration has been estimated for many drugs used in anesthesia, analgesia, and sedation. For example, a propofol target concentration of 3 mg/L or 3 μg/mL in a typical patient can be achieved using preprogrammed target-controlled infusion devices. In teenagers, a BIS monitor can provide feedback to guide the infusion rate to achieve a desired target effect in the particular individual. The luxury of such a feedback system is not available for most drugs and unfortunately may be of little value in neonates and infants.

A target concentration of 10 μg/L may be used for morphine analgesia. Observations in children after cardiac surgery found that steady-state serum concentrations greater than 20 μg/L resulted in hypercarbia (PaCO₂ [partial pressure of carbon dioxide in arterial blood] >55 mm Hg) and flattened CO₂ response curves. During wash-out, morphine concentrations in excess of 15 μg/L caused hypercarbia in 46% of children, whereas concentrations less than 15 μg/L were associated with hypercarbia in only 13%. No age-related differences in the respiratory effect occurred at the same serum concentration of morphine.[211] Observation or self-reporting pain scales are used as part of the feedback loop for dose incremental changes.

The target concentration may vary depending on the desired target effect. The target concentration for ketamine analgesia (0.25 mg/L) differs substantially from that of anesthesia (2 mg/L), and BIS monitoring would be totally useless because ketamine causes central excitation, thereby increasing bispectral monitoring numbers.[253–256]

Drug Interactions

There are many common examples of drug interactions that increase or decrease responses mediated through either PK or PD routes. Phenobarbital induction of CYP3A4 metabolism and consequent increased ketamine requirements for radiologic sedation[143] is an example of a PK interaction. PK interactions are often dealt with in mixed-effects modeling by including the effect of a second drug as a covariate on affected PK parameters such as those describing clearance (CL), volume of distribution (Vd), or bioavailability (F). The midazolam-propofol PK interaction has been investigated by adjusting midazolam CL and V using propofol plasma concentrations included in an exponential covariate model—that is,

$$CL_{IND} = CL_{POP} * \exp^{(cov(C_{PROP} - Median\ C_{PROP}))}, \quad \text{Eq. 7.21}$$

where CL is clearance from the central compartment, for the population (CL_{POP}) and the individual (CL_{IND}). Here, the effect of plasma propofol concentration (C_{PROP}) on the CL parameter is estimated (the parameter "cov") and scaled to the population median C_{PROP}.

Interactions may also occur at entry into the effect site. An increase in the $T_{1/2}keo$ of d-tubocurarine with increasing inspired concentrations of halothane has been reported.[257] Halothane is a negative inotrope[258] and reduces skeletal muscle blood flow,[259] so it is reasonable to interpret changes in $T_{1/2}keo$ as a result of changes in organ blood flow.

Competitive antagonists reduce receptor availability by competing for occupancy at the same receptor site. Drugs that elicit an effect are called agonists, while those that do not are called antagonists, so the occupancy of some receptors by the antagonists results in less effect. In general, competitive antagonists shift the effect-concentration curve to the right by altering the C_{50}. The Emax equation (Eq. 7.19) can then be expressed as

$$Effect = E0 + \frac{Emax \cdot Ce^N}{\left(\left(EC_{50}^N \cdot \left[1 + \dfrac{A}{EA_{50}}\right]\right) + Ce^N\right)} \quad \text{Eq. 7.22}$$

where Ce is the concentration in the effect site, and A and EA_{50} represent ligand A concentration and potency. Noncompetitive antagonists shift the observed maximum effect (Emax) rather than the C_{50}:

$$Effect = E0 + \frac{Emax \cdot \left(1 - \dfrac{A}{A + EA_{50}}\right) \cdot Ce^\gamma}{Ce^\gamma + C_{50}^\gamma} \quad \text{Eq. 7.23}$$

PD interactions are not restricted to same-site binding interactions; some proteins have multiple binding sites, and ligands binding at these sites can also alter the above relationship (i.e., through changes in protein conformation that lead to downstream changes or modulate agonist-receptor affinity). These are referred to as

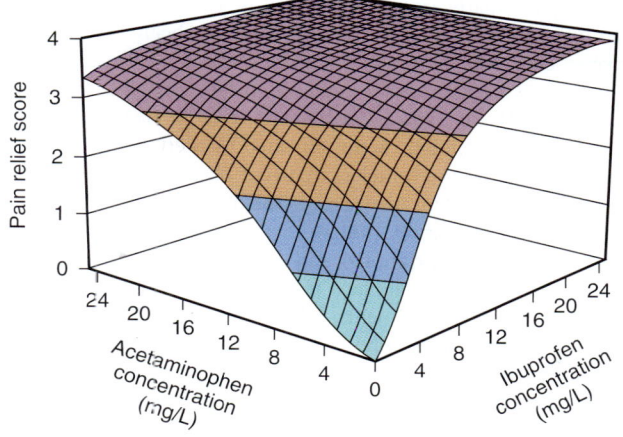

FIGURE 7.13 The response surface of analgesic effect for acetaminophen and ibuprofen. Concentrations are those in the effect compartment. The concentration response for acetaminophen is plotted on the x-y axis, while that for ibuprofen is on the z-y axis. The "surface" is that plotted between these axes. Each point on the surface is a measure of the pain relief provided by acetaminophen and ibuprofen combination. (From Hannam J, Anderson BJ. Explaining the acetaminophen-ibuprofen analgesic interaction using a response surface model. *Paediatr Anaesth.* 2011;21(12):1234–1240, with permission.)

"allosteric" interactions. Action at a receptor level may be studied in vivo. Several techniques exist for evaluating pharmacodynamic interactions in vivo.

Anesthetic drug interactions traditionally have been characterized using isobolographic analysis or multiple logistic regression. Minto[260] and Greco[261] proposed models based on response-surface methodology (see Chapter 8). Computer simulations based on interactions at the effect site predicted that the maximally synergistic three-drug combination (midazolam, propofol, and alfentanil) tripled the duration of effect compared with propofol alone. The response surface for ibuprofen and acetaminophen is shown in Fig. 7.13. The addition of acetaminophen to ibuprofen improved analgesia when the dose of ibuprofen was less than 100 mg (5 mg/kg) in a 5-year-old child.[262] Response surfaces can describe anesthetic interactions, even those between agonists, partial agonists, competitive antagonists, and inverse agonists.[260,263]

Inhalation anesthetic agents can prolong the duration of block, and this effect is agent specific. When compared with halothane, sevoflurane potentiates the effects of vecuronium to a greater extent. When compared with balanced anesthesia, sevoflurane and halothane decrease the dose requirements of vecuronium by 60% and 40%, respectively.[264]

Surface modeling techniques have been used to demonstrate strikingly synergistic effects from sevoflurane with alfentanil[265] and remifentanil with propofol[266,267] on respiration in adults.[265,266,268,269] It is little wonder that the use of three or more sedating medications is associated with significantly more adverse outcomes than the use of one or two medications.[266]

The Drug Approval Process, the Package Insert, and Drug Labeling

A great concern has been the general lack of regulatory approval of many of the medications for populations of pediatric patients.

This is particularly ironic because most of the changes in legislation pertaining to pharmaceuticals have been the result of adverse events in infants and children. The 1938 Federal Food, Drug, and Cosmetic Act[270] replaced the original Federal Food and Drugs Act of 1906 (Wiley Act)[271] because nearly 100 individuals, mostly children, were poisoned by diethylene glycol (an antifreeze analog for vehicles) that had been added to an elixir of sulfanilamide. This new legislation prohibited the addition of poisonous substances (unless they were demonstrated to be safe in small concentrations) and instituted other measures to protect the consumer. The next major piece of legislation was the Kefauver-Harris Amendments, which were passed in 1962 after the thalidomide catastrophe.[272] This legislation strengthened the safety standards by requiring the drug company to demonstrate effectiveness before marketing. The U.S. FDA then allowed drugs to be marketed to adults as *"safe and effective,"* but now the drug label was required to indicate that *"safety and effectiveness had not been established in children"* because no trials in children had been carried out. This had an enormous negative impact on drug development for children and led Shirkey to coin the now common expression *"therapeutic orphans"* when referring to drug development for children.[273]

Until the late 1990s, nearly 80% of approved medications contained language within the drug label (package insert) that excluded children of varying ages; it should be noted that the legislation described later in the text has now resulted in some pediatric labeling in ~60% of marketed medications, which is an unequivocal victory for drug safety in children.[274] The majority of the drugs used in the operating room (OR) and the intensive care unit (ICU) today have similar language.[275] Common examples of disclaimers for drugs used in our daily practice include those for bupivacaine (*"Until further experience is gained in children younger than 12 years, administration of Sensorcaine [bupivacaine HCl] injection is not recommended"*)[269] and for fentanyl (*"The safety of SUBLIMAZE in children younger than two years of age has not been established"*).[276] Such disclaimers are placed in the package insert because the contents of the package insert must, by law, be based on *"adequate, well controlled studies involving children."*[272,277-279] Any use of a drug that is not specifically described in the package insert is considered *"unapproved"* or *"off label."* The reason for the lack of labeling for children is that the appropriate controlled clinical trials were never supported by industry and the FDA did not have the legislative power to force the pharmaceutical companies to perform pediatric studies.[280] In 1994, the FDA passed a new interpretation of the original Food, Drug, and Cosmetic Act[270,278,281] that allowed manufacturers to review the published medical literature and submit these data to the FDA to support revised pediatric labeling.[279] This led to additional changes in the drug label for 48 medications. Unfortunately, for drugs that were no longer under patent protection, there was no financial incentive to force the issue, so many drugs remained unlabeled for children despite many publications that outlined their safe use in children of all ages.

During the early stages of the AIDS epidemic, there was great pressure placed on the FDA to reduce the time for the drug approval process. New legislation was passed to raise funds to pay for additional consultants and experts to help the FDA with this process (The Prescription Drug User Fee Act [PDUFA]).[282] This legislation was renewed in 1997, 2002, 2007, and 2012 and was redrafted for the sixth time (PDUFA VI) and signed into law in August 2017, thus providing "stable and consistent funding during fiscal years 2018–2022."[282a,282b] The PDUFA regulations have three components: (1) an application fee when a new drug

or biologic is submitted to the FDA, (2) an annual product fee for nongeneric marketed drugs, and (3) an annual fee for each manufacturing site for nongeneric drugs.[282c] The goals of the new legislation are to further enhance scientific expertise and processes for regulatory decisions, improve patient perspectives in drug development, and provide longer stability of the PDUFA initiative. The monies from these fees greatly reduce the time from a New Drug Application (NDA) or Biologic License Application (BLA) to be marketed. The most recent iterations have expanded funding to support marketing safety and pharmacoepidemiology activities, as well as increased inspection of non–USA-based pharmaceutical manufacturing facilities. Approximately 72% of NDAs or BLAs were approved on the first application under PDUFA V compared with ~55% under PDUFA IV.[283,284]

Additional changes at the FDA occurred in the late 1990s when the Food and Drug Administration Modernization Act[268] and the Final Rule were passed.[285] Tacked onto this legislation was the Better Pharmaceutical Act for Children, which granted 6 months of patent extension in exchange for pediatric studies of drugs that were still patent protected. This was later replaced with the Best Pharmaceutical Act for Children (BPCA) in 2002, which earmarked money for the National Institutes of Health (NIH) to support study of drugs no longer patent protected.[286] This was subsequently challenged as giving excessive legal power to the FDA, but further legislation reinstituted the legal power to the FDA to now require drug companies to conduct research in children if the drug would have use in children (the Pediatric Research Equity Act).[287] PDUFA IV was a much larger bill entitled the Food and Drug Administration Amendments Act of 2007. This bill renewed PDUFA IV, the Medical Device User Fee and Modernization Act, and BPCA.[288] Of importance to researchers was the new requirement for registration of all clinical trials with an archive of thousands of trials that is easily searchable for clinicians as well as the public.[289] Many journals now will not publish clinical pharmaceutical trials that have not been registered. Since the first legislation for children passed in 1998, there has been an explosion of pediatric drug trials (>1000 requested or carried out since 1997) and new drug labels have been created for 703 drugs; between 2005 and 2017 patent extension has been granted to at least 79 medications (https://www.accessdata.fda.gov/scripts/sda/sdNavigation.cfm?sd=labelingdatabase).[290] Unfortunately, the money that was supposed to be earmarked to the NIH for generic drug trials has not been fully provided, so deficiencies in labeling for older drugs persist.[291]

It is important for clinicians to appreciate that despite language on the label regarding use in children, they are perfectly within their medical and legal rights to use these drugs based on their judgment. *"Unapproved use does not imply an improper use and certainly does not imply an illegal use."*[292,293] The use of a drug in a child is the decision of the individual physician and may be based on the available literature, despite the fact that formal FDA approval and labeling have not been achieved.[277,278] The Committee on Drugs of the American Academy of Pediatrics is very clear on this issue: *"Lack of approval for a specific use should not prevent physicians from prescribing an available drug in the best interest of their patients."*[292,293]

Inhalation Anesthetic Agents

PHYSICOCHEMICAL PROPERTIES

The potent inhaled anesthetics are ether-based anesthetics with either a methyl ethyl (enflurane, isoflurane, and desflurane) or a methyl isopropyl (sevoflurane) polyhalogenated ether skeleton (E-Table 7.1). The single exception in chemical structure is halothane, which is a polyhalogenated alkane. Of the methyl ethyl ether anesthetics, isoflurane and enflurane, are constitutional isomers. Desflurane differs from isoflurane in the single atomic substitution of a fluoride for a chlorine atom on the α-carbon of isoflurane. Sevoflurane differs from isoflurane in the substitution of a trifluoromethyl group for the chlorine atom, resulting in a methyl isopropyl structure. Although the general chemical structures of the four ether agents are similar, the single atomic substitutions confer substantially different physicochemical and pharmacologic properties described in later text and contrasted to the properties of halothane (see E-Table 7.1).

In comparison to the potent inhaled anesthetics, nitrous oxide and xenon exist in gaseous form under atmospheric conditions. Nitrous oxide is a by-product of chemical processes, whereas xenon is a naturally occurring element (0.05 ppm in the atmosphere), produced by fractional distillation of atmospheric gas. Environmentally, nitrous oxide depletes the ozone layer, whereas xenon is environmentally inert. There is a wealth of data on the pharmacology of nitrous oxide in humans but far less on xenon in adults and none, to date, in children.

PHARMACOKINETICS OF INHALED ANESTHETICS

The rate of increase or equilibration of the partial pressures of alveolar to inspired anesthetic (also known as the wash-in) is a function of the rate of delivery of anesthetic to and uptake from the lungs. Six factors determine the wash-in of inhaled anesthetics (Table 7.3)[294]: the first three determine the delivery of anesthetics to the lungs, and the second three determine their rate of removal (uptake) from the lungs. The wash-in, defined as the ratio of the alveolar to inspired anesthetic partial pressures (F_A/F_I, or fractional alveolar to fractional inspired partial pressures), increases from zero to a value of unity (1), when the inspired and alveolar partial pressures have equilibrated (Fig. 7.14). Although not shown in the figure, the wash-in of xenon should be the most rapid of all inhaled anesthetics based on its physicochemical properties (see E-Table 7.1).[295] For the F_A/F_I to increase toward equilibration, the rate of delivery of anesthetic to the lungs must substantially exceed its uptake from the lungs.

The rates of increase of F_A/F_I of halothane (as well as isoflurane, enflurane, and nitrous oxide) in infants and children are more rapid than those in adults (Fig. 7.15).[296-298] The more rapid rate of increase of F_A/F_I in neonates compared with adults has been attributed to four factors (Table 7.4); the order in the table reflects their relative contributions to the rapid wash-in. Based on these factors and their physical chemical properties, we speculate that the wash-in of sevoflurane and desflurane in neonates and infants will be comparable to those in adults. This amounts to a safety factor for the latter anesthetics that was not previously afforded with halothane.

TABLE 7.3	Determinants of the Wash-In of Inhalational Agents

- Inspired concentration
- Alveolar ventilation
- Functional residual capacity
- Cardiac output
- Solubility
- Alveolar to venous partial-pressure gradient

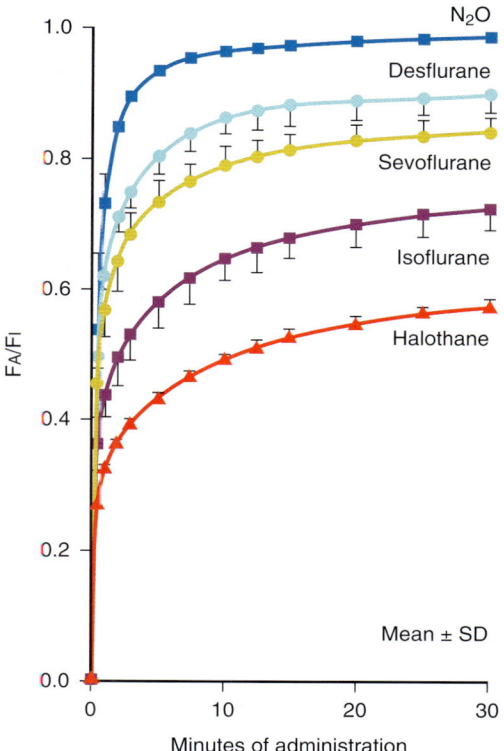

FIGURE 7.14 Wash-in (or F_A/F_I) of N_2O, desflurane, sevoflurane, isoflurane, and halothane in adults. The order of wash-in (N_2O > desflurane > sevoflurane > isoflurane > halothane) is inversely related to their solubilities in blood. F_A, fractional alveolar partial pressure of anesthetic; F_I, fractional inspired partial pressure of anesthetic; N_2O, nitrous oxide; SD, standard deviation. (Redrawn from Yasuda N, Lockhart SH, Eger EI 2nd, et al. Comparison of kinetics of sevoflurane and isoflurane in humans. *Anesth Analg.* 1991;72(3):316–324.)

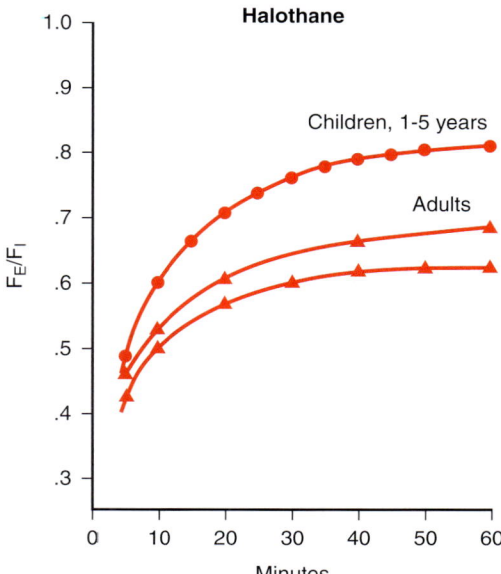

FIGURE 7.15 Rate of rise of expired to inspired fractional partial pressures (F_E/F_I) of halothane in children and adults. (Redrawn from Salanitre E, Rackow H. The pulmonary exchange of nitrous oxide and halothane in infants and children. *Anesthesiology* 1969;30(4):388–394.)

TABLE 7.4	Determinants of the Rapid Wash-In of Inhalational Agents in Infants Compared With Adults
Greater ratio of alveolar ventilation to functional residual capacity	
Greater fraction of the cardiac output distributed to the vessel-rich group	
Reduced tissue/blood solubility	
Reduced blood/gas solubility	

Factors Affecting Delivery of Inhaled Anesthetics to the Lungs

Inspired Concentration

The effect of the inspired concentration on the FA/FI of anesthetics relates only to those that are administered in large concentrations (i.e., nitrous oxide). The greater the FI of nitrous oxide, the more rapid the increase of FA/FI.[299] This effect, known as the concentration effect (second gas effect), depends on both a concentrating effect and an increase in alveolar ventilation that results from an increased uptake of nitrous oxide.[294] Hence, agents that depend on alveolar ventilation for their wash-in (i.e., the more soluble anesthetics) will have a more rapid wash-in when administered with nitrous oxide. This effect diminishes as the solubility of the anesthetic decreases and as time passes.[300–302]

Alveolar Ventilation and Functional Residual Capacity

The ratio of alveolar ventilation (Va) to functional residual capacity (FRC), Va/FRC, is the primary determinant of the rate of the delivery of inhaled anesthetics to the lungs. The greater the Va/FRC ratio, the more rapid the FA/FI (E-Fig. 7.5). However, the ratio does not affect all anesthetics similarly: Va/FRC affects more soluble anesthetics (e.g., halothane) to a greater extent than less soluble anesthetics (i.e., sevoflurane and desflurane). In the case of soluble anesthetics (e.g., halothane), their increase in FA/FI depends substantively on a large Va/FRC ratio since their uptake from the lungs is great (because of their solubilities), and this limits the rate of increase in FA/FI. Changes in the Va/FRC directly affect the FA/FI of anesthetics in proportion to their blood solubilities.

In terms of age-related effects of FA/FI, the Va/FRC ratio accounts for most of the differences between the FA/FI of anesthetics in neonates and adults (see Table 7.4). The Va/FRC ratio is approximately 5 : 1 in neonates compared with only 1.5 : 1 in adults. The greater Va/FRC ratio in neonates may be attributed to the 3-fold greater metabolic rate and, therefore, 3-fold greater Va/FRC in neonates compared with adults. This is true for both spontaneous and controlled ventilation, depending on the settings used during controlled ventilation.

Factors Affecting the Uptake (Removal) of Inhaled Anesthetics From the Lungs

Cardiac Output

The rate of increase in FA/FI is inversely related to changes in cardiac output; that is, the smaller the cardiac output, the more rapid the increase in FA/FI and vice versa (E-Fig. 7.6). As cardiac output diminishes, less anesthetic is removed from the lungs, thus increasing the rate of equilibration of FA/FI. A patient in heart failure who receives an inhalational induction may achieve greater anesthetic concentrations in the lungs more rapidly than expected compared with a patient with a normal cardiac output. This very serious problem may be exacerbated if the "overpressure" technique has been used, because it may cause acute anesthetic-induced myocardial depression and decompensation in cardiac

output. Conversely, in a high cardiac output state (as in the case of anxiety), the greater blood flow through the lungs removes more anesthetic from the alveoli, thus reducing the alveolar partial pressure of anesthetic, which slows the rate of equilibration of FA/FI. The impact of changes in cardiac output on FA/FI depends, in part, on the solubility of the anesthetic: the less soluble the anesthetic (sevoflurane and desflurane), the less this effect and vice versa.[294] This represents yet another safety feature of the less soluble anesthetics currently in use.

Paradoxically, the greater cardiac index in neonates actually speeds the increase in FA/FI. This has been attributed to the preferential distribution of the cardiac output to the vessel-rich group (VRG) of tissues (brain, heart, kidney, splanchnic organs, and endocrine glands) in neonates. The VRG receives a greater proportion of the cardiac output in neonates compared with adults because the VRG constitutes 18% of the body weight in the former compared with only 8% in the latter. As a result of the increased blood flow to the VRG, the partial pressures of anesthetics in the VRG equilibrate with those in the alveoli more rapidly in neonates than in adults. Because the uptake of anesthetic by tissues other than those in the VRG in neonates is small, the rapid increase in FA/FI in the VRG and blood suggests that the partial pressure of anesthetic in venous blood returning to the lungs rapidly equilibrates with that in the alveoli. Uptake of anesthetic from the lungs then diminishes. The net effect of the greater cardiac output in neonates is paradoxical in that it speeds the equilibration of anesthetic partial pressures in the VRG and thus speeds the equilibration of FA/FI. This also explains the "downward spiral" that occurs when an excessive concentration of inhaled agent (particularly the soluble anesthetic halothane) is administered to a neonate or infant during controlled ventilation, as discussed later.

Solubility

Inhalational agents partition into two compartments in body fluids and tissues: (1) an aqueous phase and (2) a protein/lipid phase. This partitioning is analogous to the distribution of gases such as oxygen in blood between the aqueous phase (dissolved fraction) and hemoglobin (bound fraction). Because inhaled anesthetics move along partial pressure gradients (and not concentration gradients) within and between fluids and tissues, the rate of increase of FA/FI and, therefore, the anesthetic partial pressure in blood determines how rapidly anesthetics move in and out of tissues and affect organ function (e.g., central nervous and cardiac systems).

The rate of increase of FA/FI of inhalational anesthetics, which varies inversely with the solubility of the anesthetic in blood, follows the order: nitrous oxide > desflurane > sevoflurane > isoflurane > enflurane > halothane > methoxyflurane (see E-Table 7.1 and Fig. 7.14).[294,303] Although the solubilities of nitrous oxide and desflurane are similar, the rate of increase in FA/FI of nitrous oxide is more rapid than that after desflurane because of the concentration effect from administering 70% nitrous oxide. After a stepwise change in the inspired partial pressure of less soluble anesthetics, the alveolar partial pressure equilibrates rapidly with the new inspired partial pressure. Because the wash-out of these anesthetics is equally rapid (see later), the alveolar partial pressure can be adjusted to previous values rapidly by decreasing the inspired partial pressure. Thus anesthetic depth can be adjusted more rapidly with a less soluble (i.e., desflurane or sevoflurane) than with a more soluble inhalational anesthetic (i.e., halothane).

Age is an important determinant of the solubility of inhalational anesthetics in blood. The blood solubilities of halothane, isoflurane, enflurane, and methoxyflurane are 18% less in neonates than in adults (E-Fig. 7.7; see also E-Table 7.1).[304] Serum cholesterol and proteins (including albumin) account for these age-related differences in blood solubilities.[304,305] In contrast, the blood solubility of the less soluble anesthetic sevoflurane is similar in neonates and adults.[305] Factors that do not significantly affect the blood solubility of most inhaled anesthetics include age-related differences in hemoglobin, serum concentration of α_1-acid glycoprotein, and prematurity.[304,305]

The tissue/gas solubilities of the inhaled anesthetics in the VRG in neonates are approximately one-half those in adults (E-Fig. 7.8).[306] The reduced tissue solubilities in neonates are attributable to two differences in the composition of tissues: (1) greater water content and (2) decreased protein and lipid concentrations. In terms of the uptake and distribution of inhaled anesthetics in tissues, the tissue/blood solubilities determine the speed of equilibration of anesthetics in tissues. The reduced tissue solubilities of inhaled anesthetics reduce the time for partial pressure equilibration of anesthetics (see time constant discussion, later). Although the partial pressures of inhaled anesthetics in tissues cannot easily be measured in vivo, they may be estimated by their concentrations in the exhaled or alveolar gases. The solubilities of these anesthetics in the brain of adults vary approximately 50% from desflurane to halothane (see E-Table 7.1). In the case of neonates, the reduced tissue solubilities of inhaled anesthetics speed the rate of increase in FA/FI compared with the rates in adults. In the cases of sevoflurane and desflurane, their respectively small but similar blood solubilities and likely similar tissue solubilities in neonates and adults offer a safety factor in neonates compared with adults, because tissue equilibration of these relatively insoluble inhalational anesthetics should be similar in both age groups. In contrast, the reduced tissue solubility of halothane in neonates leads to a more rapid and unexpected anesthetic effect compared with the time course in adults.

We can estimate the time to equilibration of the partial pressures of inhaled anesthetic in tissues by calculating the time constant for equilibration in tissue. For example, the time constant (tau τ) for equilibration of anesthetic partial pressure in the brain is based on the expression:

$$\tau_{brain} = \frac{\text{Volume of the brain (mL)} \times \text{Brain/blood solubility}}{\text{Brain blood flow (mL/minute)}},$$

Eq. 7.24

where one time constant is the time for 63% equilibration of brain to blood anesthetic partial pressures. If the blood flow to the brain is approximately 50 mL/minute per 100 g of brain tissue and the brain/blood solubility ratio for an inhalational anesthetic is 2.0 (assuming the density of brain tissue is 1 g/mL), then the time constant is:

$$\tau_{brain} = \frac{100 \text{ mL} \times 2}{50 \text{ mL/minute}} = 4 \text{ minutes}$$

Knowing that four time constants achieve 98% equilibration, then the time to 98% equilibration is 16 minutes. If the brain/blood solubility ratio were halved to 1.0, as it might be in the case of the neonate, then the time to 95% equilibration would decrease by 50% to 8 minutes. *Thus the time to equilibration of anesthetic partial pressure within the brain of the neonate would be approximately one-half that of the adult but still requires 8 minutes.* This holds true for the more soluble anesthetics, such as halothane, whose tissue solubility in neonates is diminished compared with adults[306] but not for the less soluble anesthetics, such as desflurane

and sevoflurane, whose tissue solubilities may be similar in neonates and adults.

Whereas the PK of inhalational anesthetics during the first 15 to 20 minutes depends primarily on the characteristics of the VRG, the PK during the subsequent 20 to 200 minutes depends primarily on the characteristics of muscle.[294] The solubility of inhalational anesthetics in skeletal muscle varies directly with age in a logarithmic relationship.[306] Thus the lower solubility of inhalational anesthetics in the muscle of neonates and the smaller muscle mass speed the increase in FA/FI during this period compared with that in adults. This effect of age on the solubility of anesthetics in muscle has been attributed to age-dependent increases in protein concentration (i.e., muscle bulk) during the first 5 decades of life and in fat content during the subsequent 3 decades of life.[306] Overall, the reduced solubility combined with the reduced muscle mass in neonates (and infants) decreases uptake by the muscle group, leaving the FA/FI to equilibrate more rapidly in neonates compared with adults.

Alveolar to Venous Partial Pressure Gradient

The difference in the anesthetic partial pressures between the alveolar and venous blood returning to the heart is a measure of the driving force of inhalational anesthetics from the alveoli into the bloodstream. As the anesthetic partial pressures in the VRG, muscle group, and others approach equilibration and less anesthetic is taken up by those tissues, the anesthetic partial pressure in the blood returning to the heart is similar to that when it left the alveoli. Thus the driving force for anesthetics to move along a partial pressure gradient from the alveoli to the blood is diminished. This reduces the partial pressure gradient and diminishes the uptake of anesthetic from the alveoli.

Second Gas Effect

When two anesthetics are administered simultaneously, the wash-in of the anesthetic administered in a small concentration may be increased if the uptake of the second anesthetic is relatively large.[294] Nitrous oxide is the only anesthetic for which the uptake may be relatively large compared with that of the potent inhalational anesthetics, as described earlier. There is evidence, however, that casts doubt on the clinical relevance of the second gas effect.[307,308] These data suggest that the concentrating effect, if it exists in humans at all, is a small and weak effect.

Induction

The more rapid increase in FA/FI of insoluble anesthetics compared with soluble anesthetics is generally thought to result in a more rapid induction of anesthesia. However, the speed of induction of anesthesia depends not only on the wash-in (PK) but also on (1) the potency or MAC of the agent, (2) the rate of increase of the inspired concentration, (3) the maximum inspired concentration, and (4) respiration (including airway irritability and the mode of ventilation [spontaneous or controlled]). It is the combination of these four factors that determines the relative rate of induction of anesthesia.

The rate of wash-in of inhalational anesthetics into the lungs varies inversely with their solubilities in blood. Although anesthetics that are less soluble (e.g., sevoflurane and desflurane) wash into the lungs more rapidly than more soluble anesthetics (e.g., halothane), the more rapid increase in FA/FI of less soluble anesthetics is offset by their greater MAC (see E-Table 7.1). To ensure that induction of anesthesia is as rapid with less soluble anesthetics as it is with more soluble anesthetics, two criteria must be satisfied.

First, the inspired concentration of the less soluble anesthetic must be increased in greater increments (based on the relative MAC values and wash-in profile, where the MAC is defined as the minimum alveolar [or end-tidal or end-expiratory] concentrations of anesthetic at which 50% of subjects do not move in response to a noxious stimulus) than the more soluble anesthetic and, second, the maximum inspired concentration of the less soluble anesthetic must provide an alveolar concentration that is equipotent with that of the more soluble anesthetic. Theoretically, the overpressure technique should provide rapid and similar rates of induction of anesthesia with anesthetics of differing solubilities. However, if the maximum inspired anesthetic concentrations from the vaporizers preclude the delivery of equipotent end-tidal concentrations or if airway irritability (as in the case of coughing and breath-holding) interrupts the smooth delivery of anesthetic, induction of anesthesia will not be comparable.

To illustrate this, contrast the steep wash-in of F_A/F_I for sevoflurane and halothane during the first few minutes of induction of anesthesia (see Fig. 7.14). The F_A/F_I for halothane in adults reaches 0.35 in the first few minutes, whereas that in children reaches ~0.45.[296] This corresponds with an alveolar concentration in a child of 2.25% or ~2.25 MAC multiples. Contrast this to the wash-in of sevoflurane during the same time frame; the F_A/F_I for sevoflurane in adults and children both reach ~0.5. This corresponds to an alveolar concentration in children of ~4% or 1.6 MAC multiples, 25% less than that achieved with halothane.

A similar but more clinically important case can be made for neonates with an MAC for halothane of ~0.87% and sevoflurane of 3.3%. With halothane the alveolar concentration reaches 2.9 MAC multiples, whereas with sevoflurane it reaches only 1.2 MAC multiples, 60% less depth of anesthesia. Thus it is difficult to rapidly induce a deep level of anesthesia with sevoflurane in spontaneously breathing neonates and infants but at the same time, more difficult to cause an anesthetic overdose during induction with sevoflurane compared with halothane in a neonate.

These two examples illustrate several extremely important features of the pharmacology of sevoflurane that distinguish it from halothane. First, it may be difficult to rapidly achieve a deep level of anesthesia with sevoflurane in children (as was previously achieved with halothane) when sevoflurane is the sole anesthetic. Hence, inserting an IV catheter or performing laryngoscopy and tracheal intubation or bronchoscopy immediately after induction of anesthesia with sevoflurane may result in a physiologic or motor (withdrawal) response or physiologic sequelae (bronchospasm), even if the inspired concentration remains at 8%. We caution against decreasing the inspired concentration of sevoflurane (and nitrous oxide) as soon as the eyelash reflex is lost or the child appears to have lost consciousness, because a deep level of anesthesia has not been achieved (despite theoretical fears of epileptiform brain activity, see later text). In such cases, supplemental IV anesthetics may be effective to rapidly deepen the level of anesthesia. Second, these examples illustrate an important safety feature of sevoflurane. With the current vaporizer design, anesthetic overdose with sevoflurane is not easily accomplished in neonates and infants because their large MAC values more than offset their reduced solubilities. These insights contribute to the cardiovascular safety profile of sevoflurane and explain why the morbidity and mortality associated with sevoflurane in children appear to be less than with halothane.[309] It should be noted that halothane vaporizers allow administration of many more MAC multiples than sevoflurane vaporizers, and this factor may also contribute to anesthetic overdose (see later text).

CONTROL OF ANESTHETIC DEPTH

Two feedback responses modulate the depth of anesthesia during inhalational anesthesia: (1) a negative-feedback respiratory response and (2) a positive-feedback cardiovascular response. The feedback responses refer to the relationships between the inspired concentration of anesthetic and depth of anesthesia. After an increase in the inspired concentration, a negative feedback response refers to a decrease in the depth of anesthesia, whereas a positive-feedback response refers to an increase in the depth of anesthesia. Two examples that follow are used to illustrate the importance of these responses in clinical pediatric anesthesia practice.

During spontaneous respirations, as the partial pressure of inhaled anesthetics increases, alveolar ventilation decreases, thereby limiting both the wash-in of anesthetics and the depth of anesthesia achieved (E-Fig. 7.9A).[310] This negative-feedback response is a protective mechanism that permits the safe use of inspired concentrations of inhalational anesthetics that are severalfold greater than MAC (overpressure technique) during spontaneous respirations. Excessive depth of anesthesia cannot normally be achieved during spontaneous respirations (irrespective of the inspired concentrations of anesthetics, even if multiple anesthetics are administered simultaneously) because of the negative-feedback effect such anesthetic concentrations have by depressing minute ventilation. As alveolar ventilation decreases and the wash-in of anesthetics slows, the uptake of anesthetic by blood slows and the delivery of anesthetics to the VRG slows. When the partial pressure of anesthetics in the VRG exceeds that in blood, anesthetics move along their partial pressure gradients from the VRG into blood and other tissues, thus decreasing the depth of anesthesia. As the depth of anesthesia decreases, alveolar ventilation again increases and uptake of anesthetic from the alveoli resumes. *Thus spontaneous ventilation protects against an anesthetic overdose by virtue of its negative feedback effect to decrease respiration.*

In contrast to the negative-feedback response of spontaneous ventilation, the positive-feedback effect of controlled ventilation relentlessly delivers inhaled anesthetic to the alveoli, increasing both F_A/F_I and the depth of anesthesia, which in turn decreases cardiac output that, if unabated, may lead to cardiac arrest (E-Fig. 7.9B).[310] For a specific minute ventilation in a neonate, the risk of profound cardiovascular collapse occurring is reflected in part by the maximum number of MAC multiples the vaporizer can deliver; halothane and isoflurane ≫ sevoflurane and desflurane (Table 7.5). With sevoflurane and desflurane, the number of MAC multiples that can be administered (~2.5) is less than with halothane (~6), building in a safety margin with these two anesthetics.

The safety of spontaneous versus controlled ventilation during inhalational anesthesia is predicated on the feedback loops. This

TABLE 7.5	Minimum Alveolar Concentration Multiples for a Neonate Allowed by Current Vaporizers		
Agent	Maximum Vaporizer Output (%)	MAC (%)	Maximum Possible MAC Multiples
Halothane	5	0.87	5.75
Isoflurane	5	1.20	4.2
Sevoflurane	8	3.3	2.42
Desflurane	18	9.16	1.96

See text for further discussion.
MAC, minimum alveolar concentration.

has been illustrated in anesthetized dogs that all survived when they breathed halothane at 4% to 6% spontaneously, but died in a dose response when ventilation was controlled.[310] This concept is of particular importance in neonates and small infants who are more susceptible to the cardiodepressant effects of inhaled agents.[294]

Shunts

Two types of shunts exist in the lungs and heart: left-to-right or right-to-left. Left-to-right shunts refer to conditions in which blood recirculates through the lungs (usually via an intracardiac defect, such as a ventricular septal defect). In general, left-to-right shunts do not significantly affect the PK of inhalational anesthetics (they may affect IV medications), provided cardiac output remains unchanged. In contrast, right-to-left shunts refer to conditions in which venous blood returning to the heart bypasses the lungs as in an intracardiac shunt (cyanotic heart disease) or intrapulmonary shunt (pneumonia or an endobronchial intubation). With these shunts, the equilibration of FA/FI can be markedly delayed. The magnitude of the delay depends on the solubility of the anesthetic: the FA/FI of less soluble anesthetics is delayed to a greater extent than that of the more soluble anesthetics.[294] These effects are independent of the location of the shunt: intracardiac or intrapulmonary.

To understand the effects of right-to-left shunts on the PK of inhalational anesthetics, consider a simplified model of a right-to-left shunt using an endobronchial intubation to mimic the shunt. In this model, each lung is represented by one alveolus and each is perfused by one pulmonary artery (Fig. 7.16). When the tracheal tube is positioned with its tip at the mid-trachea level (Fig. 7.16A), ventilation is divided equally between both alveoli (lungs), thereby yielding equivalent anesthetic partial pressures in both pulmonary veins ($P\bar{v} = 1$). However, if the tip of the tracheal

tube is advanced into the right main-stem bronchus (equivalent to a right-to-left shunt) (Fig. 7.16B), all of the ventilation is delivered to one alveoli (lung); that is, the ventilation to that alveoli (lung) is doubled and ventilation to the nonventilated lung is nil. Under these conditions, total ventilation remains unchanged. For the remainder of this discussion, it is important to recognize that with a right-to-left shunt, the end-tidal and blood anesthetic partial pressures will differ, with the magnitude of the difference dependent on the solubility of the anesthetic.

With a more soluble anesthetic (e.g., halothane), when the tracheal tube that is positioned in the right main-stem bronchus (to model a right-to-left shunt) doubling the ventilation to that lung speeds the increase in FA/FI (effect of changes in ventilation on the wash-in of soluble anesthetics) (see E-Fig. 7.5) such that the augmented ventilation increases the FA/FI sufficiently to compensate, for the most part, for the absence of ventilation to the contralateral lung (see Fig. 7.16B).[294] The more soluble the anesthetic, the closer the partial pressure of anesthetic in the combined pulmonary vein that drains both the ventilated and nonventilated lungs approximates the partial pressure from delivering the anesthetic to lungs without a right-to-left shunt. The net effect of a right-to-left shunt on the FA/FI of a more soluble inhalational anesthetic is thus minimal.

In contrast, when a less soluble anesthetic (e.g., sevoflurane or desflurane) is administered in the presence of such a right-to-left shunt, doubling the ventilation to the lung minimally increases the FA/FI, because ventilation has a limited effect on the speed of increase of FA/FI of less soluble anesthetics (see E-Fig. 7.5 and Fig. 7.16C).[294] Consequently, the increase in FA/FI in the ventilated lung is insufficient to offset the lack of anesthetic in the blood draining the nonventilated lung. The *net effect is to almost halve* the anesthetic partial pressure in the combined pulmonary vein. The

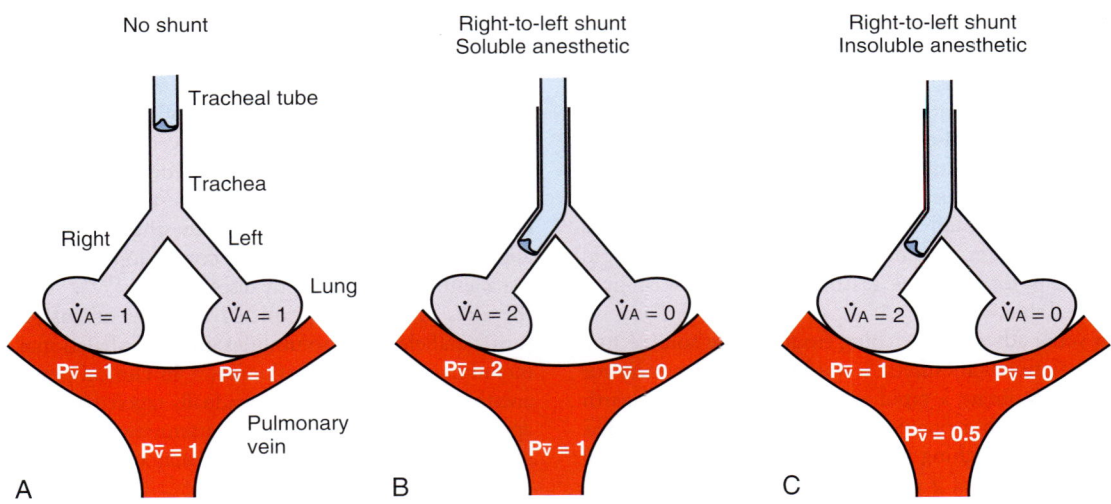

FIGURE 7.16 Effect of a shunt on the rate of increase of anesthetic partial pressure in blood using a model. **A,** Normal situation with no shunt, equal alveolar ventilation ($\dot{V}_A$) to both lungs, and normocapnia. **B,** The effect of a right-to-left shunt (via an endobronchial intubation) with a more soluble anesthetic (e.g., halothane). Ventilation and therefore normocapnia are maintained, and hypoxic pulmonary vasoconstriction is negligible. In this case, the increased ventilation to the ventilated lung speeds the increase in FA/FI (wash-in) and offsets the effect of the shunt. Results in terms of the mixed pulmonary venous partial pressure of the anesthetic ($P\bar{v} = 1$) are similar to those in **A. C,** The effect of a shunt with a less soluble anesthetic (e.g., desflurane or sevoflurane). Because the increase in alveolar ventilation does not increase FA/FI in the ventilated lung there is a dramatic reduction in the anesthetic partial pressure in the blood ($P\bar{v} = 0.5$). *FA,* Fractional alveolar partial pressure of anesthetic; *FI,* fractional inspired partial pressure of anesthetic. (Redrawn from Lerman J. Pharmacology of inhalational anaesthetics in infants and children. *Paediatr Anaesth.* 1992;2:191–203.)

less soluble the anesthetic, the greater the discrepancy between the anesthetic partial pressure in the pulmonary vein that drains the ventilated and nonventilated lungs and the partial pressure when the tube is in the trachea. The overall effect of a right-to-left shunt is to slow induction of anesthesia or even limit the depth of anesthesia that can be achieved with less soluble anesthetics.[311,312]

Few studies have documented the clinical importance of such a shunt.[311,312] Clinical situations that have posed challenges with these shunts include children with right-to-left cardiac shunts and infants with chronic lung disease. In the case of halothane, the most soluble anesthetic available, anesthesia remained quite effective in children with right-to-left shunts even though the ratio of arterial to inspired partial pressures lags behind the ratio when the shunt is closed.[312] The most likely explanation for this is that the 5% inspired concentration of halothane from the vaporizer permitted delivery of a 5 × MAC overpressure effect. Although the ratios of the arterial to inspired partial pressures of sevoflurane and desflurane have not been measured in children with right-to-left shunts, we theoretically expect that they will pose even greater difficulties than halothane, particularly with their limited overpressure effect (i.e., the maximal inspired concentrations of the vaporizers are limited to 3 × MAC or less [see Table 7.5]). Our experience suggests that when we use these less soluble anesthetics in such circumstances (e.g., bronchoscopy for a bronchial foreign body), IV anesthetics may be needed to achieve an adequate depth of anesthesia in infants and younger children.

Wash-Out and Emergence
The wash-out of inhalational anesthetics follows an exponential decay (the inverse of the wash-in curves, see Fig. 7.14) and during emergence, this is achieved by setting the inspired concentration to zero.[303] The speed of the wash-out (and speed of emergence) of the inhalational anesthetics parallels their blood solubilities: desflurane > sevoflurane > isoflurane > halothane > methoxyflurane (see E-Table 7.1).[303,313] For most inhalational anesthetics, metabolism does not contribute substantively to the wash-out. Halothane is the one exception; its wash-out is as rapid as that of isoflurane, likely because its metabolism is 15- to 20-fold greater than that of isoflurane (see later discussion). The order of the wash-out of anesthetics in children should be similar to that in adults, whereas the wash-out in neonates and infants is likely to be more rapid than that in adults for the same reasons the rate of wash-in is more rapid (see Table 7.4).

Although some advocate switching from a more soluble to a less soluble inhalational anesthetic toward the end of surgery for economy and to facilitate a rapid emergence, there is a dearth of data to support such a practice in children. In adults, it has been suggested that switching from isoflurane to desflurane 30 minutes before the end of a 2-hour anesthetic does not speed emergence.[314]

A number of other strategies have been used to speed emergence and recovery from anesthesia. In adults, discontinuing nitrous oxide accelerates the wash-out of and emergence from inhalational anesthesia.[315] Most recently, charcoal filters added to anesthesia breathing circuits adsorb anesthetics and have been shown to speed emergence.[316] Hypercapnic hyperventilation with a charcoal filter to adsorb the inhaled anesthetic has been shown to speed emergence from isoflurane, sevoflurane, and desflurane anesthesia in adults by about 60%.[317,318] Similar data in children are lacking.

When comparing the speed of recovery after anesthesia, the results are heavily influenced by the study design. Studies in which the anesthetic concentration is maintained at a fixed MAC multiple until the end of surgery usually demonstrate a pattern of recovery that parallels the solubilities of the anesthetics in blood, at least during the early recovery period: halothane > isoflurane > sevoflurane > desflurane (see earlier).[319-323]

However, when the inspired concentrations of inhalational anesthetics are tapered toward the end of surgery, this attenuates the differences reported with the fixed MAC technique. Second, differences in the speed of recovery among anesthetics parallels the duration of anesthesia; for example, differences will be less for brief surgery and greater for surgery of greater duration.[320,324–326] Third, failure to prevent or treat pain before emergence will trigger a much more rapid and stormy emergence after less soluble than after more soluble anesthetics.[320,323] A more sophisticated approach to the wash-out of inhalational anesthetics is to use the CSHT, which is a measure of the time required for the anesthetic partial pressure to decrease by 50%. Using a computer model and PK data from adults, the CSHTs of the potent inhalational anesthetics enflurane, isoflurane, sevoflurane, and desflurane were similar (<5 minutes) and were unaffected by the duration of the anesthetic.[327] The 80% decrement times were similar for desflurane and sevoflurane (<8 minutes), whereas those for isoflurane and enflurane were greater (30 and 35 minutes, respectively). However, after 6 hours of simulated anesthesia, the 90% decrement times differed substantially: 14 minutes for desflurane, 65 minutes for sevoflurane, 86 minutes for isoflurane, and 100 minutes for enflurane. These data suggest that the early recovery (up to 80% decrement in partial pressure) after inhalational anesthesia is similar among these four anesthetics (although sevoflurane and desflurane are more rapid), but after 6 hours (i.e., prolonged anesthesia) 90% decrement is achieved much more rapidly with desflurane than with the remainder.

In animal models, recovery of motor function (a metric for more complete recovery than the expired anesthetic concentrations) parallels the speed of wash-out of inhalational anesthetics from fastest to slowest: desflurane > sevoflurane > isoflurane > halothane.[328] Notably, the time to recover increases in parallel with the duration of anesthesia.[328] In pediatric studies in which the recovery times after two or more anesthetics were compared, the end-tidal concentrations of the anesthetics were maintained at approximately 1 MAC until the conclusion of surgery, after which the anesthetics were abruptly discontinued.[319,320,329] In this paradigm, the rates of recovery paralleled the rates of wash-out, which in turn paralleled the solubilities of the inhalational anesthetics, including xenon and desflurane.[330] In clinical practice, however, anesthetic concentrations are gradually tapered as the end of surgery approaches. This practice may attenuate the differences in the speed of recovery among inhalational anesthetics.

PHARMACODYNAMICS OF INHALED ANESTHETICS
Minimum Alveolar Concentration
MAC is defined as the minimum alveolar (or end-tidal or end-expiratory) concentration of anesthetic at which 50% of patients do not move in response to a noxious stimulus. The classic stimulus for MAC in humans is skin incision; throughout the remainder of this chapter, MAC will refer to this stimulus. MAC has also been determined in response to other stimuli, including tracheal intubation, insertion of a laryngeal mask airway, tracheal extubation, and awake responsiveness (see Table 7.6). The MAC response to tracheal intubation during sevoflurane anesthesia in children is

TABLE 7.6	MAC Values in Children	
	MAC (%)	**References**
Tracheal intubation	Halothane: 1.33	2036
	Enflurane: 2.93	2037
	Sevoflurane: 2.69, 2.66, 2.83	341, 357, 2038
Tracheal extubation	Isoflurane: 1.4	2039
	Sevoflurane: 1.70, 2.3	2040, 2041
	Desflurane: 7.7	2042
LMA insertion	Sevoflurane: 2.0	2038
LMA extubation	Sevoflurane 1.84	2043
	Desflurane (with 1–1.3 μμg/ kg Fentanyl): 3.56%	2044
Tracheal intubation/ skin incision ratio[a]	Halothane, enflurane, sevoflurane: 1.33	Calculated from MAC data
MAC awake	Sevoflurane: 0.66 (2–5 years) and 0.43 (5–12 years)	2045

LMA, Laryngeal mask airway; *MAC,* minimum alveolar concentration.
[a]Calculated using the above MAC data.

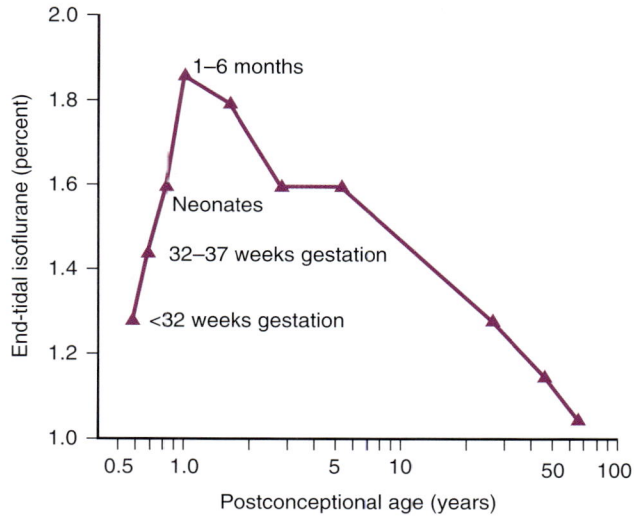

FIGURE 7.17 MAC (minimum alveolar concentration) of isoflurane in preterm and full-term neonates, infants, and children. MAC increased with gestational age in infants younger than 32 weeks gestation (1.3%), reaching a zenith in infants 1 to 6 months of age of 1.87%, and decreased thereafter with increasing age to adulthood. Postconceptional age is the sum of the gestational age and postnatal age in years. (Data from Cameron CB, Robinson S, Gregory GA. The minimum anesthetic concentration of isoflurane in children. *Anesth Analg.* 1984;63(4):418–420 and LeDez KM, Lerman J. The minimum alveolar concentration (MAC) of isoflurane in preterm neonates. *Anesthesiology* 1987;67(3):301–307.)

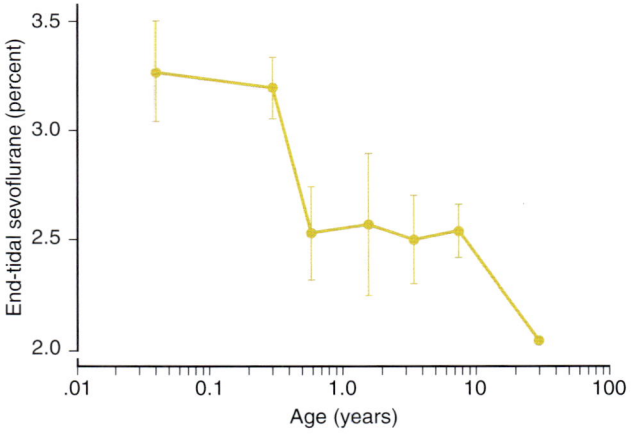

FIGURE 7.18 The MAC (minimum alveolar concentration) of sevoflurane in neonates, infants, and children. MAC is greatest in full-term neonates (3.3%), less in infants 1 to 6 months of age (3.2%), and then decreases 25%, to 2.5%, for all infants and children 6 months to 10 years of age. (The thin vertical yellow bars are standard deviations.) Age is postnatal age in years. The MAC of sevoflurane in adults, 30 years of age, is shown for completeness. All MAC measurements were performed with sevoflurane in 100% oxygen using a single skin incision. (Data from Lerman J, Sikich N, Kleinman S, Yentis S. The pharmacology of sevoflurane in infants and children. *Anesthesiology* 1994;80(4):814–824.)

attenuated in the presence of adjuvants, such as clonidine (see E-Table 7.2).[331] Conflicting evidence exists regarding the relative potencies of isomers or enantiomers of chiral inhalational anesthetics.[332–334] Studies in animals suggest that the $S(+)$ optical enantiomer may be more potent than the $R(-)$ enantiomer, as evidenced by its ability to enhance potassium conductance in neurons.[332,335] In adults, the $R(-)$ enantiomer of isoflurane was nominally (17%) more potent than the $S(+)$ enantiomer.[334]

The difference in the potency (or MAC) of inhalational anesthetics varies inversely with lipid solubility; that is, as the lipid solubility decreases, the potency decreases in parallel (i.e., MAC increases) (see E-Table 7.1).

In children, MAC varies significantly with age. For example, the MAC of halothane increases as age decreases, reaching a maximum value in infants 1 to 6 months of age (1.20% ± 0.06%) and then decreases by about 30% to (0.87 ± 0.03%) in full-term neonates.[335,336] Similar relationships hold true for isoflurane and desflurane (Figs. 7.17 and E-Fig. 7.10).[337,338] However, the relationship for sevoflurane differs substantively from that of the other inhalational anesthetics in that the MAC of sevoflurane does not increase steadily as age decreases (Fig. 7.18).[339] In fact, the MAC of sevoflurane in neonates and infants younger than 6 months of age is 3.3%, whereas in older infants and children it is 2.5%.[339–341] The explanation for this different relationship for sevoflurane remains unclear.

The MAC of inhalational anesthetics in preterm neonates has been determined only for isoflurane (see Fig. 7.17). The (mean ± standard deviation [SD]) MAC of isoflurane in preterm neonates younger than 32 weeks gestation (1.28% ± 0.17%) is 10% less than it is in neonates of 32 to 37 weeks gestational age (1.41% ± 0.18%), which in turn is 12% less than it is in full-term neonates (1.60% ± 0.03%).[218] The etiology of these age-dependent changes in MAC remains elusive. Several possible causes have been proposed, including maturational changes in the CNS and neurohumoral factors, but none of these have been confirmed.

Several other factors are known to affect MAC. The presence of the melanocortin-1 receptor gene affects the MAC of desflurane. That is, 90% of adults who are either homozygous or heterozygous for mutations of this gene (i.e., redheads) require 20% more

anesthesia than those who have no mutations (brunettes).[342] A similar relationship is likely to hold true for children with these mutations. Hypothermia decreases MAC; in children 4 to 10 years, the MAC of isoflurane decreases 5% per degree Celsius.[343]

Cerebral palsy and severe cognitive impairment reduce the MAC of halothane approximately 25% compared with healthy children.[344] Although tetanic stimulation was used to elicit the pain response, this stimulus underestimates the MAC compared with skin incision.[345] Nonetheless, the MAC of halothane in healthy children was similar to published data with skin incision.[336] Chronic anticonvulsant therapy decreased the MAC of halothane in handicapped children by 15%, compared with those without anticonvulsants, from 0.71% ± 0.10% to 0.62% ± 0.03%.[344] Several factors may account for this decrease in MAC, including central sensory impairment, increased pain threshold or insensitivity, and a disequilibrium of inhibitory and excitatory regulatory neurons within the spinal cord in these children.[346,347] Although the acute administration of barbiturates and benzodiazepines decreases MAC,[348,349] chronic administration of similar medications does not.[350] The effects of specific anticonvulsants, such as valproic acid and phenytoin, on the MAC of inhalational anesthetics in children remain unclear.

The MAC for nitrous oxide has been estimated to be 104% in adults[351]; comparable data do not exist in children. The additivity of MAC fractions of nitrous oxide with inhalational anesthetics is well established. The concept of additivity has been confirmed in adults for nitrous oxide with all inhalational anesthetics, including sevoflurane and desflurane,[352,353] although in children, it holds true only for halothane or isoflurane.[354,355] When nitrous oxide is combined with sevoflurane or desflurane in children,[199,200,214] 60% nitrous oxide decreases the MAC of sevoflurane only 20% and that of desflurane 26% (see Table 7.7).[338,339,356] The MAC response to tracheal intubation during sevoflurane anesthesia in children is also attenuated by nitrous oxide.[357] The explanation for the differential additivity effect of nitrous oxide remains unclear.

The MAC for xenon in middle-aged adults is about 70%[358,359]; the MAC of xenon in children has not been determined.

Central Nervous System

All potent inhalational anesthetics depress the central nervous system (CNS), as evidenced by dose-dependent decreases in the cerebral vascular resistance and the cerebral metabolic rate for oxygen ($CMRO_2$). The decrease in vascular resistance causes a reciprocal increase in CBF that begins at approximately 0.6 MAC.[360] The extent of the increase in CBF, however, depends on the inhalational anesthetics: halothane > enflurane ~ desflurane > isoflurane > sevoflurane.[360-363] In adults, the cerebral vasculature remains responsive to CO_2 under general anesthesia but decreases

with increasing MAC, disappearing at 1.5 MAC in the case of desflurane.[364] The net effect of inhalational anesthetics is a dose-dependent increase in the ratio of the CBF to $CMRO_2$.

The effects of inhalational anesthetics on the CNS in children have not been fully elucidated. Autoregulation of CBF does not appear to vary with age in children up to 1.5 MAC sevoflurane.[365,366] CBF velocity in children varies directly with the end-tidal CO_2 ($ETCO_2$) during halothane and isoflurane anesthesia.[367] CBF velocity increases as the concentrations of halothane[368] and desflurane[369] increase. Compared with halothane, however, sevoflurane does not increase CBF velocity, suggesting it may be the preferred anesthetic.[370] Based on current evidence, sevoflurane and isoflurane remain the preferred inhalational anesthetics for neuroanesthesia in children at small MAC values (<1 MAC) and in the presence of mild hyperventilation (see Chapter 26).

In children, the EEG activity during halothane anesthesia differs substantially from that of sevoflurane. In the case of halothane, the EEG is characterized by slow waves superimposed on fast rhythms (α and β waves), whereas in the case of sevoflurane, the EEG is characterized by mainly sharp slow waves.[371] Furthermore, the shift of power of the EEG from low (1–4 Hz) to medium frequencies (8–30 Hz) is greater with halothane than it is for sevoflurane. The clinical relevance of these EEG differences remains unclear at this time, but may explain in part the inconsistencies reported with processed EEG monitoring in children anesthetized with various inhalation anesthetics (see later discussion).

Both myoclonic movement of the extremities and transient spike-and-wave complexes on EEGs have been reported during sevoflurane anesthesia in children.[371-375] Diffuse spike-and-wave complexes were noted on EEGs at 5% and 7% inspired concentrations in two children with histories of epilepsy.[373] In a third child without a history of seizures, a 30-second burst of spike-and-wave complexes was recorded during sevoflurane anesthesia but was identified only after the event resolved.[376] The EEG data were analyzed in children who were premedicated with midazolam and then anesthetized with halothane or sevoflurane. There was no evidence of seizure activity.[371] Cortical epileptiform EEG activity has been reported during 1 to 2 MAC sevoflurane in adults with one episode of seizures that occurred with a partial pressure of carbon dioxide (PCO_2) of 34 mm Hg.[377] This prompted some to recommend limiting the depth of anesthesia with sevoflurane to minimize epileptiform EEG activity or even clinically evident seizure activity.[378] However, the coadministration of other anesthetic medications, such as midazolam, nitrous oxide, and opioids, may attenuate epileptiform EEG activity.[377] Furthermore, the notion of limiting the depth of sevoflurane anesthesia by reducing the concentration of sevoflurane as soon as the eyelash reflex is lost has not been shown to benefit children, and may actually increase the risk of awareness and physiologic responses (see later discussion).

The association between myoclonic movement and seizures during induction of sevoflurane anesthesia remains tenuous. To prevent involuntary movements during induction, we recommend increasing the inspired concentration of sevoflurane in a single stepwise manner from 0% to 8% (see Induction, earlier). If apnea occurs, ventilation should be gently assisted, while avoiding hyperventilation.

Awareness during inhalational anesthesia has been reported to occur with an incidence of 0.2% to 1.2% during sevoflurane anesthesia in children,[379-381] which exceeds that in adults. The studies suggest that children who experience awareness did not develop long-term sequelae.[382] However, the reason for this discrepancy remains elusive. Concerns regarding awareness during

TABLE 7.7	Percent MAC Reduced in 2-Year-Olds With 60% Nitrous Oxide		
Agent	MAC With Oxygen (%)	MAC With 60% Nitrous Oxide	Percent MAC Reduced
Halothane	0.91	0.37	65
Desflurane	8.67	6.4	26
Sevoflurane	2.5	2.0	20

MAC, minimum alveolar concentration.
From Gregory GA, Eger EI 2nd, Munson ES. The relationship between age and halothane requirements in man. Anesthesiology 1969;30(5):488–491; Taylor RH, Lerman J. Minimum alveolar concentration of desflurane and hemodynamic responses in neonates, infants, and children. Anesthesiology 1991;75(5):975–979; Lerman J, Sikich N, Kleinman S, Yentis S. The pharmacology of sevoflurane in infants and children. Anesthesiology 1994;80(4):814–824; Murray DJ, Mehta MP, Forbes RB, Dull DL. Additive contribution of nitrous oxide to halothane MAC in infants and children. Anesth. Analg. 1990;71(2):120–124; Fisher DM, Zwass MS. MAC of desflurane in 60% nitrous oxide in infants and children. Anesthesiology 1992;76(2):354–356.

anesthesia have increased interest in the use of processed EEG monitoring in children.[383] The most widely studied monitor to date is the BIS monitor, which displays the value on a scale between 0 and 100 (see Chapter 52). In adults, BIS readings less than 60 may be associated with a small risk of awareness and recall, whereas readings greater than 70 are associated with a greater risk for awareness. The BIS value has been studied in children to a limited degree to date, but its validity and role in the anesthetic management of infants and children younger than 5 years of age remain in question. One concern is that the EEG algorithm in current BIS software is derived from adult EEG data, not from children. Despite use of an algorithm derived from adults, BIS measurements in older children appear, for the most part, to track the depth of anesthesia, and these values correlate with the end-tidal concentration of the anesthetic. However, several unexplained curiosities have been reported. The BIS readings for halothane in children exceed those for isoflurane, desflurane, and sevoflurane at equal MAC values.[246,247,384] This has been attributed to the differential effects of anesthetics on the EEG. In addition, the BIS values for a specific sevoflurane concentration decrease with increasing ages.[243,246,385] Paradoxically, the BIS values actually increase as the sevoflurane concentration increased between 3% and 4%, an observation that has been attributed to the unique EEG during sevoflurane anesthesia in children.[385]

A further concern is the enormous interindividual variability in processed EEG monitoring, making it difficult to define thresholds for awareness or lack thereof.[385] Interestingly, spontaneous respirations increase the variability in the BIS readings.[386] The issue is further complicated by the fact that ketamine, nitrous oxide, and opioids do not depress the EEG in a dose-dependent manner. Discrepant BIS readings have been reported from the right and left sides of the brain[387] as well as in the prone position.[388] The BIS values in children with cognitive impairment were 28 points less than those who were unaffected at the same anesthetic concentration, although the MAC reduction for cognitive impairment was not accounted for.[389] Had the reduced MAC been accounted for in cognitively impaired children,[344] the BIS readings may not have differed. With the State Entropy monitor, entropy increases in the presence of nitrous oxide, rendering the readings misleading. The aggregate of this evidence undermines the validity of processed EEG monitoring during inhalational anesthesia in children (see Chapter 52).

Cardiovascular System

Inhalational anesthetics (with the exception of xenon) affect the cardiovascular system either directly (by depressing myocardial contractility [calcium channel blockade], altering the conduction system, or by dilating the peripheral vasculature) or indirectly (by affecting the balance of parasympathetic and sympathetic nervous systems and neurohumoral, renal, or reflex responses). The cardiovascular responses to inhalational anesthetics in children are further complicated by maturational changes in the cardiovascular system and responsiveness to these anesthetics. When all of these developmental changes are taken in aggregate, there is a reduced margin of safety between adequate anesthesia and severe cardiopulmonary depression in infants and children compared with adults. The salient features of the immature cardiovascular system in infants and children at both the macroscopic and microscopic levels have been reviewed elsewhere.[390]

Assessment of cardiovascular variables in infants and children presents a challenge for clinicians. Although BP and electrocardiography are standard monitors of hemodynamics in infants and children of all ages, measures of cardiac output and myocardial contractility are much more difficult to quantitate accurately. Two-dimensional echocardiography and impedance cardiometry have been used to estimate cardiac output and myocardial contractility in infants and children,[391–394] although the echocardiographic measurements are subject to variability depending on the preload and afterload. Load-independent–derived echocardiographic variables (stress-velocity and stress-shortening indexes) have improved the accuracy of echocardiographic estimates of myocardial function and are used with increasing frequency.[395] Transesophageal echocardiography is used much more frequently in children, although its use is limited to children with congenital heart disease undergoing cardiac surgery. Future studies using continuous noninvasive cardiac output estimates obtained using bioimpedance may shed further light on this issue in the future.[396–400]

In children, several factors determine the BP responses to inhalational anesthetics, including the particular anesthetic studied, the dose, the administration of a premedication, the level of preoperative anxiety, and the systemic pressure measured: systolic, diastolic, or mean. Most studies demonstrate modest, dose-dependent decreases in BP with all of the inhalational anesthetics, although the magnitudes of the changes vary. In a direct comparison of sevoflurane and halothane, systolic BP decreased 7.5% at 1 MAC sevoflurane and 12.5% at 1 MAC halothane, but returned to awake values at 1.5 MAC with both anesthetics.[395] In children older than 1 year of age, systolic BP decreased 0% to 11% at 1 MAC sevoflurane, and 22% to 28% at 1 MAC desflurane, compared with awake values.[338,339] At 1 MAC, mean BP in children decreased 15% to 25% with isoflurane and sevoflurane.[392,394] All of the inhalational anesthetics (in concentrations up to 1.5 MAC) modestly depress the systolic BP in children.

Myocardial contractility decreases to a greater extent during halothane (up to 1.5 MAC) than during isoflurane or sevoflurane anesthesia, as evidenced by decreases in cardiac output and ejection fraction in healthy children.[393,394,401] Cardiac index decreases to similar extents with halothane and sevoflurane at 1 and 2 MAC: 10% at 1 MAC and 20% to 35% at 2 MAC.[394] Ejection fraction decreases 30% at 0.5 and 1.5 MAC halothane compared with awake values, but is unchanged at equipotent concentrations of isoflurane.[392] The addition of nitrous oxide to halothane or isoflurane in infants and small children depresses myocardial function to a similar extent as equipotent anesthetic concentrations of halothane or isoflurane in oxygen.[401] In children, halothane decreases myocardial contractility in a dose-dependent manner and to a greater extent than the ether anesthetics. Isoflurane and sevoflurane decrease myocardial contractility to a lesser extent than halothane and are preferred for children with limited cardiovascular reserves. IV atropine restores the decrease in myocardial function, in part, associated with halothane anesthesia,[401–404] whereas IV balanced salt solution restores the decrease in myocardial function associated with isoflurane anesthesia.[393]

The mechanism by which inhalational anesthetics depress myocardial function remains controversial. Studies in both animal and human myocardial cells suggest that halothane, isoflurane, and sevoflurane directly depress myocardial contractility by decreasing intracellular calcium ion (Ca^{2+}) flux. Inhalational anesthetics decrease the Ca^{2+} flux by their action on the calcium channels themselves, ion exchange pumps, and the sarcoplasmic reticulum.[390] Evidence suggests that inhalational anesthetics attenuate contractility of ventricular myocytes via voltage-dependent L-type calcium channels (which are responsible for release of large amounts of calcium from the sarcoplasmic reticulum).[405,406]

That neonates and infants are more sensitive to the depressant actions of inhalational anesthetics than are older children is supported by experimental evidence of maturational differences between neonatal and adult rat, rabbit, and feline myocardium.[406–409] Structural differences that may account, in part, for the changes in myocardial sensitivity to inhalational anesthetics with age include a reduction in contractile elements, immature sarcoplasmic reticulum, and functional differences in calcium sensitivity of the contractile elements, calcium channels, and the sodium-calcium pump in the neonatal myocardium.[390,405–407,409–412] The determinants of Ca^{2+} homeostasis in neonatal ventricular myocardial cells depend on transsarcolemmic Ca^{2+} flux to a far greater extent than on the sarcoplasmic reticulum.[390] This is based on a growing body of experimental evidence that includes the finding that the concentration of the Na^+-Ca^{2+} exchange protein in the neonatal myocardium, a protein that regulates transsarcolemmic flux of Ca^{2+}, exceeds that in adult cells by 2.5-fold and that its concentration decreases with age as the concentration of L-type voltage-dependent calcium channels increases.[407] Furthermore, halothane reversibly inhibits the Na^+-Ca^{2+} exchange protein in immature myocardial cells.[407] The sarcoplasmic reticulum is poorly developed in neonatal myocardial cells, and this finding weighs heavily against the sarcoplasmic reticulum being the major source of Ca^{2+} required for myocardial contractility. Further research is required before the contribution of each aspect of Ca^{2+} homeostasis to myocardial contractility in the neonate can be confirmed.

Ever since the introduction of halothane into clinical practice, clinicians have been aware of a greater incidence of hypotension and bradycardia in neonates who were anesthetized with halothane than in adults. However, this was not the case when *equipotent* concentrations (approximately 1 MAC) of halothane[336,403] were administered to neonates and older infants 1 to 6 months of age. Subsequent studies demonstrated that isoflurane,[413] sevoflurane,[339] and desflurane[338] all decreased systolic pressure in neonates to similar extents as in older infants 1 to 6 months of age. Interestingly, systolic BP decreased 30% in response to 1 MAC sevoflurane in neonates and infants 1 to 6 months of age, which was substantially greater than the 5% decrease in older infants and children up to 12 years of age.[339] In the case of desflurane, systolic BP decreased 30% in response to 1 MAC desflurane across all age groups.[338] These data suggest that systolic BP decreases up to 30% in response to 1 MAC of all inhalational anesthetics in infants and children, and that caution should be exercised when administering these anesthetics to infants and children who are at risk for hemodynamic instability, or in whom greater concentrations of inhaled anesthetics are required. On the basis of echocardiographic determinations, cardiac output and ejection fraction decrease in a dose-dependent fashion from awake to 1.5 MAC halothane and isoflurane in neonates and infants.[391] In a comparison of sevoflurane and halothane up to 1.5 MAC in infants, sevoflurane maintained cardiac index but decreased BP and systemic vascular resistance.[414] Myocardial contractility decreased in a dose-dependent manner with halothane as well as with sevoflurane, although the decrease with the former exceeded that with the latter.

The baroreceptor reflex response is also depressed in infants with either halothane[415] or isoflurane,[416] albeit to a greater extent with halothane. In view of the greater incidence of hypotension in neonates and infants than older children, an intact baroreceptor reflex could offset, in part, the cardiovascular consequences. However, inhalational anesthetics blunt this response, leaving the infant vulnerable to the direct cardiodepressant actions of the anesthetics. Prophylactic anticholinergics augment the cardiac output by increasing the heart rate.

Two studies evaluated the effects of inhalational anesthesia on the hemodynamics of children with congenital heart disease undergoing cardiac surgery.[417,418] Sevoflurane maintained cardiac index and heart rate with less hypotension and negative inotropic effect than halothane. Isoflurane maintained cardiac index and ejection fraction, increased heart rate, and caused less depression of mean arterial pressure than halothane.[417] Sevoflurane was also associated with fewer episodes of severe hypotension and reduced need for vasopressors and chronotropes during emergence than halothane.[418]

Inhalational anesthetics also vary in their effect on cardiac rhythm. Halothane slows the heart rate, in some cases leading to junctional rhythms, bradycardia, and asystole. This response is dose dependent. Three mechanisms have been proposed to explain the genesis of halothane-associated dysrhythmias: a direct effect on the sinoatrial node, a vagal effect, or an imbalance in the parasympathetic and sympathetic tone. It has also been suggested that the etiology of the bradycardia during halothane anesthesia may be a withdrawal of sympathetic tone. Bradycardia is particularly marked in the neonate, presumably because parasympathetic influences predominate over the sparse sympathetic innervation of the myocardium in this age group. Junctional rhythms are also common during halothane anesthesia. Atrial or ventricular ectopic beats and brief episodes of ventricular tachycardia are rare, except in the presence of hypercapnia.[419] In infants and children anesthetized with halothane, 10 µg/kg atropine increases heart rate by 50% or more and promotes sinus rhythm.[420] This dose of atropine also increases BP in infants and children 2 years of age and older.

Sevoflurane has limited effect on heart rate, at 1 MAC and during induction of anesthesia, generally maintaining or increasing the heart rate. The heart rate may slow transiently during the first 3 minutes of induction of anesthesia but the rate usually recovers spontaneously without treatment. Heart rate remained stable during studies with 1 MAC sevoflurane. However, children with Down syndrome are at increased risk for bradycardia during induction of anesthesia. The bradycardia usually resolves by decreasing the inspired concentration of anesthetic. Heart rate is usually unaffected by the administration of desflurane unless the inspired concentration is increased suddenly in the absence of opioids, a phenonmenon reported in adults.

Halothane also sensitizes the myocardium to catecholamines, particularly in the presence of hypercapnia and "light anesthesia."[419] Halothane decreases the threshold for ventricular extrasystoles during epinephrine administration threefold.[421–423] In contrast, isoflurane, desflurane, and sevoflurane maintain or increase heart rate during the early induction period of anesthesia,[a] although a transient slowing of the heart rate, usually preceeded by a nodal rhythm, has been reported during induction of anesthesia with sevoflurane.[427] When bradycardia occurs in an anesthetized child, hypoxia must be considered first before other causes, such as a direct drug effect (i.e., high concentration of halothane). Isoflurane, desflurane, and sevoflurane do not sensitize the myocardium to catecholamines to the same extent as does halothane, and ventricular arrhythmias are rare.[421,422,428] Nonetheless, sevoflurane may cause transient bradycardia during induction of anesthesia. The bradycardia usually resolves spontaneously, without requiring any

---

[a]References 320, 338, 339, 392, 394, 413, 414, and 424–426.

interventions. In children with Down syndrome, bradycardia during induction of anesthesia with sevoflurane occurs three to four times more frequently than in children without Down syndrome, irrespective of whether a congenital heart defect is present.[429,430] Bradycardias in children with Down syndrome were treated with an anticholinergic twice as frequenty as children who were unaffected.

The mechanism by which the sinus node controls automaticity is incompletely understood but may include potassium ion (K^+) currents, hyperpolarization-activated current, and T and L forms of Ca^{2+} currents.[390] Moreover, developmental changes in these channels likely account, in part, for the differential effects of inhalational anesthetics on heart rate with age.[410]

Recent concerns of a relationship between inhalational anesthetics and prolonged QT interval that progressed to induce cardiac arrest or torsades de pointes have emerged. Although the ether inhalational anesthetics prolong the QTc interval (with >500 milliseconds being abnormal),[431,432] this alone appears to be insufficient to induce torsades de pointes. Torsades de pointes also requires the transmural dispersion of repolarization. This is defined as the variability in the rate of repolarization across the myocardium, from epicardium to endocardium. The rate of repolarization may be estimated by the interval in the peak to end of the T wave on a 12-lead electrocardiogram. Evidence has demonstrated that the risk of torsades de pointes during sevoflurane anesthesia is minimal because the transmural dispersion of repolarization is limited.[433]

Paroxysmal increases in BP (both systolic and diastolic pressures) and heart rate have been reported in adults and observed by one of the authors (CJC) in children after a rapid increase in the inspired concentration of isoflurane or desflurane.[434] This occurs as a result of a massive sympathetic response, mediated by norepinephrine and/or epinephrine, that culminates in tachycardia and hypertension.[435,436] Further increases in the inspired concentration of the inciting anesthetic while attempting to attenuate the tachycardia and hypertension are ineffective and may perpetuate or augment the response. To restore vital signs to normal, the inciting anesthetic should be discontinued and replaced with another anesthetic. Repetitive small increases (1%) in the inspired concentration of the putative anesthetic produce transient but attenuated catecholamine bursts and cardiovascular responses compared with larger increases in concentration.[437,438] Fentanyl (2 µg/kg), esmolol, and clonidine have all been shown to be effective in preventing, attenuating, or eliminating these responses.[439–441] The origin of these responses is unknown, although the rapidity of the response points to the lung.[442] Others, however, dispute this notion, contending that two sites must be responsible for triggering the sympathetic discharge—the lung and the VRG[443]—with the latter mediating the greater response.[443,444] Neuroexcitatory responses have not been reported in children with isoflurane, desflurane, or sevoflurane.[445]

Xenon offers an immense advantage over the ether-based inhalational anesthetics in that it maintains circulatory stability. However, the cardiovascular effects of xenon in children have not been studied. Although the MAC of xenon in adults is very large (see E-Table 7.1), the MAC for xenon in children may be even greater. If the MAC exceeds the adult values, this may limit not only the dose that may be administered to children (e.g., much less than 1 MAC), but it may also limit the inspired concentration of oxygen as well. Notwithstanding the MAC of xenon in children, this anesthetic will certainly be much less effective in children with cyanotic congenital heart disease, as it is the least soluble anesthetic and its large MAC restricts the MAC multiples that may be administered.

Respiratory System

During spontaneous ventilation, both tidal volume and respiratory rate vary with the specific anesthetic, depth of anesthesia, and nociception. The increased respiratory rate during inhalational anesthesia in children has been attributed to sensitization of the stretch receptors within the lung as well as possible central effects. Inhalational anesthetics significantly affect respiration in infants and children in a dose-dependent fashion via effects on the respiratory center, chest wall muscles, and reflex responses. Halothane depresses minute ventilation by decreasing tidal volume and attenuating the response to CO_2.[446–449] This depression is offset, in part, by an increase in the respiratory rate.[446,449] These ventilatory responses to halothane are age dependent; minute ventilation in infants decreases to a greater extent than in children.[448] In infants and young children anesthetized with halothane, intercostal muscle activity is attenuated before the diaphragm.[446,450] This effect is most pronounced in preterm and full-term neonates and infants and when a tracheal tube is used in place of a laryngeal mask airway.[451] The movement of the chest and abdomen during the respiratory cycle is one of synchronized protrusion of the abdomen and collapse of the chest wall during inspiration (with some intercostal indrawing) and indrawing of the abdomen and flattening of the chest wall during expiration. This is commonly referred to as the "rocking horse" movement of the chest (similar to the phenomenon that occurs during upper airway obstruction in infants and children). This results in loss of FRC and is of particular concern in infants younger than 2 years of age who have decreased type I muscle fibers in both the diaphragm and intercostal muscles (see Fig. 14.11). This explains why infants fatigue easily and why positive end-expiratory pressure is useful in this age group. Isoflurane, enflurane, sevoflurane, and desflurane also depress ventilatory drive, decrease tidal volume, and attenuate the response to CO_2.[447,449,452–458] The increase in respiratory frequency that follows respiratory depression (decreased tidal volume) may not restore minute ventilation to preanesthetic levels.

Sevoflurane depresses respiration to a similar extent as halothane up to 1.4 MAC but depresses respiration to a greater extent at concentrations greater than 1.4 MAC.[452] This results from a direct effect of sevoflurane on respiratory frequency.[455] Although respiratory effort may decrease rapidly during sevoflurane or desflurane anesthesia, the low blood solubilities and rapid wash-out profiles of these drugs in part ensure that this is a self-limiting phenomenon during spontaneous respirations. Sevoflurane decreases the tone of the intercostal muscles to a lesser extent than halothane.[450,454] The compensatory changes in respiratory rate differ among the anesthetics; respiratory rate increases at 1.4 MAC or more with halothane, is unchanged with isoflurane, but decreases at 1.4 MAC or less with sevoflurane and enflurane.[447,449] This inadequate compensatory response to respiratory depression with sevoflurane and enflurane suggests that when children are anesthetized with those anesthetics, spontaneous ventilation must be monitored carefully to avoid hypopnea or apnea. Sevoflurane maintains or decreases airway resistance in children with normal airways and those with asthma or a recent upper respiratory tract infection. Insertion of a tracheal tube during sevoflurane anesthesia increases airway resistance without sequelae.[459,460]

Desflurane depresses respiration in children during spontaneous respirations at greater than 1 MAC by decreasing tidal volume.[458] However, desflurane increases airway resistance in children with asthma and respiratory tract infections to a greater extent than sevoflurane.[460] Desflurane is probably best avoided in these children.

Studies of the upper airway in children anesthetized with inhalational anesthesia have sought to explain the pathophysiology of airway obstruction. Sevoflurane at 1 MAC causes more upper airway obstruction than halothane.[461] In escalating doses between 0.5 and 1.5 MAC, sevoflurane decreased the cross-sectional area of the airway by one-third, predominantly in the anteroposterior dimension.[462] This effect primarily results from pharyngeal wall collapse, which can be easily offset with positive end-expiratory pressure (see Chapter 14).

Renal System

Potent inhalational anesthetics may affect renal function via four possible mechanisms: cardiovascular, autonomic, neuroendocrine, and metabolic. Although the first three mechanisms pose no direct threat to renal function, the fourth mechanism, metabolic, is a serious clinical concern that has resulted in renal dysfunction after inhalational anesthesia.

Inhalational anesthetics are metabolized in vivo by the CYP isozyme system to varying extents (see E-Table 7.3). Metabolism of inhalational anesthetics may release both inorganic and organic fluoride moieties.[463] It is the inorganic fluoride that is released from these ether anesthetics that has stimulated interest in renal dysfunction after inhalational anesthesia.

Isoflurane and desflurane undergo limited metabolism in vivo, resulting in very small plasma concentrations of inorganic fluoride even after 131 MAC hours of isoflurane.[464] In contrast, halothane is metabolized to a substantially greater extent but releases most of the fluoride in an organic form, trifluoroacetate. Trifluoroacetate has, however, been linked to halothane hepatitis (see later discussion). The metabolism of enflurane, sevoflurane, and methoxyflurane yields greater plasma concentrations of inorganic fluoride than isoflurane. The metabolism of sevoflurane yields both inorganic and organic fluoride moieties.[465] The organic form, hexafluoroisopropanol, is rapidly conjugated and excreted by the kidneys[465] and poses no threat to humans. Peak plasma concentrations of inorganic fluoride after exposure to inhalational anesthetics follow an order similar to that in E-Table 7.3: methoxyflurane > sevoflurane > enflurane > isoflurane > halothane $\cong$ desflurane.[466–470] In the case of methoxyflurane, two metabolites are produced: inorganic fluoride and oxalic acid. Both were implicated in the pathogenesis of renal dysfunction, although clinically, the renal injury was more consistently associated with inorganic fluoride.[471] Subsequent studies demonstrated that subclinical nephrotoxicity occurred after more than 2.5 MAC hours of methoxyflurane, provided the plasma concentration of inorganic fluoride exceeded 50 μmol/L. Nephrotoxicity occurred after more than 5 MAC hours if the concentration of inorganic fluoride exceeded 90 μmol/L.[472] These clinical concerns led to the voluntary withdrawal of methoxyflurane from clinical practice.

That the plasma concentrations of inorganic fluoride in children who were anesthetized with sevoflurane were similar to or greater than those after enflurane[473–475] raised concerns about possible renal dysfunction after prolonged exposure. However, inorganic fluoride concentrations after relatively brief anesthetics in children are similar to those in adults: less than 20 μmol/L after about 1 MAC hour, which decreases to less than 10 μmol/L by 4 hours after discontinuation of anesthesia.[457] Nonetheless, the peak plasma concentrations of inorganic fluoride paralleled the MAC hour exposure to sevoflurane in both children and adults.[475] Concerns

regarding the risk of renal dysfunction after sevoflurane were heightened after reports that the peak plasma concentration of inorganic fluoride in some adults exceeded the purported threshold for nephrotoxicity (50 μmol/L).[476] Despite the large plasma concentrations of inorganic fluoride after sevoflurane anesthesia, there was no evidence of renal dysfunction. These reports, together with a dearth of evidence in the toxicology literature, suggest that fluoride-mediated nephrotoxicity may be independent of the plasma concentration of inorganic fluoride.

Kharasch and colleagues postulated that inhalational anesthetic-induced nephrotoxicity might be anesthetic specific. They determined that the primary isozyme responsible for the degradation of enflurane, isoflurane, sevoflurane, and methoxyflurane anesthetics was CYP2E1,[463,477–479] with secondary isozymes including CYP2A6 and CYP3A.[480] Subsequently, they reported large quantities of CYP2E1 not only within the liver but also within the kidneys.[477] They also noted that the affinity of renal CYP2E1 for methoxyflurane was 5-fold greater than it was for sevoflurane.[480] This provided further evidence that the renal dysfunction after ether inhalational anesthetics resulted from the local production of inorganic fluoride within the renal medulla rather than extrarenal production, and that certain anesthetics were more prone to release of inorganic fluoride than others (e.g., methoxyflurane much more so than sevoflurane). Because CYP2E1 has a greater affinity for methoxyflurane than sevoflurane, we now understand why renal dysfunction occurs after methoxyflurane and not after sevoflurane.[480] The lack of an association between sevoflurane, plasma inorganic fluoride concentration, and renal dysfunction in children and adults supports this new understanding of the mechanism of renal dysfunction after inhalational anesthesia. Consequently, the risk of renal dysfunction after sevoflurane is independent of the duration of exposure to sevoflurane. Sevoflurane does not pose any greater risk for perioperative renal disease than other maintenance anesthetics.[481] A second theoretical cause of sevoflurane-associated renal dysfunction is compound A, a product of alkaline hydrolysis of sevoflurane in the presence of CO_2 absorbents (see later discussion).

Hepatic System

In vivo metabolism of inhalational anesthetics varies with age, increasing to adult values within the first 2 years of life. The developmental changes in metabolism may be attributed to several factors, including reduced activity of the hepatic microsomal enzymes, reduced fat stores, and more rapid elimination of inhalational anesthetics in infants and children compared with adults. Halothane, isoflurane, enflurane, sevoflurane, and desflurane have all been associated with postoperative liver dysfunction and/or liver failure in adults, although the relationship between sevoflurane and desflurane and liver dysfunction remains tenuous.[482–485] In children, halothane and sevoflurane have been associated with transient hepatic dysfunction.[486–489] Indeed, several pediatric cases of transient postoperative liver failure and one case of fulminant hepatic failure and death have been attributed to "halothane hepatitis" that was confirmed serologically with antibodies to halothane-altered hepatic cell membrane antigens.[486] The exact mechanism of the hepatic dysfunction after halothane exposure remains unclear, although some clinicians have speculated that it is caused by an immunologic response to a metabolite of halothane. This putative toxic metabolite, a trifluoroacetyl halide compound, is produced during oxidative metabolism of halothane. It is thought that this compound induces an immunologic response in the liver by binding covalently to hepatic microsomal proteins, thereby forming an immunologically active hapten. A subsequent exposure to halothane then incites an immunologic response in the liver.[490] Hepatic enzymes may also be induced by previous administration of drugs, such as barbiturates, phenytoin, and rifampin. Although some have admonished clinicians for administering repeat anesthetics with halothane in children, it is our opinion that, in view of the millions of uneventful repeat halothane anesthetics in infants and children worldwide, insufficient evidence exists to support such an admonition.

CLINICAL EFFECTS
Induction Techniques
Although the physicochemical characteristics of the ether series of anesthetics would predict that anesthesia could be induced smoothly and more rapidly with these agents than with halothane,[304,306] this has not proved to be the case. All of the ether anesthetics except sevoflurane irritate the upper airway in children, resulting in a high incidence of breath-holding, coughing, salivation, excitement, laryngospasm, and hemoglobin–oxygen desaturation.[424,491–500] Clinical studies with desflurane in children demonstrated a high incidence of breath-holding, laryngospasm, and desaturation during inhalational induction (~50%).[424,500] As a result, a "black box" warning was issued against the use of desflurane for induction of anesthesia in infants and children. Before the introduction of desflurane, some advocated inducing anesthesia in children with isoflurane.[493–497] For example, it has been suggested that the quality and speed of induction of anesthesia with isoflurane in oxygen in infants and children is similar to that with halothane.[494] However, airway reflexes were commonly triggered with isoflurane despite the use of a number of strategies to attenuate them,[498,500,501] including slowly increasing the inspired concentration and using scented masks. Given the smooth induction characteristics, economy, and availability of sevoflurane, there are no reasons to consider other anesthetics for induction of anesthesia in infants and children.

In contrast to the noxious effects of the methyl ethyl ether series of anesthetics on the airway, sevoflurane does not irritate the upper airway and is well tolerated when administered by mask to infants and children at any concentration.[a] The introduction of sevoflurane has challenged and displaced halothane as the induction agent of choice in children in most countries. The incidences of coughing, breath-holding, laryngospasm, and hemoglobin–oxygen desaturation during induction with sevoflurane, whether by slow incremental increases in concentration or a single breath, are similar to those that occur during halothane (there was a significantly greater incidence of breath holding with halothane compared with sevoflurane but a greater incidence of induction excitement with sevoflurane compared with halothane) (see E-Table 7.4). The observation that the airway reflex responses are infrequent after a single-breath induction with 8% sevoflurane or 5% halothane casts doubt on the adage that large concentrations of inhalational anesthetics trigger airway reflex responses.[506–508] In fact, the induction is so smooth with sevoflurane that adjuvants, such as a premedication, concurrent use of nitrous oxide, or other strategies to prevent airway reflex responses, are generally unnecessary.

Induction of anesthesia with xenon has not been studied in children. In adults, inhalational induction with xenon at equi-MAC with sevoflurane resulted in a more rapid induction with stability

of respirations.[509] These data suggest that xenon may be an excellent induction anesthetic in children, provided its characteristics are upheld in well-designed clinical trials.

There is no single ideal approach to induce anesthesia by inhalation for all children. However, we advocate empowering children as much as possible to minimize fear. After appropriate preoperative preparation (involving premedication or parental presence or distraction techniques), the child is seated on the bed and encouraged to breathe through a face mask scented with a favorite flavor (to disguise the plastic odor of the mask) that is held over the nose and mouth. A fresh gas composed of 70% nitrous oxide in oxygen is breathed (while the pop-off value is completely open for 1 to 2 minutes). As soon as the child becomes "silly" or ceases to respond verbally, 8% sevoflurane is administered. Induction of anesthesia with halothane was performed with stepwise increments in the inspired concentration of 0.5% to 1.0% every three to four breaths until an adequate depth of anesthesia was achieved. This slow increase in the inspired concentration of halothane was thought to attenuate the incidence of airway reflex responses, although this is not evidence based. In fact, when a single-breath vital capacity induction was performed in children older than 6 years of age with 5% halothane, the incidence of airway reflex responses was surprisingly small.[506] Initially, sevoflurane was also administered in slow increments of 1% to 1.5% until 8%, but this caused transient agitation and involuntary movement of the extremities, frequently and sometimes violently, particularly in adolescents.[339] This was attributed to an exaggerated excitement phase. To minimize the excitement phase, we recommend that the inspired concentration of sevoflurane be increased as rapidly as possible, from 0% to 8% in a single-step increase.[506] This is based on a study of single-breath induction with 8% sevoflurane and 5% halothane in which the incidence of involuntary movement and the need for restraint were significantly less with sevoflurane than with halothane.[506] Recently, induction of anesthesia with 12% sevoflurane was reported to be more rapid than with 8%.[510] This is not a surprising finding, although 12% sevoflurane vaporizers should not be used in clinical practice because inspired concentrations of sevoflurane (in a laboratory setting) of 11% in oxygen and 10% in nitrous oxide support combustion.

Although some studies report more rapid induction of anesthesia with sevoflurane than with halothane, others have not. This inconsistency in the relative speed of induction reflects differences in study design that likely failed to take advantage of the 8% sevoflurane vaporizer and the differences in MAC. For children who are unable to perform a single-breath vital capacity induction, a rapid increase in the inspired concentration of sevoflurane has been a very effective alternative, with results comparable to the single-breath technique.[324,504–506]

Sevoflurane does not trigger airway reflex responses either alone or in combination with other agents, such as nitrous oxide. One study suggested that sevoflurane is the least irritating to the airway of all the inhalational anesthetics.[511] Previous studies suggested that airway irritability and excitement during sevoflurane anesthesia were similar whether nitrous oxide was present or absent, although others have disputed these findings.[506,512] The lack of effect of nitrous oxide on the speed of induction in the single-breath study was attributed to its concentration-reducing effect on sevoflurane.[506]

Although halothane has been the preferred agent for induction of anesthesia because of its lack of airway irritability, arrhythmias occur more frequently during halothane anesthesia than during anesthesia with the ether anesthetics. Halothane-induced arrhythmias occur more frequently during spontaneous ventilation and

---

[a]References 320, 321, 324, 325, 329, 339, 425, 502–506.

in association with high levels of circulating catecholamines or hypercarbia.[419] Most of these arrhythmias are unifocal or multifocal premature ventricular beats, nodal rhythm, bigeminy, or supraventricular arrhythmias.[325,419,499] Despite their appearance, most of these arrhythmias are benign and preserve the BP; ventricular tachycardia, however, may cause hypotension. Management of arrhythmias during halothane anesthesia includes inflating the lungs with large tidal volumes, hyperventilation to decrease the arterial CO_2 tension, increasing the concentration of halothane if there is evidence of "light" anesthesia (i.e., sweating, hypertension), and substituting another inhalational anesthetic for halothane.[419,513] Lidocaine has no role in the treatment of these arrhythmias because the myocardium is not intrinsically irritable. Moreover, a rapid IV bolus of lidocaine (2 mg/kg) may cause profound bradycardia.[514] Arrhythmias are rare during anesthesia with the ether series of anesthetics, but when they occur they are usually nodal in origin.[a] Arrhythmias during anesthesia with the ether anesthetics are usually self-limiting, resolving spontaneously or with parenteral administration of an anticholinergic. If the arrhythmias persist, then a cardiology consultation should be sought, particularly in a child with a history of congenital heart disease. Both IV and inhalational anesthetics have been used for induction and maintenance of anesthesia in children with congenital heart disease. (See the earlier cardiovascular section and Chapter 23 for a more detailed discussion.)

Once an adequate depth of anesthesia has been achieved, it is prudent to maintain spontaneous respirations with the maximal inspired concentration of sevoflurane tolerated until IV access has been achieved. If hypopnea or apnea occurs, then ventilation should be assisted. The reason to recommend this practice is to prevent awareness from occurring in the early induction period.[379,380] Discontinuing or decreasing the inspired concentration of nitrous oxide or sevoflurane individually or together may predispose to awareness, particularly if the child is stimulated at a light plane of anesthesia. This may occur in situations when anesthesia is induced in one location (induction room) and the child is then transferred to another (OR) without continuously supplying sevoflurane. Appreciating the limited solubility of nitrous oxide and sevoflurane will help to understand how rapidly these anesthetics egress from the body, particularly after a brief exposure. Once IV access is established, some practitioners administer propofol or another IV anesthetic before discontinuing the nitrous oxide to facilitate insertion of a laryngeal mask airway or tracheal intubation. The concentration of sevoflurane can then be decreased.

Emergence

Emergence or recovery has been arbitrarily divided into early (extubation, eye opening, following commands) and late (drinking, discharge time from postanesthesia care unit or hospital). Although most studies have demonstrated a more rapid early recovery after less soluble anesthetics,[321-323,326,329] few have demonstrated a more rapid late recovery.[320,329,515,516]

The speed of emergence and recovery from anesthesia are discussed in earlier text. The incidence of complications, such as airway reflex responses and vomiting during emergence from anesthesia, after mask anesthesia or tracheal intubation, are similar with most inhalational agents.[b] However, the incidence of airway responses of any severity after desflurane was significantly greater

than after isoflurane. Moreover, the incidence of airway adverse responses after removing a laryngeal mask airway (LMA) deep during desflurane anesthesia was significantly greater than was the incidence after removal of an LMA after recovery from desflurane (awake) or after isoflurane anesthesia.[518]

Emergence Delirium

Emergence delirium (ED) is defined as a dissociated state of consciousness in which children are inconsolable, irritable, uncompromising, and/or uncooperative (see Videos 47.1 and 47.2).[519,520] Children who experience ED often demand that all monitors, IV lines, and bandages be removed and that they be dressed in their own clothing. Many of these children fail to recognize and respond appropriately to their parents. Parents who witness this transient state usually volunteer that this behavior is unusual and uncustomary for their child. The core behaviors identified in association with ED after anesthesia in children include nonpurposeful action and averting eyes or staring.[521]

ED is not a new phenomenon; it was first reported in 1961[522] and was reported repeatedly after the introduction of almost every new anesthetic, including most inhalational anesthetics,[c] as well as IV agents, including midazolam, remifentanil, and propofol.[525,526] The incidence of ED after inhalational anesthesia in children ranges from 2% to 80%.[321,323,326,516,519]

The incidence of ED is greatest in children 1 to 5 years of age, similar after all inhalational anesthetics except halothane, reduced in the presence of adjuvant medications (e.g., opioids), increased in the presence of pain, and quite variable when a non-validated assessment scale is used.[519,520,527-530] These episodes have an average duration of 10 to 20 minutes and resolve spontaneously without sequelae. The mechanism by which ED occurs remains unknown.

ED has been reported in adults as well as infants, although the incidence is much less in both age groups than in children. Diagnosing ED after anesthesia and surgery has been complicated by our inability to distinguish it from pain. In one study, ketorolac decreased the incidence of ED 3-fold to 4-fold after myringotomy with either halothane or sevoflurane anesthesia.[517] Because ketorolac does not sedate children, it is likely that pain was confused with ED. Subsequent studies in children demonstrated that ED occurs after sevoflurane anesthesia even in the presence of neuraxial blocks.[519,530] The frequency of ED is independent of the speed of awakening from anesthesia,[531,532] the duration of a deep level of anesthesia,[533] the duration of general anesthesia,[534] and the presence of parents.[529]

The definitive study regarding the incidence of ED was undertaken in healthy children who required anesthesia for magnetic resonance imaging (MRI) and who did not undergo surgery.[529] The incidence of ED was 2-fold greater after sevoflurane than it was after halothane.

However, in most published studies, the metric used to diagnose ED had not been validated. To address this deficiency, the **P**ediatric **A**nesthesia **E**mergence **D**elirium (PAED) scale was developed (see Table 47.4).[520] The threshold PAED score to diagnose ED was thought to be greater than 10, but more recently a value greater than 12 was suggested.[535] When the PAED scale was compared with two nonvalidated scales,[535] the three appeared to be comparable, although the comparison was biased because the PAED scale was assessed first, followed by the other two scales (Table 7.8).

---

[a]References 325, 415, 416, 496, 499, 506, and 515.
[b]References 321, 323, 324, 326, 416, 493, 494, 516, and 517.

[c]References 319, 320, 323, 326, 517, and 523–525.

TABLE 7.8 Development and Psychometric Evaluation of the Pediatric Anesthesia Emergence Delirium Scale

1. The child makes eye contact with the caregiver.
2. The child's actions are purposeful.
3. The child is aware of his or her surroundings.
4. The child is restless.
5. The child is inconsolable.

Items 1, 2, and 3 are reverse scored as follows: 4 = not at all, 3 = just a little, 2 = quite a bit, 1 = very much, 0 = extremely. Items 4 and 5 are scored as follows: 0 = not at all, 1 = just a little, 2 = quite a bit, 3 = very much, 4 = extremely. The scores of each item were summed to obtain a total Pediatric Anesthesia Emergence Delirium (PAED) scale score. Emergence delirium is diagnosed if the total score is ≥10 or ≥12.

From Sikich N, Lerman J. Development and psychometric evaluation of the pediatric anesthesia emergence delirium scale. *Anesthesiology* 2004;100(5):1138–1145.

Pharmacologic interventions to prevent and treat ED have been summarized (see Table 47.6).[527,536] Effective treatment included fentanyl,[537] ketamine,[538] a propofol infusion or a bolus at the end of anesthesia, clonidine,[539,540] and dexmedetomidine.[541] In contrast, a single dose of propofol at induction of anesthesia, midazolam, and flumazenil were all ineffective.[536,542–546] Additional studies using assessment with a validated delirium scale are needed to clarify the contribution of anesthetics to ED during pain-free surgery.

Neuromuscular Junction

All inhalational anesthetics potentiate the actions of nondepolarizing muscle relaxants[547–549] and decrease neuromuscular transmission[550]; the latter, however, occurred only at increased concentrations. The mechanism of the reduced neuromuscular transmission is unknown but is likely attributable to actions of these anesthetics at the synaptic junction rather than PK or CNS effects. The potentiation of action of nondepolarizing relaxants follows the following order: isoflurane ~ desflurane ~ sevoflurane > enflurane > halothane > nitrous oxide–opioid technique.[547,551] However, this potentiation may depend on the type of nondepolarizing relaxant studied (longer-acting relaxants are affected to a greater extent than intermediate-acting relaxants),[547,548,552] and the concentration of anesthetic (reduced concentrations may yield small or no differences between anesthetics, whereas greater concentrations may demonstrate substantive differences).[548] In two parallel studies of atracurium infusions in children,[552,553] halothane and isoflurane decreased the atracurium requirements similarly in the first, whereas enflurane markedly decreased the requirements compared with halothane in the second. These observations suggest that inhalational anesthetics potentiate both intermediate-acting and long-acting NMBDs.

Malignant Hyperthermia

All potent inhalational anesthetics, except xenon,[554] trigger malignant hyperthermia (MH) reactions in susceptible adults and children.[555–564] Studies indicate that the relative capabilities of the four inhalational anesthetics to augment caffeine-induced contractures in MH-susceptible muscle in vitro are halothane > enflurane > isoflurane > methoxyflurane.[565] Using the surrogate marker of the time interval from administration of anesthesia until a reaction was detected to estimate the relative potency of the modern anesthetics to trigger MH, the order was halothane > sevoflurane > isoflurane ~ enflurane.[566] Currently, all inhalational anesthetics should be avoided in children who are MH susceptible (see Chapter 41).

The wash-out of inhalational anesthetics from anesthetic machines before anesthetizing a child with MH requires an understanding of the PK of these anesthetics in the specific anesthetic workstation. See Chapter 41 for a full discussion.

Stability and Toxicology of Breakdown Products

Inhalational anesthetics may be degraded via several pathways in the presence of most CO_2 absorbents to form several potentially toxic by-products. Enflurane, isoflurane, and desflurane (but not halothane and sevoflurane) react with desiccated soda lime to produce carbon monoxide. Halothane and sevoflurane react with soda lime to yield several organic compounds that are potentially organ toxic. In contrast, xenon is completely inert with CO_2 absorbents, thereby posing no risk from the genesis of metabolites or degradation products in humans.

Two strategies to address the clinical risks associated with the degradation of ether inhalational anesthetics are molecular sieves[567] and new CO_2 absorbents.[568–572] While molecular sieves were thought to have great promise, they have not reached the market for clinical use. In contrast, a number of new CO_2 absorbents have been developed to absorb CO_2 from the breathing circuit without degrading inhalational anesthetics to carbon monoxide and compound A (E-Table 7.5).[568,569] The previous generation of CO_2 absorbents differed in their composition and, therefore, in their affinity to degrade inhalational anesthetics. Soda lime contained 95% calcium hydroxide, either sodium or potassium hydroxide, and the balance as water. Baralyme, which is no longer available, contained 80% calcium hydroxide, 20% barium hydroxide, and the balance as water. E-Table 7.5 compares the compositions of the older with the newer CO_2 absorbents, which do not contain a strong base. Most recently, Amsorb Plus (Armstrong Medical, Coleraine, UK), Drägersorb Free (Dräger, Lubeck, Germany), and Yabashi lime (Yabashi product, Gifu, Japan) were formulated for minimal degradation of inhalational anesthetics, as well as to address efficient CO_2 absorption.[573]

Carbon monoxide may be produced when a methyl ethyl ether inhalational anesthetic is incubated with a desiccated CO_2 absorbent (most commonly soda lime or Baralyme). The absorbent within a CO_2 canister may become desiccated if dry fresh gas flows through the canister at a rate sufficient to remove most of the moisture (i.e., >5 L/minute continuously through the absorbent canister for 24 hours or longer while it is not in service). If the circuit reservoir bag is detached from the canister while fresh gas is flowing, then fresh gas may flow retrograde through the canister and exit primarily where the reservoir bag is normally placed. This cannot occur in anesthetic machines in which the fresh gas enters distal to the inspiratory flow valve. If the fresh gas flows retrograde through the canister for a sufficient time, it desiccates the absorbent and increases the risk of degradation of subsequently administered inhalational anesthetics. If one of the methyl ethyl ether inhalational agents (desflurane, isoflurane, or enflurane) is administered through a desiccated absorbent, carbon monoxide may be generated.[572,574,575] The magnitude of the carbon monoxide CO_2 production for a specific absorbent follows the order: desflurane = enflurane > isoflurane ≫ halothane = sevoflurane. Other factors that determine the magnitude of the carbon monoxide concentration produced include the concentration of the inhalational agent, the dryness of the absorbent, the type of absorbent (Baralyme > soda lime > newer absorbents), and the temperature of the absorbent.[574] The newer absorbents remove the strong alkalis, sodium hydroxide (NaOH) and potassium hydroxide (KOH), which are essential for the production of carbon monoxide, virtually eliminating this risk (E-Table 7.5).[576]

Small concentrations of carbon monoxide (up to 18 ppm) have been detected in children who were anesthetized with desflurane or sevoflurane using fresh CO_2 absorbent that included KOH and NaOH.[577] Carbon monoxide concentration correlated closely with the fresh gas flow to minute ventilation ratio (<0.68) and weakly with the type of anesthetic agent (desflurane) and age.[577] Carbon monoxide has been detected in concentrations up to 3 ppm during and after anesthesia, even spinal anesthesia.[578] One may question whether a minimum fresh gas flow with desflurane and other nonsevoflurane anesthetics is warranted. The presence of carbon monoxide in the exhaled breath has been attributed to heme metabolism, inflammation, and sepsis, although the authors did not use fresh soda lime in their breathing circuits.[578]

Carbon monoxide is not detectable by any freestanding anesthetic agent analyzer, pulse oximetry, or blood gas analyzer (with the exception of co-oximeters), although it is detectable by mass spectrometry. A carbon monoxide analyzer is currently marketed for use during anesthesia. The solution to this problem is prevention: turn off the anesthetic machine at the end of the day, disconnect the fresh gas hose to the absorbent canister, always have the reservoir bag connected to the canister, and avoid passing desflurane, enflurane, and isoflurane through a desiccated absorbent. Others have suggested that high-flow anesthesia should be avoided whenever a circle circuit is used to prevent inadvertent desiccation of absorbent. If the absorbent is desiccated, some have suggested "rehydrating" the absorbent, although this, too, is fraught with potential problems (including clumping of the absorbent).[579] If there is suspicion that the absorbent is desiccated, we strongly recommend replacing the absorbent before introducing an inhalational anesthetic. Alternatives to conventional absorbents, such as the molecular sieve and the newer absorbents, may very well obviate degradation of the ether anesthetics, provided the absorbent is not desiccated.[568,569,571,572] When methyl ethyl ether anesthetics are incubated with desiccated Amsorb, carbon monoxide is not produced, although it may be produced with other desiccated absorbents (E-Table 7.6).[568,569,572] The incidence of carbon monoxide poisoning during anesthesia remains extremely rare even when soda lime is used as the absorbent. In contrast, the potential for carbon monoxide poisoning is zero if Amsorb or one of the absorbents that does not include strong metal alkali is used.

Halothane is degraded in the presence of CO_2 absorbents to the unsaturated vinyl compound, 2-bromochloroethylene, which is lethal in mice.[580] Although 2-bromochloroethylene is potentially nephrotoxic, it poses very little risk in humans, even under low-flow conditions, because its maximal concentration in the circuit is less than 3% of its lethal concentration (LC_{50}).[581]

Sevoflurane is both absorbed and degraded via the Cannizzaro reaction in the presence of absorbent, resulting in five degradation products.[582,583] Although the degradation of sevoflurane by the absorbent was initially posited to delay its wash-in, evidence suggests that this effect is trivial.[584] Of the five degradation products produced when sevoflurane is degraded in either soda lime or Baralyme, compounds A and B appear in the greatest concentrations. Compound A, fluoromethyl-2,2-difluoro-1-(trifluoromethyl) vinyl ether, is nephrotoxic in rats at concentrations of 100 ppm or greater and has an LC_{50} of 1100 ppm. Compound B, a methoxyethyl ether compound that is minimally volatile at room temperature, is present in closed circuits at less than 5 ppm and poses no serious risk to animals or humans. The remaining three metabolites, compounds C, D, and E, are present in such low

concentrations in the breathing circuit that they are inconsequential. In a low-flow closed-circuit model with an inspired concentration of 2.5% sevoflurane, the concentration of compound A peaks at 20 to 40 ppm after several hours of anesthesia.[584–588] In children, compound A concentrations reach 16 ppm after 5.6 MAC hours of sevoflurane in a semi-closed circuit with 2-L/minute fresh gas flow.[589] Factors that are known to increase the production of compound A include an increase in the inspired concentration of sevoflurane, Baralyme greater than soda lime, and an increase in the temperature of the absorbent.[583,584] The newer formulation of CO_2 absorbents degrade sevoflurane to a lesser degree compared with the previous absorbents (see E-Tables 7.5 and 7.6). As in the case of carbon monoxide production, monovalent bases are important ingredients for the degradation of sevoflurane to compound A and their absence reduced the extent of degradation of sevoflurane.[570,576,590] In rats under low-flow conditions, compound A is nephrotoxic.[591–593] In contrast, studies in humans have been far from conclusive.[585–587,594] Commonly used indicators, such as albuminuria, have yielded inconsistent evidence of renal dysfunction.[585–588,594] One mechanism to explain compound A–induced nephrotoxicity is the β-lyase–dependent metabolism to nephrotoxic fluorinated compounds. However, this has been the subject of intense debate.[595,596] If compound A–associated nephrotoxicity were proven to depend on the β-lyase metabolic pathway, the limited concentration of this enzyme system in the renal cytoplasm and mitochondria of humans would make nephrotoxicity an unlikely outcome. Indeed, the inconsistency in the evidence of nephrotoxicity associated with compound A between rats and humans has been attributed to an 8- to 30-fold greater concentration of β-lyase in rats compared with humans.[597] To date, there have been no reported complications related to compound A and kidney damage in humans.

At the present time, sevoflurane is the only inhalational agent for which some federal authorities have recommended a minimum fresh gas flow when it is administered in a closed circuit with soda lime or Baralyme. The minimum fresh gas flow is 1–2 L/minute for 2 MAC-hours in the USA, although this limitation has not been universally adopted.

NITROUS OXIDE

Nitrous oxide confers several properties that differ substantively from the potent inhalational anesthetics that merit consideration. Nitrous oxide has a very limited solubility in blood, with a blood/gas partition coefficient ($\lambda_{blood/gas}$) value of 0.47. The MAC for nitrous oxide is 104% in adults; MAC has not been determined in children. Its chemical structure is N–N–O.

Nitrous oxide diffuses into gas cavities that are filled with nitrogen more rapidly than nitrogen egresses because it is 34 times more soluble in blood than nitrogen ($\lambda_{blood/gas}$ for nitrogen 0.014). Consequently, the volume of the cavity expands. However, the magnitude of the increase in the volume of the cavity depends, in part, on the concentration of nitrous oxide administered, as determined by the formula $100/(100 - \%N_2O$ [nitrous oxide]). The rate at which the cavity expands also depends on the source of the blood supply: those cavities in which the blood supply decreases as the volume of the cavity increases (e.g., a loop of obstructed bowel) will expand slower and to a smaller overall volume than a cavity in which the blood supply is independent of the cavity volume (e.g., a pneumothorax). By using a model of these conditions the time to double the volume of a loop of obstructed bowel with nitrous oxide was estimated to be 120 minutes, whereas the time to double the volume of a pneumothorax was 12 minutes.[598] Any gas-filled cavities within the body are vulnerable for expansion if nitrous oxide is administered; expansion can occur with obstructed bowel,[598] pneumothorax, gas cavities within the eye, endotracheal tube cuffs,[599] laryngeal mask airways,[600,601] bubbles in veins,[602] and pneumoencephalography.[603] Theoretically, nitrous oxide should be avoided during laparoscopic surgery to avoid expanding CO_2 bubbles that reach the venous circulation (see Chapter 29).

Inhalational anesthetics confer a low risk for postoperative nausea and vomiting. In contrast, nitrous oxide is considered to be an emetogenic anesthetic. In a large meta-analysis of the impact of nitrous oxide on the incidence of postoperative nausea and vomiting in adults, the authors determined that for emetogenic surgery, eliminating nitrous oxide was salutary (number needed to treat of six), whereas for nonemetogenic surgery there was no benefit from omitting nitrous oxide.[604] Hence, avoiding nitrous oxide in surgery that is emetogenic is reasonable. At the same time, the authors of that study noted that the number needed to harm, in the form of intraoperative awareness when nitrous oxide was omitted from the anesthetic, was 46, or more than 2%. A recent Cochrane review failed to establish whether the presence of nitrous oxide has an impact on the incidence of awareness in adults after general anesthesia.[605]

A number of studies have investigated the contribution of nitrous oxide to postoperative vomiting in children. Although there is some evidence that avoiding nitrous oxide reduces the incidence of postoperative vomiting in children,[606] the preponderance of evidence fails to show any benefit.[607–611] In part, this may be attributed to the multiplicity of factors that contribute to postoperative vomiting, as well as the salutary effects of other factors, such as the use of propofol and/or antiemetics. Evidence from adults indicates that the contribution of nitrous oxide to postoperative vomiting increases with the duration of exposure.[612] Similar data in children have not been forthcoming. In none of the studies in children where nitrous oxide was omitted was awareness reported.

The inclusion of nitrous oxide in remifentanil-propofol anesthesia in children has been associated with a reduction in postoperative hyperalgesia.[613]

ENVIRONMENTAL IMPACT

The National Institute for Occupational Safety and Health (NIOSH) recommendations currently limit the chronic exposure to nitrous oxide to 25 ppm and to inhalational anesthetics to 10 ppm. The basis for these recommendations is uncertain but may be attributed to the risk of teratogenicity and end-organ dysfunction. In pediatric anesthesia, mask anesthesia and/or uncuffed tracheal tubes and laryngeal mask airways in children leak inhalational anesthetics into the environment. As a result, there is local exposure to inhaled anesthetics during anesthesia in children that should be considered.

Concern over the pollution of the stratosphere and ozone layer depletion by polyhalogenated anesthetics has raised further questions for the long-term use of these agents and the need to fully recycle or adsorb the waste gases.[614] The polyhalogenated anesthetics are produced in extremely low concentrations and although they have a large molecular weight, atmospheric winds likely facilitate their transfer up to the stratosphere, where they cause global warming and decrease the ozone layer. However, the most compelling data of their limited impact on the environment relate to their half-lives. The half-lives of these polyhalogenated anesthetics in the stratosphere are approximately 5 years. Contrast

these to nitrous oxide, a compound with a very small molecular weight, which is administered in large concentrations (50%–70%) and has a half-life in the stratosphere of 120 years. Nitrous oxide is a known greenhouse gas that also depletes the ozone layer. The case for banning the polyhalogenated anesthetics pales in comparison with the enormous potential environmental impact of nitrous oxide. Although nitrous oxide is a serious greenhouse pollutant, agriculture and industry account for the vast majority of the nitrous oxide released into the atmosphere, with medical sources accounting for a trivial, unidentified fraction.[615] To preserve the ozone layer, all anesthetic providers should strive to limit the fresh gas flow and concentrations of inhalational anesthetics and nitrous oxide.

Oxygen

The concentration of oxygen for each anesthetic should be carefully titrated to the child's needs. Requirements are monitored by inspired oxygen concentration measurement, oxygen-hemoglobin saturation (pulse oximetry), and arterial blood gas determinations. Oxygen is often liberally administered in excess of the child's metabolic needs. However, potential dangers in this excess should be noted,[616] particularly in two areas. (1) Pulmonary oxygen toxicity is well documented; despite the fact that it develops slowly, general recommendations are to use an air/oxygen combination for prolonged procedures when nitrous oxide is contraindicated.[617] (2) Of additional concern is the remote possibility of adverse effects on the immature neonatal retina leading to retinopathy of prematurity (ROP).[618–629] Several cases of ROP have been reported in infants whose only known exposure to supplemental oxygen occurred in the OR; it should be noted that no new cases related to OR management have been reported since 1981![630,631] Many factors contribute to the development of ROP; it has been reported in children with cyanotic congenital heart disease, infants not exposed to exogenous oxygen, and even in stillborn infants.[632,633] A possible relationship of the development of ROP to arterial CO_2 variations, hypercarbia, hypotension, candida sepsis, inflammatory response, red blood cell transfusions, corticosteroid therapy, duration of ventilation, elevated blood glucose values, low gestational age, chronic lung disease, a deficiency of insulin-like growth factor, and vascular endothelial growth factor, as well as hypoxemia and fluctuating levels of oxygen, have all been suggested.[634–654] Other factors, such as exogenous bright light, maternal diabetes, maternal chorioamnionitis, and maternal antihistamine use within 2 weeks of delivery, are risk factors; the evidence for vitamin E deficiency is less convincing.[655–658] The possibility of a genetic predisposition—that is, a genetic polymorphism altering control of neovascularization—has also been proposed.[648,659–661] The use of continuous transcutaneous oxygen tension monitoring was not found to reduce the risk of ROP in infants weighing less than 1000 g, compared with controls.[662] It appears the major risk factor for developing ROP is extreme prematurity; *oxygen therapy represents only part of this complex problem*.[621,622,624] The incidence of ROP is predominantly limited to infants weighing 1000 g or less, but it is a concern in infants with a birth weight less than 1500 g born at less than 28 weeks gestation.[663–665] It should be noted that new treatments may involve systemic administration of propranolol (which improves neovascularization) and intravitreal injections of anti–vascular endothelial growth factors; both of these treatments may have anesthetic implications.[666,667] The evidence implicating hyperoxia as contributing to the development of ROP must be recognized but placed in perspective. Although it was thought that tight control of oxygen saturation and minimizing exposure to exogenous oxygen would reduce the incidence of ROP,[668] a multicenter study, the **S**upplemental **T**herapeutic **O**xygen **P**rethreshold for **R**etinopathy of **P**rematurity study (STOP-ROP), failed to support that hypothesis.[669] In fact, the conclusion reached stated, *"Although the relative risk–benefit of supplemental oxygen for each infant must be individually considered, clinicians need no longer be concerned that supplemental oxygen, as used in this study, will exacerbate active prethreshold ROP."*[669] This study suggests that anesthesiologists should take practical precautions to protect an infant's retinas from hyperoxemia without unnecessarily endangering the infant. No comprehensive epidemiologic studies have yet examined anesthetic risk factors, but given the many cofactors that are associated with this entity, it appears that anesthesia management, although very important, is a small piece of this puzzle.

Bearing in mind the possible role of hyperoxia and hypercarbia, intraoperative management must include careful monitoring of inspired oxygen and expired CO_2 concentrations. Maintaining the oxygen saturation at 93% to 95% results in an arterial partial pressure of oxygen (PaO_2) of approximately 70 mm Hg, with values exceeding 80 mm Hg on occasion.[623,670,671] Unfortunately, individual oximeters may vary considerably in terms of their accuracy, so practitioners must be familiar with their equipment.[672] The use of air blended with oxygen can be used to further reduce the inspired oxygen concentration. A transport system equipped with an air–oxygen blender is desirable to continue the titration of oxygen therapy from the OR to the ICU. (When using portable oxygen tanks, a good rule of thumb to determine the capacity of an E-cylinder is as follows: the minutes of oxygen delivery left in the tank = pounds of pressure [in pounds per square inch] × 0.3 divided by gas flow [in liters per minute].) While avoiding hyperoxia, one must never lose sight of the importance of *avoiding hypoxemia; hypoxemia is life-threatening whereas hyperoxia is not.* One cannot be faulted if ROP should occur, provided a reasonable and safe approach to oxygen administration and ventilation has been made.

Intravenous Anesthetic Agents

The anesthetic effects of IV agents are primarily reflected by brain concentrations (the effect site). To achieve anesthesia, it is necessary to obtain an adequate cerebral blood concentration that equilibrates with the effect size. Each drug administered is rapidly redistributed from vessel-rich well-perfused areas (brain, heart, lung, liver, kidneys, and endocrine glands) to muscle, and finally to vessel-poor less well-perfused areas (bone, fat). Thus termination of the effect of a single drug dose is primarily determined by redistribution. The much slower tertiary distribution to relatively underperfused tissues of the body is noted with long-term drug infusions. Protein binding, body composition, cardiac output, distribution of cardiac output, metabolism, and excretion all alter the PK and PD of IV drugs. Anesthetic depth may be altered if a constant cerebral blood concentration is not maintained. The changes in body composition and the BBB that occur during maturation may also greatly affect the duration of action of IV drugs, especially in neonates. In addition to perinatal circulatory changes (e.g., ductus venosus, ductus arteriosus), there are maturational differences in relative organ mass and regional blood flow while a symptomatic patent ductus arteriosus (PDA) may also result in differences in distribution. Blood flow, as a fraction of the cardiac output, to the kidney and brain increases with age, whereas that to the liver decreases

through the neonatal period.[673] Cerebral and hepatic mass, as proportions of body weight in the infant, are much greater than in the adult.[96] Whereas onset times are generally faster for neonates than adults (a size effect), reduced cardiac output and cerebral perfusion in neonates means that the expected onset time after an IV induction is slower in neonates, although reduced protein binding may counter this observation for some drugs. Offset time is also delayed because redistribution to well-perfused and deep underperfused tissues is more limited.

BARBITURATES

Methohexital

Methohexital (Brevital) is a short-acting barbiturate for IV induction of anesthesia (1–2 mg/kg). Administered intravenously as a 1% solution (10 mg/mL), it produces pain at the injection site; hiccups, apnea, and seizure-like activity may also be occasionally observed.[674,675] Methohexital has minimal effects on cardiovascular function (increased heart rate) in children.[676] Methohexital may be contraindicated in children with temporal lobe epilepsy.[674] Slow IV titration averts apnea. A possible advantage of methohexital (clearance 0.76 L/minute per 70 kg) over thiopental (clearance 0.24 L/minute per 70 kg) is that its mature rate of metabolism is greater while the volumes of distribution at steady state are similar (170 L/70 kg),[677] suggesting a more rapid recovery when large doses have been administered.[678-680] Anesthesia is achieved at plasma concentrations of 3.12 ± 0.99 mg/L.[681]

Rectal methohexital in a 10% solution (20–30 mg/kg) is a safe and atraumatic method of induction with an acceptably small incidence of undesired adverse effects (hiccups 13%, defecation 10%),[682] although this technique is no longer commonly used. It was particularly suited for brief radiologic procedures in children 3 months to 6 years of age, such as computed tomography (CT) scans, with a single rectal administration of a 10% solution given through a well-lubricated catheter.[683,684] Absorption by this route is quite variable and may account for an occasional child with slow or rapid onset of sedation.[678,685] It is also an alternative for children who are still in diapers and who are not candidates for other premedicants, such as midazolam (e.g., a child taking erythromycin).[686,687]

Oxygen desaturation occurs in approximately 4% of cases and is usually related to airway obstruction, which is readily corrected by repositioning the head[682,688]; methohexital should be administered only under the supervision of a physician trained in airway management to ensure adequacy of the airway because airway obstruction, seizures, or apnea may rarely occur.[689] *Children must not be left unobserved after administration.*

THIOPENTAL

The most likely anesthetic mechanism of action of thiopental is via binding to $GABA_A$ receptors, which increases the duration of GABA-activated chloride channel opening. The median effective dose (ED_{50}) of thiopental varies with age: 3.4 mg/kg in neonates, 6.3 mg/kg in infants, 3.9 mg/kg in children aged 1 to 4 years, 4.5 mg/kg in children 4 to 7 years, 4.3 mg/kg in children 7 to 12 years, and 4.1 mg/kg in adolescents aged 12 to 16 years.[690,691] The ED_{95} in children is 5 to 6 mg/kg and further increased to 7–8 mg/kg in children recovering from burn injuries.[692-694] Children aged 13 to 68 months given rectal thiopental (44 mg/kg) 45 minutes before surgery were either asleep or adequately sedated with plasma concentrations above 2.8 mg/L.[695] The effect-site concentration of thiopental for induction of anesthesia in neonates may be less than that in infants because the neonate has relatively immature cerebral cortical function, rudimentary dendritic arborization, and relatively few synapses.[696]

The hypotensive response in neonates given thiopental appears not as dramatic as that associated with propofol, although it still may occur with reversion to fetal circulation.[697,698] Thiopental has little direct effect on vascular smooth muscle tone. Cardiovascular depression is centrally mediated by inhibition of sympathetic nervous activity and direct myocardial depression through effects on transsarcolemmic and sarcoplasmic reticulum calcium flux. Although doses of 6 mg/kg have been given before intubation in term infants without physiologic consequences,[699] the mean dose required for satisfactory induction in neonates is less, at 3.4 ± 0.2 mg/kg.[690]

The duration of the clinical effect of thiopental depends primarily on redistribution rather than metabolism (10% per hour). As a result, repeated doses of thiopental may accumulate, causing prolonged sedation. Children 5 months to 13 years of age, however, metabolize thiopental almost twice as rapidly as adults when expressed as per kilogram (see E-Fig. 7.3).[700–702] The elimination half-life of thiopental in neonates is greater than that in adults and children[703,704] because of reduced clearance. Clearance, expressed using a ¾ allometric model, at 26 weeks PMA was 0.015 L/minute per 70 kg and increased to 0.119 L/minute per 70 kg by 42 weeks PMA.[182] Maturation of the CYP2C19 pathway increases rapidly after birth in term neonates,[705] and the mature clearance of 0.24 L/minute per 70 kg is achieved within 3 months of age.

Acute tolerance to thiopental may occur.[706] A total IV dose of 10 mg/kg is generally the upper limit; however, with this dose it is common to have a prolonged period of sedation after brief procedures. Thiopental is a weak vasodilator and a direct myocardial depressant; both of these effects may cause significant systemic hypotension in the *hypovolemic* state (e.g., dehydration resulting from prolonged fasting or trauma).[707]

Thiopental in a 10% solution (20–30 mg/kg) may also be used for induction of anesthesia by rectal instillation when methohexital is contraindicated (temporal lobe epilepsy).[674] The period of sedation may be greater for thiopental than for methohexital, partly because of the reduced rate of metabolism.[708]

Thiopental has also been used in the pediatric critical care setting as a continuous high-dose infusion (~2–4 mg/kg per hour) to control intracranial hypertension. Monitoring the blood concentration of thiopental may be useful during such therapy to avoid depressing myocardial function. The elimination of thiopental after a continuous infusion may be markedly prolonged compared with that after a single bolus (11.7 vs. 6.1 hours) because of zero-order elimination (Michaelis-Menten kinetics).[701,702] The maximum rate of metabolism (V_{max}) increased from 11 mg/hour per 70 kg at 25 weeks PMA to 172 mg/hour per 70 kg at term. The adult estimate for V_{max} was 402 mg/hour per 70 kg with a Michaelis constant of 28.3 mg/L.[182,709] Slower elimination reported in neonates may, in part, be attributed to the underlying illness (e.g., hypoxic insult) and intercurrent drug treatment.

PROPOFOL

Propofol (Diprivan) is a sedative-hypnotic agent useful for both the induction and maintenance of anesthesia.[710] Diprivan is formulated with 1% propofol, 10% soybean oil, 1.25% egg yolk phosphatide (ovolecithin), 2.25% glycerol, EDTA (ethylenediaminetetraacetic acid), and sodium hydroxide to maintain a pH of 7.0 to 8.5. This formulation has a white milky appearance because it is a lipid macroemulsion with average droplet size of 0.15 to 0.3 μmol/L (where 5 to 7 μmol/L is required to pass through capillaries).[711] These droplets remain distinct in suspension owing to the negative surface charges on the phosphate moieties in the ovolecithin phospholipids in the aqueous outer layer. These droplets may coalesce if the negative surface charges on the emulsion droplets dissipate, which is a slow, naturally occurring process, but which may also be precipitated by physical maneuvers (freeze-thawing, high temperatures, or agitation) or by changes in the chemical composition of the emulsion, such as by decreasing pH or the addition of electrolytes (i.e., sodium, potassium, calcium, or magnesium) or medications (i.e., lidocaine [see later discussion]).[711] Soybean oil is composed of long-chain triglycerides (LCT), defined by the 12 to 22 carbon atoms in their skeletons: linoleic acid (54%), oleic acids (26%), linolenic acid (7.8%), and stearic acid (2.6%). EDTA was added to Diprivan after 1998 as an antimicrobial agent. Generic formulations of propofol are available; these contain sulfites or metabisulfite as the antimicrobial agent.

Propofol is a very lipophilic drug that is rapidly distributed into vessel-rich organs, accounting for its rapid onset and usefulness as an induction agent. Termination of this effect is achieved by the combination of rapid redistribution and rapid hepatic and extrahepatic clearance.[712–714] The rapidity of the redistribution from vessel-rich organs accounts for its brief action and the need for repeated small boluses or a constant infusion to maintain a stable plane of anesthesia and sedation. PK studies demonstrated a larger Vdss (9.7 L/kg) in children compared with adults, and more rapid redistribution, but a clearance (34 mL/minute per kilogram) similar to or greater than that reported in adults (see Chapter 8 for a review of PK parameter sets used to describe propofol disposition).[715–718] Clearance, standardized to a 70-kg person using allometry, is immature in preterm neonates (0.4 L/minute per 70 kg at 30 weeks PMA); there is rapid maturation around term (1 L/minute per 70 kg), achieving 90% of mature clearance (1.8 L/minute per 70 kg) by 5 months postnatal age (see Fig. 7.11).[174,719–722] Clearance is limited by hepatic blood flow and is consequently reduced in children in low cardiac output states.[723] Although interindividual variability in the PK in neonates is large, the reduced clearance suggests that recovery after propofol in neonates may be prolonged and that repeat doses may not be required as frequently as in older children and adults. Propofol is conjugated to a water-soluble glucuronide in the liver and excreted in the urine.[715] Propofol also undergoes extrahepatic metabolism (in lung, kidney), as evidenced by the similar PK in infants with biliary atresia and healthy controls.[724]

Integrated PK–PD studies in neonates are lacking, partly because of a lack of consistent effect measures. However, studies in children are increasing (see Chapter 8).[55–57] The equilibration half-time ($T_{1/2}$keo) for the effect compartment is smaller (< 2 minutes) than in adults (3 minutes).[725,726] Reduced GABA$_A$ receptor numbers in the neonatal brain may contribute to a reduced target concentration, but this hypothesis remains untested. A circadian night-rhythm effect has been noted in an investigation of infant propofol sedation after major craniofacial surgery,[727] but such an effect is unlikely in neonates who do not have established day–night sleep cycles.[728]

Although measuring the concentration of propofol in blood has been the sole means to assess its disposition in vivo, alternate noninvasive techniques have been sought to provide online measurements. Mass spectrometry of the exhaled breath from adults and children, a technique similar to end-tidal gas monitoring of inhalational anesthetics, has proven to provide stable estimates of the concentration of propofol in blood.[729,730] It may soon be possible to guide administration of propofol in the OR by the measurement of expired propofol.[731-734]

In children who have not been premedicated, the dose of propofol (per kilogram) required for loss of the eyelash reflex generally increases with decreasing age.[735-739] The ED_{50} for loss of the eyelash reflex in infants (1–6 months) is 3 ± 0.2 mg/kg, which decreases in children (1–12 years) to 1.3 to 1.6 mg/kg, and increases in older children (10–16 years) to 2.4 ± 0.1 mg/kg. A more linear decrease in propofol dosing with increasing age between infants and children 12 years of age was determined in Chinese children.[738] A 10% decrease in the propofol dose for the ED_{95} between children younger than age 2 years, 2 to 5 years, and 6 to 12 years was noted. The ED_{90-95} for loss of eyelash reflex for all age groups is 50% to 75% greater than the ED_{50}.[735,736] Larger doses may be required for acceptance of the face mask.[736,740] The dose of propofol in neonates has not been clearly established but appears to be slightly less on the first day of life; the mean dose was 3.3 ± 1.2 mg/kg with 15% of neonates requiring additional medication.[741] In one study, a dose of 2.5 mg/kg permitted tracheal intubation in the majority of neonates, although the exact dose used was not specified.[742] In neonates, the ED_{50} for tracheal intubation ranged from 0.72 to 1.3 mg/kg, although only 58% were successfully intubated on the first attempt.[743] In infants 1 to 4 months, the intubating conditions 1 minute after a (median) propofol dose of 3 mg/kg and remifentanil 2 µg/kg were poor in almost one-third[744]; the addition of rocuronium 0.2 mg/kg did not improve their success rate. After induction of anesthesia with sevoflurane and nitrous oxide, excellent conditions for tracheal intubation are achieved with 1.5 to 2 mg/kg in children.[745-748] In contrast to the propofol doses needed for tracheal intubation with inhalation agent, successful insertion of a laryngeal mask airway (LMA) in unpremedicated children requires an even larger dose of propofol (5.4 mg/kg [4.7–6.8 mg/kg, 95% confidence interval (CI)]).[749]

Propofol is widely used as a continuous infusion or in intermittent doses in children undergoing brief radiologic procedures, during medical procedures such as oncology and gastroenterology, and for children with MH.[24,750-753] Although early evidence suggested that 100 µg/kg per minute propofol was required after a halothane induction to maintain immobility during MRI,[750] subsequent studies showed that much larger doses are required in unpremedicated children or after sevoflurane inductions.[24] Specifically, initial infusion rates of propofol of 200 to 250 µg/kg per minute (12–15 mg/kg per hour) or even greater may be required (up to 500 µg/kg per minute for the first 15 minutes and then tapered) to prevent nonpurposeful limb movement during scans. The initial rate may have to be increased for younger children (e.g., infants)[754] and for those who are cognitively impaired, but there is no difference for children with attention deficit disorder.[755] Midazolam premedication may reduce the propofol requirements, but it delays emergence after brief procedures. Once movement has abated, the infusion rate of propofol may be titrated approaching 200 µg/kg per minute in infants and 150 µg/kg per minute in older children. If minor movement can be tolerated (e.g., medical procedures), then intermittent boluses may be preferred for brief procedures, whereas if immobility is required (radiation oncology and radiologic procedures), then infusions are preferred. Repeated sedation with propofol over a prolonged period such as radiation oncology has not demonstrated the development of tolerance.[756] Propofol may offer advantage over dexmedetomidine sedation for MRI in terms of rapidity of onset, emergence, and parental satisfaction.[757]

Propofol affects a number of organ system responses in vivo. Systolic BP decreases approximately 15% in children,[716,740,758,759] which is similar to what occurs in adults.[760] Most studies reported similar decreases in BP after propofol and thiopental in children.[759,761] A study of preterm infants (29–32 weeks gestational age) enrolled in the **IN**tubation **SUR**factant **E**xtubation (INSURE) study found unacceptable hypotension after low-dose propofol (1 mg/kg) 10 minutes after propofol administration (mean arterial pressure 38 mm Hg reduced to 24 mm Hg); the authors concluded that *"propofol should be used with caution in very preterm infants with respiratory distress during the first hours of life."*[697] The incidence of apnea after an induction bolus of either propofol or thiopental is similar.[740,758,759,761] The major clinical disadvantage of propofol in children is pain when it is injected intravenously into a small vein.[762] This pain can be diminished by using any one of a number of strategies, including injecting propofol into a large vein; pretreatment with IV lidocaine (0.5 mg/kg), meperidine, nitrous oxide, metoprolol, dexmedetomidine, low-dose ketamine or tramadol; and combining a small dose of lidocaine (0.5–1.0 mg/kg) with the propofol.[a] The most effective method to eliminate pain in adults is to apply a "mini-Bier block" by manually occluding the IV flow by squeezing the extremity proximal to the IV site for 45 to 60 seconds and injecting IV lidocaine (0.5–1.0 mg/kg).[762] As soon as the Bier block is released, the desired dose of propofol is administered painlessly (E-Fig. 7.11). The average number of patients who need to be treated to benefit from this maneuver to prevent pain (*number needed to treat*) in adults is less than two,[766] indicating that this technique is extremely effective.[762] Some advocate that the use of IV lidocaine should be routine practice,[771] but the tourniquet may cause discomfort in some children. In children, IV lidocaine 2 mg/kg before propofol (without a tourniquet) dramatically reduced the pain.[771] In a meta-analysis, IV lidocaine effectively reduced pain before propofol although in most of the studies, lidocaine (10–20 mg) was admixed with the propofol immediately before administration.[772] Pretreatment of lidocaine with a tourniquet may be of greater benefit to prevent injection pain of propofol LCT/medium-chain triglycerides (MCT) compared to a premixed injection with lidocaine (see Chapter 8).[773]

The mechanism by which IV propofol causes pain has been attributed to the nociceptive effects of trace concentrations of propofol (15–20 µg/mL) in the outer aqueous layer of the Diprivan soybean-oil micelles. When the concentration of propofol in the outer layer was reduced (i.e., by increasing the concentration of MCT in the formulation or IV lidocaine), irritation of the nociceptive nerve endings in the veins and the severity of the pain during injection were attenuated.[774]

Indicators for recovery from anesthesia, such as time to eye opening and time to extubation, are more rapid in children when anesthesia was induced with propofol compared with thiopental.[775-780] Recovery of psychomotor function is more rapid after a propofol induction and maintenance of anesthesia compared with thiopental–isoflurane anesthesia.[781] Recovery room stay and time to hospital discharge are reduced with propofol.[775,777] ED rarely occurs after propofol anesthesia in children, and small doses at the end of inhalation anesthesia have been shown to reduce ED.[782-784] Propofol reduces the incidence of nausea and vomiting when used as an induction agent or when used for the maintenance of anesthesia.[777,785-791] However, there have been conflicting results for particular procedures, such as strabismus repair and

---

[a]References 716, 736, 740, 759, 761, and 763–770.

tonsillectomy, and when the drug is combined with opioids.[792–795] Nausea and vomiting may be considered surrogate endpoints for serious adverse outcomes after surgery in children. No studies have demonstrated clinically important abbreviated times to discharge or decrease in overnight admission rate for vomiting and/or dehydration in children treated with propofol. Short-term infusions of propofol for surgical or medical procedures have shown that the depth of sedation is easily controlled by adjusting the infusion rate while still ensuring rapid and complete recovery.[796–800] Propofol compromises airway patency and respiration in children; the upper airway narrows particularly in the hypopharyngeal region, but it does remain patent.[801] If airway obstruction occurs, the chin lift maneuver augments the patency of the upper airway.[802,803] Theoretically, collapse of the upper airway increases in parallel with the dose of propofol by direct inhibition of genioglossus muscle activity, as well as an inhibition of centrally mediated airway dilatation and airway reflexes.[804] All of these upper airway changes are reversed on emergence from anesthesia.[805] When propofol is given as an IV bolus, transient apnea may occur.[738,745,759]

Diprivan and the current lipid-based generic formulations of propofol must be handled with aseptic techniques because the lipid is a culture medium.[806] Propofol 1% can support the growth of at least four well-known organisms: *Staphylococcus aureus*, *Pseudomonas aeruginosa*, *Escherichia coli*, and *Candida albicans*.[807–809] When Diprivan was first introduced, it was prepared (as are all lipid emulsions) under strict aseptic conditions, with a layer of nitrogen above the liquid emulsion in each vial.[711] Once opened, external contamination of the vials, however, resulted in severe sepsis and several deaths before bacteriostatic or bacteriocidal agents were mandated to be included in the propofol formulations to prevent or retard bacterial growth. In very small concentrations, EDTA inhibits bacterial growth by chelating vital trace metals without affecting the emulsion droplet size or stability. Other formulations of propofol contain sulfite or metabisulfites, which release sulfur dioxide that prevents bacterial growth. Sulfites are more effective at reduced pH values, but there is a limit to how acidic the emulsion can become because this destabilizes the emulsion droplets. To further prevent any risk of bacterial contamination, all opened vials of propofol should be discarded after 12 hours.

Long-term propofol infusions were used extensively for sedation in ICUs after recognizing that its favorable PK would facilitate a rapid wake-up.[712] However, a report of five deaths in infants and children (4 weeks to 6 years of age) who were sedated with Diprivan raised serious doubts about the safety of such a practice.[810] The syndrome, now known as propofol infusion syndrome (PRIS), occurs primarily, but not exclusively, in children who are sedated for prolonged periods in ICUs.[810–814] Clinical experience indicates that PRIS is most common when propofol is infused continuously at more than 5 mg/kg per hour (70 µg/kg per minute) for more than 48 hours. Manifestations of PRIS include the insidious onset of lipemia, metabolic acidosis, hyperkalemia, and rhabdomyolysis that may precipitously transform into profound myocardial instability and cardiovascular collapse refractory to all resuscitative efforts. Manifesting signs may be subtle, with the sudden onset of bradycardia refractory to the usual interventions. PRIS was suspected in a 5-year-old undergoing an arteriovenous malformation resection when an unexplained metabolic acidosis was detected after a 7-hour infusion of propofol.[815] When propofol was discontinued, the signs of PRIS abated. In an adult neurosurgical ICU where propofol sedation was used, a retrospective review

determined that for every 1 mg/kg per hour that the propofol infusion exceeded 5 mg/kg per hour, the odds ratio of death was 1.93.[816] After a total of at least 28 deaths in children and 14 adults, the FDA cautioned against the use of propofol for long-term sedation. Predisposing risk factors include concomitant catecholamine inotrope infusions or high-dose corticosteroids and sepsis. In addition, some have cautioned against using propofol for extended periods of time in children with mitochondrial disorders.[817] Mortality currently ranges from 30% to 80%; institution of hemodialysis, partial exchange transfusion, and extracorporeal membrane oxygenation may improve survival.[818,819]

Despite PRIS risk, infusion at rates greater than 5 mg/kg per hour continue to be used in the ICU.[820] Unraveling factors that predispose to PRIS has proved to be difficult. Early investigations noted that during PRIS, the blood concentrations of malonylcarnitine and C5-acylcarnitine increased. These compounds are known to inhibit carnitine palmitoyl transferase and the transfer of LCT into mitochondria.[821,822] Propofol may also directly inhibit carnitine palmitoyl transferase to impede flux of LCT into mitochondria. Within the mitochondria, propofol uncouples the β-oxidation spiral at complex II in the respiratory chain, which in turn inhibits transmembrane flux of LCT into mitochondria, strangling the mitochondria from a much needed source of energy. One trauma center reported their experience with adult patients and correlated PRIS with duration of infusion and increasing triglyceride levels and suggested that the latter might be a useful biomarker for PRIS.[823]

The safety of propofol in the neonatal period has raised concerns after reports of profound episodes of cardiorespiratory collapse in neonates.[824,825] In these cases, precipitous and severe decreases in systolic BP, heart rate, and oxygenation were observed after a single induction dose of propofol (1–7 mg/kg) in neonates without evidence of congenital heart defects or cardiomyopathy. Resuscitation was extremely difficult in all cases despite intervention with both inotropic and chronotropic agents. A myriad of causes of bradycardia associated with propofol administration have been proposed.[826] In a comprehensive review of bradycardia after propofol in children and adults, the authors concluded that "propofol carries a finite risk for bradycardia with potential for major harm."[827] Whether these responses reflect acute right-to-left shunting, a return to fetal circulation, or another, as yet undisclosed cause in neonates has not been confirmed; caution should be exercised when propofol is used to induce anesthesia in neonates.[698]

Although anaphylactoid reactions have been reported after propofol administration in children, specific causes for the allergic reaction have not been identified.[828] In some instances, the "reactions" were primarily respiratory and attributed to preservatives, such as metabisulfites.[829] However, 13 of 14 adults who developed anaphylactoid reactions after their first exposure to propofol displayed a hypersensitivity response to propofol with at least one test during immunologic testing.[830] Similar findings in children have not been reported. It has been proposed that first-exposure reactions suggest a previous sensitization, possibly arising from isopropyl epitopes similar to propofol in cosmetics, detergents, and cough medicines.

Some clinicians avoid propofol in patients with egg, soy, or peanut allergies out of concern that cross-sensitivity with trace components in propofol may trigger perioperative anaphylactoid reactions. Both a case series and a recent review concluded that there is no evidence to eschew propofol in patients with egg, soy, or peanut allergies.[831,832]

The package insert for Diprivan cautions against its use in all patients with "egg allergy." However, children with egg allergy (including severe allergy) have received the measles-mumps-rubella vaccine, which is derived from eggs, without untoward experience,[833–835] although isolated reactions have been reported. In the past 2 decades, no immunologically verified anaphylactic reactions have been reported in children with egg allergy who received Diprivan.[832] In fact, Diprivan contains egg lecithin, which is derived from heated egg yolk. Egg lecithin is a phospholipid and has not been reported to trigger allergic reactions, although trace concentrations of egg yolk, of which only 2 of 9 proteins present (Gal d 5 and Gal d 6) are possibly immunogenic. When propofol was given 43 times to 28 children with egg allergy, only one experienced a mild nonanaphylactoid reaction, which led to the recommendation to avoid propofol only in children with documented anaphylaxis to eggs.[832] There is little evidence for present practice of choosing alternatives to propofol in patients with egg allergy.[831]

Soy protein allergy is primarily a gastrointestinal allergy that dissipates by 5 to 6 years of age because most foods consumed contain soy protein, resulting in natural desensitization. Very rarely is soy allergy a systemic disease. Although propofol is a soy-based emulsion, the AstraZeneca website states that all protein moieties are removed during the manufacturing process, rendering soy an exceedingly unlikely epitope to trigger an immunologically based anaphylactic reaction, although one case has been reported[836] in an adult not known to be soy-allergic. The reader should note that there is an approximately 5% cross-reactivity between soy and peanut allergy.[837] In children with both soy allergy and peanut anaphylaxis, it may be prudent to avoid propofol, especially if administering generic formulations. However, there is little evidence for the present practice of choosing alternatives to propofol in patients with peanut or soy allergy.[831]

In an effort to divest propofol of its lipid carrier and pain during IV administration, alternate formulations of propofol have been under development for parenteral use. New formulations of propofol must satisfy a number of conditions: easy to administer, stable formulation, no or minimal pain on injection, no infectious risk, no adverse organ effects including anaphylaxis and rapid PK. Unfortunately, most formulations to date have failed in one or more of the previous criteria.

Some have recommended replacing LCT in propofol with MCT to reduce the risk of PRIS and pain during injection. When 1% propofol with LCT was compared with the same with MCT, both with 1 mL of 2% lidocaine, the frequency of pain and its intensity during injection were similar.[838]

KETAMINE

Ketamine (Ketalar) is a derivative of phencyclidine that similarly antagonizes the N-methyl-D-aspartate (NMDA) receptor.[839] Its action is related to central dissociation of the cerebral cortex, and it also causes cerebral excitation. The latter property may be responsible for precipitating seizures in susceptible children and the reason that processed EEG monitoring devices do not work with ketamine sedation or anesthesia.[254–256,840,841]

Ketamine is available as a mixture of two enantiomers; the $S(+)$ enantiomer has four times the potency of the $R(-)$ enantiomer. $S(+)$-ketamine has approximately twice the potency of the other enantiomer. The metabolite norketamine, has a potency that is one-third that of its parent compound. Plasma concentrations associated with anesthesia are approximately 3 µg/mL,[842] whereas concentrations for hypnosis and amnesia during surgery are reported to be 0.8 to 4 µg/mL; awakening usually occurs at concentrations

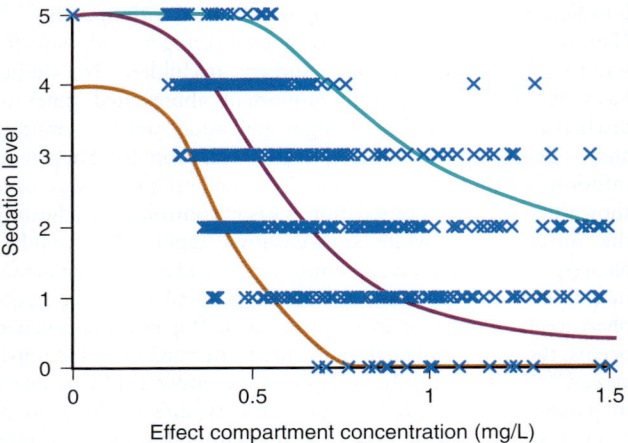

FIGURE 7.19 The relationship between effect compartment concentration and level of ketamine sedation (*purple line*). The concentration producing 50% of the maximum effect (EC_{50}) was 0.562 mg/L. Categorical data are shown as crosses. The *brown* and *blue lines* demonstrate the 5% and 95% confidence intervals. (Reproduced with permission from Herd DW, Anderson BJ, Keene NA, Holford NH. Investigating the pharmacodynamics of ketamine in children. *Paediatr Anaesth.* 2008;18(1):36–42.)

less than 0.5 µg/mL. Pain thresholds are increased at 0.1 µg/mL.[843] The concentration-response curve for ketamine sedation is steep.[66,844] This means that small serum concentration changes will have dramatic effect on the degree of sedation observed (Fig. 7.19).

Ketamine is very lipid soluble with rapid distribution and the onset of anesthesia after IV administration is approximately 30 seconds. This is usually heralded by horizontal or vertical nystagmus (Video 7.1).[845,846] Studies separating equivalent anesthetic doses of ketamine isomers identified a reduced incidence of adverse effects, more potent analgesia and rapid onset, and fewer cardiovascular effects with the dextro isomer rather than the levo isomer[113,845,847–849]; acute tolerance has been reported.[850] Children require greater doses of ketamine (per kilogram) than adults because of greater clearance (per kilogram); however, there is considerable patient-to-patient variability.[253,843,845,847]

Ketamine undergoes N-demethylation to norketamine. It is metabolized mainly by CYP3A4, although CYP2C9 and CYP2B6 also have a role. Elimination of racemic ketamine is complicated by the $R(-)$-ketamine enantiomer, which inhibits the elimination of the $S(+)$-ketamine enantiomer.[851] Clearance is immature in neonates but matures to reach adult rates (80 L/hour per 70 kg; that is, liver blood flow) within the first 6 months of life, when described using allometric size models.[852] Clearance in neonates is reduced (26 L/hour per 70 kg),[853–855] while Vdss is increased (3.46 L/kg at birth, 1.18 L/kg at 4 years, 0.75 L/kg at adulthood).[853] This larger Vdss in neonates contributes to the observation that neonates require a 4-fold greater dose than 6-year-old children to prevent gross motor movement.[856]

Bioavailability after IM administration is approximately 93% in adults and even greater in children.[843,857,858] There is a high hepatic extraction ratio, and the relative bioavailability of oral, nasal, and rectal formulations is 20% to 50% (Table 7.9).[128,858,859] Children presenting for burn surgery had slow absorption (absorption half-time [$T_{1/2}$abs] of 59 minutes) with large between-subject variability.[128]

Ketamine is an excellent analgesic and amnestic; the recommended dose for induction of anesthesia is 1 to 3 mg/kg

TABLE 7.9	**Ketamine Equivalency by Route of Administration[a]**

Route	Approximate Bioequivalence (mg/kg)
Intravenous	2
Intramuscular	2.15
Nasal	4
Rectal	8
Oral	11.75

[a]Note that these are estimates and that there is extreme patient-to-patient variability.

Extrapolated from data from Grant IS, Nimmo WS, McNicol LR, Clements JA. Ketamine disposition in children and adults. *Br J Anaesth*. 1983;55(1):1107–1111; Grant IS, Nimmo WS, Clements JA. Pharmacokinetics and analgesic effects of i.m. and oral ketamine. *Br J Anaesth*. 1981;53(8):805–810; Clements JA, Nimmo WS, Grant IS. Bioavailability, pharmacokinetics, and analgesic activity of ketamine in humans. *J Pharm Sci*. 1982;71(5):539–542.

intravenously or 5 to 10 mg/kg intramuscularly.[849,860] The duration of action of a single IV dose is 5 to 8 minutes, with an α-elimination half-life of 11 minutes and a β-elimination half-life of 2.5 to 3.0 hours.[861–863] Further supplementary doses of 0.5 to 1.0 mg/kg are administered when clinically indicated. Atropine or another antisialagogue accompanying the initial dose diminishes the production of copious secretions that may occur with ketamine.[864–866] Ketamine may also be administered in very low doses intravenously (0.25–0.5 mg/kg) or intramuscularly (1–2 mg/kg), either alone or in combination with low-dose midazolam (0.05 mg/kg [50 μg/kg]), along with atropine (0.02 mg/kg) for sedation, for a variety of procedures, such as oncology evaluations, suture of lacerations, or radiologic interventions.[849,860,867–872] If an antisialagogue is not administered, there is a greater risk for laryngospasm,[873] although guidelines for emergency departments suggest that supplementation with atropine or a benzodiazepine may not be necessary with doses of 1 to 1.5 mg/kg.[874–876] Larger doses of ketamine will produce a state of general anesthesia.[877–879] Even after small doses there is potential for apnea or airway obstruction, particularly when combined with other sedating medications.[877,880,881]

Ketamine has also been administered orally, nasally, and rectally, both as a premedication before general anesthesia and for procedural sedation.[882–900] Oral ketamine administered as a premedicant has also been reported to reduce ED; there is conflicting evidence regarding the efficacy of ketamine to reduce pain scores after tonsillectomy.[901–904]

There are concerns regarding both rectal and nasal drug administration. Rectal administration can result in very irregular and less predictable times of onset and peak sedation, just as with rectal barbiturates. Nasal drug administration may result in drug entering directly into the CNS by tracking along neurovascular tissue of the nasal mucosa (E-Fig. 4.2),[905–909] although this remains unproven in humans. Because the preservative in ketamine has been shown to be neurotoxic, there is the theoretic possibility of CNS toxicity because of the preservative.[910,911] These theoretical concerns have not been evident in clinical practice. The bioavailability of both S(+)-ketamine and racemic ketamine administered by nasal spray was ~36% with a peak blood level occurring at ~8.5 minutes.[113,118] A ketamine-sufentanil combination nasal administration provided rapid onset of analgesia for a variety of painful procedures with few adverse effects and has promising features for use in pediatric procedural pain management.[118]

Ketamine has also been administered as a means of providing caudal epidural analgesia.[860,912–917] There is risk of neurotoxicity during neuraxial administration of ketamine: *epidural ketamine must not be administered unless it is preservative free.*

The use of ketamine is increasing for postoperative pain management when administered in small doses as an opioid-sparing drug.[849,860,918–921] Although a recent meta-analysis documented reduced pain scores and nonopioid-sparing effects, it failed to substantiate its efficacy in opioid-sparing (see later discussion). Ketamine has also been used topically to treat mucositis and other painful conditions.[287,922–928] Ketamine increases heart rate, cardiac index, and systemic BP; it also increases pulmonary artery pressure in adults but has a small effect on respiration.[845,929] In children, there is apparently no effect on pulmonary artery pressure provided that ventilation is controlled.[930] If a child is sedated with ketamine but allowed to breathe spontaneously, increases in ETCO$_2$ could increase pulmonary artery pressures.[931] Ketamine sedation has been shown to maintain peripheral vascular resistance, thus affecting intracardiac shunting less than propofol in children sedated for cardiac catheterization.[932] However, the combination of ketamine and propofol[933,934] might be superior to either drug alone in this circumstance.[935,936] Ketamine has negative inotropic effects in those who depend on vasopressors.[937] The effect of ketamine on the musculature of the upper airway differs from that of midazolam; in adults, ketamine does not cause airway obstruction, whereas midazolam does.[938] Ketamine has one of the best safety profiles of any anesthetic agent. After unintended overdoses as great as 56 mg/kg IM and 15 mg/kg IV,[939] the duration of sedation persisted for 3 to 24 hours; respiratory depression occurred in four children, whereas tracheal intubation was required in two. When the children who received an overdose were monitored and their airways were maintained, recovery occurred without incident. This report, combined with the minimal effect of ketamine on airway patency, may explain, in part, the successful widespread use of this anesthetic by nonanesthesiologists. However, there remains a small but consistent incidence of adverse airway-related events, such as laryngospasm, apnea, and airway obstruction associated with ketamine, underscoring the need to ensure that the personnel responsible for administering ketamine are trained in advanced airway management. Ketamine also relaxes the smooth musculature of the airway stimulated by histamine[940]; treatment of acute asthma with subanesthetic doses has yielded mixed results.[941–946]

The most common adverse reaction to ketamine is postoperative vomiting, which occurs in up to 33% of children depending on the route of administration.[846,882] Intraoperative and postoperative dreaming and hallucinations occur more commonly in older than in younger children.[846] The incidence of these latter adverse effects may be reduced when ketamine is supplemented with a benzodiazepine.[947,948] One clinical report described 2 children, each 3 years of age, who had recurrent nightmares and abnormal behavior persisting for 10 months after a single ketamine administration.[949] A soporific environment may reduce the incidence of emergence phenomena.[950]

Ketamine is useful for children who are developmentally delayed or those who become combative because they are too frightened to come to the OR. IV ketamine can be used in very low doses (0.25–0.5 mg/kg) for short-term procedures, such as diagnostic spinal punctures and bone marrow aspiration, and in larger doses for angiography and cardiac catheterization. Ketamine may be particularly valuable for changes of burn dressings, suture removal, induction of anesthesia in hypovolemic children, children for whom application of a face mask may prove hazardous (such as those with epidermolysis bullosa), and children who require invasive monitoring before induction of general anesthesia.[845,847,951–953] Ketamine has been successfully used even in neonates with less apparent cardiovascular depression than occurs with halothane or isoflurane.[554] Oral ketamine given to children suffering burns is slowly absorbed owing to delayed gastic emptying. However, formation of the active metabolite (norketamine) contributes to analgesia and facilitates IV cannulation for subsequent IV administration in the OR.[128]

The role of ketamine for postoperative pain has been reviewed in a meta-analysis. Administration of ketamine in the OR was associated with decreased postoperative pain intensity and nonopioid analgesic requirement in the postoperative care unit, but it failed to exhibit a postoperative opioid-sparing effect in the subsequent 6 to 24 hours.[955,956] While postoperative low-dose infusion (0.02–0.25 mg/hour per kilogram) is ineffective in reducing opioid consumption after pediatric spinal surgery, it has been shown effective after adult abdominal surgery.[957]

Ketamine may produce increases in intracranial pressure (ICP) as a result of cerebral vasodilation; it also increases CMRO$_2$. Ketamine may be contraindicated in children with intracranial hypertension.[958,959] This concern regarding ICP has been challenged[960,961]; adult patients whose lungs were mechanically ventilated and who were sedated with a ketamine infusion demonstrated a decrease in ICP after bolus doses of 1.5, 3.0, and 5.0 mg/kg.[962] The caveat is that the tracheas were already intubated, ventilation was controlled, and they were sedated. There may be a use for ketamine sedation in the ICU, where there is meticulous attention to airway management and control of ventilation.[961]

A 30% increase in intraocular pressure (IOP) has also been noted; thus ketamine may be potentially dangerous in the presence of a corneal laceration.[963] In children with active upper respiratory tract infections, copious secretions caused by ketamine may well exacerbate an already irritable airway and result in laryngospasm.[864,873] Ketamine may cause an incompetent gag reflex and thus should not be administered in anesthetic induction doses to children with a full stomach without appropriate airway management. Ketamine may not be useful as the sole anesthetic agent in any surgical procedure in which total control of the child's position is necessary, because purposeless movements frequently occur. Ketamine may be inappropriate in any child with a history of psychiatric or seizure disorder because of its psychotropic and epileptogenic effects.[840,845]

In addition, studies in newborn rodents and nonhuman primates correlated ketamine treatment with increased neuronal apoptosis during rapid synaptogenesis.[839,964,965] Infusions of ketamine (20–50 µg/kg per hour) to neonatal rhesus monkeys yielded apoptosis after 24 hour but not after 3-hour infusions.[966] The clinical importance of these findings is unclear since it is unknown if these data can be extrapolated from animals to developing humans (see Chapter 25).

Although the administration of ketamine appears simple, its adverse side effects are potentially dangerous. *Ketamine must be administered only by physicians experienced with managing a compromised airway.* We urge that it not be used as a premedication unless given in the presence of continuous supervision by properly trained personnel.

ETOMIDATE

Etomidate (Amidate) is a steroid-based hypnotic induction agent metabolized principally by hepatic esterases. Concentrations associated with anesthesia are 300 to 500 µg/L. As with most induction agents, offset of effect is by redistribution. Etomidate PK have been studied in children with a median age of 4 years (range 0.53–13.21 years) and weight 15.7 kg (7.5–52 kg). The estimates of PK parameter (standardized to a 70-kg adult) for typical 4-year-old children were CL 1.50 L/minute per 70 kg; Q2 1.95 L/minute per 70 kg; Q3 1.23 L/minute per 70 kg; V1 9.51 L/70 kg; V2 11.0 L/70 kg; and V3 79.2 L/70 kg.[967] Similar to propofol, younger children require a larger bolus dose of etomidate than older children to achieve equivalent plasma concentrations.[968] Etomidate clearance is reduced in neonates and infants (postnatal age 0.3–11.7 months) with congenital heart disease. A two-compartment model with allometric scaling to a 70-kg adult revealel a CL 0.624 L/minute per 70 kg and Q2 0.44 L/minute per 70 kg; central (V1) and peripheral distribution volume (V2) were 9.47 L/70 kg and 22.8 L/70 kg, respectively. Children also require a 30% increased bolus dose because of an increased V1.[969]

Etomidate is painful when administered intravenously. However, concerns regarding the risks of anaphylactoid reactions and suppression of adrenal function (which lasts for ~24 hours)[970,971] have resulted in most anesthesiologists avoiding this agent in routine cases.[972] Etomidate is useful in children with head injury and those with an unstable cardiovascular status, (e.g., cardiomyopathy) because of its lack of effect on cardiac function.[973,974] It is often used by emergency physicians for management of the airway.[975–978] Usual doses include 0.2 to 0.3 mg/kg before administration of a low-dose opioid and a muscle relaxant. Etomidate is often used to facilitate tracheal intubation in critically ill children—that is, those in whom it would seem to offer the most advantage. Because a very large proportion of critically ill children, particularly those resistant to vasopressors, suffer from relative adrenal insufficiency, corticosteroid supplementation may be indicated in such patients in whom etomidate is deemed necessary for their airway management.[979,980]

New etomidate formulations that are very short-acting and not associated with adrenal suppression are in development (Fig. 7.20).[981–985] An additional ester group on methoxycarbonyletomidate (MOC-etomidate) rendered this compound vulnerable to nonspecific esterases. MOC-etomidate showed very rapid degradation in vitro as well as in animals (E-Fig. 7.12). In animals, the righting reflex recovers more rapidly after MOC-etomidate treatment than after treatment with the parent compound. Adrenal suppression was addressed by substituting a pyrrole group in place of the imidazole group to preclude the binding of etomidate to 11-β-hydroxylase in the synthesis of adrenal hormones. As a consequence, carboetomidate did not bind well to 11-β-hydroxylase and therefore did not suppress adrenal hormone synthesis (E-Fig. 7.13). However, the slow onset of action of MOC-carboetomidate has not led to clinical trials.

Neuromuscular Blocking Drugs

NEUROMUSCULAR MONITORING

The measurement of evoked responses after an electrical stimulus is the standard method for evaluating neuromuscular function. This method allows nearly instantaneous evaluation of the degree of neuromuscular blockade in the unconscious individual. The force of contraction of the thumb, the accelerometer, or the electromyogram may be used to make this assessment.[986] Twitch tension measurements use the force of contraction of the adductor pollicis. This muscle is the only thumb muscle supplied by the ulnar nerve; measurements therefore approach the single-muscle precision of the experimental nerve muscle preparation.[547] The

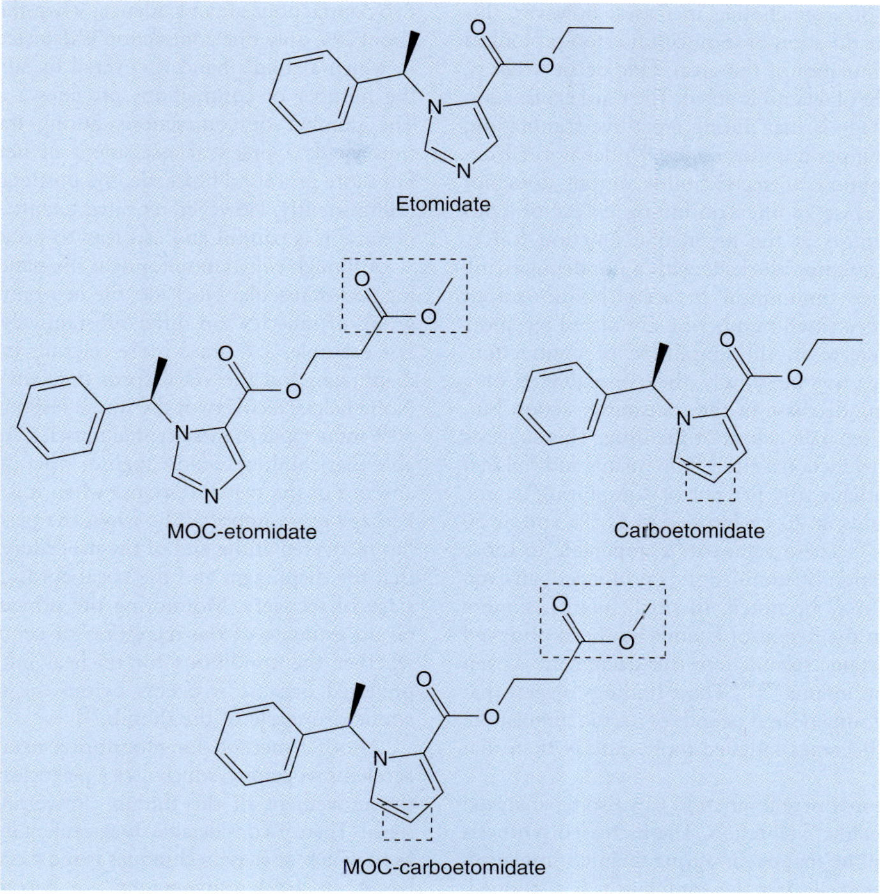

FIGURE 7.20 Molecular structures of etomidate (parent compound), methoxycarbonyl-etomidate *(MOC-etomidate)* (the doubly substituted ester side chain), carboetomidate (the imidazole ring has been replaced by a pyrrole ring), and MOC-carboetomidate (in which both the double ester and the pyrrole-for-imidazole ring substitutions are present). MOC-carboetomidate has a brief duration of action, does not suppress adrenal hormone synthesis, and appears to share similar potency with etomidate. (Reproduced with permission from Pejo E, Cotton JF, Kelly EW, et al. In vivo and in vitro pharmacological studies of methoxycarbony -carboetomidate. *Anesth Analg.* 2012;115(2):297–304.)

evoked tension of the adductor pollicis in response to stimulation of the ulnar nerve can be recorded by a force displacement transducer (E-Fig. 7.14A). With the electromyogram, the compound muscle action potential is recorded by surface or needle electrodes applied to any muscle, usually the adductor pollicis brevis, the abductor digiti minimi, or the first dorsal interosseous muscle of the hand (see E-Fig. 7.14B). To achieve reproducibility and to ensure full activation of all stimulated nerve and muscle fibers, the stimuli should be supramaximal in intensity, square wave in nature, and no longer than 0.2 milliseconds in duration.

Clinically, three types of stimulation are used (E-Fig. 7.15):
1. Single twitch (0.1 to 0.25 Hz [cycles/second])
2. Train-of-four (2 Hz for 2 seconds)
3. Tetanus (50 Hz, usually for 5 seconds)

Single-twitch rates are useful whenever there is an observable control response. By comparing the percentage change of twitch tension before and after administration of the neuromuscular blocking agent, one can assess the degree of paralysis. Single stimuli detect relatively profound degrees of neuromuscular blockade. In fact, depression of the twitch response can be observed only if more than three-fourths of the postsynaptic receptors are blocked.[987]

The *train-of-four* is the most commonly used method for assessing nondepolarizing neuromuscular blockade. It consists of four supramaximal stimuli applied to the ulnar nerve at a frequency of 2 cycles/second. The ratio of the amplitude of the fourth twitch to the first is an indicator of the degree of neuromuscular blockade. The main advantage of the train-of-four is that it does not require a control measurement. Furthermore, the train-of-four technique can be repeated every 10 seconds, thus allowing rapid changes in neuromuscular blockade to be closely monitored.[547] In general, when the train-of-four is zero, the conditions for tracheal intubation are satisfactory (excellent or good).[988] Preterm infants younger than 32 weeks PCA have reduced train-of-four fourth-response values ($83\% \pm 2\%$) compared with more mature neonates (E-Fig. 7.16).[989] In full-term infants younger than 1 month of age, the height of the fourth evoked response of the train is about 95%.[990] The change to the greater value during the first month of life probably indicates maturation of the myoneural junction. In children 2 months of age and older, all components of the train-of-four are nearly equal (100%).[989]

Tetanic stimulation is usually obtained by supramaximally stimulating the nerve for 5 seconds or more. During tetanic stimulation, synthesis of acetylcholine increases; however, this increase is limited. If the duration of stimulation is too prolonged or the frequency of stimulation is too great, fade occurs—that is, a decrement in the height of tetanus is noted. The usual explanation for the occurrence of fade is that during repetitive stimulation, the acetylcholine output-per-impulse wanes. Under normal circumstances, the diminution of acetylcholine output does not affect transmission because of the continuing excess of both acetylcholine and receptors at the myoneural junction (safety factor). During partial receptor blockade with a nondepolarizing relaxant, the progressive diminution of acetylcholine output eventually results in a decreased number of stimulated receptors and a consequent decrease in the amplitude of contraction. Alternatively, fade may not be simply the consequence of a spontaneously occurring decrease in the transmitter action but, in fact, a different and separate action of the drug. This suggests that the relaxant has a prejunctional effect.[991] In infants and children anesthetized with halothane, the percent of fade during tetanic stimulation for 5 seconds at 20 cycles/second is 5% and at 50 cycles/second it is 9%.[990] These values are comparable to those for adults.[992] If the duration of stimulation is prolonged, an even greater degree of fade may be noted. In small infants, a more than 50% decrement in the height of tetanus has been observed during 15 seconds of tetanic stimulation; this decrement is even more marked in preterm infants.[993,994] These findings suggest that small infants can indeed sustain short periods of tetanic stimulation, but their musculature becomes fatigued more quickly than that of older children.

The integrity of the myoneural junction can also be analyzed by evaluation of posttetanic facilitation. The increased synthesis and release of acetylcholine that occur during tetanic stimulation continue for a short interval after the stimulation has stopped. This increased production normally does not result in facilitation because all the muscle fibers are excited by the stimulus. In the presence of nondepolarizing (competitive) neuromuscular blockade, however, the increased posttetanic acetylcholine release stimulates a greater number of muscle fibers, producing the characteristic posttetanic facilitation.[992]

The posttetanic count has been used to evaluate intense neuromuscular blockade in children.[995,996] This is a measure obtained by applying a 50-cycle/second tetanic stimulus to the ulnar nerve for 5 seconds, followed by single-twitch stimulation at 1 cycle/second; the number of twitches observed in the posttetanic period is known as the posttetanic count (E-Fig. 7.17). Because tetanus and posttetanic responses are indicators of deep neuromuscular blockade, they can usually be elicited during recovery before the reappearance of the train-of-four. At very deep levels of blockade, no tetanus or posttetanic effect can be seen; as the patient recovers, a single posttetanic response eventually manifests itself. The number of posttetanic counts increases as recovery proceeds until, at posttetanic counts of six to seven, the first twitch of the train-of-four reappears. It has been shown that during recovery, the first posttetanic response precedes the first response of the train-of-four by 5 to 10 minutes with intermediate relaxants and by 20 to 30 minutes with long-acting relaxants.[995,996] In a clinical situation in which neuromuscular recording instruments are not available, the number of contractions during train-of-four are counted. This technique depends on the fact that the number of twitches in the train-of-four usually correlates well with the degree of blockade. When the height of the first twitch is about 21% of control, three contractions are usually detected during train-of-four stimulation; at a single-twitch height of 14% of control,

two contractions are in evidence; when the single-twitch height is about 7%, only one contraction is detected.[997] During procedures in which a child's hand is covered by surgical drapes, palpating the number of contractions provides a satisfactory alternative. The number of contractions during train-of-four stimulation thus yields a practical assessment of neuromuscular blockade. For more profound blockade, the posttetanic counts can be used intermittently. However, repeated tetanic stimulation is not ideal because it is painful and can lead to posttetanic exhaustion.

Although twitch monitoring is the standard method of evaluating neuromuscular blockade, the neuromuscular blockade in one group of muscles can differ substantively from that in another. For example, 1.7 times more relaxant is required to block the diaphragm and the vocal cords than the adductor pollicis.[998,999] Nonetheless, recovery of the twitch response is also approximately 50% more rapid in these central muscles. Accordingly, it is conceivable that children could cough or react during intubation in the absence of the twitch response when it is measured peripherally. Perhaps more importantly, when the peripheral twitch response has recovered at the end of the procedure, it is a clear indication that the diaphragm and the vocal cords are in a more advanced stage of recovery. Monitoring the orbicularis oculi contraction (as an estimate of the relaxation of central muscles) to predict whether the conditions for tracheal intubation are suitable is preferred because it occurs before the twitch response of the adductor muscle of the thumb.[1000]

Another method for monitoring neuromuscular blockade is acceleromyography, which uses a piezoelectric sensor to quantitate the movement of the thumb, converting this to an electrical signal. There is considerable disagreement in the published literature as to which of these techniques is most accurate.[1001-1003] Monitors based on acceleromyography are becoming more commonly available; however, these are not "user friendly" and are difficult to use in infants because of the small arc of the displaced thumb. Some consider this monitor to be more accurate than standard mechanomyography-based train-of-four monitors.[1004,1005] Others think that mechanomyography is more accurate because it is "less influenced by external disturbances"—that is, it does not go out of calibration.[1006] Therefore at present, for clinical purposes in infants and children, mechanomyography still seems to be the simplest and most helpful clinical monitor during the use of nondepolarizing competitive blockers.

NEUROMUSCULAR JUNCTION

Adult postjunctional acetylcholine receptors possess five subunits—two α and one β, δ, and ϵ subunits. Preterm neonates (<31 weeks PMA) have a γ subunit instead of an ϵ subunit in their neuromuscular receptor.[1007] Fetal receptors have a greater opening time than adult receptors, allowing more sodium to enter the cell, with a consequent larger depolarizing potential. The resulting increased sensitivity to acetylcholine is at odds with the observed increased sensitivity to NMBDs, but may compensate for reduced acetylcholine stores in the terminal nerve endings.[1008]

Neuromuscular transmission is immature in neonates and infants until the age of 2 months.[990,1009] Neonates deplete acetylcholine vesicle reserves more quickly than do infants older than 2 months, in response to tetanic nerve stimulation.[990] Data from phrenic nerve–hemidiaphragm preparations from rats aged 11 to 28 days suggest this is the result of a low quantal content of acetylcholine in neonatal endplate potentials.[223] Neonates display an increased sensitivity to NMBDs. An alternative proposal to explain this increased sensitivity is based on NMBD synergism observations.[1010,1011] Neonates display poor synergism and this has been explained on the basis that NMBDs occupy only one of the two α-subunit receptor sites in neonates as opposed to two in children and adults.[1011] If this is true, then neonates may use NMBDs more efficiently than children.

Preterm infants tolerate respiratory loads poorly. The diaphragm in the preterm neonate contains only ~10% of the slowly contracting type I fibers (see Fig. 14.11). This proportion increases to ~25% at term and to ~55% by 2 years of age.[225] A similar maturation pattern has been observed for the intercostal muscles.[225] Type I fibers tend to be more sensitive to NMBDs than type II fibers, and consequently the diaphragmatic function in neonates may be better preserved and recover earlier than peripheral muscles.[999,1012–1014]

Total body water and extracellular fluid (ECF)[1015] are greatest in preterm neonates and decrease throughout gestation and postnatal life, whereas fat as a percentage of body weight increases with postnatal age. Muscle contributes only ~10% of body weight in neonates and ~33% by the end of childhood. Polar drugs, such as depolarizing and nondepolarizing NMBDs, distribute rapidly into the ECF, but enter cells more slowly. Consequently, a larger initial dose of such drugs is required in infants compared with children or adults. Increasing the muscle bulk contributes new acetylcholine receptors. This greater number of receptors requires a greater amount of drug to block activation of receptor ion channels.

PHARMACODYNAMICS

There is age-related variability in the dose required to achieve a predetermined level of neuromuscular blockade during balanced thiopental–N$_2$O–fentanyl anesthesia. The ED$_{95}$ of vecuronium was 47 ± 11 μg/kg in neonates and infants, 81 ± 12 μg/kg in children between 3 and 10 years of age, and 55 ± 12 μg/kg in children aged 13 years or older (Fig. 7.21).[1016]

Similar profiles have been reported for other NMBDs.[335,999,1017–1019] In addition, duration of neuromuscular blockade is greater in neonates than in children.[1020] The reduced dose requirement in neonates is attributable to immaturity of the neuromuscular junction. The increased Vd from an expanded ECF in neonates means a similar initial dose (per kilogram) is given to neonates

and teenagers. Children tend to require larger doses than adults; the reason for the larger dose requirement in children is unclear but it may be the result of increased muscle bulk.

Investigation of concentration–response relationships is more revealing. The plasma concentration required in neonates to achieve the same level of neuromuscular block as in children or adults is 20% to 50% less, consistent with immaturity of the neuromuscular junction.[86,1021–1024] Plasma concentration requirements are reduced by inhaled anesthetic agents.[552,1025,1026]

The onset time for NMBDs in neonates is faster than it is in older children and adults. Onset time (time to maximal effect) after vecuronium 70 μg/kg was most rapid for infants (1.5 ± 0.6 minutes) compared with that for children (2.4 ± 1.4 minutes) and adults (2.9 ± 0.6 minutes).[1020] These observations are similar to those reported for other intermediate- and long-acting NMBDs.[1014] The more rapid onset of these drugs in neonates has been attributed to a greater cardiac output seen with the per-kilogram model.[1014]

Cardiac output is used as a surrogate measure for muscle perfusion. Onset time is a function of size. An onset time standardized to a 70-kg person using an allometric ¼-power model is around 3 minutes for most long-acting NMBDs. In children with low cardiac output or decreased muscle perfusion, onset times are prolonged. The onset time of neuromuscular paralysis is proportional to T$_{1/2}$keo. An old study demonstrated an increase in the T$_{1/2}$keo of *d*-tubocurare with increasing inspired halothane concentrations[257]; a possible explanation for the delayed action of tubocurarine may be that halothane is a negative inotrope[258] and decreases muscle blood flow.[259]

PHARMACOKINETICS

The dose of NMBDs at different ages depends on the complex interweaving of PD and PK factors. The Vd mirrors ECF changes and can be predicted using either an allometric ¾-power model or the surface area model (⅔-power model), both of which approximate ECF changes with weight.[68]

The clearance of *d*-tubocurarine, standardized to an allometric or surface area model, is reduced in neonates and infants compared with older children and adults.[86] These age-related clearance changes follow age-related maturation of glomerular filtration in the kidney,[171] which is the elimination route of *d*-tubocurarine. Total plasma clearance of other nondepolarizing muscle relaxants cleared by renal (alcuronium) and/or hepatic pathways (pancuronium, pipecuronium, rocuronium, and vecuronium) are all reduced in neonates.[1021,1023,1027–1029] In contrast, the clearances of atracurium and cisatracurium are neither renal- nor hepatic-dependent but rather depend on Hofmann elimination, ester hydrolysis, and other unspecified pathways.[1030] Clearance of these drugs is increased in neonates when expressed as per kilogram.[1031–1033] When clearance is standardized using allometric ¾-power scaling, the clearances for atracurium and cisatracurium are similar throughout all age groups. The clearance of succinylcholine, expressed as per kilogram, also decreases as age increases.[189,190] Succinylcholine is hydrolyzed by butyrylcholinesterase. These observations are consistent with that observed for the clearance of remifentanil,[39] which is also cleared by plasma esterases. These clearance pathways are mature at birth.[40]

Conversion of *d*-tubocurarine half-times from chronologic time to physiologic time is revealing. T$_{1/2}$α increases with age in chronologic time, but in physiologic time it is the same at all ages, as we would expect from a distribution phase standardized by allometry. T$_{1/2}$β decreases with age in physiologic time, consistent

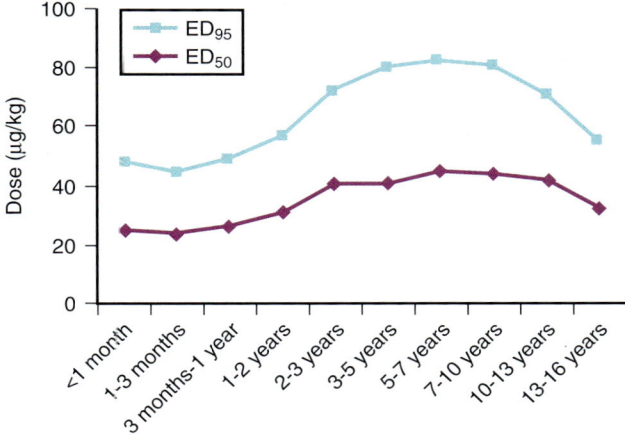

FIGURE 7.21 Dose changes with age for vecuronium during balanced anesthesia. *ED$_{50}$* is the dose that achieves 50% of the maximum response; *ED$_{95}$* is the dose that achieves 95% of the maximum response. (Data extracted from Meretoja OA, Wirtavuori K, Neuvonen PJ. Age-dependence of the dose-response curve of vecuronium in pediatric patients during balanced anesthesia. *Anesth Analg.* 1988;67(1):21–26.)

with reduced clearance related to the greater Vd in the very young. The $T_{1/2}$keo is large in neonates and infants, reduced in children, and further reduced in adults, possibly because of increased muscle bulk and concomitant increased muscle perfusion in children and young adults.

Depolarizing Neuromuscular Blocking Drugs

SUCCINYLCHOLINE

Succinylcholine is the only depolarizing relaxant used in children. Infants are more resistant to its neuromuscular effects than adults.[1034] Early studies demonstrated that the degree of neuromuscular blockade achieved by 1 mg/kg IV in infants is about equal to that produced by 0.5 mg/kg in older children.[1035] The increase in dose requirement in younger children is thought to result, in part, from the drug's rapid distribution into the infant's large ECF volume (E-Table 7.7 and Table 7.10).

Succinylcholine remains the NMBD with the most rapid onset. The onset time of a paralyzing dose (1.0 mg/kg) of succinylcholine is 35 to 55 seconds in children and adolescents; the onset time after 3 mg/kg in neonates is faster (30–40 seconds).[1036] Onset time is dependent on both age and dose; the younger the child and the greater the dose, the shorter the onset time.

As in adults, administration of a continuous infusion of succinylcholine in infants and children can result in tachyphylaxis (increased requirement). In addition, Phase II block may be produced, as evidenced by a train-of-four less than 50% (blockade similar to that produced by nondepolarizing muscle relaxants). In children, tachyphylaxis generally develops after administration of about 3 mg/kg of succinylcholine, and Phase II block develops during tachyphylaxis after 4 mg/kg.[190,1037]

Succinylcholine is effective when administered by the IM route; in this instance, complete paralysis is achieved in 3 to 4 minutes. Evidence of relaxation of the respiratory muscles, as manifest by decreased positive pressure required to ventilate by face mask, can be detected before the abolishment of the twitch response. A dose of 2 mg/kg IM does not achieve satisfactory relaxation in all children, whereas the larger dose of 3 mg/kg IM produces a mean twitch depression of 85%; 4 mg/kg produces profound relaxation in all children, but its effects may last up to 20 minutes.[1038] In infants younger than 6 months of age, a dose of 5 mg/kg IM is required to achieve profound relaxation; maximal twitch depression occurred a mean of 3.3 ± 0.4 minutes.[1039] Recovery

TABLE 7.10	Suggested Standard Intubating IV Doses of Commonly Used Relaxants in Infants and Children	
	Infants (mg/kg)	Children (mg/kg)
Succinylcholine	3	1.5–2
Cisatracurium	0.1	0.1–0.2
Atracurium	0.5	0.5
Rocuronium[a]	0.25–0.5	0.6–1.2
Pancuronium	0.1	0.1
Vecuronium	0.07–0.1	0.1

See text for source data.

[a]Low-dose rocuronium (0.3 mg/kg) allows tracheal intubation after 3 minutes during inhalational anesthesia in children, but then is easily antagonized in about 20 minutes. Large-dose rocuronium (1.2 mg/kg) may be used as a substitute for succinylcholine for rapid intubation in children in less than one minute.

from the neuromuscular effect of IM succinylcholine is faster in infants than in children. Changes in the heart rate after IM succinylcholine are not pronounced. Consequently, routine IM administration of atropine with IM succinylcholine is not generally indicated.[1040] Succinylcholine has also been administered intralingually.[1041,1042] One study examined the time to clinical apnea in 60 children younger than 10 years of age. Succinylcholine (1.1 mg/kg) resulted in apnea in 75 ± 4 seconds when administered intralingually, in 35 ± 1 seconds when administered intravenously, and in 210 ± 17 seconds when administered intramuscularly.[1042] In that study, 8 of 10 children given intralingual succinylcholine who did not receive concomitant atropine developed an arrhythmia (primarily bradycardia).

In an emergency, an alternate route for administration of succinylcholine (3 mg/kg) when an IV line is not in place should offer a fairly rapid onset of relaxation. Intralingual administration with an onset of 133 seconds, is significantly more rapid than after IM injection, 295 seconds.[1041] Caution should be exercised, however, when administering sublingual or intralingual medications. To preclude an intralingual hematoma, it is advised that a 25-gauge needle be used and the blood vessels on the undersurface of the tongue identified to minimize the risk of puncture. Sublingual succinylcholine is an alternative to the IV route, but it should be preceded by a vagolytic agent to avoid arrhythmias. The submental approach would seem to avoid the potential for causing bleeding from the tongue.

Cholinesterase Deficiency

Plasma cholinesterase (pseudocholinesterase) is a circulating glycoprotein that metabolizes succinylcholine into succinylmonocholine. The activity of plasma cholinesterase may be increased or decreased as a result of genetic inheritance (see Chapter 6).

Activity of plasma cholinesterase may decrease as a result of a congenital enzyme variant or an acquired cause. This enzyme codes at the E1 locus of the long arm of chromosome 3. Ninety-six percent of the population is homozygous for the "usual" cholinesterase enzyme and 4% are homozygous or heterozygous for the variant alleles.[1043] Five alleles code for the majority of cholinesterase enzyme: (1) normal cholinesterase enzyme, which is designated by "usual" (E^u); (2) decreased cholinesterase activity or quantity, which is designated as atypical (E^a) (homozygote in $1:3000–1:10,000$); (3) fluoride-resistant allele (E^f) (homozygote in $1:150,000$); (4) silent allele (E^s) (homozygote $1:10,000$); and (5) the Cynthiana (C_5) or Neitlich variant, which is associated with an increase in (or rapid) cholinesterase activity.[1044] Variations on the silent gene have been detected in Eskimo populations with three variants labeled: S for silent, T for trace, and R for residual. The duration of succinylcholine in children who are homozygous for the silent gene may be up to 6 to 8 hours. Additional genetic variants of pseudocholinesterase have been identified, including types H, J, and K, which represent a 60%, 66%, and 30% reduction in enzyme activity, respectively.[1043] Evidence suggests that the K variant occurs in 13% of the population and that the K/K homozygous variant may be present in $1:63$, one of the most common variants with a duration of prolonged blockade of less than 1 hour. Moreover, the K variants have occurred in the presence of other mutations suggesting that multiple mutations may be present in the same patient.

Heterozygote atypical (E^uE^a), which occurs in $1:30$ of the population, may prolong neuromuscular blockade by only a few minutes and may go undetected. In contrast, homozygote atypical (E^aE^a), which occurs in approximately $1:3000$ population, may cause paralysis for up to 1 hour after a single dose of succinylcholine. Of the genetic variants of cholinesterase, the silent gene (E^s) confers the least plasma cholinesterase activity and therefore the most prolonged duration of paralysis. Homozygote (E^sE^s) occurs in 1:10,000 population and may result in 8 hours of paralysis.

Plasma cholinesterase activity is more often diminished when a genetic variant is present, but a number of clinical conditions may also reduce its activity. These include severe liver disease, malnutrition, organophosphate poisoning, severe burns, renal failure, plasmapheresis, and medications (cyclophosphamide, echothiophate iodide, oral contraceptives).[1043,1045,1046] Several conditions are associated with increases in plasma cholinesterase activity, including thyroid disease, obesity, nephrotic syndrome, and cognitively challenged children.[1043,1047-1049]

Plasma cholinesterase activity is determined by the percent inhibition of benzyl choline degradation by the amide local anesthetic dibucaine when it is incubated with a sample of plasma. With the homozygous normal allele (E^uE^u), dibucaine profoundly inhibits plasma cholinesterase activity (approximately 80%), whereas with the homozygous atypical allele (E^aE^a), it inhibits the activity by only 20%. When fluoride is added to the plasma, fluoride inhibits E^uE^u by 60% but inhibits E^fE^f by only 36%. Thus a low dibucaine number indicates a deficiency of plasma cholinesterase.

Adverse Effects of Succinylcholine
Temporomandibular Joint Stiffness
IV succinylcholine is infrequently associated with an increase in masseter muscle tone that limits mouth opening (trismus), particularly when given during halothane anesthesia. The incidence of isolated trismus when IV succinylcholine is administered during halothane anesthesia is 0.3% to 1%; it is severalfold greater than that after IV thiopental and succinylcholine, 0/4457 (upper 95% confidence interval of 7/10,000).[1050,1051] The increase in masseter muscle tone after succinylcholine is transient, lasting for only a few minutes and occurring despite abolition of the evoked twitch response in the masseter and peripheral muscles. The increase in masseter muscle tone is usually mild and can be overcome by manually distracting the mandible.[1052] However, on rare occasions, the increase in muscle tone may be so severe that mouth opening is impossible, thus interfering or preventing tracheal intubation. Whether this marked increased tone is related to the so-called "jaws of steel" (see Fig. 41.2) encountered in children with MH remains a matter of debate.[1053] Prospective studies designed to evaluate masseter muscle tone have failed to demonstrate a child with a marked increase in masseter tone who later developed evidence of MH.[1054,1055] In several retrospective reports, however, a number of children experienced severe trismus and did develop or have a positive test response for MH.[1056-1058] These studies failed to clarify how best to proceed when severe trismus occurs. Some advocate canceling the surgical procedure, treating the child as susceptible to MH, and recommending a muscle biopsy.[1058,1059] This recommendation is based on a 50% incidence of positive muscle biopsies for MH in children who developed severe trismus after succinylcholine. Others advocate continuing the procedure, avoiding further exposure to triggering agents by changing the anesthetic technique to one that is free of triggers, observing for signs of MH (e.g., increased CO_2 production or tachycardia), and, if indicated, initiating arterial and central venous blood gas sampling, as well as early treatment.[1060,1061] Finally, others have advocated continuing with the original triggering anesthetic while monitoring for signs of MH.[1050] For the

most part, this entire issue has become moot because sevoflurane has supplanted halothane as the primary inhaled anesthetic in children, and the FDA issued a black box warning regarding the routine use of succinylcholine for tracheal intubation in children. Curiously, the now widespread use of nondepolarizing relaxants has generated several purported reports of masseter muscle rigidity after use of these agents. Whether these cases actually represent nondepolarizing relaxant–induced masseter spasm or a combination of light anesthesia and incomplete muscle relaxation is unclear.[1062-1064]

Arrhythmias
The molecular structure of succinylcholine resembles that of two acetylcholine molecules joined by an ester linkage. The consequent stimulation of cholinergic autonomic receptors can be associated with cardiac arrhythmias, increased salivation, and bronchial secretions. Changes in heart rate are frequently observed after treatment with succinylcholine. Heart rate usually increases transiently, and this response appears to be more pronounced in the presence of sevoflurane than halothane.[1065] Succinylcholine-associated arrhythmias are rarely a result of ventricular irritability. Prior IV administration of a vagolytic agent (e.g., atropine) markedly decreases, but does not completely abolish, the incidence of these arrhythmias.[1066] As in adults, the incidence and severity of these irregularities in heart rate increase after a second dose.[1042,1067] Of greater concern is the occasional bradycardia and asystole after a single dose in children.[1066] Accordingly, it is recommended that a vagolytic agent precede the IV administration of succinylcholine unless there is a contraindication to such medications.

Hyperkalemia
Succinylcholine-induced muscle fasciculation is also associated with mild hyperkalemia, increased intragastric and intraocular pressures, and skeletal muscle pains; rhabdomyolysis and myoglobinemia may occur in patients with neuromuscular disorders. These disorders are not always diagnosable in neonates. Congenital myotonic dystrophy, for example, may present with mild respiratory dysfunction or feeding difficulty in the neonate. The response to succinylcholine in these neonates, however, remains dramatic, with sustained muscle contraction.[1068]

The serum potassium concentration increases 1 mEq/L or less after IV succinylcholine in normal children; this increase does not cause arrhythmias.[1069] However, life-threatening hyperkalemia can occur after a single IV dose of succinylcholine in children with burns (>8% body surface area), those who are immobile, or who have chronic infections (including intraabdominal sepsis and *Clostridium*), upper motor neuron lesions (e.g., paraplegia, encephalitis), lower motor neuron lesions (e.g., tetanus, neuropathy complicating nephropathy), crush injuries, and neuromuscular diseases (including Werdnig-Hoffmann disease).[1070-1077] In these situations, direct denervation injury or a pseudo-denervation state (immobilization) leads to a proliferation of extrajunctional normal acetylcholine receptors, as well as proliferation of immature (containing γ subunits) and nicotinic (neuronal) acetylcholine receptors, along the muscle membrane such that the entire muscle becomes capable of releasing potassium during depolarization.[1077] These immature and nicotinic acetylcholine receptors release more intracellular potassium, and for a longer period after the channels open, than do the usual acetylcholine receptors. The presence of extrajunctional receptors has been documented within several hours of injury, although clinically significant hyperkalemia does not seem to occur until 1 to 3 days after injury. Thus administration of succinylcholine to children with these injuries may result in a massive efflux of intracellular potassium, leading to a cardiac arrest.[1078] In contrast to these acquired conditions, children who are born spastic quadriparetic from cerebral palsy or those with a myelomeningocele respond with a normal increase in serum potassium concentration (<1 mEq/L) after IV administration of succinylcholine.[1078-1080] Another recent concern is the possible fatal interaction of β-blockade–induced hyperkalemia and succinylcholine.[1081,1082]

The definitive treatment of succinylcholine-induced hyperkalemia is IV calcium (10 mg/kg calcium chloride or 30 mg/kg calcium gluconate or more). This restores the gap between the resting membrane potential of the cardiac cells and the threshold potential for depolarization. Repeated doses of calcium may be required, together with cardiopulmonary resuscitation, epinephrine, sodium bicarbonate, hyperventilation, inhaled albuterol (salbutamol) (or the IV formulation), or glucose and insulin, until the arrhythmias abate. Defibrillation of the heart has no role in this circumstance. Successful treatment of hyperkalemia might require a very prolonged resuscitation. Sodium polystyrene sulfonate by nasogastric or rectal administration may be required for leaching potassium after acute redistribution between extracellular and intracellular spaces by the above measures (see Chapters 9, 12, 28, and 40).

Biochemical Changes
Serum creatine kinase concentrations were reported to increase after administration of succinylcholine in the presence of inhalational agents, especially halothane,[1083] an effect that was more pronounced in children with neuromuscular diseases.[1084] After an MH reaction, creatine kinase reaches its peak 12 to 18 hours after the onset of the reaction. It may also be found in association with a jaws of steel response to succinylcholine.

Rhabdomyolysis
Rhabdomyolysis can occur after halothane or sevoflurane,[1085] even in the absence of succinylcholine as in the case of Duchenne and Becker muscular dystrophy.[1086,1087] Isolated rhabdomyolysis or rhabdomyolysis in combination with hyperkalemia, as in the case of Duchenne muscular dystrophy, requires hyperhydration and osmotic diuresis with alkalinization of the urine to prevent acute tubular necrosis from deposition of myoglobin.

Myoglobinemia
Myoglobinemia, another sensitive indicator of muscle injury, may occur after succinylcholine treatment but rarely leads to myoglobinurea (i.e., "cola"-colored urine).[1088] If it occurs, it should be aggressively treated as described previously for rhabdomyolysis.

Fasciculations
Fasciculations are usually observed in adolescents and children but rarely in infants; in children 1 to 3 years old they are described as gross muscle movements.[1083,1089] Pretreatment with small doses of succinylcholine (100 μg/kg), pancuronium (20 μg/kg), fentanyl (1–2 μg/kg), or alfentanil (50 μg/kg) may decrease the frequency and intensity of the fasciculations and the resulting increase in intragastric pressure.[1083,1089-1092] This increase in intragastric pressure, however, is more than offset by the increase in skeletal muscle tone of the crura of the diaphragm, with a net effect of increasing the barrier to regurgitation.

Intraocular Pressure
Intraocular pressure increases transiently in children after IV succinylcholine independent of the presence of fasciculations.[1093] The exact mechanism of this increase in IOP is not clear. Initially, the increase in IOP was attributed to tonic contractions of extraocular muscles, but it is probably because of the cycloplegic action of succinylcholine, with deepening of the anterior chamber and increased outflow resistance. The IOP usually increases by about 10 mm Hg, peaks in 2 to 3 minutes, and then returns to baseline in 5 to 7 minutes.[1093] It is advisable to perform applanation tonometry before succinylcholine or to wait at least 7 minutes after succinylcholine before performing tonometry in children. Although the use of succinylcholine in children with open-eye injuries has not resulted in further damage to the eye,[1094] it is nonetheless prudent to refrain from its use in situations of penetrating ocular wounds unless the eye is not salvageable. High-dose rocuronium (1.2 mg/kg) is a reasonable substitute for succinylcholine rapid-sequence intubation in these circumstances.[1095]

Clinical Uses of Succinylcholine
The use of succinylcholine for routine surgical procedures in children has been abandoned, primarily because of the rare but life-threatening possibility of cardiac arrest in male children with undiagnosed muscular dystrophy.[1096,1097] On the other hand, succinylcholine does have the most rapid onset and the briefest duration of action of all currently available muscle relaxants. Consequently, succinylcholine is desirable for rapid-sequence tracheal intubation for brief procedures and for the treatment of laryngospasm.[1036,1098,1099] Because the rapidity of onset is dose related, 1.5 to 2.0 mg/kg IV succinylcholine should be administered to children to depress the neuromuscular twitch 95% within 40 seconds; the smaller dose of 1.0 mg/kg would achieve the same degree of depression in about 50 seconds.[1036,1098] In infants younger than 1 year of age, 3 mg/kg IV would be an appropriate dose because of the larger Vd. These doses provide excellent intubating conditions in all children.[1036] To decrease the incidence of arrhythmias after succinylcholine (particularly after a second dose), atropine 0.01 to 0.02 mg/kg IV should precede the succinylcholine.

In 1993 the FDA issued a black box warning against the routine use of succinylcholine in children and adolescents except for emergency airway management. This was based on several case reports of hyperkalemic cardiac arrests, primarily in children with undiagnosed Duchenne muscular dystrophy.[1100] The disturbing observation about this complication was the staggering mortality rate of 55%. Almost all of these cases, however, occurred in male children 8 years old and younger. In many instances the arrhythmias were misdiagnosed as MH and not treated with IV calcium in a timely manner. Subsequently, the FDA and the manufacturer revised the product label (package insert) to read as follows:

> "Since there may be no signs or symptoms to alert the practitioner to which patients are at risk, it is recommended that the use of succinylcholine should be reserved for emergency intubation or in instances where immediate securing of the airway is necessary, e.g., laryngospasm, difficult airway, full stomach, or for intramuscular use when a suitable vein in inaccessible."

In cases in which the child has a full stomach and is at risk for a hyperkalemic response to succinylcholine, a standard rapid-sequence intubation with equivalent intubation conditions may be performed using high-dose rocuronium (1.2 mg/kg)[1095] or a large dose of propofol with an opioid (e.g., propofol/remifentanil).[1101] The main disadvantage of using a large dose of nondepolarizing relaxant is that the duration of blockade may exceed the duration of the planned procedure. Less likely is the disadvantage of an ensuing "cannot intubate, cannot ventilate" situation in which the dose of the relaxant cannot be antagonized. The availability of sugammadex allows rapid intubation with rocuronium, even for brief emergency procedures, while avoiding the need to use succinylcholine (see later discussion).[1102–1105] In an emergency, the cost of sugammadex may be tolerated, but it is currently too expensive to use routinely for antagonizing nondepolarizing relaxants.

Intermediate-Acting Nondepolarizing Neuromuscular Blocking Drugs

ATRACURIUM

Chemically, atracurium (Tracrium) is an imidazoline bisquaternary compound that undergoes spontaneous decomposition into inactive metabolites. At physiologic (alkaline) pH, it undergoes enzymatic hydrolysis independent of plasma cholinesterase (Hofmann elimination), ester hydrolysis, and other unspecified pathways.[1030] In blood and other tissue fluids, the quaternary ammonium compound breaks down primarily into laudanosine and a related quaternary acid (methylacrylate). The elimination half-life of atracurium is similar in infants and children (14–20 minutes). The steady-state plasma concentration resulting in 50% neuromuscular block (EC_{50}) does not differ between infants, children, or adults (363, 444, or 436 ng/mL, respectively).[1022]

For intubating purposes, two to three times the ED_{95} (300–600 µg/kg) is given to produce effective blockade in most children.[1106,1107] Such doses provide satisfactory conditions for intubation within 2 minutes. The period of absence of twitch response after an intubating dose of atracurium usually lasts 15 to 30 minutes. Hence, in clinical situations an intubating dose should provide complete neuromuscular blockade for such an interval, followed by another 20 minutes of intermediate blockade (twitch height 5%–25%); complete recovery usually occurs within 40 to 60 minutes. Comparison of data from children and adults demonstrates that children require more atracurium per kilogram and generally recover faster. This difference, however, is relatively small and is masked in most cases by the wide range of individual patient responses.

Because atracurium is degraded spontaneously and its metabolites do not have neuromuscular blocking properties, it can be easily administered by continuous infusion. The infusion requirement to maintain 90% to 99% twitch depression in children is 6 µg/kg per minute during isoflurane anesthesia, 7 to 8 µg/kg per minute with halothane, and 9 µg/kg per minute with an $N_2O:O_2$ opioid technique.[552,553] No significant differences in the Vd, clearance, or half-lives have been detected for atracurium between normal infants and children with impaired hepatic function.[1031] Plasma laudanosine concentrations tend to be greater in children with hepatic impairment than in children with normal hepatic function.[1031]

The side effects of atracurium are minimal; at doses of up to 600 µg/kg, there are no significantly changes in the heart rate or BP in children. Mild cutaneous flushing reactions are sometimes observed.[1106] Extremely rare instances of anaphylactoid reactions or bronchospasm have been reported.

CISATRACURIUM

Cisatracurium (Nimbex) is one of the 10 stereoisomers of atracurium (1R-cis, 1′R-cis). Cisatracurium is three times more potent than atracurium, with the same duration of action.[1108] Similar to other nondepolarizing relaxants, its onset can be accelerated by increasing the dose (see E-Table 7.7 and Table 7.10); as with the other relaxants, this will increase the duration of the action. Cisatracurium, like atracurium, is a noncumulative agent with recovery occurring during the elimination phase rather than during the distribution phase.

Cisatracurium has a slightly slower onset of action than atracurium, consistent with its relative potency. Twice the ED_{95} dose (80 µg/kg) of cisatracurium leads to complete suppression of the twitch response in 2.5 minutes. The recovery to 25% and 95% of control response occurs in 31 and 53 minutes, respectively.[1108–1111] Its histamine-releasing effects are minimal; its duration and recovery profile are similar to atracurium.

The distribution and elimination half-lives of cisatracurium in children are 3.5 and 23 minutes, respectively. The Vdss and the total body clearance of most drugs in children are greater (expressed as milligrams per kilogram; see the example of dexmedetomidine Fig. 7.5) than in adults, thus explaining the faster recovery in children.[1032] In adults with renal failure, the clearance of cisatracurium is reduced by 13%; plasma laudanosine levels were greater but were only about 10% of those reported with atracurium.[1112] The duration of action of cisatracurium in patients with renal failure is not significantly prolonged.[1113] It should be noted that patients receiving chronic anticonvulsant therapy (carbamazepine or phenytoin) can develop a moderate resistance to the action of cisatracurium.[1114]

VECURONIUM

Vecuronium is the monoquaternary homologue of pancuronium in which the methyl group of the 2β-nitrogen atom is absent. The Vd is greater in infants than in children (357 ± 70 vs. 204 ± 116 mL/kg), whereas plasma clearances are similar (5.6 ± 1.0 vs. 5.9 ± 2.4 mL/kg per minute).[1021]

Its primary advantage is the absence of any adverse cardiovascular effects even in doses several times greater than the usually recommended clinical doses (see E-Table 7.7 and Table 7.10).[1115] Vecuronium is primarily metabolized by the liver and excreted in bile.[1116] Dose requirements according to age groups are much more pronounced (>50%), with a biphasic distribution of the dose requirement and duration of action; infants younger than 1 year of age are significantly more sensitive to the action of vecuronium than older children. As adolescence is reached, the requirement diminishes to that of adults.[1016,1020,1117,1118] However, on rare occasions there may be resistance to vecuronium in neonates.[1119]

Neuromuscular blockers are often administered to critically ill children. Vecuronium has been popular because of the absence of cardiovascular side effects and because its metabolites do not seem to have CNS effects. However, adult and pediatric patients in ICUs have had residual weakness after the discontinuation of vecuronium, possibly contributed by active 3-OH metabolite or its steroid-like structure.[1120–1122] In one study in which the rate of infusion was adjusted by accelerometry, all children recovered within 1 hour. Of note in these children, the requirements of neonates and small infants were 45% less than those of older children.[1123] In this respect, cisatracurium may offer advantage because its recovery from prolonged infusion is faster than vecuronium.[1124]

ROCURONIUM

Rocuronium (Zemuron) is a monoquaternary steroidal muscle relaxant similar to vecuronium. It has the fastest onset of action of the intermediate-acting nondepolarizing relaxants because of its low potency and greater dose requirements.[1125] The onset time of rocuronium is 1 to 1.5 minutes after a dose of $2 \times ED_{95}$; this is 20 to 70 seconds faster than vecuronium, although its duration of action is similar.[1126] Rocuronium is eliminated primarily by the liver; the kidney excretes about 10%.[1127-1132] Renal failure does not affect the onset of rocuronium-induced neuromuscular blockade in adults or children. However, it may prolong the duration of action of rocuronium in adults, a finding not shared for children older than 1 year of age.[1127,1129,1132]

Rocuronium has an ED_{95} of 303 μg/kg in children during halothane anesthesia,[1133] with slightly greater doses required during $N_2O:O_2$ opioid anesthesia.[1134-1136] After the administration of 600 μg/kg rocuronium ($2 \times ED_{95}$), 90% and 100% neuromuscular block occurred in 0.8 and 1.3 minutes, respectively (see E-Table 7.7 and Table 7.10). At this dose, heart rate increased by approximately 15 beats/minute in children. The mean time to recover to 25% of control was approximately 28 minutes, and recovery to 90% of control was 46 minutes.[1136]

For brief cases in which children are anesthetized with 8% inspired sevoflurane, 0.3 mg/kg rocuronium yields satisfactory intubating conditions within 2 to 3 minutes.[1137] This dose of rocuronium can be antagonized within approximately 20 minutes of administration.[1132] The intubating conditions after rocuronium (600 μg/kg) have been compared with those after vecuronium (100 μg/kg), atracurium (500 μg/kg), and succinylcholine (1 mg/kg). It was found that tracheal intubation could be performed within 60 seconds in all the children who had received rocuronium or succinylcholine, but not until 120 seconds after vecuronium and 180 seconds after atracurium.[1138,1139] The time for intubating conditions is shortened by increasing the dose[1140]; at a dose of 1.2 mg/kg (3 to $4 \times ED_{95}$), the intubating conditions are similar to those after treatment with succinylcholine.[1095,1136] At the larger doses, heart rate increases transiently, while systolic and diastolic pressures are unchanged.[1133,1141] It is unclear whether this increase in heart rate after rocuronium is the result of pain on injection or an inherent chronotropic effect.[1104] Dosing studies in infants 2 to 11 months of age demonstrated a slightly faster onset of neuromuscular blockade than in older children with the same dose (600 μg/kg). The times to 90% and 100% twitch depression were 37 and 64 seconds, respectively. In infants, the rate of onset of neuromuscular blockade 60 seconds after rocuronium is comparable to that after succinylcholine.[1133,1142] Neonates appear to be more sensitive to rocuronium than older infants.[1143] In neonates, the duration of action of 600 μg/kg is approximately 90 minutes, and there is marked patient-to-patient variability. Consequently, 450 μg/kg rocuronium provides adequate intubating conditions, with a duration of action of approximately 1 hour.[1143]

In a PK study, the clearance of rocuronium in infants was less than in children (4 vs. 7 mL/kg per minute), whereas the Vd was greater in infants. The mean residence time was 56 minutes in infants versus 26 minutes in children, thus explaining the prolonged duration of action of rocuronium in infants compared with children. In a steady-state target-controlled infusion study, the potency of rocuronium was greatest in infants, least in children, and intermediate in adults.[1144] The greater plasma clearance and smaller Vd of rocuronium in children compared with infants and adults result in a markedly smaller mean residence time and a

decreased duration of neuromuscular blockade.[1023] Consistent with the dose-response effects of curare and vecuronium in infants, smaller plasma concentrations of rocuronium are required in the effect compartment in infants than in children to produce the same degree of neuromuscular blockade.[86] Sevoflurane markedly potentiates the effects of rocuronium.[1145]

If an IV route is unavailable, the IM route for rocuronium is a reasonable alternative; IM rocuronium (1.8 mg/kg, $3 \times$ the IV intubating dose) provided poor intubating conditions 4 minutes after administration in most children. Neuromuscular blockade (>98%) was achieved in 6 to 8 minutes.[1146] The bioavailability of IM rocuronium at these doses is approximately 80%.[1147] IM rocuronium appears to be a viable alternative to IM succinylcholine, although the time of onset of neuromuscular blockade is very slow and would not be appropriate for emergent situations. The duration of IM rocuronium effect (approximately 80 ± 22 minutes) is much greater than that after IM succinylcholine.[1146]

CLINICAL IMPLICATIONS WHEN USING SHORT- AND INTERMEDIATE-ACTING NEUROMUSCULAR BLOCKING DRUGS

Short- and intermediate-acting NMBDs have great utility in infants and children because of the large number of brief surgical procedures performed. Because of their short duration of action, these drugs can be given in one intubating dose (atracurium [500 μg/kg]; cisatracurium [200 μg/kg]; vecuronium [100 μg/kg]; rocuronium [600 μg/kg]), and a light anesthetic level is maintained throughout the procedure. If more than 45 minutes elapse after the last dose of these neuromuscular blockers, one may reasonably assume that neuromuscular function has nearly recovered, but safe practice would recommend confirming *recovery of neuromuscular integrity by clinical signs or by assessment with a neuromuscular blockade monitor. We recommend antagonism in all neonates and infants despite clinical signs of recovery.*

The benzylisoquinoliniums and organosteroidal NMBDs are acidic compounds (pH 3–4) that can precipitate thiopental (pH 10–11) if admixed.[1148] Consequently, when these drugs are administered in tandem, the IV tubing should be thoroughly flushed between the thiopental and these relaxants. Vecuronium and rocuronium are painful when administered intravenously in a small vein during the light stages of anesthetic. This pain is usually demonstrated by withdrawal of the hand. Pain can be attenuated by deepening the level of anesthesia or pretreating with fentanyl, lidocaine, or ketamine.[1149,1150]

Long-Acting Nondepolarizing Neuromuscular Blocking Drugs

For almost half a century the mainstay of NMBDs was curare (*d*-tubocurarine). After the development of intermediate-acting NMBDs, its use diminished because its duration of action was too great for most surgeries, and large doses released histamine. Curare is no longer available.

After the introduction of curare, several long-acting NMBDs with minimal adverse effects were developed. These included metocurine, pipecuronium, and doxacurium, which are 2, 4, and 10 times as potent as curare, respectively. The only long-acting relaxant that is still used in some institutions is pancuronium.

PANCURONIUM

Pancuronium bromide (Pavulon) is a bisquaternary ammonium steroidal compound with nondepolarizing neuromuscular blocking properties. Pancuronium undergoes partial (15%–20%) hepatic deacetylation to produce 3-OH, 17-OH, and 3,17-di-OH metabolites. A prolongation of effect can be expected in patients with renal or hepatic failure because a major proportion of pancuronium is excreted in the urine (40%–60%) and in the bile (11%). Vd (203 ± 36 mL/kg) and plasma clearance (1.7 ± 0.2 mL/kg per minute) of pancuronium are associated with a prolonged elimination half-life (103 ± 23 minutes) in children (3–6 years) under halothane anesthesia.[1151] It induces mild tachycardia by blocking presynaptic noradrenaline uptake (increased cardiac output in infants) but has no histamine-releasing properties, so systolic BP tends to increase.[1152] Pancuronium (100 μg/kg) provides satisfactory conditions for tracheal intubation in 70% to 90% of infants and children within 150 seconds of administration. Increasing the initial dose to 150 μg/kg provides satisfactory intubating conditions in all children within 80 seconds (see E-Table 7.7 and Table 7.10).[1098,1153]

Pancuronium is frequently advocated for cardiac surgery and other high-risk procedures in infants and children. The anesthetic technique of combining a high-dose opioid with air–oxygen–pancuronium is well tolerated by infants, from a cardiovascular perspective. The vagolytic effect (tachycardia) of pancuronium counteracts the vagotonic effect (bradycardia) of potent opioids, and its relaxant properties counteract opioid-induced chest wall and glottic rigidity.[1154] Pancuronium has been used to facilitate ventilation in preterm infants in neonatal ICUs.[1155] Because pancuronium increases the heart rate, BP, and plasma epinephrine and norepinephrine levels in neonates, there is some concern that it may contribute to the risk of an intracerebral hemorrhage.[1156] Accordingly, it would seem prudent to administer pancuronium with either general anesthesia or with adequate sedation to blunt adverse cardiovascular responses. Vecuronium may offer an advantage over pancuronium because it does not significantly increase the BP.[1157–1161] Nasotracheal intubation or intratracheal suctioning in neonates who are paralyzed with pancuronium results in smaller increases in intracranial pressure than in neonates who are not paralyzed.[1161,1162] By abolishing fluctuations in CBF through the use of muscle relaxants, the incidence and severity of intraventricular hemorrhages should theoretically be reduced.

Antagonism of Neuromuscular Blocking Drugs

GENERAL PRINCIPLES

In children and especially infants, oxygen consumption is greater than in adults. Therefore a slight diminution in respiratory muscle power may lead to hypoxemia and CO_2 retention. Consequently, it is very important that neuromuscular function is returned to normal at the end of the surgical procedure. Neonates are at greater risk for residual neuromuscular blockade than adults for several reasons, including (1) immaturity of the neuromuscular system, (2) greater elimination half-life of relaxants, (3) the reduced number of type I muscle fibers in the ventilatory musculature (thus being more susceptible to fatigue [see Chapter 14, Fig. 14.11]),[225] and (4) the closing lung volume of a neonate overlaps with the tidal volume (i.e., airway closure occurs at the end of expiration) (Fig. 2.5).[1163] If respiration is mildly impaired as a result of residual muscle paralysis, even more alveoli will collapse. The result may be hypoxemia as well as hypercarbia and acidosis, which may potentiate and prolong the duration of action of the muscle relaxant, thus creating a vicious cycle.

When monitoring neuromuscular blockade in infants and children, train-of-four monitoring of the adductor pollicis overestimates the degree of neuromuscular blockade in the diaphragm.[999] Larger doses of muscle relaxants are required to block the diaphragm than the adductor pollicis train-of-four would suggest. Therefore if the train-of-four of the adductor has fully recovered, one can assume that the diaphragm has fully recovered.

Clinical evaluation of the adequacy of antagonism in infants is more difficult than in children or adults. Neither grip strength nor voluntary head lifting can be elicited; rather, it is important when working with infants to observe the clinical conditions preoperatively (muscle tone, depth of respiration, vigor of crying) and to aim for a comparable level of activity in the postantagonism period. Useful clinical signs that the neuromuscular blockade has been antagonized include the ability to flex the hips, flex the arm, lift the legs, and the return of abdominal muscle tone.[1164] Inspiratory force may be measured; a negative force of −25 cm H_2O or greater indicates adequate antagonism.[1165] A crying vital capacity greater than 15 mL/kg indicates an adequate respiratory reserve. The train-of-four is a valuable aid because it can be used in the smallest of infants in whom the force of contraction can easily be palpated (four equal contractions indicating adequate antagonism).

Although edrophonium may establish a faster onset of effect, final recovery is invariably greater with neostigmine, which is why the latter is recommended for routine pediatric practice.[1166,1167] The distribution volumes of neostigmine are similar in infants (2–10 months), children (1–6 years), and adults (Vdss 0.5 L/kg), whereas the elimination half-life is less in children.[1168] Clearance decreases as age increases (13.6, 11.1, 9.6 mL/minute per kilogram in infants, children, and adults 29–48 years, respectively).[1168] The dose requirement of anticholinesterase agents to antagonize neuromuscular blockade in children is less than in adults.[1168] However, the speed of antagonism depends on the extent of neuromuscular blockade at the time of the antagonism, as well as the type and dose of antagonizing agent. In the presence of train-of-four responses with fade, 20 to 25 μg/kg of neostigmine, preceded by 10 to 20 μg/kg of atropine or 5 to 10 μg/kg of glycopyrrolate, is sufficient to achieve full recovery of muscle strength. This dose of neostigmine can be repeated if required (up to 70 μg/kg). Doses of neostigmine in excess of 100 μg/kg may induce a paradoxical weakness from excessive acetylcholine at the neuromuscular junction. The dose of edrophonium for children is greater than it is for adults; at least 0.3 mg/kg is needed, but 0.5 to 1.0 mg/kg is most common.[1167,1169–1172]

Some have suggested that it is not necessary to antagonize intermediate-acting NMBDs, particularly if a lengthy time interval has elapsed since the last dose. With the advent of reliable neuromuscular monitors and their use in conjunction with clinical observations and measurements of respiratory adequacy, clinicians are more confident that antagonism is not always required. This may be appropriate for the short- and intermediate-acting NMBDs, particularly atracurium or cisatracurium, which are hydrolyzed in plasma. Children have the additional advantage of recovering from neuromuscular blockade more rapidly than adults.[1171,1172] In infants, the elimination of all muscle relaxants might be delayed, necessitating antagonism of any NMBD; if there is any concern that some degree of neuromuscular blockade persists, then the blockade must be antagonized.

Hypothermia potentiates the action of most nondepolarizing muscle relaxants and delays their elimination.[1173] This effect can create a special problem at the end of a surgical procedure when the children attempt to resume spontaneous respirations. Shivering increases oxygen consumption and augments the load on the respiratory system. If the respiratory muscles are unable to match this increased load, hypoxemia and CO_2 retention may occur, which in turn may lead to acidosis, which, again, may potentiate the relaxant. To avoid the extra cardiorespiratory load in a postsurgical infant, it is reasonable to warm the infant if the temperature is less than 35°C (95°F). Once the core temperature is above this level, antagonism of neuromuscular blockade may be attempted.

Theoretically, all antibiotics have neuromuscular depressing properties when administered in association with relaxants.[1174] Among the antibiotics, aminoglycoside derivatives, such as gentamicin, tobramycin, and neomycin, have the greatest effect. A single clinical dose of antibiotic will likely have minimal effect on the neuromuscular blockade.[1175] This factor alone does not rule out the possibility that large concentrations of antibiotics, especially in the presence of other potentiating factors, may augment the neuromuscular blockade. The clinical importance of the interaction of antibiotics with NMBDs to prolong neuromuscular blockade has diminished with the introduction of intermediate-acting NMBDs.

Magnesium also relaxes muscles and may also potentiate neuromuscular blockade. When magnesium was administered after paralysis from rocuronium was antagonized by sugammadex in an adult, plasma magnesium concentrations of 2.67 mM caused recurarization that resolved after 45 minutes.[1176]

SUGAMMADEX

Sugammadex (Org 25969), a member of the cyclodextrin family, is a cyclic oligosaccharide[1177] with hydrophobic molecules within the center (Fig. 7.22).[1178,1179] This compound encapsulates rocuronium, and vecuronium to a lesser degree, and forms a stable complex that prevents further action of the relaxants; the complex is then excreted unchanged by the kidneys. The chemical encapsulation decreases the plasma concentration of rocuronium, thus promoting the dissociation of rocuronium from the acetylcholine receptor, speeding recovery of muscle strength. Three minutes after 0.6 mg/kg rocuronium produced profound neuromuscular block in adult volunteers, a single dose of sugammadex, 2 mg/kg or greater, reversed the neuromuscular block within 2 minutes.[1180] An early sugammadex study in children suggested that sugammadex, at 2 mg/kg, reverses a rocuronium-induced moderate neuromuscular blockade in infants, children, and adolescents.[1103] The average time to recover a train-of-four ratio of 0.9 at the time of appearance of the second twitch response was ~1.2 minutes in children, adolescents, and adults. Recent studies have demonstrated much more rapid times to extubation and recovery after sugammadex compared with

neostigmine in children with similar side effects.[1181,1182] Clinical trials confirm the safety and efficacy of this new concept, and studies in children demonstrate safety and efficacy.[1182a,1182b] Sugammadex may be effective in antagonizing large doses of rocuronium rapidly, efficiently, and soon after the onset of neuromuscular blockade in children.[1183–1187] Sugammadex rapidly antagonizes even intense neuromuscular blockade in adults, in whom no twitches were observed.[1184,1188] The rapidity of the reversal depends on both the intensity of the block and the dose of sugammadex.[1102,1104,1189] Under these circumstances, rocuronium might then supplant succinylcholine in many circumstances, including rapid-sequence intubations for brief procedures in children.[1105,1190] Sugammadex is cleared through the renal system, and the elimination kinetics of rocuronium are known to be prolonged in renal failure.[1127] Although GFR is immature in neonates, this is unlikely to be of consequence. Sugammadex has been used in patients with end-stage renal failure [1191–1193] with reversal characteristics similar to those with normal renal function.

Two impediments delayed the introduction of sugammadex in the United States. First, there was some evidence that sugammadex may trigger allergic or anaphylactic reactions.[1194] Second, sugammadex is exceedingly expensive. The expense of sugammadex has put this medication out of financial practicality for routine use in nearly every health care facility in the world (E-Table 7.8).[1195] This renders sugammadex a rescue drug only. Data suggest that this drug could be used for rescue of a cannot intubate–cannot ventilate situation after administration of a rapid intubating dose of rocuronium (1.2 mg/kg) within 2 minutes, compared with the time for the effects of succinylcholine to abate.[1105,1184] This great expense is quite unfortunate, as the incidence of hyperkalemia or MH induced by succinylcholine would likely have decreased to near zero if we could routinely substitute high-dose rocuronium for succinylcholine without fear of prolonged neuromuscular blockade.

If neuromuscular blockade must be reinstituted after administration of sugammadex, the dose of rocuronium that would be required for neuromuscular blockade is unclear[1151]; it would seem prudent to switch to a benzylisoquinolinium muscle relaxant that is unaffected by the presence of sugammadex.

Neuromuscular Blocking Drugs in Special Situations

Of the many drug combinations possible, that of succinylcholine after a halothane induction seems to be most likely to trigger MH[1196] (see Chapter 41). The use of depolarizing neuromuscular

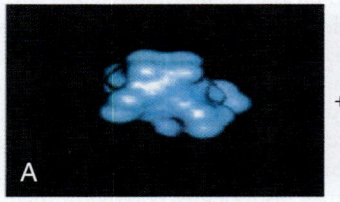 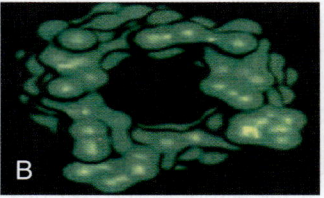 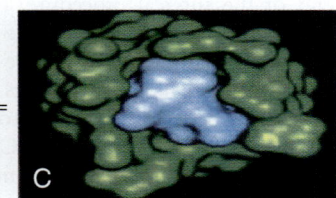

FIGURE 7.22 X-ray crystallography of **(A)** the rocuronium molecule (shown in *blue*) and **(B)** sugammadex (*green ring*). **C,** The 3-D conformation of the rocuronium molecule complements the conformation of the inner ring of sugammadex. The rocuronium–sugammadex complex is stable, without a dissociation constant, and is excreted unchanged via the kidneys. (Redrawn from Gijsenbergh F, Ramael S, Houwing N, van Iersel T. First human exposure of Org 25969, a novel agent to reverse the action of rocuronium bromide. *Anesthesiology* 2005;103(4):695–703.)

blocking agents in combination with halogenated agents should be avoided in children at risk for this syndrome.[1197] The safest general anesthetic technique for children at risk for MH is an opioid plus N_2O plus O_2 combination, together with benzodiazepines, propofol, and a nondepolarizing relaxant. Nondepolarizing agents devoid of cardiovascular side effects may offer an advantage in not causing tachycardia, an early sign of MH.[1198,1199] There has been some concern of the potential association between mitochondrial disease and MH. A major review, along with evidence from pathology specimens from patients who had a family member with MH, suggest that this is not at all clear and may be a case of "fortuitous association."[1200] Because many of these children are bedridden, it would seem prudent to avoid succinylcholine, although there are *"inadequate data to support the recommendation … that the anesthetic plan for patients with mitochondrial disease should routinely include MH precautions."*[1201]

The use of NMBDs in children with neuromuscular and mitochondrial diseases has been the subject of debate.[1199,1202,1203] Rhabdomyolysis has been reported after succinylcholine in children with Duchenne and Becker muscular dystrophy (see Chapters 24 and 41). It is prudent to avoid succinylcholine in any child with a suspicious neuromuscular or mitochondrial disease (see earlier). The response of children with neuromuscular disease to nondepolarizing relaxants is variable. Most are relatively sensitive to the NMBDs, particularly those with muscular dystrophy, because of muscle wasting.[1199,1204,1205] The duration of neuromuscular blockade is often prolonged. Rarely, resistance may be evident as a result of chronic immobilization. Of all the nondepolarizing relaxants, we recommend cisatracurium because of its multiple sites of degradation that are independent of organ function.[1206–1208] The dose requirement of atracurium in children with Duchenne muscular dystrophy is similar to that in unaffected children, although the duration of action may be prolonged.[1206] The dose response of rocuronium in children with Duchenne muscular dystrophy shows marked prolongation of both the onset and recovery times (two to three times normal).[1209] Thus NMBDs should be administered with caution in children with severe preexisting respiratory dysfunction, because even a small dose of a NMBD may cause profound muscle weakness and the need for ventilatory support. Similarly, it is important to antagonize any residual neuromuscular blockade at the end of surgery. *If there is any doubt about the competence of the neuromuscular junction, the trachea should remain intubated until muscle strength has recovered.*

Succinylcholine can cause hyperkalemia in children with burns, which may cause a cardiac arrest.[1210] The more extensive the burn, the more likely and the greater the hyperkalemic response. An 8% burn is the smallest burn that has been associated with hyperkalemia. Although most instances of cardiac arrest have occurred 20 to 50 days after the burn injury, exaggerated increases in the plasma concentration of potassium after succinylcholine can occur within a few days of the burn. However, hyperkalemia after succinylcholine has not been reported in the first 24 hours after a burn. Hyperkalemia is thought to result from the upregulation of acetylcholine receptors along the surface of the muscle membrane in the postburn phase (see Chapter 36).[1211]

Children with burns may require two to three times the usual IV dose of nondepolarizing relaxants. This resistance peaks about 2 weeks after the burn, persists for many months in those with major burns, and decreases gradually as the burns heal. The degree of resistance appears to correlate with both the extent of the burn and the period of healing. The resistance can be explained, in part, by an increase in the Vd of the relaxant (including binding

to an increased plasma concentration of α_1-acid glycoprotein) and an increase in number, sensitivity, and type of extrajunctional acetylcholine receptors (see Chapter 36).

Opioids

MORPHINE

Morphine is the most frequently used opioid to treat postoperative pain in children and is the standard against which all other opioids are compared. Morphine's main analgesic effect is by supraspinal μ_1-receptor activation. The μ_2-receptor in the spinal cord plays an important analgesic role when the drug is administered by the intrathecal or epidural route.[1212] Morphine is soluble in water, but poorly soluble in lipids compared with other opioids.

Pharmacodynamics

Target analgesic plasma concentrations are thought to be 10 to 20 ng/mL after major surgery in neonates and infants.[1213,1214] No concentration-response relationship has been described in children.[1215] The large PK and PD variability suggests that morphine be titrated to effect using small incremental IV doses (0.02 mg/kg) in neonates and infants with postoperative pain.[1216,1217] Both sex and genetics have major impacts on PD.[1218] There is polymorphism A118G of the human mu-opioid receptor gene controlling response.[1219] Inflammatory cytokines, mood and adrenergic response also impact on PD (see Chapter 6).[1220]

Morphine's low oil–water partition coefficient of 1.4 and its pKa of 8 (10%–20% un-ionized drug at physiologic pH) contribute to its delayed onset of peak action, with slow CNS penetration. The $T_{1/2}$keo for morphine is approximately 17 minutes in adults[1221] but is estimated to be 8 minutes in the full-term neonate.[1222]

Pharmacokinetics

Morphine is primarily metabolized by the hepatic enzyme UGT2B7 to morphine-3-glucuronide (M3G) and morphine-6-glucuronide (M6G); both have pharmacologic activity. Sulfation and renal clearance are minor pathways in adults but are more dominant in neonates. Contributions to both the desired effect (analgesia) and the undesired effects (nausea, respiratory depression) of M6G are the subject of clinical controversy.[1223] It has been suggested that M3G antagonizes morphine and contributes to the development of tolerance.[1224]

Clearance increases from 3.2 L/hour per 70 kg at 24 weeks PMA to 19 L/hour per 70 kg at term, reaching adult values (80 L/hour per 70 kg) at 6 to 12 months (see Fig. 7.11).[45,48,1225] These developmental factors for morphine metabolism explain in part the prolonged duration of action in neonates. The maturation profile also suggests that older infants are able to exceed the reported clearance (in liters per hour per kilogram) of morphine in adults. Clearance is perfusion-limited, with a high hepatic extraction ratio. Oral bioavailability is approximately 35% because of this first-pass effect.[1226] The metabolites are cleared by the kidney and, in part, by biliary excretion. Impaired renal function leads to M3G and M6G accumulation.[1227] Clearance is reduced in critically ill neonates compared with healthier cohorts and in those undergoing cardiac surgery (Fig. 7.23).[45–47,1213]

Morphine PK parameters show large interindividual variability contributing to the range of morphine serum concentrations observed during constant infusions.[1228] A large number of covariates contribute to PK variability. For example, African America children have a more rapid clearance of morphine than Caucasian children after tonsillectomy.[1229] Variability in clearance is influenced by

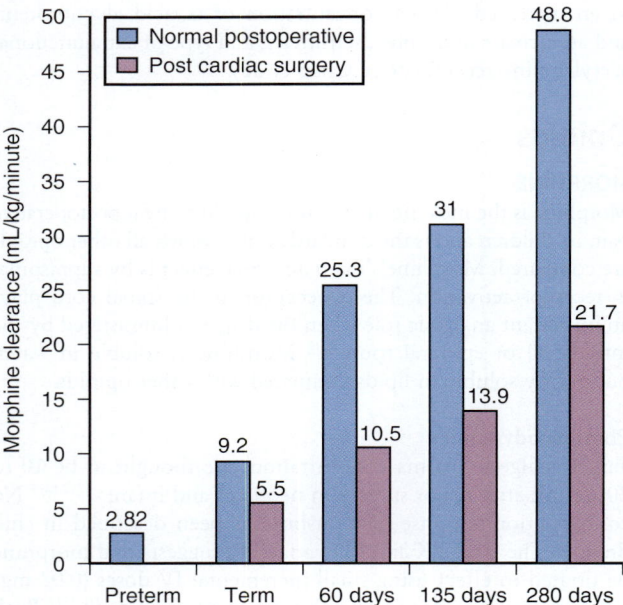

FIGURE 7.23 Morphine clearance versus postconception age in normal postoperative infants and infants undergoing cardiac surgery. Note that there is a rapid increase in an infant's ability to metabolize morphine in the first several weeks of life and that some infants achieve adult values by 1 month of age. Also note that after cardiac surgery infants have a marked impairment of morphine metabolism, which may reflect the use of vasopressors and/or decreased cardiac output to the liver. There is extreme patient-to-patient variability at all ages; preterm infants have the lowest clearance of any age group. (Data from Lynn A, Nespeca MK, Bratton SL, et al. Clearance of morphine in postoperative infants during intravenous infusion: the influence of age and surgery. *Anesth Analg.* 1998;86(5):958–963 and Mikkelsen S, Feilberg VL, Christensen CB, Lundstrøm KE. Morphine pharmacokinetics in preterm and mature newborn infants. *Acta Paediatr.* 1994;83(10):1025–1028.)

genetic factors controlling the UGT enzyme system[1220]; even the patient's domicile (e.g., high altitude) could have an impact (see also Chapter 6).[1230,1231]

Routes of Administration

Although morphine is usually administered intravenously to neonates, other routes have been used. A large variability in the analgesic effect of morphine has been observed after rectal administration[1232]; however, delayed absorption with multiple doses causing respiratory arrest has been reported so **this route is not recommended**.[108] Morphine administered orally also has considerable absorption variability (F 0.3, coefficient of variation [CV] 36%; absorption half-time [$T_{1/2}abs$] 0.71 hour; CV 55%), contributing to wide prediction intervals for observed concentrations.[1233] Morphine (25–50 µg/kg) can also be given via the caudal route and subarachnoid spaces (see Chapters 42 and 44). Although systemic absorption is slow, morphine spreads within the CSF to the brainstem, where it may cause respiratory depression lasting from 6 to more than 18 hours.[1223]

Morphine may be administered IV by intermittent bolus, continuous infusion, or patient-controlled analgesia (see Chapter 44).[1234–1236] The usual initial IV dose is 0.05 to 0.2 mg/kg. A reduced dose is indicated in neonates, children who are critically ill, those who are receiving supplemental analgesics or hypnotics, and/or those who have nocturnal hemoglobin desaturation (<85%) during obstructive sleep apnea (OSA).[1237–1239]

Adverse Effects

The major risk associated with opioid use in infants and children is respiratory depression.[99,1205] Morphine infusion rates of 10 to 30 µg/kg per hour provide adequate postoperative analgesia without respiratory depression in children.[1240] Postoperative analgesia is achieved at reduced infusion rates in infants 4 weeks of age or older (~5 µg/kg per hour for neonates, ~8.5 µg/kg per hour at 1 month, ~13.5 µg/kg per hour at 3 months, ~18 µg/kg per hour at 1 year, and slightly less than 16 µg/kg per hour for 1- to 3-year-olds).[213] Respiratory depression may occur at plasma concentrations of 20 ng/mL in infants and children,[211] but concentration-response relationships in neonates, particularly in preterm neonates who are prone to physiologic apnea, are unknown. When respiratory depression from morphine occurs, it results from both diminished tidal volume and respiratory rate. Whether morphine causes a parallel shift in the CO_2 response curve or a change in the slope, as well as a parallel shift, has not been clearly established. Morphine appears to depress respirations in neonates to a greater extent than meperidine,[1241] although the mechanism behind this is uncertain and may relate to altered PK, an immature BBB,[203] altered regional blood flow, or an increased cerebral uptake. In neonatal rats, the brain uptake of morphine is two to three times that in adult rats.[203] This may explain the 5-fold reduced LD_{50} of morphine in neonatal versus adult animals.[201–203] This immaturity of the BBB may account, in part, for the increased sensitivity of the premature neonate to morphine compared with meperidine or fentanyl; because of their lipophilicity, the latter two opioids rapidly cross an adult's or infant's BBB—that is, there is essentially no BBB.[1242]

Alternatively, reduced clearance could lead to drug accumulation in some infants given repeat doses of morphine.[167] Another possibility is a maturation of the PD effects on respiration rather than altered PK—that is, a maturation of the sensitivity of the respiratory center to morphine, rather than a change in brain equilibrium.[1243] Whether one or more of these mechanisms is relevant, morphine must be used with caution in preterm infants and in infants younger than 1 year of age. Significant histamine release may follow a rapid IV bolus of morphine and, on rare occasions, result in systemic hypotension.[1244] Urticaria over the course of the vein in which morphine was infused is a local, not systemic, allergic reaction.

M6G can also contribute to respiratory depression in children with renal failure. M6G has a $T_{1/2}keo$ of 6.7 hours (range 4–8 hours) for both analgesic effect and for respiratory depression. The EC_{50} for morphine and M6G of 16.9 ng/mL (range 10–18 ng/mL) and slope parameter (n = 2.35) are also similar.[1245]

The incidence of postoperative nausea and vomiting (PONV) is related to the morphine dose; doses in excess of 0.1 mg/kg are associated with a greater than 50% incidence of vomiting in children.[1246,1247] For unclear reasons, Latino children have a 4-fold greater incidence of pruritus and a 7-fold greater incidence of vomiting with similar morphine and morphine metabolite values.[1248] Gender may also be a factor as another study of children undergoing tonsillectomy found a significantly greater incidence of PONV in Caucasian females compared with Caucasian males (P = 0.001) as well as a prolonged stay in the postanesthesia care unit (P = 0.01).[1249]

Withdrawal symptoms may be observed in neonates after cessation of a continuous morphine infusion for more than 2 weeks, and after infusion periods less than 2 weeks if the morphine infusion rate is greater than 40 µg/kg per hour. Strategies to prevent withdrawal from morphine include the use of neuraxial analgesia, nurse-controlled sedation management protocols, ketamine or

TABLE 7.11	Relative Comparison of Commonly Used Oral and Parenteral Opioids in an Adult		
Drug	Parenteral Dose (mg)	Oral Dose (mg)	Half-Life (Hours)
Morphine	10	30–40	2.0–3.5
Hydromorphone	1.5–2.0	6.0–7.5	2–4
Oxycodone		15–30	2–4
Methadone	7.5–10.0	15	22–25
Meperidine	75–100	300	3–5
Codeine	120–130	200	3
Fentanyl	0.1	0.1	0.5

Adapted from Lugo RA, Kern SE. Clinical pharmacokinetics of morphine. *J Pain Palliat Care Pharmacother.* 2002;16(4):5–18.

naloxone mixed with morphine infusion, and the use of alternate agents (e.g., methadone) with lower potential for tolerance.[1250,1251] Table 7.11 summarizes the relative doses of opioids administered to adults via the parenteral and oral routes.

The use of oral morphine for tonsillectomy pain and other chronic painful conditions is increasing after the safety issues regarding codeine were promulgated by the FDA and the American Academy of Pediatrics.[1226,1252–1254] There are limited data available in children.[1234,1255] A starting dose of 1.5 to 2 mg/kg per day has been suggested for children with chronic pain.[1256] These doses may be excessive for children with acute pain, particularly those sensitized by OSA. Conversion from IV to oral morphine is estimated at 3 to 6 mg equivalent to 1 mg IV and oral morphine solutions are available in multiple concentrations. Extended-release tablets are also available again with limited pediatric data and are likely only useful for teenagers with chronic pain.

MEPERIDINE

Meperidine (pethidine, Demerol) has been traditionally considered a potent opioid to treat severe pain; meperidine is no longer indicated as an analgesic (because of its adverse effects and metabolites). Because repeated doses of meperidine may result in the accumulation of normeperidine, which causes seizures,[1257,1258] this drug has been removed from the formulary in many children's hospitals. We do not recommend the use of this opioid other than for a single-dose administration. Meperidine is a weak opioid, primarily a μ-receptor, agonist that has a potency approximately one-tenth that of morphine. The analgesic effects are detectable within 5 minutes of IV administration, and peak effect is reached within 10 minutes in adults ($T_{1/2}$keo of approximately 7–8 minutes).[1259,1260] Meperidine is metabolized by N-demethylation to meperidinic acid and normeperidine. Meperidine clearance in infants and children is approximately 8 to 10 mL/minute per kilogram.[1261,1262] Elimination in neonates is greatly reduced, and elimination half-time in neonates who have received meperidine by placental transfer may be 2 to 7 times greater than that in adults.[1263] The elimination half-life of meperidine in children after IV administration is approximately 3 ± 0.5 hours,[1261] with a very variable half-life in neonates between 3.3 and 59.4 hours.[1262] The Vdss in infants, 7.2 (3.3–11) L/kg,[1262] is greater than that in children 2 to 8 years (2.8 ± 0.6 L/kg).[1261]

In children, meperidine is indicated only to stop shivering, not for analgesia. Although its onset time is more rapid than morphine, the risk of seizures after repeated dosing in children

has all but removed it from routine clinical use. The dose of meperidine is 1 to 2 mg/kg (see Table 7.11), although reduced doses should be used in critically ill children. Peak plasma values after IV, IM, and rectal administration are 5 minutes, 10 minutes, and 60 minutes, respectively.[1264,1265] Rectal administration of meperidine in children results in wide variations in systemic bioavailability (32%–81% of administered dose) and **is not recommended**.[1261]

In infants, respiratory depression after meperidine is less than that after morphine; the larger Vd of meperidine may contribute.[1241] The LD$_{50}$ of meperidine in the neonatal animal is only 20% less than in the adult animal, corresponding with the human clinical response.[201] This is consistent with the reduced respiratory depression with meperidine compared with the equivalent dose of morphine. As with any opioid, the use of meperidine in very young infants must be accompanied by careful observation for respiratory depression and airway obstruction because the PK vary considerably.[1262] Meperidine was used for a number of years as a component of various "lytic cocktails" that provided sedation. The safety of these admixtures is dubious, and its use in sedation mixtures is not indicated.[1266]

HYDROMORPHONE

Hydromorphone (Dilaudid) is a semisynthetic congener of morphine with a potency of around 5 to 7.5 times that of morphine.[1267] The IV and IM dose is 10 to 20 μg/kg with a continuous IV infusion of 1 to 4 μg/kg per hour. Its bioavailability is about 55% after nasal and oral (30–80 μg/kg every 3 to 4 hours) administration and about 35% after rectal administration (not recommended)[1268–1270]; there is extensive first-pass metabolism.[1271] A clearance of 51.7 (range, 28.6–98.2) mL/minute per kilogram is reported in children, with a half-life of 2.5 ± 0.9 hours.[1268,1272] Hydromorphone is metabolized to hydromorphone-3-glucuronide (95%) and to other metabolites and does not appear to present added risk caused by polymorphisms.[1273]

Hydromorphone is commonly used when prolonged analgesia is required.[1274–1277] Morphine is often changed to hydromorphone to reduce the adverse effects or because of concern of accumulation of morphine metabolites, particularly in the presence of renal failure.[1278] Hydromorphone is commonly administered intravenously, orally, epidurally, and intranasally.[1267,1274,1275,1279–1282] Hydromorphone is used for chronic cancer pain, and plasma concentrations of around 4.7 ng/mL (range 1.9–8.9 ng/mL) relieve mucositis in children given patient-controlled analgesia devices.[1267,1272] Some may require greater plasma concentrations (10–30 ng/mL) to control severe pain. Oral extended-release formulations are available, and a pediatric trial of children 7 to 17 years of age is in progress (FDA.gov).

OXYCODONE

Oxycodone (OxyContin) is a long-acting semisynthetic opioid that is usually administered orally and is available in controlled-release formulations.[1283–1285] Metabolism is through CYP3A-mediated N-demethylation to noroxycodone and CYP2D6 O-demethylation to oxymorphone and noroxymorphone; these pathways are immature in neonates.[1286,1287] Extremely preterm neonates have a median elimination half-life of 8.8 hours (range 6.8–12.5 hours); the half-life in preterm neonates is 7.4 hours (4.2–11.6 hours) and in older neonates it is 4.1 hours (2.4–5.8 hours). Infants aged 6 to 24 months have a smaller half-life of 2.0 hours (1.7–7.2.6 hours). Median renal clearance is fairly constant in all age groups, whereas nonrenal clearance increases markedly with age.[1286–1289]

Clearance matures within the first year of life. Maturation aspects of clearance in children 6 months to 7 years are adequately described using allometric models; CL/F = 55 × (Wt/70)$^{0.87}$ L/hour/70 kg, Vd/F = 86 × (Wt/70)$^{1.16}$ L/70 kg.[1288] Clearance is similar in children 5.4 years (range 2–9 years) given oxycodone hydrochloride (0.1 mg/kg) by IV bolus after ophthalmic surgery. Mean values of drug clearance and volume of distribution (Vdss) are 46 L/hour per 70 kg and 147 L/70 kg.[1290] As with many medications, interindividual variability in the elimination half-life of oxycodone in the neonate is extreme.[1288] In children, the elimination half-life after IV, buccal, IM, or orogastric administration is 2 to 3 hours.[1289] Clearance may be decreased in patients with liver dysfunction.[1291]

The relative bioavailability in adults of intranasal, oral, and rectal formulations is approximately 50% that of the IV route. The buccal and sublingual absorption of oxycodone is similar in young children.[1272] The bioavailability after various routes is IM, 68%; buccal, 55%; and orogastric, 37%.[1289,1292] Oxycodone may also be administered rectally, with a similar bioavailability, although absorption can be prolonged; **this route is not recommended**.[1293] The IV formulation of oxycodone significantly depresses respiration; 0.1 mg/kg in children after ophthalmic surgery caused greater ventilatory depression than other opioids.[1288,1290,1294,1295] Maximum mean ETCO$_2$ concentration and minimum mean ventilatory rate occurred 8 minutes after administration of oxycodone IV in children, but the minimum mean peripheral arteriolar oxygen saturation occurred at 4 minutes.

CYP2D6 catalyzes O-demethylation producing oxymorphone, which accounts for 10% of the circulating oxycodone metabolites and is 14 times more potent than oxycodone because of its 40-fold greater affinity for the mu-opioid receptor compared with oxycodone. Consequently, "fast metabolizers" who are breastfeeding mothers may expose their infants to excessive opioids.[1290,1296] Clearance may also be decreased in patients with liver dysfunction.[1291] This opioid is commonly used to transition from patient-controlled analgesia and to treat chronic painful conditions (see Chapters 44 and 45).[1290] The therapeutic concentration range is broad: 10 to 100 ng/mL.[54,1297]

HYDROCODONE

Hydrocodone is also metabolized by the CYP2D6 enzyme system to the active metabolite hydromorphone (see also Chapter 6). One study of adult females after cesarean section found that 60% were extensive metabolizers, 30% intermediate, 3% poor, and 7% ultrarapid. This genotypic variability can have profound effects on effectiveness and the potential for toxicity with ultrarapid metabolism.[1298] A pediatric study of African American children treated for sickle cell disease found a similar distribution of metabolic conversion from hydrocodone to hydromorphone.[1299] Thus caution is advised as both inadequate analgesia and potential overdose are possible with this opioid.[1300-1302] This drug is frequently provided in combination with acetaminophen in fixed doses (e.g., Lortab elixir); therefore it is essential to avoid adding other acetaminophen-containing analgesics when it is prescribed. The dose should be based on ideal body weight.[1303] The dose should be reduced by 33%–50% for children at risk for OSA. The therapeutic concentrations are 10 to 40 ng/mL.[1304]

METHADONE

Methadone is a synthetic opioid with an analgesic potency similar to that of morphine but with a more rapid distribution and a slower elimination. Methadone is used as a maintenance drug in opioid-addicted adults to prevent withdrawal. Methadone might have beneficial effects because it is a long-acting synthetic opioid with a very high bioavailability (80%) by the enteral route. It also has NMDA receptor antagonistic activity and this may be beneficial in chronic pain treatment because agonism of this receptor is associated with opioid tolerance and hyperalgesia. Methadone is a racemate, and clinical effect is a result of the R-methadone isomer. Methadone is 2.5 to 20 times more analgesic than morphine.[1305]

The primary indication for methadone in children is to wean from long-term opioid infusions to prevent withdrawal, and to provide analgesia when other opioids have failed or have been associated with intolerable side effects.[1306] Oral administration has been recommended as the first-line opioid for severe and persistent pain in children.[1307] It seems also to be a safe enteral alternative for IV opioids in palliative pediatric oncologic patients.[1308]

IV methadone has been shown to be an effective analgesic for postoperative pain relief. The minimum effective analgesic concentration of methadone in opioid-naïve adults is 58 μg/L,[1309] while no withdrawal symptoms were observed in neonates suffering opioid withdrawal if plasma concentrations of methadone exceeded 60 μg/L.[1310] The racemate of methadone, which is commonly used in pediatric and anesthetic care, is metabolized to EDDP (2-ethylidene-1,5-dimethyl-3,3-diphenylpyrrolidine) and EMDP (2-ethyl-5-methyl-3,3-diphenylpyrroline).

Methadone is cleared by the cytochrome P450 mixed oxidase (CYP3A4, CYP2B6, and CYP2D6) enzyme systems, all of which are immature at birth. CYP3A7 may contribute to clearance in the neonate.[1311,1312] Methadone has high lipid solubility with a large Vd of 6 to 7 L/kg in children and adults.[1313,1314] Pharmacokinetic parameters, standardized to a 70-kg adult using allometry, have been estimated using a three-compartment linear disposition model. Population parameter estimates (CV, between subject variability) were central volume (V1) 21.5 (29%) L/70 kg; peripheral volumes of distribution V2 75.1 (23%) L/70 kg; V3 484 (8%) L/70 kg; clearance (CL) 9.45 (11%) L/hour per 70 kg; and intercompartment clearances Q2 325 (21%) L/hour per 70 kg, Q3 136 (14%) L/hour per 7 kg. EDDP formation clearance was 9.1 (11%) L/hour per 70 kg; formation clearance of EMDP from EDDP was 7.4 (63%) L/hour per 70 kg; elimination clearance of EDDP was 40.9 (26%) L/hour per 70 kg; and the rate constant for intermediate compartments was 2.17 (43%) per hour.[1315] These parameter estimates in children and neonates are consistent with those reported by others in neonates,[1251] children,[1314] adolescents,[1316] and adults.[1317] There was no clearance maturation with age. Neonatal enantiomer clearances were also similar to those described in adults.[1315]

An IV regimen of 0.2 mg/kg 8 hourly in neonates achieves a target concentration of 60 μg/L within 36 hours. Infusion, rather than intermittent dosing, should be considered if this target is to be achieved in older children after cardiac surgery. Analgesic responses in adults on chronic methadone programs suggests a steep concentration-response relationship for pain relief (Hill = 4.4 ± 3.8) with very rapid equilibration between plasma methadone concentrations and the sites mediating pain relief. Consequently, the drug rapidly loses effect as concentrations decrease to less than EC$_{50}$. A single dose of 0.2 mg/kg will contribute little analgesia after a few hours. An infusion (Fig. 7.24) has been suggested for analgesia in adolescents after spinal instrumentation surgery,[1316] and consideration could be given to this technique after cardiac surgery in children. It should be noted that methadone, like other opioids, has large between-subject PK variability that could result in drug accumulation and possible fatal outcomes with long-term administration.[1318]

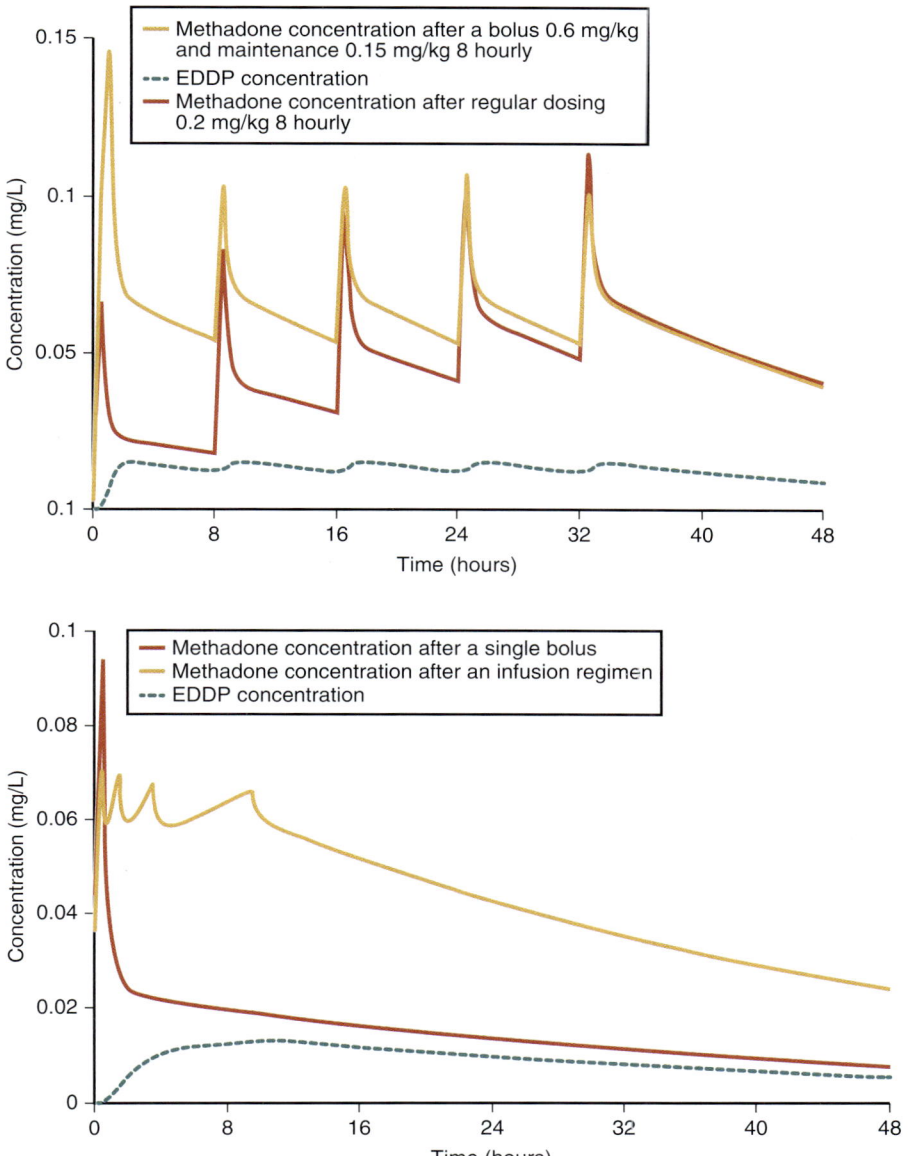

FIGURE 7.24 The upper panel shows a simulation for a 3.5-kg neonate given a methadone loading dose of 0.6 mg/kg followed by a maintenance dose of 0.15 mg/kg 8 hourly. EDDP concentrations track parent drug concentrations. The methadone target concentration of 0.06 mg/L is achieved rapidly compared with the neonate given 0.2 mg/kg 8 hourly without a loading dose. A single dose of methadone 0.2 mg/kg given for postoperative analgesia in a child is unlikely to achieve long duration of analgesia because concentrations are below 0.03 mg/kg within 1.5 hours (lower panel). An infusion may be a better option. A regimen consisting of a methadone bolus of 0.15 mg/kg followed by 0.15 mg/kg per hour for 1 hour, 0.075 mg/kg per hour for 2 hours, and 0.025 mg/kg per hour for 6 hours maintains a concentration of 0.06 mg/L. EDDP concentrations after this infusion regimen are also shown. *EDDP,* 2-ethylidene-1,5-dimethyl-3,3-diphenylpyrrolidine. (From Ward RM. The pharmacokinetics of methadone and its metabolites in neonates, infants, and children. *Paediatr Anaesth.* 2014;24(2):591–601, with permission.)

FENTANYL

Fentanyl (Sublimaze) offers greater hemodynamic stability than morphine, a rapid onset ($T_{1/2}$keo of 6.6 minutes in adults), and a short duration of effect. Its relative increased lipid solubility and small molecular conformation enables efficient penetration of the BBB and redistribution. It is the most commonly used opioid during general anesthesia in infants and children. It is particularly effective in the care of high-risk preterm and term neonates, as well as in infants and children during cardiac surgical

procedures. High doses of fentanyl (10–100 µg/kg) are often administered to maintain cardiovascular homeostasis.[1154,1319–1329] Fentanyl may be administered intravenously, intramuscularly, intranasally, as a supplement to epidural analgesia, orally, oral transmucosal absorption, and transdermally—both passively and by iontophoresis.[1330–1337]

Fentanyl is metabolized by oxidative *N*-dealkylation (CYP3A4) into norfentanyl and hydroxylated. All metabolites are inactive and a small amount of fentanyl is eliminated via the kidneys unchanged. Compared with term neonates, the clearance of fentanyl in preterm infants is markedly reduced (mean elimination half-life is 17.7 ± 9.3 hours), contributing to prolonged respiratory depression in preterm neonates. Clearance matures with gestational age; 7 mL/minute per kilogram at 25 weeks PMA, 10 mL/minute per kilogram at 30 weeks PMA, and 12 mL/minute per kilogram at 35 weeks PMA.[1338] The clearance of fentanyl is 70% to 80% of adult values in term neonates and, when standardized to a 70-kg person, reaches adult values (~50 L/hour per 70 kg) within the first 2 weeks of life.[852] Clearance of fentanyl in older infants (>3 months of age) and children is greater than that in adults when expressed per kilogram (30.6 mL/kg per minute vs. 17.9 mL/kg per minute, respectively), resulting in a reduced elimination half-life (68 minutes vs. 121 minutes, respectively).[1319,1322,1339–1341]

The Vdss of fentanyl is approximately 5.9 L/kg in term neonates and decreases with age to 4.5 L/kg during infancy, 3.1 L/kg during childhood, and 1.6 L/kg in adults.[1342] This increased Vdss results in a smaller blood concentration after bolus administration in neonates and infants.[1343] Administration of fentanyl 3 μg/kg by slow IV push in term infants (1–7 months of age) intraoperatively neither depressed respiration nor caused hypoxemia in placebo-controlled trials.[1344,1345] Slow administration and both an increased Vdss and an increased clearance (per kilogram) in this age group contributed to these results. Fentanyl clearance may be impaired with decreased hepatic blood flow (e.g., from increased intra-abdominal pressure in neonatal omphalocele repair), although a maldistribution of blood away from regions of concentrated cytochrome enzyme activity in the liver may also play a role.[1346]

Infants with cyanotic heart disease had reduced Vdss and greater plasma concentrations of fentanyl with infusion therapy.[1321] These greater plasma concentrations resulted from a reduced clearance (34 L/hour per 70 kg), which was attributed to hemodynamic disturbance and consequent reduced hepatic blood flow.[1347] Hypothermia also reduces fentanyl clearance.[1348] Profound hypotension has been reported after a bolus of midazolam in neonates in whom fentanyl was infused and vice versa.[1349] Other drugs metabolized by CYP3A4 (e.g., cyclosporine, erythromycin) may compete for clearance and result in increased fentanyl plasma concentrations.

Fentanyl is a potent μ-receptor agonist with a potency 70 to 125 times greater than that of morphine. A plasma concentration of 15 to 30 ng/mL is required to provide total IV anesthesia in adults, whereas the EC50, based on EEG evidence, is 10 ng/mL.[1350,1351] Fentanyl has been shown to effectively prevent preterm neonates from surgical stress responses and to improve postoperative outcomes.[1352] Single doses of fentanyl (3 μg/kg) can reduce the physiologic and behavioral measures of pain and stress associated with mechanical ventilation in preterm infants.[1353] Fentanyl has similar respiratory depression in infants and adults when plasma concentrations are similar.[1354]

The PK of fentanyl in critically ill children receiving long-term infusions is also quite variable, with a mean terminal elimination half-life of 21 hours and a range of 11 to 36 hours.[1355,1356] The infusion rates of fentanyl that are required to achieve a similar level of sedation and analgesia may vary as much as 10-fold.[1355] This variability in PK and PD strongly reinforces the need to titrate the dose to effect and to be prepared to provide postoperative ventilatory support as needed. Children receiving a long-term infusion of fentanyl are at risk of rapidly developing tolerance with a doubling of opioid dose more likely to occur after 7 days[1357]; on discontinuation of the infusion, these children may demonstrate signs of withdrawal. Continuous infusions of fentanyl in

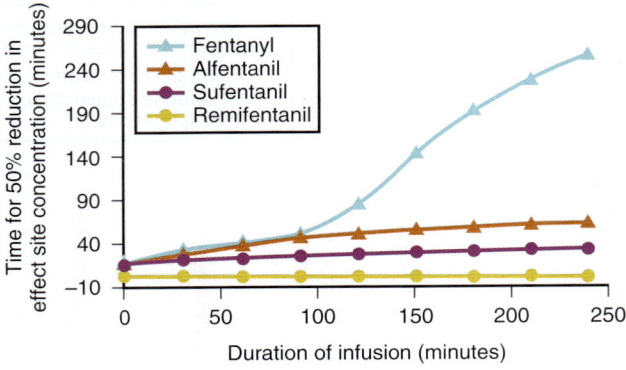

FIGURE 7.25 This figure is a simulation of the time required for a 50% reduction in the effective site concentration of remifentanil (*yellow circles*), sufentanil (*purple circles*), alfentanil (*brown triangles*), and fentanyl (*blue triangles*) after an infusion (duration of 240 minutes) designed to maintain a constant effect-site concentration. Note that there is a completely flat curve for remifentanil, suggesting that a plateau effect is rapidly reached with remifentanil compared with the other opioids, such that even after a long infusion, the time to 50% reduction in effect-site concentration is still less than 4 minutes. (Redrawn and modified with permission from Westmoreland CL, Hole JF, Sebel PS, Hug CC Jr, Muir KT. Pharmacokinetics of remifentanil [GI87084B] and its major metabolite [GI90291] in patients undergoing elective inpatient surgery. *Anesthesiology* 1993;79(5):893–903.)

mechanically ventilated preterm infants combined with intermittent boluses have been shown to reduce acute pain compared with bolus dosing alone.[1358] All long-term infusions should be tapered slowly over days rather than discontinuing them abruptly.[1340,1359,1360]

With low-dose fentanyl, the termination of action is primarily a combination of redistribution and rapid clearance by the liver.[1340,1361] The CSHT after a 1-hour infusion of fentanyl is approximately 20 minutes, which increases to 270 minutes after an 8-hour infusion in adults (Fig. 7.25).[23] Although the CSHT is reduced in children, there are no data in neonates.[1341] High-dose fentanyl, accumulates in muscle and fat and is therefore released (recirculated) more slowly, thus accounting in part for the prolonged respiratory depression after large doses. There is no evidence of dose-dependent kinetics—that is, there is no tissue or enzyme saturation in the clinically used ranges.[1361] In some respects, the pharmacology of opioids is very similar to that of barbituates: at low doses their clinical effect is terminated by redistribution, whereas at large doses their clinical effect is terminated by metabolism.[1354,1361–1364]

The usual initial dose of fentanyl is 1 to 3 μg/kg, a dose that may be supplemented as clinically indicated. Fentanyl is very lipid soluble and rapidly crosses the BBB. This characteristic may, in part, explain why the LD50 for fentanyl in neonatal animals is 90% of that in adult animals. Continuous intraoperative and postoperative infusions of fentanyl are common in children of all ages.[1321,1364,1365] Fentanyl is also used to provide patient-controlled analgesia (see Chapter 44).[1366,1367]

Chest wall and glottic rigidity have been reported after IV administration of opioids, although most often after fentanyl. The reason for this is not clear.[1368–1373] Glottic rigidity may account for the inability to ventilate by bag and mask after IV fentanyl.[1373,1374] This adverse response can be minimized by administering the opioid slowly, and it can be reversed by administering either a muscle relaxant or naloxone.[1374] Another concern is the rare association of increased vagal tone with bolus administration;

bradycardia may have profound effects on the cardiac output of neonates. Additionally, fentanyl markedly depresses the baroreceptor reflex control of heart rate in neonates.[1375] It is for these reasons that pancuronium (with its vagolytic effect) is often combined with high-dose fentanyl and why atropine is administered before a fentanyl-succinylcholine combination for neonatal intubation.[1376]

Oral transmucosal fentanyl (Fentanyl Oralet) was approved by the FDA for premedication of children but is no longer marketed. A new formulation (Actiq) has been approved for adults and children 16 years of age or older, but it has been used off-label in children for the treatment of cancer breakthrough pain.[1377-1379] This route of administration provides more rapid onset of analgesia than buccal immediate-release tablets but is slower in onset than nasal administration.[1379] Fentanyl is rapidly absorbed through the oral mucosa, which bypasses the liver.[794,1331,1332,1380-1384] Nonetheless, approximately half the absorption is gastrointestinal. The bioavailability of this formulation in children (33%) is less than that in adults (50%).[1331,1332] Uptake continues for a period of time after consumption, which potentially can provide analgesia for several hours.[794,1331,1332]

The fentanyl patch was developed to provide an extended release of fentanyl similar to that provided with a continuous IV infusion.[1330,1385-1394] *This formulation was not designed to be administered to treat postsurgical pain, but rather for those who require opioids chronically.* This fentanyl transdermal therapeutic system (TTS) is available with a drug release rate of 12.5 µg/hour and matches the smaller dosing requirements of cancer pain control in children.[1395] An approximate conversion factor of 45 mg/day oral morphine to 12.5 g/hour fentanyl TTS is used for initial dose estimation in children receiving long-term morphine therapy. This is conservatively low to avoid respiratory depression. In adults, uptake of fentanyl begins within 1 hour and achieves therapeutic levels within 6 to 8 hours and peak levels at 24 hours.[1391,1394,1396] In children, the peak occurs earlier, at about 18 hours.[1397] The skin acts as a reservoir, and even after removal of the patch, uptake continues for several hours, with a consequent apparent elimination half-life of 14.5 ± 6 hours.[1397] Fentanyl uptake is markedly affected by skin blood flow, skin thickness, location of the patch, and adherence to the skin.[1395,1398-1400] Alterations in skin blood flow (e.g., fever) may increase absorption.[1401] Alterations to skin blood flow caused by warming devices (increased absorption) or hypothermia (decreased absorption) during anesthesia should be considered in children with chronic pain who present with TTS fentanyl.

The use of TTS medication should be limited to pain specialists who are familiar with the unusual PK of this drug delivery system.[1402] One study suggests that the PK of fentanyl by this route in children and adult patients are similar.[1397] A multicenter study in children 2 to 16 years of age reported satisfactory long-term analgesia. However, it should be noted that the data submitted to the FDA revealed plasma concentrations of fentanyl in children 1.5 to 5 years of age that were twice those in adults.[1403] These data are consistent with another study that found a negative correlation between fentanyl concentrations and age—that is, greater concentrations in younger children.[1397] Children may be particularly vulnerable to the rapid drug absorption compared with adults because they have thinner skin and better skin blood flow.[905] Accordingly, it seems prudent to begin with the smallest size patch and gradually increase as indicated (see Chapters 44 and 45). All patches, including those that have already been used, contain large amounts of fentanyl that may cause a fatal intoxication if accidentally or intentionally ingested or improperly applied.[1404-1406] Proper disposal of these opioid-containing patches is required.

Epidural fentanyl is often combined with an amide local anesthetic for provision of postoperative analgesia; pruritus, nausea, and vomiting may be exacerbated by the addition of fentanyl. Spread beyond the site of administration is dose dependent but limited, and respiratory depression is uncommon.[1283,1407] It should be noted, however, that plasma concentrations may increase for a period of time after cessation of epidural fentanyl, thus prolonging the potential for respiratory depression for several hours.[1337]

ALFENTANIL

Alfentanil (Alfenta) is a fentanyl analog whose main advantage is its reduced lipid solubility and smaller Vd compared with fentanyl.[1408] It has a rapid onset ($T_{1/2}$keo of 0.9 minutes in adults), a brief duration of action, and one-fourth the potency of fentanyl. A target plasma concentration of 400 ng/mL is used in anesthesia. Metabolism is through oxidative *N*-dealkylation by CYP3A4 and *O*-dealkylation and then conjugation to metabolites that are excreted renally.[1409] Studies indicate that brain concentrations of alfentanil are 7-fold to 9-fold less, the Vd is four times less, and protein binding is greater than fentanyl.[1410]

Alfentanil is more rapidly eliminated from the body than fentanyl, thus necessitating more frequent dosing. Clearance in neonates (20–60 mL/minute per 70 kg) is one-tenth that in adults (250–500 mL/minute per 70 kg) with rapid maturation.[68] In preterm neonates, the half-life is as long as 6 to 9 hours.[1411,1412] The Vd in children and adults are similar but are increased in preterm neonates (Vd 1.0 ± 0.39 vs. 0.48 ± 0.19 L/kg). Clearance is greater in children, expressed as per kilogram (11.1 ± 3.9 mL/kg per minute vs. 5.9 ± 1.6 mL/kg per minute). As a result, the elimination half-life in children is less (63 ± 24 vs. 95 ± 20 minutes).[1413-1416] The Vd and elimination half-life in infants 3 to 12 months of age and older children are similar.[1415] Because clearance is markedly diminished in children with hepatic disease, clinical effects are prolonged in those with reduced hepatic blood flow (e.g., children with increased intraabdominal pressure, children receiving vasopressors, and those with some forms of congenital heart disease).[1408,1417,1418] Renal failure has little effect on its elimination.[1419] Because less alfentanil is bound to α_1-acid glycoprotein in preterm infants (65%) than in term infants (79%), an increased unbound fraction of alfentanil is available for biologic effect in the former.[80]

The PK and PD of alfentanil suggest potential applications for the rapid control of analgesia and awakening from anesthesia. Alfentanil (10 µg/kg) has been combined with propofol (2.5 mg/kg) for tracheal intubation without an NMBD.[1420] High-dose alfentanil is also used for cardiac procedures. Alfentanil should be used with caution without NMBDs in neonates because of the frequency of chest wall or glottic rigidity.[1262,1421]

SUFENTANIL

Sufentanil (Sufenta) is a potent synthetic opioid that in many respects is similar to fentanyl and alfentanil. Sufentanil is 5 to 10 times more potent than fentanyl, with a $T_{1/2}$keo of 6.2 minutes in adults.[1422] A concentration of 5 to 10 ng/mL is required for total IV anesthesia, and 0.2 to 0.4 ng/mL for analgesia. PD differences are suggested in neonates. The plasma concentration of sufentanil at the time of additional anesthetic supplementation to suppress hemodynamic responses to surgical stimulation was 2.51 ng/mL in neonates, significantly greater than the concentrations of 1.58, 1.53, and 1.56 ng/mL observed in infants, children, and adolescents, respectively.[1423]

Elimination of sufentanil is by *O*-demethylation and *N*-dealkylation in animal studies. As with fentanyl and alfentanil, the CYP3A4 enzyme is responsible for the *N*-dealkylation.[1424] The majority of studies of IV sufentanil in children have focused on those undergoing cardiac surgery. Evidence has shown age-dependent PK in which neonates have a larger Vdss, reduced clearance, and a greater and more variable elimination half-life than older children and adults (E-Fig. 7.18).[1423,1425,1426] Clearance in neonates undergoing cardiovascular surgery (6.7 ± 6.1 mL/kg per minute) is reduced compared with values of 18.1 ± 2.7, 16.9 ± 3.2, and 13.1 ± 3.6 mL/kg per minute in infants, children, and adolescents, respectively,[1423] which is consistent with rapid development of hepatic metabolic pathways.[1425] Clearance maturation standardized to a 70-kg person using allometry is similar to that of other drugs that depend on CYP3A4 for metabolism (e.g., levobupivacaine, fentanyl, alfentanil) (see Fig. 7.11).[1427] Clearance rates in infants (27.5 ± 9.3 mL/kg per minute) were greater, expressed per kilogram, than those in children (18.1 ± 10.7 mL/kg per minute) in another study of children undergoing cardiovascular surgery.[1426]

Clearance in healthy children (2–8 years) was greater (30.5 ± 8.8 mL/kg per minute) than in those undergoing cardiac surgery.[1428] Decreased hepatic blood flow reduces clearance.[1428] The elimination of sufentanil is unaffected by renal failure but markedly altered by factors that influence hepatic blood flow; cirrhosis apparently has little effect on its elimination.[1408,1429,1430] The Vdss was 4.15 ± 1.0 L/kg in neonates, greater than the values of 2.73 ± 0.5 and 2.75 ± 0.5 L/kg observed in children and adolescents, respectively.[1423,1428]

Bradycardia and asystole have been observed after a bolus administration of sufentanil, suggesting that pretreatment with a vagolytic agent (atropine, glycopyrrolate, or pancuronium bromide) may be sensible.[1431,1432]

Nasal sufentanil may have a role for sedation/analgesia in children undergoing painful procedures,[118] although data in neonates are lacking and there are concerns about the risk of respiratory depression.[1433-1438] Several studies demonstrated that children are more likely to accept nasal sufentanil compared with nasal midazolam, although there was a greater incidence of vomiting after sufentanil and several children experienced decreased chest wall compliance after or during induction of anesthesia. The dose of sufentanil that is most effective when administered intranasally is 2 to 3 µg/kg.[1434,1436] Epidural sufentanil (0.7–0.75 µg/kg) has been effective in children, lasting more than 3 hours, although pruritus can be bothersome.[1439-1441] If administered as a continuous epidural infusion, it should be noted that sufentanil is slowly eliminated. Plasma concentrations may continue to increase even after discontinuation, which could potentially lead to respiratory depression.[1442] Nasal sufentanil 0.5 µg/kg had a maximum plasma concentration (C_{max}) of 0.042 µg/L at 13.8 minutes.[118]

REMIFENTANIL

Remifentanil (Ultiva) is the newest in the family of synthetic opioids.[1443,1444] Its brief elimination half-life of 3 to 6 minutes requires that it be given as an infusion.[185,1445-1447] This opioid is unique because blood and tissue esterases rapidly terminate its action by degrading an ester linkage in the molecule to a carboxylic acid metabolite.[1448] Metabolism is unaffected by hepatic or renal function.[1449] The active metabolite of remifentanil that is eliminated by the kidneys has approximately 1/300th to 1/1000th the opioid activity of the parent compound and, theoretically, could accumulate and cause clinical manifestations in children with impaired renal function.[1450] One study in adults failed to demonstrate any residual opioid effects after a 12-hour infusion in patients with renal failure.[1451] Perhaps the most important characteristic of remifentanil is its very brief half-life and the associated rapid recovery within about 10 minutes. Clearance in patients with butyrylcholinesterase deficiency is unaffected. The nonspecific blood esterases that metabolize remifentanil are mature at birth.[40]

A target plasma concentration of 2 to 3 µg/L is adequate for laryngoscopy, 6 to 8 µg/L for laparotomy, and 10 to 12 µg/L might be sought to ablate the stress response associated with cardiac surgery (see Chapter 8 for remifentanil use in total IV anesthesia).[1452] Analgesic concentrations are 0.2 to 0.4 µg/L. The $T_{1/2}keo$ is 1.16 minutes in adults,[184] but the neonatal $T_{1/2}keo$ has not been reported. Analgesic alternatives should be available when the short-duration analgesic effects from remifentanil are dissipating. Reports of a rapid development of µ-receptor tolerance with remifentanil are in conflict; activity at δ-opioid receptors may contribute.[1453] Remifentanil clearance can be described in all age groups by simple application of an allometric model.[39] This standardized clearance of 2790 mL/minutes per 70 kg is similar to that reported by others in children[185,1454] and adults.[184,1444] The smaller the child, the greater the clearance when expressed as milliliters per minute per kilogram. Clearance decreases with increasing age, with rates of 90 mL/kg per minute in infants younger than 2 years of age, 60 mL/kg per minute in children 2 to 12 years of age, and 40 mL/kg per minute in adults (Fig. 7.26 and Table 7.12).[39,185,1454]

The Vdss was greatest in infants younger than 2 months of age (452 mL/kg) and decreased to 308 mL/kg in children 2 months to 2 years, and to 240 mL/kg in children older than 2 years of age.[185] The elimination half-life appears to be constant, approximately 3 to 6 minutes, independent of dose or duration of the infusion,[185,1445] and the CSHT is constant (see Fig. 7.25).[1450] For example, when the infusion rates of remifentanil differed as much as 20-fold, the time to return to spontaneous respirations varied by only 1 to 3 minutes.[1449,1455] As an opioid, the effect of remifentanil on respiration is an excellent reflection of its PD effects.[1456] After 3-hour infusions of alfentanil and remifentanil in adults, the elimination half-lives were 47.3 ± 12 minutes for alfentanil, compared with 3.2 ± 0.9 minutes for remifentanil. The time to recover 50% of the minute ventilation, a PD effect of opioids, was 54.0 ± 48.1 minutes for alfentanil, compared with 5.4 ± 1.8 minutes for remifentanil.[1456]

Although covariate effects, such as cardiac surgery, appear to have a muted effect on PK, cardiopulmonary bypass (CPB) does have an impact. Remifentanil dosage adjustments are required during and after CPB because of marked changes in its Vd.[1457] Other PK changes during CPB are consistent with adult data in which a decreased metabolism occurred with a reduced temperature[1458] and with reports of greater clearance after CPB (increased metabolism) compared with during CPB.[1454]

Respiratory depression is concentration dependent.[1459,1460] Vocal cord closure, commonly interpreted as muscle rigidity, remains a concern with bolus doses above 3 µg/kg used for intubation in neonates.[1461] Induction with propofol (4 mg/kg) and either remifentanil (3 µg/kg) or succinylcholine (2 mg/kg) for intubation was similar, with no bradycardia, hypotension, or chest wall rigidity.[1462] The initial loading dose of remifentanil may cause hypotension and bradycardia,[1463] prompting some to target the plasma rather than effect-site concentration when initiating an infusion. This hypotensive response has been quantified in children undergoing cranioplasty surgery. A steady-state remifentanil

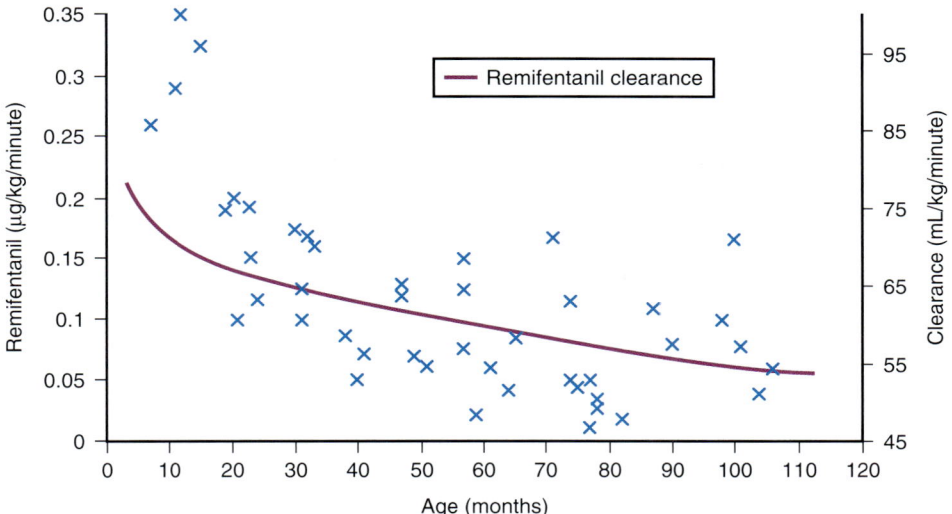

FIGURE 7.26 The effect of age on the dose (infusion rate) of remifentanil tolerated during spontaneous ventilation under anesthesia in children undergoing strabismus surgery.[248] Superimposed on this plot is the estimated remifentanil clearance determined using an allometric model.[76] There is a mismatch between clearance and infusion rate for those individuals still in infancy. The larger infusion rates recorded in those infants can be attributed to greater suppression of respiratory drive in this age group than with the older children during the study; a respiratory rate of 10 breaths/minute in an infant is disproportionately slow compared with the same rate in a 7-year-old child, suggesting excessive dose. (Reproduced with permission from Anderson BJ. Pediatric models for adult target-controlled infusion pumps. *Paediatr Anaesth.* 2010;20(3):223–232; Rigby-Jones AE, Priston MJ, Sneyd JR, et al. Remifentanil-midazolam sedation for paediatric patients receiving mechanical ventilation after cardiac surgery. *Br J Anaesth.* 2007;99(2):252–261; and Barker N, Lim J, Amari E, Malherbe S, Ansermino JM. Relationship between age and spontaneous ventilation during intravenous anesthesia in children. *Paediatr Anaesth.* 2007;17(10):948–955.)

TABLE 7.12	Remifentanil Pharmacokinetics by Age					
	0–2 Months	**2 Months–2 Years**	**2–6 Years**	**7–12 Years**	**13–16 Years**	**16–18 Years**
C_{max}	24.2 ± 10.2[a]	25.4 ± 3.7[a]	34.8 ± 8.2	42.5 ± 13.7	35 ± 10.2	42.7 ± 12.9
Vdss	452.8 ± 144.7[a]	307.9 ± 89.2	240.1 ± 130.5	248.9 ± 91.4	223.2 ± 30.6	242.5 ± 109.2
CL (mL/minute per kilogram)	90.5 ± 36.8[a]	92.1 ± 25.8[a]	76 ± 22.4	59.7 ± 22.5	57.2 ± 21.1	46.5 ± 2.1
Half-life (minutes)	5.4 ± 1.8	3.4 ± 1.19	3.6 ± 1.19	5.3 ± 1.4	3.7 ± 1.1	5.7 ± 0.7

CL, clearance; C_{max}, peak plasma concentration; Vdss, volume of distribution at steady state.
[a]Significantly different from other groups.
Data extracted from Ross AK, Davis PJ, Dear G, et al. Pharmacokinetics of remifentanil in anesthetized pediatric patients undergoing elective surgery or diagnostic procedures. *Anesth Analg.* 2001;93(6):1393–1401.

concentration of 14 μg/L would typically achieve a 30% decrease in mean arterial pressure. This concentration is twice that required for laparotomy but is easily achieved with a bolus injection. The $T_{1/2}keo$ of 0.86 minutes for this hemodynamic effect[58] is less than remifentanil-induced spectral edge frequency changes described in adults ($T_{1/2}keo$ of 1.34 minutes).[184,1464]

One theoretical concern associated with the long-term administration of remifentanil is the development of acute tolerance. In a study of adult volunteers, the analgesic threshold was one-fourth of the peak values within 3 hours.[1465] A study of adolescents undergoing spinal instrumentation for scoliosis has also demonstrated acute tolerance.[1466] Another prospective randomized trial in children 1 to 5 years of age undergoing laparoscopic procedures that compared three remifentanil infusions of 0, 0.3, 0.6, and 0.9 μg/kg per minute found that those who received 0.6 or 0.9 μg/kg per minute required more postoperative fentanyl at 24 hours than those who received 0 or 0.3 μg/kg per minute, suggesting that large doses of remifentanil may cause tolerance.[1467]

Remifentanil has an important role in providing safe analgesia to children of all ages, but particularly in very sick preterm infants and children.[1458-1472] Its main advantage is the ability to provide an intense opioid effect with cardiovascular stability during the procedure, and then transition to a less intense opioid effect, allowing for early extubation.[1468,1473] *Remifentanil is the only opioid for which there is a greater rather than a reduced clearance (per kilogram) in neonates (see Fig. 7.26), and the reason that it is so valuable in this age group.*[1474-1481] These pharmacologic differences have important clinical implications because they translate into the ability to rapidly titrate the opioid effect, without regard to prolonged sedation. *This opioid should be administered only by continuous infusion. If an IV line becomes interrupted, kinked, or disconnected, the opioid effect will rapidly dissipate and the child will show evidence of pain.* Therefore this drug should be "piggybacked" into a continuous infusion carrier as close to the IV cannula as possible to provide smooth constant drug delivery. In neonates, a more dilute concentration is useful (e.g., 5 μg/mL). This also means that at the end of a procedure, the anesthetic plan must include a transition to some other form of analgesia, including another longer acting opioid or a regional block.[1482]

Although remifentanil can be administered as a loading dose, 0.1 to 0.25 μg/kg, the risk of hypotension and the rapidity of achieving steady-state analgesia (0.05–0.15 μg/kg per minute) with an infusion renders a loading dose unnecessary. However, if a loading dose is used, then the plasma concentration, rather than effect-site concentration, is commonly targeted.[733] The infusion may be titrated to effect with little fear of producing an "overdose" because of the very favorable PK. As with many synthetic opioids, severe bradycardia and hypotension may occur after bolus administration, especially at large doses.[185,1483] Remifentanil may have a direct negative chronotropic effect; therefore the concomitant use of a vagolytic or pancuronium may prevent this adverse cardiac response.[1484,1485] The negative chronotropic effect and the concomitant decrease in BP at large concentrations (e.g., 15–20 ng/mL) may also be used to induce controlled hypotension.[1486,1487]

Remifentanil would seem to be the ideal opioid to provide a deep analgesic effect that allows spinal cord–evoked motor and sensory monitoring.[1488,1489] Nonetheless, anesthesia is not produced by opioids alone. An anxiolytic must be administered to ensure that amnesia occurs. The half-lives of all anxiolytics exceed that of remifentanil, and this needs to be considered during recovery.

Remifentanil has also been used to supplement propofol to facilitate endotracheal intubation without the use of an NMBD.[1490] Several dose-response studies found that about 3 μg/kg of remifentanil combined with ~3 to 4 mg/kg of propofol provided the best intubating conditions, similar to those with an NMBD. Remifentanil 2 μg/kg did not produce satisfactory intubating conditions.[744] Resumption of spontaneous respirations after a remifentanil–propofol combination was similar to that after succinylcholine.[1462,1491,1492] This combination is a reasonable alternative to succinylcholine to facilitate tracheal intubation in children.

BUTORPHANOL AND NALBUPHINE

Butorphanol (Stadol) and nalbuphine (Nubain) are synthetic opioid agonist-antagonist analgesics that are equianalgesic.[1493-1496] They are effective through κ-receptor agonism and partial μ-receptor antagonism, have 0.5 to 0.7 times the potency of morphine, and an antagonist effect 25 times weaker than naloxone. An appealing PD effect is sedation, particularly when compared with midazolam.[1493,1496-1499] The elimination half-life of nalbuphine is significantly smaller in children 1.5 to 5 years of age (0.9 hours) than in children 5 to 8.5 years of age (1.9 hours) and in adults (2.3 hours). A half-life of 4 hours has been reported in neonates, reflecting immaturity of hepatic glucuronide metabolism. The half-life of butorphanol is similar to that of nalbuphine at about 3 hours in adults.[1496,1500-1502] Nalbuphine PK have been reported using allometric scaling in children 1 to 10 years: CL 130 L/hour per 70 kg, Q 75.6 L/hour per 70 kg, V1 210 L/70 kg, and V2 151 L/70 kg.[1502]

Both of these drugs can be administered orally with bioavailability in young adults of 12% to 17%, but this dramatically increases to about 80% when administered to the nasal mucosa.[1501,1503-1505] The claimed advantage of this family of drugs is adequate analgesia with a ceiling on respiratory depression[1493,1494,1506-1508]; thus there is some popularity for use in children,[1509-1515] although a systematic review reported that quantitative analysis of nalbuphine compared with other analgesics for postoperative pain management was lacking.[1516] The administration of butorphanol by the nasal route may offer particular advantage for children without IV access.[1509,1517-1520] One report suggested that the frequency of postoperative vomiting after butorphanol was less than with morphine.[1510] Another describes the use of rectal administration; as expected, the authors found irregular absorption, but peak blood levels were relatively rapidly achieved (25 ± 11 minutes), and the elimination half-life was 2.7 ± 0.7 hours.[1521] **We do not recommend the rectal route of administration.** What must be remembered is that these agents may reverse μ-receptor–mediated analgesic effects of the more potent opioids and should therefore be used as the initial or the sole opioid.

This family of drugs has had mixed results in reversing or preventing opioid-induced pruritus.[1522,1523] Nalbuphine does not reverse respiratory depression after morphine,[1524] but may be effective after fentanyl.[1525] Butorphanol has also been administered by the caudal epidural route (25 μg/kg).[1526,1527]

CODEINE

Codeine, or methylmorphine, is a morphine-like opioid with 10% of the potency of morphine. It is mainly metabolized by glucuronidation, but minor pathways are by N-demethylation to norcodeine and O-demethylation to morphine. However, a full accounting of the metabolism of codeine has remained elusive. Approximately 10% of codeine is metabolized to morphine. As the affinity of codeine for opioid receptors is very low, the analgesic effect of codeine is a result of its morphine metabolite.[1528] Evidence suggests that up to 11% of codeine is metabolized to hydrocodone,[1529] which may provide an alternate mechanism of analgesia to its metabolism to morphine. The continued use of this minor opium alkaloid for pediatric analgesia remains baffling because it is effectively a prodrug analgesic and is highly subject to genomic variations resulting in either no analgesia or potential drug overdose (see further text and Chapters 6 and 33); most children's hospitals have removed this drug from their pharmacy because of safety concerns.[1157,1530-1533] The American Academy of Pediatrics recommended a better understanding of the dangers of this drug and the need for alternative methods for analgesia, particularly in obese children with the potential for OSA.[1534] In 2013 the U.S. FDA issued a black box warning against the use of codeine in children after tonsillectomy and adenoidectomy (T&A) surgeries after a number of deaths were attributed to overdoses associated with undiagnosed ultrarapid polymorphisms; this has resulted in a sharp reduction in the prescriptions of codeine after T&A surgery (see Chapters 6 and 33). The FDA recently extended this warning to obese children and those with OSA or lung disease who are less than 18 years of age undergoing T&A.[1534a] St. Jude's Research Hospital, however, addressed the CYP2D6 polymorphism issue by identifying the CYP2D6 polymorphisms in hundreds of children with sickle cell disease and obviating the use of codeine in those with the poor and ultrarapid polymorphisms.[1535] The remainder of the children were successfully managed with codeine for their sickle cell disease.

The primary routes for delivery of codeine are the oral and IM routes, although the rectal route has also been advocated.[1536] The dose of codeine by all three routes is similar, 0.5 to 1.5 mg/kg. IV codeine was used in the past, but serious life-threatening adverse effects, including transient but severe cardiorespiratory depression[1537-1539] and seizures,[1540] led to proscription of this route of delivery.

Codeine's popularity as a perioperative analgesic in children is based in part on its favorable PK. When given orally, it is rapidly and completely absorbed, with 50% undergoing first-pass hepatic metabolism. Bioavailability after oral codeine is 90%, although after surgery the bioavailability may be quite variable.[1528,1541] Blood concentrations after oral codeine reach a peak by 1 hour. Its terminal elimination half-life is 3 to 3.5 hours. When given by the IM and rectal routes, peak blood concentrations are achieved rapidly, within 0.5 hours, with the blood concentrations after the rectal route being less than after the IM route. The duration of action after these two routes of administration is 1 to 2 hours. The elimination half-life after rectal administration in children is approximately 2.6 hours in children, but 4.6 hours in infants,[1542] suggesting the need for a much greater interval between subsequent doses in infants. A Vd of 3.6 L/kg and a CL of 0.85 L/hour have been described in adults, but there are few data detailing the developmental changes in children.

In vivo, 5% to 15% of codeine is excreted unchanged in the urine. The remaining 85% to 95% undergoes metabolism in the liver by one of three routes: glucuronidation (principal route), O-demethylation, and N-demethylation.[1528] Five percent to 15% of codeine undergoes O-demethylation to morphine. This metabolic pathway depends on CYP2D6, an enzyme responsible for the metabolism of more than 20% of prescribed medications. The N-demethylation pathway depends on the CYP3A enzyme system.

The wide array of CYP2D6 polymorphisms of codeine may be summarized into three broad categories: poor metabolizers (PM, negligible morphine produced), extensive metabolizers (EM, normal), and ultrarapid metabolizers (UM, rapid production and large amounts of morphine produced). Up to 10% of Caucasians and 30% of Hong Kong Chinese are PM, rendering codeine an ineffective analgesic for these children.[1528] Alternately, 29% of the Ethiopian and 1% of Swedish, German, and Chinese populations are UM.[1528] Recent evidence suggested that the frequency of CYP2D6 polymorphisms, particularly in children who are PM, may be more common and more varied than previously thought. Children with these polymorphisms who also have upregulated opioid receptors as a result of long-term intermittent nocturnal hypoxia may be particularly vulnerable to a mishap after a usual or subclinical dose of codeine.[1253,1254] Consequently, the wide clinical response to a standard (or less than standard) dose of codeine necessitates careful monitoring in those with compromised cardiorespiratory status or with obesity and possible OSA. Several deaths or near-deaths have been reported with "standard" doses of oral codeine in children later found to be UM.[1253,1532,1543-1545]

Codeine may be effective for pain control, although its limited conversion to morphine likely makes it suitable for only mild and moderate forms of pain. The limited conversion to morphine and fewer adverse effects of codeine have made it popular for infants and young children, particularly when a single dose is involved. There is some evidence that codeine is associated with less nausea and vomiting than morphine.[1546] Codeine is often used in combination with acetaminophen or NSAIDs. The addition of codeine to acetaminophen has been shown to improve postoperative pain relief in infants.[1547] One study found that the analgesic effect of the combination of acetaminophen (10–15 mg/kg) and codeine (1–1.5 mg/kg) was comparable to that of ibuprofen (5–10 mg/kg) in children after tonsillectomy.[1548]

In PM, codeine confers little or no analgesia, although adverse effects persist.[1549] In ultrarapid metabolizers on the other hand, a large incidence of adverse effects might be expected, including apnea, because of large plasma morphine concentrations. Administration (especially of codeine preparations with an antihistamine and a decongestant) in the neonate may cause intoxication.[1252,1534,1550] A mother who ingested codeine while breastfeeding is thought to have transferred morphine in the breast milk, resulting in a fatality in her neonate. The mother, an UM, produced morphine more rapidly from the codeine, which resulted in respiratory depression in the neonate.[1543,1551] Because of the unpredictable variability in converting codeine to morphine, we recommend alternative medications.[1552] We no longer recommend codeine unless the child's blood is tested for CYP2D6 polymorphisms; if the child is a PM, he or she will receive very little analgesia with codeine. If a child is an UM, he or she could sustain a life-threatening event because of increased conversion to morphine.[1553]

TRAMADOL

Tramadol (Ultram) is a weak opioid with minimal effects on respiration and causes monoaminergic spinal cord inhibition of pain.[1554-1557] This formulation is structurally related to morphine and codeine.[1557] Two enantiomers provide analgesia; one is a opioid μ-receptor agonist, and the other inhibits neuronal reuptake of serotonin and inhibits norepinephrine uptake, thus producing "multimodal antinociception."[1557] It is primarily metabolized into O-desmethyltramadol (M1) by CYP2D6. PM have both reduced analgesia and reduced nausea.[1558,1559] Unfortunately, the identification of genotype does not predict phenotype. Those classed as PM may have normal clearance (see Fig. 6.2). The active M1 metabolite has a μ-receptor affinity approximately 200 times greater than tramadol. Tramadol provides analgesia both from the parent compound (target concentration 100 ng/mL) and from its M1 metabolite (target concentration 15 ng/mL).[1560]

Tramadol clearance increases from 25 weeks PCA (5.52 L/hour per 70 kg) to reach 84% of the mature value (8.58 L/hour per 70 kg) by 44 weeks PMA.[1561] A target concentration of 300 μg/L is achieved after a bolus of tramadol hydrochloride of 1 mg/kg, and can be maintained by an infusion of tramadol hydrochloride at 0.09 mg/kg per hour at 25 weeks, 0.14 mg/kg per hour at 30 weeks, and 0.18 mg/kg per hour at 40 weeks PMA.[1561] CYP2D6 activity was observed as early as 25 weeks PCA.[1561] Clearance in children is similar to that in adults, using standardized allometric models.[1562] Tramadol has been shown to be effective for moderate to severe pain in a variety of pediatric populations and may offer some advantage for the treatment of pain after tonsillectomy in children with OSA.[1563-1571] Because of the metabolism by CYP2D6 polymorphisms, the FDA has issued a similar contraindication for use in children <18 years of age undergoing T&A.[1534a] Apnea is associated with a 10-fold dosing error in children (>9 mg/kg).[1572] One formulation is prescribed in drops rather than in milliliters and this can confuse caregivers and result in an accidental overdose.[1573]

Tramadol (1.5–2 mg/kg) has been administered rectally with peak plasma concentrations occurring at approximately 2 hours.[1574] Tramadol has also been administered in the caudal epidural space[1277] with longer-lasting analgesia than when administered intravenously.[1575] Caudal epidural tramadol (5%, 2 mg/kg) was also compared with caudal epidural bupivacaine (0.25%, 2 mg/kg) and found to provide superior analgesia.[1576] *Caudal administration is not recommended until further clarification of potential neurotoxicity.*[1563,1577] Tramadol has also been very useful as a transition to oral analgesics after IV therapy (see Chapter 44). The low incidence of respiratory depression and constipation, fewer controls on use, and similar frequency of nausea and vomiting (10%–40%) compared with other opioids make tramadol an attractive alternative.[1578]

TAPENTADOL

Tapentadol (Nucynta, Palexia, and Tapal) is an oral opioid analgesic in the benzenoid class with a dual mechanism of action that is similar to tramadol; it is a μ-opioid receptor agonist and also inhibits the reuptake of norepinephrine. Its advantage over tramadol is that it has only weak effects on the reuptake of serotonin and is a more potent opioid with no known active metabolites.[1579] We might anticipate better analgesia than following tramadol in those children who are PM of CYP2D6. It is generally regarded as a weak-moderate strength opioid that can be reversed with naloxone.

Tapentadol is cleared by glucuronide conjugation in the liver and, although not reported, it is anticipated that clearance maturation will be similar to other drugs cleared by this route (acetaminophen, morphine). Experience in children is limited. Adverse effect profiles (nausea, dizziness, vomiting, and somnolence) appear similar to those described for tramadol.[1580] Tapentadol produces both nociceptive and neuropathic pain relief, but there are concerns about abuse and dependence. Caution with the use of tapentadol within 14 days after cessation of monoamine oxidase inhibitors is advised because of fear that serotonin syndrome could occur.[1581]

Acetaminophen

Acetaminophen (Tylenol, paracetamol) is widely used in the management of pain, but lacks antiinflammatory effects. Prostaglandin H_2 synthase (PGHS) is the enzyme responsible for metabolism of arachidonic acid to the unstable prostaglandin H_2. The two major forms of this enzyme are the constitutive PGHS-1 (COX-1) and the inducible PGHS-2 (COX-2). PGHS has two sites, a cyclooxygenase (COX) site and a peroxidase (POX) site. The conversion of arachidonic acid to prostaglandin G_2, the precursor of the other prostaglandins (E-Fig. 7.19), depends on a tyrosine-385 radical at the COX active site. Acetaminophen acts as a reducing cosubstrate on the POX site. Alternatively, acetaminophen effects may be mediated by an active metabolite (p-aminophenol). p-Aminophenol is conjugated with arachidonic acid by fatty acid amide hydrolase and exerts its effect through cannabinoid receptors.[1582]

The ED_{50} for rectal acetaminophen to reduce the need for supplemental opioids after day-stay surgery is 35 mg/kg.[1583] Further studies are required before regular doses greater than 40 mg/kg can be recommended because of concerns about hepatotoxicity,[1583–1585] which can occur after single doses of 250 mg/kg.[1586] Time delays of approximately 1 hour between peak concentration and peak effect have been reported.[1587,1588] An estimate of a maximum effect was 5.17 (the greatest possible pain relief [Visual Analog Scale (VAS) 0 to 10] would equate to an Emax of 10 out of 10 pain units) and an EC_{50} of 9.98 mg/L. The $T_{1/2}keo$ of the analgesic effect compartment was 53 minutes.[1587,1589] A target effect compartment concentration of 10 mg/L was associated with a pain reduction of 2.6/10.[1589]

The relative bioavailability of rectal to oral acetaminophen formulations (rectal/oral) is approximately 0.5 in children but the relative bioavailability is greater in neonates and approaches unity.[106] There are two IV acetaminophen formulations available, and caution must be exercised with the choice of formulation.[1590] One is an acetaminophen formulation,[1591] whereas the other, propacetamol (N-acetyl-para-aminophenoldiethyl aminoacetic ester), is a water-soluble prodrug of acetaminophen that can be administered intravenously over 15 minutes. It is rapidly hydroxylated into acetaminophen (1 g propacetamol = 0.5 g acetaminophen).[1592]

The $T_{1/2}abs$ of acetaminophen from the duodenum is rapid (4.5 minutes) in children who were given acetaminophen as an elixir.[1593] The $T_{1/2}abs$ in infants younger than 3 months was delayed (16.6 minutes), consistent with delayed gastric emptying in young infants.[106,1593] In contrast, rectal absorption is slow and erratic with large variability. For example, absorption parameters for the triglyceride base were a $T_{1/2}abs$ of 1.34 hours (CV = 90%) with a lag time before absorption began of 8 minutes (CV = 31%). The $T_{1/2}abs$ for rectal formulations was prolonged in infants younger than 3 months (1.51 times greater) compared with older children.[1594]

Sulfate metabolism is the dominant route of elimination in neonates, whereas glucuronide conjugation (via UGT1A6) is dominant in adults. A total body clearance of 0.74 L/hour per 70 kg at 28 weeks PMA and 4.9 L/hour per 70 kg (CV = 38%) in full-term neonates after enteral acetaminophen has been reported using an allometric ¾-power model.[1594,1595] Clearance increases over the first year of life (see Fig. 7.11) and reaches 80% of that in older children (16 L/hour per 70 kg) by 6 months postnatal age.[106,169] Similar clearance estimates are reported in neonates after IV formulations of acetaminophen.[1595,1596] The relative bioavailability of the oral formulation is 0.9.

The Vd for acetaminophen is 49 to 70 L/70 kg. The Vd decreases exponentially, with a TM_{50} of 11.5 weeks, from 109.7 L/70 kg at 28 weeks PCA to 72.9 L/70 kg by 60 weeks PMA, reflective of fetal body composition and water distribution changes over the first few months of life.[106]

The toxic metabolite of acetaminophen, N-acetyl-p-benzoquinone imine (NAPQI), is formed by CYP2E1, 1A2, and 3A4. This metabolite binds to intracellular hepatic macromolecules to produce cell necrosis and other damage. Infants younger than 90 days postnatal age have decreased expression of CYP2E1 activity in vitro compared with older infants, children, and adults,[1597] CYP3A4 appears during the first week after birth, whereas CYP1A2 appears later.[1] Neonates can produce hepatotoxic metabolites (e.g., NAPQI), but the reduced activity of CYP in neonates may explain the rare occurrence of acetaminophen-induced hepatotoxicity in neonates.[1598,1599] Nonetheless, two massive 10-fold overdoses of acetaminophen were reported in infants and underscore the need for extreme care when administering IV forms of acetaminophen.[1600] Neither infant progressed to acute liver necrosis and both recovered fully.

Acetaminophen is useful as an adjunct to spare opioids.[59,1583,1601–1606] Acetaminophen can be administered orally before induction of anesthesia to achieve a therapeutic blood concentration at the time of emergence, even after brief surgery, such as myringotomy and tube insertion. For procedures of greater duration, rectal administration of acetaminophen at the beginning of surgery provides therapeutic blood concentrations at the time of emergence and before the child would be likely to tolerate oral medications.[1607] The current maximum 24 hour dosing of oral acetaminophen varies around the world between 75 and 90 mg/kg per day in hospitalized children, although the total daily dose should be reduced in neonates.[1608] Suppository doses of 35 to 40 mg/kg followed by 20 mg/kg every 6 hours have been proposed for children for the first 24 hours,[1608] consistent with reduced bioavailability and slower absorption of rectal formulations.[1609]

A review of acetaminophen-associated toxicity revealed 76 children with hepatic injury and 26 deaths after repeated administration in children younger than 6 years of age; no deaths or injury occurred when the total daily dose was less than 75 mg/kg in children.[1610] It is difficult to assess those prone to hepatotoxicity after routine dosing. Liver function changes during therapy are commonly transitory and may not reflect hepatotoxicity.[1611]

Nonsteroidal Antiinflammatory Agents

The NSAIDs are a heterogeneous group of compounds that share common antipyretic, analgesic, and antiinflammatory effects. NSAIDs act by reducing prostaglandin biosynthesis through inhibition of the COX site of the PGHS enzyme (see E-Fig. 7.19).

The prostanoids produced by the COX-1 isoenzyme protect the gastric mucosa, regulate renal blood flow, and induce platelet aggregation. NSAID-induced gastrointestinal toxicity, for example, is likely mediated through blockade of COX-1 activity, whereas the antiinflammatory effects of NSAIDs are likely mediated primarily through inhibition of the inducible isoform, COX-2.

The NSAIDs are commonly used in children for antipyresis and analgesia. The antiinflammatory properties of the NSAIDs have, in addition, been used in such diverse disorders as juvenile idiopathic arthritis, renal and biliary colic, dysmenorrhea, Kawasaki disease, and cystic fibrosis. The NSAIDs indomethacin and ibuprofen are also used to treat delayed closure of PDA in preterm infants.[1612–1615] One prospective study found paracetamol to be as effective as indomethacin and ibuprophen for ductal closure, but conferring fewer side effects on renal function, platelet count, and bleeding events.[1617]

NSAID-associated analgesia has been compared with analgesia from other analgesics or analgesic modalities (e.g., caudal blockade, acetaminophen, or morphine) in children. These data confirm that NSAIDs in children are effective analgesic drugs, improving the quality of analgesia, but the effects are poorly quantified.[1618] Data from adults given ibuprofen after dental extraction suggest a similar Emax to that described for acetaminophen (1.54 on a scale 0 to 3), with an EC_{50} of 10.2 mg/L.[1619] The $T_{1/2}$keo of 28 minutes was less than the 53 minutes reported for acetaminophen.[1589] In addition, the slope (reflected by the Hill coefficient, see Fig. 7.6) of the concentration-response curve was steeper than that for acetaminophen (Hill = 2 for ibuprofen, Hill = 1 for acetaminophen), indicating a more rapid onset of analgesia. Parameter estimates for acetaminophen and some common NSAIDs using a sigmoid Emax model are shown in Table 7.13.

NSAIDs are rapidly absorbed in the gastrointestinal tract after oral administration in children. The relative bioavailability of oral preparations approaches unity. The rate and extent of absorption after rectal administration of NSAIDs, such as ibuprofen, diclofenac, flurbiprofen, indomethacin, and nimesulide, are less than after the oral routes.

Diclofenac, 2-[(2,6-dichlorophenyl) amino] benzene acetic acid, has an approximate relative COX-1/COX-2 specificity ratio of 1. Formulations may be administered orally, topically, intraocularly, intraarticularly, intravenously, intramuscularly, and rectally. Diclofenac is metabolized by P450 (CYP2C9, 3A4, and 3A5) phase I hydroxylation and phase II conjugation. The principal metabolite in humans is the 4′-hydroxyl derivative of diclofenac (D4OH), metabolized by CYP 2C9. The 4′-hydroxyl metabolite has 30% of the antiinflammatory and antipyretic activity of diclofenac.[1620] Diclofenac is rapidly absorbed when administered rectally; the $T_{1/2abs}$ of the suppository formulations is 35 minutes, with a lag time (T_{LAG}) of 11 minutes.[1621]

There are few IV NSAID formulations available. Parecoxib sodium is an IV NSAID with increased use in pediatric practice despite limited data concerning PK and PD in this population.[1622–1624] Parecoxib is a prodrug that is rapidly and completely converted to valdecoxib (the active metabolite) within 0.5 to 1 hour. Valdecoxib acts by specifically inhibiting COX-2–mediated prostaglandin synthesis. Onset of analgesia in adults was 7.14 minutes with a peak effect within 2 hours and duration of analgesia that ranged from 6 to 24 hours. Valdecoxib is extensively metabolized by the liver through the cytochrome P450 pathways (CYP3A4 and CYP2C9). The Vd of most NSAIDs is small in adults (<0.2 L/kg) but larger in children. Preterm neonates (22–31 weeks gestational age) given IV ibuprofen had a Vd of 0.62 ± 0.04 L/kg.[1625] One paper reported a dramatic reduction in ibuprofen central volume after closure of the PDA in preterm neonates (0.244 vs .0171 L/kg).[1626] The NSAIDs, as a group, are weakly acidic, lipophilic, and highly protein bound. The impact of altered protein binding is probably minimal with routine dosing, because NSAIDs cleared by the liver have a low hepatic extraction ratio.[82]

NSAIDs undergo extensive phase I and phase II enzyme biotransformation in the liver, with subsequent excretion into urine or bile. Renal elimination is not an important elimination pathway for the commonly used NSAIDs. PK parameter variability is large, in part attributable to covariate effects of age, size, and pharmacogenomics. Ibuprofen, for example, is metabolized by the CYP2C9 and CYP2C8 subfamily. Considerable variation exists in the expression of CYP2C activities among individuals, and functional polymorphism of the gene coding for CYP2C9 has been described.[1627] CYP2C9 activity is low immediately after birth (21% of adult values), subsequently increasing progressively to reach a peak activity within 3 months, when expressed as milligrams per hour per kilogram.[1628]

Clearance (liters per hour per kilogram) is generally greater in children than it is in adults, as we might expect when the linear per-kilogram model is used. Ibuprofen clearance maturation follows the similar pattern to other drugs (e.g., Fig. 7.5). Clearance increases from 2.06 mL/hour per kilogram in extreme preterm neonates 22 to 31 weeks PMA,[1625] to 9.49 mL/hour per kilogram in preterm neonates 28 weeks PMA,[1626] peaking at 140 mL/hour per kilogram in preschool children, before decreasing again during late childhood and adolescence (71 mL/hour per kilogram).[1629] Similar data exist for indomethacin.[1612,1630,1631]

Many NSAIDs exhibit stereoselectivity.[1632] Ibuprofen stereoselectivity is reported in preterm neonates (<28 weeks gestation). R- and S-ibuprofen half-lives were about 10 hours and 25.5 hours, respectively. The mean clearance of R-ibuprofen (12.7 mL/hour) was about 2.5-fold greater than that of S-ibuprofen (5.0 mL/hour).[1633]

During pregnancy, there is relatively little transfer of NSAIDs from maternal to fetal blood. Very small quantities of NSAIDs are secreted into breast milk. Similarly, infant exposure to ketorolac via breast milk is estimated to be only 0.4% of maternal exposure.[1634]

TABLE 7.13	Parameter Estimates for the Sigmoid Emax Equation for Some Common NSAIDs and Paracetamol			
Parameter	Paracetamol	Ibuprofen	Ketorolac	Diclofenac
Emax (0–10)	5.2	5.1	8.5	4.89
EC_{50}	9.8 mg/L	10.2 mg/L	0.37 mg/L	1.2 mg/L
N	1	2	1	1
$T_{1/2}$keo	53 minutes	28 minutes	24 minutes	14 minutes
Reference	1609	1619	1664	1649

From Anderson BJ, Hannam JA. Considerations when using PKPD modeling to determine effectiveness of simple analgesics in children. *Expert Opin Drug Metab Toxicol.* 2015;11(9):1393–1408, with permission

NSAIDs undergo drug interactions through altered clearance and competition for active renal tubular secretion with other organic acids. A large fractional protein binding has been proposed to explain drug interactions between NSAIDs and oral anticoagulant agents, oral hypoglycemics, sulfonamides, bilirubin, and other protein-bound drugs. The classic example is that of the coadministration of warfarin and phenylbutazone (an NSAID). Both the plasma warfarin concentration and the prothrombin time were increased.[1635] However, even though phenylbutazone displaces warfarin from its albumin binding sites in vitro, this observation does not explain the changes in prothrombin time. The increased prothrombin time has been attributed to increased serum warfarin concentrations, which stems from its reduced clearance, and not from changes in protein binding.[82] Both warfarin and phenylbutazone compete for similar protein binding sites; they also compete for similar clearance pathways. NSAIDs have the potential to cause gastrointestinal irritation, blood clotting disorders, renal impairment, neutrophil dysfunction, and bronchoconstriction, effects attributed to COX-1/COX-2 ratios, although this concept may be an oversimplification.

Ibuprofen reduces the GFR by 20% in preterm neonates, affecting aminoglycoside clearance, an effect that appears to be independent of gestational age.[1636] No significant difference in the change in cerebral blood volume, change in cerebral blood flow, or tissue oxygenation index was found between administration of ibuprofen or placebo in neonates.[1637] The risk of acute gastrointestinal bleeding in children given short-term ibuprofen was estimated to be 7.2/100,000 (CI 2–18 per 100,000), a prevalence not different from children given acetaminophen.[1638,1639] The incidence of clinically significant gastropathy in children with juvenile arthritis given NSAIDs is comparable to that in adults given long-term NSAIDs, but the prevalence of gastroduodenal injury may be greater, depending on the assessment criteria applied (e.g., abdominal pain, anemia, endoscopy).[1640,1641] Aspirin- or NSAID-exacerbated respiratory disease (ERD) occurs more frequently in adults, although instances in children and teenagers have been reported.[1642] These cases are countered by reports that the symptoms of asthma improved when ibuprofen was administered for antipyresis. One study concluded that a benefit is likely to occur in younger children with mild episodic asthma and that aspirin-ERD is a concern in one in three teenagers with severe asthma and coexistent nasal disease.[1643] COX-2 inhibitors are reported to be safe in NSAID-ERD.[1643]

The commonly used NSAIDs have reversible antiplatelet effects, which are attributable to the inhibition of thromboxane synthesis. Bleeding time is usually slightly increased, but remains within normal limits in children with normal coagulation systems. Neonates given prophylactic ibuprofen to induce PDA closure did not have an increased frequency of intraventricular hemorrhage.[1644] A Cochrane review has established that even after tonsillectomy, NSAIDs did not cause any increase in bleeding that required a return to the operating room in children. There was significantly less nausea and vomiting with NSAIDs compared with alternative analgesics, suggesting their benefits outweigh their negative aspects.[1645,1646] Recent concerns with OSA-associated deaths from opioids for postoperative pain management have resulted in several studies examining alternating doses of ibuprofen and acetaminophen; this regimen provided adequate analgesia with no increase in the incidence of posttonsillectomy bleeding requiring surgical intervention.[1647,1648] Combination therapy achieves the same maximal response (Emax), but this response is achieved using smaller doses of each drug, and the duration of effect is greater.[262,1649]

KETOROLAC

Ketorolac (Toradol) is an NSAID with very potent analgesic properties.[1650–1653] The analgesic properties of ketorolac are similar to those of low-dose morphine for posttonsillectomy analgesia.[1653,1654] Its major use in pediatric anesthesia is as an adjuvant to opioid analgesia or for the treatment of mild to moderate pain where there is a desire to reduce the potential for respiratory depression or for nausea and vomiting.[1652,1655–1660] It is an important adjuvant to the treatment of postoperative pain, especially for children who require prolonged pain management or those at risk for OSA.[1661] It is particularly useful for the transition from IV to oral therapy. Ketorolac may also be administered nasally, although pediatric perioperative data are limited.[117,1662,1663] Data from adult patients (n = 522) given a single oral or IM administration of 10, 30, 60, or 90 mg ketorolac for postoperative pain relief after orthopedic surgery, revealed an Emax of 8.5/10 (VAS 0-10), EC_{50} 0.37 mg/L, and $T_{1/2}keo$ 24 minutes.[1664] This Emax (see Fig. 7.6) is greater than that of acetaminophen or ibuprofen (see Table 7.13) and may be attributed to the population cohort of adult women suffering pain from bone fractures.

The PK, standardized using allometry, are similar in adults and children (E-Table 7.9). The terminal elimination half-life in children 4 to 8 years of age is approximately 6 hours, although there is considerable variability.[1665–1667] PK may also be influenced by chronobiology,[728] and many NSAIDs exhibit stereoselectivity. Ketorolac is supplied and administered as a racemic mixture that contains a 1:1 ratio of the R(+) and S(–) stereoisomers. Pharmacologic activity resides almost exclusively with the S(–) stereoisomer.[1632,1668] Clearance of the S(–) enantiomer was four times that of the R(+) enantiomer (6.2 vs. 1.4 mL/minute per kilogram) in children 3 to 18 years.[1669] Terminal half-life of S(–)-ketorolac was 40% that of the R(+) enantiomer (107 vs. 259 minutes), and the Vd of the S(–) enantiomer was greater than that of the R(+) form (0.82 vs. 0.50 L/kg). Recovery of S(–)-ketorolac glucuronide was 2.3 times that of the R(+) enantiomer. Because of the greater clearance and shorter half-life of S(–)-ketorolac, PK predictions based on racemic assays may overestimate the duration of pharmacologic effect.[1669]

One of the major concerns with ketorolac is the inhibition of platelet function through inhibition of cyclooxygenase, and the consequent potential for postsurgical bleeding. Ketorolac has been shown to have minimal effect on prothrombin and partial thromboplastin times but has been shown to cause modest increases in the bleeding time.[1652,1670–1673] Unlike aspirin, the ketorolac antiplatelet effect is reversible and, therefore, the effect depends on the presence of ketorolac within the body.[1674] This effect on platelet function has been of most concern in children undergoing adenotonsillectomy.[1675–1678] In the studies reporting posttonsillectomy bleeding, most involved administration of the ketorolac during or at the beginning of the surgical procedure, before hemostasis was achieved. In addition, the increased incidence of bleeding appears to be primarily during the first 24 hours, which corresponds to the several half-lives it would take to eliminate ketorolac from the body. The incidence of bleeding after the first 24 hours does not appear to be different.[1679] It would therefore be reasonable to not administer this medication until the end of surgery, after hemostasis is achieved. Some practitioners eschew this issue altogether and administer ketorolac only when the potential for a life-threatening hemorrhage is less.[1519] Concerns regarding the possibility of postoperative hemorrhage appear to be valid, but the true frequency of life-threatening bleeding exclusively the result of ketorolac administration is quite small.[1659,1680–1683] There is a dose-response relationship for this bleeding propensity; the risk associated with the drug was larger and clinically important when ketorolac was used in larger doses, in older subjects, and for more than 5 days.[1684] A systematic review found an increased risk for bleeding in adults but not in children younger than 18 years of age after tonsillectomy.[1685] Safety assessment showed no changes in renal or hepatic function tests, surgical drain output, or continuous oximetry between groups given placebo, 0.5 mg/kg, or 1 mg/kg ketorolac at 6 to 18 hours after surgery.[1632,1668] Many clinicians discuss the possible use of ketorolac with the surgeon before administering it and document the conversation in the anesthesia record. Ketorolac can be used to treat pain after congenital heart surgery without an increased risk of bleeding complications.[1681] A retrospective report of 1451 pediatric neurosurgical patients reported no increase in the incidence of bleeding with short-term therapy.[1686] Ketorolac has been safely used to provide analgesia for preterm and term infants, but the PK in this age group has not been described.[1687]

Another concern is the potential for adverse effects on bone healing, particularly spinal fusion.[1688,1689] Evidence suggests that nonunion of the spine is associated only with large-dose and not small-dose ketorolac. However, ketorolac has been used safely to provide analgesia for other types of orthopedic conditions with no evidence of delayed union or nonunion of fractures.[1690–1693] One other concern is the report of sudden and profound bradycardia after rapid IV administration of ketorolac.[1694] Although the mechanism of this response is unclear, ketorolac should be administered slowly when given intravenously.

Benzodiazepine Sedatives

These drugs produce anxiolysis, amnesia, and hypnosis. They are commonly used as adjuncts to both local and general anesthesia. Benzodiazepines bind to $GABA_A$ receptors, resulting in increased cellular chloride entry. This renders these receptors resistant to excitation because they are hyperpolarized.

MIDAZOLAM

Midazolam (Versed) is a water-soluble benzodiazepine that offers significant clinical advantages over diazepam. It is not painful when administered intravenously or intramuscularly. Midazolam is only one of a few medications that are approved as premedicants in children, and it is the only benzodiazepine approved by the FDA for use in neonates including preterms.

PK–PD relationships have been described for IV midazolam in adults. When an EEG signal is used as an effect measure, the EC_{50} is 35 to 77 ng/mL, with a $T_{1/2}keo$ of 0.9 to 1.6 minutes.[67,1695,1696] Duration of effect persists despite decreasing plasma concentrations (Fig. 7.27). The $T_{1/2}keo$ is increased in the elderly and in low cardiac output states. PK–PD relationships are more difficult to describe after oral midazolam because the active metabolite, 1-hydroxymidazolam, has approximately half the activity of the parent drug.[1697]

Sedation in children is more difficult to quantify. No PK–PD relationship was established in children, age 2 days to 17 years, who were given a midazolam infusion in the ICU. Midazolam dosing could, however, be effectively titrated to the desired level of sedation, assessed by the COMFORT distress scale (see Table 44.5).[1698] Consistent with this finding, desirable sedation in children after cardiac surgery was achieved at mean serum concentrations between 0.1 and 0.5 mg/L.[1699–1701] Plasma concentrations of 0.3 to

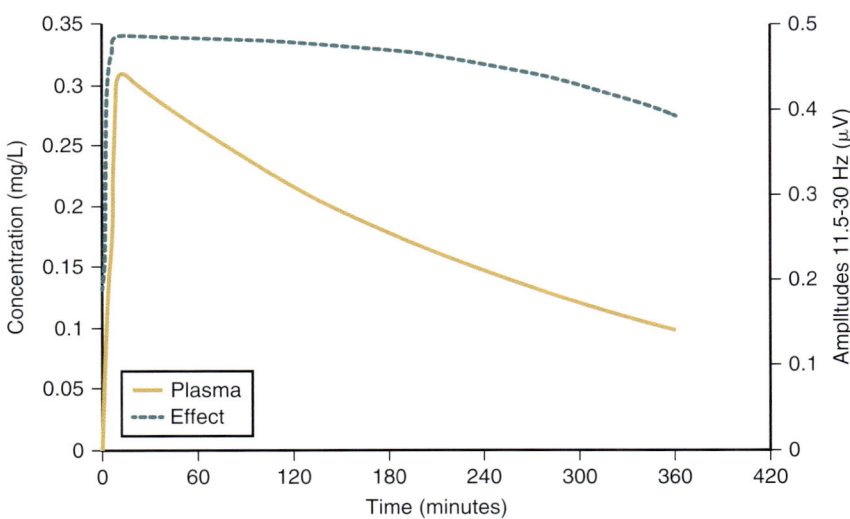

FIGURE 7.27 Plasma concentrations and effect in a neonate given midazolam bolus (0.1 mg/kg) on two early occasions (5-minute interval) to achieve sedation. Plasma concentration declines slowly because of immature clearance. Sedation recovery lags way behind the decline in plasma concentration even though a maintenance infusion was not even given. (Pharmacodynamic parameter estimates are from Mandema J, Tuk B, van Steveninck AL, Breimer DD, Cohen AF, Danhof M. Pharmacokinetic-pharmacodynamic modeling of the central nervous system effects of midazolam and its main metabolite alpha-hydroxymidazolam in healthy volunteers. *Clin Pharm Ther.* 1992;51(6):715–728.) (From Wolf A, Blackwood B, Anderson BJ. Tolerance to sedative drugs in PICU: can it be moderated or is it immutable? *Intensive Care Med.* 2016;42(2):278–281.)

0.4 mg/L are associated with anesthesia in adults.[1702,1703] A target concentration for sedation (arouses to command) in adults is 0.1 mg/L.[170]

Midazolam is metabolized mainly by hepatic hydroxylation (CYP3A4).[1704] These hydroxylated metabolites are glucuronidated and excreted in the urine. CYP3A7 is the dominant CYP3A enzyme in utero and in the neonate; it is expressed in the fetal liver and appears to have activity from as early as 50 to 60 days after conception. CYP3A4 expression increases dramatically after the first week of life, reaching 30% to 40% of adult expression by 1 month.[1427] Midazolam has a hepatic extraction ratio in the intermediate range of 0.3 to 0.7. Metabolic clearance depends on both liver perfusion and enzyme activity.

Clearance is reduced in neonates (0.8–2.2 mL/minute per kilogram, 60 mL/minute per 70 kg) (E-Fig. 7.20),[1705-1712] but increases rapidly (Hill coefficient = 3) after 39 weeks PMA,[1709] to reach 90% mature clearance at 1 year of age.[1712] Mature clearance was 523 mL/minute per 70 kg. The TM_{50} was 73.6 weeks.[1710,1712] Central Vd is related to weight (V1 = 0.591 ± 0.065 L/kg), whereas peripheral Vd remained constant (V2 = 0.42 ± 0.11 L) in 187 neonates weighing 0.7 to 5.2 kg.[1709] It has been suggested that midazolam induces its own clearance.[1699] The latter observation, from infants after cardiac surgery, likely results from the improved hepatic function after the insult of CPB. Neonates have an increase in Vdss during extracorporeal membrane oxygenation therapy (0.8 L/kg–4.1 L/kg), caused by sequestration of midazolam by the circuitry, although clearance (1.4 ± 0.15 mL/minute per kilogram) was unchanged.[1713]

Clearance may be reduced in the presence of clinical illness.[1714,1715] A reduced clearance of midazolam has been reported after circulatory arrest for cardiac surgery.[1716] Covariates, such as renal failure, hepatic failure,[1701] and concomitant administration of CYP3A inhibitors,[686,687] are important predictors of altered midazolam and metabolite PK in pediatric intensive care patients.[1717] The clearance of midazolam was reduced by 30% in neonates receiving sympathomimetic amines, probably as a consequence of the underlying compromised hemodynamics.[1709]

The suggested infusion rate of midazolam is 0.5 µg/kg per minute for preterm infants younger than 32 weeks gestational age and 1.0 µg/kg per minute for infants more than 32 weeks gestational age. Any factor that impairs hepatic blood flow (e.g., CPB, vasopressors) may decrease midazolam elimination, although cirrhosis only minimally affects its elimination in adults.[1716-1719] Midazolam offers the best PK profile for neonates because the active metabolite has a half-life similar to the parent compound, but with minimal clinical activity.[1341] *Bolus administration to preterm and term neonates has been associated with profound hypotension; the likelihood may be greater if fentanyl is also administered.*[1350] *Likewise, a neonate who is receiving a midazolam infusion is more likely to suffer profound hypotension with a bolus of fentanyl.* Rapid IV and nasal administration have also been associated with myoclonic activity.[1720] Midazolam has been administered as a continuous infusion, both in the OR as an adjunct to general anesthesia and in the ICU.[854,1721-1723] Prolonged administration leads to tolerance, dependency, and benzodiazepine withdrawal.[1724,1725] Long-term infusions, particularly in neonates, should be tapered over days while carefully monitoring for signs of withdrawal (vomiting, agitation, sweating, bowel distention, seizures, change in neurologic status).[1360,1726,1727] A theoretical concern associated with midazolam is benzyl alcohol toxicity with the development of metabolic acidosis and gasping respirations.[1728,1729] The 24-hour dose of benzyl alcohol in midazolam when administered according to recommended dosing guidelines should not cause toxicity.

Midazolam is the most commonly used benzodiazepine in pediatric anesthesia. It is administered orally, nasally, buccally, rectally, intravenously, and intramuscularly. Buccal and sublingual administration (0.3 mg/kg [maximum 10 mg]), like the nasal route, offer ease of administration, rapid systemic absorption, and avoidance of hepatic first-pass metabolism. The buccal route is popular for emergency seizure control. It is better than rectal diazepam (relative risk 1.14; 95% CI, 1.06–1.24).[120]

The desired clinical effects for anesthesia include antegrade amnesia (approximately 50%),[1730-1732] as well as sedation and anxiolysis before induction of anesthesia or a medical procedure.[899,1733-1739] One study suggested that its amnestic properties may be superior to those of diazepam.[1740] The clinical endpoint with midazolam may differ somewhat when compared with diazepam. Midazolam produces a general calming effect with minimal sedation and little effect on speech. In contrast, diazepam frequently causes obvious sedation and slurring of speech.

When midazolam was first introduced, a number of deaths were attributed to respiratory depression. These deaths were probably the result of combining large doses of midazolam with other medications, particularly opioids. An important pharmacologic difference between the benzodiazepines is that the time to achieve peak CNS effect with IV midazolam, 4.8 minutes, is almost 3-fold greater than with diazepam, 1.5 minutes (see Fig. 48.7).[67,1741] This is because of the greater fat solubility of diazepam and therefore a more rapid transit into the CNS.[1742] **Accordingly, one must wait sufficient time between doses of midazolam (3–5 minutes) to achieve the peak CNS effects before considering supplemental doses or other medications.**[1743] IV midazolam depresses the response to hypoxemia, an effect that is exaggerated in the presence of a potent opioid, such as fentanyl. This combination (0.1 mg/kg midazolam and 6 µg/kg fentanyl IV) has been associated with a respiratory arrest in an infant.[1744,1745] Children with sleep-disordered breathing who were premedicated with oral midazolam (0.5 mg/kg) experienced only a small incidence (1.5%) of transient desaturation.[1746] However, IV midazolam (0.1 mg/kg) has been shown to cause both central apnea as well as upper airway obstruction, the latter by reducing pharyngeal muscle tone.[1747] In addition, the combination of oral midazolam (0.5 mg/kg) and nitrous oxide (50%) may cause partial upper airway obstruction four times more frequently in children with large tonsils than in those with normal-sized tonsils.[1748] Interestingly, mouth opening may increase upper airway collapse, thus increasing the airway obstruction in children sedated with midazolam for dental procedures.[1749]

One final concern relates to the administration of drugs that interfere with the cytochrome isoforms that metabolize midazolam (CYP3A4). Examples of such drugs and foods are grapefruit juice, erythromycin, calcium channel blockers, and protease inhibitors.[a] The net effect is to prolong the duration of action of midazolam.

Midazolam has been used as an induction agent, but it is not as satisfactory as other agents.[1750,1752] One author (CJC) has administered as much as 1.0 mg/kg intravenously to a child without producing unconsciousness. The same dose given orally produces rapid onset of sedation and anxiolysis.[1753] Commonly used doses and routes of administration are presented in Table 7.14. The nasal route has some proponents[1733]; with an onset of sedation that may be more rapid than the oral route.[1754] There is a direct

---

[a]References 138, 661, 662, 1736, 1737, 1750, and 1751.

TABLE 7.14	Dosing and Onset Times of Midazolam in Infants and Children (Excluding Neonates)		
Route	Dose (mg/kg)	Time of Onset (Minutes)	Time to Peak Effect (Minutes)
Intravenous	0.05–0.15	~1	3–5
Intramuscular	0.1–0.2	3–5	10–20
Oral	0.25–0.75	5–30	10–30
Nasal	0.1–0.2	3–5	10–15
Rectal	0.75–1.0	5–10	10–30

See text for details.

connection with the CNS at that level (see E-Fig. 4.2),[905] and because the preservative in midazolam is neurotoxic when applied directly to neural tissue,[911] there is the theoretical risk of CNS toxicity.[905] In addition, 85% of children who receive nasal midazolam cry and complain of a bitter aftertaste.[125,1438] It would seem prudent to avoid this route of administration because the oral route appears to be equally effective and without risk.

DIAZEPAM

Diazepam (Valium) (0.2–0.3 mg/kg) is rapidly absorbed after oral administration, with peak plasma concentrations at 30 to 90 minutes; the absorption rate is more rapid in children than in adults.[1755,1756] It has been used extensively as a premedication, as an adjunct to balanced anesthesia, and for sedation, amnesia, and control of seizures. IM administration is painful and results in irregular absorption; plasma concentrations are only 60% of those obtained with a similar oral dose.[1757–1759] Rectal diazepam (0.2–0.5 mg/kg) is used for prehospital treatment of pediatric status epilepticus. The recommended IV dose is 0.1 to 0.2 mg/kg. Diazepam has been administered rectally to children for sedation in doses ranging from 0.3 to 1.0 mg/kg with satisfactory results.[1760–1763] One study found a more rapid uptake during the first 2 hours after administration when given in liquid rather than suppository form.[1760] Bioavailability after nasal administration in adults is 70% to 90% with maximal blood concentrations at ~45 minutes.[1764]

Diazepam is highly plasma bound, with a serum half-life varying from 20 to 80 hours. Its half-life is reduced in younger adults and children (~18 hours).[1760] Hepatic disease may also decrease the elimination of diazepam.[1765] Studies in neonates who received diazepam transplacentally just before delivery demonstrate prolonged drug effects and serum half-lives (40–100 hours) a result of immature hepatic excretory mechanisms and reduced hepatic blood flow (see E-Fig. 7.20).[1755,1766,1767] Diazepam undergoes oxidative metabolism by demethylation (CYP 2C19). Its active metabolite, desmethyldiazepam, has potency similar to the parent compound and a half-life as great or greater than the parent compound, thus emphasizing that caution is required when administering this benzodiazepine to neonates.[1755,1768,1769]

The preservative benzyl alcohol is present in many formulations of diazepam. This preservative should be avoided in neonates because it is difficult to metabolize, is associated with kernicterus, and can cause a metabolic acidosis.[1770–1772] The amount of benzyl alcohol that accompanies a usual dose of diazepam would likely be insufficient to cause harm to the neonate.[1773] Diazepam has respiratory depressant effects that are quite variable, especially when combined with opioids.[1774]

Diazepam is useful as an oral premedication, although midazolam has overshadowed this role. Its main disadvantage when given intravenously is pain. Administering IV lidocaine before the diazepam and administering the diazepam slowly through a rapidly flowing IV catheter minimizes this pain. Diazepam is avoided in neonates and infants because of the prolonged half-life of the drug and its metabolites. Finally, diazepam should not be administered intramuscularly because of the pain and erratic absorption.

Other Sedatives

CLONIDINE

Clonidine is also commonly used in pediatric anesthesia practice as a premedicant, as an adjunct to anesthesia and analgesic agents, to reduce ED, as an antiemetic, to prevent postoperative shivering, to supplement regional blockade, and to reduce the stress response secondary to tracheal intubation and surgery.[1775] Clonidine can be administered by the IV, IN, IM, transdermal, oral, rectal, and epidural routes.[127,1776,1777]

The clonidine target concentration depends on the effect sought. A plasma clonidine concentration range of 0.3 to 0.8 µg/L has been estimated as satisfactory for preoperative sedation in children 1 to 11 years.[1773] Fifty percent of children achieve a modified Ramsay sedation score of 3 (appears asleep, purposeful responses to verbal commands at conversation level) at a concentration of 0.79 µg/L, and 90% of children achieve this at 0.95 µg/L. The concentration required for 50% of children to achieve a sedation scale of 4 (appears asleep, purposeful responses to verbal commands but at louder than usual conversation level or requiring light glabellar tap) is slightly more at 0.85 µg/L, and 90% of children achieve this at 1.15 µg/L.[1779] A BIS of less than 60 in adults is associated with adequate anesthesia, and this is achieved with a concentration of 4 µg/L[1780]; the target concentration for analgesia in adults is greater than that for sedation. Reduction of morphine use of up to 30% is reported when clonidine is added to analgesic regimens[1780,1781] with a plasma clonidine concentration of 1.5 to 2 µg/L.[1782,1783] The biphasic hypotensive/hypertensive BP response, reported with dexmedetomidine (see later text[1784]), has also been demonstrated with clonidine. Decreases in BP were related to plasma concentration of 1.5 to 2 µg/L, but at greater concentrations the hypotensive effect was attenuated.[1785]

Approximately 50% of clonidine is eliminated unchanged by the kidney. The exact amount of clonidine that undergoes hepatic biotransformation is uncertain, but has been reported to be between 40% and 60% after IV administration.[1785–1788] The major metabolite of clonidine is p-hydroxyclonidine, formed by hydroxylation of the phenol ring, which accounts for less than 10% of the concentration in the urine.[1786] Cytochrome P450 2D6 is involved in this process.

Clearance estimates in children who are not infants are similar to those described in adults when standardized for size using allometric scaling (CL 12.8–16.7 L/hour per 70 kg). Population parameter estimates (between subject variability) for a two-compartment model were CL 14.6 (CV 35.1%) L/hour per 70 kg; central Vd (V1) 62.5 (71.1%) L/70 kg; intercompartment clearance (Q) 157 (77.3%) L/hour per 70 kg; and peripheral Vd (V2) 119 (22.9%) L/70 kg. Clearance at birth was 3.8 L/hour per 70 kg and matured with a half-time of 25.7 weeks to reach 82% of the adult rate by 1 year of age. Clearance in neonates is approximately one-third that described in adults, consistent with immature elimination pathways.[1777] The volumes of distribution, but not clearance, were increased after cardiac surgery (V1 123%, V2 126%). There was a lag time (T$_{LAG}$) of 2.3 (CV 73.2%) minutes before absorption began in the rectum. The absorption half-life (Tabs) from the epidural space was slower than that from the rectum (0.98 hours CV 24.5% vs. 0.26 hours CV 32.3%). The relative bioavailability of epidural, nasal, and rectal clonidine was unity (F = 1).[1776,1777] Oral bioavailability is reduced in children (F = 0.55).[127]

DEXMEDETOMIDINE

Dexmedetomidine (Precedex), the *dextro* optical isomer of medetomidine, is a pharmacologically selective α_2-agonist with sedative, anxiolytic, and analgesic properties. Dexmedetomidine is in the same class as clonidine but differs from clonidine in its eightfold greater affinity for α_2- compared with α_1-receptors than with clonidine. In anesthesia and intensive care, dexmedetomidine is currently being administered for procedural sedation and as an anesthetic adjunct.

Dexmedetomidine exerts its effects on numerous organ systems via α-adrenoceptors. These sympathetic adrenoceptors are categorized as either α_1- or α_2-receptors, based on receptor selectivity.[1789] The latter are further subdivided into three subtypes: α_{2A}-, α_{2B}-, and α_{2C}-adrenoceptors according to ligand binding. The α_2-agonists, such as dexmedetomidine, bind all three receptor subtypes, although the receptor subtype binding may vary with the dose of dexmedetomidine. The α_2-adrenoceptors trigger responses by activating G proteins. The common path for the effector response to dexmedetomidine is sympatholysis (suppression of the sympathetic nervous system). Depending on the specific receptor that is activated, α_2-agonists may cause hypotension, bradycardia, sedation, analgesia, attenuation of shivering, and a number of other physiologic responses. Consequently, dexmedetomidine use in neonates and children has expanded to include prevention of ED, postoperative pain management, invasive and noninvasive procedural sedation, and the management of opioid withdrawal.[751,1790–1798]

The α_2-adrenoceptors are located ubiquitously throughout the body. In the CNS, they are located primarily in the locus coeruleus, spinal cord, and autonomic nerves. The CNS manifestations of α_2-agonists include sedation and anxiolysis, both of which are mediated through the locus coeruleus. Sedation may also be mediated by α_2-agonist inhibition of the ascending norepinephrine pathways. Analgesia is mediated primarily via the spinal cord, although there is evidence that supraspinal and peripheral nerves may contribute to this effect as well. Cardiovascular manifestations of α_2-adrenoceptors include actions on the heart and on peripheral vasculature. The primary action of α_2-adrenoceptors on the heart is a chronotropic effect in which it slows heart rate by blocking the cardioaccelerator nerves as well as by augmenting vagal activity. In infants, dexmedetomidine-induced bradycardia may be exacerbated by the coadministration of digoxin. Decreasing the dose of dexmedetomidine restores the heart rate to normal values.[1799] The α_2-agonist action on the autonomic ganglia includes decreasing sympathetic outflow, which can lead to hypotension and bradycardia. Actions on the peripheral vasculature depend on the dose of dexmedetomidine: vasodilatation is the result of sympatholysis, which occurs at low doses, and vasoconstriction is the result of direct action on smooth muscle vasculature at large doses (Fig. 7.28).

In the peripheral nervous system, α_2-adrenoceptors are located at both the presynaptic and postsynaptic junctions.[1789] The presynaptic and postsynaptic effects of α_2-agonists diminish norepinephrine release and inhibit sympathetic activity. Other manifestations of α_2-adrenoceptors include inhibition of shivering as well as promotion of diuresis, although their mechanisms remain elusive.[1789,1800]

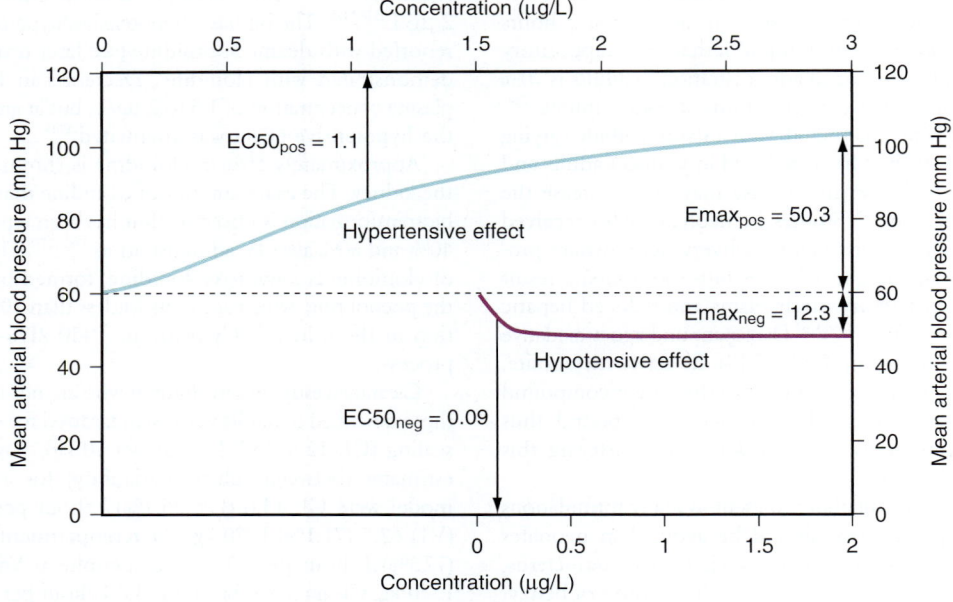

FIGURE 7.28 Composite Emax model showing the hypertensive and hypotensive effect of dexmedetomidine on mean arterial blood pressure in children after cardiac surgery. The vasoconstrictor effect occurred with minimal time delay, whereas an equilibration half-time (T$_{1/2}$keo) of 9.66 minutes was estimated for the sympatholytic response.[2035] *EC50*, concentration that produces half the maximal effect. (Reproduced with permission from Potts AL, Anderson BJ, Holford NH, Vu TC, Warman GR. Dexmedetomidine hemodynamics in children after cardiac surgery. *Pediatr Anesth.* 2010;20(5):425–433.)

A plasma concentration in excess of 0.6 μg/L is estimated to produce satisfactory sedation in adult ICU patients,[1801] and similar target concentrations are estimated in children who require sedation in the ICU after cardiac surgery.[1802] Hypotension has been described in children after cardiac surgery[1784] and in children presenting for sedation during radiologic procedures. In infants and children sedated with large-dose dexmedetomidine, the incidence of hypertension was 5%, affecting a larger fraction of those younger than 1 year of age and those who required an additional bolus dose to maintain sedation.[1803] These adverse cardiovascular effects of dexmedetomidine generate some concern. Dexmedetomidine also decreases heart rate in a dose-dependent manner in children.[1792,1804–1807] This effect is attributed to a centrally mediated sympathetic withdrawal, which results in unregulated cholinergic activity. With large doses of dexmedetomidine (2–3 μg/kg over 10 minutes followed by 1.5–2 μg/kg per hour), 12 children younger than 6 years of age experienced heart rates less than 50 beats/minute although their BPs were maintained.[1807] Administration of anticholinergics or other medications to increase the heart rate during dexmedetomidine-induced bradycardia has not been required, but it should be noted that severe and persistent hypertension has been reported when glycopyrrolate was used to treat large-dose dexmedetomidine-induced bradycardia.[1808] Dexmedetomidine 0.5 μg/kg IV has resulted in several episodes of bradycardia 30 seconds or longer with an unrecordable systolic BP in two children during strabismus surgery (without anticholinergic pretreatment) when the surgeon pulled gently on the extraocular muscle (personal communication, JL, 2017). Vital signs were restored after administration of ephedrine 0.1 to 0.2 mg/kg IV.

Less favorable results have been noted in the electrophysiology laboratory. Heart rate decreased and arterial BP increased significantly after 1 μg/kg IV over 10 minutes followed by a 10-minute continuous infusion of 0.7 μg/kg per hour. Both sinus and atrioventricular node function were depressed. The use of dexmedetomidine may not be prudent during electrophysiology studies and may be associated with adverse effects in patients at risk for bradycardia or atrioventricular nodal block.[1809] However, dexmedetomidine did not interfere with the conduct of pediatric electrophysiologic studies for supraventricular tachycardia and the successful ablation of such arrhythmias, this despite a greater need for isoproterenol when dexmedetomidine was used.[1810] Conduction delay caused by dexmedetomidine has been used to decrease the incidence of junctional ectopic tachycardia after tetralogy of Fallot repair.[1811]

Population parameter estimates for a two-compartment model were clearance of 42.1 L/hour per 70 kg (CV = 30.9%), central Vd of 56.3 L/70 kg (CV 61.3%), intercompartment clearance of 78.3 L/hour per 70 kg (CV 37.0%), and peripheral Vd of 69.0 L/70 kg (CV 47.0%).[1802] Clearance increases from 18.2 L/hour per 70 kg at birth in a full-term neonate to reach 84.5% of the mature value by 1 year postnatal age (see Figs. 7.4 and 7.11). The clearance of dexmedetomidine after an infusion after cardiac surgery was reduced (83.0%) compared with the clearance after a bolus in a noncardiac surgical population.[1802] Similar parameter estimates, including a reduced clearance in children who received a dexmedetomidine infusion after cardiac surgery, have been described by others[1812]; this trait has also been described for morphine, fentanyl, and midazolam.

The preferred route of administration of dexmedetomidine is the IV route, although others have been studied. The PK of dexmedetomidine have also been studied after parenteral (IM),

buccal, and oral administration.[1813] Parenteral delivery yielded kinetics similar to the IV route, buccal administration yielded an 82% bioavailability, and orogastric delivery yielded only a 16% bioavailability. Data from adults indicate limited effects of renal failure on the kinetics of dexmedetomidine.[1814] Dexmedetomidine is metabolized extensively in the liver (UGT enzymes), with 40% metabolized by CYP2D6 isozyme.[1800] After metabolism to methyl and glucuronide conjugates, 95% of dexmedetomidine is eliminated via the kidneys.[1815] There appears to be no evidence that dexmedetomidine interferes with the PK of other medications that are substrates for CYP2D6 metabolism.[1815] Dexmedetomidine is 93% protein-bound in children.[1800,1806]

Dexmedetomidine is formulated as a concentrated solution in a 2-mL vial (100 μg/mL). After diluting it with normal saline, lactated Ringer's solution, or 5% dextrose in water to an appropriate concentration, dexmedetomidine can be delivered by syringe pump. Current dosing recommendations for dexmedetomidine begin with a loading dose followed by an infusion, although some skip the loading dose during general anesthesia and administer only an infusion.[1792,1806,1816] The recommended loading dose is 1 μg/kg dexmedetomidine infused over 10 minutes, although loading doses between 0.5 and 3.0 μg/kg have been reported.[751,1792,1803,1816–1818] The purpose of infusing the loading dose over 10 minutes (as opposed to a rapid IV bolus) is to attenuate the severity of the hypertension that can occur with bolus dosing. After completing the loading dose, dexmedetomidine should be infused at 0.5 to 1 μg/hour per kilogram.[751,1792,1816–1818] (*Note*: dexmedetomidine is infused in *micrograms per kilogram per hour, not micrograms per kilogram per minute.*) In the United States, dexmedetomidine is approved only for infusion up to 24 hours, although data exist attesting to hemodynamic stability even after infusions of greater duration.[1819] One reservation concerning dexmedetomidine is the fear of a withdrawal from dexmedetomidine itself after prolonged use (>24 hours). Up to 80% of children (0–17 years) in intensive care experienced withdrawal symptoms after infusion (0.42 ± 0.17 μg/kg per hour).[1820,1821]

When compared with propofol for sedation during MRI, dexmedetomidine provides adequate sedation during the scan but has a slower onset and recovery profile.[1819,1822] It is our experience, and that of others, however, that sedation with the recommended maximal doses of dexmedetomidine generally require the addition of other sedatives, such as midazolam, for a child to remain motionless for a procedure such as an MRI.[751,1823,1824]

One of the major advantages of dexmedetomidine over other sedatives is its minimal respiratory depression in adults and children.[1804–1806,1816,1825–1827] Although dexmedetomidine blunts the CO_2 response curve,[1828] it does not lead to extreme hypoxia or hypercapnia. Indeed, respiratory rate, CO_2 tension, and oxygen saturation are generally maintained during dexmedetomidine sedation in children.[751,1806,1817] In children without OSA, increasing doses of dexmedetomidine (1–3 μg/kg) result in small changes in the upper airway and are not associated with clinical signs of airway obstruction. Even though these changes are small, all precautions to manage airway obstruction should be taken when dexmedetomidine is used for sedation.[1829] In children with suspected OSA, significantly less frequent artificial airway support was required when dexmedetomidine (2 μg/hour per kilogram) was used for sedation for MRI sleep studies, compared with propofol for sedation.[1830]

Quantifying the MAC-sparing effect of dexmedetomidine has proven difficult. Three studies have estimated the MAC of isoflurane or sevoflurane in adults at two concentrations of dexmedetomidine–high (0.6–0.7 ng/mL) and low (0.36–0.3 ng/mL).[1805,1831,1832] The MAC-sparing effect of large-dose dexmedetomidine concentration ranged from 17% to 50% and that of low-dose dexmedetomidine concentration from 0% to 35%. Accordingly, it is difficult to predict the exact MAC-reducing effect of dexmedetomidine on sevoflurane and isoflurane in adults. Similar data in children have not been forthcoming.

Dexmedetomidine provides an interesting quality of sedation that permits arousal with gentle stimulation.[1806] The lack of respiratory depression distinguishes this sedative from opioids, benzodiazepines, and other sedatives. It has been studied for sedation in children for a number of different purposes, including radiologic procedures such as MRI.[751,1792,1816,1817]

Dexmedetomidine provides a modest degree of analgesia, reducing the need for, but not totally supplanting, opioids and other analgesics. Several studies demonstrated that it spares opioid requirements during surgery.[1800,1833,1834]

The CNS effects of dexmedetomidine have been addressed in animals and, in part, in humans.[1835] The data suggest that dexmedetomidine decreases CBF directly by vasoconstricting the smooth muscle of the cerebral blood vessels, and indirectly through a reduction in arterial BP and cardiac output. In humans, dexmedetomidine decreases CBF by 30%, as determined by positron emission tomography, as well as Doppler measurements of the middle cerebral artery. Interestingly, using Doppler measurements of the cerebral blood vessels in adult volunteers, both the CO_2 response and autoregulation of CBF were preserved. When dexmedetomidine was infused before introducing an inhalational anesthetic, dexmedetomidine attenuated the cerebral vasodilatation induced by the inhalational anesthetic.

Dexmedetomidine depresses sensory-evoked potentials but, for the most part, the potentials are adequate for evaluations.[1836] Similarly, motor-evoked potentials are reduced in a dose-dependent manner during dexmedetomidine infusion but are measurable nonetheless.[1837] There are contrasting reports about the degree of evoked potential suppression, but most report successful spinal cord monitoring during scoliosis surgery.[1838–1841]

ED occurs in 15%–30% of children after most inhalational anesthetics particularly in the 3–5 year age range.[1825] A number of medications attenuate the incidence of delirium after anesthesia, including dexmedetomidine.[1795] Dexmedetomidine decreases the incidence of ED after sevoflurane anesthesia: after an infusion of dexmedetomidine (0.2 µg/kg per hour), recovery was not prolonged,[1842] whereas after a single dose of 0.5 µg/kg administered 5 minutes before the end of surgery, emergence was prolonged.[1843] Further studies are required to assess the cost/benefit ratio for this indication.

The interaction between dexmedetomidine and neuromuscular blockade has been studied during balanced anesthesia with propofol and alfentanil.[1844] In adults, dexmedetomidine decreased the twitch response after sevoflurane 7%, although this was not deemed to be clinically important. Current evidence does not substantiate any clinically significant interaction between dexmedetomidine and neuromuscular blockade.

At present, this medication seems to offer specific advantages for awake fiberoptic intubation, awake craniotomy, sedation in the ICU (opioid-sparing), and perhaps for reducing the incidence of ED.[1796,1845–1848] However, high-dose dexmedetomidine is associated with adverse effects on the heart rate and BP, and unpredictable effects with anticholinergics.[1808,1849] Additional research in children is required before recommendations can be made regarding appropriate dosing and drug interactions.[1809,1850,1851] There are

conflicting data regarding its safety in children with congenital heart disease.[1809,1852–1854]

CHLORAL HYDRATE

Chloral hydrate is one of the oldest and, in the past, most widely used sedatives in infants and children, exerting its sedation effect by enhancing the GABA receptor complex. Like many other sedatives, it has no analgesic properties. Its primary use in pediatrics is for sedation for noninvasive procedures and as a premedication. Its principal advantage is that it may be administered orally or rectally, with excellent absorption and relatively good sedation, within 30 to 45 minutes, and the infrequent need to supplement the sedation with other sedatives. The usual dose is 20 to 75 mg/kg orally or rectally, although total doses up to 100 mg/kg (maximum 2 grams) have been used alone or in combination with other sedatives.

Chloral hydrate used to be the most commonly used sedative for infants undergoing a variety of nonpainful procedures[1855–1859]; however, chloral hydrate liquid production ceased in the United States in May 2012 (https://www.drugs.com/drug-shortages/chloral-hydrate-oral-solution-and-capsules-902 [accessed September 29, 2017]). Since this drug is no longer commercially available in the United States, individual hospital pharmacies must reformulate it with reconstituted crystals. One study reported that the duration of sedation was less, the frequency of supplemental sedatives greater, and the incidence of sedation failures greater with compounded chloral hydrate compared with the commercial preparation.[1860]

Chloral hydrate has minimal effects on respiration[1861]; however, it has caused airway obstruction and desaturation, particularly in children with enlarged tonsils.[1862–1864] In addition, apnea, airway obstruction, bradycardia, and hypotension have been reported in a series of infants younger than 6 months of age who were sedated for echocardiograms; this report emphasized that this is not the benign drug that many previously thought.[1865] Indeed, arrhythmias have been reported after chloral hydrate, attributed to its primary metabolite, trichloroethanol. After a single dose of 30 mg/kg, sedation was evident for up to 12 hours after administration in former premature nursery graduates. Bradycardia (as slow as 60 beats/minute) was also observed in these neonates.[1866] Deaths after chloral hydrate overdose when given for sedation have also been reported.[1257,1867,1868]

Chloral hydrate has several disadvantages. It has a bitter taste and is known to cause vomiting.[1869] This drug should not be administered for long periods of time because theoretically (1) its metabolites may be carcinogenic, (2) it may cause severe gastritis (possibly related to its metabolism to trichloroacetic acid), and (3) drug metabolites may accumulate.[1870,1871] In addition, it may interfere with the binding of bilirubin to albumin and toxic metabolites may accumulate, leading to metabolic acidosis, renal failure, and hypotonia in neonates.[1872]

Chloral hydrate is metabolized in the liver and erythrocytes by alcohol dehydrogenase to an active metabolite, trichloroethanol, which has a half-life of 9.7 ± 1.7 hours in toddlers but 39.8 ± 14.3 hours in preterm infants (see Fig. 48.3).[1873] Trichloroethanol is cleared by UGT (see the sections on morphine, acetaminophen, and dexmedetomidine), which is immature in neonates. These very long half-lives imply that residual drug effect will be present long after any procedure requiring sedation.[1874–1876] Because of the long half-life, there is a real risk for prolonged sedation, resedation after leaving medical supervision, and death.[1868,1877–1880] It is for this reason that *chloral hydrate is not generally recommended for premedication before surgery* and that a prolonged period of observation is recommended after sedation for a procedure. If nitrous oxide is administered to children who have received chloral hydrate, a state of deep sedation or general anesthesia may occur.[1881]

Antihistamines

DIPHENHYDRAMINE

Antihistamines are often used in pediatric anesthesia both for their histamine 1 (H_1)-receptor inhibition and for their sedative properties. Diphenhydramine (Benadryl) is one of the more commonly used antihistamines. It is rapidly absorbed when administered orally (at a dose of 1.25 mg/kg) with a duration of effect that lasts anywhere from 3 to 6 hours. Clearance is through CYP2D6 (see the section on codeine and Chapter 6). It is often administered as a premedicant or as an in-hospital sedative. Caution is advised for children with respiratory problems because diphenhydramine dries secretions, causing difficulty expectorating. The IV dose to treat an allergic reaction is 0.5 mg/kg.

CIMETIDINE, RANITIDINE, AND FAMOTIDINE

Cimetidine (Tagamet) was the first generation of potent, very hydrophilic, competitive inhibitors of H_2-receptor–mediated histamine reactions, which was later followed by ranitidine and famotidine. This class of drugs increases gastric-fluid pH and reduces gastric fluid residual volume.[1882] Indications for an H_2-receptor antagonist include a history of gastroesophageal reflux, hiatus hernia, previous esophageal surgery, obesity, or an anticipated difficult intubation that will require prolonged laryngoscopy, as well as, perhaps, high-risk patients (American Society of Anesthesiologists classes 3 and 4). Cimetidine is likely the most studied of this category of drugs, but its use has diminished because of serious drug interactions through its effects on the cytochrome oxidase system. Cimetidine partially inhibits numerous CYP enzymes (CYP1A2, CYP2C9, CYP2C19, CYP2D6, CYP2E1, and CYP3A4), which prolongs the half-lives of many drugs, including phenytoin, phenobarbital, theophylline, cyclosporine, carbamazepine, benzodiazepines that do not undergo glucuronidation, calcium channel blockers, propranolol, quinidine, sulfonylureas, mexiletine, warfarin, and tricyclic antidepressants, such as imipramine.[1883] The elimination half-life of cimetidine is prolonged in neonates and infants compared with older children.[1884] The kidney is the primary clearance organ in children. Renal clearance in children 4 to 13 years constituted 70% of total body clearance, more than double that of adults. As expected, children have a greater total body clearance (11.6 mL/minute per kilogram) than do adults (7.0 mL/minute per kilogram), a larger Vd (1.24 vs. 0.80 L/kg), and a shorter elimination half-life (83 vs. 122 minutes).[1885]

Although ranitidine (Zantac) also weakly reduces CYP activity, *it does not increase the half-life of other medications significantly* when administered at the usual therapeutic doses.[1886-1889] Ranitidine has been administered by intermittent bolus (2–4 mg/kg in four divided doses), or as a loading dose (0.5 mg/kg) followed by an infusion of 0.05 mg/kg per hour.[1890-1892] The peak effect occurs between 2 and 4 hours after administration.[1495] The elimination half-life of ranitidine is 3 ± 1.35 hours. When a dose of 1.5 mg/kg per 8 hours was administered, ranitidine maintained the gastric fluid pH greater than 4.[1891] Reduced doses have met with less success in controlling the gastric fluid pH.[1890]

Famotidine (Pepcid) is about eight times more potent than ranitidine and about 40 times more potent than cimetidine.[1893] Famotidine has been well studied, including in neonates. Because famotidine is primarily excreted by the kidneys, dosing depends on the maturity of the renal function. Infants younger than 3 months of age have reduced clearance and require 24 hours between doses (0.25 mg/kg IV or 0.5 mg/kg orally), whereas infants older than 3 months are similar to older children and adults and require 12 hours between doses.[1884,1894,1895] There is some evidence to suggest decreased responsiveness to famotidine (a weaker effect in altering gastric acid pH and volume) with long-term administration.[1896] Famotidine increases gastric fluid pH, although it does not reduce gastric residual volumes when administered before anesthesia.[1897]

Antiemetics

METOCLOPRAMIDE

Metoclopramide (Reglan) has been used in children for its antiemetic and gastric emptying properties.[1898] The antiemetic properties result from its direct effects on the chemoreceptor trigger zone. Gastric emptying is a result of the antagonism of the neurotransmitter dopamine, which stimulates gastric smooth muscle activity.[1899,1900] A dose of 0.15 mg/kg at the end of surgery effectively reduces emesis after strabismus surgery and tonsillectomy, although the magnitude of its effectiveness may be limited.[1901] Metoclopramide is less effective than 5-hydroxytryptamine type 3 (5-HT_3) receptor inhibitors, but does offer an alternative rescue medication.[1902] As with many other medications cleared by sulfate and glucuronide conjugation, the elimination half-life in neonates is prolonged compared with older children, thus necessitating a 6-hour interval between oral doses (0.15 mg/kg).[1903] Clearance in infants (0.9–5.6 months) was 0.67 ± 0.13 L/hour per kilogram with Vdss 4.4 ± 0.6 L/kg.[1904]

5-HYDROXYTRYPTAMINE TYPE 3–RECEPTOR ANTAGONISTS

Antagonists to the 5-HT_3 receptor include ondansetron (Zofran), granisetron (Kytril), dolasetron (Anzemet), tropisetron (Navoban), and palonosetron (Aloxi). These agents have proven to be an effective preventive and therapeutic measure for PONV. Notwithstanding their widespread usage, these drugs have been the subject of much debate regarding which is the most effective, which has the better side-effect profile, which lasts the longest, which is best combined with other agents, which costs too much, and so on.[1905-1917] Because ondansetron was the first in this class of serotonergic receptor antagonists that effectively reduced the incidence of nausea and vomiting in children, it forms the basis for discussion of measures to prevent PONV after pediatric surgery.[1918-1927] Some studies report that ondansetron (0.1 mg/kg) is superior to metoclopramide (0.15 mg/kg) for the prophylactic control of postoperative vomiting in children undergoing tonsillectomy.[1928] Most pediatric anesthesiologists limit their routine use to children undergoing procedures known to have a substantial incidence of PONV, such as strabismus repair, tonsillectomy, or middle ear surgery, and to children with a known history of motion sickness or previous nausea and vomiting after surgery.[1929-1937] Ondansetron is effective in preventing nausea and vomiting, as well as in reducing the severity of established nausea and vomiting. The usual recommended dose is 100 to 150 µg/kg every 6 hours. One clinical trial found efficacy in children as young as 1 month of age; however, the PK were different in the infants younger than 4 months of age, suggesting the need for a greater interval between dosing.[1938] This is not surprising, given that clearance is by hydroxylation, followed by glucuronide or sulfate conjugation in the liver. A mature clearance of 541 mL/minute per kilogram is reported, but ondansetron clearance was reduced by 31%, 53%, and 76% for the typical 6-, 3-, and 1-month-old infant, respectively. Clearance matured with a TM_{50} of 4 months.

Simulations showed that an ondansetron dose of 0.1 mg/kg in children younger than 6 months produced exposure similar to a 0.15-mg/kg dose in older children.[1939] One further concern with this class of drugs is the potential for ventricular tachyarrhthmias (e.g., Torsades de pointes) in patients with long QT syndrome, particularly when they are anesthetized with potent inhalation agents such as sevoflurane.[1940,1941] However, concentrations reached after routine dosing are well below the inhibitory concentration of 50% (IC_{50}) reported for inhibition of Na channels in healthy individuals.[1907]

A number of studies in children demonstrated that the antiemetic effect of drugs from this class can be improved if they are combined with dexamethasone or other anesthetic techniques known to reduce vomiting.[1922,1923,1925,1942,1943] An oral disintegrating tablet of ondansetron is also available.[1944]

Other agents in this class (e.g., granisetron, dolasetron, tropisetron) have all been shown to be effective in ameliorating PONV, which is further improved when combined with other antiemetic modalities.[1918,1936,1945–1952] Granisteron and tropisteron have more prolonged half-lives (7.8 hours) and coincident duration of effect than ondanstron (4 hours); these may be better suited to chemotherapy-induced nausea and vomiting. Tropisteron is metabolized by CYP2D6, which renders its termination susceptible to polymorphisms and an extended elimination half-life of 40 hours is reported in poor metabolizers (PM). CYP3A4 is the predominant enzyme pathway for ondandestron and granisteron metabolism.[1907]

Palonosetron is a new 5-HT_3 receptor antagonist that differs from the 5-HT_3 receptor antagonists described previously in that it allosterically inhibits the receptor rather than physically binding to the receptor.[1953] Because it takes 30 to 40 hours for the receptor to restore its normal conformation, the agent may be metabolized (and is susceptible to polymorphisms of CYP2D6, but that does not affect its antiemetic effect as the receptor remains deformed for the duration. Palonosetron effectively reduces PONV in adults.[1954] In a dose-finding study in children, 0.5 μg/kg palonosetron was as effective as 1 and 1.5 μg/kg for PONV for 48 hours after strabismus surgery.[1955] A double-blind, double dummy study of 502 pediatric patients undergoing emetogenic chemotherapy found non-inferiority for 20 μg/kg 6 hourly compared with ondansetron 150 μg/kg 8 hourly; it is now approved by the FDA and European Medicines Agency for this indication in children as young as 1 month of age.[1956]

NEUROKININ 1 AND OTHER ANTIEMETICS

Despite the introduction of 5-HT_3 receptor antagonists along with dexamethasone to treat PONV, PONV has continued. It has been known that the receptor for substance P, the neurokinin 1 (NK1) receptor, in the brainstem (area postrema and nucleus tractus solitarius) may hold the key to the persistence of PONV.[1957,1958] The first NK1 receptor antagonist is aprepitant (Emend), which has proven effective in reducing nausea and vomiting in adults after chemotherapy and surgery and in children after chemotherapy.[1959,1960] Aprepitant is an oral drug, fosaprepitant is the parenteral formulation of aprepitant, and several others are under development for use (and dosing) in PONV in combination with 5-HT_3 receptor antagonists and dexamethasone.[1961]

Anticholinergics

ATROPINE AND SCOPOLAMINE

Atropine (0.02 mg/kg) and scopolamine (0.01 mg/kg) both have CNS effects, although the sedating effect of scopolamine is 5 to 15 times greater than atropine. Scopolamine possesses two to three times more potent antisialagogue action than atropine. Atropine and scopolamine decrease the ability to sweat, and thus may cause a slight increase in temperature.[1962] Atropine and scopolamine have equipotent cardiovascular accelerator properties. The dose for both anticholinergics in infants to speed the heart rate is greater per kilogram than in adults.[1963] Anticholinergics are appropriate in specific situations, such as to diminish secretions preoperatively, to block laryngeal and vagal reflexes, to treat or prevent the bradycardia associated with succinylcholine, to treat the bradycardia of anesthetic-induced myocardial depression, the muscarinic effects of neostigmine, and the oculocardiac reflex. Atropine is painful when administered intramuscularly. When it is administered as a premedicant, it does not block laryngeal reflexes; it is more effective in blocking laryngeal reflexes when it is given by the IV route. Although some data suggest that children with trisomy 21 are more susceptible to the cardiac effects of atropine,[1964] our clinical experience and that of others do not support this notion.[1965,1966] Because some children with trisomy 21 have narrow-angle glaucoma, atropine must be administered cautiously because it might worsen the glaucoma.[1965,1966] Atropine may be administered orally, rectally, and via the trachea. Oral atropine may blunt the hypotensive response to potent inhalation agents during induction of anesthesia in infants younger than 3 months of age.[1967] When administered via the trachea, atropine is rapidly absorbed, producing physiologic effects.[1968–1971]

Atropine is metabolized in the liver by N-demethylation followed by conjugation with glucuronic acid[1972]; both processes are immature in the neonate. Half the drug is also eliminated by the kidneys. An old technique to diagnose atropine poisoning was to place a small aliquot of the victim's urine into the eye of a cat and observe for mydriasis!

It is anticipated that clearance is reduced in the neonatal age range because of an immaturity of renal and hepatic function, but data remain elusive. Children younger than 2 years have an increased Vdss compared with those older than 2 years (3.2 ± 1.5 vs. 1.3 ± 0.5 L/kg).[1973] Clearance was similar in those younger than 2 years (6.8 ± 5.3 mL/minute per kilogram) and those older than 2 years (6.5 ± 1.6 mL/minute per kilogram). The elimination half-life in healthy adults is 3 ± 0.9 hours, whereas that in term neonates is 4 times this.[1973,1974]

PD characterization is similarly lacking in neonates. Some have held that the minimum dose of atropine in neonates and infants is 0.1 mg; recent evidence has demonstrated that 5-μg/kg IV atropine in young infants 1 to 12 months does not increase heart rate or cause bradycardia.[1975] Infants younger than 6 months require a larger dose to increase heart rate than older children.[420] A dose of 5 μg/kg had no impact on heart rate and does not cause bradycardia in young infants 4 to 6 months age.[1975] Systolic BP did not change for any dose of atropine (5–40 μg/kg) in this neonatal cohort.[420]

In clinical practice, scopolamine is usually limited to those situations in which its sedative effect, combined with that of morphine, will be most advantageous, such as during cardiac surgery. It is also very useful as an adjuvant to ketamine anesthesia because of its antisialagogue and central sedative effects. The central sedative effects of both atropine and scopolamine may be antagonized with physostigmine. Most centers no longer routinely administer anticholinergic medications as part of the premedication because they are painful, the optimal effect may not coincide with induction of anesthesia, and current potent inhalation agents produce fewer secretions and infrequent bradycardia.

Scopolamine is a tertiary amine with greater CNS effects than atropine, causing sedation and amnesia. It has moderate antiemetic activity.[1976] To minimize the relatively large incidence of side effects, the transdermal dosage form has been developed for nausea and vomiting; however its use is generally limited to teenagers to avoid potential toxicity.[1977-1979] Scopolamine patch–induced delirium has been reported and is more likely in younger patients.[1980] Unequal pupils have also been reported.[1981]

Scopolamine has a distribution volume of 1.4 L/kg in adults.[1969] Glucuronide conjugation, sulfate conjugation, and hydrolysis by the CYP3A family are involved in its clearance.[1977] Both glucuronidation and the CYP3A enzyme systems are immature at birth and clearance is anticipated to be reduced.[1969]

GLYCOPYRROLATE

Glycopyrrolate (0.005–0.01 mg/kg) is a synthetic quaternary ammonium compound with potent anticholinergic properties. It offers some advantage over atropine and scopolamine because it minimally penetrates the BBB and thus causes few CNS effects. Several studies have demonstrated that glycopyrrolate is superior to atropine because its anticholinergic effects are more prolonged, lasting several hours.[1982,1983] The heart rate changes minimally after IV administration, causing fewer arrhythmias and offering an advantage when tachycardia might be detrimental.[1984,1985] It should be noted that prolonged and severe hypertension has been reported when glycopyrrolate was used to treat dexmedetomidine-induced bradycardia[1808]; the mechanism for the hypertension is unknown. Further pretreatment of children before administration of dexmedetomidine demonstrated no value in blunting bradycardia and resulted in greater increases in systolic BP compared with no pretreatment (~20% vs. ~10%).[1986] In some children, gastric fluid volume and acidity are reduced after glycopyrrolate administration.[1987,1988] The drug remains popular for antagonizing the parasympathomimetic effects of neostigmine and is as effective as atropine for preventing the oculocardiac reflex.[1989]

There is poor absorption from the gastrointestinal tract (10%–25%).[1990] Clearance in infants younger than 1 year (n = 8) was 1.01 (range 0.32–1.85) L/kg per hour and Vdss of 1.83 (range 0.70–3.87) L/kg,[1990] but there are no neonatal data available. However, the renal system accounts for 85% of elimination,[1982] and clearance is anticipated to be reduced in neonates because renal function is immature.[171]

Antagonists

NALOXONE

Naloxone (Narcan) is a pure opioid antagonist with a greater affinity for the μ-receptor compared with the κ- and δ-receptors. When given intravenously, naloxone has a very rapid onset of antagonism of the opioid receptors (within 30 seconds to 1 minute). Naloxone undergoes glucuronidation in the liver, with minimal bioavailability after oral administration. In adults, the elimination half-life is 1 to 1.5 hours, whereas in neonates it is 3 hours. When administered intramuscularly, the apparent elimination half-life is prolonged from 80 minutes to 6 hours in adults because of the depot effect.[1991]

Naloxone is effective for reversing opioid-induced adverse effects, including respiratory depression, chest-wall and glottic rigidity, nausea and vomiting, pruritus,[1992] urinary retention, and constipation. It may be administered via any route, including parenteral, neuraxial, tracheal, and oral. For children who are ventilating and not in extremis, but in whom opioid-induced respiratory depression needs antagonism in the perioperative period, it is reasonable to initiate antagonism with a very small dose of IV naloxone (0.25–0.5 μg/kg). This is similar to the dose recommended in one large review of 10 to 20 μg of naloxone in children in the perioperative period.[1993] If the response is inadequate, the same dose may be repeated until ventilation improves. The same cumulative total IV dose of naloxone can then be administered as an IM injection to ensure that recrudescence of the respiratory depression does not occur. *For children in extremis or in whom a potential opioid overdose has occurred (including neonatal resuscitation), a larger dose of 10 to 100 μg/kg IV of naloxone may be indicated.* The American Academy of Pediatrics simplified the naloxone dosing for infants and children up to 5 years of age, recommending 100 μg/kg, and for children older than 5 years (20 kg), 2 mg naloxone.[1994] This is based, in part, on concerns that smaller doses of naloxone may not be uniformly effective. However, it is equally important to recognize that overzealous dosing of naloxone will not only reverse the opioid analgesic effect but could also lead to profound systemic hypertension, cardiac arrhythmias (including ventricular fibrillation), and pulmonary edema (noncardiogenic).[1995] Evidence suggests that pulmonary edema may not be a dose-dependent response to naloxone, because it has been reported after as little as a single dose of 100 μg. A retrospective review of the management of 195 children and adolescents who received naloxone postoperatively, in the emergency department, or in the pediatric ICU revealed an IV dosing range of 1 to 500 μg/kg; this resulted in resolution of the respiratory depression, systolic hypertension in 17% of children, and one case (incidence of 0.5%) of pulmonary edema.[1993] A continuous infusion of naloxone may be required to treat severe opioid-induced respiratory depression.[1996] *Any child who receives naloxone for antagonism of opioid-induced respiratory depression must be observed in a monitored environment for a minimum of 2 hours to ensure that there is no recrudescence of the respiratory depression.*

The recommended dose of naloxone during neonatal resuscitation far exceeds that in older children. Doses as great as 400 μg/kg have been used without ill effects.[1997] In a systematic review of naloxone use in neonates, evidence demonstrated that naloxone increased alveolar ventilation, although there was no evidence that outcome, in terms of assisted ventilation or admission to a neonatal ICU, was affected by the use of naloxone.[1998] Caution is recommended when administering naloxone to an infant of a mother who has chronically abused opioids because seizures have been reported.[1999]

Naloxone has also been administered via infusion at low doses (≥ 1 μg/kg per hour)[2000] concomitantly to ameliorate adverse effects from opioids, including nausea and vomiting, pruritus, urinary retention, and constipation.[2001] Evidence is mixed regarding the beneficial effect of such a practice,[2002,2003] although double-blind, randomized controlled trials have provided a significant reduction in morphine-associated nausea and pruritus during patient-controlled analgesia when administered as a separate infusion.[2004] When administered for this indication, there is a need to balance antagonism of the opioid-induced side effects with the antagonism of the pain relief.

NALTREXONE

Naltrexone (Depade, ReVia) is an oral opioid antagonist that also has a greater affinity for the μ- rather than κ- and δ-receptors. The activity of naltrexone is thought to be a result of both the parent and its 6β-naltrexol metabolite (via hepatic dihydrodiol dehydrogenase). The mean elimination half-lives for naltrexone and 6β-naltrexol in adults are 4 hours and 13 hours, respectively. Naltrexone has a good oral bioavailability, with an elimination half-life of up to 8 hours in children, which is similar to adults.[2005] This opioid antagonist has also been used in the management of autism.[2006,2007] Children displaying self-injurious behavior or hyperactivity have been noted to have high CSF endorphin concentrations and decreased pain sensitivity. Some opioid-induced behavior in animals and opioid addicts resembles that seen in autistic children. Naltrexone reduces self-injurious behavior.[2006]

Although naltrexone reverses opioid-associated adverse effects, its use for this purpose has not become popular.[1998] Naltrexone and its primary metabolite, 6β-naltrexol, are excreted, albeit in low concentrations, in breast milk from a lactating female.[2008] Care should be taken when managing infants of opioid-addicted mothers.

METHYLNALTREXONE

Methylnaltrexone (Relistor) is the first quaternary ammonium opioid antagonist that has very limited ability to penetrate the BBB.[2009] It is prepared in an oral as well as in a parenteral formulation for subcutaneous and IV administration. Doses of 0.45 mg/kg have been administered intravenously to adults. Because methylnaltrexone does not cross the BBB, it is suited to reverse the peripheral adverse side effects of opioids without attenuating the central analgesic effect. Opioid-induced side effects, including gastric emptying, urinary retention, postoperative ileus, and chronic constipation,[2010] improve after administration of methylnaltrexone.[2011–2015] There are few pediatric data available. If the preliminary adult safety and efficacy data are also demonstrated in children, this drug may offer the benefit of improving our ability to provide opioid-induced analgesia, while eliminating many of the peripheral adverse effects, thus improving the comfort of children. The drug is used currently for opioid-induced constipation in children with cancer and those in palliative care.[2016]

FLUMAZENIL

Flumazenil (Romazicon) is a specific GABA$_A$ receptor–competitive antagonist that reverses the effects of benzodiazepines. Flumazenil has been administered by rectal, nasal, IM, and IV routes.[2017–2020] After a single IV dose, flumazenil shows limited protein binding (40%) with an elimination half-life of approximately 1 hour in adults, owing primarily to rapid and extensive metabolism by hepatic carboxylesterases.[2021–2023] In adults with severe liver disease, elimination of flumazenil is reduced.[2024] In children, the elimination half-life after a single IV dose of 10 μg/kg flumazenil followed by an infusion of 5 μg/kg per minute is 35 minutes.[2025] The rectal dose required is greater (e.g., 50 μg/kg). The PK of intranasal flumazenil (40 μg/kg) were determined in healthy children with a median age of 4 years. The elimination half-life was 2 hours.[2017] Oral flumazenil is also available, but its bioavailability is only 16% owing to the first-pass effect in the liver.[2023]

In adults, a dose of 17 μg/kg of flumazenil has antagonized benzodiazepine-induced sedation; studies in children have found doses of 24 μg/kg to be clinically effective without evidence of re-sedation.[2025] There is a limited role for flumazenil in clinical pediatric anesthesia, although specific indications are warranted, including benzodiazepine overdose, wake-up test during scoliosis

surgery, treatment of a comatose child, and paradoxical response to benzodiazepines.[2026,2027] *With its brief elimination half-life, re-sedation after the initial response has been reported in children 1 to 5 years of age, thus necessitating close observation for at least 2 hours after antagonism of benzodiazepine-induced sedation.*[2028,2029] Caution should be taken in administering larger doses of flumazenil because seizures have been reported.[2030]

PHYSOSTIGMINE

This tertiary ammonium is a reversible cholinesterase inhibitor used to treat central cholinergic syndrome and delirium, and to antagonize the actions of atropine and scopolamine in the peripheral nervous system and CNS.[2031–2033] It is not generally used to antagonize neuromuscular blockade because its nonionized ammonium group facilitates transfer across the BBB, causing CNS effects. After an IV dose, its elimination half-life is 20 to 30 minutes with a duration of action that may exceed 1 hour, depending on the cholinesterase activity. Physostigmine is hydrolyzed at the ester linkage by cholinesterase. The usual single IV dose of physostigmine in children is 10 to 30 μg/kg.[2034] To treat intoxication by long-acting drugs, an infusion of physostigmine may be required at an infusion rate of 30 μg/kg per hour. Side effects of physostigmine include cardiac arrhythmias (bradycardia), cholinergic crisis, and seizures.[2034] Accordingly, physostigmine should be administered with electrocardiographic monitoring.

ANNOTATED REFERENCES

Anderson BJ, Holford NHG. Mechanism-based concepts of size and maturity in pharmacokinetics. *Annu Rev Pharmacol Toxicol.* 2008;48:303-332.
A review explaining the fundamentals of allometric theory and its application to pharmacology.
Görges M, Zhou G, Brant R, Ansermino JM. Sequential allocation trial design in anesthesia: an introduction to methods, modeling, and clinical applications. *Paediatr Anaesth.* 2017;27(3):240-247.
Sequential allocation trial design is commonly used in anesthesia to determine the MAC of inhalation agents, impact of other drugs, and minimal effective dose. The authors explain the theory behind this methodology and its limitations and offer practical examples.
Hannam JA, Anderson BJ. Pharmacodynamic interaction models in pediatric anesthesia. *Paediatr Anaesth.* 2015;25:970-980.
A review paper explaining interpretation of drug interaction models commonly used in anesthesia.
Kearns GL, Abdel-Rahman SM, Alander SW, et al. Developmental pharmacology—drug disposition, action, and therapy in infants and children. *N Engl J Med.* 2003;349(12):115-167.
This article explains the complex interactions that come into play to shape developmental pharmacology.
Upton RN, Foster DJ, Abuhelwa AY. An introduction to physiologically-based pharmacokinetic models. *Paediatr Anaesth.* 2016;26(11):1036-1046.
Physiological based pharmacokinetic (PBPK) models can be used to predict pediatric PK. PBPK models require detailed physiological data. Data on the ontogeny of individual clearance pathways, derived from measurements of enzyme expression and activity in post-mortem livers, and from in vivo data from drugs that are cleared by similar pathways are useful. Information concerning genetic, physiological, organ and tissue size and composition, protein binding, demographic and clinical data has progressively improved their prediction ability.

A complete reference list can be found online at ExpertConsult.com.

Total Intravenous Anesthesia and Target-Controlled Infusion

BRIAN J. ANDERSON AND JAMES HOUGHTON

THE MOST COMMON INDICATIONS for total intravenous anesthesia (TIVA) techniques in children are as follows: those at risk for malignant hyperthermia (in whom inhalational agents are contraindicated); children with a high risk of postoperative nausea and vomiting, brief radiologic or painful procedures when rapid recovery is needed (e.g., magnetic resonance imaging, bone marrow aspiration, gastrointestinal endoscopy); frequent repeated anesthesia (e.g., radiation therapy); major surgery to control the stress response; neurosurgical procedures to assist with control of intracranial pressure and for cerebral metabolic protection; spinal instrumentation requiring evoked motor and auditory brain potentials; and children in need of airway procedures (e.g., bronchoscopy).[1-3] Total intravenous (IV) sedation and anesthesia are used in pediatric intensive care, but propofol is contraindicated for prolonged use in very sick or young children because of the risk of developing propofol infusion syndrome (PRIS).[4-13]

Pharmacokinetic and Pharmacodynamic Principles

The goal of pharmacologic treatment is a desired response, known as the target effect. An understanding of the concentration-response relationship (i.e., pharmacodynamics [PD]) can be used to predict the target concentration required to achieve this target effect in a typical child.[14] Pharmacokinetic (PK) knowledge (e.g., clearance [CL], volume [V]) then determines the dose that will achieve the target concentration. Calculation of the dose for a drug where the PK disposition can be described using a one-compartment model with first-order elimination can be readily calculated:

$$Loading\ dose = V \times Target\ Concentration$$

$$Maintenance\ Dose = CL \times Target\ Concentration$$

However, most drugs used in anesthesia require two or more compartments to describe their disposition and although the principles for drug dosing calculation are the same, calculations are complicated by two or more clearances and volumes (see below).

Although the parameters used in PK and PD equations (known as models) for many drugs are published, the values may vary substantively from child to child. Several covariates have been identified to more accurately predict the dose for a particular child, including weight, age, sex, pathology, drug interactions, and pharmacogenomics. Current pumps used for TIVA incorporate weight and age to predict the typical drug dose and infusion rate for a specific patient.[15]

The use of TIVA for propofol is a good example of "pharmacology in action." The target effect (level of general anesthesia) for propofol has been defined (e.g., bispectral index [BIS] 50–55), the target (plasma) concentration to achieve this level of anesthesia is known (e.g., propofol 4 mg/L) and its PK in children is well described. Advanced concepts in PK modeling and computer technology have led to sophisticated delivery systems that facilitate anesthesia given by the IV route. Further advances involving feedback from receptor organs have also been developed for children.[16,17] Target-controlled infusion (TCI) devices or "smart pumps" are an example of a sophisticated delivery system that may be directed at either plasma (Cp) or effect-site (Ce) drug concentration. These computerized pumps are a considerable advance over earlier manual techniques for children[18,19] that targeted only the Cp of the drug. However, they require input of both PK and PD parameters and a lack of robust PK-PD estimates and variability in the parameter estimates limit the current accuracy of TCI in children under 3 years of age.[20]

PEDIATRIC PHARMACOKINETIC PARAMETER SETS

TCI techniques use propofol and remifentanil as the principal drugs for induction and maintenance of anesthesia. Popular pediatric programs used for propofol infusion targeting a plasma concentration are based on data from Marsh[21] and Gepts,[22] Kataria,[19] Short,[23] Rigby-Jones,[24] Schuttler,[25] Murat,[26] Saint-Maurice,[27] Coppens[28] or Absalom (Paedfusor).[29] These parameter sets are commonly termed "models" and named after the author who

Parameter	Kataria et al.[19]	Marsh[21] & Gepts[22]	Paedfusor[29]	Short et al.[23]	Schuttler & Ihmsen[25]	Rigby-Jones et al.[24]	Murat et al.[26]	Saint Maurice et al.[27]	Coppens et al.[28]
V1 (L)	10.4	4.56	9.16	8.64	7.68	11.68	20.6	14.44	3.48
V2 (L)	20.2	9.28	18.98	10.8	20.74	26.68	19.4	35.6	4.68
V3 (L)	164	58.04	116.58	69.4	264.82	223.86	121.74	168	19.02
CL (L/minute)	0.68	0.542	0.568	0.836	0.56	0.444	0.98	0.62	0.78
Q2 (L/minute)	1.16	0.51	1.044	1.22	1.036	0.32	1.34	1.24	2.04
Q3 (L/minute)	0.52	0.192	0.384	0.34	0.46	0.268	0.4	0.22	0.66

TABLE 8.1 Propofol Parameter Estimates for a 20-kg Child

Performance of these models differed markedly during the different stages of propofol administration. Most models underestimated propofol concentration 1 minute after the bolus dose, suggesting an overestimation of the initial volume of distribution. Not all models tested were within the accepted limits of performance (median performance error, bias <20% and median absolute performance error, precision <30%). The model derived by Short and colleagues performed best[32] in children 3 to 26 months.

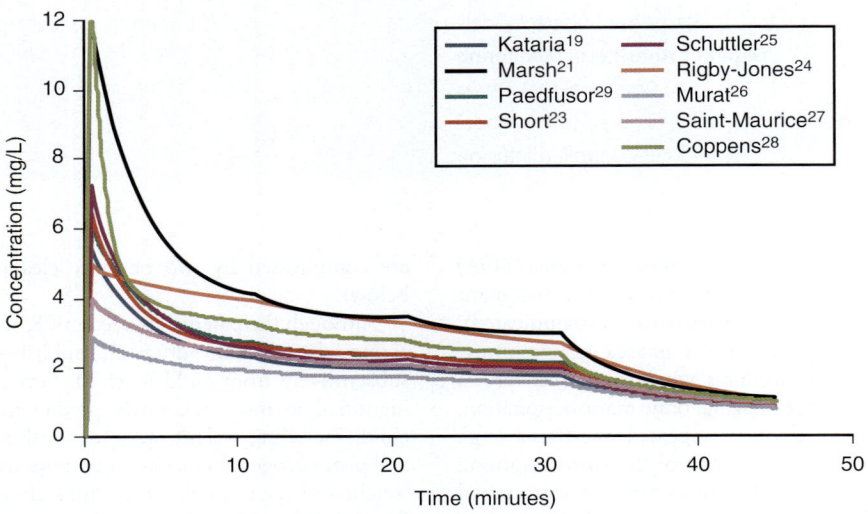

FIGURE 8.1 Simulated time-concentration profiles for propofol using differing parameter sets are shown. A 3-mg/kg bolus was administered and the infusions were administered as for an adult (10-8-6 regimen, see text). (From Anderson BJ. Pharmacology of pediatric TIVA. *Rev Colomb Anestesiol.* 2013;41:205-214. Used with permission.)

reported them (e.g., the Kataria model). Parameter estimates (e.g., CL; intercompartment clearance, Q; central volume of distribution, V1; peripheral volume of distribution, V2) are different for each parameter set (Table 8.1). Although parameter estimates are different for each author, most predict similar concentrations for the same infusion regimen (Fig. 8.1).

Covariate influences that contribute variability to the parameters, such as the severity of illness are often unaccounted for—for example, the volume of the central compartment is increased in children after cardiac surgery.[24] Even weight or age, the most common sources of variability,[30] may be omitted from parameter estimates. Both the administration method (IV bolus or infusion)[31] and the collection of venous blood for assay rather than arterial blood will influence the PK parameter estimates in the early phase when the drug is moving into the effect-site compartment. Time-concentration profiles and context-sensitive half-lives will differ depending on which parameter set is used.[32]

There is a paucity of validation studies for these differing parameter sets.[28] The Paedfusor model[29] is reported to have a median performance error, bias (MDPE) of 4.1% and a median absolute performance error, precision (MDAPE) of 9.7% in children between 1 and 15 years of age.[29] A more recent study concluded

that all parameter sets except that based on the Marsh model performed acceptably in children between 3 and 26 months.[32] Others have described a poor fit for the Kataria model, despite the fact that it is the most widely used model.[33] However, clearance (expressed as liters per hour per kilogram) decreases with age and MDPE is minimized at low CL and exaggerated at greater values. Evaluating models outside the age range in which their parameter sets were determined will increase the bias and worsen the precision of the model.

Adult remifentanil PK parameters[34] continue to be used in TCI devices for patients of all ages, despite an increasing knowledge regarding the pharmacology of this drug in children.[35] There is an element of safety with this approach because both volume of distribution[36] and clearance (expressed as milliliters per minute per kilogram)[37] decrease with increasing age and the elimination half-life is small with a constant context-sensitive half-life. The greater volume of distribution in children reduces the peak concentrations of remifentanil after bolus dosing; the increased clearance in children results in a smaller plasma concentration when infused at adult rates expressed as mg/minute per kilograms. Remifentanil PK can be described in all age groups by simple application of an allometric size model (see Chapter 7).[37] This

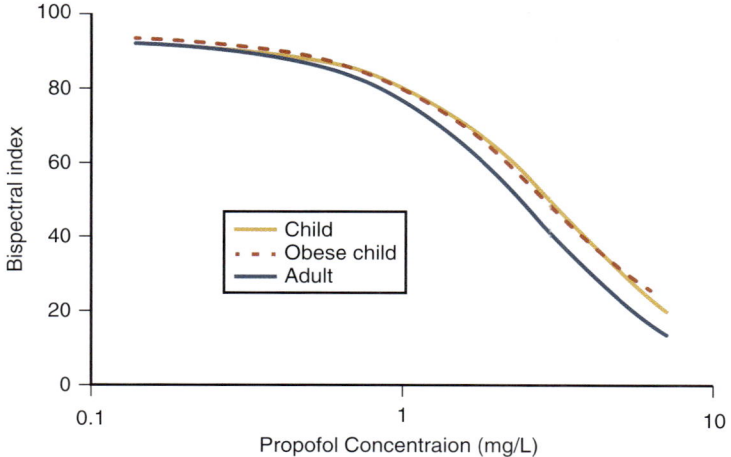

FIGURE 8.2 The propofol concentration and its relationship with bispectral index in children and adults. (Data from Coppens MJ, Eleveld DJ, Proost JH, et al. An evaluation of using population pharmacokinetic models to estimate pharmacodynamic parameters for propofol and bispectral index in children. *Anesthesiology* 2011;115:83-93; and Chidambaram V, Venkatasubramanian R, Sadhasivam S, et al. Population pharmacokinetic-pharmacodynamic modeling and dosing simulation of propofol maintenance anesthesia in severely obese adolescents. *Pediatr Anesth.* 2015;25:911-923.)

standardized clearance of 2970 mL/minute per 70 kg is similar to that reported by others in children[36,38] and adults.[34,39] The smaller the child, the greater the clearance when expressed as milliliters per minute per kilogram. Owing to these enhanced clearance rates, smaller (younger) children will require larger infusion rates of remifentanil than larger (older) children and adults to achieve equivalent blood concentrations.

THE TARGET CONCENTRATION

The target concentration is the concentration desired at the effect site. The plasma and effect-site concentrations are the same at steady state. The target concentration depends on the desired effect. This effect is determined by an understanding of the concentration-response relationship of the drug. This will differ with age, pathology, drug interactions, and stimulus. The target concentration may vary depending on the magnitude of the desired effect. A remifentanil target of 2 to 3 µg/L is adequate for laryngoscopy, 6 to 8 µg/L for laparotomy and 10 to 12 µg/L might be sought to ablate the stress response associated with cardiac surgery.[40]

A propofol concentration of 2 to 3 mg/L is an appropriate target for sedation and 4 to 6 mg/L is adequate for anesthesia. The target effect-site propofol concentrations for both the loss and return of consciousness in children, 2.0 ± 0.9 mg/L and 1.8 ± 0.7 mg/L, respectively, (mean ± standard deviation) are similar to those reported in adults.[41,42] The relation between drug concentration and effect is commonly described by the Hill equation (see Eq. 7.19)[43]:

$$Effect = E0 - \frac{Emax \cdot Ce^N}{(EC_{50}^N + Ce^N)} \qquad \text{Eq. 8.1,}$$

where $E0$ is the baseline level of consciousness (e.g., BIS = 100), $Emax$ is the maximum response, EC_{50} the concentration at half this maximum response, Ce the concentration in the effect compartment, and N defines the steepness of the slope.

Jeleazcov et al.[44] have described propofol PD in children 1 to 16 years using BIS where $E0$ was estimated as 93.2, $Emax$ 83.4, EC_{50} 5.2 mg/L, and N 1.4. This relationship is very similar to that described in obese children.[45] The equilibration rate constant (keo) between the plasma and effect compartment was 0.6/minute ($T_{1/2}keo$ 1.15 minutes). Children may have a slightly lower sensitivity to propofol than adults (Fig. 8.2),[33] although this difference may be due to PK rather than PD factors.[46] The Kataria parameter set is known to underpredict concentration as age increases, consistent with allometric scaling. When this parameter set is used to estimate PD parameters, older children appear to require a smaller concentration to maintain anesthesia[47]; this is a PK effect and not a PD effect.[48]

Maintenance infusion requirements for propofol in neonates differ substantively from those in older infants and children. These may be attributed to differences in PK and/or PD. In terms of the kinetics, the clearance of propofol in neonates is reduced compared with older infants; clearance decreases with decreasing postmenstrual age owing to immature enzyme clearance systems.[49] To develop a dosage scheme for propofol infusion rates in infants and children, the adult dosage scheme was adapted to the requirements in the younger population by observing the total number and time of administration of boluses and time to awakening from propofol in infants younger than 3 years (n = 2271) (Table 8.2).[50] The predicted infusion rates for the first 10 minutes in neonates are large (24 mg/kg per hour; 400 µg/kg per minute), values that should be used cautiously because of the danger of an overdose if the infusion continues beyond 10 minutes. Delayed awakening, hypotension, and an increased incidence of bradycardia have been reported in neonates and infants.[50] Propofol can cause profound hypotension in neonates and PK-PD relationships in this age group remain elusive.[51]

LINKING PHARMACOKINETICS WITH PHARMACODYNAMICS

A simple situation in which drug effect is directly related to concentration does not mean that drug effects parallel the time

TABLE 8.2	Propofol Dose Requirements in Children Younger Than 3 Years of Age				
Time (minutes)	0-3 months	3-6 months	6-9 months	9-12 months	1-3 years
0–10	24.3	19.7	15.3	14.8	12.1
10–20	20.4	15.2	12.3	11.9	9
20–30	15.1	12	9	9	6
30–40	12	9	6	6	6
40–50	9	6	6	6	6
50–60	6	6	6	6	6

Infusion rates are expressed as milligrams per kilogram per hour.
(Adapted from Steur RJ, Perez RS, De Lange JJ.. Dosage scheme for propofol in children under 3 years of age. *Paediatr Anaesth*. 2004;14:462-467.)

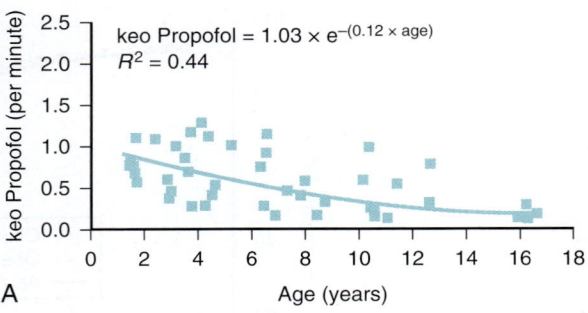

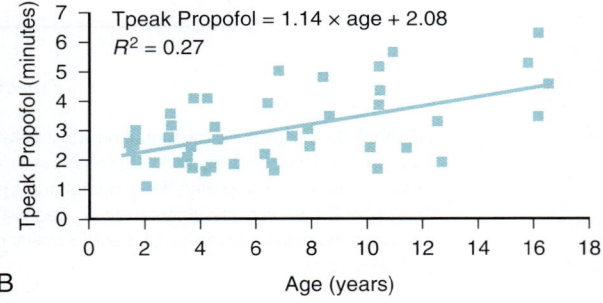

FIGURE 8.3 This figure shows the equilibration rate constant of propofol and time to peak propofol concentration as a function of age. The keo decreases with age; that is. the $T_{1/2}$keo increases with age. This results in a later time to peak concentration (Tpeak) as age (and weight) increases. (Data from Jeleazcov C, Ihmsen H, Schmidt J, et al. Pharmacodynamic modelling of the bispectral index response to propofol-based anesthesia during general surgery in children. *Br J Anaesth*. 2008;100:509-516.)

course of concentration. This occurs only when the concentration is low in relation to EC_{50}. In this situation, the half-life of the drug may correlate closely with the half-life of drug effect.

A plasma concentration-effect plot can form a hysteresis loop because of a delay in effect. Hull et al.[52] and Sheiner et al.[53] introduced the effect compartment concept for muscle relaxants. A single first-order parameter ($T_{1/2}$keo) describes the equilibration half-time:

$$T_{1/2}keo = \frac{Ln(2)}{keo}$$ Eq. 8.2

This mathematical trick assumes the concentration in the central compartment is the same as that in the effect compartment at equilibrium, but that a time delay exists before drug reaches the effect compartment. The concentration in the effect compartment is used to describe the concentration-effect relationship.[54]

Adult $T_{1/2}$keo values are well described—for example, morphine 16 minutes; fentanyl 5 minutes; alfentanil 1 minute; propofol 3 minutes. This $T_{1/2}$keo parameter is commonly incorporated into TCI pumps to achieve a rapid effect-site concentration.

There are few estimates of the $T_{1/2}$keo for propofol in children using simultaneous PK-PD modeling. An estimate of 1.86 min (95% confidence interval [CI] 1.16–2.31) was reported in healthy children 2 to 12 years,[55] and 1.2 minutes (95% CI 0.85–2.1) in obese children.[45] We might expect a smaller $T_{1/2}$keo with decreasing age based on size models.[56] Faster half-times in children can be accounted for by considering the physiologic time that scales to a power of $1/4$:[57]

$$T_{1/2}keo_{Child} = T_{1/2}keo_{ADULT} \times \left(\frac{WT}{70}\right)^{1/4}$$ Eq. 8.3

An increasing $T_{1/2}$keo with age (linked to weight) has been described for propofol in children (Fig. 8.3).[44] Similar results have been demonstrated for sevoflurane and BIS in patients 3 to 71 years.[58] If unrecognized, this will result in excessive dose in a young child if the effect site is targeted and peak effect (Tpeak) is anticipated to be later than it actually is because it was determined in a teenager or adult (Fig. 8.4).

When both PK and PD data are collected simultaneously and parameters for both models are estimated together, then the model is described as "integrated." PK estimates should not be used in conjunction with PD estimates from a different data set without a few "fudge factors." Tpeak methodology (see Chapter 7) is commonly used to estimate $T_{1/2}$keo that then links separate PK and PD data sets. Tpeak will increase with age (see Fig. 8.3). Model

dependence of the $T_{1/2}$keo was demonstrated by an estimate of 1.7 min with the Kataria[19] parameter set and 0.8 minute with the Paedfusor model (Graseby Medical Ltd., Hertfordshire, UK) parameter set.[29]

Pharmacodynamic Interaction Models

Drugs may interact with each other at multiple levels. These are discussed in Chapters 6 and 7. Drug interactions for those drugs used in TIVA are commonly described using PD interaction models.

TRADITIONAL METHODS

Traditional methods of evaluating PD interactions include using isoboles (graphs illustrating equi-effective combinations of drugs), shifts in dose (or concentration) response curves (see Chapter 7), or interaction indexes based on parameters of potency derived from separate monotherapy and combination therapy analyses. Such methods provide an estimation of the magnitude of effect for dose or concentration combinations, but they do not inform us on the time course of that effect or its associated variability.

Competitive antagonists reduce receptor availability by competing for occupancy at the same receptor site. Drugs that elicit an effect are called agonists, whereas those that do not are called antagonists, so the occupancy of some receptors by the antagonists results in less effect. In general, competitive antagonists shift the effect-concentration curve to the right by altering the EC_{50}. Noncompetitive antagonists shift the observed maximum effect (Emax) rather than the EC_{50}.

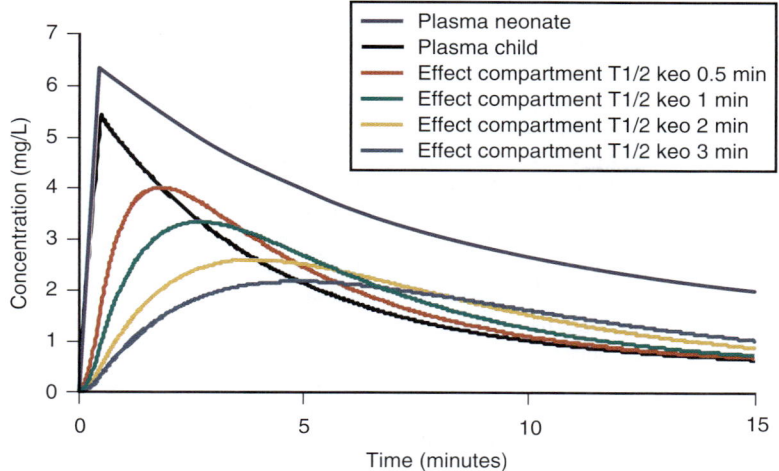

FIGURE 8.4 This figure shows simulated plasma time-concentration profiles for a typical 20-kg child given propofol 3 mg/kg using the Kataria parameter set. The $T_{1/2}$keo used will affect predicted effect-site concentrations—that is, the greater the $T_{1/2}$keo, the longer it takes to achieve the target concentration.

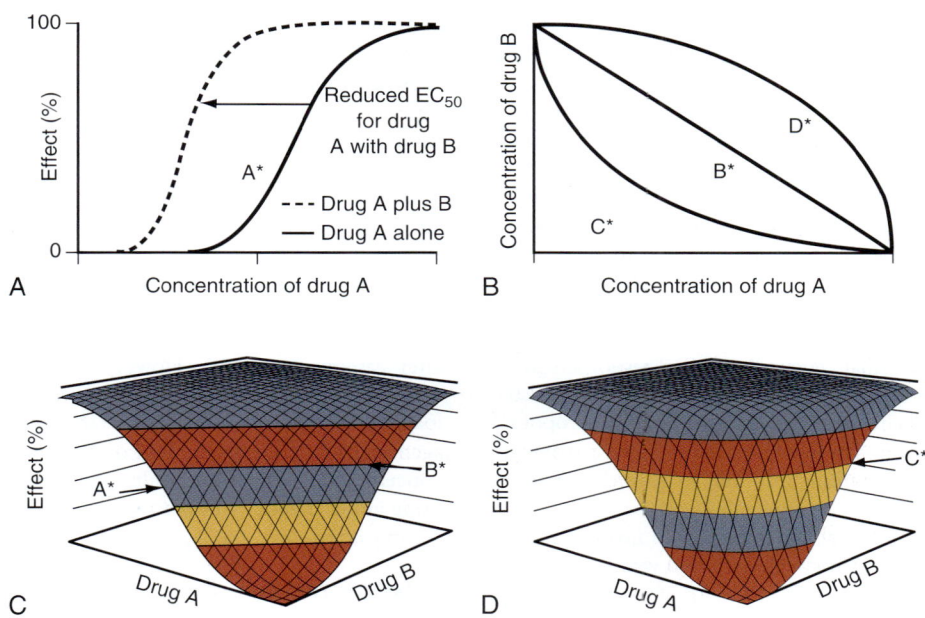

FIGURE 8.5 Methods of investigating interactions. **A,** Shift in response curve analyses involve plotting the concentration (or dose)-effect relationship for one drug alone and in the presence of steady-state concentrations of a second drug. **B,** Isoboles are constructed using iso-effect lines with curves derived from observations assessed against the expected (or "additive") response line (B*). Supra-additivity is depicted by curves bowing toward the plot origin (C*), while infra-additivity is shown with outward curves (D*). Information from both methods is represented within response surfaces with isoboles displayed as horizontal planes and individual concentration-response curves as vertical slices (indicated by *arrows* on surfaces for A* single concentration-response curve drug A, B* additive isobole, and C* supra-additive isobole). **C** shows the additive response surface for two drugs. **D** shows the synergistic response surface for two drugs, with synergy depicted through outward bowing of the surface. (Data from Hannam JA, Anderson BJ. Pharmacodynamic interaction models in pediatric anesthesia. *Pediatr Anesth.* 2015;25:970–980.)

RESPONSE SURFACE MODELS

Emax models for individual drugs can be combined and extended to incorporate PD interactions between two or more drugs. The "response surface" models are an extension of empirical, single-drug models that can be used to describe and predict the combined effects between two or more drugs (Fig. 8.5). Horizontal lines within the response surface hold equivalent information to that given by isoboles. Surface parameters are estimated using data points pertaining to all areas of the concentration and effect range for both drugs simultaneously (as opposed to considering individual concentration pairs or effect levels in isolation, as is done with isobolographic analyses). Resulting

PD models can be used to characterize the type of interaction across the entire range of concentrations and responses and make predictions about response (effect) for any ratio of the studied drugs.[59]

Two equations are commonly used: those of Greco et al.[60] and Minto and Vuyk[61] (see Chapter 7). The Greco equations have been used to describe additive effects for propofol, remifentanil, and fentanyl on BIS response in children aged 1 to 16 years undergoing general surgery.[44] These authors reported EC_{50} estimates of propofol 5.20 μg/mL, remifentanil 24.1 ng/mL, and fentanyl 8.6 ng/mL, and suggested a propofol and remifentanil pair of 2.3 μg/mL and 4.3 ng/mL, respectively, to maintain hemodynamic parameters and sedation scores within ranges suitable for surgery. The Greco model has also been used to describe loss of response to various noxious stimuli under propofol-remifentanil anesthesia.[62] Synergistic surfaces for sedation and response to laryngoscopy were reported.

The Minto equations have been used to assess synergy for hypnosis among three commonly combined drugs for anesthesia: propofol, midazolam, and alfentanil.[63] Computer simulations based on interactions at the effect site predicted that a synergistic three-drug combination (midazolam, propofol, and alfentanil) tripled the duration of effect compared with propofol alone. Response surfaces can describe anesthetic interactions, even those among agonists, partial agonists, competitive antagonists, and inverse agonists.[63]

Synergism between propofol and alfentanil has been demonstrated using response-surface methodology. Remifentanil alone had no appreciable effect on response to shaking and shouting or response to laryngoscopy, whereas propofol could ablate both responses. Modest remifentanil plasma concentrations dramatically reduced the concentrations of propofol required to ablate both responses.[64] When comparing the different combinations of midazolam, propofol, and alfentanil, the responses varied markedly at each endpoint assessed and could not be predicted from the responses of the individual agents.[65] Similar response-surface methodology has been used to investigate the combined administration of sevoflurane and alfentanil[66] and remifentanil and propofol[67] on control of ventilation. These combinations have a strikingly synergistic effect on respiration, resulting in severe respiratory depression in adults.

The ability of propofol to ablate responses to noxious stimuli has been studied in children between 3 and 10 years undergoing esophagogastroduodenoscopy.[68] The EC_{50} for 50% probability of no response was reduced from a propofol concentration of 3.7 μg/mL to 2.8 μg/mL when it was combined with a remifentanil infusion at 0.025 μg/kg per minute. Remifentanil infusions at greater infusion rates did not further reduce the propofol requirements, but they did increase the risk of remifentanil-related adverse respiratory events. The concurrent administration of opioids during TIVA techniques in children has a significant "propofol-sparing" effect while providing analgesia and stress control.[68,69] It is sensible to take advantage of this synergism to avoid excessive propofol dosing and long-chain triglyceride loads, particularly with concerns about PRIS during prolonged surgeries or sedations. *Remifentanil provides the most effective propofol-sparing effect, but fast recovery means alternative techniques of analgesia must be well established before the remifentanil is discontinued.* Other analgesics and anesthetics are also effective in reducing the propofol dose required. Fentanyl, alfentanil, and sufentanil are effective, as are local and regional analgesia techniques, once the block becomes established. Nitrous oxide as well as low concentrations of inhalational anesthetics also act synergistically with propofol and opioids to attenuate the dose required.

Depth of Anesthesia Monitoring

A common effect measure used to assess depth of anesthesia is the electroencephalogram (EEG) or a modification of detected EEG signals (spectral edge frequency, BIS, entropy). Physiologic studies in adults and children indicate that EEG-derived anesthesia depth monitors can provide an imprecise and drug-dependent measure of arousal. Although the outputs from these monitors do not closely represent any true physiologic entity, they can be used as guides for anesthesia and in so doing have improved outcomes in adults. In older children the physiology, anatomy, and clinical observations indicate the performance of the monitors may be similar to that in adults. The BIS showed a close relationship with the modeled effect-site propofol concentration and serves as a measure of anesthetic drug effect in children older than 1 year.[44] Their use in infants anesthetized with propofol cannot yet be supported in theory or in practice.[70,71] During anesthesia, the EEG in infants is fundamentally different from the EEG in older children; there remains a need for specific neonate-derived algorithms if EEG-derived anesthesia depth monitors are to be used in neonates.[72,73]

Depth of anesthesia monitors were used in 1% of all general anesthetics in the United Kingdom in 2015. However, these monitors were used in 33% of children undergoing general anesthesia using a TIVA technique with a neuromuscular blocking drug, but not at all in infants.[74] Despite limitations in infants, BIS is useful in older children, particularly when neuromuscular blocking drugs are used in conjunction with TIVA; modified EEG has also been successfully used for closed-loop anesthesia.[16,20] These systems may prove superior to open-loop systems that rely on a calculated effect Ce that are associated with large variability.

Awareness has been more commonly reported after TIVA than after gaseous anesthesia. However, many reports of awareness occur after the switch from gaseous anesthesia to TIVA where a loading dose was not given.[75] Clearance of the gaseous anesthesia agent occurs before attainment of effective steady-state propofol concentrations. The future ability for point-of-care propofol assay using either breath[76,77] or plasma[78–80] may be useful to reduce this complication.

COMMON TIVA DRUGS

The commonly used medications include propofol, remifentanil, alfentanil, and sufentanil; ketamine is occasionally used but has a long context-sensitive half-time with consequent delayed awakening.[81] Delivery can be achieved using either a manual infusion scheme (Table 8.3) or PK model–driven infusion devices with software developed specifically for use in children. Unfortunately, the commercially available software packages usually limit the applicable age to 1 to 3 years or older or weight to 10 to 15 kg or greater, and the PK parameters are derived from studies of a relatively few healthy children. Propofol programs that allow for age-, weight- and gender-related changes in central compartment volume, clearance, and distribution have been developed and perform well in healthy children.[82,83] However, there are considerable gaps in knowledge for some drugs, for ill children, and for young children, infants, and neonates. Consequently, caution is needed when applying such programs to these populations. The anesthesiologist can use these preprogrammed devices as a basis for initiating a TIVA technique but must also use skill, knowledge,

TABLE 8.3	Manual Infusion Schemes		
Drug	**Loading Dose**	**Maintenance Infusion**	**Notes**
Propofol[84]	1 mg/kg	10 mg/kg per hour for 10 minutes, then 8 mg/kg per hour for 10 minutes, then 6 mg/kg per hour thereafter	Adult regimen to achieve blood concentration of 3 µg/mL Underdelivers to children and achieves lower blood concentration of 2 µg/mL
Propofol[69]	1 mg/kg	13 mg/kg per hour for 10 minutes, then 11 mg/kg per hour for 10 minutes, then 9 mg/kg per hour thereafter	Concurrently with alfentanil infusion
Alfentanil[85]	10–50 µg/kg	1–5 µg/kg per minute	Results in blood concentration of 50–200 ng/mL
Remifentanil[8e]	0.5 µg/kg per minute for 3 minutes	0.25 µg/kg per minute	Produces blood concentrations of 6–9 ng/mL
Remifentanil[8e]	0.5–1.0 µg/kg over 1 minute	0.1–0.5 µg/kg per minute	Produces blood concentrations of 5–10 ng/mL
Sufentanil[86,87]	0.1–0.5 µg/kg	0.005–0.01 µg/kg per minute	Results in blood concentration of 0.2 ng/mL for sedation and analgesia
Sufentanil[86,87]	1–5 µg/kg	0.01–0.05 µg/kg per minute	Results in blood concentrations of 0.6–3.0 ng/mL for anesthesia
Fentanyl[85]	1–10 µg/kg	0.1–0.2 µg/kg per minute	
Ketamine[85]	1–2 mg/kg	0.1–2.5 mg/kg per hour	Smaller dose and infusion rate for analgesia and sedation. Larger dose and infusion rate for anesthesia titrated to effect
Midazolam[85]	0.05–0.1 mg/kg	0.1–0.3 mg/kg per hour	

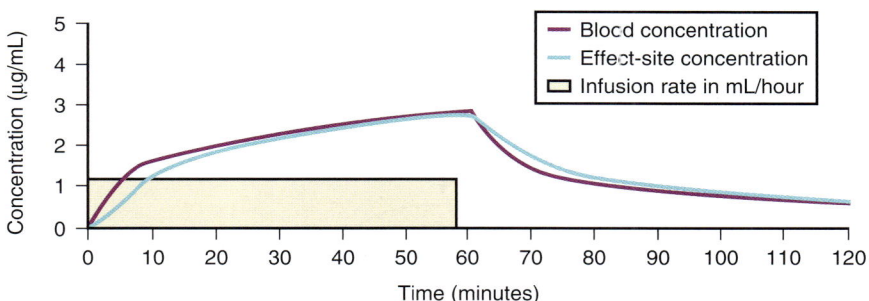

FIGURE 8.6 A fixed-rate infusion of propofol at 10 mg/kg per hour with no bolus dose in a healthy 10-kg, 1-year-old infant. Note that a steady state is not reached even after 1 hour. There is a lag of effect-site concentration behind blood concentration both during infusion and after stopping infusion. Effect-site concentration reaches blood concentration at about 1 hour. The context-sensitive half-time is 9 minutes (simulated using Tivatrainer; available at http://www.eurosiva.org/TivaTrainer/tivatrainer_main.htm).

and experience to titrate the IV agents to effect to avoid awareness, pain, and adverse effects.

ACHIEVING THE TARGET CONCENTRATION IN A MULTICOMPARTMENT MODEL

For a fixed infusion rate in a single-compartment model, it takes five half-lives to reach a steady-state concentration (>96% of the target) in the blood (Fig. 8.6). A loading dose is required to more rapidly achieve the target concentration. This dose rapidly fills the volume of distribution, after which the calculated infusion maintains the blood concentration (Fig. 8.7). Calculation of the loading dose is relatively easy for a simple one-compartment model. Unfortunately, drugs such as propofol require two- or three-compartment models to describe their disposition. A loading dose may be too large if calculated using the volume of distribution at steady state (Vss, where Vss = V1 + V2 + V3 for a three-compartment model) for a drug that is described by multiple compartments because it is initially administered into the smaller central compartment (V1) to effect the desired response: loss of consciousness. A loading dose based on the Vss will cause adverse

effects, hemodynamic instability, and/or toxicity. Even a remifentanil bolus should be administered over several minutes to reduce the risk of bradycardia, hypotension, and/or difficult mask ventilation. An anticholinergic drug may prove useful if remifentanil 3 µg/kg is used for rapid-sequence intubation.

To more clearly understand the disposition of drugs after an IV dose, it is useful to consider a three-compartment model (Fig. 8.8, Table 8.4). The drug is delivered and eliminated from a central compartment V1 (which includes the blood) but also distributes to and redistributes from two peripheral compartments, one representing well-perfused organs and tissues (fast compartment, V2) and the other representing more poorly perfused tissues such as fat (slow compartment, V3). The transfer of the drug between V1 and the two peripheral compartments (V2, V3), in addition to the elimination of the drug from V1, is described by a series of clearances (CL, Q2, Q3) indicating the distribution back and forth between paired compartments, such as V1 to V2 and then V2 back to V1. The primary target organ that intravenous anesthetic agents affect is the brain. Therefore, an additional rate constant is added to describe the equilibration between the central

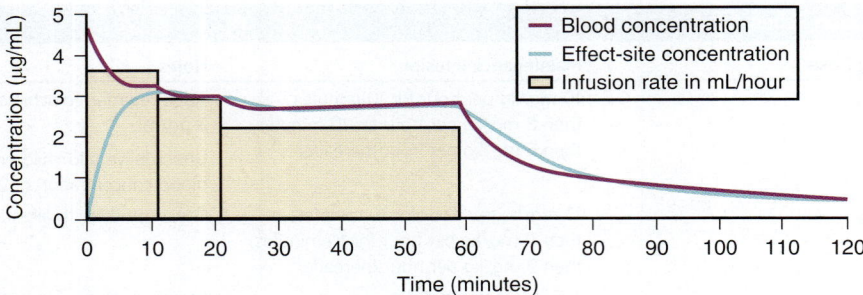

FIGURE 8.7 This figure illustrates the manual infusion technique in a healthy 70-kg 40-year-old. Note the importance of the early higher initial infusion rates to ensure that the target concentration is more constant. (Data from the Diprifusor pharmacokinetic data set.) Bolus dose (propofol 1%) was 1 mg/kg, then 10 mg/kg per hour for 10 minutes, 8 mg/kg per hour for 10 minutes, then 6 mg/kg per hour thereafter until 60 minutes when the infusion is discontinued. The maximum blood concentration is 4.5 μg/mL. Effect-site concentration reaches 3 μg/mL after around 10 minutes but drifts down to around 2.6 μg/mL and then very gradually rises. The context-sensitive half-time after 1-hour infusion is 7 minutes.

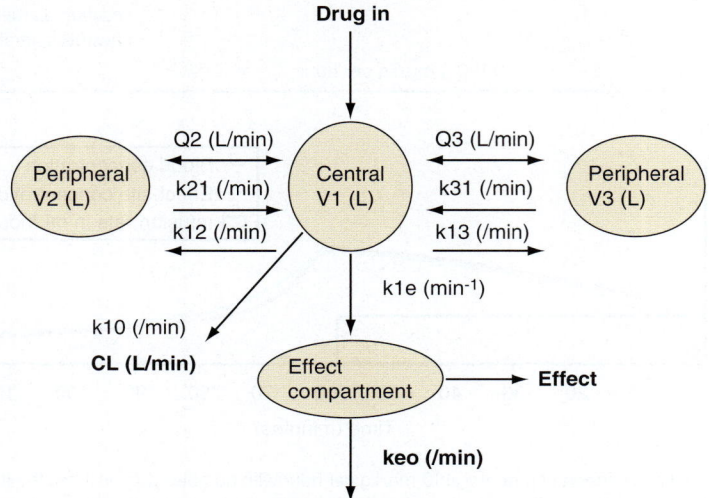

FIGURE 8.8 A three-compartment model with an additional compartment used to describe concentration in the effect compartment. A single first-order parameter (k1e = keo at steady state) describes the equilibration rate between the central (V1) and effect compartment. This compartment model is conceptualized in Fig. 8.9, where hydraulics are used to illustrate compartment interactions. The *arrows* in this figure could be considered "pipes" that deliver drug into the central compartment, out rapidly to V2 (and back to V1) and out more slowly to V3 (and back to V1) and are then eliminated through simultaneous clearance. k1e is the rate constant describing drug movement from compartment 1 to the effect compartment.

compartment and the effect site in the brain (keo = k1e at equilibrium). This compartment is not represented by a volume but rather by the time required to equilibrate. Consequently, there is a time lag before changes in the blood concentration are reflected in the effect site (shown on Figs. 8.6 and 8.7).

A hydraulic model is useful for understanding these concepts. The central compartment is connected to the peripheral compartments and effect site by a series of pipes of different diameters and also a drainage pipe to represent elimination (Fig. 8.9A-F). The height of the columns of fluid, which represents the concentration of drug, illustrates the gradient down which the drug travels between the central and peripheral compartments; this can be animated over time to show filling and emptying of compartments relative to each other. The diameter of the interconnecting pipes between the central and peripheral compartments represents the intercompartment clearances (Q2, Q3), and the size of the drainage

channel represents elimination (CL). This hydraulic analogy is used in the TIVA Trainer simulation program.[88]

Fixed Infusion Rate and a Three-Compartment Model

When a fixed infusion rate is started (see Fig. 8.6), the blood concentration will increase but, almost simultaneously, distribution of the drug to the fast compartment and elimination both begin. Distribution of drugs throughout the body contributes more to the removal of drug from blood than elimination for most medications. Remifentanil is an exception; it has extremely rapid esterase clearance and elimination of this drug is far greater than redistribution from the central compartment. As the concentrations within each compartment equilibrate, the concentration gradient between compartments lessens (slowing drug transfer between compartments) but distribution to the slow compartment continues along with elimination. The net effect is that the blood concentration continues to increase, albeit at a slower rate. As the blood concentration increases toward equilibrium, elimination becomes relatively more important; Fig. 8.6 illustrates how far behind the effect-site concentration lags. Eventually, after several hours (or in some cases, days), a steady state is reached where the infusion rate is directly proportional to clearance.

Bolus and Variable Rate Infusion in a Three-Compartment Model

A loading dose can start to fill the central compartment and ideally should attempt to create an effect-site concentration at a specific target concentration without overshoot. Then the rate of infusion should decrease in a stepwise manner to maintain a constant effect-site concentration until a steady state is reached. As drug is delivered into the central compartment, it continuously distributes to the peripheral compartments while it is also continuously eliminated. The infusion rate must vary because it has to match the concurrent changes in the contribution of distribution and elimination with time (Figs. 8.10 and 8.11). When the infusion is stopped, then elimination will continue to drain the central compartment, and drug will continue to distribute to V2 and V3 along concentration gradients from V1 for some time. Equilibrium may be reached, but the drug now begins to move back from the peripheral compartments into the central compartment, maintaining the central compartment drug concentration. This can continue for a protracted interval, particularly for highly lipid-soluble drugs that have a very large slow compartment V3 contributing a reservoir or depot effect (e.g., fentanyl; see Fig. 8.9F). Eventually the central compartment concentration will decrease. For most anesthetics, the longer the duration of an infusion, the more the drug has distributed into the peripheral compartments and the larger the reservoir of drug to be redistributed back into the central compartment and eliminated once the infusion ceases. The half-time of the decrease in drug concentration in blood is related to the duration of the infusion for most drugs (except remifentanil). This is termed the *context-sensitive half-time (CSHT)*, where the context is the duration of the infusion and relates to a pseudo-steady state maintained by a TCI. For an individual drug in an individual patient, CSHTs can be plotted against the duration of the infusion (Fig. 8.12A and B). The CSHT will eventually asymptote and this is when the pseudo-steady state becomes a true steady state. At that time, the infusion has become context *in*sensitive. This pattern is observed for nearly all IV anesthetics. In the case of propofol, the slope of the context-sensitive half-life with time increases from adults to children to infants to full-term and then preterm neonates, with preterm neonates having the greatest half-life of all age groups. The exception is remifentanil, whose half-time becomes context insensitive almost immediately after initiation of the infusion because its elimination is rapid and complete; the capacity of the red cell, plasma, and tissue esterase enzyme systems are enormous.

PK parameters for remifentanil, alfentanil, and sufentanil are summarized in Table 8.5.[86] The differences in context-sensitive

TABLE 8.4	Nomenclature for TCI Systems	
Term	**Meaning**	**Units**
TCI	Target-controlled infusion	
Vc or V1	Central compartment volume	L
V2	Fast compartment volume (vessel-rich group) = $V1 \times k_{12}/k_{21}$	L
V3	Slow compartment volume (vessel-poor group) = $V3 \times k_{13}/k_{31}$	L
Cl 1 or CL	Elimination clearance = $V1 \times k_{10}$	L/hour
Cl 2 or Q2	Clearance between V1 and V2 = $V2 \times k_{21}$	L/hour
Cl 3 or Q3	Clearance between V1 and V3 = $V3 \times k_{31}$	L/hour
Cp	Blood concentration	
Ce	Effect-site concentration	
T	Target concentration	
CALC	Concentration calculated by TCI software	
MEAS	Concentration measured	
k_{10}	Elimination rate constant	/minute
keo	Rate constant for equilibration between blood and effect-site	/minute
$T_{1/2}keo$	Half-time for equilibration between blood and effect site $$T_{1/2}keo = \frac{L_N(2)}{keo}$$	minutes
k_{12}, k_{21}	Rate constants for movement between V1 and V2	/minute
k_{13}, k_{31}	Rate constants for movement between V1 and V3	/minute

TABLE 8.5	Pharmacokinetic Parameters for Short-Acting Opioids		
	Remifentanil[34,89,90]	**Alfentanil[91]**	**Sufentanil[92]**
V1	$5.1 - 0.0201 \times (age - 40) + 0.072 \times (LBM - 55)$	Male: $0.111 \times weight$ Female: $1.15 \times 0.111 \times weight$	$0.164 \times weight$
V2	$9.82 - 0.0811 \times (age - 40) + 0.108 \times (LBM - 55)$	12.0	$0.359 \times weight$
V3	5.42	10.5	$1.263 \times weight$
k_{10}	$2.6 - 0.0162 \times (age - 40) + 0.0191 \times (LBM - 55)/V1$	$0.356/V1$	0.089
k_{12}	$2.05 - 0.0301 \times (age - 40)/V1$	0.104	0.35
k_{21}	$2.05 - 0.0301 \times (age - 40)/V2$	0.067	0.16
k_{13}	$0.076 - 0.00113 \times (age - 40)/V1$	0.017	0.077
k_{31}	$0.076 - 0.00113 \times (age - 40)/5.42$	0.0126	0.01
keo	$0.595 - 0.007 \times (age - 40)$	0.77	0.12

Age in years; weight in kilograms.
LBM, lean body mass.
From Absalom AR, Struys MMRF. *An Overview of TCI and TIVA.* Ghent, Belgium: Academia Press; 2005.

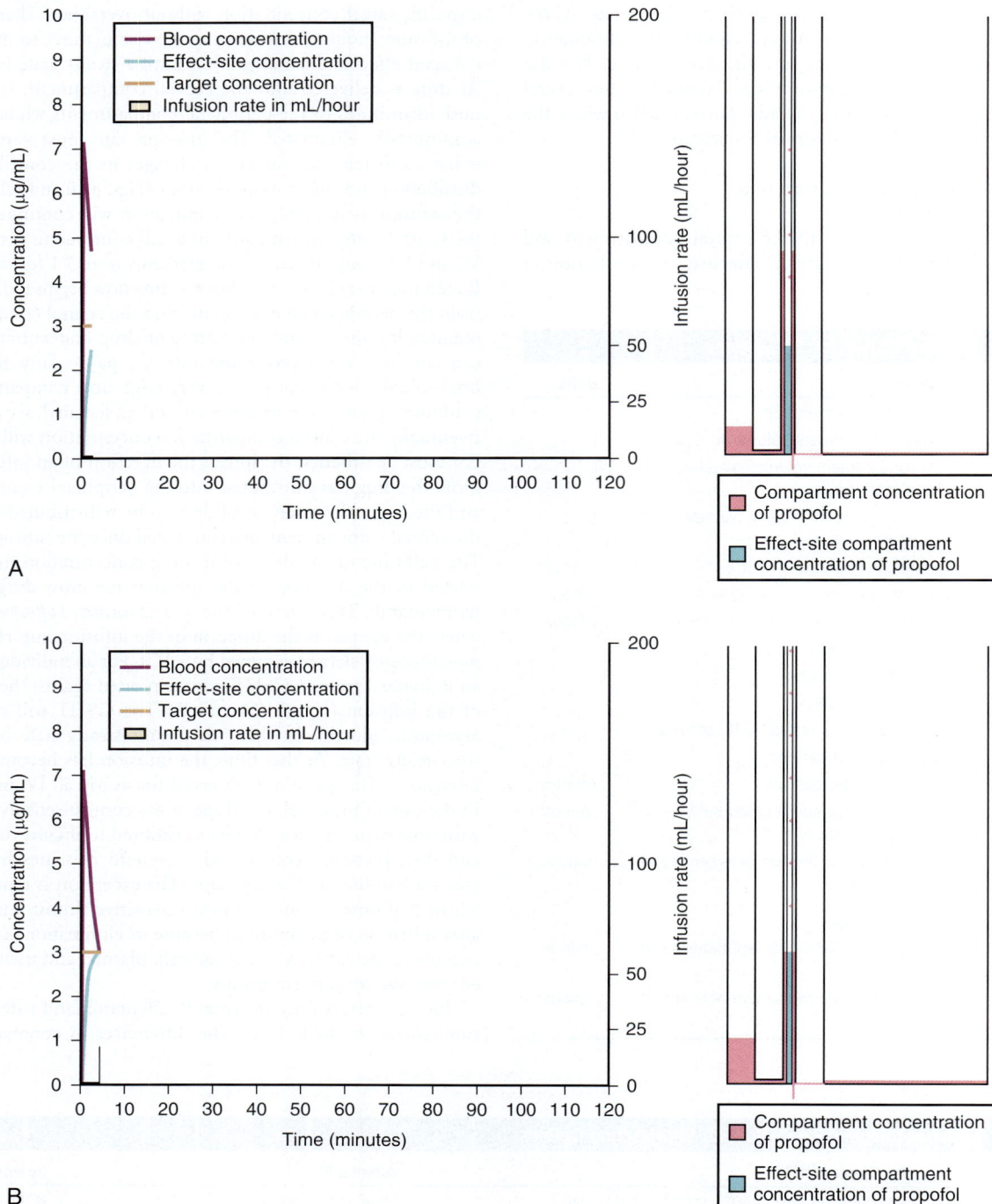

FIGURE 8.9 A, Hydraulic model representation of effect-site TCI. Compartment volumes and intercompartmental clearance values for the Paedfusor model in a healthy 10-kg, 1-year-old infant. In the first few minutes the central compartment to effect-site concentration gradient is marked to "overpressure" the transfer of propofol to the effect site. The peak blood concentration is 7.1 µg/mL. Distribution from the central compartment (C1) to the first peripheral compartment (C2) occurs rapidly also, which slows the rise in effect-site concentration and blood concentration. Elimination from C1 and distribution from C1 to the second peripheral compartment (C3) is also occurring. **B,** At 4.5 minutes, the effect-site concentration has reached the target of 3 µg/mL and has equilibrated with the concentration in C1. The infusion device, which has been off after the initial loading infusion, now switches back on to maintain the effect-site target concentration at 3 µg/mL.

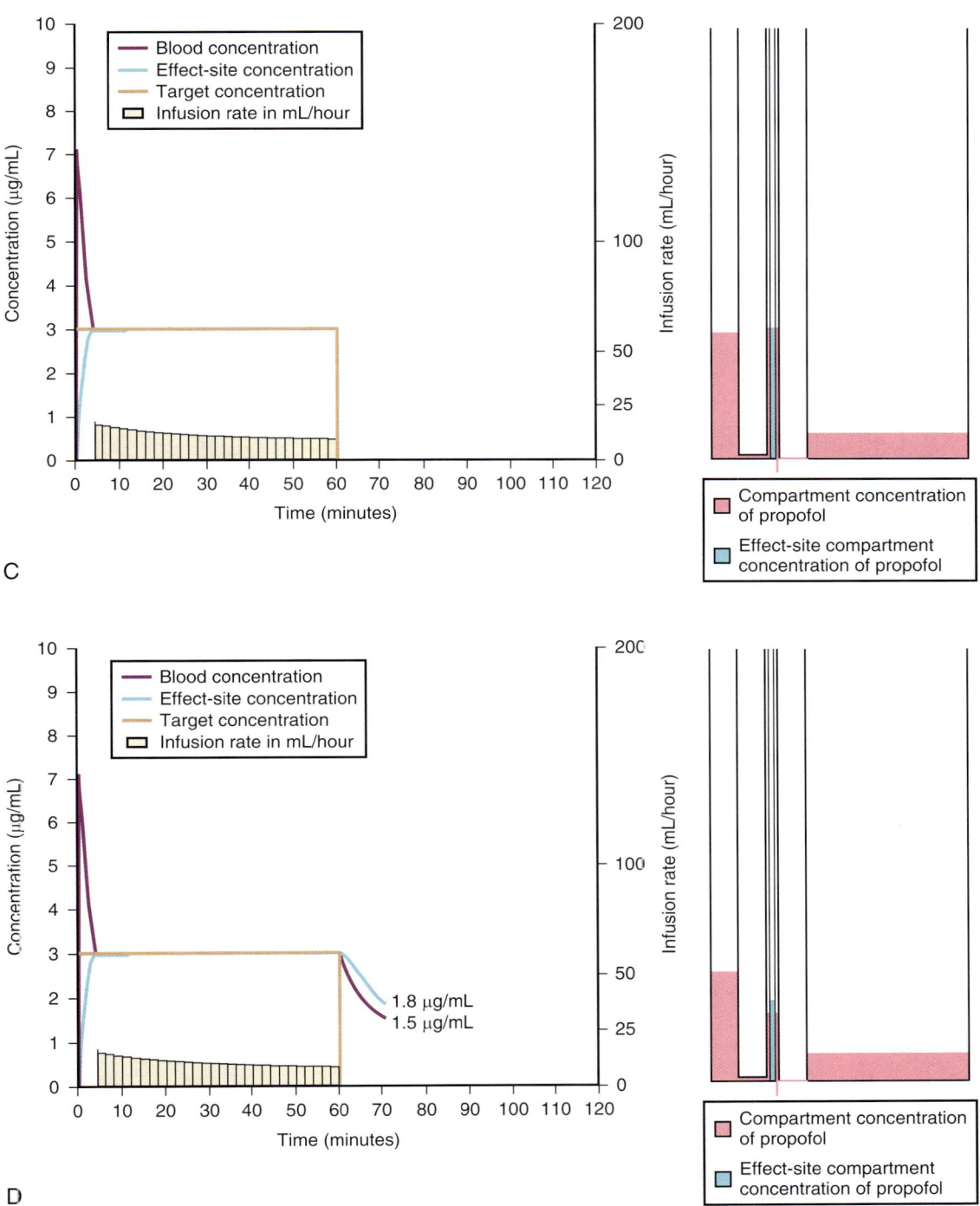

C

D

FIGURE 8.9, cont'd C, After 1 hour of maintenance at an effect-site concentration of 3 μg/mL, the target is set to 0 μg/mL and the pump switches off. A total of 14 mL of propofol (1%) has been administered, or 14 mg/kg. There is now a considerable accumulation of propofol in C2 and C3, while C1 and the effect site are still in equilibrium. **D,** Approximately 10 minutes after the effect-site target concentration is set to 0, the blood concentration has halved; thus the context-sensitive half-time is 10 minutes. The lag in the decline in effect-site concentration is clearly seen, and there is now a gradient between effect site and C1. There is now also a concentration gradient from C2 to C1 and to C3 and this slows the decline in the concentration in C1.   *Continued*

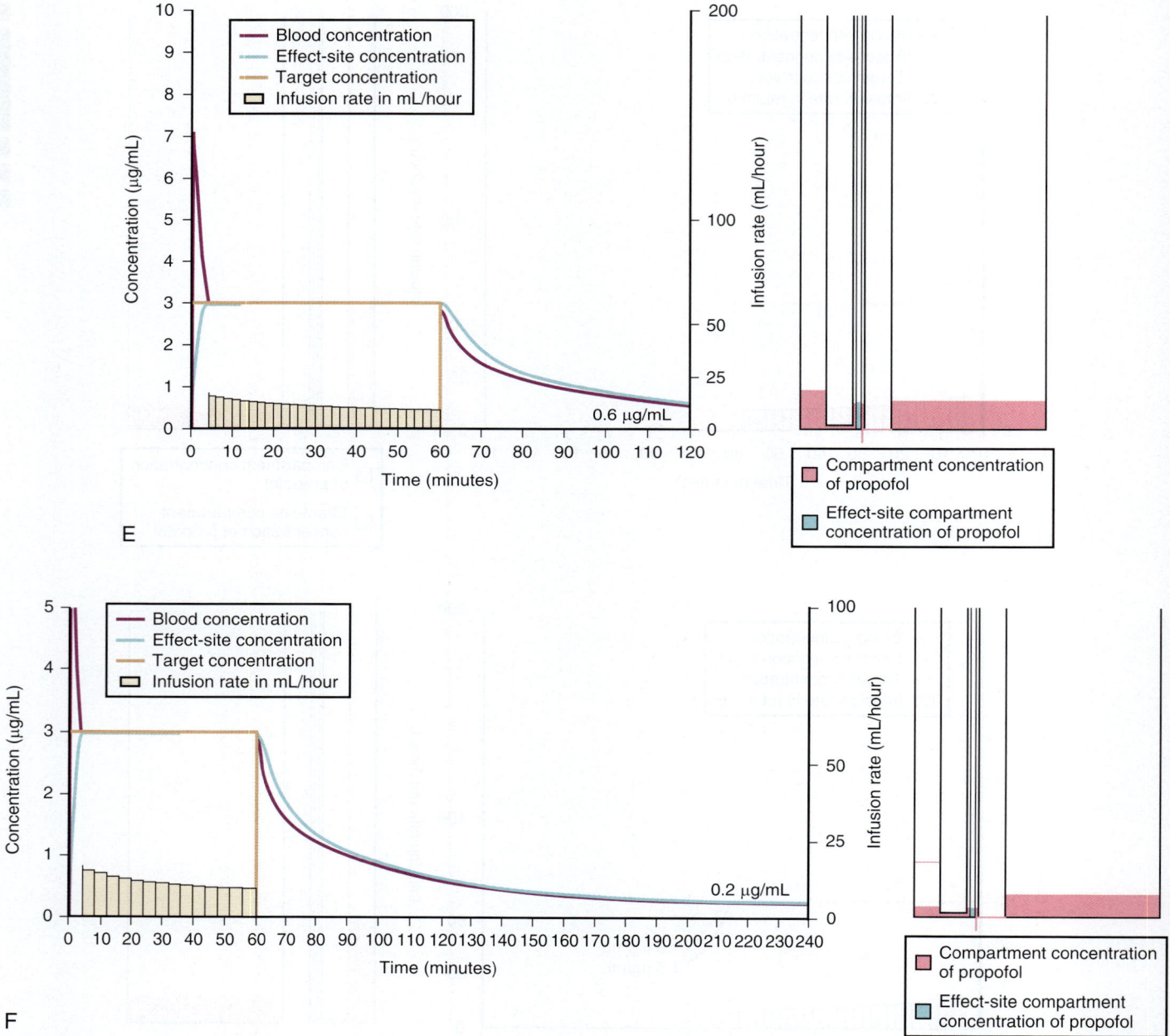

FIGURE 8.9, cont'd E, One hour after the infusion is stopped, the blood and effect-site concentrations have fallen to ⅕ of the maintenance effect-site concentration. There are still considerable quantities of propofol in compartments C2 and C3 that slow the decline of the concentration of C1 and effect-site concentrations. **F,** Even after 4 hours, the depot of propofol in C2 and C3 is considerable, although blood and effect-site concentrations are extremely low. However, these low concentrations may still be exerting significant antiemetic and anxiolytic effects (data from the Paedfusor pharmacokinetic data set).

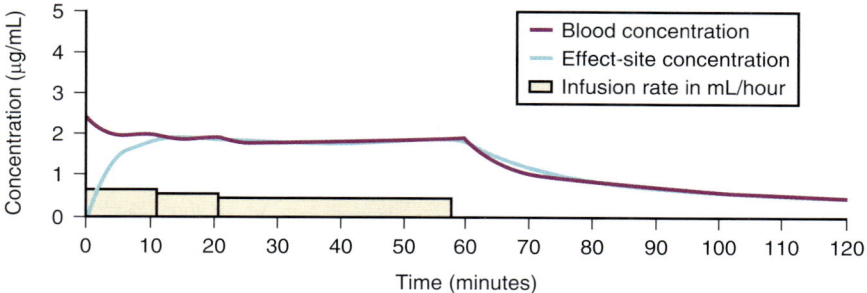

FIGURE 8.10 This figure illustrates the manual infusion technique of propofol in a healthy 1-year-old, 10-kg child. Note the importance of the early higher initial infusion rates to ensure that the target concentration is more constant. The adult dose regimen is illustrated. The figure shows a bolus dose of 1 mg/kg, then 10 mg/kg per hour for 10 minutes, then 8 mg/kg per hour for 10 minutes, then 6 mg/kg per hour thereafter. The infusion was stopped at 60 minutes. The effect-site concentration dose does not equilibrate until 11 minutes. The blood and effect-site concentrations stabilize around 1.8 µg/mL. However, this is unlikely to represent a sufficient depth of anesthesia for surgery. The context-sensitive half-time after 1 hour infusion is 9 minutes (data from the Paedfusor pharmacokinetic data set).

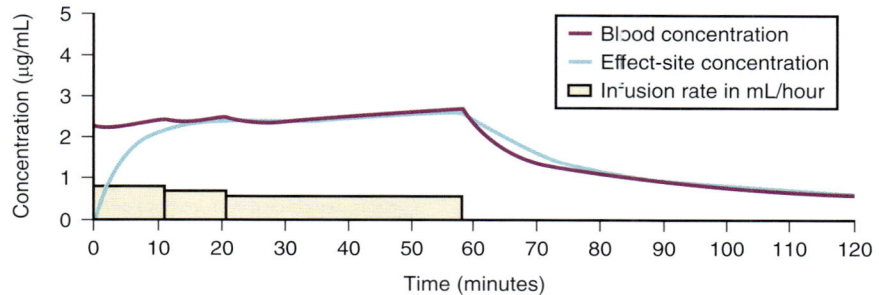

FIGURE 8.11 Manual infusion of propofol in 1-year-old, 10-kg child. The figure shows a bolus dose of 1 mg/kg, then 13 mg/kg per hour for 10 minutes, then 11 mg/kg per hour for 10 minutes, then 9 mg/kg per hour thereafter. The infusion was stopped at 60 minutes. The effect-site concentration does not equilibrate until 20 minutes. The blood and effect-site concentrations stabilize around 2.4 µg/mL but gradually rise over the next hour to 2.6 µg/mL. This concentration is larger than that achieved using the adult 10-8-6 regimen but may still be inadequate. Larger infusion doses are required in a 1-year-old child. (Data from the Paedfusor pharmacokinetic data set.)

half-times are illustrated in Table 8.6 and Fig. 8.12A and B. Fentanyl has a small CSHF when given by infusion for a short time, but this dramatically increases as the duration of the infusion increases. Alfentanil's CSHF reaches a plateau after approximately 90 minutes.

THE TARGET-CONTROLLED INFUSION

A TCI is accomplished by a computer that performs rapid sequential calculations every 8 to 10 seconds to estimate the infusion rate required to produce a user-defined drug concentration in the blood or at the effect site of action of the drug in the brain in an open-loop system.[86] *Thus TCI may be blood targeted or effect-site targeted.* The standard nomenclature for TCI systems is listed in Table 8.4. Modern TCI systems are computer-controlled syringe drivers capable of infusion rates up to 1200 mL/hour with a precision of 0.1 mL/hour. They incorporate a user interface and display a range of safety alarms, monitoring functions, and warning systems. For most programs, the user has to choose a drug and its concentration from a menu and also select a PK parameter set (referred to as a model). The models suitable for use in children are quite limited, and some models are not suitable for all age groups. Others may be suitable but have not been validated in younger

children; neonatal and infant models are quite rare. Experience with the various models may be gained by running the simulation programs such as Tivatrainer (http://eurosiva.org/; European Society for Intravenous Anaesthesia [EuroSIVA; Amsterdam, The Netherlands) or Rugloop (http://www.demed.be/rugloop.htm; Demed, Temse, Belgium) on a personal computer. Tivatrainer now allows uploading of new models via a central website and server and contains details and simulations of pediatric models for propofol and neonatal and pediatric models for sufentanil, in

TABLE 8.6	Context-Sensitive Half-Times (minutes) of Opioids in Children				
	Infusion Duration (minutes)				
Opioid	**10**	**100**	**200**	**300**	**600**
Remifentanil	3–6	3–6	3–6	3–6	3–6
Alfentanil	10	45	55	58	60
Sufentanil		20	25	35	60
Fentanyl	12	30	100	200	

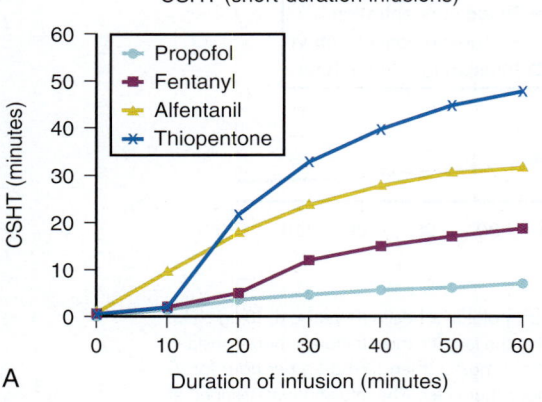

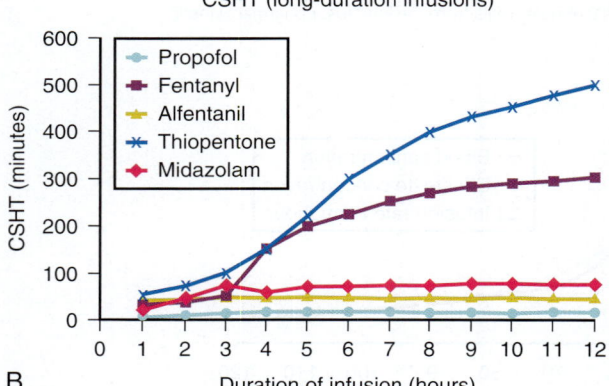

FIGURE 8.12 A, Context-sensitive half-times *(CSHTs)* after short-duration infusions. **B,** CSHTs after longer-duration infusions. For very lipid soluble drugs such as fentanyl and propofol, V3 is very large compared with V1. Intercompartmental clearance between V1 and V3 is given by the equation V1 χ k_{13} = V3 χ k_{31}, which implies that if V1 is much smaller than V3, rapid distribution from V1 to V3 is associated with very slow redistribution from V3 to V1. This is indeed seen with propofol and fentanyl, which have a slow offset of effects after prolonged infusions. Propofol has a CSHT that varies between approximately 3 minutes for a short-duration infusion to approximately 18 minutes after a 12-hour infusion. This is because elimination is quite rapid compared with the rate of redistribution from V3. For alfentanil, the concentration of the un-ionized form is 100 times greater than that of fentanyl (pKa alfentanil 6.4, fentanyl 8.5). Alfentanil therefore has a more rapid onset time and shorter half-life keo, a smaller V1, lower volume of distribution at steady state, and lower clearance than fentanyl. Fentanyl does, however, have a shorter CSHT than alfentanil after a short-duration infusion lasting less than 2 hours **(A)**; but for longer-duration infusions, alfentanil reaches a maximum CSHT after about 90 minutes, whereas for fentanyl the CSHT continues to increase after 12 hours **(B)**. This is because fentanyl has a huge V3, and redistribution back to V1 maintains the blood concentration when the infusion stops. (Simulated using Tivatrainer; available at www.eurosiva.org/TivaTrainer_main.htm.)

TABLE 8.7 — Paedfusor Propofol Pharmacokinetic Parameters

1–12 years	V1 = 0.4584 × weight; V2 = V1 × k_{12}/k_{21}; V3 = V1 × k_{13}/k_{31}
	k_{10} = 0.1527 × weight$^{-0.3}$
	k_{12} = 0.114; k_{21} = 0.055
	k_{13} = 0.0419; k_{31} = 0.0033
	keo = 0.26
13 years	V1 = 0.400 × weight
	k_{10} = 0.0678
	(other constants as above)
14 years	V1 = 0.342 × weight
	k_{10} = 0.0792
	(other constants as above)
15 years	V1 = 0.284 × weight
	k_{10} = 0.0954
	(other constants as above)
16 years	V1 = 0.22857 × weight
	k_{10} = 0.119
	(other constants as above)

k_{10}, Elimination rate constant; k_{12} and k_{21}, rate constants for movement between V1 and V2; k_{13} and k_{31}, rate constants for movement between V1 and V3; keo, effect site equilibration rate constant; V1, central compartment volume; V2, fast compartment volume; V3, slow compartment volume.
Note: The k_{10} value in the age group 1–12 years is a negative power function of weight that reflects the increasing clearance values in younger children.
Data from Marsh B, White M, Morton N, Kenny GN. Pharmacokinetic model driven infusion of propofol in children. *Brit J Anaesth*. 1991;67:41-48; Rigby-Jones AE, Nolan JA, Priston MJ, et al. Pharmacokinetics of propofol infusions in critically ill neonates, infants, and children in an intensive care unit. *Anesthesiology* 2002;97:1393-1400; Murat I, Billard V, Vernois J, et al. Pharmacokinetics of propofol after a single dose in children aged 1-3 years with minor burns. Comparison of three data analysis approaches. *Anesthesiology* 1996;84:526-532.

TABLE 8.8 — Comparison Between Paedfusor and Kataria Models for Propofol in Children

	Paedfusor[93,94,97,98]	Kataria[99]
V1	0.458 × weight	0.41 × weight
V2	0.95 × weight	0.78 × weight + 3.1 × age
V3	5.82 × weight	6.9 × weight
k_{10}	0.1527 × weight^{-03}	0.085
k_{12}	0.114	0.188
k_{21}	0.055	0.102
k_{13}	0.0419	0.063
k_{31}	0.0033	0.0038
keo	0.26[a]	N/A[a]

[a]This is the value for adults, but Munoz et al.[101] have studied these two models to define a more accurate keo for children age 3–11 years, and the values are 0.91 for the Paedfusor model and 0.41 for the Kataria model. Jeleazcov et al.[102] have derived age-related keo values by the formula keo = 1.03 × e$^{-0.12 × age}$.

addition to a wide range of adult models for propofol, alfentanil, remifentanil, fentanyl, ketamine, and midazolam. The simulation shows animated graphs of blood and effect-site concentrations against time, infusion rates, volumes, compartment sizes, and many other features.

The models within TCI systems are derived from studies of small numbers of healthy patients and are only a guide to drug administration for an individual patient.[83] The accuracy of TCI propofol has been assessed in children.[83,93] TCI propofol has

been incorporated into a modified version of the commercial Diprifusor device and is known as the Paedfusor,[94] which has been evaluated clinically and performs well (Table 8.7).[93,95,96] In children undergoing cardiac surgery, the model performed significantly better than the adult model in adults.[94,97,98] Parameter estimates for the Kataria model are similar (Table 8.8) and it also performs reasonably well,[83,99] but all models have shortcomings.[100] Experience shows that clinicians need to learn how to use each model to optimize levels of anesthesia, ensure stability during

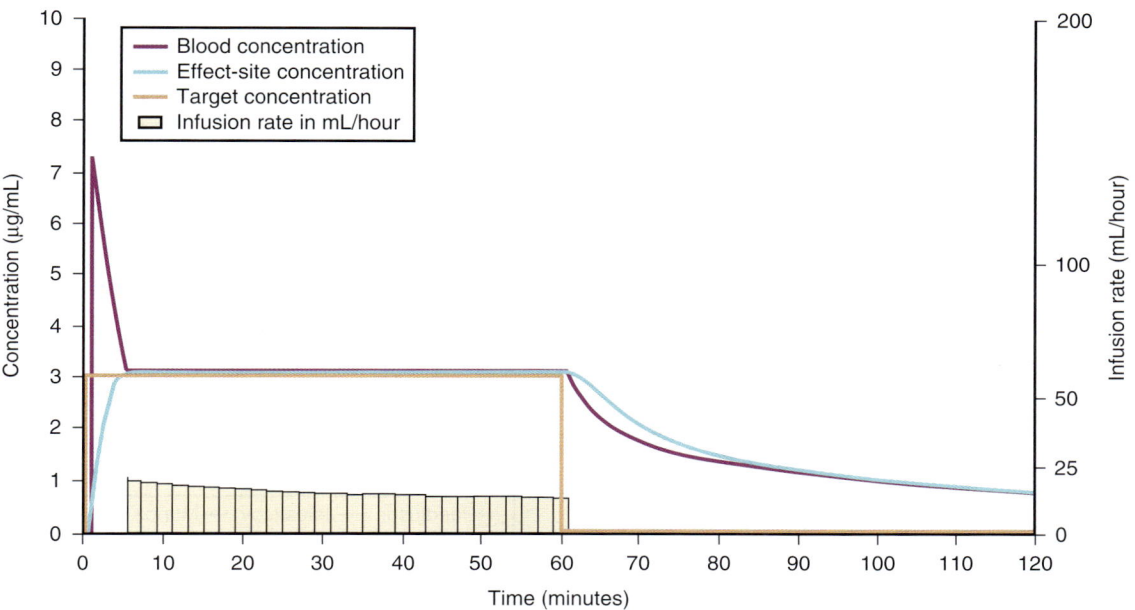

FIGURE 8.13 Target-controlled infusion modeled using the Paedfusor pharmacokinetic data set. Effect-site–targeted infusion of propofol in a healthy 1-year-old, 10-kg child. The effect-site target is 3 µg/mL. The figure shows a bolus dose of 3.4 mg/kg delivered at 45.5 mL/hour to accentuate the gradient from blood to effect site, then the infusion switches off for 4 minutes. Peak blood concentration after bolus dose is 7.1 µg/mL. Stepwise-reducing the infusion from 15.7 mg/kg per hour to 9.5 mg/kg per hour for 1 hour was done. The infusion was stopped at 60 minutes (i.e., effect-site target is set for 0 µg/mL). The effect-site concentration reaches 3 µg/mL at 3 minutes 39 seconds. The total dose of propofol is 14 mg/kg. The context-sensitive half-time is 10 minutes 37 seconds.

induction and maintenance phases, and enhance recovery speed and quality. Most pediatric models overestimate the initial volume of distribution, which risks too large an initial bolus dose.[83] The Paedfusor model makes an allowance for the increased clearance with age (per kilogram) in younger children; particularly those below 30 kg in weight (see Tables 8.7 and 8.8, Fig. 8.13). The minimum age and weight limits for each model also differ with age 1 year and 5 kg for the Paedfusor system and 3 years and 15 kg for the Kataria system. Below a weight 12.5 kg and age 2 years, the second compartment becomes negative with the Kataria model, which means that model cannot be used clinically in such young patients. For simulation using the Paedfusor data set, the adult value for keo of 0.26/minute ($T_{1/2}$keo 2.7 minutes) can be used (see Table 8.8). This means effect-site targeting may be simulated with the Paedfusor model (Table 8.9), and it may be possible to display an effect-site predicted concentration while using a pump in blood-targeted TCI mode, as with Diprifusor. Attempts have been made to define a more accurate keo for children in an ingenious study using auditory evoked responses with both the Paedfusor and Kataria models.[101] For children age 3 to 11 years, the median extrapolated keo values for the Paedfusor models was 0.91/minute ($T_{1/2}$keo 0.8 minutes) and for the Kataria model 0.41/minute ($T_{1/2}$keo 1.7 minutes). The BIS was used to derive a value for the time to peak effect, and hence, keo.[87,102,103] It was concluded that the time to peak effect after a bolus dose was shorter in children than adults as the extrapolated $T_{1/2}$keo values were considerably smaller.[100] Similar findings were reported by Hahn et al. using state entropy monitoring.[104] This approach has enabled calculation of an age-specific range of values for the keo (see Fig. 8.3), which should allow more accurate effect-site targeting using propofol in the future. It must be stressed that compartmental values are highly specific to a single model and are

TABLE 8.9	Example of Target-Controlled Infusion (Propofol 5 µg/mL) Based on Calculated Blood-Concentration Targeting Compared With Calculated Effect-Site Concentration Targeting for a Healthy 1-Year-Old (10 kg), Using the Paedfusor Pharmacokinetic Data Set

	Blood Concentration Targeting	Effect-Site Concentration Targeting
Loading dose	1.7 mg/kg	5.7 mg/kg[a]
Maximum blood target reached	5 µg/kg	12 µg/kg[a]
Total propofol infused after 60 minutes	23.2 mg/kg	23.3 mg/kg
Time to achieve effect site target of 5 µg/mL	17.5 minutes	4.5 minutes[b]

[a]Potential for hemodynamic changes due to high peak blood concentration from larger bolus dose.
[b]Very much shorter time to achieve effect-site target.

not interchangeable.[83,100] It can be argued that these calculations and extrapolations are a trick to sidestep imperfect PK values.[83,100] Integrating pharmacokinetic and pharmacodynamics into models appropriate for use in children is challenging, not the least because of doubts about the sensitivity and specificity of the depth of anesthesia monitoring in children.[33,104–106]

Some pumps display predicted plasma or effect site concentrations from the programmed PK model and are invaluable as an educational tool for demonstrating the intricacies of TIVA. TCI pumps do not have current FDA approval within North America,

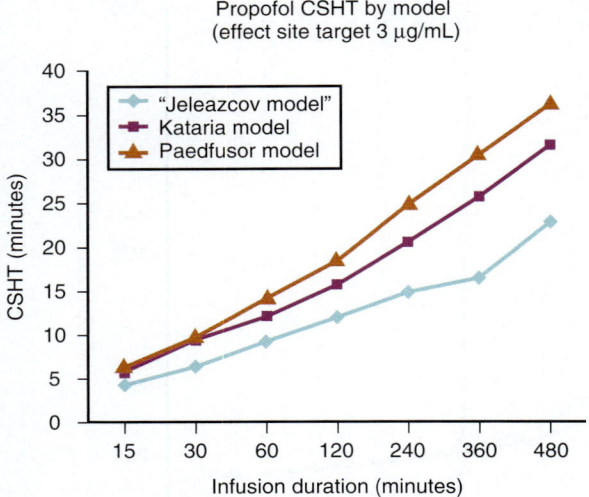

Propofol CSHT by model
(effect site target 3 μg/mL)

FIGURE 8.14 The predicted context-sensitive half-time (CSHT) of propofol depends on the pharmacokinetic model. Effect-site targeting can result in higher propofol doses if the keo is incorrect. The Jeleazcov model uses age-appropriate keo values and this results in the shortest predicted CSHTs for all infusion durations. This has clinical importance as it predicts a shorter recovery time for a given target concentration. (Data from Limb J, Morton NS. Age specific effect-site TCI in children; modelling using Tivatrainer. *Anaesthesia* 2010;65:542; and Absalom A, Vereecke HE, Eleveld DJ. A hitch-hiker's guide to the intravenous PK/PD galaxy. *Paediatr Anaesth.* 2011;21:915-918.)

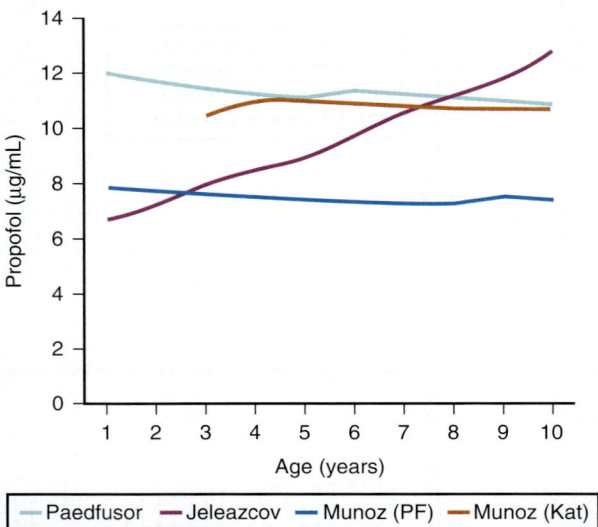

FIGURE 8.15 The peak plasma concentrations attained in simulations in Fig. 8.14 for an effect-site target of 5 μg/mL are shown. A large bolus dose does not necessarily equate to high peak plasma concentrations because of the variable volumes of distribution in the pediatric models at different ages. Even though more drug may be administered when using effect-site targeting if the keo is inappropriate, this may not mean an increase in peak plasma concentration because the peripheral volumes of distribution may be increased in any one model. More drug is redistributed. (Data from Limb J, Morton NS. Age specific effect-site TCI in children; modelling using Tivatrainer. *Anaesthesia* 2010;65:542; and Absalom A, Vereecke HE, Eleveld DJ. A hitch-hiker's guide to the intravenous PK/PD galaxy. *Paediatr Anaesth.* 2011;21:915-918.)

but it is anticipated that approval will be granted in the near future.

Effect-site targeting offers the advantages of more rapid achievement of desired depth of anesthesia and less titration of the target depth in practice, but while it has been used in research in children, it has yet to become a clinical tool.[107] Table 8.9 shows how the behavior of the TCI infusion differs between blood and effect-site targeted infusion using the adult keo of 0.26/minute ($T_{1/2}$keo 2.7 minutes). It can be expected that effect-site targeting may have more profound cardiovascular and respiratory effects than blood targeting owing to the larger initial bolus doses with resultant higher peak blood propofol concentrations attained.[107] It is known that slower administration of propofol preserves spontaneous respiration in children,[108] and the use of an age-appropriate $T_{1/2}$keo value and careful titration from a low initial target value may ameliorate some adverse effects. Without such titration, adverse effects may be more marked in infants (Fig. 8.14).[102,107] Although the use of BIS remains uncertain in children,[109] particularly those younger than age 1 year, the use of age- or weight-appropriate $T_{1/2}$keo values in TCI systems provides the prospect of more accurate and efficient propofol delivery to children.[107] This has safety implications in terms of reducing lipid load and clinical utility by increasing speed of recovery (Fig. 8.15).

A Practical Approach in Children

Mastery of TIVA requires familiarity with the technique. Such familiarity can be gained by practice with older children before progressing to those younger and beginning with children who present for elective, nonurgent surgery where a known stimulus will be applied. Cooperation from surgical colleagues is always advantageous when mastering the use of TIVA.

DRUG DELIVERY

Secure IV access is essential to safely administer TIVA. A dedicated line is not necessarily required as long as there is access to the IV cannula being used. Syringes that screw into infusion sets reduce the risk of poor or leaky connections. Infusion lines should be placed as close as possible to the venous cannula.[110] The setup should prevent retrograde infusion of propofol up the IV infusion set if resistance to flow into the cannula is greater than that in the fluid line. This is optimally achieved using one-way, nonreturn valves to prevent backflow up the IV fluid line. Percutaneous intravenous central catheters (PICC) may be unsatisfactory because high infusion rates are not possible. Combined infusions into a single vein run the risk of an inadvertent bolus of a companion drug. Anesthesia for major surgery may be best served using central venous access, diminishing the risk of unintended subcutaneous infusion. The infusion site is not always readily accessible in small children whose limbs may be covered in surgical drapes, and inadvertent dislodgment, obstruction, or subcutaneous tissue infiltration may occur. Common drug delivery problems are listed in Table 8.10.

Although closed-loop anesthesia is currently impractical because effect measures are poor in infants and neonates, changes in cerebral effect measures with changes of dose may at least confirm that the infusion is not disconnected or subcutaneous. Pump performance characteristics (e.g., lag time), IV tubing dead space, and syringe size and type all contribute to the observed response (see also Chapter 52). The more dilute the solution, the faster the syringe plunger travels with a better matched delivery to change the drug delivery prescription.[110] Dilution is especially important

TABLE 8.10 | **Potential Problems With Drug Delivery From Intravenous Anesthesia Pumps[a]**

Problem	Prevention/Detection/Solution
IV cannula disconnect/out of vein	Venous access should be visible and accessible during procedure
Disconnection of infusion tubing from pump or cannula	Pump and tubing connections should be visible
	Use Luer-lock syringes
Pump power supply failure or pump paused	Ensure pump has an audible alarm
Occlusion of IV cannula or tubing	Pump high-pressure alarm
Occlusion alarm because of small cannula or long infusion tubing (e.g., PICC)	Ability to alter alarm threshold
"Backtracking" of propofol into intravenous fluid infusion tubing	Use of one-way valves
Drug disparity between settings and drug used (e.g., different concentration)	Keep only one concentration of propofol in hospital. Double-check drug dilution concentrations (or dispense from pharmacy premixed)
	A dedicated IV with a constant carrier solution for TIVA is the ideal
Wrong drug programmed into pump (remifentanil rather than propofol)	Prominent pump displays with the drug name.
	Color coding of the pump LCD displays and syringe labels
	Bar coding

[a]Adapted from Nimmo AF, Cook TM. Accidental awareness during general anesthesia in the United Kingdom and Ireland. In: Pandit JJ, Cook TM, eds. *National Audit Project*, ed 5. Royal College of Anaesthetists and the Association of Anaesthetists of Great Britain and Ireland, 2014:151-158. *PICC*, percutaneous intravenous central catheters.

TABLE 8.11 | **Possible Weight-Based Propofol Regimes in Children**

Weight	Infusion Scheme
>35 kg	Schneider effect-site concentration model
15–35 kg	Kataria plasma concentration model *or*
	McFarlan manual plasma concentration regimen
<15 kg	Steur manual infusion regimen

in improving the accuracy of delivery in infants and neonates. Modified EEG monitoring (e.g., BIS) is not necessary in the spontaneously breathing patient but should be considered in the patient who is receiving TIVA and neuromuscular blockade. The BIS is reasonably valid for children as young as approximately 3 years of age with propofol, but there are very limited data for other medications. It is essential to appreciate that in younger children the BIS number may not be reliable, but some interpretation can be made from BIS number changes rather than the absolute BIS number displayed.

TCI parameter sets (models) available for use in children generate different plasma propofol concentrations. It is important to be aware of these differences; this is especially so with regard to the initial loading dose. Consequently, it is important to be aware of the performance of the infusion pump being used, the particular parameter set installed, and its appropriateness for a given clinical scenario. The immature neonate, the critically ill child, or the child with major organ failure needs a smaller dose of IV anesthetic agent; care is particularly needed in children receiving vasoactive medication and those with congenital heart disease.[111] Titration is advisable to allow for between-subject variability of PK and PD parameters.

Pumps should be serviced regularly. Unrecognized pump failures can occur with subsequent patient awareness or overdose so vigilance is required. If problems with anesthesia occur, then the prudent thing to do may be to convert to an inhalational anesthetic technique if clinically appropriate.

INFUSION REGIMES

In general, the TCI pumps deliver propofol more accurately than manual regimes, result in better hemodynamic stability, use a lower induction dose, and result in improved recovery time. If a dedicated TCI pump is available, then it should be preferred over a manual regime. Surgical anesthesia is generally obtained with a propofol effect site concentration of 4 to 6 µg/mL. This will be achieved more rapidly with an effect-site target model than with plasma-targeted models because of equilibration between the plasma concentration and effect-site concentration.

Most TCI programs (models) are inaccurate for some ages within their specified age ranges[28–30] or when parameter estimates have not been tested (e.g., intensive care patients or children with neuromuscular disease undergoing scoliosis surgery).[80] Clearance (per kilogram) is increased as age decreases in children (allometric theory). The Kataria parameter set is known to underpredict concentration as age increases, consistent with allometric scaling. When this parameter set is used to estimate PD parameters, it appears that the older children require lower concentrations to maintain anesthesia[47]; this is a PK effect and not a PD effect.[48]

The adult Schnider[112] model may be more accurate than either the pediatric Kataria,[19] pediatric Marsh[21] or Schuttler[25] models in children weighing more than 35 kg.[33] The Schnider effect-site–targeted model has also been shown to have better accuracy in adults.[113] The Kataria TCI model is plasma targeted and is valid for children from 3 to 15 years weighing 15 to 65 kg. For children younger than 3 years, Steur et al.[50] have produced a manual regime (see Table 8.2). Neonates are susceptible to hypotension with propofol[51] and it is advisable to gradually increase infusion rate until anesthesia is achieved rather than starting at a high infusion rate.[114] Manual regimes have also been produced to mimic Kataria plasma targeted infusion for 3 to 6 µg/mL.[18,115] One approach to the use of propofol regimes in children for TIVA is shown in Table 8.11.

The Obese Child

Problems with drug dosing in obese adults are also common in children. The size metric varies with both drug and infusion type. The initial bolus may depend on the lean body mass, whereas the infusion rate may depend on another size metric. For example, propofol infusion rates relate best to total body weight scaled using allometry,[45,116] whereas lean body weight is a better metric for remifentanil infusions. A further complication is that the calculator program[117] of the pump used to estimate lean body mass fails in short obese people.[118] Solutions to this problem include setting limits on maximum weight,[119] inventing a fictitious height,[120] or creating a new metric[121]; use of a better metric such as fat-free mass might be the best solution.[118] Investigations using normal fat mass[122] as a size metric suggest that the appropriate "size" may differ for each drug. These dose calculation problems can be circumvented by reducing the target concentration (e.g., propofol 4 µg/mL rather than 6 µg/mL) and then titrating to effect. The use of a cerebral function monitor such as BIS can be helpful.

Remifentanil as an Adjunct

Remifentanil is very useful as an adjunct.[123,124] It adds a degree of "smoothing" even in those children who require sedation only (e.g., radiologic imaging). Propofol is not an analgesic and the addition of remifentanil reduces movement in response to surgical stimulation[125]; there is approximately 30% more movement with propofol compared with an inhalational anesthetic. Remifentanil also reduces the propofol target concentration.[67,126] The consequent propofol dose reduction can be useful when anesthesia duration is prolonged because the concomitant context-sensitive half-life of propofol increases over time and concomitant remifentanil adjunct allows earlier awakening. Remifentanil is also useful to reduce pain during limb procedures where a tourniquet is used.

Most children will maintain spontaneous respirations with a remifentanil-propofol combination. Fig. 7.26 demonstrates the remifentanil infusion rates that will maintain a spontaneous respiration rate of 10 breaths/minute. Use of the adult Minto parameter set for remifentanil infusion in children confers a degree of safety because concentrations measured will be lower than those predicted because of the higher clearance (expressed as per kilogram) in children. Occasionally some respiratory support may be required; that is easily done using the pressure support ventilation mode. Controlled ventilation is required when high target concentrations of remifentanil are used. High effect-site remifentanil concentrations (>10 ng/mL) are associated with hypotension (Fig. 8.16) and this property can be used advantageously during some neurosurgical procedures or spinal instrumentation.[127]

Fixed propofol-remifentanil combinations (mixed together in the same syringe) are frowned upon by some because (1) they do not allow separate titration of analgesia and sedation and (2) targeting a propofol concentration can result in a relatively large bolus of remifentanil. However, they remain widely used—for example, propofol 10 mg/mL with remifentanil 5 µg/mL. If a combination is used with a TCI pump then a propofol target concentration of 3 µg/L usually allows spontaneous breathing, whereas a propofol

target of 6 µg/mL requires ventilatory support. Although such mixtures are widely used, remifentanil in such mixtures may become unstable and has a limited life span in the syringe. The weaker the mixture, the less stable it is. This is due to a pH effect on the rate of ester hydrolysis of the remifentanil.[128]

Injection Pain With Propofol

The pain associated with IV injection of propofol is problematic. This is especially common when given through the small veins in the hands or feet. Perhaps the best approach to reduce injection pain is to place a larger-bore cannula in a large vein. Lignocaine 1 mg/kg placed in the IV with a proximal tourniquet (or just manual compression of the arm to stop the IV from flowing) applied for 30 to 60 seconds effectively attenuates this pain. Opioid or ketamine administered IV before propofol injection is also helpful. This can be best done by beginning the remifentanil infusion first and running it at a Cp of approximately 2 to 3 ng/mL for 2 minutes (using the Minto model) before starting the propofol infusion; most children and adults will continue to maintain spontaneous respirations through this short period. Alternatively, a bolus of fentanyl 1 µg/kg or remifentanil 1 µg/kg through the IV cannula is effective.

ESTABLISHING TIVA AFTER AN INHALATIONAL INDUCTION

Inhalational induction is standard in many pediatric centers. Propofol TIVA can start once gaseous induction has been performed and IV access obtained. The use of a fixed infusion rate only is frowned upon because steady-state concentrations will not be established before 3 to 4 elimination half-lives (see Fig. 8.6). While end-tidal inhalational agent partial pressure decreases, it is reasonable to target a reduced propofol concentration of 3 µg/mL as an initial target and then titrate against clinical response. If using a manual regimen, then reduce the initial bolus, especially if spontaneous respirations is required; a bolus of propofol 1 mg/kg is usually satisfactory.

PRACTICAL APPROACHES FOR SOME CLINICAL SCENARIOS

Spontaneously Breathing Diagnostic Procedures (Radiology Investigations)

Anesthesia and spontaneous respiration will generally be maintained at a target of 4 to 6 µg/mL in the absence of opioids or other

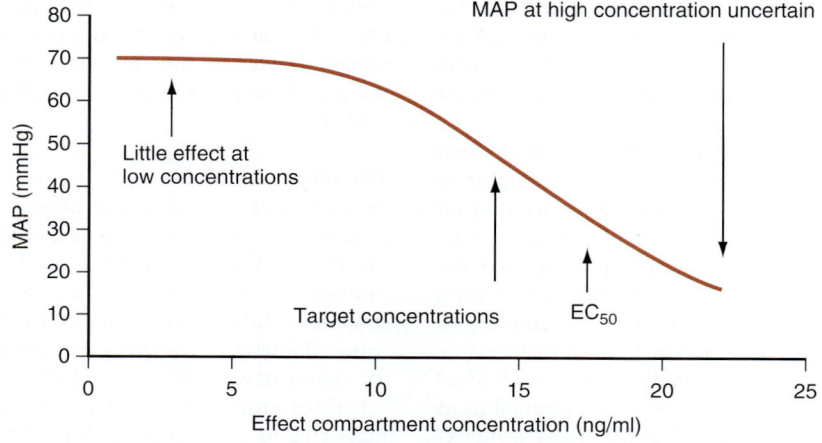

FIGURE 8.16 The relationship between remifentanil concentration and mean arterial blood pressure (MAP) in infants (4 months to 1 year) undergoing cranioplasty surgery. A steady-state remifentanil concentration of 14 µg/L would typically achieve a 30% decrease in mean arterial blood pressure. *EC50*, concentration is that at half maximum response. (From Anderson BJ, Holford NH. Leaving no stone unturned, or extracting blood from stone? *Paediatr Anaesth.* 2010;20:1-6. Used with permission.)

adjuncts. Pressure-supported respirations using either an endotracheal tube (ETT) or a laryngeal mask airway (LMA) will generally maintain normal or near normal $PaCO_2$. In the absence of pressure support ventilation, $PaCO_2$ will increase.

Spontaneously Breathing Airway Procedures Without an Endotracheal Tube (Flexible Respiratory Bronchoscopy, Rigid Laryngobronchoscopy)

Anesthesia may be induced by either inhalational or IV means. If induction is inhalational, then an initial propofol target of 3 μg/mL is reasonable to maintain desired spontaneous respirations and this target can then be titrated against response. If IV induction is used, then a plasma target of 4 to 6 μg/mL is reasonable but induction should be slow, especially if using an effect target model, because the relatively larger propofol bolus used to rapidly obtain the target Ce may cause apnea.

Remifentanil helps dampen airway reactivity and is a useful adjuvant. A remifentanil bolus of 1 μg/kg followed by an infusion at a low dose of 0.02 to 0.03 μg/kg per minute is effective. The remifentanil infusion can then be titrated to maintain a normal respiratory rate. If using the Minto Ce TCI model, then starting at an initial target of 1 μg/mL can be titrated to effect.

Laryngoscopy and topicalization with lidocaine can be carried out following induction. Generally laryngoscopy is tolerated more quickly if inhalational induction has been performed first. If using an IV induction, it pays to bide your time before performing laryngoscopy and topicalization; this allows effect-site equilibration.

Once the procedure has commenced, reactivity can be addressed by slow increments of propofol (1 μg/mL Cp or Ce if using TCI or 1 mg/kg bolus if using a manual regimen) and by increasing the remifentanil infusion. Further topicalization may be useful. It is generally best to avoid large boluses of propofol as this may induce apnea.

Spontaneously Breathing Procedures With an Endotracheal Tube (Adenotonsillectomy)

Induction may be either inhalational or IV. Intubation can be performed once the desired Cp or Ce has been achieved or after a bolus dose has been administered. The most stimulating part of the procedure is often mouth gag (e.g., Boyle-Davis) placement. Propofol can be increased in anticipation of this response to gag stimulation. This may cause apnea but once surgery has commenced, propofol can be slowly reduced until spontaneous respirations return.

Spontaneously Breathing Surgical Procedures With an LMA (Orthopedic and Peripheral Surgical Procedures)

Induction can be inhalational or an IV technique can be used. Commence propofol with an appropriate bolus if using a manual regimen. Remifentanil is a very useful adjunct, especially with peripheral orthopedic procedures where regional local anesthesia blockade has not been placed, to prevent movement in response to surgical stimulation.

BIS monitoring is a useful adjunct to titrate the propofol dose. Generally children will maintain spontaneous respirations with a BIS score in the 40 to 60 range and a remifentanil infusion of 0.1 to 0.2 μg/kg per minute or an effect concentration of 3 μg/mL Ce using the Minto model. Spontaneous respirations may not be adequate to provide CO_2 clearance and respiratory support may be required. Remifentanil remains a useful agent even if regional blockade has been used. It facilitates rapid induction and ready performance of the block without response to needle placement. Furthermore, it provides analgesia while the block takes effect and reduces any response to tourniquet pain. With the absence of surgical stimulation owing to a functional block, the propofol dose can generally be reduced. The remifentanil infusion or target concentration can also be reduced to assess block function.

Remifentanil is not necessarily useful if central blockade is used. However, it is still helpful for induction and during airway management and block placement. Infusion rate or target concentration can then be reduced or stopped once the block is established.

Major Invasive Procedures With Intubation (General, Thoracic, Neurosurgical, or Major Orthopedic Surgery (e.g., Posterior Spinal Fusion)

Commencement of TCI or a manual regimen can be followed by neuromuscular blockade and airway management. Remifentanil blunts the intubation response. Modified EEG monitoring in such patients undergoing major surgery is prudent. This may be achieved using the actual BIS score or the processed EEG waveform if the patient is younger than 3 years of age. Remifentanil is useful to reduce the total propofol dose and avoid delayed awakening at the end of the procedure. Analgesia can be managed with multimodal analgesia schemes and/or regional or neuraxial blockade.

Toward the later stages of the procedure, the propofol infusion may be reduced by titration against the EEG. This allows for a more rapid return of consciousness. One approach at the end of the procedure is to reverse residual neuromuscular blockade and stop both propofol and remifentanil infusions. Generally by the time the remifentanil effect has worn off, spontaneous respirations will have returned and anesthesia is still deep, attributable to propofol's prolonged CSHT; extubation can then proceed safely.

A Neonate Having Combined Anesthesia and Regional Blockade

There are concerns that some anesthetic drugs may cause neuronal apoptosis in the developing brain of a human neonate (see also Chapter 25) because drugs that bind to γ-aminobutyric acid-A ($GABA_A$) receptors cause neuronal apoptosis and other neurodegenerative changes in animal models ranging from rodents to primates.[129] Dexmedetomidine[130,131] and remifentanil[130,131] may be alternative options because their action is not mediated through $GABA_A$ receptors and they do not cause neuronal apoptosis or other neurodegenerative effects in rodents and primates. Dexmedetomidine also attenuates isoflurane-induced neurocognitive impairment in neonatal rats.[132] One regimen consists of IV premedication of glycopyrrolate 5 μg/kg followed by a dexmedetomidine 1-μg/kg loading dose over 10 minutes and remifentanil 1 μg/kg over 1 to 2 minutes. The dexmedetomidine infusion 1 μg/kg per hour can be started and titrated up or down within 50% of starting doses as needed, although it is crucial to appreciate that dexmedetomidine is not a complete general anesthetic. Similarly, a remifentanil infusion 0.1 μg/kg per minute can be titrated up or down (maximum infusion 0.5 μg/kg per minute). Airway management may require an ETT or LMA and ventilation assisted to maintain normocapnia.

COMMON MANUAL PROPOFOL INFUSION SCHEMES
Adults

A simple scheme was devised to maintain a blood concentration of propofol in healthy adults of 3 μg/mL.[133] A bolus IV dose of 1 mg/kg is followed by a continuous infusion of 10 mg/kg per hour for 10 minutes, then 8 mg/kg per hour for 10 minutes, then 6 mg/kg per hour (Fig. 8.17).[133] When this "10-8-6" regimen is modeled and verified using the Marsh model for an adult patient, the

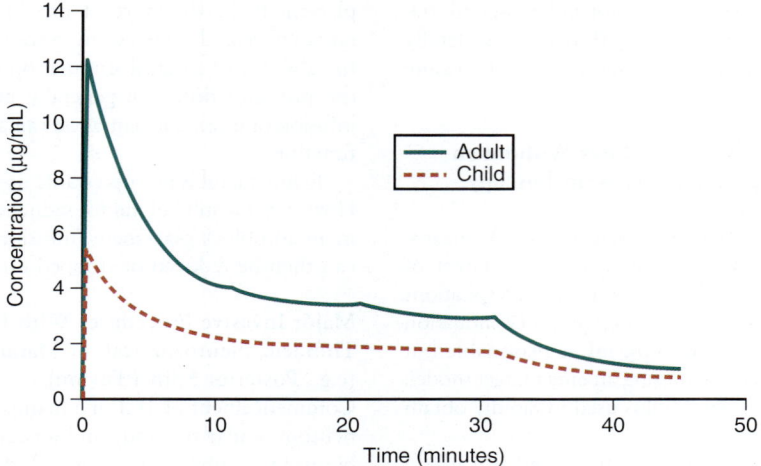

FIGURE 8.17 Simulated time-concentration profiles for propofol using a pediatric parameters set and an adult set. A 3 mg/kg bolus was administered and the infusions were administered as for an adult (10-8-6 regimen). Peak concentrations in the child are lower because of an increased volume of distribution. Increased clearance (expressed per kilogram) in children means subsequent concentrations also remain lower.

estimated blood concentration slightly exceeds 3 µg/mL but remains reasonably stable.[93]

Adolescents

Adolescents can generally be grouped as small adults and the 10-8-6 regimen can be used (see Table 8.3).[133]

Children

Children require larger infusion rates of propofol than adults to maintain clinical anesthesia (Fig. 8.17) because clearance (expressed per kilogram) is greater in children than in adults (Table 8.12). Parameter estimates reported by Kataria[19] were used to determine infusion regimens that maintain a steady-state blood concentration of 3 µg/mL in children aged 3 to 11 years. A loading dose of 2.5 mg/kg followed by an infusion rate of 15 mg/kg per hour for the first 15 minutes, 13 mg/kg per hour from 15 to 30 minutes, 11 mg/kg per hour from 30 to 60 minutes, 10 mg/kg per hour from 1 to 2 hours, and 9 mg/kg per hour from 2 to 4 hours was proposed. The CSHT in children was greater than in adults, increasing from 10.4 minutes at 1 hour to 19.6 minutes at 4 hours compared with adult estimates of 6.7 minutes and 9.5 minutes, respectively.[18] Subsequent clinical assessment of the infusion regimen's performance proved acceptable.[115]

This increased dose requirement for propofol in children can cause problems because it is formulated as a lipid emulsion and the lipid load can be considerable, particularly in young infants (Fig. 8.18). Propofol formulations are now available in some countries in concentrations varying from 5 mg/mL to 20 mg/mL (0.5%–2%); the most effective "lipid-sparing" strategy for infusions is to use 20 mg/mL propofol (2%) as this immediately halves the lipid load.

Infants

With the clearance of propofol reduced in infants, one might anticipate infusion rates at steady state reduced to similar extents. However, infusion rates for children younger than 3 years of age based on clinical experience from a pilot study of 50 patients were actually increased. This experience was used to develop dose regimens that were then evaluated in 2271 children undergoing

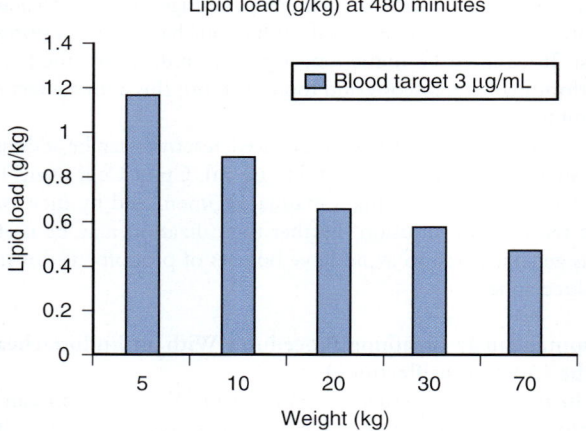

FIGURE 8.18 Lipid load after 480 minutes of a blood targeted propofol 1% infusion (formulated in vehicle containing 0.1 g/mL lipid) with target concentration of 3 µg/mL. Note the smaller infants have almost twice the lipid load and so 2% propofol is recommended to halve the relative lipid exposure and other propofol-sparing and lipid-sparing measures should be used. (Simulated using Tivatrainer; available at http://www.eurosiva.org/TivaTrainer/tivatrainer_main.htm.)

TABLE 8.12	Differences Between Adult and Pediatric Propofol Pharmacokinetic Parameters		
Age	Vd (mL/kg)	Elimination Half-Life (minutes)	Clearance (mL/minute per kg)
1–3 years	9500	188	53
3–11 years	9700	398	34
Adult	4700	312	28

Notes: The apparent volume of distribution (Vd) of propofol in the child is twice that of adults. The clearance of propofol in young children is twice that of adults and elimination is much more rapid.
Data from Absalom A, Struys MMRF. *An Overview of TCI and TIVA*. Gent, Belgium: Academia Press; 2005.

anesthesia with mechanical ventilation. Infusion changes were every 10 minutes, similar to that proposed by Roberts et al. in adults.[133] These are shown in Table 8.2. Few adverse effects were recorded—(bradycardia (12%), blood pressure decrease (8%), oxygen saturation decrease (1%)—all of which were easily countered by routine measures.[50]

COMMON MANUAL OPIOID INFUSION SCHEMES

Simple manual infusion regimens can be used for the opioids fentanyl, alfentanil, remifentanil, and sufentanil. The manual infusion regimens for these opioids in children are summarized in Table 8.3. Maintenance analgesia after infusions of these opioids should be planned, and it is important that adequate doses of systemic analgesics are given well before the infusion is discontinued. Transitioning is somewhat smoother after sufentanil than after alfentanil or remifentanil in children. The problem of acute tolerance to ultra-short-acting opioids (see Chapter 7) has been noted after use of remifentanil in surgery for pediatric scoliosis.[134]

READY MIXES

Individual anesthesia practitioners, like good chefs, often have their own recipes using fixed drug mixes for some clinical scenarios.

These have the advantage of simplicity but lack the versatility of separate infusions. Sterile infusions are prepared by the pharmacy in some centers, although there can be reluctance to prepare such infusions because of concerns about stability and the lack of clinical studies documenting the safety and efficacy of these mixtures. A common example used for endoscopy is shown in Table 8.13.

Ketofol is a mixture of ketamine and propofol (1:1) that is finding a niche for procedural sedation in the emergency room.[135] Stable hemodynamics, analgesia, and good recovery are reported.[136] The additive interaction for anesthesia induction in adults has been reported.[137] These data have been used to simulate effect in children[138]; an optimal ratio of racemic ketamine to propofol of 1:5 for 30 minutes of anesthesia and 1:6.7 for 90 minutes of anesthesia was suggested (Fig. 8.19).[138] The "ideal mix" for sedation will depend on the duration of sedation and the degree of analgesia required. The CSHT of ketamine increases with the duration of the infusion, resulting in delayed recovery.[139]

ACKNOWLEDGEMENT

We wish to thank Neil Morton, Frank Ebers, Grace Lai-Sze Wong, and James Limb for prior contributions to this chapter.

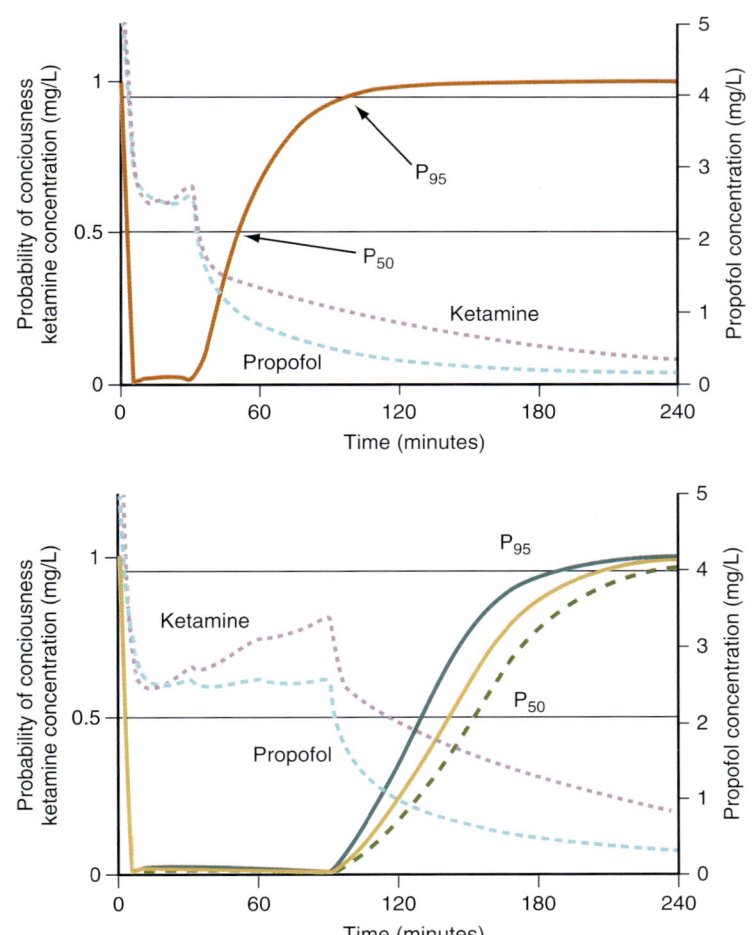

FIGURE 8.19 The upper panel shows the probability of consciousness during anesthesia using a propofol/ketamine ratio of 5:1. The loading dose for induction of anesthesia was 2.5 mg/kg propofol and 0.5 mg/kg of ketamine. The infusion rate was 67% of that suggested by McFarlan, Anderson, and Short[18] for propofol alone. Ketamine time-concentration profile is shown as a purple dotted line. Propofol time-concentration profile is shown as a blue dotted line. The lower panel shows simulation results for a 90-minute infusion. This panel also shows the probability of consciousness as age increases from a 2-year-old *(solid blue line)*, to a 5-year-old *(solid orange line)*, and a 10-year-old *(green dashed line)* child. The younger children have greater clearance and regain consciousness earlier than older children. P_{50} is the probability of consciousness in 50% of children; P_{95} is the probability of consciousness in 95% of children. (From Coulter FL, Hannam JA, Anderson BJ. Ketofol simulations for dosing in pediatric anesthesia. *Pediatr Anesth.* 2014;24:806-12. Used with permission.)

TABLE 8.13	A Recipe for Gastrointestinal Endoscopy Using a Propofol-Remifentanil Mixture

Age >10 Years

50 μg remifentanil in 19 mL propofol (2.5 μg/mL remifentanil)

Start propofol mix at 175 μg/kg per minute

Age <10 Years

100 μg remifentanil in 18 mL propofol (5 μg/kg remifentanil)

Start propofol mix at 150 μg/kg per minute

If a higher remifentanil concentration is used in teenagers, then they breathe at 2–4 breaths/minute and have systolic blood pressure of approximately 75 mm Hg. If a lower remifentanil concentration is used, they breathe at 8–10 breaths/minute and have a systolic blood pressure of 76–84 mm Hg. Those aged <10 years generally do not usually require any up or down change in the rate of infusion and breathe at normal rates.

ANNOTATED REFERENCES

Absalom A, Amutike D, Lal A, et al. Accuracy of the "Paedfusor" in children undergoing cardiac surgery or catheterization. *Br J Anaesth*. 2003;91:507-513.

The other widely used parameter set (children 1-15 years) programed into target-controlled infusion pumps is the Paedfusor model. This parameter set is one of the few whose performance has been validated.

Holford NHG, Sheiner LB. Understanding the dose-effect relationship: clinical application of pharmacokinetic-pharmacodynamic models. *Clin Pharmacokinet*. 1981;6:429-453.

This classic study explains use of the Hill equation to explain the concentration-response relationship. The equation and its variants are used to relate both vapors and drugs to anesthesia depth using such monitors as BIS.

Kataria BK, Ved SA, Nicodemus HF, et al. The pharmacokinetics of propofol in children using three different data analysis approaches. *Anesthesiology*. 1994;80:104-122.

Population modeling was used to determine a propofol parameter set in children 3 to 11 years. This parameter set is known as the Kataria model and is programmed into many target-controlled infusion pumps.

Minto CF, Schnider TW, Egan TD, et al. Influence of age and gender on the pharmacokinetics and pharmacodynamics of remifentanil. I. Model development. *Anesthesiology*. 1997;86:10-23.

This is an important study that characterized remifentanil pharmacokinetics in adults. The parameter set is also used in children. There is an element of safety with this approach because both volume of distribution and clearance decrease with increasing age. The greater volume of distribution in children reduces the peak concentrations of remifentanil after bolus dosing; the increased clearance in children results in a smaller plasma concentration when infused at adult rates expressed as milligrams per minute per kilogram.

Roberts FL, Dixon J, Lewis GT, et al. Induction and maintenance of propofol anaesthesia. A manual infusion scheme. *Anaesthesia*. 1988;43(suppl):14-17.

The authors describe a manual infusion regimen for propofol that uses a decreasing infusion rate change every 10 minutes to account for compartment kinetics. This 10-8-6 rule is still widely used and the principle has been adopted by others for use in children administered drugs such as propofol, ketamine, and methadone.

Steur RJ, Perez RS, De Lange JJ. Dosage scheme for propofol in children under 3 years of age. *Paediatr Anaesth*. 2004;14:462-467.

This analysis yielded one of the few infusion regimens available for neonates. Data are limited in this age group, who are prone to an increased incidence of adverse effects, and practitioners are advised to use caution with this technique. Dose-response relationships for hypotension are lacking and the impact of postmenstrual age on clearance and infusion regimens or combination therapy that retains spontaneous respiration are awaited.

A complete reference list can be found online at ExpertConsult.com.

Fluid Management

CRAIG D. MCCLAIN AND MICHAEL L. MCMANUS

ELECTROLYTE DISTURBANCES ARE COMMON in children because of their small size, large ratio of surface area to volume, and immature homeostatic mechanisms. As a result, fluid management can be challenging. On the ward, in the operating room, or in the intensive care unit (ICU), additional difficulties may result when fluid management is not tailored to the individual or when therapeutic decisions are based on extrapolations from adult data. To better understand the former and to limit the latter, this chapter reviews the basic mechanisms underlying fluid and electrolyte regulation, the developmental anatomy and physiology of fluid compartments, and the management of selected pediatric disease states relevant to anesthesia and critical care.

Regulatory Mechanisms: Fluid Volume, Osmolality, and Arterial Pressure

Water is in thermodynamic equilibrium across cell membranes, and it moves only in response to the movement of solutes (E-Fig. 9.1). Movement of water is described by the Starling equation:

$$Q_f = K_f [(P_c - P_i) - \sigma(\pi_c - \pi_i)],$$

where Q_f is fluid flow; K_f is the membrane fluid filtration coefficient (a proportionality constant); subscripts c and i refer to capillary and interstitial; P_c and P_i are hydrostatic pressures and π_c and π_i are osmotic pressures on either side of the membrane; and σ is the reflection coefficient for the solute and membrane of interest. The reflection coefficient gives a measure of a solute's permeability and, consequently, its contribution to osmotic force after equilibration. Across the blood-brain barrier, for example, the σ for sodium approaches 1.0,[1] whereas in muscle and other cell membranes, σ is on the order of 0.15 to 0.3.[2] Therefore, when isotonic sodium-containing solutions are given intravenously, usually only 15% to 30% of administered salt and water remains in the intravascular space, whereas the remainder migrates to the interstitium.[3,4] In contrast, hypertonic solutions permit greater expansion of circulating blood volume with smaller fluid loads and less fluid in the interstitium (e.g., as edema).[5-7]

Both the amount and the concentration of solute are tightly regulated to maintain the volumes of intravascular and intracellular compartments. Because sodium is the primary extracellular solute, this ion is the focus of homeostatic mechanisms concerned with maintenance of intravascular volume. When osmolality is held constant, water movement follows sodium movement. As a result, total body sodium (although not necessarily serum Na$^+$) and total body water (TBW) generally parallel one another. Because sodium "leak" across membranes limits its contribution to the support of intravascular volume, this compartment also critically depends on large, impermeable molecules such as proteins. In contrast to sodium, albumin molecules, for example, follow the Starling equilibrium with a reflection coefficient in excess of 0.8.[8] Soluble proteins create the so-called *colloid oncotic pressure*, approximately 80% of which is composed of albumin.

Although the presence of albumin supports intravascular volume, protein leak into the interstitium (and consequent water movement) may limit its effectiveness. It has been observed, for example, that the reflection coefficient for albumin decreases by as much as one-third after mechanical trauma.[9] Furthermore, because of ongoing leakage, a slow continuous infusion of albumin is superior to bolus administration for increasing the serum albumin concentration in critically ill individuals.[10]

Potassium is the primary intracellular solute, with approximately one-third of cellular energy metabolism devoted to Na^+/K^+ exchange. Sodium continuously leaks into cells along its concentration gradient, yet it is rapidly extruded in exchange for potassium. As the cell is exposed to varying osmolarity, water movement occurs, causing cell swelling or shrinkage. Because stable cell volume is critical for survival, complex regulatory mechanisms have evolved to ensure that stability is maintained.[11,12] The processes by which swollen cells return to normal size are collectively termed *regulatory volume decrease* processes, and those returning a shrunken cell to normal are termed *regulatory volume increase* processes (Fig. 9.1). With sudden, brief changes in osmolality, regulatory volume increase or decrease processes are activated after small (1%–2%) changes in cell volume, returning cell volume to normal primarily through transport of electrolytes. If anisosmotic conditions persist, chronic compensation occurs through the accumulation or loss of small organic molecules termed *osmolytes* or idiogenic osmoles. These osmogenic agents can also be cytoprotective under stress and include polyols, sorbitol, myoinositol, amino acids and their derivatives (e.g., taurine, alanine, proline), and methylamines (e.g., betaine, glycerylphosphorylcholine).

Like intracellular volume, circulating blood (intravascular) volume is also tightly controlled. Increases in intravascular volume result from increases in sodium and water retention, whereas decreases in intravascular volume result from increases in excretion of sodium and water. As noted earlier, serum osmolality must be maintained within a very narrow range if serum sodium is to be an effective focus of intravascular volume control. Serum osmolality is usually maintained between 280 and 300 mOsm/L; changes in osmolality as small as 1% trigger compensatory mechanisms.

Serum osmolality is primarily regulated by arginine vasopressin (AVP), thirst, and renal concentrating ability. Because the indirect aim of osmolar control is actually volume control, these same osmoregulatory mechanisms are also influenced by factors such as blood pressure (BP), cardiac output, and vascular capacitance.[13,14] In pathologic conditions such as ascites or hemorrhage, intravascular volume preservation takes precedence over osmolality and osmoregulatory mechanisms operate to restore intravascular volume, even at the expense of disrupting solute balance.

AVP is released from neurons within the supraoptic and paraventricular nuclei of the hypothalamus.[15] Microelectrode recordings suggest that different subpopulations of neurons are responsive to osmotic input, baroreceptor-mediated input, or both. Osmoresponsive cells react to osmolar fluctuations in cell size, so solutes that readily permeate cell membranes (such as urea) increase the serum osmolality without triggering the release of antidiuretic hormone (ADH). Infusion of solutes with large actual or effective cell membrane reflection coefficients (σ) (e.g., sodium, mannitol) elicit a robust AVP release. Typically, AVP release begins when the serum osmolality reaches a threshold of approximately 280 mOsm/L. In keeping with our understanding of cell volume regulation, rapid increases in osmolality lead to greater release of AVP rather than slow increases. Meanwhile, baroreceptors on the arterial side of the circulation (left ventricle, carotid sinus, aortic arch, and juxtaglomerular apparatus) provide tonic inhibition of nonosmotic AVP release. Hypovolemia and hypotension diminish this inhibition, release AVP stores, and increase the overall "gain" of the system (E-Fig. 9.2). Thus, in a volume-depleted or hypotensive child, brisk AVP release occurs even in the presence of plasma osmolalities as low as 260 to 270 mOsm/L. On balance, baroreceptor signals always override osmotic signals so that water is retained as needed to maintain circulatory homeostasis.

Intravascular fluid volume, salt and water intake, electrolyte balance, and cardiovascular status are interrelated at several levels.[16] For example, as the veins and arteries distend with fluid and the systemic BP increases, AVP release decreases, and both *pressure diuresis* and *natriuresis* begin.[17] The resulting relationship between urine output and arterial pressure is termed the *renal function curve* and its intersection with salt and water intake determines the *equilibrium point* at which arterial BP ultimately stabilizes (Fig. 9.2). Equilibrium (chronic) BP is influenced only by shifts of the

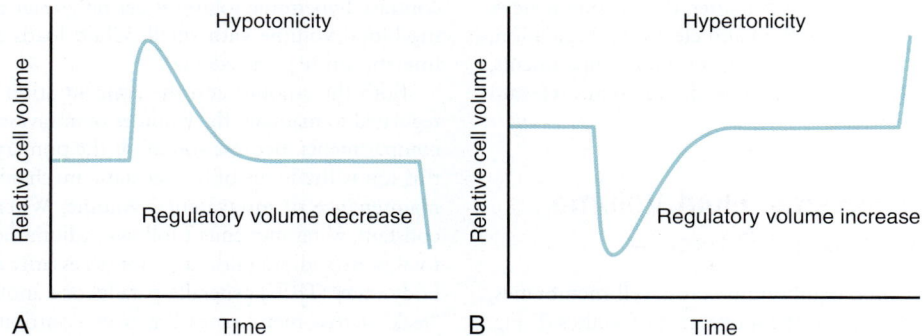

FIGURE 9.1 Activation of mechanisms regulating cell volume in response to volume perturbations. Volume-regulatory losses and gains of solutes are termed *regulatory volume decrease* **(A)** and *regulatory volume increase* **(B)**, respectively. The course of these decreases and increases varies with the type of cell and experimental conditions. Typically, however, a regulatory volume increase mediated by the uptake of electrolytes or a regulatory volume decrease mediated by the loss of electrolytes and organic osmolytes occurs over a period of minutes. When cells that have undergone a regulatory volume decrease **(A)** or increase **(B)** are returned to normotonic conditions, they swell above or shrink below their resting volume. This is caused by volume-regulatory accumulation or loss of solutes, which effectively makes the cytoplasm hypertonic or hypotonic, respectively, as compared with normotonic extracellular fluid. (From McManus ML, Churchwell KB, Strange K. Regulation of cell volume in health and disease. *N Engl J Med.* 1995;333:1260–1266. ®Massachusetts Medical Society.)

renal function or fluid intake curves. Transient changes in arterial pressure secondary to peripheral vascular resistance changes are always resolved by opposing shifts in total body salt and water.

In response to a decreasing arterial pressure, the renin-angiotensin system is also activated. With decreased renal perfusion, juxtaglomerular cells release renin, which in turn converts renin substrate (angiotensinogen) to angiotensin I. Angiotensin I is then rapidly converted to angiotensin II by angiotensin-converting enzyme present in lung endothelium. Angiotensin II supports arterial pressure in three ways: (1) direct vasoconstriction, (2) increased salt and water retention (via renal vasoconstriction and decreased glomerular filtration), and (3) stimulation of aldosterone secretion (Fig. 9.3).

AVP, pressure diuresis, and the renin-angiotensin system permit wide ranges in salt and water intake while maintaining the BP and volume status within narrow ranges; all serve to support the systemic circulation when threatened and to complement the more immediate activity of the sympathetic nervous system. In addition to high-pressure sensors such as aortic arch and carotid sinus baroreceptors, intravascular volume information is provided by low-pressure thoracic sensors. For this reason, effective increases or decreases in intrathoracic blood volume may mimic changes

in whole-body volume status and produce natriuresis, diuresis, or fluid retention. Intravascular volume may also be sensed by atrial muscle fibers; as the fibers stretch, atrial natriuretic peptide (ANP) is released.[18] Although its complete physiologic role is uncertain, ANP may serve to "fine-tune" the volume status by vasodilating modestly, gently increasing the glomerular filtration rate (GFR), and decreasing reabsorption of sodium. The combination of complex autoregulatory mechanisms with complementary actions operating on varying time scales, all responding to different, yet interrelated, effector stimuli, yields an elegant system by which the mature individual may maintain circulation amid a variety of challenges. In this context, it is interesting to observe that successful heart transplant recipients, despite general cardiovascular stability, typically manifest fundamental derangements in body fluid homeostasis.[19]

Maturation of Fluid Compartments and Homeostatic Mechanisms

BODY WATER AND ELECTROLYTE DISTRIBUTION

Much of our understanding of the development of body water compartments is derived from deuterium oxide dilution studies performed in the 1950s.[20] In a series of 21 neonates, TBW was found to be approximately 78 ± 5% of body weight. Subsequent measurements in fewer subjects showed that TBW decreased to approximately 60% in the second 6 months of life with most of the loss being extracellular. A smaller decrease (to about 57%) is observed late in childhood (Fig. 9.4).

The importance of the extracellular compartment, its relationship to the intracellular space, and much of the chemical anatomy of both were first described by Gamble in educational monographs issued during the first part of the 20th century (E-Fig. 9.3).[21,22] The chemical compositions of mature body fluid compartments are provided in Table 9.1.

CIRCULATING BLOOD VOLUME

The blood volume in neonates was determined to be 82 ± 9 mL/kg using an iodine 121–labeled human serum albumin technique, although substantial variability may result from the degree of placental-fetal transfusion.[23] In low–birth-weight (LBW), preterm, or critically ill infants, values as high as 100 mL/kg have been measured.[24] Blood volume increases slightly during the first few months of life, reaching its zenith at 2 months of age (approximately 86 mL/kg), then returns to near 80 mL/kg and finally stabilizes at 70 mL/kg by the end of the first year of life. In general, the

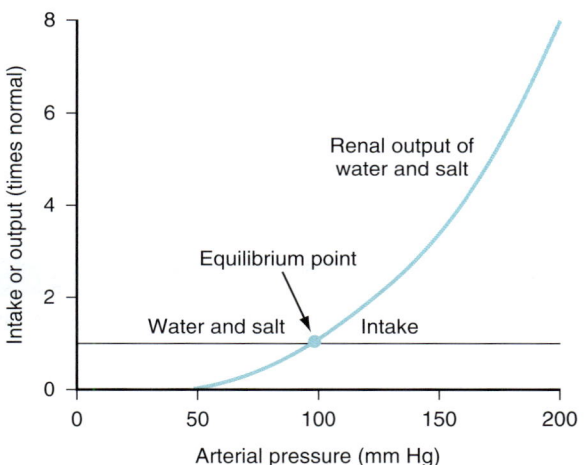

FIGURE 9.2 Analysis of arterial pressure regulation by equating the renal output curve with the salt and water intake curve. The equilibrium point describes the level to which the arterial pressure will be regulated. (That portion of the salt and water intake that is lost from the body through nonrenal routes is ignored in this figure.) (From Guyton AC, Hall JC, eds. *Textbook of Medical Physiology*. Philadelphia: WB Saunders; 1996;221–237.)

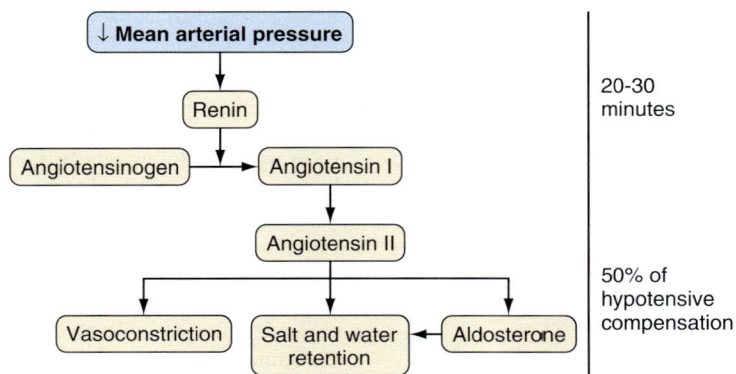

FIGURE 9.3 Physiologic responses to hypotension.

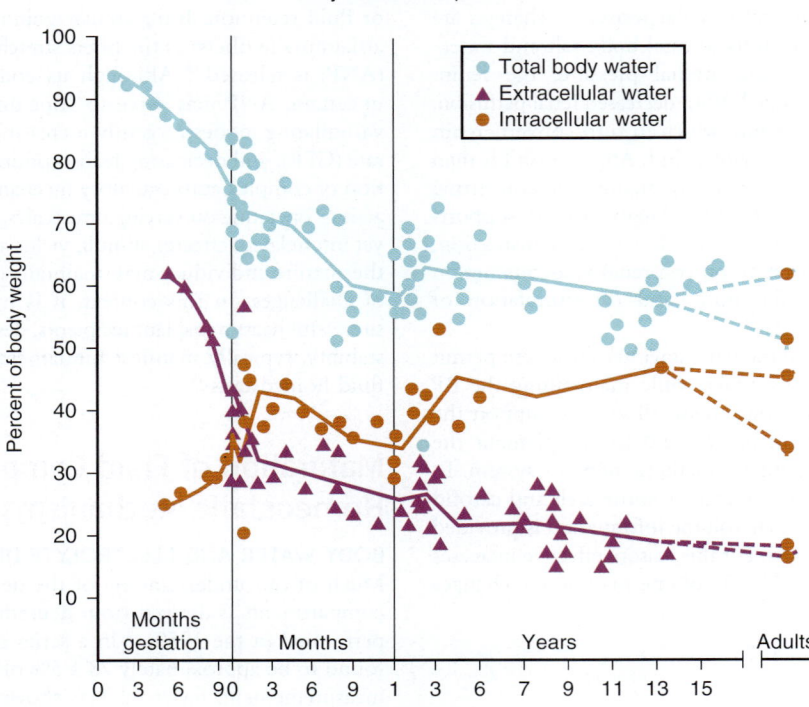

FIGURE 9.4 Total body water *(blue circles)*, extracellular water *(purple triangles)*, and intracellular water *(orange circles)* as percentages of body weight in infants and children, compared with corresponding values for the fetus and adults. (From Friis-Hansen B. Body water compartments in children: changes during growth and related changes in body composition. *Pediatrics* 1961;28:169–181.)

TABLE 9.1	Composition of Body Fluid Compartments	
	Extracellular Fluid	**Intracellular Fluid**
Osmolality (mOsm)	290–310	290–310
Cations (mEq/L)	**155**	**155**
Na$^+$	138–142	10
K$^+$	4.0–4.5	110
Ca^{2+}	4.5–5.0	—
Mg^{2+}	3	40
Anions (mEq/L)	**155**	**155**
Cl$^-$	103	—
HCO$_3^-$	27	—
HPO$_4^{2-}$	—	10
SO$_4^{2-}$	—	110
PO$_4^{2-}$	3	—
Organic acids	6	—
Protein	16	40

TABLE 9.2	Estimate of Circulating Blood Volume
Age	**Estimated Blood Volume (mL/kg)**
Preterm infant	100
Full-term neonate	90
Infant	80
School age (5 years)	70
Adults	70

of nephrons is in place by about the 38th week. In the outermost regions of the renal cortex, postnatal nephron differentiation may continue for several weeks to months. In the early stages of gestation, renal blood flow is approximately one-fifth of normal. Initially this is related to structural immaturity, and later it is caused by increased renovascular resistance. By 38 weeks of gestation, renal blood flow is approximately one-third of normal. High renovascular resistance protects the developing nephron from both pressure and volume overload. The resulting renal contribution to metabolic homeostasis in utero is limited.

As with the pulmonary bed, vascular resistance in the kidney decreases after birth, leading to abrupt increases in renal blood flow and GFR. In utero, despite a low GFR, urine output is brisk, owing to poor reabsorption of salt and water. Plasma renin activity is increased in utero, decreases immediately after birth, and then increases again as excess extracellular water is mobilized and excreted. Aldosterone levels are increased in cord blood and are maintained at this level for the first 3 days of life. The increased aldosterone may be necessary for sodium retention during periods of increased anabolism early in life.

ratio of blood volume to weight decreases with growth. The most accurate basis for prediction of blood volume is lean body mass, the consideration of which removes any male/female variation even into adulthood.[25] An estimate of the circulating blood volume is presented in Table 9.2.

MATURATION OF HOMEOSTATIC MECHANISMS

Renal development begins at approximately 5 weeks of gestation and continues in a centrifugal pattern until the full complement

Intrarenal gradients of NaCl and urea are less steep in the immature kidney, and full nephron length has yet to be achieved. Consequently, urine-concentrating ability is limited in neonates, with maximum urine osmolality being about half that of the adult (700–800 mEq/L vs. 1300–1400 mEq/L). In part, this also relates to low circulating ADH levels and decreased renal responsiveness to ADH. Although overall ADH production is not impaired, excessive secretion may occur in some disease states. Limited urine-concentrating ability necessitates large urine volumes for elimination of large solute loads.

Renal plasma flow and GFR (based on body surface area or allometry) are 30% of adult values in neonates. Both increase during the first year, reaching 50% of adult values by 6 months age (350 and 70 mL/minute per meter squared, respectively, and 90% by approximately 1 year[26] see Figs. 7.11 and 7.12).[27] At birth, the serum creatinine reflects the maternal concentration, which may be increased in term and preterm infants, but normalizes in the second month after birth, reflecting creatinine production. Fractional excretion of sodium (FE_{Na}) is markedly increased in preterm infants, decreases somewhat by term, and stabilizes at adult rates by the second month of life. Although the adult kidney may easily achieve FE_{Na} values as small as 0.5%, the 34-week-gestation infant is limited to no less than 2%.

These maturational features limit the ability of the preterm or young infant to handle large fluctuations in fluid and solute loads. Both sodium conservation and regulation of extracellular fluid volume are impaired in comparison with the older child and adult. Limited GFR makes excretion of a fluid challenge difficult. Excessive urinary sodium loss leads to increased maintenance requirements; hyponatremia is common. Conversely, diminished concentrating ability increases free water losses during excretion of a solute load, whereas the high ratio of surface area to volume increases evaporative water loss. Consequently, fluid requirements are relatively high, and dehydration is common. Any errors in fluid management are poorly tolerated. As a rule, the most severe impairment exists in preterm infants, and the majority of homeostatic mechanisms are fully developed after the first year of life.

Fluid and Electrolyte Requirements

Holliday summarized the evolution of contemporary hydration therapy.[21] In 1831, Latta first reported the use of intravenous (IV) fluids in the resuscitation of patients dehydrated by cholera.[28] In 1918, growing information on the subject permitted Blackfan and Maxcy to successfully treat nine infants by intraperitoneal injection.[29] In 1923, Gamble and associates detailed the anatomy of fluid and electrolyte compartments, introducing the use of milliequivalents to clinical practice.[22] This paved the way for the development of the "deficit therapy" regimen of Darrow.[30]

In subsequent decades, various recipes to replace the extracellular and intracellular fluid losses were suggested. For the most part, these failed because of excessive potassium and insufficient sodium content. Hyponatremia was common. When the focus of the treatment shifted to replacing the extracellular fluid deficit, rapid restoration of extracellular fluid volume using solutions with sodium concentrations similar to those in blood became commonplace. This, along with oral rehydration, is the preferred method of treatment today.

The concept of "maintenance fluids" is a complex subject. Although water and salt are required to sustain life, it is fair to say that for an individual child at any particular time, the precise amounts necessary are unknown (and perhaps unknowable). Instead,

fluids and electrolytes, like anesthetics, are titrated to effect with general guidelines provided by clinical assessment, basic physiologic principles, and limited published data. The term *maintenance fluids* is often more limiting than helpful, and in all cases it is less precise than other terms familiar to anesthesiologists, such as *minimum alveolar concentration* (MAC) or *median effective dose* (ED_{50}).

Holliday and Segar provided calculations for a first approximation of *"the maintenance need for water in parenteral fluid therapy"* in 1957.[31] Integrating the relevant known physiology at that time, these authors observed that *"insensible loss of water and urinary water loss roughly parallel energy metabolism and do not parallel weight."* However, because water utilization parallels energy metabolism, energy metabolism follows surface area, and surface area follows weight, it should be possible to estimate water requirement from weight alone. The authors then proceeded under a series of assumptions to extrapolate from limited data to a *"relationship between weight and energy expenditure that might easily be remembered."*

Assuming energy requirements of *"hospitalized patients"* to be *"roughly midway between basal and normal levels,"* they constructed a curve of caloric requirement versus weight.[31] This curve could be seen as consisting of three linear sections: 0 to 10 kg, 10 to 20 kg, and 20 to 70 kg (Fig. 9.5). Viewing the curve in this manner, the authors reasoned that *"fortuitously, the average need for water, expressed in milliliters, equals energy expenditure in calories"*: 100 mL/kg per day for weights to 10 kg, an additional 50 mL/kg per day for each kilogram from 11 to 20 kg, and 20 mL/kg per day more for each kilogram beyond 20 kg. In anesthetic practice, this formula has been further simplified, with the hourly requirement referred to as the "4-2-1 rule" (4 mL/kg per hour for the first 10 kg of weight, 2 mL/kg per hour for the next 10 kg, and 1 mL/kg per hour for each kilogram thereafter; Table 9.3).

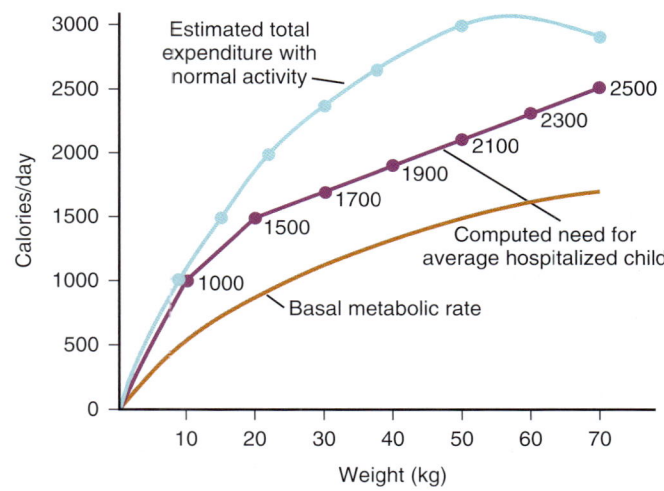

FIGURE 9.5 The upper and lower curves were plotted from data from the study by Talbot.[32] Weights at the 50th percentile level were selected for converting calories at various ages to calories related to weight. The computed line for the average hospitalized child was derived from the following equations:
- 0–10 kg: 100 kcal/kg.
- 10–20 kg: 1000 kcal + 50 kcal/kg for each kg over 10 kg
- ≥20 kg: 1500 kcal + 20 kcal/kg for each kg over 20 kg

(From Holliday MA, Segar WE. The maintenance need for water in parenteral fluid therapy. *Pediatrics* 1957;19:823–832.)

TABLE 9.3 | Relationship Between Weight and Hourly or Daily Maintenance Fluid Requirements of Children as per the 4-2-1 Rule

| Weight (kg) | MAINTENANCE FLUID REQUIREMENTS | |
	Hour	Day
<10	4 mL/kg	100 mL/kg
10–20	40 mL + 2 mL/kg for every kg >10 kg	1000 mL + 50 mL/kg for every kg >10 kg
>20	60 mL + 1 mL/kg for every kg >20 kg	1500 mL + 20 mL/kg for every kg >20 kg

TABLE 9.4 | Normal Water Losses for Infants and Children

Cause of Loss	Volume of Loss (mL/100 kcal)
Output	
• Urine	70
• Insensible loss	
Skin	30
Respiratory tract	15
Hidden intake (from burning 100 calories)	15
Total	100

TABLE 9.5 | Perioperative Causes of Increased ADH Release

Nonosmotic
Pain
Inflammation
Stress, catecholamines
Surgery; laparoscopic surgery
Vomiting
Hypoxia
Hypercapnia
Medications (e.g., opioids, amiodarone, vincristine)
Respiratory diseases (e.g., asthma, pneumonia, atelectasis)
Central nervous system disorders (e.g., head injury, tumors)
Osmotic
Fasting
Hypovolemia
Hypertonicity
Hypotension
Renal insufficiency
Hepatic insufficiency

For decades, the simplicity and elegance of the Holliday and Segar formula has made it the starting point for fluid management in healthy children. Until recently, the majority of consultant anesthetists in the United Kingdom administered hyponatremic glucose-containing solutions intraoperatively and postoperatively to children undergoing elective surgery.[33] However, the uncritical use of these solutions was never intended, and their blind application in the operating room, or in any clinical situation, resulted in instances of hyponatremia, aspiration, and death.[34–36] Further, as Holliday has since pointed out, their original approach involved hyponatremic glucose-containing solutions rather than near-isotonic solutions such as 0.9% saline or lactated Ringer's solution (LR).[37] In addition, these requirements were assessed at a basal metabolic state and not when the child was acutely ill or under physiologic stress during which increased levels of ADH were present. As the authors cautioned, *"understanding of the limitations and of exceptions to the system [is] required. Even more essential is the clinical judgment to modify the system as circumstances dictate."* General water losses for infants and children are summarized in Table 9.4.

More recently, Holliday and colleagues revised the approach to fluid therapy in children that he and Segar enshrined with several caveats.[38] In a related commentary, he pointed out several problems with applying the original 4-2-1 rule to acutely ill children.[39] Namely, dysregulation of ADH is a hallmark of critical illness because ADH secretion is affected by a variety of nonosmotic factors such as pain, stress, mechanical ventilation, and medications (Table 9.5).[40] As a result, the choice of IV fluid and the rapidity of deficit replacement must be approached with care. The authors recommended a relatively simple strategy for healthy children undergoing elective surgery (including outpatients) to turn off ADH secretion and prevent perioperative water retention and subsequent hyponatremia. When a child (who is without significant heart or kidney disease) presents with marginal to moderate hypovolemia (e.g., after fasting for surgery), 20 to 40 mL/kg of isotonic fluids should be given during the surgery and postanesthesia care unit stay (as rapidly as 10–20 mL/kg per hour). Clinical judgment

must always allow for modification of these recommendations if indicated for an individual child.[37,41] If hypovolemia is more severe (e.g., after an extensive bowel preparation), 40 to 80 mL/kg may be necessary during the perioperative period. Some have expressed concern that such volumes of fluid could cause volume overload even in healthy children. However, evidence suggests that children handle crystalloid volumes much more efficiently than adults.[42]

Postoperative IV fluid therapy should consist of an isotonic solution infused to replace ongoing fluid losses plus about half the rate described in the original 4-2-1 fluid regimen (i.e., 2 mL/kg for the first 10 kg, 1 mL/kg for the next 10 kg, and 0.5 mL/kg for each additional kilogram thereafter). Historically, when a child is unable to tolerate oral intake postoperatively, routine maintenance fluid therapy has been resumed with hypotonic saline solution (e.g., 0.45% saline). Although this regimen was believed to limit the ADH response and reduce the risk of postoperative hyponatremia and hypernatremia,[37,38,41] pain and surgical stress can maintain increased ADH levels and risk the development of hyponatremia with seizures and encephalopathy.[35,36,43,44] In the postoperative setting therefore, an isotonic salt solution is a better choice for maintenance[45] at a rate of 2 : 1 : 0.5 rule for the first 12 hours then returning to the 4 : 2 : 1 rule thereafter, until the child tolerates oral fluids.[36,46,47] Regardless of the fluids administered, it remains prudent to serially monitor plasma electrolyte concentrations until the child is drinking normally and homeostasis is restored.[45,48,49]

NEONATAL FLUID MANAGEMENT

In the first few postnatal days, isotonic losses of salt and water cause the healthy neonate to lose 5% to 15% of body weight. Although GFR increases rapidly, urine output is initially minimal, and renal losses are modest. Day 1 fluid requirements of the wrapped neonate, therefore, are relatively small. Over the next few postnatal days, losses and fluid requirements increase. In the poorly feeding infant, progression to hypernatremia and dehydration are common. When intake is appropriate, the term infant will regain body weight during the first week.

9

Three distinct phases of fluid and electrolyte homeostasis have been described in LBW[50] and very low–birth-weight (VLBW)[51] infants. In the first postnatal day, there is minimal urine output, and body weight is stable despite limited fluid intake. In the second phase, days 2 and 3 of life, diuresis occurs irrespective of the amount of fluid administered. By the fourth and fifth days, urine output begins to vary with changes in fluid intake and state of health.

Prematurity increases neonatal fluid requirements substantively. Fluid requirements are therefore estimated and then titrated to the infant's changing weight, urine output, and serum sodium concentration.

No less important is glucose homeostasis. In the ninth month of gestation, the fetus begins to form glycogen stores at a rate of more than 100 kcal/day. In the unstressed, term infant, hepatic glycogen stores are 5% of body weight. Immediately after birth, glycogenolysis depletes most of these stores within the first 24 to 48 hours. Gluconeogenesis must then proceed to yield glucose at a rate of approximately 4 mg/kg per minute.

At birth, the serum glucose concentration in the fetus is 60% to 70% of the maternal value. This may decrease within the first postnatal hours before recovering but should exceed 45 mg/dL to avoid neurologic injury. Symptoms of hypoglycemia may include jitteriness, lethargy, temperature instability, and convulsions. Ten percent dextrose in water ($D_{10}W$) may be given as a bolus of 2 to 4 mL/kg followed by a continuous infusion (using a pump) at 4 to 6 mg/kg per minute. The serum glucose concentration is then analyzed frequently and the infusion adjusted as necessary to prevent hypoglycemia and hyperglycemia. Alternately, neonatologists are switching to a 40% dextrose gel that is applied to the buccal mucosa for rapid absorption and resolution of hyponatremia.[52,53] This obviates the need for IV access if one has not been established by this time. It is important that the amount of glucose being provided be calculated in milligrams per kilogram per minute to avoid errors during fluid changes and to facilitate the diagnosis of persistent hypoglycemia.

Typical *day 1* infant fluid orders recommend 70 to 80 mL/kg of $D_{10}W$. Because $D_{10}W$ contains 10 g of glucose per deciliter, this regimen provides

$$10 \text{ g/dL} \times 70 - 80 \text{ mL/kg per day} = 7 - 8 \text{ g/kg per day}$$
$$= 0.333 \text{ g/kg per hour}$$
$$\cong 5 \text{ mg/kg per minute}$$

On *day 2*, fluids are routinely increased to at least 100 mL/kg per day, and sodium is added at 2 to 3 mEq/dL. After urine output is established, potassium is added at 1 to 2 mEq/dL. The final solution, containing 30 mEq Na^+ and 10 to 20 mEq K^+ per liter, approximates the 0.2% saline "maintenance" solution commonly used previously in older children.

In the neonatal ICU, fluid management focuses on provision of adequate nutrition, maintenance of electrolyte balance, and limitation of fluid overload. The last factor is of particular concern because plasma oncotic pressure is reduced in preterm infants and the whole-body protein reflection coefficient is less than that in adults.[54] VLBW infants are at particular risk for fluid and electrolyte imbalances.[55] Even modest fluid overload may exacerbate pulmonary edema, prolong ductal patency, and more readily produce congestive heart failure. This perspective typically accompanies the infant to the operating room, where the primary considerations are routinely quite the opposite: restoration of circulating blood volume after third-space accumulation, maintenance of intravascular volume amid ongoing blood loss, replacement of potentially massive evaporative losses, and maintenance of BP despite anesthetic-induced vasodilatation and increased venous capacitance. During surgery, these concerns must take precedence, yet unnecessary administration of fluid is best avoided.

Intraoperative Fluid Management

INTRAVENOUS ACCESS AND FLUID ADMINISTRATION DEVICES

In infants and children, the first step toward intraoperative fluid management is often the most challenging: that is, establishing IV access. In general, simple procedures in healthy children are successfully approached using a single peripheral IV line. Although preferences vary among anesthesiologists, establishing IV access is most easily accomplished after induction of anesthesia. In young children, anesthesia is often induced by inhalation, and a catheter is inserted by an assistant into a hand or foot vein. In older children, or when IV access is desirable before anesthesia is induced, IV access may be facilitated by the use of topical anesthesia (e.g., EMLA [eutectic mixture of local anesthetics] cream, amethocaine, lidocaine infiltration) or sedation or both.

Complex surgeries in sicker children usually require at least two large-bore catheters. In pediatrics, however, "large-bore" is a relative term, with 22-gauge catheters typically providing sufficient access in infants. Preferred sites for larger catheters include the antecubital and saphenous veins (see Fig. 49.1). In cases in which access to the central circulation is required (as for pressure monitoring, infusion of vasoactive medications, or prolonged access), longer catheters may be placed via the femoral, subclavian, or internal jugular vein (the latter usually via a high, anterior approach; see Figs. 49.2–49.5).[56] Although secure access may also be obtained via the external jugular vein, it is often difficult to negotiate the J-wire or catheter tip into the central circulation.[57] Peripherally inserted central catheter (PICC) lines have become common among hospitalized children. Although they represent a long-term means of delivering IV fluids and medications to those who need them, their intraoperative utility is very limited for several reasons. First, modern patient safety practices prohibit repeated access to central lines and practitioners must maintain strict sterile technique whenever entering them. Second, flow resistance is great within long, small-diameter catheters, precluding their use for large-volume resuscitation. Finally, PICCs are often placed for delivery of hyperalimentation or other solutions, which may be incompatible with anesthetic needs. For these reasons and others, separate IV access is often required and secure larger-bore shorter IV catheters with much lower resistance must always be placed if large fluid shifts or significant blood loss is anticipated.

In selecting the appropriate IV catheter, it is useful to consider the relative effects of catheter length and diameter on solution flow rates. Longer catheters offer more resistance to flow than shorter ones and are therefore less desirable when rapid infusion of a large volume of fluids is necessary (see E-Figs. 52.1, 52.2, and Fig. 51.1). In vitro, catheters designed for peripheral venous access had 18% to 164% greater flow rates compared with the same-gauge catheters designed for central venous use. Under pressure, as might be used during emergent volume resuscitation, rates differed up to 17-fold.[58] Although this seems to suggest that short peripheral catheters should be preferred, in vivo data are more complex. In animal models, overall catheter flow rates are less than in vitro rates, and central access presents somewhat less resistance to flow than peripheral access.[59] Finally, when the risks and benefits of central versus peripheral access are compared, central administration of resuscitation medications may provide little practical advantage compared with peripheral administration.[60]

Intraosseous devices are now commonly used in the initial resuscitation of critically ill or injured children (see E-Figs. 49.1 and 49.6 and 49.7).[61,62] Flow rates via these devices depend less on needle diameter than on resistance in the marrow compartment.[63] In the operating room, the intraosseous route has been used for both induction and maintenance of anesthesia.[64–66] However, onset of drug effect is less predictable, and the device is more easily dislodged than an IV catheter. Potential complications include compartment syndrome[67–69] and, very rarely, damage to the growth plate.[62,70] Such devices are probably best considered an emergency or last-resort option.[65]

To prevent accidental volume overload, the amount of IV fluid available to administer to a child at any one time should not exceed the child's calculated hourly requirement. Particularly in infants, a volumetric chamber should be used to limit the amount of fluid available for infusion. Similarly, a microdrip infusion set limits the rate of fluid administration and permits much greater control. Although a fluid infusion pump provides the most precise mode of regulating the rate of fluid administration (and is therefore very useful in providing supplemental fluids or medications), such devices are impractical on primary access lines because they hinder the ability to administer drugs and fluids rapidly. In addition, the clinician should be mindful that pumps may continue to infuse through dislodged catheters, giving misleading reassurance that adequate IV access is present and fluids are being administered. Administering large volumes of fluid and drugs interstitially will not deliver the anticipated results. Moreover, if an identification or allergy bracelet is on a limb proximal to the IV insertion site, it may act as a tourniquet if the IV is interstitial, possibly causing ischemia to digits. Therefore access to the IV site is important in children, as well as removing all bracelets proximal to ipsilateral IV insertion sites.

In neonates and small infants, when rapid infusion of resuscitation solutions or blood products is anticipated, many practitioners insert a stopcock manifold into the IV infusion. Additional fluids may be prepared in syringes and warmed separately; during periods of sudden blood loss, stored syringes may then be inserted into the manifold and a fluid volume rapidly infused.

Finally, in prolonged surgeries or when volume replacement is great, all IV infusions may be warmed to maintain thermal homeostasis. Also, in younger infants and children in whom communication exists between the right and left sides of the circulation (e.g., patency of the foramen ovale), an in-line "bubble" filter is desirable.

CHOICE AND COMPOSITION OF INTRAVENOUS FLUIDS

In the early 1960s,[71] simultaneous measurements of plasma and extracellular fluid volumes demonstrated that, during surgery, plasma volume is supported at the expense of the extravascular space. At the same time, it was classically observed that isotonic resuscitation fluids temporarily redistribute from the intravascular spaces to what was originally believed to be a third, nonfunctional space. However, when the endothelial glycocalyx is perturbed, as can occur with surgical trauma, fluid may shift from the intravascular to interstitial space. Therefore the historical "third space" may simply represent the reversible expansion of the interstitium. Because of the differences in fluid distribution and renal function in infants compared with older children, it was at first unclear that these findings could be extended to infancy. Thus fluid restriction remained the standard of care until careful studies specifically demonstrated that fluid and electrolyte requirements are often extremely large in neonates who are undergoing major surgical procedures.[72–74]

Historically, hypotonic fluids were used as the maintenance solutions throughout the hospital, but this is no longer the practice. Isotonic solutions are preferred intraoperatively for several reasons. First, most ongoing volume losses are isotonic, consisting of shed blood and interstitial fluids. Second, large volumes of hypotonic solutions may rapidly diminish serum osmolality, producing very low concentrations of electrolytes (in particular, sodium) and undesirable fluid shifts. Indeed, even large volumes of "isotonic" fluids significantly decrease the serum osmolality in adult volunteers.[75] Third, as discussed earlier, the plasma volume expansion that is necessary in response to diminished vascular tone under anesthesia is difficult to achieve even with isotonic fluids. Finally, increases in ADH levels and other elements of intraoperative physiology retain free water in excess of sodium if inadequate amounts of the latter are provided.

The compositions of commonly used IV solutions are presented in Table 9.6. Assuming normal plasma osmolality is 275 to 290 mOsm/L, 0.9% NaCl (normal saline, NS) is theoretically hypertonic to plasma but is effectively isotonic when the in vivo activities of its constituents are considered.[76] For dextrose-containing solutions, the osmolality decreases rapidly as sugar is metabolized, resulting in increased volumes of free water. Therefore, administration of 5% dextrose in water is ultimately equivalent to administering free water.

Controversy regarding the perioperative use of colloid versus crystalloid fluid replacement remains unresolved. Colloid solutions carry the theoretical benefit of more effective expansion and retention of intravascular volume. Crystalloid solutions are much less expensive, easier to store, and carry few side effects. Although an initial meta-analysis of adult studies suggested worse outcomes

TABLE 9.6	Composition of Extracellular Fluid and Common Intravenous Solutions								
		CATIONS (mEq/L)					ANIONS (mEq/L)		
	mOsm/L	Na⁺	K⁺	Ca²⁺	Mg²⁺	NH₄⁺	Cl⁻	HCO₃⁻	HPO₄⁻

	$mOsm/L$	Na^+	K^+	Ca^{2+}	Mg^{2+}	NH_4^+	Cl^-	HCO_3^-	HPO_4^-
Extracellular fluid	280–300	142	4	5	3	0.3	103	27	3
Lactated Ringer's (LR) solution	273	130	4	3			109	28	
0.45% NaCl	154	77					77		
0.9% NaCl (normal saline)	308	154					154		
PlasmaLyte A[a]	294	140	5		3	1.6	98	98	
3% NaCl	1024	513					513		

[a]PlasmaLyte is a trademark of Baxter International Inc., its subsidiaries or affiliates. (Plasmalyte also contains acetate 27 mEq/L and gluconate 23 mEq/L.)

after albumin resuscitation,[77] this was not confirmed in a subsequent randomized controlled trial.[78] However, subgroup analyses from the latter trial suggested that some patients, such as those with head injury,[79] may be harmed by albumin, whereas others, such as those with septic shock,[80] may realize some benefit. Thus the choice of solution may depend on the underlying medical conditions and remains a matter of clinical judgment.

It is worth noting that aside from 5% albumin, synthetic colloids are gaining popularity among pediatric practitioners. One reason for this is the development of newer synthetic colloids with a more favorable side effect profile. Hydroxyethyl starches (HES) are synthetic colloids that are simply modified polysaccharides. Circulating amylases quickly degrade natural polysaccharides, but HES solutions are not quickly degraded because the solutes contain hydroxyethyl groups in place of hydroxyl groups at carbon positions C-2, C-3, and C-6, rendering the molecules resistant to hydrolysis. These compounds are characterized by three attributes: average mean molecular weight (MW), molar substitution (MS), and the C-2/C-6 ratio, which relates to the relative positions of hydroxyethyl groups on the polysaccharide molecule.

HES solutions with a greater MW/MS ratio remain in the intravascular space for longer periods than those with smaller ratios. However, they also are prone to more adverse effects including hypocoagulability. Newer, low MW/low MS solutions have much less effect on hemostatic mechanisms than older, higher MW/higher MS solutions. The precise mechanism by which HES compounds affect coagulation remains unclear, although it has been attributed to interference with von Willebrand factor, factor VIII, and platelet function. A greater C-2/C-6 ratio is responsible for a slower degradation of the starch by amylase with fewer adverse effects.[81] When renal function is normal, newer HES solutions (e.g., HES 130/0.42/6 : 1) are safe for children undergoing elective surgery, since they maintain hemodynamic stability and produce only mild to moderate changes in acid-base status.[82] Synthetic colloids such as these can therefore be considered in surgical patients who demonstrate the need for aggressive intraoperative fluid resuscitation (see also Chapter 12). Use of these solutions in cardiac surgery remains controversial given the effects on coagulation factors and platelet function induced by the cardiopulmonary bypass circuit.

The routine intraoperative use of glucose-containing solutions has also been a subject of debate. As a rule, operative stress evokes physiologic responses that increase serum glucose. In practice, therefore, hypoglycemia is seldom a problem in healthy, fasted children when glucose is omitted from perioperative IV fluids.[83,84] Indeed, the risk should be particularly small if the period of fasting is limited to less than 10 hours.[84] At the same time, rapid administration of dextrose solutions may certainly produce acute hyperglycemia and hyperosmolality.[83,84] Therefore, glucose-containing electrolyte solutions should not be used to replace fluid deficits, third-space losses, or blood losses, but they may be used as a background electrolyte maintenance solution.[85] Some populations, such as debilitated infants,[86] children who are malnourished, neonates and infants younger than 6 months of age,[83,87,88] and those undergoing cardiac surgery, are at risk for intraoperative hypoglycemia.[89,90] The use of glucose-containing solutions (1%–2.5% dextrose),[83,85,87,91] along with intraoperative glucose monitoring, may be beneficial in these children.

HYPERALIMENTATION

It is now common practice that critically ill children arrive in the operating room with hyperalimentation solutions infusing.

TABLE 9.7	Common Contents of Parenteral Nutrition Solutions[a]
Carbohydrates	
10%, 12.5%, 20%, 25%, 30% Dextrose	
Limited to D_{10} or $D_{12.5}$ if through a peripheral catheter	
Protein	
In the form of amino acids	
0.5, 1.0, 1.5, 2.0, 2.5, or 3.0 g/kg per day	
Lipids	
10%, 20% Lipids	
Standard Additives	
Sodium: 30 mEc/L	
Potassium: 20 mEq/L	
Calcium: 15 mEq/L	
Magnesium: 10 mEq/L	
Phosphorus: 10 mmol/L	
Heparin	

[a]Common contents of parenteral nutrition solutions containing dextrose, protein, lipids, and standard additives such as electrolytes. These values represent standard starting points that may be modified based on individual patient needs.

Common contents of hyperalimentation solutions are shown in Table 9.7. In general, children require 0.5 to 3.0 mg/kg per day of protein, 6 to 9 mg/kg per minute of glucose, and 0.5 to 3 g/kg per day of fat. Children receiving parenteral nutrition preoperatively should continue to receive those infusions separately, and a corresponding volume should be deducted from isotonic operative fluids. Hyperalimentation typically consists of two infusions: fat (e.g., Intralipid, Fresenius Kabi AB, Uppsala, Sweden) and a concentrated glucose/protein solution. It is prudent to discontinue the Intralipid solution during surgery, but if that is not possible, then every effort should be made to avoid accessing any ports in the line to reduce the risk of contaminating the Intralipid. Conversely, the concentrated glucose/protein solution should be continued at the same rate (because circulating insulin concentrations have acclimated accordingly). Because of hyperglycemic responses to the stress of surgery and reduced metabolism related to anesthesia and hypothermia, some practitioners routinely decrease hyperalimentation infusion rates by one-third to one-half. If the latter practice is followed, clinicians should consider checking serum glucose concentrations at regular intervals to monitor for hypoglycemia. Under no circumstances should concentrated glucose solutions (such as D_{10} or D_{20}) be abruptly discontinued, because high concentrations of circulating insulin may cause a precipitous and profound decrease in the serum glucose concentration.

Concerns regarding the routine intraoperative use of dextrose-containing solutions increased with recognition that hyperglycemia may exacerbate neurologic injury after an ischemic or hypoxic event. As a result, many clinicians now elect to avoid dextrose-containing solutions during routine surgery. When dextrose-containing solutions are used, appropriate monitoring is advised to avoid serum glucose extremes. Many practitioners administer glucose-containing solutions as a separate piggyback infusion using an infusion pump or other rate- or volume-limiting device to avoid accidental bolus administration. Alternatively, evidence indicates that isotonic solutions that contain reduced glucose concentrations (e.g., 1% or 2.5% vs. 5%) are safe alternative solutions for intraoperative use.[92] In the United States, several Food and Drug Administration (FDA)-approved solutions containing 2.5% dextrose are available but none with concentrations lower than 2.5%. In Europe, 1% dextrose electrolyte solutions are available.[87,92] Because intraoperative administration of solutions containing 5% dextrose (D₅LR) frequently causes hyperglycemia, prudent anesthesiologists should selectively administer dextrose-containing solutions to those who are at particular risk for intraoperative hypoglycemia (i.e., neonates, chronic malnourished children, and cachectic children). In these instances, it may be sensible to administer solutions with a reduced dextrose concentration.[81,87]

FASTING RECOMMENDATIONS

The goal of fasting is to minimize the volume of gastric contents and thereby lessen the risk of vomiting and aspiration during induction of anesthesia. In children, as opposed to adults, this is of particular concern because in many institutions induction in children is more often accomplished by inhalation than by IV anesthesia and the period of vulnerability to regurgitation is potentially protracted compared with an IV induction.

At issue is the effectiveness of fasting in reducing a child's gastric volume and the benefits of this effect when weighed against the added discomfort and risk of dehydration. Numerous studies of gastric volume and pH have convincingly demonstrated that clear liquids are rapidly emptied from the stomach and the stimulated peristalsis actually serves to decrease gastric volume and acidity. Taking this together with the benefits of improved hydration and mental status, it is clear that prolonged *nil per os* (NPO) status is unwarranted. Clear fluids are emptied from the stomach with a half-life of ~20 minutes,[93] depending, in part, on the volume of sugar fluid ingested.[94] Recent evidence indicates that an NPO time of 1 hour for clear fluids does not increase the risk of pneumonitis if aspiration occurred in healthy children presenting for elective anaesthesia.[95,96] NPO guidelines currently in use in many institutions are included in Table 4.1.[97] As described earlier, for the vast majority of children, 20 to 40 mL/kg of LR given intraoperatively will provide adequate fluid deficit replacement.

ASSESSMENT OF INTRAVASCULAR VOLUME

Once the child is anesthetized, many clinical clues to volume status are lost or confounded by operative events. For example, although tachycardia is a fairly reliable indicator of volume status in the quietly resting preoperative child, a number of factors besides the intravascular volume status may increase the heart rate. Systolic BP (SBP) also reflects the volume status intraoperatively; fluid resuscitation should take priority over administering vasopressors and other inotropes and chronotropes. It is the challenge of the anesthesiologist to view the entire clinical picture, consider the possibilities, integrate them into a hypothesis, and then test the hypothesis.

Assessment of intravascular volume begins with knowledge of age-related norms for heart rate and BP (see Tables 2.7 and 2.8). Is the heart rate persistently increased or does it vary only with surgical stimulation? Is the pulse pressure (PP) narrow or, more ominously, is the BP reduced for age? Does it vary with positive-pressure breaths? Are the extremities warm? Is capillary refill brisk? What is the urine output? Are these variables changing? What is the rate of the change?

Measurement and continuous monitoring of central venous pressure (CVP) is commonly taken as both a direct measure of cardiac preload and an indirect measure of circulating volume (see Figs. 49.2 to 49.5). In addition to traditional central lines introduced into the superior vena cava or left atrium, animal[98] and limited clinical[99] data suggest that femoral lines that terminate in the abdominal vena cava may also be useful. In one study of infants and children, mean end-expiratory pressure measurements of venous pressure in the right atrial and inferior vena cava differed by less than 1 mm Hg.[99] Unfortunately, CVP as a static measure of volume status is confounded by many factors, including right ventricular compliance, positive end-expiratory pressure, abdominal pressure, and so on. In sum, these confounders render the CVP a relatively poor predictor of preload and volume status.[100]

Dynamic assessments best reflect the volume status and "volume responsiveness" (>10%–15% increase in stroke volume after a bolus) best indicates the volume for administration.[101] The respiratory cycle produces cyclic changes in stroke volume that are augmented when the ventricle is underfilled. This is particularly true under positive-pressure ventilation (PPV). As a result, SBP, diastolic BP (DBP), and pulse pressure (SBP-DBP, PP) variation is readily apparent on the arterial waveform of a hypovolemic child (see Fig. 12.10). PP variation may be quantified as $(PP_{max} - PP_{min})/[PP_{max} + PP_{min}/2] \times 100$, and volume responsiveness inferred from decreasing PPV. With this guidance, volume has been administered by some in 5- to 10-mL/kg test challenges until SBP and PPV no longer respond.[100] However, the usefulness of variability to determine volume status in children continues to be debated and should be performed carefully.[102–104]

ONGOING LOSSES AND THIRD-SPACING

During all surgical procedures, fluid loss from the vascular space is primarily the result of three simultaneous physiologic processes. First, whole blood is shed at various rates and must be replaced. Second, capillary leak and surgical trauma result in extravasation of isotonic, protein-containing fluid into interstitial compartments (the so-called third space). Third, anesthetic-induced relaxation of sympathetic tone produces vasodilatation (increased capacitance) and relative hypovolemia (a virtual loss). In very small infants, a fourth source of losses, direct evaporation, must also be considered. These ongoing losses are often difficult to quantitate (or even estimate). Although these losses occur in children of all sizes, the small circulating blood volume of an infant (e.g., for a 5-kg infant, 80 mL/kg × 5 kg = 400 mL) leaves little room for error. Faced with uncertainty, the prudent response is constant vigilance and reliance on general principles.

As a rule, 1 mL of shed blood is replaced with 1 mL of colloid (5% albumin or blood) or about 1.5 mL of isotonic crystalloid such as LR.[78,91] Isotonic crystalloid is also used to replenish third-space losses. Surgical procedures that involve only mild tissue trauma may entail third-space losses of 3 to 4 mL/kg per hour. More extensive surgical procedures involving moderate trauma may require replacement equivalent to 5 to 7 mL/kg per hour to adequately support intravascular volume. In small infants undergoing very large abdominal procedures, the losses may approach 10 mL/kg per hour or more.[72,74] In neonates, fluid requirements for emergent abdominal surgery for necrotizing enterocolitis have been estimated at up to 50 mL/kg per hour.[91] These "losses" include both evaporation and redistribution of fluid to the interstitium. The latter must be considered most carefully because it is exacerbated by the hemodilution and increased capillary pressures that results from excessive fluid administration.

Although necessary intraoperatively, third-space accumulation represents whole-body salt and water overload that will need to be mobilized postoperatively. The price of unchecked fluid administration is generalized anasarca, pulmonary edema, bowel swelling, and laryngotracheal edema. In the healthy child, this relative fluid overload is well tolerated, with most excess fluid excreted over the first 2 postoperative days. In children with impaired pulmonary, cardiac, or renal function, however, such fluid excess may result in clinically important postoperative morbidity.

Postoperative Fluid Management

GENERAL APPROACH

Well-planned postoperative fluid management complements the intraoperative plan and accounts for evolving physiology as the child recovers from anesthesia. Both fluid deficits and ongoing losses are replaced. The child is repeatedly reassessed, adjusting the intake until normal fluid and electrolyte homeostasis are present. To aid in decision making, trends in vital signs are identified, all sources of fluid intake and output are quantitated, urine specific gravity is monitored, daily weights are obtained, and serum electrolytes are measured.

In simple outpatient surgeries, discharge from the hospital is possible after fluid deficits have been replaced. In complex cases, replacement fluids may require hourly readjustment based on the prior hour's intake and output. Rather than reacting to isolated variables, such as low urine output, one must discern overall patterns. High urine output and low urine specific gravity may indicate overhydration or diabetes insipidus. Oliguria may suggest hypovolemia when it is accompanied by high urine specific gravity and clinical signs of dehydration or low cardiac output when it is accompanied by signs of poor perfusion. In the well-hydrated child, oliguria may represent renal failure if the urine specific gravity is normal (or dilute) but increased concentrations of ADH if the urine is concentrated. A careful physical examination is necessary; in many cases, certainty in diagnosis requires simultaneous measurement of serum and urine electrolytes.

Frequently, losses via surgical or gastric drains are large in both real and relative terms. For example, a neonate with a nasogastric tube may lose more than 100 mL/kg per day (normally 20–40 mL/kg per day) in gastric fluid. Therefore, in determining the volume and composition of replacement fluids, it is sometimes helpful to consider the electrolyte content of various losses (Table 9.8).

POSTOPERATIVE PHYSIOLOGY AND HYPONATREMIA

Children retain salt and water postoperatively, in part as a result of neuroendocrine activation by stress, continued capillary leak with third-space accumulation, nonosmotic stimulation of ADH (see Table 9.5) and hypovolemia-induced renin secretion. As outlined earlier, depleting the intravascular volume is a potent nonosmotic signal to retain fluid that may override osmotic signals under a variety of clinical circumstances.

At the same time, ongoing fluid and electrolyte losses after surgery via chest tubes, nasogastric suction, weeping incisions, and even continued slow bleeding may be substantial. Postoperatively, children often depend entirely on IV fluids to replace these and other losses.

Therefore, unless isotonic, sodium-containing fluids are provided, postoperative children are universally at risk for developing hyponatremia.[105,106] In a retrospective review of 24,412 surgical admissions to a large children's hospital, the incidence of significant postoperative hyponatremia was 0.34%, with a substantial mortality rate (8.4%) in these previously healthy children.[34] If this measured incidence were extended to the entire U.S. population, 7448 children would present annually with postoperative hyponatremia and 626 would die from an entirely avoidable cause. Mortality rates as great as 40% to 60% have been reported after hyponatremia, although it may only be a surrogate marker for a disease with a poor prognosis rather than the actual cause of the death.[107,108]

In reviewing the etiology of hyponatremia, two factors stand out: extensive extrarenal loss of electrolyte-containing fluid and IV replacement with hypotonic fluids.[34] In addition, delay in recognition often plays a major role in associated morbidity. The solution seems a simple one: (1) administration of hypotonic fluids without a specific indication should be avoided postoperatively, (2) ongoing losses should be replaced in a timely fashion, and (3) serum electrolytes should be measured routinely in children exhibiting potential symptoms of hyponatremia (see later discussion).

POSTOPERATIVE PULMONARY EDEMA

Children who receive large volumes of fluid intraoperatively are at risk for development of pulmonary edema as operative fluids are mobilized. Usually, fluid begins to be mobilized on the second postoperative day and continues through day 3 or 4. Although this is less common in children than in the elderly, it occurs occasionally in children with burn injuries[109] or in pediatric patients receiving large amounts of fluid during resuscitation from trauma or sepsis. In one review,[110] 13 patients (11 adults and 2 children) developed postoperative pulmonary edema; all began to exhibit symptoms within 36 hours after surgery and had total net fluid retention in excess of 67 mL/kg postoperatively.

TABLE 9.8	Composition of Body Fluids					
Source	Na⁺ (mEq/L)	K⁺ (mEq/L)	Cl⁻ (mEq/L)	HCO₃⁻ (mEq/L)	pH	Osmolality (mOsm/L)
Gastric	50	10–15	150	0	1	300
Pancreas	140	5	0–100	100	9	300
Bile	130	5	100	40	8	300
Ileostomy	130	15–20	120	25–30	8	300
Diarrhea	50	35	40	50		
Sweat	50	5	55	0	Alkaline	
Blood	140	4–5	100	25	7.4	285–295
Urine	0–100ᵃ	20–100ᵃ	70–100ᵃ	0	4.5–8.5ᵃ	50–1400ᵃ

ᵃVaries considerably with fluid intake.
From Herrin J. Fluid and electrolytes. In: Graef JW, ed. *Manual of Pediatric Therapeutics*. 6th ed. Philadelphia: Lippincott-Raven; 1997:63–75.

Pathophysiologic States and Their Management

FLUID OVERLOAD AND EDEMA

Edema is essentially a "sodium disease," representing sodium and water overload with excessive fluid residing in the extracellular space. Although intracellular volume changes can sometimes be substantial, prolonged cell swelling represents failure of essential volume regulatory functions and is likely a preterminal event. In fluid-overload states, plasma volume is generally increased unless the balance of Starling forces is disturbed, as in nephrotic syndrome or lymphatic obstruction. Edema formation is opposed by (1) low compliance of the interstitial compartment, (2) increased lymphatic flow, (3) osmotic washout of interstitial proteins, and (4) impedance and elasticity of the proteoglycan gel. The differential diagnosis of fluid overload and edema formation is presented in Table 9.9. Principles of therapy for fluid overload states include the following:

- Fluid restriction
- Salt restriction
- Diuresis, dialysis
- Salt-poor albumin for diminished plasma volume

DEHYDRATION STATES

Dehydration states are common in children. The extent of dehydration is best assessed by weight, because clinical signs such as tachycardia, capillary refill, and skin elasticity,[111] although often reliable, may be influenced by factors other than hydration status. A capillary refill time of 1.5 to 3.0 seconds, for example, suggests a fluid deficit of between 50 and 100 mL/kg, yet this sign is extremely dependent on ambient temperature.[112] Similarly, poor skin elasticity reflects significant volume loss, yet elasticity may be well preserved in children with hypernatremic dehydration.[111] Clinical signs associated with varying levels of dehydration are presented in Table 9.10.

As a first approximation, correction of most dehydration states in older children is most readily achieved with administration of a simple bolus of NS, LR, or PlasmaLyte 148 (balanced crystalloid solution). In infants or children with unusual, prolonged, or severe dehydration, however, management must be more precise. A 5-point questionnaire to assess the severity of dehydration may help develop an appropriate treatment strategy[113]:

1. *Does a volume deficit exist and, if so, how great is it?*

   As noted previously, assessment of volume deficit is best made by weight, yet rough estimates of 5% (mild), 10% (moderate), and 15% (severe) may be made in infants based on clinical signs (see Table 9.10).

2. *Does an osmolar disturbance exist?*

   Is it acute or chronic? An osmolar imbalance is determined by measuring the serum sodium concentration. The majority of clinically encountered dehydration states (~80%) are isotonic (Na^+ = 130–150 mEq/L). These isotonic losses are easily managed by almost any strategy.

   Approximately 15% of dehydrated children present with hypertonic dehydration (Na^+ >150 mEq/L). These children are at greatest risk and have usually experienced the greatest fluid losses for a given set of clinical signs.[114] If the condition is chronic, they may require extensive, slow rehydration over prolonged periods.[115]

   Five percent of children present with hypotonic dehydration (Na^+ <130 mEq/L). For a given fluid deficit, these individuals are often more symptomatic than others, and their requirement for sodium replacement is greatest. Surprisingly, rapid improvement in clinical condition often results after the first fluid bolus.

   In general, states of acute dehydration (<24 hours) may be corrected rapidly, whereas states of chronic dehydration must be corrected slowly. This difference in treatment plan is attributed to the speed at which the cell volume equilibrates: acutely through gain or loss of electrolytes

TABLE 9.9	Differential Diagnosis of Fluid Overload and Edema Formation
Condition	**Differential Diagnosis**
Imbalance of intake and output	Salt poisoning
	Formula dilution errors
	Intravenous infusion errors
	Drugs given as sodium salts
Steroid excess with normal sodium intake	Congenital adrenal hyperplasia
	Exogenous steroids
Perceived decreases in effective plasma volume	↓ MAP → baroreceptors → ↑ sympathetic tone, ADH, renin, aldosterone
	Vasodilators
	Congestive heart failure
	Cirrhosis
	Nephrotic syndrome
Impaired sodium excretion	Chronic renal failure
	Acute glomerular disease (↓ GFR with normal tubular function)
	Nonsteroidal antiinflammatory drugs (↓ PGE_2 and RBF)
Water excess	SIADH
	Hypotonic infusion
	Stress (↑ ADH)

ADH, antidiuretic hormone; *GFR,* glomerular filtration rate; *MAP,* mean arterial pressure; *PGE_2,* prostaglandin E_2; *RBF,* renal blood flow; *SIADH,* syndrome of inappropriate antidiuretic hormone secretion.

TABLE 9.10	Clinical Signs and Symptoms for Estimation of Severity of Dehydration in Infants

	DEGREE OF DEHYDRATION		
Clinical Signs	**Mild**	**Moderate**	**Severe**
Weight loss (%)	5	10	15
Behavior	Normal	Irritable	Hyperirritable to lethargic
Thirst	Slight	Moderate	Intense
Mucous membranes	May be normal	Dry	Parched
Tears	Present	Normal to reduced	Absent
Anterior fontanel	Flat	Possibly sunken	Sunken
Skin turgor	Normal	Slightly increased	Increased
Urine output	Normal	Oliguric	Anuric

Modified in part from Herrin J. Fluid and electrolytes. In: Graef J, ed. *Manual of Pediatric Therapeutics.* 6th ed. Philadelphia: Lippincott-Raven; 1997:63–75.

(which are transported rapidly across membranes) or chronically through gain or loss of organic osmolytes (which are transported more slowly).[11] Reequilibration of brain cell volume during correction of hypertonicity can be very slow, mandating patience in correction of chronic fluid deficits. Similarly, rapid correction of hyponatremic disturbances can be hazardous,[34] even when seemingly safe isotonic solutions are infused.[116]

3. *Does an acid-base abnormality exist?*

Quantitation of the child's acid-base status gives useful, although limited, information in terms of the severity of dehydration. When evaluating acid-base status, it is important to recall that bicarbonate reabsorption and urine acidification are limited in preterm and young infants, leaving even the normal infant in a state of mild metabolic acidosis (pH, 7.3; serum bicarbonate 20–21 mEq/L [normal 22–26 mEq/L]). Although slow, spontaneous correction of acid-base status is typically observed on rehydration, rapid fluid boluses in poorly perfused children may result in a transient "reperfusion acidosis" as returning circulation washes the products of anaerobic metabolism out of the tissues. In this setting, or when renal insufficiency exists, blood-buffering capacity is such that children with serum bicarbonate concentrations less than 8 mEq/L or pH less than 7.2 may benefit from administration of supplemental base (sodium bicarbonate) (Fig. 9.6).[113]

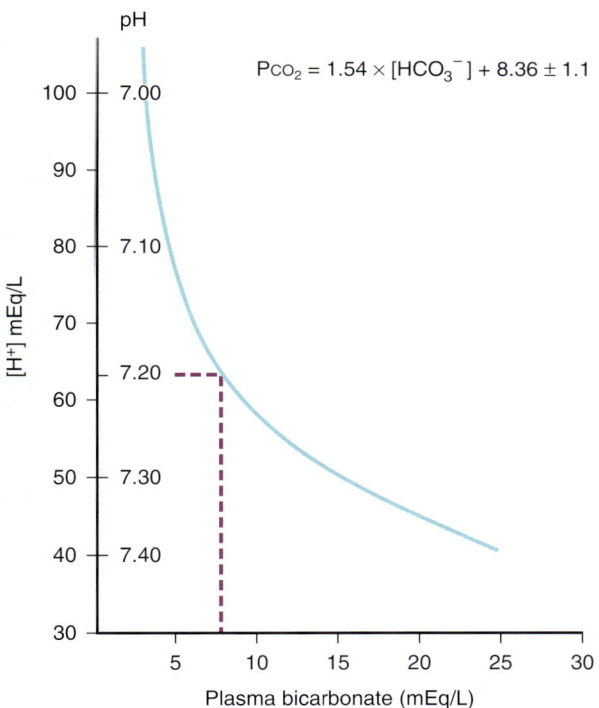

FIGURE 9.6 Data from children with metabolic acidosis[117] were used to depict the displacement of pH as serum bicarbonate declines. The zone of rapid pH displacement (pH <7.20) has a slope that is several times greater than the zone of gradual pH displacement (pH ≥7.20). As the pH moves through the zone of rapid pH displacement, a further decline of serum bicarbonate of as little as 1 or 2 mEq/L produces a highly leveraged further decrease of pH. $[H]^+$, hydrogen ion concentration; $[HCO_3^-]$, bicarbonate ion concentration; PCO_2, carbon dioxide tension. (From Kallen RJ. The management of diarrheal dehydration in infants using parenteral fluids. *Pediatr Clin North Am.* 1990;37:265–286.)

Rapid bedside evaluation of acid-base status uses the following general relationships: a pH decrease of 0.1 unit accompanies a base excess (BE) of approximately 6 mEq/L or an increase in carbon dioxide tension (PCO_2) of 10 to 12 mm Hg. The total replacement base required is then determined by the following equation:

$$\text{Dose (mEq)} = 0.3 \times \text{Weight (kg)} \times \text{BE (mEq/L)}$$

Clinically, a smaller sodium bicarbonate dose (1–2 mEq/kg) is given initially, the response is verified by blood gas analysis, and the remaining doses are titrated to effect.

4. *Is renal function impaired?*

Initial evaluation includes the timing of the last urine void and recent urine output, measurement of urine specific gravity, and serum levels of blood urea nitrogen and creatinine. If uncertainty persists, measurement of serum and urine electrolytes for comparison and calculation of the FE_{Na} are indicated (see Chapter 28).

FE_{Na} values of less than 1% imply prerenal conditions causing renal dysfunction, whereas FE_{Na} values greater than 2% to 3% suggest renal insufficiency. In prematurity, however, values as large as 9% have been recorded in otherwise normal infants.

5. *What is the state of potassium balance?*

Potassium homeostasis is critical to life, and serum potassium concentrations are generally maintained within a very narrow range. Nonetheless, serum potassium concentrations do not reflect whole-body stores and substantial potassium depletion may exist in the presence of modest changes in serum potassium concentration (K^+_{serum}). Gastrointestinal losses or metabolic acidosis is usually accompanied by a potassium deficit, whereas other dehydration states are not. Rapid fluid boluses or pH correction, or both, may acutely reduce K^+_{serum},[118] and refractory hypokalemia may occur in children deficient in magnesium.[119] In all cases, adequate renal function should be present before administration of potassium, and complete repletion should span 48 to 72 hours. Once the nature and severity of dehydration have been determined, the clinician may proceed using any of a variety of correction strategies. In one approach, moderate to severe dehydration deficits may be estimated, as in Table 9.10. Fluid and electrolyte repair may then proceed according to a three-phase approach wherein circulating plasma volume, perfusion, and urine output are restored rapidly using isotonic crystalloid or colloid solution and remaining deficits are corrected over 24 hours as follows[120]:

- Emergency Phase: 20 to 30 mL/kg isotonic crystalloid/colloid bolus
- Repletion Phase 1: 25 to 50 mL/kg over 6 to 8 hours. Anions: Cl⁻ 75%, acetate 25%
- Repletion Phase 2: remainder of deficit over 24 hours (isotonic) or 48 hours (hypertonic). Include calcium replacement as necessary.

SEPTIC SHOCK

Both the Pediatric Advanced Life Support (PALS) recommendations from the American Heart Association and the "Surviving Sepsis" campaign from the Society of Critical Care Medicine have long emphasized fluid administration as the cornerstone of successful resuscitation. As a Ib recommendation, the original "Surviving Sepsis" campaign called for "a minimum of 30 mL/kg of crystalloid," whereas PALS guidelines directed "20 mL/kg of isotonic crystalloid over 5 to 20 minutes" repeated as needed with expectations for "at least 60 mL/kg" during the first hour.[121,122] Since these guidelines have been widely adopted, fluid overload has been associated with poor outcome in a variety of settings including certain populations of children with sepsis.[123-127] Alternative views now hold that administration of large crystalloid volumes (20–30 mL/kg) is unphysiologic and, ultimately, counterproductive in sepsis and cardiac arrest since little stays in the circulation, saltatory effects dissipate rapidly, and resulting edema can exacerbate circulatory and respiratory derangements.[128] Recent PALS recommendations acknowledge this controversy and call for a less aggressive approach; an initial fluid bolus of 20 mL/kg is "reasonable" but "should be undertaken with extreme caution" with "individualized patient evaluation."[129] Meanwhile, "Surviving Sepsis" consensus bundles now call for 30 mL/kg of crystalloid "for hypotension or lactate ≥4 mmol/L" and redefine "septic shock" as a severe subset of "sepsis."[130] Anesthesiologists are accustomed to continually reassessing circulatory homeostasis, and so in the setting of septic shock, should feel comfortable pursuing standard physiologic endpoints with judicious fluid administration complemented with inotropes and vasopressors.

HYPERNATREMIA AND HYPONATREMIA

As previously detailed, disorders of sodium equilibrium are primarily marked by disturbances of fluid balance and are corrected according to the principles outlined earlier. Serious hypernatremia or hyponatremia is accompanied by neurologic symptoms whose severity is determined by the degree and rate of change of Na^+_{serum}.

Hypernatremia

In contrast to its rareness in adults, acute hypernatremia is common in children. A mortality rate greater than 40% for the acute disorder and 10% for the chronic disorder has been quoted (serum sodium >160 mEq/L).[107,131] Mortality and permanent neurologic injury are even more common in infants. Depending on the degree and duration, neurologic findings include irritability and coma; seizures may be a presenting symptom, but are more commonly encountered after the start of therapy. Children with acute conditions are usually symptomatic, whereas those with chronic conditions (acclimated individuals) are typically asymptomatic. General principles for treatment of hypernatremia are as follows:

- In the setting of circulatory collapse, colloid or NS bolus should be administered. Although the assertion is debatable, a colloid bolus provides the theoretical benefit of sustained hemodynamic support with a smaller fluid load. Saline, in contrast, rapidly reequilibrates, necessitating repeated boluses while adding to the total salt burden.
- Once a stable circulation has been restored, fluid deficit should be assessed as accurately as possible and corrected over 48 to 72 hours. Cautious correction of the serum sodium concentration is required. The serum sodium concentration and osmolality should be continuously reassessed during fluid administration, aiming for a correction of no more than 1 to 2 mOsm/L per hour. After as little as 4 hours of hypernatremia, idiogenic osmoles (e.g., trimethylamines) appear in the brain to prevent cerebral volume depletion. Rapid administration of free water could induce cerebral edema, seizures, and death. Therefore free water should be administered slowly. Because of possible associated hypoglycemia, some solutions should

be glucose-containing, and serum glucose levels should be monitored.
- Vigilance for seizures, apnea, and cardiovascular compromise is essential because appropriate and timely treatment of such complicating factors can be the primary determinants of successful outcome.

Hyponatremia

Hyponatremia is also common in infants and children; increasing prevalence owing to erroneous formula dilution has intermittently been reported.[132,133] In the practice of anesthesiology, mild hyponatremia is a common postoperative condition after surgery of any severity[134-136]; in neurosurgical patients, hyponatremia may represent cerebral salt wasting or syndrome of inappropriate antidiuretic hormone secretion (SIADH).[137] In general, symptomatic patients are acutely hyponatremic and asymptomatic individuals are chronically hyponatremic.[138] After surgery, acutely hyponatremic children may present with nonspecific symptoms that are often erroneously attributed to other causes. Early central nervous system symptoms include headache, nausea, weakness, and anorexia. Advancing symptoms include mental status changes, confusion, irritability, progressive obtundation, and seizures. Respiratory arrest (or irregularity) is a common manifestation of advanced hyponatremia.

When planning to correct hyponatremia, the presence of symptoms must be considered a medical emergency, whereas asymptomatic children do not require rapid intervention. Chronic hyponatremia must be corrected slowly and by no more than 0.5 mEq/L per hour to avoid neurologic complications that include central pontine myelinolysis.[139] The best treatment for acute hyponatremia is early recognition and intervention. Because hypoxia exacerbates the neurologic injury, the simple ABCs of resuscitation are attended to first, and the airway is secured in the child who has seizures or respiratory irregularity. Hyponatremic seizures may be quieted by relatively modest (3–6 mEq/L) increases of serum sodium.[140] In several series,[133,141,142] such limited, rapid correction of symptomatic hyponatremia with hypertonic saline (514 mEq/L NaCl) was well tolerated. It should be emphasized, however, that complete correction is unnecessary and unwise.[143] Initial therapy is aimed at increasing the Na^+_{serum} no more than is necessary to stop seizure activity (usually 3–5 mEq/L). Further, the correction takes place over several days. Hypertonic saline may be used for the correction until the Na^+_{serum} increases to greater than 120 mEq/L. Remembering that TBW may range from 75% in infancy to 60% or less in older children, total sodium deficit is estimated as follows:

$$\text{Sodium change (mEq/L)} \times \text{fraction TBW (L/kg)} \times \text{weight (kg)}$$
$$= \text{mEq sodium}$$

$$(\text{Desired } [Na^+]_{serum} - \text{observed } [Na^+]_{serum}) \times 0.6 \times \text{weight (kg)}$$
$$= \text{mEq sodium required}$$

For example, in a 25-kg child, to correct a serum sodium concentration of 110 mEq/L to 125 mEq/L using hypertonic saline (514 mEq/L), infuse

$$(125 \text{ mEq/L} - 110 \text{ mEq/L}) \times 0.6 \times 25 = 225 \text{ mEq total}$$

or

$$225 \text{ mEq}/514 \text{ mEq/L} = 0.44 \text{ L over 48 hours} = 9 \text{ mL/hour}$$

Because such calculations involve estimates, frequent measurement of the Na^+_{serum} is necessary during correction. As with hypernatremia, much of the morbidity and mortality associated with hyponatremia relates to complicating factors such as seizures and hypoxia that may occur during therapy. Therefore, children undergoing therapy should be cared for in a monitored setting. When overzealous correction has occurred, there may be value in acutely relowering Na^+_{serum} using hypotonic fluids,[138] although such therapy is not without its own hazards.

General principles for treatment of hyponatremia are as follows:
- Asymptomatic hyponatremia in and of itself need not be rapidly corrected. Associated cardiovascular compromise caused by volume depletion may be addressed by colloid bolus or administration of isotonic saline (1 L/m² per day). Provision of sodium is accompanied by free water restriction.
- Symptomatic hyponatremia is a medical emergency and may sometimes reflect irreversible neurologic injury. Correction should be rapid, yet limited, as discussed previously. A dose of 2 to 3 mL/kg of 3% saline (514 mEq/L) may be administered over 20 to 30 minutes to halt seizures.
- Subsequent correction is accomplished through calculation of the sodium deficit and provision of sodium so as to slowly correct at a rate not to exceed 0.5 mEq/L per hour or 12 to 25 mEq/L (total) in 24 to 48 hours.
- If the attendant fluid load is excessive or if oliguria is present, diuretics may be useful.

DISORDERS OF POTASSIUM HOMEOSTASIS

Hyperkalemia

Hyperkalemia is occasionally the presenting finding in conditions such as congenital adrenal hyperplasia. More commonly, it results from acute renal insufficiency, massive tissue injury, acidosis, or iatrogenic mishaps. In the operating room, acute hyperkalemia may follow the use of succinylcholine in children with myopathies, burns, upper and lower motor neuron lesions, chronic sepsis, or disuse atrophy and occasionally during massive, rapid transfusion of red blood cells or whole blood (see Chapter 12).[144] It may occur with rhabdomyolysis or as a late sign in malignant hyperthermia (see Chapter 41).

Although neurologic status is the main concern for children with abnormal Na^+_{serum}, cardiac status (rate and rhythm) determines the care of children with hyperkalemia. In children with hyperkalemia, the appearance of peaked T waves is followed by lengthening of the PR interval and widening of the QRS complex until P waves are lost. Finally, the QRS complex merges with its T wave to produce a sinusoidal pattern (Fig. 9.7). Successful treatment traditionally uses the following approach:
- Emergent therapy is first directed toward antagonism of the cardiac effects of potassium by cautious administration of IV calcium (chloride 20 mg/kg, or 60 mg/kg of calcium gluconate as a 10% solution) over 3 to 5 minutes to avoid bradycardia. Calcium does not decrease the serum potassium concentration but rather reestablishes the gradient between the resting membrane potential, which is increased in the presence of hyperkalemia, and the threshold potential, which is determined by the calcium concentration. It also increases the refractory period of the action potential, the net effect being the prevention of spontaneous depolarization.
- Serum potassium is then reduced by returning potassium to the intracellular space. This is achieved by correcting the acidosis by administering sodium bicarbonate (1–2 mEq/kg) intravenously, a β-agonist, and mild to moderate hyperventilation.

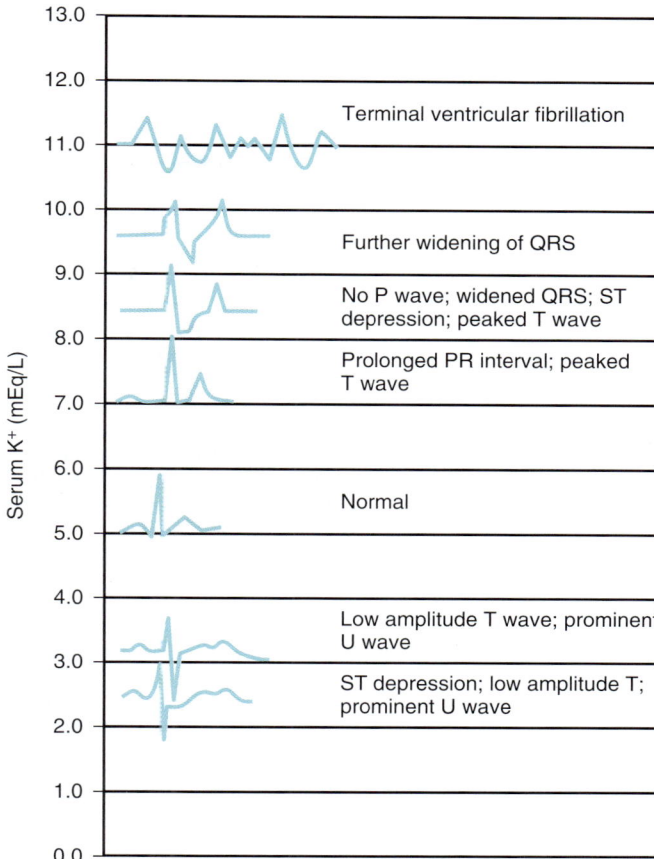

FIGURE 9.7 Electrocardiographic changes associated with hypokalemia and hyperkalemia. (From Williams GS, Klenk EL, Winters RW. Acute renal failure in pediatrics. In: Winters RW, ed. *The Body Fluids in Pediatrics: Medical, Surgical, and Neonatal Disorders of Acid-Base Status, Hydration, and Oxygenation.* Boston: Little, Brown; 1973;523–557.)

- To maintain potassium in the intracellular space, glucose and insulin are administered by infusion (0.5–1 g/kg glucose with 0.1 U/kg insulin over 30 to 60 minutes).
- After stabilizing the K^+_{serum}, attention is directed toward removal of the whole-body potassium burden (sodium polystyrene sulfonate [Kayexalate], furosemide, dialysis) and correction of the underlying cause (Fig. 9.8).

The knowledge that β-adrenergic stimulation modulates the translocation of potassium into the intracellular space[145,146] prompted the consideration of β-agonists in the treatment of acute hyperkalemia.[147–150] In children, a single infusion of an IV β-agonist such as salbutamol (5 μg/kg over 15 minutes) effectively reduces serum potassium concentrations within 30 minutes. Because of the rapidity, efficacy, and safety of salbutamol in children, it has become the first-choice treatment for hyperkalemia.[147] In addition to IV therapy, salbutamol[151] (also known as albuterol[150]) by inhalation effectively reduces the serum potassium concentration. The inhalation route has the significant advantages of being readily available in emergency departments and not requiring IV access. However, the observation that a paradoxical exacerbation of hyperkalemia sometimes occurs on initiation of treatment,[151] together with concerns regarding the possibility of associated arrhythmias,[152] suggests that more experience is required before such therapy can be considered the standard of care. Inhalation of salbutamol during such an event in the operating room may

Treatment Algorithm for Hyperkalemia

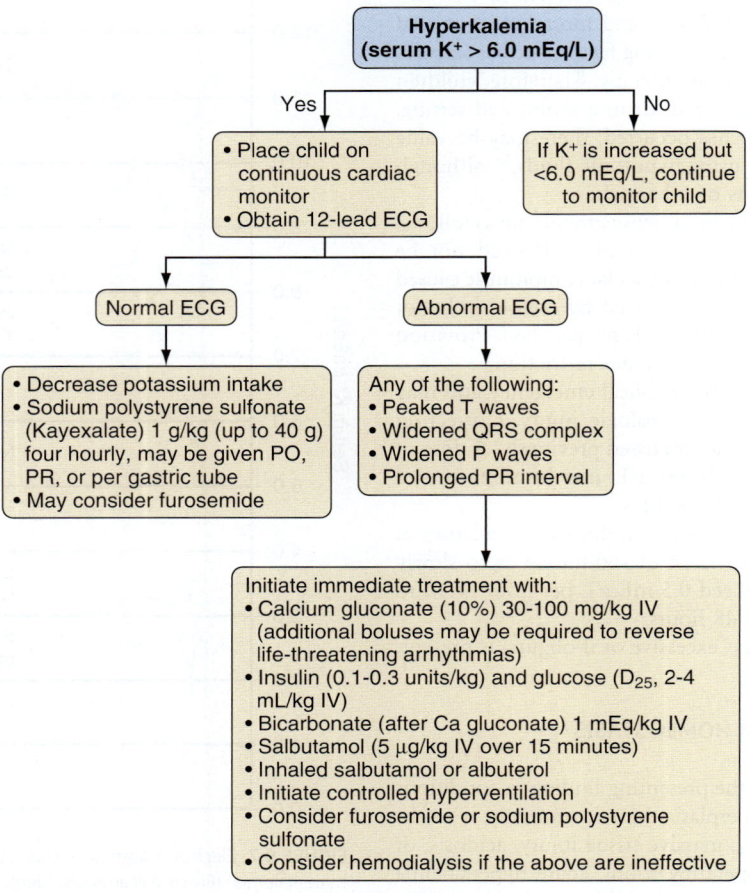

FIGURE 9.8 Algorithm for treatment of hyperkalemia. After stabilization, attention is directed toward removal of the whole-body potassium burden (Kayexalate, dialysis) and correction of the underlying cause. D_{25}, 25% dextrose; *ECG*, electrocardiogram; *IV*, intravenous; *PO*, orally; *PR*, per rectum.

speed the reduction in serum potassium while other methods of treatment are instituted.

Hypokalemia

Hypokalemia is most common in children as a complication of diarrhea or persistent vomiting associated with gastroenteritis. Muscle weakness is the most common sign in hypokalemia and has been correlated with the serum potassium concentration.[153] In the operating room or ICU, hypokalemia may also accompany a wide variety of other conditions, including diabetes, hyperaldosteronism, pyloric stenosis, starvation, renal tubular disease, chronic steroid or diuretic use, and β-agonist therapy. Severe hypokalemia can also be accompanied by electrocardiographic changes, including QT prolongation, diminution of the T wave, and appearance of U waves (see Fig. 9.7).

As noted previously, the K^+_{serum} does not accurately reflect total potassium homeostasis, and low serum concentrations may or may not be associated with significant depletion of total body potassium. Indeed, the extracellular fraction of potassium is only a tiny proportion (approximately 3%) of the entire body store. For these reasons, the precise point at which to begin replacement therapy is controversial, and total replacement requirements are impossible to calculate. In general practice, serum potassium values

(K^+_{serum}) between 2.0 and 2.5 mEq/L are corrected before surgery on the assumption that further decreases may predispose the child to muscular weakness, arrhythmias, and hemodynamic instability.

Potassium replacement is best accomplished orally over an extended period while the underlying cause is evaluated and treated. When IV correction is required, concentrations up to 40 mEq/L should be given slowly *(not to exceed 1 mEq/kg per hour)* in a monitored setting. Because such solutions often cause phlebitis, large-bore or central catheters are preferred. In the setting of hypochloremia and hypokalemia, chloride deficits must first be replaced, usually by administration of normal saline.

SYNDROME OF INAPPROPRIATE ANTIDIURETIC HORMONE SECRETION

Many nonosmotic factors are capable of stimulating ADH release, and these can occasionally override osmotic control priorities. When this occurs, clinicians have historically deemed the increased ADH concentrations "inappropriate" because control of the serum osmolarity is lost (see Chapter 28). As detailed earlier, however, intravascular depletion is the most potent stimulus for vasopressin release, and it is hardly *inappropriate* that defense of circulation takes priority over defense of serum sodium levels. Pain, surgical stress, critical illness, sepsis, pulmonary disease, central nervous system injury, drugs, and a variety of other factors may all stimulate ADH release above and beyond that necessary to maintain osmolar balance (see Table 9.5).

SIADH is common in children yet it is often overlooked. Minor head trauma, for example, may elicit spikes in ADH levels, although infrequently to the extent that it produces serious hyponatremia and seizures.[154] Urine output after spinal fusion is often reduced because of increased concentrations of ADH, which usually return to normal within 24 hours without therapy.[155] Infants with bronchiolitis and hyperinflated lungs frequently demonstrate markedly increased plasma ADH concentrations and exhibit fluid retention, weight gain, urinary concentration, and plasma hypoosmolality until their illness begins to resolve.[156] Hyponatremia to the point of seizures, however, is only occasionally observed.

The diagnosis of SIADH rests on the identification of impaired urinary dilution in the setting of plasma hypoosmolality. Hyponatremia (Na^+ <135 mEq/L), serum osmolality less than 280 mOsm/L, and urine osmolality greater than 100 mOsm/L in the absence of volume depletion, cardiac failure, nephropathy, adrenal insufficiency, or cirrhosis are generally considered sufficient for diagnosis. Therapeutic principles are similar to those for hyponatremia and depend on the following:

- Restriction of free water
- Repletion of sodium deficits (if present)
- Administration of diuretics to offset the effects of vasopressin

DIABETES INSIPIDUS

In the operating room and the ICU, diabetes insipidus is most commonly associated with the care of neurosurgical patients.[157–159] Diabetes insipidus is also caused by neuroendocrine failure in brain death and management may be necessary if organ donation is planned.[160,161] Diabetes insipidus results from decreased secretion of, or renal insensitivity to, vasopressin (see Chapter 27). Manifestations include massive polyuria, volume contraction, dehydration, and plasma hyperosmolality. Dilute polyuria (<250 mOsm, >2 mL/kg per hour) in the presence of hypernatremia (Na^+ >145 mEq/L) with hyperosmolality (>300 mOsm/L) is the hallmark. In central diabetes insipidus, administration of desmopressin concentrates the urine although water deprivation does not. Postoperative diabetes insipidus may initially be difficult to distinguish from mobilization of operative fluids.

Children with craniopharyngioma or a similarly situated pathologic lesion may not manifest vasopressin deficiency early in the disease but become symptomatic preoperatively after steroid administration or intraoperatively during surgical manipulation. Postoperative diabetes insipidus typically begins on the evening after surgery and may resolve in 3 to 5 days if osmoregulatory structures have not been permanently injured. An often-confusing triphasic response may also occur wherein postoperative diabetes insipidus appears to resolve, fluid status normalizes, or SIADH appears and then vasopressin secretion ceases and diabetes insipidus returns. It is hypothesized that this pattern reflects nonspecific vasopressin release from degenerating neurons in the hypothalamic supraoptic and paraventricular nuclei.

Attempts have been made to develop protocols for perioperative management of diabetes insipidus.[162] Because vasopressin is difficult to titrate to urine output, our practice involves maximal antidiuresis and fluid restriction. In this setting, volume status must be monitored closely, because urine output is no longer a marker of renal perfusion. Children who need close perioperative monitoring for the development of diabetes insipidus include those with preexisting diabetes insipidus as well as those who are undergoing resection of craniopharyngiomas or pituitary lesions or other procedures that involve resection or manipulation of the pituitary stalk.[163]

HYPERCHLOREMIC ACIDOSIS

Administration of large amounts of NS can lead to excess serum chloride.[164] NS-induced acidosis has been attributed to the Stewart physicochemical approach to acid-base balance.[165,166] In this framework, plasma pH is determined by its "strong ion difference" (SID), or the concentration differences between dominant cations and anions ([SID] = $[Na^+]$ + $[K^+]$ + $[Ca^{+2}]$ + $[Mg^{+2}]$ − $[Cl^-]$). Because electroneutrality must be preserved, the SID must always be balanced by additional negative charges arising collectively from weak acids and HCO_3^-. Since the mass of weak acids is relatively fixed and $[HCO_3^-]$ is an immediately responsive buffer, acute changes in SID translate directly to acute changes in [HCO3]. *Increases* in the SID therefore *increase* [HCO3−] to yield plasma *alkalinization*, whereas *decreases* in the SID *decrease* [HCO3−] to yield plasma *acidification*. Since administration of saline in large volumes produces hyperchloremia, this must be accompanied by a decrease in [HCO3−]. Typically, the SID is ~40 to 42 mEq/L (example, 140 + 4 + 4.5[a] + 2[b] − 110). Increasing $[Cl^-]$ can be expected to increase the base deficit by an equivalent amount.

A simpler explanation of NS-induced acidosis is that it arises through dilution of [HCO3]. When plasma volume is expanded by saline, its primary buffer system (CO_2/$[HCO_3^-]$) is diluted. Because it is an open system, respiration holds the buffer acid (CO_2) constant while the buffer base ($[HCO_3^-]$) decreases. This physicochemical behavior and the resulting base deficit acidosis can be reproduced in model systems.[167]

Regardless of the source, it is clinically apparent that administration of large NS volumes is accompanied by metabolic acidosis related to both the amount and rate of infusion. In healthy women undergoing gynecologic surgery, 35 mL/kg NS over 2 hours produced acidosis, whereas similar infusions of LR did not.[164] In a study of children undergoing craniofacial surgery, 80% of those who received NS (40% to pH ≤ 7.25) and 37% of those who received Ringer lactate (8% to pH ≤ 7.25) developed an acidosis.[168] The clinical significance of the saline-associated acidosis is still being clarified, although one large study observed less postoperative morbidity in adults receiving balanced solutions, other than saline, for replacement of losses during abdominal surgery.[169]

HYPOCHLOREMIC METABOLIC ALKALOSIS

Infants with pyloric stenosis and other children with chronic vomiting may develop a hypochloremic metabolic alkalosis. In both of these conditions, chronic vomiting results in large losses of hydrogen and chloride ions and water. This leads to an alkalotic, dehydrated state. In the absence of IV fluid therapy, the renal response is to conserve water by retaining sodium through upregulation of aldosterone, in which hydrogen ions (which are already in short supply because of the vomiting) and potassium ions are excreted in the urine in exchange for sodium. Excretion of the remaining hydrogen ions in exchange for sodium exacerbates the existing alkalosis or prevents resolution of the alkalosis. It also leads to the unusual syndrome of paradoxical aciduria in the presence of a metabolic alkalosis.

---

[a]Normal Ca = 8-10 mg/dL = 4-5 mEq/L (mg/dL × 10 × 2 Eq/mol × 1/40 g/mol, so multiply by 0.5).
[b]Normal Mg = 2 mg/dL = 1.6 mEq/L (mg/dL × 10 × 2 × 1/24 g/mol, so multiply by 0.83).

The potassium loss leads to hypokalemia. Although hypokalemia between 3.4 and 4.4 mEq/L may appear trivial because the concentration is within the normal range, chronic hypokalemia equilibrates throughout all bodily fluids including the intracellular fluid volume. The intracellular potassium concentration, 135 to 145 mEq/L, is 30- to 40-fold greater than the extracellular concentration. Hence, a chronic decrease of 1 mEq/L in extracellular potassium, which is only 1% to 2% of the total body potassium, may reflect an enormous deficiency in total body potassium stores, on the order of 100 to 200 mEq K^+ in an adult. However, potassium loss from the extracellular fluid is not linearly related to the total body potassium (owing to interference from Na^+/K^+ pumps and other electrolyte-stabilizing mechanisms). With an extracellular K^+ concentration less than 3.5 mEq/L, this small loss in extracellular potassium translates into a huge loss of total body potassium, whereas with an extracellular K^+ concentration greater than 4 mEq/L, extracellular potassium losses exert an attenuated effect on the total body potassium.

In infants and children with chronic hypokalemic, hypochloremic, metabolic alkalosis, correction of the electrolyte abnormalities and hypovolemia is optimally achieved using NS with 20 mEq/L K^+ infused at a rate of 10 to 20 mL/kg per hour through a peripheral IV line until the potassium level is greater than 3.0 mEq/L, the chloride concentration is greater than 95 mEq/L, and the clinical signs of hypovolemia are resolved. In the case of pyloric stenosis, this may take 24 to 48 hours depending on the severity of the electrolyte and fluid imbalance.

CEREBRAL SALT WASTING

Cerebral salt wasting (also known as renal salt wasting) is a hyponatremic syndrome of unclear etiology. Most commonly recognized in neurosurgical patients, it is a primary natriuresis probably related to dysregulation of brain or atrial natriuretic peptides. The condition has been increasingly recognized, and an incidence as great as 5% has been reported in children with brain tumors.[170] Cerebral salt wasting can sometimes be difficult to distinguish from SIADH but the former is marked by hyponatremia, natriuresis, and *hypovolemia*, unlike the latter, which features hypervolemia. Initial therapy consists of fluid resuscitation with isotonic solutions and ongoing correction of intravascular volume depletion with sodium-containing solutions. Although spontaneous resolution is the norm, persistent cases may require mineralocorticoid therapy.

ACKNOWLEDGMENT
The authors acknowledge the contributions of Letty M. P. Liu to previous editions of this chapter.

ANNOTATED REFERENCES

Arieff AI, Ayus JC, Fraser CL. Hyponatraemia and death or permanent brain damage in healthy children. *BMJ*. 1992;304:1218-1222.

Much concern has been displayed in recent years about iatrogenic hyponatremia caused by administration of hypotonic solutions. This study highlights the grave consequences of such errors.

Constable PD. Hyperchloremic acidosis: the classic example of strong ion acidosis. *Anesth Analg*. 2003;96:919-922.

This review is an excellent description of alternative methods of evaluating acid-base status. The focus of this paper is on the physiology behind the acidosis created by large, rapid administration of normal saline.

Holliday MA, Friedman AL, Segar W, et al. Acute hospital-induced hyponatremia in children: a physiologic approach. *J Pediatr*. 2004;145:584-587.

This update to the authors' classic 1957 article addresses the problems associated with applying the original formula (4-2-1 rule) to perioperative fluid management. The authors present an alternative approach to perioperative fluid management with a focus on attenuating the antidiuretic hormone response to perioperative stress.

Oh GJ, Sutherland SM. Perioperative fluid management and postoperative hyponatremia in children. *Pediatr Nephrol*. 2016;31:53-60.

This thorough review traces the history of fluid management in the perioperative period with a focus on the development of postoperative hyponatremia. The review is evidence-based, analyzing how the composition of common perioperative electrolyte solutions may contribute to hyponatremia in the face of perioperative upregulation of ADH.

Sümpelmann R, Becke K, Brenner S, et al. Perioperative intravenous fluid therapy in children: guidelines from the Association of the Scientific Medical Societies in Germany. *Pediatr Anesth*. 2017;27(1):10-18.

The Scientific Working Group for Paediatric Anaesthesia updated its 2006 guidelines for perioperative intravenous fluid therapy in children. The recommendations highlighted as brief a fasting interval as possible preoperatively, balanced isotonic electrolyte solution with 1% to 2.5% glucose as a background maintenance solution and a glucose-free balanced electrolyte solution to maintain circulatory homeostasis. Colloid solutions may be administered in place of balanced electrolyte solution to replace ongoing fluid losses when blood products are not indicated. Monitoring electrolyte concentrations should be undertaken serially when intravenous fluids are continued postoperatively to ensure electrolyte and glucose homeostasis.

A complete reference list can be found online at ExpertConsult.com.

Essentials of Hematology

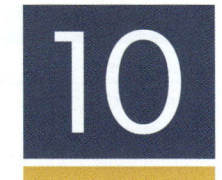

TREVOR L. ADAMS, GREGORY J. LATHAM, MICHAEL J. EISSES, M.A. BENDER, AND CHARLES M. HABERKERN

HEMATOLOGIC DISORDERS IN CHILDHOOD may present to an anesthesiologist in many ways. They may be the primary cause for a surgical procedure, such as hereditary spherocytosis (HS) in a child requiring splenectomy, or a factor complicating a common surgical procedure, such as sickle cell disease in a child undergoing tonsillectomy. Questions about hematologic problems, such as anemia, thrombocytopenia, decreased or increased coagulation, childhood cancer, and hematopoietic stem cell transplantation (HSCT), are often raised in the perioperative setting.

In this chapter, we address hematologic diseases and considerations that are of significance and interest to pediatric anesthesiologists. We highlight priorities of the hematologist that the anesthesiologist should incorporate in the care of a child during the perioperative period.

The Basics

LABORATORY VALUES AND DIAGNOSTIC TESTS

What is a normal hematocrit or platelet count for an infant or child who comes to the operating room? Red blood cell (RBC), white blood cell, platelet, and coagulation indexes evolve in various ways through late gestation, the neonatal period, infancy, and childhood (Table 10.1).

A term neonate has relative polycythemia, reticulocytosis, and leukocytosis compared with an older child. Neonatal platelet counts are similar to those of adults. Although in vitro function may be impaired for the first postnatal month, most in vivo assays of platelet function indicate normal or accelerated function. Both the prothrombin time (PT) and activated partial thromboplastin time (aPTT) are prolonged in preterm and term neonates because of a relative deficiency in vitamin K–dependent and contact activation factors, respectively; however, concentrations of factor VIII and von Willebrand factor (vWF) are increased.[1] The average

international normalized ratio (INR), a normalized PT, is 1.0 for all age groups. Fibrinogen concentrations are comparable between term neonates and adults, although neonatal fibrinogen is qualitatively dysfunctional. The plasma concentrations of many anticoagulant factors (i.e., tissue factor pathway inhibitor, antithrombin, vitamin K–dependent glycoproteins, and proteins C and S) are decreased in preterm and term neonates. The quantity and quality of plasminogen are decreased in neonates, a condition that increases the risk for thrombosis, especially in a compromised infant.[1,2] Most of these differences between the neonate and older child or adult persist for 3 to 6 months postnatally.

After the immediate neonatal period, preterm and term infants experience physiologic anemia, presumably the result of the downregulating effect of increased oxygen supply in extrauterine life on erythropoiesis and the dilutional effect of a rapidly increasing blood volume. Preterm infants reach their nadir hemoglobin of 7 to 9 g/dL at 3 to 6 postnatal weeks, and term infants reach their nadir hemoglobin concentration of 9 to 11 g/dL at 8 to 12 postnatal weeks. Most hematologic values reach adult norms by the end of infancy (i.e., first postnatal year), although some continue to change gradually into the second decade. All of these changes underscore the importance of age-adjusted standards accompanying laboratory results for infants and children.

There is no ideal single screening test to assess the *bleeding risk* of a child in the perioperative period. *Bleeding time* appears to be greater in the infant and child (and less in the neonate) than it is in the adult, but the range of values is wide and overlapping (Table 10.1). Although bleeding time is potentially helpful in predicting posttonsillectomy and adenoidectomy hemorrhage,[3] as well as hemorrhage after percutaneous renal[4] and liver[5] biopsy, there is little evidence to support its use as a screening test to predict bleeding in the presence of a careful, inclusive clinical history.[6–8]

TABLE 10.1	Hematology Values at Different Ages					
Measurement[a]	Preterm 28–32 Weeks	Preterm 32–36 Weeks	Term Neonate	1-Year-Old	Child	Adult
Hemoglobin (g/dL)	12.9	13.6	16.8	12	13	15
Hematocrit (%)	40.9	43.6	55	36	38	45
Reticulocyte count (%)	—	—	5	1	1	1.6
White blood cell count (/mm³)	5160	7710	18,000	10,000	8000	7500
Platelet count (/mm³)	255,000	260,000	300,000	300,000	300,000	300,000
Prothrombin time (seconds)	15.4	13	13	11	11	12
International normalized ratio (INR)	—	1	1	1	1	1
Activated partial thromboplastin time (seconds)	108	53.6	42.9	30	31	28
Fibrinogen (mg/dL)	256	243	283	276	279	278
Bleeding time (minutes)	—	3.5	3.5	6	7	5

[a]All values expressed as the mean. Age in weeks refers to gestation.
Data from Andrew M. The relevance of developmental hemostasis to hemorrhagic disorders of newborns. *Semin Perinatol.* 1997;21:70–85; Andrew M, Vegh P, Johnston M, et al. Maturation of the hemostatic system during childhood. *Blood* 1992;80:1998–2005; Goodnight SH, Hathaway WE. *Disorders of Hemostasis and Thrombosis: A Clinical Guide.* 2nd ed. New York: McGraw-Hill; 2001:31–38; Ohls RK, Christensen RD. Development of the hematopoietic system. In: Behrman RE, Kliegman RM, Jenson HB, eds, *Nelson Textbook of Pediatrics.* 17th ed. Philadelphia: WB Saunders; 2004:1599–1604.

In contrast to the standard historical laboratory tests, point-of-care testing using viscoelastic tests such as the thromboelastogram (TEG), rotational thromboelastometry (ROTEM), and Sonoclot (Sienco, Inc., Boulder, CO) allow the practitioner to receive data about the bleeding patient more quickly. The advantage of point-of-care viscoelastic testing is that it provides information of the entire clotting process from fibrin formation to clot retraction and fibrinolysis at the bedside. These tests also use whole blood, which allows the interaction of plasma derived coagulation factors with red cells and platelets, thereby providing information on platelet function. Viscoelastic point-of-care coagulation devices require trained personnel to maintain strict quality control procedures, as well as strict standardization procedures, to ensure optimal accuracy and reliability.[9] The TEG has been used to investigate the coagulation status of children undergoing spinal fusion,[10] neurosurgical procedures,[11] cardiopulmonary bypass for cardiothoracic procedures[12,13] and trauma.[14] Although the TEG may provide useful information in the surgical setting to evaluate fibrinolysis, hypercoagulability, and other coagulation perturbations, its use is usually limited to clinical scenarios with dynamic coagulation changes, such as open-heart surgery with cardiopulmonary bypass and liver transplantation.

The platelet function analyzer (PFA-100; Siemens, AG, Erlangen, Germany) is increasingly used to assess platelet abnormalities. It has the benefit of avoiding some of the difficulties of obtaining a bleeding time in children. Although several studies suggest PFA-100 analysis is equivalent or superior to the bleeding time for detecting bleeding abnormalities, there is no consensus about its role in preoperative screening.[15] Current evidence does not identify a single screening tool sensitive or specific enough to predict bleeding disorders or surgical bleeding risk in children. However, the PFA-100 analysis had the greatest probability of detecting a bleeding disorder in children.[16] With the increasing use of newer agents that modify platelet function (e.g., platelet G protein–coupled receptor P2Y12 antagonists, glycoprotein GPIIb/IIIa complex antagonists), clinicians must understand that the TEG, PFA-100, and other methods that assess platelet function may vary in their ability to monitor the effects of these agents and those of cyclooxygenase inhibitors.[17]

GUIDELINES FOR TRANSFUSION

Critical analyses of the risks and benefits of transfusions in infants and children in the perioperative period have resulted in fewer transfusions. Even for infants and children in intensive care, a restrictive transfusion threshold (i.e., 7 g/dL) reduces transfusions without increasing morbidity compared with a liberal threshold (i.e., 9.5–10 g/dL).[18,19] Data from the U.K.'s national audit of clinical transfusion, the Serious Hazards of Transfusion (SHOT), indicate that infants and children younger than 18 years of age are at greater risk for adverse transfusion-related reactions (37 and 18 in 100,000, respectively) than are adults (13 in 100,000). Most events were error related, including administrative, laboratory, clinical judgment, and handling errors.[20]

Guidelines for RBC transfusion in infants and children in the perioperative setting should be consistent with those established by the American Society of Anesthesiologists Task Force on Blood Component Therapy, which proposed that transfusion is not indicated for hemoglobin concentrations greater than 10 g/dL but is indicated for concentrations less than 6 g/dL.[21,22] When the concentration is between 6 g/dL and 10 g/dL, packed red blood cells (PRBCs) should be transfused based on the child's vital signs, adequacy of oxygenation and perfusion, acuity and degree of blood loss, and other physiologic and surgical factors.[23,24] When the concentration exceeds 10 g/dL, the decision to transfuse PRBCs should be based on the same physiologic and surgical factors. In a neonate or infant, this decision should also take into account increased baseline concentrations of hemoglobin in this population; increased oxygen consumption; increased affinity of residual fetal hemoglobin (hemoglobin F) for oxygen; and absolute blood volume (i.e., ~85 mL/kg for a term neonate and ~100 mL/kg for a preterm neonate). The threshold for transfusing a healthy neonate may be 7 g/dL in some clinical settings, but it may be 12 g/dL or greater for a neonate in other settings, such as significant lung disease requiring mechanical ventilation, chronic lung disease, cyanotic congenital heart disease, or heart failure.[23,25,26] For a preterm infant, the risks of hypovolemia, hypotension, acidosis, and postoperative apnea are magnified in the setting of operative blood loss and anemia. It is impossible to address all of the guidelines in this chapter, but many pediatric hematology and oncology consultants have clearly defined transfusion

TABLE 10.2	Commonly Used Triggers for Platelet Transfusion
Medical Condition or Procedure	**Platelet Count (/mm³)**
Stable hematology-oncology or chronically thrombocytopenic patient	10,000–20,000
Lumbar puncture in stable leukemic child	10,000
Bone marrow aspiration or biopsy	20,000
Gastrointestinal endoscopy in cancer patient	20,000–40,000
Disseminated intravascular coagulation	20,000–50,000
Fiberoptic bronchoscopy in hematopoietic stem cell transplantation patient	20,000–50,000
Neonatal alloimmune thrombocytopenia	30,000
Major surgery	50,000
Dilutional thrombocytopenia with massive transfusion	50,000
Spinal anesthesia	50,000
Cardiopulmonary bypass	50,000–60,000
Liver biopsy	50,000–100,000
Nonbleeding preterm infant	60,000
Obstetric epidural anesthesia	70,000–100,000
Neurosurgery	100,000

Data from references 27, 28, 32, 35, 36.

TABLE 10.3	Indications for Leukocyte-Reduced Red Blood Cell Units

Prevention of Alloimmunization

Congenital hemolytic anemias (including sickle cell disease and thalassemia)

Hypoproliferative anemias likely to need multiple transfusions
  Aplastic anemia
  Myelodysplasia/myeloproliferative syndrome
  Plasma cell dyscrasias
  Hematopoietic stem cell transplants
  Hematopoietic malignancies

Therapy for Preexisting Conditions

Recurrent, severe febrile hemolytic transfusion reactions

Known HLA alloimmunization

Possible Uses

Alternative to cytomegalovirus-seronegative components (see Table 10.5)

Human immunodeficiency virus–infected patients

Modified from Simon TL, Alverson DC, AuBuchon J, et al. Practice parameter for the use of red blood cell transfusions: developed by the Red Blood Cell Administration Practice Guideline Development Task Force of the College of American Pathologists. Arch Pathol Lab Med. 1998;122:130–138.

thresholds for their patient populations that should be reviewed preoperatively.

Consensus committees from France, the United Kingdom, and the United States have published guidelines for platelet transfusion; these reports are based on available evidence that has been gathered and critically reviewed (Table 10.2).[21,22,27–31] Without evidence that platelet function is significantly different in the healthy infant and child, these guidelines should be applicable to these patients. The decision to transfuse platelets must take into account underlying medical conditions, platelet transfusion history, current medications, surgical bleeding, surgical interventions (e.g., cardiopulmonary bypass), and all other factors that may affect platelet function and turnover.[32–36] Sevoflurane and propofol have been reported to both suppress[37] and enhance platelet aggregation in vitro.[38] Despite these effects on platelet aggregation, no change in the bleeding time has been reported, suggesting that the possible inhibitory effects of these agents do not impair hemostasis in vivo.[39]

Transfusion guidelines for other blood products, including fresh frozen plasma (FFP) and cryoprecipitate, have been established[21,22,35,40] and are discussed later in the context of coagulation disorders. Indications[41] for transfusing FFP are usually limited to the following:

1. Replacement of documented congenital or acquired coagulation factor deficiency when a specific sterilized or combined factor concentrate is unavailable, especially in the setting of anticipated or active bleeding
2. Acquired coagulopathy resulting from massive transfusion
3. Immediate reversal of warfarin's effect when prothrombin complex concentrate (PCC) is unavailable
4. Coagulation support in disease processes such as disseminated intravascular coagulation (DIC) and thrombotic thrombocytopenic purpura
5. A source of antithrombin III for children deficient of this inhibitor who require heparin

Cryoprecipitate should be administered only for anticipated or active bleeding in children with congenital fibrinogen deficiencies or von Willebrand disease who are unresponsive to desmopressin acetate (DDAVP) or for patients with acquired hypofibrinogenemia (<80–100 mg/dL) associated with massive transfusion.

Guidelines have been established by the College of American Pathologists and other transfusion study groups for leukocyte reduction of RBC units[25] and irradiation (x-ray or γ-ray) of cellular blood components (Tables 10.3 and 10.4).[42] These guidelines are valuable when determining the specific choice of blood components that should be ordered and administered in the perioperative setting. For hematologic patients receiving chronic RBC transfusions, an extended phenotypic crossmatch and leukocyte reduction can decrease the risk of developing alloantibodies and transfusion reactions, especially in children of African descent if the local donor pool is primarily derived from Caucasian populations of Northern European descent.[43] For oncology patients, updated specific requirements for blood products including leukocyte reduction and irradiation are often indicated and should always be reviewed with oncology specialists. To reduce the risk of cytomegalovirus (CMV) transmission in susceptible patients, donated seronegative CMV blood, leukoreduced blood, or both can be used. However, the risk cannot be completely eliminated because supposed seronegative donors could be in the initial stages of viremia at the time blood is collected (Table 10.5).[44]

Hemolytic Anemias

Hemolytic syndromes are a group of disorders in which lysis of erythrocytes often leads to anemia. Although RBCs in these disorders may be characterized by abnormal morphology and shorter life span, these indices may be normal at baseline. Clinical signs of a hemolytic syndrome include anemia, splenomegaly, and jaundice, signs that may be apparent chronically or only during acute exacerbations of a disease process. Hemoglobinuria may be

TABLE 10.4   Indications for Irradiation of Cellular Blood Components

Well-Defined Indications

Hematopoietic stem cell transplantation

Actual or anticipated congenital cell-mediated immunodeficiency

Intrauterine transfusion or after intrauterine transfusion

Directed donation from blood relative or HLA-matched donor

Hodgkin disease

Acute lymphocytic leukemia

Immunocompromised organ transplant recipient

Probable Indications

Malignancy and organ transplantation treated with immunosuppressive therapy

Exchange transfusion in neonate

Extracorporeal membrane oxygenation in neonate

Low–birth-weight neonate (<1200 g)

Human immunodeficiency virus–infected patient with opportunistic infection

Possible Indications

Term neonate (<4 months)

Human immunodeficiency virus–infected patient

Modified from Simon TL, Alverson DC, AuBuchon J, et al. Practice parameter for the use of red blood cell transfusions: developed by the Red Blood Cell Administration Practice Guideline Development Task Force of the College of American Pathologists. *Arch Pathol Lab Med.* 1998;122:130–138; Treleaven J, Gennery A, Marsh J, et al. Guidelines on the use of irradiated blood components prepared by the British Committee for Standards in Haematology blood transfusion task force. *Br J Haematol.* 2010;152:35–51.

TABLE 10.5   Indications for Cytomegalovirus-Seronegative or Leukocyte-Reduced Red Blood Cells for Prevention of Virus Transmission

Well-Defined Indications

Low–birth-weight neonate (<1200 g)

Human immunodeficiency virus–infected patient

Recipient of seronegative allogeneic organ or hematopoietic stem cell transplant or prospective recipient

Pregnant woman

Intrauterine transfusion

Possible Indications

Hodgkin disease or non-Hodgkin lymphoma

Recipient of immunosuppressive therapy

Candidate for autologous hematopoietic stem cell transplantation

Hereditary or acquired cellular immunodeficiency

Probable Absence of Indications

Seronegative term infant

Seropositive pregnant woman

Modified from Simon TL, Alverson DC, AuBuchon J, et al. Practice parameter for the use of red blood cell transfusions: developed by the Red Blood Cell Administration Practice Guideline Development Task Force of the College of American Pathologists. *Arch Pathol Lab Med.* 1998;122:130–138.

a late finding if massive hemolysis has occurred. Although not well studied, in theory any hemolytic disorder may alter nitric oxide (NO) metabolism.

Many of the hemolytic anemias important to the anesthesiologist result from intracellular defects and can be classified as erythrocyte membrane defects, such as HS; enzymatic defects, such as glucose-6-phosphate dehydrogenase (G6PD) deficiency; and qualitative and quantitative defects of hemoglobin, such as sickle cell disease and thalassemia. Other hemolytic anemias that may be encountered in the operating room are largely extracellularly mediated, such as transfusion-related hemolysis and other immune-mediated anemias (alloimmune or autoimmune); this group of anemias is not reviewed here.

HEREDITARY SPHEROCYTOSIS

HS, the most common cause of inherited chronic hemolysis in North America and Northern Europe, has a prevalence of approximately 1 to 2 cases per 5000 people if mild forms of the disease are included.[45,46] First described in 1871, HS is present in many ethnic populations but is rare in African Americans. Because 75% of children inherit the disease in an autosomal dominant pattern, there is often a family history of the disorder, although autosomal recessive mutations, de novo mutations, and incomplete penetrance have been reported.[46]

Pathophysiology

Abnormalities in any of several erythrocyte membrane proteins, including the β subunit of spectrin, ankyrin, and band 3, can lead to HS. The variety of proteins affected and mutations observed in each gene account for the clinical heterogeneity of the disorder.[45] When the erythrocyte loses surface area, it changes from a biconcave disk to a sphere, which alters its stability and flow pattern through the capillaries. The deformity leads to a more rigid membrane, which predisposes it to rupture, a condition that is worsened if the membrane surface area decreases by more than 3%.[46] Damaged erythrocytes are sequestered in the splenic capillaries, which can lead to splenomegaly. The combination of intravascular and extravascular hemolysis can result in anemia, which induces extramedullary erythropoiesis. The life span of the erythrocyte is reduced from 120 days to just a few days when the RBC membrane has been deformed. If large numbers of damaged erythrocytes are lysed, unconjugated bilirubin is released, which causes jaundice and possibly gallstones in as many as 60% of children.[45] Membrane fragments from hemolytic reactions can lead to DIC. Pulmonary hypertension may occur in the HS population, presumably as a result of hemolysis-induced alterations in NO metabolism.

Clinical and Laboratory Features

Children may present at any age with the triad of anemia, splenomegaly, and jaundice that often is aggravated by concomitant viral infection. Mild, moderate, and severe forms of HS occur and are characterized by variations in laboratory results and clinical correlates. HS can manifest soon after birth and should be considered in infants who are jaundiced after the first postnatal week; resulting hyperbilirubinemia can sometimes necessitate an exchange transfusion. Mild disease occurs in 20% of children with HS; these children only occasionally present with symptomatic bilirubinate gallstones before adolescence. Approximately 5% of children have severe HS characterized by chronic anemic (hemoglobin concentration <8 g/dL) and the need for chronic transfusions. The course of this disease may be complicated by viral infections such as parvovirus B19 infection, which can suppress reticulocyte production[46] and precipitate aplastic crises.

HS is most commonly suspected when numerous spherocytes with loss of central pallor appear on a peripheral smear. A complete blood cell count usually reveals a reduced hemoglobin and increased reticulocyte count. Osmotic fragility (OF) was regarded as the gold standard for the diagnosis of HS, but this test produces age-related results and must be performed by experienced laboratory technicians in a timely fashion. The OF test is known to give false-negative results in 10%–20% of patients, as well as false-positive results in patients with autoimmune hemolytic anemia. The updated guidelines for the diagnosis and management of HS no longer recommend the OF test as a first-line screening tool.[47] Increasingly, flow cytometry using eosin-5′-maleimide is being used to confirm the diagnosis because it requires little blood and can be performed after overnight storage.[48] In addition, as a direct result of chronic hemolysis, unconjugated bilirubin and serum lactate dehydrogenase concentrations increase, and serum haptoglobin concentrations decrease. Thrombocytopenia may develop as a result of hypersplenism.

Perioperative Considerations

Anemia, thrombocytopenia, and splenomegaly are the major considerations for a child with HS undergoing surgery. The most common disease-related operations performed in children with HS are splenectomy and cholecystectomy, individually or in combination, and these procedures may be performed by laparotomy or laparoscopy.

Splenectomy significantly increases red cell survival in most cases and reduces the severity of the anemia and jaundice. It is usually reserved for more severe cases of HS, characterized by severe anemia that require frequent RBC transfusions, poor growth, chronic fatigue, or evidence of extramedullary hematopoiesis (e.g., frontal bossing). Splenic enlargement in a child interested in participating in contact sports is another indication.[46] Splenectomy is ideally performed after the age of 6 years because of the increased risk of overwhelming infection by encapsulated organisms such as *Streptococcus pneumoniae*, *Neisseria meningitidis*, and *Haemophilus influenzae* type B in splenectomized younger children.[49] Preoperative vaccination against these organisms is essential unless surgery is required emergently.[50] Guidelines for the indications and duration of postoperative penicillin prophylaxis vary among institutions.[45]

Splenectomy in children is more frequently performed laparoscopically than by open laparotomy because the former is associated with decreased pain, quicker return of bowel function, shorter hospital stay, and improved cosmetic result. Conversion from laparoscopic to open splenectomy is necessary in fewer than 10% of cases.[51] Partial splenectomies are increasingly performed because they allow retention of some immune function against bacterial infections in younger children while reducing the sequestration of spherocytes. However, residual splenic tissue can increase in size and necessitate total splenectomy at a later time.[52,53] If anemia recurs after splenectomy, it may indicate the presence of accessory splenic tissue that was unrecognized initially. Transient postsplenectomy thrombocytosis marked by dramatic increases in platelet counts may also occur in children,[54] in addition to a general increase in the risk of thromboembolic disease.

Gallstones occur in 21% to 63% of children with HS, but cholecystectomy is usually performed only when children are symptomatic with cholelithiasis. Children who undergo splenectomy and who also have radiographically identified gallstones may undergo concurrent cholecystectomy, regardless of whether

TABLE 10.6	Perioperative Concerns for Patients With Hereditary Spherocytosis
Preoperative Considerations	
Hemoglobin, reticulocyte count, platelet count	
History of transfusions and special blood requirements (e.g., extended phenotypic matching, leukocyte reduction)	
History of infections, aplastic crises, and presplenectomy vaccinations	
Presplenectomy antibiotic prophylaxis and immunization when indicated	
Intraoperative Considerations	
Appropriate antibiotic coverage	
Attention to physiologic effects of laparoscopy on circulatory and respiratory function	
Potential for significant blood loss (unusual in splenectomy and cholecystectomy)	
Judicious use of regional anesthesia, intramuscular medications, nasogastric tubes, nasal intubation, and other methods when platelet count is low	
Limited use of medications with potential bleeding risk (e.g., ketorolac)	
Postoperative Considerations	
Sequential hemoglobin determinations and platelet counts	
Potential thrombocytosis: management as recommended by hematology consultants	
Infection risk	

the stones are symptomatic.[55–57] Table 10.6 summarizes the clinical features and important perioperative considerations for the child with HS undergoing incidental or disease-related surgical procedures.

GLUCOSE-6-PHOSPHATE DEHYDROGENASE DEFICIENCY

G6PD deficiency causes hemolysis in the presence of oxidative stressors. It is the most common enzyme deficiency in humans, affecting approximately 400 million people worldwide. This enzyme deficiency is inherited in an X-linked, recessive fashion. Although males are most commonly affected, females (heterozygous or homozygous for the gene) may have clinical manifestations of the disease. More than 100 variants have been described, including a relatively mild form that affects about 10% of African American males (i.e., G6PD A–) and a more severe form that affects Italians, Greeks, and other populations in the Mediterranean, African, and Asian regions (i.e., G6PD Mediterranean).[58–60] This deficiency is prevalent in geographic areas where the incidence of malaria is high, presumably because G6PD deficiency may attenuate the severity of malarial infections.

Pathophysiology

G6PD plays an important role in the hexose monophosphate/pentose phosphate shunt, which is essential for normal energy metabolism in erythrocytes. G6PD generates the reduced form of nicotinamide adenine dinucleotide phosphate (NADPH). NADPH maintains glutathione in the reduced form, which reduces peroxides and protects cells from oxidative damage in the course of normal biochemical events or in the event of excess free oxygen radical generation. Superoxide ion or hydrogen peroxide, or both, can oxidize hemoglobin, which then precipitates as insoluble membrane inclusions. These inclusions, together with the oxidative damage to cell membranes, lead to cell damage in the G6PD-deficient child. Erythrocytes are particularly sensitive to oxidative damage because of their lack of synthetic activity. In the presence of oxidants and free radicals (e.g., produced by infection or by ingestion of certain medications and foods), this cascade of events may precipitate hemolysis in the G6PD-deficient child.[58,60]

Clinical and Laboratory Features

Clinical symptoms of G6PD deficiency may be deceptively variable, and they may occur in the neonatal period or in older age groups as episodic or chronic hemolytic anemia. Presenting signs include anemia and jaundice; in severe cases, these signs can be followed by lumbar and abdominal pain and by renal failure. Acute illness such as diabetic acidosis or ingestion of a variety of substances may precipitate a hemolytic event (Table 10.7). Fava beans, also known as broad beans, contain high concentrations of vincine and convincine, which are nonvolatile glucosides that can trigger hemolysis.[61] On a global basis, favism is likely the most common form of acute hemolytic anemia associated with G6PD deficiency.[62] Hemolysis may range from benign and transitory to severe and life-threatening; the latter situation is more likely if the triggering agent is not eliminated or controlled. Laboratory findings include normocytic anemia, increased reticulocyte count and serum bilirubin concentration, and the presence of Heinz bodies in the peripheral blood smear.

TABLE 10.7	Agents That May Precipitate Hemolysis in Patients With Glucose-6-Phosphate Dehydrogenase Deficiency
Antibiotics	
Sulfonamides	
Trimethoprim-sulfamethoxazole (Bactrim, Septrin)	
Dapsone	
Chloramphenicol	
Nitrofurantoin	
Nalidixic acid	
Antimalarials	
Chloroquine	
Hydroxychloroquine	
Primaquine	
Quinine	
Mepacrine	
Other Medications	
Aspirin	
Phenacetin	
Sulfasalazine	
Methyldopa	
Vitamin C (large doses)	
Hydralazine	
Procainamide	
Quinidine	
Chemicals	
Moth balls (naphthalene)	
Methylene blue	
Food	
Fava (broad) beans	

Perioperative Considerations

In the perioperative setting, G6PD deficiency does not usually cause problems. The most effective management strategy centers on avoiding oxidative stressors (such as pain and anxiety) and avoiding the triggering agents (Table 10.8). Treating or eliminating precipitating causes such as infection is also paramount in safely anesthetizing G6PD-deficient patients. Monitoring for and treatment of possible complications are appropriate; transfusion is rarely required.[63]

Administration of large or excessive doses of medications such as prilocaine, benzocaine, and sodium nitroprusside may trigger hemolysis in G6PD-deficient children in the perioperative setting.[58,60,64,65] Although these children can reduce methemoglobin that is normally produced by these agents, G6PD-deficient children may not tolerate large amounts of potent oxidizing agents (i.e., superoxide ion and hydrogen peroxide) produced by methemoglobin. Infants may be particularly susceptible to symptomatic methemoglobinemia (because of their low NADPH dehydrogenase activity) and to methemoglobin-induced hemolysis if they are G6PD deficient. Treatment of methemoglobinemia with methylene blue is contraindicated in these infants because the agent itself may precipitate hemolysis[53]; there is a relative contraindication to methylene blue in all G6PD-deficient patients. G6PD-deficient patients lack the enzymes necessary to reduce methylene blue to an inactive form, leukomethylene blue. Methylene blue might also add to the oxidative hemolysis.[66] Hemolysis has occurred during cardiopulmonary bypass in G6PD-deficient children,[65,67] and methemoglobinemia has occurred in a child with partial G6PD deficiency after application of EMLA (eutectic mixture of local anesthetics) cream.[68]

HEMOGLOBINOPATHIES

Sickle Cell Disease

First identified by Herrick about 100 years ago, sickle cell disease is a group of inherited hemoglobinopathies with a diverse worldwide prevalence. The disease affects about 1 in 365 African Americans and 1 in 16,300 Hispanic births.[69] The spectrum of the disease includes sickle cell anemia (HbSS), which accounts for about 70% of the American sickle cell disease population; sickle cell/hemoglobin C disease (HbSC), accounting for about 20%; sickle cell/β-thalassemia (HbSβ-thalassemia), accounting for about 10%; and a host of other, uncommon sickle variants whose prevalence is increasing over time.[70] HbSβ-thalassemia includes HbSβ[0]- and

TABLE 10.8	Perioperative Concerns for Patients With Glucose-6-Phosphate Dehydrogenase Deficiency
Preoperative Considerations	
History of hemolysis and precipitating factors	
Hemoglobin concentration, reticulocyte count	
Intraoperative Considerations	
Avoidance of triggering agents	
Caution in use of high doses of agents that increase methemoglobin, especially in infants	
Hemoglobin and urine output in high-risk settings (e.g., cardiopulmonary bypass)	
Postoperative Considerations	
Hemoglobin concentration, reticulocyte count, urine output if hemolysis occurs	

HbSβ⁺-thalassemias. The distinction between the two is the absence of normal HbA in the former versus decreased amount of HbA in the latter; even a small amount of HbA present in the latter partially mitigates the severity of disease. While there are large phenotypic variations among the many forms of sickle cell disease, in general HbSS and HbSβ⁰-thalassemia are clinically similar and more severe than HbSC and HbSβ⁺-thalassemia. Sickle cell trait (HbAS), in which approximately 40% of hemoglobin is hemoglobin S, occurs in about 8% of African Americans and in a much smaller percentage of Hispanic and other subpopulations.[69] The sickle gene is found commonly in sub-Saharan Africa, the Mediterranean, the Arabian Peninsula and India, where sickle cell trait provides a significantly increased fitness in malaria-endemic regions. Sickle hemoglobinopathies have many implications for perioperative care because they increase perioperative morbidity and mortality.

Pathophysiology

Hemoglobin A is composed of two α- and two β-globin chains. Hemoglobin S results from a single base-pair mutation in the β-globin gene on chromosome 11, which results in the replacement of a negatively charged, hydrophilic glutamate residue with a noncharged, hydrophobic valine residue. This hydrophobic valine is exposed when HbS is deoxygenated and is stabilized by binding the same hydrophobic valine pocket on other HbS molecules, thereby leading to polymerization of HbS, precipitation and hemolysis.[71]

In contrast to prior simplistic models in which sickled cells were simply thought to block flow through the microcirculation, the pathophysiology of sickle cell disease is now understood to be considerably more complex. This understanding is, in turn, leading to more therapeutic interventions.[71-73] Any factor that promotes hemoglobin crystallization (e.g., hypoxia, acidosis, and cellular dehydration) or prolongs capillary transit time (e.g., dehydration, hypothermia, leukocytosis, thrombosis, and inflammation) increases HbS polymerization and formation of sickled cells. Inflammation, vascular endothelial adhesion abnormalities, platelets, and coagulation cascade activation all contribute to vasoocclusive episodes. The sickle red cell membrane becomes compromised by exposure to destructive oxidizing effects of precipitated HbS, thereby leading to altered permeability to sodium, potassium, and calcium, causing dehydration of the cell and irreversible sickling.[74] Membrane abnormalities of phospholipid content also contribute to its deformability, and exposure of phosphatidyl serine facilitates activation of the clotting cascade. These and other factors lead to entrapment of irreversibly sickled red cells in the microcirculation, activation of coagulation and inflammatory pathways, ischemia, and infarction of tissue. At the same time, chronic intravascular hemolysis decreases production of NO, while increased scavenging decreases the bioavailability of NO. The resulting NO deficiency causes endothelial dysfunction and disease complications, such as pulmonary hypertension, priapism, and skin ulceration.[74,75]

Clinical and Laboratory Features and Treatment

Sickle cell disease is a multisystem process involving most organs of the body and at times necessitating surgical intervention. While there is considerable variation in disease severity, all patients have a progressive clinical course. Therapeutic interventions and genetic factors account in large part for the differences in outcome. Children with persistence of hemoglobin F (which itself protects against the effects of deoxygenation on red cells) and those with HbSC or HbSβ⁺ have fewer complications than those with HbSS or HbSβ⁰.

Early diagnosis and treatment of sickle cell disease have been facilitated by the widespread use of universal neonatal screening, which was first used in the state of New York in 1975. Most screening programs for sickle cell disease use isoelectric focusing of an eluate from dried blood spot samples, a technique that is also used to screen for other disorders. A few programs use high-performance liquid chromatography. Because a small percentage of children with sickle cell disease are not African American (i.e., Native American, Hispanic, and Caucasian),[76] selective screening may not detect all affected infants. As of 2006, all 50 states and the District of Columbia screen neonates for sickle hemoglobinopathies. Families of infants diagnosed with sickle trait (HbAS) on neonatal screening may not be made aware of the diagnosis, but reports of perioperative complications suggested to be associated with sickle cell trait are exceedingly rare. Affected children born within the United States before universal neonatal screening and those born outside the United States without routine health care may not have received diagnosis and appropriate care before surgery. Notwithstanding the controversy over the utility of nonselective preoperative screening,[77] children at risk whose hemoglobin status is unknown preoperatively should have a sickle-screening test, followed by a hemoglobin electrophoretic evaluation if screening is positive. However, infants younger than 6 months of age may have a false-negative screening test result because of the presence of fetal hemoglobin, although electrophoresis is diagnostic at all ages. Children older than 10 years of age with a normal hemoglobin value, standard peripheral blood smear, and unremarkable clinical history are at low risk of having a clinically significant hemoglobinopathy.[78]

Common clinical symptoms of sickle cell disease in children include chronic hemolytic anemia, pain crises secondary to recurrent vasoocclusive episodes, acute chest syndrome (ACS), infection, renal insufficiency, osteonecrosis, and cholelithiasis. Pulmonary hypertension, priapism, and skin ulcerations may also occur and are related to the degree of red cell hemolysis.[79] Chronic pulmonary and neurologic disease (e.g., stroke) are additional causes of significant morbidity and mortality.[70] In the perioperative period, the most common complications in sickle cell children include ACS (about 10%), fever or infection (about 7%), vasoocclusive episodes (about 5%), and transfusion-related events (about 10%).[80]

Chronic hemolytic anemia is a hallmark of HbSS disease. It is characterized by a baseline hemoglobin value of 5 to 9 g/dL (often more than 9 g/dL in HbSC disease), reticulocytosis (5% to 10%), and a distinctive red cell morphology observed on a peripheral blood smear.[73] Red cell fragility and chronic hemolysis are associated with anemia, increased red cell turnover, and a propensity to form biliary stones. The anemia may be complicated by other events, such as acute splenic sequestration, typically occurring in infants and young children after a viral illness; or an acute cessation of red cell production, the equivalent of transient erythroblastopenia of childhood and typically associated with parvovirus B19 infection. For some children, chronic and acute severe anemia are managed with RBC transfusions, although these children are prone to develop alloantibodies to RBC antigens, and untreated iron overload resulting from recurrent transfusions can lead to life-threatening cirrhosis and cardiac failure. Most children are maintained on chronic folic acid therapy to prevent megaloblastic erythropoiesis that can result if increased demands for purine synthesis from red cell production are not met.

Vasoocclusive episodes in sickle cell disease occur as a result of episodic microvasculature occlusions at one or more sites. The occlusive process occurs most commonly in the phalanges (i.e., dactylitis or hand-foot syndrome), long bones, ribs, sternum, spine, and the pelvis; it also can occur in the mesenteric microvasculature, producing abdominal pain that may mimic a surgical acute abdomen. Pain associated with vasoocclusive episodes should be managed with a multidimensional approach including reversal of potential triggers (via warming, hydration, and ambulation), distraction, psychological and behavioral interventions, and complementary modalities in addition to analgesic medications. Initial pharmacologic management often entails scheduled antiinflammatory agents because inflammation is central to the vasoocclusive process, and these agents synergize with opioids to provide analgesia. It is essential to foster an ideal environment for pain control (e.g., calm, pleasant distractions, supportive personnel and objects). Hydroxyurea is used to prevent vasoocclusive episodes and end-organ damage, and it is now widely recommended for all patients with HbSS and HbSβ[0]. Although grossly underused,[81] hydroxyurea is a safe and effective component of chronic management in decreasing the frequency of events through several mechanisms; inhibiting hemoglobin precipitation by increasing fetal hemoglobin concentrations; reducing white blood cell count; modifying the inflammatory response; and facilitating NO metabolism.[75,81–83] Inhaled NO or precursors of NO may prove to be effective therapy for vasoocclusive episodes.[84]

ACS is characterized by acute respiratory symptoms concurrent with new infiltrate(s) observed on chest radiograph.[85] ACS frequently occurs 2 to 3 days after a vasoocclusive episode, and although its clinical presentation varies, it often includes any, or all, of the following: fever, tachypnea, cough, and hypoxemia. The process may be self-limited over a period of a few days, or it may progress to respiratory failure (15%) and even death. The inconsistent presentation in part reflects the complex and variable pathogenesis of ACS. An episode may have a single or multiple causes, including infection (i.e., bacteria or atypical bacteria [often *Chlamydia* or *Mycoplasma*], viruses, or a combination of agents), pulmonary fat embolism, pulmonary infarction, and pulmonary hemorrhage.[86] Acute management includes supportive care and oxygen, antibiotics that treat encapsulated and atypical organisms, bronchodilators, pain control, ventilatory support as needed, and transfusion. Incentive spirometry or continuous positive airway pressure can be helpful, especially in the perioperative setting. Hydroxyurea therapy and chronic transfusion therapy decrease the frequency of ACS, whereas inhaled NO, NO precursors, and antioxidants (e.g., arginine and glutamine) may attenuate the process acutely.[75,81,84,87–89] Airway reactivity is also common in children with sickle cell disease, in part due to NO deficiency, and it is responsive to bronchodilator therapy.[90,91] In later life, children with sickle cell disease may develop restrictive lung disease and pulmonary hypertension as a result of repeated ACS-induced lung injury and chronic inflammation. NO deficiency, the result of decreased production, increased consumption, or altered metabolism, may also play an important role in these processes.[79,85,92]

Infections are common because of deficits in the immune system and the specific effects of splenic atrophy and dysfunction that occur over the first few years of life.[72] As a result of susceptibility to overwhelming infection by *S. pneumoniae* and *H. influenzae* type B, young children receive penicillin prophylaxis until 6 years of age and bacteria-specific immunizations in addition to those routinely administered to children. A host of infectious organisms have been implicated in ACS, and infection with gram-negative organisms (e.g., osteomyelitis caused by *Salmonella*) is common in older children and adults.[86]

Stroke is a potentially devastating complication that occurs in about 10% of children; as high as 40% have silent infarcts and 10% have overt strokes.[93] One-fourth of children have motor or cognitive deficits at the time of presentation for surgery.[94,95] A child's first stroke often appears as early as 2 to 5 years of age.[96,97] Risk factors include reduced hemoglobin concentration, increased concentration of HbS, increased leukocyte count, and a history of dactylitis. Pain episodes, ACS, and infection may precipitate strokes.[98] Children suffering an acute stroke are managed supportively with emergent exchange transfusion to reduce the concentration of HbS to less than 30%, followed by chronic transfusions and hydroxyurea administration to minimize the risk of recurrence.[99] The thrust of the current management of stroke is prevention. Yearly screening with transcranial Doppler starting at age 2 identifies most children at high risk, and subsequent management with chronic transfusion and hydroxyurea therapy may minimize the risk of a future stroke.[100–103]

Renal abnormalities can include proteinuria, hematuria, hyposthenuria, and renal tubular acidosis. Acute and chronic renal failure may develop, and angiotensin-converting enzyme (ACE) inhibitors may be of benefit of resulting hypertension.[104,105] Renal dialysis and transplantation have proven successful interventions for renal complications of the disease.[106]

HbAS is usually benign, although it may be characterized by microhematuria and hyposthenuria,[106,107] and sickling may occur under extremely altered physiologic circumstances (e.g., cardiopulmonary bypass).[108,109] There is also a small but significant risk of pulmonary embolism. An increased risk of rhabdomyolysis with exercise, as well as sudden death with extreme exertion in individuals with HbAS, has led to the controversial mandate to offer trait testing to all National Collegiate Athletic Association (NCAA) Division I athletes.[110]

Children with HbSC disease usually have a greater baseline hemoglobin concentration and fewer complications than those with HbSS disease. Because splenic function is often preserved, the risk for infection in early childhood is reduced.[78] Children with HbSC disease are more likely to have proliferative retinopathy and avascular necrosis of long bones.[72]

Children with HbSβ[0] (i.e., one sickle globin allele and one thalassemic allele expressing no β-globin) have a course identical to that of HbSS, whereas those with HbSβ[+] (i.e., one sickle globin allele and one thalassemic allele expressing β-globin at a reduced level) tend to have a more benign course that is proportional to the amount of normal β-globin expression. The coexistence of hemoglobin S with α-thalassemia produces a variable clinical picture, but it may predispose children to a significant incidence of pain episodes.[78]

Many additional approaches to sickle cell care are being investigated and are notable for targeting multiple aspects of the complex physiology. These include administration of short-chain fatty acids such as butyrate or demethylating agents such as decitabine to induce production of hemoglobin F; small molecules to interfere with polymerization; antibodies to alter cell adherence; ion channel inhibitors to decrease cellular dehydration; NO-related compounds and precursors; and manipulation of inflammatory pathways. New therapeutic targets such a BCL11A, a zinc finger protein that plays a key role in the silencing of fetal globin genes, is being targeted by multiple mechanisms.[111] HSCT is increasingly used as a curative intervention for sickle cell disease. While cure rates with HLA-matched sibling donors exceed 80%, the lack of such donors for most patients has led to the increasing use of cord blood units as well as unrelated and haplo-identical donors. To circumvent many complications of transplantation, gene therapy protocols using a child's own modified stem cells are underway, and multiple gene editing approaches are being pursued.

Perioperative Considerations

Perioperative morbidity and mortality are greater in children with sickle cell disease than in the general population. These children often require surgical procedures. The most common include cholecystectomy[112]; ear, nose, and throat procedures[113]; and orthopedic procedures (especially hip procedures for osteonecrosis).[114] Placement of long-term vascular access for transfusions, antibiotics, analgesia, and other therapies is frequently performed. The Cooperative Study of Sickle Cell Disease reported that 7% of all deaths among children with this disease were related to surgery.[70] Early reviews reported perioperative mortality rates as great as 10% and morbidity rates as great as 50% for children with sickle cell disease.[115–118] Studies published in the 1990s indicated that the 30-day mortality rate was about 1%.[119] In a group of more than 600 patients managed according to standard guidelines of care and prospectively studied, the incidence of any complication was about 30%, and the incidences of ACS and vasoocclusive pain episodes were 10% and 5%, respectively.[80] Patient factors (e.g., age, history of pulmonary disease, number of prior hospitalizations) and surgical factors (i.e., invasive vs. superficial) appear to affect the incidence of complications. The impact of newer interventions and technologies (e.g., laparoscopic and robotically assisted cholecystectomy and splenectomy)[120–122] on perioperative morbidity and mortality rates is unclear, although more recent reports cite reduced rates of complications than in the past.[123] Although multiple anesthesia and surgical approaches are under investigation, there is a dearth of comparative studies identifying optimal perioperative care for these children.

The principles of optimal perioperative care are based on maintaining optimal physiologic parameters throughout the perioperative period, avoiding factors that may precipitate a sickle crisis, optimizing pain management, and close consultation among hematologists, surgeons, and anesthesiologists (Table 10.9).[124] The child with sickle cell disease who is undergoing surgery should be viewed and managed primarily as a hematology patient whose care is being shared with, rather than assumed by, the surgeon and anesthesiologist during the perioperative period. Avoiding unnecessary and potentially dangerous surgical procedures (e.g., exploratory laparotomy to rule out appendicitis in a child who is experiencing an abdominal pain crisis) and minimizing perioperative complications should be the focus of the multidisciplinary care team. Based on a survey of perioperative management of sickle cell disease among anesthesiologists in North America, most anesthesiologists consult with hematologists in all cases or on a case-by-case basis.[125]

Although there is no evidence to support or refute many of the long-standing guidelines for perioperative care and individual practices vary widely,[125] it seems prudent to avoid those factors that may promote intravascular sickling: hypoxia, acidosis, hyperthermia, hypothermia, and dehydration.[71] Meticulous attention to pain management is also essential because perioperative vasoocclusive pain is common and is associated with ACS. Monitoring vital signs throughout the perioperative period is mandatory, especially monitoring oxygenation with pulse oximetry. Oxygen saturation as determined by pulse oximetry may underestimate measured oxygen saturation in patients with sickle cell disease, although this is usually clinically insignificant.[126,127] Because ACS, a common (10%)

TABLE 10.9	Perioperative Concerns for Patients With Sickle Cell Disease

Preoperative Considerations

Screening if unknown status in at-risk children

Primary management by hematology service (in most circumstances)

History of acute chest syndrome, vasoocclusive pain crises, hospitalizations, transfusions, transfusion reactions

Neurologic assessment (e.g., strokes, cognitive limitations)

History of analgesic and other medication use

Hematocrit

Oxygen saturation (on room air), chest radiograph

Pulmonary function tests (when appropriate)

Practice incentive spirometry at home

Work with child-life specialist if indicated

Echocardiography (when appropriate)

Neurologic imaging (for recent changes)

Renal function studies

Transfusion crossmatch (e.g., antibody-matched, leukocyte-reduced, sickle-negative)

Transfusion to correct anemia (in most circumstances)

Parenteral hydration for *nil per os* (NPO) status

Pain management

Aggressive bronchodilator therapy

Appropriate antibiotic therapy, including presplenectomy antibiotics and immunizations (as indicated)

Intraoperative Considerations

Maintenance of oxygenation, perfusion, normal acid-basis status, temperature, hydration

Availability of appropriately prepared blood (as indicated)

Replacement of blood loss

Anesthetic technique appropriate for procedure and postoperative analgesic requirements

Attention to physiologic effects of laparoscopy on circulatory and respiratory function

Appropriate antibiotic therapy

Judicious use of tourniquets, cell saver, and cardiopulmonary bypass

Postoperative Considerations

Management by hematology service

Monitoring for complications, especially acute chest syndrome and vasoocclusive pain crises

Maintenance of oxygen saturation monitoring and supplementation as needed, including prophylactic supplemental oxygen the first 24 hours regardless of oxygen saturation

Appropriate hydration (oral plus parenteral)

Appropriate antibiotic therapy

Aggressive pain management—must ensure ability to breathe deep and do incentive spirometry

Early mobilization

Incentive spirometry (possibly with continuous or bilateral positive airway pressure) and bronchodilator therapy

and potentially life-threatening complication of surgery, occurs 1 to 3 days postoperatively, it is important to extend adherence to guidelines of care into the postoperative period, regardless of the apparent well-being of the child.[80] In light of the renal-concentrating defect found in these patients, perioperative hydration is important to maintain and may require in-hospital preoperative care, although one must be aware that overhydration may compromise vulnerable cardiovascular and respiratory physiology.

Transfusion in the perioperative period remains a controversial subject despite several studies suggesting its benefit.[80,128,129] Transfusion of non-HbS RBCs to a child with sickle cell disease has several beneficial effects: correction of anemia; dilution of HbS red cells; compensation for blood loss; and prevention of some complications (e.g., stroke). However, transfusion is not without risks, including alloimmunization,[43,130] transfusion reactions (about 7% in the perioperative period),[80] infection, iron overload, time, and expense. Although there have been many reports of surgery performed safely in children with sickle cell disease without preoperative transfusion,[131] uncontrolled studies indicate that preoperative transfusion does decrease the rate of perioperative complications.[112,119] The Preoperative Transfusion in Sickle Cell Disease Study Group demonstrated prospectively in 604 operations (70% were cholecystectomies and otolaryngologic and orthopedic operations) that simple transfusion (i.e., correction of preoperative anemia to 10 g/dL with simple transfusion) was as effective as aggressive transfusion (i.e., lowering the preoperative HbS level to <30%, often with exchange transfusion) in preventing perioperative complications and was associated with less alloimmunization and fewer transfusion-related complications in children.[80]

To directly determine if transfusion prevents perioperative complications in the current era of surgical and anesthesia practices, an international randomized trial was initiated, the Transfusion Alternatives Preoperatively in Sickle Cell Disease (TAPS) trial. However, this trial was halted early during the recruitment process as a result of an excessive number of complications in the non-transfusion group. This led to the continued recommendation of transfusion for moderate and complicated operations in sickle cell patients.[81,129] It is currently recommended that most children with HbSS undergoing most surgical procedures receive preoperative correction of anemia with a "simple" (i.e., direct) transfusion targeting a hemoglobin concentration of 10 g/dL. Children maintained on chronic transfusion programs (e.g., for stroke prevention or acute chest) should continue such management preoperatively, and common sense dictates performing surgery soon after a scheduled transfusion. Children with sickle cell disease who are undergoing magnetic resonance imaging (MRI) and other examinations under sedation/anesthesia without prior transfusion do not have increased complications.[132] Recommendations for children with HbSC disease are less clear because these children typically maintain a baseline hemoglobin concentration at about 10 g/dL. For HbSC children who have a history of ACS, frequent pain crises, underlying pulmonary disease, or other complications, it is recommended that they receive selective preoperative exchange transfusion to reduce the HbS concentration without increasing total hemoglobin.[133] Because of the high risk of alloimmunization in the sickle cell population, blood for these patients should undergo the following preparation: extended phenotype matching, including Rh, Cc, D, Ee, and Kell in addition to ABO[81,102,134]; leukocyte reduction; and screening for sickle cell hemoglobin. Directed donation of blood from family members should be avoided if the child is an HSCT because it can lead to alloimmunization and later graft rejection.

Anesthetic agents and techniques do not have a clear effect on perioperative outcomes for children with sickle cell disease.[135] Inhalational anesthetics do not affect the sickling process, although there is experimental evidence suggesting that halothane may increase the viscosity of sickled blood.[136] Pharmacokinetics of some agents commonly used with general anesthesia such as atracurium may be altered in this population.[137] Regional anesthesia has been associated with an increased risk of postoperative complications in one retrospective study,[119] but it has not been shown to affect perioperative outcome in others.[112,114] The vasodilatory and analgesic properties of regional anesthesia can be effective in the management of vasoocclusive episodes and priapism and in providing perioperative anesthetic care.[138,139]

Other aspects of anesthetic care of sickle cell disease patients merit consideration. Hyperventilation should be avoided because of its potential to reduce cerebral perfusion in children at an increased risk for stroke.[140] The use of a tourniquet in HbSS and HbAS diseases has been questioned.[141–143] However, tourniquets have been applied intraoperatively for up to 2 hours without complication, and the predominance of evidence supports their safe use as long as they are used carefully and selectively in combination with general guidelines of perioperative care.[144–147] Intraoperative blood salvage with cell saver devices has been used safely in sickle cell patients,[148] although there is some evidence that the salvage device itself may produce sickling in the processed blood, even sickle trait blood.[149] Cardiopulmonary bypass seems to present conditions that are favorable toward sickling, given the cold, hypoxic, acidotic, and stagnant environment created. Although there are reports of bypass surgery conducted in children with HbSS or HbAS with standard bypass procedures without transfusion,[150–153] these children usually are managed with aggressive exchange transfusion before or during bypass.

While comparative studies that specifically address optimal postoperative care, understanding of the pathophysiology of the disease and studies of sickle cell pain suggest that postoperative care should minimize postoperative pain to allow deep inspirations, use of incentive spirometry, and encouraging early ambulation to prevent ACS. Maintaining euvolemia, normal body temperature, and sufficient oxygenation should minimize the risk of vasoocclusive pain at this time of increased risk due to anesthesia and postoperative inflammation.

Thalassemias

Thalassemia disorders are among the most common genetic disorders worldwide. They are characterized by a perturbation of the normal 1:1 ratio of α- to β-globin polypeptide chains, usually due to reduced synthesis of one polypeptide, but also possibly due to excess genes (e.g., triplicated α-globin genes). The clinical severity of the disease is proportionate to the degree of chain imbalance, ranging from an asymptomatic carrier state to profound ineffective erythropoiesis with transfusion dependence to fetal death due to hydrops fetalis. Both α- and β-thalassemia primarily affect children of Mediterranean, African, and Southeast Asian descent. Whereas neonatal assay screening for HbS can detect many forms of α-thalassemia, these tests typically detect only profound forms of β-thalassemia. The concomitant presence of qualitatively abnormal hemoglobins (e.g., HbS, HbE) affects the clinical course of thalassemia disorders. The primary ineffective erythropoiesis and hemolytic anemia, as well as resultant disease therapy, may affect perioperative care.

Pathophysiology

Anemia in thalassemia is the result of hemolysis and ineffective erythropoiesis; the latter results, in turn, from accelerated cell apoptosis triggered in part by excess deposition of unpaired globin chains in erythroid precursors.[154] Unpaired globin subunits are oxidized and form hemichromes, whose degree of formation affects the degree of hemolysis. Precipitation of hemichromes leads to a complex process that includes release of toxic agents and formation of reactive oxygen species; alteration of red cell membranes causes cells to become aggregates that lead to embolic complications and activation of the coagulation process. As a result of chronic anemia and ineffective erythropoiesis, bone marrow expansion and extramedullary hematopoiesis may develop in the liver and spleen. Marrow space expansion may occur at sites such as the cranium and paravertebral areas, thereby causing pathologic fractures, disfiguring bony changes, and pain. Erythroid hyperplasia and ineffective erythropoiesis lead to inappropriately low hepcidin expression (a polypeptide that inhibits iron absorption by binding to the ferroportin in the gut wall and macrophages), resulting in increased iron absorption from the gastrointestinal tract and iron overload, even in the absence of transfusion iron overload. Iron overload and deposition lead to fibrosis and cirrhosis with concomitant organ dysfunction and eventual failure. While there are many target organs for iron overload, the most relevant are liver, pancreas, heart, and pituitary; the extent of iron deposition in each can be accurately and sequentially monitored by MRI.

Clinical and Laboratory Features and Treatment

Disease severity in α-thalassemia typically reflects the complete loss of expression of between one and all four of the α-globin genes. A four-gene globin deletion typically results in hydrops fetalis with in utero or perinatal death unless diagnosed early and supported with in utero transfusions. A three-gene deletion, or hemoglobin H (HbH) disease, is relatively benign, characterized by chronic hemolytic anemia, which may be exacerbated by exposure to stress and oxidants.[155,156] The few patients with profound anemia or requiring intermittent transfusion therapy often have a two-gene deletion along with a hemoglobin Constant Spring (HbCS) mutation (HbH-Constant Spring).[155,156] A two-gene deletion alone is benign, manifest by a mild, clinically insignificant microcytic anemia. A one-gene deletion results in a silent carrier state with no anemia or microcytosis.

In contrast to α-thalassemia, β-thalassemia reflects partial or complete loss of expression of the β-globin genes. The broad spectrum of disease results from the number of genes affected and the degree to which each gene is affected. When only one β-globin gene is affected (i.e., β-thalassemia trait), mild microcytic anemia is the primary clinical manifestation. When both β-globin genes are affected, the clinical picture may be mild to moderate, potentially requiring intermittent, but not chronic transfusions (thalassemia intermedia), or severe, requiring chronic transfusions (thalassemia major or Cooley's anemia). Children with hemoglobin E (HbE)/β-thalassemia manifest a dramatic range of severity ranging from very mild to severe and transfusion-dependent.

The clinical problems in thalassemia are those associated with chronic anemia, the physiologic response to ineffective erythropoiesis, iron overload from transfusions and paradoxical increased iron absorption, as well as chelation therapy.[154] Clinical problems include transfusion-associated alloimmunization and infection, splenomegaly, bone abnormalities (due to extramedullary hematopoiesis, chelation therapy, and other factors), endocrine dysfunction (including hypogonadism, hypopituitarism, and diabetes mellitus), short stature, pulmonary hypertension, venous thrombosis and thromboembolism, and cardiomyopathy (primarily due to iron overload). Thalassemia patients also may be hypercoagulable,[157] a condition that may be exaggerated after splenectomy.[157,158]

The approach to moderate to severe disease is to balance transfusion to treat the underlying anemia and suppress erythro-poiesis while minimizing and aggressively treating iron overload. Phenotypic matching and leukocyte reduction of transfused blood can reduce immune complications, and careful surveillance for end-organ damage and endocrine management is essential. When an appropriate donor is available, HSCT is recommended before severe liver damage occurs because it provides a potential cure for thalassemia. To ameliorate the course of the disease, other therapies are being investigated, including administration of erythropoietin, fetal hemoglobin modifiers (e.g., hydroxyurea, butyrate), and antioxidants. Of particular excitement is the modulation of ineffective erythropoiesis by manipulating erythropoietin gene signaling via inhibition of the JAK2-STAT5 pathway.[159] Increasing numbers of gene therapy trials are currently underway and proving successful, and gene editing approaches similar to those with sickle cell disease are being pursued.

Perioperative Considerations

Children with moderate or severe thalassemia may require cholecystectomy and vascular access placement for frequent transfusions.[160] While splenectomy can aid transfusion support, it is avoided if possible (particularly for thalassemia intermedia) because of the increased risk of embolic disease after splenectomy. If splenectomy is performed, short-term antithrombotic prophylaxis with unfractionated or low-molecular-weight heparin should be considered during and after surgery. Pneumococcal vaccination protocols, as well as prophylactic antibiotic protocols for asplenic patients, should be followed.[161] Patients with thalassemia who have undergone splenectomy should be considered at high risk for thrombosis and should be administered appropriate prophylaxis therapy when exposed to transient thrombotic risk factors such as surgery, pregnancy, and immobilization.[158,162] Demineralized long bones may be prone to fracture, and older children may require osteotomies for bony deformities.

Perioperative management for thalassemia has not been extensively studied. It is important to consult with a hematologist to define transfusion parameters and the optimal preoperative hemoglobin level. In addition, one should be aware of the risk of the possible complications of iron overload in these patients: liver dysfunction; diabetes; pituitary dysfunction; and cardiac dysfunction (the latter an indication for preoperative electrocardiogram and echocardiogram).[163] Bony abnormalities of the maxillofacial area may render securing the airway challenging.[164] Similarly, extramedullary erythropoiesis can lead to paravertebral masses potentially interfering with epidural or other nerve blocks. Laparoscopic and robotic techniques for cholecystectomy[165] and splenectomy have been used successfully in children with thalassemia, although perioperative hypertension may be a common problem in laparoscopic splenectomy.[166,167] Perioperative considerations and concerns for children with thalassemia, especially for those with thalassemia major, are listed in Table 10.10.

Thrombocytopenia

PLATELET DISORDERS AND BLEEDING

Platelets are an essential component of hemostatic regulation. Platelets are distributed between the bloodstream (two-thirds) and spleen (one-third). Their normal life span is 7 to 10 days. In children, the platelet number may decrease as the result of decreased production or increased consumption, or they may have abnormal function. Bleeding typical of platelet disorders often involves skin and mucous membranes. Although there are many causes of primary and secondary thrombocytopenia in infants and

TABLE 10.10	Perioperative Concerns for Patients With Thalassemia

Preoperative Considerations

Hemoglobin concentration

Transfusion crossmatch if appropriate (antibody-matched, leukocyte-reduced source for frequently transfused children)

Evaluation for endocrine dysfunction (e.g., diabetes mellitus, hypopituitarism)

Cardiac function, including echocardiogram (when appropriate)

Hepatic function, awareness of risk of cirrhosis and iron- or virus-induced damage

Airway evaluation, preparation for possible difficult airway

Presplenectomy antibiotics and immunizations (when appropriate)

Intraoperative Considerations

Careful positioning of demineralized extremities

Attention to cardiovascular function, including postsplenectomy hypertension

Attention to physiologic effects of laparoscopy on circulatory and respiratory function

Prophylaxis for thromboembolism

Postoperative Considerations

Monitoring of cardiac function

Prophylaxis for thromboembolism

TABLE 10.11	Perioperative Concerns for Patients With Idiopathic Thrombocytopenia Purpura

Preoperative Considerations

Hemoglobin concentration, platelet count

History of platelet transfusions

History of corticosteroid use

History of infections

Presplenectomy antibiotic prophylaxis and immunizations (when appropriate)

Discussion with a hematologist regarding medical therapy and platelet transfusion for a platelet count <30,000/mm³

Discontinuation of any platelet-inhibiting medication (e.g., aspirin)

Intraoperative Considerations

Appropriate antibiotic coverage

Stress corticosteroid coverage

Medical therapy and platelet transfusion as above (platelets ideally administered after clamping of the splenic artery during splenectomy)

Judicious use of regional anesthesia, intramuscular medications, nasogastric tubes, nasal intubation, and other methods

Limited use of medications with potential bleeding risk (e.g., ketorolac)

Attention to physiologic effects of laparoscopy on circulatory and respiratory function

Postoperative Considerations

Hemoglobin concentration, platelet count

Infection

Corticosteroid coverage

Pain management

children, this discussion focuses on idiopathic thrombocytopenic purpura (ITP).

IDIOPATHIC THROMBOCYTOPENIC PURPURA

ITP is the most common cause of acute-onset thrombocytopenia in the otherwise healthy child, and it commonly manifests in the operative setting. ITP has an estimated incidence of about 4 per 100,000 children, and it is usually a benign, self-limited disorder affecting children between the ages of 2 and 10 years.[54] Primary ITP has no clear predisposing cause, but secondary ITP is triggered by a drug or medical disorder. Diagnosis is by exclusion, the differential list is extensive, and response to ITP-specific treatment usually solidifies the diagnosis.

Pathophysiology

ITP is characterized by antibody-mediated clearance by tissue macrophages, resulting in thrombocytopenia (platelet count <100,000/mm³) and shortened platelet survival. Antibodies may also suppress megakaryocytes and platelet development. Platelet autoantibodies may exist alone or as part of immune complexes, and they usually are immunoglobulin G (IgG) in type. They often show specificity for platelet membrane glycoproteins IIb/IIIa and Ib/IX.[168] Thrombocytopenia develops when the reticuloendothelial system, typically the spleen, destroys the antibody-covered platelets.

Clinical and Laboratory Features and Treatment

Usually, ITP in children is a benign process occurring after a viral illness or immunization that manifests as petechiae of mucosal surfaces or purpura over bony prominences, thrombocytopenia, and a normal to increased mean platelet volume with increased megakaryocytes in the marrow. This process resolves within weeks or months regardless of therapy. ITP is classified as newly diagnosed (<3 months), persistent (3–12 months), and chronic (>12 months).[169]

Although platelet function in children with ITP is usually increased, treatment is often initiated only when the counts are less than 10,000 to 20,000/mm³.[168] Observation with avoidance of activity that may lead to head trauma is an increasingly accepted treatment plan. Medical treatment most commonly consists of agents that decrease monocyte/macrophage-mediated destruction of antibody-coated platelets (e.g., steroids, intravenous immunoglobulin, anti-D immunoglobulins, vinca alkaloids). Agents that decrease antibody production (e.g., cyclophosphamide, anti-CD20 antibody) and investigational agents that stimulate the thrombopoietin receptor are reserved for those who demonstrate an inadequate response to initial therapy.[170] Platelet transfusions are recommended only for life-threatening emergencies. Splenectomy removes a major site of platelet destruction and is recommended as an option only in chronic, symptomatic ITP, or acute, life-threatening ITP unresponsive to medical treatment.[171,172] This procedure, which is commonly performed noninvasively, has a success rate of about 75%.[173–175]

Perioperative Considerations

In view of the clinical and laboratory features of ITP, the anesthesiologist providing care for the child with ITP who is undergoing splenectomy or incidental surgery should consider the concerns listed in Table 10.11. A hematologist should be consulted to assess the need for medical therapy, including platelet transfusion, before surgery.

Coagulation Disorders

Children may present for surgery with a personal or family history suggesting a bleeding disorder. The anesthesiologist must decide expeditiously whether to postpone surgery to further evaluate or treat the child A careful medical history, physical examination, and family history, followed by laboratory evaluation in consultation with a hematologist, are important elements in screening for, diagnosing, and treating a bleeding disorder in the perioperative setting.

SCREENING

The clinical history of the child and family is the most essential screening tool. The family history should identify family members who have been labeled as "bleeders," who have required blood transfusion unexpectedly during surgery, or who returned to surgery for unexpected postoperative bleeding. A history of maternal menorrhagia may also be significant. Suggestive signs and symptoms in a child's medical history are easy bruising, mucosal bleeding, and in older girls, menorrhagia. Although diagnosing easy bruising is subjective, the clinician should suspect bleeding tendencies if skin bruising occurs in nontraumatized sites (e.g., trunk) or is unusually large without evidence of previous trauma. Mucosal bleeding includes epistaxis and gingival bleeding. Occasional nosebleeds can be common in children, but their clinical significance is enhanced by increased frequency, duration, bilaterality, and coexistence with abnormal bleeding from other sites. Gingival bleeding is common after tooth brushing or flossing, but its clinical significance is enhanced by spontaneous occurrence or chronicity, especially in the presence of good dental hygiene.[176] A history of prolonged or excessive bleeding is important when associated with umbilical cord stump dehiscence, dental work (especially extractions), and circumcision. Although mouth injuries can produce impressive blood loss acutely in any individual, recurrent or persistent bleeding from such an injury may indicate an underlying disorder.

Consultation with a hematologist and laboratory evaluation should be considered for children with a clinical history and physical examination result that suggest a bleeding diathesis, especially for children scheduled to undergo procedures associated with large blood loss or that make particular demands on hemostasis, such as tonsillectomy. Laboratory evaluation of all children, regardless of history or type of surgery, may result in false-positive results that lead to costly workups and potentially unnecessary cancellation of operations, both of which can contribute to greater health care inefficiencies and expense. Bleeding owing to medications should be distinguished from an actual bleeding disorder.

When a bleeding disorder is strongly suspected, a set of laboratory tests that include a platelet count, PT, INR, aPTT, thrombin time (TT), and fibrinogen concentration should be ordered. The PT test is most sensitive to deficiencies in factors II, V, VII, and X, and it is useful for differentiating a vitamin K deficiency from other causes. The PT is most often used to monitor the anticoagulant effects of warfarin; it is not sensitive to the effects of heparin. The aPTT test is most sensitive to deficiencies in factors VIII, IX, and XI and less sensitive to deficiencies of factor V, factor X, prothrombin, and fibrinogen. The aPTT is also prolonged in deficiencies of the contact or kallikrein/kinin system proteins, factor XII, prekallikrein, and high-molecular-weight kininogen, but these deficiencies are not associated with bleeding. Because aPTT reagents vary in sensitivity for detection of deficiencies of each factor, it is inappropriate to make a general statement about the ability of this test to detect a specific abnormality; abnormal results require discussion with a hematologist or laboratory medicine physician. Although a prolonged aPTT may be caused by a deficiency in one or more factors, it can also result from inhibition by heparin or a plasma inhibitor, such as lupus anticoagulant. Correction of a prolonged aPTT after mixing the child's plasma with normal plasma (1 : 1 mix) suggests a factor deficiency. The TT test, which determines the amount of time it takes for blood to clot, is useful for determining deficiencies or abnormalities in fibrinogen and is very sensitive to heparin contamination. Bleeding time, a TEG, and platelet function screens (e.g., PFA-100) are probably not appropriate as first-line screening tests.

Children with an upper limit of normal aPTT test result and a strongly suspicious personal or family history for a bleeding disorder may have an abnormality (e.g., von Willebrand disease). These children require further evaluation in consultation with a hematologist. Whether a procedure should be delayed for the consultation depends on several factors, including the patient's history, site and urgency of surgery, potential bleeding risks associated with the planned procedure, and results of previously discussed set of screening tests.

VON WILLEBRAND DISEASE

Von Willebrand disease (vWD) is one of the most common bleeding disorders, although studies suggest that the prevalence may be as low as 1 case per 1000 people.[177] Initially named *pseudohemophilia* because of an inheritance pattern that is different from that of hemophilia, vWD is the result of an abnormal amount, structure, or function of the vWF.[178]

Pathophysiology and Classification

The glycoprotein vWF serves two main roles in the coagulation cascade: adhering platelets to damaged subendothelium and carrying factor VIII in plasma. vWF exists as small and large multimers. Large multimers play a more active role in the binding of platelets to subendothelium than do small ones and are, therefore, necessary for platelet adhesion, whereas binding to factor VIII is independent of multimer size. The two aspects of vWF make it an essential part of primary hemostasis (through platelet binding) and secondary hemostasis (as carrier of factor VIII to sites of injury).

Classification of vWD is essential for understanding and management of this disorder. The current classification was developed by a subcommittee on vWD through the International Society on Thrombosis and Haemostasis.[179,180] The two general types are categorized as quantitative abnormalities (types 1 and 3) or qualitative abnormalities (type 2, including subtypes A, B, M, and N). All types are inherited in an autosomal dominant pattern, except types 2N and 3, which are autosomal recessive.

Because vWD is heterogeneous, clinical definitions have been proposed using categories such as mild, moderate, and severe, categories based on bleeding history (i.e., number of bleeding episodes) and laboratory measurement of factor concentration and activity.[181] As the molecular basis of vWD becomes better understood, classification of this disease likely will change to reflect the new data. For example, Rodeghiero and colleagues proposed a practical approach to diagnosing and categorizing patients with vWD to provide optimal management. Their approach includes a standardized bleeding history score, focused laboratory analysis, and a trial infusion of DDAVP in certain subtypes.[182] Better categorization of patients with vWD may predict clinical outcomes and allow better management in the perioperative setting.[183]

Clinical and Laboratory Features and Treatment

Children with vWD may exhibit many of the clinical features associated with bleeding disorders in general, although there is a notable absence of joint bleeding. The typical symptoms of vWD reflect poor platelet adhesion and include bruising, epistaxis, and menorrhagia.

Children with vWD have traditionally been described as having prolonged bleeding times and aPTTs, but those with mild disease often have normal values. The aPTT is prolonged only if factor VIII activity is at, or below, a concentration that is determined by the sensitivity of the particular assay at an institution (often below 30%–35%). The platelet functional assay (PFA-100) has better sensitivity and specificity (both near 90%) for diagnosis of the disease.[184,185] The PFA-100 test, which measures closure time of an aperture on a membrane coated with collagen and adenosine diphosphate (ADP) or epinephrine, depends on vWF activity and platelet function. Because this test has some variability, its interpretation should be used in conjunction with results of other tests.[186] Platelet count is typically normal in all types of vWD except type 2B.

Other laboratory tests used to delineate vWD include the following: vWF antigen (vWF:A), which is a measure of the total level of vWF; vWF activity, often measured as a ristocetin cofactor activity (vWF:R), itself a measure of vWF binding to platelets through GPIb receptors; factor VIII coagulant activity; and vWF multimer analysis. Certain disease states have been associated with "acquired vWD" and include lymphoproliferative disorders or gammopathies (marked by antibodies to vWF), chronic renal failure, hypothyroidism, Wilms tumor, and certain congenital heart disease (characterized by proteolysis of vWF multimers).[187] Treatment focuses on increasing concentrations of endogenous vWF with administration of DDAVP when possible or on replacement of factors with factor concentrates.[188] DDAVP is usually effective in type 1 but less so in types 2A and 2M. DDAVP may have little or even undesired effects in some children: it may increase abnormal vWF in types 2A, 2M, and 2N; it can exacerbate thrombocytopenia in type 2B; and its repeated administration may lead to tachyphylaxis. DDAVP usually is not administered to very young children because of the risk of free water retention, hyponatremia, and central nervous system pathology, including seizures. Similarly, intravenous fluids may need to be limited after its administration to any child. Factor concentrates (including factor VIII and vWF [Humate-P (CSL Behring, King of Prussia, Pennsylvania) or Alphanate (Grifols, Barcelona, Spain)]) typically are required for types 2B, 2N, and 3. Cryoprecipitate may be used when vWF-containing concentrates are unavailable, but it is not recommended as first-line therapy because it is not virus free, and vWF in solvent or heat-treated cryoprecipitate may be abnormal.[189] Because of the complexity of response to therapies in this disease and the ever-changing availability of replacement products, determination of appropriate treatment in conjunction with a hematologist before surgery is crucial.[182,190]

Perioperative Concerns

The major preoperative concerns in children with confirmed vWD are directed toward appropriate preoperative treatment, avoidance of medications that may interfere with coagulation, and anticipation of intraoperative and postoperative bleeding (Table 10.12).[191,192]

TABLE 10.12	Perioperative Considerations for Patients With von Willebrand Disease
Preoperative Considerations	
Consultation with hematologist: establish correct diagnosis and response to desmopressin (DDAVP); administer DDAVP *or* viral attenuated factor concentrates containing factor VIII and von Willebrand factor (vWF) such as Humate-P for severe vWD or for those types not responsive to DDAVP[186]	
Determination of actual and desired factor concentrations and expected duration of postoperative therapy[191]	
Discontinuation of any platelet-inhibiting medication (e.g., aspirin)	
Intraoperative Considerations	
Judicious use of regional anesthesia, intramuscular medications, nasogastric tubes, nasal intubation, and other procedures that may cause bleeding	
Limited use of medications with potential bleeding risk (e.g., ketorolac)	
Coagulation profiles, including platelet counts for more invasive surgeries	
Treatment of bleeding with appropriate blood products	
Consider use of antifibrinolytic agents (i.e., ε-aminocaproic acid, tranexamic acid)[190]	
Possible use of recombinant factor VIIa for severe bleeding episodes in severe vWD type 3 or patients with inhibitors	
Postoperative Considerations	
Follow factor concentrations (i.e., factor VIII and vWF)	
Availability of blood products and factors	
Appropriate treatment of bleeding episodes	
Monitor for thromboembolism in children receiving multiple concentrates or antifibrinolytic agents, or both[186]	

Although regional anesthesia for these children usually is contraindicated, there are reports of its use without complications.[193]

HEMOPHILIA

Hemophilia was first reported in the *Talmud*, in which there are descriptions of 8-day-old boys exsanguinating after ritual circumcision. Widespread public attention was drawn to this disease after members of Queen Victoria's family developed sequelae from hemophilia in the late 19th and early 20th centuries. The discovery of multiple forms of hemophilia was first made in 1944 when blood from two hemophiliacs was mixed and found to clot. In 1952, hematologists explained their earlier finding by noting that a 10-year-old boy, Stephen Christmas, exhibited a type of hemophilia, factor IX deficiency, which differed from the classic form, factor VIII deficiency.

Hemophilia is a group of congenital bleeding disorders caused by deficiency in factor VIII (i.e., hemophilia A, or classic hemophilia), factor IX (i.e., hemophilia B, or Christmas disease), or factor XI (i.e., hemophilia C). During the 10-year period from 1982 through 1991, the incidence of the more common varieties, hemophilia A and B, was 1 per 5032 live male births in the United States within a six-state surveillance area; the prevalence of hemophilia A was 10.5 cases per 100,000 male births, and that of hemophilia B was 2.9 cases per 100,000 male births.[194] Because of X-linked recessive inheritance of hemophilia A and B, family history is very important in establishing the diagnosis. Although boys are usually affected, girls may rarely inherit the disorder if their fathers are affected and their mothers are carriers or in instances of extreme lyonization (inactivation of an X chromosome). The daughter of an affected father is an obligate carrier with a 50% chance of passing it on to any of her sons. De novo mutations are relatively common (about one-third of hemophilia A and B cases) and suspected in male patients lacking a family history.[176] Hemophilia C, affecting primarily Ashkenazi Jews, is a mild form of hemophilia. It is also known as plasma thromboplastin anteced-ent (PTA) deficiency or Rosenthal syndrome. In the United States, its incidence is 1 : 100,000 adults, or 10% the incidence of hemophilia A. It is distinguished from the other two forms of hemophilia by an autosomal recessive inheritance pattern (the gene for factor XI is located on chromosome 4), lack of joint bleeding, and infrequent need for treatment. Affected female patients may notice heavy menses, and affected male patients may have frequent nosebleeds and occasionally have excessive bleeding during surgery.

Pathophysiology

Normal in vivo hemostasis initiates at sites of endothelial disruption through interaction of activated factor VII (FVIIa) and tissue factor (TF) to form a complex that activates factor IX and factor X directly. Activated factor IX in conjunction with factor VIII further activates factor X, which with factor V converts prothrombin to thrombin. Both factor VIII and factor IX are required for sufficient hemostasis, as evidenced by the severe bleeding that occurs if either is completely deficient. Factor XI activates factor IX, but its precise role in the hemostatic pathway is not completely understood.

Clinical and Laboratory Features and Treatment

The wide range of clinical features is similar for hemophilia A and B (Table 10.13). The severity of bleeding in these children directly relates to the degree of their deficiency.[184] Children with mild or moderate hemophilia may bleed excessively only after a hemostatic challenge such as trauma or surgery, whereas children with severe hemophilia may bleed spontaneously (e.g., hemar-throses).[195] Female carriers on average have 50% of normal factor concentrations and usually are asymptomatic, although they occasionally present with a clinical picture similar to that of mild cases of hemophilia.[184]

Results of a general coagulation screen are typically normal except for the aPTT, which is prolonged in proportion to the concentration of factors in the blood. The diagnosis is confirmed by measuring the specific factor concentrations.[196] If hemophilia is suspected but there is no family history, testing for vWD is prudent, especially for the types that may mimic hemophilia (i.e., types 2N and 3). Because of the variable sensitivity of the aPTT to specific factor deficiencies, the ability of this test to detect carriers varies between laboratories; diagnosis of a carrier state usually requires specific factor assays.

Hemophilias A and B are treated by replacing the deficient factor concentrations. These factor concentrations should be maintained at specified levels to prevent sequelae (Table 10.14). Exposure to plasma products should be minimized. The duration of treatment should be tailored to the severity of disease. DDAVP may be effective in selected mild cases by increasing factor VIII concentrations through the release of endogenous stores. Because tachyphylaxis limits the prolonged use of DDAVP, it is typically recommended only for minor operations.[197] For most cases, especially for those who require increased factor concentrations to be maintained for effective hemostasis, factor concentrates should be used. Although recombinant forms are preferable because they do not carry infectious risk, substitution with plasma-derived forms may be needed when supplies are limited.[184,197] For the rare patient with hemophilia C who has excessive surgical bleeding, treatment with recombinant factor XI or FFP may be required. It is essential to consult with a hematologist to determine a custom-ized factor treatment plan for every child with hemophilia.

Children who have developed inhibitors to factor concentrates pose a challenge in the perioperative period. For years, they were denied surgery unless it was absolutely necessary, at which point they were often managed with increased concentrations of factors or a desensitization regimen. However, recently there has been improved management in these patients with the use of bypassing agents that treat bleeding by stimulating thrombin generation through pathways that do not require the missing factors (VIII or IX). Such agents include recombinant factor VIIa (rfVIIa, NovoSeven RT, Novo Nordisk Inc., Plainsboro, NJ) and activated prothrombin complex concentrates, such as FEIBA (anti-inhibitor coagulant complex; Shire, Massachusetts, USA), that have shown efficacy greater than 80%. Specific factor concentrates are preferred, however, unless patients have significantly elevated inhibitors.[198]

Perioperative Concerns

The perioperative concerns in hemophilia focus on prevention and treatment of bleeding, similar to the management of patients

TABLE 10.13	Clinical Manifestations of Hemophilia A			
Clinical Manifestations	Mild (>10%)[a]	Moderate (2%–10%)[a]	Severe (<2%)[a]
Age at first hemorrhage	3–14 years or older	<2 years	<1 year
Signs in neonatal period	None	Postcircumcision bleeding	Postcircumcision bleeding, intracranial hemorrhage
Musculoskeletal bleeding	Unusual except with severe trauma	Joint and muscle bleeding with minor trauma	Spontaneous
Central nervous system bleeding	Rare except with severe trauma	Less prevalent than severe	Prevalence, 3% Mean age, 14 years
Postsurgical bleeding	Wound hematomas and oozing	Wound hematomas and oozing	Usually frank bleeding
Trauma-related bleeding	Hematomas and deep bleeding with significant trauma	Muscle and joint bleeding with minor trauma	Common with minor trauma
Dental bleeding	Often	Common	Usual
Inhibitors present	Rarely	<3%	Prevalence, 15%–20%

[a]Percent factor VIII activity. Modified from DiMichele D: Hemophilia A (FVIII deficiency). In: Goodnight SH Jr, Hathaway W, eds. *Disorders of Hemostasis and Thrombosis*. New York: McGraw-Hill; 2001:127–139.

TABLE 10.14	Treatment Targets for Hemophilia A and B			
Type of Hemorrhage	Desired Plasma Factor Levels (IU/DL) for Hemophilia A[a]	Desired Plasma Factor Levels (IU/DL) for Hemophilia B[a]	Duration (days)[b]	
Muscle				
Superficial	40–60	40–60	2–3	
Deep (initial)	80–100	60–80	1–2	
Deep (maintenance)	30–60	30–60	3–5	
Joint	40–60	40–60	1–2	
Gastrointestinal Tract				
Initial	80–100	60–80	7–14	
Maintenance	50	30		
Oral mucosa	30–50	30–50	2–3	
Epistaxis	30–50	30–50	2–3	
Renal	50	40	3–5	
Surgery (major)				
Preoperative	80–100	60–80	1–3	
Postoperative	30–80	30–80	4–14	
Surgery (minor)				
Preoperative	50–80	50–80	1–5	
Postoperative	30–80	30–80	1–5	
Central Nervous System				
Initial	80–100	60–80	1–7	
Maintenance	50	30	8–21	

[a]Recommended targets when there are no product constraints. Targets may be adjusted lower when products are constrained.
[b]May be increased or reduced depending on clinical circumstances and severity of disease.
Modified from Brown DL. Congenital bleeding disorders. *Curr Probl Pediatr Adolesc Health Care.* 2005;35:38–62; and Srivastava A, Brewer AK, Mauser-Bunschoten EP, et al. Treatment Guidelines Working Group on behalf of the World Federation of Hemophilia. Guidelines for the management of hemophilia. *Haemophilia.* 2013;19:e1–e47.

TABLE 10.15	Perioperative Concerns for Patients With Hemophilia

Preoperative Considerations

Consultation with hematologist, establishment of correct diagnosis

Determination and testing of treatment plan, including use of desmopressin or factors (concentrates or recombinant)

Consideration of multiple procedures performed together to reduce factor exposure

Discontinuation of any platelet-inhibiting medication (e.g., aspirin)

Intraoperative Considerations

Judicious use of regional anesthesia, intramuscular medications, nasogastric tubes, nasal intubation, and other procedures that may cause bleeding

Limited use of medications with potential bleeding risk (e.g., NSAIDs)

Follow coagulation profiles, especially factor levels (factors VIII and IX)

Anticipate and treat bleeding with appropriate blood products

Consider recombinant activated factor VII (rFVIIa) for severe bleeding

Postoperative Considerations

Maintain factor concentrations for specified time period as recommended by the hematologist

Ensure availability of blood products and factors from the blood bank

Anticipate and treat bleeding episodes

NSAIDs, nonsteroidal antiinflammatory drugs.

for those who are asymptomatic, even those with a positive family history.[203]

Evidence-based guidelines for children are lacking with regard to screening and prophylactic treatment of those with suspected hypercoagulability. Current evidence suggests pharmacologic prophylaxis in the nonoperative setting is recommended only in children receiving long-term home total parenteral nutrition (TPN) and those with specific complex cardiac lesions (e.g., Fontan patients).[204] However, children who present for surgery with a strong family history of thromboses may benefit from screening and referral to a hematologist for management and consideration of pharmacologic prophylaxis, such as enoxaparin administered postoperatively. The use of nonpharmacologic prophylaxis, including early mobilization after surgery, adequate hydration, and compression stockings, is left to the discretion of individual providers and to institutional practice based on the child's medical history, family history, and risk factors for VTE.

Studies on the use of antifibrinolytic medications for preventing blood loss in high-risk surgeries (e.g., scoliosis, craniosynostosis) for patients with thrombophilia or a family history of thrombophilia are lacking. A risk/benefit discussion with the patient, family, and surgeon for each individual patient and surgery is recommended.

Hematologic Malignancies

Unlike in adults, hematologic malignancies are very common in children, accounting for over 40% of all new cancer diagnoses, the majority of which are leukemia.[205] Childhood malignancy occurs within any blood cell lineage. Each of the hematologic malignancies is a heterogeneous disease with multiple distinct biologic subtypes and thus multiple treatment options and survival rates. The hematologic malignancies are often categorized as listed in Table 10.16, which lists the groups and most common subtypes.

with vWD (Table 10.15). Many consider regional anesthesia to be contraindicated for patients with hemophilia, but there are reports of its use without complications as long as factor concentrations are maintained.[199]

HYPERCOAGULABILITY

A hypercoagulable state is a condition in which the development of thrombus is favored (i.e., thrombophilia). The condition results in an increased risk for abnormal clot formation and venous thromboembolic events (VTEs), which often are the presenting symptoms at the time of diagnosis. Thrombophilia can be acquired or congenital. The incidence of VTE among children is less than in adults, even in those with known congenital thrombophilic conditions,[200] although neonates and adolescents are at relatively high risk in the pediatric population.[201] Congenital thrombophilic conditions include factor V Leiden disorder, prothrombin gene mutation, protein C and S deficiencies, and antithrombin III deficiency.[202] Risk factors for acquired thrombophilia include the presence of a central venous catheter, infection, malignancy, surgery, or trauma.[201] Preoperative screening of nonoperative children with suspected hypercoagulability is controversial and not recommended

However, recent advances have demonstrated overlapping pathogenesis and features between some subgroups, leading to recent changes to some categorizations.[206] Fig. 10.1 illustrates the incidence of pediatric hematologic cancers by age. Acute lymphoblastic leukemia (ALL) has a spike of diagnosis between 2 and 5 years of age, acute myelogenous leukemia (AML) has a steady incidence throughout childhood, and lymphoma has a steadily rising incidence throughout childhood and adolescence. As such, children of all ages are at risk for a newly diagnosed hematologic malignancy, and each can present unique and challenging considerations during anesthetic care.

All hematologic malignancies stem from genomic alterations within a certain blood cell lineage in either the immature progenitor stage or mature stage of cellular differentiation. Leukemia is a malignant transformation of lymphoid or myeloid progenitor cells in the bone marrow, whereas lymphoma is malignant transformation of progenitor lymphoid cells (or less commonly, mature lymphocytes) in lymph nodes or other lymphatic tissues. Several subtypes of leukemia and lymphoma are very closely related and thus challenging to differentiate both clinically and histologically, especially if marrow and lymph involvement are both present at diagnosis. Histiocytoses are a group of malignant disorders characterized by abnormal function of dendrocytes, monocytes, or macrophages. Myelodysplastic syndromes and myeloproliferative neoplasms are rare malignant disorders of pluripotent hematopoietic stem cells that result in aberrant proliferation of one or more hematopoietic cell lineages and suppression of the rest.

ACUTE LYMPHOBLASTIC LEUKEMIA

ALL is the most common childhood malignancy, accounting for 25% of all pediatric cancers and 76% of all leukemias.[207] Continued evolution of treatment protocols has led to an overall survival rate of 90% in children and adolescents in Western countries, some subgroups reaching survival rates as high as 95%.[211,212] Subgroups with lower 5-year survival rates include infant diagnosis (53% survival), adolescent diagnosis (76%), T-cell immunophenotype (82%), and a so-called high-risk categorization group (83%).[211] The incidence of ALL diagnosis peaks between the ages of 2 and 5 years and quickly declines thereafter (see Fig. 10.1).

Pathophysiology

ALL is a heterogeneous malignancy caused by mutation of lymphocyte progenitor cells at an early phase of differentiation, called lymphoblasts. The mutation arises either in B-cell or T-cell lymphoblasts in the bone marrow. Approximately 85% of ALL cases are of the pre–B-cell lineage (B-ALL), and the remaining 15% of cases originate from a progenitor T-cell lineage (T-ALL).[213] Both B-ALL and T-ALL can be further classified into several distinct genetic subtypes that influence the approach to treatment and subsequent outcomes. Leukemic potential commonly arises from a series of gene alterations that include chromosomal translocations and changes to chromosomal number. Subsequent additional genetic alterations then trigger the ultimate conversion to leukemia via inappropriate suppression or activation of regulatory proteins. These acquired genetic alterations lead to clonal proliferation and accumulation of immature blast cells in the bone marrow.[214–216]

TABLE 10.16	Incidence of Hematologic Malignancies in Childhood (Ages 0–14 Years)	
Cancer	**Incidence per 1,000,000**	**5-Year Survival (%)**
Leukemias	54.1	85
Acute lymphoblastic leukemia	41.2	89
Acute myelogenous leukemia	8.4	65
Lymphomas	16.7	93
Hodgkin lymphoma	6.0	98
Non-Hodgkin lymphoma	7.5	89
Histiocytosis	–	–
Langerhans cell histiocytosis	5	85–100
Myelodysplastic syndromes	2	50

Data from references 207–210.

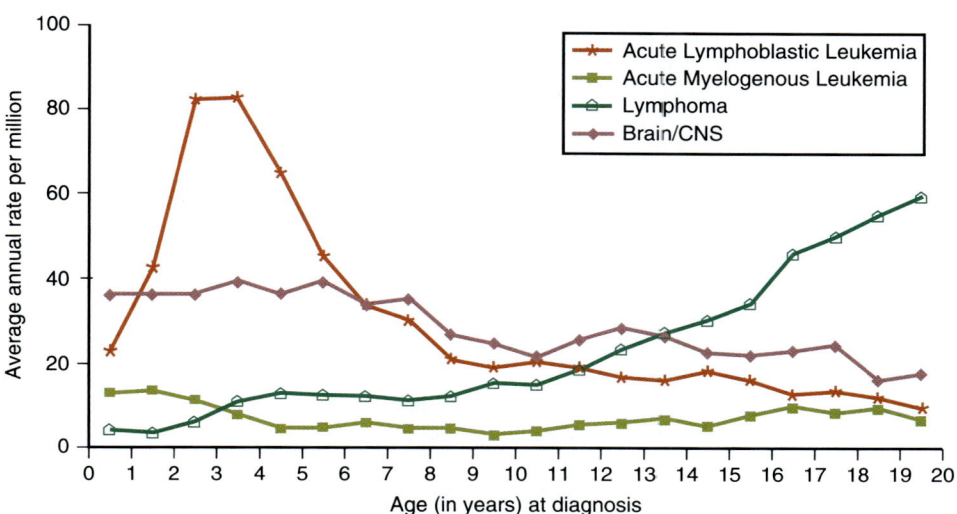

FIGURE 10.1 Age-Specific Incidence Rates for Childhood Cancer by International Classification of Childhood Cancer (ICCC) Group, All Races, Both Sexes, SEER 1986–94. (From Ries LAG, Percy CL, Bunin GR. Introduction. In: Ries LAG, Smith MA, Gurney JG, et al., eds. *Cancer Incidence and Survival among Children and Adolescents: United States SEER Program 1975-1995*. Bethesda, MD: National Cancer Institute, SEER Program, 1999. NIH Pub. No. 99-4649.)

Rapid expansion of blast cells crowds the marrow space and leads to ineffective hematopoiesis and peripheral cytopenias. Over time, leukemic cells invade other organs and tissues.

Few risk factors for developing ALL have been identified. Generally accepted risks include prior exposure to radiation (including in utero), inherited genetic polymorphisms, and genetic syndromes (e.g., Trisomy 21, Bloom syndrome, ataxia telangiectasia, and Fanconi anemia).[217,218] Children with Trisomy 21 have an 18-fold increased risk of developing leukemia during childhood, and two-thirds of the leukemic diagnoses are ALL. Survival of children with Trisomy 21 and ALL is less than in the non–Trisomy 21 population because of the frequencies of relapse and treatment-related mortality.[219,220]

Clinical and Laboratory Features and Treatment

The presenting signs and symptoms of childhood ALL are usually nonspecific in the early stages. The extent of bone marrow suppression and cytopenias influences the severity of presenting symptoms, which often include frequent upper respiratory infections, fevers, fatigue, malaise, pallor, petechiae, easy bruisability, lymphadenopathy, hepatosplenomegaly, pain in extremities, and refusal to walk.[221] When a complete blood cell count (CBC) is first obtained, it is often suggestive of leukemia. The initial CBC will typically show leukocytosis in half of children, anemia in 80% of children, neutropenia, and thrombocytopenia.[221–223] Often the child will appear pale and tired but otherwise healthy. However, children with advanced disease and a large tumor burden with extramedullary spread at diagnosis might be decidedly sicker; they can present with hyperuricemia, renal insufficiency, calcium and phosphorus abnormalities from skeletal invasion, liver dysfunction from leukemic infiltration, and mild coagulopathy.[223] At diagnosis, the presence of central nervous system (CNS) leukemia or an anterior mediastinal mass is uncommon in B-ALL; however, half of children with T-ALL have an anterior mediastinal mass, one-half have hyperleukocytosis and risk for vascular stasis, and 10% to 15% have CNS leukemia at diagnosis.[221,222,224] A bone marrow aspirate provides the definitive diagnosis, and immunophenotyping and cytogenetic studies confirm the ALL subtype and genetic characteristics that guide the child's therapy. Usually under the same anesthetic, a lumbar puncture is performed to assess the presence of lymphoblasts in the cerebrospinal fluid (CSF).

Because ALL is a heterogeneous disease, genomic data from the child's specific leukemia cells guide estimates of survival probability, response to treatments, and optimal treatment protocol.[216,225] In most pediatric oncology centers, treatment occurs in five phases: induction, consolidation and CNS preventive therapy, interim maintenance, delayed intensification, and maintenance. The intensity and time interval of each therapy is tailored to the child's risk category, which is determined by the risk of relapse of the specific tumor subtype. Of note, cranial radiation is seldom used for newly diagnosed ALL in children; outcomes are similar without it, and radiation risks chronic neurocognitive dysfunction and secondary tumors.[226,227]

Induction begins soon after diagnosis, and the goal is to administer intensive systemic and intrathecal chemotherapy to eradicate more than 99% of leukemic cells and restore normal hematopoiesis. In standard-risk ALL, three-drug treatment includes a glucocorticoid, vincristine, and asparaginase. Those at increased risk typically receive a fourth agent such as an anthracycline.[212] Remission at the end of the 4- to 6-week induction is defined as less than 5% blasts in the marrow and recovery of normal blood counts. Submicroscopic depth of remission can be further quanti-

fied by minimal residual disease (MRD) detection, typically by flow cytometry. The child's rapidity of response to induction and degree of MRD at the end of this cycle are important predictors of outcome and influence therapy in subsequent stages.[228] Although most children achieve remission at the end of induction, relapse is inevitable without continued therapy.[212] The overall health of the child during this phase is variable.[229]

Thereafter, consolidation, interim maintenance, and delayed intensification are used for 6 to 9 months depending on the treatment protocol. This phase uses high-dose intrathecal and intravenous chemotherapy to continue leukemic cytoreduction in all tissues and maintain remission. The pharmacologic regimen, duration, and intensity vary per treatment protocol. The recent addition of targeted antitumor agents (e.g., imatinib for Philadelphia chromosome–positive leukemia) has improved outcomes for children at increased risk during this phase of treatment.[225] Significant myelosuppression and toxicities of therapy are common during this period and often limit and delay chemotherapy dosages, particularly the presence of severe neutropenia. Alopecia, mucositis, anorexia, vomiting, significant infections, and fatigue are common during this period.[224] While outpatient management is usual, hospitalization is often required during intensive stages or at any time to manage sequelae of this aggressive phase. Supportive care with blood transfusions, nutritional support, infection precautions, and medications to counter toxicity are crucial.[230] The final phase is maintenance for 1.5 to 2.5 years, and this phase is managed with oral chemotherapy (methotrexate, mercaptopurine, ± additional agent) in the outpatient setting. Children at this stage often lead near-normal lives outwardly. However, some may require short-term hospitalization for neutropenic infections or deterioration of their clinical status, and many continue to suffer chronic therapy-related dysfunction, including pain, neuropathies, depression, and psychosocial dysfunction.[229]

Up to 20% of children will relapse; survival rates are significantly reduced with relapse, especially if it occurs during treatment rather than after treatment.[231] Because of increasingly poor outcomes in relapsed disease, therapies with greater toxicity or investigative therapies are often used. HSCT is a frequently used modality in relapsed children, whereas HSCT is uncommonly used during initial diagnosis, save for those at greatest risk.[232] Investigational therapies, such as adoptive T-cell therapies discussed in Chapter 11, are showing considerable promise as well.[233] The overall clinical status of children during relapse is broad, ranging from outpatient to intensive care management.

Perioperative Considerations

The newly diagnosed child with ALL will present soon after diagnosis for long-term central venous access under anesthesia to facilitate frequent intravenous chemotherapy and blood draws. Before the first anesthetic, the presence of an anterior mediastinal mass must be ruled out (see also Chapter 15), given that more than half of children with T-ALL will have a mass at the time of diagnosis, although only a minority will be symptomatic.[222] During induction and consolidation stages of therapy (in the first 6–9 months), the child will undergo multiple bone marrow aspirations and lumbar punctures. Other surgical procedures during ALL treatment are not particularly common, with the exception of revision of malfunctioned or infected central venous access. Before any anesthetic, a CBC should be reviewed. Table 10.2 lists commonly recognized minimal safe platelet counts before invasive procedures, but institutional protocols may vary for lumbar puncture and bone marrow aspiration. Strict adherence to aseptic

10

TABLE 10.17	Perioperative Concerns in Pediatric Cancer and Hematopoietic Stem Cell Transplantation

Preoperative Considerations

Consultation with service primarily responsible for child's care

Complete blood cell count (when appropriate)

Echocardiogram or chest radiograph, or both (when appropriate)

Transfusion crossmatch with specifications (e.g., cytomegalovirus seronegativity, leukocyte reduction, irradiation) determined in consultation with oncology service

Determination of blood typing requirements for all stem cell transplant recipients

History of acute and chronic pain medication use

Infection prophylaxis with antibiotics

Avoidance of any marrow-suppressive medications in stem cell transplant patients

Observation of indicated isolation precautions

Sterile technique with central line access

Intraoperative Considerations

Attention to skin, teeth, eyes, and joints; careful positioning and padding

Careful airway instrumentation in the setting of mucositis

Sterile technique with central line access

Full-stomach precautions (when appropriate, as in graft-versus-host disease)

Appropriate hydration and maintenance of urine output

Continuation of total parenteral nutrition (and other parenteral fluids with high glucose concentration)

Avoidance of high fraction of inspired oxygen (FIO_2) and restriction of hydration if prior treatment with bleomycin

Judicious use of cardiac depressants in patients with compromised cardiac function

Nausea and vomiting prophylaxis: avoid corticosteroids for antiemesis unless discussed with oncology

Administer stress dose steroids when indicated, after consultation with oncology

Regional anesthesia when safe and indicated

Postoperative Considerations

Patient-appropriate opioid and other analgesic administration

Sterile technique with central line access

Observation of indicated isolation precautions

protocols is imperative, especially for neutropenic children, as is attention to friability of oral mucosal tissue during laryngoscopy in patients with mucositis. Indiscriminant use of parenteral steroids should be avoided, especially before the diagnosis is confirmed and a treatment plan is prescribed, as it may (1) complicate the diagnosis by causing tumor cell necrosis, (2) cause tumor lysis syndrome, and/or (3) affect treatment randomization. Table 10.17 lists general perioperative considerations for all children with hematologic malignancies, and additional detailed anesthetic considerations are discussed in Chapter 11.

ACUTE MYELOGENOUS LEUKEMIA

Although far more prevalent in older adults, AML is the second most common leukemia in childhood, representing 18% of leukemias in children but 50% of all leukemic deaths in children.[207,234] The incidence of AML in children is biphasic, with a greater incidence of diagnosis before age 3 and after age 14 years (see Fig. 10.1). The increasing incidence in adolescence reflects the gradual increased prevalence throughout all of adulthood.[207] The 5-year survival of childhood AML has improved dramatically in the past several decades to 65% to 70%, but nearly half of all children diagnosed with AML eventually relapse and die from the disease. AML remains one of the major groups of childhood cancer with the worst overall survival rates, and the mortality rate increases with increasing age at diagnosis.[207,234,235]

Pathophysiology

AML is a heterogeneous malignancy of undifferentiated myeloid precursor cells. AML can arise as a de novo disease or as a secondary disease from previous cytotoxic exposures (e.g., previous cancer therapy) or myelodysplastic syndromes. Like ALL, AML is further categorized based on subtypes of tumor cytology, and as such, treatment protocols and outcomes differ among the subtypes.[236] The genesis of AML appears to be due to a series of genetic mutations that lead to rapid clonal proliferation and accumulation of maturation-arrested myeloid cells.[237] Marrow crowding and eventual infiltration of extramedullary sites lead to the development of the symptomology seen at presentation.[236]

Inherited risks are an important component in the development of childhood AML. Some of the more common risk factors include Trisomy 21, Fanconi anemia, Bloom syndrome, ataxia telangiectasia, Shwachman-Diamond syndrome, and familial monosomy 7.[238] Trisomy 21 is the most common of these syndromes and has a 10- to 20-fold increased risk of development of AML.[239] Environmental risks are not well understood in childhood AML, with the exception of the greatly increased risk of AML in children exposed to high radiation (e.g., survivors of atomic bombs in 1940s' Japan). Prior exposure to chemotherapeutics, especially topoisomerase inhibitors, and acquired marrow suppression conditions are an important cause of secondary AML.[236]

Clinical and Laboratory Features and Treatment

Clinical symptoms prior to diagnosis are usually nonspecific but often include pallor, bleeding, easy bruising, and infections, all as a result of pancytopenia. Depending on the degree of marrow suppression at the time of diagnosis, anemia and thrombocytopenia are present in the majority of patients.[236,240] The white blood cell count may range from low to high, but neutropenia is common, which predisposes to severe infections. Hyperleukocytosis (>100,000/mm^3) is present in 20% of patients with AML at diagnosis.[241] Approximately 14% of children are at risk of bleeding and thrombosis as a result of thrombocytopenia, platelet dysfunction, and anticoagulant or procoagulant factors released from tumor cells; this is particularly an issue in acute promyelocytic leukemia.[242] Extramedullary manifestations are uncommon, found in about 10% of children at diagnosis, and they most commonly occur in skin (leukemia cutis), head, neck, brain (leptomeningeal), and spinal cord.[243] When AML is suspected, a bone marrow aspiration and biopsy is diagnostic. Cytogenetic evaluation of leukemic cells in the marrow influences the treatment protocol and estimation of survival.[244]

The goal of induction is remission of leukemic cell burden, for which cytarabine, daunorubicin, and etoposide are standardly used. Compared with ALL induction, AML induction is significantly more intense with a much higher risk of life-threatening complications including infection. Although postinduction remission rates have risen over time to approximately 85% to 90%, treatment-related morbidity and mortality continue to be problematic.[245] Substantial myelosuppression is usual, and supportive care is crucial, including hospitalization through induction therapy and aggressive management of neutropenic infections.[246] Tumor lysis syndrome is also a risk in children with high tumor burden.[247] Up to 4% of children develop early significant cardiomyopathy after daunorubicin or other anthracycline therapy.[248] CNS involvement is present in 10% to 10.30% of children; thus lumbar punctures with intrathecal chemotherapy are routine.[249,250] Like ALL, additional therapy is required after induction to avoid universal relapse of disease. Many treatment protocols use three to four cycles of intensification therapy after induction, which attempt to balance optimal tumor suppression with avoidance of severe toxicity. The role of HSCT in newly diagnosed childhood AML is typically reserved for children with high-risk AML in postremission therapy.[228] Chronic health conditions in survivors of AML are present in 55%, particularly those treated with HSCT.[251] With the high risk of relapse in pediatric AML, many children will then undergo more intensive treatment protocols, including HSCT. Thus these children are at risk for greater morbidity and mortality through this treatment.[252]

Several subtypes of AML are important to mention. Acute promyelocytic leukemia (APL) represents 5% to 10% of AML and is a form of AML in which the predominant cells are promyelocytes with specific mutation to the retinoic acid receptor gene.[253] When APL cells were found to be exquisitely sensitive to all-*trans*-retinoic acid (ATRA) and ATRA was added to treatment protocols, survival in childhood APL improved to approximately 90%, which is significantly better than AML overall.[254] The current therapy for APL omits all chemotherapy other than ATRA and arsenic trioxide; thus the toxicity profile and chronic morbidity are dramatically different than that of other AML therapy. Of note, severe coagulopathy is often present at the time of diagnosis, and the risk of bleeding and thrombosis is multifactorial, in part due to high rates of DIC and hyperleukocytosis.[242,255,256]

Children with Trisomy 21 are at significant risk of myeloid malignancies. De novo AML in Trisomy 21 has an excellent overall survival, allowing reduction of chemotherapy intensity.[257] This lower intensity chemotherapy reduces the risk of treatment-related morbidity seen in children with Trisomy 21 in the past, including a 17% incidence of early, symptomatic cardiomyopathy and 3% mortality from cardiomyopathy.[258] Transient abnormal myelopoiesis (TAM), which is currently classified as a myeloproliferative disorder rather than a myeloid leukemia, is present in at least 4% to 10% of neonates with Trisomy 21. TAM shares some similarities with AML, yet it usually undergoes spontaneous remission. Progressive cases can require chemotherapy to achieve remission and survival. Approximately 16% to 20% of these children will subsequently develop AML after remission of the myelopoietic disorder.[259,260]

Therapy-related AML (t-AML) occurs in 1% to 2% of children treated with chemotherapy or radiotherapy for a malignant or nonmalignant condition, and this subtype represents 10% to 20% of childhood AML. The onset of t-AML occurs 2 to 10 years after exposure to the causative chemotherapy drug. Prognosis is very poor overall, although the use of HSCT in early remission may improve outcomes.[261]

Perioperative Considerations
As in ALL, children with AML present soon after their diagnosis is confirmed for a surgically placed central venous access and serial bone marrow aspirates and lumbar punctures. Newly diagnosed children should be screened for hyperleukocytosis, retinoic acid syndrome, an anterior mediastinal mass, and the

sequelae of pancytopenia. Because anthracycline chemotherapeutics are routine during AML therapy, the presence of cardiomyopathy must be assessed, and serial echocardiograms should be performed throughout the treatment. Aseptic technique should always be observed. In children with mucositis, care should be taken during laryngoscopy to minimize any trauma to friable oral mucosal tissue. Indiscriminant use of parenteral steroids should be avoided, especially before the diagnosis and treatment determination, as it may (1) cause tissue necrosis impairing diagnosis, (2) cause tumor lysis syndrome, and (3) affect the treatment randomization. Additional detailed anesthetic considerations are discussed in detail in Chapter 11, including recommendations for those with cardiomyopathy and post-HSCT.

HODGKIN LYMPHOMA
Hodgkin lymphoma (HL) is the eighth most common pediatric cancer and constitutes 40% to 50% of all pediatric lymphoma cases. In economically advantaged countries, the incidence of HL has a bimodal age distribution, with the first peak between 15 and 35 years and the second after the age of 55 years. As such, infantile HL is rare, but the steady rise in incidence with age leads to HL being the most common childhood cancer among 15- to 19-year-olds. Onset of disease in earlier childhood is more prevalent in developing countries.[207,262,263] Survival rates for pediatric HL are excellent; 5-year survival exceeds 97% in the United States.[207] Because of excellent survival, the current focus of treatment protocols has shifted to minimizing lifelong morbidity while maintaining these survival rates.[264,265]

Pathophysiology
HL is a B-cell lineage malignancy characterized by clonal proliferation of malignant Hodgkin/Reed-Sternberg (HRS) cells. The HRS cells accumulate within lymph nodes and other lymphatic tissues and are joined by a significant infiltrate of variable inflammatory cells, which constitute 99% of the tumor volume.[266] Established risk factors for childhood HL include immunodeficiency states, infection with Epstein-Barr virus (EBV), and family history of HL. Depending on age of diagnosis and geographic location, up to 40% to 50% of pediatric HL cases are associated with latent EBV infection, as determined by EBV[+] tumor cells.[267,268] HL is subclassified into classical HL and nodular lymphocyte predominant HL; although the prevalence of each subtype varies across age groups, classical HL constitutes approximately 80% to 90% of pediatric cases and has slightly less favorable outcomes compared with the nodular lymphocyte predominant subclass.[269]

Clinical and Laboratory Features and Treatment
Splenomegaly and painless lymphadenopathy of the cervical, supraclavicular, axillary, and occasionally inguinal lymph nodes are the presenting signs in 80% of children. Mediastinal involvement is common; 55% to 65% have a mediastinal mass with the possibility of cardiopulmonary compromise (see also Chapter 15), and 5% have pericardial involvement with the possibility of effusion at presentation. Up to 10% of children present with constitutional "B" symptoms, which include fever, drenching night sweats, and weight loss greater than 10% within 6 months before diagnosis. The presence of B symptoms has important implications for staging and prognosis.[270–272] Laboratory evaluation at diagnosis is often nonspecific, including leukocytosis, lymphopenia, eosinophilia, and monocytosis. RBC and platelet counts are usually normal except in the setting of severe metastatic disease. However,

immune suppression is often already present at the time of diagnosis.[271]

Diagnostic evaluation includes physical examination and imaging studies. A chest x-ray rapidly screens for mediastinal disease, and CT of the neck, chest, abdomen, and pelvis evaluates the extent of adenopathy. Diagnostic staging and interim assessment with positron emission tomography (PET) is increasingly used.[273] Definitive diagnosis requires an excisional lymph node biopsy because it provides the only means to obtain the scarce HRS cells for histologic confirmation.[274]

The treatment protocol depends on the child's risk stratification from the biopsy and imaging studies. Decades ago, treatment protocols with high-dose radiation therapy and chemotherapy led to excessive chronic toxicity in survivors of childhood HL. Current strategies focus on less toxic combined modality therapy that includes low doses of multiple chemotherapeutics and low-dose or even elimination of radiation therapy.[274,275] When used, the low-dose involved field radiation administered in pediatric HL is usually well tolerated, and most acute affects are transient and reversible.[275] Outcomes in relapsed HL remain favorable, and as such, children with low-risk relapse can often be cured with conventional-dose chemotherapy and radiation therapy. However, high-risk relapse often requires high-dose chemotherapy and HSCT.[276]

Perioperative Considerations

Excisional lymph node biopsy and long-term central venous access are usually performed with the patient under anesthesia soon after presentation. At least two-thirds of children will have mediastinal lymphadenopathy at diagnosis, and one-half of those will have a symptomatic anterior mediastinal mass larger than 30% of the cardiac silhouette,[270,272,277] which places them at risk of death during anesthesia.[278] Any child with significant lymphadenopathy should be suspected of having a lymphoma and be assessed for the presence of an anterior mediastinal mass before beginning anesthesia, as discussed in Chapters 11 and 15. With large, compressive mediastinal masses, the risks of general anesthesia even for minor procedures such as excisional node biopsy may warrant that the procedure be performed with the patient under local anesthesia with or without sedation.

Although chemotherapy protocols vary, most patients will be treated with a four- to seven-drug combination of a vinca alkaloid (e.g., vincristine), anthracycline (e.g., doxorubicin), bleomycin, cyclophosphamide, corticosteroid, methotrexate, procarbazine, and etoposide, as well as possible radiation therapy.[279] Thus, significant myelosuppression and toxicities of therapy may occur during treatment. Children who receive bleomycin are at risk for developing pulmonary dysfunction and acute respiratory failure, particularly after high concentrations of oxygen. Recent evidence has questioned the role of oxygen in the pathogenesis of bleomycin-induced lung injury, and the risk in children has never been confirmed (see also Chapter 11).[280–282] Among survivors of childhood cancer, those with HL have one of the greatest burdens of chronic disease, especially those treated with both chemotherapy and radiation. The rate of cardiac disease during and after treatment with anthracyclines and chest radiation is of particular concern, and survivors must be screened for cardiac disease; however, most cardiac-related mortality does not occur until years later.[283–286] As usual, attention to sterile technique, awareness of possible friability of oral mucosal tissue during laryngoscopy, and indiscriminant use of parenteral steroids should be avoided. Additional detailed anesthetic considerations are discussed in Chapter 11.

NON-HODGKIN LYMPHOMA

Non-Hodgkin lymphoma (NHL) accounts for 7% of all childhood cancers, making it the fifth most common pediatric cancer. NHL is rarely diagnosed in infancy, and the incidence increases steadily through each year of childhood. There is a clear male predominance, especially in the preadolescent age group. Among the lymphomas, NHL is more common in children younger than 10 years of age, and HL is more common in those older than 10 years. The 5-year survival of children from birth to age 19 years at diagnosis of NHL is 87%, which is considerably less than HL and nearly identical to ALL.[207]

Pathophysiology

NHL is a heterogeneous group of neoplasms that derive from lymphocyte B-cell progenitors, T-cell progenitors, mature B cells, or mature T cells and accumulate predominantly in lymph nodes and lymphoid tissues. However, up to 40% of NHL tumors arise in nonlymphatic extranodal tissues, which may create a diagnostic challenge.[287,288] Compared with HL, NHL is both a more systemic malignancy that disseminates from lymphoid tissues to extranodal tissues (and vice versa, and aggressive at the time of diagnosis.[274,289] Multiple subtypes of NHL occur in children, the most common being Burkitt lymphoma, lymphoblastic T-cell or B-cell lymphoma, diffuse large B-cell lymphoma, and anaplastic large cell lymphoma; other subtypes are rare.[274,290] A congenital or acquired immunodeficiency state is the leading risk factor for the development of NHL, which include Wiskott-Aldrich syndrome, ataxia telangiectasia, X-linked lymphoproliferative syndrome, AIDS, and posttransplant or other iatrogenic immunosuppressed states. Inherited conditions, however, predispose less than 2% of pediatric cases.[291,292]

Clinical and Laboratory Features and Treatment

Clinical presentation of NHL is similar to that of HL; most children present with painless but rapidly expanding masses, which can produce a symptomatic mass effect of surrounding tissues and structures. As such, clinical emergencies from compression of vital structures are common in NHL, including an anterior mediastinal mass, spinal cord compression, CNS involvement in 6% of children, pericardial tamponade, thromboembolism, and intestinal intussusception or obstruction.[289,293] The most common sites of primary tumor in all children with NHL are the abdomen, mediastinum, and peripheral lymph nodes, especially of the head and neck.[294] In Burkitt lymphoma, which is the most common form of pediatric NHL, the most common primary sites of disease are the head, neck, and then abdomen; however, tumor masses may also be found in bone, bone marrow, skin, testes, and CNS. Advanced disease with bone marrow and CNS involvement is present in 25% of children.[289,295]

Results of initial laboratory evaluation are variable. The CBC can be normal, but pancytopenia is present when there is extensive marrow invasion. Thrombocytopenia and anemia are signs of splenic sequestration and internal bleeding, respectively. About 20% of children experience tumor lysis syndrome at induction of treatment as a result of the high metabolic rate of rapidly proliferating NHL tumor cells. A significant percentage of these children may require dialysis.[296,297] Initial CT imaging of the neck, chest, abdomen, and pelvis evaluates the extent of disease. Because extranodal spread of noncontiguous tumor is common in childhood NHL, PET scanning has become an integral part of baseline, interim, and posttreatment staging; however, the role of PET to influence treatment protocols remains under investigation.[273,298,299]

MRI scans are usually limited to evaluation of specific tissue involvement, such as bone or brain.[290] Definitive diagnosis is made by pathologic evaluation of a lesion biopsy, and then bilateral bone marrow aspiration and biopsy and CSF cytology provide further disease staging.[289]

Treatment of pediatric NHL is focused on chemotherapy protocols that vary with the subtype of NHL and clinical staging. The advent of targeted therapies, such as rituximab, are playing an increasing role for some subtypes of NHL.[300-302] Overall, treatment cycles of many stages of pediatric NHL are very short, using high-dose pulses of chemotherapy drugs with intensive supportive care. The use of prophylactic radiation therapy has become exceedingly uncommon in pediatric NHL as it risks lifelong toxicity and has not been shown to appreciably improve outcomes in most subtypes. As such, it remains in some therapy protocols only for those with documented CNS involvement at the time of diagnosis or those with incomplete response to chemotherapy.[302-304] The usual sequelae of chemotherapy are seen during treatment, including myelosuppression, infections, mucositis, nausea and vomiting, cardiac toxicity, and neurobehavioral complications.

Perioperative Considerations

Like most pediatric hematologic malignancies, surgery during therapy is mostly limited to the initial diagnostic biopsy, placement of central venous access, and treatment of any complications of therapy. Complete resection of localized tumors is uncommonly indicated, and debulking surgery of large tumor masses is no longer indicated.[305] However, tumor invasion and destruction of the bowel or other vital organs may require urgent surgical attention. Lumbar punctures with cerebrospinal cytology and intrathecal methotrexate may be indicated as prophylaxis in some subtypes of NHL and in children with CNS disease at diagnosis.[289]

The primary anesthetic considerations specific to children with newly diagnosed NHL include anterior mediastinal mass, mass effect of tumor on the upper airway, and tumor lysis syndrome. Because of the considerable risks of anesthesia in the presence of an anterior mediastinal mass, all children with suspected NHL must receive a thorough physiologic and radiographic evaluation prior to anesthesia (see also Chapter 15). NHL lesions of the upper airway may obstruct the airway or bleed during airway management.[306,307] Although tumor lysis syndrome most frequently occurs during chemotherapy induction, it can occur spontaneously, during anesthesia and surgery, or with a dose of corticosteroids.[308] Additional discussion of anterior mediastinal mass, tumor lysis syndrome, and anesthetic considerations not specific to NHL are discussed in detail in Chapter 11.

LANGERHANS CELL HISTIOCYTOSIS

Histiocytic disorders are a group of disorders of "histiocytes," which is an archaic term for dendrocytes, macrophages, and monocytes. Histiocytosis is generally divided into Langerhans cell histiocytosis (LCH) and non-Langerhans histiocytosis. Given the rarity of the non-Langerhans subtypes, the subsequent focus of this section will be on LCH only.

The etiology and epidemiology of LCH remain poorly understood. It is an uncommon and predominantly childhood disorder with an incidence of 4 to 9 cases per million children per year, similar in incidence to Hodgkin lymphoma or AML. The usual age at diagnosis is 1 to 6 years.[208,309-311] The spectrum of childhood LCH ranges from single-system focal lesions to life-threatening multisystem disease. The overall survival rate of the more common

low-risk focal disease is 99%, but high-risk disseminated disease has a survival of approximately 85%.[208,209]

Pathophysiology

LCH is an inflammatory neoplasia of myeloid dendritic cell precursors. Although the etiology is poorly understood, malignant transformation of dendritic cells leads to clonal proliferation and accumulation into lesions. The lesions are accompanied by a host of inflammatory cells that release a local cytokine storm, leading to the symptomatic destruction of surrounding tissues.[312]

Clinical and Laboratory Features and Treatment

Most childhood LCH presents with single-system focal lesions. About 30% of children present with multisystem disease, and this form is most common in the youngest of children.[309,311,313] The lesions can form in any organ system; however, nearly 80% of cases present with lytic bone lesions, followed by papular skin lesions in 40%.[314] Involvement of bone marrow, liver, lung, or spleen portends a poor prognosis. Physical symptoms depend on the site and extent of tissue lesions. Laboratory values are most notable for evidence of an inflammatory state, although anemia is common.[309,311]

LCH can be difficult to diagnose because its clinical presentation is often insidious and representative of a broad differential diagnosis. The exception is in the subset of neonates who present with a rapidly progressive disseminated disease.[208] Biopsy of a lesion, usually skin or bone, confirms the diagnosis. The histology demonstrates LCH cells surrounded by a substantial volume of inflammatory cells. Subsequent radiologic imaging with skeletal survey, CT, and PET confirm the extent of disease and influence the approach to treatment.[315] Unless the liver, spleen, or pituitary gland are directly involved, laboratory analysis is usually normal.

Treatment of childhood LCH is widely variable depending on the extent of disease and organs involved. Isolated bone lesions may be treated with surgical curettage and intralesional steroids with excellent results, but reactivation of disease can occur. Isolated cutaneous disease can be resolved with topical medications only or may regress on its own, but subsequent progression to multisystem disease may be fatal in young children. Thus most children are treated with a combination of steroids and relatively low-dose chemotherapy for 6 to 12 months. Surgical removal of lesions may be indicated in some cases, and radiation is sparingly used for invasion of critical organs or structures (e.g., CNS).[314,316-319]

Perioperative Considerations

Depending on the clinical staging, treatment administered, and presence of disease relapse, 3% to 50% of children will have diabetes insipidus before, during, or especially after treatment.[309,319] Children with polyuria and polydipsia should be fully evaluated prior to elective surgery, and children with previously diagnosed diabetes insipidus should be managed after consultation with the oncology team, as optimal treatment with desmopressin and fluid management varies among children.[320] Chemotherapy protocols are generally less toxic than in other childhood hematologic cancers, and major toxicity is less common. However, liver and lung fibrosis can occur and can be at least mildly symptomatic.[317]

MYELODYSPLASTIC AND MYELOPROLIFERATIVE DISORDERS

Myelodysplastic and myeloproliferative disorders are rare hematologic malignancies that are categorized into three distinct groups: myelodysplastic syndromes (MDS), juvenile myelomonocytic leukemia (JMML), and Trisomy 21–specific diseases. Transient abnormal myelopoiesis of Down syndrome and myeloid leukemia of Trisomy 21 were discussed with AML and are not being discussed here.

The MDSs are a rare form of myeloid malignancy in children, accounting for just 4% of hematologic malignancies in children; the median age at diagnosis is 7 years.[206,210] Recognition of MDS is important because of its frequent evolution to pediatric AML. Five-year survival is variable (approximately 50%) and depends on the disease characteristics.[321] JMML is a rare myeloid malignancy of young children, with an average age of onset at 2 years of age.[206] Approximately 13% of patients with JMML eventually progress to AML.[322] Five-year survival is approximately 40% but specific survival is variable based on disease characteristics.[321]

Pathophysiology

MDSs are clonal hematologic disorders, characterized by abnormal proliferation and differentiation of hematopoietic stem cells. Mutation of hematopoietic stem cells early in the cell line leads to chronic cytopenia of all cell lines but with varying severity, and as such, MDS may appear similar to aplastic anemia or bone marrow failure disorders. MDS is subclassified into three groups: refractory cytopenia, refractory anemia with excess blasts (RAEB), and refractory anemia with excess blasts in transformation (RAEB-t).[206,323] Inherited bone marrow failure syndromes are associated with childhood MDS in 20% of children, including Fanconi anemia, Kostmann syndrome, Shwachman-Diamond syndrome, Diamond-Blackfan anemia, Trisomy 8 mosaicism, familial MDS, and aplastic anemia. Prior chemotherapy and radiation are important acquired factors.[206,322,324]

JMML is also a potentially lethal malignant disorder of myeloid stem cell proliferation, but in this disorder, differentiation and maturation of monocytes is not blocked, leading to isolated monocytosis.[325] Neurofibromatosis type 1 (NF1) is the primary risk factor for JMML; more than 10% of children with JMML have NF1, and another 20% have mutation of the tumor suppressor *NF1* gene.[326]

Clinical and Laboratory Features and Treatment

Children presenting with MDS are typically pancytopenic, and hepatosplenomegaly is very common.[322] Initial treatment is dependent on the severity of cytopenia. Some children, especially those with refractory cytopenia or mild RAEB, have mild disease for months or even years with only infrequent need for blood transfusions, while others present with severe disease. Regardless of presentation, progression is inevitable and the only cure for MDS is HSCT. Recent data suggest that outcomes improve in children who do not receive pre-HSCT chemotherapy and who advance to HSCT shortly after diagnosis.[327,328] Preconditioning regimen-related mortality and HSCT-related mortality are high, and survival rates in children who relapse after HSCT are dismal.[206]

In children with JMML, anemia, thrombocytopenia, and monocytosis are seen on initial laboratory studies; RBC evaluation demonstrates Hgb F in a majority of children.[322,325] Clinical presentation usually includes fever, respiratory symptoms, skin rash, adenopathy, and hepatosplenomegaly, which may be severe in advanced disease. Peripheral blood tests can confirm the diagnosis, but bone marrow studies are usually performed.[329] The clinical course can be rapidly progressive or indolent; regardless, JMML is resistant to treatment with chemotherapy, and without HSCT, survival is short with only 6% surviving 10 years.[330] Thus all patients are treated with HSCT. Despite advances in HSCT and supportive care, half of these children will not survive 5 years, and within that time period, up to 15% will progress to AML.[331]

Perioperative Considerations

Anesthetic considerations for children with MDS or JMML are similar to those discussed previously for children with AML. As most of these children will undergo HSCT, Chapter 11 details the anesthetic considerations for children before and after HSCT.

ANNOTATED REFERENCES

Allen CE, Kelly KM, Bollard CM. Pediatric lymphomas and histiocytic disorders of childhood. *Pediatr Clin North Am.* 2015;62(1):139-165.
This review article summarizes the biology, treatment, and complications of pediatric lymphomas and histiocytic disorders.

Cooper SL, Brown PA. Treatment of pediatric acute lymphoblastic leukemia. *Pediatr Clin North Am.* 2015;62(1):61-73.
This review article summarizes the risk stratification, treatment, and complications of pediatric ALL.

Guzzetta NA, Miller BE. Principles of hemostasis in children: models and maturation. *Paediatr Anaesth.* 2011;21:3-9.
This review article summarizes the fundamentals of hemostasis and highlights the differences in thrombosis and coagulopathy from the preterm neonate through childhood. The impact of disease states on hemostasis is also discussed.

Key NS, Derebail VK. Sickle-cell trait: novel clinical significance. *Hematology.* 2010;2010:418-422.
This review discusses sickle cell trait as a risk factor for adverse outcomes, focusing on its impact on exercise, renal function, and venous thromboembolism.

Latham GJ, Greenberg RS. Anesthetic considerations for the pediatric oncology patient—part 1: a review of antitumor therapy. *Paediatr Anaesth.* 2010;20:295-304.
This article briefly reviews the current principles of cancer therapy and the general mechanisms of toxicity to the child, focusing on the impact to perioperative care and decision-making.

Latham GJ, Greenberg RS. Anesthetic considerations for the pediatric oncology patient—part 2: systems-based approach to anesthesia. *Paediatr Anaesth.* 2010;20:396-420.
A systems-based approach is used to assess the impact of the tumor and its treatment on children, and relevant anesthetic considerations are discussed.

Morley SL. Red blood cell transfusions in acute paediatrics. *Arch Dis Child Educ Pract Ed* 2009;94:65-73.
The risks and benefits of blood product transfusion in children are considered on the basis of current evidence from adult and pediatric studies.

Vichinsky EP, Haberkern CM, Neumayr L, et al. A comparison of conservative and aggressive transfusion regimens in the perioperative management of sickle cell disease. The Preoperative Transfusion in Sickle Cell Disease Study Group. *N Engl J Med.* 1995;333:206-213.
This multicenter study found that a conservative transfusion regimen was as effective as the aggressive strategy in patients with sickle cell disease, and the conservative regimen resulted in one-half as many transfusion-associated complications.

A complete reference list can be found online at ExpertConsult.com.

11 Perioperative Management of the Oncology Patient

FAITH J. ROSS AND GREGORY J. LATHAM

ALTHOUGH CHILDHOOD CANCER is not particularly common, it is the second most common cause of death in children younger than 15 years of age.[1,2] The most common malignancies affecting children are different from those affecting adults. Leukemia, brain tumors, lymphomas, and sarcomas of tissue and bone are the most common pediatric cancers and account for over 50% of all pediatric malignancies (Table 11.1). Embryonal tumors (e.g., neuroblastoma, Wilms tumor, retinoblastoma, medulloblastoma) are unique to early childhood, which underscores the need for these children to be cared for in pediatric centers with sufficient expertise in their management. Survival rates for most pediatric cancers have improved significantly in the past several decades; more than 80% of children diagnosed with a childhood malignancy will become 5-year survivors of their cancers,[3,4] and 5-year survival rates for acute lymphoblastic leukemia (ALL) have now increased to nearly 90%.[5] The great improvements in survival for many malignancies of childhood are directly related to advances in diagnostic modalities and the large percentage of children treated in cooperative clinical trial protocols.[5,6] Treatment options in these protocols include chemotherapy, radiation therapy, biologic modifiers, hematopoietic stem cell transplantation (HSCT), and adoptive T-cell therapies.

Children with cancer typically undergo many surgical procedures that require anesthesia. The procedures may occur before or during the cancer therapy, years into remission, or during terminal stages of the disease. Certain considerations apply to this population, including the direct effects of the tumor, effects of the chemotherapy and radiation therapy, impact of the surgical procedure, pain syndromes, and psychological vulnerabilities of the child and family. Children undergoing active treatment for cancer range from gravely ill to relatively healthy with excellent functional capacity. Survivors of childhood cancer experience various long-term and often debilitating sequelae after completion of cancer therapy. In one report, 62% of survivors of childhood cancer reported at least one chronic health condition from cancer, and 28% reported a severe or life-threatening condition.[4] These chronic health conditions may impact nearly every organ system and have considerable bearing on any anesthetic plan years into remission. The field of pediatric oncology is extensive, complicated, and ever-changing. Multidisciplinary communication in the perioperative period is crucial to ensure the safe care of these complex patients.

Principles of Cancer Therapy

Most pediatric cancers are treated with an aggressive multimodal approach that may include surgical resection, radiation therapy, and chemotherapy for control of local and metastatic disease. Equally important is supportive care to ensure minimization of toxicity from the tumor and treatment therapy, including nutritional, emotional, and psychological support. A brief review of these therapies with pertinence to the perioperative period follows,

TABLE 11.1	Incidence of Pediatric Cancer by Age				
	INCIDENCE (%) BY AGE GROUP				
Type of Cancer	0–4 years	5–9 years	10–14 years	15–19 years	0–19 years
Leukemias	36.1	33.4	21.8	12.4	25.2
Central nervous system tumors	16.6	27.7	19.6	9.5	16.7
Lymphomas	3.9	12.9	20.6	25.1	15.5
Carcinomas and other malignant epithelial tumors	0.9	2.5	8.9	20.9	9.2
Soft tissue sarcomas	5.6	7.5	9.1	8.0	7.4
Germ cell, trophoblastic, and other gonadal tumors	3.3	2.0	5.3	13.9	7.0
Malignant bone tumors	0.6	4.6	11.3	7.7	5.6
Sympathetic nervous system tumors	14.3	2.7	1.2	0.5	5.4
Renal tumors	9.7	5.4	1.1	0.6	4.4
Retinoblastoma	6.3	0.5	0.1	0.0	2.1
Hepatic tumors	2.2	0.4	0.6	0.6	1.1
Other and unspecified malignant neoplasms	0.5	0.3	0.6	0.8	0.6

From Latham CJ, Greenberg RS. Anesthetic considerations for the pediatric oncology patient—part 1: a review of antitumor therapy. *Pediatr Anesth.* 2010;20:295–304. Used with permission.

but additional sources are available concerning the current indications, side effects, and precautions of the available chemotherapeutic drugs.[7–9]

CONVENTIONAL CHEMOTHERAPEUTICS

Conventional chemotherapeutics, along with radiation therapy, have been the mainstay of pediatric antitumor treatment for decades. In the modern era of multidrug combination chemotherapy, molecularly targeted therapies, radiation therapy, rescue therapies, and HSCT, anticipation of precise toxicities from any given therapy in an individual patient is difficult. However, treatment protocols include a potentially vast array of antitumor agents with widely divergent mechanisms of action and toxicity profiles, and the average child with cancer will be at risk for focal or widespread toxicity to nearly every organ system.[10] Most chemotherapeutic agents are cytotoxic to rapidly dividing cells via several mechanisms. Because these agents lack specificity to tumor cells alone, the impact to healthy tissues is unavoidable and often limits effective chemotherapy dosing schedules. Concurrent administration of several chemotherapeutics with non-overlapping toxicity profiles and at lower doses lessens the additive toxicity while also increasing the simultaneous cytotoxic attack on tumor cells.[11] Regardless, bone marrow suppression, immunosuppression, myocardial toxicity, pulmonary toxicity, and dysfunction of nearly every other organ system are possible in children with cancer[12] and must be thoroughly considered when evaluating and caring for these children. These toxicities range from short-term to lifelong effects.

Several chemotherapeutic agents are of specific interest to the anesthesiologist caring for a child with cancer. Anthracycline chemotherapeutics (e.g., doxorubicin, daunorubicin, idarubicin, and epirubicin) and mitoxantrone cause cardiomyopathy in a dose-dependent fashion, an effect exacerbated by mediastinal irradiation. L-Asparaginase is associated with a 1% to 2% risk of hemorrhage or thrombosis owing to deficiencies in fibrinogen, plasminogen, antithrombin III, and von Willebrand factor, as well as hepatic dysfunction and acute hemorrhagic pancreatitis.[13–15] Bleomycin may cause acute pneumonitis with progression to pulmonary fibrosis.[16] Cisplatin and ifosfamide may cause renal tubular damage that can lead to Fanconi syndrome with electrolyte wasting.[17,18] In large doses, methotrexate (>1 g/m²) may cause renal failure.[19,20] Corticosteroids may be directly cytotoxic to some hematopoietic tumors by inducing apoptosis, as well as causing adrenal suppression, hypertension, thromboembolism, and obesity. Specific toxicities of chemotherapeutic agents pertinent to anesthesia are discussed in detail below; Table 11.2 provides a brief list of major toxicities of the traditional chemotherapy agents. E-Table 11.1 provides a comprehensive list of traditional chemotherapeutic agents, molecularly targeted agents, and adjuvant medications used in children, with their corresponding toxicities.

Several non-chemotherapy adjunct medications and therapies are used to provide supportive care and to attenuate the toxicities of chemotherapy. With adequate treatment of toxic adverse effects, larger doses and/or additional chemotherapeutic agents can enhance the rate of remission. Such therapies include antiemetics, hematopoietic growth factors, HSCT, transfusion of blood products, and a number of medications that lessen or block organ-specific toxicity. Many of these therapies also pose acute and chronic risks to children; these risks must be balanced against their benefits.[11]

TARGETED ANTITUMOR AGENTS

Commensurate with the growing understanding of cancer biology is the recent development of "targeted" strategies that are directed specifically at cancer cells and thus limit direct toxicity to healthy cells. A commonly known example of these types of agents is the use of tyrosine kinase inhibitors (e.g., imatinib) in BCR-ABL (Philadelphia chromosome)–positive leukemia. As a result of less toxicity, oncologists can combine targeted therapies with full-dose standard chemotherapy for improved outcomes.[21–23] Targeted agents include antiangiogenic therapies, immunomodulatory therapies, gene therapies, and humanized antibodies.[23,24] Monoclonal antibodies are targeted to specific, unique tumor cell surface antigenic proteins. Small-molecule drugs, which are designed to target specific genetic signatures and biologic pathways critical to cancer growth and progression, have been developed that target tumor cell apoptotic pathways, histone deacetylation, protein farnesyl-transferases, proteasome action, angiogenesis, and inhibition of the epidermal growth factor receptor tyrosine kinase.[21,23,25]

Although toxicities of these agents as a whole appear to be far less than those of traditional chemotherapeutic agents, rash, fatigue, alterations to skeletal growth plates (antiangiogenic agents), nausea, diarrhea, hypotension, and anaphylaxis have been reported.[26] The use of investigational and novel targeted antitumor agents amplifies the importance of reviewing cases with the oncologist.

RADIATION THERAPY

One quarter of all children newly diagnosed with cancer will require radiation as frontline therapy.[27] Photons (e.g., x-rays) and particle radiation (e.g., electrons, protons, neutrons) are the two major types of ionizing beam radiation. Regardless of the

TABLE 11.2	Therapy-Related Adverse Effects and Toxicity
Drug	**Adverse Effects**
L-Asparaginase	Hyperglycemia, hypersensitivity, hepatic dysfunction (secondary hypoalbuminemia and coagulopathies), pancreatitis, thrombosis, stroke
Bischloroethyl nitrosourea (BCNU)	Encephalopathy, hepatotoxicity, pulmonary toxicity
Bleomycin	Anaphylactoid reactions, fever, hyperpigmentation, nausea, vomiting, oxygen toxicity, pulmonary fibrosis
Busulfan	Encephalopathy, hepatotoxicity, pulmonary toxicity
Carboplatin	Myelosuppression, nausea, vomiting, nephrotoxicity, neurotoxicity, ototoxicity
Cisplatin	Nausea/vomiting, nephrotoxicity, ototoxicity, peripheral neuropathy
Corticosteroids	Adrenal suppression, avascular necrosis, cataracts, edema, gastritis, hyperglycemia, hypertension, myopathy, osteoporosis, obesity, osteopenia, tumor lysis syndrome, tumor necrosis, psychosis
Cyclophosphamide (Cytoxan)	Cardiotoxicity, hemorrhagic cystitis, myelosuppression, nausea, vomiting, syndrome of inappropriate secretion of antidiuretic hormone (SIADH)
Cyclosporine	Cortical blindness, electrolyte disturbances, encephalopathy, gingival hyperplasia, hemolytic uremia, hepatotoxicity, hyperlipidemia, hypertension, hirsutism, myositis, paresthesias, tremor
Cytarabine	Myelosuppression, mucositis, hepatitis, nausea/vomiting, neurotoxicity
Dactinomycin (Actinomycin D)	Nausea/vomiting, mucositis, myelosuppression, radiation recall?[a]
Daunorubicin (Daunomycin) Doxorubicin (Adriamycin) Idarubicin (Idamycin)	Cardiomyopathy, mucositis, myelosuppression, red-orange urine
Etoposide	Hypotension, mucositis, myelosuppression, nausea, vomiting
Ifosfamide	Hemorrhagic cystitis, myelosuppression, nephrotoxicity, neurotoxicity
Melphalan	Mucositis
Methotrexate	Hepatotoxicity, mucositis, myelosuppression, renal failure, neurotoxicity
Mercaptopurine (6-MP)	Hepatotoxicity, myelosuppression
Mycophenolate mofetil (CellCept)	Electrolyte disturbance, gastrointestinal toxicity, hypercholesterolemia, myelosuppression, rash
Procarbazine	Myelosuppression
Sirolimus	Hyperlipidemia, myelosuppression
Tacrolimus (Prograf)	Anemia, anorexia, back pain, encephalopathy, diarrhea, hyperglycemia, nephrotoxicity, pleural effusion, rash
Thiotepa	Neurotoxicity, mucositis
Thioguanine (6-TG)	Hepatotoxicity, myelosuppression
Total body irradiation	Dental/bony maldevelopment, gastrointestinal toxicity, hepatotoxicity, pulmonary toxicity
Vinblastine (Velban)	Myelosuppression, neurotoxicity, SIADH
Vincristine (Oncovin)	Neurotoxicity, SIADH

[a]Radiation recall: the "recalling" by skin of previous radiation exposure in response to the administration of certain response-inducing drugs.
Modified from Carpenter PA, Mielcarek M, Woolfrey AE. Hematopoietic cell transplantation. In: Irwin S, Rippe JM, eds. *Intensive Care Medicine*. 6th ed. Philadelphia: Lippincott Williams & Wilkins; 2008:2150–2168.

particle source, ionizing radiation leads to cell death by damaging cellular DNA. Toxicity from the effects of radiation therapy to surrounding healthy tissues is unavoidable, and the developing tissues of children are particularly susceptible to the acute and late effects of irradiation. The susceptibility of normal tissues depends on the total and fractional dose received, the inherent sensitivity of the tissue to the dose of radiation, the volume of tissue irradiated, and time course of treatment (Table 11.3).[28] Overall, normal host cells have a greater capacity to repair the damaging effects of radiation than cancer cells but require time to recover. To allow sufficient time for the healthy tissue to repair, the total dose of radiation is usually divided into a series of fractional doses over time.[29] Recent technological advances have led to three-dimensional conformal radiotherapy, which closely conforms the radiation dose to the tumor shape and minimizes radiation to the surrounding tissues.[30–32] Despite these advances to reduce the toxicity of radiation therapy to healthy tissues, children remain at risk for acute and chronic complications. Furthermore, concurrent chemotherapy may potentiate the radiation toxicity, increasing the tissue damage.

Proton radiation therapy (PRT) is a newer modality in pediatric radiation oncology and has become an established alternative to traditional photon therapy; however, PRT centers remain relatively uncommon (two dozen in the United States in 2016 [http://www.proton-therapy.org/map.htm]), which limits rapid access to frontline PRT for many children worldwide. In contrast to the destructive impact to all tissues in the path of a traditional photon beam, the specifically charged velocities of the proton beams are targeted to the calculated depth and shape of the tumor. By modulating the energy of the proton beam to become maximally energized at a specific depth of tissue, the relative dose to the healthy tissues in the plane of entry is as low as 20% to 30%, increases to 100% at the depth of tumor, and then decays to nearly no further penetration beyond the tumor (Fig. 11.1).[33] As such, the advantages of PRT include limited damage to healthy tissues surrounding the tumor and enhanced cell killing of the

TABLE 11.3	Late Effects of Radiation Therapy	
Radiation Field	Late Effects	Risk Factors
Cranial	Neurocognitive deficits	>18 Gy, IV/IT methotrexate
	Leukoencephalopathy	>18 Gy with IT methotrexate
	Growth hormone deficiency	>18 Gy
	Panhypopituitarism	>40 Gy
	Large vessel stroke	>60 Gy
	Second cancers	Variable
	Dental problems	>10 Gy
	Cataracts	>2–8 Gy single dose, 10–15 Gy fractionated dose
	Ototoxicity	>35–50 Gy
Chest	**Cardiac disease**	
	Coronary artery disease	>30 Gy
	Cardiomyopathy	>35 Gy, >25 Gy with anthracyclines
	Valvular disease	>40 Gy
	Pericardial disease	>35 Gy
	Arrhythmias	Unknown
	Thyroid disease	
	Hypothyroidism	>20 Gy local, >7.5 Gy TBI
	Hyperthyroidism	>20 Gy local, >7.5 Gy TBI
	Thyroid nodules, cancer	Any dose
	Pulmonary disease	
	Pulmonary fibrosis	>15–20 Gy
	Restrictive lung disease	Unknown
	Obstructive lung disease	Unknown
Abdomen/ Pelvis	Chronic enteritis	>40 Gy
	Gastrointestinal malignancy	Unknown
	Hepatic fibrosis/cirrhosis	>30 Gy
	Renal insufficiency	>20 Gy
	Bladder disease	
	Fibrosis	>30 Gy prepubertal, >50 postpubertal
	Hemorrhagic cystitis	Enhances cyclophosphamide and ifosfamide effect
	Bladder cancer	Unknown
	Gonadal dysfunction	
	Ovarian failure	4–12 Gy
	Testicular failure	>1–6 Gy
Any Radiation	Skin cancer	
	Musculoskeletal changes	
	Bone length discrepancy	>20 Gy
	Pathologic fractures	>40 Gy
TBI	All the above	

Gy, gray; *IT*, intrathecal; *IV*, intravenous; *TBI*, total body irradiation.
From Latham GJ, Greenberg RS. Anesthetic considerations for the pediatric oncology patient—part 1: a review of antitumor therapy. *Pediatr Anesth.* 2010;20:295–304. Used with permission.

targeted tumor tissues.[34] Despite these beneficial physical properties, the overall advantage of PRT over conventional radiation therapy is not yet uniformly supported by clinical trials, randomized pediatric trials are lacking, and long-term outcomes are yet to be realized.[27,35–38] However, there are recent reports suggesting decreased neurotoxicity, improved health-related quality of life, and reduced neuroendocrine deficits with PRT compared with historical data with conventional photon radiation therapy.[36–39]

Preoperative Considerations by Organ System

AIRWAY

Though primary tumors of the airway are rare in children,[40] various cancer treatment regimens can cause airway changes that challenge the anesthesiologist. Both chemotherapy and radiation treatment can cause mucositis and xerostomia, first appearing soon after initiating treatment.[41,42] Severe mucositis causes painful and friable oral mucosa and may threaten the airway as a result of pseudo-membrane formation, supraglottic edema, bleeding, or aspiration of blood and secretions.[43,44] Graft-versus-host disease (GVHD) after HSCT may also cause significant mucositis, with up to 30% of those children developing a difficult airway.[44] Chronic radiation therapy to the head and neck may cause fibrosis, which distorts facial tissues and renders them less mobile.[45] Children who have undergone chronic radiation therapy may present a challenge during laryngoscopy, with difficult glottic visualization, poor laryngeal mask airway seal, and subglottic stenosis.[45,46]

Anesthesiologists caring for children who have undergone chemotherapy, HSCT, or radiation therapy should perform a thorough preoperative airway history and physical examination focusing on symptoms of airway compromise, prior anesthetic history, visualization of oral mucosa, and external assessment of the degree of distortion and immobility of face and neck tissues.

CARDIAC

Primary cardiac tumors are uncommon in children, but when they occur (e.g., in children with tuberous sclerosis), they are usually benign and resolve spontaneously.[47] However, cancer-related compromise of the cardiovascular system may occur and includes the effects of chemotherapy and/or radiation-induced treatment, pericarditis, and anterior mediastinal masses.

Anthracycline chemotherapeutic agents (doxorubicin, daunorubicin, idarubicin, and epirubicin) as well as the unrelated agent mitoxantrone, are well known for their cardiotoxic effects.[48,49] Cyclophosphamide, fluorouracil, vinca alkaloids, cytarabine, cladribine, L-asparaginase, paclitaxel, trastuzumab, etoposide, teniposide, and pentostatin have also been associated with cardiac toxicity.[49,50] Anthracycline toxicity primarily affects the myocardium, leading to cardiomyopathy and arrhythmias. Acute or subacute toxicity presents with symptoms ranging from only electrocardiographic (ECG) changes to fulminant heart failure shortly after the initial dose. Most children recover from acute toxicity with supportive therapy. Chronic progressive dilated or restrictive cardiomyopathy may develop within a year of treatment. The onset of symptoms can be delayed, and children may present with cardiac failure 20 or more years after treatment.[51–53] Overall, one in eight survivors of childhood cancer who received both anthracyclines and chest radiation develop a serious, chronic cardiac disease.[54] The risk of cardiotoxicity increases with increasing anthracycline doses, especially when the cumulative dose exceeds

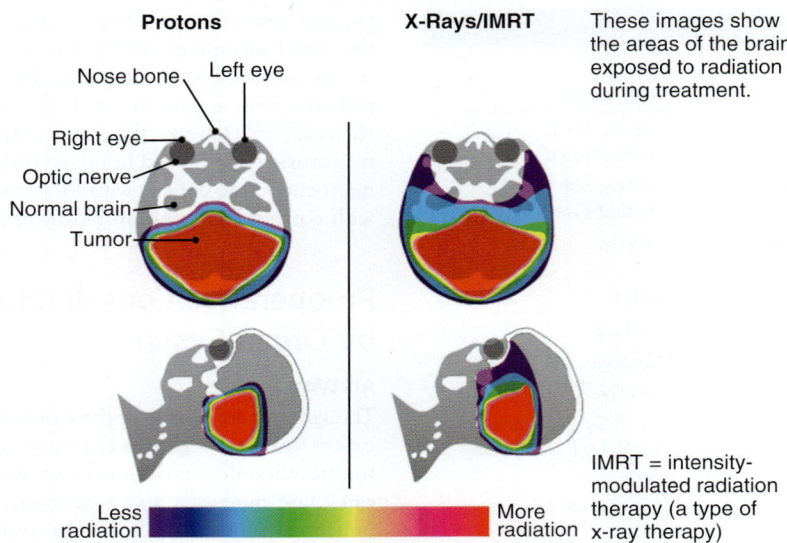

FIGURE 11.1 Rendering of the difference between photon (x-ray) and proton beam therapies for posterior fossa radiation. As radiation passes from posterior to anterior, the entry dose of radiation to healthy tissues of the posterior skull is similar. However, the exit radiation dose is markedly different: the protons lose their energy at a calculated depth, resulting in no radiation to sensitive tissues beyond the tumor (eyes, pituitary, and so on). (From SCCA Proton Therapy Center, Seattle, WA. Used with permission.)

250 to 360 mg/m^2.[53] However, there is no "safe" threshold dose for anthracyclines, as doses less than 240 mg/m^2 have resulted in cardiac damage.[55] Preventative measures include the use of newer anthracycline analogs, antioxidants, iron chelators, and alterations in the dose.[51] The cardiotoxic effects of chemotherapy are significantly compounded (perhaps tripled) by concurrent chest irradiation.[53,54,56]

Unlike anthracycline toxicity that primarily affects the myocardium, radiation therapy can damage all components of the cardiovascular system. Complications from mediastinal radiation include cardiomyopathy, pericardial effusions, pericarditis, valvular fibrosis, conduction disturbances, and accelerated arteriosclerosis.[51,56] Radiation-related myocardial fibrosis can induce a progressive restrictive cardiomyopathy, leading to pulmonary vascular disease and pulmonary hypertension. Systolic and/or diastolic dysfunction may be present. Premature arteriosclerosis affects the coronary arteries as well as the carotid arteries, pulmonary arteries, renal arteries, and aorta.[54] Fatal myocardial infarction has been reported in children 6 to 22 years of age after mediastinal radiation.[57] Valvular heart disease is predominately characterized by progressive mitral and aortic stenosis and insufficiency. Conduction disturbances range from atrial and ventricular arrhythmias, to right bundle branch block, and occasionally complete heart block requiring pacemaker placement. Radiation damage to autonomic nerves in proximity to the heart can result in tachycardia and loss of phasic respiratory variability similar to a denervated heart. Autonomic denervation can attenuate the perception of anginal pain, so providers should have a low threshold for suspicion of myocardial ischemia in those who have undergone mediastinal radiotherapy in infancy and childhood. With low doses of radiation (<25-30 Gy), short-term radiation toxicity is limited, but late toxicity occurs even at these low doses.[54,56,58,59]

Symptomatic acute heart failure after cardiotoxic cancer therapy is uncommon in childhood; however, the potential for cardiovascular compromise in the setting of major surgical stress and anesthesia should be considered. Children who have undergone cardiotoxic chemotherapy or mediastinal radiation should be examined preoperatively for clinical evidence of impaired cardiac function or arrhythmia, including history and physical examination, chest radiography, and ECG. A preoperative or recent echocardiographic evaluation is recommended for the children receiving the following[60]:

- Cumulative anthracycline dose >240 mg/m^2
- Any dose of anthracycline during infancy
- Chest irradiation >40 Gy (or >30 Gy with concomitant anthracycline treatment)
- Unknown doses of chemotherapy and radiation

ANTERIOR MEDIASTINAL MASS

Children with Hodgkin or non-Hodgkin lymphoma often have mediastinal involvement at the time of diagnosis, and half have respiratory symptoms.[61] Less common oncologic causes of anterior mediastinal mass include neuroblastoma, germ cell tumors, and ALL.[62] These children may require anesthesia for biopsy or resection of the mass, intravenous line placement, or radiologic procedures.

Children with clinical findings of superior vena cava syndrome or airway compression from anterior mediastinal mass are at the greatest risk for life-threatening perioperative complications (Table 11.4). Symptoms of orthopnea, upper body edema, stridor, nighttime cough, the need to sleep on one preferred side or position, or wheezing should alert the anesthesiologist of the need for further evaluation. Radiographic or ultrasound evidence of airway or great vessel compression, pulmonary artery outflow obstruction, ventricular dysfunction, or pericardial effusion are particularly concerning findings that necessitate a discussion about the utility of preoperative treatment to reduce the size of the mass.[63] Pretreatment is controversial because either corticosteroids or radiation may alter the tumor histology by causing tumor necrosis and render the precise diagnosis more difficult. However, diagnosis may still be possible in 95% of children after a 5-day course of

TABLE 11.4	Strongest Risk Factors for Acute Perioperative Cardiorespiratory Complications in Children With an Anterior Mediastinal Mass
Clinical signs and symptoms	
Orthopnea	
Upper body edema (signs of SVCS)	
Stridor	
Wheeze	
Night cough	
Sleeping in odd or only one position	
Diagnostic imaging findings	
Tracheal, bronchial, or carinal compression	
Great vessel compression	
SVC obstruction	
Pulmonary artery outflow obstruction	
Ventricular dysfunction	
Pericardial effusion	

SVC, superior vena cava; *SVCS,* superior vena cava syndrome.
From Latham GJ, Greenberg RS. Anesthetic considerations for the pediatric oncology patient—part 2: systems-based approach to anesthesia. *Pediatr Anesth.* 2010;20(5):396–420. Used with permission.

corticosteroids.[64] A multidisciplinary discussion of the risks and benefits with anesthesia, surgery, and oncology will clarify the optimal management for these children.

Anesthetic considerations for children with an anterior mediastinal mass are presented in detail in Chapter 15. In brief, local anesthesia and sedation are preferred. However, if general anesthesia is required, crucial perioperative considerations include maintaining spontaneous ventilation (i.e., avoiding paralysis) and being prepared to secure the airway with a tracheal tube and turn the child to the left lateral decubitus or prone position for resuscitation in the face of cardiopulmonary collapse.[65,66]

PULMONARY

Primary and metastatic lung malignancies are uncommon in children.[67] Pulmonary compromise as a direct effect of pediatric tumors is more often the result of a pleural effusion, pulmonary infiltrates, pulmonary embolus, chylous effusions, anterior mediastinal mass, or hyperleukocytosis-induced pulmonary leukostasis.[68]

Therapy-related symptomatic pulmonary dysfunction or abnormal pulmonary function tests occur in 6% of children treated with chemotherapy alone, 20% treated with both chemotherapy and radiation, and 25% after HSCT.[51] Several chemotherapeutic agents—most notably bleomycin—have the potential to cause acute or chronic lung injury, including pneumonitis, pulmonary fibrosis, or noncardiogenic pulmonary edema.[16,69] Pneumonitis presents insidiously with nonproductive cough, progressive dyspnea, and rales. Although the symptoms usually resolve with completion of the treatment, in some children pneumonitis progresses to irreversible pulmonary disease.[16,70] In adults, bleomycin-induced pneumonitis occurs in up to 46%, with a 3% mortality. The incidence of pneumonitis in children is less well established.[71,72]

Pulmonary fibrosis may present acutely during treatment or as a late sequela of chemotherapy, radiation treatment, or GVHD and may be associated with severe morbidity and mortality.[52] The administration of large concentrations of oxygen to children with bleomycin-induced pulmonary fibrosis can acutely or chronically exacerbate their restrictive lung disease.[73,74] Thus the concentration of inhaled oxygen should be adjusted to the minimum concentration required to ensure adequate tissue oxygen delivery in the perioperative period. Overall, it is important to assess the clinical and functional status of these children for symptomatic or occult pulmonary disease before administering anesthesia.[63] A thorough assessment of baseline pulmonary status is particularly important to assess the need for postoperative ventilatory support or tolerability of thoracoscopy. It is reasonable to seek preoperative pulmonary function testing in those with clinical evidence of pulmonary dysfunction, bearing in mind that formal pulmonary function testing may be a challenge in young children.

RENAL

Wilms tumor is the most common primary renal tumor in children, followed by clear cell sarcoma of the kidney, malignant rhabdoid tumor, congenital mesoblastic nephroma, and renal cell carcinoma.[75,76] Each of these tumors can directly impact renal function. Similarly, extrarenal tumors, such as neuroblastoma, can impact the renal system by infiltrating the kidneys, obstructing urinary flow, or compressing the renal vasculature.[76]

Most chemotherapeutic drugs are directly nephrotoxic in a dose-dependent manner or lead to physiologic conditions that impair renal function (e.g., sepsis, dehydration, tumor lysis syndrome [TLS]). Cisplatin, carboplatin, and ifosfamide are notorious nephrotoxic chemotherapeutic agents in children and adults, especially when combined.[77] Cisplatin causes a dose-dependent nephrotoxicity and hypomagnesemia.[18] Ifosfamide causes subclinical glomerular toxicity in up to 90% of patients, with clinically apparent toxicity occurring in 30%. Ifosfamide can also induce Fanconi syndrome in up to 7% of children, with a delayed presentation possible up to 18 months after therapy.[17,77] Methotrexate has the potential to cause severe acute renal failure in children.[19] Many other chemotherapeutic drugs cause nephrotoxicity at large doses. The syndrome of inappropriate antidiuretic hormone (SIADH) is associated with multiple chemotherapeutic agents. Many non-chemotherapeutic drugs (such as antibiotics and diuretics) commonly used in children with tumors also contribute to nephrotoxicity.[76]

Focal abdominal radiation or total body irradiation as preconditioning for HSCT can cause radiation nephritis, which presents with azotemia, proteinuria, anemia, and hypertension.[78] The cumulative dose that leads to renal damage in children has not been established.[79] After HSCT, the incidence of acute renal failure in children is as great as 40%, with chronic renal failure in 18% to 54%.[80–82]

Anesthesia providers should be aware of the size and location of renal or juxtarenal tumors to determine the risk of significant intraoperative bleeding or great vessel obstruction, particularly in tumors that involve the renal vasculature. Preoperative evaluation of children who have undergone chemotherapy or abdominal radiation treatment should focus on identifying clinical and subclinical renal dysfunction, electrolyte disturbances (hypomagnesia, hypophosphatemia), fluid overload, anemia, and hypertension. The need for preoperative dialysis should be considered in those with profound renal dysfunction. Nonsteroidal antiinflammatory drugs (NSAIDs) should be used with caution in children with renal dysfunction as NSAID-related restriction of renal perfusion may exacerbate any preexisting renal dysfunction.

HEPATIC

Primary liver tumors comprise only 1% of childhood cancers, and up to 20% of these are associated with a genetic syndrome, such as Beckwith-Wiedemann syndrome. In young children, hepatoblastomas are the most prevalent primary hepatic tumor, followed by sarcomas, germ cell tumors, and rhabdoid tumors. Hepatocellular carcinoma is occasionally found in older adolescents.[83]

Methotrexate, actinomycin D, 6-mercaptopurine, and 6-thioguanine are associated with acute hepatic toxicity, which can present hours to weeks after a chemotherapeutic dose. Hepatic impairment is typically transient and reversible.[63] Radiation typically causes self-limited acute toxicity, but chronic hepatic fibrosis may follow large doses of radiation (>40 Gy).[52] Most concerning is the potential to develop sinusoidal obstruction syndrome (SOS) in children after HSCT. SOS is characterized by portal hypertension, liver failure, and multiorgan system failure affecting the heart, lungs, and kidneys. Up to 60% of children develop SOS after HSCT, with an associated mortality rate of 19% to 50%.[84,85]

Both acute and chronic liver disease may be found in children with cancer, associated with a coagulopathy and/or impaired drug metabolism. The dose and timing of drugs that undergo significant hepatic elimination should be adjusted accordingly. Potentially hepatotoxic medications (e.g., acetaminophen) should be used with caution in children who are particularly vulnerable to further hepatic insult. Children exhibiting chronic liver failure may have coexisting genetic syndromes, such as Beckwith-Wiedemann syndrome, which present additional anesthetic challenges.[63]

GASTROINTESTINAL

Primary gastrointestinal (GI) tumors are uncommon in children; however, various intraabdominal malignancies can affect the GI tract by intestinal obstruction, intussusception, erosive perforation, intraabdominal hemorrhage, biliary obstruction, venous or arterial obstruction, and massive hepatomegaly.[63,86] The most common GI concern in children with cancer pertains to adverse effects of the chemotherapy and radiation treatment.

As chemotherapy and radiation treatments target rapidly proliferating tissues, the gastrointestinal mucosa is particularly vulnerable. Chemotherapeutic agents are well known to cause nausea and vomiting but may also cause more serious GI pathology such as diarrhea, mucositis, stomatitis, and neutropenic enterocolitis.[87] These adverse effects may exacerbate the malnutrition and dehydration that are often found in children with cancer. Similarly, radiation doses in excess of 20 to 30 Gy can cause inflammation and edema of GI tissues.[88] Importantly, acute and chronic GVHD after HSCT (discussed in detail below) commonly impacts the GI tract, although the majority of cases are mild in the current era of prophylaxis with calcineurin inhibitors plus methotrexate or mycophenolate. The incidence of moderate to severe gut GVHD after HSCT is approximately 10%, and the mortality rate is substantial without prompt treatment.[89]

Before induction of anesthesia, children who have been treated for their cancer may have chronic nausea and vomiting or delayed gastric emptying, both of which are exacerbated by opioids. These children may be at increased risk for aspiration and should be managed accordingly. Children with GI dysfunction may also present with malnutrition, dehydration, and electrolyte imbalances that warrant correction before embarking on elective surgical procedures.

CENTRAL NERVOUS SYSTEM

Primary intracranial tumors such as astrocytomas, ependymomas, primitive neuroectodermal tumors, and gliomas represent 17% of all childhood malignancies.[2] Signs and symptoms of the tumor itself depend on the size and location of the tumor and the local mass effect on adjacent neurologic structures. Symptoms may include irritability, lethargy, macrocephaly, and vomiting. Increased intracranial pressure, herniation, stroke, seizure, or leukemic meningitis may herald acute decompensation.[62] Primary spinal tumors are uncommon but may present with acute spinal cord compression requiring immediate surgical treatment.[90] Furthermore, 3% to 5% of children with metastatic disease have some degree of spinal cord compression, often at initial diagnosis.[91,92] Detailed discussion and perioperative management of children with brain tumors is covered in Chapters 24 and 26.

Platinum chemotherapeutic agents (cisplatin, carboplatin, oxaliplatin), L-asparaginase, ifosfamide, methotrexate, cytarabine, etoposide, vincristine, and cyclosporine A may cause neurologic toxicity.[93,94] Acute toxicity is characterized by altered mental status, seizures, stroke, encephalopathy, ototoxicity, and peripheral nerve dysfunction.[11] These symptoms are often reversible with cessation of the drug. Chronic toxicity usually manifests as neurocognitive and psychiatric dysfunction, which are discussed below. Brain irradiation can also have profound neurologic effects. Radiation doses in excess of 50 Gy can cause severe focal tissue damage, myelitis, stroke, and optic toxicity. Smaller doses, less than 18 Gy, are associated with subtler neurocognitive dysfunction.[88]

As discussed in detail in Chapters 24 and 26, children who present for resection of an intracranial tumor should undergo a thorough neurologic evaluation focusing on the signs and symptoms of increased intracranial pressure (ICP) and existing neurologic deficits. The benefits of sedative premedications must be balanced against their risks in children with increased ICP. As timely postoperative neurologic examination is important in these children, the choice of anesthetic agents and timing of extubation should be tailored to facilitate as early an assessment as circumstances allow.

ENDOCRINE

Primary endocrine tumors account for less than 5% of childhood cancers.[95] Gonadal germ cell tumors (testicular, ovarian, and extragonadal tumors), thyroid adenomas and carcinomas, and pituitary tumors (craniopharyngiomas and pituitary adenomas) account for the vast majority of these childhood endocrine tumors.[96]

Most chemotherapeutic agents have minimal effect on endocrine function, and chronic endocrine dysfunction is very uncommon in survivors of childhood cancer.[97,98] However, the use of glucocorticoids leads to a dose-dependent adrenal suppression. Studies in children with cancer have demonstrated that although a majority of children with ALL recover adrenal function in 2 weeks after cessation of chronic steroid therapy, some remain suppressed to various degrees of severity for 2 to 8 months.[99] It has thus been recommended that stress-dose steroids be administered before stressful procedures in the first 1 to 2 months after cessation of therapy.[99] If the anesthesiologist considers intraoperative stress-dose steroids or steroids for antiemesis, this must first be discussed with the child's oncologist; steroids are active anticancer drugs that may cause tumor necrosis or TLS in some tumors, cause immune suppression, impact the cancer treatment protocol, and constitute grounds for a study violation.[63]

Unlike the minimal chronic endocrine suppression of chemotherapy drugs, total body irradiation (TBI) preconditioning for HSCT and focal cranial radiotherapy, especially to regions in proximity to the hypothalamus, can cause significant, chronic neuroendocrine dysfunction.[97] Cumulative radiation doses as small as 18 to 20 Gy can cause growth hormone and gonadotropin deficiency, and doses greater than 35 to 40 Gy can cause panhypopituitarism.[100] Hypothyroidism can occur at doses of 20 Gy, typically manifesting 2 to 4½ years after therapy.[101]

HEMATOLOGY

Myelosuppression is commonplace during pediatric cancer treatment, both as a consequence of the tumor effect itself and subsequent treatment of disease. Several cancers present with anemia at first diagnosis, including neuroblastoma, rhabdomyosarcoma, Hodgkin disease, Ewing sarcoma, osteosarcoma, and leukemia.[102,103] Thrombocytopenia is common in children with hematologic cancers as well as solid tumors invading the bone marrow.[104] The presenting leukocyte count in children with leukemia is variable. Neutropenia is typical at presentation in some children with ALL, but hyperleukocytosis (>100,000/mm³) may be present in 20% of children with acute myelogenous leukemia. Hyperleukocytosis can cause hyperviscosity and potentially fatal leukostasis as tissue perfusion is impaired by plugging of leukocytes in the vasculature.[105]

Both chemotherapy and radiation therapy can have profound effects on myeloid cell production. Chemotherapy-related myelosuppression is common and is often dose limiting. Although radiation has the potential to completely suppress myeloid cell production, this typically requires exposure of a significant percentage of marrow sites to cause clinically significant suppression. However, TBI for HSCT preconditioning, by design, results in complete destruction of the host hematopoietic cells to prepare the marrow space for new cells. TBI doses of only 3 to 5 Gy to all marrow sites are fatal if new cells are not transplanted. Recovery of hematopoiesis after HSCT follows a predictable pattern: granulocytes recover first, followed by platelets, lymphocytes, and lastly erythrocytes. During recovery, the child is susceptible to infections, bleeding, and anemia.[106] Reducing the dose of chemotherapy or stopping radiation allows cell counts to recover; however, owing to the life span of hematologic cells and the time to produce new cells, pancytopenia typically requires 4 weeks to resolve.[107,108] For prophylaxis or chronic treatment of cytopenia, both erythropoietin and recombinant human granulocyte-macrophage colony-stimulating factor may minimize anemia and neutropenia.[109]

Children with neutropenia are at increased risk for life-threatening infections. Providers should be vigilant about patient isolation and strict aseptic technique during invasive procedures or access of existing lines. Administration of medications and placement of temperature probes in the rectum can cause bacteremia and should be avoided. Similarly, catheterization of the urinary tract should also be used sparingly.[110]

COAGULATION

Abnormal bleeding in cancer patients may result from a number of factors, including thrombocytopenia, clotting factor deficiency, circulating anticoagulants, and defects in vascular integrity.[111] Even in the presence of adequate platelet numbers and function, the presence of any of these other coagulopathic defects may increase the risk of procedural bleeding. Hematologic cancers, especially any of the subsets of leukemia, often present with unexplained bleeding and a coagulopathy.[112] Disseminated intravascular coagulation may be present at the time of diagnosis of acute promyelocytic leukemia and less commonly of acute myelogenous leukemia and T-cell ALL. Patients may have lupus anticoagulant syndrome with subsequent thrombophilia or factor VIII inhibitors, leading to acquired hemophilia. Up to 8% of children with Wilms tumor have acquired von Willebrand syndrome at the time of diagnosis.[113,114]

Chemotherapy can cause a significant coagulopathic response. L-Asparaginase may be associated with up to a 2% risk of hemorrhage or thrombus via induced deficiencies in plasminogen, fibrinogen, antithrombin III, and von Willebrand factor.[13] Vitamin K deficiency in the setting of hepatic dysfunction or severe malnutrition also contributes to coagulopathy.[115] Sepsis, disseminated intravascular coagulation, hepatic failure, acute or chronic anticoagulant usage, platelet sequestration with splenomegaly, and the burden of chronic disease may also contribute to the increased risk of perioperative hemorrhage.

Venous thromboembolism (VTE) is rare in children in general but considerably more common in those with malignancy as a result of coagulation dysfunction and frequent use of long-term indwelling vascular access. Nearly 8% of children with cancer experience VTE, with the greatest incidence among those with sarcoma and hematologic malignancies.[116] The optimal timing to stop anticoagulants before surgery in children with VTE warrants discussion with both the surgical and hematology-oncology teams. These children are at risk for perioperative thrombosis,[117] and their management must strike a delicate balance between provoking additional thrombus formation and an increased risk of surgical bleeding.

PAIN

Both acute and chronic pain are common sequelae of cancer and cancer therapy. In one survey of 160 children undergoing cancer treatment, 87% of inpatients and 75% of outpatients rated their pain as moderate to severe.[118] In a survey of survivors of pediatric cancer, the single most painful experience during their treatment was a painful medical procedure or surgery.[119]

The use of general anesthesia for painful procedures, such as lumbar puncture and bone marrow biopsies, is one of the most effective techniques for reducing pain; anesthesiologists have a central role in optimizing patient comfort and parental stress during this difficult period.

Just as with other sources of chronic pain, children with cancer are often opioid tolerant and may benefit from a multimodal approach to analgesia. Regional anesthesia can be advantageous, but the benefits must be carefully weighed against the risks in those with a coagulopathy or significant chemotherapy-induced neuropathy. A multidisciplinary discussion with anesthesia, surgery, oncology, and pain service providers is essential to ensure an optimal balance between comfort and safety for these complex patients.

NEUROPSYCHOLOGY

Up to 40% of childhood cancer survivors suffer neurocognitive impairment in at least one of several areas, including academic achievement and executive function.[120,121] Intrathecal methotrexate and cranial irradiation appear to be particularly detrimental; thus children with ALL, central nervous system (CNS) tumors, and head and neck sarcomas are at the greatest risk for cognitive impairment.[122] The increasing availability of proton beam radiotherapy and its precise targeting of malignant tissue has been shown to reduce collateral tissue injury, and it may result in improved neurocognitive outcomes.[39,123–125]

The psychological response to cancer diagnosis and treatment is extremely age and individual dependent. Young children are often distressed by parental separation and anticipation of painful procedures. Many of these children benefit from an honest discussion of upcoming procedures to allow them a greater sense of control in their treatment. The placement of central access devices and topical anesthetic creams have greatly reduced the anxiety associated with many interventions required in their treatment. Role-playing and desensitization can be particularly helpful in this age group.[126] Older children and adolescents are in many ways more profoundly affected by the psychosocial stress associated with cancer treatment. Compliance with medical treatment can be problematic in adolescents, who have difficulty coping with their diagnosis. To the extent that it is possible, adolescents should be actively involved in their own care, and assent from adolescent patients should be sought for anesthesia and invasive procedures.[60,126] Children and adolescents with cancer become isolated from peers because of school absences and the rigors of the treatment schedule, despite the natural need for peer interactions for healthy coping and adjustment. Feeling "alone" with their disease can worsen the sense of isolation from their healthy peers. As such, opportunities for peer engagement and interactions should be encouraged and provided. Peer interactions may include the child's choice of peers, as well as formal socialization or mentorship from other children with cancer or cancer survivors. Camps, group interventions, or formal coaching by childhood cancer survivors are highly effective.[127]

TUMOR LYSIS SYNDROME

Children with rapidly proliferating cancers, particularly ALL and non-Hodgkin lymphoma, are at risk for developing potentially fatal TLS. TLS has been reported in more than 40% of patients with non-Hodgkin lymphoma, although the rate of serious TLS was only 6% in one study.[128] Nonhematologic malignancies with rapid proliferation, large tumor burden, and high sensitivity to chemotherapy are also subject to TLS after initiation of therapy. TLS occurs when rapid destruction of tumor cells yields a massive release of intracellular contents, resulting in hyperuricemia, hyperkalemia, hyperphosphatemia, hypocalcemia, and acid-base derangements. The cellular outpouring most commonly precipitates acute renal failure, but arrhythmias, cardiac failure, seizures, multiorgan failure, and death may occur. TLS can present suddenly with induction of chemotherapy, radiotherapy, fever, surgery, or anesthesia but most often occurs 1 to 3 days after initiation of cytotoxic therapy.[128,129] In the current era, the incidence of severe TLS has decreased with the institution of appropriate preventative measures in high-risk children. The occurrence of perioperative TLS requires prompt and aggressive management, including hydration and diuresis, rasburicase (a uric acid–reducing agent), and allopurinol to ameliorate organ damage as well as aggressive measures to treat life-threatening arrhythmias owing to hyperkalemia (see Chapter 9; see also Fig. 9.7).[128] The cytotoxic effects of corticosteroids such as dexamethasone have been associated with TLS, and alternative perioperative antiemetics should be used in those at risk.

RETINOIC ACID SYNDROME

Retinoic acid syndrome (also referred to as differentiation syndrome) is a potentially life-threatening complication found in 2% to 27% of children treated for acute promyelocytic leukemia (APL) with all-*trans* retinoic acid (ATRA). The exact mechanism of this condition is unknown but is believed to be related to the release of inflammatory cytokines from APL cells during ATRA treatment. Retinoic acid syndrome typically occurs around 7 days after beginning treatment and is characterized by respiratory distress, fever, pulmonary infiltrates, and weight gain. Pericardial effusion, hypotension, cardiac failure, and renal failure can also occur. Thus children who were recently managed with induction therapy with ATRA for APL should be screened for pulmonary,

cardiac, and renal abnormalities before undertaking general anesthesia.[130,131]

Hematopoietic Stem Cell Transplant

BACKGROUND

The first attempts to use bone marrow to treat malignancy took place over 50 years ago,[132] and the first successful pediatric transplant occurred almost 40 years ago.[133] HSCT is a potentially curative treatment for a wide range of malignant and nonmalignant pediatric disorders. HSCT is used in the treatment of many forms of leukemia, Hodgkin and non-Hodgkin lymphoma, and many types of solid tumors, including germ cell tumors, some sarcomas, neuroblastoma, Wilms tumor, and some malignant brain tumors. Additionally, it is used to treat many nonmalignant diseases, including myelodysplasia, aplastic anemia, hemoglobinopathies (including sickle cell disease and thalassemia), and congenital immune and metabolic deficiencies.[134–137] Because of the prevalence of ALL in the pediatric population, it is the primary indication for HSCT in many centers.

Hematopoietic stem cells used for transplantation can be obtained from bone marrow, "mobilized" peripheral blood, or umbilical cord blood. The source of the cells may be the child (autologous), an identical twin (syngeneic), or another individual (allogeneic). Allogeneic donor cells are commonly derived from human leukocyte antigen (HLA)-identical siblings (available in about 25% to 30% of patients), but advances in matching and supportive care have improved outcomes with HLA-matched unrelated and mismatched donors.[138,139]

CLINICAL FEATURES AND TREATMENT

The process of HSCT involves several steps:
1. The preparative or conditioning regimen, during which high-dose chemotherapy with or without irradiation or immunomodulating agents eradicates malignancy (where present), clears marrow space for incoming stem cells, and suppresses the recipient's immune system
2. Transplantation through infusion of hematopoietic stem cells
3. Transplant engraftment (>30 days after transplantation)
4. Early engraftment (30–100 days after transplantation)
5. Late engraftment (>100 days after transplantation)

Cumulative toxicity associated with HSCT is the result of the underlying illness and complications of past therapy, the transplant-conditioning regimen, complications from long-term myelosuppression, and GVHD and its treatment. The incidence of transplant-related morbidity and mortality depends on the child's age, primary disease, comorbidities, and histocompatibility between donor and recipient.[140] Overall, 100-day mortality is 5% to 20% from sibling donors and 10% to 40% from unrelated donor allogeneic HSCT.[141]

HSCT-related toxicity can involve every organ of the body through the direct and indirect effects of irradiation and chemotherapy, as discussed previously. Immunologic and physical host defenses are impaired throughout the transplantation process. Infections are among the most important causes of transplant-related morbidity and mortality.[142] Children are vulnerable to a wide range of routine and opportunistic pathogens, including bacteria, fungi, and viruses. Mucositis is common and may increase the risks of aspiration and airway compromise.[44,143] SOS, previously called venooclusive disease, occurs in 10% to 60% of children after HSCT. Mortality rates in the setting of SOS-induced hepatorenal failure and subsequent multiple-organ failure range from

19% to almost 50%.[144] Hepatorenal syndrome and fluid retention associated with SOS mandate careful attention to fluid balance, sodium administration, and the presence of acquired coagulopathy, including thrombocytopenia that is refractory to platelet transfusions.[84,144,145] Other gastrointestinal complications include hemorrhage, infections, and opioid-induced abdominal pain and distention (i.e., opioid-associated bowel syndrome).[146] Acute pulmonary complications, which occur in 30% to 60% of children after HSCT, include infection, hemorrhage, edema, bronchiolitis obliterans, acute respiratory distress syndrome, and idiopathic pneumonia syndrome, a noninfectious inflammatory lung process.[147-149]

In the early phase after HSCT, significant cardiomyopathy and arrhythmias are uncommon (5%), but sepsis, heart failure, and cardiovascular collapse are common admitting diagnoses in 10% to 40% of children who require intensive care after HSCT.[147,150,151] Late cardiac complications depend on the dose of radiation and the cardiotoxic chemotherapeutic agents used during the conditioning regimen. Acute renal failure occurs in 30% to 50% of children and warrants judicious use of fluids[80,81,152]; hemorrhagic cystitis is also common.[153] A process of thrombotic microangiopathy similar to hemolytic uremic syndrome may occur in as many as 25% of children who were treated with cyclosporine or the calcineurin inhibitor, tacrolimus.[154] CNS complications may include infection, hemorrhage, encephalopathy, and peripheral neuropathy owing to metabolic and chemotherapeutic effects.[155]

In contrast to the myeloablative procedures described previously, pediatric centers are increasingly using reduced-intensity preconditioning regimens and even nonmyeloablative preconditioning to reduce morbidity and mortality after hematologic malignancies.[156,157] Use of these regimens is based on the observation that in some instances, minimal myelotoxicity in conjunction with profound and prolonged immunosuppression leads to successful donor engraftment.[158] This modality is mostly used in children with nonmalignant hematologic conditions, marrow failure, and immunodeficiency syndromes but is increasingly used in pediatric hematologic malignancies.

GRAFT VERSUS HOST DISEASE

GVHD is the clinical manifestation that donor T cells recognize recipient alloantigens. Acute GVHD occurs in 20% to 80% of children within the first 100 days after HSCT. The incidence depends on the histocompatibility of the donor and recipient, as well as the stem cell source.[159] It is characterized by inflammatory dermatitis, enteritis, and hepatitis. Chemoprophylaxis (cyclosporine or tacrolimus with short-course methotrexate) is crucial as the outcomes after the onset of acute GVHD are disappointing. Treatment includes continuation of immunosuppression, the addition of corticosteroids, and the introduction of salvage therapy with profound immunosuppression. These children are at very high risk of succumbing to opportunistic infections.[159]

Chronic GVHD occurs in 6% to 50% of children 100 days or more after HSCT. This broad range of incidence depends on the age of the donor and recipient, gender matching, and degree of matching between donor and recipient.[160] Chronic GVHD has many features of autoimmune diseases, impacting nearly every organ of the body (e.g., sclerodermatous changes; dry mouth and conjunctivae; esophagitis; pulmonary dysfunction, including bronchiolitis obliterans; contractures or fasciitis of extremities and soft tissue; liver dysfunction; alopecia; thrombocytopenia). The pulmonary system is involved in 30% to 60% of children. Significant cardiac and renal disease is rare in chronic GVHD.

Opportunistic infections are common during chronic GVHD, in part, as a result of the immunosuppression associated with GVHD. Hemolysis is an additional manifestation of alloantigenicity, the result of major and minor blood group incompatibilities between donor and recipient.[161]

Adoptive T-Cell Therapies in Children

Along with the use of newer, small immunologic molecules and monoclonal antibodies mentioned at the start of this chapter, investigation into and use of adoptive immunotherapy using an infusion of T cells genetically engineered to express receptors targeting a specific tumor antigen (e.g., CD19 in ALL) has been growing rapidly. Pediatric indications are expanding, but most applications in children are associated with relapsed cancer or residual tumor after HSCT. Briefly, autologous T cells are removed through a central venous catheter, genetically engineered ex vivo to express receptors to the desired antigen, and then reinfused into the proband. After infusion, the cells engraft, multiply, and eradicate tumor cells for months or years.[162-164] However, sufficient engraftment and expansion depend on prior lymphodepletion, which requires significant immunosuppression with TBI and chemotherapy, with all the associated risks discussed above.[165] Trials of T cell infusion therapies in children with neuroblastoma, B cell ALL, glioma, osteosarcoma, and disialoganglioside GD2 sarcoma are underway.[162]

Three points should be understood when caring for these children before and after T-cell infusions. First, akin to children receiving HSCT, these children are immunosuppressed and at significant risk for infections. Isolation and meticulous use of sterile technique must be observed. Second, T-cell and other cellular forms of adoptive cellular therapy constitute a rapidly changing field that requires effective communication between the oncologist and the perioperative team to ensure the safe and optimal management of the child. Third, this therapy is accompanied by potentially significant morbidity and mortality. In addition to the toxicity of the preconditioning regimen, the modified T cells occasionally trigger an autoimmune response. Cytokine-release syndrome is the most serious toxicity, resulting from supraphysiologic levels of immune cell activation and the subsequent massive release of inflammatory cytokines. Mild cases manifest as fevers and myalgias, but severe cases may lead to cardiorespiratory failure, multiorgan dysfunction, and possible death if not treated early.[162-164]

Preoperative Laboratory Testing and Evaluation

As is the case for children without cancer, there is insufficient evidence to recommend any routine preanesthetic testing in children with cancer. Instead, preoperative laboratory or radiologic testing should be based on the child's history, physical exam, concurrent illnesses, and surgical procedure. Tests should be ordered only if they have the potential to influence the surgical risk or the child's perioperative management.[166] In complex patients, these tests should be ordered in advance to (1) permit corrective action to be taken and satisfactory responses recognized and (2) allow communication with the oncology team before commencing the anesthetic plan. It is helpful for the oncology service to provide up-to-date information regarding hemoglobin, platelet counts, absolute neutrophil counts, coagulation studies, the most recent echocardiogram and pulmonary test results, as well as any other

TABLE 11.5	Risk Factors for Hematologic Abnormalities in Children With Cancer

Children at Risk for Anemia
- New diagnosis of leukemia (50%–80% incidence) or lymphoma
- Recent chemotherapy, radiation therapy, or hematopoietic stem cell transplant
- Children with cancer and age less than 6 months

Children at Risk for Hyperleukocytosis Include Any New Diagnosis of Leukemia (>20% Incidence)

Children at Risk for Leukopenia and Neutropenia Include Any Child Receiving Aggressive Chemotherapy or Irradiation

Children at Risk for Thrombocytopenia Include the Following:
- New diagnosis of leukemia
- Any child receiving aggressive chemotherapy or irradiation
- Disseminated intravascular coagulation
- Splenomegaly

From Latham GJ, Greenberg RS. Anesthetic considerations for the pediatric oncology patient—part 3: pain, cognitive dysfunction, and preoperative evaluation. *Pediatr Anesth.* 2010;20(6):479–489. Used with permission.

TABLE 11.6	Risk Factors for Coagulopathy, Electrolytes, and Renal Dysfunction in Children With Cancer

Risk Factors for Coagulopathy

Sepsis

Vitamin K deficiency or malnutrition

Anticoagulant therapy

Hyperleukocytosis

L-Asparaginase treatment

Diagnosis of T-cell acute lymphoblastic leukemia, myelomonocytic leukemia, or acute promyelocytic leukemia

Recent hematopoietic stem cell transplant

Prior splenectomy

Risk Factors for Electrolyte Abnormalities

Syndrome of inappropriate antidiuretic hormone (SIADH)

Hypercalcemia (bone tumors and neuroblastoma)

Intracranial disorder with altered level of consciousness

Dehydration or malnutrition

Aggressive hydration

Renal dysfunction

Recent tumor lysis syndrome (hyperkalemia, hyperphosphatemia, hypocalcemia)

Risk Factors for Renal Disease

Renal or ureteral compression by newly diagnosed neuroblastoma or Wilms' tumor

Sinusoidal obstructive syndrome

Tumor lysis syndrome

Nephrotoxic antitumor therapy (ifosfamide, cisplatin)

Recent hematopoietic stem cell transplant

From Latham GJ, Greenberg RS. Anesthetic considerations for the pediatric oncology patient—part 3: pain, cognitive dysfunction, and preoperative evaluation. *Pediatr Anesth.* 2010;20(6):479–489. Used with permission.

information that might affect anesthetic management. Possible factors that may require preoperative laboratory testing in the child with cancer are further discussed in the following text.

A complete blood cell count is not routinely required before anesthesia in children with cancer. However, it may be warranted based on the condition of the child, presence of comorbidities, proposed surgical procedure and potential blood loss, potential thrombocytopenia, attendant risk of prolonged bleeding, and known or suspected anemia (Table 11.5).[60]

Preoperative coagulation testing is not routinely indicated in children with cancer. A preoperative platelet count is frequently obtained for children who are scheduled for lumbar puncture, neuraxial anesthesia, surgical procedures with risk of significant blood loss, or neurosurgical procedures. If the platelet count is sufficient for the surgical procedure and the regional anesthetic plan and there is no further clinical evidence of bleeding, then additional coagulation studies are probably unwarranted. However, any history of abnormal coagulation in the setting of an appropriate platelet count does warrant further investigation.[60] Known conditions in the pediatric oncology population in which coagulopathy, renal dysfunction, or electrolyte derangements occur are listed in Table 11.6.

Perioperative Considerations

CHILDREN WITH CANCER
The perioperative complication rate after anesthesia in 177 children undergoing 3833 radiotherapy sessions was 1.3%, an incidence comparable to that for children without cancer anesthetized with propofol.[167] However, many children with cancer who present to the operating room are gravely ill with limited physiologic reserves and susceptible to relatively small changes to their physiology. Most children with standard risk leukemia in clinical remission receiving maintenance chemotherapy live a near normal lifestyle with good physical capacity; however, a significant number of children with cancer, especially those immediately before and after HSCT, can have multiorgan dysfunction and require intensive support in the hospital. It is imperative that the anesthesiologist carefully stratifies the risk of each child with cancer who presents for surgical or procedural intervention. All of the previously described considerations regarding the possible effects of pediatric cancer and its treatment on each organ system must be considered preoperatively. Prior anesthesia experiences, plus current information regarding the child's treatment protocol, cumulative chemotherapy or radiation therapy doses, major side effects, recent echocardiogram, current laboratory values, and organ dysfunction must be readily available. When all of this current information is not readily available in the electronic medical record where the child is being anesthetized, the authors recommend that an updated data summary sheet be provided by the oncology team to the anesthesiologists prior to anesthesia (Fig. 11.2).

Children with cancer undergo a host of procedures that require anesthesia during acute and chronic phases of disease. Included among these are diagnostic tumor or lymph node biopsy, tumor resection, placement and replacement of chronic indwelling venous catheters for treatment and nutrition, diagnostic and monitoring procedures (e.g., lumbar puncture, bone marrow aspirate and biopsy, lung and liver biopsy, skin biopsy, bronchoalveolar lavage, esophagogastroduodenoscopy), radiologic procedures, radiation therapy, and placement of pain management devices (e.g., indwelling epidural catheters). Splenectomy is performed as part of staging or management of some pediatric malignancies, and the procedure

CANCER TREATMENT SUMMARY

Name:	MRN:	DOB:
Oncologist:	Oncologist contact info:	

CANCER DIAGNOSIS
Cancer diagnosis:
Date of diagnosis:
Stage and site(s):
Relapse(s):

CHEMOTHERAPY PROTOCOL		
Protocol:	Initiated:	Completed:
Description:		

CHEMOTHERAPY DRUGS		
Drug	Route	Cumulative dose/complications

OTHER MEDICATIONS

RADIATION THERAPY			
Site/volume	Dates of treatment	Cumulative dose	Complications

THERAPIES
Surgeries:
Hematopoietic cell transplant:

DIAGNOSTIC STUDIES - Echo, CT, PFTs, etc.

NOTES, COMPLICATIONS, OTHER ILLNESSES

FIGURE 11.2 Example of a cancer data sheet that should be made available to the anesthesiologist when the child's current key information is not readily available from electronic or paper records. (From Latham GJ, Greenberg RS. Anesthetic considerations for the pediatric oncology patient—part 3: pain, cognitive dysfunction, and preoperative evaluation. *Paediatr Anaesth*. 2010;20:479–489. Used with permission.)

may be associated with increased risk of postoperative infection, postoperative thrombocytosis, and thrombocytopenia.[168]

Lumbar puncture and bone marrow aspiration procedures are commonly performed in children with cancer, especially those with hematologic malignancies. The use of short-acting medications for a brief general anesthetic ensures complete comfort during the procedure while permitting a rapid recovery and discharge from the hospital. Propofol and a short-acting opioid or low-dose ketamine, for instance, are commonly used to achieve this goal.[169–173] The anesthesiologist must be fastidious with sterile technique when accessing central venous sites, regardless of whether the child is immunosuppressed, to avoid catheter-related infections. *It is of paramount importance that systems are in place to avoid the inadvertent administration of vincristine chemotherapy into the intrathecal space during lumbar punctures.* Intrathecal vincristine causes severe neurologic consequences and may have contributed to nearly 100 fatalities in children with otherwise curable hematopoietic tumors.[174] *Intravenous chemotherapy should be excluded from any procedure room where lumbar punctures and intrathecal chemotherapy are performed.*

Radiation beam therapy is used in frontline treatment of many pediatric brain tumors and some extracranial solid tumors. The duration of radiation therapy varies depending on tumor type but typically occurs daily over 4 to 8 weeks, frequently concurrent with chemotherapy.[28] The goal of modern radiation therapy—both conventional photon beam and the newer proton beam therapies—is to accurately conform radiation to the tumor while minimizing radiation of healthy surrounding tissues. As such, immobility is crucial and requires general anesthesia in younger children.

Radiation treatment planning begins with a simulation, which requires anesthesia in those who will need anesthesia for the subsequent treatments. The child is ideally positioned as he or she will be for treatment, computed tomographic imaging of the tumor is obtained, and appropriate custom-made molds or masks are formed that will allow reproducible positioning during daily treatments (Fig. 11.3). For PRT, custom brass and/or acrylic molds are later fabricated that will be used to tightly shape and focus the proton beam as required to conform precisely to the tumor

mass (Fig. 11.4). Provision of anesthesia in the radiation oncology suite presents key challenges. Many radiation therapy centers, especially PRT centers, are freestanding outpatient facilities separate from a hospital or children's hospital; it is therefore obligatory that all necessary equipment and medications are available to handle any potential anesthesia-related emergency, including rapid transport to a pediatric hospital. Children may suffer physical and emotional stress from daily anesthetics, procedures, diagnostics tests, chemotherapy, and previous or upcoming surgery. As much as possible, parent and child education, peer-to-peer support, distraction techniques, and reward systems may be used to ease

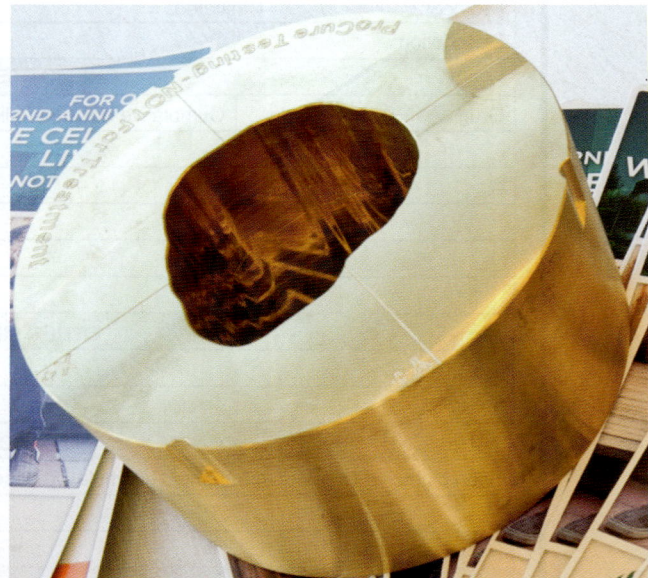

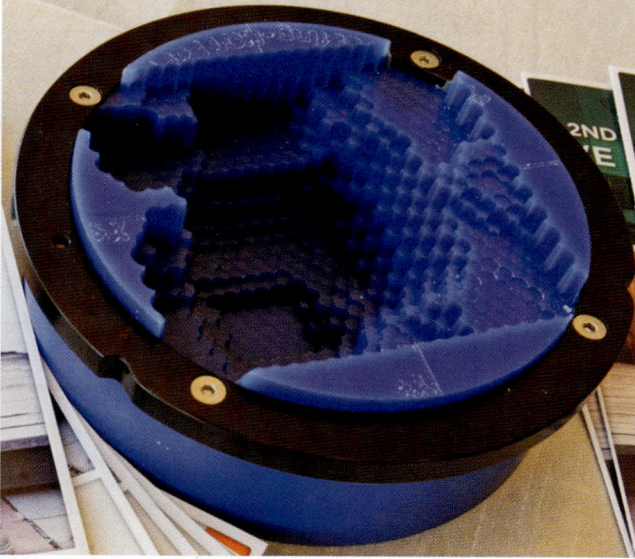

FIGURE 11.4 Upper image: an aperture made from brass composite shapes the lateral borders of the proton beam to shield healthy tissues lateral to the tumor. Lower image: a compensator made of wax or acrylic is used to control the active depth of the protons along the distal border of the tumor. Use of the aperture and compensator together shapes the lateral and distal treatment field accurately, leaving primarily entry path radiation to healthy tissues. (Photo courtesy SCCA Proton Therapy Center, Seattle, WA. Used with permission.)

FIGURE 11.3 A custom-made mask holds this anesthetized child's head in the repeatable, exact position required for cranial radiation therapy. A nasal canula provides supplemental oxygen and end-tidal CO_2 monitoring during a total intravenous anesthetic with propofol. (Photo courtesy Andrew Pittaway, BM, BS.)

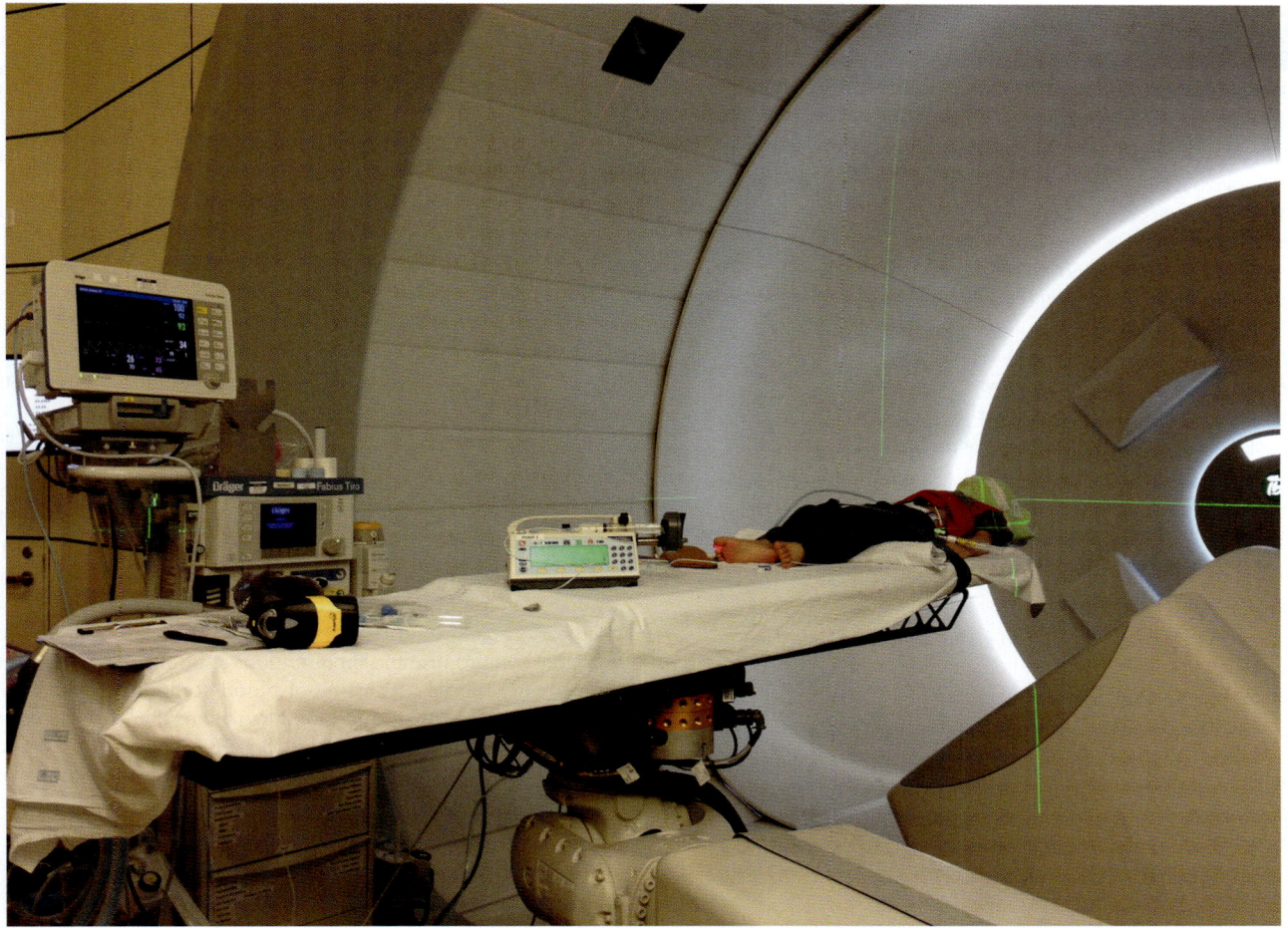

FIGURE 11.5 An anesthetized child in a proton therapy vault. The head mold positions the child's head, and a nasal cannula provides oxygen and CO_2 monitoring. Propofol total intravenous anesthesia is used, and an anesthesia machine and rescue medications are immediately available. Video feeds in a shielded control room allow the anesthesia and radiation teams to view the patient, the propofol pump, and vital signs continuously. (Photo courtesy Karen Wong, MB, BS.)

the child's anxiety.[127,175] The parents and anesthesia team cannot remain in the treatment vault during irradiation; therefore multiple video feeds of the child and anesthesia equipment/monitor are essential for the safe care of the child under anesthesia (Fig. 11.5).

Most children will have an indwelling central venous catheter, which facilitates intravenous induction and maintenance of anesthesia. Strict aseptic technique is mandatory to avoid sepsis and the need for catheter removal, both of which risk morbidity and delays in treatment.[176] Port-a-catheters may be accessed on Monday (topical anesthetic cream may be used) and left accessed until Friday to lessen the anxiety of daily percutaneous port access. A standing anesthesia consent is used in some centers to ease the burden of daily consents, but such consent does not negate the need to evaluate the child prior to each anesthetic. The risk of anesthetizing a child with mild to moderate respiratory infection must be considered in conjunction with the risk of missing a treatment. A key consideration in choosing the anesthetic regimen includes the use of short-acting medications to allow quick recovery from anesthesia, and to this end, various anesthetic techniques have been described in the literature.[167,176–178] Total intravenous anesthesia with propofol is commonly used as it provides rapid

onset of anesthesia, excellent immobility during radiation, rapid emergence from anesthesia, and theoretic antiemetic properties. Although adjunct medications such as opioids and benzodiazepines can be added, they are often unnecessary and may increase respiratory events.[167,179] A nasal cannula provides supplemental oxygen and the ability to monitor end-tidal CO_2 as a surrogate of effective ventilation via remote monitoring (see Fig. 11.3). Sevoflurane anesthesia with a laryngeal mask airway is another option with a low rate of complications.[177] If an invasive airway is needed routinely in a child receiving cranial radiation, then the head mold must be modified to allow access to the airway.

Surgical intervention may be required for acute and potentially life-threatening emergencies in children with cancer, and the effects of specific tumors may complicate the anesthesia care. Wilms tumor may be accompanied by an acquired von Willebrand condition,[113] and anterior mediastinal masses may produce superior vena cava obstruction, pulmonary artery compression, and tracheal obstruction.[180] Neuroblastoma may be accompanied by pheochromocytoma-like signs and symptoms (3% of cases),[181] venous obstruction, and in advanced stages, it may cause massive hepatic enlargement, making the potential for massive rapid blood

TABLE 11.7	Perioperative Concerns in Pediatric Cancer and Hematopoietic Stem Cell Transplantation

Preoperative Considerations

Consultation with service primarily responsible for child's care

Complete blood cell count, serum electrolytes (when appropriate)

Echocardiogram or chest radiograph, or both (when appropriate)

Transfusion cross-match with specifications (e.g., cytomegalovirus seronegativity, leukocyte reduction, irradiation) determined in consultation with oncology service

Determination of blood typing requirements for all stem cell transplant recipients

History of acute and chronic pain medication use

Anxiolytic and analgesic therapy (when appropriate)

Infection prophylaxis with antibiotics

Avoidance of *any* marrow-suppressive medications in stem cell transplant patients

Observation of indicated isolation precautions

Sterile technique with central line access

Use of support services (when appropriate)

Intraoperative Considerations

Attention to skin, teeth, eyes, and joints; careful positioning and padding

Sterile technique with central line access

Full-stomach precautions (when appropriate, as in graft-versus-host disease)

Appropriate hydration and maintenance of urine output

Continuation of total parenteral nutrition (and other parenteral fluids with high glucose concentration)

Avoidance of high fraction of inspired oxygen (FiO_2) and restriction of hydration if prior treatment with bleomycin

Judicious use of cardiac depressants in patients with compromised cardiac function

Nausea and vomiting prophylaxis

Stress corticosteroids (when appropriate)

Regional anesthesia when safe and indicated

Postoperative Considerations

Patient-appropriate opioid and other analgesic administration

Sterile technique with central line access

Observation of indicated isolation precautions

---

loss a significant risk. Spinal tumors may cause acute spinal cord compression, and tumor or hemorrhage in the brain may cause acute intracranial hypertension. In view of the complexity of pediatric oncologic disease, there are many considerations for the perioperative period[63] (Table 11.7).

HEMATOPOIETIC STEM CELL TRANSPLANTATION RECIPIENTS

Surgical and procedural interventions are common throughout the transplantation process and are similar to those described previously for children with cancer. Harvesting of hematopoietic stem cells from the recipient or another individual is an integral component of HSCT. Harvesting of bone marrow in children usually requires general anesthesia, although the procedure can be performed safely with the child under spinal anesthesia if required.[182] The donor is usually placed in a prone position to

extract approximately 10 mL/kg (recipient weight) of marrow from the posterior iliac crests. When stem cells are obtained from peripheral blood, sedation or general anesthesia is usually required to establish vascular access. There is little evidence to support the avoidance of nitrous oxide for harvesting procedures, a concern raised in the past because nitrous oxide affects methionine synthase activity and DNA synthesis.[183]

In view of the wide range of possible complications at the time of HSCT, the many issues outlined earlier for children with cancer must be considered for children undergoing HSCT (see Table 11.7). Radiation, glucocorticoids, mucositis, and chronic GVHD may contribute to an airway that is friable and a neck that is scarred, thereby increasing the risks of airway trauma, dental injury, and difficult tracheal intubation. Chemotherapy and GVHD may affect the skin and make venous access difficult. Chronic GVHD can lead to sclerodermatous changes, which can profoundly restrict range of motion, and sicca syndrome, which may necessitate use of artificial tears. GVHD may alter gut motility and delay gastric emptying. Immune compromise increases the risk of infection from vascular access lines and therefore mandates meticulous technique at all times. Chemotherapy may compromise cardiac and pulmonary function, alter hepatic metabolism of medications, and limit renal excretion of medications and fluids. Immune compromise and modifications resulting from transplantation require special processing of blood components, as recommended by hematology and blood bank consultants, as described in the following text and in Tables 10.3, 10.4, and 10.5. It is critical to coordinate the choice of blood products with the transplant service.

Transfusion Considerations

RED BLOOD CELLS

Anemia is very common in children with cancer, with an incidence that ranges from 51% to 74% in children with solid tumors or Hodgkin disease, greater than 50% of children with Wilms tumor and osteosarcoma,[102] greater than 80% of children receiving chemotherapy, and 97% of children with leukemia.[184] There is limited evidence regarding the optimal transfusion thresholds for children with cancer, and guidelines have not been established. Accordingly, current practice patterns stem from adult oncology studies, data from other pediatric populations (e.g., intensive care), and individual institutional practice patterns.[185] The threshold for red blood cell transfusion in adults with cancer is a hemoglobin concentration of 7 to 9 g/dL in asymptomatic individuals and 8 to 10 g/dL in symptomatic individuals.[186] Whether these thresholds are appropriate for children with cancer, who range in age from infancy to adolescence and with conditions ranging from leukemia to brain tumors, is unknown. Nonetheless, these values have been adopted empirically in children.[187] In practice, pediatric oncology patients usually receive transfusions when their hemoglobin concentrations decrease to 5.5 to 8 g/dL.[184]

Several factors should be considered when determining the need for blood transfusion, including the overall clinical condition of the child, symptoms of anemia, the presence of cardiopulmonary dysfunction, the stress and anticipated blood loss of the surgical procedure, the risk of increased intraoperative hemorrhage owing to coexisting coagulopathy, and the ability of the child to tolerate a volume load. Finally, blood products should be administered cautiously in those with hyperleukocytosis as the added viscosity can trigger leukostasis.[188] Thus sound clinical judgment and attention to the greater clinical context are warranted in each case.[189]

THROMBOCYTOPENIA

Thrombocytopenia occurs commonly in association with marrow suppression from chemotherapy, radiation, or even marrow replacement by hematologic malignancy. Additional effects on platelets include consumption during infections or disseminated intravascular coagulation, platelet sequestration with splenomegaly, and platelet dysfunction from medications.[187] The platelet count is not the sole indicator of the risk of bleeding in children with cancer, as evidenced by the occurrence of major bleeding at any platelet count[190]; treatment- or cancer-induced damage to vascular epithelium and alterations anywhere in the coagulation cascade pose additive risks for hemorrhage. Regardless, platelet transfusions play an important role in avoiding the risk of catastrophic hemorrhage in children.[191] Of note, the risk/benefit of perioperative platelet transfusion in the immediate post-HSCT period must be discussed with the oncology team, as transfusions during this time may impact the transplant engraftment.[191]

The optimal prophylactic platelet transfusion strategy in pediatric oncology remains complicated and controversial. As noted previously, the risk of bleeding is neither solely dependent on nor inversely proportional to the platelet count.[190] However, in the absence of adequate prospective trials, most practice guidelines continue to recommend a platelet count >50,000/μL for invasive procedures to >100,000/μL for CNS procedures, and 10,000-20,000/μL for lumbar punctures.[192] Despite the knowledge that these thresholds may not be appropriate for every age of child and cancer diagnosis, they remain our best guide at this time for children presenting for surgery.[191]

COAGULATION FACTOR DEFICIENCY

Perioperative administration of fresh frozen plasma or factor components is reasonable if the child with cancer has documented prolongation of prothrombin or partial thromboplastin time, verified factor deficiency, or surgical bleeding despite normal platelet levels and function. The invasiveness of the surgical procedure also should be taken into account. Cryoprecipitate and coagulation factor concentrates may also be necessary in the setting of abnormal laboratory studies and clinical coagulopathy.[189] It should be noted that fresh frozen plasma is ineffective in reversing the coagulopathy associated with L-asparaginase.[193]

BLOOD PRODUCT PREPARATION

Immunocompetent white blood cells in donor blood can elicit a profound immune response and other complications in the recipient, especially immunocompromised children. Leukoreduction by filtration eliminates greater than 99% of donor leukocytes. Most blood products in the United States and all blood products in Canada and Europe are routinely leukoreduced,[187] and leukoreduced products should be used in children with cancer. Tables 10.3 and 12.8 provides a complete list of indications for leukoreduced products. Leukoreduction reduces the rate of platelet alloimmunization, transfusion-related immunomodulation, febrile transfusion reactions, and transfusion-related infections, including cytomegalovirus (CMV) infection.[194,195] Although leukoreduction may be sufficient to prevent donor-related CMV infection, CMV-negative donor blood is recommended for CMV-negative infants and children with cancer, especially children undergoing HSCT (Table 10.5 and E-Table 12.1).[196]

Donor lymphocytes contained in the component blood products can replicate and engraft in the host, leading to a transfusion-associated graft-versus-host disease (TA-GVHD), especially in immunocompromised patients. TA-GVHD manifests days to weeks after transfusion, is resistant to treatment, and is often fatal. Leukoreduction alone is insufficient to eliminate the risk of TA-GVHD. As a result, irradiation of platelets and red blood cells is mandatory for immunosuppressed patients, including children with cancer (Table 10.4 and E-Table 12.2).[194,197,198] Irradiation of blood products can lead to cell membrane destabilization, leading to ongoing leakage of intracellular potassium and a shortened shelf life; thus irradiation optimally occurs immediately before use of the blood to avoid hyperkalemia.[197]

Children who have undergone HSCT may represent a challenge for blood typing. Major and minor ABO mismatch, as occurs in the setting of allogeneic HSCT, potentiates a shift in the ABO/Rh status of the recipient, the degree of which depends on the timing and engraftment status of the transplant. Preoperative communication with the blood bank and oncologist is warranted for all children who have recently undergone HSCT and are at risk for requiring perioperative transfusion of blood products.[199]

Effects of Anesthetic Agents on Perioperative Immunomodulation

Recent research has focused on the potential impact of multiple perioperative factors on immunomodulation and the risk of tumor recurrence. To date, research has been in vitro or in retrospective adult studies; thus some or all of the findings may not be directly applicable to children.[200,201] Theoretically, a whole host of perioperative factors could potentially suppress the host immune system or even directly augment the cancer cells, leading to the growth of minimally residual tumor cells and recurrence of cancer.[201,202] Some studies have reported potentially harmful immunosuppression or cancer cell augmentation after anesthesia with volatile anesthetics, ketamine, opioids (particularly morphine), and benzodiazepines.[200-202] Propofol has shown mixed results, and nitrous oxide, while harmful in vitro, has not been linked to cancer recurrence in adults. The use of regional anesthesia has been shown to confer protection against recurrence in some but not all studies.[201,203] Multiple other factors have shown intermittent association with poor outcomes, including surgical stress response, hypotension, hypothermia, hyperglycemia, blood transfusions, glucocorticoids, and NSAIDs.[200] In summary, data are insufficient to support altering the anesthetic plan in children on the basis of reducing the risk of tumor recurrence.

Summary

Children with cancer present a host of challenges for the anesthesiologist as virtually every organ system may be dysfunctional as a result of the underlying malignancy, the toxicity of treatment, or both. Those in cancer remission often suffer varying degrees of chronic effects of cancer treatment that impact their anesthetic care decades later. As treatment options for pediatric cancer have expanded, it has become increasingly important for providers who care for these children to maintain an open line of communication with the surgical and oncology teams. An understanding of the physiologic and psychological aberrations in this population is essential in providing safe perioperative care for these vulnerable and complex patients.

ANNOTATED REFERENCES

Bindra RS, Wolden SL. Advances in radiation therapy in pediatric neuro-oncology. *J Child Neurol.* 2016;31(4):506-516.

This paper presents an update of the recent advances in radiation technology and treatment protocols for children with cancer.

Latham GJ, Greenberg RS. Anesthetic considerations for the pediatric oncology patient—part 1: a review of antitumor therapy. *Paediatr Anaesth.* 2010;20:295-304.

This article briefly reviews the current principles of cancer therapy and the general mechanisms of toxicity to the child, focusing on the impact to perioperative care and decision-making.

Latham GJ, Greenberg RS. Anesthetic considerations for the pediatric oncology patient—part 2: systems-based approach to anesthesia. *Paediatr Anaesth.* 2010;20:396-420.

A systems-based approach is used to assess the impact of the tumor and its treatment on children; relevant anesthetic considerations are discussed.

Latham GJ, Greenberg RS. Anesthetic considerations for the pediatric oncology patient—part 3: pain, cognitive dysfunction, and preoperative evaluation. *Paediatr Anaesth.* 2010;20:479-489.

This paper discusses the psychosocial impact of cancer and pain syndromes that should be considered in the perioperative period. A discussion of preanesthetic testing and evaluation in children with cancer follows.

Mackall CL, Merchant MS, Fry TJ. Immune-based therapies for childhood cancer. *Nat Rev Clin Oncol.* 2014;11(12):693-703.

This review excellently summarizes the rapidly growing field of immunotherapeutics used in the common forms of pediatric cancer.

A complete reference list can be found online at ExpertConsult.com.

Strategies for Blood Product Management, Reducing Transfusions, and Massive Blood Transfusion

CHARLES J. COTÉ, ERIC F. GRABOWSKI, AND CHRISTOPHER P. STOWELL

DESPITE ADVANCES IN PEDIATRIC SURGERY, infants and children may sustain major operative blood loss, but little information is available about when coagulation defects will begin to appear in children.[1,2] Most studies of massive blood transfusions have involved adult patients, with little evidence from children to build a massive transfusion strategy.[3]

A rational blood transfusion strategy is imperative in children because there is limited blood available and transfusions can cause complications. In countries with sophisticated health care systems, the most common fatal hazards of transfusion are hemolytic transfusion reactions related to ABO incompatibility (usually as a result of a transfusion error), transfusion-associated circulatory overload (TACO), and transfusion-related acute lung injury (TRALI).[4] In developing countries, the risk of infectious disease transmission may be greater because of endemic infections (e.g., Dengue, Chikungunya, malaria) and the technical or logistic limitations of donor screening.[5] Recently, the neurotropic Zika virus has become of great interest because of its marked association with microcephaly in the newborn,[6] and arthrogryposis in infants, and in adults, to Guillain-Barré syndrome and cognitive dysfunction.[7] RNA testing of blood donors in areas with high prevalence rates such as Brazil and Puerto Rico was instituted in the summer of 2016, and by late 2016 in the United States.[8] In nonendemic areas, donors are currently being screened for recent travel to countries where infection is prevalent. Children suffer from noninfectious complications of transfusion more frequently than adults. A review of 133,671 transfusions found 108 adverse events in children and 277 in adults; in children there was an increase in allergic reactions (2.7 vs. 1.1/1000), febrile reactions (1.9 vs. 0.47/1000) and hypotension (0.29 vs. 0.078/1000); unlike adults, reactions were twice as likely in male children (7.9 vs. 4.3/1000).[9]

Nothing changed the use of blood products more than the threat of AIDS.[10–12] Fortunately, the risk of infection with human immunodeficiency virus (HIV), hepatitis C virus (HCV), and Hepatitis B virus (HBV) by blood transfusion today is extremely rare. Implementation of donor education programs, improved health history screening, new tests, and new test technologies (Table 12.1) have markedly altered the spectrum of transfusion-transmitted infectious agents in the developed world. The risks of some of the infectious and noninfectious hazards of transfusion are summarized in Table 12.2.

Despite marked reductions in the transmission of HIV, HCV, and HBV, transfusions can produce other deleterious effects.[13,14] Every transfusion must be medically justified and its benefits weighed against the potential infectious, immunologic, and metabolic risks.[15] It is in the child's best interest to transfuse with a clear clinical goal and in the anesthesiologist's best interest to document the reason for each transfusion. It is not acceptable medical practice to administer a transfusion when it is of questionable benefit.

Blood Volume

The circulating blood volume of the child should be estimated before induction of anesthesia. The blood volume of a preterm infant (90–100 mL/kg) constitutes a greater proportion of body weight than that of a term neonate (80–90 mL/kg), an infant between 3 months and 1 year of age (70–80 mL/kg), and an older child (70 mL/kg). Body habitus affects the blood volume calculation since the latter is normalized to body weight. For example, an obese child has a smaller blood volume per kilogram, 60–65 mL/kg, than a nonobese child of the same weight. Using the estimated

TABLE 12.1	Current Blood Screening Tests Used on Donated Blood in the United States

Hepatitis B surface antigen (HBsAg)

Hepatitis B core antibody (anti-HBc)

Nucleic acid amplification testing for HBV DNA

Hepatitis C virus antibody (anti-HCV)

Nucleic acid amplification testing for HCV RNA

Human immunodeficiency virus type 1 (HIV-1) antibody (anti-HIV-1)

HIV-2 antibody (anti-HIV-2)

Nucleic acid amplification testing for HIV-1 RNA

Human T-lymphotropic virus type 1 (HTLV-I) antibody (anti-HTLV-I)

HTLV-II antibody (anti-HTLV-II)

Serologic test for syphilis (*Treponema pallidum*)

Nucleic acid amplification for West Nile virus (WNV) RNA[a]

Trypanosoma cruzi antibody (Chagas disease)[b]

Nucleic acid testing for Zika virus RNA

Screen for bacterial contamination—Platelets only

[a]This test depends on the incidence in the geographic area.
[b]At first donation or after residence in endemic area.
From American Association of Blood Banks. Blood FAQ. Available at http://www.aabb.org/tm/Pages/bloodfaq.aspx (accessed April 2016).

TABLE 12.2	Estimated Frequency of Complications per Number of Units Transfused	
Category	Complication	Frequency
Noninfectious	Allergic (urticarial)	1:100
	Febrile, nonhemolytic	1:100
	Transfusion-associated circulatory overload	1:1000
	Delayed hemolytic	1:1600
	Transfusion-related acute lung injury	1:10,000
	Acute hemolytic	1:50,000
	Fatal acute hemolytic	1:500,000
Infectious	Hepatitis B virus	1:1,000,000
	Hepatitis C virus	1:1,700,000
	Human T-lymphotropic virus type I	1:2,700,000
	Human immunodeficiency virus type 1	1:1,900,000
	Bacterial contamination of red blood cells	1:50,000
	Bacterial sepsis of red blood cells	1:500,000
	Bacterial contamination of platelets	1:2000
	Bacterial sepsis of platelets	1:75,000

Data from Galel SA. Infectious disease screening. In: Fung MK, et al. (eds.). *Technical Manual*. Bethesda, MD: AABB Press; 2014:194; Mazzei CA, Popovsky MA, Kopko PM. Non-infectious complications of transfusion. In: Fung MK, et al. (eds.). *Technical Manual*. Bethesda, MD: AABB press; 2014:684.

TABLE 12.3	Estimated Predicted Blood Loss and Recommended Monitoring and Equipment	
Predicted Blood Loss	Recommended Monitors or Equipment
<0.5 blood volume	Routine monitoring
0.5–1.0 blood volume	Routing monitoring + urine catheter
1.0 blood volume or more	Routine monitoring + urine catheter + CVP + arterial line
1.0 blood volume or more with potential for rapid blood loss	Routine monitoring + urine catheter + CVP + arterial line + large-bore IV line + rapid-infusion device
Severe head injury	Routine monitoring + urine catheter + CVP + arterial line + large-bore IV line
Major trauma with unknown severity	Routine monitoring + urine catheter + CVP + arterial line + large-bore IV line (preferably in upper extremity or central) + rapid-infusion device

CVP, central venous pressure; *IV*, intravenous.

demand depends on a number of factors, including the oxygen content of blood, cardiac output and its regional distribution, and metabolic needs. Rheologic considerations (e.g., ensuring adequate hepatic artery blood flow in liver transplant recipients) may also affect the optimal hematocrit. A child with severe pulmonary disease or cyanotic congenital heart disease often requires a greater hematocrit than a healthy child to satisfy oxygen demands. Preterm infants may require a greater hematocrit to prevent apnea, reduce cardiac and respiratory work, and possibly improve neurologic outcomes,[16] although the data are not clear.[17,18] If there is uncertainty about the need to transfuse these infants, the neonatologist should be consulted.[16,19,20] A healthy child readily tolerates a hematocrit well below 30%. It is our practice not to transfuse otherwise healthy infants up to about 3 months old until their hematocrits have decreased to 25% and hematocrits of older children have decreased to 20% if there is little potential for postoperative bleeding. *The circulating blood volume must be maintained in every case.* Observing the operative field to estimate blood loss and monitoring the vital signs, hematocrit, urine output, and the central venous pressure (CVP) help to assess the adequacy of volume replacement. If a procedure is expected to result in significant blood loss or fluid shifts, the anesthesiologist should strongly consider the use of a urine catheter, a central venous line, and invasive arterial monitoring. The child's size or age should not deter one from the use of a central venous catheter (Table 12.3). The introduction of noninvasive cardiac output monitors may further clarify the need for and response to transfusion and volume replacement (see also Chapter 52).[21]

There are three approaches for estimating the MABL: an approximation of circulating RBC mass, a modified logarithmic equation, and a simple proportion.[22,23] All three approaches yield clinically similar estimates of the MABL. The most straightforward method is to estimate the MABL by simple proportion.[22] For purposes of discussion, we use a hematocrit of 25% as the minimum acceptable hematocrit:

$$\text{MABL} = \frac{\text{EBV} \times (\text{Child's hematocrit} - \text{Minimum acceptable hematocrit})}{\text{Child's hematocrit}}$$

blood volume, the initial hemoglobin or hematocrit, and the minimum acceptable hematocrit, we can *estimate* the maximum allowable blood loss (MABL) before red blood cell (RBC) transfusion is indicated.

The minimum acceptable hematocrit varies according to an individual child's need. The balance between oxygen supply and

For example, a 10-kg child has an estimated blood volume of 10 (kg) × 70 (mL/kg), or 700 mL. If the child's hematocrit is 42, the MABL is calculated as follows:

$$MABL = \frac{700 \times (42 - 25)}{42}$$
$$= \frac{700 \times 17}{42}$$
$$= 285 \text{ mL}$$

These calculations only estimate the MABL. The actual hematocrit varies with the child's preexisting medical conditions, the rapidity of the blood loss, and the rate of concurrent crystalloid replacement.

It should be noted that commonly used crystalloid solutions for volume replacement actually consist of two solutions: normal saline and balanced electrolyte solutions. These are not identical solutions. Normal saline is slightly hyperosmolar (sodium concentration of 154 mEq/L [308 mOsm/L]) and may produce a non–anion gap hyperchloremic metabolic acidosis when given in large quantities (in polyvinyl bags the pH is 4.5–7.0). Balanced electrolyte solutions comprise a group of solutions that are slightly hypoosmolar (273 mOsm/L), contain one of several bases (lactate, gluconate, or acetate), and a pH of 5 to 8 (see also Chapter 9).

Initial therapy is directed at replacing fluid deficits and providing maintenance requirements (see Chapter 9). Additional fluid administration is directed at replacing blood loss and third space fluid losses. There seems to be little danger in replacing the entire MABL with crystalloid provided that the child is healthy and that postoperative oozing will not exceed the MABL. Historically, the consensus has been to replace each milliliter of shed blood with 2 to 3 mL of crystalloid.[24,25] However, more recent evidence suggests to replace each milliliter of shed blood with a smaller volume of crystalloid (i.e., 1–2 mL).[26] Colloid replacement is expensive and without clear evidence that it is superior to crystalloid, but it may be used to replace blood loss as 1 mL of 5% albumin per milliliter of shed blood.[27,28] New starch volume expanders have been introduced that may hold promise in the future for use in children, but the long-term safety implications for their use are as yet unclear.[29,30]

In our example of the 10-kg child with a 700-mL blood volume and a 285-mL MABL, the child's blood volume can be restored by administering either 570 mL of isotonic crystalloid or 285 mL of 5% albumin. However, if the blood loss exceeds the MABL or if the hematocrit decreases to 20% to 25% (particularly if additional blood loss is expected during or after surgery), then transfusion with packed red blood cells (PRBCs) or whole blood (if available) is indicated. If postoperative bleeding is likely to occur (e.g., posterior spinal fusion, open heart operations, burn wound excision and grafting), it is reasonable to transfuse to a level greater than the minimum acceptable hematocrit. This is especially true if a greater hematocrit can be achieved without exposing the child to additional units of blood. If a unit of blood has been started, it is reasonable to give the child an additional 5% to 10% volume rather than a fraction of a new unit postoperatively. It is our practice to administer as much of the unit as can be safely tolerated rather than expose the child to another unit of blood postoperatively. Blood banks often prepare several aliquots from one unit of blood, especially for neonates and infants. In this manner, a single donor unit can be assigned to a particular child with each aliquot infused as needed at different times.

If PRBCs are used to replace the shed RBCs, then the volume of PRBCs needed to restore a specific hematocrit may be calculated quite simply. For example, if the hematocrit of a 10-kg child has decreased to 23% and the intraoperative blood loss is expected to continue postoperatively, then the anesthesiologist can use the following formula to estimate the volume of PRBCs needed to achieve a final hematocrit of 35% as follows:

Volume of PRBCs =

$$\frac{(\text{Desired Hct} - \text{Present Hct}) \times \text{Estimated Blood Volume (70 mL/kg} \times 10 \text{ kg)}}{\text{Hematocrit of PRCBs}}$$
$$= \frac{(35 - 23) \times (70 \times 10)}{60}$$
$$= 140 \text{ mL PRBCs}$$

Because this volume is less than 1 unit, it may be reasonable to transfuse more volume than calculated—that is, up to a hematocrit of 40% (~200 mL PRBCs) to allow an additional margin of safety for postoperative blood loss. A prospective study by the American College of Surgeons National Quality Improvement Program–Pediatrics involving 50 institutions found that there were significant differences in transfusion practices among institutions and that transfusions were more likely in infants and children 2 years of age or younger (odds ratio [OR]) 5.9–3.4), ASA class IV (OR 3.2), preoperative septic shock (OR 14.5), and preoperative cardiopulmonary resuscitation (OR 8.1).[31]

Blood Components and Alternatives

In countries with well-developed health care systems, most whole blood collected from donors is fractionated into components. A unit of whole blood can provide 1 unit of PRBCs, 1 unit of whole blood–derived platelets, and 1 unit of fresh frozen plasma (FFP). Apheresis technology can be used to collect any one of these three components selectively. Separation of the individual components from blood allows each to be stored under conditions that optimally preserve its function—for example, at refrigerator temperature (4°–10°C) for PRBC, at less than −18°C for FFP, and at room temperature (20°–24°C) for platelets. Most children with specific disease states (e.g., anemia, clotting factor deficiencies, thrombocytopenia) require only one of these fractions, which is why use of component therapy is widespread.

RED BLOOD CELL–CONTAINING COMPONENTS

Blood components containing RBCs are indicated for the treatment of symptomatic deficits of oxygen-carrying capacity.[32,33] PRBCs are the most widely available RBC-containing blood component, although in settings where the collection facilities do not have the capability to make components, whole blood may be the only component available. Donor whole blood is collected in a preservative-anticoagulant solution that contains citrate, phosphate, dextrose (glucose), and adenine (CPDA) or just citrate, phosphate, and dextrose (CPD). In the latter case, the platelet-rich plasma is removed after centrifugation of the whole blood unit, and a solution containing adenine, dextrose, and occasionally mannitol is added to the PRBCs. The additive-solution systems permit storage for 42 days (compared with 35 days for CPDA) and better preservation of 2,3-diphosphoglycerate (DPG) levels. The characteristics of the CPDA and additive-solution PRBCs and of whole blood at the time of outdate are shown in Table 12.4; the hematocrit is reduced in the additive-solution PRBCs and the total volume is increased, but the red cell mass remains the same.

RBCs carry glycoconjugate antigens of the ABH histo-blood group system on the cell surface that are determined by three common alleles at the ABO locus on chromosome 9.[34] During

TABLE 12.4 Composition of Components Containing Red Blood Cells at Outdate

Parameter	CPDA-1 Whole Blood[a]	CPDA-1 RBC[a]	Additive Solution RBC[b]
Storage time (days)	35	35	42
Volume RBC (mL)[c]	203	203	203
Residual plasma (mL)[c,d]	248	50	30
Hematocrit (%)	40	72	53
pH	6.98	6.71	6.6
Adenosine triphosphate (% of day 1)	56	45	60
2,3-DPG (% of day 1)	<10	<10	<10
Total supernatant K$^+$ (mEq/unit)	5–7	5–7	5–7

CPDA, citrate, phosphate, dextrose, and adenine solution; DPG, 2,3-diphosphoglycerate; RBC, red blood cell.
[a]Outdated at 35 days.
[b]Outdated at 42 days.
[c]Based on collection of 450 mL of whole blood with a hematocrit of 45%.
[d]The concentration of factors V and VIII is reduced to 20% to 50% of normal levels (0.2 to 0.5 units/mL). The other clotting factors are quite stable.

TABLE 12.5 ABO Compatibility of Blood Components

Recipient ABO Group	ACCEPTABLE COMPONENT ABO GROUPS (SECOND CHOICE)			
	Whole Blood	PRBC	FFP/Cryo	Platelets
O	O	O	O (A, B, AB, plasma)	O (A, B, AB)
A	A	A (O)	A (AB)	A (AB)[a]
B	B	B (O)	B (AB)	B (AB)[a]
AB	AB	AB (A, B, O)	AB	AB[a]

Cryo, cryoprecipitate; FFP, fresh frozen plasma; PRBC, packed red blood cells.
[a]Can come from group apheresis platelets (or whole blood–derived platelets for small child) if plasma is removed or replaced.

TABLE 12.6 Rh(D) Compatibility of Blood Components

Recipient Rh(D) Type	ACCEPTABLE COMPONENT Rh(D) TYPES (SECOND CHOICE)			
	Whole Blood or PRBCs	FFP/Cryo	Apheresis Platelets	Whole Blood–Derived Platelets
Positive	Rh-positive (Rh-negative)	Any	Any	Rh-positive (Rh-negative)
Negative	Rh-negative (Rh-positive)[a]	Any	Any	Rh-negative (Rh-positive)[a,b]

Cryo, cryoprecipitate; FFP, fresh frozen plasma; PRBCs, packed red blood cells.
[a]Depending on inventory, the blood bank may switch to Rh(D)-positive, particularly for male patients or postmenopausal females.
[b]Consider Rh immune globulin for females with childbearing potential receiving whole blood–derived platelets from Rh(D)-positive donors.

TABLE 12.7 Common Initial Doses of Blood Components and Expected Effects in Children

Component	Dose	Effect
Packed red blood cells	10–15 mL/kg	Increase hemoglobin by 2–3 g/dL[a]
Platelets[b]	5–10 mL/kg	Increase platelet count by 50,000–100,000/mm^3
Fresh frozen plasma	10–15 mL/kg	Factor levels increase by 15%–20%
Cryoprecipitate	1–2 units/kg	Increase fibrinogen by 60–100 mg/dL
Fibrinogen concentrate	70 mg/kg	Increase in fibrinogen level of 120 mg/dL

[a]Note that the hematocrit of PRBCs varies from ~60% to 70% for packed red blood cells in citrate, phosphate, dextrose (glucose), and adenine (CPDA) versus ~55% for packed red blood cells in additive-solution systems; the total volume of packed red blood cells is, however, the same.
[b]This recommendation may be reduced pending the impact of the prophylactic platelet dose (PLADO) trial, as published for all age groups[35] and for the pediatric age range.[36]

the first year of life, infants begin to elaborate alloantibodies to whichever A or B antigens they lack. These isoagglutinins are invariably present after a few months and constitute a formidable immunologic obstacle to transfusion or transplantation across this ABO barrier. The RBCs for transfusion must be compatible with the ABO isoagglutinins of the intended transfusion recipient. Similarly, components with a large volume of plasma (e.g., whole blood, FFP, apheresis platelets) must be compatible with the A or B surface antigens expressed on the recipient's RBCs. PRBCs must be ABO *compatible* with the recipient, whereas whole blood must be ABO *identical* because of the larger volume of donor plasma and, hence, AB isoagglutinins. Table 12.5 summarizes the permissible combinations.

Only RBCs express the Rh(D) antigen. Rh(D)-positive patients may receive Rh(D)-positive or Rh(D)-negative RBCs. Rh(D)-negative patients are routinely given Rh(D)-negative RBCs for any elective transfusions, but in the setting of massive transfusion it may be necessary to switch to Rh(D)-positive RBCs to preserve the supply of Rh(D)-negative RBCs. The blood bank usually determines when to make this substitution based on the inventory and does so more quickly for a patient who is a male or a postmenopausal female (Table 12.6). The objective is to avoid exposing a female with childbearing potential to Rh(D)-positive RBCs and possibly triggering the production of the anti-D alloantibody, which is responsible for the most severe forms of hemolytic disease of the newborn. Table 12.7 shows the common initial volume of PRBCs needed to increase the hemoglobin level by 2 to 3 g/dL.

The changes that occur to RBCs during storage under conventional blood bank conditions have been well described.[37] These observations have generated physiologically plausible hypotheses about how such changes may impair the function of the banked RBCs in vivo. The reduced hemoglobin level of 2,3-DPG and its corresponding decrease in the P_{50} value may reduce the ability of stored RBCs to relinquish bound O_2 compared with 2,3-DPG–replete RBCs. The depletion of nitric oxide (NO) may reduce the vasodilatory properties of the RBCs, hence impairing their ability to maintain the patency of the small vessels in the microcirculation and blood flow to the tissues.[38] Numerous changes in the composition and behavior of the RBC plasma membrane, including the loss and oxidation of membrane lipids and proteins and the rearrangement of some membrane constituents,[39] correlate with changes in the shape and elasticity of the RBC membrane.[40-42] The loss of elasticity in particular can impede the rapid movement of the RBCs through the microcirculation.

These hypotheses and some supportive data from animal models[43] have led to a number of observational clinical studies (mostly in trauma, critical care, colorectal surgery, and cardiac surgery) of outcomes after using stored PRBCs, but the results have been inconclusive.[44-46] One prospective, observational study from 30 North American Centers in 296 children younger than 18 years of age who received blood stored 14 days or longer reported increased multiple organ dysfunction (OR 1.87) and increased pediatric intensive care unit (PICU) stay (~3.7 days) but no difference in mortality.[47] A small study of pediatric cardiac surgical patients found that children who received blood older than 3 days required additional RBC and FFP transfusions but this study was underpowered.[48] About half of such observational studies found a statistical association between an unfavorable clinical outcome measure and the transfusion of RBCs that had been stored for a greater time. However, no such association was reported in the other half of the studies, including two that were extensions of previous studies with positive findings. A small number of randomized, controlled trials (RCTs) addressed this issue without statistically significant differences in outcomes between patients receiving RBCs stored for different amounts of time,[49] although two of them were underpowered.[50,51] Knowing that RBCs change during storage raises the question of whether these changes affect children in a clinically meaningful way, a question that remains unanswered by the observational studies.[52]

In the past few years, several RCTs have addressed these issues in four different patient populations, two of which were in pediatric cohorts. A multicenter RCT conducted in Canada randomized low–birth-weight neonates in ICUs to receive PRBCs stored 8 days or less or the standard of care, which was to provide aliquots from one unit of PRBCs to each infant until transfusion was no longer required or the donor unit was depleted.[48] There were no differences in the incidence of infections, bronchopulmonary dysplasia, necrotizing enterocolitis, death, or the composite between the two groups. Children in Uganda between the ages of 6 months and 6 years who presented with severe anemia (hemoglobin <5 g/dL) and lactic acidosis (lactate >5 mmol/L) were randomly assigned to receive PRBCs stored 10 days or less or 35 days longer.[49] There were no differences in lactate clearance, left ventricular strain, as assessed by β-naturietic peptide or, in a subset of patients, correction of cerebral tissue oxygen saturation as measured by near-infrared spectroscopy. Two studies in adults compared clinical outcomes after transfusion with PRBCs stored for different periods of time. Patients 12 years of age or older undergoing complex cardiac surgery and very likely to require PRBC transfusion were randomly assigned to receive PRBCs stored 10 days or longer or 28 days or less.[50] No differences were observed in the change in the Multiple Organ Dysfunction Score (MODS) or mortality at 7 or 28 days, in length of ICU or hospital length of stay, or in the frequency of serious adverse events. Adult patients in ICUs in Canada were randomly assigned to receive PRBCs stored 8 days or less versus the standard of care, which was to issue the oldest units first.[51] No differences were found for 30- or 90-day mortality, ICU or hospital length of stay, changes in MODS, or several other clinical endpoints. There is no apparent clinical benefit derived by transfusing units of PRBCs, which have been stored for a period of time that is substantially shorter than that of the PRBCs routinely supplied by our current inventory practices for these vulnerable populations.

PLATELETS

Platelets may be obtained from a unit of whole blood or collected by apheresis. Platelets from whole blood are separated by centrifugation and suspended in 40 to 60 mL of plasma at a concentration that is two to four times greater than in the circulation. Each unit contains a minimum of 5.5×10^{10} platelets and is stored at 20°C to 24°C with gentle continuous agitation for a maximum of 5 days. One unit of whole blood–derived platelets can be expected to increase the platelet count in an 18-kg child by 15,000/mm^3 and in a 70-kg adult by 5000 to 10,000/mm^3.[41,53] A unit of platelets obtained by apheresis contains at least 3×10^{11} platelets in 200 to 400 mL of plasma, or the equivalent of approximately 6 units of whole blood–derived platelets. A common dose for children is 0.1 to 0.3 unit/kg of body weight, or 10 to 15 mL/kg (see Table 12.7); this dose usually produces an increment of 30,000 to 90,000/mm^3. However, in several prophylactic platelet dose trials for medical causes of bleeding, doses equivalent to the standard dose of 1 pheresis unit (or 6 units of whole blood–derived platelet concentrates) per meter squared, half of this dose and double this dose were compared in 1272 adult and children who received at least 1 platelet transfusion.[54,55] Blood losses were determined with the World Health Organization (WHO) bleeding scale: grade 0 = no bleeding, grade 1 = petechiae, grade 2 = mild blood loss, grade 3 = gross blood loss, and grade 4 = debilitating blood loss. No differences were observed in bleeding outcomes (WHO grade ≥2) among the three doses. The subset of 200 children were found to have a greater risk for bleeding than adults for unknown reasons, but bleeding in this age group also did not differ by platelet dose received and was seemingly unrelated to platelet counts.[42] The recommended platelet dose may be reduced in the near future, but this change awaits further discussion by the blood transfusion and hemostasis community.[56-58] This trial assessed the use of platelets to prevent bleeding events and did not address patients undergoing surgical procedures with ongoing bleeding.

In the setting of dilutional thrombocytopenia with ongoing blood loss or a consumptive coagulopathy (e.g., disseminated intravascular coagulation), larger doses (≥0.3 unit/kg) may be required to boost the platelet count above 50,000/mm^3. Because platelets are suspended in plasma that contains the anti-A and anti-B isoagglutinins, they should be ABO compatible with the recipient's RBCs. Some blood donors have high-titer isoagglutinins that can produce hemolysis in transfusion recipients if a large enough volume of plasma is given.[59] The transfusion of plasma-incompatible, whole blood–derived platelets to adult recipients does not produce clinically significant hemolysis because the volume of plasma given is so small relative to the plasma volume of an adult. However, apheresis platelets (and whole blood–derived platelets for small children) should be ABO compatible with the recipient's RBCs. Matching for Rh(D) antigen is not necessary for apheresis platelets because platelets do not express Rh antigens and they contain virtually no RBCs. However, whole blood–derived platelets may contain enough RBCs to provoke Rh alloimmunization, so platelets from Rh(D)-negative donors are given preferentially to Rh(D)-negative recipients with childbearing potential. If a premenopausal female receives whole blood–derived platelets from an Rh(D)-positive donor, Rh immune globulin (Rhogam) can be administered within 72 hours to prevent alloimmunization. Platelets should never be withheld in an emergency situation because of Rh(D) incompatibility.

Platelets are essential to hemostasis associated with the vascular injury of surgery and are necessary for the control of surgical bleeding. Platelets are also required for the maintenance of an intact endothelial barrier to spontaneous blood loss. The number of platelets required to provide adequate hemostasis in the surgical setting is much greater than the number needed to provide prophylaxis against spontaneous hemorrhage. A platelet count of 40,000 to 50,000 /mm³ is considered adequate to prevent spontaneous bleeding or bleeding from minor invasive procedures (e.g., lumbar puncture, line placement) in an otherwise stable child. If overt signs of bleeding are present or a more significant hemostatic challenge in the form of a surgical procedure is imminent, sustaining a level of 30,000 to 50,000/mm³ for several days may be required.[60-64] A target level of 50,000/mm³ is appropriate in the setting of massive transfusion.[61,65-67] Platelets may also be required for children with adequate counts but in whom platelet function is impaired in some forms of congenital heart disease and following cardiopulmonary bypass.[68,69] Many medications (e.g., aspirin; other nonsteroidal antiinflammatory agents, including ibuprofen and naproxen; dipyridamole; platelet P2Y12 receptor blockers such as clopidogrel or prasugrel; or glycoprotein IIa/IIIb receptor inhibitors such as abciximab, eptifibatide, or tirofiban; serotonin uptake antagonists such as Zoloft) and some medical conditions (e.g., renal failure with blood urea nitrogen levels above 60 mg/dL) cause abnormal platelet function, which may interfere with surgical hemostasis, in which case it may be necessary to maintain the platelet count at a somewhat greater concentration, at least until the effect of the medication dissipates or the child's platelets have largely been replaced by banked platelets.[70,71] In a few settings, such as intracranial, ophthalmic, and otologic surgery, even greater concentrations (100,000/mm³) may be sought, although the appropriate threshold in these settings has not been examined in detail.

There is no clear-cut threshold value below which the platelet count predicts clinical bleeding in the perioperative period. Each child must be individually assessed by constantly observing the surgical field for evidence of abnormal bleeding.[72] Unfortunately, we lack a well-validated bedside tool to assess platelet function. The utility of the thromboelastogram and other devices to measure platelet function under controlled flow conditions, such as microfluidic flow devices[73,74] and the platelet function analyzer (PFA-100), are currently under investigation but are not at this time able to predict risk for hemorrhage.[75-78] The standard technique for diagnosis and evaluation of thrombocytopathies remains Born-O'Brien platelet aggregometry, but it is not useful in the intraoperative or intensive care setting.[79] Most commonly, dilutional thrombocytopenia rather than a newly acquired platelet function defect is the cause in the operative setting and in massive transfusion.

A child occasionally presents for surgery with a previously characterized platelet dysfunction that may be associated with bleeding. If the child has a normal platelet count, it is reasonable practice to ensure that the blood bank has an adequate platelet supply available for the operating room and to withhold transfusion of platelets until pathologic bleeding occurs.

Several additional points should be considered[80]:

1. Not all hospitals have platelets in the inventory. Unless the need is anticipated before surgery, platelets may not be available when they are required. Therefore, a preemptive request for platelets may have to be arranged.

2. For children who are thrombocytopenic before surgery, platelets should be infused just before the surgical procedure to ensure the greatest concentrations during the time of peak demand. The start of the procedure should *not* be delayed to obtain the results of a posttransfusion platelet count.

3. Platelets should be filtered only by large-pore filters (≥150 μm) or leukocyte-reduction filters (if indicated). Micropore filters may adsorb large numbers of platelets, thereby diminishing the effectiveness of the platelet transfusion.

4. Platelets are suspended in plasma, which may help to replenish coagulation factors other than factors V and VIII, which are labile, and factor VII, which has an especially brief half-life.

5. Platelets should not be refrigerated or placed in a cooler with ice before administration, because cold-exposed platelets are rapidly cleared from the circulation.

SPECIAL PROCESSING OF CELLULAR BLOOD COMPONENTS

Leukocytes collected with whole blood donations partition into both the platelet and the PRBC components; few intact leukocytes are present in FFP. Passenger leukocytes are responsible for most febrile, nonhemolytic transfusion reactions, human leukocyte antigen (HLA) alloimmunization, and transmission of cytomegalovirus (CMV). To prevent the complications from these leukocytes, blood components should be passed through leukocyte-reduction filters that effectively remove leukocytes (by a 2–3 log reduction) immediately after collection (prestorage leukoreduction) or at the bedside (pretransfusion). This technique is superior to washing or freezing-deglycerolizing, which was used in the past. Table 12.8 lists those patients who may benefit from leukocyte-reduced cellular components (i.e., PRBCs or platelets). It should be noted that anaphylaxis may very rarely occur when using white-cell reduction filters.[81]

CMV transmission can also be reduced by screening donors for CMV exposure (testing for antibody to CMV), although leukocyte reduction is the more widely used approach. Even though primary CMV infection is benign in children with intact immune systems, some pediatric populations are at risk for developing systemic disease and should be protected from blood-borne CMV transmission. Only patients who have not previously been infected with CMV (i.e., CMV-seronegative) are at risk. Children who are particularly vulnerable to systemic CMV infections are listed in E-Table 12.1.

Transfused lymphocytes may mediate a graft-versus-host process in some recipients with impaired cellular immunity. Because this process involves the bone marrow as well as the usual targets (i.e., skin and gastrointestinal tract), the fatality rate is substantial. Transfusion-associated graft-versus-host disease (TA-GVHD) can be prevented by exposing cellular blood components to gamma irradiation that disables the donor lymphocytes.[82] Children who are considered to be at risk for TA-GVHD and who should receive irradiated cellular components are listed in E-Table 12.2. This complication can also occur in children with intact immune

TABLE 12.8	Indications for Leukocyte-Reduced Cellular Blood Components

- To prevent further febrile, nonhemolytic transfusion reactions in a child with a history of such reactions
- To prevent human leukocyte antigen alloimmunization in a child who may require long-term platelet transfusion support (e.g., leukemia, lymphoma)
- To prevent human leukocyte antigen alloimmunization in a transplant recipient
- To prevent cytomegalovirus infection and disease in a susceptible child

systems in the unusual circumstance when the transfusion donor is homozygous for an HLA haplotype that is shared with the recipient. In this case, the recipient's immune system, although fully functional, cannot recognize the donor lymphocytes as foreign. The donor lymphocytes mount a GVHD attack on the recipient's tissues, recognizing the mismatched haplotype. This situation is more likely to occur when the donor is a blood relative of the recipient. It is for this reason that blood and HLA-matched platelets donated by family members are routinely irradiated.

Because irradiation damages the cell membrane, irradiated RBCs lose K^+ at a greater rate than usual. As a result, the shelf life of irradiated RBC is only 28 days (from a maximum permitted of 42 days). The problem of increased amounts of circulating K^+ can be obviated by irradiating units close to the time of issue or washing the unit if it was irradiated early in the storage period.

FRESH FROZEN PLASMA

FFP represents the fluid portion of whole blood that is separated and frozen within 8 hours of collection. After thawing at 37°C, which usually requires 30 minutes, it may be administered within 24 hours if stored at 1°C to 6°C. The volume of 1 unit varies from 180 to 300 mL and represents 7% to 10% of the coagulation factor activity in a 70-kg patient. It contains all of the clotting factors and regulatory proteins at approximately the native concentration, but after 6 hours at 1°C to 6°C, the concentrations of the labile factors V and VIII begin to diminish, as does that of the short-lived factor VII.[83] FFP does not provide functional platelets, nor does it contain leukocytes or RBCs. Thawed FFP may be used for transfusion up to 7 days after thawing; however, it must be labeled as thawed plasma to indicate that it has reduced levels of factors V, VII, VIII, and protein S.

FFP should be ABO compatible with recipient red cells because it contains the anti-A and anti-B isoagglutinins appropriate to the donor's ABO blood group. If the recipient's blood type is not known, plasma from a donor with blood type AB, which contains neither anti-A nor anti-B, may be administered. Because the citrate anticoagulant is present in the plasma, rapid administration of FFP is more likely to be associated with citrate toxicity than the transfusion of components with smaller volumes of plasma (e.g., PRBCs).

FFP is all too often administered without justification by evidence-based medicine.[84] One major surgical indication for FFP is to correct the coagulopathy associated with massive blood transfusion (see Table 12.7). Other indications include correction of a prolongation in the prothrombin time (PT) before surgery or in the setting of bleeding, the emergency reversal of warfarin, or the presence of a specific congenital or acquired coagulation protein deficiency for which a factor concentrate or a recombinant factor is not available (e.g., for factor X deficiency).[85] Administration of vitamin K should not be overlooked in children with hepatic insufficiency, who have been exclusively breastfed,[86–88] who have been treated with warfarin, broad-spectrum antibiotics (which often eliminate normal vitamin K–producing gastrointestinal flora), or total parenteral nutrition for inadequate oral caloric intake, or who have had a prolonged hospitalization. Correction of a mild increase in the PT (e.g., international normalized ratio [INR] <1.5) is rarely necessary. Fig. 12.1 shows the relationship between the level of coagulation factors and the in vitro clotting time—in this case, the PT. Relatively modest levels of coagulation factors can support normal hemostasis, even though the PT is prolonged. When the PT is markedly increased (see Fig. 12.1, point A), the transfusion of 1 unit of FFP, which increases the coagulation factor levels by 7% to 10% in an adult, dramatically decreases the PT. When the PT is only mildly prolonged, as at point C, where factor levels are already adequate for hemostasis, infusion of 1 unit of FFP (in an adult) decreases the PT to a much smaller

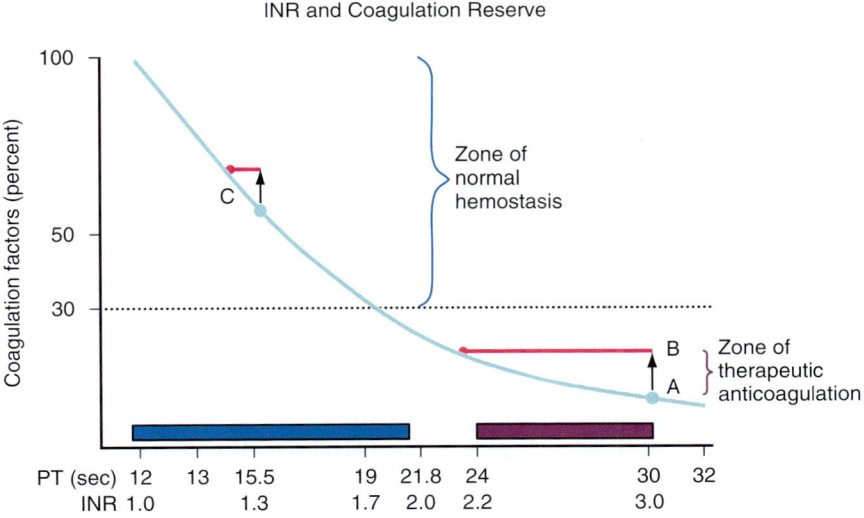

FIGURE 12.1 Nonlinear relationship between levels of coagulation factor and clotting test results. Decreases in clotting factor levels to about 30% of normal prolong the clotting test times but still support normal hemostasis. Treating an adult or child at point **A** with fresh frozen plasma to raise the level of coagulation factors to point **B** has a marked effect on the prothrombin time and the international normalized ratio (INR). The same amount of fresh frozen plasma administered to an adult or child at point **C**, however, has only a minor effect on the prothrombin time (PT). (Modified from Dzik WH, Stowell CP. Transfusion and coagulation issues in trauma. In: Sheridan RL, ed. *The Trauma Handbook of Massachusetts General Hospital.* Philadelphia: Lippincott Williams & Wilkins; 2004:139.)

extent. This small decrease in the PT does not clinically improve hemostasis.

CRYOPRECIPITATE

Cryoprecipitate is prepared by thawing FFP at 4°C to 10°C and removing most of the plasma, leaving behind precipitated protein that is then resuspended in a small volume of residual plasma (15–25 mL) and refrozen. This component contains 20% to 50% of the factor VIII from the original unit of plasma. It also contains von Willebrand factor (vWF), fibrinogen (approximately 250 mg), and factor XIII. Cryoprecipitate is indicated for the treatment of factor XIII deficiency, dysfibrinogenemia, and hypofibrinogenemia (see Table 12.7).[89-98] It has not been used for the treatment of von Willebrand disease or hemophilia A since the advent of clotting factor concentrates and recombinant factor VIII. Plasma concentrates of factor XIII and fibrinogen have been licensed in the United States for use in patients with these congenital deficiencies.

PATHOGEN INACTIVATION/REDUCTION

Techniques to inactivate or reduce the level of infectious agents have been in place for plasma derivatives such as intravenous (IV) immunoglobulin and plasma-derived clotting factors for over 20 years. More recently, pathogen inactivation technologies have been applied to RBCs, FFP, and platelets with the goal of eliminating a wide range of infectious organisms.[99] There are several potential advantages of these technologies over screening by donor history and testing for specific organisms, particularly for those pathogens that frequently cause asymptomatic infection, have a long serologic "window" period before screening tests become positive, are newly emerging, or are completely new and unrecognized.[100]

There are two general approaches to pathogen inactivation: methods that disrupt lipid membranes (solvent detergent treatment[101] and methylene blue plus visible light exposure[102]) and methods that target RNA and DNA (or nucleic acid techniques) [amotosalen[103] or riboflavin[104] plus ultraviolet (UV) light exposure, or UV light exposure alone].[105] The nucleic acid–targeted techniques also inactivate leukocytes and eliminate the risk of transfusion-transmitted graft versus host disease, which may make gamma irradiation of cellular components for susceptible patients unnecessary.[106]

However, these techniques do have limitations. Even though inactivation techniques can achieve a 5 or 6 log reduction in infectious particles, they may not be completely effective in components with high pathogen loads.[107] In addition, the lipid-targeted techniques do not inactivate nonlipid enveloped viruses such as hepatitis A virus, hepatitis E virus, and parvovirus B19, and none of the techniques inactivates prions. These procedures also damage or deplete plasma proteins[108,109] and platelets, which may reduce their effectiveness.[110] Although there is no evidence to date of major adverse effects,[111] there is the potential for toxicity such as the formation of plasma or membrane protein neoantigens,[101] or from long-term effects of exposure to amotosalen. Finally, these treatments are relatively complex and expensive.

In the United States, several pathogen-inactivated component systems have been licensed by the Food and Drug Administration (FDA): plasma[112] and platelets[113] treated with amotosalen and UV-A light; plasma treated with riboflavin and UV light[104]; and solvent/detergent-treated plasma.[101] There are currently no licensed systems for pathogen inactivation of RBCs, although several are under investigation.

PLASMA-DERIVED FACTOR CONCENTRATES AND RECOMBINANT FACTORS

The most commonly administered factor concentrate is factor VIII, used in the treatment of hemophilia A. Children with hemophilia can have many problems related to their disease, including splenomegaly, abnormal liver function, and joint disease related to hemarthrosis. In the past, the use of pooled plasma products was associated with very high rates of transmission of viral hepatitis (especially HCV) and HIV.[114-116] The use of more rigorous viral removal and inactivation processes and the introduction of recombinant factor VIII and IX products[117-121] have greatly reduced these problems.[89-96,122] Initial concerns that there may be an increased incidence of inhibitors in children who receive recombinant therapy compared with plasma-derived factor therapy have been confirmed by the SIPPET trial (Survey of Inhibitors in Plasma-Product Exposed Toddlers),[123] which showed that toddlers treated with plasma-derived factor VIII containing VWF had a nearly twofold lower incidence of inhibitors than those treated with recombinant factor VIII. However, the study failed to show a significant difference with regard to high-titer inhibitors and did not include any of the newer concentrates that have appeared since the trial started in 2010. Therefore, final conclusions regarding the use of recombinant factors remain unclear. Mild hemophilia A usually responds well to desmopressin (1-deamino-8-D-arginine vasopressin [DDAVP]) therapy.[124,125]

New extended half-life factor concentrates are now available for both hemophilia A and B. For factor VIII and factor IX concentrates, these include fusion to either albumin or the monomeric Fc fragment of immunoglobin G1 (IgG1). Conjugation with polyethylene glycol (glycosylation) is another modification technique.[126] The optimal use of these concentrates is under current investigation.

Von Willebrand disease is routinely treated with DDAVP or plasma-derived factor VIII concentrates that are also rich in vWF, such as Humate-P, Alphanate, Koate DVI, and Wilate,[127] with dosing in ristocetin cofactor units per kilogram, not factor VIII units. A newly available alternative is a recombinant VWF,[128] although this product is so far only approved for those 18 years or older. In children who have von Willebrand disease and are resistant to DDAVP or for whom DDAVP is contraindicated (e.g., central nervous system [CNS] bleeding, allergic reaction, brain tumor, recent CNS surgery), it is reasonable to withhold treatment with blood-derived products until surgery has begun unless surgery is performed in an area where even minor bleeding can produce serious complications. These children often do not demonstrate pathologic bleeding. Adjunctive therapies that can further limit hemorrhage include use of the antifibrinolytic agent ε-aminocaproic acid (Amicar) and tranexamic acid (Cyklokapron), a competitive inhibitor of plasminogen, both being administered orally or intravenously, and topical hemostatic agents, including topical collagen and fibrin glues.

Children with hemophilia B (i.e., Christmas disease or factor IX deficiency) are managed with recombinant human factor IX and highly purified factor IX (preparations with various amounts of factors VII, X, and prothrombin) that are treated to inactivate or remove viruses.[91,92,94,129-142] Careful planning of any surgical procedure for these children includes close communication with the child's hematologist to ensure optimal therapy while reducing unnecessary transfusions (see Chapter 10).

PROTHROMBIN COMPLEX CONCENTRATES

Prothrombin complex concentrates (PCC) have been used to rapidly reverse vitamin K–based anticoagulants in the setting of significant hemorrhage, especially in the CNS. They consist of either three-factor (II, *low VII*, IX, and X, proteins C and S) or four-factor (II, *high VII*, IX, and X, proteins C and S) human plasma-derived products. These have been primarily used in adults; pediatric experience is limited.[143] The advantages appear to be a more rapid reversal than the administration of FFP or vitamin K (without, however, any difference in clinical outcomes) and for some patients, reduced volume of administration.[144–147] One systematic review concluded that four-factor PCC more reliably corrected the INR than three-factor PCC, whereas another suggested that protocols based on body weight offer an advantage over individual physician decisions.[148,149] However, in the setting of intracranial bleeding in patients taking warfarin, four-factor PCC has not proven superior to FFP. The efficacy of PCCs in the operating room setting to treat perioperative coagulopathy is unclear.[150]

DESMOPRESSIN

DDAVP, a synthetic analog of vasopressin, can increase the levels of factor VIII:C (i.e., coagulant activity) and factor VIII:vWF in children with mild hemophilia A or von Willebrand disease.[125,151–156] An IV dose of 0.3 μg/kg (maximum 20 μg; a subcutaneous preparation is available in Europe) increases the levels of both factors twofold to threefold within 30 to 60 minutes, with a half-life of 3 to 6 hours.[152] Intranasal DDAVP is also effective, but onset is less rapid and, in younger children for whom a sustained inhalation may be more difficult, part of the dose may find its way into the gastrointestinal tract, bypassing nasal blood vessels. Between 80% and 90% of children with von Willebrand disease are responders,[157,158] and affected children should be tested for their responsiveness to IV DDAVP. This treatment is best suited to treat bleeding from surgical procedures, which ceases within 2 to 3 days. When bleeding continues beyond this period, as is the case with some orthopedic procedures, daily IV Humate P (or Alphanate or Koate DVI) can obviate possible tachyphylaxis with DDAVP. Products rich in the vWF allow better control over peak concentrations of factor VIII. When in excess of 200%, factor VIII predisposes to postoperative deep venous thrombosis and pulmonary embolism.

DDAVP has been used to treat the coagulopathy associated with platelet dysfunction, uremia, and cirrhosis.[159,160] It may reduce elective surgical bleeding when the potential for blood loss is substantial, such as in cardiac surgery and spinal fusion.[125,161–166] Although initial reports apparently demonstrated a benefit in patients who did not have a preexisting coagulopathy, other controlled studies failed to show an effect despite increases in factor VIII:C and vWF, and its use for these indications has largely been abandoned.[167–169] Because of the potential for hyponatremia from water retention, use of DDAVP is avoided in children younger than 2 years, in children with CNS lesions, including a brain tumor, history of CNS irradiation, or recent neurosurgery or CNS trauma.[170]

ALBUMIN, DEXTRANS, STARCHES, AND GELATINS

Solutions of several high–molecular-weight molecules (i.e., colloids) have been used for volume replacement, although systematic reviews have determined they offer no advantage over crystalloid solutions. These colloids include albumin, dextrans, starches, and gelatins.

Albumin has the longest track record and the fewest adverse effects.[171,172] In the past, dextrans (i.e., high– and low–molecular-weight glucose polymers) were administered for volume expansion

and hemodilution in children,[173,174] but currently their primary use is for antithrombosis, although their value for even this indication is questionable.[175]

Starches are branched polysaccharide polymers available in high–, medium–, and low–molecular-weight ranges (480,000-70,000 Da). Although they expand blood volume, they also alter hemostasis by diluting clotting factors and impairing platelet function and the coagulation cascade.[176,177] In addition, starches accumulate in the reticuloendothelial system and carry the potential for unknown long-term adverse effects.[178] Minor coagulation changes have been reported when the dose exceeded 20 mL/kg.[179–181] A 6% hydroxyethyl starch (HES 130/0.4) yielded clinical and physiologic profiles similar to those for 5% albumin in volumes up to 16 mL/kg in noncardiac surgery and in volumes up to 50 mL/kg in cardiac surgery, although at smaller cost.[182,183] A meta-analysis of randomized controlled trials of hydroxyethyl starch concluded that mortality, creatinine, and blood loss did not increase, although platelet counts and the duration of ICU stay significantly decreased. The authors recommend against their use in pediatric patients.[184] Several major reviews regarding the use of starches and gels in adult patients who are critically ill have raised substantive concerns regarding adverse effects on coagulation[185,186] and renal function,[187,188] and they found inadequate overall safety data, even for the third-generation products.[26,189] If these concerns have been raised in adult populations, we should hold even greater concern about their use in children.

Gelatins are polypeptides derived from bovine collagen that seem to have a minimal effect on coagulation and provide reasonable plasma volume expansion. However, life-threatening anaphylactic or anaphylactoid reactions have been reported, and their use in children remains somewhat limited.[171,190–194] A systematic review identified a lack of safety and efficacy data in neonates and children.[195]

RED BLOOD CELL SUBSTITUTES

Blood substitutes offer the promise of agents with universal compatibility, minimal infectious risks, and prolonged shelf life (years rather than days) to carry oxygen to vital organs.[196] Early efforts to develop these products involved human, bovine, and genetically engineered hemoglobin polymer solutions, perfluorocarbons, and lipid-encapsulated hemoglobin. Most failed in clinical trials because of severe complications such as renal failure, stroke, and vasoconstriction.[197,198] The last of the hemoglobin-based oxygen carriers under investigation, Hemospan (Sangart, Inc., San Diego, CA), failed in clinical trials and is no longer being investigated.[199–201] Liposome-encapsulated hemoglobin[202] is currently under investigation as a means to carry oxygen to compromised tissues such as cerebral infarction.[203] At this juncture, none of these attempts at investigation of blood substitutes have reached the pediatric population.

Massive Blood Transfusion

Massive blood transfusion may be defined as replacement of a patient's entire blood volume one or more times or as more than 30 mL/kg PRBC transfused in less than 4 hours with ongoing uncontrolled bleeding (see http://www.surgery.med.umich.edu/pediatric/trauma/protocols/MassiveTransfusionProtocol4113.pdf [Last downloaded 8/26/2016]). In a retrospective study of 1113 combat trauma injuries in children younger than 18 years, those children who received 40 mL/kg or more in the first 24 hours had a greater risk for mortality compared with those who received

TABLE 12.9	Approximate Time for Expedited Release of Red Blood Cells			
ABO Group	Crossmatch	Preparation in Blood Bank (minutes)	Risk of Incompatibility
O	None	5	RBC alloantibody
ABO specific	None	15	RBC alloantibody
ABO specific	Abbreviated	30	Screen negative = none
			Screen positive = RBC alloantibody
ABO specific	Full	60	None

RBC, red blood cell.
Modified with permission from Dzik WH, Stowell CP. Transfusion and coagulation issues in trauma. In: Sheridan RL, ed. *The Trauma Handbook of the Massachusetts General Hospital.* Philadelphia: Lippincott Williams & Wilkins; 2004:128–147.

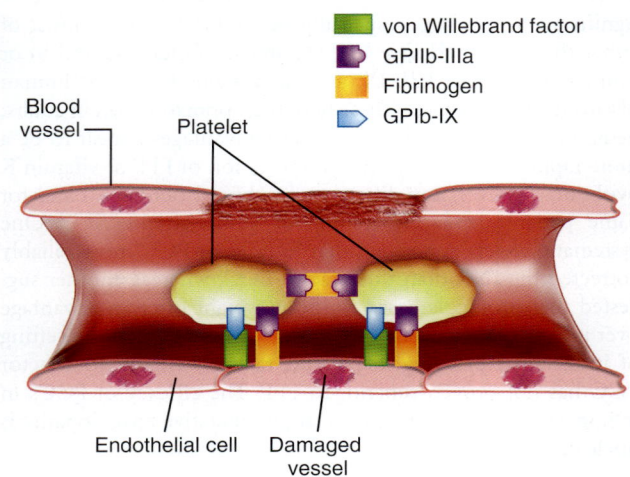

FIGURE 12.2 A blood clot forms when platelets adhere to one another through the GPIIb-IIIa complex (*purple*), which serves as a receptor for the adhesive protein fibrinogen (*orange*). Platelet interaction with an injured vessel wall requires synergy between the GPIb-IX (*blue*) and GPIIb-IIIa complexes and the adhesive proteins of von Willebrand factor (*green*) and fibrinogen, respectively. In high-velocity gradients, the efficacy of GPIb-IX interaction with the von Willebrand factor is significantly impaired.

less than 40 mL/kg.[204] There are few other published pediatric data.[205] In children, the anesthesiologist must think in terms of percent of blood or blood volumes lost rather than units of blood transfused. The composition of each blood component must be considered to anticipate problems and determine at what stage of a massive transfusion these problems may occur (see Table 12.3). Transfusion of large quantities of blood components may seriously affect coagulation, potassium and calcium concentrations, acid-base balance, body temperature, oxygen-hemoglobin dissociation, and hematocrit (i.e., oxygen-carrying capacity).

Most blood banks have a system for the expedited or "emergency" release of blood products, when there is inadequate time to perform complete serologic testing, including the crossmatch. Group O Rh-negative blood can be transfused into any child without the need for a crossmatch; group O Rh-positive blood may be transfused into male patients. After the blood bank has a sample of the child's blood, then switch to group-specific blood and then to blood that has completed standard compatibility testing. Table 12.9 illustrates the process and risks associated with expedited release of RBCs.[206] This switch usually occurs "behind the scenes" in the blood bank but underscores the critical importance of getting a properly labeled patient specimen as quickly as possible and before the patient's blood is substantially diluted by banked group O RBCs and accurate testing is compromised. Many institutions also have developed massive transfusion protocols that incorporate the mechanism in place for abbreviated serologic testing as well as the expedited provision of specific blood components (E-Fig. 12.1).

With massive blood loss, infusing crystalloid solutions alone or in large quantities may worsen the underlying coagulopathy, such as from trauma-induced bleeding, and may result in increased ICU stay.[207] Protocols using fixed ratios of PRBCs, FFP, and platelets (1:1:1) have been used in combat situations but have not been systematically examined or proven to offer advantage compared with standard component approaches in noncombat associated adults or children.[208-210] Additionally there are likely differences between controlled massive bleeding compared with massive rapid bleeding which add to the difficulty of systematic study. The approach to trauma patients has been termed "damage control," which means correcting hypothermia, maintaining adequate perfusion, and early administration of clotting factors and platelets to correct coagulopathy; systematic pediatric trauma studies are lacking.[211]

COAGULOPATHY

The coagulation system involves platelets, coagulation proteins, and localized tissue factor, which initiate all steps of hemostasis. Fig. 12.2 shows that an initial step is platelet adhesion to a wound or site of vessel wall injury, with adhesion being mediated by the vWF through its receptor on the platelet, the glycoprotein Ib–glycoprotein IX complex (GPIb-IX), and fibrinogen through the fibrinogen receptor on the platelet, the glycoprotein IIb–glycoprotein IIIa complex (GPIIb-IIIA). In flowing blood, initial platelet attachment is facilitated by vWF, whereas platelet spreading and more secure (shear stress-resistant) platelet-platelet aggregation is driven by fibrinogen and by the GPIIa-GPIIIa complex. However, there is also evidence that platelets attach even to intact endothelium, which has an activated phenotype, as after inflammatory cytokine exposure or sepsis. Platelets attach to the endothelium through high-molecular-weight von Willebrand multimers. Fibrinogen is attached to endothelium through upregulated integrins and selectins.

Initial platelet hemostasis (i.e., platelet plug formation) is accompanied by the local generation of fibrin, which is the end product of at least three surface-active enzyme complexes. Clotting is initiated by the tissue factor/factor VIIa surface-active enzyme complex and amplified by the factor VIIIa/IXa/X and factor II/Va/Xa complexes. A mural platelet thrombus, which includes platelets and fibrin, then forms a scaffold on which healing of the vessel wall can take place. The fibrin component of a platelet thrombus forms beneath, not above aggregating platelets,[212] as was previously thought. The scaffold is removed when it is no longer needed by thrombolysis and the effects of macrophages.

The surface-active enzyme complexes (Fig. 12.3) are active on the phospholipid surfaces provided by platelets, leukocytes, and endothelial cells but not in the bulk of the blood. Initially it was believed that formation of the tissue factor/factor VIIa complex, as shown, was critical for the action of recombinant FVIIa (rFVIIa) and for activation of factors X and IX. However, the high doses of rFVIIa necessary to achieve clinical hemostasis are far in excess

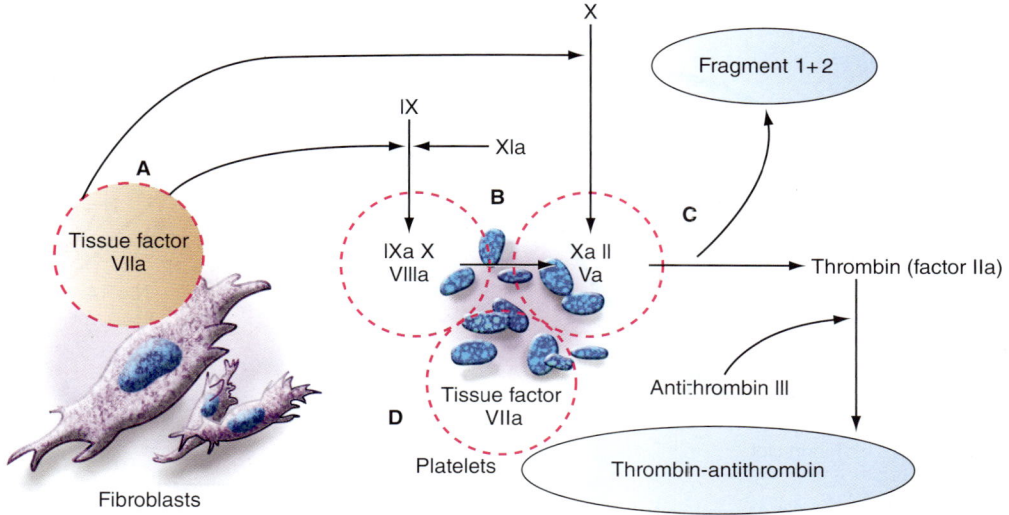

FIGURE 12.3 The key clotting factor enzyme complexes in coagulation. Tissue factor **(A)** (shown on the surface of a fibroblast) initiates coagulation, leading to the activation of clotting factors IX and X (shown on the surface of a platelet) and the processing of prothrombin (factor II) to form thrombin (factor IIa). Factor XIa has a contributory role in factor IX activation. Key to this cascade are three surface-active enzyme complexes: **(A)** the complex of tissue factor and factor VIIa; **(B)** the complex of factor IXa, factor VIIIa, and factor X; and **(C)** the complex of factor Xa, factor Va, and factor II (where the letter "a" denotes the activated form of a factor). Prothrombin fragment 1 + 2 and thrombin-antithrombin complexes are markers of the generation of thrombin. Fragment 1 + 2 is an inactive fragment formed during the processing of prothrombin; thrombin-antithrombin complex is formed when antithrombin III binds to thrombin, resulting in the inactivation of thrombin. In addition, **(D)** high doses of rFVIIa are able to generate thrombin in the presence of platelet-associated recombinant FVIIa and recombinant FVIIa can contribute to the assembly of the IXa-X-VIIIa complex via the activation of factor IX. Not shown in this diagram is the important influence of blood flow; for example, arteriolar and arterial velocity gradients, along with the presence of red cells, promote collisions between platelets and, consequently, platelet aggregation. (Modified with permission from Grabowski EF. The hemolytic-uremic syndrome toxin, thrombin, and thrombosis. *N Engl J Med.* 2002;346:58–64.)

of those required to saturate available tissue factor, suggesting that rFVIIa must also operate in large part independent of tissue factor,[213] especially in view of the observation that rFVIIa can bind to platelets directly via platelet anionic phospholipid[214] or via platelet GPIb.[213] In this regard, the conventional coagulation cascade shown in Fig. 12.4 is oversimplified, although it is a convenient approach to understanding the PT and partial thromboplastin time (PTT). All of the steps must be considered in the milieu of flowing blood, such that the high-velocity gradients of arterioles (i.e., mucous membranes of the uterus, gastrointestinal tract, upper respiratory tract, oral cavity, and gums) and arteries favor thrombi with a greater proportion of platelets (i.e., white thrombi), and low-velocity gradient states, such as those found in stasis or blood accumulation within a body cavity, favor a greater proportion of red cells (i.e., red thrombi). This explains why a patient with von Willebrand disease, characterized by a defect in the protein that allows blood platelets to adhere to a wound, tends to bleed from mucous membranes, sites of high-velocity (arteriolar) gradients, whereas hemophiliacs tend to bleed into joint spaces and muscle planes, sites of low- or near-zero–velocity gradients.

The coagulopathy associated with massive blood transfusions is usually attributable to the dilution of clotting factors or platelets, or both. The point at which the deficiency in clotting factors is sufficient to produce a coagulopathy depends on the volume of blood lost and the type of blood component transfused (i.e., PRBCs or whole blood). Dilutional thrombocytopenia sufficient

to cause clinical bleeding depends on the starting platelet count and the volume of blood replaced (Fig. 12.5). In some cases, the cause of bleeding is a consumptive coagulopathy such as fibrinolysis or disseminated intravascular coagulation (DIC).[65,215–235] In other scenarios, bleeding is caused by hypothermia, severe metabolic acidosis, poor tissue perfusion, and the release of tissue factors. Body temperature should be maintained by using efficient blood-warming devices, acidosis should be treated, and normovolemia and cardiac output should be restored to prevent a coagulopathy from developing.[222,236–239]

DILUTIONAL THROMBOCYTOPENIA

In an effort to formulate a plan to manage children who require massive blood transfusions, we must rely on our clinical experience and data extrapolated from adults and limited pediatric studies. A study of adult trauma patients during the Vietnam War reported that the onset of clinical bleeding occurred after about 15 units of whole blood or 1.5 blood volumes had been transfused. The incidence of coagulopathy was unrelated to an abnormal PT or PTT but correlated closely with a platelet count of less than 65,000/mm[3].[65,240] Studies of massive blood loss with *whole blood* replacement also support the conclusion that the coagulopathy at these levels of blood loss results from thrombocytopenia rather than a clotting factor deficiency.[65,222–231] Fig. 12.6 compares the calculated reduction in platelet count with the observed decline in platelet count in adults and children; when normalized for blood volumes shed, the observed changes were nearly identical.

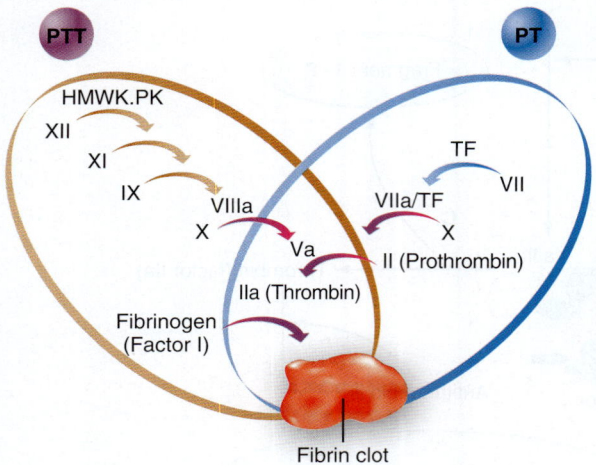

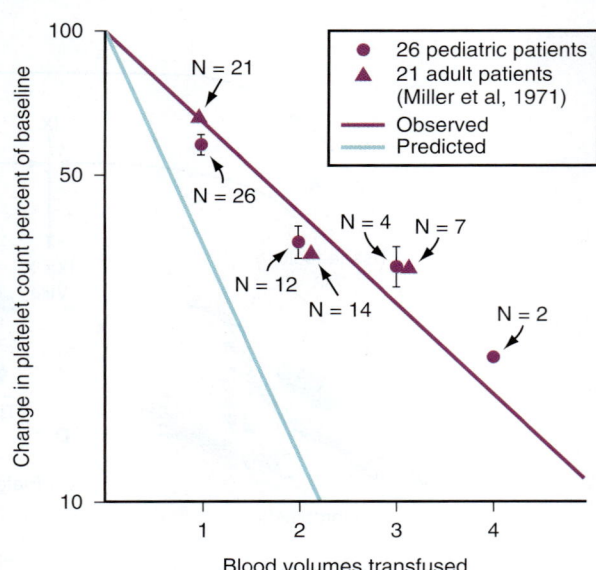

FIGURE 12.4 The conventional activated partial thromboplastin time (aPTT) is considered to be a measure of the intactness of the intrinsic coagulation system, which includes clotting factors XII, XI, IX, VIII, V, X, II, and I (fibrinogen). The prothrombin time (PT) is a measure of the intactness of the extrinsic coagulation system and encompasses tissue factor–bearing membrane surfaces and microparticles and factors VII, X, II, and I. In the PTT test, the blood clots without the need for an exogenous agent and comprises an *intrinsic* or complete clotting system. In practice, an agent such as diatomaceous earth is added to speed the reaction in the laboratory, and the term *activated* is added to the designation (aPTT). In the PT test, the blood clots by virtue of an *extrinsic* activator (i.e., tissue factor). This view in the diagram obscures the central role of tissue factor in clot initiation. Tissue factor circulates in an inactive form in the blood and is no longer considered only an extrinsic factor to the blood itself.

FIGURE 12.6 Percent of change in platelet count versus blood volumes transfused in young healthy adults and children.[65,66] The adult estimates assumed that these were ideal 70-kg men with a blood volume of 70 mL/kg such that 10 units of whole blood was estimated to be equivalent to 1 blood volume. The *magenta line* represents observed values, whereas the *blue line* represents calculated values. This difference suggests increased bone marrow production and/or splenic recruitment of platelets during massive transfusion. (From Miller RD, Robbins TO, Tong MJ, Barton SL. Coagulation defects associated with massive blood transfusions. *Ann Surg.* 1971;174:794–801; Coté CJ, Liu LM, Szyfelbein SK, et al. Changes in serial platelet counts following massive blood transfusions in pediatric patients. *Anesthesiology* 1985;62:197–201.)

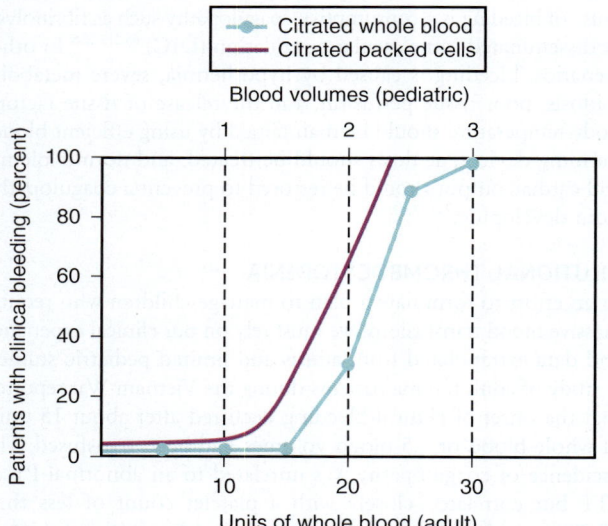

FIGURE 12.5 A study that considered the use of citrated whole blood (*blue line*) in adults found that bleeding in most cases resulted from dilutional thrombocytopenia. The *magenta line* represents estimated points of dilutional clotting factor deficiency if solely citrated packed cells are transfused. (Modified from Miller RD. Transfusion therapy and associated problems. *ASA Refresher Courses in Anesthesiology* 1973;1:107.)

The observed and calculated decrements differ because platelets are mobilized from the bone marrow, spleen, lungs, and lymphatic tissues. The platelet count usually does not decrease to concentrations that may cause bleeding in children until 2.0 to 2.5 blood volumes have been shed[66] or until 20 to 25 units of whole blood are transfused in adults.[66,229,241] Clinical bleeding does not usually occur in children whose platelet counts exceed 50,000/mm³, despite blood losses as great as 5.0 blood volumes (Fig. 12.7A).[66] Consequently, children should be monitored for thrombocytopenia and possible transfusion of platelets or clotting factor deficiency (see further) after the loss of the first 1.0 to 1.5 blood volumes. After the platelet count has decreased to 50,000/mm³, it is likely that approximately one platelet dose (i.e., 6 units for an adult or 10-15 mL/kg for a child) will be required for each blood volume replaced. If a coagulopathy develops earlier than expected (i.e., before a 1.0-blood volume loss), a search should be initiated for other causes of bleeding, such as increased arterial or venous pressure in the surgical field or DIC.

The starting platelet count is important for estimating how much blood loss can be tolerated before critical thrombocytopenia occurs. For example, with a starting platelet count of 600,000/mm³, dilutional thrombocytopenia is unlikely to occur until 4.0 or more blood volumes have been shed, whereas with a starting count of 100,000/mm³, dilutional thrombocytopenia should be anticipated after 1.0 blood volume has been lost (see Fig. 12.7B). Prophylactic transfusion of platelets typically is not indicated without documented evidence of dilutional thrombocytopenia, visible microvascular bleeding, and ongoing blood loss, although

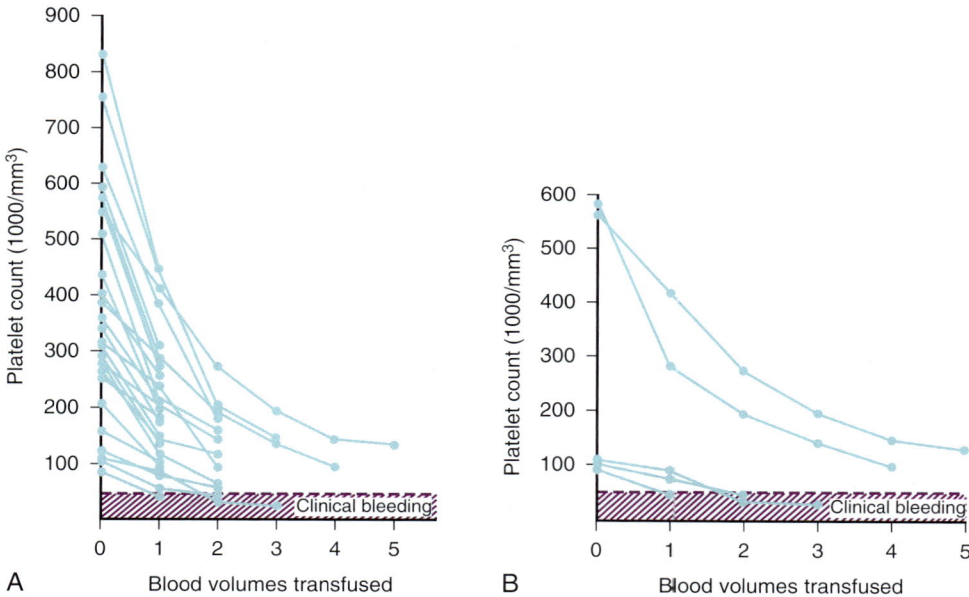

FIGURE 12.7 A, Serial changes in platelet counts are plotted for 26 pediatric patients whose blood loss was 1 to 5 blood volumes. Most of the children suffered from severe thermal injuries, and many had relatively large platelet counts at baseline. Clinically evident signs of coagulopathy appeared when the platelet count decreased to less than 50,000/mm³. **B**, Platelet counts of five children abstracted from **A**. The baseline platelet count is invaluable in estimating potential platelet needs in relation to blood volumes transfused. A low initial count suggests the need for early exogenous platelet transfusion, whereas a high initial platelet count indicates that exogenous platelets may not be required until several blood volumes or more have been lost. The three children who developed a coagulopathy began surgery with a relatively low platelet count, whereas the two children with a very high platelet count did not require platelet transfusion despite the loss of 4 and 5 blood volumes. (It should be noted that these children received sufficient FFP so as to maintain the PT and PTT within a normal range.) (Reproduced with permission from Coté CJ, Liu LMP, Szyfelbein SK, et al. Changes in serial platelet counts following massive blood transfusions in pediatric patients. *Anesthesiology* 1985;62:197–201.)

it should be anticipated based on the starting platelet count and the volume of blood lost.[66,72,218,222,242]

Although the primary platelet defect in massive transfusion is thrombocytopenia, some data suggest that platelets may not function normally (i.e., thrombocytopathy) after massive trauma or in the presence of hypothermia.[238,243,244] This has not been our experience in the children we studied whose temperature remained within the normal range.[66,223] The only simple test to assess platelet function is the bleeding time. However, this test is also sensitive to thrombocytopenia and its predictive value is of equivocal utility.[218,243,245] The PFA-100 test shows less potential as a rapid screening tool than it once did, because the device uses citrated blood warmed to 37°C and is relatively insensitive to milder defects in platelet-vessel wall interaction, such as that in mild von Willebrand disease. There remains a critical need for a point-of-care device or simple test to assess platelet function, as noted previously. Currently, the platelet count is our best indication for the need for platelet transfusions in situations involving rapid blood loss.[246] Other devices such as thromboelastography to measure whole blood clotting have been used to guide transfusion therapy, but their efficacy in improving outcomes has not been established.[247]

In several in vitro and animal model systems, recombinant factor VII (rFVIIa) activates factors IX and X on the surface of activated platelets, probably through the binding of rFVIIa to the platelet membrane (from which rFVIIa can also be taken up into storage sites within the platelet) and subsequent recruitment of circulating tissue factor. Although this has significantly improved

hemostasis in hemophiliacs with inhibitors to factor VIII, there is limited evidence that rFVIIa reduces mortality for off-label use, as in cardiovascular surgery, trauma, and intracerebral hemorrhage. Dosing in children appears to be greater than in adults, but this has not been systematically examined and is anecdotal.[248] This factor increases the risk of thromboembolism, hence its use should also consider the possibility of this sequela.[249]

Basic clotting studies (e.g., PT, PTT, fibrinogen, platelet count) should be performed before elective surgery when major blood loss can be anticipated to determine the cause of underlying coagulopathies and provide adequate quantities of blood components.

FACTOR DEFICIENCY

Laboratory results for developing deficiencies in clotting factors are integral when managing component therapy in massive transfusions. The PT (for the extrinsic system) measures the adequacy of factors VII, X, and V; prothrombin; and fibrinogen,[65] whereas the PTT (for the intrinsic system) measures the adequacy of factors XII, XI, IX, VIII, X, and V; prothrombin; and fibrinogen (see Fig. 12.4). Banked whole blood contains normal plasma concentrations of all of the clotting factors and regulatory proteins, with the exception of factors V and VIII (20%–50% of normal at the time of outdate), as well as factor VII. For a coagulopathy to develop because of a clotting factor deficiency, factor VIII must be less than 30% of the normal concentration and factor V less than 20% of normal.[223] For these to occur, at least 3.0 blood volumes must be exchanged with *whole blood*. In this scenario, the first coagulation test that is abnormal is the PTT because factor VIII is diluted to less than 30%.[219]

If blood loss is replaced with PRBCs, as is the current practice with modern blood banking techniques, the amount of plasma that is transfused is minimal because ~70% was sequestered in the FFP fraction when it was separated. Massive replacement of blood loss with PRBCs and no other blood products quickly dilutes all of the clotting factors, including fibrinogen (see Fig. 12.4).[3,218–222,228,230,231,250–252] Data have confirmed that the PT and PTT are prolonged in children with multiple clotting factor deficiencies (e.g., during massive transfusion) at concentrations of clotting factors that are greater than in children with single clotting factor deficiencies (e.g., congenital coagulopathies).[230,231] This was also documented in adult patients who were transfused exclusively with PRBCs and crystalloid; the dilution of multiple clotting factors correlated with the volume of blood and crystalloid transfused.[197] Replacing 1.0 to 1.5 blood volumes with PRBCs and crystalloid exclusively dilutes clotting factors to approximately 30% of normal. Because moderately prolonged PT and PTT values exist without overt signs of clinical bleeding,[230] administration of FFP should be initiated with the onset of a clinical coagulopathy. However, the anesthesiologist should anticipate that PRBCs and crystalloid solutions or albumin will dilute the concentration of clotting factors so that FFP is begun after ~1.0 blood volume of blood loss has been replaced to avoid falling behind in the clotting indexes. Documented deficiency of fibrinogen (<80 mg/dL) may also be corrected by transfusing FFP, but marked deficiency, particularly in the presence of a consumptive coagulopathy (e.g., DIC, fibrinolysis), may require the addition of cryoprecipitate (0.2 to 0.4 unit/kg).[3,252–255]

Our experience with 26 children (12 ± 4 years old, weight of 41.9 ± 15.8 kg) who underwent 22 Harrington rod procedures, three tumor excisions, and one Whipple procedure received no FFP or whole blood despite losing between 0.5 and 1.0 blood volume. They exhibited no clinical signs of coagulopathy. Slight prolongations of the PT or PTT occurred when the blood loss was equal to 1.0 blood volume or less (Table 12.10). Two children who lost 1.5 to 2.0 blood volumes exhibited prolonged PT and PTT values. The only child who developed signs of a clinical coagulopathy lost 2.0 blood volumes.[256,257]

The magnitude of the increase in PT or PTT that is predictive of a clinical coagulopathy is not well defined. However, the consensus panel of the National Institutes of Health and others suggest that when either clotting index exceeds 1.5 times normal (or INR >2.0), it should be considered pathologic.[72,225,229,258–261] Our studies suggest that the PT and PTT are prolonged to more than 1.5 times normal when the blood loss is 1.5 blood volumes or more and the blood loss has been replaced with only PRBCs and crystalloid or 5% albumin.[256,257] Our clinical practice is to initiate FFP after 1.0 blood volume blood loss (Table 12.11). At that point, FFP is administered in a ratio of 1 unit for every 2 units of PRBCs transfused. The indications for and timing of FFP depend on which blood product has been transfused, the volume of that transfusion as it relates to the child's blood volume, and whether the blood loss will continue perioperatively. The PT, PTT, fibrinogen concentration, and platelet count should be measured after each blood volume has been replaced and used to guide the need for additional FFP and platelets.

Recombinant factor VIIa (rFVIIa; NOVOSeven) is approved for use in the United States for hemophiliac patients with high-titer inhibitors and congenital factor VII deficiency. Anecdotal reports describe its effectiveness in controlling hemorrhage in a variety of other settings including congenital heart disease.[1,2,262–266] However, in several randomized clinical trials during partial hepatectomy, liver transplantation, prostate surgery, pelvic (orthopedic) surgery, trauma, and upper gastrointestinal tract bleeding rFVIIa failed to confer any benefit.[267–272] In a large randomized clinical trial of rFVIIa in children with intracranial hemorrhage, the largest-dose group showed only a small improvement in hematoma expansion, and 10% also experienced thromboembolic complications. In adults who received rFVIIa, the frequency of major thromboembolic complications was 1.4% to 10%, including acute myocardial infarction and stroke.[273] Until controlled trials demonstrate a clear benefit for its use, rFVIIa should be used with great caution for off-label indications,[263,267–272,274,275] and even then only for life-threatening bleeding.

Several studies[272,276] have compared transfusion strategies in adults for treating trauma incurred during combat in the Middle East. A consensus conference and other reviews on massive transfusion concluded that the evidence did not support the up-front use of a 1:1:1 ratio of units of PRBC, FFP, and platelets, but it did support the early use of an antifibrinolytic medication (i.e., tranexamic acid).[208–211,276] The consensus conference also recommended an integrated approach to managing massive transfusion that included rapid provision of PRBCs, the use of antifibrinolytics, and a foundation ratio of blood components

TABLE 12.10	Changes in Prothrombin and Partial Thromboplastin Times During Massive Blood Transfusions in Children			
PT and PTT Times (sec)	Baseline[a] (n = 26)	0.5[b] (n = 16)	0.75[b] (n = 12)	1.0[b] (n = 10)
Prothrombin Time				
Mean ± SD	10.9 ± 0.96	12.5 ± 0.77	13.2 ± 0.76	13.6 ± 0.98
Range	9.3–12	11.4–14.0	11.4–14.2	11.9–15.8
Partial Thromboplastin Time				
Mean ± SD	31.8 ± 4.4	38.0 ± 4.9	40 ± 5.4	45.1 ± 13.1
Range	25–45.9	28.1–59.6	33–51.5	25.6–60.0

PRBCs, packed red blood cells; *PT*, prothrombin; *PTT*, partial thromboplastin.
[a]Baseline normal values for blood volume may be greater in infants younger than 3 months.
[b]Blood volume loss. NOTE: Not all children in this subset lost a half blood volume or more.

TABLE 12.11	Minimal Fresh Frozen Plasma Recommendations According to the Type of Blood Product Transfused and the Volume of Blood Lost		
Type of Blood Replaced	FFP Indicated		Volume FFP to Be Transfused
Whole blood	After 2.0–3.0 blood volumes lost and each blood volume thereafter		25%–33% of each blood volume lost
PRBCs	After 1.0 blood volume lost and each blood volume thereafter		1 unit FFP/2 units PRBCs

FFP, fresh frozen plasma; *PRBCs*, packed red blood cells.

directed by the results of standard coagulation testing (e.g., PT, PTT, platelet count, fibrinogen) or clot viscoelasticity, or both.[276]

The dilutional coagulopathy associated with massive blood transfusion is reasonably predictable. When using whole blood, dilutional thrombocytopenia usually develops first and may occur as early as after the first blood volume has been replaced (if the initial platelet count is <50,000/mm³). In most cases, clotting factors (particularly factors V and VIII) are not diluted until the blood loss exceeds three blood volumes. On the other hand, when PRBCs are used to replace blood loss, all the clotting factors and platelets may be diluted after as little as 1.0 blood volume is lost. However, the predictable coagulopathy of dilution is only an approximate guide. The PT, PTT, fibrinogen, and platelet count should be assessed during massive transfusions to guide replacement therapy.

DISSEMINATED INTRAVASCULAR COAGULATION AND FIBRINOLYSIS

DIC and fibrinolysis are frequently associated with shock, trauma, and other forms of tissue damage, with release of procoagulants (e.g., tissue factor) and fibrinolytics (e.g., tissue plasminogen activator). In the presence of massive blood loss, these processes must be differentiated from dilutional coagulopathy. Differentiation may be difficult, because both are associated with pathologic oozing of blood in the surgical field and each may result in prolongation of the PT and PTT, as well as thrombocytopenia.[277–280] With massive replacement using whole blood or PRBCs and *adequate* FFP, the fibrinogen concentration should remain normal; with uncompensated (acute) DIC, it may be decreased. However, replacing the blood loss with PRBCs, albumin, and crystalloid also leads to a reduction in fibrinogen.

The most helpful test for DIC and fibrinolysis is documentation of a significant increase in the level of D-dimer, a small peptide fragment generated during the digestion of fibrin by ongoing thrombolysis (i.e., through plasmin), along with evidence on the peripheral blood smear of schistocytes and helmet cells (i.e., microangiopathic hemolytic anemia).[281–283] Abnormal RBCs and RBC fragments are believed to arise from the slicing action of immobilized fibrin strands in the microcirculation, although the precise mechanism remains unknown. A scoring system to screen for potential DIC has been developed but not evaluated in the operating room setting.[284] If pathologic oozing in the surgical field is observed and 1.0 blood volume or less has been lost in a child who had a normal platelet count and PT and PTT values preoperatively, the child may have developed a consumptive coagulopathy.

The most effective treatment for DIC is to eliminate the cause, such as correcting shock, acidosis, or sepsis.[279,280] Heparin therapy remains controversial even in children with thrombotic manifestations of DIC. It is not advisable in children with active bleeding, especially in the operative setting.[278,282,283,285]

HYPERKALEMIA

RBCs leak potassium into the extracellular fluid during storage, particularly as the units of PRBCs age. The concentration of adenosine triphosphate (ATP) decreases, and the ATPase-driven Na^+/K^+ pump activity decreases. At the point when the unit of packed RBCs reaches its maximum shelf life, approximately 5–7 mEq of K^+ are present in the extracellular fluid of each unit. Since the volume of extracellular fluid is different for whole blood and packed RBCs collected in CPDA-1 or Additive-Solution systems, the concentration of K^+ is the highest in CPDA-1 packed RBCs and the lowest in CPDA-1 whole blood units (E-Table 12.3). The

K^+ leak is doubled and more rapid from RBCs that have been irradiated.[82,286] To avoid the accumulation of large amounts of extracellular K^+, irradiated RBCs may be stored for a maximum of 28 days (vs. 35 or 42 days for whole blood or PRBCs).

Although extracellular K^+ is present in banked RBCs, clinically important hyperkalemia has not been reported after the slow transfusion of blood through peripheral IV lines but has occurred in children undergoing rapid transfusion particularly through a central venous line.[287–293] A study of serum potassium in neonates after exchange transfusion with PRBCs documented a decrease in serum potassium concentrations.[294] A retrospective study of children undergoing massive intraoperative but slow transfusion with PRBCs documented transient, but not life-threatening, hyperkalemia.[295] It appears that clinically important hyperkalemia does not usually occur when PRBCs are administered *at normal, slow infusion rates through peripheral IV access*.[296,297] This may be explained by the combination of the small absolute amount of K^+ (~6 mEq); its rapid reabsorption into the potassium-depleted, transfused RBCs; the large volume of distribution; and dilution with crystalloid or albumin during administration. Hyperkalemia in the setting of massive transfusion is usually the consequence of extensive tissue injury, extremely rapid transfusion, acidemia resulting from inadequate tissue perfusion, hypothermia, and hypocalcemia.[298]

The need to relate the size of the patient to the rate of blood replacement is infrequently a problem in adults, but it is vitally important to consider in an infant or small child. An alert from the Society for Pediatric Anesthesia[299] described 4 deaths among 11 children who developed hyperkalemia during transfusion; 8 were younger than 1 year, and 6 were younger than 6 months old. The Perioperative Cardiac Arrest Registry reported eight hyperkalemic cardiac arrests related to blood transfusion.[299,300] Hyperkalemia may become a problem when large volumes of whole blood or PRBCs are administered very rapidly in adults (rates ≥120 mL/minute) and in infants and children undergoing rapid blood transfusion, particularly through a central venous catheter.[301] A rapid transfusion rate of 120 mL/minute in a 70-kg adult is equivalent to 1.5 to 2 mL/kg per minute of blood, which is relatively easy to infuse in an infant or small child using a pressure bag or a rapid-transfusion device. An adult sustained a cardiac arrest and died after receiving Adsol-preserved PRBCs with a supernatant potassium concentration of 24 to 34 mEq/L at a transfusion rate of 6.4 mL/kg per minute through a rapid infusion device (see Chapter 52).[302] Similar and greater transfusion rates are possible in infants and children without such devices.[292,295,303,304]

The principle is to avoid falling behind in replacing the blood loss and to avoid a situation in which a rapid and massive infusion of blood is required. Warming the blood and administering it through a peripheral IV line (rather than a central venous catheter) reduce the risks of hyperkalemia on the cardiac conduction system.[305] When the rate of infusion of whole blood or PRBCs exceeds 1.5 to 2.0 mL/kg per minute, the electrocardiogram (ECG) must be closely monitored. If ventricular arrhythmias occur with peaked T waves in the setting of hyperkalemia (see Fig. 9.7), appropriate treatment should be instituted (e.g., calcium chloride or calcium gluconate, hyperventilation, sodium bicarbonate, albuterol, glucose and insulin; see Tables 9.8 and 28.6); Kayexalate is the slowest and least effective intervention in this situation and is not recommended as an acute intervention. Intraoperative washing of PRBCs with autotransfusion devices has been recommended to avoid hyperkalemia in pediatric patients who require rapid, massive blood transfusion.[306]

Rapid, massive transfusion of whole blood or PRBCs to a neonate, particularly blood that has been stored for several weeks, can cause hyperkalemic cardiac arrest. It is common practice to administer RBC-containing components that are relatively young to avoid hyperkalemia in neonates requiring massive blood transfusion. If relatively young units are not available and time permits, it may be possible to wash the PRBCs to reduce the potassium concentration. However, RBC transfusion to an actively bleeding infant should not be delayed to obtain less than 7-day-old PRBCs or to wash the units. Similarly, blood for intrauterine transfusion, exchange transfusion, or for neonates should be relatively young (usually <7 days).

These practices are consistent with the recommendations from the Society for Pediatric Anesthesia Wake Up Safe quality improvement initiative, which suggests that anesthesiologists anticipate the blood loss, transfuse early, and cautions that transfusing the hypovolemic child slowly and through a peripheral IV catheter rather than rapidly through a central venous catheter.[299] If the infant requires irradiated RBC blood components, it is preferable to transfuse them soon after irradiating the blood to minimize the potassium concentration.

HYPOCALCEMIA AND CITRATE TOXICITY

Citrate works as an anticoagulant for stored blood components by chelating ionized calcium (iCa^{2+}). As citrate in the blood component is transfused, it is rapidly taken up and metabolized by nucleated cells in the body, although the primary site for clearance is the liver. During massive transfusion, particularly of whole blood or FFP, the influx of citrate may temporarily overwhelm the capacity of the recipient to clear it, resulting in its accumulation, which causes the plasma concentration of iCa^{2+} to decrease.[205,307-311] The residual plasma fraction in a unit of PRBCs, which contains the citrate, is a much smaller volume than in a unit of whole blood or FFP. Clinically, it is rare for the iCa^{2+} level to decrease unless the transfusion rate is very rapid; in adults, this rate must be 1.0 or more units of whole blood or FFP in 3 to 4 minutes.[307] This effect on the iCa^{2+} concentration has been reported in neonates undergoing exchange transfusion and is more likely to occur in more-premature and lower-weight infants. Pulseless electrical activity has been reported in two preterm infants who developed hypocalcemia during dilutional transfusion with FFP.[311,312] In adult cardiac surgical patients who received whole blood at 1.5 mL/kg per minute, the ventricular function curve did not improve (i.e., cardiac output did not increase although the iCa^{2+} decreased). When a similar volume of heparinized blood was administered at the same rate, the Frank-Starling response to volume loading was normal (i.e., cardiac output increased, but iCa^{2+} level did not change).[313] These case reports and the adult cardiac surgical study confirm that a decrease in iCa^{2+} concentration of clinical importance (i.e., decreased cardiac contractility) may be expected when the rate of infusion of citrated whole blood exceeds 1.5 to 2.0 mL/kg per minute.[307,313]

The change in the iCa^{2+} concentration after transfusion of large volumes of PRBCs is less than that observed with whole blood or FFP. Although measurable decreases in the iCa^{2+} concentration have been observed during rapid transfusion, they have only rarely been associated with cardiac toxicity in adults. The rates of infusion of citrated whole blood that produce hypocalcemia and hyperkalemia are almost identical, whereas the cardiac electrophysiologic effects produced by hypocalcemia and hyperkalemia are opposite. It is important to observe the ECG for abnormalities, especially widening of the QRS complex, prolonged QT interval, and peaking of the T wave.[223,314]

Both hypocalcemia and hyperkalemia are treated by the administration of exogenous calcium. Evidence from healthy animals and children with extensive thermal injuries demonstrated that calcium chloride and calcium gluconate dissociate at similar rates; hepatic metabolism of the gluconate moiety is not necessary (Fig. 12.8).[315] Studies during the anhepatic phase of liver transplantation reported a similar degree of ionization of calcium chloride and calcium gluconate, confirming that hepatic metabolism is not required to ionize calcium from calcium gluconate.[316] Calcium chloride and calcium gluconate are both indicated to treat acute ionized hypocalcemia, with the caveat that calcium gluconate, which contains one-third of the ionizable calcium of calcium chloride (by weight), be administered at a threefold greater dose (milligrams per kilogram) than the latter. Frequent, small boluses are as effective as single large boluses and result in smaller fluctuations in plasma iCa^{2+} values.[315] Ideally, both forms of calcium should be slowly administered through a large peripheral or central vein, because both are sclerosing medications.

The volume of plasma and therefore the absolute amount of citrate in a unit of FFP are slightly less than the amounts in a unit of whole blood. However, the citrate load can be more rapidly delivered in FFP because it can be infused more rapidly owing to its low viscosity. It is easy to give a large citrate load in a brief period. Caution is urged when FFP or whole blood is rapidly infused, especially if the child already has a low iCa^{2+} concentration or impaired hepatic function (e.g., neonates and children undergoing liver transplantation).[312] Fig. 12.9A shows the changes in iCa^{2+} concentrations that occurred in children who had extensive thermal injuries and who received rapid FFP infusions at 1.0 to 2.5 mL/kg per minute for 5 minutes. The maximum decrease in iCa^{2+} levels occurred between the fourth and fifth minutes with a similar nadir in the iCa^{2+} concentration in the three fastest rates of FFP infusion.[317]

If exogenous calcium is administered *during* rapid FFP transfusion, large decreases in the iCa^{2+} level can be avoided (see Fig. 12.9B). We transfused FFP at 2 mL/kg per minute for 10 minutes (equivalent to an average adult receiving 1400 mL FFP over 10 minutes) in six children with extensive burn injuries and despite very significant decreases in iCa^{2+} levels, found no consistent adverse circulatory changes. However, because these children had extensive burn injuries, we presumed they were hypermetabolic and therefore able to more rapidly metabolize the excess citrate, which limited our ability to extrapolate these data to children without burn injuries (see Chapter 36).[317]

In dogs anesthetized with halothane, we determined that citrate-induced ionized hypocalcemia caused significantly greater cardiovascular depression as the expired concentration of halothane increased.[318] These findings are consistent with the combined myocardial depression caused by ionized hypocalcemia and calcium channel blockade caused by the halothane.[319,320] Although halothane exerts the greatest calcium channel blocking activity of the inhalational anesthetics, all inhalational anesthetics depress the myocardium through this mechanism to some extent as well as through other mechanisms involving calcium flux, which augments the myocardial dysfunction associated with citrate-induced ionized hypocalcemia.[321-324]

The adverse cardiac effects of citrate-induced hypocalcemia may be increased if FFP is rapidly administered through a central venous catheter because there is less time to dilute the FFP and metabolize the citrate before it enters the heart and coronary vessels. FFP may be more safely administered through a peripheral IV line. Calcium should be administered *during* rapid transfusion of FFP (>1 mL/kg per minute) to attenuate this transient but

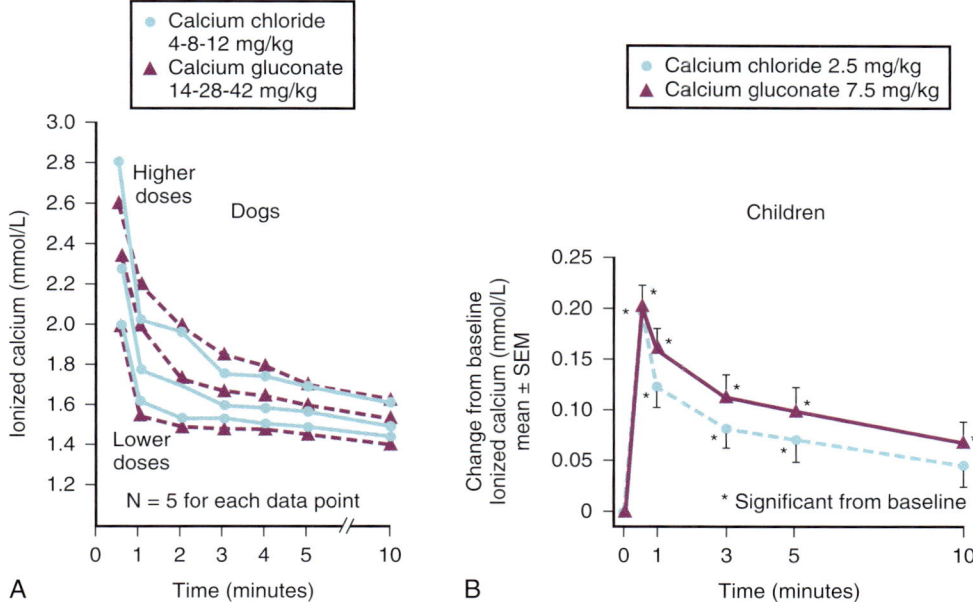

FIGURE 12.8 A, Changes in arterial iCa²⁺ levels in dogs after three equal elemental calcium doses of calcium chloride (4, 8, and 12 mg/kg) or calcium gluconate (14, 28, and 42 mg/kg). The rate of change in the iCa²⁺ concentration was identical for each form of calcium at each dose. There was no significant difference between the largest and smallest doses after 2 minutes, suggesting that frequent small doses are equally effective and perhaps safer than large boluses of exogenous calcium. **B,** Changes in arterial iCa²⁺ levels in children who received equal elemental doses of calcium chloride and calcium gluconate. At 30 seconds, both forms of calcium dissociated equally; these data indicate that hepatic metabolism of the gluconate moiety is not required to liberate ionized calcium from calcium gluconate. (From Coté CJ, Drop LJ, Daniels AL, Hoaglin DC. Calcium chloride versus calcium gluconate: comparison of ionization and cardiovascular effects in children and dogs. *Anesthesiology* 1987;66:465–470.)

potentially dangerous citrate toxicity, especially in the presence of potent inhalational anesthetics.[318–322] Neonates and small infants are particularly vulnerable to developing citrate toxicity because it is easier to administer a relatively large volume of FFP or platelets over a brief period and because citrate may not be eliminated as rapidly (i.e., first-pass effect through the liver) in infants.[312] In addition to thermally injured patients, children undergoing liver transplantation and cardiac surgery are likely to require FFP and develop hypocalcemia.[325,326] Liver transplantation recipients are particularly susceptible to decreased iCa²⁺ levels during the anhepatic phase and the pre-anhepatic phase of surgery because of impaired hepatic blood flow and the reduced ability to metabolize citrate.[327–331] An IV preparation of calcium should always be available when a major transfusion with FFP is anticipated.

ACID-BASE BALANCE

Massive transfusions usually occur in one of two situations: severe trauma with shock or major surgery with massive blood loss. In the first situation, severe metabolic acidosis may occur because of low cardiac output and diminished oxygen delivery. Correction of the acidosis may be a necessary part of the resuscitation, along with blood volume replacement. In this situation, impaired coagulation may occur because of the acidosis.[220,236,332–334] In the operating room, intravascular volume is usually maintained, and because most instances of massive blood loss are anticipated, replacement of acute blood loss is more controlled. Even with repeated massive blood loss, metabolic acidosis is not usually a problem provided severe hypovolemia is avoided.[335–337] Sodium bicarbonate therapy must be governed by the child's acid-base

status because metabolic acidosis does not usually occur with massive transfusion unless accompanied by severe hypovolemia, low cardiac output, or hypoxemia.

After a massive blood transfusion, a moderate to severe metabolic alkalosis caused by the large volume of transfused citrate and its conversion to bicarbonate is common.[308,326,338–340] Thus it is important to determine the acid-base status *before* administering sodium bicarbonate to avoid overcorrecting the pH and shifting the oxyhemoglobin dissociation curve further to the left.

HYPOTHERMIA

Hypothermia may contribute to problems associated with major blood loss and its replacement. Although hypothermia decreases oxygen consumption and reduces oxygen demand, it may also increase oxygen consumption if the child shivers and decrease tissue delivery of oxygen by a leftward shift of the oxygen-hemoglobin dissociation curve as well as induce a refractory ventricular tachycardia in the presence of severe hypothermia (about 32°C).[223,341] Hypothermia may also profoundly compromise platelet function and impair the coagulation cascade.[220,236–238,332,333,342–344]

Prevention of hypothermia by all available means is considered an essential part of damage-control resuscitation of trauma patients.[345–348] Hypothermia (<34°C in adults) by itself is an independent risk factor for mortality.[349] Banked blood products are stored between room temperature and 4°C, depending on the blood component. In the setting of large transfusion volumes, all blood products should be infused through a blood warmer. No other method should be considered (e.g., storing blood in a warming cupboard, immersing in hot water, microwave) because

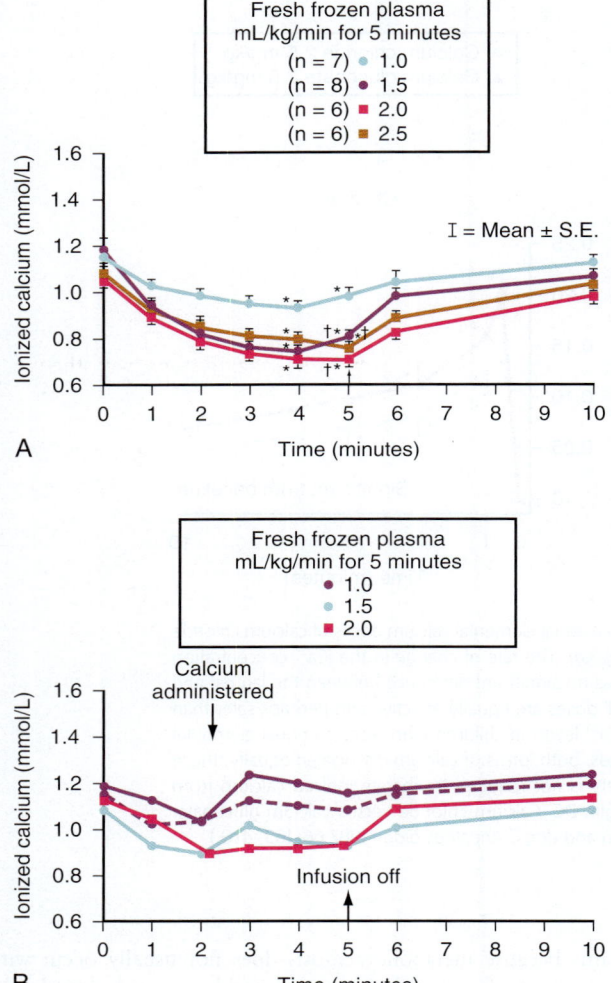

FIGURE 12.9 A, Changes in arterial iCa^{2+} levels in children with severe thermal injuries during infusions of fresh frozen plasma at a rate of 1.0 to 2.5 mL/kg per minute for 5 minutes through an infusion pump. Notice the dangerous although transient decrease in the iCa^{2+} concentration, with the nadir occurring between the fourth and fifth minutes. Ionized hypocalcemia occurs when the infusion rate equals or exceeds 1 mL/kg per minute. **B,** Changes in iCa^{2+} levels occurred in four thermally injured children who received calcium chloride (*arrow*) after 2 minutes of fresh frozen plasma infusion. There were no sharp increases or decreases in iCa^{2+} levels. (From Coté CJ, Drop LJ, Hoaglin DC, et al. Ionized hypocalcemia after fresh frozen plasma administration to thermally injured children: effects of infusion rate, duration, and treatment with calcium chloride. *Anesth Analg.* 1988;67:152–160.)

RBCs hemolyze readily with prolonged warming or overheating (>42°C). Warming blood and all other IV infusions with a high-capacity blood warmer, using hot air warming blankets and radiant warmers, placing plastic wrap around extremities, inserting a heated humidifier in the anesthesia circuit, covering the child's head, and maintaining a warm to hot operating room contribute to maintaining thermal neutrality. Rapid-transfusion devices markedly improve the rapidity of transfusion and the thermokinetics involved.[350-356] In one case, one author (CJC) and two nurses transfused more than 50 L of blood products and crystalloid in less than 1 hour, while maintaining the child's temperature at 34.5°C or greater.[350]

MONITORING DURING MASSIVE BLOOD TRANSFUSION

If massive blood loss can be anticipated, adequate monitoring should be instituted *before* surgery begins so that baseline information can be recorded. Large-bore peripheral IV access is preferable (E-Fig. 12.2) because these catheters have reduced resistance and they deposit blood products into the peripheral circulation for dilution (avoiding hypothermia and hyperkalemia in the heart), unlike a CVP line. If a child arrives in the operating room in shock (e.g., trauma patient), the physician must be careful to differentiate hypovolemia from other causes of shock (e.g., tension pneumothorax, cardiac tamponade) (see Chapters 39 and 40); invasive monitoring may assist in diagnosing the cause of the child's volume status. Our philosophy is one of aggressive invasive monitoring to provide maximum data for evaluation and management of a critically hypovolemic child.

1. Routine monitoring includes an ECG, blood pressure cuff, stethoscope, temperature, pulse oximetry, and expired carbon dioxide; a pulse oximeter placed on the tongue may be particularly valuable in special circumstances when a child is vasoconstricted, hypothermic, or without peripheral pulses.[357,358] Hypovolemia may occasionally manifest as pulsus paradoxus, identified with a pulse oximeter.[359]

2. A urinary catheter allows quantitation of urine output and assessment of organ perfusion and intravascular volume status.

3. An arterial catheter enables continuous blood pressure monitoring, arterial blood gas measurements, and determinations of hematocrit, glucose, calcium, potassium, and clotting parameters. The adequacy of the circulating blood volume may be inferred from the shape of the arterial waveform, presence of the dicrotic notch, and absence of exaggerated respiratory variation (Fig. 12.10).

4. A CVP line provides critical information, and its ease and safety of insertion have been demonstrated for children of all sizes[360]; ultrasound may improve the success and safety of insertion.[361,362] CVP readings vary depending on the location of the catheter tip and whether there is rapidly running fluid in the same catheter.[363,364] In the latter case, the infusions should be interrupted intermittently to obtain accurate readings. It is our clinical impression that in healthy, anesthetized, supine children, a very small change in CVP (2–3 mm Hg) may represent a change of as much as 10% to 15% of a child's blood volume. In most children, right-sided pressures correlate well with left-sided pressures; the right atrial CVP usually is an accurate indicator of cardiac filling pressures of both ventricles. A CVP line provides access for blood sampling and a reliable site for IV administration of medications, fluid, and blood. However, a CVP line cannot always be relied on as a volume administration line because resistance is large through the long, narrow lumen. A centrally placed introducer is a reliable volume line; however, it is preferred to give rapid transfusions through a peripheral catheter as to reduce the potential for hyperkalemic, hypocalcemic, or hypothermia-induced cardiac arrest.[299,305]

5. Continuous noninvasive cardiac output devices may provide further clinical guidance (see Figure 52.10).[21]

Monitors and the data they generate are helpful, but anesthesiologists must rely on more than numbers. It serves no purpose to have sophisticated monitoring if the data provided cannot be interpreted and related to clinical events. The final monitor is ultimately the anesthesiologist's attention and judgment.

Thromboelastography provides a standardized means of quantitating the rapidity and quality of clot formation and a means for identifying fibrinolysis.[365,366] This device was first used primarily

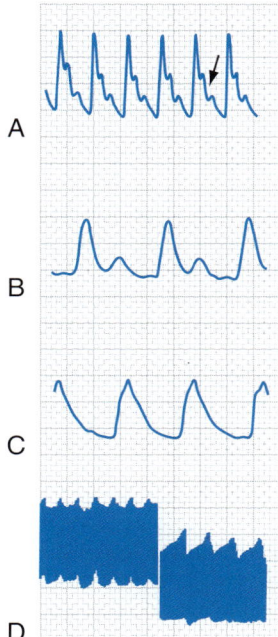

FIGURE 12.10 Changes in the contour of an arterial tracing with hypovolemia. **A,** The normal tracing shows a sharp upswing of the arterial pulse wave and position of the dicrotic notch. **B,** There is movement of the dicrotic notch and widening of the pulse wave. **C,** The pulse wave widens further. **D,** There is further widening of the pulse wave and loss of the dicrotic notch. An exaggerated ("picket fence") respiratory variation of pulse wave is shown in the *right* tracing compared with the *left*. Factors other than hypovolemia, such as hypothermia, deep anesthesia, vasodilator therapy, or damped tracing (e.g., clot, air bubble), may produce artifactual changes in the shape of the arterial waveform.

during massive blood transfusion situations related to liver transplantation, trauma, and cardiac surgery.[345,347,365–376] Some studies have found that thromboelastographic screening was not useful in predicting bleeding after cardiac surgery and was associated with a large percentage of false-positive results.[377,378] The use of heparinase improves the accuracy of the results by eliminating the effects of heparin, although this requires two machines to simultaneously sample blood (with and without heparinase) to have results within a useful period.[379] This monitor may also be used to guide the effectiveness of antifibrinolytic therapy.[372,373,380] The exact role of thromboelastography in the routine care of pediatric cardiac surgical patients, liver transplant recipients, and children who have had massive blood loss with ongoing coagulopathy has not been established.[247] Tables 12.10 and 12.11 summarize the expected changes in various blood components when administered on a per kilogram basis and the estimated FFP requirement.

INFECTIOUS DISEASE CONSIDERATIONS

It is important to use basic precautions when administering blood products and contacting body fluids to minimize the risk to anesthesiologists. Blood and body fluids, even in infants, may transmit hepatitis B, hepatitis C, and HIV through parenteral exposure (e.g., cuts, needlestick), mucous membrane contact, or exposure to nonintact skin.[10,381–390] Accidental needlesticks are

the most common means of exposure to anesthesiologists in the operating room. The introduction of safe IV needles, a needleless IV system, the use of stopcocks, and never recapping used needles has reduced the incidence of this problem.[391–394] The incidence of HIV seroconversion after needle puncture is estimated to be 0.2% to 0.5% (~1 in 300), although the conversion rate is much greater after a needlestick injury from individuals with hepatitis.[10,381,387–389,395,396] All institutions should have needlestick, mucous membrane, or nonintact skin exposure to blood protocols to immediately evaluate and institute treatment (see also Chapter 50).[397–400]

Anesthesiologists must practice universal blood and body fluid precautions (e.g., gloves, goggles) and should minimize the use of needles, especially the practice of recapping needles. The management of infants may be less than optimal with the use of three-way stopcocks because of the fluid required to flush the system and the ease of introducing air into the IV line. In these infants, single-use needles without recapping or needleless systems are recommended. If an anesthesiologist is exposed to an HIV-positive patient or is punctured by a needle of unknown origin, the need for immediate institution of prophylactic medical therapy should be determined.[394,396] Early institution of drug therapy is recommended to reduce the potential for seroconversion (see Tables 50.6 and 50.7).

Methods to Reduce Patient Exposure to Allogeneic Blood Components

Public awareness of the infectious hazards of transfusion, particularly from HIV and the hepatitis viruses, generated considerable interest in the 1980s and 1990s in developing techniques to avoid allogeneic transfusion. These techniques can minimize transfusions and the associated risks, assuaging the fears of parents and sparing the blood supply for patients for whom these options were not suitable. Within the medical community, awareness of the hazards of transfusion prompted a more thoughtful approach to transfusion, greater tolerance of asymptomatic anemia, more attention to medical treatment of anemia, and greater focus on surgical hemostasis. The amount of blood transfused for many surgical procedures has decreased steadily during the past 20 years. During the same period, the risks associated with transfusions have also dramatically decreased. After the HIV and hepatitis C viruses were identified, sensitive tests, some based on amplification technology for viral RNA, were developed to screen the donor population. Transfusions are associated with other deleterious effects, but two of the most significant risks, bacterial infection and mistransfusion, do not differ materially between banked allogeneic and autologous blood. As the risk differential between allogeneic transfusion and its alternatives narrows, a balanced appraisal of the benefits and untoward effects of each is appropriate.

ERYTHROPOIETIN

Use of recombinant erythropoietin to promote endogenous RBC production can reduce the need for allogeneic RBC transfusions and has proved useful in many populations, including preterm infants, children receiving chemotherapy, children with renal failure, children of Jehovah's Witnesses, and children undergoing elective major reconstructive surgery, spinal surgery, liver transplantation, or cardiac surgery.[401–406] Coordination with the hematology department, blood banking, and the primary patient care team is required to take full advantage of this form of therapy.[402,407–425] Although usually well tolerated, erythropoietin should be used with careful monitoring in patients with hypertension. Erythropoietin is available in a lyophilized (freeze-dried form for reconstitution) or in a dilute albumin solution; some members of the Jehovah's Witness faith prefer the lyophilized formulation.

PREOPERATIVE AUTOLOGOUS BLOOD DONATION

Donation and storage of blood before elective surgery have reduced the use of allogeneic RBCs.[408,421,426–440] Banked units of PRBCs may be stored for 35 to 42 days in the liquid state,[441,442] permitting the donation of several units and the time required for the patient (usually teenagers) to regenerate the RBC mass before surgery. Children unable to mount an erythropoietic response to phlebotomy may only succeed in making themselves anemic, so administration of iron, vitamin C, and folate is important, as is monitoring for reticulocytosis to ensure that the bone marrow is replenishing the donated RBCs. Autologous donation should not be attempted in children with significant cardiac ischemic disease (e.g., hypertrophic cardiomyopathy) or those with an active infection because bacteria can seed the collected unit and overgrow during storage. Autologous donation should be discouraged before procedures for which RBC transfusion is unlikely. Donated blood that is not used by the donor is usually discarded rather than entered into the general blood bank inventory as it is not screened for infectious agents.

Patients or family of pediatric patients may wish to obtain blood from family members or friends (i.e., directed donation). Despite the perception that this donor pool may be safer than the pool of volunteer, allogeneic donors, there is no evidence that this is true. Directed donors are considered to be allogeneic donors and are screened and tested in the same manner as any volunteer donor. Because there is a greater risk of transfusion-associated GVHD with cellular components from a donor who is a blood relative, these units are irradiated to eliminate the possibility of this fatal complication of transfusion.[443–445]

INTRAOPERATIVE BLOOD RECOVERY AND REINFUSION: AUTOTRANSFUSION

Recovery of blood from an operative site and reinfusion after some form of processing has been applied to major vascular, cardiac, and multiple trauma situations for many years.[432,437,438,446–458] The common techniques used wash the recovered blood in a centrifuge so the product consists of the child's RBCs suspended in saline at a hematocrit of 50% to 60%.[448,455] Cellular debris, excess citrate or heparin, free hemoglobin, activated clotting factors, and clotted blood are almost completely removed. Autotransfusion avoids the infectious and immunologic risks of allogeneic transfusion and, if reinfusion is carried out in the operating room, minimizes the opportunity for mistransfusion.[447,455,456,459]

Intraoperative blood recovery is not widely used in infants and children.[407,408,458,460–462] The equipment is designed for adults, although some manufacturers have adapted standard devices for pediatric use.[463,464] We have found blood recovery to be a useful adjunct to minimize allogeneic blood transfusion during scoliosis surgery. This technique may also be used in conjunction with preoperative autologous blood donation, further reducing the need for allogeneic RBC transfusions.[446,451,452,461] The capital investment for the devices and the costs for the disposables and a trained operator, however, are significant. Nonetheless, these expenses can be offset if 2 to 3 fewer units of allogeneic RBCs are transfused. Development of pediatric-sized equipment has made this technique more widely used and more cost-effective even in smaller children.[465]

Indications

Indications include any major surgical procedure in which the use of more than 2 units of banked PBCs is likely or in which massive blood loss is occurring; children with rare blood types; and multiple trauma with massive hemorrhage.

Contraindications

Major contraindications to blood-recovery devices include contamination of the operative field by bacteria (e.g., bowel trauma, abscess), cancer, and sickle cell disease (e.g., sickling in the device). Recovered blood should not be processed for reinfusion if the surgical field contains topical clotting agents, some topical antibiotics (e.g., polymyxin, neomycin), or other foreign materials (e.g., methylmethacrylate). Surgery for a malignancy is considered to be a relative contraindication because of the theoretical concern that malignant cells may be recovered and reinfused; this can be avoided by discarding blood recovered from the operative field while the tumor is being manipulated.[466–468]

CONTROLLED HYPOTENSION

Controlled hypotension has long been used to reduce intraoperative blood loss or to provide a relatively bloodless operating field.[407,462,469–481] Hypotensive anesthesia may be accomplished with many techniques, including continuous infusion of vasodilators, β-adrenergic blockade, deep inhalational anesthesia, and large-dose opioid infusions (e.g., remifentanil).[470,481–485]

Controlled hypotension is reserved for older children and teenagers undergoing major reconstructive (e.g., craniofacial surgery) or orthopedic surgery. The choice of technique and the degree of induced hypotension depend on the surgical procedure. For procedures in which a dry surgical field is the endpoint with little potential for rapid blood loss, a technique that may take some time for recovery is acceptable (e.g., deep inhalational agent with or without β-blockade). If surgery carries the possibility of rapid or massive blood loss, a technique that is rapidly reversed (e.g., nitroprusside, nitroglycerin, remifentanil) is probably safer. Controlled hypotension with mean arterial pressure (MAP) of 55 to 60 mm Hg is used much less in recent years than in the past, especially for patients cared for in the prone position. Moderate hypotensive techniques with a MAP of 65 to 70 mm Hg are a more common practice and are likely associated with less risk, although no studies have been published in this regard.[425] The main concern regarding the use of this technique is reported cases of blindness after surgery performed with the patient in the prone position[486–490]; risk factors for blindness include duration of anesthesia, extensive blood loss, anemia, large crystalloid fluid administration, and others (see also Chapters 32 and 34).

General Concepts

All potent inhalational anesthetics decrease the cerebral metabolic rate for oxygen consumption ($CMRO_2$) and increase cerebral blood flow. Isoflurane appears to offer the greatest advantage because it induces the greatest depression of $CMRO_2$, and it has been used as the sole hypotensive agent.[491–497] One of the most important considerations of any hypotensive technique is its effect on cerebral blood flow. Brain ischemia has been documented in adults when a MAP of 55 mm Hg is combined with hypocarbia; we would not recommend this degree of hypotension in prone procedures. Maintenance of normal arterial carbon dioxide tension ($PaCO_2$) is vitally important to ensure adequate cerebral blood flow; the relationship of cerebral blood flow to $PaCO_2$ is described in greater detail in Chapter 26. To optimize cerebral blood flow, we typically maintain the MAP at 65 to 70 mm Hg or greater and the $PaCO_2$ at 35 to 45 mm Hg.

Because hypotensive anesthesia with inhalational anesthetics depresses myocardial function and requires time to wash out, a rapid offset is difficult to achieve; we advocate alternative strategies (e.g., vasodilating agents, remifentanil) that provide more precise control of blood pressure without depressing the heart.

If β-blockade is to be used safely, the clinician must understand the differences in half-lives. Esmolol is very short acting, with a half-life in children of approximately 3 minutes[498]; nonanesthetized children have a greater requirement (in micrograms per kilogram) than adults.[459] In nonanesthetized children, a loading dose of 500 µg/kg per minute is followed by a maintenance infusion at a rate of 25 to 200 µg/kg per minute. Because there is limited published experience using esmolol in children under anesthesia, a smaller starting dose (25–50 µg/kg per minute) and titration of dose every 3 to 5 minutes (increase by 12.5–25 µg/kg per minute) are suggested. Labetalol[500-503] and propranolol[504,505] have longer half-lives, greater time to peak effect, and the effects are less controllable and not recommended. Acute β-blocker toxicity can be reversed with high-dose IV glucagon (50 µg/kg followed by an infusion of 0.3–3.0 µg/kg per minute [extrapolated from adult data])[506-508] and possibly with vasopressin.[509] Intralipid rescue has also been proposed for propranolol toxicity but may not be effective for less fat-soluble β-blockers.[510-512]

Pharmacology

Sodium Nitroprusside

Sodium nitroprusside has a very rapid onset of action (seconds), brief duration of action (minutes), and minimal side effects when used in the recommended dose range.[513] This agent must be administered by an infusion pump through a separate IV site and with a second pump to provide a continuous, uninterrupted, and stable infusion rate.

DOSAGE. The initial infusion rate for sodium nitroprusside is 0.5 to 1.0 µg/kg per minute.[514,515] The rate can be increased as needed to achieve the desired MAP.[516,517] A satisfactory reduction in systemic perfusion pressure can usually be obtained well below the recommended maximum rate of 10 µg/kg per minute.

TOXICITY. Cyanide toxicity is characterized by an unexplained metabolic acidosis, increased blood lactate, and an increased mixed venous oxygen content.[517,518] The nitroprusside radical interacts with the sulfhydryl groups of erythrocytes, releasing cyanide. If the amount of cyanide released overwhelms the capacity of the rhodanese system, cyanide toxicity (i.e., binding to the cytochrome electron transport system) results. This produces a change to anaerobic metabolism, metabolic acidosis, an increase in mixed venous oxygen content, and eventually death[517,519-523]; several pediatric anesthetic-related deaths have resulted from cyanide toxicity and its treatment.[520-522]

Three responses to sodium nitroprusside infusion may herald impending cyanide toxicity: more than 10 µg/kg per minute required for a response, tachyphylaxis developing within 30 to 60 minutes, and immediate resistance to the drug.[518] If any of these occur, sodium nitroprusside should be discontinued and the child investigated for possible cyanide toxicity. Treatment of cyanide poisoning is directed at reversal of the binding of cyanide to the cytochrome enzymes. This can be accomplished by producing methemoglobinemia with amyl nitrite. Methemoglobin has a greater affinity for cyanide than it does for the cytochrome system, forcing the reaction in the direction of forming cyanmethemoglobin. The breakdown of cyanmethemoglobin is promoted by administering thiosulfate, which reacts with the cyanide to form nontoxic thiocyanate, which is then excreted by the kidneys. Hydroxocobalamin may prevent toxicity by formation of cyanocobalamin (see also Chapter 18).[524]

Sodium nitroprusside is a safe medication if doses remain within guidelines established by various investigators.[525-527] For children, this is a maximum of 50 µg/kg per minute for 30 minutes and 8 to 10 µg/kg per minute for 3 hours, with frequent blood gas analyses.[517,527] The potential for toxicity and the availability of less toxic vasodilators have decreased its use for controlled hypotension; it is most commonly used for short-term control of blood pressure in special situations.

Nitroglycerin

The main advantages of nitroglycerin are its relatively rapid onset of action (minutes), lack of tachyphylaxis and toxicity, and brief duration of action (minutes); the major disadvantage is the limited achievable reduction in blood pressure.

DOSAGE. Nitroglycerin is administered by an infusion beginning at a rate of 1 µg/kg per minute; the dose is increased until the desired response is obtained. Resistance to the hypotensive effects of nitroglycerin may occur in children. However, in view of the reduced potential for toxicity compared with nitroprusside, nitroglycerin appears to be a reasonable alternative.

TOXICITY. Nitroglycerin is relatively free of toxic side effects in the usual doses applied during hypotensive anesthesia.[477,528,529] However, several reports have described nitroglycerin-induced methemoglobinemia.[530,531] Pulse oximetry may be of value in making the initial diagnosis (i.e., decreased saturation). However, if this occurs, accurate saturation determinations are not possible because of the interference in light absorbance caused by methemoglobin at both ends of the absorbance spectrum used by pulse oximeters.[532,533] The use of other adjuncts (e.g., potent inhalation agents, other vasodilators, β-adrenergic blockade, or opioids) reduces the total dose of nitroglycerin administered.

Remifentanil

Remifentanil-induced hypotension is increasing in popularity because of its relative safety, ease of administration, and titratability, particularly if a patient must be awakened during spinal fusion. Administration should be the same as for any other vasoactive anesthetic agent. It requires dedicated IV access, with the infusion as close to the IV catheter as possible and with a separate pump to avoid fluctuations in the rate of administration. The half-life of this drug is so brief that interruptions while changing IVs or boluses when giving other medications need to be avoided. We have found that the combination of a low-dose inhalational agent, low-dose propofol, and a remifentanil infusion provides excellent operating conditions. Systemic arterial pressure can be controlled by the rate of opioid infusion without fear of residual opioid effect at the end of the procedure, and this combination does not significantly interfere with sensory and motor potential monitoring. If an intraoperative wake-up is needed, a longer-acting opioid such as fentanyl should be administered before awakening.

DOSAGE. For most children, the starting dose is 0.1 µg/kg per minute, which is then increased or decreased depending on the child's response and the degree of surgical stimulus.[514] A steady-state blood concentration of remifentanil of 14 µg/L would typically achieve a 30% decrease in MAP.[534,535]

The anesthesiologist should expect variable opioid requirements during spinal fusions (doses as great as 2 µg/kg per minute and as small as 0.05 µg/kg per minute). Analgesic doses of a long-acting opioid such as morphine or hydromorphone should be administered approximately 10 minutes before discontinuation to provide adequate analgesia on awakening. This technique often allows a smooth but rapid extubation despite a very long surgical procedure.

General Concepts of Hypotensive Anesthesia

Before using controlled hypotension, it is important to understand the rationale for using this technique.[536] If it is used to reduce surgical blood loss, the preparation and monitoring of a child are different from the approach in a procedure in which the main objective for reducing the perfusion pressure is to improve operating conditions (e.g., microsurgical techniques). In the former case, direct assessment of circulating blood pressure and volume with an arterial line and central venous catheter is important, whereas in the latter case, only a direct means of measuring blood pressure (arterial line) is needed.

Anesthetic Management

All inhalational anesthetic agents have been used as a single drug to produce controlled hypotension, but profound cardiovascular depression may be difficult to control.[493-495,537,538] We do not advocate hypotensive anesthesia using potent inhalational agents as the sole hypotensive agent because the cardiovascular depression is not rapidly reversed if a problem arises. However, small to moderate concentrations of inhalational anesthetic reduce the amount of vasodilator, β-blocker, or opioid necessary to reduce blood pressure.[539]

Short-acting β-adrenergic blockers offer an alternative method to decrease MAP by directly depressing cardiac output. However, β-adrenergic blockade removes a valuable guide to the depth of anesthesia and volume status. Because the cardiac output in children approximately 2 years old or younger depends on heart rate (see Chapter 18), β-adrenergic blockade is not recommended in this age group. Low-dose, short-acting β-adrenergic blockade may be a reasonable adjunct to hypotensive anesthesia with inhalational anesthetics as a means of reducing the concentration of the anesthetic or as a supplement to reduce the vasodilator requirements.[540] A rapid-acting β-blocker such as esmolol may be the best compromise because its half-life is brief (3 minutes) and it is administered as an infusion.

Monitoring and Management Principles

The following baseline parameters are monitored: oxygen saturation and expired carbon dioxide, ECG, temperature, hematocrit, blood glucose, arterial blood gases, acid-base status, MAP, and CVP. Arterial pressure is measured using an arterial line.

When the desired MAP has been attained, a new baseline CVP should be measured and maintained at this level or a slightly greater level than the new reduced CVP value throughout the procedure. To use any hypotensive technique safely, normovolemia is maintained at all times. This means that even small (1- or 2-mm Hg) decreases in the CVP prompt an appropriate fluid response. A small change in cardiac filling pressures in a healthy, supine, anesthetized pediatric patient may represent a significant reduction in circulating blood volume. Even during hypotensive anesthesia, the kidneys should produce 0.5 to 1.0 mL/kg of urine per hour. The failure to detect urine output frequently is caused by obstruction or kinking of the urinary catheter. If the catheter is patent, an IV fluid challenge should be considered.

After hypotension has been induced and the surgical field is bloodless, the MAP should be slowly increased in 5- to 10-mm

Hg increments until increased bleeding is observed in the surgical field. At that time, the MAP can be again reduced by approximately 5 mm Hg to achieve optimal conditions. With this method, it is sometimes necessary to reduce the MAP only 10% to 20% from baseline to achieve satisfactory hemostasis with hypotensive anesthesia.

POSITION. Make the operative field the highest point of the child's body to take advantage of gravitational forces to help reduce blood pressure and minimize any possible impedance to venous drainage that may contribute to blood loss. If the head is the surgical site, the arterial transducer must be calibrated at head level rather than heart level to ensure adequate cerebral perfusion pressure.[529,541]

LABORATORY VARIABLES. An adequate hemoglobin must be maintained to have sufficient oxygen-carrying capacity; we maintain the hemoglobin at 9 to 10 g/dL during controlled hypotensive anesthesia. This is important for children undergoing spinal instrumentation, in which traction on the spinal cord may alter spinal cord blood flow and to prevent possible blindness.

Arterial blood gases must be carefully evaluated on a 30- to 60-minute basis to diagnose changes in oxygenation, ventilation, or perfusion or the development of drug toxicity (e.g., metabolic acidosis with nitroprusside) or adverse anesthesia events.[542-544] A large difference between arterial and expired carbon dioxide values may indicate a pulmonary shunt or air embolization. An increase in mixed venous oxygen content may signal cyanide toxicity. Adequate PaO_2 must be maintained at all times. Normocarbia should be maintained to ensure cerebral perfusion.[513,545,546] Although we do not advocate the routine use of β-adrenergic blockade, blood glucose values should be measured serially because β-adrenergic blockade inhibits glycogenolysis and has resulted in unsuspected hypoglycemia in children.[475,547,548]

Contraindications

The risks of hypotensive anesthesia are significant.[549] The risk/benefit ratio must always be considered on an individual basis, particularly with neurosurgical patients and those undergoing spinal instrumentation; any systemic disease compromising the function of a major organ is a relative contraindication. Most reported complications are related to inexperience of the practitioner, inappropriate patient selection, unfamiliarity with the drugs involved, or inattention to details such as blood volume status, pH, $PaCO_2$, blood glucose, or not using infusion pumps to carefully titrate medications. If a child is healthy and meticulous attention is paid to all the physiologic variables, the benefits of improved surgical technique, reduced surgical time, and decreased need for blood transfusion may outweigh the potential risks.

NORMOVOLEMIC HEMODILUTION

Intentional isovolemic hemodilution is a useful strategy for reducing allogeneic blood transfusions.[407,408,432,462,550-560] Two basic methods can be applied:

1. Allow the surgical blood loss to continue until the child's hematocrit value is in the high teens and maintain that hematocrit value until near the end of the procedure. At that time, the hematocrit can be increased to the desired value by transfusing PRBCs. This technique allows surgical bleeding to occur at a reduced hematocrit value, resulting in reduced loss of RBC mass.

2. Blood can be removed from a child at the beginning of the operation while replacing the volume with crystalloid solution

and then returning the blood at the end of the procedure or when significant bleeding occurs.

The latter technique is preferable because it reserves a quantity of the child's own blood, which can be returned at the end of the surgical procedure. For a Jehovah's Witness, this technique often conforms to religious guidelines if direct continuity is maintained with the child's circulation.[550,561-568]

During acute normovolemic hemodilution under anesthesia, the distribution of blood flow improves with the reduced hematocrit. Improved blood rheology is the major compensatory mechanism for maintaining oxygen delivery despite a reduced hematocrit. Oxygen extraction increases in the presence of an inadequate circulating blood volume or when the hematocrit decreases to less than 20%. If the hematocrit decreases to less than 15%, subendocardial myocardial ischemia may develop.[569-572] At this extreme level of anemia, dissolved oxygen begins to assume a more important role in oxygen delivery.[573] In several reports, extreme acute normovolemic hemodilution (hemoglobin as low as 2 g/dL) was well tolerated;[569,574-577] we cannot endorse the use of this technique in children because it is impossible to assess the effects of such an extreme hemoglobin concentration on the long-term cognitive ability. Nonetheless, these reports[569,577] indicate that healthy children can tolerate these extreme hematocrit concentrations provided they are anesthetized, normovolemic, slightly hypothermic, and ventilated with 100% oxygen. We limit the absolute minimum hematocrit to 15%, but we prefer to maintain the hematocrit closer to 20% at all times; if the surgery involves the prone position, then a greater hematocrit might be safer.[486-490]

Technique and Key Concepts

Arterial blood is collected from the arterial line into sterile blood bags that contain the appropriate anticoagulant. Each bag is weighed before any blood is transferred and then continuously during filling by placing it on a scale. The bag is frequently but gently agitated to ensure an even distribution of the anticoagulant. The total volume of blood to be withdrawn should be calculated preoperatively to reduce the hematocrit to the 20% to 25%. Care must be taken to replace the blood removed with 5% albumin milliliter for milliliter or 1.5 to 2 mL of lactated Ringer solution for each milliliter of blood removed. Sometimes, an even greater volume of replacement fluid is needed.[557] A reasonable estimate of the adequacy of replacement is to obtain a baseline CVP and then maintain the same CVP as blood is withdrawn and replaced. It is preferable to hemodilute before the surgical incision to monitor changes in hemodynamic indices, although it can be performed during the initial phases of surgery. The major concern is to maintain a normal circulating blood volume and provide adequate oxygen-carrying capacity. It is important to make an educated guess about how much blood loss is anticipated during the surgery so that autologous blood can be reinfused in place of homologous blood. Because a small-pore filter (20-µm) traps many more platelets than a large-pore filter (≥150 µm), the former is best avoided at this juncture.

Indications

Hemodilution may be indicated in any procedure in which blood loss is expected to exceed one-half of the child's blood volume.

Contraindications

Hemodilution is contraindicated in children with sickle cell disease, septicemia, cyanotic cardiac disease, or compromised function of any major organ that may be significantly affected by changes in perfusion and oxygenation. We do not recommend combining extreme hemodilution (hematocrit <25%) with controlled hypotension. Children with moderate anemia are not good candidates because not enough units can be removed to make the technique effective.

Complications

The major complications of hemodilution are related to blood volume status, hemoglobin content (i.e., removing too much blood), and coagulopathy (i.e., dilution of clotting factors). Anesthesiologists must pay meticulous attention to blood volume replacement. As long as normovolemia is maintained and the hematocrit exceeds 20%, problems with organ perfusion or oxygenation should not occur. Sepsis becomes a concern if strict sterile techniques are not followed during the collection process.

Advantages

The benefits of normovolemic hemodilution are that the units of blood collected at the beginning of the procedure pose no risk of infection (unless contaminated by bacteria during the collection process) or mistransfusion (if they are not removed from the operating room) when they are returned to the child at a later time. It yields a net saving in loss of RBC mass because the surgical losses occur at a hematocrit of 20% rather than 40% to 45%. The net use of banked PRBCs may be reduced if 2 or 3 units can be removed at the beginning of the procedure. This technique is generally reserved for teenagers undergoing spinal instrumentation; however, with the association of blindness and anemia, fewer anesthesiologists feel comfortable with this technique.

The Jehovah's Witness Patient

The children of Jehovah's Witnesses present a particular medical and legal dilemma.[578-581] Transfusion management of anyone with a religious objection to transfusion depends in part on the urgency of the surgical procedure and underlying medical condition of the child. If not emergent, a meeting with the patient (or the parents or guardian if a minor), the patient's spiritual advisor (if the child so chooses), and representatives of the team that will be caring for the child should be held to allow the child to clearly articulate his or her wishes with respect to the refusal of transfusion and its consequences and to discuss possible alternatives, including the use of erythropoietin, iron therapy, acute normovolemic hemodilution, intraoperative cell recovery and reinfusion, and the use of antifibrinolytic medications.[575,576,582-585] Specific inquiries should be made about each child's beliefs regarding the use of albumin, plasma, cryoprecipitate, platelets, and intraoperative cell recovery and reinfusion if the circuit is not continuously connected to the child and, in particular, what the child's response would be if a life-threatening event occurred while he or she was under anesthesia.[561,586] These discussions should be carefully documented in the child's record and informed consent signed beforehand. Not all hospitals or physicians are willing to participate in these cases, in which case arrangements should be made to transfer the child to the care of institutions or physicians who are willing to work within these constraints.

The courts have consistently ruled that the adult patient or emancipated minor has a right to refuse transfusion.[562,587] Physicians have the moral and legal obligations to respect those beliefs if an adult or teenager has made an informed decision and understands that he or she may die or suffer permanent injury without a transfusion if a life-threatening situation occurs. However, in the case of a minor child, the Supreme Courts in the United States and Canada have ruled that the fate of the minor child cannot be determined by the parents' religious convictions. The most important issue is full and open discussion of the effort that will be made to respect the person's religious beliefs and avoid blood transfusions. Optimizing the child's hemoglobin concentration is paramount for elective surgery where blood loss is anticipated. In the case of minor children about whom a mutual understanding cannot be reached on avoiding blood transfusions, a court order can be obtained to save the child's life. The parents should be informed about this possibility beforehand.[588] The ethics of this issue are discussed in Chapter 5.

ACKNOWLEDGMENT

The authors wish to thank Richard M. Dsida for his prior contributions to this chapter.

ANNOTATED REFERENCES

Dhabangi A, Ainomugisha B, Cserti-Gazdewich C, et al. Effect of transfusion of red blood cells with longer vs shorter storage duration on elevated blood lactate levels in children with severe anemia: the TOTAL randomized clinical trial. *JAMA.* 2015;314:2514-2523.

This study of children with severe anemia demonstrated that longer-stored RBCs were just as efficacious in delivering option and correcting lactic acidosis as RBCs stored for a short time and thus complements the ARIPI study that showed equivalent clinical outcomes (see Fergusson paper later in list).

Dzik WH, Stowell CP. Transfusion and coagulation issues in trauma. In: Sheridan RL, ed. *The Trauma Handbook of the Massachusetts General Hospital.* Philadelphia: Lippincott Williams & Wilkins; 2004:128-147.

This chapter discusses the issues and complications of massive transfusion and provides a practical guide for management of this difficult clinical situation.

Fergusson DA, Hébert P, Hogan DL, et al. Effect of fresh red blood cell transfusions on clinical outcomes in premature, very low-birth-weight infants: the ARIPI randomized trial. *JAMA.* 2012;308:1443-1451.

This RCT is one of four demonstrating that the duration of RBC storage does not affect patient outcomes.

Lacroix J, Hébert PC, Hutchinson JS, et al. Transfusion strategies for patients in pediatric intensive care units. *N Engl J Med.* 2007;356:1609-1619.

This landmark multicenter clinical trial compared outcomes in pediatric patients randomly assigned to red blood cell transfusion thresholds of 9.5 g/dL or 7 g/ dL. There were no differences with respect to new or progressive multiple-organ failure, mortality, or other clinical outcomes between the two groups, which highlights the capacity of even acutely ill pediatric patients to tolerate anemia.

Ness PM, Cushing MM. Oxygen therapeutics: pursuit of an alternative to the donor red blood cell. *Arch Pathol Lab Med.* 2007;131:734-741.

This review provides a comprehensive and balanced summary of the development of synthetic oxygen carriers and the current challenges they face in making the transition from the laboratory to the clinic.

Slichter SJ, Kaufman RM, Assmann SF, et al. Dose of prophylactic platelet transfusions and prevention of hemorrhage. *N Engl J Med.* 2010;362:600-613.

This paper presents new data regarding platelet transfusion for nonoperative, thrombocytopenic patients including 200 children.

A complete reference list can be found online at ExpertConsult.com.

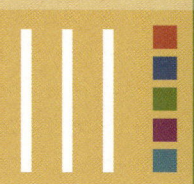

Essentials of Pulmonology

13

PAUL G. FIRTH AND T. BERNARD KINANE

RESPIRATORY PROBLEMS ARE COMMON in children. The anesthesiologist often encounters pulmonary complications ranging from mild acute respiratory tract infections to chronic lung disease with end-stage respiratory failure during perioperative consultations, intraoperatively, or in the intensive care unit. This chapter discusses the basics of respiratory physiology, how to assess pulmonary function, and the practical anesthetic management of specific pulmonary problems. Airway and thoracic aspects pertinent to ventilation are discussed in Chapters 14 and 15; pulmonary issues specific to neonates, intensive care, and various disease states are addressed in the relevant chapters.

Respiratory Physiology

The morphologic development of the lung begins at several weeks after conception and continues into the first decade of postnatal life.[1] Intrauterine gas exchange occurs via the placenta, but the respiratory system develops in preparation for extrauterine life, when gas exchange transfers abruptly to the lungs at birth.

Development of the lung, which begins as an outgrowth of the foregut ventral wall, can be divided into several stages (Fig. 13.1). During the embryonic period, in the first few weeks after conception, lung buds form as a projection of the endodermal tissue into the mesenchyme. The pseudoglandular period extends to the 17th week of life, during which rapid lung growth is accompanied by formation of the bronchi and branching of the airways down to the terminal bronchioli. Further development of bronchioli and vascularization of the airways occurs during the canalicular stage of the second trimester. The saccular stage begins at approximately 24 weeks, when terminal air sacs begin to form. The capillary networks surrounding these air spaces proliferate, allowing sufficient pulmonary gas exchange for extrauterine survival of the premature neonate by 26 to 28 weeks. Formation of alveoli occurs by lengthening of the saccules and thinning of the saccular walls and has begun by the 36th week after conception in most human fetuses. The vast majority of alveolar formation occurs after birth, typically continuing until 8 to 10 years postnatally. At birth, the neonatal lung usually contains 10 to 20 million terminal air sacs (many of which are saccules rather than alveoli), one-tenth the number in the mature adult lung. After birth, growth of the lungs occurs primarily as an increase in the number of respiratory bronchioles and alveoli rather than an increase in the size of the alveoli.

The abrupt transition to extrauterine gas exchange at birth involves the rapid expansion of the lungs, increased pulmonary blood flow, and initiation of a regular respiratory rhythm. The development of a respiratory rhythm, detectable initially by intermittent rhythmic fetal thoracic movements, begins well before birth and may be necessary for normal anatomic and physiologic lung development. Interruption of umbilical blood flow at birth initiates continuous rhythmic breathing. Amniotic fluid is expelled from the lungs via the upper airways with the first few breaths, with residual fluid draining through the lymphatic and pulmonary channels in the first days of life. Changes in the partial pressures of oxygen (PO_2) and carbon dioxide (PCO_2) and in hydrogen ion concentration (pH) cause an acute decrease in pulmonary vascular resistance and a consequent increase in pulmonary blood flow. Increased left atrial and decreased right atrial pressures reverse the pressure gradient across the foramen ovale, causing functional closure of this left-to-right one-way flap valve. Ventilatory rhythm is augmented and maintained in part by the increased arterial oxygen relative to the prior intrauterine levels.

Breathing is controlled by a complex interaction involving input from sensors, integration by a central control system, and output to effector muscles.[2] Afferent signaling is provided by peripheral arterial and central brainstem chemoreceptors, upper

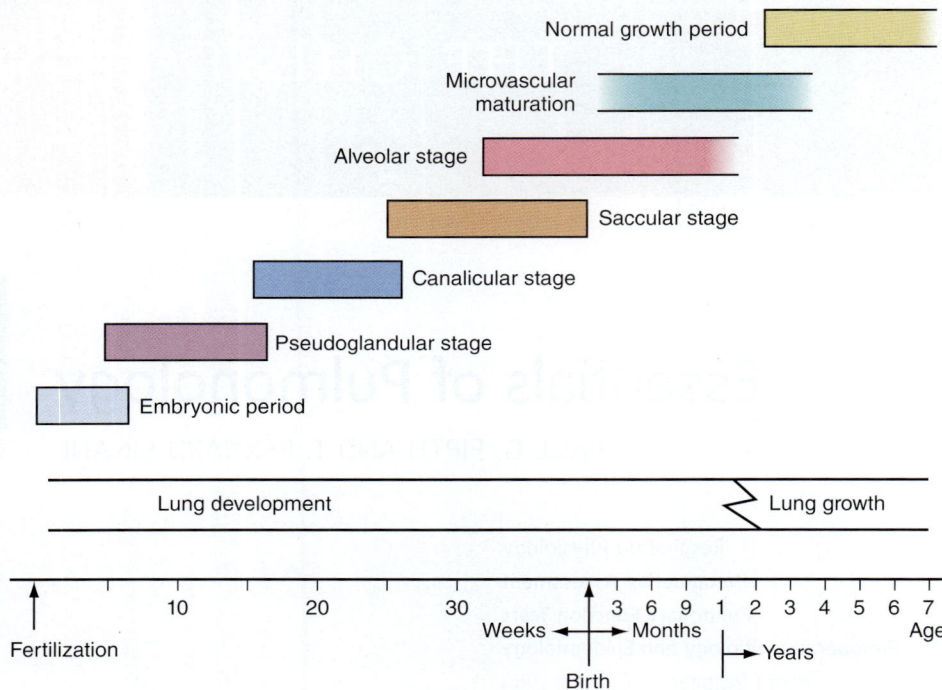

FIGURE 13.1 Timetable for lung development. (Modified with permission from Guttentag S, Ballard PL. Lung development: embryology, growth, maturation, and developmental biology. In: Tausch HW, Ballard RA, Gleason CA, eds. *Avery's Diseases of the Newborn.* 8th ed. Philadelphia: WB Saunders; 2004:602.)

airway and intrapulmonary receptors, and chest wall and muscle mechanoreceptors.

The peripheral arterial chemoreceptors consist of the carotid and aortic bodies, with the carotid bodies playing the greater role in arterial chemical sensing of both arterial O_2 tension (Pao_2) and pH. The central chemoreceptors, responsive to arterial CO_2 tension ($PaCO_2$) and pH, are thought to be located at or near the ventral surface of the medulla.

The nose, pharynx, and larynx have a wide variety of pressure, chemical, temperature, and flow receptors that can cause apnea, coughing, or changes in ventilatory pattern. Pulmonary receptors lie in the airways and lung parenchyma. The airway receptors are subdivided into the slowly adapting receptors, also called pulmonary stretch receptors, and the rapidly adapting receptors. The stretch receptors, found in the airway smooth muscle, are thought to be involved in the balance of inspiration and expiration. These receptors may be the sensors in the Hering-Breuer reflexes, which prevent overdistention or collapse of the lung. The rapidly adapting receptors lie between the airway epithelial cells and are triggered by noxious stimuli such as smoke, dust, and histamine. Parenchymal receptors, also known as juxtacapillary receptors, are located adjacent to the alveolar blood vessels; they respond to hyperinflation of the lungs, to various chemical stimuli in the pulmonary circulation, and possibly to interstitial congestion. Chest wall receptors include mechanoreceptors and joint proprioreceptors. Mechanoreceptors in the muscle spindle endings and tendons of respiratory muscles sense changes in length, tension, and movement.

Central integration of respiration is maintained by the brainstem (involuntary) and by cortical (voluntary) centers. Although the precise mechanism of the neural ventilatory rhythmogenesis is unknown, the pre-Bötzinger complex and the retrotrapezoid nucleus/parafacial respiratory group, neural circuits in the ven-

trolateral medulla, are thought to be the respiratory rhythm generators.[3] These neuron groups fire in an oscillating pattern, an inherent rhythm that is moderated by inputs from other respiratory centers. Involuntary integration of sensory input occurs in various respiratory nuclei and neural complexes in the pons and medulla that modify the baseline pacemaker firing of the respiratory rhythm generators. The cerebral cortex also affects breathing rhythm and influences or overrides involuntary rhythm generation in response to conscious or subconscious activity, such as emotion, arousal, pain, speech, breath-holding, and other activities.[2]

The effectors of ventilation include the neural efferent pathways, the muscles of respiration, the bones and cartilage of the chest wall and airway, and elastic connective tissue. Upper airway patency is maintained by connective tissue and by sustained and cyclic contractions of the pharyngeal dilator muscles. The diaphragm produces the majority of tidal volume during quiet inspiration, with the intercostal, abdominal, and accessory muscles (sternocleidomastoid and neck muscles) providing additional negative pressure. The elastic recoil of the lungs and thorax produces expiration. Inspiration is an active and expiration a passive action in normal lungs during quiet breathing. During vigorous breathing or with airway obstruction, both inspiration and expiration become active processes.

Another effect of age is a change in chest wall compliance. In adults the end-expiratory volume is equivalent to the functional residual capacity (FRC). In infants the chest wall is more compliant, so the tendency of the lung to collapse is not adequately counterbalanced by chest wall rigidity. Infants stop expiration at a lung volume greater than FRC, with the inspiratory muscles braking expiration. When this braking mechanism is impaired, as occurs with general anesthesia, the infant has a tendency to develop atelectasis.

Preoperative Assessment

The preoperative assessment of the respiratory system in a child is based on the history, physical examination, and evaluation of vital signs. Because ventilation is a complex process involving many systems besides the lung, the pulmonary appraisal must also include an assessment of airway, musculoskeletal, and neurologic pathology that might affect gas exchange under anesthesia or in the postoperative period. The potential impacts of esophageal reflux and cardiac, hepatic, renal, or hematologic disease on gas exchange and pulmonary function should be considered. Further investigations, such as laboratory, radiographic, and pulmonary function studies, may be indicated if there is doubt as to the diagnosis or severity of the pulmonary disease.

Because children may be unwilling or unable to give a reliable history, parents or caregivers are often the sole source or an important supplemental source of information during initial evaluation. Risk factors in the history that are associated with an increased risk of perioperative events include a respiratory tract infection within the preceding 2 weeks, wheezing during exercise, more than three wheezing episodes in the past 12 months, nocturnal dry cough, eczema, and a family history of asthma, rhinitis, eczema, or exposure to tobacco smoke.[1,4] Viral upper respiratory tract infections (URIs) are common in children, and the time, frequency, and severity of infection should be established. If wheezing is present, the precipitating causes, frequency, severity, and relieving factors should be determined. Chronic pulmonary diseases often have a variable clinical course, and the details of acute exacerbations of chronic problems should be elicited.

In younger children the gestational age at birth, the current postmenstrual age, neonatal respiratory difficulties, and prolonged intubation in the neonatal period are particularly important to ascertain. Apneic episodes, subglottic stenosis, and tracheomalacia are possible complications of prematurity and prolonged intubation that may be exacerbated in the perioperative period. Whereas congenital lesions often manifest at birth, symptoms of airway collapse or stenosis may become evident only later in life.

Physical examination begins when you enter the room. Particularly with young children, your best opportunity to observe them before they react to your presence is from across the room, and inspection from a distance can provide useful information. The respiratory rate is a sensitive marker of pulmonary problems, and scrutiny of the rate before a young child becomes agitated and hyperventilates is an important metric. Pulse oximetry is a useful baseline indicator of oxygenation. Nasal flaring, intercostal retractions, and the marked use of accessory respiratory muscles are all signs of respiratory distress. General appearance is also important. Apathy, anxiety, agitation, or persistent adoption of a fixed posture may indicate profound respiratory or airway difficulties, and intense cyanosis can also be detected from a distance. Weight may relate to pulmonary function; children with chronic severe pulmonary disease are often underweight owing to retarded growth or malnourishment, whereas severe obesity can produce airway obstruction and sleep apnea. Inspection of the chest contour may reveal hyperinflation or thoracic wall deformities.

Closer physical examination adds further information. Atopy and eczema may be associated with hyperreactive airways. Auscultation may reveal wheezes, rales, fine or coarse crepitus, transmitted breath sounds from the upper airway, altered breath sounds, or cardiac murmurs. Chest percussion can provide an estimate of the position of the diaphragm and serve as a useful marker of hyperinflation. Patience, a gentle approach, and warm hands improve diagnostic yield and patient satisfaction.

Pulmonary Function Tests

Further pulmonary investigations include chest imaging, measurement of hematocrit, arterial blood gas analysis, pulmonary function tests, and sleep studies. Special investigations are not routinely indicated preoperatively and should be reserved for cases in which the diagnosis is unclear, the progression or treatment of a disease needs to be established, or the severity of impairment is not evident. In most cases a comprehensive history and careful physical examination are adequate to establish an appropriate anesthetic plan. Before requesting a new investigation, the clinician should have a clear idea of the question the test is expected to answer and how the answer will modify anesthetic management and outcome. Many tests are difficult to perform in children who have short attention spans and who cannot sit still for any length of time. Judgment must be exercised when ordering these tests for young children, and due consideration must be given to the child's age and level of maturity and the influence of the parents.

Pulmonary function tests include dynamic studies, measurement of static lung volumes, and diffusing capacity. Pulmonary function tests enable clinicians to (1) establish mechanical dysfunction in children with respiratory symptoms, (2) quantify the degree of dysfunction, and (3) define the nature of the dysfunction as obstructive, restrictive, or mixed obstructive and restrictive.[5] Table 13.1 presents common indications for pulmonary function testing in children.

The dynamic studies, which are the most commonly used tests, include spirometry, flow–volume loops, and measurement of peak expiratory flow. Spirometry measures the volume of air inspired and expired as a function of time and is by far the most

TABLE 13.1	Uses of Pulmonary Function Studies in Children

- To establish pulmonary mechanical abnormality in children with respiratory symptoms
- To quantify the degree of dysfunction
- To define the nature of pulmonary dysfunction (obstructive, restrictive, or mixed obstructive and restrictive)
- To aid in defining the site of airway obstruction as central or peripheral
- To differentiate fixed from variable and intrathoracic from extrathoracic central airway obstruction
- To follow the course of pulmonary disease processes
- To assess the effect of therapeutic interventions and guide changes in therapy
- To detect increased airway reactivity
- To evaluate the risk of diagnostic and therapeutic procedures
- To monitor for pulmonary side effects of chemotherapy or radiation therapy
- To aid in predicting the prognosis and quantitating pulmonary disability
- To investigate the effect of acute and chronic disease processes on lung growth

Modified with permission from Castile R. Pulmonary function testing in children. In: Chernick V, Boat TF, Wilmott RW, Bush A, eds. *Kendig's Disorders of the Respiratory Tract in Children* 7th ed. Philadelphia: Elsevier Saunders; 2006:168. Reproduced from National Asthma Education and Prevention Program. Full report of the expert panel: guidelines for the diagnosis and management of asthma (EPR-3). Bethesda, MD: National Heart, Lung, and Blood Institute, National Institutes of Health; 2007.

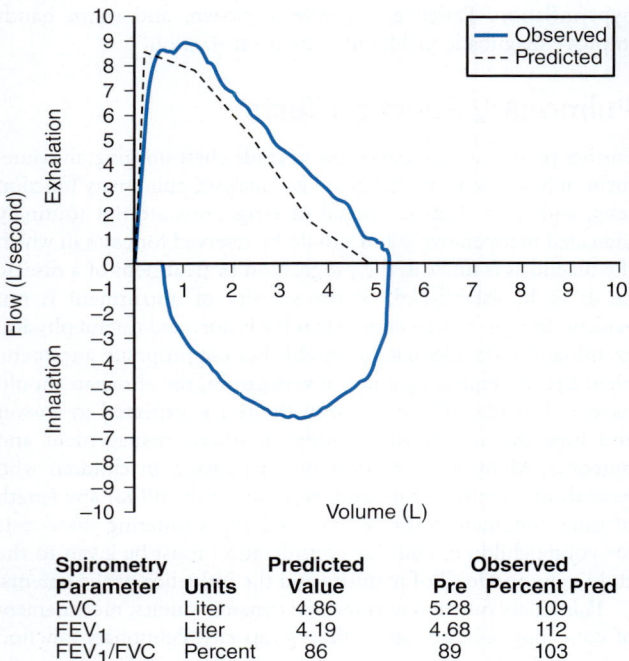

Spirometry Parameter	Units	Predicted Value	Observed Pre	Observed Percent Pred
FVC	Liter	4.86	5.28	109
FEV$_1$	Liter	4.19	4.68	112
FEV$_1$/FVC	Percent	86	89	103

FIGURE 13.2 Normal pulmonary function test. The normal flow–volume curve obtained during forced expiration rapidly ascends to the peak expiratory flow (highest point on curve), then descends with decreasing volume, following a reproducible shape that is independent of effort. In this normal flow–volume curve, the forced vital capacity (FVC), forced expiratory volume in 1 second (FEV$_1$), and FEV$_1$/FVC ratio are all within the normal range for this child's age, height, gender, and race. The shapes of both the inspiratory and expiratory limbs are normal as well. *Pre*, prebronchodilator; *Pred*, predicted value.

TABLE 13.2 | Characteristics of Obstructive and Restrictive Patterns of Lung Disease

	DISEASE CATEGORY	
Measurement	Obstructive	Restrictive
FVC	Normal/decreased	Decreased
FEV$_1$	Decreased	Decreased
FEV/FVC	Decreased	Normal

FEV$_1$, forced expiratory volume in 1 second; *FVC*, forced vital capacity.

frequently performed test of pulmonary function in children. With a forced exhalation after a maximal inhalation, the total volume exhaled is known as the forced vital capacity (FVC), and the fractional volume exhaled in the first second is known as the forced expiratory volume in 1 second (FEV$_1$). Fig. 13.2 illustrates a normal pulmonary function test (normal flow–volume loop and spirometry parameters).

An obstructive process is characterized by decreased velocity of airflow through the airways (Fig. 13.3), whereas a restrictive defect produces decreased lung volumes (Fig. 13.4). Examination of the ratio of airflow to lung volume assists in differentiating these components of lung disease. Normally, a child should be able to exhale more than 80% of the FVC in the first second. Children with obstructive lung disease have decreased airflow in relation to exhaled volume. If the volume exhaled in the first second divided by the volume of full exhalation (FEV$_1$/FVC) is less than 80%, then airway obstruction is present (Table 13.2; Fig. 13.3).

The FEV$_1$ needs to be interpreted in the context of the FVC. A small FEV$_1$ alone is insufficient evidence on which to make a diagnosis of airflow obstruction. Those with restrictive lung disease have both decreased FEV$_1$ and FVC–decreased flow rate and reduced total exhaled volume. Restrictive lung disease is associated with a loss of lung tissue or a decrease in the lung's ability to expand. A restrictive defect is diagnosed when the FVC is less than 80% of normal with either a normal or an increased FEV$_1$/FVC (see Table 13.2 and Fig. 13.4).

Most children with respiratory problems have an obstructive pattern; isolated restrictive diseases are far less common. Asthma

is the most common obstructive pulmonary disease in children. Rare causes of obstruction include airway lesions, congenital subglottic webs, and vocal cord dysfunction. Restrictive lung disease can arise from limitations to chest wall movement, such as chest wall deformities, scoliosis, or pleural effusions, or from space-occupying intrathoracic pathology such as large bullae or congenital cysts. Alveolar filling defects (e.g., lobar pneumonia) also reduce lung volume and can be considered as restrictive processes. Although the diseases arise from specific isolated genetic disorders, children with cystic fibrosis (CF) and sickle cell disease (SCD) can have highly variable pulmonary pathologic processes with both obstructive and restrictive components of lung disease. Bronchopulmonary dysplasia may also result in both obstructive and restrictive pathology.

Pulmonary function tests can also be used to differentiate fixed from variable airway obstruction and to localize the obstruction as above or below the thoracic inlet (Figs. 13.5 through 13.7, E-Fig. 13.1). This information can be gleaned from distinctive changes in the configuration of the flow–volume loop, a graphic representation of inspiratory and expiratory flow volumes plotted against time. A fixed central airway obstruction, such as a tumor or stenosis, may obstruct both inspiration and expiration, flattening the flow–volume curve on both inspiration and expiration (see Video 14.1). The child with tracheal stenosis, for example, has flattening of both inhalation and exhalation curves (see Fig. 13.6). A variable obstruction tends to affect only one part of the ventilatory cycle. On inhalation, the chest expands and draws the airways open. On exhalation, as the chest collapses, the intrathoracic airways collapse. Variable extrathoracic lesions tend to obstruct on inhalation more than exhalation, whereas variable intrathoracic lesions tend to obstruct more on exhalation. This produces the characteristic flow–volume patterns.

In addition to diagnostic uses, spirometry is used to assess the indication for, and efficacy of, treatment. For example, the obstruction in patients with asthma is usually reversible, either gradually over time without intervention or much more rapidly after treatment with a short-acting bronchodilator. An improvement in FEV$_1$ of 12% and 200 mL in adults or approximately 3 mL/kg is considered a positive response. In addition to confirming the diagnosis of asthma, the degree of airflow obstruction, as indicated by the FEV$_1$, is one measure of asthma control. A low FEV$_1$ or an acute decrease from baseline may indicate a child whose asthma is not under good control and therefore who potentially is at greater risk for a perioperative exacerbation (see Fig. 13.3).

Because it measures the amount of air entering or leaving the lung rather than the amount of air in the lung, spirometry cannot provide data about absolute lung volumes. Information about FRC and lung volumes calculated from FRC, such as total lung capacity and residual volume, must be obtained by different means, such as gas dilution or body plethysmography. Gas dilution is based

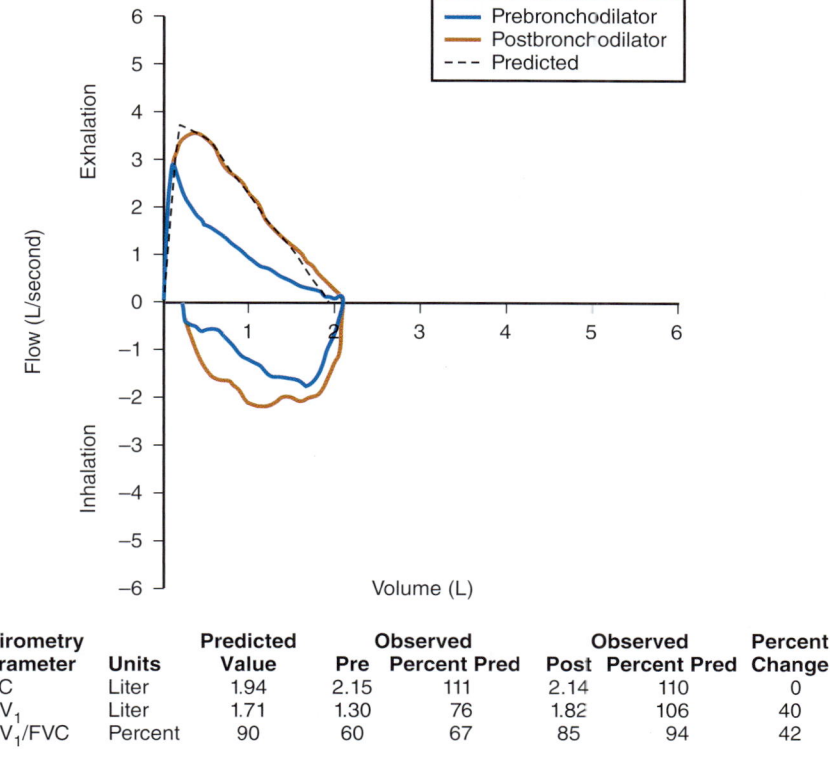

Spirometry Parameter	Units	Predicted Value	Pre	Observed Percent Pred	Post	Observed Percent Pred	Percent Change
FVC	Liter	1.94	2.15	111	2.14	110	0
FEV$_1$	Liter	1.71	1.30	76	1.82	106	40
FEV$_1$/FVC	Percent	90	60	67	85	94	42

FIGURE 13.3 This flow–volume curve demonstrates a reversible obstructive defect. The forced expiratory volume in 1 second (FEV$_1$) as a percentage of forced vital capacity (FVC), or total volume exhaled, is decreased in patients with airway obstruction. The observed curve shape before bronchodilator use *(blue curve)* is scooped. After administration of a short-acting bronchodilator, the observed curve shape *(brown)* appears normal, and there is an increase in both FEV$_1$/FVC and FEV$_1$. This child has asthma and demonstrates a marked (40%) increase in FEV$_1$ after treatment with a short-acting bronchodilator. Reversible airflow obstruction is one of the hallmarks of asthma. *Post,* postbronchodilator; *Pre,* prebronchodilator; *Pred,* predicted value.

on measuring the dilution of nitrogen or helium in a circuit in closed connection to the lungs, whereas body plethysmography calculates lung gas volumes based on changes in thoracic pressures.

Perioperative Etiology and Epidemiology

Respiratory problems account for most of the perioperative morbidity in children[6,7] and cause almost one-third of perioperative pediatric cardiac arrests.[8] Adverse events include laryngospasm, airway obstruction, bronchospasm, hemoglobin oxygen desaturation, prolonged coughing, atelectasis, pneumonia, and respiratory failure.[4,9-11] The incidence of perioperative adverse respiratory events in one study of 755 children was 34%,[9] whereas in another observational study of 9297 children it was 15%.[4] The triggers of these problems included airway manipulation, alteration of airway reflexes by anesthetic drugs, surgical insult, and depression of breathing caused by anesthetic and analgesic medications. Various pulmonary diseases common among children can further affect the frequency of perioperative respiratory complications; one retrospective study identified obesity as an additional risk factor.[11]

Studies have consistently reported greater respiratory morbidity among younger compared with older children.[4,6,7,11-14] In particular, neonates are sensitive to respiratory problems for many reasons. Although the FRC approaches adult capacity (in liters per kilogram) within days after birth, a persistently large closing capacity increases

the likelihood of alveolar collapse and intrapulmonary shunt. Residual patency of the ductus arteriosus can also contribute to shunting. The greater metabolic rate of the infant increases oxygen requirements and decreases the time to arterial desaturation after an interruption to ventilation and gas exchange. The work of breathing is also greater in young infants as a result of high-resistance, small-caliber airways, increased chest wall compliance, and reduced lung parenchymal compliance.

UPPER RESPIRATORY TRACT INFECTION

Upper respiratory tract infections (URIs) are a common problem among young children. Children are typically infected several times a year, possibly even more frequently if they are in day care. Viruses cause the majority of URIs, with rhinoviruses constituting approximately one-third to one-half of etiologic species[15,16]; other common childhood respiratory viruses include adenoviruses and coronaviruses.

Although most URIs are short-lived, self-limited infections and are by definition limited to the upper airway, they may increase airway sensitivity to noxious stimuli or secretions for several weeks after the infection has cleared. The mechanisms probably involve a combination of mucosal invasion, chemical mediators, and altered neurogenic reflexes.[15] URIs may also impair pulmonary function by decreasing FVC, FEV$_1$, peak expiratory flow, and diffusion capacity.[17,18]

Children with a recent or current URI have an increased incidence of perioperative laryngospasm, bronchospasm, arterial hemoglobin desaturation, severe coughing, and breath holding compared with uninfected children (Table 13.3).[4,13,14,19-22] However, most complications can usually be predicted and successfully managed without long-term sequelae by suitably experienced and prepared clinicians.[15,20,22-25] An approach to the child with a URI is to detect the pathologic process and associated comorbidity, establish the acuteness and severity of the URI, and then decide whether to modify the anesthetic technique or postpone surgery (Table 13.4, Fig. 13.8).

The basis for diagnosing a URI is a careful history and physical examination, with further investigations in limited situations. Because they are usually familiar with their child's state of health, the parents or caregivers can provide helpful insight into the presence and severity of a URI. The child should be evaluated for fever (defined as a temperature >100.4°F [38°C]), change in demeanor or behavior, dyspnea, productive cough, purulent sputum production, nasal congestion, rales, rhonchi, and wheezing. A chest radiograph may be considered if the pulmonary examination is questionable, but because the radiographic changes lag behind clinical symptoms, it is typically of limited value. Although laboratory tests may confirm the diagnosis of a viral or bacterial URI, they are not cost-effective or practical in a busy surgical setting.

For children with symptoms of an uncomplicated URI who are afebrile with clear secretions and who are otherwise healthy, anesthesia may proceed as planned, because the problems encountered are typically transient and easily managed.[4,15,20,22-25] Elective surgery is usually postponed for children with more severe symptoms that include at least one of the following: *mucopurulent secretions*; *lower respiratory tract signs* (e.g., wheezing) that do not clear with a deep cough; *pyrexia* >100.4°F (38°C); or a *change in sensorium* (e.g., not behaving or playing normally, has not been eating properly).[15,25]

The decision to proceed with surgery becomes much more difficult when the signs of the URI are between the extremes of mild and severe. For these intermediate URIs, other considerations play a greater role in assessing the risk/benefit ratio. These include the presence of comorbidities such as asthma, cardiac disease, or obstructive sleep apnea; a history of prematurity; the frequency of URIs; prior cancellations; the type, complexity, duration, and urgency of the surgery; the age of the child; and the socioeconomic implications for the family. The comfort level and experience of the anesthesiologist may also be an underestimated but important factor in the decision to proceed with or postpone surgery, because less experienced anesthesiologists have a greater incidence of complications.[4] The need to admit a child postoperatively because of anesthetic complications or an exacerbation of the URI may expose other children to a contagious illness.

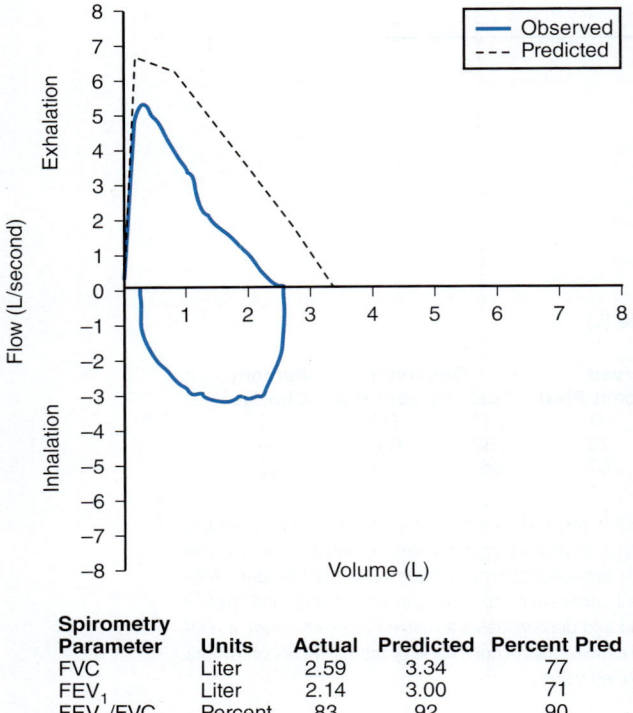

Spirometry Parameter	Units	Actual	Predicted	Percent Pred
FVC	Liter	2.59	3.34	77
FEV_1	Liter	2.14	3.00	71
FEV_1/FVC	Percent	83	92	90

FIGURE 13.4 Flow–volume curve demonstrating a restrictive defect. The flow–volume curves in children with restrictive defects are near-normal in configuration but smaller in all dimensions. The ratio of forced expiratory volume in 1 second (FEV_1) to forced vital capacity (FVC) is normal, but both FEV_1 and FVC are reduced. The curve shape appears normal. This child has interstitial lung disease. *Pred*, predicted value.

| TABLE 13.3 | Incidence of Common Upper Respiratory Tract Infection—Associated Perioperative Adverse Events |

Study	LARYNGOSPASM (%) URI	LARYNGOSPASM (%) No URI	BRONCHOSPASM (%) URI	BRONCHOSPASM (%) No URI	HEMOGLOBIN DESATURATION (%) URI	HEMOGLOBIN DESATURATION (%) No URI
Tait and Knight, 1987[134]	1.3	1.2				
DeSoto et al., 1988[135]					(<95%) 20.0	0[a]
Cohen et al., 1990[12]	2.2	1.7				
Levy et al., 1992[136]					(<93%) 63.6	59.0
Rolf and Coté, 1992[22]	5.9	3.3	13.3	0.6[a]	(<85%) 13.3	10.5
Tait et al., 1998[137]	7.3		12.2		(<90%) 17.1	
Tait et al., 2001[20]	4.2	3.9	5.7	3.3	(<90%) 15.7	7.8[a]
von Ungern-Sternberg et al., 2007.[14]	7.6	3.1[a]		0.9[a]	19.3	11.4[a]

[a]$P < 0.05$ versus corresponding URI group.
URI, upper respiratory tract infection.
Data in parentheses under hemoglobin desaturation are the limits for desaturation in each study.
Modified from Tait AR. Anesthetic management of the child with an upper respiratory tract infection. *Curr Opin Anaesthesiol.* 2005;18:603–607.

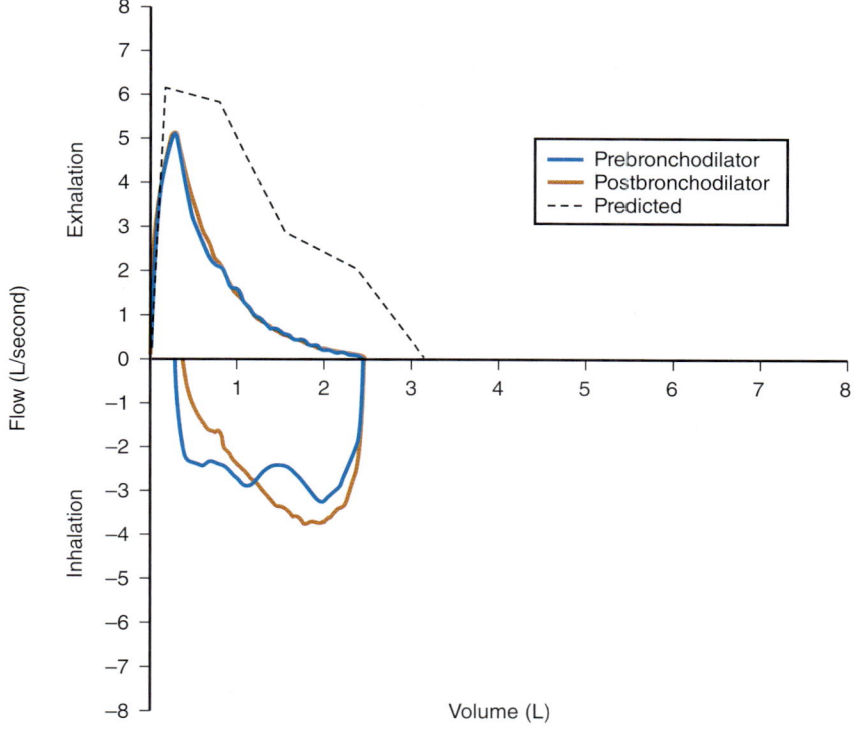

Spirometry Parameter	Units	Predicted Value	Pre	Observed Percent Pred	Post	Observed Percent Pred	Percent Change
FVC	Liter	3.16	2.50	79	2.45	78	−2
FEV₁	Liter	2.82	1.56	55	1.56	55	0
FEV₁/FVC	Percent	91	62	68	64	70	3

FIGURE 13.5 Pulmonary function test demonstrating a nonreversible obstructive defect. The ratio of forced expiratory volume in 1 second *(FEV₁)* to forced vital capacity *(FVC)* is decreased, as is the FEV₁. After administration of a short-acting bronchodilator, there is no significant improvement in the FEV₁, in contrast to the pattern in Fig. 13.3. This child has cystic fibrosis with a nonreversible obstructive defect. *Post,* postbronchodilator; *Pre,* prebronchodilator; *Pred,* predicted value.

If the decision is to proceed with general anesthesia, management is directed toward avoiding stimulation of the potentially sensitized airway. Use of an endotracheal tube (ETT) should be avoided, when possible, because it increases the risk of complications, especially in younger children.[4,20] Although managing the airway with a face mask holds the smallest frequency of airway complications,[4] it may be inappropriate for certain cases. The laryngeal mask airway (LMA) is associated with fewer episodes of respiratory events than the ETT, but its use may similarly be contraindicated by the type of surgical procedure and the need to protect the airway from pulmonary aspiration of gastric contents.

Whichever airway technique is chosen, it is essential that the depth of anesthesia be adequate to obtund airway reflexes during placement of an airway device. The optimal depth of anesthesia at which to remove an airway device is less clearly defined. The frequency of emergence complications after awake and deep extubation appears to be similar in children with and without an URI.[4,14,20,26] In contrast the incidence of arterial oxygen desaturation and coughing after removal of the ETT or LMA in awake children was greater.[27,28]

The optimal time when an anesthetic can be given to a child after a URI without increasing the risk of adverse respiratory events remains contentious, but most clinicians wait 2 to 4 weeks after resolution of the URI before proceeding.[4,14,29] This reflects a balance of three critical factors: the time interval to diminish both upper and lower airway hyperreactivity; the perioperative respiratory risk, which includes a recurrence of the URI; and the need to perform the procedure.

The incidence of laryngospasm after maintenance of anesthesia with propofol was significantly less than with sevoflurane in an observation study of more than 9000 children.[4] One might attribute this finding to a differential effect of propofol versus sevoflurane on airway reflexes.[30] The effects of spraying the vocal cords with lidocaine on the incidence of laryngospasm and bronchospasm are unclear.[4] However, after applying topical lidocaine gel lubricant to the LMA in children with URIs, the frequency of adverse airway events was significantly less than without lidocaine lubricant.[31] Prophylactic treatment with glycopyrrolate, ipratropium, or albuterol does not affect the incidence of URI-related adverse events,[32,33] although one observational study reported that prophylactic salbutamol reduced perioperative airway sequelae in children with URIs.[34] Nasal vasoconstrictors (such as phenylephrine or oxymetazoline nose drops) have been recommended for reducing oropharyngeal secretions in children with URIs, but their efficacy remains anecdotal.[25]

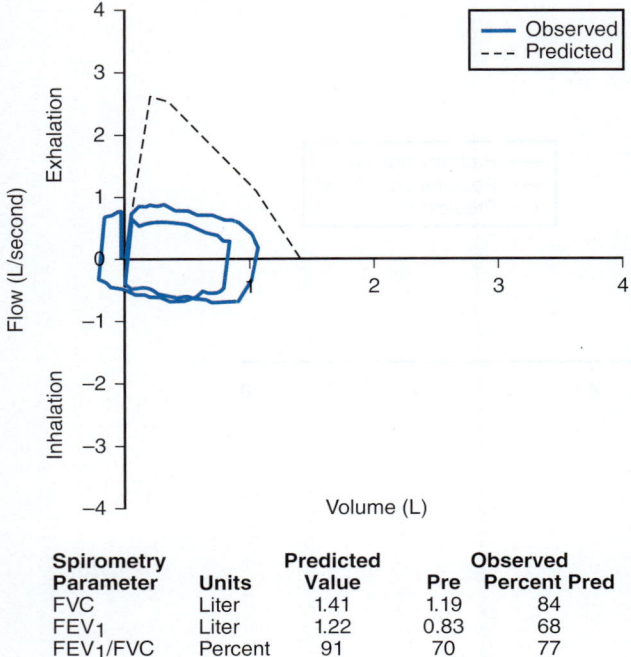

Spirometry Parameter	Units	Predicted Value	Pre	Observed Percent Pred
FVC	Liter	1.41	1.19	84
FEV$_1$	Liter	1.22	0.83	68
FEV$_1$/FVC	Percent	91	70	77

FIGURE 13.6 Pulmonary function test showing an extrathoracic airway obstruction; both the inspiratory and expiratory limbs of the flow–volume curve are flattened. This child has subglottic stenosis that developed at the site of her tracheotomy 2 years after the tracheostomy was removed. *FEV$_1$,* forced expiratory volume in 1 second; *FVC,* forced vital capacity; *Pred,* predicted value.

LOWER AIRWAY DISEASE

Acute lower respiratory tract infections in infants and children may result in rapid deterioration necessitating aggressive intervention, including tracheal intubation and ICU admission. Many children are treated with antibiotics on the presumption that the infection is bacterial. However, many may be affected by viruses. In infants and children up to 18 months of age, respiratory syncytial virus is a very serious and common viral infection that infects the lower respiratory tract.[35] Other viruses that also infect the lower respiratory tract include parainfluenza virus, adenovirus, and human metapneumovirus.[36] Acute inflammation of the small airways may result in bronchiolitis with edema of the small airways leading to desaturation, hypercapnia, and acute respiratory failure. Bronchiolitis management can involve several days of continuous positive airway pressure (CPAP), high-flow nasal prongs, or tracheal intubation until the acute infection has resolved.

Croup or laryngotracheobronchitis, defined as acute inflammation of the airway (below the vocal cords), has been attributed primarily to parainfluenza virus as well as to adenovirus.

Asthma is one of the most common chronic diseases of childhood, affecting an estimated more than 6 million children in the United States.[37,38] A history of wheezing is associated with an increased risk of perioperative bronchospasm.[4] Rare perioperative complications associated with asthma include anaphylaxis, adrenal crisis, and ventilatory barotrauma such as pneumothorax or pneumomediastinum.[39] An anesthetic approach to children with asthma should include a basic understanding of the disease, an assessment of the child's current state of health, modification of anesthetic technique as appropriate, and recognition and treatment of complications if they occur.

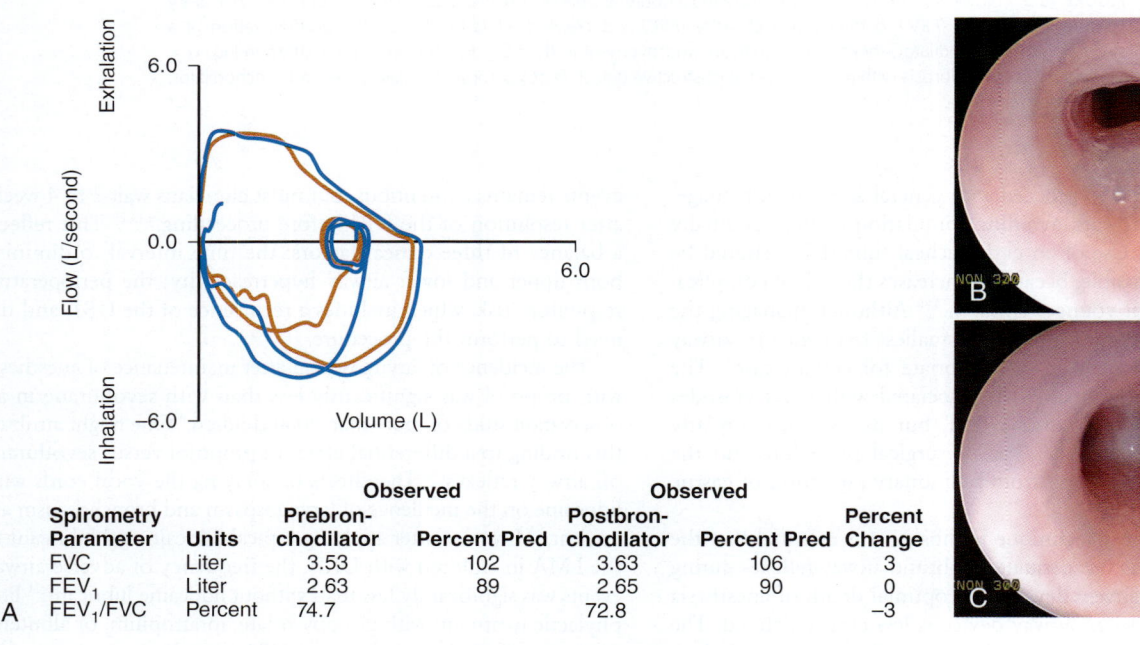

Spirometry Parameter	Units	Observed Prebron-chodilator	Percent Pred	Observed Postbron-chodilator	Percent Pred	Percent Change
FVC	Liter	3.53	102	3.63	106	3
FEV$_1$	Liter	2.63	89	2.65	90	0
FEV$_1$/FVC	Percent	74.7		72.8		−3

FIGURE 13.7 A, Pulmonary function test from a child with an intrathoracic airway obstruction (vascular ring). The flow–volume curves suggest a fixed expiratory obstruction. The shape of the inspiratory link is normal; the expiratory flow limb is flattened on both the prebronchodilator *(brown)* and postbronchodilator *(blue)* flow–volume curves. **B,** Slit-like tracheal compression before repair. **C,** Marked improvement in the tracheal lumen after division of the vascular ring. (See E-Fig. 13.1 for a magnetic resonance imaging angiogram of a vascular ring.) *FEV$_1$,* Forced expiratory volume in 1 second; *FVC,* forced vital capacity; *Pred,* predicted value. (Photographs **B** and **C** courtesy Christopher Hartnick, MD.)

TABLE 13.4	Risk Factors for Perioperative Adverse Events in Children With Upper Respiratory Tract Infections		
Study	URI Status	Factors	RR/OR
Parnis et al., 2001[19]	URI and no URI	ETT	
		Child has a "cold"	
		Child snores	
		Passive smoker	
		Anesthetic agent	
		Sputum production	
		Anticholinesterase given	
		Nasal congestion	
Tait et al., 2001[20]	URI	Copious secretions	3.9 RR
		ETT in child <5 years	1.9
		Prematurity (<37 weeks)	2.3
		Nasal congestion	1.4
		Passive smoker	1.6
		Reactive airway disease	1.8
		Surgery of airway	1.8
Bordet et al., 2002[13]	URI and no URI	Age <8 years	1.8 OR
		LMA	2.3
		Respiratory infections	3.7
Mamie et al., 2004[9]	No URI	Nonpediatric anesthesiologist	1.7 OR
		ENT procedure	1.8
		ETT without relaxants	1.2
von Ungern-Sternberg et al., 2010[4]	URI and no URI	Positive respiratory history	3.05–8.46 RR
		Symptomatic URI	2.05
		URI within previous 2 weeks	2.34
		Family history of asthma, atopy, or smoking	
		Anesthetic agent	
		Nonpediatric anesthesiologist	

ENT, ear, nose and throat; *ETT*, endotracheal tube; *LMA*, laryngeal mask airway; *OR*, odds ratio; *RR*, relative risk; *URI*, upper respiratory tract infection.
Modified from Tait AR. Anesthetic management of the child with an upper respiratory tract infection. *Curr Opin Anaesthesiol.* 2005;18:603–607.

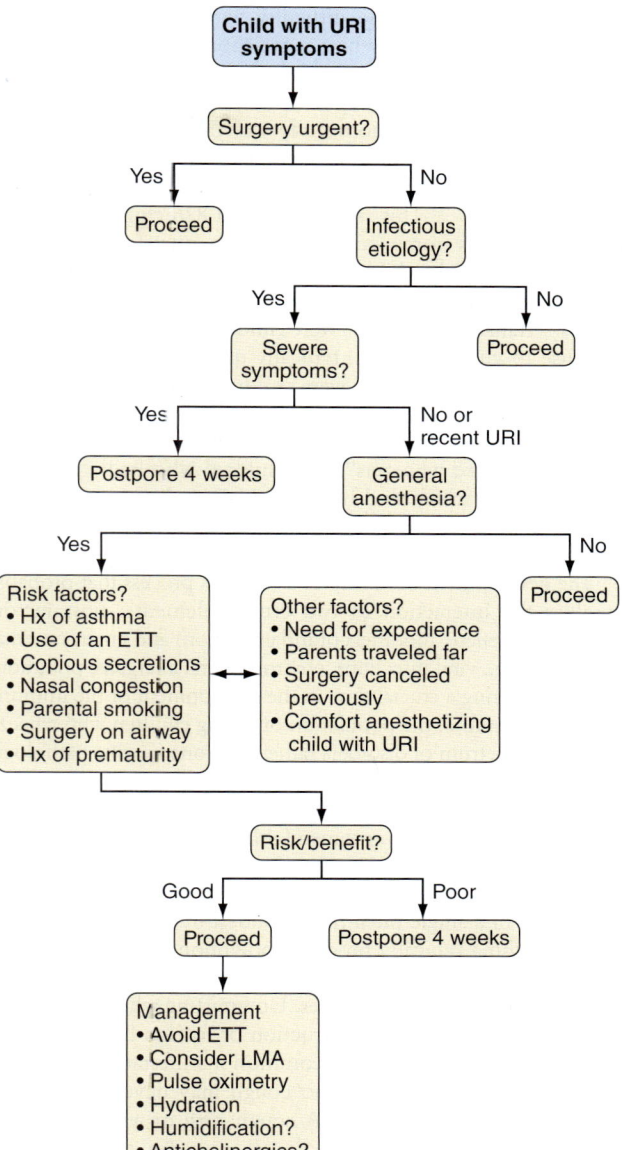

FIGURE 13.8 Suggested algorithm for assessment and management of the child with an upper respiratory tract infection (URI). *ETT*, endotracheal tube; *Hx*, history; *LMA*, laryngeal mask airway. (Modified from Tait AR, Malviya S. Anesthesia for the child with an upper respiratory tract infection: still a dilemma? *Anesth Analg.* 2005;100:59–65.)

It is difficult to define asthma with precision because the exact pathophysiology remains unclear. The word *asthma* derives from the Greek *aazein*, which means "to breathe with open mouth or to pant."[40] A working definition of asthma is a common chronic disorder of the airways that is complex and characterized by variable and recurring symptoms, airway obstruction, inflammation, and hyperresponsiveness of the airways.[37]

Clinical expressions of asthma include wheezing, chest tightness or discomfort, persistent dry cough, and dyspnea on exertion. Severe respiratory distress can occur during acute exacerbations and may be characterized by chest wall retraction, use of accessory muscles, prolonged expiration, pneumothorax, and progression

to respiratory failure and death. In some children the development of chronic inflammation may be associated with permanent airway changes, referred to as *airway remodeling*, that are not prevented by or fully responsive to current available treatments. There is a strong association between asthma and atopy, or immunoglobulin E (IgE)-mediated hypersensitivity.[37]

The diagnosis of asthma can be challenging because cough, wheezing, and bronchospasm may arise from many disease processes. Asthma itself is unlikely to be a single disease entity, and the disease process is markedly modified by various genetic and environmental factors.[37,40] Many young children wheeze, and there is no definitive confirmatory blood, histologic, or radiographic diagnostic test. Given the difficulty with diagnosis, the label "preschool wheezers" may be a more appropriate description for young children with reversible airway obstruction than a diagnosis of "asthma."[40]

The Tucson birth cohort study was the largest longitudinal study in the United States to attempt to differentiate wheezing or asthma phenotypes in children who did not subsequently develop asthma.[41-43] This study examined 826 children at ages 3 years and 6 years from a cohort of 1246 neonates. By the age of 6 years, 48.5% of the children had experienced at least one documented episode of wheezing and were categorized into three groups. "Transient wheezers" were children who wheezed only in response to viral infections, typically during the first 3 years of life. "Non-atopic wheezers" were children who wheezed beyond the first few years of life, often in response to viral infections, but who were less likely to persistently wheeze in later childhood. "Atopy-associated wheezers" were children who had a reversible wheeze together with a tendency toward IgE-mediated hypersensitivity; they had the greatest risk of persistent symptoms into late childhood and adulthood.[41]

The development of asthma is a complex process that probably involves the interaction of two crucial elements: host factors (specifically genetic modifiers of inflammation) and environmental exposures (e.g., viral infections, environmental allergens, pollution) that occur during a crucial time in the development of the immune system.[37] Therefore, the population of young children who wheeze includes a spectrum of disorders rather than one specific pathologic process.

Asthma must be differentiated from other distinct causes that produce similar symptoms (Table 13.5). Tracheomalacia or bronchomalacia may produce wheezing, but this tends to be present from birth (which is unusual for asthma), and the wheezing is commonly of a single pitch heard loudest in the central airways, whereas asthma typically produces polyphonic sounds from the lung periphery. Breathing difficulties owing to chronic aspiration are often related to feeding times. Unremitting wheeze or stridor is often caused by a fixed obstruction or foreign body.

Chronic cough is the most common manifestation of asthma in children. Many children who cough may never be heard to wheeze but still have asthma. A cough with or without wheeze may be caused by a viral infection, whereas a persistent, productive cough may suggest suppurative lung disease such as CF.[39] A positive response of the cough to asthma medications suggests the diagnosis of asthma.

The exact incidence of perioperative complications in the pediatric asthma population is difficult to ascertain because of variations in the definition of asthma, the definition and detection of complications, the presence of coexisting diseases, overlap with adult populations, and changing anesthetic management techniques.

A retrospective review of 706 adult and pediatric patients with a rigorous definition of asthma reported an incidence of documented bronchospasm in the perioperative period of 1.7% and no instances of pneumonia, pneumothorax, or death.[44] Of 211 children younger than 12 years of age, none developed bronchospasm at the time of surgery. A retrospective review of more than 136,000 computer-based anesthesia records found a 0.8% incidence of bronchospasm in patients with asthma.[45] By contrast, older studies from the 1960s reported that 7% to 8% of asthmatic patients wheezed.[46,47] A blinded, prospective study of 59 asthmatic patients detected transient wheezing after tracheal intubation in 25% of cases; however, most events were brief and self-limited.[48] An observational study of 9297 children reported an overall incidence of 2% for bronchospasm; in the subgroup of 2256 children with a history of respiratory problems, the incidence was 6%.[4,39] An editorial review of the subject of asthma and anesthesia concluded that, although the true incidence of major complications is small, severe adverse outcomes do result from bronchospasm, and children with asthma are at heightened risk for severe morbidity.[49]

Both the severity and the control of asthma must be established preoperatively. These two aspects of the current disease state should be clearly differentiated.[50] For example, asthma may be severe yet well controlled, whereas even mild asthma may be poorly controlled. Both situations may present a heightened potential for perioperative complications, because even the child with intermittent but poorly controlled asthma can have a severe exacerbation.

Severity and control of asthma may be assessed by the frequency of symptoms, limitation of effort tolerance, night awakenings, medication use, emergency department attendance, hospitalizations, and need for ventilatory support. An approach to assessment of severity and control in children aged 5 to 11 years is outlined in E-Tables 13.1 through 13.3. A history of a nocturnal dry cough, more than three wheezing episodes in the past 12 months, or a history of past or present eczema is associated with an increased risk of bronchospasm.[4]

Maintenance treatment of asthma is based on a stepwise approach, so that the type of therapy is often an indication of severity. Short-acting inhaled β-agonists are first-line therapy, with inhaled corticosteroids for those patients with persistent symptoms poorly managed by bronchodilators as the preferred second step. Alternative treatments at this step include a leukotriene receptor antagonist, a mast cell stabilizer such as cromolyn sodium or nedocromil, and a methylxanthine bronchodilator such as theophylline. The third step in therapy involves increasing the dose of inhaled corticosteroid or adding an alternative treatment to a smaller dose of corticosteroid; a long-acting β-agonist, a leukotriene receptor antagonist, or theophylline may be considered. Step 4 involves a medium dose of corticosteroid together with a long-acting β-agonist. The final steps of therapy involve a high dose of inhaled corticosteroid or commencing an oral corticosteroid (E-Fig. 13.2). Recently biologics directed at the basic pathophysiology of asthma offer the hope of personalized medicine.[51] Such medicines include

TABLE 13.5	Causes of Wheezing in Children
Acute	
Bronchiolitis	Pneumothorax
Asthma	Endobronchial intubation
Foreign body	Herniated ETT cuff
Inhalation injury	Aspiration
	Anaphylaxis
Recurrent or Persistent	
Bronchiolitis	Mediastinal mass
Asthma	Tracheomalacia/bronchomalacia
Foreign body	Vascular ring
Bronchopulmonary dysplasia	
Cardiac failure	Tracheal web/stenosis
Cystic fibrosis	Bronchial stenosis
Recurrent aspiration	Roundworm infestation
Sickle cell disease	

ETT, endotracheal tube.

omalizumab which is directed against IgE and mepolizumab and reslizumab directed against interleukin 5.

Most children with asthma have disease that is intermittent or persistent but mild and will be treated with inhaled short-acting β-agonists on an as-needed basis, alone or in combination with low-dose inhaled corticosteroids or an adjunctive therapy. Poor control may relate to poor compliance with medication, inadequate inhaler technique, or incorrect diagnosis. Severe asthma is diagnosed when symptom control is poor despite high doses of corticosteroids (see steps 5 or 6 in E-Fig. 13.2). A small group of children have "brittle asthma" that is difficult to control despite optimal therapy and may lead to life-threatening respiratory compromise. A history of severe attacks or admission to intensive care is particularly ominous.

Special investigations are not routinely indicated but may be useful in specific circumstances. A chest radiograph is not usually helpful to assess the severity of asthma but can help diagnose a superimposed infection, pneumothorax, or pneumomediastinum during an acute exacerbation. Pulmonary function tests are important in monitoring long-term responses to therapy but are of little use in the immediate, routine preoperative workup of cases at a stable clinical baseline. Measurements of nitric oxide and various inflammatory markers are primarily of use as research tools at present, but their role in asthma management is evolving.[52]

Although an assessment of disease severity is essential, an important caveat is that many asthma deaths in the community setting occur not in those with severe disease but in those with what was thought to be mild or moderate disease. Asthma is often undertreated,[53] so the sensitivity of medication prescription as a marker of disease activity must be viewed with some caution. Some studies have found a poor correlation between assessment of disease severity and the occurrence of perioperative broncho-spasm. However, disease *activity*, as noted by recent asthma symptoms, use of medications for symptom treatment, and recent therapy in a medical facility for asthma, is significantly associated with perioperative bronchospasm.[44]

Children should continue their regular medications before anesthesia. Midazolam has been reported to be a safe premedication for asthmatics.[53] Corticosteroids may help prevent postintubation bronchospasm in adults,[54] although controlled clinical data to substantiate this practice in children are lacking.[39] Inhaled β-agonists before or shortly after induction of anesthesia attenuate the increases in airway resistance associated with tracheal intubation.[55,56] Ketamine is the traditional choice of intravenous (IV) induction agent in children with severe asthma, although its superiority over other agents has not been substantiated in clinical trials.[57,58] Propofol

is typically preferred over thiopentone because it causes less bronchoconstriction.[48,59] Desflurane is associated with an increased risk of bronchospasm compared with sevoflurane or isoflurane, and because it can increase airway resistance in children, should be avoided in asthmatics.[4]

Tracheal stimulation is a potent stimulus for bronchospasm.[4] In children with a URI, in whom the airways may be acutely hyperactive, the avoidance of tracheal intubation is associated with a reduced incidence of pulmonary complications.[4,19] There are inadequate clinical outcome data on the perioperative manage-ment of asthma to make definitive recommendations about airway management. Nevertheless, avoidance of tracheal and vocal cord stimulation by use of a face mask or an LMA instead of an ETT whenever possible seems a sensible approach. If tracheal intubation is mandatory, a deep plane of anesthesia is preferred to blunt airway hyperreactivity. Similarly, unless contraindicated by other factors, deep extubation is preferred for the same reason. Surgical stimulation is another trigger of bronchospasm, and anesthetic depth and analgesia should be adequate to prevent this response.

Intraoperative bronchospasm is characterized variously by polyphonic expiratory wheeze, prolonged expiration, active expira-tion with increased respiratory effort, increased airway pressures, a slow upslope on the end-tidal CO_2 monitor waveform (Fig. 13.9), increased end-tidal CO_2, and hypoxemia. Other causes of wheezing must be excluded, such as partial obstruction of the ETT (secretions or herniation of the cuff causing obstruction), main-stem intubation (deep endobronchial intubation), aspiration, pneumothorax, or pulmonary edema. Mechanical obstruction of the circuit or ETT must also be excluded.

First-line treatment for bronchospasm involves removing the triggering stimulus if possible, deepening anesthesia, increasing the fraction of inspired oxygen (FIO_2) if appropriate, decreasing the positive end-expiratory pressure (PEEP), and increasing the expiratory time to minimize alveolar air trapping. In severe status asthmaticus, ventilation strategy focuses primarily on achieving adequate oxygenation, rather than attempting to normalize $PaCO_2$ at the potential cost of inducing pulmonary barotrauma. All children who experience anything more than minor bronchospasm should also receive corticosteroids, if they have not already done so.

Inhaled β-agonists can be delivered by nebulizer or by a metered-dose inhaler down the airway device with specially designed adaptors (Fig. 13.10). Alternatively, a 60-mL syringe can be used to deliver doses of the nebulizer into the breathing circuit (E-Fig. 13.3). However, the efficiency of delivery through an inhaler that is actuated at the elbow of the breathing circuit is poor, especially in small-diameter ETTs.[60] To improve the delivery efficiency of

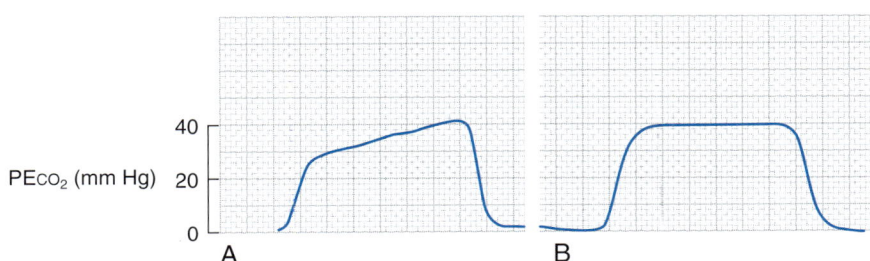

FIGURE 13.9 A, Tracing of expired carbon dioxide ($PECO_2$) in a child with acute bronchospasm. Notice the slowly rising $PECO_2$ value. **B,** Tracing from the same patient after administration of inhaled albuterol. Note that the $PECO_2$ waveform now has a flat plateau, indicating relief of the bronchospasm and efficient elimination of CO_2 from all areas of the lungs.

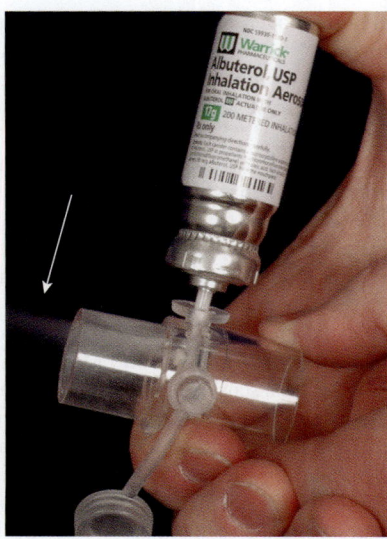

FIGURE 13.10 Adaptor that allows administration of albuterol through an endotracheal tube (ETT) and timing of that dose with inspirations to provide maximum delivery; notice that the nebulized albuterol is directed down the ETT (arrow). Use of a long intravenous catheter that extends to the tip of the ETT is an alternative method to further improve drug delivery.

the aerosol in pediatric-size ETTs, the inhaler may be actuated 10 to 20 times at the elbow or once or twice into a narrow-gauge catheter that is passed to the end of the ETT.[60,61]

If IV salbutamol (albuterol) is available, the IV route is preferred over tracheal administration. Onset of bronchodilation in a child with acute symptoms should be rapid with good effect at a plasma salbutamol concentration of 1 µg/L.[62] Salbutamol (10 µg/kg IV) may be repeated, followed by an infusion of 5 to 10 µg/kg per minute for the first hour until there is an improvement in the bronchospasm. Thereafter, salbutamol should be infused at 1 to 2 µg/kg per minute until the bronchospasm resolves. Epinephrine (0.05-0.5 µg/kg per minute) is also an effective bronchodilator.

The anesthesiologist may be involved in the management of status asthmaticus when consulted to assist a child in the emergency department or on the wards. A drowsy, silent child with a quiet chest on auscultation despite therapy is in imminent danger of respiratory arrest and requires emergent tracheal intubation by an experienced practitioner. Signs and symptoms to assess the severity of an asthma exacerbation are outlined in Table 13.6, and an algorithm for management issued by the American National Heart, Lung and Blood Institute is presented in E-Fig. 13.4.

Oxygen is recommended for most children to maintain the oxygen saturation at greater than 90%. Repetitive or continuous administration of short-acting β-agonists is first-line therapy for all children and is the most effective way of reversing airflow obstruction. The addition of ipratropium to a β-agonist may produce additional bronchodilation and may have a modest effect to improve outcome. Systemic corticosteroids should be given to those who do not respond completely and promptly to β-agonists. For severe exacerbations unresponsive to the treatment listed earlier, IV magnesium may decrease the likelihood of intubation, although the evidence is limited. Current recommended drug doses are listed in E-Table 13.4.

There is much debate about the role of methylxanthines such as aminophylline in the management of acute exacerbations of asthma. In some countries, aminophylline is considered a first-line treatment for asthma, whereas in others it is considered second-line or used less frequently. The difference in practice may be attributed to its equivocal clinical efficacy in the treatment of acute exacerbations of asthma and to complications from toxicity (including vomiting).[63-66]

Antibiotics are not recommended except for comorbid conditions. Aggressive hydration is not recommended in adults or older children, although it may be indicated in younger children who become dehydrated as a result of decreased oral intake and increased respiratory rate. In general, chest physical therapy and mucolytics are also not recommended.

Children with severe atopy-associated asthma are possibly at greater risk for developing anaphylaxis in response to neuromuscular blocking drugs, antibiotics, and latex.[39] Bronchospasm caused by anaphylaxis is differentiated from that due to asthma; it produces additional systemic signs such as angioedema, flushing, urticaria, and cardiovascular collapse.

Adrenal crisis during major surgical stress is a potential complication associated with severe asthma caused by iatrogenic suppression of the hypothalamic-pituitary-adrenal axis.[39] Adrenal suppression should be considered in any child who is taking significant doses of corticosteroids for a prolonged period. Short courses of prednisolone used to treat acute flares of asthma may affect function for up to 10 days, but prolonged dysfunction is unlikely. Large doses, prolonged therapy for more than a few weeks, and evening dosing may suppress adrenal function for up to 1 year. Prophylactic corticosteroid administration may be indicated for those receiving prolonged systemic corticosteroids, when their corticosteroid regimen is interrupted by the surgical schedule, or for those who have received high-dose inhaled corticosteroids in the recent past (see Chapter 27).

CYSTIC FIBROSIS

CF is an autosomal recessive disorder that is caused by one of more than 1500 mutations in the gene coding for the CF transmembrane conductance regulator (located on chromosome 7), a protein that regulates chloride and other ion fluxes at various epithelial surfaces.[67,68] The different gene defects may variously impact the protein's translation, cellular processing, or function as a chloride channel gating. The incidence of CF is approximately 1 of every 2000 births in Caucasians, making it the most common fatal inherited disease in this population.

The disruption of electrolyte transport in the epithelial cells of the sweat ducts, airways, pancreatic ducts, intestine, biliary tree, and vas deferens causes increased sweat chloride concentrations, viscous mucus production, lung disease, intestinal obstruction, pancreatic insufficiency, biliary cirrhosis, and congenital absence of the vas deferens. The clinical outcome is widely variable, even among children with identical mutations at the CF locus. Absence of the gene influences expression of several other gene products, including proteins important to the inflammatory response, ion maturational processing, transport, and cell signaling. These other proteins are potential modifiers of the phenotype and may help explain the substantial differences in clinical severity.

Lung disease is the main cause of morbidity and mortality in CF, and consequently it is the focus of anesthetic concern. The pathophysiology involves mucus plugging, chronic infection, inflammation, and epithelial injury.[69-71] Mucus clearance defends the lung against inhaled bacteria. The mucociliary transport system requires two fully functioning layers to be effective. The base layer of ciliary epithelia bathed in a watery liquid (sol) is overlaid by a more viscous gel (mucus) that is responsible for transporting

TABLE 13.6 | Formal Evaluation of Asthma Exacerbation Severity

	Mild	Moderate	Severe	Subset: Respiratory Arrest Imminent
Symptoms				
Breathlessness	While walking Can lie down	While at rest (infant—softer, shorter cry, difficulty feeding) Prefers sitting	While at rest (infant—stops feeding) Sits upright	
Talks in	Sentences	Phrases	Words	
Alertness	May be agitated	Usually agitated	Usually agitated	Drowsy or confused
Signs				
Respiratory rate[a]	Increased	Increased	Increased	
Use of accessory muscles; suprasternal retractions	Usually not	Commonly	Usually	Paradoxical thoracoabdominal movement
Wheeze	Moderate, often only end expiratory	Loud; throughout exhalation	Usually loud; throughout inhalation and exhalation	Absence of wheeze
Pulse/minute[b]	Slightly increased	Increased	Tachycardia	Bradycardia
Pulsus paradoxus	Absent <10 mm Hg	May be present 10–25 mm Hg	Often present >25 mm Hg (adult) 20–40 mm Hg (child)	Absence suggests respiratory muscle fatigue
Functional Assessment[c]				
PEF (% of predicted or of personal best)	≥70%	Approx. 40%–69% or response lasts <2 hours	<40%	<25% (PEF testing may not be needed in very severe attacks)
Pao_2 (while breathing room air)	Normal (test not usually necessary)	≥60 mm Hg (test not usually necessary)	<60 mm Hg: possible cyanosis	
Pco_2	<42 mm Hg (test not usually necessary)	<42 mm Hg (test not usually necessary)	>42 mm Hg: possible respiratory failure (see text)	
Sao_2% (while breathing room air) at sea level	>95% (test not usually necessary)	90%–95% (test not usually necessary)	<90%	

[a]Guide to rates of breathing in awake children: at age <2 months, normal rate is <60 breaths/minute; at 2–12 months, <50/minute; at 1–5 years, <40/minute; at 6–8 years, <30/minute.
[b]Guide to normal pulse rates in children: at age 2–12 months, normal rate is <160 beats/minute; at 1–2 years, <120/minute; at 2–8 years, <110/minute.
[c]Pao_2 or Pco_2 or both may be tested. Hypercapnia (hypoventilation) develops more readily in young children than in adults and adolescents.
Pao_2, arterial oxygen tension; Pco_2, partial pressure of carbon dioxide; PEF, peak expiratory flow; Sao_2, oxygen saturation.
Modified from National Asthma Education and Prevention Program. Full report of the expert panel: guidelines for the diagnosis and management of asthma (EPR-3). Bethesda, MD: National Heart, Lung, and Blood Institute, National Institutes of Health, 2007.

particles along the tips of the cilia. Normally, mucus is transported at about 10 mm/minute, expelling foreign particles and pathogens from the lungs. The efficacy of clearance depends on adequate hydration of the mucus.[72] Lack of regulation of sodium absorption and chloride secretion decreases liquid on the airway luminal surfaces, slows mucus clearance, and promotes the formation of adherent plugs in the airway.[73] Increased secretions, viscous mucus, and impaired ciliary clearance contribute to airway impaction, providing a nidus for infection.

At birth, the lung structure is almost normal.[67] However, chronic and recurrent bacterial infections occur early in life, assisted by the pooling of secretions and impaired neutrophil bacterial killing on airway surfaces.[69,74] Repeated and persistent infections stimulate a chronic neutrophilic inflammatory response, ultimately destroying the airway walls. Early pathogens include *Staphylococcus aureus* and *Haemophilus influenzae*. *Pseudomonas aeruginosa* typically invade later in life, acquire a mucoid phenotype, and form a biofilm in the lung, an event that is associated with accelerated decline in pulmonary function. The invasion of the lung by antibiotic-resistant pathogens such as certain strains of *Burkholderia cepacia* is often devastating, markedly increasing the death rate from lung disease.

Various insults such as bacteria, viruses, and airborne irritants can cause acute exacerbations of respiratory symptoms of cough and sputum production. This is often accompanied by systemic manifestations such as weight loss, anorexia, and fatigue. These changes from baseline are termed *pulmonary exacerbations*.[75]

Recurrent exacerbations are associated with progressive airway obstruction, bronchiectasis, emphysema, ventilation/perfusion mismatching, and hypoxemia. Growth of blood vessels with advancing bronchiectasis predisposes to hemoptysis. Bronchial hyperreactivity and increased airway resistance are common, whereas bullae formation can lead to pneumothorax.

Pulmonary function abnormalities typically have an obstructive pattern[76] and include increased FRC, decreased FEV_1, decreased peak expiratory flow rate, and decreased vital capacity (see Fig. 13.5). Compensatory hyperventilation typically produces a reduced $PaCO_2$, although hypercapnia may supersede in end-stage pulmonary pathology. End-stage cor pulmonale may lead to cardiomegaly, fluid retention, and hepatomegaly.

Malnutrition is a common problem in CF that follows from pancreatic insufficiency, failure of enzyme secretion, impaired gastrointestinal motility, abnormal enterohepatic circulation of bile, increased caloric demand owing to severe lung disease, and anorexia of chronic disease.[67] Low weight and body mass index are closely associated with, and can predict, poor lung function.

CF-related diabetes arises from progressive pancreatic disease and scarring that compromises the pancreatic islets. More than 12% of teenagers older than 13 years with CF have insulin-dependent diabetes, and the incidence increases with age. Evidence is accumulating that diabetes contributes to the lung disease and worse outcome.[69-71] In addition, classic diabetic complications occur in older CF patients. Hepatic dysfunction decreases plasma cholinesterase and clotting factors II, VII, IX, and X, whereas malabsorption of vitamin K may also contribute to coagulation issues.[77]

When CF was first distinguished from celiac syndrome in 1938, life expectancy was approximately 6 months. Since then, substantial advances in sustained multidisciplinary supportive care have increased the median survival time to 35 years (E-Fig. 13.5).[67,78] Currently almost half of the CF population are adults.[77]

The pillars of treatment include nutritional repletion, relief of airway obstruction, and antibiotic therapy for lung infection. Organ transplantation, and in particular lung transplantation, has been used in an attempt to improve quality of life and prolong survival, but a clear benefit remains to be demonstrated.[78]

Corrector and potentiator therapies are recently developed treatments that are directed at the molecular defects in the CF transmembrane conductance regulator.[79,80] Correctors are principally targeted at cellular misprocessing, while potentiators aim to correct channel's function. Ivacaftor was the first developed drug in this area, and it is a potentiator that targets a number of mutations in cystic fibrosis transmembrane conductance regulator (CFTR) gene, including the G551D mutation.

The multisystem nature of the disease and changing demographics mean that children present for a wide variety of surgical procedures. The most common indications for anesthesia in children are nasal polypectomy and ear, nose, and throat surgery, as a result of the frequency of upper airway pathologic processes such as chronic sinusitis and nasal polyps (Table 13.7).[81,82] The investigation or correction of gastrointestinal disorders is the next most common procedural category that requires anesthesia in the CF population. Other indications for anesthesia include bronchoscopy and pulmonary lavage, gastrointestinal endoscopy, sclerosing injection of varices resulting from portal hypertension, insertion of venous access devices, and incidental surgical problems.[82-84]

Because of the increasing longevity of this population, the pediatric anesthesiologist may also be involved in the care of adults.[77] Surgical procedures in adults typically include treatment of recurrent pneumothorax, cholecystectomy, and lung or cardiac transplantation. Consultation may also be requested for obstetric cases as increasing numbers of patients survive to adulthood.

Pulmonary disease is the predominant concern when planning anesthesia for these patients. Historically, morbidity and mortality from pulmonary complications were significant—for example, in 1964, a retrospective study reported a perioperative mortality rate of 27%,[85] but by 1972, this incidence had decreased to 4%.[81] More recent studies have confirmed low mortality but an appreciable rate of morbidity after general anesthesia for lung lavage; bronchoscopies; and ear, nose, and throat surgery in children with CF. With a combined cohort of 700 children, the frequency of perioperative complications was between 5% and 13%.[82,86-89] In a study of 18 patients with CF undergoing anesthesia for pleural surgery, the risks for this surgery were considered substantial, although the anesthetic hazards of CF could be minimized with careful management.[90] The effects of anesthesia on pulmonary function in children with CF are unclear. In a small study of children undergoing injection of esophageal varices, pulmonary function test results deteriorated 48 hours after general anesthesia.[91] In contrast, in almost 100 children in two studies, no difference in pulmonary function tests measured before compared with after a variety of surgical procedures was observed.[82,92] Although acute pulmonary morbidity may pose challenges, the effects of the anesthetic management techniques on pulmonary function tests are difficult to predict.

An assessment of the severity, current state, and progression of pulmonary disease should guide anesthetic planning. Fitness is a positive predictor of survival,[67] and exercise tolerance is a useful marker of pulmonary function. The quality and quantity of secretions, recent and chronic infections, use and effectiveness of bronchodilators, and number of hospitalizations are also important points to elucidate in the history. Examination of the cardiopulmonary systems should aim to detect compromise of cardiac, pulmonary, and hepatic function. Special investigations are not routinely indicated but may quantify organ dysfunction in end stages of the disease. Arterial blood gas analysis, chest radiography, pulmonary function tests, electrocardiography, echocardiography, and liver function tests may assist the planning of anesthetic technique in selected children.[84]

Children are often emotionally vulnerable, not simply because of the usual preoperative anxieties but because of the psychological consequences of progression of an ultimately fatal disease. A preoperative visit should aim to allay distress; oral benzodiazepines have been successfully used as anxiolytics.[82,89] Prophylactic use of osmotic laxatives may be indicated if opioid-induced ileus is anticipated.[84]

Because desiccation of mucous secretions is a central pulmonary issue in CF, general anesthesia poses specific problems. During spontaneous ventilation under normal conditions, inspired gases are warmed to body temperature and saturated with water vapor, reaching this state at the isothermic saturation point just distal to the carina.[93,94] This ensures that the lower airways are kept moist and warm. The alveolar environment in optimal circumstances has a saturated water vapor pressure of 47.1 mm Hg and an absolute humidity of 43.4 g/m^3 at 98.6°F (37°C).

The inspiration of cold, desiccated anesthetic gases and vapors can impair the warming and humidification of the airways. The use of any airway device (oropharyngeal airway, laryngeal mask, or ETT) bypasses the nasal and oropharyngeal passages and delivers cold, dry gas farther down the airway.[95] This shifts the isothermic saturation point distally, forcing bronchi that normally function in optimal conditions to take part in heat and gas exchange.[94]

TABLE 13.7	Most Frequent Indications for Anesthesia in Cystic Fibrosis	
Neonates	**Children/Teenagers**	**Adults**
Meconium ileus	Nasal polypectomy	Esophageal varices
Meconium peritonitis	Intravenous access	Recurrent pneumothorax
Intestinal atresia	Ear/nose/throat surgery	Cholecystectomy
		Lung (liver) transplantation

Modified from Della Rocca G. Anaesthesia in patients with cystic fibrosis. *Curr Opin Anaesthesiol.* 2002;15:95–101.

These parts of the airway are less adapted to moisture exchange and tend to dehydrate more rapidly, thereby impairing the mucociliary escalator and predisposing to impaction of secretions.[96,97] By directly impairing mucociliary motion as well as blunting the cough response and ventilatory drive, inhalational anesthetics can exacerbate this problem.

It is therefore particularly important to minimize mucus desiccation in the perioperative period. Inhalation of hypertonic saline (7% sodium chloride) accelerates mucus clearance, increases lung function, and improves quality of life[98-100]; this is now typically part of the routine maintenance management of CF. Nebulized saline treatments should continue up to the start of anesthesia and recommence after the procedure. Inhaled gases should be humidified, or an artificial "nose" should be inserted into the circuit to conserve airway moisture and minimize the risk of inspissating secretions. Although removal of pulmonary secretions is considered important in principle, a small prospective trial of intraoperative bronchial wash-out and physical therapy reported an acute increase in airway resistance with no significant long-term benefit in measures of lung function.[101]

At the conclusion of surgery, complete reversal of neuromuscular blockade should be confirmed. Whenever possible, the trachea should be extubated and the child encouraged to breathe spontaneously. A 30- to 40-degree head-up position assists movement of the diaphragm and ventilation. Postoperatively, physiotherapy, airway humidification, carefully titrated analgesics, and early mobilization should enhance clearance of secretions and minimize atelectasis. The use of neuraxial, regional or local anesthesia, as well as nonopioid analgesics, are useful strategies to avoid respiratory depression.[102,103] Ambulatory surgery is optimal, if feasible, because it minimizes disruption to the patient's schedule and decreases exposure to nosocomial infection.

SICKLE CELL DISEASE

SCD is an inherited hemoglobinopathy that results from a point mutation on chromosome 11 (see also Chapter 10). The mutant gene codes for the production of hemoglobin S, a mutant variant of the normal hemoglobin A. This leads to widespread and progressive vascular damage.[104,105] Clinical features of the disease include acute episodes of pain, acute and chronic pulmonary disease, hemorrhagic and occlusive stroke, renal insufficiency, and splenic infarction, with mean life expectancy shortened to just over 3 decades.[106] Perioperative problems and management are covered in more detail in Chapter 10; the discussion here is limited to a brief review of the pulmonary pathology of SCD.

Acute chest syndrome (ACS) is an acute lung injury caused by SCD. Diagnostic criteria include a new pulmonary infiltrate involving at least one lung segment on the radiograph (excluding atelectasis) combined with one or more symptoms or signs of chest pain, pyrexia greater than 101.3°F (38.5°C), tachypnea, wheezing, or cough.[107-109] Precipitants include infection, fat embolism after bone marrow infarction, pulmonary infarction, and surgical procedures.[109-111] Potential risk factors for the development and severity of perioperative ACS may include a history of lung disease, recent clustering of acute pulmonary complications, pregnancy, increased age, and the invasiveness of the surgical procedure.[104] ACS was associated with younger-age patients, reduced body temperature, and greater blood loss in a study of 60 children with SCD undergoing laparoscopic surgery.[112]

The risk of ACS is small (<5%) after minor surgeries such as inguinal hernia repair and distal extremity surgery, whereas it is severalfold greater (10% to 15%) after intraabdominal and major

joint surgery.[111,113,114] Although the overall perioperative mortality from SCD is quite small, <1%,[111,115] ACS can prolong postoperative hospitalization, and cause respiratory failure and death. ACS typically develops about 3 days postoperatively and persists for approximately 8 days, with a 3.3% mortality.[110]

SCD also causes chronic lung damage, known as sickle cell lung disease (SCLD).[116] Because lung function has not yet been assessed longitudinally in a cohort from early childhood to adulthood, the precise pathology of and relationship between the obstructive and restrictive patterns of lung disease is unclear.[117] Children appear to develop a predominantly obstructive pattern,[118] whereas adults develop a more restrictive pulmonary defect.[116,119,120] In the later stages of lung damage, both vital and total lung capacities decrease, gas diffusion is impaired, and pulmonary fibrosis, pulmonary artery hypertension, right-sided cardiomyopathy, and progressive hypoxemia may occur.[116,120] The development of pulmonary artery hypertension, which can precede clinically apparent lung damage, is a particularly ominous sign of disease progression and is associated with a heightened risk of sudden death.[119] Recurrent ACS is an independent risk factor for the development of end-stage SCLD, but subtle evidence of parenchymal and vascular damage commonly precedes clustered episodes of ACS.[116]

Assessment of lung function should include a history of the occurrence, frequency, severity, and known precipitants of ACS and a search for progression of chronic lung damage. A recent chest radiograph can serve as a baseline for comparison if postoperative radiographs are needed and can also delineate lung pathology. Early features of lung damage include decreased distal pulmonary vascularity and diffuse interstitial fibrosis, whereas later stages are characterized by pulmonary fibrosis, pulmonary hypertension, and right ventricular hypertrophy.[116,121] Pulmonary function testing can reveal the need for bronchodilators and the presence of obstructive or restrictive lung disease.

Although the risk of developing ACS in the perioperative period is increased, distinct genotypes, wide variation in disease severity, differing chronic treatment protocols, varied surgical procedures, and logistical complexities have made research into the optimal perioperative management difficult. Well-delivered anesthetic and postoperative care may be the best guarantor of a good outcome.[104,105]

Perioperative management frequently includes red blood cell transfusion in an effort to decrease the risk of perioperative ACS. The Transfusion Alternative Perioperatively in Sickle Cell Disease study prospectively enrolled 67 patients undergoing low- and medium-risk surgery with or without preoperative transfusion.[122] Although limited by early closure of the study, the small sample size, and too few patients enrolled in the low-risk surgery group to allow for subgroup analysis, the prevalence of clinically important events, including ACS, in the nontransfused group exceeded that in the transfused group. The authors concluded that preoperative transfusion may reduce the risk of ACS in patients with a homozygous HbSS genotype.

If preoperative transfusion is performed to attenuate SCD exacerbations, an exchange transfusion aimed at decreasing the concentration of hemoglobin S to 30% is no more effective than simply correcting the anemia to a hematocrit of 30%. However, exchange transfusion is more likely to lead to transfusion-related complications including the development of uncommon antibodies such as Kell and Duffy antibodies.[110] Consequently, if a decision is made to transfuse in the hope of preventing ACS, the target should be a hematocrit of 30% rather than a specific dilution of hemoglobin S.

The risk of ACS after low-risk surgeries or procedures without transfusion appears to be small.[123] A study of patients undergoing magnetic resonance imaging (MRI) with deep sedation reported an incidence of ACS of 1.2% within 1 month of the MRI,[124] whereas nontransfused patients undergoing minor surgery in the Cooperative Study of Sickle Cell Disease had a similar incidence of ACS of 1.4%.[110] A survey of North American pediatric anesthesiologists found that most clinicians do not transfuse children who are at low risk for perioperative complications after minor procedures, whereas a greater number transfuse sicker children undergoing more invasive procedures.[125]

The one group of children with SCD who are at high risk for complications are those who have experienced or are at risk for a stroke. Risk factors for strokes include low hemoglobin, hypertension, and male gender as well as three single-nucleotide polymorphisms.[126,127] Serial transcranial Doppler ultrasound and MRI of the brain have been used to detect pathologic changes in blood flow or subclinical strokes, respectively, and in these children blood transfusion has been effective in reducing subsequent strokes.[128,129] Silent cerebral strokes have been detected in up to 30% of asymptomatic children with SCD.[126] To reduce the risk of stroke, these children have transfusions at regular intervals, based on the results of the serial investigations. However, this approach raises concern about iron overload and other complications associated with repeated blood transfusions. A recent study to limit the number of transfusions in those at risk for a stroke had to be stopped prematurely because two strokes occurred despite serial transcranial Doppler monitoring.[130] Chronic hydroxyurea therapy has also been shown to be effective in reducing the risk of stroke.[131] The perioperative management of children with a history of stroke continues to evolve.

Children with SCD frequently develop postoperative atelectasis. It is unclear whether this relates to an underlying sickle cell lung disease, difficulty with analgesia, other causes, or a combination of factors. Pain management can be difficult in these children. Large doses of opioids can depress ventilation and cause atelectasis.[132] ACS tends to involve the lower segments of the lung,[109] suggesting an association between atelectasis and ACS; incentive spirometry can prevent the development of atelectasis and pulmonary infiltrates.[133] Regional analgesia, supplemental nonopioid analgesics, prophylactic incentive spirometry, early mobilization, and good pulmonary toilet may decrease the incidence of atelectasis and ACS.

Treatment of ACS is focused on supporting gas exchange. Supplemental oxygen, noninvasive ventilatory support such as CPAP, or intubation and mechanical ventilation are indicated by the degree of dysfunction. Bronchodilators, incentive spirometry, and chest physiotherapy may be useful in preventing disease progression. In the presence of a significant ventilation/perfusion mismatch, correction of anemia can improve arterial oxygenation. Erythrocyte transfusion increases oxygen-carrying capacity, decreases fractional peripheral tissue extraction, and increases returning venous oxygen levels. Because the mean arterial oxygen content in the presence of a shunt is significantly affected by the oxygenation of blood returning from nonventilated parts of the lung, increasing venous oxygen levels can improve arterial oxygen content. Although transfusion has not been directly linked to improved outcomes, both exchange and simple transfusions can improve oxygenation.[109]

Summary

Pulmonary complications are a major cause of perioperative morbidity in the pediatric population. Although preexisting pulmonary pathologic processes in children can present significant challenges to anesthetic delivery, a thorough assessment of the problem combined with meticulous anesthetic management allows most children to undergo surgical interventions without long-term adverse sequelae. Consultation with a pediatric pulmonologist is indicated when appropriate for specific problems as outlined in this chapter; a team approach may markedly improve operative and postoperative outcomes.

ANNOTATED REFERENCES

Bishop MJ, Cheney FW. Anesthesia for patients with asthma: low risk but not no risk. *Anesthesiology.* 1996;85:455-456.
A thoughtful editorial on the implications, dangers, and practical implications of asthma.

Davis PB. Cystic fibrosis since 1938. *Am J Respir Crit Care Med.* 2006; 173:475-482.
A succinct discourse on the evolution of management of cystic fibrosis.

Firth PG, Head CA. Sickle cell disease and anesthesia. *Anesthesiology.* 2004;101:766-785.
A comprehensive review of anesthetic management of sickle cell disease.

Howard J, Malfroy M, Llewelyn C, et al. The Transfusion Alternatives Preoperatively in Sickle Cell Disease (TAPS) study: a randomised, controlled, multicentre clinical trial. *Lancet.* 2013;381(9870):930-938.
A prospective randomized trial of the effect of perioperative red blood cell transfusion.

Huffmyer JL, Littlewood KE, Nemergut EC. Perioperative management of the adult with cystic fibrosis. *Anesth Analg.* 2009;109:1949-1961.
An updated review of anesthetic implications of advanced cystic fibrosis.

National Asthma Education and Prevention Program. *Full report of the expert panel: guidelines for the diagnosis and management of asthma (EPR-3).* Bethesda, MD: National Heart, Lung, and Blood Institute, National Institutes of Health; 2007.
An extensive review of current evidence on the pathophysiology, diagnosis, and management of asthma.

Tait AR, Malviya S. Anesthesia for the child with an upper respiratory tract infection: still a dilemma? *Anesth Analg.* 2005;100:59-65.
A broad review of the data on perioperative upper respiratory tract infections and suggested approaches to management.

von Ungern-Sternberg BS, Boda K, Chambers NA, et al. Risk assessment for respiratory complications in paediatric anaesthesia: a prospective cohort study. *Lancet.* 2010;376:773-783.
A large prospective observational study of perioperative adverse respiratory events and predictive risk factors.

A complete reference list can be found online at ExpertConsult.com.

The Pediatric Airway

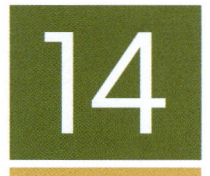

JOHN E. FIADJOE, RONALD S. LITMAN, JULIA F. SERBER,
PAUL A. STRICKER, AND CHARLES J. COTÉ

THE DIFFERENCES BETWEEN THE pediatric and adult airways are important determinants of the anesthetic technique. Knowledge of normal developmental anatomy and physiologic function is required to understand and manage both the normal and the pathologic airways of infants and children (Video 14.1). Techniques and principles to assist in this management are reviewed in this chapter.

Developmental Anatomy of the Airway

The classic works by Negus, Eckenhoff, and Fink and Demarest shaped the foundation of our knowledge about the structure and function of the pediatric and adult airways.[1-3] They suggested that there are five major anatomic differences between the neonatal and adult airways, which are outlined in this section, although recent studies suggest that not all of these long-held beliefs are valid.[2-4] In addition, the relatively large head of an infant offsets the need to place anything under the head to achieve a proper "sniffing position." Older children have airway features that represent a transition between the neonatal and adult anatomy.

TONGUE

It is generally held that the tongue of the neonate and infant is relatively large in proportion to the rest of the oral cavity and therefore more easily obstructs the airway, especially in the neonate. However, magnetic resonance imaging (MRI) studies demonstrated that in children 1 to 11 years of age,[5] there is proportional growth of the tongue and other soft tissues in relation to the bony structures of the oral cavity although that study did not examine neonates and infants (who are 1-12 months of age).

The contribution of the tongue to upper airway obstruction with sedation or induction of anesthesia is relatively minor; much of the obstruction in older children is more likely attributable to the collapse of the nasopharynx and epiglottis, although the tongue may still contribute to obstruction in all age groups.[6,7]

POSITION OF THE LARYNX

The larynx in the infant is more cephalad than in the adult, classically described at the level of C3-4 in the former compared with C4-5 in the latter (Fig. 14.1). MRI and computed tomography (CT) have confirmed the more cephalad position of the larynx in children and demonstrated that the hyoid bone is at the level of C2-3 in infants and children up to 2 years of age.[8] Consequently, the distances between the tongue, hyoid bone, epiglottis, and roof of the mouth in infants are less than those in older children or adults.

The proximity of the tongue base to the more superior larynx also makes visualization of laryngeal structures more difficult because it produces a more acute angle between the plane of the tongue and the plane of the glottic opening. It is for this reason that a straight laryngoscope blade, which lifts the tongue from the field of view during laryngoscopy, facilitates visualization of an infant's larynx. This anatomic relationship is further complicated in certain conditions such as the Treacher Collins anomaly and other syndromes associated with mandibular and midfacial hypoplasia that make direct visualization of the glottis difficult and sometimes impossible with direct laryngoscopy (Fig. 14.2). The reason for this difficulty is that with mandibular and midfacial hypoplasia, the base of the tongue is positioned more caudally (known as glossoptosis), in closer proximity to the laryngeal inlet than normal. The result is a more acute angle between the plane

Glottic Opening Relative
to Cervical Vertebra (C)

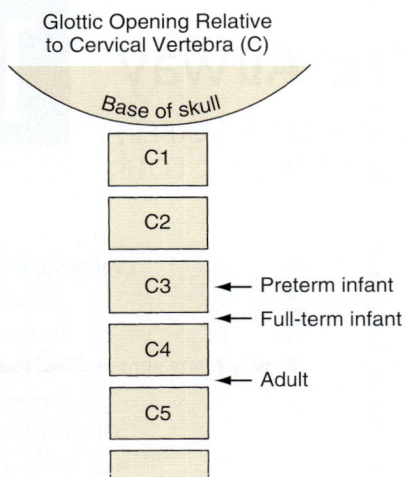

Base of skull

C1

C2

C3 ← Preterm infant
    ← Full-term infant

C4
    ← Adult

C5

FIGURE 14.1 In a preterm Infant, the larynx is located at the middle of the third cervical vertebra (C3); in a full-term infant, it is at the C3-4 interspace; and in an adult, it is at the C4-5 interspace. (Adapted from Negus VE. *The Comparative Anatomy and Physiology of the Larynx.* Oxford: Butterworth-Heinemann; 1949.)

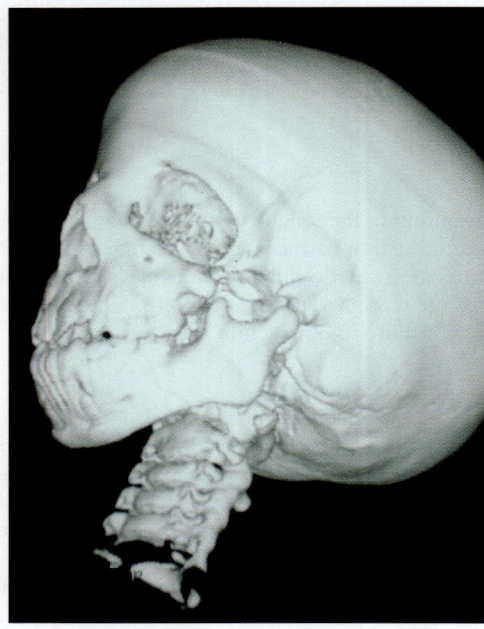

FIGURE 14.2 Three-dimensional reconstruction of a child with the Treacher Collins anomaly demonstrates the retrognathic and more posterior position of the mandible, the midfacial hypoplasia, and the closer proximity and exaggerated angle between the base of the tongue and the laryngeal inlet (almost 90 degrees), which makes direct visualization of the larynx difficult.

of the tongue and the plane of the laryngeal inlet (often 90 degrees) (Fig. 14.3). In this situation, conventional rigid laryngoscopy provides excellent visualization of the esophageal inlet rather than the laryngeal inlet, necessitating the use of special equipment or special techniques to intubate the trachea.

EPIGLOTTIS

The epiglottis in the infant is narrow, omega shaped, and angled away from the axis of the trachea, which contrasts with that in the adult, which is flat and broad, and its axis is parallel to the trachea (Figs. 14.4 and 14.5). This shape allows the epiglottis to approach the uvula during infant breastfeeding; separating breath from fluid and allowing respiration at the same time as swallowing. The shape of epiglottis makes it more difficult to directly lift in the neonate and infant with the tip of a laryngoscope blade.

VOCAL FOLDS

The vocal folds (cords) in an infant are angled such that the anterior insertion is more caudad than the posterior insertion, whereas the axis of the folds in the adult is perpendicular to that of the trachea (compare Fig. 14.4A with Fig. 14.5A). This anatomic feature alters the angle at which the tracheal tube approaches the laryngeal inlet and occasionally leads to difficulty with tracheal intubation, especially with the nasal approach. In the latter case, the tip of the endotracheal tube (ETT) may be held up at the anterior commissure of the vocal folds.

SUBGLOTTIS

Classic teaching holds that the narrowest part of an infant's larynx is the cricoid cartilage; in an adult, it is the rima glottidis. This teaching was supported by an MRI and CT studies in young children (<2 years of age) who were sedated with oral medications and breathing spontaneously.[8,9] In contrast, another study in children 2 months to 13 years of age undergoing MRI with propofol sedation and spontaneous respirations reported that the narrowest portions of the pediatric larynx were the glottic opening and the immediate sub–vocal cord level and that this finding did not change relative to the dimensions of the cricoid ring throughout childhood.[10] These observations contradict the classic observations of autopsy specimens dating back to 1897[11] and other subsequent anatomic autopsy studies.[12-17] The most likely reason for these apparent contradictory observations is that the more recent studies were conducted in spontaneously breathing children with variable portions of the respiratory cycle and that soft tissue collapse gives the appearance of a narrower airway above the cricoid cartilage. Nonetheless, when a relatively large-diameter tube is inserted into the glottic aperture, the tube readily passes through the distensible vocal cords but may meet resistance below the cords (e.g., the nondistensible cricoid ring region). Although these studies demonstrate in vivo dynamic, physiologic relationships, the cricoid cartilage is *functionally* the narrowest portion of the upper airway.

Growth of the subglottic airway occurs rapidly during the first 2 years of life; thereafter, growth of the airway is linear.[17] The cricoid and thyroid cartilages reach adult proportions by 10 to 12 years of age, thus eliminating both the angulation of the vocal cords and the narrow subglottic area.

In adults, the rima glottidis is the narrowest part of the airway,[18] and an ETT that traverses the glottis passes into the trachea without resistance. However, in about 70% of adult cadavers, the narrowest portion of the airway was identified in the subglottic region.[19] The range in diameter for adult females is 10 to 16 mm, and for adult males it is 13 to 19 mm. The likely reason that ETTs pass easily through the rima glottidis into the trachea of an adult is that overall, the narrowest portion of the airway is still larger than the most commonly used ETT sizes. The apparent subglottic narrowing in adults is generally not evident unless there is the need to pass a larger-diameter ETT such as a double-lumen tube. In contrast, in a child, it is common for an ETT to pass easily through the vocal folds (glottic opening) but not through the subglottic region (Fig. 14.6; see Video 14.1). The larynx in both

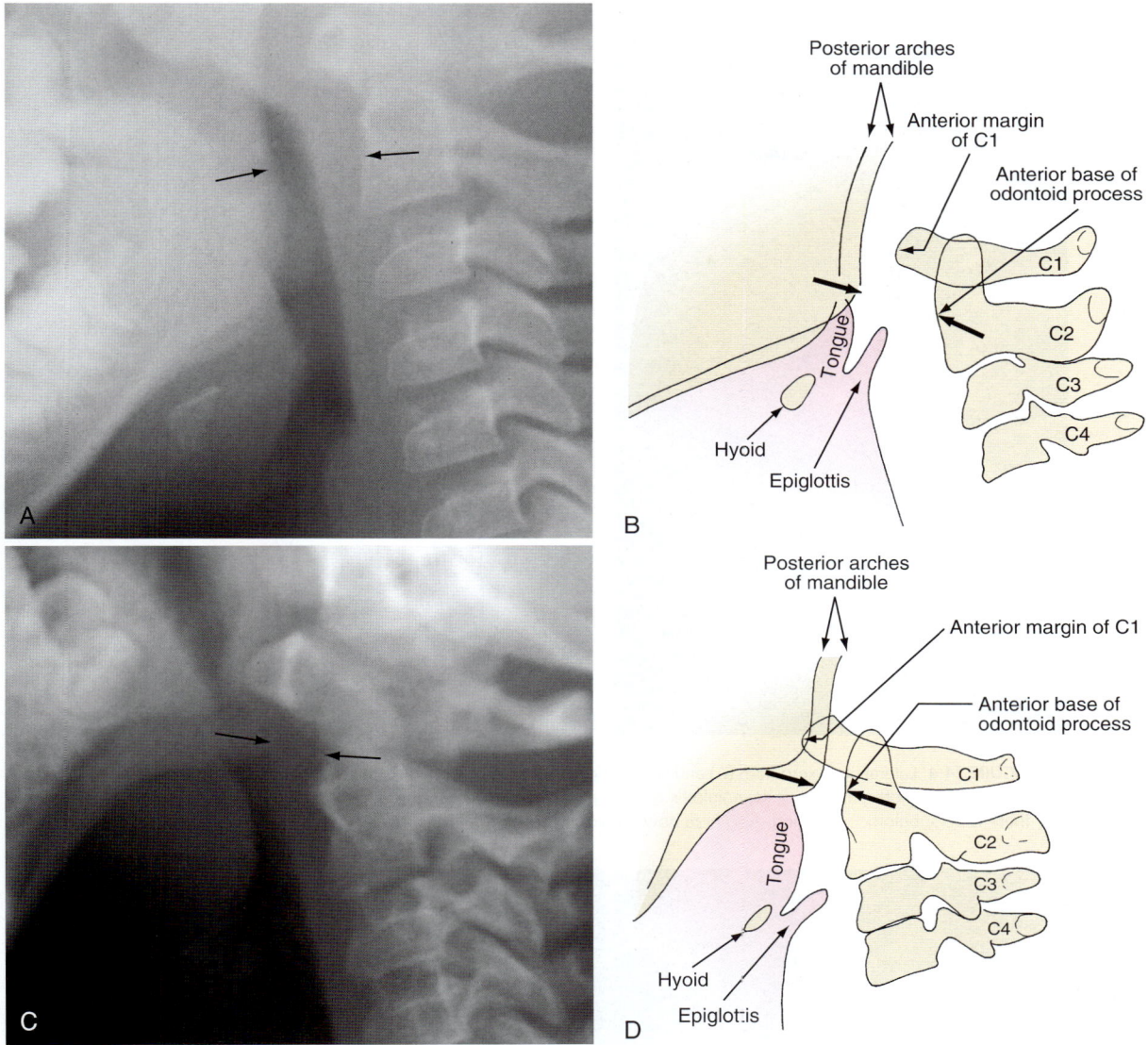

FIGURE 14.3 The larynx in children with mandibular hypoplasia is located more posteriorly than in children with normal anatomy. **A,** Lateral radiograph of the upper airway including the base of the skull and cervical spine of a normal 7-year-old child; the *arrows* denote the posterior border of the ramus of the mandible and the anterior border of the second cervical vertebra. **B,** Diagrammatic representation of the normal anatomy in **A. C,** The same radiographic projection in a 6-year-old child with Treacher Collins syndrome; the *arrows* again denote the posterior border of the ramus of the mandible and the anterior margin of the second cervical vertebra. **D,** Diagrammatic representation of the anatomy in **C**. Notice the significantly smaller space between the ramus of the mandible and the second cervical vertebra, compared with the normal anatomy; the anterior margin of the first cervical vertebra overlaps the posterior margin of the mandible. This extreme posterior location of the tongue and larynx makes direct visualization of the laryngeal inlet almost impossible in many children with this anomaly because of the acute angulation between the base of the tongue and the laryngeal inlet. (Radiographs courtesy Donna J. Seibert, MD; John A. Kirkpatrick, Jr., MD; and Robert H. Cleveland, MD.)

children and adults should be considered funnel-shaped, although this configuration is exaggerated and is of greater importance in infants and young children than in adults.

The cricoid is the only complete ring of cartilage in the laryngotracheobronchial tree; as such it is nondistensible. Because the mucosa that lines the upper airway is loose-fitting pseudostratified columnar epithelium, pressure on the mucosa may cause reactive edema that encroaches on the diameter of the lumen. A tight-fitting ETT that compresses the tracheal mucosa at this level may cause inflammation and edema when it is removed, reducing the luminal diameter and increasing the airway resistance at the time of extubation (e.g., postextubation croup). Because the subglottic region in the infant is smaller than in the adult, the same degree of airway edema results in greater resistance in the infant. For example, assuming that the diameter of the cricoid ring in the infant is 4 mm and the diameter of the adult cricoid ring or trachea is 8 mm, 1 mm of edema circumferentially within the airway (i.e., reduction of the diameter of the airway by 2 mm) would decrease the cross-sectional area of the airway in the infant by approximately 75% (to 2 mm), whereas the area in the adult

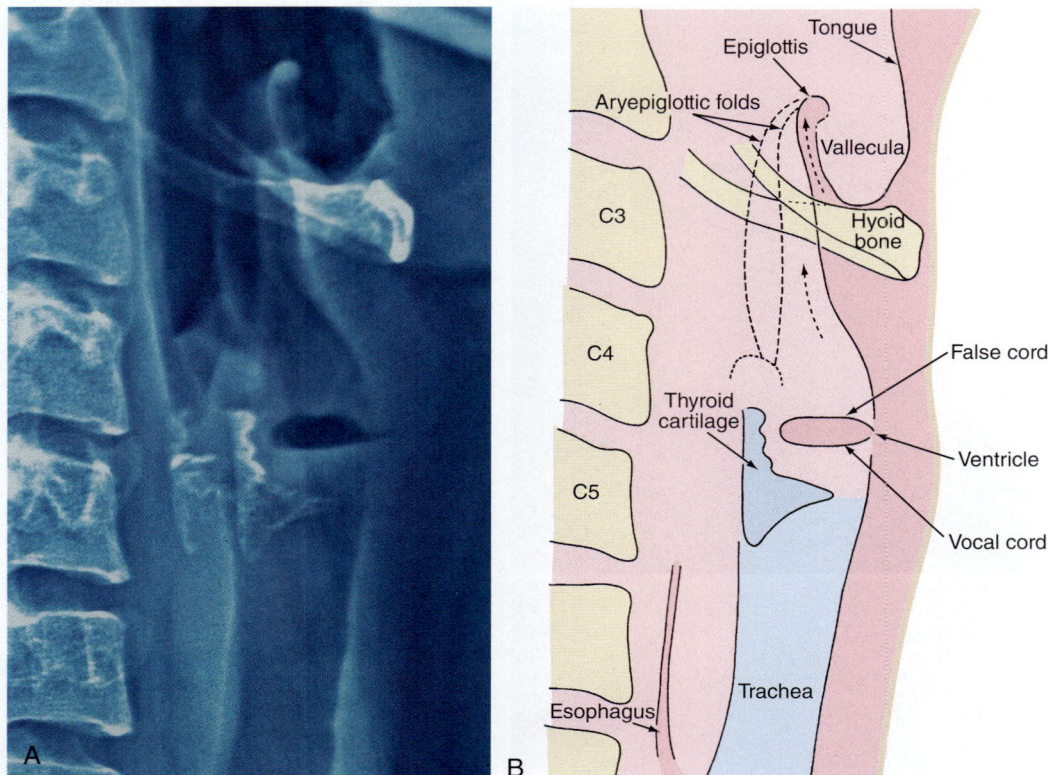

FIGURE 14.4 Lateral neck xerogram **(A)** and schematic diagram **(B)** of the larynx in an adult. Notice the relatively thin, broad epiglottis, the axis of the epiglottis which is parallel to the trachea. The hyoid bone "hugs" the epiglottis; there is no subglottic narrowing. Also note how the vocal cords are perpendicular to the axis of the trachea.

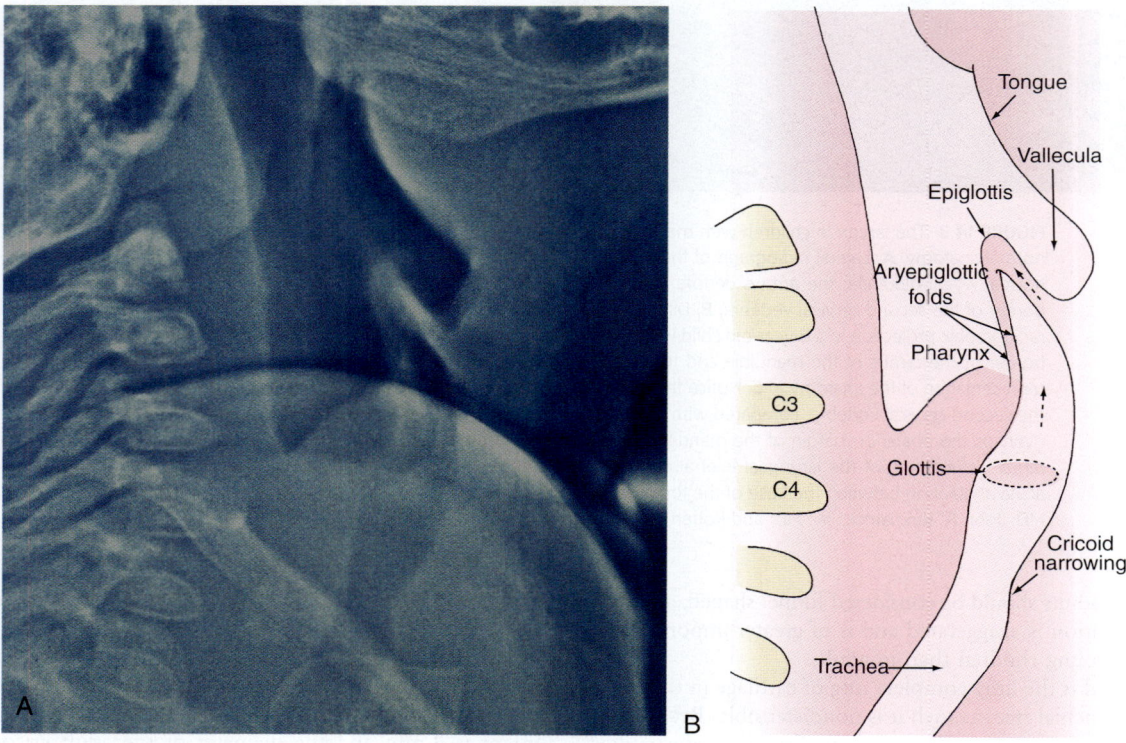

FIGURE 14.5 Lateral neck xerogram **(A)** and schematic diagram **(B)** of an infant's larynx. Notice the angled epiglottis and the narrow cricoid cartilage. Also note that the vocal cords are angled with a higher attachment anteriorly than posteriorly compared with the perpendicular position of the vocal cords in adults.

would decrease by only 44% (to 6 mm). Physiologically, because the resistance to airflow in the upper airway is turbulent, this reduction in diameter of the upper airway would increase the resistance to flow by the *radius to the fifth power*, or 32-fold, in the infant, compared with 5-fold in the adult. (Fig. 14.7).[2]

The Larynx

Understanding the anatomy and function of the larynx is critical to knowledgeable, safe, and successful airway management.

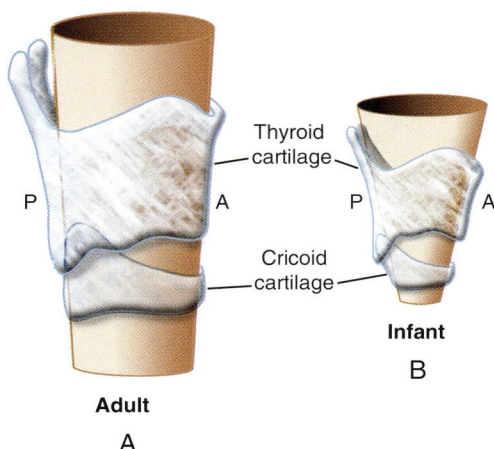

Adult

A

FIGURE 14.6 Configuration of the larynx of an adult **(A)** and an infant **(B)**. Notice that both larynxes are somewhat funnel shaped, but this shape is exaggerated in the infant and toddler. The adult laryngeal structures are of such size that most endotracheal tubes pass easily into the trachea. In infants and toddlers, it is common for the endotracheal tube (ETT) to pass easily through the vocal cords but to become snug at the level of the nondistensible cricoid cartilage. Concern for causing edema at this point resulted in the classic teaching that uncuffed ETTs should be used in young children (see text for more details). *A*, anterior; *P*, posterior.

ANATOMY
Structure

The larynx is composed of 1 bone (hyoid) and 11 cartilages (the single thyroid, cricoid, and epiglottic cartilages and the paired arytenoid, corniculate, cuneiform, and triticeal cartilages). These cartilages are suspended by ligaments from the base of the skull. The body of the cricoid cartilage articulates posteriorly with the inferior cornu of the thyroid cartilage. The paired triangular arytenoid cartilages rest on top of, and articulate with the supero-posterior aspect of the cricoid cartilage. The arytenoid cartilages are protected by the thyroid cartilage (Fig. 14.8). The triticeal cartilages are rounded nodules of cartilage, approximately the size of a pea in adults, located in the margins of the lateral thyrohyoid ligament.

Tissue folds and muscles cover these cartilages. In contrast to adults, but comparable to most mammals, the cartilaginous glottis accounts for 60% to 75% of the length of the vocal folds in children younger than 2 years of age.[17] Contraction of the intrinsic laryngeal muscles alters the position and configuration of these tissue folds, thus influencing laryngeal function during respiration, forced voluntary glottic closure (Valsalva maneuver), reflex laryngospasm, swallowing, and phonation (Fig. 14.9).

The laryngeal tissue folds consist of the following:
- Paired aryepiglottic folds extending from the epiglottis posteriorly to the superior surface of the arytenoids (the paired cuneiform and corniculate cartilages lie within for support and reinforcement, much like the metal stays in a shirt collar)
- Paired vestibular folds (false vocal cords) extending from the thyroid cartilage posteriorly to the superior surface of the arytenoids
- Paired vocal folds (true vocal cords) extending from the posterior surface of the thyroid plate to the anterior projection or vocal process of the arytenoids
- A single interarytenoid fold (composed of the interarytenoid muscle covered by tissue) bridging the arytenoid cartilages
- A single thyrohyoid fold extending from the hyoid bone to the thyroid cartilage

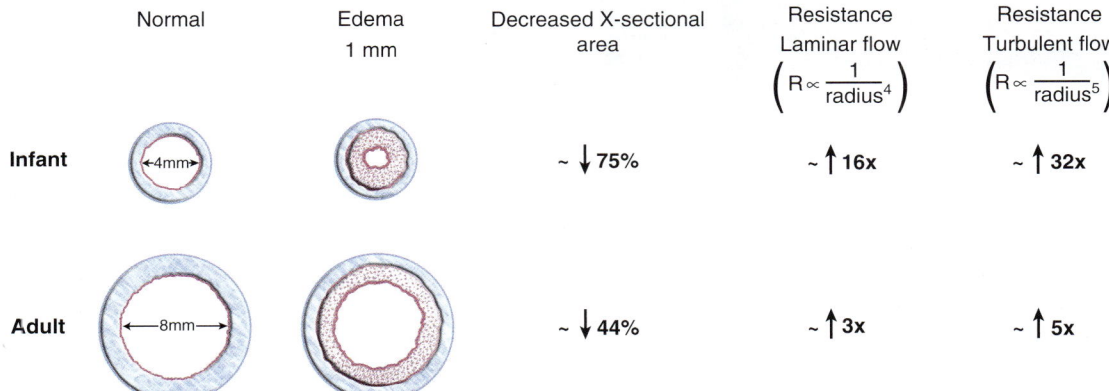

	Normal	Edema 1 mm	Decreased X-sectional area	Resistance Laminar flow $\left(R \propto \dfrac{1}{radius^4}\right)$	Resistance Turbulent flow $\left(R \propto \dfrac{1}{radius^5}\right)$
Infant	←4mm→		~ ↓75%	~ ↑16x	~ ↑32x
Adult	←8mm→		~ ↓44%	~ ↑3x	~ ↑5x

FIGURE 14.7 Relative effects of airway edema in an infant and an adult. The normal airways of an infant and an adult are presented on the left. Edematous airways display 1 mm of circumferential edema, reducing the diameter of the lumen by 2 mm. Notice that resistance to airflow is inversely proportional to the radius of the lumen to the fourth power for laminar flow (beyond the fifth bronchial division) and to the radius of the lumen to the fifth power for turbulent flow (from the mouth to the fourth bronchial division). The net result in an infant with a 4-mm diameter airway is a 75% reduction in cross-sectional area and a 16-fold increase in resistance to laminar airflow, compared with a 44% reduction in cross-sectional area and a 3-fold increased resistance in an adult with a similar 2-mm reduction in airway diameter. With turbulent airflow (upper airway), the resistance increases 32-fold in the infant but only 5-fold in the adult.

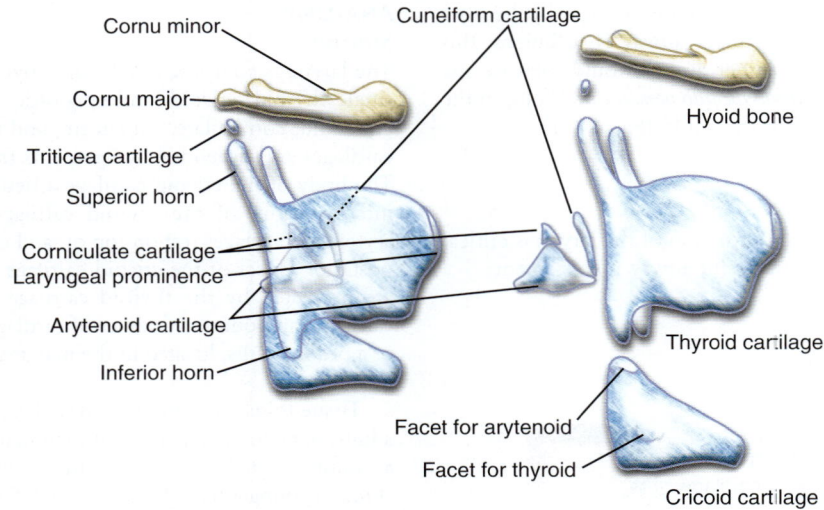

FIGURE 14.8 Laryngeal cartilages. The natural positions of the laryngeal cartilages are presented on the left, with the individual cartilages separated on the right. (Reprinted by permission from Fink BR, Demarest RJ. *Laryngeal Biomechanics*. Cambridge, MA: Harvard University Press, © 1978 by the President and Fellows of Harvard College.)

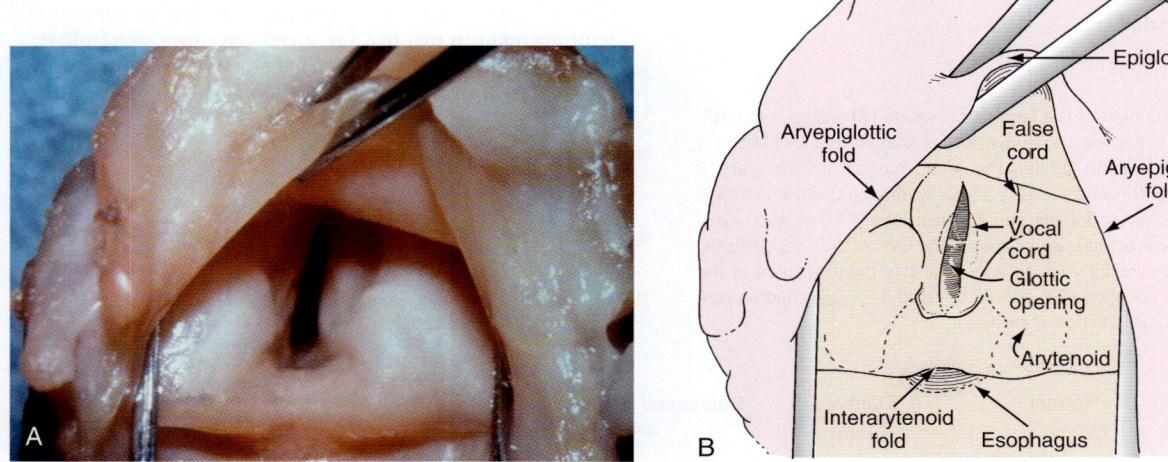

FIGURE 14.9 Photograph **(A)** and schematic diagram **(B)** of the larynx of a premature infant.

Histology

The highly vascular mucosa of the mouth is continuous with that of the larynx and trachea. This mucosa consists of squamous, stratified, and pseudostratified ciliated epithelium. The vocal cords are covered with stratified epithelium. The mucosa and submucosa are rich in lymphatic vessels and seromucous-secreting glands, which lubricate the laryngeal folds. The submucosa consists of loose fibrous stroma; therefore the mucosa is loosely adherent to the underlying structures in most areas. However, the submucosa is scant on the laryngeal surface of the epiglottis and the vocal cords, so the mucosa is tightly adherent in these areas.[20,21] Most inflammatory processes of the airway above the level of the vocal cords are limited by the barrier formed by the firm adherence of the mucosa to the vocal cords.[21] For example, the inflammation of epiglottitis is usually limited to the supraglottic structures, and the loosely adherent mucosa explains the ease with which localized swelling occurs (see Figs. 33.22 and 33.23). In a similar manner,

an inflammatory process of the subglottic region (laryngotracheobronchitis [croup]) results in significant subglottic edema in the loosely adherent mucosa of the airway below the vocal cords, but it does not usually spread above the level of the vocal cords (see Fig. 33.21C).[20]

Sensory and Motor Innervation

Two branches of the vagus nerve, the recurrent laryngeal and the superior laryngeal nerves, supply both sensory and motor innervation to the larynx. The superior laryngeal nerve has two branches: the internal branch, which provides sensory innervation to the supraglottic region, and the external branch, which supplies motor innervation to the cricothyroid muscle. The recurrent laryngeal nerve provides sensory innervation to the subglottic larynx and motor innervation to all other laryngeal muscles.[21,22] Local anesthetic agents injected to block the superior laryngeal nerve result in anesthesia of the supraglottic region down to the inferior margin of the epiglottis and motor blockade of the cricothyroid muscle, which causes relaxation of the vocal cords. Translaryngeal injection of local anesthetic through the cricothyroid membrane or a specific recurrent laryngeal nerve block is required for infraglottic and tracheal anesthesia.[23–25]

Blood Supply

Laryngeal branches of the superior and inferior thyroid arteries provide the blood supply to the larynx. The recurrent laryngeal nerve and artery lie in close proximity to each other, which accounts for the occasional vocal cord paresis after attempts to control bleeding during thyroidectomy.[26]

FUNCTION

Inspiration

During inspiration, the larynx is pulled caudad by the negative intrathoracic pressure generated by the descent of the diaphragm and contraction of the intercostal muscles. Thus, the larynx is stretched longitudinally, increasing the distance between the aryepiglottic and vestibular folds as well as between the vestibular and vocal folds. When the intrinsic muscles within the larynx contract, the arytenoids move laterally and posteriorly (rocking backward and rotating laterally), increasing the interarytenoid distance and separating as well as stretching the paired aryepiglottic, vestibular, and vocal folds. Overall, inspiration enlarges the laryngeal inlet, both longitudinally (like opening a telescope) and laterally, allowing the passage of greater quantities of air through the airway per unit time.

Expiration

At the end of expiration, the larynx reverts to its resting position, with longitudinal shortening of the distance between the aryepiglottic, vestibular, and vocal folds (like closing of a telescope). The arytenoids return simultaneously to their resting position by rotating medially and rocking forward, thus decreasing the interarytenoid distance and reducing the tension on the paired aryepiglottic, vestibular, and vocal folds and causing them to thicken.

Forced Glottic Closure and Laryngospasm

Glottic closure during forced expiration (forced glottic closure or Valsalva maneuver) is voluntary laryngeal closure and is physiologically similar to involuntary laryngeal closure (laryngospasm). Forced glottic closure occurs at several levels. Contraction of the intrinsic laryngeal muscles results in (1) marked reduction in the interarytenoid distance; (2) anterior rocking and medial movement of the arytenoids that causes apposition of the paired vocal, vestibular, and aryepiglottic folds; (3) longitudinal shortening of the larynx that obliterates the space between the aryepiglottic, vestibular, and vocal folds (like complete closing of a telescope). Contraction of an extrinsic laryngeal muscle, the thyrohyoid, pulls the hyoid bone caudad and the thyroid cartilage upward (cephalad), leading to further closure.[1,3,4,27–30]

Closure of the larynx during laryngospasm is similar to, but not identical to that described for voluntary forced glottic closure. There are two important differences. First, laryngospasm is accompanied by an inspiratory effort, which longitudinally separates the vocal from the vestibular folds. Second, in contrast to forced glottic closure, neither the thyroarytenoid muscle (an intrinsic muscle of the larynx) nor the thyrohyoid muscle contract; thus, apposition of the aryepiglottic folds and median thyrohyoid folds is minimal. These two differences allow the upper portion of the larynx to be left partially open during mild laryngospasm, resulting in the hallmark high-pitched inspiratory stridor (see Video 14.1).[1,27] Anterior and upward displacement of the mandible (jaw thrust applied at the condyle of the ascending ramus of the mandible) longitudinally separates the base of the tongue, the epiglottis, and the aryepiglottic folds from the vocal folds, helping to relieve laryngospasm.[28]

Swallowing

Glottic closure during swallowing is also similar to that which occurs during forced closure of the glottis. Protection of the glottic opening is achieved primarily by apposition of the laryngeal folds and secondarily by upward (cephalad) movement of the larynx. The upward movement of the larynx brings the thyroid cartilage closer to the hyoid bone, resulting in folding of the epiglottis over the glottic opening.[1,27,29,30] With loss of consciousness or deep sedation, the normal protective mechanism of the larynx may be lost or obtunded, thus predisposing to pulmonary aspiration of pharyngeal contents.

Phonation

Phonation is accomplished by alteration of the angle between the thyroid and cricoid cartilages (the cricothyroid angle) and by medial movement of the arytenoids during expiration.[1,22,31] These movements result in fine alterations in vocal fold tension during movement of air, causing vibration of the vocal folds. Lesions or malfunctions of the vocal folds (e.g., inflammation, papilloma, paresis) therefore affect phonation. Phonation is the only laryngeal function that alters the cricothyroid angle.[1] Therefore, despite significant airway obstruction during inspiration, it may still be possible to phonate.

Physiology of the Respiratory System

OBLIGATE NASAL BREATHING

Infants are considered obligate nasal breathers.[32,33] Obstruction of their anterior or posterior nares (nasal congestion, stenosis, choanal atresia) can cause asphyxia.[34–36] Immaturity of coordination between respiratory efforts and oropharyngeal motor and sensory input accounts in part for obligate nasal breathing.[37] Furthermore, because the larynx is more cephalad in the neck of an infant and oropharyngeal structures are closer together, the tongue rests against the roof of the mouth during quiet respiration, resulting in oral airway obstruction.[33] Multiple sites of pharyngeal airway obstruction may also contribute to airway obstruction when the infant attempts to breathe against a partially obstructed upper airway or with relaxation of upper airway muscle tone after sedation or induction of anesthesia.[38–42]

The ability to coordinate breathing and swallowing improves as the infant matures. The larynx enlarges and moves more caudad in the neck as the cervical spine lengthens and the infant begins to breathe adequately through the mouth. This matures by age 3 to 5 months. The ability to breathe through the mouth when the nares are obstructed is age dependent: 8% of preterm infants of 31 to 32 weeks postconception age were able to breathe through the mouth in response to nasal occlusion compared with 28% of more mature preterm infants of 35 to 36 weeks postconception age[43]; approximately 40% of full-term infants can switch from nasal to oral breathing.[44] However, the ability of premature neonates to breathe through the mouth may not be as poor as these early reports suggested. Slow and fast nasal occlusion applied to 17 healthy preterm infants (gestational age, 32 ± 1 weeks; postnatal age, 12 ± 2 days) led to a switch from nasal to oral breathing.

These improved results were attributed to the more extended observation period (>15 seconds) in the later study.[45] The presence of a nasogastric tube may also affect the infant's breathing if the "unobstructed" nasal passage has an existing underlying obstruction.

TRACHEAL AND BRONCHIAL FUNCTION

Tracheal and bronchial diameters are a function of elasticity and of distending or compressive forces (Fig. 14.10). The larynx, trachea, and bronchi in the infant are quite compliant compared with those in the adult and therefore are more subject to distention and compression forces.[32,46,47] The intrathoracic trachea is subject to stresses that are different from those in the extrathoracic portion.[46] During expiration, intrathoracic pressure remains slightly negative, maintaining patency of the intrathoracic trachea and bronchi (see Fig. 14.10B). During inspiration, a greater negative intrathoracic pressure dilates and stretches the *intrathoracic* trachea and bronchi.[48] The *extrathoracic* trachea at the thoracic inlet is slightly narrowed by dynamic compression that results from the differential between intratracheal and atmospheric pressures. However, the cartilages of the trachea, along with the muscles and soft tissues of the neck, maintain patency of the airway (see Fig. 14.10A).

Obstruction of the extrathoracic upper airway that can occur with epiglottitis, laryngotracheobronchitis, or an extrathoracic foreign body alters normal airway dynamics. Inspiration against an obstruction results in more negative intrathoracic pressure, further dilating the intrathoracic airways. Clinically, the net effect is a dynamic collapse of the extrathoracic trachea below the level of the obstruction. This collapse is maximal at the thoracic inlet, where the greatest pressure gradient exists between negative intratracheal and atmospheric pressures. As a result, inspiratory stridor is prominent (see Fig. 14.10C and Video 14.1).[46–53] With intrathoracic tracheal obstruction (e.g., foreign body, vascular ring) (see Video 14.1), stridor may occur during both inspiration and expiration.[54–57] In lower airway obstruction (e.g., asthma, bronchiolitis), significant intrathoracic tracheal and bronchial collapse may occur as a result of the prolonged expiratory phase and greatly increased positive extraluminal pressure (see Fig. 14.10D).[58] In addition, because the airways in children are very compliant, they may be more susceptible to closure during bronchial smooth muscle contraction (e.g., with reactive airway disease). Preterm and term infants may experience airway closure even during quiet respiration.

Avoiding dynamic airway collapse is particularly important. The very compliant trachea and bronchi of an infant or child are prone to collapse, particularly at the extremes of transluminal pressures that may occur when a child is crying vigorously. The susceptibility of a child to these dynamic forces on the airway is inversely related to age, with preterm infants being most susceptible and adults being least susceptible.[59] For this reason, it is essential that children with airway obstruction remain calm. Skill and understanding are required on the parts of the parents, nursing staff, and physicians. *Sedatives and opioids should be used with caution before insertion of an ETT, because they may depress or ablate the life-sustaining voluntary efforts to breathe, resulting in significant morbidity or mortality.*

WORK OF BREATHING

Work of breathing (WOB) may be defined as the product of pressure and volume. It may be analyzed by plotting transpulmonary pressure against tidal volume. The WOB per kilogram body weight is similar in infants and adults. However, the oxygen consumption of a full-term neonate (5–7 mL/kg per minute) is several times that of an adult (2-3 mL/kg per minute).[60] This greater oxygen consumption (and greater carbon dioxide production) in infants accounts in part for their increased respiratory frequency compared with older children. In preterm infants, the oxygen consumption related to breathing is three times that in adults.[61]

The location of airway resistance within the tracheobronchial tree differs between infants and adults. The nasal passages account for 25% of the total resistance to airflow in a neonate, compared with 60% in an adult.[33,62] In infants, most resistance to airflow occurs in the bronchi and small airways. This results from the relatively smaller diameter of the airways and the greater compliance of the supporting structures of the trachea and bronchi.[32,63,64] In particular, the soft cartilaginous chest wall of a neonate is very compliant; the ribs provide less support to maintain negative intrathoracic pressure. This lack of negative intrathoracic pressure combined with the increased compliance of the bronchi can lead to functional airway closure with every breath.[65–67] In infants and children, therefore, small-airway resistance accounts for most of the WOB, whereas in adults, the nasal passages provide the major proportion of flow resistance.[33,65,66,68–73]

In the presence of increased airway resistance or decreased lung compliance, an increased transpulmonary pressure is required to produce a given tidal volume, and therefore the WOB is increased. Any change in the airway that increases the WOB may lead to respiratory failure. Recall that the WOB (resistance to air flow) is inversely proportional to the fourth power of the radius of the lumen during laminar flow (beyond the fifth bronchial division) and to the fifth power of the radius during turbulent flow (upper airway to the fifth bronchial division). Because the diameter of the airways in infants is smaller than in adults, pathologic narrowing of the airways in infants exerts a greater adverse effect on the WOB. Increase in the WOB may also occur with a long ETT of small diameter, an obstructed ETT, or a narrowed airway. All of these situations increase oxygen consumption, which in turn increases oxygen demand.[74] The increased oxygen demand is initially addressed by an increase in respiratory rate, but the increased WOB may not be sustainable. The end result may be exhaustion, which leads to respiratory failure (CO_2 retention and hypoxemia) (Fig. 4.9).

The difference in histology of the diaphragm and intercostal muscles of preterm and full-term infants compared with older children contributes to increased susceptibility of infants to respiratory fatigue or failure. Type I muscle fibers permit prolonged repetitive movement; for example, long-distance runners through repeated exercise increase the proportion of type I muscle fibers in their legs. The percentage of type I muscle fibers in the diaphragm and intercostal muscles increases with age (preterm infants < full-term infants < 2-year-old children) (Fig. 14.11). Any condition that increases the WOB in preterm and full-term neonates may fatigue the respiratory muscles and precipitate respiratory failure more readily than in an adult.[75–77]

AIRWAY OBSTRUCTION DURING ANESTHESIA

Airway obstruction during anesthesia or loss of consciousness appears to be most frequently related to loss of muscle tone in the pharyngeal and laryngeal structures rather than apposition of the tongue to the posterior pharyngeal wall.[38,78,79] The progressive loss of tone with deepening anesthesia results in progressive airway obstruction primarily at the level of the soft palate and the epiglottis.[38,39,42,78,80,81] In children, the pharyngeal airway space decreases

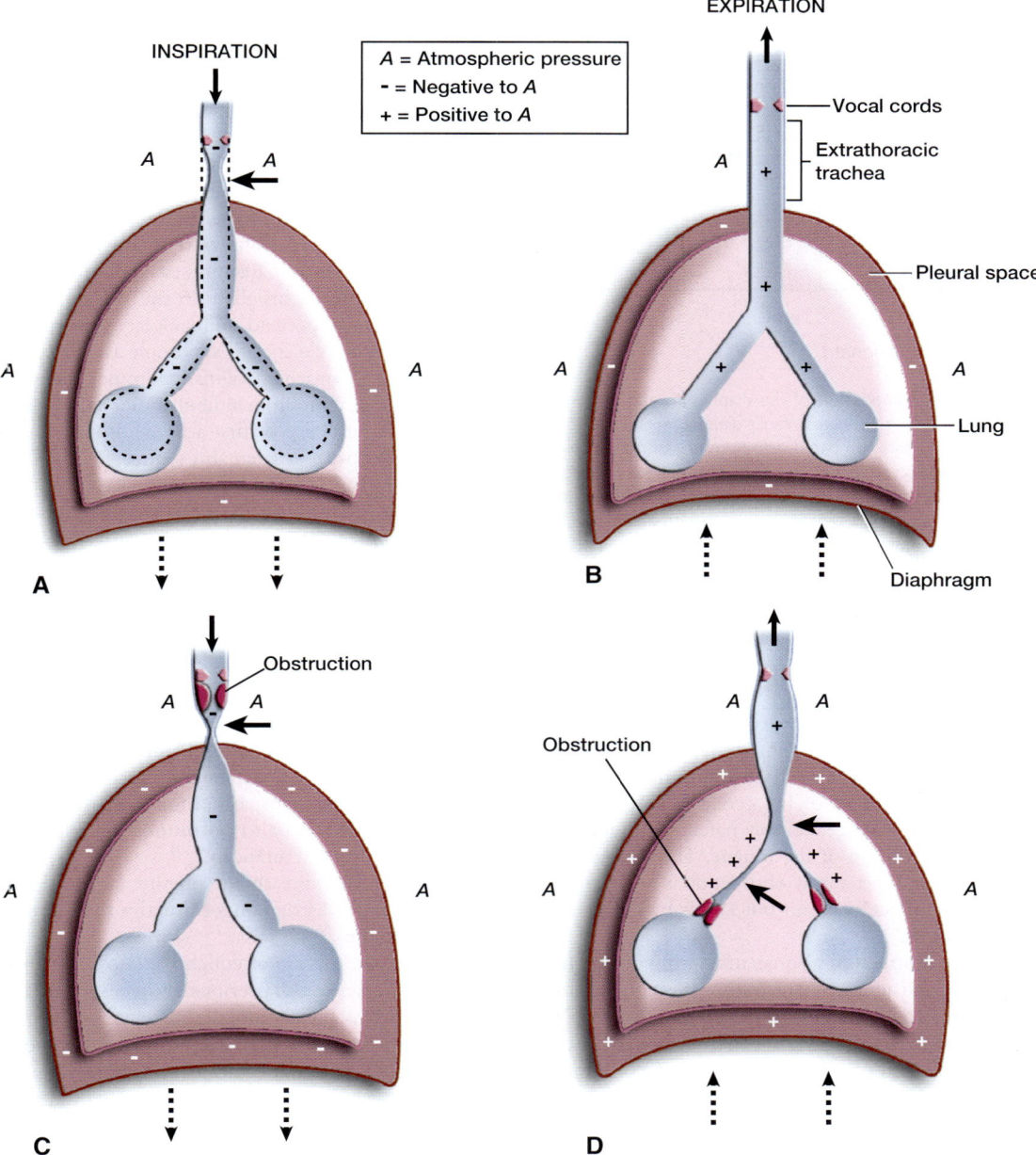

INSPIRATION

EXPIRATION

A = Atmospheric pressure
- = Negative to A
+ = Positive to A

Vocal cords

Extrathoracic trachea

Pleural space

Lung

Diaphragm

A

B

Obstruction

C

Obstruction

D

FIGURE 14.10 A, With descent of the diaphragm and contraction of the intercostal muscles, a greater negative intrathoracic pressure relative to intraluminal and atmospheric pressure is developed. The net result is longitudinal stretching of the larynx and trachea, dilatation of the intrathoracic trachea and bronchi, movement of air into the lungs, and some dynamic collapse of the extrathoracic trachea (*arrow*). The dynamic collapse is due to the highly compliant trachea and the negative intraluminal pressure in relation to atmospheric pressure. **B,** The normal sequence of events at end-expiration is a slight negative intrapleural pressure stenting the airways open. In infants, the highly compliant chest does not provide the support required; therefore airway closure occurs with each breath. Intraluminal pressures are slightly positive in relation to atmospheric pressure, with the result that air is forced out of the lungs. **C,** Obstructed extrathoracic airway. Notice the severe dynamic collapse of the extrathoracic trachea below the level of obstruction. This collapse is greatest at the thoracic inlet, where the largest pressure gradient exists between negative intratracheal pressure and atmospheric pressure (*arrow*). (Extrathoracic upper airway obstruction is characterized by inspiratory stridor.) **D,** Obstructed intrathoracic trachea or airways. Notice that breathing against an obstructed lower airway (e.g., bronchiolitis, asthma) results in greater positive intrathoracic pressures, with dynamic collapse of the intrathoracic airways (prolonged expiration or wheezing [*arrows*]).

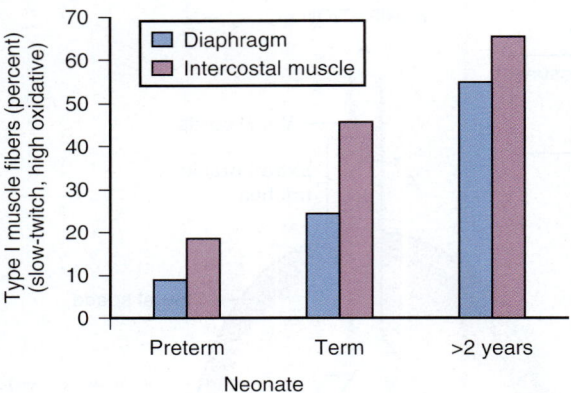

FIGURE 14.11 Muscle fiber composition of the diaphragm and intercostal muscles related to age. Note that a preterm infant's diaphragm and intercostal muscles have fewer type I fibers compared with term newborns and older children. The data suggest a possible mechanism for early fatigue in preterm and term infants when the work of breathing is increased. (Data from Keens TG, Bryan AC, Levison H, Ianuzzo CD. Developmental pattern of muscle fiber types in human ventilatory muscles. *J Appl Physiol.* 1978;44:909–913.)

in a dose-dependent manner with increasing concentrations of both sevoflurane and propofol anesthesia.[82–84] This reduction in pharyngeal space has been observed mainly in the anteroposterior dimension. As the depth of propofol anesthesia in children increases, upper airway narrowing occurs throughout the entire upper airway but is most pronounced in the hypopharynx at the level of the epiglottis. Extension of the head at the atlantooccipital joint with anterior displacement of the cervical spine (sniffing position) improves hypopharyngeal airway patency but does not necessarily change the position of the tongue. This observation supports the concept that upper airway obstruction is not primarily caused by changes in tongue position but rather by collapse of the pharyngeal structures.[40–42]

Pharyngeal airway obstruction also occurs during obstructive sleep apnea in children and adults.[37,85] The sniffing position increases the cross-sectional area and decreases the closing pressure of both the retropalatal and the retroglossal space in anesthetized adults with obstructive sleep apnea.[86] The application of continuous positive airway pressure (CPAP) is a common method to overcome such airway obstruction (see Figs. 33.10 and 33.11). During propofol anesthesia in children, CPAP works primarily by increasing the transverse dimension of the airway.[83] This occurs despite the fact that anesthesia obstructs the airway mostly by narrowing the anteroposterior dimension. Chin lift and jaw thrust also improve airway patency in anesthetized children with adenotonsillar hypertrophy.[87–89] Lateral positioning (also known as the "recovery or tonsillectomy position") dramatically enhances the effects of these airway maneuvers[88,89]; lateral positioning alone improves airway dimensions.[6] Compared with chin lift and CPAP, the jaw thrust maneuver is the most effective means to improve airway patency and ventilation in children undergoing adenotonsillectomy[87] (see Video 14.2).

Evaluation of the Airway

A history and physical examination with specific reference to the airway should be performed in all children who require sedation or anesthesia. In particular, a history of a congenital syndrome or physical findings of a congenital anomaly (e.g., microtia,

which has been associated with difficult laryngoscopy)[90] should alert the practitioner to the possibility of difficulties with airway management. In special situations, radiologic and laboratory studies are required to further evaluate and clarify a disorder revealed by the history and physical examination. Although many methods exist for evaluating and predicting the difficult airway in adults,[91–95] no comparable methods have been forthcoming in children.[96,97] Large neck circumference correlated with other issues, such as snoring, asthma, hypertension, and diabetes in children as well as adverse perioperative respiratory events, but not with difficult laryngoscopy.[98] Routine evaluation of the airway in all children often sheds insight into the risk of a difficult airway. Characteristics that portend a difficult laryngoscopy and intubation include diagnosis of a specific syndrome associated with a difficult intubation (e.g., Treacher Collins syndrome), the inability to open the mouth (e.g., temporomandibular joint ankylosis, micrognathia Pierre Robin sequence or first arch syndrome), massive glossoptosis (e.g., Beckwith-Wiedemann syndrome), fused cervical spine (e.g., Klippel-Feil syndrome), or oropharyngeal space occupying lesions (e.g., cystic hygroma or glossopharyngeal tumors). For some syndromes, the airway improves with age (e.g., Pierre Robin sequence), whereas with others (e.g., Treacher Collins), the airway becomes progressively more difficult with age.

CLINICAL EVALUATION
Medical History
The *medical history* (both present and past) should investigate the following signs and symptoms; a positive history should alert the practitioner to the potential problems noted in parentheses.

- Presence of an upper respiratory tract infection (predisposition to coughing, laryngospasm, bronchospasm, and desaturation during anesthesia or to postintubation subglottic edema or postoperative desaturation)[99–104]
- Snoring, noisy breathing, obesity (adenoidal hypertrophy, upper airway obstruction, obstructive sleep apnea, pulmonary hypertension)[105]
- Presence and nature of cough ("croupy" cough may indicate subglottic stenosis or previous tracheoesophageal fistula repair; productive cough may indicate bronchitis or pneumonia; chronicity affects the differential diagnosis [e.g., the sudden onset of a persistent cough may indicate foreign-body aspiration; a night cough may indicate tracheal compression from a thoracic mass])
- Past episodes of croup (postintubation croup, subglottic stenosis)
- Inspiratory stridor, usually high-pitched (subglottic narrowing [see Video 14.1], laryngomalacia [see Video 14.1], macroglossia, laryngeal web [Video 14.3], extrathoracic foreign body or extrathoracic tracheal compression)
- Hoarse voice (laryngitis, vocal cord palsy, papillomatosis [see Video 14.1], granuloma [see Video 14.1])
- Asthma and bronchodilator therapy (bronchospasm)
- Repeated pneumonias (incompetent larynx with aspiration, gastroesophageal reflux, cystic fibrosis, bronchiectasis, residual tracheoesophageal fistula, pulmonary sequestration, immune suppression, congenital heart disease)
- History of foreign-body aspiration (increased airway reactivity, airway obstruction, impaired neurologic function)
- History of aspiration (laryngeal edema [Video 14.3], laryngeal cleft)
- Previous anesthetic problems, particularly related to the airway (difficult intubation, difficulty with mask ventilation, failed or problematic extubation)

- Atopy, allergy (increased airway reactivity)[104]
- History of smoking by primary caregivers (increased airway resistance, increased propensity to desaturation)[104,106]
- History of a congenital syndrome (many are associated with difficult airways)
- History of prematurity (subglottic stenosis, bronchopulmonary dysplasia, apnea, desaturation)

Physical Examination

The *physical examination* should include the following observations:

- Facial expression
- Presence or absence of nasal flaring
- Presence or absence of mouth breathing
- Color of mucous membranes
- Presence or absence of retractions (suprasternal, intercostal, subcostal [see Video 14.1])
- Respiratory rate
- Presence or absence of voice change
- Mouth opening (Fig. 14.12A)
- Size of mouth
- Size of tongue and its relationship to other pharyngeal structures (Mallampati Score)[107]
- Loose or missing teeth (see Fig. 14.12B)
- Size and configuration of palate
- Size and configuration of mandible
- Location of larynx in relation to the mandible (see Fig. 14.12C)
- Presence of stridor and, if present:
  - Is stridor predominantly inspiratory, suggesting an upper airway (extrathoracic) lesion (epiglottitis, croup, extrathoracic foreign body)?
  - Is stridor both inspiratory and expiratory, suggesting an intrathoracic lesion (aspirated foreign body, vascular ring, or large esophageal foreign body)? (see Video 14.1)
  - Is the expiratory phase prolonged or stridor predominantly expiratory, suggesting lower airway disease?
- Baseline oxygen saturation in room air
- Microtia (underdeveloped pinna): bilateral but not unilateral microtia is associated with difficulty in visualizing the laryngeal inlet (grade 3 or 4 in the Cormack-Lehane classification, see Fig. 14.22 later).[90] Five (42%) of 12 children with bilateral microtia were found to have a difficult laryngeal view compared with 2 (2.5%) of 81 children with unilateral microtia and 0 of 93 children without microtia.[90] Microtia may represent a mild form of hemifacial microsomia and its associated mandibular

hypoplasia. The advantage of understanding this association is that ear deformity is often a more easily recognized clinical finding than mandibular hypoplasia.

- Global appearance: Are there congenital anomalies that may fit a recognizable syndrome? *The finding of one anomaly mandates a search for others.* If a congenital syndrome is diagnosed, specific anesthetic implications must be considered (see E-Table 14.1).

DIAGNOSTIC TESTING

Routine evaluation of the airway usually requires only a careful history and physical examination. In the presence of airway pathology, however, laboratory and radiologic evaluation can be extremely valuable. Radiographs of the upper airway (anteroposterior and lateral films and fluoroscopy) may provide evidence about the site and cause of airway obstruction. When necessary, MRI, CT, and three-dimensional (3-D) modeling provide more detailed information.[108–129] *Radiologic airway examination in a child with a compromised airway may be undertaken only if there is no immediate threat to the child's safety and only in the presence of skilled and appropriately equipped personnel able to manage the airway.* Securing the airway through tracheal intubation must not be postponed to obtain a radiologic diagnosis when the child has severely compromised air exchange. Blood gas analysis is occasionally of value for assessing the degree of physiologic compromise, especially with chronic airway obstruction and compensated respiratory acidosis. Performing an arterial (or venous) puncture for blood gas analysis may provide helpful information, but it is often upsetting to the child and may risk aggravation of the underlying airway obstruction through dynamic airway collapse. Candidates for blood gas analysis must be carefully selected and the procedure skillfully performed.

Endoscopic evaluation (flexible fiberoptic endoscopy) of the airway before tracheal intubation can be useful in infants and in cooperative older children if a glottic pathologic process is suspected or if difficulty is anticipated when visualizing the glottis. Ultrasound can also be used to examine the airway. It can be used to determine the internal diameter of the trachea, which can help with the selection of the optimal ETT size.[130]

Airway Management: The Normal Airway

MASK VENTILATION

Face masks are available in many sizes and shapes. We commonly use disposable, clear plastic masks with an inflatable cushioned

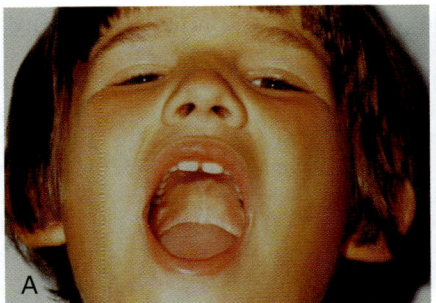
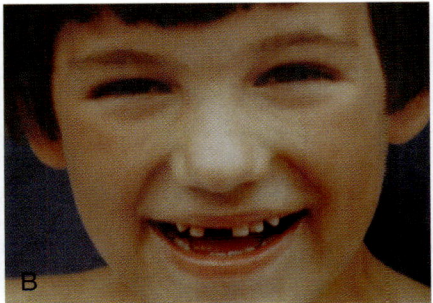
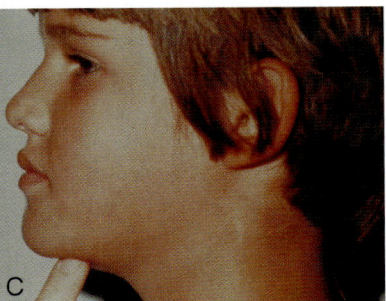

FIGURE 14.12 A, How far can a child open his or her mouth? Are there any abnormalities of the mouth, tongue, palate, or mandible? **B,** Are any teeth loose or missing? **C,** Is the mandible of normal configuration? How much space is there between the genu of the mandible and the thyroid cartilage? This space is an indication of the extent of the superior and posterior displacement of the larynx; there should normally be at least one finger breadth in a newborn and three finger breadths in an adolescent.

rim. The inflatable rim molds to the contour of the face to provide an atraumatic seal. The use of clear plastic in the cone of the mask allows visualization of humidity (indicating air exchange), secretions, vomitus, and lip color. The appropriately sized mask should rest on the bridge of the nose (avoiding the eyes) and extend to the mandible. Although mask anesthesia appears to be easy, it is one of the most difficult skills to master. The most common error during mask ventilation is to tightly compress the submental triangle with fingers placed below the mandibular ridge, thereby partially occluding the airway. Minimal pressure is required, and the fingers should rest on the mandible. Another common problem arises when the mouth is completely closed while the face mask is being applied. The upper airway may become completely obstructed, with ventilation becoming impossible both spontaneously and by manual control. In such a circumstance, the fingers should be removed from the mandible and face and a single digit applied gently to the condyles of the mandible (for a brief period), while lifting toward the hairline, until a patent upper airway is established.[131] This maneuver subluxes the temporomandibular joint, thereby opening the mouth and pulling the tongue and other soft tissues off the posterior pharyngeal wall. A hand should be on the reservoir bag at all times to monitor the effectiveness of ventilation and to provide CPAP if needed to maintain a patent airway. An alternative method is to partially close the adjustable pressure-limiting valve to inflate the reservoir bag and provide CPAP. Insertion of an oral airway may also relieve upper airway obstruction (although care must be taken as the inserted airway may also obstruct breathing if the size is excessive or too small; Figs. 14.13D and F.). If these maneuvers do not clear the upper airway, then the vocal cords may be closed or the child is apneic. Additional interventions may then be required.

Admonitions against extreme positions of the infant's head during bag-and-mask ventilation are intended to minimize the risk of stretching and thus narrowing and obstructing the very compliant infant trachea. However, a study of 18 healthy, full-term infants younger than 4 months of age showed that the tracheal dimensions did not change when the head position changed.[132] Therefore, stretching of the trachea may not result in narrowing of the tracheal lumen in otherwise healthy infants (Video 14.4). This study did not examine the effects of these head positions on the supraglottic airway or in the preterm infant. It is possible that these maneuvers (head extension) could result in supraglottic airway obstruction in some children. One study investigated the incidence of unanticipated difficult mask ventilation in children from birth to 8 years and reported an incidence of 6.6%.[133]

OROPHARYNGEAL AIRWAYS

An infant's tongue may obstruct the airway during induction of anesthesia or loss of consciousness. An oropharyngeal airway of appropriate size (or a supraglottic airway [SGA] such as the laryngeal mask airway [LMA; LMA North America, San Diego, CA]) may be inserted to relieve the obstruction. By holding the oral airway as shown in Fig. 14.13, one can estimate the appropriate size for the child; airways one size larger and one size smaller should be readily available as well. A tongue depressor may be inserted over the tongue to facilitate insertion of an oral airway and prevent downfolding of the tongue, which could impair venous and lymphatic drainage, causing tongue swelling and airway obstruction. If the airway device is too long, it may push the epiglottis into the glottic aperture, creating an additional

site of airway obstruction or causing traumatic epiglottitis, or the tip may impinge on the uvula, causing uvular swelling and airway obstruction (see Fig. 14.13C, D).[134,135] If the airway device is too short, it may rest against the base of the tongue, forcing it posteriorly against the roof of the mouth, further aggravating airway obstruction (Fig. 14.13E, F). Oral airways should not be considered panaceas for upper airway obstruction. Care must be taken to avoid trauma to the lips and tongue, which may be caught between the teeth and the flange of the airway. An oral airway is also used to protect an ETT from compression by the child's teeth, and it serves to separate the mandible and maxilla to facilitate oropharyngeal suctioning.

NASOPHARYNGEAL AIRWAYS

Nasopharyngeal airways (also known as Robertazzi nasopharyngeal airways [SunMed, Grand Rapids, MI]) are occasionally used in children to relieve upper airway obstruction; the distance from the naris to the angle of the mandible approximates the proper length. Commercial airways are available in sizes 12F to 36F (Rüsch Inc., Duluth, GA). Some have an adjustable flange that enables manipulation of the airway to the appropriate length. Alternatively, for infants and small children, a shortened ETT may be used, although this is not as soft and pliable as a commercially available non-latex nasopharyngeal airway and may be more likely to cause trauma with insertion. Softening the tip of the ETT by immersion in hot water before insertion has not been shown to reduce the incidence of bleeding during nasotracheal intubation in children.[136] The nasopharyngeal airway may be better tolerated in the lightly anesthetized child than an oropharyngeal airway. Nasopharyngeal airways are usually avoided to prevent trauma to, and bleeding from, hypertrophied adenoids, and they are more commonly used to relieve residual airway obstruction on emergence from anesthesia.

TRACHEAL INTUBATION
Technique
The techniques used to intubate the trachea in infants and children differ from those in adults.[1–4,28–30,113,137,138] The risk of obstruction with trauma to the airway structures is increased in infants because the dimensions of the pediatric airway are smaller than in children. Advancing the blade into the esophagus and then slowly withdrawing it to visualize the larynx is a technique that should be avoided if possible. *This maneuver may result in laryngeal trauma when the tip of the blade scrapes the esophageal mucosa, arytenoids, and aryepiglottic folds.*

There are several approaches to exposing the glottis in infants with a Miller blade. One approach consists of advancing the laryngoscope blade under constant vision along the surface of the tongue, placing the tip of the blade directly in the vallecula, and then using this location to pivot or rotate the blade to the right to sweep the tongue to the left and adequately lift the tongue to expose the glottic opening. This technique avoids trauma to the arytenoid cartilages. Lifting the base of the tongue lifts the epiglottis, exposing the glottic opening. If this technique is unsuccessful, the epiglottis may be lifted directly with the tip of the blade (see Video 14.1). Another approach is to insert the Miller blade into the mouth at the right commissure over the lateral bicuspids/incisors as originally described by Miller (now known as the paraglossal approach).[139,140] The blade is advanced down the right gutter of the mouth, aiming the blade tip toward the midline while sweeping the tongue to the left. Once the blade is under the epiglottis, the epiglottis is lifted with the tip, exposing the glottic aperture. By

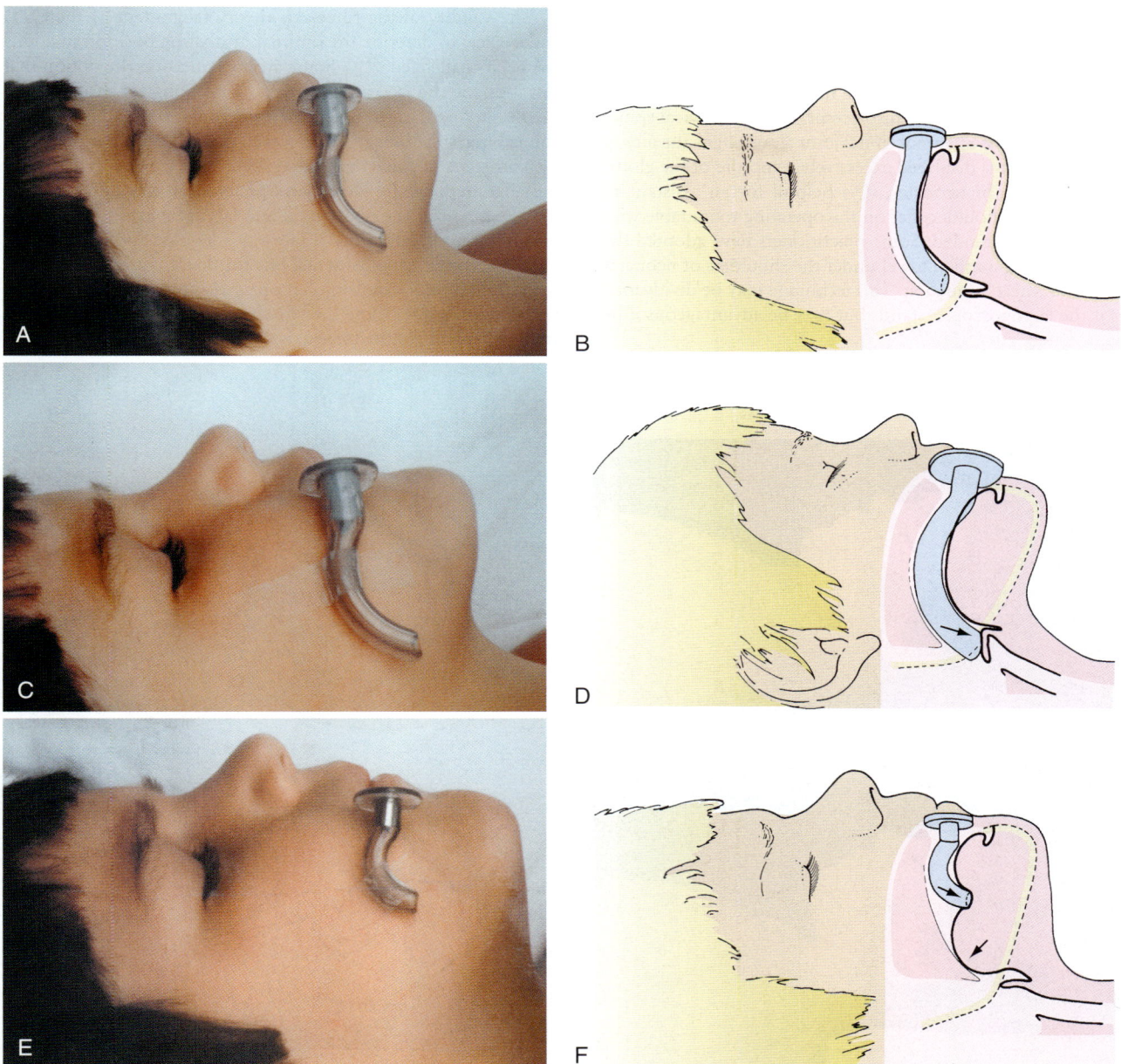

FIGURE 14.13 Correct airway selection. An artificial airway of proper size should relieve airway obstruction caused by the tongue without damaging laryngeal structures. The appropriate size can be estimated by holding the airway against the child's face: the tip of the airway should end just cephalad to the angle of the mandible (**A**). Use of the correct size should result in proper alignment with the glottic opening (**B**). If too large an oral airway is inserted, the tip will line up posterior to the angle of the mandible (**C**) and obstruct the glottic opening by pushing the epiglottis down (**D**, *arrow*). If too small an oral airway is inserted, the tip will line up well above the angle of the mandible (**E**) and exacerbate airway obstruction by kinking the tongue (**F**, *arrows*).

approaching the mouth over the bicuspids/incisors, damage to the maxillary central incisors is precluded. This is a particularly effective approach for the infant or child in whom intubation appears to be difficult. Whichever approach is used, care must be taken to avoid using the laryngoscope blade as a fulcrum through which pressure is applied to the teeth or alveolar ridge. If there is a substantive risk that pressure will be applied to the teeth, a plastic tooth guard may be applied to cover the teeth at risk (the central incisors of the maxilla).

Optimal positioning for laryngoscopy changes with age. The trachea of older children (≥6 years) and adults is most easily exposed when a folded blanket or pillow is placed beneath the occiput of the head (5- to 10-cm elevation), displacing the cervical spine anteriorly.[141] Extension of the head at the atlantooccipital joint produces the classic sniffing position.[113,142,143] These movements align three axes: those of the mouth or oral (O), pharynx (P), and trachea (T). Once aligned, these three axes permit direct visualization of laryngeal structures. They also result in improved hypopharyngeal patency.[40,42,78,86,142,143] Fig. 14.14 demonstrates maneuvers for positioning the head during airway management. In infants and younger children, it is usually unnecessary to elevate the head because the occiput is large in proportion to the trunk, resulting in adequate anterior displacement of the cervical spine; head extension at the atlantooccipital joint alone aligns the airway axes. If the occiput is displaced excessively, exposure of the glottis may be hindered. In neonates, it is helpful for an assistant to hold the patient's shoulders flat on the operating room table with the head slightly extended. Some practitioners have adopted the practice of placing a rolled towel under the shoulders of neonates to facilitate tracheal intubation. This technique may be disadvantageous if the laryngoscopist stands but may be advantageous if he or she is seated.

The validity of the three-axis theory (alignment of the O, P, and T axes) to describe the optimal intubating position in adults has been challenged.[144-147] Some authors question the notion that elevation of the occiput improves conditions for visualization of the laryngeal inlet based on evidence from both MRI and clinical investigations.[144,146] However, one MRI study in children with an LMA in place found that slight head extension improved the alignment of the glottic and pharyngeal axes but worsened the alignment of the pharyngeal and laryngeal axes.[148] In a study of adults, neck extension alone was adequate for visualization of the larynx in most patients, but for obese patients and those with limited neck extension, an optimal intubating position was not determined.[144] Others favor the sniffing position but with varying support for the three-axis theory.[149-155] Even if the tracheas

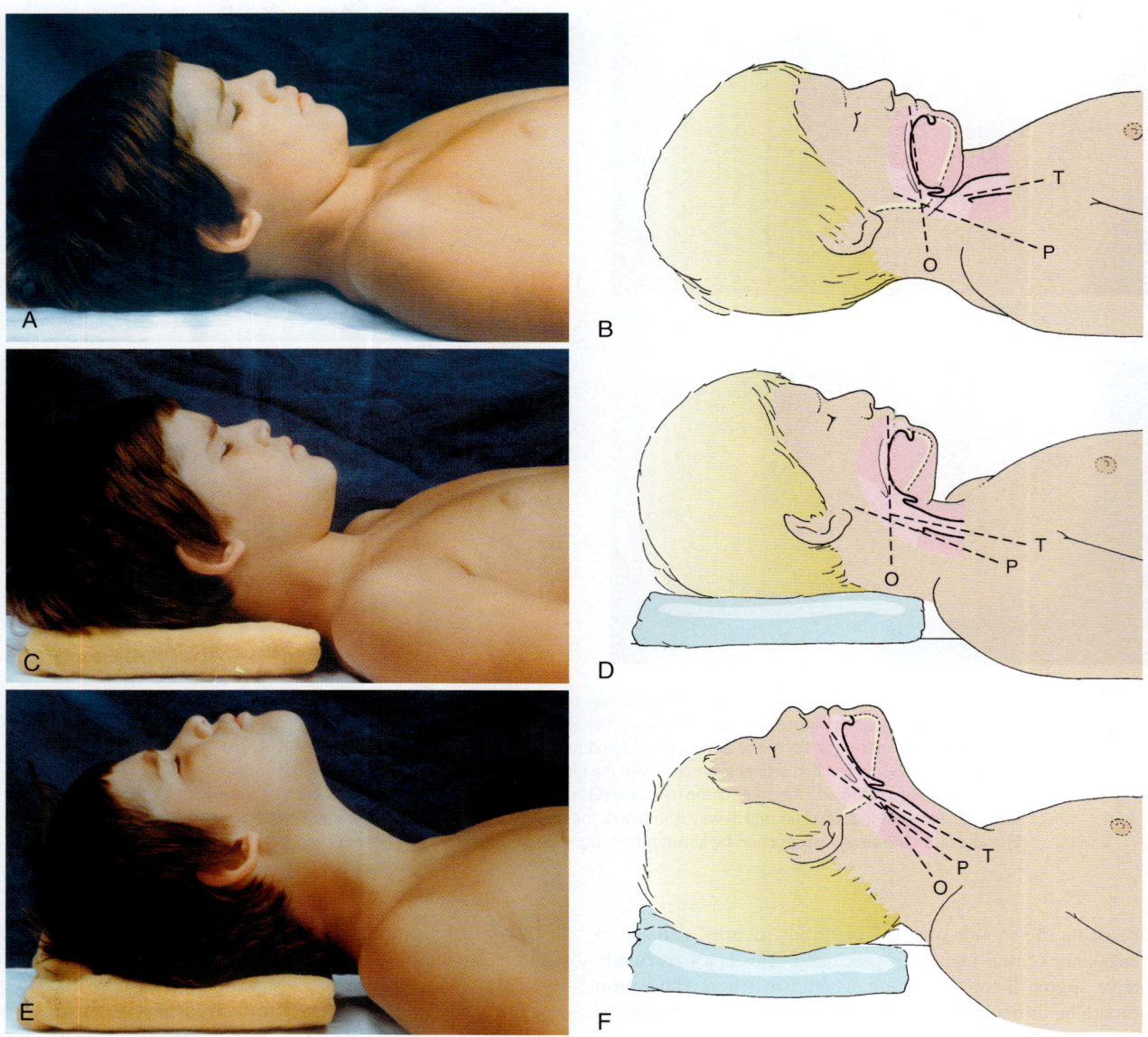

FIGURE 14.14 Correct positioning for ventilation and tracheal intubation. When a patient is lying flat on the bed or operating table **(A),** the oral (*O*), pharyngeal (*P*), and tracheal (*T*) axes pass through three divergent planes **(B)**. A folded sheet or towel placed under the occiput of the head **(C)** aligns the *P* and *T* axes **(D)**. Extension of the atlantooccipital joint **(E)** results in alignment of all three axes **(F)**.

of only a few patients are intubated more easily when placed in the sniffing position compared with simple head extension, the current routine application of the sniffing position appears to be the best clinical practice.[156]

Laryngoscopy can be performed while the child is awake, anesthetized, and breathing spontaneously, or anesthetized and paralyzed. Most tracheal intubations in children who are awake are performed in neonates, an approach that is not usually feasible or humane in older awake and uncooperative children. Awake intubation in the neonate is generally well tolerated if it is performed smoothly and rapidly; however, an international consensus group and others have cautioned against this practice unless intravenous (IV) access is not available or there is a life-threatening situation.[157–150] Preterm and term infants are better managed with sedation and paralysis to minimize adverse hemodynamic responses.[161–165]

Selection of Laryngoscope Blade

A straight blade has been adopted for use in infants and young children for decades because it was thought to elevate the base of the tongue to expose the glottic opening better than a curved blade. However, the laryngeal view with the Miller blade was never compared with the curved blade. Recently, two studies demonstrated in young children younger than 2 years of age that both the Miller and Macintosh blades provide excellent laryngeal views if the former is used to elevate the epiglottis, and the latter to elevate the tongue. However, if the Macintosh blade is used to lift the epiglottis, the laryngeal view is inferior because the curve of the Macintosh blade partially obscures the view of the vocal cords.[166,167] The blade size chosen depends on the age and body mass of the child and the preference of the anesthesiologist; Table 14.1 presents the ranges commonly used.

Endotracheal Tubes

All materials used in the manufacture of ETTs have been subjected to rabbit muscle implantation testing in accordance with the standards promulgated by the Z79 Committee of American National Standards Institute since 1967.[168] If the material causes an inflammatory response in the rabbits, it cannot be used in the manufacture of ETTs. This has resulted in the elimination of organometallic constituents, which were used in the manufacture of red rubber ETTs.

Selection of the proper size of an ETT depends on the individual child.[169] The only size requirement for a manufacturer is a standardized inner diameter (ID). The external (outer) diameter (OD) varies among manufacturers, depending on the material from which the ETT is constructed. This diversity in OD mandates checking for proper ETT size and leakage around the tube. An

appropriately sized uncuffed ETT may be approximated according to the child's age and weight (Table 14.2).[170]

ETTs sized 0.5-mm ID greater or less than the anticipated size should be available because of variability in the size of the airway. Use of the diameter of the terminal phalanx of either the second or fifth digit is unreliable.[171] Children with Down syndrome often require an ETT with a diameter smaller than that predicted by the child's age,[172] whereas children with cardiac disease often require a larger size cuffed ETT than that predicted by the child's age.[173] There are several means to identify whether the tube size is adequate. One holds that after using a standard formula to estimate the tube diameter, if the tube passes the subglottic region without meeting resistance, the tube size is not excessive. After the tube is stabilized, a sustained inflation pressure of 20 to 25 cm H_2O (short-term intubation perhaps as high as 35 cm H_2O) should be applied to detect an audible or auscultated air leak over the glottis. If no leak is detected, the ETT size is excessive and it should be exchanged for one with an ID 0.5 mm smaller. An air leak at this pressure is recommended because it is believed to approximate the capillary pressure of the adult tracheal mucosa. If lateral wall pressure exceeds this amount, ischemic damage to the subglottic mucosa may occur.[174] Be aware, however, that if the trachea has been intubated without neuromuscular blockade, laryngospasm around the ETT may prevent any gas leak and mimic a tight-fitting ETT.[175] If such a situation is suspected, the anesthetic depth should be increased before auscultating for an air leak. Changes in head position may also increase or decrease the leak.[175] These maneuvers are important for making the occasional diagnosis of unrecognized subglottic stenosis (see Fig. 37.8, and Video 14.1).

Traditional teaching has advocated the use of uncuffed ETTs for children younger than 8 years because an uncuffed ETT with an air leak exerts minimal pressure on the internal surface of the circular cricoid cartilage and thus poses potentially less risk for postextubation edema (croup).[170,174,176] An uncuffed ETT also allows insertion of a tube with a larger ID, resulting in less airway resistance, although this is only relevant for a spontaneously breathing child.[177] However, more recent clinical data and clinical practice have challenged these assumptions[178–187]; a number of studies demonstrated no differences in the incidence of postextubation complications after cuffed and uncuffed tubes when used for anesthesia,[178,183,188] except possibly with Microcuff tubes in neonates and former preterm infants.[189,190] Cited advantages of cuffed ETTs include decreased numbers of laryngoscopies and intubations to determine the appropriate size for the ETT, reduced

TABLE 14.1	Laryngoscope Blades Used in Infants and Children		
	BLADE SIZE		
Age	Miller	Wis-Hipple	Macintosh
Preterm	0	—	—
Neonate	0	—	—
Neonate–2 years	1	—	—
2–6 years	—	1.5	1 or 2
6–10 years	2	—	2
>10 years	2 or 3	—	3

TABLE 14.2	Endotracheal Tubes (ETTs) Used in Infants and Children	
Age	Size (mm ID) Uncuffed	Size (mm ID) Cuffed
Preterm		
1000 g	2.5	
1000–2500 g	3.0	
Neonate–6 months	3.0–3.5	3.0–3.5[a]
6 months–1 year	3.5–4.0	3.0–4.0
1–2 years	4.0–5.0	3.5–4.5
>2 years	(Age in years + 16)/4	(Age in years/4) +3

[a]In some neonates, a cuffed ETT may not have a leak below 30 cm H_2O, and therefore an uncuffed ETT may be more appropriate.
ID, inner diameter.

subglottic pressure, reduced operating room pollution and costs of anesthetic agents, decreased risk of aspiration, accurate control of carbon dioxide tension (PCO_2), better ability to accurately measure the sophisticated physiologic respiratory functions of modern ventilators, absolute ability to deliver increased airway pressures in children with restrictive lung disease, the ability to control cuff pressure, and no or minimal increased risk of postextubation stridor.[178-184,188,191-193]

A drawback of cuffed tubes is the greater variability in functional OD compared with uncuffed tubes because of differences in cuff shape, size, and inflation characteristics.[194] In general, if a cuffed ETT is inserted, an ETT with a smaller ID should be selected to compensate for the ETT cuff. One study found a 99% rate of appropriate cuffed tube size selection for full-term infants through children 8 years of age using the following formula[183]:

$$ID (mm) = (age [years]/4) + 3$$

To overcome the shortcomings of the many pediatric cuffed tubes, the Microcuff ETT (Microcuff, PET, I-MPEDC; Microcuff GmbH, Weinheim, Germany, distributed by Kimberly-Clark USA) was designed with a high-volume/low-pressure elliptically shaped cuff that is more distally placed along the shaft of the ETT to better accommodate the anatomy of the airway in infants and children (Fig. 14.15).[195] The ultrathin polyurethane cuff (10 µm) allows tracheal sealing at low pressures and provides a uniform and complete surface contact with minimal formation of cuff folds.[185,191,195-198] At 20 cm H_2O inflation pressure, the

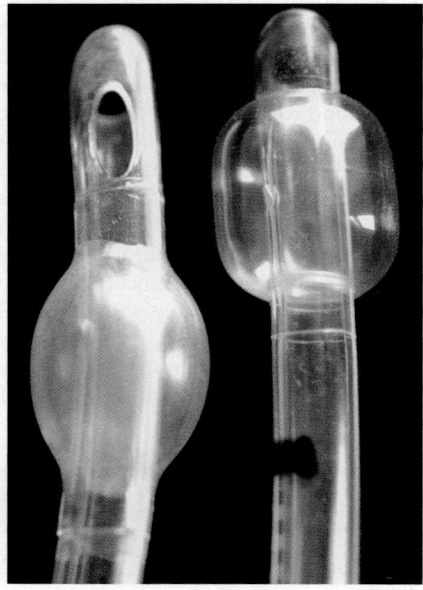

FIGURE 14.15 The MICROCUFF endotracheal tube (MICROCUFF, PET, I-MPEDC; MICROCUFF GmbH, Weinheim, Germany) (*right*) is designed with an ultrathin polyurethane (10 µm) high-volume/low-pressure cuff that has a more distal position along the shaft of the tube to better accommodate pediatric anatomy. In contrast to more traditional pediatric cuffed endotracheal tubes (*left*), the elimination of a Murphy eye allows a more distal position of the upper cuff border. The location of the cuff on the shaft of the tube helps to ensure cuff placement below the subglottis; perhaps with the advantage of less risk for endobronchial intubation or intralaryngeal cuff position. An anatomically based depth mark on the surface of the tube helps to guide correct placement.

cuffs have a cross-sectional cuff area of approximately 150% of the maximal internal tracheal cross-sectional area. Uninflated, the cuff adds only a minimal amount to the OD of the ETT. Shortened cuffs and the elimination of a Murphy eye allow a more distal position of the cuff, thereby theoretically reducing the risk of pressure being applied to the cricoid ring and adjacent mucosa.[199] The location of the cuff on the shaft of the tube helps to ensure cuff placement below the subglottis, perhaps with the advantage of less risk for endobronchial intubation or intralaryngeal cuff position. An anatomically based depth mark on the surface of the tube helps to guide correct placement. A report of neonatal stridor after Microcuff use in a neonatal intensive care unit has suggested previously unknown complications with this device.[190]

An investigation of this specially designed ETT for children used the following guidelines to select cuffed ETT sizes[191]:
- For children ≥2 years, ID (mm) = (age [years]/4) + 3.5
- For children 1 to 2 years of age, ID 3.5 mm
- For neonates ≥3 kg and infants ≤1 year, ID 3.0 mm

Use of these formulas resulted in the need to reintubate to change tube size in 1.6% of children (6/500).[191] The incidence of postintubation croup was 0.4% (2/500 children). In a randomized, multicenter study of 2246 young children (mean age, 1.9 years), investigators reported similar findings for cuffed (Microcuff) and uncuffed tubes: postextubation stridor, 4.4% and 4.7%, respectively, and ETT exchange, 2.1% and 30.8%.[193] However, in a cost/benefit analysis of the Microcuff ETT (three to six times that of standard ETTs), the reduction in anesthetic cost offset the cost of the Microcuff ETT.[192]

As a rule, if a cuffed ETT is chosen, the cuff should be inflated to the minimal pressure that seals the air leak; with the Microcuff ETT, this is approximately 10.6 cm H_2O.[191,193,200,201] The cuff pressure should be reevaluated throughout the anesthetic if nitrous oxide is used because the latter may diffuse into the cuff, and with the Microcuff ETT, the ultrathin-walled cuff has greater permeability for nitrous oxide than conventional ETTs. The net effect may be excessive tracheal mucosal pressure, although this may be offset in part, as the cuff with Microcuff ETTs seals at a low pressure, ~10 cm H_2O.[200-202] The time interval to reach 25 cm H_2O cuff pressure with the Microcuff ETT is greater than with conventional cuffed ETT.[203] Routinely checking cuff pressure throughout the use of the anesthetic or filling the cuff with nitrous oxide is recommended.[204] A pressure relief valve that can be connected to the pilot balloon of a cuffed ETT to limit cuff pressures to 20 cm H_2O when nitrous oxide is used has been described.[205]

Endotracheal Tube Insertion Distance

The length of the trachea (vocal cords to carina) in neonates and children up to 1 year of age varies from 5 to 9 cm.[48] In most infants 3 months to 1 year of age, if the 10-cm mark of the ETT is placed at the alveolar ridge, the tip of the tube rests above the carina. In preterm and full-term infants, the distance is less. In children 2 years old, 12 cm is usually appropriate. An easy way to remember these lengths is **10** for a newborn, **11** for a 1-year old, and **12** for a 2-year old. After 2 years of age, the correct length of insertion (in centimeters) for oral intubation may be approximated by formulas based on age or weight (Table 14.3)[206-209]:

$$[Age (years)/2] + 12$$
$$[Weight (kg)/5] + 12$$
$$ID of ETT \times 3$$

TABLE 14.3	Distance for Insertion of an Oral Endotracheal Tube by Patient Age

Age	Approximate Distance of Insertion (cm) Even With Alveolar Ridge
Preterm <1000 g	6–7
Preterm 1000–2000 g	7–9
Term newborn	9–10
1 year	11–12
2 years	12–13
6 years	15–16
10 years	17–18
16 years	18–20
20 years	20–22

Some practitioners suggest using anatomic markers to choose the appropriate depth for the tube in the trachea in neonates.[210,211] An advantage of anatomic measurements is that the infant's weight may not be available immediately after birth or in sick neonates who present to the emergency department with urgent respiratory or cardiac compromise. One study that used chest radiographs to evaluate final ETT position determined that the length of the foot was as accurate as weight-based formulas to determine the depth of insertion for a nasotracheal tube (44% vs. 56% rate of optimal placement and 83% vs. 72% satisfactory placement).[211] Alternatively, the nasal-tragus length (the distance from the base of the nasal septum to the tip of the tragus) or the sternal length (the distance from the suprasternal notch to the tip of the xiphoid process) predicted the depth of insertion of the ETT. Either distance plus 1 cm accurately estimated oral ETT tube insertion distance; either distance plus 2 cm accurately estimated nasotracheal tube insertion distance.[210] Both measurements compared favorably with weight-based formulas when tube position was verified by chest radiography. It has also been suggested that a body surface area formula optimizes the position of the ETT. Chest radiography was used in that study to confirm the position of the ETT. The results showed that the depth of the tracheal tube had to be corrected in 20.3% of intubations when body surface area diagrams were used compared with 37% of intubations when an age-based formula was used for children older than 1 year of age and a weight-based formula was used for infants younger than 1 year of age.[212]

Preformed tracheal tube length often poorly matches the child's anatomy.[213] Seven brands of oral preformed ETTs were compared for the same size ID tube; the distance from the bend to the tip varied by 0 to 1 cm for cuffed tubes but 0 to 4 cm for uncuffed tubes. The greatest gap between cuffed and uncuffed oral preformed ETTs of the same size for a specific manufacturer was 2 to 3 cm for Portex (Smiths Medical, St. Paul, MN) sizes between 5.0 and 7.5 mm ID. Of greater concern was the variability in the distance from the bend to the tip of preformed nasal tubes; cuffed tubes varied by 0 to 5.5 cm and uncuffed varied from 2 to 9 cm (bend to tip) among manufacturers. The gap between cuffed and uncuffed nasal preformed ETTs of the same size ETT between 4.0 and 7.5 mm ID was 5 to 9 cm for all manufacturers. Thus the risk for endobronchial intubation varies substantively among manufacturers, and is greatest with nasal ETTs if they are inserted to the bend; some brands may be unsuitable for use in children.

After the ETT has been inserted and the first strip of adhesive tape has been applied to secure it, one must observe for symmetry of chest expansion and auscultate for equality of breath sounds in the axillae and apices (not on the anterior chest wall). The anterior chest wall in the child is not used to verify tracheal intubation because breath sounds may reverberate across the precordium in small children, obscuring the diagnosis of an endobronchial intubation. A CO_2 monitor confirms intratracheal positioning but does not confirm that the tip of the ETT is not in an endobronchial position. A capnogram that diminishes during the first few breaths suggests an esophageal intubation. Unexpectedly increased airway pressures, persistent desaturation, and asymmetrical chest wall movement all suggest an endobronchial intubation. Visible humidity on the walls of the ETT during expiration also confirms tracheal placement, but the humidity may not be visible in younger infants. It is also important to auscultate over the stomach and to observe for desaturation or cyanosis. Once a satisfactory position is achieved, a second strip of tape ensures secure fixation (Fig. 14.16).

We have observed a number of children whose ETT moved into a mainstem bronchus after initial correct position during repositioning for the surgical procedure; this manifested as a slight but persistent decrease in oxygen saturation (e.g., from 100% to a range of 93% to 95%). Several studies have demonstrated that simple flexion or extension of the neck can move the ETT sufficiently to cause an endobronchial intubation or dislodgment of the tube from the trachea, respectively.[214–216] *When a small but persistent decrease in oxygen saturation is noted, rather than increase the inspired oxygen concentration (FIO_2), one must first investigate the cause and reassess the position of the ETT.*[217]

Complications of Tracheal Intubation
Postintubation Croup
Perioperative postintubation croup (also referred to as postextubation croup) occurs in 0.1% to 1% of children.[184,191,218,219] Factors associated with increased risk of croup include an ETT with an OD that is too large for the child's airway (no leak at >25 cm H_2O pressure or resistance at the time of insertion), changes in position during the procedure, a position other than supine, repeated attempts at intubation, traumatic intubation, patient age between 1 and 4 years, duration of surgery greater than 1 hour, coughing on the ETT, and previous history of croup.[203,204] Concurrent upper respiratory infection has been variously reported as a risk factor and as unrelated.[99,219]

Treatment of postintubation croup consists of nebulized epinephrine and dexamethasone. The rationale for this treatment is based primarily on experience with the treatment of infectious croup.[220–229] Caution should be exercised when translating treatments from one type of croup to another, because the two types of croup are not identical processes, and efficacy of the interventions for the treatment of postintubation croup has not been proved in controlled trials.[230] Studies that examined the effect of dexamethasone given before extubation in children with prolonged intubation are conflicting.[231–234] Methylprednisolone given intramuscularly for the same indication has been reported to reduce postintubation stridor.[235]

Laryngotracheal (Subglottic) Stenosis
The frequency of subglottic stenosis has decreased over the past several decades to its current level of 0% to 2%.[236] Ninety percent of acquired subglottic stenoses are the result of tracheal intubation, particularly prolonged intubation (see Videos 14.1 and 14.5).[237–242] The incidence of subglottic stenosis after prolonged intubation in preterm neonates is reduced because the cricoid cartilage is relatively immature. At this age, the cartilage structure is hypercellular and

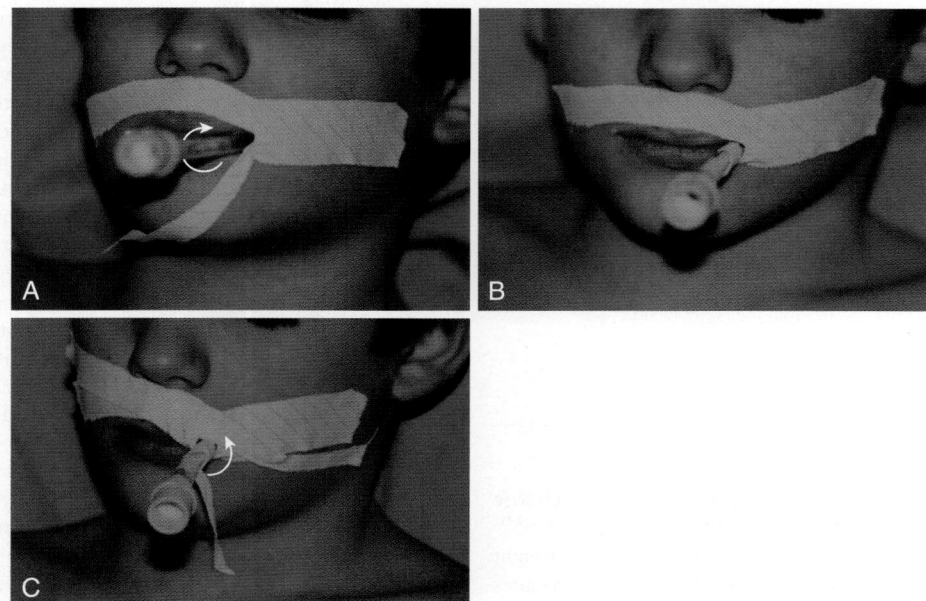

FIGURE 14.16 Securing the endotracheal tube (ETT). After insertion of the oral ETT and examination for proper position, the area between the nose and upper lip and both cheeks is coated with tincture of benzoin. **A,** After the benzoin is dry, tape that has been split up the middle is applied to the cheek, and the ETT is placed at the division of the split tape. **B,** One half is wrapped circumferentially around the tube, and the other half is applied to the space above the upper lip. **C,** A second piece of tape is applied in similar fashion from the opposite direction. A nasal ETT may also be secured with this technique.

the matrix has a large fluid content, making the structures more resilient and less susceptible to ischemic injury.[243]

The pathogenesis of acquired subglottic stenosis is ischemic injury secondary to lateral wall pressure from the ETT. Ischemia results in edema, necrosis, and ulcerations of the mucosa. Secondary infection results in exposure of the cartilage. Within 48 hours, granulation tissue begins to form within these ulcerations. Ultimately, scar tissue forms, resulting in narrowing of the airway (Fig. 14.17).[244-246] Specimens obtained from partial cricotracheal resection in children were found to have severe and sclerotic scarring with squamous metaplasia of the epithelium, loss of glands and elastic mantle fibers (tunica elastica), and dilation of the remaining glands with formation of cysts.[246] Also, the cricoid cartilage was affected on the internal and external side, with irreversible loss of perichondrium on the inside and resorption by macrophages of cartilage on both sides.[228]

Factors that predispose to subglottic stenosis include use of an ETT that is too large, laryngeal trauma (e.g., traumatic intubation, chemical or thermal inhalation, external trauma, surgical trauma, gastric reflux),[247-249] prolonged intubation (particularly greater than 25 days), repeated intubation,[250] hypotension, sepsis and infection, chronic illness, and chronic inflammatory disease.[240,251,252]

LARYNGEAL MASK AIRWAY

The LMA has become a standard alternative for airway management during general anesthesia.[253-258] A number of types of LMAs (also known as supraglottic devices [SGAs]) have been introduced into practice since the development of the original LMA, which is now referred to as the LMA Classic (Fig. 14.18).[259] These new types include the disposable LMA Unique, the ProSeal LMA (PLMA, described later), the Flexible LMA, the LMA Supreme

(discussed later), and the intubating LMA Fastrach. The Fastrach is available only in sizes 3, 4, and 5 and is described for use in children who weigh more than 40 kg.[260] The LMA Classic is made of medical-grade silicone and consists of a large-bore tubular structure (barrel) with a 15-mm adapter at its proximal end and an elliptical, mask-like device that fits over the laryngeal inlet at its distal end. All masks are inflated by means of a valved pilot tube and balloon. The LMA Classic and the PLMA can be sterilized for reuse up to 40 times. The LMA Classic is available in eight sizes. Guidelines for selecting the appropriate mask for children are based on weight (see Table 14.4). A number of other manufacturers have developed similar devices; however, there is a dearth of comparative data available for children,[259] although there are numerous studies comparing one device with another.[261-266]

The LMA has been used for many different surgeries but it was developed to replace the face mask in adults during maintenance of anesthesia.[267] Some suggest that an LMA can be used for any case in which spontaneous ventilation is appropriate or any case that might reasonably be managed by face mask. The LMA offers several advantages over the face mask including that it frees the anesthesiologist's hands for other tasks and that it may be associated with less operating room pollution compared with mask ventilation.[268,269] The use of controlled ventilation with the LMA Classic has also been described.[270,271] However, this practice is more controversial than its use in spontaneously breathing children because of the risk of insufflation of ventilated gas into the stomach and resultant regurgitation.[272-274] Insufflation of gas into the stomach is more likely to occur when high ventilation pressures are used or required (i.e., pressures greater than the pressure that produces an audible air leak).[270,275] Clinically

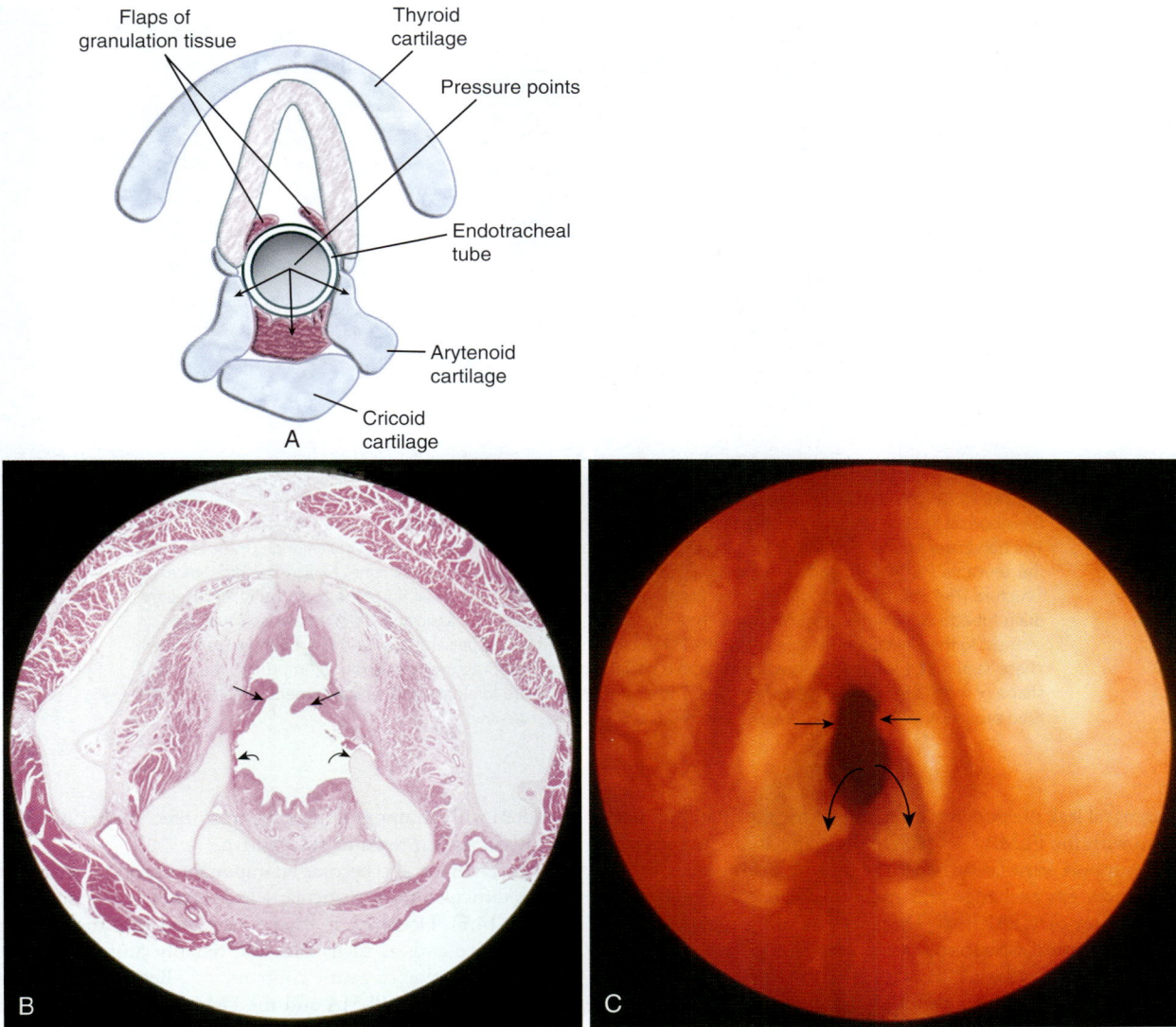

FIGURE 14.17 The pathogenesis of intubation injuries. **A,** Schemata of a cross section through the glottis. Pressure necrosis causes ulcerations at the vocal processes of the arytenoids with exposed cartilage. Flaps of granulation tissue are present anterior to these ulcerations. **B,** Cross section of the glottis at this same level; *straight arrows* indicate flaps of granulation tissue, and *curved arrows* indicate the absence of mucosa and ulcerations with exposed cartilage on the vocal processes of the arytenoids. **C,** Intubation injury to a 2-month-old infant; *straight arrows* indicate granulation tissue, and *curved arrows* indicate an area of ulcerations (*white area*). The most severe area of injury is usually at the level of the cricoid cartilage, resulting in subglottic stenosis. (Reproduced with permission from Holinger LD, Lusk RP, Green CG. *Pediatric Laryngology and Bronchoesophagology.* Philadelphia: Lippincott-Raven; 1997.)

undetected LMA Classic malpositioning has been reported to be a significant risk factor for gastric air insufflation in children between 3 and 11 years of age undergoing positive-pressure ventilation, especially at peak inspiratory pressures greater than 17 cm H$_2$O.[276] Controlled ventilation with an LMA (with or without neuromuscular blockade) is easily accomplished and less likely to cause adverse events when the seal is relatively good and the lung inflation pressures are less than 17 cm H$_2$O.

The PLMA was designed to improve sealing pressures and to provide a conduit for evacuation of stomach contents and comes is seven sizes; these features make it more appealing for use with positive-pressure ventilation.[277] In sizes 3 and larger,

there is a second dorsal cuff to increase the seal pressure of the glottic mask. The dorsal and ventral cuffs communicate, allowing simultaneous inflation by a single pilot balloon. In the smaller sizes, there is no second dorsal cuff but the profile of the mask has been altered to improve sealing. The PLMA is easy to insert, allows greater airway pressures with positive-pressure ventilation, and better protects against gastric insufflation.[278,279] A number of studies support the efficacy of the PLMA in children for both spontaneous and controlled ventilation.[279–283] In children, the PLMA and the LMA Classic are similarly easy to insert, have their proper position confirmed by fiberoptic visualization, and yield similar frequencies of mucosal trauma. The advantage is that

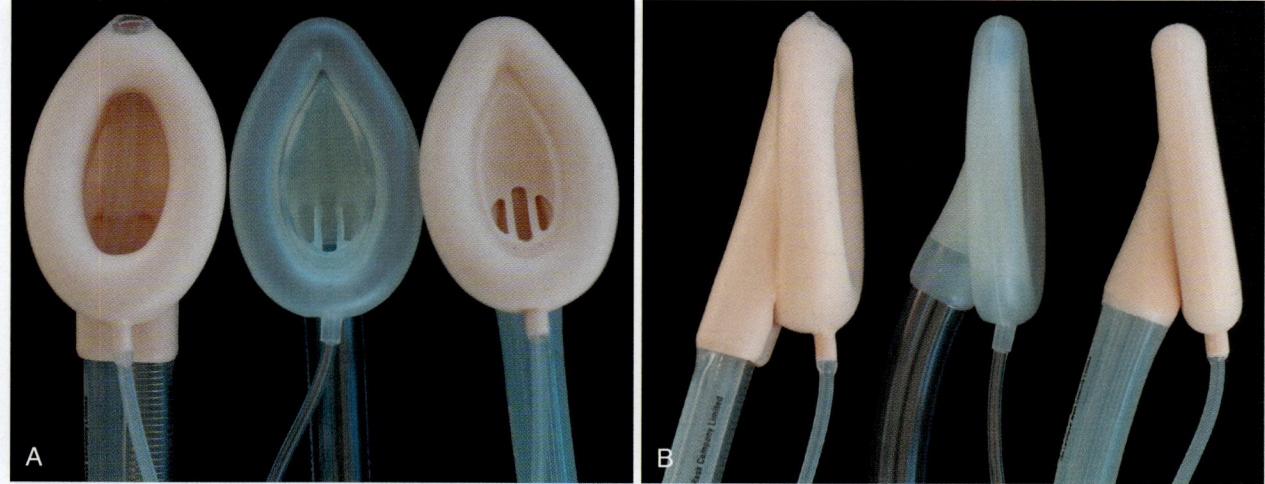

FIGURE 14.18 Three types of laryngeal mask airway (LMA) are available in pediatric sizes: the reusable LMA Classic, the disposable LMA Unique, and the ProSeal LMA (PLMA). Displayed are pediatric size 2 LMAs of each type. **A,** The transparent material of the disposable LMA Unique (*center*) is medical-grade polyvinylchloride (PVC), whereas the reusable PLMA (*left*) and LMA Classic (*right*) are made of medical-grade silicone. Notice the differences in structure. The drainage tube outlet of the PLMA can be seen at the most distal tip of the cuff. The PLMA uses the drain tube to elevate the epiglottis away from the larynx, whereas the Classic and Unique have aperture bars. In contrast to the Classic and Unique LMAs, the PLMA cuff is softer, has a special shape, and has a deeper mask bowl. These features of the PLMA allow for improved sealing for positive-pressure ventilation. **B,** In profile, the distinct shape of the PLMA (*left*) can be appreciated. The dual-tube structure (drainage and airway lumens) creates a larger tube profile (**A** *left*) that incorporates a bite block and improves stability.

oropharyngeal leak pressure is greater and gastric insufflation is less common with the PLMA.[279–283] In children, the ability to provide pressure support ventilation with the PLMA during anesthesia also improves gas exchange and reduces WOB compared with the application of CPAP.[284,285] The greater sealing pressure may also protect against aspiration, as reported in a 5-year-old child after inguinal hernia repair.[286] Pediatric gastroscopy is quicker and involves fewer airway complications when performed around the PLMA compared with nasal cannulas and with a conventional approach using an anesthetic technique in which children breathed a sevoflurane-air-oxygen mixture spontaneously with 1-mg/kg IV boluses of propofol.[287]

Flexible diagnostic and therapeutic bronchoscopy, radiation therapy, radiologic procedures, ear/nose/throat surgeries, and ophthalmologic procedures are the most commonly described pediatric indications for the LMA.[258,267,288–291] An advantage of the LMA for securing the airway in ophthalmologic surgery is that it is associated with no increase in intraocular pressure, in contrast to tracheal intubation.[292] The advantage of the LMA for diagnostic and therapeutic flexible bronchoscopy is that it provides a conduit for oxygenation and ventilation while allowing a larger bronchoscope to be used than can be passed through an age-appropriate ETT.[289,290,293,294] It also allows visualization and evaluation of the laryngeal structures. Some LMAs may provide better bronchoscopic conditions than others owing to their material or preconfigured shape.[295] For children who require frequent anesthetics over a brief period, as in radiation therapy, the LMA provides a secure airway without the trauma of repeated intubation.[258] The LMA has also been advocated for use in place of intubation in children who are at increased risk for bronchial airway reactivity (e.g., upper respiratory tract infection, history of reactive airway disease).[296–299] However, caution is required in

children with an upper respiratory tract infection because the risk of laryngospasm remains substantive.

The LMA has also become an important tool in the management of the difficult airway, particularly in neonates (see later discussion) (Video 14.6). However, it should be noted that the LMA is an SGA device and, as such, does not reliably protect against pulmonary aspiration of gastric contents.[272–274] Because of their gastric access lumens, the PLMA and the LMA Supreme may be better alternatives in this setting, but formal study in children has not been performed.[300]

The recommended insertion technique for the LMA is the same for children as for adults (Video 14.6). The correct technique mimics deglutition or swallowing of food.[301] The cuff is completely deflated, and the posterior surface of the mask is well lubricated. These actions mimic lubrication of a food bolus with saliva and formation of a soft, flattened, wedge-shaped bolus. The child is placed in the age-appropriate intubating position. Induction may proceed by inhalation of halothane or sevoflurane or by IV propofol (3 to 5 mg/kg).[267,302] The nondominant hand is used to extend the head and flex the neck (sniffing position). This head position mimics the elevation of the larynx, neck flexion, and head extension that occurs with swallowing. The LMA is inserted with the mask aperture facing anteriorly (toward the tongue). The index finger of the insertion hand should be placed in the cleft between the mask and the barrel. With the index finger, the LMA is pushed upward and backward, toward the top of the child's head. This flattens the mask against the palate. Continued backward pressure (toward the top of the child's head) guides the LMA along the palate and down into the upper esophageal sphincter. It is essential that pressure be applied to force the LMA against the roof of the mouth. The mask is advanced along the palate until some resistance is felt. These actions mimic the propulsion of a food bolus into

TABLE 14.4 Size Selection and Recommended Cuff Volumes for the Laryngeal Mask Airway

Mask Size	Patient's Weight	Maximum Cuff Volume (mL)	Largest Endotracheal Tube (ID, mm), LMA Classic	Largest Endotracheal Tube (ID, mm), LMA Unique[a]	Largest Endotracheal Tube (ID, mm), ProSeal LMA[a]
1	Neonate/infants up to 5 kg	4	3.5	3.5	N/A
1.5	Infants 5–10 kg	7	4.0	4.0	4.0, some manufacturers 3.5
2	Infants/children 10–20 kg	10	4.5	4.5	4.0
2.5	Children 20–30 kg	14	5.0	5	4.5
3	Children/small adults 30–50 kg	20	6.0, cuffed	5.0, cuffed	5.0
4	Adolescents/adults 50–70 kg	30	6.0, cuffed	5.5, cuffed	5.0, cuffed
5	Large adolescents/adults 70–100 kg	40	7.0, cuffed	6.0, cuffed	6.0, cuffed
6	Anyone >100 kg	50	7.0 cuffed	N/A	N/A

[a]These sizes differ from the manufacturers' recommendations but have been found by the authors to be the better alternatives to ensure easy passage of the endotracheal tube through the LMA. In some cases the tubes listed are smaller; in some cases a cuffed alternative is given as an option rather than an uncuffed tube.
ID, inner diameter; LMA, laryngeal mask airway; N/A, not applicable.

the hypopharynx caused by tongue pressure, first upward and backward, then downward in an arc. When resistance is felt, air is injected into the mask cuff (see Table 14.4 for size recommendations and maximum recommended inflation volumes).

Inflation of the cuff causes the end of the airway to move out of the mouth about 1 cm and forms a loose seal around the esophageal inlet, thereby directing gas flow into the trachea. *If no outward movement is observed with inflation of the mask, the LMA may not be properly positioned.* Proper position can be ascertained further by auscultation of breath sounds, movement of the anesthesia bag, measure of expired CO_2, the ability to provide gentle assisted ventilation, and, if necessary, by direct visualization with rigid or fiberoptic laryngoscopy. If the lungs cannot be gently ventilated (peak airway pressure <20 cm H_2O) or no breath sounds are heard, the LMA must be immediately removed because it has not been properly positioned, or the child's airway might be obstructed. After proper placement is confirmed, the LMA may be secured with tape and a soft bite block (e.g., a rolled gauze) inserted.

Several reports claim that when the traditional insertion technique is used in children, the LMA frequently hangs up in the posterior pharynx, making proper positioning difficult.[303,304] Therefore other insertion techniques have been described. The rotational or reverse technique for children has been advocated to be simpler and more successful than the traditional placement technique.[305] The LMA is placed in the mouth with the cuff facing the hard palate (the opposite of the traditional technique). It is then advanced and rotated into position simultaneously (Video 14.7).[303,304,306] A partial mask inflation technique has also been advocated as more successful than the traditional (mask-deflated) technique.[306–309] The LMA is left partially inflated to smooth the edges of the mask and then is inserted in the usual manner,[307,308] or in a lateral manner and then rotated and advanced,[309] or with a complete 180-degree rotation.[306] For placement of the PLMA, the rotational technique was found to have no advantage over the standard technique in children.[310] A jaw thrust maneuver and the use of a rigid laryngoscope have also been advocated to assist in placement of the LMA Classic.[311]

Regardless of insertion method, the most common cause of failure is use of a wrong size LMA. An LMA that is too large will not pass beyond the posterior pharynx. An LMA that is too small will pass easily but may not seal against the laryngeal inlet. Another common mistake when using the traditional insertion method is

to try to press the LMA *down* into the pharynx. Pressure should be directed *back*, toward the pharyngeal wall, so that the airway will follow the natural curve of the pharynx and seat correctly in the esophageal sphincter without kinking. Attempting to place the LMA when the child is inadequately anesthetized may make advancement impossible or result in laryngospasm.

LMA use can result in injuries to upper airway structures[312–314] and in damage to the recurrent laryngeal[315] or the hypoglossal nerves.[316] The incidence of sore throat may be equal to or greater than that seen with tracheal intubation.[317–319] LMA use in infants requires special caution. A review of the use of the size 1 LMA in 50 infants found that the LMA sometimes migrated over time, even after apparent correct initial placement; delayed airway obstruction occurred in 12 infants after apparent successful placement.[320] Vigilance is required to prevent loss of the airway.

Evaluation of a large dataset determined factors associated with LMA failure in children.[321,322] They included prolonged surgical duration, procedures of the head and neck, non-outpatient admission status, congenital airway abnormalities, and a category the authors called "patient transport," which consisted primarily of moving a patient's position or anesthetizing location with the laryngeal mask in situ.

LMA placement has been used successfully for neonatal resuscitation[323–325]; it may be an easier skill to acquire than bag-and-mask ventilation.[326,327] Given the recognition[328] that chest compressions are the most important factor in successful outcomes after cardiac arrest and the need to avoid interrupting compressions during cardiopulmonary resuscitation, the LMA may assume a greater role in airway management in cardiac arrest in the neonate.[329] The LMA has also been used to deliver surfactant to neonates with respiratory distress syndrome,[330] for longer-term intensive care management of neonates with difficult airways,[331–333] and for intrahospital transport of neonates with difficult airways.[334]

The LMA Fastrach was specifically designed to allow the blind passage of an ETT in an emergent situation in which direct laryngoscopy is not possible or in patients with cervical spine immobilization.[210,335–337] This is a rigid device with a fixed angulation designed primarily for adults (available in sizes 3, 4, and 5). It requires special, flexible ETTs with an ID of 6.0 to 8.0 mm.

The timing for removal of the LMA in children is controversial. Both "awake" and "deep" removal has been advocated.[338–343] Awake removal ensures return of protective reflexes but with the attendant problems of airway reactivity. Deep removal avoids excessive airway reactivity and potential laryngospasm but may increase the risk of aspiration or airway obstruction (or both) as the child emerges from anesthesia later in the recovery room. One author suggested leaving the cuff inflated until the child begins swallowing or is able to open the mouth on command as a means for reducing the potential for laryngospasm. The proposed mechanism is that secretions are swept away from the larynx, reducing the stimulus for laryngospasm.[343] Lubrication of the cuff with 2% lidocaine jelly or the addition of an intravenously administered opioid to the anesthetic may reduce coughing and laryngeal stimulation on emergence.[307]

The LMA Supreme is a single-use, curved laryngeal mask with an elliptical airway tube and an integrated drain tube that extends to the tip of the mask bowl. The proximal end of the airway tube consists of a bite block, which should lie between the teeth when the mask is properly positioned. A fixation tab allows the mask to be secured to the face (Fig. 14.19). The deflated mask is held at the fixation tab and is inserted along the palate into the pharynx in a fashion similar to that used for the LMA Classic. Once in place, the cuff is inflated and the mask position is confirmed to be appropriate with the use of simple confirmatory tests. An appropriately positioned mask forms a leak-free seal with the glottis, and the mask tip is embedded in the upper esophageal sphincter. A simple test to confirm the position of the mask is the suprasternal notch test, wherein a small amount of water-soluble lubricant is applied to the drain tube of the airway. Application of slight pressure in the suprasternal notch should result in a slight up-and-down movement of the applied lubricant on the drain tube. This confirms that the drain tube is contiguous with and adequately sealed in the upper esophageal sphincter. The ability to easily place a gastric tube through the drain tube further confirms correct positioning of the airway. Suction should not be applied to the gastric tube until it has been advanced into the stomach; this prevents collapse of the drain tube and potential injury to the upper esophageal sphincter. The LMA Supreme is available in all pediatric sizes. A study comparing the LMA Supreme with the PLMA and the Classic LMAs in a neonatal manikin

model demonstrated higher inflation pressures and shorter insertion times with the LMA Supreme.[344] Although the LMA Supreme has been found to be effective in adult populations,[345-348] there are few evaluations of the pediatric sizes.[349,350]

OTHER SUPRAGLOTTIC AIRWAY DEVICES

Many other manufacturers have created their own versions of an SGA device similar to the LMA Classic. Some of these devices have design features that make them better conduits for tracheal intubation than the LMA Classic. Some have larger-diameter airway tubes that allow passage of larger (and cuffed) ETTs, lack glottic aperture bars (which can impede ETT advancement during an intubation attempt), and shorter airway tubes. Some devices also offer advantages in terms of cost.[351-353] Since there are now so many variations available, below we discuss only those SGAs with a different design and different mechanism for maintaining the airway.

The Laryngeal Tube

The Laryngeal Tube (LT; VBM Medizintechnik GmbH, Sulz, Germany) is designed to secure a patent airway during either spontaneous breathing or controlled ventilation. This device is available with a single lumen for ventilation only or with a double-lumen tube that also allows suction of gastric contents. This system seals the esophagus at the distal end with a small cuff attached at the tip (distal cuff), and a larger balloon cuff at the middle part of the tube (proximal cuff) stabilizes the device and blocks the oropharynx and nasopharynx. The two openings that lie between the cuffs are positioned so that the more distal opening faces the glottis. The cuffs are inflated through a single pilot tube and balloon, through which cuff pressure can be monitored. There are three black lines on the tube near a standard 15-mm connector that indicate adequate depth of insertion when aligned with the teeth. The nondisposable device is made of silicone (latex-free) and is reusable up to 50 times after sterilization in an autoclave. There are four variations: (1) standard single-lumen, reusable (LT); (2) single-lumen, disposable (LT-D); (3) double-lumen with drain tube, reusable (LT-suction II, or LTS II); and (4) double-lumen with drain tube, disposable (LTS-D) (E-Fig. 14.1).[354] It is available in six sizes, suitable for neonates up to large adults (Table 14.5).

The LT should be inserted while the child's head and neck are placed in the sniffing or neutral position. The tip of a well-lubricated LT is placed against the hard palate behind the upper incisors. The device is then slid down the center of the mouth until resistance is felt or the device is almost fully inserted. After connection to the anesthesia circuit, proper placement is confirmed by assessing ease of ventilation. Some adjustment (usually slight withdrawal) may be required to provide optimal ventilation. Care should be taken not to push the tongue backward into the posterior pharynx.

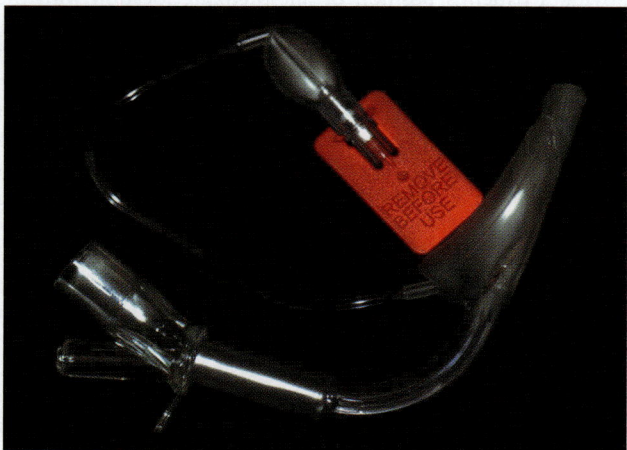

FIGURE 14.19 The LMA Supreme offers the advantages of a built-in suction port and a built-in bite block. This design may be particularly useful for tonsillectomy, because the ventilating tube is molded in a caudad direction and the bite block offers protection against distortion by a mouth gag or the child's biting on it during emergence.

TABLE 14.5	Size Selection and Recommended Cuff Volumes for the Laryngeal Tube		
Tube Size	**Body Weight or Height**	**Recommended Cuff Volume (mL)**	**Connector Color**
0 Newborn	<5 kg	10	Clear
1 Infants	5–12 kg	20	White
2 Children	12–25 kg	35	Green
3 Adults: small	<155 cm	60	Yellow
4 Adults: medium	155–180 cm	80	Red
5 Adults: large	>180 cm	90	Purple

Ease of insertion of the standard LT is reported to be comparable to that of the LMA Classic, although the LT may require more readjustments of its position to obtain a clear airway.[355,356] The incidence of complications with the two devices appears to be similar.[355] The LT may provide a better seal than the Classic LMA.[357] Compared with the PLMA, the LT may be less effective and more difficult to insert.[358-360] Although the LT-suction device may have similar success to the PLMA,[361] there are scant data in children.[362-367] An initial report of its use in children ages 2 to 12 years found a successful placement rate of 96% (77/80 children). Complications occurred in two children; one had laryngospasm that resolved with deepening of the anesthetic, and the other complained of mild difficulty with swallowing postoperatively.[363] A study comparing the LT with the LMA found it to be less effective for either spontaneous or assisted ventilation and for fiberoptic evaluation of the airway in children younger than 10 years of age.[362] A study of 70 children using sizes 0 to 3 reported failure to place the LT in 12% of children. Failures were caused by inability to ventilate, hypoxemia, gastric insufflation, cough, and laryngospasm or stridor, particularly for children weighing less than 10 kg; therefore, the LT was not recommended for children of this size.[364] Although the manufacturer states that a flexible fiberoptic bronchoscope (FOB) may be passed through the device, the openings are of insufficient size to permit passage of an ETT.

The Cobra Perilaryngeal Airway

The Cobra Perilaryngeal Airway (CobraPLA; Engineered Medical Systems, Indianapolis, IN) is a disposable SGA that is marketed for the same indications as the LMA Classic but creates a seal more cephalad in the hypopharynx using a cylindrical inflatable cuff. The distal end of the device sits over the larynx, but the distal end is not inflatable (E-Fig. 14.2).[352,368,369] An initial report that compared the CobraPLA with the LMA Classic reported that the insertion time, airway adequacy, and number of repositioning attempts were similar. Peak airway sealing pressure was significantly greater with the CobraPLA; the authors concluded that the CobraPLA has better airway sealing capabilities than the LMA Classic.[370] A more recent group of investigators studying the CobraPLA in adults raised concerns about both the design and the safety of this device, particularly during controlled ventilation. After studying 29 patients, investigations were suspended and later stopped after two cases of significant pulmonary aspiration occurred in patients while using the CobraPLA.[371] The device is available in eight sizes and can be used in infants as small as 2.5 kg (Table 14.6).[368] The distal grill has a long center slit that is specifically designed to allow passage of an FOB and ETT (the size 0.5 neonate CobraPLA allows easy passage of a 3.5 uncuffed ETT). In a pediatric study, the orientation of the larynx as viewed through the CobraPLA using video was obtained in 45 infants and children. An acceptable view of the airway was obtained in all subjects, but the laryngeal view was mostly obstructed or completely obstructed by the folding of the epiglottis over the glottic opening in 77% of children weighing less than 10 kg; a similar problem was encountered in approximately 80% of children managed with the LMA Classic.[372] The investigators suggested extra vigilance to prevent airway obstruction in small children. Also, because the grill bars of the CobraPLA were closely opposed to the epiglottis and supraglottic structures in almost all subjects, it was suggested that removal of the device in a deeper plane of anesthesia may minimize laryngeal stimulation. In a comparison of the Cobra device with the Air-Q (Cookgas LLC, Mercury Medical, Clearwater, FL) for fiberoptic intubation in children 1 to 6 years of age, the fiberoptic view was comparable with both devices. The researchers also reported that the time to achieve intubation was greater, the seal was better, and the incidence of bleeding and sore throat were greater with the Cobra.[373] Further study of this device in children, particularly infants, is needed to define its role compared with various LMAs.[374-376] The Cobra-PLUS has a distal curve for easier placement and a thermistor on the pharyngeal cuff to measure temperature that reliably trends intraoperative temperatures.[377]

The i-gel

The i-gel SGA (Intersurgical, Liverpool, NY) consists of a dual-channeled, noninflatable laryngeal mask made from a gel-like thermoplastic elastomer (Fig. 14.20). It has a built-in bite block and is available in sizes 1, 1.5, 2, 3, 4, and 5 (Table 14.7). One channel functions as the airway tube while the second channel exits at the tip of the device and provides gastric access when seated properly. The lubricated posterior surface of the i-gel is inserted along the palate into the posterior pharynx. An observational study in 50 children reported easy insertion in all patients with a mean leak pressure of 25 cm H_2O; gastric access was successfully obtained in all children.[378] When the i-gel was compared with the Ambu AuraOnce laryngeal mask (Ambu, Glen Burnie, MD), the leak pressures were greater and the times to insert the device greater with the i-gel. The authors noted a tendency for the i-gel to slide out and recommended taping it in place to prevent dislodgment intraoperatively.[379] When compared with the LMA Supreme, the airway leak pressures were greater with the i-gel.[380]

Summary

A variety of SGAs are currently available. Some are imitators of the LMA Classic but they are available at a reduced cost, whereas others are completely new designs. Many of the new devices have designs that assist in the management of normal and difficult airways in children, but there are insufficient data to clearly declare one device or one manufacturer superior to the other. Each institution must determine which devices fit best in its practice to assist in managing the pediatric airway.

Airway Management: The Abnormal Airway

CLASSIFYING THE ABNORMAL PEDIATRIC AIRWAY

It is important to recognize circumstances that may cause airway obstruction or difficult laryngoscopy. Conditions that predispose

TABLE 14.6	Suggested CobraPLA Size, Weight, Cuff Volume, and Endotracheal Tube Sizes			
Size	Patient Weight (kg)	Cuff Volume (mL)	Inner Diameter (ID, mm)	Maximal Size of Endotracheal Tube (mm ID)
0.5	>2.5	<8	5.0	3.0
1	>5	<10	6.0	4.5
1.5	>10	<25	6.0	4.5
2	>15	<40	10.5	6.5
3	>35	<65	10.5	6.5
4	>70	<70	12.5	8.0
5	>100	<85	12.5	8.0
6	>130	<85	12.5	8.0

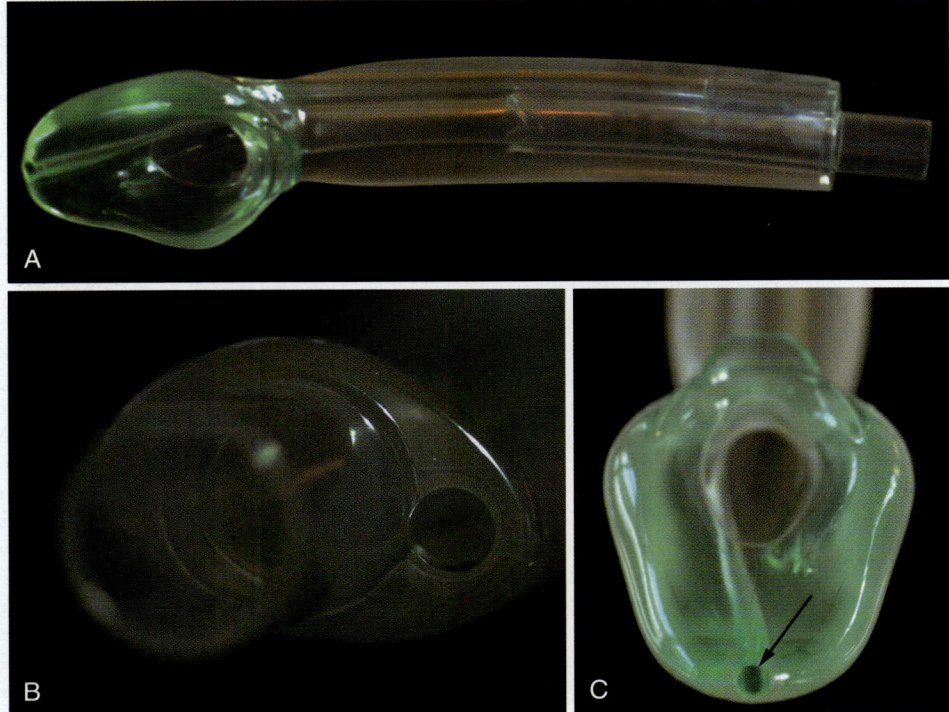

FIGURE 14.20 The i-gel supraglottic device **(A)** consists of a malleable non–latex-containing, noninflatable cuff that is designed to seal over the laryngeal inlet after insertion. The stem of the i-gel contains a "buccal cavity stabilizer," which is designed to resist accidental rotation after insertion and is made from a hard polymer that resists biting. The i-gel also contains a gastric suction channel next to the 15-mm connector **(B)**, with which practitioners may evacuate gastric contents when the device is in the correct inserted position. **(C)**, The distal position of the suction port *(arrow)*.

Size	Patient Weight (kg)	ID (mm)	Maximal Size of Endotracheal Tube (mm ID)[a]	Maximal Size of Nasogastric Tube (Fr)
1	2–5	5.6	3	
1.5	5–12	6.8	4	10
2	10–25	8.8	5	12
2.5	25–35	10.2	5	12
3	30–60	11.2	6	12
4	50–90	12.3	7	12
5	>90	12.5	8	14

TABLE 14.7 Suggested i-gel Supraglottic Device Size, Inner Diameter, Endotracheal Tube Size, and Nasogastric Tube Size

[a]May depend on outer diameter specifications of endotracheal tube manufacturer.
ID, inner diameter.

to airway problems may be grouped according to anatomic location and may result from congenital, inflammatory, traumatic, metabolic, or neoplastic disorders. Tables 14.8 and 14.9 list the more common pediatric airway problems according to anatomic location. E-Table 14.1 lists the more common pediatric syndromes and associated anesthetic considerations; more complete information may be obtained elsewhere.[381-384] For optimal management of the airway in obese children, the reader is referred to Chapter 29.

MANAGEMENT PRINCIPLES

For any laryngoscopy, but in particular for the difficult airway, an extensive array of equipment to assist with the difficult airway must be available. We advocate the creation of a difficult airway cart stocked with equipment useful in the management of the difficult airway for children of all sizes and ages. Suggestions for contents are listed in Table 14.10. The approach to a difficult airway, as described earlier, must include a careful history and physical examination and, when indicated, radiologic evaluation. In the past, lateral neck xerograms were useful in delineating anatomic aberrations; however, ultrasound, MRI, and CT imaging have supplanted this modality.[109-111,113-124,143,385-390] Ultrasound can be useful in the identification of subglottic stenosis; there may also be a role for use of ultrasound to help with the prediction of difficult tracheal intubations and for the examination of children with known difficult airways.[130] Ultrasound can also be used to intubate the trachea quickly as it can be used as a visualization tool for the lighted stylet technique and may be particularly beneficial when blood or secretions impair visualization with traditional methods.[391]

In addition to the airway pathology, the pathophysiology of the congenital syndrome or associated disease process must be fully evaluated. The safest approach to managing a difficult airway is to formulate a plan that includes several contingencies for failure or loss of the airway and to have skilled help available, especially a surgeon who is experienced in performing pediatric bronchoscopy and tracheostomy. To maximize success and safety, a skilled assistant should help to position the child, facilitate

TABLE 14.8 Pediatric Airway Pathology Related to Anatomic Site

Anatomic Site	Etiology	Clinical Condition
Nasopharynx	Congenital	Choanal atresia, stenosis,[34,35,664–668] encephalocele[669–675]
	Traumatic	Foreign body, trauma[676–678]
	Inflammatory	Adenoidal hypertrophy,[676–678] nasal congestion[36]
	Neoplastic	Teratoma[679–681]
Tongue	Congenital	Hemangioma, Down syndrome, glossoptosis[682]
	Traumatic	Burn, laceration, lymphatic/venous obstruction[134,135,676,683–689]
	Metabolic	Beckwith-Wiedemann syndrome[585,690–696] hypothyroidism,[697] mucopolysaccharidosis,[628,698–719] glycogen storage disease,[720–730] gangliosidosis,[731–734] congenital hypothyroidism
	Neoplastic	Cystic hygroma,[735–739] cystic teratoma
Mandible/maxilla	Congenital hypoplasia	Pierre Robin syndrome,[485,560,562,600,740–757] Treacher Collins syndrome,[411,561,586,758–772] Goldenhar syndrome,[390,481,614,773–780] Apert syndrome,[781–783] achondroplasia,[564,784–788] Turner syndrome,[789–793] Cornelia de Lange syndrome,[794–797] Smith-Lemli-Opitz syndrome,[798–800] Hallermann-Streiff syndrome,[801] Crouzon syndrome[802,803]
	Traumatic	Fracture,[804–806] neck burn with contractures[688,689,807]
	Inflammatory	Juvenile rheumatoid arthritis[808–814]
	Neoplastic	Tumors, cherubism[815–817]
Pharynx/larynx	Congenital	Laryngomalacia (infantile larynx) (see Video 14.1),[676,818–821] Freeman-Sheldon syndrome (whistling face),[822–835] laryngeal stenosis,[676,836] laryngocele,[818] laryngeal web,[818,837–839] hemangioma[840,841]
	Traumatic	Dislocated/fractured larynx,[676,806,842–849] foreign body,[54,55,676,850–858] inhalation injury (burn),[683–686,688,807,859] postintubation edema/granuloma/stenosis,[860–874] swelling of uvula,[134,875] soft palate trauma, epidermolysis bullosa[876–888]
	Inflammatory	Epiglottitis,[50–52,889–894] acute tonsillitis,[895] peritonsillar abscess,[896,897] retropharyngeal abscess,[898] diphtheritic membrane, laryngeal papillomatosis[899–907]
	Metabolic	Hypocalcemic laryngospasm[47]
	Neoplastic	Tumors
	Neurologic	Vocal cord paralysis, Arnold-Chiari malformation[908–911]
Trachea	Congenital	Vascular ring,[56,57,912,913] tracheal stenosis or complete tracheal rings (Video 14.18),[914–916] tracheomalacia (see Video 14.1)[818,836,870,917–919] congenital tracheal web, hemangioma[920–923]
	Inflammatory	Laryngotracheobronchitis (viral),[49,52,53,219,924–926] bacterial tracheitis
	Neoplastic	Mediastinal tumors: neurofibroma,[927] paratracheal nodes (lymphoma)[928–934]

TABLE 14.9 Cervical Spine Anomalies[a]

Etiology	Clinical Condition
Congenital	Down syndrome,[935–944] Klippel-Feil malformation,[945–950] Goldenhar syndrome,[390,481,614,773–779,951] Pierre Robin,[952] torticollis
Traumatic	Fracture, subluxation,[805,806,842–846,953–956] neck burn contracture[689]
Inflammatory	Rheumatoid arthritis[808–814]
Metabolic	Mucopolysaccharidosis (Morquio syndrome)[698–713,957]

[a]Abnormalities of the cervical spine may limit extension and flexion, thereby contributing to the difficulties of airway management; a significant percentage of infants with Down syndrome have atlantoaxial instability.[958]

airway management, and observe the monitors and the child's vital signs. To direct an assistant, there should be clear communication about the airway management plan and specific details about maneuvers needed to facilitate the process. Familiarity with difficult airway algorithms and difficult airway management reviews can help the practitioner formulate a reasonable plan and ensure that no viable management options are missed.[392–398]

Certain principles apply to the care of any child in whom difficulty with airway management is anticipated. In most circumstances, an awake or mildly sedated approach would be the primary management strategy for the anticipated difficult airway if airway concerns were considered in isolation. However, often a practitioner using the awake approach may encounter difficulty in obtaining the child's cooperation. Assisted spontaneous ventilation during general anesthesia is the preferred technique when abnormal airway anatomy is present and difficulty with patient cooperation is anticipated; it provides adequate oxygenation while the airway is evaluated for the appropriate approach to tracheal intubation. Therefore the first choice for management of a potential difficult airway, whether the child is sedated or under general anesthesia, is to *maintain spontaneous ventilation*.[393,398] There are two reasons for maintaining spontaneous gas exchange. First, neuromuscular blockade may result in total airway obstruction owing to loss of tone of the tongue, pharyngeal and laryngeal muscles, and suspensory ligaments. This obstruction may not be easily alleviated with manual ventilation of the lungs. Neuromuscular blockade should not be used if airway obstruction or the potential for airway obstruction exists.[42] Second, if a child is paralyzed, the loss of spontaneous breath sounds eliminates a valuable guide to locating the glottis. For example, in children with craniofacial anomalies or cervical burn contractures, one may be able to visualize only the tip of the epiglottis with standard rigid laryngoscopy. In such cases, if specialized airway management equipment is unavailable, shaping the ETT tip into a 90-degree angle with a stylet (Fig. 14.21), placing the tip behind the epiglottis (or the center of the base of the tongue if the epiglottis is not

TABLE 14.10	Items to Consider for an Emergency Intubation Cart

Drawer 1

LMA Classic (disposable)—sizes 1, 1.5, 2, 2.5, 3, 4, 5

LMA ProSeal (disposable)—sizes 1.5, 2, 2.5, 3, 4, 5

LMA Fastrach—sizes 3, 4, 5

ETTs for Fastrach—sizes (mm ID) 6, 6.5, 7, 7.5, 8

ETT stabilizers for Fastrach

Size or weight charts for LMA

Drawer 2

Transtracheal jet-ventilation catheters[a] (VBM)—infant (16 gauge), child (14 gauge), adult (13 gauge)

Emergency Transtracheal Airway Catheter (Cook)

Magill forceps—adult and pediatric sizes

Aillon tube bender

Miller blades—sizes 0, 1, 2, 3, 4

Macintosh blades—sizes 1, 2, 3, 4

Phillips blades—sizes 1, 2

Wis-Hipple blades—sizes 1, 1.5

Oxyscope blades—sizes 0, 1 (with oxygen tubing)

Handles (Medium and Short)

C batteries × 2

Oxygen Y-connector

Albuterol adapters for metered-dose administration (3)

Syringes (5 each)—5 mL, 10 mL

Intravenous catheters, 10 of each commonly used sizes (24 ga, 22 ga, 20 ga, 18 ga, 16 ga)[a]

Swivel adapters (Portex, Sontex)

No. 3 straight connectors × 2

Drawer 3

Preparation forceps or tongue-grabbing forceps

Safety glasses

Lens paper

Surgical lubricant

2% Lidocaine jelly[a]

4% Lidocaine solution[a]

Atomizer to spray topical lidocaine

Suction catheters—sizes 8, 10, 14F

Yankauer suction tubes—pediatric and adult sizes

Defogger

Silicone spray

Halogen light bulb

Disposable teeth guards

Drawer 4

Face masks—neonate, infant, toddler, child, adult (small/medium/large)

Frie endoscopy mask—infant, child, adult

Bronchoscopy airways[a]—infant, child, adult

Bite blocks—infant, child, adult

Ovassapian airways (2)

Nasal trumpets[a]—sizes 2 to 34 F

Oral airways—sizes 90, 80, 70, 60, 50, 00, 000

Drawer 5

Self inflating bag (Ambu) with reservoir

Enk Oxygen Flow Modulation set (Cook, Inc.)

Jet ventilator

Stylets—pediatric and adult

ETT exchange catheters with both Luer-Lok and 15-mm OD adapters—sizes (mm OD) 3, 4, 5, 7

Retrograde catheter with extra guidewire

Extension cord with converter from Hubble to three-prong plug

Other equipment to consider: lighted stylets and optical stylets (see text)

[a]Items with outdates.

Cook, Cook Critical Care, Bloomington, IN; *ETT,* endotracheal tube; *F,* French; *ga,* gauge; *ID,* inner diameter; *LMA,* laryngeal mask airway, LMA North America, San Diego, CA; *OD,* outer diameter; *VBM,* VBM Medizintechnik GmbH, Sulz, Germany.
Modified from Department of Pediatric Anesthesiology. The difficult airway cart. Lurie Children's Hospital, Chicago.

visible), and then listening for breath sounds with the ear near the proximal end of the ETT or tracking the capnogram often allows the practitioner to "blindly" locate the glottic opening and trachea. Despite the rich history of the "spontaneous ventilation" approach to the difficult airway, there has been a shift in practice of late to paralyzing children with difficult airways with nondepolarizing muscle relaxants, particularly with rocuronium because of the availability of sugammadex to reverse the paralysis should an emergency situation arise (see airway registry below).

If the child is able to cooperate while mildly sedated, there are several options for airway management. An opioid-benzodiazepine combination will blunt airway reactivity, decrease discomfort, and provide anxiolysis and amnesia. These combinations, particularly fentanyl and midazolam, are effective for sedation of adolescents and mature preteens.[399] Dosing is based on weight and is guided by clinical parameters, including preexisting medical conditions. However, benzodiazepine-opioid sedation may not suffice for a frightened young child because the dose requirement for sedation may exceed the dose that causes apnea. Alternatively, ketamine, which provides both hypnosis and analgesia, may be used alone or in conjunction with midazolam.[399] Ketamine usually preserves adequate spontaneous ventilation and upper airway patency[400] while preventing laryngeal reactions to airway manipulation. Ketamine and midazolam should be slowly titrated to effect to avoid oversedation and apnea.[401] Midazolam takes almost 5 minutes to achieve peak electroencephalographic effects, necessitating adequate time between incremental doses (see Fig. 48.7).[402,403] Ketamine is usually titrated in doses of 0.25 to 0.5 mg/kg IV every 2 minutes. Although there is a large incidence of psychomimetic emergence reactions in adults, these reactions are less common in children, particularly if ketamine is combined with midazolam. Ketamine may increase secretions that enhance airway reactivity and interfere with video-based airway management; antisialagogue administration may mitigate these effects. In addition, the anticholinergic effect of atropine or glycopyrrolate will blunt reflex bradycardia that can occur with airway manipulation. Dexmedetomidine may be administered as the sole sedating agent or combined with reduced doses of other sedatives or opioids to be effective for sedation while maintaining spontaneous respirations during fiberoptic intubation in adults and children.[404–411]

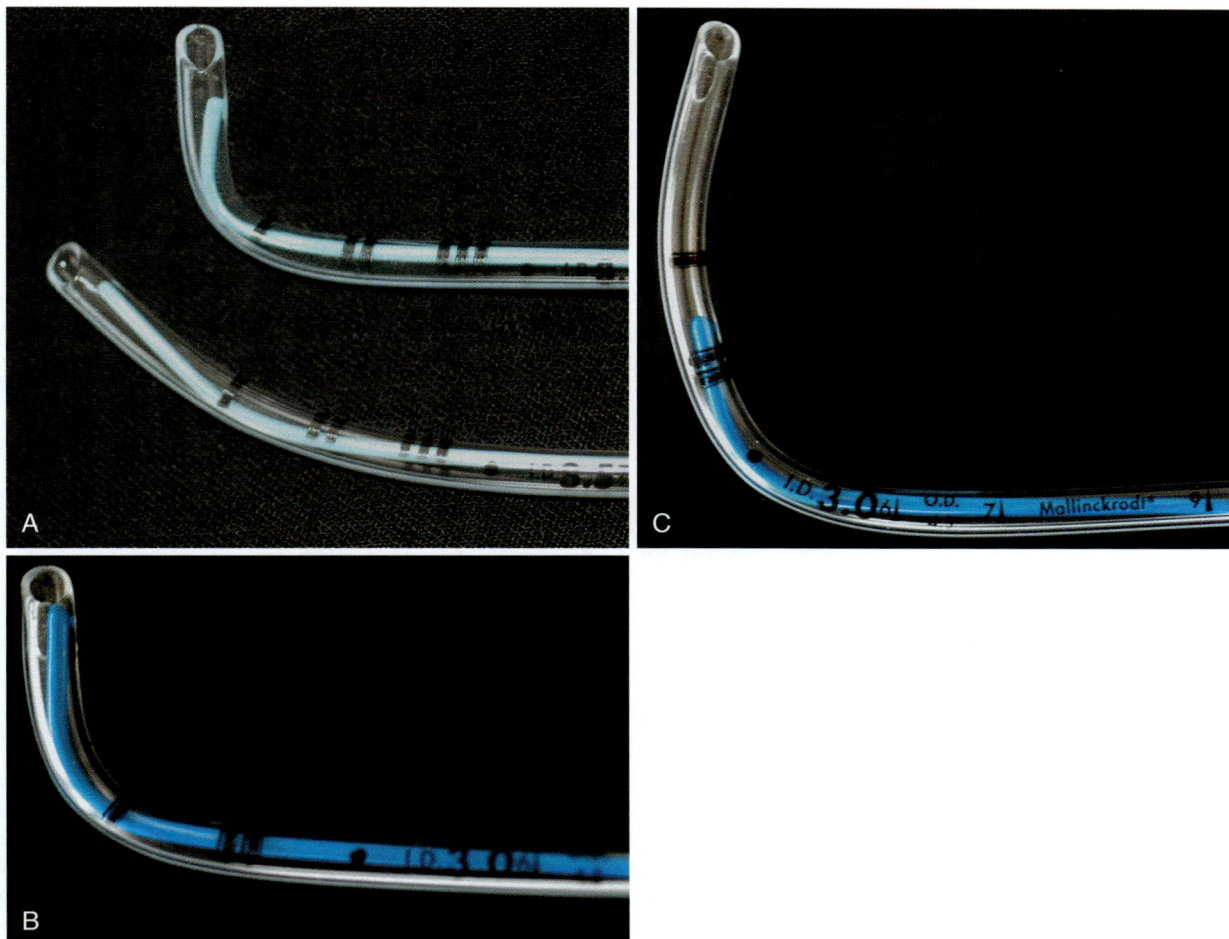

FIGURE 14.21 A stylet placed within an endotracheal tube (ETT) often facilitates placement. **A,** The "hockey-stick" configuration. **B,** In children with midfacial hypoplasia syndromes, in which the anatomic relation of the base of the tongue to the laryngeal inlet is abnormal, a stylet with a 90-degree bend 1 to 2 cm from the tip allows placement of the ETT behind the epiglottis and at the laryngeal inlet. Breath sounds audible at the 15-mm connector confirm appropriate location. **C,** Maintaining the position of the stylet while advancing the ETT frequently allows successful "blind" endotracheal intubation around the base of the tongue even without the use of special airway equipment.

A multicenter registry, the Pediatric Difficult Intubation (PediDI) registry,[412] was developed to examine the risk factors for a difficult intubation, examine the success rates of various intubation techniques, and assess the complications that occur in children with difficult tracheal intubations. Data from this registry demonstrate that children with difficult airways were often paralyzed for their airway management after confirming easy mask ventilation. This is likely because of the fear of airway activation (laryngospasm, bronchospasm, coughing) during the airway management. Performing a 5-second jaw thrust in an unparalyzed anesthetized child is a reliable test to assess the risk of airway activation when the airway is instrumented. Absence of movement, tachypnea, and tachycardia in response to the jaw thrust suggests a small risk of triggering a response to airway instrumentation. The depth of anesthesia, however, needs to be maintained during the airway manipulation, particularly if the intubation attempt is prolonged.

Topical anesthesia may be used in conjunction with sedation or general anesthesia to blunt airway reactivity in those children in whom spontaneous ventilation is preserved. Useful methods for providing topical anesthesia to the airway include (1) nebulized lidocaine; (2) topical application of local anesthetic sprays, jellies, or ointments; (3) translaryngeal delivery of lidocaine; (4) "spray as you go" with lidocaine injected onto the surface of the larynx and vocal cords through the channel of an FOB usually used for suctioning or administering oxygen; and (5) superior laryngeal nerve block.[399] Caution is required to avoid delivering a toxic dose of local anesthetic. Maximum doses of the local anesthetic are based on the patient's weight and should be calculated in advance (see Table 42.2). Lidocaine seems to have the best safety profile; we limit our maximum dose to 4 mg/kg.[412a] We do not recommend the use of benzocaine (Cetacaine) local anesthetic spray in children weighing less than 40 kg, because it is associated with methemoglobinemia and it is difficult to titrate or limit the administered dose.[96,413]

Strategies to maintain oxygenation vary according to the technique (spontaneous respiration vs. paralyzed). For infants who are breathing spontaneously, the Oxyscope (Heine Optotechnik, Herrsching, Germany) is a Miller 1 laryngoscope blade with an insufflation channel along its length so that it may be attached to an oxygen source (E-Fig. 14.3).[414–416] Other strategies include the use of high-flow nasal cannula,[417] insufflation into the hypopharynx via a nasal trumpet or shortened preformed airway RAE tracheal tube, or intubation through an LMA. For the nonbreathing patient preoxygenation with 100% oxygen is vital.

Many techniques and devices for managing a difficult airway have been recommended; these are reviewed in detail later. Previous experience in normal airways can render these devices valuable adjuncts in difficult airway management. *If one is unable to secure tracheal intubation, it is important to recognize the limits of one's ability. Do not hesitate to seek assistance from a colleague or request the surgeon to perform a tracheostomy or bronchoscopy. As an alternative, the child can be awakened and referred to a major pediatric center. In an urgent, life-threatening situation, placement of an SGA device or percutaneous cricothyroidotomy can be lifesaving* (see "The Unexpected Difficult Intubation").[255,293,294,418,419]

Cognitive biases may play a role in airway management and knowledge of these thinking patterns may help clinicians select the appropriate choices when things go wrong. Some examples of biases that may occur with airway management include loss aversion, framing, and anchoring. Loss aversion is the idea that we dislike a loss more than we like an equivalent gain, which leads us to make irrational choices. An example would be a patient with a recognized difficult airway and a known history of difficult mask ventilation. A clinician may recognize the need for an awake or sedated approach but because of a lack of familiarity with performing the awake technique and fear of failure and the associated negative perception from peers, they may decide to proceed with inhaled induction. The loss of reputation and negative perception (loss aversion) influenced the clinician to make an inappropriate choice for the patient. Anchoring occurs when a starting point influences or biases subsequent decisions; an example would be a patient who is easy to mask ventilate after induction of anesthesia but subsequently becomes impossible to ventilate. A clinician may fixate on the fact that ventilation was easy before and continue to try interventions to improve ventilation and delay definitive treatment such as a surgical airway because of anchoring to the previous condition. The cognitive frame of the clinician plays a critical role in his or her next steps and framing has been shown to influence choices in many situations. A lay example is labeling of food as 90% fat-free versus 10% fat. Though both labels communicate the same information, the former is more desirable and consumers choose that option more often. In the patient described earlier who went from being easy to mask ventilate to becoming impossible to ventilate, two thinking patterns are common in the clinician's mind. One frame could be *"This is very bad, this patient may need a surgical airway, I will be sued."* Another frame could be *"This patient needs a surgical airway, this will be lifesaving."* Clearly the latter frame results in the most favorable action, whereas the former may lead to inaction or delays.[420]

Documentation

Documentation of the difficult airway and its management is essential to provide useful information for the next time that the child requires sedation or anesthesia. A note in the anesthesia record should clearly address the following issues:

1. Whether mask ventilation was attempted, and if so, whether there was any difficulty
2. Special maneuvers that were required for successful mask ventilation
3. Special maneuvers that were not helpful with mask ventilation
4. Any difficulty with tracheal intubation
5. Special techniques that were required for successful intubation
6. Special techniques that were not helpful for intubation
7. Grade of the laryngoscopic view of laryngeal structures during direct laryngoscopy (Fig. 14.22)

In addition to discussion with the family and the child (when age appropriate), a letter should be given to the family and child outlining the difficulties with the airway, describing how the airway was managed, and referring them to the MedicAlert Foundation registry.[371] This should be copied and circulated to the medical record and to the MedicAlert registry. In the United States, the MedicAlert registry for difficult airway/difficult intubation can be reached by telephone at 1-888-633-4298. Similar registries are also being formed internationally.[421] The MedicAlert registration form asks for clinical details about the type of airway difficulty, as well as which maneuvers were successful in management and those which were not. Any practitioner who provides airway management to the registered patient can update this information

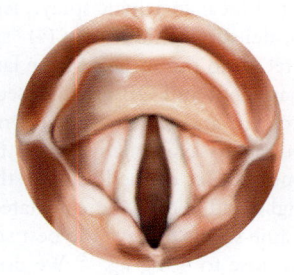

Grade I

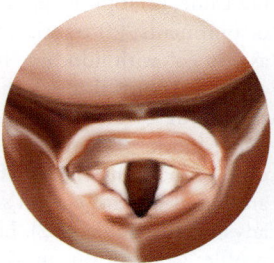
Grade II

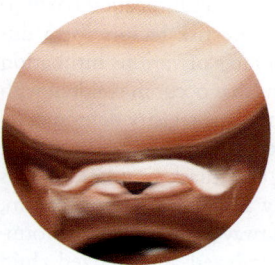
Grade III

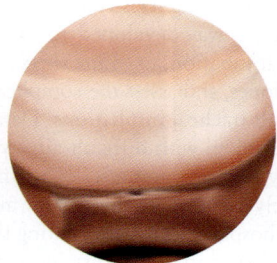
Grade IV

FIGURE 14.22 The laryngoscopic grading system of Cormack and Lehane offers a reasonable means of describing visualization of the larynx. It is useful to grade the degree of visualization during laryngoscopy and how that visualization was achieved (e.g., external cricoid pressure or laryngeal manipulation, the size and configuration of the laryngoscope blade). This provides useful information for the next person attempting laryngoscopy so that he or she has some degree of knowledge regarding what to expect. Grade I is visualization of the complete laryngeal opening; grade II, visualization of just the posterior area; grade III, visualization of just the epiglottis; and grade IV, visualization of just the soft palate. (Reproduced with permission from Cormack RS, Lehane J. Difficult tracheal intubation in obstetrics. *Anaesthesia* 1984;39:1105–1111.)

at any time. Although scoring systems used in adults[91-95] have not been thoroughly investigated in all age groups,[96,422] it is useful to describe in detail the view of the larynx that was achieved and how it was achieved (e.g., blade type, size, external laryngeal manipulation, GlideScope [Verathon, Seattle, WA]).

The Unexpected Difficult Intubation

With careful preoperative evaluation and planning, the unexpected pediatric difficult airway should be a rare occurrence. However,

the practitioner should always be prepared for this potentially life-threatening event. Because the unexpected difficult airway occurs after the anesthesia (plan A) has been initiated, many of the management decisions required for the anticipated difficult airway have already been made. Of primary importance is maintaining adequate oxygenation while a definitive course of action is pursued (i.e., plan B, plan C, and so on). A reasonable pediatric decision tree, based on the difficult airway algorithm of the American Society of Anesthesiologists (ASA), is presented in Fig. 14.23. An

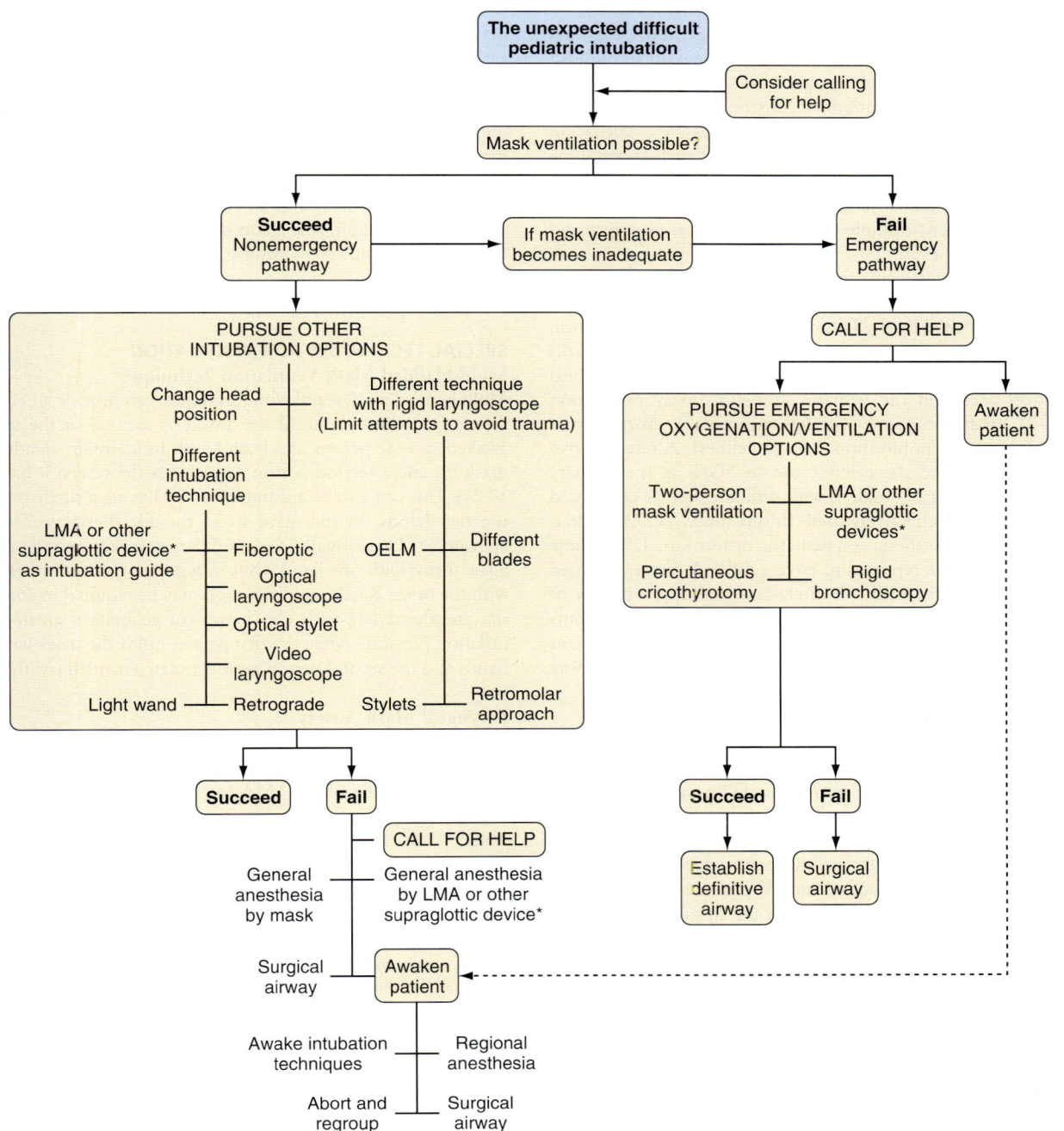

FIGURE 14.23 A proposed algorithm for management of the unexpected difficult pediatric airway. *LMA,* laryngeal mask airway; *OELM,* optimal external laryngeal manipulation; *PLMA,* ProSeal LMA. *Consider using PLMA if the child is at risk for aspiration or if high inflation pressures are needed. (Modified with permission from Wheeler M. Management strategies for the difficult pediatric airway. *Anesth Clin North Am.* 1998;16:743–761.)

important difference between infants and adults should be noted in this scenario. Because infants have an increased metabolic rate and decreased functional residual capacity, the time between the loss of the airway and resultant hypoxemia with potential secondary neurologic injury is significantly diminished compared with adults.[423] In a mathematical model, the approximate time to zero oxygen saturation from an FIO_2 of 90% is 4 minutes in a 10-kg child, whereas the same process in a healthy 70-kg adult takes almost 10 minutes.[421,424]

The PediDI registry demonstrated that more than two direct laryngoscopy attempts in children with difficult tracheal intubation was associated with a high failure rate and an increased incidence of severe complications.[412] These findings suggest that the following strategies should be considered: (1) minimize the number of direct laryngoscopy attempts, and transition to an indirect technique (videolaryngoscope/fiberoptic bronchoscope) when direct laryngoscopy fails, and (2) consider a means for passive oxygenation of the lungs during tracheal intubation attempts such as high-flow nasal cannula and the modified nasal trumpet (Video 14.8).[425] A similar registry of pediatric intensive care units confirmed the association between multiple tracheal intubation attempts and associated adverse events.[426]

SGAs can be effectively used and are often the key initial step for safe management of the difficult airway. The pediatric airway guidelines published by the Difficult Airway Society/Association of Paediatric Anaesthetists of Great Britain and Ireland (APAGBI) suggest the use of an SGA, if feasible, when failed tracheal intubation occurs in the pediatric difficult airway population (APAGBI Paediatric Airway Guidelines, available from http://www.apagbi.org.uk/publications/apa-guidelines). A retrospective study that examined the elective use of SGAs as the primary airway management in children with difficult airways concluded that they could be effectively used. In this study, 77,272 children received general anesthesia at a pediatric institution; 459 of these patients (0.6%) were reported to have a difficult airway (defined as either a history of a difficult direct laryngoscopy, a history of difficult mask ventilation, or both) and 109 of those patients received general anesthesia with an SGA for primary management with a success rate of 96%. (In four patients, an alternative airway was required.)[427]

Extubation of the Child With the Difficult Airway
Preparation for extubation begins shortly after the airway is secured. Equipment used to secure the airway should be rechecked, quickly returned to functional status, and then left in the operating room until successful safe extubation. Children who had prolonged attempts at intubation or who will have procedures that may lead to airway edema may benefit from IV dexamethasone (0.5 to 1 mg/kg, up to 20 mg).[232–234] If significant airway edema is suspected, consider leaving the child intubated postoperatively until it resolves. The child must be fully awake and have full return of strength and adequate ventilatory effort before extubation is attempted.

A Cook airway exchange catheter with Rapi-Fit adapter (Cook Critical Care, Bloomington, IN) is a hollow plastic guide with holes on its distal end that may be useful as a bridge to extubation because the adapter on its proximal end allows the placement of either a Luer-Lok connector for connection to a jet ventilator or a 15-mm adapter for connection to a standard anesthesia ventilating system (E-Fig. 14.4)[428–431] It is available in a variety of sizes to allow the exchange of ETTs with 3.0-mm ID or larger. This can be used for oxygenation and ventilation and as a guide to reinsertion of the ETT if the child's ventilatory efforts are inadequate or if airway obstruction occurs.[432] However, caution is required when using this device for jet ventilation, because significant barotrauma has been reported.[433,434]

An alternative to jet ventilation is the Enk Oxygen Flow Modulation set (Cook Critical Care), which allows flow from a standard low-pressure flow meter to be adjusted by occluding holes in the delivery system with the thumb and forefinger (E-Fig. 14.5, Top). As a potential substitute for the Enk device, one could cut a side hole in the plastic oxygen delivery tubing to create a similar low-pressure oxygen delivery system (see E-Fig. 14.5, Bottom). Pneumothorax, pneumomediastinum, and deaths have occurred when jet ventilation was used with an airway exchange catheter.[435] One report suggested that only insufflation or gentle manual ventilation should be used initially and that jet ventilation should be reserved for situations in which these techniques are ineffective. These authors also recommended that the optimal management was reintubation.[436]

If the child remains intubated for a prolonged period of time after surgery, it is advisable to return the child to the operating room for extubation. A surgeon who is prepared to perform rigid bronchoscopy and tracheostomy and an anesthesiologist who is familiar with the techniques used for the previously successful airway management should be in attendance.

SPECIAL TECHNIQUES FOR VENTILATION
Multi-Handed Mask Ventilation Techniques
Multi-handed mask ventilation techniques can provide an effective temporizing measure until the airway is secured or the child is awakened. One person uses both hands to maintain an adequate mask fit, and a second person compresses the reservoir bag (Fig. 14.24). This can also be accomplished by having a single provider use two hands on the mask while the anesthesia ventilator is activated.[437] Occasionally, a second person is required to perform a jaw thrust with one hand while compressing the anesthesia bag with the other. Rarely, a third person may be required to compress the anesthesia bag with two hands (to generate a greater peak inflation pressure) while the first person holds the mask with two hands and the second person performs a two-handed jaw thrust.[437]

Laryngeal Mask Airway
The LMA has revolutionized difficult airway management in children. Numerous case reports and extensive clinical experience attest to the value of the LMA for establishing an airway when both ventilation and intubation are extremely difficult or impossible.[395,438–440] The LMA has been described as a tool for use in both the nonemergency pathway (*cannot intubate, can ventilate*) and the emergency pathway (*cannot intubate, cannot ventilate* [CICV]) of the ASA difficult airway algorithm.[393,395] Use has been described in the awake child (LMA insertion in awake infants with Pierre Robin syndrome [Robin sequence])[441,442] (Video 14.9) and in the anesthetized child with a known or suspected difficult airway. It can be used as the definitive airway in some circumstances, as a conduit for intubation, or as a temporizing airway while other options are pursued (e.g., a surgical airway). There are now many other SGA devices reported to be useful in the management of the child with a difficult airway (see above discussion), but comparative studies in pediatrics are lacking.[300,443]

Percutaneous Needle Cricothyroidotomy
The American Heart Association changed its recommendations for emergency airway management to a percutaneous needle

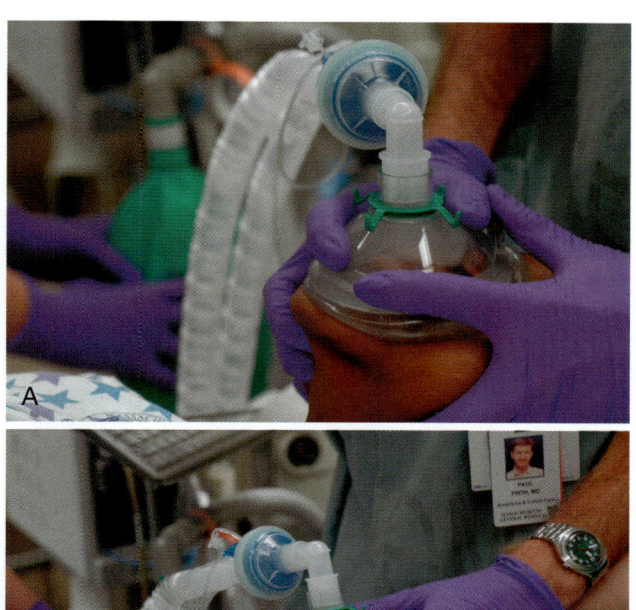

FIGURE 14.24 A, The two-handed technique for mask ventilation may be useful to improve mask fit and therefore ventilation when the traditional technique is inadequate. One person holds the mask while a second person squeezes the ventilation bag. **B,** Occasionally, a third person is required to perform a two-handed jaw thrust (see text for details).

cricothyroidotomy over a surgical cricothyroidotomy in 1992 because it was believed that the former entails less risk of injury to vital structures such as the carotid arteries or jugular veins, particularly in the hands of nonsurgical trained practitioners. In addition, most practitioners can more rapidly perform the percutaneous procedure. However, the cricothyroid membrane has a relatively small width in infants and children younger than 5 years of age. Attempts at cricothyroidotomy may readily damage cricoid and thyroid cartilages, resulting in laryngeal stenosis and permanent damage to the speech mechanism. Therefore, this procedure should be reserved for use only under emergency circumstances.[444,445] More studies are needed but at this time, needle cricothyroidotomy is still the technique of choice in the *"cannot intubate, cannot oxygenate"* (CICO) situation in infants (APAGBI Pediatric Airway Guidelines [see discussion below] available from http://www.apagbi.org.uk/publications/apa-guidelines).

Because percutaneous needle cricothyroidotomy is rarely used in infants and children, it is recommended that experience be gained with patient simulators or in animal models, because success in the hands of the inexperienced is not assured.[446–449] A schema of this procedure is presented in Fig. 14.25. A commercial product called the Jet-Ventilation-Catheter (VBM Medizintechnik GmbH) is available in three sizes: 16, 14, and 13 gauge. It consists of a slightly curved puncture needle within a Teflon, kink-resistant cannula nearly identical to an IV catheter (Fig. 14.26A). This cannula has two lateral eyes at its distal end and a combined Luer-Lok and

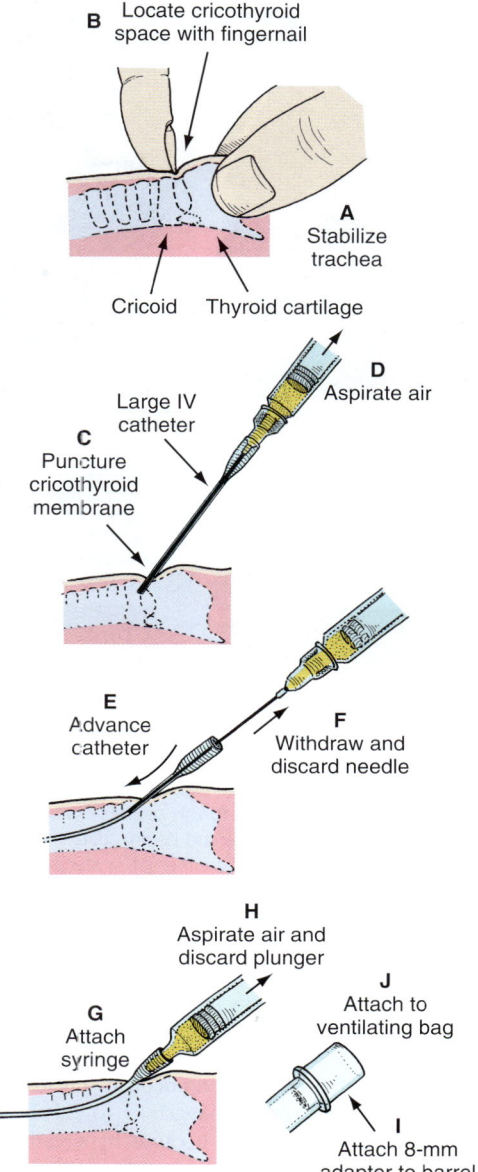

FIGURE 14.25 Percutaneous cricothyroidotomy. Extend the head in the midline with a rolled towel or folded sheet beneath the shoulders. **A,** Standing to the left of the child, stabilize the trachea with the right hand. **B,** The cricothyroid membrane is located with the index fingertip of the left hand between the thyroid and cricoid cartilages. This space is so narrow (1 mm) in an infant that only a fingernail can discern it. The trachea is then stabilized between the middle finger and thumb of the left hand while the fingernail of the index finger marks the cricothyroid membrane. **C,** A large intravenous (IV) catheter (12- to 14-gauge) is then inserted through the cricothyroid membrane, and air is aspirated **(D).** The catheter is advanced into the trachea through the membrane, and the needle is discarded; an intraluminal position is reconfirmed by attaching a 3-mL syringe **(E)** and aspirating for air **(F).** A 3-mm adapter from a pediatric endotracheal tube can be attached to any intravenous catheter **(G).** Ventilation is accomplished by attaching to a breathing circuit with a standard 22-mm connector **(H).** An alternative would be to leave the barrel of the 3-mL syringe attached to the IV catheter, insert an 8-mm endotracheal tube adapter to the syringe barrel **(I),** and then attach to a ventilating system with a standard 22-mm adapter **(J).** (From Coté CJ, Eavey RD, Todres ID, Jones DE. Cricothyroid membrane puncture: oxygenation and ventilation in a dog model using an intravenous catheter. *Crit Care Med.* 1988;16:615–619, © by Williams & Wilkins.)

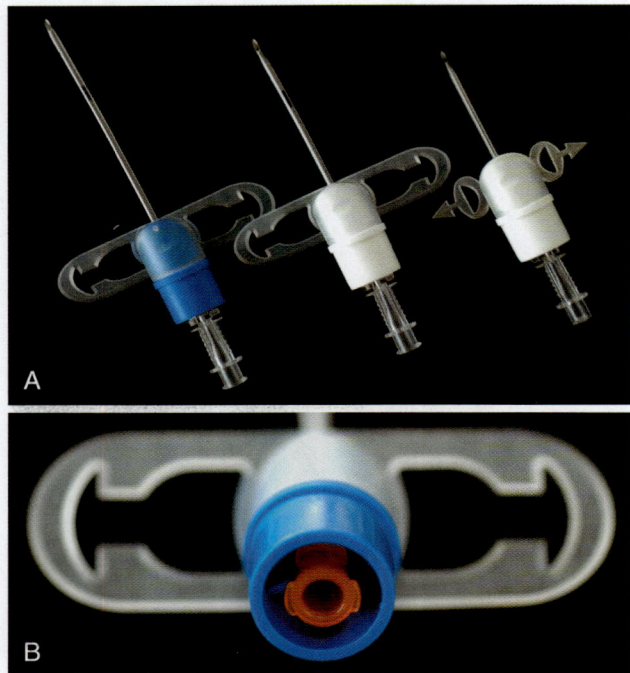

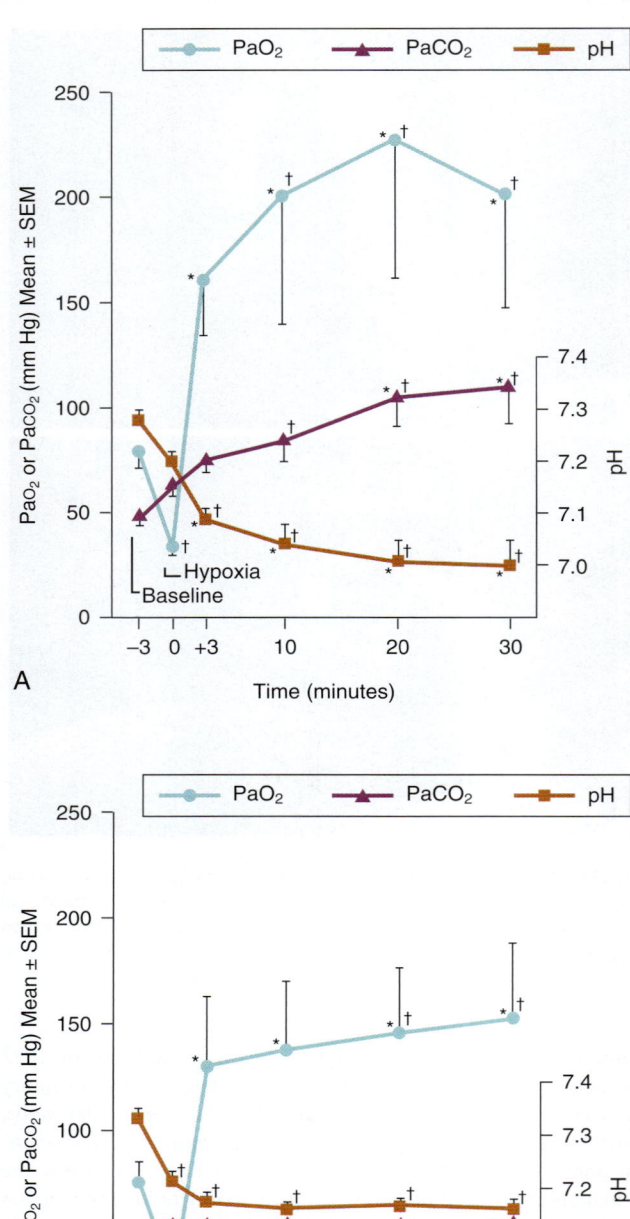

FIGURE 14.26 A, The Jet-Ventilation-Catheter (VBM Medizintechnik GmbH, Sulz, Germany) is available in three sizes: From left to right: 13 gauge (adult), 14 gauge (child), and 16 gauge (infant). It consists of a slightly curved puncture needle within a Teflon, kink-resistant cannula. The procedure for insertion is similar to that described in Fig. 14.25. **B,** This cannula has two lateral eyes at its distal end and a combined Luer-Lok and 15-mm adapter (surrounding the Luer-Lok) at its proximal end, allowing either jet or standard ventilation. It also has a fixation flange and foam neck tape to secure the airway.

15-mm adapter at its proximal end (see Fig. 14.26B). It also has a fixation flange and foam neck tape to secure the airway.

Percutaneous needle cricothyroidotomy provides only a means for oxygen insufflation and does not reliably provide adequate ventilation. In the spontaneously breathing patient, simple delivery of intratracheal oxygen (1 to 2 L/minute) may be sufficient in the short term, because hypercarbia is generally well tolerated by healthy children.[444,450,451] A number of children with arterial CO_2 values well above 150 mm Hg have survived neurologically intact when adequate oxygenation was maintained.[451] Therefore simple oxygenation without attempts at ventilation may be all that is required to sustain life (Fig. 14.27). For the child without respiratory effort, there is a need to provide ventilation in addition to oxygenation. An Ambu bag with the pop-off disabled can provide limited ventilation through a percutaneous catheter, but these devices will be ineffective at standard pop-off pressures.[444,452] Extremely high ventilating pressures are required, but mid-tracheal pressures are significantly less (10 to 16 cm H_2O).[444] A percutaneous cricothyroidotomy catheter can also be used with a jet ventilation system. Jet ventilation via a catheter passed through a narrow glottic opening has also been described.[453–456]

If upper airway obstruction is present (e.g., after multiple unsuccessful attempts at rigid laryngoscopy), there will be a limited pathway for the egress of air and oxygen, and barotrauma may result from insufflation of oxygen or attempts at ventilation. Very serious morbidity and mortality may result from massive subcutaneous emphysema or tension pneumothorax.[457,458] Therefore,

FIGURE 14.27 A, Changes in arterial blood gases and pH are plotted over time for six dogs with spontaneous ventilation; baseline values in room air are plotted at time −3; values after 2 to 3 minutes of hypoxemia as a result of airway obstruction are plotted at time 0. Marked, sustained increases in arterial oxygen tension (PaO2) follow cricothyroid membrane puncture with delivery of only 1.0 L/minute oxygen. **B,** Changes in arterial blood gases and pH are plotted over time for five dogs that were not making spontaneous ventilatory efforts. Both oxygenation and ventilation were achieved with a self-inflating bag attached via a 3.0 ID adapter to an IV cannula introduced through the cricothyroid membrane. PaCO2, carbon dioxide tension; SEM, standard error of the mean; Sig., significant difference. (From Coté CJ, Eavey RD, Todres ID, Jones DE. Cricothyroid membrane puncture: oxygenation and ventilation in a dog model using an intravenous catheter. Crit Care Med. 1988;16:615–619, © by Williams & Wilkins.)

jet ventilation must be used with extreme caution in infants and children.[459]

Another IV catheter–type emergency airway device is the Emergency Transtracheal Airway Catheter (Cook Critical Care), which consists of a 6F reinforced catheter that is advanced over a 15-gauge needle similar to the devices described earlier (E-Fig. 14.6). One study simulated use of the Enk Oxygen Flow Modulation set with a variety of IV cannulae and the Emergency Transtracheal Airway Catheter. The investigators concluded that the device worked best when all holes on the Enk device were occluded simultaneously and that minimum flow should never be less than 1 L/minute. They also suggested that initial fresh gas flow be set to 1 L/minute and then adjusted up or down to effect.[460] Successful ventilation with uncuffed devices may depend on the patency of the upper airway (i.e., the greater the patency, the less the effectiveness of ventilation in the nonbreathing patient).[461] None of these devices has been examined in controlled trials to confirm efficacy, in part because these events are so rare. Therefore, we recommend training on simulators so that each practitioner can determine what device is best in his or her hands.

Several percutaneous emergency airway devices are available that use a short but large-diameter needle or a needle, guidewire, and dilator to aid insertion of a percutaneous airway.[446,462–464] The Quicktrach (Rüsch) is a device that consists of a tapered 2- or 4-mm catheter with a fixation flange for securing with cloth tape. A removable plastic stopper is designed to limit the depth of needle insertion. This device requires several steps: puncture of the skin, aspiration for air, removal of the stopper, removal of the needle/syringe, and attachment to standard 22-mm connector. A flexible connector is also provided (E-Fig. 14.7). A rabbit model to simulate infant cricothyroidotomy found success in all attempts but 2 of 10 attempts resulted in fracture of the cricoid cartilage and 1 resulted in damage to the mucosa of the posterior tracheal wall.[465] Conversely, this device has been shown to allow more rapid establishment of an airway than other devices that use a Seldinger technique[466,467]; a larger, cuffed adult model is now available (E-Fig. 14.8).

Other devices that use the Seldinger technique (i.e., needle, guidewire, scalpel incision of the skin, and passage of a dilator and tracheostomy tube) are the Arndt and Melker devices (Cook Critical Care).[468] These devices provide a 3.0-mm ID airway that is sufficient for ventilation as well as oxygenation (E-Fig. 14.9). However, the time required to insert such devices may be longer than for simpler devices and may be inappropriate for immediate rapid establishment of an airway.[446,466,467] In contrast, a porcine cadaver study found greater comfort with this technique compared with a scalpel technique.[469] These devices are useful for elective percutaneous tracheostomy.[470]

Another device, Pertrach (Engineered Medical Systems), uses a split needle on a syringe to puncture the cricothyroid membrane (E-Fig. 14.10). A skin incision is made, and an introducer with tracheostomy tube (3.0-mm ID) is directed into the trachea, splitting the needle, which is removed. The introducer is then removed and the airway is secured with tracheostomy tape. There are no case reports in the literature to determine the ease or difficulty of insertion in children, but the multiple steps required suggest that it may be a device for elective tracheostomy rather than emergent establishment of a surgical airway.

Another percutaneous tracheostomy device is the Bivona Pedia-Trake kit (Smiths Medical) (E-Fig. 14.11). A skin incision is made with a scalpel, and a large needle is introduced with a skin dilator, which in theory opens the incision sufficiently to allow passage of an obturator and a 3.0-, 4.0-, or 5.0-mm ID tracheostomy tube (with or without cuff). This device appears sufficiently complicated to not be useful in a CICV emergency; it might be better suited when there is an urgent but not emergent need to establish surgical access to the airway.

Other devices with limited pediatric use[462] are kits designed to place a full-sized tracheostomy tube, such as the Nu-Trake (International Medical Devices, Northridge, CA) and Abelson (Gilbert Surgical Instruments, Bellmawr, NJ) devices. They may potentially cause tracheal or laryngeal injury in small patients because of the relatively large size of the needle; again, little experience in children has been published.[463,464,471]

Laryngeal Mask Airway Versus Percutaneous Needle Cricothyroidotomy and Transtracheal Jet Ventilation

The LMA Classic has proved to be an extremely useful device in airway emergencies. In contrast to percutaneous needle crico-thyroidotomy, it is an effective device for ventilation as well as a conduit for intubation.[472] The LMA is easily inserted and requires a relatively low level of skill, as demonstrated in numerous studies comparing this technique with other airway management skills (e.g., mask ventilation, endotracheal intubation). More importantly, in contrast to transtracheal jet ventilation, the complication rate with the LMA Classic is exceedingly low.[473] However, if glottic or subglottic obstruction to ventilation is present, the SGA will be ineffective and a surgical airway with or without transtracheal jet ventilation is still the emergency technique of choice. Since the introduction of the LMA, clinical experience suggests that if glottic or subglottic pathology is not suspected, LMA placement to establish ventilation may be appropriately attempted as the first step at airway rescue.[395]

Surgical Airway

An emergent surgical airway is viewed by some as an alternative to needle cricothyroidotomy.[447,474] It previously fell under the purview of the surgeon, in particular the pediatric otolaryngologist.[447,448,474–476] However, with training, it can be performed quickly by anesthesiologists.[477,478] A CICO situation event in children is extremely rare. Very few practitioners have ever performed a surgical cricothyroidotomy in a child or an adult. There is very little clinical evidence to support any surgical versus needle technique. Randomized trials are ethically impossible and case series in children are not available because of underreporting. Guidelines are based largely on animal studies and expert opinion. Both needle cricothyroidotomy and the surgical scalpel bougie technique are difficult in infants because the trachea is small and mobile[474]; the surgical emergent airway is best performed in those older than 5 years. In nonemergent airway management for children, a tracheostomy is preferred to a cricothyroidotomy because of fewer long-term complications and better results with later decannulation of the airway.[446,479]

Anterior Commissure Scope and Rigid Ventilating Bronchoscope

Two pieces of equipment used by otolaryngologists that can assist in visualizing the larynx and providing a method of ventilation are the anterior commissure scope and the rigid ventilating bronchoscope. The anterior commissure scope is a rigid, tubular, straight-blade laryngoscope with a light at the tip. The technique to place the anterior commissure scope and the advantages for visualization are similar to those described later for the straight blade used with the retromolar approach.[140]

SPECIAL TECHNIQUES FOR INTUBATION
Rigid Laryngoscopy

The rigid laryngoscope is the most familiar and most universally available piece of airway equipment; therefore it is critical for the practitioner to become familiar with its use and to know a variety of techniques. Some suggestions are reviewed here. It is reasonable to take a second look with the rigid laryngoscope after an unexpected failed intubation; however, a good rule is to always change something about the approach that may improve visualization. In the past, awake rigid intubation was the traditional approach to the problematic neonatal airway, but this approach should be used only in an extreme emergency or when IV access is not available.[157–160] Some anatomic features are completely unfavorable for success with the rigid laryngoscope, regardless of technique. Repeated unsuccessful attempts should be avoided because this can lead to airway trauma and edema. Because infants and children already have smaller airway structures, they are uniquely susceptible to a rapid progression from "cannot intubate, *can ventilate*" to the CICV scenario.

Whether the child has a normal or an abnormal airway, it is essential to ensure correct positioning and to use age-appropriate equipment. The following maneuvers have been found to be helpful in achieving successful intubation of the child with a difficult airway.

Optimal External Laryngeal Manipulation

Pressure can be applied externally to the larynx during the intubation to maximize visualization of the larynx.[480] Optimal external laryngeal manipulation (OELM) is particularly helpful for children with immobile or shortened necks and for infants. Either an assistant or the laryngoscopist can perform OELM. When the laryngoscopist performs the maneuver, the assistant either can pass the ETT into the glottis while the laryngoscopist maintains OELM or OELM can be assumed by the assistant to allow the laryngoscopist to pass the ETT.[480] OELM may also be used in conjunction with other, more advanced airway devices such as the GlideScope (discussed later).[481–483]

Intubation Guides

Intubation guides include plastic-coated, flexible metal stylets and the gum elastic bougie. These can be used for blind placement of the ETT under the epiglottis. A flexible stylet is placed inside the ETT and preformed to shape the ETT tip to one that will optimize intubation success (see Fig. 14.21). A hockey-stick configuration is frequently useful, particularly if only the epiglottis or the most posterior portion of the glottis can be visualized. The gum elastic bougie has a preformed, angled tip. It is placed alone and then the ETT is threaded over it and into the trachea (E-Fig. 14.12). When the bougie is successfully placed in the trachea, one can detect the subtle "bumpy" feel of the bougie making contact with the anterior tracheal rings. This device may also be used to facilitate intubation through an LMA or as an adjunct to other airway devices.[484–487]

Dental Mirror

The authors of one report used a short-handled dental mirror (no. 3, Storz Instrument Company, Manchester, England) to assist in the indirect visualization of the larynx of a 10-week-old infant. Laryngoscopy was impossible with a size 1 Miller blade. The infant was returned to spontaneous ventilation, a size 1 Macintosh blade was used to expose the pharynx, and the mirror was used to visualize the larynx. A styleted ETT was then passed into the glottis under indirect vision.[488]

Retromolar, Paraglossal, or Lateral Approach Using a Straight Blade

Use of a straight blade in a retromolar approach may allow glottic visualization when the classic rigid intubation technique fails, particularly if the difficulty is secondary to a large tongue or small mandible (Fig. 14.28).[140,482,485,489–493] With the child's head turned slightly to the left, a no. 1 Miller blade is introduced into the extreme right side of the mouth. It is advanced in the space between the tongue and the lateral pharyngeal wall; the tongue is swept completely to the left and is essentially bypassed. It is very helpful to have an assistant pull back the right corner of the mouth with a small retractor (e.g., Senn retractor) to increase the space for ETT placement. The blade is advanced while staying to the right, overlying the bicuspids and lateral incisors until the epiglottis or the glottis is visualized. When the epiglottis comes in view, it is lifted with the blade tip to expose the glottic opening. It is extremely unlikely that pressure from the laryngoscope blade on the bicuspids and lateral incisors could loosen these teeth, because they have two roots or their roots are deeper than the central incisors.

At this juncture in the laryngoscopy, it may be possible to move the proximal end of the blade toward the midline of the mouth to increase room for ETT placement and manipulation, although care must be taken to avoid applying pressure on the central incisors of the maxilla, lest they become loosened. If the glottis is not visualized, the head can be rotated farther to the left and the blade can be kept lateral to improve visualization. The ETT should be styletted and formed into a 90-degree bend configuration to assist in placement (see Fig. 14.21), particularly if the view of the glottis is only partial. A shorter-length blade (usually a size 1 Miller, even in older children) than that used in the traditional midline approach is chosen because the distance to the glottis with this method is greatly shortened.

Several mechanisms are responsible for the improved view of the glottis with the retromolar approach to laryngoscopy. First, there is a reduced need for soft tissue displacement and compression because the lateral placement of the blade bypasses the tongue. This approach to an improved view of the glottic opening is particularly useful for children with micrognathia.[482,485,490,492,493] In such children, the space available to displace the tongue is reduced compared with the traditional midline approach to rigid laryngoscopy. Second, there is an improved line of visualization because the incisors and maxillary structures are bypassed by lateral blade placement and by shifting of the head to the left. Third, the use of a straight blade avoids the possible intrusion of a curved blade into the line of sight.[140,489–491] Finally, both the angle and the distance from the insertion of the straight blade at the right commissure of the mouth are reduced, facilitating an easier view of the glottic opening, particularly during a difficult intubation, compared with inserting the blade in the midline.

Fiberoptic Laryngoscopy

An advantage of using the FOB for intubation of the child with a difficult airway is that it does not require extensive head or neck manipulation and is therefore useful in children who have cervical inflexibility (Klippel-Feil syndrome) or cervical instability (Down syndrome, achondroplastic dwarfism, trauma) (see Videos 14.10 and 14.11). The technique is also versatile because the flexible instrument conforms to a variety of abnormal airways; it is well tolerated by the sedated, spontaneously breathing child.[399,494–496]

Its disadvantage is that the fiberoptic bundle is small, permitting only a limited field of vision. For this reason, the presence of blood or copious secretions may render the FOB ineffective. In

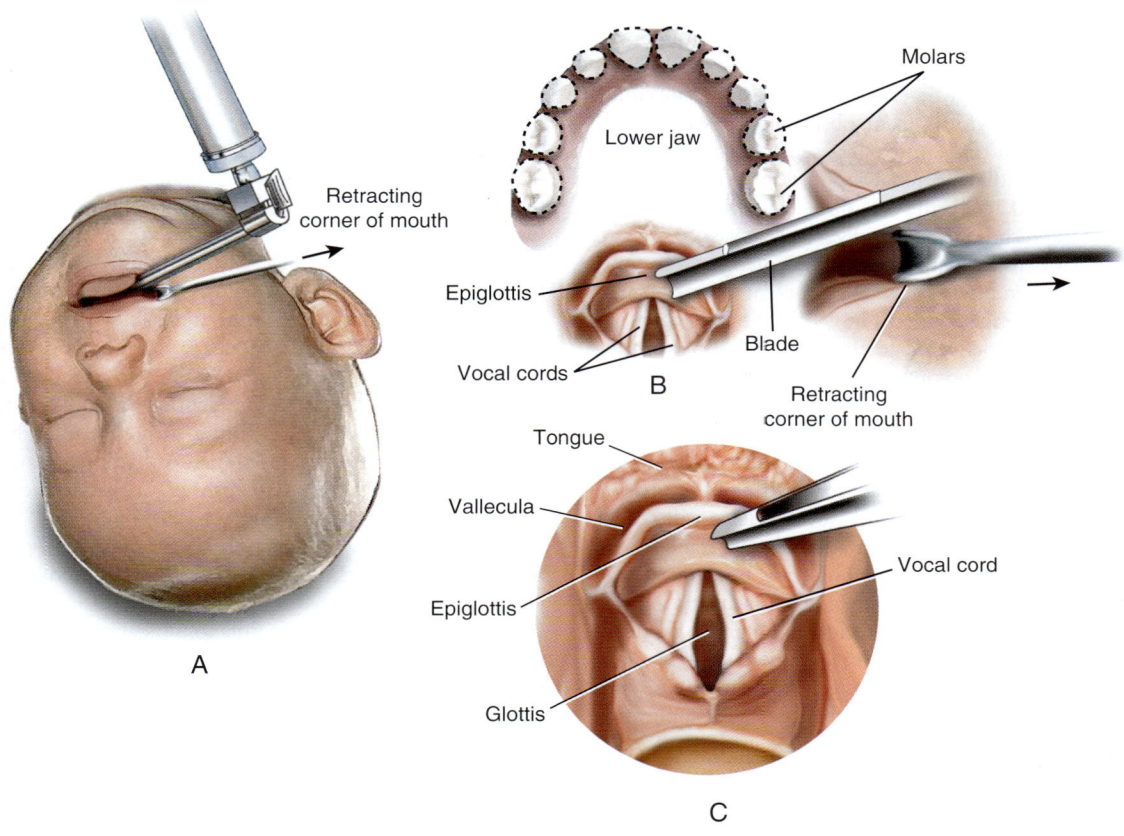

FIGURE 14.28 **A** through **C,** The retromolar, paraglossal, or lateral approach to rigid laryngoscopy using a straight blade. Notice that the child's head is turned to the left and that the laryngoscope blade is inserted over the molars toward the glottic opening (see text for details).

addition, use of the FOB requires extensive experience and practice in normal airways first. Our experience suggests that each size of available FOB should be used in at least 20 normal airways before use is attempted in an abnormal airway.[497] Practice with all available sizes of FOBs is important because the manual skills required for each size differ somewhat. Also, FOBs are fragile and expensive. Great care must be taken when using and storing FOBs to prevent breakage of the fiberoptic bundles and the adjustable tip mechanism. They must also be sterilized between uses to maintain the patency of the working channel and clear, bright vision through the fiberoptic bundles and to avoid transmission of infection.

Equipment
FOBs with directable tips are available in various sizes; the smallest, 2.2 mm in diameter (Olympus LFP; Olympus, Tokyo), can fit through a 2.5-mm ID ETT with or without the 15-mm adapter removed. However, unlike most of the larger FOBs, this scope has no working channel for suctioning or administration of oxygen or topical anesthesia. FOBs with the light source incorporated into the body of the scope are now available; these increase the portability of the instrument, making its use both outside and inside the operating room more simple and convenient.

Ancillary Equipment
Endoscopy masks can be used to provide oxygen to the spontaneously breathing child and to ventilate the paralyzed child during fiberoptic laryngoscopy. The Frei endoscopy mask (VBM Medizintechnik GmbH [E-Fig. 14.13]) and the Patil-Syracuse endoscopy mask (Anesthesia Associates, San Marcos, CA) are commercially available.[498,499] Patil-Syracuse masks are available in a child size but are too large for most children younger than age 4 years.[96] The Frei mask configuration allows the FOB to be placed in a central position, overlying the nose and mouth, which is more favorable for tracheal intubation. The clear membrane with the hole for the bronchoscope can be rotated to allow either oral or nasal approaches. Alternatively, a disposable facemask can be combined with a bronchoscopic swivel adapter.[500] The FOB can then be passed through the diaphragm of the adapter while ventilation is maintained via the anesthesia circuit. There are two types of commercially available adapters. One type attaches directly to an anesthesia mask. The other type is designed to attach to the ETT and can be modified to fit on the anesthesia mask using a 15- to 22-mm adapter.

Commercial oral airways designed for use in bronchoscopy are available for pediatric patients (IMD Inc., Park City, UT); however, there are only three sizes (infant, child, and adult), and no studies have evaluated their usefulness in assisting fiberoptic intubation in children. Guedel airways can also be modified for use as oral intubation guides.[500] A strip is cut from the convex surface of the airway to create a channel for placement of the FOB. This modified airway may be used to maintain a midline approach to the glottis; however, it is ineffective as a bite block.

Direct Technique

The optimal position of the child for fiberoptic bronchoscopy is different from the position for rigid laryngoscopy. The head should be flat on the table and slightly extended at the atlantooccipital joint to prevent the epiglottis from obstructing a view of the glottic opening.[501] If an oral approach is selected, it is vital that the FOB pass in the midline. A nasal approach may make midline placement simpler and avoids the risk of the child biting the FOB or ETT. One useful technique is to apply a topical vasoconstrictor (e.g., oxymetazoline) to the naris, place a lubricated nasal trumpet into the naris, and then insert a 15-mm connector from a tracheal tube into the nasal trumpet (Video 14.8). This allows oxygen and inhalation agent to be delivered to the child while performing standard fiberoptic laryngoscopy (see Videos 14.10 and 14.11). However, the oral approach offers several advantages over the nasal approach, including avoidance of shearing adenoidal tissue and nasal bleeding. The oral approach may also be less stimulating and better tolerated than the nasal approach. If nasal intubation is chosen in a young child, a topical vasoconstrictor will reduce the risk of bleeding. With both approaches, an assistant should perform a jaw thrust to open the posterior pharyngeal and supraglottic spaces. Alternatively, a bite block or intubating airway may be used. Occasionally, the best view is obtained by direct traction on the tongue, which optimally opens the posterior pharynx. This can be accomplished by grasping the tongue with a gauze, plastic forceps, a stitch through the tongue, or application of high suction to the underside or tip of the tongue (Fig. 14.29).[502]

The tip of the FOB should be introduced behind the tongue and gradually advanced in the midline under direct vision until a recognizable structure is observed. It is essential that the FOB be kept rigid so that when the direction of the tip is altered, it remains in the same plane as the handle of the FOB. When the FOB is rotated, the tip should be slightly bent to provide a panoramic view. In general, the tip of the FOB is passed into the trachea before any attempts are made to pass the ETT through the nose or oropharynx. Because the distances in the oropharynx in children are less than in adults, the most common initial error when using this technique is to advance the FOB too deeply and

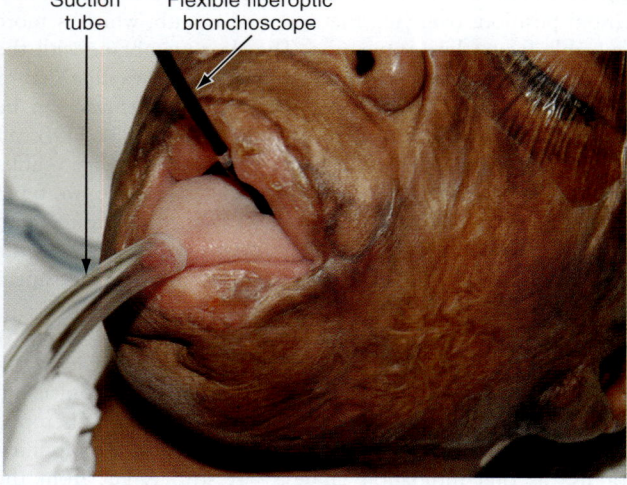

FIGURE 14.29 Suction can be applied to the tip of the tongue to facilitate pulling it forward to improve glottic visualization. This technique is particularly useful when the tongue is slippery due to secretions or if the mouth opening is small and prevents direct grasping of the tongue with a dry gauze.

into the esophagus. To avoid this pitfall, the FOB should be advanced only toward identifiable airway structures.

Once the FOB is introduced into the airway, a common problem is resistance to passage of the ETT. To minimize this occurrence, the ETT should be loaded onto the scope with the bevel facing down (Murphy eye up) for oral intubation and bevel facing up for nasal intubation.[503,504] This can be remembered by the mnemonic *UNDO*: bevel **U**p for **N**asal intubation, **D**own for **O**ral intubation.[505] If persistent resistance is encountered while attempting to pass the ETT past the glottic opening, the ETT should be rotated 90 to 180 degrees to place the bevel in a more favorable orientation for passage through the vocal cords. One study demonstrated that a 90-degree counterclockwise rotation of the ETT before advancement resulted in a smooth passage of the ETT into the larynx.[506] The depth of anesthesia or sedation as well as oxygen saturation (pulse oximetry) must be carefully monitored throughout the procedure. Arrhythmias may be avoided by providing an adequate depth of analgesia/anesthesia and ensuring a patent airway.

Fiberoptic laryngoscopy techniques should be perfected on manikins and on children with normal anatomy before such techniques are attempted on children with difficult airways.[507–513] In a study that compared the time to intubation and complications in 40 infants with the Miller size 1 laryngoscope blade or the Olympus LFP FOB, the time to intubation was slightly greater with the FOB (22.8 vs. 13.6 seconds), whereas the complication rate was similar.[514] The authors concluded that routine use of the FOB for intubation in normal infants is a safe and reasonable method to gain and maintain skills with this technique.[514] For children, video-assisted fiberoptic intubation appears to offer advantages over fiberoptic intubation using a traditional eyepiece. These include faster mastering of this skill and an overall improved success rate when compared with the traditional method.[497,515]

Staged Techniques

Staged methods of fiberoptic intubation can be used in infants and small children when the available FOBs are too large to pass through the appropriately sized ETT.[516] One method requires an FOB with a working channel and a cardiac vascular catheter with guidewire. The guidewire is passed through the working channel of the FOB to within 1 inch of its tip. The FOB is then introduced into the mouth and positioned above the vocal cords. The guidewire is advanced under direct observation through the glottis into the trachea. The FOB is removed, leaving the guidewire in place. The lungs are ventilated by mask while an assistant passes the cardiac catheter over the guidewire (to stiffen the guidewire and facilitate passage of the ETT). The ETT is threaded over the catheter/guidewire combination, which is then removed, leaving the ETT in place.[516–518] Some authors report that threading of the cardiac catheter over the guidewire is unnecessary. A modification of this technique when the FOB has no working channel has also been described.[519] An 8F red rubber catheter was attached by waterproof tape to the insertion cord of the FOB proximal to the flexible tip. The larynx was visualized with the FOB, and a guidewire was threaded through the rubber catheter into the trachea. With the guidewire in position, the FOB (with the red rubber catheter) was withdrawn, and an ETT was passed over the guidewire into the trachea.

Another alternative for intubation when the FOB is too large to pass through the appropriately sized ETT is intubation under fiberoptic observation.[520–522] The FOB is introduced through one naris to visually aid the placement of the ETT that is passed through the other naris and manipulated into the glottis. Alternatively, if the observed ETT is not easily passed into the glottis, a small catheter may be more easily manipulated into the glottis and used as a stylet to pass the ETT into the trachea. Spontaneous ventilation is preserved, and oxygen can be administered via the ETT during the intubation. This technique was used successfully in two neonates, one with congenital fusion of the jaws and a second with Dandy-Walker syndrome associated with Klippel-Feil syndrome, micrognathia, hypoplasia of the soft palate, and anteversion of the uvula.[520,521] More recently, an adult video-FOB was used to intubate the trachea of a toddler with temporomandibular joint ankyloses.[523] If the available FOB is both too large and lacks a working channel, another staged fiberoptic intubation technique can be used. The FOB is loaded with an ETT that is larger than the larynx of the infant. The larynx is visualized with the FOB, and the ETT is advanced and positioned just above the vocal cords. The FOB is then removed, and an ETT changer or catheter is advanced into the trachea through the larger ETT. The larger ETT is then removed, and the appropriately sized ETT for the child is threaded over the tube changer or catheter into the trachea. This technique was used successfully in a 6-month-old infant whose operation had previously been canceled because of failure to intubate.[524]

Lighted Stylet

A lighted stylet (Light Wand) is a useful adjunct for managing the pediatric difficult airway (E-Fig. 14.14).[525–529] A number of these devices are available: Surch-Lite Lighted Intubation Stylet (Bovie Medical Corporation, Purchase, NY), Light Wand (Vital Signs, Mexicali, Mexico), and Trachlite (Rüsch, Tuttlingen, Germany). These devices essentially comprise a malleable stylet with a high-intensity light at the tip; the stylet is shaped into a curve similar to that anticipated for successful passage into the laryngeal inlet (45 to 90 degrees). To begin, an ETT is passed over a well-lubricated lighted stylet. The tip of the stylet should remain within the tip of the ETT to minimize the potential for airway trauma. The room lights should be dimmed at this time to ensure that the stylet is visible when the wand is in the mouth. The lighted stylet is then introduced into the mouth while the proximal end of the stylet is flat against the cheek. As the stylet is inserted into the mouth, the proximal end of the handle is rotated counterclockwise until it is upright. The stylet continues to pass through the oropharynx, following the curvature of the tongue. If the tip of the lighted stylet is not in the proper position (e.g., in the esophagus), a diffuse light or no light will be observed on the surface of the neck. Proper position is usually ensured when a sharp, well-defined, bright circle or cone of light is observed transilluminating the neck directly in the midline at the level of the cricothyroid membrane (see E-Fig. 14.14). Once proper position is ensured, the ETT is gently advanced and the stylet is removed.[528,530]

This technique is useful in those children in whom there is no intrinsic laryngeal or airway pathology but in whom visualization is anticipated to be difficult. The lighted stylet may also be of value in children with a fracture of the cervical spine, because tracheal intubation can be accomplished with minimal movement of the neck.[531] The hemodynamic response to intubation with this technique is similar to that observed with rigid laryngoscopy.[527] The limitations of this technique are that it is a blind technique, the diameter of the device limits it use to larger-sized ETTs, and it may require multiple attempts; however, the success rate markedly increases with experience.[528,530] The most common cause of difficulty

in passing the ETT is that the tube hangs up on the epiglottis. When this occurs, the lighted stylet may be withdrawn and its position slightly adjusted more posterior to allow passage behind and beyond the epiglottis. Alternatively, the ETT can be rotated along the long axis of the stylet so that the bevel is facing up. Our advice for using this technique is similar to that for bronchoscopy: it should be used in children with normal anatomy to gain the necessary experience required for managing children with abnormal airway anatomy. This adjunct has also been combined with an LMA to guide the stylet into the trachea.[532]

Bullard Laryngoscope

The Bullard laryngoscope is now rarely used for direct visualization of the laryngeal inlet in children with airway pathology (E-Fig. 14.15). It is available in three sizes: adult, pediatric, and pediatric long. This instrument combines fiberoptic bundles and mirrors. It is positioned within the larynx like a laryngoscope blade, and the direction of force used to displace the tongue is similar to that used with a standard laryngoscope, although this is not intuitively obvious from its configuration. It is designed to provide visualization around a 90-degree bend at the tip (i.e., around the base of the tongue). This configuration may be helpful for direct visualization of the larynx in children with mandibular hypoplasia syndromes (e.g., Robin sequence, Treacher Collins syndrome,[533] Goldenhar syndrome, cervical fracture restricting motion), when the acute angulation of the base of the tongue to the glottic opening is exaggerated, and in children with congenital trismus (Hecht syndrome).[534] The technique used in children is different from that used in adults. Once the laryngeal inlet is visualized, a styleted ETT, with a bent configuration similar to the curve of the Bullard laryngoscope (see Fig. 14.21B), is inserted just to the side of the Bullard laryngoscope blade and advanced under direct vision into the trachea. Success with this instrument is directly proportional to the experience of the anesthesiologist, because the perspective seen through this laryngoscope, the method of visualization, and the indirect method of ETT placement are so different from standard laryngoscopy.[535,536]

Despite the availability of pediatric Bullard laryngoscopes,[537] adult scopes have also been successfully used in children.[538,539] Although tracheal intubation in children 1 to 5 years of age with a Bullard laryngoscope takes more time than with a Wis-Hipple 1.5 blade, the adult Bullard laryngoscope complements the Wis-Hipple 1.5 blade. Occasionally, the Bullard laryngoscope provides a superior laryngeal view and thus allows successful intubation when a failure with the Wis-Hipple blade occurs. When multiple passes of the tube off the adult Bullard laryngoscope were required, this is usually because of contact with the right aryepiglottic fold or anterior vocal cord. The latter appears to be more problematic when the adult laryngoscope is used in children.[538,539]

Additional limitations of the Bullard laryngoscope are that the ETT can partially obstruct the view of the larynx during insertion and that it can be used only for oral intubation.[537] An advantage is that there appears to be minimal motion of the cervical spine in patients with cervical spine disarticulations.[540–542]

Retrograde Wire-Guided Intubation

The technique of retrograde wire-guided intubation uses transtracheal passage of an IV catheter through the cricothyroid membrane into the larynx and retrograde passage of a guidewire from a Seldinger vascular cannulation set to create a guide for intubation.[416,543–549] A commercial kit is available for use with ETTs that are 5 mm ID or larger (Cook Critical Care). This technique is rarely used in children because of the greater compressibility of the trachea and the increased risk of posterior tracheal wall perforation by the catheter in children compared with adults.

Video and Indirect Intubating Devices

Advances in technology have led to the reduction in size of video cameras and optical lenses. The integration of these devices into various laryngoscopes and stylets has produced several enhanced tools for securing the airway in children.[550] Several of these new scopes improve visualization during laryngoscopy[484,551–557] and perform better than traditional laryngoscopy in children with difficult direct laryngoscopy.[558–564] However, they are often associated with prolonged time to intubation compared with direct laryngoscopy, and their utility is limited in the presence of blood and secretions. These new devices can be categorized as (1) video laryngoscopes, which incorporate a video camera into the tip of the device; (2) optical laryngoscopes, which use a series of mirrors, prisms, or both to transmit the image from the tip of the device; and (3) optical stylets, which incorporate video or optical systems into a rigid or malleable stylet.

Videolaryngoscopes

Videolaryngoscopes are quickly becoming ubiquitous in anesthesia practice and will inevitably become the standard of care. They offer unique advantages over standard direct laryngoscopy such as an improved view of the glottis, a shared view of the airway that facilitates guidance of a trainee and less force required to perform the intubation. Although the term videolaryngoscope is loosely used to describe a large number of laryngoscopes with video and optical cameras, these devices can be very different with unique design characteristics. Videolaryngoscopes can be classified in two broad categories—those with angulated blades and those with standard curved blades. The videolaryngoscopes with angulated blades may perform better in patients with difficult airways, while those with standard blades may be best suited for patients with normal airways. Although angulated blades offer a better view of an "anterior" airway, passing the tube may be more challenging because of the acute angles made between the camera line of sight and the plane of the trachea. Videolaryngoscopes with standard blades are less likely to be associated with this difficulty but may not offer as optimal a view as angulated blades in the difficult airway patient. Videolaryngoscopes with conventional blades can be used to teach traditional laryngoscopy and therefore help trainees to maintain their skill with that technique while having the advantage of direct feedback from an instructor monitoring the camera screen. Videolaryngoscopes have been associated with higher first-attempt success and success rates in adults compared with direct laryngoscopy and have been shown to have improved views of the airway in children as well.[552,565–567] A retrospective cohort study in a pediatric emergency department compared videolaryngoscopy with the C-MAC video laryngoscope (Karl Storz Gmbh & Co. KG, Tuttlingen, Germany) with direct laryngoscopy and found no differences in first-attempt intubation success (adjusted odds ratio = 1.23, 95% confidence interval [CI] = 0.78-1.94), complication rates, or intubation success rates.[568] A meta-analysis of randomized controlled trials in children (993 participants) that compared video laryngoscopes with direct laryngoscopes concluded that the use of videolaryngoscopy improved glottic visualization but prolonged the time to intubation and was associated with increased failures. They found similar first-attempt success between video laryngoscopy and direct laryngoscopy (relative risk 0.96; 95% CI 0.92-1.00; $I^2 =$

67%).[569] The report of increased failures is not consistent with our experience and is in fact doubtful with modern videolaryngoscopes. A careful examination of their meta-analysis shows that most of the failures occurred in a single study that examined the Bullard laryngoscope in which 50% of first attempts failed in a cohort of 2- to 10-year-old children with simulated restricted neck mobility.[569] Many evaluations of videolaryngoscopes are conducted in manikins; although this should be the first step to evaluate a new device, we encourage researchers to conduct clinical studies to expand our knowledge about the real-world performance of these devices. One study demonstrated that although trainees performed tracheal intubation with a variety of videolaryngoscopes expeditiously in a manikin, they took significantly longer in children younger than 2 years of age.[570]

GLIDESCOPE. The GlideScope (Verathon, Bothell, WA) (E-Fig. 14.16) consists of a hypercurved blade that incorporates a high-resolution camera with a built-in antifog system. It is available in six sizes (0, 1, 2, 2.5, 3, 4) that accommodate all sizes of patients, including as small as approximately 1 kg. Before clinical use, the GlideScope is switched on to allow the antifog system to warm up. A styletted ETT is necessary for successful intubation, and the stylet's curvature should mimic that of the selected GlideScope blade. The manufacturer markets a GlideScope-specific rigid stylet, but a standard malleable stylet has been shown to be equally effective.[571] Unlike traditional direct laryngoscopy, sweeping the tongue to the left of the blade is unnecessary because of the distally located camera. The GlideScope blade is ideally placed in the midline or slightly to the left in the pharynx (Video 14.12). This position maximizes the space available for introduction of the ETT. The blade tip is placed in the vallecula, and slight elevation of the blade exposes the glottis. The epiglottis may be elevated if placement of the blade tip in the vallecula does not result in optimal visualization. A poor view may occur if the blade size is inappropriate or if the blade is inserted too deeply in the pharynx. OELM may also be used to facilitate laryngeal visualization.[551,567]

Once the best view is obtained, the styletted ETT is inserted under direct vision alongside the GlideScope blade until it just passes the palatoglossal arches and is in full view on the GlideScope monitor. The technique of sequentially visualizing the ETT directly and then on the monitor and creating space by inserting the GlideScope slightly to the left in the pharynx helps minimize the risk of injury to the soft tissues of the airway during advancement of the ETT.[572–576] Children with severely obstructing tonsils may be vulnerable to injury if the laryngoscopist focusses their attention only on the screen and ignores the styletted tube as it is brought into view.[577]

When the ETT is visible on the monitor, the tip is directed into the glottic inlet. The stylet should be pulled back once the ETT tip is inserted through the cords, because this facilitates the advancement of the ETT down the trachea. Difficult ETT insertion despite a good view of the glottic opening is an occasional problem encountered with the GlideScope and other video and optical laryngoscopes. This is because of the indirect approach to intubation and the need for good hand-eye coordination. These skills can be acquired by frequent use of the device in children with normal airways.[578–582] The GlideScope Cobalt was successfully used for intubation in a cohort of 121 infants. The average intubation time was 30 seconds, and 95% of the intubations were successful on the first two attempts.[583] It has also been used to facilitate intubation in children with craniofacial abnormalities.[481,584–586] When compared with direct laryngoscopy, the GlideScope provided superior laryngeal views in children with baseline limited views of the glottic opening.[587]

STORZ VIDEO LARYNGOSCOPE. The Storz Video Laryngoscope (Karl Storz GbmH) integrates a camera into Miller- and Macintosh-type blades. This design allows the operator to perform laryngoscopy in the traditional fashion as the Miller-type blade with the video view available if necessary. The video view has been shown to provide one Cormack-Lehane grade improvement over the direct line-of-sight view because of the angulation of the video camera at the tip.[588] It has no antifog mechanism, so use of an antifog solution is needed for unimpaired visualization. Intubation with the Miller video blade can be performed without a stylet, although a styleted ETT with a slight bend at the tip facilitates intubation (E-Fig. 14.17). The Storz Video Laryngoscope is inserted in a fashion similar to insertion of the GlideScope. The tip of the blade can be placed in the vallecula; however, because of the magnified lens of the camera, the epiglottis often obstructs the camera view. If this occurs, the blade tip is best used to lift the epiglottis to expose the glottis. Once optimal visualization is obtained, the ETT is placed directly along the shaft of the video blade, which guarantees immediate visualization of the ETT in the magnified field of view of the camera and avoids injury to airway soft tissues.

When the Storz Video Laryngoscope was compared with the GlideScope in a pediatric manikin model with normal and difficult airway configurations, the times to intubation and the visual analog scale scores for field of view and ease of use of the two devices were similar.[589] In a small trial of 10 children younger than 2 years of age, the time to successful tracheal tube positioning was greater with the Storz instrument compared with the Airtrach (Prodol Meditec, Guecho, Spain) but the success rate was similar.[590] In another infant manikin study, the Storz Video Laryngoscope was associated with better views, more successful intubations, and similar intubation times as the standard Miller laryngoscope.[588] The Storz Video Laryngoscope has been successfully used to intubate infants and newborns with difficult and normal airways.[588,591] As with all video laryngoscopes, good hand-eye coordination is necessary for successful intubation. In addition, the operator must develop the skills necessary to manipulate the ETT indirectly and on a magnified scale. This magnification effect makes subtle movements of the ETT appear large on the video monitor and adds an additional challenge to intubation with these devices. Practice on children with normal airway anatomy is recommended before use on children with abnormal airways.[550]

MULTIVIEW SCOPE. The MultiView Scope (Medical Products International, Tokyo) is a video laryngoscope system that integrates a camera into Miller- and Macintosh-style blades (E-Fig. 14.18). The handle of the device has a mounted video screen that displays the image from the blade tip. The image from the screen can be transmitted to an external monitor wirelessly, using a manufacturer-supplied attachment (AirView). Aside from being magnified, the direct line-of-sight view is identical to the camera view, making this an ideal tool for teaching direct laryngoscopy. The MultiView Scope also comes with a malleable stylet attachment that provides the ability to insufflate oxygen through the mounted ETT.

Optical Laryngoscopes

AIRTRAQ. The Airtraq (Prodol Meditec SA, Vizcaya, Spain) is a single-use, curved plastic laryngoscope that uses lenses and prisms to transmit the image from its distal tip to an eyepiece. It may reduce the incidence of esophageal intubation and may offer greater success rates, particularly in the hands of the inexperienced laryngoscopist.[592] It has a molded channel into which the ETT is inserted (Fig. 14.30), thereby eliminating the need to manipulate the ETT independently during intubation as is required with the GlideScope, Truview (Teleflex Medical, Netanya, Israel), and Storz Video Laryngoscope. The manufacturer offers a wireless monitor for use with the device. The device should be turned on 30 seconds before use to allow the built-in antifog system to warm up. A disadvantage is that a minimum mouth opening of 16 mm is required for insertion of the Airtraq.

The selected ETT and guide channel of the Airtraq are lubricated, and the cuff of the ETT is fully deflated to avoid cuff damage during advancement of the tube in the channel.[593,594] The appropriately sized ETT is loaded into the guide channel of the device, and the child's head is placed in a neutral position. The Airtraq is inserted in the midline in the pharynx and is advanced along the tongue base into the vallecula (Video 14.13). The epiglottis may be elevated to optimize the view, if necessary. Once in position, the Airtraq is gently lifted to obtain optimal glottic exposure, the glottis is centered in the viewfinder by rotating the entire device slightly clockwise or counterclockwise as necessary, and the ETT is advanced after the optimal centered view is obtained. On occasion, the ETT is directed below the glottic opening; if this occurs, the Airtraq should be withdrawn slightly and the advancement attempted again. The guide channel deflects the ETT slightly leftward (an effect that is more pronounced in infants and neonates); this tendency may be countered by rotating the device slightly clockwise as needed.[595,596] Once the trachea is intubated, the Airtraq is separated from the ETT by holding the tube at the mouth and moving it laterally from the guide channel. The Airtraq is then rotated gently out of the oropharynx.

A suboptimal view with the Airtraq is often a result of inserting the device past the glottis. If this happens, the device should be withdrawn slowly until the larynx comes into view. As with other optical and video-enhanced laryngoscopes, the Airtraq has been associated with airway soft tissue injury. A tonsillar injury in a 4-year-old child was attributed to the width of the guide channel of the device.[597] Care should be taken when using the device in small children, given its size relative to the pharyngeal space. An Airtraq devoid of the guide channel is available for nasal intubations; the intubation may be facilitated with the use of Magill forceps or a gum elastic bougie.[598] The Airtraq has been successfully used for intubation in children with normal and difficult airways; however, despite its having a guide channel, some reports have noted difficulty with directing the ETT in neonates and infants.[484,552–554,599–601] The Airtraq is easy to learn and use.[602,603] As with many optical and video devices, there remains a learning curve to using the device,[604] particularly the manipulation of the tracheal tube into the glottis in small patients.[550]

TRUVIEW. The Truview EVO2 Infant device (Teleflex Medical, Netanya, Israel) is an optical laryngoscope with an angulated, stainless steel blade that transmits a magnified image from the tip of the device to an eyepiece using lenses (E-Fig. 14.19). A camera is available for connection to the eyepiece to allow the image to be viewed on a monitor. A side port is integrated into the blade to allow oxygen insufflation to clear the lens during intubation; however, caution should be exercised when insufflating oxygen in neonates and infants because of the rare risk of gastric insufflation and rupture.[605–607] Because of the indirect view afforded by the device, a stylet is necessary for successful intubation; a preformed stylet is available from the manufacturer. As with the GlideScope, the ETT should be shaped in a curve similar to the

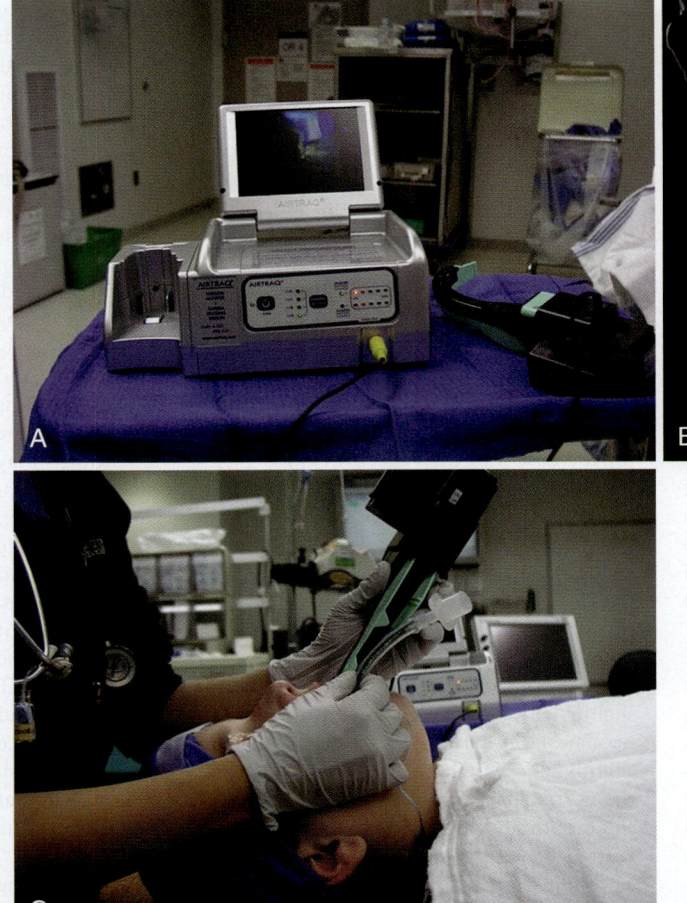

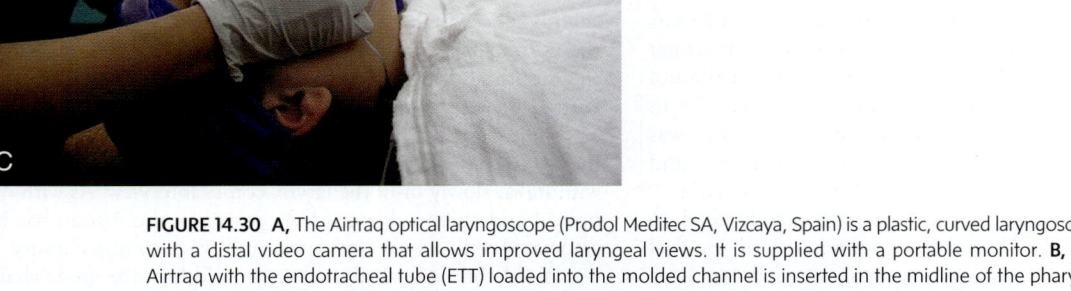

FIGURE 14.30 A, The Airtraq optical laryngoscope (Prodol Meditec SA, Vizcaya, Spain) is a plastic, curved laryngoscope with a distal video camera that allows improved laryngeal views. It is supplied with a portable monitor. **B,** The Airtraq with the endotracheal tube (ETT) loaded into the molded channel is inserted in the midline of the pharynx. **C,** The ETT is held laterally from the Airtraq after intubation, and the Airtraq is then rotated away from the operator and out of the pharynx.

Truview blade. The blade is placed centrally along the tongue in the pharynx to the vallecula, and slight elevation should expose the vocal cords. The ETT is then passed alongside the device, taking care to look in the mouth during initial insertion to make sure the airway soft tissues are not injured. The Truview EVO₂ has been compared to laryngoscopy with a Miller blade in children, with results showing improved views of the larynx but longer intubation times.[556] If the patient's head is in the neutral position as for cervical spine instability, application of OELM will improve the view.[608] A study in adults found an improved laryngeal view compared with standard laryngoscopy without the need to align the oral, pharyngeal, and tracheal axes.[609] Once again, there is a learning curve with this device, and practice should shorten intubation times and minimize injury to soft tissues.[550] The Truview PCD Pediatric is the most recent iteration of the original Truview design; it is available with four pediatric blade sizes (0, 1, 2, 3) for newborns from 800 gm to large teenagers. A recent assessment of the Truview PCD in 86 consecutive children with normal airways found that 79 patients were successfully intubated on the first attempt while 4 patients required 2 attempts. Tracheal intubation time was 30 (27.9–37) seconds.[610]

Optical Stylets

Use of optical stylets, unlike FOB intubation, allows the operator to visualize the ETT as it enters the glottis. This is because the stylet is located just within the distal tip of the ETT, providing the operator with a view of the leading edge of the ETT. This view allows immediate recognition of impediments to ETT advancement such as the right arytenoid and enables negotiation of the stylet around these obstacles. The Shikani and the Bonfils are two optical stylets available for pediatric use. Secretions, fogging, and airway soft tissue can impede intubation with optical stylets because of their small lenses and limited depth of view. Impairment of visualization by airway soft tissue can be addressed by combining these devices with direct laryngoscopy. The direct laryngoscope allows the creation of space for visualization with the optical stylet but may require two operators for successful intubation. Optical stylets may be easier to learn and maneuver than FOBs, although some have questioned the utility of these devices in the pediatric population, particularly in the presence of copious secretions.[611,612]

SHIKANI OPTICAL STYLET. The Shikani Optical Stylet (SOS; Clarus Medical, Minneapolis, MN) is a malleable, J-shaped fiberoptic stylet that transmits the image from its distal tip to an eyepiece (E-Fig. 14.20). It has an adjustable tube stop to secure the tube and a port for oxygen insufflation, which should be used with caution in small children.[607,613] The nondominant hand is used to perform a jaw thrust, elevating the epiglottis from the posterior pharyngeal wall, and the stylet is then inserted in the midline in the pharynx (Video 14.14). The tongue base, uvula, and epiglottis are visualized in succession, and the tip is placed just above or just into the glottic inlet. The ETT is then advanced while the SOS is held steady. The SOS is a useful adjunct in the management of the pediatric difficult airway.[614,615]

STORZ BONFILS OPTICAL STYLET. The Bonfils Optical Stylet (Karl Storz) is a rigid fiberoptic stylet with a fixed 40-degree curvature (E-Fig. 14.21). It delivers a higher-quality image than the SOS but is not malleable. Although the manufacturer recommends a retromolar approach to intubation, a midline approach similar to that of the SOS has been found to be successful in children.[616] The Bonfils is available in pediatric and infant sizes and can be coupled to a portable monitor (available from the manufacturer). The use of an antisialagogue and suctioning greatly improves visualization when intubating with optical stylets. When the Bonfils was compared with direct laryngoscopy in a cohort of children with normal airways, the Bonfils was associated with better views but had a greater incidence of intubation failure.[611,612,617] In a comparison of the Bonfils, standard direct laryngoscopy, and GlideScope, the Bonfils resulted in a significantly improved laryngeal view and shorter intubation times.[618] Another study that compared the Bonfils with standard FOB found a shorter time to intubation (52 ± 22 seconds vs. 83 ± 24 seconds) and better image quality with the Bonfils, although all children were successfully intubated.[619] A case report describes its successful use in an infant with massive macroglossia and multiple hemorrhagic lymphangiomata compressing the airway, wherein it converted a grade 4 laryngoscopic view to a grade 1 view.[620]

SHIKANI VERSUS STORZ BONFILS OPTICAL STYLETS. Both devices consist of a metal stylet containing a fiberoptic illumination fiber and a fiberoptic vision fiber that are connected to an eyepiece or a video monitor. The light source may be external or battery powered and attached to the housing at the base of the eyepiece; the latter version allows easy transport in an emergency outside the traditional operating room location (see E-Figs. 14.20 and 14.21).[621,622] These devices are described for use either with or without rigid laryngoscopy. There are slight differences between them. Both provide an adapter to hold the ETT that allows delivery of oxygen through the tip of the ETT, but the SOS requires removal of the 15-mm adapter, whereas the Storz Bonfils device uses the 15-mm adapter to hold the tube in place. The pediatric SOS is slightly malleable and can accommodate a 3.0-mm ID ETT; a 2.5-mm ID ETT fits but is tight. The Storz device is not at all malleable but readily accommodates a 2.5-mm ID ETT.[614,621,623,624] One further difference is that the quality of light (on battery mode) seems a bit brighter with the Storz device.

Laryngeal Mask Airway as a Conduit for Intubation

Numerous case reports affirm the usefulness of the LMA as a conduit for intubation.[472] Multiple methods for placing the ETT through the LMA have been described: blind, FOB assisted, stylet- or bougie-assisted, and retrograde-assisted.[419,625–631] Because of the high occurrence in children of the epiglottis overlying the laryngeal inlet,[372] even with apparently correct placement as judged by ability to ventilate, a visual technique for ETT placement (i.e., FOB-assisted) may be the best method. However, because the LMA and conventional ETTs have similar lengths, all intubation methods are complicated by the inability to stabilize the ETT position as the laryngeal mask is withdrawn; that is, LMA removal over the ETT may cause simultaneous withdrawal of the ETT.[632–635] Proposed solutions are leaving the LMA in place,[635–637] splitting the LMA,[335] cutting and shortening the LMA,[634,638,639] using longer ETTs,[640] and using two ETTs in sequence (tube on a tube), but each technique has disadvantages. Leaving the LMA in place makes securing the ETT difficult and precarious. Modifying the LMA may adversely affect its function, and removing a split LMA can easily dislodge the ETT. Longer ETTs may not be readily available. When an FOB is used to place the ETT, the LMA may be withdrawn first over the scope. The ETT is then grasped, passed through the LMA, and threaded over the FOB into the trachea.[628,641,642] An alternative is to telescope two identical ETTs end to end or to use two that differ in size by 0.5-mm ID, either larger or smaller (E-Fig. 14.22 and Video 14.15).[643–645] These ETTs are then threaded onto the FOB. The upper tube is used to maintain the lower tube in position as the LMA is withdrawn.[439,646] The upper ETT is then removed, the 15-mm adapter is replaced on the lower tube, and the correct position is confirmed by exhaled CO_2 and auscultation. Placing two ETTs on the FOB allows removal of the LMA, but the 15-mm adapter needs to be replaced, which can be difficult if the ETT is covered with lubricant. The apnea time from insertion of the fiberscope into the LMA until the ETT has been advanced into the trachea can be minimized by using continuous ventilation through a swivel adapter attached to the LMA or ETT.[632,647,648]

It has been suggested that smaller-sized, cuffed ETTs should be used for easier passage and then the cuff can be inflated to eliminate leaks. However, the pilot balloon of a cuffed ETT does not pass through the internal lumen of pediatric LMA sizes of 1.0 to 2.5 (Video 14.16). In larger LMAs, the ETT pilot balloon connection may be too short, so that the pilot balloon can become stuck within the LMA during withdrawal.[649] The largest ETT that will pass through each size of LMA is listed in Table 14.4. For the pediatric-sized LMA Unique and PLMA, even smaller ETTs must be used. The LMA Fastrach is available only in sizes 3, 4, and 5.

The air-Q

The air-Q Mask Laryngeal Airway (Mercury Medical, Clearwater, FL) is an oval-shaped laryngeal mask with a shortened, wide, hypercurved airway tube (Fig. 14.31). The air-Q intubating laryngeal mask is available in smaller sizes for younger children and offers some advantages over traditional laryngeal masks when used as an intubation conduit in children. It has a wider airway tube that accommodates cuffed ETTs and its length is shorter, facilitating removal of the mask after tracheal intubation. The air-Q performs well as a conduit for tracheal intubation and has been successfully used in children with difficult airways.[650–654] The air-Q is supplied with a red tag attached to the pilot balloon of the mask. This tag equalizes the pressure in the mask to atmospheric pressure, and the mask should be inserted with the tag attached. The manufacturer recommends light lubrication of the back of the mask and the tip of its inner surface.

The air-Q is held in the operator's dominant hand by its airway tube and is inserted into the pharynx at an angle (Video 14.17). The mask is advanced along the tongue base until slight resistance is encountered; a jaw thrust is then performed with the nondominant hand, and the mask is inserted slightly farther until it becomes seated in the airway. When the air-Q is used as a conduit for intubation, the ETT and its cuff should be checked

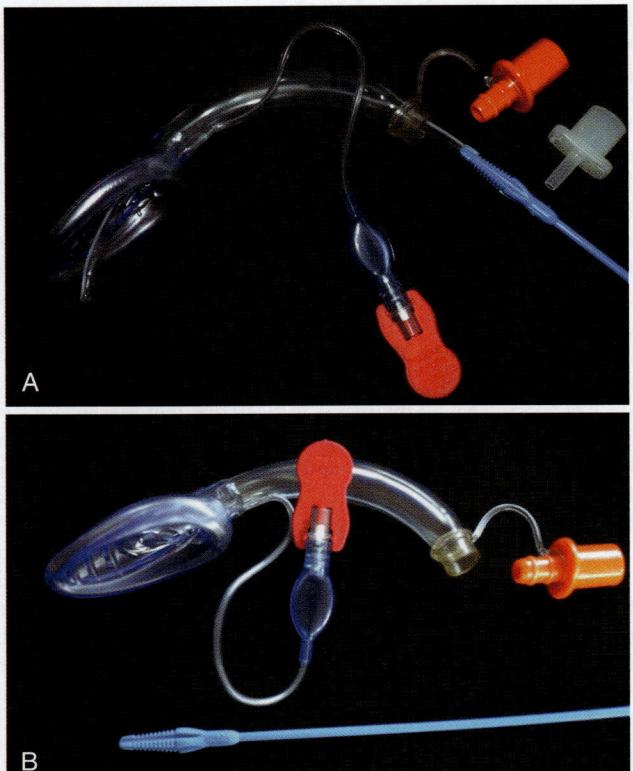

FIGURE 14.31 A, The air-Q Intubating Laryngeal Airway (Mercury Medical, Clearwater, FL) offers some advantages over traditional laryngeal masks when used as an intubation conduit in children. It has a wider airway tube that accommodates cuffed endotracheal tubes (ETTs), and its length is shorter, which facilitates removal of the mask after tracheal intubation. Before the intubation attempt, one should check that the ETT and its cuff will easily pass through the laryngeal airway size to be used. The 15-mm adapter of the air-Q is removed, the trachea is intubated with a bronchoscope, and the ETT is advanced into the trachea. B, When correct tracheal position is ensured, a special stylet (coudé-tip Tracheal Tube Introducer, available in three sizes for pediatric-sized ETTs) is inserted into the lumen of the ETT, the cuff of the air-Q is deflated, and with slight advancing pressure the ETT is held in place while the air-Q is gently withdrawn.

before the intubation attempt to be sure they will easily pass through the size to be used. The external surface of the ETT should be liberally lubricated. The 15-mm adapter of the air-Q is removed, the trachea is intubated with a bronchoscope, and the ETT is advanced into the trachea. When correct tracheal position is ensured, a special stabilizer (available in three sizes for pediatric-sized ETTs) is inserted into the lumen of the ETT. The cuff of the air-Q is deflated, and with slight advancing pressure the ETT is held in place with the stabilizer while the air-Q is gently withdrawn (Video 14.17). Proper ETT position is then reconfirmed, and the ETT is taped in place.

The air-Q was compared with the LMA Unique in a cohort of 50 children aged 6 to 36 months. The air-Q had higher airway leak pressure and a superior fiberoptic grade of view than the LMA Unique.[655] In another study that evaluated the air-Q as a conduit for tracheal intubation in infants, the mean oropharyngeal leak pressure was 18.5 ± 1.8 cm H_2O, and the mean insertion time was 13.3 ± 3.9 seconds; tracheal intubation was successful in 19 of 20 infants.[656] Another study compared the air-Q with an i-gel;

the i-gel provided a greater leak pressure but the air-Q provided better fiberoptic views in children.[657] The successful use of the air-Q as a conduit for tracheal intubation has also been reported in infants with difficult direct laryngoscopy.[654,658]

Combined Techniques

Retrograde Wire and the Flexible Fiberoptic Bronchoscope
A case series reported the use of a combined retrograde wire and FOB technique in 20 children aged 1 day to 17 years.[659] Equipment required includes a ventilating endoscopic mask, equipment for retrograde wire intubation, an FOB with a working channel, and grasping forceps. The technique begins similarly to retrograde wire-guided intubation. A venous cannula is passed through the cricothyroid membrane in a cephalad manner. The needle is removed, and lidocaine is injected to provide topical anesthesia. Aspiration is done first; detection of air confirms correct placement of the cannula within the lumen of the trachea. A guidewire of suitable length is passed through the cannula and advanced cephalad into the pharynx until it can be retrieved with the forceps from the mouth. The wire is then passed into the working channel of an FOB in a retrograde manner starting at the tip of the FOB (some FOBs may require removal of tip components to allow the wire to pass). An appropriately sized ETT should already be threaded onto the FOB. The FOB is then advanced along the wire while the laryngoscopist looks for familiar anatomic structures. After placement of the FOB tip below the vocal cords is confirmed, the wire is removed in the caudad direction from the IV cannula. The FOB is further advanced to the mid-trachea, and the ETT is threaded into place.

Tips for success with this technique are to preserve spontaneous ventilation and to remove the guidewire in the caudad direction, because this tends to pull the FOB farther into the airway rather than out of the airway, which might occur if it is removed in the opposite direction. This technique may improve success over retrograde techniques alone, because the FOB allows direct visualization and is a stiffer guide for the ETT than the wire alone. It also may improve success over the FOB alone, because the glottis is more readily identified even in the presence of blood or secretions.

Rigid Laryngoscopy and the Flexible Fiberoptic Bronchoscope
The rigid laryngoscope blade may be used to facilitate exposure so that an FOB can be used to visualize the larynx.[660]

Flexible Fiberoptic Bronchoscope Used in a Retrograde Manner
An FOB was used in a retrograde manner in a 4-year-old child with Nager syndrome who presented for tracheocutaneous fistula closure after decannulation of a tracheostomy. After failed attempts at rigid and direct fiberoptic ETT placement, a FOB was placed in a retrograde fashion, using direct vision, through the fistula, past the vocal cords, into the nasopharynx, and out the naris. It was then used as a stylet for ETT placement.[661] The clinical scenario was unusual, but the technique was successful for this child.

Retrograde Light–Guided Laryngoscopy
Retrograde light-guided laryngoscopy (RLGL) describes a method by which a light-emitting diode flashlight is placed externally in the area of the cricothyroid membrane. Direct laryngoscopy is then performed with a laryngoscope blade with the light source switched off. The glottis is illuminated by the retrograde transmission of light and the vocal cords glow red. This bright intense light provides a discrete target for the laryngoscopist to insert the

breathing tube. When compared with traditional direct laryngoscopy, use of RLGL improved first-attempt intubation success rate, time to successful intubation, and incidence of sore throat.[662,663]

ACKNOWLEDGMENTS

We wish to thank Melissa Wheeler for her prior contributions to this chapter and I. David Todres posthumously.

Many manufacturers have graciously provided us samples of airway devices so that we could illustrate examples of commonly available equipment. There is insufficient room to illustrate all available devices. Lack of illustration of a device should not be construed as lack of efficacy, nor should illustration of a device be interpreted as endorsement. Practitioners are encouraged to use all equipment available and to make their own educated decision about what devices provide the greatest safety and efficacy in their hands.

ANNOTATED REFERENCES

Crawford MW, Arrica M, Macgowan CK, Yoo SJ. Extent and localization of changes in upper airway caliber with varying concentrations of sevoflurane in children. *Anesthesiology.* 2006;105:1147-1152.

Crawford MW, Rohan D, Macgowan CK, et al. Effect of propofol anesthesia and continuous positive airway pressure on upper airway size and configuration in infants. *Anesthesiology.* 2006;105:45-50.

These two papers by Crawford and colleagues clarify how anesthetics produce airway obstruction in children. Airway obstruction during anesthesia or loss of consciousness appears to be primarily related to loss of muscle tone in the pharyngeal and laryngeal structures rather than apposition of the tongue to the posterior pharyngeal wall. This reduction in pharyngeal airway space decreases in a dose-dependent manner with increasing concentrations of either sevoflurane or propofol anesthesia.

Fiadjoe JE, Nishisaki A, Jagannathan N, et al. Airway management complications in children with difficult tracheal intubation from the Pediatric Difficult Intubation (PeDI) registry: a prospective cohort analysis. *Lancet Respir Med.* 2016;4(1):37-48.

This registry reviewed 1018 difficult intubation encounters in children. Complications were associated with more than two attempts at tracheal intubation, weight less than 10 kg, short thyromental distance, and three direct laryngoscopy attempts before an indirect technique. The most frequent complication was temporary hypoxemia, but 15 children suffered cardiac arrest. The authors concluded that limiting the number of direct laryngoscopy attempts and quickly transitioning to an indirect technique when direct laryngoscopy fails would enhance patient safety.

Fiadjoe JE, Stricker P. Pediatric difficult airway management: current devices and techniques. *Anesthesiol Clin North Am.* 2009;27:185-195.

This review paper is a comprehensive summary of the newer devices and techniques with which to manage the difficult pediatric airway.

Litman RS, McDonough JM, Marcus CL, et al. Upper airway collapsibility in anesthetized children. *Anesth Analg.* 2006;102:750-754.

This study used an innovative method to measure the propensity of the upper airway to collapse and demonstrated that halothane is a better anesthetic agent than sevoflurane for keeping the upper airway patent during general anesthesia.

Litman RS, Wake N, Chan LM, et al. Effect of lateral positioning on upper airway size and morphology in sedated children. *Anesthesiology.* 2005;103:484-488.

This study used cross-sectional magnetic resonance images of the upper airway to demonstrate that when sedated children are placed in the lateral position, upper airway patency improves, mainly at the level of the epiglottis.

Practice guidelines for management of the difficult airway: an updated report by the American Society of Anesthesiologists. Task force on management of the difficult airway. *Anesthesiology.* 2013;118(2):251-270.

The most recent guidelines from the American Society of Anesthesiologists for management of the patient with a difficult airway, whether anticipated and unanticipated. Although geared for adult anesthesia, the approach outlined in the algorithm may be applied to children.

Rolf N, Coté CJ. Diagnosis of clinically unrecognized endobronchial intubation in paediatric anaesthesia: which is more sensitive, pulse oximetry or capnography? *Paediatr Anaesth.* 1992;2:31-235.

This paper determined that pulse oximetry is more sensitive than capnography in detecting endobronchial intubation. It recommends that when a small but persistent change in oxygen saturation is noted, rather than increase the inspired oxygen concentration, one must first investigate the cause and reassess the position of the endotracheal tube.

Shi F, Xiao Y, Xiong W, et al. Cuffed versus uncuffed endotracheal tubes in children: a meta-analysis. *J Anesth.* 2016;30(1):3-11.

This meta-analysis of two randomized controlled trials and two prospective cohort studies including 1979 children intubated with cuffed endotracheal tubes versus 1803 with uncuffed endotracheal tubes. Cuffed endotracheal tubes reduced the need for tracheal tube exchanges and did not increase the risk for post extubation stridor.

Weiss M, Dullenkopf A, Gysin C, et al. Shortcomings of cuffed paediatric-tracheal tubes. *Br J Anaesth.* 2004;92:78-88.

This paper compares the physical characteristics of the most commonly available pediatric endotracheal tubes (ETTs). It also underscores the shortcomings in ETT design that may affect airway-related patient complications and that should be considered in choosing ETTs for children.

Wheeler M, Roth AG, Dsida RM, et al. Teaching residents pediatric fiberoptic intubation of the trachea: traditional fiberscope with an eyepiece versus a video-assisted technique using a fiberscope with an integrated camera. *Anesthesiology.* 2004;101:842-846.

Lack of proficiency using fiberoptic equipment for pediatric airway management remains a concern. This paper supports two important points: (1) one can achieve a satisfactory proficiency with a pediatric fiberoptic system with relatively few intubations, and (2) a video system can both improve the speed of skill acquisition and shorten the time required for successful intubation.

A complete reference list can be found online at ExpertConsult.com.

Anesthesia for Thoracic Surgery

GREGORY B. HAMMER

General Perioperative Considerations

A thorough preoperative evaluation is essential when caring for the child who is scheduled for thoracic surgery. Appropriate imaging and laboratory studies should be performed according to the lesion involved. Guidelines for fasting, choice of premedication, and preparation of the operating room (OR) are the same as for other infants and children scheduled for major surgery. After induction of anesthesia, placement of an intravenous (IV) catheter, and tracheal intubation, arterial catheterization should be considered for children undergoing thoracotomy as well as those with severe lung disease having thoracoscopic surgery. For thoracoscopic procedures of relatively brief duration in children without significant lung disease, an arterial catheter may not be required. The arterial catheter facilitates monitoring of systemic blood pressure during manipulation of the lungs and mediastinum as well as arterial blood gas tensions during single-lung ventilation (SLV). Placement of a central venous catheter is generally not indicated if peripheral IV access is adequate for projected fluid and blood administration.

Inhalational anesthetic agents are commonly administered in 100% O_2 during maintenance of anesthesia. The delivery of high concentrations of oxygen may have deleterious effects, however, including the formation of free radicals.[1] It is prudent for the practitioner to target a range of oxygen saturation values (e.g., 90% to 95%) and minimize the FiO_2 accordingly, though greater concentrations may be appropriate in anticipation of surgical maneuvers that are likely to increase intrapulmonary shunt and decrease oxygen saturation. Isoflurane may be preferred because it attenuates hypoxic pulmonary vasoconstriction to a lesser extent than other inhalational agents, although this has not been studied in children[2]; nitrous oxide is avoided. IV opioids have a sparing effect on the concentration of inhalational anesthetics required, and therefore may limit the attenuation of hypoxic pulmonary vasoconstriction. Alternatively, total IV anesthesia may be used (see Chapter 8).

A variety of approaches have been described to prevent and treat pain after videoscopic procedures. Infiltration of the incision sites with bupivacaine before skin incision decreases postoperative pain.[3,4] Infiltration with bupivacaine was found to be superior to IV fentanyl or tenoxicam for reducing postoperative pain.[5] The combination of general anesthesia with regional anesthesia that also contributes to postoperative analgesia is particularly desirable for thoracotomy, but may also be beneficial for thoracoscopic procedures. This is especially true when thoracostomy tube drainage, a source of significant postoperative pain, is used after surgery. In addition, regional blockade for postoperative analgesia facilitates deep breathing and coughing, which may limit atelectasis and pneumonia. A variety of regional anesthetic techniques have been described for intraoperative anesthesia and postoperative analgesia, including intercostal and paravertebral blocks, intrapleural infusions, and epidural anesthesia (see Chapters 42, 43, and 44).

VENTILATION AND PERFUSION DURING THORACIC SURGERY

Ventilation is normally distributed preferentially to the dependent regions of the lung, so that there is a gradient of increasing ventilation from the least to the most dependent lung segments. Because of gravitational effects, perfusion normally follows a similar distribution, with increased blood flow to dependent lung segments; therefore ventilation and perfusion are normally well matched. In infants, however, ventilation is normally distributed to the nondependent areas of the lung and perfusion is more evenly distributed because of their smaller anteroposterior distance that mitigates the effect of gravity. These two effects result in increased ventilation/perfusion ($\dot{V}/\dot{Q}$) mismatch. During thoracic surgery, several factors act to further increase $\dot{V}/\dot{Q}$ mismatch. General anesthesia, neuromuscular blockade, and mechanical ventilation may decrease functional residual capacity of both lungs. Compressing the dependent lung in the lateral decubitus position may cause atelectasis. Surgical retraction and/or SLV collapse the operative lung. Hypoxic pulmonary vasoconstriction, which diverts blood flow away from underventilated lung, minimizes $\dot{V}/\dot{Q}$ mismatch, which may be diminished by inhalational anesthetic agents and other vasodilating drugs. These factors apply equally to infants, children, and adults. The overall effect of the lateral decubitus position on $\dot{V}/\dot{Q}$ mismatch in infants, however, differs from that with older children and adults.

In adults with unilateral lung disease, oxygenation is optimal when the patient is placed in the lateral decubitus position with the healthy lung in the dependent ("down") position and the diseased lung in the nondependent ("up") position.[6] Presumably, this is related to an increase in blood flow to the dependent, healthy lung and a decrease in blood flow to the nondependent, diseased lung because of the hydrostatic pressure (or gravitational) gradient between the two lungs. This phenomenon promotes $\dot{V}/\dot{Q}$ matching in the adult patient undergoing thoracic surgery in the lateral decubitus position.

In infants with unilateral lung disease, however, oxygenation is improved with the healthy lung "up."[7] Several factors account for this discrepancy between adults and infants. Infants have a soft, easily compressible rib cage that cannot fully support the underlying lung. Therefore functional residual capacity is closer to residual volume, making airway closure more likely in the dependent lung even during tidal breathing.[8] When the adult is placed in the lateral decubitus position, the dependent diaphragm has a mechanical advantage because it is "loaded" by the abdominal hydrostatic pressure gradient. This pressure gradient is reduced in infants, thereby reducing the functional advantage of the dependent diaphragm. The infant's small size also reduces the hydrostatic pressure gradient between the nondependent and dependent lungs. Consequently, the favorable increase in perfusion to the dependent, ventilated lung is attenuated in infants.

Finally, the infant's increased oxygen requirement, coupled with a small functional residual capacity, predisposes to hypoxemia. Infants normally consume 6 to 8 mL of O_2/kg per minute compared with adult rates of 2 to 3 mL of O_2/kg per minute.[9] For these reasons, infants are at an increased risk of significant hemoglobin desaturation during surgery in the lateral decubitus position.

A modest increase in $PaCO_2$ may be beneficial in children during thoracoscopic procedures. In a study of 12 children undergoing video-assisted thoracoscopic surgery for patent ductus arteriosus closure, hypercapnea targeting $PaCO_2$ values between 50 and 70 mm Hg increased cardiac output, central venous, and arterial oxygen tension.[10] Ventilating patients during SLV to a greater PCO_2 target also results in less volutrauma and barotrauma—that is, lung injury related to use of large tidal volumes and increased inflating pressures (see below).

THORACOSCOPY

With the miniaturization of instruments, progress in video technology, and growing experience among pediatric surgeons, video endoscopic surgery of the chest, or thoracoscopy, is being performed for an increasing number of pediatric surgical indications (Table 15.1). Advantages of thoracoscopy include smaller chest incisions, reduced postoperative pain, and more rapid postoperative recovery compared with thoracotomy (Table 15.2, Fig. 15.1).[11,12] Endoscopes can be passed through a needle and trocar system and digital video signals can be electronically modified to yield sharp, detailed, color images with a minimum light intensity. Digital cameras are designed to maintain an image in an upright orientation regardless

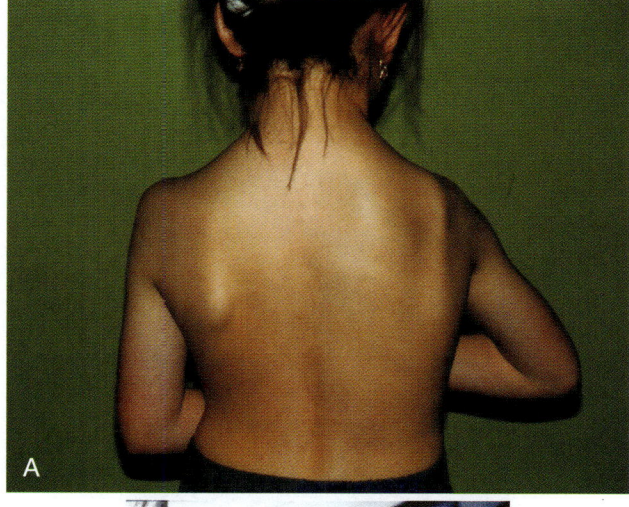

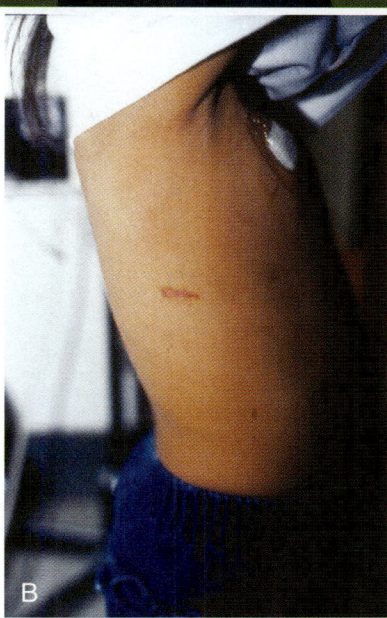

FIGURE 15.1 **A,** Significant chest deformity may occur with growth after thoracotomy. **B,** Smaller incisions associated with thoracoscopic surgery result in minimal musculoskeletal changes.

TABLE 15.1	Thoracoscopic Procedures in Infants and Children
Diagnostic inspection	
Lung biopsy	
Lobectomy	
Sequestration resection	
Cyst excision	
Lung decortication	
Foregut duplication resection	
Thymectomy	
Patent ductus arteriosus ligation	
Thoracic duct ligation	
Esophageal atresia repair	
Sympathectomy	
Aortopexy	
Mediastinal mass excision	
Anterior spinal fusion	

TABLE 15.2	Advantages of Thoracoscopic Versus Open-Chest Surgery
Improved surgical visualization	
Decreased pain	
Decreased surgical stress	
Decreased ileus/earlier return to feeding	
Quicker return to normal activity (parents and child)	
Shorter hospitalization	
Fewer long-term complications	
Cosmetically superior	

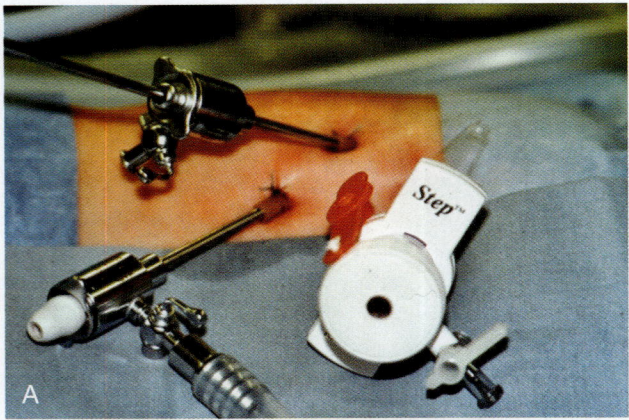

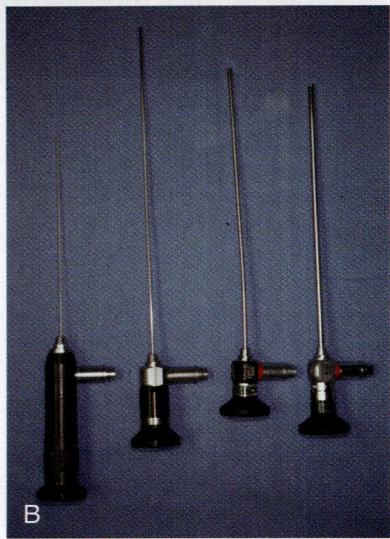

FIGURE 15.2 **A,** Thoracoscopic instruments in situ in an infant. **B,** Telescopes for use in infants range from 1.2 to 4.0 mm in diameter.

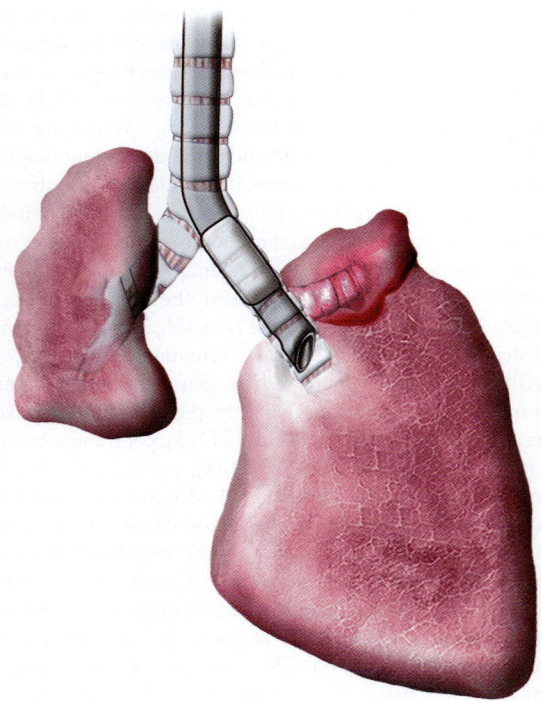

FIGURE 15.3 Placement of a single-lumen endotracheal tube (ETT) for left-sided single-lung ventilation results in obstruction of the upper lobe orifice if the distance from the proximal cuff to the tip of the ETT is longer than the main-stem bronchus.

of how the telescope is rotated. They are also equipped with an optical or digital zoom to magnify the image or give the illusion of moving the telescope closer to the object of interest. The smallest of telescopes use fiberoptics and are less than 2 mm in diameter (Fig. 15.2). Two-millimeter disposable ports, mounted on a Veress needle, are used for introduction of these small instruments. Larger instruments and ports are used in larger children and for more complex cases.

A second area of major advance in video endoscopic surgery is the development of the endoscopic suite, in which all necessary cables and wiring are located within equipment booms, ceilings, and walls. The manipulation of digital images is controlled by voice or touchscreen command either from the operative field or at a conveniently located station nearby. High-quality digital images are displayed on flat-panel monitors that can be positioned within a comfortable viewing range. Remote-controlled cameras can direct any view in the room to any of the monitors or to a remote site. Digital radiographs can be routed from the radiology department to the OR, and consultants in remote locations can be viewed on monitors in the OR so that the surgeon can see to whom he or she is speaking. An additional feature of newer endoscopy suites is voice-controlled bed positioning. Robotic tools can be vocally directed to position telescopes in the surgical field

for optimal viewing; these surgical "telemanipulators" facilitate microsurgery in confined spaces, even for small infants. Other endoscopic robots are being developed for a wide range of surgical applications.

Thoracoscopy can be performed while both lungs are being ventilated using CO_2 insufflation and placement of a retractor to displace lung tissue in the operative field. However, SLV is extremely desirable during thoracoscopy because lung deflation improves visualization of thoracic contents and may reduce lung injury caused by the use of retractors.

TECHNIQUES FOR SINGLE-LUNG VENTILATION IN INFANTS AND CHILDREN

Use of a Single-Lumen Endotracheal Tube

The simplest means of providing SLV is to intentionally intubate the ipsilateral main-stem bronchus with a conventional single-lumen endotracheal tube (ETT).[13] When the left bronchus is to be intubated, the bevel of the ETT is rotated 180 degrees and the child's head is turned to the right.[14] The ETT is advanced into the bronchus until breath sounds on the operative side disappear. A fiberoptic bronchoscope (FOB) may be passed through or alongside the ETT to confirm or guide placement. Alternatively, fluoroscopy may be used to guide and position the ETT.[15] When a cuffed ETT is used, the length of the cuff must be less than the length of the main-stem bronchus, and the proximal cuff must be placed just beyond the carina so that the right upper lobe orifice is not occluded (Fig. 15.3).[16] This technique is simple and requires no special equipment other than an FOB. This may be the preferred technique of SLV in emergency situations, such as airway hemorrhage or contralateral tension pneumothorax.

Problems can occur when using a single-lumen ETT for SLV. If a smaller, uncuffed ETT is used, it may be difficult to provide an adequate seal of the intended bronchus. This may prevent the operative lung from adequately collapsing or fail to protect the healthy, ventilated lung from contamination by purulent material or blood from the contralateral lung. Also, one is unable to suction the operative lung using this technique. Hypoxemia may occur as a result of obstruction of the upper lobe bronchus, especially when the short right main-stem bronchus is intubated.

Variations of this technique have been described, including intubation of both bronchi independently with small ETTs.[17–20] One main-stem bronchus is initially intubated with an ETT, after which another ETT is advanced over an FOB into the opposite bronchus. The disadvantages of these techniques include technical difficulties and trauma to the tracheal and bronchial mucosa. Even after successful bilateral bronchial intubation, the inner diameters of the tubes will be small, limiting gas flow and impeding suctioning of the airways.

Use of Balloon-Tipped Bronchial Blockers

A Fogarty embolectomy catheter or an end-hole, balloon wedge catheter (e.g., 5F Arndt Endobronchial Blocker (AEB; Cook Medical, Bloomington, IN) may be used for bronchial blockade to provide SLV (Fig. 15.4).[21–24] Placement of a Fogarty catheter is facilitated by bending the tip of its stylet toward the bronchus on the operative side. An FOB may be used to reposition the catheter and confirm appropriate placement. Various techniques for placing an end-hole catheter outside the ETT have been described. Using one such method, the bronchus on the operative side is initially intubated with an ETT[21]; a guidewire is then advanced into that bronchus through the ETT, the ETT is removed, and the blocker advanced over the guidewire into the bronchus. An ETT is then reinserted into the trachea alongside the blocker catheter. The

catheter balloon is positioned in the proximal main-stem bronchus under fiberoptic guidance. The guidewire may be removed to allow oxygen insufflation via the catheter lumen.

A variety of other techniques for placing the blocker outside the ETT have been described.[25] Alternatively, if an FOB small enough to pass through the indwelling ETT is not available, fluoroscopy may be used to visualize the blocker balloon and facilitate placement just distal to the carina (Fig. 15.5). With an inflated blocker balloon the airway is completely sealed, providing more predictable lung collapse and better operating conditions than with an ETT in the bronchus.

One potential problem with this technique is dislodgment of the blocker balloon into the trachea, blocking ventilation to both lungs and/or preventing collapse of the operative lung. The balloons of most catheters currently used for bronchial blockade have low compliance properties (i.e., low volume, high pressure). They require 1 to 3 mL of air or saline to fully inflate. Overdistention of the balloon can damage or even rupture the airway.[26] One study, however, reported that bronchial blocker cuffs produced lower "cuff-to-tracheal" pressures than double-lumen tubes.[27] The operative lung cannot be suctioned and continuous positive airway pressure (CPAP) cannot be provided to the operative lung if needed when closed-tip bronchial blockers are used.

When a bronchial blocker is placed outside the ETT, care must be taken to avoid injury caused by compression and resultant ischemia of the tracheal mucosa. The sum of the catheter diameter and the outer diameter of the ETT should not significantly exceed the tracheal diameter. Outer diameters for pediatric-size ETTs are shown in Table 15.3. These numbers provide an estimate of the predicted tracheal diameter, which should approximate the size of the uncuffed ETT predicted to produce a seal in the trachea.

Adapters have been developed that facilitate ventilation during placement of a bronchial blocker through an indwelling ETT.[28,29]

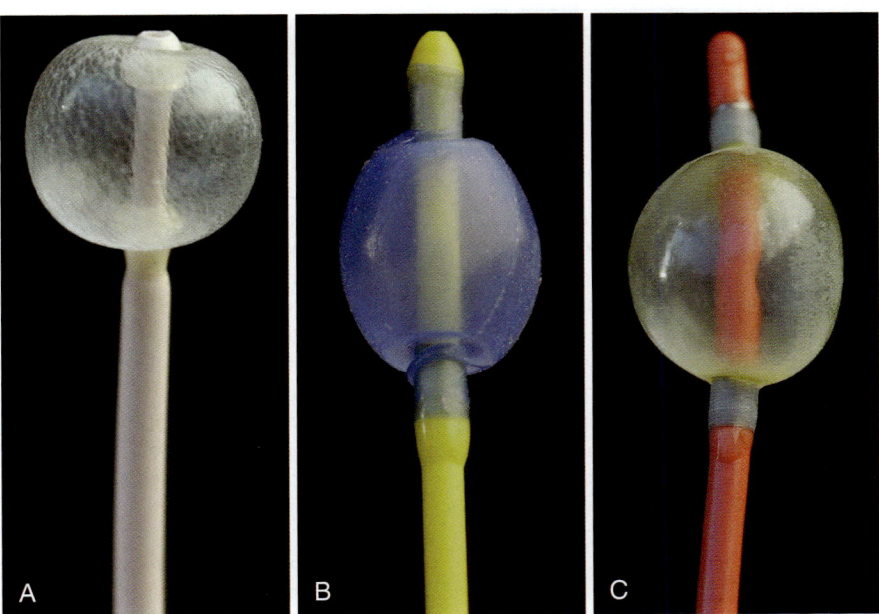

FIGURE 15.4 A variety of balloon-tipped catheters have been used for single-lung ventilation, including an Arrow balloon wedge catheter **(A)** (Arrow International, Inc., Reading, PA), a Cook pediatric bronchial blocker **(B)** (Arndt blocker, Cook Medical, Inc., Bloomington, IN), and a Fogarty embolectomy catheter (Edwards Lifesciences Corp, Irvince, CA) **(C)**. (Photographs by Michael Chen, MD.)

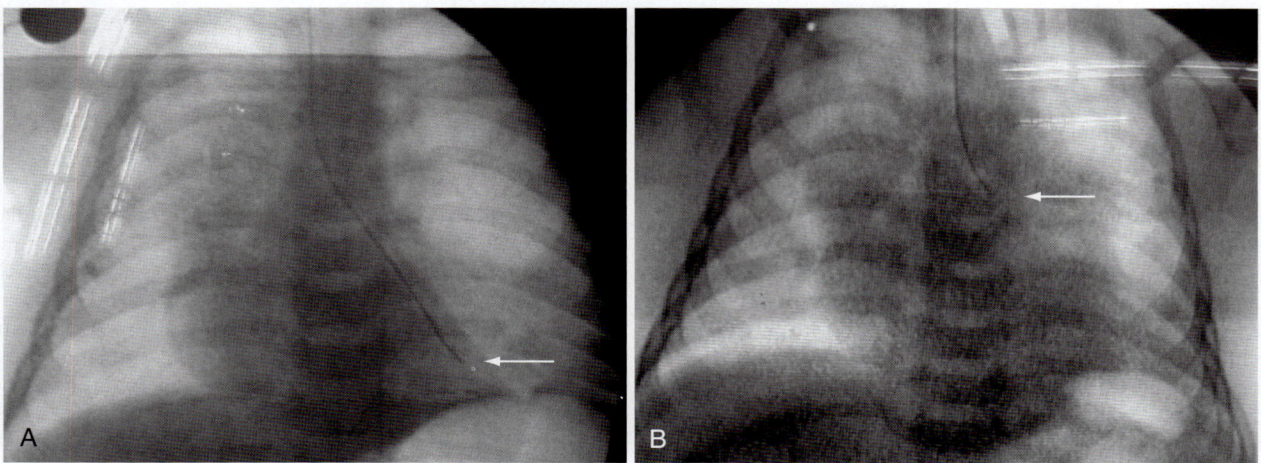

FIGURE 15.5 A bronchial blocker (*arrow*) is placed in a distal left bronchus **(A)** and withdrawn into the proximal left main-stem bronchus (**B**, *arrow*) under fluoroscopic guidance.

TABLE 15.3	Single-Lumen Uncuffed Tracheal Tube Diameters	
ID (mm)[a]	**OD (mm)**	**Equivalent French Size**[b]
3.0	4.3	13
3.5	4.9	15
4.0	5.5	17
4.5	6.2	19
5.0	6.8	21
5.5	7.5	23
6.0	8.2	25
6.5	8.9	27
7.0	9.6	29
7.5	10.2	31
8.0	10.8	32

Note: Cuffed tubes have approximately 0.5-mm additional outer diameter. The external diameter may also vary by manufacturer.
[a]Sheridan tracheal tubes (Hudson Respiratory Care Inc., Arlington Heights, IL).
[b]French (F) gauge is $\pi \times$ OD (~3 × OD) (mm).
ID, internal diameter; *OD,* outer diameter.

A 5F endobronchial blocker with a multiport adapter has been designed for use with an FOB in children (Cook Medical).[30] The balloon is elliptical so that it conforms to the bronchial lumen when inflated. The blocker catheter has a maximum outer diameter of 2.5 mm (including the deflated balloon), a central lumen with a diameter of 0.7 mm, and a distal balloon with a capacity of 3 mL. The balloon has a length of 1.0 cm, corresponding to the length of the right main-stem bronchus in children approximately 2 years of age.[31] The blocker is placed coaxially through a dedicated port in the adapter, which also has a port for passage of an FOB and ports for connection to the anesthesia breathing circuit and ETT (Fig. 15.6). The FOB port has a plastic sealing cap, whereas the blocker port has a Tuohy-Borst connector (B. Braun, Bethlehem, PA) that locks the catheter in place and maintains an airtight seal. Because oxygen can be administered during passage of the blocker and FOB, the risk of hypoxemia during blocker placement is diminished. Insufflation of oxygen via the blocker lumen decreases intrapulmonary shunt, improves oxygenation, and therefore allows delivery of a lower FiO₂ to the ventilated lung to minimize oxygen

toxicity. The blocker may be repositioned with FOB guidance during surgery.

When an FOB is used to place a bronchial blocker, both the blocker catheter and FOB must pass through the indwelling ETT. The smallest ETT through which the catheter and FOB can be passed must be larger than the sum of the outer diameters of the two. The 5F Cook bronchial blocker and an FOB with a 2.2-mm diameter, for example, may be inserted through an ETT with an internal diameter as small as 5.0 mm; for children with an indwelling ETT smaller than this, a blocker catheter can be positioned under fluoroscopy (see Fig. 15.5).[32]

Use of a Univent Tube

The Univent tube (Fuji Systems Corporation, Tokyo) is a conventional ETT with a second lumen containing a small blocker catheter that can be advanced into a bronchus (Fig. 15.7).[33,34] A balloon located at the distal end of this small tube serves as a blocker. Univent tubes require an FOB for successful placement. Univent tubes are now available in sizes with internal diameters as small as 3.5 and 4.5 mm for use in children older than 6 years of age.[35] Because the blocker tube is firmly attached to the main ETT, the Univent blocker balloon is less likely to be displaced than when other blocker techniques are used. The blocker tube has a small lumen that allows egress of gas and can be used to insufflate oxygen or suction the operated lung.

One disadvantage of the Univent tube is the large cross-sectional area occupied by the blocker channel, especially in the smaller size tubes. Therefore, Univent tubes have a large outer diameter with respect to their inner (luminal) diameters (Table 15.4). Smaller Univent tubes have a disproportionately high resistance to gas flow.[36] The Univent tube's blocker balloon has low-volume, high-pressure characteristics, predisposing to mucosal injury during normal inflation.[37,38]

Use of Double-Lumen Tubes

All double-lumen tubes (DLTs) are essentially two tubes of unequal length molded together. The shorter tube ends in the trachea, and the longer tube ends in the bronchus (Fig. 15.8). DLTs for older children and adults have cuffs located on the tracheal and bronchial lumens. The tracheal cuff, when inflated, allows positive-pressure ventilation. The inflated bronchial cuff allows ventilation

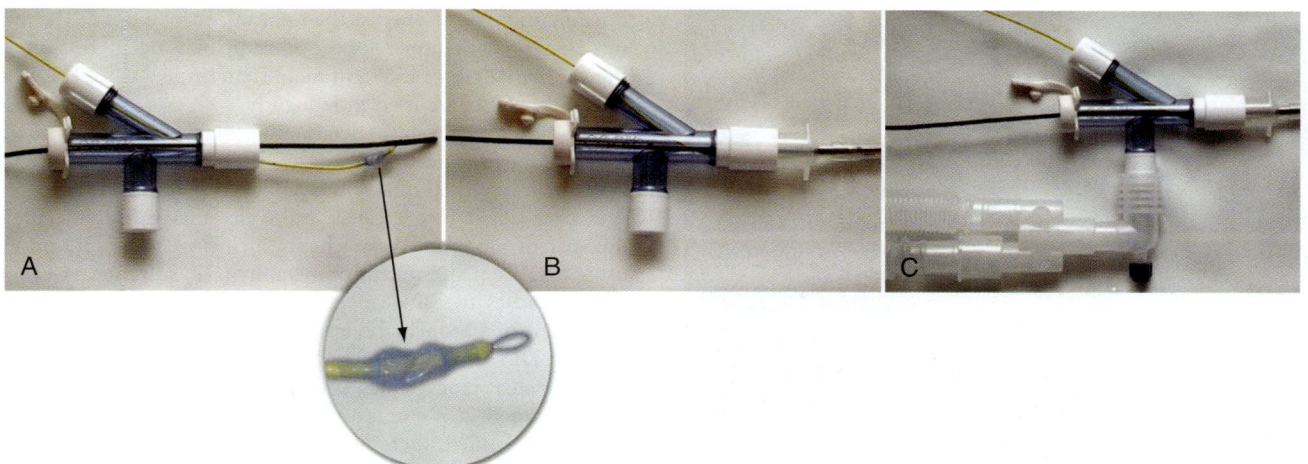

FIGURE 15.6 The Cook 5F endobronchial catheter is shown inserted in the multiport adapter. **A,** The adapter has four ports for connection to the breathing circuit, fiberoptic bronchoscope (FOB), endobronchial catheter, and endotracheal tube. After the FOB and endobronchial catheter have been inserted through the multiport adaptor, the FOB is placed through the monofilament loop at the distal end of the catheter (*arrow*). The multiport adaptor is then attached to the indwelling endotracheal tube **(B)** and the breathing circuit **(C)**. The FOB is directed into the main-stem bronchus on the operative side. The catheter is then advanced until the monofilament loop slides off the end of the FOB into the bronchus. (Photographs by Elliot Krane, MD.)

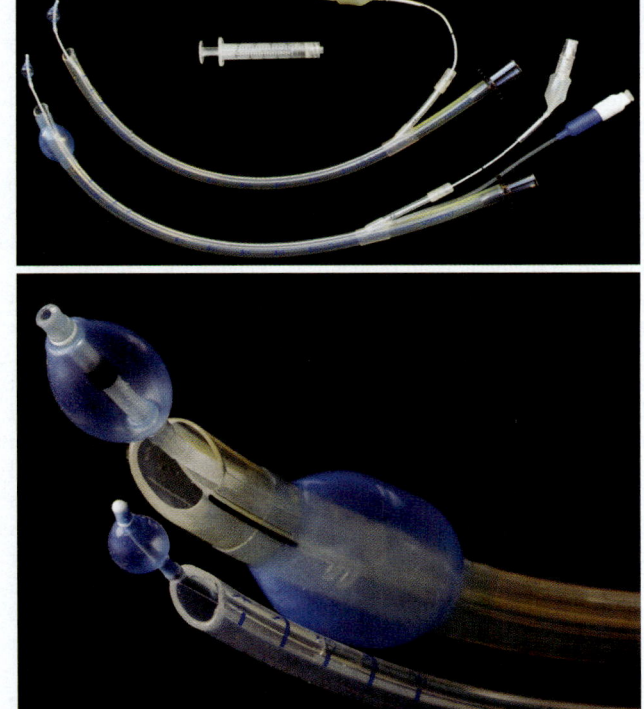

FIGURE 15.7 The Univent tube is available in a variety of adult sizes, as well as 3.5-mm internal-diameter and 4.5-mm internal diameter sizes for use in children (*top*). The adult tubes have a tracheal cuff and an end-hole bronchial blocker, allowing administration of oxygen and suction (*bottom*). The pediatric tubes are uncuffed and have a closed-tip blocker. (Photographs by Michael Chen, MD.)

TABLE 15.4	Univent Tube Diameters
ID (mm)	**OD (mm)**[a]
3.5	7.5/8.0
4.5	8.5/9.0
6.0	10.0/11.0
6.5	10.5/11.5
7.0	11.0/12.0
7.5	11.5/12.5
8.0	12.0/13.0
8.5	12.5/13.5
9.0	13.0–14.0

[a]Sagittal/transverse.
ID, internal diameter; *OD,* outer diameter.

to be diverted to either or both lungs and protects each lung from contamination from secretions, purulent material, or blood originating from the contralateral side.

Marraro described a bilumen tube for infants.[39] This tube consists of two separate uncuffed tracheal tubes of different lengths attached longitudinally. This tube is not available in the United States. The smallest cuffed DLT commercially available in the United States is a 26F size (Teleflex Medical, Research Triangle Park, NC). This DLT may be used in children as young as 8 years old. DLTs are also available in sizes 28F and 32 F (Nellcor brand [Covidien, Mansfield, MA]); these are suitable for children 10 years of age and older. Numerous manufacturers produce clear, disposable, polyvinyl chloride Robertshaw-design (P³ Medical, Briston, England) DLTs, which are available in sizes 35F to 41F (Table 15.5). Essentially, they consist of similar features with small modifications in cuff shape and location. A colored bronchial cuff, commonly blue, permits

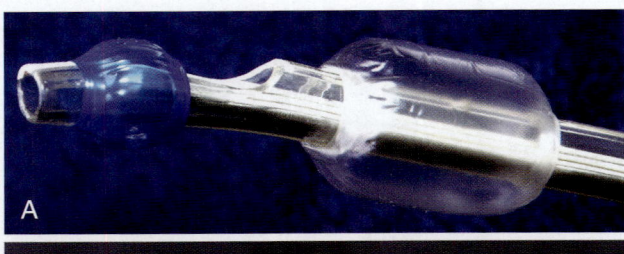

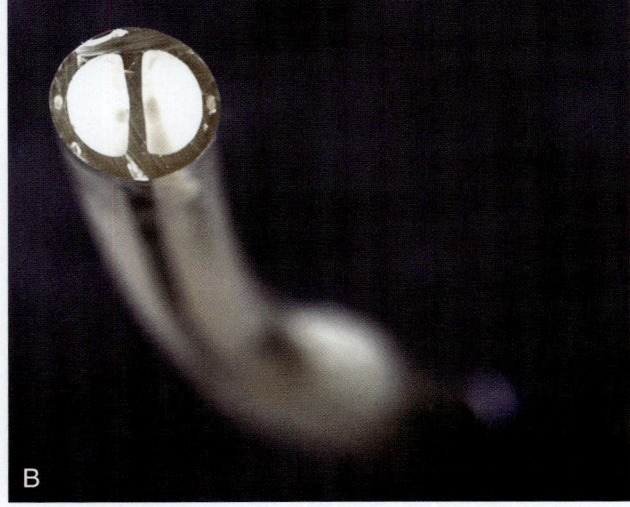

FIGURE 15.8 Although the bronchial lumen of a double-lumen tube appears to be round **(A)**, both the bronchial and tracheal lumens are D-shaped, as evident in a cross-sectional view **(B)**. Their actual lumens have restricted limiting diameters. (Photographs by Michael Chen, MD.)

TABLE 15.5	Double-Lumen Tube Dimensions		
Size (Fr)	Main Body OD (mm)	Limiting Diameter Tracheal Lumen (mm)	Limiting Diameter Bronchial Lumen (mm)
26[a]	8.7	N/A	N/A
28[b]	9.4	3.1	3.2
32[b]	10.6	3.5	3.4
35[b]	11.7	4.5	4.3
37[b]	12.4	4.7	4.5
39[b]	13.1	4.9	4.9
41[b]	13.7	5.4	5.4

Note: The limiting diameters correspond to the largest suction catheter or fiberoptic bronchoscope that can be placed via the lumen under ideal circumstances (e.g., adequate lubrication).
French (F) gauge is $\pi \times$ OD (~3 $\times$ OD) (mm). Comparing data in this table to those in Table 15.3, the OD of the DLTs corresponds to the following tracheal tubes: 26F DLT is equivalent to that of a 6.0- to 6.5-mm ID tracheal tube; a 28F is equivalent to a 6.5- to 7.0-mm ID; and a 32F is equivalent to an 8.0-mm ID. Cuff thickness is 0.049 mm; therefore a cuff adds 0.10 mm to overall OD of tube.
[a]Teleflex Medical, Research Triangle Park, NC.
[b]Covidien, Mansfield, MA.
DLT, double-lumen tube; *ID,* internal diameter; *OD,* outer diameter.

easy identification by fiberoptic bronchoscopy. In general, the cuffs used in DLTs are high-compliance cuffs that are designed to exert less pressure on the tracheal and bronchial mucosa compared with low-compliance cuffs. For right-sided DLTs, the endobronchial cuff is donut shaped and allows the right upper lobe ventilation

opening to be positioned at the right upper lobe orifice. Despite this design, right upper lobe occlusion may occur because of the shorter length of the right main-stem bronchus.[2,40] Therefore right-sided DLTs are used infrequently.

A novel mechanism for determining whether the child's airway is large enough to accommodate a DLT and, if so, what size DLT is optimal, is printed three-dimensional (3D) airway modeling.[41,42] It is now possible to create a full-scale, anatomically accurate, transparent model of the tracheobronchial tree on a 3D printer using data from computed tomography (CT) scanning. A variety of approaches to SLV can be tested on the model, including placement of a bronchial blocker inside or outside of an ETT as well as a DLT. For the former approach, the appropriate size ETT and bronchial blocker may be selected. If a recent CT scan has been obtained, as is common among patients for whom thoracic surgery is planned, there may be no additional imaging cost or radiation exposure required to create a 3D printed model. As 3D printers become more widely available and the cost of creating 3D printed models of an individual patient's tracheobronchial tree decreases, this technique may be more widely used for planning SLV as well as for training anesthesiologists how to perform these procedures more effectively.

DLTs are inserted in children using the same technique as in adults, and left DLTs are almost exclusively used.[43] The tip of the tube is inserted just past the vocal cords, and the stylet is withdrawn. The DLT is rotated 90 degrees to the appropriate side and then advanced into the bronchus. After intubation, the tracheal cuff is inflated first and equal breath sounds should be confirmed. To prevent mucosal damage from excessive pressure applied by the bronchial cuff, the cuff is inflated with incremental volumes to seal air leaks around the bronchial cuff into the trachea. Inflation of the bronchial cuff seldom requires more than 2 mL of air. After inflation of the bronchial cuff, bilateral breath sounds should be rechecked to confirm that the bronchial cuff is not herniating across the carina to impede contralateral lung ventilation. Fiberoptic bronchoscopy can be used to directly visualize the proximal edge of the bronchial cuff in the left bronchus, just distal to the carina. One simple way to verify that the tip of the bronchial lumen is located in the designated bronchus is to clamp the tracheal lumen at the level of the connector and then observe and auscultate left and right lungs. Usually, inspection will reveal unilateral movement of the ventilated hemithorax. With the tracheal lumen clamped, auscultation of the chest will demonstrate air entry in the left lung and no ventilation in the right lung. After auscultation and release of the tracheal clamp, the bronchial lumen is clamped and the tracheal lumen is ventilated to confirm movement and breath sounds of the right lung. Whenever a right-sided DLT is used, ventilation of the right upper lobe must be verified. This can be accomplished by careful auscultation over the right upper lung field or, more accurately, by fiberoptic bronchoscopy. When a left-sided DLT is used, the risk of occluding the left upper lobe bronchus by advancement of the bronchial tip into the distal left main bronchus should be considered.

DLTs may be malpositioned in up to 48% of cases despite careful inspection and auscultation.[44] The simplest way to evaluate proper positioning of a left-sided DLT is to perform fiberoptic bronchoscopy through the tracheal lumen. The carina is then visualized, and only the proximal edge of the bronchial cuff should be identified just distal to the carina. Herniation of the bronchial cuff over the carina to partially occlude the contralateral main-stem bronchus should be excluded. Fiberoptic bronchoscopy should then be performed via the bronchial lumen to identify the patent left upper lobe orifice. When a right-sided DLT is used, the right upper lobe bronchial orifice must be identified while the bronchoscope is passed through the right upper lobe ventilating slot.

The use of an FOB to facilitate positioning of DLTs in children depends on the availability of small instruments. FOBs with an external diameter of 3.6 mm are commonly available and will pass through a 35F DLT. Smaller FOBs are needed when 26F, 28F, and 32F DLTs are used (see Table 15.5 for "limiting diameters").

In the adult population, the depth of insertion of the DLT is directly related to the height of the patient.[45] No equivalent measurements are available as yet in children. Fortunately, there are very few reports in children of airway damage from DLTs.

The high-volume, low-pressure cuffs should not damage the airway, provided that the cuffs are not overinflated with air or distended with nitrous oxide. Alternatively, saline may be used to inflate the cuffs.

A disadvantage of DLTs is the need to change the DLT to a single-lumen ETT if mechanical ventilation is required after surgery. This is a particular problem for children in whom tracheal intubation was difficult initially because of anatomic or functional limitations. Even when an airway was not classified as difficult preoperatively, it may become difficult secondary to facial and supraglottic edema, the presence of secretions and/or blood in the airway, and laryngeal trauma from the initial intubation. The use of an ETT exchange catheter may facilitate the exchange of a DLT for a single lumen ETT.[46] These devices are commercially available in a variety of sizes (Cook Medical) and allow oxygen insufflation and jet ventilation (see E-Fig. 14.3A-H).

Several important caveats should be considered before using an ETT exchange catheter. First, it must be small enough to pass through the tracheal lumen of the DLT. This should be tested in vitro before the procedure is performed in vivo. Second, it should never be advanced against resistance, and the clinician must always be cognizant of the depth of insertion; perforations of the tracheobronchial tree have been reported.[47] Third, a jet ventilator should be immediately available in case the new ETT does not follow the exchange catheter into the trachea and oxygenation via the exchange catheter is needed. The jet ventilator should be preset to a peak inspiratory pressure of 25 psi (172 kPa) by an inline regulator. When passing an ETT over an ETT exchange catheter, a laryngoscope should be used to facilitate passage of the ETT into the trachea. It should be noted that the tip of the ETT may hang up on the laryngeal inlet and may require a 90-degree rotation clockwise or counterclockwise to successfully pass, should this occur.

General Considerations in the Management of Single-Lung Ventilation

Once the ETT, bronchial blocker, or DLT is in place, airway pressures should be confirmed during SLV. If peak airway pressure is 20 cm H_2O during two-lung ventilation with a given tidal volume, inflating pressure should not exceed 40 cm H_2O in SLV when the same tidal volume is delivered during SLV. In general, smaller tidal volumes with increased respiratory rates are used to deliver somewhat reduced minute ventilation with SLV as with two-lung ventilation. Some degree of permissive hypercapnia is targeted to minimize lung trauma.

After the child has been placed in the lateral decubitus position, proper ETT, bronchial blocker, or DLT position should be reconfirmed, because displacement may occur when turning the patient. Two-lung ventilation should be maintained for as long as possible before switching to SLV. When SLV is required, the minimum FIO_2 needed to maintain an acceptable oxygen saturation should be used. Assuming an intact hypoxic pulmonary vasoconstriction response, PaO_2 during SLV and an FIO_2 of 1.0 should be between 150 and 210 mm Hg.[48] The lungs should be initially ventilated with a tidal volume of 6 to 8 mL/kg at a ventilatory rate that maintains the $PaCO_2$ between 45 and 60 mm Hg, unless this degree of hypercapnia cannot be tolerated because of other physiologic factors (e.g., concomitant metabolic acidosis). Inadequate tidal volumes may lead to atelectasis in the ventilated lung (reduced functional residual capacity), and increased intrapulmonary shunting, resulting in hypoxemia. Large tidal volumes may force blood to the nondependent lung (similar to the application of positive end-expiratory pressure), thereby increasing the intrapulmonary shunt.[49,50]

After the institution of SLV, PaO_2 may continue to decrease for up to 45 minutes. Should hypoxemia develop, proper positioning of the indwelling blocker or tube should be reconfirmed by fiberoptic bronchoscopy, if possible. Several techniques can be used to improve oxygenation. The most effective maneuver for improving PaO_2 is the application of CPAP to the nondependent lung.[51] Insufflation of oxygen to achieve a CPAP of 10 cm H_2O, for example, produces alveolar inflation and decreases intrapulmonary shunt fraction. Usually this can be accomplished without significant expansion of the lung or interference with surgical conditions. If the PaO_2 continues to decrease despite the application of CPAP to the deflated lung, a malpositioned bronchial blocker or tube should be considered. This may be signaled by a sudden increase in the inflation pressure, a decrease in tidal volume, and/or a change in the capnogram. When a DLT is in place, the surgeon may aid repositioning. The surgeon can palpate the bronchi and manually occlude the main bronchial lumens, thereby guiding the tip of the DLT into the correct position. When the cause of the hypoxemia and/or hypercarbia cannot be readily identified, the balloon or cuff should be deflated and both lungs ventilated after informing the surgeon of the problem.

SLV may be associated with substantial lung injury, and measures should be undertaken to minimize adverse effects of SLV on the lung. Collapse and subsequent reexpansion of lung tissue during SLV has been associated with an increase in proinflammatory markers and alveolar damage.[52,53] In a study of 28 children undergoing SLV for thoracic surgery, a preoperative dose of methylprednisolone 2 mg/kg IV decreased both interleukin 6 levels and respiratory resistance, and increased the serum concentrations of tryptase and the antiinflammatory cytokine, interleukin 10. Three of 15 children in the placebo group and none of the 13 in the treatment group experienced clinically significant intraoperative and postoperative respiratory complications.[54]

A potentially therapeutic intervention to mitigate lung injury associated with SLV is the administration of surfactant. Surfactant instilled into the subsequently deflated lung reduced the concentration of inflammatory cytokines in a piglet model of SLV.[55] A more clinically practical method of reducing lung injury during SLV is to minimize the FIO_2 and use a lung protective strategy during the procedure. The use of 50% O_2 caused less lung injury in animals subjected to SLV for 3 hours than 100% O_2.[56] Young pigs that were mechanically ventilated with a lung protective strategy using a tidal volume of 5 mL/kg and a positive end-expiratory pressure (PEEP) of 5 cm H_2O demonstrated less lung injury than those ventilated with a tidal volume of 10 mL/kg and no PEEP.[57] Anesthesiologists should consider the use of the minimum FIO_2 needed to maintain an acceptable oxygen saturation, as well as small tidal volumes and adequate levels of PEEP, in the ventilated lung

TABLE 15.6	Tube Selection for Single-Lung Ventilation in Children			
Age (years)	ETT (ID)[a]	BB (F)	Univent[b]	DLT (F)
0.5–1	3.5–4.0	2[c]		
1–2	4.0–4.5	3[c]		
2–4	4.5–5.0	5[d]		
4–6	5.0–5.5	5[d]		
6–8	5.5–6.0	5[d]	3.5	
8–10	6.0 cuffed	5[d]	3.5	26[e]
10–12	6.5 cuffed	5[d]	4.5	26[e]–28[e]
12–14	6.5–7.0 cuffed	5[d]	4.5	32[e]
14–16	7.0 cuffed	5, 7[d]	6.0	35[e]
16–18	7.0–8.0 cuffed	7, 9[d]	7.0	35, 37[e]

[a]Sheridan tracheal tubes, Hudson Respiratory Care Inc., Arlington Heights, IL.
[b]Fuji Systems Corporation, Tokyo.
[c]Edwards Lifesciences LLC, Irvine, CA.
[d]Cook Medical, Inc., Bloomington, IN.
[e]Covidien, Mansfield, MA.
BB, bronchial blocker; *DLT*, double-lumen tube; *ETT*, endotracheal tube; *F*, French size; *ID*, internal diameter.

during SLV to minimized lung injury. Preoperative administration of corticosteroids should also be considered.

Guidelines for selecting appropriate tubes (or catheters) for SLV in children are shown in Table 15.6. There is considerable variability in overall size and airway dimensions in children, particularly in adolescents. The recommendations shown in Table 15.6 are based on average values for airway dimensions. Larger DLTs may be safely used in large adolescents.

SURGICAL LESIONS OF THE CHEST
Neonates and Infants
A variety of congenital intrathoracic lesions for which surgery is required may occur in the neonatal or infancy period. These include lesions of the trachea and bronchi, lung parenchyma, and diaphragm, as well as vascular abnormalities.

Tracheal stenosis may be acquired or congenital. Tracheal stenosis occurs most commonly because of prolonged tracheal intubation, often in preterm infants with respiratory distress syndrome. Ischemic injury of the tracheal mucosa may occur as a result of a tight-fitting ETT at the level of the cricoid cartilage, which becomes scarred and constricted after a period of time. *Subglottic stenosis* may develop, resulting in stridor and respiratory distress after a trial extubation. Nasal CPAP with high-flow oxygen may be used to maintain the oxygen saturation early after extubation. If oxygen desaturation and hypercarbia persist despite the CPAP, tracheal reintubation may be required.

Tracheal and/or esophageal compression may occur as a result of a variety of lesions in the chest, including vascular rings and slings (see also Chapters 14 and 33).

An FOB is used to evaluate the severity of the stenosis and exclude other causes of stridor (e.g., vocal cord paralysis or laryngomalacia). When general anesthesia is required, inhalational anesthesia may be administered via a face mask, with the FOB inserted through an adapter in the mask and into the nasopharynx. This is usually performed while the infant breathes spontaneously.[58] Noninvasive imaging studies are being increasingly used for the diagnosis of a variety of congenital airway lesions, including vascular rings.[58] Bronchography and "virtual" CT scanning may also be useful.[59,60]

A cricoid split procedure may be performed for infants with acquired subglottic stenosis. After diagnostic bronchoscopy, the trachea is either intubated with an ETT or a rigid bronchoscope is left in place during the operation. Anesthesia may be maintained with inhalational agents or an IV anesthetic technique, such as with propofol and remifentanil.[61] Typically, an ETT ID 0.5 mm larger than the original ETT is placed after the repair.

For infants with severe *congenital tracheal stenosis,* a laryngotracheoplasty may be performed. This procedure involves the placement of a costal, auricular, or laryngeal cartilage graft into the anterior and/or posterior trachea.[62] In some cases, a stent may be positioned within the trachea. These infants may require a tracheal tube and mechanical ventilation for a variable period of time postoperatively. In these cases, sedation, analgesia, and at times neuromuscular blockade are maintained after surgery.

Pulmonary sequestrations result from disordered embryogenesis, producing a nonfunctional mass of lung tissue supplied by anomalous systemic arteries. Children may present with cough, pneumonia, and failure to thrive; these signs often occur during the neonatal period, and usually before 2 years of age. Diagnostic studies include CT of the chest and abdomen, and arteriography. Magnetic resonance imaging may provide high-resolution images, including definition of the vascular supply, which may obviate the need for angiography. Surgical resection is performed once the diagnosis is confirmed. Nitrous oxide should be avoided in these cases. Positive-pressure ventilation does not usually expand pulmonary sequestrations.

Congenital cystic lesions in the thorax may be classified into three categories.[63] *Bronchogenic cysts* result from abnormal budding or branching of the tracheobronchial tree. They may cause respiratory distress, recurrent pneumonia, and/or atelectasis because of lung compression. *Dermoid cysts* are clinically similar to bronchogenic cysts but differ histologically because they are lined with keratinized, squamous epithelium rather than respiratory (ciliated columnar) epithelium. They usually manifest later in childhood or adulthood. *Cystic adenomatoid malformations* are structurally similar to bronchioles but lack associated alveoli, bronchial glands, and cartilage.[64] Because these lesions communicate with the airways, they may become overdistended as a result of gas trapping, leading to respiratory distress in the first few days of life. When they are multiple and air filled, cystic adenomatoid malformations may resemble congenital diaphragmatic hernias radiographically. Treatment is surgical resection of the affected lobe. As with congenital diaphragmatic hernias, prognosis depends on the amount of remaining lung tissue, which may be hypoplastic because of compression in utero.[65]

Congenital lobar emphysema often manifests with respiratory distress shortly after birth.[66] This lesion may be caused by "ball-valve" bronchial obstruction in utero, causing progressive distal overdistention with fetal lung fluid. The resultant emphysematous lobe may compress lung tissue bilaterally, resulting in a variable degree of hypoplasia. Congenital cardiac deformities are present in about 15% of children with congenital lobar emphysema.[67] Radiographic signs of hyperinflation may be misinterpreted as tension pneumothorax or atelectasis on the contralateral side (Fig. 15.9). Positive-pressure ventilation may exacerbate lung hyperinflation. Nitrous oxide is contraindicated, and isolation of the lungs during anesthesia is desirable (see also Chapter 37, Fig. 37.10).

Congenital diaphragmatic hernia is a life-threatening condition that occurs in approximately 1 in 2000 live births. Failure of a

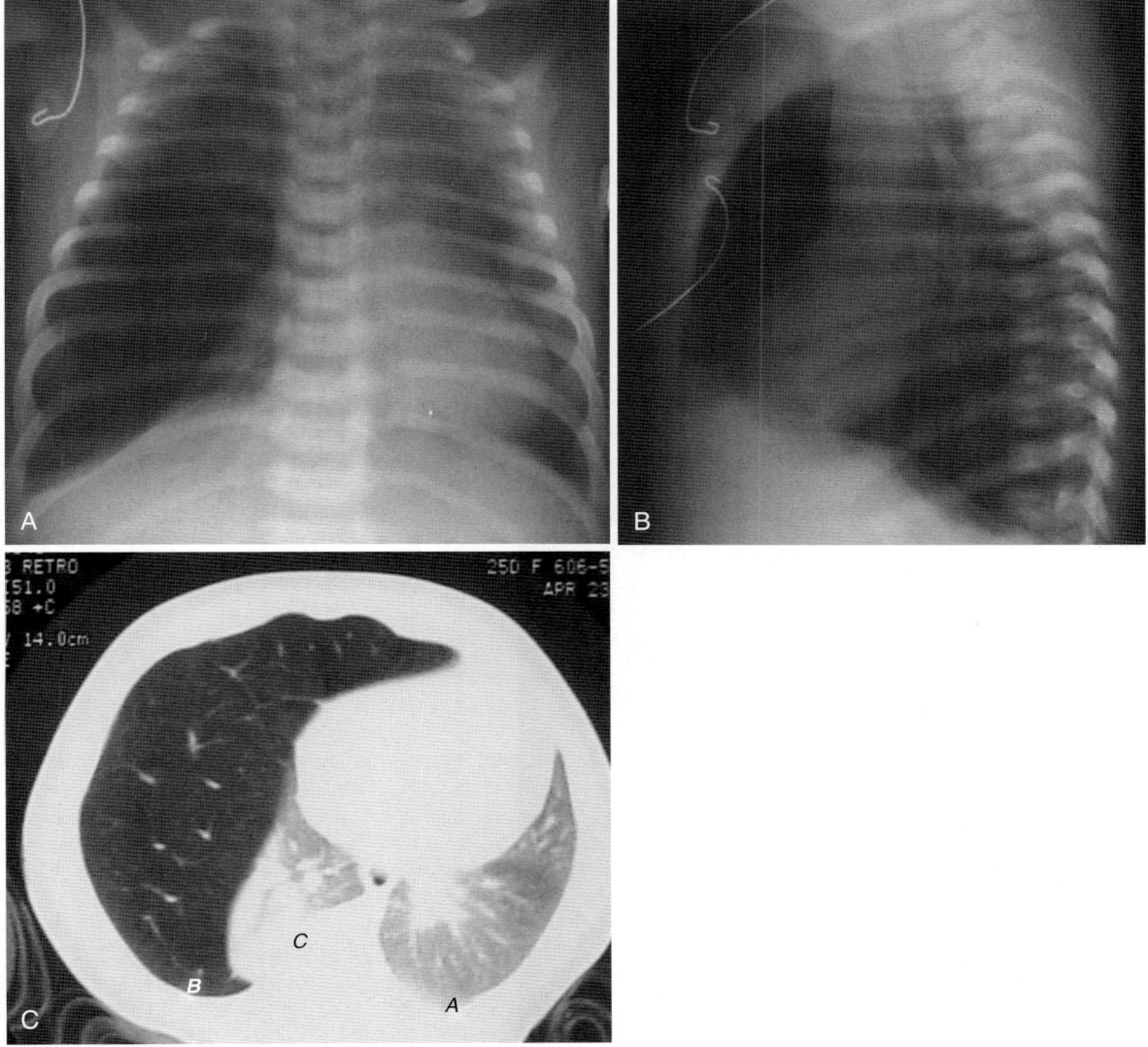

FIGURE 15.9 Congenital lobar emphysema of the right lower lobe. Plain radiography illustrates hyperlucency of the right lung on the anteroposterior image **(A)** and posterior displacement of the heart and mediastinum on the lateral image **(B)**. The computed tomography scan **(C)** demonstrates compression of the left lung *(A)* and right upper lobe *(C)* as well as hyperinflation of the right lower lobe *(B)*.

portion of the fetal diaphragm to develop allows abdominal contents to enter the thorax, interfering with normal lung growth. In 80% to 90% of diaphragmatic defects, a portion of the posterior diaphragm fails to close, (80%–85% of cases on the left side), forming a triangular defect known as the *foramen of Bochdalek*. Hernias through the foramen of Bochdalek that occur early in fetal life usually cause respiratory failure immediately after birth owing to pulmonary hypoplasia. The diagnosis is often made prenatally, and fetal surgical repair has been described.[68] Neonates present with tachypnea, a scaphoid abdomen, and absent breath sounds over the affected side. Chest radiography typically shows bowel in the left hemithorax, with deviation of the heart and mediastinum to the right and compression of the right lung (Fig. 15.10). Right-sided hernias (see Fig. 15.10C) may occur late and manifest with milder signs. In the presence of significant respiratory distress, bag-and-mask ventilation should be avoided and immediate

tracheal intubation should be performed (see also Chapter 37). Distention of the thoracic gut postnatally with aggressive bag-and-mask positive pressure further compresses the inflated lungs, rendering ventilation and oxygenation more difficult.

Because pulmonary hypertension with right-to-left shunting contributes to severe hypoxemia in neonates with congenital diaphragmatic hernia, a variety of pulmonary vasodilators have been used to increase oxygenation. These include tolazoline, prostacyclin, dipyridamole, and nitric oxide.[69-73] High-frequency oscillatory ventilation has been used in conjunction with vasodilator therapy to improve oxygenation before surgery.[74] Occasionally, prostaglandin E_1 is used to maintain a patent ductus arteriosus and reduce right ventricular afterload. In cases of severe lung hypoplasia and pulmonary hypertension refractory to these therapies (e.g., PaO_2 <50 mm Hg with FiO_2 of 1.0), extracorporeal membrane oxygenation (ECMO) should be initiated early to

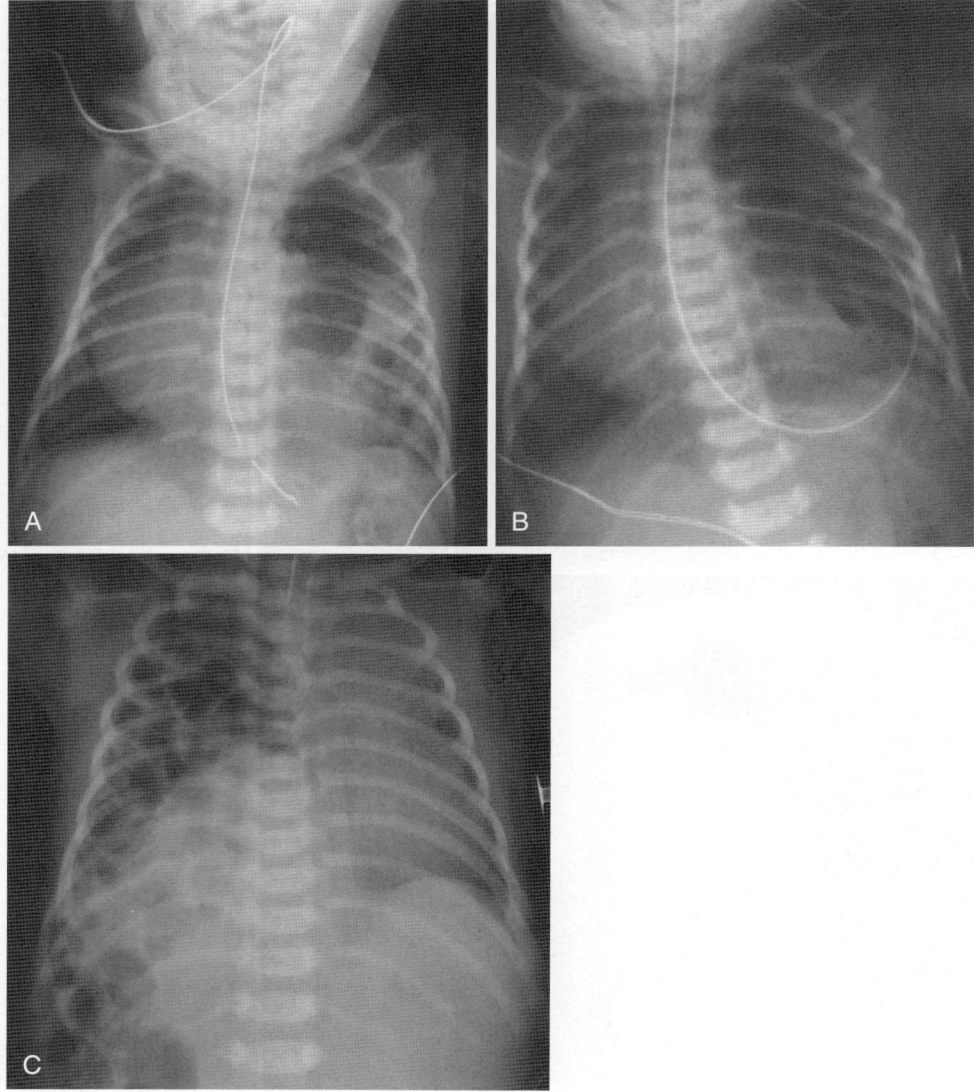

FIGURE 15.10 The majority of congenital diaphragmatic hernias are left sided. **A,** Chest radiography demonstrates the presence of bowel in the left hemithorax. **B,** A nasogastric tube has been advanced into the stomach. **C,** Congenital diaphragmatic hernias may also occur on the right side.

avoid progressive lung injury. Improved outcomes have been associated with early use of ECMO followed by delayed surgical repair.[75]

A particularly poor prognosis is predicted if congenital diaphragmatic hernia is associated with cardiac deformities, preoperative alveolar-to-arterial oxygen gradient greater than 500 mm Hg, or severe hypercarbia despite aggressive ventilation strategies.[76,77] Prognosis has also been correlated with pulmonary compliance and radiographic findings.[78,79]

Surgical correction via a subcostal incision with ipsilateral chest tube placement may be performed before, during, or immediately after ECMO.[80,81] In neonates undergoing surgical repair without ECMO, pulmonary hypertension is the major cause of morbidity and mortality. Hyperventilation to induce a respiratory alkalosis and 100% oxygen may be administered to decrease pulmonary vascular resistance. The anesthetic should be designed to minimize sympathetic discharge, which may exacerbate pulmonary

hypertension (e.g., a high-dose opioid technique). The lungs of these infants should be ventilated with small tidal volumes and low inflating pressures to avoid a pneumothorax on the contralateral (usually right) side. Both nitric oxide and high-frequency oscillatory ventilation have been used during surgical repair.[82,83] A high index of suspicion of right-sided pneumothorax should be maintained, and a thoracostomy tube should be placed in the event of acute deterioration of respiratory or circulatory function. It is also imperative that normal body temperature, intravascular volume, and acid-base status be maintained. Mechanical ventilation is continued postoperatively in nearly all infants because lung compliance is markedly reduced after surgery (a consequence of returning the thoracic gut to the abdomen and the increased abdominal pressure on the diaphragm).

Failure of the central and lateral portions of the diaphragm to fuse, comprising *10%–15% of cases of diaphragmatic hernias*, results in a retrosternal defect known as the *foramen of Morgagni*. This usually manifests as signs of bowel obstruction rather than respiratory distress. Repair is usually performed via an abdominal incision (see also Chapter 37).

Tracheoesophageal fistula and/or *esophageal atresia* occur in approximately 1 in 4000 live births. In 80% to 85% of afflicted infants, this lesion includes esophageal atresia with a distal esophageal pouch and a proximal tracheoesophageal fistula.[84,85] The fistula is usually located one to two tracheal rings above the carina. Affected neonates present with spillover of pooled oral secretions from the pouch and may develop progressive gastric distention and tracheal aspiration of acidic gastric contents via the fistula. A common association is the **VACTERL** complex, consisting of **v**ertebral, **a**norectal, **c**ardiac, **t**racheal, **e**sophageal, **r**enal, and/or **l**imb defects.[86] Esophageal atresia is confirmed when an orogastric tube passed through the mouth cannot be advanced more than about 7 cm (Fig. 15.11). The proximal pouch tube should be secured and continuous suction applied, after which a chest radiograph is diagnostic (see also Chapter 37).

Mask ventilation and tracheal intubation are avoided before surgery if possible, because they may exacerbate gastric distention and further compromise respirations. Once the trachea is intubated, it is occasionally necessary to occlude the tracheal orifice of the fistula with the tracheal tube. The tip of the tracheal tube is positioned just above the carina by auscultation of diminished breath sounds over the left axilla as the tube is advanced into the right main-stem bronchus, after which the tube is retracted until breath sounds are increased over the left chest (Fig. 15.12A). A small FOB may be passed through the tracheal tube to confirm appropriate placement. Rarely, an emergency gastrostomy is performed because of massive gastric distention. Placement of a balloon-tipped catheter in the fistula via the gastrostomy may be performed under guidance with an FOB, to prevent further gastric distention and/or enable effective positive-pressure ventilation in cases of significant lung disease or very large fistulas (see Fig. 15.12B).[87] "Antegrade" occlusion of a tracheoesophageal fistula

has also been reported with a balloon-tipped catheter advanced through the trachea into the fistula (see Fig. 15.12C).[88] Preoperative evaluation should be performed to diagnose associated anomalies, particularly cardiac, musculoskeletal, and gastrointestinal defects, which occur in 30% to 50% of affected infants.[89] A poor prognosis for infants with tracheoesophageal fistula and esophageal atresia has been associated with prematurity and underlying lung disease, as well as the coexistence of other congenital anomalies.[90]

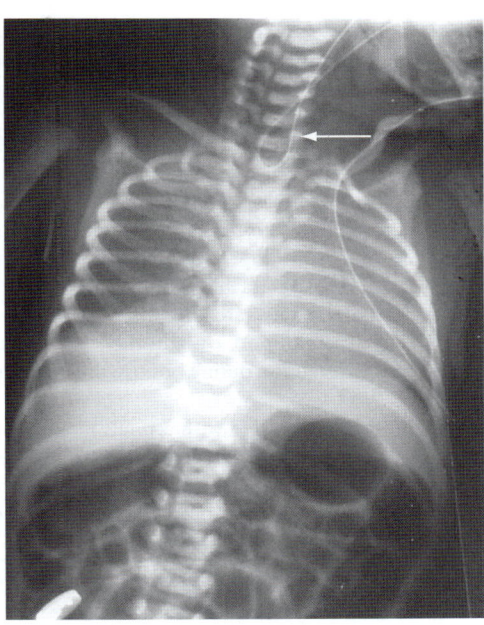

FIGURE 15.11 Tracheoesophageal fistula with esophageal atresia. Note the feeding tube coiled in the esophageal pouch (*arrow*) and the presence of a large volume of gas in the abdomen.

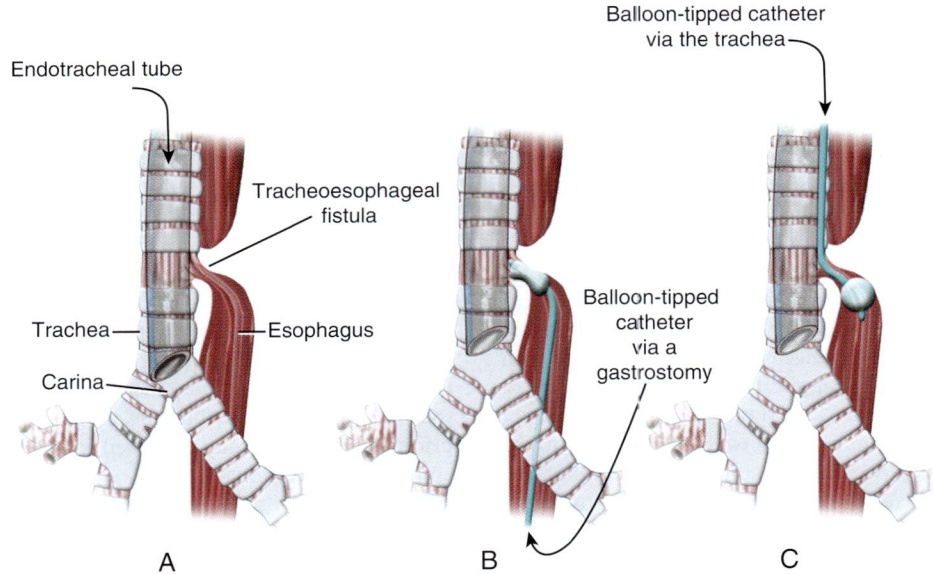

FIGURE 15.12 Methods for minimizing gastric insufflation in infants with a tracheoesophageal fistula. The tip of the ETT may be placed distal to the fistula in cases in which the fistula is well proximal to the carina **(A)**. Alternatively, a balloon-tipped catheter may be placed in the fistula via a gastrostomy **(B)** or via the trachea **(C)**.

Surgical repair has generally involved a right thoracotomy and extrapleural dissection of the posterior mediastinum, although a thorascopic approach has become more common recently. In most cases, the fistula is ligated and primary esophageal anastomosis is performed ("short gap atresia"). In cases in which the esophageal "gap" is long, the proximal segment is preserved for subsequent staged anastomosis, with or without intestinal interposition.[85] The trachea may be intubated with the infant breathing spontaneously, or during gentle positive-pressure ventilation with small tidal volumes to avoid gastric distention. If a gastrostomy tube is in place, occlusion of the fistula may be confirmed by cessation of bubbling via underwater tubing connected to the gastrostomy or the appearance of CO_2 in the end-tidal gas.[65] Alternatively, the tracheal tube may be positioned in the main-stem bronchus, opposite the side of the thoracotomy incision, until the fistula is ligated.

Esophageal atresia without connection to the trachea occurs much less commonly. These lesions are generally diagnosed by radiography after inability to pass an orogastric tube, at which time an absence of gas in the abdomen may be noted (see Fig. 37.9). So-called H-type tracheoesophageal fistula without esophageal atresia is relatively rare. Infants with H-type lesions may present later in childhood or adulthood with recurrent pneumonias or gastric distention during positive-pressure ventilation (see E-Fig. 37.2).[91,92]

Persistent symptoms associated with aspiration and respiratory distress after fistula ligation warrant investigation. Radiographic investigations including a barium swallow and/or rigid bronchoscopy with a 30-degree scope may be needed to identify a persistent fistula or a second fistula.[93]

Childhood

Some of the lesions described earlier may not be diagnosed until childhood. These include pulmonary sequestration, cystic lesions, and lobar emphysema. Other disorders for which thoracic surgery is performed in children, either for definitive treatment or diagnostic purposes, include neoplasms, infectious diseases, and musculoskeletal deformities.

Anterior mediastinal masses include neoplasms of the lung, mediastinum, and pleura. These tumors may be primary or metastatic. Perhaps the most common primary tumors are *lymphoblastic lymphoma*, a form of non-Hodgkin lymphoma, and *Hodgkin disease*. Less commonly, teratomas (germ cell tumors), thymomas, as well as thyroid, parathyroid, and mesenchymal tumors may manifest as anterior mediastinal masses.[94] Signs and symptoms that result from vascular and/or airway compression may include dyspnea, orthopnea, pain, coughing, pleural effusion, and/or superior vena cava syndrome (swelling of the upper arms, face, and neck).[95,96]

Preoperative evaluation should include CT, echocardiography, and flow-volume studies whenever feasible (see Fig. 13.7). Tracheal, bronchial, and/or vascular (superior vena cava or pulmonary outflow tract) compression, as detected by CT, is associated with a high incidence of serious complications during induction of anesthesia.[96] However, CT scans are static pictures that may not identify dynamic compression of an airway or vascular outflow tract. These tumors may occur as extrathoracic or intrathoracic, variable obstruction or fixed obstruction. Echocardiography identifies compression of the superior vena cava or pulmonary outflow tract. Flow-volume loops may be effective in detecting dynamic compression of the airways, although their utility in adult patients has been questioned[97] (see Chapter 13 and Figs. 13.6 and 13.7).

Establishing the correct diagnosis often requires a tissue biopsy. More often than not, there is an urgency to secure the tissue for diagnosis, because T-cell–type non-Hodgkin lymphoblastic lymphomas, which constitute 30% to 40% of non-Hodgkin lymphoma, have a 12-hour doubling time.[98] A rapid diagnosis and chemotherapy prescription may prevent widespread dissemination of the tumor. Indeed, today, the 5-year survival of Hodgkin and non-Hodgkin lymphoblastic lymphoma exceeds 80%. Every effort should be made to secure a tissue diagnosis by lymph node or bone marrow biopsy using local anesthesia or sedation, thereby precluding the need for general anesthesia and facilitating early treatment.[99] If peripheral tissue diagnosis cannot be obtained and signs of severe airway and/or circulatory compromise are present, careful consideration should be given to administering a 12- to 24-hour burst of corticosteroids, initiating chemotherapy, and/or treating with limited radiation to decrease the size of the tumor and reduce the risk of life-threatening compression of the airway or major vessels under anesthesia. The risk is that any or all of these interventions may cause involution of the tumor and compromise the tissue diagnosis; thus some oncologists prefer to avoid such interventions prebiopsy.[100,101] Corticosteroids effect a reduction in tissue mass (i.e., tumor lysis) of lymphomas by inducing apoptosis in the tumor via a number of mechanisms.[102] One study found that four features were predictive of perianesthesia complications in these children: orthopnea, upper body edema, great vessel compression, and main-stem bronchial compression (odds ratio of 5.1 to 8).[103] A second study found that the extent of vascular and airway compression, according to radiologic investigations, was predictive of perianesthesia complications.[99] It must be emphasized that adolescents and adults have different risk factors than children younger than 8 years of age. In adults, for example, intraoperative complications have been associated with pericardial effusions diagnosed by CT scans, whereas postoperative respiratory complications have been associated with greater than 50% tracheal compression on preoperative CT.[104] Great care must be taken to properly prepare these children and the families for general anesthesia, together with the attendant risks.

Induction of anesthesia in children with anterior mediastinal masses may be associated with severe airway obstruction and circulatory collapse.[99] This may occur even in children without signs or symptoms of respiratory or cardiovascular compromise.[105,106] Therefore a preoperative assessment of what position provides the most reliable and consistently good gas exchange should be sought from the child or the parents (nocturnal sleep position). Recommended anesthetic techniques for children with anterior mediastinal masses include inhalation induction or a slow IV induction (with ketamine or propofol), with maintenance of spontaneous respirations. The latter offsets the effect of gravity, which pulls the tumor onto the pulmonary artery, superior vena cava, and/or tracheobronchial tree, causing life-threatening cardiopulmonary consequences.[98,101,107] The use of CPAP while maintaining spontaneous respirations maintains functional residual capacity that is otherwise reduced under anesthesia.[108] In adolescents and adults, neuromuscular blockade is commonly used to facilitate tracheal intubation and prevent coughing associated with DLT placement. The morbidity associated with neuromuscular blockade appears to be minimal as long as appropriate precautions are taken. The actual risks in young children, however, have not been studied.[104] Keeping the head of the bed elevated may decrease the deleterious effects of supine positioning, including cephalad displacement of the diaphragm and secondary reduction of thoracic volume.[109] Placing the child in a partial or even full left lateral decubitus position may help to maintain airway patency and reduce cardiovascular and/or tracheal compression.[98] Performing tracheal

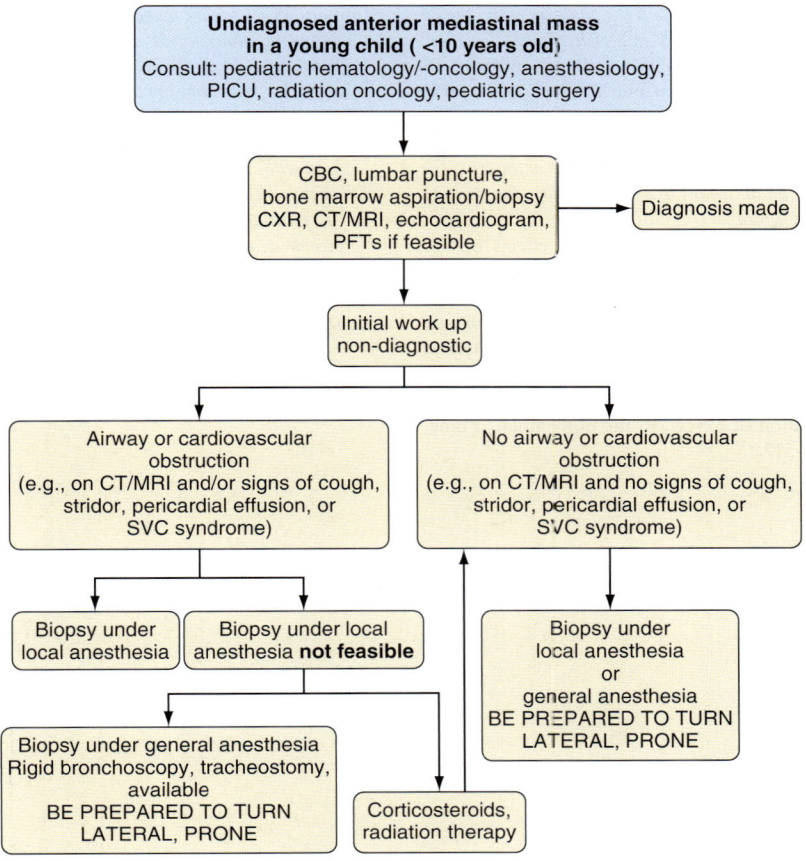

FIGURE 15.13 Algorithm for management of a child with a mediastinal mass. *CBC*, complete blood cell count; *CPB*, cardiopulmonary bypass; *CT*, computed tomography; *CXR*, chest radiograph; *LP*, lumbar puncture; *MRI*, magnetic resonance imaging; *PFTs*, pulmonary function tests; *PICU*, pediatric intensive care unit; *SVC*, superior vena cava.

intubation while the patient is deeply anesthetized, without the use of muscle relaxants and positive-pressure ventilation, preserves the normal transpulmonary pressure gradient and improves flow through conducting airways.[110–112] The loss of negative intrathoracic pressure associated with neuromuscular blockade increases the risk of severe airway compression and reduction in pulmonary blood flow (i.e., cardiac output).[113] As an alternative to tracheal intubation, use of a laryngeal mask airway has been described.[114] However, this could be a hazardous airway should the child need to be turned prone to restore cardiac output. The use of a helium-oxygen (70%/30%) mixture has been recommended to decrease the resistance to breathing and to increase hemoglobin saturation when an anterior mediastinal tumor compresses the trachea and/or bronchi (where turbulent gas flow exists).[114] It should be remembered that at least 70% helium is needed to substantively increase the flow in the airway; this concentration limits the inspired concentration of oxygen. In the event of tracheal or bronchial collapse or the sudden disappearance of the capnogram (signaling a loss of pulmonary outflow) under anesthesia, lateral or prone positioning and/or rigid bronchoscopy may be lifesaving.[98] Alternatively, towel clips or similar devices may be placed in the xiphoid cartilage and sternal notch to lift the sternum and restore patency of the collapsed structure while a longer-term solution is planned. Performing a median sternotomy and cardiopulmonary bypass in this situation has been recommended but is impractical unless access for partial bypass

has been established before induction of anesthesia.[101] Institutions should have an algorithm in place for the evaluation of children with anterior mediastinal masses that includes a multidisciplinary approach (Fig. 15.13).

Summary

The anesthesiologist caring for infants and children undergoing thoracic surgery faces many challenges. An understanding of the primary underlying lesion as well as associated anomalies that may affect perioperative management is paramount. Preoperative and intraoperative communication with the surgeon is also essential. A working knowledge of respiratory physiology and anatomy in infants and children is required for the planning and execution of appropriate intraoperative care. Familiarity with a variety of techniques for single-lung ventilation suited to the child's size will provide optimal surgical exposure while minimizing trauma to the lungs and airways.

ANNOTATED REFERENCES

Capan LM, Turndorf H, Patel C, et al. Optimization of arterial oxygenation during one-lung anesthesia. *Anesth Analg.* 1980;59:847-851.

Fisher AO, Hussain K, Wolfson MR, et al. Hyperoxia during one lung ventilation: inflammatory and oxidative responses. *Pediatr Pulmonol.* 2012;47(10):979-986.

This is an important article describing the adverse effects (e.g., inflammation) caused by using high concentrations of oxygen for SLV in a piglet model.

Hammer GB, Harrison TK, Vricella LA, et al. Single lung ventilation in children using a new paediatric bronchial blocker. *Paediatr Anaesth.* 2002;12:69-72.

This article is the first to describe the use of the Cook 5F pediatric endobronchial blocker. This is now the most commonly used bronchial blocker in children. The characteristics of the catheter and the details of the methodology for insertion and proper placement are highlighted.

Heaf DP, Helms P, Gordon MB, Turner HM. Postural effects on gas exchange in infants. *N Engl J Med.* 1983;28:1505-1508.

Changes in ventilation and perfusion of the lung associated with body position were first described in adults. This paper describes such relationships in infants, highlighting the important differences in this population that have significant clinical relevance during thoracic anesthesia.

Rees DI, Wansbrough SR. One-lung anesthesia and arterial oxygen tension during continuous insufflation of oxygen to the nonventilated lung. *Anesth Analg.* 1982;61:507-512.

These articles describe the maneuvers of choice for increasing oxygenation in patients during single-lung ventilation. Oxygen desaturation is common during single-lung ventilation, especially in children. It is essential that practitioners have an algorithm for addressing this problem promptly during surgery.

Wilson CA, Arthurs OJ, Black AE, et al. Printed three-dimensional airway model assists planning of single-lung ventilation in a small child. *Br J Anaesth.* 2015;115(4):616-620.

Although published as a single case report, this article highlights the utility of using 3D printing for planning the use of SLV in an individual child. This may become an important technique going forward as 3D printing becomes more widely available and cost-effective.

A complete reference list can be found online at ExpertConsult.com.

16

Essentials of Cardiology

WANDA C. MILLER-HANCE AND RALPH GERTLER

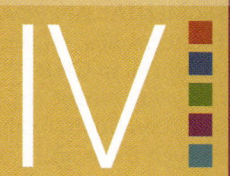

Congenital Heart Disease

INCIDENCE

Congenital heart disease (CHD) is the most common congenital anomaly, affecting approximately 1% of live births.[1] Although CHD represents the leading cause of neonatal mortality, advances in medical and surgical management over the past several decades, including significant contributions related to anesthesia care, now allow for survival of most affected infants.[2,3]

A bicuspid aortic valve is the most common cardiac defect, occurring in up to 1% of the population (Video 16.1).[4,5] Intra-

cardiac communications, including ventricular septal defects (VSDs; Video 16.2) and atrial septal defects (ASDs; Video 16.3) represent the next most common congenital pathologies.[6,7] Among cyanotic lesions, tetralogy of Fallot (TOF) predominates, affecting almost 6% of children with CHD (Fig. 16.1).[8] In the first week of life, D-transposition of the great arteries is the most frequently encountered cause of cardiac cyanosis (Fig. 16.2); TOF may not be detected until later in life because in some infants cyanosis is absent or only mild arterial desaturation is present.

SEGMENTAL APPROACH TO DIAGNOSIS

The segmental, sequential approach is the essence of diagnostic assessment in CHD.[9-11] It assumes a stepwise, systematic examination of all cardiac structures or segments and their relationships (i.e., connections or alignments between segments) by navigating through the heart in the direction of blood flow. The principle of this scheme is that specific cardiac chambers and vascular structures have characteristic morphologic properties that determine their identities, rather than their positions within the body.[12]

The approach starts by determining the cardiac position within the thorax, the direction of the cardiac apex, and the arrangement or situs of the thoracic and abdominal organs. The cardiac position can be described as the spatial location of the majority of the cardiac mass within the thorax, using the sternum as the midline reference (Fig. 16.3). The cardiac orientation refers to the alignment from the base (great arteries) to the apex (ventricular apex). In most cases, the cardiac position and base-to-apex orientation are in agreement, meaning that both are aligned in the same direction. Thus, for simplicity the following terms are frequently used in clinical practice: *levocardia* if the heart is in the left hemithorax and the ventricular apex is directed toward the left (as is case of the normal heart); *dextrocardia* if the heart is located in the right hemithorax and the apex is toward the right; and *mesocardia* if the heart and apex are in midline position. An abnormal location of the heart within the thorax (i.e., cardiac malposition) can result from displacement by adjacent structures or underlying noncardiac malformations (e.g., diaphragmatic hernia, lung hypoplasia, scoliosis).

The visceral situs, or sidedness, of the abdominal organs (i.e., liver and stomach) and atrial situs are considered independently (Fig. 16.4). Visceral situs is classified as *solitus* (i.e., normal arrangement of viscera, with the liver on the right, stomach on the left, and a single spleen on the left), *inversus* (i.e., inversion of viscera, with the liver on the left and stomach on the right), or *ambiguous* (i.e., indeterminate visceral position). Abnormal arrangements or sidedness of the abdominal viscera, heart, and lungs, as seen in heterotaxy syndromes, are associated with a high likelihood of complex cardiovascular disease. The atrial situs, atrioventricular (AV) connections, ventricular looping (i.e., position of the ventricles as a result of the direction of bending of the straight heart tube

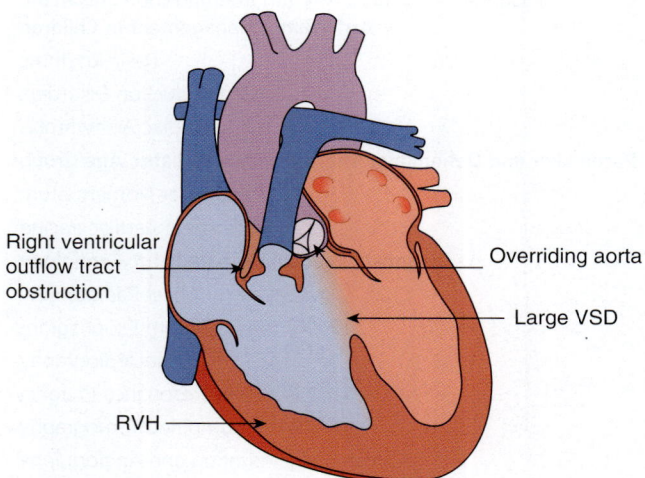

FIGURE 16.1 The anatomic features of tetralogy of Fallot are depicted, consisting of right ventricular outflow tract obstruction (may occur at any or a combination of valvar, subvalvar, and supravalvar levels), a large ventricular septal defect (*VSD*), aortic override, and right ventricular hypertrophy (*RVH*). The purple color in the aorta represents arterial desaturation from intracardiac right to left shunting. Note the infundibular narrowing and the hypoplastic pulmonary arteries.

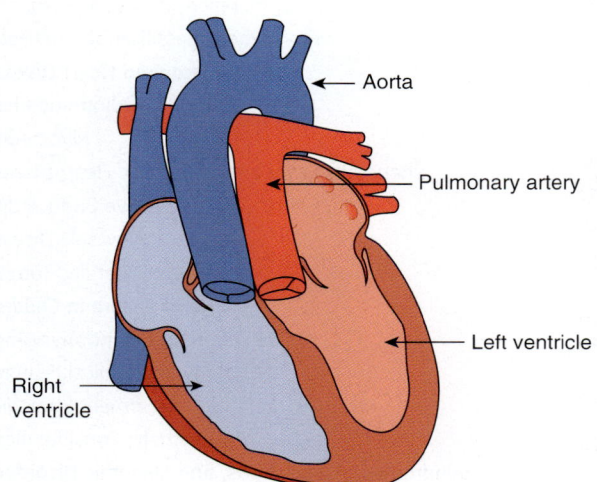

FIGURE 16.2 Diagrammatic representation of D-transposition of the great arteries displaying the discordant ventriculoarterial connections. In this lesion the right ventricle ejects blood into the aorta and the left ventricle ejects blood into the pulmonary artery. Intercirculatory mixing is essential for survival in this anomaly.

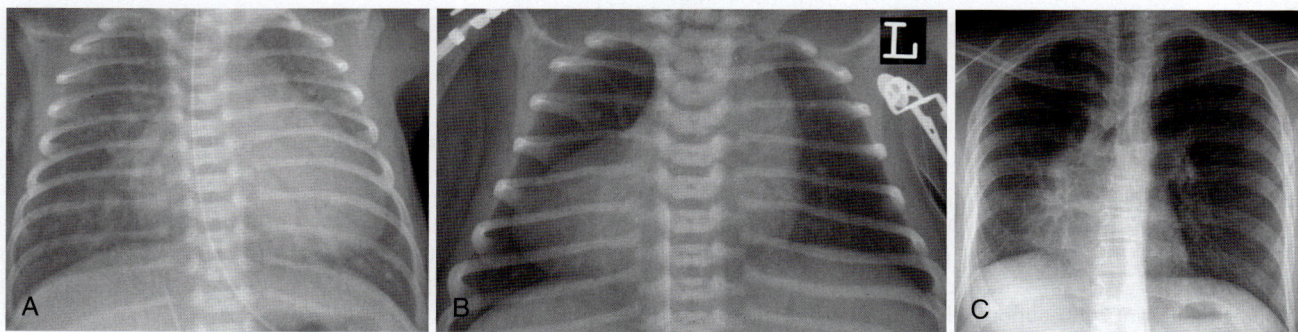

FIGURE 16.3 Chest radiographs demonstrate various cardiac positions within the thorax. **A,** Levocardia (left-sided position). **B,** Dextrocardia (right-sided position). **C,** Mesocardia (centrally located cardiac mass).

Types of visceroatrial situs: atrial localization

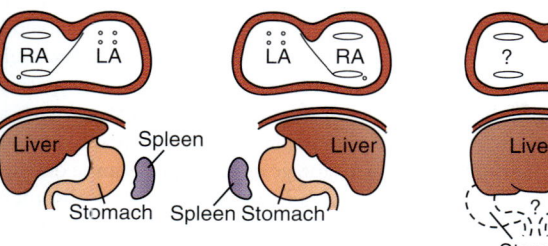
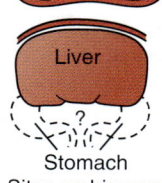

FIGURE 16.4 Three types of visceroatrial situs are shown. *Situs solitus* indicates a normal arrangement of the viscera and atria, with the right atrium (*RA*) on the right side and the left atrium (*LA*) on the left side. The stomach and spleen are on the left, and the liver is on the right. *Situs inversus* indicates inverted arrangement of viscera and atria, with the RA on the left side and the LA on the right side, as in a mirror image of *situs solitus*. In visceral *situs inversus*, the stomach and spleen are on the right, and the liver is on the left. *Situs ambiguous* denotes that the visceroatrial situs is anatomically uncertain or indeterminate because the anatomic findings are ambiguous. (From Park. Chamber localization and cardiac malposition. In: *Park's Pediatric Cardiology for Practitioners*, Sixth Edition. Philadelphia: Elsevier; 2014:314–318.)

TABLE 16.1	Physiologic Classification of Congenital Heart Disease (Representative Lesions)
Volume Overload Lesions	
Atrial septal defect	
Ventricular septal defect	
Atrioventricular septal defect	
Patent ductus arteriosus	
Truncus arteriosus	
Obstruction to Systemic Blood Flow	
Aortic stenosis	
Coarctation of the aorta	
Interrupted aortic arch	
Hypoplastic left heart syndrome	
Obstruction to Pulmonary Blood Flow	
Pulmonary stenosis	
Tetralogy of Fallot	
Pulmonary atresia	
Parallel Circulation	
D-Transposition of the great arteries	
Single-Ventricle Lesions	
Tricuspid atresia	
Double-inlet left ventricle	
Unbalanced atrioventricular septal defect	
Intrinsic Myocardial Disorders	
Cardiomyopathy	
Myocarditis	

during early development), ventriculoarterial connections, and the relationship between the great vessels are then delineated. Additional goals of the complete morphologic evaluation in CHD include, among other aspects, interrogation of structures such as the branch pulmonary arteries, aortic arch, and coronary arteries.

Associated malformations are described, including number, size, and location of septal defects, valvar pathology, and great vessel abnormalities. Whereas many types of congenital defects fall neatly into well-known classification schemes, others, such as those associated with heterotaxy syndromes where there is malposition of the heart and abdominal organs, are often more difficult to precisely define.

PHYSIOLOGIC CLASSIFICATION OF DEFECTS

The wide spectrum of cardiovascular malformations in the pediatric age group presents a challenge to the clinician who does not specialize in the care of these children. Even for those with a focus or interest in cardiovascular disease, the range of structural defects and the varied associated hemodynamic perturbations can be overwhelming (see Chapter 23).

Several classification schemes have been proposed to characterize and categorize the various congenital cardiac defects, including some that categorize structural defects into simple or complex lesions, consider the presence or absence of cyanosis, or recognize whether pulmonary blood flow is increased or decreased.[13–15] A physiologic classification system can facilitate understanding of the basic hemodynamic abnormalities common to a group of congenital or acquired lesions and assist in patient management (Table 16.1).[16,17] The following approach sorts pediatric heart disease into six broad categories according to the underlying physiology or common features of the pathologies.

Volume Overload Lesions

Volume overload lesions typically are caused by left-to-right shunting at the level of the atria, ventricles, or great arteries. If the location of the shunt is proximal to the mitral valve (e.g., ASD, partial anomalous pulmonary venous return, unobstructed total anomalous pulmonary venous return), right heart dilation occurs. Lesions distal to the mitral valve (e.g., VSD, patent ductus arteriosus [PDA], truncus arteriosus) lead to left heart dilation. Children with AV septal defects, also known as AV canal or endocardial cushion defects, also fit into this category. The magnitude of the shunt and resultant pulmonary-to-systemic blood flow ratio ($\dot{Q}_{pulm}/\dot{Q}_{sys}$) dictate the presence and severity of the symptoms and guide medical and surgical therapies. Diuretic therapy and afterload reduction are beneficial in controlling pulmonary overcirculation and ensuring adequate systemic cardiac output. Surgical interventions or transcatheter approaches may be required to address the primary pathology associated with ventricular volume overload (see Chapter 22).

Obstruction to Systemic Blood Flow

Several lesions are associated with systemic outflow tract obstruction. Conditions characterized by ductal-dependent systemic blood flow in the neonate include critical aortic stenosis, severe aortic coarctation, aortic arch interruption, and hypoplastic left heart syndrome. Prostaglandin E_1 therapy maintains ductal patency and ensures adequate systemic blood flow until surgical or transcatheter intervention is performed in the first few days of life to relieve the systemic outflow obstruction. Inotropic and/or mechanical ventilatory support are often necessary in the affected neonate/small infant. These children frequently also have significantly increased pulmonary blood flow with a large $\dot{Q}_{pulm}/\dot{Q}_{sys}$ ratio, requiring diuretic therapy and manipulation of the systemic and pulmonary vascular resistances to control blood flows.

Obstruction to Pulmonary Blood Flow

Defects with pulmonary outflow tract obstruction include those with ductal-dependent pulmonary blood flow. Critical pulmonary valve stenosis and pulmonary atresia with intact ventricular septum, for example, are anomalies that rely on patency of the ductus arteriosus for pulmonary blood flow. Affected infants frequently require prostaglandin E_1 infusions for management of their cyanosis until the pulmonary outflow obstruction is relieved or bypassed.

Parallel Circulation

In the neonate with D-transposition of the great arteries, the pulmonary and systemic circulations operate in parallel rather than in the normal configuration in series. In this condition, the right ventricle ejects deoxygenated blood into the aorta, and the left ventricle ejects oxygenated blood into the pulmonary arteries. Mixing of blood in this setting can occur at the atrial, ventricular, or ductal levels (see Fig. 16.2). Although prostaglandin E_1 therapy maintains ductal patency and enhances intercirculatory mixing, balloon atrial septostomy to create or enlarge an existing restrictive interatrial communication, allowing for or augmenting mixing, is necessary in some infants. Mixing at the atrial level is considered much more effective than at the ventricular or ductal levels.

Single-Ventricle Lesions

This category is the most heterogeneous group, consisting of defects associated with AV valve atresia (i.e., tricuspid atresia), heterotaxy syndromes, and many others.[18] In some cases, both atria empty into a dominant ventricular chamber (i.e., double-inlet left ventricle), and although a second rudimentary ventricle can be present, the physiology is that of a single-ventricle or univentricular heart. Other cardiac malformations with two distinct ventricles (i.e., unbalanced AV septal defect) can also be considered in the functional single-ventricle category because of associated defects that may preclude a biventricular repair. A common feature of these lesions is complete mixing of the systemic and pulmonary venous blood at the atrial or ventricular level. Another frequent finding is aortic or pulmonary outflow tract obstruction.

An important goal in single-ventricle management involves optimization of the balance between the pulmonary and systemic circulations early in life. This is a critical issue because low pulmonary vascular resistance and limitation of the ventricular volume load are prerequisites for later palliative strategies and optimal outcomes in these children. These considerations are also relevant for anesthesia management during noncardiac surgery (see Chapter 23).[19-23] The child with single-ventricle physiology represents a high-risk group for adverse events during noncardiac surgery.[24]

Intrinsic Myocardial Disorders

Children with primary cardiomyopathies or myocarditis have intrinsic diseases of cardiac muscle. They frequently have impaired systolic and/or diastolic ventricular function and benefit from therapies tailored to their particular disease process.

Acquired Heart Disease

CARDIOMYOPATHIES

The term *cardiomyopathy* refers to diseases of the myocardium associated with cardiac dysfunction.[25,26] They have been classified as primary and secondary forms.[27] Primary forms are those predominantly involving the heart owing to genetic mutation, including ion channelopathies, acquired disease, or mixed. The most common types in children are hypertrophic, dilated or congestive, and restrictive cardiomyopathies. Other forms include left ventricular noncompaction[28-30] and arrhythmogenic right ventricular dysplasia.[31-33] Secondary forms of cardiomyopathies are those with systemic involvement in other organ systems as seen in association with neuromuscular disorders such as Duchenne muscular dystrophy, glycogen storage diseases (i.e., Pompe disease), hemochromatosis or iron overload, and mitochondrial disorders. Chemotherapeutic agents such as anthracyclines can result in dilated cardiomyopathy.[34] It is important to understand the hemodynamic processes behind the myocardial disease and implications for acute and chronic management.

Hypertrophic cardiomyopathy (HCM) is characterized by ventricular hypertrophy without an identifiable hemodynamic cause that results in increased myocardial wall thickness.[35] This accounts for almost 40% of cardiomyopathies in children.[36-38] The condition represents a heterogeneous group of disorders, and most of the identified genetic defects exhibit autosomal dominant inheritance patterns.[39,40] This is the most common cause of sudden cardiac death (SCD) in athletes.[41,42] Some children with HCM have systemic outflow tract obstruction (i.e., obstructive cardiomyopathy). It is unclear whether the few with hypertrophic obstructive cardiomyopathy, previously known as idiopathic hypertrophic subaortic stenosis, are at increased risk for SCD compared with children without obstruction.

Most children with HCM present for evaluation of a heart murmur, syncope, palpitations, or chest pain. Occasionally, an abnormal electrocardiogram (ECG) leads to referral. An accurate family history is essential. An apical impulse is often prominent. Auscultation may reveal a systolic ejection outflow murmur that becomes louder with maneuvers that decrease preload or afterload (e.g., standing, Valsalva maneuver) or increased contractility. The murmur decreases in intensity with squatting and isometric hand grip. A mitral regurgitant murmur can also be present. The ECG meets criteria for left ventricular hypertrophy in most children (Fig. 16.5). In some, the electrocardiographic findings can be striking (Fig. 16.6). A hypertrophied, nondilated left ventricle is a diagnostic feature as determined by two-dimensional echocardiography (Video 16.4 A and B). In many children, the hypertrophy can be asymmetric (Video 16.5A and B). Echocardiography is the preferred imaging tool for long-term assessment of ventricular wall thickness, chamber dimensions, presence and severity of obstruction, systolic and diastolic function, valve competence, and response to therapy. Other diagnostic approaches such as cardiac catheterization and magnetic resonance imaging (MRI) can add helpful information in some cases.

The care of children with HCM includes maintenance of adequate ventricular preload, particularly in those with dynamic obstruction. Diuretics are not indicated and can be detrimental to the hemodynamic state by reducing left ventricular volume and increasing the outflow tract obstruction. Drugs that augment myocardial contractility (e.g., inotropic agents, calcium infusions) are not well tolerated. Patients usually undergo continuous electrocardiographic monitoring (i.e., Holter recording) and exercise testing for risk stratification.[43] β-Blockers and calcium channel blockers are the primary drugs for outpatient therapy.[44] Therapies range widely and include longitudinal observation with medical management of heart failure and arrhythmias, implantation of cardioverter-defibrillators, surgical myotomy or myectomy, transcatheter alcohol septal ablation, and cardiac transplantation.

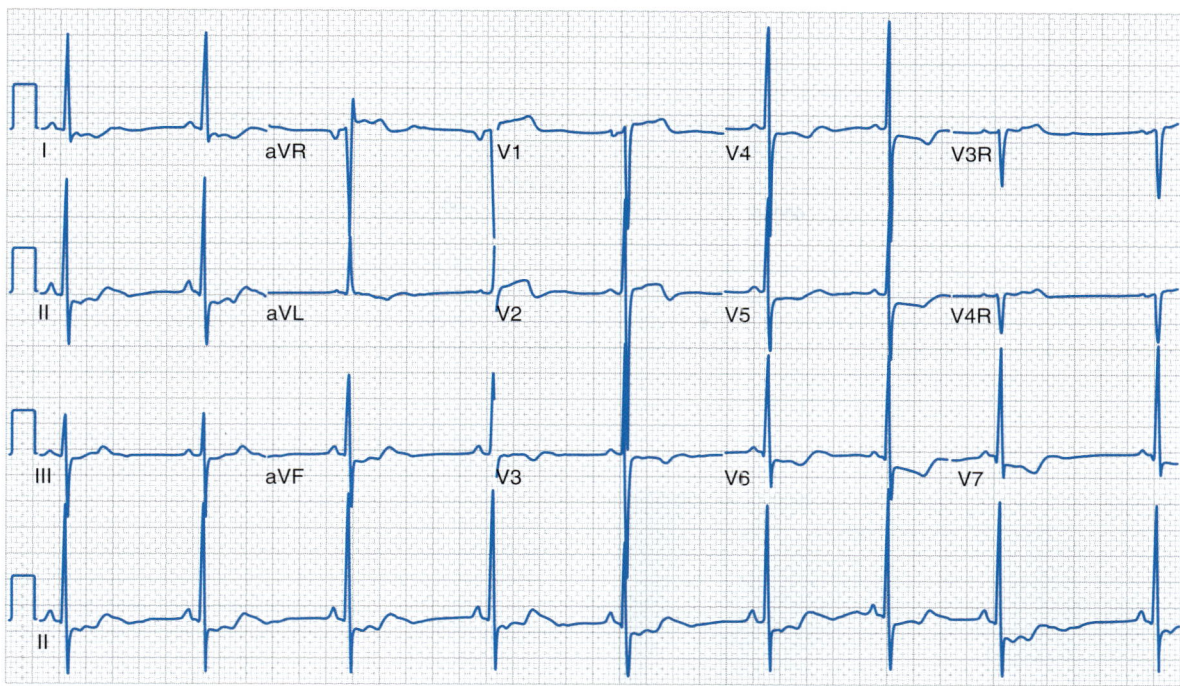

FIGURE 16.5 The electrocardiogram from an adolescent with hypertrophic cardiomyopathy demonstrates left ventricular hypertrophy (i.e., deep S wave in V₁ and tall R waves over the left precordial leads). The ST-segment depression and T-wave inversion over the left precordial leads are related to repolarization changes associated with left ventricular hypertrophy, also known as a *strain pattern*. Reciprocal ST-segment elevation can be seen over the right precordial leads. This recording is consistent with sinus bradycardia (heart rate average of 50 beats/minute).

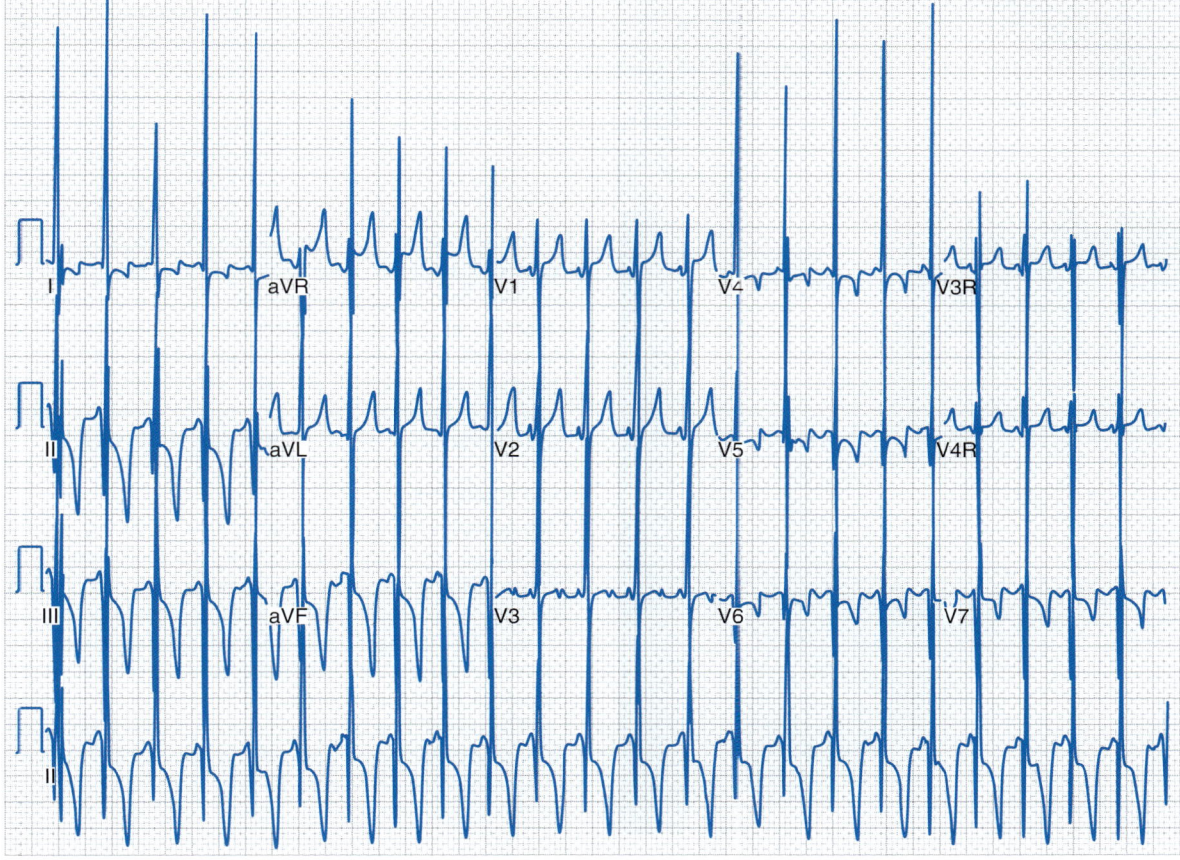

FIGURE 16.6 Pompe disease is an inherited disorder characterized by the accumulation of glycogen in cells. The electrocardiographic tracing for an infant with this glycogen storage disease and a severe form of hypertrophic cardiomyopathy displays dramatic right and left ventricular voltages, in addition to ST-segment and T-wave abnormalities. The recording is displayed at full standard (10 mm/mV), meaning that the electrocardiogram was not reduced in size to fit on the paper.

Dilated cardiomyopathy (DCM), also known as congestive cardiomyopathy, is characterized by thinning of the left ventricular myocardium, dilation of the ventricular cavity, and systolic functional impairment.[45–47] The broad number of etiologies range from genetic or familial forms to those caused by infections, metabolic derangements, toxic exposures, and degenerative disorders.[48,49] Chronic tachyarrhythmias can also lead to DCM that may or may not improve after control of the rhythm disturbance.[50,51]

Most children with DCM present with signs and symptoms of congestive heart failure (e.g., tachypnea, tachycardia, gallop rhythm, diminished pulses, hepatosplenomegaly). The chest radiograph typically demonstrates cardiomegaly, pulmonary vascular congestion, and in some cases, atelectasis (Fig. 16.7). The ECG can identify

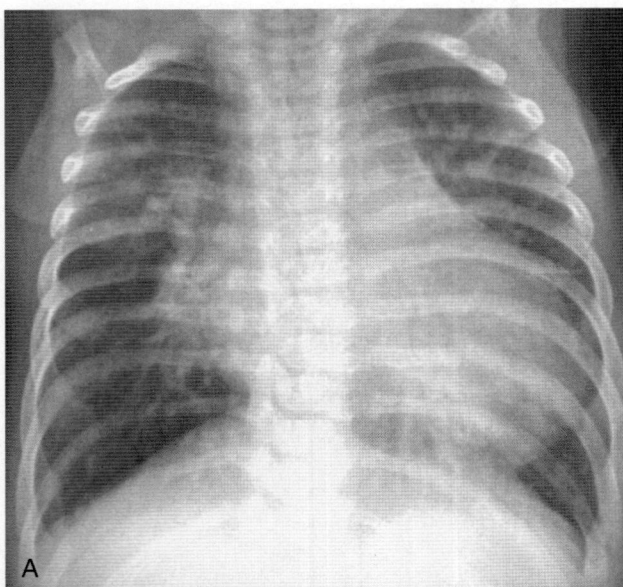

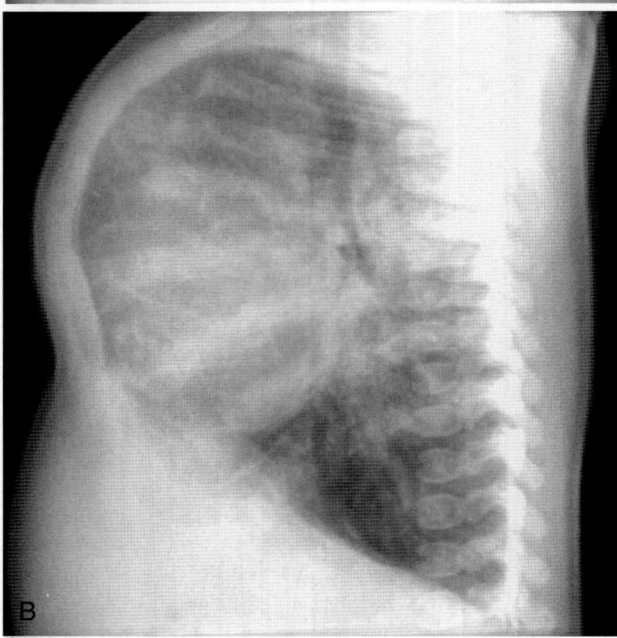

FIGURE 16.7 Chest radiographs of a young child with dilated cardiomyopathy in the posteroanterior **(A)** and lateral **(B)** projections demonstrate moderate to severe cardiomegaly and pulmonary vascular congestion.

the likely cause of the cardiac dysfunction in those with cardiomyopathy caused by rhythm disorders or anomalous origin of the left coronary artery from the pulmonary artery (ALCAPA). The ECG can confirm the diagnosis by demonstrating a dilated left ventricle with decreased systolic function (Video 16.6A and B). Therapy in the acute setting is supportive and aimed at stabilization. Management includes afterload reduction, inotropic support, and mechanical ventilation. Unlike children with HCM, those with DCM have a volume-loaded, poorly contractile ventricle. Gentle diuresis is beneficial. The infusion of large fluid boluses is poorly tolerated and can result in hemodynamic decompensation and cardiovascular collapse. The outcomes of children with dilated cardiomyopathy vary. For most, either the extent of cardiac dysfunction remains unchanged or recovery of left ventricular systolic function occurs, but others eventually require cardiac transplantation.[52,53] A subset of children with severe disease may require mechanical circulatory support as a bridge to recovery or cardiac transplantation (Fig. 16.8A and B) (see Chapter 21).[54–56]

Restrictive cardiomyopathy (RCM) is the least common of the major types of cardiomyopathies (5%) and portends a poor prognosis when it manifests during childhood.[57–59] The disorder is characterized by diastolic dysfunction related to a marked increase in myocardial stiffness resulting in impaired ventricular filling; most cases are thought to be idiopathic. Presenting symptoms are nonspecific and primarily respiratory. Occasionally, the diagnosis is made after a syncopal or sudden near-death event. The physical examination can demonstrate hepatosplenomegaly, peripheral edema, and ascites.

The echocardiographic hallmark of RCM is that of severe atrial dilation and normal or small-sized ventricles (Video 16.7). The marked diastolic dysfunction leads to increased end-diastolic pressures, left atrial hypertension, and secondary pulmonary hypertension. Children with RCM are prone to thromboembolic complications and anticoagulation therapy is frequently recommended. This is an important consideration during perioperative care because adjustments in the anticoagulation regimen may be necessary. Atrial and ventricular tachyarrhythmias can also occur. Optimal medical treatment is controversial because no specific agents or strategies have been shown to significantly alter outcomes.[60] Similar to children with HCM, diuretics often cause a decrease in the needed preload with detrimental effects on hemodynamics. Inotropic agents are not indicated because systolic function is preserved and the arrhythmogenic properties of inotropic drugs can induce a terminal event. In many centers, cardiac transplantation has been effectively used.[61]

MYOCARDITIS

Myocarditis is defined as inflammation of the myocardium, often associated with necrosis and myocyte degeneration.[62–64] In the United States, it is most often caused by a viral infection. Over the past 20 years, the spectrum of viral pathogens causing myocarditis has changed, such that adenovirus, enteroviruses (e.g., coxsackievirus B), and parvovirus have become the most frequent causes of fulminant disease.

The overall true incidence of myocarditis is unknown because it is frequently underdiagnosed and unrecognized as a nonspecific viral syndrome. A large, 10-year, population-based study on cardiomyopathy found an annual incidence of 1.24 cases per 100,000 children younger than 10 years of age; only a fraction of cases represented those with myocarditis.[65] The diagnosis is made using clinical history, physical examination, and imaging modalities. Myocarditis is highly suspected when a child presents

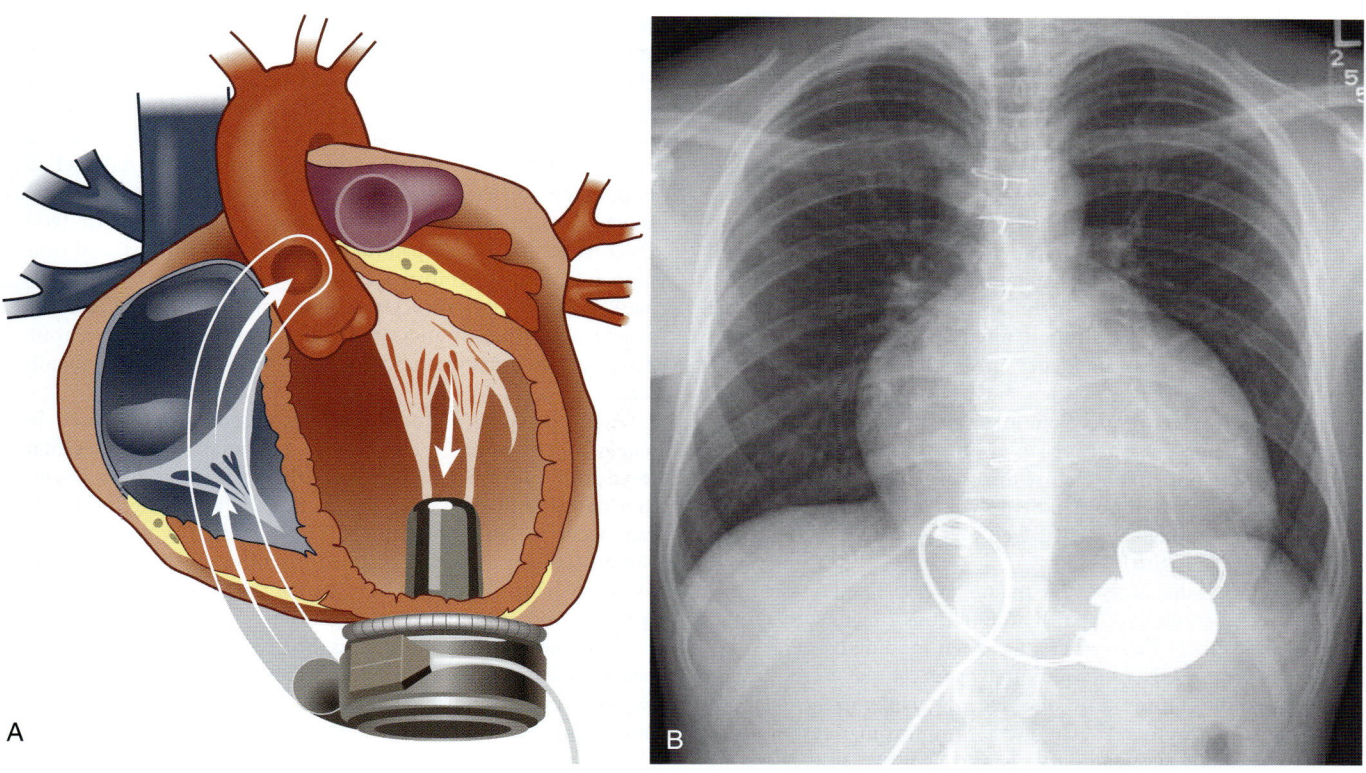

FIGURE 16.8 Mechanical circulatory support may be required in children with dilated cardiomyopathy (DCM) and severe cardiac dysfunction. **A,** HeartWare ventricular assist system (HeartWare LVAD, Framingham, MA). This miniaturized implantable device consists of a small continuous-flow pump with integrated inlet cannula placed in the left ventricle, an outflow graft placed in the aorta (not radiopaque), and a driveline that connects to an external controller with a power source. **B,** Chest radiograph of a child with end-stage DCM after placement of HeartWare ventricular assist device for circulatory support as a bridge to cardiac transplantation. (Illustration **A** printed with permission from Texas Children's Hospital.)

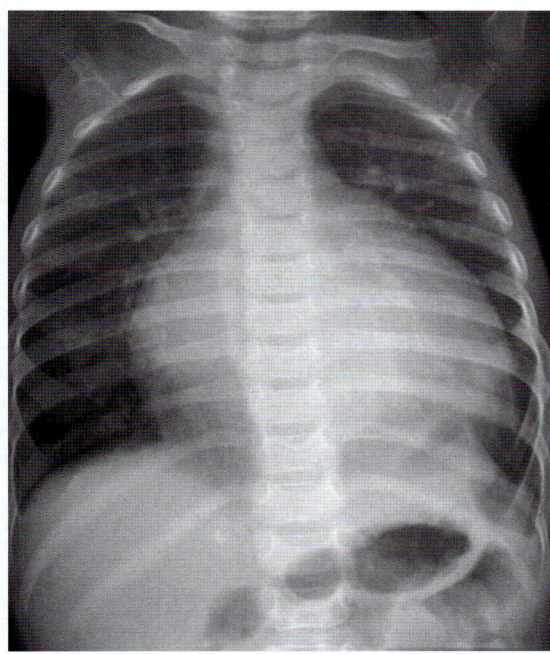

FIGURE 16.9 The chest radiograph of a child with acute myocarditis shows severe cardiomegaly and mildly increased pulmonary vascularity.

with new-onset congestive heart failure or ventricular arrhythmias without evidence of structural heart disease. The ECG typically demonstrates low-voltage QRS complexes with tachycardia, which sometimes is ventricular in origin. Chest radiography often shows cardiomegaly with pulmonary vascular congestion (Fig. 16.9). Echocardiography displays ventricular dilation with decreased systolic function, similar to DCM, and it is useful in the exclusion of alternative diagnoses, such as pericardial effusion or coronary artery anomalies. Myocarditis is a clinical diagnosis because definitive confirmation requires the analysis of tissue obtained through myocardial biopsy in the catheterization laboratory or the operating room (rarely performed).

Many children with myocarditis have subclinical or mild clinical disease, whereas others progress to overt heart failure or arrhythmias, or both. Among children with heart failure, approximately one-third will regain full ventricular function, one-third will recover but continue to demonstrate impaired systolic function, and one-third will require cardiac transplantation.[66,67] A subset of children, not all of whom initially manifest severe symptoms in the acute period, will progress to develop DCM.

Although no specific therapies have been identified to directly treat the myocardial injury, a variety of strategies have been used.[68,69] The current paradigm includes diuresis and afterload reduction to improve myocardial performance without placing a large burden on an already failing heart. Rhythm disturbances are treated appropriately. Therapy with immune modulation or suppression with intravenous (IV) immunoglobulin is the standard of care at many centers.[70,71] Mechanical circulatory support may be required in fulminant disease (see Chapter 21).[72,73]

RHEUMATIC FEVER AND RHEUMATIC HEART DISEASE

Acute rheumatic fever and rheumatic heart disease are leading causes of death related to acquired cardiac disease in developing countries and still occur, albeit infrequently, in developed countries.[74,75] The availability of antibiotic therapy for streptococcal tonsillopharyngitis (strep throat) has markedly reduced the incidence of this disease in the United States, but sporadic cases still occur.[76] The peak incidence in children occurs between 5 and 14 years of age.

Rheumatic fever results from infection by particular strains of group A β-hemolytic *Streptococcus* or *Streptococcus pyogenes* leading to a multisystemic inflammatory disorder. The incubation period for most strains of group A β-hemolytic *Streptococcus* is typically 3 to 5 days, although some children present with a more remote history of pharyngitis.

The clinical diagnosis of rheumatic fever is based on the Jones criteria. The combination of manifestations (major and minor) necessary to meet these criteria has been modified several times over the years. The most recent revision of the Jones criteria considered the contributions of echocardiography in the diagnosis of cardiac involvement.[77] The most common manifestations of acute rheumatic fever are carditis and arthritis; thus these are considered major criteria for diagnosis. Cardiac involvement or carditis occurs in 50% of children with their first attack of rheumatic fever. Rheumatic heart disease represents a sequela of the acute process, and it most frequently affects the mitral and aortic valves. The polyarticular arthritis has a migratory pattern, typically affecting large joints.

Primary prevention of rheumatic fever and rheumatic heart disease begins with prompt recognition and appropriate treatment of the initial streptococcal infection.[78] Penicillin is considered the treatment of choice for most patients. Secondary prevention with antibiotic prophylaxis is aimed at avoiding recurrences in individuals with a known history of rheumatic fever as they are considered at high risk. The duration of prophylaxis depends on several factors. Intramuscular injections of penicillin every 3 to 4 weeks is recommended. Current AHA guidelines no longer propose infective endocarditis (IE) prophylaxis for patients with rheumatic heart disease, except for those few instances where a prosthetic valve has been inserted or prosthetic material used in valve repair (refer to the following section).[79] In these cases, an alternate to penicillin is used because of the potential development of drug resistance.

Elective or emergent surgery may be required in a subset of children with severe cardiac involvement.[80] Mitral valve regurgitation is often the cause of congestive symptoms; medical management therefore has limited efficacy. Valve repair is always preferred to replacement.

INFECTIVE ENDOCARDITIS
Causes and Treatment
CHD has become the primary risk factor for IE in children in developed countries.[81,82] The risk is largely based on the nature of the cardiac condition. The infection results from deposition of bacteria or other pathogens on tissues in areas of abnormal or turbulent blood flow. The diagnosis of IE is made clinically by applying the modified Duke criteria.[83,84] Major criteria include

demonstration of microorganisms (two positive blood culture results) and evidence of pathologic lesions by echocardiography. The presentation of the disease can be acute or subacute. New or changing heart murmurs can indicate the development of regurgitation or obstruction on an affected valve. Physical findings of systemic embolization (i.e., minor criteria) include splinter hemorrhages (i.e., linear streaks under the nail beds), Janeway lesions (i.e., painless macules on the hands or feet), Osler nodes (i.e., small, painful nodules on the fingers), and Roth spots (i.e., retinal hemorrhages with clear centers). Inflammatory markers, such as erythrocyte sedimentation rate and C-reactive protein, are typically increased, albeit nonspecific. Microscopic hematuria, as a manifestation of renal involvement, is frequently seen.

Acute bacterial endocarditis is most commonly caused by *Staphylococcus aureus*.[85] The clinical presentation includes high fevers, chills, myalgias, fatigue, and lethargy. Some children present in a critically ill state or in shock. Both left- and right-sided IE can occur in children with CHD.[86] Children with indwelling venous catheters have an expanded spectrum of pathogens known to cause acute IE, including coagulase-negative staphylococcal species or other nonbacterial organisms.

Subacute bacterial endocarditis (SBE) often has a more indolent course and presentation. Children present with low-grade fever, malaise, anemia, and somatic complaints such as fatigue or weakness. Most frequently, one of the *Viridians streptococcus* group and *Enterococcus* species is the underlying pathogen.

Initial evaluation for bacterial endocarditis includes serial blood cultures obtained from separate sites before initiation of antimicrobial therapy. The temporal frequency of cultures depends on the clinical scenario and stability of the child. In up to 20% of children with evidence of IE, a pathogen cannot be isolated (i.e., negative-culture endocarditis), requiring empirical treatment throughout. Transthoracic echocardiography is routinely performed to evaluate for evidence of vegetations or other abnormalities.[87] Although visualization of a vegetation establishes the diagnosis, a negative study does not exclude the diagnosis. Depending on how strongly the diagnosis is suspected, further imaging, including transesophageal echocardiography, may be necessary (Video 16.8A and B).[88] These imaging modalities are also valuable during follow-up.

Parenteral antibiotics are initiated after blood cultures are collected. Broad-spectrum agents are used initially, and after a pathogen has been identified, the antibiotic regimen is narrowed. Daily blood cultures are obtained until they remain sterile, confirming the adequacy of treatment. A prolonged course of antibiotics (i.e., 4–6 weeks) is required in all children. This can be facilitated by placement of a peripherally inserted central catheter (PICC). Home therapy for IE is feasible in some patients, but it depends on many factors, including clinical status, initial response to antibiotics, sensitivity of the organism to antimicrobial therapy, and the ability of infrastructure to support outpatient treatment of a serious infection (e.g., parental or family member's ability, home health care provider).

In some cases, children with IE require surgical intervention. Failure of medical therapy (i.e., inability to clear the bacteremia), abscess formation, refractory heart failure, large vegetation, and serious embolic phenomenon are indications for surgical intervention. Typically, the procedures involve resection of a vegetation, tissue debridement, or repair of consequent cardiac abnormalities. These children should subsequently receive endocarditis prophylaxis for at-risk procedures for the rest of their lives.

A high level of suspicion for IE must be maintained when evaluating a child with known heart disease and persistent bacteremia (or fungemia) or a fever of unknown origin. The same holds true for any child with foreign material in the heart or vascular tissue, such as indwelling central venous catheters, transvenous pacemakers or defibrillators, and closure devices.

Endocarditis Prophylaxis

The risk for developing IE from transient bacteremia is extremely small in children with normal intracardiac anatomy; however, as previously discussed, certain cardiac conditions are predisposed to acquiring endocarditis. The American Heart Association guidelines do not recommend antibiotic prophylaxis based exclusively on an increased lifetime risk of endocarditis. They propose that it should be restricted to those at greatest risk for an adverse outcome resulting from IE. Children in this category include those with specific congenital heart defects or after certain interventions, prosthetic cardiac valves, a history of IE in the past, and cardiac transplant recipients with valvular disease (Table 16.2).[79] Since the implementation of these guidelines in 2007, a review of 1157 cases of IE from 37 pediatric institutions reported no change in the incidence of this condition between 2003 and 2010, supporting the current prophylaxis guidelines.[89]

Transient bacteremia can occur during dental procedures that involve the gingival tissues or the periapical region of teeth or perforation of the oral mucosa.[90] Although several respiratory tract procedures are associated with transient bacteremia, no definitive data demonstrate a cause-and-effect relationship between these procedures and IE. Caution may be warranted for children at high risk undergoing invasive procedures of the respiratory tract that involve incision or biopsy of the mucosa. In contrast to previous guidelines, routine prophylactic administration of antibiotics solely to prevent IE is not recommended for those undergoing genitourinary or gastrointestinal tract procedures. However, for specific clinical scenarios, antibiotic prophylaxis may be considered.[91] Routine endoscopy or transesophageal echocardiography does not merit routine antibiotic administration. Prophylaxis is not considered necessary for cardiac catheterization; and although many practitioners routinely administer antibiotics during transcatheter placement of devices, there is insufficient evidence to support this practice.

The guidelines recommend the administration of antibiotic prophylaxis 30 to 60 minutes before the procedure to achieve adequate tissue concentrations of antibiotics before bacteremia occurs (Table 16.3). The standard prophylactic regimen for children is for oral amoxicillin. For the child who is allergic to penicillin or ampicillin, oral alternatives include cephalexin, clindamycin, azithromycin, or clarithromycin. In children who are unable to ingest oral medications, alternative antibiotics include ampicillin, cefazolin, and ceftriaxone by an IV or intramuscular route. Since IV access is obtained in the majority of children who present for elective surgery or medical procedures after induction of anesthesia, it is prudent to administer the antibiotics as soon as IV access has been established to achieve adequate tissue levels of antibiotic before skin incision or other sources of bacteremia. If the child is allergic to penicillin or ampicillin and unable to swallow oral medications, cefazolin, ceftriaxone, or clindamycin can be used.

Although there was initial hesitation to alter the practice regarding endocarditis prophylaxis for patients with CHD undergoing gastrointestinal or genitourinary procedures following the most recent guidelines, many health care providers have now adopted the updated recommendations.[92,93]

KAWASAKI DISEASE

Kawasaki disease (i.e., mucocutaneous lymph node syndrome) is a fairly common and potentially fatal form of systemic vasculitis of unknown origin.[94] It is a condition seen predominantly in

TABLE 16.2	Indications for Endocarditis Prophylaxis by the American Heart Association

- Congenital heart disease
  - Unrepaired cyanotic congenital heart defect, including palliative shunts and conduits
  - Completely repaired congenital heart defect with prosthetic material or device (whether placed at surgery or by transcatheter intervention, during the first 6 months after the procedure)
  - Repaired congenital heart defect with residual defect(s) at the site or adjacent to the site of a prosthetic patch or device
- Prosthetic cardiac valve
- Prior history of infective endocarditis
- Cardiac transplant recipient with valvular disease

From American Heart Association, Inc.

TABLE 16.3	American Heart Association Guidelines for Prevention of Infective Endocarditis: Antibiotic Regimens

| Situation | Antibiotic | DOSE[a] | |
		Children	Adults
Able to take oral medication	Amoxicillin	50 mg/kg	2 g
Unable to take oral medication	Ampicillin	50 mg/kg IM or IV	2 g IM or IV
	or		
	Cefazolin or ceftriaxone	50 mg/kg IM or IV	1 g IM or IV
Allergic to penicillins or ampicillin and able to take oral medication	Cephalexin[b,c]	50 mg/kg	2 g
	or		
	Clindamycin	20 mg/kg	600 mg
	or		
	Azithromycin or clarithromycin	15 mg/kg	500 mg
Allergic to penicillins or ampicillin and unable to take oral medication	Cefazolin or ceftriaxone[c]	50 mg/kg IM or IV	1 g IM or IV
	or		
	Clindamycin	20 mg/kg IM or IV	600 mg IM or IV

IM, intramuscular; IV, intravenous.
[a]Single dose to be administered 30 to 60 minutes before the procedure. **The total pediatric dose should not exceed the adult dose.**
[b]Alternatively, another first- or second-generation oral cephalosporin is administered in an equivalent pediatric or adult dosage.
[c]Cephalosporins should not be used in an individual with a history of anaphylaxis, angioedema, or urticaria to penicillins or ampicillin.
From American Heart Association, Inc.

infants and young children. The disease can affect the coronary arteries resulting in dilation and aneurysmal formation.[95,96]

The diagnosis relies on clinical features. To meet criteria, a child must have persistent fevers and at least four of the following findings [97]:

- Polymorphous exanthem
- Peripheral extremity changes (e.g., erythema, desquamation, edema of the hands or feet)
- Bilateral, nonexudative conjunctivitis
- Cervical lymphadenopathy (often unilateral)
- Oral changes (i.e., strawberry tongue; red, dry, or cracked lips)

Nonspecific findings can include irritability, hydrops of the gallbladder, sterile pyuria, arthritis, and aseptic meningitis. Acute-phase reactants and thrombocytosis are usually present.

Intravenous gamma globulin (IVIG) and high-dose aspirin are recommended during the acute phase of the disease. In some cases, additional antiinflammatory therapy is needed. The incidence of coronary artery aneurysms is significantly reduced if high-dose IVIG is administered within the first 10 days of the illness. The presence of coronary artery aneurysms is considered diagnostic for Kawasaki disease (Fig. 16.10). In children with coronary artery aneurysms, low-dose aspirin therapy is administered, in some cases in combination with anticoagulants or antiplatelet drugs.[98] Myocardial ischemia and infarction, although uncommon, are important potential complications.[99] Anesthetic care in these children requires careful consideration regarding myocardial oxygen demand and supply; on rare occasions, coronary revascularization may be necessary.

CARDIAC TUMORS

Cardiac tumors are rare in children. The natural history and optimal treatment strategies are often determined from limited case series and small studies.[100–102] Atrial myxomas represent more than 90% of cardiac tumors in adults, but in children, they tend to be rhabdomyomas or fibromas.[103,104] Less common types include hemangiomas, myxomas (Video 16.9), Purkinje cell tumors, and teratomas. In adults, most tumors are found in the left atrium, but cardiac tumors in children can occur in any cardiac chamber. Malignant primary tumors are rare, and data on their outcomes are limited. Other nonprimary cardiac tumors, such as neuroblastoma, can invade vascular structures and extend into the heart.

Rhabdomyomas are the most common primary cardiac tumors in children.[105] They often involve the ventricular septum and left ventricle, and in most cases there are multiple tumors. Although they are considered benign, children can present with cardiomegaly, congestive heart failure, arrhythmias, or sudden death. The significance of a rhabdomyoma is determined largely by its size and any obstruction it may cause. Tumors of this type tend to regress over time or completely resolve; surgery is not indicated unless symptoms are present. Many children with cardiac rhabdomyomas have associated tuberous sclerosis.

Cardiac fibromas are the second most common type of pediatric primary cardiac tumors.[106] They are typically single and involve the ventricular free wall. In a subset of fibromas, the tumor can invade the conduction system. Surgery or cardiac transplantation may be required. The tumors can be very large, and complete surgical resection can alter cardiac function.

The primary concerns in the perioperative care of children with cardiac tumors are the impact of the mass on hemodynamics and the associated abnormalities of cardiac rhythm.[107]

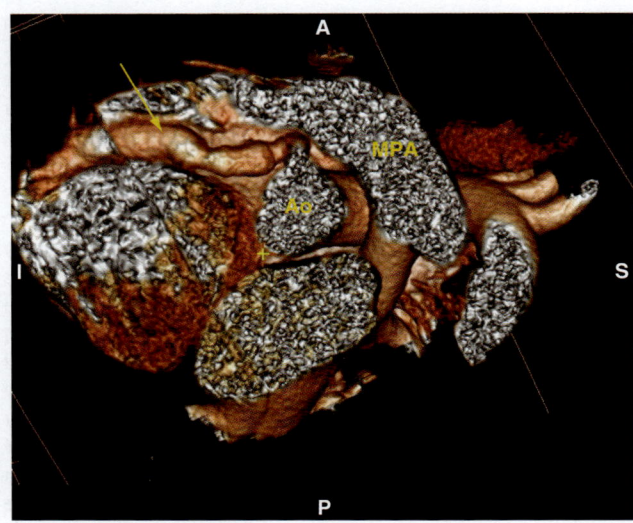

FIGURE 16.10 Magnetic resonance reconstruction at the level of the great vessels in a child with Kawasaki disease demonstrates a large, fusiform coronary artery aneurysm (*arrow*). *A,* anterior; *Ao,* aorta; *I,* inferior; *MPA,* main pulmonary artery; *P,* posterior; *S,* septal.

Heart Failure in Children

DEFINITION AND PATHOPHYSIOLOGY

Heart failure is a major field of interest and investigation in pediatric cardiology and the subject of various publications, scientific meetings, and several textbooks.[108–111] The cellular basis of heart failure, compensatory mechanisms, and therapeutic strategies in children have received the most attention. The following discussion highlights key concepts as they relate to anesthetic practice.

Heart failure is considered to be a pump and circulatory failure involving neurohumoral aspects of the circulation. Several conditions may ultimately compromise the ability to generate an adequate cardiac output to meet the systemic circulatory demands. This disease state does not necessarily imply impairment of ventricular systolic function. Diastolic heart failure is an increasingly recognized clinical entity.

ETIOLOGY AND CLINICAL FEATURES

Pediatric heart failure results from markedly different etiologies from those reported in adults.[112] The causes of heart failure in children vary with age. In the perinatal period, cardiac dysfunction can be related to birth asphyxia or sepsis or constitute an early presentation of CHD. The neonate with heart failure frequently presents with clinical signs of a low cardiac output state. Causes include left-sided outflow obstruction (e.g., aortic stenosis, aortic coarctation, hypoplastic left heart syndrome), severe valve regurgitation (e.g., Ebstein anomaly), or absent pulmonary valve syndrome.

During the first year of life, heart failure is predominantly caused by structural heart disease. Other causes include cardiomyopathies owing to inborn errors of metabolism or acute events such as myocarditis. In infants with heart failure, tachypnea, dyspnea, tachycardia, feeding difficulties, and failure to thrive are prominent features. The physical examination can display grunting respirations, rales, intercostal retractions, a gallop rhythm, and hepatosplenomegaly. Frequently, a mitral regurgitant murmur is present.

Beyond the first year of life, heart failure is a consequence of previous surgical interventions, unpalliated or unrepaired cardiovascular disease, cardiomyopathies, myocarditis, or anthracycline therapy for a malignancy. Occasionally, a child may present with severe ventricular systolic impairment related to ongoing myocardial ischemia as a result of a coronary artery anomaly or rarely because of acquired pathologies such as Kawasaki disease. Older children with heart failure exhibit exercise intolerance, fatigue, and growth failure, whereas adolescents have symptoms similar to those of adults (Table 16.4).

TREATMENT STRATEGIES

Therapy is tailored to the cause of the cardiac dysfunction and may include supportive care, mechanical ventilation, inotropic support, afterload reduction, prostaglandin E_1 therapy to maintain pulmonary or systemic blood flow, maneuvers to balance the systemic and pulmonary circulations, catheter-based interventions, and/or surgery.[113–116] The main goal of therapy for acute heart failure is to maintain organ perfusion. Pharmacologic agents include inotropes (used on a very-short-term basis, if necessary) and inodilators. Favored agents for use in children are diuretics, including aldosterone antagonists, angiotensin-converting enzyme inhibitors, and β-blockers.[117,118] Other drugs that have received attention in the management of pediatric heart failure include nesiritide (a recombinant form of human B-type natriuretic peptide) and carvedilol (a third-generation β-blocker).[119–121] An overview of diagnostic strategies and available therapies for pediatric heart failure can be found in Fig. 16.11.

ANESTHETIC CONSIDERATIONS

Anesthesia for children with heart failure can be quite challenging. The severity of the condition and degree of baseline decompensation can influence the likelihood of an untoward event and the potential for hemodynamic instability and a poor outcome. Several publications have addressed the risks associated with anesthesia in this setting.[122–124] It is important to first reexamine the risk/benefit ratio in these patients before going forward with the planned procedure. In most surgical settings, tracheal intubation and mechanical ventilation are indicated. The need for invasive monitoring should be based on the clinical situation, anticipated nature of the procedure, and impact on hemodynamic state.

Syndromes, Associations, and Systemic Disorders: Cardiovascular Disease and Anesthetic Implications

16

Many disorders, including those resulting from chromosomal abnormalities, single-gene defects, gene deletion syndromes, known associations (i.e., nonrandom occurrence of defects), and teratogenic exposure, can manifest as cardiovascular disease. The coexistence of frequently associated multiple organ system comorbidities with cardiovascular disease presents several challenges to the anesthesia care provider.

CHROMOSOMAL SYNDROMES

Trisomy 21

Trisomy 21 (Down syndrome) is the most common chromosomal anomaly, occurring with a frequency of 1 per 800 live births. The incidence increases sharply with advanced maternal age. Down syndrome results from Trisomy 21 in most children, but it may occur from a balanced or unbalanced chromosomal translocation or mosaicism. The phenotypes are indistinguishable. Affected children are typically smaller than normal for age. Craniofacial features include microbrachycephaly, short neck, oblique palpebral fissures, epicanthal folds, Brushfield spots, small and low-set ears, macroglossia, and microdontia with fused teeth. Mandibular hypoplasia and flattened facial features are common. A narrow nasopharynx with hypertrophic lymphatic tissue (e.g., tonsils, adenoids) in combination with generalized hypotonia frequently leads to obstructive sleep apnea. Other conditions include developmental delay, cervical spine disorders with vertebral and ligamentous instability (i.e., subluxation risk), thyroid disease, leukemia, obesity, subglottic stenosis, and gastrointestinal problems, particularly duodenal atresia.[125]

The preoperative assessment of children with Down syndrome should include a comprehensive evaluation and management plan to minimize risks.[126] The intellectual disability of these children may require the use of premedication or sedatives. Specific issues of concern include the potential for upper airway obstruction caused by a large tongue, postextubation stridor, and cervical spine injury.[127–130] Vascular access can be challenging. Subjectively, children have small and abnormal radial vessels, vascular hyperreactivity, fragile tissue consistency, and an increased risk for complications after arterial cannulation.[131]

Cardiovascular defects occur in 40% to 50% of children with Down syndrome, and it has been recommended that they all should undergo screening for CHD in early infancy.[132] The most common lesions include AV septal defects (Video 16.10), VSDs, TOF, and PDA. Bradycardia under anesthesia occurs commonly, although the mechanism is poorly understood.[133,134] Pulmonary hypertension can result from the cardiac pathology or from chronic hypoxemia caused by upper airway obstruction (i.e., obstructive sleep apnea) and should be considered in their management. Reduced nitric oxide bioavailability has been reported in patients with Down syndrome, leading to endothelial cell dysfunction and possibly explaining the observed increased pulmonary vascular reactivity.[135]

TABLE 16.4	Symptoms Characteristic of Heart Failure in Children	
	Commonly Encountered	**Less Commonly Encountered**
Infants and young children	• Tachypnea • Feeding difficulty (reflux, vomiting, feeding refusal) • Diaphoresis • Pallor	• Cyanosis • Palpitations • Syncope • Facial edema • Dependent edema • Ascites
Older children and adolescents	• Fatigue • Effort intolerance • Dyspnea • Orthopnea • Abdominal pain • Nausea • Vomiting	• Palpitations • Chest pain • Dependent edema • Ascites

Reproduced with permission from from Kantor PF, Lougheed J, Dancea A, et al. Presentation, diagnosis, and medical management of heart failure in children: Canadian Cardiovascular Society guidelines. *Can J Cardiol.* 2013;29(12):1535–1552.

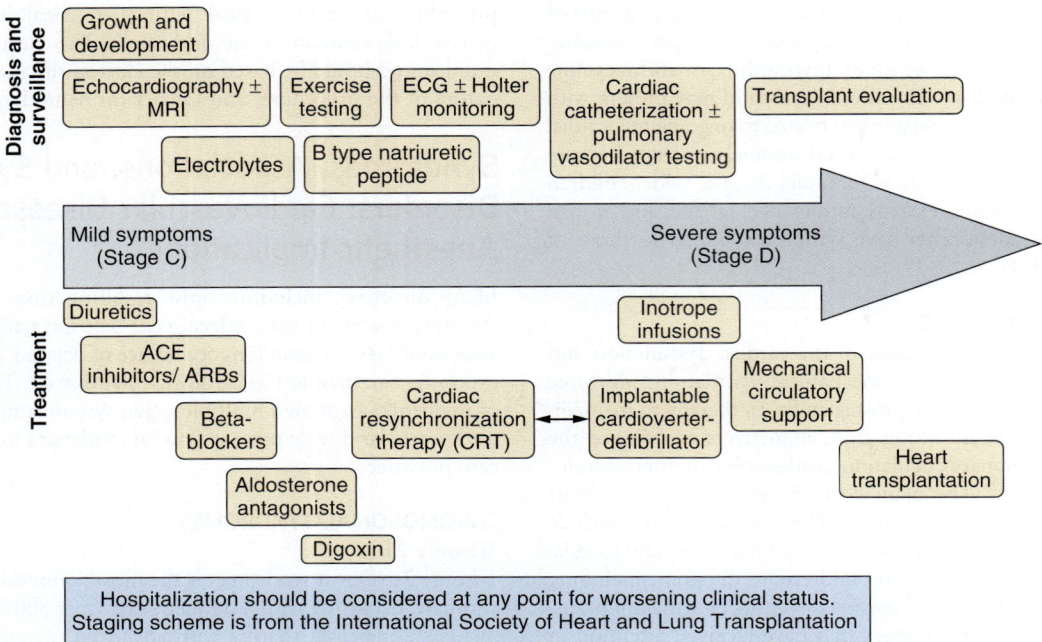

FIGURE 16.11 Outline of diagnostic and therapeutic strategies in pediatric heart failure. *ACE*, angiotensin converting enzyme; *ARBs*, angiotensin receptor blockers; *ECG*, electrocardiogram; *MRI*, magnetic resonance imaging. (Reproduced with permission from O'Connor MJ, Rosenthal DN, Shaddy RE. Outpatient management of pediatric heart failure. *Heart Fail Clin.* 2010;6(4):515–529.)

Trisomy 18

Trisomy 18 (Edwards syndrome) is recognized as the second most common chromosomal trisomy (1 per 3500 live births). Most children exhibit microcephaly, delayed psychomotor development, and developmental delay.[136] Characteristic craniofacial features include micrognathia or retrognathia and microstomia, which can affect airway management, as well as malformed ears, and microphthalmia.[137–139] Skeletal anomalies include clenched fingers and severe growth retardation. Neurologic problems include hypotonia and central nervous system malformations. Their high mortality rate is related to cardiac and renal problems, feeding difficulties, sepsis, and apnea caused by neurologic abnormalities.

Cardiovascular disease, consisting primarily of VSDs and polyvalvular disease, is present in most children with trisomy 18.[140,141] Implications for anesthesia care include the increased risk of congestive heart failure and aspiration pneumonia.[137] These children can require interventions to address associated gastrointestinal or genitourinary anomalies.

Trisomy 13

Trisomy 13 (Patau syndrome) is an uncommon autosomal trisomy with an incidence that ranges from 1 per 5000 to 12,000 live births. Major features include cleft lip and palate, holoprosencephaly, polydactyly, rocker-bottom feet, microphthalmia, microcephaly, and severe developmental delay.[142,143] Almost all children have associated cardiovascular defects, including PDA, septal defects, valve abnormalities, and dextrocardia.[140] The overall prognosis for these children is extremely poor.

Turner Syndrome

Turner syndrome is a genetic disorder characterized by partial or complete X chromosome monosomy.[144] The estimated incidence is 1 per 5000 live-born female infants. Spontaneous miscarriages occur commonly in affected fetuses. Features of this syndrome include webbed neck, low-set ears, multiple pigmented nevi and micrognathia, lymphedema, short stature, and ovarian failure.[145] Systemic manifestations include cardiac defects (notably aortic coarctation and bicuspid aortic valve), hypertension, hypercholesterolemia, renal anomalies, liver disease, and inflammatory bowel disease. Obesity is common in older children, together with an increased incidence of endocrine abnormalities such as hypothyroidism and diabetes.[144,146]

GENE DELETION SYNDROMES

Williams Syndrome

Williams syndrome (also known as Williams-Beuren Syndrome) is a congenital disorder with an incidence of 1 per 10,000–20,000 live births. In most cases, it results from a deletion in the long arm of chromosome 7, altering the elastin gene.[147] Features of Williams syndrome are elfin facies, hypersocial personality, endocrine abnormalities (including hypercalcemia and hypothyroidism), developmental delay, growth deficiency, and altered neurodevelopment. Structural cardiovascular abnormalities, which occur in 80% of these children, most commonly include valvar and supravalvular aortic stenosis (Fig. 16.12) and aortic coarctation.[148,149] The arteriopathy, manifested as stenosis, can also involve the pulmonary arteries, origins of the coronary arteries, or other vessels (e.g., aortopathy). Diffuse narrowing of the abdominal aorta can be associated with renal artery stenosis.

Several reports have described acute hemodynamic deterioration, cardiovascular collapse, and death during anesthesia.[150–152] Two conditions can increase morbidity and the potential for anesthesia and sedation-related cardiac arrest: coronary artery abnormalities, leading to myocardial ischemia, and severe biventricular outflow

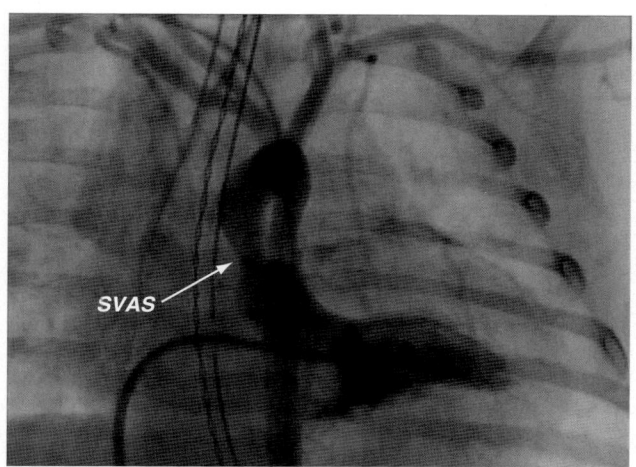

FIGURE 16.12 The angiogram displays the classic angiographic appearance of supravalvar aortic stenosis (*SVAS, arrow*) in a child with Williams syndrome.

tract obstruction. A comprehensive cardiac evaluation of all children is advisable because the spectrum of disease and the potential for devastating implications in affected individuals vary.[153] Children undergoing sedation or anesthetic care occasionally require further studies and even management changes before proceeding with a planned procedure. Even asymptomatic children and those without evidence of clinical cardiovascular disease might be at risk for major morbidity and death during situations associated with hemodynamic stress. Extreme vigilance and particular attention to signs of myocardial ischemia is warranted, as is a plan of action in the event of acute decompensation. This syndrome is one of the leading causes of cardiac arrest in the Pediatric Perioperative Cardiac Arrest (POCA) registry and requires the consideration of specific management issues.[154]

In view of these concerns and the fact that resuscitative efforts are frequently unsuccessful and refractory to aggressive efforts in children with elastin arteriopathy, the following measures have been proposed: (1) careful risk/benefit assessment of the planned procedure should be undertaken, (2) children should be cared for by personnel with expertise in this patient population and potential challenges that may be encountered, and (3) the care should be delivered at institutions with the resources to support the need for an acute intervention and an aggressive resuscitation.[152]

Children with Williams syndrome can exhibit some degree of muscular weakness, and the cautious use of neuromuscular blocking drugs has been recommended.[155] Associated neurodevelopmental delay, attention-deficit disorder, and autistic behavior often require a premedication. Subclinical hypothyroidism is common in these children.[156] Renal manifestations include renovascular hypertension, reduced function, and hypercalcemia-induced nephrocalcinosis.

Chromosome 22q11.2 Deletion Syndrome: DiGeorge and Velocardiofacial Syndrome

The 22q11.2 deletion syndrome, with an estimated incidence of approximately 1 per 3000 live births, encompasses DiGeorge, conotruncal face, and velocardiofacial syndromes. The syndrome is also known as CATCH 22, a mnemonic for **c**ardiac defects, **a**bnormal facies, **t**hymic hypoplasia, **c**left palate, and **h**ypocalcemia, all of which are commonly present. Cardiac malformations, speech delay, and immunodeficiency are the most common

features of the chromosome 22q deletion syndromes.[157] Because no single feature is overwhelmingly associated with the deletion, the diagnosis should be considered for any child with a conotruncal anomaly, neonatal hypocalcemia, or any of the less common features when seen in association with dysmorphic facial features.

Cardiac malformations are often described as conotruncal anomalies; however, outflow tract problems are also common.[158] The remainder of the cardiac defects encompass an enormous spectrum of pathologies, leaving only a minority with a normal cardiovascular system. As a consequence of thymic hypoplasia, children can have diminished T-cell numbers and function. Their immunodeficiency requires the use of irradiated blood products and strict aseptic precautions during vascular access. Neurodevelopmental features include primarily speech delay and attention-deficit disorders. Psychiatric disorders are well described in these individuals.[159]

SINGLE-GENE DEFECTS
Noonan Syndrome

Noonan syndrome, an autosomal dominant disorder of variable expression, occurs with a frequency of 1 per 1000 to 2500 live births. The syndrome is one of a group of related conditions, collectively known as RASopathies or developmental syndromes of Ras/mitogen-activated protein kinase (MAPK) pathway dysregulation. Dysmorphic features in Noonan syndrome include neck webbing, low-set ears, chest deformities, hypertelorism, and short stature. The diagnosis is suspected from key clinical features.[160] In neonates, the facial features may be less apparent; however, generalized edema and excess nuchal folds can be present as in Turner syndrome. The facial features are more difficult to detect in later adolescence and adulthood.

The disorder is associated with a high incidence of cardiovascular involvement (about 80%-90%) and pulmonary valve dysplasia or stenosis is the most common feature.[161] HCM can develop during the first few years of life in some children.[162] Clinical problems can also include developmental delay and bleeding diathesis.[163]

Marfan Syndrome

Marfan syndrome is a multisystem disorder with variable expression resulting from a mutation in the fibrillin gene, a connective tissue protein, located on chromosome 15. Clinical manifestations typically involve the cardiovascular, skeletal, and ocular systems.[164,165] Cardiovascular pathology includes mitral valve prolapse and regurgitation, ascending aortic dilation (Fig. 16.13), and main pulmonary artery dilation. The risk of aortic dissection increases considerably as the aortic size increases, but it can occur at any point in the course of the disease.[166] Cardiac arrhythmias can be related to valvular heart disease, cardiomyopathy, or congestive heart failure.

Medical therapy with either β-blocker or angiotensin receptor blocker is standard therapy and blood pressure control in children with aortic root dilation should be continued perioperatively.[167] Aortic root replacement in Marfan syndrome has been associated with a greater risk of repeat dissection and recurrent aneurysm compared with other children who have undergone similar interventions.[168] It is wise to maintain hemodynamics near baseline values in the perioperative period. After aortic root surgery, some individuals can require chronic anticoagulation therapy. Preoperative hospitalization may be necessary to adjust the anticoagulation regimen in anticipation of surgery in these children. In emergency

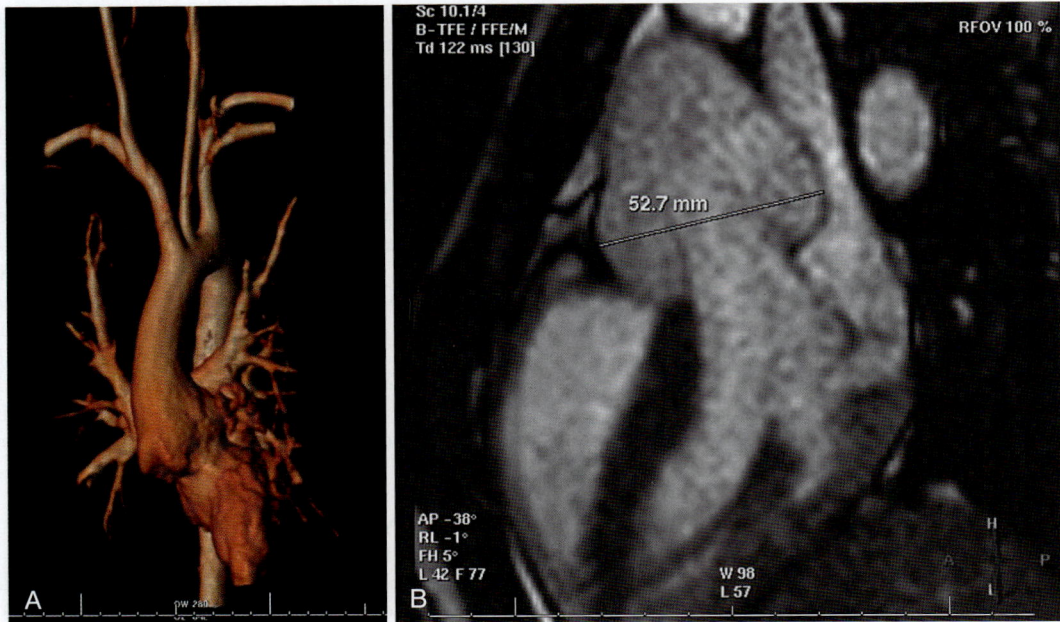

FIGURE 16.13 A severely dilated aortic root as displayed by magnetic resonance imaging in a patient with Marfan syndrome. The three-dimensional reconstruction **(A)** and sagittal view **(B)** demonstrate the aneurysmal appearance of the aortic root.

cases, administration of coagulation factors and other blood products may be required. In addition to vascular pathology, children with Marfan syndrome have a predisposition for ventricular dilation and abnormal systolic function.[169,170]

Several factors can result in pulmonary disease in these children.[171] Chest wall deformities and progressive scoliosis can contribute to restrictive lung disease. The fibrillin defect can affect lung development and homeostasis, impairing pulmonary function. Development of a spontaneous pneumothorax is relatively common.

CHARGE Syndrome

CHARGE syndrome is a genetic disorder characterized by congenital anomalies that include **c**oloboma, **h**eart defects, choanal **a**tresia, **r**etardation of growth and development, **g**enitourinary problems, and **e**ar abnormalities.[172] Most affected patients have mutations on the *CHD7* gene (chromodomain helicase DNA-binding protein), located on chromosome 8q12. The syndrome is estimated to occur at a rate of 1 per 8000 to 10,000 live births. Cardiac defects occur in as many as 50% to 70% of children and commonly include conotruncal and aortic arch anomalies.[173] Delayed growth and development usually results from cardiac disease, nutritional problems, and/or growth hormone deficiency. Most children have some degree of cognitive impairment. The anesthetic implications, in addition to those related to the cardiac defects, focus on the airway. In a retrospective review, upper airway abnormalities other than choanal atresia and cleft lip and palate were reported in 56% of children.[174] A high risk of postoperative airway events has also been reported in affected patients.[175]

ASSOCIATIONS

VACTERL (or VATER) Association

VACTERL association is an acronym given to describe a series of nonrandom anomalies that include **v**ertebral, **a**nal, **c**ardiovascular, **t**rache**o**esophageal, **r**enal, and **l**imb defects.[176] Up to 75%

of children with VACTERL association have CHD. The most common lesions include VSDs, ASDs, and TOF. Complex pathology such as truncus arteriosus and transposition of the great arteries occur less frequently.

Vertebral and tracheal anomalies can complicate airway management and regional anesthesia. Approximately 70% of children with VACTERL have vertebral anomalies, usually consisting of hypoplastic vertebrae or hemivertebra, that predispose to scoliosis. Anal atresia or imperforate anus is reported in about 55% of cases. These anomalies often require surgery in the first days of life. Esophageal atresia with tracheoesophageal fistula occurs in a large number of affected infants. Low birth weight (<1500 g) and associated cardiac pathology are independent predictors of mortality in infants undergoing surgery for esophageal atresia or tracheoesophageal fistula (see Chapter 37). The presence of a ductal-dependent cardiac lesion further increases perioperative morbidity and mortality.[177] Limb defects occur in most children, potentially affecting vascular access and monitor placement. Renal defects occur in about 50% of children.

OTHER DISORDERS

Tuberous sclerosis is a rare genetic disease with an autosomal dominant inheritance pattern and an incidence of approximately 1 per 25,000 to 30,000 births.[178] It can be attributed to spontaneous mutations in most children. This systemic disease primarily manifests as cutaneous and neurologic symptoms, but cardiac and renal lesions are frequent findings.

The presence of upper airway nodular tumors, fibromas, or papillomas in affected children can interfere with airway management. Developmental delay, autism, attention-deficit disorder, and aggressive behavior are common. Brain and renal tumors (60% to 80%) can produce significant comorbidities. Cardiac pathology includes cardiac rhabdomyoma in 60% of children and coexisting CHD in 33% of cases.[179,180] Cardiac abnormalities with obstruction to blood flow, heart failure, arrhythmias, conduction

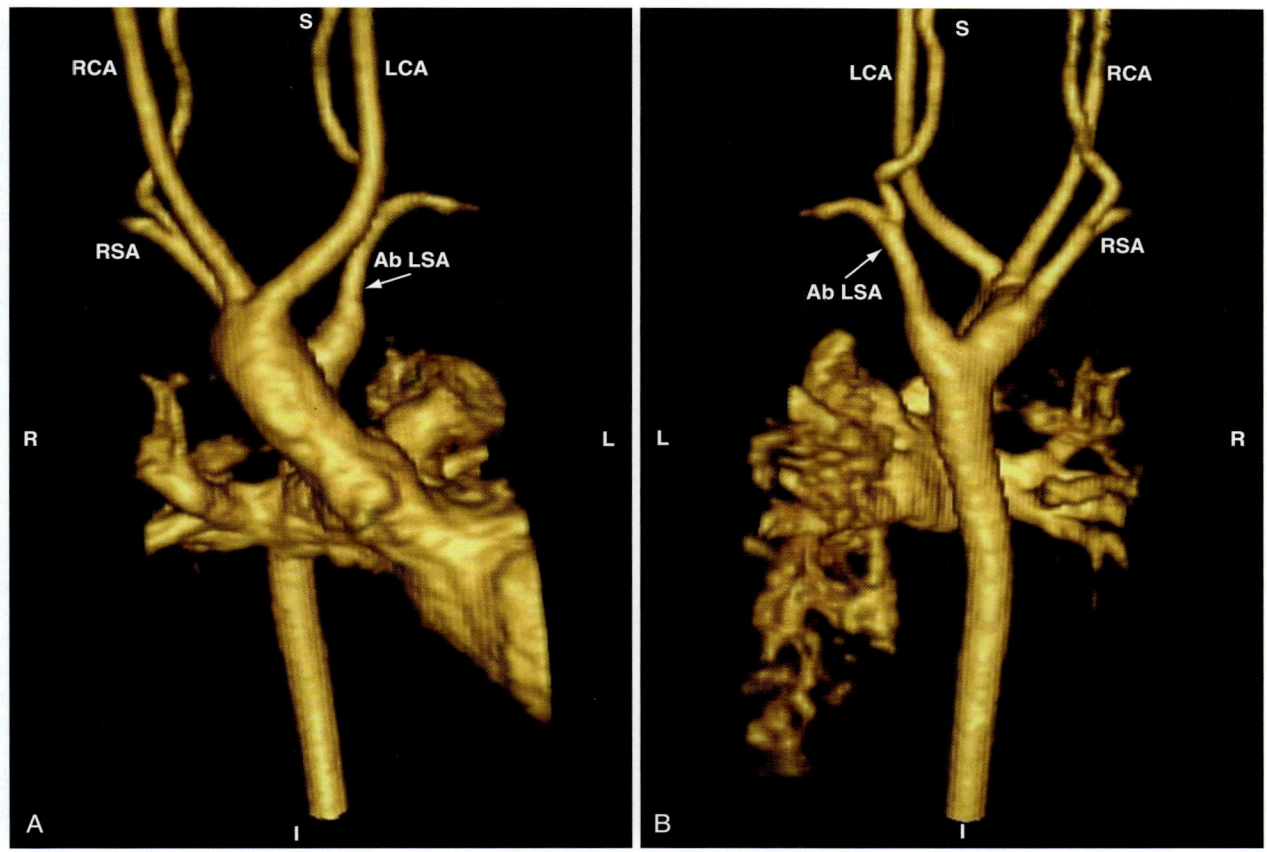

FIGURE 16.14 Three-dimensional reconstruction of a vascular ring obtained by magnetic resonance imaging. The images display an anterior **(A)** and posterior **(B)** orientation of a right aortic arch with an aberrant left subclavian artery (*Ab LSA*). The first arch vessel is the left carotid artery (*LCA*), followed by the right carotid artery (*RCA*), and right subclavian artery (*RSA*). The Ab LSA is the most distal branch originating from the descending aorta and coursing posterior to the esophagus toward the left arm. This vessel can be compressed by a transesophageal echocardiographic probe. *I*, inferior; *L*, left; *R*, right; *S*, superior.

defects, or preexcitation can affect the selection of anesthetic agents. Preoperative evaluation in most cases should include an ECG to evaluate for arrhythmia, conduction defects, or preexcitation.[181,182] Blood pressure and renal function should also be assessed. Anticonvulsants should be optimized and continued until the morning of surgery. Baseline medical treatment should be resumed as soon as possible because seizures are the most common postoperative complication.

Selected Vascular Anomalies and Their Implications for Anesthesia

ABERRANT SUBCLAVIAN ARTERY

An aberrant or anomalous subclavian artery in the classic setting arises from the descending aorta as a separate vessel distal to the usual last subclavian artery, in a posterior location. In a left aortic arch, this arrangement is as follows: the first branch is the right carotid artery, the second is the left carotid artery, and the third is the left subclavian artery. The aberrant right subclavian artery, rather than arising proximally from the innominate artery as the first arch vessel, originates distal to the left subclavian artery as the fourth branch and courses behind the esophagus toward the right arm. This branching variant is one of the most common aortic arch anomalies, occurring in 0.4% to 2% of the general population. It may or may not be associated with CHD.[183] This anomaly has a high incidence among children with Down syndrome and is associated with VSDs, TOF, and other cardiac lesions. In a right aortic arch, the anomalous left subclavian artery originates distal to the origin of the right subclavian artery (Fig. 16.14). This anomaly can be seen in the context of conotruncal malformations. The diagnosis of an aberrant subclavian artery is made by most currently available imaging modalities.

This variant has several implications:

- It can influence the location of placement of a systemic-to-pulmonary artery shunt.
- It should be considered in the selection of a site for arterial line placement if transesophageal echocardiography is planned during surgery. The aberrant vessel can be compressed along its retroesophageal course by the imaging probe, resulting in inaccurate recordings.[184] Regardless of the site of arterial line placement, it may be wise to monitor the arm supplied by the anomalous vessel by pulse oximetry or other methods during esophageal instrumentation.

- It is sometimes a component of a vascular ring.
- Rarely, older children with an aberrant subclavian artery and without the findings of a complete vascular ring can complain of mild dysphagia (i.e., dysphagia lusoria).

PERSISTENT LEFT SUPERIOR VENA CAVA TO THE CORONARY SINUS

A persistent left superior vena cava (LSVC) is a form of anomalous systemic venous drainage identified in 4.4% of children with CHD, most frequently those with septal defects.[185] It represents a venous remnant that typically involutes during development. If it persists, it remains patent and drains through an enlarged coronary sinus into the right atrium. Bilateral superior vena cavae can be present (Fig. 16.15), or the right superior vena cava can be absent. Bilateral superior vena cavae can communicate through an innominate or bridging vein. This anomaly has several implications:

- In the absence of an innominate vein, a catheter placed in the left arm or left internal jugular vein and advanced into the central circulation can rest within the coronary sinus, a potentially undesirable location in a small infant. On chest radiography, an unusual course is identified as the catheter courses along the left aspect of the mediastinum and can be mistaken for intracarotid, intrapleural, or mediastinal locations.
- An LSVC can be of relevance during venous cannulation for cardiopulmonary bypass to ensure adequate venous drainage and optimal operating conditions.
- The presence of an LSVC is important in patients with single-ventricle physiology undergoing palliation involving a cavo-pulmonary (Glenn) connection.
- The anomaly can be associated with a dilated coronary sinus. On echocardiography, it can be confused with other defects, including an ostium primum ASD (i.e., one that lies in the inferior aspect of the atrial septum) or anomalous pulmonary venous return to the coronary sinus.
- On occasion, an LSVC can drain to an unroofed coronary sinus or directly into the left atrium, in which case a right-to-left shunt is present. It can be identified by injection of agitated saline into a left arm or left neck vein while performing an echocardiogram, and it can be associated with systemic arterial desaturation. This constitutes a risk for paradoxical systemic embolization.
- During cardiac surgery, an enlarged coronary sinus can interfere with the administration of retrograde cardioplegia.
- It can confound transvenous placement of a pulmonary artery catheter in some cases.

Evaluation of the Child With a Cardiac Murmur

The finding of an incidental murmur during the perioperative period can result in significant distress to the child or family; trigger additional diagnostic studies, including a cardiology consultation; and has the potential to delay the scheduled procedure when identified preoperatively. Although cardiac auscultation is a challenging skill that takes many years of practice to master,[186] it is important for the anesthesiologist who routinely cares for children to recognize the main physical findings that may distinguish an innocent cardiac murmur from a pathologic one. Knowledge of several core concepts and red flags can help avoid overlooking potentially important diagnoses.

About 90% of normal children have a murmur at some point in their lives. It is most commonly identified during the neonatal

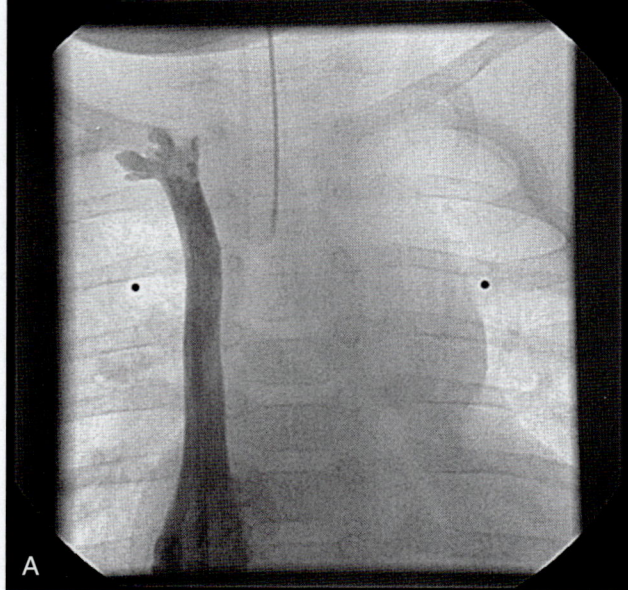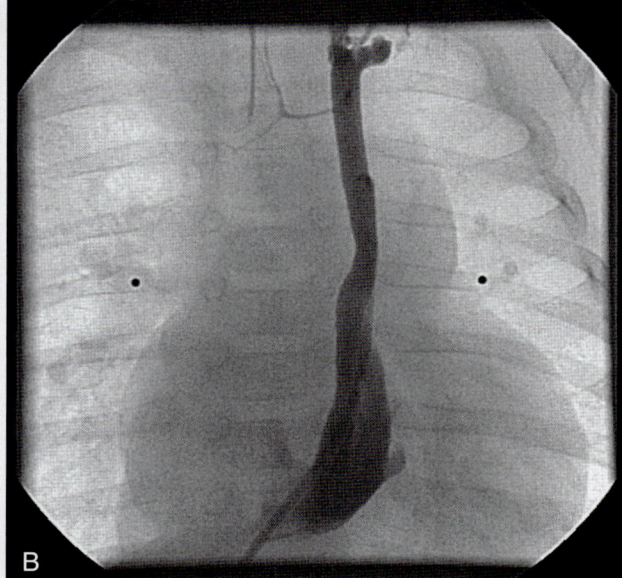

FIGURE 16.15 Bilateral superior vena cavae can exist separately or communicate through an innominate or bridging vein. **A,** The angiogram depicts the superior vena cava, normally a right-sided structure, as it drains into the right atrium. **B,** In the same patient, an angiogram shows drainage of a large left superior vena cava into the coronary sinus. The catheter courses from the inferior vena cava into the right atrium, coronary sinus, and left superior vena cava. Contrast injection into the left superior vena cava demonstrates no innominate vein between the two cavae. The coronary sinus is dilated as it receives the systemic venous blood from the left superior vena cava.

period and early school years. Most murmurs are functional, considered innocent in nature, and require no special treatment. This diagnosis is based on physical findings consistent with the benign nature of the specific murmur.

Although a complete discussion of cardiac murmur evaluation is beyond the scope of this chapter, it is important to review those findings that help to distinguish innocent from pathologic murmurs.[187,188] The basic systematic approach to assessing a heart murmur is the same as when evaluating any child's cardiovascular system.[189,190] The chest should be auscultated with both the diaphragm and bell of the stethoscope in the positions of the four primary cardiac valves in a quiet environment. Innocent murmurs in infancy and childhood include pulmonary flow murmur, a Still murmur, physiologic pulmonary branch stenosis, venous hum, and carotid bruit. Innocent murmurs are usually of low intensity (grades I and II of VI) and associated with a normal cardiovascular examination (e.g., normal precordial activity, first and second heart sounds, peripheral pulses, capillary refill). Innocent murmurs, such as those associated with peripheral pulmonary branch stenosis, right ventricular outflow murmurs, and Still murmurs, are usually soft, systolic ejection type, and not holosystolic in duration. Physiologic murmurs often resolve by changing the child's hemodynamic state with maneuvers such as lying down or sitting up or with temporal changes such as resolution of fever and improvement in anemia. Diastolic or continuous murmurs are typically pathologic, with the exception of a venous hum. This murmur is thought to be related to turbulent flow of systemic venous return in the jugular veins and superior vena cava and is best heard at the base of the neck. *Murmurs accompanied by a palpable thrill are always pathologic.*

When there is doubt regarding the benign or pathologic nature of a murmur, consultation with a pediatric cardiologist is indicated. A chest radiograph and ECG, although thought by some to add minimal value in the initial diagnostic assessment of a cardiac murmur and to not be cost-effective, can be helpful when considering if further consultation is indicated.[191]

Basic Interpretation of the Electrocardiogram in Children

Despite the increasing applications of imaging modalities in the structural and functional assessment of pediatric heart disease, electrocardiography continues to play a significant role in the diagnosis and management of these children. An ECG is considered an integral part of the evaluation of most children with congenital or acquired cardiovascular pathology.

Although the characteristic features of a normal ECG in infants and children were described many decades ago, it is surprising that it continues to be one of the most often misinterpreted screening tests in pediatric medicine.[192] This is largely because of the developmental changes that occur in the normal individual as he or she progresses from the neonatal period through childhood, adolescence, and adulthood.[193] Normal values for children of different ages have been established.[194] Knowledge of normal configurations and values for various ages of children is essential for accurate interpretation.[195] Immediately after birth, there is a predominance of right ventricular forces represented by tall R waves in the right precordial leads (V_1 and V_2) (Fig. 16.16).[196] Over the first several years, the ECG changes to a more familiar left heart–dominant configuration with larger S waves in the right precordial leads and a gradual RS progression with tall R waves

in the left precordial leads (V_5 and V_6) (Fig. 16.17). The predominance of right heart forces and the need to evaluate for dextrocardia are the primary reasons that pediatric ECGs should include the V_3R and V_4R leads, which are not routinely obtained in adult studies. These electrodes are placed in the corresponding V_3 and V_4 locations over the right hemithorax.

Clinical information of relevance in the interpretation of an ECG includes the child's age, gender, suspected or documented diagnosis, and indications for the examination. Several requirements are essential for accurate interpretation, including appropriate skin preparation, electrode placement, and an artifact-free recording. The approach to the pediatric ECG should be systematic and organized. Determination of the rate and rhythm, with evaluation of the P-wave vector and the relationship between each P wave and QRS complex, is the first step. It is important to consider the influences of age, autonomic nervous system, level of physical activity, medications, pain, and temperature on the child's heart rate. The P wave should be upright or positive in leads I and aVF, indicating that the sinus node is the pacemaker of the heart (i.e., sinus rhythm) (see Fig. 16.17). Normally, the P wave should precede the QRS complex. Next, the QRS electrical axis should be determined. The QRS frontal plane axis is determined by identifying the most isoelectric lead, which is perpendicular to the direction of ventricular depolarization. Alternatively, the direction of depolarization in leads I and aVF can be examined to roughly estimate the axis. As with all other components of the evaluation, the physiologic changes that occur with growth are responsible for the change in normal values for the QRS axis based on age. Regardless of age, QRS axes that lie in the northwest quadrant (between 180 and 270 degrees with an S-wave–dominant pattern in leads I and aVF) are always abnormal and merit further investigation. This is a classic finding in children with AV septal defects. Evaluating the T wave, or repolarization axis, is also important, because a difference of greater than 90 degrees between the QRS and T-wave axes can represent strain on the ventricle, a potential finding in ventricular hypertrophy (see Fig. 16.5).

After the evaluation of rhythm and axes is complete, each component of the cardiac cycle as reflected by the ECG should be examined.[197] The P wave represents atrial systole, and its morphology, with particular interest in leads II and V_1, can demonstrate right atrial (P-wave amplitude >2.5 mm or 3.0 mm based on age) or left atrial (P-wave duration >100-120 msec based on age) enlargement (Fig. 16.18). The PR interval represents the time required for passage of an impulse from the sinoatrial node until ventricular depolarization and is largely composed of the AV nodal delay. A prolonged PR interval, which is age specific, indicates first-degree AV block. A short PR interval should prompt evaluation of the QRS duration for signs of preexcitation (i.e., Wolff-Parkinson-White syndrome), although a short PR interval can also reflect a low right atrial pacemaker (Fig. 16.19).

The QRS complex represents ventricular depolarization. The QRS duration should be examined in a lead with a Q wave present (often lead V_5 or V_6) for signs of conduction delay. Age-dependent normal values are important, because the upper limit of normal QRS duration is only 80 msec in neonates. The presence of a wide QRS complex with an RSR′ pattern in V_1 indicates a right bundle branch block, whereas a QS pattern in V_1 and a tall notched R wave in V_6 is consistent with a left bundle branch block. Other conditions associated with prolongation of the QRS duration include ventricular preexcitation and ventricular pacing.

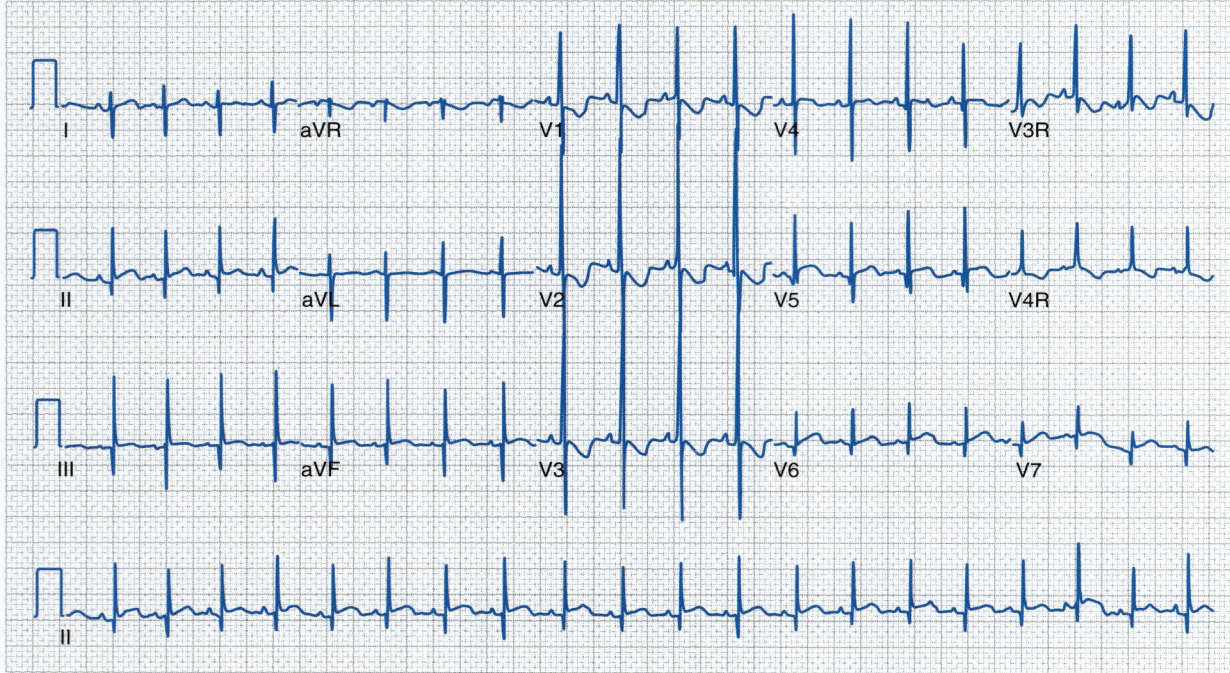

FIGURE 16.16 Normal electrocardiogram for a 2-day-old neonate shows the expected predominance of right ventricular forces during this period (i.e., tall R waves in the right precordial leads, V_1, and V_2). The inverted T waves in V_{1-3} are normal for this age.

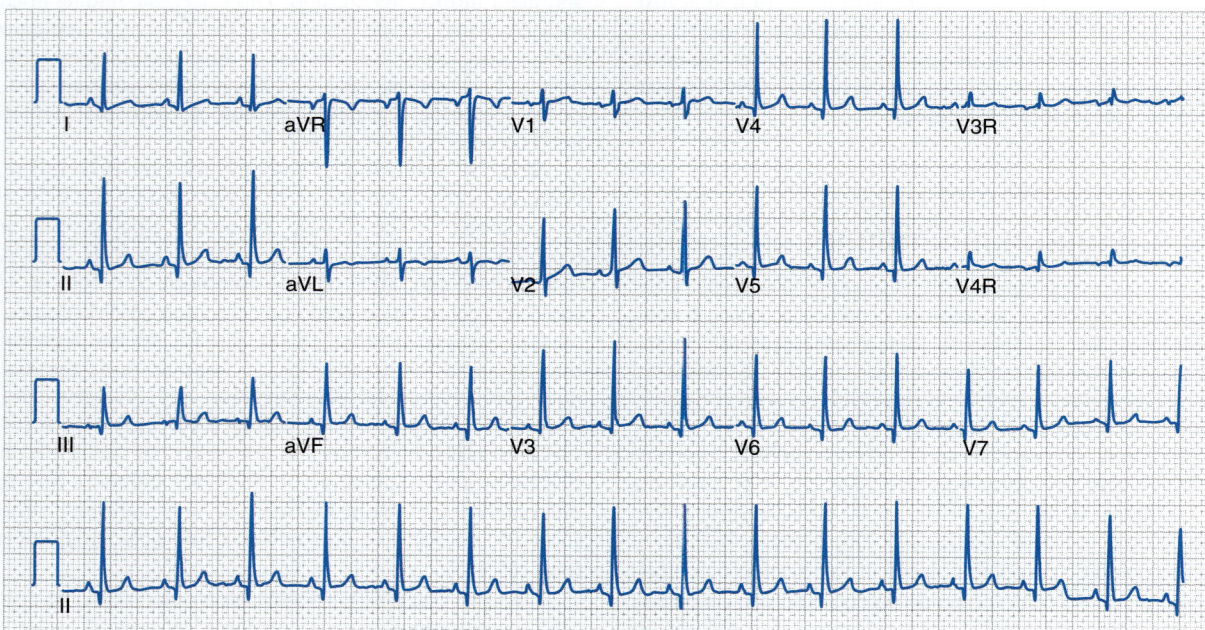

FIGURE 16.17 The normal electrocardiographic tracing was recorded for a 10-year-old child. The typical left heart–dominant configuration of children this age is characterized by gradual RS progression with tall R waves in the left precordial leads (V_5 and V_6). This contrasts with the right ventricular–dominant pattern seen during infancy and early childhood. The tracing demonstrates normal sinus rhythm as indicated by positive P waves in leads I and aVF.

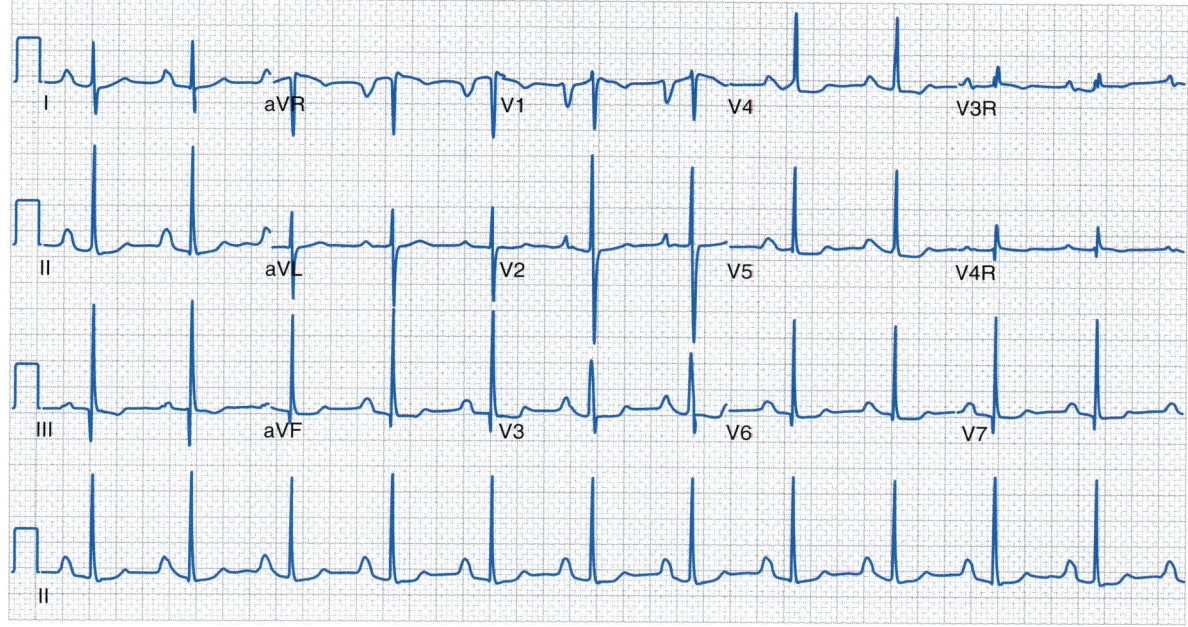

FIGURE 16.18 The tracing was obtained in the emergency room for a patient subsequently found to have restrictive cardiomyopathy. Biatrial enlargement is reflected by the tall and wide P waves in leads II and V₁, respectively.

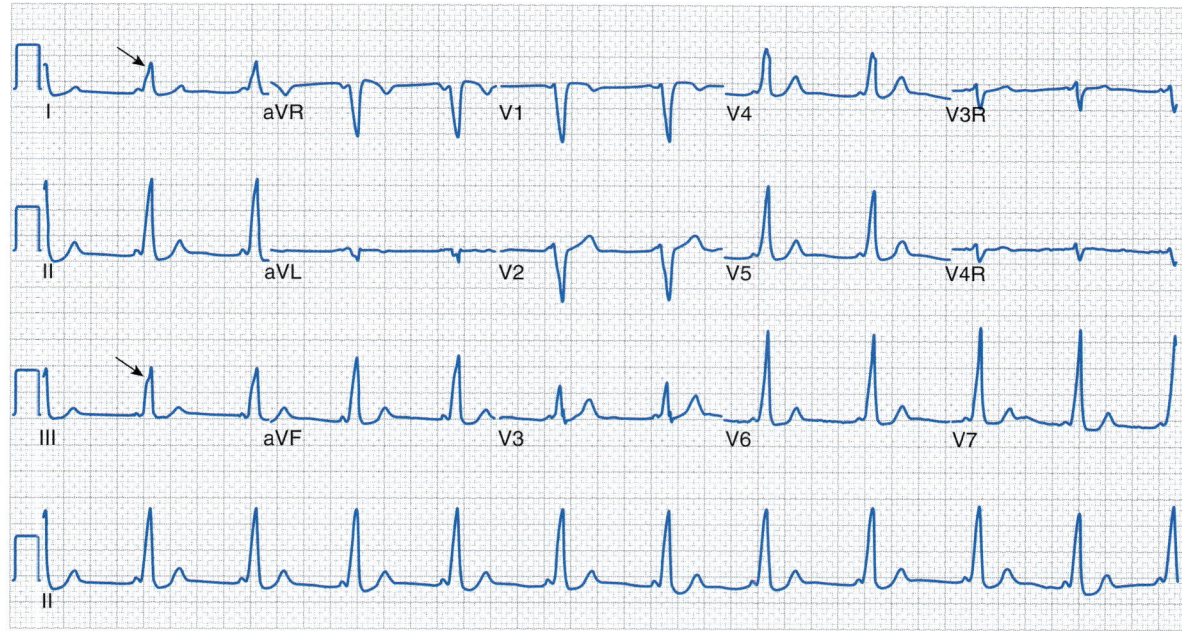

FIGURE 16.19 The tracing demonstrates the typical electrocardiographic features of Wolff-Parkinson-White syndrome: short PR interval, delta wave (*arrows*), and prolongation of the QRS interval.

In addition to the QRS duration, the components of the QRS complex should be examined. Q waves are often present in the lateral and inferior leads and in lead aVR, but they should be narrow (<40 msec) and shallow (age-dependent but usually <5-mm deep). Deep or wide Q waves suggest myocardial ischemia and require further evaluation. An uncommon but crucial finding occurs in infants with ALCAPA. Classically, the ECG in this lesion demonstrates deep, wide Q waves in leads I and aVL with ST-segment and T-wave changes in the anterior distribution

(V_2 to V_4) consistent with compromised myocardial blood flow (Fig. 16.20). The QRS amplitudes are also important in assessing left and right ventricular hypertrophy. Conditions associated with increased QRS voltages that likely require echocardiographic assessment include HCM, left ventricular noncompaction, and Pompe disease (see Figs. 16.5 and 16.6).

ST segments should be flat and should not be depressed more than 0.5 mm or elevated more than 1 mm in any lead. The major exception to this rule is when there is gradual upsloping of the

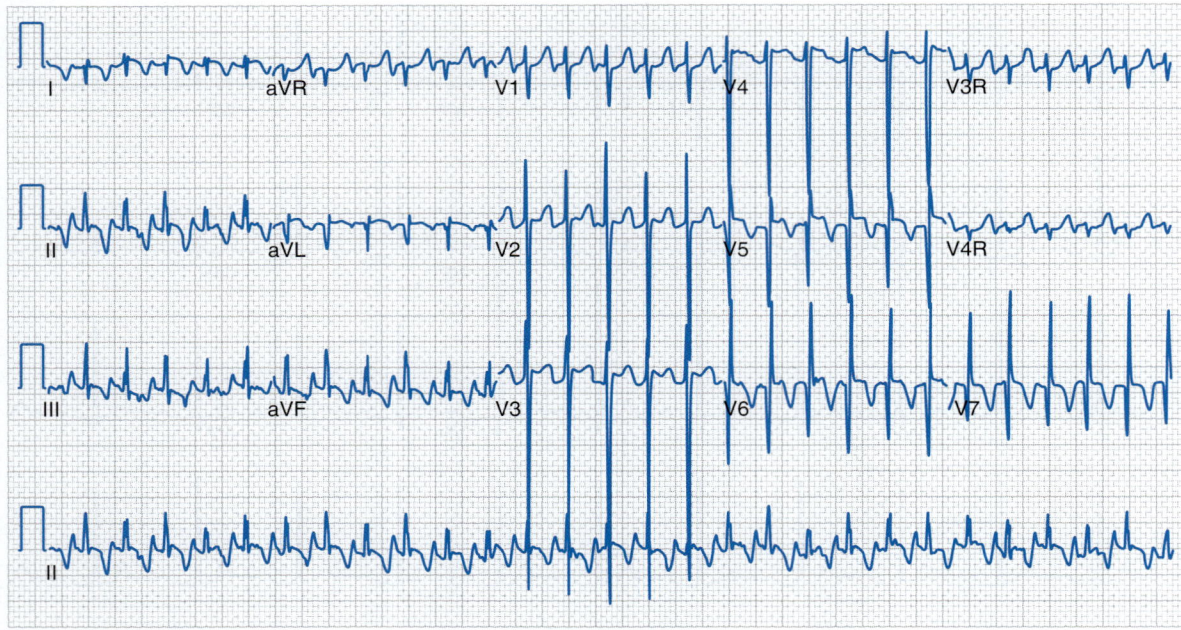

FIGURE 16.20 Electrocardiographic tracing for an infant with poor ventricular function who was found to have anomalous origin of the left main coronary artery from the pulmonary root. The presence of Q waves in aVL and the diffuse ST-T wave changes suggest ischemia and are classic for this anomaly.

ST segment in the mid-precordial leads, as seen in early repolarization. T waves represent ventricular repolarization and should all be upright in the precordial leads at birth. Within 1 to 3 days they become inverted, initially in V_1 and eventually in V_2, V_3, and sometimes in V_4. Starting at several years of age, the T waves return to the upright position in the reverse order. In normal adolescents and adults, the T wave in lead V_1 can be upright or inverted. The only limb lead that typically displays an inverted T wave is aVR.

An aspect of the cardiac cycle that must be examined on any ECG is the QT interval, the time from the onset of ventricular depolarization (marked by the onset of the QRS complex), until the completion of repolarization (marked by the end of the T wave). It represents the duration of electrical activation and recovery of the ventricular myocardium, and it is measured as follows:

$$\text{Corrected QT (QTc)} = \frac{\text{Measured QT interval}}{\text{Square root of preceding R-Rinterval}}$$

A QTc that exceeds 470 msec is considered abnormal, regardless of age. All QTc values that exceed normal values for age merit further investigation. Medications that prolong the QT interval should be avoided until the child has been evaluated by a cardiologist.

Although a detailed organized approach to interpretation of a pediatric ECG is necessary, there are occasions when particular conditions or circumstances cause global electrocardiographic changes that must be quickly recognized. One such case that can occur in the operating room is related to the electrocardiographic changes associated with hyperkalemia. As the potassium level increases, the T-wave amplitude increases. This is followed by widening of the QRS duration (see Figs. 9.7 and 16.21) owing to an intraventricular conduction delay and by AV block and arrhythmias, including ventricular tachycardia and fibrillation. Other electrolyte disturbances can result in characteristic changes on the ECG:

- Hypokalemia: decreased T-wave amplitude, ST-segment depression, and the presence of U waves
- Hypercalcemia: shortening of the QT interval, sinus rate slowing, and sinoatrial block
- Hypocalcemia: lengthening of the QT interval
- Hypomagnesemia: enhanced effects of hypocalcemia

Essentials of Cardiac Rhythm Interpretation and Acute Arrhythmia Management in Children

Rhythm abnormalities can be seen during the preoperative assessment, in the operating room, or in the postoperative period. Considerations usually include identification of the rhythm disorder, establishing the need for acute therapy, deciding whether to consult a pediatric cardiologist, and conveying pertinent information to the consultant to assist in the characterization of the rhythm disturbance and to establish a management plan.[198] The following principles should be considered in addressing these issues:

1. Operating room, bedside, or transport monitors and strip recordings facilitate the recognition of rhythm disorders, but in most cases, they are inadequate for definitive diagnosis. A 15-lead surface ECG and rhythm strip should be obtained for all children when feasible.

2. Clinicians caring for children should have a basic knowledge of cardiac rhythm interpretation. Although a comprehensive discussion of arrhythmia interpretation is beyond the scope of this chapter, a brief overview of the characteristic features of normal and abnormal cardiac rhythms in the pediatric age group is presented in the following section.

3. The need for acute therapy for a rhythm disturbance should be based primarily on the nature of the disorder, urgency of

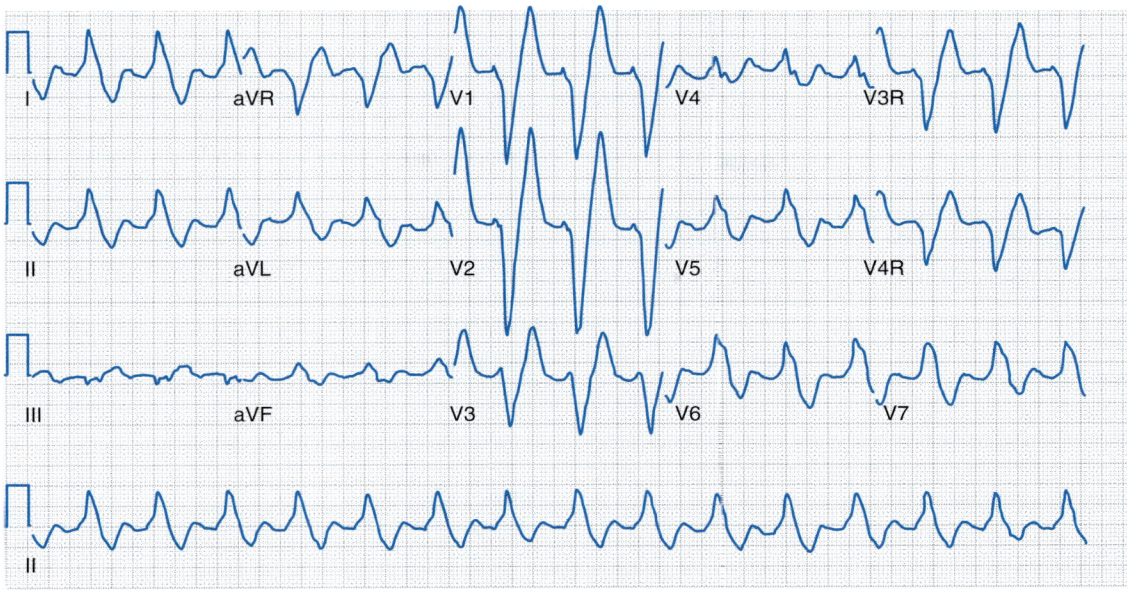

A   25 mm/sec 10 mm/mV 100 Hz

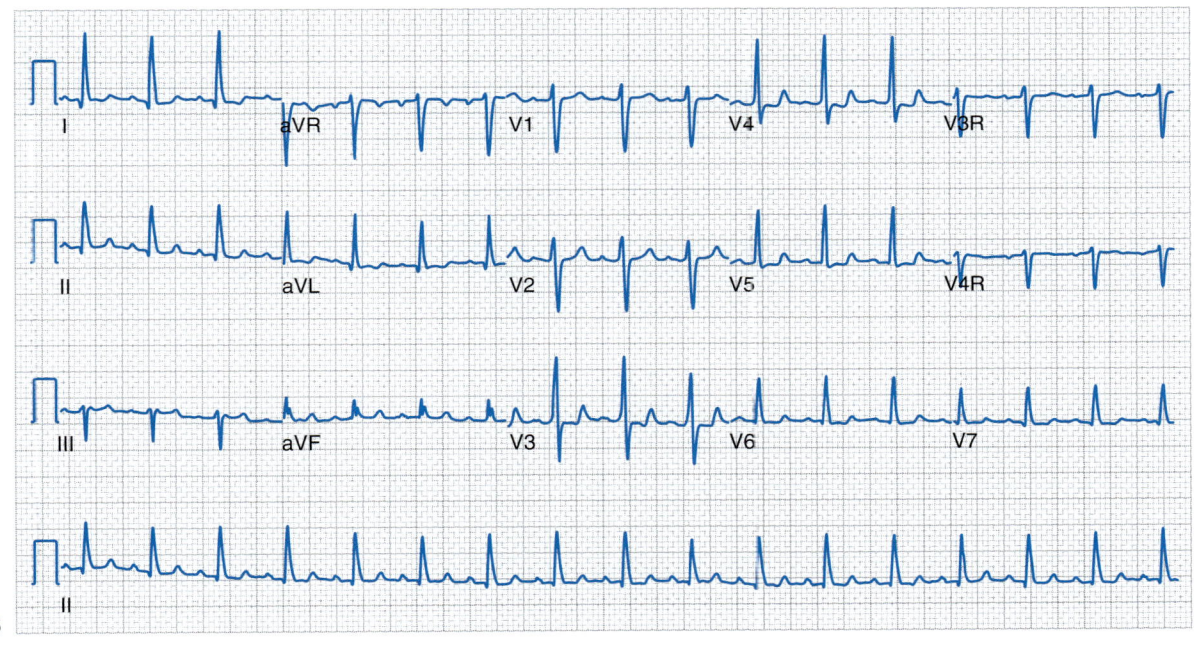

B

FIGURE 16.21 These electrocardiographic changes can result from hyperkalemia. **A,** Marked widening of the QRS complexes is associated with peaked T waves. If untreated, this condition may progress to ventricular fibrillation and asystole. **B,** A tracing obtained several hours after treatment of the electrolyte disturbance in the same patient demonstrates resolution of the electrocardiographic changes.

the situation, and the likelihood that this abnormality would or would not be tolerated beyond the immediate short-term period. The guidelines established by the American Heart Association for Pediatric Advanced Life Support should be followed in all patients.[199] In otherwise healthy children and in contrast to ventricular arrhythmias, supraventricular tachyarrhythmias are rarely life-threatening.

4. The degree of comfort in the characterization and management of pediatric cardiac arrhythmias is likely to be quite variable among anesthesia care providers. For arrhythmias caused by respiratory compromise, electrolyte imbalance, or metabolic derangements, consultation with a pediatric cardiologist is probably not required. This is also the case for variants or benign rhythm disturbances such as sinus arrhythmia, low atrial rhythms, or occasional premature atrial beats. Consultation is appropriate for most children with known structural or acquired cardiovascular pathology, in those with a history of a cardiac rhythm disorder under the care of a cardiologist, and in most of those with acute arrhythmias, particularly when initiation of antiarrhythmic drug therapy is contemplated.

5. Information that may be helpful to a consultant includes pertinent details regarding the child's history, clinical diagnosis, nature of the procedure/intervention, relevant laboratory values, description or characterization of the rhythm abnormality, associated hemodynamic parameters, circumstances surrounding the event (including the presence or absence of an intracardiac catheter), review of the pharmacologic agents administered (including anesthetic agents), and other therapies if applicable. The specialist should assist in the characterization of the rhythm disorder, advise about whether further evaluation is indicated, make recommendations for treatment, and facilitate diagnostic/therapeutic interventions as necessary.

BASIC RHYTHMS

Sinus Rhythm

Sinus rhythm is characterized by a P wave that precedes every QRS, a QRS that follows every P wave, and an upright P wave in leads I and aVF (see Fig. 16.17).

Sinus Arrhythmia

Sinus arrhythmia represents cyclic changes in the heart rate during breathing. This is a normal finding in healthy children (Fig. 16.22).

Sinus Bradycardia

Sinus bradycardia is characterized by sinus rhythm with heart rates below normal for age (see Fig. 16.5). Slow heart rates can be observed during sleep or at times of high vagal tone. When there is significant sinus bradycardia, a slow junctional escape rhythm or a slow atrial rhythm originating from an ectopic focus can be present. Certain forms of CHD may be prone to slow heart rhythms (i.e., heterotaxy syndromes).

In the intraoperative setting, particularly during induction of anesthesia, sinus bradycardia can occur with laryngoscopy, tracheal intubation, and tracheal suctioning. Sinus bradycardia can also result from drug administration (i.e., opioids) or increased parasympathetic tone. This type of sinus bradycardia rarely poses significant hemodynamic compromise and, if necessary, can be easily treated with removal of the stimulus, administration of a vagolytic agent (e.g., glycopyrrolate and atropine), or with chronotropic drugs such as epinephrine. Sinus bradycardia can also result from hypoxemia, hypothermia, acidosis, electrolyte imbalance, or increased intracranial pressure. Bradycardia related to hypoxemia should be treated promptly with the administration of supplemental oxygen and appropriate airway management (see Chapter 40). The approach to other secondary forms of sinus bradycardia should focus on addressing the underlying cause. For worrisome slow heart rates, particularly in small infants, or for clinical evidence of compromised hemodynamics, pharmacologic therapy (i.e., epinephrine, atropine, or isoproterenol infusion) or temporary pacing should be considered.

Sinus Tachycardia

During sinus tachycardia the heart rate is above normal for age (Fig. 16.23). In the perioperative setting this is often the result of surgical stimulation, stress, pain, hypovolemia, anemia, fever, medications (i.e., inotropic agents), or a high catecholamine state. Treatment is directed at the underlying cause. Sustained sinus tachycardia can be detrimental as it may impair diastolic filling time, reduce ventricular preload, and compromise cardiac output. Children at risk for hemodynamic decompensation include those with significant degrees of ventricular hypertrophy or diastolic dysfunction, aortic stenosis, and HCM.

Junctional Rhythm

A junctional rhythm is characterized by QRS complexes of morphology identical to that of sinus rhythm without preceding P waves. This rhythm is slower than the expected sinus rate. When this rhythm completely takes over the pacemaker activity of the

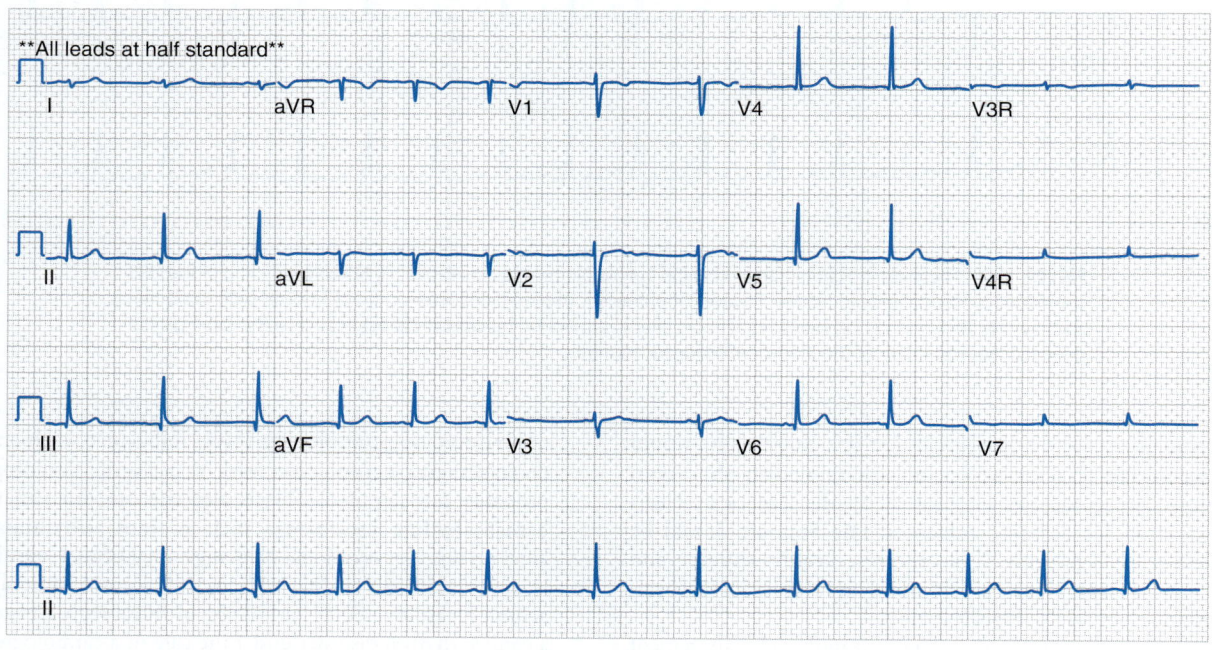

FIGURE 16.22 The rhythm tracing displays the normal heart rate variability with respiration. There is a normal increase in heart rate during inspiration. This sinus arrhythmia is a natural response and is more commonly seen in children than adults.

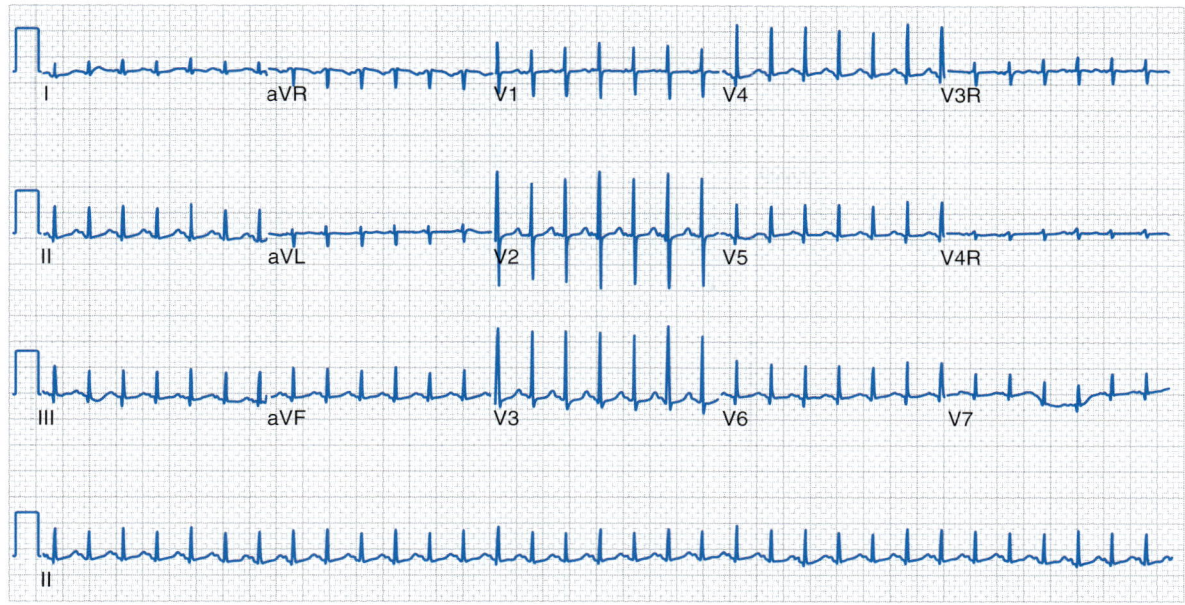

FIGURE 16.23 Electrocardiogram for a febrile infant with sinus tachycardia, characterized by a heart rate above normal for age and QRS complexes of normal appearance preceded by P waves, which are upright in leads I and aVF.

heart, retrograde P waves and AV dissociation can be seen. Junctional rhythm during cardiac surgery is frequently the result of manipulation or dissection near the right atrium. The central venous pressure contour typically demonstrates prominent cannon *a* waves (i.e., right atrial pressure wave at the end of systole) owing to the loss of AV synchrony (Fig. 16.24). The lack of atrial contribution to ventricular filling can result in decreases in the systemic arterial blood pressure.

CONDUCTION DISORDERS
Bundle Branch Block

Incomplete right bundle branch block pattern (rSR' in the right precordial leads with near-normal QRS duration) occurs in children with right ventricular volume overload (e.g., those with ASDs). Complete right bundle branch block (QRS complex >100 msec for infants, 120 msec for older children) is frequently seen in children after surgical procedures that involve the right ventricular outflow tract. This is characterized by an rSR' wave pattern in V_1, an inverted T wave, and a wide and deep S (slurred) wave in V_6. Left bundle branch block is an uncommon finding in the pediatric age group that can result from cardiac interventions along the left ventricular outflow tract. Criteria for this conduction disorder include a prominent QS or rS complex in lead V_1 and tall, wide, and often notched R wave in leads I, aVL, and V_6.

Atrioventricular Block
First-Degree Atrioventricular Block

In first-degree AV block, there is prolongation of the PR interval beyond the normal range for age. Each P wave is followed by a conducted QRS. This may be found in healthy individuals but can also be seen in various disease states. First-degree AV block is a benign condition requiring no specific treatment.

Second-Degree Atrioventricular Block

There are several forms of second-degree AV block. Mobitz type I (Wenckebach) and Mobitz type II are the two predominant types. They are characterized by a periodic failure to conduct atrial impulses to the ventricle (i.e., P wave without following QRS complex). In a type I, second-degree AV block, there is a gradual lengthening of the PR interval with eventual failure of conduction of the next atrial impulse to the ventricle. The RR intervals concomitantly shorten. The degree of AV block is expressed as the ratio of P waves to QRS complexes (i.e., 2:1, 3:2). This can occur during periods of high vagal tone or in the postoperative setting. It is usually a benign phenomenon that requires no therapy. In the less frequent type II second-degree AV block, there is a relatively constant PR interval before an atrial impulse that fails to conduct. This is considered a more serious conduction disturbance and merits further investigation.

Third-Degree Atrioventricular Block

Third-degree (complete) AV block is characterized by total failure of conduction of atrial impulses to the ventricle. It can be congenital or acquired. There is complete AV dissociation, with more atrial than ventricular contractions, and the ventricular rate is usually slow and regular (Fig. 16.25). Temporary pacing may be indicated in the acute setting.

CARDIAC ARRHYTHMIAS
Supraventricular Arrhythmias
Premature Atrial Contractions or Beats

Isolated premature atrial contractions (PACs) are relatively common in infants and small children. On the ECG, the early P waves exhibit a morphology and axis that are different from those in normal sinus rhythm. Premature atrial contractions can be conducted to the ventricles normally, blocked at the AV node, or conduct aberrantly (i.e., abnormal QRS morphology). They are usually benign and require no therapy. If a central venous catheter is present, the tip position should be evaluated.

Supraventricular Tachycardia

Supraventricular tachycardia (SVT) is the most common significant arrhythmia in infants and children.[200,201] It is characterized by a regular tachyarrhythmia (tachycardia heart rate is age dependent

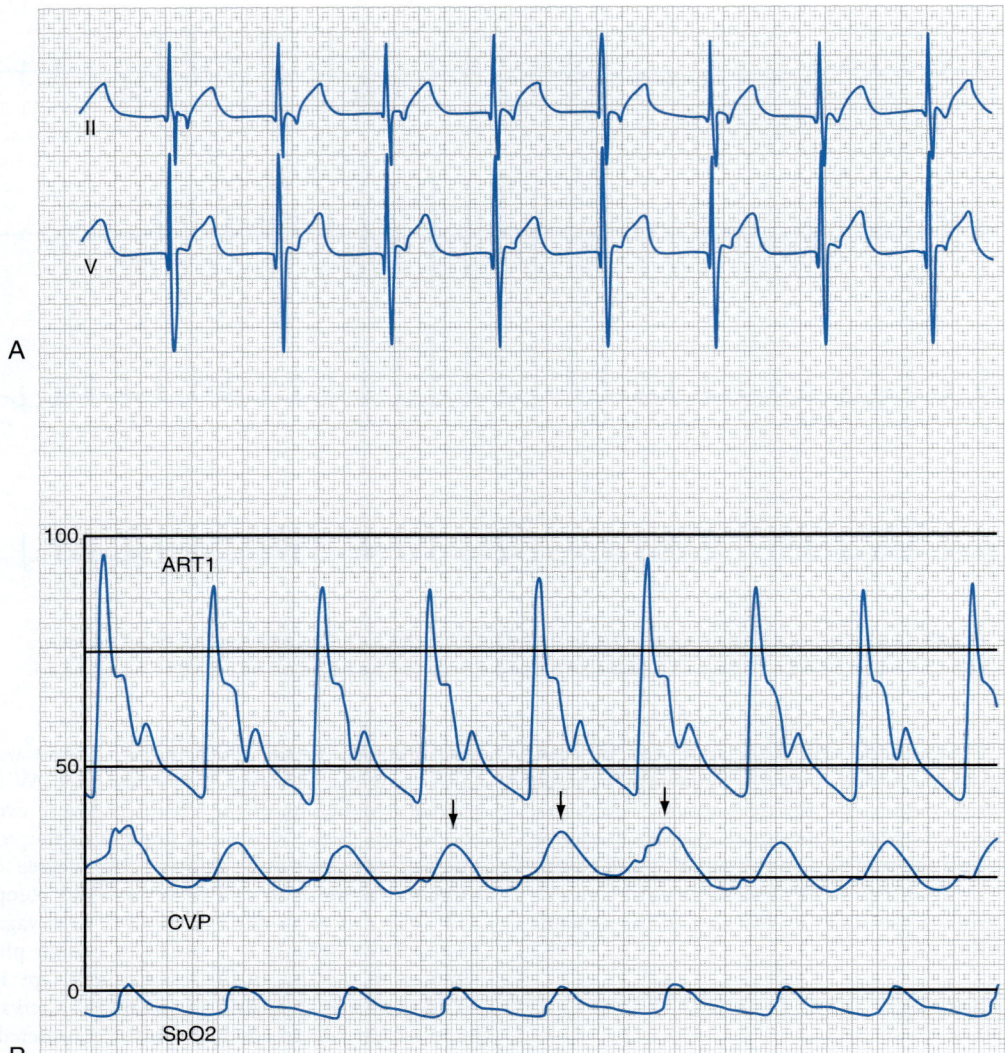

FIGURE 16.24 A, The tracing obtained during cardiac surgery at the time of right atrial dissection demonstrates the features of a junctional rhythm. Retrograde P waves are identified after the QRS complexes. **B,** The central venous pressure (*CVP*) tracing demonstrates prominent cannon *a* waves (*arrows*) related to the loss of atrioventricular synchrony (scale of 0–30 mm Hg for CVP).

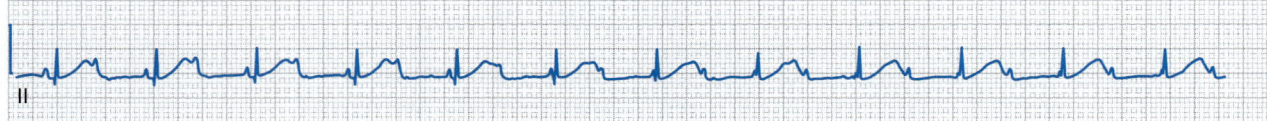

FIGURE 16.25 Rhythm strip demonstrates independent atrial and ventricular activity (i.e., atrioventricular dissociation) and failure of any atrial impulses to conduct to the ventricles. These features characterize a complete atrioventricular block.

but typically exceeding 230 beats/minute in children) with a narrow or usual complex QRS morphology. Supraventricular tachycardia can occur in structurally normal hearts and in various forms of CHD. *Usual complex* implies that the QRS morphology in tachycardia is similar to that in normal sinus rhythm (Fig. 16.26). Occasionally, widening of the QRS in SVT can result from bundle branch block or related to the tachycardia mechanism (i.e., SVT with aberrancy). A wide QRS complex can make the distinction between supraventricular and ventricular tachycardia difficult.

The two types of SVT are automatic and reentrant. They can be differentiated by assessing characteristics of the tachycardia, usually assisted by the input from a specialist. The evaluation of a tachyarrhythmia should include a surface 15-lead ECG and continuous rhythm strip to document onset and termination. If

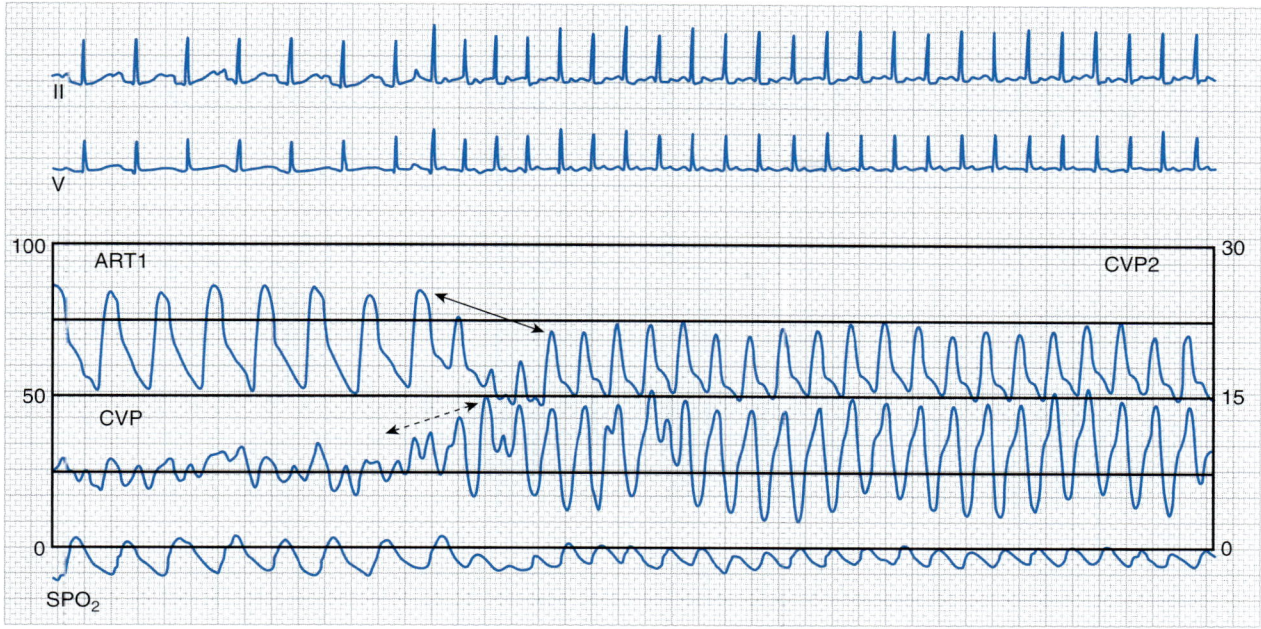

FIGURE 16.26 The initial portion of the intraoperative recording demonstrates normal sinus rhythm. A premature atrial beat initiates a narrow complex tachycardia (i.e., QRS morphology is the same as in sinus rhythm). The supraventricular tachycardia is associated with hemodynamic changes such as a decrease in the systemic arterial pressure (ART 1, scale of 0-100 mm Hg) (*solid arrow*) and increase in the central venous pressure (CVP, scale of 0-30 mm Hg) (*broken arrow*). SpO_2, oxygen saturation.

a medication such as adenosine has been administered, a recording of the response to the drug or pacing maneuvers should be obtained. The management of SVT depends on the clinical status of the child, type of tachycardia, and precise electrophysiologic mechanism. General management principles include the following:

- Hemodynamic stability should be determined. Synchronized direct current cardioversion (0.5-1.0 J/kg) should be performed for hemodynamic instability.
- Antiarrhythmic therapy is based primarily on the clinical condition and suspected tachycardia mechanism. Vagal maneuvers can be considered but should not delay treatment. Adenosine is the drug of choice in the acute setting for diagnosis and termination of most supraventricular tachycardias.[202] β-Blockers are most often used for chronic therapy.
- Others measures include treatment of fever (if present), sedation, correction of electrolyte disturbance, and decreasing or withdrawing medications associated with sympathetic stimulation (i.e., inotropic agents) or with vagolytic properties.
- In addition to pharmacologic therapy, atrial pacing or cardioversion may be required.

Ventricular Arrhythmias

Premature Ventricular Contractions or Beats

Premature ventricular contractions (PVCs) are characterized by prematurity of the QRS complex, a QRS morphology different from that in sinus rhythm, usually a prolongation of the QRS duration for age, abnormalities of the ST segment and T wave, and premature ventricular activity not preceded by a premature atrial beat. PVCs of a single QRS morphology (i.e., uniform), without associated symptoms, and in children with structurally normal hearts are considered benign. An ECG during sinus rhythm should allow careful measurement of the QT interval. Further

investigation and consultation are warranted in the presence of PVCs of multiple morphologies (i.e., multiform), if they occur with moderate frequency or in succession (i.e., couplets or runs) and are associated with symptoms or a structurally abnormal heart.

Ventricular ectopy in the perioperative period can be the result of profound hypoxemia, electrolyte disturbances, or metabolic derangements. Other causes include the use of recreational drugs, myocardial injury, poor hemodynamics, and prior cardiac surgical intervention.

Ventricular Tachycardia

Ventricular tachycardia (VT) is relatively uncommon in children. It is defined as three or more consecutive ventricular beats occurring at a rate greater than 120 beats/minute (Fig. 16.27). The QRS morphology in VT is different from that in sinus rhythm, and the QRS duration is typically prolonged for age. ECG features that support this diagnosis include AV dissociation, intermittent fusion (i.e., QRS complex of intermediate morphology between two other distinct QRS morphologies), QRS morphology of VT similar to that of single PVCs, and tachycardia rate in children usually below 250 beats/minute.

Acute onset of VT in pediatric patients can be caused by hypoxia, acidosis, electrolyte imbalance, or metabolic problems. Ventricular tachycardia can also occur in the context of depressed ventricular function, halothane anesthesia with or without hypercarbia, poor hemodynamics, prior surgical interventions, cardiomyopathies, myocardial tumors, acute injury (e.g., inflammation, trauma), and prolonged QT syndromes.[203]

Long QT Syndrome

Long QT syndrome (LQTS) (Fig. 16.28) is an electrical cardiac disturbance that can predispose children to arrhythmias that include

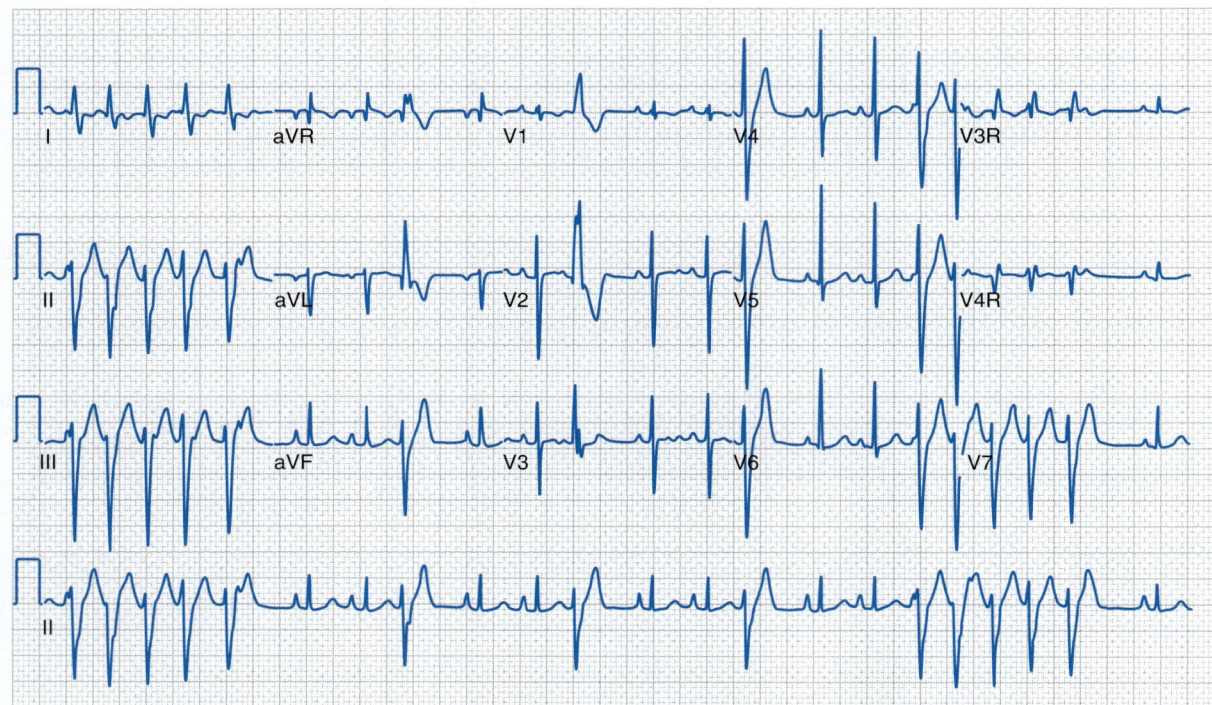

FIGURE 16.27 The tracing demonstrates frequent, uniform premature ventricular beats and episodes of nonsustained, monomorphic ventricular tachycardia.

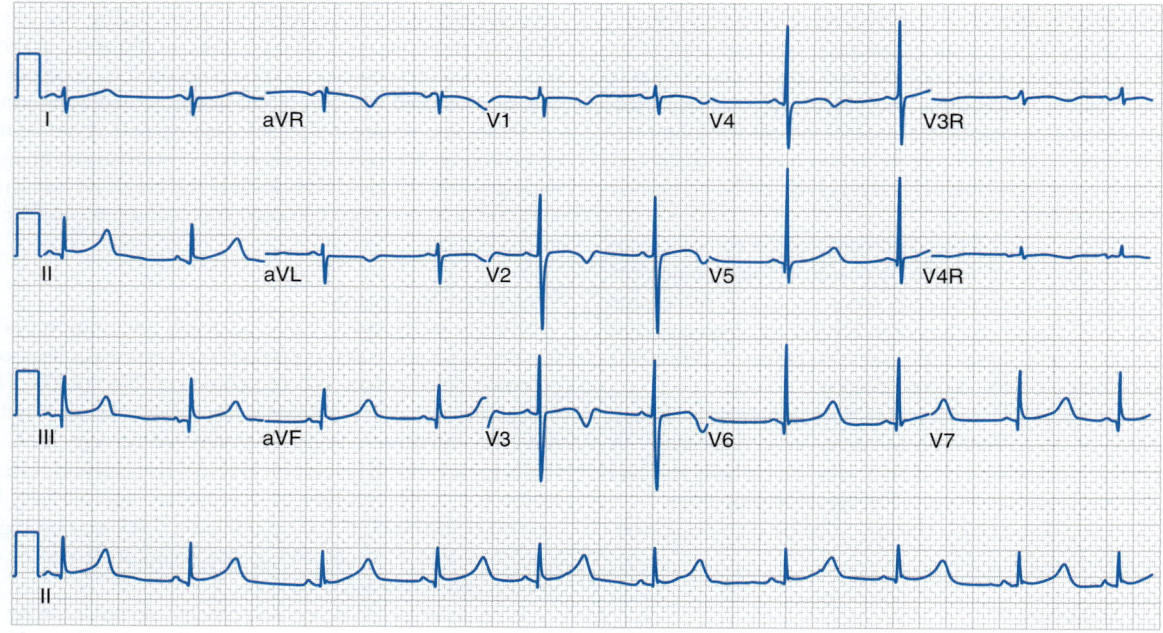

FIGURE 16.28 For a patient with long QT syndrome, the electrocardiogram demonstrates prolongation of the QT interval.

torsades de pointes ventricular tachycardia (Fig. 16.29), ventricular fibrillation, and bradyarrhythmias; any of these can result in syncope, cardiac arrest, or sudden death.[204] It occurs with an incidence of 1 per 2500 births; congenital and acquired forms have been described. The congenital varieties are likely the result of genetic defects in the ion channel proteins responsible for maintaining electrical homeostasis.[205] The Romano-Ward form of LQTS accounts for 90% of pediatric cases; it has an incidence of 1 per 10,000 births and an autosomal dominant pattern of inheritance. The Jervell Lange-Nielsen syndrome has an incidence

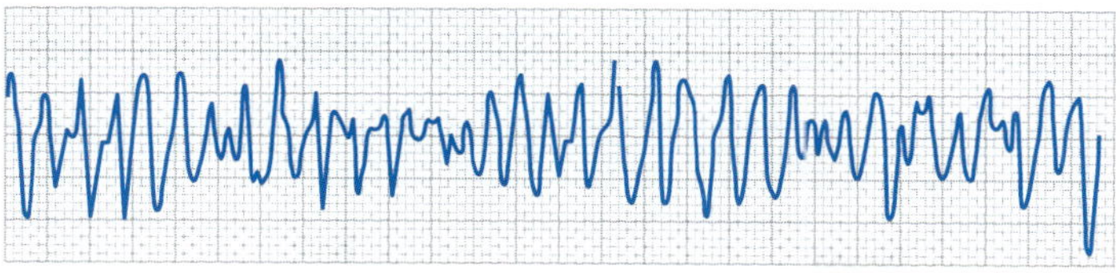

FIGURE 16.29 The rhythm strip displays positive and negative oscillation of QRS complexes, which is characteristic of torsades de pointes ventricular tachycardia.

16

of 1 per 1,000,000 births, an autosomal recessive pattern of inheritance, and an association with deafness. Diagnostic criteria for LQTS include electrocardiographic findings, clinical history (e.g., deafness, syncope), and family history. Prolongation of the QTc on the resting ECG is the hallmark of this syndrome but may not always be present.

An important consideration in the care of children with LQTS is ensuring adequate β-adrenergic blockade preoperatively and minimizing adrenergic stimulation.[206] The risk for developing torsades de pointes from the many drugs known to trigger it is almost unpredictable; these drugs have been divided into several groups that are listed and updated online at https://crediblemeds.org.[207]

In a retrospective study of children with LQTS, three adverse events were reported during emergence from anesthesia immediately after administration of ondansetron and anticholinesterase medications; one was described as torsades de pointes.[208] These arrhythmias resolved quickly with IV β-blockers, lidocaine, or the administration of both agents. The report suggests that children with LQTS are at risk for arrhythmias during periods of enhanced sympathetic activity (i.e., during emergence), particularly in the presence of drugs that prolong the QT interval. Conditions (e.g., hypothermia) and drugs that are known to prolong the QT interval should not be combined if possible. Despite the fact that most IV medications and inhalational agents routinely administered during anesthesia prolong the QT interval, adverse events are rare. This may be attributed in part to the need for a second abnormality beyond a prolonged QT interval to be present to trigger arrhythmias (e.g., increased dispersion of repolarization). Fortunately, most anesthetics do not increase the dispersion of repolarization.

Torsades de pointes is a rare but potentially life-threatening arrhythmia. To trigger torsades, a second phenomenon must occur (e.g., increased dispersion of repolarization). Dispersion of repolarization refers to the variance in the rate of repolarization; in this case, it is a circumscribed region in the heart muscle (i.e., transmurally from the epicardium to the endocardium). There is much debate over how to quantify an increased dispersion of repolarization from surface ECGs. Some suggest the dispersion is the QTc-max to QTc-min, whereas others recommend measuring the duration of the T wave from its peak to the end; in both instances the upper limit of normal is 65 msec and abnormal values exceed 100 msec.

Prolongation of the QT interval and genesis of torsades de pointes occur more commonly in the presence of several conditions and drugs: electrolyte derangements (e.g., hypokalemia, hypocalcemia, hypomagnesemia), combination drug therapies (e.g., antibiotics, antiarrhythmic agents, class III antiarrhythmics such as amiodarone and procainamide), antipsychotic drugs, neurologic or endocrine abnormalities (e.g., hypothyroidism), 5-HT$_3$ receptor–blocking drugs (except palonosetron), neostigmine, stress (including induction of and emergence from anesthesia and laryngoscopy), female gender, bradycardia, and coronary artery disease. Although

many anesthetics prolong the QT interval, few affect the dispersion of repolarization (as in the case of sevoflurane), and the risk of torsades de pointes during general anesthesia in children is rare.[209]

Management of ventricular tachycardia requires the following considerations:

1. Although some atypical forms of supraventricular tachyarrhythmias may mimic VT, a wide QRS tachycardia should always be considered to be of ventricular origin.
2. The initial approach in the setting of an acute ventricular rhythm disturbance consists of prompt evaluation of clinical status and hemodynamic stability. Sustained ventricular arrhythmias are poorly tolerated and require immediate attention. In the unstable child, cardiopulmonary resuscitation should be instituted while preparing for cardioversion. Expert consultation is advisable when advanced drug therapy is contemplated. Potential pharmacologic interventions include lidocaine, amiodarone, and procainamide. The latter two should not routinely be administered during torsades de pointes owing to QT prolongation.
3. Magnesium sulfate is considered the first-line treatment of torsades de pointes. Procainamide and amiodarone are contraindicated owing to prolongation of the QT interval. Isoproterenol and overdrive pacing can be effective for bradycardia. Electrical cardioversion (1-2 J/kg) should be performed only if the arrhythmia is refractory to pharmacologic treatment.
4. LQTS should be treated with β-blockade (not overdrive pacing); some forms of the LQTS may require the implantation of a cardioverter-defibrillator.

Ventricular Fibrillation

Ventricular fibrillation (VF) is an uncommon arrhythmia in children. It is characterized by chaotic, asynchronous ventricular activity that fails to generate an adequate cardiac output. The ECG during VF demonstrates low-amplitude, irregular deflections without identifiable QRS complexes. A loose ECG electrode can mimic these surface electrocardiographic features, therefore immediate clinical assessment should be performed and adequate pad contact ensured when VF is suspected.

Management of VF includes the following considerations:

1. This is a lethal arrhythmia if untreated.
2. Immediate defibrillation (initial dose of 2 J/kg) is the definitive therapy. Cardiopulmonary resuscitation, beginning with chest compressions, should be immediately instituted and continued for 2 minutes. If defibrillation is unsuccessful, the energy dose should be doubled (4 J/kg) and repeated. Pediatric paddles (2.2 cm in diameter) are recommended for children weighing less than 10 kg. Adult paddles (8 to 9 mm in diameter) are suggested for children weighing more than 10 kg to reduce impedance and maximize current flow.
3. Adequate airway control and chest compressions should be rapidly instituted while preparing for defibrillation or between

TABLE 16.5	The Revised NASPE/BPEG Generic Pacemaker Codes[a]				
Position Number and Category					
I	II	III	IV	V
Chamber(s) Paced	**Chamber(s) Sensed**	**Response to Sensing**	**Rate Modulation**	**Multisite Pacing**
A = Atrium	A = Atrium	I = Inhibited	R = Rate modulation	A = Atrium
V = Ventricle	V = Ventricle	T = Triggered		V = Ventricle
D = Dual (A + V)	D = Dual (A + V)	D = Dual (I + T) response restricted to dual-chamber devices		D = Dual (A + V)
O = None	O = None	O = None	O = None	O = None

[a]The pacemaker mode, specified by a code, describes the mode in which the pacemaker is operating.
Reproduced with permission from Bernstein AD, Daubert JC, Fletcher RD, et al. The revised NASPE/BPEG generic code for antibradycardia, adaptive-rate, and multisite pacing. *Pacing Clin Electrophysiol.* 2002;25:260–264, with minor modifications.

shocks if several defibrillation attempts are needed. Resuscitative drugs and amiodarone should be considered without delaying defibrillation.

Pacemaker and Defibrillator Therapy in the Pediatric Age Group

PACEMAKER NOMENCLATURE

Pacemaker nomenclature follows the guidelines of the North American Society of Pacing and Electrophysiology and the British Pacing and Electrophysiology Group (Table 16.5)[210]:

- First letter: chamber(s) paced (A = atrium, V = ventricle, D = dual or both, O = none)
- Second letter: chamber(s) sensed (A = atrium, V = ventricle, D = dual or both, O = none)
- Third letter: pacemaker response to sensing (I = inhibited, T = triggered, D = dual response, O = none)
- Fourth letter: rate modulation (R = rate modulation, O = none)
- Fifth letter: multisite pacing (A = atrium, V = ventricle, D = dual or both, O = none)

The most common pacing modes are listed in Table 16.6.

PERMANENT CARDIAC PACING

Indications

The updated guidelines for device-based therapy of cardiac rhythm abnormalities were published in 2013.[211] In general terms, indications for permanent cardiac pacing in children include symptomatic sinus bradycardia, bradycardia-tachycardia syndromes, congenital third-degree AV block, and advanced second- or third-degree AV block.[211,212]

Perioperative Considerations

It is essential for anesthesia providers involved in the care of patients with a cardiac implantable electronic device (CIED) to understand basic aspects such as indications for placement, functionality, and potential issues that may be encountered perioperatively.[213] Device interrogation is an essential part of the preoperative evaluation in all patients with an implanted pacemaker.[214,215] Results of a recent 15-lead ECG should be reviewed if available. Familiarity with unit type, settings, date of and indications for implantation, device location, and underlying cardiac rhythm is highly recommended. If records are not available and there is no identification card providing details about the unit implanted, a radiopaque marker on a chest radiograph can assist

TABLE 16.6	Most Common Pacing Modes
Single-Chamber Pacing	
AAI: atrial demand pacing (atrial pacing and sensing, inhibited on sensed beat)	
AAIR: atrial demand pacing (atrial pacing and sensing, inhibited on sensed beat), rate responsiveness	
VVI: ventricular demand pacing (ventricular pacing and sensing, inhibited on sensed beat)	
VVIR: ventricular demand pacing (ventricular pacing and sensing, inhibited on sensed beat), rate responsiveness	
Asynchronous Pacing (No Sensing)	
AOO: fixed-rate atrial pacing	
VOO: fixed-rate ventricular pacing	
DOO: fixed-rate AV pacing	
Dual-Chamber Pacing	
DDD: paces and senses both chambers	
DDDR: paces and senses both chambers, sensor-driven rate responsiveness	

in the identification of the device. Major pacemaker manufacturers can also be contacted by telephone at any time because they maintain computerized records of all implanted devices.

Reprogramming may be required before the planned procedure to avoid potential problems with pacemaker malfunction related to electrocautery. This represents one of the most common potential sources of electromagnetic interference in children with implanted cardiac devices. Recommendations for the perioperative management of the patient with a cardiac pacemaker include the use of bipolar cautery rather than a unipolar configuration if possible, avoiding cauterization near the site of the generator, and positioning the indifferent plate (dispersive pad) for electrocautery as far away as possible from the pacemaker so that the device is not between the electrocautery electrodes.[216] Devices such as the harmonic scalpel and battery-operated, hot wire, handheld cautery units do not interfere with implanted cardiac devices. Rate-responsive features of pacemakers should be deactivated in most cases.

Chronotropic drugs and alternate pacing modalities should be readily available in the event of pacemaker malfunction and compromising underlying rate. Although inserting a transvenous pacemaker has been recommended for children with complete AV block who were undergoing pacemaker implantation, a 10-year review indicated no benefit to routine preoperative temporary pacing.[217] Capture thresholds can be affected by pharmacologic agents, and this should be considered if pacing is required in the child receiving antiarrhythmic drug therapy.

Perioperative conditions can also influence pacing thresholds. A magnet should be accessible to allow asynchronous pacing if required. Most generators respond to magnet application by pacing at a fixed rate asynchronously (i.e., AOO, VOO, or DOO). A potential problem is that the specific magnet rate, as determined by the manufacturer for the particular device, can be different from the desirable or optimal pacing rate. The use of a magnet should not be considered a substitute for preoperative pacemaker interrogation/programming. In addition to perioperative electrocardiographic monitoring, additional modalities that confirm pulse generation during pacing (e.g., esophageal stethoscope for assessment of heart sounds, pulse oximetry, invasive arterial blood pressure monitoring) are strongly encouraged. The device should be tested and reprogrammed after the procedure is completed.

Transcutaneous Pacing

Several devices that combine defibrillation and cardioversion capabilities with external pacing features are available. Emergency transthoracic pacing can be considered as a temporizing measure for children with symptomatic bradycardia,[218] but this has not been effective in the treatment of asystole in children.[219] Pacing electrode size should be selected according to patient size (e.g., smaller adhesive pads for weight <15 kg). Device settings typically include pacing rate and power output. Sedation may be necessary to tolerate soft tissue discomfort. Prolonged periods of transcutaneous pacing can result in local cutaneous injury. In addition to monitoring for pacemaker capture by ECG, ongoing clinical assessment of the adequacy of cardiac output should be undertaken.

Implantable Cardioverter-Defibrillators

The primary goal of an implantable cardioverter-defibrillator (ICD) is the prevention of sudden death. Children with long QT syndrome, HCM, history of near-death events, arrhythmogenic right ventricular dysplasia, and operated CHD with a history of malignant arrhythmias represent potential candidates for device implantation.[211,212] The capabilities of these units include pacing and defibrillation. It may be feasible to terminate tachyarrhythmias by pacing.

As more children have received implantable devices in the past few years, an increasing number of them may require anesthetic care. The main considerations associated with intraoperative care of patients with these devices relate to monitoring, managing issues with potential for electromagnetic interference, and performing emergent defibrillation, cardioversion, or heart rate support.[213–215] Perioperative consultation with a cardiologist or electrophysiologist is essential in most, if not all, cases. These devices should be interrogated and likely require programming before and at the conclusion of the planned procedure.

Diagnostic Modalities in Pediatric Cardiology

CHEST RADIOGRAPHY

The standard posteroanterior and lateral chest radiographs provide clues to a child's underlying cardiovascular anatomy; however, plain radiographs are an insensitive screening tool for cardiac disease.[220] Children with numerous types of significant CHD can have initially normal-appearing radiographs; alternatively, an infant

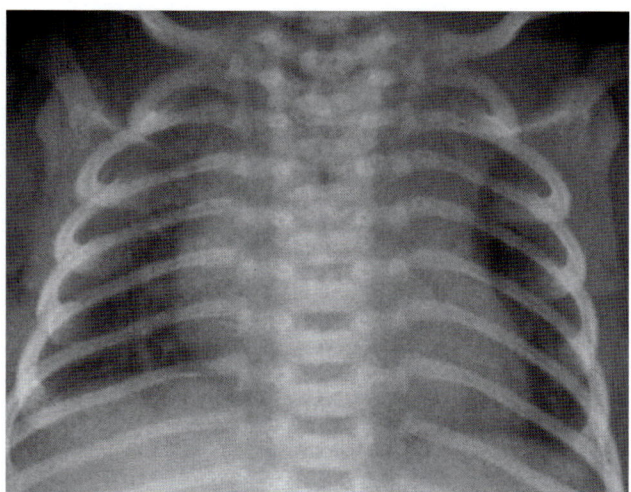

FIGURE 16.30 For a neonate with apneic episodes undergoing evaluation for potential cardiac disease, the radiograph demonstrates a poor inspiratory effort resulting in a large cardiothymic silhouette, making interpretation of cardiac size difficult. No evidence of cardiac disease was identified in this child.

with a poor inspiratory effort and the presence of a large thymus can give the appearance of cardiomegaly and have normal intracardiac anatomy (Fig. 16.30).

Interpretation of a chest radiograph begins with identification of the patient's name and ensuring that the right-left orientation of the radiograph is correct. All catheters and tubes should be followed to verify their location, course, and likely site of termination. The bones and soft tissues should be inspected for evidence of sternal wires, fractures, vertebral anomalies, or wide intercostal spaces, suggesting a prior thoracotomy. Sidedness, including the location of the gastric bubble, liver, and position and orientation of the cardiac mass, should be observed. The lung parenchyma should be examined for evidence of focal consolidation, such as pneumonia or atelectasis, and for pulmonary vascular markings.

The cardiac silhouette and great vessels should be assessed. In young children, the thymus can obscure the superior portions of the cardiac shadow. Careful inspection of the cardiac silhouette includes an assessment of overall size and evidence of individual chamber or vessel dilation. The size of the main pulmonary artery segment can provide further evidence of the degree of pulmonary overcirculation in children with left-to-right shunt lesions. The tracheal indentation can usually be seen and is useful in determining aortic arch sidedness, although in a young child with a prominent thymus, this can be difficult to assess.

More useful than an individual radiograph as a diagnostic tool are serial chest films obtained to monitor a child's cardiovascular status over time. In a young child with a volume overload lesion, the physical examination and growth parameters coupled with the degree of cardiomegaly and pulmonary overcirculation are more helpful than more advanced imaging techniques. A plain chest radiograph can also guide initiation and titration of pharmacologic therapy and the timing of a surgical intervention.

BARIUM ESOPHAGRAM

The current applications and uses of barium esophagram (swallow) studies in the diagnosis of CHD are limited. This modality has been largely replaced by MRI and chest tomography. In some

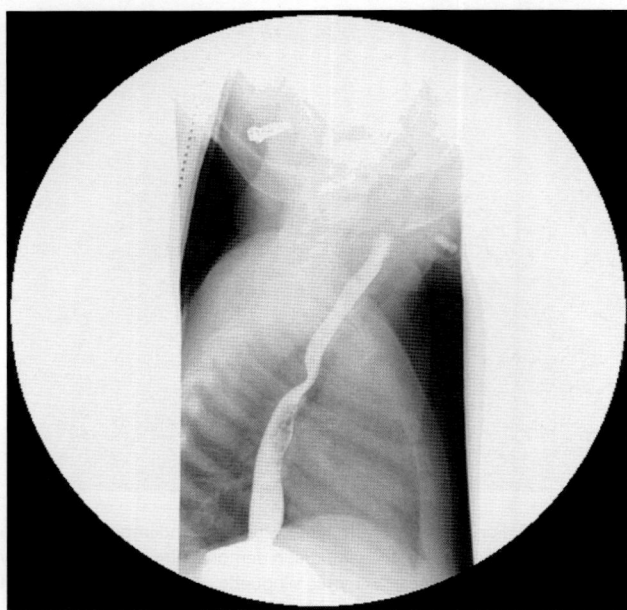

FIGURE 16.31 Barium swallow in a child with respiratory symptoms demonstrates an indentation posteriorly in the mid-esophagus, which is consistent with a vascular ring (in this particular case was caused by an aberrant subclavian artery with a retroesophageal course).

cases, a barium esophagram is used as an initial screening tool when there is concern about the presence of a vascular ring, usually because of airway symptoms or, less likely, feeding or swallowing difficulties.[221,222] Most common types of vascular rings in children are (1) a double aortic arch and (2) a right aortic arch with an aberrant left subclavian artery and left-sided ligamentum arteriosus. The indentation pattern in the barium column is suggestive of the specific vascular anomaly (Fig. 16.31).

ECHOCARDIOGRAPHY

Echocardiography is the gold standard for the initial evaluation and serial assessment in most types of pediatric heart disease.[223] Ultrasound transducers are used to acquire real-time images of cardiovascular structures. Various echocardiographic modalities are available, including transthoracic, transesophageal, fetal, epicardial, intracardiac, and intravascular ultrasound.[224–229] Each plays an important role in the evaluation and management of children with suspected or known cardiovascular disease.

Advantages of echocardiography include its noninvasive nature, provision of excellent temporal and spatial resolution, generation of portable real-time images, cost-effectiveness, and ease of use. As with any type of ultrasound, these waves are transmitted well through homogeneous tissues and fluid but poorly through air and bone. Another limitation of echocardiography is related to limited acoustic windows in certain patient groups, such as those who have undergone multiple prior cardiothoracic procedures, older individuals, or children with a significant amount of soft tissue or body fat. For this reason cardiovascular MRI is being increasingly used for noninvasive imaging. Additional challenges of echocardiography include the need to obtain serial two-dimensional tomographic images by sweeping the transducer scan in multiple planes to reconstruct these into three-dimensional structures in one's mind and to achieve expert interpretation.

Despite these limitations, echocardiography remains the main diagnostic imaging modality for most children. Many medical and surgical management strategies are primarily based on the findings allowed by this approach.

A standard transthoracic study consists of a two-dimensional examination, M-mode imaging, and Doppler evaluation (i.e., color flow, pulsed-wave, or continuous-wave modalities). Two-dimensional imaging provides structural assessment of the heart and vasculature. Cross-sectional images are obtained from several windows that allow excellent anatomic detail in multiple planes (Video 16.11). In most cases, this is adequate for a detailed segmental evaluation of the cardiac anatomy as described earlier. M-mode echocardiography allows one-dimensional imaging of the heart with excellent temporal resolution (Fig. 16.32). It is known as an *ice pick view* of the heart in real time and is primarily used in the assessment of ventricular dimensions and function.

Color flow Doppler techniques allow evaluation of directionality and velocity of blood flow. In addition to detecting flow across cardiac valves and vessels, color flow imaging allows demonstration of subtle lesions such as small septal defects that can be difficult to identify by standard two-dimensional imaging alone. Traditionally, flow toward the transducer is displayed in red, and flow away is represented as blue. Turbulent blood flow is associated with increased Doppler velocities and can be readily identified as a mosaic of colors; it typically has a greenish tint (Video 16.12).

Pulsed- and continuous-wave Doppler represent spectral modalities that complement the color flow data and provide quantitative information. Pulsed-wave interrogation localizes specific sites of stenosis or turbulence but is limited in the magnitude of velocities it can detect. Continuous-wave Doppler allows quantification of much higher velocities (see Video 16.12). Velocities obtained with spectral Doppler provide estimates of pressures within various cardiac chambers by applying the simplified Bernoulli equation. It states that the difference in pressure between two locations is approximately four times the square of the velocity of the jet of flow between them:

$$\text{Pressure gradient (in mm Hg)} = 4 \times V^2$$

The applications of three-dimensional echocardiography continue to evolve, including in patients with CHD.[230–232] This approach can provide clear and useful volumetric assessments when the images are adequate. A significant advantage of this modality is that it is able to display cardiovascular structures and their interrelationships in detail, in many cases facilitating the understanding of pathologic conditions over two-dimensional imaging. The technology is particularly helpful in cases of complex anatomy. Three-dimensional echocardiography can also be useful when interventions are planned.

Interpretation of an Echocardiographic Report
Measurements of Cardiac Chambers and Vessel Dimensions
Several measurements are routinely obtained during an echocardiographic examination. They include left ventricular end-diastolic (LVED) and left ventricular end-systolic (LVES) dimensions, thickness of the interventricular septum and left ventricular posterior wall, measurements of valve annular sizes and great artery dimensions, and left atrial volume. To determine whether these are appropriate for the child being examined, the measurements are referenced to values obtained in normal children matched for body surface area. This is accomplished by reporting the measured value and a z score, representing standard deviations of measured values from the mean in a comparative population.

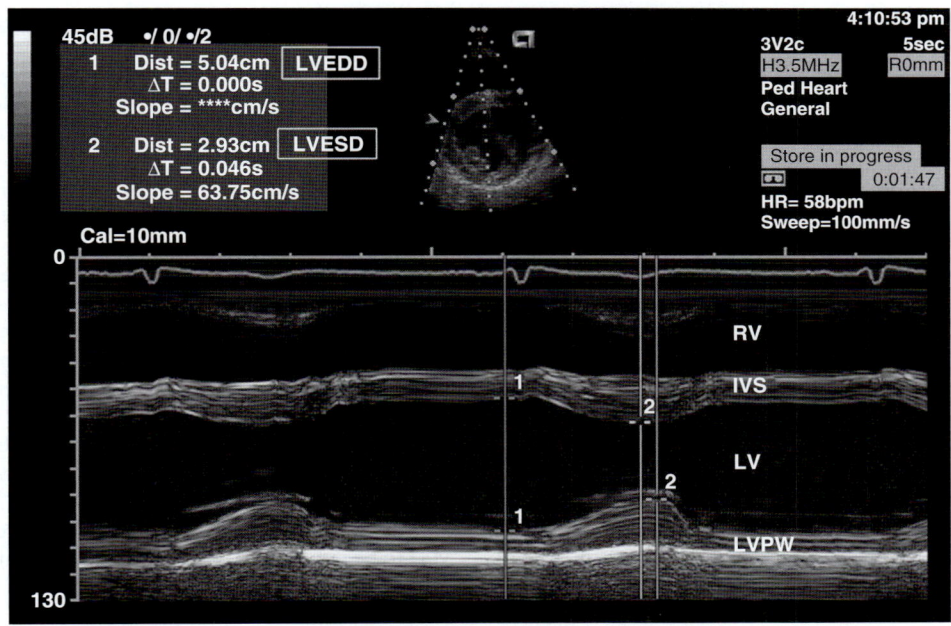

45dB   •/ 0/ •/2
1   Dist = 5.04cm   LVEDD
    ΔT = 0.000s
    Slope = ****cm/s

2   Dist = 2.93cm   LVESD
    ΔT = 0.046s
    Slope = 63.75cm/s

Cal=10mm

4:10:53 pm
3V2c   5sec
H3.5MHz   R0mm
Ped Heart
General

Store in progress
                  0:01:47
HR= 58bpm
Sweep=100mm/s

RV
IVS
LV
LVPW

FIGURE 16.32 An M-mode echocardiogram enables determination of left ventricular dimensions and calculation of left ventricular shortening fraction. *IVS*, interventricular septum; *LV*, left ventricle; *LVEDD*, left ventricular end-diastolic dimension; *LVESD*, left ventricular end-systolic dimension; *LVPW*, left ventricular posterior wall; *RV*, right ventricle.

Assessment of Ventricular Function

Several echocardiographic techniques are able to provide information regarding ventricular performance. Two of the most commonly reported indexes of ventricular systolic function are shortening fraction and ejection fraction. Shortening fraction (SF) represents the percent of change in left ventricular diameter during the cardiac cycle. This is calculated using the following equation:

$$SF (\%) = (LVED\ dimension - LVES\ dimension / LVED\ dimension) \times 100$$

Values range from 28% to 44%, with a normal mean value of 36%. This index, however, depends on ventricular preload and afterload.

Ejection fraction (EF) is the fraction of blood ejected by the ventricle (stroke volume) relative to its end-diastolic volume. This represents the percentage of blood ejected from the left ventricle with each heartbeat. EF is derived by volumetric analysis of the left ventricle by means of the following equation:

$$EF (\%) = (LVEDV - LVESV / LVEDV) \times 100$$

In the equation, LVEDV is the left ventricular end-diastolic volume, and LVESV is the left ventricular end-systolic volume. Normal values range between 56% and 78%. A low EF is associated with impaired systolic function; however, cardiac dysfunction can also occur in the presence of a normal EF, as in the case of diastolic heart failure.

Although these functional indexes are routinely and easily obtained, they have significant limitations. Estimation of EF is based on geometric assumptions for the elliptical left ventricle, and this may not be applicable to a systemic right ventricle or other types of ventricular geometries (e.g., single ventricle). This accounts for an ongoing interest in alternative approaches that may provide more sensitive and comprehensive information regarding ventricular performance, even in the absence of clinical disease.

These techniques include the myocardial performance index, also known as the Tei index, which combines systolic and diastolic intervals to assess global ventricular function,[233,234] Doppler tissue imaging (DTI), which is used to evaluate intramural myocardial velocities,[235] and strain and strain rate imaging to quantitate the rate of segmental myocardial deformation.[236] Although values in normal children have been established for these imaging modalities and alterations in the presence of pathologic conditions have been described, additional studies documenting their clinical applications in specific types of cardiovascular pathology are needed.

Estimation of Pressures

The peak velocity of a tricuspid regurgitant jet can be used to estimate right ventricular systolic pressure, which should equal pulmonary artery systolic pressure in the absence of pulmonary stenosis or outflow tract obstruction (Video 16.13). For example, if a peak regurgitant velocity of 3 m/second is recorded across the tricuspid valve using the simplified Bernoulli equation, the pressure gradient or difference between the right atrial and right ventricular systolic pressures can be estimated to be $4 \times 3^2 = 36$ mm Hg. If a normal right atrial pressure is assumed (4–6 mm Hg), it would predict a right ventricular systolic pressure of approximately 40 mm Hg. Similarly, if the peak or maximal flow velocity across a VSD is measured at 4.5 m/second, it predicts a pressure gradient of $4 \times 4.5^2 = 81$ mm Hg between the ventricles, implying that the defect is pressure restrictive and the right ventricular and pulmonary artery systolic pressures are relatively low.

Evaluation of Gradients

Estimation of a peak instantaneous gradient is the most clinically useful method for quantifying the severity of obstructions across semilunar valves and outflow tracts. It is derived by application of the simplified Bernoulli equation. When these gradients are measured across the pulmonary valve, they tend to correlate more closely with catheterization peak-to-peak gradients than with those measured across the aortic valve, for which mean gradients (obtained by automated integration of the velocities under a spectral Doppler tracing) have been shown to correlate more closely.[237] The mean rather than peak gradient determined by Doppler echocardiography is considered a better metric of the severity of the obstruction across AV valves and other low-flow venous pathways.

Evaluation of Regurgitant Lesions

Evaluation of the severity of regurgitant lesions in most pediatric cardiac centers remains largely a qualitative assessment. It is usually characterized as mild, moderate, severe, or a combination thereof when there is overlap among these categories. Serial echocardiographic assessments and comparative data are clinically more meaningful than an isolated report.

MAGNETIC RESONANCE IMAGING

Cardiovascular MRI-angiography has emerged as a complementary technology to the other imaging modalities (Videos 16.14 and 16.15). Benefits have been reported in the assessment of complex pathology, delineation of systemic and pulmonary vascular anomalies, evaluation of global and regional ventricular function, assessment of myocardial viability, and characterization of pulmonary blood supply in children with structural alterations of the pulmonary vascular tree.[238-244] Additional applications that may further expand the utility of cardiovascular MRI include the quantification of left-to-right shunts and measurement of blood oxygen saturation.[245-247] MRI is also beneficial for guiding interventions in pediatric heart disease.[248,249]

Although the temporal resolution of MRI is inferior to echocardiography, new sequences and techniques allow real-time acquisition similar to that of fluoroscopy. An important aspect in the acquisition of MRI data with high spatial resolution is the use of cardiac and respiratory gating to allow sampling during only specific portions of the cardiac and respiratory cycles. Slow heart rates and low respiratory rates facilitate this process. In contrast to computed tomography (CT), MRI does not expose the child to radiation; this makes it preferable for serial examinations that many young children with cardiovascular pathology require. However, this may be associated with the need for multiple

encounters that require deep sedation/anesthesia and their inherent risks.

Because of the nature of the magnetic fields generated in MRI, the presence of several types of metal, including pacemakers, ICDs, cerebrovascular clips/coils, and recently implanted intracardiac or intravascular coils and devices, are considered contraindications. Titanium hardware can minimize the artifact produced by the foreign material; stainless steel generates significant artifacts within the MRI study.

An additional limitation of MRI is the need for the child to remain immobile during long examinations to optimize the image quality. For small children, this usually necessitates the use of deep sedation or general anesthesia.[250-252] For infants with complex and often cyanotic CHD, specialists are often asked to provide care during these radiologic procedures. The severity of the cardiovascular disease and the need for breath-holding can add to the challenges presented to the anesthesia care provider in a remote location.[253] The lengthy nature of the studies and the significant time requirements to perform postprocessing of the images cause MRI to be much more time intensive for the interpreting physician than other noninvasive imaging modalities.

As MRI technology improves with faster scans, increasing availability, and decreasing cost, it will continue to play an increasing role in the diagnosis and longitudinal follow-up of congenital and acquired pediatric heart disease.

COMPUTED TOMOGRAPHY

CT, with or without electrocardiographic gating, represents an option among the various cardiovascular imaging modalities (Fig. 16.33).[254,255] The major advantage of CT over MRI is the very rapid scan times, and for most children, sedation is minimal or not required. A significant drawback of CT is the large radiation burden, although it typically is estimated to be similar to or slightly greater than a diagnostic cardiac catheterization, and the likely need for iodinated contrast agents with their concomitant risks. It should be noted that radiation dose varies among institutions. Optimizing the dose of radiation while maintaining an adequate diagnostic image quality continues to be an ongoing area of investigation.[256]

Cardiac CT is not as accurate as MRI to delineate intracardiac anatomy, but it provides excellent spatial resolution and

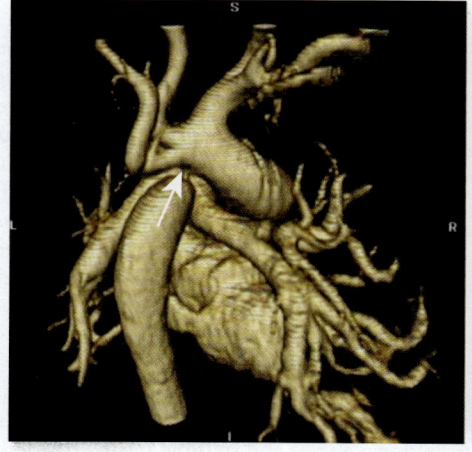 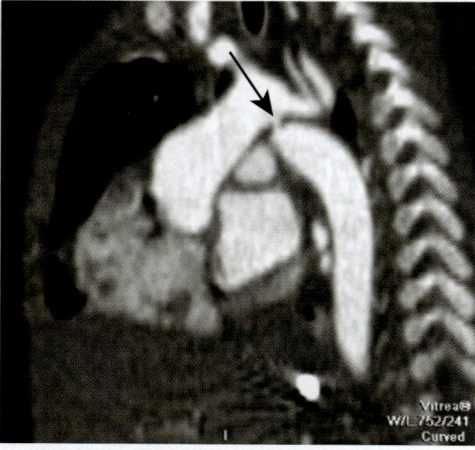

FIGURE 16.33 Computed tomography images show the detailed anatomy in an infant with severe aortic arch obstruction (*arrows*).

information on extracardiac structures. CT has been beneficial in the evaluation of aortic arch anomalies and vascular rings and for defining systemic and pulmonary venous returns. Additional applications of this technology include assessing abnormalities of the coronary arteries (congenital and acquired) and evaluating cardiovascular disorders associated with airway pathology where dynamic recordings and three-dimensional reconstructions provide detailed information.

CARDIAC CATHETERIZATION AND ANGIOGRAPHY

Cardiac catheterization invasively measures intracardiac and vascular pressures and blood oxygen saturation coupled with angiography to assess cardiac anatomy and hemodynamics (Figs. 16.34 and 16.35). Before the era of two-dimensional echocardiography,

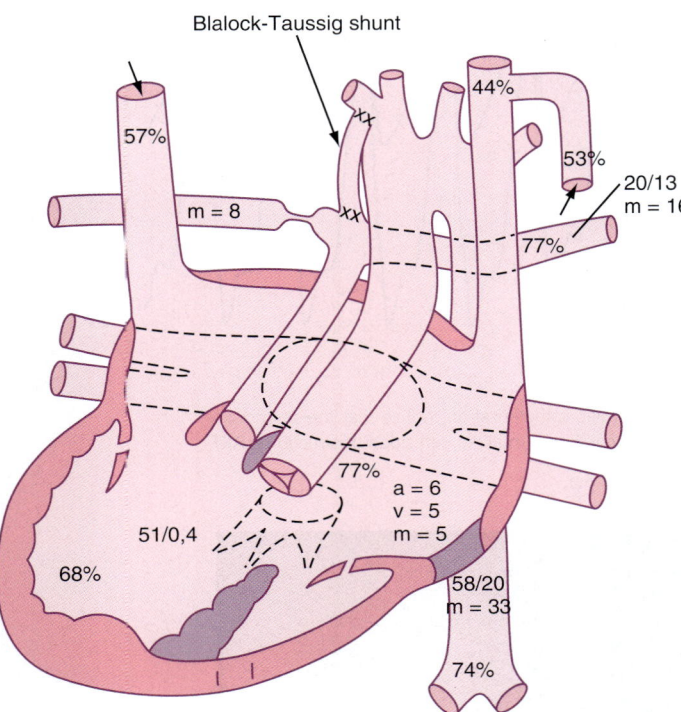

Weight 3.3 kg

Diagnosis
1. Heterotaxy
2. Dextrocardia
3. Complete atrioventricular canal
4. Double-outlet right ventricle
5. Pulmonary stenosis, severe
6. L-Transposition of the great arteries
7. Interrupted inferior vena cava with azygous continuation
8. After innominate to main pulmonary artery shunt
9. Right pulmonary artery isolation

FIGURE 16.34 A cardiac catheterization diagram is valuable when caring for patients with structural anomalies, such as this child with complex congenital heart disease. Data routinely obtained at cardiac catheterization are shown, including oxygen saturation determinations (in %), pressure measurements (in mm Hg), and hemodynamic calculations. Catheter courses are indicated by *arrows*. The atrial pressures are given for the *a* wave *(a)*, which is generated during atria systole; *v* wave *(v)*, which results from passive filling of the atrium before atrioventricular valve opening; and mean *(m)* (all in mm Hg). Refer to section "Interpretation of a Cardiac Catheterization Report."

cardiac catheterization was frequently used for diagnostic purposes. With the advances in noninvasive imaging, diagnostic procedures represent a relatively small proportion of these studies. Current indications for cardiac catheterization at most centers include the assessment of physiologic variables such as pressure and resistance data, measurements of shunt ratios, anatomic definition when other diagnostic modalities are inadequate, need for electrophysiologic testing or treatment, and when catheter-based interventions are anticipated.

Most catheterizations are performed for interventions including endomyocardial biopsies; angioplasties and stenting of stenotic vessels, dilation of valves, and conduits; and occlusion techniques for native defects (Video 16.16), fistulous connections, and surgically created communications no longer considered necessary (Fig. 16.36) (see also Chapter 22). In some cases, such as critically ill neonates with complex heart disease, catheter-based interventions such as balloon atrial septostomy and other procedures can be lifesaving.

Access to the central circulation is usually accomplished percutaneously through a femoral approach. Most examinations involve hemodynamic evaluation with recording of pressure data through catheters positioned at various sites of interest. Oxygen saturation data are obtained by reflectance oximetry or blood gas measurement from various cardiac chambers and vessels. In contrast to the oxygen saturation calculations derived from a blood gas analysis, reflectance oximetry provides measured values. This allows determination of oxygen content (i.e., total amount of hemoglobin in the blood) and, when combined with values of oxygen consumption, assessment of blood flows and other calculations (e.g., shunts).[257] Additional data that can be obtained include pressure gradients, cardiac output, and parameters for deriving vascular resistances and valve areas. Although basal measurements would ideally be performed under conditions that mimic an awake state, this is not feasible in children and in most cases requires the use of deep sedation or general anesthesia. Baseline hemodynamic assessment and oximetric data calculations are optimally obtained under conditions of normocarbia while the inspired oxygen concentration is kept low and relatively constant.

Fluoroscopy and cineangiography are essential components of most cardiac catheterization studies. Of the two, cineangiography accounts for most of the radiation exposure as images are recorded during the injection of contrast material, typically at 15 or 30 frames per second. Consequently, there is concern about radiation dose and risk during cardiac catheterization.[258] Most angiograms are obtained during biplane imaging by positioning the equipment to obtain optimal views allowing for delineation of the pathology in question (i.e., axial angiography) (Video 16.17, A and B).[259]

Although cardiac catheterization has evolved over the years, providing an improved margin of safety, it remains an invasive procedure involving risks.[260-263] They include excessive blood loss, vascular complications, infection, arrhythmias, vascular or cardiac perforation, systemic air embolization, myocardial ischemia, and those associated with the administration of contrast agents. These complications are more likely to occur in neonates and infants rather than the older child.[264] Interventional catheterizations, by the nature of the procedures, are associated with a greater rate of complications and potential for morbidity and mortality. However, as transcatheter interventions become safer and more effective, an increasing number of infants and children may obviate the need for surgery, often undergoing procedures on an outpatient basis.[265] Evolving approaches in this field include percutaneous implantation of valves, strategies that combine cardiac catheterization and surgical

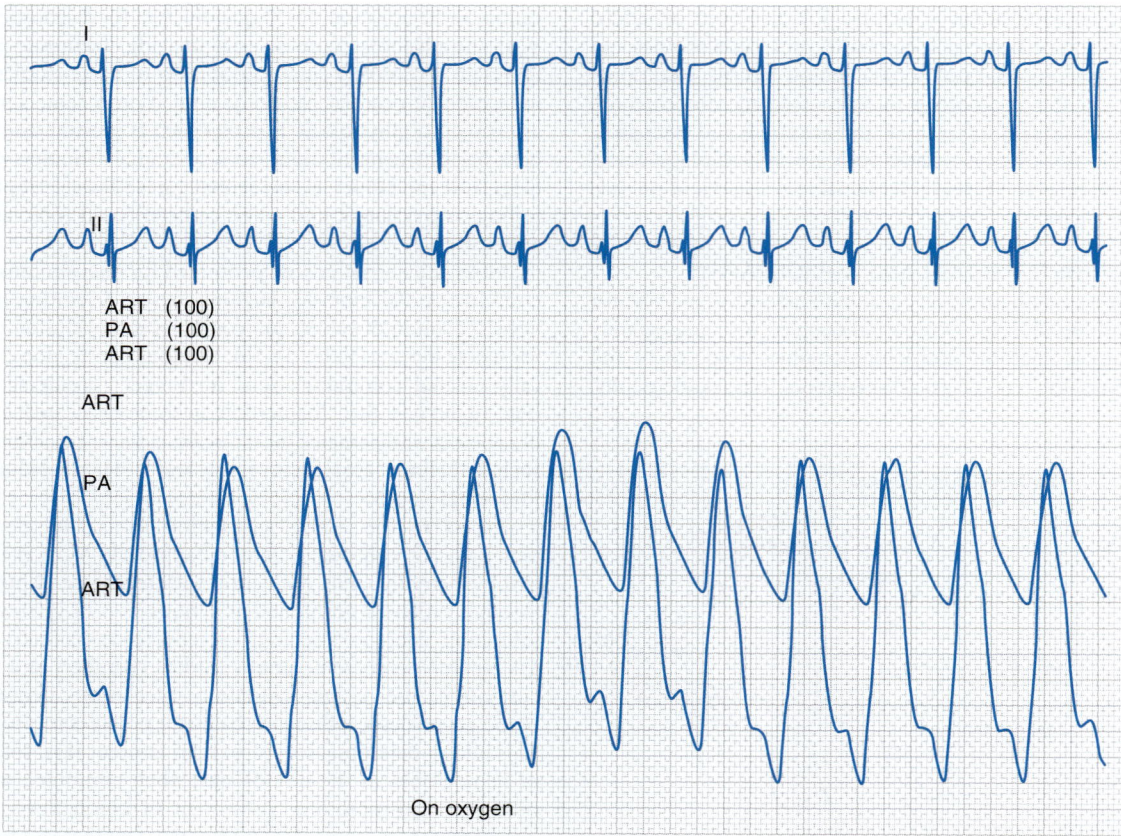

FIGURE 16.35 In the hemodynamic tracing obtained during cardiac catheterization, notice that the pulmonary artery systolic pressure (100 mm Hg) is at systemic levels in this child with multiple, left-sided obstructions. *ART*, systemic arterial pressure; *PA*, pulmonary artery pressure.

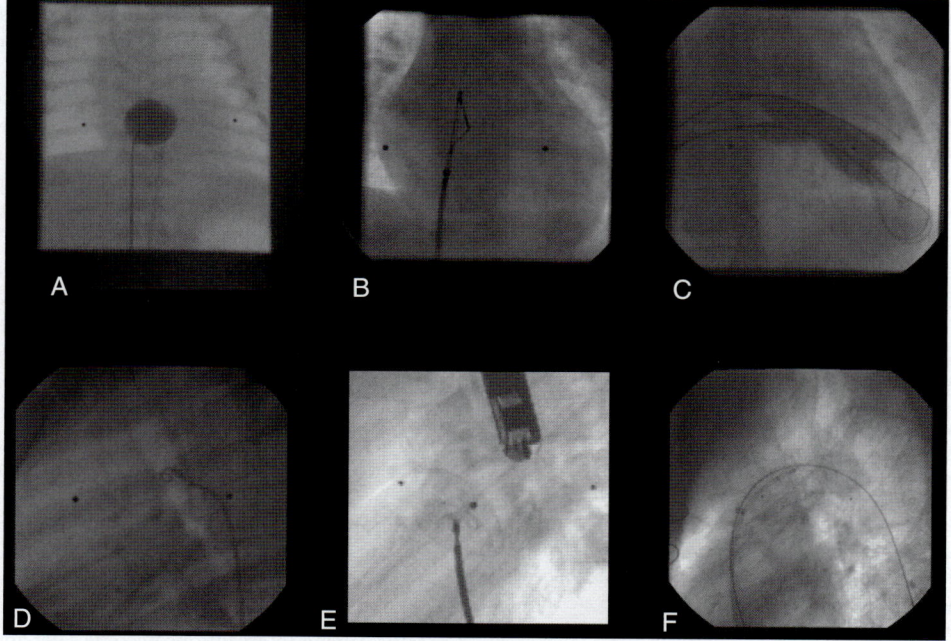

FIGURE 16.36 Several types of interventions are performed in a pediatric cardiac catheterization laboratory. **A,** Balloon atrial septostomy. **B,** Blade atrial septostomy. **C,** Double-balloon mitral valvuloplasty. **D,** Placement of a ductal coil occluder device. **E,** Transcatheter closure of a secundum atrial septal defect. **F,** Pulmonary artery dilation with stent placement.

intervention (hybrid procedures), and catheter-based interventions during fetal life.[266–270]

Interpretation of a Cardiac Catheterization Report

Pressure Data

Atrial pressure tracings are characterized by several waves (*a*, *c*, and *v* waves) and descents (*x* and *y*). Reported values correspond to the *a* and *v* waves and the mean pressures. The right atrial pressure is typically *a* wave dominant. The mean right atrial pressure is normally less than 5 mm Hg. The left atrial pressure tracing is typically *v* wave dominant. The mean left atrial pressure rarely exceeds 8 mm Hg. Abnormal pressure waveforms are often associated with AV valve stenosis, regurgitation, rhythm disturbances, and pericardial disease.

Ventricular pressures are recorded and reported during systole, at end systole, and at end diastole. For the right ventricle, systolic pressure is normally 25 to 30 mm Hg, with end-diastolic pressures of 5 to 7 mm Hg. The systolic pressure in the left ventricle increases with age and should equal the systolic arterial pressure. The end-diastolic pressure is typically less than 10 mm Hg.

The pulmonary artery pressure is reported in terms of systolic, diastolic, and mean pressures. The systolic pulmonary artery pressure in a normal child should be equal to the right ventricular systolic pressure, and the mean pulmonary artery pressure should not exceed 20 mm Hg. The pulmonary artery wedge pressure is obtained by advancing a catheter into a distal vessel until it is occluded, reflecting the left atrial pressure.

The aortic pressure and contour of the tracing depend on the site of interrogation. Typically, there is an increase in the systolic pressure as the catheter navigates toward the peripheral circulation. This phenomenon is known as *pulse wave amplification*.

Pressure gradients, or the pressure differences between two distinct sites, can be measured in several ways (i.e., mean gradient and peak gradient). It is important to consider that several factors may affect their determination. This is significantly influenced by the severity of the obstruction and the ventricular function. Smaller gradients can be seen in patients under sedation or anesthesia.

Shunt Calculations

Shunts are characterized in terms of their direction (e.g., left-to-right, right-to-left, bidirectional) and magnitude. Left-to-right shunts can be quantified based on the pulmonary ($\dot{Q}_{pulm}$) to systemic ($\dot{Q}_{sys}$) blood flow ratio. In the equation, $S_{sys}aO_2$ is the systemic arterial O_2 saturation, $S\bar{v}O_2$ is the mixed venous O_2 saturation, $S_{pulm}vO_2$ is the pulmonary venous O_2 saturation, and $S_{pulm}aO_2$ is the pulmonary arterial O_2 saturation.

$$\frac{\dot{Q}_{pulm}}{\dot{Q}_{sys}} = \frac{(S_{sys}aO_2 - S\bar{v}O_2)}{(S_{pulm}vO_2 - S_{pulm}aO_2)}$$

A $\dot{Q}_{pulm}/\dot{Q}_{sys}$ shunt ratio that exceeds 3 : 1 is considered significant, although smaller ratios can be associated with considerable symptoms.

Cardiac Output Determinations

The volume of blood ejected by the heart into the systemic circulation, or cardiac output, can be derived in several ways. Thermodilution measurements use saline as an indicator to measure pulmonary blood flow. In the absence of intracardiac shunts, this is equivalent to cardiac output (expressed as liters per minute). In the Fick method, oxygen is used as an indicator, and cardiac output is obtained by the application of the following formula:

$$\dot{Q}_{sys} = (L/minute) = \frac{VO_2 (L/minute)}{C_{sys}O_2 - C\bar{v}O_2}$$

In the equation, $\dot{V}O_2$ is the oxygen consumption (assumed or measured), $C_{sys}O_2$ is the systemic arterial O_2 content, and $C\bar{v}O_2$ is the mixed venous O_2 content. The O_2 content = O_2 saturation × $(1.36 \times 10 \times$ hemoglobin concentration).

Vascular Resistances

Resistance represents the change in pressure in the systemic or pulmonary circulation with respect to flow. It is expressed in Wood units (in mm Hg/L per minute) and is usually normalized for body surface area. The systemic vascular resistance (SVR) and pulmonary vascular resistance (PVR) are derived as follows:

$$SVR = (aortic\ mean\ pressure - right\ atrial\ mean\ pressure)/\dot{Q}_{sys}$$
$$PVR = (pulmonary\ artery\ mean\ pressure - pulmonary$$
$$capillary\ wedge\ pressure\ or\ left\ atrial\ pressure)/\dot{Q}_{sys}$$

Perioperative Considerations for Children With Cardiovascular Disease

GENERAL ISSUES

Anesthesia for children with heart disease can be both challenging and daunting because of the following[271]:

- The remarkable spectrum of disease
- The wide range of congenital lesions and their underlying physiologic consequences
- The numerous interventional and surgical options in CHD (Table 16.7), in addition to their hemodynamic implications
- The fact that many parents are unaware of the full extent or details of the child's lesion or abnormalities

To optimally care for these children, the following objectives should be met:

- Familiarity with the cardiovascular defects
- Understanding of the physiologic abnormalities and available therapies
- Recognition of signs of limited reserve, compensatory mechanisms, and perioperative risks[272]
- Ability to identify the potential impact of the proposed intervention/surgical procedure on the child's underlying condition, anticipate if/how it will be tolerated, and be prepared to manage any problems that may arise

This combination of formidable challenges and difficult objectives can be intimidating even for the most experienced clinician. When caring for children with complex cardiovascular disease, an interdisciplinary approach is recommended, allowing for the formulation and execution of optimal individualized management plans. If available, consultation with the child's cardiologist or primary care physician should include inquiries about the details of the child's disease, overall clinical status, past and current medical treatment, prior catheterization or surgical interventions, and presence of residual pathology. The interaction between members of the perioperative team should allow an exchange of information, discussion of concerns, and recommendations that can facilitate patient care and the development of comprehensive care plans.[273] This is particularly important in the management of children with complex pathology.

A complete medical history and focused examination is essential during the preoperative assessment. In addition to evaluating the child's disease processes, overall clinical status, and functional

TABLE 16.7	Surgical Procedures for Congenital Heart Disease	
Procedure	**Description**	**Goal or Result**
Arterial switch (Jatene) operation	Arterial trunks transected above the level of the semilunar valves, relocated to their appropriate respective ventricles, coronary arteries reimplanted into the neoaortic root	Establishes the normal ventriculo-arterial connection (right ventricle to pulmonary artery and left ventricle to aorta) in D-transposition of the great arteries
Atrioventricular septal defect (atrioventricular canal/endocardial cushion defect) repair	Patch closure of atrial and ventricular communications, reconstruction of atrioventricular valves, closure of cleft in left-sided atrioventricular valve	Eliminates the intracardiac shunts
Blalock-Taussig shunt	Communication between innominate or subclavian artery and pulmonary artery; "modified" implies placement of a graft	Allows for or augments pulmonary blood flow
Central shunt, Waterston shunt, Potts shunt, Mee shunt	Communication between the systemic and pulmonary circulations	Allows or increases pulmonary blood flow
Closure of septal defect	Patch or primary closure of communication at the atrial or ventricular level	Eliminates an intracardiac shunt
Coarctation repair	Relief of aortic arch obstruction (various approaches)	Establishes patency across the aortic arch
Damus-Kaye-Stansel procedure	End-to-side anastomosis of main pulmonary artery onto the aorta; necessitates reestablishing pulmonary blood flow through an alternative route (graft from a systemic artery into the pulmonary artery or a right ventricular to pulmonary artery conduit)	Allows unobstructed systemic outflow in the context of single ventricle associated with obstruction to aortic flow or other settings
Division or ligation of patent ductus arteriosus	Obliteration of the communication at the level of the ductus arteriosus	Eliminates shunting at the level of the great arteries
Fontan procedure	Connection that directs inferior vena cava blood into the pulmonary circulation	Separates the pulmonary and systemic circulations in patients with single ventricle physiology; usually the final step in the single-ventricle palliation pathway
Glenn anastomosis (cavopulmonary connection)	Anastomosis between superior vena cava and pulmonary artery (bidirectional implies flow from superior vena cava into both pulmonary arteries)	Provides pulmonary blood flow while unloading the single ventricle; may be the first or intermediate step in the single-ventricle palliation pathway
Konno-Rastan procedure (aortoventriculoplasty)	Enlargement of the left ventricular outflow tract and aortic annulus; defect created in the ventricular septum to enlarge the outflow tract repaired with a large patch	Alleviates subvalvar and valvar aortic obstruction; when the aortic root is replaced by an autologous pulmonary root, it is referred to as a Ross-Konno procedure. Alternatively, cryopreserved homograft tissue can be used in the form of an extended aortic root replacement.
Nikaidoh procedure	Involves reconstruction of left ventricular outflow tract with translocation of aortic root after division of outlet septum and excision of the pulmonary valve, patch closure of ventricular communication, and completion of right ventricular to pulmonary artery anastomosis with pericardial patch	For management of transposition of the great arteries with pulmonary stenosis and a ventricular septal defect.
Norwood procedure (stage I palliation)	Involves aortic reconstruction, an atrial septectomy, and placement of a systemic-to-pulmonary artery shunt (modified Blalock-Taussig shunt) or right ventricular to pulmonary artery conduit (Sano modification)	Addresses systemic outflow tract obstruction by allowing the right ventricle to eject into a reconstructed aorta. Atrial septectomy provides unobstructed drainage of the pulmonary venous return into the right atrium. The systemic-to-pulmonary artery connection supplies the pulmonary blood flow.
Pulmonary artery banding	Constrictive band placed around the main pulmonary artery	Limits excessive pulmonary blood flow
Rastelli operation	Creation of an intracardiac tunnel that allows left ventricular output into the aorta while closing a ventricular septal defect, and placement of a right ventricular conduit to pulmonary artery	Allows the left ventricle to eject solely into the aorta, abolishes intracardiac shunting at the ventricular level, and provides unobstructed pulmonary blood flow. The procedure results in separation of the pulmonary and systemic circulations.
Sano modification of the Norwood procedure	Placement of graft between the right ventricle and main pulmonary artery as an alternative to a modified Blalock-Taussig shunt in the Norwood operation	Provides pulmonary blood flow
Senning or Mustard procedure (atrial switch)	Intraatrial baffle procedure	Allows pulmonary venous blood to be rerouted through the tricuspid valve into the right ventricle (as the systemic chamber that ejects into the aorta). Systemic venous return is channeled across the mitral valve into the left ventricle, which pumps into the main pulmonary artery.

TABLE 16.7	Surgical Procedures for Congenital Heart Disease—cont'd	
Procedure	**Description**	**Goal or Result**
Tetralogy of Fallot repair	Closure of ventricular septal defect and relief of right ventricular outflow tract obstruction	Eliminates intracardiac shunting at the ventricular level and addresses right ventricular outflow tract obstruction (often at several levels)
Truncus arteriosus repair	Closure of the ventricular septal defect and establishment of right ventricular to pulmonary artery continuity (usually with a homograft)	Abolishes intracardiac shunting and restores the normal connection between the ventricles and great arteries
Valvectomy	Valve excision	Relieves valvar obstruction
Valvotomy	Opening of stenotic valve	Relieves valvar obstruction
Valve replacement	Placement of bioprosthetic or mechanical valve	Addresses valvar pathology (obstruction and regurgitation)
Valvuloplasty	Valve repair	Relieves valvar regurgitation and stenosis
Yasui operation	Channels blood from the left ventricle across the ventricular septal defect into a reconstructed aorta (using the native pulmonary valve as the neoaortic valve). Establishes right ventricular to pulmonary artery continuity by means of a conduit.	Provides for a biventricular repair in infants with two adequately sized ventricles and obstruction to systemic outflow.

reserve, this allows appraisal of issues that may affect anesthesia management (e.g., limited vascular access, difficult airway, gastroesophageal reflux, manipulations of pulmonary and systemic blood flow and pressures). Available diagnostic studies (e.g., ECG, chest radiograph, echocardiogram, Holter monitor, cardiac catheterization, MRI, CT) should be reviewed. Depending on the nature of the procedure, complexity of the disease, and potential impact on perioperative outcome, additional evaluation and diagnostic studies may be warranted. In many cases, the anesthesiologist as a perioperative physician plays a major role in determining whether the available information is adequate.

A fundamental goal in the preoperative evaluation is the identification of children who are at increased risk because of cardiac and pulmonary limitations imposed by their cardiovascular disease. After the preoperative visit, the anesthesiologist caring for a child with CHD should understand the pathophysiology of the cardiac defect and implications of any previous interventions. Abnormal indexes that should raise potential concerns include hypoxemia (SpO$_2$ <75%), $\dot{Q}_{pulm}/\dot{Q}_{sys}$ exceeding 3 : 1, outflow tract gradients greater than 50 mm Hg, pulmonary hypertension (i.e., mean pulmonary artery pressure >25 mm Hg), increased pulmonary vascular resistance index (>2 Wood units/m^2), or polycythemia (i.e., hematocrit >60%). Several clinical states may place children at significant risk for severe cardiopulmonary decompensation during anesthesia and surgery: recent congestive heart failure, uncontrolled arrhythmias, severe ventricular dysfunction, unexplained syncope, substantial exercise intolerance, single-ventricle physiology, supravalvular aortic stenosis (Williams syndrome), or any condition associated with significantly impaired cardiac or pulmonary function. For some children, a planned admission to the intensive care unit following the procedure should be discussed with the parents, child, and care team preoperatively.

CLINICAL CONDITION AND STATUS OF PRIOR REPAIR

Children with CHD may require anesthesia care before or after palliation or following definitive procedures. Corrective procedures are those that result in a normal life expectancy and full cardiovascular reserve, and children undergoing these interventions usually require no further medical or surgical treatment. In the strict sense, only a few procedures fulfill these criteria: ligation, division, or occlusion of a PDA and closure of an isolated secundum ASD. Other interventions or surgical procedures can result in repair or correction but not necessarily in normal hemodynamics or life expectancy. The clinician should assume potential limitation in cardiovascular reserve, a need for follow-up, further medical management, and in some cases, additional catheter-based interventions or surgical therapies. In other cases, as in children with palliated CHD, the circulation may still be abnormal. These individuals have been reported to be at greater risk for adverse perioperative events.[24,274–277] Published data from the POCA registry examined anesthesia-related cardiac arrests in children with congenital and acquired heart disease.[154] Cardiac arrests occurred more frequently in children with heart disease than in those children without heart disease. Causes were primarily cardiovascular in nature. These events occurred more frequently in the general operating room, usually during the surgical maintenance phase. The most common anatomic substrate in this setting was that of a single ventricle, particularly those early in the palliation pathway. The overall mortality rate for children with heart disease was greater than those without heart disease, with the greatest mortality rate occurring in children with aortic stenosis (Williams syndrome) and cardiomyopathy.

The effects of previous procedures on the heart and other systems require careful consideration. Problems that can remain or develop after surgical intervention include residual shunts, valvar stenoses or outflow tract obstruction, valvar regurgitation, pulmonary hypertension, arrhythmias, and ventricular dysfunction. Children who require a detailed appraisal of perioperative risks are those with residual significant pathology, suspected or known pulmonary hypertension, single-ventricle physiology, and those after outflow conduit placement, valve replacement, or cardiac transplantation (see Chapters 17, 18, and 22).

Summary

Caring for children with heart disease is a major aspect of pediatric anesthesia practice. The spectrum of cardiovascular disease includes a wide range of structural defects and varied congenital or acquired diseases. The ability to provide optimal perioperative care heavily relies on a clear understanding of the basic pathophysiology of the lesions, familiarity with the commonly used diagnostic modalities and their clinical applications, and medical and surgical treatment options available to affected individuals. In this chapter, we have presented basic concepts in cardiology that can enhance the overall knowledge of the practicing anesthesiologist in pediatric cardiovascular disease.

ACKNOWLEDGMENT

We wish to recognize Dr. Timothy C. Slesnick for his contributions to this chapter in a prior edition.

ANNOTATED REFERENCES

Bai W, Voepel-Lewis T, Malviya S. Hemodynamic changes in children with Down syndrome during and following inhalation induction of anesthesia with sevoflurane. *J Clin Anesth.* 2010;22:592-597.

The retrospective study evaluated whether children with Down syndrome are at increased risk for bradycardia and hypotension during and after sevoflurane induction. The investigation reported a significantly higher prevalence and degree of bradycardia in children with Down syndrome. Despite these findings, there were no differences between Down syndrome and control groups in the prevalence of hypotension or pharmacologic interventions.

Brown ML, DiNardo JA, Odegard KC. Patients with single ventricle physiology undergoing noncardiac surgery are at high risk for adverse events. *Paediatr Anaesth.* 2015;25(8):846-851.

The retrospective chart review examined outcomes of anesthetics in children with single ventricle physiology undergoing noncardiac surgery. There was no mortality in a high-risk subgroup of palliated children; however, adverse events associated with anesthetic care occurred in almost 12% of children.

Cordina RL, Celermajer DS. Chronic cyanosis and vascular function: implications for patients with cyanotic congenital heart disease. *Cardiol Young.* 2010;20:242-253.

This excellent article reviews the effects of chronic cyanosis and associated alterations in blood vessel structure and function, with an emphasis on the endothelium and important implications for patients with cyanotic congenital heart disease.

Matisoff AJ, Olivieri L, Schwartz JM, et al. Risk assessment and anesthetic management of patients with Williams syndrome: a comprehensive review. *Paediatr Anaesth.* 2015;25(12):1207-1215.

The article provides an overview of the clinical manifestations of Williams syndrome, proposes a method to estimate anesthetic risk, and outlines recommendations for periprocedural care of affected children.

Rossano JW, Shaddy RE. Heart failure in children: etiology and treatment. *J Pediatr.* 2014;165(2):228-233.

This comprehensive manuscript addresses important aspects of pediatric heart failure, including epidemiology, diagnosis, risk stratification, and current therapies.

A complete reference list can be found online at ExpertConsult.com.

Anesthesia for Children Undergoing Heart Surgery

17

ANGUS MCEWAN AND VASCO LAGINHA ROLO

Preoperative Evaluation

Congenital heart disease (CHD) accounts for nearly one-third of major congenital abnormalities, with an estimated worldwide birth prevalence of 9.1 cases per 1000 live births.[1] In the United States, this represents the birth of 40,000 babies with CHD each year.[2] Although CHD can occur in isolation, it is often associated with other cardiovascular and extracardiac malformations.[3] The incidence of CHD is increased in the presence of other congenital abnormalities, in children with chromosomal disorders such as trisomy 21, as well as in siblings of other children with CHD.[4] As diagnostic techniques have improved, many children with CHD are diagnosed antenatally or early postnatally.[5,6] In association with improvements in diagnostic ability, surgical techniques, and perioperative care, most centers have shifted their practices to definitively repair the defects earlier, with many undergoing corrective surgery as neonates.[7,8] Overall, about one-half of all children with CHD undergo cardiac surgery in the first year of life, and about 25% undergo surgery in the first month of life.[9,10]

The perioperative management of children with complex cardiac defects requires a dedicated team of surgeons, cardiologists, anesthesiologists, intensivists, perfusionists, and nurses. Professionals caring for these children are challenged by some of the greatest physiologic aberrations encountered in clinical medicine. The anesthesiologists responsible for the care of these children require a comprehensive understanding of cardiac anatomy, physiology, and pathophysiology and must be able to adapt to each nuance of rapidly changing pathophysiology as it is encountered.

In addition to treating children with CHD, the pediatric cardiac anesthesiologist may also be responsible for the care of adults with CHD, whose underlying cardiac problems differ substantially from those in children.[11] The success of pediatric cardiac surgery has resulted in an ever-increasing population with "grown-up CHD" (GUCHD), as most children with CHD are now expected to survive into adulthood.[12] The ideal approach for this group of patients is to care for them in specialist units.[13,14] Although these GUCHD centers are increasing in number and capacity, they are currently unable to provide universal coverage. In the meantime, the care of these patients falls to the most qualified physicians, including the pediatric cardiac anesthesiologist. Along with their underlying CHD, these patients often present with comorbidities of old age, thus presenting additional challenges.

When assessing children with complex cardiac defects, we rely to a large extent on echocardiography and magnetic resonance imaging (MRI) to acquire diagnostic data. Although fewer children are subjected to diagnostic angiography today, more interventional cardiac catheterization procedures are being performed. Many conditions such as patent ductus arteriosus (PDA), atrial septal defects (ASDs), and ventricular septal defects (VSDs) that would previously have been treated surgically are now treated in the angiography suite by interventional cardiologists. Other interventions include dilating arteries with balloon catheters with and without stents and coiling of aberrant or excessive collateral vessels. The pulmonary artery is commonly balloon dilated and stented, and coarctation of the aorta is treated similarly by balloon dilation. Stenotic valves are also commonly dilated. These procedures have led to the risk of patients being transferred emergently from the angiography suite to the operating room.[15] For the individual child, there has been a dramatic decrease in morbidity as increasing numbers of conditions are treated in the angiography suite, but the risks of complications that occur in the angiography suite have increased as more complex procedures are performed (see Chapter 22).

THE PREOPERATIVE VISIT AND EVALUATION

The preoperative visit is an important part of the overall management of anesthesia for children with CHD.[16] The preoperative visit has several aims:

- Medical assessment
- Prescribing premedication
- Providing information
- Creating a relationship with the child and family
- Formulating an anesthetic plan

Medical Assessment

The anesthesiologist must have a clear and detailed understanding of the cardiac anatomy and pathophysiology, the surgery to be undertaken, as well as any associated congenital abnormalities or medical conditions. The medical assessment includes collation of information from the history, physical examination, and review of imaging and laboratory data. Most diagnostic information is obtained from the medical record. Particular attention should be paid to the echocardiographic, angiographic, MRI, and other imaging data; the chest radiograph; and the electrocardiogram. Many centers have joint cardiac conferences where decisions about treatment are discussed in a multidisciplinary forum. Reports from these meetings are valuable in the preoperative assessment.

In addition to gathering this specific diagnostic information, a directed history and physical examination should be performed to assess the overall condition of the child. Attention should focus upon assessing the presence and degree of cardiac failure, cyanosis, or risk of pulmonary hypertension. Information about previous surgical procedures should also be sought, as it may alter access to the central circulation and placement of invasive monitors. The general nutritional state of the child should be assessed; poor growth and development may be a sign of severe CHD. Other information should be sought that may have a bearing on the anesthetic plan. For example, repeat surgery and redo sternotomy may indicate the need to establish peripheral cardiopulmonary bypass (CPB) before surgically accessing the heart and great vessels for central CPB cannulation. This has a bearing on line placement because either jugulo-carotid or femoro-femoral bypass may be required; the appropriate area should be preserved for CPB cannulation and avoided for line placement. If the child received aprotinin within the preceding 12 months, another dose should not be given because the risk of anaphylaxis is increased within this period (Trasylol package insert: Bayer Pharmaceuticals Corporation, West Haven, CT. December 2006).[17]

The type of surgery to be performed is important. For example, if a Blalock-Taussig shunt is placed on the left, the arterial line should not be placed in the left arm because the trace will be lost or distorted during subclavian cross-clamping. If a superior cavopulmonary anastomosis (Glenn shunt) is planned, a short internal jugular catheter can be useful to monitor pulmonary artery pressure, but it should be removed early in the postoperative period so as not to risk the formation of thrombosis in the superior vena cava (SVC), with its potential disastrous consequences.

Good veins should be sought and marked for the application of local anesthetic cream. This is useful in sick children even if an inhalational induction is planned because it allows placement of a venous cannula during a very light plane of anesthesia and avoids myocardial depression from large concentrations of inhalation anesthetics.

Prescribing Premedication

The use of sedative premedication can be useful, but this practice varies widely. Numerous medications and routes of administration may be used, and ample recommendations exist, but the use of premedication is often dictated by local preferences and not always evidence-based. There is heightened awareness and increasing concerns about the possibility of postoperative behavioral problems resulting from inadequate preparation and handling the uncooperative child preoperatively.[18] It is important for of the pediatric anesthesiologist to reduce perioperative anxiety in children by both nonpharmacologic and pharmacologic methods.[19] While prescribing premedication is best assessed on an individual basis, some general considerations apply to most children who present for pediatric heart surgery. Premedication for infants younger than 6 months of age is usually unnecessary. Premedication for older, healthy children who show little anxiety and with whom good preoperative rapport can be established is also often unnecessary. However, older children, particularly those who have undergone previous surgery, have fears about anesthesia and surgery. Although it is important to address their fears, sedative premedication may play a pivotal role in achieving adequate anxiolysis for parental separation and a smooth induction. Premedication in children with severe congestive heart failure is probably best used judiciously, if at all, as the effects of the usually prescribed doses may be unpredictable. On the contrary, children with dynamic obstruction to the left or right ventricular outflow tracts often benefit from sedative premedication because crying and struggling during induction may worsen obstruction. Cyanotic children (e.g., those with tetralogy of Fallot [TOF]), may develop increasing cyanosis if agitated during induction. However, it is important to monitor cyanotic children after premedication and provide supplemental oxygen as needed because they exhibit a blunted ventilatory response to hypoxia.[20,21] In the United States, supplemental premedication is sometimes administered under the direct supervision of the anesthesiologist in the preoperative facility, providing for a calm child and gentle separation from the parents. In the United Kingdom, where induction of anesthesia takes place in a dedicated anesthesia room, parents are present until after the induction, often making additional premedication unnecessary.

The most common premedication is oral midazolam (0.5-1.0 mg/kg).[22] However, the effect of midazolam may be unpredictable as it may cause paradoxical reactions, with agitation and dysphoria instead of anxiolysis and sedation. Numerous other medications including ketamine, clonidine, temazepam, chloral hydrate, and dexmedetomidine have been effective premedications in children with CHD.[23]

Giving Information

Providing information to the parents and to the child in a manner that is nonthreatening and appropriate to the child's age and developmental stage is a key element of the preoperative visit. This information includes the use of sedative premedication, fasting times, the type of induction, the type and likely position of invasive lines, the need for a stay in an intensive care unit (ICU) postoperatively, and the expected length of that stay. The use of other monitors such as transesophageal echocardiography (TEE) should be outlined and any contraindications identified, along with the probability that a blood transfusion may be necessary. Questions about the risk of anesthesia and surgery should be addressed to the satisfaction of the parents (see Chapter 4).

Creating Rapport With the Child and Family

By creating a good relationship with the family, the anesthesiologist can reduce the anxiety of the child and the parents. The family develops a sense of trust, which can improve their hospital experience. A good rapport with the child may also facilitate a smoother anesthetic induction, and the use of specific nonpharmacologic techniques of reducing perioperative anxiety can be tailored to the child's individual preferences and possible previous experiences.

Formulating an Anesthetic Plan

After assessing the child, it is possible to formulate a detailed anesthetic plan. The anesthesiologist should have acquired a complete understanding of the child's heart defect and its hemodynamic consequences, as well as any comorbidities. The detailed anesthetic plan consists of a choice of anesthetic agents, techniques, ventilatory management and inotropic/vasoactive support to attain a set of appropriate hemodynamic goals for the individual patient.

UPPER RESPIRATORY TRACT INFECTION AND CARDIAC SURGERY

Otherwise healthy children undergoing elective noncardiac surgery in the presence of an upper respiratory tract infection (URI) are more likely to suffer respiratory complications (Table 17.1). These complications typically are minor, are easily managed, and usually result in minimal morbidity[24-26]; the decision to proceed with noncardiac surgery in a child with a URI is made on an individual basis (see Chapter 4).[27-29]

The decision to proceed with cardiac surgery in children with a URI may be difficult. Although children with cardiac failure are prone to multiple URIs, they may also have signs that can mimic URIs. Surgery may be relatively urgent, and postponing surgery could increase the risk to the child. Cardiac surgery in children with URIs is likely to increase the duration of stay in the ICU and prolong the duration of mechanical ventilation, although overall hospital stay may not be prolonged. Proceeding with surgery increases the incidence of atelectasis and postoperative bacterial infections. However, neither the mortality rates (4.2% with URIs vs. 1.6% without URIs) nor long-term sequelae in children with URIs who undergo cardiac surgery are significantly increased.[30] The children with URIs were significantly younger and smaller, which may account in part for the greater but statistically insignificant increased mortality rate; this should be taken into

TABLE 17.1	Diagnosis of Upper Respiratory Tract Infection

At least two of the following signs plus confirmation by a parent:
  Rhinorrhea
  Sore or scratchy throat
  Sneezing
  Nasal congestion
  Malaise
  Cough
  Fever >100.4°F (38°C)

Data from Schreiner MS, O'Hara I, Markakis DA, Politis GD. Do children who experience laryngospasm have an increased risk of upper respiratory tract infection? *Anesthesiology* 1996;85:475–480.

consideration when contemplating whether to proceed with surgery. Children who are scheduled for a Glenn shunt or completion of the Fontan circulation may be at particular risk because an increase in pulmonary vascular resistance (PVR) can adversely affect surgical outcome. It is prudent to postpone surgery in a child with a URI who is scheduled for elective cardiac surgery. If the surgery is urgent, discussion with the surgical team is required to correctly assess the risks and benefits to the child.

Perioperative Challenges in Pediatric Cardiac Anesthesia

CYANOSIS

Cyanotic children compensate for chronic hypoxia with increased erythropoiesis, increased circulating blood volume, vasodilation, and metabolic adjustments of factors such as the circulating concentration of 2,3-diphosphoglycerate (2,3-DPG). These changes facilitate greater delivery of oxygen to tissues. The increase in blood viscosity with polycythemia increases vascular resistance and sludging, which may result in renal, pulmonary, and cerebral thromboses, especially in dehydrated children.[31-33] Long periods without oral intake preoperatively and postoperatively should be avoided in children with polycythemia, unless adequate intravenous (IV) hydration is provided.

PVR increases more than systemic vascular resistance (SVR) when the hematocrit increases, further decreasing pulmonary blood flow in children who already have a compromised pulmonary circulation. Coagulopathies are common in children with cyanotic CHD and may adversely affect surgical hemostasis.[34,35] Furthermore, chronic hypoxemia can cause important changes in vascular function and structure, some of which are maladaptive and probably contribute to impaired cardiovascular performance.[36] When the hematocrit exceeds 65%, excessive viscosity impairs microvascular perfusion and outweighs the advantages of increased oxygen-carrying capacity. Reduction of red blood cell volume can correct the coagulopathy and improve hemodynamics when increases in hematocrit are extreme.[37] However, treatment of hyperviscosity in patients with cyanotic heart disease is controversial[38,39]; guidelines for managing adults with CHD suggest the judicious use of phlebotomy and address the issue of potential complications.[40]

INTRACARDIAC SHUNTING

In CHD, much of the pathophysiology involves communications between chambers or vessels that are normally separate, resulting in shunting of blood between ventricles, atria, the great arteries, or a combination of these, depending on the nature of the lesion. Management of shunting during anesthesia is a major concern that requires an understanding of the factors that control shunting.

Restrictive and Unrestrictive Shunts

When communications are small, the size of the defect limits shunting and considerations of relative PVR and SVR become correspondingly less important in determining the degree of shunting. When there is a large pressure differential at the same level of the circulation on either side of a communication, the communication is restrictive. Flow is limited across the defect, and other factors that determine shunt flow become less important. This is usually the situation in children with mild heart disease that is asymptomatic or minimally symptomatic, such as small ASDs and VSDs or a small PDA.

Dependent Shunting During Anesthesia

In children with dependent shunts, the direction and degree of intracardiac shunting are determined by the circulatory dynamics. Control of circulatory dynamics to minimize the shunt is a major goal of anesthesia management. Because shunting depends on the relationship between SVR and PVR, anesthesia management often revolves around control of relative vascular resistances.

In children with dependent right-to-left shunts, the shunt increases when SVR decreases or PVR increases. In children with dependent left-to-right shunts, the shunt increases when SVR increases and PVR decreases. In children with bidirectional or balanced shunting, changes in vascular resistance increase the net shunt away from the side with increased vascular resistance.

For practical purposes, acute increases in left-to-right shunts during anesthesia are of clinical importance in several situations. A substantial steal of systemic blood flow by the pulmonary circulation can occur in conditions with unrestrictive, significant, left-to-right shunting such as atrioventricular (AV) canal, truncus arteriosus, and hypoplastic left heart syndrome. Left-to-right shunting is well tolerated, except when pulmonary steal leads to systemic hypotension, increasing acidosis from poor systemic end-organ perfusion or insufficient coronary perfusion. Shunting from right to left, because it is accompanied by at least some degree of arterial oxygen desaturation, is more frequently a problem during anesthesia.

IMPAIRED HEMOSTASIS

Hemostasis is impaired after bypass in infants and children to a greater extent compared with adults. The initiation of CPB triggers contact activation of the hemostatic systems, with ongoing coagulation and fibrinolysis, as well as the initiation of a systemic inflammatory response, both contributing to the coagulopathy. In infants and children, these effects are further compounded by a larger size of the CPB circuit relative to patient size. In this patient population, impaired hemostasis after bypass results from a combination of immature coagulation factor synthesis, hemodilution after bypass, and a complex interaction involving consumption of clotting factors and platelets. At birth, the levels of vitamin K–dependent coagulation factors in healthy, full-term neonates are only 40% to 66% of adult values. During the first month of life, these levels increase to 53% to 90% of adult values (see also Chapter 2).[41,42] However, in children with CHD, especially those with cyanosis or systemic hypoperfusion, coagulation factors often continue to be depressed owing to impaired hepatic protein synthesis. Although antithrombin III levels are also low, true heparin resistance is rare in infants because of parallel decreases in coagulation factors.

At the onset of CPB, the introduction of the prime volume, which is two to three times greater than the child's blood volume, dilutes the clotting factors, particularly fibrinogen to 50% and platelets to 30% of their prebypass values. This degree of dilution occurs even when the pump circuit is primed with whole blood. Greater dilution may occur when packed red blood cells (PRBCs) are used in the priming volume. At the conclusion of neonatal bypass, the activity of clotting factors is often extremely low, the fibrinogen concentration is frequently less than 100 mg/dL, and the platelet count is only 50,000 to 80,000/mm^3.[43-45] In addition to these quantitative changes, functional changes in the platelets occur during bypass. Extracorporeal circulation causes a loss of platelet adhesion receptors, activation of platelets, and formation of leukocyte-platelet conjugates. Platelet adhesion receptors in cyanotic children are depressed to a greater extent than in those with

acyanotic cardiac defects. Heparin also impairs platelet function independent of CPB.[46,47]

Cardiac surgery is associated with significant activation of the fibrinolytic system.[48,49] Inadequate heparin concentrations during CPB may also contribute to postoperative bleeding because inadequate anticoagulation may allow continued activation of the hemostatic pathways. Ongoing activation of the coagulation cascade causes the consumption of platelets and clotting factors. The standard measurement of anticoagulation for bypass, the activated clotting time (ACT), shows a poor correlation with heparin concentrations (usually measured using the surrogate, anti-Xa) in children undergoing CPB.[50] In one study, the use of individualized heparin monitoring and heparin titration was associated with larger doses of heparin but smaller doses of protamine for antagonism.[51] Activation of the clotting cascade using that heparin-protamine regimen is also reduced, thus potentially decreasing bleeding in the postoperative period.[51-53] As a result of this multifactorial coagulopathy, blood loss is a greater problem in children than in adults and is a particular problem in neonates and small infants (see Chapter 19).[54]

Strategies to Reduce Bleeding After Bypass

In an effort to normalize factors and platelets to effective concentrations, some medical centers use fresh whole blood in the cardiopulmonary circuit prime. In adult patients and in an in vitro aggregation study, transfusion of fresh whole blood provided equal or greater hemostatic and functional benefit when compared with transfusion of platelet concentrates. In children, transfusion with fresh whole blood less than 48 hours from harvest reduced the blood loss compared with transfusion of reconstituted whole blood (e.g., packed erythrocytes, fresh frozen plasma [FFP], and platelets).[55] Other studies have shown that the use of fresh whole blood in the prime in neonatal and pediatric cardiac surgery reduced transfusion requirements[56,57] and improved outcomes.[58] However, the benefits of using fresh whole blood to prime the CPB circuit have been questioned in at least one study, which showed no advantage from its use and an increased length of stay in the ICU, as well as increased perioperative fluid overload in the group treated with fresh whole blood.[59] It is possible that different pediatric patient populations (e.g., age, cyanotic vs. noncyanotic CHD) derive different benefits from the use of fresh whole blood. Until this matter is clarified, it is difficult to make clear recommendations about its use in pediatric cardiac surgery. Moreover, fresh whole blood is often difficult to obtain. The units must be refrigerated for 24 to 48 hours while donor screening is performed, and storage causes significant platelet injury. Insistence on fresh whole blood places tremendous pressures on the transfusion service and donor center to coordinate the matching of donor types with recipient needs. Furthermore, in the presence of suitable, simpler alternatives to this blood component management strategy, it is likely that a considerable number of centers will continue to use individual blood component administration to treat bleeding and coagulopathy in children undergoing heart surgery.

Therefore individual component therapy remains the standard of practice in most institutions. In neonates and small infants with dilutional coagulopathy, platelets should be given in combination with cryoprecipitate to correct the defect in clotting. An initial dose of platelets (10 mL/kg) may need to be repeated. Platelets are usually administered if bleeding persists and the platelet count is less than 100,000/mm^3.[60] Cryoprecipitate contains high concentrations of fibrinogen, factor VIII, von Willebrand factor, and factor XIII. Fibrinogen and von Willebrand factor are required for platelet adhesion and aggregation to occur. Platelet adhesion and aggregation are the fundamental first steps in primary hemostasis (see Chapters 10 and 12). The subsequent step of platelet degranulation switches on the entire coagulation cascade and cannot take place without adhesion and aggregation.[61] Administration of FFP, which is not evidence-based for this type of coagulopathy, may excessively dilute the red cell mass and platelets.[62]

Transfusion guidelines have been described for adults and have been shown to reduce postoperative bleeding and transfusion requirements.[63,64] Although similar guidelines have not been as forthcoming for children in whom the practice frequently seems to be more empirical, there is a growing body of evidence that point-of-care (POC) monitoring of hemostasis is useful to guide specific blood component therapy in children undergoing heart surgery.[65] In a surgical context, the time it takes to return routine coagulation tests is often too long for clinical decision making. Consequently, POC platelet count and viscoelastic monitoring of coagulation such as thromboelastography and thromboelastometry are being increasingly used to make timely informed decisions about blood product administration.[66] The use of transfusion algorithms in pediatric cardiac surgery has reduced blood product requirements and bleeding[67,68]; however, further work is needed to produce well-validated guidelines for monitoring and treating bleeding in children undergoing heart surgery.

Antifibrinolytics

The antifibrinolytics used in pediatric cardiac surgery include aprotinin, ε-aminocaproic acid (EACA) and tranexamic acid (TXA). EACA and TXA are lysine analogs that reduce bleeding after cardiac surgery in adults and children,[69,70] with apparent similar efficacy and safety.[71–73] Doses of EACA and TXA for pediatric cardiac surgery have yet to be clearly established. Furthermore, in view of the disproportion between circulating blood volume and CPB prime volume, a drug target concentration that differs between neonates and children, as well as other differences in pharmacokinetics, suggest that different dosing schemes should be used in neonates and smaller children compared with older children.[74–76]

Aprotinin is a serine protease inhibitor no longer available in many countries, and with only very limited availability in others, after its marketing license was withdrawn because of safety concerns. In fact, despite having been studied thoroughly in adults, its use remains a cause for great concern. Early evidence demonstrated that aprotinin reduces bleeding, reduces the time taken to extubation, shortens ICU stay, and reduces overall mortality rates.[77] However, subsequent studies have contradicted these earlier findings.[78] The same volume of evidence has not been published for children, although several studies suggest that it is effective in reducing bleeding and that it reduces the duration of postoperative mechanical ventilation.[34,79–81] An increased risk of renal failure or stroke in adults undergoing revascularization surgery has been reported.[82] The same investigators reported an increase in the 5-year mortality rate for adults after the use of aprotinin in revascularization surgery, mostly resulting from stroke and myocardial infarction.[83] Aprotinin has increased the 30-day mortality rate by as much as one-third compared with TXA or EACA.[78] However, it appears that the early data regarding increased death rates have not been supported by a subsequent study and that the benefits may outweigh risks in specific populations.[84] While aprotinin use in adults is still surrounded by significant controversy, taking into account the differences in pathophysiology and underlying risk factors, it seems plausible that data about

increased mortality from stroke and myocardial infarction have only limited relevance for the pediatric population. Similarly, it appears unlikely that the risk of renal failure associated with the use of aprotinin in children is the same as it is in adults, despite some concerns about its propensity to cause acute kidney injury (AKI) in children,[85] which another study failed to demonstrate.[86] An important additional safety consideration pertains to the risk of severe hypersensitivity reactions. The reported incidence of side effects in children varies. Even though anaphylaxis seems to be infrequent in pediatric patients after primary exposure, the risk of such a severe reaction is increased after reexposure, particularly if it occurs within 12 months after the most recent prior aprotinin exposure.[17,87] This has led the manufacturer to issue a black box warning for aprotinin reexposure within 1 year of a prior exposure. The Food and Drug Administration (FDA) has also recommended that aprotinin should be administered only in the operative setting when CPB can be started quickly, in the event of a severe reaction. Uncertainty about the relative safety profiles of aprotinin and the lysine analogs is met with similar considerations about the effectiveness of these different drugs. Whereas there is some evidence that EACA or TXA are at least as effective as aprotinin,[88,89] research has also suggested that aprotinin use may decrease the output of the chest drain,[90] effect superior blood-sparing effect,[91] as well as confer differences in other outcomes such as cytokine activation or early indexes of postoperative recovery.[92] In fact, it appears that aprotinin may have unique antiinflammatory properties, which may benefit pediatric patients.[93] Further research is needed to clarify issues concerning safety and relative effectiveness of the two classes of drugs, as well as proving benefits and improve effective dosing schemes in specific patient populations (see Chapter 20).

Topical Agents

The use of topical agents to promote clot formation and reduce bleeding after cardiac surgery is common. The most frequently used topical agents are fibrin sealants. Fibrin sealants mimic the stages of the blood coagulation process. Unlike the synthetic adhesives, they are biocompatible.[94] Fibrin sealants are usually sourced from plasma components, and most contain virally inactivated human fibrinogen and thrombin with different quantities of factor XIII, antifibrinolytic agents, and calcium.[95] When the fibrinogen and thrombin are mixed during the application process, the fibrinogen is converted to fibrin monomers. This results in the formation of a semirigid fibrin clot. By mimicking the later stages of the coagulation process, these sealants stop bleeding and assist in wound healing.[94] They have significantly reduced bleeding in children undergoing heart surgery.[96]

Ultrafiltration

Ultrafiltration is a process that results in the production of an ultrafiltrate by means of convection forces and a hydrostatic pressure gradient across a semipermeable membrane. Thus free water and low–molecular-weight substances are removed from a child during and after CPB. It provides many benefits, including increasing the hematocrit, concentrating the clotting factors and platelets, increasing blood pressure, reducing PVR, and removing inflammatory mediators in the ultrafiltrate. It has significantly reduced bleeding after cardiac surgery in children.[97-99]

Desmopressin

Desmopressin acts by increasing plasma concentrations of factor VIII and von Willebrand factor (see also Chapters 10 and 12). It has been effective in reducing bleeding after CPB in adult cardiac surgery[100] and its use is indicated in specific subgroups of patients.[101-103] Unfortunately, studies in children failed to demonstrate a similar effectiveness in reducing bleeding or transfusion requirements.[104]

Anesthesia Management for Surgery Requiring Cardiopulmonary Bypass

MONITORING

Noninvasive monitoring during pediatric cardiac surgery includes pulse oximetry, five-lead electrocardiography, an automated blood pressure cuff, a precordial or esophageal stethoscope, continuous airway manometry, inspired and expired capnography, anesthetic gas and oxygen analysis, multiple-site temperature measurement, and volumetric urine collection. The pulse oximeter is especially important when managing children with congenital cardiac disease. At least two probes should be placed on different limbs in the event that one fails during the procedure. In children with cyanotic heart disease, conventional pulse oximetry overestimates arterial oxygen saturation as saturation decreases[105-108]; this error tends to be exacerbated in the presence of severe hypoxemia.[109] When monitoring children with a shunt across the ductus arteriosus, a probe should be placed on the right upper limb to measure preductal oxygenation, and a second probe should be placed on a toe to measure postductal oxygenation (children with a right-sided aortic arch may require the probe to be placed on a left upper limb). Children undergoing repair of coarctation of the aorta should be monitored with a pulse oximeter on the right upper limb, because it may be the only reliable monitor during the repair, and blood pressure cuffs should be placed before and after the coarctation. These two cuffs may be cycled and the differential documented before and after surgical correction.

Monitoring end-tidal carbon dioxide tension ($PETCO_2$) is of value in most children. However, in children with cyanotic-shunting cardiac lesions, the $PETCO_2$ measurement may be less reflective of $PaCO_2$ because of ventilation-perfusion mismatching.[110-112] Arterial blood gases are the most accurate measure of the adequacy of ventilation and oxygenation. To provide rapid decision making, it is helpful to have the blood gas analysis machine located in or near the cardiac operating room.[113,114]

Monitoring ionized calcium concentrations is essential during surgical procedures in which significant quantities of citrated blood are infused rapidly or when entire blood volumes are replaced. Neonates are particularly prone to disturbances in their ionized calcium concentration when citrated whole blood, FFP, or platelets are infused. Those with limited cardiac reserve tolerate ionized hypocalcemia poorly because of their greater sensitivity to the myocardial effects of citrate infusion (see Chapter 12).[115] In isolation, the total serum calcium concentration is misleading.

Temperature monitoring during CPB is a critical guide to adequate brain cooling and to appropriate rewarming before separation from bypass. Because it is not practical to measure brain temperature directly, surrogate measuring sites including the tympanic membrane, nasopharyngeal, and rectum have been used. The nasopharyngeal site most closely matches true brain temperature and is the site at which temperature is most often monitored. The tympanic and rectal sites tend to overestimate the brain temperature.[116] Measurement of skin temperature gives an indication about peripheral perfusion and provides information about adequate peripheral rewarming.

After induction of anesthesia, an arterial catheter should be placed in children who will undergo CPB. The radial artery may be percutaneously cannulated with relative ease, even in infants. In neonates, the femoral arteries are frequently used for arterial access, and the axillary arteries may also be used. The radial, femoral, and axillary arteries all seem to constitute suitable sites for arterial cannulation and invasive blood pressure monitoring, with complication rates similar to those in adults.[117,118] The brachial artery is generally avoided because it is an end artery, lacking collateral circulation, although one retrospective series of 200 children reported complication rates similar to other arterial sites.[119] Catheters placed in the dorsalis pedis or posterior tibial artery often provide inaccurate hemodynamic data, especially after separation from bypass, and it may become difficult to sample blood for laboratory testing. In the rare circumstance that peripheral arterial cannulation cannot be accomplished percutaneously, consideration should be given to obtaining arterial access by the cutdown method; alternatively, the surgeon may place a catheter in the internal mammary artery after sternotomy, and a sterile monitoring line may be passed over the drapes.

Central venous catheters are very useful for both central venous pressure monitoring and as a safe, reliable route for the administration of inotropes or vasopressors as well as potentially venoirritant solutions. For cardiac surgical procedures, there are two commonly used methods of obtaining central access. The decision of which to use may be determined in part by institutional bias. In the first method, the cardiac surgeons expose the heart quickly and have it available for inspection and estimation of filling pressures. Central lines can be readily established from the surgical field and handed off to the anesthesia team. These transthoracic central lines are useful but carry a small amount of risk.[120,121] The second method is percutaneous insertion of central venous lines via the subclavian or internal jugular vein.[122-124] This route is particularly useful for long, complex procedures, especially when access to the infant is limited or the heart is not exposed. It is important to appreciate that the internal jugular or subclavian route may fail or be associated with pneumothorax, hemorrhage, and hematoma formation after puncture of major arteries.[125,126] Cannulation of the external jugular vein may avoid some of these serious complications when the catheter can be successfully threaded into the central circulation.[127] Increasingly, ultrasound-guided techniques are being used to establish central venous access (see also Chapter 49). In the United Kingdom, the use of ultrasound for the placement of these lines is recommended by the National Institute of Clinical Excellence (NICE); ultrasound is used routinely for the placement of central lines.

In children with unrestrictive VSDs or ASDs, including hearts with a single ventricle or single atrium, central venous pressure is identical to left ventricular filling pressure. Cannulation of vessels that drain into the SVC should be approached with caution in children with univentricular anatomy who may undergo the Fontan procedure, because thrombosis of the SVC can be a devastating complication. In these children, the femoral veins may be the preferred sites for central venous access. Left-sided central venous lines in the SVC territory should also generally be avoided in cardiac patients. There is a greater risk of erosion and perforation from central venous catheters placed through the left internal jugular or left subclavian veins. Furthermore, in up to 10% of patients with CHD, these veins join a persistent left SVC that most often drains into the coronary sinus or left atrium, both undesirable locations for a central venous catheter tip.[128-130]

Percutaneously inserted pulmonary arterial catheters in children with intracardiac defects usually provide information that is not substantively different from that of a simple central line, are difficult to insert without fluoroscopy, and may not provide meaningful measurements of cardiac output. As a result, they are rarely used in pediatric cardiac patients. In circumstances that would be deemed useful, it is probably preferable to insert them surgically. In some complex CHDs and procedures in which postoperative left ventricular dysfunction is expected, it may be valuable to have continuous monitoring of pressures in the left heart. Such measurements are usually obtained via an LA pressure monitoring line inserted by the surgical team.[131-133]

Transesophageal Echocardiography

Use of perioperative echocardiography has become the standard of care in the United States for both adults[134-137] and children undergoing heart surgery.[138-140] In adult practice, anesthesiologists usually perform the transesophageal echocardiography (TEE), but in children, the TEE is more commonly performed by a pediatric cardiologist. This may reflect the increased complexity of congenital lesions and the difficulty in accurately assessing these lesions and their repairs. TEE is cost-effective[141] since its use can have a significant impact on surgical and medical management. In one study, a second bypass run was undertaken in 7.3% of cases based on the findings of the TEE, surgical alteration in the management in 12.7% and medical alteration in 18.5% of cases. Pediatric cardiac anesthesiologists usually can perform TEE before and after bypass if they have received adequate training.[142]

The introduction of small probes with multiplane capability has greatly increased the use of TEE, even in infants and neonates.[143,144] In 1999, a survey of centers in the United States indicated that 93% used intraoperative echocardiography and that all but one used TEE.[145] The American Society of Echocardiography and the Society of Cardiovascular Anesthesiologists have published guidelines for performing a comprehensive intraoperative TEE in adults[137] and children.[139]

Although the use of TEE in children is generally safe, complications do occur and may be more common in small infants.[146] Complications include damage to the mouth, tongue, oropharynx, esophagus, and stomach. Other complications include hemodynamic disturbance as a result of compression of the left atrium or other structures; erroneous invasive blood pressure monitoring may result if the compressed structure is an artery proximal to the arterial line insertion site. Interference with the airway also occurs in a small number of cases. This includes inadvertent extubation, right main-stem bronchus intubation, and compression of the tracheal tube. However, the overall incidence is small, approximately 2%.[147] Information gathered from the TEE examination takes place before and after bypass and may be divided broadly into two categories: hemodynamic assessment with monitoring and structural diagnostic information. Hemodynamic information includes information about ventricular function and filling.[148] Diagnostic information relates to confirmation of preoperative findings and assessment of the surgical repair.

Near-Infrared Spectroscopy

Near-infrared spectroscopy (NIRS) allows real-time monitoring of tissue oxygenation. This technology is based on the principle of optical spectrophotometry, making use of the fact that body tissues are relatively transparent to light in the near-infrared wavelength range. The majority of NIRS monitors use reflectance-mode NIRS, in which a region underlying the sensor is interrogated by a transmitter optode and a receiving sensor. The value obtained is a reflection of the underlying heterogeneous tissue area, composed of arteries, veins, and capillaries, as well as other nonvascular tissues. Even though there are several reports of the applicability of this technology to monitor other tissue beds[149,150] such as the renal and splanchnic circulations, cerebral NIRS has received the most attention in the context of pediatric cardiac surgery. This noninvasive monitoring is becoming widely used during CPB in children to assess the adequacy of oxygen delivery to the brain.[151-153] This may lead to improved neurologic outcomes after cardiac surgery, although there is no clear evidence for target based NIRS values in humans. One algorithm suggested that a 20% drop from baseline bilaterally was significant and should trigger efforts to increase the cerebral saturation, such as optimizing the neck position, increasing mean arterial pressure, increasing arterial CO_2, or increasing the hematocrit. If the change was unilateral, it may be related to incorrect aortic cannula positioning.[154] To be most accurate, baseline readings should be undertaken prior to the induction of anesthesia as anesthesia itself may result in changes (see Chapter 52).

INDUCTION OF ANESTHESIA

In the United Kingdom, most children are anesthetized in an anesthesia induction room, which is a small room immediately adjacent to the operating room, and in most cases, the parents are present at the induction. Anesthesia is commonly induced while the child is sitting with or being held by a parent. It is possible to engage some older children to hold the mask themselves during the first stages of induction; alternatively, some parents can hold the mask for the child as he or she is anesthetized. After the child is asleep, he or she is transferred to the anesthetic trolley, where venous and arterial access is secured and the trachea is intubated. This contrasts with the practice in most centers in North America, where induction of anesthesia usually occurs in the operating room.

The method of induction, either intravenously or by inhalation, should be tailored to the child and the cardiac defect. When an IV induction is selected (e.g., mask induction is refused) but IV access appears to be difficult, ketamine may be given intramuscularly or orally to sedate the child during the attempts. Application of a local anesthetic cream such as EMLA (eutectic mixture of local anesthetics; AstraZeneca, Wilmington, DE) or Ametop Gel (Smith-Nephew, Mississauga, ON, Canada) also reduces the pain of injection. However, this requires close communication in that suitable veins should be identified during the preoperative visit and clear instructions are given to the parents or nursing staff regarding where and when the cream should be applied (1 hour for EMLA and 30 minutes for Ametop). When IV access is already present, an IV induction is preferred. In severely ill children, it is generally advisable to secure IV access before induction of anesthesia.

Sevoflurane is the most commonly used inhalational induction agent in children. Sevoflurane is very rapid acting and should be used with care in the child with CHD because high concentrations can produce bradycardia, hypotension, and apnea if not titrated carefully. Concentrations should be rapidly reduced after an adequate depth of anesthesia is achieved (remembering that the minimum alveolar concentration [MAC] in children is 2.5%) to limit myocardial depression. To facilitate establishing IV access when the concentration of sevoflurane must be restricted, application of local anesthetic cream is helpful because it allows cannulation at a much lighter plane of anesthesia. In children who are cyanotic with a right-to-left shunt and reduced pulmonary blood flow, inhalational inductions are slow. Moreover, in neonates and young infants with large right-to-left shunts, the desired depth of anesthesia may not be achieved; the end-tidal concentration does not accurately reflect the blood and brain partial pressures. Many include nitrous oxide during inhalational inductions for two reasons. First, it is odorless; therefore it can be started before the introduction of the sevoflurane to sedate the child before the stronger-smelling anesthetic is introduced. Second, it allows a smoother and more rapid induction compared with sevoflurane alone. Concentrations up to 70% nitrous oxide can be used to smooth induction of anesthesia even in cyanotic children, but the nitrous oxide should be replaced with air and oxygen or 100% oxygen as soon as IV access is obtained and a muscle relaxant is given. Some children do not want an inhalational induction out of fear of the mask. To address this problem, we put the mask aside and begin the induction by cupping our hands with the elbow of the breathing circuit between two fingers and slowly bringing our hands toward the face from under the chin (this gas mixture is heavier than air). It is important to warn the child about each event before it occurs (such as a mask applied to the face) and, when possible, to demonstrate the action on yourself, a parent, or a toy animal to avoid startling or scaring the child. Some children prefer to hold the mask themselves, or if the child is accompanied by a parent and unable to hold the mask, the parent may hold it. Good premedication often aids this process (see also Chapter 4).

For sick children in whom an IV induction is preferable, several options are available. In neonates, for example, those with coarctation of the aorta or with hypoplastic left heart syndrome who are not ventilated before coming to the operating room, one approach is to administer fentanyl in a dose of 2 to 3 μg/kg, followed by pancuronium and then by a very low dose (i.e., sedative dose) of sevoflurane or isoflurane. Fentanyl obtunds the hypertensive response to intubation, and the pancuronium maintains cardiac output by maintaining the heart rate. The very-low-dose inhalational agent provides the sedation or anesthesia. In older children, etomidate is an excellent choice as an induction agent, providing stable hemodynamics, although it does cause pain on injection. Ketamine is also widely used for IV induction in neonates and older children. Ketamine maintains or increases blood pressure, heart rate, and cardiac output. The exact mechanism of these effects of ketamine is unknown; ketamine may stimulate the release of endogenous stores of catecholamines, although it is a negative inotrope in the denervated heart.[155] This negative inotropic effect may make ketamine a poor choice in children in whom catecholamine stimulation may already be maximal, such as in severe cardiomyopathy.[156] It may also be a poor choice if tachycardia is undesirable, such as in the case of aortic stenosis.

Monitors should ideally be applied before induction begins, although applying monitors can upset the child, which can be detrimental (e.g., the child with TOF who begins to cry and precipitates a tet spell). A pulse oximeter probe may be the only monitor applied before induction of anesthesia. Sevoflurane and other halogenated agents may provide another advantage by offering a degree of ischemic preconditioning to the heart and to other organs, particularly the brain and kidney. In fact, sevoflurane use has decreased biochemical markers for myocardial and renal injury in coronary artery bypass grafting in adults.[157] Current evidence suggests a role of inhalational anesthetic agents in improving outcomes after cardiac surgery, in particular for some subsets of patients.[158–160] Further research is needed to clarify their protective role in different organs and systems, in noncoronary and noncardiac surgery, as well as recommended doses and timing of administration.[161] It is thought that the same effect is observed in children. Sevoflurane, but also midazolam and propofol, protect against myocardial injury in pediatric cardiac surgery when using cardiac troponin T as a marker of such damage.[162] One study has demonstrated definite cardioprotective effects from inhalational agents in children,[163] although these effects do not seem to be universally applicable to all children undergoing heart surgery, suggesting the need for further investigations.[164]

MAINTENANCE OF ANESTHESIA

Maintenance of anesthesia in children with CHD depends on the preoperative status and the response to induction of anesthesia. Whether inhalational agents, additional opioids, or other IV agents are used for maintenance depends on the tolerance of the child and postoperative plans for ventilation. If a primary opioid-based anesthetic is chosen, additional opioid should be administered on initiation of CPB to offset dilution from the pump prime and to maintain adequate opioid plasma concentrations. Awareness during adult cardiac surgery has been reported when amnestic agents were not used. Although small children may be unable to describe such events, the potential for awareness during pediatric cardiac surgery should not be underestimated. In effect, while it is unclear whether the incidence of awareness in children is more or less than in adults,[165,166] anesthesiologists should be cognizant of the possibility of intraoperative awareness in pediatric anesthesia, and mindful of the potential short- and long-term psychological effects of such a complication.[167–169] Recently, a national audit project in the United Kingdom (NAP5) suggested strategies to minimize the risk of awareness in pediatric cardiac surgery[170] that in part may depend on the several factors, including the child's age, hemodynamic stability, predicted duration of surgery and CPB, and plans for postoperative ventilation. The choice of a specific strategy is often dictated by institutional or personal preferences. Different agents, singly or in combination, may prevent awareness: an inhalational agent may be administered through the membrane oxygenator with an anesthetic vaporizer; IV midazolam (0.2 mg/kg) may be administered at the institution of CPB; propofol may be given by infusion during the bypass period. More recently, the use of a dexmedetomidine infusion has been proposed to attenuate awareness as it attenuates the hemodynamic and neuroendocrine responses to surgical stress and CPB in pediatric cardiac surgery.[171] Other benefits include decreased intraoperative anesthetic requirements and postoperative opioid consumption,[172] which suggest it may have a role in reducing the possibility of awareness. However, dexmedetomidine is *not* a general anesthetic (conferring 0.5 MAC equivalence) and its effectiveness in preventing awareness has not been established.[173] In one study, dexmedetomidine conferred a protective effect in the heart, brain, kidney, and lungs; the administration of dexmedetomidine may contribute to improved outcomes, a decrease in postoperative mortality, and a reduced incidence of complications and delirium in adults undergoing cardiac surgery.[174] Dexmedetomidine also slows sinus and AV node conduction[175]; this may prove useful in those with junctional ectopic tachycardia (JET).

INSTITUTION AND SEPARATION FROM BYPASS

Before initiation of CPB, the surgeon requests heparin to be given; after administration (preferably flushed through a central venous catheter) but *before the initiation of bypass*, the ACT should be determined. By convention, the ACT measurement should be at least three times greater than the baseline value or greater than 480 seconds. Despite significant interindividual variations in heparin dose requirements and multiple problems associated with its use, heparin remains the anticoagulant of choice for CPB.[176,177] In fact, achieving an adequate balance between the appropriate amount of heparin to minimize the risk of thrombosis and platelet activation while reducing the risk of bleeding from overanticoagulation may be particularly challenging in children.[50] Similarly, the use of the ACT as the sole metric of anticoagulation may hold a number of inaccuracies, based on the inconsistent relationships between plasma heparin concentrations, thrombin inhibition, and coagulation tests.[178] Individualized management of anticoagulation and its reversal seem to result in less activation of the coagulation cascade, less fibrinolysis, and reduced blood loss and transfusion requirements. However, until further research defines the clinical impact of these findings, it is likely that the use of heparin and ACT measurement for anticoagulation management will remain the standard of care in most centers (see also Chapter 19).[51] When bypass is started, additional anesthetic drugs should be administered to counteract the effects of dilution and adsorption by the CPB circuit. Ventilation should cease. Both hypertension and hypotension may complicate bypass. Blood pressure may be controlled within an appropriate range to ensure end-organ perfusion by using α-adrenergic agonists or blockers such as phenylephrine and phentolamine. The child is usually cooled at this stage, guided by the nasopharyngeal temperature. If the heart is to be stopped, cardioplegia is given by the perfusionist after the aorta is cross-clamped to provide myocardial protection during the period of ischemia.[179,180] Cardioplegia is usually repeated every 20 to 30 minutes, although it is not required if the surgery is performed while the heart is beating. Myocardial damage is related to the duration of the aortic cross-clamping and the effectiveness of the myocardial protection.[181]

At an appropriate time during the surgery, the cross-clamp is removed, and perfusion to the heart is restored. The heart usually starts to beat in normal sinus rhythm, although this is not always the case. In the early phase of reperfusion, it is possible for various degrees of heart block to occur. However, these are usually short-lived and as the effects of cardioplegia wear off, normal sinus rhythm is usually restored. Persistent heart block may result from damage to the conducting system during surgery.

After release of the cross-clamp, any inotropes or vasodilators that are required are usually started. Rewarming may have begun before release of the cross-clamp, but more commonly, the child is rewarmed after release of the clamp.

When the child has adequately rewarmed, as reflected by (1) a normal core and minimal core-peripheral temperature gradient, (2) inotrope(s) infusion as needed, (3) restoration of satisfactory heart function, and (4) the adequate ventilation of the child's lungs, the child is ready to be weaned from CPB. If a TEE probe is in place, the heart should be scanned for the presence of air. If air is present, additional attempts to de-air the heart should be attempted before separating from bypass. In the initial stages after coming off bypass, additional volume can be administered through the aortic cannula by the perfusionist, usually under the direction of the surgeon or anesthesiologist. Many centers institute modified ultrafiltration at this point, which involves taking arterial blood from the aortic cannula and passing it through the ultrafine filter. This blood, which is oxygenated and warm, is then reinfused into the right atrium. As previously discussed, reported benefits from the use of modified ultrafiltration include increasing the hematocrit, concentrating the clotting factors and platelets, increasing blood pressure, reducing PVR, and removing inflammatory mediators from the patient. When this process is complete, a thorough TEE examination can be undertaken.

When the team is satisfied with the TEE result, the perfusionist and the surgical team should be informed that protamine will be administered soon. The surgeon should remove any pump suckers from the field, and the perfusionist should stop all pump suction. This is done to ensure that no protamine enters the bypass circuit in case it is necessary to reestablish bypass for any reason, especially if this needs to be done in an emergency situation. Once these preliminary activities are complete, the surgeon asks for protamine to be administered to antagonize the circulating heparin. At this point, a blood gas analysis is performed and the ACT repeated; the ACT should return to prebypass levels. Required blood products may be given during modified ultrafiltration or after the administration of protamine, usually while the surgeons are achieving hemostasis. As soon as reasonable stability is achieved and the chest is closed (or the decision to leave the chest open has been made), the child can then be transferred to the ICU.

Control of Systemic and Pulmonary Vascular Resistance During Anesthesia

In some children with hypoplastic left heart syndrome (HLHS) who present for a Norwood procedure, excessive blood flow to the lungs resulting from a relatively low PVR and a relatively high SVR steals blood from the systemic circulation, leading to hypotension, poor tissue oxygen delivery, myocardial ischemia, and progressive acidosis. However, when the reverse occurs and the PVR is greater than the SVR, the child develops progressive excessive desaturation.[182,183] Similar pathophysiology exists with other duct-dependent circulations and to some extent with other shunting lesions. It may prove difficult to manipulate the SVR and PVR predictably because control of PVR is poorly understood, vasoactive drugs usually are distributed on both sides of the circulation, and pharmacologic attempts to modify the degree and direction of shunting have produced unpredictable results.[184,185] Despite these problems, several techniques have proved useful in manipulating the relative PVR and SVR. Increasing inspired oxygen to 100% and by hyperventilation to a pH of 7.6 or greater decreases the PVR in children. Positive end-expiratory pressure, acidosis, hypothermia, and the use of 30% or less inspired oxygen can increase PVR. Potent inhalational anesthetics reduce SVR more than PVR. Etomidate does not change the pulmonary blood flow in children with TOF, whereas ketamine increases the flow in children with limited cyanosis (presumably by dilating the pulmonary artery) and decreases the flow in children with moderate cyanosis (by constricting the pulmonary artery).[186] Because vasoconstrictors such as phenylephrine increase SVR more than PVR, they are effective acutely in reducing right-to-left shunting and increasing left-to-right shunting in the operating room.

During cardiac surgical procedures, a direct method of selectively increasing PVR or SVR is to have the surgeon place partially obstructing tourniquets around pulmonary arteries or the aorta to increase resistance so that flow to the opposite side of the circulation increases. Although these are only temporary measures, they may reestablish a better relative balance of resistances and a more normal physiology in a deteriorating clinical situation.

Anesthetic Drugs Used in Pediatric Cardiac Anesthesia

INHALATIONAL AGENTS

Sevoflurane

Sevoflurane is the induction agent of choice for inhalational inductions in pediatric anesthesia.[187,188] It is associated with little myocardial depression or dysrhythmias,[189–191] and there is a reduced likelihood of precipitating airway hyperreactivity than that observed with other inhalational agents. It has specific advantages over halothane when used in children with CHD, particularly in children younger than 1 year of age and in cyanotic children.[192,193] In contrast to halothane, sevoflurane causes no reduction in heart rate at 1.0 and 1.5 MAC in healthy children compared with awake values.[194] However, at greater concentrations, it can slow the heart rate and depress respiration. Both features are important in children with CHD because a slow heart rate reduces cardiac output and hypoventilation leads to hypercarbia and hypoxia, which can increase PVR. In the absence of nitrous oxide, sevoflurane depresses myocardial contractility to a lesser extent than halothane during induction of anesthesia. However, it does decrease left ventricular systolic function to a limited extent as well as SVR, but in common with halothane and isoflurane, it does not alter the degree of left-to-right shunting through an ASD or VSD at concentrations of ~1 MAC in 100% oxygen.[195] Sevoflurane causes bradycardia in specific subsets of patients (e.g., trisomy 21)[196,197] and conduction abnormalities in susceptible children,[198] which may be clinically significant in children with marginal cardiovascular reserve. Sevoflurane should also be used with great caution in children with severe ventricular outflow tract obstruction.[199]

Isoflurane

Isoflurane is not recommended for induction of anesthesia because the frequency of laryngospasm is greater than 20%.[200] The inability to ventilate whether due to laryngospasm or other causes quickly leads to hypoxemia and hypercarbia, both of which increase PVR. This increase in PVR and the resulting pulmonary hypertension is poorly tolerated in small children with heart disease, especially in the presence of right-to-left shunting (see Chapter 7). Even though isoflurane depresses the hemodynamics in healthy neonates and infants to a similar extent as halothane at equipotent concentrations,[201,202] isoflurane may hold an advantage in children with CHD, as it depresses myocardial contractility to a lesser extent than halothane.[203,204]

Halothane

In the United States, Canada, and the United Kingdom, the use of halothane has all but ceased, but it is still widely used in other parts of the world. It is included here for completeness. Uptake of halothane in infants younger than 3 months of age is more rapid than it is in adults. This also is the case for the uptake of halothane by the myocardium.[205] Although the precise effects of halothane on the human neonatal myocardium are unknown, young rodents have a reduced cardiovascular tolerance for halothane but require greater amounts for anesthesia.[206] Studies in infants with normal cardiovascular systems have demonstrated a significant incidence of hypotension with bradycardia during induction with halothane.[207] During induction of anesthesia in normal infants, halothane decreases the cardiac index to 73% of awake values at 1.0 MAC and to 59% at 1.5 MAC.[202] The MAC

for halothane in infants 1 to 6 months of age is the greatest of any age group.[208] This increased anesthetic requirement in infants, combined with the immaturity of their cardiovascular system, explains in part the relative cardiovascular intolerance of halothane by infants. In fact, hemodynamic depression associated with halothane has been shown to be inversely related to age in pediatric patients.[209] When compared with induction of anesthesia with sevoflurane, halothane decreased heart rate and systolic blood pressure in children of different age groups.[187] As such, atropine intramuscularly before induction and IV atropine during anesthesia partially offset the myocardial depression by halothane by attenuating the severity of the bradycardia and hypotension and increasing cardiac output. Despite the hypotension caused by halothane, it increases the arterial saturation in children with cyanotic CHD.[210]

A careful induction with sevoflurane is usually well tolerated in children with mild to moderate heart disease. However, large concentrations of potent inhalational agents may be an unwise choice for induction in young infants with severe cardiac disease. In children of any age with marginal cardiovascular reserve and in those with severe desaturation of systemic arterial blood due to right-to-left shunting, inhalational anesthetic-induced myocardial depression and systemic hypotension are poorly tolerated. A more appropriate use of these anesthetic agents in children with severe heart disease is the addition of low concentrations of the inhalational agent to provide amnesia and hypnosis, as well as to control possible hypertensive responses after an IV induction (see Chapter 7).

Nitrous Oxide

Nitrous oxide should be avoided for maintenance of anesthesia in children with CHD because of the risk of enlarging intravascular air emboli and the potential to increase the PVR. Nitrous oxide may expand microbubbles and macrobubbles, increasing obstruction to blood flow in arteries and capillaries. In all children with right-to-left shunts, there is a potential for these bubbles to be shunted directly into the systemic circulation and coronaries, a phenomenon designated by paradoxical embolization. The passage of air bubbles from the right to left sides is possible even in patients with predominantly left-to-right shunts, as the direction of shunting may transiently change under the influence of multiple factors during anesthesia and surgery. Consequently, care must be taken to ensure that no air bubbles are accidentally injected into the veins. Adverse outcomes after coronary air embolism are exacerbated by nitrous oxide.[211] The hemodynamic effects of venous air embolism are increased by nitrous oxide, even without paradoxical embolization.[212] In children with preexisting right-to-left shunts, paradoxical air embolism is clearly a potential problem; but even those with large left-to-right shunts can transiently reverse their shunts, as mentioned previously. This is particularly true during coughing or a Valsalva maneuver, when the normal transatrial pressure gradient is reversed. Right-to-left shunting of microbubbles of air after injection of saline into the right atrium has been demonstrated during these maneuvers.[213–215] Because coughing and Valsalva maneuvers may occur during anesthesia induction, even the most rigorous attention to removing air bubbles from IV lines may not prevent small amounts of air from reaching the systemic circulation. Microbubbles have also been observed after CPB.[216]

Nitrous oxide can increase PVR in adults.[217,218] However, in a 50% inspired concentration, it does not appear to affect PVR or pulmonary artery pressure in infants.[219] Nitrous oxide mildly decreases cardiac output at this concentration.[220] Avoidance of its use has been suggested in children with limited pulmonary blood flow, pulmonary hypertension, or depressed myocardial function. In the well-compensated child who does not require 100% inspired oxygen, nitrous oxide (usually at concentrations of 50%) may be used during induction of anesthesia but discontinued before tracheal intubation. If a reduced inspired oxygen concentration is indicated to maintain an appropriate balance between PVR and SVR after tracheal intubation, air may be added to the inspired gas mixture.

INTRAVENOUS INDUCTION AGENTS

Ketamine

Ketamine is a dissociative anesthetic agent that is a good analgesic. It increases blood pressure, heart rate, and cardiac output. Although the mechanism responsible for these responses is incompletely understood, it is thought to result from its ability to stimulate the release of endogenous catecholamines.[221-223] Ketamine exerts a negative inotropic effect on isolated human myocardium in vitro,[224-226] which is dependent on the underlying adrenergic tone.[227,228] Consequently, the net effects of ketamine in vivo are likely to reflect the balance between its direct myocardial depressant effects and its ability to cause sympathetic stimulation. As such, it may be a poor choice for children in whom sympathetic stimulation may already be maximal, such as in those with severe cardiomyopathy. It is also a poor choice if tachycardia is undesirable, such as in a child with aortic stenosis. Ketamine is thought to have minimal effects on PVR in children with CHD as long as the airway and ventilation are well preserved.[229,230] These likely clinically insignificant effects on PVR seem to be applicable to children with normal[231,232] and increased[186,233,234] pulmonary artery pressures, although it has been shown to occasionally cause an increase in PVR, as well as a decrease in pulmonary blood flow in certain subsets of patients with CHD.[235] Ketamine is quite a versatile anesthetic that may be administered intramuscularly and orally when IV access is difficult or an inhalational induction is contraindicated. The usual IV dose of 1–2 mg/kg produces a very predictable response, and an intramuscular dose of 4 to 10 mg/kg (possibly combined with intramuscular midazolam) is less predictable. The oral dose of ketamine is 5 to 6 mg/kg. The use of ketamine varies greatly from one institution to another, with some units using it extensively and others using it rarely (see Chapter 7).

Etomidate

Etomidate is an imidazole derivative short-acting anesthetic without any analgesic properties. It is a very safe drug, with a median lethal dose (LD$_{50}$)/median effective dose (ED$_{50}$) ratio of 26 in animal models,[236] which indicates that the lethal dose (LD) is 26 times greater than the effective dose (ED). Etomidate has little effect on systemic blood pressure, heart rate, and cardiac output after a single dose in healthy children[237]; it also appears to have minimal hemodynamic effects in children with CHD.[237,238] It has a favorable hemodynamic profile even when used in children in shock and appears to have a low risk of clinically important myoclonus or status epilepticus, pain on IV injection, and nausea and vomiting.[239,240] The major concern regarding etomidate is the increased mortality rates reported when it is administered as a continuous infusion. This grave adverse effect has been attributed to adrenal suppression.[241-243] The inhibition of steroid synthesis occurs after a prolonged infusion and after a single dose of etomidate, and this has created controversy regarding its use as an anesthetic agent, particularly in the ICUs in some jurisdictions.[244] The decrease in plasma cortisol and ACTH concentrations in children undergoing heart surgery after etomidate may persist for 24 hours or longer[245,246]

and may be potentiated by the use of other anesthetic agents.[247] The notion that etomidate causes adrenal suppression is well established, but what remains unclear is whether patient outcomes differ after a single bolus dose for induction of anesthesia.[248] Newer analogs of etomidate have addressed these deficiencies and may lead to a surge in its use in the future (see also Chapter 7).

Propofol

Propofol is a rapidly acting IV hypnotic agent that may be administered as a single dose or by continuous infusion. It has no analgesic activity, but it possesses antiemetic properties, even in subhypnotic doses.[249-253] It is effective for prophylaxis against emergence agitation in young children.[254,255] Its short duration of action is the result of rapid redistribution and metabolism, which also allows the drug to be given by continuous infusion with limited accumulation. Induction doses decrease SVR, blood pressure, and cardiac output; the effect on heart rate varies. The ED$_{50}$ for propofol in infants and small children is greater than it is in adults.[241-244,249,256-258] If propofol is given very slowly, smaller doses are required to achieve the anesthetic state, although the induction time increases. A slower infusion also results in more stable hemodynamics.[259] Pain on injection and involuntary movement after IV propofol have been concerns that have been overcome (see Chapter 7). However, there remain significant concerns about its potential to trigger a propofol-related infusion syndrome (PRIS). This rare but potentially lethal syndrome is characterized clinically by acute bradycardia progressing to asystole; it is frequently associated with progressive metabolic acidosis, hemodynamic instability, myocardial failure, and rhabdomyolysis, with or without the presence of hepatomegaly or lipemia after 4 mg/kg per hour infused for 48 hours.[260-263] The symptoms of PRIS may develop rapidly and often are refractory to aggressive pharmacologic treatment, requiring hemodialysis or hemoperfusion, with cardiorespiratory support as extracorporeal membrane oxygenation in some cases.[264-266] These concerns about propofol have led to recommendations to maintain close vigilance for developing signs indicative of PRIS, as well as limiting dose rates and duration when propofol is used as a continuous infusion.[267] Although propofol can be used safely in children with CHD, it is typically avoided as an induction agent in those with severe CHD, especially in those with a fixed cardiac output such as severe aortic or mitral stenosis; in these patients, it may cause severe hypotension due to its effects on SVR and blood pressure. It can be used by continuous infusion during CPB to reduce awareness and may be particularly useful if an early extubation is planned (see also Chapter 7).[268,269]

OPIOIDS

Fentanyl

As in adults with severe cardiac disease, an IV induction with fentanyl combined with pancuronium and 100% oxygen or air and oxygen provides hemodynamic stability even in very sick children with CHD, although it is not amnestic. Inclusion of IV midazolam or another amnestic agent is strongly urged to avoid awareness. In neonates and infants, the use of high-dose opioid anesthesia provides excellent hemodynamic stability, with suppression of the hormonal and metabolic stress responses.[270,271] When fentanyl or other opioids are combined with nitrous oxide, the negative inotropic effects of nitrous oxide may be evident, particularly in sicker children.[272] The high-dose fentanyl technique is effective in preterm neonates undergoing ligation of a PDA.[273] In high-risk, full-term neonates and in older infants with severe CHD, the high-dose fentanyl technique in doses of up to 75 μg/kg, combined with pancuronium, maintains stable hemodynamics during induction, tracheal intubation, and surgical incision.[274] Oxygen saturation is well maintained and often improves during induction, even in cyanotic children.[275] The cardiac index, SVR, and PVR in infants given 25 µg/kg of fentanyl do not change substantively.[276] Combining pancuronium with fentanyl is desirable because the vagolytic effects of pancuronium offset the potential vagotonic effects of fentanyl. The hemodynamic stability reported in infants with the combination of high-dose fentanyl and pancuronium may not be replicated when other muscle relaxants are used (see Chapter 7).[277]

Sufentanil

Sufentanil (5 to 20 µg/kg), an alternative to fentanyl, is 5 to 10 times more potent than fentanyl but has a large margin of safety.[278,279] It is highly lipophilic and is rapidly distributed to all tissues. It is infrequently used in infants and children with CHD.

Remifentanil

Remifentanil is an ultra-short-acting opioid that is rapidly metabolized in the plasma and tissue by nonspecific esterases to an inactive metabolite. It has a very brief elimination half-life, with a context-sensitive half-life of only 3 minutes, independent of the duration of infusion (see Fig. 7.24). In pediatric cardiac surgery, it is an attractive alternative to fentanyl that provides intense analgesia during the most stimulating parts of surgery but facilitates rapid awakening and weaning from mechanical ventilation without residual opioid effect. Its pharmacodynamics are unaffected by CPB.[280] It provides stable hemodynamic conditions in children, although there is a tendency toward bradycardia and systemic hypotension.[281-283] It has no negative inotropic effect, even in the failing heart.[284]

A significant concern is the development of acute tolerance with increasing analgesic requirements after discontinuing remifentanil.[285-287] One study suggested that this is not clinically important.[288] Strategies to prevent tolerance to remifentanil have included nitrous oxide as well as IV magnesium infusions.[289,290] Remifentanil is also used for prolonged sedation of children in the ICU. Many units have moved toward early extubation and discharge from the ICU after cardiac surgery (i.e., fast tracking), and remifentanil is a useful drug in this setting (see also Chapter 7). Consideration must be given to transitioning to a longer-acting opioid before discontinuation of remifentanil.

NEUROMUSCULAR BLOCKING DRUGS

Pancuronium has been studied in depth in children with CHD.[291] When administered over a 60- to 90-second interval, pancuronium maintains heart rate and blood pressure.[292,293] An intubating bolus dose of pancuronium may produce tachycardia and increase cardiac output. This bolus dose effect is sometimes desirable to support cardiac output in infants in congestive heart failure because their stroke volume is fixed. Pancuronium may be the neuromuscular blocking drug (NMBD) of choice when high-dose opioid techniques are used to offset the vagotonic effects of opioids such as fentanyl. Other NMBDs are also widely used, particularly if patients are to be extubated in the operating room or early in the ICU.

LONG-TERM NEUROCOGNITIVE-DEVELOPMENTAL OUTCOMES ASSOCIATED WITH ANESTHESIA

Concerns have been raised about the possibility that many of the anesthetic agents such as inhalational anesthetics, propofol, ketamine, and midazolam may cause long-term neurocognitive-developmental problems in neonates and young infants.[294-297] This effect is thought to result from the neuronal apoptosis caused by these agents in newborn rodents and primates. Neither opioids nor dexmedetomidine have been implicated in these changes at the present date.[298,299] There is no evidence to directly link anesthetic exposure in infancy to long-term neurocognitive defects.[300] There is much ongoing research in this area (see Chapter 25), including an interest in elucidating the potential contributive role of different anesthetic techniques in determining neurodevelopmental outcomes in children undergoing heart surgery.[301-303] In fact, many full-term children with CHD have been shown to have widespread brain abnormalities with small brain volumes similar to those of preterm infants prior to any surgery or CPB.[304-306]

Regional Anesthesia

The use of regional anesthesia to provide pain relief during and after cardiac surgery in adults also reduces the stress response to surgery and may reduce morbidity and mortality. In adults undergoing cardiac surgery, the benefits of regional analgesia or anesthesia techniques, whether in isolation or combined with general anesthesia, include earlier extubation, fewer respiratory complications, a reduction in renal failure, fewer strokes, and less myocardial damage after CPB.[307-312] In animals, thoracic epidural anesthesia reduces myocardial damage after coronary occlusion.[313] Similar effects in improving blood flow, thus reducing coronary ischemia and myocardial damage, have been shown in humans by the use of thoracic epidural anesthesia in adults undergoing coronary bypass graft surgery.[314,315] The same benefits may be achieved by using intrathecal (spinal) analgesia.[316] For example, high spinal anesthesia using bupivacaine reduces the stress response to CPB and β-adrenergic dysfunction and improves cardiac performance after cardiac surgery in adults.[317]

Research into regional anesthesia and analgesia in pediatric cardiac surgery is limited. Caudal morphine has been used to provide postoperative analgesia and has produced good analgesia for about 6 hours while reducing analgesic requirements for up to 24 hours.[318] Two retrospective studies in children[319,320] included a variety of neuraxial regional anesthetic techniques. Most children were extubated in the operating room, although approximately 4% required reintubation within 24 hours. Adverse effects included emesis (39%), pruritus (10%), urinary retention (7%), postoperative transient paresthesia (3%), and respiratory depression (1.8%). The rate of adverse effects was less with a thoracic catheter epidural approach compared with various caudal, lumbar epidural, and spinal approaches.[320] Hospital duration of stay was unaffected by the presence of regional anesthesia complications. Although this study appears to indicate that regional analgesia is safe, the numbers in the study are too small to conclude that regional analgesia is safe for pediatric cardiac surgery.

The use of neuraxial regional anesthesia in children undergoing heart surgery remains controversial.[321,322] The main concern is the risk of bleeding and the potential for disastrous neurologic complications. The risks may be greater in children than in adults because of the presence of collateral vessels, increased venous pressure, coagulopathy related to cyanosis, and the use of aspirin. There remain many unanswered questions regarding neuraxial block in children, such as the true incidence of epidural hematoma, the time delay required between placement of the epidural catheter and full anticoagulation, and the correct management of a bloody tap, even though a considerable research effort has been made to address these issues.[319,323-325] The estimated risk of epidural hematoma during cardiac surgery in adults is 1 case per 1000 patients and 1 case per 2400 patients for spinal and epidural block, respectively.[326] Whether the risks are similar or greater in children cannot be determined because the numbers of children reported thus far are too small. A large, randomized, prospective study to evaluate a true risk/benefit ratio without bias is needed; until such data are available, various commentators have advised great caution with the use of regional analgesia for cardiac surgery, and some have suggested that it may not be possible to perform the study required because of ethical considerations.[321]

More recently, there has been an increasing interest in bilateral thoracic paravertebral blocks (PVB) as a means of providing good-quality regional analgesia while possibly minimizing complications associated with neuraxial techniques. While their use in thoracic surgery has been shown to result in equally effective pain control and a better side-effect profile compared with thoracic epidurals in both adults[327,328] and children,[329,330] their use in cardiac surgery remains controversial. In fact, similar considerations about anticoagulation and neuraxial analgesia techniques in cardiac bypass procedures may apply to PVB, although the risk of serious neurologic complications resulting from bleeding and subsequent hematoma formation is, at least theoretically, reduced by the use of non-neuraxial analgesia. These concerns have been addressed in the literature in adult cardiac surgery,[331,332] and although PVB have been used for analgesia in children undergoing heart surgery and recommended by some authors; the evidence for their use in children is limited.[333–335] However, it is likely that hesitations in their routine use will persist until concerns about safety are completely clarified by a methodologically sound, large, randomized, prospective study.

Fast Tracking

Fast tracking refers to abbreviating the perioperative period of children undergoing cardiac surgery. Fast track programs, otherwise known as enhanced recovery programs, can be defined as protocols developed to reduce physiologic stress and postoperative organ dysfunction by optimizing all aspects of perioperative care. These protocols consist of a multimodal package of techniques designed to improve postoperative recovery, hence expediting return to health and functional status and reducing hospital length of stay. Fast track surgery programs improve the standardization of medical care and have been shown to result in improved outcomes and lower health care costs. Enhanced recovery programs for children undergoing heart surgery should include every phase of the child's journey from referral and preoperative evaluation to less invasive surgery, early weaning from respiratory support, extubation, and discharge from the ICU and hospital. In this context, the term "fast tracking" is generally used to designate extubation shortly after arrival to the intensive care unit, most commonly in the first 6 hours, whereas the term "ultra-fast" tracking usually refers to extubation of the trachea in the operating room immediately after surgery.

Early extubation of pediatric patients after cardiac surgery offers advantages in terms of cost and reduced morbidity associated with longer ICU stays.[336–340] The success of this approach depends on the close teamwork of a multidisciplinary team, with every member of the team working toward the same goal. Successful fast tracking usually requires the development of care pathways to ensure that the quality of patient care is not compromised.[341] Early extubation and discharge from the ICU requires preplanning and the adoption of a technique that facilitates this goal. The use

of very large doses of fentanyl is not appropriate; alternative techniques have been used, including smaller doses of fentanyl in combination with inhalational agents[342,343] or the use of remifentanil in combination with inhalational agents or with propofol. Others have advocated regional anesthesia as a means of speeding extubation, but this approach remains controversial. It is important to choose a NMBD with a shorter duration of action than pancuronium to ensure that it is easy to reverse the neuromuscular block at the end of surgery. Other important considerations to ensure that early extubation is a success include adequate pain relief (e.g., IV paracetamol can be useful), patient-controlled or nurse-controlled analgesia, and antiemetics because nausea appears to be more of a problem in children who are extubated early.

Some clinicians advocate extubating the trachea in the operating room, whereas others advocate waiting until the child is in the ICU. Delaying the extubation until the child is in the ICU may save operating room time and may reduce the risks of cardiovascular instability, bleeding, and hypothermia.[344] Despite these concerns, the tracheas of many children are extubated in the operating room with good outcomes. While currently available evidence does not allow for a definitive evidence-based recommendation about early extubation in children undergoing heart surgery, data available at the present date attest its role in improving outcomes and reducing hospital length of stay. It is reasonable to conclude that fast track programs, possibly including tracheal extubation in the operating room, have now demonstrated their efficacy, safety, and feasibility in low- to medium-risk pediatric congenital cardiac surgery patients.[345–347]

Cardiopulmonary Bypass

CPB is discussed in Chapter 19.

Stress Response to Cardiac Surgery

Cardiac surgery and CPB are altered physiologic conditions associated with an amplified stress response characterized by the release of numerous hormonal and metabolic substances. This constitutes part of the systemic reaction to injury, which consists of a broad variety of hematologic, immunologic, and neuroendocrine effects. Substances released as part of the stress response include catecholamines, cortisol, growth hormone, glucagon, glucose, insulin, prostaglandins, complement, β-endorphins,[270,271,348,349] as well as oxidative stress mediators[350–352] and many others.[353–355] The cause of the elaboration of these substances is likely to be multifactorial: contact of blood with foreign surfaces, nonpulsatile flow, low perfusion pressure, anemia, hypothermia, myocardial ischemia, and possibly low levels of anesthesia. Other factors that contribute to the increase in stress hormones are delayed renal and hepatic clearance and exclusion of the pulmonary circulation during extracorporeal circulation.[356]

Neonates of all viable gestational ages, older infants, and children have nociceptive systems that are sufficiently developed and integrated with brainstem cardiovascular control centers to trigger humoral and circulatory responses to pain and stress.[357–360] Substantial humoral, metabolic, and cardiovascular responses to painful and stressful stimulation during surgery have been documented in neonates of all gestational ages and in older infants.[361,362] Hormonal stress responses in neonates subjected to cardiac and noncardiac operations are threefold to fivefold greater than those in adults after similar surgeries. Circulatory responses to stressful stimuli in children include systemic and pulmonary hypertension.

Humoral stress responses are particularly extreme during and after cardiac surgery. These responses are characterized by increases in a number of circulating regulatory substances, including catecholamines, cortisol, insulin, glucagon, growth hormone, and β-endorphins; circulating concentrations of catecholamines may increase by as much as 400% over baseline preoperative concentrations. This is evidence of a massive activation of sympathetic outflow in response to surgical stimulation. Some of these responses may continue for several days postoperatively.[363]

It has been suggested that such extreme stress responses and neuroendocrine activation may be associated with greater morbidity and mortality. In adults, intraoperative adrenergic levels 50% above baseline are associated with significant postoperative alterations in β-adrenergic receptor function, including increased β-receptor density and decreased receptor affinity. Mortality among adults with severe congestive failure is associated with increased levels of hormones regulating cardiovascular function, including aldosterone, epinephrine, and norepinephrine.[364] In neonates undergoing cardiac surgery, increased concentrations of stress hormones may be associated with increased mortality rates.[363]

The metabolic response to stress in children includes increased oxygen consumption, glycogenolysis, gluconeogenesis, and lipolysis, which causes substantial intraoperative and postoperative catabolism. The metabolic response is usually related to changes in plasma cortisol, catecholamines, and other counterregulatory hormones such as glucagon and growth hormone. The most prominent clinical effects that result from activation of these processes are perioperative hypoglycemia and hyperglycemia, lactic acidemia, and negative nitrogen balance extending well into the postoperative period. Neonates and infants tolerate such metabolic derangements poorly. Their impaired tolerance is the result of a relative lack of endogenous reserves of carbohydrates, fat, and proteins; the large metabolic cost of rapid growth; a high obligate requirement for glucose by the relatively large brain; the immature hormonal control of intermediary metabolism; and the limited functional capabilities of immature enzyme systems in the metabolic organs. Severe stress responses superimposed on the normal neonatal and infant physiology may be poorly tolerated. However, it remains unclear whether these metabolic alterations may provide some beneficial effects for mobilizing the bodily resources to provide a metabolic milieu for healing tissues or they are purely maladaptive, resulting in detrimental effects on postoperative outcome.

Another factor is the potential effect of stress-induced hyperglycemia on the neurologic outcome. Neonates and young infants are capable of substantial rates of glucose production, mainly from glycogenolysis and gluconeogenesis during surgical stress that can result in hyperglycemia. Such hyperglycemic responses may be associated with poorer neurologic outcomes, particularly after a period of cerebral ischemia.[365] The use of high doses of fentanyl (>50 μg/kg) has reduced the hormonal stress response and resultant hyperglycemia and may lessen the risk of neurologic injury.[366]

In sufficient doses, opioids can blunt the stress responses in neonates, infants, and adults.[356,367,368] This blunting results in a more normal, homeostatic humoral and metabolic milieu in the circulation by reducing neuroendocrine activation and levels of regulatory hormones. In infants, the use of high-dose opioids for major surgical procedures and postoperative sedation substantially attenuates the neuroendocrine response to surgically induced pain and stress. Catecholamine release from intraoperative stress responses may predispose the vulnerable myocardium to dysrhythmias. In neonates with HLHS, sudden ventricular fibrillation occurred in 50% during surgical manipulation under halothane anesthesia. This incidence was dramatically reduced when high doses of fentanyl were introduced as the primary analgesic/sedative.[369] With the use of high-dose opioids, intraoperative ventricular fibrillation has virtually disappeared as a problem in this group of neonates.[370] Opioids increase the ventricular fibrillation threshold in isolated cardiac Purkinje fibers and alter action potential duration similar to that with class III antiarrhythmic agents.[371] Even electrophysiologic events in the neonatal heart, in addition to humoral and hemodynamic responses, may be altered by using high-dose fentanyl anesthesia to attenuate the effects of pain and stress.

REDUCING THE STRESS RESPONSE TO SURGERY AND BYPASS

Corticosteroids

Corticosteroids are used in many centers in an attempt to reduce the inflammatory response to surgery and bypass and improve outcomes after cardiac surgery.[372] However, there is huge variability in the formulation of the corticosteroids used, the doses administered, the timing of administration, and the indications for their use. Although several small studies in humans and animals suggest prophylactic corticosteroids in cardiac surgery may confer a benefit,[373,374] their routine use in children undergoing heart surgery is not supported by currently existing evidence.[375,376] Many investigators have called for a large multicenter study to determine the benefit of corticosteroids before bypass and the optimal dose and timing.[377]

Aprotinin

Aprotinin, which was originally used to reduce bleeding after CPB, is now also appreciated to confer significant antiinflammatory effects.[378-382] In adults, it has been shown to reduce mortality and length of ICU stay,[383] even though these effects were not replicated by later studies. In children, it improves pulmonary function in the postoperative period and reduces the time to extubation and ICU stay.[92] However, aprotinin is no longer available for routine use in the United States or continental Europe, because some grave concerns have been raised about its use increasing complications and mortality rates in adult cardiac surgery. In the United Kingdom, it is available for use on a named patient basis, but its use has been dramatically reduced as a result.

Allopurinol

Allopurinol is thought to provide protection against oxygen free radicals during reperfusion by inhibiting xanthine oxidase. It reduces oxygen free radical production and may reduce neurologic and cardiac damage after deep hypothermic circulatory arrest.[384] Analogously, it has been used in trials to prevent mortality and morbidity in neonates with hypoxic-ischemic encephalopathy.[385] This strategy does not appear to have developed widespread use, probably because of the lack of sufficient data to determine whether it has clinically important benefits and uncertainties about its effects on mortality and long-term neurodevelopmental outcomes.

Ischemic Preconditioning

The heart is capable of short-term rapid adaptation to brief ischemia such that during a subsequent, more severe ischemic insult, myocardial necrosis is delayed. Numerous animal studies have been conducted to further characterize this property of the myocardium, which could have very important clinical applications. The infarct-delaying properties of ischemic preconditioning have been observed in all species studied. An ischemic period of 5 minutes is sufficient to initiate preconditioning, and the protective period lasts for 1 to 2 hours. Laboratory experiments have demonstrated that the stimulation of adenosine receptors initiates preconditioning and the intracellular signal transduction mechanisms involve protein kinase C and adenosine triphosphate (ATP)-dependent potassium channels, although there may be some differences between species. An analysis of studies of myocardial infarction in humans has demonstrated that some adults who report having had angina in the days before infarction have a better outcome after their infarction in part owing to the ischemic preconditioning. More direct evidence has come from an investigation of adults undergoing percutaneous transluminal angioplasty in whom the ST-segment changes induced by balloon inflation were more marked during the first inflation than the second. In adults undergoing coronary artery bypass grafting, the decline in ATP content during the first 10 minutes of ischemia was reduced in those subjected to a brief preconditioning protocol.[386–390]

It may be possible to protect organs other than the heart by ischemic preconditioning. It may even be possible to protect organs remotely by producing a period of ischemia in one area such as a limb, which then confers protection to remote organs.[391] One study demonstrated that the use of a blood pressure cuff to produce short periods of limb ischemia can produce beneficial effects on the heart, lungs, and generalized inflammatory response.[392] The effects of remote ischemic preconditioning (RIPC) on children undergoing heart surgery have been inconsistent, likely reflecting heterogeneity between different studies developed to evaluate its ischemia-delaying properties.[393]

A wide variety of anesthetic agents and anesthesia adjuvants have also been found to offer protection against ischemia to the heart and other organs, particularly the brain and kidney, by ischemic preconditioning mechanisms. Inhalational anesthetics, but also midazolam and propofol, among others, protect against myocardial injury in pediatric cardiac surgery. Other studies have shown definite cardioprotective effects from inhalational agents in children, although these do not seem to be universally applicable to all children undergoing heart surgery. Further research is needed to clarify their protective role for different patient populations, to different organs and systems, as well as recommended doses and timing of administration.

Glucose-Insulin and Potassium

The use of glucose-insulin and potassium has been advocated for more than 40 years in adult cardiac surgery. It is thought to protect the myocardium from the effects of ischemia caused by aortic cross-clamping.[394–397] Its effects have not been studied in children undergoing cardiac surgery.

Anesthesia Considerations for Specific Cardiac Defects

Discussion of anesthesia considerations for repair of every form of CHD is beyond the scope of this chapter. However, a brief discussion of the problems that may be encountered during repair of the more common congenital heart lesions is presented. It is useful to group lesions together because the management principles can be applied more generally within groups (Table 17.2).

TABLE 17.2	**Classification of Congenital Heart Disease**
Simple Left-to-Right Shunt: Increased Pulmonary Blood Flow	
Atrial septal defect (ASD)	
Ventricular septal defect (VSD)	
Patent ductus arteriosus (PDA)	
Endocardial cushion defect (e.g., atrioventricular septal defect [AVSD])	
Aortopulmonary window (AP window)	
Simple Right-to-Left Shunt: Decreased Pulmonary Blood Flow With Cyanosis	
Tetralogy of Fallot (TOF)	
Pulmonary atresia	
Tricuspid atresia	
Ebstein anomaly	
Complex Shunts: Mixing of Pulmonary and Systemic Blood Flow With Cyanosis	
Transposition of the great arteries (TGA)	
Truncus arteriosus	
Total anomalous pulmonary venous connection (TAPVC)	
Double-outlet right ventricle (DORV)	
Hypoplastic left heart syndrome (HLHS)	
Obstructive Lesions	
Aortic Stenosis	
Mitral Stenosis	
Pulmonary Stenosis	
Coarctation of Aorta	
Interrupted Aortic Arch	

TABLE 17.3	**Clinical Features of Cardiac Failure in Children**
Failure to thrive	Cardiac murmur
Difficult feeding	Hepatomegaly
Breathlessness	Cardiomegaly
Recurrent chest infection	Pulmonary plethora
Tachycardia	Wheezing

SIMPLE LEFT-TO-RIGHT SHUNTS

Simple left-to-right shunts increase pulmonary blood flow. If the shunt is large, blood flow to the lungs can be as much as threefold to fourfold greater than normal, resulting in volume loading of the right heart. This can lead to right atrial and right ventricular enlargement that is potentially associated with tricuspid and pulmonary valve regurgitation. The combination of the aforementioned pathophysiologic consequences of large left-to-right shunts results in cardiac failure (Table 17.3).

Medical management of these children is primarily achieved with diuretics. If pulmonary blood flow is large and left untreated, pulmonary vascular disease begins to develop, resulting in pulmonary hypertension.[398–403] In the early stages, the changes are reversible, but in time, the changes may become irreversible. Eisenmenger syndrome refers to severe pulmonary hypertension that leads to suprasystemic pulmonary artery pressures that cause the shunt to reverse, leading to cyanosis. The previous left-to-right shunt reverses to become a right-to-left shunt. At this point, the child's condition becomes inoperable.

Increasingly, definitive surgery is being performed at a younger age to reduce the risk of developing pulmonary vascular disease. If early definitive surgery is not possible, a pulmonary artery band may be applied through a sternotomy incision but without CPB, to reduce pulmonary blood flow. This provides the infant the opportunity to grow, postponing the need for definitive surgery without increasing the risk of developing pulmonary hypertension. In the presence of substantively increased pulmonary blood flow, pulmonary vascular disease is often severe and irreversible by 1 year of age. Definitive surgery should be performed between 3 and 6 months of age to avoid this complication.

Atrial Septal Defect

ASD is a common heart defect in children, occurring in 1 of 1500 live births and accounting for approximately 10% of all CHD.[404,405] Several types of ASDs exist.

- Patent foramen ovale (PFO) is a normal fetal communication between the two atria that usually closes soon after birth. The PFO remains patent in up to 30% of people. PFO is usually left untreated in children.
- Primum ASD (Fig. 17.1A) is located in the inferior part of the atrial septum close to the AV valve and may be associated with a cleft mitral valve. This is a variant of AV septal defect (AVSD).

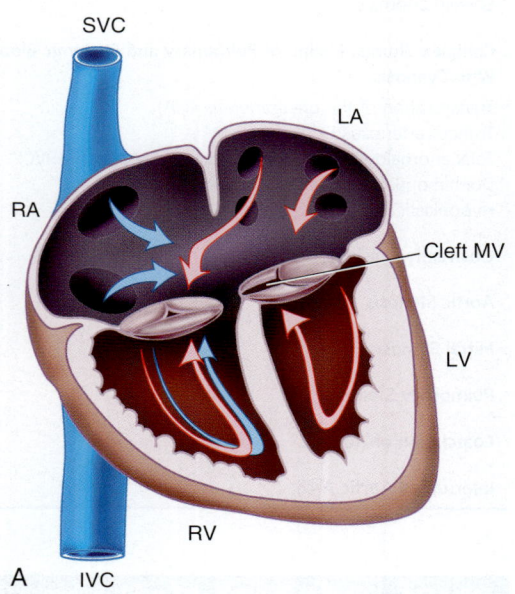

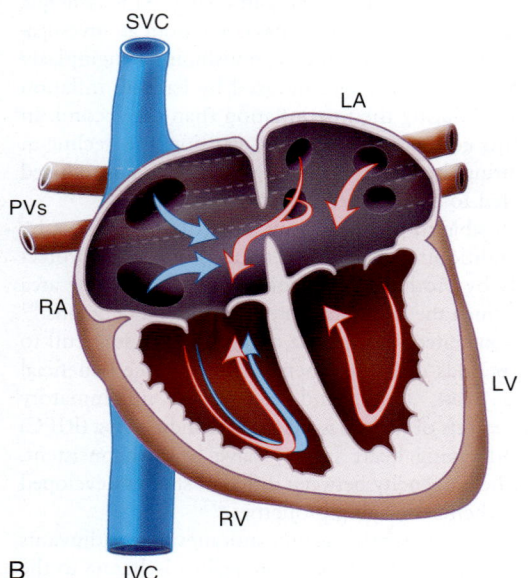

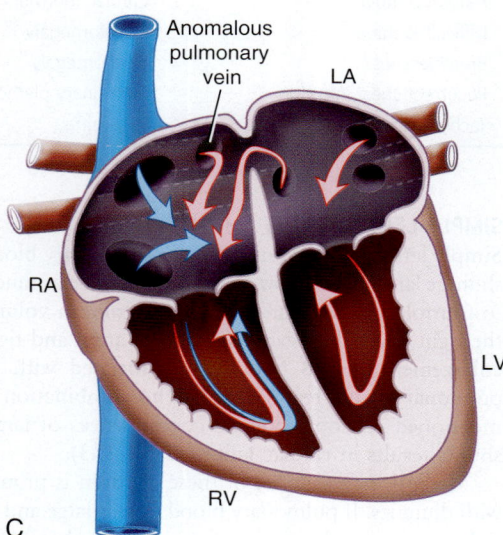

FIGURE 17.1 A, Diagram of a primum atrial septal defect (ASD) with the great vessels removed to show the left-to-right shunt through the defect and a cleft of the mitral valve (*MV*), also called a partial atrioventricular septal defect. **B,** Diagram of a secundum ASD with the great vessels removed to show the left-to-right shunt through the defect. **C,** Diagram of a sinus venosus ASD shows the left-to-right shunt through the defect close to the superior vena cava (*SVC*) and an anomalous pulmonary vein (*PV*) draining to the right atrium (*RA*). *IVC,* inferior vena cava; *LA,* left atrium; *LV,* left ventricle; *MV,* mitral valve; *RV,* right ventricle. (Modified from May LE. *Pediatric Heart Surgery: A Ready Reference for Professionals.* Milwaukee, WI: Maxishare; 2005.)

- Secundum ASD (see Fig. 17.1B) is found in the region of the fossa ovalis and results from a deficiency in the septum secundum.
- Sinus venosus ASD (see Fig. 17.1C) can be of the superior or inferior sinus venosus types, close to the opening of the SVC or inferior vena cava (IVC), respectively. It may be associated with anomalous pulmonary venous drainage.
- Coronary sinus ASD (i.e., unroofed coronary sinus) is a defect in the atrial wall that allows blood to flow from the left atrium to right atrium through the coronary sinus.
- Common atrium has a complete absence of the atrial septum. The AV valves may be abnormal or unaffected.

Many ASDs can be closed using a percutaneous, transcatheter device. PFO and secundum ASDs are most commonly closed using this technique.

Anesthesia Considerations

- These children can frequently be extubated on the operating table or early in the ICU, and smaller doses of opioids can be used. Alternatively, short-acting drugs (e.g., remifentanil) administered by infusion and possibly in combination with propofol are useful if early extubation is planned.
- The problems of postoperative pulmonary hypertension are seldom encountered.

Ventricular Septal Defect

VSD is the most common congenital defect in children, occurring in 1.5 to 3.5 of 1000 live births and accounting for more than 20% of CHD (Fig. 17.2A).[406,407] Four types are described: subarterial (5%), perimembranous (80%), inlet (5%), and muscular (10%). If the flow through the VSD is small, it is referred to as *restrictive*, but if the flow is large, it is called *unrestrictive*. A significant proportion of VSDs close spontaneously during the first few years of life. It is possible to close a small percent of VSDs in children using percutaneous, transcatheter devices.

Anesthesia Considerations

- Children who are asymptomatic preoperatively and undergo a predictably uncomplicated VSD surgical closure should be considered for fast tracking, and anesthetic management should aim to facilitate early extubation.
- Inotropic support may be required postoperatively for children in cardiac failure.
- Postoperative pulmonary hypertension may be a problem if the left-to-right shunt has been significant preoperatively or if the surgery is undertaken late.

Atrioventricular Septal Defect

AVSDs are also known as AV canal defects or endocardial cushion defects. They arise from a defect in the AV septum, with inadequate fusion of the superior and inferior endocardial cushions with the atrial septum and muscular ventricular septum, respectively. Their incidence is approximately 0.2 cases per 1000 live births, and they account for about 3% of CHD. They are commonly associated with trisomy 21, TOF, and DiGeorge syndrome (Table 17.4). It is worth noting that with a common AV valve annulus, the two separate valve orifices are referred to as the left and right AV valves, not the mitral and tricuspid valves. Three types of AVSD exist:

- Incomplete or partial AVSD usually consists of a primum ASD with a cleft in the anterior mitral valve leaflet; two separate AV valves are present and there is no VSD (see Fig. 17.1A).

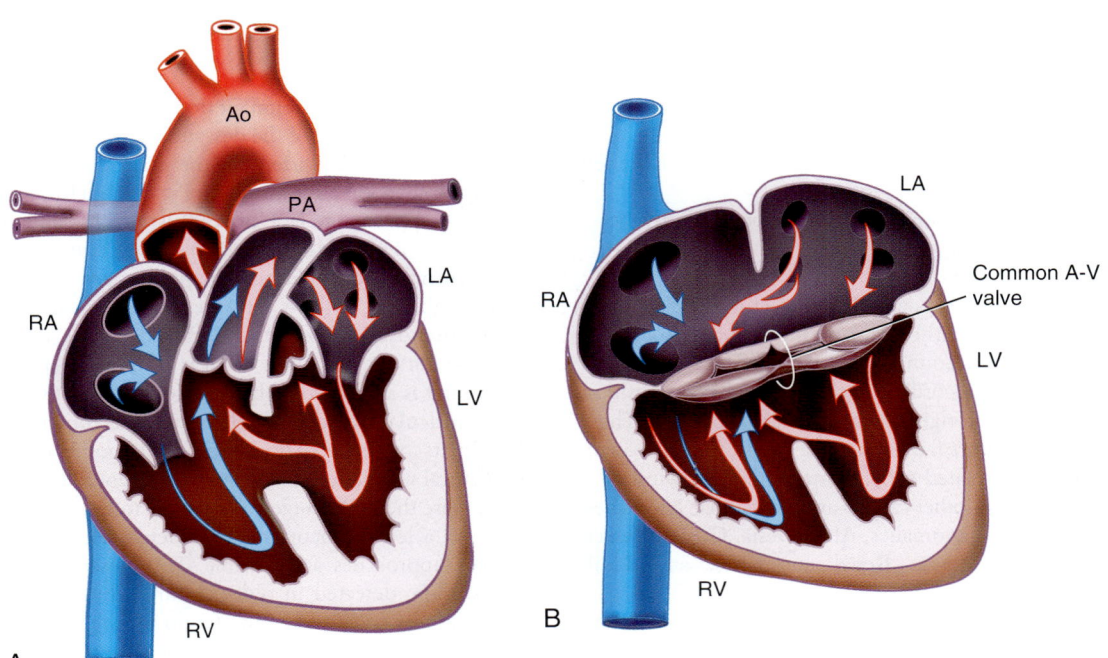

FIGURE 17.2 A, Diagram of a ventricular septal defect shows a left-to-right shunt. **B,** Diagram of a complete atrioventricular septal defect with the great vessels removed to show the left-to-right shunt through both atrial and ventricular components of the defect and a single common atrioventricular (*A-V*) valve. *Ao,* aorta; *LA,* left atrium; *LV,* left ventricle; *PA,* pulmonary artery; *RA,* right atrium; *RV,* right ventricle. (Modified from May LE. *Pediatric Heart Surgery: A Ready Reference for Professionals.* Milwaukee, WI: Maxishare; 2005.)

TABLE 17.4	Clinical Features and Concerns of DiGeorge Syndrome
Absent or small thymus	
T-cell abnormality with associated immunodeficiency	
Hypoparathyroidism with associated hypocalcemia	
Dysmorphic features, particularly a small mouth	
Increased surgical morbidity and mortality	
Irradiated blood products needed to prevent graft-versus-host disease	

- Complete AVSD consists of a large septal defect with atrial and ventricular components and a large common AV valve (see Fig. 17.2A).
- With transitional AVSD an ASD is present and the left and right AV valves may be only partially separated; the VSD may be small or moderate in size (see Fig. 17.2B).

Other descriptions of AVSD refer to balanced or unbalanced conditions, depending on the relative contributions of the two sides of the heart to the circulation. This in turn may depend on relative sizes of the two sides of the heart, but also on whether the AV valve is stenotic or atretic or if there is significant AV valve overriding (i.e., one AV valve emptying into two ventricles) or some of the valve chordae or papillary muscles are straddling (i.e., crossing to the other side of the ventricular septum). The hemodynamic effects associated with AVSD vary according to the type of defect and AV valve morphology and include shunting at the atrial or ventricular level and AV valve stenosis and/or regurgitation.

Anesthesia Considerations

- If the child has trisomy 21 or DiGeorge syndrome, the anesthesia implications of the associated comorbidities need to be managed.
- Inotropes are frequently required.
- Postoperative pulmonary hypertension may occur.
- There is often postoperative stenosis and/or regurgitation of one or both AV valves, with potential implications for hemodyamics and anesthesia management.
- TEE is particularly helpful in assessing the repair of the left AV valve.
- Heart block and dysrhythmias may occur postoperatively.

Aortopulmonary Window

Aortopulmonary window is a rare CHD defect in which there is a communication between the main pulmonary artery and the ascending aorta, and it accounts for 0.1% of CHD (Fig. 17.3). Four types are classified according to the size and exact position of the defect.[408] A left-to-right shunt is usually present. These children present with heart failure and are at risk for pulmonary vascular disease if not treated early. Aortopulmonary window is frequently associated with other cardiac and noncardiac anomalies:

- VACTERL: **V**ertebral anomalies, **A**nal atresia, **C**ardiac defect, **T**racheo**E**sophageal atresia, **R**enal anomalies, and **L**imb abnormalities
- CHARGE: **C**oloboma of the eye and central nervous system anomalies, **H**eart defects, **A**tresia of the choanae, **R**etardation of growth and development, **G**enital or urinary defects, and **E**ar anomalies
- CATCH-22 association (i.e., mnemonic for DiGeorge syndrome): **C**ardiac defect, **A**bnormal facies, **T**hymic hypoplasia, **C**left palate, **H**ypocalcemia (velocardiofacial syndrome), with 22q11 chromosome microdeletion (see Table 17.4)

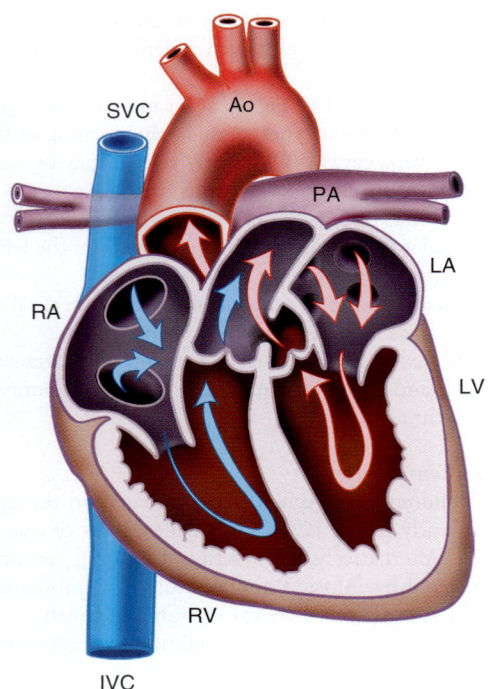

FIGURE 17.3 Diagram of an aortopulmonary window shows a left-to-right shunt through the defect. *Ao*, aorta; *IVC*, inferior vena cava; *LA*, left atrium; *LV*, left ventricle; *PA*, pulmonary artery; *RA*, right atrium; *RV*, right ventricle; *SVC*, superior vena cava. (Modified from May LE. *Pediatric Heart Surgery: A Ready Reference for Professionals.* Milwaukee, WI: Maxishare; 2005.)

Anesthesia Considerations

- Inotropes may be required.
- Postoperative pulmonary hypertension may be problematic.

Patent Ductus Arteriosus

The ductus arteriosus, a remnant from the fetal circulation, extends from the undersurface of the descending aorta, distal to the origin of the left subclavian artery, to the main pulmonary artery and usually closes soon after birth (see Fig. 18.1). However, it remains patent in approximately 1 of 2500 live births and accounts for about 10% of all CHD (Fig. 17.4). In the fetus, blood from the right ventricle is directed into the pulmonary artery, but because of the high PVR, it flows into the descending aorta through the ductus arteriosus. After birth, the PVR decreases, and blood flows from the aorta to the lungs. PDA is common in preterm infants, in whom it is associated with respiratory distress syndrome (RDS), intraventricular hemorrhage (IVH) and necrotizing enterocolitis (NEC); its presence may explain an ongoing requirement for mechanical ventilation. In these infants, should medical treatment fail to close the PDA, surgery is required to ligate or divide it, most often via a left thoracotomy approach, even though minimally invasive approaches are possible. The presence of a PDA may also only be detected in older children; but at this age, where size no longer constitutes a limitation for the use of endovascular devices, percutaneous closure by an interventional cardiologist is the preferred approach. The anesthesia implications are similar to those of other lesions described with left-to-right shunts preoperatively.

In many centers, the PDA is closed in preterm infants who weigh less than 1000 g and who are already mechanically ventilated in the neonatal intensive care unit (NICU). This avoids the need

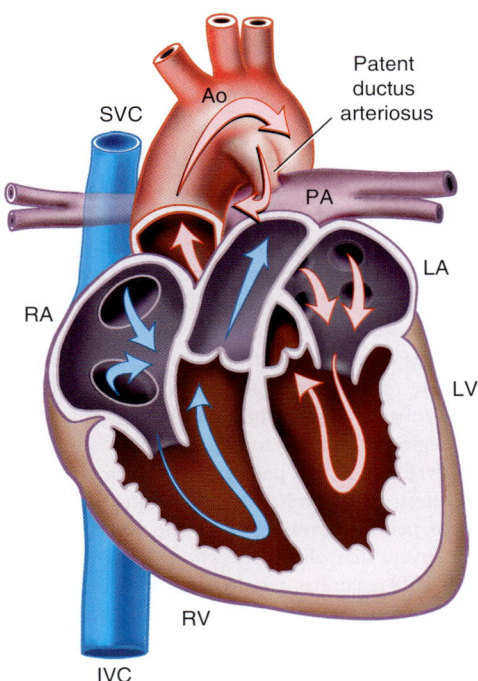

FIGURE 17.4 The diagram of a patent ductus arteriosus shows a left-to-right shunt. *Ao, aorta; IVC,* inferior vena cava; *LA,* left atrium; *LV,* left ventricle; *PA,* pulmonary artery; *RA,* right atrium; *RV,* right ventricle; *SVC,* superior vena cava. (Modified from May LE. *Pediatric Heart Surgery: A Ready Reference for Professionals.* Milwaukee, WI: Maxishare; 2005.)

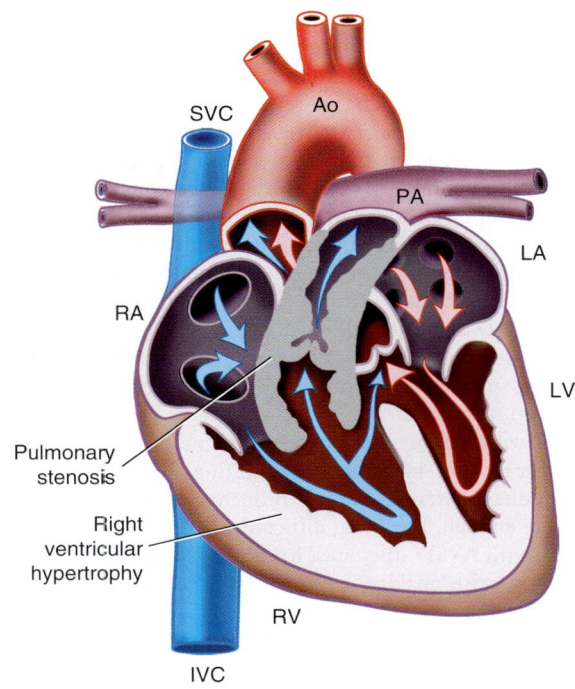

FIGURE 17.5 The diagram shows the features of the tetralogy of Fallot: ventricular septal defect, overriding aorta, right ventricular hypertrophy, and pulmonary stenosis. Pulmonary and subpulmonary obstructions are shown (*grey area*). The result is right-to-left shunting leading to cyanosis. *Ao,* aorta; *IVC,* inferior vena cava; *LA,* left atrium; *LV,* left ventricle; *PA,* pulmonary artery; *RA,* right atrium; *RV,* right ventricle; *SVC,* superior vena cava. (Modified from May LE. *Pediatric Heart Surgery: A Ready Reference for Professionals.* Milwaukee, WI: Maxishare; 2005.)

to transfer these very small infants to the operating room and the associated problems, particularly hypothermia.

Preoperative requirements include the following:

- Crossmatched blood
- Antibiotics (risk of endocarditis)
- Vitamin K
  Particular perioperative risks include the following:
- Difficulty ventilating or hemoglobin desaturation because of lung retraction
- Inadvertent ligation of the aorta or pulmonary artery
- Tearing the PDA with massive hemorrhage
- Endocarditis
- Paradoxical air embolism

Monitoring

Monitoring includes the use of all standard monitors, including end-tidal carbon dioxide assessment, and two pulse oximeters, one on the right hand and one on a lower limb, thus monitoring preductal and postductal saturations. If the pulse is lost from the lower limb during a test clamping of the duct, it may indicate that the aorta has been clamped inadvertently. At the authors' institution, all the requirements are stipulated in a protocol and monitoring and other requirements are in place before the arrival of the operating room team.

Invasive blood pressure monitoring is helpful if already established but is not usually placed if not already in place. Monitors used in non–operating room sites may not be compatible with the electrocautery equipment, resulting in loss of monitoring whenever the cautery is used.

Anesthesia Considerations

- A dedicated IV line for fluids and drugs with a long (100 to 150 cm), low-caliber extension to allow access from a distance (space around the cots in NICU is limited)
- High-dose opioids
- Muscle relaxation
- The tracheal tube should have only a small air leak. A large leak may prevent adequate ventilation during lung retraction (recheck tube size and position before the start of the procedure, as well as security and correct position of the tip of the tube after repositioning in the decubitus position, before starting surgery).
- Intercostal nerve block can be placed by surgeon at the completion of surgery
- Glucose-containing fluids maintained at basal rates

SIMPLE RIGHT-TO-LEFT SHUNTS

Tetralogy of Fallot

TOF is the most common cyanotic CHD defect accounting for 6% to 11% of all CHD. Its hallmark is the anterocephalad deviation of the outlet septum, resulting in four features (Fig. 17.5):

- VSD
- Overriding aorta
- Right ventricular outflow tract obstruction (RVOTO)
- Right ventricular hypertrophy

The RVOTO ranges from mild to severe, and the level of the obstruction also varies. Commonly, a dynamic subpulmonary infundibular obstruction is present. Dynamic narrowing of the infundibulum is frequently the cause of hypercyanotic episodes, also known as *tet spells*, in which there is an increase in the shunting of blood from right to left. However, the RVOTO may also be at the level of the pulmonary valve or main or branch pulmonary arteries (PAs). There are four main variants of TOF:

- TOF with pulmonary stenosis—the stenosis may be subvalvar, valvar, supravalvar, or any combination of the three; this represents the most common subtype of TOF.
- TOF with pulmonary atresia—severe variant, with no antegrade flow from the right ventricle into the pulmonary artery; it is commonly associated with hypoplastic pulmonary arteries with major aortopulmonary collateral arteries; if the pulmonary arteries are well developed, pulmonary blood flow is usually derived from a PDA.
- TOF with absent pulmonary valve—the pulmonary valve is dysplastic and incompetent, resulting in dilatation of the pulmonary arteries, causing bronchial compression and, if severe enough, breathing difficulties.
- TOF with AVSD—the rarest form of TOF, in which ASD and TOF coexist, making complete surgical repair particularly challenging.

The right-to-left shunt and cyanosis observed in children with TOF results from a combination of the RVOTO and VSD. The degree of hypoxemia depends on the relationship between the RVOTO and the SVR that determines the degree of right-to-left shunting across the ventricular septal defect. TOF may be associated with a large number of other cardiac and extracardiac anomalies. Extracardiac anomalies most commonly include DiGeorge syndrome (see Table 17.4) and trisomy 21.

Hypercyanotic Episodes

Hypercyanotic spells are episodes of cyanosis that occur in 20% to 70% of untreated children. They may be initiated by crying or feeding and may even occur during anesthesia. The cause of these spells is unclear, but metabolic acidosis, increased $PaCO_2$, circulating catecholamines, and surgical stimulation have all been implicated.

Management of a tet spell requires urgent intervention. Simple measures (e.g., morphine to reduce infundibular spasm, Valsalva maneuver or legs-to-knee chest position to increase SVR) may be effective. Early and aggressive use of a vasoconstrictor is essential (e.g., metaraminol or phenylephrine). Phenylephrine should be premixed and in a syringe for immediate use. Management may require any of the following:

- 100% oxygen and hyperventilation
- IV fluid bolus
- Sedation or analgesia (e.g., fentanyl, morphine) and paralysis
- Sodium bicarbonate
- Vasoconstriction
  - Phenylephrine is given as a 1-µg/kg bolus and doubled at 1-minute intervals until a satisfactory response is achieved (doses required in small preterm infants may be up to 30 µg/kg); this is followed by an infusion at 1 to 5 µg/kg per minute.
  - Norepinephrine is given at a rate of 0.01 to 0.2 µg/kg per minute, if central venous access is available.
  - β-Blockers are administered to relax infundibular spasm and reduce the heart rate.
  - Propranolol 15–20 µg/kg is given as a slow intravenous injection (max 100 µg/kg), and repeated depending on clinical effect.

- Esmolol is given as a 500-µg/kg loading dose administered over 1 minute, followed by a continuous infusion at a rate of 50 to 250 µg/kg per minute.

Surgical Management

The optimal surgical management of children with TOF remains controversial. The choice is between initial palliation with a systemic-to-pulmonary shunt followed by a complete repair when the infant is older and complete repair during the neonatal or early infant period. The current trend is toward early complete repair.[409,410] Complete repair involves closure of the VSD and relief of the RVOTO. Relief of the RVOTO may require a transannular patch (i.e., a patch extending from the right ventricular outflow tract across the pulmonary valve annulus into the supravalvar area) that involves a right ventriculotomy. If this is the case, a significant degree of pulmonary regurgitation is inevitable. Right ventricular dysfunction is a particular problem after repair, and it usually manifests as RV restrictive physiology in the immediate postoperative period; compliance of the RV is greatly reduced, resulting in severe diastolic dysfunction. Long-term follow-up of patients with TOF repair has revealed the consequences of significant pulmonary regurgitation after a transannular patch technique to be more serious than previously anticipated. In fact, late RV dilatation and dysfunction with reduced tolerance to exercise, hemodynamic compromise, dysrhythmias, and an increased risk of sudden death have led surgeons to avoid a transannular patch whenever possible, often accepting a degree of pulmonary stenosis as a trade-off.[411–413] In the immediate postoperative period, JET is a particular risk after complete correction. JET is a self-limiting, narrow QT tachycardia, arising from increased automaticity from the AV node region, which does not predispose to more severe dysrhythmias. Its importance resides in the fact that it usually occurs postoperatively in the first 24 to 48 hours, when a degree of already existing cardiac dysfunction may be further aggravated by the rapid heart rate and loss of the contribution of atrial contraction to ventricular filling.

Anesthesia Considerations

SYSTEMIC-TO-PULMONARY SHUNT. The systemic-to-pulmonary shunt typically is a modified Blalock-Taussig shunt. This is a connection between the subclavian artery to a branch pulmonary artery via the interposition of a synthetic tube graft.

- The patient is usually a neonate or small infant.
- Sedative premedication is useful to prevent crying during induction, which may provoke a hypercyanotic spell.
- There is a risk of a hypercyanotic spell during induction and surgery.
- Inhalational or IV induction are both appropriate.
- Surgery is most often performed through a thoracotomy (left or right) but may occasionally be performed through a sternotomy.
- CPB is not usually required.
- Arterial and central venous access is required.
- Tracheal tube should be snug (or use a cuffed tracheal tube), with no or minimal air leak because lung retraction during surgery can make ventilation difficult.
- The arterial line should not be in the arm on the side that the shunt will be placed because the subclavian artery will be clamped, and the arterial pressure will be lost.
- Hemodynamic and respiratory disturbance can be problematic during surgery.
- The surgeon may request a small dose of heparin.
- Bleeding may occur after clamps are released; be prepared for a blood transfusion.

- Postoperatively, the pulmonary blood supply predominantly depends on the size of the shunt. If the shunt is too small, the infant may have a low saturation level; if the shunt is too large, the infant may develop heart failure or pulmonary edema and hypotension.
- Pulmonary blood flow also depends on systemic blood pressure; the greater the blood pressure, the more blood flows to the lungs and the higher the saturation.
- Milrinone is often combined with norepinephrine because norepinephrine increases the low diastolic pressure created by the shunt by systemic to pulmonary artery runoff in diastole, but does not produce the unwanted tachycardia seen with epinephrine.
- Postoperative ventilation may be required.

COMPLETE REPAIR. If the child is scheduled for early complete correction with no previous palliation by a systemic-to-pulmonary shunt, the child is likely to be a neonate or small infant. These children remain at risk for hypercyanotic spells. However, if the child has had a shunt placed previously, he or she is likely to be older and much less likely to have a hypercyanotic episode. Some children with less severe disease may not require a shunt and may be operated on when they are a bit older because they remain asymptomatic. Good sedative premedication is important in those at risk for hypercyanotic episodes.

- Both IV and inhalational induction agents are appropriate.
- CPB is required.
- Right ventricular dysfunction and pulmonary regurgitation may be postoperative problems.
- Intense inotropic support may worsen RVOTO postoperatively by dynamic narrowing of the RVOT; norepinephrine may be preferable to epinephrine in this setting, considering its predominant α-adrenergic effects.
- Milrinone may be particularly useful owing to its lusitropic properties, promoting diastolic relaxation of the stiff right ventricle.
- Surgeons frequently measure right ventricular pressure to assess the quality of the repair.
- Perioperative echocardiography is useful in assessing repair and right ventricular function.
- Excessive β-adrenergic stimulation and pyrexia may contribute to triggering JET postoperatively.

COMPLEX SHUNTS. In complex shunts (i.e., mixing shunts), there is mixing of pulmonary and systemic blood flow, with resulting cyanosis.

Transposition of the Great Arteries

Transposition of the great arteries (TGA) is common and accounts for about 6% of all CHD. It frequently occurs as an isolated lesion and is rarely associated with extracardiac anomalies. The operation most commonly performed in these infants is the arterial switch operation (ASO), the short- and long-term results of which have improved to such an extent that children with a good repair can expect a normal life.[414]

TGA refers to the situation in which the aorta arises from the morphologic right ventricle and the pulmonary artery arises from the morphologic left ventricle (Fig. 17.6). In this ventriculoarterial (VA) discordance, the atria are related to the ventricles in the normal way (i.e., AV concordance). This results in two circulations that run in parallel rather than in series, which is the normal anatomic arrangement. Without some mixing of the two circulations, the systemic circulation would remain completely deoxygenated. However, some mixing does occur through the PDA or through a VSD that is present in approximately 25% of cases. If there is

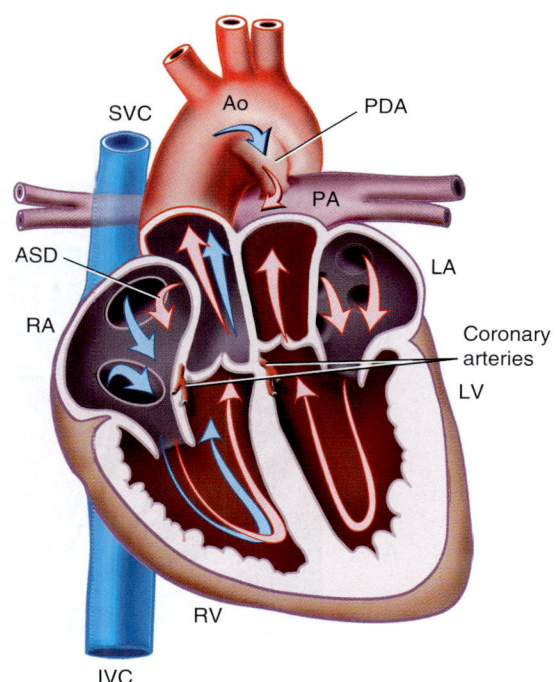

FIGURE 17.6 Diagram of transposition of the great arteries shows an intact ventricular septum. The aorta (*Ao*) arises from the right ventricle (*RV*), and the pulmonary artery (*PA*) arises from the left ventricle (*LV*). The coronary arteries arise from the aorta. These children are cyanotic. *ASD*, atrial septal defect; *IVC*, inferior vena cava; *LA*, left atrium; *PDA*, patent ductus arteriosus; *RA*, right atrium; *SVC*, superior vena cava. (Modified from May LE. *Pediatric Heart Surgery: A Ready Reference for Professionals*. Milwaukee, WI: Maxishare; 2005.)

no VSD and mixing is inadequate, ductal patency is maintained after birth with an IV prostaglandin E_1 infusion, and a balloon atrial septostomy is performed urgently in the neonatal period.

In TGA with an intact ventricular septum, the ASO should be performed early in the neonatal period, preferably in the first 2 to 3 weeks of life, because the left ventricle is exposed only to the pressure of the pulmonary circulation. The longer this situation is allowed to continue, the less the left ventricle will be able to adapt to the work required to pump blood at systemic pressure after corrective surgery. However, if there is an unrestrictive VSD, the left and right ventricle pressures equalize and both ventricles are exposed to systemic blood pressure, and the left ventricle is better conditioned to perform the work of the systemic ventricle after the ASO.

If untreated, most infants with TGA die in the first year of life of hypoxia and heart failure. Pulmonary vascular disease develops early and contributes to this high mortality rate.[415,416] The mechanism for the early development of pulmonary vascular disease is complex and not simply related to high pulmonary blood flow. However, the presence of a VSD further accelerates this process. These infants are at risk for pulmonary hypertensive crises in the postoperative period.[417]

Surgical Options

ARTERIAL SWITCH OPERATION. An ASO is the operation of choice if the intracardiac anatomy is appropriate. The ASO involves transecting the two main arterial trunks distal to their respective valves and switching them to produce VA concordance (Fig. 17.7).

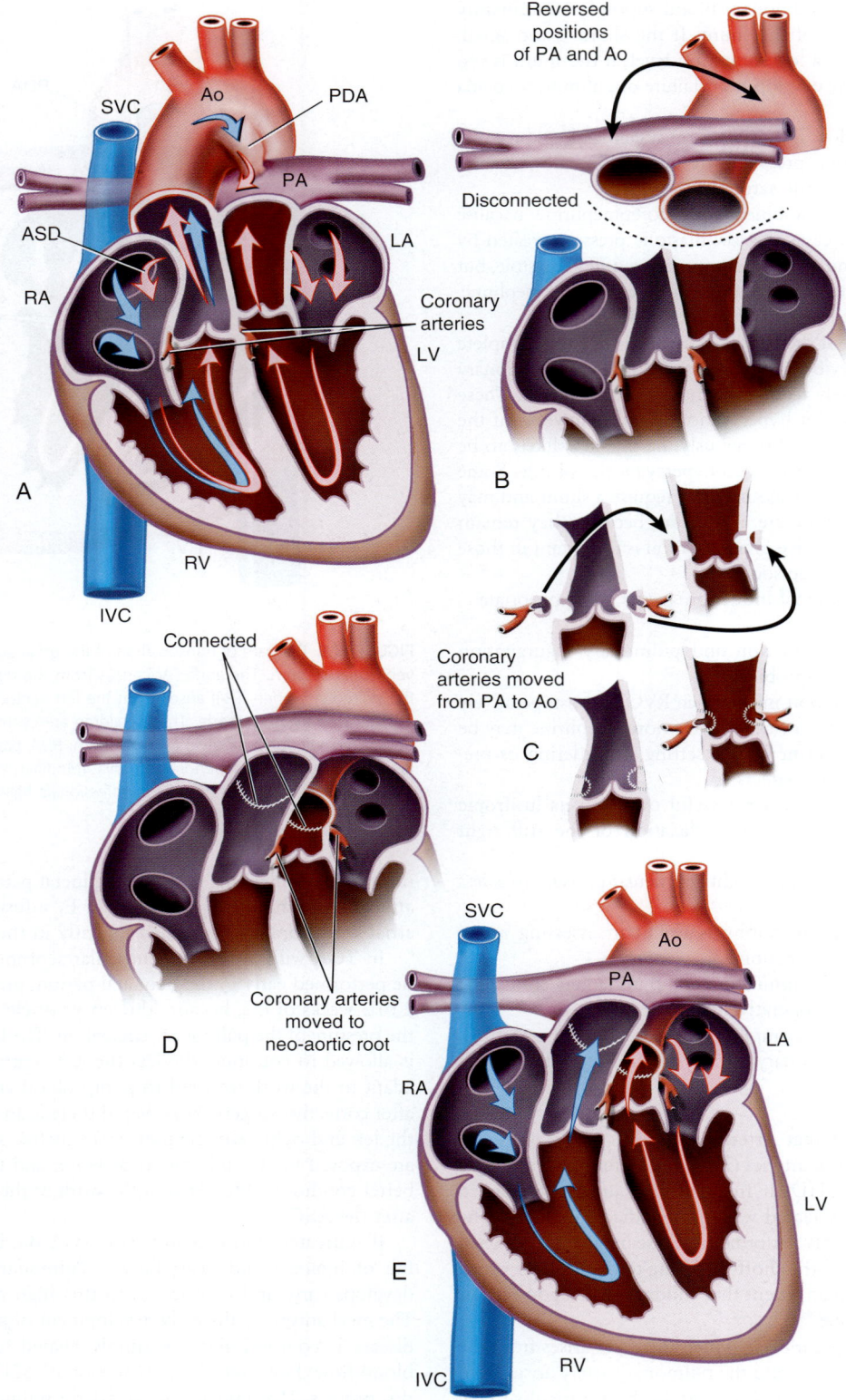

FIGURE 17.7 Diagram of an arterial switch operation. **A,** The original anatomy. The aorta (*Ao*), pulmonary arteries (*PA*), and coronary arteries are disconnected from their origins. **B,** The PA is moved anterior to the Ao. **C,** The Ao is connected to the left ventricle, and the PA is connected to the right ventricle. **D,** The coronary arteries are connected to the neoaortic root. **E,** Final configuration. *IVC,* inferior vena cava; *LA,* left atrium; *LV,* left ventricle; *RA,* right atrium; *RV,* right ventricle; *SVC,* superior vena cava. (Modified from May LE. *Pediatric Heart Surgery: A Ready Reference for Professionals.* Milwaukee, WI: Maxishare; 2005.)

It also involves disconnecting the coronary arteries from the "old" aorta and reconnecting them to the neoaorta. This restores anatomic and physiologic normality. The coronary anatomy varies widely in TGA but must be well assessed preoperatively because moving the coronary arteries to the neoaorta is difficult but crucial to a successful outcome. In some cases, the coronary arteries run in the wall of the aorta (intramural), and this poses particular difficulties for the surgeon. Ventricular function after surgery depends largely on unrestricted flow in the coronary arteries.

MUSTARD AND SENNING PROCEDURES. The Mustard and Senning procedures are atrial switch operations. They involve the use of intraatrial baffles to redirect deoxygenated blood from the venae cavae to the left atrium, left ventricle, and pulmonary artery and oxygenated pulmonary venous blood to the right atrium, right ventricle, and aorta. They create AV discordance, restore physiologic but not anatomic normality, and leave the morphologic and physiologic right ventricle as the systemic ventricle. These procedures were performed as definitive procedures before the arterial switch became successful but are rarely used today as definitive repairs. They are still used as palliation in children with TGA, VSD, and pulmonary vascular disease.[418] In these cases, the VSD is left open. Atrial switch operations are also used as definitive repairs in congenitally corrected transposition of the great arteries (ccTGA or L-TGA), a rarer form of TGA with both AV and VA discordance. In these cases, an atrial switch is combined with an ASO, thus restoring AV and VA concordance, as components of what is denominated a double-switch procedure.[419-421]

RASTELLI PROCEDURE. The Rastelli procedure is used in children with TGA, VSD, and LVOTO. The procedure closes the VSD in a way that directs blood from the left ventricle to the aorta. The pulmonary artery is ligated just distal to the pulmonary valve, and a valved conduit is inserted from the right ventricle to the pulmonary artery. The result is continuity between the left ventricle and aorta and between the right ventricle and the pulmonary artery, and the LVOTO (i.e., subpulmonary area) is bypassed. In the past, the Rastelli procedure was performed at 2 to 3 years of age, following palliation in the neonatal period by a Blalock-Taussig shunt. However, as with other forms of CHD, there is currently a trend toward neonatal Rastelli repair, thus eliminating the need for previous palliation.

Anesthesia Considerations for the Arterial Switch Procedure
- The patient is a neonate in the first few weeks of life.
- Inhalational or IV induction is possible.
- Invasive arterial and central venous lines are required.
- Myocardial ischemia occurring after the cross-clamp is removed may be related to coronary air emboli or inadequate coronary anastomoses. A generous perfusion pressure after removal of cross-clamp encourages flushing air from coronary arteries. If ischemia results from an anatomic problem with the transferred coronary arteries, they may need to be redone with a second bypass run.
- TEE or epicardial echo is useful in assessing adequate de-airing, myocardial function, and adequacy of coronary anastomoses.
- Post-CPB myocardial dysfunction may result from one or more of the following:
  - Coronary air
  - Poor coronary transference
  - Poor myocardial protection
  - Inherently poor left ventricle
- The anesthesiologist should anticipate pulmonary hypertension.

- Inotropes are almost always required. Dopamine or epinephrine can be used, and milrinone is a particularly useful agent in these cases because it is an inodilator.
- After the repair, the pulmonary artery is anterior to the aorta. Any dilation of the pulmonary artery as a result of pulmonary hypertension can lead to coronary artery compression and myocardial ischemia.
- The left ventricle is frequently noncompliant, and volume should be increased with care and in small amounts. LA pressure can rise quickly if fluid is given injudiciously.
- Coagulopathy after bypass is common.
- Antifibrinolytics are often used.

Truncus Arteriosus
Truncus arteriosus is a rare congenital heart defect that occurs in about 0.7 of 1000 live births and accounts for about 1% of all CHD. The basic lesion is that of a common arterial outlet for the aorta and pulmonary artery associated with a single valve with variable morphology (called a truncal valve) and a VSD (Fig. 17.8). The different subtypes depend on how the pulmonary arteries arise from the aorta and on the size of the aorta. Blood mixes at the arterial level with a resultant high pulmonary blood flow. This leads to heart failure and early development of pulmonary hypertension. Surgery must be performed early in life to prevent pulmonary hypertension from becoming irreversible. Truncus arteriosus has a known association with DiGeorge syndrome (see Table 17.4). In the presence of this syndrome or uncertainty about an existing 22q11 deletion, irradiated blood products should be used and calcium concentrations carefully monitored.

Surgical repair involves separating the systemic and pulmonary circulations as well as closing the VSD. The pulmonary artery or arteries are disconnected from the aorta, and the truncal valve is repaired. The pulmonary arteries are then connected to the right ventricle, usually with a valved conduit. Circulatory arrest may be required. The early postoperative mortality rate ranges from 5% to 25%. Several factors are known to influence mortality, including the presence of other cardiac abnormalities, particularly truncal valve stenosis and coronary abnormalities, as well as chromosomal anomalies and low birth weight.[422,423]

Anesthesia Considerations
- The patient is a small neonate.
- Patients may already be intubated and ventilated and may be on inotropes.
- If the child is not ventilated, premedication is probably best avoided.
- Heart failure is possible.
- Repair is a high-risk procedure.
- Risks include a postoperative pulmonary hypertensive crisis.
- Invasive lines are required.
- Circulatory arrest may be required.
- Coagulopathy may occur after bypass.
- Antifibrinolytics are often used.

Anomalous Pulmonary Venous Drainage
Anomalous pulmonary venous drainage comprises about 2.5% of CHD and may be total (TAPVD) or partial (PAPVD). In TAPVD, all four pulmonary veins insert into an anomalous site, and in PAPVD, a subset of the veins insert into an anomalous site and the remaining veins insert into the left atrium. Survival is usually good but depends on the site of insertion, with survival poorer

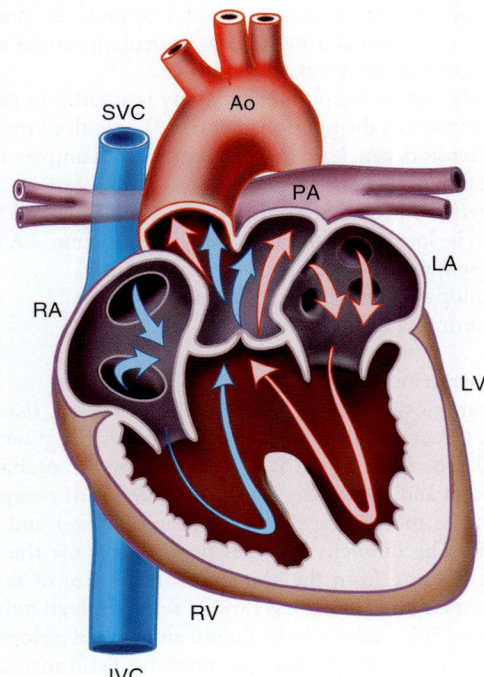

FIGURE 17.8 The diagram of a truncus arteriosus shows the common truncal valve and mixing of red and blue blood. *Ao*, aorta; *IVC*, inferior vena cava; *LA*, left atrium; *LV*, left ventricle; *PA*, pulmonary artery; *RA*, right atrium; *RV*, right ventricle; *SVC*, superior vena cava. (Modified from May LE. *Pediatric Heart Surgery: A Ready Reference for Professionals.* Milwaukee, WI: Maxishare; 2005.)

for the infracardiac than for the supracardiac and cardiac types; the size of the venous confluence at the insertion into the left atrium; and the presence or absence of obstruction. In some circumstances, even though the pulmonary veins may be appropriately connected to the left atrium, an ASD results in part of the pulmonary venous return being directed preferentially to the right atrium. Therefore it is probably more appropriate to refer to these forms of CHD as anomalous pulmonary venous drainage or return, even though the term anomalous pulmonary venous connection is also used. Four types of TAPVD exist:

- In supracardiac TAPVD, the pulmonary veins drain to the SVC territory via the left brachiocephalic vein through an ascending vertical vein (Fig. 17.9A).
- In cardiac TAPVD, the pulmonary veins connect to the right atrium through the coronary sinus (see Fig. 17.9B).
- In infracardiac TAPVD, the pulmonary veins drain to the IVC territory through a common vein, which traverses the diaphragm (see Fig. 17.9C).
- In mixed TAPVD, any combination of the previously mentioned three types may occur (see Fig. 17.9C).

Infants with obstructed anomalous pulmonary venous drainage, pulmonary hypertension, and reduced pulmonary blood supply usually present early with cyanosis and tachypnea. The degree of cyanosis depends on the size of an existing ASD and the associated right-to-left shunt, as well as on the degree of mixing of systemic and pulmonary venous blood. Children without pulmonary venous obstruction and pulmonary hypertension usually have few symptoms.

Anesthesia Considerations

- The patient may be a neonate.
- Heart failure can occur.
- Pulmonary edema may be present.
- There is a risk of pulmonary hypertension preoperatively and postoperatively; nitric oxide may be required.
- Circulatory arrest may be used, and profound hypothermia may be required.
- Coagulopathy may occur after bypass.
- Antifibrinolytics are often used.

As previously mentioned, there is a risk of pulmonary hypertension, for which inhaled nitric oxide may be necessary. However, it should be used with caution in these patients. In fact, children with obstructive lesions at the atrial level before surgery or patients with a poorly compliant left ventricle may be unable to tolerate an acute increase in pulmonary venous return; the use of inhaled nitrous oxide could thus result in paradoxical pulmonary hypertension.[424,425]

Hypoplastic Left Heart Syndrome

The incidence of HLHS in the United States is about 2 cases per 10,000 live births. In Europe, this figure is probably reduced because many mothers with a prenatal diagnosis of HLHS opt for pregnancy termination.

The anatomic features of HLHS (Fig. 17.10) include the following:

- Hypoplastic left ventricle
- Mitral stenosis or atresia
- Aortic stenosis or atresia
- Hypoplastic aortic arch
- Duct-dependent circulation

The prognosis for infants who are born with HLHS has improved dramatically. Previously, virtually all of these infants died of this condition, but in some centers, most children now survive at least into childhood.[426] The longer-term outlook has not been fully determined, and many hurdles remain.

The diagnosis of HLHS is usually made in the prenatal period, although it can be difficult and is sometimes missed. At birth, neonates present with tachypnea, tachycardia, and cyanosis, and a systolic murmur can be heard.

Surgical Palliation

The aim of surgery is to convert the anatomy of the HLHS into a single-ventricle–type circulation in which the right ventricle becomes the single systemic ventricle and the pulmonary blood flow is supplied passively from the SVC and IVC (i.e., Fontan circulation). This is done by a series of three operations known as Norwood stage I, Norwood stage II (also called superior cavopulmonary connection, bidirectional Glenn or hemi-Fontan), and Norwood stage III (Fontan).

NORWOOD STAGE I. The Norwood stage I operation is performed in the neonatal period. It involves reconstructing the aortic arch so that it arises from the pulmonary trunk. The pulmonary valve becomes the neoaortic valve. The branch pulmonary arteries are disconnected from the pulmonary trunk, and a new source of pulmonary blood supply is provided by a shunt from the subclavian artery (i.e., Blalock-Taussig shunt) or from the right ventricle (i.e., Sano modification) (Fig. 17.11).[427] If the ASD is restrictive, it is enlarged to allow for unobstructed pulmonary venous return into what becomes a common atrium, then draining across the interatrial septum through the right side into the right ventricle. The important physiologic principles of the Norwood stage I operation are

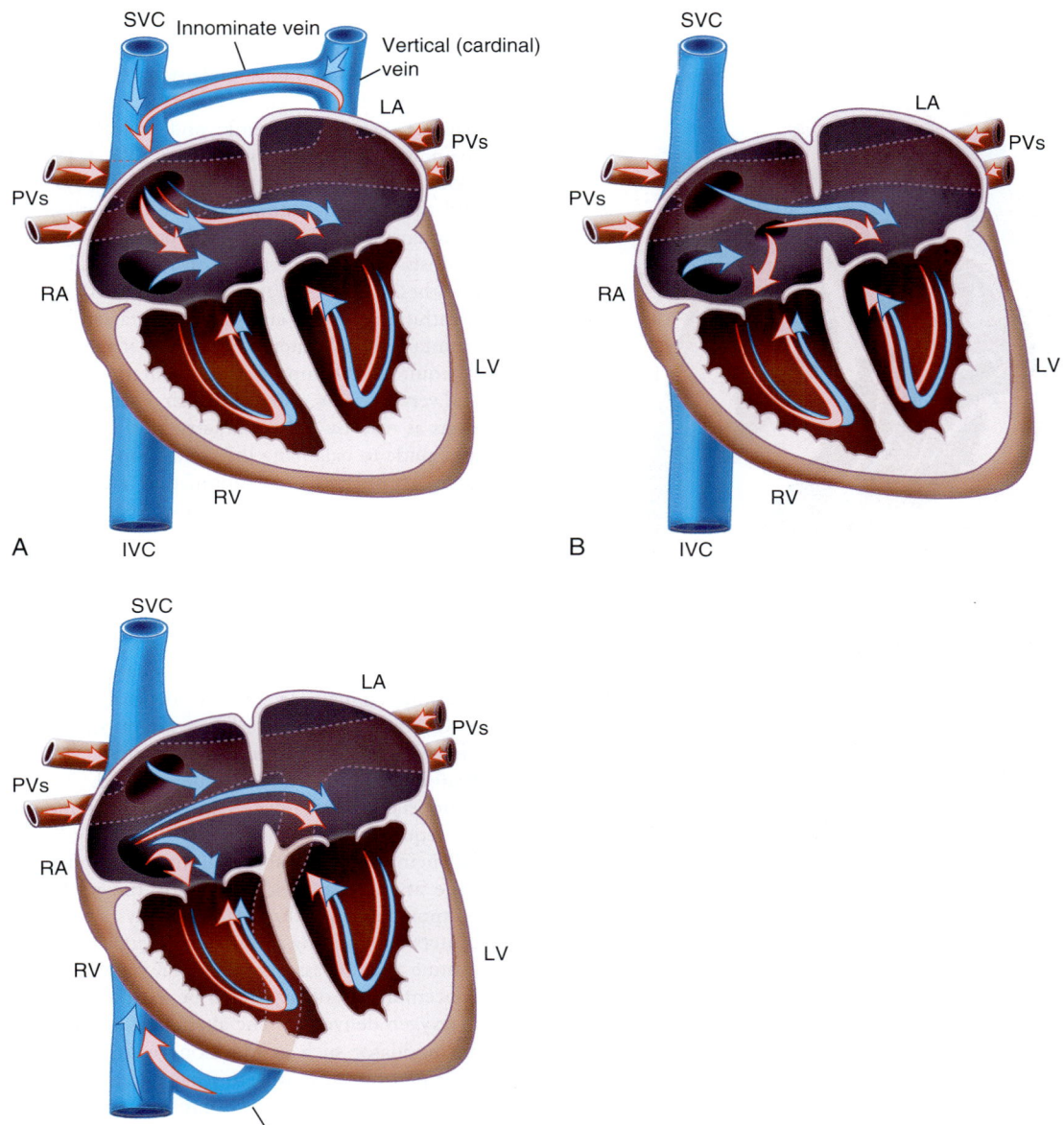

FIGURE 17.9 A, In the diagram of a supracardiac total anomalous pulmonary venous connection (TAPVC), the main arteries are removed. The pulmonary veins (*PVs*) drain through the innominate vein to the right atrium (*RA*), and there is an atrial septal defect (ASD). The result is a left-to-right shunt. These children are cyanotic. The veins may also be obstructed, leading to pulmonary hypertension. **B,** In the diagram of an intracardiac TAPVC, the PVs drain to the RA. There is a ventricular septal defect, and the effect is to create a left-to-right shunt. The veins may also be obstructed, which can lead to pulmonary hypertension. **C,** In the diagram of an infracardiac TAPVC, the PVs drain through the ductus venosus to the RA. An ASD exists, and the circulation results in a right-to-left shunt; the child is blue. The veins may also be obstructed. *IVC,* inferior vena cava; *LA,* left atrium; *LV,* left ventricle; *RA,* right atrium; *RV,* right ventricle; *SVC,* superior vena cava. (Modified from May LE. *Pediatric Heart Surgery: A Ready Reference for Professionals.* Milwaukee, WI: Maxishare; 2005.)

unobstructed pulmonary venous return with unrestrictive interatrial communication; unobstructed systemic blood flow and adequate coronary perfusion; and controlled source of pulmonary blood flow.

NORWOOD STAGE II. The Norwood stage II (superior cavopulmonary connection, bidirectional Glenn or hemi-Fontan) operation takes place at about 6 months of age. It involves taking down the shunt that was created at the first operation and creating a new connection from the SVC to the pulmonary arteries (i.e., a bidirectional or Glenn shunt). The result is a pulmonary blood supply that is provided by systemic venous blood from the SVC. Flow is passive and depends on pulmonary artery pressures remaining low, since its driving force is the pressure gradient between the SVC (connected to the pulmonary arteries, upstream from the lungs) and atrial pressure (pressure downstream from the lungs). The gradient between these two pressures is called the

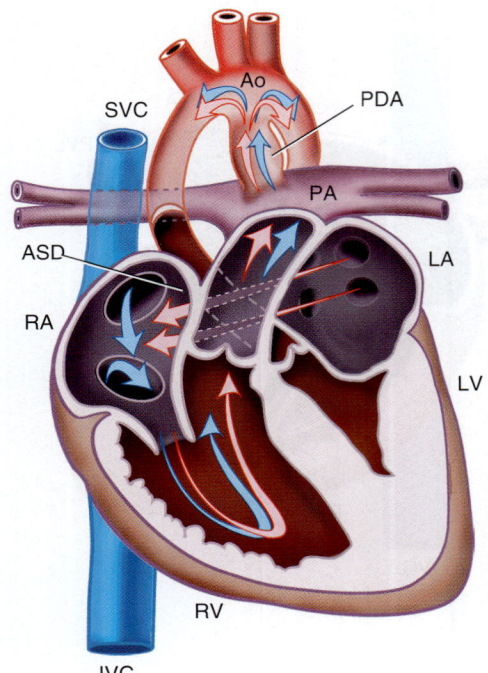

FIGURE 17.10 Diagram of hypoplastic left heart syndrome shows a very small left ventricle (*LV*), mitral valve, aortic valve, and aortic arch. Pulmonary venous blood drains to the left atrium (*LA*), then through an atrial septal defect (*ASD*) to the right atrium (*RA*), and from there through the right ventricle (*RV*) to the pulmonary artery (*PA*). A patent ductus arteriosus (*PDA*) provides blood to the systemic circulation. *Ao*, aorta; *IVC*, inferior vena cava; *SVC*, superior vena cava. (Modified from May LE. *Pediatric Heart Surgery: A Ready Reference for Professionals.* Milwaukee, WI: Maxishare; 2005.)

transpulmonary gradient, and any obstruction between these two sites (for example, pulmonary hypertension) will result in inadequate pulmonary blood flow. The infants remain cyanotic with arterial saturations in the mid-80s because desaturated blood from the IVC continues to flow into the heart and the systemic circulation (Fig. 17.12).

NORWOOD STAGE III. The Norwood stage III (Fontan) operation converts the anatomy into a Fontan circulation. The surgery involves connecting the IVC through an extracardiac or intracardiac conduit to the pulmonary artery. This creates a single-ventricle or Fontan circulation (Fig. 17.13). The single right ventricle pumps blood to the systemic circulation, and the pulmonary blood supply is provided by passive flow by systemic venous blood from the SVC and IVC. The PVR must remain low because any increase will dramatically reduce pulmonary blood flow. It is common for a small hole (i.e., fenestration) to be created between the conduit and the right atrium so that if the PVR rises, blood will be directed to the right atrium and allow cardiac output to be maintained. In this situation, the child becomes cyanotic, but cardiac output is maintained, a much safer situation than a state of low cardiac output. Postoperatively, increased systemic venous pressure may cause pleural effusions, an enlarged liver, or protein-losing enteropathy. Later, if PVR remains consistently low, the fenestration can be closed with a transvenous device.

The long-term problem for these children is that the morphologic right ventricle, which then becomes the systemic ventricle, fails over time. The only recourse is heart transplantation.[428,429]

Anesthesia Considerations

NORWOOD STAGE I.

- The anesthesiologist must understand the anatomy and physiology of HLHS.
- Balance between systemic and pulmonary circulations is maintained by balancing PVR and SVR. If the PVR decreases, blood flow will be directed away from the systemic circulation and there will be pulmonary overcirculation. This results in hypotension and systemic hypoperfusion with increasing acidosis. If PVR increases, cyanosis will increase. Before anesthesia, these infants are best managed spontaneously breathing in room air with a prostaglandin E_1 infusion to maintain ductal patency. However, if mechanical ventilation is required, it is important to maintain normal to high $PaCO_2$ and very low FIO_2, usually with air. Even though oxygen saturations as read by pulse oximetry have traditionally been used as a guide to balancing the circulation, there is evidence that, when considered in isolation, they are a poor reflection of such a balance. As such, systemic venous saturations should also be used to provide an estimate of tissue oxygen delivery.[183,185,430,431] NIRS monitoring can also be used as a continuous indicator of the adequacy of oxygen delivery to the brain.
- Air should be available for transfer to and from the ICU; alternatively, a self-inflating bag can be used.
- Venous access is gained through the femoral or umbilical veins. The internal jugular vein is avoided because narrowing of the SVC would jeopardize a future Glenn shunt.
- High-dose opioid technique is preferred.
- Profound hypothermia may be required.
- Postoperative myocardial dysfunction is common, and inotropes are required.
- Balancing systemic and pulmonary blood flow remains an issue after bypass and estimating the relative systemic and pulmonary blood flows is not always straightforward. Some centers use the long-acting α-adrenergic blocker phenoxybenzamine after bypass to reduce SVR variability, allowing greater concentrations of oxygen to be used and an overall increase in oxygen delivery.[432] The alternative approach is to combine an inodilator such as milrinone with a vasopressor such as dopamine or epinephrine to achieve a similar effect. The authors' preference is to deliver a bolus dose of milrinone (0.5 µg/kg over 20 minutes during rewarming), followed by an infusion of 0.3 µg/kg per minute, in combination with a continuous infusion of epinephrine, 0.05 to 0.1 µg/kg per minute.
- Coagulopathy is likely to occur after bypass.
- Antifibrinolytics are often used.
- The sternum is frequently left open, and closure may be delayed for several days.

NORWOOD STAGE II.

- The procedure is carried out with CPB.
- Cardioplegia is not used. The heart remains beating, and inotropes are seldom required.
- Venous access is achieved through the femoral veins. However, only a single side should be used because femoral bypass is occasionally required. A short temporary cannula is useful as an additional monitor in the internal jugular vein. It reflects the pulmonary artery pressure after anastomosis of the SVC to the pulmonary artery. It is removed early in the postoperative period to avoid any possibility of thrombosis in the SVC.
- This is repeat surgery, and external defibrillator pads should be attached.
- Antifibrinolytics may be used.

17

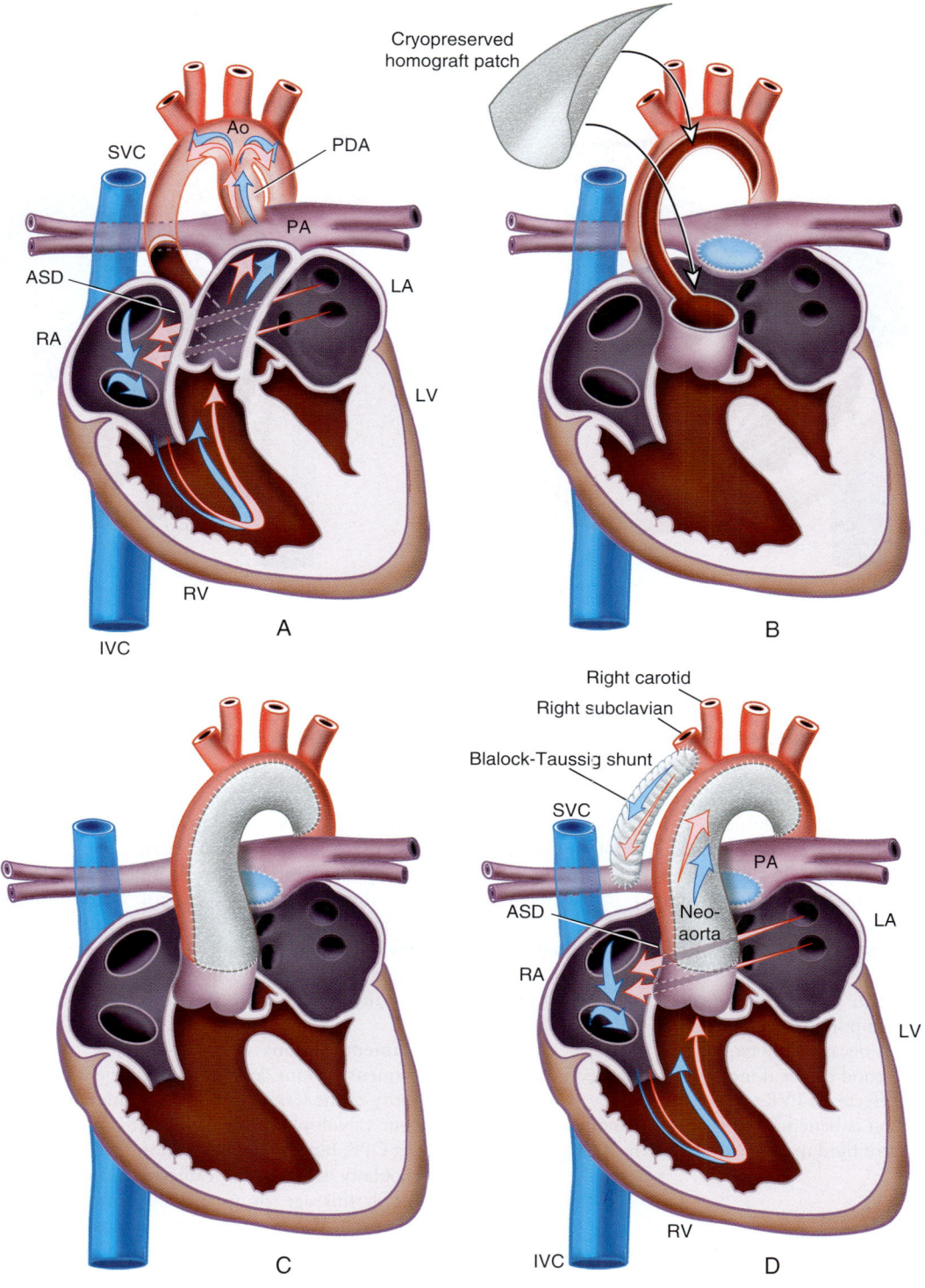

FIGURE 17.11 Diagram of the Norwood stage I operation. **A,** The main pulmonary artery (*PA*) is disconnected from the right ventricle (*RV*). **B** and **C,** The aortic arch is reconstructed with homograft and connected to the RV, which becomes a single ventricle. **D,** Pulmonary blood is then supplied by a Blalock-Taussig shunt from the subclavian artery to the PA. The children remain cyanotic. *Ao,* aorta; *ASD,* atrial septal defect; *IVC,* inferior vena cava; *LA,* left atrium; *LV,* left ventricle; *PDA,* patent ductus arteriosus; *RA,* right atrium; *SVC,* superior vena cava.. (Modified from May LE. *Pediatric Heart Surgery: A Ready Reference for Professionals.* Milwaukee, WI: Maxishare; 2005.)

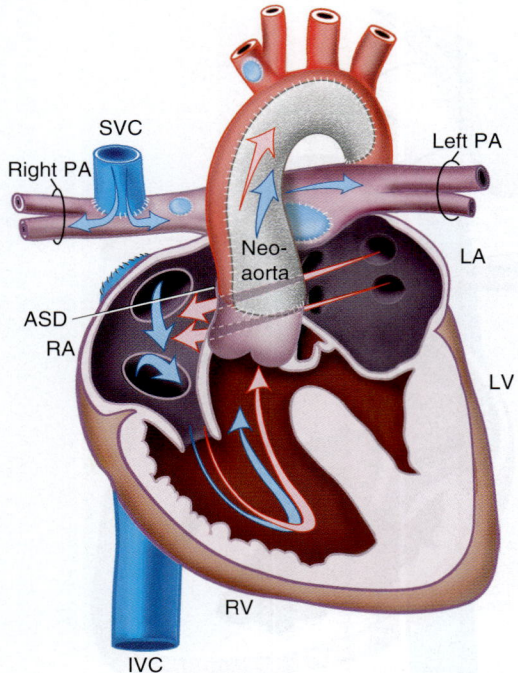

FIGURE 17.12 Diagram of Norwood stage II (hemi-Fontan) operation. The Blalock-Taussig shunt is disconnected, and a Glenn shunt is created by connecting the superior vena cava (*SVC*) to the pulmonary artery (*PA*). *ASD,* atrial septal defect; *IVC,* inferior vena cava; *LA,* left atrium; *LV,* left ventricle; *RA,* right atrium; *RV,* right ventricle. (Modified from May LE. *Pediatric Heart Surgery: A Ready Reference for Professionals.* Milwaukee, WI: Maxishare; 2005.)

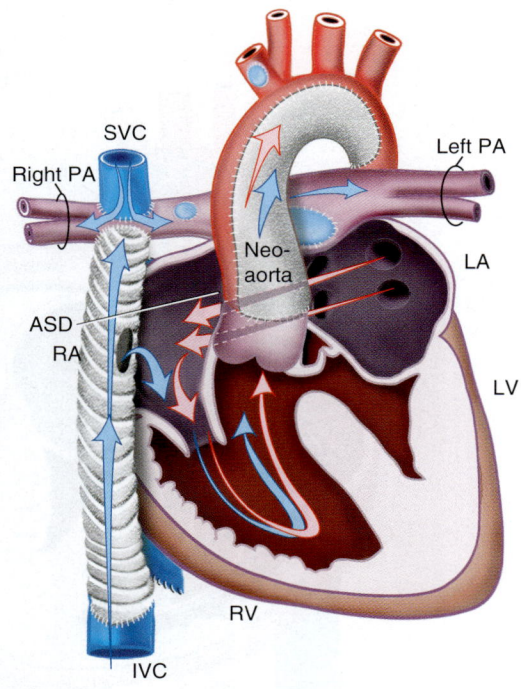

FIGURE 17.13 Diagram of Norwood stage III (Fontan) operation. The Fontan circulation is created by connecting the inferior vena cava (*IVC*) to the pulmonary artery (*PA*) with a conduit. A fenestration is shown between the conduit and the right atrium (*RA*). *ASD,* atrial septal defect; *LA,* left atrium; *LV,* left ventricle; *RV,* right ventricle; *SVC,* superior vena cava. (Modified from May LE. *Pediatric Heart Surgery: A Ready Reference for Professionals.* Milwaukee, WI: Maxishare; 2005.)

- The aim is early extubation; positive intrathoracic pressure reduces flow in the Glenn shunt.
- Infants should be nursed with the head up at 30 degrees after surgery, to improve flow in the Glenn shunt and reduce the possibility of edema in the SVC territory.

NORWOOD STAGE III.

- Surgery is carried out with CPB but usually without cross-clamping the aorta.
- PVR must remain low postoperatively, careful management of the lungs is important to minimize atelectasis, and inhaled nitrous oxide is occasionally required.[433]
- Milrinone is a good choice if inotropes are needed because of its beneficial effects on PVR.
- Early extubation is beneficial in terms of hemodynamics.
- Large amounts of fluid may be required in the early postoperative period.

AORTIC STENOSIS

Obstruction to the LVOT can occur at the valvular, subvalvular, or supravalvular areas or in various combinations, and it occurs commonly, accounting for up to 10% of CHD.[434,435] Congenital valvar aortic stenosis is frequently associated with a bicuspid valve. Severe critical aortic stenosis in neonates occurs in approximately 10% of cases and requires urgent treatment. Supravalvular aortic stenosis may be associated with Williams syndrome.[436]

Despite the many anatomic varieties of aortic stenosis, the resulting pathophysiology remains essentially the same. There is an increasing imbalance between myocardial oxygen supply and demand. Coronary blood flow is impaired due to low coronary perfusion pressure, while workload on the left ventricle is increased,

leading to subendocardial ischemia, left ventricular hypertrophy, and a risk of left ventricular failure. The risk of sudden death is always present, especially with Williams syndrome.[437] The age at which the child presents is a risk factor; younger children are most at risk. Two-thirds of those presenting in the first 3 months of life will require inotropic or ventilatory support before treatment of the stenosis.[438] Approximately 5% of Williams syndrome patients may suffer a cardiac arrest during anesthesia.[439]

Treatment Options

Treatment options depend on the patient's age and the type and severity of the lesion. In neonates with critical aortic stenosis, an urgent valvuloplasty is required. It can be performed surgically using CPB, but it typically is performed using transluminal balloon angioplasty in the cardiac catheterization laboratory.[440] Complications in this age group include ventricular fibrillation, aortic incompetence, or residual aortic stenosis.

In the older child, several surgical approaches may be used, depending on the anatomy. Transluminal balloon valvuloplasty commonly is performed in older patients. The most common complications of valvuloplasty are aortic incompetence and residual aortic stenosis. Valve replacement with a mechanical valve or bioprosthetic valve is delayed as long as possible because of the long-term problems associated with the anticoagulation needed with a mechanical valve and because of the inevitable calcification of the bioprosthetic valve. An alternative surgical option is the Ross procedure, which involves moving the pulmonary valve into the aortic valve position and using a homograft in the pulmonary position. The need for reoperation with the Ross procedure is reduced because the systemic valve (i.e., neoaortic valve) grows with the child and calcification of the homograft in the pulmonary position is slow. There is no need for anticoagulation.[441-443] More recently, there has been an interest in the possibility of aortic valve repair for aortic stenosis (rather than replacement) by use of a reconstruction technique with pericardial patch, thus avoiding the potential problems associated with valve replacement.[444-446]

Anesthesia Considerations

- A crucial aim of anesthesia is to maintain the balance of oxygen supply and demand. This involves maintaining a normal heart rate (no tachycardia or bradycardia), maintaining SVR and diastolic blood pressure to preserve coronary perfusion, avoiding hypertension, and avoiding myocardial depression.
- Anesthesia for neonates with aortic stenosis having surgery with CPB is similar to other neonatal cardiac surgery.
- For transluminal balloon valvuloplasty:
  - The catheter crossing the aortic valve and inflation of the balloon can lead to dramatic cardiovascular changes. Cardiac output decreases, myocardial ischemia occurs, and bradycardia is common. In neonates, ventricular fibrillation may occur after passing the wire across the valve. The anesthesiologist must be prepared to resuscitate the neonate quickly, and drugs, particularly epinephrine, should be immediately available.
  - It is possible the child will remain ventilated after the procedure because ventricular function can remain poor for some time.
  - Arterial access is needed by the cardiologist for the procedure, but pressure is not always displayed. An independent arterial line is very useful.
  - Occasionally, adenosine is given to slow or stop the heart at the time of balloon inflation to prevent damage to the valve by the inflated balloon being expelled through it. However, this practice is not universal.

Coarctation of the Aorta

Coarctation of the aorta is discrete narrowing of the aorta, and it accounts for about 5% of CHD. The lesion is often isolated with no other associated abnormalities. This type of lesion, however, may occur in association with other CHD, such as aortic arch, valve abnormalities, or VSD. The coarctation may be preductal, juxtaductal, or postductal, depending on the relationship to the ductus arteriosus. The most common form presenting in the neonatal period is the preductal type. Preductal coarctation is associated with minimal collateral circulation below the coarctation and requires prostaglandin to maintain ductal patency. Juxtaductal and postductal coarctations are characterized by the development of collateral vessels that supply the area below the coarctation. This is important because the spinal cord is supplied by these collaterals, which supply the spinal cord during aortic cross-clamping.

In practical terms, children with coarctation of the aorta can be classified in two groups. One group presents in the neonatal period with preductal coarctation with few collaterals, very poor left ventricular function, and possible heart failure. The second group of children (usually older than 1 year of age) have well-developed collaterals and better left ventricular function. Femoral pulses are often weak, and patients usually have a progressive acidosis. Differences between the systolic systemic blood pressures in the right arm (proximal to the stenosis) and legs (distal to the stenosis) may indicate the presence of a coarctation of the aorta.

Anesthesia Considerations

NEONATAL REPAIR.

- These infants are sick, with poor left ventricular function. They should be treated very carefully, and the anesthesiologist should not be misled by an infant who looks reasonably well.
- Some infants are already intubated and ventilated, and may be on inotropic support.
- IV access often is established to give prostaglandin E_1; this IV line can also be used to administer induction agents. The authors' preference is to give incremental doses of fentanyl (up to 5 µg/kg) and then a muscle relaxant and to supplement this with a very low dose of inhalation agent (e.g., isoflurane [0.3% to 0.5%]). This can be omitted if hypotension ensues.
- Inotropes may be required before surgery, and they should be available.
- Ideally, the arterial line should be placed in the right arm (right radial or axillary arteries) to allow continuous blood pressure measurement during arterial cross-clamping. The left subclavian may be partially obstructed during the repair. Some have advocated an arterial line below the coarctation to measure perfusion pressure during cross-clamping, but this may be very difficult in practice because femoral pulses are usually absent.
- A central venous line should be placed.
- Surgery usually takes place through a left thoracotomy without the use of CPB. The lung is retracted, and ventilation may be problematic. The endotracheal tube must fit snugly and have a minimal leak because a tracheal tube with a large leak may make ventilation very difficult. Alternatively, a cuffed endotracheal tube can be used.
- Paraplegia may occur in about 1% of cases and is thought to result from hypoperfusion during aortic cross-clamping.[447,448] To reduce the chance of spinal cord damage, infants should be cooled to 34°C or 35°C before the cross-clamp is applied, although this approach is not evidence-based. Normocarbia and upper limb blood pressure should be maintained, and the anesthesiologist should resist the temptation to lower blood pressure while the cross-clamp is applied. Low-dose anticoagulation may be requested. A short cross-clamp time is thought to be important.
- Epidural anesthesia is occasionally used but controversial, especially if anticoagulation is to be used, owing to the risk of neurologic damage.
- Postoperative hypertension may be a problem, since ventricular remodeling after relief of the obstruction is not immediate; a degree of left ventricular hypertrophy is to be expected for some weeks to months; in the immediate postoperative period, a vasodilator such as sodium nitroprusside may be required.

ANESTHESIA FOR THE OLDER CHILD.

- These children usually are not as sick as the neonates with this heart defect.
- Issues about vascular lines are similar to those in neonatal repair.
- Careful IV induction with a combination of fentanyl and an induction agent of choice is standard. Etomidate is a good anesthetic because of its cardiovascular stability.
- Although a collateral blood supply is present, the spinal cord remains at risk during the cross-clamping, and the same precautions taken with neonates should be taken with these children.
- An oral cuffed tracheal tube is useful because early extubation is the norm.
- Postoperative hypertension is a common problem, and good analgesia combined with sodium nitroprusside and β-blockers

is usually required. Up to 30% of children eventually develop long-term hypertension that will require therapy.

Some of these children are managed with balloon angioplasty with or without stent placement. Rupture of the aorta is a risk in these patients, and the institution in which the procedure is undertaken should be in a position to deal with this possibility, with a rescue plan clearly established.

Interrupted Aortic Arch

Interrupted aortic arch is a rare anomaly, accounting for less than 1% of CHD. In this condition, disruption occurs between the ascending aorta and descending aorta (Fig. 17.14). The three types depend on where the disruption takes place. It is a duct-dependent systemic circulation, since a PDA is required to supply the descending aorta. A VSD is also common. An interrupted aortic arch is frequently associated with chromosome 22q11 deletion and results in the aforementioned DiGeorge syndrome (see Table 17.4).[449]

These children are often small for gestational age and are started on a prostaglandin infusion to maintain ductal patency. They are often sick with progressive acidosis and poor cardiac output. There is increasing pulmonary blood flow as the duct closes. Surgical repair depends on the presence of associated lesions, particularly a VSD. In the single-stage repair, the arch is reconstructed and the VSD is closed. The two-stage repair involves repair of the aortic arch and banding of the pulmonary artery to limit blood flow to the lungs. The VSD is closed at a later date. Either way, deep hypothermic circulatory arrest is likely to be used. Some centers use selective regional perfusion to try and limit neurologic injury.[450] The early and late mortality rates are high. Greater mortality rates correlate with small size, preoperative acidosis, and associated cardiac lesions.[451]

Anesthesia Considerations

- The patient is a small, sick neonate.
- DiGeorge syndrome should be identified preoperatively, especially regarding the potential for hypocalcemia and the need for irradiated blood products; in case of uncertainty about 22q11 deletion status, it is prudent to proceed as if it is present.
- High-dose opioid technique is standard.
- Ideally, blood pressure should be monitored above and below the interruption, but this is often difficult in practice.
- Deep hypothermic circulatory arrest may be used.
- Coagulopathy is likely to occur after bypass.
- An antifibrinolytic is frequently used.
- Anticipate poor renal function postoperatively.
- There is a risk of postoperative pulmonary hypertensive crises.

These infants are likely to require repeat operations to deal with recurrent LVOTO, which may occur at any level. Restenosis of the repaired aortic arch can often be treated by transluminal balloon dilation.

Transport and Transfer to a Pediatric Intensive Care Unit

After surgery is completed, cardiac surgical patients need a period of intensive care. The first phase of this care is transport of the children from the operating room to the pediatric intensive care unit (PICU). This is a potentially hazardous time and requires good organization, teamwork, and appropriate equipment. Guidelines exist for the safe transport of these children.[452]

Transport to the PICU can be subdivided into a preparatory phase, transport phase, and stabilization phase.[453] During the preparatory phase, the estimated time of arrival in the PICU is communicated with the PICU. The bed space is prepared, ventilator and monitors are configured in an appropriate way, and any additional interventions that may be required are made ready. In the authors' institution, a form is sent to the PICU that indicates the child's age and weight, the ventilator settings that will be required, the number of transducers that will be required, and the infusions that are running. After arrival in the PICU, two basic tasks need to be completed: transfer of technology and transfer of information. It is better to allow the technology transfer to occur before the information handover. This includes ensuring that all the monitors are connected and working appropriately, that the ventilator is connected and delivering adequate ventilation, that all infusions are working, and that drains and urinary catheter are all in place with baseline readings documented. After this has been accomplished, a single handover of information should be done with all of the appropriate personnel present, and it should include information given by the anesthesiologist and surgeon. In our institution, a checklist is followed to ensure that no important information is omitted. It is important to avoid a large number of information handovers between individuals rather than a single, comprehensive handover with all the relevant personnel present.

ACKNOWLEDGMENT

The authors wish to thank Paul R. Hickey, Richard L. Marnach, Dolly D. Hansen, Robert W. Reid, and Frederick A. Burrows for their prior contributions to this chapter.

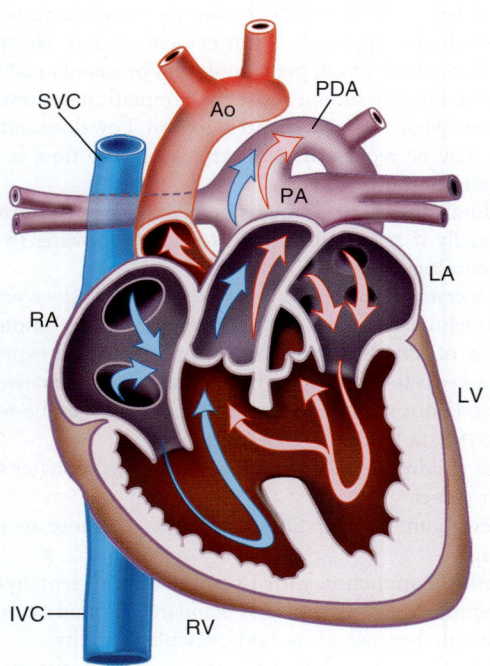

FIGURE 17.14 Diagram of an interrupted aortic arch. The patent ductus arteriosus (*PDA*) supplies the body below the interruption. *Ao,* aorta; *ASD,* atrial septal defect; *LA,* left atrium; *LV,* left ventricle; *PA,* pulmonary artery; *RA,* right atrium; *RV,* right ventricle. (Modified from May LE. *Pediatric Heart Surgery: A Ready Reference for Professionals.* Milwaukee, WI: Maxishare; 2005.)

ANNOTATED REFERENCES

Bettex DA, Pretre R, Jenni R, Schmid ER. Cost-effectiveness of routine intraoperative transesophageal echocardiography in pediatric cardiac surgery: a 10-year experience. *Anesth Analg.* 2005;100:1271-1275.

Bettex and coworkers showed in a retrospective study of 580 pediatric patients undergoing cardiac surgery that the use of routine intraoperative transesophageal echocardiography (TEE) was cost effective. They identified 33 children who required a second bypass run on the basis of the intraoperative TEE. The authors estimate that the savings per child were in the range of $690 to $2130.

Hoffman TM, Wernovsky G, Atz AM, et al. Prophylactic intravenous use of milrinone after cardiac operation in pediatrics (PRIMACORP) study. Prophylactic Intravenous Use of Milrinone After Cardiac Operation in Pediatrics. *Am Heart J.* 2002;143:15-21.

In this large, multicenter, prospective, randomized, double-blind study, it was shown that the use of milrinone in high doses (75 µg/kg bolus over 60 minutes, followed by an infusion at a rate of 0.75 µg/kg per minute) in infants undergoing complex congenital cardiac operations reduced the incidence of low cardiac output syndrome in the postoperative period.

Kern FH, Morana NJ, Sears JJ, Hickey PR. Coagulation defects in neonates during cardiopulmonary bypass. *Ann Thorac Surg.* 1992;54:541-546.

Kern and colleagues showed that hemodilution is an important factor in the development of post-bypass coagulopathy in neonates. They showed that platelets and coagulation factors were dramatically reduced as soon as the neonate was placed on cardiopulmonary bypass (CPB) and were not significantly reduced further during CPB.

Malviya S, Voepel-Lewis T, Siewert M, et al. Risk factors for adverse postoperative outcomes in children presenting for cardiac surgery with upper respiratory tract infections. *Anesthesiology.* 2003;98:628-632.

These investigators have shown that children with an upper respiratory tract infection at the time of cardiac surgery are at risk for more complications in the postoperative period and have a longer stay in the intensive care unit. These children need very careful assessment before surgery, and the risk/benefit ratio for the child must be considered.

Mangano DT, Tudor IC, Dietzel C. The risk associated with aprotinin in cardiac surgery. *N Engl J Med.* 2006;354:353-365.

Mangano and associates reported a large observational study in adult patients undergoing revascularization surgery. They reported an increase in renal failure, myocardial infarction, heart failure, stroke, and encephalopathy. This study has been criticized for not being randomized. These effects have not been shown in children, but it has created an unease about the use of aprotinin in children. It is important that well-designed, independent, large studies are carried out in children to establish the role of aprotinin.

Naik SK, Knight A, Elliott M. A prospective randomized study of a modified technique of ultrafiltration during pediatric open-heart surgery. *Circulation.* 1991;84(suppl):III422-III431.

Naik and colleagues were the first to report the use of modified ultrafiltration (MUF) after cardiopulmonary bypass in children. Beneficial effects included reduced total body water, higher hematocrit, higher blood pressure, less postoperative bleeding, and a reduced requirement for inotropes. MUF is now used in many centers worldwide and has a number of benefits.

Pasquali SK, Li JS, He X, et al. Comparative analysis of antifibrinolytic medications in pediatric heart surgery. *J Thorac Cardiovasc Surg.* 2012;143:550-557.

The Society of Thoracic Surgeons Congenital Heart Surgery Database (2004-2008) was linked to medication data from the Pediatric Health Information Systems Database. A total of 22,258 children were included in the study. Aprotinin (vs. no drug) was associated with a reduction in combined hospital mortality/bleeding requiring surgical intervention overall (odds ratio [OR], 0.81; 95% confidence intervals [CI], 0.68–0.91) and in the redo sternotomy subgroup (OR, 0.57; 95% CI, 0.40–0.80). There was no benefit in neonates and no difference in renal failure requiring dialysis in any group. In comparative analysis, there was no difference in outcome for aprotinin versus aminocaproic acid recipients. Tranexamic acid (vs. aprotinin) was associated with significantly reduced mortality/bleeding requiring surgical intervention overall (OR, 0.47; 95% CI, 0.30–0.74) and in neonates (OR, 0.30; 95% CI, 0.15–0.58). These observational data suggest aprotinin is associated with reduced bleeding and mortality in children undergoing heart surgery with no increase in dialysis. Comparative analyses suggest similar efficacy of aminocaproic acid and improved outcomes associated with tranexamic acid.

Williams GD, Ramamoorthy C. Brain monitoring and protection during pediatric cardiac surgery. *Semin Cardiothorac Vasc Anesth.* 2007;11:23-33.

This article reviews brain monitoring modalities available during pediatric cardiac surgery. Its emphasis is on ways of reducing brain injury during cardiopulmonary bypass and deep hypothermic circulatory arrest in children. Neuroprotective stategies are discussed, including selective cerebral perfusion during deep hypothermic circulatory arrest, management of acid-base balance, the degree of hemodilution, blood glucose management, and antiinfammatory therapy.

Zhou G, Feng Z, Xiong H, et al. A combined ultrafiltration strategy during pediatric cardiac surgery: a prospective, randomized, controlled study with clinical outcomes. *J Thorac Cardiovasc Surg.* 2013;27:897-902.

The combined use of ultrafiltration of the prime solution, zero-balance ultrafiltration, and a modified ultrafiltration (MUF) strategy was associated with modest improvements in pulmonary function compared with the combination of coventional and MUF strategies in the early postoperative period, but the principal clinical outcomes are similar.

A complete reference list can be found online at ExpertConsult.com

18

Cardiac Physiology and Pharmacology

ANNETTE Y. SCHURE AND JAMES A. DINARDO

THE CARDIOVASCULAR SYSTEM plays a dominant role within the human body: a centrally located "powerhouse" provides oxygen and nutrients via an extensive network of vessels and capillaries throughout the body. All other organ systems depend on its normal development and function. At birth, and especially in the first few hours of life, the heart and the vascular system have to adapt to the extrauterine conditions. Prematurity, congenital defects, complications during labor and delivery, and many other factors can prevent or delay the necessary changes and cause significant morbidity.

A thorough understanding of the fetal circulation, the changes at birth, and the age-specific characteristics is important for the safe management of neonates, infants, and especially the growing number of preterm and small-for-gestational-age (SGA) infants who come to our diagnostic suites and operating rooms. Given the complex embryology and difficult transition from fetal to extrauterine life, it is amazing that more than 90% of neonates are delivered without any special interventions and that congenital heart defects occur in only 7 to 10 of every 1000 live births.[1] (A detailed discussion of the embryologic development is beyond the scope of this chapter; the interested reader is referred to the excellent review by Van Praagh[2] or Langman's classic embryology textbook.[3])

Congenital heart defects are among the most common birth defects. In the United States, approximately 32,000 infants are born every year with congenital heart disease (CHD); a significant number require urgent interventions in the catheterization laboratory or surgical procedures during the neonatal period. In addition, CHD is often associated with other, noncardiac anomalies, and many of these children will present for procedures outside the cardiac operating room. Pediatric anesthesiologists have to be able to classify and recognize the pathophysiologic effects of

CHD on the cardiovascular system of the neonate or infant and the potential impact of anesthesia and surgical manipulations.

With recent advances in surgical techniques, critical care, and anesthesia management, 85% of all infants with CHD are now expected to reach adulthood. Anesthesiologists will increasingly encounter children with "repaired" or "palliated" CHD presenting for noncardiac procedures. Chapter 23 addresses specific long-term problems and anesthetic considerations for various repaired heart defects, but a few conditions deserve additional discussion: the basic changes in the exercise physiology of repaired heart defects, the characteristics of the Fontan physiology after single ventricle palliation, and the altered physiologic responses in the transplanted heart.

Many conditions require pharmacologic support with cardiovascular drugs, some of which can have significant age-specific effects. Well-controlled drug studies in infants and children are rare; dosing is often based on long-standing experience or extrapolation from adult data. Understanding the basic pharmacology of the most commonly used cardiovascular drugs and the special considerations for infants and children is essential for successful perioperative care. This chapter will help the pediatric anesthesiologist to understand the complexity of the neonatal cardiovascular system, the implications of CHD, basic pharmacologic considerations, and will provide the necessary tools to develop a safe management plan.

Cardiovascular Physiology

FETAL CIRCULATION

In utero, the placental gas exchange provides the fetus with poorly oxygenated blood; the partial pressure of oxygen (PO_2) in the umbilical vein is approximately 30 mm Hg, and in the umbilical arteries it is approximately 16 mm Hg. The fetal lungs are fluid filled and only minimally perfused (10%–15% of the cardiac output). The normal postnatal circulation can be described as a serial circuit: two pumps, the right ventricle (RV) and left ventricle (LV), support two different resistance systems, the pulmonary and systemic vasculatures, one after the other. In contrast, the fetal circulation is better explained by the concept of a parallel circuit: both ventricles provide systemic blood flow and a variety of fetal shortcuts or connections allow for mixing of oxygenated and deoxygenated blood (Fig. 18.1).[4,5] Oxygenated blood from the placenta returns via the umbilical vein to the portal venous system, where 30% to 50% of the blood flow is shunted across the *ductus venosus* to the inferior vena cava (IVC), bypassing the liver and thereby maintaining higher oxygenation and velocity. The rest of the umbilical venous blood passes through the hepatic microcirculation into the suprahepatic IVC.

The IVC blood entering the right atrium (RA) is a mixture of bloodstreams with different velocities and saturations: the low-velocity, deoxygenated venous return from the lower body and hepatic veins and the high-velocity, oxygenated umbilical venous blood from the ductus venosus. Valve-like tissue in the RA (eustachian valve) and the Chiari network preferentially direct the high-velocity bloodstream from the IVC across the *foramen ovale* into the left atrium (LA), bypassing the RV and pulmonary vessels. In the LA, the oxygenated blood mixes with the minimal amount of venous return from the pulmonary circulation and is then ejected by the LV into the ascending aorta and the major vessels of the aortic arch. This blood, with a saturation of 65% to 70%, provides the oxygenation for the growing heart and brain.

Most of the venous return from the superior vena cava (SVC) and about 20% of the IVC blood flow (mainly the low-velocity,

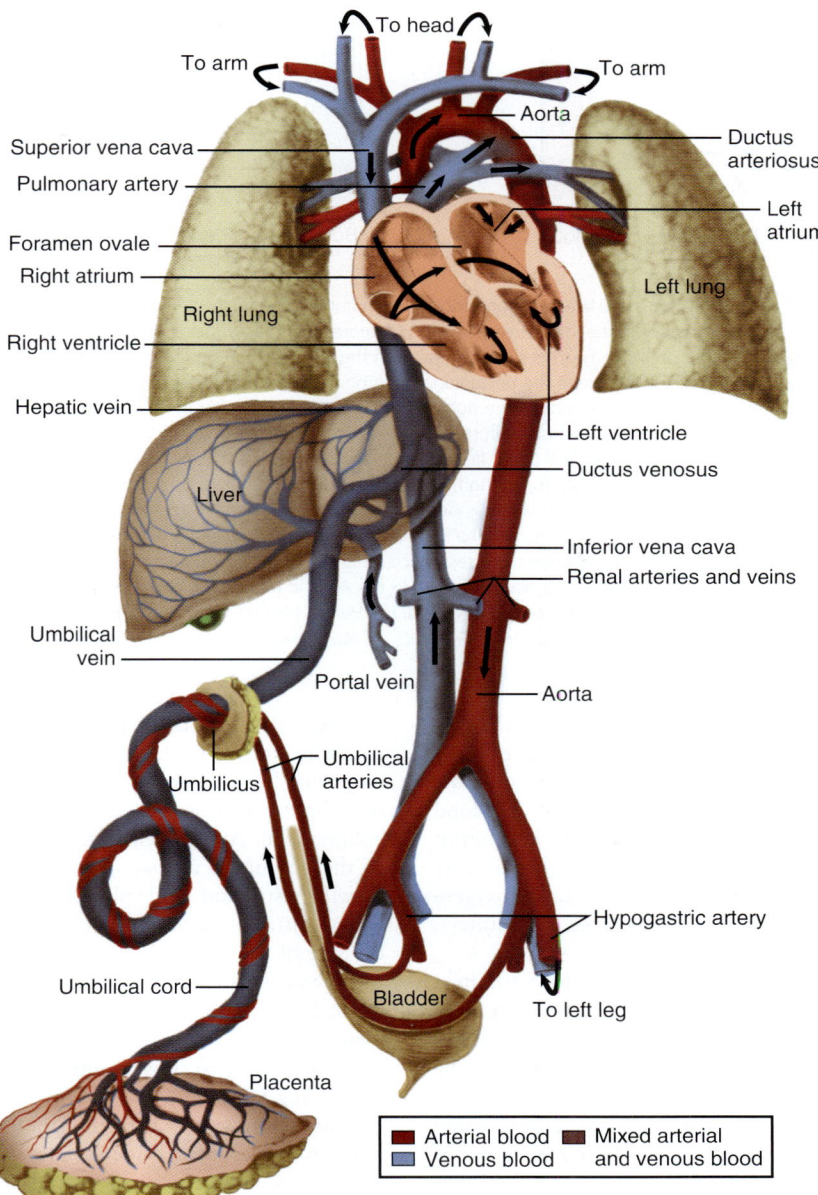

FIGURE 18.1 Course of the fetal circulation in late gestation. Notice the selective blood flow patterns across the foramen ovale and the ductus arteriosus. (From Greeley WJ, Berkowitz DH, Nathan AT. Anesthesia for pediatric cardiac surgery. In: Miller RD, ed. *Anesthesia*. 7th ed. Philadelphia: Churchill Livingstone; 2010, Fig. 83.1.)

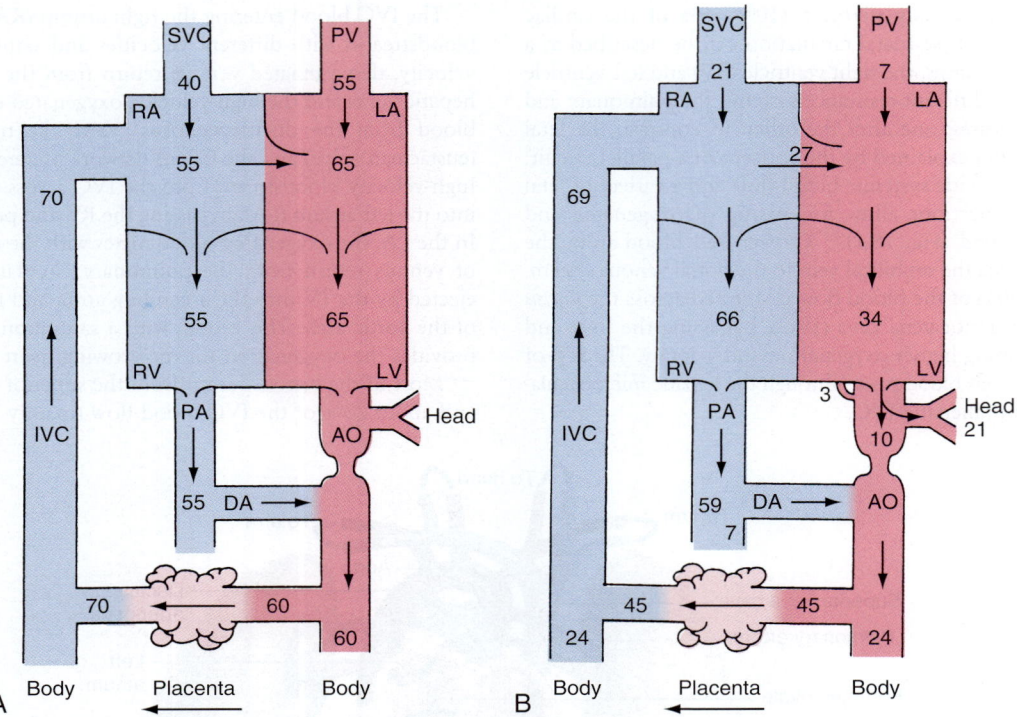

FIGURE 18.2 Fetal circulation in the late-gestation lamb. **A,** The numbers indicate the percentage of oxygen saturation. Oxygen saturation is greatest in the inferior vena cava *(IVC)*, representing flow that is primarily from the placenta. The saturation of the blood in the heart is slightly greater on the left side than on the right side. **B,** The course of the circulation. The numbers represent the percentage of combined ventricular output. Some of the return from the IVC is diverted by the crista dividens in the right atrium *(RA)* through the foramen ovale into the left atrium *(LA)*, where it meets the pulmonary venous return *(PV)*, passes into the left ventricle *(LV)*, and is pumped into the ascending aorta. Most of the ascending aortic flow goes to the coronary, subclavian, and carotid arteries, with only 10% of combined ventricular output passing through the aortic arch (indicated by the narrowed point in the aorta) into the descending aorta *(AO)*. The remainder of the IVC flow mixes with return from the superior vena cava *(SVC)* and coronary veins (3%), passes into the RA and right ventricle *(RV)*, and is pumped into the pulmonary artery *(PA)*. Because of the increased pulmonary resistance, only 7% of the blood passes through the lungs *(PV)*, with the rest passing through the ductus arteriosus *(DA)* to the AO and then to the placenta and lower half of the body. (Modified from Rudolph AM. *Congenital Diseases of the Heart.* Chicago: Year Book Publishers; 1974:1-48; and from Freed MD. Fetal and transitional circulation. In: Fyler DC, ed. *Nadas' Pediatric Cardiology.* Philadelphia: Mosby-Year Book; 1992:57-61.)

deoxygenated part) reach the RV and are pumped into the pulmonary artery (PA), where the high pulmonary resistance in the nonexpanded lung redirects 90% of the blood flow into the descending aorta via the *ductus arteriosus*. The bulk of the blood flow in the descending aorta is generated by the RV, with minor contributions from the LV. The blood has a saturation of only 55% to 60%; two-thirds of it returns to the placenta for oxygenation, and the rest is distributed to the intestines, the kidneys, and the lower part of the body (Fig. 18.2).

The fetal circulation has to support a growing fetus in a relatively cyanotic atmosphere (highest oxygen saturation, 65% to 70%). This difficult task is further complicated by the parallel circuit, which creates increased workload for the RV, and the limitations of the fetal shortcuts, which add additional volume load by incomplete shunting of oxygenated and deoxygenated blood. Initially, our understanding of the fetal circulation was based mainly on experimental animal data, but recent advances in ultrasound technology have facilitated assessment and monitoring of fetal cardiovascular parameters, especially stroke volume and cardiac output, under various conditions throughout the gestational period. RV stroke volume has been found to increase from about

0.7 mL at 20 weeks to 7.6 mL at 40 weeks, and LV stroke volume increases from 0.7 mL to 5.2 mL. The combined fetal cardiac output of both ventricles is estimated to be 400 to 425 mL/kg per minute, with an RV dominance because of the increased volume load. At 38 weeks, the RV provides approximately 60% of the combined cardiac output (E-Table 18.1).[6–8] Intrauterine growth restriction and placental compromise are associated with redistribution of cardiac output and relative changes in the size of the foramen ovale.[9] A functional placenta, the fetal cardiovascular high-output state, greater hemoglobin concentrations, and additional alterations in oxygen binding and release (hemoglobin F, increased 2,3-diphosphoglycerate [2,3-DPG]) are all necessary to provide adequate tissue oxygenation for the developing fetus.

Until recently, CHD was thought to be relatively well tolerated in utero, but growing evidence suggests that fetal cardiovascular defects can induce intrinsic autoregulatory changes in cerebral perfusion and thereby compromise brain development.[10–12] Ultrasound and magnetic resonance imaging demonstrate that 25% to 40% of neonates with CHD have neurologic abnormalities before any surgical intervention.[13,14]

TRANSITIONAL CIRCULATION

At birth, a variety of humoral, biochemical, and physiologic changes occur abruptly. First, the placental circulation is eliminated shortly after the lungs expand. Second, expansion of the lungs to a normal functional residual capacity (FRC) results in an optimal geometric relationship of the pulmonary microvasculature. Third, air entering the lungs causes the alveolar PCO_2 to decrease and the alveolar PO_2 to increase. These three factors act in concert to markedly reduce pulmonary vascular resistance (PVR).[5,15,16] The net effect is a considerable increase in pulmonary blood flow, which augments pulmonary venous return to the left heart. Along with elimination of the placenta and the low-resistance umbilical circulation, the LV is suddenly subjected to increased volume and afterload (Table 18.1). Typically, LV end-diastolic pressure, and thus LA pressure, increases enough to exert hydrostatic pressure on the septum primum, resulting in functional closure of the foramen ovale. In contrast to the increased stress for the LV, the RV is relatively unloaded by the transition to extrauterine life.

The three fetal connections (ductus arteriosus, ductus venosus, and foramen ovale) close over a variable period after birth. The ductus arteriosus functionally (but not anatomically) closes in 58% of normal full-term infants by day 2 after birth and in 98% by day 4.[17] Although many substances (such as eicosanoids) have been implicated in initiating constriction of the ductus, initial constriction probably occurs primarily in response to the increased arterial oxygen tension[18,19] and the reduction in circulating prostaglandins that follow separation of the placenta.[20] The response to oxygen is age dependent: term neonates usually demonstrate effective constriction of the smooth muscles in the ductal tissue when exposed to oxygen, whereas preterm infants respond poorly and often require medical (prostaglandin inhibitor) or even surgical therapy. Additional catecholamine-induced changes in PVR and systemic vascular resistance (SVR) and other substances such as acetylcholine contribute to ductal closure. Within 2 to 3 weeks, functional constriction is followed by a process of ductal fibrosis, leaving a band-like structure, the ligamentum arteriosum.[21,22] With ligation of the umbilical vein, the portal pressure falls, triggering functional closure of the ductus venosus. This process rarely requires more than 1 to 2 weeks; by 3 months only fibrous tissue, the ligamentum venosum, is left.

The foramen ovale is functionally closed when the LA pressure exceeds the RA pressure, but it remains anatomically patent in most infants, in 50% of children younger than 5 years of age, and in 25% to 30% of adults.[23] Echocardiographic studies have confirmed right-to-left shunting via the foramen ovale in healthy infants emerging from general anesthesia, and this can be a significant cause of persistent arterial desaturation at that time despite ventilation with 100% oxygen.[24]

NEONATAL CARDIOVASCULAR SYSTEM

Compared with the adult, the neonatal myocardium is immature and incompletely developed (Table 18.2). Differences in cytoarchitecture and metabolism account for many of the functional limitations. The neonatal heart contains fewer muscle cells and more connective tissue than the adult myocardium. Contractile elements represent only 30% of the total cardiac mass, in contrast to 60% in the adult.[25] The ratio of surface area to mass and water to collagen content are greater in neonates than older children. There are fewer myofibrils within the muscle cells, and they tend to be less organized (i.e., not parallel to the long axis of the cell). The sarcoplasmic reticulum and the T-tubule network, both important components of rapid and effective calcium regulation, are incompletely developed, and the immature myocardium relies substantially on the calcium flux through the sarcolemma to initiate and terminate contraction.[26-28] One practical consequence

TABLE 18.1	Hemodynamic Changes at Birth
Right Ventricle	**Left Ventricle**
Decreased Afterload:	**Increased Afterload:**
Decreased pulmonary vascular resistance	Placenta eliminated
Ductal closure	Ductal closure
Decreased Volume Load:	**Increased Volume Load:**
Eliminated umbilical vein return	Increased pulmonary venous return
Output diminished 25%	Output increased almost 50%
	Transient left-to-right shunt at ductus

TABLE 18.2	Characteristic Differences Between the Immature and the Adult Myocardium	
	Immature Myocardium	**Adult Myocardium**
Cytoarchitecture	Fewer mitochondria and sarcoplasmic reticula Poorly formed T-tubules Limited contractile elements and increased water content Dependence on extracellular calcium for contractility	Organized mitochondrial rows, abundant SR Well-formed T tubules Increased number of myofibrils with better orientation Rapid release and reuptake of calcium via SR
Metabolism	Carbohydrates and lactate as primary energy sources Increased glycogen stores and anaerobic glycolysis for ATP Decreased nucleotidase activity, retained ATP precursors Better tolerance to ischemia with rapid recovery of function	Free fatty acids as primary source for ATP Limited glycogen stores and glycolytic function Increased 5'-nucleotidase activity, rapid ATP depletion Less tolerance to ischemia
Function	Decreased compliance Limited CO augmentation with increased preload Decreased tolerance to afterload Immature autonomic innervation: parasympathetic dominance, incomplete sympathetic innervation	Normally developed tension Able to improve CO with increased preload and to maintain CO with increasing afterload

ATP, adenosine triphosphate; *CO*, cardiac output; *SR*, sarcoplasmic reticulum.
Data from Mossad EB, Farid I. Vital organ preservation during surgery for congenital heart disease. In: Lake CL, Booker PD, eds. *Pediatric Cardiac Anesthesia.* 4th ed. Philadelphia: Lippincott, Williams & Wilkins; 2005:266–290; and DiNardo J, Zwara DA. Congenital heart disease. In: DiNardo J, Zwara DA, eds. *Anesthesia for Cardiac Surgery.* 3rd ed. Malden, MA: Blackwell Publishing; 2008:167–251.

of this disorganized and immature myocardium is a greater degree of contractile dysfunction in the infant exposed to substances that decrease extracellular ionized calcium, such as citrate (blood products) and albumin; there is also increased sensitivity to inhalational anesthetics and calcium channel blockers.

Reduced numbers of underdeveloped mitochondria and maturational differences in various signaling pathways and related messenger systems are also characteristic of the neonatal myocardium. Immature mitochondrial enzyme activity for fatty acid transport may explain the primary use of carbohydrates and lactates as energy sources and might be a reason for the greater anaerobic tolerance and faster recovery after periods of ischemia. A variety of developmental changes in contractile proteins occur from fetal through early postnatal life, including changes in pH, calcium sensitivity, and adenosine triphosphate (ATP) hydrolyzing activity. The key features of the immature cardiac function are summarized in Table 18.2.

The increased amount of noncontractile tissue in the neonate decreases ventricular compliance and limits the response to an increased preload. Compliance of both ventricles progressively increases during fetal life and the postnatal period, so that maximal stroke volume occurs at a significantly reduced atrial pressure in the neonate compared with the fetus (Figs. 18.3 and 18.4).[29–31] The high metabolic rate of the neonate (oxygen consumption, 6-8 mL/kg per minute, compared with 2-3 mL/kg per minute in the adult) requires a proportional increase in cardiac output. The neonatal heart meets this demand, in part, by a greater heart rate (HR).[32,33] The cardiac output is commonly described as depending primarily on HR owing to a fixed stroke volume, but echocardiographic studies in human fetuses and neonates have demonstrated the capacity to increase stroke volume (Fig. 18.5)[34] In fact, the neonate uses both tachycardia and stroke volume adjustments to meet metabolic demand. On the other hand, neonates exhibit exquisite sensitivity to pharmacologic agents that produce negative inotropic or chronotropic effects. At birth, both ventricles are equal in mass and connected via a common septum. Increased pressures in one ventricle shifts the septum, decreasing compliance of the other ventricle. The net effect is a reduction in cardiac output. Neonates and infants often present with biventricular failure as a result of this interventricular dependence.

Immature autonomic regulation of cardiac function persists throughout the neonatal period. Both sympathetic and parasympathetic innervation of the heart can be demonstrated at birth. However, evidence suggests that development of the sympathetic nervous system is incomplete at both the postganglionic nerve-receptor level and the receptor-effector level.[35] The sympathetic system reaches maturity by early infancy, whereas the parasympathetic system reaches maturity within a few days after birth.[36] The relative imbalance of these two components of the autonomic nervous system at birth may account for the clinical observation that neonates are predisposed to marked vagal responses to a variety of stimuli.

PULMONARY VASCULAR PHYSIOLOGY

At birth, pulmonary vascular development is incomplete. Lung sections demonstrate a diminished number of arterioles, and the arterioles exhibit thick medial muscularization (Fig. 18.6).[37–39] The pulmonary vasculature matures during the first few years of life. During this period, arterioles proliferate faster than alveoli, and the medial smooth muscle thins and extends more distally in the vascular tree. PVR continues to decrease as long as pulmonary

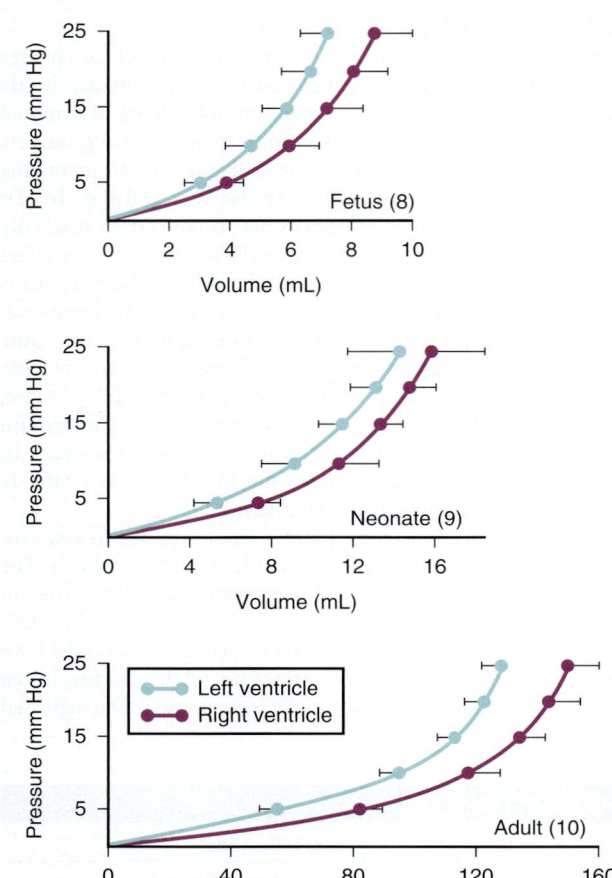

FIGURE 18.3 Comparison of ventricular pressure–volume curves for fetal, neonatal, and adult sheep. Differences between ventricles are significant only in adult sheep. Notice that the right and left ventricles have similar compliance curves in the neonates, making the physiologic relationship between ventricles more intimate (i.e., infants tend to develop biventricular failure). (From Romero T, Covell J, Friedman WF. A comparison of pressure-volume relations of the fetal, newborn and adult heart. *Am J Physiol.* 1972;222:1285–1290.)

mechanics and alveolar gas composition remain favorable, with a significant decrease occurring immediately after birth as the result of lung expansion and oxygenation. Progressive remodeling of the pulmonary vasculature facilitates further decreases in PVR (assuming normal physiology) during the first 2 to 3 months of life; by 6 months of age, the PVR has almost reached adult levels.[39]

The fetal pulmonary vasculature is extremely reactive to a number of stimuli. Hypoxia, acidosis, increased levels of leukotrienes, and mechanical stimulation (e.g., coughing on an endotracheal tube) can cause significant and prolonged increases in PVR (e.g., reactive pulmonary hypertension). On the other hand, acetylcholine, histamine, bradykinin, prostaglandins, β-adrenergic catecholamines, and nitric oxide (NO) are strong vasodilators.[37] In the first days after birth, many pathophysiologic conditions can trigger severe and sustained increases in PVR[40,41] and prevent the normal adjustment to extrauterine life (E-Table 18.2). The acute load imposed on the RV can induce diastolic dysfunction and promote right-to-left shunting via the foramen ovale. Once PVR exceeds the SVR, a right-to-left shunt develops through both the ductus arteriosus and the foramen ovale. This situation is called *persistent fetal circulation*,[42] and it can result in a life-threatening hypoxemia

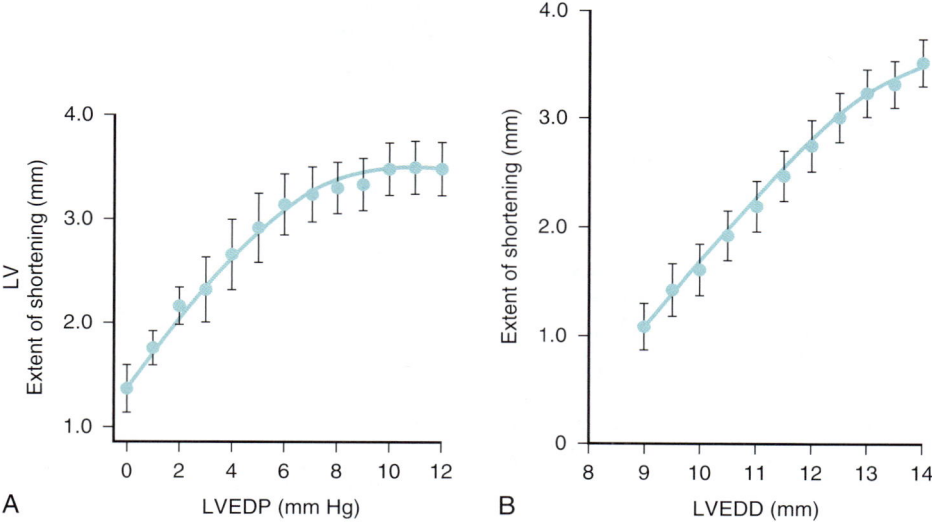

FIGURE 18.4 Frank-Starling relationship in fetal lamb model (gestational age, 135 ± 5 days). **A,** The relationship between left ventricular end-diastolic pressure *(LVEDP)* and shortening in a chronically instrumented fetal lamb model. Although myocardial performance improves with increasing LVEDP, the effect achieves a plateau at 10 mm Hg. **B,** In the same model, the relationship between left ventricular end-diastolic diameter *(LVEDD)* and left ventricular shortening. Taken together, these experiments support the capacity, albeit blunted, of the fetal heart to change stroke volume on the basis of volume loading conditions. Each point and vertical bars represent mean ± standard error. (From Kirkpatrick SE, Pitlick PT, Naliboff J, et al. Frank-Starling relationship as an important determinant of fetal cardiac output. *Am J Physiol.* 1976;231:495–500.)

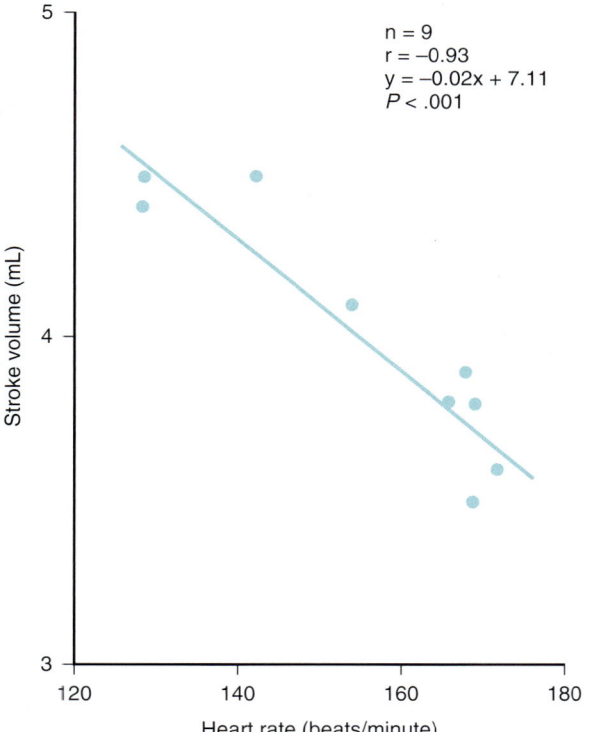

FIGURE 18.5 Doppler echocardiographic comparison of the effect of spontaneous changes in heart rate on stroke volume in a normal human fetus in utero, illustrating decreased stroke volume with increased heart rate. These observations confirm the ability of the fetal heart to change stroke volume under normal physiologic conditions. (From Kenny J, Plappert T, Doubilet P, et al. Effects of heart rate on ventricular size, stroke volume, and output in the normal human fetus: a prospective Doppler echocardiographic study. *Circulation* 1987;76:52–58.)

that may require inhaled NO,[43–47] sildenafil,[48] or extracorporeal support (i.e., extracorporeal membrane oxygenation)[49,50] (see Chapter 21) to provide oxygenation and sustain life.

Pulmonary vascular occlusive disease (PVOD) describes the structural changes in the pulmonary vasculature after long-standing exposure to abnormal pressures and flow patterns in utero and after birth. Lung biopsies demonstrate thickened muscle layers in the small pulmonary arteries, intimal hyperplasia, scarring, and thrombosis as well as a decreased number of distal (intraacinar) arteries.[38] Over time, these changes lead to a progressive and ultimately irreversible obstruction to pulmonary blood flow with increases in PVR and PA pressures. The very muscularized pulmonary arteries are also extremely sensitive to pulmonary vasoconstrictors, which can easily trigger a pulmonary hypertensive crisis.

Many cardiac defects are associated with abnormal pulmonary flow patterns and can be categorized into three basic groups:

- *Exposure of the pulmonary vasculature to systemic arterial pressures and high flow:* The classic example is a large, nonrestrictive ventricular septal defect (VSD) with rapid progression of PVOD.
- *Exposure of the pulmonary vasculature to high flow without increased pressure:* Large atrial septal defects (ASDs) and small, restrictive patent ductus arteriosus (PDA) defects fall into this category. PVOD develops much more slowly in this setting.
- *Obstruction of pulmonary venous drainage resulting in increased PA pressures:* Pulmonary vein stenosis (e.g., total anomalous pulmonary venous return [TAPVR], cor triatrium) or increased LA pressures (e.g., mitral atresia, congenital aortic stenosis, severe coarctation) can cause backpressure in the pulmonary vasculature and induce PVOD.

The muscle tone in the pulmonary arteries is regulated by numerous factors, and various therapeutic interventions can be used to manipulate the PVR (Table 18.3)[16]:

- *Arterial oxygen tension (PaO₂):* Alveolar as well as arterial hypoxia increases PVR. A PaO₂ value less than 50 mm Hg, especially

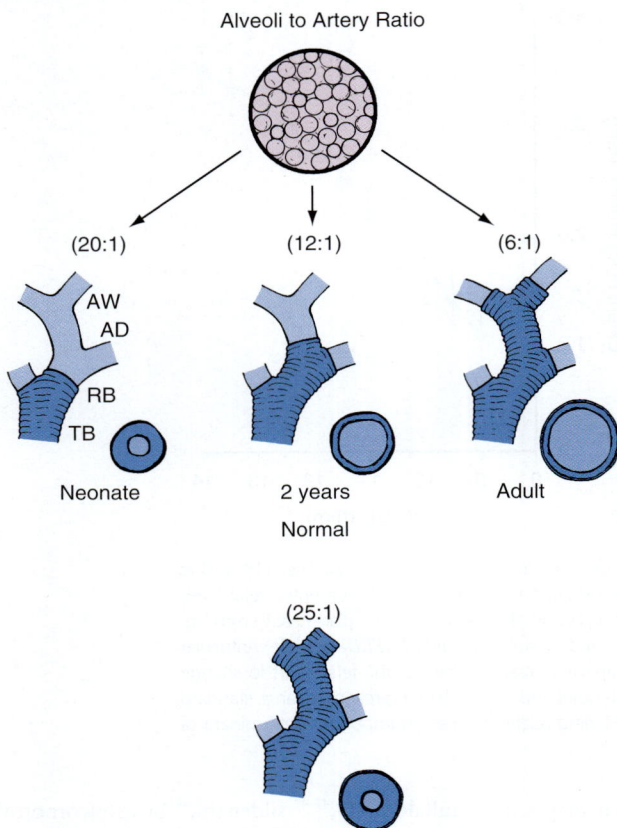

Alveoli to Artery Ratio

(20:1)   (12:1)   (6:1)

AW
AD

RB

TB

Neonate   2 years   Adult

Normal

(25:1)

VSD 2 years
(high pressure, high resistance)

FIGURE 18.6 Peripheral pulmonary artery development. The normal pattern of pulmonary vascular development and that of a 2-year-old child with pulmonary vascular changes accompanying a large ventricular septal defect (VSD). Rabinovitch and colleagues characterized the pulmonary vasculature morphometrically in three respects: vessel thickness, muscular extension, and the ratio of alveoli to arteries seen on lung biopsy specimens. The normal neonate exhibits thick vascular smooth muscle, but this extends only as far as the arterioles accompanying the respiratory bronchiole. In neonates, the alveoli/artery ratio is 20:1. In the first few months of life, the vessels thin substantially and proliferate relative to the alveoli, so that by the age of 2 years, the normal child has an alveoli/artery ratio of 12:1 and thin muscles extending to the arteries associated with alveolar ducts. In the normal adult, the alveoli/artery ratio is 6:1 and muscle extends all the way to the arteries in the alveolar wall. In contrast, in the 2-year-old child with a large VSD, the vessel numbers are markedly diminished (alveoli/artery ratio, 25:1), and persistent neonatal muscle thickness extends all the way to the alveolar wall. *AD,* artery at alveolar duct; *AW,* artery at alveolar wall; *RB,* respiratory bronchiole; *TB,* artery at terminal bronchiole. (From Steven JM, Nicolson SC. Congenital heart disease. In: Miller RD, series editor. *Atlas of Anesthesia.* Vol 7. In: Greeley WJ, volume editor. *Pediatric Anesthesia* Orlando, FL.: Harcourt Publishers; 1998:6.6; modified from Rabinovitch M, Haworth SG, Castaneda AR, et al. Lung biopsy in congenital heart disease: a morphometric approach to pulmonary vascular disease. *Circulation.* 1978;58:1107–1122.)

when associated with an acidic pH (<7.4), leads to significant pulmonary vasoconstriction. On the other hand, increased inspired oxygen can lead to pulmonary vasodilation and overcirculation.

■ *Arterial carbon dioxide tension (PaCO₂):* Hypercapnia increases PVR, independent of the blood pH. In contrast, hypocapnia induces alkalosis and thereby decreases PVR. Reliable pulmonary

TABLE 18.3	Manipulations of Pulmonary Vascular Resistance
Increasing PVR	**Decreasing PVR**
PEEP	No PEEP
High airway pressures	Low airway pressures
Atelectasis	Lung expansion to FRC
Low FiO₂	High FiO₂
Respiratory and metabolic acidosis	Respiratory and metabolic alkalosis
Increased hematocrit	Low hematocrit
Sympathetic stimulation	Blunted stress response (deep anesthesia)
Direct surgical manipulation	Nitric oxide
Vasoconstrictors: phenylephrine	Vasodilators: milrinone, prostacyclin, others

FiO₂, fraction of inspired oxygen; *FRC,* functional residual capacity; *PEEP,* positive end-expiratory pressure; *PVR,* pulmonary vascular resistance.

vasodilation can be achieved with a PaCO₂ of 20 to 33 mm Hg and a pH of 7.5 to 7.6.

■ *pH:* Respiratory and metabolic acidosis increase PVR; alkalosis reduces PVR.

■ *Lung volumes:* PVR is optimized at a lung volume close to the FRC; larger volumes compress small intraalveolar vessels, and smaller volumes can cause atelectasis and vascular collapse.

■ *Stimulation of the sympathetic nervous system:* Catecholamine surges from stress, pain, or light anesthesia can trigger significant increases in PVR.

■ *Vasodilators:* Most intravenous (IV) agents used for pulmonary vasodilation also affect the systemic circulation and induce hypotension. Alternatively, inhaled substances such as NO or prostacyclin can provide a more selective pulmonary vasodilation (see "Cardiovascular Pharmacology").

In summary, the pulmonary vasculature undergoes a complex maturation process that can be influenced by a multitude of external factors and congenital heart defects. Persistent fetal circulation and PVOD are examples of inadequate adaptation and development. In cases of increased PVR, ventilator strategies using greater inspired oxygen concentrations, lung volumes close to the FRC, and interventions aiming for a PaO₂ greater than 60 mm Hg, a PaCO₂ of 30 to 35 mm Hg, and a pH of 7.5 to 7.6 can improve pulmonary blood flow.

Incidence and Prevalence of Congenital Heart Disease

CHD can be defined as *"a gross structural abnormality of the heart or intrathoracic great vessels that is actually or potentially of functional significance."*[51] This definition covers a wide array of defects, which are among the most common congenital malformations. However, the precise incidence of CHD, both collectively and by individual anatomic subset, varies depending on definition, method of case identification, and epoch (E-Table 18.3). Including all categories of CHD, large epidemiologic surveys place the prevalence between 4 and 50 cases per 1000 live births.[52–55] When stratified according to trivial, moderate, and severe forms, the incidence for moderate and severe forms of CHD has been relatively consistent, at about 6 per 1000 live births.

Anatomic diagnoses within the population of infants with CHD vary according to the method used to identify cases. In 2002, Hoffman and Kaplan compiled 62 epidemiologic studies published after 1955 and investigated the potential causes for the wide variability in the reported incidence of CHD.[56] More recent studies based mainly on prenatal and postnatal echocardiographic screening data often include a large number of trivial lesions (e.g., tiny VSDs, nonstenotic bicuspid aortic valve, "silent" PDA) for which no interventions may be required; other data collections, such as the New England Regional Infant Cardiac Program (NERICP), a registry of children with CHD who died or required catheterization or surgery during the first year of life, are clearly biased toward more severe forms of CHD.[1]

The increasing availability of prenatal diagnostic methods may influence the relative prevalence of reported lesions as well as their outcome. When fetal echocardiography is used, the apparent shift toward more complex lesions may reflect technical limitations in identifying simple defects.[57] In addition, evaluation in utero skews the results because it includes fatally malformed fetuses that will not survive to term. The prevalence of CHD among spontaneous abortions reaches 20% and remains as large as 10% among stillborn infants.[58] In one study, 50% of women whose children were given a prenatal diagnosis of CHD elected to terminate the pregnancy, particularly when presented with complex heart lesions.[57]

On the other hand, female infants with severe CHD have a mortality rate that is 5% less than similarly affected male infants,[1] and with increased survival rates more females will reach childbearing age, where they continue to have reduced mortality.[59] The recurrence risk of CHD for their offspring is about 3% to 4%.[60,61]

A study from Canada examined the changing epidemiology of CHD with respect to prevalence and age distribution in the general population between 1983 and 2010.[62] The prevalence of all categories of CHD in 2010 was ~13 per 1000 in children (<18 years of age) and ~6 per 1000 in adults. For the subcategory of severe CHD, the prevalence was ~1.8 per 1000 in children and ~0.62 per 1000 in adults. In 2010, 60% of all patients with severe CHD were adults, compared with 49% in 2000 and 35% in 1985. Between 1983 and 2010 the prevalence of CHD has been steadily increasing for both children and adults but at a different pace: from 1985 to 2000 the increase for severe CHD was 85% in adults and 22% in children compared with 57% for adults and 11% for children from 2000 to 2010. The median age of all patients with severe CHD was 11 years in 1985, 17 years in 2000 and 25 years in 2010, reflecting the fact that more children with CHD were surviving to adulthood (E-Fig. 18.1). Improved survival may be attributed to improved prenatal care, early diagnostic imaging, and major advances in pediatric cardiac care, particularly for those with severe CHD; these improved outcomes will continue to influence the future demographic profile. The growing number of adolescents and adults with CHD will require long-term follow-up with experienced cardiologists and access to specialized care facilities; this will require a thorough understanding of their underlying pathophysiology by all members of the adult care team, including anesthesiologists.

Pathophysiologic Classification of Congenital Heart Disease

CHD consists of an almost endless array of anatomic and functional variants. Many different classification systems have been introduced, some using a segmental approach to anatomic features, others by examining the amount of pulmonary blood flow (cyanotic versus acyanotic) or the common physiologic characteristics (e.g., volume versus pressure overload).[63–73] Several of these classifications are discussed in Chapter 16. However, certain defects are better described using the concepts of shunting (physiologic, anatomic, simple or complex), intercirculatory mixing, and single ventricle physiology, which are presented in the following sections.

SHUNTING

Shunting occurs when blood return from one circulatory system (systemic or pulmonary) is recirculated to the same system, completely bypassing the other circulation. For example, if deoxygenated blood from the systemic veins flows directly to the aorta, the result is a right-to-left shunt with recirculation of deoxygenated blood in the systemic circulation. In contrast, redirection of oxygenated blood from the pulmonary veins to the PA causes a left-to-right shunt with recirculation of oxygenated blood within the pulmonary circulation. The terms *physiologic* and *anatomic* are often used to describe shunting. Basically, any kind of recirculation of blood within one circulatory system is called *physiologic shunting*. In most cases, physiologic shunting is caused by an anatomic shunt (i.e., a communication between the cardiac chambers or the great vessels), but physiologic shunting can also exist by itself, as in the classic transposition physiology.

To really understand the pathophysiology of shunting and its implications, it is important to introduce the concepts of effective and total systemic/pulmonary blood flows. *Effective blood flow* is the quantity of venous blood from one circulatory system that reaches the arterial system of the other circulatory system. Effective *pulmonary* blood flow is the volume of systemic venous blood reaching the pulmonary circulation, whereas effective *systemic* blood flow is the volume of pulmonary venous blood reaching the systemic circulation. Effective pulmonary blood flow and effective systemic blood flow are always equal, no matter how complex the lesions. *Total blood flow*, on the other hand, is the sum of recirculated and effective blood flow and a measure of the workload of the circulatory system. Total systemic and pulmonary blood flows are not equal. Even in healthy patients there is a small amount of normal physiologic shunting (e.g., thebesian cardiac veins, bronchial vessels), but with CHD the difference can be quite substantial. Physiologic shunting or recirculation should be viewed as a noneffective, superfluous load added to the essential nutritive blood flow (effective blood flow).

Anatomic shunts are communications between the two circulatory systems, either within the heart or at the level of the great vessels. They can be divided into simple and complex shunts, depending on the presence of additional outflow obstructions. In *simple shunts* without any additional outflow obstruction, the size of the communication (the so-called shunt orifice) determines the flow characteristics. For small orifices (restrictive shunts) with large pressure gradients across the communication, the size of the opening essentially regulates the amount of shunting. Changes in SVR or PVR have little influence. In contrast, for large orifices or nonrestrictive shunts (also classified as *dependent shunts*), the quantity and direction of blood flow are controlled by the respective outflow resistances (i.e., the ratio of SVR to PVR) (Table 18.4 and Fig. 18.7).

Complex shunts are defined by an additional outflow obstruction, which can be at various levels within the ventricle, valves, or great vessels and is often described as subvalvular, valvular, or supravalvular. These obstructions can be fixed (e.g., valvular stenosis) or variable (e.g., dynamic infundibular obstruction by muscle bundles). Shunt flow and direction are determined by the combined resistance across the outflow obstruction and the pulmonary/systemic vascular beds. For severe obstructions downstream, SVR or PVR will have little influence on the shunt. Tetralogy of Fallot (TOF) is a good example of a complex shunt lesion. The amount of right-to-left shunt and therefore the amount

TABLE 18.4	Characteristics of Simple Shunts (Without Additional Outflow Obstruction)	
	Restrictive (Small Shunt Orifice)	**Nonrestrictive (Large Shunt Orifice)**
Examples	Small ASD, VSD, or PDA; modified Blalock-Taussig shunt	Large VSD, PDA, CAVC
Pressure gradient across shunt	Large	Small or none
Direction and magnitude of shunt	Independent of PVR/SVR	PVR/SVR dependent
Influence of pharmacologic and ventilatory interventions	Minimal	Large

ASD, atrial septal defect; *CAVC,* common atrioventricular canal; *PDA,* patent ductus arteriosus; *PVR,* pulmonary vascular resistance; *SVR,* systemic vascular resistance; *VSD,* ventricular septal defect.
Modified from DiNardo J, Zwara DA. Congenital heart disease. In: DiNardo J, Zwara DA, eds. *Anesthesia for Cardiac Surgery.* 3rd ed. Malden, MA: Blackwell Publishing; 2008:167–251.

of cyanosis are influenced by the degree and type of right ventricular outflow tract obstruction (RVOTO). This is especially evident in the setting of a dynamic infundibular obstruction, where changes in preload, contractility, and HR can lead to significant decreases in pulmonary blood flow and increased shunting (Table 18.5).

INTERCIRCULATORY MIXING

The concept of intercirculatory mixing is often used to explain the unique physiology in children with transposition of the great arteries (TGA). In this cardiac defect, the aorta arises from the RV, transporting deoxygenated blood back to the right heart, and the PA originates from the LV, returning oxygenated blood to the pulmonary circulation (see Fig. 17.6). Unless there is some mixing of blood via an ASD, VSD, or PDA, this defect will result in a complete separation of the two systems, a parallel circulation with 100% physiologic shunting, or recirculation of oxygenated and deoxygenated blood that is incompatible with life once the fetal ductus arteriosus has closed. Effective pulmonary blood flow (i.e., deoxygenated blood reaching the pulmonary vascular bed for oxygenation) has to be provided by some form of right-to-left shunt; effective systemic blood flow (i.e., oxygenated blood returning to the systemic circulation) must be achieved by a left-to-right shunt. Intercirculatory mixing is the combined systemic and pulmonary effective blood flow and is only a small portion of the total blood flow. The bulk of the respective systemic and pulmonary total blood flows consists of recirculated blood (Fig. 18.8). Usually the total blood flow and the volume in the pulmonary system are two to three times greater than in the systemic circulation.

The arterial saturation (SaO_2) is influenced by the volumes and saturations of recirculating and effective systemic blood

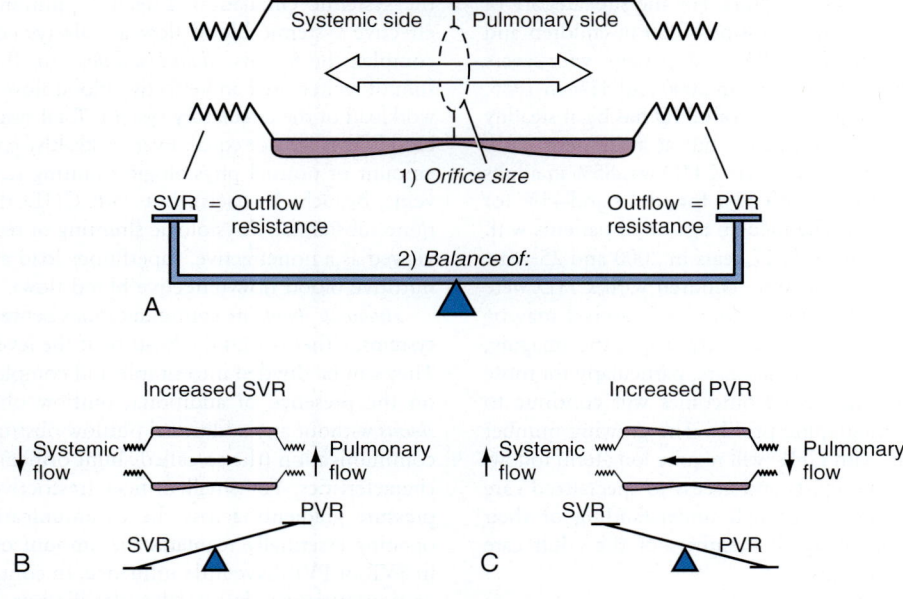

FIGURE 18.7 Influence of orifice size and the ratio of pulmonary vascular resistance *(PVR)* to systemic vascular resistance *(SVR)* on the magnitude and direction of a simple shunt. **A,** PVR and SVR are balanced, resulting in equal pulmonary and systemic blood flows. **B,** PVR is reduced relative to SVR, resulting in an increase in pulmonary blood flow and a decrease in systemic blood flow. **C,** PVR is elevated relative to SVR, resulting in a decrease in pulmonary blood flow and an increase in systemic blood flow. (Modified from DiNardo J, Zwara DA. Congenital heart disease. In: DiNardo J, Zwara DA, eds. *Anesthesia for Cardiac Surgery.* 3rd ed. Malden, MA: Blackwell Publishing; 2008:167–251.)

flows and can be calculated with the use of the following equation:

$$\text{Aortic saturation} = [(\text{Systemic venous saturation} \times \text{Recirculated blood flow}) + (\text{Pulmonary venous saturation} \times \text{Effective blood flow})] \div [\text{Total systemic venous blood flow}]$$

TABLE 18.5	Characteristics of Complex Shunts (With Additional Outflow Obstruction)	
	Partial Outflow Obstruction	Complete Outflow Obstruction
Examples	TOF, VSD/PS, VSD/ coarctation	Tricuspid or mitral atresia, Pulmonary or aortic atresia
Shunt magnitude and direction	Relatively fixed	Totally fixed
Dependence on PVR/SVR ratio	Inversely related to obstruction	Independent
Pressure gradient across shunt	Dependent on shunt orifice and degree of obstruction	Dependent only on shunt orifice

PS, pulmonary stenosis; *PVR*, pulmonary vascular resistance; *SVR*, systemic vascular resistance; *TOF*, tetralogy of Fallot; *VSD*, ventricular septal defect.
Modified from DiNardo J, Zwara DA. Congenital heart disease. In: DiNardo J, Zwara DA, eds. *Anesthesia for Cardiac Surgery*. 3rd ed. Malden, MA: Blackwell Publishing; 2008:167–251.

Increasing the intercirculatory mixing will improve the arterial saturations, and in severely cyanotic neonates with TGA, intact ventricular septum, and inadequate atrial communication, a balloon atrial septostomy (balloon dilation of an existing patent foramen ovale or small ASD, either echo-guided at the bedside or under fluoroscopy in the catheterization laboratory) can be lifesaving. Additional measures to improve systemic and pulmonary venous saturations (e.g., blood transfusion, inotropic support, ventilatory strategies) can help to stabilize the arterial saturation.

SINGLE VENTRICLE PHYSIOLOGY

Single ventricle physiology defines the circulation present in a wide variety of complex cardiac defects. It is characterized by complete mixing of systemic and pulmonary venous blood return at either the atrial or the ventricular level; the mixed blood is then distributed to both systemic and pulmonary circulations in parallel. The defects can consist of one anatomic single ventricle with severe hypoplasia and inflow or outflow obstruction of the other one (hypoplastic left heart syndrome [HLHS] or pulmonary atresia with intact ventricular septum) or even two well-developed ventricles with atresia of the outflow tract or severe obstruction (TOF with pulmonary atresia, interrupted aortic arch). In some lesions, a PDA is the only source of systemic or pulmonary blood flow; these are called duct-dependent circulations. In others, intracardiac communications provide adequate blood flow to both circulations (Table 18.6).

Irrespective of the anatomic features, in single ventricle physiology the ventricular output (delivered by one or two ventricles)

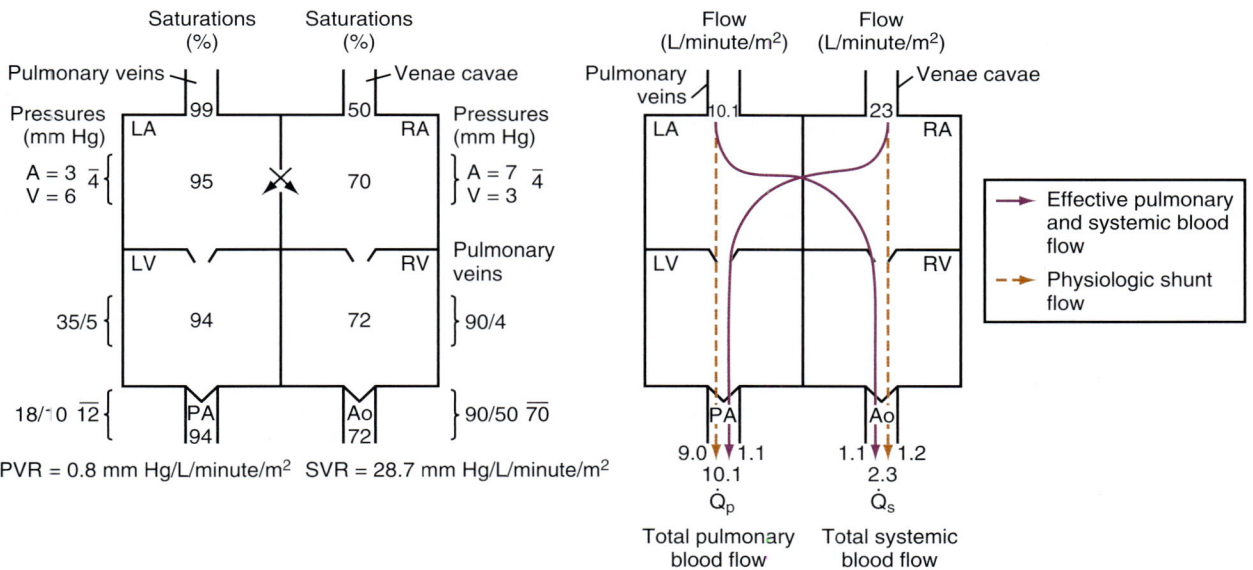

FIGURE 18.8 Saturations, pressures, and blood flows in transposition of the great arteries with a nonrestrictive atrial septal defect and a small left ventricular *(LV)* outflow tract gradient. Intercirculatory mixing occurs at the atrial level. Effective pulmonary and effective systemic blood flows are equal (1.1 L/minute per m²) and are the result of a bidirectional anatomic shunt at the atrial level. The physiologic left-to-right shunt is 9.0 L/minute per m²; this represents blood recirculated from the pulmonary veins to the pulmonary artery *(PA)*. The physiologic right-to-left shunt is 1.2 L/minute per m²; this represents blood recirculated from the systemic veins to the aorta *(Ao)*. Total pulmonary blood flow ($\dot{Q}_P = 10.1$ L/minute per m²) is almost five times greater than the total systemic blood flow ($\dot{Q}_S = 2.3$ L/minute per m²). The bulk of pulmonary blood flow is recirculated pulmonary venous blood. In this depiction, pulmonary vascular resistance *(PVR)* is low (approximately 1/35 of systemic vascular resistance [*SVR*]) and there is a small (17 mm Hg peak to peak) gradient from the LV to the PA. These findings are compatible with the high pulmonary blood flow depicted. *LA*, left atrium; *RA*, right atrium; *RV*, right ventricle. (From DiNardo J, Zwara DA. Congenital heart disease. In: DiNardo J, Zwara DA, eds. *Anesthesia for Cardiac Surgery*. 3rd ed. Malden, MA: Blackwell Publishing; 2008:167–251.)

TABLE 18.6	Examples of Single Ventricle Physiology	
Congenital Heart Defect	**Aortic Blood Flow From**	**Pulmonary Blood Flow From**
Hypoplastic left heart syndrome	PDA	RV
Neonatal critical aortic stenosis	PDA	RV
Interrupted aortic arch	Proximal LV, distal PDA	RV
Tetralogy of Fallot with pulmonary atresia	LV	PDA, MAPCAs
Pulmonary atresia with intact septum	LV	PDA
Tricuspid atresia 1B (VSD and PS)	LV	LV through VSD to RV
Truncus arteriosus	LV and RV	Aorta
Double inlet left ventricle, no TGA	LV	LV through VSD to bulboventricular foramen

LV, left ventricle; *MAPCAs*, major aortopulmonary collateral arteries; *PDA*, patent ductus arteriosus; *PS*, pulmonary stenosis; *RV*, right ventricle; *TGA*, transposition of the great arteries; *VSD*, ventricular septal defect.
Modified from DiNardo J, Zwara DA. Congenital heart disease. In: DiNardo J, Zwara DA, eds. *Anesthesia for Cardiac Surgery.* 3rd ed. Malden, MA: Blackwell Publishing; 2008:167–251.

is the sum of the pulmonary and systemic blood flows. The distribution of the respective flows depends on the relative outflow resistances into the two parallel circulations. Oxygen saturations in the aorta and PA are equal. The severity and location of anatomic obstructions and the ratio of PVR to SVR determine the balance of flows to the two circulations

The following equation illustrates the various factors that influence the arterial saturation (SaO_2) in a single ventricle physiology:

$$\text{Aortic saturation} = [(\text{Systemic venous saturation} \times \text{Total systemic venous blood flow}) + (\text{Pulmonary venous saturation} \times \text{Total pulmonary venous blood flow})] \div [(\text{Total systemic venous blood flow} + \text{Total pulmonary venous blood flow})]$$

Accordingly, three major variables determine arterial saturation and the initial management options for patients with single ventricle physiology:

- *The ratio of pulmonary to systemic blood flow* ($\dot{Q}_{pulm}/\dot{Q}_{sys}$). With high $\dot{Q}_{pulm}/\dot{Q}_{sys}$, a greater percentage of the blood in the ventricle (or ventricles) is oxygenated because more fully saturated pulmonary venous blood is entering the heart to mix with desaturated systemic venous return. Saturations greater than 85% can be achieved only by significant pulmonary overcirculation. $\dot{Q}_{pulm}/\dot{Q}_{sys}$ can be influenced by careful manipulations of the PVR/SVR ratio.
- *Systemic venous saturation* ($S_{sys}vO_2$): For a given $\dot{Q}_{pulm}/\dot{Q}_{sys}$ and pulmonary venous saturation ($S_{pulm}vO_2$), any decrease in $S_{sys}vO_2$ causes a decrease in arterial saturation. Oxygen delivery and consumption are the basic determinants for SvO_2. Adequate oxygen delivery depends on cardiac output and arterial oxygen content and thus on hemoglobin levels and arterial saturation. All measures that increase oxygen delivery (e.g., transfusion to increase the hematocrit to 0.45-0.50 or decrease oxygen consumption (e.g., adequate analgesia and sedation during painful procedures) improve arterial saturations.

- *Pulmonary venous saturation* ($S_{pulm}vO_2$): Normally the blood in the pulmonary veins should be fully saturated ($S_{pulm}vO_2 = 100\%$) on room air, but lung disease, $\dot{V}/\dot{Q}$ mismatch, or large intrapulmonary shunts can cause pulmonary venous desaturation. $\dot{V}/\dot{Q}$ mismatch usually responds to therapy with increased inspired oxygen, whereas intrapulmonary shunts are refractory to oxygen therapy. Pulmonary venous desaturation will decrease arterial saturations.

Special Situations

EXERCISE PHYSIOLOGY IN THE CHILD WITH REPAIRED CONGENITAL HEART DISEASE

Children with CHD, including those with lesions considered repaired, exhibit an array of abnormalities elicited during exercise testing consistent with reduced exercise capacity (E-Table 18.4). It is worthwhile to review the various exercise testing abnormalities to gain insight into the limitations imposed by the presence of congenital heart lesions.

Oxygen consumption ($\dot{V}O_2$) is equal to the product of cardiac output and O_2 extraction. O_2 extraction is equal to the arterial-venous oxygen content difference. Peak $\dot{V}O_2$ is the greatest measure of $\dot{V}O_2$ obtained during a progressively more difficult exercise test. $\dot{V}O_2$ at rest is defined as 1 metabolic equivalent energy expenditure unit or 1 MET (approximately 3.5 mL O_2/kg per minute).[74] A typical elite endurance athlete can reach 20 to 22 METs, or 70 to 77 mL O_2/kg per minute, at peak exercise. Activities of daily living require at least 4 METs or 14 mL O_2/kg per minute. Peak $\dot{V}O_2$ is the best overall assessment of the capabilities of the cardiovascular system, but determination of normal values is difficult owing to the effects of age, gender, effort, and body composition (e.g., adipose tissue) on peak $\dot{V}O_2$. Nonetheless, peak $\dot{V}O_2$ has been demonstrated to be a reliable predictor of hospitalization and mortality in patients with a wide variety of congenital heart lesions.[75]

During exercise, the HR normally increases linearly with increases in $\dot{V}O_2$. Normal peak HR is generally defined (in beats per minute [beats/minute]) as 220 minus age in years. In children with chronotropic incompetence, which is defined as the inability to increase HR to greater than 80% of the predicted value at peak exercise, the relationship between HR and $\dot{V}O_2$ is depressed. Chronotropic incompetence is an indicator of poor prognosis and is most commonly the result of sinus node dysfunction. By comparison, well-trained endurance athletes have a normal peak HR and a depressed HR/$\dot{V}O_2$ relationship, because they can generate a larger-than-normal stroke volume increase as exercise progresses. The inability to increase stroke volume (discussed later) during exercise results in an increased HR/$\dot{V}O_2$ relationship as a compensatory mechanism.

The *oxygen pulse* is the quantity of oxygen delivered per heartbeat. The peak O_2 pulse is calculated by dividing the peak $\dot{V}O_2$ by the peak HR. Because peak $\dot{V}O_2$ = cardiac output × O_2 extraction and because O_2 extraction remains remarkably constant over a wide range of exercise, O_2 pulse is proportional to stroke volume. Determination of normal peak O_2 pulse is hampered by the same factors that confound determination of normal peak $\dot{V}O_2$. In addition, O_2 pulse overestimates stroke volume in the presence of erythrocytosis and underestimates it in the presence of anemia or reduced arterial O_2 saturation. O_2 pulse is reduced in patients with impaired ventricular function, severe valvular regurgitation, or pulmonary vascular disease.[75] It is also uniformly reduced in those with Fontan physiology as a consequence of the inability of this circulation to augment systemic ventricular preload during exercise.[76]

The *respiratory exchange ratio* (RER) is defined as the ratio $\dot{V}CO_2/\dot{V}O_2$ (ratio of the volume of CO_2 produced per minute to the volume of oxygen consumed per minute). A normal resting RER is between 0.67 and 1.0, depending on the precise composition of protein, carbohydrates, and fat in the diet. As exercise intensifies, anaerobic metabolism commences and the lactate threshold is reached; buffering of lactic acid with bicarbonate causes the carbon dioxide production ($\dot{V}CO_2$) to increase out of proportion to oxygen consumption ($\dot{V}O_2$), resulting in an increased RER. An RER of 1.09 or greater is thought to indicate the onset of anaerobic metabolism and to be consistent with a good effort.[74,75] Because RER increases only if anaerobic metabolism occurs, exercise limitation and low $\dot{V}O_2$ owing to musculoskeletal problems or poor effort are associated with an RER less than this threshold.

The *ventilatory anaerobic threshold* (VAT) is used to identify the onset of anaerobic metabolism that occurs before $\dot{V}O_2$ peaks and is relatively effort and motivation independent. As aerobic exercise progresses, minute ventilation ($\dot{V}_E$) increases in direct proportion to $\dot{V}CO_2$ and $\dot{V}O_2$. When anaerobic metabolism commences and CO_2 production increases as lactic acid is buffered, $\dot{V}_E$ increases accordingly. VAT is the point at which $\dot{V}_E/\dot{V}O_2$ and $\dot{V}_E/\dot{V}CO_2$ diverge, with $\dot{V}_E$ increasing in proportion to $\dot{V}CO_2$ but out of proportion to $\dot{V}O_2$. An important characteristic of successful endurance athletes is the ability to reach and sustain effort at an anaerobic threshold that is a large percentage (80%–85%) of peak $\dot{V}O_2$.

Ventilation efficiency can be assessed with the use of the $\dot{V}_E/\dot{V}CO_2$ slope. This relationship is defined as $863 \cdot \dot{V}CO_2/[PaCO_2 \cdot (1 - V_D/V_T)]$, where V_D/V_T is the ratio of physiologic dead space to tidal volume.[77] The $\dot{V}_E/\dot{V}CO_2$ slope can be thought of as the number of liters of ventilation required to eliminate 1 L of CO_2. Normal children have a $\dot{V}_E/\dot{V}CO_2$ slope of less than 28.[75] To maintain a normal $PaCO_2$ during exercise, children with increased V_D/V_T and reduced ventilatory efficiency have a greater than normal increase in $\dot{V}_E$ and therefore a steeper $\dot{V}_E/\dot{V}CO_2$ slope. Increased V_D/V_T is the consequence of either reduced V_T in the setting of a normal V_D or pulmonary flow maldistribution and subsequent $\dot{V}/\dot{Q}$ mismatch that increases V_D. The latter is the major source of inefficient ventilation and steepening of the $\dot{V}_E/\dot{V}CO_2$ slope in children with cardiac disease.

In children with PA stenosis, (e.g., repaired TOF), pulmonary hypertension, or increased LA pressure from any cause (e.g., LV systolic or diastolic dysfunction, mitral valve disease), an increase in the $\dot{V}_E/\dot{V}CO_2$ slope is associated with increased mortality. When pulmonary stenosis is corrected in children with TOF, the $\dot{V}_E/\dot{V}CO_2$ slope and peak $\dot{V}O_2$ improve.

Children with Fontan physiology also exhibit an increase in $\dot{V}_E/\dot{V}CO_2$ slope. These children have inherent nonhomogeneous pulmonary perfusion at rest owing to the lack of pulsatile pulmonary blood flow. In addition, there is poor recruitment of the distal pulmonary vasculature during exercise. The presence of a Fontan fenestration further contributes to this increase in the $\dot{V}_E/\dot{V}CO_2$ slope by allowing mixed venous blood high in CO_2 to be shunted into the systemic circulation. This produces, via central chemoreceptor stimulation, an increase in $\dot{V}_E$ out of proportion to $\dot{V}CO_2$.[78] Fontan fenestration closure eliminates this right-to-left shunt and reduces the $\dot{V}_E/\dot{V}CO_2$ slope but does not improve the peak $\dot{V}O_2$.[78] The reason is that the primary limitation to increases in $\dot{V}O_2$ during exercise in Fontan patients is the inherent inability of the pulmonary vascular bed to substantially increase surface area, flow, and preload delivery to the systemic ventricle.

FONTAN PHYSIOLOGY

Francis Fontan, a French cardiac surgeon, described a new treatment for complex cardiac malformations with only one ventricle in 1971.[79] To decrease the chronic volume overload for the single ventricle and normalize oxygenation, he separated the systemic and pulmonary circulations by directly connecting the systemic venous return (SVC and IVC) to the PA, without a pumping chamber. This created a circulation wherein pulmonary blood was driven solely by a nonpulsatile pressure gradient across the pulmonary vascular bed, with the single ventricle being the sole source of kinetic energy. All other shunt connections were interrupted. The original indication was tricuspid atresia, but over the years the classic Fontan technique has been modified in many ways and is now used for various complex cardiac lesions with single ventricle physiology, such as HLHS, double-inlet RV, and pulmonary atresia with intact septum (see also Chapters 17 and 23).[80-85]

It is impossible to create a Fontan circulation at birth; high PVR and small vessel sizes prevent adequate pulmonary blood flow. In the neonatal period, palliative procedures such as stage I Norwood operation with aortic arch reconstruction, atrial septostomy, and aortopulmonary shunts (modified Blalock-Taussig shunt) or the Sano modification of the Norwood procedure (RV-to-PA conduit) aim for balanced systemic and pulmonary blood flows, allowing the infant to grow for several months despite cyanosis and volume load on the ventricle. At the age of 3 to 6 months, an intermediate procedure called the bidirectional Glenn operation or superior cavopulmonary anastomosis, is performed. The SVC is connected directly to the PA, providing nonpulsatile pulmonary blood flow, whereas the IVC remains connected to the heart. As a result, the volume load on the ventricle is significantly reduced, but oxygenated and deoxygenated blood still mix and the saturations remain in the low 80% range. By the age of 1 to 5 years, most of these children are ready for the Fontan circulation. With adequate growth and maturation of the pulmonary vascular bed, the resistance should be small enough to allow the complete separation of the systemic and pulmonary flows. The IVC is now also connected to the PA, most often via a lateral tunnel in the atrium or an extracardiac conduit, with or without a small fenestration (small opening in the baffle or conduit connecting the systemic venous return with the common atrium of the single ventricle). The fenestration can provide a residual right-to-left shunt in case of sudden increases in PVR, maintaining ventricular preload and function. This seems to facilitate the adaptation to the new loading conditions, shorten the recovery time, and decrease the incidence of early complications. The fenestration often occludes spontaneously, or it is closed during a cardiac catheterization and hemodynamic evaluation with a special device (Fig. 18.9; see also Figs. 17.11 through 17.13).[86-89]

The Fontan operation has dramatically improved the mortality rates for children with single ventricles, but the success comes at a price: chronic systemic venous hypertension and congestion have been implicated in a multitude of potential early and long-term complications, including arrhythmias, residual right-to-left shunts, coagulopathies with increased risk for thrombosis and stroke, lymphatic dysfunction with pleural effusions, and protein-losing enteropathy.[90-95] Late cardiac failure and poor functional outcome remain risks for patients with Fontan circulations. The anatomy of the single ventricle and the type of Fontan connection influence the duration of freedom from complications. Children with systemic RVs and the classic atriopulmonary Fontan procedure (RA directly anastomosed to the PA) tend to have a shorter duration of freedom from complications than those

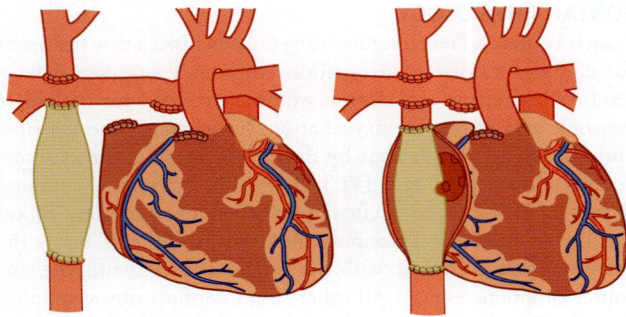

FIGURE 18.9 Fontan modifications: extracardiac conduit *(left)* and lateral tunnel with fenestration *(right)*. (Courtesy of Children's Hospital of Boston.)

with systemic LVs and newer Fontan modifications (E-Figs. 18.2 and 18.3).[96]

Inherent limitations of the Fontan circulation, such as altered control of cardiac output with decreased hemodynamic response to stress and reduced exercise tolerance, have been documented (Fig. 18.10).[97–105] Even at rest, cardiac output is usually only 70% (range, 50%-80%) of normal for body surface area. Cardiac output is classically determined by four factors: preload, contractility, HR, and afterload. Over a physiologic range, cardiac output improves with increased preload, contractility, and HR and with decreased afterload. For the Fontan circulation, the determinants of cardiac output are more complex (Fig. 18.11).[100,106,107] The classic determinants of cardiac output are less effective, while other factors, such as transpulmonary gradient and PVR, must be considered. The following mechanisms regulate cardiac output in children with Fontan physiology.

- *Preload:* The RV usually provides the kinetic energy to distend the pulmonary vasculature and create a preload reservoir for the LV, thereby enabling an increase in cardiac output up to fivefold or greater with exercise.[106,108] The lack of a pre-pulmonary pump leads to a significant decrease in available pulmonary blood volume and, consequently, reduced or absent LV preload reserve.[100,109,110]
- *Contractility:* During the staged palliation, the single ventricle typically develops from a volume-overloaded and dilated ventricle to a hypertrophied, underfilled ventricle.[111,112] Although the contractile response to β-adrenergic stimulation seems to be preserved, the resulting increase in cardiac output is diminished, most likely owing to limited preload reserve.[103,110]
- *Heart rate and rhythm:* Within the physiologic range, atrial pacing at different HRs does not alter cardiac output because there is a simultaneous decrease in stroke volume.[113] Normalization of HR increases the reduced cardiac output associated with severe bradycardia or tachycardia.[114] During exercise testing, Fontan patients demonstrate chronotropic incompetence, a blunted HR response to exercise. This is likely the result of autonomic dysfunction or abnormal reflex control. In contrast to the HR, cardiac rhythm is of utmost importance. Ectopy or loss of atrioventricular (AV) synchronization compromises ventricular filling and decreases the transpulmonary gradient.[115]
- *Afterload:* The Fontan circulation is characterized by increased afterload, which is a physiologic response to decreased cardiac output and occurs because a single ventricle is ejecting into

two large resistance beds (systemic and pulmonary vascular) arranged in series.[100,110,116,117] Autonomic regulation and activation of various endocrine systems increase the systemic venous resistance and help to maintain adequate perfusion pressures and venous tone. Because of the limited preload reserve, attempts at afterload reduction often result in significant hypotension. On the other hand, excessive afterload, such as that which occurs with residual aortic arch obstruction, is poorly tolerated.

- *Transpulmonary flow:* Transpulmonary flow is directly proportional to the gradient between the systemic venous pressure (usually between 10 and 15 mm Hg, rarely >20 mm Hg) and the preventricular atrial pressure, which is determined by the functional status of the AV valve, the ventricle, the rhythm, and the potential presence of outflow obstruction. Transpulmonary flow is inversely proportional to the resistance over the Fontan circuit. This resistance is largely determined by PVR, but mechanical obstruction such as stenosis or thrombosis may also play a role. The geometry of the cavopulmonary connections is also important in that turbulent flow produces energy loss and a reduction in effective driving pressure. It has been suggested that PVR is the key determinant of transpulmonary flow, delivery of pulmonary venous flow to the systemic ventricle, and, consequently, cardiac output (Fig. 18.12).[100,118–128]

In conclusion, the Fontan circulation can be described as a serial circulation with a single kinetic energy pump. Increased systemic venous pressures are necessary to create the transpulmonary pressure gradient that drives flow across the pulmonary vascular bed; however, these increased pressures simultaneously increase the ventricular afterload. Cardiac output depends on an adequate preload and low PVR. Decreased cardiac output at rest and limited exercise tolerance are characteristics of the Fontan circulation.

PHYSIOLOGY OF THE TRANSPLANTED HEART

According to the International Society for Heart and Lung Transplantation (ISHLT), children younger than 18 years of age account for about 13% of all heart transplantations. Every year, approximately 450 cardiac transplants in children are reported to this voluntary registry, mainly from centers in Europe and North America.[129] Major indications are cardiomyopathies, CHD, and a growing number of retransplantations, especially in older children. The median survival time (the time at which 50% of recipients are still alive) has improved over the years, mainly because of reduced early posttransplant mortality. Survival time is currently 20.6 years for infants, 17.2 years for children aged 1 to 5 years, 13.9 years for children aged 6 to 10 years, and 12.4 years for teenagers. Ninety-four percent of transplant recipients describe a normal functional status with no limitations during physical activity.[129]

As survival continues to improve, more and more children with transplanted hearts will present to operating rooms and sedation suites for diagnostic studies and general procedures. A basic understanding of the physiologic changes in the transplanted heart and the implications of current immunosuppressive therapy are important for safe management.

Physiology of the Denervated Heart

After transplantation, the function of the surgically denervated heart depends primarily on an intact Frank-Starling mechanism and stimulation from circulating catecholamines. The classic Frank-Starling mechanism describes the ability of the cardiac muscle to increase contractility in response to stretch or tension

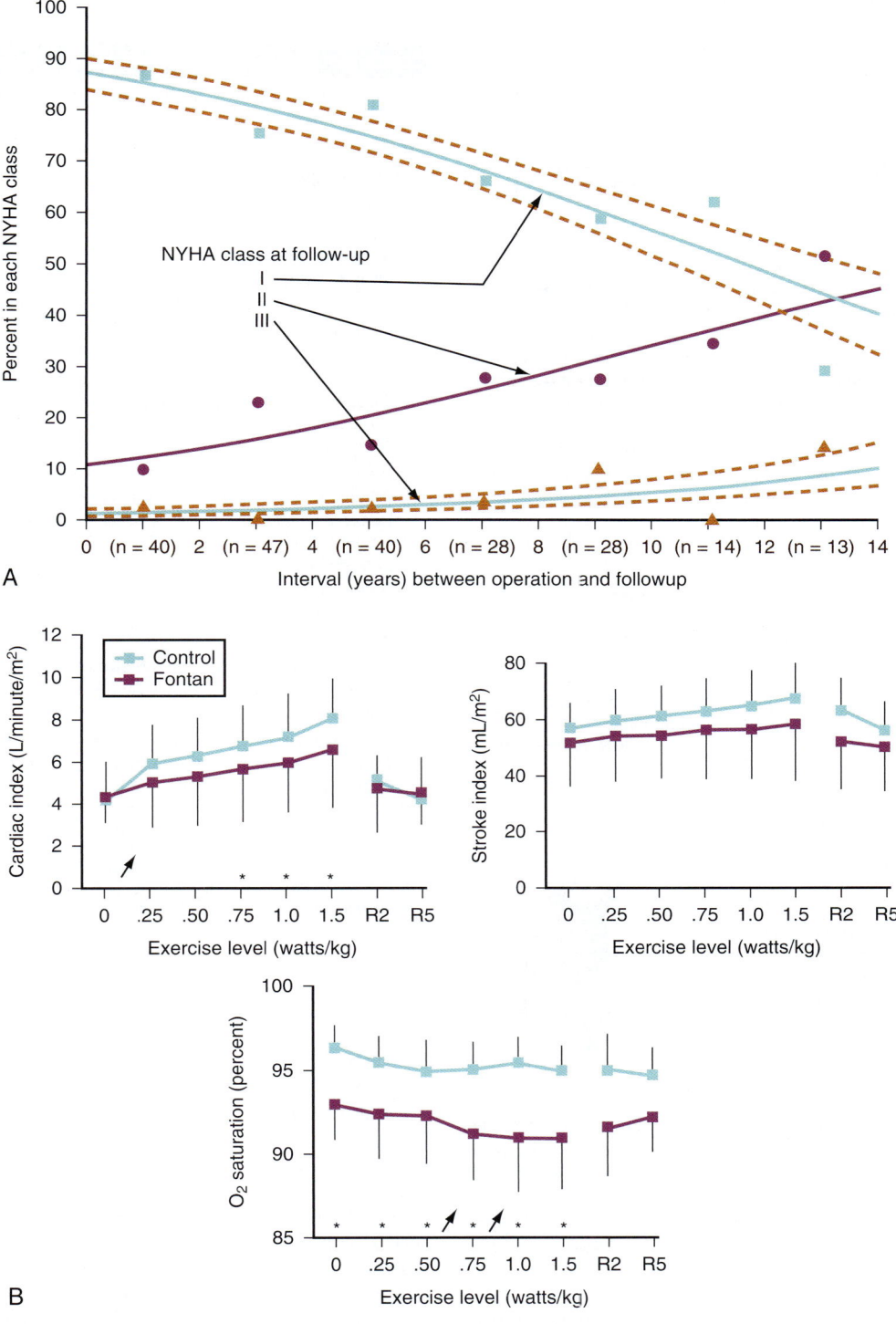

FIGURE 18.10 A, Symptomatic outcomes of 334 survivors of Fontan operations who were monitored for 1 month to 20 years. The graph illustrates the changes since surgery in patients assessed as New York Heart Association (NYHA) classification I *(blue squares),* II *(purple circles),* or III *(brown triangles).* Although most children exhibited good functional status (NYHA class I) immediately after surgery, mild functional limitations evolved over time. Broken lines indicate 70% confidence intervals. **B,** Results of exercise studies (cardiac index, stroke index, and oxygen saturation vs. exercise level) of 42 children after Fontan operation *(purple squares)* compared with normal control subjects *(blue squares).* Although the protocol was designed to achieve modest targets, significant differences emerged in the capacity of Fontan children to increase cardiac output with exercise, and systemic arterial oxygen saturation remained below normal throughout. The primary reason for the inability to increase cardiac output appears to be an inability to increase pulmonary blood flow and, consequently, systemic ventricular filling. Potential reasons for decreased arterial saturation include intrapulmonary shunting owing to arteriovenous malformations and ventilation/perfusion imbalance. *Arrows* indicate a significant difference *(P < .05)* in values between consecutive exercise levels. **(A** from Fontan F, Kirklin JW, Fernandez G, et al. Outcome after a "perfect" Fontan operation. *Circulation* 1990;81:1520–1536; **B** from Gewillig MH, Lundstrom UR, Bull C, et al. Exercise responses in children with congenital heart disease after Fontan repair: patterns and determinants of performance. *J Am Coll Cardiol.* 1990;15:1424–1432. Reprinted with permission from the American College of Cardiology.)

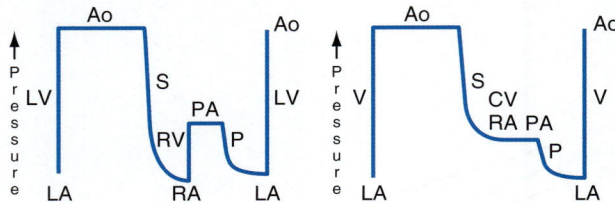

FIGURE 18.11 In the normal cardiovascular circulation *(left)*, the pulmonary circulation *(P)* is connected in series with the systemic circulation *(S)*. The right ventricle *(RV)* maintains a right atrial *(RA)* pressure that is lower than the left atrial *(LA)* pressure and provides enough energy for the blood to pass through the pulmonary resistance. In the Fontan circuit *(right)*, the systemic veins are connected to the pulmonary artery *(PA)* without a subpulmonary ventricle or systemic atrium (the RV is not present on the right). In the absence of a fenestration, there is no admixture of systemic and pulmonary venous blood, but the systemic venous pressures are markedly increased. *Ao,* aorta; *CV,* caval veins; *LV,* left ventricle; *V,* single ventricle. (From Gewillig M, Brown SC, Eyskens B, et al. The Fontan circulation: who controls cardiac output? *Interact Cardiovasc Thorac Surg.* 2010;10:428–433.)

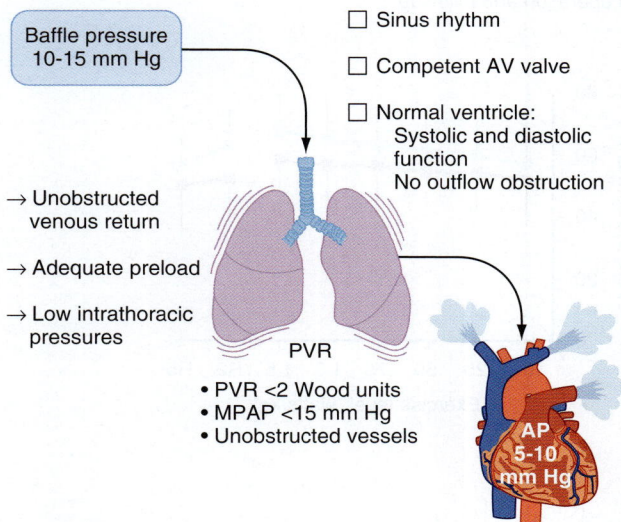

FIGURE 18.12 Several factors determine the transpulmonary gradient in the Fontan circulation. These include unobstructed venous return, adequate preload, and low intrathoracic pressure on the venous side; low pulmonary vascular resistance *(PVR)*, and unobstructed pulmonary vessels; and, on the atrial side, adequate ventricular function, competent atrioventricular valves, normal sinus rhythm, and no evidence of outflow obstruction. *AP,* atrial pressure; *MPAP,* mean pulmonary arterial pressure. (Courtesy A. Schure.)

TABLE 18.7	Physiology of the Transplanted Heart

Increased filling pressures (LVEDP 12 mm Hg 4–8 weeks after transplantation)

Low-normal left ventricular ejection fraction

Restrictive physiology (stiff heart)

Increased afterload

Afferent denervation
  No angina during ischemia
  Altered cardiac baroreceptors and mechanoreceptors
  Less stress-induced increase in systemic vascular resistance
  Increased blood volume due to decreased natriuresis and diuresis

Efferent denervation
  Resting tachycardia (loss of baseline vagal tone)
  Impaired chronotropic response to stress (dependent on circulating catecholamines)

Altered response to medications
  No heart rate response to atropine, glycopyrrolate, and digitalis
  Possible severe bradycardia or cardiac arrest with neostigmine
  Exacerbated response to calcium channel blockers, β-blockers, adenosine
  Exacerbated response to direct acting sympathetic agents
  Decreased response to indirect-acting agents such as dopamine and ephedrine

Electrophysiology
  High incidence of sinus node dysfunction in immediate postoperative period, normal AV node
  Shift to β₂-receptors

Possible sympathetic reinnervation: timing and extent variable
  Enhanced contractile response and exercise tolerance
  Higher peak heart rates during exercise

AV, atrioventricular; *LVEDP,* left ventricular end-diastolic pressure.
Data from Schure AY, Kussman BD. Pediatric heart transplantation: demographics, outcomes, and anesthetic implications. *Pediatr Anesth.* 2011;21:594–603; and Cotts WG, Oren RM. Function of the transplanted heart: unique physiology and therapeutic implications. *Am J Med Sci.* 1997;314:164–172.

(e.g., increasing cardiac output with increases in venous return). Afferent and efferent denervation has multiple effects on circulatory control mechanisms and leads to physiologic changes, including an increase in the resting HR and a blunted response to stress and exercise. Despite excellent physical activity, exercise testing easily demonstrates that heart transplant recipients can usually achieve only 60% to 70% of normal capacity. In the transplanted heart, exercise-induced increase in cardiac output is initially caused by an increase in stroke volume, a highly preload-dependent process. Tachycardia occurs only later, in response to circulating catecholamines.[130] Further details of the altered physiology are summarized in Table 18.7.[130] The incidence, timing, and extent of sympathetic reinnervation are still being investigated, but the positive effects on cardiac performance have been clearly demonstrated.[131] During standardized exercise testing, transplant recipients with evidence of reinnervation show improved endurance with greater peak HRs and better contractile function.

Chronic denervation also causes an altered response to many medications. Atropine, glycopyrrolate, digoxin, and pancuronium have no chronotropic effect on the denervated heart. Sympathomimetics that act indirectly, such as ephedrine and dopamine, have a blunted response, whereas direct-acting adrenergic agents, such as epinephrine, isoproterenol, and dobutamine, can cause exaggerated effects and should be carefully titrated.[132] A single-center retrospective study did not find any negative effects of neostigmine in patients with heart transplants,[133] but several case reports have described profound bradycardia and even cardiac arrest after neostigmine was used for reversal of neuromuscular blockade.[134–137] Neostigmine has been shown to produce an atropine-sensitive, dose-dependent bradycardia in both recent (<6 months) and remote (>6 months) cardiac transplants. Direct stimulation of postganglionic nicotinic cholinergic receptors with denervation hypersensitivity, a direct effect of the old sinoatrial node on the pacemaker cell of the new sinoatrial node, and parasympathetic reinnervation have been postulated as potential mechanisms.[138–140] Avoidance of neuromuscular blockade, use of short-acting neuromuscular blocking agents without reversal, and use of edrophonium for reversal have all been suggested.[136,137] Edrophonium seems to have less effect on the HR in this population than neostigmine.[141]

The denervated heart is also extremely sensitive to adenosine. The magnitude and duration of the effects on the AV node are three to five times greater, and the initial and subsequent doses should be reduced by 50%.[142] Calcium channel blockers and β-blockers are associated with exaggerated bradycardia and hypotension. The lack of reflex tachycardia can also lead to profound hypotension with the use of direct vasodilators such as nitroglycerine, nitroprusside, or hydralazine; therefore initial doses of these medications should also be reduced.

Transplant Morbidity

Children who have undergone cardiac transplantation continue to experience morbidity associated with immunosuppressive therapy. Rehospitalization for treatment of infections and episodes of rejection is common, especially during the first year (~42%). Acute rejection episodes are a major threat. With the latest immunosuppressive regimens, the incidence has decreased from almost 30% during the first year in 2008 to 15% in 2014.[129] Rejection is thought to be associated with the development of cardiac allograft vasculopathy (CAV) or coronary artery disease, which is a major cause of morbidity and graft failure. Indeed, 10 years after transplantation, ~16% of infants, ~27% of children 1 to 10 years of age, and ~37% of adolescents have CAV.[129] Most centers include annual coronary angiography or intravascular echocardiography as a part of regular rejection surveillance. Children with CAV present the same anesthetic challenges as adults with severe coronary artery disease and ischemic heart disease. Aggressive immunosuppressive therapy with induction and maintenance regimens carries its own risks.[143] A detailed discussion is beyond the scope of this chapter but, in general, monoclonal or polyclonal T-cell antibodies (OKT3, ATG) and specific interleukin-2 receptor antagonists (basiliximab, daclizumab) are used for the induction phase and various combinations of corticosteroids, calcineurin inhibitors (cyclosporine, tacrolimus, FK506), mechanistic target of rapamycin inhibitors (mTOR inhibitors: sirolimus, everolimus) and antiproliferative agents (azathioprine, mycophenolate mofetil) are used for maintenance. Adverse effects are common and include neurotoxicity with seizures, hypertension, liver and renal dysfunction, hyperlipidemia, diabetes, gingival hypertrophy, hypertrichosis, bone marrow suppression, and posttransplantation lymphoproliferative disease.[144]

Several excellent review articles describe the anesthetic management of children with heart transplants (see also Chapter 23).[145–148] A thorough preoperative evaluation with attention to episodes of rejection, presence of coronary artery disease, and organ dysfunction; a detailed medication history with investigation of major side effects; consideration of the denervated physiology; and appropriate choice of anesthetic drugs and other medications are essential components of a sensible anesthetic plan for those with a transplanted heart.

Cardiovascular Pharmacology

RATIONAL USE OF VASOACTIVE DRUGS

Many factors influence the selection of appropriate inotropic and vasopressor therapies, including the clinical situation, underlying cardiac abnormalities, and perfusion requirements of other organs. The major goal is to improve tissue oxygenation. Oxygen delivery is principally dependent on cardiac output and oxygen content. In addition to an increased cardiac output (i.e., optimal HR, preload,

contractility, and afterload), adequate hemoglobin concentration and oxygen saturation values are important components. On the other hand, a careful balance of pulmonary and systemic blood flows can be crucial for certain congenital heart defects.

Catecholamines and catecholamine-like agents remain the most commonly used inotropic and vasoconstrictor drugs. It is likely that improvements in cardiac output in neonates in response to drugs such as dopamine or dobutamine are the result of increases in both HR and contractility. Some evidence exists in infants and young children after cardiac surgery that the increases in cardiac output produced by dopamine and dobutamine may be more related to a positive chronotropic effect than to an increase in the intrinsic contractile state.[149–151] With few exceptions, drugs that primarily increase afterload, such as α-adrenergic agonists, have limited use in children. Large increases in afterload without corresponding improvements in contractile state are often poorly tolerated by infants and children, particularly in the context of significant underlying contractile dysfunction.

PRACTICAL CONSIDERATIONS FOR THE USE OF VASOACTIVE AGENTS

Commonly used drugs, their doses, and a summary of their effects on selected cardiac functions are presented in Table 18.8; most of this information has been empirically derived from studies in adults. Limited direct information regarding the effects of commonly used vasoactive drugs in children at different ages and in various pathophysiologic states is available. Neonates, infants, and small children demonstrate unique responses to inotropic and vasoactive drugs primarily because of age-specific pharmacokinetics; differences in receptor types, number, and function; and a variability in drug delivery. Important variations in the volume of distribution and measured plasma concentrations have been observed in children receiving inotropic agents. As much as a 10-fold range in plasma concentration has been reported for a given infusion rate.[152–154]

Substantial pharmacodynamic variability (i.e., variability in the serum concentration required to produce the desired effect) can also be observed. Some of these differences are related to receptor maturation and function. For example, it appears that β-adrenergic receptors have a high density in the term neonate and young infant but their coupling to adenyl cyclase may be incomplete.[35,155] In addition to developmental changes, which are to some extent controlled by thyroid hormone, β-receptor, and adenyl cyclase activities are diminished in response to sustained administration of exogenous β-agonists and also as a result of increased endogenous catecholamine concentrations, which are often seen as a complication of moderate to severe heart failure and other forms of severe stress (e.g., sepsis).[156–158]

In the neonatal myocardium, chronic catecholamine exposure may upregulate adrenergic receptor number or function, or both, perhaps mimicking the normal developmental program of increasing sympathetic nervous system activity as term approaches.[159] With further maturation in early postnatal life, β-adrenergic receptor density declines. The impacts of various pathophysiologic states on these processes have been incompletely identified. For example, congestive heart failure, cardiopulmonary bypass (CPB), and ischemic reperfusion all lead to decreased β-receptor and adenyl cyclase expression and activity.[160–163] On the other hand, the myocardium of infants with TOF exhibits increased β-receptor density and greater receptor-stimulated adenyl cyclase activity with increased gene and protein expression.[164,165]

One must pay particular attention to technical issues when administering vasoactive infusions to infants. Infusions are often

TABLE 18.8 | Inotropics and Vasopressors

Agent	Intravenous Dose	Comments
Dopamine	2–20 µg/kg per minute infusion	Primary effects at β_1, β_2, and dopamine receptors, somewhat related to dose; lower doses (2–5 µg/kg per minute) can increase contractility and can also have a direct dopaminergic receptor effect to increase splanchnic and renal perfusion; increasing doses increase contractility via β-effects and increase likelihood of α-mediated vasoconstriction; effects depend on endogenous catecholamine stores.
Dobutamine	2–20 µg/kg per minute infusion	Relatively selective β_1 stimulation; also potential β_2 stimulation, tachycardia, and vasodilation, especially at higher doses (>10 µg/kg per minute); may be less potent than dopamine, especially in immature myocardium; no significant α-adrenergic effects; tachydysrhythmias perhaps more likely than with dopamine; effects are independent of endogenous catecholamine stores.
Epinephrine	0.02–2.0 µg/kg per minute infusion	Primary β-effects to increase contractility and vasodilation at lower doses (0.02–0.10 µg/kg per minute); increasing doses (>0.1 µg/kg per minute) are accompanied by increased contractility and increased α-mediated vasoconstriction; may be best choice to augment contractility and perfusion, especially in situations of severely compromised ventricular function, shock, or anaphylaxis.
Isoproterenol	0.05–2.0 µg/kg per minute infusion	Pure, nonselective β-agonist; significant inotropic, chronotropic (β_1 and β_2), and vasodilatory (β_2) effects; may be an effective pulmonary vasodilator in some children; tachycardia and increased myocardial oxygen consumption may be dose limiting; tachydysrhythmias may also occur; bronchodilator.
Norepinephrine	0.05–2 µg/kg per minute infusion	Primary effects on α_1-, α_2-, and β_1-receptors, no significant clinical effects on β_2. Increased systemic blood pressure and cardiac output (α_1 and β_1) as well as improved pulmonary blood flow (α_2). Less tachycardia. Mainly used for treatment of septic shock and pulmonary hypertension.
Phenylephrine	1–10 µg/kg bolus, 0.1–0.5 µg/kg per minute infusion Preterm and term infants may require as much as a 30 µg/kg bolus (see Chapter 17)	Pure α-mediated vasoconstriction; no increase in contractility.
Vasopressin	0.0003–0.002 U/kg per minute	Induces intense vasoconstriction via V_{1a} receptors in the vascular endothelium. May cause vasodilation via V_2 receptors in specific tissues (release of nitric oxide and vasodilating prostaglandins). Used for the treatment of vasodilatory shock, refractory hypotension, and pulmonary arterial hypertension. Careful when programming syringe pumps: multiple dosing forms (U/minute, U/kg per hour, U/kg per minute, or mU/kg per minute).
Amrinone	0.75–1 mg/kg repeated twice, maximum 3 mg/kg Neonates and infants may require loading doses of 2–4 mg/kg and infusions of 10 µg/kg per minute	Increases cyclic adenosine monophosphate by phosphodiesterase inhibition; positive inotropy, positive lusitropy, and smooth muscle vasorelaxation; hypotension; reversible thrombocytopenia.
Milrinone	50–75 µg/kg loading dose, 0.5–1.0 µg/kg per minute infusion	Similar to amrinone (antiplatelet effects may be less).
Calcium chloride Calcium gluconate	10–20 mg/kg per dose (slowly) 30–60 mg/kg per dose (slowly)	Positive inotropic and direct vasoconstricting effects; inotropy is significant only if ionized calcium is low and/or ventricular function is depressed by other agents; can slow sinus node; increases electrophysiologic abnormalities from hypokalemia and digoxin.
Digoxin	Total digitalizing dose (TDD): Premature: 20 µg/kg Neonate (1 mo): 30 µg/kg Infant (<2 yr): 40 µg/kg Child (2–5 yr): 30 µg/kg Child (>5 yr): 20 µg/kg Maintenance: 2.5–5 µg/kg q12 hour	TDD given in divided doses: ½ TDD followed by ¼ TDD q8–12 hour ¾ × 2; increases cardiac contractility; slows sinus node and decreases atrioventricular (AV) node conduction; long half-life (24–48 hours) that is prolonged by renal dysfunction; numerous drug interactions; toxicity includes supraventricular tachycardia, AV block, ventricular dysrhythmias; symptoms include drowsiness, nausea, vomiting; toxicity exacerbated by hypokalemia.

specifically prepared as very concentrated, nonstandardized solutions to minimize the amount of volume infused; hence, the potential for dose or concentration error is substantial. One study at a tertiary care children's hospital demonstrated that the actual concentration of prepared solutions varied significantly.[166] Because of the high concentration of these drugs relative to the child's size, small errors (either in calculation or in infusion pump flow rate) can have a large impact on the actual amount of drug delivered. The extremely small infusion rates can also lead to a delay in drug delivery and effect (see Chapters 8 and 52). Confirming that the pump drive mechanism is actually delivering drug at the distal end of the infusion tubing, connecting the infusion tubing as close to the child as possible, and using a carrier infusion to "push" the medication at a constant rate are important steps to ensure the safety and effectiveness of drug infusions. The rate of the carrier infusion is also crucial. Most standard infusion setups require rates in excess of 5 mL/hour to effect rapid (less than ~10 minutes) changes in the concentration of drug delivered to the infant and therefore preclude all attempts of fluid restriction.

VASOACTIVE DRUGS

Dopamine

Dopamine continues to be the most frequently used inotropic agent in neonates, infants, and children. It has activity at α-, β-, and dopaminergic receptors. Dopamine augments cardiac contractility through two mechanisms. First, it directly stimulates cardiac β_1-receptors and provokes norepinephrine release from cardiac sympathetic nerve terminals. Second, circulating concentrations of endogenous epinephrine and norepinephrine increase during dopamine infusions, leading to the suggestion that at least some of the effects of a dopamine infusion are indirectly mediated via induced release of endogenous catecholamines.[167] Because of its indirect effects, particularly the release of myocardial norepinephrine stores, the response to dopamine may be diminished in children with congestive heart failure or other relatively long-standing forms of hemodynamic stress.

Activity at dopaminergic receptors in the kidney and gastrointestinal tract can lead to improved perfusion of these organ systems. The evidence that dopamine specifically and selectively improves renal perfusion via stimulation of renal dopaminergic receptors (i.e., as opposed to a nonspecific and generalized improvement in cardiac output that might occur with any positive inotrope) is conflicting.[168–172] Regardless of the mechanism, most evidence indicates that renal blood flow and perfusion are increased by dopamine, even at very large doses.

As in the case with other inotropes, pharmacokinetic studies of dopamine have shown wide variability in serum concentration in neonates and children.[173,174] Because of variability in the plasma concentration for a given infusion rate, as well as the wide range of serum concentrations necessary to produce a given effect, doubling or halving a dopamine infusion rate may be a logical approach to bracketing the optimal dose. The frequent practice of changing the infusion rate by small proportions (i.e., 5% to 10%) may be inconsistent with our current understanding of the pharmacokinetics and pharmacodynamics of most inotropes.

Neonates have classically been considered to have a greater dependence on HR, a reduced myocardial compliance, and a relative resistance to inotropic effects of exogenous catecholamines. Nonetheless, there is substantial echocardiographic evidence that small dopamine infusion rates (≤5 µ/kg per minute) increase myocardial contractility before significant increases in HR.[175,176] Evidence regarding the effects of dopamine in sick preterm infants is also somewhat controversial.[169,177–181] There may be a relative dissociation between its effects on the renal and mesenteric beds in these infants, such that a portion of the increase in arterial blood pressure during a dopamine infusion may result from mesenteric vasoconstriction and an actual decrease in mesenteric blood flow.

Although it is generally accepted that large infusion rates (>10 to 15 µg/kg per minute) of dopamine cause substantive vasoconstriction, studies have shown that both cardiac output and renal blood flow improve, even at very large doses (≥20 µg/kg per minute) in neonates and infants.[182,183]

The effects of dopamine on PVR are variable. Both minimal effect and increased PVR have been observed.[151,184–190] The effects of dopamine on PVR most likely depend on the dose as well as the underlying state of the vascular endothelium and smooth muscle. Vasoconstriction may be more likely after ischemia-reperfusion and in the presence of hypoxia. Conversely, the presence of vasodilators, such as nitroprusside, or α-adrenergic blockers, such as phenoxybenzamine, can prevent increased PVR in response to dopamine.[191,192] Overall, dopamine remains the drug of choice in most infants and children, owing to its beneficial effects on mesenteric and renal blood flow, lesser chronotropic effects than some other agents, and a somewhat reduced arrhythmogenic potential.

Dobutamine (Dobutrex)

Dobutamine is a structural analog of isoproterenol. It was developed to provide relatively selective β-adrenergic receptor stimulation. Its inotropic and α-adrenergic effects are somewhat less potent than those of dopamine. Dobutamine does possess significant β_2-adrenergic receptor agonist properties, accounting for its peripheral vasodilatory properties. Substantial vasodilation and tachycardia occur at larger infusion rates (≥10 µg/kg per minute).[150,193–196] The tendency toward tachycardia and tachyarrhythmia may be greater in neonates than in older children or adults. There is some evidence from immature animal models that the efficacy of dobutamine is reduced, perhaps because of greater circulating catecholamine concentrations and alterations in β-receptor expression and function.[149,150,197–199]

Because the actions of dobutamine do not depend on endogenous catecholamine stores, the drug may be more effective in increasing cardiac output in patients with severe congestive heart failure or cardiogenic shock.[200,201] In children with normal LV function, dobutamine increases LV relaxation. It also improves diastolic relaxation by decreasing end-systolic wall stress.[202] Evidence indicates that dobutamine improves LV contractility in neonates with LV dysfunction, dispelling the notion that there is relative resistance in neonates.[203] Dobutamine does not selectively improve renal or mesenteric blood flow independently of its effect on increasing cardiac output. The improvement in cardiac output with dobutamine is related to both an increased contractility and decreased SVR via vasodilation. Pulmonary vasodilation in the presence of an increased PVR may also occur.[199]

As is the case with dopamine, exponential increases in serum concentrations are required to produce linear improvements in cardiac index. There is also substantial pharmacokinetic variability in the plasma concentrations of dobutamine.[153,204,205] Tolerance may occasionally develop.[206] In one animal study, high-dose dobutamine infusion was associated with significant dysfunction of platelet aggregation after hypoxia and reoxygenation.[207]

Isoproterenol (Isuprel)

Isoproterenol is a pure, nonselective β-adrenergic agonist.[208] It increases HR and contractility and vasodilates mesenteric and renal vessels and skeletal muscle. Isoproterenol is also a fairly effective vasodilator of the pulmonary circulation.[209] The tachycardia, which almost always accompanies its use, and greater contractility cause an increase in myocardial oxygen consumption, which is usually well tolerated. However, these changes may be limiting in compromised hearts. The pulmonary vasodilation produced by isoproterenol may be useful in settings in which tachycardia is either unimportant or somewhat beneficial.[210] Systemic vasodilation induced by isoproterenol can be sufficiently profound as to cause systemic hypotension.[189,211] The positive chronotropic effects of isoproterenol may be useful in children with bradycardia.[212] The drug is increasingly used in electrophysiology suites to facilitate the detection of abnormal conduction pathways in infants and children under general anesthesia.[213] Isoproterenol is also a potent bronchodilator. Prolonged use or large doses of isoproterenol and other catecholamines may be associated with the development of myocardial fibrosis.[214]

Epinephrine (Adrenaline)

Epinephrine has α-, β_1-, and β_2-adrenergic agonist effects. Data derived mainly from studies in adults indicate that lower doses of 0.02 to 0.1 µg/kg per minute are associated with predominantly β-adrenergic effects. In this range, increases in HR and systolic blood pressure and reduced diastolic blood pressure owing to skeletal muscle vasodilation predominate. Doses between 0.1 and 0.2 µg/kg per minute have mixed α- and β-effects. At larger doses, α-adrenergic–induced vasoconstriction is significant, and hence there is reduced skin, muscle, renal, and mesenteric blood flow. Compared with pure α-agonists, epinephrine provides significant inotropic effect. The effects of epinephrine do not depend on endogenous tissue catecholamine stores. Based on experience, epinephrine seems to be effective in children who do not respond to dopamine or dobutamine, particularly those with significant dysfunction of the systemic ventricle in the immediate postoperative period. The addition of moderate vasoconstriction to increased contractility may be advantageous to maintain myocardial perfusion and may also increase both systemic and pulmonary blood flow in children with shunt-dependent circulations. Important adverse effects include dysrhythmias (usually ventricular) and, at larger doses, regional ischemia and hypoperfusion as the result of vasoconstriction.

Pharmacokinetic studies have shown a linear relationship between serum concentration and infusion rate, but again there is significant variability in the individual response to a specific concentration.[215,216] In infants and children with postoperative low cardiac output syndrome, increased concentrations of glucose and of lactate have been reported after 1 to 2 hours of an epinephrine infusion of 0.1 µg/kg per minute.[215]

Norepinephrine (Levophed)

Norepinephrine is often indicated as a first- or second-line treatment for severe hypotension associated with septic shock, but it has also been used in the treatment of persistent pulmonary hypertension of the newborn and other forms of pulmonary hypertension.[217–222] This endogenous adrenergic agent activates both α- and β-receptors. Compared with epinephrine, it seems to be equally effective on β_1-receptors, slightly less on α_1-receptors, and has no clinically significant effects on β_2-receptors. Norepinephrine has been shown to increase systemic blood pressure as well as cardiac output, oxygen delivery, and splanchnic perfusion in animal models and clinical studies.[223,224] It causes less tachycardia than epinephrine. Through activation of α_2-receptors and release of NO, norepinephrine reduces PVR and can improve pulmonary blood flow.[184,225–228] Norepinephrine has a very rapid onset of action with a duration of effect of only 1-2 minutes. It is metabolized by catechol-O-methyltransferase and monoamine oxidase, the inactive metabolites are eliminated in the urine. Pharmacokinetic data are mainly derived from adult studies; the few available pediatric reports emphasize the wide interindividual variability and the need for careful titration. The initial dose of 0.05 to 0.1 µg/kg per minute has to be slowly increased to the desired effect, usually in a range of 0.1 to 2 µg/kg per minute. In a small prospective observational study in term neonates, the majority responded to a mean dose of 0.5 ± 0.4 µg/kg per minute, with a range of 0.2 to 7.1 µg/kg per minute.[219] A retrospective study in children in septic shock reported mean initial doses of 0.5 ± 0.4 µg/kg per minute to 2.5 ± 2.2 µg/kg per minute, with a maximum individual dose of 10.5 µg/kg per minute.[217] Norepinephrine may be administered via peripheral venous access (and is recommended to avoid delays in treatment) until central access can be established, but some institutions report IV infiltrates in up to 15% of children on vasoactive infusions especially during transport. Accordingly, ongoing vigilance is important.[229] Other side effects include arrhythmias and hypertension, which usually respond to dose reductions.

Phenylephrine (Neosynephrine)

Phenylephrine is a pure α-adrenergic agonist. As such, its major function is to cause peripheral vasoconstriction. It has no β-adrenergic or inotropic effect and therefore does not increase contractility. It may be temporarily used to improve afterload, systemic blood pressure, and, therefore, critical organ blood flow. But without concurrent inotropic support, an isolated acute increase in afterload is often poorly tolerated, particularly by a compromised ventricle. There are a at least three situations in which phenylephrine can be extremely useful. The first is to increase systemic afterload and decrease right-to-left shunting in children with TOF and dynamic RVOTO (tet spell). This pure α-adrenergic effect is particularly important in this situation, since any additional increase in contractility would worsen the outflow obstruction. Second, phenylephrine is also beneficial in cyanotic children who depend on a systemic-to-PA shunt for pulmonary blood flow and adequate oxygenation. The increased afterload may increase flow across the shunt and improve pulmonary blood flow. Third, acute hypotension in children with hypertrophic obstructive cardiomyopathy or critical aortic stenosis increases the outlet obstruction; phenylephrine increases afterload attenuating the severity of the obstruction.[230–233]

Vasopressin (Pitressin)

Arginine vasopressin is a peptide secreted by the pituitary gland. Secretion is promoted by angiotensin II and increased stimulation from hypothalamic osmoreceptors; increased activity from cardiopulmonary baroreceptors and increased levels of natriuretic peptide inhibit the secretion of vasopressin. Vasopressin acts at the tissue level by binding to specific receptors. It causes vasoconstriction via vasopressin$_1$ (V_{1a}) receptors and renal reabsorption of water, renal secretion of renin, and synthesis of renal prostaglandins via vasopressin$_2$ (V_2) receptors. In addition, vasopressin may mediate vasodilatation via V_2 receptors by increasing the release and synthesis of NO and vasodilating prostaglandins. Vasopressin also sensitizes baroreceptors and therefore may cause vasodilatation by decreasing sympathetic activity. Normally, vasopressin acts primarily via V_2 receptors in the kidney to promote water retention. However, during extreme hypotension, vasopressin may act via V_{1a} receptors in the vascular endothelium to induce intense vasoconstriction.

In adults, vasopressin has been shown to be beneficial in the treatment of vasodilatory shock and during cardiopulmonary resuscitation.[234] A few pediatric case reports and small observational studies have demonstrated improved blood pressure and accelerated weaning of inotropic support with low-dose vasopressin.[235–238] However, a multicenter, randomized, controlled trial in children with vasodilatory shock did not confirm these findings. Low-dose vasopressin (0.0005-0.002 U/kg per minute) had no beneficial effects compared with placebo; there was even a suggestion of increased mortality.[239] Further studies are necessary to establish the effectiveness and safety of vasopressin in children. Currently its role as a "rescue" medication for the treatment of catecholamine-resistant vasodilation during or after congenital cardiac surgery[240,241] and for refractory hypotension in extremely low–birth-weight (ELBW)[242] infants is being investigated. In 2013, a Cochrane Review found no eligible studies to analyze the effects of vasopressin and its analogues on refractory hypotension in neonates.[243] All available evidence for a role of vasopressin in children is based on case reports, small case series and three randomized controlled trials in older children.[239,244,245] A small pilot study in 20 infants, published in 2015, compared vasopressin and dopamine as the primary treatment for hypotension in ELBW infants. Vasopressin appeared to be safe and effective, but this interpretation must be tempered by the small sample size.[223,246,247] The prophylactic use of low dose vasopressin (0.0003 U/kg per minute) in the early postoperative phase after the Norwood or arterial switch procedure has been reported to decrease catecholamine and fluid requirements.[248] Refractory pulmonary hypertension is another potential indication for vasopressin and its analogues. In animal studies and in vitro experiments with human tissue, vasopressin causes pulmonary vasodilation via endothelium-dependent release of NO or by direct activation of smooth muscle receptors.[249–252] This vascular response seems to be age and disease specific and could explain the conflicting results in the literature. Several case reports and case series describe the successful use of vasopressin for this indication, but further studies are necessary to assess appropriate dosing and safety.[253–256] Extrapolated from adult data, pediatric dosing algorithms currently range from 0.0003 to 0.002 U/kg per minute. Careful attention to the infusion rate is important, especially when programming syringe pumps. The literature and common reference tools often cite the doses in units per minute (U/minute), units per kilogram per hour (U/kg per hour), units per kilogram per minute (U/kg per minute), or even milliunits per kilogram per minute (mU/kg per minute), which can be quite confusing and readily lead to dosing errors.

Phosphodiesterase Inhibitors

Phosphodiesterase inhibitors, which include amrinone, milrinone, and enoximone, are the most commonly used non–catecholamine-mediated inotropic agents. Their mechanism of action is also relatively straightforward. Phosphodiesterases degrade cyclic adenosine monophosphate (cAMP) to 5′-AMP. Phosphodiesterase inhibitors prevent this degradation and therefore increase levels of cyclic nucleotides, primarily cAMP. The increased concentration of this secondary messenger leads to an increase in calcium availability and thus increased contractility. Because the response is related to an increase in cAMP and not purely to inhibition of phosphodiesterase, the greatest effect occurs if initial levels of cAMP exceed normal values. In this way, synergy exists with β-agonists.[257] The absence of adrenergic stimulation minimizes effects on HR, rhythm, and dependency on endogenous tissue catecholamine stores. In addition to positive inotropic effects, these drugs also have significant lusitropic properties (i.e., diastolic relaxation) and promote peripheral vasodilation.[258–260] Phosphodiesterase drugs may also have substantial antiinflammatory properties that are currently not well understood.[261–263]

Amrinone (Inocor, Wincoram, Cordemcura)

Amrinone produces significant increases in myocardial contractility and reduces ventricular afterload.[259,264,265] As with all phosphodiesterase inhibitors, there has been an ongoing debate about the relative contribution of systemic vasodilation and afterload reduction relative to the increased cardiac contractility as the primary underlying mechanism for improving cardiac output. Amrinone improved cardiac performance in neonates and infants after cardiac surgery such as the arterial switch procedure and in older children after the Fontan operation.[260,264,266] Pharmacokinetic data in children suggest that the loading and infusion doses for amrinone need to be approximately twice those reported for adults.[267] In addition to differences in volume of distribution and clearance (both greater in infants), binding of amrinone to the oxygenator membrane needs to be considered if the loading dose is administered during CPB.[268] Overall, these data suggest that loading doses of 2 to 4 mg/kg and infusion rates starting in the range of 10 μg/kg per minute may be indicated in the neonate and infant.[268] Large bolus doses of amrinone can cause significant systemic hypotension, particularly in the period immediately after cardiac surgery. From a practical standpoint, it may be best to administer the loading dose of amrinone slowly over 1 hour. Caution is also indicated because the elimination half-life of amrinone is large (3–15 hours). Other side effects include thrombocytopenia, which is reversible, occasional drug-related fever, and increased hepatic enzymes.[269]

Milrinone (Primacor)

Several studies have demonstrated improved cardiac output and outcome from the use of milrinone after cardiac surgery in neonates and infants and with other states associated with ventricular dysfunction.[270–275] Renal clearance is the primary route of elimination and the maturation of milrinone clearance closely follows that of the glomerular filtration rate. A clearance of 9 L/hour per 70 kg is reported in adults with congestive heart failure and we might anticipate that clearance in premature neonates is reduced to 10% of this value because of a corresponding immaturity of renal function in this cohort. This has been confirmed in 26-week postmenstrual age infants who had a clearance of 0.96 L/hour per 70 kg.[276] Milrinone has a larger volume of distribution and greater clearance (expressed per kilogram) in children compared with adults; adjustments to bolus dosing and infusion rates have therefore been recommended.[270,275] Unlike amrinone, milrinone does not bind to the CPB circuit and has less deleterious effect on platelet function. Loading doses of 50 to 100 μg/kg (typically 75 μg/kg) and initial infusion rates of 0.50 to 1.0 μg/kg per minute have been recommended.[270,273] Neonates with HLHS who underwent stage I palliation exhibited reduced renal clearance in the immediate postoperative period, and dose adjustments should be considered (i.e., infusion rates of 0.2 μg/kg per minute).[277] Milrinone increases cardiac output, reduces cardiac filling pressures, and reduces afterload; its effects are typically not associated with tachyphylaxis and are independent of β-adrenergic receptor density or activity. An initial multicenter, double-blind, placebo-controlled trial demonstrated that prophylactic use of high-dose milrinone significantly reduced the development of low cardiac output syndrome relative to placebo after cardiac surgery in high-risk pediatric subjects.[272] In 2011, a survey of European hospitals performing open heart surgery showed that milrinone was used in 70% of all drug regimens.[278] Several limited small studies reported that milrinone and the calcium sensitizer, levosimendan, were equally effective in preventing low cardiac output syndrome.[279–281] In addition, a recent Cochrane Review found no significant mortality advantage for prophylactic milrinone in the available literature (only five eligible studies).[282] Milrinone is also increasingly used to improve oxygenation in neonates with persistent pulmonary hypertension who are unresponsive to therapy with NO.[283,284] Animal studies have shown that IV or inhaled milrinone enhances the response of the pulmonary vasculature to iloprost and prostacyclin.[285,286] Potential side effects of milrinone include hypotension, tachycardia, tachyarrhythmias, and platelet dysfunction.[287]

Enoximone (Perfan)

Enoximone is a phosphodiesterase inhibitor that has been used extensively in Europe but is not currently available in the United States. Its properties are similar to those of the other members of its class.[258,288] Improvements in indirect indexes of cardiac function, such as mixed venous oxygen saturation, ventricular filling pressures, and systemic arterial blood pressure, were observed in infants treated with enoximone after cardiac surgery. In addition, the length of hospital stay was reduced.[289] Enoximone was also useful to support cardiac function and potentially reduce PVR in children after cardiac transplantation.[290]

Digoxin (Digitek, Digox, Lanoxicaps, Lanoxin)

Digoxin can act as an inotropic agent; however, its effectiveness in children with congestive heart failure caused by large left-to-right shunts has been questioned. The clinical picture in such children often improved without echocardiographic evidence of increased contractility, and frequently progressive ventricular dilatation was observed.[291,292] Use of digoxin to improve RV dysfunction owing to pulmonary hypertension or as part of a multimodal therapy during the interstage phase for infants with single ventricle physiology has also been debated.[293]

Digoxin has both direct and indirect effects. Its direct effects are mediated by inhibition of the membrane sodium-potassium adenosine triphosphatase (ATP) and thereby outward sodium ion flux. The resulting increased intracellular sodium concentration stimulates the membrane sodium-calcium exchanger, producing increased intracellular calcium and positive inotropic effect. The indirect effects of digoxin are mediated by stimulation of the parasympathetic nervous system. The parasympathetic effects of digoxin result in slowing of atrial and AV node conduction. The drug can also be used to slow down the ventricular response in atrial flutter and atrial fibrillation and to treat supraventricular tachycardia (SVT) (see later discussion).

Because digoxin has a slow distribution phase after oral administration and a long elimination half-life (up to 1–2 days in neonates and young infants), a loading dose is usually administered (see Table 18.8). Renal dysfunction can significantly prolong the elimination half-life. Therapeutic digoxin concentrations are between 0.5 and 2.0 ng/mL. IV and oral dosing regimens are the same, although the onset of electrophysiologic effects from IV dosing is much more rapid (5–20 minutes).

Many drugs interact with digoxin and influence its pharmacokinetics. It should be assumed that almost any drug administered along with digoxin can affect the absorption and clearance, usually necessitating a reduction in dose.[294,295] The likelihood of digoxin toxicity increases with serum concentrations greater than 3 ng/mL.[296,297] Symptoms of toxicity include drowsiness, nausea, and vomiting. Various conduction abnormalities and SVT are the most frequent cardiac rhythm manifestations of digoxin toxicity in infants and young children. Older children and adults are more likely to experience AV block, ventricular dysrhythmias, junctional tachycardia, and premature ventricular contractions. Hypokalemia, specifically intracellular potassium depletion (often a result of long-standing diuretic use), exacerbates the proarrhythmogenic effects of digoxin.

CALCIUM

The role, mechanisms of action, and potential for deleterious consequences of IV calcium continue to be controversial.[298] It is the ionized calcium concentration that is important for myocardial function. Calcium is a positive inotrope, particularly when administered in the presence of ionized hypocalcemia. It may also improve ventricular contractility when LV function is depressed by inhalational agents, β-adrenergic blockade, or disease (e.g., sepsis).[299,300] In the presence of a normal myocardium and normal ionized calcium concentrations, the effects of IV calcium on contractility are much more modest.[301] Extracellular calcium levels also play an important role in the regulation of peripheral vascular resistance. A calcium-sensing receptor has been identified on vascular cell walls.[302]

There is evidence in adults that the primary effect of calcium administered after cardiac surgery is to increase SVR and mean arterial pressure with little or no effect on intrinsic myocardial contractility.[298,303] In fact, the increase in afterload, if not accompanied by a corresponding increase in contractility, may only serve to decrease stroke volume and cardiac output. Calcium may cause or exacerbate reperfusion injury and cellular damage by mechanisms that include activation of calcium-dependent proteases and phospholipases and organelle damage caused by cellular calcium overload.[304,305] These concerns are particularly relevant in children immediately after cardiac surgery. IV calcium may also attenuate the β-adrenergic effects of concurrently administered epinephrine.[298]

The role of IV calcium administration in neonates and young infants, both alone and after cardiac surgery, is more complicated. Preterm and term neonates have erratic calcium handling and are prone to ionized hypocalcemia.[306,307] The neonatal myocardium is more sensitive to ionized hypocalcemia than the adult myocardium, owing to reduced intracellular calcium stores, immaturity of sarcoplasmic reticulum calcium-handling mechanisms, and greater dependency on transmembrane calcium flux for excitation-contraction coupling.[308] Furthermore, the need to administer substantial volumes of citrated and albumin-containing blood products (both of which bind calcium) and other fluids after CPB increases the likelihood of ionized hypocalcemia.[309] The most prudent approach includes awareness of the greater dependency of the immature myocardium on extracellular calcium, monitoring of ionized calcium concentrations, and careful administration to maintain normal, or at most mildly increased, ionized calcium concentrations. This approach is particularly needed in neonates and in those with diminished LV function. Administration of large bolus doses of calcium immediately on reperfusion of the heart after a period of ischemia is probably ill-advised because of the potential to exacerbate reperfusion injury and even to cause myocardial contracture.

Extravasation of calcium can cause local venous irritation and significant tissue necrosis. Although it has been suggested that calcium gluconate may cause less harm in this regard than calcium chloride, we recommend that both forms be administered via a centrally positioned catheter whenever possible. Both forms of calcium increase ionized calcium concentrations similarly when equal amounts of elemental calcium are administered (3 : 1 calcium gluconate to calcium chloride).[310] Calcium may cause significant slowing of AV conduction and should be administered cautiously in children with sinus bradycardia or junctional rhythm. Care must also be exercised when administering calcium to children who are receiving digoxin, particularly in the presence of concurrent hypokalemia, because IV calcium exacerbates the potential for digoxin-induced dysrhythmias in this setting.

TRIIODOTHYRONINE (THYROXINE)

Triiodothyronine hormone (T_3) is essential for the maturation of sarcolemmal calcium channels, myosin, actin, and troponin. In addition, hypothyroid rats demonstrate reduced numbers of β-receptors and reduced density of stimulatory secondary messenger protein with an increase in inhibitory secondary messenger protein density. T_3 is mostly produced by monodeiodination of thyroxine. This process is inhibited by surgery, hypothermia, catecholamines, propranolol, and amiodarone; therefore postoperative T_3 levels are often reduced.[311-313]

T_3 replacement therapy acts via two pathways, intranuclear and extranuclear. Intranuclear effects include an increase in mitochondrial density and respiration, an increase in contractile protein synthesis, and an upregulation in β-adrenoceptors. Extranuclear effects include an improvement in glucose transport, increased stimulation of L-type calcium channels with subsequent calcium mobility, and increased efficiency in calcium reuptake with subsequent improvement in diastolic relaxation.

Endocrine function is compromised after cardiac surgery. Infants younger than 3 months of age with low T_3 concentrations on intensive care admission after cardiac surgery have a more complicated intensive care course. Low cortisol concentration is common in the early postoperative period but is not associated with postoperative complications.[314] A randomized, double-blind, placebo-controlled study of T_3 administration in children undergoing simple or complex cardiac surgery demonstrated that myocardial function was better and length of stay in the intensive care unit was decreased in the T_3 group.[315] T_3 improved contractility without any associated increase in oxygen consumption. In addition, the T_3 group demonstrated no delay in recovery of thyroid function secondary to exogenous administration. The dose of T_3 used was 2 μg/kg on day 1 followed by 1 μg/kg on days 2 through 12. A randomized, double-blind, placebo-controlled study of T_3 administration in neonates undergoing the Norwood procedure or repair of interrupted aortic arch and VSD closure demonstrated only more rapid achievement of negative fluid balance.[316] Many follow-up studies have been flawed by small numbers and significant patient heterogenicity; thus routine postoperative T_3 replacement therapy remains controversial.[317-320]

CALCIUM-SENSITIZING AGENTS

Levosimendan (Simdax, Simendan)

Calcium-sensitizing agents represent a relatively new class of drugs with inotropic properties. Levosimendan has been in clinical use since 2000 and is one of the best studied drugs in this class. It provides positive inotropy, lusitropy, vasodilation and cardioprotection via two distinct mechanisms: calcium sensitizing and opening of K⁺-channels. Levosimendan binds to troponin C and seems to maintain the calcium-binding site of troponin C in its active conformation. This shifts the calcium binding–concentration relationship toward increased binding (i.e., more binding at reduced intracardiac calcium concentrations). Contraction is thereby enhanced for a given cytosolic calcium concentration. In contrast to other types of inotropic agents, myocardial contractility is greater with minimal increase in oxygen demand. The concept of increasing the sensitivity to calcium rather than the cellular calcium concentration is also attractive because it reduces the deleterious effects of increased calcium concentrations on oxygen consumption, mitochondrial function, and activation of various calcium-dependent proteases and phospholipases (e.g., during ischemia-reperfusion).

Levosimendan has also been shown to stimulate membrane and mitochondrial ATP-sensitive potassium (K_{ATP}) channels; the former dilates the coronary, pulmonary, and the systemic vasculature. Opening mitochondrial K_{ATP} channels is likely to be an important mechanism of pharmacologic (and anesthetic) preconditioning and potential cytoprotection. Interestingly, and for reasons that are not entirely clear, levosimendan has either no effect or a positive effect on lusitropy (diastolic relaxation). At much larger doses than clinically used, it does inhibit phosphodiesterase III. Compared with other inotropic agents (e.g., dopamine, amrinone, milrinone), its effectiveness as a positive inotrope is maintained in the depressed myocardium.[287,321,322] The safety of levosimendan has been well established in adults; headaches, hypokalemia, and tachycardia are the most common side effects. A reported possible increased incidence of atrial fibrillation is controversial.[323,324]

Clinical effects include improved cardiac output, reduced ventricular filling pressures, and decreased PVR during the acute treatment of adult patients with either stable or decompensated heart failure.[323-326] However, initial mortality studies failed to show any improvements in short- or long-term prognosis for acute heart failure with levosimendan compared with dobutamine or placebo[327]; a meta-analysis of 45 studies in a wide variety of settings reported potential advantages.[328] Other investigations demonstrated improved cardiac performance after cardiotomy and bypass, including beneficial responses in adult patients who appeared to be poorly responsive to other inotropes.[329-334] Beneficial effects were also found with levosimendan pretreatment directly before bypass.[335]

Current recommendations suggest a 6- to 12-μg/kg loading dose followed by an infusion of 0.05 to 0.2 μg/kg per minute for 24 hours. Although the elimination half-life is approximately 1 hour, effects are mediated through changes in structural calcium sensitivity that may last for 7 to 9 days. At least one metabolite (OR-1896) has prolonged (approximately 80 hours) effects and this may, in part, account for observations of sustained benefit after drug discontinuation.[336]

There are limited data available regarding the use of levosimendan in children or immature animal preparations. Most of the evidence in children stems from observational studies, case reports, or registry inquiries.[279,337-349] These reports suggest that levosimendan is well tolerated, improving cardiac output and reducing afterload in children with low cardiac output syndrome.[337] Only a few randomized controlled trials have been published: two studies compared levosimendan with milrinone in children after congenital cardiac surgery and concluded that levosimendan is safe and at least as effective as milrinone.[279,280] Another study compared levosimendan with a standard treatment with milrinone and dopamine and came to the same conclusion.[350] The most recent investigation examined pulmonary artery pressures and the response to levosimendan or dobutamine during pediatric cardiac surgery. The results showed that levosimendan was superior.[351] These early data and the drug's mechanism of action suggest the need for further studies in children and a likely indication for use in infants and children with decreased myocardial performance from cardiac surgery, myocarditis, and sepsis.[287,337,352] Its widespread clinical application is significantly limited due to the high cost of the drug and the restricted availability. Currently levosimendan is only approved in 12 European countries, Asia, South America, and Australia. The use in children (<18 years) is off-label, under compassionate care, and requires informed consent.[287]

B-TYPE NATRIURETIC PEPTIDE AND NESIRITIDE (NATRECOR)

B-type natriuretic peptide (BNP) and its N-terminal precursor (NTpBNP) are members of the natriuretic peptide family. These peptides are released from the heart in response to pressure and volume overload and play an important role in maintaining fluid balance and hemodynamic stability. BNP is secreted from cardiac ventricles in response to increased stimulation of cardiac stretch receptors and increased wall tension. It acts mainly via natriuretic peptide receptors (NPRs) that are present in large vessels and kidneys. Once stimulated, NPRs promote diuresis, natriuresis, and vasodilation and inhibit the renin-angiotensin-aldosterone system. BNP is used as a marker for heart failure in adults and as a monitor for the response to anticongestive heart failure therapies.[353] These markers are also increasingly used to diagnose cardiovascular disease in neonates, infants, and children. The concentrations of NTpBNP are often markedly increased immediately after birth but decrease during the first week of life. Age-adjusted cut points and reference values have been suggested.[354,355] Post hoc analysis of a large multicenter heart failure trial (Pediatric Carvedilol Trial) tried to establish prognostic cutoff values. In children with moderately symptomatic heart failure from cardiomyopathy or CHD, a BNP greater than or equal to 140 pg/mL was associated with worse outcomes.[356] Disease-specific cutoff points and their prognostic value, especially for congenital heart defects, are still under investigation.[357-359]

Nesiritide is a recombinant form of BNP and therefore acts via NPRs to promote diuresis, natriuresis, and vasodilation. Early investigations in the adult population suggested that nesiritide may be beneficial for patients with decompensated heart failure; it seemed to improve cardiac output, reduce pulmonary capillary occlusion pressure, and dilate arterial and venous vessels with only minimal increase in HR or myocardial oxygen consumption.[360-362] However, a large multicenter study found no significant advantages of nesiritide and only recommended its use as an individualized case-based therapy.[363] Empirical perioperative nesiritide or milrinone infusions were not associated with improved early clinical outcomes after Fontan surgery.[364] Although nesiritide reduces mean arterial pressure in children after cardiac surgery and has been used as adjunct therapy in children with biventricular failure, more extensive studies are required before its usefulness and safety in children can be determined.[365-372]

β-BLOCKING AGENTS

There are several indications for the use of β-blockers in children, including control of hypertension (both acutely in a perioperative period and chronically), treatment of cyanotic spells and RVOTO in TOF, reduction of left ventricular outflow tract obstruction (LVOTO) in hypertrophic cardiomyopathy, control of HR in thyrotoxicosis and pheochromocytoma, and control of SVT (see later discussion).[373-377] In contrast to the situation in adults, the use of β-blockers to treat chronic heart failure in children is controversial.[378] Important distinctions include β-receptor subtype selectivity, variability in half-life and metabolism, and intrinsic sympathomimetic activity. Even "selective" β-blockers lose their selectivity at increased plasma concentrations. Although the mechanism is incompletely understood, β-blocker use in children is associated with hypoglycemia.[379] Consequently, vigilance should be exercised during periods of fasting and illness as reflex adrenergic responses to hypoglycemia may be blunted.

Propranolol (Inderal, InnoPran)

Propranolol is one of the most frequently used β-blockers in children. Typical oral doses start at 0.25 to 0.5 mg/kg every 6 hours, titrated every 3 to 5 days; the usual dose is 2 to 4 mg/kg per day. A sustained-release form is available for older children who are able to swallow pills. IV propranolol is administered at doses of 0.01 to 0.1 mg/kg over several minutes; this may be increased if necessary (maximum dose 1 mg in infants, 3 mg in children). Sinus bradycardia and hypotension can be serious complications, particularly in infants or after IV administration. Propranolol may also cause conduction disturbances at the AV node and worsen pump function in congestive heart failure. Other important adverse effects include fatigue, depression, and lethargy. Interactions with the β2-receptor may also exacerbate broncho-spasm.[380] Propranolol is primarily metabolized in the liver. Significant population variability in its kinetics has been noted. Metabolism is also affected by factors that alter hepatic blood flow because it has perfusion limited clearance. Its major metabolite, 4-hydroxypropranolol, is also active.[374]

Atenolol (Tenormin)

The use of atenolol has been increasing in children.[377,381,382] Compared with propranolol, it is more selective for the β1-adrenergic receptor subtype; the elimination half-life is 8 to 12 hours. There is little hepatic biotransformation, and there are no active metabolites. The typical starting dose is 0.8 to 1.5 mg/kg per day in one or two doses daily, with an upper limit in the range of 2 mg/kg per day. No IV form is available. Atenolol does not cross the blood-brain barrier, so some of the limiting adverse effects common to propranolol are absent. At large doses, β1 selectivity is probably lost, leading to the potential to exacerbate bronchospasm and hypoglycemia.

Esmolol (Brevibloc)

Esmolol is a relatively selective β1-adrenergic blocker with several unique features. Its onset is fast, it can easily be titrated to a desired endpoint, and its effects are rapidly terminated through metabolism by red blood cell and plasma esterases.[383,384] The drug has been particularly useful for the acute control of perioperative hypertension and for treatment of SVTs (see later discussion). Loading doses between 100 and 500 μg/kg given over 1 to 5 minutes are followed by maintenance infusions of 50 to 100 μg/kg per minute. If the desired response is not achieved, the infusion rate is then doubled every 5 minutes until a desired response is achieved.

Specific data on pediatric dosing are limited at present.[385] One study investigated the pharmacokinetics of esmolol therapy after an episode of stimulated or spontaneous SVT. The results were similar to the findings in the adult population.[386] Esmolol has been investigated to control blood pressure immediately after coarctation repair using 3 different bolus doses: 125 μg/kg, 250 μg/kg, and 500 μg/kg IV infused over 10 to 20 seconds, each followed by an infusion that consisted of the same dose as in the bolus every minute.[387] Blood pressure response and adverse events were similar among the groups. Clearance in neonates was twice that in older children (281 mL/kg per minute vs. 126 mL/kg per minute), consistent with other drugs cleared by plasma esterases (e.g., remifentanil).[387] The current maximum loading dose recommended is 500 μg/kg followed by an infusion rate of 25 to 300 μg/kg per minute.[388] A major potential adverse effect of esmolol is hypotension, particularly during bolus therapy. As noted earlier, esmolol rapidly distributes and has a very small elimination half-life (7-10 minutes) that is unaffected by organ blood flow or disease. Therefore, hypotension is usually short-lived, but therapy with vasopressors may occasionally be required until it resolves.[389,390]

Labetalol (Normodyne, Trandate)

Labetalol has nonselective β-adrenergic blocking properties and is also a selective α-adrenergic receptor blocker. The ratio of α- to β-blockade efficiency is 1:3 and 1:7 after oral and IV administration, respectively. The primary use of labetalol in children is to control hypertension. The drug has been given by IV to treat hypertensive crisis, to control hypertension after aortic coarctation repair, and as an adjunct to induce controlled hypotension during surgery.[391-394] Typical doses are 0.1 to 0.4 mg/kg given every 5 to 10 minutes until the desired effect is achieved with infusions of 0.25 to 1 mg/kg per hour. The elimination half-life of labetalol is 3 to 5 hours.

Carvedilol (Coreg)

Carvedilol is a nonselective β-blocker with additional vasodilator and some antioxidant properties.[395,396] The ratio of α_1 to β_1 blockade is 1:1.7. It is primarily used for the treatment of heart failure. In adults, significant benefit has been demonstrated, including reduced mortality, reduced hospital stay, improved New York Health Association (NYHA) functional class, and a somewhat reduced progression of the clinical disease.[397] However, a randomized, double-blind, placebo-controlled, multicenter study of children and adolescents with symptomatic systolic heart failure found no significant differences in outcome between carvedilol and placebo during an 8-month follow-up period.[398] Nevertheless, carvedilol is often prescribed after an episode of acute decompensation in patients with cardiomyopathy.[399] Carvedilol may have differential effects based on ventricular morphology, and further studies are necessary.[400-403] A retrospective review of the initial experience with carvedilol therapy in children showed that adverse effects—mainly dizziness, headaches, and hypotension—were common (>50%) but well tolerated.[404] The ideal dose in children has not yet been determined. Pharmacokinetic simulation studies suggest that larger doses[405] than those used in adults are warranted, although clinical experience in small patient populations favors smaller doses and gradual dose adjustments with frequent echocardiographic and BNP monitoring.[403]

VASODILATORS

Vasodilators are used in children to control blood pressure during and after surgery, to treat systemic and pulmonary hypertension, and to decrease afterload on either the systemic or the pulmonary ventricle, thereby improving pump function. Vasodilators are also administered during CPB to reduce SVR, improve regional perfusion, and facilitate rapid and even core cooling and rewarming.

Vasodilators can be divided into pharmacologic groups. Direct-acting nitrosovasodilators such as sodium nitroprusside (SNP) and nitroglycerin (NTG) are the most commonly used cardiovascular medications. These drugs relax vascular smooth muscle to cause vasodilation by directly (SNP) or indirectly (NTG), releasing NO that subsequently activates smooth muscle soluble guanylyl cyclase to form cyclic guanosine monophosphate (cGMP). Nicardipine is a dihydroxypyridine calcium channel blocker that is highly selective for calcium channels in the coronary and peripheral vasculature. It is an effective vasodilator with minimal effects on HR and contractility and is often used as a longer-acting alternative to SNP. Hydralazine is another direct-acting smooth muscle vasodilator that is occasionally given to children to reduce blood pressure. Selective α-adrenergic blockers, such as phentolamine and phenoxybenzamine, are occasionally used to reduce blood pressure and SVR in the perioperative period. The classic indication is the treatment of pheochromocytoma, but they are also frequently given during hypothermic CPB.

Ventricular "remodeling" and long-term blood pressure control is often achieved with angiotensin-converting enzyme (ACE) inhibitors. Prostaglandin E_1 (PGE_1) is a direct-acting vasodilator primarily used to maintain the patency of the ductus arteriosus in duct-dependent circulations. In contrast, prostacyclin and inhaled NO are vasodilators with relatively selective effects on the pulmonary vasculature. Commonly used vasodilators and antihypertensive agents are summarized in Table 18.9.

Sodium Nitroprusside (Nipride, Nitropress)

The primary indication for SNP is the rapid and reliable reduction of afterload and blood pressure before, during, and after a wide variety of procedures. For example, it is used to control intraoperative and postoperative hypertension in children with aortic coarctation and other forms of LVOTO. The reduction in afterload may improve performance of a dysfunctional ventricle, particularly in combination with a positive inotropic agent.[406,407] The ability of nitroprusside to successfully treat pulmonary hypertension is variable and may be age dependent.[408-412]

SNP is an extremely potent vasodilator that acts directly on smooth muscle to cause dilation.[413,414] Its effects reduce cardiac preload as well as afterload. Onset of effect is fast (within minutes), and offset is similarly rapid; the effect ends within 1 to 2 minutes after termination of the infusion. Because of its potency, it should always be administered using an infusion pump in conjunction with continuous direct arterial pressure monitoring. The starting dosage is 0.3 to 1 μg/kg per minute. This can be increased or decreased to achieve the desired effect. The titration of nitroprusside to achieve specific blood pressure goals can be rather frustrating and often results in large blood pressure swings.[415] A recent multicenter, randomized, double-blinded dose-ranging trial developed a population-based pharmacokinetic/pharmacodynamic model and presented dosing guidelines. A starting dose of 0.3 μg/kg per minute, small dose adjustments, and slow weaning are recommended to avoid significant hypotension or rebound hypertension.[416,417] The hypotensive effects of nitroprusside are potentiated by hypovolemia, inhalation anesthetics, and drugs that inhibit the reflex responses to direct vasodilation (e.g., increase in sympathetic tone, renin release), such as propranolol and ACE inhibitors.

Adverse effects of SNP include cyanide and thiocyanate toxicities, rebound hypertension, inhibition of platelet function, and increased intrapulmonary shunting via attenuation of hypoxic pulmonary vasoconstriction. Rebound hypertension is most likely caused by activation of the aforementioned reflex mechanisms. This effect is minimized by slowly tapering the infusion rather than abruptly discontinuing it. Toxicity may occur when more than 10 μg/kg per minute of SNP is administered, if tachyphylaxis develops within 30 minutes, or if there is immediate resistance to the drug. A blood cyanide concentration of approximately 500 μg/dL has been linked to a death in a child,[418] but subsequent studies showed that increased concentrations of cyanide were not necessarily associated with the clinical signs of cyanide toxicity.[419,420] Cyanide and thiocyanate toxicities are rare but may be more likely in neonates and young infants and in those with impaired hepatic or renal function.[418,421]

Cyanide is produced from the metabolism of SNP. Free cyanide is then conjugated with thiosulfate by rhodanase in the liver to produce thiocyanate. A major mechanism of cyanide toxicity is binding to cytochrome oxidase in the mitochondrial electron transport chain, which prevents mitochondrial respiration and ATP production. Signs of toxicity include tachyphylaxis and an increase in mixed venous oxygen saturation and metabolic acidosis. In children who have received prolonged (>24 hours)

TABLE 18.9	Antihypertensives and Vasodilators[a]	
Drug	**Intravenous Dose**	**Comments**
Propranolol	0.01–0.1 mg/kg slowly	Nonselective β-blockade; bradycardia, hypotension, worsening of myocardial pump function; atrioventricular block; hypoglycemia; bronchospasm; depression; fatigue
Labetalol	0.1–0.4 mg/kg per dose; 0.25–1.0 mg/kg per hour infusion	Nonselective β-blockade; selective α-blockade; ratio of α- to β-blockade is 1:7 for intravenous form; doses (0.1 mg/kg) can be repeated every 5–10 minutes until desired effect is achieved; side effects are similar to those of propranolol.
Esmolol	100–500 µg/kg loading dose (over 5 min); 50–250 µg/kg per minute infusion	Relatively selective β-blockade; short elimination half-life (7–10 minutes); hypotension, especially during bolus administration; if less than desired response after 5 minutes, can repeat or double bolus dose, followed by doubling infusion rate; non–organ-based metabolism by plasma and red blood cell esterases; infusion concentrations >10 mg/mL may predispose to venous sclerosis; dilute infusion at high rates increases risk of volume overload.
Sodium nitroprusside	Start at 0.3–1.0 µg/kg per minute infusion; maximum 6–10 µg/kg per minute	Potent direct smooth muscle relaxation; dilates both arteriolar resistance and venous capacitance vessels; hypotension potentiated by hypovolemia, inhalation anesthetics, other antihypertensives; variable pulmonary vasodilation; potential cyanide toxicity; reflex tachycardia; check cyanide and thiocyanate levels if >4 µg/kg per minute is infused or drug is used longer than 2–3 days.
Nitroglycerin	0.5–10 µg/kg per minute infusion	Direct smooth muscle relaxation; predominantly dilates venous capacitance vessels, modest effects on arterial resistance at larger doses; weak antihypertensive effects; variable pulmonary vasodilation; used to facilitate cooling and rewarming during cardiopulmonary bypass.
Nicardipine	Start at 0.5–1 µg/kg per minute infusion; maximum 4–5 µg/kg per minute	Dihydroxypyridine calcium channel blocker: primary effects on coronary and peripheral vasculature, predominantly vasodilation, minimal effects on heart rate and contractility. Hypotension potentiated by inhalational agents. Potentiation of neuromuscular blockers. Prolonged effects after discontinuation.
Phentolamine	0.05–0.1 mg/kg dose; 0.5–5 µg/kg per minute infusion	Selective α-blocker, produces mainly arteriolar vasodilation; some direct vasodilation with mild venodilation.
Enalaprilat	5–10 µg/kg per dose q8–24 hours	Long duration of effect; angioedema, renal failure, hyperkalemia; potential problematic hypotension with anesthetic agents (see text).
Hydralazine	0.1–0.2 mg/kg bolus q6 hours	Maximum 20 mg/dose; direct-acting smooth muscle (predominantly arteriolar) vasodilation; long effective half-life; tachyphylaxis; reflex tachycardia; lupus-like syndrome; drug fever; thrombocytopenia.
Prostaglandin E1	0.05–0.1 µg/kg per minute infusion	Direct smooth muscle relaxation, relatively specific for ductus arteriosus; variable pulmonary and systemic vasodilation; apnea in neonates.

[a]All drugs should be started in the lower dose range and titrated to effect.

or large-dose infusions of nitroprusside and in those with organ dysfunction, it may be advisable to measure blood cyanide concentrations.[420,422–425] Serum thiocyanate concentrations may also be measured. Thiocyanate concentrations may increase if renal function is abnormal. Central nervous system (CNS) dysfunction can occur when thiocyanate concentrations reach 5 to 10 mg/dL. Treatment of cyanide toxicity consists of IV infusion of sodium nitrite, 6 mg/kg (maximum dose 300 mg) over 5 minutes, and sodium thiosulfate, 250 mg/kg or 7 g/m^2 (maximum dose 12.5 g) over 15 minutes. In children with abnormal renal function in whom stimulating the production of thiocyanate from thiosulfate may be contraindicated, administration of hydroxocobalamin has been recommended.[426,427]

Nitroglycerin (Nitronal, Nitro-Bid)

Nitroglycerin is primarily a venodilator that acts on venous capacitance vessels. It has a substantially smaller effect on arteriolar smooth muscle, and its ability to attenuate an increased PVR is variable. Compared with nitroprusside, it is a poor antihypertensive agent. It has a brief half-life and no significant toxic metabolites. Similar to nitroprusside, it may increase intrapulmonary shunting and cause platelet dysfunction. Nitroglycerin is typically administered in doses of 0.5 to 3.0 µg/kg per minute. Effects occur within 2 minutes after nitroglycerin is started and resolve within

5 minutes after discontinuation. Mild decreases in blood pressure may be observed at doses exceeding 2 to 3 µg/kg per minute. In case of prolonged simultaneous infusions of nitroglycerin and nitroprusside, methemoglobin and cyanmethemoglobin levels can accumulate.[428]

Nitroglycerin is frequently used during CPB to facilitate rapid and effective cooling and rewarming and to improve tissue blood flow. Nitroprusside and nitroglycerin differ substantially with regard to their effects on the microcirculation. Because nitroprusside primarily reduces arteriolar tone and dilates precapillaries, it decreases microvascular blood flow and tissue perfusion more than nitroglycerin does, particularly in the presence of reduced arterial blood pressure (e.g., during CPB).[429] In contrast, nitroglycerin dilates precapillaries and postcapillaries with equal efficacy, thereby maintaining stable or enhanced capillary perfusion.[430,431]

Nicardipine (Cardene)

Nicardipine was the first available IV dihydroxypyridine calcium channel blocker and has been used to treat hypertension in children of all ages for over 20 years. Compared with nifedipine, nicardipine has a greater selectivity for calcium channels in the coronary and peripheral vasculature, resulting in predominant vasodilation and only minimal effects on HR and contractility.[432,433] Many adult studies investigated nicardipine for perioperative blood pressure control,[434–437] but only limited pediatric data are available, derived mainly from small case series and observational reports.[438–441] Nicardipine has been successfully used to control hypertension in preterm infants and neonates.[439,442,443] Given as a continuous infusion at an initial rate of 0.5 to 1 μg/kg per minute, the rate is slowly increased every 15 to 30 minutes until the target blood pressure is reached. Usual doses range from 1 to 3 μg/kg per minute, with a maximum dose of 4 to 5 μg/kg per minute[438,444,445]; 50% of the maximum change occurs within 45 minutes. In one retrospective study in children, it took an average of 2.7 ± 2.1 hours (range 0.5–9 hours) to achieve blood pressure control with this dosing regimen.[438] An alternative high-dose approach has been described, starting with an initial dose of 5 to 10 μg/kg per minute and followed by a smaller maintenance dose of 2 to 3 μg/kg per minute (range 1–5 μg/kg per minute) once the blood pressure is well controlled.[446,447] Nicardipine is extensively metabolized in the liver (cytochrome P450, isoenzyme CYP3A4) and excreted in urine and feces. An adult two-compartment pharmacokinetic model revealed an α-half-life of 2.7 minutes, a β-half-life of 44.8 minutes, and a slow terminal phase (γ-half-life) of 14.4 hours, contributing to the prolonged effects of nicardipine. After discontinuing the infusion, the antihypertensive effects decrease by 50% within the first 30 minutes but can be present for up to 50 hours. Clearance is affected by hepatic dysfunction. Commonly seen adverse effects are mild reflex tachycardia, flushing, nausea and vomiting, or phlebitis at the infusion site.[438] In contrast to nitroprusside, there is no tachyphylaxis, and nicardipine can be administered for extended periods of time without accumulation of toxic metabolites. Interactions with inhalational anesthetic agents and neuromuscular-blocking drugs should be considered during intraoperative use.[448] Inhalational anesthetics blunt the baroreflex mediated increase in HR and increase the hypotensive effects of nicardipine[449]; the effects of depolarizing and nondepolarizing neuromuscular-blocking drugs will be potentiated by the calcium channel blocker and should be closely monitored.[450] In the United States, due to the limited availability and high costs of nitroprusside, nicardipine is increasingly used as a substitute.

Phentolamine (Regitine, OraVerse) and Phenoxybenzamine (Dibenzyline)
Both phentolamine and phenoxybenzamine are α-adrenergic blocking agents with little selectivity for α-receptor subtypes. Their primary effect is to decrease resistance on the arterial side of the circulation, although both possess weak venodilating capabilities. Phentolamine is usually administered by infusion at 0.5 to 5 μg/kg per minute, whereas phenoxybenzamine is administered orally initially 0.2 mg/kg once daily, then slowly increased every 4 days by 0.2 mg/kg per day. The usual maintenance dose is 0.4 to 1.2 mg/kg per day divided in three doses. The elimination half-life of phenoxybenzamine is much greater than that of phentolamine. Some cardiovascular centers have found the potent arteriolar-dilating effects of phenoxybenzamine and its prolonged elimination half-life to be advantageous, especially to provide adequate vasodilation during deep hypothermic CPB.[451–455]

Angiotensin-Converting Enzyme Inhibitors
ACE inhibitors are administered to children with increasing frequency.[456–458] In the perioperative setting, they are given to control blood pressure after aortic coarctation repair or to relieve LVOTO. In addition, ACE inhibitors are given on a more long-term basis to reduce afterload on the systemic ventricle and to improve ventricular performance in children with congestive heart failure

or single ventricle physiology.[293,399,459] Among the growing number of ACE inhibitors, captopril, enalapril, and lisinopril are most often used in children, although data in children are scant. Adverse effects common to all ACE inhibitors include angioedema, acute renal failure, and hyperkalemia; case reports of substantive complications have been published.[460–462] Cyanosis and coadministration of furosemide are independent risk factors for acute kidney injury in children undergoing cardiac surgery who were treated with ACE inhibitors.[463]

The contribution of ACE inhibitors to anesthetic-induced hypotension remains controversial.[464–468] Angiotensin receptor–blocking agents such as losartan and lisinopril can produce significant and refractory hypotension with standard anesthetic induction techniques.[469] Because of the potential risk for substantive refractory hypotension that is usually unresponsive to volume expansion and requires substantial vasoconstrictor treatment, it is our practice to discontinue long-acting ACE inhibitors 1 day before surgery.

Captopril (Capoten)
Captopril has a relatively brief elimination half-life (<2 hours); clearance is by metabolism in the liver (captopril-cysteine disulfide and the disulfide dimer) and excretion by the kidney.[470] Oral dosing in neonates is 0.05 to 0.1 mg/kg every 8 to 24 hours, titrated up to 0.5 mg/kg every 6 to 24 hours. Infants initially receive 0.15 to 0.3 mg/kg every 6 to 8 hours. This can be titrated toward a maximum dose of 6 mg/kg per day in four divided doses. Oral dosing in older children is 0.3 to 0.5 mg/kg every 6 to 12 hours. The brief duration of effect, necessitating more frequent dosing, has led to increased use of the longer-acting ACE inhibitors (enalapril and lisinopril) in children.

Enalapril (Vasotec, Epaned)
Enalapril is metabolized in the liver to its active form, enalaprilat. Enalapril is the only ACE inhibitor currently available in the United States that has an IV formulation. It can be given orally, once or twice daily, with daily doses ranging between 0.1 and 0.5 mg/kg. The IV dose is 0.005 to 0.01 mg/kg per dose, one to three times a day.[456] Both enalapril and lisinopril are eliminated by the kidney. The duration of their hypotensive actions averages 24 hours but can extend to 30 hours.

Losartan (Cozaar)
Losartan blocks selectively angiotensin II type 1 (AT1) receptors. In children, it is used mainly in the treatment of proteinuria and hypertension associated with renal disease and seems to be well tolerated.[471–475] Lorsartan may also help to slow the rate of aortic root dilation in patients with Marfan syndrome.[476]

Hydralazine (Apresoline)
In the past, hydralazine was frequently used for long-term blood pressure control in children, but has been largely replaced by ACE inhibitors. In contrast to its effect in adults, its ability to decrease pulmonary hypertension in children was disappointing.[477] Hydralazine directly relaxes smooth muscle without known effects on receptors. It reduces cardiac afterload but may cause significant reflex tachycardia. With long-term use, it may also cause fluid retention, requiring concurrent administration of a diuretic. Oral dosing is in the range of 0.75 to 1 mg/kg per day divided in 2 to 4 doses and is slowly increased over 3 to 4 weeks to a maximum dose of 5 mg/kg per day for infants and 7.5 mg/kg per day for children. In the perioperative setting, it is occasionally used by

the IV route to control blood pressure and reduce afterload. IV doses are administered as a bolus of 0.1 to 0.2 mg/kg not to exceed 20 mg. The effects of IV hydralazine on PVR are variable.[477,478] Tachyphylaxis to the antihypertensive effects of IV hydralazine may occur. Important adverse effects include a drug-related fever, rash, pancytopenia, and lupus-like syndrome. The elimination half-life of the drug is approximately 4 hours, but the effective biologic half-life may be substantially longer because of significant binding of the drug to vascular smooth muscle.[479]

Prostaglandin E₁ (Alprostadil, Prostin)

The major indication for PGE₁ is to establish or maintain patency of the ductus arteriosus in neonates. It is best able to reopen a closing ductus in neonates up to 1 to 2 weeks of age but may occasionally be effective even in older infants.[21,480]

Ductal patency is important and often lifesaving for duct-dependent circulations—those in which either the lower body is supplied by right-to-left ductal flow (e.g., interrupted aortic arch, critical aortic stenosis, HLHS) or the PDA is the sole provider of pulmonary blood flow (e.g., pulmonary atresia, tricuspid atresia, severe TOF). Adverse effects of PGE₁ include systemic hypotension, apnea, increased risk of infection, leukocytosis, gastric outlet obstruction, and CNS irritability.[481–483] PGE₁ infusions usually start at 0.05 μg/kg per minute and may be increased to 0.1 μg/kg per minute or more; maintenance infusions range from 0.003 to 0.01 μg/kg per minute.[484,485] The risk of apnea may be related to the infusion rate. Tracheal intubation and ventilation are often required with infusion rates greater than 0.05 μg/kg per minute.[486,487] Prophylactic treatment with aminophylline was found to be effective in reducing the apnea risk.[488] Caffeine may also prove useful for those with apnea. PGE₁ has also been used to treat primary or acquired pulmonary hypertension with varying degrees of success.[489–492]

Inhaled Nitric Oxide (Inomax)

An important development in the treatment of pulmonary hypertension is inhaled NO gas, which can be delivered directly to the pulmonary circulation. NO is an endothelium-derived relaxing factor that acts on guanylate cyclase in vascular smooth muscle.[493] Endogenous NO is produced by endothelial cell NO synthase. NO synthases convert the amino acid L-arginine into NO and the by-product L-citrulline. NO then diffuses into the subjacent vascular smooth muscle. It produces relaxation by acting on smooth muscle guanylate cyclase to produce cGMP, which acts on a series of protein kinases and reduces intracellular calcium levels to inhibit muscle contraction (see Fig. 37. 3A and B). Diffusion of NO in the other direction from the endothelial cell into the blood vessel lumen can decrease the adhesiveness of white blood cells and platelets. NO in the blood is rapidly bound by oxyhemoglobin, which is then oxidized to methemoglobin. From this reaction, NO is inactivated and nitrite and nitrate are released in the blood. Red blood cell methemoglobin is subsequently reduced back to hemoglobin. The rapid binding and inactivation of NO in the blood means that inhaled NO has a minimal effect on the systemic circulation and functions as a very specific pulmonary vasodilator.

Significant reductions in PVR from inhaled NO have been demonstrated in adults with mitral stenosis, in neonates with persistent pulmonary hypertension of the neonate, in lung transplant recipients, and in children after surgical repair of a variety of CHDs.[494–498] The efficacy of inhaled NO is in large part related to the ability to deliver it into the alveolus, which is in close proximity to the pulmonary vascular smooth muscle.

Inhaled NO has found several indications in children with CHD. In the cardiac catheterization laboratory, it is used to assess the reactivity of the pulmonary vasculature in children with pulmonary hypertension. This can help distinguish between children with fixed pulmonary vascular obstructive disease and those with a reversible component to pulmonary hypertension, thereby facilitating therapeutic management and operative planning.[499–501]

In the postoperative period after the repair of CHD, NO can be used to reduce PVR and improve cardiopulmonary performance.[502–504] Experience thus far suggests that children with two ventricles who have increased LA pressure or its pathophysiologic equivalent (e.g., mitral stenosis, severe congestive heart failure, cardiomyopathy, large left-to-right shunt, TAPVR) are more likely to respond to NO in the postoperative period. Some children who do not respond to NO immediately after CPB in the operating room demonstrate significant reductions in PVR with NO several hours later. NO is administered in concentrations of 1 to 80 ppm in oxygen via a special delivery device attached to the ventilator or oxygen delivery system. Inspired gas is monitored for toxic nitrogen oxides; during long-term therapy with NO, blood methemoglobin concentrations should be assessed on a regular basis.[505]

Prostanoids

Members of the prostacyclin and prostaglandin families are often classified as *prostanoids*. All prostanoids are potent vasodilators and inhibitors of platelet aggregation. Since the 1980s, they have been used in the treatment of PA hypertension and are part of the official treatment guidelines (E-Fig. 18.4, E-Table 18.5),[506–509] even though they are not selective pulmonary vasodilators. Common adverse effects include flushing, hypotension, headache, jaw pain, skin rash, nausea and diarrhea, and nonspecific musculoskeletal pains. Tolerance can develop over time, requiring increasing doses.[510] In the United States, only three prostanoids are currently approved by the Food and Drug Administration (FDA): epoprostenol (Flolan), treprostinil (Remodulin), and iloprost (Ventavis). Beraprost is an oral prostacyclin analog licensed in Japan and still being investigated.

Epoprostenol (Flolan, Veletri)

Continuous IV infusion of epoprostenol has been used effectively for many years in children with PA hypertension of any cause. It improves hemodynamics by reducing PA pressure, increasing cardiac output, increasing oxygen transport, and improving symptoms such as exercise capacity and dyspnea.[511] It has been used with excellent results in the treatment of primary pulmonary hypertension and irreversible acquired pulmonary hypertension in CHD; in children awaiting heart, lung, or heart-lung transplantation; in children with primary pulmonary hypertension; in neonates with persistent pulmonary hypertension; and in pulmonary hypertensive crises.[512–520] The fact that children who were initially nonresponders may respond after prolonged use of NO suggests that its mechanism of action involves a degree of remodeling, although no absolute mechanism has been elucidated.

Unfortunately, epoprostenol is chemically unstable at room temperature and has a half-life of 6 minutes or less; it requires cooling for storage, continuous IV infusion via a central venous catheter, and a specific delivery system. Rapid and unintended decreases in the rate, dislodgments or occlusions of the central venous catheter, or pump malfunctions can lead to severe and life-threatening rebound pulmonary hypertension.[521,522] The infusion is usually started at 1 to 2 ng/kg per minute and gradually increased over several months to doses between 30 and 80 ng/kg per minute.

In patients with pulmonary venous disease, IV epoprostenol can worsen the pulmonary edema; it can also increase the ventilation/perfusion mismatch in patients with pneumonia and thereby negatively affect oxygenation. In the acute setting, epoprostenol is increasingly used in the inhaled form to benefit from the selective pulmonary vasodilation and reduction of ventilation/perfusion mismatch.[510,523-525] Some centers have used inhaled epoprostenol as an alternative to the rather expensive NO, although the currently available delivery systems are far from ideal and may alter the delivered tidal volumes.[510]

Treprostinil (Remodulin)

Treprostinil was first introduced in 2002, initially only for continuous subcutaneous infusion, but later also for IV infusion in patients who could not tolerate the pain at the subcutaneous infusion site. The hemodynamic effects are similar to those of epoprostenol, with fewer adverse effects.[526-529] IV infusions of treprostinil are started at 1 to 2 ng/kg per minute and slowly increased over several weeks to 40 ng/kg per minute, occasionally even higher doses (80-120 ng/kg per minute) are used. One pediatric study confirmed the effectiveness of IV treprostinil in children.[530] Since 2009, inhaled treprostinil has been used for long-term outpatient management. Because of the relatively short half-life, it must be administered every 6 hours.[531-534] More recently a sustained release oral form of treprostinil has been investigated. In adults, it showed some promising effects in treatment-naïve patients but failed to demonstrate significant long-term improvements in more advanced disease stages.[535-538] Side effects were common and included headaches, nausea, diarrhea, and flushing. The initial dose for adults is 0.25 mg every 12 hours or 0.125 mg every 8 hours. If more than two doses are missed (prolonged NPO status owing to gastrointestinal symptoms or surgical procedure), appropriate treatment with subcutaneous or IV treprostinil has to be initiated. Pediatric data are not yet available.

Iloprost (Ventavis)

Iloprost, approved by the FDA in 2004, is another prostaglandin I_2 analog that can be delivered by IV or via an ultrasonic nebulizer. It has a very brief elimination half-life of only 7 to 9 minutes, although its clinical efficacy is greater, with a half-life of 20 to 25 minutes. Frequent nebulized treatments (6 to 9 times each day) are required.[539] In adult studies, iloprost was shown to be beneficial in patients with PA hypertension of any cause, idiopathic PA hypertension, or chronic thromboembolic pulmonary hypertension. These patients demonstrated improvements in hemodynamics and in subjective parameters such as quality of life scores.[540-542] Studies in children are scarce and have involved only small numbers of patients, although numerous case reports are encouraging.[510,543-550] Long-term effects and compliance are still under investigation.[551] When iloprost and NO were compared in children with CHD, the two agents produced similar effects.[552] In one study, combination therapy using both systemic and inhaled prostacyclin analog showed promise.[553] It has also been successfully used in the perioperative management of CHD patients with pulmonary hypertension[554] and for the postoperative transition from inhaled NO to an inhaled prostacyclin.[555] A study in lambs demonstrated an enhanced effect of prostacyclin and iloprost when combined with milrinone.[286]

Beraprost (Careload)

Beraprost sodium is an oral prostacyclin analog that is chemically more stable and has a prolonged elimination half-life but nevertheless requires dosing three to four times per day, reaching its peak blood concentration at 30 minutes. Two double-blind studies showed no significant long-term benefit, but there may still be a role for this drug in combination therapy, because improvements have been observed in the exercise capacity of children with idiopathic PA hypertension.[556,557] Case reports of successful long-term treatment with beraprost and of combination therapy using oral beraprost and inhaled prostacyclin have been published.[553,558-560] Another case series described the use of beraprost for the treatment of persistent pulmonary hypertension in newborns.[561]

Endothelin Receptor Antagonists

Endothelin 1 is a potent vasoconstrictor that is thought to be a key factor in the pathogenesis of PA hypertension. There are two known receptors on which it acts: endothelin A and endothelin B. Endothelin A receptors are present on smooth muscle cells, and agonist action causes vasoconstriction; endothelin B receptors are present on endothelial cells, and agonist action causes both relaxation and vasoconstriction through different pathways. In addition, endothelin B receptors are involved in the clearance of endothelin.

Bosentan (Tracleer)

Bosentan is an oral, nonselective endothelin-receptor antagonist. Adult studies have shown long-term benefit in patients with PA hypertension. It can also improve exercise capacity in adolescent and adult patients with a Fontan circulation.[562] Bosentan can cause abnormal liver function test results, although no severe liver dysfunction has been reported in adults.[563-567] Two studies in children showed both short-term reduction in PA pressure and PVR and longer-term improvement in symptoms and stabilization of the disease process.[511,568] In addition, three studies have suggested that the dose for children weighing more than 10 kg could largely follow adult guidelines, with the total daily dose not exceeding 125 mg. There is growing evidence, although few controlled studies, suggesting that bosentan is an effective and well-tolerated therapy in children.[569-571] Compared with the results in adult studies, hepatic dysfunction was less frequently reported but was still the most common adverse effect.[572-575]

Ambrisentan (Letairis)

Ambrisentan is a selective endothelin A receptor antagonist that has been extensively studied in the adult population.[576-578] It seems to be associated with an increased incidence of peripheral edema but a lower risk for liver dysfunction.[579,580] The pediatric experience is limited but ambrisentan could be a safe and effective treatment alternative for some children with pulmonary arterial hypertension.[581]

Sildenafil (Viagra)

Sildenafil is a selective inhibitor of phosphodiesterase type 5, the isoform that is responsible for hydrolysis of cGMP in the pulmonary vasculature. By preventing the breakdown of cGMP, sildenafil increases cGMP concentrations and potentiates the pulmonary vasodilation caused by endogenous NO.[582-584] Sildenafil can also have positive effects on the ventricular contractility in patients with pulmonary hypertension because phosphodiesterase type 5 is highly expressed in the hypertrophied human right ventricle.[585] It has a long-standing track record in the adult population.[586-591] In the pediatric population, sildenafil is currently used as an adjunctive agent during weaning from NO, in the treatment of PA hypertension, for patients with congenital diaphragmatic hernia, for the perioperative management of patients after cardiac surgery, and also for persistent pulmonary hypertension of the newborn.[48,592–603] The benefit of combining oral sildenafil with inhaled iloprost for the treatment of severe pulmonary hypertension has also been demonstrated.[604] Most of the pharmacokinetic data for sildenafil are derived from adult studies with oral dosing. Sildenafil is rapidly absorbed; the bioavailability is 38% to 41% in the fasted state; and the maximum plasma concentration is achieved after 0.5 to 2.5 hours. It is highly metabolized in the liver into active metabolites. With a half-life of only 2 to 4 hours, sildenafil is relatively short-acting. Clearance decreases in patients with severe renal or hepatic dysfunction. Compared with healthy volunteers, patients with pulmonary hypertension have reduced clearance and greater bioavailability.[605–610] In adult patients, a 10-mg IV bolus and a 20- mg oral tablet have comparable effects.[611] According to in vitro studies, plasma concentrations of 50 to 400 ng/mL are necessary to provide a 50% to 90% inhibition of phosphodiesterase 5 activity.[612,613] Only a few pediatric pharmacokinetic studies are available. Children (1–17 years of age) with PA hypertension given oral sildenafil had a relatively high oral clearance.[614] Investigations in neonates demonstrated a larger volume of distribution, greater elimination half-life, and a rapidly increasing age-dependent metabolic clearance over the first month of postnatal life.[615,616] Oral therapy usually begins with 0.25 to 0.5 mg/kg every 4 to 6 hours with increasing doses as tolerated.[598,617,618] The IV use of sildenafil has been investigated in premature infants, neonates with persistent pulmonary hypertension, and children after congenital cardiac surgery.[48,619–622] Case reports of sublingual use of sildenafil have also been published.[623] Sildenafil seems to be well tolerated; the most commonly reported adverse effects are headache, fever, respiratory infections, vomiting, and diarrhea,[614] but serious adverse events such as pulmonary hemorrhage, stridor or hypotension have been occasionally observed.[572,614,624] In 2012, the results of a randomized, double-blind, placebo-controlled clinical trial (STARTS-1) investigating three different dose regiments of oral sildenafil for treatment-naïve children with pulmonary arterial hypertension were published. Body weight–adjusted groups were treated for 16 weeks with placebo, small- (10 mg tid), medium- (10-40 mg tid), or large-dose (20-80 mg tid) sildenafil. The effect was greater with the medium- and large-dose ranges.[614] A follow-up study (STARTS-2) after 2 years of treatment found an increased risk of mortality for the large-dose group,[625] which triggered the release of an FDA warning against the chronic use of sildenafil for children aged 1 to 17 years. The European Medicines Agency warned only against the use of large doses. The current controversy among pediatric cardiologists regarding the safety of sildenafil was fueled by several publications, which questioned the START-2 results.[624,626–628] In 2014, the FDA issued another statement clarifying that the risk-benefit profile of sildenafil might be acceptable for selected children in special situations. Oral phosphodiesterase 5 inhibitors are currently still part of the treatment guidelines for pulmonary hypertension in children.[506,508]

Cialis is another selective phosphodiesterase 5 inhibitor. Compared with sildenafil, it has a greater duration of action, which permits once-daily dosing. The initial experience in pediatric patients is promising.[629,630]

ANTIARRHYTHMIC AGENTS

Antiarrhythmic agents have been traditionally categorized according to the Vaughan Williams classification, which is based on the presumed primary mechanism of action. For example, class I agents are sodium channel blockers. They are also called membrane-stabilizing agents because of their ability to decrease the excitability of the plasma membrane. Class I drugs can be subdivided into class IA, IB, or IC agents depending on their effects on the cardiac action potential (Table 18.10). Many antiarrhythmic drugs have multiple mechanisms of action and are therefore difficult to classify. Commonly used IV antiarrhythmic agents for children are described in Table 18.11.

Procainamide (Pronestyl)

Procainamide is one of the most commonly used class IA agents in children. It has sodium channel and moderate potassium channel blocking activities (class III effect). Its major effect is to delay repolarization. This effect is more pronounced at faster HRs. IV procainamide is used to treat SVT associated with the Wolff-Parkinson-White syndrome, atrial flutter, and ventricular dysrhythmias unresponsive to lidocaine.[631–634] It may also be effective in postoperative junctional ectopic tachycardia.[635,636] In addition, electrophysiologists use it as a "procainamide challenge" to unmask the characteristic electrocardiographic changes of Brugada syndrome.[637]

Procainamide is the only class IA agent that is still clinically used in children, mainly for short-term IV therapy. A loading dose of 3 to 10 mg/kg is given over 30 to 60 minutes to infants

TABLE 18.10	Vaughan Williams Classification of Antiarrhythmic Drugs	
Class	**Mechanism**	**Examples**
I	Sodium channel blockers	
IA	Increase length of action potential	Procainamide Quinidine Disopyramide
IB	Decrease length of action potential	Lidocaine Mexiletine Phenytoin
IC	No effect on length of action potential	Flecainide Propafenone
II	β-Blockers	Propranolol Atenolol Metoprolol Esmolol
III	Potassium channel blockers	Amiodarone Sotalol Bretylium Ibutilide Dofetilide Dronedarone
IV	Calcium channel blockers	Verapamil Diltiazem
V	Other or unknown mechanism	Adenosine Digoxin Magnesium sulfate

Data from Vaughan Williams EM. A classification of antiarrhythmic actions reassessed after a decade of new drugs. *Clin Pharmacol*, 1984;24:129–147; and Fuster V, Ryden LE, Cannom DS, et al. ACC/AHA/ESC 2006 guidelines for the management of patients with atrial fibrillation: a report of the American College of Cardiology/American Heart Association Task Force on Practice Guidelines and the European Society of Cardiology Committee for Practice Guidelines (Writing Committee to Revise the 2001 guidelines for the management of patients with atrial fibrillation). Developed in collaboration with the European Heart Rhythm Association and the Heart Rhythm Society. *Circulation* 2006;114:e257–354.

TABLE 18.11 | Intravenous Antiarrhythmic Agents

Agent (Vaughan Williams Class)	Dose	Comments
Procainamide (IA; sodium ± potassium channel blockade; antivagal effects)	Infant (<1 year): 3–10 mg/kg loading dose over 30 minutes Child (>1 year): 5–15 mg/kg loading dose over 30 minutes All ages, infusion rate: 20–80 µg/kg per minute	Used to treat SVT due to WPW, atrial flutter, junctional ectopic tachycardia (with patient hypothermia), lidocaine-resistant ventricular dysrhythmias; hypotension and negative inotropy; lupus-like syndrome.
Lidocaine (IB; sodium channel blockade; speeds repolarization)	1 mg/kg bolus; then 20–50 µg/kg per minute	Used for ventricular dysrhythmias; CNS toxicity (apnea, seizures, abnormal sensations).
Phenytoin (IB)	1–3 mg/kg q5 minutes up to 15 mg/kg loading dose, then 5–10 mg/kg divided q6 hours	Drug must be infused slowly (>30 minutes) due to potential hypotension; antidysrhythmic profile similar to that of lidocaine; may be useful to treat digoxin-induced dysrhythmias.
Propranolol (II; β-adrenergic blockade; sodium channel blockade also)	0.01–0.1 mg/kg slowly	Nonselective β-blockade; used mainly to treat SVT; bradycardia, hypotension, worsening of myocardial pump function; AV block; hypoglycemia; bronchospasm; depression; fatigue.
Esmolol (II; B-receptor blockade)	100–500 µg/kg loading dose (over 5 minutes); 50–250 µg/kg per minute infusion	Used to treat SVT; relatively selective β₁ blockade; short elimination half-life (7–10 minutes); hypotension, especially during bolus; if less than desired response after 5 minutes, can repeat or double bolus dose, followed by doubling infusion rate; non–organ-based metabolism by plasma and red blood cell esterases; infusion concentrations >10 mg/mL may predispose to venous sclerosis; dilute infusion at high rates increases risk of volume overload.
Amiodarone (III; prolongs repolarization; adrenergic and calcium blockade)	1–2.5 mg/kg bolus over 5–10 minutes (total loading dose up to 5–6 mg/kg); 5–15 mg/kg per 24-hour infusion	Used for resistant reentrant atrial and ventricular dysrhythmias; may be useful for postoperative junctional ectopic tachycardia; hypotension with bolus IV administration; bradycardia; AV block; rare proarrhythmia and torsades de pointes; pulmonary fibrosis; hypothyroidism; controversial association with acute perioperative lung injury.
Verapamil (IV; calcium channel blockade)	0.1–0.3 mg/kg bolus (maximum 5 mg)	Used for SVT in older children and adults; potential for hypotension and asystole contraindicates use in children <1 year of age; bradycardia; AV block; may increase ventricular response rate in some children with WPW.
Adenosine	0.05–0.1 mg/kg rapid bolus followed by flush; may repeat with doses increasing in increments of 0.05 mg/kg q2 minutes (maximum dose 0.25 mg/kg or 12 mg, whichever comes first)	Increases potassium channel flux and inhibits slow inward calcium current; causes transient sinus bradycardia and AV block; transient hypotension; rarely causes ventricular ectopy or atrial fibrillation; bronchospasm; used to terminate SVT; used diagnostically to transiently produce AV block. Reduce dose by 50% in heart transplant patients or if given through a central line.
Digoxin	Total digitalizing dose (TDD)ᵃ: Premature: 15–25 µg/kg Neonate (<1 month): 20–30 µg/kg Infant (<2 years): 30–50 µg/kg Child (2–5 years): 25–35 µg/kg Child (>5 years): 15–30 µg/kg Child (>10 years): 8–12 µg/kg	TDD given in divided doses: ½ TDD followed by ¼ TDD q8-12 hours × 2; slows sinus node and decreases AV node conduction; used to slow ventricular response in atrial flutter and fibrillation and may also treat junctional tachycardia or SVT; variable effect on accessory pathways; long half-life (24–48 hours) that is prolonged by renal dysfunction; numerous drug interactions; toxicity includes SVT, AV block, ventricular dysrhythmias; toxicity symptoms include drowsiness, nausea, vomiting; toxicity exacerbated by hypokalemia.
Magnesium sulfate	25–50 mg/kg bolus; maximum single dose 2 g; 30–60 mg/kg per 24-hour infusion	May be first-line therapy for torsades des pointes; also used for refractory ventricular tachycardia and ventricular fibrillation; hypotension and respiratory depression may accompany IV bolus dosing—IV calcium is an antidote.

ᵃDaily maintenance dose varies by age; consult pharmacy or cardiologist.
AV, atrioventricular; *CNS*, central nervous system; *IV*, intravenous; *SVT*, supraventricular tachycardia; *WPW*, Wolff-Parkinson-White syndrome.

younger than 1 year of age. Older children receive IV bolus doses of 5 to 15 mg/kg given over 30 to 60 minutes. After the bolus dose, an infusion is usually started at 20 to 80 µg/kg per minute. Infusion rates in excess of 100 µg/kg per minute are occasionally necessary, particularly in infants. Infusion rates are adjusted to achieve procainamide plasma concentrations of 4 to 10 µg/mL.[638] The first concentration should be measured 6 to 20 hours after initiation of the infusion. It is recommended to stop the infusion

if hypotension occurs or the QRS widens by more than 50%. Procainamide can have substantial negative inotropic effects, which may be more pronounced in the ischemic/reperfused or otherwise damaged myocardium.

The clearance of procainamide depends 50% on hepatic (phase II acetylation) metabolism and 50% on the renal clearance of the unchanged drug. Metabolism in the liver to *N*-acetyl procainamide (NAPA), which has significant class III antiarrhythmic effects,[639] depends on the individual's genetic polymorphism of N-acetyltransferase-2 as a slow or fast acetylator. In the past, procainamide and NAPA serum concentrations were added, with a therapeutic goal of 10 to 30 μg/mL. Today, only procainamide plasma concentrations are monitored. Oral procainamide therapy is complicated by unreliable absorption, the need for frequent dosing, potential proarrhythmogenic effects, and a wide spectrum of adverse effects. Typical doses are 15 to 50 mg/kg per day, divided every 4 to 6 hours. A sustained-release form (administered every 8–12 hours) is available for older children.

The majority of procainamide-related adverse effects depend on the plasma concentration and the duration of therapy. A systemic lupus erythematosus–like syndrome is common, manifested as fevers, pleural effusions, pericarditis, arthralgias, myalgias, and rashes. A considerable number of children demonstrate positive antinuclear antibodies with chronic therapy, but they do not necessarily require discontinuation of the therapy.

Lidocaine (Xylocaine)

Lidocaine is a member of the class IB antiarrhythmic agents, which include mexiletine and phenytoin. Proarrhythmogenia is less common with class IB agents. In addition to blocking fast sodium channels, they also reduce the duration of both the action potential and repolarization.[638] As with class IA agents, the effects of these agents may be greater at faster HRs. Lidocaine primarily affects cells inferior to the AV node. It produces its greatest effects on cells with the action potentials with the greatest duration and thereby balances ventricular repolarization.

Because of its rapid hepatic metabolism, lidocaine is available only in an IV formulation. It is indicated for the emergency treatment of ventricular dysrhythmias. Lidocaine is initially administered as an IV bolus of 1 mg/kg that can be repeated once within 5 to 10 minutes. Standard lidocaine infusion rates range from 20 to 50 μg/kg per minute.

The major adverse effects of lidocaine administration are well known to anesthesiologists. They primarily consist of CNS toxicity, which typically occurs at plasma concentrations in excess of 6 to 8 μg/mL. Mental status changes, abnormal taste or other sensations, apnea, and seizures may occur. Lidocaine doses should be reduced in children with reduced cardiac output because it has perfusion limited clearance. The administration of lidocaine to children with atrial tachydysrhythmias or a prolonged QT interval can increase the ventricular response rate.[640]

Phenytoin (Dilantin)

Phenytoin shares many similarities to lidocaine in terms of its antiarrhythmic effects, which are also restricted primarily to tissues inferior to the AV node and the bundle of His. Phenytoin primarily binds to sodium channels, maintaining them in the inactivated state. Very large concentrations may also affect calcium channels and automaticity. This drug is useful in treating refractory ventricular arrhythmias and especially digoxin-induced dysrhythmias.[641,642]

IV loading with phenytoin is achieved by a bolus dose of 1 to 3 mg/kg. For treatment of status epilepticus, larger loading doses (10–15 mg/kg) are used. IV maintenance is 5 mg/kg day divided into two to three doses. IV phenytoin must be administered extremely slowly (>30 minutes) owing to its potential to cause hypotension. The oral dose in infants and older children is 5 mg/kg per day given every 12 hours, after a total loading dose of 15 mg/kg that has been divided over 6 hours. Other typical adverse effects are well described from its use as an antiepileptic medication and include gingival hyperplasia, aplastic anemia, ataxia, and nystagmus.

Phenytoin should be avoided in patients who are pregnant or who may become pregnant because of its significant teratogenic profile (fetal hydantoin syndrome).

Flecainide (Tambocor) and Propafenone (Rythmol)

Flecainide and propafenone are class IC agents. As such, they have potent sodium channel blocking activity. In adults, flecainide is used to treat various tachyarrhythmias, and it has a special role in the pharmacologic cardioversion of recurrent atrial fibrillation in patients with normal hearts ("pill in a pocket").[643,644] Flecainide has also been extensively evaluated in children in whom it is frequently used in the treatment and prevention of supraventricular tachyarrhythmias.[645-653] It blocks activated slow sodium channels but exerts less of an inhibitory effect on potassium channels. It appears to reduce the refractory time and decrease the automaticity in His-Purkinje cells. In contrast, the duration of the action potential and refractory period is prolonged in ventricular muscle, resulting in a greater duration of the QRS complex.

Clearance is achieved via renal excretion of the unchanged drug and by hepatic metabolism by CYP2D6; both are immature in neonates. Neonatal dosing starts at 2 mg/kg per day orally, divided every 12 hours and titrated to clinical response; monitoring of serum concentration is also advised. Infants over 1 month of age require 3 to 6 mg/kg per day. Oral dosing of flecainide may be more reliable when it is calculated on the basis of body surface area. Typical dosages in infants are in the range of 80 to 90 mg/m² per day, given in two divided doses (40–45 mg/m² every 12 hours). Older children receive 100 to 110 mg/m² per day (50–55 mg/m² every 12 hours). Loading doses are not used. Serum elimination half-life is age dependent: approximately 1 day in neonates, 12 hours in infants younger than 6 months of age, and 8 to 12 hours in older children and adults. Therapeutic trough concentrations are believed to be in the range of 200 to 1000 ng/mL. Alterations in diet can markedly affect drug absorption with oral dosing. IV flecainide is available outside the United States. A dose of 1 to 2 mg/kg given over 5 to 10 minutes has been used. Continuous infusions are not given because of its prolonged elimination half-life.

Flecainide has mild to moderate negative inotropic effects. Substantial proarrhythmogenic effects have been observed in children with atrial tachydysrhythmias or significant abnormalities of myocardial anatomy and function. Proarrhythmia was considerably increased in adult patients who received flecainide after myocardial infarction.[654] In children and adults with paroxysmal SVT, a slow but incessant SVT may result on initiation of therapy. As a result, it is recommended to closely monitor these patients when initiating therapy with flecainide. The efficiency and safety of class IC antiarrhythmic agents in children with an abnormal or damaged myocardium are unclear; many pediatric electrophysiologists would avoid these drugs in children with severe myocardial dysfunction, myocardial injury (e.g., immediately postoperatively), right- or left-sided hypertrophy (e.g., TOF), or aortic stenosis.[632,655] Nevertheless, a retrospective cohort study based on an administrative database from 43 pediatric tertiary care hospitals in the United States reported a trend towards increased use of flecainide in patients with CHD or cardiomyopathies (8.7% in 2011 compared with 4.6% in 2004) with a cardiac arrest rate comparable to other antiarrhythmic medications.[656]

The effects and risks of propafenone are similar to those discussed for flecainide. Propafenone can also control dysrhythmias that arise from automatic mechanisms and can be used to treat postoperative junctional ectopic tachycardia. Oral propafenone is administered at 200 to 600 mg/m² per day divided into three doses (for children under 15 kg, 10–20 mg/kg per day and for children over 15 kg, 7–15 mg/kg per day). IV propafenone is not available in the United States. An IV loading dose of 0.2 to 1.0 mg/kg should be given slowly over 10 minutes. The initial dose may be doubled to achieve a maximum 2-mg/kg total loading dose. Infusion rates of 4 to 7 μg/kg per minute have been reported.[657-662]

Significant hypotension can occur with a bolus of propafenone. Hypotension has been attributed primarily to its negative inotropic effects. Like flecainide, propafenone is probably contraindicated in children with significant structural or metabolic myocardial abnormalities, such as those related to severe pressure or volume overload, ischemia-reperfusion, or myocardial infarction. In addition, propafenone has the potential for proarrhythmogenic effects. Propafenone is extensively metabolized in the liver, with significant interindividual variability. Its reported elimination half-life ranges from 4 to 18 hours. Serum concentrations of propafenone do not correlate well with the clinical response.[663]

β-Blockers

β-Blockers are class II antiarrhythmic agents. Mechanism of action, relevance of subtype selectivity, metabolism, and other features are described in the section on vasoactive drugs. Here we focus on their indications as antiarrhythmic agents. In children, propranolol, atenolol, and esmolol are the most frequently used β-blockers.[377]

Propranolol (Inderal)

Propranolol is probably the most widely studied β-blocking agent in children.[664] Its primary indication is the treatment and prophylaxis of SVT. Even infants seem to tolerate high-dose propranolol (up to 4 mg/kg per day) but require frequent weight-based dose adjustments to maintain effect.[665,666] In addition to nonselective β-blockade, propranolol has effects on the sodium channels and at high concentrations on calcium channels as well. It seems that conduction tissues of neonates are more sensitive to the drug than those of older children and adults.[642,667]

Atenolol (Tenormin)

Atenolol is a commonly used, longer-acting β-blocker[645,668,669] It has more selective effects on β-adrenergic receptors, although the risk of bronchospasm may not be completely eliminated with this drug. Atenolol does not cross the blood-brain barrier, which may be a reason for its lower incidence of depression, fatigue, and malaise compared with propranolol.[382,670]

Esmolol (Brevibloc)

Esmolol is increasing in popularity for the control of perioperative tachydysrhythmias in children.[632] Esmolol acts predominantly on the sinus and AV nodes. It does not appear to have significant antiarrhythmic effects in the His-Purkinje or ventricular conducting tissues. Pharmacokinetics and the efficacy to terminate SVTs were found to be similar in children and adults.[386]

Class III Agents

The primary class III agents are amiodarone, sotalol, and ibutilide. They prolong depolarization and therefore increase refractoriness. All of these drugs have numerous other properties, including membrane-stabilizing effects, calcium channel blockade, and adrenergic blockade.

Amiodarone (Cordarone, Pacerone)

In addition to prolonging refractoriness, amiodarone has sodium channel blocking and noncompetitive α- and β-adrenergic receptor blocking properties. It may also interfere with potassium channels and inhibit the release of myocardial norepinephrine. Oral amiodarone is absorbed quite slowly from the gastrointestinal tract and is metabolized in the liver to an active metabolite, desethylamiodarone. Because of its high lipid solubility and large volume of distribution, tissue concentrations are maintained for 2 to 3 months after discontinuation of therapy. There are increasing data demonstrating the efficacy and safety of oral and IV amiodarone for the treatment of dysrhythmias in infants and children.[671-675] In addition to resistant reentrant atrial and ventricular dysrhythmias, amiodarone may be effective in treating postoperative junctional ectopic tachycardia.[676-678] Amiodarone, in a dose of 5 mg/kg IV push, is also indicated for shock-resistant arrhythmias during cardiopulmonary resuscitation in infants and children.[679]

The loading dose for oral amiodarone is 10 to 15 mg/kg per day for 5 to 10 days. After the loading dose, long-term oral dosing is 2 to 5 mg/kg once daily. IV amiodarone is usually given in boluses of 1.0 to 2.5 mg/kg, reaching a total of 5 to 6 mg/kg, with each bolus administered over 5 to 10 minutes. In children with resistant dysrhythmias, the average loading dose was 6.3 mg/kg, with 50% of children requiring a continuous amiodarone infusion of 10 to 15 mg/kg per day.[673,680,681]

Hypotension is the most significant acute adverse effect of IV amiodarone therapy. The effects of amiodarone may be synergistic with those of other agents that depress sinus node and AV node function. Important cardiac dysrhythmias include bradycardia and AV block. Proarrhythmogenic effects and torsades de pointes may occasionally occur. Long-term oral amiodarone therapy can lead to progressive and irreversible pulmonary fibrosis; all patients taking amiodarone chronically are usually monitored with pulmonary function tests at regular intervals.[682-684] The high iodine content of amiodarone can affect thyroid function, resulting in either hyperthyroidism or hypothyroidism; therefore thyroid function tests are indicated periodically or at least annually. Other effects include drug deposits in the cornea, skin photosensitivity, and chemical hepatitis with increased liver transaminases. Coadministration of amiodarone with other antiarrhythmic agents may result in significant increases in the plasma concentrations of the other drugs.[671,673]

The incidence of perioperative organ dysfunction in children who receive either acute or long-term amiodarone therapy is controversial. A syndrome with similarities to the adult respiratory distress syndrome has been described, particularly in children exposed to high inspired oxygen concentrations who are undergoing thoracic surgery or CPB.[685-688] This finding led to the recommendation that amiodarone be discontinued for several weeks before elective surgery.[689] Subsequent studies failed to demonstrate a significantly increased incidence of injury to lungs or other organs in children undergoing surgery while receiving amiodarone. Because it is most frequently given to children with severe and life-threatening cardiac rhythm disturbances, the current recommendation is to continue amiodarone up to the time of surgery. However, it may be wise to attempt to limit the inspired oxygen concentration and other factors that may predispose the children receiving amiodarone to free radical and inflammatory injury.[690]

Dronedarone (Multaq)

Dronedarone is a non-iodinated analog of amiodarone that was developed to reduce the iodine-associated adverse effects of chronic amiodarone therapy. Like amiodarone, it inhibits sodium, potassium, and calcium currents. It is mainly indicated for maintenance of sinus rhythm in patients with atrial fibrillation but is still undergoing investigations regarding its long-term safety profile.[643,691-693] After the initial drug approval, a high incidence of serious adverse events has been reported, including several cases of severe hepatocellular injury, which prompted the FDA to issue a warning in 2011.[694,695] Pediatric data are not yet available.

Sotalol (Betapace, Sorine, Sotylize)

Sotalol, a newer agent available in the United States, is a class III antiarrhythmic that also acts as a nonselective β-blocker. At small doses, the β-adrenergic blocking effects predominate; at larger doses, the class III effects become more important. Sotalol is indicated for a number of refractory tachydysrhythmias, including fetal supraventricular tachyarrhythmias.[696] Current oral dosing recommendations for children start at target doses of 2 and 4 mg/kg in neonates, 3 and 6 mg/kg for children up to 6 years, and 2 and 4 mg/kg, divided into three doses, for children older than 6 years of age.[697] The major adverse effects of sotalol include mild cardiodepression owing to its β-blocking ability and prolongation of the QT interval and torsades de pointes owing to its class III effects.[698] It should be avoided in children with asthma, heart failure, renal dysfunction, or QT interval prolongation. Sotalol may be used as an alternative to amiodarone in some children who are unable to tolerate the adverse effects associated with amiodarone. Adult studies have shown that sotalol is not as effective for pharmacologic conversion of atrial fibrillation compared with other strategies or medications, but it can be indicated for maintenance of sinus rhythm after an episode of atrial fibrillation, especially for patients with coronary artery disease.[644] It has also been recommended as an alternative to amiodarone for postoperative atrial fibrillation in cardiac patients, but for prophylaxis and rate control pure β-blockers are still preferred.[699-701] The pediatric experience with sotalol is steadily increasing, but most studies have been limited by small numbers.[377,632,702-706]

Ibutilide (Corvert)

Ibutilide is one of the more recently released intravenous class III antiarrhythmic drugs. It prolongs repolarization by increasing the slow inward sodium current and by blocking the late rectifier current. It can be given intravenously and has a fast onset. Ibutilide is currently indicated for the rapid pharmacologic conversion of atrial fibrillation and atrial flutter, although it may be more efficacious for the latter. As with other class III drugs, ibutilide can prolong the QT interval and can cause associated polymorphic ventricular tachycardia (torsades de pointes, which occur in 5%–8% of adults).[707,708] Because the elimination half-life of ibutilide is approximately 6 hours, the current recommendation is to observe children for several hours after an IV administration of this drug. Studies to date have used a bolus dose of 10 to 25 µg/kg administered over 10 minutes, which may be repeated once. Ibutilide has been successfully used in neonates,[709] children with CHD,[710] and in children with accessory pathways.[711]

Dofetilide (Tikosyn)

Dofetilide is another new class III antiarrhythmic drug that has been approved for treatment of atrial fibrillation and flutter.[644] It prolongs the effective refractory period by selectively blocking the rapid component of the delayed rectifier potassium current. The major adverse effect is the potential for torsade de pointes as a result of QT prolongation.[712,713] Dofetilide is currently available only for oral administration; IV formulations are still under investigation. It has been successfully used in adult patients with CHD, but pediatric data are still lacking.[714]

Verapamil (Calan, Covera, Isoptin, Verelan)

Verapamil is a member of the class IV antiarrhythmic agents, the calcium channel blockers. Its primary action is depression of sinus node and AV node function.[715] Oral doses range from 4 to 8 mg/kg per day divided into three doses. A sustained-release preparation is available for older children. IV doses range from 0.1 to 0.3 mg/kg with a maximum dose of 5 mg. The most important side effect of verapamil occurs in children younger than 1 year of age, in whom IV administration can cause severe hypotension and asystole.[716] In fact, the drug is now contraindicated in infants (<1 year of age) because of this complication. Other side effects include bradycardia, AV block, and increased ventricular response in some children with Wolff-Parkinson-White syndrome.

Verapamil has been shown to be effective in terminating most SVTs in older children and adults.[632,717,718] Verapamil is also used to relieve outflow obstruction in hypertrophic cardiomyopathy[719] and as an antihypertensive in some children. The negative inotropic and AV conduction effects of verapamil are potentiated by β-blockers and anesthetic agents.[720,721] IV calcium and β-adrenergic drugs such as isoproterenol have been given to reverse the depressive effects of verapamil and other calcium channel antagonists.[722,723]

Adenosine (Adenocard, Adenoscan)

IV adenosine has markedly changed the therapy for SVTs. Its electrophysiologic effects are multiple and include increased potassium channel flux and decreased slow inward calcium current. These effects result in sinus bradycardia and transient AV block and are mediated primarily by stimulation of the A1-purinergic receptor subtype. Its onset of action is within 10 to 20 seconds. Bradycardia, AV block, and hypotension last an additional 10 to 30 seconds.

The best response to adenosine is achieved when it is rapidly administered into the central circulation. The initial central venous dose is 50 µg/kg and the initial peripherally administered dose is 100 to 150 µg/kg given as a rapid bolus, followed by a fluid bolus given via a syringe to flush the medication into the circulation. If this is unsuccessful or the effect is not sustained, the procedure can be repeated with a double dose (up to a maximum of 300 µg/kg). In adults, the starting dose is 6 to 12 mg.[724,725] Adenosine can also be used as a diagnostic tool to differentiate between SVT and other dysrhythmias. The slower HR caused by the transient AV conduction block often allows the recognition of specific electrocardiographic features, such as delta waves in Wolff-Parkinson White syndrome.[726]

Other than the noted electrophysiologic changes, the major adverse effect from adenosine is transient hypotension. In children with an antegrade-conducting accessory pathway, adenosine can induce atrial fibrillation with a rapid ventricular response. Therefore it should be used only in an appropriate setting with electrocardiographic monitoring and available resuscitation equipment.[727] Dipyridamole and diazepam may inhibit the metabolism or cellular redistribution of adenosine. Either drug can significantly potentiate the effects of adenosine, resulting in more prolonged hypotension and AV node blockade.[728] Children with transplanted hearts can demonstrate prolonged bradycardia and asystole in response to adenosine. **The denervated heart is extremely sensitive to the AV node–blocking effects. It is recommended that the initial dose be reduced by 50% in these children.[142] This can be very important in the cardiac catheterization laboratory, where wire-induced supraventricular arrhythmias are common during surveillance biopsies.** Adenosine has been reported to cause bronchospasm in children both with and without known reactive airway disease. It is usually mild and, if necessary, can be treated with IV aminophylline, which directly counteracts the receptor-mediated effects of adenosine.

Digoxin (Digitek, Digox, Lanoxicaps, Lanoxin)
Digoxin has antiarrhythmic as well as positive inotropic effects. Its basic pharmacology and therapeutic dosing were discussed earlier in the section on vasoactive drugs. As an antiarrhythmic agent, digoxin slows both atrial and AV node conduction. It slows the ventricular response in atrial flutter and fibrillation and may be used to treat children with junctional tachycardia and SVT.[377,632] Digoxin can have an unpredictable effect on the refractory period of accessory pathways[729,730] and is therefore relatively contraindicated in children with Wolff-Parkinson-White syndrome or other forms of SVT with accessory pathways. Digoxin easily crosses the placenta and remains the primary treatment for termination of fetal SVT.[731–733]

The dosing of digoxin in infants and children must be undertaken with care. Infants have greater myocellular concentrations of digoxin than adults.[291,734–736] The dosing schedule of digoxin, based on age, is shown in Tables 18.8 and 18.11. IV and oral dosing are essentially the same. The onset of effect is more rapid with IV dosing (5–10 minutes) than with oral dosing (1–2 hours). The elimination half-life of digoxin is prolonged, approaching 1 to 2 days in young infants. Significant renal dysfunction and congestive heart failure can extend the elimination half-life. There are no active metabolites of digoxin. Therapeutic digoxin concentrations are 0.5 to 2.0 ng/mL. To properly measure the blood concentration of digoxin, blood should be obtained either just before a dose or at least 6 hours after the preceding dose.

Cardiac injury (e.g., ischemia-reperfusion, myocarditis) may increase the sensitivity to digoxin. Toxicity is more likely in children whose plasma concentrations exceed 3 ng/mL.[296] Signs of toxicity include proarrhythmia, nausea, vomiting, and drowsiness. Infants and young children frequently manifest digoxin toxicity as SVT and AV node conduction disturbances, whereas adults are more prone to ventricular arrhythmias, premature ventricular contractions, AV blocks, and junctional tachycardias. Hypokalemia exacerbates the risk of digoxin toxicity. Many drugs interact with digoxin. As a rule, the administration of other drugs may require a reduction in the digoxin dosing.

Magnesium Sulfate
Magnesium plays an important role in many biologic processes. The catalytic actions of more than 300 enzymes, including those for ATP and DNA synthesis, depend on the presence of the Mg^{2+} ion, the physiologically active form. Myocardial conduction and contractility, transmembrane calcium flux, potassium transport, vascular smooth muscle tone, coronary reactivity, and NO synthesis are all regulated by magnesium. Only 1% of the total body magnesium is extracellular; 60% is found in bones and 39% is intracellular, especially in muscle cells. This distribution explains why serum concentrations of magnesium may be normal despite an underlying intracellular deficiency. Of the extracellular magnesium, 55% is in the active ionized form. Ionized magnesium is a better predictor of the intracellular magnesium status; age-specific reference values have been published.[737,738]

Magnesium sulfate is currently used for the correction of hypomagnesemia, for management of seizures and hypertension, for bronchodilation during status asthmaticus, and in the treatment of life-threatening arrhythmias. It is especially valuable in the treatment of long QT syndromes and torsades de pointes.[739,740] More recently, prophylactic magnesium supplementation during pediatric CPB has been advocated to reduce the incidence of postoperative junctional ectopic tachycardia.[741,742] The IV dose is usually 25 to 50 mg/kg over 10 minutes (0.2–0.4 mEq/kg), with a maximum single dose of 2 g. This dose can be repeated every 6 to 8 hours depending on renal function and serum concentrations. Because magnesium is excreted solely by the kidneys, renal insufficiency requires increasing the intervals between doses to avoid toxicity. The normal serum concentration of magnesium is 1.5 to 2.5 mEq/L. Concentrations greater than 5 to 7 mEq/L can lead to increasing CNS and cardiac depression, initially manifested as loss of deep tendon reflexes and muscle weakness, potentially leading to respiratory depression and cardiac arrest (at levels >15–20 mEq/L). IV calcium directly antagonizes magnesium-induced toxicity.

ACKNOWLEDGMENTS
We wish to thank Avinash C. Shukla, James M. Steven, Francis X. McGowan, Jr., Paul R. Hickey, Robert K. Crone, and Susan L. Streitz for their prior contributions to this chapter.

ANNOTATED REFERENCES
Baum VC, Palmisano BW. The immature heart and anesthesia. *Anesthesiology.* 1997;87:1529-1548.
Review article describing the developmental changes in the immature heart and the implications for anesthesia on a physiologic, structural, and molecular level.
Cotts WG, Oren RM. Function of the transplanted heart: unique physiology and therapeutic implications. *Am J Med Sci.* 1997;314:164-172.
Classic article describing the physiologic changes in the denervated heart.
Hoffman JL, Kaplan S. The incidence of congenital heart disease. *J Am Coll Cardiol.* 2002;39:1890-1900.
Interesting literature review looking into the reasons for the wide range of incidence data on congenital heart disease.
Jolley M, Colan SD, Rhodes J, DiNardo J. Fontan physiology revisited. *Anesth Analg.* 2015;121(1):172-182.
Review article discussing the fundamental characteristics of the Fontan circulation.
Kiserud T. Physiology of the fetal circulation. *Semin Fetal Neonatal Med.* 2005;10:493-503.
Review article with a thorough description of the fetal circulatory physiology and the implications of placental compromise.
Latus H, Delhaas T, Schranz D, Apitz C. Treatment of pulmonary arterial hypertension in children. *Nat Rev Cardiol.* 2015;12(4):244-254.
Review article summarizing the current treatment options for pediatric pulmonary hypertension.
Rhodes J, Tikkanen AU, Jenkins KJ. Exercise testing and training in children with congenital heart disease. *Circulation.* 2010;122:1957-1967.
Original article describing the exercise limitations in children with repaired congenital heart disease.

A complete reference list can be found online at ExpertConsult.com.

19 Cardiopulmonary Bypass and Management

RALPH GERTLER, ERIN A. GOTTLIEB, AND DEAN B. ANDROPOULOS

THIS CHAPTER REVIEWS THE equipment and strategies for cardiopulmonary bypass (CPB) in infants and children, focusing on how they differ compared with CPB in adults. We review the effects of CPB on the key organ systems and discuss specific management issues that occur in daily practice.

Basic Aspects of Cardiopulmonary Bypass

The basic principles of CPB remain unchanged from when they were first introduced in the 1950s: the CPB machine assumes the functions of the heart and lungs during the time necessary to complete either an intracardiac or an extracardiac repair. A basic bypass circuit (Fig. 19.1) consists of an oxygenator, heat exchanger, and venous reservoir; pump heads for perfusion, cardiotomy suction, and cardioplegia; and appropriate tubing, cannulas, and monitoring and alarm devices.[1] Major differences exist between pediatric and adult CPB, stemming from anatomic, metabolic, and physiologic differences in these age groups (Table 19.1).

THE CIRCUIT AND CANNULAS

Unfortunately, the circuit size cannot be reduced proportionately to the patient's size; this disproportion commonly leads to hemodilution and dilutional coagulopathies in children. Surgical procedures require extremes of temperature, hemodilution, and changes in flow rates. Because of the smaller vascular structures and greater flow rates (150–200 mL/kg per minute) in infants and children compared with flow rates of 2.2 to 2.4 L/minute per meter squared in adults, selection of appropriately sized cannulas is critical to maintain these flows. Shear stress is significant in small cannulas and several-fold greater than needed for activation of blood cells and platelets, leading to a disproportionately exaggerated systemic inflammatory response syndrome (SIRS).

Bypass Circuit

Technical advances in the field of oxygenator construction and size, including the reduction of priming volumes to as small as 45 mL for neonatal oxygenators, have allowed marked reductions

19

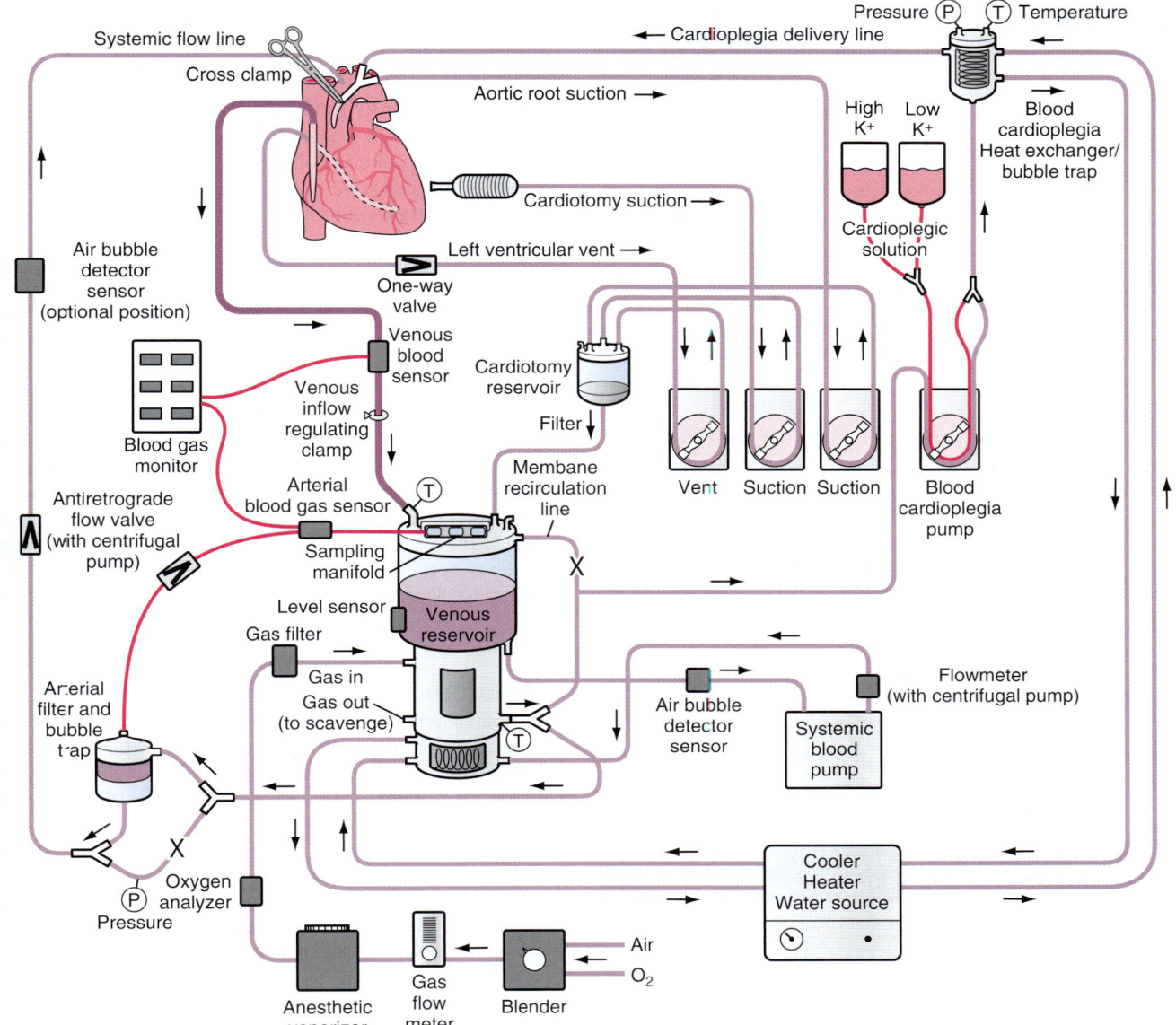

FIGURE 19.1 Schematic diagram of a cardiopulmonary bypass circuit. This scheme depicts a membrane oxygenator with integral hard-shell venous reservoir and external cardiotomy reservoir. Many circuits have the cardiotomy reservoir, venous reservoir, and oxygenator integrated into one single unit. The systemic blood pump may be either a roller or centrifugal pump. Most pediatric venous cannulations are bicaval with two separate venous cannulas instead of the single venous cannula depicted here. Carbon dioxide can also be added to the inspired gas to facilitate pH-stat blood gas management. *Arrows* indicate direction of flow; *P*, pressure sensor; *T*, temperature sensors; *X*, placement of tubing clamps. (From Hessel EA, Hill AG. Circuitry and cannulation techniques. In: Gravlee GP, Davis RF, Kurusz M, Utley JR, eds. *Cardiopulmonary Bypass: Principles and Practice*. 2nd ed. Philadelphia: Lippincott Williams & Wilkins; 2000:69–97.)

of circuit volumes over the past decade. Also, tubing sizes can be reduced to $\frac{3}{16}$-inch diameters, which in combination with shorter length tubing, can allow the reduction of priming volumes to the range of 100 to 150 mL for neonates. A summary of the Texas Children's Hospital sizing chart is shown in Table 19.2.

Heparin-Coated Versus Noncoated Circuits

Young children are more susceptible to the adverse effects of CPB than adults, and the inflammatory response to CPB may

have serious consequences for neonatal and pediatric patients.[2,3] This is in part related to the surface area of the CPB circuit, which is large relative to the infant and child's blood volume. For example, a 3-kg neonate with a blood volume of 90 mL/kg has a total blood volume of approximately 270 mL, and with an average priming volume in many centers of 350 mL (120% of the neonate's estimated blood volume), the CPB circuit volume thus causes greater than 100% dilution. A 70-kg adult with 70-mL/kg blood volume has an approximately 5000-mL blood volume, and

TABLE 19.1 Comparison of Pediatric Versus Adult Cardiopulmonary Bypass

	Child	Adult
Hemodilution	3–15 × adult	Moderate
Perfusion pressure	30–40 mm Hg	Moderate (>50–80 mm Hg)
	Wide flow rates (0–200 mL/kg per minute)	Narrow range (CI 2.0–2.4 L/m² per minute)
Blood gas management	pH-stat (PCO₂ 20–80 mm Hg or greater)	α-stat (PCO₂ 30–45 mm Hg)
Cannulation techniques	Variable	Predictable
Aortopulmonary collaterals		Uncommon
Temperature ranges	Variable	DHCA occasionally
Glucose management		Predictable
Inotropic response	Negative	Positive
Perfusion circuit	Per kilogram weight	Standard
Parameters	Hematocrit often >55%–60%	
	Po₂ 40–80 mm Hg	±
	Sao₂ 75%–85%	
	Ultrafiltration (MUF/CUF)	± Ultrafiltration

CI, cardiac index; *CUF*, conventional ultrafiltration; *DHCA*, deep hypothermic circulatory arrest; *MUF*, modified ultrafiltration.

TABLE 19.2 Cardiopulmonary Bypass Circuit Prime Volume and Constituents at Texas Children's Hospital

Patient Weight	Prime Volume	Prime Constituents
<8 kg	350 mL	Whole blood or PRBC + FFP + crystalloid prime[a]
8–15 kg	650 mL	100 mL albumin 25% ± PRBC + crystalloid prime[a]
15–25 kg	900 mL	100 mL albumin 25% + crystalloid prime[a]
15–25 kg	1200 mL	Crystalloid prime[a]

FFP, fresh frozen plasma; *PRBC*, packaged red blood cells.
[a]Crystalloid prime: ½ normal serum + PlasmaLyte + CaCl₂ + KCl.

with a CPB circuit prime of 1500 mL, this results in less than 33% dilution. Contact of blood with the surface of the circuit also plays an important role for activation of coagulation and fibrinolysis. Heparin-coated biocompatible bypass systems reduce this activation in children weighing less than 10 kg undergoing CPB.[4] They also reduce the activation of factor XII and the complement system.[5,6] This results in less production of kallikrein and bradykinin, which in turn reduces the secretion of tissue plasminogen activator from endothelial cells. One study has documented more bleeding with a conventional, non–heparin-coated circuit compared with a heparin-coated circuit.[6] Overall, children who underwent surgery while supported with heparin-coated circuits have significantly less

inflammatory mediator release and fewer consequences thereof, such as prolonged postoperative ventilation and duration of stay in the intensive care unit (ICU).[7]

CARDIOPULMONARY BYPASS PUMPS

The two pumps used most commonly for CPB are roller pumps and centrifugal pumps. Roller pumps have the advantages of simplicity, low cost, ease and reliability of flow calculation, and the ability to pump against increased resistance without reducing flow.[8] Disadvantages include the need to assess occlusiveness, spallation or fragmentation of the inner tubing surface (potentially producing particulate arterial emboli), potential for pumping large volumes of air, and ability to create large positive and negative pressures. Compared with roller pumps, centrifugal pumps offer the advantages of less air pumping potential, less ability to create large positive and negative pressures, less blood trauma, and virtually no spallation. Disadvantages of centrifugal pumps include a greater cost, the lack of occlusiveness (creating the possibility of accidental patient exsanguination), and afterload-dependent flow that requires constant flow measurement. In the setting of short-term CPB for cardiac surgery, it remains uncertain whether the selection of a roller pump over a centrifugal pump, or of any specific centrifugal pump over another, has clinical importance. Pulsatile perfusion may prove to be beneficial in the future, but further outcome data and technical improvements are needed.[9]

CARDIOPULMONARY BYPASS PRIME

The optimal priming fluid in cardiac surgery is a topic of enduring debate. Crystalloid solutions, colloids, and mixtures of both are used. Children appear to benefit from a colloid prime. If crystalloid is used for priming, it should not contain lactate or dextrose because CPB induces a metabolic acidosis[10] that is iatrogenic, not splanchnic, in provenance.[11] The addition of lactate to the prime increases the serum concentration of lactate postoperatively and should be avoided.[12] Hyperchloremic metabolic acidosis is the second contributing component of a metabolic acidosis on CPB. This is often only detected by measuring the strong ion difference via the Stewart approach to the acid-base homeostasis.[13] Both acidifying events are attenuated by the dilutional hypoalbuminemia induced by the pump prime. Because a hyperchloremic acidosis of a mild degree seems to be well tolerated and not associated with a poor outcome, no intervention seems necessary. Understanding the nature of CPB-associated acidosis, however, is likely to prevent unnecessary investigations or interventions.

The avoidance of dextrose is especially important during complex repairs using deep hypothermic cardiac arrest in which the risk of neurologic injury is substantive. The additives in banked blood, namely, glucose in citrate-phosphate-dextrose (CPD) storage solutions, also need to be considered as a source of glucose (together with the increased plasma concentrations of potassium in stored blood). We use a balanced electrolyte solution, such as PlasmaLyte, for the crystalloid component of our prime.

The proportionally large volume of the bypass circuit compared with the child's blood volume has a significant impact on the coagulation factors and cellular components. Platelet count decreases and coagulation factors, including fibrinogen, are diluted after bypass thereby contributing to a coagulopathy. The fibrinogen concentration at the end of bypass correlates with the 24-hour chest drainage in children who weigh less than 8 kg.[14] This occurs more frequently in infants and neonates in whom the plasma concentrations of hemostatic proteins decrease postoperatively by 56% immediately upon initiation of bypass[15]; younger age represents the single most important risk factor for coagulopathy and bleeding complications.[16]

One approach to offset this dilutional coagulopathy is the addition of whole blood to the circuit prime. Proponents cite two theoretical advantages: (1) improved hemostasis and (2) decreased SIRS with less edema formation and less organ dysfunction. However, one study challenged these perceived advantages when the researchers reported that the use of fresh whole blood actually increased perioperative fluid requirements, leading to a more prolonged duration of mechanical ventilation and ICU stay than in the single component group.[17] The only advantage of whole blood prime was fewer donor exposures, a problem we obviate by matching packed red blood cells (PRBCs) and fresh frozen plasma (FFP) from the same donor.[18] One retrospective analysis of donor exposures using fresh whole blood concluded that donor exposures were reduced in patients younger than 2 years of age compared with published reports using component therapy.[19] Unfortunately, fresh whole blood is frequently unavailable. However, when a commitment to use fresh whole blood for pediatric cardiovascular surgery exists, it is possible to build a sustainable operating protocol to provide this resource. An alternative approach is to use FFP in the prime.[20] Some investigators determined that the use of FFP led to greater fibrinogen concentrations at the end of surgery. On average, children in the FFP group needed 1.3 fewer donor exposures and tended to need fewer PRBCs. The reduced donor exposure was primarily the result of fewer transfusions of cryoprecipitate.[20] FFP may be safely substituted by 5% albumin in the prime in children with less complex repairs and acyanotic lesions.[21] Whenever possible, we prefer fresh blood that is less than 5 days old. Fresh PRBCs are presumably more balanced metabolically than stored PRBCs; the former contain less potassium, greater concentrations of glucose, reduced concentrations of lactate, and a greater pH.[22] Also, postoperative morbidity increases with increasing age of red blood cells.[23] Pulmonary complications, acute renal failure, and increased infection rates were among the main complications associated with increased red blood cell storage time. As far as potassium concentrations and acid-base balance are concerned, PRBC priming can be safely performed with stored PRBCs if the priming solution is circulated for 20 minutes before the initiation of CPB.[24]

Depending on the size and age of the child and the complexity of the repair, a target hematocrit is chosen. Based on the child's blood volume and the prime volume, homologous blood is added using the following calculation:

$$\text{Prime PRBC volume (mL)} = [\text{Target hematocrit}]$$
$$\times [\text{Patient blood volume (mL)}]$$
$$+ \text{Prime volume (mL)}]$$
$$- [\text{Patient PRBC volume (mL)}]$$

The average prime volume of the circuits in use at Texas Children's Hospital is shown in Table 19.2. Other prime additives are heparin, antifibrinolytics, antiinflammatory agents (corticosteroids), antibiotics, vasodilators, and, sometimes, diuretics (mannitol, furosemide). At the end of the case and before separation from bypass, a blood gas sample should be analyzed to ensure the electrolytes (including calcium and magnesium ions), glucose, and hematocrit are within a desired range. Acid-base changes and sodium concentration are corrected with sodium bicarbonate and wash solutions, and residual lactate is washed out using hemofiltration.

ANTIFIBRINOLYTIC AGENTS
Aprotinin
Inhibitors of serine proteases regulate and prevent uncontrolled activation of thrombin, coagulation factors, complement products, kallikrein, trypsin, elastase, and cathepsin among others of these potent enzymes (see Chapter 20). Of the serine protease inhibitors, the broad-spectrum agent aprotinin is the most widely studied in both experimental and clinical settings. Aprotinin is derived from bovine lung. It inhibits plasmin, kallikrein, trypsin, and other proteases, resulting in both antiinflammatory and antifibrinolytic effects and maintenance of glycoprotein homeostasis.

The first use of aprotinin in pediatric cardiac surgery was reported in 1990[25]; a high-dose regimen was administered to 28 children that included those undergoing a reoperation or surgery for transposition of the great arteries or endocarditis. No reduction in blood loss or drainage was observed; there were no adverse effects, and the time to chest closure from the end of cardiopulmonary bypass was reduced.

Despite the expense of aprotinin, follow-up studies reported more favorable results. Its use has reduced overall costs, from a reduced number of blood products used, operative time, duration of postoperative ventilation, and hospitalization.[26,27] This was confirmed in a comparative analysis among antifibrinolytic medications.[28] However, this benefit was observed only in complex repairs and the use of a high-dose regimen.[29] The lesser effect of a low-dose regimen may be attributable to the dilutional effects in pediatric surgery compared with the adult population.[30] Pediatric lung transplantation has been studied as a potential target group for the use of aprotinin.[31] As in most high-risk groups, a significant benefit was found for children with repeat operations (defined as repeat sternotomies or repeat transplantations), either with a high- or a low-dose regimen. This is consistent with our experience. Also, in general, infants younger than 6 months of age and those with repeat sternotomies benefit from a high-dose regimen of aprotinin[32] compared with reduced doses, despite greater drug costs. Economic studies have shown a cost-effective benefit of aprotinin in repeat cardiac procedures.[26,27]

Aprotinin influences the inflammatory response to CPB in children.[33] There has been a decrease in the duration of postoperative mechanical ventilation[34] and an improved PaO_2/FIO_2 (ratio of arterial oxygen concentration to the fraction of inspired oxygen, or P/F ratio), as an indicator of an attenuated reperfusion injury of the lung.[35] The clinical relevance of its antiinflammatory action remains unclear but points toward significant antiinflammatory properties.

Although a standard dosing regimen has yet to be defined in children, pediatric studies have demonstrated decreases in operative time after CPB, in exposure to donor blood products, and in postoperative chest tube drainage.[34] In vitro plasma concentrations of aprotinin have been related to antifibrinolytic and antiinflammatory activity at concentrations of 50 to 125 kallikrein inhibitor units (KIU)/mL and 200 KIU/mL, respectively.[26,36,37] Anaphylactic and anaphylactoid reactions may occur with aprotinin, and a test dose should be given before administration of the loading dose or addition of aprotinin to the CPB circuit. In a retrospective review of 681 children, reactions occurred in 1% of first exposures, 1.3% of second exposures, and 2.9% of more frequent exposures.[38]

We used aprotinin for complex neonatal repairs, such as arterial switch operations or Norwood procedures, as well as for most reoperative procedures and organ transplantations.[39,40] The drug is currently unavailable in the United States and Europe because of safety concerns in adults, who presented with a different profile of complications after cardiac surgery than children. Aprotinin has been shown to be safe and effective in the neonate.[41] Furthermore, serious questions have been raised regarding the statistical method used in the sentinel study that questioned the safety of aprotinin. Aprotinin continues to be used in Australia and New Zealand and has been reintroduced for adult coronary artery bypass graft surgery in Canada. Our dosing regimen is based on a 60,000 KIU/kg loading dose by the intravenous (IV) route and in the pump prime. The aprotinin infusion (7000 KIU/kg per hour) is started before skin incision. This infusion rate maintains the blood concentrations until the end of surgery at which time it is discontinued, just before leaving the operating room. Regimens based on body surface area are also used, along with a CPB prime dose that is based on the priming volume designed to achieve a plasma level above 200 KIU/mL. An example of one such calculation is a 0.85 to 1.7×10^6 KIU/m^2 loading dose both into the patient and the bypass prime, and an infusion of 2.0 to 4.0 $\times$ 10^5 KIU/m^2 per hour.[26]

The Lysine Analogs: Aminocaproic Acid and Tranexamic Acid

Despite meticulous surgical technique, it is still frequently difficult to achieve adequate hemostasis after CPB, particularly in neonates. ε-Aminocaproic acid (EACA) and tranexamic acid (TXA) are analogs of the amino acid lysine that exert their antifibrinolytic effects by interfering with the binding of plasminogen to fibrin, thereby preventing the activation of the active plasmin (see Chapter 20). TXA may also improve hemostasis by preventing plasmin-induced platelet activation. Both EACA and TXA exercise some antiinflammatory properties, but not to the same extent as aprotinin. In one study, EACA reduced bleeding postoperatively in 25 of 71 children undergoing cardiac surgery on CPB but only benefited children with cyanotic heart disease.[42] The empirical EACA loading dose was 75 mg/kg followed by an infusion of 15 mg/kg per hour, with an additional 75 mg/kg was added to the CPB prime. A larger loading dose of 150 mg/kg that was followed by an infusion of 30 mg/kg per hour of EACA has also been studied. In the latter case, intraoperative blood loss was reduced, although postoperative blood loss did not differ between the treatments.[43] Blood coagulation measured with a thromboelastograph showed less fibrinolysis with EACA. The clearance of EACA is reduced in neonates compared with children and adults; dosing requirements in neonates were approximately half of those for children and adults. A regimen of 40 mg/kg as a loading dose, 30 mg/kg per hour infusion, and a pump prime concentration of 100 mg/L effectively maintained the plasma concentration in excess of 50 mg/L in 90% of neonates undergoing cardiac surgery using cardiopulmonary bypass.[44] Dosing regimens for EACA at Texas Children's Hospital are displayed in Table 19.3. A recent meta-analysis established the efficacy of EACA in pediatric cardiac surgery.[45]

TXA compares favorably with EACA but confers a particular benefit in children with cyanotic heart disease alone.[46] Those with acyanotic defects and those who required repeat sternotomies did not benefit from TXA, although that dosing regimen only included a single 50 mg/kg loading dose before incision. In children, the TXA plasma concentration between the peak of the loading dose and the end of CPB decreased 80% when it was not followed by a continuous infusion.[47]

Although less efficient than aprotinin, EACA and TXA are equally effective in reducing perioperative blood loss in pediatric cardiac surgery.[48] Given their safety profile, they may be even more appealing in the future. Further studies are needed to delineate

TABLE 19.3	ε-Aminocaproic Acid Dosing (Texas Children's Hospital)		
Age (Weight)	**Loading Dose to Patient**	**Infusion Dose**	**Loading Dose to Bypass Circuit**
<30 days (3.5 kg)	40 mg/kg	30 mg/kg per hour	0.1 mg/mL of CPB prime volume
1 months–12 years (3.5–40 kg)	75 mg/kg	15 mg/kg per hour	75 mg/kg
>12 years (>40 kg)	5 g	1 g/hour	5 g

Neonatal dose from Eaton MP, Alfieris GM, Sweeney DM, et al. Pharmacokinetics of epsilon-aminocaproic acid in neonates undergoing cardiac surgery with cardiopulmonary bypass. *Anesthesiology* 2015;122(5):1002–1009.
Child dose from Ririe DG, James RL, O'Brien JJ, et al. The pharmacokinetics of epsilon-aminocaproic acid in children undergoing surgical repair of congenital heart defects. *Anesth Analg.* 2002;94(1):44–49.

their pharmacokinetic profiles and their efficacy. We use EACA based on simulation results from a study in children and adults.[49] An initial loading dose of 75 mg/kg over 10 minutes followed by an infusion rate of 15 mg/kg per hour complemented a 75-mg/kg dose in the pump to maintain serum concentrations in excess of the therapeutic concentration (assumed to be 130 μg/mL) in more than 95% of children.

Special Coagulation and Hematologic Problems

HEPARIN-INDUCED THROMBOCYTOPENIA

The use of unfractionated heparin for anticoagulation for CPB in adults produces antiheparin antibodies in 25% to 50% of patients within 10 days postoperatively. In a small minority of these patients, high-titer immunoglobulin G (IgG) platelet-activating antibodies form and make immune complexes with heparin and platelet factor 4 (PF4).[50] This results in activation of platelets (via their Fc receptors) and formation of procoagulant platelet microparticles, leading to thrombin generation and thrombosis. Thus the major problem in heparin-induced thrombocytopenia (HIT) is thrombocytopenia that occurs several days after heparin exposure accompanied by thrombosis, often in major vessels or structures. HIT appears to be less common, of milder course, and probably underrecognized in neonates and children. About 1% of children exposed to CPB have PF4 antibodies when tested before their second exposure to CPB, and actual HIT is much less common.[51] When HIT is suspected, either PF4 enzyme-linked immunosorbent assay or a functional assay for HIT can be used to make the diagnosis; if positive, no further heparin should be given. If CPB is necessary, alternatives to heparin, such as the direct thrombin inhibitors argatroban, lepirudin, and bivalirudin, may be used. None of these agents is approved for use in children for anticoagulation for CPB, but case reports and small series have documented their successful use when HIT is diagnosed.[52–54] The partial thromboplastin time (PTT), activated clotting time (ACT), and a specialized clotting time called the *ecarin clotting time* can be used to follow anticoagulation with these agents, but there is no reversal agent for them. Thus, treatment of post-CPB bleeding involves only administration of blood products and coagulation factors.

ANTITHROMBIN III DEFICIENCY

Heparin produces anticoagulation by combining in a 1:1 ratio with antithrombin III (ATIII), which then binds to and inhibits thrombin, leading to anticoagulation. Of adult patients, 4% to 13% have a resistance to normal doses of heparin for CPB; most instances occur because of a partial deficiency of ATIII, rendering heparin less effective at producing anticoagulation.[55] In children this is often unknown, and the first suspicion of ATIII deficiency may occur when the standard heparin dose of 300 to 400 units/kg fails to adequately anticoagulate before CPB; that is, the ACT remains less than 300 seconds. The usual response is to apply another dose of heparin from a different vial and remeasure the ACT, but if the ACT is still not adequately prolonged, a diagnosis of ATIII deficiency may be suspected. Infants younger than 6 months of age and children with congenital heart disease have decreased ATIII concentrations.[56] Therefore heparin may not achieve adequate anticoagulation, and disorders in hemostasis and thrombosis and an exaggerated inflammatory response may occur. In this case, blood can be sent for ATIII levels, but to proceed with CPB, the ATIII must be increased. This can be accomplished in two ways: (1) by supplementing ATIII with 75 units/kg of recombinant ATIII and ensuring that the ACT is adequately prolonged before proceeding with CPB, or (2) by adding FFP (which has ample concentrations of ATIII) to the CPB prime or administering it to the child before bypass.[55,57]

In the presence of reduced baseline concentrations of ATIII, the total dose of heparin, the amount of thrombin that was generated during bypass, and the fibrinogen that was consumed and fibrinolysis that was produced increased in infants undergoing cardiac surgery with CPB. This can exacerbate after bypass coagulopathy and transfusion requirements.[58,59]

RECOMBINANT FACTOR VIIA FOR MASSIVE HEMORRHAGE

Recombinant factor VIIa (rFVIIa) was originally approved for use in patients with hemophilia who possess inhibitors to factors VIII or IX, and was shown to be effective in treating bleeding in these patients with doses of 90 μg/kg (see also Chapter 10).[60] Endogenous factor VII circulates at small concentrations in the plasma. At a site of tissue or blood vessel injury, tissue factor (TF) is exposed, and the extrinsic coagulation pathway is activated by the binding of factor VII to TF, resulting in the activation of factor X to factor Xa, leading to the generation of thrombin from prothrombin, with further activation of platelets and the coagulation cascade.[61] Large concentrations of rFVIIa activate the extrinsic pathway at the site of injury, theoretically without inducing systemic hypercoagulability. However, thrombotic complications are increased after its use. rFVIIa also activates platelets, adding to the potential benefit of this agent in significant hemorrhage. Thus this therapy seems appropriate for the treatment of surgical bleeding; a very complete review of the off-label uses of rFVIIa in pediatric cardiac surgery patients found no evidence to support the routine or prophylactic use of the therapy.[61a] However, rFVIIa may be beneficial as a rescue therapy for severe life-threatening refractory bleeding; the authors caution against the use of rFVIIa in children at risk for thromboembolic complications.[62] A dose of 45 to 90 μg/kg, repeated every 2 hours, has been used. rFVIIa cannot produce hemostasis alone and should only be administered after the transfusion of sufficient amounts of platelets, plasma, and fibrinogen to form the substrate for hemostasis.

FIBRINOGEN CONCENTRATE

Fibrinogen concentrate is an alternative to cryoprecipitate to replace fibrinogen after CPB. Compared with cryoprecipitate, fibrinogen concentrate, which is lyophilized and purified human plasma fibrinogen, has an improved safety profile because it has undergone viral inactivation and is devoid of microparticles that can cause vasoreactivity. In addition, fibrinogen concentrate contains a known amount of fibrinogen, and cryoprecipitate varies in the amount of fibrinogen per unit. One randomized pilot trial found no difference in the safety and efficacy of fibrinogen concentrate compared with cryoprecipitate when managing bleeding in children undergoing CPB.[63] The dose of fibrinogen concentrate may be empiric (70 mg/kg), based on either the laboratory fibrinogen concentration or thromboelastometry.

SICKLE CELL DISEASE

Sickle cell disease (SCD), one of the most common hemoglobinopathies among patients of African American or West Indian origin (with a prevalence of 0.2%–0.3% in that population), is the result of the substitution of valine for glutamic acid in position 6 of the β-hemoglobin chain. Normal adult hemoglobin is referred to as HbA, whereas hemoglobin containing the mutant β-hemoglobin chains is referred to as HbS. SCD is represented by a homozygous genotype (HbSS) with fractional concentrations of HbS in the range from 70% to 90%. Sickle cell trait, on the other hand, is a heterozygous manifestation (HbAS) with a prevalence of 8% to 10% in the same population. The definitive diagnosis of any sickle cell hemoglobinopathy is confirmed by hemoglobin electrophoresis (see Chapter 10).

Children with SCD are at particular risk for perioperative complications.[64,65] Sickling can be triggered by hypoxia, dehydration, acidosis,[66] hypothermia, stress, and infections. Hypoxia opens a Ca^{2+}-activated K^+ channel (Gardos channel) that causes intracellular dehydration.[67] Chain formation occurs that leads to increased blood viscosity with vasoocclusion. Opening of the Gardos channel, which is an important mechanism of sickle cell dehydration, depends on temperature, with greater potassium efflux at reduced temperatures.[68] Shrinkage of sickle erythrocytes may also result from activation of a K^+/Cl^- cotransport pathway under acidotic conditions.[69] Activation of this pathway can be blocked by increasing the abnormally low level of intracellular magnesium in sickled erythrocytes. The use of magnesium and hydroxyurea in the perioperative period therefore seems to be reasonable.[70]

CPB, particularly for more complex surgical procedures, may involve periods of low flow or even circulatory arrest, as well as hypothermia with consequent local vasoconstriction, hypoxemia, and acidosis. There is some evidence that CPB can be safely undertaken in SCD.[71] Flow conditions are an important determinant of sickle erythrocyte adherence to endothelium. Under low-flow conditions, the adhesion of sickled cells to endothelium increases with contact time in the absence of endothelium activation or adhesive proteins, whereas under low-flow conditions in venules, sickle cell adhesion occurs only after endothelial activation. During CPB, both low-flow conditions and endothelial activation may occur. Multiple triggers of sickling are likely to occur during CPB, and close attention should be paid to the conduct of all aspects of bypass.

In the past, routine exchange transfusion has been recommended to prevent these complications.[72] More recent experience provides evidence that not all children require an exchange transfusion.[73] The growing evidence of the harmful effects of blood transfusion adds to the need to carefully reconsider routine exchange transfusion.[74] For uncomplicated bypass surgery without periods of cardiac arrest, the omission of exchange transfusion has led to good outcomes.

Guidelines have been proposed for the perioperative management of children with sickle cell disorders.[73] It is essential to avoid hypothermia using tepid or warm CPB in its stead; blood transfusion only for a decrease in hematocrit to less than 20%; maintenance of intravascular volume and body temperature while on CPB; the avoidance of vasopressors; the use of postoperative multimodal pain therapy; and early incentive spirometry to prevent pulmonary complications.[75] In our practice, we use cerebral near-infrared spectroscopy (NIRS) to help determine an acceptable lower limit of hemoglobin for the individual child.

For children undergoing hypothermia, successful management with[76] and without[77] partial or complete exchange transfusion on bypass has been reported. Exchange transfusion can be performed preoperatively or on initiation of CPB.[78] For exchange transfusion during CPB, the extracorporeal circuit is primed with blood and the usual components. When CPB is commenced, the child's blood volume is drained into storage bags and separated. The platelet-rich plasma is reinfused at the end of CPB, and the concentrated sickle cells are discarded. Platelet and plasma sequestration in conjunction with exchange transfusion reduces the need for postoperative transfusion and protects the platelets from the negative effects of CPB.[79]

There seems to be no consensus as to a suitable target concentration of HbS. Reducing the absolute level of HbS may provide a greater benefit than targeting a particular ratio of HbA to HbS because the remaining sickle cells are still 100% at risk for sickling.[80] In SCD, exchange transfusion has been shown to favorably affect cerebral tissue oxygenation.[81] Exchange transfusion decreases both the proportion and absolute amount of HbS, but it does not remove every cell that may sickle. It may also improve hypoxic pulmonary vasoconstriction.[81] In this context, these children may benefit from continuous hemofiltration to reduce inflammatory mediators and improve pulmonary recovery.[82] Inhaled nitric oxide also has been recommended as an adjunct to prevent sickle cell crisis. It may improve the binding of oxygen, thereby reducing the formation of sickle cells; reduce pulmonary hypertension; and improve pulmonary function without adverse effects on normal hemoglobin.[83]

A Perspective on Blood Preservation: Cardiopulmonary Bypass in Jehovah's Witness Patients

Jehovah's Witnesses differ from other religious groups in their conscious objection to the therapeutic infusion of blood and blood components. They uniformly refuse the transfusion of red blood cells, and some individuals also refuse platelets and plasma, as well as predonated autologous blood. Individual choices that can be made are the acceptance of fractions of blood, such as albumin and globulins, dialysis, cell savage, and acute isovolemic hemodilution (see Chapters 5 and 12).

Acute isovolumic reduction of hemoglobin to a concentration of 5 g/dL has been well tolerated in healthy children under anesthesia in one study and does not appear to reduce tissue oxygenation significantly.[84] Reduction of oxygen delivery to 7 to 8 mL/kg per minute under resting conditions does not increase the oxygen debt. This degree of anemia is compensated for, in part, by an increased extraction, an increase in cardiac index, and a subsequent decrease in systemic vascular resistance.[85,86] In a retrospective study of the morbidity associated with reduced concentrations of hemoglobin in Jehovah's Witness patients, the hemoglobin concentration of those who died was less than 5 g/dL.[87] A safe limit of hemodilution in children has not been established. Hemodilution in acyanotic children up to 50% appears

to be well tolerated and safe,[88] although in cyanotic children, hemodilution probably should not exceed 40%. If this level of hemodilution is exceeded, hemodynamic instability and inadequate oxygen delivery can occur. Evidence suggests that hematocrit concentrations of 21.5% in infants on CPB significantly increase adverse psychomotor developmental outcomes compared with concentrations of 27.8%.[89]

The most important and simplest strategy to avoid transfusion in the setting of cardiac surgery is to limit blood loss. Unnecessary and reduced amounts of blood removed for testing and sampling reduce the blood loss.[90] Pharmacologic agents, such as aprotinin, TXA and EACA, reduce the risk of perioperative blood loss.[91] The administration of erythropoietin in the cardiac surgery setting has been shown to reduce the risk of exposure to allergenic blood.[92] Preoperative recombinant erythropoietin is an acceptable strategy to Jehovah's Witnesses to augment the red cell concentration. This strategy requires that oral iron (2–6 mg/kg of elemental iron in 2–3 divided doses) and vitamin C are started about 6 weeks before surgery followed by twice weekly erythropoietin (50–100 IU/kg) intramuscularly about 3 weeks before surgery. Hemoglobin concentrations should be tracked to ensure that the concentration does not exceed 15 to 20 g/dL as venous thromboembolism may occur. Some Jehovah's Witnesses refuse albumin, a constituent in the preparation of erythropoietin that is supplied in glass ampoules. In the latter case, a lyophilized preparation of erythropoietin, which is albumin-free, may be used. The cost of erythropoietin can be substantial, and one cost analysis suggested that its use in cardiac surgery is not cost-effective.[93]

Intraoperative recovery of blood with a cell salvage device is also acceptable to many Jehovah's Witnesses. This involves the removal by suction of blood from the operative field followed by washing, filtering, and return of red blood cells to the patient. A randomized controlled trial of intraoperative cell salvage in cardiothoracic surgery demonstrated a reduction in RBC transfusion and an increase in postoperative hemoglobin.[94]

Acute normovolemic hemodilution involves the preoperative removal of a volume of blood from the patient with the simultaneous administration of crystalloid or colloid to maintain circulating volume.[95] The collected blood is then reinfused during the operation. Some Jehovah's Witnesses find this process acceptable, especially if the blood remains in continuity with the patient throughout. Acute normovolemic hemodilution has other advantages, including lower costs, because the blood does not need compatibility testing; reduced the possibility of administrative error; and achieved patient time-saving (see also Chapters 10 and 12). The development of artificial red cell substitutes could potentially obviate the need for compatibility testing, as well as vastly reduce infection risks, with none of the immunomodulatory side effects of allogeneic blood.[96] Some of these products would also be acceptable to Jehovah's Witness families. Substitutes include perfluorocarbons, hemoglobin solutions, intramolecular cross-linked hemoglobin, and liposome-encapsulated hemoglobin. None of these has reached clinical practice. Lastly, autologous retrograde priming has been used in Jehovah's Witness patients and can further reduce the hemodilutional effects of the prime.[95,97] For this purpose, priming of the arterial line of the CPB circuit is accomplished with the patients' own blood.

Modern bypass circuits reduce the priming volumes to less than 200 to 300 mL. Main components that are amenable to volume reduction on a regular circuit are the size and length of the lines, small oxygenators and arterial filters, and priming the hemofilter for modified ultrafiltration with blood from the venous line after

CPB. Line volumes, for example, may vary from 1.73 mL per 10 cm of a $\frac{3}{16}$-inch tubing to 0.75 mL per 10 cm of a $\frac{1}{8}$-inch tubing. The limiting factor, however, is the necessary flow. For a $\frac{3}{16}$-inch arterial line, a maximum flow of 1.8 L/minute was established as the point at which the Reynolds number reaches a critical value indicating turbulent flow, which may damage RBCs. Modified ultrafiltration at the end of CPB through a fluid warmer line to prevent heat loss or continuous ultrafiltration has been used. The venous line and the reservoir are emptied before discontinuation of bypass, the field is suctioned, and all blood is retransfused through the arterial line. Decannulation is achieved and protamine is given as usual. Crystalloid cardioplegia solution should be evacuated from the field by an external sucker to prevent dilution of the pump volume.

Postoperative care involves minimal blood sampling, and only on special indications. Noninvasive monitoring allows uncomplicated weaning from the ventilator.[98] The first report of successful outcomes in Jehovah's Witness children with congenital cardiac defects was in 1985[99]; 110 children older than 6 months of age successfully underwent operation, with a perioperative mortality rate of 5.3%. Only one death was attributed to blood loss. A weight less than 5 kg is considered by some as a contraindication for open-heart surgery and palliative procedures were advocated in the past.[100] For some lesions, however, no palliation is possible. The development of miniaturized circuits, preoperative optimization, use of antithrombolytic drugs, vacuum-assisted drainage to allow smaller tubing and cannula sizes, as well as the use of modified ultrafiltration, enabled the safe expansion of surgery into the neonatal population. Individualized heparin level–based anticoagulation management further results in a reduction of coagulation problems, blood loss, and transfusion requirements.[101] The addition of desmopressin, 0.3 µg/kg, is thought by some to improve platelet activity and stimulate the release of von Willebrand factor after protamine infusion, although this is not evidence-based.

In one study, when center-specific blood conservation strategies were used, bloodless cardiac surgery was most successful in children greater than 18 kg in weight, followed by those 6 to 18 kg in weight. All 73 patients less than 6 kg in weight had transfusions during their hospitalization.[102]

All of the aforementioned considerations are important in approaching the Jehovah's Witness patient; however, at Texas Children's Hospital, Jehovah's Witness children are not treated differently with regard to blood transfusion practice than any other child. Cerebral NIRS is used to help determine the safe hemoglobin level for the individual child at all phases of surgery. Consent for blood transfusion in this situation is a complicated issue, because the legal status of children differs from that of an adult. Each institution must develop a legal informed consent process for blood transfusion for Jehovah's Witness children, in consultation with local legal authorities, social work and ethnic groups, and representatives of the Jehovah's Witness faith (see Chapter 5). Currently, we have a release of liability form for the parents to sign stating that he or she requests that no blood products be used, but acknowledges they may be needed to treat his or her child. The parent further agrees to release and hold harmless the physicians and hospital for any liability associated with blood transfusion. This form was developed in conjunction with the local Jehovah's Witness church representatives, and in our practice this has been accepted by more than 95% of parents and has obviated the need for more extreme measures, such as temporary child protective services custody during the perioperative period, which was our former practice.

Myocardial Protection

Myocardial protection during cardiac surgery has evolved over the years, and the concept of chemical cardioplegia was introduced in 1955.[103] Before the popular use of chemical cardioplegia, topical cardiac hypothermia was used. In the late 1970s and early 1980s, the concept of cold hyperkalemic blood cardioplegia was introduced.[104] Potassium concentrations in cardioplegic solutions ranging from 12 to 30 mEq/L are typically used to achieve cardiac standstill within 1 to 2 minutes under hypothermic conditions, with greater concentrations or induction times required for normothermic conditions. Myocardial edema after bypass and global ischemia can be reduced by a number of strategies that involve modifying the conditions of delivery and composition of cardioplegia solutions as they affect the movement of intracellular and interstitial fluid. In contrast to studies in adults, most studies conducted in neonates have shown little difference between blood and crystalloid cardioplegia.[105,106] Hypothermia also decreases myocardial oxygen consumption. The benefits of this approach appear to be optimal at myocardial temperatures between 24°C and 28°C. However, there is growing evidence that warm, intermittent blood cardioplegia may be advantageous to either cold crystalloid or cold blood cardioplegia.[107] The benefits of blood cardioplegia are more pronounced in younger, cyanotic children who require longer aortic cross-clamping. For acyanotic children, the cardioplegic technique is probably not as critical.[108] Avoidance or reduction of myocardial edema occurs by limiting the pressure of cardioplegia infusions and by providing moderately hyperosmolar cardioplegia solutions that contain blood. Buffering the acidosis that results from ischemia is achieved by including tromethamine, histidine-imidazole, or both in the cardioplegia solution. Close management of myocardial calcium balance to avoid extremes of intracellular hypercalcemia or hypocalcemia, especially during reperfusion, is very important.[109,110] The addition of magnesium may solve this dilemma by preventing damage from greater cardioplegic calcium concentrations by its action as a calcium antagonist.[110,111] This prevents mitochondrial calcium overload as a consequence of reperfusion injury. Magnesium also prevents the influx of sodium into the postischemic myocardium, which is exchanged for calcium during reperfusion.

Every cardiac program has its own philosophy regarding cardioplegia and myocardial protection. At Texas Children's Hospital, plain crystalloid cardioplegia is used. The prime blood gas and electrolytes should mimic physiologically the child's arterial blood gas as closely as possible. If whole blood or packed cells are added to the prime, the target hemodilution range should be 28% to 30%; the prime should be recirculated continuously and warmed between 35.0°C and 36.5°C before initiation of bypass. In neonates and infants, albumin is added to the cardioplegic solution to maintain an appropriate colloid osmotic pressure. This may decrease edema formation of the arrested heart. In children undergoing circulatory arrest, long cross-clamp times, and large pump suction return cases, 20 mg/kg methylprednisolone is used, up to a maximum of 500 mg, to reduce the production of inflammatory mediators that result in myocardial dysfunction. Table 19.4 summarizes the Texas Children's Hospital protocols for cardioplegia and myocardial protection.

Phases of Cardiopulmonary Bypass

Surgical cases requiring CPB are divided into several basic phases.

TABLE 19.4 | Cardioplegia Solution

CARDIOPLEGIA BASE SOLUTION (385 ML)

Concentration		Contents	
Sodium chloride BP	3.54 g/L	Sodium	23 mmol
Anhydrous glucose BP	6.65 g/L	Potassium	15 mmol
Potassium chloride	2.92 g/L	Calcium	0.35 mmol
Mannitol	6.54 g/L	Chloride	39 mmol
Calcium chloride	135 mg/L	Glucose	2.52 g
		Mannitol	2.48 g
		Approximate pH 4.5	
		275 mOsm/L	

CARDIOPLEGIA BUFFER SOLUTION

Concentration		Contents	
Sodium carbonate	9.37 g/L	Sodium carbonate	0.28 g
Sodium bicarbonate	27.0 g/L	Sodium bicarbonate	0.81 g

USES OF CARDIOPLEGIA SOLUTION DURING CARDIOPULMONARY BYPASS

Children Weighing <10 kg

385 mL Cardioplegia base solution

26 mL Cardioplegia buffer solution

100 mL 25% Albumin

Note: This is usually delivered at a pressure of 30 mm Hg for newborns and 30–40 mm Hg for older infants.

Children weighing >10 kg

385 mL Cardioplegia base solution

100 mL 0.9% Sodium chloride

10 mL 25% Mannitol

5 mL 8.4% Sodium bicarbonate

Note: This is usually delivered at a pressure of 30–60 mm Hg. A good guide is to note the end-diastolic pressure of each child before bypass. This will be a guide to the normal filling pressure of the coronary arteries. When aortic incompetence is present, the CPS flow may need to be increased.

ADMINISTRATION OF CARDIOPLEGIA SOLUTION

For All Patients:

Temperature	8°C–12°C
Initial dose	110 mL/m² per minute for 4 minutes
Subsequent doses	110 mL/m² per minute for 2 minutes

Note: Following the initial dose, cardioplegia is delivered every 20 minutes during the cross-clamp period unless otherwise indicated by the surgeon. The perfusionist will remind the surgeon of the need for cardioplegia and keep track of the time. Because of the nature of the surgical procedure, it may be necessary to deliver cardioplegia directly into the coronary ostia via a handheld delivery system. In this case, the surgeon will direct the perfusionist. Close attention should be paid to the delivery line pressures.

EXAMPLES OF PRIMES

Neonate: Whole Blood, if Available, Otherwise Reconstituted

Whole blood	225 mL
PlasmaLyte A	50 mL
0.45% NaCl	125 mL
Heparin	2500 units
NaHCO₃	5 mEq
CaCl₂	250 mg

Pediatric: Packed Red Blood Cells

PRBCs	250 mL
Plasmalyte A	300 mL
0.45% NaCl	75 mL
25% Albumin	100 mL
Heparin	3500 units
NaHCO₃	20 mEq
CaCl₂	300 mg

Adult: Crystalloid Prime

PlasmaLyte A	700 mL
0.45% NaCl	600 mL
25% Albumin	100–200 mL (volume varies depending on the size of the patient)
5% Dextrose	40 mL
Heparin	5000 units
NaHCO₃	40 mEq
CaCl₂	300 mg
KCl	2.4 mEq

BP, the material conforms to the specifications and procedures outlined in the British Pharmacopoeia; *CPS*, cardioplegia solution; *PRBCs*, packed red blood cells.

PREBYPASS PERIOD

This phase begins with surgical incision and lasts through initial dissection and preparation for cannulation. During this period transesophageal echocardiography (TEE) is performed to confirm the diagnosis and establish a basis for postbypass comparison.

CANNULATION AND INITIATION OF BYPASS

After sternotomy and mediastinal dissection, the aorta is cannulated, along with either the right atrium, if single venous drainage is planned, or the superior and inferior venae cavae for bicaval venous drainage. After a large dose of heparin (300-400 units/kg) is administered intravenously, the adequacy of the anticoagulation is measured using the ACT *before initiating CPB*. The target ACT is usually 480 seconds. High ACTs are maintained during CPB with the addition of heparin to the prime as needed, because larger doses of heparin lead to a reduced degree of consumptive coagulopathy, which translates into reduced blood product requirements.[101] Other methods of measuring anticoagulation include the Hepcon system (a plasma heparin concentration assay), which may allow for more accurate titration of heparin and protamine dosages since ACT is prolonged by hypothermia, hemodilution, platelet dysfunction, and low coagulation factor levels.[112,113] The thromboelastogram may also be used as a baseline measure of the coagulation system and then repeated during and after bypass, with heparinase added to more objectively assess each child's anticipated need for coagulation factors.[114,115] An improved preservation of the hemostatic system with subsequent reduction in blood loss and transfusion requirements has been demonstrated after maintenance of high heparin levels during CPB.[116] The additional maintenance of high ATIII concentrations may further contribute to a reduction of hemostatic activation.[117]

In most centers, bicaval cannulation is used for all but the smallest children (<2 kg) to prevent venous return from interfering with the surgical field. A gradual transition to full CPB is then performed to minimize myocardial stress, using a prime that has essentially the same composition as the child's blood with regard to temperature, pH, calcium, potassium, and hematocrit. CPB flows of 150 mL/kg per minute are used for infants weighing less than 10 kg, and 2.4 L/minute per meter squared is used for children weighing more than 10 kg. Flow rates may be reduced during periods of hypothermia (see later), although many centers now prefer to maintain greater flows throughout the bypass period. Misplaced cannulas can lead to significant morbidity. Obstruction of the inferior vena cava (IVC) by a misplaced IVC cannula can lead to increased venous pressure, which causes ascites and decreased perfusion pressure in mesenteric, hepatic, and renal vascular beds. Misplacement of the cannula in the superior vena cava can result in cerebral edema from inadequate venous drainage and a subsequent reduction in cerebral blood flow, potentially resulting in ischemia. Arterial cannula misplacement can also occur. If the cannula inadvertently slips beyond the takeoff of the right innominate artery, preferential perfusion to the left side of the brain can be observed. This can be detected on the NIRS monitor, which may be an important monitor, particularly in pediatric cardiac surgery.[118]

The presence of any anomalous systemic-to-pulmonary shunts can lead to shunting of blood away from the systemic circulation, through the pulmonary circuit, and then through the venous cannula to the CPB machine. Thus, the systemic perfusion is shunted away from the body in a futile circuit back to the CPB machine. Anatomic lesions where such shunting can occur include an unrecognized patent ductus arteriosus and large aortopulmonary collaterals, as found in pulmonary atresia. Bypass flow needs to be increased to compensate for these shunts until they can be controlled.

COOLING PHASE
Systemic cooling is used frequently in pediatric cardiac surgery, but normothermia is used with increasing frequency in modern practice for selected cases.[119] Hypothermia is classified as mild (30°C–36°C), moderate (22°C–30°C), or deep (17°C–22°C). In general, the coldest temperatures are used for more complex operations that carry a greater potential for requiring periods of low-flow bypass or circulatory arrest. Cooling is primarily achieved extracorporeally through the heat exchanger in the bypass circuit; some surgeons may request that ice be applied to the head to prevent brain rewarming during circulatory arrest.

AORTIC CROSS-CLAMPING AND INTRACARDIAC REPAIR PHASE
The aorta is cross-clamped, with the heart then rendered asystolic after infusion of cardioplegia solution into the aortic root.

DEEP HYPOTHERMIC CIRCULATORY ARREST OR SELECTIVE CEREBRAL PERFUSION PHASE
If circulatory arrest is to be used, it is initiated after a slow cooling period of at least 20 minutes, and an attempt is made to limit the total duration of deep hypothermic circulatory arrest (DHCA) to less than 40 minutes. Special bypass techniques (see later) have been developed to avoid the necessity of using DHCA and may also be performed during this time.

REMOVAL OF AORTIC CROSS-CLAMP AND REWARMING PHASE
After completion of the intracardiac repair and de-airing of the heart, the aortic cross-clamp is removed, allowing reperfusion of the myocardium. Optimally, normal sinus rhythm and myocardial contractility are restored during this time, while the child is slowly rewarmed. During rewarming, surgery is completed, inotropic and vasoactive agents are started, the trachea is suctioned, and ventilation begins. Hemofiltration and blood transfusion are used to achieve the desired hematocrit. Left atrial and/or pulmonary artery monitoring lines, if indicated, are placed at this time, as are temporary atrial and ventricular pacing wires. If the child is incompletely rewarmed before separation from CPB, a significant afterdrop with precipitous postbypass reduction in core body temperature can occur. This can lead to vasoconstriction, shivering, increased oxygen consumption, and acidosis. However, postischemic hyperthermia can lead to delayed neuronal cell death.[120] Mild degrees of hypothermia and certainly the avoidance of hyperthermia are essential in the perioperative period.[121] In children, rectal temperature mostly reflects peripheral temperature. One study showed that the temperature of the foot was more sensitive than the temperature of the hand.[122] Another study revealed that for anatomic or physiologic reasons, temperature gradients in the toes develop more readily than those in the fingers.[123] Several endpoints have been proposed, such as nasopharyngeal temperatures greater than 35.0°C, bladder temperature greater than 36.2°C, or skin temperatures greater than 30°C[124,125]; we use an endpoint of 35.5°C rectal temperature.[126]

SEPARATION FROM BYPASS
The child's core body temperature, hematocrit, and metabolic variables should be optimized before attempting separation from CPB. Careful observation for air in the systemic ventricle, confirmation with the TEE, and concurrent inspection of electrocardiogram (ECG) changes should continue throughout the weaning process, with the child in the Trendelenburg position and the aortic root vented. While fluid volume is gradually added to the child by reducing the outflow to the venous reservoir until optimal filling pressures are achieved, CPB flow is then slowly reduced to zero. If inotropic support is anticipated to separate from CPB, infusions should be initiated before beginning separation.

POSTBYPASS PERIOD
This phase lasts until chest closure and transfer to the ICU have been accomplished. During this time, modified ultrafiltration (MUF) may be performed for 10 to 15 minutes after cessation of CPB. Cardiac function and the quality of the surgical repair are assessed using TEE, and if found to be satisfactory, protamine is administered to neutralize residual heparin. The usual dose of protamine is 1.0 to 1.3 mg/100 units of heparin given at the onset of bypass. Limiting protamine to this dose prevents an overdose with its associated effects on platelet function (reduction of the interaction of glycoprotein Ib receptor interaction with von Willebrand factor).[127] If the ACT remains increased or prime blood is given back to the child, an additional 10% of the initial dose of protamine is added and the ACT is rechecked, keeping in mind that high ACT values after bypass may be related to factors other than the presence of residual heparin.[128]

Early use of heparinase-assisted thrombelastography or protamine titration ACT will allow a diagnostic separation of residual heparin effect. However, particularly in infants, the administration of protamine and the persistent treatment of a suspected incomplete heparin reversal should not distract and delay the treatment of other commonly associated postbypass coagulopathies, such as thrombocytopenia, platelet dysfunction, hypofibrinogenemia, and other coagulation factor deficiencies. The child should be transferred to the ICU only after adequate hemostasis has been established since ongoing bleeding increases surgical mortality.[129]

Protamine reactions occur much less frequently in children younger than 16 years of age, approximately 1.8% to 2.9%.[130] Independent risk factors are a female gender, a larger protamine dose, and smaller heparin doses. Type I reactions or effects during administration are rare and adding calcium does not change the hemodynamic consequences of injection.[131] Fortunately, severe anaphylactic reactions (type II) or catastrophic pulmonary vasoconstriction (type III) are rare but have been observed.[132] Administering the protamine over 5 or more minutes reduces the severity and precipitous nature of any protamine reaction.

Unstable neonates and small infants may have their sternums temporarily left open, with surgical closure planned 24 to 72 hours later when cardiac function has improved and myocardial edema has diminished.

Because CPB can have a multitude of adverse physiologic effects, attempts are made to minimize both the duration of CPB and ischemic (aortic-clamp) time; thus, as much of the surgery as possible is performed outside of these phases. In general, physiologic responses to bypass are more extreme with decreasing age and size of the child. The neonate experiences a greater degree of hemodilution and colder temperatures on bypass and frequently requires longer aortic cross-clamp times, all of which can result in a greater inflammatory response. Table 19.5 summarizes clinical management issues during the major phases of CPB.

Particular Aspects of Management on Cardiopulmonary Bypass

PH-STAT VERSUS α-STAT MANAGEMENT

Some degree of hypothermia is used for nearly every cardiac operation to slow the metabolism and oxygen consumption of all organs, particularly the brain and heart.[133] During cooling, the carbon dioxide contained in blood becomes more soluble and its partial pressure decreases. The $PaCO_2$ sensed by the body decreases as body temperature decreases, with the result that at a core temperature of 17°C to 18°C, if pH and $PaCO_2$ have not been corrected for temperature, the body experiences a pH of about 7.6 and $PaCO_2$ of 15 to 18 mm Hg (Fig. 19.2).[134] This very low $PaCO_2$ causes cerebral vasoconstriction, particularly during the cooling phase of bypass, which in turn leads to less cerebral blood flow, less efficient brain cooling, and less cerebral protection at a given temperature.[135] Because blood samples are normally heated to 37°C before measurement of pH, $PaCO_2$, and PaO_2, the use of pH-stat management indicates that blood gases are being corrected for the child's actual body temperature by increasing the $PaCO_2$ during bypass, as it is measured at 37°C, so that the body experiences a $PaCO_2$ of approximately 40 mm Hg and a pH of 7.4 at all temperatures. Conversely, α-stat management means not correcting the blood gases for temperature, as if the child's blood was always at 37°C, with the goal of pH 7.4 and $PaCO_2$ 40 mm Hg. In the early days of CPB, pH-stat was used to preserve cerebral blood flow at all ages.[134] Subsequently, in

TABLE 19.5	Checklist for Bypass Management

Before CPB

1. Check temperature; maintain normothermia during induction and preparation.
2. Supplement premedication.
3. Ensure noninvasive monitoring: blood pressure, ECG, pulse oximetry, stethoscope.
4. Perform inhalational induction after preoxygenation; intravenous induction, if cannula is in place.
5. Peripheral intravenous placement(s)
6. Neuromuscular blockade and ventilation
7. Intubation and mechanical ventilation according to shunt lesion (CO_2, O_2 control)
8. Monitoring:
   a. Arterial line and central venous line
   b. ECG electrodes
   c. Bladder catheter
   d. Temperature probes
   e. TEE probe (in infants >3 kg)
9. Positioning
10. Deepening of anesthetic level
11. Antifibrinolytics and corticosteroids, as indicated
12. Heparin, 300–400 units/kg, before arterial cannulation
13. Check activated clotting time 400–480 seconds.
14. Supplement anesthetics on initiation of bypass.

During CPB

1. Stop ventilation and drips when full flow is reached.
2. Inspect head perfusion.
3. Evaluate quality of perfusion (perfusion pressure, central venous pressure, diuresis, arterial blood gases, temperature gradient).
4. Prepare for separation.
   a. Drips (inotropic drugs, calcium)
   b. Pacemaker
   c. Blood products
5. Set and control temperature and rewarming (heating blanket, room temperature).
6. Zero transducers
7. Check arterial blood gases in preparation for discontinuation of CPB; correct abnormalities.
8. Suction and ventilate.

After CPB

1. Separate when
   a. Temperature >35.5°C
   b. Stable rhythm or pacing
   c. Heart contracting well
2. Fine-tune blood pressure; consider direct blood pressure measurement for hypotension at the aortic cannula; volume ± drips.
3. Consider modified ultrafiltration.
4. Check arterial blood gases.
5. Evaluate with transesophageal echocardiography for residual defects and intracardiac air bubbles.
6. Give protamine, 1–1.3 mg/100 IU of initial heparin.
7. Check activated clotting time and arterial blood gases.
8. Chest closure and recheck arterial blood gases.
9. Transport to the intensive care unit.

CPB, cardiopulmonary bypass; *ECG*, electrocardiogram; *TEE*, transesophageal echocardiography.

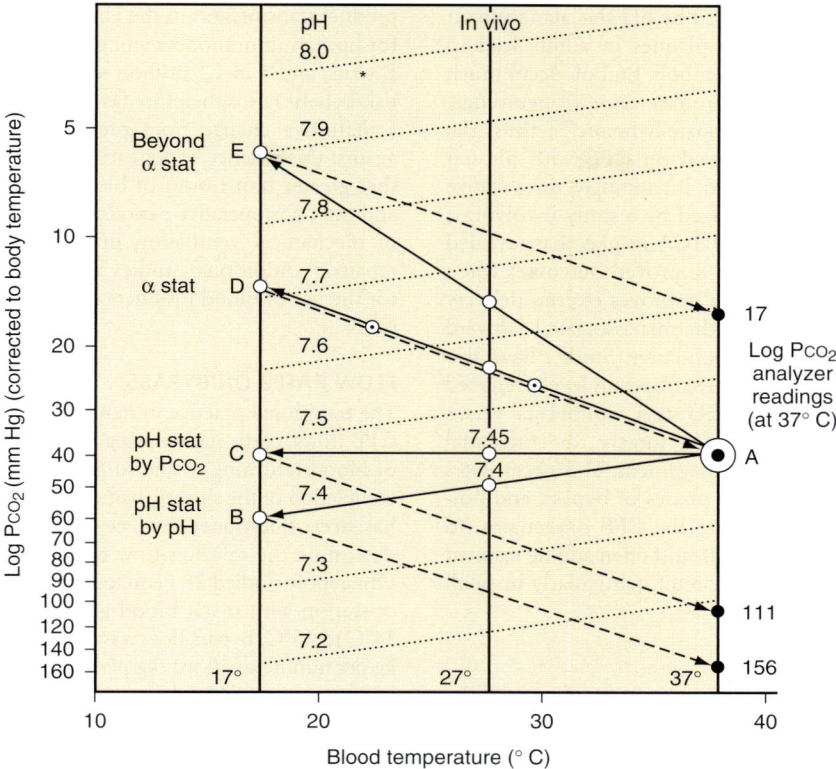

FIGURE 19.2 pH and P_{CO_2} changes when blood temperature is varied between 17°C and 37°C. Point **A** is the starting point, with pH 7.4 and P_{CO_2} 40 mm Hg at 37°C. Points **B, C, D,** and **E** are the conditions the brain experiences at 17°C with various blood gas management strategies. pH-stat management (correcting the pH and P_{CO_2} for temperature) results in an acid-base environment that is neutral, whereas α-stat management (not correcting for temperature) results in a very alkalotic environment at 17°C. Warming the blood sample (as is done for blood gas measurement) results in very high P_{CO_2} values when pH-stat is used. The pH of blood becomes slightly more alkalotic with cooling, owing to the decreased dissociation of hydrogen ions. (From Jonas RA. Carbon dioxide, pH, and oxygen management. In: Jonas RA, DiNardo J, Lawson PC, et al, eds. *Comprehensive Surgical Management of Congenital Heart Disease.* London: Arnold Publishers; 2004:151–160.)

the 1970s and 1980s, randomized controlled studies in adults confirmed that acute, post-CPB neurologic problems were worse with pH-stat management.[136] α-Stat management was, therefore, adopted for both adult and pediatric CPB. However, studies in a neonatal pig model have challenged this conclusion, proving that neurologic outcomes, both behavioral and neuropathologic, are significantly worse when α-stat management is used in infants.[135,137]

Advantages of pH-stat CPB have been shown to include:

- A decreased brain metabolic rate[138]
- An increased rate of brain cooling and reperfusion,[139] thereby providing better protection through more even and faster cooling and rewarming secondary to increased CBF[139,140]
- Molecular effects of altered PaO_2 and pH, including changes in cerebral oxygenation and brain enzyme activity, as well as decreased brain electrical activity[140-142]
- Decreased oxyhemoglobin affinity[143]
- Increased cortical oxygenation before arrest (through hypercapnic capillary vasodilation) and decreased oxygen metabolic rate, providing slower deoxygenation compared with α-stat management (~10 vs. ~7 minutes).[135,144] Cortical anoxia occurs at 36 minutes with pH-stat management versus 24 minutes for α-stat management.

In cyanotic infants with aortopulmonary collaterals, pH-stat management significantly improves brain oxygenation as measured by NIRS oximetry.[145] A retrospective study of 16 infants revealed worse neurodevelopmental outcomes with α-stat management.[146] In a randomized prospective trial of pH- versus α-stat management in 182 infants younger than 9 months of age, there was a strong trend toward improved outcomes with pH-stat management, including earlier return of electroencephalographic activity, fewer seizures, and improved psychomotor development index.[147] Another study examined the effects of α-stat and pH-stat on developmental and neurologic outcomes after deep hypothermic CPB in infants.[148] Psychomotor Development Index scores of 110 patients did not differ significantly between the groups (P = 0.97). The results of the Mental Development Index scores were dependent on diagnosis. In all but the ventricular septal defect subgroup, the pH-stat group did not have statistically greater Mental Development Index scores. Abnormalities on the electroencephalogram (P = 0.77) and neurologic examination (P = 0.70) were similar with the two methods of blood gas management. The authors concluded that the use of α-stat or pH-stat strategy is not consistently associated with improved or impaired early neurodevelopmental outcomes in infants undergoing deep hypothermic CPB.[148] One reason for the differing results between pediatric and adult studies is that the increased cerebral blood flow produced by pH-stat management and the presence of atherosclerotic plaques in adults lead to microcerebral atherosclerotic plaque emboli. Emboli occur much less frequently in children, and the primary cause of neurologic injury from CPB in children is hypoxic-ischemic[149]; thus, the increased cerebral blood flow observed on CPB with pH-stat management lessens this risk in children. Interestingly, this putative mechanism has been recently challenged by a study involving a controlled microembolic load and DHCA in pigs that revealed that pH-stat was still associated with improved outcomes when compared with α-stat.[150] pH-Stat also improves oxygen delivery by counteracting the pH- and hypothermia-associated leftward shift in the oxyhemoglobin dissociation curve. Studies have also revealed a decrease in peak postoperative troponin levels, reduced ventilator dependence, and reduced ICU stays with pH-stat versus α-stat.[151] Most programs specializing in surgery for congenital heart defects currently use pH-stat management. This necessitates careful attention to $PaCO_2$ during all phases of bypass, and possibly reducing the sweep gas flow into the CPB oxygenator (to decrease the efficiency of CO_2 removal), and often adding inspired CO_2 to the sweep gas of the bypass circuit, particularly in small infants.

HEMATOCRIT ON BYPASS

The relatively small total blood volume in infants, along with the volume required to prime the CPB circuit, means that adding blood to the CPB prime is mandatory. However this practice is institution specific; many centers add either whole blood, PRBCs with FFP (for children <8 kg), or PRBCs alone (for children <12 to 15 kg) to ensure that the hematocrit on bypass is not less than 20%. As a result of increased transfusion-related concerns from bloodborne viral disease transmission during the 1980s and 1990s, and given that a low hematocrit is thought to be necessary to ensure adequate blood flow through capillary beds (because the blood viscosity increases at low temperatures), hematocrits of 20% or less on CPB with deep hypothermia were frequently tolerated.[152] There is increasing evidence that the practice of extreme hemodilution is detrimental to neurologic outcome in children. In a newborn pig model, one group of investigators determined that the incidence and degree of hypoxic-ischemic brain injury after a period of DHCA was significantly greater with a hematocrit of 20% versus one of 30%, regardless of whether pH- or α-stat strategy was used.[153] In another newborn pig model, using intravital microscopy of pial capillaries during deep hypothermic CPB, a hematocrit of 30% did not impair cerebral microcirculation when compared with a hematocrit of 20%.[154] Finally, in a prospective randomized trial of CPB hematocrit of 20% versus 30% at Boston Children's Hospital, children in the lower hematocrit group demonstrated significantly reduced psychomotor development index scores 1 year after surgery.[89] In a follow-up study of hematocrit 25% versus 35%, the same group did not observe a difference in neurodevelopmental outcomes.[155] However, when they combined all children from both hematocrit trials, they found that a hematocrit less than 24% was associated with poorer psychomotor index scores 1 year after surgery.[156] The hypoxic-ischemic damage most likely occurs during the cooling and rewarming phases of bypass, when cerebral oxygen metabolism is not suppressed, yet hematocrit and, thus, oxygen delivery, are reduced. Therefore, many centers are now maintaining greater hematocrits on CPB (at least 25%), which either means using more donor blood products or using hemofiltration to increase the hematocrit during bypass. The current quantifiable risk of viral transmission through blood product transmission in the United States is 1 in 1.9 million units for human immunodeficiency virus, 1 in 1,000,000 for hepatitis B virus, and 1 in 1.7 million units for hepatitis C virus.[157,158] The risk/benefit ratios therefore favor the greater hematocrit approach, a definitive change from previous practice patterns. Balanced against this practice of a greater hematocrit on CPB is the finding that greater transfusion of blood products in the intraoperative and early postoperative periods is associated with a greater duration of mechanical ventilation in infants undergoing two-ventricle repairs.[159] Additional studies are required to optimize strategies for the use of blood products in infants and children undergoing CPB.

FLOW RATES ON BYPASS

The traditional practice in many institutions has been to decrease CPB flows, particularly during hypothermia, to reduce the volume of blood returning to the surgical field and allow more efficient completion of the surgery, particularly in small infants. This concept has been questioned in recent years owing to the inability to determine the safe low-flow bypass rate in the individual child. One report studied 28 neonates who underwent the arterial switch operation with α-stat blood gas management during CPB.[160] At 14°C to 15°C, bypass flow was sequentially reduced from 150 mL/kg per minute to 50 mL/kg per minute, and then further decreased in increments of 10 mL/kg per minute until circulatory arrest was initiated (to 0 mL/kg per minute). All neonates had detectable cerebral blood flow by transcranial Doppler (TCD) at CPB flows above 20 mL/kg per minute, but one had no detectable perfusion at 20 mL/kg per minute, and eight had none at 10 mL/kg per minute, leading the authors to conclude that 30 mL/kg per minute was the minimum acceptable flow in this population. A neonatal pig model determined that, at normothermia, bypass flows of at least 150 to 175 mL/kg per minute were necessary to ensure full oxygenation of all end organs and tissues.[161] Clinical studies of a high-flow bypass strategy, which included flows of 150 mL/kg per minute at all phases of bypass except during DHCA, minimal use of DHCA, and α-adrenergic receptor blockade with phenoxybenzamine to produce long-duration systemic vasodilation, demonstrated excellent short- and long-term clinical and neurodevelopmental outcomes; no child scored outside normal ranges for testing performed at a mean age of 9 years.[162] This strategy also has led to excellent early results for the Norwood operation, with an early perioperative survival of 83% for cases carried out from 1993 to 1999.[163] During the same era, one report documented that 26.7% of children who had arterial switch procedures had neurologic abnormalities, and 55% had at least one abnormal area on neurodevelopmental testing (performed at a mean of 10 years) when DHCA and low-flow bypass had been used.[163]

Vasoconstriction and increased vascular resistance, resulting in uneven regional organ perfusion, are among the undesired side effects of CPB. Endogenous catecholamine production and the alkaline α-stat CPB technique, if used, are responsible for these effects. To be able to run full flow during hypothermic CPB without significant hypertension, vasodilators are often used. Agents currently used to provide systemic vasodilation and more even cooling and rewarming include phentolamine, nitroprusside, or nitroglycerin. Phenoxybenzamine, which is no longer available, was used as part of a treatment strategy after stage 1 palliation for hypoplastic left heart syndrome and has been associated with improved outcomes.[164,165] Phenoxybenzamine was more effective than sodium nitroprusside in improving peripheral circulation, as shown by temperature gradients intraoperatively.[166] Greater

CPB flows are associated with an improved oxygen delivery, which can improve patient outcome.[167]

Phentolamine is a nonselective competitive α_1 and α_2 catecholamine receptor blocker. It has a half-life of 19 minutes and is eliminated mainly by the kidneys. Through postsynaptic α_1 and α_2 receptor inhibition it has a vasodilating and hypotensive effect that can improve cardiovascular variables and metabolic acidosis during CPB management.[168] In children receiving phentolamine, increasing lactate concentrations at the end of the CPB period show a steady state toward the end of the surgery, whereas lactate continues to increase in patients who did not receive phentolamine.[169] These findings suggest that the use of phentolamine limits lactic acid production during the hypothermic period and aids the disposal of lactic acid from tissues. Seelye and associates called the physiologic state after hypothermia the "oxygen debt repayment" period in infants.[169] Although it has a beneficial effect on CPB management, the potential harmful effects of phentolamine, especially on the brain, have still not been fully elucidated. One study provided evidence that phentolamine increases S100B protein and a parameter indicative of altered cerebrovascular resistance, the pulsatility index in the middle cerebral artery, in infants given phentolamine during open-heart surgery.[170]

Nitroprusside has been used as an easily titratable agent with direct arterial smooth muscle relaxant properties through production of nitric oxide and enhancement of the cyclic guanosine monophosphate (GMP) pathway. One study examined the effect of perioperative sodium nitroprusside in 25 neonates undergoing an arterial switch operation.[171] In comparison to the prebypass values, a similar increase in the concentration of S100B protein was found 2 hours after the termination of CPB in the sodium nitroprusside–treated and nontreated neonates, which decreased over the subsequent 48 postoperative hours. However, reduced postbypass serum levels of S100B protein were found in the sodium nitroprusside–treated group after 24 and 48 hours of treatment.

Nitroglycerin has been used with the same success. The only proven benefit over other agents is its nitric oxide donation capacity.[172] In Japan, high-dose chlorpromazine has been used as part of a low-resistance strategy during CPB for the Norwood procedure.[173]

We routinely use phentolamine, 0.1 to 0.2 mg/kg, to provide normal CPB flow and mean arterial pressure in the range of the diastolic pressure. If hypotension develops during bypass, the flow should be increased up to 150% of predicted; also one should examine the acid-base status in conjunction with cerebral oxygenation and mixed venous saturations. Often, severe hemodilution with oxygen debt is the cause and should be treated as such. After exclusion, we treat the hypotension carefully with vasoconstrictors, knowing that normal systemic pressures will not restore splanchnic hypoperfusion[174] and that vasoconstrictors will often lead to a greater base excess. Excessive α-adrenergic receptor blockade can be antagonized by vasopressin.[175] One study demonstrated that vasoconstrictor treatment results in the administration of more sodium bicarbonate to treat the acidosis and is associated with a later time to extubation and return of bowel function.[176] In conclusion, α-adrenergic receptor blockade during bypass should be considered because of its benefits for tissue perfusion, but carefully executed and balanced against potential drawbacks afterwards.

CONVENTIONAL ULTRAFILTRATION AND MODIFIED ULTRAFILTRATION

Ultrafiltration involves placing a hemofilter (similar to that used for continuous arteriovenous or venovenous hemofiltration in the ICU) in the CPB circuit and has become the standard of care for nearly all programs that specialize in surgery for congenital heart defects.[177] Conventional ultrafiltration (CUF) is performed during CPB, with the filter placed between the arterial and venous sides of the CPB circuit. The hemofilter has thousands of fibers with pores, which allow water, electrolytes, and small molecules to be filtered out of the blood. Suction is applied to the hemofilter on CPB, and an ultrafiltrate of plasma is produced. Advantages of ultrafiltration include the ability to increase the hematocrit, fibrinogen, plasma proteins, and platelet count,[178,179] without necessitating further blood transfusion, the ability to remove excess free water and sodium (which contribute to excess intravascular volume, tissue edema, pulmonary and myocardial edema), as well as the ability to correct acid-base and electrolyte imbalances and to remove small molecules, such as interleukins and tumor necrosis factor-α (TNF-α) in particular,[180] which are involved in the postbypass inflammatory process.[181,182] This improves systolic and diastolic function of the myocardium and reduces endothelial dysfunction in the systemic and pulmonary vasculature.[182,183] Pulmonary function is better preserved, probably owing to a slight reduction in interleukin 6 (IL-6) and thromboxane B_2,[184] even though this is not a consistent finding.[185,186] Endothelin-1, another mediator of pulmonary damage and hypertension, is not reduced by any filtration method.[186] Clinically, however, any ultrafiltration method seems to benefit children, especially those undergoing complex repairs, neonates, and children with preexisting pulmonary hypertension.[185]

MUF is performed for 10 to 15 minutes immediately after the conclusion of CPB. It can be performed in an arteriovenous manner with a hemofilter placed between the aortic cannula and the IVC cannula, or in a venovenous fashion using bicaval cannulation or an internal jugular venous catheter.[187] It was developed in 1991[188] as an alternative method to reduce the side effects of CPB. CUF during bypass is often limited by the minimal venous reservoir levels and requires the addition of crystalloid or colloid to be able to continuously remove cytokines during ultrafiltration. During MUF, blood passes out of the aorta, through the hemofilter, and is returned through the IVC cannula. The theoretical advantage of MUF over CUF is that only the child's blood volume is filtered, yielding a more efficient system for achieving the goals outlined previously. The disadvantages are that the child remains heparinized, and body temperature may decrease during the process (unless the circuit is modified to include the heat exchanger).[189] It also requires extra time, an aortic cannula is needed that can obstruct the aorta in small infants, and acute intravascular volume shifts may occur at a time when the child is prone to hemodynamic instability. Opposite to the expected effects of fluid removal, MUF actually increases arterial pressures despite decreasing filling pressures and improving myocardial performance.[190]

There is increasing evidence that the use of ultrafiltration reduces bypass-related postoperative morbidity. Outcome studies have demonstrated that ultrafiltration improves myocardial and pulmonary function, lessens tissue edema, allows faster weaning from mechanical ventilation, and decreases the need for inotropic support.[191] In that aspect it may be as efficient as the perioperative application of steroids.[192] Unfortunately, the reduction of inflammatory transmitters is only temporary, because the levels of cytokines are similar after 24 hours.[193]

Although each method has its proponents, and some centers perform both techniques in the same children, controlled comparative studies revealed no difference in outcome between MUF and CUF.[191,194] We routinely use a balanced ultrafiltration technique for all cases on CPB because it removes fluids and cytokines, as well as reduces lactate, which can aggravate reperfusion injury.[195]

Prebypass Anesthetic Management

The objectives of the anesthetic management of children before bypass include maintenance of normal sinus rhythm and ventricular function and avoidance of extreme increases in heart rate, ventricular contractility, and pulmonary vascular resistance (PVR). Special attention should be given to maintaining adequate coronary perfusion. Methods for accomplishing these objectives are lesion-specific and may include the maintenance of PVR with controlled hypoventilation and delivery of a low fraction of inspired oxygen to avoid pulmonary overcirculation, diastolic runoff, and coronary hypoperfusion in patients with a large left-to-right shunt (truncus arteriosus, aortopulmonary window, large patent ductus arteriosus, central shunt). Vasoactive and inotropic infusions and temporary snaring of the pulmonary artery may be required to achieve these goals. The duration of the prebypass period varies greatly, particularly in children who have had previous surgery, and maintaining hemodynamic stability for prolonged periods of time can be challenging. Adequate anesthetic depth should be ensured to avoid increases in sympathetic stimulation and hypercyanotic spells, and temperature homeostasis should be maintained to avoid cardiac arrhythmias, especially when the duration of the pre-CPB surgical dissection is protracted. For children undergoing repeat sternotomy, blood products with an appropriate-capacity blood warmer should be readily at hand in case of emergent need.

Neonates and children who have been receiving total parenteral nutrition preoperatively receive an infusion of 5% or 10% dextrose before CPB, with frequent monitoring of glucose concentrations to avoid hypoglycemia or hyperglycemia. Older children receive PlasmaLyte, a balanced electrolyte solution, at a reduced maintenance rate, allowing the administration of 5% albumin, if necessary, for volume augmentation.

The placement of purse-string sutures before cannulation, as well as the actual cannulation of the great vessels before CPB, can often precipitate arrhythmias, hypotension, and arterial desaturation, especially in small infants and children. It is common for volume replacement to be necessary during placement of the cannula; if the aortic cannula is already in place, it is our practice to coordinate the administration of fluid volume between the anesthesiologist and perfusionist while the surgeon completes cannulation. Calcium chloride (10 mg/kg) is also frequently useful to support hemodynamics at this time.

Anesthesia on Cardiopulmonary Bypass

CHANGES IN PHARMACOKINETICS

The initiation of CPB introduces additional volume to the intravascular space (hemodilution). Hemodilution and altered protein concentrations greatly affect drug distribution and consequent plasma concentrations. Plasma protein binding,[196] hypotension, hypothermia,[197] pulsatility,[198] isolation of the lungs from the circulation, altered hepatic and renal function, ultrafiltration, and uptake of anesthetic drugs by the bypass circuit are other major factors that affect pharmacologic responses.[199,200] Drugs in the blood exist in the free (unbound and therefore the active form) or plasma-bound (inactive form bound to protein, e.g., albumin) forms and therefore are subject to marked changes with alterations in plasma protein levels. CPB alters all these factors,

which makes description of pharmacokinetic parameters during CPB problematic. The greatest changes occur within 5 minutes of initiation of CPB. The addition of the prime volume immediately reduces the protein concentration, and the ratio of bound-to-free drug in the circulation changes. Hemodilution occurs, and free drug concentrations are also reduced owing to dilution; this reduces the amount of drug available for interaction with the receptors. Most studies show a reduction in total drug concentration in plasma with little change in unbound drug concentration over time, whereas on CPB other than the transient (<5 minutes) reduction at initiation of CPB,[201] it would appear that the greatest risk for unwanted "lightening of anesthesia" is within this time frame, and additional doses of fentanyl, muscle relaxant, and midazolam are generally administered just before or with the onset of CPB. The explanation for why unbound drug concentrations are sustained during CPB is that the volume of distribution for most anesthetic agents is large relative to the volume of the CPB prime and serves as a huge reservoir for drug after IV administration. A decrease in the plasma concentrations of medications as a result of hemodilution shifts drugs down their concentration gradient from tissue to plasma. Hypothermia contributes to the changes in plasma concentrations, primarily by depressing enzyme function and slowing drug clearance by approximately half for every 10°C reduction in temperature. When normothermia is reestablished, reperfusion of tissues might lead to washout of drug sequestered during the hypothermic CPB period. This may explain the secondary increases in plasma concentrations of opioids reported during the rewarming phase. pH-stat management also affects the degree of ionization and protein binding of certain medications, leading to increased unbound drug. During CPB, the lungs are out of circuit and medications that are taken up by the lungs (e.g., opioids) are sequestered during CPB. These medications are released when systemic reperfusion is established and concentrations are transiently increased. The volume of distribution of many drugs is expanded because of the priming volume of the bypass circuit, especially with neonates and small infants, where the priming volume is often greater than the child's blood volume. Medications may be taken up by various components of the CPB circuit itself. Renal dysfunction associated with CPB reduces the clearance of drugs such as cephalosporin antibiotics, TXA, EACA, and milrinone.

CHANGES IN PHARMACODYNAMICS

The pharmacodynamic effects of anesthetic agents are affected primarily via the central nervous system, which undergoes major changes during CPB. For example, hypothermia during CPB reduces anesthetic requirements. Hypothermia causes a host of other effects, including decreases in receptor affinity (e.g., decreased opioid receptor affinity[202] and nicotinic acetylcholine receptor sensitivity[203]), enhanced effects of neuromuscular receptor blocking drugs at the neuromuscular junction,[204,205] and alterations in tissue blood flow that may affect the response to catecholamines.[206]

CPB also affects the degree of ionization and protein binding (hence free or unbound drug concentrations) of weak acids and bases, as well as the electrolyte balance achieved by the blood gas management strategy used during CPB. Plasma concentrations of calcium, magnesium, and potassium decrease during CPB,[207,208] and these changes may lead to muscle weakness, dysrhythmias, and digitalis toxicity. The number of receptors available for interaction with a ligand will determine the subsequent magnitude of a drug effect. A reduction in the number of cardiac receptors has been observed in congestive heart failure, and defects in receptor transduction, as well as impairment of synthesis and reuptake of norepinephrine occur.

Administration of β-adrenergic agonists in this condition has been associated with further reductions in β-receptor numbers, with diminished pharmacologic effect. Removal of β-adrenergic blockade may lead to β-adrenergic receptor upregulation and increased adrenergic responsiveness.[209] Changes in receptor density and function may occur very quickly and have been observed to occur during cardiac surgery. Many perfusionists, under the direction of the anesthesiologist, can also administer inhalation agents via a separate vaporizer mounted on the bypass machine. Alternatively, a propofol infusion can be used during bypass to maintain anesthetic depth. Anesthetic requirements decrease with systemic hypothermia,[210] but as rewarming is initiated, additional anesthetic drugs, including a benzodiazepine, are added to the bypass circuit to ensure that amnesia is maintained. Further work is required to elucidate the mechanisms and clinical implications of these acute changes in receptor density and function.

Special Techniques

MANAGEMENT OF DEEP HYPOTHERMIC CIRCULATORY ARREST

In the early days of cardiac surgery and CPB, hypothermia was used to improve intracardiac surgical exposure. In 1950, Bigelow and colleagues were the first to show that hypothermia decreases the metabolic rate.[211] Since then, we have discovered other advantages of hypothermia, including decreases in the inflammatory response of CPB,[212] decreases in blood loss,[213] myocardial protection,[214] and neuroprotection.[215] The last effect relates primarily to the decrease in the metabolic rate (by approximately 64%) that is achieved by cooling from 37°C to 27°C. The disadvantages of deep hypothermic circulatory arrest (DHCA) include a prolongation of CPB duration and a greater tendency toward postoperative bleeding.[216] Postoperative recovery, however, is not prolonged by hypothermia.[217] The rate of wound infection is uninfluenced by hypothermic bypass.[218]

Hypothermia during cardiac surgery gained widespread acceptance only after the 1959 development of a heat exchanger that could be integrated into the CPB machine.[219] DHCA involves cooling the child's body temperature during CPB to 17°C to 18°C, stopping the bypass machine, draining the blood from the child into a venous reservoir, and removing the cannulas from the heart. After the first reports of DHCA in the 1960s, this technique gained popularity in the 1970s and 1980s because of the bloodless field it provided, thus facilitating complex intracardiac and aortic repairs in neonates and small infants,[220] as well as reducing myocardial edema. However, it soon became evident that DHCA was associated with neurologic morbidity. Choreoathetosis, seizures, coma, and hemiparesis were all noted, especially with prolonged (>60-minute) DHCA. The incidence of these acute morbidities seemed to increase when α-stat management became the widely accepted standard. Long-term adverse neurodevelopmental outcomes have also been associated with long periods of DHCA, including abnormalities in mental development and in fine and gross motor skills.[221] The Boston Circulatory Arrest Study is a remarkable achievement in which 155 neonates undergoing the arterial switch operation from 1988 to 1992 were studied, with follow-up complete to 8 years of age.[222] The CPB protocol in those years included α-stat management, routine hemodilution to a hematocrit of 20%, and the absence of an arterial filter on the CPB circuit. A DHCA time longer than 40 minutes was associated with a significant increase

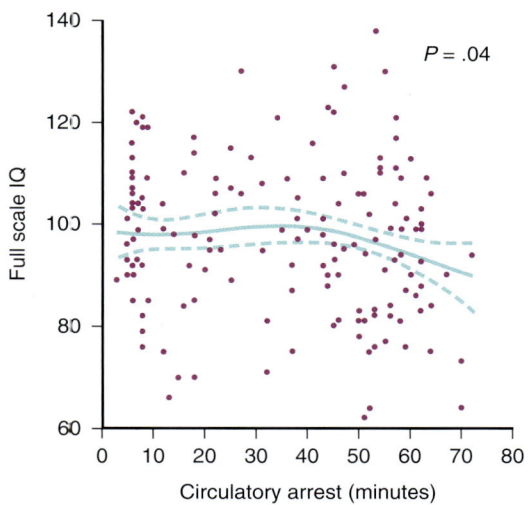

Variable	Cut-point estimate (minutes)	95% lower confidence limit (minutes)
Full-scale IQ	42	27
Verbal IQ	41	23
Performance IQ	47	31
Average achievement	43	4
Grooved pegboard	35	13
Mayo test for apraxia	40	29
Combined analysis (overall six outcomes)	41	32

FIGURE 19.3 Safe duration of circulatory arrest. From the Boston Circulatory Arrest Study, 155 8-year-olds who underwent arterial switch operation for D-transposition of the great arteries as neonates. Bypass protocol used α-stat pH management, with hematocrit of 20% and temperature of 18°C. Above 40 minutes DHCA, both mental and physical performance test scores at 8 years of age decreased significantly. (From Wypij D, Newburger JW, Rappaport LA, et al. The effect of duration of deep hypothermic circulatory arrest in infant heart surgery on late neurodevelopment: the Boston Circulatory Arrest Trial. *J Thorac Cardiovasc Surg.* 2003;126:1397–1403.)

in adverse long-term neurologic outcomes (Fig. 19.3). Although the 40-minute cutoff is now well accepted in surgery for congenital heart defects, a number of changes have subsequently been made to bypass protocols. Results from animal experiments using a neonatal pig model of DHCA, as well as data from the Boston Circulatory Arrest Study, led to the following recommendations for increasing the child's safety margin when using DHCA:

- Hematocrit of 30% should be the target.[89]
- Systemic hypothermia should be achieved slowly, over no less than 20 minutes.[223]
- pH-stat blood gas management should be used, at least for cooling (Fig. 19.4).[135,137]
- Core body temperatures of 17°C to 18°C should be used, and ice bags should be applied to the head.[224]
- DHCA should be divided into periods of less than 20 minutes, allowing a reperfusion period of at least 2 minutes between each segment of DHCA, to improve neurologic outcome.[225]
- Low-flow CPB is better than DHCA. Selective regional cerebral perfusion may be better than full-body low-flow CPB.[226]
- Normoxia should be maintained to decrease exacerbation of brain injury after DHCA.[227]

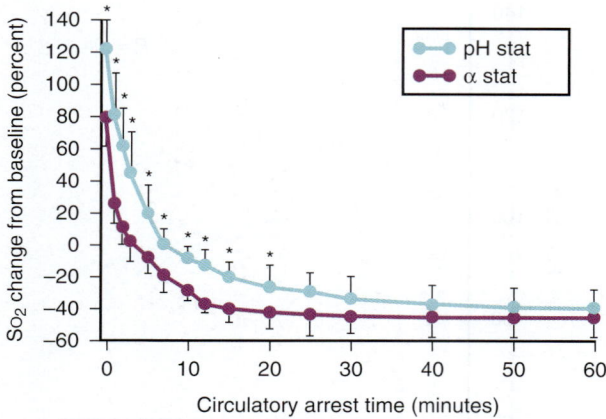

FIGURE 19.4 Cortical oxygen saturation (So_2) during deep hypothermic circulatory arrest in pH-stat and α-stat groups. The cortical So_2 half-life during arrest was significantly greater in the pH-stat than in the α-stat group. Mean ± SD, eight animals per group. *$P < 0.05$ between groups. (From Kurth CD, O'Rourke MM, O'Hara IB. Comparison of pH-stat and alpha-stat cardiopulmonary bypass on cerebral oxygenation and blood flow in relation to hypothermic circulatory arrest in piglets. *Anesthesiology* 1998;89:110–118.)

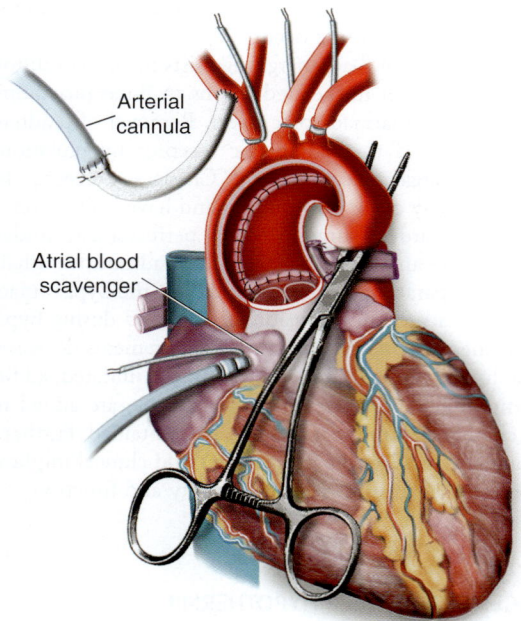

FIGURE 19.5 Selective cerebral perfusion for the Norwood stage 1 palliation for hypoplastic left heart syndrome. Arterial inflow for bypass is provided by a small polytetrafluoroethylene graft sewn to the right innominate artery. Instead of deep hypothermic circulatory arrest, flow is provided to the brain at low rates, while the brachiocephalic vessels and descending thoracic aorta are snared, providing a bloodless operating field. (From Pigula FA, Nemoto EM, Griffith BP, Siewers RD. Regional low-flow perfusion provides cerebral circulatory support during neonatal aortic arch reconstruction. *J Thorac Cardiovasc Surg.* 2000;119:331–339.)

Neurologic monitoring (see later discussion) may be useful in the individual child to aid in determining the safe duration of DHCA.[135,228]

Although there are situations in which DHCA must be used, many surgeons are avoiding it whenever possible, minimizing its duration and dividing the periods of its use, or using alternate methods, such as selective cerebral perfusion (see the following discussion).

REGIONAL CEREBRAL PERFUSION

Several novel CPB techniques have been developed to avoid the use of DHCA. The purpose of these techniques is to allow perfusion of the brain during critical periods of surgery, such as aortic reconstruction during the Norwood operation.[229,230] These techniques are collectively referred to as selective cerebral perfusion. Regional cerebral perfusion (RCP) is one variation in which a small Gore-Tex graft (W.L. Gore and Associates, Flagstaff, AZ) of 3 to 4 mm is sewn onto the innominate artery before initiation of CPB and is then used as the aortic cannula during CPB (Fig. 19.5). During aortic reconstruction, snares are placed around the brachiocephalic vessels and CPB flow is decreased, with the brain receiving perfusion only via the right carotid artery. In this way, a bloodless operative field is achieved, just as if DHCA was being performed, yet the brain is still receiving blood flow and oxygen, theoretically increasing protection from hypoxic ischemic brain injury. Another potential advantage of this technique occurs in neonates, who frequently have extensive arterial collaterals between the proximal branches of the aorta and the lower body via the internal mammary and long thoracic arteries. In this instance, the use of selective cerebral perfusion also provides some blood flow to the lower body, protecting renal, hepatic, and gastrointestinal systems from hypoxic damage as well.[231] This protection is, however, incomplete and RCP at 25°C is no more protective than DHCA.[232] Also, the ongoing perfusion prolongs the effective bypass time, leading to more cytokine release and capillary leakage, with worse pulmonary function, more weight gain, and decreased right ventricular function.[233]

One study described a cohort of 57 neonates undergoing RCP for stage 1 palliation of hypoplastic left heart syndrome and other aortic arch reconstructions.[234] Mean RCP time was 71 ± 28 minutes and flow rate 57 ± 11 mL/kg per minute (38% of normal full CPB flow). Postoperative brain MRI revealed no differences in patients undergoing RCP versus standard CPB. Twelve-month neurodevelopmental outcomes assessed with the Bayley Scales of Infant Development-III revealed Cognitive Score of 100 ± 15, Language Score of 87 ± 15, and Motor Score of 88 ± 17. Increasing duration of RCP was not associated with adverse neurodevelopmental outcomes. Neurologic monitoring, consisting of NIRS and TCD measurements, was used to adjust the flow rate during RCP.[235,236] Radial arterial pressures of 30 to 40 mm Hg were maintained during RCP.[235]

Effects of Cardiopulmonary Bypass

CARDIAC EFFECTS

In addition to myocardial ischemic injury secondary to aortic cross-clamping, several other factors can contribute to perioperative myocardial dysfunction. The first is entrainment of air into the coronary arteries, which frequently occurs during weaning from bypass.[237] Despite meticulous de-airing of the heart, air may enter the right coronary artery, producing ischemia that is heralded by a pale myocardium, poor contractility, and ST-segment elevation of the ECG. Should this occur, appropriate management involves remaining on CPB, increasing perfusion pressure, and "milking" the air through the coronary arteries, allowing time for recovery of the ECG and ventricular function before attempting to wean from bypass. Surgical factors, such as reimplantation of coronary arteries with possible resultant ischemia or residual surgical defects, can also occasionally contribute to myocardial dysfunction.

The inflammatory response to CPB (see later discussion) has important implications for cardiac function.[238] This systemic response results in a capillary leak syndrome, which in turn leads to accumulation of edema fluid in interstitial and extravascular spaces, including the myocardium.[239] Myocardial edema can contribute to post-CPB myocardial dysfunction by impairing diastolic function and causing mechanical limitation of cardiac filling and outflow in small infants whose sternums have been closed. Additionally, myocardial edema has been implicated as a causative factor in the frequent decline in myocardial function that occurs 6 to 12 hours after conclusion of CPB. Inflammatory mediators also affect the responsiveness of the myocardium to catecholamines by interfering with their binding to the cell surface receptors,[240] rendering exogenously administered drugs, such as dopamine and epinephrine, as well as the child's endogenous catecholamines, less effective at augmenting cardiac function perioperatively.

Mechanisms for prevention and treatment of myocardial dysfunction include the use of ultrafiltration and antiinflammatory drugs, such as corticosteroids and aprotinin.[241,242] The prophylactic use of noncatecholamine inotropic agents, such as milrinone, has also been shown to prevent low cardiac output syndrome in infants, even if cardiac function is adequate in the immediate postoperative period.[243]

SYSTEMIC AND PULMONARY VASCULATURE EFFECTS

The inflammatory response to CPB often produces mediators that directly increase pulmonary and systemic vascular resistance. These include interleukins, leukotrienes, and endothelin.[244] Indeed, when pulmonary artery pressure is measured directly, it is often significantly increased immediately after bypass, even if surgical results are optimal. This increase can be extremely detrimental in children with large left-to-right shunts, those undergoing cardiac transplantation secondary to dilated cardiomyopathy, and those undergoing bidirectional cavopulmonary anastomosis, where right ventricular output depends on maintaining low PVR. Prevention and treatment of increases in PVR include maintaining an adequate depth of anesthesia, ventilating with 100% oxygen, and judicious use of hyperventilation. Milrinone will increase right-sided cardiac output via its actions as both an inotropic agent and a pulmonary vasodilator. When PVR is significantly increased, inhaled nitric oxide is often used to assist in the early postoperative period.[245] Although effective, its cost is not inconsequential, and because PVR almost always decreases with time, inhaled nitric oxide is generally reserved for selected cases of pulmonary hypertension. Other simpler, less expensive treatments include oral or IV sildenafil[246,247] and inhaled nebulized prostacyclin.[248]

PULMONARY EFFECTS

The lungs are not ventilated during CPB and are usually totally collapsed by intention, with the ventilator circuit disconnected, especially in small infants. This leads to significant atelectasis and lung function can be improved by continuation of ventilation even on bypass.[249] The lungs are also at least partially ischemic during the bypass period, resulting in decreased production and reduced alveolar levels of surfactant after CPB.[250] In addition, reperfusion injury (pulmonary edema or hemorrhage after a sudden increase in pulmonary flow) can also occur after creation of a

systemic-to-pulmonary artery shunt or pulmonary artery unifocalization. Inflammatory mediators liberated by the bypass run also predispose to increases in smooth muscle tone and resistance and can result in bronchospasm.[251]

In addition to complement, endotoxins and certain cytokines can also activate neutrophils and attract them toward sites of inflammation.[252] In animal studies, endotoxin-induced lung injury can lead to rapid (within 45 minutes) accumulation of neutrophils within lung capillaries. Activation of neutrophils, with upregulation of adhesion molecules, neutrophil adhesion to the endothelium of lung vessels, and endothelial damage through proteases, appears to be the main step of the underlying pathophysiologic mechanism (Fig. 19.6). Macrophages play an important role in the evolution of the inflammatory acute lung injury through the secretion of cytokines, cytotoxic metabolites, and chemoattractants for leukocytes. At the clinical level, acute respiratory distress syndrome (ARDS) is often only one part of multiorgan failure, and lung injury should be seen as part of a more general state of systemic inflammation. The reported prevalence of ARDS after CPB in adults is 0.5% to 1.7%; the incidence in children is unknown. Interestingly, general hypothermia at 28°C failed to prevent the loss of ATP and the accumulation of lactate in lungs.[253] Other methods that aim to protect the lungs during CPB, such as continuous lung perfusion, pneumoplegia, and inhaled nitric oxide ventilation at lung reperfusion, prevent more severe hemodynamic deterioration and preserve reactivity of the pulmonary vasculature, but fail to prevent pulmonary dysfunction.

The severity of pulmonary dysfunction after CPB can be measured via changes in the alveolar-arterial oxygenation gradient, intrapulmonary shunt, degree of pulmonary edema, pulmonary compliance, and PVR. Treatment of pulmonary atelectasis includes careful reinflation of the lungs when weaning from bypass (by administering several vital capacity breaths), gentle but thorough suctioning of the tracheal tube, and prophylactic use of inhaled bronchodilators before separation from CPB. Using these measures, pulmonary function has been shown to improve immediately in most children with large left-to-right shunts, with the duration of CPB seemingly having little effect on pulmonary outcomes.[254] Thus, CPB itself has little effect on pulmonary function in most children. There is still an occasional child, however, who experiences classic "pump lung" ARDS, caused by the factors noted earlier. Treatment is supportive as for anyone with ARDS.

NEUROLOGIC MONITORING AND EFFECTS OF CARDIOPULMONARY BYPASS ON THE BRAIN

Cerebral monitoring can help to detect those children who are at risk for neurologic sequelae after bypass, promptly recognize and treat changes in cerebral blood flow/oxygenation, evaluate the effect of therapeutic interventions on cerebral physiology, optimize brain protection during the vulnerable periods of CPB, and potentially improve short- and long-term neurologic outcomes.[255] However, one must recognize that there is an increased frequency of congenital structural CNS abnormalities in association with complex CHD that appear to be present at birth in nearly half of these neonates and cannot be reversed. Further damage can be prevented using specific management strategies during the perioperative period.[255a]

The cerebral NIRS monitor measures brain tissue oxygenation (see Chapter 52). This device noninvasively measures the cerebral tissue oxygen saturation and displays a numerical value for the regional cerebral oxygen saturation (rSO_2), the ratio of oxyhemoglobin to total hemoglobin in the light path. Regional

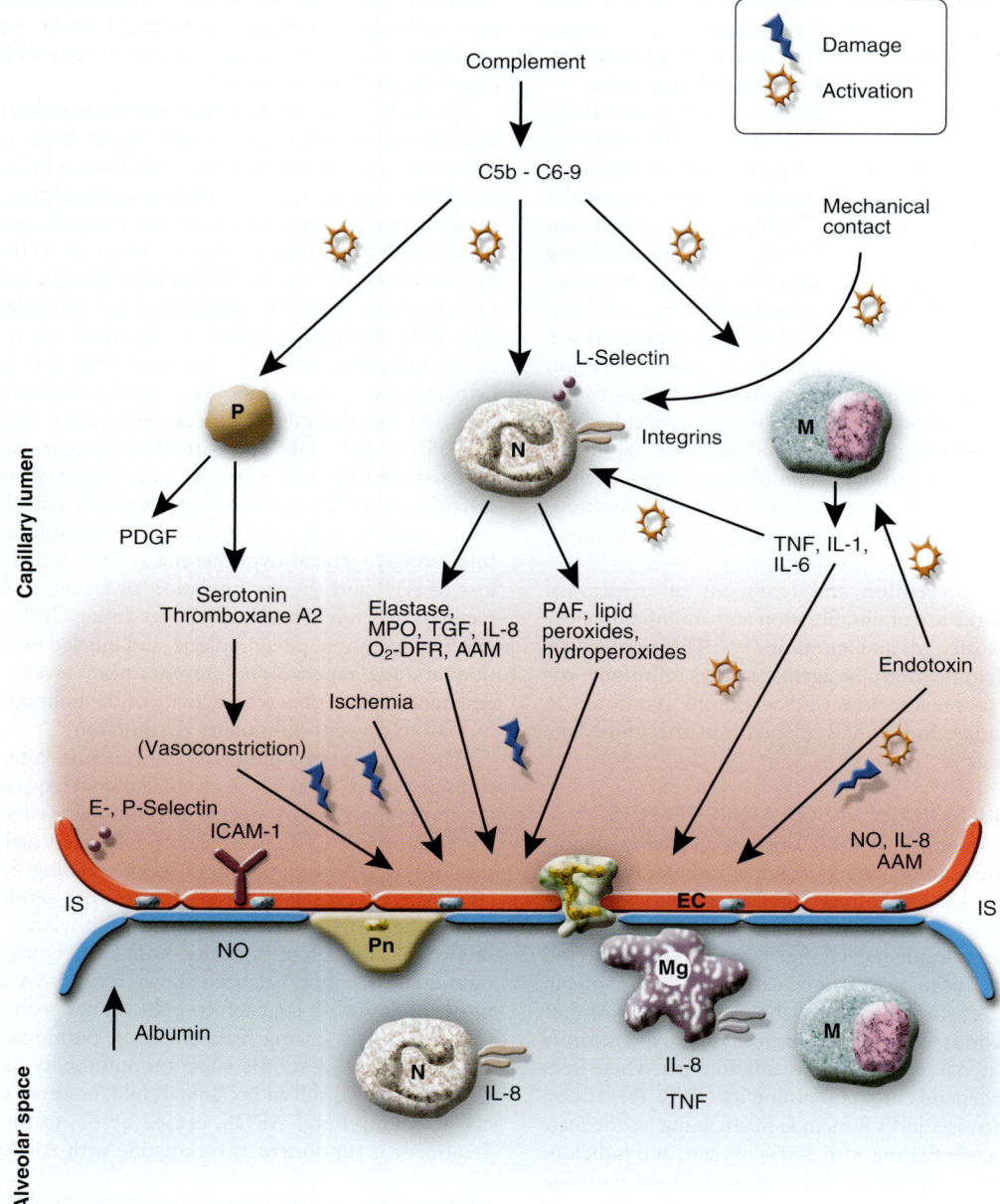

FIGURE 19.6 Leukocytes, endothelial cells (*EC*), and humoral inflammatory mediators have been shown to play an important role in the cardiopulmonary bypass-induced lung injury. Complement (*C*) activation and complement-independent mechanical injury activates leukocytes, which, in turn, secrete several inflammatory mediators, such as proteases and cytokines. Complement, cytokines, and ischemia-reperfusion also activate endothelial cells. Endotoxin, probably released from intestinal bacteria, exerts similar effects on leukocytes and endothelium. This process leads to disruption of endothelial and epithelial integrity and allows albumin, plasma, and activated leukocytes to enter the interstitial and alveolar spaces, causing tissue edema and reducing pulmonary compliance and blood oxygenation. *AAM*, arachidonic acid metabolites; *ICAM-1*, intercellular adhesion molecule 1; *IL*, interleukin; *IS*, interstitial space; *M*, monocyte; *Mg*, macrophage; *MPO*, myeloperoxidase; *N*, neutrophil; *NO*, nitric oxide; O_2-*DFR*, oxygen-derived free radicals; *P*, platelet; *PAF*, platelet-activating factor; *PDGF*, platelet-derived growth factor; *Pn*, pneumocyte; *TGF*, tumor growth factor; *TNF*, tumor necrosis factor. (From Asimakopoulos G, Smith PL, Ratnatunga CP, Taylor KM. Lung injury and acute respiratory distress syndrome after cardiopulmonary bypass. *Ann Thorac Surg*. 1999;1107–1115.)

cerebral oxygen saturation is a measure of local microcirculatory oxygen supply-and-demand balance and is reported on a scale from 15% to 95%. It has been assumed from anatomic models that 75% of the cerebral blood volume in the light path is venous and 25% is arterial. One study verified this in children with congenital heart disease by directly measuring the jugular venous bulb and arterial oxygen saturations and comparing these with the cerebral oxygen saturation measured with NIRS.[256] The actual ratio in children varied widely, but on average the venous to arterial ratio was 85:15. All devices measure both the arterial and venous blood oxygen saturations. Accordingly, this device does not provide a measure of the jugular venous bulb oxygen saturation ($SjvO_2$). A corollary of this is that maneuvers that increase arterial oxygen saturation (e.g., increasing FIO_2) increase cerebral oxygenation as measured by these devices, although the $SjvO_2$ may remain unchanged. In a study of 40 infants and children with congenital heart disease who were undergoing cardiac surgery or catheterization, NIRS correlated poorly with $SjvO_2$ measurements, except in infants younger than 1 year of age.[257] In contrast, in a study of 30 children undergoing cardiac catheterization, NIRS correlated very well with $SjvO_2$ ($r = .93$).[258] These data suggest that NIRS is a useful indicator of trends in cerebral oxygenation in individual infants and children who have a stable FIO_2, hemoglobin, and carbon dioxide. NIRS values also correlate with long-term neurodevelopmental outcomes after infant heart surgery. In a prospective study of 104 two-ventricle repairs, low rSO_2 in the intraoperative period did not correlate with death or major morbidity.[259] However, when these children underwent neurodevelopmental testing at 1 year of age, lower average and minimum rSO_2 in the 60-minute period immediately after CPB correlated with worse psychomotor development index scores. Low rSO_2 also correlated with remote ischemic changes on brain MRI at 1 year of age.[260]

Neurologic Monitoring for Low-Flow Hypothermic Bypass

TCD ultrasonography has been used to determine the threshold of detectable cerebral perfusion during low-flow CPB. *TCD velocities reveal trends or changes in cerebral blood flow and not absolute values.* One report studied 28 neonates undergoing the arterial switch operation using α-stat blood gas management.[160] Their study suggested that NIRS and TCD may be useful to determine the minimum acceptable bypass flow rate for an individual neonate during low-flow hypothermic bypass. Blood flow becomes insufficient at bypass flow rates less than 30 mL/kg per minute.[160,261] Inadequate blood flow to the brain during this technique could be undetected without such monitoring, and low-flow bypass may confer no advantage to the brain over DHCA in some children. Long-term outcome studies of this monitoring strategy are not available.

Neurologic Monitoring for Deep Hypothermic Circulatory Arrest

Despite clinical and experimental evidence that periods of DHCA that exceed approximately 40 minutes are associated with an increased risk of adverse long-term neurologic and developmental outcomes, this technique is still widely used in surgery to correct congenital heart defects. Recent recommendations for improving outcomes after DHCA, based on both animal and clinical studies, were described previously. During DHCA, rSO_2 predictably decreases to a nadir 60% to 70% (relative change) below baseline values obtained before bypass. The nadir is reached at 10 to 20 minutes, after which there is no further decrease.[262] At this point,

it appears that there is no additional oxygen uptake by the brain. Several studies suggest the potential for NIRS to determine the safe conduct and duration of DHCA in the individual child. In a study of infants and children undergoing surgery with bypass and DHCA, three children with low rSO_2 developed acute postoperative neurologic changes—seizures in one and prolonged coma in two.[262] In these three children, the increase in rSO_2 after the onset of CPB was much less (average 3% relative increase vs. 33% increase in children without neurologic deficit), and the duration of cooling before DHCA was less than in the remaining 23 children who did not develop neurologic changes. In a neonatal pig model, the timing of the nadir of rSO_2 values during DHCA correlated with neurologic outcome: a more prolonged period without oxygen uptake by the brain correlated with a greater incidence of adverse neurologic outcomes. The maximum safe duration at 17°C without additional brain oxygen uptake was 30 minutes.[153] Interestingly, this time period correlates with clinical and experimental studies, suggesting that 40 minutes is the safe duration for circulatory arrest (see Fig. 19.3). When circulatory arrest is initiated at warmer temperatures (e.g., 25°C), the rSO_2 decreases more rapidly, and the nadir is achieved sooner, than at cooler temperatures.[263] Reperfusion results in an increase in rSO_2 to levels observed at full bypass flow before DHCA, with a subsequent decrease during rewarming. Based on these data, our current practice is to reperfuse after the NIRS nadir has been reached for a period of 20 to 25 minutes.

Neurologic Monitoring for Regional Cerebral Perfusion

RCP (also known as selective cerebral perfusion or antegrade cerebral perfusion) uses a polytetrafluoroethylene (PTFE) graft or a small aortic cannula as arterial inflow to the right innominate artery for neonatal aortic surgery, such as the Norwood stage 1 operation or aortic arch advancement. The other brachiocephalic vessels and descending thoracic aorta are snared, resulting in a bloodless operating field. The brain is perfused through the right innominate and right vertebral arteries only. This approach significantly reduces or eliminates the use of DHCA for these operations and preserves brain perfusion, potentially improving neurologic outcome. Initial descriptions of this technique used the pressure in the radial artery or a predetermined bypass rate of 25 to 30 mL/kg per minute as an estimate for the bypass flow during RCP without neurologic monitoring. When flow rate was estimated on the basis of NIRS monitoring in individual children, it was determined that 20 to 25 mL/kg per minute was required.[229] However, NIRS was applied only to the right side of the skull (i.e., the right side of the brain), the same side as the sole arterial inflow. Using a pH-stat blood gas strategy for RCP, we noted that the majority of our children had an rSO_2 of 95% (the maximum reading on the rSO_2 scale) when we used the left radial artery pressure of 20 to 25 mm Hg as the target for bypass flow. These children were theoretically at risk for excessive cerebral perfusion. Therefore we performed a study using both NIRS and TCD of the right cerebral hemisphere to determine if TCD could be used as a guide to RCP flow rate.[235] The bypass flow rate was adjusted to achieve a cerebral blood flow volume within 10% of baseline (e.g., TCD was used to determine necessary flow). The estimated flow rate, 63 mL/kg per minute (range, 24–94 mL/kg per minute), proved to be significantly greater than that estimated in the earlier studies. This flow rate did not correlate with the pressure in the right or left radial artery. The rSO_2 was well maintained in all children, leading us to conclude that TCD was a useful monitor to ensure adequate but not excessive cerebral blood flow during

RCP. Because RCP perfuses the brain through a single arterial inflow vessel, questions have arisen about the adequacy of cerebral blood flow and oxygenation to the left cerebral hemisphere. Although the circle of Willis is expected to be intact without stenoses in neonates, 10% of healthy full-term neonates exhibit deviations from normal flow patterns. Two studies concluded that although cerebral blood flow and oxygenation were adequate to both cerebral hemispheres in neonates during RCP, bilateral monitoring, at least of NIRS, may be warranted.[235,264]

SYSTEMIC INFLAMMATORY RESPONSE SYNDROME

In cardiac surgery, SIRS is thought to result from four main sources of injury: (1) contact of the blood components with the artificial surface of the bypass circuit, (2) ischemia-reperfusion injury, (3) endotoxemia, and (4) operative trauma. Inflammatory cytokines, together with endothelial activation and endothelial-leukocyte interactions, appear to play an important role in the induction of this systemic inflammatory response.

Exposure of blood to the artificial materials in the bypass circuit—plastics, polypropylene oxygenator fibers, and metal suction devices—initiates a cascade of inflammatory responses, including activation of the complement system, the kallikrein system, and the coagulation system.[239] As a result, interleukins, TNF, endotoxin, heat shock protein, and many other inflammatory mediators are released into the circulation. Leukocyte activation also results in secretion of inflammatory mediators, such as proteases and cytokines (e.g., TNF-α and IL-1), which are secreted early in the evolution of the inflammatory process. This chemokine-mediated increased leukocyte activation constitutes an important link in the chain of the propagation of the inflammatory response (see Fig. 19.6).

This inflammatory response is counterbalanced by a complex system of inhibitors, such as IL-10 and soluble cytokine receptors.[265] Also, the inflammatory response of the neonate may be more exaggerated than that of the infant or older child,[266] justifying a more aggressive approach to its modulation in the neonate (see later discussion).

A number of novel treatments have been studied, including monoclonal antibodies for inflammatory products, such as complement, endotoxin, and TNF. Although theoretically attractive, no clinical difference has been noted with any of these treatments.

Effective treatments used every day in the operating room and ICU include:

- Use of corticosteroids[267]
- Ultrafiltration[241] (see earlier discussion)
- Aprotinin (if available)[242] (see earlier discussion)
- Leukocyte depletion[268]: leukocyte-depleted blood in prime and in-line arterial filter
- Initiate bypass using normoxic management (FiO$_2$ of 21%) in severely cyanotic infants.

Corticosteroids interrupt the inflammatory response at several levels by entering cell nuclei and changing the rate of transcription of inflammatory molecules. Increasing evidence suggests that glucocorticoids act by regulating transcription or translation of antiinflammatory cytokines, such as IL-10, and altering expression of other proteins, such as endothelin-1 and inhibitor NF-κβ.[269,270] Because these processes take time to develop, the effects of corticosteroids are not immediate, taking up to several hours.[271] Thus the common practice of adding corticosteroids to the CPB prime will not fully prevent the inflammatory response[272]; to be effective, corticosteroids may need to be administered 4 or more hours before the onset of CPB.[273]

Despite these theoretical advantages of using corticosteroids to modulate the inflammatory response, the benefit is still unproven.[274] A recent large discharge database review of more than 46,000 infants and children, in which 54% received corticosteroids, demonstrated no difference in mortality. Using propensity score matching, the authors concluded that corticosteroids were associated with greater length of hospital stay, greater rate of infection, and greater use of insulin. There was no difference in duration of ventilation. Steroids conferred no significant benefit; conversely, in the simpler surgery categories, there was increased morbidity with these drugs.[275] Although inflammatory activation from CPB definitely occurs, and it would seem intuitive that this would lead to worse outcomes in those patients with excessive inflammation, in contemporary practice, the correlation of the magnitude of this response and length of ICU stay and blood product administration is statistically significant, but clinically modest, accounting for only 4% to 9% of the difference in these variables, in a large study of infants undergoing two-ventricle repairs.[276]

COAGULATION EFFECTS

Blood coagulation is frequently abnormal after CPB for several reasons. The inflammatory cascade activates the coagulation system, resulting in factor consumption and fibrinolysis, which, in turn, breaks down existing blood clots, leading to increased bleeding.[16] Treatment is adequate heparinization, reversal with protamine, and the use of an antifibrinolytic to inhibit fibrinolysis and improve platelet function.[34] In addition, the smaller the child, the greater the dilution of clotting factors by the bypass prime, and the greater the risk for low concentrations of clotting proteins and fibrinogen postoperatively. Platelets are also degranulated and consumed by the CPB circuit, leading both to low platelet counts and nonfunctioning platelets.[16] The smaller the infant, the greater the duration of bypass, and the more complicated the surgery, the greater the incidence of coagulopathy after bypass. Efforts to minimize the postbypass coagulopathy in infants include priming the CPB circuit with fresh whole blood for small infants, if available, or packed cells plus FFP if fresh whole blood cannot be obtained.[20,277] Treatment often involves administration of platelets to small infants as the first line of therapy, followed by the replacement of fibrinogen and FFP to replace clotting factors. If these factors are repleted and studies are normal, then surgical bleeding may be the cause and surgical reexploration may be warranted.[278] Coagulation can be monitored intraoperatively with thromboelastography (TEG), rotational thromboelastometry (ROTEM), or laboratory coagulation studies. TEG has been shown to be a cost-effective monitor to decrease the amount of transfusions.[279] rVIIa has also been used as a last resort in children who have significant postbypass bleeding unresponsive to standard measures.[61] Current interest exists in the use of factor concentrates such as fibrinogen concentrate and three- or four-factor prothrombin complex concentrates for correction of coagulopathy in children undergoing cardiac surgery (see also Chapter 12). Fig. 19.7 presents the intraoperative coagulation monitoring and blood product and factor transfusion algorithm used at Texas Children's Hospital.

HEPATIC, RENAL, AND GASTROINTESTINAL EFFECTS

The liver, kidneys, and gastrointestinal tract, like the brain and heart, may be rendered ischemic by prolonged CPB, DHCA, or low cardiac output syndrome. Renal function is compromised on CPB. This is manifested by the appearance of proteinuria and impaired tubular cellular function immediately after CPB. Renal

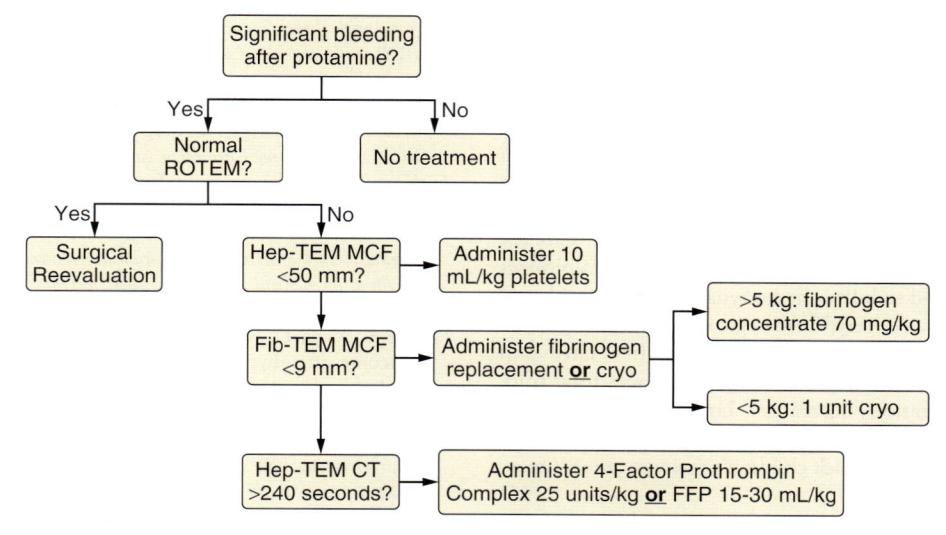

CV Operating Room Transfusion Pathway

1. Identify patients at risk for postbypass coagulopathy. If none of the following patient or procedural factors are identified, there is a low risk for post-CPB bleeding, and no ROTEM is needed.

   a. Patient factors
      □ Young age, low weight
      □ Cyanosis/polycythemia
      □ Preoperative anticoagulant or antiplatelet therapy
      □ History of VAD or ECMO support

   b. Procedural factors
      □ Multiple reoperation
      □ Use of deep hypothermia
      □ Complex surgery; extensive high-pressure suture lines

2. If patient has one or more of the above factors, confirm availability of all blood products and pharmacologic factors.
3. Send ROTEM upon rewarming to guide postbypass factor replacement.
4. Evaluate clinical bleeding and ROTEM results.

Significant bleeding after protamine? → Yes → Normal ROTEM? → Yes → Surgical Reevaluation
Significant bleeding after protamine? → No → No treatment
Normal ROTEM? → No → Hep-TEM MCF <50 mm? → Administer 10 mL/kg platelets
Fib-TEM MCF <9 mm? → Administer fibrinogen replacement **or** cryo → >5 kg: fibrinogen concentrate 70 mg/kg / <5 kg: 1 unit cryo
Hep-TEM CT >240 seconds? → Administer 4-Factor Prothrombin Complex 25 units/kg **or** FFP 15-30 mL/kg

5. If clinically indicated, send second ROTEM after treatment.
6. If bleeding continues, consider use of recombinant Factor VIIa 90 µg/kg unless four-factor prothrombin complex has been given due to high risk of thrombosis.

FIGURE 19.7 Texas Children's Hospital Coagulation Monitoring and Blood Product and Coagulation Factor Transfusion Algorithm. *CPB,* cardiopulmonary bypass; *cryo,* cryoprecipitate; *ECMO,* extracorporeal membrane oxygenation; *Fib-TEM MCF,* fibrinogen-thromboelastometry maximum clot firmness; *FFP,* fresh frozen plasma; *Hep-TEM CT,* heparinase thromboelastometry clotting time; *Hep-TEM MCF,* heparinase-thromboelastometry maximum clot firmness; *ROTEM,* rotational thromboelastometry; *VAD,* ventricular assist device.

dysfunction from ischemia is also common. Low urine output may occur secondary to secretion of antidiuretic hormone, a response to surgical stress. However, the latter appears to be transitory and usually resolves spontaneously.[280] The incidence of acute renal dysfunction after surgery with bypass to correct congenital heart defects is 17%, ranging from 0.7% for atrial septal defect closure to 59% for arterial switch operations.[281] Deep hypothermic cardiac arrest subjects the kidney to additional ischemia reperfusion injury.[282] Acute renal failure after CPB is uncommon in children, with fewer than 3% requiring dialysis perioperatively.[281,283] Infants who undergo cardiac surgery routinely receive diuretics or a peritoneal dialysis catheter, the latter prophylactically in some instances.[284,285] Although some have attributed the improved survival with early peritoneal dialysis to the prevention of fluid overload, others have attributed it to a more rapid clearance of CPB-induced proinflammatory cytokines.[286] Further

study is required to clarify the mechanism of action of early peritoneal dialysis. In our center, neonates and children with a complex heart defect usually receive peritoneal dialysis immediately postoperatively to prevent fluid overload and decrease inflammatory cytokines. The use of aminophylline has been tested as an alternative but without success.

Recovery of hepatic and gastrointestinal function follows hemodynamic recovery but may require several days. Therapy is mainly supportive. Splanchnic and renal perfusion can be monitored noninvasively using somatic oximetry. Somatic oxygenation may predict renal dysfunction and predict organ failure. Interventions based on the somatic NIRS may improve outcome.[287]

IMMUNE SYSTEM EFFECTS

Leukocytes are activated by the CPB circuit, although their numbers may be depleted by leukocyte filters, which are sometimes used to attenuate the inflammatory response. Despite the theoretical possibility that this may increase the risk of infection or neutrophil dysfunction, this has not been observed in published studies or clinical practice.[288]

ENDOCRINE SYSTEM EFFECTS

The magnitude of the inflammatory and endocrine responses after cardiac surgery depends in part on the duration of the surgical procedure and CPB.[289] In children undergoing brief operating times, postoperative blood concentrations of cortisol, adrenocorticotropic hormone, and β-endorphins are significantly greater than those in children undergoing prolonged operation times. In contrast, the serum concentrations of the proinflammatory cytokines IL-6, IL-1β, and TNF-α are similar in the two groups. Adrenocorticotropic hormone and cortisol concentrations correlated positively with the blood concentrations of IL-1β, IL-6, and TNF-α in the group of children with prolonged operation times.

The plasma concentrations of both epinephrine and cortisol increase after cardiac surgery.[290] In children, prebypass and postbypass cortisol and norepinephrine increase significantly during isoflurane anesthesia when 2 µg/kg of fentanyl is used rather than 25, 50, 100, or 150 µg/kg.[291] No significant increase in the blood concentrations of these hormones occurred with any of the fentanyl doses of 25 µg/kg or greater. In addition to cardiovascular stability, continued use of larger doses of opioids during bypass minimizes the stress responses and stabilizes hemodynamics during and after bypass, but may delay recovery.[292] Also, growth hormone, glucose and insulin, lactate, glutamate, aspartate, and free fatty acid concentrations increase after cardiac surgery, whereas total triiodothyronine concentrations decrease.[293] Limiting the amount of opioids balances the negative effects of inflammation and stress with the opportunity to fast-track children's recovery after surgery for congenital heart disease.[294,295]

Transport to the Intensive Care Unit

Extreme vigilance is required during transfer of the child from the cardiac operating room to the ICU. Monitoring of ECG, arterial, venous, and atrial pressures, and end-tidal CO_2 and pulse oximetry must be maintained continuously; the battery charge of the monitor and the infusion pumps should be checked beforehand to prevent monitor failure and interruption of infusions of vasoactive medications. Resuscitation drugs, airway equipment, and blood products should accompany the child to the ICU. Before leaving the operating room, a report should be given to the ICU staff. Children who are transported with tracheal tubes in situ are usually ventilated manually during transport using the Jackson-Rees modification of the Ayres T-piece circuit, with either 100% oxygen or, for those who require an F_{IO_2} less than 1.0, an oxygen-air blender. For children who require nitric oxide, a respiratory therapist should assist with transport to ensure that no interruptions in therapy occur and that a smooth transfer occurs in the ICU as well. On arrival in the ICU, vital signs are confirmed, all monitoring devices are transferred sequentially to the ICU monitors and rechecked to ensure they are in working order, and a detailed report is given to the ICU staff.

Summary

CPB is a necessary technique for intracardiac and major extracardiac surgery on the great vessels. CPB induces a multitude of physiologic and inflammatory derangements, but, through extensive experience and research, these ill effects can be largely mitigated by a number of evidence-based strategies. Therefore, outcomes after CPB have improved dramatically, and CPB is no longer a barrier to accomplishing complex surgery to correct congenital heart defects, even in neonates.

ANNOTATED REFERENCES

Andropoulos DB, Easley RB, Brady K, et al. Neurodevelopmental outcomes after regional cerebral perfusion with neuromonitoring for neonatal aortic arch reconstruction. *Ann Thorac Surg.* 2013;95(2):648-654; discussion 654–655.

Fifty-seven neonates were studied using MRI and 12-month neurodevelopmental outcome after neonatal aortic arch reconstruction using regional cerebral perfusion (RCP). Pre- and postoperative MRI revealed new injuries in 40% of all patients. However, cognitive outcomes were comparable to a population norm with slightly reduced language and motor outcomes than the reference. RCP can be considered an effective and safe method to support intraoperative cerebral perfusion.

du Plessis AJ, Jonas RA, Wypij D, et al. Perioperative effects of alpha-stat versus pH-stat strategies for deep hypothermic cardiopulmonary bypass in infants. *J Thorac Cardiovasc Surg.* 1997;114:991-1000.

In this study, 182 neonates and infants were randomized to pH-stat or α-stat CPB strategy. Important trends or statistically significant improved outcomes were seen with pH-stat management for deaths, electroencephalographic (EEG) seizures, return of EEG activity, acidosis, hypotension, inotropic support, and length of mechanical ventilation. These improvements were most significant for arterial switch operation patients.

Jonas RA, Wypij D, Roth SJ, et al. The influence of hemodilution on outcome after hypothermic cardiopulmonary bypass: results of a randomized trial in infants. *J Thorac Cardiovasc Surg.* 2003;126:1765-1774.

One hundred thirteen infants randomized to a target hematocrit of 20% (actual 21.5%) versus 30% (actual 28%) on CPB had lower neurodevelopmental outcome scores on the Psychomotor Development Index of the Bayley Scales of Infant Development with 82 for the low hematocrit versus 90 for the high hematocrit group at 1 year of age. The children with lower target hematocrit also had a greater incidence of scores more than 2 SD below the mean (29% vs. 9%).

Manlhiot C, Gruenwald CE, Holtby HM, et al. Challenges with heparin-based anticoagulation during cardiopulmonary bypass in children: impact of low antithrombin activity. *J Thorac Cardiovasc Surg.* 2016;151(2):444-450.

Antithrombin III is an important co-factor for heparin to work particularly in neonates who have lower values leading to a lower heparin efficacy and less suppression of thrombin generation. Recognizing risk factors and individually treat these can improve anticoagulation during pediatric cardiac surgery.

Miller BE, Mochizuki T, Levy JH, et al. Predicting and treating coagulopathies after cardiopulmonary bypass in children. *Anesth Analg.* 1997;85:1196-1202.

This is the classic article describing the reasons for post-CPB bleeding in infants and children. Platelet defects are the most important cause and the first blood product to administer; hypofibrinogenemia is the second most important, and fibrinogen is the next most important blood product, with fresh frozen plasma ineffective or possibly worsening bleeding.

Newburger JW, Jonas RA, Soul J, et al. Randomized trial of hematocrit 25% versus 35% during hypothermic cardiopulmonary bypass in infant heart surgery. *J Thorac Cardiovasc Surg.* 2008;135:347-354.

Perioperative hemodynamics during hypothermic cardiopulmonary bypass and developmental outcome and brain magnetic resonance imaging at 1 year were evaluated. Hemodilution to hematocrit levels of 35% compared with those of 25% had no major benefits or risks overall among infants undergoing two-ventricle repair. Developmental outcomes at 1 year of age in both randomized groups were below those in the normative population.

Odegard KC, Zurakowski D, DiNardo JA, et al. Prospective longitudinal study of coagulation profiles in children with hypoplastic left heart syndrome from stage I through Fontan completion. *J Thorac Cardiovasc Surg.* 2009;137(4):934-941.

Coagulation profiles throughout staged repair of the hypoplastic left heart syndrome were studied. In general, pro- and anticoagulatory factors were lower than the norm and patients after the Fontan operation presented with significantly higher F VIII levels. This could potentially increase the risk of thrombosis.

Pasquali SK, Li JS, He X, et al. Comparative analysis of antifibrinolytic medications in pediatric heart surgery. *J Thorac Cardiovasc Surg.* 2012;143(3):550-557.

Comprehensive review on antifibrinolytic therapy in pediatric cardiac surgery.

Withington DE, Fontela PS, Harrington KP, Lands LC. Perioperative steroids in pediatric cardiopulmonary bypass: we still do not have all the answers. *Pediatr Crit Care Med.* 2016;17(5):475.

This paper discusses the perioperative use of steroids in pediatric cardiac surgery 2016.

Wypij D, Jonas RA, Bellinger DC, et al. The effect of hematocrit during hypothermic cardiopulmonary bypass in infant heart surgery: results from the combined Boston hematocrit trials. *J Thorac Cardiovasc Surg.* 2008;135:355-360.

In this combined review of 271 infants, analysis was undertaken of the effects of hematocrit level at the onset of low-flow cardiopulmonary bypass. A hematocrit level at the onset of low-flow cardiopulmonary bypass of approximately 24% or higher was associated with higher Psychomotor Development Index scores and reduced lactate levels.

Wypij D, Newburger JW, Rappaport LA, et al. The effect of duration of deep hypothermic circulatory arrest in infant heart surgery on late neurodevelopment: the Boston Circulatory Arrest Trial. *J Thorac Cardiovasc Surg.* 2003;126:1397-1403.

Neurodevelopmental outcomes were assessed with a battery of 6 tests in 155 8-year-olds who had a neonatal arterial switch operation using α-stat bypass management, hematocrit of 20% on bypass, and varying duration of DHCA at 18°C. Neurodevelopmental outcomes were not adversely affected for the group as a whole until the DHCA time exceeded 41 minutes (95% lower confidence limit 32 minutes).

Yamamoto T, Wolf HG, Sinzobahamvya N, et al. Prolonged activated clotting time after protamine administration does not indicate residual heparinization after cardiopulmonary bypass in pediatric open heart surgery. *Thorac Cardiovasc Surg.* 2015;63(5):397-403.

A prolonged activated clotting time after pediatric cardiac surgery is a common finding. At a closer look, this does not represent residual heparin concentrations but rather low concentrations of coagulation factors.

A complete reference list can be found online at ExpertConsult.com.

20 Medications for Hemostasis

PHILIP ARNOLD

BLEEDING IS AN INEVITABLE CONSEQUENCE of surgery and trauma. Provided the coagulation processes are normal, a meticulous hemostatic surgical technique is usually adequate to achieve hemostasis for most surgical procedures. However, if the degree of injury is more extensive, major blood loss can occur, particularly if there is a coexistent deficiency of the normal coagulation process. Since the early part of the 20th century, it has been appreciated that transfusion of fluids and human (allogeneic) blood can prevent many of the adverse effects of blood loss. Despite this, it is important to appreciate the risks and limitations of transfusion: packed red blood cells (PRBCs) will fail to correct any existing coagulopathy and immunologic and pathophysiologic adverse effects of exogenous stored blood products may occur.

This chapter examines the specific interventions to correct coagulopathy and reduce the requirement for transfusion of blood products by encouraging hemostasis. Although similar, these objectives are not synonymous. During many types of surgery, in vitro tests may demonstrate only mild coagulation defects, and yet the use of hemostatic medications may reduce blood loss and obviate the need to transfuse PRBCs.[1,2] In the absence of these medications, bleeding itself is often unlikely to be life-threatening. In comparison, severe coagulopathic bleeding is, by its nature, life-threatening. Transfusion of blood products cannot be avoided and the hemostatic medications used are often the blood products themselves. The balance of risk and benefit is very different in these two situations. In the former case, benefit will occur if the risk reduction associated with the avoidance of blood products is greater than the risk from the medication itself. In the latter case, the use of medications that carry a high risk of causing adverse effects is more acceptable if the aim is to prevent death from uncontrolled bleeding.

Avoiding the transfusion of human blood products seems to be a fundamentally good notion. However, many common ideas about the potential harm of transfusion may be mistaken. An audit of the Serious Hazards of Transfusion (SHOT) organization in the United Kingdom reported 3239 adverse events over a 10-year period; this is only 0.013% of all blood transfusions.[3] These adverse events were more common in infants but were reported in only 0.037% of infants who had transfusions. The true incidence of events is likely to be more common because of underreporting, though many of these "events" were procedural errors not associated with actual harm. It is clear that the risk of immediate harm directly attributable to transfusion is exceptionally low. The risk of direct transmission of infection (the most feared risk in the public perception) is particularly small; the risk of transmission of HIV from transfusion of blood in the United Kingdom is 1 in 5 million.[3] The greatest hazard of immediate harm is transfusion of incompatible blood.[4] However, subtle negative effects of transfusion on children's outcomes may be considerably more important.[5] Transfusion of blood may lead to deterioration in pulmonary function and immunologic effects that predispose children to infection. In addition, if the objective of transfused red cells is to boost tissue oxygenation by improving oxygen-carrying capacity, then transfused blood is less effective than the child's own blood for this purpose.[6] Additional considerations include the increasing costs of transfused blood products, the logistical difficulties of maintaining a secure blood supply (in both well-resourced and less well-developed health systems), substantially greater risks of transfusion in poorly developed health systems, and the possibility of new, unrecognized, infective agents entering the blood supply.

There are 2.3 million transfusions each year (37 per 1000 population) in the United Kingdom; 4.2% are given to children younger than 18 years of age (7.1 per 1000) and 1.7% to infants less than one year of age (52 per 1000). An audit of pediatric blood transfusion from Australia revealed 41% of blood transfused was given perioperatively,[7] and blood was transfused during 6.3% instances of anesthesia. The majority of units were used during heart surgery (58% of perioperative use), while a very small minority, 4%, were used during major trauma surgery. Heart surgery (on and off bypass), craniosynostosis surgery, and liver transplantation were all commonly associated with blood transfusion. The epidemiology of major bleeding is less certain. Reports of blood use may be misleading (e.g., neonates undergoing cardiac surgery to correct congenital defects may receive few blood units despite significant bleeding), and blood is also used for purposes such as priming the bypass circuit. Observational studies have reported very heavy blood loss associated with heart surgery in children, with increased (per kilogram) blood loss in smaller children and more complex surgery.[8,9] Cardiac surgery can probably be considered the main cause of major blood loss in children and account for most severe bleeding events in children younger than 1 year.

Aprotinin, recombinant factor VIIa (rFVIIa), and fibrinogen concentrate have all been proposed as "magic bullets" able to restore hemostasis at some stage. However, all of these agents have proved to have limitations; each is of value when they address a specific deficit in coagulation. In many respects, the management of severe bleeding has not greatly changed in recent years. Newer approaches are now emerging, although at the time of writing, robust evidence of their risks and benefits for children is not available. Optimal management of severe bleeding requires the following:

- Good surgical hemostasis
- Adequate preparation, including availability of blood products and the means to administer them
- Targeting of coagulation defects that are either likely (given the clinical context) or have been identified by appropriate coagulation tests
- Avoidance (and recognition) of hypothermia, acidosis, and electrolyte disturbance

Physiology of Coagulation

The understanding of coagulation has shifted greatly in the past few years. The "traditional" model, which emphasizes the importance of a cascade of proteolytic enzymes, has given way to the "cell-based" model of coagulation that emphasizes the importance of cellular elements in coagulation and presents coagulation as a complex web of interactions rather than a linear process.[10,11] This complexity can be confusing and abstract compared with the decisions made in clinical care. However, there are lessons that can be drawn from this, and a basic knowledge of current models of coagulation is of value.

To achieve effective hemostasis, a platelet plug must form at the site of vessel injury. To prevent widespread thrombosis, this process needs to remain localized to the injured site. This is achieved through changes at the cell surface and localization of the procoagulant reactions on the surfaces of specific cells. Different cells possess different procoagulant and anticoagulant properties; these are incompletely understood, but platelets and cells bearing

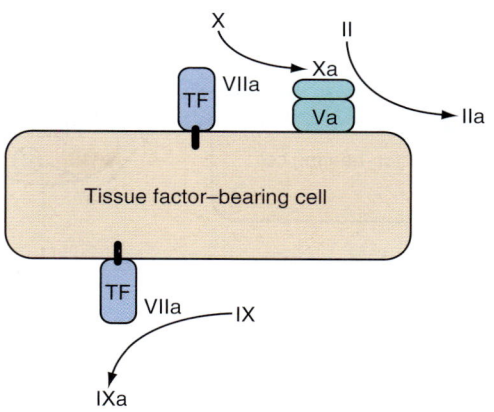

FIGURE 20.1 Initiation. The tissue factor (TF)/VIIa complex on the TF-bearing cell activates factors IX and X. The factor Xa/Va complex, known as the "prothrombinase" complex, forms small amounts of thrombin (factor IIa). (Reproduced from Hoffman M. Remodeling the blood coagulation cascade. *J Thromb Thrombolysis.* 2003;16:17–20.)

tissue factor (TF) are central to the process. Endothelium is vital to inhibition of coagulation, both by forming a physical barrier between components of the coagulation system (principally preventing activated factor VII and platelets from contacting collagen and TF bearing cells) and by playing a more active role in the expression of inhibitory proteins such as thrombomodulin (TM). The phases of coagulation are often described as initiation, amplification, and propagation,[11] though in reality there is considerable overlap.

INITIATION

Coagulation is initiated by an interaction between circulating factor VIIa and TF (a membrane-bound lipoprotein expressed on subendothelial cells such as fibroblasts). A complex is formed between TF and factor VIIa (TF/VIIa), which activates factors IX and X. Factor Xa, in association with cofactor Va, also forms "prothrombinase" complexes on the surface of the TF-bearing cell, which activates a small amount of thrombin (factor IIa)[11] (Fig. 20.1), leading to activation of platelets and factors V and VIII.

This low level of thrombin production occurs constantly and is not sufficient to initiate widespread clot formation. Inhibitors, such as TF pathway inhibitor (TFPI) and antithrombin (AT), provide a localizing function on factor Xa by inhibiting any factor Xa that becomes dissociated from the TF-bearing cell.

AMPLIFICATION

More extensive damage to the vasculature allows greater interaction between TF and factor VIIa and contact between platelets and extravascular components (including collagen and von Willebrand factor [vWF]).[10] There is a strong positive interaction between these two processes that leads to recruitment of further platelets and production of thrombin in large quantities.

Small quantities of thrombin are generated on the TF-bearing cells. This sets up the subsequent propagation phase, during which thrombin is generated in larger quantities (Fig. 20.2). This thrombin has several functions:

- Activation of platelets, exposing receptors and binding sites for clotting factors
- Activation of cofactors V and VIII on the activated platelet surface, thereby releasing vWF to mediate additional adhesion and aggregation at the injury site
- Activation of factor XI to XIa[12]

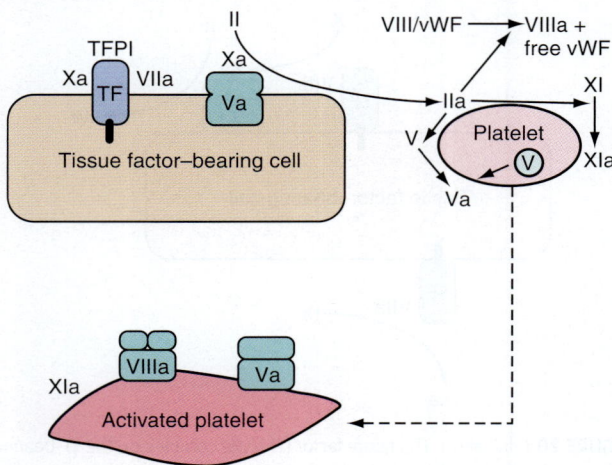

FIGURE 20.2 Amplification. Small amounts of thrombin (factor IIa) set the stage for large-scale generation of thrombin in the propagation phase. Small amounts of thrombin activate platelets, as well as other important coagulation enzymes and cofactors. *TF*, tissue factor; *TFPI*, tissue factor pathway inhibitor; *vWF*, von Willebrand factor. (Reproduced from Hoffman M. Remodeling the blood coagulation cascade. *J Thromb Thrombolysis.* 2003;16:17–20.)

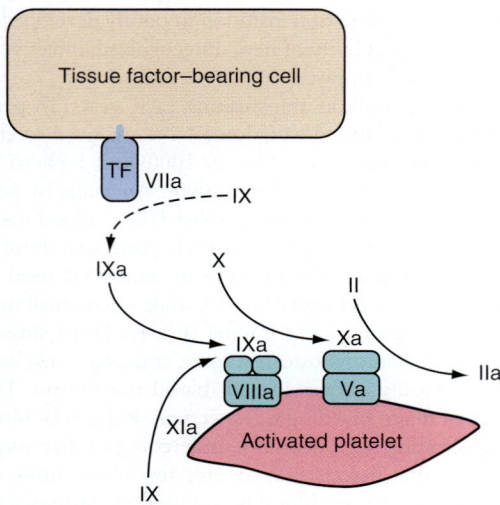

FIGURE 20.3 Propagation. Factor Xa is formed locally by the VIIIa/IXa complex on the surface of the activated platelet. The resulting Xa/Va prothrombinase complex causes a burst of thrombin (factor IIa) generation. *TF*, tissue factor. (Reproduced from Hoffman M. Remodeling the blood coagulation cascade. *J Thromb Thrombolysis.* 2003;16–20.)

- Activation of factor XIII (fibrin-stabilizing factor) and promotion of fibrin cross-linking
- Cleaving fibrinopeptides A and B from fibrinogen (forming fibrin)

The concept of platelet activation is important. Circulating platelets are discoid in shape. Upon activation, they change shape dramatically to increase their surface area, increase expression of a variety of receptors and binding proteins, and release a series of chemicals (including clotting factors and platelet activators). These complex intracellular changes are central to normal coagulation and alterations in this process are central to the coagulopathy seen during surgery and major bleeding.[13,14] Once formed into a clot, the platelets will undergo a further change spreading out to form a physical plug.

PROPAGATION

Propagation occurs on the surface of activated platelets that are recruited to the site in large numbers. Activated factor IX (from both initiation phase and provided by factor XI on the platelet) binds to factor VIIIa. The resultant IXa/VIIIa complex activates factor X on the platelet surface. This factor Xa associates with factor Va and forms the prothrombinase complex. The prothrombinase complex causes a "burst" of thrombin generation to cause clotting via fibrinogen (Fig. 20.3).[10] An inability to form the IXa/VIIIa complex and therefore produce this sustained burst in thrombin production explains the bleeding tendency of children with hemophilia A.[10]

Traditional models of coagulation have also described an alternative pathway initiated by contact factors (XII, XI, prekallikrein, and high–molecular-weight kininogen [HMWK]). This pathway is of no physiologic importance in terms of coagulation activation; however, it provides important acceleration loops through feedback activation of factors VIII, IX, and XI[15] and is important in fibrinolytic and inflammatory pathways.[16]

CLOT INHIBITION

The clot is confined to the site of injury by direct and indirect thrombin inhibitory systems. The direct system consists of AT,

α_2-macroglobulin, and heparin cofactor II (HCII). AT and HCII activities are accelerated in the presence of heparin.

Several indirect systems inhibit thrombin, including the protein C-protein S-TM system and TFPI. Thrombin binds to TM on the surface of intact endothelial cells and can no longer cleave fibrinogen to form fibrin. The TM/thrombin complex is neither able to activate platelets nor activate factors V and VIII. Instead, this complex activates protein C, which binds to the cofactor protein S and inactivates factors Va (on the surface of endothelial cells and platelets) and VIIIa.[10,15]

FIBRINOLYSIS

Fibrinolysis, the breakdown of fibrin into soluble degradation products, is mediated by the proteolytic enzyme, plasmin. Plasmin is formed from an inactive zymogen, plasminogen, which is produced in the liver. This process is controlled by activators and inhibitors. The principal intravascular plasminogen activator is tissue plasminogen activator (tPA).[17] The main inhibitory proteins are plasminogen activator inhibitor-1 (PAI-1), antiplasmins (α_2-PI and α_2-macroglobulin), and thrombin-activated fibrinolysis inhibitor (TAFI) (Fig. 20.4).[18]

In addition to cleaving fibrin, plasmin metabolizes a number of other proteins, including the platelet receptor for fibrinogen (glycoprotein IIb/IIIa) and fibrinogen.[19] Furthermore, plasmin accelerates its own production by metabolizing the conversion of single-chain plasminogen activators to more active two-chain versions. The action of plasmin on fibrin produces a series of degradation products, some of which convey anticoagulant properties; this effect is achieved by preventing polymerization of fibrinogen and by inhibition of platelet function.

tPA is released by vascular endothelium of small blood vessels. Release is increased in the presence of stimuli such as trauma, endotoxins, ischemia, or normal exercise. This effect is mediated via contact activation (through the kallikrein system) and by a series of other substances, including thrombin. Once released, tPA is rapidly metabolized by the liver with a half-life of approximately 5 minutes.[20] Fibrin binds both plasminogen and tPA and

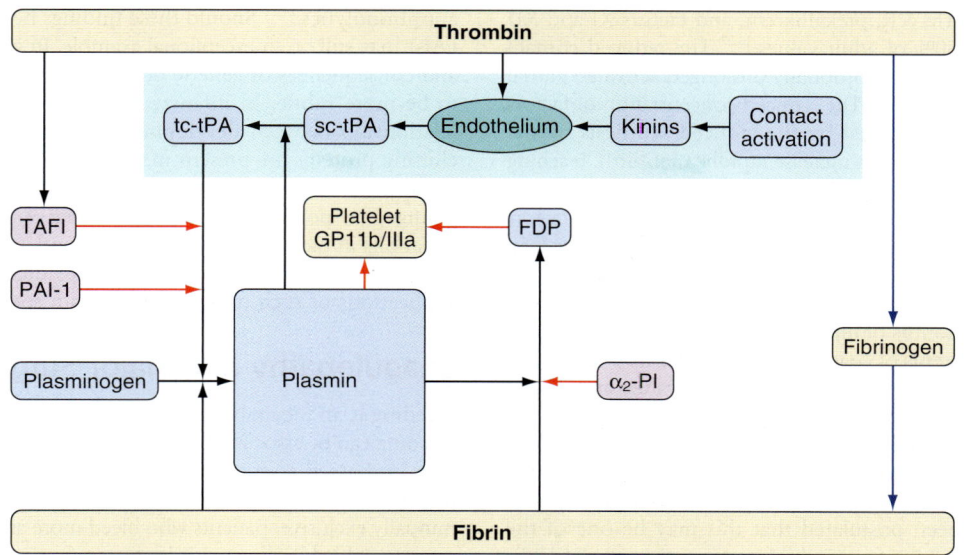

FIGURE 20.4 The main fibrinolytic pathway, leading to the breakdown of fibrin into fibrin degradation products *(FDP)*. It is initiated by release of tissue plasminogen activator *(tPA)* from endothelial cells in response to contact activation *(shaded area)*. Plasminogen needs to be bound to fibrin in order to allow conversion to plasmin. *sc-tPA* and *tc-tPA* refer to single- and (more active) two-chain tPA, respectively. Endogenous fibrinolysis inhibitors are shown in *blue boxes*. Interactions with the coagulation system are shown by *red arrows*. *TAFI*, thrombin-activated fibrinogen inhibitor; *PAI-1*, plasminogen activator inhibitor; *GP*, glycoprotein; α_2-*PI*, α_2-plasmin inhibitor.

greatly accelerates the conversion of plasminogen to plasmin (facilitating its own degradation, but also localizing the process to areas of clot). An alternative mechanism for plasminogen activation by tPA exists through binding to receptors expressed by certain cells (endothelium, white cells, and some tumor cells); the importance of this is unclear.

Excessive fibrinolysis can directly result from excess production of fibrin, as in disseminated intravascular coagulation. This is termed secondary hyperfibrinolysis and in this context, the fibrinolysis is considered beneficial because it prevents widespread vascular occlusion. Therapy is directed at replacement of consumed clotting factors, inhibition of excessive coagulation, and treatment of the underlying cause. Primary hyperfibrinolysis can occur during cardiac bypass, massive blood loss, trauma, and liver transplantation.[20] During the anhepatic stage of liver transplant surgery, there is hyperfibrinolysis because of failure to metabolize tPA. On reperfusion of the liver, a further surge of tPA occurs that can take several hours to return to normal. In coagulopathic patients, reduced thrombin formation may lead to reduced production of TAFI (important in inhibition of membrane-bound plasmin), whereas conversion of single- to two-strand tPA by plasmin may further sustain the process. Individual susceptibility is likely to be important and may have a genetic component.[21,22]

Two groups of drugs are used clinically to inhibit fibrinolysis:
1. Synthetic lysine analogs—for example, tranexamic acid (TXA) and ε-aminocaproic acid (EACA)
2. Protease inhibitors (e.g., aprotinin)

Synthetic lysine analogs are specific inhibitors of plasminogen activation, working by competitively binding to lysine-binding sites on the plasminogen molecule (see Fig. 20.5). This blocks the binding of plasminogen to fibrin, a required step for the conversion of plasminogen to plasmin by plasminogen activators.[23] At larger doses, they may have additional effects through direct inhibition

of plasmin; this includes inhibition of the plasmin-mediated effects on platelets.

Aprotinin is a less specific inhibitor of proteolytic enzymes; it has actions on the kallikrein-kinin (contact) system, as well as the enzymes involved in coagulation and fibrinolysis. In addition, aprotinin may be associated with greater preservation of platelet function, as well as an antiinflammatory effect. This wider spectrum of effects from aprotinin may have additional benefits over the antifibrinolytic lysine analogs.

Developmental Coagulation

The hemostatic system in the neonate rapidly matures toward that of the adult (see also Chapter 10).[24–26] Understanding the rate at which the coagulation system matures with age in childhood is necessary to correctly interpret coagulation tests and to select appropriate interventions to manipulate hemostasis in vivo.

All fetal coagulation factors are produced independently of the mother; fibrinogen starts to be formed as early as 5.5 weeks gestation, and blood can clot at 11 weeks. The development of microassay techniques in the 1980s facilitated the determination of reference ranges for the coagulation factors beginning at 19 weeks gestational age.[15,24,25] In general, there are four fundamental differences between the coagulation systems in the infant and the adult[27]:

- Concentrations of components of the hemostatic system
- The turnover rate of coagulation proteins
- The rate of synthesis
- Differences in the overall ability to generate and regulate the key enzymes: thrombin and plasmin

The concentration of vitamin K–dependent factors II, VII, IX, and X in the neonate are only 50% those of adult values; this leads to a slightly prolonged prothrombin time (PT) or international normalized ratio (INR).[15] Similarly, the concentrations of contact factors HMWK, prekallikrein, and factors XI and XII are approximately 50% of adult values.[15,27] The reduced contact factors account for a disproportionally prolonged activated partial thromboplastin time (aPTT). The reduced concentration of factors at birth is probably explained by the reduced synthesis by the liver; however, concentrations increase rapidly after birth, reaching approximately 80% of adult values by 6 months of age.[15,28]

In contrast, the plasma concentrations of fibrinogen and factors V and VIII at birth are similar to those in adults, although the fetal form of fibrinogen differs in structure from that in the adult; the physiologic significance of this is not clear.[29] Concentrations of vWF in the first 2 months of life are greater than those in adults.[30]

The inhibitor systems of coagulation also differ from adults. At birth, plasma proteins C and S are 35% of adult values and do not reach adult values until adolescence. Neonatal concentrations of AV and HCII are 50% of adult values; they reach adult concentrations by 6 months of age. The concentration of α_2-macroglobulin, however, is increased at birth and remains increased throughout childhood. It has been postulated that this may be one of the mechanisms that protects young children from thromboembolic complications.[31] Thrombin generation in vitro is reduced in children to approximately 75% of adult values.

Despite reduced plasma concentrations of many procoagulant and anticoagulant proteins in infants, there still appears to be an effective hemostatic balance; healthy fetuses, neonates, and children do not suffer excessive hemorrhage in the presence of minor challenges. This is consistent with the thromboelastogram (TEG) studies of healthy children younger than 2 years of age; no defects in coagulation were noted using this test compared with adults, indicating an intact hemostatic system.[32] A further study, conducted using TEG, reported that infants younger than 1 year with complex congenital heart disease have an intact and balanced coagulation-fibrinolytic system but at a "lower level" than healthy children.[33]

GENETICS OF BLEEDING

The hemophilias are a group of genetic diseases that cause excessive bleeding, often in response to minor trauma. Hemophilia A and von Willebrand disease are the most common variants (see also Chapters 10 and 12), associated with low levels of factor VIII and vWF, respectively. A wide range of single-gene defects resulting in deficiencies of single clotting proteins or regulatory proteins has now been described. A further group of single-gene disorders may result in thrombophilic disorders, associated with abnormalities of inhibitory proteins.

Unexplained variation has been observed in bleeding between apparently similar patients in the absence of specific factor deficiency. The causes of this variation are likely to be multifold, according to nuances of surgical technique and subtle difference in disease process and therapy. It might appear counterintuitive that genetic factors have a significant role in acquired bleeding resulting from surgery; however, recently there has been increased interest in the interplay of genetic and environmental factors in the progress of acquired diseases. The genetics of most clotting proteins has been described, and common variations within populations have been revealed for some. Of these, a common polymorphism of PAI-1 has been well described. PAI-1 is an important endogenous inhibitor of fibrinolysis, and deficiency is associated with increased bleeding.[34] The G5/G5 polymorphism is common (about 20% in European populations) and is associated with reduced concentrations of PAI-1. It has been linked (though not consistently) to bleeding after heart surgery and to increased benefit from use of antifibrinolytics.[21,22] Should these findings be substantiated, then PAI-1 may still be an exceptional example. In general, the influence and consequences of genetic determinants of bleeding are likely to be more subtle. In infancy, an additional factor may be the relationship between developmental and genetic factors. Many clotting proteins are present in infants as isoforms distinct from those in adults; this implies a different gene expression in the young. It is possible that understanding genetically determined variations in bleeding will increase our understanding of bleeding and allow us to guide therapy for the individual child. The practical applications of such observations remain speculative.

Coagulopathy and Major Surgery

Bleeding is an inevitable consequence of invasive surgery. Severe bleeding can be associated with derangement of coagulation, which may increase the severity of bleeding or, alternatively, may put the child at risk for thrombosis. These two adverse events are not mutually exclusive: patients who bleed more and who demonstrate coagulopathic bleeding may also be at increased risk of thrombosis.

Coagulation changes during major surgery and bleeding are complex[35] and depend on the clinical context in which bleeding occurs. Coagulation changes that occur in surgical patients have some similarities to those who present after severe trauma. However, the balance of pathophysiologic factors is likely to be very different. The factors underlying these coagulation changes include the following:

- *Dilution.* Components of the coagulation system are lost in shed blood. The volume of blood lost is then replaced by crystalloid, colloid, or blood products that lack these components, leading to progressively smaller concentrations of these coagulation components. To some degree such changes are balanced as the concentration of coagulation inhibitors also decreases. In addition, coagulation components may be produced or released in response to trauma, which limits the reduction in concentration. To complicate this issue, a reduction in the concentration of one component of the coagulation system may not have the same clinical effect as the same reduction of another component. For example, substantial decreases in the concentration of many clotting proteins will not result in severe bleeding, whereas even modest decreases in the number of platelets or the fibrinogen concentration may cause clinically noteworthy bleeding (see also Chapters 10 and 12).
- *Effect of tissue damage.* Extensive interactions occur between inflammatory and coagulation pathways. Inflammation following trauma to tissues can be linked to excess activation of fibrinolytic pathways (resulting in excess bleeding) and to activation of procoagulant pathways (resulting in increased risk of thrombosis).
- *Physiologic derangement associated with blood loss.* Acidosis, hypothermia, and hypocalcemia are associated with excess bleeding.[36] Hypothermia slows proteolytic enzyme activity, reduces fibrin synthesis, and reduces platelet function. These effects are largely reversible on rewarming. Acidosis markedly reduces the activity of coagulation proteins.[37] These effects are not fully reversed by correcting acidosis. Dilution and the effect of citrate (contained in many blood products) cause the plasma calcium concentration to decrease. During major bleeding, the concentration of calcium ions should be monitored and replaced as needed. Cryoprecipitate and fresh frozen plasma (FFP) contains high concentrations of citrate and rapid

administration may cause a precipitous decrease in the plasma concentration of calcium (Fig. 12.9).

- *Effects of treatment.* The use of some synthetic colloids may worsen bleeding to an extent greater than might be expected by dilution. The use of hydroxyethyl starch increases the risk of coagulation abnormalities and of acute kidney injury when compared with albumin, gelatins, or crystalloids.[38] Whether differences exist in coagulation effects of different starches is controversial.[39–41] Concerns about safety of starch solutions have limited their use in adults and children.
- *Use of specific techniques during surgery.* The important effects of cardiac bypass and anticoagulation are discussed later. Liver transplant surgery (see also Chapter 31) and major trauma (see also Chapter 39) are discussed in detail elsewhere in this book.

Alterations in Hemostasis During Pediatric Cardiac Surgery

ROUTINE ANTICOAGULATION

Without anticoagulation, blood will rapidly form thrombi on the artificial surface of the cardiopulmonary bypass (CPB) circuit. The major mechanism for activation of the coagulation cascade during CPB is thought to be the "extrinsic" TF pathway, which is activated as a result of surgical trauma and inflammation.[42–45] Inflammatory mediators induce expression of TF on endothelial cells and monocytes. The "intrinsic" coagulation system is also activated when factor XII is adsorbed onto the surface of the CPB circuit, causing activation of complement, neutrophils, and the fibrinolytic system via kallikrein.[42] Although the intrinsic system has little role in initiating coagulation, activations of kinins will lead to increased fibrinolysis and inflammation.[16]

Heparin

Heparin remains the most effective anticoagulant used to facilitate CPB.[46] The binding of heparin to lysine sites on AT causes a conformational change in AT. This results in an increase in AT potency; the inhibition of thrombin and factors IXa, Xa, XIa, and XIIa is increased by a factor of 1000.[42,47] In infants, AT concentrations are low until 3 to 6 months of age and other heparin cofactors may have greater importance. However, neonates who require surgery for congenital heart disease have unusually reduced concentrations of all major heparin cofactors, and this may be one reason for the greater concentrations of thrombin produced in these patients.[48]

Heparin therapy is most frequently guided by the activated clotting time (ACT). The ACT is an inexpensive and rapid on-site test in which a small sample of blood is mixed with a coagulation activator such as celite, kaolin, or diatomaceous earth. The ACT is the time to produce a stable clot, with a normal value being between 80 and 140 seconds. A value greater than 400 seconds is required for CPB.

There are limitations to the use of the ACT. First, the ACT is altered by hypothermia, hemodilution, platelet activation, activation of the hemostatic system, and aprotinin therapy.[49,50] Accordingly, it does not accurately reflect the heparin concentrations. One study reported that the heparin concentration decreased by 50% as soon as the children went on CPB, even though the ACT doubled.[51] The decrease in the heparin concentration was attributed to hemodilution. Second, in the bleeding child, the ACT is unable to differentiate bleeding because of excess heparin from that of other acquired hemostatic defects.[51] The gold standard

for measurement of heparin concentration is the antifactor Xa assay; however, this test remains too cumbersome for routine clinical use. An alternative point-of-care test is protamine titration (Medtronic Hepcon HMS Plus, Medtronic, Minneapolis, MN). In adult patients, use of this system reduces thrombin formation.[52] Reduced bleeding and reduced thrombin generation in children, as well as reduced thrombin formation in infants, have also been demonstrated with this system.[23,53] However, the accuracy of the device has been questioned[54] and a trial, in infants, was terminated early when increased bleeding and increased length of stay were demonstrated in children in whom the Hepcon device was used.[53] The device underestimated heparin concentration in this group, leading to excess dosing of heparin and inadequate reversal with protamine. After modification of their protocol, use of the device demonstrated reduced bleeding, length of stay, and reduced thrombin formation compared to standard treatment.[53] Agreement between protamine titration, measures of heparin concentration, and laboratory measures has been demonstrated.[55]

A common feature of the pediatric studies using the Hepcon device is increased heparin use compared with regimens based on units per kilogram kg dosing or ACT. This is consistent with other studies of traditional dosing regimens. Using common pediatric heparin regimens (300 units/kg before CPB, then 100 units/kg to keep the ACT above 450 seconds), 50% of children on CPB had low levels of heparin (<2 units/mL).[51] It is suggested that reduced heparin concentrations during CPB is a major factor responsible for activation of coagulation and fibrinolysis. It is likely that widely used regimens for dosing of heparin in children lead to inadequate dosing, and that units per kilogram kg dosing fails to allow for important pharmacokinetic (PK) and pharmacodynamic (PD) differences in children.

Even effective dosing of heparin does not completely abolish the production of thrombin. Low-grade ongoing thrombin production leads to ongoing activation of the coagulation cascade, platelets, fibrinolysis, and the endothelium. The continued thrombin generation and activity during CPB reflects the inability of the heparin/AT complex to inactivate fibrin-bound thrombin or to inhibit thrombin-induced platelet activation.[56] Theoretically, direct thrombin inhibition may be free of these limitations. Practically, the use of the current generation of thrombin inhibitors (such as hirudin and bivalirudin) is limited because of a lack of effective monitoring and reversal. Currently few reports exist of the use of thrombin inhibitors in children, although they would be indicated when heparin use is not possible.[57–62]

Adverse effects of heparin are uncommon; hypotension can result from a reduction in calcium ions or, rarely, anaphylaxis. A benign transient decrease in the platelet count can occur. Heparin-induced thrombocytopenia is a rare but life-threatening prothrombotic condition.[60,63–68]

Reversal of Anticoagulation With Protamine

Protamine is a positively charged polypeptide derived from salmon sperm. It neutralizes heparin by forming an ionic bond with heparin. The resultant complex is removed by the reticuloendothelial system. The most appropriate dosing regimen has yet to be determined. Current dosing used in pediatric practice fails to take into account the range of concentrations of heparin that occur in infants and children.[46,53] The administered heparin dose is often used to guide the dose of protamine; however, it is unclear how this should be modified by various factors, such as additional doses of heparin administered (to prime or during bypass), duration of bypass, ultrafiltration, or developmental coagulation differences in children.[69]

Excessive protamine has been associated with catastrophic pulmonary hypertension and hemorrhagic pulmonary edema.[70,71] It is also known that protamine can be associated with coagulation abnormalities; an increasing ACT occurs at a protamine/heparin ratio of 2.6 : 1, and platelet aggregation occurs with a minimal excess in protamine.[72] Although some studies of regimens to titrate protamine in adults demonstrated encouraging results in terms of reduced bleeding,[73] others failed to demonstrate differences in transfusion requirements.[74]

The clearance of protamine is greater than that of heparin, and "heparin rebound" is described when tissue-bound heparin redistributes.[46] The diagnosis of residual heparin effect or heparin rebound is challenging. The ACT is not a specific measure of excessive heparin and is also poor at detecting heparin at low concentrations (<0.5 unit/mL).[75] The aPTT and PT are similarly nonspecific and may be increased after CPB in the absence of heparin.[76] An unmodified TEG does not reliably detect heparin rebound if the heparin concentration is small.[77] The sensitivity of these tests may be improved by performing similar tests in parallel and comparing the results, such as a reptilase time (unaffected by heparin), or by eliminating residual heparin in vitro with heparinase or protamine. Protamine titration can be used to guide the protamine dose in children; however, in infants, protocols will require modification (50% greater than the calculated dose).[53] In practice, most anesthesiologists continue to give protamine empirically at a protamine/heparin ratio of between 1 and 1.3 to 1. The author's current practice is to give a standard dose of protamine (4 mg/kg) regardless of heparin dose and to give a further 2 mg/kg in the presence of continued bleeding or unusually high ACT. In the presence of continued bleeding, a TEG is run both with and without heparinase to exclude residual heparin.

FAILURE OF HEMOSTASIS ASSOCIATED WITH CARDIAC SURGERY

Complex abnormalities occur in the coagulation system during cardiac surgery owing to the profound surgical insult, hypothermia, acid-base disturbance, blood transfusion, anticoagulants, and use of cardiac bypass. In addition, children and infants with congenital heart disease may have preexisting coagulation defects or be taking medications that affect coagulation before surgery (Table 20.1). The common preoperative and intraoperative risk factors for excessive bleeding are summarized in Table 20.2.

Antiplatelet drugs such as aspirin or clopidogrel may exacerbate bleeding. The clinician must balance the risk of perioperative bleeding against the risk of drug discontinuation when deciding if, and when, to withhold the drug before surgery. In most cases, aspirin can be safely discontinued 5 days before surgery. Prostaglandin E1 can inhibit platelet aggregation at clinically relevant concentrations,[78] although this effect is too subtle to detect in vitro using the TEG.[33] For elective surgery in children receiving oral anticoagulant therapy, it is usually possible to stop the drug before surgery, but "bridging" the patient with heparin may be necessary. An INR of less than 1.5 is usually considered acceptable for surgery. If urgent correction of anticoagulants is required, prothrombin complex concentrates, together with vitamin K, are more effective than FFP.[79] FFP should be used only if prothrombin complex concentrates are not available.

In children with cyanotic congenital heart disease, hemostasis is impaired because of polycythemia, low platelet count and altered function, reduced factors V, VII, and VIII, and increased

TABLE 20.1 Causes of Excessive Bleeding After Pediatric Cardiac Surgery

Preoperative Causes
Liver immaturity
Congenital coagulopathy
Poor nutrition
Cyanotic congenital heart disease
Drugs: prostaglandin E1, aspirin, clopidogrel

Intraoperative Causes
Surgical insult
Inadequate surgical hemostasis before bypass
Inflammatory cascade, fibrinolysis, and so on

Cardiopulmonary bypass
Inflammatory cascade
 Ongoing fibrinolysis
 Increased vascular permeability
 Capillary damage

Hemodilution
 Platelet reduction
 Clotting factor reduction
 Fibrinogen reduction
Complement activation
Platelet abnormality
Disseminated intravascular coagulation

Postcardiopulmonary Bypass
Inadequate surgical hemostasis
Acidosis
Hypothermia
Hypocalcemia
Excessive blood transfusion and clotting factor dilution
Inadequate reversal of heparin with protamine
Excess protamine
Inadequate reversal of heparin in transfused pump blood

TABLE 20.2 Common Predictive Factors for Bleeding

Preoperative	Intraoperative
Age <1 year or weight <8 kg	Individual surgeon
High hematocrit	Complex surgery
Congestive heart failure	Low platelet count during CPB
Repeat sternotomy	Prolonged CPB
Congenital and preoperative acquired coagulopathy	Duration of hypothermia on CPB
Cyanotic congenital heart disease	Deep hypothermic cardiac arrest

CPB, cardiopulmonary bypass.
Data from Williams GD, Bratton SL, Ramamoorthy C. Factors associated with blood loss and blood product transfusions: a multivariate analysis in children after open-heart surgery. *Anesth Analg.* 1999;89:57–64.

fibrinolysis.[33,80] The degree of derangement is related to the degree of cyanosis.[81] Preexisting coagulopathy may also occur in children with severe underlying illness or poor nutritional status.

Despite improvements in the design and materials of equipment, CPB and associated techniques still pose a considerable challenge to the coagulation system. Children are particularly vulnerable because of their small size (relative to the size of the circuit), the complexity of many surgeries, and a lack of reserve owing to developmental differences in the coagulation system.[82] As soon as CPB is established, there is a decrease in the concentration of all hemostatic protein concentrations with a commensurate decrease in platelet numbers as a result of dilution.[51,83] This effect is exacerbated owing to organ sequestration, mechanical disruption, and adhesion to the circuit.[84] Despite anticoagulation, there will be further platelet consumption resulting from activation of coagulation (and particularly platelets) on the surface of the bypass circuit and the contact of "spilt" blood with the pericardium or air (and returned via pump suction). In addition to acquired deficiencies, it is likely that substances that interfere with coagulation accumulate during bypass (e.g., degradation products of fibrin and activators of fibrinolysis). The risk of greater coagulopathy (and of severe bleeding) is increased by smaller patients, more complex surgery, longer bypass, and use of deep hypothermic circulatory arrest.[9,85,86]

A further feature of coagulopathy after heart surgery is platelet dysfunction.[13,14,51,87] As described previously, platelets exert many functions initiated by a range of different activators. Assessing this function in vitro can be difficult. Recent studies have used "multi-plate platelet aggregometry" to access platelet function.[88–90] Platelet adhesion to an electrode is detected in response to specific agonists, with different agonists chosen to detect different pathways within the platelet. When assessing the effect of drugs used to inhibit individual pathways, the application of this is logical and relatively straightforward. It is less clear how this relates to a "global" measure of platelet function during coagulopathy. In a study conducted in children after heart surgery, three of these measures do appear to alter in tandem, suggesting a global change in platelet function. Recovery is observed at 24 hours, despite persistence of thrombocytopenia, with early signs of recovery seen by the time the patient is admitted to the intensive care unit.[14] The speed at which recovery to restore adequate hemostasis occurs, or whether this recovery will occur in patients during active bleeding, is unclear. More widely available testing using TEG demonstrated an inconsistent relationship to "platelet function" measured in this way.[13] In the period soon after bypass it should be assumed that platelet function is abnormal, especially in the patient with active bleeding.

Medications Used for Hemostasis

The pathophysiology of coagulopathies and bleeding in children during surgery is complex, with a multifactorial etiology (see Table 20.1). No single blood component or drug treatment can reverse the abnormal clotting profile. Initially, an attempt should be made to identify the causes of bleeding that may be remedied by surgical interventions. The anesthesiologist should attempt to ensure adequate reversal of heparin and restore normal physiologic variables, such as body temperature, serum calcium concentrations ($[Ca^{2+}]$), and acid-base balance. In the postoperative period, platelets and other blood products, such as FFP and cryoprecipitate, remain the mainstays of treatment for excessive bleeding.[91] Blood products (see also Chapter 12) are briefly discussed here, primarily within the context of pediatric heart surgery.

BLOOD PRODUCTS

It is frequently necessary to administer blood products on a largely empirical basis; laboratory tests describe only parts of

the coagulation process[33] and it often takes too long to obtain results that guide the anesthesiologist in real time as to the requirement for blood components. The TEG is a dynamic whole-blood test that is frequently used as a near-patient test to assess clot elasticity properties and more precisely delineate the bleeding and homeostasis profile. The role of TEG during pediatric heart surgery has been reviewed.[92–95] The use of treatment algorithms based on TEG can limit transfusion of blood products in adults[96–100] and children.[101] In children, it may not be appropriate to use protocols originally designed for adults; alternative approaches have been proposed.[92]

PLATELETS

Platelet dysfunction and thrombocytopenia are common after cardiac bypass in infants. Hence, in the presence of bleeding, transfusion of platelets is logical. Coagulation variables that relate to platelet number and function (such as TEG maximum amplitude) are corrected by infusion of platelets, and clinical experience indicates that platelet transfusion reduces bleeding. This has been confirmed in a small study of children after cardiac surgery.[32] A platelet count of less than 108,000/mm^3 has been identified as a predictor of bleeding, whereas clot strength measured by TEG reduces steeply at platelet counts below 120,000/mm^3. It would appear sensible to follow the common current practice by targeting a platelet count of approximately 100,000/mm^3 during bleeding after heart surgery.[102] In the absence of bleeding, platelet transfusion is generally not indicated unless thrombocytopenia is profound.[103] It would also appear reasonable to use platelets for the initial treatment of presumed coagulopathic bleeding (in the absence of specific clotting tests).

FRESH FROZEN PLASMA

The case for the use of FFP, either as empirical treatment of bleeding or guided by coagulation tests, is considerably weaker than for platelets. The use of FFP in cardiac surgery is based on the observation that the concentration of clotting factors is often reduced in bleeding patients, especially in the period after bypass. The PT (with its derived measure, INR) is the most common test used to detect the presence and gauge the severity of clotting factor deficiency. Unfortunately, observation studies have shown that (1) the PT correlates poorly with clinical bleeding and (2) transfusion of plasma often achieves neither measurable change in the INR nor provides a clinical benefit (particularly if the INR was only marginally raised to <1.7; see also reference 104 and Fig. 12.1). Despite this, FFP is frequently transfused in the absence of either bleeding or significantly increased PT.[105] Administration to patients with greater PT values is more effective in correcting clotting test results; however, large volumes may be required[104] even in the absence of ongoing loss of clotting factors. The situation is further complicated in that initially normal coagulation test results deteriorate during severe bleeding.

Systematic reviews of the use of FFP to treat or prevent bleeding resulting from acquired coagulopathy failed to demonstrate benefit, although the trials examined were small, used a wide range of outcomes, and were conducted in heterogeneous populations.[106,107] In a small observational study of children undergoing heart surgery, a number of patients had coagulopathic bleeding after transfusion of platelets; if these patients were then given FFP, the bleeding increased, whereas if cryoprecipitate was given, bleeding decreased.[32]

It is possible that the lack of efficacy may be related to the dose of FFP used. The dose of FFP most frequently recommended (10–15 mL/kg)[105,108] may be inadequate to restore factor concentrations.[104] Modeling of FFP administration in major trauma suggests that larger doses (30–40 mL/kg) may be required to increase or maintain factor concentrations[109]; however, administration of such a large volume is often undesirable in the absence of severe ongoing bleeding. Addition of FFP to the bypass circuit or during modified ultrafiltration may allow administration of much larger doses but benefit appears to be confined to small infants.[110,111]

CRYOPRECIPITATE

Not all coagulation factors are of equal importance during bleeding. Fibrinogen is present in much greater concentrations than other clotting factors, and while other factors are mainly involved in initiating or amplifying thrombin formation, fibrinogen is the substrate for the production of fibrin. Deficiencies of fibrinogen are reflected in reduced strength of clot and increased bleeding.[112] Cryoprecipitate is the most concentrated fibrinogen replacement widely available, with a fibrinogen concentration four to eight times that of FFP. However, a unit of cryoprecipitate contains less fibrinogen than a unit of FFP, and multiple cryoprecipitate units are required in larger patients. One cryoprecipitate unit for each 10 kg should increase the fibrinogen concentration by 0.5 to 1.0 g/L. Cryoprecipitate is also a source of vWF and factors VIII and XIII, although the clinical significance of this to prevent bleeding is unclear. Cryoprecipitate has been effective in treating bleeding resistant to platelet concentrates alone during pediatric heart surgery.[32]

FRACTIONATED HUMAN BLOOD PRODUCTS

Products such as FFP or cryoprecipitate can be considered crudely purified blood products. It is possible to produce more refined products containing greater concentrations of a single clotting protein or relatively standardized concentrates of selected proteins. Examples of these are prothrombin complex concentrates and fibrinogen concentrate (e.g., RiaSTAP, Haemocomplettan P, CSL Behring GmbH, Marburg, Germany). These products are human blood products produced from pooled plasma; they are presented as a powder requiring reconstitution for use. They do not require freezing or cross-matching, which simplifies their supply, storage, and administration. Risk of viral transmission should be small[113] because of sourcing of plasma from low-risk populations, pooling of plasma from many individual donors (reducing viral load resulting from a single infected donor), and pasteurization. Although the effect of pasteurization on prion infection is less certain, the risk of transmission would be expected to be similarly low. Recombinant factor concentrates (as opposed to factor concentrates of human origin) are increasingly available and avoid cross infection. One such agent, rFVIIa, is discussed later in this chapter (see also Chapter 12). Although the agents discussed in this section are used in a manner similar to traditional factor supplementation to reestablish near-physiologic concentrations, rFVIIa is used very differently to produce factor levels greatly in excess of "normal."

Prothrombin Complex Concentrates

Prothrombin complex concentrates (PCCs) are mixtures of coagulation proteins and inhibitors whose production depends on vitamin K. Initially developed for treatment of hemophilia B (now superseded by the development of factor IX concentrates[114]), PCCs are now most commonly used for rapid reversal of oral anticoagulants,[115] although there is increasing interest in their use to treat other forms of abnormal coagulation.[116–120]

Factor concentrations in different preparations of PCC differ and the production of PCCs has also varied over time.[121] All PCCs contain large concentrations of factors II (PT), IX, and X. They differ in the degree of activation of the factors, the addition of heparin and coagulation inhibitors (such as AT, proteins C and S) and the concentration of factor VII. Those with reduced concentrations of fVII are referred to as three-factor PCCs, while those with greater concentrations as four-factor PCCs. Four-factor PCCs have only recently become available in the United States (KCentra [CSL Behring, King of Prussia, PA], essentially identical to Beriplex or Confidex marketed in other countries). These differences affect both the risks of administration (largely thrombotic risk) and efficacy. Thrombotic risk is associated with low concentrations of inhibitors, high concentration of activated factors (principally VIIa), and possibly with greater activity of prothrombin (essentially owing to accumulation when given repeatedly).[122] Three-factor PCCs are considered less effective at reversing the effects of oral anticoagulants and presumably also in the reversal of other causes of abnormal coagulation.[121,123]

PCCs should be regarded as the agent of choice when rapid reversal of warfarin is required.[79] FFP is indicated (for this indication) only when PCCs are not available. They should be used only when rapid reversal is required (because of bleeding or the need for urgent surgery). In other cases, discontinuation of the anticoagulant is preferred. Vitamin K should be given simultaneously, as the duration of effect of the anticoagulant will exceed that of the PCC (and repeat administration may lead to increased risk of thrombosis). Oral anticoagulants are given to patients at risk of serious complications of thrombosis; when PCCs are given, there should be a clear plan about the timing of surgery and the need for continuing anticoagulation. Dosing depends on the PCC used, on the patient's INR, and on the target INR. Oral anticoagulants other than warfarin are rarely used in children, although such use can be expected to increase. PCCs may be used for reversal of the effects of some of these drugs (e.g., dabigatran, apixaban[124]); however, this can be a complex problem, the management of which is uncertain and such cases should be discussed with a hematologist.

The use of PCCs in cases of severe coagulopathy (not associated with oral anticoagulants) has been described. These agents have been used for some time in some European countries. The scientific rationale is that coagulopathy can result from low concentrations of clotting proteins leading to a failure of adequate thrombin production and failure to initiate and maintain coagulation. Agents such as FFP allow the administration of these clotting proteins but only in a dilute form (reflecting normal population concentrations but no greater). As described earlier, FFP may lack efficacy in reversing established coagulation defects. PCCs may help to restore thrombin production by providing (as inactive zymogens) those clotting factors most critical to coagulation: principally in restoring prothrombin concentration. This is supported by experimental research[125] and observational studies.[116–120] One study conducted ex vivo used plasma from children after cardiac bypass, in which a three-factor PCC was more effective than rFVIIa in restoring thrombin generation.[125] European Society of Anaesthesiology (ESA) guidelines on management of massive bleeding support the use of PCCs (at a dose of 20–30 IU/kg) in adults.[126] It is acknowledged, however, that the evidence for this approach is limited and the associated risks are uncertain. It would be wise to confine use to management of life-threatening bleeding when there is evidence of slow initiation of clotting (a long PT or latent period on TEG) and only after failure of more established therapies. Risk of thrombosis is unclear[127]; however, the risk benefit in this situation is likely to support measures that prove effective in reducing bleeding. Risk should also be compared with other therapeutic options in this situation. The dose in this situation (especially in children) is uncertain. The author has only rarely used these agents and would use a dose of 20 to 40 units/kg.

Fibrinogen Concentrate

The importance of fibrinogen depletion in coagulopathy and bleeding has been increasingly appreciated.[128,129] It has also been recognized that traditional cutoff values for supplementation of fibrinogen during bleeding (1.0 g/L) may be too low and that further advantage can be gained from greater targets, possibly as large as 2.0 g/L. This may be difficult to achieve with traditional blood products. FFP contains only physiologic concentrations of fibrinogen and only modest increases may be achieved, whereas cryoprecipitate requires administration of product from several donors to achieve significant increases in fibrinogen concentration (especially in larger patients). Human fibrinogen concentrate has been available in continental Europe for some time and has recently been licensed within the United Kingdom and the United States for treatment of congenital fibrinogen deficiency. Unlike cryoprecipitate, fibrinogen concentrates contain only fibrinogen and a direct comparison in other forms of coagulopathy has not been made.

Initial reports on the use of fibrinogen concentrate to manage bleeding were largely positive.[130,131] This was supported by two systemic reviews[132,133]; however, the variable quality of early studies was noted. Three recent larger randomized trials reported a lack of efficacy in the management of postpartum hemorrhage,[134] prevention of bleeding after heart surgery,[135] and management of bleeding after adult cardiac surgery.[136] In all three studies the fibrinogen concentration was within the "normal" range (>1.5 g/L) in the majority of patients. The later study (the REPLACE [Randomized Evaluation of fibrinogen versus PLACEbo] trial)[136] is of particular note. Patients were recruited if they demonstrated clinical evidence of significant bleeding shortly after bypass. A low fibrinogen concentration was not required for recruitment, though dosing of the drug (or placebo) was based on the FIBTEM assay (Instrumentation Laboratory, Bedford, MA). The median fibrinogen concentration at recruitment was almost 2 g/L with a narrow interquartile range. Transfusion of allogenic blood products was actually increased in the group receiving fibrinogen.

Several descriptions report individual children receiving fibrinogen concentrates with apparently good effect.[101,137,138] A small trial that compared fibrinogen concentrates with cryoprecipitate in children after heart surgery reported no difference.[139] The role of this agent, therefore, remains uncertain and initial enthusiasm should be tempered by more recent findings.[140] Further trials that may provide a clearer picture are under way in both adults[141] and children. Current use should be confined to the treatment of established bleeding in the presence of a low fibrinogen concentration. The decision to use fibrinogen concentrates in place of cryoprecipitate is likely to be dictated by their availability in different locations, cost, and logistical factors rather than presumed efficacy or safety. The optimal fibrinogen concentration in the presence of bleeding of different severities, and the means by which the fibrinogen concentration is measured, remain issues for further investigation.[142] Inadequate fibrinogen concentration is likely to be a common feature of severe bleeding in children and efforts to maintain concentrations within the normal range are required.

Factor XIII Concentrate

Deficiency of factor XIII during and after CPB has been described, although the importance of this finding is uncertain.[143–146] Supplementation with human or recombinant factor XIII has been demonstrated to reduce bleeding after adult heart surgery, although possibly only in the presence of factor deficiency.[145,147,148] A study in children after heart surgery (in which FFP had been added to the prime) did not demonstrate clinically significant deficiency or correlation between low concentrations and bleeding.[149] The action of factor XIII is to catalyze the formation of cross-bridges between fibrin molecules. High concentrations of factor XIII can be administered as cryoprecipitate, human factor XIII, and recombinant factor XIII. There is insufficient evidence to support its use in acquired bleeding.

PHARMACEUTICAL AGENTS TO REDUCE BLEEDING

Blood products (including fractionated products of human origin) are, in most cases, effective in treating coagulopathic bleeding, but they may be associated with deleterious effects on the patient. An alternative is to use pharmaceuticals to reduce bleeding and blood product requirements. The most commonly used agents are antifibrinolytic drugs are synthetic lysine analogs TXA and EACA and protease inhibitors (aprotinin). Other classes of drugs include recombinant factor VIIa (rFVIIa), used as rescue therapy for severe bleeding, and the hormone analog desmopressin.

Antifibrinolytic Drugs During Pediatric Heart Surgery

Fig. 20.5 summarizes the data currently available on the efficacy of antifibrinolytics during heart surgery in children (to reduce postoperative blood loss).[150–169] Overall almost 2000 children have been recruited into studies of these drugs. Some caution is required in the interpretation of these data. The majority of trials are small, trial methodology is of variable quality; the studies examine a diverse population, use variable dosages, and are statistically heterogeneous. Data from adult cardiac surgical patients are included in Fig. 20.6 for comparison.[169] While these adult studies are also primarily small and of variable quality, they include almost 10,000 patients (in studies reporting postoperative blood loss) and 7 trials with more than 200 participants. Given the available data on efficacy of antifibrinolytic drugs (e.g., tranexamic acid [TXA], ε-aminocaproic acid [EACA], and aprotinin) in children undergoing heart surgery and the evidence of efficacy in different but similar patient populations, it is reasonable to conclude that these drugs are effective (compared with placebo) in reducing blood loss after heart surgery in children. In addition, the three drugs (TXA, EACA, and aprotinin) can all be shown to reduce blood loss individually.

Efficacy is not the only consideration when choosing whether to use a drug. To further define the benefit, it is necessary to consider whether the reduction in blood loss is of a magnitude likely to produce a clinical benefit, whether any benefits are offset by adverse effects, how other outcomes are affected, if the drug also works in important subgroups of patients, and whether the benefits can be better realized by use of other medications. From the earlier analysis, a crude estimation of the expected reduction in bleeding (in children) can be made at 7.7 (3.9–11.6) mL/kg. while the mean blood loss across these studies is 28 mL/kg. This is a potentially useful reduction in blood loss. In a previous meta-analysis, the mean volume of red cell transfusion was also reduced, although only by relatively small volumes.[2] The use of these drugs has not affected the avoidance of transfusion, life-threatening bleeding, surgical reexploration (for bleeding), or

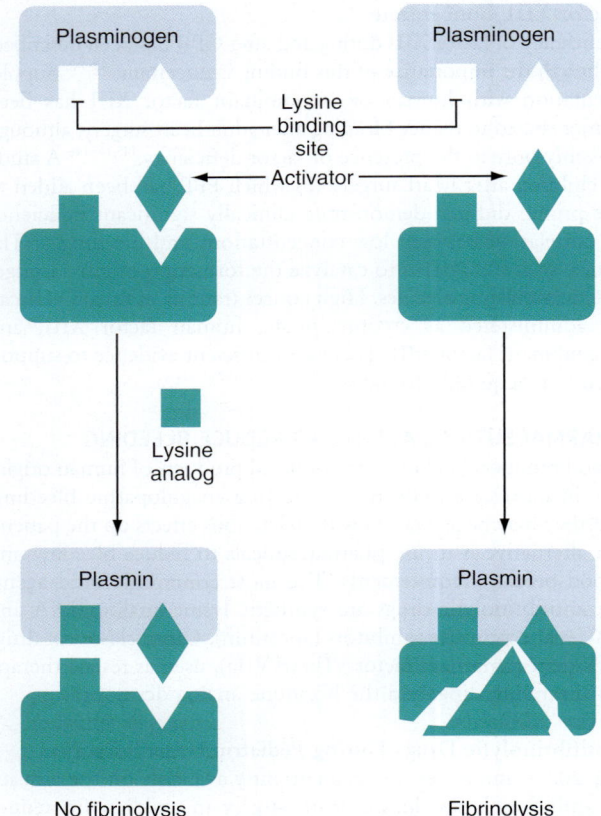

FIGURE 20.5 Diagrammatic representation of the mode of action of the synthetic lysine analogs tranexamic acid and ε-aminocaproic acid. (Reproduced from Mahdy AM, Webster NR. Perioperative systemic haemostatic agents. *Br J Anaesth.* 2004;93:842–858.)

mortality in children. In adults undergoing heart surgery, exposure to transfused blood and surgical reexploration is reduced, although the impact on mortality is unclear.

Children undergoing heart surgery represent a heterogeneous group. Efficacy may be affected by the presence (or absence) of chronic hypoxemia and polycythemia (owing to excessive fibrinolysis in cyanotic patients) or might differ in neonates as opposed to older children (owing to developmental differences in the coagulation system and its response to surgery). Studies of synthetic antifibrinolytic drugs have been undertaken mainly in children with cyanotic heart disease and most studies originate from a single institution (the All India Institute of Medical Science)[152,153,159,160,170] undertaking late correction of cyanotic heart disease. From studies of TXA, data on 6-hour blood loss were available for 144 acyanotic children. No significant reduction in bleeding (mean reduction 1. 8 mL/kg, 95% confidence interval [CI] of −0.8 to 4.5 mL/kg) was demonstrated.[150,151,155]

The fibrinolytic system of neonates differs from that of older children. Plasminogen concentrations are about 50% of adult values, and plasminogen activation occurs more slowly, while levels of inhibitor (PAI-1) are normal.[26] Reduced concentrations of TXA are required to inhibit fibrinolysis in cord blood.[171] Deficiency of substrate (fibrinogen and platelets) may be a greater risk factor for bleeding in neonatal patients than fibrinolysis and it cannot therefore be assumed that inhibition of fibrinolysis will be equally effective.[112] Among studies of synthetic antifibrinolytics, only one recruited infants younger than 2 months of age[150] and it is not

possible to identify any effect specific to this group of patients. In a study of use of aprotinin in children undergoing arterial switch procedures, reduced blood loss, exposure to allogeneic blood products, and reexploration for bleeding was demonstrated.[166] A further randomized trial of aprotinin in neonates was terminated early (because of the concerns about toxicity in adults) and did not show any advantage in indexes of bleeding or postoperative recovery.[168]

Adverse Effects of Synthetic Lysine Analogs

As with any drug used to promote hemostasis, the most worrisome complication is thrombosis. This is likely to be a particular concern in cardiac surgical patients because of vascular anastomoses, conduits, and indwelling vascular lines. Thrombosis is also a potential concern for those patients receiving extracorporeal support.

After any major surgery or trauma patients can be hypercoagulable and at risk of thrombosis. The lysine analogs (TXA or EACA) have not shown an increased risk of renal, cardiac, or cerebral events in adult cardiac surgery patients.[172] Several meta-analyses in adults concluded that prophylactic lysine analogs in cardiac surgery did not increase the incidence of thromboembolic complications.[173-175] However, thrombosis has been reported in nonsurgical hypercoagulable states.[176] Despite isolated case reports, there is no clear-cut evidence that the incidence of thrombosis is increased with either of the lysine analogs. Both TXA and EACA have a very low incidence of anaphylaxis.

The most common acute adverse effect of EACA is hypotension, usually associated with rapid intravenous (IV) administration. Rash, nausea, vomiting, weakness, myopathy, and rhabdomyolysis have been less frequently reported and are associated with longer-term use.[177] EACA is teratogenic and therefore contraindicated in pregnancy. Rapid IV administration of TXA can cause hypotension. Oral administration can be associated with gastrointestinal adverse effects. In an adult study, prolonged infusion was associated with renal dysfunction.[178]

Concern has been raised that both TXA[179-182] and EACA[183] may be associated with an increased risk of seizures in a dose-dependent fashion. Possible mechanisms have been recently reviewed.[184] TXA crosses the blood-brain barrier[185] and causes seizures when applied directly to the brain of animals. The most probable mechanism is antagonism of (inhibitory) glycine receptors.[180] A similar effect can be observed with EACA at equivalent concentrations.[180] This effect is inhibited by general anesthetic agents including propofol and inhalational agents but not by sedatives commonly used during intensive care. A recent large randomized trial in adults undergoing coronary surgery demonstrated an increase in the incidence of seizures in those treated with TXA compared with placebo (0.7% vs 0.1%).[186] A meta-analysis of observational studies of TXA in adults demonstrated a 2.3% incidence of seizures with an odds ratio (compared with no exposure to TXA) of 5.4 (3.3–8.9).[182] This association has also been described in children undergoing heart surgery.[187] A strong publication bias is likely and this may be an overestimate the true size of this effect.

Adverse Effects of Aprotinin

There has been much controversy regarding the adverse effects of aprotinin, largely after the publication of an observational study in adults with acute coronary syndromes that concluded that rates of renal failure, serious intravascular thrombosis (myocardial infarction and stroke), and death at 5 years were increased if aprotinin was used.[172,188] The rate of these complications was not increased with the use of synthetic antifibrinolytics, whereas all

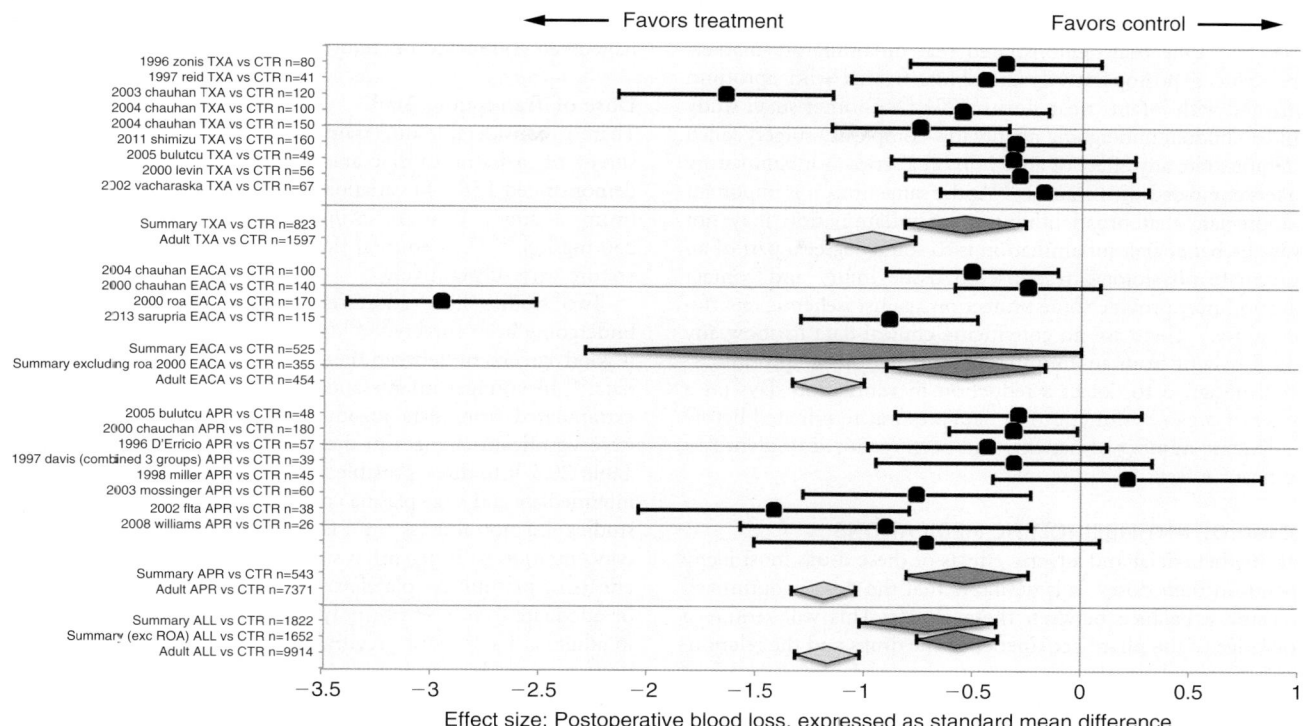

FIGURE 20.6 Efficacy of antifibrinolytic medications in reducing postoperative blood loss compared with control. Results of studies are shown as a standardized mean difference (the size of the treatment effect divided by the standard deviation of the outcome); the outcome used is expressed as milliliters per kilogram over the first 24 postoperative hours. Standardized mean difference is given to allow studies with similar but different outcome measures to be included and to allow a comparison with adult studies. The effect size expressed in this way is generally smaller than that seen in adults, indicating that other causes for variation in bleeding have a greater impact. All three drugs perform better than control. *APR*, aprotinin; *EACA*, ε-aminocaproic acid; *TXA*, tranexamic acid.

agents appeared effective for reducing bleeding. This was followed by the early termination of a large randomized trial (the Blood conservation using Antifibrinolytics: Randomized Trial [BART]) comparing synthetic antifibrinolytics and aprotinin (in "high-risk" adults undergoing heart surgery), when interim analysis showed an increased mortality in the group treated with aprotinin.[189] Excess deaths appeared to result from heart failure and myocardial infarction. Rates of renal failure were not increased in those treated with aprotinin, although an increase in plasma creatinine was common. The relative risk of death in adults treated with aprotinin compared with those treated with synthetic antifibrinolytics was 1.53 (95% CI 1.06–2.22). Data on bleeding in this study were inconclusive, although they suggested a small benefit for aprotinin in preventing severe bleeding. The conclusion of these papers was that aprotinin should not be used in the patient populations studied and led to the drug being effectively unavailable in several countries. Subsequently there has been a reevaluation of the evidence regarding adult patients, pointing at potential shortcomings in the BART study, and the availability of aprotinin has once more increased.

The implication of these studies for children and young adults with congenital heart disease is uncertain. The use of aprotinin in children has reduced dramatically within the United Kingdom.[190] The main cause of death reported in adult patients was from stroke and myocardial infarction. Although thrombotic complications do occur in children, the pathogenesis and underlying risk factors are very different from those in adults. Renal failure occurs in

children after high-risk operations and may share pathogenic factors with postoperative renal failure in adults; aprotinin accumulates within renal tissue and affects local autoregulation of blood flow in response to ischemia. Whether aprotinin causes any more than temporary derangement of renal function tests in adults or children remains unclear. A number of retrospective studies have attempted to examine the link between aprotinin and renal failure in neonates and in children[191–197] with contradictory results. In a large retrospective study, the use of aprotinin was not associated with an increased risk of either renal failure or death.[198] In a further study on an overlapping data set, aprotinin was again not associated with increased risk relative to no antifibrinolytic; however, risks of dialysis or death were lower in those treated with TXA.[199]

Of greater concern is the association between aprotinin and the risk of anaphylaxis.[200,201] The risk is small in children during primary exposure, but the risk increases with repeated exposure (estimated as 2.4%).[202] Therefore, administration of a test dose before the full dose is wise.

Secondary Benefits of Aprotinin
While synthetic antifibrinolytics are selective inhibitors of fibrinolysis, aprotinin is a less specific inhibitor of proteolytic enzymes.[16] Proteolytic enzymes are important mediators of inflammation via contact activation and the complement system; it is postulated that aprotinin may exert a beneficial antiinflammatory effect. A number of studies have demonstrated a reduction in inflammatory

markers, although other studies have failed to corroborate this effect.[203-205] One trial demonstrated that inflammatory markers were reduced postoperatively in infants treated with aprotinin compared with infants treated with TXA.[206] Another small study in older children undergoing mainly low-complexity surgery failed to demonstrate any effect of aprotinin on a series of inflammatory markers compared with control.[204] At the same time, it is important to appreciate that broad inhibition of inflammation may not always be beneficial: inflammation is to some degree a part of an appropriate physiologic response to tissue injury and contact activation may provide some protection against ischemic reperfusion injury.[16] There are no convincing clinical data to show any clinical benefit from an antiinflammatory action of aprotinin.[204] A trial designed to detect a reduction in ventilation days (as a marker of organ dysfunction) in neonates was terminated before an adequate number of patients had been recruited to identify a significant effect.[168]

DOSING OF ANTIFIBRINOLYTIC MEDICATIONS

Both the beneficial and adverse effects of these drugs most likely depend on their doses. It is desirable that the dose is optimized to ensure a balance between these effects. This will require a knowledge of the pharmacokinetics of the drugs and the relationship between their plasma concentration and both effect and toxicity. Regimens based on a single dose have performed less well than those based on infusions or repeated intermittent dosing.[152,161] A reasonable approach is to aim to maintain effective concentration of the drugs throughout surgery and such regimens are best informed by pharmacokinetic studies.[207-213] Experiments conducted in vitro can identify the concentration required to produce the intended biochemical effect (inhibition of fibrinolysis); however, these may vary with the concentration required to produce the intended clinical effect in vivo. The gold standard would be properly conducted dosing studies, using a PK/PD design based on clinically relevant outcomes. As yet only limited dosing studies have been conducted in children.[152,161,214,215]

Dose of Tranexamic Acid

There is considerable uncertainty regarding the dose of TXA. A survey of pediatric cardiac anesthetists in the United Kingdom demonstrated a 50-fold variation in TXA dose used during surgery (from a single dose of 5 mg/kg to a cumulative dose of 250 mg/kg).[190] Furthermore, the doses recommended in the literature vary substantively.

Two studies have addressed the PKs of TXA in children undergoing heart surgery.[210,211] In children older than 1 year, there is good agreement between these studies and suitably scaled adult data.[208] In younger infants and neonates, the PKs could not be extrapolated from data in adults or older children, and there were significant changes in the PKs during the first year of life. Table 20.3 lists three possible dosing schedules that target low, intermediate and large plasma concentrations. Unfortunately, these studies did not address the PD effect of blood loss. In vitro, a concentration of 20 µg/mL is sufficient to inhibit fibrinolysis and effects of plasmin on platelets.[171,216] Smaller concentrations may be adequate to inhibit fibrinolysis in neonatal plasma. However, in adult cardiac patients, regimens that targeted larger concentrations may produce an improved clinical effect.[217] Factors such as bleeding and administration of large volumes of IV fluid may also affect the PKs the drug. The author's practice is to routinely administer a dose similar to the intermediate concentration described (i.e., 60 µg/mL); although more drug is given during severe bleeding.

Dosing of EACA

Two small PK studies can be used to inform the dose of EACA in children[207] and neonates.[218] A larger dose is required to maintain target concentrations assumed to be therapeutic in children older

TABLE 20.3	Three Possible Dosing Schedules Targeting Plasma Concentrations of Tranexamic Acid in Children			
		TARGET TXA CONCENTRATION		
Age		**Low (20 µg/mL)**	**Intermediate (60 µg/mL)**	**High (150 µg/mL)**
0–2 months	Loading dose (mg/kg)	15	50	120
	Infusion (mg/kg per hour)	2.5	7	17
	CPB prime dose (µg/mL prime)	20	60	150
2–12 months	Loading dose (mg/kg)	9 (6–12)[a]	26 (20–30)[a]	65 (45–85)[a]
	Infusion (mg/kg per hour)	2	6	14
	CPB prime dose (µg/mL prime)	20	60	150
>12 months ≤20 kg	Loading dose (mg/kg)	4	13	31
	Infusion (mg/kg per hour)	2	5.5	14
	CPB prime dose (µg/mL prime)	20	60	150
Adults[a,b]	Loading dose (mg/kg)	8	12.5	30
	Infusion (mg/kg per hour)	4	6.5	16
	CPB prime dose (mg/kg prime)	0.6	1	2

Suggested dosing regimen for tranexamic acid during heart surgery to achieve target concentrations of 20, 60, and 150 µg/mL . A dose is added to the circuit prime to prevent dilution on initiation of bypass. This is calculated according to the size of the circuit rather than the patient.

CPB, cardiopulmonary bypass; *TXA*, tranexamic acid.

[a]The required loading dose in children aged 2 months to 1 year alters rapidly with age. The larger relative dose in the range is appropriate for infants close to 2 months while a smaller dose (relative to body size) is appropriate for children closer to 1 year.

[b]Adult low, intermediate, and high dosing would aim for target concentrations of 33 µg/mL, 52 µg/mL, and 126 µg/mL, respectively. The prime dose is in milligrams per kilogram rather than micrograms per milliliter. Pediatric dosing estimations from Wesley MC, Pereira LM, Scharp LA, et al. Pharmacokinetics of tranexamic acid in neonates, infants, and children undergoing cardiac surgery with cardiopulmonary bypass. *Anesthesiology* 2015;122(4):746–758. Adult dosing estimations from Dowd NP, Karski JM, Cheng DC, et al. Pharmacokinetics of tranexamic acid during cardiopulmonary bypass. *Anesthesiology* 2002;97(2):390–399.

than 9 months compared with adults. A dose of 75 mg/kg at induction and repeated on bypass combined with an infusion of 75 mg/kg per hour was recommended.[207] This dose was more effective than two divided doses of 100 mg/kg in a study of patients undergoing late repair of tetralogy of Fallot.[161] A dose of 40 mg/kg, followed by 30 mg/kg per hour and a prime concentration of 100 mg/mL added to the prime, should be adequate to maintain a plasma concentration of 50 μg/mL in neonates.[218] This is, however, a smaller concentration than targeted by the earlier study in children. As with TXA, the concentration required to produce an optimal clinical effect is uncertain. Generally, potency is around 10 times less than TXA and lower concentrations are effective in vitro using neonatal plasma.

Dosing of Aprotinin

Aprotinin rapidly redistributes into the extracellular space after IV administration. It is metabolized in the proximal renal tubules and eliminated in a biphasic pattern: a distribution half-life of 40 minutes and an elimination half-life of 7 hours.[219,220] A PK study of aprotinin in children undergoing CPB examined aprotinin concentrations after administration of weight-based dosing (25,000 KIU/kg bolus before CPB, 35,000 KIU/kg in CPB prime, and 12,500 KIU/kg per hour infusion).[221] There was considerable variation in plasma concentration of aprotinin, with the lowest concentration seen in the smallest patients. This study may help to explain inconsistent results from aprotinin trials in children. Using a dose-per-weight regimen, the smaller children may fail to achieve therapeutic concentrations of aprotinin, in terms of plasmin inhibition and antiinflammatory effects (a concentration of aprotinin <200 KIU/mL would be insufficient to inhibit contact activation on the CPB circuit). This is consistent with greater clearance (expressed as per kilogram) in children (see also Chapter 7, Fig. 7.5). A further PK study of aprotinin in neonates also demonstrated rapid clearance and suggested that considerably larger doses are required to maintain therapeutic concentrations: a 50,000-KIU/kg bolus, 40,000 KIU/kg for CPB priming, and continuous infusion of 54,000 KIU/kg per hour for 3.4 hours and 10,000 KIU/kg per hour for 3.4 hours. Calculation of the dose using nonlinear functions (e.g., body surface area or an allometric ¾-power model; see Chapter 7), as opposed to the linear dose per kilogram may provide more effective dosing. This would result in a 2.5 times greater doses in neonates than would otherwise be given.[54]

WHICH ANTIFIBRINOLYTIC DRUG FOR PEDIATRIC CARDIAC SURGERY?

A meta-analysis of trials in adult patients demonstrated no difference between EACA and TXA. Aprotinin was more effective than either TXA or EACA, and although that effect was marginal, only aprotinin reduced the risk of reoperation.[173] Direct comparisons between TXA and EACA demonstrated no differences in their effects in children.[170,222] Low-dose aprotinin (10,000 KIU/kg followed by 10,000 KIU/kg per hour) has been compared with EACA (100 mg/kg on induction, 100 mg/kg in the pump prime, and 100 mg/kg on weaning from CPB).[159] There was a reduction in postoperative blood loss and transfusion requirements in both groups compared with control, but no significant difference between the two drugs. More recently, TXA (100 mg/kg before, during, and after CPB) was compared with aprotinin (30,000 KIU after induction, 30,000 KIU in the pump, and 30,000 KIU after weaning off bypass). There was a reduction in the time to sternal closure, transfusion requirements, and blood

loss compared with control but there was no significant difference between the two drugs. When the two drugs were combined at the same doses, they showed no additional benefit.[156] A further small trial demonstrated no difference in outcomes between aprotinin and TXA.[223]

Retrospective studies have examined a number of outcomes related to efficacy and adverse effects. Results have been contradictory; some studies reported greater benefit with aprotinin,[192,195,224] whereas others showed no significant effect.[225] One study reported reduced bleeding with aprotinin, but greater creatinine concentrations and more prolonged postoperative ventilation.[193] A large multicenter study (>22,000 patients) demonstrated a benefit with all these drugs; however, mortality and reexploration were least in those who received TXA.[198]

In the absence of convincing evidence of improved efficacy for any drug, the choice of antifibrinolytic depends on the adverse effects and cost. The incidence of important adverse effects is also uncertain. Both mechanistically and from the available data, it would appear that the recent "safety" concerns about aprotinin in adults are not applicable to children. A more certain risk of aprotinin is anaphylaxis with repeated exposure. This is a concern because many pediatric cardiac patients undergo repeat surgery. The greater cost of aprotinin is also difficult to justify in the absence of a clear advantage over lysine analogs. In the absence of further studies, it is the author's conclusion that if an antifibrinolytic is indicated, lysine analogs are preferred over aprotinin.

USE OF ANTIFIBRINOLYTIC DRUGS IN NONCARDIAC SURGERY

There is a trend toward increased use of antifibrinolytic drugs (especially TXA) during noncardiac surgery; principally major orthopedic surgery (e.g., spinal instrumentation, see also Chapter 32) and craniofacial surgery (see also Chapter 35). Aprotinin is less commonly used because of reduced availability and the safety concerns discussed previously.

A total of 27 trials have examined the use of TXA during orthopedic surgery in adults[173]; they report a 50% reduction in the relative risk of requiring a blood transfusion. In 20 of these trials, there was a reduction in the incidence of total blood loss of more than 400 mL. Almost all these studies were conducted in adults undergoing major joint replacement surgery. In one study of adults (n = 147) undergoing posterior spinal fusion, TXA reduced total blood loss by 25%; however, the reduction in blood products transfused was not statistically significant.[226] The popularity of antifibrinolytic use during scoliosis surgery in children and adolescents is reflected in two surveys, which show use in 70% to 80% of hospitals.[227,228] It is unclear whether this use is mostly confined to higher-risk cases; however, in the author's institution, TXA is currently used during all scoliosis surgery as part of a program aimed at reducing the use of blood products. Two meta-analyses and a further systematic review have examined this question (reviewing 6 and 7 studies, respectively); no single prospective study included more than 45 patients.[2,229,230] These meta-analyses concluded that antifibrinolytic drugs reduce bleeding and the volume of red cells transfused. To date there has been no single prospective trial comparing different antifibrinolytics. A retrospective comparison of TXA and EACA appeared to show a superiority of TXA but the doses used were not comparable.[231] The two meta-analyses failed to establish any difference between the drugs.[2,229] It is also not possible to determine whether reported benefits hold for all children undergoing scoliosis repair. Bleeding is greater in children with nonidiopathic scoliosis (including patients with Duchenne muscular dystrophy),[232] those with hemostatic disorders, and in those undergoing more extensive surgery; therefore, in these groups a greater advantage in terms of bleeding reduction might be expected. At least one study examined children with idiopathic scoliosis and demonstrated a reduction in blood loss with aprotinin (see also Chapter 32).[233] As with cardiac studies there is a considerable range in the dose of drug used; in a survey of practice in the United Kingdom, the TXA dose ranged from 3-fold to 5-fold, whereas in published trials the dose varied 10-fold.[227]

Antifibrinolytics are also used widely in craniosynostosis surgery.[234-236] In a survey of North American practice, they were used in 20% of hospitals for strip craniotomy, increasing to 30% for more complex repairs.[237,238] Four small trials—three using TXA[239-241] and one using aprotinin[242]—(a total of 141 children) have addressed the use of these agents for this indication. All of these trials demonstrated reductions in blood transfused and in bleeding. A recent publication demonstrated a greater than 50% reduction in the volume of blood transfused and in the proportion of children transfused (70% vs. 37%).[239] Although all these studies were relatively small, it would appear likely that antifibrinolytics produce a useful reduction in blood loss during craniosynostosis surgery.

A further trend has been the use of antifibrinolytic drugs during surgery not commonly associated with transfusion.[243-246] The objective is to prevent uncommon, but potentially life-threatening, bleeding. Even if these drugs are beneficial in this circumstance, it is likely that very large numbers of patients would require treatment to realize this benefit. In this context, even rare adverse effects may outweigh any advantage.

ANTIFIBRINOLYTIC MEDICATION AND TRAUMA

There is no evidence in children that antifibrinolytic medications should be used to treat massive hemorrhage after trauma. The Clinical Randomization of an Antifibrinolytic in Significant Hemorrhage 2 (CRASH-2) study (a blinded randomized control trial of more than 20,000 patients) demonstrated a reduction in mortality with TXA in adult trauma patients with, or at risk for, significant hemorrhage; mortality was reduced from 16% to 14.5%.[247] Mortality related to bleeding was reduced from 5.7% to 4.9%. No difference was reported in the rates of vascular occlusive events. Despite the size and complexity of the study, it appears that it was properly randomized and blinded. One nonrandomized study of 766 children younger than 18 years of age who were victims of trauma in Afghanistan evaluated 66 children who received TXA; the study found that TXA administration was independently associated with decreased mortality.[248] In the absence of prospective well-controlled studies in children and in the absence of definite evidence of toxicity, it would seem reasonable to consider TXA as part of the treatment for *severe* bleeding from trauma or surgery. Some caution is required and its use should be reserved for severe bleeding—for example, bleeding requiring treatment with non–red cell blood products. A dose of 15 mg/kg followed by 2 mg/kg per hour has been recommended for use in trauma.[249] This represents a simple per kilogram scaling of the dose used in the CRASH-2 study. The dose in children should probably be modified in line with the previous discussion regarding cardiac surgery. A further caveat is that administration more than 3 hours after injury in adults appeared to increase mortality.[250] The significance of this is unclear; however, such late administration should be avoided.

AUTHOR'S RECOMMENDATIONS FOR USE OF ANTIFIBRINOLYTICS

Many children and adults have been recruited for studies of antifibrinolytic drugs. As a consequence, it is reasonable to use these drugs during cardiac surgery, during other surgeries likely to require blood transfusion, and in the management of trauma associated with severe bleeding. Considerable uncertainty remains, however: the dose remains uncertain, the incidence of important adverse effects is unclear, the choice of drug is open to question, and their effectiveness in different patient subgroups and clinical situations is debatable. Any further studies should be designed very carefully to address these questions. In the absence of these data, it is not possible to make solid recommendations. The author's current practice is as follows:

- Antifibrinolytics are used routinely during heart surgery in children with cyanotic heart disease, especially in the presence of polycythemia, reduced saturations for a prolonged period, or iron deficiency.
- Antifibrinolytics are used during cardiac procedures in other children as part of a strategy to reduce transfusion. Greater benefit is likely (but not proven) in children with a greater tendency to bleeding, including smaller children, when bypass times is likely to be long and during repeat surgery.[151,162]
- Antifibrinolytics are given during other major surgical procedures in children including scoliosis repair, multilevel joint surgery, and craniosynostosis repair.
- Synthetic antifibrinolytics are used in preference to aprotinin.
- TXA is used in high dose: 30 to 50 mg/kg bolus followed by 15 mg/kg per hour infusion. Additional drug is given to the CPB circuit. Infusion is continued until significant bleeding has stopped up to 4 hours postoperatively. A larger bolus dose is administered to smaller infants.
- EACA is not used by the author; however, an appropriate dose would be a 75-mg/kg bolus followed by 75 mg/kg per hour (plus, if cardiac bypass is used, an additional 75 mg/kg to the CPB circuit).
- These drugs are used together with other measures to reduce bleeding and transfusion.

DESMOPRESSIN

Desmopressin acetate (1-desamino-8-D-arginine [DDAVP]) is a synthetic analog of vasopressin. The production of desmopressin involves alteration in the chemical structure of naturally occurring vasopressin. In the process, the antidiuretic effect is enhanced and the vasopressor effect is virtually eliminated. Desmopressin is more resistant to enzymatic cleavage, and hence the duration of action is prolonged to 6 to 24 hours.[177] Desmopressin potently causes endothelial release of factor complexes VIII/protein C and VIII/vWf. It has been used in mild hemophilia, von Willebrand disease, coagulopathy of uremia, liver failure, and in adults undergoing cardiac and spinal fusion surgery (see also Chapter 12). The maximum effect of desmopressin is observed at a dose of 0.3 µg/kg. It must be given *after* cessation of the extracorporeal circuit to prevent unwanted platelet activation.[54]

Several meta-analyses of the use of DDAVP in adults have been published. The most recent showed that desmopressin was associated with a small reduction in blood loss, but had no benefit in terms of repeat sternotomy, proportion of patients requiring transfusion, or mortality.[174] It was also associated with a 2.4-fold increase in risk of myocardial infarction.

In children, desmopressin at 0.3 µg/kg failed to demonstrate any benefit for both non–high-risk[251] and high-risk cardiac surgery.[252]

Younger children are not as capable of releasing vWf from endothelial storage sites as older children, and the maximal release of vWf caused by the operative stimulus cannot be enhanced by desmopressin.[253] Potential adverse sequelae from desmopressin include fluid retention, hyponatremia, tachyphylaxis, tachycardia, and mild hypotension.[254] Desmopressin is not currently recommended in pediatric surgery,[82] although one could postulate that it could be reserved for those with ongoing bleeding with evidence of platelet function abnormalities, such as prolonged bleeding time or decreased maximum amplitude values on a TEG.[255]

RECOMBINANT FACTOR VIIA

Recombinant activated factor VII (rFVIIa) is known to be safe and effective for treatment and prevention of hemorrhage in children with hemophilia who have circulating inhibitors to replacement factors (see also Chapters 10 and 12). It is also used in patients with Glanzmann thrombasthenia refractory to platelet transfusion and in patients with factor VII deficiency. Regulatory approval has been granted in Europe and the United States for these indications.

Off-label use of this drug has grown steadily and now accounts for 97% of in-hospital use (Fig. 20.7).[256] This has encompassed a number of indications involving treatment or prevention of acquired bleeding or coagulopathy of varying severity.[257-269] The most common off-label indications are treatment of bleeding related to cardiovascular surgery, trauma, and intracranial bleeds. Off-label use in children is also widespread. One retrospective study recorded 3655 administrations (in 39 U.S. pediatric hospitals over a 7-year period); 46% of uses were in children admitted to a surgical specialty or to a pediatric intensive care unit and more than 20% to cardiac surgery or cardiology. Administration was most common in children younger than 1 year. Another report from a single U.S. hospital reported use in 148 patients over 3 years. This is approximately 7% of cardiac surgeries in children performed at that hospital.[270]

The therapeutic effects of factor rFVIIa begin at doses up to 10 times greater than physiologic concentrations of the endogenous factor. It is therefore not simply a "replacement" therapy of a deficient factor.[271] For rFVIIa to exert a beneficial action, it must generate a burst of thrombin at the site of injury. Two mechanisms likely work in synergy to produce this: first, the TF pathway described previously is stimulated to augment generation of factor Xa; second, high concentrations of rFVIIa bind directly to the surface of activated platelets, again activating factor Xa, leading to thrombin production (Figs. 20.8 and 20.9).[272] Sufficient concentrations of substrate are needed to produce a clot. Measures should be taken to ensure adequate fibrinogen concentration and platelet numbers before giving rFVIIa. In addition, factors such as acidosis and hypothermia reduce the efficiency of rFVIIa.[273] Adequate circulating concentration of prothrombin is also required and a synergy between administration of prothrombin concentrates and rFVIIa has been suggested. Given the expense of rFVIIa, in addition to doubts over its safety, it appears wise to use more established measures before administration.

Evidence that rFVIIa reduces bleeding comes mainly from case reports. Numerous anecdotes appear to demonstrate dramatic reductions in bleeding in apparently catastrophic situations. Demonstrations of even occasional success, in the face of an otherwise hopeless situation, might themselves be taken as a good reason to use the drug. However, rFVIIa is often used for patients at much lower risk of bleeding to death. Reported cases of off-label use in anesthesiology and surgical practice range from truly prophylactic use (in high-risk populations before evidence of severe bleeding), use to control prolonged or severe (but not immediately life-threatening) bleeding, to compassionate use in immediately life-threatening bleeding after exhaustion of all conventional

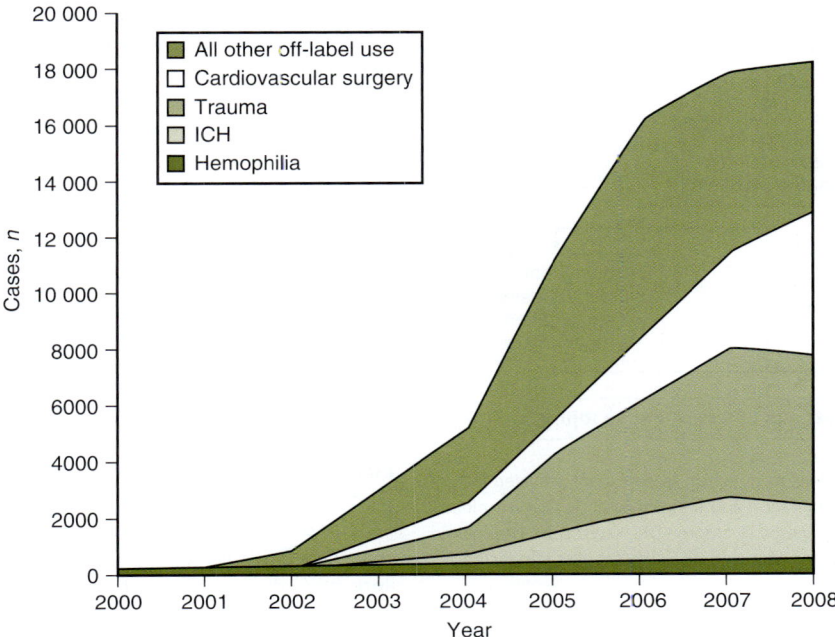

FIGURE 20.7 Use of rFVIIa during hospitalizations in a sample of U.S. hospitals. Data from 12,644 hospitalizations in children and adults. "Off-label" use has grown substantially, while use for hemophilia has remained largely constant. (From Logan AC, Yank V, Stafford RS. Off-label use of recombinant factor VIIa in U.S. hospitals: analysis of hospital records. *Ann Intern Med.* 2011;154(8):516–522.)

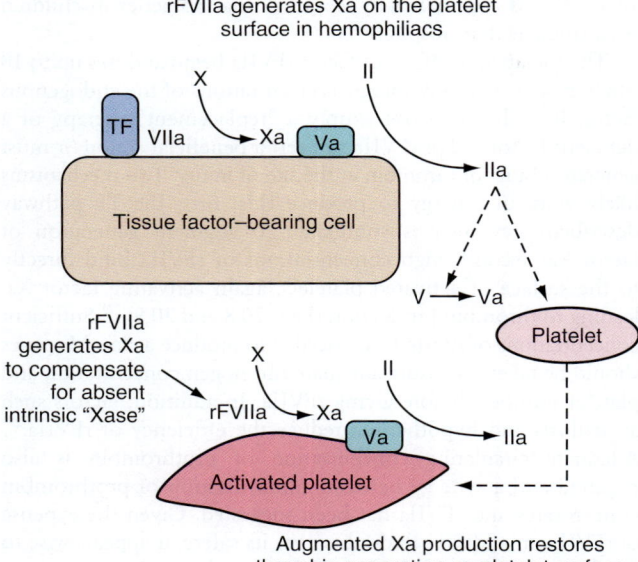

FIGURE 20.8 Schematic representation of the cell-based coagulation model and the proposed mechanism of how recombinant activated factor VII (rFVIIa) can potentially improve coagulation in hemophiliacs. At supraphysiologic concentrations, rFVIIa can bind to the phospholipid membranes of activated platelets, where it activates factor X independent of the tissue factor (TF) pathway, causing a large rise in thrombin at the platelet surface. It can therefore compensate for a lack of factor VIII or IX, a possible explanation for its effectiveness in platelet function disorders. (From Welsby IJ, Monroe DM, Lawson JH, Hoffmann M. Recombinant activated factor VIIa and the anaesthetist. *Anaesthesia* 2005;60:1203–1212.)

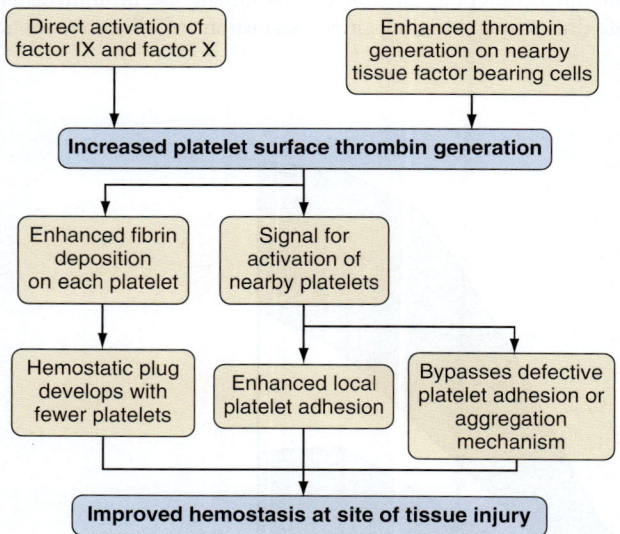

FIGURE 20.9 Theoretic mechanisms by which recombinant activated factor VII could increase thrombin generation and fibrin deposition that may lead to improved hemostasis. (From Welsby IJ, Monroe DM, Lawson JH, Hoffmann M. Recombinant activated factor VIIa and the anaesthetist. *Anaesthesia* 2005;60:1203–1212.)

treatments. The balance of risk and benefit will vary widely within these differing clinical scenarios.

Most controlled trials of rFVIIa have focused on prophylactic use or use in less severe bleeding. Twenty-six randomized controlled trials have examined off-label use of rFVIIa and five have focused

on surgical use.[220,274–277] A meta-analysis of these trials demonstrated no reduction in mortality and only relatively modest reductions in bleeding and transfusion.[278] A study that examined patients with moderately severe bleeding (>200 mL/hour or >2 mL/kg for 2 consecutive hours) after heart surgery in adults demonstrated a reduction in reexploration, bleeding, and in transfusion requirements.[275] The objective of the trial was to examine the safety of using rFVIIa. Unfortunately, the trial was terminated early and although a trend to increased adverse effects was seen, the result was inconclusive. The authors of this study cautioned against wider use before further trials. A single randomized trial (n = 76) that examined prophylactic rFVIIa administration (40 µg/kg) in infants undergoing heart surgery[276] demonstrated neither efficacy nor toxicity in this group. A small trial of patients undergoing neurosurgical procedures appeared to demonstrate a dose-dependent reduction in bleeding.[279] The use of rFVIIa in children has been reviewed.[280]

Concerns about adverse effects of this drug have grown. Two studies have systematically reviewed the data on toxicity.[281,282] In the first study, the rate of thrombosis was greater (10.2% vs. 8.7%) in those treated with rFVIIa. In the second study, data from observational trials reported that mortality was unaffected by treatment with rFVIIa, although the risk of thrombosis increased in some groups (including adult cardiac patients). Both reviews combined data from studies on very different patient populations; thus some caution is required in their interpretation. The risk of thrombosis in children is uncertain and data are inconclusive.[280] In a large multicenter registry, thrombotic complications occurred in 10.8% of children who received off-label rFVIIa and the overall mortality rate in those receiving rFVIIa was 34%.[283] In a further series of children receiving rFVIIa for severe bleeding, the reported rate of thrombosis was low; however, only events believed by the reporter to be directly related to use of rFVIIa or events with a fatal outcome, were reported.[284] Neonates treated with either FFP or rFVIIa for similar indications had a similar incidence of thrombosis (7%),[285] and administration of very large repeated doses in preterm infants did not produce thrombosis.[286] It is clear that both thrombotic complications and mortality are common in patients with bleeding serious enough to warrant use of this drug. Use of rFVIIa is likely to increase the risk of thrombosis, although the impact of this—and the benefit of the drug—vary in different clinical situations. The risk of thrombosis may be further increased in highly proinflammatory states resulting from damage to endothelium and expression of TF on circulating monocytes and platelets. For this reason, rFVIIa should be used very cautiously in patients supported by extracorporeal membrane oxygenation[280] and avoided when there is evidence of widespread activation of coagulation (disseminated intravascular coagulation). The importance of this to patients soon after separation from bypass is unknown.

The dosing regimen for off-label use of rFVIIa is not yet firmly established. One of the difficulties is that there is no satisfactory laboratory test to monitor its effectiveness,[287,288] and factor VII activity does not always predict efficacy.[289] Although it is known that the PT, aPTT, and TEG improve after rFVIIa is given in liver surgery,[290] they cannot reliably be used to determine a dosing regimen. If the main effect of rFVIIa is at the site of injury, clinical observation still remains the best indication of effect.[287] The dose used often closely relates to the dose indicated in hemophilia patients (90 µg/kg), although in practice doses are often rounded to the nearest vial.[290] Although a lower dose of 40 to 60 µg/kg has been proposed,[280] a dose of 40 µg/kg has been shown to have no effect.[276] Larger doses of 60 to 90 μg/kg may prove more effective. Differences in the pharmacokinetics may be a justification for use of larger does in children (clearance is 67 mL/kg per hour in children vs. 37 mL/kg per hour in adults).[291,292]

It would appear that rFVIIa can be effective for the treatment of severe bleeding refractory to other treatments, but it is not universally effective. A detailed review of the off-label use of rFVIIa concluded that evidence of efficacy across a wide range of indications was poor.[293] The risk of thromboembolic complications is substantial in those recovering from severe bleeding, and rFVIIa is likely to increase this risk.[294] There seems to be no reason to think that these considerations do not apply to children, although the balance of risk and benefit may be very different. It is the author's view that rFVIIa should be used only to treat life-threatening bleeding that has proved refractory to other treatments. Outside of properly conducted trials, it should not be used to prevent bleeding, for treatment of less severe bleeding, or as an alternative to blood products. Its use should not delay surgical reexploration if indicated. Every attempt should be made to ensure an adequate platelet count, adequate fibrinogen concentration, correction of acidosis, and near-normothermia before use.

New Drug Development

Much of the previous discussion has concerned use of drugs (and blood products) that have been available for many years. Development of medications for treatment of bleeding is largely driven by a desire to improve long-term treatment of congenital hemophilias.[295] In the past this has led to new therapies for acute bleeding and acquired coagulopathy, and this may be the case in the future. A novel area of research that may be more directly applicable to management of surgical bleeding is development of novel inhibitors of fibrinolysis.[296]

Summary

This chapter began with a review of the mechanism of coagulation and how this is altered during normal development and disease. This understanding of coagulation has led to the development of new treatments, most notably rFVIIa.[11] Complex systems such as the coagulation system behave in unanticipated ways and while mechanisms can be found to justify many interventions, not all interventions will result in a clinically useful improvement for the patient. The coagulation model becomes more complicated when the interactions between coagulation and other systems (noticeably the kinin-kallikrein system[16] and other proinflammatory cascades) are considered in addition to the effects of transfusion of allogeneic blood products. Mechanistic justifications for use of any treatment are therefore limited. Direct evidence that a specific treatment provides a benefit to the child is required. Although the evidence available is still lacking, and at times appear contradictory, I have aimed to give clear advice to the practicing anesthesiologist when possible.

The problems associated with conducting research on this subject are demonstrated by the aprotinin studies. Despite relatively large numbers of patients (including children) recruited into trials, many important questions remain incompletely resolved. Concerns over safety in adults led to the effective withdrawal of this drug. Reappraisal of this evidence (without further studies) has led to its reintroduction in many countries. Regardless of the pros and cons

of using this drug in children, its use has been dictated by factors other than the interests of this population. For therapies aimed at treatment rather than prevention of bleeding, the challenges of conducting well-designed trials are even greater. Currently, several therapeutic approaches are proposed (rFVIIa, fibrinogen concentrates, transfusion protocols based on TEG) that differ from traditional treatment. The requirement for well-conducted trials, with meaningful outcome measures, remains greater than ever.

ACKNOWLEDGMENT

I thank Andrew Wolf and Adam Skinner for their prior contributions to this chapter.

ANNOTATED REFERENCES

Faraoni D, Goobie SM. New insights about the use of tranexamic acid in children undergoing cardiac surgery: from pharmacokinetics to pharmacodynamics. *Anesth Analg.* 2013;117:760-762.

This editorial summarizes the challenges in optimizing the use of antifibrinolytic medications for use in children. It offers an insight into the problems of translating drugs widely used in adults to use in children and how pharmacokinetic, in vitro, and clinical studies can be used to make logical recommendations about dosing.

Faraoni D, Goobie SM. The efficacy of antifibrinolytic drugs in children undergoing noncardiac surgery: a systematic review of the literature. *Anesth Analg.* 2014;118(3):628-636.

A balance review of the evidence regarding use of antifibrinolytic drugs in children during noncardiac surgery.

Guzzetta NA, Miller BE. Principles of hemostasis in children: models and maturation. *Paediatr Anaesth.* 2011;21:3-9.

An excellent review of the changes in coagulation with development, with a particular emphasis of the relevance of this to the use of rFVIIa in pediatric practice. This is part of an issue of Paediatric Anesthesia *themed around topics related to coagulation.*

Hoffman M. Remodeling the blood coagulation cascade. *J Thromb Thrombolysis.* 2003;16:17-20.

Hoffman explains the difficulties associated with the "old model" of coagulation cascade. The paper contains an excellent step-by-step discussion of the cellular based model of coagulation.

New HV, Berryman J, Bolton-Maggs PH, et al. British Committee for Standards in Haematology. Guidelines on transfusion for fetuses, neonates and older children. *Br J Haematol.* 2016;175:784-828.

Extensive and informative guidelines produced in the United Kingdom covering aspects of transfusion in the child, infant, and fetus. While written to reflect U.K. practice, the guidelines are informative for readers from other locations.

Rahe-Meyer N, Levy JH, Mazer CD, et al. Randomized evaluation of fibrinogen vs placebo in complex cardiovascular surgery (REPLACE): a double-blind phase III study of haemostatic therapy. *Br J Anaesth.* 2016;117:41-51.

The REPLACE trial is an important trial conducted in adult cardiac surgical patients. The findings cast doubt on the effectiveness of fibrinogen concentrates in the management of bleeding serving as a further warning that there is no "magic bullet" in the treatment of severe bleeding. Rather, there is a need for good surgical hemostasis and a methodical approach based on an understanding of the physiology and pathophysiology of coagulation.

Warren OJ, Rogers PL, Watret AL, et al. Defining the role of recombinant activated factor VII in pediatric cardiac surgery: where should we go from here? *Pediatr Crit Care Med.* 2009;10:572-582.

A thorough review of the use of rFVIIa in pediatric heart surgery.

Welsby IJ, Monroe DM, Lawson JH, Hoffmann M. Recombinant activated factor VIIa and the anaesthetist. *Anaesthesia.* 2005;60:1203-1212.

This is a very good overview of the mechanisms and use of rFVIIa.

A complete reference list can be found online at ExpertConsult.com.

21

Mechanical Circulatory Support

ADAM C. ADLER, KELLY L. GROGAN, AND LAURA K. BERENSTAIN

THE NUMBER OF INFANTS and children who are hospitalized each year with cardiorespiratory collapse that requires artificial support is substantive. Despite maximal medical therapy, failure of the cardiac and/or respiratory systems to provide adequate end-organ perfusion and oxygenation often results in the need for mechanical support of the circulation, either as an adjunct to cardiopulmonary resuscitation (CPR) or as a bridge to recovery or transplantation. The number of pediatric patients requiring support has been increasing yearly, especially for those with primary cardiac dysfunction. Improved recognition, management, and surgical and perioperative survival of those with congenital heart disease (CHD) has significantly increased the number of children with impaired ventricular function.[1] In addition, with earlier recognition and more aggressive medical management, children with cardiomyopathies are surviving the initial phase of their illness. As a result, there are nearly 15,000 admissions for pediatric heart failure in the United States each year. These admissions carry a mortality of approximately 10%, although 10% to 15% result in the institution of mechanical circulatory support (MCS).[2,3]

The prevalence of heart failure in adults is greater than in the pediatric population, and the development of MCS for adults with end-stage heart failure has correspondingly grown and matured at a faster pace than in children. First-generation ventricular assist devices (VADs) came into routine use in adults in the 1980s.[4] The use of VADs in children began with the application of adult devices in adolescents. Expansion of their use in the children has proceeded more slowly as technologic challenges of effectively "miniaturizing" adult devices to accommodate pediatric weight ranges has resulted in fewer VAD options for children compared with the number and types of devices available for adults. Potential differences between the adult and pediatric patient population include physiologic and anatomic variations, a dissimilar immunologic response to blood transfusions, and a greater thromboembolic risk owing to an immature coagulation cascade.[5,6] Finally, regulatory constraints of device evaluation in a small and heterogeneous patient population[7] also make advances more challenging. Although the number and type of MCS devices available for children remains comparatively limited, particularly for children weighing less than 20 kg in the United States, the use of extracorporeal life support (ECLS) in this population has continued to grow. Initiatives by the National Heart, Lung, and Blood Institute (NHLBI) supporting the development of MCS devices for infants and children offer promising future alternatives.[8]

Mechanical support can be provided either in the form of extracorporeal membrane oxygenation (ECMO) for cardiopulmonary support or in the form of VADs to support cardiac function and maintain perfusion.

Indications for Mechanical Circulatory Support

It is important and often difficult to choose the appropriate time for initiation of MCS. As ECMO has become safer, it is generally agreed that MCS should be initiated early to avoid prolonged low cardiac output states and organ hypoperfusion. Early institution of support better preserves end-organ function and maximizes the opportunity for recovery or bridge to transplantation. Indications for MCS in children can be divided primarily into cardiac and noncardiac indications (Table 21.1). The following criteria for implementation of MCS have been used in one institution: (1) cardiac index less than 2 L/minute per square meter with inotropic dependence; (2) poor peripheral perfusion with metabolic acidosis and mixed venous oxygen saturation less than 40%; (3) signs of impending respiratory, renal, or hepatic failure; and (4) increased or rapidly increasing B-type natriuretic peptide (BNP) concentrations (Table 21.2).[9]

In general, with the exception of pulmonary hypertension and isolated respiratory failure, either ECMO or VAD can be used for all indications. Each device has pros and cons, with the optimal device depending on the acuity of the illness, patient comorbidities, potential for recovery, and anticipated duration of support.[10] Table 21.3 summarizes the numerous patient and device characteristics that must be considered when choosing a strategy for mechanical

TABLE 21.1 Indications for Mechanical Circulatory Support

Preoperative Stabilization

Severe cyanosis/hypercyanotic spells

Pulmonary hypertensive crises

Myocardial dysfunction/cardiac arrest

Malignant dysrhythmias

Sepsis

Postcardiotomy Patients

Heart failure

Early: inability to wean from cardiopulmonary bypass

Late: prolonged low cardiac output syndrome

Procedure related

Stage I palliation for hypoplastic left heart syndrome

After ALCAPA[a] repair

Persistent malignant dysrhythmias

Bridge to Myocardial Recovery

Acute myocarditis

Cardiomyopathy

Acute cardiac transplant rejection

Bridge to Transplantation

Direct bridge to transplantation

Bridge to bridge (short- to long-term support)

Noncardiac Indications

Respiratory failure of oxygenation and/or ventilation

Near-drowning

Severe hypothermia

Drug toxicity

Critical airway (tracheal stenosis)

Sepsis/shock

Extracorporeal Cardiopulmonary Resuscitation

Refractory Cardiopulmonary Arrest

[a]ALCAPA, anomalous origin of the left coronary artery from the pulmonary artery.

TABLE 21.2 Suggested Clinical Criteria for Mechanical Cardiac Support Implementation

Rapid Circulatory Deterioration (CI <2 L/minute per meter squared)

Inotropic dependence

High or rapidly increasing B-type natriuretic peptide

Critical Peripheral Perfusion

Development of metabolic acidosis

Mixed venous oxygen saturation <40%

Signs of Renal, Hepatic, and Respiratory Failure

Ventilatory support with increasing FIO_2

Critically Impaired Myocardial Function on Echocardiography.

CI, cardiac index; FIO_2, fraction of inspired oxygen.

Modified from Hetzer R, Potapov EV, Alexi-Meskishvili V, et al. Single-center experience with treatment of cardiogenic shock in children by pediatric ventricular assist devices. *J Thorac Cardiovasc Surg.* 2011;141(3):616–623; and Potapov EV, Stiller B, Hetzer R. Ventricular assist devices in children: current achievements and future perspectives. *Pediatr Transplant.* 2007;11:241–255.

support. In patients with cardiac failure, the primary goal is to allow the myocardium to rest and recover function (bridge to recovery). In the absence of myocardial recovery, heart transplantation is often considered. However, considering the paucity of available organs, the patient may be transitioned with long-term mechanical support while awaiting a suitable organ (bridge to transplant). Primarily in the adult patient population, a large patient subset exists who are not expected to have myocardial recovery nor are they considered transplant candidates. Use of MCS in this population is designated as destination therapy and is extremely rare in the pediatric population, with the possible exception of a small group of children with Duchenne muscular dystrophy who have undergone VAD placement.[6,11] It is expected that this population will continue to grow because of strong advocacy by these patients and their families. Other pediatric patients who may ultimately benefit from destination therapy include children with chemotherapy-induced cardiomyopathy with ongoing malignancy and unlikely long-term remission, and children with cardiac dysfunction accompanied by multiple comorbidities or impairment that might preclude transplantation.

A critical early decision point in the deployment of VAD support in children is determining whether left ventricular (LV) support alone will suffice. For a left ventricular assist device (LVAD) to provide satisfactory support, adequate right ventricular (RV) function is crucial to allow for adequate LV function and, ultimately, LVAD filling. Unlike heart failure in adults, pediatric heart failure is commonly associated with biventricular failure and/or elevated pulmonary vascular resistance (PVR), both of which may limit LV diastolic filling. Limited data suggest that biventricular VAD (BiVAD) support is more common in pediatric patients, with 29% requiring BiVAD support in a large single-center trial[12] and 35% in the Berlin Heart Investigational Device Exemption (IDE) trial.[13] This contrasts with 9% in a large analysis of the United Network for Organ Sharing (UNOS) data from adult MCS patients listed 1A for heart transplantation and 7% in data from the Interagency Registry for Mechanically Assisted Circulatory Support (INTERMACS).[14] BiVAD support has been associated with increased mortality in both adults and children, likely reflecting the severity of disease in patients requiring such intensive support.

Preoperative cardiopulmonary stabilization may be required in children with profound hypoxemia and/or cardiovascular collapse resulting from hypercyanotic spells, pulmonary hypertensive crises, obstructed total anomalous pulmonary venous return, occlusion of systemic-pulmonary shunts, or cardiogenic shock (see Table 21.1). Preoperative ECMO was used as a bridge to surgical repair or palliation in 26 children, with 62% surviving to discharge and no observed differences in outcome between single-ventricular and biventricular patients.[15] ECMO has also been successfully used to stabilize children with refractory dysrhythmias.[16–18] In a retrospective study, ECMO was used in nine infants with a variety of tachy- or bradydysrhythmias, with all nine surviving to discharge.[19] ECMO has also been used to stabilize children in the cardiac catheterization laboratory, both preemptively before high-risk interventional procedures and as a rescue technique for catheter-induced complications, persistent low cardiac output, or hypoxemia.[20,21]

Failure to wean from CPB after congenital heart surgery is the most common cardiac indication for mechanical support.[22,23] It is estimated that 2% to 5% of all children require ECMO after congenital heart surgery.[24] Postcardiotomy myocardial dysfunction can manifest as either early (inability to wean from CPB) or late

TABLE 21.3 Characteristics of Commonly Used Pediatric Support Devices

Device	Patient Size Restrictions	Duration of Support	Type of Support	Pump Type	Flow	Advantages	Disadvantages	FDA Approval
Short-Term Support Devices								
ECMO	None	<3 weeks	Cardiac/Pulmonary	Continuous	Variable	• Central or peripheral cannulation • Extensive experience in all age groups • Rapid rescue capability • Can be placed at bedside • Less expensive • Easy decannulation	• Higher levels of anticoagulation needed • Increased neurologic complications • Increased bleeding/transfusions • No/limited patient mobility • Usually remain intubated • Need for trained personnel and continuous monitoring	Yes
BioMedicus BP-50 (Medtronic)	None	Days/weeks	Univentricular or biventricular	Continuous centrifugal		• Simpler setup than ECMO • Requires less anticoagulation than ECMO	• No respiratory support • No/limited patient mobility • Generally remain intubated • Direct cannulation of the heart via sternotomy	Yes (6 hours)
CentriMag (Thoratec)	None		Univentricular or biventricular	Continuous centrifugal		• Better ventricular unloading than ECMO		
PediMag (Thoratec)	<20 kg, BSA <1.3 m²		Univentricular or biventricular	Continuous centrifugal	Up to 1.5 L/minute			
Jostra RotaFlow (Maquet)	None		Univentricular or biventricular	Continuous centrifugal	Up to 10 L/minute			
TandemHeart (CardiacAssist)	>40 kg, BSA >1.3 m²	Days	Univentricular or biventricular	Continuous centrifugal	Up to 5 L/minute	• Percutaneous placement possible • Extubation possible	• Transseptal puncture necessary • Risk of thromboembolism • Risk of pump dislodgment	
Impella (AbioMed)	BSA >0.93 m²	Days	Univentricular	Continuous axial	2.5–5 L/minute	• 3 pump sizes • Percutaneous placement possible • Improved unloading of ventricle • Extubation possible	• Pump migration may occur	
Long-Term Support Devices								
Berlin Heart Excor	>3 kg, BSA 0.2–1.3 m²	Months-years	Univentricular or biventricular	Pneumatic, pulsatile	Varies with pump size	• Extubation, ambulation possible • Less anticoagulation than ECMO	• Sternotomy required for implantation	Yes for BTT
HeartWare HVAD	>15 kg or BSA >0.65 m²	Years	Univentricular or biventricular	Continuous centrifugal	Up to 10 L/minute	• Reduced anticoagulation requirements compared with older VADs	• Device exchange may be necessary	Yes for BTT
HeartMate II	>30 kg, BSA >1.4 m²	Years	Univentricular	Continuous axial	>2.5 L/minute	• Discharge home possible		Yes for BTT and DT
SynCardia TAH	BSA >1.2 m² (50 mL) BSA >1.7 m² (70 mL)	Years	Biventricular	Pneumatic, pulsatile	Up to 9.5 L/minute			Yes for BTT

BSA, body surface area; BTT, bridge to transplantation; DT, destination therapy; ECMO, extracorporeal membrane oxygenation; FDA, U.S. Food and Drug Administration; TAH, total artificial heart.

(sustained postoperative low cardiac output syndrome) failure with poor end-organ function, persistently increased plasma lactate concentrations, low mixed venous saturations (<40%), reduced cerebral saturation (>20% below baseline), and escalating inotropic support. It is essential to rule out the presence of residual surgical lesions, coronary insufficiency secondary to surgical manipulation, and mechanical problems (e.g., cardiac tamponade) before initiating MCS.[25] Again, it is crucial to reiterate that early initiation of mechanical support leads to better outcomes. In a study of 81 children, those who had ECMO initiated in the operating room (OR) had a survival rate of 64% compared with 29% in those who had initiation of ECMO in the intensive care unit (ICU).[26] Patients with single-ventricle physiology or cyanotic heart disease are more likely to require mechanical support after CPB. According to the 2015 Extracorporeal Life Support Organization (ELSO) registry,[27] hypoplastic left heart syndrome (HLHS) is the most frequent type of CHD requiring ECMO in neonates. Certain centers have advocated the routine use of MCS to optimize postoperative cardiac output following stage I Norwood procedures.[28] Both ECMO and LVADs have been used for postoperative ventricular support in infants with anomalous origin of the left coronary artery from the pulmonary artery trunk (ALPACA), either as a bridge to recovery or transplant.[29,30]

In children without CHD, viral myocarditis is the most common cause of acute heart failure and ECMO has been successfully used as a bridge to either subsequent VAD therapy or recovery in this population.[31] Other cardiac pathophysiologic processes, such as coronary ischemia, graft rejection after cardiac transplantation, or end-stage heart failure owing to chronic cardiomyopathies, dysrhythmias, or congenital heart defects, may also warrant the use of MCS. ECMO has been used for patients with early and late ventricular dysfunction after cardiac transplantation. In cardiac transplant recipients, 10% required venoarterial (VA) ECMO within the first 2 days of surgery.[32] ECMO is usually the initial modality of choice for support because of the speed of application, familiarity of use, and the ability to manage situations in which RV failure and/or high pulmonary artery vascular resistance are present.[33]

Patients with pulmonary hypertension of varying etiologies may be considered as candidates for ECMO support. Both perioperative patients with reversible pulmonary hypertension (for example, patients with total anomalous pulmonary venous drainage, whose increased PVR should improve after surgical intervention) and those experiencing pulmonary hypertensive crises may benefit from ECMO support. Patients with severe medically refractory pulmonary hypertension may also require VA-ECMO as a bridge to lung or heart-lung transplant. Novalung (Novalung GmbH, Hechingen, Germany) has recently developed a paracorporeal pumpless interventional lung assist device using a low-resistance hollow fiber oxygenator that has been used in patients with cardiogenic shock secondary to pulmonary hypertension. Cannulas are placed in the pulmonary artery and left atrium and the high pulmonary pressures drive the blood through the oxygenator, removing carbon dioxide and improving oxygenation, without the need for a mechanical pump. This allows pulmonary pressures to decrease, off-loading the failing right ventricle and thus facilitating recovery. Four infants and children, 23 days to 23 months of age, were bridged from ECMO to a pumpless paracorporeal lung assist device while awaiting lung transplantation for chronic lung disease and pulmonary hypertension. Three of the four were extubated while supported by the device. One was bridged to recovery, one to transplant, and two died supported by the device while awaiting transplant.[34] One potential advantage of the device is its small size; as it is much smaller than an ECMO circuit, it may allow for easier patient transport during device utilization.

Multiple noncardiac indications exist for the use of ECMO, most importantly respiratory failure. Data from the 2012 ELSO Registry Report show that nearly 50% of patients receiving ECMO have been neonates with respiratory failure.[23] In neonates, the most common indications for ECMO are congenital diaphragmatic hernia, meconium aspiration syndrome, and persistent pulmonary hypertension of the newborn, with an overall survival rate of more than 70%.[23,35] With the H1N1 influenza pandemic, the number of pediatric patients supported by ECMO for respiratory failure increased dramatically.[23,36–38] ECMO can also provide short-term respiratory support for tracheobronchial reconstruction in infants and children with critical airways when conventional mechanical ventilation is either not feasible or has not been successful.[39] Other noncardiac indications for MCS include hypothermia, drug toxicity, and near-drowning. Although septicemia was initially considered a contraindication to MCS, a review of 45 children who required ECMO for hemodynamic support because of septic shock found that almost half survived to discharge.[40] In fact, utilization of ECMO as a bridge to recovery in children with refractory acute respiratory distress syndrome (ARDS) or pneumonia has become widely accepted.[23] ECMO can provide a bridge to lung transplantation or retransplantation, and after transplantation it can be used in cases of severe primary graft dysfunction, although survival in these patient groups remains lower overall than for other indications.[41–43]

ECPR, or extracorporeal CPR, was suggested by the American Heart Association Pediatric Advanced Life Support (AHA PALS) 2010 guidelines for use during refractory CPR during in-hospital cardiac arrests resulting from potentially reversible causes.[44] The AHA 2015 evidence summary continues to support the use of ECPR in pediatric patients, showing improved survival compared with CPR alone. Outcomes after ECPR for children with underlying cardiac disease have been better than for children without underlying heart disease. AHA 2015 guidelines recommend that ECPR be used for children with an underlying cardiac diagnosis who suffer in-hospital cardiac arrests in centers with ECMO protocols.[45]

Contraindications

Contraindications to implementation of MCS should be considered on a case-by-case basis but may include advanced multisystem organ failure, active infection, significant neurologic damage or intracranial hemorrhage (ICH), and severe coagulopathy. Extreme prematurity, very low birth weight, certain chromosomal defects, and/or multiple congenital anomalies may also be considered contraindications.[46] Neonates with low birth weight, extreme prematurity, and pre-existing ICH pose a particular risk when considered for ECMO because of the risk of developing or worsening ICH. Most bleeds occur within the first 72 hours of birth so, in theory, the risk of hemorrhage or extension of existing hemorrhage may be less after 3 days of age. Most ECMO exclusion criteria include patients with grade 3 or 4 ICH, and many consider a birth weight of less than 1.6 kg as a reasonable contraindication to ECMO, as a regression analysis suggested that a minimum weight of 1.6 kg was necessary to achieve a 40% survival in noncardiac ECLS.[47]

For children who require MCS secondary to a cardiac etiology, due consideration should be given to the likelihood of myocardial recovery before instituting support; and if it is unlikely, whether the child is a suitable candidate for cardiac transplantation. While there are no true contraindications, there are some common anatomic issues that should be considered before initiating MCS. These include the thickness of the ventricles, semilunar valve regurgitation, and presence of intracardiac shunts. Thick ventricles, such as in hypertrophic cardiomyopathy, can prevent proper filling of the device. In some patients with a large atrium, atrial cannulation may allow proper filling of the VAD. Significant aortic or pulmonary valve insufficiency will not permit adequate ventricular emptying. Instead, blood recirculates through the regurgitant valve, occasionally necessitating closure or repair of the valve at the time of VAD implantation.[48] Intracardiac defects will also need to be closed at the time of device placement to prevent embolization of thrombus, air, or right-to-left shunting.

The Devices

A variety of devices are available to provide mechanical support for the cardiopulmonary circulation in children. Devices are discussed sequentially based on the type and duration of support provided.

Extracorporeal Membrane Oxygenation

Whereas adults generally have isolated LV failure, children more often require cardiopulmonary support because of hypoxemia,

pulmonary hypertension, or concurrent RV failure. For infants and children who require short-term or urgent cardiopulmonary support, ECMO remains the modality of choice. Initially reported for the treatment of cardiac failure in children in the 1970s, ECMO was subsequently used for mechanical support during interhospital transport.[49,50] Currently the most common cardiac indications for ECMO are failure to wean from CPB, emergent support after cardiac arrest with failure of conventional resuscitation, and early graft failure after cardiac transplantation. Since the ELSO registry began in 1989, ECMO has been the MCS modality with the most pediatric usage, with more than 7500 usages in neonates and children for cardiac indications and more than 26,000 usages in neonates for respiratory support.[23,51]

A typical ECMO circuit is composed of a pump (either a roller pump with a servoregulatory mechanism for controlling circuit flow or a centrifugal pump); a hollow fiber or membrane oxygenator; a heat exchanger; and cannulas (either venous, arterial or both) (Fig. 21.1). A modified ECMO circuit composed of a heparin-coated circuit, Bio-Medicus centrifugal pump (Medtronic, Minneapolis, MN), hollow fiber membrane oxygenator, flow probe, and hematocrit/oxygen saturation monitor, allowing the circuit to be set up and primed in 5 minutes for rapid resuscitation, has been described.[52] Most hospitals supporting such a service have readily available trained personnel to assist with implementing and

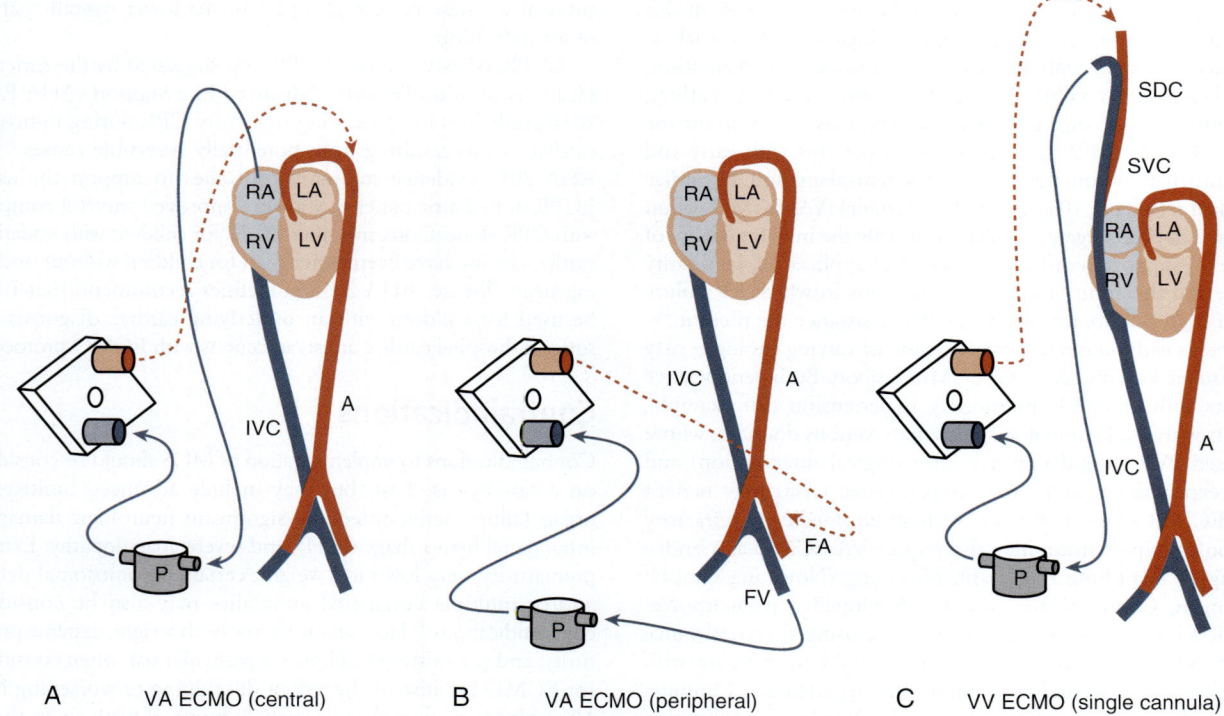

A   VA ECMO (central)   **B**   VA ECMO (peripheral)   **C**   VV ECMO (single cannula)

FIGURE 21.1 Schematic diagram of extracorporeal membrane oxygenation (ECMO) circuit configurations. *Dotted red arrow:* oxygenated blood. The *solid blue arrow* designates deoxygenated blood. **A,** venoarterial (*VA*) central ECMO. The dual venous cannula (right atrium [*RA*] and interior vena cava [*IVC*]) drain blood toward a pump (*P*) that pushes the blood through an oxygenator (*O*) with an integrated heat exchanger before returning via an aortic cannula placed in the ascending aorta (*A*). **B,** VA peripheral ECMO. The venous drainage via a cannula in the femoral vein (*FV*) is pumped through the oxygenator and returned into the femoral artery (*FA*). **C,** Veno-veno (*VV*) ECMO: single dual-chamber (*SDC*) venous cannulation strategy. One chamber has the distal orifice in the inferior vena cava (*IVC*) and the proximal orifice in the superior vena cava (*SVC*). Together they drain blood into the pump/oxygenator; blood returns through an outflow exit orifice into the RA. *LA,* left atrium; *LV,* left ventricle; *RA,* right atrium; *RV,* right ventricle. Alternatively, this can be accomplished through cannulae in both femoral veins. (From Martinez G, Vuylsteke A. Extracorporeal membrane oxygenation in adults. *Continuing Education in Anaesthesia, Critical Care & Pain* 2012;12(2):57–61.)

maintaining ECMO therapy. Versatility and suitability for rapid implementation are advantages of ECMO; venoarterial cannulation in postcardiotomy patients may be either transthoracic via the right atrial appendage and aorta, transcervical via the right internal jugular vein and common carotid artery, or femoral via the femoral artery and vein in larger patients. Heparin-bonded circuitry is often used to minimize surface-induced complement activation, platelet dysfunction, and anticoagulation requirements.[53] A dry circuit can be kept ready for rapid deployment, with crystalloid prime used during initiation of support and addition of blood products (packed red blood cells [PRBCs] and fresh frozen plasma [FFP]) as soon as they become available. Alternatively, use of non–cross-matched blood (O negative) can be used, especially in neonates, until type-specific blood becomes available. During resuscitative efforts, before institution of mechanical support, multiple doses of vasoconstrictors should be avoided if possible, acidosis should be corrected, and the infant's head should be packed in ice to facilitate cerebral protection. Ultimately, the restoration of cardiac output, even with a low hematocrit, is the most important factor for successful resuscitation and long-term survival.[54,55]

Other advantages of ECMO include the ability to institute support in the ICU, provide ultrafiltration or hemodialysis for children during mechanical support, and provide biventricular cardiopulmonary support even in very small neonates.

ECMO CIRCUIT CONFIGURATIONS

Three common configurations exist for ECMO circuits (see Fig. 21.1). The most commonly used configuration, venoarterial ECMO (VA ECMO), is similar to cardiopulmonary bypass (CPB). A venous cannula is placed centrally via the superior or inferior vena cava and an arterial cannula is placed in either the aorta (open chest), femoral, or carotid artery. Blood is drained from the venous cannula, bypassing the heart and lungs, and replaced into the patient via the arterial cannula. VA ECMO can provide gas exchange and hemodynamic support without assistance from the native heart. VA ECMO decreases myocardial work and oxygen consumption and can be used to "rest" the native heart, especially in cases of myocarditis. If there is minimal ventricular ejection, care must be taken to avoid ventricular overdistention, which may necessitate placement of a left atrial vent.

Veno-veno ECMO (VV ECMO) can be accomplished either with a double-lumen catheter or two venous cannulas placed in large veins (femoral, internal jugular). Blood is drained from the patient, gas and/or heat exchange occurs, and the blood is returned to the patient's venous circulation. VV ECMO can provide gas and/or temperature exchange and is primarily used for primary respiratory failure in patients with preserved cardiac function, since VV ECMO requires adequate function of the native heart. Although VV cannulation is technically more difficult and may be associated with a greater frequency of flow issues and cannulation site bleeding, CNS injury is seen less frequently than with VA ECMO.[56]

In arterial-venous ECMO (AV ECMO), both arterial and venous cannulas are placed. The patient's own blood pressure and native heart function pump the blood through the ECMO circuit specifically for gas exchange.

Cannulation in infants and small children is generally performed either directly through the chest (especially postoperatively) or via the neck (carotid and jugular) vessels, as in small patients the ability to provide adequate flow is often unachievable through the femoral vessels. While they are supported by ECMO, patients generally remain continuously ventilated to allow for surfactant production and circulation and for mobilization and extrusion of secretions to avoid infection. "Lung rest" settings, with minimal inspiratory pressure and inspired oxygen and addition of positive end-expiratory pressure to prevent atelectasis, have been suggested.[35]

In a small series of 27 children who underwent VA ECMO for cardiac indications, both nonsurgical and postcardiotomy, the overall survival rate was 59%; of these, 56% required CPR at the time ECMO support was instituted. Of the latter group, 73% survived.[57] Hemodynamic benefits of ECMO include decreased RV preload and pulmonary artery pressures. Owing to reentry of blood into the aorta, an increase in afterload often occurs and may require pharmacologic afterload reduction therapy such as milrinone.

Several management options exist for children with single-ventricle physiology and shunt-dependent pulmonary circulation who require ECMO support. The survival rate of 10 children who underwent single-ventricle palliation and subsequently required ECMO support was greater in those in whom the aortopulmonary shunt was left open during ECMO.[58] Adequate alveolar ventilation must be provided, however, and greater ECMO flow rates are generally required to maintain adequate pulmonary and systemic circulations. In children with low PVR, pulmonary blood flow may prove to be excessive and limitation of shunt flow with surgical clips may become necessary. Although overall children with single-ventricle physiology have comparable survival rates after ECMO support compared with other cardiac patients,[57] in neonates who required ECMO after stage I palliation for HLHS survival to hospital discharge was only 36%, with reduced body weight, duration of support, and renal failure associated with greater mortality.[59] ECMO has been successful in treating children with single-ventricle physiology who develop acute shunt thrombosis or transient depression of ventricular function.[60] Of 44 children with single-ventricle physiology and shunts who required ECMO support, the indication for support was the strongest predictor of survival to discharge, with 81% of those cannulated for hypoxemia surviving, but only 29% of those cannulated for hypotension surviving to discharge.[61] Patients with Fontan physiology who require ECMO have a significantly greater mortality rate (65%), possibly the result of long-standing ventricular dysfunction that is not easily reversible.[62]

ECMO for primary respiratory failure in larger pediatric patients and young adults was heavily used during the H1N1 pandemic starting in 2009. The H1N1 influenza pandemic resulted in a significant number of pediatric patients with respiratory failure and ARDS that proved refractory to conventional and advanced modes of ventilation. According to the ELSO database, use of either VV ECMO or VA ECMO achieved a 60% survival rate in patients refractory to medical therapy.[23]

Disadvantages of ECMO include complex circuitry, the need for greater levels of systemic anticoagulation than required by VADs, the necessity for both blood prime and frequent transfusions, and decreased pulmonary blood flow. Compared with other support modalities, ECMO circuitry is complex and requires full-time supervision by trained personnel. Left atrial decompression may occasionally be inadequate, requiring either the placement of a left atrial vent or an atrial septostomy. Inadequate unloading of the left atrium can lead to mitral regurgitation and pulmonary edema or hemorrhage, and can also minimize the chances of myocardial recovery when the left ventricle is not sufficiently unloaded. Most often moderate levels of ventilatory support must be maintained to ensure that well-oxygenated blood is provided to the coronary arteries, requiring tracheal intubation and sedation throughout the

ECMO period.[63] However, there are recent case reports of awake or ambulatory ECMO (VV or VA) in children.[64]

Although it is effective for rapid rescue and short-term support, ECMO support is generally maintained only for 1 to 3 weeks before the risk of significant complications limits its usefulness.[65] In children who require postcardiotomy ECMO support, the need for prolonged support, renal failure, and low pH in the first 24 hours of support have been associated with a greater mortality.[56] A review of combined data between 2004 and 2009 from the ELSO registry and the Organ Procurement Transplant Network database showed that more than half the children bridged with ECMO to heart transplant failed to survive to hospital discharge, illustrating that ECMO is not able to reliably provide intermediate to long-term mechanical support to bridge children safely to transplantation.[67] Survivors of ECMO support also have greater risk of neurologic impairment than those supported with VADs, with poorer outcomes noted in younger children with more complex disease.[68]

Ventricular Assist Devices

VADs are used for cardiovascular support and are designed to reduce the work of the left ventricle, right ventricle, or both ventricles and to restore adequate cardiac output. They can be classified based on the duration of support, the mechanism by which they propel blood, and the indication for therapy (as discussed earlier). Commonly used devices in children are shown in Fig. 21.2. The length of support is generally divided into short-term use (typically <2 weeks) and long-term use (>2 weeks). Forward flow of blood can be achieved with a rotational device (e.g., centrifugal pumps), a pneumatic pusher plate (e.g. Berlin Heart [Berlin Heart GmbH, Berlin, Germany]), or axial flow (e.g., HeartMate II [Thoratec Corp., Pleasanton, CA]) (see Table 21.3).

Compared with ECMO circuits, VAD circuits have reduced priming volume owing to the lack of an oxygenator and shorter tubing and cause less trauma to blood cells. VAD circuits are composed of an inflow and outflow cannula, a pump (intracorporeal or extracorporeal), a power source with a driveline, and a system controller. Because they do not have an oxygenator and heat exchanger, they require reduced systemic anticoagulation compared with an ECMO circuit. For the LVAD, blood travels from the inflow cannula in the left atrium or the left ventricle, through the device, and into the aorta via the outflow cannula. For the right-sided VAD (RVAD), blood travels from the inflow cannula in the right atrium or the right ventricle, through the device, and into the pulmonary artery via the outflow cannula. In general, inflow cannulas in the ventricle achieve better unloading of the heart, thereby reducing wall stress and allowing for better ventricular recovery and a reduced incidence of thrombotic events.

SHORT-TERM DEVICES

Most commonly used short-term devices are centrifugal pumps providing continuous flow. They include the Bio-Medicus Biopump (Medtronic), CentriMag and PediMag (Thoratec), RotaFlow (Maquet Cardiovascular, Wayne, NJ), and TandemHeart (CardiacAssist, Pittsburgh, PA). The Impella (Abiomed, Danvers, MA) is a continuous-flow axial device. The term *centrifugal pump* is not always synonymous with VAD because a centrifugal pump may also be used with an oxygenator to construct an ECMO circuit. Centrifugal pumps offer the advantage of excellent ventricular unloading and decreased wall stress, optimizing the chances of myocardial remodeling and recovery. Unloading the left ventricle can also decrease LV size and improve septal configuration, resulting

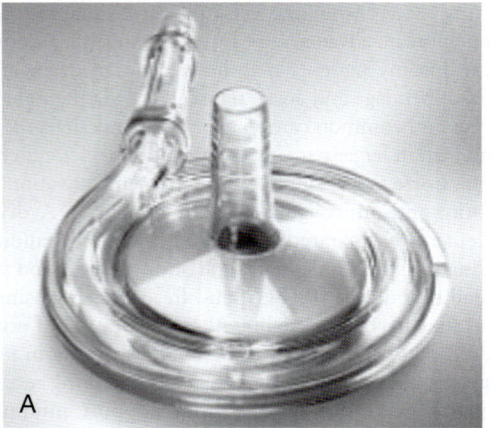

A

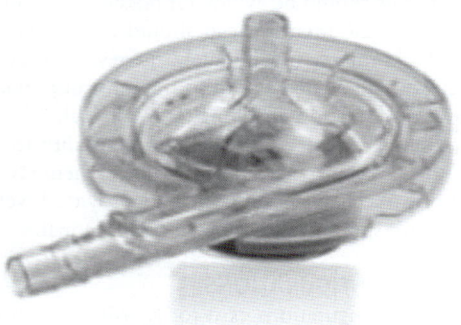

B

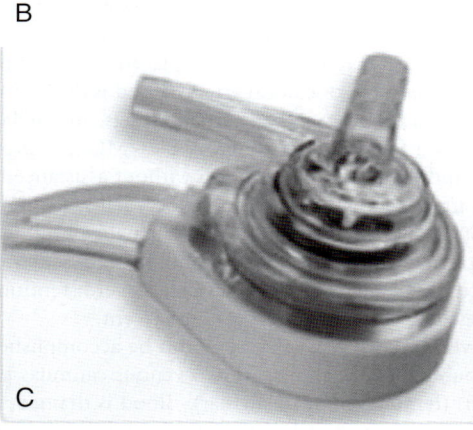

C

FIGURE 21.2 Ventricular assist devices. **A,** RotaFlow assist device. **B,** PediMag assist device. **C,** TandemHeart assist device. (Modified from Mascio CE. The use of ventricular assist device support in children: the state of the art. *Artif Organs.* 2015;39(1):14–20.)

in improved tricuspid valve function and RV inflow.[69] Decreased trauma to red blood cells and a less pronounced systemic inflammatory response are also observed compared with roller pumps.[70] A centrifugal pump spins, creating a vortex, with negative pressure at the inlet drawing blood into the cone and positive pressure at the outlet allowing nonpulsatile ejection at the base. Cardiac output from a centrifugal pump depends on preload, afterload, and the rotational speed of the pump. A flow probe is necessary because increases or decreases in preload and afterload can affect pump flow without changes in rotational speed. Excessive negative inlet pressures (hypovolemia) must be avoided because air can be entrained into the circuit. The main limitation of centrifugal pumps is the inability to provide long-term support related to issues with thrombosis, bleeding, and infection

The RotaFlow pump (see Fig. 21.2A) is an extracorporeal, centrifugal, continuous-flow device that has a rotating mechanism levitated in three magnetic fields with one point bearing, allowing laminar flow and reducing mechanical friction, heat production, and clotting potential compared with the Bio-Medicus pump.[71] It can be used in patients of all sizes, irrespective of body surface area (BSA), and can flow up to 10 L/minute. It has a small priming volume (32 mL), surface area, and passage time, minimizing hemodilution and blood trauma, and can be used along with a membrane oxygenator as an ECMO circuit. It is approved by the U.S. Food and Drug Administration (FDA) for up to 6 hours of use. However, one report described 2 months of support using the RotaFlow in an infant with a dilated cardiomyopathy.[72]

The PediMag (see Fig. 21.2B) is the pediatric version of the CentriMag. It is an extracorporeal, centrifugal, continuous-flow device for children who weigh less than 20 kg. The device has a bearingless, magnetically levitated technology with no points of contact. It has a priming volume of only 14 mL and can provide up to 1.5 L/minute of flow. The PediMag is approved by FDA for up to 6 hours of support and is also commonly used as part of an ECMO circuit.[73]

The TandemHeart is an extracorporeal, centrifugal, continuous-flow device with a priming volume of 10 mL and is capable of flows up to 5 L/minute, with a hydrodynamic fluid bearing supporting the spinning rotor (see Fig. 21.2C). Although size requirements (>40 kg) preclude its use in most children, it is advantageous because it can be placed percutaneously through the femoral vessels in either the OR or the cardiac catheterization laboratory, with a transseptal extended-flow cannula allowing entry from the femoral vein into the left atrium. The arterial cannula can be placed directly into the femoral artery in larger patients, and in patients who weigh less than 80 kg, a vascular graft to the femoral artery may be cannulated to avoid lower extremity vascular compromise.[74] It is FDA approved for up to 6 hours of support.

The Impella is a microaxial continuous-flow device contained in a single-pigtail catheter with three pump sizes: 2.5 L/minute (Impella 2.5 via 12F), 3.3 L/minute (Impella CP via 14F), and 5 L/minute (Impella 5.0 via 21F), respectively (Fig. 21.3). The smaller pump is designed for use in adults requiring partial LV support during high-risk cardiac catheterizations and ablation procedures.[74a] It can also provide full LV support in pediatric patients. The Impella is inserted retrograde through a femoral artery; with the device inlet zone resting in the LV cavity where blood is collected and propelled into the aorta, the deployment is performed under direct vision by fluoroscopy and transesophageal echocardiography (TEE). It has been placed into the ascending aorta in smaller patients via a sternotomy. Pediatric experience is limited to small case series, and the smallest patient reported to be supported was 10 years old, weighing 21 kg with a BSA of 0.93 m².[75]

LONG-TERM DEVICES
Pulsatile Pumps
Pulsatile pumps are VADs facilitating long-term support of the circulation while also allowing tracheal extubation, enteral nutrition, and ambulation for the child. They are paracorporeal and either pneumatically or electromechanically driven. Like centrifugal pumps, pulsatile VADs enjoy several advantages over ECMO: they are simpler in design, less expensive, require lower levels of anticoagulation, and may be used for left, right, or biventricular support of the circulation. Unlike the previously discussed devices, pulsatile pumps are suitable for long-term MCS, but until the advent of the Berlin Heart Excor (BHE), their use in infants and children was severely limited by patient size constraints.

At the time this chapter was written, the BHE is the most popular pediatric long-term support device. First used in adults in 1987, the BHE is a pulsatile, paracorporeal pump currently manufactured in several different pump sizes (10, 15, 25, 30, 50, and 60 mL) (Fig. 21.4).[76] Smaller pumps are appropriate to support neonates and infants, while the 25- and 30-mL pumps will support children weighing up to 20 to 25 kg. The pediatric version was first used in 1992 and has since been successfully used in neonates and infants with a BSA as low as 0.2 m².[77,78] An investigational device exemption (IDE) trial was begun in the United States in 2007; before this, the BHE was used nearly 100 times in North America at 29 different institutions under compassionate use regulations. A review of 73 of these initial patients (weight 3–87.6 kg) revealed a 77% success rate in bridging to either transplant or recovery, with a median support time of 1.6 months. Younger age and the need for BiVAD support were risk factors for increased mortality.[79] The BHE received FDA approval in 2011.

The BHE consists of a pneumatically driven translucent polyurethane pump, trileaflet polyurethane inlet and outlet valves, and silicone inflow and outflow cannulas (see Fig. 21.5). The cannulas exit the skin to the paracorporeal location through the upper abdominal wall. One advantage to the external location is the ability to change the device if thrombus formation is identified.

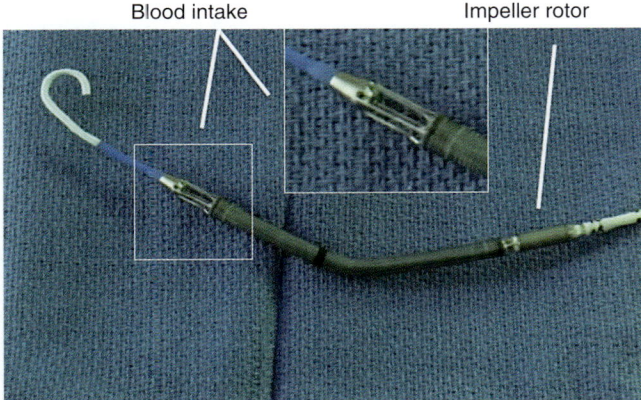

FIGURE 21.3 Impella microaxial continuous-flow device pigtail catheter. The pigtail end with the blood intake is inserted into the left ventricle. The impeller rotor is positioned in the aortic root/ascending aorta and is electromagnetically powered, generating suction and driving blood through the outflow into the aorta.

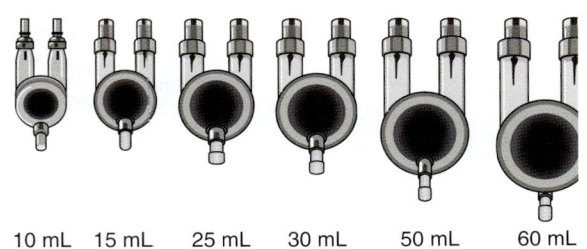

10 mL   15 mL   25 mL   30 mL   50 mL   60 mL

FIGURE 21.4 Berlin Heart EXCOR sizes 10, 15, 25, 30, 50, and 60 mL. (Adapted from Vanderpluym C, Fynn-Thompson F, Blume E. Ventricular assist devices in children: progress with an orphan device application. *Circulation* 2014;129: 1530–1537.)

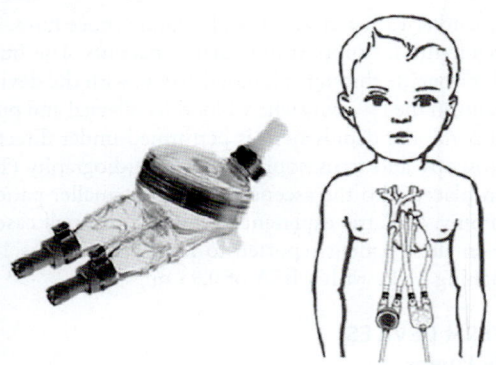

FIGURE 21.5 Illustration of a HeartWare ventricular assist device in situ. (From Adachi I, Burki S, Zafar F, et al. Pediatric ventricular assist devices. *J Thorac Dis.* 2015;7(12):2194–2202.)

All blood-contacting surfaces, including the polyurethane valves, are heparin-coated (Carmeda AB, Upplands Väsby, Sweden). A flexible diaphragm in three layers divides the pump chamber into an air chamber and a blood chamber (Fig. 21.6B), with the two diaphragm layers facing the air chamber serving as driving membranes and the third seamless blood membrane passively moved by the driving membranes.[80] In diastole, blood enters the pusher-plate polyurethane chamber through an inlet valve and negative pressure is generated to aid in pump filling. In systole, the blood-filled chamber is compressed from an air-filled chamber, creating pulsatile systolic flow ejected through the outlet valve into the aorta. Mechanical valves direct the flow, and there is no direct contact between the pumping mechanism and blood. The pump rate can be adjusted to between 30 and 150 beats/minute. The BHE has been successfully used to provide univentricular (left or right) or biventricular support, even in infants, and may be operated in a synchronous, asynchronous, or fill-to-empty mode. A rechargeable battery is available that can provide up to 5 hours of independent power supply for adult-sized pumps, but power requirements are greater for pediatric pump operation,

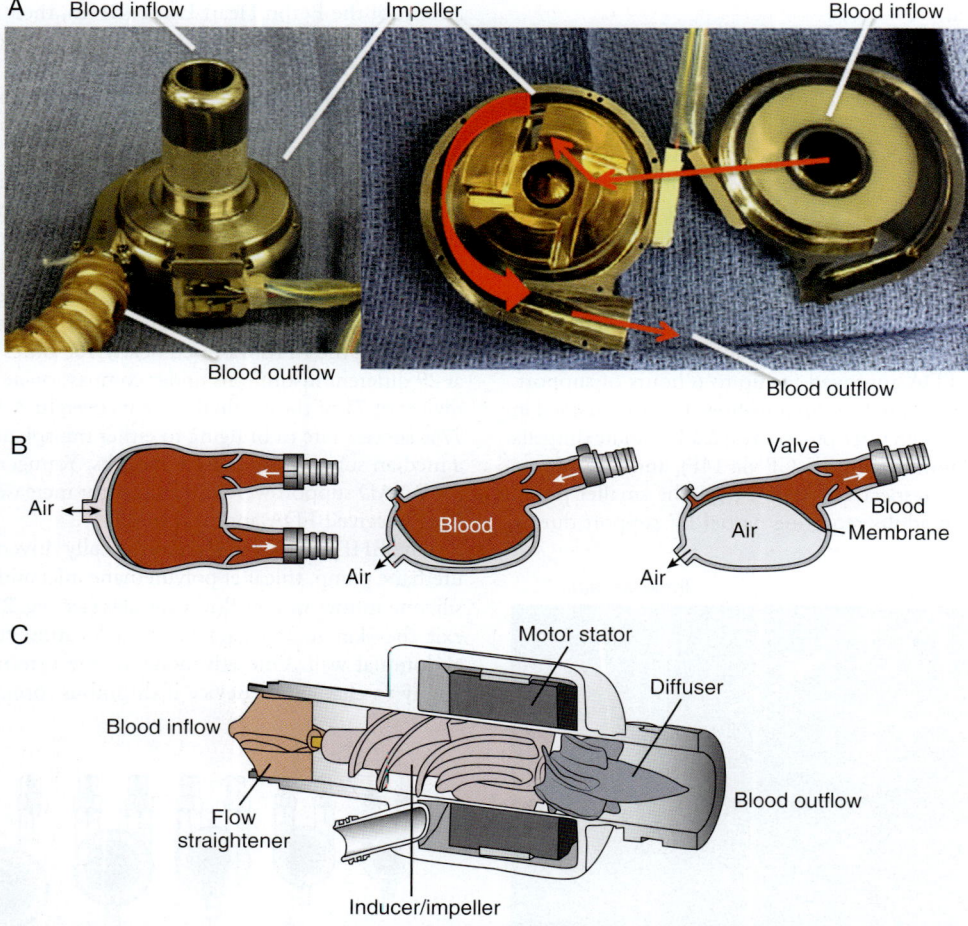

FIGURE 21.6 Illustration of ventricular assist device internal functionality. **A,** In the HeartWare device, the inflow cannula is placed in the ventricle while an internal electromagnetically driven impeller creates suction driving blood through the outflow into the aorta (blood pathway shown by *red arrows*). **B,** In the Berlin Heart Excor, a flexible diaphragm in three layers divides the pump chamber into an air chamber and a blood chamber. **C,** MicroMed DeBakey Child ventricular assist device (MicroMed Cardiovascular, Inc.; Houston, TX). (**A** and **B** from Hetzer R, Potapov E, Stiller B, et al, Improvement in survival after mechanical circulatory support with pneumatic pulsatile ventricular assist devices in pediatric patients. *Ann Thorac Surg.* 2006;82:917–925. **C** Images provided courtesy MicroMed Cardiovascular, Inc.)

owing to the greater flow resistance with small-diameter cannulas and greater pump rates.[81] A newer-generation pneumatic driver is under development that will permit discharge from the hospital for pediatric patients.[46]

Major benefits of BHE support include the ability to extubate the trachea, encourage enteral nutrition, and optimize patient mobility during long-term support. In addition, the transfusion of blood products during MCS is less in children supported with the BHE compared with those supported with ECMO. In a study comparing 30 children receiving BHE support with 34 children supported by ECMO, transfusion requirements for platelets, PRBCs, and FFP were significantly less in BHE patients. The overall mortality rate was also noted to be lower in BHE patients.[82] Anticoagulation is currently initiated with unfractionated heparin, maintaining the activated thromboplastin time (aPTT) at 60 to 80 seconds. Thromboelastography (TEG) is also used, along with platelet aggregation tests, to monitor the use of aspirin and dipyridamole. Antithrombin III (AT III) concentrations are closely monitored and substituted if the concentrations fall below 70%.[80] Low–molecular-weight heparin (LMWH), with monitoring of anti–factor Xa concentrations, has been used since 2007.[9] Pump exchange may be necessary if thrombus formation occurs in the valves, although one group reported no complications from this procedure during 15 years of adult and pediatric experience.[83]

Continuous-Flow Pumps

The increased risk of thromboembolic events with the BHE and the current absence of an option for hospital discharge prompted interest in the pediatric application of adult continuous-flow devices despite patient–device size mismatch. Continuous-flow pumps can be either axial or centrifugal, depending on the design of the impeller, and are designed to limit the interaction of moving parts. Like a centrifugal pump, axial pump function depends on the preload and afterload. Decreases in preload can cause emptying and collapse of the ventricle ("suction events"), whereas increases in afterload initially result in reductions in forward flow and ultimately can lead to regurgitant flow. Axial pumps offer several advantages over pulsatile pumps, including their small blood-to-device interface, the lack of a compliance chamber or artificial valves, and fewer moving parts. They are quieter than pulsatile pumps, which is a decided advantage for the child. Axial pumps can also allow some pulsatile flow to occur as the ventricle recovers, and cardiac output can increase in response to increased patient activity. The major disadvantages for children are the continuing size limitations for placement and the fact that the device provides only LV support.

The HeartMate II (Thoratec; Fig. 21.7) is an implantable, intracorporeal, axial flow device that is FDA approved for use as bridge-to-transplant and destination therapy and has been used in more than 10,000 adults[73]; it is an option for children with a BSA greater than 1.3 m². The device is placed in a pocket developed by dissecting the diaphragm away from the abdominal wall. It uses an electrical motor accelerating the blades of a rotating impeller to propel blood entering the device and has only one moving part and no unidirectional valves. The HeartMate II has a lower thromboembolic risk compared with other devices, and anticoagulation is managed using vitamin K antagonism and antiplatelet therapy (aspirin and dipyridamole). The portable system controller is also small enough to wear on a belt, allowing unencumbered movement for several hours, and even discharge home.[84,85] One group reported a bridge-to-transplant rate of more than 90% with use of the HeartMate II in their pediatric population.[86]

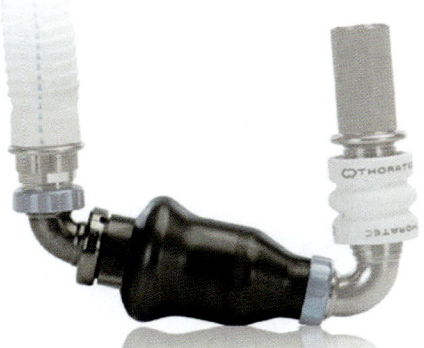

FIGURE 21.7 HeartMate II device. (From Adachi I, Burki S, Zafar F, et al. Pediatric ventricular assist devices. *J Thorac Dis.* 2015;7[12]:2194–2202.)

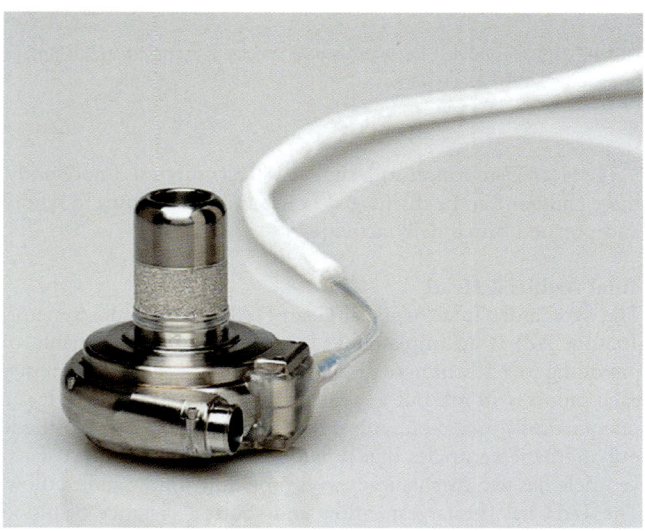

FIGURE 21.8 HeartWare Ventricular Assist System. (From Adachi I, Burki S, Zafar F, et al. Pediatric ventricular assist devices. *J Thorac Dis.* 2015;7[12]: 2194–2202.)

The HeartWare Ventricular Assist System (HVAD) (HeartWare Systems, Framingham, MA) is a continuous-flow device with a centrifugal pump directly attached to the inflow cannula (Fig. 21.8). It can provide up to 10 L/minute of flow. Although recommended for use in patients with a BSA greater than 1.5 m², it is clear from the literature that multiple groups are using these devices off-label in smaller children[87–89]; use has been reported in a toddler weighing 13 kg with a BSA of 0.65 m².[85] The HVAD is a small pump with a rotating impeller forcing blood through the device via hydrodynamic and centrifugal forces (see Fig. 21.6A) It can be placed either adjacent to the heart in the pericardial space or in a small pocket created above the left hemidiaphragm (Fig. 21.9, Video 21.1).[90] The HeartWare Left Ventricular Assist Device for the Treatment of Advanced Heart Failure (ADVANCE) trial[91] provided the data for FDA approval for bridge-to-transplant therapy, and it is anticipated that the HeartWare will be approved for destination therapy as well. In this trial, 140 patients receiving HeartWare were compared with a control group (n = 499) from the INTERMACS database, most of whom had received the HeartMate II device. Less bleeding and infection were observed

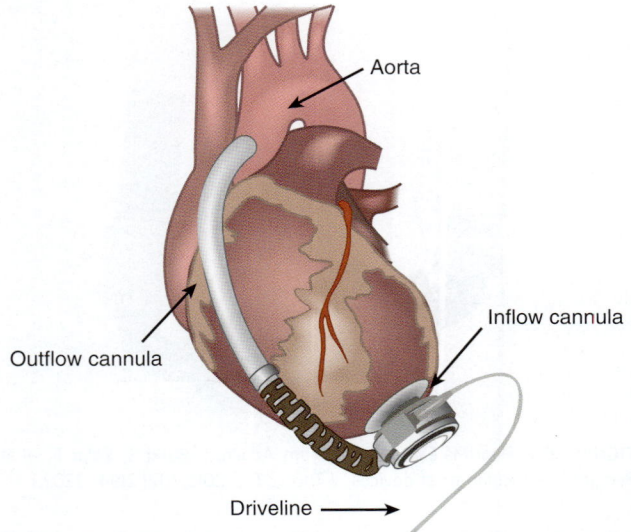

FIGURE 21.9 Illustration of a HeartWare ventricular assist device in situ. (Image provided courtesy HeartWare.)

in the HeartWare cohort with similar 180-day survival. Importantly, these children can be discharged home and often return to school and pursue normal daily activities.[85]

Total Artificial Heart

The SynCardia Total Artificial Heart (TAH) (SynCardia Systems, Tucson, AZ) is an implantable biventricular device capable of providing to 9.5 L/minute of pulsatile flow (Fig. 21.10). Currently each pump is 70 mL but a 50-mL version is in FDA trials. It is a pneumatically driven pulsatile device designed with two prosthetic polyurethane ventricles that provide biventricular support. Each ventricle has two mechanical valves providing inflow and outflow. The TAH has the largest inflow and shortest distance of blood traveled of all available VADs. The large valves and short blood path provide little resistance, thereby decreasing stasis and thrombosis.[92,93] The 50-mL version would allow application of the TAH in patients down to a BSA of 0.9 m^2 or in patients in whom virtual fit has determined that size is appropriate.[94] It is FDA approved for bridge to transplant and more than 1200 implants have occurred worldwide. Major advantages of the TAH include immediate elimination of concern regarding right heart failure, atrioventricular or aortic valve issues, dysrhythmias, LV clot, and intracardiac shunts.[46] Its use has also been described in patients with chronic graft dysfunction who are immunocompromised, as use of the TAH eliminates the need for immunosuppressive therapy.[95] A recent review of the SynCardia database showed that the TAH was used in 24 patients with CHD, or 2.2% of total implants.[96] Six of the 24 patients were adolescents (age 12–18 years) and this subgroup had 100% survival. For the entire CHD cohort, survival was 62%.

Perioperative Management of Mechanical Circulatory Support

Successful management of critically ill children receiving MCS requires multidisciplinary expertise. The Hospital for Sick Children, Toronto, Ontario, developed an Interprofessional VAD Support

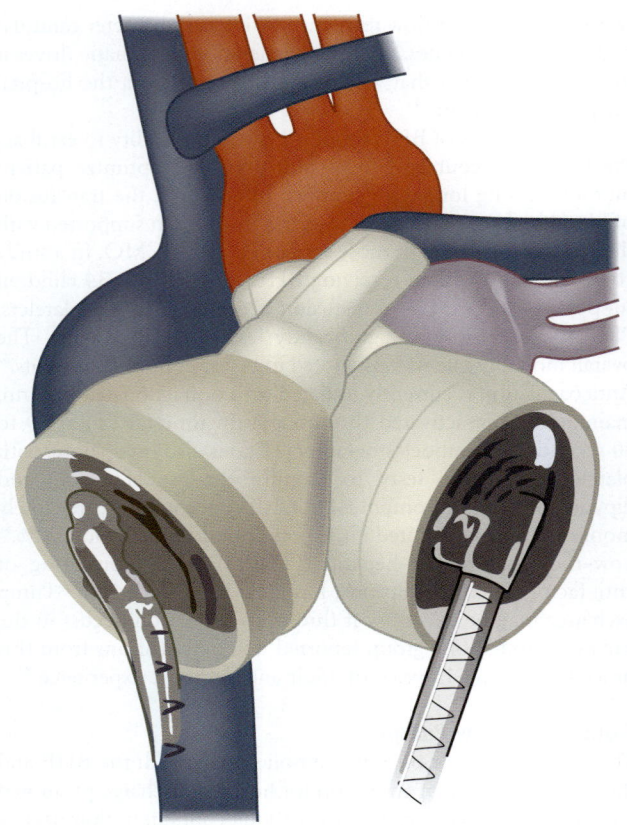

FIGURE 21.10 SynCardia Total Artificial Heart. (From Vanderpluym C, Fynn-Thompson F, Blume E. Ventricular assist devices in children: progress with an orphan device application. *Circulation* 2014;129:1530–1537.)

Team involved in clinical care, education, and family support for patients receiving Berlin Heart Excor MCS. In addition to physicians (cardiac surgeons, cardiac intensivists, heart failure and transplant cardiologists, hematologists, and psychiatrists) and nurses (cardiac and critical care), team members include pharmacists, respiratory therapists, dieticians, social workers, physiotherapists, biomedical engineers, and perfusionists.[97] Development of a team approach and use of interdisciplinary guidelines for care of these children can enhance communication, family support, and outcomes.[98]

HEMODYNAMICS

During ECMO support, central venous pressure (CVP) should remain low to ensure adequate venous drainage. Left atrial pressure should be closely monitored using echocardiographic evaluation of atrial septal position. An increase in left atrial pressure may indicate incomplete unloading of the left atrium and ventricle, potentially requiring a blade and/or balloon atrial septostomy or surgical placement of a left atrial vent.[99] Anatomic issues, such as the presence of aortopulmonary collateral vessels, aortic insufficiency, or a patent ductus arteriosus, can also result in a persistently increased left atrial pressure.

Increased arterial pressures and systemic vascular resistance during ECMO can be due to large pump flows, but other causes, such as unrecognized seizure activity, inadequate pain or sedation management, and hypothermia, should also be considered. High systemic vascular resistance (SVR) during ECMO support can be pharmacologically managed. In general, mean arterial pressures should be maintained at a level appropriate to the child's size and body weight.

Unlike ECMO support, LVAD support requires maintenance of effective RV output to provide adequate LV preload. RV failure, pulmonary hypertension, and arrhythmias can all limit LV filling and must, therefore, be aggressively treated.[100] Other potential causes of inadequate LV filling include cannula malposition or low intravascular volume. CVP can be used to evaluate volume status. Serial echocardiograms are useful to assess RV function and estimate RV and pulmonary artery pressures. Clinical signs of right-sided heart failure include increased central venous or right atrial pressures, hepatomegaly, peripheral edema, and decreasing hemoglobin-oxygen saturations. RV function can be augmented pharmacologically with drugs such as milrinone or isoproterenol. Increased pulmonary artery pressures are best initially treated by ensuring adequate alveolar ventilation, and subsequently by using inhaled nitric oxide if necessary. Mechanical issues, such as cardiac tamponade, can also negatively affect hemodynamics. These can be diagnosed at the bedside using echocardiography. Inadequate LV decompression can increase left atrial and pulmonary artery pressures and may be treated by augmenting LVAD flow; if necessary, biventricular or ECMO support can be initiated.[101]

Children supported by VADs often require vasodilators to maintain the low SVR necessary for optimal pump function. Frequently used vasodilators include milrinone, hydralazine, β-blockers, angiotensin-converting enzyme (ACE) inhibitors, and clonidine. Left atrial pressure is optimally maintained at 3 to 4 mm Hg, while allowing some ventricular ejection to avoid stasis. Systemic mixed venous hemoglobin-oxygen saturation, either continuously via in-line monitoring with a centrifugal VAD, or intermittently with a paracorporeal pulsatile VAD, is a useful metric to monitor the adequacy of cardiac output.

RESPIRATORY CONSIDERATIONS

Although ECMO can provide full cardiopulmonary support, tracheal intubation and mechanical ventilation help to avoid atelectasis and optimize oxygenation of blood returning to the left atrium that will provide coronary artery blood flow. Modest ventilator settings are generally recommended: (1) 6 to 8 mL/kg tidal volume, (2) 5 to 10 cm H_2O of positive end-expiratory pressure, (3) a rate of 10 to 12 breaths/minute, and (4) a fractional inspired oxygen value of 0.4 or less (to avoid oxygen toxicity). Recently "awake" VA ECMO has been reported in pediatric patients, including allowing the tracheas to be extubated during support.[102] Maintenance of adequate ventilation is particularly important in children with single-ventricle physiology with an open systemic-pulmonary shunt. Because of the complexity of the ECMO circuit, mechanical issues, such as oxygenator malfunction, must be considered when increasing hypoxemia occurs. After ruling out oxygenator failure, ECMO flow may be increased or the membrane size may be increased to improve systemic oxygenation.

Children supported by VADs receive only cardiac support. With centrifugal VAD support the trachea generally remains intubated and the lungs mechanically ventilated, while paracorporeal pulsatile VADs and implantable VADs, on the other hand, allow children to be weaned to extubation. Anatomic issues, such as an atrial septal defect, should be recognized as potential causes of hypoxemia from right-to-left shunting.[103] Children who receive LV support via either a centrifugal or pulsatile VAD may also

require inhaled nitric oxide to decrease PVR and augment RV function.

HEMATOLOGIC CONSIDERATIONS

Anticoagulation management continues to be one of the most challenging clinical issues in caring for children who require MCS, in part owing to age-based differences in the coagulation cascade.[104] Patients with MCS are at substantive risk for hemorrhage and/or thromboembolic complications.[105] Ongoing hemorrhage around cannulation sites is a frequent issue, particularly with ECMO support. Of greater concern are gastrointestinal (GI), pulmonary, or, more devastatingly, ICH; infarctions or thromboembolic events may also occur. Serial ultrasonography of the head may be used to monitor for intracranial bleeding in infants and neonates, and, when possible, computed tomography may be used in older children.

Contact with the non-endothelial surfaces in an ECMO circuit can activate hemostatic agents, including platelets, factor XII, tissue factor, and von Willebrand factor (vWF). There is also a tendency toward fibrinolysis as well as release of proinflammatory cytokines. This leads to both a state of hypercoagulability and coagulopathy in ECMO patients. These effects are more pronounced in neonates and infants because of their lower blood volume relative to circuit size.[106] Destruction of platelets and coagulation factors and an increase in fibrinolysis can cause bleeding around cannula sites and, more detrimentally, in intracavitary spaces. Activation of tissue factor and the inflammatory system contribute to hypercoagulability, which can cause both internal and circuit thrombosis. It is the role of the ECMO team to balance this precarious state of coagulation.

Unfractionated heparin is the first-line drug for maintenance of anticoagulation during ECMO therapy. Heparin binds to ATIII, producing anticoagulation via inhibition of activated factors IXa, Xa, XIa, XIIa, and, to a lesser extent, IIA (thrombin). Infants tend to have reduced ATIII concentrations and can rapidly develop acquired ATIII deficiency during MCS, which is reflected by the need for increased supplementation of ATIII to provide adequate levels in this age group.[107,108] The anticoagulation effect of heparin is most commonly monitored with the activated clotting time (ACT), a real-time bedside test that measures whole blood clotting after exposing the blood to either kaolin or celite activators. Although ECMO protocols vary, ACTs are generally maintained between 180 and 220 seconds using heparin infused at 10 to 50 units/ kg per hour. The use of heparin-bonded tubing can reduce the need for greater ACTs. There are numerous concerns regarding the reliability of ACT monitoring and its correlation with heparin concentration in pediatric patients on ECMO. Many factors, including hemodilution, temperature, reduction in coagulation factors, and platelet dysfunction, may alter ACT results. Some centers rely on alternative monitoring tests including aPTT, anti-Xa concentration assays, anti-Xa range, TEG, and rotational TEG.[109]

Hematocrit is generally maintained between 40% and 50%, although efforts are made to limit transfusions because most children are potential candidates for cardiac transplantation. When necessary, leukocyte-reduced, cytomegalovirus-negative, irradiated PRBCs are administered. Platelet counts greater than 100,000/ mm^3 and fibrinogen concentrations greater than 100 mg/dL are maintained to minimize bleeding complications.[110] In the presence of continued bleeding, cryoprecipitate and/or FFP may be added to the circuit prime. TEG may assist in determining which blood products are appropriate. In cases of persistent hemorrhage refractory to blood component administration, recombinant activated factor VII significantly decreases bleeding and aids in normalizing the TEG profile, although disastrous clotting of circuitry has also been reported with its use.[111-114] Hemolysis may be monitored by measuring of plasma-free hemoglobin, with increasing concentrations potentially representing the development of thrombus in the circuit. Antifibrinolytic agents have also been used in pediatric patients receiving ECMO therapy, albeit with limited available data. In one study of 298 patients, the frequency of thrombotic events or ICH was increased with the use of ε-aminocaproic acid.[115]

Without an oxygenator in the circuit, anticoagulation requirements are not as stringent for children on VADs, and ACTs may be maintained between 140 and 180 seconds. A percutaneously placed VAD, such as the TandemHeart, requires a target ACT greater than 180 seconds. Most long-term VADs, such as the BHE, are placed while the patient is supported by CPB and under full anticoagulation. Once weaned from bypass, the heparin is fully reversed with protamine. In the first 24 hours after VAD placement, there is a high incidence of reoperation to achieve hemostasis. After the immediate postoperative period, the risk of bleeding decreases while the risk of thrombosis increases. Unfractionated heparin infusions are used with a target aPTT of 1.5 times normal. The ATIII levels are also monitored and maintained in excess of 70% to avoid thrombotic complications. The use of argatroban (a small molecule direct thrombin inhibitor) has been described in children with heparin-induced thrombocytopenia type II.[116]

While a recent study examining trends in coagulation therapy in pediatric patients with assist devices revealed wide variability of in-hospital anticoagulation management,[117] currently most institutions follow the Edmonton antithrombotic protocol once the patient is discharged from the ICU. This protocol involves a three-drug regimen: aspirin, dipyridamole, and either warfarin (for patients ≥12 months of age) or enoxaparin (for patients <12 months of age). Enoxaparin is used more frequently in infants because warfarin is difficult to manage, as infants are more likely to use vitamin K–containing formulas and have significant changes in diet during their growth. There is also a lack of robust data on which to base the dose of warfarin in infants and no appropriate formulations (i.e., suspensions) are available. The use of LMWH requires the use of anti–factor Xa activity monitoring.[118,119] After normalizing the platelet count and function, aspirin and dipyridamole are started, using TEG and platelet aggregation tests to monitor clotting tendency, with a target activation of 30%. Once an appropriately aged child is tolerating enteral feedings, a transition to warfarin may commence. Although embolic and bleeding complications remain problematic, with this management strategy a marked increase in survival has been noted in children undergoing BHE support compared with earlier regimens.[120]

Although hemolysis and thrombosis may be less frequent with continuous-flow devices, acquired von Willebrand syndrome has been frequently described in adult patients, most likely secondary to the shear stress of the pump, with unfolding and cleavage of the high–molecular-weight multimers of vWF. This is also thought to account for the increased incidence of GI bleeding noted in these patients, though not all patients with documented acquired von Willebrand syndrome display increased bleeding tendencies.[121,122]

PREVENTION OF INFECTION

Infection is a constant concern, particularly in children requiring intermediate- to long-term ECMO and VAD support. Devices with larger surface area and areas of turbulent flow are associated with greater infection rates owing to increased adherence of blood-borne pathogens. As a result, smaller, fully implantable devices and devices with improved flow dynamics may decrease

the incidence of infection.[123,124] Devices such as the BHE allow for removal of tracheal tubes, indwelling catheters, and intravenous lines; minimize the need for blood transfusions; and offer a reduced risk of device-related infections.[82,125] Deep wound complications of inflow and outflow cannulas have been successfully treated with vacuum-assisted wound closure systems.[126] The fact that children with the HeartMate II and HeartWare devices can be discharged home may also decrease the incidence of infection.

The use of MCS can result in immunologic dysfunction, further increasing infection risk.[127] Signs and symptoms of infection can be subtle, and a need for increasing inotropic support to maintain mean arterial pressure can often be a harbinger of infection. Endogenous reactions to infection can also result in activation of the coagulation cascade, increasing the difficulty of anticoagulation management.[128] Many children prophylactically receive antibiotics with gram-positive coverage, as well as oral nystatin for fungal prophylaxis.

ANESTHETIC CONSIDERATIONS

In preparing for the anesthetic care of infants and children, either when ECMO or VAD support is being used or when implementation of MCS is imminent, initial planning centers on two main areas of concern: the child's current status and the location of the proposed procedure (Table 21.4). The need for emergency surgery, the child's condition at the time of surgery, the presence of preoperative multiorgan failure, and the need for CPB with cross-clamping of the aorta have all been shown to increase perioperative risk.[129]

A comprehensive preoperative evaluation is essential, with knowledge of the underlying pathology necessitating MCS and the length of the child's illness, along with evaluation of other potential multiorgan dysfunction, including neurologic, hematologic, renal, hepatic, and pulmonary issues. Review of current drug therapy, particularly the duration and degree of current inotropic support, anticoagulation protocols, sedation regimens, cardiac function, intravascular volume status, and the presence and degree of preoperative hemorrhage, is also necessary. Physical examination should encompass the airway and both current vascular access and the availability of sites for potential vascular access. In infants, ultrasonography of the head is useful before considering institution of MCS, as significant intraventricular hemorrhage is a relative contraindication to MCS. Similarly, infants on ECMO, especially those younger than 35 weeks gestation, are at high risk for intraventricular hemorrhage and are often monitored by daily head ultrasound.[130]

Preoperative laboratory evaluation should include a complete blood cell count (CBC) with platelet count, electrolytes, blood urea nitrogen and creatinine concentrations, prothrombin time and partial thromboplastin time, and liver function tests. Concentrations of BNP, produced in the myocardium, serve as a marker of ventricular overloading and have been shown in adult and children with CHD to correlate with the degree of ventricular dysfunction.[131,132] Serial BNP concentrations in children supported with ECMO have also been used to predict clinical outcomes, with greater BNP concentrations noted after termination of ECMO support in nonsurvivors than in children who ultimately survived.[133]

Useful preoperative coagulation data includes recent TEG results, fibrinogen concentrations, and platelet function tests, if available. The most recent echocardiography data and chest radiograph should be reviewed. Blood products, including PRBCs, platelets, cryoprecipitate, and FFP, should be available at the bedside or in the OR, with provision for a continuing supply of

TABLE 21.4 Anesthetic Considerations

Preoperative Assessment	Intraoperative Management
History	*Availability of blood products*
Etiology and duration of cardiac failure	*Monitoring*
Review of system/end-organ dysfunction	Standard ASA monitors
Pulmonary	Electrocardiogram
Renal	Noninvasive blood pressure
Hepatic	End-tidal CO_2
Neurologic	Ttemperature
Medications	Peripheral oxygen saturation
Inotropic/vasoactive support	Assess need for invasive arterial or central venous monitoring
Angiotensin-converting enzyme inhibitors	Urine output
Antiarrhythmic therapy	
Anticoagulation protocols	*Transesophageal echocardiography*
Analgesic/sedative drugs	Presence of septal defects
Antibiotics	Aortic insufficiency
Planned surgical procedure	Mitral stenosis
Timing of procedure: elective/urgent/emergent	Cardiac de-airing
	Ventricular function
Laboratory	
Hematology	*Management principles*
Complete blood cell count	Maintain adequate intravascular volume/preload for ventricular assist device
Platelet count	Avoid abrupt decreases in preload
Serum chemistries	Support right ventricular function, reduce pulmonary vascular resistance
Electrolytes	Nitric oxide availability
Liver function studies	Maintain adequate ventilation
Blood urea nitrogen, creatinine	Inotropic support: milrinone, prostaglandin E_1
B-type naturietic peptide concentration	Hypotension can be treated with volume or α-adrenergic agonists
Coagulation studies	
Prothrombin time/partial thromboplastin time	**Postoperative Issues**
Fibrinogen concentration	Transport to intensive care unit
Activated clotting time	Control of ongoing hemorrhage
Thromboelastogram	Timing of extubation
Physical examination	
Airway	
Vascular access, both existing and available	
Neurologic status	
Evidence of ongoing hemorrhage	
Assessment of intravascular volume status	

products as needed. PRBCs should preferably be cytomegalovirus-negative, leukocyte-reduced, and irradiated, because all of these children should be considered potential transplant candidates (note that the potassium concentration of irradiated PRBCs may be greatly increased, resulting in acute hyperkalemia if administered rapidly). Appropriate antibiotic prophylaxis should be discussed with the surgeon.

Standard American Society of Anesthesiologists monitoring should be used before induction of anesthesia. Depending on the child's condition and the type of surgery planned, the use of arterial and central venous lines should be considered. In children who have been in the ICU for a prolonged time or those undergoing current resuscitation, securing additional vascular access lines can be quite challenging and may occasionally require surgical assistance. For children already supported by mechanical support device, it is important to know that VAD ejection is usually asynchronous with the child's underlying heart rate, yielding a discrepancy between the observed electrocardiographic and the arterial line waveform. Multiple peripheral intravenous lines are

useful for the administration of volume and blood products. If RVAD support is being used, special care must be taken not to entrain air if the great veins are accessed.

For patients undergoing VAD placement, etomidate is generally an advantageous drug for induction of anesthesia because it does not depress myocardial contractility at clinically relevant concentrations, even in children with severely compromised ventricular function.[134] Judicious doses of opioids and benzodiazepines may be used. The choice of a neuromuscular blocking agent is usually based on the presence of hepatic or renal dysfunction. Adequate depth of anesthesia should be ensured before tracheal intubation to avoid abrupt increases in PVR, particularly in children with marginal RV function. In children undergoing device placement, induction drugs should be given incrementally as the onset time may be abnormally slow owing to depressed ventricular function. Children may be less responsive to β-adrenergic agonists owing to depletion of myocardial catecholamines.[135] Hypotension on induction of anesthesia and decreased responsiveness to catecholamines may also be observed in children receiving long-term ACE inhibitors for afterload reduction preoperatively.[136-138] Opioids, benzodiazepines, and neuromuscular blocking agents are generally used to maintain anesthesia before ECMO cannulation or initiation of CPB for VAD implementation, with the express goal of maintaining adequate cardiac output and resultant systemic perfusion to end organs. Serial serum lactate concentrations, mixed venous hemoglobin-oxygen saturations, and the presence or absence of metabolic acidosis are useful indexes to evaluate the adequacy of cardiac output.

Unless contraindicated, a TEE probe should be placed after the induction of anesthesia for use throughout the procedure. Initial TEE examination is important for determining the presence of any intracardiac shunts that would require closing before initiation of MCS. Aortic valve competence should also be evaluated, because greater than trivial insufficiency can recirculate blood through an LVAD. The mitral valve should also be examined for significant stenosis that could limit LV inflow. After device placement, TEE ensures that adequate cardiac de-airing has occurred, evaluates ventricular function, monitors the orientation of intracardiac cannulas, and evaluates whether the left atrium and ventricle have been decompressed after pump activation.

For children undergoing LVAD placement, as the venous line from the CPB circuit is occluded, the pump speed is gradually increased. If LVAD flow (and rate when fill-to-empty mode is used) is less than desired, the major areas of concern center on hypovolemia or poor RV function. The RV should be monitored closely for signs of dysfunction or failure. In children with pre-existing RV dysfunction, pulmonary vasodilatory agents, such as milrinone, prostaglandin E_1, or nitric oxide, should be aggressively used to optimize right-sided heart function. Children with low pressures and signs of vasodilatory shock may require infusions of vasopressin, epinephrine, or norepinephrine to support the circulation. In addition, adequate volume loading and VAD output should be ensured.

Tracheal extubation is not generally an option for those undergoing ECMO or centrifugal VAD support, but children receiving pulsatile VADs or axial pumps may be considered candidates for extubation. Timing of the extubation depends on the child's preoperative condition, degree of preexisting pulmonary dysfunction, duration of the surgical procedure, extent of postoperative bleeding, and maintenance of appropriate hemodynamic parameters.

Poorly predictable drug pharmacokinetics is another important consideration in patients undergoing VAD or ECMO placement. These patients often have altered hepatorenal perfusion and function, drug interactions, reduced protein binding, and may additionally be receiving renal replacement therapy. ECMO in particular complicates drug pharmacokinetics related to the volume of the circuit, the polymer components, and altered perfusion and drug eliminations. At the time of commencing ECMO, the volume of fluid within the membrane oxygenator and tubing increases the circulating blood volume by 200 to 300 mL depending on the circuit. This has little effect on drugs with large volumes of distribution, such as fentanyl, which show little change in plasma concentration. However, drugs with smaller volumes of distribution, such as nondepolarizing neuromuscular blocking agents and the antibiotics gentamycin and vancomycin, have larger changes in plasma concentration and may therefore have a prolonged elimination half-life. Hemodilution with ECMO may also be associated with reduced concentrations of plasma proteins, which in turn would increase the free fraction of highly protein-bound drugs. Significant drug absorption can occur on the large surface area of the tubing or the membrane oxygenator of the circuit, further increasing the volume of distribution of drugs.

The opposite may occur when a drug is discontinued; it is then released back into the circulation, adding further unpredictability to its disposition and potential prolongation of its effect.[139] The degree of this sequestration depends on both the materials used in the circuit and the nature of the drugs. In general, drugs that are lipophilic, such as opioids, propofol, and benzodiazepines, are more likely to adhere to the tubing. Drug clearance may improve in children supported by ECMO, coincident with better organ function as oxygenated blood flow to those organs improves.[140] Multiple factors in this patient population make accurate prediction of drug doses extremely challenging and understanding of the issues involved is essential.

Anesthesia for the VAD Patient for Noncardiac Surgery

With the steadily increasing use of VAD support in infants and children, a growing demand for anesthesia for noncardiac surgeries during the period of support has occurred. While these patients should generally be cared for in centers with personnel and resources accustomed to caring for children with VADs, the increasing number of children discharged to home while receiving MCS raises the possibility that these patients require emergent care at other institutions. As these patients require significant care coordination, it is prudent to conduct a preoperative discussion with all perioperative team members to discuss the specifics and concerns related to caring for a patient with a VAD. The patient's baseline VAD flow parameters should be identified to readily identify any deviations from the new physiologic "normal." When possible, assistance from the perfusion or VAD management team should be sought. Temporary conversion from warfarin or LMWH to an unfractionated heparin infusion should be discussed with the team caring for the patient, including the hematologist, prior to surgery, and appropriate blood products should be ordered. As previously discussed, VADs depend on adequate preload for filling and an afterload that is not excessive so as to impede forward flow. For children with VAD support, appropriate pump function continues independently of the induction drugs used, provided adequate preload is maintained and no acute changes occur in SVR. When preload may be inadequate, it may be prudent to administer blood or fluids before induction of anesthesia. In a series of children with in situ BHE support undergoing noncardiac surgeries, anesthesia induced with ketamine was less likely to induce hypotension that required treatment with a fluid bolus or α-adrenergic agonists.[141] As continuing function of an LVAD relies on adequate right heart function, measures to maintain or increase right heart output may be required. Care should be taken to avoid increases in PVR, as RV failure is the likeliest cause of decompensation in such patients. Nitric oxide and appropriate vasoactive drugs should be readily available for use. When possible, the use of spontaneous ventilation is thought to enhance venous return and hemodynamic stability.[74,142] Before induction of anesthesia, defibrillation pads should be applied as rhythms other than sinus may reduce VAD inflow. The VAD should be connected to wall power whenever possible.

Noninvasive blood pressure monitoring can be challenging in patients with VADs, particularly in those with continuous-flow devices. Blood pressure may be difficult to measure noninvasively. Sampling errors and the ability to obtain reliable cuff pressures should be established before induction. Placing an arterial line is often warranted to continuously measure mean arterial blood pressure. Intraoperative use of transthoracic or transesophageal echocardiography may be helpful to continuously assess volume status, monitor inflow cannula patency, and to help diagnose any disruptions in VAD output. The use of minimal insufflation pressures should be discussed with the surgical team in cases involving laparoscopic surgery as excessive pressures can adversely affect VAD filling conditions. Additionally, extreme positioning maneuvers such as steep reverse Trendelenburg may affect VAD preload, resulting in hemodynamic changes. Whenever possible, consultation with an anesthesia provider experienced in caring for these patients should be sought.

Outcomes and Complications

OUTCOMES

Regardless of the type of MCS chosen, it has become increasingly apparent that the indication for and timing of initiation of support are major factors in determining outcome. Although the majority of pediatric patients with cardiac disease have structural CHD, only 20% of children undergoing VAD implantation have structural disease.[143] Universally, survival has been greater in children who required support secondary to acute myocarditis or dilated cardiomyopathy compared with children who received support because of congenital heart defects or postcardiotomy failure.[144–146] Patients presenting with long-standing cardiomyopathy who require VAD support as a result of gradual or acute decompensation represent a much different cohort than those who have CHD and require salvage VAD support postoperatively. The latter group has a significantly greater mortality rate, particularly if they also require ECMO to bridge them to VAD support.

When feasible, VAD support offers several major advantages over ECMO. First, the lack of an oxygenator simplifies the circuit, lessening anticoagulation requirements and trauma to blood elements. Second, ECMO-supported patients suffer greater rates of neurologic deficits than those supported with VADs, particularly in younger children with more complex heart disease,[68] although the frequency of neurologic complications with VV ECMO is less than with VA ECMO.[147,148] Additionally, evidence suggests that VAD support provides superior ventricular decompression and physiologic rest, promoting myocardial recovery in children with acute myocarditis or dilated cardiomyopathy by normalizing the ventricular geometry and reverse remodeling.[149–151] Children with chronic heart failure who are waiting for transplantation and who experience progressive multiorgan dysfunction benefit from the use of pulsatile VADs with recovery of pulmonary, renal, and hepatic function.[152]

In some children, transition to VAD support may follow initial ECMO support.[79,145] Patients supported with ECMO may require transition to a VAD if they do not achieve adequate myocardial recovery and cannot be weaned from ECMO. Most often these patients are supported with ECMO after congenital heart surgery or cardiopulmonary support. Rarely, children previously listed for transplantation deteriorate rapidly requiring emergent institution of MCS and thus are initially supported by ECMO. In evaluating VAD usage and outcomes, one review reported that 21% of 187 children with VADs had prior ECMO support.[145] Regardless of diagnosis, the use of ECMO to bridge patients to VAD is associated with significantly decreased survival; children in whom ECMO was initiated for cardiac failure after cardiac surgery and who required VAD support for continued cardiac dysfunction had particularly poor survival rates.

A review of 55 pediatric patients revealed significantly increased survival rates in children who received BHE support compared with those who received ECMO, despite a mean duration of support that was nearly three times as great in the BHE group.[153]

The first multiinstitutional study reviewing the outcomes of 99 children bridged to cardiac transplantation with MCS compared them with 2276 children listed for transplantation during the same era (1993–2003) who did not require MCS. Significant findings included a lack of difference in survival rates between VAD-supported and non–VAD-supported children, along with similar survival rates for children who required BiVAD support versus LVAD support. An increasing trend in the number of children undergoing transplantation who required pretransplantation VAD support was also observed, with an increase in the use of long-term MCS devices in the most recent era. Children with long-term devices were more likely to survive to transplantation than those with short-term devices. Ten children were "double bridged" from ECMO to VAD support before transplantation, with nine then undergoing successful transplantation. Not surprisingly, smaller, younger patients and those with CHD had poorer outcomes.[154]

Single-center reports of the use of BHE in children in the United States increased in the early 2000s, with markedly improved transplant wait-list survival.[79,153] This resulted in the NHLBI-sponsored randomized, controlled trial of the BHE VAD in 2006, with results published in 2012.[13] This study, notable for being the first controlled trial of a VAD in children, led the FDA to issue IDE approval for the Berlin Heart Excor. Using strict inclusion criteria, 48 patients were enrolled, 24 with BSA less than 0.7 m^2 and 24 with BSA 0.7 to 1.5 m^2. The prospectively enrolled patients were compared with a historical control group of patients who received ECMO support. Survival to transplantation occurred in a substantially greater proportion of patients supported with the BHE VAD compared with patients receiving ECMO, while the time receiving support without catastrophic neurologic events was significantly greater in the BHE VAD group.

Outcomes of all children with an implanted BHE VAD between May 2007 and December 2010 (n = 204) showed a 12-month survival of 75%, including 6% who underwent device explantation after recovery and 5% who continued with the device in place at the end of the study.[155] In multivariate analysis, smaller patient size, renal impairment, greater total bilirubin, and the use of biventricular support were associated with a greater mortality rate. Patients weighing less than 5 kg experienced particularly high mortality (64%). The incidence of stroke, 29%, was identical to the incidence in the IDE study and notable as the largest cause of death.

In a multicenter analysis of the BHE in children weighing less than 10 kg, major risk factors for mortality during support included a diagnosis of CHD and increased bilirubin, likely reflecting more severe right heart failure.[156] Outcomes were especially poor in infants with CHD, in whom mortality exceeded 90%. ECMO was identified as a univariate predictor of mortality in patients weighing less than 10 kg. No children who weighed less than 5 kg with CHD supported by ECMO survived after transplant. The challenges involved in improving survival in the smallest patients with CHD are especially daunting because of their complex physiology and hemodynamics, immature coagulation systems, infection risk, and previous surgical correction. Pump size in relation to BSA has been shown to have a major impact on the rate of thromboembolic events. Children supported with large pumps (>50 mL/m^2) had significantly more thromboembolic events compared with those supported with small- or normal-for-BSA–sized pumps.[157] This was initially observed when adult VADs were implanted in older children who subsequently developed complications such as arterial hypertension and cerebral vascular accidents,[158] possibly owing to pumping large stroke volumes into anatomically small aortas.[159] In 2013 a new 15-mL BHE designed especially for children with a BSA of 0.3 to 0.5 m² was introduced. This 15-mL pump has the potential to substantially reduce the risk of thromboembolic events in the subset of pediatric patients for whom the 10-mL device was too small and the 25-mL device was too large.[157]

INTERMACS, an NHLBI-sponsored registry for FDA-approved durable MCS devices in the United States, began data entry on adult and pediatric durable device implants in June 2006. As part of this project, a dedicated pediatric component was developed to collect data on MCS devices and outcomes in the pediatric population. This database, the Pediatric Interagency Registry for Mechanical Circulatory Support (PediMACS) national registry, began registering patients on September 19, 2012. Through April 2015, 36 institutions had enrolled 251 devices in 216 patients receiving temporary or long-term MCS devices. This registry focuses on capturing data elements unique to pediatric patients, evaluating special issues in pediatric MCS, chronicling the variety of devices applied in the pediatric population, and identifying the particular cohort in whom therapy is most effective. Goals of this registry are to delineate the best support strategies for VAD therapies, refine patient selection of VAD therapies, develop "best practices" by analyzing outcomes, and facilitate and guide the development and clinical evaluation of pediatric devices. Between September 19, 2012, and December 31, 2014, nearly 50% of implants in children younger than 5 years of age were pulsatile LVADs. Fifty-six percent of implants in children 6 to 10 years of age and nearly 90% of those 11 to 18 years of age were continuous-flow LVADs. Among patients with continuous-flow devices, the overall actuarial 6-month survival has approached 90%, with 66% of children undergoing transplantation by 12 months.[160]

The Effect of MCS on Wait-List Survival

Of all patients wait-listed for organ transplantation in the United States, children listed for heart transplantation face one of the largest mortality rates on a waiting list, regardless of age.[161] Every year, approximately 500 additional pediatric candidates are added to the transplant waiting list, with approximately 17% dying each year while awaiting a donor heart.[162] The impact of MCS on cardiac transplantation is evident when considering the evolution of the proportion of patients supported by MCS devices at transplant. In 2000, fewer than 5% of patients were supported by durable devices at transplant, but by 2013 the frequency had increased to greater than 20%.[163] For critically ill children, the presence of a pediatric VAD program decreases the wait-list mortality by as much as 50%, despite the increased waiting time.[164] Importantly, the increased proportion of pediatric patients supported by MCS devices at the time of transplant has not adversely affected posttransplant survival.[165] Not only has the wait-list mortality decreased, many patients are actually stabilizing and rehabilitating, making the posttransplant period easier.

The UNOS database from 1999 to 2012 identified 5532 pediatric candidates (age ≤18 years) actively listed for pediatric heart transplant; 2191 were listed between 1999 and 2004 (Era 1) and 3341 were listed between 2005 and 2012 (Era 2). Wait-list mortality rates were less in Era 2 (8%) versus Era 1 (16%). VAD therapy was used more frequently in Era 2 (16%) than in Era 1 (6%) and was associated with improved wait-list survival (P <.001). Independent predictors of wait-list mortality included weight less than 10 kg, congenital heart diagnosis, ECMO, mechanical ventilation, and renal dysfunction. Independent predictors of survival on the wait-list included VAD therapy, cardiomyopathy diagnosis, blood type A, and being listed in Era B. Despite an increase in the number of children listed as status 1A, wait-list mortality decreased more than 50% during Era B. Irrespective of other factors, those supported with a VAD were four times more likely to survive to transplant.[164]

The first multi-institution study to evaluate outcomes of VAD support in pediatric patients revealed that 77% of children bridged to transplant survived.[166] Risk factors for mortality in the VAD cohort in this study included earlier era and CHD. There was no difference in 5-year survival after transplantation for patients with VADs at the time of transplant compared with those not requiring VAD support.[154] In addition, a study that evaluated posttransplant outcomes after VAD support in children using the UNOS database found that posttransplant survival was improved in VAD patients compared with patients supported with ECMO or those without mechanical support. VAD support is likely superior to ECMO for several reasons: increased need for sedation and mechanical ventilation with ECMO, the need for greater levels of anticoagulation, the persistent inflammatory response, and the possibly deleterious effects of nonpulsatile flow on renal perfusion in small children.[5,13,146] Although the use of ECMO as a bridge to transplant continues to be necessary in selected cases, especially for those whose congenital anatomy is not amenable to VAD support, every effort should be made to avoid its use when other methods of mechanical support are possible. Less favorable outcomes with the use of extracorporeal VADs were also observed, suggesting that conversion to other modes of support may improve posttransplant outcomes. Consistent with adult data,[167] the researchers found that the poor survival with extracorporeal VADs extended to the posttransplant period. They acknowledge that although the use of extracorporeal devices to stabilize children may be necessary in some situations, there should be a timely conversion to an implantable device to improve outcomes. A retrospective study comparing children who received multimodality MCS before transplant with those who received single-modality MCS showed similar survival to transplant and discharge between groups, despite the greater duration of support required in patients with multimodality MCS.[168]

Of 259 children who were listed for isolated heart transplantation at Texas Children's Hospital between 1995 and 2013, the proportion of patients who received MCS while on the wait-list increased significantly from 13% before 2005 (i.e., before BHE when only ECMO and centrifugal pumps were available for those <20 kg) to 37% after 2005 (P = .0001). Among the 70 patients who received MCS, a temporary device was used as an initial therapy in 27 (ECMO = 14 and short-term VAD = 13), whereas long-term VAD was the first device in 43 patients. Wait-list mortality before 2005, 25%, decreased significantly after 2005, 11% (P = .0006). Median MCS duration before 2005, 12 days, also increased compared with after 2005, 78 days (P = .004). Kaplan-Meier estimates showed weak evidence (P = .08) for improved survival after bridge-to-transplant both at 1 year (70% before 2005 and 88% after 2005) and at 5 years (60% and 78%, respectively).[169] This reduction in wait-list mortality is likely attributable to both the increased use of MCS as well as improvements in medical management and the maturation and experience of their program.

Mechanical Circulatory Support and Single-Ventricle Physiology

Not surprisingly, children with CHD who require VAD support are often anatomically more challenging to support and have a greater mortality rate compared with children with cardiomyopathy.[155,170,171] In multiple studies, CHD has been identified as a risk factor, with those with single-ventricle physiology at greatest risk.[172] Based on data from the Pediatric Heart Transplant Study (PHTS) and Cardiac Transplant Research Database, single-ventricle anatomy is the most common cardiac lesion necessitating heart transplantation from age 6 months to adulthood. Unfortunately, outcomes after VAD support have been disappointing in the growing population of patients with failed single-ventricle palliations, with only 50% survival compared with overall pediatric VAD survival rates of 70% to 86%.[79,154,171] Because most patients who have undergone palliative cavopulmonary connections ultimately develop heart failure, the Mechanical Support as Failure Intervention in Patients with Cavopulmonary Shunts (MFICS) registry has been developed to improve the quality of care in this population.[170]

Infants who require ECMO support after stage I palliation for HLHS experience significant mortality. In a recent review of the ELSO database from 1998 to 2013, only 36% of children survive to hospital discharge for this population.[59] An analysis of ELSO data from 1999 to 2012 reported a 41% survival to hospital discharge in those who had undergone superior cavopulmonary anastomosis.[173] Of patients with single-ventricle physiology who required VV ECMO for oxygenation/ventilation, the majority of whom had stage I physiology, 48% survived.[174]

Although MCS has been used after all stages of single-ventricle palliation, a multiinstitutional analysis of BHE use in patients with functional single-ventricle physiology reported particularly poor outcomes in neonates who required support after stage I palliation for HLHS and successful bridge to transplant in only 40% of patients overall.[172] Only 11% of those who received an implant after stage I palliation survived, whereas 58% to 60% of patients after stage II or III palliation survived. Difficulty in selecting the correct pump size for patients with parallel circulations, extra sources of collateral pulmonary blood flow, and difficulty in balancing systemic and pulmonary circulations may all contribute to the high mortality after stage I palliation.

Supporting the patient with failing Fontan circulation presents unique barriers for MCS. Two basic physiologic subsets exist, which importantly affect support options. When heart failure symptoms develop because of a failing systemic ventricle (primary ventricular dysfunction), either pulsatile or continuous mechanical support is quite feasible, typically including inflow from the systemic ventricle and pump outflow to the ascending aorta. If right-sided pressures have been markedly increased, fenestration can be added at the time of implant.[175] When increased PVR or increased cavopulmonary resistance exists (failing Fontan physiology), successful support is more difficult to achieve and may require the addition of a pump from the systemic venous to the pulmonary circulation, requiring revision of the Fontan pathway to separate systemic venous and pulmonary circulations. When ventricular function is preserved and PVR is the predominant issue, pump outflow can be directed toward the pulmonary artery, providing isolated right-sided MCS. In circumstances in which a patient has significant diastolic dysfunction or residual structural lesions, a SynCardia TAH may be the most viable option for support[176]; successful use has been described in a teenager with failing Fontan circulation.[177]

VAD implantation is also technically difficult after previous sternotomies. Cannulation of the systemic right ventricle can be complicated secondary to dense trabeculations and septal positioning, predisposing to "suction" events in which the cannula is too closely opposed to the septum. After device implantation, Fontan patients generally have more bleeding and thrombotic complications related to inherent protein C and S deficiencies, resulting in coagulopathy.

Predicting the Need for BiVAD Support

The pathology leading to left heart failure in the pediatric population is also more likely to lead to RV failure than the typical adult ischemic cardiomyopathy.[178] As a consequence, BiVAD support is more often necessary in pediatric patients, with reports of BiVAD use in 25% to 45% of patients.[79,179,180] Multiple studies have shown that patients who receive BiVAD support have reduced rates of survival.[155,180–182] This may be related to the pathophysiology necessitating BiVAD support, or the fact that use of multiple devices can lead to an increased risk of adverse events including infection, bleeding, and clot formation. Outcomes are also worse in patients who have delayed RVAD placement.[183] RV dysfunction was assessed in 57 patients who underwent BHE implantation for bridge-to-transplant; 25% required BiVAD support and an additional 17% had RV dysfunction (defined as CVP >16 mm Hg with inotropic therapy and/or inhaled nitric oxide for >96 hours). Preoperative variables such as younger age; use of ECMO; and increased urea, creatinine, and bilirubin were associated with RV dysfunction and increased urea and need for ECMO were risk factors for BiVAD placement. Patients who developed RV dysfunction with LVAD support had complicated postoperative courses but excellent survival (100%) comparable with those with preserved RV function (91%). Survival of those patients who required BiVAD support was only 71%.[180] Another study demonstrated that patients who required biventricular support had a significantly greater postoperative mortality and that preoperative milrinone therapy decreased the risk of severe RV failure necessitating RVAD insertion and improved postimplantation survival.[12]

ECMO for Cardiac Arrest

Emergent use of ECMO for children during in-hospital cardiac arrest with failure of conventional resuscitation methods has become increasingly common. An analysis of data from the National Registry of CardioPulmonary Resuscitation (NRCPR) database of outcomes from children younger than 18 years of age who received ECPR for cardiac arrest refractory to conventional CPR demonstrated a 43.7% survival to discharge. Preexisting septicemia, pneumonia, and/or renal insufficiency correlated with an increased risk of mortality. Children with a cardiac-related diagnosis exhibited slightly improved odds of survival to discharge when compared with children without cardiac disease.[184] In a review of pediatric cardiac patients from the ELSO registry who received ECPR, single-ventricle physiology and a history of more complex cardiac surgery were negative predictors of survival.[185] Renal dysfunction, pulmonary hemorrhage, neurologic injury, and the need for additional CPR during ECMO have also been associated with increased mortality.[186]

Acceptable neurologic outcomes have been described in children after CPR of up to 3 hours in duration before institution of ECMO.[187] The duration of CPR before ECMO cannulation was similar in survivors and nonsurvivors.[188] Of the children in the ELSO registry who received ECPR, 22% of the 682 developed an acute neurologic injury, with an in-hospital mortality rate of 89%. The risk of neurologic injury in children with cardiac disease in this cohort was reduced.[189]

COMPLICATIONS

VAD use is associated with neurologic, hematologic, GI, and immunologic complications, with the frequency and severity of many of these complications being device specific. The profiles of adverse events differ between pulsatile devices and currently used continuous-flow pumps.

Stroke is the most feared complication related to MCS, occurring more commonly with pulsatile-flow than continuous-flow devices.[190] Strokes may be hemorrhagic in nature or ischemic owing to embolism from ventricular clot or device thrombus, the latter being more common. Of 3517 cardiac surgical patients who received ECMO support between the years 2002 and 2013, neonatal status, smaller weight for age, and greater duration of ECMO were associated with a greater risk of stroke risk.[191] In the BHE trial, stroke occurred in 29% of supported patients, with thromboembolic strokes occurring eight times more often than hemorrhagic strokes.[13] Temporally, neurologic events were more common during the first month of support and, overall, was the leading cause of death after pump implantation. Mortality was 42% among patients with at least one neurologic event versus 18% in the absence of this event (P = .0006). Patients weighing less than 10 kg have the greatest incidence of stroke.[166,192] Increased institutional experience and appointment of a single physician to manage a patient's anticoagulation therapy can decrease the risk of stroke.[193]

Bleeding is quite common after ECMO and VAD device placement and is usually most severe in the early postoperative period. One-third of patients in the Pediatric Heart Study assist device multiinstitutional study and up to 50% of those in the Berlin Heart Trial had bleeding requiring reoperation.[154] Major bleeding was also the most commonly encountered complication in patients enrolled in the randomized Berlin Heart Pediatric VAD study, occurring in 42% of the low-BSA and 50% of the high-BSA cohorts.[13]

Infection is a relatively common complication and occurs in 50% to 69% of patients,[13,194] with infection attributable to the prolonged hospitalizations and exposure to multiple invasive therapies. The potential also exists for VAD-specific (driveline, hardware, or pump pocket) or VAD-related (mediastinitis, endocarditic, or bloodstream) infections. Commonly implicated organisms include *Staphylococcus aureus*, coagulase-negative staphylococci, *Pseudomonas aeruginosa*, and *Candida* spp.[194] Aggressive antibiotic and/or antifungal therapy, in addition to source control, is crucial, particularly in the setting of antirejection medications at the time of transplantation. Patients with driveline infections are often maintained with suppressive oral antibiotic therapy until 2 weeks after cardiac transplantation.

Immunologic complications related to VAD support involve the formation of antibodies against human leukocyte antigens (anti-HLA antibodies), a process that has been consistently observed. The mechanism of antibody formation is complex and likely involves factors specific to the device itself as well as clinical events occurring during VAD support, particularly blood product transfusion.[195] After taking into account the blood product usage, some studies still reported an increase in panel reactive antibodies.[196] The presence of HLA antibodies is of significant concern as their presence in significant numbers may limit the suitability of a donor organ should the donor have preformed anti-HLA antibodies against specific HLA antigens. Although the adult sensitization rates of patients supported with a VAD have been reported to be as great as 60% on modern devices,[197] the true incidence of anti-HLA antibody formation in children supported with VADs is difficult to ascertain. In one study, there was a decrease in survival approximately 5 years after transplantation for patients who received VAD support[166]; the authors postulated that this could be related to increased risk of graft failure, secondary to increased allosensitization in VAD patients. The smaller surface area and materials used to make the newer continuous-flow devices appear to decrease the incidence of anti-HLA antibody formation.

Increased rates of both aortic insufficiency and aortic valve leaflet fusion exist with continuous-flow devices, thought to be due to an increased gradient across the aortic valve and increased strain on valve leaflets.[198] An increased rate of pulmonary hypertension and GI bleeding in the adult population has also been reported with continuous-flow devices.[199] GI bleeding occurs from a combination of factors, including anticoagulation, acquired vWF deficiency and decreased pulsatility, leading to the formation of arteriovenous malformations.[121] Although this has not been described in the pediatric population, acquired vWF deficiency has been described and is attributed to the destruction of the large vWF multimers by the rotor.[88] The risk of GI bleeding may become an issue in pediatric VAD patients as more of them receive continuous-flow devices for longer durations.

VAD therapy is also associated with other GI complications, including the need for peritoneal disruption as part of implantation. It is estimated that 55% of adult patients experience abdominal complications with VAD support, with problems such as wound/pocket infection, *Clostridium difficile* infection, hepatic dysfunction, and pancreatitis.[200] The incidence of such complications in the pediatric population is unknown.

The Future

In the face of an increasing need for advanced circulatory support in the pediatric patient population, the NHLBI developed a Pediatric Circulatory Support Program in 2004 that matured into the Pumps for Kids, Infants, and Neonates Program (PumpKIN) in 2010. Although a prospective, randomized trial of two implantable pumps was designed (PumpKIN trial) for 22 centers, the FDA suspended the study before it started after in vitro studies revealed an excessive degree of hemolysis with the Jarvik 2000 device (Jarvik Heart, Inc., New York, NY).[201] Additional in vitro studies failed to reveal the source of hemolysis. Since then a slightly larger version of this pump, the Jarvik 2015 (with 40% larger inflow cannula) was designed and in vitro studies reported an acceptable level of hemolysis. Further in vitro studies are planned before proceeding with the clinical trial.[163]

Both Thoratec (HeartMate III device) and HeartWare (MVAD device) have new, smaller continuous-flow devices entering U.S. clinical trials. These devices, especially the MVAD, will be rapidly applied to the pediatric population as an off-label indication as soon as FDA approval occurs.[163]

Minimally invasive pulmonary replacement devices are also now in development; devices such as the Biolung[202] and others are being developed as an alternative to ECMO for gas exchange and may become available in the near future.

ANNOTATED REFERENCES

Adachi I, Fraser C. Mechanical circulatory support for infants and small children. *Semin Thorac Cardiovasc Surg Pediatr Card Surg Annu.* 2011;14:38-44.
This review article summarizes currently available devices for support of children with acute heart failure.

21

Almond C, Singh T, Gauvreau K, et al. Extracorporeal membrane oxygenation for bridge to heart transplantation among children in the United States: analysis of data from the Organ Procurement and Transplant Network and Extracorporeal Life Support Organization Registry. *Circulation.* 2011;123:2975-2984.

The authors review data from two major databases, evaluating outcomes of children undergoing ECMO as a bridge to heart transplantation in the United States between 1994 and 2009.

Baldwin J, Borovetz H, Duncan B, et al. The National Heart, Lung, and Blood Institute Pediatric Circulatory Support Program: a summary of the 5-year experience. *Circulation.* 2011;123:1233-1240.

This paper presents a summary of the progress made and devices under development in the United States from the Pediatric Circulatory Support Program.

Barrett C, Bratton S, Salvin J, et al. Neurological injury after extracorporeal membrane oxygenation use to aid pediatric cardiopulmonary resuscitation. *Pediatr Crit Care Med.* 2009;10:445-451.

This is a retrospective cohort study of data from the Extracorporeal Life Support Organization registry, evaluating neurologic injury in children undergoing ECPR.

Blume E, Naftel D, Bastardi H, et al. Outcomes of children bridged to heart transplantation with ventricular assist devices: a multi-institutional study. *Circulation.* 2006;13:2313-2319.

This paper presents a multiinstitutional review of children undergoing heart transplantation, evaluating outcomes in those who required VAD support as bridge to transplantation.

Hetzer R, Potapov E, Alexi-Meskishvili V, et al. Single-center experience with treatment of cardiogenic shock in children by pediatric ventricular assist devices. *J Thorac Cardiovasc Surg.* 2011;141:616-623.

The authors offer a review of management strategies and outcomes in 94 patients with Berlin Heart EXCOR support, between 1990 and 2009.

Jefferies J, Price J, Morales D. Mechanical support in childhood heart failure. *Heart Fail Clin.* 2010;6:559-573.

This is a comprehensive review of indications for MCS and currently available devices for children of all ages.

Mascio CE. The use of ventricular assist device support in children: the state of the art. *Artif Organs.* 2015;39(1):14-20.

The author provides an excellent overview of the commonly used ventricular assist devices in children.

Maslach-Hubbard A, Bratton SL. Extracorporeal membrane oxygenation for pediatric respiratory failure: history, development and current status. *World J Crit Care Med.* 2013;2:29-39.

The authors provide a comprehensive review of the use of extracorporeal membrane oxygenation for respiratory failure in children.

Mossad E, Motta P, Rossano J, et al. Perioperative management of pediatric patients on mechanical cardiac support. *Paediatr Anaesth.* 2011;21:585-593.

The authors review the demographics of children requiring MCS and perioperative management concepts for their care.

Rais-Bahrami K, Van Meurs KP. Venoarterial versus venovenous ECMO for neonatal respiratory failure. *Semin Perinatol.* 2014;38(2):71-77.

The authors provide a good brief review of ECMO in neonates complete with cannulation pictorial.

Sani A, Spinella PC. Management of anticoagulation and hemostasis for pediatric extracorporeal membrane oxygenation. *Clin Lab Med.* 2014;34:655-673.

The authors provide a thorough review of various methods for anticoagulation and monitoring for patients on ECMO support.

A complete reference list can be found online at ExpertConsult.com.

22

Interventional Cardiology

ELLEN RAWLINSON AND NATALIE FORSHAW

THE USE OF CATHETERIZATION in the care of children with congenital heart disease (CHD) was first described by Dexter and colleagues in 1947[1] with the first interventional procedure, balloon atrial septostomy, subsequently described by Rashkind and Miller in 1966.[2] Over the intervening decades the discipline of pediatric interventional cardiology has vastly expanded within the field of pediatric cardiovascular medicine.

Technologic advances have increased the scope of pediatric cardiac catheterization procedures. As echocardiography, computed tomography (CT), and magnetic resonance imaging (MRI) diagnostic capabilities have increased, the need for purely diagnostic cardiac catheterization has waned.[3] There has been a transition from diagnostics toward more therapeutic interventions, with interventional procedures now accounting for more than two-thirds of all pediatric cardiac catheterizations.[4] Interventional cardiology has afforded patients a wider range of nonsurgical options for the management of CHD, postponing or replacing the requirement for surgery. Hybrid procedures, combining interventional cardiology with cardiac surgery, have enabled the management of more complex cardiac lesions.[5] As more children with CHD survive into adulthood, there has been a shift in patient demographics. Children presenting for interventional cardiology represent a diverse group from premature neonates to older adolescents, with simple to complex pathophysiology, requiring procedures of varying complexity. Catheterization laboratories are often remote sites and can be challenging environments. Anesthesiologists providing care to children undergoing cardiac catheterizations must have a good understanding of the patient's pathophysiology and tailor anesthesia to the patient- and procedure-specific requirements. Adverse events are common during catheterization procedures. The anesthesiologist must be able to anticipate, prevent, and treat complications that may arise in this high-risk population.

In this chapter, we outline the main procedures performed in interventional cardiology, describe the challenges and complications faced by anesthesiologists, and address the principles and details of anesthetic techniques.

Types of Procedures Performed

DIAGNOSTIC CATHETERIZATION

Diagnostic catheterization allows accurate documentation of pressure and oxygen content from different regions of the circulation. Interpretation of these hemodynamic data allows quantification of the degree of intracardiac shunting and calculation of vascular resistances. This information is necessary to guide critical decisions, such as the suitability of a child to undergo palliative or reparative surgery for congenital heart lesions, and to direct medical therapy. Consistent and reproducible physiologic conditions are required during the procedure to allow correct interpretation and comparison of results. Expected values for hemodynamic variables are listed in Table 22.1. There are no absolute values for these variables, which vary with the age of the child. The use of angiocardiography during catheterization to define complex cardiac anatomy is waning because of the increased use and capabilities of noninvasive imaging modalities such as echocardiography, CT, and MRI.[6]

INTERVENTIONAL CATHETERIZATION

Interventional procedures now account for approximately two-thirds of all cardiac catheterization cases in children of all ages.[7]

Atrial Septostomy

Atrial septostomy involves passing a balloon-tipped catheter across the atrial septum, typically through the membranous foramen

22

ovale. The balloon is inflated and pulled back through the septum creating a larger intraatrial communication that improves mixing of oxygenated and deoxygenated blood at the atrial level. The procedure is most commonly performed in neonates with D-transposition of the great vessels (D-TGA) as an emergency procedure. Children with D-TGA have systemic and pulmonary circulations in parallel rather than in series; the right ventricle pumps deoxygenated blood to the aorta, and the left ventricle pumps oxygenated blood to the main pulmonary artery. Atrial septostomy allows critical mixing of oxygenated and deoxygenated blood, thereby increasing systemic oxygen saturation. The procedure can be performed in the catheterization laboratory under fluoroscopic guidance or undertaken at the bedside in the intensive care unit using echocardiographic guidance.[8] Other indications for atrial septostomy include tricuspid atresia, mitral atresia, and pulmonary atresia with intact ventricular septum. The major risks associated with the procedure are vessel injury, paradoxical embolism, arrhythmia, and cardiac perforation. More recent concerns of an association with increased brain injury do not seem to have been evidence-founded.[9]

Atrial Septal Defect Closure

With the development of specifically designed closure devices, atrial septal defect (ASD) closure has become one of the most commonly performed endovascular procedures. The technique is intended for closing secundum ASDs, which are defects located in the region of the fossa ovalis. Defects falling outside this area, such as sinus venosus and primum ASDs, are generally not suitable for percutaneous closure.

To warrant closure, children need to demonstrate clear evidence of volume loading of the right heart structures and a defect that is unlikely to close spontaneously in the short to medium term. Devices have evolved from the early bulky meshes and a wide variety of sizes and designs are now available. The choice of closure device depends on the size and margins of the defect, but brand selection depends more on the clinician's preference than objective performance (Fig. 22.1).[10] Daily aspirin in a dose of 3 to 5 mg/kg is recommended for a minimum of 6 months after the procedure. The main perioperative complications associated with ASD device closure include vessel injury, cardiac arrhythmia, cardiac perforation, and device embolization. In the long term, devices are well tolerated with atrial arrhythmias the most common problem, although life-threatening complications such as cardiac erosion have been reported.[11] ASD closure devices can also be used to close surgically created fenestrations when they are no longer required, such as between the atrium and venous conduits after a Fontan operation.

Ventricular Septal Defect Closure

Ventricular septal defect (VSD) closure presents a technically greater challenge than ASD closure and is associated with a greater incidence of complications. Defects of the midmuscular septum or apex are most suitable for device closure, although perimembranous VSDs may also be closed percutaneously.[12,13] A combined surgical and interventional approach may be appropriate for certain cases, such as the small infant with an anterior apical VSD that is difficult to reach surgically.[14]

When using a device to close a VSD, a snare is placed in the right side of the heart to capture a guidewire that has been passed across the VSD from the left ventricle. The guidewire is brought outside the body via the venous access to form an arteriovenous rail. The delivery sheath for the VSD device is then advanced over the wire to approach the VSD from the right side of the heart. For anterior and high muscular defects, the wire is best snared and exteriorized through a femoral vein approach, whereas for defects in the middle to low muscular septum, the wire is best snared and exteriorized through a jugular venous approach (Fig. 22.2).

TABLE 22.1	Normal Values in Diagnostic Cardiac Catheterization
Structure	**Value (mm Hg)**
Right atrium	3–5 (mean)
Right ventricle	20–25/3–5 (systolic/end-diastolic)
Pulmonary artery	12–15 (mean)
Left atrium	7–10 (mean)
Left ventricle	65–110/3–5 (systolic/end-diastolic)
Aorta	65–110/35–65 (systolic/diastolic)

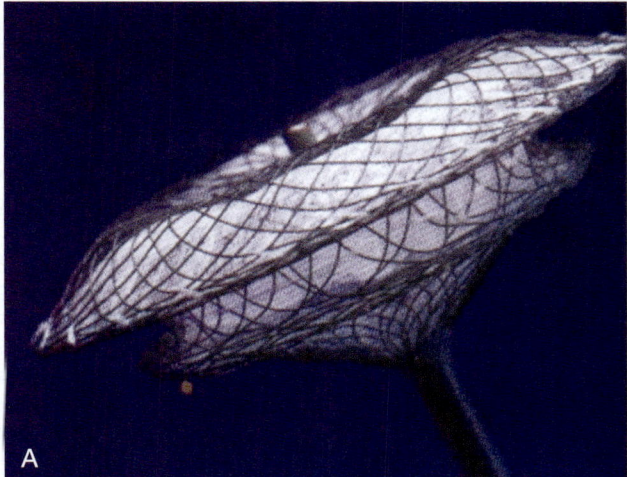
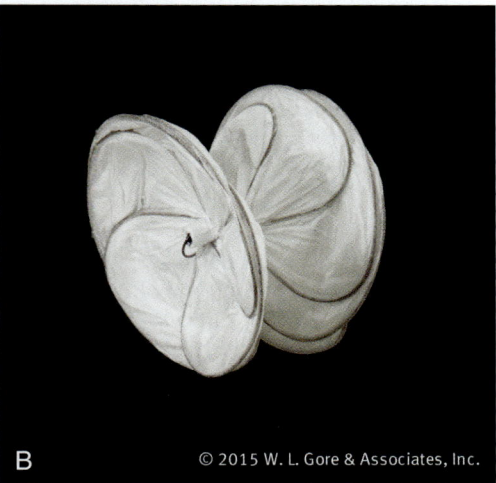

© 2015 W. L. Gore & Associates, Inc.

FIGURE 22.1 Devices for closure of an atrial septal defect. **A,** The Amplatzer (St. Jude Medical, St. Paul, MN) Septal Occluder. **B,** Gore CARDIOFORM Septal Occluder. (**A,** Courtesy AGA Medical Corporation, Golden Valley, MN. **B,** Courtesy W.L. Gore & Associates, Flagstaff, AZ.)

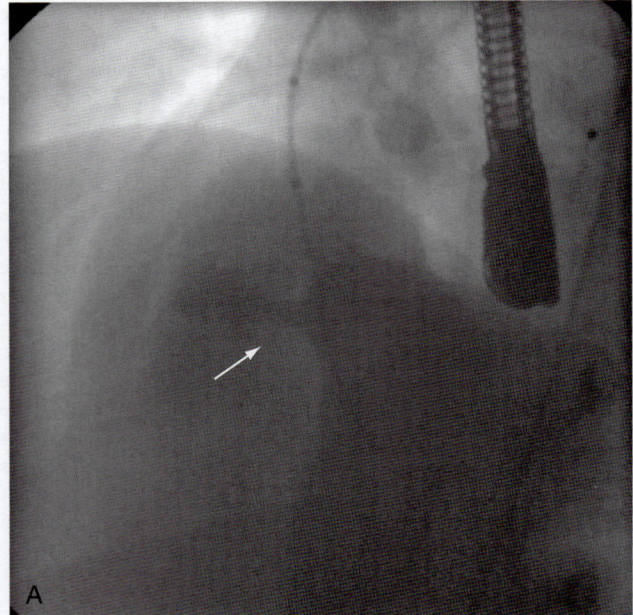

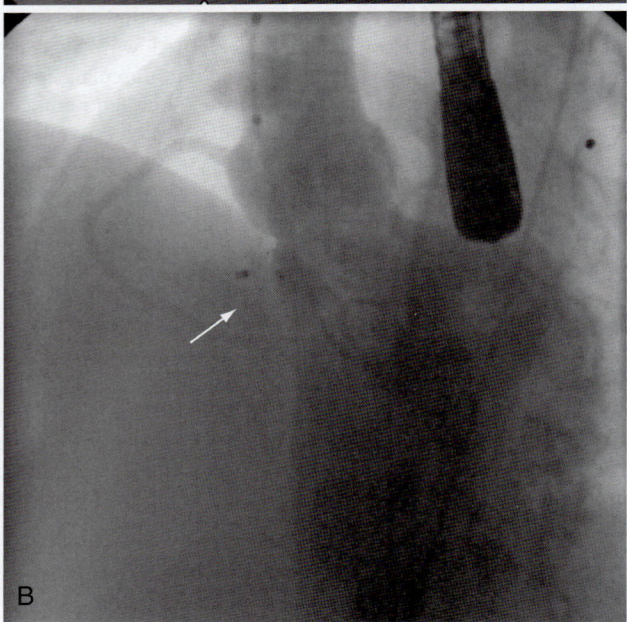

FIGURE 22.2 A, Angiography of a ventricular septal defect (VSD) device before deployment. Contrast agent passes through the perimembranous VSD (*arrow*). **B,** Appearance of same region (*arrow*), no contrast agent after deployment of the device.

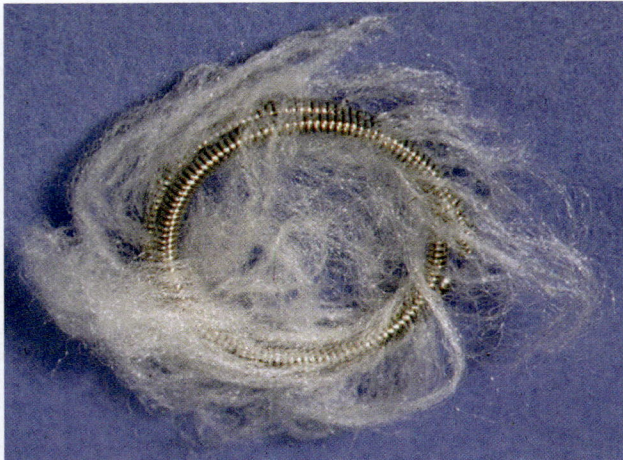

FIGURE 22.3 The coil is used for closure of a patent ductus arteriosus.

Complications include dysrhythmias, blood loss, valve dysfunction, low cardiac output state, and device embolization.[15,16] Device closure of perimembranous VSDs in particular has been associated with an increased incidence of complete heart block and aortic valve disruption owing to the close proximity of conduction pathways and the aortic valve apparatus. This has led to some controversy in their use, with many centers considering the risk unacceptable, given the good outcomes following surgical VSD closure.

Patent Ductus Arteriosus Closure

Transcatheter closure of patent ductus arteriosus (PDA) was the second specific intervention developed for children with CHD, and the procedure continues to be performed using techniques similar to the original methods pioneered by Rashkind and associates.[17] The procedure has a high occlusion rate with the smallest incidence of adverse events of all interventional procedures and is indicated in any child with evidence of left ventricular overload. PDA morphology varies from short and broad to narrow and tortuous, so the customary approach is to perform an aortogram to define the size and geometry. For closure of small and moderate PDAs, stainless steel coils (e.g., Gianturco, Cook Medical, Bloomington, IN) are most commonly used, whereas for larger PDAs, occluder devices (e.g., Amplatzer, St. Jude Medical, St. Paul, MN) are more appropriate.[18,19] Devices can be deployed with a retrograde or anterograde approach. Embolization of the device at the point of deployment is a risk but there are several techniques that can help control device release. Embolization may also be delayed, so proper follow-up is required; the other major risk associated with this procedure is vessel injury. Despite impressive technical evolution over the years, PDA device closure in premature or low body weight infants remains prohibitively challenging and further catheter design is required in this area.[20] These techniques can also be used to close other unwarranted vascular connections such as major aortopulmonary collateral arteries (MAPCAs) and Blalock-Taussig (BT) shunts that are no longer required (Figs. 22.3 and 22.4).

Balloon Dilation and Stent Implantation

Balloon angioplasty techniques are used to dilate stenotic valves, most commonly pulmonary and aortic, as well as stenotic segments of the aorta or pulmonary arteries and surgically placed shunts or pulmonary artery bands. Neonatal membranous pulmonary atresia can be treated using this technique, crossing the pulmonary valve membrane with the stiff end of a guidewire or with radiofrequency catheters[21] before subsequent dilatation of the valve annulus. Balloon valvuloplasty of isolated pulmonary stenosis in older infants and children is often a curative procedure, whereas neonates with critical pulmonary stenosis or atresia often require further interventions to supplement pulmonary blood flow such as ductal stenting or a BT shunt.[22] Inflation of the balloon temporarily arrests right ventricular output and is often accompanied by transient hypotension but is generally well tolerated.[23] Paradoxically, those with tighter stenosis and little antegrade flow may maintain

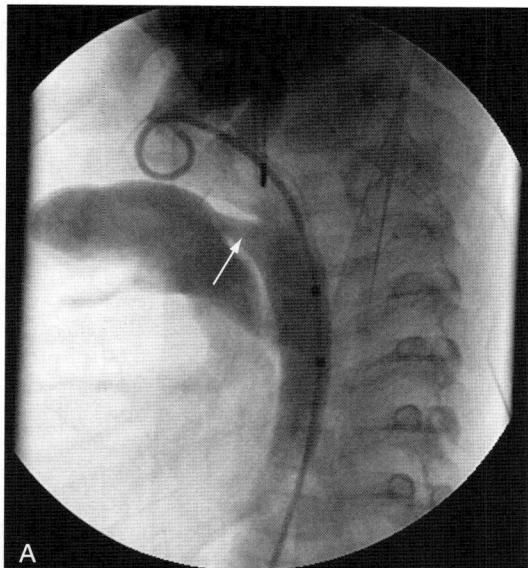

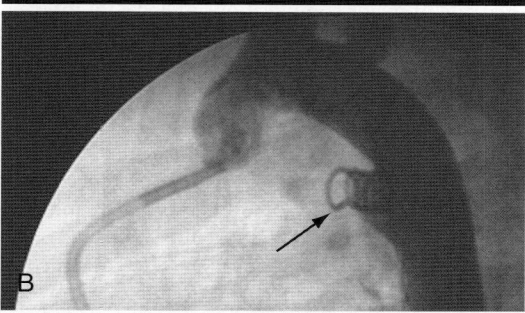

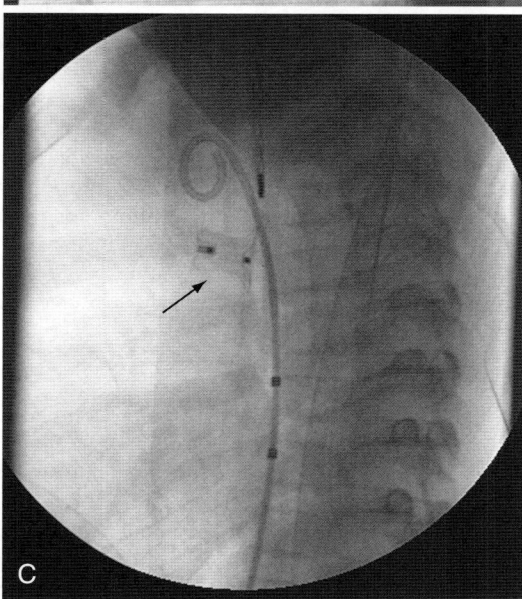

FIGURE 22.4 A, Lateral angiography demonstrates a patent ductus arteriosus (PDA) (*arrow*). The PDA lies between aorta and pulmonary artery (*arrow*). The angiography catheter is in the proximal aorta. **B,** Lateral angiography after closure of the PDA with a coil (*arrow*). **C,** Lateral fluoroscopy after closure of the PDA with the Amplatzer TM Duct Occluder device. The device (*arrow*) is in the PDA.

hemodynamic stability better, particularly if the duct is still open, as cardiac output is less disrupted.

The role of balloon valvuloplasty for critical aortic stenosis remains controversial; in some centers, it remains the treatment of choice, whereas others prefer a primary surgical approach. Concerns relate to longer-term outcomes and the rate of surgical intervention required in those treated initially with valvuloplasty.[24,25] When performed, balloon dilation of aortic stenosis in the neonate is a particularly high-risk procedure. These infants often present in a low–cardiac output state requiring ventilation, inotropic support, and prostaglandin E_1 (PGE_1) infusion to maintain ductal patency. Catheterization can be complicated by arrhythmias (including asystole), the development of significant aortic regurgitation (which may require surgical intervention), and sudden death resulting from acute coronary ischemia.[26] The complication rate in older children is less than in younger children, yet transient hypotension, bradycardia, and left bundle branch block are commonly reported.

Stents are sometimes implanted across focal areas of persistent stenosis in the systemic and pulmonary circulations or within surgically placed shunts.[27] The technique of implantation requires great precision for correct positioning of the stent, and the cardiac interventionalist needs to take into account the inevitable shortening that occurs with stent implantation when selecting a device for a particular lesion. There is also a risk of stent malposition with the potential for dislodgment. Although rare, late aneurysm formation has been reported after stenting the aorta for coarctation.[28]

Nonsurgical Pulmonary Valve Replacement

Bonhoeffer and colleagues[29] first described the technique of replacing a dysfunctional valve in a right ventricle to pulmonary artery (RV-PA) conduit with a catheter-implanted valve in 2000. The Melody valve (Medtronic Inc., Minneapolis, MN) is one such device that has been approved for use in surgically placed RV-PA conduits meeting specific requirements.[30] Studies have confirmed a high procedural success rate and satisfactory short-term and medium-term valve function after implantation of the Melody valve.[31] The need for careful patient selection and for adequate relief of right ventricular outflow tract (RVOT) obstruction at the time of valve implantation are paramount in achieving results comparable to those of surgical replacement of dysfunctional conduits. Off-label use has additionally demonstrated promising results with implantation of Melody valves in children with native RVOTs.[30] Unfortunately, most children who are managed with transannular patch repair of tetralogy of Fallot are currently unsuitable for transcatheter valve replacement because of an aneurysmal RVOT. New hybrid procedures are, however, emerging to circumvent this, allowing more options for patients with tetralogy of Fallot, many of whom are likely to require recurrent interventions over their lifetime.[32] Alternative devices are also being developed to reduce the size of the delivery systems to enable use of these technologies in younger and smaller children. As with surgical valve replacements, thrombus formation and infective endocarditis are concerns after transcatheter valve implantation.[31]

ELECTROPHYSIOLOGIC CATHETERIZATION

Endocardial catheters that record an electrocardiogram first became available in the early 1960s. Intracardiac electrograms, supplemented by external electrocardiogram leads, record electrical activity in the heart, and programmable stimulators aim to induce and terminate tachyarrhythmias. This allows arrhythmia mechanisms to be defined and arrhythmogenic foci to be mapped. Ablation catheters can then be guided to deliver local energy to the endocardium to destroy the source of the arrhythmia or interrupt aberrant conduction pathways. Ablation can be delivered as radiofrequency, cryoablation, laser therapy, or direct currents. Ablative procedures are indicated for the treatment of cardiac arrhythmias, particularly atrial tachyarrhythmias.

The procedures are complex, requiring specialized equipment, specially trained staff, and use of multiple catheters to measure electrical signals. These procedures are often of greater duration than other catheterization procedures. Ablation of ectopic foci has a good success rate and small complication rate.[33,34] The main risks with this procedure are heart block, cardiac perforation, vessel injury, and stroke.

Choice of Vessel Access

The most common approach for cardiac catheterization is the femoral route. Femoral venous catheterization avoids the risk of pneumothorax and the vessel is often easier to access than the internal jugular vein in the unanesthetized child. In children who are likely to have a cavopulmonary shunt placed surgically for palliation, avoiding routine cannulation of the internal jugular vein may decrease the risk of compromising the superior vena cava. Internal jugular vein access, however, is sometimes required, such as during some VSD closures, investigation of cavopulmonary connections in children, and when the cardiac interventionalist is unable to obtain femoral access. In neonates, the umbilical vein may be used, although difficulty can be encountered attempting to cross the ductus venosus to access the inferior vena cava. Patency of the ductus venosus can be assessed by ultrasound before the procedure to avoid unnecessary manipulation of the umbilical vein. An alternative route is transhepatic puncture. This route has been used for temporary access during catheterization and for long-term vascular access.[35]

Complications and Limitations of Procedures

The pediatric cardiac catheterization laboratory is a high-risk environment associated with significant morbidity and mortality. Of the 373 anesthesia-related cardiac arrests reported in the Pediatric Perioperative Cardiac Registry, 34% occurred in children with cardiac disease and 17% of these occurred in the catheterization laboratory.[36] Additionally, there are complications directly attributable to the procedures. Successful practice in this setting requires a thorough understanding of pathology, vigilance, excellent communication between team members, and appropriate backup from surgeons and other specialties. Standard procedures for predictable emergencies should be in place. An intensive care bed should be available for high risk procedures. The facility for cardiopulmonary bypass or extracorporeal membrane oxygenation (ECMO) for high-risk patient groups or procedures may be beneficial,[16] although this type of therapy may not be available everywhere. Local policies on appropriate case mix should be based on experience and infrastructure and clear referral pathways for high-risk cases should be established.

OVERALL MORTALITY AND MORBIDITY

Recent studies of pediatric catheterization have reported mortality rates in the immediate perioperative period (in theatre or recovery) of between 0.05 and 0.28%.[18,30] However, the **IM**proving **P**ediatric and **A**dult **C**ongenital **T**reatment (IMPACT) database of more than 16,000 pediatric catheterizations reports all-cause mortality for children undergoing catheterization during their admission as 2.1%, with the majority of deaths occurring within 14 days of the procedure.[4] Despite the increasing complexity of both patients and procedures being undertaken, the mortality rate is decreasing.

Adverse events occur in 8.8% to 10.6% of catheterization procedures overall.[4,37] Morbidity may be classified as either major or minor. Major complications are life-threatening events requiring immediate medical or surgical intervention (e.g., cardiac arrest, removal of an embolized device) or which result in a significant permanent lesion (e.g., embolic stroke, vessel aneurysm). These types of adverse events occur during 1% to 2% of procedures. Minor complications are transient and resolve with specific treatment (e.g., tolerated dysrhythmias, transient arterial thrombosis). Complication rates have remained largely constant despite technologic advances, reflecting the changing nature of the patient population and interventions.

Certain patient and procedural characteristics confer increased risk of complications. Neonates are particularly vulnerable, with a reported rate of major complications of 4.7% for interventional catheterization, which may be explained by reduced physiologic reserve, presence of uncorrected or partially palliated congenital heart defects, and an increased risk of obstruction to great vessels and cardiac chambers by wires and devices.[23] Age younger than 1 year and low body weight have been identified as independent risk factors for complications.[38] Specific cardiac lesions are also associated with greater risks of both morbidity and mortality, notably single ventricle physiology, whether unrepaired or palliated, and significant left ventricular outflow tract obstruction (e.g., Williams-Beuren syndrome and hypertrophic cardiomyopathy).[39] The presence of pulmonary hypertension, particularly with an idiopathic etiology and suprasystemic pulmonary artery pressures, increases perioperative risk substantially.[40] With respect to procedural risk, interventional procedures have greater complication rates than diagnostic procedures for all age groups except neonates, in whom the complication rates are similar.[4,23] Specifically, high-risk procedures include VSD device closure; atrial septostomy where the septum is restrictive; balloon interventions for the mitral valve, pulmonary vein, pulmonary artery, and neonatal aortic valve; and stent placement in surgical shunts.[41,42] At the other end of the spectrum, PDA and ASD device closures have the least risks of complications.[23]

VASCULAR COMPLICATIONS

Vascular complications are the most common complication of pediatric catheterizations, accounting for almost a third of the total.[43] They may be acute, leading to unexpected hemodynamic instability, or delayed, leading to longer-term morbidity. Many factors may contribute to unexpected hemodynamic instability, including blood loss, balloon- or catheter-induced interruptions in blood flow or coronary perfusion, arrhythmias, tamponade, vessel rupture, acute valve dysfunction, and device malposition.

Arterial Thrombosis and Occlusion

Arterial thrombosis is common after pediatric cardiac catheterization, with a reported incidence in two large studies of 4.3% and 11.4%.[44,45] However, diagnosis based on clinical assessment of pulses is likely to lead to underestimation; when measured by Doppler ultrasound, 32% of infants had compromised arterial blood flow to the leg.[46] Young age, small size, larger sheath size, and repeated arterial catheter exchanges are independent risk factors for thrombosis; polycythemia and dehydration may increase risk further.

Prophylactic heparin reduces but does not remove the risk of arterial thrombosis[47]; and despite widespread use, there is no consensus on the appropriate dose. Common schedules prescribe 50 to 100 IU/kg; larger doses do not appear to add additional benefit. Most cases of reduced or absent pulse will resolve either spontaneously or with additional heparin anticoagulation. Thrombolysis is a viable next step, but surgical intervention will be needed for thrombosis resistant to medical therapy, arterial tears or avulsion, and pseudoaneurysms. Percutaneous thrombectomy may be suitable in older children.[48,49] Occasionally, a pulse may be persistently reduced in a clinically well-perfused limb despite intervention. The long-term concern is delayed limb growth; cases have been reported but one small study failed to demonstrate limb-length discrepancy after median follow up of 3½ years. Currently there is no means to identify those at risk.[48,50]

Venous Thrombosis and Occlusion

Isolated cases of femoral or iliofemoral venous occlusions with limb edema have been published as part of large series,[37] but two small prospective observational studies found an incidence of 0% and 1.6%, respectively.[51,52] All affected children responded to heparin therapy without the need for further intervention. Using the smallest catheter necessary and heparin prophylaxis should assist in limiting the incidence.

Vessel Rupture, Perforation, and Dissection

Vessel rupture can occur at the site of vessel entry or at the site of intervention. It is a rare but potentially catastrophic event. One death caused by intraabdominal hemorrhage after rupture of a femoral vein in a neonate was reported in a series of 4454 catheterizations.[23] Arterial or venous perforations were responsible for four major complications and six minor complications in a series of 4952 procedures, and significant groin hematoma occurred in 25 cases.[37]

Vessel rupture appears most common during balloon dilation of branch pulmonary arteries and during RVOT valve implantation procedures, but it has also been reported along the ascending aorta and arch after dilation on the aortic valve.[53] Occasionally, arterial dissection, aneurysm, and pseudoaneurysm formation may occur. Rupture may cause hemopericardium or hemothorax, or both; pulmonary artery disruption after balloon dilation may manifest as hemoptysis.[48] If rupture and hemorrhage occur, hypertension should be avoided, the trachea should be intubated (if the airway is not already secured), and any circulating heparin should be reversed. In extremis, blood from pericardial or pleural drains may be returned directly to the patient via femoral cannulae until surgical intervention can be achieved.

Cardiac Perforation and Tamponade

Perforation of the myocardium during catheterization procedures is relatively common, with the atrial appendage and RVOT the most common sites. Procedures associated with a greater risk include atrial septostomy, balloon dilation of the mitral valve, and attempted radiofrequency perforation of membranous pulmonary atresia.[48] Signs that suggest a perforation include wires appearing in unexpected places, atypical contrast appearance, lack of a return to baseline blood pressure after catheter-induced tachycardia, narrow pulse pressure, and hemodynamic instability. Echocardiography should always be immediately available to confirm a suspected perforation or tamponade. Perforation is often well tolerated and frequently can be managed conservatively, but the **C**ongenital **C**ardiac **C**atheterization **P**roject on **O**utcomes (C3PO) database of nearly 9000 cases recorded 5 neonatal deaths resulting from cardiac perforation during atrial septostomy.[54]

Cardiac tamponade is an uncommon complication of cardiac catheterization with an incidence reported at 0.1% to 0.2%.[4] In one series of 4952 patients, tamponade was responsible for 2 deaths: one neonate after a balloon atrial septostomy and one 4-year-old child after a recent Fontan procedure for stent insertion in a branch pulmonary artery.[37] Tamponade may be treated by needle pericardiocentesis, insertion of a pericardial drain, or occasionally, by the formation of a pericardial window by cardiac surgeons.

DAMAGE OR DYSFUNCTION OF A VALVE

Damage to a valve is uncommon but most commonly occurs with balloon valvuloplasty rather than with other procedures. The primary complication is creation of excessive regurgitation. The hemodynamic consequences of such a defect are more significant on the systemic side of the circulation than on the pulmonary side.[48] The mechanism of injury is most commonly leaflet avulsion during dilation, although the leaflet can be inadvertently perforated by the guidewire and then further damaged as the catheter wire is manipulated. Emergency repair is occasionally required.[48] Direct injuries to atrioventricular valves are rare, but placement of wires and large sheaths across atrioventricular valves and septal defects can cause severe, albeit temporary, hemodynamic disturbance. This is particularly true during implantation of VSD occlusion devices.[15] ASD and PDA occlusions are less likely to produce significant hemodynamic disturbance.[26]

BLOOD LOSS

Blood loss may be sudden with rupture of vessels, but more often, it is slow and insidious owing to multiple blood samples and blood loss associated with catheter exchanges, exacerbated by systemic heparinization. Noteworthy blood loss is more likely to occur during device placement procedures because of the necessity of larger catheters and multiple catheter exchanges. Preoperative blood measurements of hematocrit and a current blood type and screen are advisable. For procedures with a greater risk of blood loss, a crossmatch should also be requested. Access to emergency blood and blood administration equipment should be readily available for unexpected bleeding.

DYSRHYTHMIAS AND THE CATHETERIZATION LABORATORY

Cardiac dysrhythmias are common during cardiac catheterization. Most are mechanically induced and repositioning the wire or catheter usually results in rapid resolution. Other causes of rhythm abnormality include coronary air embolism, electrolyte imbalance, and hypercarbia. Although most are minor and self-limiting, dysrhythmias can cause significant hemodynamic instability and are a common cause of major complications.[23,43] Young age and a prolonged duration of the procedure are both risk factors for developing dysrhythmias. Treatment may include defibrillation, pacing, or medical therapy and should be managed in collaboration with the cardiologist. The relevant equipment should always be available in the catheterization suite.

Types of Dysrhythmias

Dysrhythmias may originate from the atria, ventricle, or involve the conduction system with varying degrees of block. Atrial tachyarrhythmias are generally considered the most common but frequently resolve with adjustments to the catheterization technique or spontaneously. However, they may be poorly tolerated by children with single ventricle physiology, mitral stenosis, or poor myocardial function and these children may need intervention earlier than others. Catheter-induced complete heart block (CIHB) has been reported between 0.3% and 2.2% of cases; the latter study retrospectively searched specifically for CIHB from a database of more than 6000 pediatric catheter cases.[43,55] In this series, 96% of CIHB resolved spontaneously shortly after the procedure, but six children required pacemaker insertion. First- or second-degree atrioventricular block is well tolerated at all ages. Device closure for VSD may cause severe junctional bradycardia or complete heart block in up to 10% of cases, and almost half of these children require pacing or isoproterenol.[15]

The overall incidence of ventricular tachycardiac or fibrillation is around 0.3% but these are the most common rhythms causing major complications.[43] Children undergoing VSD device placement had ventricular arrhythmias that required lidocaine or cardioversion in 8.5% of cases.[15]

Children with obstructions to systemic flow (e.g., hypertrophic obstructive cardiomyopathy or aortic stenosis) are at a greater risk of developing ventricular fibrillation secondary to myocardial ischemia.

CARDIOVERSION

Histologic injury to the myocardium is rare when the starting power for cardioversion is set at 0.5 J/kg.[26] Systemic and pulmonary emboli are rare in children compared with adults, for whom the incidence is 1% to 2%. All forms of dysrhythmia may occur after cardioversion; factors that influence the incidence include the underlying pathology, electrolyte disturbance, residual drugs, and the strength of shock. Children with implantable pacemaker devices requiring cardioversion require special consideration. Electrode pads should be placed a distance from the generator and the pacemaker circuits, and pacemaker programming mode should be checked after the procedure.

DESATURATION

Arterial desaturation or cyanosis in the pediatric patient undergoing cardiac catheterization may be respiratory or circulatory in origin. A systematic approach is required to diagnose and treat the underlying cause. A transesophageal echocardiographic (TEE) probe can cause desaturation by compressing the bronchi or vessels, compressing on the trachea, or precipitating bronchospasm. These events are more common in children weighing less than 10 kg.[26] Pneumothorax is rare but possible during cardiac catheterization. Hypercarbia, acidosis, excessive positive-pressure ventilation, contrast media, and hypoxia can increase pulmonary vascular resistance, which may lead to increased shunting and cyanosis. Hypercyanotic episodes are frequently observed,[37] particularly in infants with uncorrected tetralogy of Fallot. In one study, 12% of children with tetralogy of Fallot exhibited a hypercyanotic episode within 12 hours of catheterization despite adequate hydration, sedation, and the use of nonionic contrast media.

EMBOLIZATION

Introduced devices, native tissues, and air can all result in embolization. Children with aberrant connections between the right and left circulations are at risk of embolization to the systemic circulation, with cerebral and coronary vessels at particular risk.

Device, Balloon, Thrombus, or Dislodged Material

Embolization of devices including coils, duct umbrellas, occlusion devices, and endovascular stents have all been reported, although improvements in device design (particularly in retrieval techniques) have reduced these risks.[4,37] Similarly, the incidence of balloon rupture has decreased with technical improvements in materials and design. Use of an inflation device with an attached manometer is recommended to ensure that the inflation pressure does not exceed the burst pressure of the balloon. Thrombus may be dislodged from devices or catheters, and balloon dilation may dislodge calcium, intimal lining from conduits, and thrombus from surgical systemic-pulmonary shunts.

Air Embolism

Gas emboli may originate from sheaths, catheters, burst balloons, or anesthetic infusion lines. The many wire and catheter exchanges required during interventional procedures make air embolism an ever-present risk.[26] Balloons are dilated with a weak contrast mixture and, in view of the occasional balloon rupture, it is important to ensure all gas bubbles are eliminated from the contrast mix syringe and catheter before dilation is undertaken. All intravenous (IV) lines, injections, and infusions should also be free of air bubbles. Balloons used for flotation tip catheters should ideally be filled with carbon dioxide rather than air to minimize the potential embolic effect if the balloon bursts. Nitrous oxide should be avoided because it may expand air bubbles.

CONTRAST TOXICITY

Adverse reactions to intravascular media are relatively uncommon, but accurate recognition and management by the anesthesiologist is critical. Idiosyncratic reactions may be acute or delayed, but the pathophysiologic mechanisms underlying these responses are complex, varied, and remain to be fully elucidated. Unless formal allergy testing has been undertaken, hypersensitivity is an appropriate term that does not misattribute a mechanism.[56] Both acute and delayed reactions can occur with first exposure to contrast media, and all grades of severity including anaphylaxis are possible.[57]

Acute Reactions

Acute reactions to contrast agents can range from mild to severe; symptoms include tachycardia, bronchospasm, flushing, urticaria, laryngeal edema, and cardiovascular collapse. Replacing high-osmolar (ionic) contrast solutions with isomolar or low-osmolar (nonionic) solutions has reduced the incidence substantively. In one series of more than 11,000 administrations of nonionic iodinated contrast media to children, acute reactions were noted in 20 (0.18%) cases; 16 were mild, 1 moderate, and 3 severe.[58] Reactions appear to be more common when contrast medium is given through an arterial access compared with venous access. Acute reactions should be managed in accordance with standard anaphylaxis protocols (i.e., oxygen, IV fluid, epinephrine, corticosteroids, and histamine 1- and histamine 2-antagonist therapy). If there is a history of an acute reaction to contrast agents, then prophylaxis with corticosteroids and antihistamines can be considered if further exposure is proposed. However, breakthrough reactions of all severity grades have been observed in up to 40% of all pretreated patients, so alternative agents or imaging modalities should be strongly considered.[56]

Delayed Reactions

Delayed reactions have a much broader spectrum of clinical symptoms including: headache, heat feeling, skin redness, fixed drug eruptions, drug reaction with eosinophilia and systemic symptoms (DRESS) and Stevens-Johnson syndrome. With the increasing trend to day-case treatment, many such reactions occur once the child has left hospital. It is therefore important that a specific history is taken from children presenting for catheterization of any previous exposure and reactions to contrast media.

Renal Adverse Reactions and Prevention

The term contrast media nephrotoxicity (CMN) refers to an increase in serum creatinine concentration by more than 25% or 0.5 mg/dL within 3 days of receiving IV contrast media in the absence of another cause.[59] The underlying mechanism of injury is unclear, although it is thought that contrast can reduce renal perfusion and is toxic to tubular cells. CMN occurs more frequently but not exclusively in children with preexisting renal damage; additional risk factors include dehydration, cardiac failure, and the subclinical renal insufficiency seen in cyanotic children. It has been suggested that infants and children who receive more than 5 mL/kg of nonionic contrast agent are at increased risk for CMN.[60] Contrast for angiography does not increase the risk of postbypass acute kidney injury[61] and most CMN appears to resolve without intervention. However, a recent study of 233 heterogeneous children receiving contrast for CT scanning found an association between CMN and unfavorable outcome, suggesting the process may not be as benign as previously hoped.[62] Many interventions have been given prophylactically to prevent CMN; preliminary studies with N-acetylcysteine (NAC) have been promising but no interventions have been more effective than normal saline hydration.[63] Currently, the only modifiable risk factors are hydration status and dose of contrast used. When possible, potentially nephrotoxic drugs should be stopped at least 24 hours before the procedure. Gadolinium-based contrast materials are considered nonnephrotoxic in the normal MRI dose of up to 0.3 mmol/kg. However, there is some evidence that the increased doses required for cardiac angiography may confer adverse renal effects.[64] Most radiologic contrast media have significant osmotic diuretic effects. During procedures requiring large volumes and/or repeated doses of contrast media, a significant diuresis may occur, causing concealed fluid losses and potential hypovolemia. Additional IV fluid may be required to avoid dehydration. Occasionally, bladder distention and retention can also occur, which should be considered in a child with unexplained postoperative distress.

NEUROLOGIC EVENTS

Central and peripheral neurologic damage can occur as a complication of the catheterization procedure. In one prospective study, 0.38% of children suffered a neurologic complication, and the incidence was significantly greater after interventional than diagnostic procedures.[65]

Central Nervous System

Ischemic cerebrovascular events may occur because of embolization, damage to the carotid artery, or acute low–cardiac output states causing hypoxic-ischemic encephalopathy. Thrombotic emboli may originate from any site in which there is endovascular or endocardial damage from the inner surface of the catheter or an implanted device. Factors that increase the risk during interventional procedures include large catheter size, more numerous vascular punctures, and procedures of increased duration. The most common complications after an embolic stroke are convulsions and hemiplegia, but children with this type of stroke often make a good recovery. The outcome is more guarded after hypoxic-ischemic

encephalopathy occurring after a period of reduced cardiac output.[65]

Peripheral Nervous System

During catheterization procedures, the arms are frequently extended above the head to improve the lateral radiologic views of the heart; in these circumstances the brachial plexus may be injured.[66] Reduced cardiac output states associated with cardiac catheterization can augment this risk. To reduce the risk of injury, the elbows should be flexed with the hands up and the elbows then adducted a minimum of 15 cm above the table (many adduct the elbows until they are positioned directly above the shoulders and taped in position), while maintaining the head/neck in a neutral position.[66] At-risk positions should be adopted only when necessary, for the briefest time possible, and all precautions documented.[67]

RADIATION

Cardiac catheterization procedures deliver some of the largest radiation doses owing to the requirement for rapid-sequence screening and/or prolonged screening.[68] Complex interventional procedures require long fluoroscopy times with multiple angiographic or fluoroscopic acquisitions. This poses a risk to both the patient and staff. Radiation overexposure can lead to scarring and skin injury, cellular injury, gene mutation, cell death, radiation-induced cancers, and birth defects. The acronym ALARA (or ALARP), which means "as low as reasonably achievable (or practical)," is a principle for radiation exposure that should be applied in the context of obtaining adequate diagnostic images.[69]

Radiation Exposure of Patients

Children are especially vulnerable to the oncogenic effects of radiation; their actively growing tissue and organs are more sensitive to radiation, a greater proportion of their bodies are irradiated during procedures, and procedures are often longer because of smaller vessel size and difficulty cannulating target vessels. Many children with CHD will require more than one catheterization procedure and, with improvements in long-term outcomes, a longer life span to develop radiation-related problems.[70]

Oncogenic effects of radiation require a long latent time, often decades. When estimating the lifetime risk of cancer from radiation exposure, the child's age and weight need to be considered along with the duration and effective dose of radiation exposure. The risk for adult coronary angiography is 6% per sievert (Sv), and the average dose is about 10 mSv, which gives an increased risk of 0.06%. In contrast, infants require smaller exposures because of their reduced body weights, but they have an increased sensitivity. An infant has a lifetime cancer risk of 11% to 15% per sievert. If an infant is exposed to approximately 20 mSv (e.g., 1 hour of fluoroscopy and 7 digital acquisition runs), the lifetime cancer risk is estimated as 0.03%.[71,72]

Radiation Exposure of Staff

Most radiation exposure to staff comes from scatter from the beam entry point on the patient. Lesser amounts come from the x-ray tube and intensifier. The need for staff protection is well established and is accomplished by wearing lead aprons, thyroid shields, goggles, and suspended mobile glass lead screens for the head and neck. In addition, staff should aim to keep a maximal possible distance from the radiation source and minimize exposure time. All personnel working regularly in the catheterization suites should wear dosimeters to monitor cumulative radiation exposure.

HYPOTHERMIA AND HYPERTHERMIA

Catheterization procedures are often prolonged, increasing the need for close temperature monitoring. Hypothermia can exacerbate blood loss or dysrhythmias and hyperthermia may exacerbate any neurologic injury. External body and fluid warming devices should be used for all but the briefest procedures and central temperature should be measured.

ENDOCARDITIS

Under current recommendations, routine endocarditis prophylaxis is not indicated for cardiac catheterization procedures; however, the CHD patient population undergoing the procedures may warrant prophylaxis because of their increased risk of endocarditis.[73] Children with acquired valvular disease, hypertrophic cardiomyopathy, and previous infective endocarditis are at increased risk. Clinical practice varies between centers. Prophylactic antibiotics should be administered before any devices are implanted, and some centers continue to recommend endocarditis prophylaxis for a minimum of 6 months after implantation. Diagnostic or routine angioplasty procedures do not usually warrant antibiotic prophylaxis, but there is usually a residual flow disturbance after angioplasty procedures that some consider warrants preventive therapy.

OVERCOMING LIMITATIONS

The main limitation in the use of catheterization techniques in younger or smaller children has been the delay in development of equipment of appropriate size. To overcome this difficulty, clinicians have developed hybrid procedures to permit current catheter-based techniques to be used in infants and small children. Examples of this collaborative approach between surgeon and interventional cardiologist include periventricular closure of muscular ventricular septal defects[74] and hybrid stage 1 palliation for hypoplastic left heart syndrome (i.e., off-pump placement of a PDA stent and creation of an unrestricted ASD).[75]

The next great challenge is to develop equipment and techniques that can be used in conjunction with MRI.[76] This would minimize radiation exposure to children and staff. However, there are significant technical obstacles that need to be overcome before this approach can fully replace catheterization laboratories using ionizing radiation.

Anesthesia

WHO AND HOW?

The aims of anesthesia care for pediatric interventional cardiology are to ensure the child is not distressed, to provide optimal conditions for accurate diagnostic measurements and successful interventions, and to manage any complications or alterations in the child's cardiovascular physiology during the procedure. These aims often require general anesthesia but occasionally may be met with deep sedation.

The choice of sedation or general anesthesia and the seniority of the anesthetic provider should match the complexity of the procedure and the child's cardiac pathology. Deep sedation can easily merge into general anesthesia; therefore children undergoing sedation should be cared for by someone skilled at providing both and who possesses the ability to manage and resuscitate children with CHD.[77] This person must not be the proceduralist. Full standard patient monitoring should be available for all cases, and there must be adequate facilities for postprocedural recovery and emergency resuscitation.

Increasingly, there are fewer diagnostic procedures and more interventional procedures. This change is reflected in a shift from sedation to general anesthesia and the expanding role of specialized pediatric cardiac anesthesiologists.[78] Anesthesia providers for these children must have a high level of experience in pediatric anesthesia and a thorough understanding of pediatric cardiology and CHD. They must understand the physiology, the procedure, and the potential complications and have the ability to anticipate, diagnose, and respond to any hemodynamic changes or deteriorations.

PREPROCEDURAL ASSESSMENT AND MANAGEMENT

Children scheduled for elective interventional cardiology are often admitted to the hospital on the day of the procedure. Ideally, all children should have an anesthesia assessment at the same time as their preprocedural cardiologic workup. An efficient and complete anesthesia assessment requires good coordination and communication between cardiology and anesthesia units. The anesthesia preoperative assessment should establish the cardiac anatomy and details of any previous surgery, interventions, and investigations. Current functional status should be elicited, as should any signs of worsening function, cyanosis, or heart failure. Baseline observations for heart rate, blood pressure, and oxygen saturation should be recorded.

Up to 25% of children with CHD have syndromes or other anomalies that may affect their anesthesia care. Children with CHD are likely to have undergone previous procedures and anesthetics, and the family may be well informed about the child's condition, hospital process, and anesthesia. It is important that discussions include sedative premedication, parental presence, and the mode of induction of anesthesia (see Chapters 1 and 4). Sedative premedication may be particularly beneficial in children where anxiety and associated sympathetic activation and tachycardia are best avoided, such as those with left ventricular outflow tract obstruction or with sympathetically induced arrhythmias.

Interventional cardiology procedures may involve considerable physiologic trespass, and some children may have limited cardiac reserve. They should be in optimal health whenever possible. Intercurrent illness or infection may bias cardiorespiratory diagnostic values, increase the risk of endocarditis, and increase the risk of anesthesia-related complications. Respiratory illness in particular may lead to detrimental increases in pulmonary vascular resistance. The urgency and extent of the procedure must be carefully balanced against the cardiovascular status of the child before proceeding in a child with intercurrent illness.

ANATOMY AND FUNCTION

When assessing the anatomy and function, answers to four primary questions may affect anesthesia management:

- Where does the blood go?
- What is the ventricular function?
- How reactive is the pulmonary circulation?
- Is there a fixed or dynamic stenosis?

Answers to these and other questions can help the anesthesiologist determine the optimal approach to management:

- How well will hyperoxia or hypoxia be tolerated?
- What is the likely effect of increased sympathetic stimulation, vasodilation, or a reduction in myocardial contractility?
- What are the likely causes of cardiovascular collapse, and how should they be managed?

Most primary questions can be answered from the record, details of previous surgery, and recent echocardiographic results. However, an index of suspicion is always required: while very poor function may be readily detected, moderate levels of dysfunction may not be acknowledged or as easily detected clinically.

Preoperative blood tests may include hematocrit and a type and hold or crossmatch. Sedative premedication may consist of oral midazolam (0.5 mg/kg) or ketamine (up to 5 mg/kg). Larger doses of sedative premedications may be used to provide more reliable or greater sedation if required, but they may cause delayed recovery or considerable sedation after the procedure. Topical anesthesia creams facilitate venous cannulation if IV induction is planned. Care should be taken that these children do not become excessively dehydrated. In selected children, preprocedure IV fluids should be considered (e.g., BT shunts).

THE ENVIRONMENT

The cardiac catheterization suite can be a challenging environment for the anesthesiologist. Ideally, catheterization suites should be located near cardiac operating rooms to facilitate rapid availability of ECMO support for high-risk cases. In practice, laboratories are often remotely located from the main operating room complex, limiting availability of immediate assistance and additional resources. Limited functional space may hinder access to the child during procedures and during emergency resuscitation. Blood gas analyzers should be readily available, and blood should be immediately accessible for urgent transfusion for interventional procedures such as balloon dilation and device insertion.

Lateral and anterior-posterior cameras used for imaging are in close proximity to the patient during procedures and, in combination with sterile drapes, limit access to the patient and his or her airway during procedures. Blind manipulation under the drapes can dislodge monitoring or the tracheal tube. X-ray cameras are liable to move during procedures to acquire different fields and magnifications, which risk dislodging airway devices, breathing circuits, and IV fluid lines. Meticulous care must be taken to ensure all monitoring, airway devices and IV lines are well secured prior to draping and positioning of cameras. IV line extensions are required to enable easy drug administration during the procedure. The catheterization laboratories are often cooled and temperature should be monitored in all patients. Small children will likely require active warming to maintain normothermia. Lighting is often subdued to enhance viewing of the radiographs (Fig. 22.5).

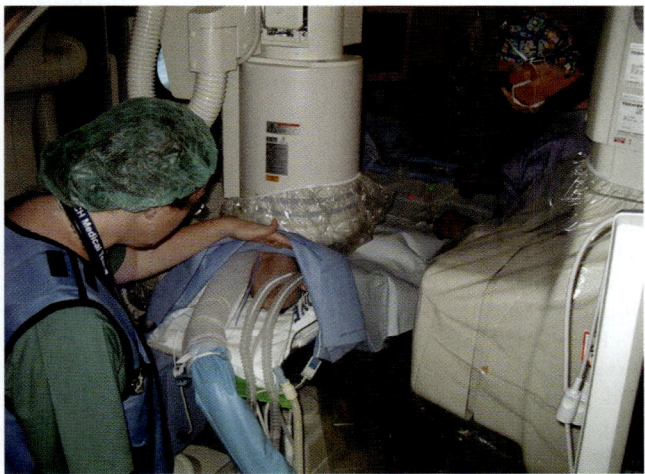

FIGURE 22.5 Typical setup of a catheterization laboratory showing limited access to a child.

THE CARDIAC PATIENT

The management of anesthesia for children with CHD is discussed further in Chapters 16 to 18. Important considerations include the potential for myocardial dysfunction and identifying limited functional reserve. This may be a particular problem in children with hypertrophied right ventricles operating at near-systemic pressures or with volume-loaded dilated ventricles. Another important consideration is the status and reactivity of the pulmonary vasculature. Difficulties may be anticipated in the following circumstances:

- Increased reactivity of the pulmonary vasculature, such as neonates, or children with primary pulmonary hypertension
- Established pulmonary hypertension with irreversible, chronically increased pulmonary artery pressures and consequent right heart dysfunction
- Circulations that require balancing (e.g., BT shunts or duct-dependent situations), in which increases or decreases in pulmonary vascular resistance may lead to spiraling hypoxia or systemic ischemia and acidosis
- Circulations that rely on low pulmonary vascular resistance to function correctly (e.g., cavopulmonary shunts or after Fontan surgery)

CHOICE OF ANESTHESIA

Many anesthetic agents and techniques have been used safely in pediatric interventional cardiology; thus the choice of technique should be guided by the patient's pathophysiology and procedural requirements. There is no specific anesthetic method that is appropriate for all children undergoing cardiac catheterization; what is important is that the operator understands the benefits and limitations of the choices he or she makes.[39]

Sedation

The difference between deep sedation and general anesthesia is imprecise and controversial, especially for small children in whom consciousness and memory are harder to measure (see Chapters 46 and 48). When considering the suitability of sedation or general anesthesia, several issues are important:

- Does immobility need to be guaranteed?
- What level of stimulation is expected?
- Do oxygen and carbon dioxide tensions need to be controlled?
- What are the cardiovascular effects of the anesthetic agents?
- How likely is significant physiologic trespass?
- What is the anticipated duration of the procedure?

Sedation is often advocated to avoid the potential effects of general anesthesia on diagnostic measurements; spontaneous ventilation may maintain a more natural intrathoracic physiology promoting the acquisition of more accurate hemodynamic data. However, sedation can be associated with substantial respiratory changes and hypoxia and can have as much effect on the circulation as general anesthesia, altering hemodynamics and intracardiac shunts and thus limiting the theoretical advantages.[79–81] Diagnostic studies require controllable, reproducible physiologic conditions, such as consistent arterial carbon dioxide tension with manipulation of inspired oxygen concentrations. Such conditions may be difficult to achieve and/or reproduce in the sedated child. Many modern diagnostic and interventional techniques require the patient to be absolutely still for prolonged periods of time and may require breath-holds. Sedation can be associated with a degree of patient movement that makes procedures such as device placement or balloon dilation potentially difficult or dangerous. However, despite these concerns, sedation remains the technique of choice in some institutions, with evidence of a comparable safety record compared to general anesthesia. Reports from the C3PO database including more than 13,000 pediatric catheterizations reported 31% were performed with a spontaneous ventilation technique with a safety profile comparable to those managed with an artificial airway. In this series, 2% required conversion to general anesthesia with younger age and higher-risk procedures and pressor/inotrope requirements predictive of sedation failure. The eight institutions participating in C3PO had clearly established practice preferences, with two centers undertaking most cases under sedation and the remaining six using general anesthesia as their primary strategy.[82] If sedation is used, full standard monitoring should be undertaken, including monitoring of their airway and end-tidal carbon dioxide (ETCO$_2$), and provisions must be in place for rapid and expert transition to general anesthesia.

Sedation techniques have evolved over the past few decades, resulting in much more effective and titratable strategies today. In the past, the classic lytic cocktail of intramuscular meperidine, promethazine, and chlorpromazine was the standard for sedation. Rectal formulations that included thiopentone or methohexitone were also popular. However, these cocktails had a high incidence of failure and oversedation, and intramuscular routes were associated with sterile abscess formation. Oral ketamine and midazolam provide more reliable sedation, but occasionally respiratory support is required.[79] In theory, IV ketamine is an excellent choice for sedation because it provides a stable or increased heart rate and blood pressure and has little or no effect on pulmonary vascular resistance. However, prolonged recovery, vomiting, and dysphoric reactions may be problematic. The performance of IV ketamine has been improved by combination with midazolam or propofol, allowing lower doses of each agent and mitigating some of the unwanted side effects.[83] Propofol is also widely used for sedation, but compared with ketamine, it causes a greater reduction in systemic blood pressure and systemic vascular resistance, with no effect on pulmonary vascular resistance. This may increase a right-to-left shunt, or in diagnostic procedures, it may attenuate the gradient across a stenosis, making the decision to dilate the stenosis more difficult.[84] Compared with propofol sedation, a combination of ketamine with propofol produces similar sedation with less cardiovascular depression.[85] Relative combinations can be tailored to the degree of stimulus anticipated.[86] Dexmedetomidine has been proffered for sedation of children undergoing cardiac catheterization, although it may not provide sufficient sedation by itself.[87] Dexmedetomidine combined with ketamine was inferior to propofol and ketamine.[88]

Local anesthetic infiltration at cannulation sites at the start of the procedure will help reduce painful stimulation for the sedated patient, such as during catheter insertions and exchanges. Spinal anesthesia has been described as an alternative to sedation or general anesthesia in high-risk infants younger than 6 months of age when the procedure is expected to take less than 90 minutes.[89]

General Anesthesia

In the pediatric population, more than 80% of catheterization procedures are performed with patients under general anesthesia.[4] General anesthesia with controlled ventilation has several advantages, including establishing a secure airway without the risk of obstruction and hypoventilation, the ability to control arterial carbon dioxide and inspired oxygen accurately, and ensuring immobility. In addition, many patients prefer general anesthesia for fear of being awake; as many children require repeat procedures, patient satisfaction with the whole process is important. However, there are also disadvantages. The increased intrathoracic pressure associated with positive-pressure ventilation may decrease preload to the pulmonary and systemic atria, increase afterload on the right ventricle, and decrease afterload on the left ventricle. These effects may be particularly pronounced in patients with right ventricular failure or those dependent on passive pulmonary blood flow (Fontan physiology). Spontaneous ventilation through a supraglottic airway device facilitates venous return and pulmonary blood flow, although the degree of hypoventilation often seen in this situation can result in respiratory acidosis and altered pulmonary vascular resistance. This may be particularly troublesome in patients with pulmonary hypertension. The choice of tracheal intubation or supraglottic airway depends on patient factors, the length of procedure, the requirement for TEE, and whether the neck vessels will need to be accessed by the cardiology team.

A variety of general anesthetic agents have been used successfully for interventional cardiology, with no ideal agent identified. There are arguments for and against inhalational and IV anesthesia, but no outcome studies have provided strong evidence to recommend one technique over another. Great care should be taken to avoid myocardial depression or systemic vasodilation associated with excessive doses of either inhalational or IV anesthetic agents. Due to the low patient stimulation during most catheterization procedures, sufficient depth of anesthesia can often be maintained at low minimum alveolar concentration (MAC) values or plasma concentrations, particularly when supplemented with opioids and paralyzing agents, thereby mitigating some of the negative depressant effects of general anesthesia.

Inhalational agents can be used safely for both induction and maintenance of anesthesia for cardiac catheterization. Sevoflurane has a safe hemodynamic profile and isoflurane maintains cardiac output; both reduce hypoxic pulmonary vasoconstriction and increase ventilation-perfusion ($\dot{V}/\dot{Q}$) mismatch.[90] These changes may affect cardiac output calculations using the Fick principle (equations shown in Table 22.2).

While nitrous oxide does not appear to affect the pulmonary vasculature in children (in contrast to its effects in adults), it can cause expansion of gas bubbles, which is an important consideration in children at risk of paradoxical air embolus. Its use is therefore usually limited to facilitation of inhalation induction rather than routine use in the maintenance of anesthesia.[91]

Propofol has been safely and extensively used for maintenance of anesthesia in pediatric cardiac catheterization procedures. It has no effect on pulmonary vascular resistance, but dose-dependent reductions in cardiac contractility and systemic vascular resistance are well recognized. Care must be taken in patients with limited myocardial reserve, aortic stenosis, systemic-to-pulmonary shunts or pulmonary hypertension. However, there was no change in shunt fraction or pulmonary-systemic flow (Qp/Qs) ratio with doses of 100 μg/kg per minute.[92] Propofol causes loss of airway reflexes and causes respiratory depression but has the advantage of reduced postoperative delirium and postoperative nausea and vomiting compared with volatile agents.

Ketamine produces dissociative anesthesia while preserving airway reflexes and ventilation. It produces stable hemodynamics and, provided carbon dioxide is controlled, has no significant effect on pulmonary vascular resistance or pulmonary artery pressure in patients with pulmonary hypertension.[93] Disadvantages include dysphoria, nausea, prolonged recovery, and salivation. Furthermore, ketamine maintains cardiac output through stimulation of the sympathetic nervous system. A direct myocardial depressant

TABLE 22.2	Hemodynamic Calculations Using Cardiac Catheterization Data	
Hemodynamic Variable	**Equation**	**Normal Values**
Oxygen consumption	$\dot{V}O_2 = (CO \times CaO_2) - (CO \times CvO_2)$	Age-, heart rate-, gender-dependent[a]
Flow		
Pulmonary	$Q_P = \dfrac{\dot{V}O_2}{(S_{PV}O_2 - S_{PA}O_2) \times Hgb \times 1.36 \times 10}$	L/minute per m²: 3.5–5
Systemic	$Q_S = \dfrac{\dot{V}O_2}{(S_{AO}O_2 - S_{MV}O_2) \times Hgb \times 1.36 \times 10}$	3.5–5
Shunt flow ratio	$\dfrac{Q_P}{Q_S} = \dfrac{S_{AO}O_2 - S_{MV}O_2}{S_{PV}O_2 - S_{PA}O_2}$	1:1
Resistance		Wood units:
Pulmonary	$PVR = \dfrac{PAP - LAP}{Q_P}$	Newborns: 8–10 Older children: 1–3
Systemic	$SVR = \dfrac{AoP - RAP}{Q_S}$	Newborns: 10–15 Older children: 15–30

[a]LaFarge equation for $\dot{V}O_2$:
Boys $\dot{V}O_2 = 138.1 - [11.49 \times \log_e (\text{age in years})] + 0.378$ (heart rate)
Girls $\dot{V}O_2 = 138.1 - [17.04 \times \log_e (\text{age in years})] + 0.378$ (heart rate)

AO, aorta; *AoP*, aortic pressure; *CaO₂*, arterial oxygen content; *CO*, cardiac output; *CvO₂*, venous oxygen content; *Hgb,* hemoglobin; *LAP,* left atrial pressure; *MV*, mixed venous; *Oᵥ,* pulmonary flow; *Qₛ,* systemic flow; *PA,* pulmonary artery; *PAP,* pulmonary artery pressure; *PV,* pulmonary vein; *PVR,* pulmonary vascular resistance; *QP,* pulmonary blood flow; *Qs,* systemic blood flow; *RAP,* right atrial pressure; *SₐₒO₂,* aortic oxygen saturation; *SₘᵥO₂,* mixed venous oxygen saturation; *SO₂,* oxygen saturation; *SᵥₒO₂,* pulmonary venous saturation; *SVR,* systemic vascular resistance; *V̇O₂,* oxygen consumption.
Modified from Lam JE, Lin EP, Alexy R, Aronson LA. Anesthesia and the pediatric catheterization suite: a review. *Paediatr Anaesth.* 2015;25(2):127–134.

effect may be seen when it is administered to children whose sympathomimetic responses are already maximally stimulated.[94]

Opioids are a useful anesthetic adjunct that reduces both the required dose of other anesthetic agents and the pulmonary vascular response to noxious stimuli. Appropriate dosing should avoid the side effects of respiratory depression and hypercarbia. In general, these are not painful procedures; longer-acting opioids, however, may confer postprocedure sedation in addition to analgesia, as the children must remain recumbent for several hours to preclude bleeding from the femoral access sites. Remifentanil may offer an advantage in long catheterization procedures compared with other opioids as the short, context-sensitive half-time allows for rapid clearance and awakening. Bradycardia may be prevented by prophylactic administration of glycopyrrolate.[95] Local anesthetic infiltration around vessel cannulation sites can significantly limit the degree of procedural stimulus and further reduce anesthetic requirements. Maximum safe doses should be calculated according to the child's weight and communicated to the interventionalist to reduce the risk of local anesthetic toxicity (see Table 22.2).

Radiofrequency ablation procedures may be protracted, require immobility, and precipitate arrhythmias requiring defibrillation. For these reasons, general anesthesia is usually preferred, but many anesthetic agents affect cardiac conduction and may prevent the generation of preexcitation and automatic tachycardia. Dexmedetomidine has useful sedative, anxiolytic, and analgesic properties without effects on respiratory drive. It depresses sinus and atrioventricular nodal function, and avoiding its use in electrophysiology settings has been recommended.[96] However, a study using the different techniques of anesthetists at one institution has recently challenged this. Induction and ablation of arrhythmias was not inhibited using dexmedetomidine, although slightly higher doses of isoproterenol were required in the higher-dose group.[97] Controversy has surrounded the use of inhalational agents for the maintenance of anesthesia during ablation procedures but sound clinical data are scant. It appears that for preexcitation,

isoflurane and sevoflurane have little effect at less than 1 MAC, whereas propofol and opioids have no demonstrable effects at any dose. In contrast, automatic tachycardia may be suppressed by large doses of propofol and opioids. In a prospective, randomized trial, isoflurane- and propofol-based anesthesia resulted in a similar duration of anesthesia and effectiveness of ablation.[98] Reducing the dose of anesthesia may limit some of the unwanted effects on conduction.

Principles of Technique

The most important principle of anesthesia in this setting is that the anesthetic practitioner has a sound knowledge and experience of CHD physiology and procedures and that the techniques used are reliable and are ones with which he or she is familiar. Attention to detail is critical for the provision of safe anesthesia. Consideration of preprocedural anxiolysis, fluid management, full monitoring, expert assistance, and choice of anesthetic technique is critical, in addition to generating a functional interaction with the rest of the catheterization team.

Careful attention to volume status is very important. Prolonged preoperative fasting can cause significant dehydration, particularly in small infants, and should be actively avoided. Hypovolemia is poorly tolerated in most children with CHD, particularly those with shunt-dependent circulations and those who are preload dependent such as children with single ventricle physiology. Prolonged procedures can be associated with gradual hypovolemia secondary to blood sampling, bleeding, and diuretic effects of contrast media. Volume overload is also a risk with liberal fluids and high-dose contrast, which may be poorly tolerated in children with congestive heart failure. Cyanotic patients or those with single ventricles are usually accustomed or benefit from a higher hematocrit, which needs to be taken into consideration when replacing fluid losses. Significant fluid replacement during diagnostic catheterization may affect filling pressures, gradient, and flow and should be communicated to the cardiologist.

Difficult IV access is prevalent in this patient population but reliable IV access is essential in case rapid resuscitation is required. Availability of ultrasound may facilitate access and intraosseous access should be available for emergency access (see Chapter 49). IV lines should ideally be placed in the upper extremities, as the femoral vessels are most commonly accessed for procedures in young children, and the presence of catheters may prevent reliable IV drug and fluid administration. Similarly, pulse oximetry and noninvasive blood pressure cuffs may be less reliable if placed on a limb used for cardiology access. Invasive central or arterial monitoring may be indicated for high-risk cases to monitor and treat any perioperative instability. During procedures to dilate the aortic arch or aortic valve, it may be prudent to have an arterial line (preferably a right radial line) to allow continuous blood pressure monitoring during the dilatation. If continuous arterial monitoring is not required from induction, arterial access obtained by the cardiologist for the procedure can sometimes be transduced for anesthetic monitoring using either a second stopcock or a slave monitor.

Problems associated with anesthesia-induced myocardial depression and hypotension are well recognized but inadequate anesthesia can create its own problems. Hemodynamic consequences of light anesthesia, such as hypoxia owing to laryngospasm, are poorly tolerated in children with pulmonary hypertension. Hypoxia or hypercapnia may lead to increasing pulmonary vascular resistance, which may increase cardiac shunts and further worsening hypoxia. Increased pulmonary hypertension may also lead to significant decreases in pulmonary compliance, further increasing hypoxia and precipitating a downward spiral.

Catheterization procedures often involve long periods of very little painful stimulation with discrete periods of increased painful stimuli, such as during dilation of arterial and venous vessels, sheath changes, or balloon dilation. By maintaining good communication between the cardiologist and anesthesiologist, these periods can be anticipated and the depth of anesthesia or sedation analgesia adjusted accordingly.

TEE is increasingly being used during diagnostic procedures and to guide intracardiac catheter placement. TEE insertion can be very stimulating and often requires a deeper plane of anesthesia with the addition of opioids, neuromuscular blockade, or both. A tracheal tube is required to ensure a patent airway during TEE, and care must be taken to avoid dislodging the tracheal tube during manipulations of the TEE probe.

Procedures in the catheterization laboratory can often be lengthy with limited access to the patient. Extra care should be taken to ensure careful positioning of the patient to avoid pressure areas and potential nerve injury. Patients' arms are frequently placed above the head to reduce image interference, and care must be taken to avoid excessive stretching, which can lead to brachial plexus injury.

Coughing and straining on extubation may increase the risk of hematoma formation. For this reason, deep extubation may be preferred. The advantages of deep extubation must be balanced against the risks of hypoxia, hypercapnia, and loss of airway control or laryngospasm that may ensue if the tracheal tube is removed before the child is fully awake.

Catheterization procedures are usually minimally invasive and are not associated with high levels of postprocedural pain. Simple analgesics, such as paracetamol, combined with local anesthetic infiltration are usually adequate. Opioids are rarely required for postoperative analgesia and may contribute to postoperative nausea and vomiting. Emergence delirium and postoperative restlessness may increase the risk of bleeding at catheter puncture sites. Additional analgesia or sedatives may occasionally need to be administered by the anesthesiologist in recovery to gain control of an agitated patient and prevent such complications.

Effective teamwork is critical to the safe and effective pediatric cardiac catheterization procedure. This is particularly important for high-risk children and complex procedures that may involve many multidisciplinary professionals. Good communication between the interventional cardiologist (and surgeon in hybrid procedures) and anesthesiologist should be maintained before and throughout the procedure to (1) plan and modify anesthesia and (2) anticipate any hemodynamic changes or adverse events. Often treatment of complications, such as bleeding or dysrhythmias, involves interventions using both cardiology and anesthesiology techniques. A good team approach is key to achieving the best possible patient outcomes.

FUTURE OF ANESTHESIA IN INTERVENTIONAL CARDIOLOGY

Anesthesia for interventional cardiac catheterizations will become more challenging as new interventions are developed for sicker children and more procedures are performed in combination with open surgery or MRI. As is often the case in pediatric practice, technologic advancements in cardiac catheterization have lagged behind those for the adult population. Focused development of smaller pediatric-appropriate devices will continue to expand the scope of pediatric interventional cardiology; promising potential for wider applications of transcatheter valve replacements is already on the horizon. More children are likely to require general anesthesia, and specialist pediatric cardiac anesthesiologists will be spending an increasing proportion of their time in interventional cardiology suites.

The ability to risk stratify children and procedures prospectively to accurately predict and potentially prevent adverse events is key to improving patient safety in the catheterization laboratory.[39] Significant progress has been made in this area with the development of the **C**atheterization **RIS**k **S**core for **P**ediatrics (CRISP) score (available online at http://www.pmidcalc.org/?sid=26527119&newtest=Y), which uses patient demographics, current physiologic status and procedural risk to predict the risk of adverse events for an individual child.[99] This ability is potentially invaluable both for assessing the level of resources and expertise required and informing anesthetic strategies to minimize risk of harm to the children we seek to care for.

ACKNOWLEDGMENT

We thank Drs. Geoffrey K. Lane and Adam Skinner for their previous contributions to this chapter.

ANNOTATED REFERENCES

Feltes TF, Bacha E, Beekman RH III, et al. Indications for cardiac catheterization and intervention in pediatric cardiac disease: a scientific statement from the American Heart Association. *Circulation.* 2011;123(22):2607-2652.
The American Heart Association has provided a comprehensive overview of the subject.
Lam JE, Lin EP, Alexy R, Aronson LA. Anesthesia and the pediatric catheterization suite: a review. *Paediatr Anaesth.* 2015;25(2):127-134.
This is a good review of anesthesia for pediatric cardiac catheterization.
Odegard KC, Vincent R, Baijal RG, et al. SCAI/CCAS/SPA expert consensus statement for anesthesia and sedation practice: recommendations

for patients undergoing diagnostic and therapeutic procedures in the pediatric and congenital cardiac catheterization laboratory. *Anesth Analg.* 2016;123(5):1201-1209.

A comprehensive review of anesthetic concerns in the pediatric catheterization laboratory.

Taylor CJ, Derrick G, McEwan A, et al. Risk of cardiac catheterization under anaesthesia in children with pulmonary hypertension. *Br J Anaesth.* 2007;98(5):657-661.

This investigation examined the important high-risk subgroup of patients with pulmonary hypertension.

Vincent RN, Moore J, Beekman RH, et al. Procedural characteristics and adverse events in diagnostic and interventional catheterisations in pediatric and adult CHD: initial report from the IMPACT Registry. *Cardiol Young.* 2016;26(1):70-78.

This paper describes complications in pediatric cardiac catheterization from the currently largest dataset.

A complete reference list can be found online at ExpertConsult.com.

22

23

Anesthesia for Noncardiac Surgery in Children With Congenital Heart Disease

WANDA C. MILLER-HANCE

THE NATURAL HISTORY OF CONGENITAL HEART DISEASE (CHD) has been favorably altered over the past several decades by remarkable advances in medical and surgical care. These refinements have resulted in decreased morbidity and improvement in long-term outcomes in affected children. As survival rates further improve and life expectancy continues to increase, an escalating number of children with CHD will present for noncardiac surgery or other procedures unrelated to their heart disease. The care of these children is becoming more common in all diagnostic and surgical settings.[1] As the trend for earlier palliation and corrective surgery for congenital cardiovascular malformations continues, children who have undergone these interventions represent the main patient group that an anesthesiologist is likely to encounter during elective, urgent, and emergent noncardiac surgery. In some cases, children may require noncardiac surgery before undergoing procedures to address their cardiovascular disease. In others, the cardiac condition may not require or be amenable to surgical intervention.

A variety of extracardiac anomalies have been described in children with CHD[2-6] and the reported prevalence of associated malformations ranges between 10% and 33%.[7-9] The organ systems most often affected include musculoskeletal, central nervous, renal-urinary, gastrointestinal, and respiratory. Although many extracardiac malformations are relatively minor and have limited or no clinical implications, a considerable number of children with CHD have significant noncardiac comorbidities.[10] These pathologic and disease processes may necessitate surgical intervention. Other routine ailments may affect these children, requiring diagnostic procedures and/or surgical care. In addition, chromosomal syndromes and genetic disorders, well known to be associated with CHD, may lead to conditions that necessitate anesthesia care.

The challenges of caring for children with CHD for noncardiac surgery are magnified by the wide range of structural malformations, each with specific physiologic perturbations, hemodynamic consequences, and severity. This is further complicated by the variety of medical and surgical strategies available for management of these conditions. Many children, but particularly those with more than mild disease, require an individualized approach to anesthesia care.[11,12]

Clinical outcomes for CHD depend on the nature of the structural abnormalities and the possibility of successful palliation or correction.[13] The primary goal of palliative surgery is to favorably influence the natural history of the defect and decrease the likelihood of the severe consequences of the disease. However, these children continue to have abnormal cardiovascular anatomy and physiology, and their abnormal circulation is associated with an increased risk of perioperative adverse events.[14–17] Reparative, corrective, or definitive procedures are expected to improve hemodynamics and cardiac function while minimizing long-term ill effects of an abnormal circulation, improving the overall clinical outcome. Although the pathology might have been surgically treated, the cardiovascular system should not be considered normal. Therefore, repair of a congenital cardiac lesion should not be equated with a cure for many children.

Despite these considerations, for children with good hemodynamic results, the risks associated with noncardiac surgery may not be significantly different from those of others without CHD. These children are considered to be doing well clinically, have a good functional status, require few or no medications, have no exercise restrictions, and undergo routine surveillance. They require minimal or no adjustment in perioperative care compared with that provided to children without CHD. In others, however, residual abnormalities exist. In some who are less fortunate, a pathologic process may remain or develop after cardiac surgery that is related to the primary disease or therapy. This may lead to severe cardiovascular or pulmonary impairment. These residua and sequelae may necessitate further medical or surgical interventions and can increase perioperative morbidity during noncardiac surgery.[18] Management of these children is guided by several factors but to a significant extent by the residual problems of the disease and treatment and associated hemodynamic perturbations.[19]

Many publications have examined the implications of anesthesia for patients with CHD undergoing noncardiac surgery[11,19–37]; however, only a limited number provide data on perioperative outcomes.[38–45] In contrast to the extensive literature regarding perioperative cardiac assessment and risk stratification during noncardiac surgery in adults with heart disease, the availability of guidelines aimed at improving clinical outcomes, and the data regarding cardiac complications and cardiac risks of noncardiac surgery,[46–48] the lack of rigorous scientific data on this subject for the pediatric age group or the patient with CHD has made an equivalent effort challenging.[49]

Optimal anesthesia care for children with CHD requires a thorough understanding of the underlying cardiovascular anatomic abnormalities, pathophysiologic consequences of the defect, functional status, residua, sequelae, and expected long-term outcome, in addition to the planned procedure and potential complications. In this chapter, general principles of anesthesia practice are reviewed as they pertain to the care of children with CHD during noncardiac surgery. Unique perioperative considerations and issues applicable to high-risk patient groups are also addressed.

Preoperative Assessment

A detailed preoperative evaluation is indispensable for identifying and anticipating factors that may place a child with CHD at

TABLE 23.1	Factors That Place Children With Congenital Heart Disease at Increased Risk During Anesthesia for Noncardiac Surgery
Anticoagulation therapy	
Arrhythmias	
Congestive heart failure	
Emergent surgery	
History of implanted device (pacemaker or defibrillator)	
Hypoxemia	
Long-standing cyanosis	
Major noncardiac surgery	
Older age at the time of cardiac intervention	
Older type of cardiac surgical procedure	
Pulmonary hypertension/pulmonary vascular disease	
Significant outflow tract obstruction	
Significant sequelae or residua	
Single-ventricle physiology or complex defects	
Syncope	
Unrepaired pathology	
Ventricular dysfunction	
Young age (infancy)	

increased risk during anesthesia care (Table 23.1).[50,51] An important goal of this assessment is to gather information regarding the specifics of the cardiovascular disease and prior therapeutic interventions. A determination of functional status is based primarily on clinical data. The history and physical examination, in addition to the laboratory data and ancillary tests, provide complementary information about the structural cardiovascular malformations and hemodynamic status, enabling an overall risk assessment. Based on this clinical evaluation and consideration of the major pathophysiologic consequences of a particular condition, a systematic, detailed, organized plan is formulated for anesthesia and perioperative management. In some cases, the preoperative evaluation may establish the need to delay or defer elective noncardiac surgery, other interventions, or diagnostic procedures.

An additional important aspect of the preoperative visit is that it provides an opportunity to initiate psychological preparation of parents and children before the planned intervention. Issues regarding expectations on the day of surgery in terms of premedication, the potential need for intravenous access, plans for induction of anesthesia, the estimated duration of the procedure, and postoperative recovery can be addressed at that time. In addition to the surgeon and anesthesia providers, other teams that may be part of this preoperative assessment may include the child's cardiologist, nursing, social work, child-life specialists, and other support services.

HISTORY AND PHYSICAL EXAMINATION

As for all children undergoing anesthesia, the history and physical examination are essential components of a thorough preoperative evaluation. In addition to the details regarding the present illness and planned procedure, the history should focus on the status of the cardiovascular system. Relevant information includes the type of cardiovascular disease and comorbid conditions, medications, allergies, prior hospitalizations, surgical procedures or other interventions, anesthesia experiences, and complications. Symptoms, including tachypnea, dyspnea, tachycardia, fatigue, and those related to rhythm problems, should be sought. Feeding difficulties and diaphoresis can represent significant symptoms in infants, whereas decreased activity level or exercise intolerance may be a concern for older children. Palpitations, chest pain, and syncope should be characterized. The history should include an assessment of growth and development because these may be affected in children with CHD. Failure to thrive suggests ongoing cardiorespiratory compromise. Those with decompensated disease, complex pathologies, associated genetic defects, or other syndromes may be particularly vulnerable. Recent illnesses such as intercurrent respiratory infections or pulmonary disease may increase the potential for perioperative complications and require careful appraisal of the risk/benefit ratio in elective cases.[52,53]

The physical examination should include the child's weight and height. Vital signs, including heart rate, respiratory rate, and blood pressure, should be documented. If the child is known or suspected to have or has been treated for any form of aortic arch obstruction or has had any systemic-to-pulmonary artery shunt, upper and lower extremity and the right and left upper extremity blood pressure recordings and palpation of the quality of pulses should be documented. This assessment provides information about the patency of arterial beds and helps in the selection of blood pressure monitoring sites. The examination should explore suitable sites for vascular access (venous and arterial) and identify potential difficulties. Emphasis should be given to the airway and cardiovascular system, with particular attention to any changes from previous examination findings.

General assessment includes the child's level of activity, breathing pattern, level of distress (if any), and presence/degree of cyanosis. Respiratory evaluation focuses on the quality of the breath sounds and should indicate the presence or absence of labored breathing, intercostal retractions, wheezing, rales, or rhonchi. Abnormalities may suggest congestive symptoms or a pneumonic process. Cardiac auscultation should include assessment of heart sounds, pathologic murmurs, and gallop rhythms. The presence of a thrill, representing a palpable murmur, should be documented. The abdomen should be examined for the presence of hepatosplenomegaly. Assessment of the extremities should include examination of pulses, overall perfusion, capillary refill, cyanosis, clubbing, and edema. Noncardiac anomalies or pathology that may affect anesthesia care (e.g., specific syndrome complex, potentially difficult airway, gastroesophageal reflux) should be recorded.

An important objective of the preoperative evaluation is to identify children with functional cardiopulmonary limitations imposed by their cardiovascular disease. Symptoms and signs consistent with congestive heart failure, cyanosis, hypercyanotic episodes, and compromised functional status (i.e., significant exercise intolerance or syncopal episodes) should raise concerns about potential perioperative problems. The pediatric cardiologist should facilitate information about the nature and severity of the cardiovascular pathology, describe the child's overall clinical status, and assess prior complications. The cardiologist should identify those children who may be at increased risk and optimize their preoperative clinical condition. The perioperative care teams should be alerted to any concern that may affect the care of the child. The anesthesiologist should have a detailed understanding of the child's cardiac defect, pathophysiologic consequences, nature of the medical and surgical therapies applied, functional status, and implications for perioperative management. In patients at increased risk, pediatric anesthesia consultation is recommended before the procedure. In some cases, based on this assessment, an inpatient

setting may be favored over an outpatient surgical facility. Although the surgical team may not have an in-depth understanding of the child's cardiovascular disease, by discussing the details of the surgical plan and potential issues with the perioperative care providers, problems can be anticipated and proactively addressed.

ANCILLARY STUDIES AND LABORATORY DATA

The baseline systemic arterial saturation value should be determined by pulse oximetry (SpO_2) when the child is calm and, in most cases, while breathing room air. Acceptable values depend on many factors, including the specific cardiovascular defect(s), whether the child has a two- or a one-ventricle circulation, the preoperative versus postoperative status with respect to the cardiac pathology, and the stage in the palliative pathway for those undergoing such a strategy. Children who have undergone definitive (corrective) procedures should be expected to have normal to a near-normal SpO_2 value (at least 95%). After palliative interventions, SpO_2 values typically range between 75% and 85%.

The extent of preoperative laboratory testing largely depends on the status of the patient and the type, anticipated duration, and complexity of surgery. Studies most commonly obtained include hematocrit, hemoglobin, electrolytes, and coagulation tests. In cyanotic children, a complete blood cell count allows determination of polycythemia, anemia, and thrombocytopenia. Prothrombin time, partial thromboplastin times, and international normalized ratio (INR) provide an indication of clotting ability. Cyanotic children usually have increased red blood cell mass and relatively small plasma volumes. The collection of specimens for coagulation tests requires sampling tubes that adjust the amount or concentration of citrate to prevent artifactually prolonged values. For those receiving diuretic therapy, digoxin, or angiotensin-converting enzyme inhibitors (ACEIs), the determination of a basic metabolic panel can be useful. A comprehensive metabolic panel that assesses electrolyte and acid-base balance, the health of the kidneys and liver, as well as concentrations of blood glucose and blood proteins may be more appropriate in some cases. Blood typing and cross-matching should be performed depending on the anticipated need for blood administration.

A recent electrocardiogram (ECG) should be reviewed for any changes from prior studies (particularly regarding criteria consistent with chamber dilation or ventricular hypertrophy), the presence of rhythm abnormalities, and findings suggesting myocardial ischemia. If an arrhythmia is identified on the preoperative assessment, further evaluation is warranted because it may reflect an underlying hemodynamic abnormality that may affect the perioperative course. A continuous ECG recording (i.e., Holter monitor) and further evaluation may be indicated in the child with a history of rhythm disturbance, palpitations, or syncope or with an ECG suggesting significant ectopy or arrhythmia. An exercise tolerance test or treadmill study is warranted if there is concern about myocardial ischemia, as may be the case for the child with aortic stenosis, coronary artery anomalies, or exercise-induced arrhythmias.

Review of a recent chest radiograph, including a lateral view, provides information regarding cardiac size, chamber enlargement, and pulmonary vascularity. Prior studies such as echocardiograms, cardiac catheterizations, electrophysiologic procedures, magnetic resonance imaging, and computed tomography should be reviewed. In some cases, it may be necessary to obtain further diagnostic information before proceeding with the planned procedure if there are symptoms that merit additional investigations or issues of concern. These evaluations should be coordinated with the child's cardiologist. It is also important to consider whether the child would benefit from cardiac catheterization to undertake interventions addressing significant structural, functional, or hemodynamic abnormalities before the anticipated noncardiac procedure. In addition to providing potentially helpful information, the clinical status of the child can be substantially improved in many cases by catheter-based interventions. This may be of significant benefit when the planned procedure is of an elective nature and considered to be major.

One of the goals of the preoperative evaluation is to obtain the most diagnostic information with the fewest tests and the least risk, discomfort for the child, and expense. The anesthesiologist is particularly suited to determine which tests are appropriate for optimal perioperative planning and whether additional data are needed.

INFORMED CONSENT

The physicians involved in the care of the child should meet with the patient and family to discuss the anesthetic plan and answer any questions. The preoperative consultation provides the opportunity to alleviate patient and parental anxiety. At the same time, the possible benefits and risks involved should be discussed. Although anesthesia and surgery in children with CHD, particularly in those with uncorrected defects, may carry an increased risk, it may not be possible to define the specific contribution of each factor to the overall risk.

FASTING GUIDELINES

The optimal period of fasting for children before surgery has been the subject of debate.[54–59] However, most centers follow guidelines established by their national societies to reduce the risk of aspiration. The same principles are applicable to children with CHD with a few additional considerations. Intake of clear fluids or the intravenous (IV) administration of maintenance fluids should be considered in some children to ensure adequate hydration if the fasting period is anticipated to be prolonged. This is particularly important in small infants and in children with obstructive pathology, cyanotic disease, or single-ventricle physiology. Maintenance of adequate hydration and ventricular preload may minimize potential detrimental hemodynamic changes associated with anesthesia and surgery.

MEDICATIONS

Children with CHD may be taking medications on a regular basis. Although there may be an occasional exception, such as diuretic, vasodilator (e.g., ACEI), or anticoagulation therapy, there is usually no need to discontinue long-term medications before surgery. It is often important to continue these drugs until the time of surgery, and in most centers, children are allowed to take scheduled oral medications with small sips of water preoperatively.

Intraoperative Management

Anesthesia and surgery impose additional stresses on the cardiovascular system and provoke compensatory mechanisms to maintain homeostasis. It is important to assess the child's physiology and cardiovascular reserve to anticipate his or her ability to increase cardiac output to meet metabolic demands and procure optimal oxygen delivery. This information, along with the nature and complexity of the surgery, affects the extent of monitoring required and the selection of anesthetic agents and techniques. Prompt intervention is imperative if decompensation

occurs. Good communication among the surgeon, cardiologist/intensivist, anesthesiologist, and nursing teams during the entire perioperative period is essential in treating children with complex disease.

GENERAL CONSIDERATIONS

Anesthesia Care Provider and Health Care Facility

Anesthesia care should be provided by individuals who are familiar with children with CHD, the planned operative procedure, and the surgeon's usual approach. Although many specialized centers that care for children have dedicated pediatric cardiac anesthesiologists, they may not be available at all facilities. Even if these providers are available, the number might be limited and they may not be able to support all noncardiac cases; in some instances, this type of advanced expertise may not be required. The most important factor that an anesthesiologist can offer a child with CHD is a comprehensive understanding of the anatomic abnormalities, pathophysiology of the cardiac malformation, and how this may be affected by the anesthetic and surgical procedure. Familiarity with the most likely residua and sequelae is essential.[18] Adequate communication among all physicians involved enhances the likelihood of the best possible outcome.

Recent publications have addressed one of the ongoing controversies in CHD—namely, which medical facility should provide care for these patients during noncardiac surgery.[36,60,61] Data regarding this specific issue and support for a strong recommendation are otherwise extremely limited. It has been suggested that high-risk children should be cared for at specialized centers.[36,60] A recent outcome review concluded that procedures requiring general anesthesia could be performed safely in children from any of the three risk groups in a noncardiac center with the caveat that this requires close communication and careful planning among the various specialties.[61] Further data in this regard are necessary.

Premedication

The use of premedication provides sedation and anxiolysis before most surgical procedures because some degree of fear or anxiety is expected. This facilitates parental separation, entry into the operating room, placement of monitors, and induction of anesthesia.

Commonly used premedications include oral or IV benzodiazepines, opioids, and small amounts of hypnotic agents. Drugs such as barbiturates and ketamine are occasionally used. Alternative routes for premedication include intramuscular, intranasal, and rectal. The cardiorespiratory effects of premedication in children can be influenced by the underlying systemic disease.[62–66] Children with marginal clinical status or hemodynamic decompensation may require little or no premedication. Caution should also be exercised in children with a history of cardiovascular pathology associated with pulmonary hypertension because hypoventilation and hypoxemia can be detrimental. Conversely, children susceptible to hypercyanotic episodes or those with catecholamine-induced arrhythmias can benefit from heavy premedication. In selected children, for example those affected by cyanotic heart disease, oxygen saturation monitoring after premedication should be considered with the administration of supplemental oxygen as needed.[63]

Intravenous Access

Secure IV access is mandatory for administration of fluids and medications during anesthesia care in children with CHD. In most, IV access is established after an inhalational induction. In those considered at great risk, such as children with severe ventricular outflow tract obstruction, moderate to severe cardiac dysfunction, pulmonary hypertension, or potential for hemodynamic compromise, consideration should be given for placement of IV access before induction of anesthesia or very early in the process. The size of the IV catheter should be determined by the anticipated fluid/transfusion requirements. If peripheral access is poor, central venous access may be necessary, particularly if there is potential for large intravascular volume shifts and to allow monitoring of central venous pressure. Placement of a central venous catheter is assisted by two-dimensional ultrasound imaging or audio Doppler (see Chapter 49). In the small infant with single-ventricle physiology, central venous cannulation with catheter placement in the superior vena cava may be undesirable in view of concerns about potential vascular complications that may affect pulmonary blood flow or subsequent surgical palliation. In these children, a small catheter or alternative approach (e.g., femoral venous access) should be considered. In children with an existent or potential right-to-left shunt, all air must be removed from IV infusion tubing. Air filters can be difficult to use in the operating room because they potentially restrict the rate at which IV fluids or blood may be administered in emergency situations. They can be more useful in the preoperative and postoperative periods.

Emergency Drugs

Hemodynamic instability can occur in children with CHD under any circumstance and at any time. Therefore drugs for emergency situations should be prepared in advanced or be immediately available to the anesthesiologist providing care.

MONITORING

A fundamental principle of intraoperative monitoring is to use techniques or devices that provide useful information to facilitate clinical decision making and to avoid monitors that are distracting or redundant. Basic monitoring involves observation of the child, including skin color, capillary refill, respiration, pulse palpation, events on the surgical field, and color of shed blood. Standard noninvasive monitors used during most surgical interventions include oscillometric blood pressure assessment, electrocardiography, pulse oximetry, capnography, and temperature recordings. A precordial stethoscope can be extremely helpful for monitoring changes in heart tones that may suggest early hemodynamic compromise. In the child with CHD, relatively sophisticated and invasive monitoring may be needed.

Arterial Blood Pressure Assessment

Blood pressure monitoring begins with pulse palpation. An automated blood pressure measurement is used in most children. The selection of monitoring site is influenced by vascular anomalies (e.g., aortic arch pathology, aberrant origin and course of aortic arch vessels) or prior surgical interventions (e.g., Blalock-Taussig shunt, arterial cutdown). Direct blood pressure monitoring by an indwelling arterial catheter may be necessary for beat-to-beat assessment and for blood gas analysis. In most children, this is accomplished after induction of anesthesia. Percutaneous arterial cannulation can be achieved in most cases with a low risk of complications (see Chapter 49). The radial artery usually is preferred over the ulnar artery because avoiding the ulnar artery allows preservation of a larger contributor of blood supply to the hand. The ulnar artery often is the larger vessel and it can be cannulated if required. However, some centers have a policy that the ulnar artery should never be cannulated. This policy ensures that there is always at least one vessel (ulnar artery) available to perfuse the hand should the radial vessel be compromised. Ultrasound guidance with two-dimensional imaging or audio Doppler can facilitate cannulation. The need for invasive monitoring is largely based on the child's clinical condition and nature of the surgical procedure.

Electrocardiography

The ECG provides a surface recording of the electrical myocardial activity and is used to monitor heart rate, cardiac rhythm, and ST-segment analysis. One or multiple leads typically are displayed. Arrhythmias can occur because of hypoxia, electrolyte imbalances, acid-base abnormalities, intravascular or intracardiac catheters, and surgical manipulations near or around the thorax. Ischemia may be evident on direct examination of the ECG or ST-segment analysis.[67,68] Although in adults this is associated with worsened outcome, the implication for the pediatric population is unknown.[67,69]

Pulse Oximetry

Placement of an oximeter probe is well tolerated, even by uncooperative children, and it is usually one of the earliest monitors applied during induction of anesthesia. Monitoring arterial oxygen saturation by pulse oximetry is particularly useful in infants, cyanotic children, and those with complex anatomy or significant hemodynamic compromise. In addition to providing continuous assessment of oxygen-hemoglobin saturation and heart rate, the pulse oximeter waveform can indicate the adequacy of peripheral perfusion and cardiac output.[70,71] Other parameters that can be reflected by the SpO_2 include intracardiac or great artery–level shunting and pulmonary blood flow.

Capnography

Capnography confirms proper tracheal tube placement, helps to assess the adequacy of ventilation, and aids in the recognition of pathologic conditions such as bronchospasm, airway obstruction, and malignant hyperthermia. Capnography is also useful in spontaneously breathing, sedated children receiving supplemental oxygen through a nasal cannula; a prospective, observational study in children undergoing cardiac catheterization with sedation administered by nonanesthesiologists found that exhaled carbon dioxide values ($P_{ET}CO_2$) provided a reasonable estimate of arterial blood CO_2 values.[72] Although the absolute value for $P_{ET}CO_2$ may not be as reliable as in the presence of a tracheal tube, the capnograph waveform confirms the presence or absence of respirations and air exchange. End-tidal CO_2 monitoring also provides a gross index of pulmonary blood flow. In children with cyanotic heart disease, $P_{ET}CO_2$ values can underestimate arterial carbon dioxide tension ($PaCO_2$) measurements owing to altered pulmonary blood flow and ventilation-perfusion mismatch.[73,74]

Temperature Monitoring

Temperature should be routinely monitored during most procedures. Although temperature swings are usually not profound, some children, particularly small neonates, may become hypothermic because of the large body surface area/body weight ratio and decreased amount of subcutaneous tissue. This can influence oxygen delivery (i.e., increased oxygen consumption) and emergence from anesthesia, cause detrimental changes in hemodynamics, and affect hemostasis. The neonate or small infant with CHD can be particularly vulnerable to the effects of hypothermia.

Urinary Output Measurements

The production of urine is a useful index of the adequacy of renal perfusion and cardiac output. Urine output is usually monitored during cases involving major fluid shifts or blood loss or when the surgical procedure is expected to be prolonged. No specific value for intraoperative urine output is predictive of good renal function in the postoperative period.

Echocardiography

Numerous publications have documented the utility of transesophageal echocardiography in general anesthesia practice[75] and as a monitoring device in high-risk adults undergoing noncardiac procedures.[76–88] Sporadic reports have demonstrated the utility of this imaging approach in children undergoing noncardiac surgery.[89–92] However, the application of this imaging modality in the pediatric age group or contributions in this particular setting has not been well defined and deserves further investigation.

Newer Technologies

Of significant interest over the past several years has been the use of point-of-care ultrasonography in various settings, including the perioperative period.[93,94] This is an evolving field that is receiving increasing attention during noncardiac surgery.[95] Continuous noninvasive cardiac output assessment represents an area of ongoing investigation in children using a variety of techniques.[96–98] These monitoring modalities are likely to further enhance the practice of pediatric anesthesia in the future.

SELECTION OF TECHNIQUES AND AGENTS

Several anesthetic regimens have been used in children with CHD undergoing noncardiac surgery and studies or procedures that require deep sedation or immobility. Although no single formula or protocol is recommended, the anesthetic techniques and agents used for a particular situation should be selected in consideration of the procedure, the child's disease process and functional status, and the impact of the hemodynamic effects of the anesthetic and procedure on the pathophysiologic process. Factors such as age, physical characteristics, and preferences of the anesthesiologist must be considered. The primary goals of anesthesia management with respect to the cardiovascular system are to optimize systemic oxygen delivery, maintain myocardial performance within expected parameters for the patient, and ensure the adequacy of cardiac output. A potentially limited cardiovascular reserve, reduced tolerance for perioperative stress, and detrimental alterations of the balance between pulmonary and systemic blood flow during anesthesia and surgery should be considered. A carefully titrated anesthetic, regardless of the specific agent or drug, should be the goal.

Anesthesia Technique

General anesthesia has the advantages of wide acceptance, ease of application, and certainty of effect. It is the appropriate choice for most children undergoing noncardiac surgery. Disadvantages include a greater potential for wide fluctuations in the hemodynamics and a prolonged recovery period. The IV route allows for rapid induction of anesthesia. If IV access is not available, inhalational induction can be performed. Inhalational anesthetics dilate vascular beds and reduce sympathetic responsiveness. These are desirable goals for most children, even those with heart disease, because adequate myocardial function and a reactive sympathetic nervous system are usual. However, sick children, and in particular those with ventricular dysfunction, may require an increased resting sympathetic tone to maintain systemic perfusion. Potent inhalational agents in this setting can further impair myocardial function, decrease sympathetic tone, and potentially lead to cardiovascular decompensation. These children and others with a relatively fixed cardiac output frequently require a technique that combines several medications (i.e., balanced technique) to achieve anesthesia while minimizing the risk of hemodynamic compromise. A combined opioid, amnestic agent, and muscle relaxant technique minimizes myocardial depression and tends to leave sympathetic responsiveness intact while providing analgesia, amnesia, and immobility.

Regional anesthesia has been used safely and shown to be effective in children with CHD (see Chapters 42 and 43).[99–102] Advantages of regional anesthesia, such as epidural and spinal techniques, include an effect largely limited to the surgical site, decreased number of systemic medications, a potentially brief recovery period, and usually a more pleasant experience for the child. Use of these techniques, however, may not always be effective. Regional anesthesia retains the potential for hemodynamic alterations, particularly in hypovolemic children or those with a fixed cardiac output. It is also contraindicated in those with coagulation defects. The administration of agents such as local anesthetics, opioids, or other adjuvants (e.g., clonidine) into the caudal space can attenuate the sympathetic outflow associated with surgical manipulation and noxious stimuli and facilitate postoperative pain management.

The choice of technique affects the termination of anesthesia and emergence. Anesthesia performed with fewer agents is inherently simpler, usually easier, and more predictable to terminate. The availability of ultra-short-acting opioids (e.g., remifentanil) and other agents (e.g., dexmedetomidine) has avoided the need for postoperative ventilation solely related to residual effects of depressant drugs. Ventricular function and the presence of intracardiac shunts can significantly affect uptake and distribution of inhalational anesthetics and the kinetics of IV medications (see Chapter 7).

Inhalational Agents

Inhalational anesthesia has been at the forefront of pediatric anesthesia practice for many years.[103,104] Sevoflurane was introduced in the mid-1990s, replacing halothane for inhaled induction in many centers. A study on the safety and efficacy of inhaled agents in infants and children with CHD during cardiac surgery demonstrated twice as many episodes of hypotension, moderate bradycardia, and emergent drug use in those who received halothane compared with those given sevoflurane.[105] These data, combined with those from other studies that demonstrated the potential benefits of sevoflurane on hemodynamic stability and minimal impact on myocardial performance, led to sevoflurane becoming the preferred anesthetic agent for children, particularly those with heart disease.[106–110] Nonetheless, in some jurisdictions and under some conditions, halothane may remain the primary anesthetic for children. After an inhalational induction with sevoflurane, agents such as isoflurane or desflurane might be used to maintain anesthesia.

Intravenous Agents

Propofol is one of the most frequently used medications for IV sedation and general anesthesia. It has been used in children with CHD in numerous settings.[111–114] The hemodynamic effects of propofol have been investigated in children with normal hearts and in those with cardiovascular disease. An echocardiographic study in infants with normal hearts undergoing elective surgery demonstrated that propofol did not alter heart rate, shortening fraction, rate-corrected velocity of circumferential fiber shortening, or cardiac index after IV induction.[115] However, propofol decreased arterial blood pressure to a greater extent than thiopental, an effect attributed to a reduction in afterload. A comparison of propofol and ketamine during cardiac catheterization found that propofol caused a transient decrease in mean arterial pressure and mild arterial oxygen desaturation in some children.[116] In view of the significantly faster recovery, propofol was identified as a practical alternative to ketamine for elective cardiac catheterization in children.

Another investigation in 30 children with CHD undergoing cardiac catheterization demonstrated significant decreases in mean arterial blood pressure and systemic vascular resistance during propofol administration.[111] No changes in heart rate, mean pulmonary artery pressure, or pulmonary vascular resistance were observed. In children with intracardiac shunts, the net result of propofol was a significant increase in the right-to-left shunt, a decrease in the left-to-right shunt, and a decreased pulmonary/systemic blood flow ratio, resulting in a statistically significant decrease in the PaO_2 and arterial oxygen saturation (SaO_2), as well as reversal of the shunt direction from left-to-right to right-to-left in two patients. It was also shown that propofol could lead to further arterial desaturation in children with cyanotic heart disease. A recent study examined the effects of propofol on cerebral oxygenation in children with CHD.[117] Propofol sedation was associated with increased cerebral tissue oxygenation despite a significant decrease in mean arterial pressure, stroke volume, cardiac output, and cardiac index. The authors reported that the hemodynamic changes were not considered clinically relevant and none required intervention.

The effects of propofol have been examined in children undergoing electrophysiologic testing and radiofrequency catheter ablation for tachyarrhythmias. The drug has no significant effect on sinoatrial or atrioventricular (AV) node function or accessory pathway conduction in Wolff-Parkinson-White syndrome.[118,119] However, another study documented that ectopic atrial tachycardia can be suppressed during propofol administration in children.[120]

Collectively, these data support the judicious use of propofol in children with adequate cardiovascular reserve who can tolerate mild decreases in myocardial contractility and heart rate and mild to moderate decreases in systemic vascular resistance. Given the effects of propofol on the direction and magnitude of intracardiac shunts, this might be an important consideration in children with cyanotic heart disease and can influence the hemodynamic assessment of those undergoing evaluation of pulmonary/systemic blood flow ratios in the cardiac catheterization laboratory.

Sodium thiopental, a rapid-onset short-acting barbiturate, was used for many years for induction of anesthesia. The last company to market sodium thiopental in the United States stopped production of the drug in early 2011. Several investigations documented the cardiovascular responses to this agent; in children with normal hearts, the cardiac index remained unchanged, although the shortening fraction decreased along with alterations in load-independent parameters of contractility. The data regarding myocardial depressant properties of barbiturates and its effects on venodilation and peripheral blood pooling suggested that the administration of thiopental in a subset of children could cause hemodynamic instability. Thus it was recommended that thiopental should be used with caution, particularly in those with limited reserve or increased sympathetic tone.

Etomidate, a carboxylated imidazole derivative, has anesthetic and amnestic properties but is devoid of analgesic effects. This agent demonstrates favorable qualities over other IV drugs because of its lack of effect on hemodynamics.[121,122] This, combined with laboratory and clinical data that support minimal effects on myocardial contractility, makes this drug a particularly desirable agent in critically ill individuals and in those with limited cardiovascular reserve.[123] Despite these benefits, several undesirable adverse effects are associated with etomidate, including pain on IV administration, myoclonic movements that may mimic seizure activity, and inhibition of adrenal steroid synthesis perioperatively.[124,125] Although used primarily as an induction agent, etomidate has been administered for sedation of children during cardiac catheterization and in other settings.[126-128]

Ketamine is a dissociative anesthetic agent administered by the IV, intramuscular, nasal, rectal, and oral routes. Because its sympathomimetic effects result in an increased heart rate, blood pressure, and cardiac output, this drug has been widely used in children with heart disease, particularly in young infants. The effects of this agent on systemic vascular resistance make it a suitable choice in children with right-to-left shunts because pulmonary blood flow is enhanced. This contrasts with inhalational agents, which by causing systemic vasodilation can decrease pulmonary blood flow in the presence of an intracardiac communication and potentially worsen the degree of cyanosis. In clinical use, however, arterial oxygen saturation typically increases with both agents. Additional favorable properties include intense analgesia at subanesthetic doses and a lack of respiratory depressant effects.

Several investigations have addressed the concern of potential detrimental changes in pulmonary vascular tone resulting from ketamine, although no significant effects have been reported on pulmonary arterial pressures and pulmonary vascular resistance at the usual clinical doses.[129-132] Regarding its effect on myocardial performance, in vitro investigations have shown a direct myocardial depressant effect in animal species and the failing adult human heart. This is considered to be the result of inhibition of L-type voltage-dependent calcium channels in the sarcolemmal membrane and may be a consideration in the critically ill infant with a severely impaired cardiac reserve. Additional undesirable effects of ketamine include emergence reactions, excessive salivation, vomiting, and increased intracranial pressure.

Dexmedetomidine is a selective α_2-adrenergic agonist agent being increasingly used in the pediatric age group. Compared with clonidine, the drug exhibits greater specificity for the α_2-adrenergic receptor over the α_1-adrenergic receptor. Favorable effects of the drug include sedation, anxiolysis, and analgesia. This medication provides hemodynamic stability, although adverse effects have been reported, including bradycardia, hypertension, and hypotension. A study of the hemodynamic effects in children undergoing dexmedetomidine sedation for radiologic imaging demonstrated modest decreases in heart rate and blood pressure. These changes in response to moderate doses were independent of age, required no pharmacologic interventions, and did not result in any adverse events; however, high-dose dexmedetomidine can be associated with significant bradycardia.[133,134] In addition, treatment of dexmedetomidine-induced bradycardia with glycopyrrolate (5 µg/kg) has been associated with severe persistent hypertension.[135]

Dexmedetomidine is used as a premedication agent during diagnostic studies and procedural sedation, to reduce emergence delirium, in the treatment of symptoms associated with opioid withdrawal, and as an adjuvant agent in the operating room and postoperative settings.[136] In children with CHD, its benefits have been reported during monitored anesthesia care, diagnostic and interventional cardiac catheterization, intraoperative sedation, after cardiac and thoracic surgery, as a primary agent during invasive procedures, and in the treatment of perioperative atrial and junctional tachyarrhythmias.[137-145] The drug has also been used in children with pulmonary hypertension with good results.[146,147]

Known electrophysiologic effects of dexmedetomidine in children include significant depression of sinus and AV nodal function.[148] Other findings include a reduction in the heart rate and increases in arterial blood pressure. Although dexmedetomidine has been described as an undesirable agent for electrophysiologic studies because it could be associated with adverse effects in patients at risk for bradycardia or AV block,[148] another study reported that dexmedetomidine was not associated with any significant or atypical ECG interval abnormalities, except for a trend toward a decrease in heart rate in children with CHD.[149] Until additional data are available, it may be prudent to exercise caution when considering the use of dexmedetomidine in children with conduction abnormalities. Although experience suggests an overall safety profile in children with CHD, fragile patients may not tolerate the heart rate and blood pressure fluctuations associated with dexmedetomidine; significant adverse effects include severe bradycardia progressing to asystole.[150]

Opioids and *benzodiazepines* are widely used medications in pediatric anesthesia practice. Opioids attenuate the neuroendocrine stress response associated with anesthesia and surgery.[151,152] After repair of CHD, these medications blunt the stress response in the pulmonary circulation elicited by airway manipulations.[153] Morphine administration can cause histamine release and vasodilation. The synthetic opioids are devoid of these effects and provide excellent hemodynamic stability with minimal changes in heart rate and blood pressure in children with CHD.[154] The primary concern about opioid administration is their central respiratory depressant effects because their primary cardiovascular manifestations are minimal. Benzodiazepines provide sedation and amnesia during the perioperative period. Midazolam may allow a reduction in the inspired concentration of inhalational anesthetic agents, which is a desirable feature in children with labile hemodynamics or in those considered at great risk for the myocardial depressant properties of inhalational anesthetics. Studies of the effects of benzodiazepines in children with CHD are limited.[155]

Neuromuscular blocking drugs facilitate tracheal intubation and prevent reflex movement during surgery if the anesthetics alone are insufficient. All inhalational anesthetics potentiate the effects of nondepolarizing muscle relaxants. These medications have various onsets and durations of action and diverse hemodynamic effects. The cardiovascular and autonomic effects of muscle relaxants have been characterized mainly in adults with acquired cardiovascular disease (see also Chapter 7).[156-159] Drug selection is based on the need to facilitate tracheal intubation and surgical relaxation, hemodynamic side effects, and the anticipated duration of surgery.

INDUCTION OF ANESTHESIA

Induction of anesthesia in children with CHD most commonly can be accomplished using the inhaled or IV route. The intramuscular route (i.e., ketamine administration) may be preferable in some cases, particularly in an uncooperative, developmentally delayed, or combative child. Less common induction techniques include subcutaneous, intranasal, and rectal administration of induction or sedative agents. These various approaches may also be used in combination (see Chapter 4).

An IV induction is preferable in some children in view of its potentially greater safety margin. In addition to the ability to titrate medications and rapidly correct hemodynamic alterations, other benefits include the speed of effect, although this may be slowed in children with large left-to-right shunts owing to recirculation of the drug in the lungs. Left-to-right shunting decreases the concentration of anesthetic agents reaching the brain and delays its onset of action. In contrast, right-to-left shunts speed IV inductions because a significant portion of the medication bypasses the lungs (where it is degraded) and directly enters the systemic circulation, reaching the brain more rapidly than with an intact circulation.

If IV access is not available, an inhalational induction is performed in most cases. A carefully titrated inhalational induction and early placement of an IV catheter usually is safe, even in children with moderate hemodynamic disturbances, particularly after premedication has been given. This produces loss of consciousness, with acceptable conditions for establishing IV access. Inhalational induction can be delayed in cyanotic children and those with right-to-left shunts, particularly for anesthetics with reduced blood solubility, because the decreased pulmonary blood flow limits the rate of increase in the concentration of the anesthetic in the systemic arterial blood. The rapidity of an inhalational induction is increased in the presence of a reduced cardiac output because the anesthetic partial pressure in the alveoli increases more rapidly as less anesthetic is removed by the smaller pulmonary blood flow (see Chapter 7). Left-to-right intracardiac shunts have limited effects on the speed of induction of inhaled anesthetics.

MAINTENANCE OF ANESTHESIA

After induction, anesthesia can be maintained using an inhalational, IV, or combined inhalational and IV technique. In children with CHD, anesthesia can result in hemodynamic changes regardless of the technique, agents, or experience of the anesthesiologist. Some children may not tolerate even minor alterations in hemodynamics. Factors that may lead to cardiovascular collapse in the marginally compensated child include hypovolemia, relative anesthetic overdose, increased vagal tone, positive-pressure ventilation, hypoxemia, airway obstruction, alterations in $PaCO_2$ or other factors that influence the balance between systemic and pulmonary blood flow, myocardial ischemia, arrhythmias, and anaphylaxis. The anesthesiologist should be prepared to manage these rare but occasionally unavoidable occurrences at any time.

EMERGENCE FROM ANESTHESIA

Most children undergoing noncardiac surgical interventions are expected to awaken immediately at the completion of the procedure or shortly thereafter. This usually involves reducing and then discontinuing IV or inhalational anesthetics, antagonizing neuromuscular blockade, and extubating the trachea. Ensuring the return of protective reflexes and monitoring the adequacy of the airway and respirations are important considerations.

Postoperative Care

The postoperative management of the child with CHD involves many of the same physiologic principles applicable to intraoperative care. The extent of the postoperative care, optimal place for recovery, and need for monitoring and hospitalization depend in large part on the child's clinical condition and type and extent of the procedure. Immediately after surgery, most children awaken from anesthesia and recover from neuromuscular blockade, which may impose various stresses and hemodynamic changes. Adequate oxygenation and ventilation along with airway protection must be ensured and may need to be provided if the child cannot manage these functions on his or her own. Significant hypoventilation must be avoided during this time because it may negatively affect pulmonary vascular tone and overall hemodynamics in vulnerable children with CHD. Adequate pain control and, sometimes, sedation are important postoperatively. This may be a challenging issue for the child who requires noncardiac surgery soon after a prolonged hospitalization in view of the increased likelihood for tolerance to analgesic and sedative drugs.

Observation and physical examination provide much information about the child's respiratory status, cardiac function, and systemic perfusion during the postoperative period. Adequacy of oxygenation and ventilation can also be assessed with noninvasive monitoring and blood gas analysis. Monitoring urine output can be helpful.

Hemoglobin or hematocrit values are monitored as a measure of oxygen-carrying capability in cases in which significant blood loss or the administration of fluids might have occurred. Serum electrolytes are screened if fluid shifts have taken place during the surgical and/or postoperative periods. Although digoxin is now used less frequently, attention should be given to the avoidance of hypokalemia in children receiving this drug. Serum glucose concentrations should be followed in neonates and small infants and dextrose-containing IV solutions administered as appropriate. Determination of ionized calcium (iCa^{++}) levels is indicated for patients with a history of DiGeorge syndrome because of a propensity toward hypocalcemia. Fluid replacement is dictated by the child's heart defect, type of surgery performed, and volume losses (see Chapters 9 and 12).

Perioperative Problems and Special Considerations

Several potential problems may be encountered during the perioperative period in children with CHD undergoing noncardiac interventions. This section highlights some of these issues to serve as a framework and outlines selected considerations in these children.

HYPOTENSION

Hypotension can be related to hypovolemia owing to prolonged fasting, volume loss, arrhythmia, anesthetic agents, myocardial dysfunction, or mechanical influences associated with the operative procedure. A practical diagnostic approach to the hypotensive patient is to consider factors that may affect ventricular preload, contractility, afterload, and the assessment of cardiac rhythm. Although the management of hypotension should be guided primarily by the causative factor, acutely increasing blood pressure by the administration of volume and an appropriate vasopressor, if indicated, often restores adequate perfusion while definitive therapy is instituted. Ensuring adequate intravascular volume with a fluid challenge often helps to restore perfusion and blood pressure, especially in hypovolemic patients. A pure α-adrenergic agent such as phenylephrine increases systolic blood pressure without further increases in heart rate. Some children are unable to tolerate any degree of myocardial depression or reduction in sympathetic outflow and require continuous inotropic support or vasopressor infusions throughout and after the operative procedure.

CYANOSIS

Cyanosis is a common finding in children with defects characterized by reduced pulmonary blood flow or intracardiac mixing. As surgical management strategies evolve to target the youngest of infants, the chronic effects of cyanosis may be limited in these children. However, in those requiring delayed surgery, palliation, or staged correction of their defects, the effects of cyanosis can be long lasting. Chronic hypoxemia affects all major organ systems. Compensatory mechanisms that attempt to provide adequate systemic oxygen delivery in the presence of chronic hypoxemia include polycythemia (related to secondary erythrocytosis), increases in blood volume, alterations in oxygen uptake and delivery, and neovascularization. Despite the favorable effects of the adaptive responses, these alterations can be detrimental. Polycythemia, the most significant compensatory response, is associated with increases in blood viscosity and red cell sludging. The common occurrence of iron-deficiency anemia in cyanotic children further enhances hyperviscosity and the unfavorable consequences of this condition. Several hemostatic abnormalities (e.g., thrombocytopenia, altered platelet function, and clotting factor abnormalities) have been described as a result of hypoxemia and erythrocytosis that may affect the coagulation system and increase perioperative risks.[160-165] This is compounded by increased tissue vascularity, with a larger number of blood vessels per unit of tissue.

The increased blood viscosity in children with cyanosis is associated with stasis and a risk for thrombotic events.[165a] If the hematocrit exceeds 65% preoperatively, some clinicians advocate phlebotomy to reduce the hematocrit to 60% to 65%. This limits sludging of red blood cells and increases oxygen delivery to tissues. If blood is removed by preoperative phlebotomy, it may be saved for autologous transfusion in the perioperative period.

During the perioperative period, adequate hydration should be maintained in children with cyanotic CHD, and care should be taken to avoid prolonged venous stasis. Cyanotic children are at risk for paradoxical embolic events, mandating meticulous attention to IV lines during fluid or drug administration. This is a reasonable routine approach for all children with CHD, regardless of the nature of the structural abnormalities. The use of air filters to IV tubing should not replace vigilance.

TETRALOGY SPELLS

Hypercyanotic episodes in children with tetralogy of Fallot (i.e., tet spells) may be the result of significant dynamic right ventricular outflow tract (RVOT) obstruction leading to acute reductions in pulmonary blood flow. Tet spells are rare during noncardiac surgery, probably because general anesthesia attenuates the triggers. Occasionally, however, increased cyanosis may occur without warning in response to obscure stimuli. Whatever the cause, worsening cyanosis implies increases in dynamic obstruction and exacerbation of ventricular-level right-to-left shunting. Factors that decrease systemic blood pressure and systemic vascular resistance, such as hypovolemia and extreme vasodilation, should be avoided. Therapy consists of increasing blood volume and systemic vascular tone, the latter using either a phenylephrine bolus of 5 µg/kg IV initially and if needed, 0.1 to 2 µg/kg per minute by continuous infusion, norepinephrine 0.5 µg/kg IV initially, and then 0.05 to 2 µg/kg per minute by continuous infusion or metaraminol 0.01 mg/kg IV initially and then 0.05 to 0.5 µg/kg per minute by continuous infusion. Vasopressin infusion (0.02–0.04 units/kg per hour) may be an alternative agent. Increasing the inspired oxygen concentration and reducing inspiratory ventilatory pressures may also produce clinical improvement. Additional therapies include increasing the level of sedation or anesthetic depth and β-adrenergic blockade (esmolol [starting dose 50 μg/kg per minute] has largely replaced propranolol in this setting) (see also Chapters 16 and 17). Pulmonary vascular tone does not play a major role in the physiology of hypercyanotic episodes in tetralogy of Fallot; however, it is reasonable to limit additional afterload stresses to the right ventricle.

HEART FAILURE

In infants, congestive heart failure is most often due to ventricular volume overload resulting from ventricular or great artery–level communications. Heart failure can also result from severe valvar regurgitation, obstructive disease, or intrinsic myocardial disease (e.g., cardiomyopathy). Structural defects can lead to heart failure as a result of poor myocardial contractility, compromising cardiac output and the ability of the cardiovascular system to meet systemic demands.

In children with significant pulmonary vascular congestion, positive-pressure mechanical ventilation may be necessary before and after surgery. In cases of elective noncardiac surgery, it can be of significant benefit to optimize medical therapy or address the cardiovascular defect(s) before the planned procedure.

In a retrospective review of 21 children with severe heart failure who underwent 28 general anesthetics, 10% had a cardiac arrest requiring unplanned postoperative admission to the intensive care unit, and 96% required perioperative inotropic support. The investigators concluded that general anesthesia for children with severe heart failure is associated with a significant complication rate.[166]

VENTRICULAR DYSFUNCTION

Children with CHD can have ventricular dysfunction involving the right heart, left heart, both sides of the heart, regional myocardium, or global cardiac tissue. The impairment can be of a temporary or permanent nature. In systolic dysfunction, contractile function is primarily impaired. Diastolic dysfunction is associated with abnormal cardiac relaxation or impaired ventricular compliance. Some children have both, systolic and diastolic dysfunction. Ventricular dysfunction can result from factors such as age at the time of the operation and chronicity of the cardiac workload (pressure or volume); it can also be caused by the primary disease, myocardial hypertrophy, ischemia, or cyanosis or can occur as a direct effect of surgery (e.g., ventriculotomy, cardiopulmonary bypass, ischemic time, circulatory arrest). Diseases that affect cardiac muscle (e.g., myocarditis, dilated cardiomyopathy) can be associated with congestive symptoms, whereas others (e.g., restrictive cardiomyopathy) can lead to diastolic heart failure.

In children with cardiomyopathy that was accompanied by severe ventricular dysfunction, general anesthesia for noncardiac procedures was associated with an increased frequency of complications.[167] The children often required hospital support before and after the procedure that in many cases included intensive care management. Hospital stay was prolonged for children with severe ventricular dysfunction compared with those with a lesser degree of impairment. Based on these findings, early consideration of perioperative intensive care support was recommended for monitoring and optimization of cardiovascular therapy.

VENTRICULAR VOLUME OVERLOAD

Ventricular volume overload, which manifests as increased left atrial pressure, left ventricular (LV) end-diastolic pressure, and stroke volume, is a common feature in many children with unoperated CHD. Long-standing volume overload results in atrial enlargement, ventricular dilation, and cardiomegaly. In the postoperative child, residual valvar regurgitation can be associated with altered loading conditions that, if significant, can result in congestive symptoms and ventricular dysfunction. Patients with a palliated single ventricle can be particularly vulnerable to conditions associated with ventricular volume overload (e.g., systemic-to-pulmonary artery shunts).

VENTRICULAR PRESSURE OVERLOAD

Pressure overload in the postoperative patient typically results from residual or recurrent muscular, valvar, or distal outflow obstruction or from increased pulmonary artery pressure or vascular resistance. In children with abnormal distal pulmonary arterial beds, for example, the hypoplastic vessels may not be amenable to surgical repair or other intervention, although associated defects may be satisfactorily addressed. This results in increased proximal pulmonary artery and RV pressures and compensatory myocardial hypertrophy. RV pressure can exceed systemic values and compromise LV function because septal shift can impair LV filling or result in obstruction to systemic outflow (ventricular interdependence). Abnormal pressure loads to the right ventricle can also result from progressive obstruction after procedures that involve outflow tract reconstructions. In children who have undergone outflow conduit placements, surgical interventions for successive conduit replacements are delayed as much as possible. This translates into long-standing pressure loads on the myocardium with associated wall hypertrophy and potentially some element of ischemia until the criteria for surgical intervention have been met.

Whether the altered loading conditions affect the right or left ventricle primarily, the result is an increased myocardial demand because of the increased wall tension. This implies a susceptibility of the ventricular myocardium to the supply-and-demand relationship, a reduced tolerance for factors that may alter this fine balance, and an increased risk of ischemia.

MYOCARDIAL ISCHEMIA

Several factors can cause myocardial ischemia in children with CHD. They include chronic hypoxemia, increased systolic and diastolic wall stress, and decreased coronary perfusion owing to reduced diastolic pressures in the presence of large systemic-to-pulmonary shunts. The effects of cardiopulmonary bypass, aortic cross-clamping, and surgery itself cannot be ignored. Other conditions with a propensity for myocardial ischemia include congenital coronary artery lesions, aortic stenosis, and the increased blood viscosity associated with cyanosis. The deprivation of myocardial perfusion can lead to ventricular dysfunction and eventual development of myocardial fibrosis.

ALTERED RESPIRATORY MECHANICS

Chronically increased pulmonary blood flow and pulmonary artery pressures can result in progressive pulmonary vascular changes, elevated pulmonary vascular resistance, and alterations in lung mechanics. The primary effects on respiratory mechanics are related to increased airway resistance and decreased lung compliance. These alterations can have detrimental respiratory consequences in children with inadequate palliation or residual shunts. In some children, left atrial dilation can lead to respiratory compromise (e.g., air trapping, atelectasis) caused by bronchial compression.

PULMONARY HYPERTENSION

Pulmonary hypertension is defined as a mean pulmonary artery pressure in the resting state that exceeds 25 mm Hg or more. Several factors can lead to increased pulmonary artery pressures. These include increased pulmonary blood flow, pulmonary venous pressure, and pulmonary vascular resistance, among many others.[168] Unoperated CHD represents a major cause in children. It usually is the consequence of an unrestricted pulmonary blood flow owing to a communication between intracardiac structures or at the level of the great arteries. One of the benefits of early correction is a reduction in pulmonary artery pressures and less potential for pulmonary vascular reactivity after cardiac surgery. However, in some cases, pulmonary hypertension can persist or develop after a corrective intervention.

A less common entity is that of increased pulmonary vascular resistance, which can be reactive or fixed. Pulmonary hypertension and increased pulmonary vascular resistance pose significant risks for perioperative complications in children, regardless of cause.[43,132,169,170]

An acute increase in pulmonary vascular tone, also known as pulmonary hypertensive crisis, can result in cardiac arrest. In the presence of an intracardiac communication that allows for shunting, acute increases in pulmonary artery pressure can manifest as arterial desaturation, bradycardia, and systemic hypotension. In the absence of an intracardiac communication, the acute increase in RV afterload can lead to encroachment of the left ventricle caused by unfavorable leftward shifting of the interventricular septum, compromising LV filling and decreasing cardiac output. These events can be catastrophic.

Several factors can acutely affect pulmonary vascular tone (Table 23.2). Treatment should be aggressive in the acute setting, aimed at reducing pulmonary artery pressures with interventions such as sedation, oxygen administration, hyperventilation to produce hypocarbia, and treatment of acidosis.[170–173] The use of selective pulmonary vasodilators (e.g., inhaled nitric oxide) and inotropic support of the right ventricle may be indicated. Manipulation of pulmonary hemodynamics is challenged by the difficulty of directly measuring these parameters in children. Management of critical situations requires a thorough understanding of the pathophysiologic process and experienced clinical judgment. Because of the significant morbidity and potential periprocedural mortality for children with a history of severe pulmonary hypertension, an in-depth evaluation of the risk/benefit ratio of the planned procedure and its impact on the overall quality of life is essential.

Children with pulmonary hypertensive vascular disease (PHVD) in many cases undergo initial cardiac catheterization to confirm diagnosis, assess disease severity, for vasoreactivity testing, and to gather data with prognostic implications. Subsequent studies may be performed to determine response to drug therapy. Although a setting that may mimic an awake state might be desirable, it is well recognized that spontaneous ventilation under conditions of sedation implies potential risk of respiratory depression and hypercapnia, which may influence pulmonary artery pressures and resistances. Thus most children require general anesthesia for these procedures. The consensus statement of the Pulmonary Vascular Research Institute, Pediatric and Congenital Heart Disease Task Forces indicates the following: *"we recommend the presence of an anesthesiologist familiar with the management of neonatal and childhood PHVD when either sedation or general anesthesia is used."*[174] It is noted that general anesthesia and mechanical ventilation provide stable conditions for the procedure but require the availability of a trained pediatric anesthesiologist with experience in the management of children with cardiopulmonary disease.

ENDOCARDITIS PROPHYLAXIS

The current guidelines of the American Heart Association for infective endocarditis (IE) prevention published in 2007 recommends prophylaxis only for patients with cardiac conditions associated with the highest risk of adverse outcome from IE. These recommendations represented a major change from prior guidelines significantly narrowing the indications for antibiotic prophylaxis (see Chapter 16). In accordance with the revised guidelines, only a subset of children with CHD should be offered subacute bacterial endocarditis prophylaxis for specific surgical/procedural indications (see Table 16.2).[175] The writing group considered the following cardiac conditions appropriate for IE prophylaxis:

- Prosthetic cardiac valve
- History of infective endocarditis
- Unrepaired cyanotic CHD, including palliative shunts and conduits
- Completely repaired congenital heart defect with prosthetic material or a prosthetic device, whether placed by surgery or by catheter intervention, during the first 6 months after the procedure
- Repaired CHD with residual defects at the site or adjacent to the site of a prosthetic patch or prosthetic device (which inhibit endothelialization)
- Cardiac transplant recipients who develop cardiac valvulopathy

For patients with these underlying conditions prophylaxis is recommended during (1) all dental procedures that involve manipulation of gingival tissues or periapical region of teeth or perforation of oral mucosa and (2) procedures on respiratory tract or infected skin, skin structures, or musculoskeletal tissue (Table 16.3). Antibiotic prophylaxis solely for the prevention of IE is not recommended for genitourinary or gastrointestinal tract procedures, although we advise verifying the institutional practice with local surgeons and cardiologists.

SYSTEMIC AIR EMBOLIZATION

Intracardiac communications in children with CHD have the potential for right-to-left shunting and paradoxical systemic air embolization. The increased right-heart pressures associated with many cardiovascular malformations further increase this risk. It is well recognized that arterial gas embolism can lead to catastrophic consequences; thus it is imperative to ascertain the presence of or likelihood for intracardiac or vascular shunting or to assume that this may potentially be the case in most children with CHD and consider appropriate precautions.

TABLE 23.2	Factors Associated With Increased Pulmonary Vascular Tone
Acidemia	
Atelectasis	
Hypercarbia	
Hypothermia	
Hypoxemia	
Stress response, stimulation, light anesthesia, pain	
Transmitted positive airway pressure	

ANTICOAGULATION

Anticoagulants, antiplatelet drugs, and thrombolytic agents are increasingly being used in children, particularly in those with CHD.[176-180] Decisions regarding perioperative management of anticoagulation are primarily influenced by the nature of the procedure, urgency of the intervention, specific drug therapy, and expected effects or laboratory data. The main concern relates to the potential for significant bleeding.

Low-dose aspirin does not represent a contraindication for most simple, superficial procedures, but if major surgery is planned, a discussion should take place and consideration given to discontinuing the drug for 7 to 10 days preoperatively, if appropriate. Recommendations for the management of children receiving warfarin (Coumadin) therapy vary widely.[181-183] The proposed strategies are quite heterogeneous, and the lack of consensus reflects the paucity of studies addressing this issue in a large cohort of children. The problem is further complicated by the lack of guidelines specific to pediatric practice.[184]

If the indications for anticoagulation are for native valve disease or atrial arrhythmias, the risk of a major thromboembolic event is considered relatively small, and warfarin may be discontinued 1 to 2 weeks before the day of surgery. In those with mechanical prosthetic valves, the risk of thromboembolic events is greater. Many recommend discontinuing the oral anticoagulant a few days before surgery and allowing the prothrombin time to return to within 20% of normal.[181] Administration of parenteral vitamin K, factor concentrates, or fresh frozen plasma, may be required to restore the prothrombin time within an acceptable range, especially in those with liver disease and in emergency cases. Some experts advise elective preoperative hospitalization, particularly in high-risk individuals, such as those with mitral or combined valve prostheses, to discontinue warfarin therapy and to initiate a heparin infusion, which is continued up until a few hours before surgery. Others suggest that low–molecular-weight heparin may be the better option instead of unfractionated heparin because the perioperative conversion from warfarin therapy to heparin can be accomplished without the need for hospitalization.[182]

Anticoagulation is usually reinitiated after 24 hours in children with valvular prostheses, and this may be achieved with a continuous heparin infusion or intermittent subcutaneous injections. The advantage of heparin is the ability to rapidly reverse the drug effect with protamine sulfate if bleeding complications occur. Oral anticoagulants are reinitiated 2 to 3 days after surgery if there are no bleeding concerns and the child is able to take oral medications. Although it has been suggested that there is no need to discontinue anticoagulation therapy for minor procedures, such as dental or ophthalmologic surgery in adults, guidelines for children are less clear.

The risk of bleeding from the surgical intervention versus the risk of a thromboembolism from a reduced anticoagulant dose determines to what extent and for what duration the anticoagulant therapy should be modified. In some cases, the cardiologist and surgeon may decide to temporarily use aspirin therapy before and after surgery. There is disagreement regarding whether antiplatelet therapy is preferable to anticoagulation in children with prosthetic aortic valves or after certain surgical interventions.[185-188]

CONDUCTION DISTURBANCES AND ARRHYTHMIAS

Acute rhythm disturbances can occur with the use of any anesthetic agent or technique and can be related to several factors. The administration of drugs with vagolytic or sympathomimetic properties requires consideration in patients with a prior history of or pathology associated with arrhythmias. Bradycardia can occur during induction of anesthesia, laryngoscopy, and tracheal intubation, particularly in infants and in children with Down syndrome.[189-191] In most cases, bradycardia is self-limited and requires no therapy, although if hypoxemia is the cause, it must be treated immediately.

Certain lesions can be associated with rhythm abnormalities and the potential for acute hemodynamic deterioration, increasing perioperative risks. Conduction system disorders and rhythm disturbances can occur after cardiac surgery as a direct result of the procedure or can develop owing to the inadequacy of the palliation or repair. Because cardiac arrhythmias are more prevalent among specific surgical subgroups, anticipation of their occurrence and planning for management are advocated. These cases may require prior consultation with a pediatric cardiologist or electrophysiologist, availability of specific medications, and the ability to electrically manage an acute rhythm disorder.

PACEMAKERS AND IMPLANTABLE CARDIOVERTER-DEFIBRILLATORS

An in-depth discussion of perioperative considerations related to implanted pacemakers or defibrillators can be found in Chapter 16. Consultation with a cardiologist or electrophysiologist is essential when caring for children with implanted units. Device interrogation and programming are required in most cases. The main goal is to avoid problems with hardware malfunction related to electromagnetic interference (i.e., electrocautery). Chronotropic agents and backup pacing modalities (e.g., transvenous, epicardial, transcutaneous) should be readily available and carefully considered in the event of pacemaker malfunction associated with an inadequate underlying heart rate. A magnet should be accessible to enable asynchronous pacing if required but should not be considered a substitute for preoperative device interrogation and reprogramming to the appropriate mode. Perioperative ECG monitoring is essential, as is the use of monitoring modalities that can confirm pulse generation during pacing. Implanted devices should be interrogated and reprogrammed after the procedure.

NERVE PALSIES

Surgery for CHD can be associated with transient or permanent injury to the recurrent laryngeal and phrenic nerves. Recurrent laryngeal nerve injuries can result in abnormal phonation or airway difficulties and lead to aspiration, particularly in small infants. These injuries usually occur during or in association with aortic arch surgery (e.g., patent ductus arteriosus [PDA] ligation or aortic arch reconstruction) with two-thirds resolving within 2 years. Diaphragmatic palsies resulting from phrenic nerve injuries are associated with abnormal lung mechanics and limited pulmonary reserve, both of which may account for perioperative morbidity. These injuries occur in association with bidirectional Glenn shunts, Blalock-Taussig shunts, and others.

EISENMENGER SYNDROME

Eisenmenger syndrome, rarely seen in the current era, is characterized by progressive, irreversible pulmonary vascular disease in the patient with CHD owing to pathology associated with significant left-to-right shunting. The pulmonary artery pressure in such patients reaches systemic/suprasystemic pressures from increased pulmonary vascular resistance (usually exceeding 10 Wood units). Cyanosis is the result of reversal in the direction of an intracardiac or arterial level shunt.[192,193] When seen, Eisenmenger syndrome is most likely to occur in older children, adolescents, or adults with CHD. Morbidity relates to problems associated with chronic cyanosis and erythrocytosis. Other medical issues include hemoptysis, gout, cholelithiasis, hypertrophic osteoarthropathy, and decreased renal function. These comorbidities in most cases mandate extensive preoperative preparation and testing. Laboratory studies of relevance include a hematologic profile, as well as assessment of renal and liver function. Other considerations include preoperative therapeutic phlebotomy in selected patients. The blood removed should be saved for potential subsequent autologous transfusion. It should be recognized that samples sent to the blood bank might require additional time for processing owing to the presence of antibodies from blood product exposure during prior surgical interventions.

Variables associated with poor outcome in Eisenmenger syndrome include syncope, increased RV end-diastolic pressure, and significant hypoxemia (i.e., $SaO_2 < 85\%$). Life expectancy is significantly reduced in affected individuals.[194] Most succumb suddenly, probably from ventricular tachyarrhythmias. Surgical modalities that have been advocated in selected patients include combined heart and lung transplantation[195] and lung transplantation alone.[196]

The considerable morbidity and mortality in patients with Eisenmenger syndrome during noncardiac surgery require not only expertise from the providers but also care at facilities capable of managing problems that may arise perioperatively. Despite the overall poor prognosis and the extremely high risk of untoward events, several reports have documented good outcomes with a variety of anesthetic techniques and agents.[39,197-200] In a retrospective study of institutional outcomes in patients with Eisenmenger syndrome, significant arterial hypotension was reported in 26% and arterial desaturation in 17%.[201] This finding led to the recommendation for blood pressure support with a vasopressor before or during the induction period to maintain systemic vascular tone and prevent worsening of the shunt flow. It is vital that the family and patient, if of appropriate age, understand these risks before undertaking any procedure requiring anesthesia or deep sedation.

CARDIAC TRANSPLANTATION

In some cases of end-stage cardiac pathology as a result of congenital or acquired disease, cardiac transplantation may represent the best or only option for survival.[202,203] The preoperative assessment should note indications for transplant and specifically assess transplant organ function.

An important consideration is the lack of external nerve supply of the transplanted heart (i.e., no sensory, sympathetic, or parasympathetic innervations). The physiology of the denervated heart implies that the usual autonomic regulatory mechanisms are not operational, increasing the vulnerability of children receiving heart transplants to hemodynamic alterations.[204] Compensatory responses may be delayed, further increasing the potential for compromise.

In the child with a transplanted heart, the resting heart rate is greater than normal because of the loss of parasympathetic inhibition. Critical determinants of cardiac output are the systemic venous return (preload dependence) and maintenance of an adequate heart rate. During the early posttransplantation period, the heart rate may be supported by exogenous chronotropes or pacing. Subsequently, circulating catecholamines drive the heart rate. Regardless of the time interval from transplantation, while caring for these children the following are recommended: (1) availability of medications with chronotropic properties and

drugs with direct action on the myocardium and vasculature, and (2) access to emergent cardiac pacing modalities (see also Chapter 18).

Long-term immunosuppression in children who have undergone cardiac transplantation presents several issues during noncardiac surgery. First, administration of multiple medications, particularly immunosuppressant agents, throughout the perioperative period is a concern. In most cases, immunosuppressant medications are continued, if feasible, to maintain adequate blood concentrations and limit the potential for rejection of the transplanted organ. Children receiving long-term corticosteroid therapy can be at risk for adrenal crisis during an acute illness or other stress, such as may be encountered during surgery or other minor procedures. The perioperative administration of corticosteroids ("stress-dose") should be considered based on the procedure and severity of the illness (anticipated stress). Second, immunosuppressive therapy is associated with adverse effects that may impact various organ systems. Cyclosporine administration, for example, increases systemic arterial blood pressure, potentially influencing hemodynamics. The drug is also responsible for renal dysfunction. Anesthesia management must consider potential alterations in hepatic and renal function. Third, strict aseptic technique is needed in managing a child with a compromised immune system in view of the infectious risk.

An additional concern is the potential for cardiac allograft vasculopathy (i.e., small-vessel coronary artery disease). Because older children or adolescents with ongoing myocardial ischemia may not experience angina symptoms, it is reasonable to assume that most of these children are at risk for ischemic events, particularly those who are several years after transplantation.

MECHANICAL CIRCULATORY SUPPORT DEVICES

In recent years, an increasing number of mechanical circulatory support devices have been implanted in children, in most cases, as a bridge to cardiac transplantation. These children may require sedation/general anesthesia for noncardiac procedures of a diagnostic or therapeutic nature, for placement of indwelling catheters used for long-term vascular access, and for other procedures. As the hardware is typically implanted at specialized cardiac centers, these children are usually well known to the anesthesia teams who are involved in multiple patient encounters during a usually relatively long hospital stay.

Several publications have highlighted the unique perioperative considerations in this patient group.[205-207] Key issues include familiarity with the various devices, their operation, control features, waveforms, and alarms.[208] In addition, it is important to understand factors that influence device output such as fluid status and systemic vascular tone. The functional status of the right heart influences device preload; thus it is important to minimize any increases in RV afterload that can compromise device filling and stroke volume. Hypotension has been described as a common occurrence during anesthesia, necessitating the administration of IV fluid and α-adrenergic agents. This may be the result of vasodilation and a decrease in systemic afterload under conditions of a fixed cardiac output delivered by the device. Preparation and immediate access to drugs with vasoactive properties is key. Although in adult patients a trend toward perioperative care by educated noncardiac anesthesiologists has been reported, the anesthesia care of these children is primarily the responsibility of specialty providers.[209]

PERIOPERATIVE STRESS RESPONSE

The typical physiologic response to painful stimuli in normal children consists of an increase in heart rate and blood pressure and a transient decrease in PaO_2. These normal patterns, however, may be detrimental to children with CHD. Tachycardia may shorten diastolic filling time and diminish cardiac output, and hypertension increases ventricular afterload. The reduced ability of the postoperative child with CHD to increase cardiac output in response to stimulation and their limited maximal exercise capacity have been well described.

Outcomes of Noncardiac Surgery

Limited data regarding the risks of noncardiac surgery and anesthesia in children with CHD raise concerns. A review of 110 children with CHD over a 1-year period undergoing noncardiac outpatient surgery found a 47% incidence of adverse events and more than one adverse event in a significant number of children.[210] In addition, the study reported an increased incidence for unplanned intensive care admission. Continuous monitoring of perioperative rhythm abnormalities in 70 children with CHD and a history of ventricular arrhythmias documented a 35% and 87% incidence of intraoperative and postoperative ventricular arrhythmias, respectively.[211] Other studies have reported cyanosis, treatment for congestive heart failure, poor health, and young age as risk factors.[40] A retrospective review of a large number of children reported that these risks involved major and minor interventions.[42]

Data from the Pediatric Perioperative Cardiac Arrest (POCA) registry shed further insight into this subject. Causes of cardiac arrest were primarily cardiovascular in nature, occurring more frequently in those with heart disease than those without. Events occurred more frequently in the general operating room, usually during the maintenance period. Two cardiac malformations stood out: children with single-ventricle physiology (particularly those managed early with palliation) and children with aortic stenosis. The overall mortality rate for children with heart disease was greater than for those without heart disease. Children with aortic stenosis (i.e., Williams syndrome) and cardiomyopathy had the greatest mortality rate.[212]

A study in children undergoing cardiac catheterization found an increased frequency of cardiac arrests in children undergoing cardiac catheterization[213]; the frequency of these events was greater compared with the incidence during pediatric noncardiac and cardiac surgery. A retrospective review of children with complex CHD identified children before stage II single-ventricle palliation, those undergoing more invasive procedures, and receiving inotropes, ACEIs, or digoxin to be at risk for intraoperative hemodynamic instability during noncardiac operations.[214] Another large database review noted that children with major and severe CHD undergoing noncardiac surgery have an increased risk of mortality and a greater incidence of life-threatening postoperative outcomes compared with matched controls of children without CHD undergoing comparable procedures.[45]

The overall data suggest that younger age, higher ASA status, severe heart disease, and emergency procedures represent risk factors for poor outcomes during noncardiac surgery in patients with CHD.

Specific Congenital Heart Defects

The provision of anesthesia care to children with CHD undergoing noncardiac surgery is strongly influenced by the specific nature of the cardiovascular anomalies, pathophysiology of the lesions, operative state (e.g., unoperated, prior palliative or definitive procedure), complications associated with the primary pathology or treatment, and other comorbidities.[35]

This section reviews selected cardiac defects with an emphasis on anatomic features, hemodynamic consequences, and treatment strategies. Potential residua, sequelae (Table 23.3), and long-term outcomes of these lesions are discussed, focusing on their implications for anesthesia care.

ATRIAL SEPTAL DEFECTS
Anatomy and Pathophysiology
Defects in the interatrial septum, or atrial septal defects (ASDs) (see Fig. 17.1), are among the most common congenital cardiac anomalies (30%–40% of CHD) in childhood. ASDs occur in 1 of 1500 live births. Based on their location, several types of defects are identified:

- *Ostium secundum or fossa ovalis defect* (75% of ASDs) results from a deficiency in the region of the fossa ovalis, representing a true defect in the atrial septum (see Fig. 17.1B). These defects can be associated with mitral valve prolapse and/or mitral regurgitation.[215–217]
- *Ostium primum defect* (15%–20% of ASDs) represents a form of AV septal (canal or endocardial cushion) defect (see Fig. 17.1A).[218] The malformation is characterized by a deficiency in the inferior portion of the interatrial septum and is frequently associated with a commissure or cleft in the anterior leaflet of the mitral valve and various degrees of mitral regurgitation.
- *Sinus venosus defect* (5%–10% of ASDs) typically is located at the superior aspect of the interatrial septum, at the junction of the superior vena cava and the right atrium (i.e., superior vena cava type) (see Fig. 17.1C).[219] An inferior-type defect (at the inferior vena cava) is less common. These defects are frequently associated with partial anomalous pulmonary venous drainage.[220]
- *Coronary sinus defect* (uncommon) consists of a communication between the atria through the mouth of the coronary sinus. Left-to-right shunting occurs across an "unroofed" coronary sinus. It is often associated with a persistent left superior vena cava that drains directly into the left atrium, resulting in a right-to-left shunt.[221]
- *Other entities* that may allow for interatrial shunting include a *patent foramen ovale* (PFO) at one end of the spectrum and a *common atrium* at the other. A PFO is a flap-like opening or channel between the two septa (septum primum and septum secundum) that divides the primordial single atrium into right and left atrial chambers. This structure can be identified in approximately 25% of individuals. The communication may have implications for perioperative care because of the potential for right-to-left shunting and paradoxical emboli under certain circumstances.[222,223] In a common atrium, there is complete or near-total absence of the interatrial septum. This can be seen in complex congenital cardiac pathologies.

An atrial communication allows mixing of the pulmonary and systemic venous returns. A left-to-right shunt permits pulmonary venous blood to enter the right atrium. The magnitude of shunting correlates with the size of the defect, relative ventricular compliances, and pulmonary artery pressures. A clinically significant defect results in right-sided volume overload. A pulmonary-to-systemic blood flow ratio ($\dot{Q}_{pulm}/\dot{Q}_{sys}$) that exceeds 2:1 and the potential detrimental effects of chronic right-sided volume overload are indications for intervention.

Treatment Options, Residua, Sequelae, and Long-Term Outcomes
Surgical closure of secundum ASDs in childhood provides excellent results, almost normal long-term survival, and negligible

| TABLE 23.3 | Potential Issues After Interventions for Selected Congenital Heart Defects |

Atrial Septal Defects

Residual intracardiac shunt

Persistent right ventricular dilation and abnormal motion of interventricular septum

Atrial arrhythmias, ventricular dysfunction if late repair

Pulmonary venous obstruction (sinus venosus defect associated with anomalous pulmonary venous return)

Mitral valve problems, left ventricular outflow tract obstruction (ostium primum defect with cleft mitral valve)

Development of pulmonary vascular disease (rare)

Atrioventricular Septal Defects

Mitral valve problems (regurgitation, stenosis)

Left ventricular outflow tract obstruction

Residual intracardiac shunts

Atrioventricular block, conduction abnormalities

Prior palliation with pulmonary artery banding might have resulted in inadequate protection of pulmonary vasculature or distortion of pulmonary artery anatomy

Pulmonary hypertension may persist

Coarctation of the Aorta

Systemic hypertension

Residual or recurrent obstruction

Death from untreated pathology related to heart failure, aortic rupture or dissection, infective endarteritis or endocarditis, premature coronary artery disease, or cerebral hemorrhage

Endocarditis risk with concomitant aortic valve disease

Congenitally Corrected Transposition of the Great Arteries

Residual defects (e.g., shunts, outflow tract obstruction)

Systemic (right) ventricular dilation, dysfunction, failure

Left-sided (tricuspid) valve regurgitation

Atrioventricular block or arrhythmias

Coronary artery anomalies

May go unsuspected for some time

Myocardial ischemia

Ventricular dysfunction

May present as syncope, or lead to sudden death

D-Transposition of the Great Arteries

Residual pathology (e.g., intracardiac shunts, outflow tract obstruction)

After atrial baffle procedure: baffle leak, obstruction of systemic or pulmonary venous pathways, progressive right ventricular dilation or failure, tricuspid regurgitation, sinus node dysfunction, or atrial arrhythmias

After arterial switch operation: aortic root dilation, aortic regurgitation, supravalvar stenosis (pulmonary or aortic), or coronary insufficiency

Ebstein Anomaly

Progressive tricuspid regurgitation and right-sided volume overload

Right ventricular dysfunction

Atrial tachyarrhythmias (particularly if Wolff-Parkinson-White syndrome)

Potential for paradoxical right-to-left shunting in the presence of an interatrial communication

Valve repair or replacement may be necessary

Interrupted Aortic Arch

Residual intracardiac defects

Subaortic obstruction

Residual or recurrent aortic arch obstruction

Left Ventricular Outflow Tract Obstructions

Residual or recurrent obstruction

Aortic regurgitation, aortic root dilation

Risk of endocarditis

Ventricular dysfunction

Potential subendocardial ischemia if ongoing ventricular pressure overload

Coronary ostial stenosis, diffuse arteriopathy (supravalvar aortic stenosis)

Need for reoperation in those with bioprosthetic or mechanical valves or conduits

After Ross procedure: autograft or right ventricular homograft failure, progressive aortic root dilation, or aortic regurgitation

Patent Ductus Arteriosus

Residual or recurrent shunting

Increased pulmonary vascular resistance (now rare)

Right Ventricular Outflow Tract Obstructions

Residual or recurrent obstruction resulting in ventricular pressure overload

Pulmonary regurgitation may require intervention

After right ventricle–to–pulmonary artery conduit: need for intervention or reoperation related to conduit failure

Single Ventricle

After aortopulmonary shunt: shunt stenosis with associated hypoxemia, ventricular volume overload, systemic ventricular dilation, distortion of pulmonary artery anatomy, or pulmonary hypertension

After bidirectional Glenn connection or hemi-Fontan procedure: progressive cyanosis owing to venous collaterals or other vascular communications, allowing venous pathways to bypass the pulmonary circuit or owing to development of pulmonary arteriovenous malformations (more likely with classic Glenn anastomosis)

After Fontan procedure: increased systemic venous pressures, right atrial hypertension (with atriopulmonary connection), sinus node dysfunction, atrial rhythm disturbances, atrioventricular valve regurgitation, hepatic dysfunction, thrombotic complications, coagulation defects, protein losing enteropathy, or progressive systemic ventricular dilation or dysfunction

Tetralogy of Fallot

Residual or recurrent pathology (e.g., intracardiac shunts, right ventricular outflow tract obstruction, distal pulmonary artery bed abnormalities)

Progressive pulmonary regurgitation with need for repeat intervention (e.g., right-sided heart dilation, dysfunction)

Arrhythmias associated with poor hemodynamics

Syncope or sudden death (arrhythmogenic cause)

Restrictive right ventricular physiology

Truncus Arteriosus

Residual intracardiac shunting

Revision of right ventricle–to–pulmonary artery reconstruction (for stenosis or regurgitation)

Truncal (aortic) valve stenosis or regurgitation

Ventricular Septal Defect

Potential residual defects

Risk of endocarditis (diminishes with time after repair)

Aortic regurgitation

Rarely, increased pulmonary vascular resistance may not improve postoperatively mortality.[224-227] Normal ventricular function should be anticipated after repair of these defects. Rarely, children can demonstrate persistent RV dilation and abnormal ventricular septal motion, but this may not result in a functional deficit.[228] Atrial arrhythmias and ventricular dysfunction can occur after late repairs owing to chronic volume overload. Delayed defect closure can be a risk factor for the rare development of pulmonary hypertension later in life as the result the chronic abnormally increased pulmonary blood flow.[229]

Transcatheter device occlusion is an alternative approach to surgery for closure of secundum ASDs in selected children, with excellent success rates (see Chapter 22).[230-232] Complications are rare and may be associated with the catheter-based procedure or occur at a later time.[233]

After surgical closure of ostium primum defects, morbidity manifests primarily as mitral valve dysfunction (e.g., mitral regurgitation or stenosis) and LVOT obstruction.[234-238] In most children, outcomes are favorable after repair at an early age. After closure of sinus venosus defects, potential problems include pulmonary venous obstruction and loss of sinus node function.[239-241] Repair of coronary sinus defects depends on the specific nature of the defect and associated anomalies. The intervention consists of redirection of the coronary sinus blood and possibly the associated abnormal systemic venous return to the right atrium. Patch closure of the atrial communication at the mouth of the coronary sinus may be all that is required in some cases, leaving a small right-to-left shunt as deoxygenated blood from the coronary sinus continues to drain directly into the left atrium.[242] For most children with atrial communications, significant postoperative sequelae are unlikely to occur, and outcomes are generally good.

An important consideration in the child with an interatrial communication is the avoidance of IV air in view of the potential for gas embolism. In most cases, no major repercussion from a repaired defect should be expected for future anesthesia care.

VENTRICULAR SEPTAL DEFECTS
Anatomy and Pathophysiology
Ventricular septal defects (VSDs) are the most common of all congenital cardiac anomalies, occurring in 30% to 60% of CHD (excluding a bicuspid aortic valve) with an incidence of 2 to 6 cases per 1000 live births (see Fig. 17.2A).[243] VSDs can be found in isolation or within the context of other structural malformations. Large defects require early attention for symptoms related to congestive heart failure or pulmonary hypertension. VSDs have a greater rate of spontaneous closure in childhood—about 75% closure by 6 months to 1 year.[244,245]

Various classification schemes have been proposed for VSDs based on their anatomic location, size, restrictive versus nonrestrictive nature, and hemodynamic significance.[246,247] The following scheme categorizes defects as four major morphologic types based on their anatomic location. In some cases, the boundaries of a defect extend beyond the margin of a particular region of the ventricular septum into another and these are qualified as such.

- *Perimembranous defects* (most common type) are located in the membranous region, under the septal leaflet of the tricuspid valve and just below the level of the aortic valve. They are frequently associated with redundant septal tricuspid valve tissue (e.g., aneurysmal tissue) that may limit shunting or eventually result in complete defect closure.
- *Muscular defects* are located anywhere within the trabecular (muscle-bound) component of the ventricular septum. Multiple defects give the appearance of a "Swiss cheese" septum, which complicates surgical closure.
- *Doubly committed, subarterial, conal, or supracristal defects* are found within the region of the subpulmonary infundibulum. They can be associated with aortic valve herniation or prolapse into the defect and aortic regurgitation.[248]
- *Inlet defects* are located in the posterior aspect of the ventricular septum near the AV valves. Associated anomalies of the AV valves frequently coexist.

The characterization of VSDs based on their size and likely hemodynamic importance is extremely useful when caring for unoperated children:

- *Small defect:* The pulmonary-to-systemic systolic pressure ratio is less than 0.3 and the $\dot{Q}_{pulm}/\dot{Q}_{sys}$ is less than 1.4. The defect causes negligible to minimal hemodynamic effects. Normal RV systolic pressure, pulmonary vascular resistance, and LV size are typically found.
- *Moderate defect:* The systolic pressure ratio is greater than 0.3 and the $\dot{Q}_{pulm}/\dot{Q}_{sys}$ is 1.4 to 2.2. The defect can be associated with volume overload and congestive symptoms. Some degree of left atrial and LV dilation exists, as well as elevated pulmonary artery pressures.
- *Large defect:* The systolic pressure ratio is greater than 0.3 and the $\dot{Q}_{pulm}/\dot{Q}_{sys}$ exceeds 2.2. The defect is associated with significant symptoms (e.g., failure to thrive, congestive heart failure). Cardiomegaly and increased pulmonary vascularity are usual findings.

The physiologic effects of the communications that allow for ventricular-level shunting are determined by factors such as the size of the defect, amount of shunting, and relative pulmonary and systemic vascular resistances. Physiologically, isolated defects can be classified as pressure restrictive (i.e., RV pressure < LV pressure) or nonrestrictive defects (i.e., equal or near-equal ventricular pressures). Restrictive defects often imply limited flow through the communication. This is usually the case with small VSDs in which the pressure gradient determines the magnitude of shunting. If the defect is large and nonrestrictive, the amount of shunting depends on the ratio between the pulmonary and systemic vascular resistances. A low pulmonary vascular resistance in the context of a nonrestrictive VSD leads to a large left-to-right shunt, increased pulmonary blood flow, pulmonary hypertension, and increased myocardial work, as evidenced by a volume load to the left heart. Nonrestrictive left-to-right shunts result in pulmonary congestion and abnormal respiratory mechanics characterized by decreased lung compliance, increased airway resistance, and increased work of breathing. Increases in alveolar dead space and alveolar to arterial oxygen gradients are to be expected, as well as increases in minute ventilation and potential oxygen requirements.

An important perioperative consideration for children with defects associated with increased pulmonary blood flow is the pulmonary steal phenomenon, which may result from decreases in pulmonary vascular resistance as left-to-right shunting increases at the expense of systemic blood flow. This requires an appraisal of the factors that may influence pulmonary vascular tone to prevent compromises in systemic output.

Treatment Options, Residua, Sequelae, and Long-Term Outcomes
Surgical closure of VSDs early in childhood results in excellent outcomes, usually without sequelae.[249-251] Surgical intervention in older children may lead to reduced LV function and increased LV mass.[252]

Small communications, although regarded as hemodynamically insignificant, may not be benign. This has led to ongoing controversy regarding the need for definitive intervention. Occasionally a young child with a defect of moderate size remains relatively asymptomatic until later life, when gradual decompensation may ensue related to increased end-diastolic volume and ventricular dilation. Defect closure in this setting is indicated if the magnitude of the increase in pulmonary vascular resistance is not prohibitive, which would be extremely rare. Severely increased pulmonary vascular resistance (more than 7 Wood units/m^2) increases the perioperative risks, and it may not return to normal levels after the surgical intervention.[253] If postoperative pulmonary hypertension persists, the prognosis is unfavorable, with the potential for eventual RV failure.[254] Development of Eisenmenger syndrome (i.e., pulmonary vascular obstructive disease and reversal in the direction of the ventricular level shunt) has become rare owing to early recognition and management of children with these defects.

Postoperative sequelae after VSD closure include residual or, less commonly, recurrent defects, arrhythmias or other conduction system disturbances, subaortic obstruction, and valvar regurgitation.[255] Although surgical closure is considered the gold standard, transcatheter closure by device placement is feasible for selected defects, typically muscular and postoperative residual defects.[256,257] Results to date demonstrate excellent closure rates with reduced rates of complications[258] (see also Chapter 22). Limited experience and follow-up are available with catheter-based interventions for closure of membranous communications.[259–262] In view of associated substantial risk of complete AV block with the initial occluder device, a newer-generation device (Amplatzer membranous VSD occluder, St. Jude Medical, Inc., St. Paul, MN) is favored.[263,264]

Children with a small defect or without residual pathology after undergoing VSD closure often have normal ventricular systolic function and should be expected to do well during future noncardiac procedures.

ATRIOVENTRICULAR SEPTAL DEFECTS
Anatomy and Pathophysiology
Atrioventricular septal defects (AVSDs), also referred to as AV canal defects or endocardial cushion defects, are characterized by deficiency of the AV septum and abnormal formation of the AV valves (see Fig. 17.2B).[265] These defects represent only 4% of CHD cases, although they have a high prevalence among patients with Down syndrome (25%). Although the nomenclature of AVSDs has been the subject of confusion and even controversy, in general the lesions that represent the spectrum of pathologies can be classified as follows:

1. The *complete form* (i.e., common AV canal defect) consists of an ostium primum defect and an interventricular communication at the superior aspect of the inlet or posterior muscular septum (contiguous defects), and a large common AV valve. They are frequently associated with various degrees of AV valve regurgitation.

2. The *partial form* (i.e., incomplete form) is usually characterized by an ostium primum ASD accompanied by a cleft or commissure in the left-sided AV valve. Two functionally distinct AV valvar orifices are usually identified (see "Atrial Septal Defects").

3. The *transitional or intermediate forms* represent variants of AVSDs. When considered as separate entities, a transitional defect is regarded as a partial form of the defect characterized by a primum ASD, a small inlet VSD (usually restrictive), and two distinct AV valve components. An intermediate defect refers

to a variant of the complete form of the defect characterized by a primum ASD and a nonrestrictive VSD in the setting of a common AV valve annulus and two distinct AV valvar orifices separated by a tongue of tissue.

Complete defects are associated with nonrestrictive intracardiac shunting, excessive pulmonary blood flow, congestive heart failure, and systemic RV and pulmonary artery systolic pressures. Without intervention, they can lead to early pulmonary vascular changes. The severity of AV valve regurgitation also influences the clinical presentation. Partial AVSDs are less likely to be associated with pulmonary overcirculation of sufficient severity to cause significant heart failure.

Perioperative concerns like those previously described in children with nonrestrictive ventricular communications are applicable, but they also are magnified in those with unrepaired complete defects. In children with unrepaired defects with increased pulmonary vascular resistance and a reactive pulmonary bed, issues such as airway manipulation, light anesthesia, hypoxemia, or hypercarbia can lead to acute increases in pulmonary artery pressures to suprasystemic levels and detrimental hemodynamic consequences.

Treatment Options, Residua, Sequelae, and Long-Term Outcomes
The surgical approach for complete defects has evolved from a two-stage intervention (i.e., initial pulmonary artery banding aimed at limiting pulmonary blood flow and subsequent complete repair) to a single strategy of primary repair in infancy. In the case of a complete defect, the intervention consists of patch closure of the intracardiac communications, partition of the common AV valve, and closure of the left-sided valvar cleft (otherwise known as the zone of apposition). The long-term outlook after repair is generally good, with a small likelihood of residual dysfunction.[266-268]

Postoperative problems include left AV valve regurgitation or stenosis, residual intracardiac shunting, AV block, and subaortic obstruction.[237,238] Occasionally, pulmonary hypertension persists or develops postoperatively; it is more likely in children with Down syndrome. In the remote past, uncorrected defects associated with high pressure and high flow resulted in muscular development of the pulmonary vasculature and Eisenmenger physiology, accounting for significant late morbidity and early death.[269] As mentioned, these patients are at high risk for anesthesia for any procedure.

RIGHT VENTRICULAR OUTFLOW TRACT OBSTRUCTIONS
Anatomy and Pathophysiology
Pulmonary valve stenosis is the most common pathology among children with RVOT obstruction.[270] Other lesions that result in obstruction to pulmonary blood flow include infundibular (subpulmonary) stenosis, anomalous muscle bundles within the body of the right ventricle, and structural alterations in the pulmonary arterial bed. These pathologies may be found in isolation or occur as part of more complex malformations. Such is the case in tetralogy of Fallot (discussed later), in which multiple anatomic levels of RVOT obstruction are typically encountered (see Fig. 17.5).

Although isolated valvar pulmonary stenosis is congenital in most cases, the disease can be progressive. In the uncomplicated or pure variant, an interatrial communication in the form of a PFO or secundum ASD may be identified, and the ventricular septum is intact.

The magnitude of RVOT obstruction is directly related to the degree of valvar narrowing. This imposes an afterload burden on the right ventricle, resulting in RV hypertrophy and decreased ventricular diastolic compliance. Tricuspid regurgitation may be an associated finding. In severe cases, the RV systolic pressure may exceed that of the left ventricle. Cyanosis in children with pulmonary stenosis usually reflects right-to-left interatrial shunting and reduced pulmonary blood flow. It can be associated with severe RV hypertrophy, myocardial fibrosis, or ventricular dysfunction.

Most children with mild to moderate valvar stenosis remain asymptomatic, and the pathology is relatively well tolerated chronically. Severe obstruction in older children is frequently associated with limited exercise tolerance. Subendocardial ischemia is a potential risk in children with a hypertensive, hypertrophied right ventricle. Management is directed at maintaining coronary perfusion and the inotropic state of the myocardium.

Treatment Options, Residua, Sequelae, and Long-Term Outcomes

Percutaneous balloon valvuloplasty is very effective and currently is considered the treatment of choice for isolated valvar pulmonary stenosis, replacing surgical valvotomy in most cases. Outcomes are excellent, and long-term issues are rare.[271-273] Dysplastic valves have a less favorable response to catheter-based interventions, and affected children are more likely to require surgery. Indications for repeat intervention include residual outflow tract obstruction and progressive pulmonary regurgitation.[274]

In children with significant RV hypertrophy undergoing noncardiac surgery, adequate ventricular preload and optimization of volume status are recommended. Further increases in RV afterload should be avoided in those with residual or recurrent outflow tract obstruction.

LEFT VENTRICULAR OUTFLOW TRACT OBSTRUCTIONS
Anatomy and Pathophysiology

LV outflow tract (LVOT) obstruction may occur at the level of the aortic valve, supravalvar region, or subvalvar region. It may take place in isolation or as part of complex cardiovascular disease. A *bicuspid aortic valve* is the most common of all congenital cardiac anomalies, occurring in approximately 2% of the general population.[275] Although it may not necessarily imply valvar stenosis, this abnormality can be associated with progressive obstruction or regurgitation as well as aortic root dilation. A bicuspid valve can be found in asymptomatic individuals or within the context of severe left heart obstruction. The prevalence of coexistent defects is relatively high and frequently includes PDA, VSD, aortic coarctation, and other abnormalities of the aorta and its branches.

Infants with critical aortic stenosis and those with severe obstruction require early intervention based on ductal dependency for systemic blood flow, heart failure symptoms, and the degree of ventricular dysfunction. Older children with moderate to severe obstruction can present with decreased exercise tolerance, syncopal episodes, or myocardial ischemia. Impedance to LV ejection in aortic stenosis results in elevation of LV systolic pressure and increased myocardial work. Ventricular hypertrophy is the compensatory response to the increased afterload. Contractile function is normal to increased, but diastolic impairment can occur.

In *supravalvar aortic stenosis,* the narrowing usually occurs at the sinotubular junction. The coronary arteries arise proximal to the area of obstruction and are subjected to increased systolic pressures equal to that of the left ventricle. This pathology is seen most commonly in children with Williams syndrome (also known as Williams-Beuren syndrome). Elfin facies, developmental delay,

idiopathic hypercalcemia, and other features characterize the disorder. The associated arteriopathy can involve the origin of the coronary arteries and/or other systemic and pulmonary vessels.[276] Several reports have described unexpected complications in these children, including cardiac arrest during anesthesia care.[277-281] In view of the increased risk for cardiovascular decompensation and frequently unsuccessful resuscitative efforts, careful perioperative/procedural planning is highly advised in children with Williams syndrome.[282] Care should ideally be provided by pediatric anesthesiologists familiar with the syndrome and at facilities with the infrastructure capable of providing the necessary support for these children during an acute event. Affected children should be considered at increased risk for any procedure.

Subvalvar aortic stenosis may take a variety of forms, including a discrete fibromuscular ridge or membrane, complex tunnel-like obstruction, or hypertrophy of the interventricular septum (i.e., hypertrophic cardiomyopathy). The association of LV pathology of an obstructive nature such as a bicuspid aortic valve, subaortic stenosis, aortic coarctation, and mitral valve inflow obstruction (e.g., parachute mitral valve, supravalvar mitral ring) is referred to as the *Shone complex.*

Hypoplastic left heart syndrome (HLHS) represents an extreme form of LVOT obstruction (see Fig. 17.10). It encompasses a constellation of malformations, affecting left-sided cardiac structures (e.g., mitral and aortic valves, aorta, aortic arch) (see "Single Ventricle").

Common features of the anomalies that result in obstruction to LV output include a pressure gradient across the involved region, increased LV systolic pressure, altered myocardial force, and LV wall stress. With chronic obstruction, the hypertrophied myocardium is at risk for subendocardial ischemia because of an imbalance in the ratio between myocardial oxygen supply and demand. Factors such as increases in LV afterload, inadequate hypertrophic remodeling, and decreases in myocardial systolic or diastolic performance can compromise stroke volume and contribute to cardiac dysfunction and heart failure.[283] These issues are relevant for children with more than mild obstruction, and they influence anesthesia care during noncardiac surgery or other interventions.

Treatment Options, Residua, Sequelae, and Long-Term Outcomes

Individuals with a bicuspid aortic valve can remain asymptomatic for many years but are at risk for developing aortic stenosis or regurgitation and concomitant hemodynamic alterations. Some of those requiring surgical intervention during childhood undergo reoperation for recurrent stenosis or progressive regurgitation in the next 25 years.[284] Percutaneous balloon valvuloplasty may be a treatment option for critical or severe aortic valve disease.[285] Surgical alternatives include valvotomy, mechanical or bioprosthetic valve placement, and root replacement with homograft or autograft material. In the Ross operation, the native, diseased root is replaced by a pulmonary autograft, and an extracardiac conduit establishes continuity between the right ventricle and main pulmonary artery.[286] Repeat intervention for eventual failure of the RV conduit is anticipated in these children.[287] In addition to surveillance of the RVOT, monitoring for aortic root dilation and concomitant regurgitation is an important component of follow-up.[288,289] Ascending aorta aneurysm formation, dissection, and rupture also represent long-term concerns.

Management of discrete subaortic stenosis and the timing of surgery are controversial.[290] Postoperative issues include residual or recurrent obstruction and progressive aortic regurgitation. For severe supravalvar obstruction, surgical intervention is recommended, resulting in adequate relief of the obstruction in most cases.[291]

Myocardial fibrosis and ventricular dysfunction can be a feature of severe aortic outflow obstruction in infancy. Although adequate relief of the obstruction results in significant clinical improvement, abolition of congestive heart failure symptoms, and myocardial remodeling in most children, ventricular hypertrophy or dilation persists along with various degrees of systolic or diastolic impairment in many. Other problems include myocardial ischemia, ventricular failure, and risk of sudden death.[292,293] Important concerns related to anesthesia and surgery are the potentially limited LV functional reserve and alterations of the fine balance between myocardial oxygen supply and demand. Maintenance of coronary perfusion and ventricular contractile function is key in the care of these children. Pharmacologic agents with vasoactive and inotropic properties should be readily available during anesthesia care.

PATENT DUCTUS ARTERIOSUS

Anatomy and Pathophysiology

The ductus arteriosus is an essential vascular structure in fetal life that connects the pulmonary trunk and thoracic aorta (see Figs. 17.4 and 18.1). It enables RV output into the descending aorta in the fetus, within the context of normally increased pulmonary vascular resistance. Persistent PDA can be an isolated finding or can be associated with other forms of heart disease. Prematurity is an important risk factor.

The magnitude and direction of great artery shunting depends on the size of the communication and the pulmonary vascular resistance. In children with moderate or large left-to-right shunts, the physiologic effects are those of increased pulmonary blood flow and LV volume overload.

Treatment Options, Residua, Sequelae, and Long-Term Outcomes

Children with a tiny or small PDA have a normal life expectancy.[294] Those with hemodynamically significant communications eventually develop symptoms related to LV volume overload. In some cases, this predisposes them to pulmonary hypertension. Although unlikely in the current era, in the past, the long-standing high-pressure and high-flow states associated with a moderate or large patent ductus resulted in Eisenmenger syndrome in some children.

Ductal closure can be performed by surgical ligation or division. Surgery is the favored approach in preterm infants and those with large communications.[295] Percutaneous catheter occlusion can also be accomplished with a good success rate in infants and children[296] (see also Chapter 22). Ductal ligation can also be performed using video-assisted thoracoscopic surgery.[297,298] Regardless of the approach, interruption of this vascular structure is rarely associated with long-term issues. Children can expect a normal cardiovascular reserve and should be managed accordingly during future anesthesia care.

COARCTATION OF THE AORTA

Anatomy and Pathophysiology

Coarctation of the aorta is characterized by narrowing of the aortic lumen in the thoracic region. The constriction can be discrete or diffuse. In infants, a long, narrowed aortic segment often is associated with hypoplasia of the transverse arch and aortic isthmus, in which case other structural cardiac malformations may also be present.[299] Associated defects include a bicuspid aortic valve, VSD, mitral valve abnormalities, and other types of left-sided obstructive lesions. In the neonate, if the aortic arch pathology is severe, it

can represent a ductal-dependent lesion for systemic blood flow. Hemodynamic consequences result from obstruction to systemic blood flow and increased LV afterload. During infancy, ventricular dilation and heart failure predominate.

In older children, the presentation is usually that of arterial hypertension, with a gradient between the upper and lower extremities. There is usually an element of LV hypertrophy although ventricular function is well preserved. Collateral circulation develops when the pathology is long-standing.

Treatment Options, Residua, Sequelae, and Long-Term Outcomes

Symptoms associated with severe aortic arch obstruction or concomitant cardiovascular pathology lead to early intervention.[300] In the neonate, alterations in ventricular systolic function usually resolve after relief of the obstruction. Systemic hypertension and a residual gradient that exceeds 25 to 30 mm Hg are regarded as indications for reintervention. Various catheter-based and surgical approaches have been applied to the management of this lesion; each has advantages and disadvantages[301] (see also Chapter 22).

Repair at an early age is advocated in consideration of the reduced surgical risks for the younger age group and minimization of late morbidity with an early repair.[302] Long-term issues include systemic hypertension (independent of the hemodynamic result) and residual or recurrent aortic arch obstruction.[303] LV hypertrophy may persist in some children after repair, particularly in those undergoing interventions later in childhood. Abnormalities in diastolic ventricular function have been reported after successful repair.[304] Catheter techniques (i.e., balloon angioplasty with and without stent implantation) have been effective in relieving the obstruction and normalizing blood pressure.[305] This approach may be used either as primary therapy or to address residual or recurrent disease.[306] Aortic aneurysms can occur around the area of coarctation or elsewhere in the aorta after surgical intervention or balloon angioplasty. Additional long-term problems result from coexistent defects, such as bicuspid aortic valve and premature development of coronary artery disease. Aortic coarctation has been associated with cerebral aneurysms. Most children whose arch defects have been repaired, however, have essentially normal cardiac function when presenting for noncardiac procedures.

TETRALOGY OF FALLOT

Anatomy and Pathophysiology

Tetralogy of Fallot (TOF) is the most common cyanotic cardiac lesion (see Fig. 17.5).[307] This malformation is characterized by RVOT obstruction/pulmonary stenosis, an interventricular communication, RV hypertrophy, and aortic override. There is considerable variation in the severity of the disease, accounting for the wide clinical spectrum. The subpulmonary obstruction is due to anterior deviation of the infundibular septum and typically has both dynamic and fixed components.[308] Pulmonary valve stenosis almost invariably exists, and the main pulmonary artery and distal branches often demonstrate various degrees of hypoplasia. The limitation of pulmonary blood flow and magnitude of ventricular level right-to-left shunting account for the degree of cyanosis.

Pressure overload results in hypertrophy of the RV myocardium. The large, nonrestrictive VSD and the outflow obstruction account for a RV pressure at systemic levels while the pulmonary artery systolic pressure in the classic form of TOF remains normal. Increases in the severity of the RVOT obstruction (infundibular spasm) or decreases in systemic vascular resistance exacerbate right-to-left intracardiac shunting and systemic arterial desaturation, increasing the level of cyanosis. These features characterize hypercyanctic episodes or tet spells in unoperated children. These spells are triggered by catecholamine release owing to pain, stress, and light anesthesia. In infants, the spells may be due to emotional upset. Treatment involves volume administration to augment RV preload and stroke volume, increasing the level of sedation or anesthesia, avoidance of exogenous catecholamines, and increasing systemic vascular resistance to enhance left-to-right shunting or minimize the amount of blood shunted in the right-to-left direction. Although the pulmonary vascular tone does not play a major role in this physiology, it is prudent to administer oxygen or increase the inspired oxygen concentration and limit factors that may increase pulmonary vascular tone and further impede pulmonary blood flow.

Several TOF variants are recognized, including the "pink" or mild forms at one end of the spectrum, and complex defects, such as pulmonary atresia with diminutive or discontinuous distal pulmonary artery branches, at the other. Associated cardiovascular anomalies in children with TOF include an atrial communication, right aortic arch, multiple VSDs, persistent left superior vena cava to the coronary sinus, complete AVSD, and abnormal origin or course of the coronary arteries.

Treatment Options, Residua, Sequelae, and Long-Term Outcomes

The surgical management of TOF has evolved from a strategy of a staged approach with initial palliation using a systemic-to-pulmonary shunt to a single-stage, definitive repair in infants. Ongoing controversy exists about the favored approach in the neonate or very young infant in need of an intervention.[309,310] In selected cases, percutaneous balloon pulmonary valvuloplasty has been performed as a palliative, temporizing measure.[311] The definitive repair of TOF, although a successful operation enabling most children to be free of symptoms, can be associated with significant postoperative residua.[312,313] Volume loads arise from pulmonary regurgitation, residual shunts, and the presence of aortopulmonary collaterals. Ventricular pressure loads can result from residual or recurrent obstruction of the RVOT or the pulmonary arteries. This pathology is associated with RV hypertension, myocardial hypertrophy, and reduced ventricular compliance.

Conditions that can require repeat intervention in TOF include pulmonary regurgitation, residual or recurrent pulmonary outflow tract obstruction, and hemodynamically significant residual intracardiac shunts. Catheter-based procedures can be effective in the management of obstruction of the pulmonary vasculature and have been applied to rehabilitate the vascular tree in cases of significant underdevelopment. Children who have undergone right ventricle–to–pulmonary artery reconstruction by means of placement of an extracardiac conduit eventually develop conduit failure (i.e., stenosis or regurgitation) requiring catheter interventions or reoperation.[314] Percutaneous valves that can be implanted in pulmonary position are now available, precluding the need for surgical valve replacement in some patients. Aortic root dilation can lead to increasing degrees of regurgitation and the need for surgery.

In the past, most children underwent definitive repair at an older age, consisting of an extensive right ventriculotomy to facilitate resection of the infundibular obstruction and closure of the VSD. Many were also subjected to procedures that included placement of a large patch that encompassed the subpulmonic region, valve annulus, and supravalvar region (i.e., transannular patch). Although effective in relieving the obstruction, this approach invariably resulted in pulmonary regurgitation, which was reasonably well tolerated but progressed over time.

On late follow-up, pulmonary regurgitation has been identified as a major cause of morbidity, and it may result in progressive RV dysfunction owing to volume overload, ventricular arrhythmias with their associated disabilities, and even sudden death. In recognition of the long-term morbidity linked to severe pulmonary regurgitation, the surgical strategy for this defect has undergone reappraisal and modification over the years.[315] A current method uses a transatrial approach for closure of the VSD, minimizing the size of an infundibular incision (if one is required), and avoiding or limiting the size of the transannular patch.[316,317]

Although surgical refinements have led to overall improvements in postoperative outcomes, the preoperative evaluation of these children for noncardiac surgery should include inquiries regarding exercise tolerance as an indicator of functional status and an appraisal of RV function, residual pathology, potential rhythm abnormalities, and conduction disturbances. Review of data obtained by surveillance echocardiography is important in planning an anesthetic. Magnetic resonance imaging is extremely useful in the evaluation of RV systolic function, quantitation of the severity of pulmonary regurgitation, and evaluation of the distal pulmonary vascular bed. If available, the results of these studies should also be reviewed. Electrophysiologic testing and programmed ventricular stimulation may be indicated to refine antiarrhythmic drug therapy, for ablation of arrhythmia foci, or for implantation of a cardioverter-defibrillator system.

After corrective surgery, a subset of children develops a pattern that is characterized by RV diastolic noncompliance, which is known as *restrictive RV physiology*. This may have acute and chronic consequences. In the late postoperative follow-up, it is associated with a reduced likelihood of progressive pulmonary regurgitation and RV dilation. The right ventricle operates at a greater end-diastolic pressure in this setting, and affected individuals demonstrate superior exercise performance in addition to a reduced likelihood of developing ventricular rhythm abnormalities.[318]

Perioperative goals for the child with pulmonary regurgitation and RV dysfunction include optimizing RV filling, maintaining or supporting RV function, and minimizing factors that may further increase RV work (e.g., increased pulmonary vascular resistance, increased peak inspiratory pressures). Any detrimental factor that may affect the right ventricle can also negatively affect the left ventricle owing to the phenomenon of ventricular interdependence.

D-TRANSPOSITION OF THE GREAT ARTERIES
Anatomy and Pathophysiology

In D-transposition of the great arteries (D-TGA), the aorta arises from the anatomic right ventricle, and the pulmonary artery arises from the left ventricle (see Fig. 17.6). This anomaly accounts for the most common cause of cyanotic heart disease in the neonatal period. Associated defects include VSDs, LVOT obstruction, and coronary artery anomalies.

In D-TGA, the systemic and pulmonary circulations operate in parallel rather than in series, resulting in cyanosis. Mixing at the atrial, ventricular, or ductal level is essential for survival. Initial management in most infants includes prostaglandin E_1 therapy to maintain ductal patency and to enhance intercirculatory mixing. If restrictive, the interatrial communication may require enlargement by balloon atrial septostomy.

Because most neonates with D-TGA are otherwise healthy, the concerns before surgical correction primarily are those associated with diagnostic procedures or interventions in the cardiac catheterization laboratory. Considerations for anesthetic management primarily are related to cyanosis. An inadequate communication for intercirculatory mixing results in significant hypoxemia, potentially progressing to metabolic acidosis caused by compromised tissue oxygenation. Less commonly, increased pulmonary vascular resistance may account for severe cyanosis despite prostaglandin E₁ therapy and an adequate anatomic communication.

Treatment Options, Residua, Sequelae, and Long-Term Outcomes

The approach to D-TGA many decades ago consisted of an atrial baffle (i.e., atrial switch) or redirection procedure (i.e., Mustard or Senning operations). Physiologic correction was accomplished by allowing systemic venous blood to enter the left ventricle and pulmonary artery while pulmonary venous blood was rerouted through the tricuspid valve into the right ventricle and aorta. The right ventricle remained as the chamber ejecting against systemic afterload. These procedures, while relieving cyanosis and allowing reasonably good survival,[319] led to long-term complications such as sinus node dysfunction and atrial rhythm disturbances.[320] Progressive RV dilation, tricuspid (i.e., systemic AV valve) annular dilation, associated regurgitation, and eventual RV dysfunction or failure were causes of major morbidity.[321-323] In addition to the rhythm abnormalities and conduction defects, this problem was thought to account for sudden death in some individuals later in life. Other problems included progressive obstruction of venous pathways and atrial baffle leaks with associated intracardiac shunting. Abnormal RV and LV responses to exercise have also been reported in these patients.[324]

The arterial switch operation (i.e., Jatene procedure) is considered the standard surgical approach in neonates with D-TGA. The repair establishes a normal, concordant relationship between the ventricles and their respective great arteries, achieving anatomic correction. The procedure involves transection of the arterial trunks above the level of the semilunar valves, anastomotic connections to their appropriate outflows, translocation of the coronary arteries to the neoaortic root, and closure of existing intracardiac communications (see Fig. 17.7A–E). Normal physiology is restored, enabling the left ventricle to function as the systemic chamber. This surgical procedure can be performed with excellent results, and long-term outcomes are very favorable.[325-328] Potential postoperative problems include supravalvar pulmonary or aortic obstruction. Neoaortic root dilation and aortic regurgitation can be identified on follow-up in some children. Ventricular function is normal in most cases.[329]

Anesthetic management of children after the arterial switch operation in general should be the same as in those without structural or functional cardiovascular abnormalities. However, there is some degree of concern related to late coronary artery problems that may not be evident clinically or identified by routine surveillance methods. Investigations have demonstrated postoperative regional LV wall motion abnormalities, evidence of myocardial perfusion defects, and pathologic changes in the coronary vasculature, suggesting a risk for coronary insufficiency.[330-334] Thus, cognizance of these issues in this patient group is prudent.

CONGENITALLY CORRECTED TRANSPOSITION OF THE GREAT ARTERIES

Anatomy and Pathophysiology

Congenitally corrected transposition is characterized by AV and ventriculoarterial discordance (double discordance). There is ventricular inversion and malposition of the great vessels. In this anomaly, the morphologic right atrium empties into an anatomic left ventricle, which then contracts into the pulmonary trunk. The morphologic left atrium opens into an anatomic right ventricle, which ejects into the aorta. The aorta is usually oriented in a leftward and anterior position with respect to the pulmonary artery, thus accounting for nomenclature of L-transposition of the great arteries (L-TGA) in this lesion.

Cyanosis is absent because the circulations are physiologically corrected. The anatomic right ventricle functions as the systemic pump in this lesion. Associated defects are frequently present and include pulmonary outflow tract obstruction, an interventricular communication, and tricuspid valve (left-sided) abnormalities. This pathology can remain undetected until the onset of arrhythmias or syncope owing to complete AV block or the effects of concomitant defects later in life.[335]

Treatment Options, Residua, Sequelae, and Long-Term Outcomes

Without associated defects, children with corrected transposition may do well for many years. Development of complete AV block is common with increasing age.[336] Young children with coexistent defects that maintain LV pressure at systemic levels might be suitable candidates for a surgical intervention that restores the left ventricle as the systemic chamber.[337] This complex repair, known as the double-switch operation or a variation thereof, combines redirection of the systemic and pulmonary venous flows in an atrial baffle procedure with the arterial switch operation. This strategy, however, may not affect mortality compared with conservative management.[338]

Issues that require long-term surveillance in children with congenitally corrected transposition include RV performance and tricuspid valve competency.[339] The overall long-term survival of individuals with this condition is substantially reduced compared with age-matched controls.[340,341]

TRUNCUS ARTERIOSUS

Anatomy and Pathophysiology

Truncus arteriosus is characterized by a single arterial trunk that gives rise to the aorta, pulmonary root, and coronary arteries (see Fig. 17.8). A ventricular communication is located underneath the single arterial root or truncal valve. Various anatomic types are identified based on the origin of the pulmonary arteries from the arterial trunk.[342,343] Associated findings may include a right aortic arch, aortic arch interruption, abnormalities of the truncal valve (e.g., abnormal number of cusps, stenosis, regurgitation), and coronary artery anomalies. Approximately one-third of children with truncus arteriosus have DiGeorge syndrome (see Chapter 16).

Clinical features of the neonate with this defect largely depend on the status of the pulmonary vasculature. If the resistance is increased, the infant is well compensated. The normal decrease in pulmonary vascular resistance leads to symptoms related to pulmonary overcirculation and congestive heart failure, accounting for the need for surgical intervention early in life. Truncus arteriosus is one of the structural malformations associated with a significant risk for adverse events before repair, because balancing the pulmonary and vascular resistances can be quite challenging.[344] The physiology that characterizes a reduced pulmonary vascular resistance and a significant runoff setting is that of an increased arterial oxygen saturation, reduced diastolic arterial pressures (potentially leading to myocardial ischemia), systemic hypotension, impaired cardiac output, and hypoperfusion of distal beds.

Treatment Options, Residua, Sequelae, and Long-Term Outcomes

Surgery for truncus arteriosus consists of detaching the main pulmonary artery from the truncal root, repairing the ensuing aortic wall defect, closing the VSD to allow LV output through the arterial root, and placing an extracardiac right ventricle–to–pulmonary artery conduit. Alternative approaches to establishing RV outflow continuity have been performed without the use of conduits.[345]

Neonates undergoing truncus arteriosus repair have excellent survival rates.[346-349] Late complications include conduit failure, residual or recurrent pulmonary artery obstruction, and truncal valve problems. Truncal valve dysfunction may require repair or replacement. The main issues of concern are the status of the right ventricle–to–pulmonary artery conduit and truncal root, consequences related to semilunar valve problems, and biventricular function.

EBSTEIN ANOMALY
Anatomy and Pathophysiology

The classic findings in Ebstein anomaly of the tricuspid valve include a large, sail-like anterior leaflet and apically displaced septal and posterior leaflets.[350,351] This configuration commonly results in an atrialized portion of the right ventricle and tricuspid regurgitation. Some degree of RV dysplasia is common. An interatrial communication is a frequent finding, and it can produce right-to-left shunting and clinical cyanosis. The spectrum of disease ranges from minimal or no symptoms to intractable congestive heart failure.[352] A neonatal presentation implies a major clinical problem and usually portends a poor prognosis. Symptoms in older children include cyanosis, palpitations, dyspnea, and exercise intolerance. The association of Wolf-Parkinson-White syndrome with Ebstein anomaly is well recognized. Initial presentation can be related to the development of supraventricular tachycardia (reported ~20%–25% incidence of accessory pathways).

Treatment Options, Residua, Sequelae, and Long-Term Outcomes

Children with Ebstein anomaly can be asymptomatic, requiring only conservative management and follow-up. Surgery is indicated for significant tricuspid regurgitation, closure of interatrial communications, or other associated problems. Procedures to ablate arrhythmias may be performed. In contrast to adults, children are less likely to require valve replacement.[353] A cavopulmonary or Glenn connection is performed in some cases as part of a so-called one-and-a-half ventricle approach to limit the right-sided volume load associated with severe tricuspid valve regurgitation.[354,355] Good functional outcomes and long-term survival have been reported after surgery for Ebstein anomaly.[356] Atrial arrhythmias in affected individuals are common before and after surgery.

INTERRUPTED AORTIC ARCH
Anatomy and Pathophysiology

Interrupted aortic arch is an uncommon malformation characterized by discontinuity between the ascending and descending thoracic aorta (see Fig. 17.14). Ductal patency is essential for systemic perfusion beyond the area of interruption. This anomaly is classified in terms of the site of interruption. Type A occurs distal to the left subclavian artery, type B between the left carotid and left subclavian arteries, and type C between the carotid arteries. Type B interruption is the most common variant, followed in frequency by types A and C.

Interrupted aortic arch is typically associated with a posteriorly malaligned VSD, resulting in subaortic obstruction. Associated defects include a right aortic arch, aberrant origin of a subclavian artery, and truncus arteriosus. Many children with this anomaly have DiGeorge syndrome.

Neonatal presentation of interrupted aortic arch is related to ductal closure in the setting of aortic arch obstruction (e.g., congestive heart failure, poor perfusion, cardiovascular collapse, shock) and occasionally to differential cyanosis (i.e., oxygen saturation in right hand is less than that in the foot). Stabilization of the infant and initiation of prostaglandin E_1 therapy is critical. The site of interruption and presence of coexistent anomalies can influence the selection of sites for blood pressure monitoring and pulse oximetry. An adequate response to prostaglandin E_1 therapy implies no significant gradient between the areas proximal and distal to the obstruction and an oxygen saturation differential (i.e., increased values in beds supplied proximal to the interruption, reduced values distally).

Treatment Options, Residua, Sequelae, and Long-Term Outcomes

Surgical intervention is necessary for interrupted aortic arch during the first few days of life. The goal is to establish aortic arch continuity and to address coexistent defects. The current approach favors a one-stage repair.[357-359] Survival in uncomplicated cases is excellent.[360] Problems after repair mainly involve the LVOT.[361] Reoperation may be required and in some cases consist of LVOT enlargement (i.e., Konno procedure). Eventual aortic root or valve replacement or a Ross-Konno procedure may be necessary. Aortic arch obstruction can occur in the long-term. Given that the site of obstruction has implications for monitoring, the anesthesia provider should be aware of the anatomic details and the severity of the pathology.

CONGENITAL ANOMALIES OF THE CORONARY ARTERIES
Anatomy and Pathophysiology

Congenital anomalies of the coronary arteries include an abnormal origin of one of the main branches, aberrant vascular course, or pathologic communications that involve the coronary circulation.[362,363] The most common anomalies detected during childhood include anomalous origin of the left main coronary artery from the pulmonary artery (ALCAPA), coronary artery-to-pulmonary artery fistulas, and coronary cameral fistulas (i.e., connection between a coronary artery and cardiac chamber). Although rare, anomalous origin of a coronary artery from the incorrect (contralateral) sinus of Valsalva can occur in asymptomatic children and adolescents.[364] In some instances, a major coronary artery courses between the great arteries. This situation can be associated with compromised coronary blood flow and myocardial ischemia during exercise, presumably related to dilation of the arterial roots to accommodate the increased stroke volume.

The clinical presentation varies depending on the nature of the anomaly. Infants and young children with ALCAPA typically exhibit severe ventricular dysfunction and mitral valve regurgitation, which are largely ischemic in nature. Children with fistulous coronary artery connections can present with a heart murmur or evidence of ventricular volume overload. Significant symptoms indicate congestive heart failure. Other coronary artery anomalies can manifest as myocardial ischemia, causing exertional syncope or chest pain, and in some cases, arrhythmias may lead to a near-death event.

Treatment Options, Residua, Sequelae, and Long-Term Outcomes

After surgical intervention for ALCAPA, most children demonstrate reasonable recovery of myocardial function. Others continue to exhibit alterations in myocardial performance and can develop dilated cardiomyopathy; if it is severe, they may require cardiac transplantation. A few children reach adulthood without symptoms or any intervention. Coronary artery fistulas resulting in congestive symptoms are referred for catheter-based or surgical interventions. Angina complaints, myocardial infarction, and sudden death are risks when an aberrant coronary artery courses between the arterial trunks. The risk is greater when the left coronary artery originates from the right sinus of Valsalva and courses between the aorta and the RVOT. Sudden death is most likely to occur during or immediately after strenuous exercise. The implications of anesthesia for coronary artery anomalies primarily are related to the underlying potential for myocardial ischemia, effects of ventricular volume overload, and ventricular dysfunction.

SINGLE VENTRICLE

Anatomy and Pathophysiology

The single-ventricle (i.e., univentricular heart) spectrum encompasses several congenital cardiac defects. They are characterized by abnormalities such as ventricular hypoplasia (i.e., HLHS), AV valve atresia (i.e., tricuspid atresia), or abnormal AV connections (i.e., double-inlet left ventricle). Pathologies with two distinct ventricles may also be considered in the functional single-ventricle category because of associated defects that may preclude a biventricular circulation (i.e., unbalanced AVSD).

Single-ventricle physiology is characterized by complete mixing of the systemic and pulmonary venous circulations at the atrial or ventricular levels. Aortic or pulmonary outflow tract obstruction is a common feature of these pathologies. An important management strategy early in the palliation pathway involves optimizing the balance between the pulmonary and systemic circulations.

Treatment Options, Residua, Sequelae, and Long-Term Outcomes

Surgical interventions available for children with functional single-ventricle physiology include the following procedures.

Systemic to Pulmonary Artery Shunt

Infants with limited or ductal-dependent pulmonary blood flow require the creation of a connection between the systemic and pulmonary circulations. This most commonly takes the form of a Gore-Tex graft between the right subclavian and right pulmonary arteries (i.e., modified right Blalock-Taussig shunt). The goal of the procedure is to augment or allow for pulmonary blood flow. Potential problems include shunt malfunction associated with reductions in pulmonary blood flow and congestive heart failure related to excessive pulmonary blood flow. Several factors determine blood flow across an aortopulmonary shunt, with systemic arterial pressure playing a major role.

Pulmonary Artery Band

Pulmonary artery banding results in limitation of pulmonary blood flow in children with minimal or no restriction. The intervention aims to protect the pulmonary vascular bed from increased flow and excessive pressure, an essential requirement for subsequent strategies in the child with a functional single ventricle.

Distortion of the proximal branch pulmonary arteries can result from pulmonary artery band placement. The main considerations in these children are the presence of an intracardiac communication, associated shunting, ventricular volume load, the consequences of ventricular hypertrophy developed as a response to the mechanical limitation of pulmonary blood flow, and issues associated with coexistent defects. In a few children, pulmonary artery banding can lead to ventricular dysfunction and the development of or an increase in the severity of AV valve regurgitation.

Norwood Procedure

In infants with HLHS, its variants, and other lesions with similar hemodynamic consequences, systemic blood flow largely depends on patency of the ductus arteriosus. Cerebral and coronary blood flow is usually provided in retrograde fashion across a typically hypoplastic transverse aortic arch. A key strategy in the management of these neonates before cardiac surgery is to optimize systemic perfusion and the balance between the pulmonary and systemic circulations.[365] Alteration of this balance manifests with signs of inadequate systemic output (e.g., hypotension, lactic acidosis, decreased urine output) within the context of high systemic arterial oxygen saturation, reflecting the relatively excessive pulmonary blood flow.

In this setting, maneuvers that increase pulmonary vascular resistance are indicated to improve hemodynamics, including limiting inspired oxygen concentrations, the administration of subambient gas mixtures, and increasing the partial pressure of carbon dioxide (PCO_2) by hypoventilation or the administration of inspired carbon dioxide. A comparison of hypoxia versus hypercarbia in infants with HLHS under conditions of anesthesia and paralysis demonstrated that although decreases in both conditions, inspired CO_2 was more effective than hypoxic gas mixtures at increasing parameters associated with improved systemic output.[366] The administration of inspired carbon dioxide may be favored over hypoventilation as a means of increasing pulmonary vascular resistance and improving the overall clinical condition.

The Norwood procedure is considered the first step along the three palliative stages for infants with HLHS or similar cardiac malformations.[367] The intervention, also referred to as stage I single-ventricle palliation or reconstruction, is typically performed within the first few days of life. Surgery consists of aortic reconstruction or creation of a neoaorta, establishing continuity between the native main pulmonary artery and aortic arch to provide for unobstructed systemic outflow from the right ventricle; the creation of an unrestricted atrial communication by means of an atrial septectomy; and establishing a source of pulmonary blood flow (see Fig. 17.11). Pulmonary blood flow is allowed by the creation of a modified Blalock-Taussig shunt or placement of a right ventricle–to–pulmonary artery conduit (i.e., Sano modification and variations). Although the potential benefits of one approach over the other have been debated, additional studies, with long-term follow-up, are required to provide further information in this regard.[368-373] It should be emphasized that the functional single ventricle following stage I palliation handles both the systemic and pulmonary circulations and consequently it is a volume loaded ventricle. This leads to changes in ventricular geometry that include progressive chamber dilatation and may be associated with problems such as the development of tricuspid regurgitation, systolic and/or diastolic functional impairment.

A hybrid stage I strategy has been used as an alternate approach to the Norwood procedure in the neonate. The combined effort of an interventional cardiologist and surgeon aims at delivering a stent across the ductus arteriosus under fluoroscopic guidance and banding the branched pulmonary arteries via a median sternotomy.[374-377] The interatrial communication is enlarged as needed at the same time or soon thereafter.

Outcomes after the Norwood procedure vary; good results imply operative survival for 85% to 90% of infants. Immediate postoperative problems include inadequate or excessive pulmonary blood flow and decreased myocardial performance. Monitoring of mixed venous oxygen saturation and cerebral near-infrared spectroscopy are helpful in balancing the pulmonary and systemic circulations in this setting. Occasionally, aortic arch obstruction develops, and less commonly, the atrial septum becomes restrictive. Interstage mortality accounts for attrition among Norwood survivors.[378] Among infants who have undergone placement of a right ventricle–to–pulmonary artery conduit, stenosis of the conduit associated with progressive cyanosis may account for significant interstage morbidity and often requires intervention or early second-stage palliation.[379,380]

The anticipated arterial oxygen saturation after stage I surgery is expected to be in the range of 75% to 85%. During perioperative care and in the selection of monitoring sites it should be considered that the presence of a Blalock-Taussig shunt can compromise ipsilateral subclavian artery flow and may not allow for accurate blood pressure assessment. In these infants, the right ventricle ejects into the pulmonary and systemic circulations. Although this is a more stable arrangement compared with the preoperative physiology, it remains a relatively fragile parallel circulation. These infants display little tolerance to even the most common childhood conditions, and ailments such as dehydration, febrile illnesses, or other stresses that can have catastrophic consequences. Despite these challenges, successful outcomes have been reported during noncardiac surgery for a variety of procedures, including those that may be associated with significant hemodynamic perturbations.[381]

Glenn Anastomosis or Hemi-Fontan Procedure

A cavopulmonary connection or Glenn procedure (i.e., stage II palliation) consists of the creation of a direct anastomosis between the superior vena cava and a branch pulmonary artery (see Fig. 17.12). This is considered an intermediary step in the sequential diversion of the systemic venous blood into the pulmonary vasculature in children with single-ventricle physiology. The original or classic Glenn operation consisted of an end-to-end anastomosis of the transected superior vena cava onto a disconnected right pulmonary artery. Long-term issues included decreasing arterial saturation, attributed in many cases to the development of pulmonary arteriovenous fistulae.[382] The current approach is to anastomose the superior vena cava to the right pulmonary artery in end-to-side fashion, preserving pulmonary artery continuity (i.e., bidirectional cavopulmonary anastomosis [BCPA] or bidirectional Glenn connection). Depending on the specific anatomic abnormalities, right, left, or bilateral BCPAs may be indicated.

An alternative approach in the second-stage of single ventricle palliation is the hemi-Fontan procedure. It directs superior vena cava blood to the pulmonary circulation while excluding entry of superior vena cava blood into the right atrium by placement of a patch (dam). This approach provides a step closer to lateral tunnel Fontan completion (described later). When present, a systemic-to-pulmonary artery connection (shunt or conduit) is ligated and divided as part of stage II palliation, regardless of whether a BCPA or hemi-Fontan procedure is undertaken.

The second-stage intervention requires a low pulmonary vascular resistance because of the passive nature of the pulmonary blood flow. This approach provides adequate palliation to a significant number of infants at an early age while conferring favorable

hemodynamic benefits.[383] Diverting a portion of the systemic venous return directly into the pulmonary bed reduces the output requirements of the single ventricle while decreasing the ventricular volume load and myocardial work.

One study demonstrated a 12% rate of interstage attrition between BCPA and the Fontan procedure in children with HLHS palliation.[384] Risk factors included tricuspid valve regurgitation and low body weight at the time of the BCPA. These factors can affect the anesthesia-related risks for noncardiac procedures required between these two stages of palliation.

Considerations in children who have undergone palliation include the passive nature of the pulmonary blood flow, the importance of maintaining adequate intravascular volume (i.e., minimal fasting) to enhance pulmonary blood flow, and limiting significant increases in pulmonary vascular tone. It should be noted that high peak inflation pressures or positive-end expiratory pressure (PEEP) can reduce pulmonary blood flow. Pulmonary blood flow and systemic arterial oxygenation are significantly influenced by the interplay between pulmonary artery pressure (i.e., equal to the pressure in the superior vena cava), pulmonary venous pressure, and pulmonary vascular resistance. The expected systemic arterial oxygen saturation ranges between 75% and 85%. Although factors that increase pulmonary vascular resistance can negatively influence pulmonary blood flow, the observation has been made that early after BCPA, moderate hypercapnia with respiratory acidosis improves arterial oxygenation and reduces oxygen consumption, enhancing overall oxygen transport in these children.[385] Hyperventilation can decrease cerebral oxygenation and should be avoided.[386] Postoperative issues include hypoxemia related to the development of collateral vessels that bypass the pulmonary circulation, AV valve regurgitation, and impaired ventricular function.

Fontan Procedure

The Fontan procedure is the final step (i.e., stage III reconstruction) in the separation of the pulmonary and systemic circulations in children with a functional single ventricle. This intervention allows passive blood flow from the inferior vena cava into the pulmonary vascular bed while bypassing the heart and achieves a circulation in series (see Fig. 17.13). The creation of a fenestration, or communication, between the systemic venous pathway and physiologic common atrium is favored in some cases as it allows right-to-left shunting (pop off), providing cardiac output that is not solely dependent on pulmonary blood flow. It also alleviates potential problems associated with chronically increased systemic venous pressures. Common features of the various Fontan modifications are separation of the pulmonary and systemic circulations and relief of hypoxemia.[387] Pulmonary blood flow occurs without an intervening ventricular chamber. It depends critically on the transpulmonary pressure gradient (or driving pressure across the pulmonary bed) and is influenced by pulmonary vascular resistance. This blood flow determines cardiac output, emphasizing the importance of adequate hydration and maintenance of central venous pressure.

Several anatomic and hemodynamic variables influence Fontan physiology.[388] Critical factors include unobstructed systemic venous return, status of the pulmonary vasculature, reduced intrathoracic pressures, systemic AV valve competency, systemic ventricular function, unobstructed systemic outflow, and atrial contribution to ventricular filling.[389] Long-term problems are related to sinus node dysfunction, loss of AV synchrony, atrial arrhythmias, AV valve regurgitation, ventricular dysfunction, venous pathway obstruction or thrombotic complications, and symptoms resulting from a chronic reduced cardiac output state.[390] Long-standing increases in systemic venous pressures in children after the Fontan procedure can produce hepatic dysfunction, coagulation defects, protein-losing enteropathy, rhythm disturbances, and plastic bronchitis. The quality of life after the Fontan operation can be compromised by a late decline in functional status, reoperations, arrhythmias, and thromboembolic events.[391-396] Decreased exercise tolerance in most children represents limited cardiopulmonary reserve, which manifests as an inability to increase cardiac output to meet the metabolic demands associated with increased work. In some cases, surgical revision to a more hemodynamically favorable Fontan modification is indicated.[397,398]

Several considerations are important in the perioperative care of children with Fontan circulation.[399,400] Even mild alterations in factors that influence cardiac output, such as ventricular preload, AV synchrony, contractile function, afterload, and stress response, can adversely affect hemodynamics. Ensuring the adequacy of hydration, preserving sinus rhythm, and limiting the stress response are key goals. Maintenance of adequate ventricular function may require the administration of inotropic or vasoactive agents perioperatively. Because systemic venous pressures are typically increased, the potential for bleeding and its effects on ventricular filling should be considered. The likelihood of blood loss with ensuing hemodynamic instability is exacerbated by the coagulation defects in these children.[401] The potential for end-organ dysfunction related to chronically decreased organ perfusion, particularly in the renal and hepatic systems, should be considered, and problems may require interventions to minimize perioperative morbidity. Drugs or devices appropriate for cardiac rhythm or arrhythmia management should be readily accessible.

Important principles apply to airway and ventilatory management after the Fontan operation. Although spontaneous ventilation favors phasic pulmonary flow patterns in these children, controlled ventilation is preferable in most cases. This approach minimizes the detrimental effects of factors, such as hypoventilation, atelectasis, hypoxemia, hypercarbia, and respiratory acidosis on pulmonary vascular resistance during spontaneous ventilation, limiting passive drainage of systemic venous blood into the pulmonary circulation. The pH and PCO_2 should be maintained within the normal range, and arterial oxygen saturation should remain close to baseline. The saturation level may depend on the presence or absence of a fenestration in the Fontan pathway and the degree of right-to-left shunting. Mechanical ventilation with large lung volumes can impair pulmonary blood flow because high mean intrathoracic pressures transmitted to the pulmonary vascular bed increase pulmonary artery pressures and decrease systemic venous return. Judicious use of mechanical ventilatory support is therefore warranted. Suggested parameters include smaller than usual tidal volumes and reduced PEEP times, allowing delivery of the smallest mean airway pressure possible and normal to relatively small inspiratory times (i.e., normal to slightly prolonged inspiratory/expiratory ratios). Although adequate minute ventilation may require increases in the respiratory rate, the potential detrimental effects of very fast rates should also be considered. The goals are to maintain adequate lung volumes, functional residual capacity, and optimal gas exchange. Modern modes of assisted mechanical ventilation—for example, pressure support ventilation with the ability to accurately control preset indexes—may also be suitable in this patient population.

It should be emphasized that patients with single-ventricle physiology are at high risk for complications during noncardiac surgery regardless of their stage of palliation.[44] A retrospective chart review of 70 patients with single-ventricle physiology who underwent 102 anesthetics for a variety of procedures revealed 100% 48-hour survival, although almost 12% of cases involved an adverse event associated with their anesthetic.

Several reports have documented the use of laparoscopic surgery in the patient with single-ventricle circulation.[381,402-404] Despite its benefits, a significant concern in this setting is the potential for cardiorespiratory compromise owing to the physiologic effects of the pneumoperitoneum, patient positioning (Trendelenburg or reverse Trendelenburg), and increased carbon dioxide tensions. A study assessing cardiac function by transesophageal echocardiography in single-ventricle patients reported a reversible decrease in shortening fraction during laparoscopic gastrostomy tube placement.[405] It is well recognized that in the single-ventricle patient group there is also less tolerance for complications that might be associated with the procedure (e.g., gas embolism, pneumothorax, and pneumomediastinum), resulting in increased vulnerability for untoward events. During these procedures communication between the anesthesia and surgical teams is imperative. Early consideration should be given to reducing the intraabdominal pressure by deflation of the pneumoperitoneum and possible conversion to an open procedure if hemodynamic, oxygenation, or ventilation difficulties are encountered.

Summary

Noncardiac surgery in children with CHD can usually be accomplished in a safe and effective manner. A comprehensive understanding of the child's cardiovascular anatomy, physiology, and potential hemodynamic alternations is essential to guide appropriate perioperative management and to achieve the best possible outcomes. Many children with CHD have undergone complete repair in infancy, with resultant normal or near-normal hemodynamics at the time of noncardiac surgery. Routine care is likely to be well tolerated by these children. However, special attention should be given to identify children at increased risk, particularly those with unrepaired defects or those who have undergone palliative interventions. Factors such as congestive heart failure, cyanosis, pulmonary hypertension, young age, or significant residua or sequelae increase the potential for perioperative problems.

An important objective in caring for children with a history of CHD is to diminish cardiac-related morbidity and minimize the likelihood of an adverse outcome. An interdisciplinary approach is much preferred to accomplish this goal. Application of perioperative strategies that can limit the risks of anesthesia and surgery should be a combined effort by all health care providers involved. Anticipation of these risks can decrease the potential for complications and facilitate prompt and appropriate treatment when difficulties are encountered. Good communication among the perioperative team members is essential.

ANNOTATED REFERENCES

Brown ML, DiNardo JA, Odegard KC. Patients with single ventricle physiology undergoing noncardiac surgery are at high risk for adverse events. *Paediatr Anaesth.* 2015;25(8):846-851.
This is a retrospective review of all patients who underwent single-ventricle palliation at a single institution with the goal to assess outcomes related to noncardiac surgery. The study identified 417 patients with single-ventricle physiology who underwent a palliative procedure. Of these, 70 patients (16.7%) underwent 102 anesthetics for 121 noncardiac procedures. The study observed no mortality during

or after noncardiac surgery; however, a high rate (11.8%) of intraoperative and early postoperative adverse events was identified in this patient population.

Chau DF, Gangadharan M, Hartke LP, et al. The post-anesthetic care of pediatric patients with pulmonary hypertension. *Semin Cardiothorac Vasc Anesth.* 2016;20(1):63-73.

This work presents an excellent review regarding the perioperative care of pediatric patients with pulmonary hypertension. The paper addresses topics such as current concepts related to the condition, preanesthetic preparation, risks factors for adverse events during postanesthesia care, and postanesthetic disposition.

Faraoni D, Zurakowski D, Vo D, et al. Post-operative outcomes in children with and without congenital heart disease undergoing noncardiac surgery. *J Am Coll Cardiol.* 2016;67(7):793-801.

This study compared the incidence of mortality and major adverse postoperative outcomes following noncardiac surgery in children with and without CHD using a pediatric database of the American College of Surgeons National Surgical Quality Improvement Program. The review identified 4520 children with CHD who underwent noncardiac surgery. Children in each of three subgroups consisting of minor, major, and severe CHD were matched and compared with controls without CHD who underwent noncardiac surgery of comparable complexity. It was found that children with major or severe CHD who undergo noncardiac surgery have an increased risk of mortality with a higher incidence of life-threatening postoperative outcomes compared with children without CHD.

Matisoff AJ, Olivieri L, Schwartz JM, et al. Risk assessment and anesthetic management of patients with Williams syndrome: a comprehensive review. *Paediatr Anaesth.* 2015;25(12):1207-1215.

The article is a comprehensive review addressing the clinical manifestations of Williams syndrome and proposing a protocol for risk assessment based on current literature. The paper also provides recommendations for preoperative evaluation and management of anesthesia in affected low-, moderate-, and high-risk patients.

Ramamoorthy C, Haberkern CM, Bhananker SM, et al. Anesthesia-related cardiac arrest in children with heart disease: data from the Pediatric Perioperative Cardiac Arrest (POCA) registry. *Anesth Analg.* 2010;110:1376-1382.

This is a report from the Pediatric Perioperative Cardiac Arrest (POCA) registry on anesthesia-related cardiac arrests, with a focus on children with heart disease. The data were provided by many North American institutions. Children with heart disease who suffered a cardiac arrest were sicker that those without heart disease and more likely to suffer arrest from cardiovascular causes. Mortality rates were greater for those with heart disease. The events were more likely to occur in the general operating room compared with the cardiac setting. The subset of children with a single ventricle was the most common category of heart disease to suffer cardiac arrest. Children with aortic stenosis (e.g., Williams Syndrome) and cardiomyopathy had the greatest cardiac arrest–related mortality rates.

Williams GD, Maan H, Ramamoorthy C, et al. Perioperative complications in children with pulmonary hypertension undergoing general anesthesia with ketamine. *Paediatr Anaesth.* 2010;20(1):28-37.

This is a retrospective study in children with pulmonary arterial hypertension to determine the nature and frequency of periprocedural complications and to assess whether ketamine administration was associated with complications. In this cohort (68 children), the incidence of cardiac arrest was 10% for major surgery, 0.78% for cardiac catheterization, and 1.6% for all procedures. There was no procedure-related mortality. Ketamine administration was not associated with an increased rate of complications.

A complete reference list can be found online at ExpertConsult.com.

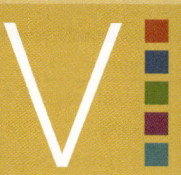

Essentials of Neurology and Neuromuscular Disorders

24

PETER M. CREAN AND SANDYA TIRUPATHI

General Considerations	**Neuromuscular Disorders**
Static Neurologic Disorders	Disorders of the Anterior Horn Cell
Cerebral Palsies	Axonal Disorders
Malformations of the Nervous System	Disorders of the Neuromuscular Junction
Disorders of Ventral Induction	Disorders of Muscle Fibers
Disorders of Cortical Development	**Epilepsy**
Progressive Neurologic Disorders	**Summary**
Primary Brain Tumors	
Metabolic Disease	

DISORDERS OF THE NERVOUS SYSTEM are common in childhood, and their diverse manifestations and complications may lead to diagnostic and surgical interventions that require anesthesia. Children with these disorders are subject to the same acute illnesses, such as acute appendicitis, as other children. Many neurologic disorders exert profound effects on other body systems that function under complex autonomic control. For example, dysfunction of bulbar musculature may predispose to regurgitation and aspiration in the perioperative period because protective reflexes may be impaired. Medications taken for chronic conditions may interact with anesthetic agents, which may have an impact on an underlying disorder in specific ways. The mechanisms of these interactions are becoming better understood with advances in molecular genetics. Anesthesiologists must have an understanding of the patient's underlying neurologic or neuromuscular condition and its influence on anesthesia management to optimize perioperative outcomes.

General Considerations

The term *neurologic disorder* encompasses a wide variety of conditions that may have extremely mild or very serious effects (Table 24.1).[1-5] These disorders are likely to be associated with a degree of physical, cognitive, or combined disabilities. Many children with severe physical disabilities have normal intelligence and are competent to make decisions about treatment options. Those with mild cognitive impairment may wish to be consulted about treatment choices; adolescents in particular must be involved in decision making.[6] This approach is especially important for managing individuals with chronic disorders who are accustomed to thinking about health issues and who often have strong and well-defined opinions about how they wish to be treated.[7]

When planning anesthesia for these individuals, physicians must become knowledgeable about them and their conditions. Assumptions should not be made about their level of comprehension or about how they and their parents' view the choices available.[8] It was formerly acceptable practice for children with chronic neurologic disorders to be excluded from the full range of therapeutic options, but it is now essential that all options are included.[9]

Parents of children with chronic disorders of all types are usually accustomed to dealing with health care situations and often have thought carefully about the implications of various treatments. They know the child best and are usually most qualified to make decisions by proxy. Widespread use of the Internet has assisted many parents in becoming knowledgeable about their child's condition and about potential interventions.[10] Their aims are usually entirely appropriate, and this knowledge may assist physicians in their collaboration with children and parents in determining optimal management. Occasionally, the information has been obtained from an unreliable source and may be inaccurate or inappropriate for a particular child.[11] Misinformation can precipitate difficult situations for professionals, especially when there is a perceived disparity between the desires of the parents and those of the child and what the clinician considers to be in the child's best interest. The surgical team members usually are most involved in the process of obtaining informed consent, but the anesthesiologist must participate in the dialogue because anesthesia may be the part of treatment that carries the greatest risk.

561

TABLE 24.1	Neurologic Disorders
Condition	**Prevalence**
Cerebral palsy: all types	2.2 per 1000 live births
Epilepsy	5–10 per 1000 all ages
Central nervous system tumors	1–5 per 1000 all ages
Neuromuscular disorders (all ages)	1 per 2900 total population
Congenital myopathy	1 per 28,600
Duchenne muscular dystrophy	1 per 3500
Myotonic dystrophy	1 per 12,000
Limb girdle dystrophy	1 per 90,000
Spinal muscular atrophy	1 per 74,000
Mitochondrial disorders	11.5 per 100,000 all ages

Children with neurologic disorders usually have a regular physician overseeing their care, and this person should participate in the decision-making process. For elective procedures, the surgeon should establish contact with the child's regular pediatric specialist and anesthesiologist as soon as surgery is contemplated, inform them about the proposed operation, and seek their opinions to optimize perioperative management. Cognitive, communication, and behavioral problems; coexisting diseases; and drug therapy that may influence management of the anesthesia for these patients should be evaluated at an early stage.[12] Some children may be receiving long-term respiratory support, including cough assist devices and home ventilation; all current therapies should be considered.

Oral communication may be difficult for some children with neurologic disorders. Use of age-appropriate assisted communication devices may help to ensure open communication between physician and patient.[12] Parents' opinions and attempts to protect their children should be respected and understood as a consequence of previous experiences, stress, frustration, anger, and probably guilt.[13] Each procedure has to be assessed in terms of morbidity, mortality, and probability of improving quality of life. All aspects must be clearly and objectively discussed with parents or guardians and informed consent forms signed.

Clinicians who are responsible for providing emergency care to children must have the knowledge and skills required to manage children with neurologic disorders. A preoperative assessment may be required on an urgent basis; a parent-held record of previous diagnoses and treatment is extremely helpful. Concurrent medications, previous reactions, and a history of complications such as respiratory insufficiency, electrolyte disturbance, or cardiac, renal, or hepatic dysfunction should be elicited before induction of anesthesia. A specific management plan for seizure medications is important for children who are likely to develop ileus postoperatively and thereby require a change from oral to intravenous (IV) medications.

Static Neurologic Disorders

CEREBRAL PALSIES

Cerebral palsies are a group of disorders of movement, muscle, or posture that are caused by injury or abnormal development of the immature brain attributed to nonprogressive causes. The prevalence of cerebral palsy is 1 case per 500 live births.[14] About 40% of these children are born premature. Eighty percent of cases are acquired prenatally and have no obvious cause, although they are associated with prematurity, low birth weight, placental insufficiency, maternal infection and pyrexia, intrauterine infections, intrauterine growth retardation, intracranial hemorrhage, and trauma. Birth complications, including asphyxia, are estimated to account for another 6% of cases. Postnatal causes of cerebral palsy (10%) usually arise from infectious causes (e.g., bacterial meningitis, viral encephalitis), trauma (e.g., motor vehicle collisions, falls, child abuse), or metabolic disturbance (e.g., hyperbilirubinemia).[15,16]

Classification depends on the severity, distribution, and the nature of the motor deficit. With the advent of modern imaging techniques, including magnetic resonance imaging (MRI), understanding the pathogenesis of cerebral palsies has advanced dramatically.[17–19] Clinical features are classified most commonly according to the type of motor deficit, its distribution, and the severity of the deficit (Table 24.2). Involvement of a single limb is referred to as *monoparesis*, of both limbs on one side of the body as *hemiparesis*, of both lower limbs as *paraparesis* or *diparesis*, of three limbs as *triparesis*, and of all four limbs as *tetraparesis* or *quadriparesis*. The motor deficit may manifest as hypotonia, spasticity, or extrapyramidal features such as choreoathetoid/dystonic movements, dyskinesia, or ataxia. A descriptive classification includes neurologic deficit, severity, and distribution (e.g., spastic paraparesis or paraplegia dystonic hemiparesis). Paresis or palsies are terms used to denote differing severities.

Children with cerebral palsies require neuroimaging to confirm the diagnosis and underlying cause of the condition. Although some centers use oral sedation (i.e., midazolam or chloral hydrate) for neuroimaging, many children require general anesthesia. They may require multiple anesthetics throughout their lifetimes because of the associated comorbidities (i.e., respiratory, gastrointestinal, neuromuscular, and orthopedic), common surgical conditions, and problems unique to cerebral palsies that require treatment.[20–22]

Many of the comorbid conditions can affect anesthesia management. Understanding the pathophysiology and comorbidities of cerebral palsies allows anesthesiologists to anticipate and prevent perioperative complications.

Multisystem Comorbidities

Most children with cerebral palsies have clinically significant oromotor dysfunction, and when associated with gastroesophageal reflux, it may lead to recurrent aspiration, decreased respiratory reserve, esophageal stenosis, and malnutrition.[23] Frequently used procedures include fundoplication, gastrostomy, and esophageal dilatation.[12] Immobility, underhydration, and poor diet predispose patients to bowel stasis and constipation and, if severe, may result in fecal impaction. Malnutrition may depress immune responses, and electrolyte imbalance and anemia are common. Preoperative assessment of these parameters is essential.

Pulmonary complications are common causes of death in cerebral palsies. Aspiration associated with gastroesophageal reflux is the leading cause, and it may be exacerbated by excessive oral secretions, bulbar dysfunction, recurrent respiratory infection, and chronic lung disease.[24,25] Scoliosis may also restrict pulmonary function, with cardiopulmonary involvement depending on the curve pattern and the severity of the curve (see Chapter 32).[12]

Orthopedic operations are the most frequently performed procedures in children with moderate to severe cerebral palsies.[12] Procedures include tendon releases to ease contractures, femoral osteotomy, and hip adductor and iliopsoas releases.[26] The trend in orthopedic surgery is to perform multiple procedures involving

TABLE 24.2 | Cerebral Palsy

Type and Cause	Motor Deficits	Distribution	Complications
Hypotonic • Syndromic • Dysgenesis • Hypoxia-ischemia	Low axial tone Variable limb tone Deep tendon reflexes usually increased	Diffuse	Learning disability Epilepsy Feeding dysfunction Hearing or vision impairment Respiratory infections
Spastic (pyramidal) • Hypoxia-ischemia • Vascular	Increased tone: pyramidal type Increased deep tendon reflexes	Monoplegia Diplegia Hemiplegia Triplegia Quadriplegia	Epilepsy Contractures Feeding difficulties Learning difficulties
Dyskinetic (extrapyrimidal) • Hypoxia-ischemia • Neonatal hyperbilirubinemia • Metabolic	Involuntary movement: often a mixture of choreoathetosis, dystonia and dyskinesia	May be diffuse involving all four limbs or confined to one or more limbs Often coexists with spasticity	Hearing impairment Contractures Intellect can be maintained
Ataxic • Cerebral dysgenesis • Rare syndromes	Usually generalized truncal and limb ataxia May coexist with spasticity	May be diffuse but often associated with diparesis	Poor balance, speech difficulties, poor fine motor skills
Mixed	Can be a combination of all above	Often diffuse	Mixture of all above

24

tenotomies or osteotomies at different levels of all extremities during a single general anesthesic, rather than staging them during multiple operations.[12,20] Scoliosis often requires surgery to prevent further deterioration in lung function and to stabilize the spine to facilitate ambulation and sitting. Spinal fusion is considered in all children with progressive curves greater than 40 to 50 degrees.[27]

Botulinum toxin is commonly used to reduce muscle spasticity in affected children, and it may be injected with or without sedation or, more commonly, in children under general anesthesia. The need for repeated treatments (every 3-6 months) and the use of a nerve stimulator to confirm correct placement of the needle should be taken into consideration when assessing the child's need for sedation or anesthesia.

Approximately 30% of children with cerebral palsies have epilepsy. It is more common in spastic hemiplegia and quadriplegia, especially with a history of neonatal encephalopathy (53% vs. 29%) and less common in the ataxic and choreoathetotic forms. Secondary generalized and focal seizures frequently occur. Anticonvulsants should be maintained until the surgery date (given the morning of surgery) and restarted as soon as possible in the postoperative period.[12,28]

Anesthesia Considerations for Cerebral Palsies

The many multisystem comorbidities and therapies specific to children with cerebral palsies must be understood to minimize perioperative complications. Risk factors include an inability to walk, severe neurologic deficit, major cognitive dysfunction, severe scoliosis, malnutrition, and the presence of a gastrostomy or tracheostomy.[20] Severely compromised children can be optimally managed postoperatively with admission to the pediatric intensive care unit to provide analgesia with comprehensive monitoring, maximum support, and aggressive respiratory care; after their conditions are stabilized, they can be transferred to a setting with less intense monitoring.

All medications that the child is receiving should be reviewed; they may include anticonvulsant, antireflux, and antispasticity agents. Baclofen should not be discontinued abruptly because it can produce acute withdrawal symptoms. Oral dantrolene has

also been used to reduce spasticity. Baclofen and dantrolene cause weakness; therefore the dose of neuromuscular blocking drugs may need to be reduced as these antispasticity drugs can delay the return of adequate respiratory effort during emergence from anesthesia.

Most of these children have above-average intelligence. They have the same emotional and cognitive concerns as others about undergoing anesthesia, including preoperative anxiety that may require premedication. Children with contractures, especially in the upper extremities, may present a challenge for establishing IV access. If gastroesophageal reflux is not controlled, consideration should be given to rapid-sequence induction. Although these children have a peripheral motor disorder, IV succinylcholine yields only a normal release of potassium,[29] despite evidence of proliferation of extrajunctional acetylcholine receptors.[30] Maintenance of and emergence from anesthesia requires special considerations, including the possibility of a reduced minimal alveolar concentration (MAC),[31] resistance to neuromuscular blocking agents,[32] and reduced bispectral index (BIS) measurements.[33] If vomiting is likely to occur, the airway must be protected.

These children have normal responses to pain, which should be managed as if they were unaffected by cerebral palsy. Caudal or epidural analgesia may be a reasonable approach for perioperative pain management if the child does not have a ventriculoperitoneal shunt.[34] Management and assessment of perioperative pain in children with neurocognitive impairment is addressed in Chapter 44.

MALFORMATIONS OF THE NERVOUS SYSTEM

Malformations are common in pediatric neurologic practice and a frequent cause of early mortality. The appearance of the neural plate shows that the central nervous system (CNS) develops very rapidly in the 2-week embryo and continues until several years after birth. The cause of CNS malformations is largely uncertain, but timing appears to be more important than the nature of the insult in producing the specific type of malformation. Causative agents include maternal drugs such as sodium valproate, which is associated with neural tube defects (NTDs); infections such as cytomegalovirus, which can cause various cerebral lesions, depending on the time in gestation of the infection; toxins such as alcohol; vitamin deficiency (e.g., folic acid), and genetic disorders. Historically, because diagnostic investigation was limited, postmortem examination was required to demonstrate the neuropathologic changes causing the clinical disorder. MRI now can provide adequate images to enable a diagnosis in many instances (e.g., cortical dysplasia).[35]

Neural Tube Defects: Cranial and Spinal Dysraphism

The fetal incidence of NTDs is 17 per 10,000 pregnancies; the live birth incidence is 5.7 to 6.7 per 10,000. NTDs are a group of birth defects presumed to have a common origin in failure of the neural tube to develop properly during the embryonic stage. NTDs include anencephaly, encephaloceles, and spina bifida.

The cause of NTDs is multifactorial, with genetic and environmental factors the most important. Approximately 10% of NTDs are caused by chromosomal abnormalities such as trisomies (i.e., 18, 13, and 21), triploidy, and 22q11 microdeletion. Some of the environmental causes include folate deficiency, maternal antiepileptic drugs (valproate, phenytoin, carbamazepine, and polytherapy), retinoins, and maternal diabetes.

Preconceptual folic acid supplementation has reduced the prevalence of NTDs by 30% to 50%.[36,37] Along with antenatal ultrasound examination, screening is done for increased maternal serum levels of α-fetoprotein, reduced human chorionic gonadotropin levels, and reduced unconjugated estriol levels; termination of pregnancy in cases with positive test results has further reduced the prevalence of NTDs.[38]

Anencephaly is a lethal disorder resulting from the neural tube failing to close between the 23rd and 26th day following conception. This leads to disorganization of neural elements and the absence of skull formation.[35] Some deep cerebral structures may remain intact, and the brainstem may develop normally. With the latter situation, normal respiration and cardiovascular functions may develop, enabling the infant to survive for hours or days after birth. Other structures in the head and brain, including the eyes, face, and pituitary gland, may not develop normally. An infant with anencephaly is usually blind, deaf, and unable to feel pain.

Encephalocele is a herniation of neural tissue and meninges out of the skull through deficient skin and bone (see Fig. 26.12A). They may be associated with other cerebral malformations. Encephaloceles found anteriorly are associated with underlying brain, orbital structures, or pituitary gland anomaly. Posteriorly, encephaloceles are associated with cerebral or cerebellar tissue that herniates through a bony defect in the posterior cranium. Intranasal encephaloceles may be difficult to detect. These defects carry a poor prognosis for long-term survival. The only treatment is reparative surgery; occasionally shunts are placed for resulting hydrocephalus. Most infants die, and in survivors, severe neurodevelopmental disability is common. Most of these children have hydrocephalus.[39]

Spina bifida refers to a group of conditions in which there is abnormal or incomplete formation of the midline structures over the back (see Fig. 26.12B).[35] Skin, bony, and neural elements may be involved singly or in combination. Congenital malformations of the spinal cord may exist in isolation or in association with brain anomalies. These defects may present at birth, as in the case of the more severe and open lesions (i.e., spina bifida) or be identified later in childhood if the skin overlying the spinal defect is intact (e.g., spina bifida occulta). Those who develop a Chiari

malformation may present with cervical cord or bulbar deficits, placing them at risk for respiratory embarrassment (see Figs. 26.13, and 26.14). Children with spinal cord lesions are at increased risk for sensory deficits, making meticulous skin care and positioning essential to prevent pressure sores and damage to neuropathic joints.

Spina bifida occulta occurs in the absence of herniation of neural tissue or coverings so that the overlying skin appears to be intact and normal. In many cases, a hairy patch or a dermal sinus (i.e., sacral dimple) may communicate with the meninges or attach to the spinal cord or a lipoma that causes a fatty swelling overlying the bony defect. The spinal cord may be tethered by internal connection to such structures, making it vulnerable to trauma at surgery and during growth, especially at puberty. The spinal cord may be abnormally formed, with cartilaginous or bony spurs that damage or divide the cord during growth as the neural tissue grows at a slower rate than the surrounding bone (i.e., diastematomyelia). These infants may not be candidates for a caudal block because the spinal cord may end at an unusually low position.

Spina bifida cystica, the most common type of spinal dysraphism, manifests as an obvious lesion on the back. The defect may be diagnosed antenatally or at birth. The abnormally developed spinal cord may be covered by a layer of meninges (i.e., meningocele) or remain uncovered (i.e., myelomeningocele). The spinal level of the lesion is the major determinant of morbidity. Myelomeningoceles need to be repaired within a few days of birth to prevent infection and further damage to the neural tissues. A cerebrospinal fluid (CSF) leak or frank dural rupture may develop, leading to intravascular volume and electrolyte abnormalities that should be treated preoperatively.

When the defect is identified at birth, it is optimally managed in a specialist center by a multidisciplinary team (i.e., pediatrician, neurologist, neurosurgeon, orthopedic surgeon, and others) who can anticipate, prevent, and treat complications and assist in the child's long-term care. Children with dysraphism often develop postoperative hydrocephalus because of disrupted CSF flow and require a ventriculoperitoneal shunt. Long-term complications, including paraparesis, neurogenic bladder and bowel, renal insufficiency, trophic limb changes, pressure sores, joint contractures, and scoliosis may require surgical repair and future intervention. Children with NTDs may acquire latex allergy if they are exposed repeatedly to latex products (they do not have a genetic predisposition toward latex allergy). To prevent latex allergy, these children should be cared for in a latex-free environment. The anesthesia considerations for NTDs are presented in Chapter 26.

Chiari Malformation

Chiari malformations of the nervous system may coexist with other anomalies and manifest in the neonatal period or later in the early decades of life (Table 24.3).

Chiari I. This is the mildest of the hindbrain malformations and is characterized by displacement of cerebellar tonsils more than 5 mm caudally through the foramen magnum. The brainstem and fourth ventricle retain a relatively normal position, although the fourth ventricle may be small and slightly distorted. Although the spectrum of Chiari I malformations is not usually associated with other cerebral abnormalities, syringomyelia is found in 20% to 70% of patients, depending on the degree and extent of disruption of normal CSF flow between the spine and cranium. Adequate surgical decompression at the foramen magnum and upper cervical spine is the treatment of choice for neuronal dysfunction,

TABLE 24.3 | Chiari Malformations

Type	Main Features	Associated Abnormalities	Neurologic Features
Chiari I	Downward displacement of cerebellar tonsils >5 mm caudally through the foramen magnum	Syringomyelia (in 20%-70%); hydrocephalus	Later onset (>age 12 years), cervical cord signs: tetraparesis, sensory deficits of upper limbs
Chiari II	Downward displacement of cerebellar tonsils, vermis fourth ventricle and brainstem with obstruction of CSF flow	Supratentorial and infratentorial abnormalities; myelomeningocele or meningocoel in virtually all	Present in neonate, macrocephaly, increased intracranial pressure, cranial nerve palsies, cord signs
Chiari III (rare)	Downward displacement of cerebellum into posterior encephalocele; elongation of fourth ventricle	Posterior defects: cervical spina bifida ± cranium bifidum	Present in neonate with signs of hydrocephalus ± brainstem and cervical cord signs
Chiari IV (extremely rare)	Cerebellar hypoplasia or primary cerebellar agenesis	Usually none	± Ataxia

24

symptomatic syrinx, or hydrocephalus. Ventriculoperitoneal shunting may be required for hydrocephalus and syringostomy or syrinx shunting for cord drainage if the craniocervical decompression alone does not relieve the pressure in the syrinx.

Chiari II. This is a more extensive and complex abnormality than the Chiari I malformation, with infratentorial and supratentorial abnormalities. It affects 0.02% of births, females twice as often as males. The cerebellar tonsils, inferior vermis, fourth ventricle, and brainstem are herniated from a shallow posterior fossa through a wide foramen magnum with obstruction to CSF flow at the exit of the fourth ventricle. Occasionally the fourth ventricle becomes "trapped" or encysted and will enlarge to appear normal or dilated. There is virtually always a meningocele or meningomyelocele present, some with associated hydrocephalus.

Chiari III. This defect is very rare. There is herniation of the posterior fossa contents into an associated occipital or high cervical cephalocele with the other features of a Chiari II malformation. These patients have severe neurologic defects and a poor prognosis.

Chiari IV. This abnormality is controversial and extremely rare. Many authors consider the features of primary cerebellar agenesis as a Chiari IV malformation, but it must be differentiated from a Chiari II malformation associated with a "vanishing" cerebellum. In primary cerebellar agenesis, there are remnants of a residual cerebellum (for example, anterior quadrangular lobule), a normal brainstem, a normal-sized posterior fossa, and a normal spine. The lack of a meningomyelocele virtually excludes a Chiari II malformation.[40]

Syringomyelia

Syringomyelia results from a glial cell–lined cavitation within the spinal cord. Diagnosis has been greatly simplified by the use of MRI, which provides images of the spinal cord and the tubular fluid-filled space within.[35] Although the spectrum of Chiari I malformations is not usually associated with other cerebral abnormalities, syringomyelia is found in 20% to 70% of patients, depending on the degree and extent of disruption of normal CSF flow between the spine and cranium. Syringomyelia manifests with dissociated sensory loss, usually in the upper limbs, causing loss or impairment of pain and temperature sensation, which may cause trophic changes in the fingers and neuropathic joints. It may progress to paralysis and hyporeflexia later in life. The lower limbs may exhibit pyramidal signs; some lesions may extend upward (i.e., syringobulbia) and produce lower brainstem signs, such as stridor and laryngospasm (i.e., vocal cord palsy).

Treatment of syringomyelia is controversial, especially if the lesion is asymptomatic. Management may focus on associated disorders as syringomyelia may progress slowly or not at all.

Adequate surgical decompression at the foramen magnum and upper cervical spine is the treatment of choice for neuronal dysfunction, symptomatic syrinx, or hydrocephalus. Ventriculoperitoneal shunting may be required for hydrocephalus and syringostomy or syrinx shunting for cord drainage if the craniocervical decompression alone does not relieve the pressure in the syrinx.

Hydrocephalus

Hydrocephalus is defined as an increase in the volume of CSF in the brain, particularly the ventricles, associated with an increase in the intracranial pressure (ICP) with classical signs and symptoms. It results from overproduction or impaired drainage of CSF from the brain.[39] In practice, overproduction is an uncommon source of hydrocephalus; these cases most often result from tumors of the choroid plexus. Obstructed drainage of CSF is the far more common source for hydrocephalus. The causes of hydrocephalus include intraventricular hemorrhage, Arnold-Chiari malformation, brain tumor, congenital obstruction, and myelomeningocele. Hydrocephalus may present with chronic or acute symptoms of ICP. Children typically present with a headache and irritability, but signs and symptoms can progress to lethargy, seizures, vomiting, and ophthalmoplegia as pressure within the brain increases. In infants, it presents as accelerated head growth, bulging fontanelle, poor feeding, sunsetting sign, and developmental delay. If left untreated, it may lead to a reduced level of consciousness, oculomotor palsies, sluggish pupillary light reactions, bradycardia, and eventually respiratory arrest. Diagnosis of hydrocephalus is confirmed by neuroimaging, often with computed tomography (CT) in the acute situation, followed by MRI.

Surgery is the definitive treatment for hydrocephalus. It usually involves inserting a drainage system to shunt CSF from the brain to another site in the body (see Fig. 26.11). After insertion of a shunt, children should be closely monitored for shunt complications; these include infection, blockage or fracture of the shunt, and overdrainage of CSF. The anesthesia considerations for treating hydrocephalus are discussed in Chapter 26. An endoscopic cerebral aqueductoplasty or third venticulostomy may be helpful for obstructive hydrocephalus.

DISORDERS OF VENTRAL INDUCTION

Holoprosencephaly is a cephalic disorder in which the forebrain of the embryo fails to develop into discrete hemispheres with normal connections.[35] There are three types:

1. Lobar: There is almost complete separation of the hemispheres, and the corpus callosum is almost absent.
2. Semilobar: The two hemispheres are divided posteriorly, with interhemispheric connections present anteriorly. The corpus callosum is absent anteriorly, and the thalami are fused in the midline.
3. Alobar: An undivided and small forebrain with a dorsal sac may contain some cortex. Severe facial defects may include cyclopia (i.e., single orbit with fused globes), cebocephaly (i.e., single nostril), and a midline cleft lip.

Associated malformations (e.g., congenital heart disease, scalp deficits, polydactyly) are common. Chromosomal anomalies may be identified, and a complex syndromic disorder may occur in some of these children. The diagnosis rests on a careful description of the external and internal morphology using MRI, followed by genetic assessment. Complications include hydrocephalus, endocrine deficits, epilepsy, and severe complex disability, usually with a shortened life expectancy.

DISORDERS OF CORTICAL DEVELOPMENT

Malformations of the cerebral cortex are many and varied. Malformations of cortical development (MCD) are increasingly recognized as an important cause of epilepsy and developmental delay. It is estimated that up to 40% of children with refractory epilepsy have a cortical malformation. MCD encompass a wide spectrum of disorders with various underlying genetic etiologies and clinical manifestations. High-resolution imaging has dramatically improved our recognition of MCD.[41] Disruptions at the various stages of development lead to characteristic MCDs. Disorders of neurogenesis give rise to microcephaly (small brain) or macrocephaly (large brain). Disorders of early neuroblast migration give rise to periventricular heterotopia (neurons located along the ventricles), whereas abnormalities later in migration lead to lissencephaly (smooth brain) or subcortical band heterotopia (smooth brain with a band of heterotopic neurons under the cortex). Abnormal neuronal migration arrest gives rise to overmigration of neurons in cobblestone lissencephaly. Lastly, disorders of neuronal organization cause polymicrogyria (abnormally small gyri and sulci). MRI has advanced the identification of these features and their classification.

Environmental agents and genetic abnormalities have been identified for many of these malformations, and genetic derangements can produce a multisystem syndrome. Some of the genes involved are the *LIS1* gene, 4p– (Wolf-Hirschhorn), and 17p– (Miller-Dieker syndrome). Intrauterine insults in early pregnancy have been implicated in cases in which autopsy is performed. Clinical effects vary, and the severity depends on the site and extent of the lesion. Survivors may have no symptoms or have profound, complex neurodisability. Children may have learning disabilities, epilepsy, focal neurologic deficits, motor dysfunction, and other system involvement.

Progressive Neurologic Disorders

PRIMARY BRAIN TUMORS

The incidence of primary brain tumors is 2.6 per 100,000 children, and they account for 15% to 20% of all childhood malignancies. The male/female ratio is equal except for a male preponderance in medulloblastoma and germ cell tumors. One-third of these tumors occur before 5 years of age, and 75% occur before 10 years of age.[42] CNS tumours are the second most common pediatric tumor, surpassed only by leukemia. Supratentorial tumors are common in the first 2 or 3 years of life, whereas infratentorial tumors predominate from ages 4 to 10 years. Two-thirds of the tumors are located infratentorially and one-third supratentorially (Table 24.4).[43] After the age of 10 years, tumors occur with equal frequency in both locations in the brain. Pathologic classification, which is based on the cell of origin and degree of malignancy, extends from grade I (benign) to grade IV (malignant).[44]

The presentation depends on the age of the child and site of the tumor. Infants are typically irritable, with increasing head circumference, failure to thrive, and developmental regression. Older children develop headaches, nausea and vomiting, seizures, gait disturbances, and visual deficits. Supratentorial tumors can present with seizures, focal neurological deficit, personality change, visual field defects (optic pathway gliomas), and endocrine dysfunction (craniopharyngiomas). Infratentorial tumors present with cerebellar ataxia (medulloblastoma, cerebellar astrocytomas), nausea and vomiting, signs of increased ICP (ependymomas), and cranial nerve and pyramidal tract signs. If the lesion is rapidly expanding and is accompanied by significant cerebral edema or obstructs CSF drainage, ICP will increase. Occasionally, a hemorrhage occurs into the tumor, causing a dramatic increase in ICP with the associated signs and symptoms, necessitating emergency treatment. Ultimately, brainstem decompensation and death ensue if the lesion is left untreated.

Diagnosis of a primary brain tumor is usually confirmed with MRI and magnetic resonance spectroscopy (MRS). Tissue diagnosis by a biopsy is always desirable, although not always achievable. Microscopy of CSF may yield tumor cells and facilitate the diagnosis. Image-guided biopsy may be possible and is preferred for appropriately sited lesions.

Surgery is the mainstay of treatment and is usually combined with radiotherapy or chemotherapy, or both. Preoperatively, cerebral edema should be treated with corticosteroids to reduce ICP, alleviate symptoms and signs, and enable correction of fluid and electrolyte abnormalities. Seizures require anticonvulsant therapy. Nutrition may be poor and necessitate aggressive management with enteral and parenteral feedings. Operative intervention for increased ICP may require CSF diversion by shunting internally or externally. Depending on the tissue diagnosis and location, total resection of the tumor may be indicated, although the timing of the surgery may depend on whether the tumor should first be treated with radiation therapy or chemotherapy. Aggressive surgery with the intent of completely resecting the tumor improves the prognosis for many tumor types but carries with it significant risks of residual neurologic deficits.

The 5-year survival rate of greater than 60% for primary brain tumors largely reflects improved imaging, aggressive surgery, and evidence-based therapy.[45] Unfortunately, children who survive CNS tumors frequently have permanent neurologic deficits, including epilepsy, learning disabilities, visual or hearing impairment, and growth and endocrine disorders. Short-term and long-term follow-up evaluations by specialist teams are required, along with careful emotional and social support for children and their families. Some children have genetic predispositions for CNS tumors, such as neurofibromatosis (i.e., schwannomas of the spinal cord, peripheral nerve tumors, skeletal deformities, carcinoid syndrome, and multiple endocrine neoplasia, including pheochromocytoma) and tuberous sclerosis (i.e., brain tumors,

TABLE 24.4 | Common Central Nervous System Tumors in Childhood

Tumor Type	Percentage of All Childhood CNS Tumors	Clinical Features	Treatment	Prognosis or Survival
Medulloblastoma	14–20	Acute ataxia ↑ Intracranial pressure	Surgical excision + radiotherapy or chemotherapy in children <2 years	75% at 5 years 50% at 10 years
Cerebellar astrocytoma (80% cystic)	15–20	Subacute-chronic ataxia Head tilt ± ↑ Intracranial pressure	Surgical excision	100% at 5 years, if totally excised
Posterior fossa ependymoma	6–10	Cranial nerve palsies Stiff neck ataxia ↑ Intracranial pressure	Surgical excision Radiotherapy	40% at 5 years but 14% if <5 years
Brainstem glioma	6–16	Cranial nerve palsies Long tract signs ↑ Intracranial pressure late	(Stereotactic) biopsy if possible Radiotherapy ± chemotherapy, depends on age and cell type	Survival variable and depends on cell type
Craniopharyngioma	6–10	Endocrine disorders ↑ Intracranial pressure Visual impairment	Surgery Hormonal therapy	Survival variable
Visual pathway glioma	3–5	Proptosis, ↓ vision Associated disorders (e.g., neurofibromatosis type I)	Controversial and individualized	Variable
Pineal region tumors	<2	↑ Intracranial pressure Loss of upward gaze	Surgery ± radiotherapy	Variable
Hemisphere glioma	25–30	α Location: ↑ intracranial pressure, seizures, focal neurologic deficit	Surgery ± radiotherapy ± chemotherapy	Depends on cell type
Meningioma	<2	↑ Intracranial pressure Seizures	Surgery	Variable
Ganglioma and dysembryoplastic neuroepithelial tumor (DNET)	1–5	Focal epilepsy	Surgery	Good May cure epilepsy
Primitive neuroepithelial tumor (PNET)	1–2	↑ Intracranial pressure, focal neurologic deficit	Surgery + radiotherapy	Poor
Intraventricular tumors, various cell types	5	↑ Intracranial pressure: hydrocephalus	Shunting and surgical excision	Variable
Basal ganglia tumors, various cell types	5	Hemiparesis, dystonia	Stereotactic biopsy Radiotherapy if malignant	Depends on cell type

CNS, central nervous system; ±, with or without; ↓, decreased; ↑, increased.

cardiac rhabdomyomas, renal abnormalities, tumors, and hepatoma) that require genetic analysis and long-term follow-up.

Tumors of the spinal cord are rare in childhood. They may be benign or malignant, sited within the cord (intramedullary) or outside (extramedullary), and are usually astrocytomas (60%) or ependymomas. Symptoms may initially be nonspecific and vague, especially in young children. These may include pain, paresthesia, paresis, sphincter disturbance, spinal deformity (astrocytomas), torticollis, and hydrocephalus (ependymoma). A diagnosis may be delayed owing to the vagueness of the symptoms, with an increased risk of spinal cord compression. Delayed decompression can cause vascular compromise, which may lead to total and irreversible paralysis of the limbs, bladder, and bowel, and permanent, severe disability. Diagnosis is best made by MRI of the cord, which provides details of the lesion and adjacent structures without the risk of further decompensation, a problem raised by the use of myelography in the past.[43]

Treatment usually involves surgery to decompress the cord and excise or biopsy the lesion. For intramedullary tumors, excision may be impossible, and biopsy may risk further damage to the spinal cord. Cell type may be determined by CSF examination. Follow-up treatment with radiotherapy may be indicated. Children with established neurologic deficits require a program of rehabilitation.

METABOLIC DISEASE

Inborn errors of carbohydrate, protein, or fat metabolism usually are genetic in origin. The molecular defects of many of these metabolic disorders have been identified. Most of these disorders are inherited as autosomal recessive.

Metabolic disorders may present differently depending on the age of the child. In the neonatal period, they present with poor feeding/suck, vomiting, hypotonia, respiratory compromise/apnea, progressive encephalopathy, and seizures, and the clinical picture may be mistaken for sepsis. It is therefore important to also consider metabolic disorders when thinking of infection as a potential cause of these symptoms in a neonate. In childhood, metabolic disorders can present with recurrent unexplained vomiting with

TABLE 24.5	Neurometabolic Disorders
Lysosomal diseases	
Mucolipidoses, sialidoses, disorders of glycoprotein metabolism	
Peroxisomal disorders	
Amino acid disorders	
Organic acid disorders	
Neurotransmitter disorders	
Urea cycle disorders	
Disorders of vitamin metabolism	
Lactic acidosis	
Respiratory chain disorders	
Mitochondrial fatty acid β-oxidation defects	
Disorders of cholesterol metabolism	
Disorders of copper metabolism	
Miscellaneous disorders	

dehydration, strokelike episodes, acute liver or renal failure, cardiomyopathy, unexplained encephalopathy, and seizures. These diseases may cause a static encephalopathy but more often produce a progressive course with loss of physical and intellectual skills. Some neurometabolic diseases are associated with intellectual deficits and some with physical deficits; systemic features may be prominent and neurologic signs are common (Table 24.5).

There are three main groups of neurometabolic diseases[46]:

1. Those with a known enzymatic defect, including disorders of amino acid metabolism (e.g., phenylketonuria), peroxisomal disorders (e.g., adrenoleukodystrophy), and lysosomal storage disorders (e.g., Tay-Sachs disease)
2. Those with abnormal storage accumulation in CNS cells, including lysosomal storage disorders and mucopolysaccharidoses
3. Those with no identified biochemical defect (e.g., Cockayne syndrome), a heterogeneous group that is shrinking as research identifies the biochemical and genetic defects.

There is considerable overlap among the three groups. All of these disorders are rare, and although some are treatable, most are relentlessly progressive and associated with early death. Many patients show a steady decline, with a gradual increase in symptoms and loss of function or a stepwise deterioration with bouts of acute illness leading to a sudden loss of function.

There are several basic laboratory tests that should be performed in every child with an acute illness in whom a metabolic disorder is a possibility. Blood glucose, ammonia, acid-base status, lactate, and urinary ketones are essential tests; other tests include plasma amino acids, urine organic acids, acylcarnitine profile, blood cell counts, liver function tests, coagulation studies, creatine kinase and uric acid. In an acute situation, the management consists of stopping feeds and starting an infusion of 10% glucose with appropriate electrolytes (150 mL/kg per day). Glucose supply at this infusion rate equates to normal hepatic glucose production. This is usually sufficient for disorders of reduced fasting tolerance, such as glycogen storage disorders or medium-chain acyl-CoA dehydrogenase deficiency (MCAD) (fatty acid oxidation disorders). Exogenous glucose may not be sufficient in disorders that are exacerbated by catabolism (organic acidurias or urea cycle disorders). However, exogenous glucose administration may be potentially dangerous in mitochondrial disorders (specifically pyruvate dehydrogenase deficiency) as a high glucose supply may enhance lactic acidosis. In most cases, the benefits of high glucose infusion

outweigh the risks; however, lactate and acid-base status should be checked regularly.[47]

Treatment is available for only a few of these diseases and consists primarily of dietary strategies, although some pharmacologic treatments are used. Started early, especially in the presymptomatic phase, treatment may prevent neurologic complications. An example is phenylketonuria, a disorder of amino acid metabolism. The prevalence varies by population, with an incidence of 1 case per 100,000 people in the United States. Screening occurs in the neonatal period, and affected children start a special diet. Those who have good dietary management throughout life may develop relatively few problems, although close monitoring by a specialist team of physicians and dieticians is essential to ensure metabolic stability. Unfortunately, treatments may be of questionable benefit for many children.

Disorders that cause lactic acidosis are the most common of these diseases, although many individuals who harbor the genetic substrate for one of these disorders may not express it or may come to diagnosis very late in life.[48] The features of these diseases are extremely varied, and, although the neuropathologic, biochemical, and imaging abnormalities are well recognized, a precise diagnosis may remain elusive.

Anesthesia Considerations for Progressive Neurologic Disorders

The risks associated with general anesthesia for children with progressive neurologic disorders include problems posed by fasting and the need to keep the patient's metabolism stable during a period of stress. Meticulous planning with the child's metabolic specialist is essential before elective procedures. In the case of emergency surgery, the children and parents should be aware of or have written instructions regarding the preferred management of nutrition and metabolic indices, or they should have a resource person to call for specific advice.

Neuromuscular Disorders

Neuromuscular disorders are caused by an abnormality of any component of the lower motor neuron system: anterior horn cell in the spinal cord, axon, neuromuscular junction, or muscle fiber (Fig. 24.1).[49] The cardinal features are weakness of skeletal muscles that is proximal, distal, or generalized in distribution; hypotonia; and reduced deep tendon reflexes. True fatigability suggests a defect of the neuromuscular junction. Neuropathy is characterized by distal weakness and sensory deficit. Joint contractures, scoliosis, and respiratory and cardiac involvement are common complications and some conditions are associated with cognitive deficits.

DISORDERS OF THE ANTERIOR HORN CELL
Spinal Muscular Atrophies

Spinal muscular atrophy (SMA) is one of the most common autosomal recessive diseases, affecting approximately 1 in 10,000 live births, and with a carrier frequency of approximately 1 in 50. SMAs are a group of disorders in which there is progressive degeneration of the anterior horn cells (lower motor neurons) of the spinal cord and brainstem nuclei, leading to death of motor neurons. Recent evidence has shed new light on the involvement of nonmotor neuronal cells both within and outside the CNS in the pathogenesis and phenotypic presentation of SMA.[50] The diagnosis of SMA is based on molecular genetic testing. Mutations in *SMN1* (survival motor neuron 1) are known to cause SMA; increases in the *SMN2* copy number often modify the

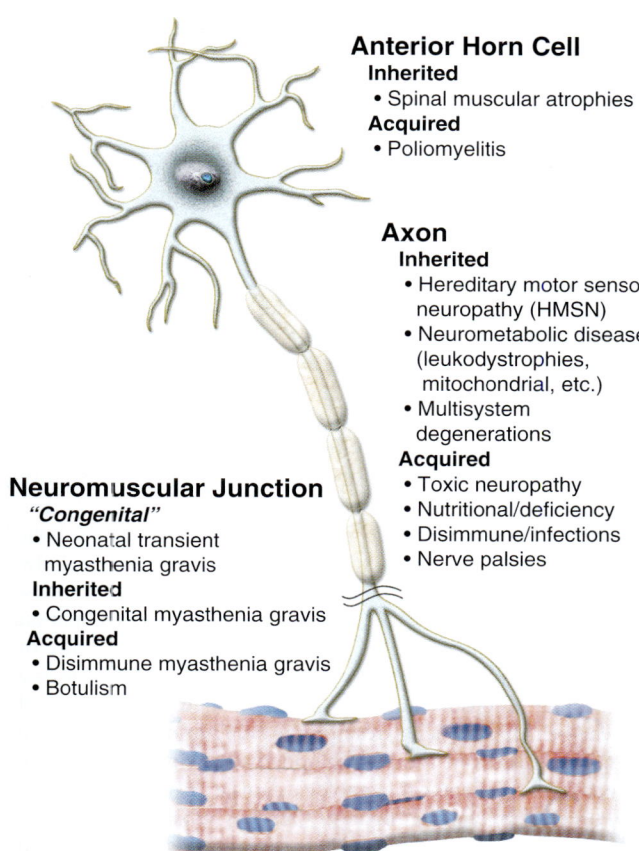

Anterior Horn Cell
Inherited
- Spinal muscular atrophies

Acquired
- Poliomyelitis

Axon
Inherited
- Hereditary motor sensory neuropathy (HMSN)
- Neurometabolic disease (leukodystrophies, mitochondrial, etc.)
- Multisystem degenerations

Acquired
- Toxic neuropathy
- Nutritional/deficiency
- Disimmune/infections
- Nerve palsies

Neuromuscular Junction
"Congenital"
- Neonatal transient myasthenia gravis

Inherited
- Congenital myasthenia gravis

Acquired
- Disimmune myasthenia gravis
- Botulism

Muscle Fiber
Inherited
- Congenital myopathies
- Muscular dystrophies
- Myotonias
- Metabolic myopathies

Acquired
- Disimmune myopathies (dermatomyositis)
- Endocrine myopathies
- Toxic (e.g., drug-induced [steroid])

FIGURE 24.1 Diagram of a lower motor neuron. (Modified from Dubowitz V. *Muscle Disorders in Childhood*. Philadelphia: WB Saunders; 1978. Courtesy A. Moosa, MD.)

phenotype. *SMN1* is the primary gene in which mutation causes SMA.

The existent classification by age of onset and maximum function achieved is useful for prognosis and management.[51,52] Subtypes include the following:

- SMA 0 (proposed), with prenatal onset and severe joint contractures, facial diplegia, and respiratory failure.
- SMA 1, with onset before age 6 months
- SMA 2, with onset between age 6 and 12 months
- SMA 3, with onset in childhood after age 12 months and ability to walk at least 25 m
- SMA 4, with adult onset

Curative treatment is not available, but much can be done to improve duration and quality of life, especially for mildly affected children.

Type 0 SMA: In the most severe forms, decreased intrauterine movements suggest prenatal onset of the disease and present with severe weakness and joint contractures at birth, have been labeled SMN 0. Some of these children may have congenital bone fractures and extremely thin ribs.

Type 1 SMA (i.e., Werdnig-Hoffmann disease) manifests at or soon after birth in most cases. The infant may appear neurologically normal at first, but the typical picture soon emerges. Parents may first notice an abnormal breathing pattern as the intercostal muscles are affected, and the respiratory pattern becomes diaphragmatic, with a bell-shaped chest observed clinically and radiographically. The infant is usually very alert and interactive but severely weak and floppy. There is good facial expression and normal eye movements, but the tongue fasciculates, and the tendon reflexes are absent. There is no cardiac involvement. Weakness, hypotonia, and bulbar involvement lead to progressive respiratory insufficiency and swallowing dysfunction, which are frequently complicated by episodes of aspiration. Most children die within the first 2 years of life, mainly owing to respiratory complications. Management is essentially palliative, with gentle physiotherapy to keep the limbs flexible and special care with feeding. Noninvasive nocturnal ventilation is increasingly used, but invasive ventilation through a tracheostomy is not considered appropriate in most medical centers. This issue has provoked considerable debate in the literature.[53]

Type 2 SMA is an intermediate form, but is the most prevalent. Because the weakness is milder, many children survive for years with meticulous multidisciplinary therapy, orthopedic and respiratory management, and care with nutrition. Onset occurs at 6 to 12 months of age. The clinical signs are similar to those of type 1 SMA, and the children are bright, intelligent, and particularly verbal. Patients with type 2 SMA usually achieve independent sitting at some stage, but these children never bear weight or walk. Respiratory infections are a particular problem, and noninvasive nocturnal respiratory support (i.e., biphasic or continuous positive airway pressure) with a face mask and portable ventilator is well tolerated. This improves well-being and enables remarkably full activity despite weakness.[54,55] Joint contractures are almost inevitable, as is progressive scoliosis, which usually appears early, and management is difficult in the very young child. Operative correction and stabilization with instrumentation is delayed as long as possible to prevent the complications of pubertal growth with a fixed spine; children usually tolerate the procedure well if they are carefully prepared and managed. Some children with type 2 SMA develop feeding difficulties because of weakness of bulbar musculature or as a complication of chronic nocturnal hypoventilation. Good nutrition is essential for health, and supplementation and gastrostomy feeding may be required.[56]

Type 3 SMA (i.e., Kugelberg-Welander disease) is a mild variant with similar signs of flaccid and areflexic weakness of lower limbs more so than upper limbs and with proximal predominance. These children attain independent walking, although it may be later than normal and tenuous. There is often deterioration around the time of puberty, when the growth spurt causes the previously precariously balanced muscle groups to become dysfunctional. Obesity and joint contracture also may affect the situation. Aggressive measures to keep the child walking are often effective and delay or prevent scoliosis and lower limb contracture.[57] Respiratory support may be necessary for nocturnal hypoventilation. Prognosis for long-term survival is good.

Type 4 SMA has been added to this classification to describe those patients with adult onset (>18 years) and mild course. This group includes patients who are able to walk in adulthood and without respiratory and nutritional problems.

Other very rare SMA variants also exist in childhood. The scapuloperoneal SMA with predominant weakness of scapuloperoneal and laryngeal muscles with autosomal dominant (AD) inheritance is due to gene defect 12q24.1-q24.31. SMA with pontocerebellar hypoplasia with brainstem and cerebellar hypoplasia that presents before 6 months with autosomal recessive (AR) inheritance is caused by gene *VRK1*. X-linked infantile SMA with arthrogryposis, presenting with contractures at birth or infancy and leading to early death, has a genetic defect in Xp11.3-q11.2 with AR inheritance. SMA with respiratory distress type 1 presents with eventration of diaphragm, distal weakness, and pes equinas and has an AR inheritance owing to immunoglobulin mu binding protein 2 (IGHMBP2). Congenital distal SMA is nonprogressive and presents with distal contractures, with AD inheritance and gene defect in 12q23-q24.[52]

Anesthesia Considerations for Spinal Muscular Atrophies

Children with SMA present for a variety of surgical and diagnostic procedures, including gastrostomy placement, tracheostomy, and spinal surgery, that will require anesthesia.[58] Rigorous preanesthesia evaluation is essential; perioperative care needs to be tailored to each child's needs, and postoperative respiratory support may be required. A variety of anesthesia techniques have been used successfully with and without muscle relaxants. Various degrees of sensitivity to nondepolarizing neuromuscular blocking drugs (NMBDs) have been described, and it seems prudent to avoid or reduce the dose of these agents. If they are used, neuromuscular function should be assessed continuously and the effect of the relaxant antagonized at the conclusion of surgery. Succinylcholine is contraindicated in these children. Spinal and epidural anesthesia and postoperative epidural analgesia have been used without adverse effects; however, the potential for respiratory depression may be increased with the addition of neuraxial opioids.

Poliomyelitis

Poliomyelitis is a highly contagious, infectious disease caused by poliovirus, a human enterovirus. Most poliovirus infections are asymptomatic. If symptomatic, it occurs in two phases: an acute, nonspecific, febrile illness followed by aseptic meningitis and acute, flaccid, lower motor neuron paralysis. It typically manifests asymmetrically and may affect any muscle group. In children with respiratory involvement, lifelong ventilation may be needed. Fortunately, this situation is almost unheard of in the Western world because polio has been almost eradicated by immunization.[59]

AXONAL DISORDERS

Hereditary Neuropathies

The hereditary neuropathies are a heterogeneous group of disorders that can be divided into two major subgroups: neuropathies in which the neuropathy is the sole or primary feature and neuropathies in which the neuropathy is part of a more generalized neurologic or multisystem disorder. There are five subgroups in the common hereditary neuropathies[60]:

- Charcot-Marie-Tooth disease (CMT): hereditary motor sensory neuropathy (HMSN)
- Hereditary neuropathy with liability to pressure palsy (HNPP)
- Hereditary sensory and autonomic neuropathy (HSAN)
- Distal hereditary motor neuropathy (dHMN)
- Hereditary neuralgic amyotrophy (HNA)

Neuropathies can also be part of a more widespread neurologic or multisystem disorder:

- Familial amyloid polyneuropathy (FAP)
- Disturbances of lipid metabolism (e.g., adrenoleukodystrophy)
- Porphyrias
- Disorders with defective DNA (e.g., ataxia telangiectasia)
- Neuropathies associated with mitochondrial diseases
- Neuropathies associated with hereditary ataxias
- Miscellaneous

Clinical presentation depends on the subtype and can occur at any age. Children usually present with disorders of gait or foot deformity, or they may come to the attention of a neurologist or geneticist through an affected parent. Clinical signs are usually confined to the lower limbs in the early years and may lead to orthopedic intervention before diagnosis. Some neuropathies are associated with multisystem involvement, including cardiac, autonomic, and respiratory systems, and a complete preoperative assessment of these children is essential.[61]

Peripheral neuropathy is a component of various neurometabolic disorders in which there is involvement of other parts of the nervous system or of other organs. For example, in the leukodystrophies (metachromatic and Krabbe disease),[62,63] demyelination affects central and peripheral axons, giving a clinical picture of combined upper and lower neuron features. Refsum disease is a peroxisomal disorder caused by the impaired α-oxidation of branched-chain fatty acids, resulting in buildup of phytanic acid and its derivatives in the plasma and tissues.[64] Individuals with Refsum disease present with neurologic damage, cerebellar degeneration, and peripheral neuropathy. Onset is most commonly in childhood/adolescence with a progressive course. In children with mitochondrial diseases, peripheral neuropathy is often found, along with myriad other features.[65]

Multisystem degenerations are often genetically determined disorders of the nervous system that rarely begin in childhood.[61] Features may include dementia, epilepsy, extrapyramidal signs, brainstem dysfunction, vision and hearing impairment, anterior horn cell involvement, and peripheral neuropathy. They tend to have a progressive course.

Acquired Disorders of the Peripheral Nerves

Acquired disorders of the peripheral nerves are rare in childhood. In clinical practice in the developed world, neuropathies complicating metabolic or nutritional disorders and treatment for cancer are the most common forms. In underdeveloped parts of the world, nutritional deficiencies, especially of vitamins E, B_1, B_6, B_{12}, niacin, and thiamine, are important. The neuropathic features may be overshadowed by the other characteristics of the disease.

Guillain-Barré Syndrome

Guillain-Barré syndrome (GBS) is an acute demyelinating disorder that causes progressive weakness, usually 2 to 4 weeks after an illness with features of a viral infection or after immunization.[38] It has an incidence of 1 to 2 per 100,000. The term acute inflammatory demyelinating polyneuropathy (AIDP) is often used synonymously with GBS. Variants with a similar/related clinical picture include acute motor axonal neuropathy (AMAN), acute motor and sensory axonal neuropathy with prominent sensory features (AMSAN, poor prognosis), and Miller Fisher syndrome (ophthalmoplegia, ataxia, and areflexia). The causal mechanism is an immunologic cross-reactivity process secondary to a prodromal illness within the previous 4 weeks, typically an upper respiratory tract infection or gastroenteritis. Implicated organisms include mycoplasma, CMV, EBV, vaccinia, variola, *Campylobacter,* vesicular stomatitis virus (VZV), measles, mumps, hepatitis A and B, rubella, influenza A and B, coxsackievirus, and echovirus. Although the precise pathologic process has not been delineated, various antibodies, immune complexes, and complement components have been found, suggesting pathologic heterogeneity.

The disorder is rare in children younger than 3 years of age, and the onset is usually sudden, although subacute presentations have been reported. The first sign is weakness in the lower limbs, which characteristically ascends the body, next affecting the trunk, the upper limbs, and occasionally the cranial nerves. It causes a flaccid paralysis, usually sparing sensory function but causing pain and areflexia at all levels. Autonomic neuropathy may develop, causing instability of blood pressure and cardiac arrhythmias. Involvement of respiratory muscles may produce acute respiratory failure or apnea that necessitates tracheal intubation.

Guillain-Barré syndrome is diagnosed clinically, and the diagnosis is reinforced by finding an increased protein concentration in the CSF (despite a normal cell count) and abnormalities on nerve conduction studies. The studies may confirm demyelination by showing lowered nerve conduction velocity with distal delay, axonal involvement by low-amplitude action potentials, and in early cases, abnormality or absence of the Hoffmann reflex, indicating absence of the spinal reflex arc. MRI of the spine may show thickening and contrast enhancement of the nerve roots and cauda equina.[66]

Pediatric Guillain-Barré is usually a disease of briefer duration and more complete recovery than in affected adults.[67] Patients with very mild symptoms that do not interfere with activities of daily living can be observed for deterioration without treatment. The natural course is improvement, generally in 2 weeks, but progressive weakness can be seen up to 4 weeks. One-third of children may have long-term sequelae, although these are usually mild. Supportive care in the intensive care unit may be needed for children with severe bulbar or respiratory weakness.[68] In those children who are nonambulatory or with respiratory failure, IV immunoglobulin with or without plasmapheresis are the current treatment options.[65] Children with axonal neuropathies usually recover motor function more slowly than those with demyelination; it is believed that early treatment with IV immunoglobulin may speed recovery.[67,69] However, corticosteroids are ineffective and may delay recovery.

Chronic Inflammatory Demyelinating Polyneuropathy

Chronic inflammatory demyelinating polyneuropathy is extremely rare in childhood, and it is usually confined to older age groups. It manifests in a subacute, chronic progressive or relapsing and remitting pattern with prominent sensory involvement. Diagnostic investigations are similar to those for acute GBS. Corticosteroids, IV immunoglobulin, and plasma exchange have been effective.[68] Although these treatments may be effective in the short term, recurrences may take place, and the usual pattern is that of a chronic, disabling, and relapsing and remitting condition that does not threaten longevity but interferes significantly with the quality of life.[70]

Nerve Palsies

Like neuropathies, nerve palsies are uncommon in childhood.[71] The most common palsy encountered in children is neonatal or congenital facial nerve palsy. Babies can present with a paucity of arm movement depending on the site of the brachial plexus injury following difficult deliveries involving traction of head and shoulders. Erb palsy (injury to C5,6), Klumpke paralysis (injury to C8, T1), or commonly an injury to the whole brachial plexus with the arm limp and an associated clavicular fracture. Cranial nerve palsies, especially those that involve the eye muscles, are usually related to intracranial disease such as increased ICP in children, but they may also be isolated findings that result from viral infections; in the latter instances, recovery is the norm.

Peripheral nerve palsies such as carpal tunnel syndrome have been reported in childhood.[72] They may complicate severe juvenile arthritis[73] or storage disorders such as mucopolysaccharidoses. Because symptoms may be difficult to elicit from children at the best of times, identifying palsies may be problematic in children with severe learning disabilities. Young children usually have difficulty with pencil grip or other fine motor tasks. In older children, symptoms may include pain, tingling, or numbness in the hands. Specialist care may require routine assessment of nerve conduction and possible surgical decompression. Concern has been expressed regarding the emergence of carpal tunnel syndrome as a type of repetitive strain injury in children owing to excessive use of video games.[74] Case reviews refer to other types of repetitive strain injury, such as basketball training and skiing, as etiologic factors.[75]

DISORDERS OF THE NEUROMUSCULAR JUNCTION
Myasthenia Gravis

Myasthenia gravis is a disorder of the neuromuscular junction. The term *myasthenia gravis* includes heterogeneous autoimmune diseases, with a postsynaptic defect of neuromuscular transmission as the common feature. The autoimmune disorder is characterized by one of several lesions of acetylcholine-mediated transmission.[76] Weakness results from antibodies that block various receptors, inhibiting the excitatory effects of acetylcholine at the neuromuscular junction. This defective transmission at the junction results in a characteristic pattern of progressively reduced muscle strength with repeated use and recovery of muscle strength after a period of rest. Myasthenia gravis can be classified according to Table 24.6.

Juvenile myasthenia gravis is the childhood form of the adult disease. It is also an autoimmune disease, with the production of antibodies that attack the acetylcholine receptor and sometimes other proteins as mentioned in Table 24.6; management is similar to that for adult myasthenia gravis.

Symptomatic treatment of myasthenia gravis with acetylcholine esterase inhibition (e.g., pyridostigmine) is usually

TABLE 24.6	Classification of Myasthenia Gravis

Based on serum antibody specificity:
1. Acetylcholine receptor (AChR) antibody–positive
2. Muscle-specific tyrosine kinase (MuSK) receptor antibody–positive
3. Low-density lipoprotein receptor–related protein 4 (LRP4) antibody–positive
4. Antibody-negative

Based on thymus histopathology:
1. Thymitis
2. Thymoma
3. Atrophy

Based on degree of involvement:
1. Only eyes: ocular myasthenia
2. Full body: generalised myasthenia
3. Mainly swallow, speech: bulbar myasthenia

combined with immunosuppression. Azathioprine remains the first choice for long-term immunosuppressive therapy, usually along with steroids.[77,78] Alternative immunosuppressive options to azathioprine include cyclosporin, cyclophosphamide, methotrexate, mycophenolate mofetil, and tacrolimus.[79] Rituximab is a promising new drug for severe generalized myasthenia gravis. Emerging therapy options include belimumab, eculizumab, and the granulocyte macrophage colony-stimulating factor. For decades, thymectomy has been performed in younger adults to improve nonparaneoplastic myasthenia gravis.[80] With optimal treatment, the prognosis is good in terms of daily functions, quality of life, and survival.[81]

Neonatal Transient Myasthenia Gravis

Neonatal myasthenia gravis is caused by placental transfer of antibodies to acetylcholine receptors from an affected or previously affected mother.[82] The infant may present with feeding difficulties or respiratory dysfunction.[83] Treatment, which involves anticholinesterase medications, must be tailored to the nature and severity of the weakness, and intensive support occasionally is required. This form of myasthenia gravis is a transient disorder for which treatment is temporary and the risk of recurrence small. It should be anticipated in the offspring of any woman who has active myasthenia gravis or a history of the disorder, because cases have been described in infants of mothers in remission from myasthenia gravis.

Congenital Myasthenic Syndromes

Congenital myasthenic syndromes (CMSs) form a heterogeneous group of genetic diseases characterized by a dysfunction of neuromuscular transmission that usually starts during childhood; this causes muscle weakness that increases with exertion. The prevalence of CMSs is estimated at 1 in 500,000 in Europe and is considered to be less common than autoimmune myasthenia. The classification of CMSs is based on where the defect occurs in the neuromuscular synapse:presynaptic, synaptic, and postsynaptic. Several genes have been identified in which mutations cause the disease. The various CMSs share a common clinical presentation and the onset is generally early. Clinical signs consist of ophthalmoplegia and ptosis, dysphonia and swallowing disturbance, facial paresis, muscle fatigability, and recurrent apneas. The occurrence of such clinical events, worsened by exertion, is characteristic of the disease. Acute respiratory failure may occur, triggered by infectious episodes, and is frequent in the first months of life. In the absence of respiratory assistance, the risk of death is high. The favorable effect of cholinesterase inhibitors is a significant argument in favor of a myasthenic syndrome. However, two types of CMS are worsened by cholinesterase inhibitors: slow channel syndrome and acetylcholinesterase deficiency.[84]

Although rare, CMSs should be considered in the differential diagnosis of any neonate or infant who presents with motor problems (e.g., weakness, hypotonia, fatigability), eye signs (e.g., ptosis, ophthalmoplegia, pupillary abnormalities), and respiratory insufficiency (e.g., recurrent apneas, ventilator dependence). Late-onset muscle weakness has been reported in adolescence or early adulthood. Diagnosis may be difficult because the classic features of myasthenia, including responses to anticholinesterase medications, may be absent.[85] A Tensilon test, electromyography with repetitive nerve stimulation, a muscle biopsy, and molecular analysis in a specialist center should be sought to confirm the diagnosis.

Anesthesia Considerations for Myasthenia Gravis

The anesthesiologist may become involved in the management of children with myasthenia gravis for several reasons[86]:

- Children may suffer a crisis requiring mechanical ventilation
- There is a need for large-bore central access to facilitate plasma exchange transfusion
- They may require thymectomy
- They may undergo elective or emergency surgery unrelated to their myasthenia

The severity of the muscle weakness and the muscle groups affected by the disease should be documented preoperatively, focusing on respiratory and bulbar function. The responses of patients with myasthenia to NMBDs depend on the type of relaxant. Decreased density of acetylcholine receptors at the motor end plate means that children with myasthenia may require up to four times the calculated dose of succinylcholine to establish a depolarizing muscle block. Because succinylcholine is metabolized by acetylcholinesterase, its metabolism is reduced and duration of action is prolonged in the setting of chronic acetylcholinesterase inhibition. For this reason, succinylcholine is best avoided in these children.

The activity of nondepolarizing NMBDs is increased through their increased duration of action. Unfortunately, the degree to which the sensitivity is increased is somewhat unpredictable and depends on an interaction between the severity of the disease (e.g., level of acetylcholine receptor antibodies) and the efficacy of treatment. Inhalational anesthetic agents inhibit neuromuscular transmission, and these effects may be exaggerated in myasthenia gravis patients. However, no clinically significant postoperative neuromuscular depression has been demonstrated with isoflurane, sevoflurane, or desflurane. These potential neuromuscular effects are not shared by propofol, making total intravenous anesthesia (TIVA), in theory at least, the technique of choice for these children. For all but the most minor surgery in the patient with stable myasthenia gravis without significant respiratory or bulbar compromise, a tracheal tube and intermittent positive-pressure ventilation are likely to be required. If possible, intubation of the trachea should be performed without the use of NMBDs. Tracheal intubation with inhalational anesthetics alone or propofol with a short-acting opioid has been described in these children.[87]

Myasthenia-Like Syndrome

The toxin of *Clostridium botulinum* produces a myasthenia-like syndrome that may occur through two mechanisms: ingestion of food contaminated by *C. botulinum* toxin, including contaminated honey, and wound infection by *C. botulinum*. Features include blurring of vision with ptosis, dilated and unresponsive pupils, cranial nerve palsies, limb paralysis with areflexia, feeding difficulty, and respiratory insufficiency. Diagnosis depends on clinical suspicion, identification of the toxin in residual food, and electromyography.

Treatment is supportive, and recovery may take weeks to months.[88] Succinylcholine is contraindicated in children with infections that affect the neuromuscular junction, including botulism and tetanus.[89]

DISORDERS OF MUSCLE FIBERS
Myopathies
Congenital Myopathies

Congenital myopathies are rare disorders that have many variations in the type and severity of features.[90] There can be significant clinical overlap between congenital myopathies and other neuromuscular disorders. including the congenital muscular dystrophies (CMDs), congenital myotonic dystrophy, congenital myasthenic syndromes (CMS), metabolic myopathies including Pompe disease, SMA, as well as Prader-Willi syndrome. They can all present in the neonatal period with marked weakness and/or hypotonia ("floppy infant"). While it may not be possible to distinguish a congenital myopathy from other disorders, the presence of prominent facial weakness with or without ptosis, generalized hypotonic ("frog-leg") posture with hyporeflexia, and weakness and dysfunction of the respiratory and bulbar muscles are suggestive of congenital myopathy. The severity of weakness and disability varies widely, ranging from profound generalized weakness in neonates to patients with more subtle weakness. This may initially develop during childhood with signs of delayed motor milestones, or even later in life with symptoms of proximal weakness. Reduced muscle bulk is usually observed. In patients with severe weakness, respiratory insufficiency is common and the most severely affected infants require continuous ventilation for survival. The diagnosis usually is confirmed by characteristic findings on muscle biopsy (Table 24.7). Genetic diagnosis, and indeed genetic panels, are now available for many of these myopathies in specialist laboratories as outlined in Table 24.7 and are largely dictated by the pathologic finding.[91] Support of respiration and nutrition may be necessary. Minimally invasive methods, such as noninvasive nocturnal ventilation by face mask, are indicated to assist with management at home. Regular passive movements and careful management of posture and positioning to prevent contractures, especially scoliosis, is essential. Meticulous care of skin, joints, bowels, and teeth help to avoid the need for more invasive management. A complete evaluation of cardiovascular and respiratory status is required before anesthesia and surgery.[92,93]

Malignant hyperthermia (MH) is a disorder of skeletal muscle that manifests in response to anesthetic triggering agents. Core myopathies (central core disease and multi-minicore disease) are closely associated with MH (see Chapter 41), with extreme variation in the severity of its features. MH and core myopathies are primarily disorders of calcium regulation in skeletal muscle. Genetic testing identifies mutations in the ryanodine receptor gene (RYR1) in most affected individuals, accounting for their susceptibility to MH.[94] The RYR1 gene encodes the channel that controls calcium release from the sarcoplasmic reticulum in skeletal muscle and, to a lesser extent, in other organ systems. RYR1 abnormalities alter the channel kinetics for calcium inactivation, and calcium buildup causes excessive skeletal muscle contraction resulting from disinhibition of the normal actin-myosin interaction. The level of adenosine triphosphate decreases, leading to anaerobic and aerobic metabolism and to acidosis. Early manifestations of MH include hypercarbia or tachypnea and tachycardia. Late signs and symptoms include fever, sympathetic nervous system activation, hyperkalemia, muscle rigidity, disseminated intravascular coagulation, myoglobinuria, and multiorgan dysfunction and failure if not treated early.

The in vitro contracture test (IVCT) was developed to confirm susceptibility to MH by studying the contracture of muscle fibers in response to triggers such as caffeine and halothane.[95] This is an invasive and expensive investigation because an open muscle biopsy is required, and very few specialized centers perform this procedure; it is generally not performed in children younger than 10 years of age because of the size of the muscle biopsy required. Most individuals with core myopathy may be susceptible to MH, as demonstrated by IVCT, which has been the only means to confirm MH susceptibility until the emergence of molecular testing.[96] DNA analysis can provide a fairly reliable test for susceptibility to MH for 60% of affected individuals who have had an IVCT but for only 20% of those who have not had an IVCT (see Chapter 41).[97] However, the complexity of the situation is such that assessment and advice by a specialist is recommended rather than immediately embarking on DNA analysis so that the child and family may benefit from appropriate investigation and interpretation.[98] Any individual with core myopathy, and his or her family, should be informed about the clinical situation, diagnosis, and possible risks and complications, including MH, and should be offered a specialized investigation. An individual who may be susceptible to MH should carry information (e.g., a medical alert bracelet) to inform medical staff in an emergency.[99] Any elective operative procedure must be meticulously planned in advance with the full involvement of the anesthesiologist.

Metabolic Myopathies

Metabolic myopathies (Table 24.8) are uncommon and complex. Most affected children have multisystem involvement of sufficient severity to mask the myopathic features. The most important concerns for the anesthesiologist are the risk of metabolic instability during surgery and the need for close liaison with the child's pediatrician to plan fluid and electrolyte balance and nutritional management.[99,100]

TABLE 24.7	Congenital Myopathies
Pathologic Findings With Genotyping	
Disorder	**Genetics**
Core myopathies (including central core disease and multi-minicore disease)	RYR1, SEPN1, ACTA1, TTN, MYH7, KBTBD13
Centronuclear myopathies	MTM1, RYR1, DNM2, BIN1
Nemaline myopathy (including cap disease and zebra body myopathy and core-rod myopathy since these appear to be pathologic variants of nemaline myopathy)	ACTA1, NEB, TPM2, TPM3, TNNT1 ,CFL2, KBTBD13, KLHL40
Myosin storage myopathy (also known as hyaline body myopathy)	MYH7
Congenital fiber–type disproportion	ACTA1, TPM3, TPM2, RYR1, SEPN1

TABLE 24.8	Metabolic Myopathies
Disorders of purine nucleotide cycle: myoadenylate deaminase deficiency	
Mitochondrial myopathies: chronic progressive external ophthalmoplegia (CPEO)	
Kearns-Sayre syndrome (CPEO, conduction disturbance, pigmentary retinopathy)	
Myo-neurogastrointestinal encephalopathy (MNGIE)	
Glycogen storage disorders: muscle phosphorylase deficiency (glycogen storage disease [GSD] type V: McArdle disease)	
Lysosomal acid maltase disease (GSD type II: Pompe disease	
Disorders of fatty acid oxidation: carnitine palmitoyl transferase I and II deficiency	

Mitochondrial Disorders Underlying Myopathies

Mitochondrial disorders are a common cause of inherited neurologic disease in children, occurring in 1 of 5000 live births. They are caused by mutations in mitochondrial or nuclear DNA. The respiratory chain is under bigenomic control: nuclear DNA codes for 85% of the proteins, and mitochondrial DNA codes for 15%. Nuclear DNA is inherited along Mendelian inheritance patterns, whereas mitochondrial DNA follows maternal inheritance patterns in a ratio of 9 to 1. Most mitochondrial disorders in children are determined by nuclear DNA, whereas those in adults are determined by mitochondrial DNA. The organs involved by mitochondrial disease are determined by the presence of defective nuclear or mitochondrial DNA in the embryo. The relative amount of defective DNA in affected tissues determines the severity of the disease. Disruption of the most fundamental cellular energy process, the mitochondrial respiratory chain, results in a diverse and variable group of multisystem disorders known collectively as mitochondrial disease. Involvement of the brain, nerves, and muscles can occur in isolation or in combination.

Diagnosis relies on characteristic clinical features, an understanding of mitochondrial genetics, and a logical, informed approach to investigations. Abnormalities of the mitochondrial genome are extremely common, and they can cause devastating phenotypes or be completely subclinical; assessment and diagnosis are challenging.[5]

Neurologic symptoms and signs are common. However, they tend to be varied and include myopathy, neuropathy, stroke-like episodes, ataxia, dementia, epilepsy, migraine, sensorineural deafness, and pigmentary retinopathy. The more common clinical scenarios in childhood are outlined in Table 24.9. Involvement of other organ systems, such as diabetes mellitus, gastrointestinal disease, and cardiomyopathy, may coexist or dominate the clinical picture. Evidence of mitochondrial dysfunction, such as lactic acidosis, increased CSF protein, and ragged red fibers on muscle biopsy, may or may not exist. Assessment of the child with atypical and otherwise unexplained features should include a search for evidence of mitochondrial abnormalities. The clinical details determine the investigative plan, which should include cerebral imaging with MRI and MRS (to detect lactate peaks), blood biochemistry (i.e., creatine kinase, lactate, and glucose levels), tests of urinary amino and organic acids, cardiologic assessment (i.e., chest radiography, electrocardiogram, and echocardiogram), electroencephalography, and exercise testing and neurophysiology, leading to mitochondrial studies of blood and muscle tissue.[101]

Muscle biopsy investigations include histopathology, electron microscopy, respiratory chain enzymology, and molecular analysis of mitochondrial DNA. Further investigation with respiratory chain enzymes and molecular genetic analysis is indicated in some cases.[102]

Treatment of mitochondrial disorders includes management of specific features such as antiepileptic therapy and efforts to maintain stability of metabolic pathways.[103,104] Vitamins and other supplements such as coenzyme Q_{10} (i.e., ubiquinone), riboflavin, thiamine, and carnitine are referred to as the *mitochondrial cocktail* and are used in most of the mitochondrial disorders.[105] Use of the cocktail is largely based on the assumption that higher doses of these agents may improve mitochondrial energy generation.[106] Arginine has been used in the treatment of patients with mitochondrial encephalopathy with lactic acidosis and strokelike episodes (MELAS).[107]

Anesthesia Considerations for Myopathies

The challenge for the anesthesiologist is to maintain metabolic stability and prevent complications. The main problems associated with anesthetizing children with mitochondrial myopathies include respiratory failure, cardiac depression, conduction defects, and dysphagia.[108] The preoperative fasting period should be kept to a minimum to avoid hypovolemia and depletion of glucose stores. Stresses that may provoke increased energy requirements, such as perioperative pain, hypothermia, or hyperthermia, must be minimized. In children prone to lactic acidosis, IV fluids that contain lactate should be avoided, whereas administration of glucose-containing solutions is essential in any but the shortest of procedures to avoid hypoglycemia.[100,109] However, those children using a ketogenic diet for seizures should not have glucose in their IV fluids. Children with Kearns-Sayre syndrome must have adequate assessment and perioperative monitoring because cardiac conduction abnormalities, as well as myopathy, diabetes, proximal renal tubular acidosis, and other multisystemic abnormalities, are prominent features.[106]

Inhalational and IV anesthesia have been used successfully in many children with mitochondrial disorders, although several cases of untoward complications have been reported in the perioperative period.[109-112] However, the relationships between specific anesthetics and serious adverse effects remain tenuous. Two retrospective reviews of perioperative complications in 180 children with mitochondrial myopathies reported no complications after general anesthesia.[100,113] There is no evidence for either of

---

TABLE 24.9	Clinical Mitochondrial Syndromes in Childhood
Syndrome	**Features**
Alper-Huttenlocher, neuronal degeneration	Catastrophic onset of epilepsy, paralysis, ataxia, dementia, visual impairment, liver disease; death usually in months
Leigh encephalomyeloneuropathy	Brainstem signs predominant; relapsing/remitting or steadily progressive to death
Infantile myopathy and lactic acidosis	Hypotonia in infancy, feeding difficulties, respiratory problems, cardiomyopathy; fatal and nonfatal forms
Leber hereditary optic neuropathy (LHON)	Progressive visual loss in childhood, cardiac arrhythmias, dystonia
Kearns-Sayre (KSS)	Progressive external ophthalmoplegia, pigmentary retinopathy, deafness, heart block, choreoathetosis and ataxia, myopathy, endocrine disorders
NARP	Neuropathy, ataxia, retinitis pigmentosa
MELAS	Mitochondrial encephalomyopathy, lactic acidosis, stroke-like episodes, dementia
MERFF	Myoclonic epilepsy, myopathy with ragged red fibers (muscle Gomori trichrome stain), ataxia
MNGIE	Myoneurogenic gastrointestinal encephalopathy

two notions in these children: that inhalational anesthetics pose a particular risk to these children or that those with mitochondrial myopathies are more susceptible to MH than normal children.[114] However, mitochondrial disorders arise from a variety of molecular changes that have varied responses to anesthetics, which precludes blanket statements about the risks of general anesthesia in the entire population of these children.[115]

All inhalational anesthetics and propofol depress mitochondrial function at several levels, including the cytochrome oxidase chain and fatty acid membrane transport.[108] It has been postulated that children who develop metabolic acidosis and myocardial failure after propofol infusions for extended periods (>5 mg/kg per hour for more than 48 hours) [known as propofol infusion syndrome (PRIS)] have a subclinical form of a mitochondrial disorder. The basis for this is thought to be impaired cytochrome oxidases in the respiratory chain and free fatty acid transport in the mitochondria. However, evidence to support this notion is lacking. In a review of 61 patients with PRIS, 7 (4 children and 3 adults) developed PRIS during anesthesia.[116] Impaired tissue perfusion (in association with sepsis) may be a common underlying mechanism. Propofol interferes with the respiratory chain and fatty acid metabolism in the mitochondria, in much the same manner as other anesthetics and medications, suggesting that its use for induction of anesthesia or for brief procedures in children with mitochondrial myopathies is reasonable, a belief that is shared widely.[21,117] However, children with mitochondrial myopathies who are treated with a ketogenic diet may be susceptible to propofol.[118] Sensitivity and resistance to nondepolarizing neuromuscular blocking agents have been reported in children with these myopathies. To ensure appropriate dosing, the drugs should be titrated judiciously while neuromuscular blockade is monitored.

Ventricular dysrhythmias have been reported after a small dose of bupivacaine in a patient who was subsequently discovered to have carnitine deficiency.[119,120] Knowing that bupivacaine inhibits carnitine-acylcarnitine translocase, patients with defects in fatty acid metabolism may be considered to be more sensitive to toxicity from this anesthetic.[120]

Evidence would suggest that any anesthesia technique might be used in children with mitochondrial myopathies. However, mitochondrial myopathies represent a wide variety of molecular defects and thus a wide range of different diseases with similar phenotypes. It is likely that some types of defects are more sensitive to inhibition by anesthetics than others, and therefore possibly more prone to untoward effects.[108] Thus *all* children with mitochondrial myopathies must be monitored closely when administering any type of anesthetic. All medications should be titrated slowly, and great care should be exercised to ensure that the effects of the anesthetic agents have largely dissipated before allowing the patient to resume spontaneous ventilation.

Muscular Dystrophies

Muscular dystrophies represent a group of more than 30 inherited disorders of muscle that may occur in infancy, childhood, or adulthood (Table 24.10). The word *dystrophy* implies a destructive progressive process, and although this is the characteristic clinical course for many of those affected by muscular dystrophies, the course is extremely slow or has no muscle strength deterioration for others.[121]

This area of neurology has undergone substantive advances in molecular genetics and, to a lesser extent, in muscle pathology. Duchenne muscular dystrophy (DMD) was the first inherited

disorder for which the causative gene and defective protein were identified.[121] Characterizing defective proteins led to advances in immunohistochemistry that can help to confirm the diagnosis using a muscle biopsy. Detection of genetic mutations enables the diagnosis to be determined using a blood specimen in most instances, removing the need for muscle biopsy in many children. The mutated gene and molecular site of the defect have been identified for most of the common disorders, enabling much more focused management in the form of new drugs, gene therapy using adeno-associated viral vectors and informed counseling of families.[122-124] The characteristic clinical features of muscular dystrophy include muscle weakness, the distribution of which varies from type to type—contractures, sluggish deep tendon reflexes, and involvement of respiratory and heart musculature. Other features often coexist, including learning disabilities, deafness, and ophthalmologic disorders. The serum creatine kinase level may be normal or increased. If it is increased, it provides an important marker for some disorders such as the dystrophinopathies, in which it may be 100 times normal. Diagnosis rests on careful clinical assessment, creatine kinase concentration, molecular

TABLE 24.10	Muscular Dystrophies
Disorder	**Genetics**
Myotonic dystrophy	
DM1 (98%), autosomal dominant	9q13.3, *DMPK* or *DM1*, dystrophia myotonica
DM2 (2%), autosomal dominant	3q21, *CNBP* (formerly *ZNF9*)
Congenital Muscular Dystrophies	
Autosomal recessive	
Fukuyama type (LGMD2M)	9q31.2, *FKTN*, fukutin
Walker-Warburg (LGMD2K)	9q34.1, *POMT1*
Merosin-negative (MDC1A)	6q22-q23, *LAMA2*
Merosin-positive (Ulrich)	21q22.3, *COL6A1, COL6A2* 2q37, *COL6A3*
X-linked recessive dystrophinopathies	
Duchenne and Becker types	Xp21.2, *DMD*, dystrophin
Emery-Dreifuss muscular dystrophy	
X-linked recessive	Xq27.3-q28, *EMD*, emerin; Xq26, FHL1
Autosomal dominant	1q22, *LMNA*, lamin A/C
Limb girdle muscular dystrophies	
Autosomal recessive (LGMD2)	25 currently characterized (2A–2Y)
Autosomal dominant (LGMD1)	8 currently characterized (1A–1H)
X-linked	4 currently characterized
Facioscapulohumeral muscular dystrophy	
Autosomal dominant	4q35, *FSHMD1A; 10qter FSHMD1B; 18p11FSHD2 (SMCHD1 gene)*
Distal myopathies	5q31.2, *MATR3*, matrin 3
Oculopharyngeal	14q11.2, *PABPN1* (formerly *PABP2*)

Data from Washington University in St. Louis, http://neuromuscular.wustl.edu/syncm .html (accessed 2016); HUGO Gene Nomenclature Committee, http://www.genenames .org (accessed 2016).

24

analysis, and muscle biopsy. Although there is no specific curative treatment for these disorders, advances in understanding the molecular genetic defect and the proteins responsible for the disease have focused the search for an effective pharmacologic treatment to reverse the clinical signs and symptoms.[124–126]

For an infant who presents with severe weakness and hypotonia, signs of facial weakness, reduced alertness, poor swallow, and reduced respiratory effort raise the possibility of a congenital myotonic dystrophy (DM1), which is usually inherited from the mother in an autosomal dominant pattern. Clinical suspicion of DM1 may be confirmed by molecular testing for the affected gene (DMPK), which codes for myotonic dystrophy protein kinase. The gene is located on the long arm of chromosome 19, expressing a protein primarily in skeletal muscle. This information negates the need for a muscle biopsy. A similar infant with good facial muscle movement, alertness, areflexia, and a diaphragmatic respiratory pattern indicating intercostal weakness is most likely to have SMA. The molecular test for the survival motor neuron is indicated to avoid the need for a muscle biopsy. Similar principles may be applied to children who present later in childhood. For example, a boy with gait abnormalities and a creatine kinase concentration 10 to 100 times normal is most likely to have a dystrophinopathy, and targeted molecular genetic testing can avoid the need for a biopsy.[127]

Myotonic Dystrophy

Myotonic dystrophy is the most common inherited neuromuscular disorder in the general population, and many more cases remain subclinical or undiagnosed.[4] All degrees of severity are possible, from the almost immobile infant with the congenital variant to the elderly adult with minimal motor weakness. Severity of the muscle weakness correlates with the molecular defect.

These children are susceptible to prolonged recovery from anesthesia. Accordingly, the dose of sedative medications and neuromuscular blocking agents should be titrated judiciously.[128] Sensitivity to succinylcholine is increased, and maximal use of regional nerve blocks or local infiltration with local anesthetic agents should be used whenever possible to minimize the need for opioids.

Most children with congenital or later-onset myotonic dystrophy have some degree of learning difficulties, which may be severe. One or the other parent is affected to a greater or lesser extent. In congenital cases (DM1), the mother is always the affected parent and, in most instances, is not aware of the disorder. The diagnosis is confirmed by the pediatrician or pediatric neurologist who examines the child.[129] The infant does not demonstrate signs of myotonia, and a muscle biopsy is not helpful to confirm the diagnosis at this age. The finding of facial weakness and clinical myotonia in the mother strongly suggests this disorder in a weak and floppy neonate.[130] The neonatal literature suggests that shaking the maternal hand (i.e., mother is unable to easily release her grip) may be sufficient to allow the pediatrician to make this diagnosis.[131] However, with the ability to confirm the diagnosis by molecular testing of blood from the infant and mother, it is no longer necessary to rely on clinical expertise in muscle strength testing. Genetic counseling is essential and should be offered to the wider family circle. It is not unusual to uncover a large kindred with previously unsuspected disease in this situation.

These infants may require intensive care in the neonatal period, including respiratory support, but they tend to improve with age. However, significant learning disability is the rule, and the input of the multidisciplinary child development team followed by special schooling is the norm. Surveillance should be in place for cardiac features that include hypotension, syncope, conduction defects, and arrhythmias. Specific conditions requiring surgery include scoliosis and joint contractures, and perioperative care must be carefully planned.[129]

Dystrophinopathies

The next most commonly encountered dystrophies are the dystrophinopathies. DMD is the more severe phenotype, and Becker muscular dystrophy (BMD) is the milder phenotype with a later age of onset (adolescence). Both dystrophies are inherited in an X-linked recessive pattern and affect boys almost exclusively.[132] These disorders are caused by a deficiency of dystrophin (i.e., less than 3% of the normal content in DMD), a muscle membrane protein essential to the skeletal and cardiac muscle cytoskeleton and to neural tissue. Dystrophin reinforces the inner strength of the myocyte during lateral stretching and is involved in signal transduction (Fig. 24.2). DMD occurs as a result of mutations, mainly deletions in the dystrophin gene (DMD, locus Xp21.2).[127]

Affected children experience a deterioration in muscle strength between the ages of 6 and 8 years that continues to progress until adolescence, at which age a wheelchair is usually required. Respiratory, orthopedic, and cardiac complications emerge with increasing age. From 10 years of age, annual or biannual echocardiograms should be performed to detect cardiomyopathy. Respiratory surveillance includes overnight sleep studies and early morning blood gas analysis to detect early nocturnal hypoventilation. As the lack of dystrophin affects the integrity of neural tissue, progressive cognitive dysfunction may occur. Also, the absence of dystrophin predisposes the muscle to tearing from normal stretching or from use of depolarizing drugs such as succinylcholine. Additional damage to skeletal muscle cells occurs from increased intracellular calcium concentrations, which may result from a defect in the sarcoplasmic reticulum. Upregulation of acetylcholine receptors has also been reported in these children. Without intervention, children with DMD usually die by a mean age of 19 years. With improvements in care, some are now surviving into the third decade. The mode of death is usually the result of underlying respiratory or cardiac failure.

Coordination of clinical care is a crucial component of DMD management. Care is best provided in a multidisciplinary setting in which the individual and family can collaborate with specialists about the required multisystem management of DMD. Depending on local services, coordinated clinical care can be provided by a wide range of health care professionals, including neurologists, rehabilitation specialists, neurogeneticists, pediatricians, and primary care physicians. The person responsible for coordination of clinical care must be aware of the available assessments, tools, and interventions to proactively manage all potential issues for the child with DMD.

Glucocorticoids are essential in the management of DMD; these agents slow the decline in muscle strength and function in the short term (up to 2 years), which reduces the risk of scoliosis and stabilizes pulmonary function.[133] Cardiac function may also improve; limited data indicate a slower decline in echocardiographic measures of cardiac dysfunction.[134,135] Prednisone is commonly used, although deflazacort is an alternative used in some countries and is probably just as effective. The most effective prednisolone regimen appears to be 0.75 mg/kg per day. International guidelines for initiation of steroids and other pharmacologic agents and the implementation of multidisciplinary care are clearly outlined by

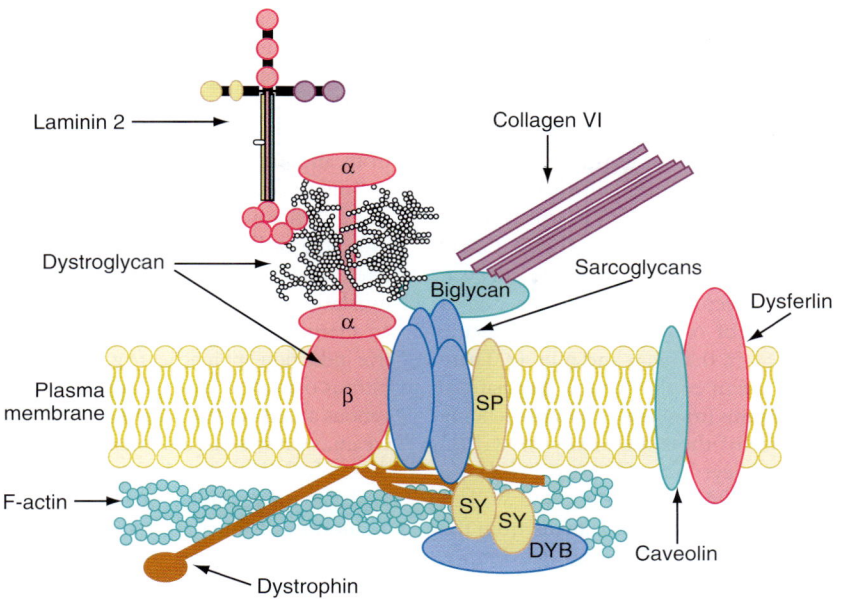

FIGURE 24.2 Schematic diagram of the proteins associated with dystrophin in skeletal muscle cells. The three key elements of the membrane skeleton and signal transduction path are laminin 2, which is the extracellular component; dystrophin-associated protein complex (DAPC) with its α- and β-dystroglycan, sarcoglycan, and cytoplasmic subunits, which is the transmembrane component; and dystrophin, which is the intracellular component. The cytoplasmic subunit of the DAPC consists of syntrophin (*SY*) and dystrobrevin (*DYB*). Sarcospan (*SP*) has four transmembrane-spanning helixes, and its expression is lost in patients with Duchenne muscular dystrophy. Dystrophin is the pivotal element that reinforces the muscle cell cytoskeleton, and it mediates signal transduction across cell membranes through its interactions with syntrophin, dystrobrevin, and neuronal nitric oxide synthase. Notice that the noncontractile F-actin binds to the N terminus of dystrophin. (From Goodwin FC, Muntoni F. Cardiac involvement in muscular dystrophies: molecular mechanisms. *Muscle Nerve* 2005;32:577–588.)

the DMD Care Considerations Working Group.[135,136] Children receiving glucocorticoids should be monitored regularly to prevent secondary complications from this therapy. They must have frequent weight measurements to prevent weight gain, regular blood pressure checks to prevent hypertension, and regular urine analysis for early detection of diabetes. They also require regular bone densitometry or dual-energy x-ray absorptiometry scans and maintenance of vitamin D levels. If there is evidence of reduced bone mineral density or presence of a vertebral fracture, they should be considered for bisphosphonate therapy. They should also be monitored for weight gain and obesity. Annual monitoring for cataracts is also advised. Early dietetic advice and, if necessary, a reduction in the dose of steroids should be undertaken. Prolonged use of steroids (beyond 2 years) does not improve strength and may result in growth failure, which warrants early referral to an endocrinologist.

If lower limb contractures exist despite range-of-motion exercises and splinting, surgery can be considered in some scenarios.[137] The approach must be strictly individualized. Surgical intervention is frequently used to treat lower limb contractures and enable rehabilitation in long leg orthoses so that the ambulatory phase may be prolonged.[138] This is usually indicated for children between 8 and 12 years of age, and it is well tolerated and successful if supported by a specialist team; however, it may increase the burden of care for parents and families.[139]

Children who are not treated with glucocorticoids have a 90% chance of developing significant progressive scoliosis[140] and a small chance of developing vertebral compression fractures caused by osteoporosis. Although glucocorticoids can reduce the risk of scoliosis,[141,142] the risk of vertebral fracture is increased.[143,144] Spinal care should involve an experienced spinal surgeon and consists of scoliosis monitoring, support of spinal and pelvic symmetry, and spinal extension by the wheelchair seating system. Corrective spinal surgery improves posture and seating options, eliminates pain from vertebral fracture resulting from osteoporosis, and slows the rate of respiratory decline.[140,145] The procedure is fraught with difficulty owing to postoperative respiratory weakness and possible cardiac dysfunction.[145] Careful preparation and liaison among the pediatrician or neurologist, surgeon, and anesthesiologist is essential; a plan for postoperative management, including the provision of intensive care, should be made.[99]

Facioscapulohumeral dystrophy (FSHD) is less often encountered in childhood, and specific surgical and anesthesia issues are limited. There are several phenotypes in childhood, including a severe neonatal form and a variably progressive childhood type that may be associated with sensorineural deafness. Irregular alignment between phenotype and genotype implies inconsistent expression of the molecular defect.[146,147] These children may benefit from surgery to fix the scapulae, which improves functionality of the upper limbs.[148,149]

Limb girdle syndromes (LGMD) (no longer a single entity; see Table 24.10) occur infrequently. Some have cardiac and respiratory implications and require preoperative assessment. In Emery-Dreifuss muscular dystrophy (EDMD), a syndrome in which cardiac conduction defects and dysrhythmias are common, syncope is usually the presenting complaint. These children are followed by a specialist team that includes a cardiologist.[99] A preoperative cardiac workup is essential before embarking on general anesthesia with these children.

CMDs are a group of muscular dystrophies that become apparent at an early age (from birth). They are slowly progressive or can be static, and can be associated with learning difficulties. The two most common forms of CMD are Ullrich congenital muscular dystrophy (owing to defective collagen VI), which affects 50% of people with CMD, and merosin-deficient CMD (CMD 1A), which affects another 25%. These do not affect the intellect. The CMDs with prominent intellectual impairment are caused by a defect in the glycosylation of α-dystroglycan, producing abnormal basal lamina formation in the brain and muscle. There is varying severity of disorganization of the cortical lamination, muscular dystrophy, and eye problems (muscle-eye-brain) depending on the genetic defect. Examples of these are Fukuyama CMD (caused by fukutin defect), muscle-eye-brain disease (caused by a protein O-mannosyltransferase 1 [POMGnT1] defect) and Walker-Warburg syndrome (due to POMT1). Diagnosis is made from the clinical picture, creatinine kinase levels, dystrophic muscle biopsy, presence or absence of cortical abnormalities, and finally, by the genetic testing. Medical care for patients with CMD remains diverse and is outlined in a Consensus Statement on Standard of Care for Congenital Muscular Dystrophies.[150]

Anesthesia Considerations for Muscular Dystrophies

The anesthesia implications for muscular dystrophies are dictated by the age of the child and severity of the disease. In early childhood, those affected by DMD undergo destruction of skeletal muscle, and when exposed to triggers that include succinylcholine and inhalational anesthetics, they have presented with severe rhabdomyolysis and hyperkalemia that resulted in cardiac arrest. Some children who were not known to have muscular dystrophy had a cardiac arrest during inhalational anesthesia as the first sign of the disorder. In contrast, during adolescence and adulthood, progressive cardiac and respiratory failure are the major concerns. The severity of DMD usually is greater than that of BMD and EDMD.

Despite extensive documentation that inhalational anesthetics or succinylcholine, or both, can trigger life-threatening rhabdomyolysis in children with muscular dystrophy, this problem persists.[151-153] Case reports have described rhabdomyolysis, hyperkalemia, and cardiac arrest with or without the use of succinylcholine in children with DMD. No single inhalational anesthetic appears to be without blame.[154,155]

The defect in dystrophinopathies results from the lack of the membrane-stabilizing protein dystrophin. It has been suggested that the addition of another destabilizing agent, such as an inhalational anesthetic, predisposes these children to mild or severe rhabdomyolysis, hyperkalemia, and death. Those most at risk for these complications are younger children, some of whom are undiagnosed until the perioperative rhabdomyolysis develops and establishes the diagnosis. Adolescents in whom muscle breakdown has waned and muscle mass has been lost and replaced by fatty infiltration have had uneventful perioperative courses when exposed to inhalational anesthetic agents and succinylcholine. Although succinylcholine is infrequently used today, the mortality rate associated with a succinylcholine-induced cardiac arrest is 30%.[155]

Although there is insufficient evidence to contraindicate inhalational anesthetics in young children (<8 years of age and males) with muscular dystrophy, total intravenous anesthesia (TIVA) has emerged as the preferred technique as an alternative to inhalational anesthetics. In the absence of a compelling reason, it seems prudent to generally avoid inhalational anesthetics in young children with known DMD.[153,156] At the same time, without knowledge of the minimum concentration of inhalational anesthetic that triggers muscle breakdown, washing out inhalational anesthetics from anesthesia workstations, as in cases of MH, is unjustified. In some specific clinical situations such as a child with DMD and a difficult airway for whom an IV technique may be contraindicated or IV access cannot be established before induction of anesthesia (or with nitrous oxide alone), a brief exposure to an inhalational anesthetic to secure the airway followed by TIVA is an alternative approach. Consideration should be given to alternative induction approaches (e.g., ketamine IV, orally, intramuscularly), nitrous oxide and/or the addition of ancillary techniques to secure venous access readily (EMLA [eutectic mixture of local anesthetics] cream, ultrasound-guided catheterization). Case reports of rhabdomyolysis during and after inhalational anesthesia[157-159] warrant vigilance for possible sequelae in these children. The child should be monitored for signs of rhabdomyolysis (i.e., urine myoglobin, serum K+ level) even if the risk is small.[156] If rhabdomyolysis occurs, the inhalational anesthetic should be discontinued and replaced with a TIVA anesthetic. The child should not be discharged home until the signs of rhabdomyolysis resolve; myoglobinuria should be managed with large volumes of IV balanced salt solutions.[156]

Rhabdomyolysis caused by anesthetic agents may mimic MH.[160] The risk of MH in children with DMD is the same as in the general population.[161] Hyperkalemic arrhythmias are most effectively reversed by rapid IV administration of calcium (10 mg/kg of calcium chloride), which may be repeated until the arrhythmias abate. Other therapies, including hyperventilation, administration of bicarbonate, albuterol, insulin and glucose, and sodium polystyrene sulfonate (Kayexalate) are also recommended. The hyperkalemia associated with acute rhabdomyolysis may be refractory to the usual treatments and may require a prolonged resuscitation (see Chapters 9 and 40).

Boys with undiagnosed DMD have been anesthetized with inhalational agents and developed rhabdomyolysis. To minimize the risk of this complication, clinicians should question family members about any history of dystrophinopathies during the preoperative evaluation, mild signs of hypotonia, and motor weakness and delayed motor milestones. However, at least 30% of children present de novo (no family history) and represent new mutations. A brief developmental and neuromuscular history should be obtained, and if there is any question or suspicion, it is reasonable to measure a random serum creatine phosphokinase concentration preoperatively.

Undiagnosed Myopathy

The child with a possible myopathy (e.g., floppy, hypotonic, motor developmental delay) but without a definitive diagnosis can pose a challenge to the anesthesiologist.[162] A careful history and physical examination should be carried out. Serum creatine kinase and lactate concentrations should be evaluated, and the child's pediatrician or pediatric neurologist contacted for advice. If a progressive muscular dystrophy cannot be excluded (in the presence of an increased creatine kinase level), it may be prudent to avoid inhalational anesthetics, although their careful use for induction may be considered. An increased creatine kinase level in an asymptomatic infant or child may suggest a progressive muscular dystrophy, and inhalational anesthetics should be used with caution unless DMD or BMD is excluded.

Epilepsy

Epilepsy is a common disorder in childhood, with a prevalence of 0.5% to 1% in the school-age population. It is defined as the tendency to have recurrent spontaneous seizures. A seizure is a sudden, excessive, uncontrolled electrical discharge of cortical neurons.[163]

Any part or all of the cerebral cortex may be involved, and the manifestations of seizures are numerous. The first and most important step in managing epilepsy is to establish a correct diagnosis by determining whether the episodes are epileptic, classifying the episodes, and identifying the epilepsy syndrome that matches the clinical features (Table 24.11).

Diagnosis of seizures is largely a clinical process, with investigations providing information to determine cause (imaging) or seizure syndrome (electroencephalography). The cause may be a cerebral lesion of any type, in which case neurologic deficits may coexist, such as in cerebral palsy, or it may be a genetic disorder with no other neurologic features.

After a diagnosis of seizures has been made, the next step is to determine the epilepsy syndrome. This is achieved by reviewing the following:

- Seizure type
- Age
- Associated features
- Electroencephalographic features
  - Interval since the last seizure
  - Current medication, timing of the last dose and blood levels

TABLE 24.11	Epilepsy
Classification of Seizure Types	
Self-limited seizures	
Generalized	
Focal	
Continuous seizures	
Status epilepticus	
Epilepsy Syndromes in Childhood (Some Examples)	
Neonatal seizures	
Benign neonatal convulsions	
Benign neonatal familial convulsions	
Early infantile epileptic encephalopathy (EIEE; Ohtahara syndrome)	
Early myoclonic encephalopathy (EME)	
Childhood syndromes	
Epileptic spasms (West syndrome)	
Benign myoclonic epilepsy of infancy	
Severe myoclonic epilepsy of infancy	
Lennox-Gastaut syndrome	
Myoclonic astatic epilepsy	
Primary generalized epilepsies	
Absence seizure syndromes (childhood absence epilepsy, myoclonic absence epilepsy)	
Generalized tonic-clonic seizure syndromes	
Juvenile myoclonic epilepsy	
Juvenile absence epilepsy	
Benign focal epilepsy syndromes	
Benign rolandic epilepsy with centrotemporal spikes (BRECTS)	
Childhood epilepsy with occipital paroxysms (CEOPS)	
Lesional focal epilepsies	
Temporal lobe epilepsy (mesial temporal sclerosis)	
Frontal lobe epilepsy (structural abnormalities)	

- Check if the patient is using alternate nondrug therapies—for example, a ketogenic diet (KD) or vagal nerve stimulation (VNS).

The details of the epilepsy syndrome can guide further investigations, help to plan treatment, and educate the family regarding the prognosis.[164]

Management is directed at treating the cause if possible and in preventing seizures using antiepileptic drugs. Medication is chosen according to the seizure type and epilepsy syndrome, taking into account the age of the child, associated disorders, and other maintenance medications.[165] Most of the current antiepileptic drugs are licensed for use in childhood, although there are limitations for some drugs, especially in younger children. The aim of the treatment is to eliminate all seizures with the least number of antiepileptic drugs at the minimum doses. When the epilepsy has failed to respond to two or more appropriate antiepileptic drugs and the child is not suitable for epilepsy surgery, the alternate therapies such as KD or VNS are offered. The American Epilepsy Society guidelines and practice parameters are available at www.aesnet.org,[166] and the U.K. Epilepsy guidelines are available at www.nice.org.uk/CG.[167]

For children with epilepsy who are undergoing surgical procedures under anesthesia, the main problems are provocation or increased frequency of seizures, which have several causes:

- Anti-seizure medication missed due to perioperative fasting
- Epileptogenic anesthetics (e.g., enflurane)
- Hypoxia
- Electrolyte disturbance (e.g., hyponatremia)
- A direct effect of neurosurgery on the brain
- Cerebrovascular instability
- Coincidental exacerbation of severe epilepsy
- Postoperative ileus resulting in poor drug absorption
- Loss of ketosis in a well-controlled child using a KD

Certain disorders that cause epilepsy may be associated with other medical conditions, such as cardiorespiratory deficits, nutritional difficulties, and learning disabilities.[168]

Preparation for surgery should include a thorough review of the child's clinical status, including consultation with the physician who manages the child's epilepsy. In addition, it is important to know if the child is using alternate therapies such as a KD or VNS. For most minor elective procedures, there is no need to miss or omit any medication in the perioperative period, and parents should be advised to give regular medications as usual on the morning of surgery and anesthesia. Careful scheduling of the time of surgery may facilitate this because many children receive antiepileptic drugs on twice-daily regimens, with doses given at 8 AM and 8 PM. If surgery is scheduled for late morning or early afternoon, no medication need be missed. For children with complex epilepsy, such as those undergoing neurosurgery for the epilepsy itself, careful preoperative assessment is imperative.[169] In managing surgery and anesthesia in children with epilepsy, the aim is to prevent seizures and enable smooth and effective treatment (Table 24.12).

To avoid interfering with epilepsy control, it would appear prudent to maintain children with a KD in the perioperative period and ensure that all IV solutions are carbohydrate free (e.g., normal saline). In one report, none of the 9 children on a KD who underwent general anesthesia for 24 surgical procedures developed complications or exacerbations of their seizure activity.[170] None of the children experienced any exacerbation of seizure activity perioperatively. Although all the children maintained stable glucose concentrations intraoperatively, they appeared to be at

TABLE 24.12 Perioperative Medication Management for Children With Epilepsy

Preoperative Management

Liaise with child's pediatrician or neurologist.

Clarify usual seizure types, frequency, and trigger factors.

Review and document regular medication regimen (ideally twice daily).

Check antiepileptic drug level (phenobarbitone, phenytoin, or carbamazepine only).

Review rescue medication regimen.

Check drug allergies and adverse reactions.

Management for Minor or Day Surgery

Schedule for early afternoon.

Allow usual morning medication.

Avoid prolonged fasting.

Aim for evening medication as usual.

Management for Major Surgery

Ensure regular medications up to fasting.

Use intravenous preparations of regular drugs (phenytoin, phenobarbitone, valproate, benzodiazepine), if possible; use same doses two or three times daily.

If regular drugs not possible, administer the following:
    Phenytoin: Give intravenous load of 15–20 mg/kg at a rate of 50 mg/minute and then give twice-daily maintenance dose of 2.5–5.0 mg/kg.
        Benzodiazepine: Give intravenously as rescue.

If enteral administration is possible, reestablish regular maintenance and wean intravenous phenytoin dose.

---

risk of developing a metabolic acidosis during anesthesia, particularly during prolonged surgery. For this reason, blood glucose, pH, and bicarbonate levels should be monitored perioperatively, especially in procedures lasting more than 3 hours. If a child develops an acidosis, IV bicarbonate should be used as clinically indicated. If the blood sugar is less than 3 mmol/L (55 mg/dL), a glucose containing IV fluid (glucose 2.5% or 5%) should be used to maintain blood glucose between 3 and 4 mmol/L (55–70 mg/dL).[171] IV fluids should be continued postoperatively until oral fluids are tolerated. Oral fluids should be appropriate for a KD and low in carbohydrate. Finally, the KD should be reintroduced as soon as possible after surgery.

In patients with a VNS implant, it is recommended to use the minimum amount of appropriate energy during each electrical current delivery and to place defibrillation pads as far removed from the generator and implanted lead as possible. Electrocautery or radiofrequency ablation may damage the generator. Although the VNS does not need to be deactivated (via magnet placement) during surgery, it is recommended to position grounding pads to prevent current flow through the system and that they be as far away from the VNS generator as possible.[172]

Summary

Neurologic disease is common in childhood. Many severely disabled children are living longer but with increasingly complex medical and social needs. The challenges for surgeons and anesthesiologists in treating them include consent, complications of anesthesia, and issues related to long-term outcomes. The key to effective management is good basic neurologic and pediatric care with careful preparation, including close liaison with parents and the child's usual clinicians.

ANNOTATED REFERENCES

Dubowitz V, Sewry CA. *Muscle Biopsy: A Practical Approach*. 3rd ed. Philadelphia: WB Saunders; 2007.
This textbook provides a comprehensive review of neuromuscular conditions and associated pathology in children.
Forsyth R, Newton R. *Paediatric Neurology (Oxford Specialist Handbooks in Paediatrics)*. 2nd ed. Oxford, UK: Oxford University Press; 2012.
An excellent handbook for practical management and up-to-date information on a wide range of topics.
Hoffmann GF, Johannes Zschocke J, Nyhan WL. *Inherited Metabolic Disease: A Clinical Approach*. Berlin: Springer-Verlag; 2010.
This textbook provides an excellent review of an extremely complex subject.
Klinger W, Lehmann-Horn F, Jurgat-Rott K. Complications of anaesthesia in neuromuscular disorders. *Neuromuscul Disord*. 2005;15:195–206.
The article reviews the topic for anesthesiologists.
Neuromuscular Disease Center, Washington University at St. Louis, St. Louis. Available at: http://neuromuscular.wustl.edu. Accessed June 2016.
This is a web-based review of all childhood neuromuscular disorders.
Swainman KF, Ashwal S., Ferraro DM, Schor NF. *Swaiman's Paediatric Neurology. Principles and Practice*. 5th ed. Philadelphia: WB Saunders; 2012.
This is an up-to-date, comprehensive textbook that is a well-illustrated, extensively referenced and searchable online text.

A complete reference list can be found online at ExpertConsult.com.

Surgery, Anesthesia, and the Immature Brain

25

ANDREAS W. LOEPKE AND ANDREW J. DAVIDSON

MILLIONS OF CHILDREN UNDERGO SURGERY with anesthesia every year.[1] During the perioperative period they are exposed to a multitude of stressors capable of interfering with normal brain development. Pain, stress, inflammation, hypoxia, and ischemia have all been shown to adversely affect the immature central nervous system (CNS). However, recent findings from animal studies have indicated that sedatives and anesthetics—the very drugs used to reduce pain and stress—may themselves undesirably influence brain development by triggering structural and functional abnormalities. In fact, this phenomenon is currently one of the most intensely investigated laboratory research fields in anesthesiology and a passionately debated topic (Fig. 25.1). To date, more than 400 animal studies have addressed the effects of anesthetics on the developing brain.[2] However, translating these laboratory findings to humans in clinical settings has been complicated.

To begin with, human epidemiologic studies have found mixed evidence for an association between surgery with general anesthesia in childhood and subsequent neurodevelopmental abnormalities. Some studies identified more frequently occurring learning disabilities in children after surgery with general anesthesia early in life, whereas others have not. Although surgery or comorbidities may affect the developing brain, the mounting laboratory data demonstrating deleterious effects of anesthetic exposure without

surgery have forced clinicians to consider the possibility that anesthetics may also play a role in this phenomenon. However, similar to the uncertainties surrounding animal studies, the interpretation of the human data is fraught with substantial limitations.

Any discussion of the long-term effects of anesthetics on the developing brain is further complicated by the fact that anesthetic drugs may be organ protective under certain conditions, and may indeed mitigate brain damage that is due to inflammatory responses, hypoxia-ischemia, or other insults that might occur during the perioperative period.

It is currently impossible to provide any definitive statements about the effects of anesthesia on human neurodevelopment. This chapter provides an overview of the current laboratory and clinical data concerning the affect of sedatives, anesthetics, and analgesics on the immature brain.

Background

About 170 years ago, William T.G. Morton conducted the first successful public demonstration in the Western hemisphere of a drug-induced, reversible coma during a surgical procedure at the Massachusetts General Hospital. After witnessing Morton's demonstration, Oliver Wendell Holmes called the phenomenon

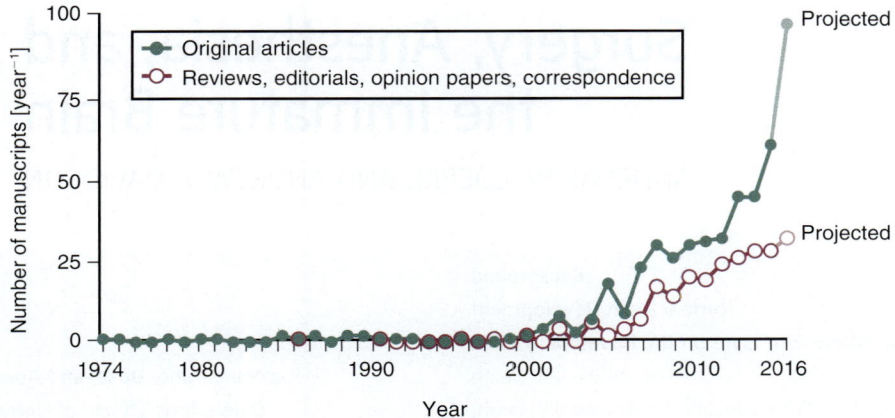

FIGURE 25.1 Research into the effects of anesthetic exposure in immature animals represents one of the most intensely investigated fields in anesthesiology and one of the most hotly debated topics. Graphical depiction of the annual publication of original articles (*solid circles*) and reviews, editorials, letters, commentaries, or opinion papers (*open circles*) spanning from 1974 to 2016, identified in a PubMed database search and screened for relevance using the terms "anesthesia or anesthetic or isoflurane or sevoflurane or desflurane or halothane or enflurane or ketamine or barbiturate or pentobarbital or benzodiazepine or midazolam or propofol or dexmedetomidine or xenon" and "neurotoxicity or apoptosis" and "neuron or brain". (From Lin EP, Lee J-R, Lee CS, et al. Do anesthetics harm the developing human brain? An integrative analysis of animal and human studies. *Neurotoxicol Teratol.* 2017;60:117–128.)

"anesthesia," from the Greek words *an-* (without) and *aisthēsis* (sensibility), and it instantaneously revolutionized the field of surgery. The inscription on Morton's tombstone, *"Inventor and Revealer of Inhalation Anesthesia: Before Whom, in All Time, Surgery was Agony; By Whom, Pain in Surgery was Averted and Annulled; Since Whom, Science has Control of Pain,"* represents a powerful testament to the tremendously positive impact that anesthesiology has made on the field of medicine. The use of general anesthetics to facilitate surgery quickly spread around the world and according to recent estimates, anesthesia currently allows more than 230 million patients of all ages worldwide to undergo major surgical procedures every year.[3] This positive impact is now tempered by the possibility that anesthetics may adversely affect normal brain development. During the first century of their use, general anesthetics were regarded with serious concern because they were combustible and carried substantial hemodynamic and respiratory adverse effects. Accordingly, up until 25 to 30 years ago, general anesthesia was rarely used in critically ill neonates because of the fear of myocardial depression and hemodynamic instability. Perioperative drug regimens were often limited to neuromuscular blocking agents and nitrous oxide. However, with the realization that unopposed pain exerts deleterious effects on the developing brain, that dramatic stress responses to painful stimulation are detectable even in preterm infants, and that modern anesthetics and analgesics can abolish these responses without substantial hemodynamic compromise, pediatric anesthesia, for the past three decades, has afforded critically ill neonates the benefits of amnesia, analgesia, and immobility during increasingly invasive surgeries. These surgical interventions have helped to save countless lives and preserve quality of life in this vulnerable population. All the while, the powerful coma induced by general anesthetics has been thought to be temporary and devoid of serious long-term adverse effects after emergence. This notion of reversibility is now being seriously questioned because of structural abnormalities detected in neonatal animals during and immediately after anesthetic

exposure and long-term cognitive abnormalities reported in animals and some children exposed to anesthesia at a young age.

Normal Brain Development

To put the effects of anesthetic exposures into context of brain development, the natural developmental processes must be taken into consideration. The human brain undergoes a complex and extended process of enormous growth in cell number, synapses, and connections during the perinatal period and beyond. Combined with this expansion of cells and connections early in life, subsequently massive regressive processes also occur during normal brain development. These expanding and regressive processes allow the brain to fully develop and eventually execute tasks, such as talking, walking, reading, writing, calculating, acquiring social skills, perfecting fine motor dexterity, and accomplishing complex functions, including learning, abstract thinking, as well as planning and executing long-term objectives.

To accommodate these functions, the human brain initially undergoes a rapid growth in size and cell number both in utero and during the early postnatal period, and is then pared back to achieve an efficient network of about 100 billion neurons in the adult brain. At birth, the size of the immature brain is one-third that of the adult brain, doubling in weight within the first year of life, and reaching 90% of its adult size by 6 years of age.[4] This dramatic growth spurt coincides with a remarkable overabundance of neurons and neuronal connections. In fact, less than half the neurons generated during development survive into adulthood.[5,6] Superfluous neurons that lose in the competition for a limited amount of trophic factors are removed by programmed cell death.[7]

After their rapid growth in number during early brain development, immature neurons subsequently form an excess of connections via synapses. Depending on the brain region, synaptic densities are maximum in infants and young toddlers between 3 and 15 months of age and will undergo a progressive reduction by about half during adolescence and into adulthood.[8] Connections that are active with continued electrical and chemical signals are sustained, whereas those with little or no activity are lost. Axons are myelinated by oligodendrocytes, leading to maturation of the CNS.

In summary, brain architecture changes rapidly and dramatically throughout early life. Neuronal density is greatest during fetal life, and excess neurons are eliminated via apoptosis or programmed cell death, predominantly in utero, during the neonatal period and throughout infancy.[9] Rapid growth of dendrites and synaptic connections occur during infancy and early childhood, and unneeded dendrites and synapses are trimmed back, predominantly during later childhood and adolescence.[8,9]

While these processes occur at slightly different stages of development for different regions of the brain, the first several years after birth represent a critical period for the entire developing CNS. Recent findings in animals suggest that exposure to anesthetics or sedatives during this period may interfere with proper neuronal development, brain architecture, and subsequent function. Although the exact molecular mechanisms by which anesthetics afford their therapeutic properties of amnesia, analgesia, and immobility are incompletely understood, their interaction with a wide variety of ion channels, such as sodium, calcium, and potassium channels, as well as several cell membrane proteins, including γ-aminobutyric acid (GABA), glycine, glutamate (N-methyl-D-aspartate [NMDA]), acetylcholine, and serotonin receptor systems, make it conceivable that anesthetics could create permanent abnormalities by interfering with important processes during critical windows of brain development. In fact, both GABA and NMDA receptors play critical roles in trophic signaling and in the regulation of neuronal maturation and programmed cell death. During early brain development, for example, GABA directs cell proliferation, neuroblast migration, and dendritic maturation.[10] In turn, developmental NMDA receptor stimulation directly fosters survival and maturation of some neurons.[11,12] It is therefore plausible that, by acting as modulators of these receptors, anesthetics might interfere with these critical developmental processes.

Effects of Anesthetic Exposure on the Developing Brain

Concerns regarding neurologic abnormalities after general anesthesia in young children were first raised more than half a century ago, when postoperative behavioral changes were observed after administration of vinyl ether, cyclopropane, or ethyl chloride for otolaryngologic surgery.[13] However, these abnormalities were regarded as psychological in nature because they were alleviated by the timely administration of preoperative sedative drugs.[13,14] Approximately two decades later the focus of research into the long-term effects of anesthetics shifted to animal models representing occupational exposure in pregnant health care workers.[15–18] Delayed synaptogenesis and behavioral abnormalities were observed in neonatal rats born to rodent dams that were chronically exposed to subanesthetic doses of halothane during their entire pregnancy. However, interest in the effects of anesthetics on brain development in children was not elicited until a seminal study observed widespread neuronal degeneration after a prolonged exposure to ketamine in neonatal rat pups.[19] This initial discovery led to numerous editorials and reviews, and more than 400 original articles (see Fig. 25.1) into the brain structural and/or functional

effects of almost every sedative and anesthetic in current clinical use in a wide variety of immature animal species.[20–67] However, no discussion about the effects of drug exposure of the developing brain would be complete without examining the effects of opioid analgesics in the developing brain.[56,57] Accordingly, this chapter examines the specific cellular effects that sedatives, anesthetics, and analgesics trigger in the immature brain.

APOPTOTIC CELL DEATH

The most widely studied deleterious structural consequence of exposure to sedatives or anesthetics in immature animals is widespread apoptosis. Although neuronal apoptosis eliminates approximately 50% to 70% of neurons throughout the brain during the entire developmental period, this natural process affects only a small fraction of cells at any particular time point. Exposure to anesthetics or sedatives briefly, but dramatically, increases the number of apoptotic neurons (Fig. 25.2). Some studies demonstrated up to a 68-fold increase in the density of degenerating neurons after a combination of anesthetics in newborn rats compared with control animals,[68] although it remained unclear what fraction of the entire neuronal population these degenerating neurons represented. In newborn mice, a 6-hour exposure to a clinically relevant dose of isoflurane triggers apoptotic cell death in 2% of neurons in the superficial cortex, a substantially affected brain region at this age. Under normal conditions, less than 0.1% of neurons undergo physiologic apoptosis in this region in unanesthetized littermates.[69] The exact mechanism and selectivity of the cell death process remains unknown as dying neurons are located immediately adjacent to seemingly unaffected neighboring cells (Fig. 25.3). Increased neuroapoptosis has now been observed after in vitro and in vivo exposures to a wide variety of sedatives and anesthetics, including chloral hydrate, clonazepam, diazepam, midazolam, nitrous oxide, desflurane, enflurane, halothane, isoflurane, sevoflurane, ketamine, pentobarbital, phenobarbital, propofol, and xenon, as well as opioid receptor agonists in a wide variety of species, including fruit flies, nematodes, chicks, mice, rats, guinea pigs, piglets, and rhesus monkeys (E-Table 25.1). Selective stains such as cupric silver and Fluoro-Jade (EMD Millipore, Billerica, MA) have confirmed the cellular demise in neurons that positively stained for activated caspase 3, the central executioner enzyme of the apoptotic cascade.

Apoptosis represents an inherent, energy-consuming process using a cascade of enzymes called caspases. Apoptosis is highly conserved among species and culminates in self-destruction and elimination of cells, even under physiologic conditions, when these cells are functionally redundant or potentially detrimental to the organism.[242] It involves an orderly breakdown of the cell that includes chromatin aggregation, nuclear and cytoplasmic condensation, and partitioning of cytoplasmic and nuclear material into apoptotic bodies for subsequent phagocytosis, without an extensive inflammatory response. That contrasts with features observed during necrosis, for example during ischemia, which includes energy failure, cellular swelling, membrane rupture, and release of cytoplasmic content into the extracellular compartment, followed by an inflammatory response.[242] However, there seems to exist substantial overlap and common pathways between cell death processes, such as apoptosis, necrosis, and autophagy, which have previously been thought to be entirely separate.[243] Apoptosis, which has also been termed cellular suicide or programmed cell death, is extensively used during tissue homeostasis, endocrine-dependent tissue atrophy, and normal embryogenesis (e.g., cardiac sculpting, ablation of tail tissue as part of tadpole metamorphosis

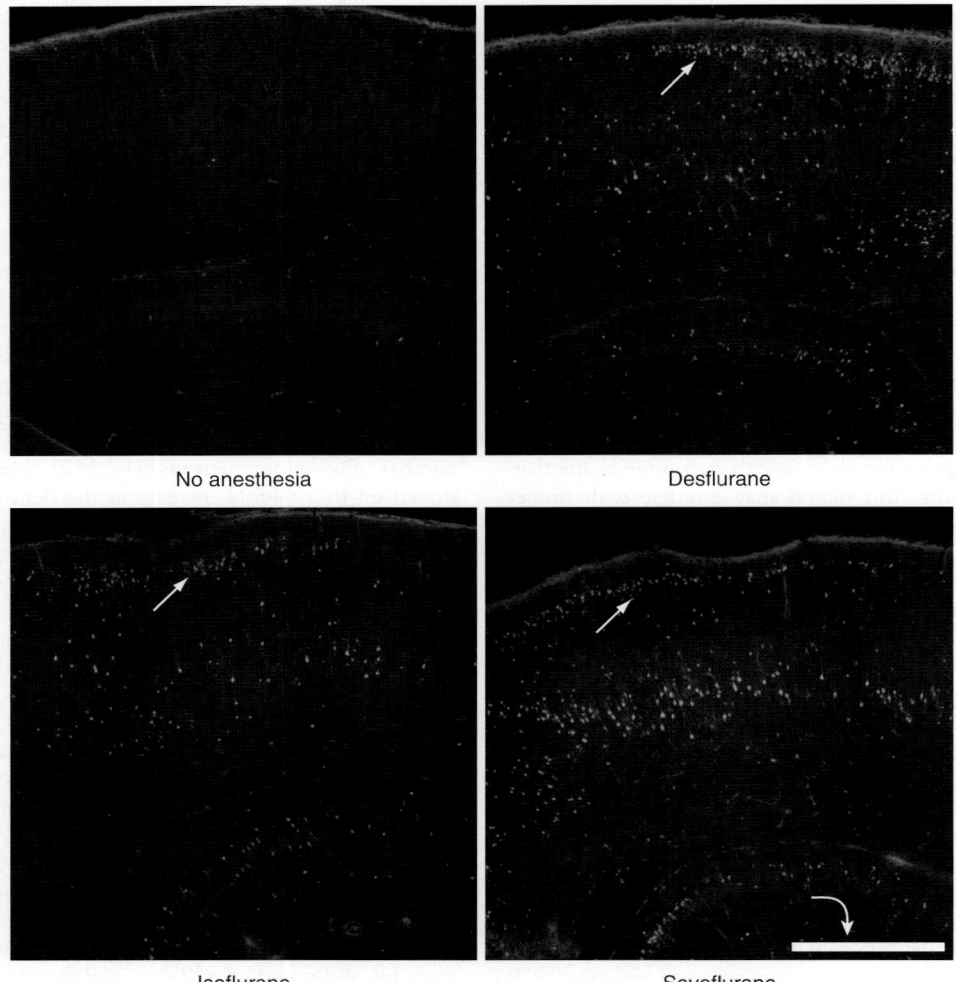

FIGURE 25.2 Prolonged exposure to anesthetics causes widespread apoptotic cell death in the developing animal brain. Representative photomicrographs of brain sections from 7- to 8-day-old mice exposed to 6 hours of equipotent doses of 7.4% *desflurane*, 1.5% *isoflurane*, 2.9% *sevoflurane* in 30% oxygen, respectively, or fasted, unanesthetized litter mates in room air (*no anesthesia*). These doses were previously determined to represent 0.6 minimum alveolar concentration for the respective anesthetics. *Arrows* mark clusters of cells in layer II/III of the neocortex that are dying from programmed cell death and are therefore labeled for the apoptotic marker, activated caspase 3 (*bright green*). Scale bar = 500 μm. (From Istaphanous GK, Howard J, Nan X, et al. Comparison of the neuroapoptotic properties of equipotent anesthetic concentrations of desflurane, isoflurane, or sevoflurane in neonatal mice. *Anesthesiology* 2011;114:578–587.)

in amphibians, or elimination of interdigital mesenchymal tissue of fingers and toes). Similarly, brain cells are produced in excess during normal brain development and are eliminated in large number during normal brain maturation in rodents, nonhuman primates, and humans.[5,6] This physiologic apoptotic cell death is critical to establish proper brain structure and function, and any disruption of this process can lead to massive brain malformations and intrauterine demise.[244] In the developing brain, apoptotic cell death can also be triggered by pathologic, extrinsic factors, such as hypoxia and ischemia.[245] It currently remains unclear whether anesthesia-induced neuroapoptosis accelerates physiologic programmed cell death or whether it eliminates cells not destined to die, as in pathologic apoptosis.

Animal studies have initially identified a narrow window of susceptibility to neuronal cell death induced by several anesthetic drugs, such as the NMDA antagonist ketamine, the GABA agonist isoflurane, or ethanol (a combined NMDA antagonist and GABA agonist). Ketamine-induced neuronal demise is most pronounced during exposure between 5 and 7 days of age in neonatal rodents or before 6 days of age in monkeys.[19,73,159] Similarly, a dramatic increase in neuronal apoptosis was detected in the cortex, thalamus, and amygdala of 3- to 10 day-old rodents after prolonged exposure to isoflurane, but minimal cell death was detected in 1-day-old animals or those older than 10 days of age.[102] However, data from the laboratory of one of the authors challenge the notion that anesthetic-induced neuroapoptosis is limited to a narrow age range. In mice, neuronal apoptosis was similarly observed in the cortex and hippocampus of neonatal animals after a prolonged exposure to isoflurane; however, vulnerability extended into adulthood in brain regions with ongoing neurogenesis, such as the dentate and

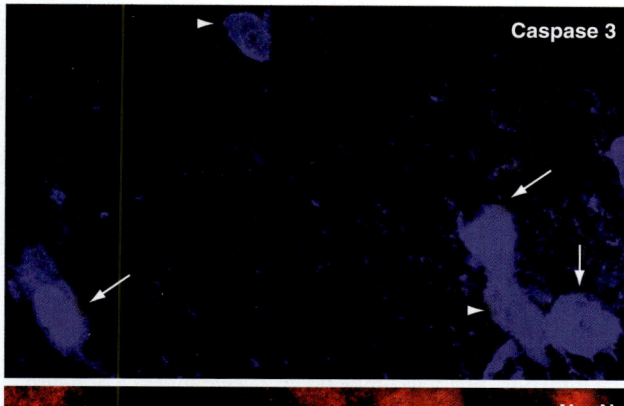
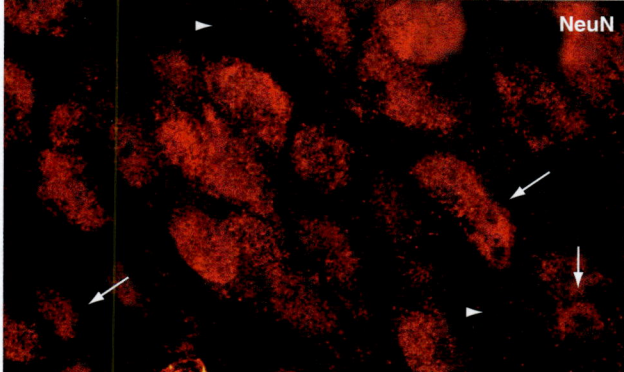
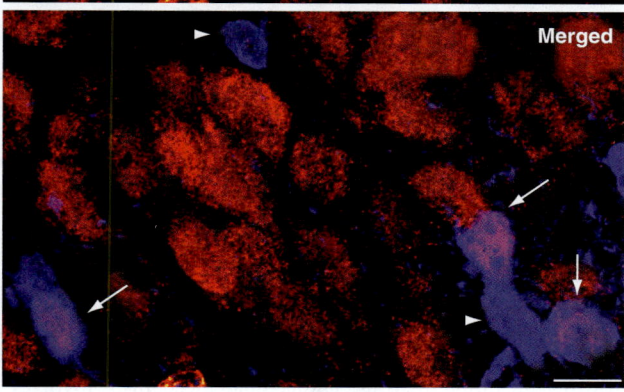

FIGURE 25.3 Neurons affected by apoptotic cell death following anesthetic exposure are surrounded by seemingly unaffected cells. Representative photomicrograph from a 7-day-old mouse following a 6-hour exposure to 1.5% isoflurane, showing neocortical cells stained for the apoptotic cell death marker activated caspase 3 (*blue, top*), the neuronal marker NeuN (*red, middle*), and a merged image of the two stains (*bottom*). The majority of dying cells are identified as postmitotic neurons, as indicated by the purple cells coexpressing activated caspase 3 and NeuN in the bottom (*arrows*), whereas some cells expressing caspase 3 are NeuN-negative (*arrowheads*). Importantly, cells affected by anesthetic-induced neuroapoptosis are surrounded by numerous, seemingly unaffected neurons. Scale bar = 10 μm. (Image courtesy Loepke Laboratory.)

olfactory bulb.[144] This finding could be explained by the fact that neurons were found particularly vulnerable to isoflurane-induced apoptosis before 14 days of cellular age and therefore would be expected to occur throughout the life of the animal in neurogenic niches containing neurons of this particular age.[142] Surprisingly, however, other studies suggest that intrauterine exposure to clinical doses of isoflurane in prenatal rats may actually decrease physiologic apoptosis and improve subsequent memory retention,[110] whereas

only supraclinical doses of isoflurane induced neuroapoptosis in this setting.[125] Whereas chronic opioid exposure in immature animal models can lead to long-term neurodegeneration,[98,97,246] a recent study found no neuronal cell death immediately after a brief exposure to morphine in newborn rats.[206] Additional research is needed to elucidate the timing of exposure on cellular demise and the differential effects of anesthetics and analgesics on brain structural integrity.

LONG-TERM BRAIN CELLULAR VIABILITY, NEUROLOGIC FUNCTION, AND BEHAVIOR

To answer the important question of whether anesthetics simply hasten natural apoptosis or whether they induce pathologic apoptosis, long-term neuronal density and neurologic function have to be assessed in adult animals exposed to anesthesia as neonates. If exposure to anesthetics or analgesics only temporarily accelerated physiologic apoptosis, one would expect normal cellular density and function in adulthood. Conversely, permanent neuronal cell loss and long-term neurocognitive impairment after anesthetic exposure early in life would suggest that anesthesia-induced neuronal apoptosis may be pathologic in nature and that the organism was unable to compensate for the neonatal cell loss by postexposure neuronal plasticity and repair. To address these questions, several studies measured neurologic function, assessed behavior, and/or determined neuronal density in adult animals after anesthetic exposure in the neonatal period. Results from these studies, however, are conflicting. A number of studies reported long-term neurocognitive or behavioral abnormalities after neonatal exposure to enflurane, halothane, isoflurane, sevoflurane, propofol, or ketamine, or to a combination of isoflurane, nitrous oxide, and midazolam.[a] Importantly, however, many of these studies only observed abnormalities in very specific tests or subsets of neurocognitive batteries, whereas many other neurobehavioral domains remained intact. For example, a 6-hour exposure to midazolam, isoflurane, and nitrous oxide in neonatal rats transiently impaired learning in a water maze task in young adulthood and in older animals, whereas in the same animals, several other tests of behavior and learning, including acoustic startle response, sensorimotor tests, spontaneous behavior in an open field, and learning and memory in the radial arms maze, remained unimpaired.[100] Similarly, after a 4-hour exposure to one minimum alveolar concentration (1 MAC) of isoflurane in 7-day-old rats, long-term memory retention was abnormal at two time points, whereas performance at several other time points, as well as in other tests of learning and memory, remained intact.[121] Accordingly, the relevance of these temporary and limited learning deficits remains unclear. Similar to humans, the performance of rodents and primates in learning tasks depends to a great extent on maternal behavior and rearing conditions, making them strong confounders during neurocognitive testing.[119,247–249] Moreover, another obvious and important factor in neurocognitive testing is the verification of similar degrees of motivation when comparing separate groups of animals. For example, a 24-hour exposure to ketamine sedation early in life impaired subsequent performance of rhesus monkeys in learning and memory tests, in addition to decreasing their motivation to perform these tasks.[178]

Studies of prolonged opioid administration in immature animals have also found evidence for long-term impairment in learning

---

[a]References 15, 16, 87, 89, 100, 117, 120, 121, 126, 131, 149, 150, 162, 164, 178, 221, 223, and 230.

tasks,[197-199,202-204] as well as altered pain responses in adult animals after exposure to morphine, fentanyl, heroin, or methadone early in life.[a]

Conversely, several other investigations have observed no neurologic abnormalities after administration of midazolam, isoflurane, sevoflurane, or ketamine, even when using complex neurologic tests in neonatal animals.[b] It remains to be determined whether these differential findings are attributable to the anesthetic doses, exposure times, species, or are related to the specific type of neurologic test used or the timing of the exposure or the assessment. Interestingly, escalating exposure times of isoflurane in neonatal rats caused neuronal apoptosis beginning at 2 hours of anesthesia, but no evidence of long-term neurologic abnormalities until 4 hours of anesthesia.[120] In another study, a 6-hour exposure to isoflurane caused significant apoptosis immediately after exposure in neonatal mice but resulted in no measurable long-term deficits in performance of complex neurologic tests as adult animals.[119] Moreover, in this study, brain neuronal density in adulthood was not diminished in regions significantly affected by anesthesia-induced neuroapoptosis compared with unanesthetized littermates.[119] Studies in mice exposed to 6 hours of isoflurane at 21 days of age did not observe subsequent diminution in dentate granule cells, despite considerable apoptotic cell death immediately after exposure.[250] These findings could either suggest that isoflurane may only accelerate physiologic apoptosis or that the developing brain's plasticity and capacity for repair can compensate for a pathologic insult early in life. Conversely, a study in similarly aged rats observed a permanent elimination of neurons, as well as neurologic abnormalities in adult animals, after exposure to isoflurane, nitrous oxide, and midazolam as neonates, suggesting that either the specific combination of anesthetic drugs (isoflurane alone vs. the combination exposure) or species differences (rats vs. mice) could affect relationships between neonatal neuroapoptosis and long-term function and neuronal density.[111] Alternatively, these conflicting results may be explained by the dissimilar testing environment because neurocognitive tests are not easily transferable among laboratories.[251] Yet another explanation holds that neonatal apoptosis may not be causally linked to adult neurocognitive performance at all, as evidenced by substantial apoptotic cell death observed immediately after carbon dioxide–induced hypercarbia in unanesthetized neonatal rats, which lacked long-term neurologic sequelae.[121]

EFFECTS ON NEUROGENESIS AND GLIOGENESIS
The generation of new neurons, or neurogenesis, as well as new astrocytes—gliogenesis—is most active in the immature brain in utero or soon after birth. Accordingly, several studies have investigated the effects of anesthetic exposure, primarily isoflurane, on progenitor viability and rates of neurogenesis. Although isoflurane did not kill neural progenitor cells in vitro, 3.4% isoflurane for 4 hours decreased the rate of neuronal proliferation and increased neuronal fate selection.[252] These findings have been confirmed as 2.8% isoflurane for 6 hours had no effect on neural stem cell viability, whereas larger doses inhibited cell proliferation.[134] In vivo studies in newborn mice failed to find significant cell death in radial glial-type progenitor cells in the dentate gyrus immediately after a 6-hour isoflurane exposure, although more

mature neuroblasts made up a substantial number of cells affected by anesthesia-induced apoptotic cell death.[142] Morphine, on the other hand, did not affect cell survival in a murine cerebellar neuronal precursor culture, although, exposure decreased DNA synthesis.[193]

Isoflurane also impairs the growth of cultured immature astrocytes and delays their maturation after a 24-hour administration of 3% isoflurane, although even this extreme exposure showed no effect on cell viability.[132] Morphine, although increasing apoptosis in neurons and microglia, did not affect astrocytes in a study involving human fetal cell cultures.[196]

ALTERATIONS IN DENDRITIC ARCHITECTURE
The immature brain accumulates an overabundance of neuronal connections in infancy, and the number of dendrites and synapses dramatically decreases after the first year of life. Several studies have examined the effects of a wide variety of anesthetics, such as propofol, isoflurane, sevoflurane, desflurane, midazolam, and ketamine on dendritic arborization and synaptic architecture.[c] A common theme in these studies is that anesthetics can affect dendritic arborization and synaptic density, and that the direction of any change, either an increase or a decrease in the number of dendritic spines, depends on the age at which the animals were exposed to anesthetics and therefore the developmental state of the brain. During the first 2 weeks of life, anesthetic exposure can lead to a decrease in synaptic and dendritic spine density in small rodents, whereas exposure beyond this age can lead to an increase in the number of dendrites.[123,222] Other studies suggest that this differential effect may depend on the maturational switch of GABA from excitation to inhibition, which is related to the switch from the immature form of the potassium-chloride-cotransporter NKCC1 to the mature KCC2. However, the permanence of these dendritic changes remains controversial because some studies have observed only a transient effect after ketamine, midazolam, or isoflurane anesthesia exposure early in life.[133,173]

DECREASE IN TROPHIC FACTORS
Isoflurane- or propofol-based anesthesia in neonatal animals has been associated with a decrease in brain-derived neurotrophic factor (BDNF),[105,122,223] a protein integral to neuronal survival, growth, and differentiation. The cellular mechanism involves a reduction in tissue plasminogen activator and plasmin, which converts proBDNF to BDNF. Accordingly, isoflurane has been found to trigger proBDNF/p75[NTR] (p75 neurotrophin receptor) complex–mediated apoptosis in neonatal mice.[122] Similarly, prolonged exposure to opioid receptor agonists early in life alters nerve growth factors in the immature brain.[70,186]

DEGENERATION OF MITOCHONDRIA
Ultrastructural morphologic abnormalities have been reported in mitochondria of pyramidal neurons in the subiculum of 7 day-old rats following 6 hours of isoflurane, nitrous oxide, and midazolam.[139] A morphometric analysis demonstrated mitochondrial enlargement, impaired structural integrity, and decreased mitochondrial density, indicating protracted mitochondrial injury after drug exposure.[253,254] Moreover, an ultrastructural examination with electron microscopy revealed increased autophagy, a form of cell death.[139]

---

[a]References 90, 96, 97, 183, 184, and 200.
[b]References 77, 110, 119, 120, 128, 130, 152, 161, 165, 188, and 221.

[c]References 74, 122, 123, 133, 156, 160, 172, 173, 187, and 222.

ABNORMAL REENTRY INTO CELL CYCLE

Ketamine induces reentry of postmitotic neurons into the cell cycle in immature rats.[175] This could be one trigger for apoptotic cell death, since postmitotic neurons lose the ability of neuronal progenitor cells to enter the cell cycle during proliferation and are committing programmed cell death when forced to reenter the cell cycle.

DESTABILIZATION OF THE CYTOSKELETON

Structural integrity of the cellular cytoskeleton is critical for proper neuronal morphology and function. Actin is one of the major components of the cytoskeleton of all eukaryotic cells and participates in important cellular processes, including cell signaling, motility, and division. It is also essential for the formation of dendritic spines. Isoflurane has been found to depolymerize actin in neurons and astrocytes, initiating cytoskeletal destabilization, impairment of astrocyte morphologic differentiation and maturation, as well as neuronal apoptosis.[132,136]

EFFECTS ON THE DEVELOPING SPINAL CORD

Most animal studies have focused on the effects of general anesthetics and sedatives on the developing brain. However, it is important to also consider the developmental impact of anesthetics on the spinal cord. One study observed increased neuroapoptosis in the lumbar spinal cord of 7-day-old rats after 6 hours of 0.75% isoflurane with 75% nitrous oxide.[114] Increased neurodegeneration was also documented in brain and spinal cord after 6 hours of 1% isoflurane in a similar model, but not after 1 hour of anesthesia or following spinal administration of bupivacaine.[137] Intrathecal ketamine can also cause neuroapoptosis in the developing spinal cord of 3-day-old rats, but not of 7-day-old rats.[177] Preservative-free ketamine caused long-term alterations in spinal cord function and gait disturbances,[177] whereas in a separate study, even high-dose intrathecal morphine produced no signs of spinal cord toxicity.[255]

Putative Mechanisms for Neurotoxicity

The exact mechanisms that trigger the previously listed effects of anesthetics and sedatives on the immature brain and spinal cord remain unresolved. Elucidating these mechanisms will be critical in establishing the relevance of these findings for pediatric anesthesia and neonatal critical care medicine, as well as for developing mitigating interventions, if necessary. The current, overarching hypothesis is that anesthetics and sedatives interfere with normal GABA$_A$ and NMDA receptor–mediated activity, which are the putative targets for unconsciousness, amnesia, and immobility,[256] and at the same time are essential for mammalian CNS development.[11,257] Administering GABA$_A$-receptor agonists and/or NMDA-receptor antagonists could potentially cause abnormal neuronal inhibition during a vulnerable period in neuronal development, triggering apoptosis in susceptible neurons, which in turn leads to neurocognitive impairment and decreased neuronal density into adulthood.[24,62,100,111] Other lines of evidence suggest that the NMDA receptor–blocking properties of ketamine may upregulate NMDA receptors, rendering neurons more susceptible to excitotoxic injury caused by endogenous glutamate action or the increased number of receptors immediately after withdrawal of the anesthetic such as proposed for ketamine.[155,159] However, several observations partly contradict both hypotheses; neuronal cell death has been reported during exposure to anesthetics and not only after their discontinuation. Moreover, several anesthetics with minimal NMDA-receptor interaction, such as propofol

and barbiturates, have demonstrated robust neurotoxic properties, whereas the neurotoxic potency of the NMDA-antagonist xenon has been found to be limited, therefore casting doubt on receptor upregulation as the sole mechanism for anesthetic neurotoxicity. In terms of abnormal neuronal inhibition being the main trigger for apoptosis in developing neurons, GABA$_A$-receptor stimulation indeed decreases neuronal activity in the mature brain; however, it also causes excitation in developing neurons,[258] thereby contradicting the inhibition hypothesis. In immature neurons, intracellular chloride (Cl⁻) concentration is high; thus GABA-induced opening of Cl⁻ channels allows this anion to exit the cell, leading to membrane depolarization. On the other hand, the intracellular Cl⁻ concentration is low in mature neurons. When anesthetics open Cl⁻ channels in mature neurons, ions enter the cell, thereby hyperpolarizing the membrane. This reversal of the cellular Cl⁻ gradient occurs as a result of a switch from the immature Na⁺-K⁺-2Cl⁻ cotransporter 1 (NKCC1) to the mature brain form, K⁺-Cl⁻ cotransporter 2 (KCC2).[259] Along these lines, studies in neonatal rats demonstrated excitatory properties in the brain and episodes of epileptic seizures during sevoflurane anesthesia.[232] Isoflurane has also been shown to cause an excessive release of Ca²⁺ from the endoplasmic reticulum via overactivation of inositol 1,4,5-trisphosphate receptors (InsP3Rs) in neonatal rats in vivo and in vitro.[260] A similar mechanism may be linked to the production of Alzheimer-associated increases in β-amyloid protein levels after anesthesia.[261] Although xenon and hypothermia cause neuronal inhibition, they do not exacerbate isoflurane-induced neuronal cell death as expected by the cumulative inhibition of neurons, but rather significantly reduce it.[108,115,239]

Importantly, evidence indicates that equianesthetic concentrations of the three contemporary inhalational anesthetics cause similar degrees of neuroapoptosis, suggesting that it is the anesthetic depth and not the specific doses or end-tidal concentrations of the anesthetics that determines cytotoxic potency.[76] However, other studies have failed to link the anesthetic and the apoptotic mechanisms. Specifically, although racemic ketamine and (S)-ketamine both elicit their anesthetic effects via NMDA-receptor blockade, (S)-ketamine induced up to 80% less cell death in vitro compared with equipotent doses of racemic ketamine.[174] Moreover, concomitant administration of the GABA$_A$-receptor antagonist gabazine failed to attenuate neuroapoptosis induced by the GABA agonist isoflurane, whereas administration of the α₂-agonist dexmedetomidine did.[79] Decreases in anesthetic-induced neuronal activity may therefore be less important than the disruption of the neuronal balance of excitation and inhibition, as demonstrated by studies that examined anesthesia-induced dendritic morphologic changes in mice.[74,172] In a mechanistic study of brain development, simultaneous blockade of excitatory and inhibitory activity with tetrodotoxin did not lead to structural changes during synaptogenesis that would have been expected from a causative relationship between neuronal inhibition and structural abnormalities; the administration of either GABA$_A$-agonistic or NMDA-antagonistic compounds alone did alter synaptogenesis.[172]

It is not entirely clear at this time whether cytotoxicity is a direct effect of the anesthetic itself, of any anesthetic by-products, or if it is related to physiologic derangements observed during anesthesia in small rodents.[119,121,262] Hypercarbia can trigger widespread neuroapoptosis, even in unanesthetized neonatal rats exposed to increased partial pressures of carbon dioxide. Whereas apoptotic cell death was quantitatively indistinguishable from neurodegeneration in isoflurane-treated litter mates, which were also hypercarbic; neurocognitive impairment in adults was observed only in the isoflurane-treated animals.[121] However, widespread apoptotic neurodegeneration observed in anesthetized nonhuman primates, where carbon dioxide tensions were controlled by tracheal intubation and ventilation, suggests that metabolic derangements may not be sufficient to explain the structural abnormalities observed in immature animal species. Lastly, experimental models of neurodegeneration have implicated reentry of postmitotic neurons into the cell cycle, leading to cell death. Ketamine exposure has been found to induce aberrant cell cycle reentry, leading to apoptotic cell death in the developing rat brain.[175] However, a causative link between neuronal degeneration immediately after exposure and subsequent cognitive abnormalities observed into adulthood have yet to be firmly established.

Specific Anesthetic and Sedative Agents

To provide a succinct overview of the available laboratory data, we briefly review the effects of each class of anesthetics separately. Although the effects of some anesthetics, such as ketamine and isoflurane, have been extensively studied in the developing brain, the effects of others, such as xenon and desflurane, have not been examined in depth. However, current data suggest that all routinely used anesthetics exert deleterious effects to some degree (see E-Table 25.1). When examining the available animal literature, it is important to appreciate that potencies for inhalational anesthetics, as measured in MAC values (a concentration measure), are largely comparable across species, whereas doses for intravenous (IV) medications are not—that is, weight-based dosing rather than concentration varies substantively. Weight-based dosing of most IV medications to effect sedation or anesthesia in animals is approximately 6- to 10-fold greater than comparable doses in humans. The dosing is further complicated by the different routes used to administer these drugs in most neonatal animal models, frequently relying on the subcutaneous (SC) and intraperitoneal (IP) routes as opposed to the oral or IV routes in humans. However, the possible importance of these interspecies pharmacodynamic differences on brain structural and functional outcomes has not yet been adequately addressed.

KETAMINE

The injectable anesthetic most frequently studied in this context is ketamine, an antagonist of the NMDA glutamate receptor that also interacts with other cell membrane proteins, such as muscarinic, nicotinic, and opioid receptors, as well as voltage-gated calcium channels. Ketamine's properties, which include potent analgesia, dissociative anesthesia, and relative hemodynamic stability, have made it a popular choice for procedural sedation and induction of anesthesia in children with concerns for hemodynamic stability, such as critical congenital heart disease or pulmonary hypertension.[263-265] However, about 17 years ago, a seminal study examining the effects of repeated IP injections of ketamine on the brain of neonatal rats observed widespread apoptotic cell death.[19] Seven injections of 20 mg/kg of ketamine, administered to 7-day-old rat pups over a 9-hour period in evenly divided intervals, caused a 3- to 31-fold increase in degenerating neurons, depending on brain region, compared with vehicle-injected control animals. This has led to speculation that these changes might contribute to subsequent neuropsychiatric disorders.[19] These initial findings for ketamine have been confirmed in more than 50 studies in small rodents, as well as nonhuman primates, both in vitro and in vivo (see E-Table 25.1). Several of these studies have identified relationships between neurodegeneration and dose, number of injections, as well as animal species and age during exposure.

Single doses up to 75 mg/kg or multiple IP injections up to 17 mg/kg per hour for 6 hours were not neurotoxic to neonatal rats.[148] In contrast, single doses between 20 and 50 mg/kg SC in neonatal mice[150,154] or six or seven repeated injections of 20 to 25 mg/kg IP consistently led to apoptosis in the neonatal rat brain.[19,148,151,169,170] Although these doses appear to be excessive compared with clinical practice and plasma concentrations in these rodents were up to 7 times greater than those in humans,[151] these doses of ketamine were required for sedation owing to increased requirements for IV anesthetics in small animals based on body weight (refer to the later section "Critical Evaluation of Animal Studies and Interspecies Comparisons." Moreover, coadministration of midazolam, diazepam, propofol, or thiopental can compound the neuronal injury caused by ketamine.[150,154,162] Studies in rats, mice, and nonhuman primates suggest that susceptibility to ketamine-induced neurotoxicity may be most pronounced during a brief period after birth, with a maximum impact between 3 and 7 days of age in small rodents and less than 35 days of age in monkeys.[19,159] In addition to neuronal apoptosis, both small rodents and nonhuman primates that were anesthetized with ketamine also exhibited impaired learning tasks later in life.[87,149,178]

In summary, ketamine is the most frequently studied anesthetic, in terms to its neurotoxic effects, and has repeatedly been shown to cause widespread apoptosis (an effect that is exacerbated by the coadministration of other anesthetics), as well as neurologic impairment in adult animals exposed early in life. Importantly, long-lasting learning impairment has also been demonstrated in nonhuman primates, the closest animal model to humans, albeit after an IV exposure of 24 hours.[178] However, this exposure time exceeds most anesthetics in humans.[178] Furthermore, it is unclear whether the observed learning abnormalities could be explained by a reduction in motivation to perform the learning tasks, as also demonstrated in the exposed animals.[178]

INHALATIONAL ANESTHETICS

Another commonly studied class of drugs is the inhalational anesthetics (see E-Table 25.1). Desflurane, sevoflurane, isoflurane, enflurane, and halothane exert their anesthetic properties predominantly by their agonistic effects on the GABA$_A$ receptor, but also to differing degrees on glycine, NMDA, acetylcholine, serotonin (5-HT$_3$), α-amino-3-hydroxy-5-methyl-4-isoxazole-propionic acid (AMPA), and kainate receptors. Whereas GABA represents the main inhibitory neurotransmitter in the adult CNS, it has excitatory properties in the developing brain,[258] which may have implications for neurotoxicity, as discussed previously. Most studies of inhalational anesthetics examined either isoflurane by itself or in combination with midazolam and nitrous oxide. This combination of GABA agonists and NMDA antagonists has been repeatedly found to cause widespread brain cell degeneration in neonatal animals.[100,102,105,106] In addition to the immediate deleterious effects on brain structure, long-term abnormalities in spatial learning tasks and decreased neuronal cell density in adult rats have also been observed after exposure to this anesthetic combination early in life.[100,111] One MAC of isoflurane administered to neonatal rats as the sole anesthetic for 4 hours led to neurocognitive deficits in rats when they matured to adults,[120,121] whereas up to 0.6 MAC for 6 hours in neonatal mice caused widespread neuronal degeneration immediately after exposure, although it failed to lead to neurocognitive deficits or decreases in neuronal density in adulthood.[119,128] These inconsistencies raise questions of whether neonatal neuronal apoptotic cell death during exposure is causatively linked to long-term behavioral and learning abnormalities observed in adult animals. In fact, similar degrees of neurodegeneration were observed in 7-day-old rats after a 4-hour exposure to either carbon dioxide or isoflurane; however, long-term neurocognitive deficits were observed only after the anesthetic exposure.[121] Importantly, widespread neuronal cell death has also been observed in neonatal rhesus monkeys after 5 hours of isoflurane in concentrations between 0.75% and 1.5%,[127] although long-term neurologic studies in this species have yet to be published.

Sevoflurane has also induced widespread neuroapoptosis in neonatal mice similar to isoflurane,[76,128,230] although the long-term effects on learning and behavior are conflicting.[77,128,230] To date, few studies have examined desflurane in this context. Desflurane causes age- and species-dependent neuronal cell death in 7-day-old mice, but not 16-day-old rats.[74,76]

Several studies have attempted to compare the neurotoxicity of contemporary inhaled anesthetics. Equianesthetic concentrations of 0.6 MAC of desflurane, isoflurane, or sevoflurane for 6 hours in neonatal mice caused a similar degree of neuronal degeneration in superficial neocortex, a brain region significantly affected in this model.[76] These results contrast with studies in which neonatal mice were exposed to much lower concentrations of sevoflurane that resulted in significantly less neuronal loss immediately compared with isoflurane, albeit no neurocognitive performance deficits were observed in adult animals with either regimen.[128] In yet another comparative mouse study, desflurane caused greater injury than isoflurane or sevoflurane, which demonstrated comparable degrees of neurodegeneration, and long-term neurologic impairment occurred only after exposure to desflurane.[77] The significance of these differential findings remains unclear but could be related to methodologic differences in the assessment of brain injury. Importantly, however, these conflicting results prohibit any clinical recommendations for choosing one particular volatile anesthetic over another.

Although largely phased out from clinical anesthesia practice, halothane and enflurane have also been shown to induce brain abnormalities. These anesthetics were initially studied in rat models of chronic occupational exposure during pregnancy, causing delayed synaptogenesis as well as behavioral and learning abnormalities.[15–18,89]

In summary, inhalational anesthetics represent one of the most frequently used classes of anesthetics in pediatric anesthesia, and their neurotoxic properties have been extensively studied. Widespread apoptosis immediately after exposure in a wide variety of animal models, including nonhuman primates, is a consistent finding. However, neurologic impairment in adult animals exposed to anesthesia early in life has not been consistently found, and in fact, some studies have observed no neurologic impairment at all. Accordingly, long-lasting learning impairment has not been convincingly linked to neonatal neuroapoptosis. Primate studies on long-term neurocognitive outcomes after inhalational anesthesia early in life have yet to be published.

NITROUS OXIDE

Nitrous oxide, an NMDA antagonist, is the oldest anesthetic still in clinical use, although its low potency (MAC of 115% in adult humans) necessitates the coadministration of other anesthetics to provide surgical anesthesia. Anesthetic combinations studied in this context have often included the GABA agonist midazolam, and the mixed GABA-agonist/NMDA-antagonist isoflurane.[a] In rats, nitrous oxide alone did not induce neuronal apoptosis,[100,102,108] whereas in an in vitro study, it caused neuronal cell death in

hippocampal slices in mice.[108] When administered in combination with other anesthetics, however, nitrous oxide exacerbated neuronal cell death induced by isoflurane and also contributed to long-term neurologic abnormalities in rats when combined with isoflurane and midazolam.[100]

XENON

Because of the cost differential between other inhalational anesthetics and this rare, colorless, and odorless noble gas, xenon has not achieved widespread clinical use, despite its NMDA-antagonistic anesthetic properties.[266] Xenon has a relatively low anesthetic potency, with a MAC measuring between 65% and 70% in adults,[267,268] but a very low blood-gas solubility that facilitates a rapid onset and emergence from anesthesia.[269] Xenon's effects on neuronal apoptosis have been examined in two in vivo studies, with slightly differing results. Although 75% xenon for 6 hours did not cause neuronal apoptosis in 7-day-old rat pups,[108] 70% xenon for 4 hours increased neuroapoptosis in 7-day-old mice.[239] Interestingly, both studies demonstrated that xenon decreased the neurodegeneration induced by isoflurane anesthesia,[108,239] which may have relevance to the phenomenon's putative mechanism (see later text). An investigation of xenon's effects on neuronal viability in hippocampal slice cultures observed neuronal cell death after exposure to more than 0.75 MAC of xenon for 6 hours.[241] In this setting, isoflurane pretreatment reduced neuronal cell death caused by 1 MAC of xenon,[241] again demonstrating the confusing finding that combinations of anesthetics can have both exacerbating and ameliorating effects related to their respective neurotoxic properties.

BENZODIAZEPINES

Benzodiazepines, such as clonazepam, diazepam, and midazolam, have been investigated regarding their effects on the immature brain, either alone or in combination with other drugs. These GABA agonists are most frequently used for anxiolysis in toddlers and older children in the perioperative setting, but they are also used in premature neonates in the critical care setting. Studies have shown that repeated exposure can increase neuronal degeneration in small-animal models, depending on the dose, region of the brain, species, and age of the animal studied. Repeated injections for a 6-hour exposure to midazolam increased neuronal cell death in neonatal rats,[189] whereas single doses of 5 mg/kg of diazepam or 9 mg/kg of midazolam IP did not.[72,100] While 5 mg/kg SC of diazepam caused neuronal cell death in some brain regions in mice, this was not associated with learning deficits in adulthood.[87] In these studies, the neuroapoptosis associated with diazepam was significantly augmented by the coadministration of other sedatives, such as ketamine.[87] The dose-dependence of neuroapoptosis observed in neonatal rats is highlighted by the fact that diazepam doses of 10 mg/kg or greater have been found to be injurious,[73,72] an effect that was prevented in one study by the coadministration of the benzodiazepine-antagonist flumazenil.[72] Two studies reported no neurocognitive learning disabilities in adult mice after they were sedated with diazepam or midazolam as neonates.[87,188] It is therefore unclear whether dose- or species-specific factors are responsible for the disparate findings.

CHLORAL HYDRATE

The sedative chloral hydrate, a chlorination product of ethanol that acts as a combined GABA agonist and NMDA antagonist, has been largely supplanted by barbiturates and benzodiazepines in pediatric clinical practice. However, it is still used in doses of up to 120 mg/kg for sedation for some imaging studies,[270] and

---

[a]References 92, 100, 102, 105, 106, 111, and 112.

its neurotoxic properties have been investigated in an animal study. Preliminary results indicate that it causes neuroapoptosis in the cerebral cortex and the caudate-putamen complex in immature mouse pups in doses of 100 mg/kg or greater.[71] The neurofunctional outcome in adult mice, however, has not as yet been investigated.

BARBITURATES

Barbiturates act primarily via the $GABA_A$ receptor but also exert effects via nicotinic acetylcholine, AMPA, and kainate receptors. Thiopental in doses of 25 mg/kg SC does not induce apoptosis in neonatal mice, although when doses as small as 5 mg/kg are combined with 25 mg/kg of ketamine SC, neuronal degeneration occurs and is associated with long-term impairment of learning and memory.[162] Pentobarbital and phenobarbital induce neurodegeneration in mouse and rat pups. Furthermore, after receiving these sedatives as neonates, long-term alterations in brain protein expression and abnormalities in learning and memory have been observed,[117,209,211] although in one study these long-term alterations may be attributed in part to hypoxia and hypercarbia during the neonatal sedation.[209] Interestingly, estradiol has been shown to attenuate phenobarbital-induced neuroapoptosis.[72,210]

PROPOFOL

Propofol predominantly acts via GABA and glycine receptor–agonistic properties, but also weakly on nicotinic, AMPA, and NMDA receptors. Its neurotoxic profile has been repeatedly studied both in vitro and in vivo. Propofol has consistently caused neuroapoptosis after single doses greater than 50 mg/kg (SC or IP) or repeated doses greater than 20 mg/kg per hour for 4 to 5 hours in neonatal rodents.[162,168,216,221] Interestingly, lithium prevents propofol-induced neuroapoptosis in neonatal mice.[168] However, after 24 hours of IV anesthesia with propofol (6 mg/kg per hour) and fentanyl (10 µg/kg per hour), no evidence of apoptosis was found in a pig model.[217] Apart from overt neuronal cell death, propofol also decreased the effect of GABAergic enzyme glutamic acid decarboxylase,[213] diminished nerve growth factors,[219,223] and caused neurite growth cone collapse in tissue culture.[215] In addition, propofol alters dendritic spine architecture in developing rats, depending on the age at the time of anesthetic exposure.[222] Specifically, dendritic spine density decreased during exposures in the first week of life, but increased if exposure took place during week 3 of life; the mechanism of these differing responses remains elusive.[222] Propofol has also been found to cause significant apoptotic degeneration of neurons and oligodendrocytes in fetal and neonatal rhesus monkeys after a 5-hour exposure.[226] Accordingly, the overall consensus of this body of literature is that propofol, in a dose- and exposure time-dependent fashion, can dramatically affect the developing brain of animals.

DEXMEDETOMIDINE

Unlike other anesthetics and sedatives, dexmedetomidine is a sedative and analgesic that does not interact with GABA, NMDA, or opioid receptors, but rather interacts presynaptically with α_2-adrenergic receptors. Given this dissimilar mechanism of action and the fact that all anesthetics acting on GABA or NMDA receptors have been found deleterious to the developing brain, there has been substantial interest in the use of dexmedetomidine as an alternative sedative since it may not cause neurocognitive dysfunction. Several initial studies that examined the brain structure after dexmedetomidine administration in rodents and monkeys reported none to minimal neurodegeneration.[79–85,228] However,

one study observed increased neuroapoptosis after a prolonged exposure to dexmedetomidine, albeit in brain regions distinct from those vulnerable to ketamine-induced apoptosis.[86] Furthermore, dexmedetomidine has been found to reduce or even ameliorate brain structural or long-term cognitive abnormalities caused by isoflurane, sevoflurane, ketamine, or propofol.[79–81,84,228] These results clearly warrant conducting additional studies comparing dexmedetomidine and standard anesthetic regimens with particular attention to comparable levels of sedation.

OPIOID ANALGESICS

Since all currently used general anesthetics can dramatically alter the structure of the developing brain, opioid analgesics represent a class of drugs that reduces anesthetic requirements and could therefore diminish the deleterious effects of anesthetics in the developing brain. To date, only one study has investigated neurotoxic properties of opioids compared with an inhalational anesthetic regimen. Mechanically ventilated, neonatal pigs, injected with an IV bolus of 30 µg/kg fentanyl followed by 15 µg/kg per hour for 4 hours, exhibited less neuroapoptosis in several regions of the brain compared with a balanced anesthetic of 1 mg/kg of midazolam, followed by 4 hours of 0.55% isoflurane and 75% nitrous oxide.[92] These initial findings are encouraging, although future neurotoxicity studies with opioid infusions need to also include adjuvants that produce amnesia as this is an expectation during clinical anesthesia. However, whether neonates and infants require the same level of amnesia as adults during surgery remains a hotly debated subject.[271,272] Finally, it is critical to confirm that equipotent anesthetic doses are used when comparing the effects of different regimens (e.g., IV versus inhalational anesthetics) on neurotoxicity.

The long-term consequences of opioid administration to the immature brain need to be elucidated before recommending such a regimen as an alternative strategy for clinical practice. Similar to GABA and NMDA receptors, opioid receptors are also intimately involved in early brain development and synaptogenesis,[273,274] which would make it plausible that opioids could similarly affect brain development during the critical period of synaptogenesis. Moreover, repeated neonatal exposures could alter long-term opioid receptor composition. Increased neuronal cell death and decreased neuronal density after perinatal exposure to µ-receptor agonists, such as morphine and heroin, have been observed in developing animals after prolonged exposures.[98,125,246] Long-term buprenorphine and methadone treatment early in life diminished the concentrations of nerve growth factors in the immature brain.[70,186] Moreover, perinatal exposure to morphine has immediately and permanently reduced µ-opioid receptor density[191,192] and may be associated with long-term impairment of memory and cognitive function in small animals,[194,197–199,202–204] as well as exaggerated nociceptive responses to a pain challenge later in life.[200,205] Stimulation of the κ-opioid receptor may amplify neuronal cell death induced by proapoptotic agents.[275] High-dose fentanyl significantly exacerbated white-matter brain lesions induced by glutamatergic overstimulation in mice.[91] However, a single morphine injection of up to 10 mg/kg in 7- or 15 day-old rats failed to affect survival or dendritic differentiation of pyramidal neurons in the medial prefrontal cortex.[206] These animal data suggest that prolonged perinatal exposure to opioid analgesics could potentially cause structural and long-term functional alterations in the developing brain and may amplify proapoptotic stimuli, whereas a brief or single exposure may not. These data support the need for further studies into the interactions of opioid analgesics and anesthetics in the developing brain.

Exposure Time, Dose, and Anesthetic Combinations

Similar to opioid analgesics, the impact of developmental anesthetic exposure seems to depend on the dose and/or duration of anesthesia for inhalational anesthetics, as well as the dose, route of administration, and number of doses (i.e., exposure time) for injectable anesthetics. Moreover, combinations of several anesthetics and sedatives have, in general, caused more neuroapoptosis and long-term cognitive changes than have single drugs. For example, combinations of midazolam, nitrous oxide, and isoflurane cause a much greater degree of neuroapoptosis in neonatal rats than isoflurane alone, even when the latter is administered at a greater inspired concentration.[100] In the case of ketamine, its neurodegenerative potency is amplified when coadministered with thiopental or propofol.[162] Anesthetic combinations of mixed GABA agonists and NMDA antagonists demonstrate exaggerated effects. This evidence supports the notion that a deeper level of anesthesia increases the neuroapoptotic injury. However, coadministration of two anesthetics, xenon and dexmedetomidine, as well as isoflurane before treatment (all of which attenuated the neurotoxic effects of isoflurane anesthesia[79,108,239]), somewhat contradict this hypothesis. The effects of muscle relaxants on neurologic outcomes, while unlikely related to their insignificant permeation of the intact blood-brain barrier, have not yet been studied. Moreover, the study of local anesthetic toxicity has been limited to the developing spinal cord and has not yet been expanded to the developing brain. This line of investigation will require greater emphasis if the use of regional anesthetic techniques are expanded in infants and young children to reduce requirements for general anesthetics.

Deleterious Effects of Untreated Pain and Stress

Given the evidence for deleterious effects of anesthetics and analgesics on the developing brain and the paucity of complete anesthetics devoid of cytotoxicity, one approach would be to reduce or even withhold potentially toxic drugs at the expense of children experiencing pain and stress during surgery. Such practice would not only be unethical, but animal and clinical research actually suggest that these recurrent stressful and painful experiences also adversely affect the developing brain. Noxious stimulation in neonatal rodents has been associated with subsequent hyperalgesia as well as hypoalgesia, depending on the type and severity of injury.[276] In human neonates, repetitive painful skin lacerations for procedures as minor as blood draws lead to long-term, local sensory hyperinnervation.[277] In immature animals, in addition to these local responses, repetitive, inflammatory pain early in life results in hyperalgesia and lasting changes in nociceptive circuitry of the adult dorsal horn.[278] Repeated painful injections into the paws of rat pups resulted in a generalized thermal hypoalgesia.[276] In addition to altered pain processing and sensory perception, repetitive or persistent pain in the neonate alters behavior and cognitive function in adulthood, decreases pain thresholds, and increases vulnerability to stress and anxiety disorders or chronic pain syndromes later in life.[161,279-282]

In addition to painful stimulation, early adverse emotional experiences can also induce long-lasting abnormalities in animals such as imbalances of the inhibitory nervous system,[283] impairment of normal development of the nociceptive system, long-term behavioral changes,[284] and persistent learning impairment.[202] Therefore fetuses, neonates, and infants subjected to pain and stresses associated with invasive procedures without adequate anesthesia and analgesia may also be at risk for long-term adverse outcomes.

Accordingly, preemptive administration of analgesics and sedatives such as morphine or ketamine has been found to ameliorate the deleterious effects of neonatal pain in some of the animal studies.[161,202,282] Either the presence of painful stimulation or 5 days of morphine administered to neonatal mice without pain independently impaired adult rewarded behavior, although the combination of pain and analgesia did not cause behavioral abnormalities.[202]

Clinical reports have also demonstrated that human neonates and infants can mount a substantial metabolic and endocrine response to perioperative stress and painful stimulation, which include surges in catecholamine, cortisol, β-endorphin, insulin, glucagon, and growth hormone levels.[285-287] Some of these markers, such as cortisol, can remain increased for more than a year after the insult, possibly as a result of cumulative stress related to multiple painful procedures early in life.[288] Inhalational anesthetics, opioid analgesics, as well as regional anesthesia, inhibit intraoperative stress and improve postoperative outcomes.[286,289,290] Moreover, adequate perioperative anesthesia reduced the incidence of other complications, such as the incidence of sepsis and disseminated intravascular coagulation, leading to a decrease in overall mortality.[291] Even less invasive procedures, such as circumcisions performed without analgesia in young boys, can exaggerate responses to painful challenges (e.g., immunizations) later in life.[292] Conversely, topical or regional anesthesia for circumcision not only mitigated the immediate humoral stress response during the procedure[293] but also blunted the pain-induced, long-term hyperalgesia.[292] In preterm neonates, painful stimulations early in life have also been associated with subsequent diminished cognition and motor function.[294] In a retrospective study of children older than 1 year of age who were born at less than 32 weeks gestational age without significant neonatal brain injury or major sensorineural impairment, an increased number of skin-breaking procedures from birth to term (including heel sticks, intramuscular injections, chest tube placements, and central line insertions) predicted poorer subsequent cognitive and motor development (as assessed using the Bayley Scales of Infant Development II) when compared with term controls. Importantly, after controlling for severity of illness, duration of morphine administration, and exposure to postnatal dexamethasone, gestational age at birth was not significantly associated with poorer cognitive or motor outcomes. These findings suggest that repetitive pain-related stressful experiences and not prematurity per se were in part responsible for the altered neurodevelopmental outcome.[294] Although this study did not examine the effects of anesthetic or analgesic administration during painful stimulation on subsequent outcome, a small, retrospective report suggested an improvement in outcome after administering anesthesia during painful stimulation.[295] In this study, painful stimulation during reduction of herniated bowel without anesthesia in infants suffering from gastroschisis tended to more frequently lead to serious adverse events, such as bowel ischemia, the need for total parenteral nutrition, and unplanned reoperation, than in infants undergoing the same procedure with general anesthesia.[295] Surprisingly, despite the persistently large numbers of painful and stressful procedures performed in vulnerable neonates, data indicate that the majority of these procedures are still not accompanied by adequate analgesia or anesthesia.[296] In clinical practice, the relative effects of anesthetic exposure or inadequate anesthesia or analgesia during painful stimulation as the potential basis for cognitive abnormalities remain open to speculation.

Together, the data from animals and humans convincingly demonstrate that pain-related stress experienced early in life is deleterious to the developing nervous system, that pain in children remains undertreated, and that analgesics and/or anesthetics may alleviate many of the degenerative effects of unopposed pain and improve outcomes. However, if anesthetics protect from the deleterious effects of painful stimulation but at the same time confer their own cytotoxic effects, the quintessential question is whether other adjuvant compounds can alleviate these adverse effects.

Potential Alleviating Strategies

Whereas the translational relevance of anesthetic-induced neurotoxicity observed in neonatal animals to humans remains unresolved, several laboratory studies have investigated strategies to alleviate some of the deleterious effects of anesthetics and sedatives in animals, which may have relevance for clinical practice. These protective strategies have been directed at both the structural effects observed immediately after anesthesia, such as neuronal cell death, as well as the long-term abnormalities, such as neurocognitive impairment and learning abnormalities. Importantly, many animal studies administered adjuvants immediately before or during anesthesia, thereby maintaining an adequate level of anesthesia and analgesia to avoid the deleterious effects of unopposed pain.

The sedative dexmedetomidine and the anesthetic xenon possess limited neurotoxic potencies themselves but seem to significantly reduce isoflurane-induced neuroapoptosis.[79–81,84,108,228,239] The coadministration of dexmedetomidine also prevented long-term memory impairment after 6-hour isoflurane exposure in rats.[79] Interestingly, preconditioning with a brief exposure of isoflurane conferred protection from the deleterious effects of a subsequent prolonged exposure to the same drug, both in vitro and in vivo.[109,145] In in vitro studies, the inositol triphosphate–receptor antagonist xestospongin C, tissue plasminogen activator, plasmin, inhibition of the neurotrophic receptor p75[NTR] or RhoA receptor, as well as prevention of cytoskeletal depolymerization with either jasplakinolide or TAT-Pep5 significantly attenuated isoflurane-mediated neuroapoptosis.[118,122,136] In addition, L-carnitine attenuated neuronal apoptosis after 6 hours of isoflurane and nitrous oxide in 7-day-old rat pups.[116] Moreover, supplementation with the naturally occurring hormones β-estradiol or melatonin prevented the deleterious effects on neuronal survival of a prolonged exposure to midazolam, isoflurane, and nitrous oxide.[102,105] Similarly, coadministration of β-estradiol significantly reduced phenobarbital-induced neuroapoptosis.[72,210] Conversely, blocking the GABA receptor with the antagonist gabazine has not been found to ameliorate isoflurane-induced neurodegeneration.[79] On the other hand, pilocarpine reduces neuroapoptosis induced by the GABA agonists isoflurane and midazolam, while augmenting the damage after administration of the NMDA antagonist phencyclidine, based on preliminary results from neonatal mice.[107] Preliminary data from the same laboratory also suggest that whole-body hypothermia with a targeted brain temperature of less than 30°C may protect from the neuroapoptotic ramifications of a 4-hour exposure to 0.75% isoflurane or to 40 mg/kg of IP ketamine in neonatal mice.[43,115] Another therapy that has been successfully tested in mouse pups as well

as nonhuman primates that either received ketamine, propofol, or isoflurane was lithium, which abolished the anesthetic-induced neuroapoptosis in cortex and the caudate-putamen complex.[147,168]

Because the applicability and extent of anesthetic neurotoxicity has not been established in humans, it seems premature to recommend any of these protective strategies for children. Moreover, the safety of many of these drugs and interventions has yet to be determined in human neonates and infants. For example, tissue plasminogen activator and plasmin promote fibrinolysis and may not be first-line treatments during invasive surgical procedures. The sex hormone β-estradiol may not be a feasible adjuvant in prepubescent boys. The safety of pilocarpine in young children may be hampered by its proconvulsant activity observed in some animal studies.[297,298] Lithium has been labeled harmful to the human fetus and may cause neurocognitive abnormalities in young children.[299–301] Whole-body hypothermia below 30°C is not a clinically feasible modality, because even mild perioperative hypothermia, at least in adults, has been causally linked to numerous complications, including increased blood loss and transfusion requirements, morbid myocardial outcomes, prolonged postanesthetic recovery and hospitalization, thermal discomfort, as well as an increased risk of surgical wound infections.[302] Therefore hypothermia to treat anesthesia-induced neurotoxicity is unlikely to play a substantive role during routine pediatric anesthesia, but it may have a role in infants undergoing hypothermic cardiopulmonary bypass for heart surgery to treat congenital defects. Unfortunately, the latter population often presents with neurocognitive abnormalities even before anesthetic exposure, which confounds the potential effects of anesthetics.[303] Xenon's scarcity renders it a very expensive adjuvant or anesthetic, although dexmedetomidine's more widespread availability and increasing familiarity among pediatric anesthesiologists makes it a more attractive option for further research into protective strategies.[304,305]

Anesthetic Neuroprotection

Complicating any discussion about the deleterious effects of anesthetics on the developing brain are their potential protective effects during noxious stimulation. Because of the limited tolerance of the brain to ischemia, even relatively brief periods of inadequate oxygen or blood flow to the brain may lead to neuronal injury and long-term neurologic impairment. Importantly, animal studies have repeatedly confirmed the protective properties of anesthetics when administered during episodes of brain hypoxia-ischemia, albeit most of these studies have been conducted in adult animals and the longevity of the protective effects are controversial.[306] In immature animal models, anesthetics have also been found to reduce neurologic injury and improve functional outcome after brain ischemia.[67] Desflurane alleviates neuronal cell death and early neurologic dysfunction in a neonatal pig model during hypothermic cardiopulmonary bypass and deep hypothermic circulatory arrest.[307,308] Isoflurane treatment before hypoxia-ischemia protects the brain and improves survival in neonatal rats and mice.[309–311] Both xenon and sevoflurane protect the immature brain during simulated hypoxia-ischemia in vitro.[312] Furthermore, sevoflurane combines with mild hypothermia to protect brain structure and function in neonatal mice during hypoxia-ischemia.[313] These findings in immature animals suggest that critically ill human neonates could potentially benefit from these protective properties during clinical scenarios of greater risk for neurologic injury, such as cardiopulmonary bypass, neurologic surgery, or perioperative cardiocirculatory arrest; these potential benefits therefore should

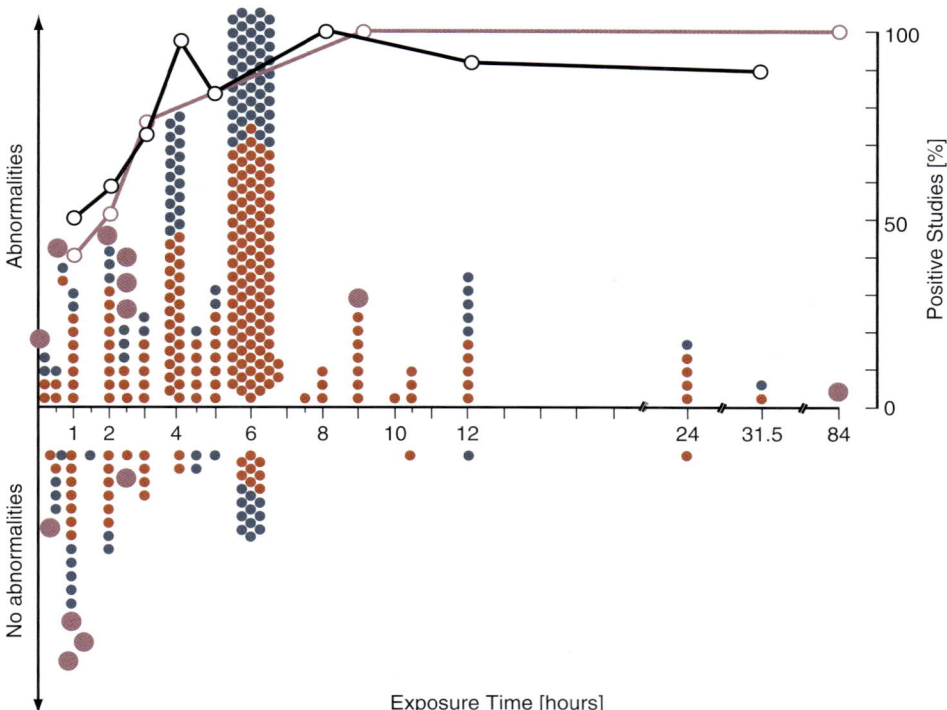

FIGURE 25.4 The majority of in vivo animal studies into the effects of anesthetic exposure on brain structure and function examine substantially longer exposure times than occurring in clinical practice. However, longer exposures trend toward more positive findings in both animal and human studies. Animal studies, inclusive of various anesthetic drugs and doses, reporting abnormal findings (above the horizontal line) or negative findings (below the horizontal line) for brain structural (*solid red circles*) or cognitive outcomes (*solid blue circles*), as a function of exposure time. *Solid purple circles* represent clinical studies of long-term cognitive outcomes in humans demonstrating abnormalities (above the horizontal line) or lack thereof (below the horizontal line). Exposure times denote all reported anesthetic durations, either single or cumulative, or estimated exposure times based on injection schedules, ranging from 10 minutes to 31.5 hours. For the purpose of analysis, results are reported separately for structural and functional outcomes, resulting in up to two circles, if both outcomes were reported, and may include opposing results, if structural and functional findings diverged. The graphs express the ratio of positive to negative studies in animals (*black*) or humans (*purple*); circles represent the percentage of positive studies for respective exposure epoch ranging from specific data point to next lower data point on the graph Note that positive studies outnumber negative studies for all exposure times in both animals and humans, except for only 40% of human studies demonstrating cognitive abnormalities following anesthetic exposures of 1 hour or less. (From Lin EP, Lee J-R, Lee CS, et al. Do anesthetics harm the developing human brain? An integrative analysis of animal and human studies. *Neurotoxicol Teratol.* 2017;60:117–128.)

Critical Evaluation of Animal Studies and Interspecies Comparisons

To determine whether findings from animal studies can inform clinical practice, it is critically important to evaluate how well animal studies represent the perioperative experience of young children.[a]

To date, no animal model exists covering all aspects of human physiology and pathophysiology during surgical procedures. The task of modeling potential vulnerabilities of the developing human brain in animals is complicated by the fact that human CNS

development is much more protracted than that of any of the model species. However, human neurocognitive performance is also much more complex compared with lower animals, and any potential neurologic injury might therefore have a greater impact on such an intricate system.

DURATION OF EXPOSURE

To elicit toxic effects, the designs of many animal studies include durations of anesthesia from 1 to 31.5 hours (Fig. 25.4). The majority of animal studies used exposure times of 6 hours—a duration extending far beyond the average time required for most routine pediatric anesthetics.[2] However, expressing the duration of anesthesia as a fraction of a subject's life span, thereby equating a 6-hour anesthetic in mice to a 2-week or greater anesthetic in humans, is probably an oversimplification. Life expectancy or even the relative duration of neurodevelopment may not be immediately relevant when considering the likelihood of injury at a cellular level. Nonetheless, the extent of the injury and its

---

[a]References 4, 25, 100, 119–121, 178, and 314–319.

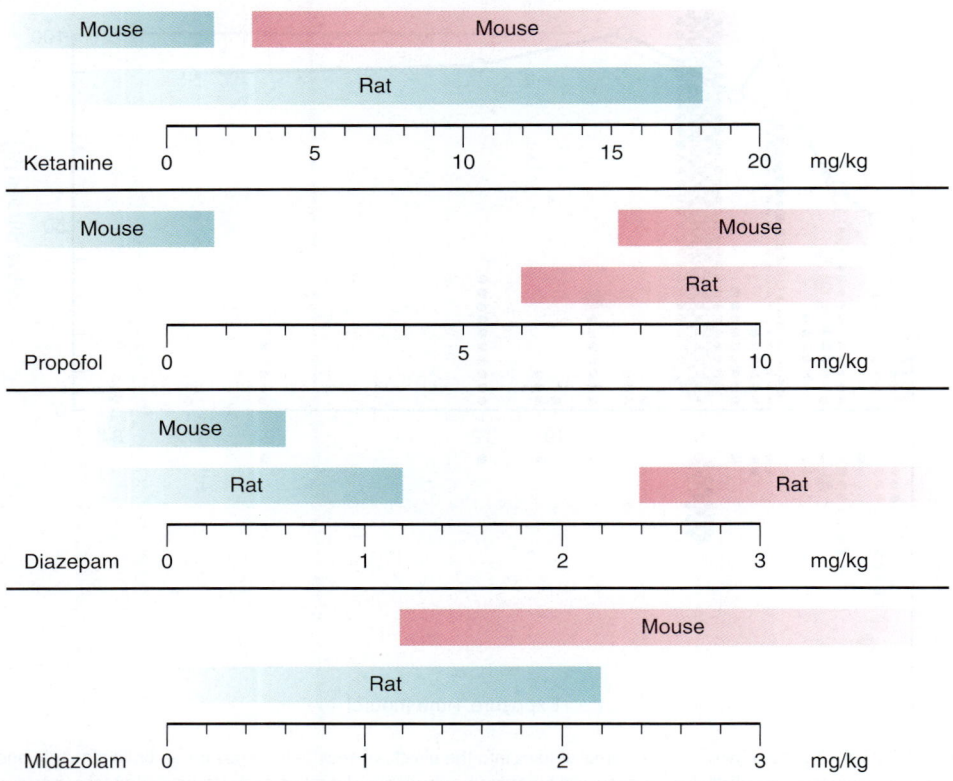

FIGURE 25.5 Neurodegenerative effects of injectable anesthetics in developing animals are dose-dependent. *Blue bars* represent doses of the respective anesthetics not causing neurodegeneration in rats and mice; *pink bars* represent doses causing neurodegeneration in animals. The figure includes only studies using single injections of anesthetics, and doses used in animals were scaled to doses for children by using an allometric scaling technique, based on calculations outlined in reference 325. Neurotoxic data are based on experiments described in references 19, 72, 73, 87, 100, 148, 151, 154, 159, 162, 171, and 219.

functional implications may potentially be related to the duration of the entire brain developmental period, even though the mechanism of anesthetic-induced neurodegeneration is unknown. Because human brain development occurs at a much slower pace than in any of the other species, similar exposure times could potentially result in differential susceptibility and ability for postexposure repair among species. For example, the brain reaches adult size at 20 days of age in rats, 3 years of age in rhesus monkeys, 7 years of age in chimpanzees, and not until 15 years of age in humans.[4,320,321] Exposure to anesthesia during a larger proportion of the period of development could result in a greater impact on total development and maturation. Similarly, given the plasticity of the developing brain, it seems conceivable that brains with slower growth rates are afforded more time for repair.[322,323] Conversely, in complex organisms, such as humans, relatively minor injuries in crucial areas or at critical times during development could have profound effects on long-term cognitive and executive function. Accordingly, cognition may be altered by briefer periods of anesthetic exposure in children, compared with animals functioning on a simpler cognitive level.

ANESTHETIC DOSES

Animals are subjected to greater weight-based doses of injectable anesthetics, sometimes by orders of magnitude, compared with doses commonly used in human clinical practice. In the discussion of whether these doses have applicability to pediatric anesthesia practice, it is important to understand that small animals require significantly greater weight-based doses of IV anesthetics to produce immobility than larger animals or humans. These differences can be explained, in large part, by the animals' smaller size, greater metabolic rate, and shorter physiologic time compared with humans.[324] Using a process called allometric scaling, which takes the differences among species into account, doses for injectable drugs in animals comparable with human doses have been estimated to be approximately 3-, 6-, or 12-fold greater for monkeys, rats, or mice, respectively (see also Chapter 7).[324,325] Whereas drug doses used in anesthetic neurotoxicity studies frequently still exceed these comparable doses calculated using allometric scaling, they do not include a significant safety margin (Fig. 25.5). Using allometrically scaled doses, plasma concentrations for ketamine, for example, were approximately 3 to 10 times greater in small rodents and monkeys than those observed during clinical human practice.[151,159] This might suggest that the neurotoxic properties observed with large doses of injectable anesthetics, such as ketamine, could potentially have direct applicability to humans only if the anesthetic and the neurotoxic effects were based on the same molecular mechanism, which has yet to be verified. Otherwise, animal studies would expose subjects to much greater plasma concentrations of potential neurotoxicants than those used during anesthesia in humans, thereby leading to an overestimation of the neurotoxic effects of IV anesthetics in laboratory studies.

Doses for inhaled anesthetics generating immobility in animals, on the other hand, are much closer to clinically used doses. Moreover, similar to human anesthesia, potency of inhaled anesthetics increases with subject age, necessitating larger doses in younger animals,[76,262,326] which could suggest closer clinical applicability of laboratory data using these compounds.

EXPERIMENTAL VERSUS CLINICAL CONDITIONS

Another important distinction between laboratory studies in animals and clinical practice in humans is the presence of significant comorbidities and underlying disease, the genetic diversity in human populations, as well as the frequent occurrence of stress and pain associated with surgical procedures. Very few laboratory studies have examined the effects of surgical stress and pain on anesthesia-induced neurotoxicity. When tail clamping or injection of caustic substances were used to model surgical stress, results have varied; one study reported no influence of the painful stimulus on anesthesia-induced apoptosis,[234] whereas a second reported that painful stimulation increased anesthetic-induced neuroapoptosis.[140] Conversely, pain-induced neurodegeneration was ameliorated by coadministration of small doses of analgesics or sedatives.[161,202] It is therefore unclear whether noxious stimuli in the perioperative setting exaggerate the anesthesia-induced toxicity or whether the two deleterious effects cancel each other out.

Studies that measured metabolic and respiratory variables during anesthetic exposure in small rodents reported significant abnormalities not routinely observed during pediatric anesthesia practice, such as extensive hypercarbia, metabolic acidosis, and hypoglycemia.[119,121,262] Tracheal intubation and mechanical ventilation do not necessarily completely obviate all of these abnormalities in rodents.[262] In stark contrast to anesthesia in children, administering clinical doses of anesthetics for periods greater than 4 hours can be lethal for up to 20% of small rodents,[119] even when intermittent painful stimuli are applied.[121] However, the growing evidence from nonhuman primate studies, in which animals were tracheally intubated, ventilated, had vital signs stringently monitored, and lacked mortality during anesthetic exposure, but still demonstrated comparable neuronal injury patterns observed in rodents,[141,181,226] suggests that the short-comings in physiologic conditions in small animal studies does not eliminate their potential biologic relevance to humans. Moreover, rearing conditions after anesthesia have a profound impact on the brain's repair mechanisms after injury. Environmental enrichment and exercise dramatically increase neurogenesis in rodents and therefore may facilitate plasticity and repair after anesthesia, compared with the customary bare cage housing environment of rodents.[327,328] Comparably, children face daily cognitive challenges in their normal "enriched" environment, substantially different from normal laboratory animal housing,[92,127,159,178] which could attenuate the postulated neurocognitive effects of anesthesia in humans. This is highlighted by recent animal studies in which environmental enrichment reversed the deleterious effects of prolonged or repeated anesthetic exposures on subsequent neurologic performance in rats.[234,329] These studies suggest that neurobehavioral outcomes depend on multiple factors, of which anesthesia represents only one of many other events important for the developing brain.

COMPARATIVE BRAIN DEVELOPMENT

A major challenge in translating any animal data to human clinical practice is properly matching brain maturational stages between model species and young children. The ongoing discussion regarding these comparisons is somewhat reminiscent of the cliché of 1 "dog year" being equivalent to 7 "human years." Because earlier animal studies have suggested that anesthesia-induced structural abnormalities may be most pronounced during very defined, early stages of development, such as neuroapoptosis in cortex and thalamus peaking between 3 and 10 days of age in small rodents[19,102] or between gestational day 120 and day 6 of life in rhesus monkeys, it becomes imperative to appropriately identify the equivalent period during human brain development to assess human applicability of the animal data and to adequately design clinical studies.

Brain architecture and development, however, both in magnitude and timing, vary widely among mammalian species. Small rodents, such as mice and rats, have a smooth (or lissencephalic) brain surface, whereas humans and monkeys exhibit the typical fissured, gyrencephalic brain surface of gyri and sulci. Overall brain size and the number of neurons differ by orders of magnitude between humans and animal species; the mature human brain contains approximately 86 billion neurons, compared with the rhesus macaque's 6 billion and the adult mouse brain's 70 million neurons.[330] Other important species differences exist in timing and duration of critical developmental events. Rodents are altricial species, meaning considerable steps of brain development occur postnatally during their first 2 to 3 weeks of life, whereas numerous critical developmental steps take place in utero in monkeys and humans.[314] Given these substantial differences, it is difficult to unequivocally associate specific ages in animals to humans. Older data based on simple species comparisons of brain growth equated the first week of life in small rodents, when the peak of vulnerability to anesthetic neuroapoptosis occurs for most brain regions, to an extended time span in humans from the third gestational trimester all the way to the third year of life.[4,24,315] However, more contemporary approaches using computational models have approximated the 7-day-old rat or mouse to be closer in brain maturity to human fetuses during the third trimester of pregnancy, whereas the immature rhesus monkey 5 to 6 days old seems closer to the postnatal human brain in infancy (Fig. 25.6).[316-318,331] According to these models, stages of brain maturity equivalent to term human neonates are not reached until after postnatal days 10 to 14 in rats or mice (online calculator available at http://www.translatingtime.net, accessed October 2016). In general, the majority of in vivo laboratory studies examine animals during developmental stages equivalent to the very immature human brain (Fig. 25.7). Importantly, in aggregate, animal data do not clearly identify a "safe" age beyond which no deleterious anesthetic effects can be observed.[2]

Interestingly, limited human data seem to suggest that postnatal brain development may be most susceptible to anesthetic or sedative exposure, whereas animal studies, including a recent nonhuman primate study,[141] demonstrate a greater degree of neuroapoptosis after exposures that model the premature human brain. However, substantial differences in brain development still exist between humans and nonhuman primates. In general, development progresses at a much slower pace in humans compared with any other model species, including nonhuman primates, and developmental stages are up to 50% longer. Even on a cellular level, remarkable differences exist between humans and all other animals; cell cycle duration during cortical neurogenesis is approximately 17 hours in mice, 28 hours in macaque monkeys, and 36 hours in humans.[323] All these differences indicate that it is not sensible to directly equate observations of anesthetic effects in the developing animal brain of any species to human clinical

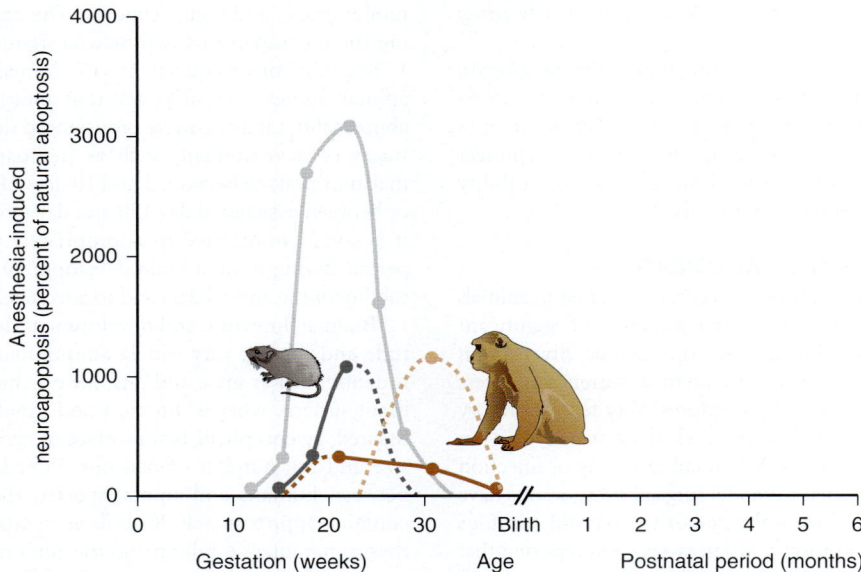

FIGURE 25.6 The degree of neuronal apoptotic cell death following anesthetic exposure is highly dependent on the age of the animal during exposure. Graphs demonstrate the percent increase of apoptotic cell death compared with natural apoptosis following an exposure to an isoflurane/nitrous oxide–based anesthetic in immature rats (*dark grey*) or very young macaque monkeys (*dark brown*) or prolonged exposure to ketamine in immature rats (*light grey*) or macaque monkeys (*tan*). *Solid lines* connect the available data points; *dashed lines* represent extrapolations of the available data. Neurotoxicity data were derived from references 19, 105, 127, and 159. To infer the potential age of anesthetic vulnerability in humans, respective brain maturity in the animal species during exposure was equated to the corresponding state of the developing human brain, and relative human ages for each data point were plotted accordingly, using a mathematical model outlined in references 317, 318, and 331, which is available in the online calculator at http://www.translatingtime.net (accessed May 2016).

anesthesia practice. The potential long-term effects of anesthetics therefore have to be carefully examined in clinical studies before accepting results obtained in animals.

ASSESSING NEUROBEHAVIORAL OR COGNITIVE OUTCOMES

Translating neurodevelopmental outcomes from animals to humans is difficult. Human cognitive performance includes the vast capacity for learning, the ability for abstract thinking, the aptitude for solving complex mathematical equations, and even the capability of inventing and operating complex machinery. Cognition is a complex process that includes such diverse processes as perception, attention, motivation, working memory, long-term memory, executive function, language, and social cognition. These brain functions are all difficult to model in animals.[319] It is therefore imperative to critically evaluate any animal model attempting to replicate human cognitive performance. Moreover, it is important to assess the validity of these models in the context of the critical period for human brain development that they are trying to represent. Current assessment of neurocognitive performance after developmental exposure largely relies on hippocampal-dependent tests administered to adult animals after anesthetic exposure early in life.[100,119–121,178] However, it remains unclear whether these are the same domains that may potentially be targeted in children during anesthesia. Brain regions maximally affected by anesthesia may depend on their state of development and therefore change with the age of the organism during exposure.[92,181] Accordingly, subsequent neurobehavioral abnormalities may vary, depending on the age at which anesthesia was administered.

This discussion, however, does not entirely discredit the results from small animal studies, but rather seriously limits the generalizability of their findings to clinical practice. More closely resembling clinical pediatric anesthesia practice, several large-animal models have used tracheal intubation and mechanical ventilation.[92,127,141,181] However, these large-animal studies have only included minor stimulation, such as skin clamping, but not surgical stimulation during the anesthetic exposure.[92,127,159,178]

Long-Term Outcome in Children Exposed to Anesthesia and Surgery

The difficulties in translating animal data to clinical anesthesia in human infants increase the importance of identifying potential clinical evidence for or against neurologic abnormalities in children after otherwise uneventful anesthesia early in life. Unfortunately, this question is not easily answered.

Examining outcomes reported for surgical cohorts, there is evidence for an association between surgery with anesthesia in early childhood and subsequent altered neurodevelopmental outcome.[39] Some human cohort studies have demonstrated an association between major surgery in the neonatal period and poor neurodevelopmental outcome.[332] Children born with esophageal atresia, for example, had a lower IQ and more frequently suffered from depression, emotional, and behavioral problems compared with the general population.[333] Children with congenital diaphragmatic hernia repair also have a high rate of neurologic sequelae.[334] Extremely premature, low–birth-weight neonates who

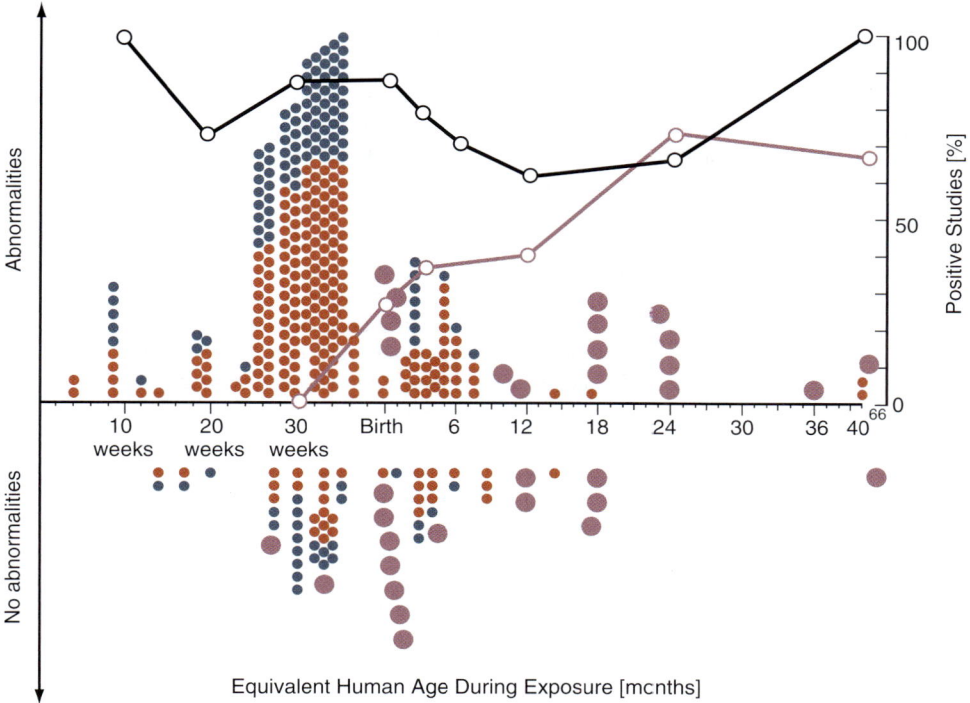

FIGURE 25.7 The majority of in vivo animal studies into the effects of anesthetic exposure on brain structure and function focus on brain developmental stages equivalent to premature neonates. Studies with negative results never outnumber those with positive results at any time point, suggesting that no age can be clearly identified at which anesthetics do not cause abnormalities. Animal studies, inclusive of various anesthetic drugs and doses, reporting abnormal findings (above the horizontal line) or negative findings (below the horizontal line) for brain structural (*solid red circles*) or cognitive outcomes (*solid blue circles*) are depicted as a function of maturational age of the animals' brain relative to the human brain during exposure. *Solid purple circles* represent clinical studies into long-term cognitive outcomes in humans. The animals' age during exposure was converted to the corresponding maturational stage of the human brain by using a computational neurodevelopmental model (www.translatingtime. net, translating "neurogenesis" for "whole brain," accessed 10/6/2016). For the purpose of analysis, reports with separate anesthetic protocols consisting of different anesthetic regimens or multiple exposure times of the same anesthetic were classified as separate studies. For repeated exposures at different ages, the equivalent mean age of the human brain is reported. The graphs express the ratio of studies with positive findings to those with negative finds in animals (*black*) or humans (*purple*); *open circles* represent the respective percentage of positive studies for age epochs ranging from specific data points to next lower data point on the graph. Note that animal studies with positive findings outnumber those studies with negative findings from conception until 40 months' equivalent age in humans, while this ratio does not turn positive for human studies until exposures between 12 and 24 months of age. (From Lin EP, Lee J-R, Lee CS, et al. Do anesthetics harm the developing human brain? An integrative analysis of animal and human studies. *Neurotoxicol Teratol.* 2017;60:117–128.)

underwent laparotomy exhibited poorer neurodevelopmental outcomes compared with matched controls.[335] A cohort of infants who underwent major surgery did not perform as well in school as a matched control group of healthy infants or with infants who had major nonsurgical medical conditions.[336] In a randomized trial of indomethacin treatment in 426 infants less than 1000 g at birth, neurologic impairment was present in significantly more of the 110 children who had undergone surgery (53%) compared with that in the 316 children who had received medical therapy (34%).[337] In a study of extremely preterm infants, the IQ of those who had undergone surgery was lower at 5 years of age and exhibited more sensorineural disability than those who had not undergone surgery.[338]

These studies all included infants with major confounding factors, such as congenital malformations or very preterm birth, which might increase the risk of poor neurodevelopmental outcome independent of surgery and anesthesia. Preoperative brain lesions

and white-matter injury have been observed in a substantial number of neonates suffering from major congenital heart disease.[339-343] Moreover, surgery itself can lead to poor outcome as a result of the perioperative neurohumoral and inflammatory response, or the hemodynamic instability associated with major surgery. Severity of illness may have also been greater in surgical patients compared with their respective control groups. Moreover, selection bias may have resulted in the sicker children being treated with surgery, while less severely ill children received medical therapy. Thus, whereas these studies suggest that some infants undergoing major surgery are at increased risk of poor neurodevelopmental outcome, none of the studies provide conclusive evidence that surgery or even anesthesia is the cause of the increased risk of poor neurodevelopmental outcome.

Several recent cohort studies and one randomized controlled trial have focused primarily on the effects of anesthesia in healthier children undergoing surgical procedures early in life. In an established population–based, retrospective birth cohort, Wilder and colleagues studied the association between anesthetic exposure before 4 years of age and the subsequent development of learning disabilities.[344] Regression was used to calculate hazard ratios (HRs) for anesthetic exposure as a predictor of learning disability, with adjustment for gestational age at birth, sex, and birth weight. Of 5357 children in the cohort, 593 had been exposed to general anesthesia before 4 years of age. Compared with those not exposed to anesthesia, a single exposure was not associated with an increased risk of learning disability (HR 1.0; 95% confidence interval [CI] of 0.79–1.27). However, children who underwent two separate episodes of anesthesia had an increased risk of a learning disability (HR 1.59; 95% CI 1.06–2.37) and those who underwent 3 or more separate anesthetics had an even greater risk (HR 2.60; 95% CI 1.60–4.24). The association between learning disability and multiple episodes of anesthesia remained after adjusting for American Society of Anesthesiologist physical status. The risk for a learning disability also increased according to the cumulative duration of anesthesia. However, this study suffered from several limitations. Because the study reported anesthetics administered between 1976 and 1982, the most common anesthetic treatment was halothane and nitrous oxide, and none of the children were monitored with pulse oximetry or capnography. It is not possible to determine in how many of these children excessive hyperventilation or unrecognized desaturation had occurred. Furthermore, the maternal birth histories were not described (e.g., magnesium may cause neuroapoptosis or be neuroprotective). Three different learning disabilities were considered with equipoise in the final analysis, and these disabilities were not tested in all children, but only when a teacher or parent requested testing. These questions limit the external validity of these data.

To reduce the impact of confounding factors, using the same population-based, retrospective birth cohort, the same group conducted further studies with a matched cohort design.[345] The researchers matched 350 children exposed to anesthesia before the age of 2 to 700 children not exposed to anesthesia. The matching was based on several known risk factors for learning disabilities: gender, mother's education, birth weight, and gestational age at birth. Outcomes of interest were learning disability, need for individualized education program for an emotional or behavioral disorder, and group-administered achievement tests. In the analysis, an adjustment was also performed for burden of illness. The primary finding was that children exposed to two or more occurrences of anesthesia (but not a single occurrence) were at increased risk for having a learning disability (HR 2.12; 95% CI of 1.26–3.54), and an amplified need for individualized education programs for speech and language impairment. However, there was not an increased need for a program for emotional or behavioral disorders. The authors also detected an association between multiple exposures to anesthesia and lower mathematical scores. The same criticisms apply to this study as to the earlier study from this institution.[344]

To investigate a potential association between perinatal exposure to general anesthesia during cesarean delivery and subsequent diagnosis of learning disability,[346] the risk of a learning disability was compared in the 193 children delivered via cesarean section with general anesthesia, the 304 delivered via cesarean section with regional anesthesia, and 4823 delivered vaginally without any anesthesia. The association between mode of delivery and learning disability was adjusted for sex, birth weight, gestational age at birth, exposure to anesthesia before 4 years of age, and maternal education. The risk of disability was similar between children delivered vaginally with no anesthesia and cesarean delivery

with general anesthesia, but risk of disability was less in children delivered via cesarean with regional anesthesia than vaginal delivery with no anesthesia (HR 0.64; 95% CI 0.44–0.92; P = .017). The results implied that brief exposure to general anesthesia during delivery was not associated with subsequent learning disability, but the reason the risk was less with regional anesthesia compared with no anesthesia is unclear, although this may suggest the possibility of substantial confounding influences. To explore the possibility that the regional blockade was protective, the authors subsequently compared those born without general anesthesia by vaginal delivery with and without regional analgesia and found no difference in risk of learning disability.[347] Using the same epidemiologic cohort, the same research group detected an increased prevalence of attention deficit hyperactivity disorder in children who had undergone repeated surgical procedures with anesthesia, compared with none or only one exposure.[348]

A small pilot study (in 314 children) to test the feasibility of using a cohort of children who had urologic surgery to test the association between age at surgery and neurobehavioral outcomes (measured with the Child Behavior Checklist)[349] found no evidence of an association between the timing of surgery and neurobehavioral outcomes.

Another retrospective cohort analysis using the New York State Medicaid records matched 383 children who underwent hernia repair before 3 years of age with 5050 children who did not undergo inguinal hernia repair.[350] After adjustment for sex, age, and complicating birth conditions (such as low birth weight), children who had hernia repair were more than twice as likely to have a subsequent diagnosis of a developmental or behavioral disorder (HR 2.3; 95% CI 1.3–4.1).

To reduce environmental confounding effects, the authors then proceeded to use the data from the New York State Medicaid program to construct a retrospective sibling birth cohort.[351] Once again, they assessed the association between exposure to anesthesia in children younger than 3 years of age and the subsequent risk of diagnosis of developmental or behavioral disorders. A total of 10,450 siblings were identified, 304 of whom underwent surgery before 3 years of age, with no history of behavioral or developmental disorders before the surgery, and 10,146 children who did not undergo surgery. The association of exposure to anesthesia with subsequent developmental or behavioral disorders was assessed with both proportional hazards modeling and pair-matched analysis. As with their previous study, they found evidence for an association between surgery and poor neurodevelopmental outcome. The incidence of developmental or behavioral disorders was 128.2 diagnoses per 1000 person-years for those who had surgery and 56.3 diagnoses per 1000 person-years for those who did not. This association persisted when adjusted for sex, history of birth-related medical complications, and clustering by sibling status; the estimated HR of developmental or behavioral disorders associated with any exposure to anesthesia was 1.6 (95% CI 1.4–1.8). The risk increased from 1.1 (95% CI 0.8–1.4) for one operation to 2.9 (95% CI 2.5–3.1) for two operations and 4.0 (95% CI 3.5–4.5) for three or more operations. The number of siblings available for a matched analysis was relatively small. There were only 138 sibling pairs. In the pair-matched study, there was no evidence of an association between surgery and poor outcome, with a relative risk of 0.9 (95% CI 0.6–1.4); however, the small numbers may limit the power of this analysis.

Even better than sibling studies are investigations involving identical twins, which may further reduce confounding environmental and genetic influences. Performing such a study, Bartels and associates examined the possible association between anesthesia exposure before 3 years of age and school performance in 1143 monozygotic twin pairs.[352] In the identical twins who were discordant for exposure to anesthesia (one twin was exposed to anesthesia and the other was not), their school performance was identical. This would suggest that surgery with anesthesia may not be the cause of poor school performance. Interestingly, the school performance in both the discordant pairs and the pairs where both twins underwent surgery was poorer than that for concordant twin pairs where neither twin was exposed to anesthesia. This finding could imply that there may exist an unknown genetic factor that increases the risk of both the need for surgery and poor school performance.

The Western Canadian Complex Pediatric Therapies Follow-Up Group published a prospective follow-up study of 95 infants at 2 years of age who underwent surgical correction for congenital heart disease at the Alberta Children's Hospital from April 2003 to December 2006.[353] A multiple logistic regression analysis of variables associated with developmental delay found that only more days of ventilatory support postoperatively and older age at surgery were associated with significant developmental delay. There was also no evidence for an association between the sedation variables and significant motor delays. However, the use of two neurocognitive assessment tools during the study period precluded an analysis of the cognitive and motor scores as continuous variables, which may have been a more sensitive way to detect subtle impairment.

Hansen and colleagues used a very large Danish birth cohort to compare academic performance in 2689 children who had inguinal hernia repair in infancy with 14,575 children who were randomly selected as an age-matched sample from the general population.[354] Those who had hernia repair performed worse at school, although after adjusting for likely confounding variables, there was no evidence of any association between surgery and school performance. A similar but smaller study conducted in Iowa[355] in which investigators reviewed school test scores in 287 children who had surgery in infancy determined that scores in surgical infants were slightly less than in the general population. However, 12% had scores in the lowest 5th centile in the general population. In a subset of 58 children with no risk factors for neurodevelopmental issues, test scores were not below the average for the population, although 14% still scored in the lowest 5th percentile. These results suggest that a subset of the population may be particularly vulnerable.

Two similar population-based Canadian cohort studies examined the association between surgery in young children and their Early Development Index (EDI). The EDI is a test of readiness for school. The 103-item questionnaire is completed by teachers when children are 5 years of age. It has five domains: physical health and well-being, social knowledge and competence, emotional health and maturity, language and cognitive development, and communication skills and general knowledge. Both studies assessed the association between surgery and their EDI using data from the entire province of Ontario. The 28,366 children who had surgery before they performed the EDI[356] were compared with 55,910 controls who did not have surgery but were matched for gestational age at birth, mother's age at birth, rurality, gender, and year and quarter of birth, and excluded children with known physical disability health-related causes of impaired development, and those with a diagnosis of behavioral, learning, or developmental disorder. The primary outcome was defined as vulnerable (scoring in the lowest 10th percentile in any domain). They also adjusted for aboriginal

status, age, and household income. Vulnerability was increased slightly in those who had surgery: 7,259/28,366 (25.6%) compared with 13,957/55,910 (25%) controls (odds ratio 1.05; 95% CI 1.01–.08). Interestingly, the odds of vulnerability were increased in those younger than 2 years at the time of surgery (odds ratio 1.05; 95% CI 1.01–1.10), whereas the odds were not increased in those older than 2 years at the time of surgery (odds ratio 1.04; 95% CI 0.98–1.10). They also found no evidence of increased vulnerability in those who had multiple surgeries. In another study, 4470 children who had surgery in Manitoba before the age of 4 were matched with 13,586 controls for gestational age at birth, mother's age at birth, rurality, income quintile, gender, and year of birth.[357] They excluded children with a diagnosis of any developmental disability. In their analysis, the authors adjusted for welfare status, gestational age, small or large for dates, mother's age at birth, child's age and Johns Hopkins Resource Utilization Band. As in the Ontario study, these investigators reported a small difference with children who had surgery performing worse than those who had not had surgery. However, the domains in which they performed poorly were not consistent with the Ontario study. Like the Ontario study, the Johns Hopkins study detected evidence for an association in children who had surgery at age greater than 2 years of age but no evidence for any association if surgery occurred at less than 2 years of age. They also found no evidence of a greater risk in those who had multiple surgeries compared with those who underwent only one surgery. While findings in these two studies may seem inconsistent with nonhuman studies, suggesting a greater risk in younger children, exposures in the older patients could have more severely affected vulnerable neuronal networks used in the later performance of the assessed tasks. Alternatively, the association seen in these cohort studies could be due to factors other than the neurotoxicity observed in animal studies.

The above studies relied on a diagnosis of a learning or behavioral disorder or school grades as an outcome measure. Although important outcomes for daily activities, these measures are not sensitive and may miss more subtle deficits in specific neurodevelopmental domains.[358] Several studies have used more detailed neuropsychological tests.

A number of investigations examined the association between surgery and neurodevelopmental outcome using the Western Australian Pregnancy Cohort (Raine). In one analysis they found an association between language and abstract reasoning deficits in 10-year-old children who were exposed to one or more anesthetics before age 3 years compared with unexposed children. After adjusting for confounders, any anesthetic before age 3 years increased the risk ratio of disability in receptive, expressive, or total language as measured by the Clinical Evaluation of Language Fundamentals (CELF-3) test, as well as abstract reasoning (Raven's Colored Progressive Matrices) to between 1.7 and 2.1 of unexposed controls, whereas other tests of vocabulary, behavior, and motor function were unaffected by exposure.[359]

The same authors performed a subsequent analysis, comparing the diverse outcome measures of neuropsychological testing, International Classification of Diseases, Ninth Revision (ICD-9)-coded diagnoses, and academic performance.[360] Of the 781 children who had all outcome measures, 211 had received an anesthetic before 3 years of age. Compared with the unexposed children, those who had received anesthesia demonstrated an increased risk of deficit in neuropsychological language assessment and an increased risk of an ICD-9-coded diagnosis of language or cognitive disorder. However, they did not demonstrate poorer academic performance. This finding highlights the limitations of using school performance as a measure of neurodevelopmental outcome. In the subset of children who were exposed at older ages (3- to 5-year-olds and 5- to 10-year-olds), there was no association between exposure and any deficit in any neuropsychological test except for children exposed between 3 and 5 years of age who demonstrated worse scores on motor function tests.[360]

Another study used an established cohort of children 5 to 18 years of age that had magnetic resonance imaging (MRI) scans as part of a large language development study.[361] The cohort did not include children with any risk factors for poor neurodevelopmental outcome. Within this cohort, they found 53 children who had undergone surgery before the age of 4 and matched these to 53 peers who had not, matching on age, gender, and socioeconomic status. All children underwent a battery of neuropsychological tests and brain MRI. Exposed children scored lower in listening comprehension and performance IQ. Exposed children did not exhibit comparably decreased grey-matter density in the thalamus or retrosplenial cortex, as previously seen in rodent studies, but instead demonstrated diminished grey-matter volumes in the occipital cortex and cerebellum, associated with lower-performance IQ.

Studies in animals have also identified deficits in recognition memory tasks after general anesthesia. Recognition is based on recollection and familiarity. To test if humans had similar deficits in recollection, investigators studied 28 children aged 6 to 11 years who had undergone anesthesia in infancy compared with 28 age- and gender-matched controls.[362] They found that scores in tests of recollection in exposed children were less than in unexposed children, but scores in tests of IQ, behavior, and familiarity were similar.

Perhaps the most important cohort study is the Pediatric Anesthesia and Neurodevelopment Assessment (PANDA) study.[363] In this bidirectional cohort study, 105 children aged 8 to 15 years who had surgery for inguinal hernia repair before 3 years of age were compared with 105 matched siblings who were of similar age at testing but did not undergo surgery early in life. Children underwent a range of well-validated neuropsychological tests. The choice of tests was based on their psychometric properties and on their relevance to animal data and previous cohort study findings. The primary outcome was full-scale IQ. The median duration of anesthesia exposure was 80 minutes. There was no evidence for a difference in any of the IQ domains. In the exposed cohort, full-scale IQ was 111, performance IQ was 108, and verbal IQ was 111, while in the unexposed siblings full-scale IQ was 111, performance IQ was 107, and verbal IQ was 111. Differences in mean IQ scores between exposed and unexposed siblings for full-scale IQ were 0.2 (95% CI, −2.6 to 2.9); performance IQ, 0.5 (95% CI, −2.7 to 3.7); and verbal IQ, −0.5 (95% CI, −3.2 to 2.2). There was also no evidence of differences in secondary outcomes that included memory and learning, motor and processing speed, visuospatial function, attention, executive function, or language. Exposed children did, however, have poorer scores in some aspects of behavior even when adjusted for gender. Subanalyses that addressed age at the time of exposure and duration of exposure reported no effects of either variable on outcome, although these analyses had limited power. This study is by far the most rigorous cohort study and provides strong evidence that approximately 1 hour of exposure to anesthesia in early childhood is unlikely to cause significant cognitive impairment at a later age.

Cohort studies are inherently limited by the risk of confounding. Adjustments in the analyses can never completely remove the risk that the association is due to a factor apart from anesthesia. Only randomized trials can reliably reduce the risk of confounding. Randomized trials are obviously difficult to perform as it is impossible to randomize to anesthesia versus no anesthesia for children undergoing surgery. It is, however, possible to randomize to two different anesthetic techniques. To date, the General Anaesthesia compared to Spinal anaesthesia trial (GAS) is the only randomized trial that has examined the effect of different anesthetic regimens in infancy on neurodevelopmental outcome.[364] In the GAS study, 722 infants younger than 60 weeks postmenstrual age were randomly assigned to awake-regional (nearly always spinal anesthesia) or sevoflurane general anesthesia for inguinal hernia repair. In this study, the median duration of sevoflurane exposure in the general anesthesia group was 54 minutes. The spinal failure rate was 19% and the loss to follow-up was 14%. The primary outcome was the Wechsler Preschool and Primary Scale of Intelligence, Third Edition (WPPSI-III) full-scale IQ at 5 years of age. These data will be available in 2018. The cognitive score of the Bayley-III scale at 2 years of age was a prespecified secondary outcome and these results have been published.[364] The Bayley-III has five domains: cognitive, language, motor, social emotional, and adaptive behavior. There was strong evidence of equivalence in all domains. In the per-protocol analysis using multiple imputation, the mean difference (awake regional − general) in the cognitive composite score adjusted for gestational age at birth was 0.17 (95% CI −2.30 to 2.64). This was within the predefined equivalence margin of 5 points. The difference in language was 1.15 (95% CI −1.59 to 3.88), motor 0.60 (95% CI −1.77 to 2.97), social emotional 1.0 (95% CI −3.12 to 5.13) and adaptive behavior −0.89 (95% CI −3.52 to 1.73). The results were similar in intent-to-treat and complete case analyses, implying spinal failure and loss to follow-up did not bias the results. However, the trial had three important limitations: first, the relatively brief anesthetic exposure (54 minutes), second, the lack of sensitivity to test higher executive function and memory with the Bayley scale at 2 years of age, and third, only one anesthetic was administered.[365] Accordingly, future studies are need to address these limitations.

Outcome After Exposure to Anesthesia Outside of the Operating Room

The operating room is not the only area where anesthetic neurotoxicity may be relevant. Ketamine and benzodiazepines are frequently administered in the emergency room and in neonatal and pediatric intensive care units. These drugs may be administered for a prolonged period of time, in theory increasing the risks of neurotoxicity.[55,57]

Unfortunately, determining the clinical relevance of any neurotoxicity in intensive care patients is even more difficult than in the operating room. The total number of children who can be examined is smaller, the children tend to be a heterogeneous population, and most importantly, they often have multiple significant confounding comorbidities including exposure to anesthesia, which could significantly affect interpretation of adverse outcomes. To date, there is mixed evidence that exposure to anesthetic or sedative drugs is associated with poorer neurobehavioral outcome in this patient population. A Cochrane review found some evidence for worsened short-term outcome in neonates who had prolonged exposures to midazolam infusions.[366] In contrast, after correction for severity of illness, another study (using the Etude EPIdémiologique sur les Petits Ages GEstationnels [EPIPAGE] cohort) found no evidence of an association between prolonged sedation and adverse neurologic outcomes.[367] In that study, however, many children received opioids for sedation rather than benzodiazepines and the study was not powered to detect performance differences of less than 10%.

Limitations of the Available Clinical Studies

There are numerous reasons the clinical data on neurobehavioral outcomes after anesthesia are difficult to interpret, and it is perhaps not surprising that the earlier clinical studies return conflicting results. Because of their retrospective nature, several of these studies require mathematical adjustments, such as multiple logistic regression analyses for confounding variables. This limits the findings to known or suspected confounders and does not address as yet unknown variables that may be more important to the outcome.

Epidemiologic studies are generally unable to separate the effects of surgery or the need for surgery from the potential anesthetic effects. As previously discussed, surgery may result in significant neurohumoral stress and/or inflammatory responses that may influence neurocognitive outcome in addition to metabolic, hemodynamic, and respiratory events that occur perioperatively. Data collection for several of the epidemiologic studies occurred before continuous pulse-oximetry and capnography monitoring were standard monitors and at a time when inhalational anesthetics with profound adverse cardiovascular effects such as halothane, were used.[344,345] Prospective studies of capnography and pulse oximetry have demonstrated that the very population considered to be at increased risk (those <2 years of age) had the greatest incidence of desaturation events, hypercarbia, and hypocarbia.[368-370]

Children undergoing surgery or diagnostic procedures early in life may suffer more frequently from concomitant chromosomal and genetic abnormalities or comorbidities such as prematurity, which have been linked to abnormal neurobehavioral outcomes. For example, children with cyanotic congenital heart disease often have abnormal neurocognitive development and some have smaller brain volumes before any surgical or anesthesia intervention.[303] The indication for surgery or for a diagnostic procedure requiring anesthesia, such as injury or infection, may artificially increase the incidence of neurodevelopmental abnormalities in the anesthetized cohort.[303] On the other hand, it has been argued that subjects suffering from underlying abnormalities adversely affecting neurodevelopment who do not receive the required surgery may be introduced into the pool of unanesthetized children, and therefore mask potentially toxic effects of anesthesia.[59]

Further complicating the interpretation of retrospective data is the substantial gap in time between exposure and neurologic assessment. The advantage of performing neurologic assessments in school-age children includes the increased precision and greater predictive value of such assessments compared with neurobehavioral testing performed for children younger than 2 years of age, for both prospective and retrospective studies.[371] However, especially in retrospective studies that cannot adequately control for confounders, the protracted time interval between surgery and the neurocognitive assessment may introduce even more "noise" into the study by increasing the time for negative influence of other environmental confounders of brain development or, conversely, the positive effects of repair mechanisms and plasticity to affect neurologic outcome.

Current animal studies do not provide sufficient guidance on the most vulnerable brain regions, the individual neurocognitive domains that may be affected, or the particular age at which the human brain may potentially be most susceptible to the neurotoxic effects of anesthetic exposure.

No consensus exists, even in the animal literature, concerning the duration of anesthesia exposure required to induce long-lasting injury. Although the anesthetic exposure may represent a much larger fraction of an animal's life than a human's, at the cellular level apoptosis is likely triggered by a more similar duration of exposure. However, both cell cycle duration and the developmental period of the brain are considerably greater in humans than in rodents. It is therefore plausible, if an anesthesia-induced increase in apoptosis does occur in humans during a prolonged anesthetic exposure, that it may be functionally less important than the same increase in apoptosis over the same period of time in a rodent. Similarly, the plasticity and capacity for recovery may differ between species. On the one hand, it can be argued that the period of development in humans is greater than it is in animals, and hence there may be more time for recovery, but on the other hand, this may extend the potentially vulnerable period in humans into adolescence. Moreover, human development and subsequent cognitive performance are far more complex than in animal species and humans may therefore be more vulnerable, even following less severe neurodegeneration than that observed in laboratory studies. Injuries during critical periods of development may have an exaggerated effect compared with the same injury outside of these periods.[314,372] Accordingly, studies that find no evidence of association with shorter exposures may not be generalizable to all applications of anesthesia.

As children grow they develop additional skills and abilities, and wider arrays of psychometric tests can be applied to evaluate these more extensive neurobehavioral domains. However, we currently lack adequate information on which specific domains to examine in humans following anesthetic exposure, complicating the interpretation of human cohort studies. Many of these studies use summary scores, such as IQ or average school grades. These outcome measures may miss subtle effects confined to specific neurobehavioral domains. Similarly, a diagnosis of developmental delay or behavioral problems may also miss more subtle changes in particular areas. In contrast, broad batteries of detailed tests are increasingly likely to find at least one association purely by chance.

The vulnerable period in humans, if it exists, has not been clearly identified. Animal data seem to suggest that anesthetic exposure may be most relevant during pregnancy or in early infancy, but it could be possible that the period of vulnerability may extend beyond infancy and young age for some brain regions with ongoing neurogenesis. These critical uncertainties not only complicate the interpretation of published studies, but they also make the design of future prospective studies very difficult.

Lastly, the possible neuroprotective effects of anesthesia complicate this conundrum even further. Infants undergoing surgery who experience major intraoperative adverse events, such as cardiopulmonary arrest, are generally expected to suffer from abnormal neurologic outcomes, irrespective of their anesthetic exposure. Neurologic abnormalities observed after an otherwise uneventful procedure are considered neurotoxic effects of anesthesia. However, because anesthetics may also, at least partially, protect from the harmful metabolic, immunologic, and humoral responses to surgery and pain,[286] an alternative explanation may be that inadequate levels of anesthesia, insufficient postoperative pain relief, or unabated inflammation may be the culprit for the neurodevelopmental abnormalities observed in epidemiologic studies. It is also possible that anesthetics may protect in major adverse settings but may be deleterious in the absence of toxic stimuli, causing injury during minor procedures but ameliorating injury during major surgery, such as complex heart surgery involving cardiopulmonary bypass.

In summary, for exposures of less than 1 hour in otherwise healthy infants, there is increasing evidence that there is no association between anesthetic exposure and poor neurobehavioral outcome in human studies. This is consistent with animal studies not detecting brain structural abnormalities or functional deficits after exposures of 1 hour or less. It is pertinent, however, to note that more prolonged exposures (up to several hours) more consistently lead to deficits in preclinical studies. Since there are no data in humans reporting the neurobehavioral effects of several hours of exposure to anesthesia, this should be addressed in future studies. However, collection of more definitive data supporting a deleterious role for anesthetics during brain development will continue to be complicated by uncertainties regarding the toxic threshold dose for anesthetics, the lack of information about the age of maximum susceptibility, and ambiguity related to the most appropriate neurobehavioral domains to examine. On the other hand, the positive associations between anesthetic exposure and learning abnormalities seen in cohort studies may be spurious because of sampling bias in selecting children in need of early-life surgery and the inability to separate anesthetic effects from those of surgery and related comorbidities.

Future Research

Further animal data will continue to provide information on the mechanisms of and susceptibility to anesthetic neurotoxicity. Understanding the mechanisms will be critical in translating the animal findings to clinical settings. Moreover, future animal work may also assist in determining which domains of neurobehavioral outcome are most likely to be affected, and this would assist in the design of human clinical trials. If neurotoxicity is found to be clinically relevant, animal data will also guide in devising prevention strategies.

Further human clinical studies must also be performed. Cohort studies will better identify children most at risk and characterize the neurobehavioral changes that occur.[373] Future cohort studies should focus on those with multiple or prolonged exposures. Because of the multiple confounding factors, cohort studies will always have great difficulty determining if the outcomes are a result of the surgery, the comorbidities, or the anesthetic exposure. Finding evidence for a lack of neurologic abnormalities in certain populations would provide some reassurance that laboratory studies in animal models lack immediate clinical relevance; however, it is important to note that such findings may not be automatically generalizable to all clinical settings.

To definitively answer this important health concern, clinical trials provide the strongest evidence. However, such trials are difficult to perform, as randomization to anesthesia or no anesthesia is impossible. It is, however, feasible to randomize to different types of anesthetic agents or approaches, such as regional versus general anesthesia. Finding a "nontoxic" anesthetic for longer procedures will be challenging. High-dose opioid with or without α_2-agonists might be a feasible nontoxic anesthetic for a trial. An international collaboration, the Trial of an alternative technique of Remifentanil and dEXmedetomidine (T-REX) study, is designed to investigate an alternative anesthetic for infants consisting of dexmedetomidine, remifentanil, and caudal anesthesia with either ropivacaine or bupivacaine for lower abdominal/extremity surgery (https://clinicaltrials.gov/ct2/show/NCT02353182). The study is

now completed with 60 patients enrolled. Data at the time of this writing are being analyzed for feasibility and safety.

Even if anesthesia-induced neuroapoptosis is found to be clinically irrelevant, it is still important to recognize that there is a strong association between major surgery in neonates and abnormal neurobehavioral outcomes. Thus the questions become which other factors may be causing the poor outcome and which perioperative interventions could be performed by anesthesiologists to improve outcomes in these children.

Recommendations for Clinical Practice

The currently available laboratory data are not sufficient to make definitive recommendations for clinical pediatric anesthesia practice. As outlined previously, numerous laboratory studies have unequivocally documented deleterious effects of anesthetic exposure on the developing animal brain, including in nonhuman primates undergoing anesthetic management closely simulating clinical practice. Although these results should not be easily dismissed, the problems in translation from animal to human are substantial. Epidemiologic studies in children are contradictory; however, there is increasing evidence suggesting that a single, short exposure does not cause significant neurodevelopmental problems. However, as mentioned earlier, essentially no data exist about the neurobehavioral effects of prolonged exposure and the evidence pertaining to multiple exposures remains mixed and of poor quality.

SmartTots, a collaboration between the U.S. Food and Drug Administration (FDA) and the International Anesthesia Research Society (IARS) has produced a consensus statement endorsed by many pediatric anesthesia societies. (http://smarttots.org/about/consensus-statement/). The statement indicates that

The effect of exposure to anesthetic drugs in young children is unknown; however, some but not all studies have suggested that problems similar to those seen in animals could also occur in infants and toddlers. It is important to recognize that the studies in children suggest that similar deficits may occur. These studies in children have limitations that prevent experts from understanding whether the harmful effects were due to the anesthetic drugs or to other factors such as the surgery or related illness.... Because there is not enough information about the effects of anesthetic drugs on the brains of young children, it is not yet possible to know whether use of these medicines poses a risk, and if so, whether the risk is large enough to outweigh the benefit of the planned surgery, procedure, or test.

The statement goes on to advise health care providers to consider that

Clearly, anesthetic drugs are a necessary part of the care of children needing any surgery, procedure, or test that cannot be delayed. Decisions regarding the timing of a procedure requiring anesthesia should be discussed with all members of the care team as well as the family or caregiver before proceeding. The benefits of an elective procedure should always be weighed against all of the risks associated with anesthesia and surgery.

Parents are advised to

Discuss the timing of planned procedures with your child's primary care physician, surgeon/proceduralist and anesthesiologist. Concerns regarding the unknown risk of anesthetic exposure to your child's brain development must be weighed against the potential harm associated with cancelling or delaying a needed procedure.

Pediatric surgery is rarely entirely elective, and in neonates may be required to preserve life, such as for critical congenital heart disease, necrotizing enterocolitis, or congenital diaphragmatic hernia. Accordingly, calls to postpone infant surgery are not easy to accommodate. Delaying surgery is also problematic, as no vulnerable or safe period has been clearly identified in animal studies to guide this practice. It might be reasonable to delay purely elective surgeries; however, these represent only a very small fraction of surgeries performed in children.

It is well documented that neonates are at an increased risk for respiratory and cardiovascular complications during anesthesia, which influences the choice of anesthetic technique and drugs used in this population. It would be very unwise to change practice based on concerns over anesthetic neurotoxicity, while potentially increasing the risks of cardiovascular or respiratory complications. Similarly, it must be stressed that insufficient anesthesia and analgesia are definitely associated with poor neurologic outcomes.

Lastly, when discussing the risks and benefits of anesthesia with parents, pediatricians, and surgeons, anesthesiologists need to be cautious not to cause undue alarm, while taking the matter of potential toxicity seriously and not hastily dismissing parental concerns.

ANNOTATED REFERENCES

Davidson AJ, Disma N, de Graaff JC, et al. Neurodevelopmental outcome at 2 years of age after general anaesthesia and awake-regional anaesthesia in infancy (GAS): an international multicentre, randomised controlled trial. *Lancet.* 2016;387:239-250.

The first human randomized trial to examine neurotoxicity comparing infants having awake regional or sevoflurane anesthesia; the authors found no evidence of a difference in neurodevelopmental outcome measured at 2 years of age.

Deng M, Hofacer RD, Jiang C, et al. Brain regional vulnerability to anaesthesia-induced neuronal cell death shifts with age during exposure and extends into adulthood for some regions. *Br J Anaesth.* 2014;113(3):443-451.

This animal study demonstrates that anesthesia-induced neuronal cell death varies by brain region, dependent on the age during exposure, and extends into adulthood in brain regions with ongoing neurogenesis.

Hofacer RD, Deng M, Ward CG, et al. Cell age-specific vulnerability of neurons to anesthetic toxicity. *Ann Neurol.* 2013;73(6):695-704.

This animal study supports the hypothesis that anesthesia-induced neurodegeneration is dependent on the age of the neuron, rather than the age of the animal,

by demonstrating that 2-week-old neurons were most vulnerable to apoptosis during anesthetic exposure.

Ikonomidou C, Bosch F, Miksa M, et al. Blockade of NMDA receptors and apoptotic neurodegeneration in the developing brain. *Science.* 1999;283:70-74.

This paper represents the first study to examine the effects of anesthetic exposure early in life on brain structure, demonstrating widespread neuronal degeneration following repeated administration of ketamine in newborn rats.

Istaphanous GK, Howard J, Nan X, et al. Comparison of the neuro-apoptotic properties of equipotent anesthetic concentrations of desflurane, isoflurane, or sevoflurane in neonatal mice. *Anesthesiology.* 2011;114:578-587.

This is the first study in animals to compare the neurodegenerative properties of equipotent doses of the three contemporary inhaled anesthetics with each other, finding no advantage of using one agent over another in regards to the degree of apoptotic neuronal cell death caused during exposure.

Jevtovic-Todorovic V, Hartman RE, Izumi Y, et al. Early exposure to common anesthetic agents causes widespread neurodegeneration in the developing rat brain and persistent learning deficits. *J Neurosci.* 2003;23:876-882.

This is a seminal study into the brain structural and long-term functional effects of a combined exposure to isoflurane, nitrous oxide, and midazolam in newborn rats, showing both increased neuroapoptosis immediately following exposure and long-term learning impairment.

Paule MG, Li M, Allen RR, et al. Ketamine anesthesia during the first week of life can cause long-lasting cognitive deficits in rhesus monkeys. *Neurotoxicol Teratol.* 2011;33:220-230.

This is the first study in nonhuman primates to link a prolonged exposure to ketamine very early in life to long-term neurobehavioral abnormalities.

Sun LS, Li G, Miller TL, et al. Association between a single general anesthesia exposure before age 36 months and neurocognitive outcomes in later childhood. *JAMA.* 2016;315:2312-2320.

This is the most definitive cohort study that compared children aged 5 to 8 years who had hernia repair before the age of 3 years with their siblings and found no evidence of a difference across a battery of neuropsychologic tests.

Wilder RT, Flick RP, Sprung J, et al. Early exposure to anesthesia and learning disabilities in a population-based birth cohort. *Anesthesiology.* 2009;110:796-804.

The authors provide one of the earliest epidemiologic studies to suggest an association between repeated exposure to surgery with anesthesia early in life to long-term neurobehavioral abnormalities in children.

A complete reference list can be found online at ExpertConsult.com.

26

Pediatric Neurosurgical Anesthesia

CRAIG D. MCCLAIN AND SULPICIO G. SORIANO

CHILDREN WHO REQUIRE NEUROSURGICAL PROCEDURES present unique challenges to pediatric anesthesiologists. In addition to addressing problems common to general pediatric anesthesia practice, anesthesiologists must consider the effects of anesthesia on the developing central nervous system (CNS) of children with neurologic disease. This chapter reviews the age-dependent physiology of the CNS of children undergoing neurosurgical procedures requiring anesthesia and addresses some of the unique situations that anesthesiologists must face when anesthetizing children for neurosurgical procedures.

Pathophysiology

INTRACRANIAL COMPARTMENTS

The skull can be compared to a rigid container with almost incompressible contents. Under normal conditions, the intracranial space is occupied by the brain and its interstitial fluid (80%), cerebrospinal fluid (CSF, 10%), and blood (10%). In pathologic states, space-occupying lesions such as edema, tumors, hematomas, or abscesses alter these proportions. The Monro-Kellie hypothesis, elaborated in the 19th century, states that the sum of all intracranial volumes is constant. An increase in the volume of one compartment must be accompanied by an approximately equal decrease in the volume of the other compartments, except when the cranium can expand to accommodate a larger volume. Gradual increases in intracranial volumes, such as a slow-growing tumor or hydrocephalus, can be compensated by the compliant nature of open fontanelles and sutures in young children; increasing head circumference can result.[1] However, herniation can occur even in children with open fontanelles if large increases in intracranial pressure (ICP) develop acutely. In the nonacute situation, the brain can compensate for pathologic increases in intracranial

volume by intracellular dehydration and reduction of interstitial fluid.[2–4]

Under normal conditions, CSF exists in dynamic equilibrium, with absorption balancing production. The rate of CSF production in adults is approximately 0.35 mL/minute or 500 mL/day.[5] The average adult has 100 to 150 mL of CSF distributed throughout the brain and subarachnoid space. Children have correspondingly smaller volumes of CSF, but the rate of CSF production is similar to that of adults.[5,6]

Production of CSF is only slightly affected by alterations of ICP and is usually unchanged in children with hydrocephalus.[6] Some drugs, including acetazolamide, furosemide, and corticosteroids, are mildly effective in transiently decreasing CSF production.[1,7,8] There is an inverse relationship between the rate of CSF production and serum osmolality; an increase in serum osmolality causes a decrease in CSF production. Choroid plexus papillomas causing overproduction of CSF are rare but are more likely to occur during childhood.

Absorption of CSF is not well understood, but the arachnoid villi appear to be important sites for reabsorption of CSF into the venous system. One-way valves between the subarachnoid space and the sagittal sinus appear to open at a gradient of about 5 mm Hg. Some resorption may occur from the spinal subarachnoid space and from the ependymal lining of the ventricles. Resorption increases with an increase in ICP. However, CSF absorption is decreased by pathologic processes that obstruct arachnoid villi or interfere with CSF flow, such as intracranial hemorrhage, infection, tumor, and congenital malformations.[9,10]

INTRACRANIAL PRESSURE

Increased ICP causes secondary brain injury by producing cerebral ischemia and ultimately causing herniation. Ischemia occurs when

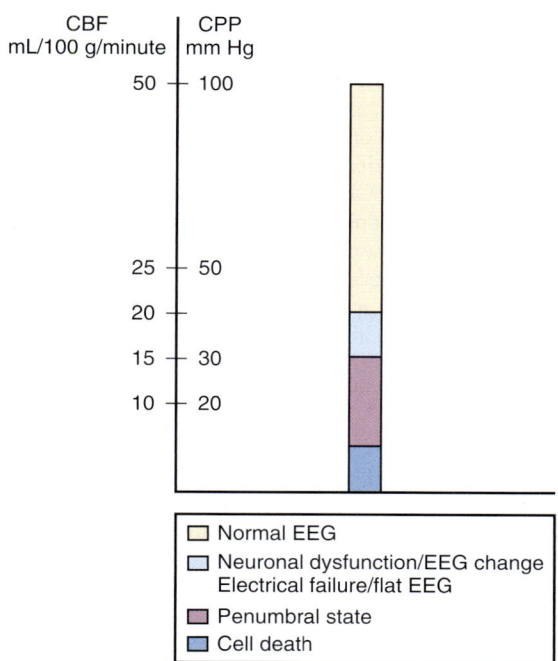

FIGURE 26.1 Cerebral blood flow (*CBF*), cerebral perfusion pressure (*CPP*), and brain ischemia. Changes in CBF and CPP affect neuronal synaptic function and cellular integrity. When CBF decreases to 15 to 20 mL/100 g per minute, there is distinct neuronal dysfunction on the electroencephalogram (*EEG*). At 15 mL/100 g per minute, the EEG is essentially flat, and electrical activity ceases to function. At 6 to 15 mL/100 g per minute, a penumbral state occurs in which there is energy for cellular integrity but insufficient energy for synaptic function. Neuronal survival is unlikely if this low CBF is allowed to persist for more than an ill-defined but critical period. At less than 6 mL/100 g per minute, there is no energy for cellular membrane integrity. Infarction occurs at this stage unless reperfusion is accomplished immediately.

ICP increases and cerebral perfusion pressure (CPP) decreases. As cerebral blood flow (CBF) and the supply of nutrients are curtailed, cell damage and death occur, leading to increased intracellular and extracellular water and further increases in ICP. When ICP increases, CPP decreases, the brain becomes ischemic, and cell death can ensue (Fig. 26.1).[11]

Herniation Syndromes

Several herniation syndromes exist. The most common is *transtentorial* herniation, in which the uncus of the temporal lobe is displaced from the supratentorial to the infratentorial space. Compression of the third cranial nerve and brainstem results in pathognomonic signs of pupillary dilatation, hemiparesis, and loss of consciousness. If this compression is not promptly relieved, apnea, bradycardia, and death occur.

In *cerebellar* herniation, the cerebellar tonsils herniate through the foramen magnum from the posterior fossa to the cervical spinal space. This can lead to obstruction of CSF circulation and ultimately to hydrocephalus. Compression of the brainstem results in cardiorespiratory failure and death.

Signs of Increased Intracranial Pressure

The clinical signs of increased ICP vary in children. Papilledema, pupillary dilation, hypertension, and bradycardia may be absent despite intracranial hypertension, or these signs may occur with normal ICP.[9,12] When associated with increased ICP, they are usually late and dangerous signs.[13] Chronic increases in ICP are often manifested by complaints of headache, irritability, and vomiting, particularly in the morning. Papilledema may not be present even in children dying as a result of intracranial hypertension.[14] A diminished level of consciousness and abnormal motor responses to painful stimuli are frequently associated with an increased ICP.[9] Computed tomography (CT) or magnetic resonance imaging (MRI) can reveal small or obliterated ventricles or basilar cisterns, hydrocephalus, intracranial masses, and midline shifts. Diffuse cerebral edema is a common finding when increased ICP is associated with closed-head injury, encephalopathy, or encephalitis.

Monitoring Intracranial Pressure

Techniques to monitor ICP in adults have been successfully used in children.[15–17] Noninvasive techniques seem to be less accurate than invasive methods.[18] Ventricular catheters are generally accepted as the most accurate and reliable means of measurement, permitting removal of CSF for diagnostic or therapeutic indications. The major risks of intraventricular catheters are infection and hemorrhage; although rare, they can lead to devastating complications. These catheters may be difficult to insert precisely when they are needed most, as in a child with severe cerebral edema and small ventricles. Compared with intraventricular catheters, subarachnoid bolts can be placed even when the ventricles are obliterated. This procedure minimizes trauma to brain tissue and poses less risk of serious infection and hemorrhage. The major disadvantages are that subarachnoid bolts may underestimate ICP, particularly in areas distant from their insertion site, and they are difficult to stabilize in infants with thin calvarias.

Epidural monitors that do not require a fluid interface can be implanted outside the dura, avoiding the risks of CSF contamination and the limitations of fluid-dependent systems.[19,20] Most epidural systems correlate well with intraventricular measurements, but they cannot be recalibrated after insertion. Epidural monitors have also been secured noninvasively to the open anterior fontanelle of infants and appear to reflect changes in ICP. Fiber optic catheters with self-contained transducers can also be used to measure ICP from intraventricular, subarachnoid, or intraparenchymal sites. These monitors avoid some of the problems of external fluid-filled transducers, but like epidural transducers, they cannot be recalibrated after insertion.

The normal ICP in children is less than 15 mm Hg. In term neonates, normal ICP is 2 to 6 mm Hg; it is probably even less in preterm infants. Children with intracranial pathology but normal ICP values occasionally exhibit pressure waves, which are considered abnormal.[9] In children with open fontanelles, the ICP may remain normal despite a significant intracranial pathologic process; increasing head circumference may be the first clinical sign. Bulging fontanelles may not develop, especially when the process evolves slowly.

Intracranial Compliance

The absolute value of ICP does not indicate how much compensation is possible. If the ICP increases significantly, compensatory mechanisms have failed. However, pathologic states may be present despite an ICP within the normal range. Intracranial compliance (i.e., the change in pressure relative to a change in volume) is a valuable concept. Fig. 26.2 is a schematic diagram of the relationship between the addition of volume to intracranial compartments and ICP. The shape of the curve depends on the time over which the volume increases and the relative size of the compartments. At normal intracranial volumes (point 1 in the figure), ICP is low,

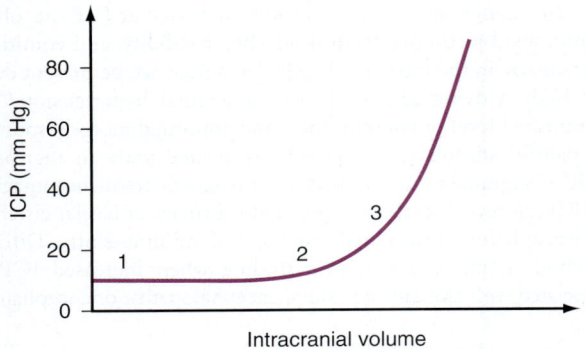

FIGURE 26.2 Idealized intracranial compliance curve for intracranial pressure (*ICP*) plotted against intracranial volume.

but compliance is high and remains so despite small increases in volume. If volume increases rapidly, compensatory abilities are surpassed, and further increases in volume are reflected as increases in pressure. This can occur when the ICP is still within normal limits but the compliance is low (point 2). If the ICP is already increased, further volume expansion causes a rapid increase in ICP (point 3). In clinical practice, compliance can be evaluated with a ventriculostomy catheter or by observing the response of ICP to external stimulation (e.g., tracheal suction, coughing, agitation).

Several physiologic and mechanical factors such as a greater percentage of brain water content, less CSF volume, and a greater percentage of brain content to intracranial capacity contribute to a relatively decreased intracranial compliance in children compared with adults.[2] Children may be at increased risk for herniation compared with adults when similar relative increases in ICP have occurred. However, infants faced with a slowly increasing ICP may have a greater compliance because of their open fontanelles and sutures.

CEREBRAL BLOOD VOLUME AND CEREBRAL BLOOD FLOW

In addition to CSF, cerebral blood volume (CBV) represents another compartment in which compensatory mechanisms influence ICP. Although the CBV occupies only 10% of the intracranial space, changes related to dynamic blood volume occur, often initiated by anesthesia or intensive care procedures. As with other vascular beds, most intracranial blood is contained in the low-pressure, high-capacitance venous system. Increases in intracranial volume are initially met by decreases in CBV. This response is apparent in hydrocephalic infants, in whom venous blood shifts from intracranial to extracranial vessels, producing distended scalp veins.[21]

In the normal adult, CBF is approximately 55 mL/100 g of brain tissue per minute.[22–24] This represents almost 15% of the cardiac output for an organ that accounts for only 2% of body weight. Estimates of CBF are less uniform for children. Normal CBF in healthy awake children is approximately 100 mL/100 g of brain tissue per minute, which represents up to 25% of cardiac output.[25,26] CBF in neonates and preterm infants (approximately 40 mL/100 g of brain tissue per minute) is less than in children and adults.[27,28] In infants, CBF is subject to modification by sleep states and feeding.[29]

Understanding CBF in neonates, infants, and other children is fundamental to being able to safely care for these most vulnerable patients during procedures requiring sedation and general anesthesia. Recent work has focused on delineating the factors that contribute to adequate CBF in children undergoing general anesthesia. Classically, teaching has focused on a variety of factors that underlie maintenance and autoregulation of CBF–mean arterial pressure (MAP), Pa_{CO_2}, and so on. While these concepts remain critical underpinnings of neurophysiology, it is also incumbent upon anesthesia providers to have a broader understanding and approach to the idea of CBF. Regulation of CBF is best understood as the nexus of different physiologic systems. These systems include the respiratory, cardiovascular autonomic, nervous, and endocrine systems, metabolic processes, and the intracranial environment itself.[30] In light of this approach, CBF is regulated by integrative processes that involve respiratory gas exchange, hemodynamic parameters and their consequent effects on cerebrovascular resistance. In adults, the cerebral metabolic rate for oxygen consumption ($CMRO_2$) is 3.5 to 4.5 mL O_2/100 g per minute; in children, it is greater.[25] General anesthesia reduces $CMRO_2$ by as much as 50%.[31] Coupling of CBF and $CMRO_2$ is probably mediated by the effect of the local hydrogen ion concentration on cerebral vessels. Conditions that cause acidosis (e.g., hypoxemia, hypercarbia, ischemia) dilate the cerebral vasculature, which augments CBF and CBV. A reduction in brain metabolism (i.e., $CMRO_2$) similarly reduces CBF and CBV. When autoregulation is impaired, CBF is determined by factors other than metabolic demand. If the CBF exceeds metabolic requirements, luxury perfusion or hyperemia exists. Many pharmacologic agents act directly on the cerebral vasculature to alter CBF and CBV.

CEREBRAL PERFUSION PRESSURE

CPP is a useful and practical estimate of the adequacy of the cerebral circulation, because CBF is neither easily nor widely measured. Defined as the pressure gradient across the brain, CPP is the difference between the systemic MAP at the entrance to the brain and the mean exit pressure (i.e., central venous pressure [CVP]). When ICP exceeds CVP, it replaces CVP in the calculation of CPP. In supine children, the mean CPP is the difference between the MAP and the mean ICP (CPP = MAP – ICP). If the brain and heart are positioned at different heights, all pressures should be referenced at the level of the head (e.g., external auditory meatus).

Alterations in cerebral perfusion under general anesthesia make anesthetizing neonates and infants a particularly challenging endeavor. Neonates already have an increased perioperative morbidity and mortality. Recent concerns for the risks of adverse neurocognitive outcomes from exposure to common anesthetic drugs have evolved into greater efforts in optimizing the physiologic management of neonates undergoing general anesthesia (see Chapter 25). It comes as no great surprise that part of this renewed effort to improve the care of neonates has focused on understanding the role of an adequate cerebral perfusion. Problems include difficulties with accurate blood pressure measurement, knowledge of appropriate hemodynamic goals, maintaining said normal hemodynamic ranges and hemodynamic goals while avoiding hypocapnia.[32,33]

CEREBROVASCULAR AUTOREGULATION
Effects of Blood Pressure

Classical teaching has maintained that, in adults, CBF remains relatively constant within an MAP range of 50 to 150 mm Hg (Fig. 26.3). There is growing evidence that this concept that blood flow is constant over this MAP range is not necessarily correct. Interpretation of a constant flow is the result of limitations to this research that include methods of measuring and the assumptions made by such methods (e.g., transcranial Doppler [TCD]

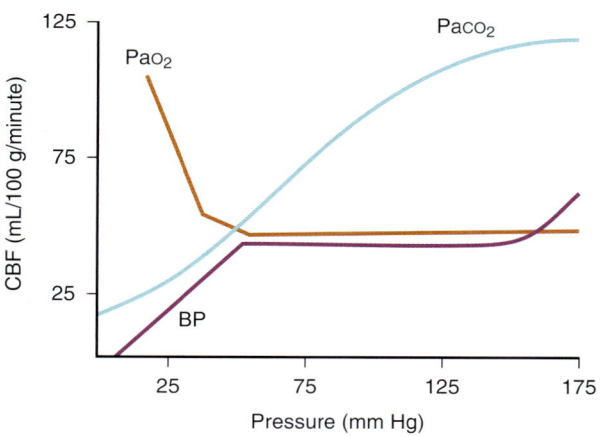

FIGURE 26.3 The effects of increasing mean blood pressure (*BP*), arterial partial pressure of oxygen (*PaO₂*), and arterial partial pressure of carbon dioxide (*PaCO₂*) on cerebral blood flow (*CBF*) in the normal brain. (From Shapiro HM. Intracranial hypertension: therapeutic and anesthetic considerations. *Anesthesiology* 1975;43:447.)

and the assumption that the diameter of the measured vessel remains constant), the manipulation of CBF pharmacologically (the influence on cerebrovascular tone is not well understood and controversial), and the confounding effect of the arterial partial pressure of carbon dioxide (PaCO₂) alterations during pharmacologic manipulations of blood pressure.[30] Despite these limited data, as clinicians we still depend on published evidence to optimize the care of our patients under anesthesia. It is useful to understand these new concepts but try to not simply disregard older, probably too basic, ideas of maintenance of CBF in our patients under anesthesia.

We can view autoregulation as a mechanism that enables brain perfusion to remain relatively stable despite changes in MAP or ICP. There is recent evidence that this relationship between MAP and CBF is likely more pressure passive than originally thought. In fact, it seems as if stricter autoregulation occurs at greater values of MAP than smaller values.[34] Autoregulation is mediated by autonomic and myogenic control of vascular resistance, although there remains considerable debate regarding the exact mechanism and exact location of this modulation. When CPP decreases, cerebral vessels dilate to maintain CBF, thereby increasing CBV. When CPP increases, cerebral vasoconstriction occurs, maintaining the CBF with a reduced CBV. When ICP and CVP are low, MAP normally approximates CPP. Beyond the range of autoregulation, CBF becomes more pressure-dependent. In children with chronic hypertension, the upper and lower limits of autoregulation are increased. Cerebral autoregulation can be abolished by acidosis, medications, tumor, cerebral edema, and vascular malformations, even at sites far removed from a discrete lesion.[22]

The limits of autoregulation for normal infants and children are unknown, but autoregulation probably occurs at lower absolute values than in adults.[35] Although the lower limit of autoregulation in adults is approximately 50 mm Hg MAP, this blood pressure may be beyond that of the neonate. Intact autoregulatory mechanisms have been demonstrated within lower blood pressure ranges in newborn animals compared with mature animals.[36] Children younger than 6 months during sevoflurane anesthesia had a decrease in CBF velocity that was not present until the MAP was 38 mm Hg.[37] That study has not been repeated, so results should

perhaps be taken with a degree of skepticism. Cerebral autoregulation may even be abolished in critically ill humans.[38]

Effects of Oxygen

CBF is constant over a wide range of oxygen tensions. When the partial pressure of arterial O₂ (PaO₂) decreases to less than 50 mm Hg, CBF increases exponentially in adults; for example, at a PaO₂ of 15 mm Hg, CBF is doubled compared with normal (see Fig. 26.3).[39] The resulting increase in CBV increases ICP when intracranial compliance is low; the lower limit for PaO₂ is probably less in neonates. Oxygen delivery is more important than the actual PaO₂. Evidence suggests that hyperoxia decreases CBF. Kety and Schmidt[40] demonstrated a 10% decrease in CBF in adults breathing 100% O₂, although decreases of 33% have been reported in neonates.[41] However, a decrease in MAP with sevoflurane anesthesia has also been reported to increase regional brain oxygenation as measured by near-infrared spectroscopy (NIRS).[42] This lends further credence to the idea that various physiologic systems have complex interactions that lead to modulation of CBF.

Effects of Carbon Dioxide

The relationship between the arterial partial pressure of carbon dioxide (PaCO₂) and CBF typically is linear (see Fig. 26.3). In adults, a 1-mm Hg increase in PaCO₂ increases CBF by approximately 2 mL/100 g per minute.[40] The direct effect of changes in PaCO₂ on CBF and the consequent effect on CBV are the basis for the fact that hyperventilation reduces ICP. Likewise, increases in PaCO₂ increase the CBF, although the limits at which this occurs in neonates differ from those in adults. In lambs and monkeys, CBF does not seem to change in response to decreased PaCO₂.[43] There are no data to suggest the lower limits of PaCO₂ effect on CBF in human infants and children. Similarly, there is little information about the extent and duration of cerebrovascular responsiveness to hyperventilation in brain-injured and critically ill children. Moderate hyperventilation has been used to rapidly reduce ICP, but several reports have demonstrated worsening cerebral ischemia in children with compromised cerebral perfusion.[44-46]

Autoregulation of CBF is impaired in regions of damaged brain.[47] Blood vessels in an ischemic zone are subject to hypoxemia, hypercarbia, and acidosis, which are potent stimuli for vasodilation. These vessels develop maximally reduced cerebrovascular tone or vasomotor paralysis. Small, localized lesions may impair autoregulation in areas far removed from the site of injury.[22] The extent of autoregulatory impairment varies in children with brain damage.

Management of Anesthesia

PREOPERATIVE EVALUATION
History

Preoperative evaluation of infants and children is discussed in Chapter 4. Children who are scheduled for neurosurgery might have been healthy until the onset of their symptoms, might have been developmentally delayed from birth, or may have impaired neuromuscular function. The anesthetic plan, including postoperative care, needs to consider the particular issues of each child and the disease state.

A history of food or drug allergies, eczema, or asthma may provide warning of an adverse reaction to contrast agents frequently used in neuroradiologic procedures. Special attention should be given to symptoms of allergy to latex products, such as lip swelling after blowing up a toy balloon or tongue swelling after insertion of a rubber dam into the mouth by a dentist, because latex anaphylaxis has been reported in some children who have undergone multiple operations, especially those with a meningomyelocele.[48] Children with latex allergy may also report allergies to fruits (e.g., kiwi, banana, avocado, strawberry, and others).[49]

Concurrent pediatric diseases and symptoms of neurologic lesions may influence the conduct of anesthesia. Protracted vomiting, enuresis, and anorexia related to intracranial lesions should prompt evaluation of hydration and electrolytes. Diabetes insipidus or inappropriate secretion of antidiuretic hormone are common. A history of the use of aspirin or aspirin-containing remedies for headaches or respiratory tract infections is information that is not usually forthcoming but may have important implications for operative and postoperative bleeding. Corticosteroids are often initiated at the time of diagnosis of intracranial tumors, and they should be continued and a pulse dose administered during the perioperative period. Therapeutic concentrations of anticonvulsants should be verified preoperatively and maintained perioperatively. Children receiving long-term anticonvulsants may develop toxicity, especially if seizures are difficult to control; this is frequently manifested as abnormalities in hematologic or hepatic function, or both. Children receiving long-term anticonvulsant therapy may also require increased amounts of sedatives, nondepolarizing muscle relaxants, and opioids because of enhanced metabolism of these drugs (see also Chapters 7 and 24).[50-52]

Physical Examination

The physical examination should encompass a brief neurologic evaluation, including level of consciousness, motor and sensory function, normal and pathologic reflexes, integrity of the cranial nerves, and signs and symptoms of intracranial hypertension. Examination of pupillary size and responsiveness can detect benign anisocoria. Preoperative respiratory assessment should include the effects of motor weakness, impaired gag and swallowing mechanisms, and evidence of active pulmonary disease, such as aspiration pneumonia. Muscle atrophy and weakness should be documented, because upregulation of acetylcholine receptors may precipitate sudden hyperkalemia after administration of succinylcholine and induce resistance to nondepolarizing muscle relaxants in the affected limbs.[53]

Laboratory and Radiologic Evaluation

In all but the most minor procedures, laboratory data should include a hematocrit determination. Blood typing and crossmatching should be performed for any major procedure. The need for additional studies, such as evaluation of coagulation parameters, serum electrolyte levels and osmolality, blood urea nitrogen and creatinine values, arterial blood gas analysis, chest radiography, or electrocardiography (ECG), is determined on an individual basis. Liver function tests and a hematologic profile should be obtained if not recently reviewed in children receiving long-term therapy with anticonvulsants. Specific neuroradiologic studies are usually obtained by the neurosurgeon and should be reviewed by the anesthesiologist. For example, the anesthesiologist should know which children with a ventriculoperitoneal shunt have "slit ventricles" because these children have special risks in the perioperative period[54] (see "Hydrocephalus"). Information on the amount of sedation needed to perform radiologic studies may also be helpful in planning the induction of anesthesia. Preoperative neurophysiologic studies, including electroencephalography (EEG) and evoked potentials, may provide a baseline for comparison of intraoperative and postoperative evaluations.

PREMEDICATION

Sedation is usually withheld from pediatric neurosurgical patients until they arrive in the preoperative area to allow titration of drug to desired effect while under direct supervision. Opioids are usually withheld preoperatively because they may cause nausea or respiratory depression, especially in children with increased ICP, and sedatives alone usually are adequate to relieve anxiety.

Sedatives are administered in the parents' presence to facilitate a smooth separation and induction. Midazolam (~0.5-1.0 mg/kg) may be given orally; it usually requires 10 to 20 minutes to take effect. Incremental doses of intravenous (IV) midazolam (0.05 mg/kg) may also be useful in children who tolerate IV placement.

MONITORING

Minimal monitoring for pediatric neuroanesthesia requires a stethoscope (precordial or esophageal), electrocardiograph, pulse oximeter, sphygmomanometer, capnograph, and thermometer. Neuromuscular blockade monitoring is also important, but nerve stimulators may give misleading information about the extent of relaxation if applied to a denervated extremity. If the child has paresis, nerve stimulation should be at a site of normal neurologic function. Precordial Doppler ultrasound is recommended in children undergoing craniotomy, especially in the head-up position, because the relatively large head size of children places them at increased risk for air emboli. Monitoring devices for ICP are used for the same indications as in adults. Intraoperative EEG and electrophysiologic monitoring require advanced coordination among the neurosurgeon, anesthesiologist, and neurophysiologist. Urinary output should be measured during prolonged procedures, in cases with anticipated large blood loss, and when diuretics or osmotic agents are administered.

An arterial catheter is placed for craniotomies in which there is a potential for sudden and severe hemodynamic changes. Small child size should not preclude the use of invasive monitoring and may actually be an indication for a more aggressive approach. An increase in the paradoxical arterial pressure waveform with positive-pressure ventilation is often an excellent indication of intravascular volume deficiency and the need for fluid replacement (see Fig. 12.10). Intraarterial catheters can be placed percutaneously in the radial, dorsalis pedis, or posterior tibial arteries even in small infants, and it is rarely necessary to resort to surgical cutdown. The arterial transducer should be zeroed at the level of the head if the head and heart positions are different so that CPP can be accurately assessed. The lateral corner of the eye or the external auditory meatus approximate the level of the foramen of Monro and either is a convenient landmark. In the first days of life, the umbilical artery and the umbilical vein can be cannulated. These catheters should be discontinued as soon as alternative access is established because of the potential for serious complications.

Percutaneous central venous cannulation (i.e., external or internal jugular, femoral, or subclavian veins) using the Seldinger technique is possible even in the smallest infants (see Chapter 49). However, in children undergoing neurosurgical resections, consideration should be given to sites other than neck veins, such as the femoral vein, thereby avoiding the Trendelenburg position during catheter insertion and the risk of accidental carotid artery puncture and hematoma formation, which may compromise CBF and intracranial venous drainage. If there is no issue with ICP, the subclavian vein is a reasonable alternative. Cannulation of antecubital veins may provide central venous access, but threading the catheter into the inlet of the right atrium may be technically difficult in small children. When rapid blood loss is a consideration in a small child in whom adequate peripheral venous access is difficult to obtain, a single-lumen, large-bore catheter is most commonly inserted in a femoral vein. Catheters inserted into the femoral veins usually are accessible to the anesthesiologist during most neurosurgical procedures. Multiple-lumen central venous catheters are inadequate for rapid blood transfusion. All central catheters should be removed as soon as possible after the procedure to minimize the risk of venous thrombosis.

INDUCTION

For children with intracranial hypertension, the primary goals during induction are to minimize severe increases in ICP and decreases in blood pressure. Most IV drugs decrease $CMRO_2$ and CBF, which consequently decreases ICP.[55] Historically, sodium thiopental (4–8 mg/kg) was the default induction agent for neurosurgical cases. However, sodium thiopental is no longer available in the United States, although it remains available in other countries. In the United States, propofol has become the IV induction agent of choice for most children. Propofol (2–4 mg/kg) appears to have similar cerebral properties and an antiemetic effect; however, its antiemetic effect is usually not relevant for lengthy procedures. Etomidate, a possible neuroprotective agent, can be used if hemodynamic stability is a concern.[56-58] Ketamine should be avoided because of its known ability to increase cerebral metabolism, CBF, and ICP. Sudden increases in ICP have been reported after ketamine administration, especially in infants and children with hydrocephalus.[59,60]

Other measures to reduce ICP during induction include controlled hyperventilation and administration of opioids (e.g., fentanyl, remifentanil, or sufentanil) and supplemental hypnotics before laryngoscopy and intubation. Lidocaine (1.5 mg/kg) limits the increase in ICP when administered intravenously just before laryngoscopy.[61]

Sevoflurane has replaced halothane for inhaled inductions because of its more rapid onset, acceptability for pediatric patients, and hemodynamic stability. Similar to isoflurane in its cerebral physiologic effects, sevoflurane with hyperventilation appears to blunt the increase in ICP related to cerebral vasodilatation from inhalational anesthetic agents alone.[62-64] Sevoflurane offers an additional advantage because it causes less myocardial depression compared with halothane.[65] As stated earlier, sevoflurane anesthesia, while decreasing MAP, can also lead to an increase in regional cerebral oxygenation.[42] However, sevoflurane when combined with hyperventilation produces epileptiform activity as measured by EEG. This may occur even in children with no history of clinical seizure activity (see Chapter 7).[66]

A common presentation is an uncooperative toddler who has an intracranial tumor and moderately decreased intracranial compliance and who is agitated and resistant to separation from parents. Some clinicians would argue that a crying, agitated child has demonstrated a tolerance to increased ICP and that an IV induction is safer. Fortunately (for the anesthesiologist, although not for the child), children who have severe intracranial hypertension typically have a decreased level of consciousness, and it becomes easier to insert an IV catheter in those situations when it is most necessary.

AIRWAY MANAGEMENT AND INTUBATION

Airway management must be effective and smooth to avoid the ICP-increasing effects of hypoxemia, hypercarbia, and coughing. Opioid administration and supplemental hypnotics before intubation improve cerebral compliance and minimize increases in ICP caused by laryngoscopy and intubation.

Either oral or nasal intubation may be appropriate. Nasotracheal intubation offers the advantage of increased stability and increased comfort for children when postoperative intubation is necessary. Nasotracheal tubes are often used for children who will be in the prone position (e.g., for a posterior fossa craniotomy), children whose airway will be inaccessible during the surgical procedure, and for smaller children. Nasotracheal tubes also offer the advantage of a decreased risk of kinking intraoperatively, especially in prone positioning of small children for whom a smaller-sized endotracheal tube is necessary. The angle is more gentle using the nasopharynx compared with the angle using an oral approach, particularly in a prone patient whose neck is flexed. In this position, it is essential that the direction of the tube is toward the chin to avoid excessive and prolonged pressure on the alae and ischemic necrosis of the ala nasae.

Contraindications to nasal intubation include choanal stenosis, possible basilar skull fracture, transsphenoidal procedures, and sinusitis. If nasotracheal intubation is planned, it is advantageous to prepare the nares with topical vasoconstrictors, recognizing that systemic hypertension can occur in response to nasally administered vasoconstrictors. Placing a few drops of 0.25% phenylephrine (Neo-Synephrine) or oxymetazoline on cotton-tipped applicators and positioning them in the nares against the nasal mucosa can prevent overdosage and help to gauge the patency of the nasal passage when anesthesia has been induced. It may also be useful to use a red rubber catheter or a nonlatex nasal trumpet (the Robertazzi nasopharyngeal airway [Rusch Nasal Airway, Teleflex, Morrisville, NC]) to gently dilate the nares and minimize the risk of a nosebleed.[67] Directly spraying the nares with 0.25% phenylephrine should be avoided as there are reports of development of lethal cardiopulmonary compromise in children after such delivery.[68] Whichever route is chosen for intubation, it is important to secure the tracheal tube with care because loss of the airway intraoperatively in a child with head pins in the prone position or a child with limited airway access can result in disaster.

In prolonged, combined neurosurgical and craniofacial reconstructions, the tracheal tube may be sutured to the nasal septum or wired to the teeth. A nasogastric or orogastric tube is inserted after intubation to decompress the stomach and evacuate gastric contents; leaving it open to gravity drainage during the case can prevent positive pressure from building up in the stomach if air leaks around an uncuffed tracheal tube. The child's eyes should be closed, lubricated with eye ointment, and covered with a large, clear, waterproof dressing.

NEUROMUSCULAR BLOCKING DRUGS

Because of its rapid onset and brief duration of action, succinylcholine is frequently used to facilitate intubation in children with a full stomach. The intubating dose is 1 to 2 mg/kg given intravenously or 4 to 5 mg/kg given intramuscularly.[69] In children, succinylcholine should be preceded with atropine (0.01–0.02 mg/kg) to prevent bradycardia. Succinylcholine does not significantly increase ICP in humans,[70] and any effect may be minimized by pretreatment with a nondepolarizing muscle relaxant.[71] However, this may make succinylcholine less effective, even when the dose of succinylcholine is increased. Succinylcholine is contraindicated when it may induce life-threatening hyperkalemia in the presence of denervation injuries related to various causes, including severe head trauma, crush injury, burns, spinal cord dysfunction, encephalitis, multiple sclerosis, muscular dystrophies, stroke, or tetanus,[72] but it has no impact on the serum potassium concentration in children with cerebral palsy.[73]

Alternatively, nondepolarizing muscle relaxants such as rocuronium, cisatracurium, or vecuronium may be used, but all have a slower onset of action than succinylcholine. However, when rocuronium is administered in sufficiently large doses (1.2 mg/kg), the onset of action approaches that of succinylcholine, with equivalent intubating conditions achieved in about 1 minute.[74]

POSITIONING

Positioning is an especially important consideration in pediatric neuroanesthesia. Children with increased ICP should be transported to the preoperative holding area and operating room with the head elevated in the midline position to maximize cerebral venous drainage.

After the child is in the operating room, the neurosurgeons and anesthesiologists must have adequate access to the child. In infants and small children, slight displacement of the tracheal tube can result in extubation or endobronchial intubation. During prolonged procedures, it is important for the anesthesiologist to be able to visually inspect the tracheal tube and circuit connections and to suction the tracheal tube when necessary. Using proper draping and a flashlight, the operator can usually create a "tunnel" to ensure access to the airway. All but very small children are placed in pins in a Mayfield head holder (Integra, Plainsboro, NJ). The direction of the tube exiting the nares should be adjusted to remove pressure and avoid the risk of ischemia, particularly for cases that will continue for several hours. Neonates and small infants have thin calvaria, so head-pinning systems are often avoided. Instead, there are a variety of non–pin-based headrests available for these children. Adequate padding should be used in such situations (Figs. 26.4 and 26.5). Extreme head flexion can cause brainstem compression in children with posterior fossa pathology, such as a mass lesion or Arnold-Chiari malformation. Extreme flexion can also cause high cervical spinal cord ischemia and tracheal tube kinking and obstruction.[75]

Extremities should be well padded and secured in a neutral position (i.e., palm supinated or neutral to avoid ulnar nerve compression). It is important to avoid stretching peripheral nerves and to prevent skin and soft tissue pressure injury because of direct contact with surgical accessories such as instrument stands and grounding wires (see Fig. 26.5). It is also important to ensure that extremities that are not directly visible to the anesthesiologist (e.g., those on the opposite side of the operating room table) cannot fall off the table during surgery, even if the table is rotated. In older children and adolescents undergoing prolonged procedures, deep vein thrombosis prophylaxis should be considered using compression or pneumatic stockings.[76,77]

Prone Position

The prone position is commonly used for posterior fossa and spinal cord surgery. The torso should be supported to ensure free abdominal wall motion because increased intraabdominal pressure may impair ventilation, cause vena cava compression, and increase epidural venous pressure and bleeding. This is achieved most easily by placing silicone rolls or rolled blankets laterally on each side of the child's chest running from the shoulders toward the pelvis. A separate silicone roll or rolled blanket under the pelvis may occasionally be necessary in larger children. These rolls must not press into the flexed hips or compress the femoral nerve or genitalia. Placing the rolls in this position should also allow a

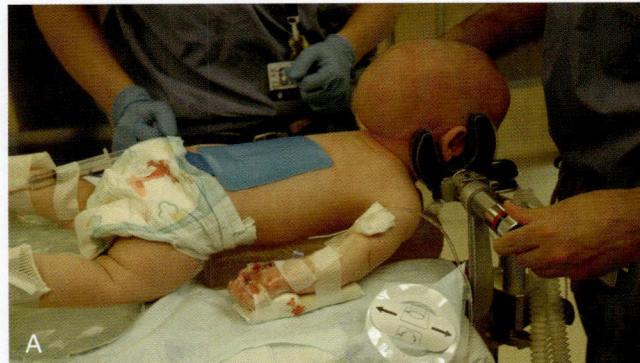
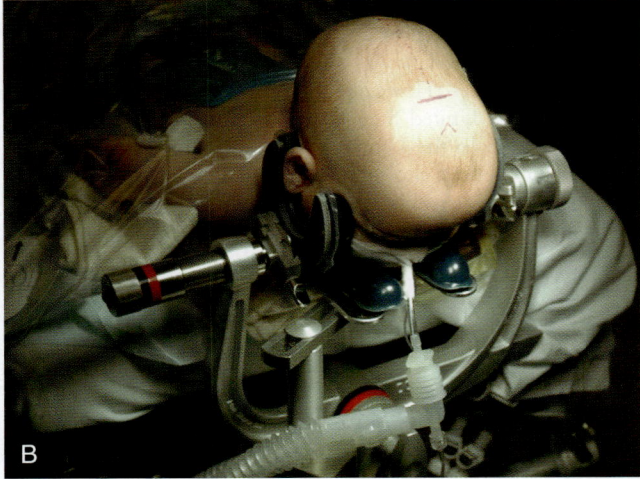

FIGURE 26.4 A, The child is positioned prone before surgery. Extreme head extension was needed for correction of craniosynostosis, but the equipment for securing the head was the same as that used for a prone craniotomy. **B,** This particular frame uses gel pads to support the chin, ears, and forehead.

precordial Doppler monitor to be easily placed on the anterior chest without undue pressure.

The head position depends on the surgical procedure. If surgery is limited to the lower spine, the head may be rotated and supported by padding, with care taken to avoid direct pressure on the eyes and nose and to keep the ears flat. For posterior fossa surgery, the head usually is suspended in pins to maintain central alignment of the head and maximal flexion. For infants and toddlers, a cerebellar head frame is another alternative when the cranium is too thin for pins. In this situation, the child's forehead and cheeks rest on a well-padded head frame, and the eyes are free in the center of a horseshoe-shaped support (see Fig. 26.4). Ensure that the tracheal tube is properly positioned (after taping) and does not migrate to a main-stem position while positioning the child prone. This can be confirmed before turning the child prone by flexing the child's head maximally onto the chest and auscultating for equal air entry bilaterally. Tape used to fix other tubes (e.g., gastric, esophageal) in place should be separate from the tape used to secure the tracheal tube so that if these other tubes are accidentally dislodged, an extubation will not occur. An emergency plan should be formulated to turn the child supine if it suddenly becomes necessary.[78]

Significant airway edema may develop in a child who is in the prone position for an extended period. Oral airways are best avoided because they can cause edema of the tongue. Alternatively,

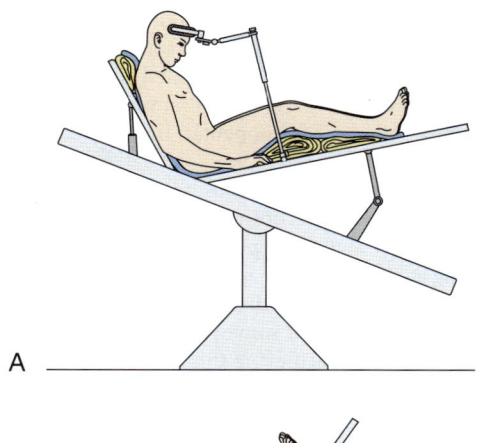

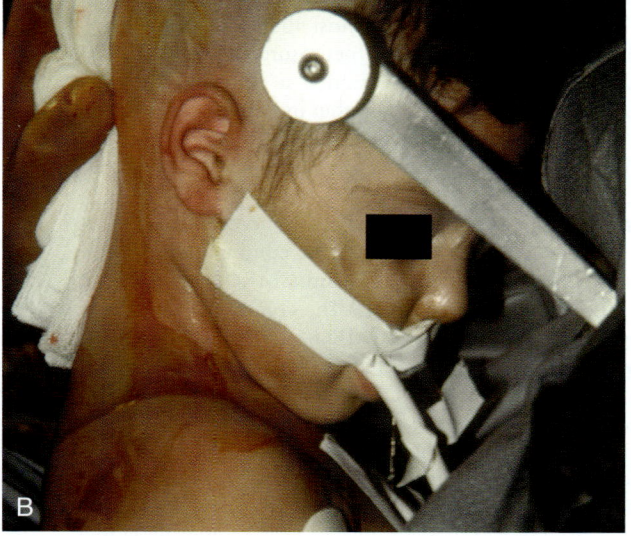

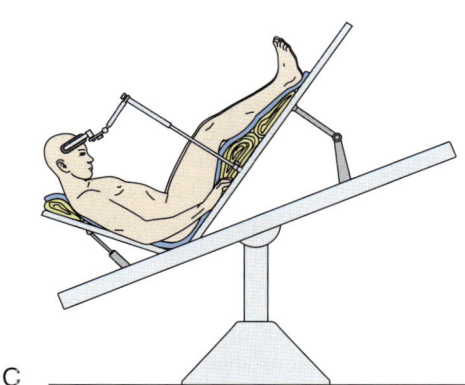

FIGURE 26.5 Resuscitation from the modified standard sitting position. The normal operative position (**A** and **B**) is compared with the resuscitation position (**C**). The position can be expeditiously changed by one control of the operating table.

a folded roll of gauze can be inserted between the lateral incisors to prevent the tongue from extruding. The latter maneuver is essential if cortical motor potentials are used intraoperatively as the nerve stimulation may trigger the child to bite his or her tongue, resulting in a bloody laceration. Rarely, prophylactic postoperative intubation may be necessary if a great deal of facial swelling has developed during a prolonged surgery. Postoperative vision loss has been linked with prolonged spine surgery in the prone position and significant blood loss.[79] Avoidance of direct pressure on the globe of the eyes, staged procedures to decrease surgical time, and maintenance of stable hemodynamics with avoidance of excessive intraoperative fluid administration should be ensured in prone children.[80]

Modified Lateral Position

Insertion or revision of ventriculoperitoneal shunts may require the child to be rotated from the supine to the semilateral position. This is achieved by placing a roll under the child's dependent axilla (to prevent a brachial plexus injury). The knees should be supported in a slightly flexed position and the heels padded. This position is also used for some temporal and parietal craniotomies.

Sitting Position

The sitting position is now used less commonly in pediatric neurosurgical procedures and is rarely used in children younger than 3 years of age. However, this position may be used for morbidly obese children who cannot tolerate the prone position because of excessive intrathoracic and abdominal pressures. When

the sitting position is used, precautions to prevent hypotension and air embolism must be followed. The lower extremities should be wrapped in elastic bandages. The head must be carefully flexed to avoid kinking the endotracheal tube, advancing it into a bronchial position, or to avoid compressing the chin on the chest, which can block venous and lymphatic drainage of the tongue. Extreme flexion can also result in brainstem or cervical spinal cord ischemia, or both. As in the prone position, nasotracheal tubes are often used because they are more secure. The child's upper extremities are supported in the child's lap. Control levers to lower the head position should be easily accessible to the anesthesiologist and unencumbered by wires and drapes (see Fig. 26.5).

LOCAL ANESTHESIA

Local anesthetic should be injected subcutaneously before a skin incision to provide analgesia, and epinephrine is included in the local anesthetic to reduce cutaneous blood loss. If 0.25% bupivacaine with 1:200,000 epinephrine is used, the dose should be limited to 0.5 mL/kg. When greater volumes are required, the solution can be diluted with normal saline. This dilute solution is still effective for vasoconstriction and provides a prolonged sensory block postoperatively. Specific blocks of supraorbital and supratrochlear nerves can provide analgesia from the frontal area to the midcoronal portion of the occiput.[81] Blockade of the great occipital nerve provides analgesia from the posterior of the occiput to the midcoronal area of the occiput, whereas block of the supraorbital nerve provides analgesia to the front of the occiput (see Figs. 42.9 and 42.10).[82,83]

MAINTENANCE OF GENERAL ANESTHESIA

General anesthesia is required for most therapeutic and many diagnostic procedures in pediatric neurosurgery. Ventilation is controlled if intracranial hypertension is a concern. Although spontaneous ventilation provides another indication of brainstem function, its disadvantages (e.g., hypoventilation, increased potential for air embolism) are usually outweighed by the safety of controlled ventilation.

Maintenance of general anesthesia can be accomplished using inhalational anesthetics, IV infusions, or a combination of these drugs. Anesthetics that decrease ICP and $CMRO_2$ and maintain CPP are most desirable (Table 26.1). The commonly used inhalational agents uncouple CBF and $CMRO_2$ such that CBF increases while $CMRO_2$ decreases. All potent inhalational agents are cerebral vasodilators, which increase both CBF and ICP. Low concentrations of isoflurane, sevoflurane, or desflurane, combined with ventilation to maintain normocarbia, minimally affect CBF and ICP.[62,63,84] Isoflurane is often the inhalational agent of choice for maintenance of neuroanesthesia. At two times the minimal alveolar concentration (MAC), this dose of isoflurane induces a level of anesthesia that is associated with an isoelectric EEG while, unlike several other inhalational agents, maintaining hemodynamic stability. Enflurane is no longer used and may be epileptogenic, especially when combined with hyperventilation.[85] Other studies have demonstrated a similar effect with sevoflurane and hyperventilation, but the clinical implications of this are yet to be defined.[86]

Practitioners debate the routine use of nitrous oxide for intracranial neurosurgical procedures. Opponents cite the increased risk of postoperative nausea and vomiting (PONV) with nitrous oxide in a surgical population already at greater risk for PONV.[87] Proponents cite studies that failed to demonstrate an increased risk of PONV.[88] Nitrous oxide can increase CBF in humans in a dose-dependent fashion through cerebral vasodilatation.[89,90] This increase in CBF can lead to an increase in ICP, which can be deleterious if the child already has reduced intracranial compliance.[91] Nitrous oxide can also suppress somatosensory and motor evoked potentials, especially when inspired concentrations exceed 50%.[92–94] Animal data have shown that nitrous oxide can counteract the protective effects of thiopental in a model of cerebral ischemia.[95]

Proponents of the use of nitrous oxide for intracranial procedures cite its long track record of safety. There are no outcome studies in humans that distinguish between using nitrous oxide or not using it. It is often of great clinical interest to obtain a neurologic assessment immediately after the conclusion of an intracranial procedure, and some practitioners prefer the use of nitrous oxide to aid in achieving this goal. Studies have demonstrated the safety of using nitrous oxide in a variety of combinations with other agents during intracranial procedures.[96] Nitrous oxide is relatively contraindicated, however, if the child has undergone a craniotomy within the past few weeks because air can remain in the head for prolonged periods after previous neurosurgery.[97]

Fentanyl is often administered as part of an opioid-based technique because it is easily titratable with minimal adverse effects. A common loading dose is 5 to 10 µg/kg, with a dose of 2 to 5 µg/kg per hour usually adequate for maintenance, recognizing that the context-sensitive half-life of fentanyl increases dramatically after 2 hours in adults.[98] Adverse effects, including hypotension, can be avoided by giving the loading dose incrementally. Practitioners commonly use other opioids such as remifentanil and sufentanil. Total intravenous anesthesia (TIVA) using propofol and remifentanil is popular when rapid emergence is required at the end of surgery (see Chapter 8). Note that the context-sensitive half-life for propofol increases with time but is particularly steep in younger age infants and children[99]; in contrast, the context-sensitive half-life of remifentanil is unchanged with time or age of the child, including neonates. Dexmedetomidine, an α_2-agonist sedative, has also been used in children for neurophysiologic

						CSF		SSEP	
TABLE 26.1 Neurophysiologic Effects of Common Anesthetic Agents									
Agent	MAP	CBF	CPP	ICP	$CMRO_2$	Production	Absorption	Amplitude	Latency
Nitrous oxide	0-↓	↑↑↑	↓	↑↑↑	↓↑	↑↓	↓↑	↓	↑-0
Inhalational Anesthetics									
Halothane	↓↓	↑↑↑	↑↑	↑↑	↓↓	↓↓	0-↓	↓	↑
Enflurane	↓↓	↑↑	↑↑	↑	↓↓	↑	↓	↓	↑
Isoflurane	↓↓	↑	↑↑	↑	↓↓↓	↓↑	↑	↓	↑
Sevoflurane	↓↓	↑	↑	↑	↓↓↓	↑	↓	↓	↑
Desflurane	↓↓	↑↑	↑	↑	↓	↑↓	↑	↓	↑
Hypnotics									
Thiopental	↓↓	↓↓↓	↑↑↑	↓↓↓	↑↑↑	↑↓	↑	↓	↑
Propofol	↓↓↓	↓↓↓	↓↓	↓↓↓	↑↓	↑	↑	↑	0-↑
Etomidate	0-↓	↓↓↓	↑	↓↓↓	↓↓↓	↑↓	↑	↑	↑
Ketamine	↓↓	↑↑↑	↓	↑↑↑	↑	↑↓	↓	↑	0
Benzodiazepine	0-↓	↓↓	↑	0-↓	↓↓	N/A	↑	↓	0-↑
Opioids	0-↓	↓	↑↓	0-↓	↓	↑↓	↑	↓	↑
Droperidol	↓↓	N/A	↑	↓	0-↓	N/A	N/A	N/A	N/A

NOTE: The relative number of arrows refers to the degree of effect on the noted parameter. For example, $CMRO_2$ is decreased much more with isoflurane than opioids. In cells with up and down arrows, there are conflicting reports on the effect of the drug.
CBF, cerebral blood flow; *CMRO₂,* cerebral metabolic rate for oxygen; *CPP,* cerebral perfusion pressure; *CSF,* cerebrospinal fluid; *ICP,* intracranial pressure; *MAP,* mean arterial pressure; *N/A,* not applicable; *SSEP,* somatosensory evoked potential; ↑, increased; ↓, decreased; 0, no change.

monitoring, for awake craniotomies, to facilitate smooth wake-ups after neurosurgical procedures, and for neuroprotection.[100-103] These pharmacokinetic limitations of IV infusion agents must be appreciated if the surgeons expect a timely arousal to ensure that the CNS is intact.

APOPTOTIC NEURODEGENERATION

Several investigators have demonstrated that commonly used anesthesia drugs accelerate programmed cell death (i.e., apoptosis) in the CNS of immature rodents and rhesus monkeys.[104-106] This laboratory observation has provoked a heated debate about its relevance to anesthetizing neonates,[107-110] which has been extended to the lay press.[111] Although these experimental paradigms have yielded some surprising findings, extrapolating these data to the practice of anesthetizing human neonates is questionable (see Chapter 25).

The animal and in vitro studies have significant limitations with respect to the experimental model, agent dosage or concentration, duration of exposure (absolute and compared with human exposures), lack of surgical stimulation, and developmental age and stage. No detectable clinical marker or syndrome is associated with early anesthesia exposure in former neonates who have undergone surgery and anesthesia at birth or in the first several years of life during rapid brain growth (i.e., synaptogenesis). In the only primate study, the degree of apoptosis after 3 hours of a ketamine infusion was similar to that of the control but significantly less than after a 24-hour infusion.[106] This occurred in the presence of blood concentrations of ketamine that were 10-fold to several hundred-fold greater than those reported after a single dose of ketamine in infants. These findings suggest that in this model, ketamine-associated neurodegeneration is a time-dependent, dose-dependent phenomenon whose limits in human neonates have not been established.

Despite the confounding effects of prematurity and coexisting congenital anomalies, clearly characterized syndromes have been associated with maternal consumption of alcohol and anticonvulsant drugs. Discrepancies in neurocognitive outcomes exist.[105,112] Most neonatal and infant surgery is urgent, and anesthesia care is essential to proceed safely. Several retrospective database studies suggest that multiple anesthesia episodes are associated with learning disabilities and cognitive dysfunction, but most of these children were anesthetized before pulse oximetry and capnography were a standard of care. Unrecognized episodes of hypoxemia or excessive ventilation with reduced CBF might have contributed. It is also unclear whether children who required more than one surgical procedure when younger than 4 years of age might have had neurocognitive developmental issues that were associated with the pathology requiring surgery and were totally separate from exposure to anesthetic agents.[110,113,114] One retrospective study demonstrated that identical twins who were discordant for general anesthesia and surgery showed no evidence of cognitive dysfunction in follow-up assessments.[115]

Two recent major, well-designed studies were published that examined the effects of exposure to general anesthesia in infants. The first of these studies, the General Anaesthesia versus Spinal anaesthesia (GAS) study, was an international, multicenter, randomized study that compared young infants (<60 weeks postconception age born at >26 weeks) requiring inguinal herniorrhaphy. The infants were randomly assigned to receive either general anesthesia with sevoflurane or awake-regional anesthesia (i.e., spinal). Neurocognitive outcomes were assessed at 2 years of age. The researchers concluded from this interim analysis that brief general anesthesia with sevoflurane (≤1 hour) resulted in no increased risk of adverse neurodevelopmental outcome compared with infants who underwent awake-regional anesthesia.[116]

The second landmark study was published in 2016: the Pediatric Anesthesia and Neurodevelopment Assessment (PANDA) study. This multicenter study examined a sibling-matched cohort across four university-based U.S. pediatric tertiary care hospitals. The researchers studied siblings within 36 months of age in whom one healthy sibling had undergone a single general anesthetic 20 to 240 minutes in duration before age 3 years. No statistical difference in a variety of metrics of neurocognitive development scores was demonstrated. The authors concluded that among healthy children with a single exposure to a general anesthesia before age 3, there was no statistically significant difference in measured neurocognitive abilities compared with unexposed children.[117]

Additionally, two large population studies of children were examined using an early development instrument tested at age 5 to 6 years.[118,119] Combined, more than 32,000 exposed children from the two studies were matched with 70,000 unexposed children. The results of the studies showed no effect of anesthesia on either a single- or multiple-anesthetic exposure in children younger than 2 years, whereas the results of both studies showed a small impairment in cognition and general language in children older than 2 years at the time of surgery.

A growing body of evidence supports the idea that some anesthetic agents are harmful to the developing brain in various species of neonatal animals. Evidence from the above studies[116,117] suggests that a short, single exposure to general anesthesia in a developing human neonate does not increase the risk of adverse neurocognitive outcomes. That said, this question is far from definitively answered. The neurocognitive effect of multiple exposures or the modulating effects of severe multisystem disease on such outcomes remain unclear. Thus, this remains an area of great interest and research.

BLOOD AND FLUID MANAGEMENT

Blood loss is difficult to estimate accurately during neurosurgery because most of the losses are absorbed by the operative drapes and the surgical field is difficult for the anesthesiologist to visualize. Accuracy can be improved if all suctioned blood is collected in calibrated containers visible to the anesthesiologist and an overhead camera provides a view of the operative field at all times. Blood loss is usually greatest at the beginning of surgery, when the scalp is incised, and when a large bone flap is removed.

Fluid and blood product management are discussed in Chapters 9 and 12. Disruption of the blood-brain barrier by underlying pathologic processes, trauma, or surgery predisposes neurosurgical patients to cerebral edema, which may be exacerbated by excessive administration of IV fluids. IV fluid management during neurosurgical anesthesia affects cerebral perfusion, cerebral edema, water and sodium homeostasis, and serum glucose concentration.

In most cases, blood transfusions are not planned and attempts are made to avoid administration of blood products with their associated risks. Crystalloid solutions are commonly administered. Lactated Ringer's solution is not considered truly isotonic because its osmolality is 273 mOsm/L (normal: 285–290 mOsm/L). Normal saline solution, which is slightly hypertonic (308 mOsm/L), is the fluid of choice because reduction of serum osmolality is not desirable. However, rapid infusion of large volumes of normal saline has been associated with a hyperchloremic non–anion gap metabolic acidosis.[120] The clinical significance of this acidosis is unclear. If there are large fluid requirements during surgery, alternating bags of lactated Ringer's solution with normal saline solution can minimize the risk of hypernatremia and acidosis and avoid hypoosmolality.

Inducing dehydration with osmotic and loop diuretics is a useful strategy to minimize cerebral edema and provide an optimal surgical field. However, hypotension and rebound effects may be associated with their use. Rapid administration of hypertonic solutions can cause profound but transient hypotension as the result of peripheral vasodilation.[121] Glucose-containing solutions are usually unnecessary during neurosurgical procedures because blood glucose concentrations are well maintained even in small children in the absence of IV glucose administration during typical (balanced) neurosurgical anesthetics. However, glucose may be indicated when hypoglycemia is a concern, such as in diabetic children, children receiving hyperalimentation, preterm and full-term neonates, and malnourished or debilitated children. In these situations, glucose solutions should be administered at or slightly below maintenance rates (by constant infusion pump) and serum glucose concentrations should be monitored periodically throughout surgery. The potential association of larger cerebral infarct size with hyperglycemia (i.e., blood glucose values >250 mg/dL) during ischemia is of particular concern.[122]

Meticulous management of fluids and blood products to minimize cerebral edema is a cornerstone of pediatric neuroanesthesia. Although cerebral hemorrhage is fortunately a rare event, when it does occur, it can be sudden and catastrophic. All children should have secure, large-bore IV access, and blood products should be available along with the means for warming the blood.

TEMPERATURE CONTROL

Because the head accounts for a large proportion of an infant's body surface area, infants are particularly susceptible to heat loss during neurosurgical procedures. Attention should be focused on maintaining normal temperature from the time the child is brought into the operating room, although moderate hypothermia during neurosurgery may be useful to decrease the $CMRO_2$. Ambient room temperature should be increased before the child enters the operating room. Infrared warming lights may be helpful for infants, and warming blankets may be useful for infants weighing less than 10 kg. Forced-air warming devices remain the most effective means to maintain body temperature in infants and children.[123]

VENOUS AIR EMBOLI

Venous air embolism (VAE) is a potential danger during intracranial procedures. The larger the pressure gradient between the operative site and the heart, the greater the potential for clinically significant entrainment of air into the central circulation.[124] For example, when the operative site is far above the heart (e.g., in a seated craniotomy) or when the CVP is low (e.g., acute blood loss during craniofacial procedures), it creates an environment for a VAE. Intracranial procedures are a particular concern because intracranial venous sinuses have dural attachments that impede their ability to collapse. Other potential air entry sites during neurosurgical procedures include bone, bridging veins, and spinal epidural veins. The sequence of events that should be followed when a VAE occurs is to identify the problem, stop further air entrainment, and support the circulation. Understanding the cause, prevention, and treatment of VAE is crucial because the consequences can be life-threatening.

When air enters the central circulation, it can accumulate in the right atrium or the right ventricular outflow tract. Cardiac output may be reduced, depending on the size of the air lock. If enough air is entrained into the circulation, the preload to the right ventricle decreases, or the right-sided heart afterload increases acutely, which can lead to cor pulmonale, acutely decreasing left ventricular preload and ultimately causing cardiovascular collapse. One study in dogs demonstrated that as little as 1 mL/kg of air could increase pulmonary artery pressure 200% to 300%.[125] Intracardiac shunts such as a patent foramen ovale, atrial or ventricular septal defects, and other congenital cardiac defects, may allow air to access the systemic circulation, including the coronaries and brain. The risk of VAE is even greater in infants and children because potential intracardiac shunts exist in many otherwise healthy infants and children. They may become clinically important if pulmonary hypertension develops acutely after a large air embolism. Some clinicians recommend preoperative echocardiographic screening for patent foramen ovale in any child being considered for a sitting craniotomy; others regard a patent foramen ovale to be an absolute contraindication to the sitting position.[126,127]

Although the incidence of VAE is greatest in the sitting position, the lateral, supine, and prone positions are not free of risk. VAE have also been observed during craniotomy for craniosynostosis, even when the operating room table is flat and rarely when the surgery involved endoscopic strip craniectomy, although most occur without clinical sequelae.[128,129] The incidence of VAE in children undergoing suboccipital craniotomy in the sitting position is not significantly different from that in adults, but children appear to have a greater incidence of hypotension and a smaller likelihood of successful aspiration of central (intravascular) air.[130]

Several techniques may be used to detect VAE. Depending on the study design, the usual order of sensitivity of detecting air in the heart is transvenous intracardiac echocardiography (0.15 mL/kg) > transesophageal echocardiography (0.19 mL/kg) = precordial Doppler probe (0.24 mL/kg) > pulmonary artery pressure (0.61 mL/kg) = end-tidal CO_2 tension (0.63 mL/kg) = arterial O_2 tension > MAP (1.16 mL/kg) = arterial CO_2 tension.[131,132] Transvenous intracardiac echocardiography is commonly used to guide catheters in cardiac ablation procedures or insertion of foramen ovale occlusion devices, but it is invasive and infrequently used in pediatric anesthesia. A precordial Doppler probe has been traditionally placed over the fourth or fifth intercostal space at the right sternal border to best monitor right heart sounds, although evidence suggests that placing the Doppler probe at the left parasternal border may be at least as sensitive (Fig. 26.6).[133,134] Appropriate Doppler positioning can be confirmed by listening for the characteristic change in sounds after rapid administration of a few milliliters of saline solution into a venous catheter. The precordial Doppler probe is particularly valuable because it is inexpensive, easy to use, benign, and noninvasive. Although transthoracic or transesophageal echocardiography is the most specific method for detecting small air emboli, it is not easily used intraoperatively, especially in children during neurosurgical procedures.[126,135,136]

Monitoring end-tidal gas tensions is important during neurosurgical procedures. When VAE occur, there is a ventilation-perfusion mismatch caused by the air blocking passage of blood through the pulmonary circulation, increasing dead-space ventilation with a sudden decrease in end-tidal CO_2 partial pressure ($ETCO_2$) and activation of complement resulting in pulmonary interstitial edema, neutrophil infiltration, and lung injury (Fig. 26.7).[131] The $ETCO_2$ remains a useful and cost-effective strategy in diagnosing massive VAE, although its sensitivity has been surpassed by other approaches (see Fig. 26.6). An increase in

AIR EMBOLISM
Relative sensitivity

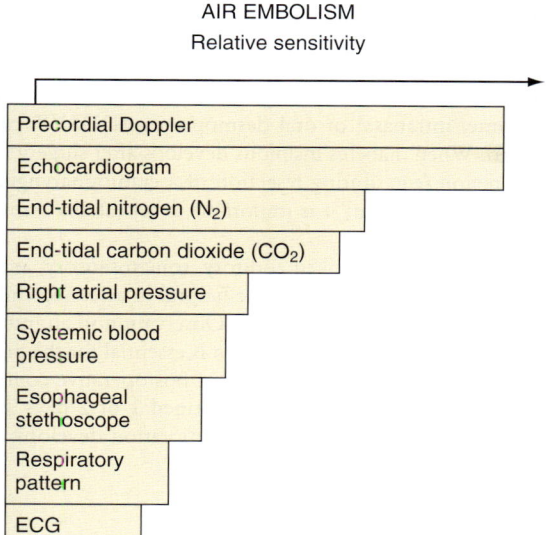

FIGURE 26.6 Relative sensitivities of air embolism–monitoring modalities. *ECG*, electrocardiogram.

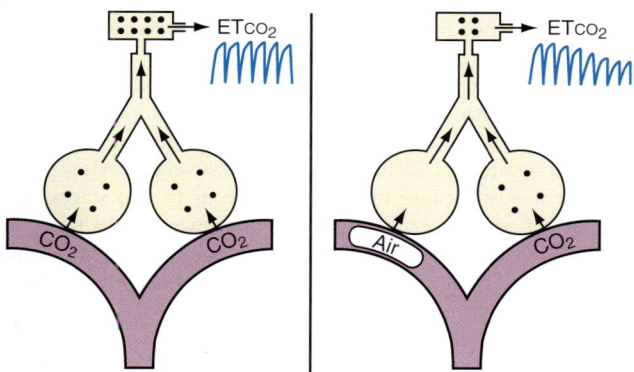

FIGURE 26.7 Mechanism of decreased end-tidal carbon dioxide (*ET*CO_2) after an air embolus. (Courtesy J. Drummond, MD.)

end-tidal nitrogen partial pressure during continuous monitoring is a specific sign of air emboli. Although slightly more sensitive than a decrease in $ETCO_2$, an increase in end-tidal nitrogen is not detected by most infrared analyzers in practice and is usually of such small magnitude that it may be difficult to detect.

Less sensitive or more invasive methods to detect VAE include ECG changes, changes in heart rate, decreases in systemic blood pressure, and increases in right atrial and pulmonary arterial pressures. Right atrial and pulmonary artery pressures increase quickly after the emboli develop (within 30 seconds). The magnitude of these increases correlates with the size of emboli, although these findings should not be relied on alone for monitoring and diagnosis.

On suspicion or diagnosis of VAE, immediate measures must be taken by the surgeons and anesthesiologists to prevent continued entrainment of air and consequent hemodynamic deterioration. The surgeon should immediately flood the field with saline solution and apply bone wax to exposed bone edges. The anesthesiologist should discontinue nitrous oxide and place the child in the

Trendelenburg position, which has the effect of increasing cerebral venous pressure, stopping entrainment of air, augmenting the child's peripheral venous return, and increasing systemic blood pressure. Occlusion of the internal jugular veins in an attempt to increase cerebral venous pressure should be done with great care because occlusion of the carotid arteries can lead to cerebral ischemia. The application of positive end-expiratory pressure increases CVP but also decreases cardiac filling pressure, cardiac output, and blood pressure; extreme increases in positive end-expiratory pressure are usually unwarranted. Chest compressions, vasopressors, and aggressive fluid resuscitation may be required.

Aspiration of air from a central venous catheter is rarely successful unless massive amounts have been entrained. When central venous catheters are necessary, such as for a child in the sitting position or when massive blood loss is anticipated, an attempt should be made to place the tip at the junction of the superior vena cava and right atrium to provide the optimal location for aspiration of entrained air. More importantly, a central venous catheter is useful to estimate maintenance of circulating blood volume and to rapidly administer fluids and resuscitative medications when necessary. The position of a central venous catheter near the heart should be confirmed by radiograph, by transducing CVPs, or with the aid of ECG monitoring (i.e., biphasic P waves develop in a lead at the tip of the catheter). The threshold for aspirating air may be increased by properly positioning a multiple-orifice central venous catheter using a transvenous intracardiac echocardiography probe.[131] Because erosion of the catheter tip through the heart causing fatal pericardial tamponade has occurred after surgery in small children, soft silicone catheters are recommended.[137,138]

EMERGENCE

Protecting the brain is a major concern during neurosurgical procedures (Table 26.2). Emergence and extubation should be smooth and controlled to prevent fluctuations in ICP and in venous and arterial pressures.[139] To avoid vomiting during emergence, a multimodal antiemetic approach is advised.[140] Despite this approach, the incidence of PONV is high, which may be attributed to several factors: blood in the CSF is a potent emetic, opioids are often used to treat postoperative pain, and headache itself can precipitate emesis.

IV lidocaine (1.0–1.5 mg/kg) given before extubation may help to suppress coughing and straining on the tracheal tube, although fentanyl appears to be equally effective and may be less sedating. Labetalol, an α- and β-adrenergic blocking agent, can be administered incrementally for the control of blood pressure during the acute period of emergence, but this is rarely necessary in children who have received adequate doses of opioids during surgery. For adolescents, IV labetalol (0.1–0.4 mg/kg given every 5 to 10 minutes until the desired effect is achieved) may be necessary, but this usually does not have to be repeated in the postoperative period. Esmolol is used by some practitioners and has been as effective as labetalol in controlling hypertension after intracranial surgery in adults.[141] However, esmolol should be used with caution in infants and smaller children because their cardiac output depends on heart rate. There are no studies evaluating the use of esmolol in children for such an application. Dexmedetomidine may be useful in facilitating a smooth emergence while still allowing evaluation of the child's neurologic status.

Neuromuscular blockade should be pharmacologically reversed because even the slightest residual weakness is poorly tolerated and may interfere with the neurologic examination. Adequate spontaneous ventilation and oxygenation and an awake mental

TABLE 26.2   Maneuvers of Neuroprotection

Goals	
	Avoid cerebral edema
	Avoid cerebral hypoxia
	Avoid cerebral hypoperfusion
	Avoid cerebral hypermetabolism
	Avoid neuronal membrane damage
Maneuvers	
Head of bed at 30 degrees in midline	Increases cerebral venous drainage while maintaining CPP
Corticosteroids	May improve outcome in spinal cord injury
	Decrease vasogenic cerebral edema in children with tumors
	Stabilize neuronal membranes
	Free-radical scavengers
Controlled ventilation	Maintain $PaCO_2$ at normal to slightly low levels: prevents both cerebral vasodilation and increased ICP
Muscle paralysis	Avoids coughing, straining, child movement, and other causes of increased ICP
Ventricular drainage	Decreases ICP
Antihypertensives	Prevent further cerebral edema, ischemia, and cerebral hemorrhage. Severe hypotension can significantly decrease CPP.
Anticonvulsants	Prevent seizure activity and increased ICP
Hypothermia	Decreases $CMRO_2$ and CMRglu consumption
Barbiturate coma	Membrane-stabilizing effect
	Decreases CBF and $CMRO_2$

CBF, cerebral blood flow; CMRglu, cerebral metabolic rate for glucose; $CMRO_2$, cerebral metabolic rate for oxygen; CPP, cerebral perfusion pressure; ICP, intracranial pressure; $PaCO_2$, partial pressure of arterial carbon dioxide.

status are required before extubation. If postoperative intracranial hypertension is possible or if the child does not meet respiratory or neurologic criteria for extubation, the tracheal tube should be left in place, sedation administered, and the child transported to an intensive care unit.

The child should be as fully alert as possible immediately after the operation to permit repeated neurologic examinations to assess recovery and to detect a deteriorating status. In unconscious children, ICP can be monitored invasively. CT scans can help to evaluate the cause of an increased ICP or deteriorating mental status.

Pain is usually not severe after a craniotomy, but it can be treated with incremental doses of opioids. Ketorolac is best avoided in the early postoperative period because of its effects on platelet function. Acetaminophen may be administered orally, rectally, or intravenously for mild pain.[142]

Diabetes insipidus or inappropriate secretion of antidiuretic hormone may complicate postoperative fluid and electrolyte management, particularly when surgery is in the region of the hypothalamus and pituitary gland (see Chapter 27). Careful observation of fluid status and repeated laboratory evaluation of blood and urine osmolality and sodium levels are important in this situation. When diabetes insipidus occurs, it can be managed with a continuous infusion of dilute aqueous vasopressin (0.001–0.01 U/kg per hour).[143] In such circumstances, large volumes of hypotonic IV solutions must be avoided because they may rapidly decrease

the serum sodium concentration and osmolality. If normal saline solution is administered in strictly limited volumes, aqueous vasopressin can control the electrolyte and fluid balances of children with diabetes insipidus until they resume oral fluids. At that time, intranasal or oral desmopressin (DDAVP) can be substituted. When diabetes insipidus develops after surgery in the pituitary region (e.g., during resection of a craniopharyngioma), it may only be transient; it is important to repeatedly assess the need for vasopressin.

Portable EEGs and evoked auditory, somatosensory, and less commonly, visual potentials may be helpful in assessing children who are deeply sedated or paralyzed. Observation in an intensive care unit capable of managing children is essential for the prevention or early detection and treatment of postoperative complications. CT and/or MRI are often performed 1 or 2 days after a craniotomy or earlier if neurologic deterioration develops.

Special Situations

TRAUMA

Head Injury

Among children, trauma is the primary cause of death, and head injuries produce most of this mortality and cause much of the morbidity in survivors.[144-146] Motor vehicle accidents continue to be the most frequent preventable cause of head injury, although domestic violence and sports-related head injury are also common in children (see Fig. 39.1). Assaults and suicide attempts have become increasingly common among adolescents.

Children with head trauma may have minimal neurologic abnormalities at the time of initial evaluation. However, increased ICP and neurologic deficits may progressively develop. They develop slowly because brain injuries occur in two stages. The primary insult that occurs at the time of impact results from the biomechanical forces that disrupt the cranium, neural tissue, and vasculature. The secondary insult is the parenchymal damage caused by the pathologic sequelae of the primary insult. These changes can result from hypotension, hypoxia, cerebral edema, or intracranial hypertension. Whereas prevention of primary injuries must be addressed in a sociopolitical forum such as through seat-belt laws, sports injury prevention, and domestic violence legislation, anesthesiologists are instrumental in preventing or minimizing secondary insults (see Chapter 39).

There are significant differences between children and adults in the pattern of CNS injuries. Although intracranial hematomas (i.e., epidural, subdural, or intraparenchymal) are common in adults, they are less common in children. In contrast, diffuse cerebral edema after blunt head trauma occurs more often in children than in adults.[147]

Scalp Injuries

One of the most common head injuries in children is the scalp laceration. Most can be managed in the emergency department, but more serious injuries may require the operating room to provide immobility and comfort. Children can lose a considerable amount of blood from a scalp injury because a larger fraction of the cardiac output perfuses the head compared with adults. Infants younger than 1 year of age may become hemodynamically unstable from blood loss from a subgaleal hematoma alone, as in a closed scalp injury, and hypovolemia should always be considered and treated before induction of anesthesia. Coexisting intracranial or other injuries must be considered, and a preoperative CT scan may be warranted.

Skull Fractures

Skull fractures are a common manifestation of head trauma in children. Most are linear and do not require surgical treatment. These fractures are of concern primarily because the force required to produce them may damage the underlying brain and vasculature. A linear fracture over a major blood vessel (e.g., middle meningeal artery) or a large dural sinus may result in intracranial hemorrhage. Most children have an uneventful course after sustaining a simple skull fracture. A few develop a leptomeningeal cyst or growing fracture that eventually requires surgical treatment. Multiple skull fractures in the absence of documented major trauma should always raise the suspicion of child abuse (see Fig. 39.2), which is also referred to as *nonaccidental trauma*.

Depressed skull fractures often require surgical repair. They may occur even in the absence of a scalp laceration. However, displacement of the inner table of the skull requires greater force than that needed to produce a simple linear fracture and has greater potential to damage underlying tissues. Approximately one-third of all depressed fractures are uncomplicated, another third are associated with dural lacerations, and the remaining third are associated with cortical lacerations. The extent of cortical injury is the primary determinant of morbidity and mortality. Surgical débridement and elevation of the depressed bone are usually performed as soon as possible after the injury (Fig. 26.8A).

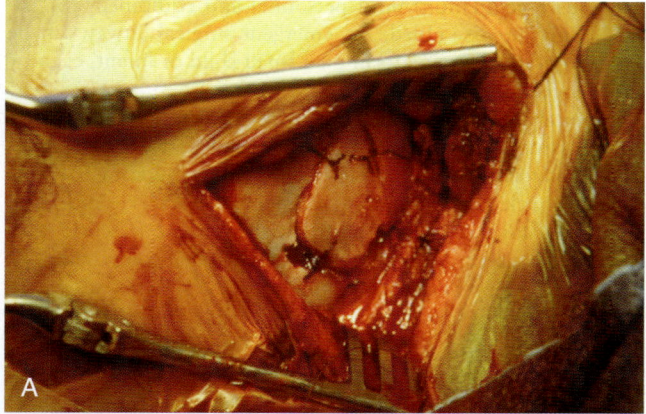

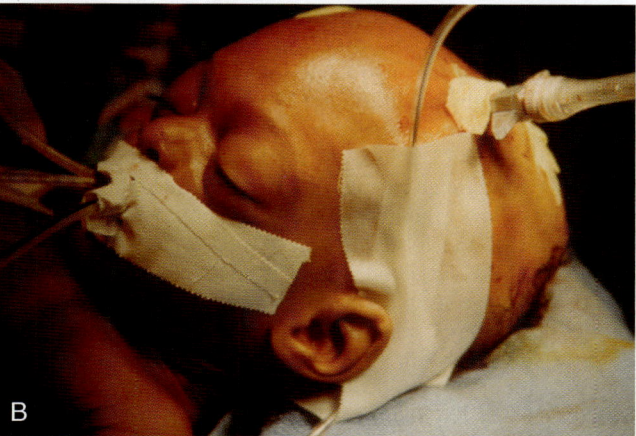

FIGURE 26.8 A, This depressed skull fracture required surgical intervention. **B,** Children with severe head trauma (in this case, a shaken baby) may present with marked increases in intracranial pressure.

Basilar skull fractures are less common in children. Despite the force needed to produce these fractures, they typically have an excellent prognosis and rarely require surgical intervention. However, the possibility of a basilar skull fracture should be considered when caring for children with altered mental status, seizures, or associated trauma requiring surgery. Findings include periorbital ecchymoses ("raccoon eyes"), retroauricular ecchymosis (i.e., the Battle sign) (see Fig. 39.2B), hemotympanum, clear rhinorrhea, or otorrhea. Unless absolutely necessary (e.g., mandibular wiring), nasotracheal intubation or passage of a nasogastric tube is best avoided because these tubes have inadvertently traversed these skull fractures and entered the cranium.[148–150] Complications of basilar skull fracture include meningitis from a CSF leak, cranial nerve damage, and anosmia.

Epidural Hematoma

Epidural hematomas most commonly develop in the temporoparietal region as a result of arterial bleeding from a severed middle meningeal artery. They can also develop in the posterior fossa as a result of bleeding from a venous sinus. Epidural hematomas are not necessarily associated with an overlying skull fracture. The classic natural history in adults is a "lucid interval" between the initial loss of consciousness and subsequent neurologic deterioration. Infants and children may not demonstrate an altered mental status in the early stages after the injury. However, as the hematoma expands, it can lead to a loss of consciousness, hemiparesis, and pupillary dilatation. This deterioration can be quite rapid once a mass effect occurs. Treatment is prompt surgical evacuation because delays are associated with increased morbidity. Medical therapy directed at decreasing ICP should be instituted as soon as a diagnosis is suspected but should not delay surgical repair (see Fig. 26.8B). Children recover well after these hemorrhages, although morbidity is usually a reflection of underlying brain injury or lengthy delay in treatment.

Subdural Hematoma

Subdural hematomas are usually associated with cortical damage resulting from direct parenchymal contusion or laceration of venous blood vessels. Acute subdural hematomas are almost always traumatic and are frequently a result of abuse, such as shaking of small children, particularly those younger than 1 year of age. Shaken baby syndrome occurs when an infant is shaken so vigorously that significant neuronal disruption occurs and tears in the cortical bridging veins cause subdural hematomas.[151–153] These infants suffer brain damage complicated by episodes of apnea and further hypoxic insult.

Subdural hematomas occasionally result from birth trauma within the first hours of life. Vitamin K deficiency, congenital coagulopathies, and disseminated intravascular coagulation are considerations in these situations. Great force is required to produce a subdural hematoma, whether by direct impact, laceration of blood vessels, or traumatic separation of the brain and overlying dura. Cerebral edema, uncontrolled intracranial hypertension, and persistent neurologic deficits often characterize the postoperative course. Chronic subdural hematomas or effusions may also develop in infancy, although these children do not usually present with acute symptoms. Children are often diagnosed because they are irritable and vomiting or have an increased head circumference. Chronic subdural hematomas can increase in size, causing slow but significant increases in ICP. Although a craniotomy is sometimes performed, most children undergo some form of hematoma drainage or shunting procedure as definitive treatment.

Intracerebral Hematoma

Intracerebral hematomas fortunately are rare but have a poor prognosis. Deep parenchymal hematomas are most often extensions of cortical contusions in a child with severe neurologic injury. Rarely, a localized hematoma may be appropriate for surgical evacuation to decompress the brain. However, intraparenchymal hematomas are not evacuated for fear of damaging viable brain tissue. Anticonvulsants are usually administered prophylactically, and it is safest in the initial period after injury to avoid any medications that interfere with coagulation (e.g., ketorolac).

Spinal Injury

Although isolated cervical spine injuries are uncommon in children, those with severe head trauma should always be managed as if they also have a cervical spine injury.[154,155] Different causes of spinal injuries are associated with specific age groups. Motor vehicle accidents produce the largest number of injuries in older children and adolescents, whereas birth injuries and falls are the most common cause in infants and young children.[156] Spinal cord injury itself may be caused by a variety of forces, including hyperflexion, hyperextension, rotation, vertical compression, flexion rotation, and shearing. The injury may involve bony, ligamentous, cartilaginous, vascular, or neural components of the spine or adjacent structures. The biomechanics and functional anatomy of the pediatric spine depend on the age of the child. Older children and teenagers are more likely to sustain injuries in the thoracolumbar region of the spine, whereas infants and younger children are more likely to suffer injuries in the high cervical region, particularly in the atlantoaxial region. The cervical spine is at greater risk in the infant and younger child because of the relatively weak and flexible neck muscles that support a proportionally large and heavy head, with the atlantooccipital area acting as a pivot point. Atlantooccipital dislocations are major neurologic injuries, leaving children neurologically devastated but not necessarily dead.

As with brain injury, spinal cord injury occurs in two phases. The primary insult results from biomechanical forces and bony fragments directly impacting the spinal cord. The secondary insult results from the pathologic sequelae of the primary insult: edema and ischemia owing to cortical compression, hypotension, or hypoxia. Inappropriate manipulation of a child with an unstable fracture can exacerbate primary and secondary injuries. Anesthesiologists who provide care for a child with a potential cervical spine injury should be aware that spinal cord injuries in children commonly occur without actual evidence of spinal bone fractures on plain cervical radiographs. These injuries are known as spinal cord injuries without radiologic abnormality (SCIWORA).[157] Injuries to the cervical spine in particular are often difficult to recognize but may be identified by odontoid displacement or prevertebral swelling on radiographs. As a result, a CT scan is frequently indicated when a spinal injury is initially suspected in a child with trauma. After a child with a potential spinal injury is determined to be medically stable, these studies should be obtained as soon as possible. The child's airway and cardiorespiratory function must be continuously and closely monitored until a spinal cord injury can be ruled out. Sometimes, as with brain injury, there can be a delay in the onset of neurologic deficits with SCIWORA injuries.[158]

Respiratory failure is the most common cause of death after isolated cervical spine injury. The level of injury determines the degree of impairment. The phrenic nerve originates primarily from C4 but receives contributions of fibers from C3 and C5.

Lesions at C5 leave partial diaphragmatic innervation but impair abdominal and intercostal accessory muscles. Lesions between C6 and T7 preserve diaphragmatic innervation but diminish accessory muscle function.

Children with a cervical spine injury may rapidly develop respiratory failure owing to decreased vital capacity, increased dead space, retention of secretions, and respiratory muscle fatigue. Resultant hypercarbia and hypoxia aggravate the secondary injury to the brain and spinal cord. Respiratory status may be further impaired by associated trauma to the chest, causing pulmonary contusion or pneumothorax, or by aspiration of gastric contents.

Prompt airway management is essential to avoid hypoxia, ensure adequate respiratory mechanics, preserve neural function, and prevent extension of spinal injury (see Figs. 39.5–39.7). The head and neck must be immediately immobilized; restraint of the extremities may also be required. Various tracheal tubes and laryngoscope blades should be available, as well as equipment and personnel for an emergency tracheostomy. Insertion of a laryngeal mask airway may be lifesaving until a more secure airway can be achieved with fiberoptic or other means.[159-164] Small fiberoptic bronchoscopes (2.2-mm diameter) can fit through infant-sized tracheal tubes. Retrograde intubation using a guidewire introduced through the cricothyroid membrane may be useful in older children or adolescents (see Chapter 14). However, an unstable infant or child whose airway cannot be secured by conventional means is probably best managed by an emergency tracheostomy. As a temporizing measure, a cricothyroidotomy can be performed (see Figs. 14.25–14.27).[165] This permits oxygenation (although inadequate ventilation) until personnel and equipment for tracheostomy are assembled. An emergent surgical airway can be extremely difficult to perform on a small child or infant, even by experienced and skilled hands.

Hemodynamic instability may be a problem owing to hypovolemia from other injuries or severe head trauma. Other sites of bleeding such as long bone fractures and abdominal trauma should be ruled out. Children with spinal shock exhibit loss of vasomotor tone or loss of normal neurocardiac function with associated bradycardia and decreased myocardial contractility; IV fluids and vasopressors may be necessary.

The use of high-dose steroids as treatment of spinal cord injury remains controversial. Many centers have abandoned such protocols because of questions of increased complications and concerns over lack of efficacy. Although there are few data for adults and children, corticosteroids are often administered to patients with spinal injuries as soon as possible after the initial trauma in the hope of reducing the neurologic injury. The most commonly used drug is methylprednisolone; 30 mg/kg is administered over the first 15 minutes, followed by an infusion of 5.4 mg/kg per hour for the next 23 hours.[166,167] Methylprednisolone is thought to be effective through multiple mechanisms, including improved spinal blood flow, inhibition of the arachidonic acid cascade, and modulation of the local immune response.[168] Some evidence suggests that GM_1 ganglioside, with or without methylprednisolone, may be advantageous in decreasing demyelination and promoting neurologic recovery if administered soon after a spinal injury.[169-175]

If the spinal cord injury is more than 24 hours old, succinylcholine should be avoided because it can result in massive hyperkalemia.[176] Physiologic changes may result from autonomic hyperreflexia, which frequently develops after cervical or high thoracic spinal lesions. Autonomic hyperreflexia can produce severe and life-threatening vasomotor instability with hypertension and arrhythmias.[177,178]

CRANIOTOMY

Tumors

Brain tumors are the most common solid tumors in children, exceeded only by the leukemias as the most common pediatric malignancy.[179,180] Between 1500 and 2000 new brain tumors are diagnosed annually in children in the United States. Unlike those in adults, most brain tumors in children are infratentorial in the posterior fossa. They include medulloblastomas, cerebellar astrocytomas, brainstem gliomas, and ependymomas of the fourth ventricle. Because posterior fossa tumors usually obstruct CSF flow, increased ICP occurs early. Presenting signs and symptoms include early morning vomiting and irritability or lethargy. Cranial nerve palsies and ataxia are also common findings, with respiratory and cardiac irregularities usually occurring late. Sedation or general anesthesia may be required for radiologic evaluation or radiation therapy.

Surgical resection of a posterior fossa tumor presents a number of anesthetic challenges. Children are usually positioned prone, although the lateral or sitting positions are used by some neurosurgeons. In any case, the head is flexed, and the position and patency of the tracheal tube must be meticulously ensured. In the event that the tracheal tube does become dislodged when the child is in a head holder and prone, successful emergent airway management has been described using a laryngeal mask airway.[181]

Arrhythmias and acute blood pressure changes may occur during surgical exploration, especially when the brainstem is manipulated or irrigated (Fig. 26.9). The electrocardiogram and arterial waveform should be closely monitored. Altered respiratory control may be masked by neuromuscular blocking drugs (NMBDs) and mechanical ventilation. Even when ICP is only marginally increased, intracranial compliance is presumed to have decreased. This warrants precautions against further increases in ICP. If ICP is markedly increased or acutely worsens, a ventricular catheter may be inserted before the tumor is resected. VAE is a potentially serious complication that is not eliminated by the prone or lateral position because head-up gradients of 10 to 20 degrees are frequently used to improve cerebral venous drainage. In infants and toddlers, large head size relative to body size accentuates this problem.

Supratentorial tumors in the midbrain include craniopharyngiomas, optic gliomas, pituitary adenomas, and hypothalamic tumors and account for approximately 15% of intracranial tumors. Hypothalamic tumors (i.e., hamartomas, gliomas, and teratomas) frequently manifest with precocious puberty in children who are large for their chronologic age. Craniopharyngiomas are the most common parasellar tumors in children and adolescents and may be associated with hypothalamic and pituitary dysfunction. Symptoms often include growth failure, visual impairment, and endocrine abnormalities.

Signs and symptoms of hypothyroidism should be sought and thyroid function measured. Corticosteroid replacement (i.e., dexamethasone or hydrocortisone) usually is administered because the integrity of the hypothalamic-pituitary-adrenal axis may be uncertain. Diabetes insipidus can occur preoperatively and is a common postoperative problem. The history usually reveals this condition preoperatively, especially if attention is focused on nocturnal drinking and enuresis. Evaluation of serum electrolytes and osmolality, urine specific gravity, and urine output is helpful because hypernatremia and hyperosmolality, along with dilute urine, are typical findings. If diabetes insipidus does not exist preoperatively, it usually does not develop until the postoperative period because there is an adequate reserve of antidiuretic hormone in the posterior pituitary gland capable of functioning for many hours, even when the hypothalamic-pituitary stalk is damaged intraoperatively.

Postoperative diabetes insipidus is marked by a sudden large increase in dilute urine output associated with an increasing serum sodium concentration and osmolality. Protocols have been developed to guide intraoperative and postoperative management of diabetes insipidus (see Chapters 9 and 27).[143] Return of

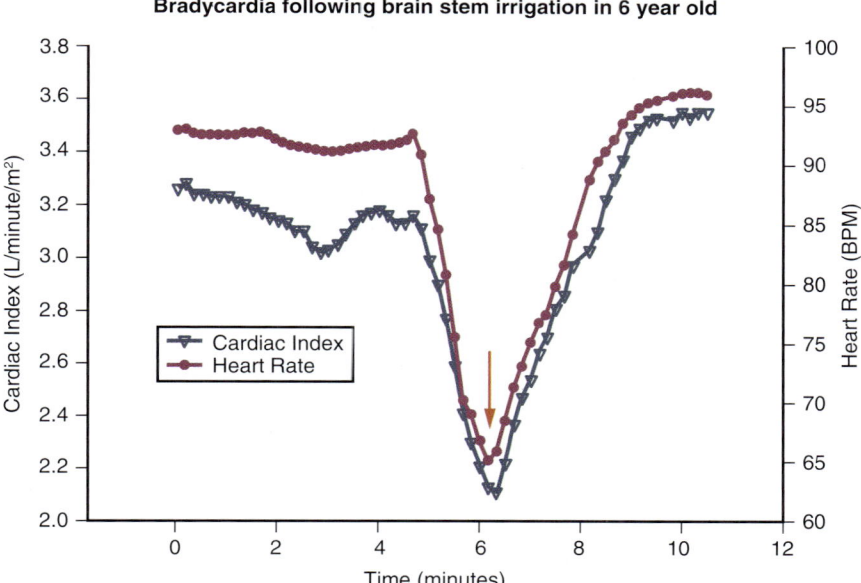

Bradycardia following brain stem irrigation in 6 year old

FIGURE 26.9 This graph illustrates the dramatic bradycardic response and accompanying decrease in cardiac index measured by a continuous noninvasive cardiac output monitor (Cardiotronic, Osypka Medical Inc., La Jolla, CA) in a 6-year-old child following brainstem irrigation. As soon as the surgeon stopped irrigation and atropine was administered, the heart rate and cardiac index were restored. (Courtesy Charles J Coté, MD.)

antidiuretic hormone activity a few days postoperatively may cause a marked decrease in urinary output, water intoxication, seizures, and cerebral edema if it is not recognized and fluid administration is not adjusted appropriately.

Transsphenoidal surgery typically is performed only in adolescents and older children with pituitary adenomas. However, it should be treated like other midbrain tumors in terms of monitoring and vascular access. Children are usually intubated orally to give the surgeon optimal access to the nasopharynx, and preparations for an emergent craniotomy should be anticipated in case unexpected massive bleeding develops. Because nasal packs are inserted at the end of surgery, the child should be fully awake before tracheal extubation.

Gliomas of the optic pathways occur with increased frequency in children with neurofibromatosis. Presenting symptoms include visual changes and proptosis; increased ICP and hypothalamic dysfunction are usually late findings. Neurofibromas tend to be highly vascular, and the anesthesiologist should be prepared for considerable blood loss.

Approximately 25% of intracranial tumors in children involve the cerebral hemispheres. They are primarily astrocytomas, oligodendrogliomas, ependymomas, and glioblastomas. Neurologic symptoms are more likely to include a seizure disorder or focal deficits. Succinylcholine should be avoided if motor weakness is present because it can cause sudden severe hyperkalemia. Nondepolarizing NMBDs and opioids may be metabolized more rapidly than usual in children who are receiving chronic anticonvulsants. Choroid plexus papillomas are rare but occur most often in children younger than 3 years of age. They usually arise from the choroid plexus of the lateral ventricle and produce early hydrocephalus as a result of increased production of CSF and obstruction of CSF flow. Hydrocephalus usually resolves with surgical resection. When lesions lie near the motor or sensory strip, a special type of somatosensory evoked potential monitoring called *phase reversal* may be used to delineate the locations.[182] If cortical stimulation is planned to help identify motor areas, NMBDs must be permitted to wear off and the anesthetic technique adjusted to achieve immobilization without paralysis.

Stereotactic biopsies or craniotomies present special concerns regarding airway accessibility. Newer head frames have adjustable anterior positions so that the airway is readily accessible (E-Fig. 26.1). They are especially useful for stereotactic neurosurgery. It is more comfortable and less distressing for the child to be anesthetized before the head frame is applied, even though this means the anesthesiologist must induce anesthesia in the radiology suite and then transport the child from the CT scanner to the operating room. The wrench that is used to apply and remove the head frame should be taped to the frame at all times so that it is always readily available if emergent removal of the head frame becomes necessary (e.g., during transport).

Vascular Anomalies
Arteriovenous Malformations
Arteriovenous malformations consist of large arterial feeding vessels, dilated communicating vessels, and large draining veins carrying arterialized blood. Large malformations, especially those involving the posterior cerebral artery and vein of Galen, may manifest as congestive heart failure (i.e., high-output heart failure, often with pulmonary hypertension) in the neonate. Consumption of coagulation factors and platelet destruction may further complicate the clinical picture. The prognosis for these types of arteriovenous malformations is quite poor. Saccular dilation of the vein of Galen

may manifest later in infancy or childhood as hydrocephalus owing to obstruction of the aqueduct of Sylvius. Malformations not large enough to produce congestive heart failure usually remain clinically silent unless they cause seizures or a stroke or until the acute rupture of a communicating vessel results in subarachnoid or intracerebral hemorrhage.[183] Intracranial hemorrhages are the most common presentation in this population, with an associated mortality rate of ~25%.

Treatment usually consists of embolization or irradiation of deep malformations, surgical excision (usually of the more superficial ones), or a combination of these modalities. Recent evidence supports surgical intervention. The surgical technique may require coordination between multiple locations and a prolonged anesthetic. However, the extra time and transport is worth the generally good outcome and avoidance of subsequent craniotomies for further resection if there is a residual arteriovenous malformation. A postoperative obliteration rate of 100% using a protocol of immediate postcraniotomy cerebral angiography to confirm obliteration has been reported.[184]

Management for elective embolic procedures involves general anesthesia. Moderate hyperventilation may enhance visualization of abnormal blood vessels that do not respond with vasoconstriction. The anesthesiologist should be knowledgeable about the types of embolic agents that can be used and their potential complications. Anticonvulsant therapy is routine. Neonates in cardiac failure may be receiving inotropic agents. Bleeding, especially from the femoral arterial puncture site (which cannot always be visualized), should always be a consideration. Fluid overload may result from the large amount of contrast agents administered, especially in a young infant who may already be in high-output cardiac failure. The anesthesiologist should be prepared for the possibility of an emergency craniotomy if a vessel ruptures.

Aneurysms
Intracranial aneurysms most often result from a congenital malformation in an arterial wall. Children with coarctation of the aorta or polycystic kidney disease have an increased incidence of these aneurysms. They usually remain asymptomatic during childhood; most ruptures that occur in childhood are fatal. Symptoms of subarachnoid or intracerebral hemorrhage frequently appear suddenly in a previously healthy young adult. When technically feasible, surgical ligation or clipping constitutes the treatment of choice.[185]

Anesthesia for surgical resection of vascular malformations and aneurysms in children presents unique challenges, especially if the diagnosis has been preceded by an intracranial hemorrhage. Blood products should be in the operating room and verified before the start of the procedure. An adequate depth of anesthesia should be ensured before any invasive maneuver to prevent precipitous hypertension. Adequate venous access to respond to sudden and massive blood loss is crucial but can wait until after induction of anesthesia. A blood-warming device, such as a rapid transfusion device, should be immediately available.

Controlled hypotension may be valuable in some situations for brief periods to reduce tension in the abnormal blood vessels and improve the safety of surgical manipulation.[186] It is not clear, however, whether the benefits of controlled hypotension are worth the risks, especially in small children (see Chapter 12). Controlled hypotension should not be used in children with increased ICP because of the risk of decreasing CPP, with resulting ischemia and further increased ICP. Although the absolute limits of acceptable hypotension are unknown, a mean blood pressure greater than 40 mm Hg for infants or 50 mm Hg for older children appears to be safe; teenagers should have a target MAP no less than 55 mm Hg. At the conclusion of the procedure, the blood pressure is returned to normal, but before closing the dura, the operative site should be inspected for bleeding.

Hemodynamic stability is important during emergence to avoid bucking, coughing, straining, and hypertension during extubation. Excessive hypertension can result in postoperative bleeding, although in most cases of aneurysm clipping, a slightly increased blood pressure may be desirable postoperatively to minimize the risk of vasospasm. After resection of an arteriovenous malformation, there can be serious postoperative complications related to cerebral edema with increased ICP or hemorrhage. This *normal perfusion pressure breakthrough* is probably caused by hyperemia of the areas surrounding the previous arteriovenous malformation site, where vessels suffer from continued vasomotor paralysis and cannot vasoconstrict. Treatment is controversial but usually involves therapy for increased ICP (e.g., diuretics, moderate hyperventilation, head elevation) in addition to judicious use of moderate hypotension (while maintaining CPP) and moderate hypothermia. When surgery is completed, it is important that children are able to cooperate with a neurologic examination and that there is careful control of blood pressure in the intensive care unit.

Moyamoya Disease

Moyamoya disease is an anomaly that results in progressive and life-threatening occlusion of intracranial vessels, primarily the internal carotid arteries near the circle of Willis.[187] An abnormal vascular network of collaterals develops at the base of the brain, and the appearance of these many, small vessels on angiography was originally described by the Japanese name *moyamoya*, which roughly translates as "puff of smoke" (Fig. 26.10A). The congenital form of the disease can involve the systemic vasculature, including pulmonary, coronary, and renal vessels; affected renal arteries are the most commonly identified angiographic lesion. The acquired variety (i.e., moyamoya syndrome) may be associated with meningitis, neurofibromatosis, chronic inflammation, connective tissue diseases, certain hematologic disorders, Down syndrome, or prior intracranial radiation.[188] Some children with neurologic symptoms from sickle cell disease may also have moyamoya.[189] Moyamoya disease appears to be more common among children of Japanese ancestry. Associated intracranial aneurysms are rare in children but may occur in more than 10% of affected adult patients. Abnormal ECG findings have been described with the syndrome in adults.

Moyamoya disease usually manifests as transient ischemic attacks progressing to strokes and fixed neurologic deficits in children. These attacks may be precipitated by hyperventilation.[190] The morbidity and mortality rates are high if the condition is left untreated. Medical management consists of antiplatelet therapy, such as aspirin, or calcium channel blockers. The most common surgical operation for correction in children is pial synangiosis, which involves suturing a scalp artery (usually the superficial temporal artery) directly onto the pial surface of the brain to enhance angiogenesis (Fig. 26.10B).[191]

Careful and continuous monitoring of ETCO2 is essential in anesthesia management.[192] Children with moyamoya disease have reduced hemispheric blood flow bilaterally, and hyperventilation may further reduce regional blood flow and cause EEG and neurologic changes.[193] *Normocapnia must be maintained throughout all phases of the procedure,* including induction of anesthesia. Adequate hydration and maintenance of baseline blood pressure are

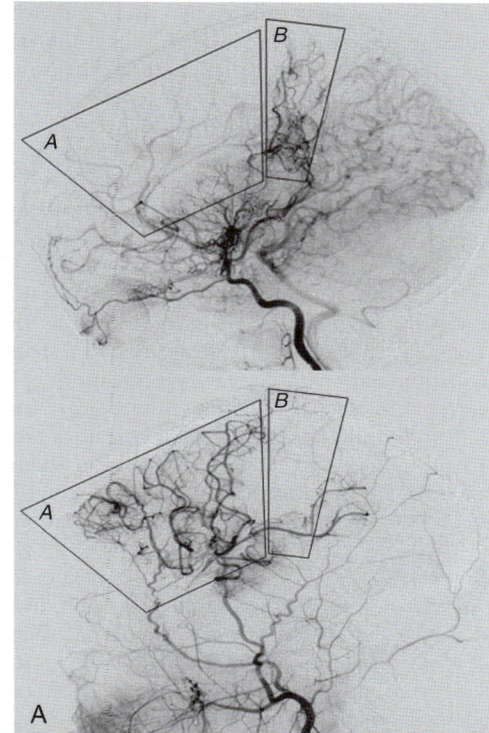

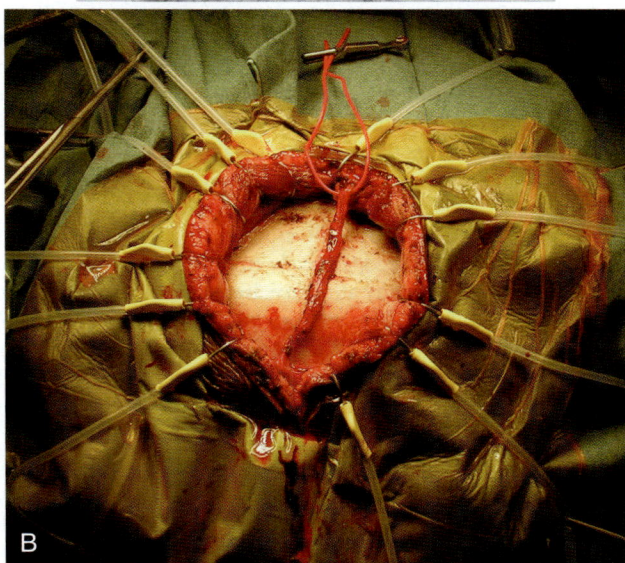

FIGURE 26.10 Moyamoya disease. **A,** The top angiogram shows the pattern of arterial filling after injection of the internal carotid artery in a child with moyamoya disease before pial synangiosis. *Area A* shows poor filling from the middle cerebral artery as a result of the disease process. *Area B* shows the characteristic hazy collaterals, or moyamoya vessels. The bottom angiogram is from the same child after pial synangiosis. The angiogram was obtained after injection of the superficial temporal artery, and it shows good filling in the middle cerebral artery distribution in *area A*. *Area B* does not fill from the middle cerebral artery. **B,** Pial synangiosis. The superficial temporal artery is prepared to be sutured to the pia of the cerebral cortex. After the craniotomy is completed, this artery can be sewn directly onto the underlying pia mater. The result of this procedure is improvement of blood flow to ischemic areas of the cerebral cortex.

indispensable. Most of these children have an IV catheter inserted the night before surgery and are given 1.5 times the amount of maintenance fluids to avoid dehydration during the perioperative period. EEG monitoring during these procedures can detect and help to treat ischemia that appears to be a result of cerebral vasoconstriction in response to direct surgical manipulation of the brain.[194] Normothermia is maintained, particularly at the end of the procedure, to avoid postoperative shivering and an exaggerated stress response. As with most neurosurgical procedures, a smooth extubation without hypertension or crying is desirable. Although scant literature exists regarding intraoperative and postoperative complications during moyamoya surgery, it appears that most complications (e.g., strokes) occur postoperatively and are associated with dehydration and crying (i.e., hyperventilation) episodes.[195] Those centers that regularly perform this surgery have better outcomes,[196] indicating that higher-volume centers are able to provide improved care and reduced mortality in children with moyamoya disease. The most marked benefit displayed was for those patients who underwent surgical revascularization.

Seizure Surgery

Epilepsy is one of the most common neurologic disorders of childhood. Despite the development of new drugs and regimens, the prevalence of pharmacologically intractable seizures remains high. Advances in neuroimaging, functional MRI, and EEG monitoring provide epileptologists anatomic targets that mediate some medically intractable seizure disorders.[197] Advances in pediatric neurosurgery have exploited these technologies and dramatically improved the outcomes for infants and children.[198]

Children presenting for surgical management of seizures take anticonvulsant medications, which can have serious adverse effects, including abnormalities of hematologic function such as abnormal coagulation, depression of red or white blood cell production, and decreased platelet counts.[199] Other problems may arise from altered hepatic function. Specific anticonvulsant concentrations should be determined preoperatively to detect subtherapeutic or toxic concentrations. Many anticonvulsants enhance metabolism of nondepolarizing NMBDs and opioids, increasing (up to 50%) the amount of these drugs needed during a surgical procedure. The preoperative evaluation should detect underlying conditions that are causing the seizures and the disabilities that can result from progressive neurologic dysfunction.

A major concern during resection of seizure foci is avoiding harming brain tissue that controls vital functions, such as motion, sensation, speech, and memory (the so-called eloquent cortex), especially if a seizure focus is adjacent to cortical areas controlling these functions. Cooperative adolescents and adults can assist in determination of the limits of safe cortical resection if they can be continually assessed during the surgical procedure. The technique of awake craniotomy is often performed in carefully selected adolescents. An awake craniotomy encompasses a wide variety of techniques whose common goal is to allow intraoperative assessment and feedback to determine if the eloquent cortex is at risk during resection.

Children are selected for this procedure on an individual basis. Most children younger than 12 years of age and many teenagers cannot tolerate an awake craniotomy. However, selected individuals may do well. The anesthesiologist should have detailed conversations with the child and parents to determine appropriateness before initiating such a procedure.

Some practitioners perform the entire procedure, including line placement, infiltration of local anesthetic, skull and dural opening, and resection, with the child completely awake or with minimal sedation. This particular approach requires an extremely motivated child. A variation on this technique uses short-acting sedatives and analgesics, such as propofol and fentanyl or remifentanil, titrated to induce unconsciousness but maintain spontaneous ventilation for instillation of local anesthetics, insertion of monitoring catheters, placement of head pins, and skull opening.[200] Subsequently, children can be allowed to awaken during surgical resection. They can then have sedatives and opioids reinstituted for the craniotomy closure.

Alternatively, some anesthesiologists use the asleep-awake-asleep technique. It consists of inducing general anesthesia and maintaining airway control with a supraglottic device (i.e., laryngeal mask airway). General anesthesia is maintained for line placement, placement of head pins, and skull and dural opening. The child is then awakened, the supraglottic airway is removed, and the surgeons proceed with resection. At the conclusion of the resection, general anesthesia is again induced and the supraglottic airway is reinserted for closure of the dura, skull, and skin. There are several disadvantages to the asleep-awake-asleep approach. One of the major concerns with this approach is airway management during emergence and induction while the child is in head pins. If the child coughs or bucks while immobilized, cervical spine injuries or scalp lacerations can occur. Brain swelling is also a concern in a child who is breathing spontaneously under general anesthesia with an inhalational anesthetic and possibly nitrous oxide.

Regardless of the technique chosen, the anesthesiologist must have an in-depth discussion with the child or adolescent about intraoperative needs and expectations.[201] The preoperative period is the time to decide whether the child is a candidate for an awake craniotomy. There are no randomized, controlled trials comparing the safety or effectiveness of the techniques described.

Younger children (<12 years of age) or uncooperative children of any age do not tolerate this approach and require general anesthesia throughout. In these circumstances, intraoperative electrophysiologic studies, such as somatosensory evoked potentials, EEG, and motor stimulation, may be used to help localize and determine the function of the site of planned resection. If EEG studies are to be performed, the anesthetic technique should be adjusted to maximize EEG signals. If direct cortical motor stimulation is planned, NMBDs must be permitted to wear off. Occasionally, a seizure focus is difficult to identify intraoperatively. In these situations, hyperventilation or methohexital (in small doses, 0.25–0.5 mg/kg) may be helpful in lowering the seizure threshold and producing EEG seizure activity.[202,203]

In some children, the site of origin of generalized seizures is difficult to determine. When this occurs, evaluation with intracranial EEG monitoring ("grids and strips") may be accomplished with direct electrocorticography (E-Fig. 26.2). The leads are placed on the surface of the cortex after a craniotomy performed with general anesthesia. Intraoperative EEG monitoring is limited during these procedures to ensuring that all leads are functional; monitoring for seizures takes place over the next several days to identify a focus that is amenable to resection. These children need to be observed carefully in the postoperative period because complications can develop from having intracranial electrodes in place. Because air frequently persists in the skull for up to 3 weeks after a craniotomy,[97] these children should not have nitrous oxide administered for a subsequent procedure (e.g., to resect a seizure focus, to remove the electrocorticography leads) until their dura has been opened to prevent the development of tension pneumocephalus.

The development of intraoperative MRI (iMRI) has aided in the surgical treatment of epilepsy. There continues to be great interest in the development of this technology to assist perioperatively with a variety of neurosurgical procedures and aid in facilitating optimal outcomes. This technology naturally lends itself to seizure surgery when a focal lesion can be identified. There is evidence in the adult literature supporting the use of iMRI in seizure surgery to facilitate higher resection volumes and consequently improved postoperative seizure outcomes.[204] A retrospective review of the role of iMRI in children undergoing resection for peri-eloquent cortical dysplasias and heterotopias has suggested that, comparison with conventional surgical approaches in these patients, iMRI led to elevated rates of gross total resection and a seizure-free postoperative course. Further, the use of iMRI in these patients led to a decrease in postoperative neurologic deficits.[205] Similar results have been published using iMRI in pediatric patients undergoing surgical resection of focal cortical dysplasia.[206]

When a focal resection is not possible, a lobectomy or corpus callosotomy may be attempted. However, children undergoing the latter procedure are often somnolent for the first few postoperative days, especially if a complete callosotomy is performed. This also occurs in children who have undergone insertion of multiple subdural grids and strips. Occasionally, small children undergo a hemispherectomy because their seizures are attributed to an abnormal hemisphere that is already severely dysfunctional, as when affected by hemiparesis. These can be challenging cases for the anesthesiologist because much blood can be lost (from one-half to multiples of the estimated blood volume).[207] This procedure is usually performed when children are very young to permit the other hemisphere to take over the function of both sides. Large-bore IV access is necessary in these cases to facilitate rapid replacement of blood, crystalloid solutions, and medications. Arterial pressure monitoring is routine, and many practitioners also use CVP monitoring.

An advance in the treatment of epilepsy has been the development of the vagal nerve stimulator. Although its exact mechanism of action is not well understood, it appears to inhibit seizure activity at brainstem or cortical levels.[208,209] It is becoming a popular form of treatment because it has shown benefit with minimal side effects in many children who are disabled by intractable seizures. Large, randomized trials are being conducted to determine the overall efficacy of this treatment. There are few published series of vagal nerve stimulation in children, but it is estimated that there is a 60% to 70% improvement in seizure control, with the best results achieved in those with drop attacks.[210,211]

The vagal nerve stimulator is a programmable device similar to a cardiac pacemaker and is placed subcutaneously under the left anterior chest wall. Bipolar platinum stimulating electrode coils, which are implanted around the left vagus nerve, are connected to the generator by subcutaneously tunneled wires. The device automatically activates for up to 30 seconds every 5 minutes. Although stimulation of the vagal nerve in this manner may affect vocal cord function, sudden bradycardia or other side effects are uncommon.[212] When children with vagal nerve stimulators return for subsequent operations, it may be appropriate to deactivate the stimulator while the child is receiving general anesthesia in order to prevent repetitive vocal cord motion.

A recently implemented technique of ablating deeper brain seizure foci such as hypothalamic hamartomas involves stereotactic placement of a laser catheter into the lesion in question and real-time thermal ablation under MR guidance. This so-called laser-induced thermal therapy (LITT) has been used for several years but its use in children is more recent. This technique offers potential for surgical treatment of lesions previously deemed too dangerous to operate on or even simply unresectable. There is some evidence of its efficacy and safety in children, especially for epilepsy surgery.[213,214]

HYDROCEPHALUS

Hydrocephalus is a condition involving a mismatch of CSF production and absorption, resulting in an increased intracranial CSF volume. It can be caused by a variety of pathologic processes, including arachnoid cysts (E-Fig. 26.3). Except for rare instances of excess CSF production, such as in choroid plexus papillomas, most cases of hydrocephalus result from some type of obstruction or an inability to absorb CSF appropriately. Commonly, this is a result of neonatal intraventricular or subarachnoid hemorrhage, congenital problems (e.g., aqueductal stenosis), trauma, infection, or tumors, especially those in the posterior fossa. Hydrocephalus can be classified as nonobstructive/communicating or obstructive/noncommunicating based on the ability of CSF to flow around the spinal cord in its usual manner.

Intracranial hypertension or decreased intracranial compliance typically accompanies untreated hydrocephalus in children. How much intracranial compliance exists and how acutely hydrocephalus develops are both factors in how severe the signs and symptoms of hydrocephalus become. If hydrocephalus develops slowly in the young infant, the skull will expand and the cerebral cortical mantle will stretch until massive craniomegaly (often with irreversible neurologic damage) occurs. However, if the cranial bones are fused or the cranium cannot expand fast enough, neurologic signs and symptoms rapidly become apparent. The child may become progressively more lethargic and develop vomiting, cranial nerve dysfunction (i.e., setting sun sign), bradycardia, brain herniation, and death.

Unless the cause of the hydrocephalus can be definitively treated, treatment usually involves surgical placement of an extracranial shunt. Most shunts transport CSF from the lateral ventricles to the peritoneal cavity (i.e., ventriculoperitoneal [VP] shunts). The distal end of the shunt occasionally must be placed in the right atrium or pleural cavity, usually because of problems with the ability of the peritoneal cavity to absorb CSF. Newer shunt systems with programmable valves reduce the need for shunt revisions.[215]

The use of a percutaneous flexible neuroendoscope through a burr hole in the skull has provided an alternative to extracranial shunt placement.[216,217] During these procedures, a ventriculostomy may be made to bypass an obstruction (e.g., aqueductal stenosis) by forming a communicating hole from one area of CSF flow to another using a blunt probe inserted through the neuroendoscope (Video 26.1). Common locations for a ventriculostomy are through the septum pellucidum (allowing lateral ventricles to communicate) or through the floor of the third ventricle into the adjacent CSF cisterns. Complications such as damage to the basilar artery or its branches or neural injuries can be life-threatening when they occur, and the anesthesiologist should be prepared for an emergency craniotomy during these procedures. Hemodynamic instability may occur intraoperatively if excessive cold irrigating solutions or large volumes are infused through the endoscope. As endoscopic techniques become more commonplace, it is important for anesthesiologists to understand the unique challenges endoscopic neurosurgical procedures present.[218]

The anesthetic plan for a child with hydrocephalus should be directed at controlling ICP and relieving the obstruction as soon as possible. Children with an increased ICP are at risk for vomiting and pulmonary aspiration. Rapid-sequence induction and tracheal intubation should be performed. Ketamine is generally avoided because of its potential to cause sudden massive intracranial hypertension[219]; however, there is some evidence that ketamine may ameliorate the increased ICP in some children.[220,221] In infants, hydrocephalus often produces large, dilated scalp veins, and they can be used for induction of anesthesia if necessary. If IV access cannot be established, induction with sevoflurane and gentle cricoid pressure may be an alternative, although less desirable, method of induction.[222] This method results in venodilation and usually facilitates establishment of IV access. After an IV catheter is inserted, the child may be paralyzed, the lungs ventilated, the trachea intubated, and the inhalational agent decreased or discontinued. The possibility of VAE during placement of the distal end of a ventriculoatrial shunt should always be considered. Postoperatively, children should be observed carefully because an altered mental status and recent peritoneal incision place them at increased risk for pulmonary aspiration after feeding begins. Analgesia may be provided with a variety of easily performed blocks of the head (see Figs. 42.9–42.11).

Anesthesiologists should be familiar with a few special situations involving shunts. Children who develop a shunt infection usually have the entire shunt system removed and external ventricular drainage established. They return to the operating room for insertion of a new shunt several days after the infection has been treated with antibiotics. While an external drain is in place, the operator must be careful not to dislodge the ventricular tubing. The height of the drainage bag should not be significantly changed in relation to the child's head to avoid sudden alterations in ICP. For example, suddenly lowering an open drainage bag can siphon CSF rapidly from the head, resulting in collapse of the ventricles and rupture of cortical veins. When transporting children with CSF drainage or when moving them from a stretcher to an operating room table, it is best to close off the ventriculostomy tubing during these brief periods.

Anesthesiologists should be aware of the condition known as slit ventricle syndrome (Fig. 26.11). This situation develops in 5% to 10% of children with CSF shunts and is associated with overdrainage of CSF and small, slit-like, lateral ventricular spaces. Children with this condition do not have the usual amount of intracranial CSF to compensate for alterations in brain or intracranial blood volume. Special attention should be paid when CT scans identify this condition. It is probably safest to avoid the administration of excess or hypotonic IV solutions in these situations in the intraoperative and postoperative periods to minimize the potential for brain swelling. Some of these children cannot

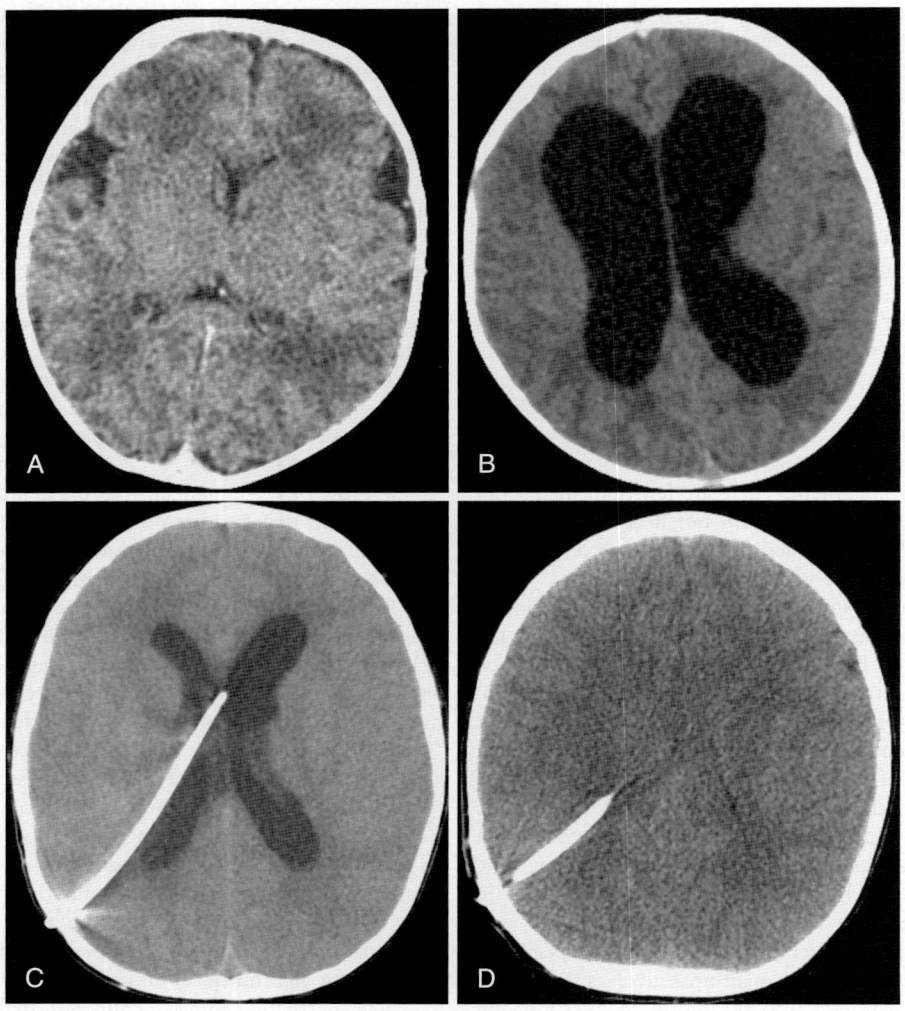

FIGURE 26.11 Computed tonographic scans of children with normal-sized ventricles **(A)**, untreated hydrocephalus **(B)**, hydrocephalus treated with a ventricular shunt **(C)**, and hydrocephalus treated with a ventricular shunt, resulting in slit ventricles **(D)**. (Courtesy Ellen Grant, MD.)

accommodate to situations that otherwise healthy children can easily tolerate. Episodes of postoperative cerebral herniation have been reported after uneventful surgical procedures.[54]

CONGENITAL ANOMALIES

Congenital CNS anomalies typically occur as midline defects. This dysraphism may occur anywhere along the neural axis, involving the head (i.e., encephalocele) (Fig. 26.12A) or spine (i.e., meningomyelocele) (Fig. 26.12B). The defect may be relatively minor and affect only superficial bony and membranous structures, or it may include a large segment of malformed neural tissue.

Encephalocele

Encephaloceles can occur anywhere from the occiput to the frontal area. They can even appear to be nasal polyps if they protrude through the cribriform plate. They are rarely filled with so much CSF that the defect can be almost as large as the head itself (see Fig. 26.12A). Large defects may present challenges to tracheal intubation. Blood loss can be severe, especially if venous sinuses are involved. Adequate IV access should be ensured and blood products readily available. If hemodynamic instability is anticipated, an arterial catheter is indicated.

Myelodysplasia

Defects in the spine are known as *spina bifida*. Meningoceles are lesions containing CSF without spinal tissue. When neural tissue is also present within the lesion, the defect is called a *meningomyelocele*. Open neural tissue is known as *rachischisis*. Hydrocephalus is usually present and is often associated with a type II Chiari malformation.

Most children with a meningomyelocele present for primary closure of the defect within the first 24 hours of life to minimize the risk of infection. Many are now scheduled electively before birth for repair because the defect is usually apparent on prenatal ultrasonography. Many neurosurgeons prefer to insert a ventriculoperitoneal shunt at the time of initial surgery. Alternatively, a shunt may be inserted a few days later or is occasionally deferred if there is no evidence of hydrocephalus at birth.

A major anesthesia consideration is positioning the neonate for induction at surgery. In most cases, tracheal intubation can be performed with the infant in the supine position and the uninvolved portion of the child's back supported with towels (or a donut ring) so there is no direct pressure on the meningomyelocele. For very large defects, it is occasionally necessary to place the infant in the left lateral decubitus position for induction and tracheal intubation. Succinylcholine is rarely needed for tracheal intubation, although it is not associated with hyperkalemia because the defect develops early in gestation and is not associated with muscle denervation.[223] Airway management, mask fit, and intubation may be difficult in infants with massive hydrocephalus or very large defects. In such cases, a sedated "awake" intubation after preoxygenation and administration of atropine occasionally may be the safest alternative. Blood loss may be considerable during repair of a larger defect when skin is undermined to cover the defect.

Children with myelodysplasia are at high risk for latex sensitivity and possibly anaphylaxis.[48] This likely results from repeated exposure to latex products encountered during frequent bladder catheterizations and multiple (usually more than five) surgical procedures, during which latex gloves have been in contact with large mucosal surfaces. These children should be managed in a latex-free environment from birth to minimize the chances for

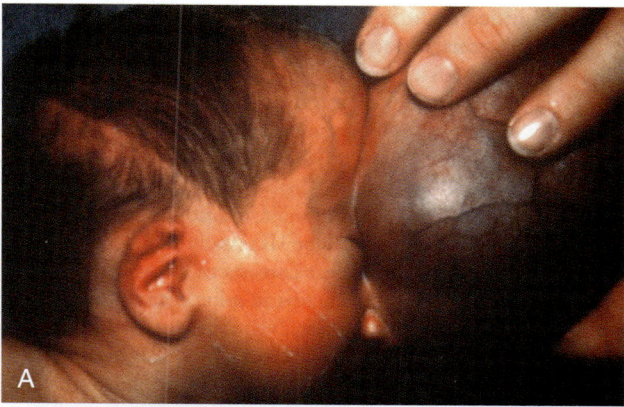

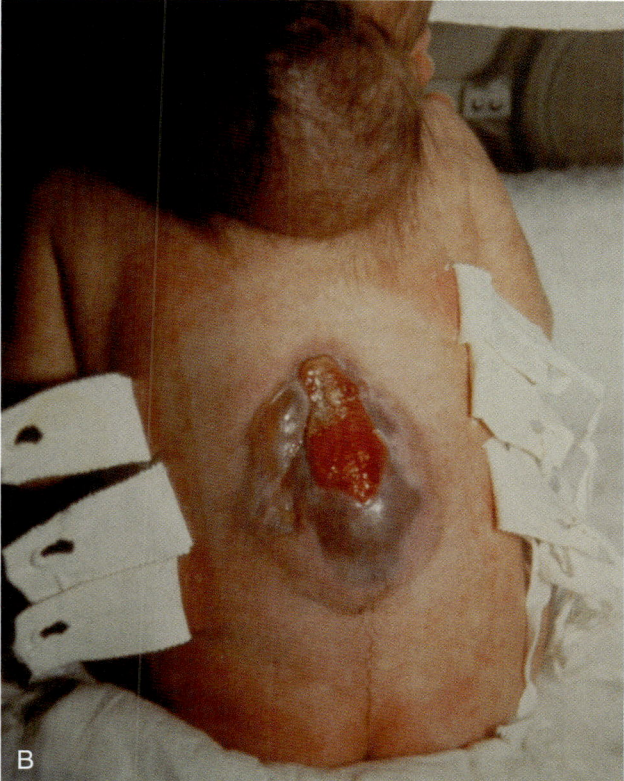

FIGURE 26.12 A, An infant with an anterior encephalocele. **B,** An infant with a posterior encephalocele and myelomeningocele defects. Notice the large exposed surface areas that make this child prone to dehydration. Difficulty may be encountered in positioning for induction of anesthesia and intubation; significant loss of blood and cerebrospinal fluid during surgical correction should be anticipated.

sensitization.[224] Latex allergy should be suspected if signs and symptoms of anaphylaxis develop during surgery. Suspected anaphylaxis should be treated with IV epinephrine in a dose of 1 to 10 µg/kg, as required. Many hospitals have replaced most or all of their latex-containing supplies with nonlatex alternatives; this has resulted in complete elimination or marked reduction of latex anaphylactic reactions during anesthesia in some institutions.[225] Children who develop latex allergy exhibit cross-reactivity with some antibiotics[226,227] and foods, especially tropical fruits such as avocados, kiwi fruit, and bananas.

Postoperatively, respiratory status should be carefully assessed. Pulse oximetry is valuable during recovery from anesthesia because breathing difficulties may occur after a tight skin closure and the ventilatory responses to hypoxia and hypercarbia may be diminished or absent when a Chiari malformation coexists.[228] Intrauterine surgery has been advocated as a way of diminishing the degree of damage caused by myelodysplasia.[229-231]

Chiari Malformations

There are several types of Chiari malformations (Table 26.3). The Arnold-Chiari malformation (type II) usually coexists in children with myelodysplasia. This defect consists of a bony abnormality in the posterior fossa and upper cervical spine with caudal displacement of the cerebellar vermis, fourth ventricle, and lower brainstem below the plane of the foramen magnum. Medullary cervical cord compression can occur (Figs. 26.13 and 26.14). Vocal cord paralysis with stridor and respiratory distress, apnea, abnormal swallowing and pulmonary aspiration, opisthotonos, and cranial nerve deficits

TABLE 26.3	Types of Chiari Malformation
Type I	Caudal displacement of cerebellar tonsils below the plane of the foramen magnum
Type II (Arnold-Chiari; associated with myelomeningocele)	Caudal displacement of the cerebellar vermis, fourth ventricle, and lower brainstem below the plane of the foramen magnum Dysplastic brainstem with characteristic kink, elongation of the fourth ventricle, beaking of the quadrigeminal plate, hypoplastic tentorium with small posterior fossa, polymicrogyria, enlargement of the massa intermedia
Type III	Caudal displacement of the cerebellum and brainstem into a high cervical meningocele
Type IV	Cerebellar hypoplasia

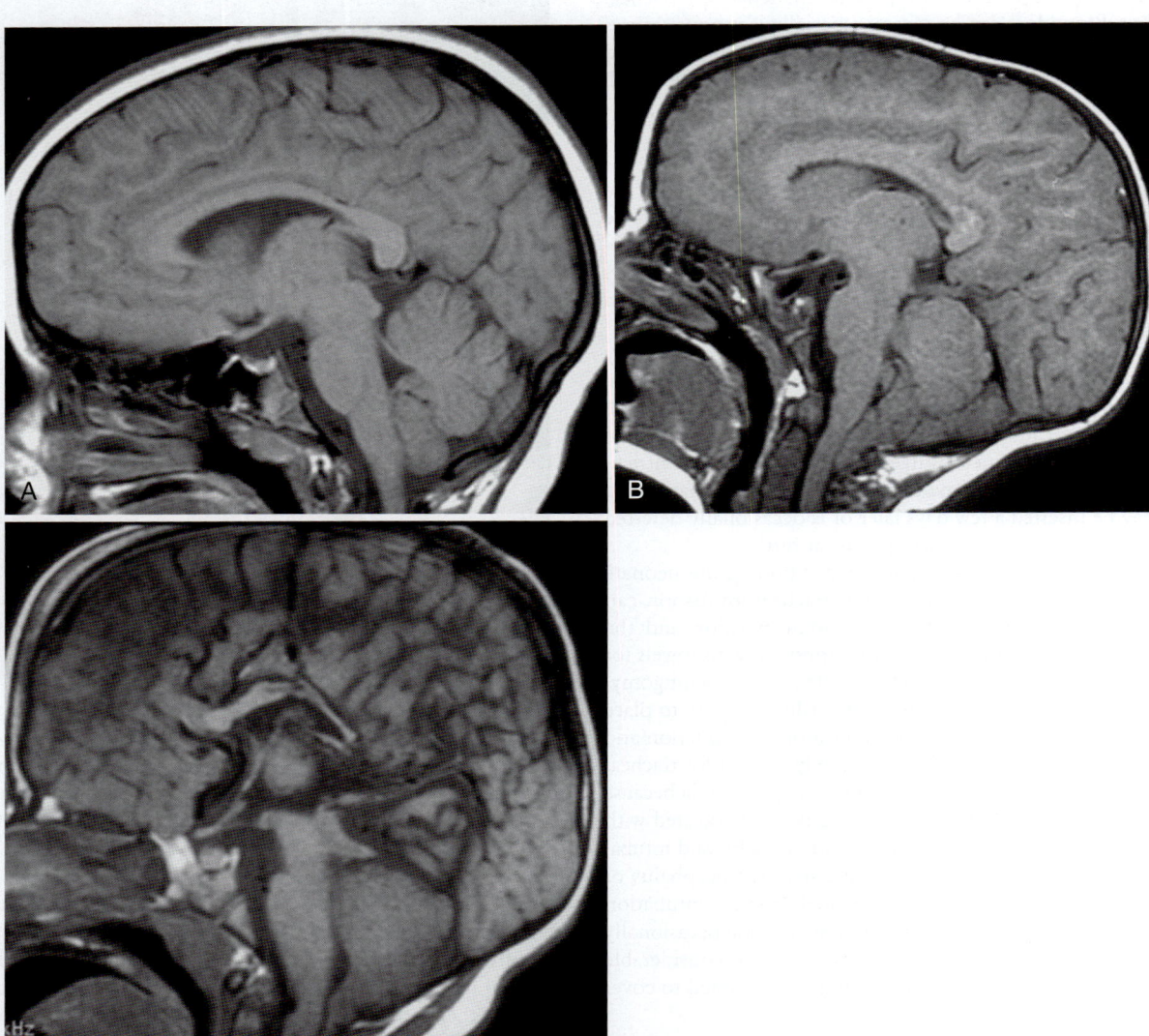

FIGURE 26.13 A, Sagittal, T1-weighted magnetic resonance imaging (MRI) of a normal child. **B,** Sagittal, T1-weighted MRI of a child with a Chiari I malformation, which consists of caudal displacement of the cerebellar tonsils at least 5 mm into the upper cervical spinal canal, often with no clinical symptoms. **C,** Sagittal, T1-weighted MRI of a child with a type II Chiari malformation, which is characterized by caudal displacement of the cerebellar tonsils, additional brain anomalies, and a meningomyelocele deformity. (Courtesy Ellen Grant, MD.)

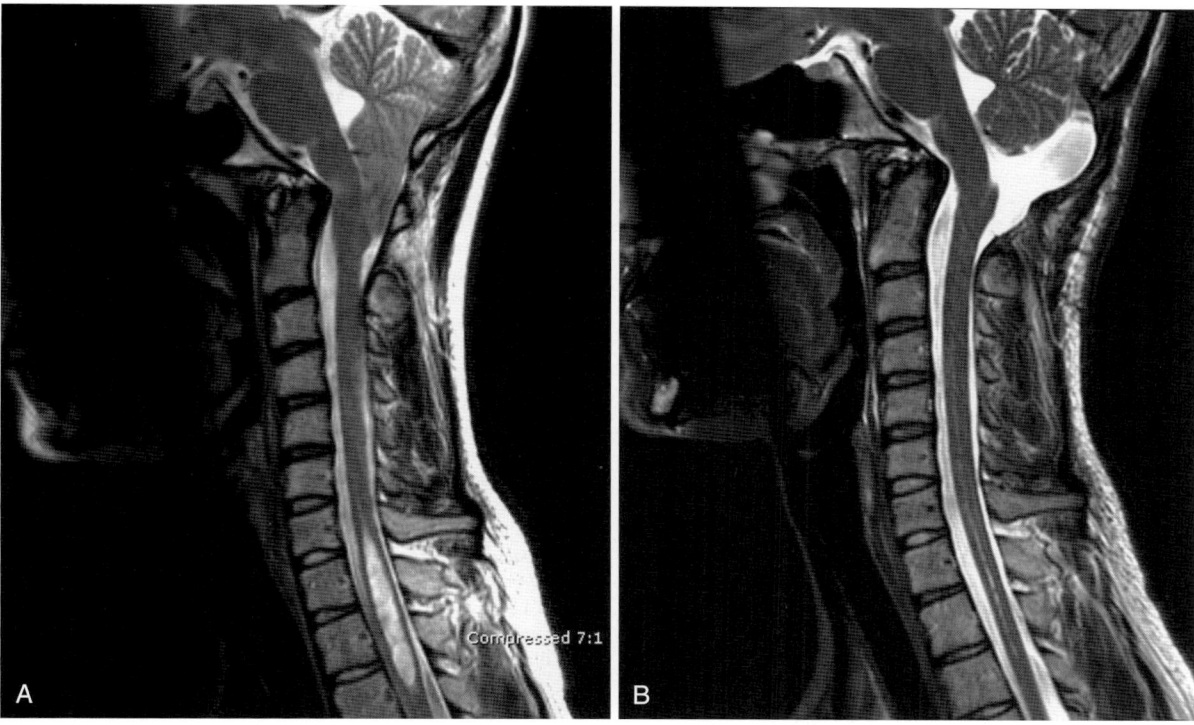

FIGURE 26.14 The images show the posterior fossa in a child with a Chiari II malformation before and after posterior fossa decompression. **A,** Notice the downward herniation of the cerebellar tonsils. **B,** Resolution of cerebellar tonsillar herniation after posterior fossa decompression.

may be associated with the Arnold-Chiari malformation and usually manifests during infancy. Children with vocal cord paralysis or a diminished gag reflex may require tracheostomy and gastrostomy to secure the airway and to minimize chronic aspiration. Children of any age may have abnormal responses to hypoxia and hypercarbia because of cranial nerve and brainstem dysfunction.[228,232] Extreme head flexion may cause brainstem compression in otherwise asymptomatic children.

Type I Chiari malformations can occur in healthy children without myelodysplasia. These defects also involve caudal displacement of the cerebellar tonsils below the foramen magnum, but children usually have much milder symptoms, sometimes manifesting only as headache or neck pain.[233] Surgical treatment usually involves a decompressive suboccipital craniectomy with cervical laminectomies.

Other Spinal Defects

Other spinal anomalies (e.g., lipomeningoceles, lipomyelomeningoceles, diastematomyelias, dermoid tracts) may manifest as tethered cords. Skin defects, typically over the lower lumbar region, may occur as dural sinus tracks or lipomeningoceles. Midline hair tufts, skin dimples, or fat pads may be associated with spinal defects. These anomalies sometimes manifest when toilet training or ambulation is observed to be abnormal or later in childhood when children complain of back pain. Children who have had a meningomyelocele repaired after birth may also develop an ascending neurologic deficit from a tethered spinal cord during growth. Early detection of a tethered cord is easily diagnosed with MRI. Prophylactic surgical untethering is common.

Anesthesia management for surgical release of a tethered cord usually entails monitoring the innervation of the lower extremities and bowel and bladder with nerve stimulators and rectal electromyelograms or manometry. Muscle relaxants should be avoided or permitted to dissipate before intraoperative assessment.

NEURORADIOLOGIC PROCEDURES

Many neuroradiologic procedures are performed in children. Anesthetic considerations for neurodiagnostic procedures (e.g., CT, MRI) are discussed elsewhere (see Chapters 46 and 48), but certain therapeutic neuroradiologic procedures are addressed here.

To improve intraoperative navigation during intracranial procedures, the concept of iMRI was introduced in the mid-1990s. The technology has advanced to include a variety of operating room suite designs that encompass MRI machines (E-Fig. 26.4). These procedures present special challenges for neurosurgeons and anesthesiologists.[234–238] As with anesthesia for diagnostic MRI scans, special monitors, infusion pumps, and an MRI-safe or MRI-conditional anesthesia machine are required. It is challenging to do surgical procedures in this environment, especially because these procedures may take many hours, they may be associated with significant blood loss, and access to the child is severely limited. Some monitoring equipment found in conventional operating rooms (e.g., precordial Doppler ultrasonography, core temperature probes, fluid warmers) is not MRI safe or conditional. Nevertheless, numerous neurosurgical procedures have been safely performed in children in these MRI operating rooms, and the equipment for these procedures is rapidly evolving.

ACKNOWLEDGMENTS

The authors wish to thank Mark A. Rockoff, Veronica Miller, MD, and Elizabeth A. Eldredge, MD, for their prior contributions to this chapter.

ANNOTATED REFERENCES

Coles JP, Fryer TD, Coleman MR, et al. Hyperventilation following head injury: effect on ischemic burden and cerebral oxidative metabolism. *Crit Care Med.* 2007;35:568-578.

Hyperventilation has a detrimental effect on brain tissue at risk after head injury. The authors refute the often-taught dogma regarding routine hyperventilation, especially after a traumatic brain injury. This article and several others on the same subject should give the anesthesiologist pause when hyperventilating children with intracranial pathology.

Cox RG, Levy R, Hamilton MG, et al. Anesthesia can be safely provided for children in a high-field intraoperative magnetic resonance imaging environment. *Paediatr Anaesth.* 2011;21:454-458.

This case series demonstrates the safety of intraoperative MRI for neurosurgical procedures in children. As this technology becomes more prevalent, pediatric neuroanesthesiologists need to be aware of the challenges in caring for patients in this unique environment.

Davidson AJ, Disma N, deGraff JC, et al. Neurodevelopmental outcome at 2 years of age after general anesthesia and awake-regional anaesthesia in infancy (GAS): an international multicenter, randomized controlled trial. *Lancet.* 2016;387:239-250.

This study and that by Sun et al. (see later) represent the current best knowledge regarding concerns of anesthetic exposure in children. Both studies demonstrated no difference in neurocognitive outcomes between the general anesthesia groups and controls. They both conclude that a single, relatively brief general anesthetic does not appear to put a child at risk of adverse neurocognitive outcomes. Both of these studies will continue to be cited and discussed frequently. It is important for pediatric anesthesiologists to be familiar with them.

Jevtovic-Todorovic V, Hartman RE, Izumi Y, et al. Early exposure to common anesthetic agents causes widespread neurodegeneration in the developing rat brain and persistent learning deficits. *J Neurosci.* 2003;23:876-882.

This extremely important paper addresses the controversies surrounding the use of common anesthetic agents in neonates. The authors present compelling animal data showing that commonly used anesthetic agents such as isoflurane cause histologically evident neurodegeneration and cause behavioral and cognition problems. This reference is commonly cited when this discussion arises. However, directly extrapolating these data to the practice of anesthetizing neonates is questionable, especially in light of recently published studies. This is an issue that will require much more research to clearly define.

Lassen NA, Christensen MS. Physiology of cerebral blood flow. *Br J Anaesth.* 1976;48:719-734.

This classic review article discusses the various physiologic mechanisms of control of cerebral blood flow.

Pollack IF. Brain tumors in children. *N Engl J Med.* 1994;331:1500-1507.

Although this review is from the 1990s, it provides a comprehensive overview of the epidemiology of pediatric brain tumors and treatment approaches. Knowledge of various treatment approaches to different histologic types of tumors can inform the anesthesiologist about the extent of the process behind the procedure and how aggressive the surgery needs to be to achieve a desired outcome.

Reasoner DK, Todd MM, Scamman FL, Warner DS. The incidence of pneumocephalus after supratentorial craniotomy: observations on the disappearance of intracranial air. *Anesthesiology.* 1994;80:1008-1012.

This well-conceived study evaluates the length of time pneumocephalus persists after supratentorial craniotomy. The take-home message is that air persists in the head for several weeks after craniotomy, and care should be taken not to exacerbate the situation during subsequent administration of anesthetics. Nitrous oxide should be avoided in these children, because tension pneumocephalus could develop.

Sun LS, Li G, Miller TLK, et al.

See annotation for the article by Davidson AJ et al. earlier in this list.

Willie CK, Tzeng YC, Fisher JA, Ainslie PN. Integrative regulation of human brain blood flow. *J Physiol.* 2014;592(5):841-859.

This is a well-referenced review article that condenses current evidence on the regulation of cerebral blood flow in humans. It makes a compelling argument that our current understanding is overly simplistic and argues that we really should be thinking about CBF regulation in terms of a multisystem approach. Finally, the authors make the point that we should rethink concepts of such tight control of CBF (autoregulation) over a variety of parameters including mean arterial pressure.

A complete reference list can be found online at ExpertConsult.com.

Essentials of Endocrinology

ELLIOT J. KRANE, ERINN T. RHODES, REBECCA E. CLAURE,
ECHO ROWE, AND JOSEPH I. WOLFSDORF

Diabetes Mellitus*

The incidence of type 1 diabetes mellitus in children is increasing worldwide,[1-3] and while type 2 diabetes in children remains a less common disorder, its prevalence is also increasing.[4,5] The use of insulin pumps and various multicomponent insulin regimens has increased the complexity of perioperative management of children with diabetes. Anesthesiologists must carefully consider the pathophysiology of the disease, as well as each child's specific diabetes treatment regimen, glycemic control, intended surgery, and anticipated postoperative course, when devising an appropriate perioperative management plan. Standardized algorithms for perioperative diabetes management improve care[6-9] without significantly increasing costs[8]; several guidelines and studies of perioperative management of children with diabetes are available in the literature and examples are included.[10-16]

CLASSIFICATION AND EPIDEMIOLOGY IN CHILDREN

Type 1 and type 2 are the most common, but not the only, forms of diabetes (Table 27.1).[17,18] Type 1 diabetes is characterized by absolute deficiency of insulin, which usually results from immune-mediated destruction of pancreatic beta cells.[18] In contrast, type 2 diabetes is characterized by a combination of insulin resistance and a relative deficiency of insulin.[17,18] Children with type 2 diabetes typically are overweight and frequently have a first- or second-degree relative with type 2 diabetes.[17] However, the high prevalence of obesity in children[19] has blurred the distinction between type 1 and type 2 diabetes. Children with phenotypic characteristics of type 2 diabetes may have pancreatic autoimmunity,[20-23] and approximately 35% of children with diabetes who require exogenous insulin at diagnosis are overweight or obese[24,25]; these data are consistent with the prevalence of childhood overweight and obesity in the general U.S. pediatric population.[19]

Other forms of diabetes are less commonly encountered (see Table 27.1). Monogenic diabetes, formerly referred to as maturity-onset diabetes of the young (MODY), occurs in approximately 2% to 3% of the pediatric diabetes population, and with improvements in care, patients with cystic fibrosis–related diabetes account for a small, but significant, fraction of the diabetes population at major pediatric medical centers. Additional modifications to

*Adapted and updated from Rhodes ET, Ferrari LR, Wolfsdorf JI. Perioperative management of pediatric surgical patients with diabetes mellitus. *Anesth Analg.* 2005;101:986–999.

TABLE 27.1	Classification of Less Common Forms of Diabetes Mellitus

Genetic Defects of Beta Cell Function

Monogenic diabetes (formerly referred to as maturity-onset diabetes of the young [MODY])

Permanent neonatal diabetes

Mitochondrial disorders

Disease of the Exocrine Pancreas

Cystic fibrosis–related diabetes

Drug-Induced Diabetes

Steroids

Chemotherapeutic Agents

Genetic Syndromes

Prader-Willi syndrome

Down syndrome

Turner syndrome

Wolfram syndrome

Endocrinopathies

Autoimmune polyglandular syndrome

Cushing syndrome

(Modified from Rhodes ET, Ferrari LR, Wolfsdorf JI. Perioperative management of pediatric surgical patients with diabetes mellitus. *Anesth Analg.* 2005;101[4]: 986–999.)

TABLE 27.2	Insulin Preparations Classified According to Their Pharmacokinetic Profiles[a]		
Insulin Type	**Onset (h)**	**Peak (h)**	**Duration (h)**
Rapid-Acting[b]			
Insulin lispro (Humalog)[c]	<0.25	0.5–2.5	≤5
Insulin aspart (Novolog)[c]	<0.25	1–3	3–5
Insulin glulisine (Apidra)[c]	<0.25	0.5–1.5	3–5
Short-Acting[b]			
Regular (soluble)	0.5–1	2–4	5–8
Intermediate- and Long-Acting[b]			
NPH (isophane)	1–2	2–8	14–24
Insulin glargine (Lantus)[c]	2–4	No peak	20–24
Insulin detemir (Levemir)[c]	1–2	3–9	Up to 24
Insulin degludec (Tresiba)[c]	1–2	No peak	>42

NPH, neutral protamine Hagedorn.
[a]Times of onset, peak, and duration of action vary within and between patients and are affected by numerous factors, including dosage, site, depth of injection, dilution, temperature, and other factors.
[b]Premixed combinations of intermediate-acting and either rapid- or short-acting insulins are available whose pharmacodynamic profiles have a bimodal pattern reflecting the two insulin components.
[c]Insulin analog developed by modifying the amino acid sequence of the human insulin molecule.
Adapted from Rhodes ET, Ferrari LR, Wolfsdorf JI. Perioperative management of pediatric surgical patients with diabetes mellitus. *Anesth Analg.* 2005;101(4): 986–999.

the perioperative treatment regimen may be necessary when diabetes is associated with genetic syndromes and/or other endocrinopathies, such as adrenal insufficiency (see later discussion).

Although the worldwide incidence of type 1 diabetes is quite variable,[26] the incidence is increasing in almost all populations.[27] The SEARCH for Diabetes in Youth Study, which began in 2000, provides the most comprehensive estimates of the prevalence and incidence of type 1 and type 2 diabetes among U.S. youth younger than 20 years of age.[28–32] Type 1 diabetes remains the most common form of diabetes observed among U.S. youth, with the greatest prevalence (2.55 per 1000) among non-Hispanic white youth.[4] The epidemic of obesity contributed to a progressive increase in the incidence and prevalence of type 2 diabetes in U.S. children.[4] In the SEARCH study, the prevalence of type 2 diabetes in 10- to 19-year-old youth ranged from 0.17 per 1000 among non-Hispanic white youth to 1.20 per 1000 among Native American youth, and the incidence ranged from 3.7 per 100,000 per year among non-Hispanic white youth to 27.7 per 100,000 per year among Native American youth.[4,31–33] Increases in the prevalence and incidence of type 2 diabetes have also been noted in other parts of the world.[5,34–40]

GENERAL MANAGEMENT PRINCIPLES

Understanding both the pharmacokinetic and pharmacodynamic properties of insulin preparations and antihyperglycemic medications is critical to developing an appropriate perioperative plan.

Type 1 diabetes always requires treatment with insulin. However, an increasing number of insulin preparations (Table 27.2) and delivery systems are available.[41] The least complex regimens consist of two or three insulin injections per day. They incorporate a combination of an intermediate-acting insulin (e.g., neutral protamine Hagedorn [NPH]) and/or a long-acting insulin (e.g., insulin detemir [Levemir] or insulin glargine [Lantus]) for basal coverage with a short- or rapid-acting insulin (e.g., regular, insulin aspart [NovoLog], insulin lispro [Humalog], or insulin glulisine [Apidra]) to provide prandial glycemic coverage. More intensive multicomponent insulin regimens are being used with greater frequency and typically consist of insulin glargine, a long-acting insulin, which provides a relatively constant 24-hour basal concentration of circulating insulin without a pronounced peak to simulate basal insulin secretion,[42] in conjunction with rapid-acting insulin administered with food. Some studies have demonstrated superior glycemic control with such regimens compared with regimens using NPH insulin and regular insulin,[43] although the ideal insulin regimen for children with type 1 diabetes remains controversial and outcomes may differ geographically.[44–46] Another long-acting insulin, insulin detemir, may be used in intensive insulin regimens and has demonstrated more predictable glucose-reducing effects than both NPH[47–49] and insulin glargine.[47] The newest long-acting insulin, degludec (Tresiba), is approved for use in adults in many parts of the world[50] and recently received FDA approval for use in children and adolescents.[51,52]

Many children with type 1 diabetes are managed with an insulin pump.[46,53,54] This device administers a continuous subcutaneous infusion of insulin (typically a rapid-acting insulin, see Table 27.2) at a basal rate that is supplemented by bolus doses of rapid-acting insulin given with meals and snacks. In appropriately selected children, pump therapy has shown superiority over injection regimens.[55–59] Standard insulin preparations are U100, meaning that there are 100 units of insulin per milliliter. However, very young patients with type 1 diabetes may require diluted insulin (e.g., U10) to achieve accurate dosing.[60–62] Parents of preschool-aged children, especially toddlers, with type 1 diabetes should be specifically questioned and educated about their use of diluted insulin.

Most children with type 2 diabetes are managed with insulin and/or oral metformin, the only oral agent approved for use in children with diabetes in the United States.[63–65] Metformin's primary action is to decrease hepatic glucose production and, secondarily, to increase insulin sensitivity in peripheral tissues. Occasionally, other oral agents including sulfonylureas, which promote insulin secretion, and thiazolidinediones, which increase insulin sensitivity in muscle and adipose tissue, are used in adolescents.[66,67] Nutritional therapy is always included in the management of children with type 2 diabetes.[65] The **T**reatment **O**ptions for Type 2 **D**iabetes in **A**dolescents and **Y**outh (TODAY) trial,[68,69] evaluated the optimal treatment for type 2 diabetes in children and adolescents, age 10 to 17 years. In the TODAY trial, monotherapy with metformin was associated with durable glycemic control in approximately 50% of children and adolescents with type 2 diabetes. The addition of rosiglitazone, but not an intensive lifestyle intervention, was superior to metformin alone.

Increasingly, other medications used to manage adults with type 2 diabetes are being evaluated for use in children, although none are yet approved in the United States.[70,71] Incretins, including glucose-dependent insulinotropic polypeptide and glucagon-like peptide-1 (GLP-1), are gastrointestinal hormones released after eating that stimulate insulin secretion and are necessary for normal glucose tolerance.[72] GLP-1 acts through a G protein–coupled receptor to promote glucose-dependent insulin secretion, suppression of glucagon secretion, slowing of gastric emptying, and reduction in food intake.[70,73] Exenatide (Byetta) is a GLP-1 receptor agonist widely used in adults with type 2 diabetes as an adjunctive therapy for those taking metformin and/or a sulfonylurea.[74] Inhibitors of dipeptidyl peptidase-IV,[75] the enzyme that degrades GLP-1, are also increasingly being used for the treatment of type 2 diabetes in adults, but have not been approved for use in children. Pramlintide acetate (Symlin) is a synthetic amylin receptor agonist that can be used as an adjunct to insulin therapy in adults with type 1 or type 2 diabetes.[76–79] Amylin, a 37-amino acid polypeptide islet hormone cosecreted with insulin from islet beta cells,[70] has three effects: delay of gastric emptying, inhibition of glucagon secretion, and modulation of satiety.[70]

METABOLIC RESPONSE TO SURGERY

Trauma of any kind, and surgery in particular, triggers a complex neuroendocrine stress response that includes suppression of insulin secretion and increased production of counterregulatory hormones (frequently referred to as "stress hormones"), particularly cortisol and catecholamines.[80,81] Insulin is the primary anabolic hormone that promotes glucose uptake in muscle and adipose tissue while suppressing glucose production (glycogenolysis and gluconeogenesis) by the liver.[82] The counterregulatory hormones, which include epinephrine, glucagon, cortisol, and growth hormone, exert the opposite effects, resulting in resistance to insulin action[83–85] and an increase in blood glucose concentration by (1) stimulating glycogenolysis and gluconeogenesis in the liver, (2) increasing lipolysis and ketogenesis, and (3) inhibiting glucose uptake and utilization in muscle and fat. Glucagon, secreted by alpha cells in the pancreatic islets, suppresses insulin secretion while stimulating hepatic glycogenolysis, gluconeogenesis, and ketogenesis.[82,83] Epinephrine, which acts via β_2- and α_2-adrenergic receptors, stimulates glucagon production, increases glycogenolysis and gluconeogenesis, stimulates lipolysis, decreases insulin secretion, and decreases glucose utilization in insulin-sensitive tissues.[82]

Cortisol stimulates gluconeogenesis, proteolysis, and lipolysis and decreases glucose utilization.[83,86] Growth hormone augments glucose production, decreases glucose utilization, and accelerates lipolysis.[87] Proinflammatory cytokines may further stimulate secretion of counterregulatory hormones and alter insulin receptor signaling.[85] These changes increase catabolism, as evidenced by increased hepatic glucose production and breakdown of protein and fat. In the patient with diabetes with absolute or relative insulin deficiency, the enhanced catabolism resulting from surgical trauma can lead to marked hyperglycemia and even diabetic ketoacidosis.[88] These metabolic effects may be exacerbated by a prolonged fast before surgery.

METABOLIC RESPONSE TO ANESTHESIA

Although adequate analgesia is essential to minimize the neuroendocrine stress response to surgery, some anesthetics may also independently contribute to perioperative hyperglycemia.[10,89] Inhalation anesthetics, such as isoflurane and sevoflurane, may cause hyperglycemia by inhibiting insulin secretion[90–92]; the hyperglycemia results from both impaired glucose uptake and increased glucose production.[89] In contrast, epidural analgesia with local anesthetics prevents this hyperglycemic effect[93,94] through an inhibitory effect on endogenous glucose production.[89] Similarly, intravenous (IV) anesthesia with opioids mitigates the hyperglycemic response to surgery[89,95,96] through its apparent neutral effect on endogenous glucose production but decrease in glucose clearance.[89] Although these differences are important to consider, the metabolic effects of anesthesia per se are relatively minor compared with the direct effects of surgery.[10]

ADVERSE CONSEQUENCES OF HYPERGLYCEMIA

Hyperglycemia can impair wound healing by hindering collagen production, which may decrease the tensile strength of the surgical wound.[97] Hyperglycemia may also have adverse effects on neutrophil function, including decreased chemotaxis, phagocytosis, and bactericidal killing.[98–101] Evidence from controlled experimental studies in rabbits demonstrated that these effects may be reversed, in part, by glycemia-independent effects of insulin.[102] However, the overall benefits of intensive insulin therapy, including a reduction in mortality, were derived mainly from maintenance of normoglycemia, whereas glycemia-independent actions of insulin exert only minor, organ-specific effects.[102]

Several pediatric clinical trials have investigated whether a strategy of tight glycemic control with IV insulin should be used to normalize blood glucose concentrations in nondiabetic children after major surgery.[103–106] Unless combined with continuous glucose monitoring, this approach increases the risk of severe hypoglycemia.[105] The preponderance of published data indicates that tight glycemic control is not recommended as standard treatment for children who have undergone cardiac surgery because it does not significantly change the infection rate, mortality, length of stay, or measures of organ failure compared with standard care.[107] Similarly, in a 35-center trial in critically ill children, excluding postcardiac surgery patients, there was no evidence of observed benefit of tight glycemic control and the possibility of harm.[107]

Clinical studies in adults with diabetes mellitus have not consistently supported the relationship between perioperative glycemic control and short-term risk of infection or morbidity.[108,109] However, several studies in adults with diabetes undergoing surgery have shown an association between postoperative hyperglycemia and infectious complications.[110,111] A meta-analysis showed that patients in surgical intensive care units (ICUs) benefit from intensive insulin therapy, whereas patients in other ICU settings do not.[112] These outcomes have obfuscated the specific glycemic targets and the means for achieving them in both critically and noncritically ill patients. A recent consensus statement[113] recommended that an insulin infusion should be used to control hyperglycemia in the majority of critically ill patients in the ICU setting, with a starting threshold of no greater than 180 mg/dL. Once IV insulin therapy has been initiated, the serum glucose concentration should be maintained between 140 and 180 mg/dL. There have been no prospective, randomized controlled trials to establish guidelines in noncritically ill patients treated with insulin. The current clinical strategy for these patients includes premeal glucose targets of less than 140 mg/dL and random blood glucose values less than 180 mg/dL, as long as these targets can be safely achieved. To avoid hypoglycemia, one should reassess the insulin regimen if the blood glucose concentration decreases below 100 mg/dL. The insulin regimen should be modified if the blood glucose concentration is less than 70 mg/dL, unless the event is easily explained by other factors (such as a missed meal).[113] These perioperative blood glucose goals are also recommended in an Endocrine Society Clinical Practice Guideline for the management of hyperglycemia in hospitalized patients in the noncritical care setting[114] and are supported by the International Society for Pediatric and Adolescent Diabetes (ISPAD) Clinical Practice Consensus Guidelines 2014 for management of children and adolescents with diabetes requiring surgery.[16]

In the 1980s and 1990s the dogma of tight glucose control replaced an era in which the mantra of caring for diabetic surgical patients was "keep them sweet," but in more recent years perioperative glucose control for patients with diabetes has become controversial and is unresolved, with conflicting evidence. A systematic review of the literature concluded that there are insufficient data regarding the best strategy or regimen to attain target blood glucose concentrations in ambulatory surgical patients with diabetes mellitus.[115] The recommended practice for subspecialties, such as cardiac, neurosurgical, and solid organ transplant surgical patients, requires still more study, and it must be highlighted that few of the published investigations and meta-analyses have focused specifically on children.

PREOPERATIVE ASSESSMENT

When feasible, children with diabetes should not undergo elective surgery until they are metabolically stable (Fig. 27.1)—that is, there is no ketosis, serum electrolytes are normal, and the glycated hemoglobin (HbA1c) value approximates the recommended goal of less than 7.5% across all age groups.[116] A more stringent target of less than 7% is recommended for young adults provided this can be achieved without excessive hypoglycemia[116]; a similar target applies for those with type 2 diabetes.[17] The preoperative consultation to assess the adequacy of metabolic control should be scheduled at least 10 days before the procedure (see Fig. 27.1). If metabolic control is poor, surgery should be delayed if possible. Both the endocrinology and anesthesiology services should participate in this assessment. Whenever possible, surgery for children with diabetes should be scheduled as the first case in the morning so that prolonged fasting is avoided and diabetes treatment regimens may be most easily adjusted.

Children who present for emergent surgery (e.g., trauma or acute surgical conditions) require a multidisciplinary preoperative assessment with collaborative involvement of both the endocrinology and anesthesiology services. Surgery often cannot be delayed even if metabolic control is poor—for example, a child requiring

emergent surgery who presents in diabetic ketoacidosis. This has implications for the intraoperative management of such children; described later under "Special Surgical Situations."

PREOPERATIVE MANAGEMENT

The regimen for managing diabetes before, during, and after a surgical or diagnostic procedure that requires the child to fast should aim to maintain near-normoglycemia—that is, a blood glucose concentration of 100 to 200 mg/dL. Blood glucose in this range reduces the risks of osmotic diuresis, dehydration, electrolyte imbalance, metabolic acidosis, infection, and hypoglycemia in the sedated child who may be unable to communicate with staff.[117] The child need not be admitted before the day of surgery, but rather early on the same morning as the surgery or procedure. Parents should receive explicit written instructions regarding appropriate modifications of their child's diabetes regimen before and for the day of surgery. On admission to the hospital, metabolic control should be assessed, including a preoperative determination of the blood glucose concentration. On the morning of surgery, no rapid- or short-acting acting insulin should be administered *unless* the blood glucose concentration exceeds 250 mg/dL. However, admission to the hospital before *major* surgical procedures in children[10] and adults has been recommended if the metabolic status needs to be optimized preoperatively.[83] If the surgery must be delayed for any reason, frequent blood glucose monitoring is mandatory to prevent perioperative hypoglycemia or hyperglycemia.

If the blood glucose exceeds 250 mg/dL and no rapid-acting insulin has been given in the prior 3 hours, a conservative dose of rapid-acting insulin (e.g., insulin lispro, insulin aspart, or insulin glulisine) is administered to restore near-normoglycemia. This is achieved using the child's usual insulin "correction factor," which refers to the decrease in blood glucose concentration expected after administering 1 unit of rapid-acting insulin. This can be calculated using the "1500 rule": divide 1500 by the child's usual total daily dose (TDD) of insulin. For example, if a child typically receives 30 units of insulin daily, this child's "correction factor" would be 1500 ÷ 30 = 50. In this example, 1 unit of rapid-acting insulin would be expected to decrease the child's blood glucose concentration by approximately 50 mg/dL. Various correction factors have been described, including a "1500 rule" for short-acting insulin (regular) and an "1800 rule" for rapid-acting insulin, such as insulin lispro.[118,119] For simplicity and because of insulin resistance caused by surgical stress, the "1500 rule" is appropriate in this setting, even with the use of a rapid-acting insulin. To then calculate an appropriate corrective dose of insulin to restore near-normoglycemia, the anesthesiologist should aim for a target blood glucose concentration of 150 mg/dL.

A "correction factor" rather than a sliding scale is also used to manage a child with hyperglycemia and restore the blood glucose concentration to 150 mg/dL. For example, if the child has a correction factor of 1 unit of rapid-acting insulin to reduce the blood glucose concentration by 50 mg/dL, and the current blood glucose value is 300 mg/dL, to reduce the blood glucose concentration from 300 mg/dL to 150 mg/dL, a total dose of (300 − 150)/50 or 3 units of insulin would be required. At the start of the procedure, the "correction" dose may be administered subcutaneously (using rapid-acting insulin) or by IV infusion using short-acting (regular) insulin in those children who will be managed with an IV insulin infusion during the procedure. For children with type 2 diabetes who do *not* require insulin (but who are, by definition, insulin resistant), an insulin dose of

27

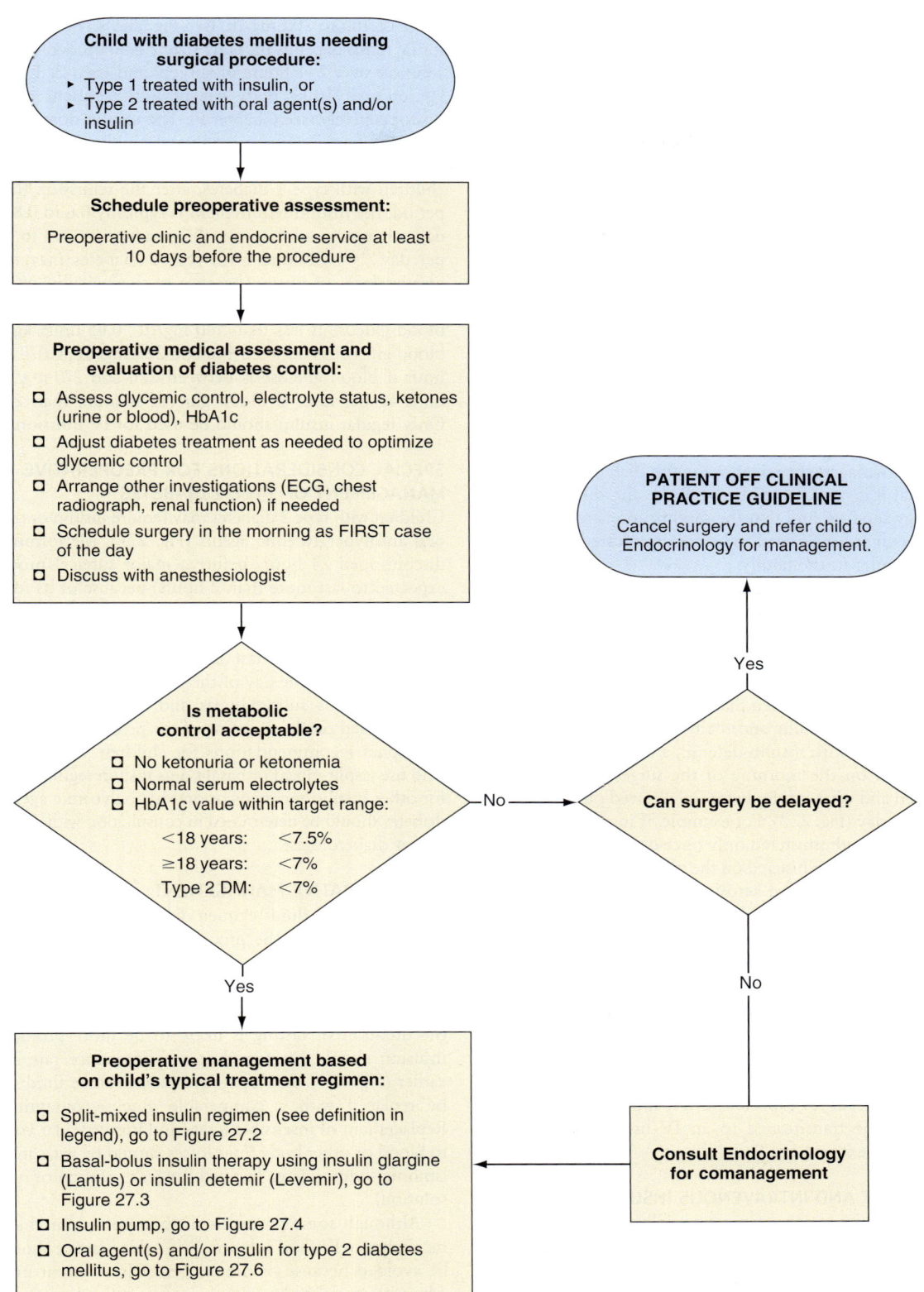

FIGURE 27.1 Clinical practice guideline for perioperative management of diabetes mellitus. Split-mixed insulin regimen refers to a regimen combining multiple daily injections of intermediate-acting insulins (e.g., neutral protamine Hagedorn) and multiple injections of rapid- or short-acting insulins (regular, insulin lispro [Humalog], insulin aspart [NovoLog], or insulin glulisine [Apidra]). *ECG,* electrocardiogram. (Modified from Rhodes ET, Ferrari LR, Wolfsdorf JI. Perioperative management of pediatric surgical patients with diabetes mellitus. *Anesth Analg.* 2005;101:986–999.)

0.1 unit/kg of rapid-acting insulin may be administered subcutaneously to correct a blood glucose concentration greater than 250 mg/dL.

More detailed preoperative recommendations must be based on the individual child's usual treatment regimen. For most children with diabetes undergoing minor outpatient surgical procedures, insulin can be provided perioperatively with subcutaneous injections. In adults, especially those with type 2 diabetes, this practice is commonly,[117] although not universally, preferred.[120] Others routinely recommend insulin infusions even for minor outpatient surgical procedures in children.[10] Several reports suggest that better glycemic control can be achieved in the perioperative period with a continuous IV infusion rather than subcutaneous insulin administration.[12,121,122] However, these studies were conducted before the availability of rapid-acting insulins whose rapid and reproducible effects after subcutaneous administration[123] may more closely match the ability to titrate IV-administered short-acting insulin. Subcutaneous insulin lispro is as effective as regular IV insulin to treat uncomplicated diabetic ketoacidosis in children.[124] Whatever the management strategy for the diabetes, it is most important that it is coordinated between the anesthesiology and endocrinology services, and that the modifications to the child's diabetes regimen at home need to be communicated clearly and in a timely manner to the family.

Split-mixed insulin regimens involve two to three injections per day with a combination of intermediate-acting insulin (NPH) plus a rapid- or short-acting insulin. For children who use such a regimen, 50% of the usual morning dose of NPH should be administered on the morning of the procedure (Fig. 27.2). For the child using a basal-bolus regimen that includes rapid-acting insulin with meals and basal insulin once-daily with insulin glargine or once- or twice-daily with insulin detemir, a dose of basal insulin may be required on the morning of the surgery based on the child's regimen and what insulin he or she received on the evening of the previous day (Fig. 27.3). For example, if insulin glargine or detemir is typically administered only once-daily in the morning, the full dose must be administered on the morning of the procedure to prevent hyperglycemia and ketosis.

Management of the child with an insulin pump depends on the duration of the surgical procedure (Fig. 27.4). Those undergoing minor procedures expected to last 2 hours or less can continue to receive their usual basal rate via their insulin pump. However, this approach requires the anesthesiologist to become familiar and comfortable with the use of an insulin pump in the operating room. Other protocols include transitioning patients who use an insulin pump to IV insulin infusion or subcutaneous insulin glargine.[83] For procedures expected to last longer than 2 hours, children should be transitioned to an IV insulin infusion, as described in the next section.

MAJOR SURGERY AND INTRAVENOUS INSULIN INFUSIONS

Children who require major surgery, especially procedures anticipated to last more than 2 hours, should have an IV insulin infusion as the preferred perioperative diabetes management plan (Fig. 27.5). Studies in children[12] and adults[6] have demonstrated that glycemic control is superior with infusions of IV insulin compared with subcutaneous injections. These children should receive their usual doses of insulin on the day before the procedure. On the morning of the procedure, an IV infusion of 5% dextrose in half-normal saline should be started at a maintenance rate, and an IV insulin infusion should also be provided to accommodate the dextrose infusion to maintain blood glucose in the target range of 100 to 200 mg/dL (see Fig. 27.5). The maintenance rate for IV fluids depends on body size: 20–40 mL/kg lactated Ringer's solution over 2–4 hours of surgery and then 2, 1, and 0.5 mL/kg for each 10 kg body weight if the patient remains NPO postoperatively (see Chapter 9). The insulin dose varies with the child's pubertal status; prepubertal children are relatively more sensitive to insulin than pubertal adolescents.[125] In prepubertal children with type 1 diabetes, after the remission (honeymoon) period, the insulin requirement is typically 0.6 to 0.8 unit/kg per day, whereas in adolescents, the requirement is 1 to 1.5 units/kg per day.[126,127] Children with type 2 diabetes may require even greater doses of insulin because of their insulin resistance. The IV insulin infusion can be started at 0.025 units/kg per hour if blood glucose is less than 140 mg/dL, 0.05 units/kg per hour if blood glucose is between 140 and 220 mg/dL, 0.075 units/kg per hour if blood glucose is between 220 and 270 mg/dL, and 0.1 units/kg per hour if blood glucose is more than 270 mg/dL.[16] Only regular insulin should be used for IV infusions.

SPECIAL CONSIDERATIONS FOR PREOPERATIVE MANAGEMENT OF TYPE 2 DIABETES

Children with type 2 diabetes may require insulin or one of several oral antihyperglycemic agents (Fig. 27.6). Metformin should be discontinued 24 hours before a major surgical procedure (e.g., expected to last more than 2 hours) because of its long duration of effect and the risk of lactic acidosis in the presence of dehydration, hypoxemia, or poor tissue perfusion.[128–131] For minor procedures, expected to last 2 hours or less, metformin may be discontinued on the day of the procedure.[16] Similarly, other oral agents, such as sulfonylureas and thiazolidinediones, may be discontinued on the morning of the procedure. Fig. 27.6 outlines additional recommendations for children with type 2 diabetes who use a split-mixed or basal-bolus insulin regimen. Adjustments for other insulin regimens or oral hypoglycemic agents in type 2 diabetes should be determined in consultation with an endocrinologist or diabetologist.

INTRAOPERATIVE MANAGEMENT

The insulin and fluid regimen during and after surgery depends on the duration of the procedure. If the procedure is likely to be brief (e.g., ≤1 hour) and one can reasonably anticipate that the child will be able to drink soon after the procedure, it may not be necessary to start a glucose-containing IV infusion. If the duration of fasting is likely to be more prolonged, an IV infusion should be started at a maintenance rate as described earlier (Fig. 27.7). Intraoperative maintenance fluid should then be replaced with a comparable glucose-containing solution. Replacement of insensible losses and intravascular volume owing to blood or other body fluid losses should be with an appropriate isotonic solution (e.g., lactated Ringer's solution or normal saline solution).

Although some protocols include potassium chloride in the maintenance IV fluid solution,[10,83,117] this practice should generally be avoided because of the danger of inadvertent intraoperative administration of large quantities of potassium during fluid resuscitation. Children undergoing a brief procedure with a baseline normal serum potassium concentration and well-controlled diabetes have a small risk of hypokalemia. Those undergoing more prolonged surgeries or emergent surgeries during which metabolic decompensation is more likely, require intraoperative assessment of electrolytes and appropriate adjustment of the electrolyte composition of their IV solution. *In all cases, blood glucose*

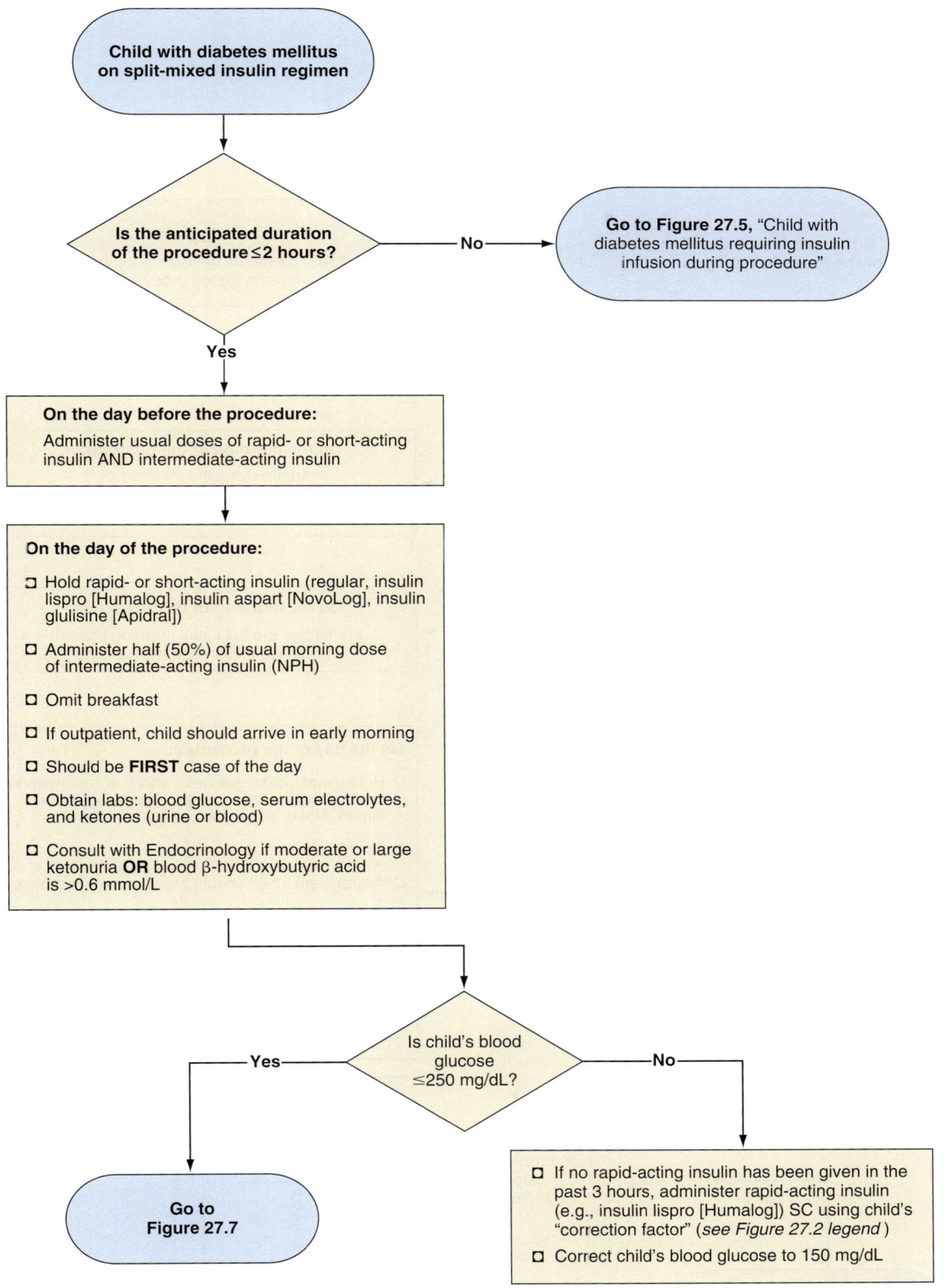

FIGURE 27.2 Preoperative management for children with diabetes mellitus on split-mixed insulin regimens. The calculation for insulin "correction factor" is as follows:

1 Divide 1500 by child's total daily dose (TDD).

2 If daily dose varies (i.e., use of sliding scales), use the *average* daily dose in the past week to determine TDD.

3 Example: If TDD = 50 units, then insulin correction factor is 1 unit insulin lispro (Humalog) to reduce blood glucose by 30 mg/dL.

NPH, neutral protamine Hagedorn; *SC*, subcutaneous. (Modified from Rhodes ET, Ferrari LR, Wolfsdorf JI. Perioperative management of pediatric surgical patients with diabetes mellitus. *Anesth Analg.* 2005;101:986–999.)

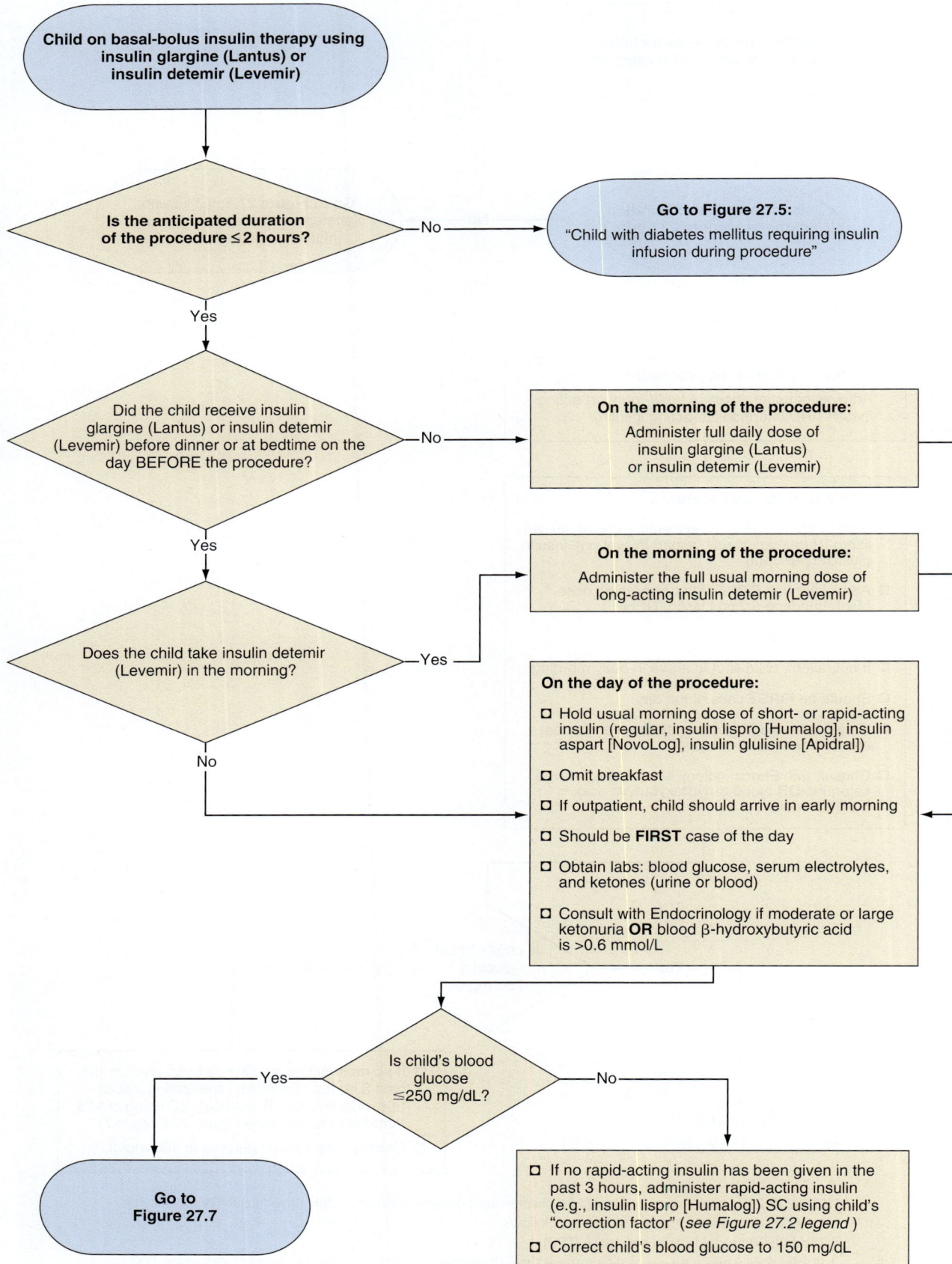

FIGURE 27.3 Preoperative management for children with diabetes mellitus using basal-bolus insulin glargine (Lantus) or insulin detemir (Levemir) regimens. Note that insulin glargine and insulin detemir should not be mixed with any other insulin. *SC,* subcutaneous. (Modified from Rhodes ET, Ferrari LR, Wolfsdorf JI. Perioperative management of pediatric surgical patients with diabetes mellitus. *Anesth Analg.* 2005;101:986–999.)

27

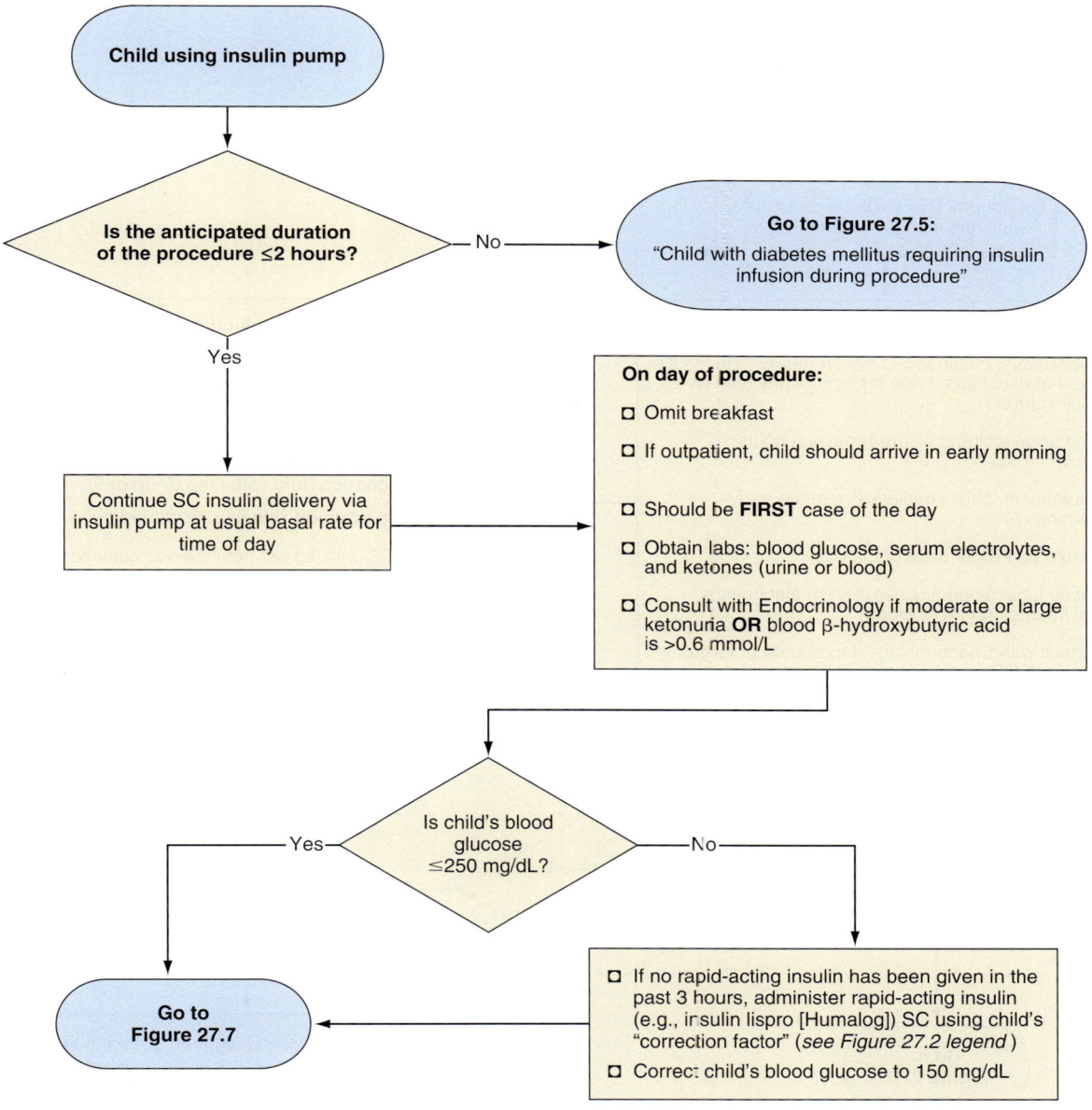

FIGURE 27.4 Preoperative management for children with diabetes mellitus who are using an insulin pump. *SC,* subcutaneous. (Modified from Rhodes ET, Ferrari LR, Wolfsdorf JI. Perioperative management of pediatric surgical patients with diabetes mellitus. *Anesth Analg.* 2005;101[4]:986–999.)

concentrations should be measured hourly and either insulin or dextrose adjusted, as necessary, to maintain blood glucose in the target range of 100 to 200 mg/dL. If the blood glucose exceeds 250 mg/dL, urine or blood ketones should also be measured (see Fig. 27.7). Either an increase in the rate of continuous insulin infusion or subcutaneous administration of a rapid-acting insulin analog is used to correct intraoperative hyperglycemia. Intraoperative IV bolus of regular insulin is not recommended because this causes a rapid supraphysiologic increase in serum insulin concentration, which, owing to insulin's short half-life (approximately 5 minutes), will have a short-lived effect on blood glucose concentration. In contrast, subcutaneously administered rapid-acting insulin analogs have a typical and reproducible pharmacologic profile.

POSTOPERATIVE MANAGEMENT

As soon as the child is able to resume drinking and eating normally, the usual diabetes regimen, including insulin and/or oral agents, may be reinstituted and the dextrose infusion discontinued (Fig. 27.8). One exception to this approach is for children with type 2 diabetes who take metformin; metformin should be withheld for 48 hours and renal function must be within normal limits before its resumption. IV dextrose and electrolyte solution should be continued until oral intake is restored. An infusion of IV short-acting insulin (regular) or intermittent subcutaneous rapid-acting insulin should be administered, not more frequently than every 3 hours, to maintain blood glucose in the target range of 100 to 200 mg/dL. Frequent blood glucose monitoring and monitoring

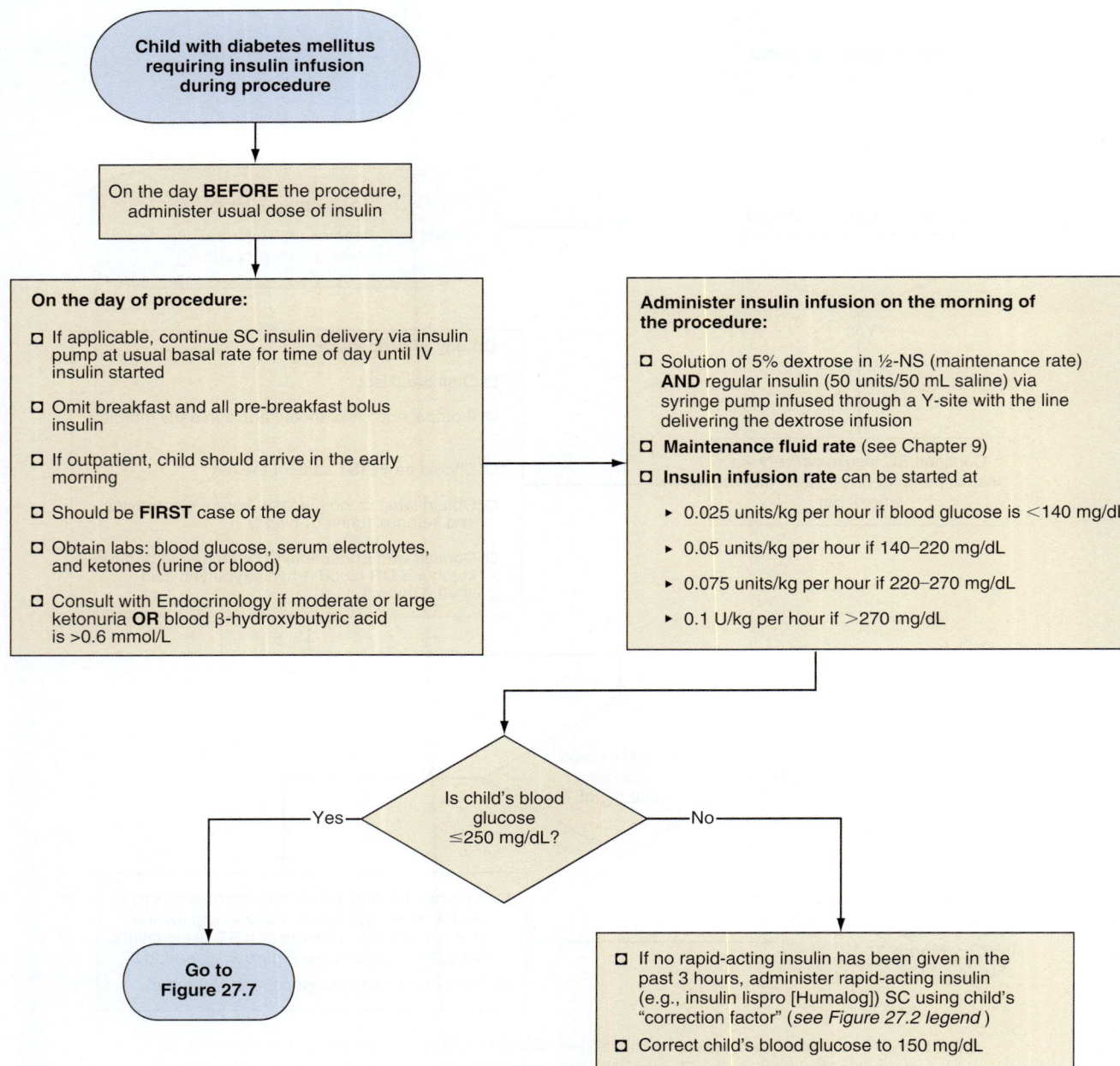

Child with diabetes mellitus requiring insulin infusion during procedure

On the day **BEFORE** the procedure, administer usual dose of insulin

On the day of procedure:

☐ If applicable, continue SC insulin delivery via insulin pump at usual basal rate for time of day until IV insulin started

☐ Omit breakfast and all pre-breakfast bolus insulin

☐ If outpatient, child should arrive in the early morning

☐ Should be **FIRST** case of the day

☐ Obtain labs: blood glucose, serum electrolytes, and ketones (urine or blood)

☐ Consult with Endocrinology if moderate or large ketonuria **OR** blood β-hydroxybutyric acid is >0.6 mmol/L

Administer insulin infusion on the morning of the procedure:

☐ Solution of 5% dextrose in ½-NS (maintenance rate) **AND** regular insulin (50 units/50 mL saline) via syringe pump infused through a Y-site with the line delivering the dextrose infusion

☐ **Maintenance fluid rate** (see Chapter 9)

☐ **Insulin infusion rate** can be started at

   ▸ 0.025 units/kg per hour if blood glucose is <140 mg/dL

   ▸ 0.05 units/kg per hour if 140–220 mg/dL

   ▸ 0.075 units/kg per hour if 220–270 mg/dL

   ▸ 0.1 U/kg per hour if >270 mg/dL

Is child's blood glucose ≤250 mg/dL?

—Yes—   —No—

Go to Figure 27.7

☐ If no rapid-acting insulin has been given in the past 3 hours, administer rapid-acting insulin (e.g., insulin lispro [Humalog]) SC using child's "correction factor" (*see Figure 27.2 legend*)

☐ Correct child's blood glucose to 150 mg/dL

FIGURE 27.5 Preoperative management for children with diabetes mellitus who require insulin infusions during surgery. *IV*, intravenous; *NS*, normal saline; *SC*, subcutaneous. (Modified from Rhodes ET, Ferrari LR, Wolfsdorf JI. Perioperative management of pediatric surgical patients with diabetes mellitus. *Anesth Analg.* 2005;101[4]: 986–999.)

blood or urine ketones is essential because of the variable effects of surgical trauma, inactivity, pain, anxiety, nausea and/or vomiting with poor oral intake, medications, and postoperative infection. At the time of discharge from the hospital, children and their parents or care providers should be given appropriate guidelines regarding these issues. Those who are admitted to the hospital overnight after surgery should be managed in consultation with the endocrinology service, if possible, to coordinate appropriate scheduling and subsequent dosing of insulin.

SPECIAL SURGICAL SITUATIONS

Children with diabetes who need urgent surgery must have a full clinical and biochemical assessment. Frequently, the problem necessitating surgery may have led to metabolic decompensation that must first be corrected and stabilized, unless the need for surgery is immediate. These children are often dehydrated; in addition to administering insulin, rehydration and electrolyte replacement is critical to address their metabolic derangements and restore normal glomerular filtration and renal function. In

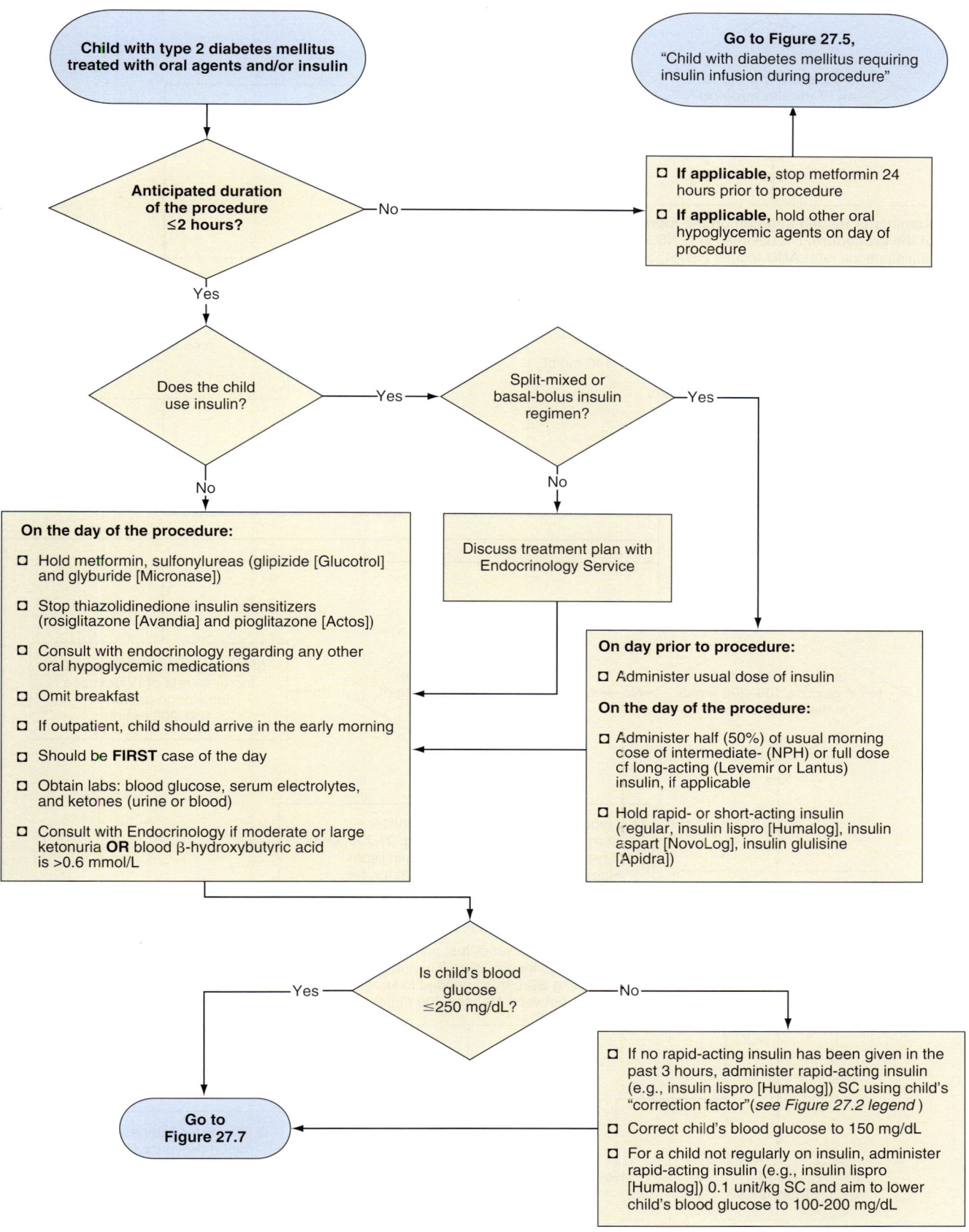

FIGURE 27.6 Preoperative management for children with type 2 diabetes who are using oral agents and/or insulin. *NPH*, neutral protamine Hagedorn; *SC*, subcutaneous. (Modified from Rhodes ET, Ferrari LR, Wolfsdorf JI. Perioperative management of pediatric surgical patients with diabetes mellitus. *Anesth Analg.* 2005;101[4]:986–999.)

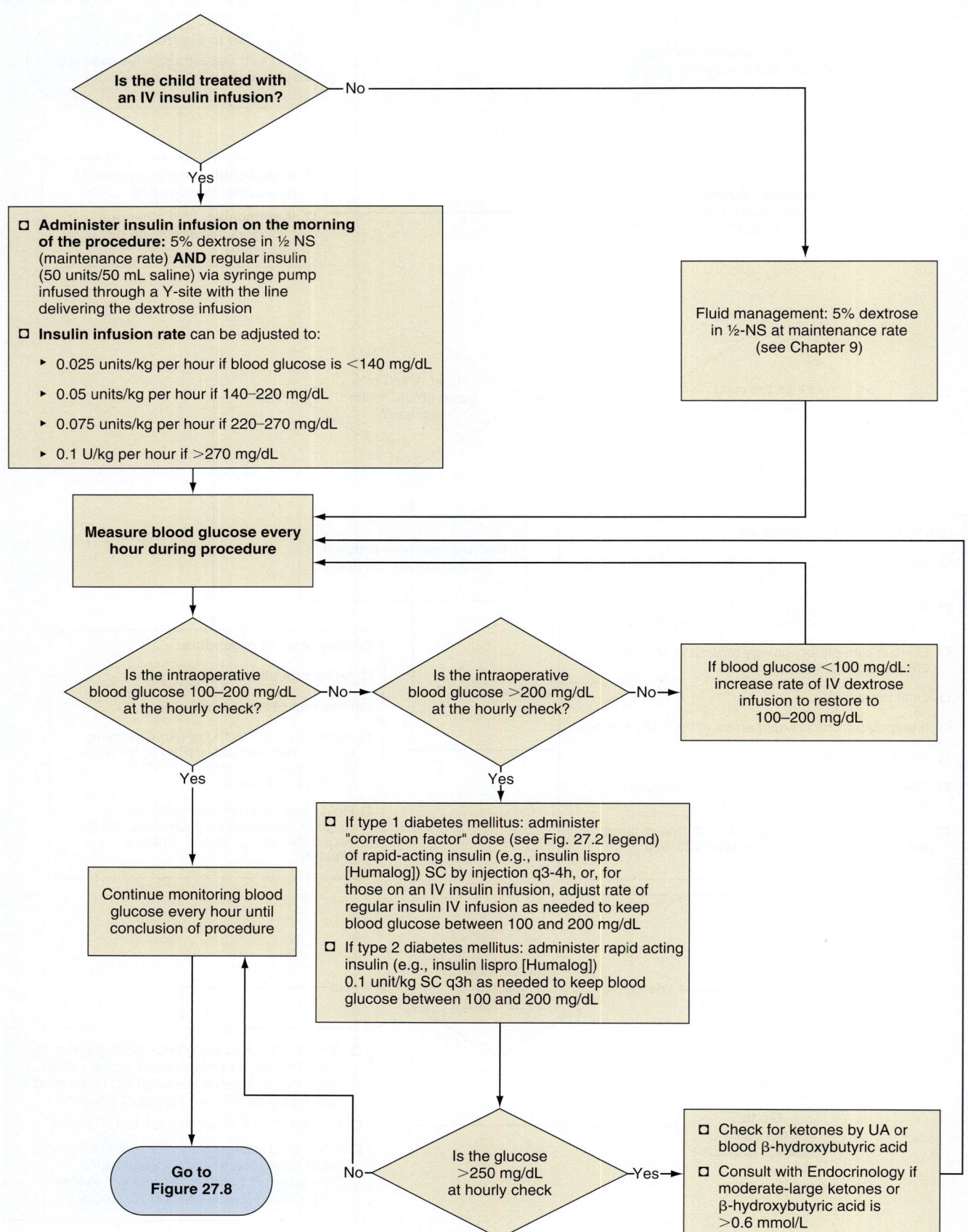

FIGURE 27.7 Intraoperative management of children with diabetes mellitus. The management goal for the child with diabetes is near-normoglycemia (100–200 mg/dL). For fluid regimen refer to page 634 and Chapter 9. *IV*, intravenous; *NS*, normal saline; *SC*, subcutaneous; *UA*, urinalysis. (Modified from Rhodes ET, Ferrari LR, Wolfsdorf JI. Perioperative management of pediatric surgical patients with diabetes mellitus. *Anesth Analg.* 2005;101[4]:986–999.)

27

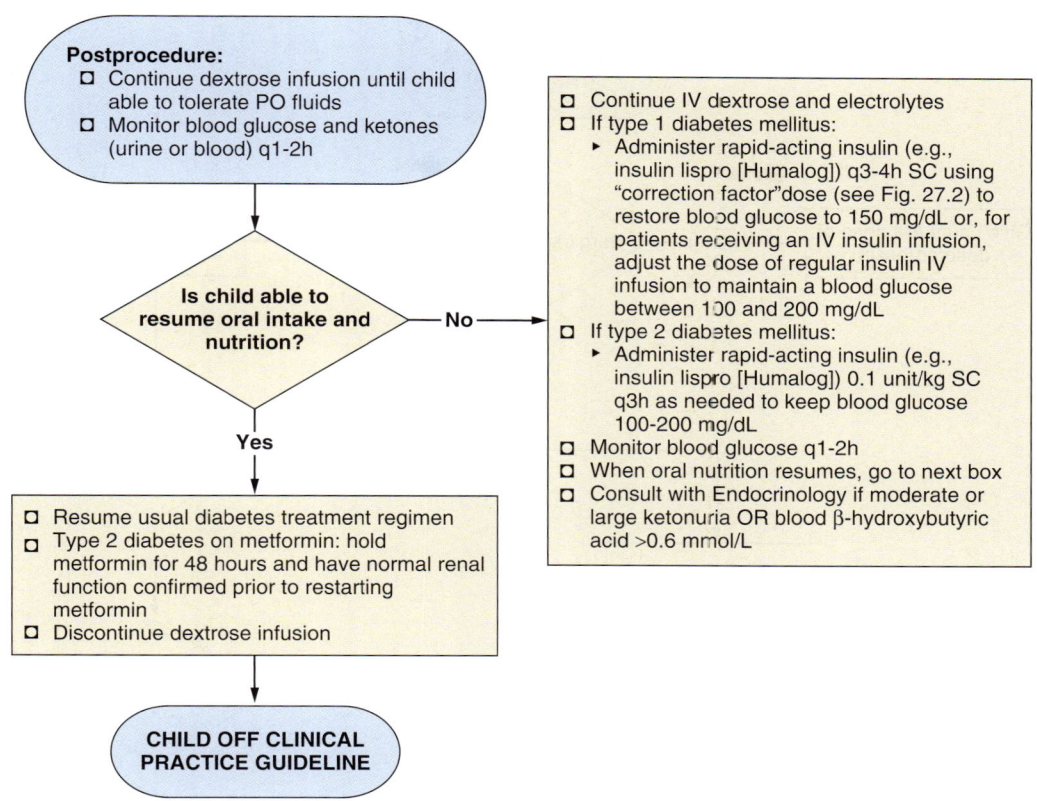

Postprocedure:
- ☐ Continue dextrose infusion until child able to tolerate PO fluids
- ☐ Monitor blood glucose and ketones (urine or blood) q1-2h

Is child able to resume oral intake and nutrition? —No→

Yes

- ☐ Resume usual diabetes treatment regimen
- ☐ Type 2 diabetes on metformin: hold metformin for 48 hours and have normal renal function confirmed prior to restarting metformin
- ☐ Discontinue dextrose infusion

CHILD OFF CLINICAL PRACTICE GUIDELINE

- ☐ Continue IV dextrose and electrolytes
- ☐ If type 1 diabetes mellitus:
  - ▸ Administer rapid-acting insulin (e.g., insulin lispro [Humalog]) q3-4h SC using "correction factor" dose (see Fig. 27.2) to restore blood glucose to 150 mg/dL or, for patients receiving an IV insulin infusion, adjust the dose of regular insulin IV infusion to maintain a blood glucose between 100 and 200 mg/dL
- ☐ If type 2 diabetes mellitus:
  - ▸ Administer rapid-acting insulin (e.g., insulin lispro [Humalog]) 0.1 unit/kg SC q3h as needed to keep blood glucose 100-200 mg/dL
- ☐ Monitor blood glucose q1-2h
- ☐ When oral nutrition resumes, go to next box
- ☐ Consult with Endocrinology if moderate or large ketonuria OR blood β-hydroxybutyric acid >0.6 mmol/L

FIGURE 27.8 Postoperative management of children with diabetes mellitus. *IV*, intravenous; *PO*, postoperative; *SC*, subcutaneous. (Modified from Rhodes ET, Ferrari LR, Wolfsdorf JI. Perioperative management of pediatric surgical patients with diabetes mellitus. *Anesth Analg.* 2005;101[4]:986–999.)

most cases, these children require emergent surgery that should be managed with an IV infusion of insulin as described earlier (see Fig. 27.5). Children with diabetic ketoacidosis require close collaboration between the anesthesiology and endocrinology services.

Diabetes Insipidus

Children undergoing neurosurgical procedures for tumors in or near the pituitary gland, especially craniopharyngioma, often require management of diabetes insipidus (DI), as do children with known DI who require anesthesia for surgical or radiologic procedures. The perioperative management of these children requires meticulous attention to fluid and electrolyte balance to prevent either overhydration or underhydration and electrolyte disturbances.

Central DI (also referred to as neurohypophyseal, neurogenic, or vasopressin-sensitive DI) is caused by a deficiency of the antidiuretic hormone, arginine vasopressin, which produces antidiuresis by stimulating V2 receptors on the principal cells of the kidney to promote reabsorption of water.[132] Central DI can be caused by disorders of vasopressin gene structure; accidental or surgical trauma to vasopressin neurons; congenital anatomic hypothalamic or pituitary defects; neoplasms; infiltrative, auto-immune, and infectious diseases affecting vasopressin neurons or fiber tracts; and increased metabolism of vasopressin. The etiology is unknown in approximately 50% of children with central DI.

DIAGNOSIS OF NEUROSURGICAL DIABETES INSIPIDUS: THE TRIPLE-PHASE RESPONSE

It is important to distinguish polyuria (>2 L/m² per day) caused by the onset of acute postsurgical central DI from polyuria resulting from diuresis of salt and fluid given during surgery. In both cases, children may have a large volume (exceeding 200 mL/m² per hour) of urine. Serum osmolality is increased, associated with inappropriately dilute urine (low urine osmolality), in DI but will be normal in the child excreting excess salt and water. In a solute diuresis, the urine osmolality is usually greater than 300 mOsmol/kg, in contrast to the dilute urine characteristic of DI. A meticulous examination of the intraoperative and postoperative records and careful bedside assessment of volume status (jugular venous distention, capillary refill) helps to distinguish between these two entities.

Of special interest is the triphasic pattern of vasopressin secretion often observed after neurosurgical procedures that interfere with the supraoptic-hypophyseal tract.[133] An initial phase of transient DI may be observed that lasts between 12 hours and 2 days after surgery. This may be explained by local edema that interferes with normal vasopressin secretion. If significant vasopressin-secreting cell damage has occurred, release of stored vasopressin from damaged neurons leads to a second phase that involves water retention. The syndrome of inappropriate antidiuretic hormone secretion (SIADH) may last up to 10 days. Finally, a third phase, permanent neurogenic DI, may follow if more than 90% of vasopressin cells are destroyed. Pronounced SIADH in

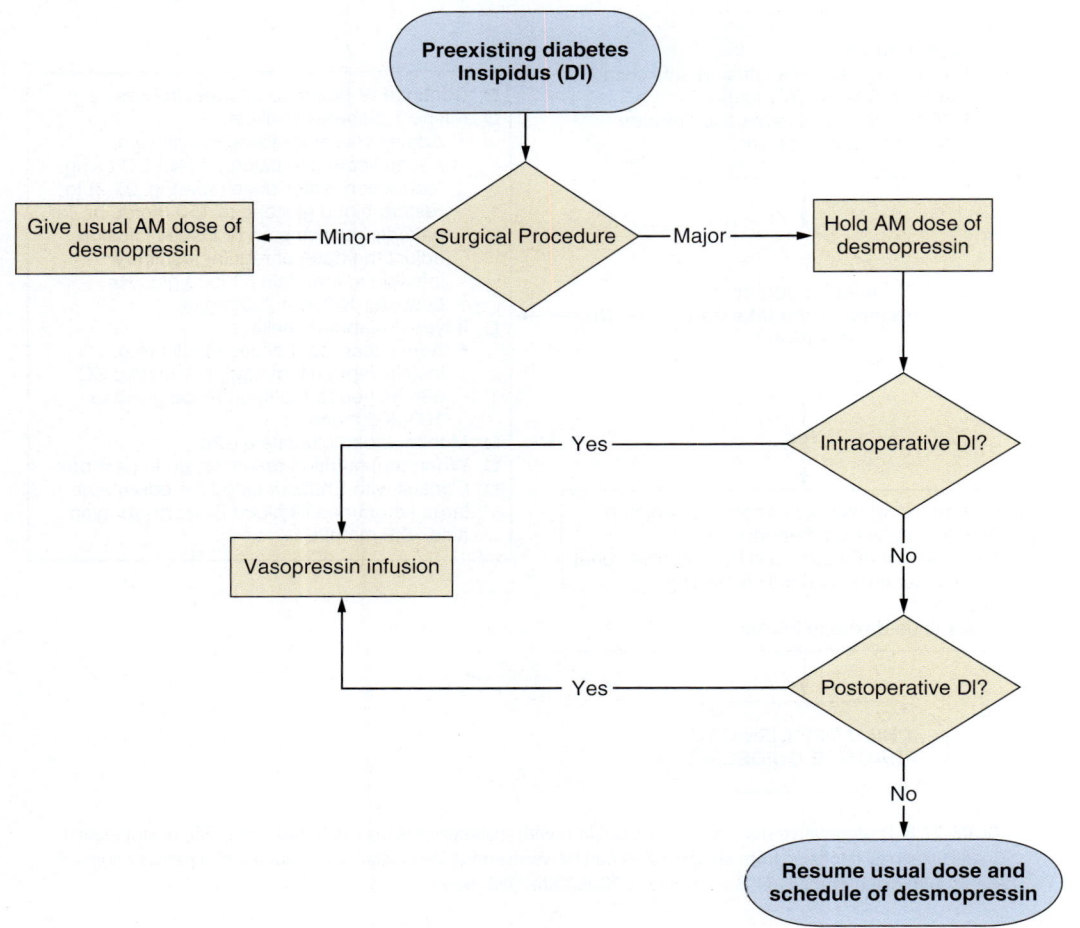

FIGURE 27.9 Perioperative management of diabetes insipidus.

the second phase generally portends permanent DI in the final phase of the triple response. In children with vasopressin and cortisol deficiency (e.g., in combined anterior and posterior hypopituitarism after neurosurgical treatment of craniopharyngioma), symptoms of DI may be masked because cortisol deficiency impairs renal free water clearance. Institution of glucocorticoid therapy may precipitate polyuria, leading to the diagnosis of DI (Fig. 27.9).

PERIOPERATIVE MANAGEMENT OF MINOR PROCEDURES

Children with preexisting DI who are scheduled for a minor procedure—that is, a procedure without significant blood loss and not followed by a period of further fasting or fluid shifts (e.g., myringotomy, radiologic imaging, peripheral orthopedic procedures)—are treated differently from those undergoing a more major procedure associated with blood loss or fluid shifts and delayed postoperative resumption of fluid intake (see Fig. 27.9).

Children undergoing minor procedures with anesthesia should receive their usual morning dose of desmopressin (DDAVP) (Table 27.3). The anesthetic technique is tailored to the procedure (e.g., IV sedation for magnetic resonance imaging [MRI], general endotracheal anesthesia for tonsillectomy). Arterial and urinary catheters are not required, and recovery takes place in the postanesthesia care unit (PACU). Once the morning dose of desmopressin has been administered, intraoperative and postoperative fluids

TABLE 27.3	Medications for Management of Central Diabetes Insipidus
Desmopressin acetate 100-, 200-µg tablets; nasal Rhinal tube 10 µg/0.1 mL; nasal spray 10 µg/0.1 mL can only deliver fixed doses of 10 µg (0.1 mL) per spray	
Oral	Dose: 100–400 µg q8–12 hours
	Oral doses are 10–20 times intranasal doses of desmopressin
	Onset of action: ~1 hour
	Duration: 6–8 hours; dose dependent (0.4 µg has antidiuretic effect up to 12 hours)
Intranasal	Dose: ~10–20 µg/dose q12–24 hours
	Onset of action: within 1 hour
	Duration: 5–21 hours
Vasopressin (Pitressin) (20 units/mL; 0.5-mL, 1-mL, and 10-mL vials). Dilute in normal saline or 5% dextrose in water	
Intravenous	Dose: 1.5 mU/kg per hour; titrate upward in 0.5 mU/kg per-hour increments to target urine output <2 mL/kg per hour
	Onset of action: rapid; maximum effect is achieved within 15 minutes of initiation of continuous infusion
	Duration: action ceases within 20 minutes of stopping intravenous infusion

should be restricted to the rate of 1 L/m² per 24 hours (~two-thirds of usual maintenance fluid requirement) to match insensible free water losses and obligatory urine output. Oral fluids may be offered once the child is awake. Although modern PACU policies often no longer require successful fluid intake before discharging the ambulatory patient, discharging the child with DI should be delayed until the child is able to freely take oral fluids without vomiting. Subsequent doses of DDAVP should be administered according to the child's usual preoperative schedule.

PERIOPERATIVE MANAGEMENT OF MAJOR PROCEDURES

A major surgical procedure is defined as an operation associated with the potential for significant blood loss; intraoperative or postoperative hemodynamic, neurologic, or respiratory instability; entry into a body cavity (e.g., craniotomy, abdominal surgery, thoracic surgery); craniofacial or airway surgery; major orthopedic surgery (e.g., spine surgery, tumor resection or amputation, major osteotomies); and/or surgery followed by delayed resumption of unrestricted fluid intake. The child with DI should be scheduled as the first case of the day. On the day before the procedure, the child treated with DDAVP should receive the usual morning dose, but only 50% of the usual evening or bedtime dose (see Fig. 27.9). On the morning of the procedure, DDAVP is withheld. The child undergoing a major procedure should receive general anesthesia with conventional monitoring, as well as insertion of arterial and urinary catheters when appropriate, and after surgery is admitted to a high-care facility (e.g., ICU). A central venous catheter for monitoring central venous pressure, although not indicated solely for the management of DI, is useful in the postoperative period.

At the start of the procedure, an infusion of aqueous vasopressin (available as Pitressin 20 U/mL in a 1-mL vial, diluted to 20 U/1000 mL to yield a final concentration of 20 mU/mL) should be started at 1.5 mU/kg per hour (0.0015 U/kg per hour). IV fluids, using normal saline with 5% dextrose, should total 1 L/m² per 24 hours to approximate insensible losses and obligate urine output. Additional IV saline, isotonic fluids, or blood products may be given to replace the blood and surgical fluid loss, to offset the third-space fluid losses, and to maintain hemodynamic stability. Fluid intake and output should be continuously monitored and serum sodium concentration measured frequently to ensure water balance is maintained. Urine output should not routinely be replaced in the child receiving a vasopressin infusion. Accidental overdoses resulting from inadequate dilution of the highly concentrated stock solution result in severe abdominal cramping, diarrhea, vomiting, and pallor owing to action at V1 receptors on smooth muscle in the gastrointestinal tract and blood vessels.

NEW PERIOPERATIVE DIAGNOSIS

The new diagnosis of intraoperative or postoperative DI is based on clinical and laboratory findings, including a serum sodium concentration greater than 145 mmol/L, polyuria (>4 mL/kg per hour) for 30 minutes or more, increased plasma osmolality (>300 mOsm/kg) in association with hypotonic urine (<300 mOsm/kg), and after excluding the presence of glycosuria and diuretic or mannitol administration as possible causes of polyuria.

When DI occurs, an infusion of aqueous vasopressin (20 U/1000 mL) is initiated at 1.5 mU/kg per hour (0.0015 U/kg per hour); because aqueous vasopressin has a brief plasma half-life (approximately 10–20 minutes), the rate of infusion is increased every 30 minutes until urine output decreases to less than 2 mL/kg per hour, indicating that antidiuresis has been achieved. Once

a urine output of less than 2 mL/kg per hour is achieved, the vasopressin infusion is maintained at a constant rate.

IV DDAVP should *not* be used in the acute management of postoperative central DI because it offers no advantage over aqueous vasopressin and because its long half-life (8–12 hours) compared with that of vasopressin, increases the risk of water intoxication and precludes dose titration.

POSTOPERATIVE MANAGEMENT

The child with DI should be cared for in an ICU after major surgery. Fluid input and output, serum electrolytes, and osmolality are monitored closely (hourly if necessary) in the intraoperative and postoperative periods. Until stability is achieved, it is important to have a urinary catheter in place to distinguish postoperative urinary retention from oliguria. The vasopressin infusion initiated intraoperatively is continued in the ICU. Fluid administration is *not* adjusted according to urine output; however, fluid deficits are replaced and blood pressure supported until antidiuresis (urine output <2 mL/kg per hour) is clearly established. In the patient with maximum antidiuresis, total (oral and IV) maintenance fluids should not exceed insensible plus obligatory urinary losses (i.e., approximately 1 L/m² per 24 hours). In the postoperative period, appropriate maintenance fluid is generally 5% dextrose in half-normal saline solution with 0 to 40 mEq/L of potassium chloride (depending on the serum potassium concentration). Blood loss should be replaced with normal saline solution, 5% albumin, or blood products, as appropriate.

Aqueous vasopressin in a dose of 1.5 mU/kg per hour results in a supranormal blood vasopressin concentration of approximately 10 pg/mL, twice that needed for full antidiuretic activity.[134] The effect of vasopressin is maximal within 2 hours after starting an infusion.[134]

After hypothalamic, but not transsphenoidal surgery, greater initial concentrations of vasopressin are occasionally required to treat acute DI. This may be attributed to the release of a substance related to vasopressin from the damaged hypothalamo-neurohypophyseal system, which acts as an antagonist to normal vasopressin activity.[135] Much greater rates of vasopressin infusions, resulting in plasma concentrations greater than 1000 pg/mL, should be avoided because they may cause cutaneous necrosis,[136] rhabdomyolysis,[136,137] and cardiac rhythm disturbances.[137]

POST–INTENSIVE CARE UNIT MANAGEMENT

Children treated with vasopressin for postneurosurgical DI should be switched from IV to oral fluid intake at the earliest opportunity. With an intact thirst mechanism and access to free water, the patient will better regulate blood osmolality. Once oral intake has been resumed without nausea and vomiting (often by the morning of the day after surgery), the vasopressin infusion should be stopped; all IV infusions should be stopped to avoid iatrogenic fluid overload, and oral fluids are permitted freely. DDAVP is then reinstituted (nasally or orally) in the child with preexisting DI or begun in the child who has new-onset DI (see Table 27.3).

Syndrome of Inappropriate Antidiuretic Hormone Secretion

SIADH is caused by the inability to excrete free water and is characterized by hyponatremia, plasma hypoosmolality (<275 mOsm/kg), inappropriately concentrated urine (>100 mOsm/kg), natriuresis in the absence of edema and volume depletion, and normal renal and adrenal function.[138–140] The dilutional hyponatremia of SIADH develops secondary to inappropriately increased levels of plasma antidiuretic hormone (ADH, also known as arginine vasopressin) relative to plasma osmolality.[140]

The major causes of SIADH are neurologic and psychiatric diseases, pulmonary disorders and interventions, malignancies, surgery, and medications (Table 27.4).[139–141] Medications that cause

TABLE 27.4	Causes of Syndrome of Inappropriate Antidiuretic Hormone Secretion
Central Nervous System Disturbances	
Head trauma	
Brain tumor	
Hydrocephalus	
Subarachnoid hemorrhage	
Stroke	
Infection (meningitis, encephalitis, brain abscess, AIDS)	
Acute psychosis	
Drugs	
Vasopressin, desmopressin	
Carbamazepine, oxcarbamazepine	
Cyclophosphamide	
Vincristine or vinblastine	
Cisplatin	
Phenothiazines	
Serotonin uptake inhibitors	
Tricyclic antidepressants	
Monoamine oxidase inhibitors	
Methylenedioxymethamphetamine ("ecstasy")	
Nicotine	
Major Surgery	
Major abdominal or thoracic surgery	
Pituitary surgery	
Pain	
Severe nausea	
Pulmonary Disease	
Pneumonia, tuberculosis	
Asthma	
Atelectasis	
Pneumothorax	
Acute respiratory failure	
Positive-pressure ventilation	
Neoplasia	
Carcinoma of lung, gastrointestinal tract or genitourinary tract	
Thymoma	
Leukemia	
Lymphoma	
Sarcoma	
Other tumors	
Miscellaneous	
Idiopathic	
Hereditary SIADH	
Gain-of-function mutation in the gene encoding vasopressin-2 receptor	

SIADH can act by stimulating the release of ADH, by enhancing the effect of ADH, or by acting as an ADH analog.[139] Although ADH secretion impairs water excretion, the other mechanisms that regulate fluid volume and sodium balance (renin-angiotensin-aldosterone system and atrial natriuretic peptide) are intact. Volume expansion activates natriuretic mechanisms (decreased proximal sodium reabsorption and decreased aldosterone production), resulting in sodium and water excretion and the restoration of near-euvolemia. With chronic SIADH, sodium loss is a more prominent feature than is water retention. Severe hyponatremia increases cell size because of entry of water into the cell along its osmotic gradient and may be associated with loss of intracellular potassium and other solutes in an attempt to restore cell volume.

Hyponatremia caused by SIADH can lead to clinical symptoms. Inappropriate infusion of hypotonic fluids in the postoperative period can exacerbate the hyponatremia caused by SIADH.[142,143] The clinical manifestations of symptomatic hyponatremia are principally neurologic. Early symptoms include headache, nausea, vomiting, weakness, confusion, altered consciousness, and lethargy. Late symptoms include seizures, coma, decorticate posturing, and death.[144] The severity of symptoms is related to both the absolute serum sodium concentration (most patients with serum sodium levels >125 mEq/L are asymptomatic) and its rate of decrease, especially if greater than 0.5 mEq/L per hour. Children are at greater risk than adults for developing hyponatremic encephalopathy because of a larger brain/skull size ratio, which limits room for brain expansion.[144,145]

PERIOPERATIVE MANAGEMENT

Many of the causes of SIADH are transient and resolve spontaneously once the underlying condition is corrected. Treatment of SIADH consists mainly of water restriction (i.e., maintaining a daily water intake that is less than daily water losses). If dilutional hyponatremia is mild and asymptomatic, therapy may not be required. In adults, both moderate and severe hyponatremia (serum sodium ≤130 mEq/L) are associated with increased mortality.[146,147]

Hyponatremic encephalopathy should be treated immediately with hypertonic (3%) saline solution. For mild to moderate symptoms with a low risk of herniation, treatment consists of 3% saline at a rate of 0.5 to 2 mL/kg per hour.[148] For severe symptoms, treatment consists of a bolus of 2 mL/kg 3% saline (to a maximum of 100 mL) over 10 minutes.[144,145,148] This may be repeated 1 or 2 times until symptoms improve, with a goal of increasing serum sodium concentration of 5 to 6 mEq/L in the first 1 to 2 hours.[144,145,148] The greater the duration of hyponatremia and the lower the serum sodium concentration, the greater the concern for brain injury secondary to overcorrection of hyponatremia. Overcorrection of chronic hyponatremia can lead to serious, permanent, and even fatal neurologic complications from osmotic demyelination (central pontine myelinolysis).[144,145,149] Recommended safe limits for the rate of hyponatremia correction vary from 6 to 15 mEq/L per 24 hours.[145,148,150–152] The hypertonic saline infusion should stop when the absolute concentration of serum sodium reaches 120 to 125 mEq/L. Hypertonic saline solution is usually combined with furosemide to limit treatment-induced expansion of the extracellular fluid volume.[151] Thereafter, treatment should consist of fluid restriction.

Thyroid Disorders

Thyroid hormones play an important role in metabolic processes, growth, and development in children.[153] The thyroid gland develops from the embryonic pharyngeal floor and descends along the thyroglossal duct to its final position in the anterior neck. Thyroid hormone production is controlled by the hypothalamic-pituitary-thyroid axis. Two principal thyroid hormones are produced, thyroxine (T_4) and triiodothyronine (T_3). Although T_4 is the predominant circulating thyroid hormone, T_3, which is primarily formed by peripheral conversion from T_4, is the major physiologically active thyroid hormone. Serum T_4 and T_3 concentrations in turn regulate hypothalamic thyrotropin-releasing hormone (TRH) and anterior pituitary thyroid-stimulating hormone (TSH) secretion via a negative feedback loop. Thyroid hormones are transported in the blood by carrier proteins, including thyroxine-binding globulin (80% of binding), prealbumin (10%–15% of binding), and albumin (5%–10% of binding). Protein-bound T_4 and T_3 are not biologically active. Only 0.03% of circulating T_4 and 0.3% of T_3 are unbound and active.[154]

HYPOTHYROIDISM

Classification and Epidemiology

Hypothyroidism, the most common thyroid disorder in children, can range from subclinical to overt disease. Subclinical hypothyroidism is characterized by a mildly elevated TSH with normal concentrations of T_4 and T_3.[155] It is usually a self-limiting problem with a low rate of progression to overt hypothyroidism, although consensus on the treatment of subclinical hypothyroidism is still a matter of debate.[156–158] Iodine deficiency continues to be the foremost cause of hypothyroidism worldwide.[159] However, the most common causes of primary hypothyroidism in the United States and other regions where iodine intake is adequate are congenital hypothyroidism and Hashimoto thyroiditis.[153] Other less frequent causes of primary hypothyroidism include sick euthyroid syndrome, hypothyroidism secondary to medications (thionamides, lithium, amiodarone), and radiation or surgery to the thyroid or neck.[153] Hypothyroidism can also be caused by disorders of the pituitary gland or the hypothalamus.

Biochemical Tests of Thyroid Function

In general, measurement of serum TSH, T_4, and unbound or free T_4 is sufficient for initial assessment of thyroid function. Free T_4 is preferable to total T_4 since it eliminates the effects of variation in protein binding. TSH is a sensitive test for diagnosing primary thyroid disorders and generally precedes noticeable changes in total T_4 and T_3 levels. In primary hypothyroidism, serum TSH is increased, whereas total T_4 and free T_4 are decreased. If the total T_4 level is reduced but free T_4 and TSH values are unchanged, thyroxine-binding globulin (TBG) deficiency is the most likely diagnosis. No treatment is required for TBG deficiency since these individuals have normal concentrations of free T_4 and are clinically euthyroid. If the hypothalamic-pituitary axis is not intact, such as in cases of secondary or tertiary (central) hypothyroidism, diagnosis and treatment is based on serum T_4 levels and clinical signs and symptoms.

Clinical Manifestations

Since thyroid hormone affects all metabolically active cells, hormone deficiency leads to a wide array of systemic abnormalities. Classic signs and symptoms of hypothyroidism in children include short stature, fatigue, weight gain, dry skin, hair loss, coarse facial features, hoarse voice, and constipation. Myxedema coma is a severe manifestation of hypothyroidism that can occur in profoundly hypothyroid individuals exposed to an external stress, such as infection, trauma, anesthesia, or cold temperature.[160] Myxedema

coma can result in severe life-threatening hypoxemia and hemodynamic instability.[160–163] Myxedema coma is rare in adults and even more uncommon in children, with only two reported cases.[163,164]

Neonatal Hypothyroidism

Congenital hypothyroidism remains the most frequent preventable cause of intellectual disability with an increased risk in neonates weighing less than 2 kg or more than 4.5 kg.[153,165] Thyroid dysgenesis or agenesis accounts for the majority of cases, whereas a smaller percentage results from thyroid dyshormonogenesis and secondary or tertiary hypothyroidism.[153,166] Since most neonates do not exhibit the classic signs or symptoms of hypothyroidism during the perinatal period owing to the transplacental passage of maternal thyroid hormones, testing via the neonatal screen is necessary to diagnose congenital hypothyroidism.[153] Screening programs may measure T_4, TSH, or both. Early detection and implementation of thyroid replacement are essential to avoid permanent neurologic sequelae. The classic syndrome of congenital hypothyroidism that develops in the first 3 months of life occurs in countries with no screening programs. The typical findings include macrosomia, enlarged fontanel, macroglossia, coarse facial features, hoarse cry, umbilical hernia, constipation, hypothermia, decreased activity, and neonatal jaundice (Fig. 27.10).[153] In general, affected children who receive adequate thyroid replacement starting early in the neonatal period lead normal lives.[167]

Treatment

The goal of thyroid replacement is to normalize T_4 within 1 to 2 weeks and TSH within 4 weeks,[168] reversing the metabolic derangements caused by hypothyroidism. In general, daily levothyroxine (LT_4) replacement normalizes T_4 concentrations within a week but normalizes TSH levels more slowly, over 4 to

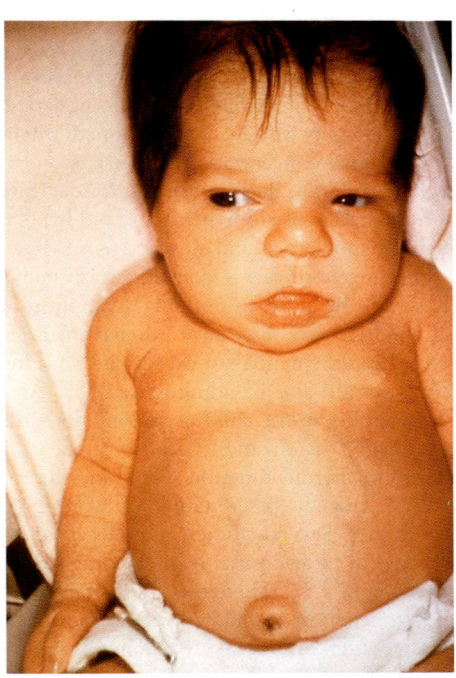

FIGURE 27.10 An infant with congenital hypothyroidism. ("Congenital hypothyroidism." Wikipedia: The Free Encyclopedia. Wikimedia Foundation, Inc., February 24, 2012, accessed March 31, 2012, http://en.wikipedia.org/wiki/Congenital_hypothyroidism.)

6 weeks.[169] The appropriate starting LT$_4$ dose varies with age and disease state. For neonates, the starting dose is 10 to 15 μg/kg per day,[153,168] which is much greater than the conventional replacement dose of 2 to 6 μg/kg per day in older children and adolescents.[153] In healthy children with acute hypothyroidism (e.g., after thyroidectomy), full LT$_4$ replacement can be started immediately. In children with severe, chronic hypothyroidism, smaller doses of LT$_4$ titrated slowly every few weeks are recommended, since these children are at risk of developing adverse effects (headaches, insomnia, hyperactivity, pseudotumor cerebri) when given a full thyroxine dose.[153,170] After stabilization of the dose, children and adolescents should continue to have regular clinical examinations and TSH monitoring owing to increased dose requirements during puberty and pregnancy.[171,172] Thyroid replacement can be given parenterally if needed. The IV dose of LT$_4$ is approximately half of the oral dose and should be given once daily.

Preoperative Management

Because thyroid hormones play a critical role in regulating metabolism, children should be clinically and biochemically euthyroid before undergoing elective surgery. Children with known hypothyroidism should have documented normal thyroid function tests before surgery. A detailed history should be obtained regarding previous thyroid disorders, head and neck radiation, radioiodine therapy, thyroid surgery, and family history of thyroid disease.[173] The majority of reported complications have occurred in patients with unrecognized hypothyroidism.[174] In addition, children with autoimmune disorders, such as type 1 diabetes mellitus and celiac disease, and children with genetic syndromes, such as trisomy 21 and Turner syndrome, are at increased risk for developing primary hypothyroidism and should be screened if symptomatic.[153,175–177]

Children with subclinical or mild hypothyroidism often must undergo urgent surgery without delay. Thyroid replacement can be started and continued with the same regimen as described in the outpatient setting. Perioperative risk in this group of children is minimally increased, but preoperative sedation should be minimized as these patients can be very sensitive to opioids and benzodiazepines.[178,179] For children with moderate to severe hypothyroidism, surgery should be postponed when possible, until thyroid hormone concentrations normalize on replacement therapy. In these children, there is concern for decreased cardiac function, abnormal response to hypercapnia and hypoxia, delayed gastric emptying, hypothermia, and increased sensitivity to anesthetics.[174,178–181] When urgent surgery is required, perioperative treatment with IV LT$_4$ should be given to minimize complications.[117,173,179] Since these children may also have adrenal insufficiency and because thyroid replacement may precipitate an adrenal crisis, glucocorticoids should also be administered.[174,179] An exception to this strategy applies to the child presenting for cardiovascular surgery or cardiac catheterization because of the concern that a rapid increase in thyroid function would increase myocardial oxygen demand, thereby precipitating or worsening unstable coronary syndromes. Several studies in adults have reported no adverse outcomes in cardiac patients undergoing surgery without thyroid replacement.[117,173,182] Therefore thyroid replacement could be initiated postoperatively in children with cardiovascular disease; however, many endocrinologists recommend starting with a minimal dose of T$_4$ in consultation with the cardiologist.[179]

Sick Euthyroid Syndrome

In sick euthyroid syndrome, abnormal thyroid test results occur in the setting of a nonthyroid illness, such as a critical illness. During times of stress or illness, increased conversion of T$_3$ to a metabolically inactive form (reverse T$_3$) occurs. With more severe illness, T$_4$ and free T$_4$ levels may be reduced. TSH levels may also be reduced because of hypothalamic-pituitary axis dysfunction.[153] Individuals are considered euthyroid if the TSH values are not increased. Controversy exists regarding possible benefits of using T$_4$ or T$_3$ therapy to treat sick euthyroid syndrome.[153,183–185]

HYPERTHYROIDISM

Classification and Epidemiology

Hyperthyroidism is a condition caused by excess circulating thyroid hormones that increases metabolic activity in the peripheral tissues. Almost all children with hyperthyroidism have suppressed serum TSH concentrations resulting from negative feedback by the increased concentrations of T$_4$ and T$_3$. Overt hyperthyroidism is characterized by both biochemical and clinical manifestations of the disease. A child with subclinical hyperthyroidism has reduced TSH concentrations but is typically asymptomatic.[186,187]

In children, hyperthyroidism occurs less frequently than hypothyroidism and is nearly always caused by Graves disease. Other causes of childhood thyrotoxicosis include autoimmune thyroiditis (Hashimoto thyroiditis), autonomously functioning thyroid nodules, infections of the thyroid gland, iodine-induced hyperthyroidism, TSH-secreting pituitary adenomas, and thyroid hormone ingestion.[188–190] Hyperthyroidism can be associated with McCune-Albright syndrome (triad of fibrous dysplasia of bone, café-au-lait skin spots, and precocious puberty).[190,191] A rare thyroid disorder that mimics the increased levels of T$_4$ and T$_3$ in hyperthyroidism is thyroid hormone resistance. However, unlike other causes of childhood thyrotoxicosis, thyroid hormone resistance should not be treated with antithyroid medications.[192,193]

Graves Disease

Graves disease is the most common cause of childhood hyperthyroidism. The pathogenesis of Graves disease is unclear but is believed to result from a complex interaction of genetic, immune, and environmental factors.[189,194] Graves disease is more frequent in children with other autoimmune diseases or with a condition associated with autoimmunity, as in Turner syndrome, trisomy 21, or DiGeorge syndrome.[195] In Graves disease, the immune system produces antibodies to the TSH receptor. These antibodies bind to and stimulate the TSH receptors found on the thyroid follicular cells, causing excessive synthesis and secretion of thyroid hormone. Most children with Graves disease have a smooth, diffusely enlarged goiter, ocular signs, as well as the systemic signs and symptoms associated with thyrotoxicosis.[189] Because few children with Graves disease enter spontaneous remission, treatment of hyperthyroidism is required. Current treatment options include antithyroid medications, radioactive iodine therapy, or surgical removal of the thyroid gland.[189,194,196] Although virtually all children enter remission during therapy with antithyroid drugs, adverse effects are relatively common (see later discussion) and the majority of children treated for 2 to 3 years relapse shortly after discontinuation of therapy.[197,198] Radioactive ablation is usually definitive and carries less risk than surgery.[199]

Thyroiditis

The term *thyroiditis* is used to describe a heterogeneous group of disorders that result in inflammation of the thyroid gland with subsequent release of preformed thyroid hormone. Hashimoto thyroiditis is the most common form of thyroiditis in children.[190] Transient hyperthyroidism can result from the initial inflammatory process, but symptoms generally last up to about 8 weeks, until preformed stored thyroid hormone is depleted. Thus the majority of children with Hashimoto thyroiditis present with a goiter but are asymptomatic.[153] In some children, antibodies that stimulate the TSH receptors on the thyroid follicular cells are present, prolonging the hyperthyroid phase by continued oversecretion of thyroid hormone.[200] In children that are symptomatic during the transient hyperthyroid phase, β-blockers should be used to control symptoms. In children with stimulating TSH receptor antibodies, antithyroid drugs are needed in addition to the β-blockers since thyroid hormone is being produced.[200] Some children develop hypothyroidism after the recovery phase because of lymphocytic infiltration of the thyroid gland and destruction of thyroid tissue.

Thyroiditis can also manifest as painful inflammation of the gland and fever secondary to bacterial or viral infection. *Haemophilus influenzae*, group A streptococci, and *Staphylococcus* are the most frequent causes of acute infectious thyroiditis, which can be complicated by thyroid gland cutaneous fistulae.[201] Viral infections of the thyroid gland are less severe. Owing to the difficulty in distinguishing bacterial from viral infections, all cases of infectious thyroiditis are treated with antibiotics. Treatment with antithyroid drugs is not indicated, but if the child is symptomatic, β-blockers should be used.

Clinical Manifestations

Most of the symptoms that children experience are the same regardless of the cause of hyperthyroidism. Classic signs and symptoms of hyperthyroidism include goiter, tachycardia, palpitations, dyspnea, fatigue, proximal muscle weakness, tremor, brisk reflexes, heat intolerance, insomnia, nervousness, increased frequency of bowel movements, and weight loss despite a normal or increased appetite.[189,194] Many children with hyperthyroidism have an inability to concentrate, resulting in poor school performance, and may be initially mistaken to have attention deficit hyperactivity disorder. Other medical conditions associated with long-standing hyperthyroidism include growth acceleration and advancement in epiphyseal maturation, delay in onset of puberty, and irregular menses.[189,202]

Children with Graves disease may develop additional autoimmune manifestations, such as ophthalmopathy. Pretibial myxedema and dermopathy are rare in children.[195] Ocular involvement in Graves disease is characterized by inflammation and edema of the retro-orbital tissue and extraocular muscles, resulting in proptosis and impaired ocular muscle function. Children with Graves ophthalmopathy often complain of eye irritation or ocular dryness because of lid retraction, which is due to increased adrenergic tone of the ocular muscles resulting in a prominent stare (Fig. 27.11). If left untreated, corneal ulceration may develop and lead to irreversible eye damage, including blindness. Once hyperthyroidism is treated, the lid retraction and "adrenergic stare" resolve quickly, but proptosis from Graves ophthalmopathy usually persists or regresses only slightly.[189,196,203]

Treatment

Since antithyroid medications are the least invasive of the treatment options for Graves disease, they remain the first line of treatment for children, even though only 25% to 40% of children with Graves disease will enter remission with treatment.[189,195] Favorable predictors of remission in Graves disease after treatment include a small thyroid gland and milder disease at time of diagnosis, older age, postpubertal status, decrease in stimulating TSH

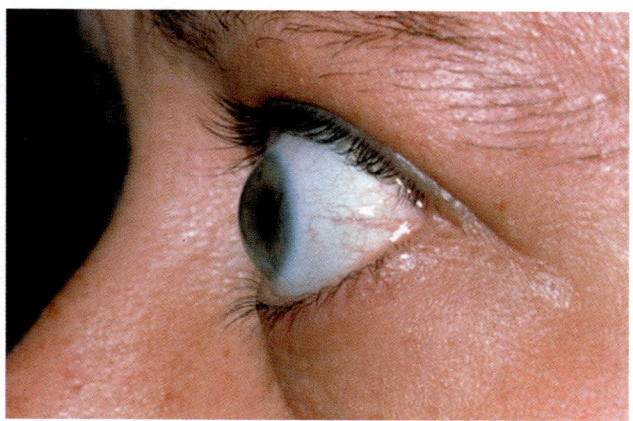

FIGURE 27.11 Proptosis of the eyes in a child with Graves disease.

receptor antibodies over time, presence of other autoimmune diseases, and duration of treatment greater than 2 years.[189,194] Methimazole is the drug of choice for children with Graves disease. Minor adverse effects occur in 14% to 25% of children treated with thioamides and include nausea, skin rash, arthralgias, myalgias, gastrointestinal problems, and neutropenia. Serious adverse effects occur in less than 2% of children and include agranulocytosis, hepatitis, liver failure, vasculitis with a lupus-like syndrome and Stevens-Johnson syndrome. Propylthiouracil is no longer recommended for treatment of Graves disease in children because of the unacceptable risk of hepatotoxicity and liver failure.[189,195]

Radioactive iodine therapy is used for adolescents who are not in remission or relapse after treatment with antithyroid medications or for those who have developed a serious adverse reaction to the medications or are noncompliant with medication use. It is also used for children who require immediate definitive therapy. Several longitudinal studies have shown that children are not at increased risk for developing thyroid cancer if appropriate ablative doses of radioiodine are used.[189,195]

Thyroidectomy is reserved for children and adolescents with a large thyroid gland, a history of failed drug therapy, severe ocular disease, or poor response to radioactive iodine therapy. Surgeons with expertise performing thyroidectomies in children should undertake the surgery because of the potential for serious complications, including hemorrhage, transient or permanent hypoparathyroidism, and vocal cord paralysis.[189,195]

Perioperative Management

Children should be euthyroid or slightly hypothyroid before surgery to minimize complications and avoid precipitation of thyroid storm. The possibility of airway compromise related to a large goiter should be considered and carefully evaluated.

In children with uncontrolled hyperthyroidism, surgery should be postponed until thyroid hormone concentrations normalize with therapy. If presenting for emergency surgery, careful preparation of the patient is essential and may include administration of antithyroid drugs, iodine, β-blockers, and corticosteroids.[179,204] Uncontrolled hyperthyroidism can be ameliorated by administering oral iodine (Lugol solution or saturated solution of potassium iodine) to block further release of thyroid hormone from the

TABLE 27.5	Management of Hyperthyroid Crisis		
Drug Class	**Recommended Drug**	**Starting Dose**	**Mechanism of Action**
Iodine	Potassium iodide (SSKI)	3–5 drops by mouth q6 hours	Blocks release of thyroid hormone from gland
	Lugol solution	4–8 drops by mouth q6–8 hours	Blocks release of thyroid hormone from gland
β-Blockers	Propranolol	Infant: 2 mg/kg per day by mouth divided q8–12 hours Child: 10–40 mg by mouth q6–8 hours	β-adrenergic blockade; decreased T_4 to T_3 conversion
	Esmolol	100–200 µg/kg per minute IV infusion	β-adrenergic blockade; decreased T_4 to T_3 conversion
Thioamide	Methimazole	0.4 mg/kg per day by mouth divided q8–12 hours	Inhibits new hormone synthesis
	Propylthiouracil	5–10 mg/kg per day by mouth divided q8 hours	Inhibits new hormone synthesis; decreases T_4 to T_3 conversion
Supportive treatment	Intravenous fluid	20–40 mL/kg normal saline	Replacement of increased insensible losses resulting from fever, diaphoresis, vomiting, and diarrhea
	Cooling blankets, ice packs	Reduce fever	
	Acetaminophen	Children 2–12 years: 15 mg/kg q6 hours or 12.5 mg/kg q4 hours; maximum daily dose: 75 mg/kg per day (≤4 g/day) Adolescents >12 years: <50 kg: 15 mg/kg q6 hours or 12.5 mg/kg q4 hours; maximum single dose: 750 mg/dose; maximum daily dose: 75 mg/kg per day (≤4 g/day) ≥50 kg: 1000 mg q6 hours or 650 mg q4 hours; maximum single dose: 1000 mg/dose; maximum daily dose: 4 g/day	Reduce fever
	Hydrocortisone	2 mg/kg IV q8 hours (maximum dose 100 mg)	Decreases T_4 to T_3 conversion; enhances vasomotor stability

SSKI, saturated solution of potassium iodide.

thyroid gland.[179,205] Excess iodine transiently inhibits thyroid hormone release (the Wolff-Chaikoff effect).[205] Iodine should not be administered before methimazole treatment as it may initially increase the amount of thyroid hormone released.[179,205]

Rarely untreated or undertreated hyperthyroidism can lead to thyroid storm, which has a reported incidence of 0.1 to 3 per 100,000 hospitalized patients.[206] Thyroid storm is usually precipitated by a second superimposed insult, such as infection, trauma, surgery, or diabetic ketoacidosis.[205] Thyroid storm may be difficult to differentiate from an acute malignant hyperthermia (MH) reaction.[207,208] However, in contrast to MH, thyroid storm has a more variable onset (usually an insidious onset 6 to 18 hours postoperatively, although it can develop precipitously during surgery), it induces a less severe metabolic acidosis than MH, and the serum creatine phosphokinase (CPK) remains unchanged. Since the serum CPK peaks at 12 to 18 hours after an MH reaction, it is a late sign to differentiate thyrotoxicosis from MH. If the presentation proves difficult to distinguish from MH (both diseases may present with tachycardia, rigidity, and fever), it is prudent to administer dantrolene sodium 2.5 mg/kg IV.[209] However, if the hypermetabolic signs abate after dantrolene, one cannot conclude that the reaction was MH, since dantrolene attenuates the hypermetabolic signs of thyroid storm as well.[208] The differential diagnosis also includes neuroleptic malignant syndrome and pheochromocytoma.[179]

Thyroid storm is an endocrine emergency and immediate, aggressive management is essential to avoid death.[161,188,207] Untreated, the mortality rate from thyroid storm is 10% to 30%.[177,210] The

recommended treatment for thyroid storm remains a multidrug approach to (1) block production and release of thyroid hormone, (2) prevent conversion of T_4 to T_3, (3) antagonize the peripheral (adrenergic) effects of thyroid hormone, and (4) control systemic disturbances with supportive therapy (Table 27.5).[162,196,205,211–215] Pharmacologic treatment includes administration of parenteral β-blockers, methimazole or propylthiouracil, glucocorticoids (which decrease conversion of T4 to T3 and prevents relative adrenal insufficiency), and antipyretics (acetaminophen).[179,204,207]

Parathyroid and Calcium Disorders

PHYSIOLOGY OF CALCIUM HOMEOSTASIS

The four parathyroid glands are usually present in two pairs on the posterior aspect of the superior and inferior poles of the thyroid gland, with the inferior pair occasionally ectopic elsewhere in the neck or chest. Parathyroid hormone (PTH) is released from secretory granules in response to a decrease in serum ionized calcium. Its secretion is inhibited by hyperphosphatemia, profound hypomagnesemia or hypermagnesemia, or increased 1,25-dihydroxyvitamin D (calcitriol). The calcium-sensing receptor in the parathyroid mediates PTH release. PTH has three primary modes of increasing serum calcium: (1) increased renal tubular reabsorption of calcium as well as decreased reabsorption of phosphate; (2) upregulation of osteoclast-mediated calcium and phosphate release from bone; and (3) renal conversion of 25-hydroxyvitamin D to the active metabolite, calcitriol. In turn, calcitriol increases absorption of calcium and phosphate from the gastrointestinal tract and has direct calcium-releasing effects on bone. Calcitonin is secreted by the thyroid C cells and has calcium-reducing properties via its own G protein–coupled receptor.

HYPOCALCEMIA

Neonatal Hypocalcemia

Neonatal hypocalcemia owing to prematurity, perinatal stress/asphyxia, and maternal diabetes is common but is typically transient.[216,217] Less common causes include maternal hyperparathyroidism, transient neonatal hypoparathyroidism, vitamin D deficiency, excessive diuretic use or phosphate load, and congenital hypoparathyroidism.[217] Maternal vitamin D deficiency remains a cause of infant hypocalcemia in the United States, regardless of the infant's dietary intake.[218,219]

The most common cause of congenital hypoparathyroidism is the DiGeorge sequence (also known as velocardiofacial syndrome or 22q11.2 deletion).[216,217] The degree of parathyroid hypoplasia in the DiGeorge sequence is variable, so hypocalcemia may present during infancy, childhood, or periods of stress.[216] Other causes of congenital hypoparathyroidism include isolated hypoparathyroidism, hypercalciuric hypocalcemia, mitochondrial disorders (Kearns-Sayre syndrome, mitochondrial encephalopathy) and metabolic syndromes (Kenny-Caffey syndrome).[216,217,220] Reduced PTH or PTH resistance (pseudohypoparathyroidism) cause hyperphosphatemia beyond the already increased normal range in neonates, whereas vitamin D deficiency or resistance is associated with low to normal serum phosphate concentrations.

Childhood Hypocalcemia

Etiologies for hypocalcemia in children include hypoparathyroidism (congenital and acquired), insensitivity to PTH (pseudohypoparathyroidism), disorders of vitamin D supply or metabolism, and calcium/phosphorus/magnesium disorders.[216,221,222] Acquired hypoparathyroidism may be due to infiltrative disease of the parathyroid gland (hemochromatosis, Wilson disease, granulomatous disease, or metastatic cancer), autoimmune hypoparathyroidism (polyglandular autoimmune disease type1), or postsurgical complications of thyroid or parathyroid surgery.

In polyglandular autoimmune disease type 1, the principal features are mucocutaneous candidiasis, hypoparathyroidism, and adrenal insufficiency.[216,221,223] Ectodermal dystrophy of the nails is often present, leading to an alternative name for this syndrome, autoimmune polyendocrinopathy-candidiasis-ectodermal dystrophy (APECED).[221,223]

Persistent hypocalcemia in infants and children can have many manifestations, including poor feeding, circumoral numbness, paresthesias, laryngospasm, tetany, seizures, myocardial dysfunction, and myopathy.[222] Initial evaluation of hypocalcemia, regardless of age, includes measurement of serum calcium, phosphate, magnesium, alkaline phosphatase, creatinine, PTH, 25-hydroxyvitamin D, and 1,25-dihydroxyvitamin D, plus urine calcium, phosphate, and creatinine. Therapy for acute hypocalcemia includes parenteral calcium, followed by oral calcium supplementation and 25-hydroxyvitamin D if reduced,[219] and calcitriol instead of synthetic PTH. The use of PTH was initially contraindicated in children because of a potential risk of developing osteosarcoma.[224] PTH is now used as an alternative to calcitriol because extensive use in adults and studies in children have not shown an increased risk.[221,224–226]

Perioperative Management

Hypocalcemia is usually managed by IV infusion of calcium in the form of calcium chloride or calcium gluconate, with frequent measurement of serum ionized calcium concentrations to guide therapy (see Chapter 12). Calcium salts release free calcium ions and should be given via a central venous catheter because their hypertonicity and the increased concentration of ionized calcium causes intense local vasoconstriction that may lead to necrosis of the skin and subcutaneous tissues and possibly gangrene of the affected limb if administered via a peripheral IV cannula that becomes interstitial. In the postoperative period after the child is tolerating oral intake, IV calcium supplementation may be converted to oral supplementation.

HYPERCALCEMIA

Hypercalcemia is an uncommon finding in children.[227,228] Parathyroid causes of hypercalcemia include neonatal hyperparathyroidism (HPT), primary HPT, parathyroid hyperplasia, familial hypocalciuric hypercalcemia (familial benign hypercalcemia), and rarely, parathyroid carcinoma.[229] Neonatal HPT is usually an adaptation to maternal hypocalcemia. In children and adolescents, 65% of HPT may be attributed to a single parathyroid adenoma that is unresponsive to increases in serum calcium level.[227]

Parathyroid hyperplasia occurs in familial forms of hyperparathyroidism, including multiple endocrine neoplasia type 1 (MEN 1), in which HPT is the presenting manifestation the majority of the time.[227,230,231] MEN 1 is also associated with pancreatic and pituitary tumors.[230,231] HPT is a less common manifestation of MEN 2A, in which medullary thyroid carcinoma and pheochromocytoma occur.[232] Mutations in the calcium-sensing receptor gene result in a greater serum calcium set point in familial hypocalciuric hypercalcemia (familial benign hypercalcemia), an incidental diagnosis that is benign.[233,234] Mutations in this calcium-sensing receptor gene can also lead to a life-threatening form of neonatal severe HPT.[227] Secondary HPT with relatively normal calcium levels is a common pediatric phenomenon that accompanies renal failure, renal tubular acidosis, and hypophosphatemic rickets.[235]

When hypercalcemia is present, the differential diagnosis includes Williams syndrome (associated with hypercalcemia in 15% cases), vitamin A intoxication, vitamin D intoxication, hypophosphatasia, granulomatous disorders, subcutaneous fat necrosis, immobility, and medications (thiazide diuretics, lithium, theophylline).[227,236] Solid tumors may secrete increased concentrations of parathyroid hormone–related protein (PTHrP). Tumors, such as leukemias, lymphomas, and others, may release excess cytokines and osteoclast-activating factors, with the hypercalcemia leading to the tumor diagnosis.[237,238]

Signs and symptoms of hypercalcemia are usually nonspecific, such as nausea and vomiting, failure to thrive, irritability, polyuria, constipation, and fatigue. Initial laboratory evaluation of hypercalcemia is similar to the evaluation for hypocalcemia given earlier.[239]

Evaluation of unexplained hypercalcemia includes additional hormone or genetic testing for MEN syndromes, measurement of PTHrP for malignancy, blood for tumor markers, bone marrow biopsy, and relevant imaging. When HPT is found, ultrasonography is helpful to assess the parathyroid glands, but MRI or technetium-sestamibi scan is more precise, especially at locating ectopic tissue.[240]

Perioperative Management

Management of acute hypercalcemia begins with discontinuing or minimizing all sources of calcium (enteral/parenteral feeds, total parenteral nutrition). Children should be aggressively hydrated with isotonic fluids. The administration of a loop diuretic, such as furosemide, increases urinary calcium excretion.[241] Calcitonin, which inhibits bone resorption, decreases the calcium concentration, although tachyphylaxis may occur within 1 or 2 days.[227] Bisphosphonates, such as pamidronate, are potent inhibitors of bone resorption. Pamidronate is preferred in children; a single dose can rapidly reduce the serum calcium concentrations with an effect that lasts 2 to 4 weeks.[227,241] Glucocorticoids may also be useful since they inhibit synthesis of 1,25-dihydroxyvitamin D₃. Definitive therapy for primary HPT is parathyroidectomy.[227,240-242] Acute management after parathyroidectomy requires careful monitoring and replacement of calcium and possibly the use of calcitriol for persistent hypocalcemia. In isolated parathyroid hyperplasia, MEN, or secondary HPT, surgeons may elect to leave a portion of one gland in the forearm to avoid permanent hypoparathyroidism, which is challenging to manage.

Adrenal Disorders

PHYSIOLOGY

Adrenal steroidogenesis begins with cholesterol as a precursor and results in three types of steroids: mineralocorticoids, glucocorticoids, and sex steroids (androgen precursors).[243] Most of the enzymes involved in adrenal (or gonadal) steroidogenesis are cytochrome P450s. The adrenal cortex consists of three zones: the outer zona glomerulosa exclusively synthesizes mineralocorticoids owing to localized expression of CYP11B2, whereas the zona fasciculata and reticularis synthesize glucocorticoid and androgens owing to localized expression of CYP17.[244] Cortisol, the end product of the glucocorticoid pathway, is the primary regulator of the hypothalamic-pituitary-adrenal axis, in which hypothalamic corticotropin-releasing hormone regulates pituitary adrenocorticotropic hormone (ACTH) secretion and downstream adrenal production of all three categories of steroid. ACTH release follows a diurnal pattern with a peak at 0400 to 0800 hours and, most importantly, markedly increases in response to trauma, acute illness, high fever, and hypoglycemia.

Mineralocorticoid production is primarily controlled by the renin-angiotensin system, in which angiotensinogen secreted by the liver is cleaved by renin to angiotensin I, which is then converted to angiotensin II.[245] The mineralocorticoid pathway is also responsive to ACTH, as demonstrated by an increase in all mineralocorticoid precursors and the end product aldosterone within minutes of exogenous ACTH stimulation. However, hypopituitarism does not lead to mineralocorticoid deficiency because an intact renin-angiotensin system independently stimulates aldosterone synthesis. Nevertheless, patients with ACTH deficiency may present with hyponatremia (glucocorticoids are required for free water excretion) and hypotension. The latter consequence of failure of the adrenal to release an adequate amount of glucocorticoid may be attributable to the role of cortisol in enhancing vascular responsiveness to catecholamines and inotropic activity.[246] This essential aspect of glucocorticoid activity is the most lethal potential consequence of both primary adrenal insufficiency and hypothalamic-pituitary deficiency and requires the utmost caution on the part of pediatrician, endocrinologist, surgeon, or anesthesiologist. When any question regarding adequacy of the hypothalamic-pituitary-adrenal axis arises, it is prudent to provide exogenous glucocorticoid, particularly perioperatively.[247]

CAUSES OF ADRENAL INSUFFICIENCY

Primary adrenal insufficiency is suspected from features such as weight loss, nausea and vomiting, poor appetite, and, specifically, the characteristic skin hyperpigmentation that is secondary to melanocyte-stimulating hormone receptor cross-stimulation by ACTH (which is present in extraordinarily large concentrations).[248] Primary adrenal insufficiency is uncommon in countries with advanced health care systems now that infectious diseases such as tuberculosis are less prevalent, but adrenal hemorrhage still causes adrenal failure.[249] Autoimmune adrenal insufficiency, sometimes as part of a polyendocrinopathy syndrome, is now the most common cause and includes both glucocorticoid and mineralocorticoid deficiency. Glucocorticoid deficiency with or without mineralocorticoid loss is characteristic of congenital adrenal hyperplasia.[250] Rare disorders causing adrenal insufficiency include adrenoleukodystrophy,[251] congenital adrenal hypoplasia, X-linked adrenal hypoplasia congenita, and ACTH receptor defects.[252]

Congenital or acquired lesions of the hypothalamus or pituitary may lead to ACTH deficiency. In general, these lesions cause other pituitary deficiencies, particularly growth hormone or TSH deficiency; isolated ACTH deficiency is rare. Both growth hormone and ACTH deficiency may cause hypoglycemia in infancy. Central nervous system malformations leading to ACTH deficiency are usually detectable by MRI. A notable central nervous system anomaly with hypopituitarism is septo-optic dysplasia,[31,253-255] which may be associated with an assortment of midline defects, such as an absent or underdeveloped septum pellucidum and optic nerve hypoplasia, but isolated pituitary agenesis or hypoplasia is more common. Acquired lesions leading to hypopituitarism include hydrocephalus, meningitis, infiltrative disorders,[256] and tumors such as craniopharyngioma or histiocytosis X.[257] Tumor resection, especially craniopharyngioma, cranial irradiation, and chemotherapy, can lead to multiple pituitary deficiencies, often evolving over many years.[168]

TESTING FOR ADRENAL INSUFFICIENCY

Serum cortisol concentrations follow a diurnal pattern, with concentrations peaking during an ACTH surge in the early morning and waning later in the day. Although a morning serum cortisol concentration of less than 5 µg/dL is less than normal and suggestive of adrenal insufficiency, it may be difficult to interpret the significance of a random cortisol concentration. A reduced concentration at any other time of day is uninformative and should not be used to test for adrenal function. In contrast, laboratory confirmation of primary mineralocorticoid deficiency by obtaining a random serum sample shows a low aldosterone concentration despite markedly increased plasma renin activity.

Primary adrenal insufficiency may be effectively assessed in two ways[258]: either by simultaneous measurement of serum cortisol and plasma ACTH concentrations or by stimulating the adrenal with exogenous ACTH (cosyntropin [Cortrosyn], the biologically active fragment of ACTH containing the first 24 amino acids). A markedly increased random plasma ACTH concentration is definitive evidence of primary adrenal insufficiency, but concentrations can be moderately increased by the stress of phlebotomy itself. Therefore blood for plasma ACTH concentrations should be obtained from an indwelling catheter to avoid false-positive values.

Hypothalamic-pituitary insufficiency is more difficult to assess. The complete absence of ACTH levels, as in the obvious case of pituitary ablation or destruction, leads eventually to adrenal atrophy and complete unresponsiveness to cosyntropin stimulation, a finding that necessitates maintenance glucocorticoid replacement. However, an "adequate" response to cosyntropin implies only tonic ACTH secretion and does not guarantee the ability to generate a normal surge of ACTH during stress. As a consequence, any patient with a central nervous system lesion that might cause hypothalamic-pituitary-adrenal axis deficiency should receive stress doses of glucocorticoid (see later discussion). In practical terms, a post–cosyntropin-treatment cortisol value of 10 to 20 µg/dL in an at-risk child suggests the need for stress coverage, whereas a value less than 10 µg/dL indicates long-term replacement.[258,259]

PERIOPERATIVE MANAGEMENT OF ADRENAL INSUFFICIENCY

Glucocorticoid Dosing

Endogenous cortisol secretion is 6 to 8 mg/m² per day. Because a fraction of oral cortisol is degraded by the liver, the typical oral replacement dose is 10 to 12 mg/m² per day. A replacement dose of hydrocortisone depends on age and body size but generally is 5.0 to 7.5 mg two to three times a day orally for an adolescent with chronic adrenal insufficiency. No dose monitoring is required, but the child's growth rate should be tracked according to age. With concomitant or isolated mineralocorticoid deficiency, replacement uses fludrocortisone (Florinef) at an approximate dose of 0.1 mg orally per day, independent of body size, with intermittent monitoring of blood pressure and plasma renin activity. When the primary goal of glucocorticoid therapy is not replacement but suppression of ACTH secretion, as in congenital adrenal hyperplasia, the daily hydrocortisone dose is generally 15 to 20 mg/m², guided by monitoring of the serum concentration of 17-hydroxyprogesterone, androstenedione, dehydroepiandrosterone sulfate, and testosterone. Alternatives to hydrocortisone include prednisone, which is four to five times more potent than hydrocortisone. Dexamethasone is 30 to 40 times more potent than hydrocortisone, but it has no mineralocorticoid activity and carries much more significant risk of adverse effects, such as osteopenia and aseptic necrosis of the femoral head, and so should not be used for long-term routine replacement therapy. Single-dose use of dexamethasone has not been associated with aseptic necrosis of the femoral head.

Conventional stress glucocorticoid coverage is 3 to 10 times the patient's usual replacement dose, depending on the severity of illness or trauma, although this practice is not evidence based.[260] There is little risk associated with the transient use of excess glucocorticoid. We recommend exogenous glucocorticoid replacement for children who are receiving oral replacement therapy with 3 to 5 times the patient's usual oral maintenance dose for intercurrent illness or fever (>101°F) and 5 to 10 times the oral maintenance dose for major surgery, during critical illness, or in major emergencies. For children who require stress glucocorticoid coverage but who do not take outpatient steroids, or who are unable to take medications by mouth, we recommend using parenteral cortisol (Solu-Cortef) at a dose of 0.5 mg/kg per every 12 hours for illness associated with nausea, vomiting, diarrhea, or fever (>101°F) and 0.5 to 1 mg/kg every 6 hours for perioperative, intensive care, or emergency department indications for up to 72 hours.[261]

Iatrogenic Adrenal Suppression and Tapering

Increased doses of exogenous glucocorticoids are used chronically for control of autoimmune disorders, suppression of transplant rejection, and control of inflammatory processes. Iatrogenic adrenal suppression depends on the duration and dose of glucocorticoid used. Periods of high-dose steroids up to 7 to 10 days do not suppress the hypothalamic-pituitary-adrenal axis. Adrenal suppressive treatments lasting 3 to 6 weeks require a taper over 1 to

TABLE 27.6	Steroid Equivalency Ratios and Doses		
Steroid	Relative Antiinflammatory Potency	Relative Mineralocorticoid Potency	Daily Replacement (mg/m²)
Hydrocortisone	1	2	10
Cortisone	0.8	2	12
Prednisone	4	1	2.5
Prednisolone	5	1	2
Dexamethasone	20–30	0	<0.5

2 weeks to allow recovery of the hypothalamic-pituitary-adrenal axis. Long-term high-dose treatment may require up to 6 to 9 months for complete return of hypothalamic-pituitary-adrenal function and necessitates a taper during that period. At the termination of the taper, a repeat cosyntropin stimulation test should be performed to confirm recovery of function, and any repeat trauma or illness during the period of taper requires short-term stress coverage.

The glucocorticoid taper has two meanings. The tempo of therapeutic tapers of prednisone by gastroenterologists, rheumatologists, nephrologists, and oncologists, and of dexamethasone by surgeons, depends entirely on their assessment of the immune or inflammatory process. As long as the glucocorticoid dose is in excess of the replacement dose, and regardless of the dose, the hypothalamic-pituitary-adrenal axis continues to be suppressed. It is only when the steroid dose is tapered down to the daily replacement dose (approximately 10 mg/m² hydrocortisone, 2 mg/m² prednisone, or <0.5 mg/m² dexamethasone) that the endocrine taper begins. At that point, the prednisone should be switched to hydrocortisone for ease of starting a gradual taper from replacement therapy to reduced doses while function of the hypothalamic-pituitary-adrenal axis is reestablished. In the perioperative period, steroid coverage should be administered if there is any concern about the integrity of the hypothalamic-pituitary-adrenal axis during a steroid taper (Table 27.6).

HYPERCORTISOLISM (CUSHING SYNDROME)

Excess cortisol, whether exogenous or endogenous, results in muscle wasting, truncal obesity, moon facies, hypertension, hyperglycemia, osteopenia, and growth deceleration.[262,263] Iatrogenic hypercortisolism is common in pediatrics,[264] whereas Cushing disease or syndrome is rare.[265] Cushing disease refers to an ACTH-secreting pituitary adenoma. Cushing syndrome refers to other conditions of excess glucocorticoid, including ectopic ACTH-secreting tumors[266] and adrenal tumors that secrete cortisol.[267] An adrenal tumor (adenoma or carcinoma) is the most likely cause of hypercortisolism in a young child. These tumors can secrete any combination of steroids and commonly cosecrete androgens, resulting in virilization.[268] A unilateral glucocorticoid-secreting tumor typically causes hypothalamic-pituitary-adrenal axis suppression, requiring careful tapering of hydrocortisone replacement after resection to reestablish normal cortisol production in the contralateral adrenal gland.[269]

In a child with signs of hypercortisolism (and not simply obesity), screening tests include an overnight small dose dexamethasone suppression test, measurement of 24-hour urinary free cortisol and creatinine, and measurement of nocturnal salivary cortisol concentrations.[270] If screening tests suggest a diagnosis of hypercortisolism, additional adrenal steroids should be measured and an adrenal computed tomographic scan or MRI obtained. In an adolescent with pure glucocorticoid effects and suspicious results of a corticotropin-releasing hormone stimulation test or longer dexamethasone suppression test[271] suggestive of a pituitary ACTH-secreting adenoma (Cushing disease), pituitary MRI is warranted.[272] Because pituitary adenomas can be very small, bilateral inferior petrosal sinus sampling may be necessary to locate the adenoma.[273]

PERIOPERATIVE MANAGEMENT OF HYPERCORTISOLISM

Therapy for Cushing disease and Cushing syndrome is surgical.[274,275] There are no specific anesthetic considerations except the supportive management of secondary manifestations, such as obesity and its attendant airway concerns, hypertension, and skin and bone fragility.

Pheochromocytoma

Pheochromocytomas and paragangliomas are rare neuroendocrine tumors that arise from neural crest–derived cells. They can occur anywhere from the base of the skull to the pelvis where paraganglia are found.[276,277] Functional tumors produce catecholamines and are known as chromaffin tumors. These tumors derive their name from the dark grey-brown immunostaining of chromogranin A by chromium salts.[278]

ETIOLOGY

Nearly 80% of functional paraganglial tumors occur in the adrenal medulla and are referred to as pheochromocytomas. The other 20% of cases arise from extraadrenal paraganglionic tissue.[276,277] The overall incidence of pheochromocytoma is estimated in the general population at approximately 0.3 cases per million per year.[278] About 10% to 20% of all pheochromocytomas are diagnosed in childhood, with an average age at the time of onset of 11 years.[276,278] In large registries of pediatric paraganglial tumors, there appears to be a male predominance in childhood, whereas during the reproductive years, this shifts to a greater female predominance with the net effect being an equal distribution in the sexes.[279] In contrast to adults, pheochromocytomas in children are more often benign, bilateral, multiple in number, and extraadrenal.[278]

While only 5% to 10% of pediatric paraganglial tumors are malignant, metastases can be widespread and have been found in the bones, lungs, lymph nodes, and liver.[276,277] The European-American Pheochromocytoma-Paraganglioma Registry reports that as many as 80% of patients diagnosed before 18 years of age had a germline mutation in one of the known susceptibility genes.[280] To date, mutations in at least 10 susceptibility genes have been linked with pheochromocytoma-associated cancer syndromes such as von Hippel-Lindau (*VHL*), multiple endocrine neoplasia (*MEN*) type 2, neurofibromatosis 1, paraganglionic syndromes types 1–4, and familial pheochromocytoma syndromes.[280,281] Additionally, tuberous sclerosis and the Carney triad have also been associated with pheochromocytomas.

CLINICAL PRESENTATION

The clinical presentation of paraganglial tumors in children can vary greatly and may be due to catecholamine secretion or from mass effect. Tumors may also be found as incidental radiologic findings or as part of screening for one of the hereditary syndromes.[278] Functional pheochromocytomas and paragangliomas can secrete different catecholamines, including epinephrine, norepinephrine, and dopamine. Norepinephrine is the most

predominant hormone secreted, whereas only 10% to 20% of tumors secrete epinephrine and dopamine. However, there is no direct relationship between circulating catecholamine concentrations and overt symptoms.

Hypertension is the most typical presenting symptom in children, but it may be sustained rather than paroxysmal as is often the case in adults,[282] and is usually not associated with tumors that primarily secrete dopamine. Another common presentation in children is regular, intermittent headaches often associated with nausea and vomiting. Other reported findings include weight loss, polyuria, visual disturbances, and anxiety.[283] Although extremely rare, epinephrine-secreting tumors can actually present as circulatory shock owing to decreased intravascular volume and myocardial depression, the result of sustained high concentrations of catecholamines.

DIAGNOSIS

Because of the deleterious consequences of a missed pheochromocytoma diagnosis, testing should be performed for any child who presents with signs suggestive of pheochromocytoma or other paraganglial tumor. Paragangliomas may be mistaken for the more common neuroblastomas because of their similar location and secretion of vanillylmandelic acid and homovanillic acid.[279] Initial screening should include biochemical testing for catecholamine excess, followed by radiologic studies to find the anatomic location of a suspected catecholamine secreting mass. Traditionally catecholamines and their metabolites are typically measured in a 24-hour urine collection; however, this is often difficult in children. Plasma free metanephrines (metanephrine and normetanephrine) are produced and secreted by tumors independent of catecholamine release caused by tumor or sympathetic responses.[284] Liquid chromatography mass spectrometry assays to detect plasma free metanephrine and normetanephrine are now available and have a reported sensitivity of 98%.[285]

Once the biochemical diagnostic tests suggest the presence of a paraganglial tumor or pheochromocytoma, additional imaging to locate the mass is warranted. The most common location in children is in the abdomen, both within and outside the adrenal gland. Both CT and MRI can be used to locate these tumors[286]; considerations such as radiation exposure and possible need for general anesthesia may influence which technique is used, depending on the age of the child. The accuracy of locating a pheochromocytoma with these two techniques is similar,[286] although both have limitations in distinguishing a pheochromocytoma from other intraabdominal lesions less than 1 cm in diameter. Another imagining test, ^{131}I-metaiodobenzylguanidine (MIBG), can be helpful for identifying small tumors outside the adrenal gland as well as metastatic disease.[287]

PREOPERATIVE MANAGEMENT

Once the diagnosis of a pheochromocytoma or paraganglioma has been established, additional workup is often needed as medical therapy is initiated before surgery. A few basic laboratory results can be helpful in detecting remote organ involvement. For example, hypokalemia may be present in the context of hyperaldosteronism, or an abnormal total and ionized calcium level may indicate parathyroid gland involvement, suggestive of MEN 2 syndrome. Excess catecholamines can also increase fasting glucose concentrations or cause an abnormal glucose tolerance test result. Long-term exposure to increased circulating catecholamine concentrations not only causes vasoconstriction and relative hypovolemia, but it can also lead to cardiomyopathy, congestive heart failure, and arrhythmias. Therefore a preoperative electrocardiogram and echocardiogram should be obtained as part of the preoperative assessment.[286]

Surgical resection of pheochromocytoma should almost always be done on an elective basis after the child's medical status has been properly investigated, medical conditions stabilized, the location of the tumor(s) determined, and therapeutic α-adrenergic receptor blockade has been established. Preoperative α-adrenergic blockade is critical to success and has reduced perioperative complications during pheochromocytoma resection from 60% to 3%.[288] Effective blockade is evidenced by normalization of blood pressures for age and resolution of other symptoms, such as palpitations and headache. It must be emphasized that β-adrenergic blockade should *never* be introduced until α-adrenergic blockade has been well established; otherwise, this could result in unopposed paroxysmal systemic hypertension, leading to acute congestive heart failure, an acute coronary event, stroke, and even death. β-Adrenergic blockade to control reflex tachycardia or arrhythmias should only be started once α-adrenergic receptor blockade has been well established.[278]

Preoperative preparation is most commonly achieved with the noncompetitive α-adrenergic blocker, phenoxybenzamine. Phenoxybenzamine irreversibly alkylates α-adrenergic receptors, reducing the risk of an α-adrenergic–mediated increase in blood pressure during surgery. Phenoxybenzamine may be administered either orally or intravenously.[281] The effective oral dose usually ranges between 0.25 and 1.0 mg/kg per day and is given in divided doses. After the initial starting dose, increases should be titrated up every 2 to 3 days (owing to the drug's long half-life) until effective α-adrenergic blockade is achieved with normalized systolic blood pressure for the child's age.[276] This may require doses as large as 2 mg/kg per day and take several weeks of therapy to establish the correct dose.[278,281]

Oral bioavailability of phenoxybenzamine is only 20% to 30% with a 24-hour onset of action.[281] Alternatively, IV phenoxybenzamine has been used to more rapidly and reliably block α₁-receptors, although this requires close monitoring for peripheral vasodilatation and decreases in blood pressure, especially in the setting of relative hypovolemia. The action of phenoxybenzamine is terminated only by synthesizing new α-adrenergic receptors. The disadvantage of irreversibly blocking α-adrenergic receptors, as conferred by phenoxybenzamine, is that reactive hypotension may follow removal of the tumor, with resistance to interventions that are intended to increase the peripheral vascular resistance. One alternative, phentolamine, has been used because it has a much shorter half-life than phenoxybenzamine and is reversible. Calcium channel blockers may also aid in normalizing blood pressure with fewer orthostatic changes, although this is more common in adults.

ANESTHETIC CONSIDERATIONS

Resection of a catecholamine-secreting tumor is one of the most challenging and rare cases in anesthetic practice. The surgical approach may be open or laparoscopic depending on the tumor location, size, and surgeon's preference. The primary goal and challenge is maintaining stable hemodynamics both before tumor removal and immediately after. This requires careful planning preoperatively and anticipating intraoperative changes. Given the high-risk nature of these patients, surgical resection ideally should be done in a center with experience in such cases.[289]

Ensuring adequate α-adrenergic receptor blockade before entering the operating room is key for both normalizing blood pressure and expanding the contracted intravascular volume.[289] Anxiolysis prior to placement of invasive monitors or induction is important to maintain circulatory homeostasis and mitigate any stressor that may trigger a catecholamine surge. If feasible, invasive monitors such as arterial catheters are placed before induction of general anesthesia. A central venous catheter is always indicated for fluid management monitoring and delivering vasoactive infusions, including both vasodilators and vasoconstrictors. In patients with evidence of myocardial dysfunction, noninvasive continuous cardiac output assessments, a pulmonary artery catheter, or transesophageal echocardiography are essential to tailor the intraoperative management.

The goal during general anesthesia induction and intubation is to limit hemodynamic stress. Depending on the age of the patient, this can be accomplished with either IV or inhalational agents. Medications that may cause histamine release and sympathomimetics, such as ketamine, morphine, curariform neuromuscular blockers, and meperidine, should be avoided. Some have suggested succinylcholine may trigger a sympathetic response via stimulation of the sympathetic ganglia or fasciculations and thus should also generally be avoided, although succinylcholine is now rarely administered in pediatric anesthesiology for other reasons.[290] Airway instrumentation should be attempted only after adequate depth of anesthesia is established, and adjuncts such as IV lidocaine may be of benefit.[289] Vecuronium or rocuronium are the preferred neuromuscular blockers owing to their lack of autonomic effects and histamine release.[291]

Hypertension can occur during the surgery, especially during manipulation of the tumor, despite α-adrenergic blockade. Measures to control the blood pressure include increasing the inspired concentration of inhalational anesthetic, sodium nitroprusside infusion, IV magnesium sulfate,[290] and in refractory cases of hypertension, nicardipine and fenoldopam have been used successfully.[292] Tachycardia may also occur; the preferred β-adrenergic blocker to control heart rate is esmolol because of its very brief duration of action.

Sudden hypotension may also occur once the tumor has been ligated as a result of the sudden removal of the source of catecholamines and irreversible α-adrenergic blockade by phenoxybenzamine. These factors, in conjunction with a contracted plasma volume, blood loss, and anesthetic agents, may lead to profound and persistent hypotension.[289] Hypotension may continue for several days postoperatively until new α-adrenergic receptors are synthesized. Supportive treatment with volume expansion and vasopressors such as epinephrine, norepinephrine, and vasopressin may be needed.[289,290] Postoperative management in an ICU is required.

Finally, reactive hypoglycemia may occur on removal of the source of catecholamines and the coexisting relative excess plasma insulin levels; thus blood glucose concentrations should be measured frequently until stabilized. Consultation with an endocrinologist and steroid replacement should be initiated if bilateral adrenalectomy has been performed.[289]

ANNOTATED REFERENCES

Baylis PH. The syndrome of inappropriate antidiuretic hormone secretion. *Int J Biochem Cell Biol.* 2003;35:1495-1499.
The author reviews the cardinal diagnostic criteria, clinical features, and pathophysiology of SIADH, which develops because of persistent detectable or elevated plasma arginine vasopressin concentrations in the presence of continued fluid intake. Inappropriate infusion of hypotonic fluids in the postoperative state is a

common cause. For symptomatic patients with chronic SIADH, the mainstay of therapy is fluid restriction.

Cameron FJ, Wherrett DK. Care of diabetes in children and adolescents: controversies, changes, and consensus. *Lancet.* 2015;385(9982):2096-2106.

A clinically focused, up-to-date review of epidemiology, pathophysiology, diagnosis, and management of diabetes in children and adolescents.

Copeland KC, Silverstein J, Moore KR, et al. Management of newly diagnosed type 2 diabetes mellitus (T2DM) in children and adolescents. *Pediatrics.* 2013;131(2):364-382.

This consensus statement provides guidance on the diagnosis and management of youth with type 2 diabetes.

LaFranchi S. Congenital hypothyroidism: etiologies, diagnosis, and management. *Thyroid.* 1999;9:735-740.

LaFranchi thoroughly reviews and discusses thyroid development and hypothyroidism in this article. He includes both embryologic and molecular defects of hypothyroidism.

Lenders JW, Eisenhofer G, Mannelli M, Pacak K. Phaeochromocytoma. *Lancet.* 2005;366:665-675.

Pheochromocytoma is a rare and dangerous disorder with many hidden problems that may complicate anesthesia. This review provides a single but most thorough analysis of the basic science and practical clinical issues needed to safely anesthetize children with this disorder and to anticipate and minimize complications and risks.

Nadeau KJ, Anderson BJ, Berg EG, et al. Youth-onset type 2 diabetes consensus report: current status, challenges, and priorities. *Diabetes Care.* 2016;39(9):1635-1642.

This report characterizes type 2 diabetes in children, describes differences between childhood and adult type 2 diabetes, describes treatment options, and describes challenges to and approaches for new therapies.

Oiso Y, Robertson GL, Nørgaard JP, Juul KV. Clinical review: treatment of neurohypophyseal diabetes insipidus. *J Clin Endocrinol Metab.* 2013;98:3958-3967.

This review summarizes information about the safety and efficacy of treatments for the types of diabetes insipidus caused by a primary deficiency of vasopressin.

Rhodes ET, Gong C, Edge JA, et al. ISPAD Clinical Practice Consensus Guidelines 2014. Management of children and adolescents with diabetes requiring surgery. *Pediatr Diabetes.* 2014;15(suppl 20):224-231.

The authors review the perioperative management of type 1 and type 2 diabetes mellitus in children who are surgical patients.

Rivkees SA. The treatment of Graves' disease in children. *J Pediatr Endocrinol Metab.* 2006;19:1095-1111.

This article reviews the pathophysiology of hyperthyroidism with particular focus on Graves disease. Rivkees outlines current treatment options for hyperthyroidism, including medical, surgical, and radioiodine ablation.

Sarlis NJ, Gourgiotis L. Thyroid emergencies. *Rev Endocr Metab Disord.* 2003;4:129-136.

A concise review article on the presentation and management of extreme thyroid disorders, myxedema coma, and thyrotoxic storm.

Seckl JR, Dunger DB, Lightman SL. Neurohypophyseal peptide function during early postoperative diabetes insipidus. *Brain.* 1987;110: 737-746.

Neurohypophyseal function, including serial measurements of plasma and urinary arginine vasopressin (AVP) and the AVP prohormone/carrier peptide neurophysin I concentrations, was investigated in 11 children undergoing pituitary or suprasellar surgery. The authors conclude that early postoperative diabetes insipidus is not a result of decreased levels of circulating AVP but may be related to the release of biologically inactive precursors from the damaged neurohypophysis. These may lead to renal refractoriness to AVP.

Silverstein J, Klingensmith G, Copeland K, et al. Care of children and adolescents with type 1 diabetes: a statement of the American Diabetes Association. *Diabetes Care.* 2005;28:186-212.

This statement provides a comprehensive review of the diagnosis of diabetes, management of type 1 diabetes, and acute and chronic complications of type 1 diabetes.

Sterns RH, Riggs JE, Schochet SS Jr. Osmotic demyelination syndrome following correction of hyponatremia. *N Engl J Med.* 1986;314: 1535-1542.

This is a description of eight patients who developed a neurologic syndrome with clinical or pathologic findings typical of central pontine myelinolysis, which developed after they presented with severe hyponatremia. Each patient's condition worsened after relatively rapid correction of hyponatremia (>12 mmol of sodium per liter per day). The data suggest that the neurologic sequelae were associated with correction of hyponatremia by more than 12 mmol/L per day. When correction proceeded more slowly, patients had uneventful recoveries. Osmotic demyelination syndrome is a preventable complication of overly rapid correction of chronic hyponatremia.

TODAY Study Group, Zeitler P, Hirst K, et al. A clinical trial to maintain glycemic control in youth with type 2 diabetes. *N Engl J Med.* 2012;366(24):2247-2256.

This is the primary report of the TODAY Study, a randomized trial of 699 adolescents with type 2 diabetes. The study found that monotherapy with metformin was associated with durable glycemic control in approximately half of children and adolescents with type 2 diabetes. The addition of rosiglitazone, but not an intensive lifestyle intervention, was superior to metformin alone.

Wolfsdorf JI, Allgrove J, Craig ME, et al. ISPAD Clinical Practice Consensus Guidelines 2014. Diabetic ketoacidosis and hyperglycemic hyperosmolar state. *Pediatr Diabetes.* 2014;15(suppl 20):154-179.

The authors review the pathophysiology of diabetic ketoacidosis in childhood and discuss currently recommended treatment protocols. Current concepts regarding cerebral edema are presented, as are strategies for prediction and prevention of diabetic ketoacidosis.

A complete reference list can be found online at ExpertConsult.com.

Essentials of Nephrology

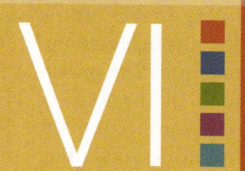

DELBERT R. WIGFALL, JOHN W. FOREMAN, AND WARWICK A. AMES

THE ANESTHESIA PRACTITIONER IS OFTEN FACED with a child who has acute kidney injury (AKI) or renal failure. Renal disease requires the practitioner to be vigilant about fluid homeostasis, acid-base balance, electrolyte management, choice of anesthetics, and potential complications. This requires a thorough understanding of the excretory and fluid homeostatic functions of the kidney, particularly in the neonate and younger child. If not managed assiduously, perioperative renal dysfunction can deteriorate into renal failure or multiorgan system failure resulting in significant morbidity or mortality. The anesthesia provider must understand renal physiology, appropriate preoperative preparation, intraoperative management, and postoperative care of the child with renal disease.

Renal Physiology

The basic functions of the kidney are to maintain fluid and electrolyte homeostasis and metabolism. The first step in this tightly controlled process is the production of the glomerular filtrate from the renal plasma. The glomerular filtration rate (GFR) depends on renal blood flow (RBF), which depends on the systolic blood pressure and circulating blood volume. The kidneys are the best perfused organs per gram of weight in the body. They receive 20% to 30% of the cardiac output maintained over a wide range of blood pressures through changes in renal vascular resistance. Numerous hormones play a role in this autoregulation, including vasodilators (i.e., prostaglandins E and I_2, dopamine, and nitric oxide) and vasoconstrictors (i.e., angiotensin II,

thromboxane, adrenergic stimulation, and endothelin). Congestive heart failure and volume contraction severely limit the ability of the kidney to maintain autoregulation.

When adjusted for body surface area (BSA) or scaled using allometric theory (see Chapter 7), both RBF and GFR double in the first 2 weeks of postnatal life and both continue to increase steadily, reaching adult values by 2 years of age (see Figs. 7.11 and 7.12).[1,2] The increases in RBF over time parallel similar increases in cardiac output and decreases in renal vascular resistance. The initial GFR and the rate of increase during the first few years correlate with the neonate's postmenstrual age at birth. For example, the GFR (corrected using BSA or allometry) of a neonate born at 28 weeks gestation is one-half of that of a full-term infant (see Figs. 7.11 and 7.12).[3] GFR may be estimated from the serum creatinine concentration and the height of the child according to the following formula[4,5]:

$$\text{GFR (mL/min/1.73 m}^2) = \text{height (cm)} \times k/\text{serum creatinine}$$

In the equation, k is a constant that varies with age; 0.413 for infants, 0.55 for children, and 0.7 for adolescent boys. The serum creatinine concentration, especially in the first days of life, reflects the maternal serum creatinine concentration and therefore cannot be used to predict neonatal renal function until at least 2 days after birth.[6]

FLUIDS AND ELECTROLYTES

The kidney regulates the total body sodium balance and maintains normal extracellular and circulating volumes.[7] The adult kidney filters 25,000 mEq of sodium per day, but it excretes less than 1% through extremely efficient resorption mechanisms along the nephron. The proximal tubule resorbs 50% to 70%, the ascending limb of the loop of Henle resorbs about 25%, and the distal nephron accounts for 10% of the filtered sodium load. Several hormones, including renin, angiotensin II, aldosterone, and atrial natriuretic peptide (ANP), and changes in circulating blood volume contribute to maintaining the sodium balance.[8]

Serum osmolality is tightly regulated through changes in arginine vasopressin (AVP) release and thirst.[9-11] AVP, also called *antidiuretic hormone,* is synthesized in the hypothalamus and stored in the posterior pituitary, where it is released in response to an increasing plasma osmolality. AVP is also released in response to decreases in the circulating blood volume and hypotension, including responses to nausea, vomiting, opioids, inflammation, and surgery. AVP binds to receptors in the collecting duct, increasing the permeability of the tubules to water and leading to increased water resorption and concentrated urine. Neonates are much less able to conserve or excrete water compared with older children, rendering the fluid management and volume issues important tasks for the anesthesiologist in this young age group.[12]

The regulation of serum potassium is managed by the kidney and depends on the concentration of plasma aldosterone. Aldosterone binds to receptors on cells in the distal nephron, increasing the secretion of potassium in the urine. Neonates are much less efficient at excreting potassium loads compared with adults, and the normal range of serum potassium concentrations is therefore greater in neonates; Table 28.1 provides the normal values.[13] Potassium regulation is affected by the acid-base status; excretion of potassium increases in the presence of alkalosis and decreases in the presence of acidosis. Causes of hyperkalemia and hypokalemia are presented in Tables 28.2 and 28.3, respectively.

ACID-BASE BALANCE

The kidney is involved in the regulation of acid-base balance and the response to the stress of illness. The kidney reclaims virtually all of the filtered bicarbonate in the proximal tubule and regenerates bicarbonate (HCO_3^-) lost in the neutralization of acid generated by the normal combustion of food, especially protein, and the formation of bone. New bicarbonate is the product of cells in the distal nephron that decompose the carbonic acid (H_2CO_3) formed from water (H_2O) and carbon dioxide (CO_2) by carbonic anhydrase. The protons (H^+) that are generated from this process are pumped into the lumen of the collecting duct, where they combine with hydrogen phosphate (HPO_4^{2-}) or ammonia (NH_3) generated by the catabolism of amino acids, mainly glutamine, in the tubule cells.

Infants, especially neonates, maintain a slightly acidotic blood (pH = 7.37) and decreased plasma bicarbonate concentration (22 mEq/L) compared with older children and adults (pH = 7.39; plasma bicarbonate = 24 to 28 mEq/L).[14] The reduced plasma concentration of HCO_3^- is the result of a reduced threshold or the plasma concentration at which HCO_3^- is incompletely resorbed by the kidney. Neonates maintain acid-base homeostasis but are limited in their ability to respond to an acid load.[15] This is especially true for preterm infants.

TABLE 28.2	Causes of Hyperkalemia
Transcellular Shifts	
Acidosis	
β-Adrenergic blockers	
Insulin deficiency	
Burns	
Tumor lysis syndrome	
Rhabdomyolysis	
Succinylcholine	
Decreased Excretion	
Renal failure	
Potassium-sparing diuretics	
Cyclosporine	
Nonsteroidal antiinflammatory drugs	
Angiotensin-converting enzyme inhibitors	
Mineralocorticoid deficiency	
Adrenal insufficiency	
Congenital adrenal hyperplasia	
Hyporeninemic hypoaldosteronism	
Primary mineralocorticoid deficiency	
Mineralocorticoid resistance	
Prematurity	
Obstructive uropathy	
Pseudohypoaldosteronism	
Increased Intake	
Potassium supplements, oral or intravenous	
Blood transfusions	
Potassium-containing antibiotics	

TABLE 28.3	Causes of Hypokalemia
Transcellular Shift	
Insulin	
β-Adrenergic agonists	
Increased Excretion	
Vomiting	
Diarrhea	
Nasogastric suction	
Laxatives	
Diuretics	
Cisplatin	
Amphotericin B	
Renal tubular acidosis	
Bartter syndrome	
Corticosteroids	
Decreased Intake	
Malnutrition	
Anorexia nervosa	

TABLE 28.1	Normal Values of Serum Potassium	
Age	Serum Potassium Range (mEq/L)
0–1 month	4.0–6.0
1 month–2 years	4.0–5.5
2–17 years	3.8–5.0
>18 years	3.2–4.8

Disease States

The causes of and differences in renal diseases between children and adults are substantive. Depending on the cause of the renal disease, management may be different. Adult renal disease usually results from long-standing diabetes mellitus or hypertension with an associated compromise in cardiovascular function. Children may also have renal failure owing to diseases such as sickle cell disease or systemic lupus erythematosus, but cardiovascular function is far less commonly compromised.

ACUTE RENAL FAILURE AND ACUTE KIDNEY INJURY

Acute renal failure (ARF) or acute renal insufficiency is defined as an abrupt deterioration in the ability of the kidneys to clear nitrogenous wastes, such as urea and creatinine. Concomitantly, there is a loss of ability to excrete other solutes and maintain a normal water balance. This leads to the clinical presentation of acute renal insufficiency: edema, hypertension, hyperkalemia, and uremia.

Acute kidney injury (AKI) has almost replaced the traditional term *acute renal failure (ARF)*, which was used in reference to the subset of patients who had an acute need for dialysis. With the recognition that even modest increases in serum creatinine are associated with a dramatic increase in mortality, the clinical spectrum of acute decline in GFR is broader. Minor deterioration in GFR and kidney injury are captured in a working clinical definition of kidney damage that allows early detection and intervention and uses AKI in place of ARF. The term ARF is preferably restricted to those with AKI who also require renal replacement therapy.[16] The prognosis of AKI is assessed in part by the use of the RIFLE criteria, which include three severity categories (i.e., **R**isk, **I**njury, and **F**ailure) and two clinical outcome categories (**L**oss and **E**nd-stage renal disease) (Table 28.4).

The term ARF has often been incorrectly used interchangeably with *acute tubular necrosis (ATN)*, which usually refers to a rapid deterioration in renal function occurring minutes to days after an ischemic or nephrotoxic event. Although acute tubular necrosis is an important cause of ARF, it is not the sole cause, and the terms are not synonymous. For the purposes of this chapter, AKI refers to the disease formerly called ARF.

Etiology and Pathophysiology

AKI is often multifactorial in origin or the result of several distinct insults. To treat AKI, it is important to understand its causes and pathophysiology. The etiologies of AKI are varied, but can be broadly classified as follows (Table 28.5):

- *Prerenal,* implying poor renal perfusion as the cause
- *Renal,* implying intrinsic renal disease or damage as the cause
- *Postrenal,* implying an obstruction to the excretion of urine as the cause

Prerenal insults comprise the majority (up to 70%) of cases of AKI. They usually result from massive losses of extracellular fluid, such as in gastroenteritis, burns, hemorrhage, or excessive diuresis, as well as in cardiac failure and sepsis. The common feature of this condition is diminished renal perfusion. In response to the reduction in RBF, there is a compensatory increase in afferent tone, which decreases the GFR and increases the retention of salt and water. The net effect of these events is a drastic reduction in urine volume, often leading to oliguria and/or anuria. If the underlying problem is recognized early and treated aggressively, progressive renal insufficiency may be averted. Nonsteroidal antiinflammatory drugs, angiotensin-converting enzyme (ACE) inhibitors, and angiotensin receptor blockers can aggravate prerenal azotemia by further reducing glomerular capillary pressure and the GFR.[17]

Parenchymal disease or injury accounts for 20% to 30% of the cases of abrupt onset of AKI. In infants, the common causes include birth asphyxia, sepsis, and cardiac surgery. In older children, the important causes of AKI include trauma, sepsis, and hemolytic uremic syndrome. Prolonged prerenal azotemia may result in overt renal injury. Similarly, intrarenal obstruction to blood flow from thrombi or vasculitis may cause renal failure. Drugs such as aminoglycosides or amphotericin B or other nephrotoxins, including radiocontrast agents, may induce AKI through tubular or interstitial injury as a result of allergic reactions, as can be seen with penicillins. Acute glomerulonephritis is another cause of AKI in children; rarely, pyelonephritis can lead to AKI.

The remaining causes of AKI result from the obstruction to urine flow. These conditions account for less than 10% of all cases of AKI and may involve obstruction of both kidneys. Sudden anuria suggests a postrenal cause for the AKI. The obstruction can occur within the collecting system of the kidney (intrarenal), in the ureter, or in the urethra (extrarenal). Intrarenal obstruction may occur with the tumor lysis syndrome with the deposition of uric acid crystals, from myoglobinuria, hemoglobinuria, or from medications such as acyclovir and cidofovir. Extrarenal obstruction can be caused by stones inspissated in the ureters or from external compression by lymph nodes or a tumor. As with other forms of AKI, prompt recognition and appropriate intervention to relieve the obstruction may facilitate full recovery of renal function and obviate a permanent reduction in renal function.

The exact pathophysiology of AKI remains unclear, but several factors have been identified.[18] In the initial phase of AKI, profound renovascular vasoconstriction reduces GFR (Fig. 28.1). Factors known to increase renal vasoconstriction include increased activity of the renin-angiotensin and the adrenergic systems and endothelial dysfunction with increased endothelin release and decreased nitric

TABLE 28.4	RIFLE Classification of Renal Failure and Kidney Injury	
RIFLE Factors	**GFR Criteria**	**Urine Output Criteria**
Risk	Increased Cr × 1.5 or decreased GFR >25%	UOP <0.5 mL/kg per hour > 6 hours	High sensitivity
Injury	Increased Cr × 2 or GFR decrease >50%	UOP <0.5 mL/kg per hour > 12 hours	
Failure	Increased Cr × 3 or GFR decrease of 75% or Cr ≥4 mg/dL Acute rise ≥0.5 mg/dL	UOP <0.3 mL/kg per hour > 24 hours or Anuria > 12 hours	
Loss	Persistent ARF: complete loss of kidney function > 4 weeks		High specificity
ESKD	End-stage kidney disease (> 3 months)		

Modified from Bellomo R, Ronco C, Kellum JA, Mehta RL, Palevsky P. Acute Dialysis Quality Initiative Workgroup. Acute renal failure—definition, outcome measures, animal models, fluid therapy and information technology needs: the Second International Consensus Conference of the Acute Dialysis Quality Initiative (ADQI) Group. *Crit Care.* 2004;8:R204–R212.
ARF, acute renal failure; *Cr,* creatinine; *ESKD,* end-stage kidney disease; *GFR,* glomerular filtration rate; *RIFLE,* Risk of renal dysfunction, Injury to the kidney, Failure of kidney function, Loss of kidney function, and End-stage kidney disease; *UOP,* urine output.

TABLE 28.5 Causes of Acute Renal Failure

Prerenal Failure	Renal Failure	Postrenal Failure
Hypovolemia	Acute glomerulonephritis	Obstruction
Volume loss	Postinfectious	Intrinsic (papillary necrosis due to diabetes, sickle
Gastrointestinal, renal losses	Membranoproliferative glomerulonephritis	cell disease, or analgesic nephropathy)
Sequestration (burns, postoperative)	Rapidly progressive glomerulonephritis	Intrarenal abnormalities, ureteral obstruction,
	Glomerulonephritis due to systemic	obstruction of the bladder or urethra
	disease (e.g., HUS, DIC, SLE)	Extrinsic (tumor compression, lymphadenopathy)
Hypotension	Acute interstitial nephritis	
Shock	Drug-induced hypersensitivity (penicillin)	
Vasodilators	Infections	
Decreased effective blood flow	Tubular disease	
Low cardiac output	ATN (ischemic, nephrotoxic)	
Cirrhosis	Intratubular obstruction (uric acid, oxalate)	
Nephrotic syndrome		
Renal hypoperfusion	Cortical necrosis	
Use of ACE inhibitors	Gram-negative sepsis	
NSAIDs	Hemorrhage	
Hepatorenal syndrome	Shock	
Vascular occlusion	Acute renal failure	
Thromboembolic phenomenon	Toxins	
Aortic dissection	Organic solvents	
Renal vein thrombosis (dehydration,	Heavy metals	
hypercoagulable state, neoplasm)	Insecticides	
	Hemoglobin	
	Myoglobin	
	Chronic renal failure	
	Chronic interstitial nephritis	
	Chronic glomerulonephritis	
	Chronic glomerulosclerosis	
	Nephrocalcinosis	
	Obstructive uropathy	
	Hypertension	

ACE, angiotensin-converting enzyme; *ATN*, acute tubular necrosis; *DIC*, disseminated intravascular coagulation; *HUS*, hemolytic uremic syndrome; *NSAIDs*, nonsteroidal antiinflammatory drugs; *SLE*, systemic lupus erythematosus.

oxide synthesis. However, therapeutic interventions to vasodilate the intrarenal vasculature, such as prostaglandin and dopamine infusions, ACE inhibitors, calcium channel blockers, and endothelin receptor antagonists, have not significantly reversed established AKI.[19]

Another factor in the pathogenesis of AKI is renal tubule cell injury, the direct result of a nephrotoxic agent or from an ischemic insult (Fig. 28.2). Cellular injury leads to sloughing of the brush border, swelling, mitochondrial condensation, disruption of cellular architecture, and loss of adhesion to the basement membrane with shedding of cells into the tubular lumen.[20] These changes, which occur within minutes of an ischemic event, contribute to the decreased GFR by obstructing the lumen of the tubule.[21] These cellular changes allow the filtrate to leak back into the peritubular blood, reducing the excretion of solutes and the effective GFR.

Some of the cellular derangements in AKI, such as a reduction in ATP concentrations,[21] cell membrane injury by reactive oxygen molecules,[22] and increased intracellular calcium concentrations from changes in membrane phospholipid metabolism, lead to cell death. Reactive oxygen molecules also stimulate the production of cytokines and chemokines that play a role in cell injury and vasoconstriction.

Neutrophils that are recruited during reperfusion injury after renal ischemia mediate parenchymal renal damage.[23] Reperfusion injury increases intracellular adhesion molecule 1 (ICAM-1) on endothelial cells promoting the adhesion of circulating neutrophils and their eventual infiltration into the parenchyma. Neutrophils then release reactive oxygen molecules, elastases, proteases, and other enzymes that lead to further tissue injury.

Diagnostic Procedures

A thorough history and physical examination can yield important insight into the likely causes of AKI. The initial laboratory assessment of a child with AKI should include the measurement of serum urea, creatinine, electrolytes, and a urinalysis. Prerenal azotemia is typically associated with a ratio of blood urea nitrogen (BUN) to creatinine that exceeds 20. In cases of renal parenchymal dysfunction, this ratio is closer to 10. Hematuria and proteinuria are consistently present in AKI, independent of the cause, although the presence of cellular casts, especially red blood cell casts, in the urinary sediment is suggestive of glomerulonephritis. Granular casts are associated with prerenal azotemia.

One test to distinguish prerenal azotemia from established renal failure from ischemia or nephrotoxins is the fractional excretion of sodium (FE_{Na}). The FE_{Na} is calculated using the following equation:

$$FE_{Na} = \frac{U_{Na} \times S_{Cr}}{S_{Na} \times U_{Cr}} \times 100\%$$

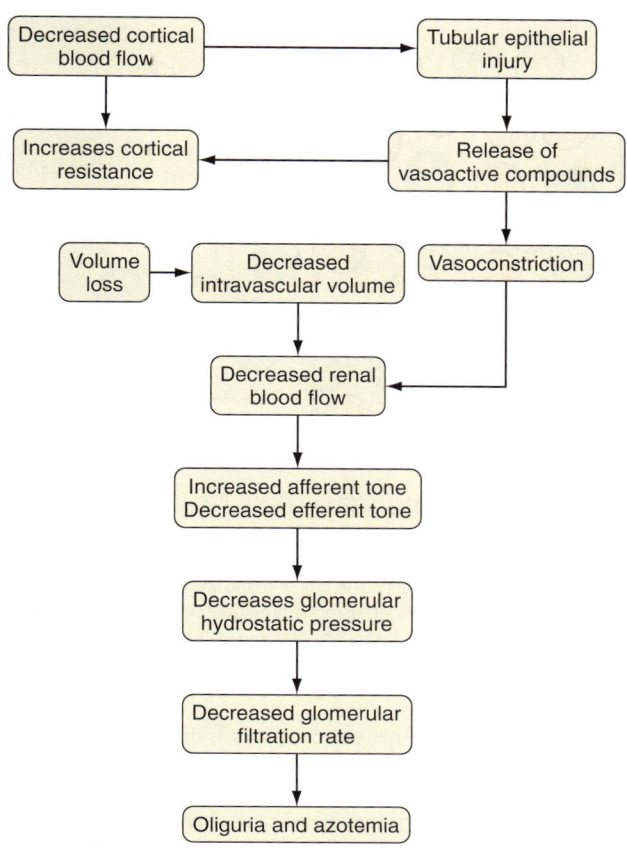

FIGURE 28.1 Hemodynamic factors in the pathogenesis of acute renal failure.

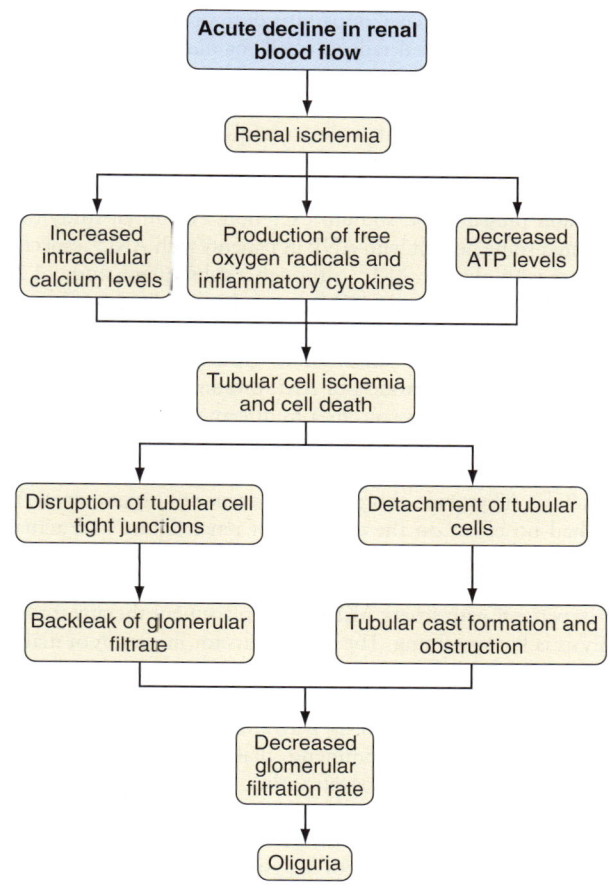

FIGURE 28.2 Influences of specific injuries on the nephron in the pathogenesis of acute renal failure. *ATP,* adenosine triphosphate.

U_{Na} and S_{Na} are urine and serum sodium concentrations, and U_{Cr} and S_{Cr} are the urine and serum creatinine concentrations, respectively. In prerenal azotemia, the FE_{Na} is usually less than 1% for adults and children and less than 2.5% for infants. In established AKI from ischemia and nephrotoxins, but not acute glomerulonephritis, the FE_{Na} usually exceeds 1%. Administration of diuretics may confound the interpretation of this test.

The initial radiologic assessment of children with AKI is ultrasonography. Renal ultrasound does not depend on renal function and can define the renal anatomy, changes in parenchymal density, and possible outlet obstruction by demonstrating dilation of the urinary tract. Doppler interrogation of the renal vessels provides information on vascular flow. Further radiographic studies, such as voiding cystourethrography, nuclear renal flow scanning, dynamic functional MRI, and abdominal computed tomography (CT), may be indicated in select children and conditions.

Therapeutic Interventions

Therapeutic interventions in children with AKI should be aimed at the underlying cause and at improving renal function and urine flow. Children with AKI caused by hypovolemia should be fluid resuscitated with at least 20 mL/kg over 30 to 60 minutes with normal saline solution or a balanced salt solution. For children with significant hypotension, an alternative choice is a colloid-containing solution. Children with oliguria caused by hypovolemia usually respond within 4 to 6 hours with increased urine output. Anecdotal reports have supported the use of low-dose dopamine in AKI. A recent clinical trial has demonstrated benefit from

dopamine in improving urine output in very low–birth-weight neonates.[24]

Diuretics have been commonly used to treat oliguric AKI. There are several theoretical reasons why mannitol, furosemide, and other loop diuretics may ameliorate AKI. First, diuretics may convert oliguric AKI to nonoliguric AKI. Second, loop diuretics decrease energy-driven transport in the loop of Henle, and this may protect cells in regions of hypoperfusion. However, neither mannitol nor loop diuretics can predictably convert an oliguric patient with AKI to a polyuric patient. Diuretics have not been shown in clinical studies to influence renal recovery, need for dialysis, or survival in patients with AKI.[25,26] Diuretics should be used only after the circulating volume has been adequately restored and should be stopped if there is no early response.

Dopamine has been widely used to prevent and manage AKI. In low doses (0.5–2.0 μg/kg per minute), dopamine increases renal plasma flow, GFR, and renal sodium excretion by activating dopaminergic receptors. Infusion rates in excess of 3 μg/kg per minute stimulate α-adrenergic receptors on systemic arterial resistance vasculature, causing vasoconstriction; cardiac β1-adrenergic receptors, increasing cardiac contractility, heart rate, and cardiac index; and β2-adrenergic receptors on systemic arterial resistance vasculature, causing vasodilatation. In a meta-analysis of 24 studies and 854 adult patients, dopamine did not prevent renal failure, alter the need for dialysis, or change the mortality rate. In a randomized clinical trial of low-dose dopamine in 328 critically ill adult patients, dopamine did not change the duration or severity of the renal failure, need for dialysis, or mortality.[27] From these data, the routine use of low-dose dopamine in patients with AKI cannot be supported.

Several other agents that were useful in experimental models of AKI have been investigated but have not shown clinical success. ANP increases GFR in animal models of AKI by increasing renal perfusion pressure and sodium excretion. An initial study demonstrated some benefit with ANP in patients with AKI,[28] especially in those with oliguric AKI,[29] although a subsequent study of 222 adult patients with oliguric AKI failed to detect a difference between patients treated with ANP and placebo in terms of the need for dialysis or mortality.[30] Insulin-like growth factor 1 has been beneficial in animal models of AKI, presumably by potentiating cell regeneration. However, in a multicenter, placebo-controlled trial in adult patients with AKI, insulin-like growth factor 1 failed to speed the recovery, decrease the need for dialysis, or alter mortality.[31] Thyroxine abbreviates the course of experimental AKI but had no effect on the duration of renal failure and actually increased mortality threefold (by suppression of thyroid-stimulating hormone).[32]

In patients with severe AKI, renal replacement therapy through dialysis is life sustaining. The indications for initiation of dialytic therapy are persistent hyperkalemia, volume overload refractory to diuretics, severe metabolic acidosis, and overt signs and symptoms of uremia such as pericarditis and encephalopathy. Many nephrologists recommend dialysis if the BUN value approaches 100 mg/dL or even earlier, especially in the oliguric patient, although this has not proved to alter outcome. A retrospective study that compared early (BUN <60 mg/dL) versus late (BUN >60 mg/dL) initiation of dialysis in adult patients suggested that early initiation improved survival.[33] However, the timing of the initiation of dialysis remains an unresolved question.

Three strategies are available to replace renal function in critically ill children and adults: hemodialysis, peritoneal dialysis, and a variation of continuous replacement therapies, such as continuous venovenous hemofiltration (CVVH), continuous venovenous hemodialysis (CVVHD), and continuous venovenous hemodiafiltration (CVVHDF). None of these strategies has been proven superior to the others. However, in the individual child, one strategy may be more practical than the others. Hemodialysis is technically more difficult than peritoneal dialysis in an infant and hemodynamically unstable children. Continuous replacement therapies appear to cause less hemodynamic instability compared with hemodialysis and offer more predictable solute and fluid removal than peritoneal dialysis. Hemodialysis and continuous replacement therapies require large-bore vascular access to achieve the large blood flows that are necessary to support these strategies.

Although these three strategies differ technically, they share similar principles (Fig. 28.3). All three strategies remove nitrogenous wastes (i.e., urea), excess fluid, and excess solutes, especially potassium. This is achieved by circulating the child's blood over a semipermeable membrane that separates the blood from a salt solution (i.e., dialysate) on the contralateral surface. The movement of solutes across the membranes occurs by diffusion (i.e., solutes move across the membrane along their concentration gradients) and ultrafiltration (i.e., osmotic or hydrostatic pressures). The rate of removal of water and solute waste depends on the characteristics of the membrane (i.e., pore size and selectivity), diffusion, and ultrafiltration.[34]

The permeability characteristics and surface areas for the membranes are known for specific dialyzers used in hemodialysis

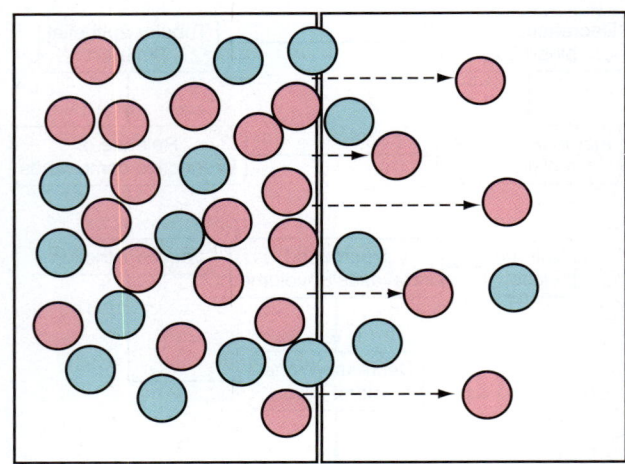

FIGURE 28.3 Principles of dialysis. Solute *(pink circles)* moves from the blood to the dialysate *(broken arrows)* in response to a concentration gradient (i.e., diffusion). The obligate passive movement of water *(blue circles)* attempts to maintain appropriate osmolarity. This flux of solute and water (i.e., ultrafiltration) may be enhanced by increased osmotic pressure (i.e., glucose in peritoneal dialysis fluid) or by increased hydrostatic pressure, which is created mechanically as transmembrane pressure in hemodialysis.

and hemofiltration. The peritoneum serves as the dialysis membrane in peritoneal dialysis and remains physically unalterable, but changes in dialysate composition and length of time the dialysate is exposed to the peritoneal membrane changes the amount of solute and water removed. In all forms of renal replacement therapy, the therapeutic prescription is individualized for the child.

Hemodialysis

Hemodialysis is very effective for AKI, being the best modality for the rapid removal of toxins, such as drug overdoses or other ingestions or metabolic toxins resulting from poisoning or inborn errors. Hemodialysis is very efficient, reducing the BUN by 60% to 70%, normalizing the serum potassium concentration, and removing fluid equal to 5% to 10% of the body weight within 3 to 4 hours. To accomplish this, large-vessel venous access is required to provide rapid blood flows (5-10 mL/kg per minute). In infants, this is achieved by inserting a double-lumen catheter into the subclavian, internal jugular, or femoral vein. In small infants, two single-lumen catheters placed in different sites may be necessary to access and return the blood. Rarely, a single-lumen catheter may be used for both outflow and return of blood. Modern hemodialysis machines have microprocessors that can accurately measure the amount of fluid removed and this should be summarized for the anesthesiologist.

Hemodialysis usually requires systemic anticoagulation with heparin, the effectiveness of which can be monitored by the activated clotting time (ACT). Hemodialysis can be undertaken without an anticoagulant in children who are at significant risk for bleeding by using a rapid blood flow rate and by frequently rinsing the blood circuit with saline. However, clotting commonly forms within the circuit with subsequent loss of the extracorporeal blood.

In addition to the risk of bleeding, hemodialysis is associated with several other adverse effects, the most common of which is hypotension. This usually results from overly aggressive removal of fluid, although it can also result from sepsis or the release of cytokines and autokines from blood passing over the surface of the hemodialysis filter. Muscle cramps, headache, nausea, and vomiting are also commonly reported. A more serious complication of hemodialysis is the disequilibrium syndrome that is related to the rapid removal of solute from the bloodstream with slow equilibration with the tissues, particularly the brain. This can cause cerebral edema, manifested by headache, obtundation, seizures, or coma. The disequilibrium syndrome is usually reported in children undergoing dialysis for the first time. This can be obviated by dialyzing for brief but frequent sessions initially, especially if the BUN concentration is increased substantially. Infection of the dialysis catheter is another common problem that can be minimized by using sterile central line techniques.

Peritoneal Dialysis

Peritoneal dialysis has a long history as renal replacement therapy in children.[35] It is relatively simple and easy to perform, even in small infants, and there is usually no hemodynamic instability. Although not as efficient as hemodialysis, optimal results are obtained if it is performed continuously to control solute and water balance. Peritoneal dialysis involves instilling dialysate fluid into the peritoneum for a set period and then draining the fluid and replacing it with fresh dialysate. This cycling removes waste products by diffusion and water by ultrafiltration as a consequence of a high glucose concentration in the dialysate. The efficacy of peritoneal dialysis depends on the volume of dialysate instilled per cycle and the number of cycles per day. Most children with acute renal failure are managed with 1- to 2-hour cycles of 5- to 30-mL/kg dwell volumes. Children with chronic renal failure are managed with greater cycle times and larger dwell volumes. The amount of fluid removed can be controlled by changing the concentration of the glucose in the dialysate. Short-term peritoneal dialysis can be accomplished with a nontunneled catheter, but should dialysis be required beyond 3 to 5 days, a subcutaneously tunneled cuffed catheter is preferred to minimize the risk of peritonitis.

The principal complications of peritoneal dialysis are infection and mechanical problems related to the catheter. It is common to find poor drainage from the catheter, usually the result of fibrin occlusion of the catheter or from omentum or bowel covering the inlet holes. The catheter may leak at its point of insertion. Hernias, especially inguinal hernias in boys, may develop as a consequence of the increased abdominal pressure from the infused dialysate. Mild hyponatremia may develop in infants because of the relatively low sodium concentration (130 mEq/L) in commercial dialysate. Less common but serious complications include bowel injury and intraabdominal hemorrhage from catheter insertion and peritonitis.

CHRONIC RENAL FAILURE

The loss of functioning renal mass results in a compensatory increase in filtration by the remaining renal tissue.[36] For example, within the first 48 hours after a unilateral nephrectomy, there is a demonstrable increase in the GFR and evidence of contralateral renal hypertrophy. By 2 to 4 weeks, the GFR has returned to 80% of normal, and there is no clinical evidence of renal dysfunction. With the loss of 50% to 75% of renal mass, there is an increase in the residual function to 50% to 80% of normal and often little evidence of clinical renal insufficiency. When the residual renal function decreases to 30% to 50% of normal, the term *chronic renal insufficiency* applies. At this point, acute illness and other stress states may result in acidosis, hyperkalemia, and dehydration. It is only when the residual function decreases to less than 30% of normal that the term *chronic renal failure* is used. At this point,

electrolyte abnormalities begin to appear, and more importantly, there is limited ability of the kidney to adjust to perturbations in volume status and electrolyte concentrations. The term *uremia* refers to the symptoms of anorexia, nausea, lethargy, and somnolence that develop as a result of chronic renal failure. Uremia ultimately leads to death unless dialysis therapy or renal transplantation is performed. Initiating dialysis or transplanting a kidney is referred to as end-stage renal disease care.

Chronic renal insufficiency and chronic renal failure are both categories within the larger schema of chronic kidney disease (CKD). Although the stages are defined by categorizing continuous measures of function (i.e., GFR) and therefore are somewhat arbitrary, they do provide a context for the evaluation and management of kidney disease. There are six stages of CKD:

Stage I: The GFR is normal (>90 mL/minute per 1.73 m^2), but there may be evidence of chronic renal disease, including an abnormal urinalysis, hypertension, or abnormal renal ultrasound.

Stage II: A GFR of 60 to 89 mL/minute per 1.73 m^2 indicates mild kidney damage and mild decrease in GFR.

Stage III: A GFR of 30 to 59 mL/minute per 1.73 m^2 is a moderate decrease in the GFR.

Stage IV: A GFR of 15 to 29 mL/minute per 1.73 m^2 is a severe decrease in the GFR, often accompanied by electrolyte or metabolic derangements.

Stage V: A GFR <15 mL/minute per 1.73 m^2 indicates kidney failure that requires renal replacement therapy.

Stage VI: Patients are undergoing dialysis or are transplant recipients.

Despite losses of up to 90% of renal function, sodium homeostasis usually is well maintained in chronic renal failure. With large decreases in the GFR, the kidney maintains normal serum sodium by increasing the FE_{Na} from less than 1% up to 25% to 30%, largely through decreases in distal tubular resorption. Some of the hormonal factors associated with this adaptation include aldosterone, ANP, and a poorly characterized natriuretic hormone that inhibits Na^+/K^+-ATPase. With chronic renal failure, the kidney loses its ability to handle a wide range of sodium intake, from 1 to 250 mEq/m^2 per day. Instead, the kidney may only be able to handle a narrow range of sodium intake of 50 to 100 mEq/m^2 per day. It may be possible to decrease this obligatory excretion of sodium to 5 to 20 mEq/m^2 per day, although it may occur only after weeks of decreasing the sodium intake slowly. Certain children with renal disease, especially those with obstructive uropathy or tubulointerstitial disease, may be unable to adjust to a decreased sodium intake and display a salt-losing nephropathy. These children are prone to dehydration with salt restriction and may need supplemental salt to ensure normal growth. In others, a regular diet may lead to sodium retention, volume overload, and hypertension; sodium intake must be individualized to fit the limitations of each child.

Water balance is also affected by chronic renal failure. There is an obligatory total osmolar excretion that limits the ability of the kidney to excrete free water. The concentrating ability of the kidney is affected, limiting its ability to make a maximally concentrated or dilute urine. These limitations may result in water retention and hyponatremia or dehydration if water is administered in amounts exceeding the kidney's capabilities. These limitations must be considered when treating children with chronic renal failure, particularly before surgery when free access to water is restricted.

In those with chronic renal failure, the serum potassium concentrations usually remain normal until the GFR is less than 10% of normal. Potassium excretion normally occurs in the distal nephron. However, in response to an increase in potassium intake or loss of renal mass, Na^+/K^+-ATPase increases in the remaining collecting tubules; this is responsible, in part, for the augmented excretion of potassium per nephron. In uremic animals, potassium is excreted from the renal tubules sixfold faster than in nonuremic animals and 1.5 times the filtered potassium load. Partial adaptation can occur in the absence of aldosterone, but aldosterone plays an important role in the maintenance of normal potassium homeostasis. This is demonstrated by the presence of hyperkalemia in children with hyporeninemic hypoaldosteronism or in those treated with the aldosterone antagonist spironolactone.

Approximately 13% of dietary potassium is excreted via the colon. This can increase to 50% by the activation of colonic Na^+/K^+-ATPase via aldosterone. An additional mechanism that plays an essential role in the adaptation to an acute potassium load is the redistribution of potassium from the extracellular to the intracellular compartment, which depends on insulin, β-adrenergic catecholamines, aldosterone, and pH. Despite the presence of total body potassium depletion in uremia, the uptake of potassium into the cells is impaired. This contributes to the intolerance to an acute potassium load in uremia despite the ability to excrete a potassium load.

Hyperkalemia is a major problem in chronic renal failure.[37] Hyperkalemia can result from an extrinsic potassium load, but it may also be caused by fasting or acidosis, in which case the source of the potassium is the intracellular compartment. This can be a particular problem when a child has fasted before surgery and can be ameliorated by an infusion of glucose and insulin. Drugs that can cause hyperkalemia in renal failure include spironolactone, β-adrenergic blockers, and ACE inhibitors. When clinically significant hyperkalemia develops in a child with chronic renal failure, the first-line therapy is to stabilize the myocardium with exogenous calcium and then to redistribute the potassium into the intracellular compartment with insulin and glucose. To deliver the same dose of ionized calcium, the dose of calcium gluconate (in milligrams per kilogram) should be three times that of calcium chloride. All doses of calcium are optimally delivered through a central venous access line because calcium infusions are irritating to peripheral veins and can cause necrosis of the skin if extravasation occurs. More definitive correction of hyperkalemia is accomplished by removing potassium from the body using dialysis or sodium polystyrene sulfonate (Kayexalate). At eight times the usual asthma dose, nebulized albuterol has been effective in redistributing potassium intracellularly, whereas sodium bicarbonate ($NaHCO_3$) administration has not been effective (Table 28.6). In contrast, significant hypokalemia is unusual in the absence of potassium restriction, alkalosis, or diuretic therapy.

Metabolic acidosis is common in those with chronic renal failure.[38] In moderate renal insufficiency, the type of metabolic acidosis is a non–anion gap acidosis, but in severe renal insufficiency, the metabolic acidosis is an anion gap acidosis, because of the presence of excess phosphate, sulfate, and organic acids. The primary cause of metabolic acidosis in chronic renal failure is the inability of the remaining proximal renal tubules to increase ammonium formation to keep pace with the loss of renal mass. The kidney becomes unable to generate the 1 to 3 mEq/kg per day of new bicarbonate that is necessary to compensate for the bicarbonate lost to buffering endogenous acids. Previous studies have suggested a major role for decreased resorption of bicarbonate by the proximal renal tubule in chronic renal failure. Although this may occur in the presence of volume overload, severe secondary hyperparathyroidism, and disorders such as Fanconi syndrome, it is not a major cause of acidosis in chronic renal failure. Except

TABLE 28.6	Treatment of Hyperkalemia
Treatment	**Dosage**
Stabilization of Myocardium	
Calcium and bicarbonate	Calcium gluconate: 10% 30–100 mg/kg IV or Calcium chloride: 10% 10–33 mg/kg IV Sodium bicarbonate: 1 mEq/kg IV if acidotic
Shifting of Potassium to Intracellular Space	
Hyperventilation	
Insulin and glucose	Insulin: 0.10–0.3 unit/kg or 0.1 U/kg per hour infusion Glucose: D_{50} 1–2 mL/kg or D_{25} 2–4 mL/kg IV or D_5 1–2 mL/kg per hour
Albuterol	Albuterol: 2.5–5 mg/mL nebulization
Decreasing Total Body Potassium	
Sodium polystyrene sulfonate (Kayexalate)	1 g/kg up to 40 g every 4 hours PO or PR
Furosemide (diuretic)	0.5 mg/kg up to 40 mg

D, dextrose; *IV*, intravenous; *PO*, per os (oral); *PR*, per rectum (suppository).

for severe phosphate depletion, decreased excretion of phosphate as a titratable acid normally does not contribute to metabolic acidosis.

One of the earliest manifestations of chronic renal failure is secondary hyperparathyroidism.[39] Secondary hyperparathyroidism, which results from inadequate formation of 1,25-$(OH)_2$ vitamin D (i.e., 1,25-dihydroxyvitamin D_3 or calcitriol), develops in moderate renal insufficiency in the presence of normal serum concentrations of calcium and phosphorus. As the renal insufficiency becomes more severe, overt hypocalcemia and hyperphosphatemia often develop. Hypocalcemia is caused by decreased calcium absorption from the gastrointestinal tract as a result of a true deficiency of 1,25-$(OH)_2$ vitamin D. Diminished release of calcium from bone occurs as a result of resistance to the action of parathyroid hormone. Calcium and phosphate may be deposited in soft tissues as a consequence of hyperphosphatemia.

The kidney plays a key role in the maintenance of phosphate homeostasis by regulating its excretion. In the presence of a normal GFR, the kidney excretes 5% to 15% of the filtered load of phosphate, whereas in chronic renal failure, the kidney can increase its fractional excretion of phosphate to 60% to 80%. Through this adaptation, the kidneys are able to maintain a phosphate balance in chronic renal failure, but they do so at an increased serum phosphate concentration. More importantly, the failing kidneys have no reserve with which to increase phosphate excretion in response to a phosphate load. In children with chronic renal failure, a large phosphate load, such as can occur with the administration of a phosphate-containing enema, can lead to life-threatening hyperphosphatemia and hypocalcemia.

Hematologic Problems

One of the most common manifestations of chronic renal failure is anemia. The anemia of chronic renal failure is the result of impaired erythropoiesis, hemolysis, and bleeding. Of these, impaired erythropoiesis is most important and usually the result of a deficiency of erythropoietin production. Erythropoietin is synthesized and secreted by the peritubular cells in the renal cortex in response to decreased tissue oxygenation. It acts on receptors on the erythroid burst-forming units and erythroid colony-forming units. With loss of renal mass, erythropoietin secretion does not respond adequately to hypoxia, and anemia ensues. Children with chronic renal failure are now treated with recombinant erythropoietin (50–150 U/kg by intravenous [IV] injection three times per week) when their hematocrit decreases to less than 30%.[40,41] When the hematocrit increases to 36%, the dose is maintained at approximately 75 U/kg with the same frequency. Erythropoietin may also be administered subcutaneously only once weekly, obviating the need for IV injections. Doses of erythropoietin in excess of 150 U/kg increase the hematocrit faster than smaller doses, but both therapies take 4 to 8 weeks to reach the target hematocrit of 33% to 36%. Children who are scheduled for erythropoietin therapy should begin oral iron, vitamin C (a cofactor for iron absorption from the gastrointestinal tract), and folic acid 2 to 3 weeks in advance to ensure adequate iron and folic acid stores to facilitate erythropoiesis. The most common cause for failure of erythropoietin, and therefore erythropoiesis, is concurrent iron deficiency. Current recommendations are aimed at maintaining serum ferritin concentrations in excess of 250 ng/mL and a transferrin saturation greater than 25%. Other causes for the failure of erythropoietin to increase or maintain the hematocrit are occult infections, hemolysis, aluminum overload, severe hyperparathyroidism, and occult bleeding. Complications of erythropoietin therapy include worsening of hypertension and a possible increased incidence of thrombosis of polytetrafluoroethylene vascular grafts.

The other major hematologic problem in chronic renal failure is bleeding. This classic and lethal complication in children with terminal uremia results from platelet dysfunction in the presence of a normal coagulation profile and normal platelet counts. The best indicator of platelet dysfunction in children with chronic renal failure is a prolonged bleeding time. The platelet dysfunction is the result of poorly described abnormalities attributed to the uremic environment, rendering platelet transfusions ineffective. Dialysis improves platelet dysfunction, as does improvement in the hematocrit with transfusions or erythropoietin therapy. Preoperative IV desmopressin acetate (1-deamino-8-D-arginine vasopressin, DDAVP) (0.3 µg/kg) improves the bleeding time in children with uremia.

Cardiovascular Complications

Hypertension is one of the most common complications of chronic renal failure and contributes significantly to the morbidity and mortality of these children. The cause is multifactorial and includes volume overload and hormonal abnormalities, such as increased secretion of renin, that result from the underlying renal disorder. In children who are undergoing dialysis, volume overload is the result of inadequate removal of volume during dialysis. The goal of ultrafiltration is to remove sufficient salt and water to achieve the dry weight that is appropriate for each child. The *dry weight* is the weight at which the child has no signs of volume overload but below which the child has hypotension. The initial response to volume overload is to increase the cardiac output. Later, the cardiac output returns to normal, but the peripheral resistance increases because of peripheral vasoconstriction, resulting in hypertension. These children may have no other signs of volume overload, such as edema, but with a reduction in total body salt and water content, the blood pressure can be controlled with little or no antihypertensive medication.

In other children, intrinsic renal abnormalities play a primary role in hypertension. Oral antihypertensive agents are often effective in controlling the severe refractory hypertension, although in some, bilateral nephrectomies may be required to control the hypertension. Of the mechanisms that cause hypertension in these children, increased renin secretion is the best understood. Renin activates the formation of angiotensin I, which is then converted to angiotensin II, a powerful vasoconstrictor. Children with renin-dependent hypertension respond poorly to control of blood pressure by salt and water removal alone but respond well to ACE inhibitors such as captopril.

Cardiovascular disease is the most common cause of death in patients undergoing long-term dialysis, including children.[42] Children with chronic renal failure can have abnormalities of the pericardium, myocardium, cardiac valves, and coronary arteries. Pericarditis was once considered a sign of the terminal phase of uremia, but it occurs in 15% of children who are undergoing dialysis and can be symptomatic or clinically silent. In uremic patients with pericarditis who are not undergoing dialysis, intensive dialysis often results in its resolution within ~2 weeks. Some children require surgical procedures such as pericardiocentesis, pericardial drainage with a catheter or through a pericardial window, or pericardiectomy.

Left ventricular failure is also a common complication of chronic renal failure. In older patients, coronary artery disease may lead to myocardial dysfunction, severely limiting cardiac output. Volume overload and hypertension, which increase preload and afterload, respectively, are important causes of heart failure. With proper fluid management and antihypertensive medication, these abnormalities can be controlled. Anemia is another contributing factor that can be controlled with the use of erythropoietin. An array of metabolic abnormalities associated with chronic renal failure, such as secondary hyperparathyroidism, electrolyte and acid-base imbalances, and the accumulation of nonspecific uremic toxins, contribute to abnormal myocardial function.

Causes of Chronic Renal Failure

The causes of chronic renal insufficiency and failure can be correlated with age (Table 28.7). The chronic renal failure that is commonly encountered in early infancy results largely from congenital anomalies or perinatal asphyxia. Later in childhood, renal failure may result from dysplasia, or acquired lesions, whereas those affected in adolescence may have deterioration of function related to acquired disease, manifestation of inherited disease, or secondary lesions resulting from other illnesses (e.g., systemic lupus erythematosus, sickle cell disease) or their treatments.

Preoperative Preparation of the Child With Renal Dysfunction

Renal disease in children is a significant cause of perioperative morbidity and mortality and thus influences the approach to general anesthesia.[43–45] The preoperative preparation of these children depends largely on the stage of the renal dysfunction and the level of severity. Whether the child has CKD, AKI, has undergone a kidney transplant, or is susceptible to an intraoperative renal insult, the approach to the preoperative and perioperative anesthesia care will change.

CKD is a multisystem disease that requires a thorough and comprehensive preoperative assessment. These children may be oliguric and at risk of fluid overload or polyuric and vulnerable

TABLE 28.7	Causes of Chronic Renal Failure and Associated Syndromes	
Infancy (Congenital Anomalies)	**Childhood**	**Adolescence**
Prune-belly syndrome	Dysplasia	Focal segmental glomerulosclerosis
Congenital obstruction	Agenesis	Membranoproliferative glomerulonephritis
Posterior urethral valves	Autosomal dominant PKD	Secondary glomerulonephritis
Multicystic dysplasia	Reflux nephropathy	Systemic lupus erythematosus
Agenesis	Obstruction	Sickle cell disease
Autosomal recessive PKD	Focal segmental glomerulosclerosis	HIV-associated nephropathy
Reflux nephropathy	Membranoproliferative glomerulonephritis	Diabetes mellitus
		Vasculitis
		Hemolytic uremic syndrome
		Henoch-Schönlein purpura
		Interstitial nephritis
		Malignancy

HIV, human immunodeficiency virus; *PKD*, polycystic kidney disease.

to dehydration. Electrolyte and acid-base disturbances are predictably common. Alterations in compartment volumes and protein binding change drug pharmacokinetics. Hypertension may be present owing to fluid overload, exacerbated by renin excretion from the failing kidney or from an autonomic hyperactivity common in CKD. Typically these children have a normocytic normochromic anemia (from reduced erythropoietin levels) and platelet dysfunction by uremia. Ascites, common in end-stage renal disease, increases the risk of aspiration and pulmonary atelectasis in the perioperative period. Children may be encephalopathic secondary to increased blood concentrations of urea and may have seizure disorders. Finally, the CKD may be part of a syndrome, with other important implications for anesthesia. Therefore careful delineation of the type of renal disease and its comorbidities should be reviewed at the time of the preoperative visit to anticipate potential problems during the anesthetic.

Perioperative renal dysfunction may also occur in any child with normal renal function who is subjected to perioperative insults. AKI after cardiopulmonary bypass (CPB) is a well-known cause of morbidity and mortality. The pathogenesis is not simply a consequence of hypoperfusion but a complex interplay of CPB-related injury, oxidative stress, and activation of a systemic inflammatory reaction.[46] Preexisting renal insufficiency compounds this risk, necessitating precautions to preserve renal perfusion. Associated risk factors include hypovolemia that leads to vasoconstriction, the administration of nephrotoxic agents such as contrast media, embolic events in cases involving arterial vessel cross-clamping, renal ischemia, and inflammation.

Consideration of associated risks is important because perioperative renal failure is associated with mortality rates of 60%–90%. It is therefore vital to avoid factors that may augment preexisting renal dysfunction.[47,48] In adult patients, 1% developed postoperative AKI after general surgical procedures[49]; those at greatest risk were older men (≥56 years old). Although these data may not be directly

applicable to children, children with congestive heart failure, hypertension, preoperative renal insufficiency, or ascites may also be at increased risk for AKI. Identification of those at risk is not a trivial exercise because postoperative AKI will increase postoperative morbidity and mortality.

PREOPERATIVE LABORATORY EVALUATION

Routine preoperative blood testing in children has become unpopular in the past few years.[50] However, several preoperative laboratory tests should be assessed in children with renal insufficiency. This allows the practitioner to determine the severity of the presenting disease and provides a baseline that may be compared with intraoperative and postoperative laboratory values to ensure proper protective renal care.

As a broad standard, a complete blood cell count, BUN, electrolytes, creatinine, and coagulation panel should be performed preoperatively. An electrocardiogram should be obtained if there is a history of hypertension and an echocardiogram if there is the suspicion of a pericardial effusion and/or cardiomyopathy.

Children with known renal failure, especially those with a significant reduction in renal function and those undergoing dialysis, require preoperative serum electrolyte analysis. Abnormal serum potassium concentrations often occur in children with renal failure; acceptable limits depend on the local laboratory standards, the child's acid-base status, and trends in the potassium concentration over time. Chronic hypokalemic or hyperkalemic states are less likely to cause cardiac manifestations than acute changes. Acute hypokalemia reduces the arrhythmia threshold and increases cardiac excitability; acute hyperkalemia may result in life-threatening arrhythmias. A child with chronic renal failure whose serum potassium concentrations are chronically 5.5 to 6.0 mEq/L does not need correction of the hyperkalemia, whereas a child with an acute increase to a potassium concentration greater than 5.5 mEq/L often requires intervention before the surgical procedure and anesthesia. Existing acidosis must be taken into consideration in determining total body potassium concentrations, understanding that acute acidosis promotes extracellular hyperkalemia at a rate of 0.5 mEq/L for every decrease in pH of 0.1 unit. There are several approaches to treating hyperkalemia and were discussed earlier (see Table 28.6). Ideally, correction of hyperkalemia is accomplished by removing potassium from the body using dialysis or sodium polystyrene sulfonate (Kayexalate). Urgent management in the operating room will include hyperventilation, nebulized albuterol and calcium, in addition to a glucose and insulin infusion.

Hypomagnesemia likewise predisposes a child to the risks of supraventricular and ventricular arrhythmias and should be corrected preoperatively. Hypermagnesemia or hypophosphatemia may cause muscle weakness and potentiate the action of neuromuscular blocking drugs (NMBDs). Administration of calcium is helpful in treating hyperkalemia or hypermagnesemia.

Hemoglobin, hematocrit, and platelet counts should be part of the preoperative evaluation. Hemoglobin levels should be measured within 24 hours of the procedure and on the morning of the procedure if the hemoglobin is labile. Morbidity and mortality in adult patients with renal failure are increased at hemoglobin concentrations less than 11 g/dL.[43,51] These were likely the effect of anemia on the incidence of left ventricular hypertrophy; in children, this relationship may not hold true. Recombinant erythropoietin reduces the risks of cardiac compromise from left ventricular hypertrophy by increasing the hemoglobin to normal values.[52,53] Blood transfusion is generally not indicated if the hematocrit is more than 25%.

The platelet count, although typically normal in children with renal failure, does not portend platelet dysfunction. The best metric to assess platelet dysfunction in children with chronic renal failure is a prolonged bleeding time. Signs of coagulopathy such as petechiae should alert the practitioner of platelet dysfunction. Platelet dysfunction does not necessarily improve with platelet transfusion. Dialysis, red blood cell transfusion, and erythropoietin improve platelet dysfunction. Desmopressin (0.3 μg/kg given by IV infusion over 15-20 minutes) can improve the bleeding time in children with uremia and can minimize hypotension when given 1 hour before surgery. It releases endothelial von Willebrand factor/factor VIII complex and improves platelet function for 6 to 12 hours.

Depending on the degree of renal failure and suspected cardiac involvement, additional testing may include an electrocardiogram, a chest radiograph, and an echocardiogram. These tests can assist the practitioner in determining evidence of left ventricular hypertrophy, arrhythmias, and the presence or absence of pericardial effusions.

Measures of renal function essentially indicate the GFR and tubular function (diluting capacity) of the kidneys. Urea and creatinine are traditional indicators of renal function, with plasma urea being a very simplistic marker of global renal function. Creatinine, being relatively constantly produced by the muscles, can be used as a guide to GFR, but lacks sensitivity and specificity. Recently, other endogenous [cystatin C, β-trace protein (BTP)] and exogenous (inulin, iohexol) biomarkers have been used to diagnose AKI after an intraoperative insult. New molecules, such as neutrophil gelatinase-associated lipocalin (NGAL), kidney injury molecule-1 (KIM-1), and netrin-1, are a few of the many new promising biomarkers that await validation in the clinical setting.[54-57]

Increasingly in the adult literature, there is evidence that specific biomarkers (such as endogenous ouabain, an adrenal stress hormone) can predict AKI in cardiac surgical patients, although to date, similar data in children have not been forthcoming.[58]

PERIOPERATIVE DIALYSIS

In the child with renal failure, dialysis prevents hyperkalemia and removes excess water. However, excessive or overly aggressive dialysis may lead to electrolyte abnormalities and hypovolemia. Accordingly, the timing of this therapy or need for the therapy should be discussed with the child's nephrologist. Ideally, children with renal failure who undergo *intermittent* hemodialysis should have dialysis on the day before surgery rather than on the day of surgery to optimize their fluid and electrolyte status and minimize problems with acute fluid shifts with hypotension, hypokalemia, and anticoagulation. To limit any effects of residual heparin, the interval between dialysis and surgery should be 4 to 6 hours. Hemodialysis can be performed without heparin if is required urgently.

Children who require peritoneal dialysis can undergo dialysis up until the day of surgery. Peritoneal dialysis should be resumed with the consideration that the child's pulmonary function must be able to tolerate the increased abdominal distention. Consultation with the child's nephrologist is recommended to optimize the child's clinical status before the procedure and to arrange the appropriate timing of the peritoneal dialysis.

MEDICATIONS

Children with renal failure may require their medications to be adjusted in the perioperative period. These medications typically include antihypertensives, and although proceeding with elective surgery with moderate hypertension may be acceptable, severe or labile hypertension should ideally be controlled before surgery. Induction of anesthesia may cause hypotension in children with chronic hypertension, although preloading with balanced salt solution may attenuate this effect. There is a temporal relationship between adults who take ACE inhibitors for blood pressure control on the day of surgery and hypotension at induction of anesthesia and cardiac arrest.[59] Moderate hypotension was significantly more frequent in those who discontinued their ACE inhibitor within 10 hours of induction of anesthesia compared with those who had not taken their medication for more than 10 hours before induction.[59] Additional studies in adults and opinion leaders recommend that ACE inhibitors should be stopped on the day before surgery to prevent hypotension after induction of anesthesia, although the hypotension can be easily managed, especially during total IV anesthesia.[60-62] All other antihypertensives, immunosuppressives, and steroids should be continued. Most other medications can be safely held until they can be resumed postoperatively. Antacid prophylaxis may be indicated for those with gastroesophageal reflux. Premedication with a benzodiazepine such as midazolam may be valuable.

Finally, a knowledge of the child's daily fluid status including output and input is important to appreciate. If and when dialysis was last performed—and therefore the child's dry weight and actual weight—should be recorded on the day of surgery. Tubular disorders, obstructive uropathy, or hypoplastic/dysplastic kidneys may have fixed polyuria and are at risk for dehydration if oral intake is restricted (NPO) for long periods. Standard fasting intervals may be followed, including clear fluids until 2 hours before the procedure, to help prevent dehydration and alleviate anxiety. Alternatively, for the inpatient, maintenance IV fluids should be continued while the child is NPO.

Intraoperative Management

STRATEGIES FOR RENAL PROTECTION

Children with chronic renal failure frequently present with serious medical problems that complicate anesthesia.[63,64] These problems stem mainly from fluid and electrolyte abnormalities, complications of chronic renal failure such as anemia and hypertension, and differences in the pharmacokinetics of anesthetic agents in children with renal failure. The most important strategies for preserving renal function are optimization of hemodynamics and intravascular volume and the avoidance or cautious use of drugs that are nephrotoxic (such as certain antibiotics, contrast agents, and nonsteroidal antiinflammatory drugs). Both the administration of isotonic saline (as compared with hypotonic saline) and, more recently, IV sodium bicarbonate before the injection of contrast agents are protective against contrast induced nephropathy.[65,66]

Strict glycemic control by titrating insulin during cardiac and vascular surgery has been associated in adults with a reduction in the incidence of AKI requiring renal replacement therapy.[65] This may not be true in children, in whom hyperinsulinemic hypoglycemia is more concerning in the critically ill child and hyperglycemia is actually better tolerated.[67]

Dopamine has long been considered renally protective, but conventional wisdom now would suggest that its actual effect is variable and difficult to predict. Fenoldopam, a selective dopamine 1–receptor agonist, increases GFR without the hypertension associated with the use of dopamine. It produces a more significant reduction in creatinine than dopamine and may therefore have a role in renoprotection. Although several empirical measures have been recommended for renal protection in the perioperative period, a Cochrane review concluded that no interventions, whether pharmacologic or otherwise, protected the kidney in the perioperative period.[68]

In a child with AKI and low urine output, it is tempting to administer diuretics to increase RBF and flush the renal tubules. However, the use of diuretics in a child with renal disease may worsen the renal failure by causing hypovolemia and decreasing renal perfusion.[69]

VASCULAR ACCESS

In addition to routine monitoring, the absolute need for arterial access should be cautiously considered because it may affect future shunt sites. Arterial access is useful to monitor blood pressure that may be labile during the perioperative period and to measure blood gases and electrolytes. However, central venous access may achieve these same goals as well as monitor volume status (as urine output is a poor metric for renal perfusion in these children), secure IV access, and ensure the safe and reliable delivery of vasoactive medications including calcium, and avoid compromising future arterial access. Serum potassium concentrations must be monitored and corrected to avoid arrhythmias or conduction problems.

ENVIRONMENT

Careful positioning of children with renal osteodystrophy and careful antiseptic techniques for vascular line placements are essential. Strategies to maintain normothermia, including increasing the room temperature and application of a forced-air warming blanket. should be considered to avoid hypothermia.

FLUIDS AND BLOOD PRODUCTS

In the child with renal insufficiency, fluid management requires a balanced approach. The child must receive adequate hydration to prevent further renal deterioration in an otherwise injured kidney. Children with renal failure and a history of hypertension are at risk for both hypotension and hypertension and require some degree of fluid resuscitation for stability. However, they also may have hypoalbuminemia with low oncotic pressure that puts them at risk for pulmonary edema. Ideally, if the child is euvolemic, standard fluid therapy based on typical surgical fluid management is preferred. Fluid overload must be avoided in all anuric children and in outpatients. Although common sense and years of practice suggest that normal saline solution is preferable to lactated Ringer's solution because of the potassium load in the latter, a series of adults who underwent kidney transplantation showed that 19% of those who received IV saline had potassium concentrations of 6 mEq/L, and 31% had a metabolic acidosis that required treatment compared with none for both the potassium concentration and metabolic acidosis in those who received lactated Ringer's solution.[70] Lactated Ringer's solution or similar balanced salt solutions should be considered for children with renal failure.

The debate over colloids versus crystalloids continues with renal function being an important endpoint. While albumin can be used in children with renal disease, it confers little advantage over saline. Hexaethyl starch, on the other hand, may cause a coagulopathy as well as renal dysfunction. In a 2013 Cochrane review, researchers found no evidence that colloids conferred any advantage over clear fluids.[71]

Children with significant renal failure are at a greater risk for bleeding in the perioperative period. As a consequence, the hemoglobin concentration should be monitored closely. This is a classic and lethal complication in children with terminal uremia that results from platelet dysfunction in the presence of a normal coagulation profile and normal platelet counts. Blood and component therapy may be used in accordance with surgical losses and to maintain the hemoglobin concentration greater than 11 g/dL. Other components that may be effective to alleviate surgical oozing or occult bleeding should be given based on the clinical need because coagulation studies may not be true indexes of the coagulation status in children with platelet dysfunction.

ANESTHETIC AGENTS

The pharmacokinetics and pharmacodynamics of anesthetic agents and perioperative medications may be altered in children with renal failure. The medications most likely to be affected are those that depend on renal excretion, such as the hydrophilic, highly ionized agents. Repeated doses of medications that depend primarily on renal excretion for elimination should be administered at greater intervals or in smaller doses than they are given otherwise. Examples of commonly used perioperative medications that primarily depend on renal elimination are penicillins, cephalosporins, aminoglycosides, vancomycin, and digoxin.

Anesthetic agents should be tailored according to the circumstances and child. For example, the duration of action of medications delivered as a single bolus depends more on redistribution than on elimination. If the volume of distribution of the medication is unchanged, the single bolus dose should be unchanged. Medications that depend only in part on renal elimination (e.g., rocuronium or vecuronium) have a normal duration of action when delivered as a bolus or short-term infusion. Many anesthetics depend in part on renal elimination, including pancuronium, vecuronium, rocuronium, atropine, glycopyrrolate, and neostigmine.

Induction of anesthesia may be carried out safely as long as the child is euvolemic and the pharmacokinetics and pharmacodynamics of the induction agent are understood and accounted for. Anesthetic agents may be affected by the presence of anemia, acidosis, and altered drug binding owing to hypoproteinemia in children with renal disease. Antihypertensives such as ACE inhibitors, particularly in combination with diuretics, may lead to profound hypotension at induction of anesthesia.[72]

The dose of propofol to induce anesthesia using the bispectral index and clinical signs to indicate the state of hypnosis in adult patients with renal failure were significantly greater than in those without renal disease.[73] This has been attributed to a larger volume of distribution in patients with renal failure, consistent with previous studies of thiopental.[74] Anemia is another contributing factor. It may indirectly cause a greater plasma volume and greater cardiac output. When propofol is delivered as an infusion, no significant differences in pharmacokinetic (principally clearance) or pharmacodynamic parameters have been observed.[75] There is also some evidence to suggest that propofol, when compared with sevoflurane, may be renoprotective as a result of its ability to attenuate the perioperative increase in proinflammatory mediators.[46]

There are insufficient data regarding the use of inhalational anesthetics for induction in children with renal impairment. For maintenance of anesthesia in adults, desflurane and isoflurane do not further impair renal function in those with preexisting renal disease.[76] Sevoflurane at low flows is associated with increased circuit concentrations of compound A, which is nephrotoxic in rats but not in humans.[77-79] In adults with normal renal function, low-flow sevoflurane anesthesia has been associated with mild, transient proteinuria but no changes in BUN, creatinine level, or creatinine clearance.[79] In adults with renal insufficiency, low-flow sevoflurane is as safe as low-flow isoflurane in terms of kidney function.[78] Overall, sevoflurane is considered safe in patients with renal disease, but low flows are best avoided. Because desflurane is minimally metabolized (rate of 0.2%) in vivo, it may be preferred even at very low flows (1 L/minute).

NMBDs have evolved over the years to provide a choice of relaxants for use in children with renal disease. Children with chronic renal failure may have existing autonomic neuropathy and associated delayed gastric emptying that puts them at risk for aspiration. Along with renal implications, aspiration should be anticipated when choosing an NMBD for airway management. Succinylcholine is often avoided in children with renal failure because of its well-known propensity for increasing serum potassium. However, succinylcholine does not increase the plasma potassium concentration in patients with renal failure any more than in patients with normal renal function (0.5–0.8 mEq/L of potassium) unless a peripheral neuropathy is present.[80,81] The plasma concentration of potassium is chronically increased in renal failure, which implies that the intracellular and extracellular potassium concentrations are in equilibrium. As a result, the usual 0.5- to 1-mEq/L increase in serum potassium after succinylcholine causes no clinical manifestations, despite the large absolute concentration of potassium. This contrasts with patients with acute hyperkalemia in whom the intracellular and extracellular potassium concentrations are in disequilibrium, which predisposes these children to ventricular arrhythmias after succinylcholine. In the latter case, succinylcholine is relatively contraindicated, whereas in the former case, it is not contraindicated.

The pharmacodynamics of NMBDs in children with renal insufficiency merit consideration. The onset time of rocuronium in children with renal failure (>2 minutes) was significantly greater than in the control children (1.5 minutes). This difference was attributed to a greater volume of distribution, decreased serum albumin concentrations, and possibly to a reduced cardiac output in children with renal failure who were taking antihypertensives. The slower onset time of rocuronium in children with renal failure must be considered when a rapid-sequence intubation is required and succinylcholine is contraindicated. On the other hand, the duration of action of rocuronium in children with normal renal function and end-stage renal disease is similar[82]; the time to recover a train-of-four ratio of 70% was 29 minutes in both groups with a 0.3-mg/kg dose. This is not surprising because elimination of rocuronium is predominantly biliary and not via the kidneys.

NMBDs such as atracurium and cisatracurium are ideal choices for children with renal insufficiency because their elimination is completely independent of the kidney. Despite the fact that both agents undergo spontaneous degradation by plasma esterase and Hofmann elimination, neuromuscular blockade should still be monitored.[83] Therefore with appropriate monitoring and dosing, atracurium, cisatracurium, vecuronium, and rocuronium are all acceptable NMBDs in children with renal disease and provide reliable durations of action after a single bolus dose.

If a prolonged neuromuscular blockade occurs, hypermagnesemia should be ruled out. In this case, calcium may be administered to help antagonize the blockade. The elimination of neostigmine may be delayed beyond elimination of atropine or glycopyrrolate, and muscarinic effects such as bradycardia, increased secretions, or bronchospasm may theoretically occur postoperatively after antagonism.

Sugammadex is a binding agent selective for aminosteroidal NMBDs such as rocuronium and vecuronium. It is entirely renally excreted with an elimination half-life of approximately 100 minutes.

As discussed elsewhere, rocuronium is metabolized almost entirely in the liver but when it is bound to sugammadex, it is both inactivated and effectively removed from the circulation; the rocuronium-sugammadex complex is eliminated by the kidney. Special consideration should therefore be given to patients with renal failure.[84] Suggamadex dosing in mild to moderate renal dysfunction is the same as in patients with normal renal function; it is not recommended for those with severe renal failure.[85] In a patient with normal renal function, rocuronium can be redosed in about 25 minutes after sugammadex administration. Because there is currently no redosing data for patients with renal failure, the use of sugammadex should be carefully considered.

Remifentanil may be a preferred choice for a maintenance opioid in the intraoperative period in children with renal insufficiency because of its rapid metabolism by nonspecific blood and tissue esterases. The pharmacokinetics and pharmacodynamics of remifentanil are not altered in patients with renal disease, but the principal metabolite of remifentanil has reduced elimination,[86,87] which is not clinically relevant. Doses of other opioids should be reduced by 30% to 50% to avoid respiratory depression in children with chronic renal failure. Active metabolites of morphine and meperidine (no longer recommended for children other than to treat shivering) can likewise accumulate in patients with renal failure, whereas those of fentanyl and sufentanil do not. Dialysis may be required to eliminate these active metabolites.[88] Hence, the latter opioids are preferred when remifentanil is not indicated.[89–93] Prolonged antagonism of opioid effects with naloxone can be expected in renal failure patients.

Dexmedetomidine, an α_2-adrenoceptor agonist, has diuretic properties via its suppression of vasopressin secretion. GFR and renal blood flow are enhanced, thereby increasing urine output. Some advocate its use in protecting against contrast-induced nephropathy, but it has also been shown to have an antiinflammatory effect. It has been shown to reduce levels of harmful inflammatory molecules such as tumor necrosis factor-α (TNF-α) and increase proteins such as bone morphogenetic protein-7 (BMP-7), thought to be protective against sepsis-induced AKI.[94] The clinical efficacy of this has yet to be established, but dexmedetomidine has been associated with improved short-term mortality in adult patients with sepsis and children after surgery for congenital heart disease. While it is metabolized in the liver, none of the renally excreted metabolites are thought to be active. The renoprotective effect of dexmedetomidine therefore may make it a logical sedation and anesthetic choice in children who are vulnerable to AKI, thereby further increasing its appeal for use in children with renal disease.[95,96]

Delayed emergence, vomiting and aspiration, hypertension, respiratory depression, and pulmonary edema are potential problems that should be anticipated with anesthetic emergence. Hyperkalemia as a consequence of tissue injury, catabolism, blood transfusion, and acidosis is common. Children with chronic renal failure usually have chronic metabolic acidosis with limited buffer reserve. Modest hypercapnia with emergence may lead to significant acidosis and hyperkalemia. Careful attention should be given to the fluid needs of the child postoperatively to minimize volume overload and pulmonary edema.

Regional anesthesia is a viable alternative to general anesthesia or an adjunct in many cases. The anesthesia team must pay particular attention to coagulation studies and signs of coagulopathy before embarking on any central block because abnormal platelet function puts the renal failure patient at risk for an epidural hematoma.

POSTOPERATIVE CONCERNS

The postoperative care of the child with renal disease must take into account the level of renal function, anemia, and preexistence of hypertension. In the child with limited ability to excrete a salt and water load, care must be given to the rate and amount of postoperative fluids administered, with consideration of the volume given during the procedure and operative losses. In children with renal insufficiency, nephrotic syndrome, or tubular disorders (especially those with concentration impairments), it is common to administer fluid volumes that approximate anticipated output and insensible needs. This volume needs to be adjusted for third spacing, ongoing losses, and the administration of blood and blood products.

For children with known renal disease, care must be taken to identify medications that need to be resumed in the immediate postoperative period. Children who have been on chronic antihypertensive medications may be able to resume oral medications when awake. It may be necessary to treat isolated hypertensive episodes with IV medications during the postoperative period. It is important to assess the contribution of pain and anxiety to increased blood pressures to avoid overtreatment.

Because of ischemic tissue injury, it is possible that preexisting metabolic acidosis and hyperkalemia may worsen in the postoperative period. In children who have renal failure, careful monitoring of electrolytes during and after the procedure may prevent untoward emergencies. When clinically significant hyperkalemia develops in a child with chronic renal failure, treatment is imperative (see Table 28.6).

Acute hypertension can be treated with a variety of IV and oral medications (Table 28.8).[97] The therapy for acute symptomatic hypertension should be directed toward rapid normalization of blood pressure. Prompt and effective therapy must be initiated, often before the cause has been discerned. The rate of change of blood pressure can be just as important as its absolute level in the pathogenesis of hypertensive emergencies. Blood pressure itself may be a poor determinant of the severity of the clinical situation and the need for aggressive parenteral therapy. The decision to use aggressive parenteral therapy should be based on an absolute number and on clinical findings that define the situation as emergent. The drugs most often chosen are potent vasodilators, such as hydralazine, diazoxide, or nitroprusside, although nitroprusside is infrequently used today. In its stead, nicardipine and labetolol have been adopted as first-line therapies for acute hypertension in children; these drugs have the advantages of IV administration, safety, and rapid onset of action.

Hemodialysis or peritoneal dialysis can be safely resumed on the first postoperative day, with the exception of children who have operative placement of a dialysis access port for more emergent therapy. In these children, the timing of renal replacement therapy must be individualized in consultation with the child's nephrologist.

Uremic encephalopathy may occur and should be considered in any child who exhibits confusion or prolonged sedation in the postanesthesia care unit. These children should be transferred to an intensive care setting for monitoring, stabilization, and airway management during further workup.

With a careful preoperative assessment and review of preexisting disease, many postoperative complications can be anticipated and avoided. Hypervigilance during the entire perioperative period allows children with renal disease to be managed in a safe manner.

TABLE 28.8	Management of Acute Malignant Hypertension	
Drug	**Dose**	**Side Effects**
Sodium nitroprusside	1–10 µg/kg per minute IV	Possible cyanide and thiocyanate toxicity, acute hypotension
Enalaprilat[a]	0.01–0.06 mg/kg IV 6 hourly	Onset 15 minutes in neonates; hypotension, angioedema, anaphylactoid reaction, and increase serum creatinine; avoid with increased plasma renin levels, AKI, and CKD
Labetalol	0.1–0.4 mg/kg per hour *or* 0.2–1 mg/kg IV every 10 minutes (maximum 40 mg)	Bradycardia; caution in children with head injuries at risk for hypotension
Nicardipine	0.5–5 µg/kg per minute IV (maximum 20 mg/hour)	Acute hypotension; possible superficial thrombophlebitis if administered through a peripheral IV.
Hydralazine	0.1–0.5 mg/kg IV or IM, not to exceed 2 mg IV 6 hourly	
Esmolol	100–500 µg/kg IV over 2 minutes LOAD 50–100 up to 300 µg/kg per minute IV infusion	Bradycardia, acute hypotension

[a]Intravenous angiotensin-converting enzyme inhibitor.
AKI, acute kidney injury; *CKD*, chronic kidney disease

ANNOTATED REFERENCES

Driessen JJ, Robertson EN, Van Egmond J, Booij LH. Time-course of action of rocuronium 0.3 mg/kg in children with and without end-stage renal failure. *Paediatr Anaesth*. 2002;12:507-510.

This study is one of the few that has specifically considered children with renal disease. It describes the differences in onset and issues related to recovery for agents used in children with renal disease.

Kheterpal S, Tremper KK, Heung M, et al. Development and validation of an acute kidney injury risk index for patients undergoing general surgery: results from a national data set. *Anesthesiology*. 2009;110:505-515.

This study is significant because it looks at patients with acute kidney injury undergoing surgery.

Petroni KC, Cohen NH. Continuous renal replacement therapy: anesthetic implications. *Anesth Analg*. 2002;94:1288-1297.

This article provides the anesthesiologist with a working knowledge of the various types of dialysis and how to manage the use of continuous renal replacement therapy in the perioperative period.

Sear JW. Kidney dysfunction in the postoperative period. *Br J Anaesth*. 2005;95:20-32.

This article reviews the significance of renal dysfunction and the associated morbidity and mortality in the perioperative period. It discusses the causes of renal dysfunction and the prevention and treatment of postoperative renal impairment.

Zaccharias M, Gilmore ICS, Herbison GP, et al. Interventions for protecting renal function in the perioperative period. *Cochrane Database Syst Rev*. 2008;(4):CD003590.

This work reports the evidence for interventions that are successful for protecting the kidney in the perioperative period.

A complete reference list can be found online at ExpertConsult.com.

General Abdominal and Urologic Surgery

29

TOM G. HANSEN, STEEN W. HENNEBERG, AND JERROLD LERMAN

ABDOMINAL SURGERY AND UROLOGIC interventions make up a large fraction of anesthetic practice for the pediatric anesthesiologist. The field is rapidly evolving, with increased use of laparoscopic surgery, including robot-assisted procedures.[1] This chapter focuses on the specific issues related to abdominal and urologic surgery, particularly in young children. The management of infants for pyloromyotomy and other neonatal abdominal procedures is discussed in Chapter 37.

General Principles of Abdominal Surgery

"THE FULL STOMACH": THE RISK FOR PULMONARY ASPIRATION OF GASTRIC CONTENTS

Many abdominal surgeries are emergent procedures that require a rapid induction of anesthesia and protection of the airway to prevent regurgitation and pulmonary aspiration. Adhering to fasting guidelines for elective surgery does not ensure that the stomachs of children with acute abdomens are empty of liquids and solids. The only metric that has been associated with gastric emptying after an acute emergency in children is the time interval between the last food ingested and the occurrence of the pathologic event or trauma.[2] However, there is no firm fasting interval after a

trauma that predicts a zero risk of regurgitation and aspiration. The presence or absence of bowel sounds is also not predictive of gastric emptying or of the risk of regurgitation. Preoperatively, some children with acute abdomens are administered oral contrast agent before abdominal ultrasonography and/or computed tomography (CT) to visualize the stomach contents and to estimate their volumes. However, these radiologic tools may not provide reliable estimates of the volume of the gastric contents.[3,4] Indeed, the absence of gastric contents in these scans does not eliminate the risk of vomiting and regurgitation. Consequently, there is no evidence that delaying the surgical procedure for the express purpose of emptying the stomach will reduce the risk of regurgitation; postponing may actually increase the risk of complications by delaying the urgently needed surgical attention to the acute abdomen.

RAPID-SEQUENCE INDUCTION

Rapid-sequence induction (RSI) is recommended for children with a full stomach to quickly secure the airway. This approach is intended to minimize the risk of aspiration, although it is not evidence-based. The strategy is to predetermine the drug doses for the child and have all the required airway equipment (age- and size-appropriate) ready to use. The predetermined drug doses are administered in a rapid sequence and when muscle relaxation has been achieved, the trachea is intubated and the cuff (if used) inflated. Many clinicians apply cricoid pressure to occlude the esophageal lumen during RSI, although not a single randomized trial has compared the frequency of regurgitation and aspiration with cricoid pressure during RSI with that with an inhalational or slow IV induction in either children or adults as summarized in a recent Cochrane review.[5] Recently, the presence of microaspirates in the tracheas of 95 adults at risk for regurgitation (obese, those with diabetes, and those with gastroesophageal reflux) was compared with and without cricoid pressure during induction of elective surgery. There was no difference in the frequency of microaspirates in the two groups.[6] This lack of evidence, combined with both theoretical and actual complications associated with RSI and cricoid pressure in children, has led to great skepticism regarding their roles in preventing pulmonary aspiration in children who are at risk, although large population-based studies are lacking.[7] Only 74% of anesthesiologists in Northern Ireland perform RSI for children scheduled for appendectomy, 78% in the United States use it for pyloromyotomy, and 83% in England use it for forearm fractures within 2 hours of eating and after recent opioid administration.[8–10] In two surveys, 16% and 28% of anesthesiologists in the United States and United Kingdom, respectively, reported that a number of children with full stomachs had experienced gastric regurgitation despite using RSI with cricoid pressure; several of them progressed to serious harm and even death.[9,11]

Despite the lack of evidence supporting the effectiveness of RSI in children with full stomachs, we continue to recommend this approach for the majority of children at risk. Whether cricoid pressure during RSI contributes substantively to preventing regurgitation performed remains unclear. Based on evidence from non-randomized controlled studies (RCTs), a recent Cochrane review concluded that cricoid pressure may not be necessary to safely achieve RSI.[5] The authors assert that well-designed and properly conducted RCTs should be encouraged to assess the safety and effectiveness of cricoid pressure in infants and children; however, because the frequency of pulmonary aspiration is so small, it would take many thousands of cases to establish a substantive outcome and likely would not be readily approved by an institutional review board.[5]

Complications of RSI, for the most part, relate to improperly performed RSI (e.g., excessive cricoid pressure distorting the anatomy of the airway,[12] causing difficulty in securing the airway) or poor selection of patients (those with a known difficult airway, where a more measured approach must take precedence over concerns for possible aspiration).

RSI in infants and children requires more planning than in older children and adults for several reasons. First, the induction drugs should be flushed into the child's veins using a separate flush syringe to ensure a rapid bolus administration of the drugs. Succinylcholine remains useful for rapid-sequence tracheal intubation for brief procedures. The introduction of intermediate-acting neuromuscular blocking drugs (NMBDs) with rapid onset, coupled with concerns about the risk of hyperkalemia after succinylcholine in children with undiagnosed neuromuscular diseases (especially males <8 years of age), has dramatically reduced the use of succinylcholine in elective surgery. With the shift from succinylcholine to nondepolarizing NMBDs for rapid paralysis in young children, inability to intubate and prolonged paralysis may present serious, possible life-threatening problems. However, with the availability of

sugammadex, the use of rocuronium (1.2 mg/kg) represents a safe alternative to succinylcholine.[13–15] Second, preoxygenation is often difficult in infants and children because they commonly resist the tight application of the face mask needed to fully denitrogenate the lungs. Failure to ventilate the lungs after induction and before tracheal intubation may result in desaturation more rapidly in young infants and children than older children, and in those with upper respiratory tract infections or other causes of a limited oxygen reserve.[16,17] During laryngoscopy and intubation, mask ventilation with 100% oxygen should begin when the saturation reaches 95%, to attenuate the nadir in oxygen saturation that follows.[16] Third, the force needed to occlude the esophagus when applying cricoid pressure to infants and children is poorly understood and poorly applied, can distort the view of the larynx during laryngoscopy, may not occlude the lumen of the esophagus, and may actually deform the lumen of the trachea if excessive force is applied.[7,12,18] For example, as little as 10-N force will distort the shape of the cricoid ring and reduce the lumen by 50% in children younger than 5 years of age.[12] Effective cricoid pressure that occludes the esophagus in children and permits bag-and-mask ventilation with up to 40 cm H_2O peak inspiratory pressure without gastric insufflation[19] is known as a modified RSI. Thus, if the first attempt at tracheal intubation fails or the child desaturates during laryngoscopy, properly maintained cricoid pressure allows bag-and-mask ventilation to restore oxygenation, without increasing the risk of regurgitation. A third technique that uses low insufflation pressures, known as the controlled RSI technique, has also been proposed.[20,21] In the United Kingdom, a recent survey of adult anesthetists that documented a large variability in how the RSI was performed[22] has prompted calls for evidence-based guidelines for RSI in infants and children.

INDICATIONS FOR PREOPERATIVE NASOGASTRIC TUBE PLACEMENT

Although there are no published guidelines for placing nasogastric tubes preoperatively, it is reasonable to insert a tube preoperatively to allow drainage of gastrointestinal fluids in cases of documented bowel obstruction (e.g., ileus, strangulated bowel, pyloric obstruction) or in other situations in which the risk of aspiration is judged to be substantial. The child may experience discomfort when a nasogastric tube is inserted preoperatively, but this must be balanced against the need to decompress the stomach and reduce the risk of regurgitation during induction of anesthesia. For every other indication, the nasogastric tube may be placed after tracheal intubation. It should be noted that the presence of a nasogastric tube may decrease lower esophageal sphincter tone, increase the risk for reflux, and reduce the ability to clear refluxed gastric contents from the distal esophagus.[23,24] Thus the anesthesiologist is faced with the dilemma of whether or not to remove the nasogastric tube that was placed before induction of anesthesia. It may be reasonable to apply suction to the nasogastric tube, evacuate all of the gastric contents, and then remove the nasogastric tube before inducing anesthesia because it is unclear whether cricoid pressure, even if properly applied, prevents wicking of gastric contents along the path created by the nasogastric tube. It should be further noted that even with a well-placed nasogastric tube, one can never guarantee that the stomach has been completely emptied.

FLUID BALANCE

Many acute abdominal emergencies are associated with pronounced and significant shifts in fluids, mainly in the form of dehydration, electrolyte losses, third-space fluid shifts, and hypovolemia. In most instances, correction of these derangements is mandatory before proceeding with anesthesia and surgery. However, when a large fraction of the bowel becomes strangulated and ischemic, large volumes of fluid may be sequestered in the bowel. In these cases, hypovolemia should be suspected and resuscitation initiated as anesthesia is rapidly induced. In some elective cases (e.g., bowel resection because of inflammatory bowel disease), fluid and electrolyte resuscitation should routinely be a focus of special interest, because the child may not be fully compensated at the time of surgery.

To date, published studies have suggested that resuscitation with crystalloid fluids and colloids have equipoise.[25] In children, initial resuscitation is usually undertaken with balanced salt solutions. A recent Cochrane review concluded that the use of isotonic intravenous (IV) fluids with sodium concentrations similar to that of plasma reduces the risk of hyponatremia.[26] Although colloids may result in less tissue edema and less volume infused, the expense may not justify their routine use. In fact, some have even questioned the use of colloids in patients with sepsis.[27]

POTENTIAL FOR STRANGULATED OR ISCHEMIC BOWEL AND SEPSIS

The need for anesthesia and surgery becomes more urgent when the bowel is potentially ischemic and/or necrotic. For example, if a volvulus is suspected, immediate action is necessary; otherwise the child is at risk for massive bowel necrosis necessitating resection of dead bowel with subsequent short bowel syndrome, a condition associated with serious lifelong medical problems or even death. Even if the child is far from optimally resuscitated, anesthesia must be induced and maintained, preferably with anesthetics that maintain circulatory homeostasis, while simultaneously correcting the dehydration (or hypovolemia) and electrolyte imbalance. The situation is somewhat less critical in the child with an incarcerated inguinal hernia, although delay of even this surgery should be minimized.

Ischemic bowel may release a host of mediators that can cause severe hemodynamic instability. Children with acute intraabdominal disease should always be regarded as being at risk for bacterial translocation and possible septicemia. Those with overt sepsis are usually easy to identify and may have already been admitted to the pediatric intensive care unit. However, children with incipient or early sepsis may not exhibit overt signs. Accordingly, the signs of sepsis should be actively sought. If septicemia is present or suspected, appropriate IV antibiotics should be administered without delay, preferably before anesthesia and surgery. Children with sepsis or presepsis can be extremely unstable and may require inotropic and/or vasoactive drugs. Immediately after induction of anesthesia vascular sympathetic tone may be attenuated, leading to sudden hemodynamic instability. Thus, when a substantial segment of the bowel becomes ischemic, the anesthesiologist must maintain anesthesia without depressing the circulation excessively, acutely resuscitate the child with appropriate fluids, correct electrolyte imbalances, particularly potential hyperkalemia, and consider the use of inotropic and/or vasoactive medications as needed. It should be noted that hemodynamic instability might acutely worsen when ischemic bowel is suddenly reperfused or immediately after the abdominal cavity is opened. In such cases, close communication with the surgeon is paramount. Furthermore, the presence of sepsis-induced acute lung injury may reduce pulmonary compliance. Thus the anesthesiologist needs to prepare for invasive monitoring (arterial and central venous pressures)

and an intraoperative ventilator that is capable of delivering high positive end-expiratory pressure (PEEP).

PRESENCE OF ABDOMINAL COMPARTMENT SYNDROME

Acute intraabdominal disease processes may lead to a critically increased intraabdominal pressure (IAP).[28] If the IAP increases above the capillary perfusion pressure of the intraabdominal organs, an abdominal compartment syndrome can develop. Organ perfusion will become compromised and ischemia and/or necrosis may develop. The most commonly affected organs in this situation are the bowels, kidneys, and liver. Abdominal compartment syndrome occurs less frequently in children than in adults.[29] Causes of abdominal compartment syndrome include burns, extracorporeal membrane oxygenation,[30] closure of gastroschisis or omphalocele (see Chapter 37),[31] abdominal trauma,[32,33] abdominal surgery,[34] and a host of other intraabdominal pathologies, including necrotizing enterocolitis, Hirschsprung enterocolitis, perforated bowel, diaphragmatic hernia, and Wilms tumor.[30,35,36] Insufficient perfusion of the bowel may cause an ileus, translocation of bacteria, lactate accumulation, and production of mediators that cause hemodynamic instability. Increased IAP can reduce liver blood flow, which will reduce hepatic function,[37] mainly manifested as an inability to metabolize lactate, impaired drug metabolism,[37,38] and, in severe cases, impaired synthesis of coagulation factors. Because the pressure is also transmitted to the retroperitoneal space, renal function may become impaired, resulting in oliguria or anuria and reduced excretion of drugs.[35] In addition, cranial displacement of the abdominal contents and splinting of the diaphragm may seriously compromise ventilation.[39]

If acute intraabdominal compartment syndrome is suspected, then the IAP should be monitored to prevent the pressures from exceeding the critical threshold of 20 to 25 mm Hg. IAP can be measured indirectly by transducing a nasogastric tube or bladder catheter.[40] Some define compartment syndrome when the vesicular (bladder) pressure exceeds 10 to 12 mm Hg.[41,42] The diagnosis of intraabdominal compartment syndrome should be suspected when the triad of (1) massive abdominal distention, (2) increased bladder pressures and increased peak inspiratory airway pressures, and (3) evidence of hepatic, renal, and/or cardiac dysfunction are present.[36,43,44]

Children with acute intraabdominal compartment syndrome are often hemodynamically unstable. Although decompression of the abdomen by a laparotomy will immediately normalize the IAP, reperfusion of the ischemic tissues almost always releases a host of biologically active substances that cause profound hypotension. These substances may also precipitate acute renal failure and lead to a disseminated intravascular coagulopathy. As in the case of sepsis, the anesthesiologist must be fully prepared to address these challenges by ensuring that blood products are present in the operating room and vasopressors are drawn up and available before induction of anesthesia. Some children will require a patch abdominoplasty as a temporizing measure to protect abdominal organs that require delayed primary closure of the anterior abdominal wall.[36,43]

PREOPERATIVE LABORATORY TESTING AND INVESTIGATIONS

Most minor elective cases (e.g., umbilical or inguinal hernia repair) do not require any preoperative workup beyond a basic history and physical examination. Many centers require a preoperative urine (or hemoglobin) screen for pregnancy in females who have reached menarche (see Chapter 4).[45] More complex elective cases may warrant additional laboratory testing, including basic hematology screening and electrolyte profile.

Preoperative laboratory testing is strongly advised in more critically ill children. Liver and renal function tests, coagulation profile, and serum albumin concentration should be assessed and blood typed and crossmatched. In children with sepsis or who have an acute intraabdominal compartment syndrome, a preoperative chest radiograph may indicate the severity of pulmonary involvement. An echocardiogram may be needed to assess myocardial contractility and volume status if cardiac dysfunction is suspected.

MONITORING REQUIREMENTS

Routine elective cases rarely require more than standard monitoring equipment. In children undergoing major intraabdominal procedures, invasive arterial and central venous blood pressure monitoring may be indicated. A multiple-lumen central venous line inserted at the beginning of the procedure will facilitate administration of inotropic and/or vasoactive drugs, in addition to measuring central venous pressure; ultrasound-guided insertion is strongly recommended.[46] These lines are of great value in the immediate postoperative period for blood sampling, drug administration, ongoing assessment of intravascular volume status, and parenteral nutrition. Transesophageal echocardiographic, transesophageal Doppler, or continuous noninvasive cardiac output (CO)[47] evaluation may provide valuable intraoperative and postoperative information regarding the child's volume status, as well as cardiac contractility (see also Chapter 52).[48-58]

A urinary catheter with a pediatric urometer (i.e., a graduated collection receptacle), which provides an accurate measure of urine output, is a useful monitor for most intraabdominal procedures. Maintaining a stable hourly urine output may safeguard against the development of hypovolemia and possibly prerenal azotemia (see the section "Laparoscopic Surgery" for discussion of changes in urine output with increased IAP).

Monitoring IAP is important during laparoscopic surgery, although it is of minimal value in omphalocele and gastroschisis surgeries, as long as the abdomen remains open. Once the abdomen is closed, however, IAP provides useful prognostic information regarding intraabdominal organ (e.g., renal) blood flow, circulatory stability, and respiratory embarrassment (see Chapter 37).[39]

CHOICE OF ANESTHETIC

The anesthesiologist may use his or her personal preference of anesthetic technique for the management of both elective and emergency intraabdominal surgery in children. However, airway management associated with intraabdominal surgery requires careful consideration. Even when the child is not at increased risk for regurgitation and aspiration, the risk of regurgitation can be increased if the surgeon positions the child in the Trendelenburg position and/or insufflates the peritoneal cavity with carbon dioxide (CO_2) during laparoscopic surgery. A particular concern arises when the surgeon decides to decompress distended bowel by creating an enterotomy and directly draining the fluid, or by "milking" or "stripping" the bowel in a retrograde direction until the contents can be vented with a nasogastric tube. The latter method can cause massive intestinal regurgitation that exceeds the capacity of the nasogastric tube causing pulmonary aspiration.[59] It is for this reason and others that a laryngeal mask airway (LMA) should not be used during intraabdominal surgery; we strongly recommend that the trachea should be intubated with a cuffed tube as standard practice in these cases.

Regional anesthetic techniques may be useful adjuncts in children undergoing both minor and major abdominal surgery. Those who have had open abdominal procedures will require IV opioids or the use of a continuous epidural infusion of local anesthetics with or without opioids for perioperative pain management (see Chapter 44). Analgesia is commonly supplemented with parenteral nonsteroidal antiinflammatory drugs and/or acetaminophen. In most children who have had laparoscopic surgery, adequate postoperative analgesia may be achieved by infiltrating local anesthetics at the port insertion sites. However, referred shoulder pain, the result of accumulated air under the diaphragm, may require IV opioids.[60] In critically unstable children or those with sepsis, the use of neuroaxial anesthesia is not recommended because sympathetic blockade may further exacerbate the hemodynamic instability and the catheter could provide a nidus for infection.

General Principles of Urologic Surgery

With the exception of acute drainage of urinary obstruction (i.e., ultrasound-guided nephrostomy or cystostomy procedures) and torsion of the testis, most pediatric urologic surgeries are elective. In the vast majority of cases, these children are otherwise healthy or have stable medical conditions that do not require more than a careful history, physical examination, and review of the child's medical record. Children who undergo urologic procedures may be suffering from emotional disturbance because of repeated interventions and sensitivity of the surgical site. This mandates special psychological attention before and after anesthesia.

Worldwide, the prevalence of latex allergy has recently been estimated to be 9.7%, 7.2%, and 4.3% among health care workers, susceptible patients, and the general population, respectively.[61] In the 1990s, the prevalence of latex allergy in children with spinal dysraphism exceeded 70%, several years later, it had decreased to less than 17%, and most recently evidence suggests the prevalence may be as small as 3% in those with dysraphism in a nonlatex environment.[62] Indeed, latex anaphylaxis is of particular concern in children with chronic urologic disorders.[63-66] In the past, children with spina bifida were prone to developing latex allergy much more often than those without spina bifida[67-70] because the former were repeatedly exposed to latex urinary catheters beginning early after birth. All children with congenital malformations of the urinary tract who were repeatedly exposed to latex via their mucous membranes beginning in the neonatal period were at significant risk for developing latex hypersensitivity until recently.[71,72] However, a widespread shift in practice to avoid exposure to all latex products in these children has been extremely (but not 100%) effective in attenuating the prevalence of this allergy.[62] The exceptions usually occur when someone unfamiliar with the child's latex allergy introduces a latex product and sensitizes the child or triggers a reaction. Thus latex-free management is highly recommended in this population.[62,73-75]

REDUCED RENAL FUNCTION

Children with chronic renal disease have impaired renal function, which may affect drug dosing and disposition, as well as cause secondary effects on the cardiovascular system. In the most severe cases, the child may require dialysis to balance fluids and electrolytes. In children with renal disease, it is essential to determine the degree of renal impairment by consulting the child's nephrologist and reviewing the serum creatinine, blood urea nitrogen, sodium, and potassium concentrations (see also Chapter 28).

Because renal impairment may also affect clotting, a coagulation profile, including platelet count, should be reviewed preoperatively if substantial blood loss is anticipated. These children are prone to fluid overload, particularly those who are anuric and dialysis dependent. Apart from clinical signs associated with fluid overload, measuring the child's weight and comparing it with their normal weight is a simple means to assess the child's current volume status. If cardiac function or volume status remains in doubt, an echocardiogram should be obtained. Children with chronic renal insufficiency often have impaired left ventricular function even before they require dialysis, so a preoperative echocardiogram may be indicated[76–80]; pericardial effusion is also a concern.[77,81,82]

For children undergoing dialysis, the most recent date of dialysis should be documented. Overhydration and/or hypervolemia and hyperkalemia should be corrected preoperatively with dialysis. Although dialysis corrects these abnormalities, and may transiently improve platelet function (peritoneal dialysis yielding more consistent improvement than hemodialysis), it is best to avoid dialysis within 12 hours of anesthesia to preclude a relative hypovolemia and to allow sufficient time for body fluids to reequilibrate (see Chapter 28).[83,84] Postdialysis laboratory indexes of serum electrolytes (particularly potassium), hemoglobin or hematocrit, renal function (creatinine and blood urea nitrogen), and the child's weight loss should be assessed. For children who undergo hemodialysis, IV access and blood pressure measurements should not be obtained in the extremity ipsilateral to the arteriovenous fistula.

SYSTEMIC ARTERIAL HYPERTENSION

Systemic hypertension is common in renal insufficiency in adults but is far less common in children. Nonetheless, some children with urologic disorders develop systemic hypertension associated with disturbances in the renin-angiotensin system.[85–88] As in adults, it is important to control systemic hypertension before induction to avoid wide swings in blood pressure. In contrast to adults, however, hypervolemia is an important cause of hypertension in children with renal insufficiency that should be considered and treated preoperatively. Children and adults are often treated with similar antihypertensive medications (see Chapter 28).[87,88] All medications should be continued up to and including the morning of surgery to maintain intraoperative and postoperative hemodynamic stability with the exception of angiotensin-converting enzyme (ACE) inhibitors. The latter drugs should be stopped 1 day before surgery to avoid intraoperative hypotension[89–91]; however, withholding this medication may also lead to rebound hypertension postoperatively. If these medications are not withheld, vasopressors may be required during anesthesia to stabilize the blood pressure.[92] Because therapy-resistant renal hypertension is an indication for nephrectomy, one should anticipate and be prepared to treat wide fluctuations in blood pressure, including severe hypertension during the first stage of the operation and profound hypotension when the responsible kidney is removed. Therefore, long-acting antihypertensive agents are best avoided during the early stages of a nephrectomy in a child.

CORTICOSTEROID MEDICATIONS

Children with renal disease may be chronically treated with corticosteroids as part of their medical management (e.g., children with proteinuria or who have undergone previous renal transplant surgery). In such cases, a stress dose of parenteral corticosteroids during surgery is indicated, with continued supplementation until the child resumes his or her normal corticosteroid medication by the enteral route. In more complex situations, consultation with a pediatric nephrologist or endocrinologist is warranted to optimize corticosteroid supplementation, although in more straightforward cases, a dose of 2.5 mg/kg of IV hydrocortisone two to three times each day is usually adequate (see Chapter 27).

INFECTION OR SEPSIS

Obstructive urinary tract disease or chronic renal insufficiency increases the risk for urinary tract infections. If treated properly, the infection should not interfere with anesthesia. However, in children with overt signs of systemic illness or septicemia, the anesthetic and postoperative courses may be difficult.

MONITORING REQUIREMENTS

Standard noninvasive monitoring is adequate for the vast majority of urologic procedures, as they are of minor or moderate magnitude (e.g., circumcision, orchiopexy, pyeloplasty, and ureter neoimplantation). The anesthetic care required for infants and children undergoing penile surgery is routine, including a forced-air heating mattress to prevent hypothermia for surgeries lasting longer than 1 hour. However, recognizing the minimal amount of skin that is exposed during this type of surgery, the child's temperature often increases, necessitating close monitoring of the child's temperature to avoid overheating.

Invasive monitors (i.e., arterial and central venous access for pressure monitoring and administration of vasoactive drugs) may be indicated in major surgical interventions, and in cases with concomitant problems (e.g., decreased renal function, significant hypertension, associated cardiac dysfunction, sepsis). If central venous access is deemed necessary, the coagulation status of the child should be evaluated because platelet function may be substantially compromised. Ultrasound guidance improves safety while securing central venous access in cases in which a coagulopathy is present or suspected on clinical grounds (see Chapter 49). In the unstable child, even more complex monitoring (e.g., esophageal Doppler monitoring, transesophageal echocardiography, or continuous noninvasive CO)[47] should be considered (see Chapter 52).

It is important to monitor urine output, although the volume of urine may not reflect renal function. During surgery that involves the bladder or in children who are anuric, urine output will not be available for part or all of the surgery. Hence, other indexes of fluid status and perfusion must be used. Heart rate and systolic blood pressure are reliable indexes of volume status and perfusion in most children, although as stated earlier central venous pressure and invasive arterial pressure measurement may be indicated in special cases. Surgeons may be heartened to observe urine flowing into the bladder after reimplantation of ureters and kidney transplantation in place of measuring it. Preloading with a balanced salt solution may be useful in such circumstances; occasionally a loop diuretic is requested.

Laparoscopic Surgery

BACKGROUND

Although laparoscopic surgery was introduced more than 80 years ago, its role in pediatric surgery has become notable only in the past 10 to 15 years. To a large extent, this has been due to improved technology in optics and miniaturization of the instruments. An increasing number of general and urologic surgical procedures (including appendectomy, cholecystectomy, and splenectomy, as well as those to treat inguinal hernia and undescended testicles) are performed either laparoscopically or using robotic techniques in children of all ages (Figs. 29.1 to 29.4).[93–101] More sophisticated

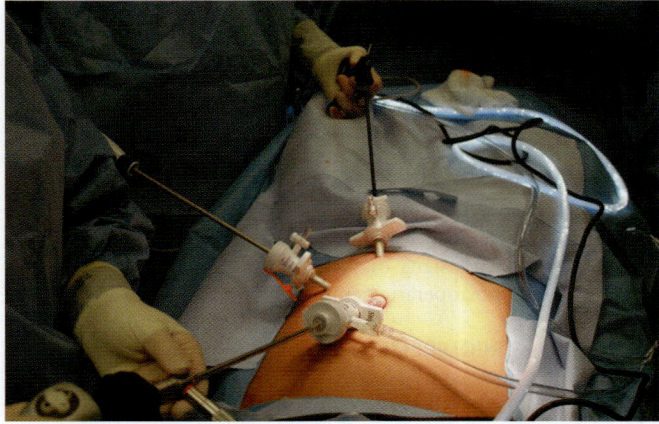

FIGURE 29.1 A child undergoing laparoscopic appendectomy, presented as a paradigm for the surgical setup for any multiple-trocar laparoscopic surgery. Three incisions were made, two in the anterior abdominal wall and the third in the umbilicus. The first two trocars carry instruments to manipulate the appendix, while the third holds the camera for viewing by all personnel in the operating room. All cables swing widely off the surgical field.

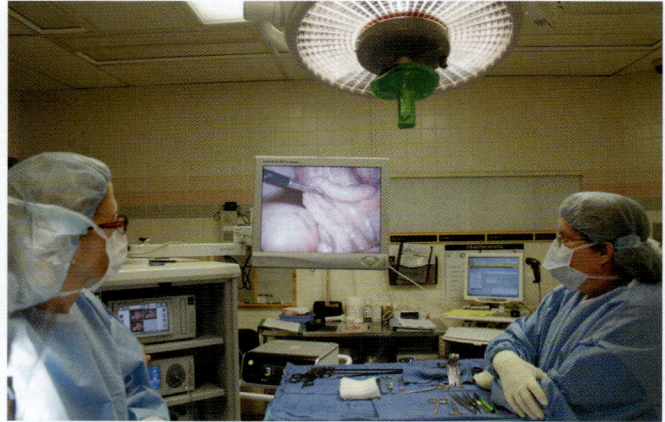

FIGURE 29.2 Wide-angle view of the operating room with surgeon and scrub nurse viewing the appendix being held by the grasper, shown on the overhead monitor.

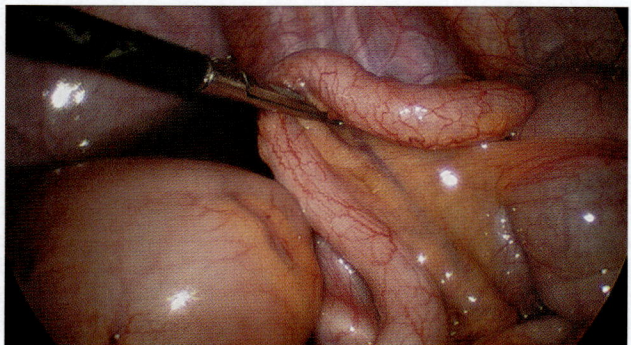

FIGURE 29.3 Inside the abdominal cavity with a view of the inflamed appendix that has been mobilized. The peritoneal attachments must be peeled off the appendix before it is ligated and removed.

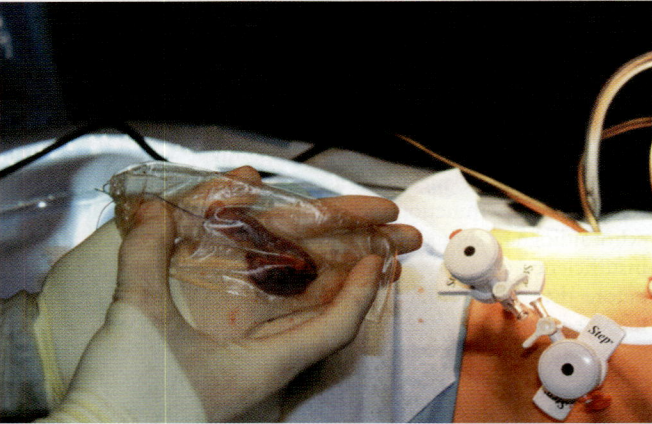

FIGURE 29.4 The appendix is ligated, inserted into a plastic container, and withdrawn, usually through the trocar or incision site without contaminating adjacent tissues. The appendix is shown in the surgeon's hand after removal.

laparoscopic techniques have enabled the performance of complex surgical procedures, including Nissen fundoplication, colectomy, pyeloplasty, bowel pull-through, and removal of large organs, including the kidney and spleen.[99,102–105] Technological advances now permit laparoscopic surgery in neonates and small infants, including those with hypoplastic left heart syndrome after stage 1 or 2 repair.[101,106–108] It must be noted, however, that laparoscopic surgery in children with cyanotic heart disease carries with it a substantial risk that exceeds most other populations having this form of surgery. Although several reports suggest that infants and children of all ages, at all stages of palliative repair of their cyanotic heart disease, tolerate laparoscopic surgery,[108–110] the risk for those with Fontan physiology undergoing laparoscopic surgery is substantial. It is essential to understand that in Fontan physiology, pulmonary blood flow is passive, and decreases in venous return (whether from increases in intrathoracic pressure or head-up positioning) or increases in pulmonary vascular resistance (because of increased CO_2 partial pressures or decreased minute ventilation) could severely reduce CO.[111] Creating a pneumoperitoneum for laparoscopic surgery and extreme positions increase IAP and arterial CO_2 tensions (increasing pulmonary artery pressure) reduces venous return and increases the risk of reducing the CO in children with Fontan physiology (see later discussion). Successful management of these children during laparoscopic surgery requires a multidisciplinary team that functions in concert to enhance the child's outcome (1) by optimizing the child's condition preoperatively and identifying any cardiac issues, (2) by recruiting surgeons who can complete the surgery quickly and efficiently, (3) by maintaining the children in the supine position throughout the surgery, (4) by maintaining normocapnia, (5) by monitoring the child with a transesophageal echo probe as needed, as well as with an arterial invasive pressure monitor for blood gas analysis, and (6) by insufflating the abdomen to the minimal (<8 mm Hg) IAP that is surgically feasible. Larger studies are required before children with cyanotic heart disease, particularly those with Fontan physiology, can routinely undergo laparoscopic surgery in any center except those with specialized teams to manage these children.

Laparoscopic surgery offers a number of advantages over open surgery, including more rapid emergence from anesthesia, faster ambulation, earlier discharge from the hospital, and reduced perioperative complications.[112–115]

Because laparoscopic surgery involves the insufflation of gas into the abdominal cavity to visualize the intraabdominal organs, the stomach should be decompressed using a nasogastric or orogastric tube for upper abdominal surgery, whereas the bladder should be emptied using a urinary catheter for lower abdominal surgery. Surgical access to the peritoneal cavity is achieved with trocars introduced through one to three small (3 to 10 mm in diameter) incisions; the laparoscopic instruments and a camera are then passed through the trocars. Laparo-endoscopic single-site (LESS), single-port, single-incision laparoscopic surgery (SILS), single-incision multiport laparoscopy (SIMPL), or "belly button" surgery has been developed, in which all instruments pass through a single incision and a single large trocar (often in the umbilicus) (E-Figs. 29.1-29.3).[116-120]

Pneumoperitoneal pressure is a major concern for all laparoscopic approaches. Experimental evidence in adult and newborn pigs demonstrated that the risks of cardiorespiratory consequences and potentially fatal emboli were directly related to the peak pneumoperitoneal pressure.[121,122] In infants and children, the optimal pneumoperitoneal pressure is the least pressure that enables adequate surgical access. CO_2 should be insufflated through one of the trocars until the IAP reaches 6 to 15 mm Hg; most surgeons currently limit the IAP in neonates and young infants to 6 to 8 mm Hg and in children to 10 to 12 mm Hg.[123] The IAP is maintained throughout the surgery by intermittently insufflating additional CO_2. Although CO_2 is most commonly used, a number of gases have been investigated (see later discussion).[124] CO_2 is the preferred gas because it does not support combustion, is rapidly cleared from the peritoneal cavity at the end of surgery, and does not expand into bubbles or spaces.[103,125,126]

Adverse Effects of Pneumoperitoneum

The increased IAP during laparoscopic surgery may cause a number of physiochemical side effects, including cardiorespiratory depression, hypothermia as the result of dry gas leakage, pneumothorax or subcutaneous emphysema, endobronchial intubation resulting from the upward shift of tracheal bifurcation, or injury resulting from paracentesis.

Carbon Dioxide

The major disadvantage of using CO_2 to insufflate the peritoneum arises from its rapid absorption from the peritoneum, with the absorption and washout of CO_2 more rapid and the peak end-tidal partial pressure of CO_2 ($P_{ET}CO_2$) greater in infants than in older children.[127,128] The inverse relationship between age and the rate of CO_2 absorption from the abdomen has been attributed to the thinner peritoneum and the reduced peritoneal fat deposits in the abdomen of infants compared with older children.[128,129] Because CO_2 is so readily absorbed, particularly in infants, both the $P_{ET}CO_2$ and $PaCO_2$ may increase 20% to 50% above baseline.[104,123,125,127,130] The resultant hypercapnia, which occurs more commonly in surgery lasting longer than 1 hour, particularly in neonates,[131] necessitates an increase in minute ventilation (from 50% to 100%) to maintain a physiologic pH.[103,132] The difference between the partial pressures of arterial and end-tidal CO_2 ($PaCO_2$–$P_{ET}CO_2$) often increases during insufflation of CO_2.[130,132] In one report, the $PaCO_2$–$P_{ET}CO_2$ gradient before and after pneumoperitoneum increased from a mean of 5.7 mm Hg to 13.4 mm Hg.[133] It should be noted that in neonates and in children with cyanotic congenital heart disease, the $P_{ET}CO_2$ may not reliably track the $PaCO_2$ during CO_2 insufflation, leading some to recommend arterial blood gas monitoring to validate the $P_{ET}CO_2$ measurements.[130,133,134]

Increased $PaCO_2$ may also trigger spontaneous respiratory efforts that could interfere with surgery. In addition, it may initiate a sympathetic response, including increases in the heart rate, blood pressure, and cerebral blood flow, as well as precipitate ventricular arrhythmias, although this occurs rarely with sevoflurane. A sudden increase in $P_{ET}CO_2$ may also suggest a diagnosis of malignant hyperthermia if accompanied with sudden onset of tachycardia.[135-137] If this diagnosis proves to be difficult to confirm or reject (in malignant hyperthermia expect venous PvO_2 <40 mm Hg; see Chapter 41), it may be necessary to desufflate the abdomen and determine if the clinical and laboratory findings suggestive of malignant hyperthermia resolve.[129,138]

Gas Emboli

Gas emboli have been reported in several laparoscopic studies, most of which were interesting curiosities of no clinical consequence, although in several, the result was profound cardiovascular collapse.[139-141] Most consider the emboli to be intravascular CO_2 bubbles, although there is evidence to suggest that some emboli contain nitrogen or air.[142] Intravascular embolization of CO_2 may occur when the insufflation pressure exceeds the venous pressure, forcing CO_2 bubbles into the venous circulation, resulting in sudden cardiovascular collapse.[140] Continuous precordial Doppler or expired CO_2 partial pressure are effective in detecting a gas embolus, although the Doppler may be overly sensitive, with numerous false-positive results. It has been suggested that many episodes of subclinical gas embolism are unrecognized because the symptoms are mild and nonspecific.[143] However, children with right-to-left shunts or potential right-to-left shunts, such as a patent foramen ovale, are vulnerable to the systemic effects of these emboli. Although CO_2 is soluble in blood and rapidly buffered, CO_2 emboli dissolve slowly in blood, taking 2 to 3 minutes to disappear.[144] Hence, large emboli may block blood flow in the heart for several minutes or more before they dissolve. The minimum rate of infusion of CO_2 into blood that triggers cardiovascular collapse in pigs is 1.2 mL/kg per minute[144]; comparable data in humans are lacking. Anesthesiologists should be aware of the high-risk conditions that predispose to CO_2 emboli (e.g., increased abdominal insufflation pressure, hypovolemia and reduced venous pressure, spontaneous respirations, and resection of vessel-rich parenchymatous organs) and communicate closely with the surgeons at all times.

Some investigators suggest that clinically important gas emboli are actually nitrogen, not CO_2 gas emboli.[140] Whereas transient emboli are thought to be composed of CO_2, emboli that persist may be nitrogen gas.[140] Nitrogen is insoluble in blood (blood/gas partition coefficient of 0.014), which explains its persistence as an embolus in blood. These emboli may arise from air, either present in or entrained by the trocar during insufflation of the peritoneum, that is forced into a transected blood vessel while the carboperitoneum is pressurized.[140] This mechanism is a rare source for gas in the circulation, which may explain, in part, why the emboli that occur during laparoscopy very rarely result in cardiovascular instability and arrest.

In contrast to CO_2, insufflation with oxygen, air, and nitrous oxide for laparoscopic surgery has been eschewed because they all support combustion. However, repeat desufflations of the pneumoperitoneal gas during laparoscopy in pigs whose lungs were ventilated with 66% nitrous oxide in oxygen prevents the concentration of nitrous oxide from exceeding 10% in the pneumoperitoneal cavity.[145] Nitrous oxide is still avoided for both insufflation and as an adjunctive anesthetic gas during laparoscopy, because it also expands into gas-filled cavities should gas emboli appear in the circulation.[125] Its use during laparoscopic surgery may distend the bowel in bowel obstruction and obscure the surgeon's view, as well as expand any CO_2 emboli that develop.

The inert gases argon and helium were also candidate gases for insufflation to create a pneumoperitoneum as they cannot be oxidized (and therefore ignited), although they are much more expensive than CO_2. When argon was used to create a pneumoperitoneum in pigs, embolization occurred more frequently than with CO_2.[146] In theory, both argon and helium can cause serious sequelae if embolized into the vascular system because they are insoluble in blood (blood/gas solubility of helium is 0.007 and argon is 0.029) and therefore likely to persist.[103,125,126,146]

RESPIRATORY EFFECTS

As the pressure within the peritoneal cavity increases, the frequency of adverse respiratory effects also increases, particularly at IAP greater than 15 cm H_2O. The respiratory manifestations of increased IAP include cephalad displacement of the diaphragm, decreased excursion of the diaphragm, and decreases in pulmonary and thoracic compliance, vital capacity, functional residual capacity, and closing volume.[147] Cephalad displacement of the diaphragm shifts ventilation to the nondependent parts of the lungs, creating a ventilation-perfusion mismatch. With a small functional residual capacity in children, cephalad displacement of the diaphragm further compresses the lungs, causing collapse of the small airways, ventilation-perfusion mismatch, and possibly hypoxemia. Other adverse pulmonary mechanics after insufflation include increased peak inspiratory pressures up to 27% and decreased compliance as much as 39%.[148] These physiologic changes are compounded by the extreme body tilting (i.e., extreme head-up or head-down positions) often requested by surgeons.[125,149] Positioning the child head down (i.e., Trendelenburg position) first decreases compliance by 17%, and second, adding a pneumoperitoneum decreases compliance by an additional 27%, requiring increases in peak inflation pressures of 19% and 32%, respectively.[150] In a recent study in which the pneumoperitoneum was created before Trendelenburg positioning in children whose lungs were ventilated using pressure control and 5 cm H_2O PEEP, a pneumoperitoneum of 12 cm H_2O decreased both dynamic compliance and tidal volume by 42%.[151] The addition of 20 degrees of Trendelenburg positioning only decreased these values by an additional 10%. All of these changes in pulmonary function can be offset by increasing minute ventilation (rate and peak inflation pressure) by as much as 50% to 100%. Pulmonary function appears to be restored more readily after laparoscopic than open surgery.[103]

Another respiratory concern is that the pneumoperitoneum and the extreme Trendelenburg position can shift the tracheal tube in a rostral direction, as far as 1.2 to 2.7 cm, possibly having an impact on the carina or passing into a bronchus.[152] With these changes, inspired oxygen concentrations in excess of 30% may be required, along with PEEP to restore adequate oxygenation. A persistent 5% decrease in oxygen saturation has been associated with partial or intermittent endobronchial intubation.[153]

Securing the airway for laparoscopic surgery requires particular attention. Cuffed tracheal tubes are preferred over uncuffed tubes to ensure effective alveolar ventilation despite the conditions described above,[134] although LMAs and ProSeal supraglottic airways (Teleflex Medical Inc.; Research Triangle Park, NC) have been used for brief procedures during laparoscopic surgery without complications.[126,154] If the child has a mature tracheotomy, the air leak around the tracheotomy must be assessed before surgery and if the leak is excessive, the tracheotomy should be replaced with a cuffed tracheotomy, a cuffed tube, or an armored (cuffed) tracheal tube. If the air leak around the tracheotomy is insignificant, then ventilation should be adequate even in the presence of increased IAP during laparoscopic surgery.

Excessive IAP may cause gas to track across the diaphragm, causing a pneumomediastinum or pneumothorax.[126] This is more common in hiatus hernia surgery and Nissen fundoplication, during which dissection of the esophagus may create passages for gas to traverse the diaphragm. Pneumomediastinum should be suspected if subcutaneous emphysema appears. If surgery creates a transdiaphragmatic passage for CO_2 to accumulate in the pleural space, the resulting pneumothorax may produce cardiorespiratory manifestations. A chest radiograph should be obtained if subcutaneous emphysema appears during or after surgery, or if there is a high index of suspicion that a pneumothorax has formed. Both pressure- and volume-controlled ventilation have been used during laparoscopic abdominal surgery in infants and children. In a single randomized study, both ventilation strategies with 5 mm Hg PEEP maintained effective ventilation and gas exchange.[155]

To avoid the cardiorespiratory compromise of a pneumoperitoneum, a gasless laparoscopic approach has been described. This requires lifting the anterior abdominal wall to create an intra-abdominal tent.[126,156] Implementation of the gasless approach in pediatric medicine has been rather slow, presumably because of technical difficulties and the scarcity of instruments for infants and children.

CARDIOVASCULAR EFFECTS

Three major factors may contribute to adverse cardiovascular responses during pneumoperitoneum: (1) IAP, (2) position (i.e., steep head-up or reverse Trendelenburg), and (3) release of neurohumoral vasoactive substances.[126,147,156] Increased IAP exerts a biphasic effect on venous return and CO. In neonatal pigs, the cardiac index (CI) decreased 55% when IAP exceeded 20 mm Hg.[126] In the animal model, the magnitude of the increase in IAP determined the degree to which the circulation was depressed.[134,157] For example, at IAP 15 mm Hg or less, blood is compressed out of the splanchnic circulation, increasing venous return, which either increases or results in no change in CO. In contrast, at IAP greater than 15 mm Hg, the inferior vena cava is compressed, reducing venous return and therefore CO. Studies in children yielded similar results; when the IAP exceeded 12 mm Hg, myocardial contractility[158] and venous return[125] decreased. In both infants and children, CO_2 insufflation to IAP 10 to 13 mm Hg decreased CI approximately 13%.[159-161] In studies in infants and children in which the CI decreased during increased IAP (10-12 mm Hg), the CI returned to preinsufflation values when the abdomen was desufflated.[158-160] Left ventricular systolic function was diminished, and septal wall motion abnormalities have been reported with an IAP of 10 to 12 mm Hg in children with a CO_2 pneumoperitoneum.[158,159] No significant changes in echocardiographic indexes of left ventricular work, preload or afterload, have been noted if the IAP is 10 mm Hg or lower during the pneumoperitoneum.[123] When standard indexes of hemodynamics were measured in infants and young children during laparoscopic Nissen fundoplication, IAP of 10 mm Hg or less yielded no significant changes in heart rate and blood pressure but a slight increase in CI.[162,163] If IAP is maintained at 10 mm Hg or less, then the impact on hemodynamics (particularly CO) should be clinically insignificant, because venous return may be enhanced as a result of displacement of blood from the splanchnic bed, and afterload is not increased.[125,134,162] Most importantly, if the IAP is less than 5 mm Hg, CI is maintained in infants during a CO_2 pneumoperitoneum[162]; these low insufflation pressures are those often used to examine the contralateral side of a hernia defect during surgery.

Body position during laparoscopic surgery may exaggerate cardiovascular changes. For Nissen fundoplication, a steep head-up position (>20-degree incline) has been used, which reduces venous return.[149] In adult pigs, laparoscopic surgery for Nissen fundoplication increased pleural and mediastinal pressures that, in turn, reduced CO episodically at an IAP of 15 mm Hg.[164] These decreases in CO were manifested by episodes of hypotension and hypoxia. When children were positioned in the steep head-up position, they developed transient hypotension and bradycardia that were reversed immediately with fluid loading and atropine.[165]

It is imperative to continuously monitor IAP to minimize the cardiorespiratory effects of laparoscopic surgery and to avoid excessive insufflation pressures. In adults, induction of anesthesia, insufflating the IAP to 14 mm Hg and a 10-degree head-up tilt decrease the CI more than 50%.[166] Some clinicians recommend a maximum IAP during laparoscopy in children of 6 to 8 mm Hg to limit the cardiorespiratory effects,[167] although most studies favor pressures of 10 to 12 mm Hg.[151,157,159,168] In neonates and infants, the maximum IAP should not exceed 6 to 8 mm Hg to minimize cardiorespiratory effects. Based on the current literature, the net cardiovascular effects of insufflating the abdomen to pressures of 12 mm Hg or less, combined with the head-up position, are likely to be well tolerated if adequate hydration is maintained and bradycardia is avoided.[165]

CENTRAL NERVOUS SYSTEM EFFECTS

Laparoscopic surgery must be carefully evaluated if planned for a child with increased intracranial pressure (ICP) or in the presence of a ventriculoperitoneal shunt. The combination of increased IAP, increased systemic vascular resistance, increased $PaCO_2$ tension, and Trendelenburg position (as in lower abdominal surgery) may dramatically increase ICP. In adults during extreme head-down position (40 degrees) for prolonged periods, such as in robot-assisted surgery in the pelvis, cerebral tissue oxygen saturation is well maintained, as evidenced by near-infrared spectroscopy.[169] Under similar surgical conditions, intraocular pressure increased 100%, and scleral edema and blurred vision may develop.[170] In anesthetized children during laparoscopic surgery, intraocular pressure increased 30% after insufflation (<15 mm Hg IAP) compared with laparotomy surgery.[171]

Patency of a VP shunt should be evaluated before the procedure to prevent sudden increases in ICP during the procedure. Children with reduced brain ventricular system compliance may sustain dramatic increases in ICP if the IAP is sufficient to attenuate the drainage of cerebrospinal fluid into the abdominal cavity. In these children, laparoscopic surgery may be relatively contraindicated.[149] The risks should be thoroughly explored and discussed with the neurosurgeon, general surgeon, anesthesiologist, and the family. Children with VP shunts have shown a range of responses to laparoscopy from dramatic increases in ICP to no change at all.[147,172,173] Accordingly, a variety of approaches have been suggested. Some advocate externalizing the shunt and clamping the distal (intraabdominal) end of the shunt before surgery to prevent CO_2 from passing retrograde up the shunt or from the laparoscopic pressure disrupting the shunt valve, although these valves are stable with an IAP up to 80 mm Hg.[174] Another approach has been to temporarily isolate the tip of the VP shunt in an Endopouch bag (Ethicon, Somerville, NJ) while insufflating

pressures to 12 mm Hg and then removing the bag at the end of the procedure.[175] Others discourage externalizing the shunt as sequelae have been reported, and instead recommend monitoring the ICP to prevent and detect increases in ICP and further recommend retraction of abdominal tissue during the laparoscopic surgery.[174] For the surgeon, using a SILS approach to laparoscopic surgery in these children reduces the risk of both traumatizing and infecting the VP shunt.[176] One retrospective review reported that laparoscopy in children with VP shunts was not associated with an increased risk of shunt infection compared with open procedures.[174] No single strategy can provide the optimal management for every child with a VP shunt undergoing laparoscopic surgery.

RENAL EFFECTS AND FLUID REQUIREMENTS

Increased IAP decreases renal blood flow, renal function (creatinine clearance and glomerular filtration rate), and urine output.[134,147,177] One study examined renal oxygenation with near-infrared spectroscopy and found no evidence of renal hypoxemia when age-appropriate IAPs were used (<6 mm Hg in neonates, <8 mm Hg in 2- to 12-month old infants, <10 mm Hg 1 to 2 years of age, <12 mm Hg 2–8 years of age). At the same time, they reported increasing cerebral oxygen saturation (likely from increased cerebral blood flow from increased arterial CO_2), heart rate, and mean arterial pressure.[178] The overall effects of IAP on renal function and renal filtration are poorly understood. Decreases in urine output during laparoscopic surgery in children vary, in part, with the age of the child: oliguria occurs in older children and anuria in infants younger than 1 year of age.[147,149,179] The etiology of the renal dysfunction and oliguria is multifactorial but includes direct and indirect effects of IAP on renal perfusion, antidiuretic hormone (ADH), endothelin, and nitric oxide (NO).[147,180] ADH concentrations increase as a result of reduced renal blood flow, resorbing water, and decreasing urine output. IAP increases renal endothelin (endothelin-1), resulting in renal venoconstriction, which reduces renal blood flow and urine output.[147,180] Inhibiting endogenous NO exacerbates the renal dysfunction during pneumoperitoneum through several mechanisms, including reduced renal perfusion and increased salt and water resorption (e.g., oliguria).[180] In theory, pretreating patients with a NO donor (such as L-arginine or nondepressor doses of nitroglycerin) may attenuate the detrimental effects of a pneumoperitoneum on renal function.[180] Renal tubular injury does not contribute to the renal dysfunction associated with increased IAP.[181] In adult donor nephrectomy patients, an overnight infusion of fluids followed by a colloid bolus immediately before the pneumoperitoneum attenuated the adverse hemodynamic effects and reduced the magnitude of changes in creatinine clearance associated with increased IAP.[182] Comparable data in children have not been forthcoming.

Fluid administration during laparoscopic surgery should be carefully monitored. Open abdominal surgery may require 10 to 15 mL/kg per hour of balanced salt solution to offset third-space fluid losses from extensive bowel manipulation. Although the existence of and manipulation of a real "third space" are debated, the conceptual fluid shift is real. During laparoscopic surgery, however, these fluid requirements are reduced because little fluid is lost and the bowels are minimally manipulated. In fact, care must be taken to avoid fluid overload. Urine output is often used as an index of preload in children undergoing abdominal surgery, but 88% of infants and 33% of children develop anuria or oliguria during laparoscopic surgery. Because these issues completely resolve within several hours of desufflation, fluid challenge is not necessary in these children as fluid overload is a real possibility.[179] Transient oliguria in children after laparoscopic surgery should not be viewed as an early indicator of impending renal dysfunction.

PAIN MANAGEMENT

Postoperative pain after open general and urologic surgery primarily results from the skin and muscle incisions. With the small incisions used during laparoscopic surgery, perioperative pain is less than with open surgery.[183–185] A systematic review of pain after laparoscopic antireflux surgery in children reported mild to moderate pain in ~20% of children and severe pain in 4%.[186] Intraperitoneal administration of local anesthetic has also been evaluated as a strategy to attenuate pain after laparoscopic surgery. A recent systematic review of this strategy in children concluded that there is some benefit from this approach although the dose of local anesthetic is limited by the child's weight. Additional studies are needed to fully assess the effectiveness of this approach.[187] To date, there have been a dearth of studies investigating pain after laparoscopic surgery in children.

Pain after laparoscopic surgery arises from several sources, including the incision sites, residual gas in the abdomen, referred pain from the diaphragm, and stretch on nerves from peculiar patient positions. A long-acting local anesthetic should be infiltrated around the incision sites at the end of laparoscopic surgery to prevent postoperative incisional pain. Some children develop pain after laparoscopic surgery, including back and shoulder tip pain. In these instances, multimodal pain therapy including acetaminophen, nonsteroidal antiinflammatory agents, and (less commonly) opioids are effective.[104,105,126] Recent evidence suggests that SIMPL for appendectomy causes less pain than surgery with a multiport system.[188]

Robot-Assisted Surgery

Robot-assisted surgery is relatively new to pediatric surgery and urology, with only limited published experience, although it has been used extensively in adults since the late 1990s to facilitate minimally invasive endoscopic surgery. Enhanced with three-dimensional magnifying views and feedback-controlled enhanced motions of human hands, robot-assisted surgery enables very fine manipulation of surgical instruments while eliminating natural human tremors. It has great potential as the future direction for pediatric surgery and urology.[1,169,189–194]

Robotic surgery was initially introduced as a tool for remote battlefield surgery. It is now available to assist pediatric surgeons in performing complex surgery, with less tissue and organ damage on extremely small surgical targets. Most of the information currently available is limited to one product (da Vinci Surgical System, Intuitive Surgical, Sunnyvale, CA) and to adult urologic procedures. However, rapid innovation and miniaturization of equipment has resulted in several pediatric centers undertaking robot-assisted laparoscopic surgery, with excellent outcomes (Videos 29.1 and 29.2). Concerns from the anesthesiologist's perspective regarding this relatively new approach are summarized in Table 29.1. Most of the perceived problems relate to the extended duration of procedures and the steep Trendelenburg position used, although numerous surgeries have been performed without this position.[169,189] Published evidence with robot-assisted surgery has yielded outcomes comparable to laparoscopic surgery in children, prompting many to question whether this new and expensive surgical venture is justified.[195–197] However, rapidly advancing technology offers enormous opportunities for robot-assisted surgery in children in

the very near future, for very fine and technical dissection in small and constrained spaces.[198]

TABLE 29.1	Issues Regarding Current Robotic-Assisted Procedures From the Anesthetist's Perspective

Dependence on Extreme Body Position, Such as Extreme Trendelenburg Position (Because of Absence of Adequate Surgical Assistance for Surgical Field Exposure), May Lead to:

Increased intracranial pressure, ocular pressure, and impairment of cerebral perfusion

Optic nerve or retinal morbidity

Cerebrofacial congestion, airway edema, vocal cord palsy, delayed awakening

Possible overstretching of nerves passing through the axilla and nerve plexus damage

Extended lithotomy leading to compartment syndrome in the lower legs

Tendency to apply greater intraabdominal pressure

Circulatory depression and respiratory depression

Carbon dioxide insufflation related complications

Absence of Touch, Traction, and Compression Sensations of Holding Instruments or Tissues:

All the manipulations are dependent exclusively on the visual sense

Inability to know the events occurring in an invisible place, overt tissue damage

Possibility of overlooking overt bleeding or tissue damage

Absence of Robot Legs and Easy Movability:

Once fixed, it is hard to change the position of the robot or the child's position

Difficulty in checking IV access sites and the airway

Unlimited and unexpected surgical approaches

Exploration of new surgical approaches and complex tasks at awkward angles

Greater surgical and setup times, hypothermia, and pressure sores

Unpredictable movement of robot and camera arms

Hitting or compressing the child's face

Organization of all tubing and cables, including intravenous tubing and breathing hoses.

Need for Emergency Undocking of the Robot in Case of Mechanical Failure or Critical Events

Specific General Surgical and Urologic Conditions

NISSEN FUNDOPLICATION

This surgery is indicated for children with documented gastric fluid reflux for whom medical management failed. It involves mobilizing the muscles around the esophagus and suturing them tightly around the esophagus at the level of the lower esophageal sphincter. This surgery requires general anesthesia and tracheal intubation and is usually performed laparoscopically, with increasing application of robot-assisted technology.[199]

Children who require a Nissen fundoplication often have a neurologic injury (i.e., cerebral palsy) that causes esophageal dysmotility. This dysmotility heralds esophageal reflux that, if severe, may result in recurrent aspiration pneumonia. If medical and gastric tube therapies fail, a Nissen fundoplication may be considered. The anesthetic considerations are few because surgery is not associated with postoperative pain, large fluid shifts, or large blood loss. Positioning a bougie within the esophagus during surgery allows the surgeons to gauge how tight to tie the muscles around the esophagus; without a bougie, the muscles around the esophagus may be overtightened, causing an esophageal obstruction. Care must be taken to avoid dislodging the tracheal tube while manipulating the bougie. At the end of the procedure, it is common for the surgeon to request that 50 to 60 mL of air be insufflated into the stomach via the gastric tube to ensure there are no anastomotic leaks. In general, surgery is completed in less than 1 hour in experienced hands, with a complication rate of about 10% and an average hospital stay of about 1.6 days. Postoperative pain is usually easily managed; however, open procedures usually require continuous analgesia for 2 to 3 days.[200,201]

PECTUS EXCAVATUM

Although this is a deformity of the chest wall, pediatric surgeons most often carry out the corrective procedure. The classic approach to correcting a pectus excavatum involves an open procedure with fracture of the sternum, removal of multiple costal cartilages, and elevating the sternum with fixation, using one or two stainless steel bars. The Nuss procedure is a less invasive technique,[202,203] whereby a U-shaped bar is blindly passed through the thorax hugging the undersurface of the sternum. Once across the chest, the bar is flipped, through which process the sternum is pushed anteriorly without fracturing it, thus avoiding the creation of a flail chest by the removal of the costal cartilages. This procedure has since been modified, whereby the bar is passed through the thorax under direct vision, using thoracoscopy to reduce possible perforation of major structures (e.g., the heart or lungs).[204-206] Although the risk of this complication is reduced when the Nuss procedure is performed under direct vision, it may still occur.[207-209] Both blind and thoracoscopic approaches cause significant postoperative pain, which may be treated with patient-controlled analgesia, a thoracic epidural catheter, or a lumbar epidural catheter and epidural morphine (see Chapters 42-45).[210-212] Because these procedures are generally performed in teenagers, the thoracic epidural is preferably placed with the teenager awake but sedated. Compliance with inserting the epidural catheter while awake may be difficult in less mature teenagers. It is unclear whether the thoracic epidural provides improved analgesia compared with standard patient-controlled analgesia for this procedure.[213] It should be noted that these children will return for removal of the pectus bar after several years. Occasionally, the bar has become adherent to the pericardium or lung, resulting in a severe, sudden, and catastrophic rupture of a major vessel or chamber in the heart when the pectus bar is removed.[214] It would be prudent to establish ample IV access to provide the means to rapidly transfuse fluids and blood should a catastrophic blood loss occur.

CIRCUMCISION

Globally, the prevalence of male circumcision is 40%, with half of these surgeries performed for religious or cultural reasons.[215] Circumcision is performed in neonates, infants, children, and adults with local, regional, or general anesthesia. The indications for circumcision include phimosis, recurrent balanitis, religious beliefs, and parental preference. Inhalational anesthesia supplemented by a regional block is preferred. Classic circumcision involves cutting the foreskin and cauterizing and suturing the skin edges. The duration of surgery is usually less than 1 hour. The type of anesthetic and airway management do not significantly affect perioperative outcomes. The most common complication arising from circumcision is bleeding.

In infants and children, circumcision is performed with the patient under general anesthesia. Multimodal pain therapy includes acetaminophen (e.g., 10–15 mg/kg orally or 30–40 mg/kg rectally before starting surgery) or 10 to 15 mg/kg IV, parenteral opioids (i.e., morphine 0.05–0.1 mg/kg), and/or local anesthetic without epinephrine (dorsal penile block, caudal block, subcutaneous ring block, and topical lidocaine-prilocaine [eutectic mixture of local anesthetics (EMLA)]) (see Chapter 42).[216] In a comparative study, suprapubic penile block provided better analgesia than subcutaneous ring block of the penis.[217] When a caudal block was compared with penile blocks and parenteral analgesics, a Cochrane review concluded that both rescue analgesia and nausea and vomiting were comparable with all three techniques, although the analysis was limited because of small numbers and poor methodology.[218,219]

HYPOSPADIAS AND CHORDEE

This congenital malformation occurs in 1 of 250 liveborn males. It often occurs in isolation, without other congenital anomalies. *Hypospadias* refers to a malposition of the meatus of the urethra: rather than opening at the distal tip of the penis, the urethra opens along the undersurface of the penis anywhere from just proximal to the glans to the scrotum (Fig. 29.5). The majority of hypospadias defects are distal, occurring near or at the glans of the penis. Between 15% and 50% instances of hypospadias have an associated chordee, whereas 8% have an undescended testis. A small number of children with hypospadias have urethral

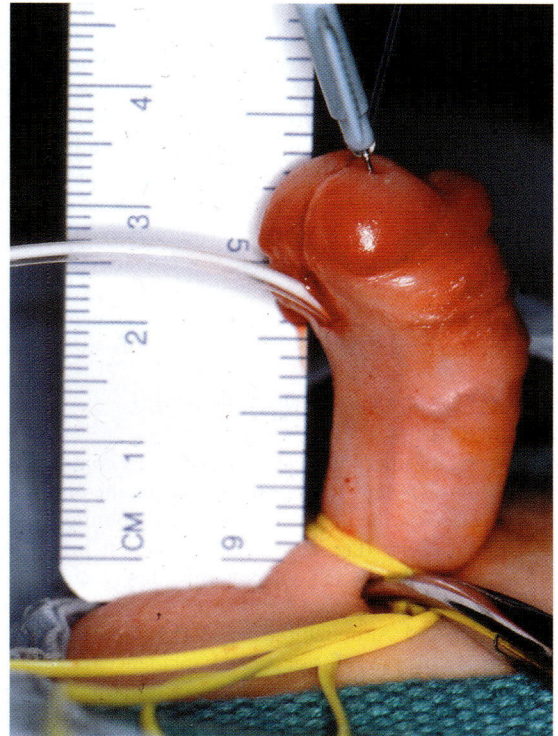

FIGURE 29.5 Classic hypospadias. Saline solution is injected to perform an erection test before surgical correction. (Courtesy Dr. P. Williot, Pediatric Urology, Women and Children's Hospital of Buffalo, Buffalo, NY.)

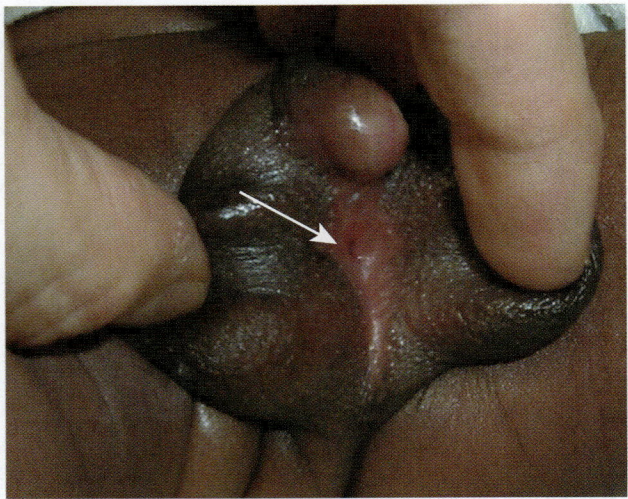

FIGURE 29.6 Scrotal hypospadias with the urethra opening in the midline of the scrotum. (Courtesy Dr. P. Williot, Pediatric Urology, Women and Children's Hospital of Buffalo, Buffalo, NY.)

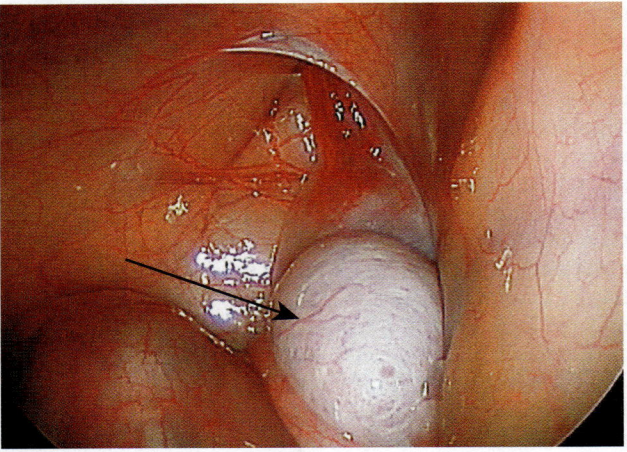

FIGURE 29.7 Intraabdominal testis in the hernia ring, discovered during laparoscopy for an undescended testicle. (Courtesy Dr. P. Williot, Pediatric Urology, Women and Children's Hospital of Buffalo, Buffalo, NY.)

openings remote from the glans of the penis, including the scrotum (Fig. 29.6; E-Figs. 29.4 and 29.5).

Surgery is undertaken with an expected duration of between 1 and 4 hours depending on the severity of the hypospadias. It is important to establish an understanding with the urologist of the type of regional block that will suit the extent of surgery: those requiring a minor hypospadias repair (single-stage procedure—that is, meatal advancement and glanuloplasty technique [MAGPI]) or Mathieu repair may be managed with a face mask, LMA, or tracheal tube. The anesthetic prescription is at the discretion of the anesthesiologist; the children are outpatients and receive either a penile block or a single-shot caudal block. Those with more extensive hypospadias who require longer surgery will require either an LMA or a tracheal tube. They may be admitted to a hospital for one to two nights and need a strategy for continuous postoperative analgesia. For the latter, either a caudal or a lumbar epidural catheter may be inserted after induction to reduce the anesthetic requirements and provide postoperative analgesia. If opioids are avoided, a caudal-epidural block consisting of only local anesthetic (e.g., bupivacaine 0.125–0.175% plain) does not delay micturition after the urinary catheter has been removed.[220]

CRYPTORCHIDISM AND HERNIAS: INGUINAL AND UMBILICAL

These surgeries, together with hydrocele repair, are common outpatient procedures. *Orchiopexy* refers to mobilizing the undescended testis that is either in the inguinal canal or, less commonly, within the abdominal cavity (Fig. 29.7), and securing it firmly in the scrotum. Approximately 33% of preterm infant males are born with one undescended testis, whereas only 3% of full-term males are similarly affected. Although the incidence of undescended testis decreases to 1% by 3 months of age, the incidence remains at 1% thereafter. Cryptorchidism usually occurs in isolation, although it is associated with a number of conditions, including Prader-Willi syndrome, Noonan syndrome, and cloacal exstrophy.

Undescended testes are categorized, based on physical examination, to include testes that are truly undescended, those that are ectopic, and those that are retracted. The retracted ones are not true undescended testes because they can be massaged into the scrotum and require no further treatment. In the case of true undescended testes, the testes must be located, mobilized, and then fixed within the scrotal sac to ensure viability. Failure to mobilize the testes out of the inguinal canal or abdomen may result in atrophy, torsion, testicular cancer, or hernias.

An *inguinal hernia* in a child is a congenital failure of the processus vaginalis to obliterate. In this case, a loop of bowel protrudes beyond the internal ring, causing a bulge in the inguinal region or scrotum. These protuberances may appear periodically, with complete resolution in the interim. On occasion, a small sac of fluid is present in the scrotum, known as a *hydrocele*, and is confused for a loop of bowel in the scrotum (E-Fig. 29.6). Hydroceles are removed electively with the same approach as for an inguinal hernia. On occasion, the loop of bowel does not reduce spontaneously from the hernia and remains trapped in the canal, necessitating a visit to the emergency department. A surgeon is often required to manually reduce the trapped bowel. In these cases, the hernia repair is then scheduled as an urgent or elective surgery, depending on whether there is suspicion of persistent or potential recurrent ischemia to the bowel. In some cases, the entrapped bowel cannot be reduced and an incarcerated hernia or obstructed bowel is diagnosed. Incarcerated hernias and bowel obstructions are surgical emergencies that require general anesthesia and muscle relaxation to reduce the strangulated bowel. The emergency nature of the surgery requires careful questioning regarding the time interval between the last meal and the onset of abdominal pain and strangulated bowel. It is usually assumed that these children have a full stomach. At the time of open reduction, if the bowel does not appear to have adequate perfusion, a segment of the ischemic or necrotic bowel may have to be resected.

Management of cryptorchidism and inguinal hernia requires general anesthesia (face mask, LMA, or tracheal tube) and a pain management strategy. When the surgeon pulls on the foreskin, hernia sac, or testis during surgery, laryngospasm may occur if the depth of anesthesia is inadequate. Anesthesia can be deepened most rapidly by an IV bolus of propofol; increasing the inspired concentration of inhalational anesthetic may also deepen the anesthetic provided gas can be exchanged. Multimodal pain therapy, as described earlier, may be used together with a regional block.

Regional blocks (ilioinguinal, iliohypogastric, scrotal block; caudal-epidural block; or transversus abdominis plane block) are used for both orchiopexy and inguinal hernia surgery, using either a landmark-based or ultrasound-guided method (see Chapters 42 and 43).[221]

An *umbilical hernia* is a 1- to 5-cm defect in the anterior abdominal wall (usually halfway between the umbilicus and the xiphisternal junction), with intermittent protuberance of bowel through the defect. This defect occurs in 15% of children, more commonly in children of African rather than European descent, and equally in both sexes. It also occurs frequently in preterm and low–birth-weight infants. Many resolve spontaneously in the first year of life, but those that persist require surgical closure. If the defect is small, then an LMA may be sufficient, provided a deep level of anesthesia is maintained when the suture needles pass through each side of the rectus muscle. If the defect is large, tracheal intubation and, depending on the surgeon, muscle relaxation may be required. A deep level of anesthesia with an inhalational anesthetic or an IV bolus of propofol (1–2 mg/kg) while the defect is closed usually provides sufficient relaxation to reduce the defect in most cases.

TORSION OF THE TESTIS

Presentation of a male with sudden onset of acute scrotal pain in the absence of trauma requires immediate investigation and possible surgery to preserve a potentially viable testis. The differential diagnosis of acute onset of torsion of the testis (Fig. 29.8) includes torsion of the testicular appendix, torsion of the spermatic cord, epididymitis, and incarcerated hernia. The majority of testes can be saved if surgery is performed within 6 hours of the onset of pain if the diagnosis is confirmed by Doppler ultrasonography or suspected on clinical grounds.[222] The salvage rate for the testis decreases to 50% if surgery is undertaken 6 to 12 hours after the onset of pain. Children with suspected acute testicular torsion should be considered "an acute abdomen" and assumed to have a full stomach and require RSI and tracheal intubation. Although pain at the time of induction of anesthesia may be intense, when the torsion is relieved, the pain abates. Hence, at the conclusion

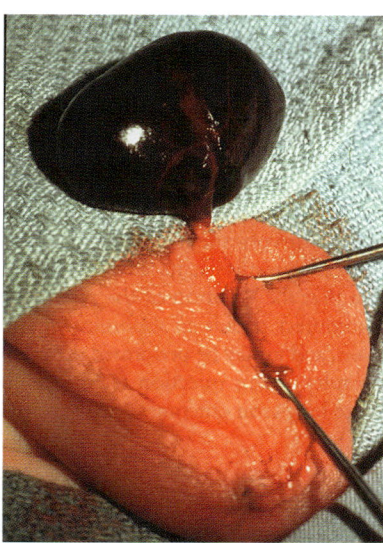

FIGURE 29.8 Torsion of the newborn testis. (Courtesy Dr. Daniel P. Doody, MD, Pediatric Surgery, MassGeneral Hospital for Children, Boston.)

of surgery many of these children no longer have substantive pain that warrants aggressive treatment.

POSTERIOR URETHRAL VALVES

Posterior urethral valves (PUV) is a spectrum of urethral obstruction that varies from mild to severe. The diagnosis is often made antenatally (preferably by 24 weeks gestation) by ultrasound identification of bladder distention, megaureters, and hydronephrosis. When PUV is diagnosed antenatally, the severity of the disease tends to be greater.[223] Decompression of the urogenital system may be achieved by a vesicoamniotic shunt in utero. Although some recommend that an intervention should be undertaken as quickly as possible to minimize the impact on renal function, evidence suggests that early intervention does not affect the outcome, because renal damage may have already occurred in utero.[224,225]

Postnatally, a lack of or decrease in urine output, urinary retention, or a poor urine stream may be the only indications of the presence of these valves.[226] Affected children can have associated renal insufficiency resulting from congenital renal dysplasia and urethral valve obstruction. Because the renal concentrating mechanism is often impaired, these infants commonly present with greater than normal urine output. Consequently, careful monitoring of urine output and balanced salt solution infusion rate is necessary. Primary valve ablation is required to decompress the urogenital system.

Several indexes have been postulated as predictors of poor long-term renal function in infants with PUV, including a creatinine value of 0.8 mg/dL or greater at birth, antenatal diagnosis, proteinuria, moderate or severe hydronephrosis, and renal dysplasia.[223,227] One study indicated that a nadir creatinine greater than 1 mg/dL and bladder dysfunction were the only independent predictors of long-term renal dysfunction.[228] Children with PUV are scheduled for elective surgery. A general anesthetic is required, with the specific management left to the discretion of the anesthesiologist; there are few special considerations needed.

PRUNE-BELLY SYNDROME

Prune-belly syndrome is a disorder that occurs predominantly (97% of the time) in males, with an incidence of 1 in 40,000 births. Affected infants present with a range of findings, from stillborn to a full-term neonate, with a host of possible organ and chromosomal abnormalities.[227,229] Affected organs may involve orthopedic in 50% (congenital hip dislocation and scoliosis), gastrointestinal in 30% (malrotation and volvulus), congenital heart disease in 10% (tetralogy of Fallot and ventricular septal defect), and chromosomal defects (trisomy 18 and trisomy 21).[227]

In utero, the child's abdomen often swells with fluid (in the presence of oligohydramnios) that is resorbed by birth, leaving the characteristic wrinkled redundant abdominal wall (Fig. 29.9 and E-Fig. 29.7). The pathophysiology of this syndrome is unclear, but it has been suggested that a urethral obstruction in utero leads to dilatation of the urethra (megaurethra is a common finding), which, combined with bladder distention and ascites, causes distention of the abdomen in utero. This ultimately leads to vesicoureteral reflux and ureteral dilatation in 80% of affected children.

Abdominal overdistention in utero causes weak rectus abdominis muscles that undermine the child's ability to exhale forcefully and to generate a strong cough to clear secretions. As a result, chronic aspiration pneumonia may contribute to an early demise. Some have suggested that aggressive intervention to correct the weak rectus muscles by plication and muscle transfer may improve

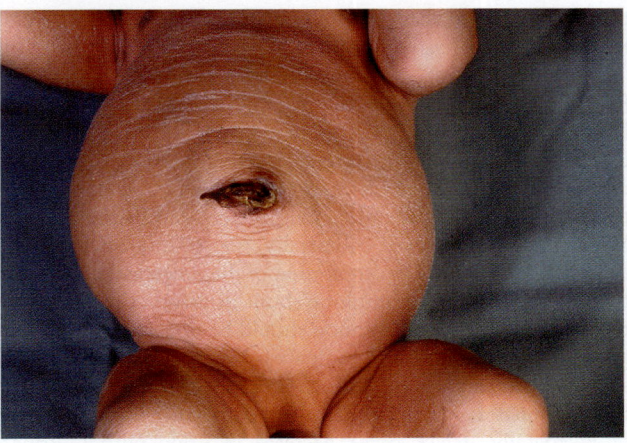

FIGURE 29.9 Prune-belly syndrome. View of the distended, weak muscled abdomen; the muscle wall is so thin that the abdominal surface is bulging in front of the bowels. (Courtesy Dr. P. Williot, Pediatric Urology, Women and Children's Hospital of Buffalo, Buffalo, NY.)

respiratory function,[230,231] reduce back strain and pain, decrease bladder volume, and arrest scoliosis.[232] However, this view is not shared by others who prefer to observe the child for signs of regurgitation and aspiration before intervening.[233] Controlling the type of feeds, preventing gastrointestinal reflux disease and constipation, and using antibiotics to treat pneumonia permit the child to grow. Pneumonia must be aggressively treated and completely resolved before entertaining surgery. Percutaneous endoscopic gastroscopy tubes are generally eschewed in these children when feeding is a problem, as abdominal wall surgery is difficult. These children often require urologic surgery to correct vesicoureteral reflux and orchiopexy. Urethral obstruction may be due to the angulation of the urethra within the prostate.

Trisomy 18, the second most common autosomal trisomy, occurs in 1 in approximately 7000 live births and is associated with prune-belly syndrome. In contrast to the simple prune-belly syndrome, 60% to 80% of these infants are female. Trisomy 18 is characterized by severe neurologic developmental problems (including microcephaly), micrognathia and/or retrognathia, microstomia, auricular abnormalities, and others. In fact, 95% die in utero, with only 5% to 10% surviving 1 year and only 1% reaching 10 years of age. Mortality results from cardiac anomalies (90% of affected children have a ventricular septal defect, valvular heart defect, atrial septal defect, hypoplastic left heart syndrome, tetralogy of Fallot, or other cardiac defect), renal anomalies, failure to thrive, and apnea.[234,235] Additional findings include pulmonary hypoplasia and gastrointestinal anomalies (including omphalocele, ileal atresia, and esophageal atresia).

General anesthesia with tracheal intubation is required for most surgeries in children with prune-belly syndrome. Controlled ventilation is recommended because of the variability in the strength of the abdominal muscles. It is prudent to suction the lungs once the trachea has been intubated to assess the severity of secretions. As little muscle relaxant as possible should be used during the surgery, with preferably no neuromuscular blocking drugs administered during the last hour, to ensure the child's muscles have had time to recover to maintain an adequate tidal volume after extubation. Opioids should be used cautiously to limit respiratory depression; regional anesthesia may be preferred

in view of their difficulty with clearing secretions from the tracheobronchial tree.[236]

URETERAL REIMPLANTATION

Vesicoureteral reflux, in which urine passes retrograde up the ureter, is a congenital disorder affecting 0.5% to 2% of children.[237] It occurs 10 times more commonly in Caucasian than African American children, is more common in male neonates but 5 to 6 times more common in females younger than 1 year of age, and more commonly occurs in red-haired children.[237] There is a genetic component to this disorder with 34% of siblings affected, although the pattern of inheritance is unknown.[238] Recurrent episodes of pyelonephritis may occur, leading to renal scarring and reduced renal function, depending on the severity of the reflux. The pathology is thought to be an anatomically abnormal insertion of the ureter into the bladder that fails to close tight when the bladder fills and contracts. A voiding cystourethrogram is the definitive test to diagnose reflux and assess its severity. Mild forms of vesicoureteral reflux are managed with daily antibiotics until the child outgrows the reflux. However, more severe forms or those who develop kidney infections despite antibiotic therapy require surgical correction. The classic surgical approach for vesicoureteral reflux is an open procedure in which the affected ureters are reimplanted into the bladder wall, re-creating a normal muscle flap valve.[239] This involves a lower abdominal incision and 2 to 4 hours of surgery. Postoperatively, the pain is often intense, necessitating 2 to 3 days of continuous infusion of local anesthetic via an indwelling caudal or epidural catheter.

More recently, laparoscopic techniques have been developed, with and without robotic control, for reimplantation of the ureters.[239] Preliminary evidence suggests an excellent success rate (>90%) for this approach,[240] although the time for the surgery is more than twice than with the open technique and more complications were identified in children with small bladders.

In the past 20 years, the search for alternatives to surgery has spawned a number of compounds to inject into the terminal submucosal tract of the ureter to prevent reflux. Initially, polytetrafluoroethylene (Teflon; Chemours, Wilmington, DE) was used but more recently a safer, more durable polymer comprised of dextranomer and hyaluronic acid (Deflux; Valeant Pharmaceuticals International, Bridgewater, NJ) supplanted Teflon. In this way, surgeons create a swelling just inferior to the opening of the ureter into the bladder that prevents urine from refluxing (Fig. 29.10, before and after injection of polymer). The technique is successful in 80% to 100% of cases of grade 1-2 reflux after one injection and in 85% of cases of grade 3-4 reflux after two injections (where the grade of reflux was related to the ureterorenal involvement).[241] Although this procedure still requires general anesthesia, its advantages far outweigh its disadvantages in that the duration of the procedure is very brief (usually 15–30 minutes), avoids an abdominal incision, causes no postoperative pain, and it may be performed as ambulatory surgery. However, the results of this injection technique continue to be monitored because long-term outcomes and sequelae have not been determined.

PYELOPLASTY

Ureteropelvic junction obstruction occurs in 0.1% to 0.2% of neonates, approximately twice as frequently in males than females. Pyeloplasty is performed to decompress the renal pelvis either because of intrinsic (congenital) or extrinsic (major vessel)

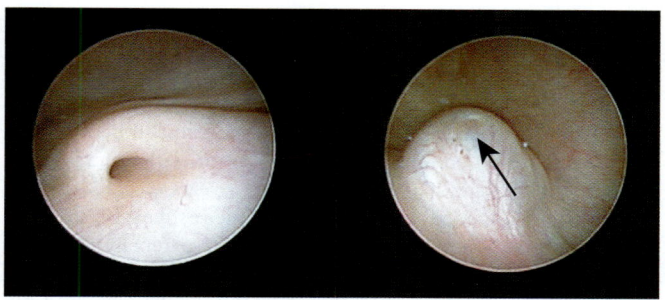

FIGURE 29.10 A child with ureteral reflux. Preinjection (*at left*) with the bladder orifice wide open with no valve to prevent the backwash of urine up the ureter. Polymer was injected into the submucosa of the bladder, raising a mound to seal off the orifice of that ureter. Postinjection (*at right*) with the orifice now appearing as a dimple on the peak of the mound (*arrow*). (Courtesy Dr. P. Williot, Pediatric Urology, Women and Children's Hospital of Buffalo, Buffalo, NY.)

compression of the ureter. A distended renal pelvis is often diagnosed antenatally and, in some instances, decompressed in utero by percutaneous nephrostomy. The ureteric narrowing often occurs at the ureteropelvic junction, where the ureter exits the renal pelvis. Surgery involves disconnecting the ureter at the renal pelvis, reshaping it, and then reinserting it into the kidney. Such surgery is often performed with the patient in the lateral or prone position, with the table jackknifed. The duration of this surgery is approximately 2 hours and has a success rate of approximately 95%. Dissection is often retroperitoneal, but the incision is placed immediately below the rib cage. This procedure has been performed laparoscopically and with the use of robotics.[115,242]

Anesthetic considerations include the prone or lateral decubitus position (complicated by placing the table in the jackknife position), postoperative pain, and adequate fluid resuscitation. IV access should be established in an upper extremity to maintain adequate atrial filling pressures. If the table is placed in the jackknife position, it is very important to measure the child's blood pressure before and after the table is jackknifed, because venous return may become severely compromised, necessitating reducing the extent of the jackknife and resuscitating the child with fluid. For postoperative pain management, an indwelling high lumbar or low thoracic epidural catheter is placed. We administer lidocaine 2% with 1:200.00 epinephrine immediately after inserting the catheter to set the block before the table is jackknifed. Thereafter a bupivacaine or ropivacaine epidural infusion may be used.

The laparoscopic approach to pyeloplasty in children is relatively new. In renal surgery, CO_2 is insufflated in the retroperitoneal space to provide surgical access.[243] Because of the anatomic differences between the retroperitoneal and intraperitoneal spaces, greater pressures may be required to provide adequate surgical visibility. A mean retroperitoneal pressure of 12 mm Hg increases PETCO$_2$ and peak inspiratory pressures, and decreases blood pressure.[244] Early evidence indicates that laparoscopic surgery yields outcomes similar to the open approach, although the duration of surgery is approximately one-third greater.[245,246] In part, this has been attributed to the learning curve of this technique. Evidence suggests that the laparoscopic approach decreases the length of hospital stay and may decrease postoperative pain[115,246] (see previous discussion of pain management after laparoscopic surgery).

NEPHRECTOMY

Indications for nephrectomy and partial nephrectomy in children include nonfunctioning kidney, dysplastic kidney, urolithiasis, Wilms or other tumor, end-stage renal failure (pretransplantation or to control hypertension), hemolytic uremic syndrome, and polycystic disease. Children who need a nephrectomy require a thorough preoperative assessment in terms of history, physical examination, and laboratory testing, depending on their underlying pathology. These children are often anemic because of chronic disease and possibly decreased erythropoietin concentrations. If the child is being staged for kidney transplant, the nephrologists may prefer to avoid blood transfusions at this time. If time is available and the patient is anemic, oral ferrous sulfate and vitamin C should be commenced 3 to 6 weeks before surgery (vitamin C increases gut absorption of ferrous sulfate) to increase the hemoglobin concentration, particularly if erythropoietin supplementation is planned.[247,248] These children are often small in size and this should be considered when preparing the anesthetic equipment.

Nephrectomies are commonly performed using a retroperitoneal approach with the child in the lateral decubitus position and the table jackknifed. The incision is usually large and located just subcostal to the twelfth rib. If an open approach is planned, an epidural catheter may be placed (see "Pyeloplasty" earlier). If, however, a laparoscopic or robotic-assisted approach is planned,[99] then a neuraxial block is not necessary but the same surgical approach occurs. Outcomes after laparoscopic nephrectomy in children are similar to those after an open procedure, according to the experience from one center,[249] although recent evidence points to less pain and earlier discharge from the hospital.[99]

NEUROBLASTOMA

The adrenal glands are located in the retroperitoneal space, adjacent to the superior pole of the kidneys. Masses that arise in the adrenal gland may be tumors, hemorrhage, infections, or cysts. The tumors in the adrenal glands may arise from the cortex (as in adenoma) or medulla (including the sympathetic chain, as in neuroblastoma or ganglioneuroma) and may be either hyperfunctioning or nonfunctioning.

Neuroblastoma is the most common extracranial solid tumor that presents in childhood, representing 10% of all tumors and 15% of all deaths from tumors.[250] It is the second most common abdominal tumor after Wilms tumor. Its incidence is approximately 1 in 100,000 children in the United States.[251,252] Neuroblastomas arise in the abdomen in 75% of cases and along the sympathetic chain anywhere from the neck to the pelvis in 25%. Only one-third of those that arise in the abdomen arise in the adrenal glands. The median age at presentation is 2 years, with up to 90% occurring in children younger than 5 years with equal sex prevalence. In some series, up to 50% of cases appear in the first month of life, with some diagnosed antenatally; reports of familial neuroblastoma are rare.[250] However, these tumors may be associated with other disorders, including Beckwith-Wiedemann syndrome, neurofibromatosis, Hirschsprung disease, and central hypoventilation syndrome.[250]

Most neuroblastomas are first detected as palpable masses in the abdomen. Symptomatic presentation may present as local pressure on adjacent organs or structures (liver, kidney, or spine), as metastases (lymph nodes, bone marrow, liver, and skin), or with manifestations of excess neurohumoral production (that is, from catecholamines [e.g., systemic hypertension] or vasoactive intestine polypeptides [e.g., diarrhea]).[250] Urinary catecholamines are increased in greater than 90% of children (>1 year of age) with neuroblastoma. In a minority of instances, the diagnosis is made through incidental examination, either by radiography or ultrasonography.

Staging of these tumors follows two protocols.[251] The International Neuroblastoma Staging System depends on tumor resectability, lymph node involvement, and metastases. However, if patients are not surgical candidates, the staging score holds little relevance. To further stage these tumors, a second scoring system was developed, the International Neuroblastoma Risk Group classification system, which is based on the preoperative radiologic findings only. Survival likelihood depends on a low score, extraabdominal (as opposed to intraabdominal) primary tumor, and younger age. Therapeutic intervention is tailored to the staging of the tumor at presentation and the size of the tumor. Those with favorable tumor biology, no distant metastases, and age younger than 18 months of age are often curable with surgical resection alone. Those with less favorable tumor biology, metastases, and a large tumor size that may present a challenge surgically are ideally treated with a combination of chemotherapy, radiation, and/or bone marrow transplantation to reduce the tumor size first and then with surgical resection. Patients with less favorable biology present a challenge for surgical resection because of local infiltration, large tumor size, and vascular extension. Debulking the tumor has been met with mixed reviews, with great success in low-risk patients but with less success when one of several other therapies in high-risk patients.[253] The most promising treatments for neuroblastomas with poor prognoses include molecular profiling of the tumor.[251] The long-term survival after treating these tumors is 88% for infants and children younger than 18 months, 49% for children 18 months to 12 years, and 10% for those 12 years and older.[254] Preoperative assessment requires a general systems review, with particular focus on the organ systems involved with the tumor. These tumors may present as a large intraabdominal mass that compromises respiration, most commonly manifested as tachypnea. Those with catecholamine-secreting tumors may also present with chronic hypertension. This is mitigated to a large extent if the tumor is shrunk preoperatively, but intraoperative hypertensive episodes still occur in 25% of the children (with urinary catecholamines) during surgery. Children with catecholamine-secreting neuroblastomas should have both α-adrenergic and β-adrenergic blockades established preoperatively (see Chapter 27) to avoid swings in blood pressure during manipulation of the tumor.[255] Less frequently, chronic diarrhea from vasoactive intestine polypeptides may cause chronic dehydration and electrolyte derangements that require correction.

The anesthetic plan depends on the nature and extent of the surgery. A general anesthetic with tracheal intubation and controlled ventilation, as well as standard anesthetic monitors, is required. These should be supplemented with invasive monitoring, including arterial and central venous access for catecholamine secreting tumors, large tumors, and those that are expected to bleed excessively. Anticipation of massive blood loss will necessitate using large-bore upper extremity IV access, blood warmers, and possibly a rapid transfusion device. No specific anesthetic regimen has been recommended for these surgeries.

Although the blood pressure may be controlled with established α-adrenergic blockade, manipulation and squeezing of the tumor during its removal may cause a surge in catecholamine release, necessitating the use of antihypertensive medications intraoperatively (see Chapter 27).[255] Labetalol may be effective in children with hypertension during resection of neuroblastomas[255]; however, it may cause paroxysmal hypertension and heart failure in children

who have only β-adrenergic blockade established because of the predominant β-adrenergic blocking action of labetalol.

WILMS TUMOR

Renal tumors represent 2.5% to 7% of tumors in children. Wilms tumor is the most common abdominal tumor, with an incidence of 1 in 100,000 children younger than 15 years of age, and the most common solid renal tumor beyond the first year of life.[252,256] These tumors arise from persistent immature parenchymal renal tissue (referred to as Wilms tumorlet cells), often in the periphery of the kidney (as opposed to the collecting ducts), enclosed by a pseudocapsule. They may achieve a large size before detection, often compressing adjacent renal parenchyma (Fig. 29.11). Histologically, the tumor often includes up to three distinct tissue cell lines: epithelial, blastemal, and stromal cells.[256] The presence of anaplastic cells (in 4% of Wilms tumors) and, more specifically, whether the cells are focal or diffuse in the tumor, and older age at the time of presentation suggest a less favorable response to chemotherapy and less favorable long-term prognosis.[256] With tailored multimodal therapy, the survival from Wilms tumor in the past several decades has increased dramatically, from 30% to ~90%.[257]

Eighty percent of the children with Wilms tumor present between 1 and 5 years of age (peaking at 3–4 years of age) with no gender or racial predominance.[252,256] Presentation of Wilms tumor is similar to that of other intraabdominal tumors in the form of an incidental mass on physical examination; approximately 6% are bilateral. Congenital anomalies coexist with Wilms tumors in 12% of children, notably genitourinary anomalies (5%), hemihypertrophy (2.5%), and aniridia (1%).[256] A number of genetic syndromes are associated with Wilms tumors (e.g., Beckwith-Wiedemann, Fanconi syndrome, and Trisomy 18).[252] Wilms tumors occur twice as frequently in children with horseshoe kidneys than in those with normal kidneys and are also more frequent in those with multicystic dysplastic kidneys.

Preoperatively, most children with Wilms tumors appear well, presenting with constitutional findings including weight loss, loss of appetite, and malaise; a palpable abdominal mass is present in 75% to 90%. Laboratory investigations before nephrectomy include routine complete blood cell count, electrolytes, renal

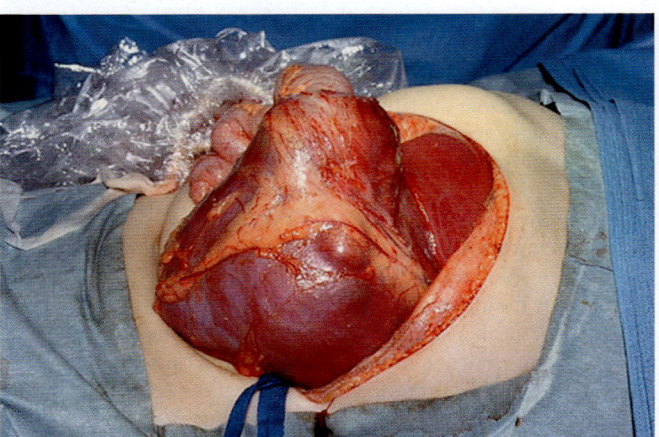

FIGURE 29.11 A Wilms tumor was mobilized and exteriorized from the abdomen. Note that it is encapsulated and contiguous with the left kidney. (Courtesy Daniel P. Doody, MD, Pediatric Surgery, MassGeneral Hospital for Children, Boston.)

function, as well as coagulation indexes. Polycythemia may be present from tumor-induced excess erythropoietin production; acquired von Willebrand disease is present in less than 10%.[252] Microscopic hematuria occurs in 25%, whereas overt hematuria is rare,[256] suggesting tumor invasion of the collecting ducts. Systemic hypertension is present in 25%, presumably as a result of hyperreninemia. Preoperative investigations should include radiography and ultrasonography, the latter highlighting hyperechogenic structures within the kidney. Tumor extension into the ipsilateral renal vein and inferior vena cava must be examined before embarking on surgery, as chemotherapy may lead to involution of these tumors (Fig. 27.12).[252] Magnetic resonance imaging and CT are valuable tools for delimiting the tumor borders within the kidney, as well as metastases in the lungs or other organs.[252] Most recent summaries of the radiologic investigations may determine the need for additional interventions, including echocardiogram and lung scan, to determine the presence of tumor in the heart and lungs, respectively. An echocardiogram may be specifically required to evaluate myocardial function if doxorubicin and other anthracycline chemotherapeutic agents have been administered.[252]

Anesthetic management of children with Wilms tumor is similar to that with neuroblastoma. No specific anesthetic regimen is preferred. The potential for massive and rapid blood loss must be anticipated and appropriate blood products should be immediately available. Invasive monitoring and large-bore IV access (upper extremities should the tumor extend into or compress the inferior vena cava) with adequate blood warming capability is mandatory; a rapid infusion device should be close at hand. Hypertension (precipitated by tumor handling), coagulopathy

(acquired von Willebrand disease), extension of the tumor into the proximal inferior vena cava or right atrium, pulmonary tumor emboli, acute right heart failure, and considerations concerning preoperative or previous treatment with chemotherapeutic drugs are anticipated potential complications during anesthesia.[252] These drugs may impair hepatic or hematopoietic function (actinomycin D), cause inappropriate antidiuretic hormone release (vincristine), or myocardial damage (anthracyclines) (see also Chapter 11).[252] Postoperative pain may be controlled using either IV opioids or regional anesthesia, though the risk of a coagulopathy must be ruled out before placing an epidural block.

BLADDER AND CLOACAL EXSTROPHY

Bladder exstrophy is a rare congenital anomaly of the genitourinary tract occurring in 1 in 50,000 births with a 2 : 1 male/female ratio, more common in Caucasians than non-Caucasians.[258,259] It occurs as a failure of the abdominal wall to close during fetal development and results in defects of the anterior wall of the bladder and overlying midline abdominal wall. Bladder exstrophy may present with a spectrum of anomalies, including widening of the symphysis pubis, and genital anomalies, such as epispadias, bifid clitoris, and undescended testes (Fig. 29.13). Some regard bladder and cloacal exstrophies as distinct entities, whereas others consider them both extremes in a continuum of antenatal defects.[260] Cloacal exstrophy includes features of bladder exstrophy, plus an omphalocele and spinal defects, and always includes imperforate anus. Because the antenatal diagnosis of bladder exstrophy using ultrasound may be technically difficult, and thus dependent on indirect signs (absence of bladder filling, a low-set umbilicus, widening of the pubic ramus, small external genitalia, or a lower abdominal mass), the diagnosis is usually confirmed at birth when the anterior abdominal wall defect with the exposed bladder mucosa are evident (Fig. 29.13).

Therapy is aimed at the surgical reconstruction of the bladder with preservation of renal function while achieving urinary continence and satisfactory appearance of the external genitalia.[261,262] In a select group of infants, surgical management may be carried out as a single-stage procedure[263]; however the majority require a staged surgical repair directed at closure of the bladder, posterior urethra, and abdominal wall.[264] In addition, a bilateral iliac osteotomy may be performed to facilitate surgical closure, decrease

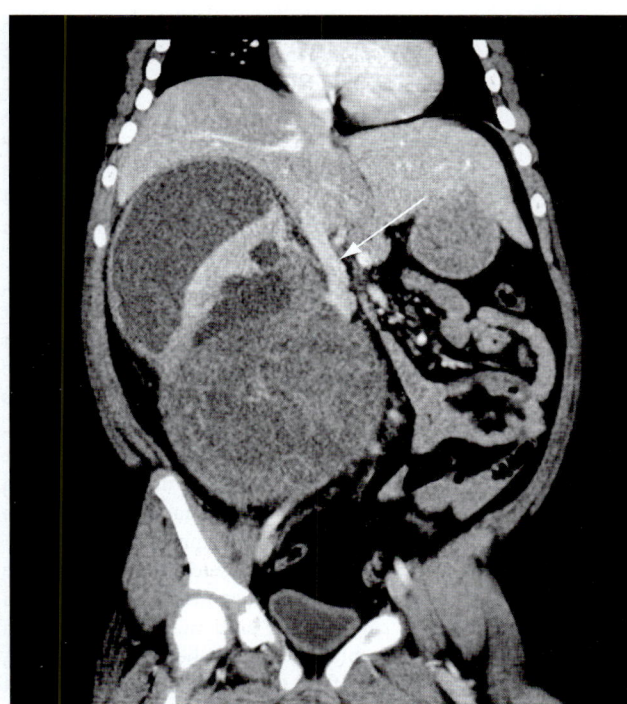

FIGURE 29.12 Coronal view of the CT scan of a Wilms tumor. Note the massive tumor enveloping the inferior vena cava, as the vena cava is only visible where it enters the liver in the upper midportion of the radiograph (*arrow*). (Radiograph courtesy Daniel P. Doody, MD, Pediatric Surgery, MassGeneral Hospital for Children, Boston.)

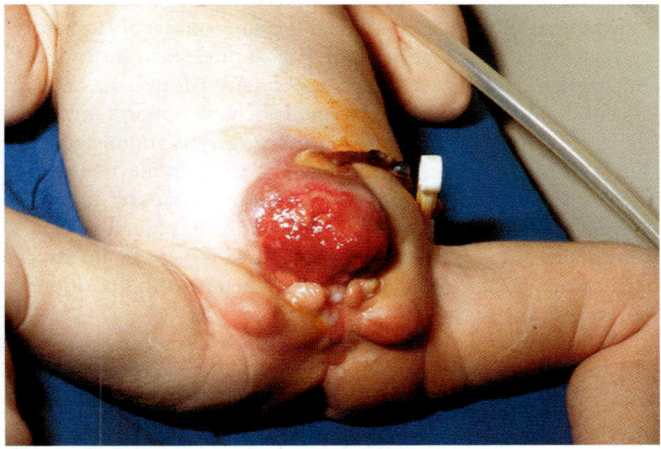

FIGURE 29.13 Bladder exstrophy in a neonate. Note the open anterior abdominal wall, protuberant bladder, distorted genitalia, and splayed hips.

the stress on the midline soft tissues, and reduce the risk of postoperative wound dehiscence.

Wound dehiscence, bladder prolapse, and multiple attempts at bladder closure are among the risk factors for decreased bladder growth and the inability for the later development of continence.[265] In addition to the immediate postoperative complications, children who have undergone surgical repair of bladder exstrophy carry an increased risk for the development of renal, bladder, and colon adenocarcinoma.[266] Children who require frequent bladder catheterizations or repeat surgeries are at risk for developing latex allergy if latex products are used[66]; fortunately most bladder catheters exclude latex.

Surgical management of the epispadias is usually performed at 6 to 12 months of age, and reconstruction of the bladder neck by 5 years, the latter to allow for bladder training.[264] After the initial surgical repair, children are immobilized for 4 to 6 weeks,[267] with a successful outcome likely when a modified Buck traction with an external fixator or a modified Bryant traction[268] and adequate postoperative analgesia are used.[269]

The preoperative assessment should evaluate the presence and severity of all congenital anomalies, particularly cardiac abnormalities. Signs or symptoms of renal insufficiency and electrolyte imbalance may be present. If the child has renal insufficiency, the dose and frequency of administration of potentially nephrotoxic drugs, as well as the commonly used anesthetic drugs, must be carefully evaluated, particularly water-soluble drugs. Typically, surgery is performed with the child in the supine and lithotomy positions. The duration of surgery is often prolonged, requiring alternating urologic and orthopedic teams for their respective segment of the surgery, and repositioning the child depending on the stage of the surgery, thus requiring judicious management of fluids, blood loss, and temperature control. It is essential to communicate with the surgical teams to ensure an optimal perioperative strategy for balanced salt solutions, colloids, and blood products; a preoperative plan for multimodal perioperative pain management and anticipation of possible postoperative ventilatory support is essential.[264] After applying the standard monitors, anesthesia may be induced either by inhalation or IV; after induction, at least one large-bore peripheral IV line should be placed. A second IV line may be placed, or a central venous catheter and possibly an arterial catheter. In general, if blood loss occurs, it is slow and steady, but if posterior iliac osteotomies are performed, the blood loss may become brisk, requiring aggressive fluid resuscitation and administration of blood products. Beat-to-beat variability of arterial blood pressure and serial laboratory evaluations are valuable during goal-directed resuscitation. Appropriate padding, a fluid warmer, and a forced-air heating system should be standard. The anesthetic prescription varies with the age of the child and whether the surgery is completed in a single or staged repair. Postoperatively, children are transferred directly to the pediatric intensive care unit for recovery.

A general anesthetic in combination with an epidural or caudal continuous infusion technique is often used if there are no associated spine abnormalities and if the catheter can be positioned out of the surgical field.[270]

Maintenance of anesthesia may be achieved using an inhalation anesthetic and small doses of opioids such as a remifentanil infusion; intermittent boluses (0.5–1 mL/kg) or continuous infusions of bupivacaine (0.125%–0.25%) or ropivacaine (0.2%) with or without epinephrine through a lumbar or caudal epidural catheter reduce the need for anesthetic agents. Caudal or epidural analgesia may be provided by advancing the catheter to the appropriate surgical dermatomal level after induction of anesthesia. In neonates, epidural infusions of bupivacaine (0.2 mg/kg per hour) provide excellent analgesia although blood concentrations of bupivacaine steadily increase by 2 days (see later text). The catheter is either secured directly to the skin or tunneled using the epidural insertion needle[271]; a continuous infusion of a local anesthetic may be maintained for several days to provide analgesia and a mild motor blockade that favors immobility. However, care must be taken to avoid systemic toxicity. Neonates are at increased risk for developing local anesthetic toxicity because of their low serum protein concentration and metabolism. Albumin and particularly α1-acid glycoprotein are reduced in this age group,[272] which reduces protein binding and increases the free fraction of bupivacaine and ropivacaine. This free form is metabolized to a lesser extent in the neonate because of immature metabolic pathways and contributes to an increased risk of cardiac and systemic toxicity.[273,274] It is for this reason that the upper limit of infusion of bupivacaine or ropivacaine is limited to 0.2 mg/kg per hour (for 48 hours), which is half that used in children older than 6 months to minimize the risk of local anesthetic toxicity.[275-277] Unfortunately, (free unbound) serum bupivacaine concentrations are difficult to assay and so lidocaine 0.1% (0.8 mg/kg per hour) or chloroprocaine may be preferable (see also Chapters 42 and 44).

The outcome of this complex surgery is determined primarily by the surgical expertise. Urologic incontinence, bladder prolapse, and epispadias revisions require additional urologic surgery. Renal function is usually well maintained throughout; complications of complete repair are reported to be similar to those of the staged repair but usually involve additional soft tissue defects.[278]

Bariatric Surgery in Children

Obesity has become a major threat to public health worldwide (http://www.un.org/en/development/desa/population/pdf/commission/2010/keynote/popkin.pdf). The prevalence of pediatric obesity has increased exponentially, affecting every country over the past few decades. In the United States, the incidence of obesity in children 2 to 19 years old has increased from ~7% in 1980 to ~18% in 2010[279]; one-third of U.S. children are either obese (BMI ≥95th percentile) or overweight (BMI between the 85th and 95th percentiles) (http://www.cdc.gov/obesity/data/childhood.html).[280] The causes of obesity are multifactorial: excess caloric intake, poor nutritional choices, and lack of exercise. However, recent evidence suggests that obese children are obese before the age of 5 years and that the underlying causes may have their provenance in early infancy and childhood.[281] Furthermore, the serious complications from obesity—for example, arterial hypertension, cardiovascular disease, fatty liver, diabetes, asthma, and obstructive sleep apnea (OSA)—are recognized earlier in childhood,[282] often serving as precursors for significant and intractable obesity in adulthood.[283] Multiple studies have reported an increase in medical/surgical complications in hospitalized obese children.[284] Thus the societal burden of obesity is enormous (estimated at $147 billion dollars in yearly health care costs)[285] and mainly driven by a number of associated comorbidities (e.g., diabetes, hypertension, sleep apnea, and depression). If left untreated, obesity may result in earlier mortality.[286,287]

The degree of obesity can be quantified using several metrics, the most common being the body mass index (BMI), defined as the weight (in kilograms) divided by the height squared (in meters squared). In adults, the degree of obesity can be defined by single BMI values (Table 29.2). However, in children the degree of obesity

TABLE 29.2 | Obesity Indexes in Adults and Children

Classification of Obesity	Adult (BMI)	Children (Percentile on BMI Growth Chart)
Normal weight	18.5–24.9	5–85
Overweight	25–29.9	85–95
Obesity	30–39.9	>95
Severe obesity	≥40	>120% of the 95th percentile

Based on http://www.cdc.gov/obesity/childhood/basics.html and Pan L, Blanck HM, Sherry B, et al. Trends in the prevalence of extreme obesity among US preschool-aged children living in low-income families, 1998–2010. *JAMA*. 2012:308(24); 2563–2565.[288]

is more difficult to quantify because BMI and other indexes of growth increase nonlinearly with age and gender. As a result, clinicians now define the degree of obesity in children based on growth charts for weight-dependent age and gender (Table 29.2).

To address these worrying statistics, bariatric surgery has emerged as one means to help the most extreme cases of adolescent obesity, especially those who are motivated toward weight loss and are psychologically prepared.[285,289] Bariatric surgery is designed to either bypass part of the small bowel to reduce caloric absorption (Roux-en-Y procedure) or to minimize the size of the stomach (laparoscopic vertical sleeve gastrectomy [LSG]). LSG has replaced the more complex Roux-en-Y gastric bypass surgery as the most commonly performed surgical procedure for obesity in the United States.[290] These surgeries have proven to be safe, cost-effective means of achieving permanent weight loss and providing partial resolution of comorbidities, especially diabetes in adolescents.[291–294]

MULTIDISCIPLINARY APPROACH TO BARIATRIC SURGERY IN ADOLESCENTS

Developing a successful approach to bariatric surgery in children requires a multidisciplinary team with collaboration from many pediatric subspecialists, including bariatric surgeons, anesthesiologists, endocrinologists, gastroenterologists, cardiologists, pulmonologists, psychologists, dietitians, and others.[295,296] Only children who are motivated to lose weight and who exhibit a positive psychological approach to this intensive process should be admitted to these programs.

ANESTHETIC IMPLICATIONS OF OBESITY IN ADOLESCENTS

Obesity is associated with a number of organ disorders including cardiovascular disease (hypertension, dyslipidemias),[297] respiratory (asthma and OSA),[298,299] renal dysfunction,[300] endocrinopathies (diabetes, metabolic syndrome), liver dysfunction (nonalcoholic fatty liver disease, and nonalcoholic steatohepatitis).[301,302] Childhood obesity is associated with early pathologic cardiovascular changes. Hypertension, previously seen most frequently in children with renal disease, is increasingly identified in obese children. The risk of hypertension in obese children is 3-fold and increases as BMI increases. Cardiac risk factors in obese children as young as 5 years of age have been described, including hypercholesterolemia, hypertension, and hyperinsulinemia. LVH has been identified in obese children as young as 10 years of age and is common in adolescents presenting for bariatric surgery. Research is underway to determine if changes in cardiac architecture and function are reversible with weight loss.

Preoperative preparation for bariatric surgery is an involved and prolonged process. A thorough and comprehensive preoperative review and investigation of these organ systems is warranted before proceeding with anesthesia. Once screening is completed, it is essential that the children learn about appropriate nutritional and attitudinal principles for achieving and maintaining weight loss. After evaluating the major organ systems and optimizing organ dysfunction, a preoperative anesthetic interview should be completed. During this evaluation, the anesthesiologist should review the investigations and laboratory results, ensure compliance of all medications and interventions (e.g., continuous positive airway pressure [CPAP] device), and then describe the anesthetic process with the patient and family in detail. Although these children appear large in size, many are psychologically immature and very anxious. Anxiolytic premedication should be offered on the day of surgery. During the interview, the airway should be assessed (see later text) and if a difficult airway is identified, supplementary airway equipment should be available. Children with CPAP devices should be advised to bring them on the day of surgery for possible use postoperatively. Routine fasting instructions and urine pregnancy testing for females who have reached menarche should be ordered or if complete, the results documented. If the child is unable to walk to the operating room, a wheelchair or stretcher rated for the child's weight should be used. The upper extremities should be examined for IV access as this may be difficult in obese patients.[303] A vein finder or ultrasound may be useful to establish venous access. In advance of undertaking bariatric surgery, appropriately sized operating room tables should be present. Operating room tables are rated for the patient's weight; for normal size patients, they may be rated for a maximum of 500 (227 kg) or 600 pounds (272 kg) and for obese patients, 1000 (454 kg) or 1200 pounds (544 kg). In all cases, the children should be strapped to the table to prevent the child from rolling off the table. Unlocking the bed and shifting the table top while the patient is on the table may cause the table to tip, even if the child's weight is within the table rating. This is more likely to occur if the table top is shifted off-center, if the child is placed in reverse orientation, or if a strong force is applied in one direction to the table (http://www.apsf.org/newsletters/html/2013/spring/07_tabletipdanger.htm).

Designing appropriate drug dosing in obese children requires an understanding of the scalars that may be used to estimate the correct dose. Total body weight (TBW) consists of two compartments: fat-free mass (FFM) and the fat mass (FM). In general, the former is the volume into which hydrophilic drugs tend to be distributed, whereas the latter is the volume into which lipophilic drugs are distributed. Because most drugs have both lipophilic and hydrophilic properties, the pharmacology of each drug (or category) must be considered to define its pharmacokinetic properties. Unfortunately, few of the drugs used for anesthesia in obese children have been studied, thus limiting the evidence on which to base drug doses. The FFM, a measure similar to lean body mass, may be considered the sum of the ideal body mass plus the additional mass required to support the physical and metabolic demands of the FM. The latter is derived primarily from an increased muscle mass as well as minor contributions from increased vessel-rich organ mass (heart, liver) and the fluid compartments. As the TBW increases, the FM increases in proportion; FFM increases steadily up to a BMI 40 but then plateaus thereafter.[304]

The ideal body weight (IBW) of a child can be obtained from tables, graphs, or simple equations.[305] Sample equations include

$$IBW = 2 \times Age\ (years) + 9\ for\ children \leq 8\ years\ and$$

$$3 \times Age\ (years)\ for > 8\ years$$

The lean body weight (LBW) may be estimated using a nomogram[305] or from a simple equation:

$$LBW = IBW + 0.3 \times (TBW - IBW)$$

Dosing is further complicated because the size metric used for a loading dose, which depends on the volume of distribution, may differ from that used for maintenance dosing or infusion rates, which depend on clearance. Most anesthetic drugs are lipophilic and are theoretically distributed in the TBW. However, drug doses for induction of anesthesia are not uniformly based on the TBW.[306] Drugs used to induce anesthesia are distributed into the central compartment and throughout the vessel-rich group of organs (e.g., brain). Even though these drugs are lipophilic, the induction dose is ideally based on the acute volume of distribution (V_d), which is more appropriately based on IBW or LBW.[307] LBW might be a good-sized metric for the dose of propofol for induction of anesthesia,[308] but TBW is better for maintenance/infusion.[309]

Other considerations in obesity include changes in plasma proteins, liver and renal functions, cytochrome enzyme activities,[310] CO, and regional blood flow.[311] Obesity may compromise organ function; dexmedetomidine clearance is reduced in obese adults.[309] The pharmacokinetics of drugs in obesity depend on the physicochemical characteristics of the drugs. For the loading dose of drugs, if the Vd/TBW ratio is reduced in obesity, then the drug is not distributed to the FM and should be based on the LBW or IBW.[304] In contrast, if the Vd/TBW ratio is unchanged or increased in obesity, then the drug is predominantly lipophilic and the dose should be based on TBW.[312,313] For drugs administered for maintenance, the dose should be based on its clearance. If the clearance in obesity is unchanged or decreased, then the dose should be based on LBW or IBW, whereas if the clearance is increased in obesity, then the maintenance dose should be based on the TBW. The use of cerebral function monitors (e.g., bispectral index in teenagers) greatly simplifies propofol infusion dosing by allowing titration of dose to a target effect.

Studies reporting the pharmacokinetics/dynamics of specific anesthetic drugs in obese children are limited.[306,314] Based on the best "available" data, a summary of the doses for induction or maintenance of anesthesia is presented in Table 29.3[315]; as more detailed evidence emerges, the basis for the dose of the drugs continues to evolve.

TABLE 29.3	Dosage of Intravenous Anesthetics in Obese Children	
Drug	**Induction Dose Based on**	**Maintenance Dose Based on**
Thiopenthal	LBW	
Propofol	LBW	TBW
Synthetic opioids (fentanyl, alfentanil, and sufentanil)	TBW	LBW
Morphine	IBW	IBW
Remifentanil	LBW	LBW
Nondepolarizing neuromuscular blockers	IBW	IBW
Succinylcholine	TBW	
Sugammadex	TBW	

IBW, ideal body weight; *LBW*, lean body weight; *TBW*, total body weight.
Reproduced with permission. Mortensen A, Lenz K, Abildstrøm H, Lauritsen TL. Anesthetizing the obese child. *Paediatr. Anaesth.* 2011;21(6):623–629.

Inhalational anesthetic agents with low blood-gas solubility are ideal in this setting. Rapid induction and emergence from anesthesia can be achieved and facilitated in this population with agents such as desflurane or sevoflurane combined with remifentanil.[316] The context-sensitive half-life of desflurane is superior to sevoflurane owing to lower solubility in blood and tissues; thus the former facilitates a more rapid recovery than the latter, particularly for surgeries longer than 2 hours when inhalation anesthetics accumulate in fat.[317] However, desflurane induces more bronchoconstriction than sevoflurane; thus in children with asthma or who smoke cigarettes, sevoflurane's bronchodilatory properties make it preferable to desflurane.

Airway management should take into consideration several basic principles. The presence of increased abdominal girth, shallow tidal volumes, and supine position predispose to rapid desaturation once anesthesia is induced. To preclude desaturation, patients should be preoxygenated in a reverse-Trendelenburg position more than 25 degrees.[318] This provides an adequate reserve of oxygen during laryngoscopy and tracheal intubation, mitigating the risk of desaturation and attenuating atelectasis. To view the glottis aperture, elevation of the head in the sniffing position should be doubled (from normal distance of 7 cm) to ~14 cm. This may be achieved by combining the ramped position with the usual head elevation (7 cm).[319] The quintessential alignment that must be ensured to successfully visualize the larynx in obese children is that the tragus of the ear is at or above the level of the sternal notch in the sniffing position.[320] If the tragus is not elevated above the sternal notch, then the head must be propped up further. An RSI is not usually required in most obese children; those who have gastroesophageal reflux are controlled medically. Gastric fluid volume is increased in obesity, but the fluid pH is not.[321] Therefore the risk of pneumonitis should aspiration occur is no greater than in a nonobese patient.

Ventilation may be a challenge in obese children, particularly during laparoscopic surgery. The pulmonary challenges from laparoscopic surgery are compounded by the large abdominal girth compressing the basal lungs. Increased inspired oxygen concentration may prevent hemoglobin desaturation but may lead to absorption atelectasis. Optimal strategies for ventilation while avoiding barotrauma include low tidal volumes (6–8 mL/kg based on LBW, not TBW), periodic alveolar recruitment maneuvers, PEEP (8–15 mm Hg), a respiratory rate to maintain normocapnia or permissive hypercapnia, particularly during pneumoperitoneum), and a sufficient inspired oxygen concentration to maintain an adequate saturation.[322–324] The ventilation mode has little bearing on the outcomes after anesthesia. At the end of surgery and after extubation, the child should be positioned in the semirecumbent position, administered oxygen by face mask, and monitored en route to the recovery room. Postoperative pain may be managed with either intermittent IV opioids or patient-controlled analgesia.

OSA is common in children who are morbidly obese. Many use nightly CPAP devices, although obese adolescents exhibit poor compliance with these devices.[325] Given the known risks of OSA causing opioid sensitivity, opioids should be administered in reduced doses ($\frac{1}{3}$–$\frac{1}{2}$ the usual doses).[326–328] Intermittent hypoxia commonly complicates the postoperative period. Hence, patients should bring their CPAP or nasal CPAP devices to the hospital for postoperative use. Children may be discharged home after uncomplicated surgery on postoperative day 3.[329–331]

Drug dosing after gastric bypass surgery is poorly understood.[332,333] After gastric bypass surgery, whether Roux-en-Y or the more popular LSG surgery, rapid weight loss occurs. This often results in the resolution of many comorbidities associated with morbid obesity such as systemic hypertension, diabetes, and so on. However, failure to adjust drug dosing in parallel with the weight loss, reduced gastric residence time, reduced exposure to intestinal cytochrome enzymes (CYP3A4; e.g., increasing atorvastatin blood concentrations), and the resolution of severity of the associated diseases may lead to relative drug overdoses and the associated consequences.[333] For example, after Roux-en-Y gastric surgery, approximately 50% of drugs taken orally have reduced area under the concentration-time curve, whereas 25% have unchanged and 25% have increased area under the concentration-time curve.[334] Oral morphine kinetics after Roux-en-Y showed dramatically increased blood concentrations within the first 2 weeks after surgery that persisted for at least 6 months.[335] The risks of an opioid overdose from the changes in pharmacokinetics not accounting for the effects of comorbidities may be substantial. In one meta-analysis, the range of postoperative to preoperative drug exposure ratio extended from a 10-fold greater ratio for penicillin to a 33% lower ratio for phenytoin and ampicillin.[333] The pharmacokinetics of midazolam after gastric bypass surgery in adults yielded similar bioavailability after oral dosing but greater clearance one year after bypass surgery.[336]

Currently, LSG surgery has eclipsed Roux-en-Y surgery in the United States in popularity, including in the adolescence age group. LSG surgery is not associated with the same extent of gastric dumping as Roux-en-Y surgery, but gastric residence time and absorption with LSG is reduced. Until practice recommendations are forthcoming, it seems prudent to titrate all parenteral drugs to effect during the period of rapid weight loss in particular and to adjust the doses of all oral drugs using therapeutic drug monitoring and individual clinical responses.

ACKNOWLEDGMENTS

The authors thank P.A. Lonnqvist, Yoichi Kondo, Yasuyuki Suzuki, Richard Banchs, Takako Tamura, Reiko Hayashi, and Katsuyuki Miyasaka for their prior contributions to this chapter.

ANNOTATED REFERENCES

Alqahtani A, Elahmedi M, Al Qahtani AR. Laparoscopic sleeve gastrectomy in children younger than 14 years: refuting the concerns. *Ann Surg.* 2016;263(2):312-319.

This retrospective study compared the outcomes after laparoscopic sleeve gastrectomy in children younger than 14 years at the time of surgery with adolescents older than 14 years. The authors concluded that sleeve gastrectomy in children younger than 14 years is both safe and effective.

Kim PH, Patil MB, Kim SS, et al. Early comparison of nephrectomy options in children (open, transperitoneal laparoscopic, laparo-endoscopic single site [LESS], and robotic surgery). *BJU Int.* 2012;109:910-915.

This up-to-date review provides comparative results of both laparoscopic techniques and robotic surgery in children.

Mortensen A, Lenz K, Abildstrøm H, Lauritsen TLB. Anesthetizing the obese child. *Paediatr Anaesth.* 2011;21(6):623-629.

This review presents the epidemiology, pathophysiology, and pharmacology of drugs used in obese children who require anesthesia.

Neira VM, Kovesi T, Guerra L, et al. The impact of pneumoperitoneum and Trendelenburg positioning on respiratory system mechanics during laparoscopic pelvic surgery in children: a prospective observational study. *Can J Anaesth.* 2015;62(7):798-806.

The authors investigated the physiologic impact of 12 mm Hg pneumoperitoneum followed by 20-degree Trendelenburg positioning. They found that both dynamic compliance and tidal volume (normalized to weight) decreased after insufflation of the pneumoperitoneum (by 42%) but decreased only 10% further after 20-degree Trendelenburg positioning. These changes could be offset by increasing the peak inspiratory pressures during pressure-controlled ventilation with PEEP in children undergoing laparoscopic surgery.

Phillip-Hohne C. Anaesthesia in the obese child. *Best Pract Res Clin Anaesthesiol.* 2011;25(1):53-60.

This review highlights the epidemiology of obesity in children, physiologic changes, and anesthetic considerations.

Walker RW, Ravi R, Haylett K. Effect of cricoid force on airway calibre in children: a bronchoscopic assessment. *Br J Anaesth.* 2010;104(1):71-74.

This investigation documents the magnitude of the external force required to distort the cricoid ring from infants until adolescents. In infants, force as little as 5 N distorts the cricoid rings. The force required to distort the ring increases with age, reaching 15 to 25 N in adolescents.

A complete reference list can be found online at ExpertConsult.com.

30 Essentials of Hepatology

JAMES E. SQUIRES, ROBERT H. SQUIRES, AND PETER J. DAVIS

Anatomy

THE LIVER AND BILIARY TREE are derived from the endoderm of the dorsal foregut during the late third to the early fourth week of gestation. By the sixth week, the fetal liver primarily serves as a hematopoietic organ, while critical biologic functions such as glycolysis, bile acid synthesis, and metabolic waste processing are managed by the maternal liver through fetoplacental circulation. Oxygenated blood is shunted from the placenta to the right atrium through the ductus venosus. Functional closure of the ductus begins immediately after birth, with complete functional closure occurring in up to 95% of infants by 2 weeks of age. Anatomic closure takes place shortly thereafter.

The functional development of the liver is reflected in the complex changes that are seen regarding hepatic enzyme efficiency and metabolic performance that occur throughout gestation. In the early gestation period, the liver is the primary site of hematopoiesis. Hepatic hematopoiesis develops in utero at 5 to 6 weeks gestation, followed closely by protein synthesis.[1] The ability to metabolize carbohydrates and lipids begins by 10 weeks gestation, followed by the development of drug-metabolizing systems. Several patterns of hepatic enzyme development have been described that correlate with the needs of the developing fetus.[2]

At the time of delivery, the liver weighs between 120 and 160 g but remains structurally and physiologically immature. Peripheral branches of the intrahepatic biliary system require an additional 4 to 8 weeks before they can be identified histologically. The liver is composed of eight structurally independent segments, each with a feeding hepatic artery, portal vein, draining hepatic vein, and bile duct. Segment 1 is the caudate lobe. Segments 2 and 3 form the left lateral segment, and with segment 4, the left lobe of the liver is defined. Segments 5, 6, 7, and 8 constitute the right lobe of the liver.

The liver receives blood from two sources: the portal vein that drains the spleen and intestine, and the hepatic artery that provides systemic oxygenated blood directly to biliary epithelium and to the hepatic sinusoids. The portal vein accounts for approximately 70% of the blood flow to the liver. In the hepatic sinusoids, the hepatic arterial and portal venous blood mix and intercalate among hepatocytes, fenestrated sinusoidal cells, and a host of resident immune cells (e.g., Kupffer cells). Sinusoids drain into terminal hepatic venules, which eventually coalesce to form the left and right hepatic veins. The veins merge into the inferior vena cava immediately before entering the right atrium. At any given time, the liver contains approximately 13% of the circulating blood volume.

During the neonatal period, liver function is immature and its ability to metabolize and clear most xenobiotics is poor. Factors believed to affect the clearance of medications include hepatic blood flow and the developmental status of hepatic transport and enzyme systems. Size alone does not account for this observed degree of immaturity, because the fetal and neonatal liver account for a greater percentage of body weight than the adult counterpart (3.6% of body weight vs. 2.4% in adults).[3] The neonatal liver contains approximately 20% fewer hepatocytes than the adult liver, and the cells are almost one-half the size of adult hepatocytes. These structural features may play some role in the functional deficiencies exhibited by infant livers. Cellular growth and hypertrophy of the liver continue at a rapid pace into young adulthood.

The structural unit of the liver parenchyma is the lobule, a hub-and-spoke structure with the central vein serving as the hub that is bordered by portal tracts, which contain a bile duct and tributaries of the portal vein and hepatic artery. While the mixed venous and arterial blood flows from the portal triad to the central vein, bile flows in the opposite direction through a canalicular matrix that then enters the bile ductule in the portal tract. The functional unit of the liver is the hepatic acinus, which is centered on the portal track and extends in three concentric zones (i.e., zones of Rappaport) outward to the central vein (Fig. 30.1). The more central zones (zones 1 and 2) are most active in oxidative processes, whereas the distal zone 3, which is closer to the central vein, depends on glycolysis and is more susceptible to ischemic and toxic injury.

Principles of Hepatic Drug Metabolism

Lipid solubility, an important and desired feature of many anesthesia drugs, allows passive diffusion across cellular membranes. Lipophilic drugs are also difficult to excrete. They have a propensity to

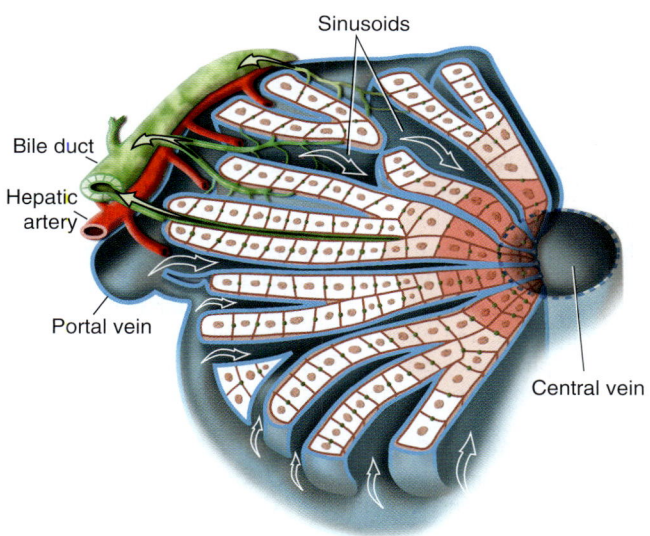

FIGURE 30.1 Blood flows from the hepatic arteries and portal vein along sinusoids toward the central vein. The hepatic triad consists of the bile duct, a branch of the portal vein, and the hepatic artery, with zone 1 *(white)* surrounding the triad, followed by zone 2 *(pink)* and zone 3 *(red)*. Cytochrome P-450 expression is higher in zone 3 with more extensive drug metabolism. (From Oinonen T, Lindros KO: Zonation of hepatic cytochrome P-450 expression and regulation. *Biochem J.* 1998; 329:17–35.)

TABLE 30.1	Major Human Liver Cytochrome P-450s		
P-450	**Substrate**	**Inhibitors**	**Inducers**
CYP1A2	Caffeine Clozapine Estradiol Theophylline	Fluvoxamine Furafylline	Omeprazole Tobacco smoke
CYP2A6	Halothane Nicotine	Methoxsalen	
CYP2C8	Rosiglitazone Taxol		Phenytoin Rifampin
CYP2C9	Diclofenac Ibuprofen Tolbutamide Warfarin	Sulfaphenazole	Rifampin Secobarbital
CYP2C19	Omeprazole	Fluvoxamine Ketoconazole	
CYP2D6	Codeine Chlorpromazine Desipramine Dextromethorphan Encainide Haloperidol Metoprolol	Fluoxetine Quinidine	
CYP2E1	Acetaminophen Halothane	Disulfiram	Ethanol Isoniazid
CYP3A4	Cyclosporin A Estradiol Indinavir Lovastatin Midazolam Nifedipine Quinidine Docetaxel	Delavirdine Erythromycin Grapefruit juice Ketoconazole Ritonavir Troleandomycin	Carbamazepine Phenobarbital Phenytoin Rifampin St. John's wort Troglitazone

Adapted from Watkins PB: The role of cytochrome P450s in drug-induced liver disease. In: Kaplowitz N, Deleve LD, eds. *Drug-Induced Liver Disease.* New York: Marcel Dekker; 2003:15–33.

accumulate in the body's fat stores and then slowly recirculate from deep compartments back into plasma. Renal and biliary excretion of lipid-soluble compounds can result in their resorption across their respective membranes. A major role of the liver is to transform lipid-soluble drugs into water-soluble compounds that become easily excreted metabolites. An interesting example of the need for this biotransformation is the anesthetic compound thiopental, which if not transformed into its less lipophilic counterpart, would have a plasma half-life of approximately 25 years.[1]

The primary family of liver enzymes assigned the task of metabolizing these exogenous substances is the cytochrome P-450 (CYP) family. *P* designates a red *pigment*, which is related to a heme molecule and absorbs light at a wavelength of 450 nm.[4] The primary reactions involved in the drug biotransformation and metabolism are hydroxylation and conjugation. Hydroxylation prepares the metabolite for conjugation (i.e., phase II reaction). The CYP family of enzymes is responsible for most phase I reactions, and the members were first thought to be chemically similar to mitochondrial cytochromes (see Chapter 7).

PHASE I REACTIONS

The CYP enzymes likely evolved as a mechanism by which the host was able to protect itself from toxins ingested from the environment. Most enzymes involved in hepatic drug metabolism are categorized in three distinct families: CYP1, CYP2, and CYP3. Each family is further divided into subfamilies that are designated with capital letters and numbered in the order in which they were discovered. The CYP enzymes are generally conserved across species, but their regulation and catalytic activity vary among species, which highlights the challenges associated with laboratory analysis of drug metabolism.[4]

Genetic and nongenetic factors contribute to the variability in the enzymatic activity seen across all CYP enzymes.[5] Genetic factors that have been shown to impact CYP variability include specific polymorphisms, gene expression regulation, and sex.[6] For example, approximately 5% of Caucasian populations lack CYP2D6 activity, which is associated with altered metabolism of some drugs.[7] A lack of CYP2D6 activity enhances the effect of drugs such as haloperidol and metoprolol that require the enzyme for efficient metabolism, whereas codeine, which is metabolized to morphine by CYP2D6, provides little analgesia in a child with CYP2D6 deficiency.[8] Furthermore, ethnicity is emerging as an important factor contributing to CYP pharmacokinetics and significant differences are now being appreciated between cohorts with differing racial makeup[9,10] (see Chapter 6).

Nongenetic factors that influence CYP activity include concomitant disease states, malnutrition,[11] and exposure to a host of pharmacologic and naturally occurring compounds. Many drugs can inhibit or stimulate the enzyme system (Table 30.1[12]). Inhibition of the CYPs occurs when drugs compete for the same enzyme. The degree to which this competition becomes clinically important depends on five factors: the relative amount of the specific CYP, the concentrations of each drug, the degree of pharmacologically active metabolite generated through this system, the importance of the enzyme in elimination of the drugs, and the therapeutic index of the drug.[4]

Enhanced CYP expression occurs after amplified transcription of the specific gene that is induced by a variety of compounds. For example, rifampin and phenytoin induce CYP3A4 by binding the cytosolic human pregnenolone-X-receptor (hPXR) or the steroid and xenobiotic receptor (SXR).[13] The activated receptor translocates into the nucleus, where it binds the regulator elements of the CYP3A4 gene and promotes increased transcription of CYP3A4, which can lead to toxic concentrations of intermediate compounds, as is the case with erythromycin, or to subtherapeutic concentrations of cyclosporine in transplant recipients.[14]

CYTOCHROME P-450 ACTIVITY

The superfamily of CYP enzymes is divided into subfamilies based on sequence homology and on demonstration of broad substrate specificities. An important example is the CYP3A subfamily, which is the most abundant group of cytochromes involved in the metabolism of xenobiotics. The three identified isoforms are CYP3A4, CYP3A5, and CYP3A7. CYP3A4 is the most abundant single enzyme in the human liver, accounting for the metabolism of approximately 50% of clinically used pharmaceuticals.[15] CYP3A5 is more commonly found in the kidneys and lungs and to a lesser degree in the liver. CYP3A7 is the predominant isoform in the neonatal liver but is replaced after birth by CYP3A4. Given its critical involvement in hepatic biotransformation of xenobiotics, the CYP3A4 family of enzymes is used to study estimated hepatic drug clearance in various age and gender groups.

Changes in the distribution and activity of the CYP enzyme systems occur with hepatic growth and maturation (Fig. 30.2). The CYP3A family is homogeneously distributed across the liver parenchyma in the fetal liver and shortly after birth. However, during postnatal growth, expression of the CYP3A protein shifts toward the periportal region of the acinus (i.e., Rappaport zone 1). By adulthood, expression of CYP2A becomes increasingly limited to the zone 1 and zone 2 hepatocytes, with sparse expression occurring in zone 3.[16] Other examples of developmental changes in the CYP system include the CYP2C and CYP 3A3/4 subfamilies, which have negligible expression in the first few weeks of life.[17,18] CYP2D6 reaches adult activity levels within 1 month chronological age; variability thereafter is determined primarily by genetic polymorphisms.[19]

Changes in activity of CYP enzyme families and subfamilies have correlated with drug clearance. For example, midazolam clearance correlates with changes in CYP3A4 activity, with decreased clearance in fetal neonatal livers and with adult clearance rates achieved by 3 months of age.[20,21] In contrast, CYP3A7 activity peaks at about 1 week postpartum and steadily diminishes during the first year of life, reaching approximately 10% of fetal liver activity by adulthood. In all, the advancements in the understanding of CYP ontogeny have led to improved integration of physiologic, developmental, and physiochemical knowledge to design more accurate pharmacokinetic modeling systems and guide optimal dosing regimens for children.[22]

PHASE II REACTIONS

Conjugation of lipophilic compounds increases their water solubility to facilitate renal excretion.[23,24] Conjugation reactions (i.e., glucuronidation, sulfation, glutathione conjugation, acetylation, and methylation) are generally decreased in infants compared with adults.[25]

Glucuronidation is catalyzed by uridine 5′-diphosphate (UDP)–glucuronosyltransferase (UGT) family of enzymes, which are derived from assimilation of proteins from separate genes or alternate splicing from single-gene transcripts.[26] UGT enzymes are responsible for the metabolism of several drugs, including phenols, estrogens, and opioids (see Chapter 7).[27] As with the CYP enzymes, individual UGT enzymes demonstrate substrate specificity and can act in concert to metabolize single compounds. Glucuronidation is not fully active in neonates because of decreased mRNA transcript production.[28] As such, this population is at risk for toxic drug accumulation (e.g., chloramphenicol causing the grey baby syndrome).[29] Hepatic UGT enzyme concentrations are reduced during fetal and early postnatal development. At 3 months of age, the levels of many UGTs are 25% of those in adults.[30]

UGT1A enzyme activity, which is involved in the conjugation of bilirubin and ethinylestradiol, is decreased in the fetus, but it increases to adult rates within 3 to 6 months after a term delivery.[31] UGT1A6, which conjugates acetaminophen and naproxen, has 10% of adult activity in the fetus and neonate, and it achieves only 50% of adult activity by 6 months of age.[25] UGT2B7 is active in the metabolism of the nonsteroidal antiinflammatory drugs (NSAIDs) naloxone, morphine, and lorazepam. Fetal activity of this enzyme approaches 10% to 20% of adult levels, with a rapid increase to adult levels by 2 months of age.[32]

Sulfation is accomplished by sulfotransferases, a family of cytosolic enzymes that are divided into two categories: catechol and phenol sulfotransferase. These enzymes conjugate inorganic sulfate from 3′-phosphoadenosine-5′-sulfophosphate (PAPS) with compounds containing functional hydroxyl groups. The catechol transferases develop earlier in fetal life than the phenol counterparts and appear to exhibit decreased activity in the developing neonate. Although specific sulfotransferase substrates require identification, the activity of these enzymes is increased in fetuses and neonates compared with adults and theorized to be an efficient conjugation pathway in this age group. Interestingly, with the obesity epidemic, UDP-UGT and sulfotransferase expression and function are altered in patients with nonalcoholic fatty liver disease.[33]

Glutathione S-transferases (GSTs) conjugate glutathione with a broad spectrum of lipophilic and electrophilic compounds. The family of GSTs is composed of up to five different groups

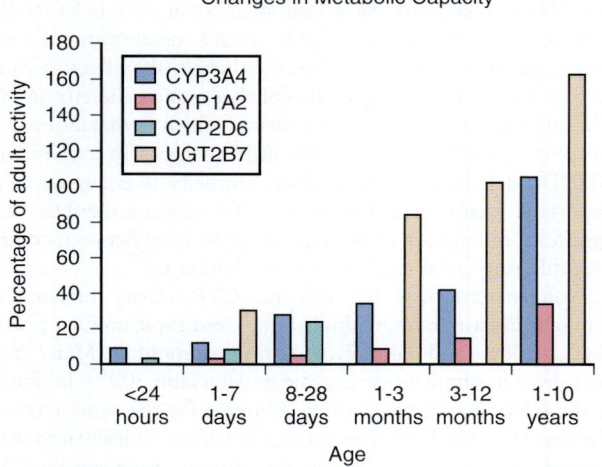

Changes in Metabolic Capacity

FIGURE 30.2 Changes in metabolic capacity versus percentage of adult activity. (Modified from Kearns G, Abdel-Rahman SM, Alander SW, et al. Developmental pharmacology—drug disposition, action, and therapy in infants and children. *N Engl J Med.* 2003;349:1157–1167.)

in various classes designated μ, α, θ, σ, and π, which are derived from at least three genetic loci.[34] Tissue-specific expression of these enzymes has been demonstrated, with the liver expressing the greatest amount of protein. Variable time-dependent expression has also been shown, with α- and π-class GSTs having enhanced expression between 16 and 24 weeks gestation, whereas only the α-class enzymes predominate in the neonate and adult liver.[35] The hepatic π-class enzymes disappear from their hepatocellular location by 6 months of age and can be found only in the epithelial cells of the biliary canaliculi. Variations in the developmental expression of this class of enzymes have made it challenging to fully appreciate what is likely a multitude of clinical interactions.[35]

Acetylation reactions are catalyzed by *N*-acetyltransferases, which transfer an acetyl group from acetyl coenzyme A to a variety of substrates (e.g., *p*-aminobenzoic acid, *p*-aminosalicylic acid, procainamide). Two genes, *NAT1* and *NAT2*, are responsible for yielding two specific enzymes with different allelic forms. Despite having 87% sequence homology, these enzymes exhibit different substrate specificities.[36] Both are cytosolic enzymes involved in the biotransformation of several drugs and the bioactivation of several human carcinogens. NAT1 is present in multiple fetal and postnatal tissues and accounts for the most *N*-acetyltransferase substrate metabolism in children younger than 1 year of age. NAT2 is located primarily in the liver and becomes the dominant acetylator after 1 year of age. NAT2 has polymorphisms with enzyme kinetics that differentiate patients with slow or rapid acetylation capabilities. Infants younger than 1 year of age usually are slow acetylators; subsequent age-dependent alterations lead an individual's targeted acetylator status.[37] Individuals who are genetically destined for rapid acetylation manifest this feature by 2 to 4 years of age.

Anesthetic Agents

INHALATION ANESTHESTC METABOLISM

Inhalational anesthetics are poorly metabolized, with 15% to 20% of halothane undergoing biotransformation. Although both oxidative and reductive pathways are involved, the primary pathway of metabolism of halothane is through oxidation to a reactive intermediate, trifluoroacetyl chloride,[38] which then undergoes glutathione conjugation.[39]

Isoflurane is metabolized by CYP2E1 to a limited extent (0.2%).[40] Isoflurane is excreted as inorganic fluoride and trifluoroacetic acid after oxidative metabolism in the liver.[41] Desflurane is the least metabolized (0.02%) of the volatile anesthetics, which is approximately 10% of the rate of isoflurane.[42] Both are metabolized in the liver along similar paths because the urinary metabolite for desflurane, trifluoroacetic acid, is the same as for isoflurane.

Only 2% to 5% of inhaled sevoflurane is metabolized in humans by means of the hepatic CYP2E1 enzyme, as occurs for the other ether anesthetics.[43] Oxidation of sevoflurane generates the intermediate formyl fluoride, a highly reactive species thought to generate liver protein adducts. Carbon dioxide and inorganic fluoride are released through this oxidative mechanism, and the final product is hexafluoroisopropanol, which undergoes glucuronide conjugation and is further excreted in the urine (see Chapter 7).[44]

NEUROMUSCULAR BLOCKING DRUGS

Neuromuscular blockade is achieved by depolarizing or nondepolarizing neuromuscular blocking drugs (NMBDs) (see Chapter 7). The only depolarizing agent still in use is short-acting suxamethonium (i.e., succinylcholine).[45] Succinylcholine is hydrolyzed completely by plasma cholinesterases, which are synthesized by the liver.[46] Enzyme activity varies with age, but it is decreased in liver disease and has been used as a metric of liver prognosis.[47,48]

Nondepolarizing NMBDs are divided into aminosteroids (i.e., pipecuronium, pancuronium, vecuronium, and rocuronium) and benzylisoquinolinium diesters (i.e., doxacurium, atracurium, and cisatracurium besylate). Renal and hepatic diseases affect their safety and efficacy.[49] Hepatic elimination depends on protein binding, hepatic blood flow, and drug extraction. The volume of drug distribution is increased in hepatic disease, leading to lower concentrations. In children with cholestatic liver disease, such as biliary atresia, uptake of these compounds by the liver is decreased, which reduces plasma clearance and prolongs their effects.[50,51] Approximately 75% of the administered dose is bound to plasma proteins, with most bound to albumin. Despite these problems, children with liver disease and a correspondingly low albumin concentration are at minimal risk for the adverse effects from this group of drugs.[52]

Rocuronium is an analog of vecuronium with a more rapid onset of action. Unlike other aminosteroids, which largely undergo renal excretion, only 12% to 22% of rocuronium is cleared through the kidney.[53] In patients with hepatic disease, the volume of distribution of rocuronium increased by 33% compared with healthy controls,[54] and patients with cholestasis exhibit prolonged duration and a longer recovery index after repeated uses.[55] In patients undergoing liver transplantation, the clearance of rocuronium was only slightly reduced by the diseased native liver compared with the functioning allograft and healthy individuals.[56] Reduced infusion requirements of rocuronium during liver transplantation may indicate graft dysfunction.[57]

Hepatic elimination of the benzyl isoquinolinium agents is poorly understood, but hepatic dysfunction has been observed to affect their effectiveness. Despite increased concentrations in biliary secretions, the pharmacokinetics of doxacurium are unchanged in the presence of hepatocellular injury, but recovery indexes are prolonged.[58] Although no longer available in the United States, mivacurium is a mixture of three stereoisomers. Clearance of the *trans-trans* and *cis-trans* isomers is reduced in patients with liver disease,[59] whereas clearance of the *cis-cis* isomer is unchanged. Prolonged recovery occurs as a result of a decrease in plasma cholinesterases in significant liver disease.[59] Clearance of cisatracurium is decreased, although patients with liver disease experience no delay in recovery and minimal delay in onset of action. Children with liver disease, regardless of cause, usually tolerate this class of compounds, and there is no observed toxicity.[60]

SEDATIVES, OPIOIDS, AND LIVER DISEASE

The commonly used sedatives midazolam, propofol, and ketamine undergo hepatic metabolism through oxidation and conjugation. These compounds are all lipid soluble, and their effects are altered by liver disease.[61] Midazolam has an extraction ratio of 0.3 to 0.5 and depends on both hepatic blood flow and intrinsic clearance. Midazolam may have an increased clearance rate if hepatic blood flow is increased. In children with cirrhosis, the clearance of midazolam is halved with a corresponding doubling of the half-life compared with healthy controls.[62,63] With 95% to 97% of midazolam bound to albumin, diseases that decrease the concentration of albumin dramatically increase the free fraction of drug, which leads to a greater effect.[29,64,65] Propofol has high intrinsic clearance and blood flow changes determine clearance. Although clearance is through a combination of both UGT and CYP enzymes (CYP2B6, 2C9, 2A6), hepatocellular injury does not alter its pharmacokinetics.[66] Ketamine is also highly lipophilic and undergoes metabolism in the liver. However, unlike the other drugs described, it does so through methylation, and its clearance is minimally affected by liver dysfunction.[67]

Clinical effects from opioids result from their binding to opioid receptors. A greater serum concentration of opioid binds a greater number of receptors, resulting in a correspondingly greater opioid effect. Hepatic clearance and protein binding govern the serum concentration of an opioid.[68] Most opioids are oxidized in the liver. However, morphine and buprenorphine undergo glucuronidation, and remifentanil is metabolized by plasma and tissue esterases, enzymes that are mature in term neonates. The ability of the diseased liver to oxidize opioids is diminished, leading to increased oral bioavailability owing to decreased first-pass metabolism and decreased drug clearance. The clearance of morphine, despite being metabolized by glucuronidation, is also negatively affected by the presence of cirrhosis.[69]

Clearance of drugs that are highly extracted by the liver, such as meperidine and morphine, depend on hepatic blood flow (i.e., perfusion limited clearance).[70,71] Clearance (CL) is a function of hepatic blood flow (Q_H) and the extraction ratio (E_H), describing the ability of the liver to efficiently remove the drug from the circulation:

$$CL_H = Q_H \times E_H$$

When E_H is greater than 0.7, as with meperidine, lidocaine, and pentazocine, CL_H approaches Q_H. Conditions that alter hepatic blood flow, such as cirrhosis, portal vein thrombosis, and portacaval shunting, significantly alter opioid clearance. Drugs with a low E_H, such as diazepam, methadone, and naproxen, do not depend on hepatic blood flow. The metabolic activity of the liver and the plasma protein-binding fraction affect the clearance to a greater degree. The hepatic clearance of these drugs is described by the following equation:

$$CL_H = CL_{INT} \times f_u$$

In the formula, f_u is the fraction of unbound drug and CL_{INT} describes the metabolic activity. When f_u is small as with methadone (<0.1), clearance is mainly affected by reduced enzyme capacity.[68]

The pharmacology of the opioids is variably affected by liver disease. The analgesic effect of codeine, obtained after its demethylation to morphine, is reduced in the presence of liver disease. Liver disease can affect glucuronidation and thereby decrease clearance and prolong the half-life of morphine.[72] The protein binding and clearance of alfentanil are reduced in the presence of hepatic dysfunction,[73,74] whereas the half-life and volume of distribution of methadone are increased.[75] The pharmacokinetics of fentanyl, remifentanil, and sufentanil are unchanged in the presence of significant hepatic dysfunction.[76–78] Because the degree of hepatic dysfunction exhibits interindividual variability, the level of adverse events of these medications also varies. Careful monitoring of children with liver disease is required when administering opioids.

Anesthetic Effects on Hepatic Cellular Functions

CARBOHYDRATES
Glucose metabolism is influenced by the availability of the substrate, the rate of entry into cells, and the ability of the target organ to convert glucose into energy or to use it to synthesize fats. In healthy individuals, hepatic glucose production accounts for most whole-body glucose production and is narrowly regulated directly and indirectly by insulin.[79] Insulin directly inhibits gluconeogenesis and glycogenolysis by binding to insulin receptors in the liver, thereby diminishing hepatic glucose production. Of the glucose available to the liver, about 50% undergoes glycolysis and is converted to energy. Between 30% and 40% is converted to fat for storage, and 10% to 20% is shunted to glycogen.[80] Anesthetics inhibit glucose uptake by hepatocytes, an action referred to as the *anti-insulin effect of anesthesia*.[81] Although all inhalational anesthetics exhibit this tendency, halothane has the greatest impact on serum glucose, with isoflurane and sevoflurane having lesser effects.[82] Inhalational anesthetics at 1 to 2 minimal alveolar concentrations (MACs) inhibit glucose uptake by up to 50%. The combined effects of anesthetics and stress from surgery or trauma increase the serum glucose concentration, which is one reason glucose-containing intravenous fluids are no longer recommended for most healthy children undergoing elective surgery.

PROTEIN SYNTHESIS
The impact of anesthesia and surgery on protein synthesis and metabolism is poorly understood. Albumin, a large, soluble, single-polypeptide protein with a molecular weight of 66 kD, is an important protein synthesized by the liver. Between 6 and 12 g of albumin are produced each day, and production can increase twofold to threefold according to the individual's needs. Albumin functions as a binding and transport protein and maintains colloid oncotic pressure. Hepatic dysfunction may result in decreased synthesis of albumin and other proteins. Anesthetics may also inhibit protein synthesis. Diethyl ether causes reversible inhibition of protein synthesis in rat hepatocytes,[83] whereas halothane and enflurane block protein synthesis in a dose-dependent manner.[84] Halothane, sevoflurane, and enflurane inhibit protein synthesis and secretion, which may be an early indicator of hepatic cytotoxic injury.

BILIRUBIN METABOLISM
Bilirubin, the end product of heme metabolism, is converted to unconjugated bilirubin by macrophages in the spleen and bone marrow and transported to the liver bound to plasma albumin. Unconjugated bilirubin is transported into the hepatocyte by bile acids and bacterial endotoxins. In the hepatocyte, bilirubin is conjugated with glucuronate, taurine, and, to a lesser extent, glucose by glucuronyl transferase. Deficiencies of glucuronyl transferase manifest clinically in Gilbert syndrome, with more severe forms in Crigler-Najjar syndrome types I and II. Gilbert syndrome affects 2% to 13% of individuals, who have increases in the unconjugated fraction of bilirubin associated with stress or fasting. Although postoperative jaundice has been described, Gilbert syndrome has not been associated with serious adverse effects in the perioperative period.[85] Patients with Crigler-Najjar syndrome can be managed safely by minimizing their exposure to drugs that may displace bilirubin from albumin and by using anesthetics that undergo minimal hepatic metabolism.[86,87]

HEPATOTOXICITY
Increases in serum aminotransferase concentrations and bilirubin up to two times the upper limit of normal occur commonly in the postoperative period.[88,89] These increases are typically self-limited and inconsequential. However, serious liver injury can be caused by anesthetics.[90,91] The Drug-Induced Liver Injury Network (DILIN), established by the National Institutes of Health in 2003, has and continues to standardize the nomenclature and causality

assessment of drug-induced liver injury (DILI).[92,93] Diagnosis of DILI is entertained when increases in alanine aminotransferase (ALT), aspartate aminotransferase (AST), alkaline phosphatase, γ-glutamyl transferase (GGT), and bilirubin occur coincident with xenobiotic exposure. Patterns of injury are classified as (1) hepatocellular, with predominantly increased ALT and AST levels; (2) cholestatic, with increases in alkaline phosphatase, GGT, and bilirubin; (3) and mixed pattern, with features of both hepatocellular and cholestatic injury. Although not specific to anesthetic medications, recent DILIN analyses conclude that mortality from DILI in individuals with preexisting liver disease or concomitant severe skin reactions is significantly greater than in patients without.[93] In April of 2012 the website LiverTox (https://livertox.nlm.nih.gov) was launched as a joint effort of the Liver Disease Research Branch of the National Institute of Diabetes and Digestive and Kidney Diseases (NIDDK) and the Division of Specialized Information Services of the National Library of Medicine (NLM), National Institutes of Health. The purpose of LiverTox is to provide up-to-date, accurate, and easily accessed information on the diagnosis, cause, frequency, patterns, and management of liver injury attributable to medications, herbals, and dietary supplements.

It is important to note that even though increases in liver-specific enzymes may reflect drug-induced injury, they are in fact poor markers of liver function. In the absence of a unique test to assess liver function, surrogate markers for liver dysfunction include a prolonged prothrombin time (PT) greater than 15 seconds or an international normalized ratio (INR) greater than 1.5, or both. Other clinical and biochemical markers, such as hypoalbuminemia, hypoglycemia, and an altered mental status, should be included in the assessment of hepatic dysfunction, but they can also result from conditions unrelated to liver function, such as malnutrition, protein-losing enteropathy or nephropathy, or medications for sedation or pain management. It is critical that in the setting of suspected drug-induced liver injury (elevated AST, ALT, bilirubin, and so on) that liver function is also determined.

An additional confounder relating to the incidence of anesthesia-induced liver injury is the increasing obesity epidemic in children. The growing disease burden associated with nonalcoholic fatty liver disease and nonalcoholic steatohepatitis have raised concerns that these children may be at increased risk for DILI.[94] Obesity and hypercholesterolemia can induce CYP2E1, which may facilitate development of liver injury.[95] Few data are available to guide the best practice of anesthesia for the obese child, and adequately powered prospective studies are needed.

Perioperative Considerations in Liver Disease

Patients with known or suspected liver disease should be assessed for hepatocellular and bile duct injury, coagulopathy, ascites, and encephalopathy. Hepatopulmonary syndrome and portopulmonary hypertension are rare but important complications in children with known chronic liver disease, and they may serve as relative or absolute contraindications to elective surgery.[96,97] Perioperative mortality is greatest among those who have acute hepatitis compared with those with chronic liver disease.[96,98,99] The physiologic stress associated with surgical procedures decreases portal blood flow. Liver disease may decrease the degree to which hepatic artery blood flow can compensate for reduced portal blood flow, which can increase the risk of developing ischemic injury.

Parenteral nutrition–associated liver disease (PNALD) occurs in children requiring parenteral nutrition for longer than 60 days. Children with short bowel syndrome are at greatest risk for PNALD. Aside from the disturbances to hepatic and portal blood flows in children with liver disease, those exposed to total parenteral nutrition (TPN) are at increased risk for perioperative glucose derangements.[100-102] Frequent perioperative glucose monitoring with adjustment of dextrose infusion appears to be the standard of care, which is associated with various rates of tapering TPN. A survey administered to members of the Study Group on Pediatric Anesthesia found that approximately 50% of respondents checked glucose levels as often as every 1 to 2 hours. They also found that 19% discontinued TPN and administered a glucose-containing solution, whereas 35% decreased the fluids to one-half of maintenance rates and 33% continued maintenance rates unchanged.[103]

ANNOTATED REFERENCES

Bjorkman S. Prediction of drug disposition in infants and children by means of physiologically based pharmacokinetic (PBPK) modeling: theophylline and midazolam as model drugs. *Br J Clin Pharmacol.* 2004;59:691-704.

This paper attempts to generate data for an age group that provides significant challenges to study and examines two very different drugs. The predicted pharmacokinetics are then thoroughly compared with the adult literature, with very reassuring results.

Chalasani N, Bonkovsky HL, Fontana R, et al. Features and outcomes of 899 patients with drug-induced liver injury: the DILIN prospective study. *Gastroenterology.* 2015;148(7):1340-1352.e7.

This paper reports the first 1257 patients enrolled in this prospective observational longitudinal study. Mortality from DILI is significantly higher in individuals with preexisting liver disease or concomitant severe skin reactions compared with patients without. Further results from ongoing enrollment are awaited.

Kharasch ED, Hankins D, Mautz D, Thummel KE. Identification of the enzyme responsible for oxidative halothane metabolism: implication for prevention of halothane hepatitis. *Lancet.* 1996;347:1367-1371.

This paper outlines a rare but serious complication of the inhaled anesthetic and provides a mechanism for its toxicity. These researchers also tested the hypothesis that the involved cytochrome enzyme was cytochrome P-450 2E1 (CYP2E1).

Watkins PB. The role of cytochrome P450s in drug induced liver disease. In: Kaplowitz N, Deleve LD, eds. *Drug-Induced Liver Disease.* New York: Marcel Dekker; 2003:15-33.

This summary of cytochrome P-450 enzymes provides a thorough review of this complex enzyme system and demonstrates their role in toxin-mediated liver disease.

A complete reference list can be found online at ExpertConsult.com.

31 Organ Transplantation

FRANKLYN P. CLADIS, BRIAN BLASIOLE, MARTIN B. ANIXTER, JAMES GORDON CAIN, AND PETER J. DAVIS

Liver Transplantation

The first successful pediatric liver transplant was performed by Tom Starzl and colleagues in 1967, but the history of liver transplantation actually began in 1955 with Stuart Welch in Albany and Jack Cannon at UCLA. Welch was the first to describe auxiliary liver transplantation in the dog and Cannon was the first to attempt orthotopic liver transplantation (OLT) in dogs. Unfortunately, none of the dogs survived the operation.[1] Francis Moore and Tom Starzl continued research with the dog model. From 1958 to 1959, they each successfully transplanted the liver, but all of the dogs died within 4 to 20 days from rejection. These deaths highlighted the barriers that prevented the first OLT application in humans.

In the early stages of animal experimentation, the main barriers to success involved surgical technique, organ preservation, and immunosuppression. The livers were initially preserved with chilled electrolyte solutions such as lactated Ringer's and normal saline; preservation time was only 5 to 6 hours. In 1987, the University of Wisconsin developed a solution that increased the preservation of livers to 18 to 24 hours. The third barrier, immunosuppression, was the most significant and likely explained most of the canine deaths. Medawar[1a] reported the role of the immune system in organ rejection. Since that time several unsuccessful attempts to deliberately weaken the immune system and control rejection had failed. It was not until an animal model demonstrated that the combination of azathioprine and prednisone were synergistic and ameliorated rejection. This combination was first used in human kidney transplants and then expanded to liver transplantation.

The first human liver transplantation was performed in 1963 in a 3-year-old boy with biliary atresia. This attempt ended in failure secondary to fatal intraoperative hemorrhage from venous collaterals. Six more attempts at three different institutions (Denver, Boston, and Paris) produced the same result. Attempts to control the intraoperative hemorrhage with coagulation factor replacement and ε-aminocaproic acid resulted in clots and fatal pulmonary emboli in the veno-venous bypass system. Inadequate immunosuppression played a significant role in these fatalities as well. At that time a self-imposed moratorium was established. In 1967, anti-lymphocyte globulin was introduced, providing lymphoid depletion and supplemented azathioprine and prednisone to provide better immunosuppression,[2] allowing Starzl to successfully transplant a liver in a 1-year-old with hepatoblastoma who survived for 13 months.

Despite the initial success of the first pediatric liver transplant, the 1-year survival rate in subsequent transplant patients remained no greater than 50%. With the introduction of cyclosporine in 1979, the 1-year patient survival increased to 70%.[3,4] In 1989, tacrolimus replaced cyclosporine[5] and the 1-year patient survival further increased to approximately 80%.

EPIDEMIOLOGY AND DEMOGRAPHICS

There has been a steady increase in the number of liver transplants performed yearly in the United States (from 1713 per year in

1988 to 7127 per year in 2015). The vast majority of this increase is attributed to adult transplants. The total number of pediatric liver transplants in 1990 was 513; this increased to 589 in 2000 and has essentially remained unchanged over the past 15 years with 580 in 2015. The increase from 1990 to 2015 is only a 13% increase compared with the 200% increase in adults (2177 in 1990 to 6547 in 2015) (United Network for Organ Sharing [UNOS] Scientific Registry, 2016; https://www.unos.org/data/).

Indications for liver transplantation in children include the presence of an underlying primary liver pathology with acute or chronic liver failure caused by cholestatic liver disease, acute hepatic failure, metabolic disorders, cirrhosis, tumors, and other derangements (e.g., Budd-Chiari syndrome) (Table 31.1). The most common cause for liver transplantation in children is cholestatic liver disease secondary to biliary atresia.[6,7] This is especially true in patients younger than 1 year of age, in whom it accounts for ≥50% of liver transplants. Biliary atresia continues to be the most common overall cause for liver transplantation and the most common cholestatic cause, but cholestatic liver disease secondary to total parenteral nutrition (TPN) has become more prominent over the past 10 years, accounting for just over 4% of all pediatric liver transplants. After cholestatic liver disease, acute hepatic failure and metabolic disorders are the next most common causes for pediatric liver transplantation. Historically, the most common metabolic disorders in decreasing frequency were α_1-antitrypsin deficiency, tyrosinemia, Wilson disease, oxalosis, and glycogen storage diseases. The most common disorders have changed. Maple syrup urine disease (MSUD) is now the most common, with cystic fibrosis the second most common metabolic indication for pediatric liver transplantation (UNOS/Organ Procurement and Transplantation Network [OPTN]; https://www.unos.org/data/).

The cause for acute or fulminant hepatic failure is not known in most pediatric patients. A viral cause (A, B, or C) may account for almost half of the acute hepatic failures in infants and children. Acetaminophen is the most common overall cause of drug- or toxin-induced liver failure.[8]

There are few absolute contraindications to pediatric liver transplantation. Children with neoplastic processes such as hepatocellular carcinoma and infections with human immunodeficiency virus (HIV) have received transplants. However, patients with acute infections from bacterial or fungal agents, metastatic neoplasm, or disease processes that are considered an immediate threat to life (severe cardiopulmonary disease, sepsis/septic shock) generally do not undergo transplantation.

Allocation of the available livers to the appropriate recipients has been a challenge. Initially liver transplant candidates were prioritized based on geographic location and medical condition defined by the Child-Turcotte-Pugh (CTP) score. Patients were ranked as status 1, 2a, 2b, or 3. Status 1 patients received the highest priority and were defined by the presence of acute liver failure of less than 6 weeks or a failed liver transplant within 1 week. Status 2a, 2b, and 3 were defined by their CTP score and time on the wait-list.[9] Efforts by the UNOS/OPTN Liver Disease Severity Scale (LDSS) committee to identify predictors of mortality in children with chronic liver disease resulted in the implementation of the Model for End-Stage Liver Disease (MELD) and the Pediatric End-Stage Liver Disease (PELD) severity score in 2002.[10] The PELD score incorporates variables for age, growth failure, serum albumin, bilirubin, and international normalized ratio (INR). PELD formerly applied to children younger than 18 years old; this was changed in 2005 to include children 12 years of age or younger. The MELD score is now used for children 13 years of

age or older.[11] Serum creatinine was incorporated into the MELD score because it predicts mortality for adult patients awaiting liver transplantation. Although serum creatinine may predict survival after liver transplantation, it does not predict mortality in the child awaiting liver transplantation.[12]

TABLE 31.1	Primary Diagnosis of Liver Disease in Pediatric Patients: 1988–2015
Primary Diagnosis	
Total	13,340
Cholestatic	52.0%
Biliary atresia	
TPN-induced cholestasis	
Alagille syndrome	
Primary sclerosing cholangitis	
Secondary biliary cirrhosis	
Familial cholestasis (Byler's, others)	
Biliary hypoplasia	
Primary biliary cirrhosis	
Neonatal cholestatic disease	
Other causes of cholestasis	
Acute hepatic necrosis	13.3%
Neonatal hepatitis	
Drug-induced	
Hepatitis A	
Hepatitis B	
Hepatitis C	
Unknown	
Other causes of hepatic necrosis	
Metabolic Disorder	12.9%
α_1-Antitrypsin	
Cystic fibrosis	
Wilson disease	
Tyrosinemia	
Oxalosis	
Glycogen storage disease	
Maple syrup urine disease	
Hemochromatosis	
Other metabolic disorders	
Cirrhosis	8.0%
Idiopathic	
Autoimmune	
Hepatitis C	
Chronic active hepatitis	
Hepatitis B	
Drug/toxin	
Hepatitis A	
Combined exposure (alcohol, hepatitis A, B, C)	
Alcoholic	
Other causes of cirrhosis	
Hepatic tumors	4.8%
Hepatoblastoma	
Hepatocellular carcinoma	
Hemangioendothelioma	
Benign tumor	
Other tumors	
Other	9%
Congenital hepatic fibrosis	
Budd-Chiari syndrome	
Graft versus host secondary to nonliver toxicity	
Trauma	
Other miscellaneous diagnoses	

The allocation of deceased liver donors has changed with the new MELD/PELD policy. Prior to this policy, organs from donors younger than 18 years were distributed only to pediatric recipients. With the new policy, the donor graft is first allocated to a status 1 pediatric recipient in the local region. If none is available, it is offered to the next status 1 adult in the region. If no status 1 adult is available, the liver is made available to pediatric patients with a greater than 50% risk of mortality. Adults with mortality risk greater than 50% are next, and then all pediatric patients are offered the liver over all other adult candidates. If there are no appropriate pediatric recipients in the region, the donor organ is offered to the national pool.[9] The introduction of the MELD/PELD score has decreased the wait time for transplantation. Analysis of pre- and post-MELD/PELD data indicate that the median time to transplant, defined as the number of days for half of the new registrants to receive organs, decreased from 981 days in 2002 to 361 days in 2007.[11]

Survival for deceased donor transplants is an age-dependent variable. Infants younger than 1 year had the lowest 3-month and 1-year survival at 88% and 83%, respectively, compared with older children. However, if the infant recipient survives the first year, the survival rate increases. In fact, the 5-year survival (84%) is the greatest for infants younger than 1 year. The 10-year survival is 77% for infants younger than 1 year, 79% for children 1 to 5 years of age, and 81% for children 6 to 11 years of age.[11]

There also appears to be a difference in recipient survival between living donor and deceased donor grafts. Children receiving a living donor organ had 10-year survival rates greater than 90%, whereas recipients of deceased donor organ had a 10-year survival rate less than 90%.[13] In addition to survival, other outcomes still need to be evaluated in children (e.g., growth and cognitive function).[14]

PATHOPHYSIOLOGY OF LIVER DISEASE

The liver is the only organ that can regenerate itself when damaged. The stigmata and multiorgan involvement from end-stage liver disease occurs because of loss of hepatocytes and the resulting fibrosis. The hepatic injury and loss of hepatocytes leads to decreased synthetic function. This cellular dysfunction results in coagulopathy, hypocholesterolemia, hypoalbuminemia, and encephalopathy. Attempts at regeneration result in fibrosis and destruction of the portal triad with increased resistance to blood flow through the liver. Portal hypertension is the final consequence of this increased resistance. Much of the characteristic features of liver disease occur because of portal hypertension, specifically varices (esophageal, bowel), hemorrhoids, ascites, spontaneous bacterial peritonitis, splenomegaly with thrombocytopenia, and hepatic encephalopathy.

Cardiac Considerations

Cardiac disturbances occur because of altered physiology, congenital heart defects, and toxic medication adverse effects. A hyperdynamic circulation with a compensatory increase in cardiac output (CO) secondary to vasodilation characterizes the altered cardiac physiology from liver disease. Vasodilation is central to the hyperdynamic circulation that accompanies portal hypertension. It likely is the result of the presence of vasoactive mediators. These mediators or gut-derived "humoral factors" (nitric oxide [NO], tumor necrosis factor [TNF]-α, endocannabinoids) enter the systemic circulation through portosystemic collaterals and bypass the hepatic detoxification that usually occurs.[15] Shunting also occurs in the skin and lungs. Mixed venous saturation is increased in patients with liver disease. Poor oxygen extraction and increased CO likely explain the increased mixed venous saturation. The arterial-venous oxygen difference is reduced because of decreased oxygen consumption and hypoxia from arterial-venous shunting.

Cardiomyopathy associated with portal hypertension is well described in adults but is not well characterized in children with liver disease. However, children with liver disease can have a cardiomyopathy for other reasons. Inborn errors of metabolism and other syndromes are associated with cardiomyopathies and cardiac anomalies. Some of the inborn errors include Wilson disease, oxalosis, glycogen storage disease type III, tyrosinemia, and Gaucher disease.[16] Tacrolimus and cyclosporine A have also been associated with hypertrophic cardiomyopathy in animal studies and in pediatric liver transplant recipients.[17-20] Other studies have demonstrated that the cardiac function is generally well preserved in pediatric liver transplant patients who are receiving tacrolimus, but there may be evidence of subtle cardiovascular changes that predispose a small percentage of patients to develop hypertrophic cardiomyopathy.[21,22] Alagille disease is commonly associated with congenital heart disease (CHD) such as pulmonary stenosis, coarctation, tetralogy of Fallot, and atrial and ventricular septal defects. Diastolic dysfunction has been associated with increased mortality after transplantation.[23]

QT prolongation of the electrocardiogram (ECG; see Chapter 16) has been described in adult patients with alcoholic liver disease and may be associated with sudden cardiac death.[24] A decrease in K^+ currents in cardiomyocytes in rats with cirrhosis may provide a possible mechanism for the QT prolongation. Children with liver failure have also been shown to have an increase in QTc interval. A QTc greater than 450 msec has been reported in 18% of children with liver disease.[25] These findings may increase the risk of ventricular arrhythmias; however, there are conflicting data regarding resolution after liver transplantation.[25,26] Nonselective β-blockade has also been shown to reduce the QT prolongation, but it is unclear if this reduces the risk of arrhythmias or improves survival.[27,28] Although previous data suggested prolonged QT did not predict survival,[29,30] more recently the presence of prolonged QT was associated with a greater PELD score and portal hypertension. Pediatric patients with chronic liver disease and prolonged QT may be at increased risk of mortality while waiting for a transplant.[31]

Pulmonary Considerations

Pulmonary hallmarks of liver disease are hypoxia and pulmonary hypertension. Hypoxia can occur for several reasons including hepatopulmonary syndrome (HPS) and $\dot{V}/\dot{Q}$ mismatch from atelectasis owing to ascites, hepatosplenomegaly, or pleural effusions. HPS is characterized by hypoxia from intrapulmonary arteriovenous shunting (caused by increased angiogenesis)[32] and intrapulmonary vascular dilatation.[33] The diagnosis is made by demonstrating either arterial hypoxia (PaO_2 <70 mm Hg) or an increased alveolar-arterial gradient greater than 20 mm Hg in the setting of pulmonary vascular dilatation. Intrapulmonary vascular dilatation can best be demonstrated using echocardiography or a lung perfusion scan with macroaggregated albumin.[34] HPS occurs in at least 15% to 20% of adults with cirrhosis.[35] HPS has been reported in infants 6 months of age and is described in 0.5% to 20% of all children with liver disease. It appears to be more prevalent in children with biliary atresia and polysplenia syndrome.[36,37] When adjusted for the severity of hepatic disease, HPS does not affect mortality.[38] A normal pulse oximetry value in children with cirrhosis does not necessarily rule out HPS. Children with normal pulse oximetry may exhibit other criteria for the diagnosis (intrapulmonary vasodilatation and alveolar-arterial gradient greater than 15 mm Hg) and may be at increased risk for morbidity and mortality.[39]

Treatment for hypoxia is long-term supplemental oxygen. Definitive treatment may occur with liver transplantation. One case series described seven children with HPS who had successful transplants; all seven children recovered from their HPS postoperatively. The average time required to correct hypoxia after transplantation was 24 weeks.[40]

Portopulmonary hypertension (PPH) is defined by the World Health Organization (WHO) as pulmonary artery hypertension (pressure >25 mm Hg) in the setting of normal pulmonary capillary wedge pressure and portal hypertension.[41] The incidence of PPH is 0.2% to 0.7% in adults with cirrhosis but increases to 3% to 9% in adults presenting for liver transplantation.[42] The number is not known in children and is limited to case reports and case series. Evidence from case series and autopsy data suggest that the incidence of PPH is 0.5% to 5% in children with portal hypertension.[43,44] Signs and symptoms on presentation were new heart murmurs, dyspnea, and syncope. Echocardiography can successfully identify pulmonary hypertension in children and adult patients with PPH.[45] The severity of PPH predicts mortality. Adult patients with mild PPH had no increase in mortality during liver transplantation. However, those patients who underwent OLT with moderate PPH (pulmonary artery pressure [PAP] = 35–45 mm Hg) had a 50% mortality rate and those with severe PPH (PAP >50 mm Hg) had a 100% mortality rate.[46]

There are no definitive guidelines for the management of children with PPH. Early identification is essential, and all children who present for liver transplantation should be evaluated for the presence of PPH with echocardiography.[43,47] If present, cardiac catheterization needs to be performed to confirm the diagnosis, measure PAPs, and assess the response to NO and epoprostenol. Children who respond to medical management may be candidates for liver transplantation.[48] Otherwise, severe PPH is generally a contraindication for liver transplantation because of the increased risk of mortality.

Neurologic Considerations

Hepatic encephalopathy (HE) is a neurologic complication of liver disease classified as either acute (seen in fulminant hepatic failure) or chronic (seen in chronic cirrhosis or chronic portal hypertension). Minimal encephalopathy, diagnosed with neuropsychological testing, may be present in as many as 50% of children with chronic liver disease.[49] The pathophysiology is not entirely known but cerebral edema is a feature of both acute and chronic HE. The cerebral edema is more severe in acute HE and can result in increased intracranial pressure (ICP). Ammonia is repeatedly implicated in the pathogenesis of HE and may participate in the process by causing astrocyte to swell, resulting in low-grade cerebral edema.[50,51] The two major sources of ammonia in humans are catabolism of endogenous protein and gastrointestinal absorption of exogenous protein. Bacterial breakdown of nitrogen-containing products in the gut results in ammonia formation, which is then absorbed in the portal circulation. Factors that can increase blood ammonia concentrations can exacerbate the signs and symptoms of HE. These typically include increased catabolism from infection or increased gut absorption from high-protein diets, constipation, and gastrointestinal bleeding. Other factors that have been implicated in the exacerbation of HE include benzodiazepines, hyponatremia, and inflammatory cytokines, which may all share a final common pathway to increase cerebral edema.

Management of HE should begin with assessing the child's ability to manage his or her airway. Children with grade 3 and 4 HE may require tracheal intubation to protect the airway to ensure adequate oxygenation and ventilation. Otherwise, management typically focuses on reducing gastrointestinal production and absorption of ammonia. Lactulose is often prescribed to create an osmotic diarrhea and to acidify the lumen of the gut to trap ammonia and minimize absorption. Antibiotics such as neomycin and metronidazole have been used to kill the gastrointestinal bacteria involved in metabolizing nitrogen products to ammonia. Other medications include sodium benzoate, which combines in the liver with ammoniagenic amino acids, such as glycine, to facilitate their excretion.[52] Ornithine aspartate may also provide a substrate to the liver for enhancing the urea cycle and glutamine synthesis and to reduce ammonia concentrations. Flumazenil has been postulated to reduce the symptoms of HE by inhibiting endogenous benzodiazepines and γ-aminobutyric acid. However, this benefit was not demonstrated in children who received 0.01 mg/kg flumazenil for HE in the setting of fulminant hepatic failure.[53]

Patients with fulminant hepatic failure can have increased ICP, which is the major cause of mortality and may be a contraindication for liver transplantation. Intracranial hypertension occurs in 38% to 81% of patients with fulminant hepatic failure.[54] ICP is often monitored in patients with fulminant hepatic failure with grade 3 to 4 HE. However, there is a risk of intracranial hemorrhage secondary to coagulopathy. This risk can be reduced by replacing clotting factors and platelets and by placing an epidural rather than a subdural ICP monitor.[55] Management strategies for patients with increased ICP should focus on maintaining a cerebral perfusion pressure greater than 60 mm Hg and an ICP less than 20 mm Hg. Often this includes tracheal intubation and ventilation. Patients should be positioned with their heads midline and slightly elevated to 30 degrees to facilitate venous drainage. Ventilation should focus on achieving a $PaCO_2$ of 30 to 35 mm Hg with minimal positive end-expiratory pressure (PEEP). Medical management to reduce ICP includes administering thiopental or propofol to minimize stimulation and to reduce ICP.[56] Mannitol can be administered if ICP remains increased. Hypothermia has also been described in a small trial with 14 patients with fulminant hepatic failure; maintaining core body temperature at 32°C to 33°C reduced ICP, but the impact on outcome is less certain.[57] Orthotopic liver transplantation is the definitive treatment for patients with acute or chronic HE.

Hematologic Considerations

Anemia is common and occurs because of a combination of gastrointestinal bleeding, poor nutritional state, and decreased erythropoietin production from renal failure. Portal hypertension can result in splenomegaly, which causes platelet sequestration and thrombocytopenia. All the coagulation factors (except factor VIII) are synthesized in the liver. As synthetic function declines, coagulation factor production diminishes. The reduction in bile salt also decreases the absorption of fat-soluble vitamins (A, D, E, K) and contributes to the deficiency of factors II, VII, IX, and X. The result is an elevated prothrombin time (PT) and partial thromboplastin time (PTT). Patients with acute or fulminant hepatic failure can present with a hematologic profile similar to disseminated intravascular coagulation (DIC).

Renal Manifestations

Renal failure is common in patients with acute and chronic liver disease and its cause is multifactorial. Renal failure can be classified as prerenal azotemia, acute tubular necrosis (ATN), or hepatorenal syndrome. Prerenal azotemia from hypovolemia occurs secondary to diuretic therapy, gastrointestinal bleeding, splanchnic pooling, and sepsis. ATN occurs because of decreased central blood volume secondary to central splanchnic pooling and decreased prostaglandin synthesis. The hepatorenal syndrome is characterized by renal failure in the setting of liver failure and portal hypertension. The incidence in adults with chronic liver disease is approximately 10% to 15%. The lower incidence in children (5%) possibly reflects the lack of criteria for the diagnosis of hepatorenal syndrome in children.[58] It occurs secondary to intense renal vasoconstriction from activation of the renin-angiotensin, arginine vasopressin, and sympathetic nervous systems. This activation is a homeostatic response to the profound splanchnic vasodilation that occurs in patients with portal hypertension.[59] Hepatorenal syndrome appears similar to prerenal azotemia (increased serum creatinine, decreased urine Na (U_{Na} <10 mM, fractional excretion of sodium [FE_{Na}] <1%]) but it is differentiated by its lack of response to a fluid challenge (see Chapter 28). Hepatorenal syndrome is classified into two types. The rate of progression of renal failure distinguishes the two types. Type 1, which has a worse prognosis, is characterized by a rapid progression of renal failure with a 100% increase in serum creatinine in less than 2 weeks. It usually occurs in acute liver failure. Type 2 progresses over weeks to months and usually occurs in children with chronic liver disease. Regardless of the type, prognosis is poor in patients with hepatorenal syndrome with a mortality rate of 80% to 95%.[58] The definitive treatment for hepatorenal syndrome is liver transplantation because the renal failure is reversible if the liver is replaced.[60]

The primary goal in the management of patients with liver disease and renal failure is to exclude treatable and reversible causes of renal failure such as nephrotoxins (e.g., nonsteroidal antiinflammatory drugs), hypovolemia (e.g., diuretics, gastrointestinal bleeding), and sepsis (e.g., spontaneous bacterial peritonitis [SBP]). All nephrotoxins should be stopped and patients should be given a fluid challenge, ideally with a colloid solution. If sepsis is suspected, extensive cultures should be obtained and non-nephrotoxic antibiotics should be started.

Pretransplant renal function predicts mortality in adults undergoing transjugular intrahepatic shunt and liver transplantation. This underscores the importance or renal function and explains why serum creatinine is used in the MELD score. Preexisting renal failure is also a major determinant of survival after liver transplantation in adults. Efforts to improve renal function pretransplant may improve posttransplantation outcome.[61] It is not clear whether serum creatinine is a predictor of mortality in children with liver disease.[12] Type 1 hepatorenal syndrome can be managed by treating reversible causes such as providing antibiotic treatment for spontaneous bacterial peritonitis before transplantation. Critically ill children may require continuous renal replacement therapy (continuous venovenous hemofiltration, continuous venovenous hemodiafiltration) and vasopressors as a bridge to transplantation.[62]

Metabolic Considerations

Metabolic derangements include glucose, ammonia, electrolyte, and acid-base disturbances. Electrolyte abnormalities include hyponatremia, hypokalemia and hyperkalemia, hypocalcemia, and hypomagnesemia. Hypoglycemia may occur in patients with fulminant hepatic failure or abrupt discontinuation of TPN, but hyperglycemia is more common in the intraoperative and post-operative period.

PREOPERATIVE EVALUATION

The preoperative evaluation begins with a history and physical examination to identify the primary cause of liver failure and to identify liver and non–liver-related alterations in physiology that may affect the anesthetic and surgical plan. A complete review of systems identifies most of the perioperative concerns (Table 31.2).

The primary cardiovascular concerns include acquired cardiomyopathies from liver disease and inborn errors of metabolism, congenital cardiac defects, and QT prolongation. Aside from a cardiovascular physical examination, the preoperative cardiac evaluation should include an echocardiogram and 12-lead ECG.

The pulmonary manifestations of concern include hypoxia and PPH. Oxygen saturation on room air and with oxygen identifies hypoxic patients and their response to oxygen. Children with significant intrapulmonary shunts from HPS will not increase their oxygen saturation significantly. HPS can be diagnosed by demonstrating intrapulmonary vascular dilatation on echocardiography with macroaggregated albumin.[34]

PPH can usually be identified on echocardiography (if a tricuspid regurgitation jet is present). Patients suspected of having PPH should undergo cardiac catheterization to define the severity of pulmonary hypertension and to assess the response to pulmonary vasodilators (NO, epoprostenol). Children with severe pulmonary hypertension (PAP >50 mm Hg) are at increased risk of perioperative mortality and liver transplantation may be contraindicated.[46]

Anemia and thrombocytopenia are common in children with liver disease and a complete blood cell count should be obtained. In addition, because of the decreased synthetic function of the liver and because of decreased vitamin K absorption, concentrations of clotting factors II, VII, IX, and X may be decreased. A PT, PTT, and platelet count should also be obtained before starting surgery.

Renal failure is common and predicts decreased survival during the posttransplant period in adults.[63] Samples for blood urea nitrogen (BUN) and serum creatinine (SeCr) testing should be obtained.

Children should be evaluated for evidence of altered mental status, particularly those with acute hepatic failure. Increased ICP is common and it is a common cause of mortality in those with fulminant hepatic failure. Altered mental status may also be caused by HE. An ammonia concentration should be obtained as part of their evaluation. Children with advanced HE (grade 3 and 4) may require orotracheal intubation to protect their airway and mechanical ventilation to control $PaCO_2$.

Baseline laboratory values should be obtained for liver function tests, sodium, potassium, calcium, glucose, and albumin. Hyponatremia and hypokalemia are common with diuretic therapy. Patients may have already received citrated containing blood products and may be hypocalcemic secondary to the chelation of calcium. Hypoglycemia occurs secondary to depleted glycogen stores in the failed liver and/or removal of long-term TPN.

A key portion of the preoperative evaluation is the preparation of the patient (child or adolescent) and the family for the anticipated risks, benefits, and clinical course. Specifically, a critically ill child will likely remain intubated and mechanically ventilated in the immediate postoperative period and may have significant facial and extremity edema. Infants and children with less severe disease or disease that does not result in portal hypertension (e.g., MSUD) may be extubated at the end of surgery. Similarly,

TABLE 31.2	Preoperative Evaluation of Liver Transplant Candidates

History and Physical Examination

Cause for liver failure

Identifiable syndrome or metabolic disorder

Past medical history: non–liver-related medical problems (e.g., asthma)

Past surgical history: portoenterostomy (Kasai), previous anesthetic concerns

Medications: diuretics, lactulose

Allergies

Family history of anesthesia-related problems

NPO history

Cardiovascular

Echocardiography: to identify cardiomyopathy, pulmonary HTN, congenital cardiac defects, and intrapulmonary vasodilation

Electrocardiogram: to identify arrhythmias and QT prolongation

Pulmonary

Oxygen saturation (possible arterial blood gas): to assess hypoxia, A-a gradient (HPS)

Chest x-ray: to identify pleural effusions and central line position

Hematology

Complete blood cell count: to assess anemia, leukocytosis/leukopenia (sepsis)

Prothrombin time and partial thromboplastin times

Platelet count

Thromboelastography

Renal

Blood urea nitrogen

Creatinine

Bicarbonate: to assess degree of metabolic acidosis

Neurologic

Assessment of increased intracranial pressure in acute/fulminant hepatic failure

Hepatic encephalopathy: ammonia level

Electrolytes

Na^+ and K^+: hyponatremia and hypokalemia secondary to diuretics

Calcium

Albumin

Magnesium

Glucose

A-a gradient, alveolar-arterial gradient; *HPS*, hepatopulmonary syndrome; *HTN*, hypertension; *NPO*, nothing by mouth.

informing the family about the potential number and location of the intravascular catheters and their associated risks can be helpful in preparing them to see their child after surgery. Informed consent should also include a discussion about the use of blood products and risks associated with prolonged positioning (peripheral nerve injury, occipital alopecia).

INTRAOPERATIVE CARE

Appropriate intraoperative care of the pediatric liver transplant patient requires an understanding of the surgical and anesthetic issues. Several factors affect the patient's physiology, including the underlying pathophysiology of liver disease, surgery, and response to anesthetic drugs. The surgical approach for OLT in children is similar to that for adults. The major difference is the smaller size of the recipient. The obstacles imposed by the size of the patient include a smaller blood volume, more challenging vascular access, size restriction of donor graft, veno-venous bypass (VVBP), and surgical complications such as hepatic artery thrombosis.

Anesthetic management begins with a thorough preoperative evaluation. Children older than 1 year will likely be anxious during the preoperative period. They can be premedicated with an anxiolytic like midazolam, which may be administered intravenously, orally, nasally, or rectally. Patients with HE should not receive premedication with midazolam.

Most children are regarded as having a full stomach because of delayed gastric emptying from ascites, gastrointestinal bleeding, HE, and the nonelective nature of most transplants. The exception may be those presenting for an "elective" transplant without any stigmata of portal hypertension (e.g., Crigler-Najjar syndrome or MSUD). Patients considered to have a full stomach should receive a rapid sequence induction (RSI). Induction agents should be tailored to meet the needs of the patient, but etomidate (0.2–0.3 mg/kg), propofol (2–4 mg/kg), or ketamine (2 mg/kg) are suitable options. Appropriate muscle relaxants for RSI include succinylcholine and high-dose rocuronium.[64] The trachea should be secured with a tracheal tube. Some children may require greater inspiratory pressures to achieve adequate ventilation in the intraoperative and postoperative period compared with unaffected children because of atelectasis from pleural effusions and ascites, surgical retractors placed on the abdominal and chest wall, and a tight abdominal closure; a cuffed tracheal tube is appropriate for these children. PEEP should be used in all patients. PEEP (10 cm H_2O) has no negative effects on liver function in donors.[65]

Children who are not at risk for aspiration may have an inhalation induction with sevoflurane and nitrous oxide. The use of nitrous oxide is not recommended after induction of anesthesia because it may distend the bowel and expand gas emboli. Anesthesia is typically maintained with an inhalational agent, an opioid, and a neuromuscular blocking drug. Isoflurane and sevoflurane are commonly used because they are readily available, undergo minimal hepatic metabolism, and have minimal adverse effects on the liver.[66,67] Desflurane also undergoes minimal hepatic metabolism and appears to be quite safe, although there are three cases reports of hepatotoxicity after desflurane exposure.[68] Sevoflurane provided more stable hemodynamics than desflurane in one study.[69] Propofol (with or without remifentanil, total intravenous anesthesia [TIVA], see Chapter 8) is also an option to maintain anesthesia during liver transplantation. It is relatively short-acting and even though the primary metabolic pathway is hepatic, there appears to be extrahepatic metabolism in the lung, kidney, and intestine.[70,71] Neuromuscular blockade can be maintained with a variety of agents. Rocuronium, vecuronium, pancuronium, atracurium, and cisatracurium have all been described. Pancuronium may have the added advantage of increased heart rate, long duration, and reduced cost. The disadvantage of pancuronium, rocuronium, and vecuronium is their partial hepatic metabolism (see Chapter 7), but this can be overcome with appropriate monitoring and dose adjustments. Dose requirements of continuous infusions of rocuronium, vecuronium, and pancuronium are reduced during the anhepatic phase of liver transplantation but return to initial infusion rates after reperfusion.[72] There is no change in the dose requirements of atracurium during the anhepatic phase.[73] Atracurium or cisatracurium may be ideal in patients with combined hepatic and renal insufficiency because they do not rely on hepatic or renal function for elimination.

The liver metabolizes all opioids, with the exception of remifentanil, which is metabolized by plasma and tissue esterases. The metabolic pathway for most opioids is oxidation, although morphine undergoes glucuronidation.[74] There is evidence that the elimination half-life and clearance of alfentanil and fentanyl are not dramatically altered in patients with cholestatic and cirrhotic liver disease.[75,76] Fentanyl, sufentanil, alfentanil, and morphine have all been described and used in children undergoing liver transplantation. Fentanyl is commonly selected and is usually administered as a bolus during induction (2–10 μg/kg) and maintained as an infusion throughout the anesthetic and the immediate postoperative period (2–5 μg/kg per hour).

Vascular access is important for resuscitation and monitoring. At least two peripheral IV catheters should be placed along with a central venous line (CVL) for administration of drug infusions, vasopressors as indicted, and assessment of volume resuscitation. The CVL can also be used to monitor trends in central venous pressure (CPV) and measure superior vena cava oxygen saturation (a surrogate marker for SvO_2). Larger patients can tolerate rapid infusion catheters. Blood loss can be significant during liver transplantation with estimates between 0.5 and 25 blood volumes (mean = 3.95 blood volumes).[77] Fluid warmers and infusion devices (Level 1 Fast Flow Fluid Warmer, Smiths Medical, Rockland, MA; Belmont Rapid Infuser, Belmont Instrument Corporation, Billerica, MA) need to be available to facilitate volume resuscitation if massive hemorrhage occurs (see Chapters 12 and 52). The early version of the Level 1 Fast Flow Fluid Warmer was associated with massive air emboli but the newer models are equipped with air detectors. Nevertheless, all air needs to be removed from the infusion bags before starting the device.[78] The Belmont Rapid Infuser is not routinely used in infants or small children (see Chapter 52). The choice of resuscitation fluids should be limited to 0.9% normal saline solution and PlasmaLyte. Lactated Ringer's solution is not recommended because the lactate will remain unmetabolized during the anhepatic stage. Many patients with liver disease are hypoalbuminemic, so the use of 5% albumin is appropriate. However, 5% albumin is hypertonic owing to a large sodium concentration and care must be taken when administering this to children with hyponatremia because it may correct the hyponatremia too rapidly and cause adverse cerebral pressure changes.

Standard monitoring should include ECG, pulse oximetry (upper and lower extremities), noninvasive blood pressure, invasive arterial blood pressure, CVP, and temperature. Other high-technology monitoring commonly used in adult liver transplantation includes transesophageal echocardiography (TEE), continuous cardiac output (CCO) catheter, bispectral index (BIS), VVBP, and more than one arterial catheter. There are limitations to the use of these monitors in children because of patient size; TEE, CCO, BIS, and VVBP are used in 0%, 7.7%, 15.4%, and 7.7% of U.S. pediatric transplant centers, respectively.[79] The recent development of continuous noninvasive or minimally invasive CO monitors such as the Cardiotronic ICON (Osypka Medical, La Jolla, CA), which simply requires four ECG pads to assess changes in bioimpedance (approved by the U.S. Food and Drug Administration [FDA] for use in neonates) or small esophageal Doppler monitors (Deltex Medical, Chichester, West Sussex, England) (FDA-approved for use in children weighing 3 kg or more) may prove to be of great value in the future (see Chapter 52).[80,81]

Hematologic and electrolyte changes are common during liver transplantation, and measurements of arterial blood gases,

sodium, potassium, calcium, magnesium, hemoglobin platelets, and coagulation parameters (PT, PTT, fibrinogen and D-dimers, thromboelastography [TEG]) need to be performed frequently throughout the procedure. Most centers use either portable devices or an operating room laboratory to obtain these data. Assessment of coagulation variables can be obtained with TEG) (E-Fig. 31.1). Point-of-care testing with TEG may reduce transfusion requirements in patients having liver transplants.[82,83] However, only 28% of U.S. pediatric transplant centers used TEG.[79]

Acid-base disturbances commonly occur during liver transplantation. Children with renal disease may have a preexisting metabolic acidosis from increased bicarbonate elimination. A metabolic acidosis is typically present during the dissection and anhepatic phase of surgery but it is usually most pronounced immediately following reperfusion. Lactic acid and citrate (from blood products) are not metabolized during the anhepatic phase and contribute to the acidosis. Cross-clamping of the inferior vena cava [IVC] and aorta alters blood flow to gut and lower extremity tissue beds and may also contribute to the development of a lactic acidosis. Once the liver graft begins to function, a metabolic alkalosis can develop as the lactate and citrate are metabolized.[77]

During the dissection and anhepatic phase there are several causes of hyperglycemia. Serum glucose will increase if there is an exogenous source or if there is altered glucose metabolism. Exogenous sources of glucose include glucose from blood products,[77] dextrose-containing IV fluids, and damaged hepatocytes from the liver graft.[84] Typically glucose concentrations will increase immediately after reperfusion. Glucose uptake is altered from the administration of methylprednisolone because of steroid-induced insulin resistance. Hepatic denervation likely results in alterations in insulin and glucose clearance during the postoperative period and may explain the frequent occurrence of impaired glucose tolerance and diabetes in liver transplant recipients.[85,86]

Positioning is critical to prevent soft tissue and peripheral nerve injuries. All extremities should be padded and all cables and wires need to be wrapped and protected from the skin. The head should be rotated and repositioned periodically to prevent the development of a pressure sore and alopecia. To minimize the risk of peripheral neuropathy, the upper extremities should not be abducted more than 90 degrees and the wrists should not be hyperextended for the arterial catheter.

SURGICAL TECHNIQUE

The surgical approach can be divided into four stages: hepatectomy, anhepatic, reperfusion, and biliary reconstruction.

Hepatectomy (Stage 1)

The initial description of OLT is referred to as the "classic" technique. In the classic approach, the liver is dissected to its vascular supply and the suprahepatic and infrahepatic vena cava (VC) are clamped along with the portal vein and hepatic artery. The liver is removed en bloc (Fig. 31.1). The disadvantage of this approach is the VC cross-clamp and the associated reduction in preload. The piggyback technique was described 1989 and is the preferred approach for pediatric transplants because there is more flexibility with the organ size and it requires only partial clamping of the VC.[87,88] The liver is dissected away from the IVC, the short hepatic veins, portal vein, and left, right, and middle hepatic vein. The infrahepatic VC of the donor is oversewn and the suprahepatic VC is anastomosed to the native hepatic veins (Figs. 31.2 and 31.3). This requires only partial clamping of the IVC. A portocaval shunt can be established for patients who do not tolerate clamping

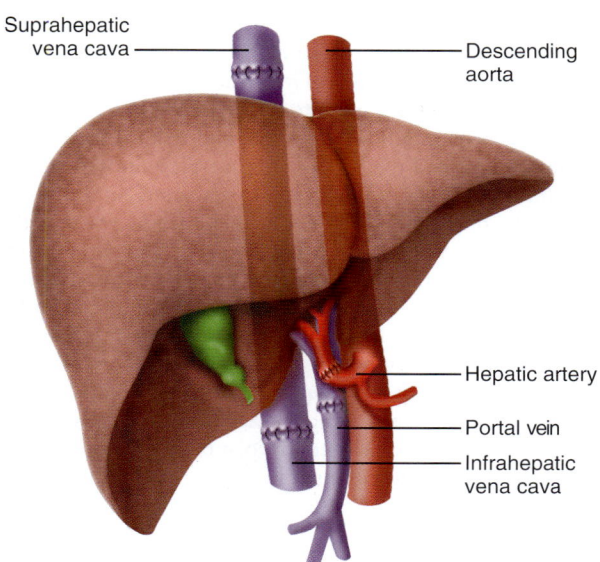

FIGURE 31.1 The classic approach for orthotopic liver transplantation. The suture lines are visible at the suprahepatic and infrahepatic anastomoses. (From Starzl TE, Iwatsuki S, Van Theil DH, et al. Evolution of liver transplantation. *Hepatology* 1982;2[5]:614–636.)

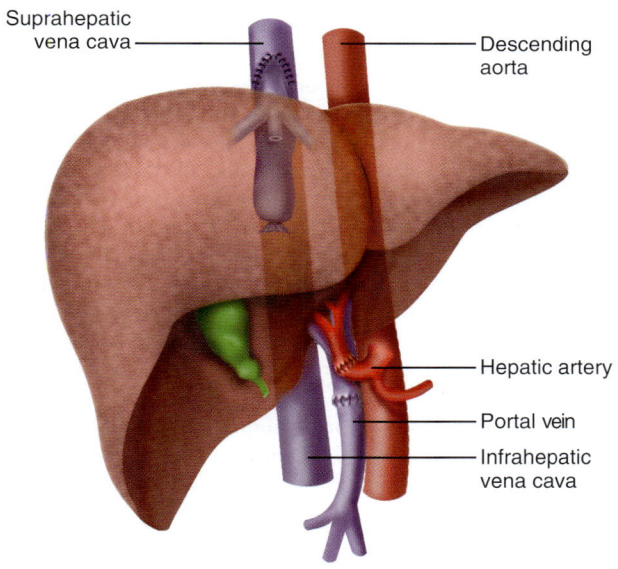

FIGURE 31.2 The piggyback technique preserves the inferior vena cava (IVC). This is the view of the liver graft after the recipient's hepatic confluence is anastomosed to the donor's IVC (the infrahepatic IVC of the donor is ligated). (From Tzakis A, Todo S, Starzl TE. Orthotopic liver transplantation with preservation of the inferior vena cava. *Ann Surg.* 1989;210[5]:649–652.)

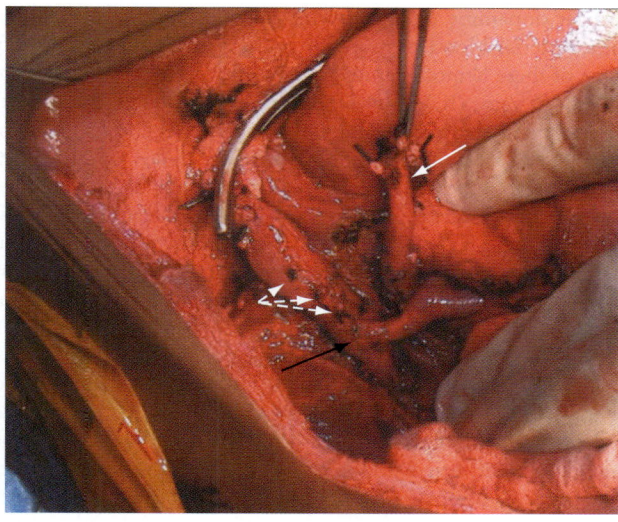

FIGURE 31.3 The native liver has been removed. There is a clamp across the right, middle, and left hepatic veins. The *black arrow* shows the portacaval shunt. The *white arrow* shows the hepatic artery. The *dashed white arrows* show the short hepatic veins. (From Kuo PC, Davis RD. *Comprehensive Atlas of Transplantation.* Philadelphia: Lippincott Williams & Wilkins; 2005:132.)

of the portal vein (see Fig. 31.3). Typically, these are patients who have not developed collateral flow secondary to portal hypertension (e.g., MSUD).

Several physiologic considerations that take place during the hepatic dissection affect the anesthetic management. Hypotension is common and can occur as the result of changes to the cardiovascular, hematologic, and metabolic systems. The most common cause of hypotension includes hypovolemia secondary to hemorrhage and third-space volume losses. Resuscitation with citrated blood products can result in hypocalcemia and surgical manipulation can cause mechanical compression of the IVC or right ventricle. Bleeding occurs from fragile collaterals, adhesions from prior surgery (e.g., Kasai procedure), and coagulopathy.[89] Blood conservation with a reduction in allogeneic blood exposure may have a significant benefit on perioperative morbidity including infections, intensive care unit (ICU) stay, and hospital stay.[90] One technique to reduce blood loss is the maintenance of low CVP (decrease of 30% from baseline) as has been described in adults. The reported benefit of a low CVP is less bleeding with subsequent decrease in allogeneic blood requirements and decreased morbidity.[88] Some studies have also suggested an overall reduction in morbidity and 1-year mortality.[91,92] The technique is controversial and the potential risks include end-organ injury, such as renal or graft failure.[93] This technique has not been described in the pediatric liver transplant population.

Hematologic abnormalities include anemia, thrombocytopenia, coagulation factor deficiency, and low fibrinogen.[94] A progressive coagulopathy can develop during this stage. Metabolic derangements including hyperkalemia, hypocalcemia, hypomagnesemia, and acidosis occur from volume resuscitation with blood products.

Anhepatic Stage (Stage 2)

The anhepatic phase begins once the hepatic veins, hepatic artery, and portal vein are cross clamped. The dissection of the recipient's liver is completed and the organ is removed. This phase ends when the hepatic and portal vein cross clamps are removed and the graft is reperfused.

Cardiovascular changes that occur during this stage can result in hypotension. This occurs from the inferior vena cava cross-clamp, which decreases the preload. Hemodynamically, CO, CVP, and PAP decrease while systemic vascular resistance increases.[89] Preload should be gently augmented to maintain mean arterial pressure (MAP) with the minimum filling pressures possible. Hypervolemia may cause hepatic congestion during reperfusion. Inotropic agents such as dopamine or epinephrine may be needed to maintain mean arterial blood pressure. A portocaval shunt may mollify some of these hemodynamic changes by preserving preload from the portal vein. (If VVBP is planned, it is initiated during this period.) Unmetabolized citrate causes hypocalcemia and hypomagnesemia since it chelates both cations. Acidosis occurs from the unmetabolized citrate, lactate, and other acids. Bicarbonate may be administered if there is a significant metabolic acidosis, although there is no evidence that this improves outcomes.[95] In fact, a mild metabolic acidosis during reperfusion may not be detrimental since it will be later offset by the metabolism of citrate, which produces bicarbonate.

Once the liver is on the surgical field warm, ischemia time begins. The time to reperfusion will be brief and steps need to be in place for reperfusion. The potassium should be low-normal and the calcium should be high-normal, hemoglobin should be maintained between 9 and 10 g/dL. If the potassium is greater than 5 mEq/L, steps need to be taken to reduce it. This includes increasing the serum pH with hyperventilation and the administration of sodium bicarbonate (1–3 mEq/kg). Glucose and insulin can be administered to acutely reduce the potassium concentration as well (see Chapters 7 and 27). Potassium-wasting diuretics such as furosemide (0.5–1 mg/kg) can also be used. Administering fresh blood or washed red blood cells will minimize the increase in potassium during transfusion therapy. β_2-Agonists may decrease potassium and can be used. Calcium and epinephrine should be immediately available for reperfusion.

Reperfusion (Stage 3)

The liver graft can be reperfused once the hepatic and portal vein anastomosis are complete. Before reestablishing hepatic blood flow, the graft is flushed to remove the preservation solution to minimize the reperfusion syndrome.

Many changes can occur acutely during the reperfusion period secondary to cardiovascular, hematologic, and metabolic derangements. Reperfusion syndrome is characterized by a decrease in MAP of greater than 30%.[96] Factors participating in this event include myocardial dysfunction, arrhythmias, and bleeding. The myocardial dysfunction is attributed to the release of NO and TNF-α.[97] Cardiovascular collapse can occur and patients may require epinephrine to correct the hemodynamic effects of reperfusion.[96] Hyperkalemia is a common event immediately following reperfusion and may cause ventricular arrhythmias.[98] Hyperkalemia should be treated with calcium chloride (10–30 mg/kg) initially to stabilize the cardiac membrane and then insulin and dextrose, hyperventilation, furosemide, β_2-agonists, and sodium bicarbonate to decrease the serum potassium concentration (see previous section). The increased potassium content of the preservation solution is the cause of hyperkalemia. The University of Wisconsin solution, a very commonly used preservation solution, contains large amounts of potassium (120 mmol/L). Histidine-tryptophan-ketoglutarate solution was introduced in 1980 as a cardioplegic solution and contains significantly less potassium (10 mmol/L) than University of Wisconsin solution.[99] A recent study comparing the two solutions found equal 1-month and 1-year graft survival with histidine-tryptophan-ketoglutarate and University of Wisconsin solution. The viscosity is reduced with histidine-tryptophan-ketoglutarate solution and may introduce itself more easily into the vascular spaces in the donor liver.[100] Although hyperkalemia is the hallmark electrolyte disturbance in the immediate reperfusion period, hypokalemia is more common in children throughout the intraoperative period and may require correction.[101]

Fibrinolysis can occur after reperfusion and in one study it occurred in 60% of children and 80% of adults.[102] This occurs from increased tissue plasminogen activator activity and decreased synthesis of fibrinolysis inhibitors. Heparin effect occurs from endogenous heparinoids from the graft and residual heparin from the preservation and the release of tissue plasminogen activator from endothelial cells of the revascularized graft. Antifibrinolytic medications blunt this process, but there is concern that there may be an association with antifibrinolytics and intraoperative thrombotic events (hepatic artery and portal vein thrombosis) in pediatric patients receiving liver transplants. Children can have a mixed coagulation picture after transplantation and may be hypercoagulable because of a decrease in protein C and antithrombin III.[103] This may result in hepatic artery thrombosis.[104-106] Tranexamic acid, ε-aminocaproic acid, and other methods to reduce transfusion needs in adult liver transplants have been advocated, but there are no pediatric transplant data to support or refute the use of tranexamic acid or ε-aminocaproic acid and the adult series have small sample sizes.[107-109]

Biliary and Hepatic Artery Reconstruction (Stage 4)

The final step is reestablishing hepatic artery blood flow and reconstructing the biliary system. The hepatic artery may require an anastomosis via a conduit to the infrarenal aorta in infants. This requires temporary cross-clamping of the aorta. Biliary reconstruction is established by either directly connecting the graft and the recipient's common bile ducts or by connecting the common duct of the graft to a Roux-en-Y limb of the recipient's jejunum.

During biliary reconstruction, metabolic and hematologic alterations are addressed. As the liver graft begins to function the citrate administered during the previous three phases is metabolized and the patient can develop a metabolic alkalosis. One of the hemodynamic goals includes maintaining a normal CVP. If the CVP is increased (>8–10 mm Hg), there is concern that the liver graft can become congested and not function normally. The risk of hepatic artery thrombosis ranges from 0% to 25% and is greater in infants and children.[105,106] This risk may be increased if the PT and PTT are corrected to normal values. Also, the viscosity from a greater hematocrit may increase the risk of hepatic artery or portal vein thrombosis. The hematocrit does not need to be corrected to normal values; maintaining the hematocrit at 8 to 9 g/dL is safe and reasonable. Surgical techniques to reduce the risk of hepatic artery thrombosis include anticoagulation with heparin, dextran, aspirin, and alprostadil.

Split Liver Techniques and Living Donor Liver Transplants

Advances in surgical technique, tissue preservation, and immunosuppression have improved the survival in patients undergoing liver transplantation. The result is more patients waiting for liver transplantation without an increase in available organs. Children are at a disadvantage because of the size limitations. Two techniques have attempted to address these issues. In 1984, Bismuth and Houssin split an adult liver and transplanted it into a child.[110] The reduced liver technique does not increase the number of available grafts and efforts were made to perform split liver techniques to make two grafts from one adult donor. The initial results were poor, with an increase in complications and mortality.[111,112] The technique has evolved and today the graft is split while still in vivo (in the heart-beating donor) compared with ex vivo (splitting performed after the graft is removed from the donor). This decreases cold ischemia time and facilitates hemostasis of the liver edge. The result is improved patient and graft survival.[113] Patient survival has increased from 60% to 70% in the 1990s to 80% to 90% in 2003. In one series, 218 split liver technique grafts were transplanted between 1995 and 2002; overall patient survival at 1 year was 81.7% and overall graft survival was 75.8%. Surgical complications that caused a return to the operating room were bleeding (9.2%), bowel perforation (8.3%), and biliary problems (7.5%). Hepatic artery complications occurred in 6.7%.[113]

Living donor liver transplantation was first described in 1989.[114] The result has been a reduction in mortality among children awaiting liver transplantation. The benefit of a living donor (especially if related) is improved posttransplant results because of better graft quality, shorter ischemic times, and better immune compatibility. One- and five-year patient survival rates were 94% and 92%, respectively.[115] The left hepatic segment is removed for pediatric recipients, whereas the right hepatic lobe is removed for adult recipients. The regenerative capacity of the liver allows the donor to regenerate the liver without hepatic insufficiency. Despite the success of this technique for the recipients, there is considerable risk to the donor. Complications include exposure to blood products, short- and long-term peripheral nerve injuries, biliary leakage, abdominal wall defects, pleural effusions, pneumonia, pulmonary emboli, and death.[115,116]

OUTCOMES

The Studies of the Pediatric Liver Transplantation (SPLIT) registry was initiated in 1995 and consists of 38 centers in the United States and Canada. These centers contributed 85% of the pediatric liver transplants in 2002. Transplants performed more recently had improved survival rates. In the past, age younger than 1 year was considered an increased risk factor for mortality, but over the past 20 years there is little difference between patients younger than 2 years and those older than 2 years. There is also no significant difference between male and female gender.[114]

Review of the MELD/PELD data indicates that survival also depends on the preoperative MELD/PELD score. Patients stratified to status 1 had a lower 1-year survival rate compared with other transplant recipients (76% vs. 87%). Adults with greater MELD scores (scores >35) demonstrated decreased 1-year patient and graft survival. Pediatric patients with greater PELD scores showed a trend toward decreased 1-year patient and graft survival but the association was not statistically significant. The overall 1-year survival rate remained excellent at >85%.[117] Cognitive outcomes appear to be reduced in pediatric recipients of liver transplants; long-term cognitive and academic deficits persist with verbal comprehension, working memory, mathematical computation, and executive deficits.[118] Factors that seemed to predict cognitive deficits included operative complications and intraoperative transfusion volume.[119] Conversely, liver transplantation improved global functioning in some children.[120]

IMMEDIATE POSTOPERATIVE CARE

At the completion of the surgery the child is transported to the ICU. Much of the preoperative pathology still exists in the postoperative period. Patients with underlying cardiac, pulmonary, and renal dysfunction will be more difficult to manage.

Patients continue to lose intravascular volume after liver transplantation because of ongoing bleeding and third-space losses. These losses need to be replaced to maintain a normal CVP and adequate urine output (0.5–1 mL/kg per hour). Replacement with a lactate-free isotonic solution (0.9% normal saline solution and PlasmaLyte) and albumin is appropriate. Particular attention should

be paid to children with underlying ventricular dysfunction or PPH because they will not tolerate fluid overload. In adults, there is some evidence that fluid overload was responsible for ICU readmission in liver transplant patients.[121] This, however, must be balanced against the risks of hypovolemia, which could cause renal failure and may increase the risk of hepatic artery thrombosis. Preexisting pulmonary hypertension does not dissipate immediately and children who previously took prostaglandins need to continue these infusions in the operating room and into the postoperative period. Systemic hypertension is common after liver transplantation and has been described in as many as one-third of the patients.[122] It is typically related to cyclosporine therapy or chronic kidney disease.[123,124]

Almost all children require tracheal intubation and mechanical ventilation in the immediate postoperative period; however, some centers extubate those who are stable immediately after surgery. Early extubation may be associated with decreased morbidity and improved graft and recipient survival.[125] It is unclear if postoperative intubation is just an association or a cause of adverse outcomes. Children who may be appropriate candidates for early extubation (extubation in the operating room) include those with reduced blood loss, hemodynamic stability, alveolar-arterial gradient less than 150 mm Hg, and absence of HE.[126] Children with significant comorbidities such as respiratory insufficiency and reoperation are more likely to require reintubation.[127]

Postoperative ventilation may be more appropriate for smaller children that have received a relatively large graft and in children with underlying lung disease (HPS). Ascites, pulmonary edema, and pleural effusions have been described after transplantation (possibly associated with the degree and duration of preoperative portal hypertension) and may necessitate prolonged mechanical ventilation.[128] Efforts to minimize atelectasis include positive-pressure ventilation with PEEP. Diuretics may be needed on the second or third postoperative day to treat edema and effusions. There is speculation that prolonged mechanical ventilation may have a negative effect on the hemodynamics of transplant patients and may contribute to overall morbidity and mortality.[129] Increased levels of PEEP may contribute to this morbidity. Some have advocated for early extubation to decrease the incidence of pulmonary complications and to facilitate discharge from the ICU.[122]

Renal failure secondary to hepatorenal syndrome usually resolves after successful liver transplantation. The goal in the immediate postoperative period is to maintain normovolemia and to avoid nephrotoxic agents. These include aminoglycoside antibiotics and immunosuppressant agents such as cyclosporine and tacrolimus. The immunosuppressant agents may need to be delayed until renal function begins to improve.

Neurologic complications after liver transplantation are also common. In the adult population these complications occur in 10% to 30% of patients.[130] Pediatric information is lacking. In adults, the complications present as encephalopathy, seizures, or coma. The causes of encephalopathy and coma include drugs (immunosuppressive agents such as tacrolimus and OKT3), infection (meningitis and brain abscess), strokes (bleeding), and hyponatremia with central pontine myelinolysis. The most common cause of seizures is an adverse drug reaction associated with immunosuppressant drugs.[131] Hyponatremia can contribute to neurologic complications and needs to be corrected. The correction should be done slowly to minimize the risk of central pontine myelinolysis. Correction no greater than 0.5 mEq/L per hour is considered safe. If the correction proceeds faster than the recommended rate, there is some evidence in the animal model that dexamethasone administered within 6 hours of the correction may minimize the risk of central pontine myelinolysis.[132]

Surgical complications that occur after transplant include vascular complications, acute rejection, and infections; frequent monitoring for their occurrence is important to ensure prompt management. Vascular complications include hepatic artery thrombosis, portal vein thrombosis, bleeding, and bowel perforation.[122,133] Hepatic artery thrombosis is identified with frequent hepatic Doppler flow imaging. Patients may undergo anticoagulation with aspirin, heparin, dextran, and alprostadil to reduce the risk of thrombosis.[133] Infections are common in immunosuppressed transplant patients and contribute to significant morbidity. The primary source for infections appears to be central venous access lines, percutaneous catheter drainage, and mechanical ventilation. Acute rejection should be suspected in patients with fever and increased liver enzymes. The diagnosis is made by histologic examination.[122]

Rejection is an immune response and efforts to understand and control this immune response lie at the heart of transplant medicine. Initial efforts to control the response involved suppressing the recipient's immune system. There has been a move away from immunosuppression to immunotolerance. Immunotolerance describes the concept of immune cells from both the recipient and the donor coexisting without attacking each other.[134] The goal of immunosuppression medication is to reach this state of tolerance. In this state of immunotolerance, minimal immunosuppression can be used. The benefits of decreasing immunosuppression include the reduced risk of infection, hypercholesterolemia, malignancy, hypertension, and diabetes mellitus. Protocols to induce tolerance include exposing patients to lymphoid-depleting agents (antilymphoid antibody) such as antithymocyte globulin before liver engraftment to reduce the antidonor response to a more controllable range and allow maintenance therapy (tacrolimus) to begin with one agent. Other agents are added if there is evidence of rejection.[135] The immunosuppressant agents currently used include calcineurin phosphatase inhibitors, such as tacrolimus and cyclosporine, that provide the mainstay of therapy. Other options include azathioprine or mycophenolate mofetil for patients who cannot tolerate the calcineurin phosphatase inhibitors because of toxicity. Adverse effects of the calcineurin phosphatase inhibitors include hypertension, tremor, and renal failure. Newer agents such as monoclonal antibodies against interleukin 2 (IL-2) are also being used.[136]

LONG-TERM ISSUES

Recipients of liver transplants return to the operating room for a variety of reasons (central line placement, wound irrigation, dental rehabilitation, bowel obstruction, cholangiogram, biliary dilation, esophagogastroduodenoscopy). A primary concern in the posttransplant patient is the adverse effects of immunosuppressant agents. Most organ systems become involved and a thorough review of systems is important.

The cardiovascular effects of immunosuppressant agents include hypertension from cyclosporine and cardiomyopathy (rare) from tacrolimus.[19,137] Renal insufficiency can occur secondary to cyclosporine, diuretics, or hypertension. Baseline BUN and creatinine should be obtained preoperatively in patients with a history of renal insufficiency, and medications or their active metabolites (e.g., morphine 6-glucuronide, aminoglycosides) that are renally cleared will need to be adjusted or avoided. Hyperkalemia may accompany renal failure and should be evaluated before induction of anesthesia.

Pediatric recipients of a liver transplant can have multiple hematologic abnormalities. Azathioprine can cause anemia, leucopenia, and thrombocytopenia. Another cause of anemia includes unrecognized gastrointestinal bleeding from steroid-induced ulcers. Patients who have been taking azathioprine should have a complete blood cell count before surgery, particularly if they are having a procedure that may involve blood loss.

The endocrine effects of chronic steroid exposure include diabetes, growth retardation, and adrenal insufficiency. Patients receiving long-term steroid therapy need stress-dose steroids during the perioperative period (see Chapter 27). Those receiving insulin for diabetes need intraoperative blood glucose monitoring and dextrose-containing IV fluids if they are hypoglycemic or are at risk of developing hypoglycemia.

Most recipients of a liver transplant have been exposed to multiple procedures and may have significant anxiety in the preoperative period. These patients should receive an anxiolytic to minimize the anxiety and to reduce the risk of postoperative behavioral changes.[138] Midazolam is an appropriate and safe medication provided there is no evidence of residual HE. Anesthesia can be induced with an inhalational technique provided the liver graft is functioning normally and no oral intake (NPO) guidelines have been followed. Children who are hospitalized, with sepsis, bleeding, encephalopathic, or rejecting should have an IV induction and their airways secured with an tracheal tube. Isoflurane, sevoflurane, and desflurane are used for maintenance of anesthesia.

Renal Transplantation

The causes of end-stage renal disease in children are different than those in adults. The main causes in adults are diabetes, hypertension, and polycystic kidney disease, whereas in children, the main causes are congenital obstructive uropathies, renal dysplasia, and acquired lesions such as glomerulosclerosis.[139] There are approximately 700 to 800 pediatric renal transplants performed yearly in the United States.[140] Both graft and patient survival have improved dramatically over the past four decades.[139–142] Improvements in immune-suppression therapies, advancements in surgical technique, improved donor selection, and a greater understanding of pediatric pharmacokinetics have all contributed substantively to improving patient survival and quality of life. Age-related changes in survival continue to exist and differ slightly from the earliest years of transplantation. Children younger than 5 years have better graft survival, whereas adolescents have the worse outcome (Fig. 31.4).[139] Graft survival from living-related donors (LDs) appears slightly better than from deceased donors (DDs): 86% versus 83%. Multivariate analysis of risk factors for graft loss include black race, history of prior transplantation, more than five transfusions, and HLA-B mismatch (Table 31.3).[141]

PATHOPHYSIOLOGY

The pathophysiology of renal disease in children involves cardiovascular, hematologic, and metabolic abnormalities. Cardiovascular changes include hypertension, coronary artery disease, dyslipidemia, left ventricular hypertrophy, and diastolic dysfunction.[143–156] Anemia occurs with a loss of renal function and as a consequence of decreased erythropoietin production.[157–159] Growth retardation is common, thought to be due to a combination of protein and calorie malnutrition, growth hormone resistance, anemia, renal bone disease, and chronic metabolic acidosis. In some instances, steroids used to treat an underlying pathology can further exacerbate growth retardation. Metabolic abnormalities and fluid and

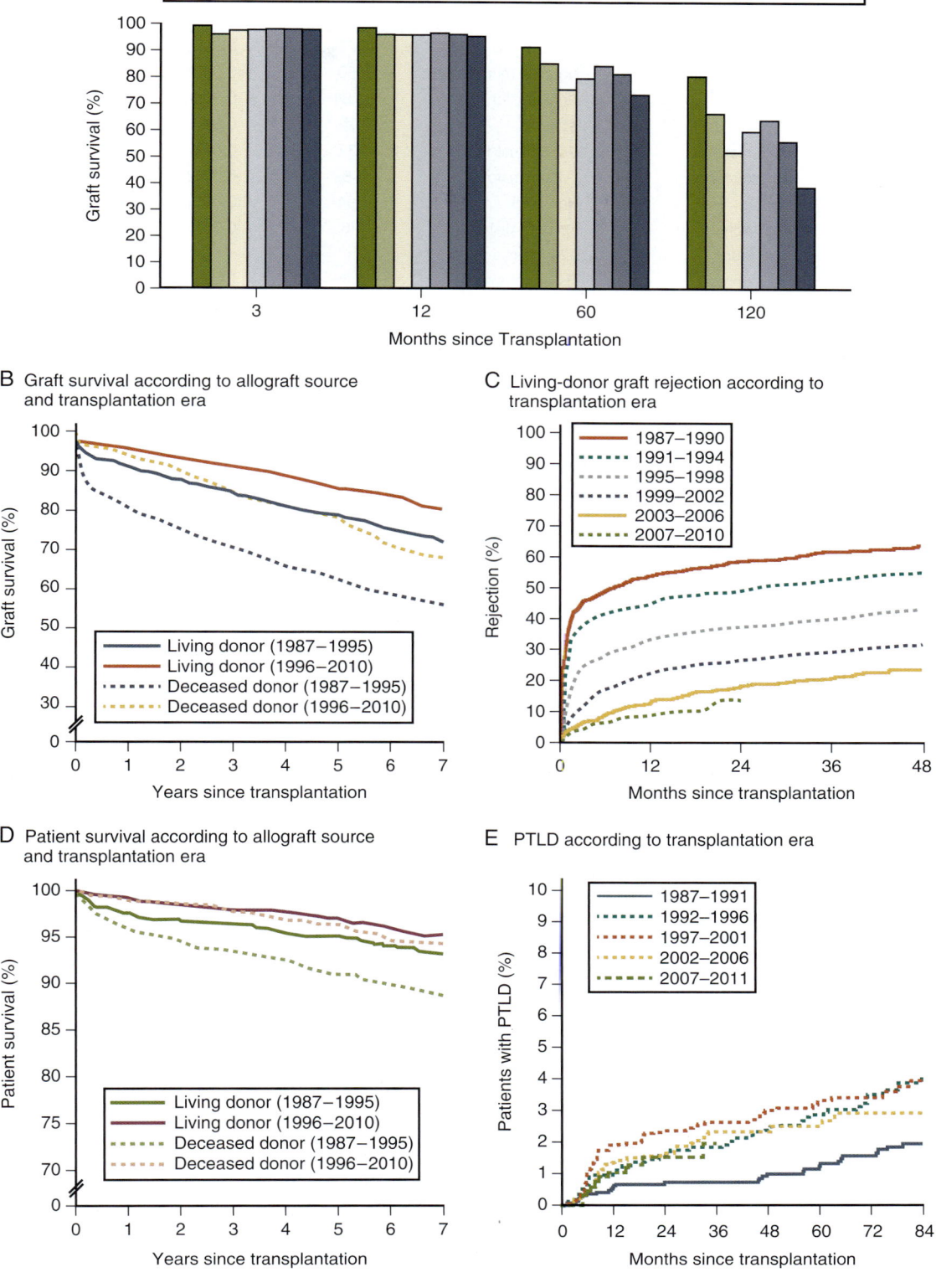

FIGURE 31.4 Pediatric graft and patient survival following kidney transplantation. **A,** Graft survival by age of recipient at time for transplantation. **B,** Graft survival by era of recipient at time of transplantation. **C,** Living-donor graft rejection by era. **D,** Patient survival according to allograft source and era. **E,** Lymphoproliferative incidence according to transplant era. *PTLD,* posttransplant lymphoproliferative disorder. (From Dharnidharka VR, Fiorina P, Harmon WE. Kidney transplantation in children. *New Engl J Med.* 2014;371(6):549–558.)

TABLE 31.3	Multivariate Model of Renal Graft Survival						
			LIVING DONOR		DECEASED DONOR	
Characteristic	Comparison Group	Reference Group	Rh	P Value	Rh	P Value
Recipient age	≥24 months	<24 months	1.23	0.0698	0.67	0.0036
Transplant history	Prior transplants	No prior transplants	1.50	<0.0001	1.45	<0.0001
Induction therapy	Induction	No induction	0.84	0.0051	0.92	0.1405
Transfusion history	>5	≤5	1.22	0.0164	1.25	0.0006
HLA-B mismatch	0 mismatches	1–2 mismatches	1.32	0.0183	1.15	0.017
HLA-DR mismatch	0 mismatches	1–2 mismatches	0.82	0.0532	1.13	0.0333
Recipient race	Black	Non-black	1.94	<0.0001	1.58	<0.0001
Dialysis history	Prior dialysis	No prior dialysis	1.16	0.0375	1.23	0.0326
Cold storage time	>24 hours	≤24 hours	—	—	1.15	0.0201
Native nephrectomy	Not removed	Tissue removed	0.86	0.0264	0.92	0.2335
Gender	Male	Female	0.88	0.0382	0.85	0.0039
Transplant year	Per year 1987–2010		0.95	<0.0001	0.94	<0.0001

Rh, relative hazard, the ratio of two hazard rates
From Smith JM, Martz K, Blydt-Hansen TD. Pediatric kidney transplant practice patterns and outcome benchmarks, 1987-2010: a report of the North American Pediatric Renal Trials and Collaborative Studies. *Pediatr Transplant.* 2013;17(2):149–157.

electrolyte disturbances are common in renal failure and are a consequence of the kidney's inability to eliminate waste products and regulate fluids and electrolytes. Hyperkalemia is a potential life-threatening complication of end-stage renal disease. Metabolic acidosis is a consequence of the failing kidney to excrete an acid load and can exacerbate hyperkalemia. Renal osteodystrophy occurs secondary to an increased concentration of parathyroid hormone and to decreased concentrations of active vitamin D. Because growth retardation and nutritional insufficiency are common in children with end-stage renal disease, cognitive function[160–165] and development can also be impaired.[160–163]

SURGICAL TECHNIQUE

The surgical techniques used in the pediatric recipient differ from those in adults and depend on the child's size and underlying preexisting abnormalities. The surgical approach to kidney transplants involves intraperitoneal or extraperitoneal approaches. The extraperitoneal approach may be more technically difficult in younger patients. Removal of native tissue can be performed either concurrently or (ideally) in advance. Native nephrectomy may be required for polycystic kidney disease, uncontrollable hypertension, urinary tract infection, or nephrotic syndrome with its associated hypoalbuminemia, malnutrition, and hypercoagulability.[166–169] Native nephrectomy at the time of transplant increases operative time, cadaveric graft ischemic time, and is also a risk factor for ATN in the grafted organ.

In children who weigh more than 20 kg, the surgical approach is similar to that in adult transplant patients. A lower-right quadrant incision is used, the kidney is placed in the iliac fossa, and the vascular anastomoses are to the common iliac vein and artery.[167,168] This extraperitoneal approach has the advantage of increased ease of future graft biopsy and ability to resume peritoneal dialysis in case of delayed graft failure.[139] In the past, the donor organs for renal transplantation in children who weighed less than 20 kg were restricted to those that were size-compatible organs. These small cadaveric donor organs presented technical challenges, sometimes resulting in a vascular thrombosis, acute rejection, and graft loss.[139,170–172] An adult-sized donor kidney is now used in infants and young children. The surgical approach may use a midline incision with mobilization of the cecum and right colon

or an alternate approach involving a right-lower quadrant incision and an extraperitoneal dissection. The donor organ may be anastomosed to either the common iliac artery and vein, or directly to the aorta and VC.[167,168,173–177]

ANESTHETIC MANAGEMENT
Preoperative Evaluation
Immediately before transplantation, the child should be hemodynamically stable and fluid/electrolyte imbalances corrected before transplantation. It is important to assess the urine output of the patient (anuric, polyuric) so that appropriate intraoperative fluid replacement can be administered before unclamping of the donor organ during surgery. Active infection is a contraindication to transplantation; any concurrent systemic disorders should be optimized. The NPO status of the child should be determined and because of the unexpected nature of cadaveric organ availability, many patients who present for cadaveric transplantation require full stomach precautions. Finally, the child's need for premedication should be assessed and either an oral or IV anxiolytic (midazolam) administered. If time permits, patients may receive immunotherapy perioperatively to assist the development of immunotolerance[178] of the implanted graft and, potentially, to delay the administration of the nephrotoxic calcineurin phosphatase inhibitors. Infusion of these induction antilymphocyte antibody agents (alemtuzumab [Campath], antilymphocyte globulin [equine] [Atgam], and antithymocyte globulin [Thymoglobulin]) cause a cytokine release. This cytokine response, which includes fever, chills, rigors, and malaise, can be attenuated by pretreatment with acetaminophen, corticosteroids, and diphenhydramine.[178,179]

Anesthetic Induction
Induction of anesthesia can involve IV or inhalational agents. Succinylcholine may be used in the absence of contraindications such as hyperkalemia (see Chapter 7). One should not assume immediate resumption of renal function by the new graft. Because renal failure affects both protein binding and volume of distribution, anesthetic agents and adjuncts should be titrated to effect. Preferential use should be made of drugs that undergo organ-independent elimination (cisatracurium, remifentanil), do not rely exclusively on the kidney for metabolism (propofol), have

metabolites that are inactive (midazolam, fentanyl), or do not depend on renal elimination (morphine-6-glucuronide). Drug metabolites that are eliminated through the kidney and are toxic (i.e., meperidine) should be avoided entirely. Although rocuronium is excreted in the urine and bile, children with renal failure do not have an increased sensitivity to the drug. The onset of action of rocuronium is delayed in renal compromise, but duration of action is similar to normal children.[180]

Monitors and Vascular Access

Standard monitors, including invasive arterial and central venous catheters if indicated, should be placed after induction of anesthesia. The need for vascular access should reflect third-spacing requirements and the potential for brisk blood loss inherent in a long intraabdominal procedure in which the surgeon will be directly accessing large vessels. Urine output may not reflect intravascular volume status secondary to native renal dysfunction, discontinuity between the grafted organ and the urinary catheter, or polyuria in the reperfused graft.[166,167] Smaller-sized children will have the most severe fluid shifts and will be the most vulnerable to graft hypoperfusion. In addition, the use of adult donors in small infants sequesters a disproportionate amount of the infant's blood volume and CO,[166,167,181,182] necessitating large amounts of fluids or blood transfusion to adequately perfuse the transplanted organ. Therefore central venous and arterial catheters to monitor intraoperative and postoperative pressures are extremely useful.[166,167,182]

Maintenance of Anesthesia

Combined general-regional techniques have been used, but they have been associated with larger intraoperative fluid requirements and the need for IV opioid supplementation in half the patients.[183] Virtually all combinations of anesthetic agents and anesthetic adjuncts have been used. A hypnotic drug supplemented with an opioid to minimize the inhalational anesthetic requirements is common. Avoiding nitrous oxide in a long intraabdominal case is prudent. One nonrandomized, single-center study of 240 patients reported similar creatinine values in patients anesthetized with sevoflurane and isoflurane with slightly greater blood urea values and reduced urine volumes in the sevoflurane patients.[184] However, no negative outcomes data exist for the use of sevoflurane in renal transplant recipients.[184,185]

The anesthetic management plan should take into account hemodynamic conditions necessary for adequate perfusion of the donor organ. Optimal hemodynamic conditions for reperfusion are more important when a large size discrepancy exists between the native organ and the graft. The extreme of this situation would be in the infant receiving an adult graft. In children, recommendations for CVP range from 8 to 12 cm H_2O to 16 to 20 cm H_2O,[175,182] with most centers using a pressure in the middle.[167] Some authors suggest a systolic blood pressure in excess of 120 mm Hg[167] and MAP greater than 65 to 70 mm Hg.[167,186] In the smaller child, blood sequestration in the graft will constitute a significant portion of the patient's total blood volume,[167,182,186] and the anastomosis will likely require the clamping, and subsequent unclamping, of the aorta. Both preload supplementation with blood, crystalloid, and colloid, and possible dopamine infusion to optimize CO may be necessary.[167,186] Furosemide and mannitol are administered at the completion of the vascular anastomoses to promote a diuresis. Sodium bicarbonate is also administered after aortic unclamping to attenuate the underlying acidosis,[166–168,187] which worsens during the procedure. Frequent monitoring of the patient's blood gas and electrolytes is essential to detect the possibility of hyperkalemia.

Hyperkalemia can be treated with hyperventilation, calcium and bicarbonate, glucose and insulin, and β-adrenergic agents. Avoidance of blood products is desirable, as patients with more than five lifetime transfusions are at increased risk of ATN, but transfusion may be necessary in an infant receiving an adult kidney. Although anemia should be avoided in the chronic management of the renal transplant patient, an optimal hematocrit in the immediate postoperative period has not been identified.

Immediate Postoperative Management

In the immediate postoperative period, maintenance of the child's blood volume remains important. Most patients can be extubated in the operating room. In small children, volume resuscitation required to adequately perfuse the graft may preclude early extubation.[168,175,182,183] Maintenance of an adequate blood volume continues into the postoperative period, where usually copious urine output is replaced milliliter for milliliter.[166–168,176,182] Prevention of graft hypoperfusion and subsequent ATN potentially prevents acute rejection,[171] as ATN in the early postoperative period is a major risk factor for graft loss.[188,189] Maintenance of the circulating blood volume continues to be important even in the late postoperative period.

LONG-TERM ISSUES

Much has been accomplished in preservation of graft function for kidney transplant patients. Unfortunately, cardiovascular morbidity, infection, and malignancy are the major long-term concerns. Almost half of renal transplant recipients die with a functioning graft.

Infection

Increased success in immunotolerance for transplant recipients places the patient at risk for opportunistic infections. After the first 5 months, infection is now a greater cause of hospitalization in the transplanted patient than acute rejection. In particular, fungal infection is a significant risk for graft loss.[189,190] Epstein-Barr virus (EBV)-related adenotonsillar hypertrophy is common in the transplant population, occurring in 11 of 16 patients in one series.[191] Risk factors for EBV-related adenotonsillar hypertrophy include young age and seronegativity at time of transplant.[192,193] Posttransplant lymphoproliferative disorder (PTLD), a result of EBV infection, is common, occurs earlier in the renal transplant population (1%–2% within the first 5 years after transplant) but is not a contraindication to later retransplantation.[194–197]

Malignancy

Malignancy is a major concern after renal transplantation in children. The incidence of malignancy is estimated to be 10 times greater than that of the general pediatric population. The crude estimate is about 2.5%, with greater than 82% lymphoproliferative in nature.[142]

Summary

Anesthetic management of the pediatric renal transplant patient may be complicated by many factors. Impaired renal function may be present before and after transplant. Comorbidities because of impaired renal function are numerous and may require altered anesthetic management. Although the renal transplant patient has a lifetime of medical issues, the continued function of the transplanted kidney allows for near-normal function, growth, and development. Therefore the ultimate goals of management are the preservation of the graft, thereby improving the quality of life.[198]

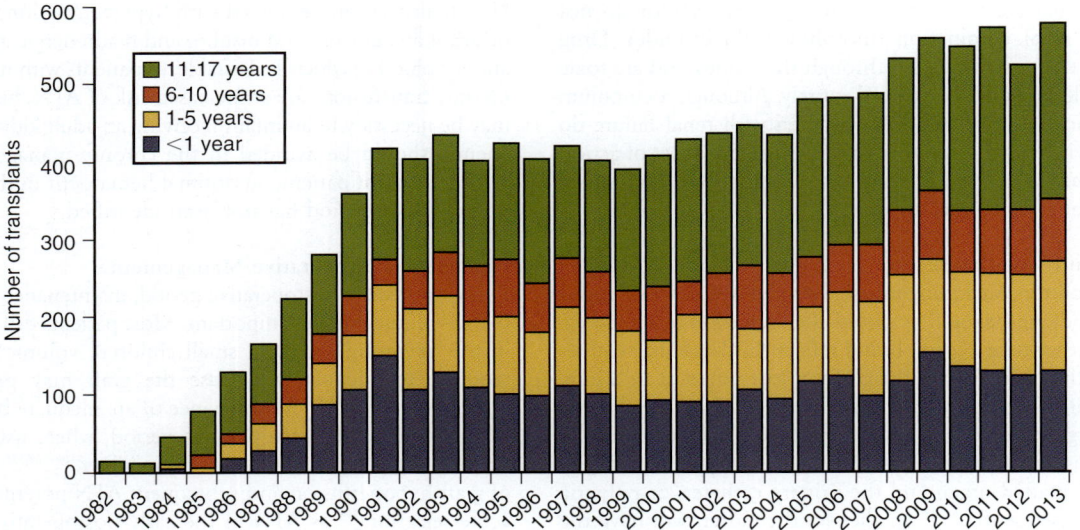

FIGURE 31.5 Age distribution of pediatric heart recipients by year of transplant. (Figure 1 from Dipchand AI, Rossano JW, Edwards LB. The Registry of the International Society for Heart and Lung Transplantation: Eighteenth Official Pediatric Heart Transplantation Report—2015; focus theme: early graft failure. *J Heart Lung Transplant.* 2015;34[10]:1233–1243.)

Cardiac Transplantation

Adrian Kantrowitz performed the first heart transplant in an infant in 1967.[199] Since that time, pediatric heart transplantation has matured considerably and is now an established treatment for children with CHD and heart failure unresponsive to other therapy. The indications for pediatric cardiac transplantation continue to evolve; however donor organ availability remains the major limiting factor.[200,201] Improved graft and child survival, fewer side effects, and an improved quality of life are the result of advancements in immunosuppression coupled with a better understanding of rejection. Unfortunately, infection, rejection, and posttransplant neoplasia continue to be the major causes of death.

DEMOGRAPHICS AND EPIDEMIOLOGY

Cardiac transplantation is a valuable treatment option for a broad range of causes of pediatric heart failure. The distribution of pediatric heart transplant recipients by age has remained stable for over 20 years with approximately 24% of the pediatric recipients younger than 1 year of age, 23% between 1 and 5 years, 15% between 6 and 10 years, and 38% between 11 and 17 years (Fig. 31.5).[202] The most common indication for transplantation in children varies by age group. In infants younger than 1 year of age, the primary indication for cardiac transplantation is a severe structural congenital cardiac defect, and the secondary indication is cardiomyopathy.[202] Cardiomyopathies represent the most common indication for heart transplant in children between 1 and 17 years of age, whereas CHD represent a decreasing proportion with increasing age (Fig. 31.6).[202]

PATHOPHYSIOLOGY OF THE DISEASE

The key to safe perioperative management of children presenting for heart transplantation requires an understanding of the basic cardiac anatomy and pathophysiology. Many transplant recipients with CHD have underlying lesions that alter the balance between systemic and pulmonary blood flow. The hemodynamic effects that accompany normal anesthetic management can radically alter this balance and thereby result in the recipient's deterioration. Other recipients have marginal CO secondary to their underlying myopathies or structural defects that hinder normal myocardial function.

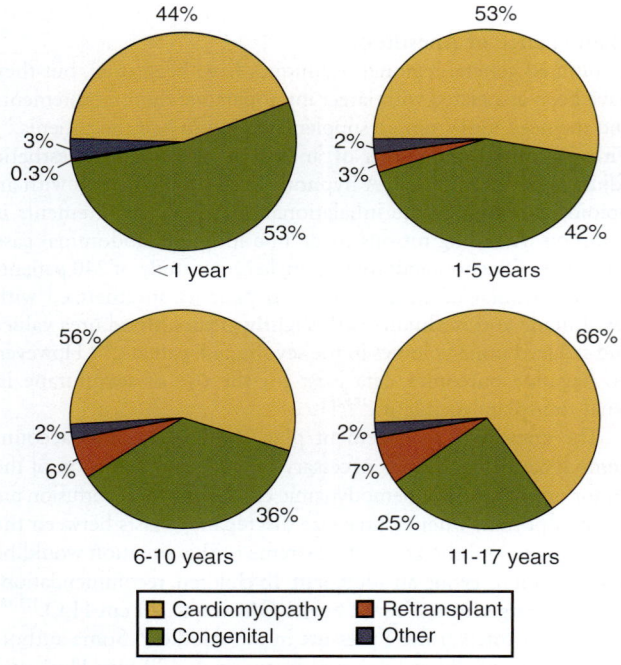

FIGURE 31.6 Diagnosis in pediatric heart transplant recipients by age group. (Figure 3 from Dipchand AI, Rossano JW, Edwards LB. The Registry of the International Society for Heart and Lung Transplantation: Eighteenth Official Pediatric Heart Transplantation Report—2015; focus theme: early graft failure. *J Heart Lung Transplant.* 2015;34[10]:1233–1243.)

CONGENITAL HEART DISEASE

This group of children includes those with complex lesions for which no option for palliation exists, children with end-stage heart failure after surgical repair of congenital heart defects, children with failed palliation for single-ventricle physiology (Fontan type), and neonates with hypoplastic left heart syndrome (HLHS). This population of patients is growing in incidence at U.S. centers that perform large-volume heart transplants, which are defined as those performing greater than 10 pediatric heart transplants per year.[202] Patients with CHD that undergo transplantation may have undergone surgical palliation with successful early results. They present later in life with dilated cardiomyopathies secondary to long-standing valvular regurgitation, ventricular outflow tract obstruction, or dysrhythmias. The majority of these children have single-ventricle physiology and are referred to as "failing the Fontan" procedure.[203-207] Although the right ventricle has been shown to be capable of adapting to work as the "systemic" ventricle in cases of HLHS or in children who have undergone an "atrial-type" switch operation for transposition of the great vessels, systemic right ventricles fail with time and develop both systolic and diastolic dysfunction. Transplantation is indicated in these children when they have acute decompensated heart failure refractory to medical therapy and not amenable to other reparative surgery or palliation.

DILATED CARDIOMYOPATHY

Dilated cardiomyopathy is the most common cardiomyopathy and reason for heart transplantation in children. The etiology is often unknown, but causes include infectious, drug-induced, ischemic, metabolic (disorders of fatty acid, amino acid, glycogen and mucopolysaccharide metabolism), or neuromuscular/genetic/mitochondrial disorders.[208,209] Dilated cardiomyopathy is characterized by systolic dysfunction and ventricular dilation with signs and symptoms of congestive heart failure. Predictors of poor outcome include a family history of cardiomyopathy, syncope, ventricular arrhythmia, left ventricular end-diastolic pressure greater than 25 mm Hg, and left ventricular ejection fraction less than 30%.

HYPERTROPHIC CARDIOMYOPATHY

Hypertrophic cardiomyopathy is a concentric thickening of the left ventricular wall not caused by a downstream obstruction that can lead to both a fixed and a dynamic obstruction to left ventricular outflow (see Chapter 16). A large septal muscular prominence can lead to mitral regurgitation secondary to abnormal systolic anterior motion of the mitral valve leaflets. The majority of hypertrophic cardiomyopathy is idiopathic (>70%), whereas inborn errors of metabolism (e.g., Pompe disease), malformation syndromes (e.g., Noonan, Beckwith-Wiedemann syndromes), and children with neuromuscular disorders account for the remainder.[210] Those who present as infants with hypertrophic cardiomyopathy have the worst outcome. If there is evidence of obstruction, more than 25% of infants will manifest congestive heart failure with symptoms of a failure to thrive and feeding intolerance. Risk factors for sudden death include a family history of sudden death,[211,212] marked concentric left ventricular wall thickness, age at presentation, and a smaller fractional shortening z score.[213] The indication for transplantation is a progression to dilated or restrictive cardiomyopathy.

RESTRICTIVE CARDIOMYOPATHY

Restrictive cardiomyopathies are uncommon disorders with generally poor prognoses that are associated with infiltration of the myocardium, such as glycogen storage disease, amyloidosis, mucopolysaccharidosis, hemochromatosis, sickle cell disease,[214] and sarcoidosis. Myocardial infiltration results in diastolic dysfunction and diminished stroke output. Endocardial fibroelastosis also causes a restrictive cardiomyopathy and an increased pulmonary vascular resistance (PVR).[215,216] The increased PVR is secondary to an increased left ventricular end-diastolic pressure with associated increases in pulmonary arterial pressure. The poor survival rates after diagnosis of restrictive cardiomyopathy prompt early consideration for transplantation.[217]

REPEAT TRANSPLANTATION

Repeat transplantation is not common in pediatrics, representing only 3.6% of all transplants in 2013[202]; the median age for retransplant is ~10 years after the primary transplant.[218] The indications for cardiac retransplantation are for patients with at least moderate graft vasculopathy with or without abnormal ventricular function.[200] Overall survival is less compared with primary transplantation.[219]

CONTRAINDICATIONS

Contraindications to pediatric cardiac transplantation include multiple severe congenital anomalies, marked prematurity (<36 weeks), low birth weight (<2 kg), ectopia cordis, diffuse pulmonary artery hypoplasia, pulmonary venous hypoplasia, active malignancy, active infection, severe metabolic disease, and irreversible noncardiac end-organ damage. These contraindications are considered by some to be relative, rather than absolute, contraindications to cardiac transplantation. For instance, combined heart/liver, heart/lung, heart/kidney transplants are not uncommonly performed,[220,221] whereas advances in HIV treatment have led to the consideration of transplantation in HIV-positive patients.[200,222] PVR, and the potential reversibility of an elevated PVR, is usually assessed during cardiac catheterization. Although the upper limit of PVR associated with successful cardiac transplantation has not been established in children, most centers generally limit transplantation to those with a PVR less than 6 Wood units/m^2 or a transpulmonary pressure gradient of 15 mm Hg or less.[223] Some centers accept an increased PVR; however, it is understood that there is a greater risk of early mortality from right ventricular failure.[224,225] Finally, severe psychosocial problems that may impede proper postoperative care, the lack of reliable caretakers, and an unstable family structure are critical factors in the decision to offer transplantation as a treatment option.

WAIT-LIST AND DONOR SELECTION

The wait-list mortality rate for pediatric heart transplant recipients was 17% in the United States between 1999 and 2006.[226] Infants experience the greatest wait-list mortality with risk factors that include weight less than 3 kg, high level of invasive support, and children with CHD requiring prostaglandin infusion.[227] Several attempts to decrease the wait-list time and mortality implemented in July 2016 by UNOS and OPTN included redefining the criteria for pediatric heart status 1A and 1B criteria, as well as criteria and allocation priority for ABO-incompatible (ABOi) heart transplants.[223] The immaturity of the infant immune system and the lack of production of ABO antibodies during the first 3 to 6 months of life provide a unique opportunity for ABOi heart transplantation. Multiple studies have documented similar survival and freedom from rejection similar to ABO-compatible donors;[229] ABOi heart transplantation has succeeded in reducing wait-list time mortality in Canada,[230] but this result has not yet been documented in the United States.[227,231] In an effort to increase infant donor heart utilization, UNOS/OPTN changed the isohemagglutinin titer to 1:16 from 1:4 or less for status 1A/1B candidates who are 1 year or older but registered before their second birthday.

Donor selection for pediatric heart transplantation is often complicated by difficult social settings associated with the death of the donor. The increasing frequency of donation after circulatory determination of death also creates a potentially controversial mechanism to increase the donor pool.[232,233] Donor size is also an important factor to consider in pediatric cardiac transplantation. Donor-to-recipient weight ratios up to 3.0 have been used successfully. In a comparison with more equally matched donor/recipient weight ratios, children who received hearts from oversized donors had no differences in ICU ventilator days, fractional shortening as assessed by echocardiography, ability to close the chest, or duration of inotropic support.[234] In contrast to the use of oversized donor organs, undersized donor organs were associated with an increased rate of donor organ failure. Recipient PVR is a major determinant for appropriate donor selection, and larger donor hearts should be considered for those with increased PVR to permit the right ventricle to compensate for the increased afterload.[235] Myocardial preservation of the donor organ is aimed at minimizing the ischemia time. Ischemic times of 6 hours were thought to be ideal, but pediatric allograft ischemic times have been extended to 8 hours with few adverse consequences.[236,237]

PREOPERATIVE EVALUATION

A comprehensive, multidisciplinary evaluation of a potential cardiac allograft recipient is required to determine the recipient's suitability for transplantation. This evaluation includes an assessment of the child's underlying cardiopulmonary, hepatic, renal, neurologic, infectious disease, and immune system status, as well as socioeconomic and psychosocial function (Table 31.4).

Assessment of cardiopulmonary function usually begins with a thorough history with attention to exercise tolerance, oxygen requirements, and need for diuretics and inotropic support. Examination of the ECG, chest radiographs, echocardiograms, and Holter monitors may be helpful in the discovery of pleural or pericardial effusions, conduction disturbances, cardiac function, and arrhythmias. Radionuclide angiography may be useful in defining systemic ventricular dysfunction in children with complex cardiac morphology. The pretransplant assessment ultimately includes cardiac catheterization with angiography. The anatomy and hemodynamics of the recipient must be carefully delineated because these factors influence anesthetic management, surgical donor harvesting, and recipient transplant technique. For instance, in children with unrepaired HLHS, the donor harvest team must harvest a large segment of donor aorta to facilitate reconstruction of the recipient aorta. Determination of the pulmonary vascular resistance index (PVRI), transpulmonary gradient (TPG), and reactivity of the pulmonary vascular bed to pharmacologic manipulation is crucial to the assessment of suitability for cardiac transplant:

$$PVRI\ (units/m^2) = PAP\ (mm\ Hg) - PAWP\ (mm\ Hg)/CI\ (L/min/m^2)$$

$$TPG\ (mm\ Hg) = PAP\ (mm\ Hg) - PAWP\ (mm\ Hg),$$

where PAP is the mean pulmonary artery pressure, PAWP is the mean pulmonary artery wedge pressure, and CI is the cardiac index.

An endomyocardial biopsy can identify acute myocarditis and myocardial infiltrates. Pulmonary function studies may be useful in older children with chronic lung disease.

Laboratory evaluation should include serum electrolytes, complete blood cell count with differential, coagulation profile,

TABLE 31.4	Routine Pre–Cardiac Transplant Evaluation
History and Physical Examination	
Age, height, weight, body surface area	
Diagnoses	
Medical history	
Medications	
Allergies	
Immunization record	
Laboratory Data	
Liver and kidney function studies	
Urinalysis	
Glomerular filtration rate	
Prothrombin time/partial thromboplastin time/INR, platelet count	
Complete blood cell count with differential	
PPD skin test	
Serologies for HIV, hepatitis, cytomegalovirus, Epstein-Barr virus, toxoplasmosis, syphilis	
ABO type	
Panel reactive antibody	
Cardiomyopathy Workup	
Thyroid function studies	
Blood lactate, pyruvate, ammonia, acyl carnitine	
Urine organic acids, acyl carnitine	
Skeletal muscle biopsy	
Karyotype	
Cardiopulmonary Data	
Electrocardiogram	
Chest radiograph	
Echocardiogram	
Radionuclide angiography	
Cardiac catheterization	
Endomyocardial biopsy	
Pulmonary function studies	
Oxygen consumption	
Psychosocial Evaluation	
History of abuse or neglect	
Parental substance abuse	
Long-term supportive care and reliability of caregivers	
Possible relocation	
Consultations as Needed	
Dental services	
Social services	
Other	

INR, international normalized ratio; *PPD*, purified protein derivative.
Adapted from Boucek MM, Shaddy RE: Pediatric heart transplantation. In: Allen HD, Gutgesell HP, Clark EB, et al, eds. *Moss and Adams' Heart Disease in Infants, Children, and Adolescents Including the Fetus and Young Adult.* 6th ed. Philadelphia: Lippincott Williams & Wilkins; 2001:295–407.

viral titers for possible latent viral infections such as cytomegalovirus (CMV) and EBV, and metabolic or genetic workups. Donor matching is based on ABO typing, although transplantation of ABOi hearts is an increasingly used option in infants[238,239] and is also being offered to older children.[240,241] The use of triple-volume exchange transfusions also minimizes the potential reaction to maternally transmitted preformed ABO antibodies.[242]

The recipient's blood is also screened for antibodies against sera of random blood donors and, if reactive, a serum crossmatch with the donor may be performed. Panel reactive antibodies are preformed circulating human leukocyte antigen (HLA) alloantibodies that, in high titers, are associated with diminished graft survival.[243-245] These antibodies arise from the use of homograft material in CHD patients and homologous blood products; thus blood products should be avoided if possible in the pretransplant period. HLA antibodies are divided into complement-fixing and non–complement-fixing antibodies, with complement-fixing antibodies more likely involved with acute allograft antibody-mediated rejection.[246] The C1q single-antigen bead (SAB) assay is a useful tool to detect only complement-fixing antibodies.[247] The presence of C1q SAB-positive donor-specific antibodies correlates with antibody-mediated rejection.[248] Treatments to reduce panel reactive antibodies have included IV immunoglobulin, cyclophosphamide, and plasmapheresis.[249] Rituximab, an anti-CD20 antibody that targets B-cells, and bortezomib, a proteasome inhibitor directed against plasma cells, can be used to reduce circulating antibodies.[250,251]

The mean time from listing for transplant to actual surgery is about 3 months but varies with the child's age, blood group, and list status. UNOS has developed allocation procedures that give priority to the most urgently ill children (Table 31.5). Status 1A patients are the most ill, and are either supported by continuous mechanical ventilation, have ductal-dependent circulation, with CHD requiring IV inotrope, or any child who requires the assistance of a mechanical circulatory support device. Status 1B patients do not qualify for pediatric status 1A but require an infusion of one or more inotropic agents or they are less than 1 year old with a diagnosis of hypertrophic or restrictive cardiomyopathy. Medical stabilization while on the wait-list frequently includes the use of diuretics, inotropic agents, arrhythmia therapy, oxygen or subatmospheric oxygen, and mechanical ventilation if warranted. β-Blockade therapy (carvedilol) is also used in the management of children with dilated cardiomyopathy and chronic heart failure.[252,253] Those with severe chamber enlargement, arrhythmias, and low

CO may require systemic anticoagulation to prevent thrombus formation and systemic embolization. Implantable defibrillators have been effective in children large enough for these devices, and biventricular pacing is showing promise as well.[254,255]

Children with end-stage myocardial failure will require mechanical circulatory support as a bridge to transplantation (see Chapter 21). The proportion of children bridged to transplant from mechanical circulatory support has steadily increased from 22% in 2005 to 34% in 2013.[202] Extracorporeal membrane oxygenation (ECMO) remains a time-limited bridge to transplant, whereas ventricular assist devices (VADs) such as the Berlin Heart EXCOR (Berlin Heart GmbH, Berlin, Germany) in infants allows for more prolonged support with fewer complications. The Berlin EXCOR regulatory database shows a median duration of support of 40 days, with 75% survival at 12 months.[256] Intracorporeal continuous flow devices such as the HeartMate II (Thoratec, Pleasanton, CA) and HeartWare HVAD (HeartWare Systems, Framingham, MA) are used for adolescents and larger children. The use of these mechanical circulatory support devices has improved survival on the wait-list; however, sepsis, neurologic injury, bleeding, and thromboembolic events are also serious complications of mechanical circulatory support.[257,258] Transplantation from ECMO continues to be associated with perioperative and early posttransplant mortality; however, children with transplantation from mechanical circulatory support devices such as a VAD have survival similar to those undergoing transplantation without mechanical circulatory support.[202,259]

CHD is the primary indication for cardiac transplantation in infants younger than 1 year of age, and many of these recipients will have HLHS. The patency of the ductus arteriosus must be maintained with prostaglandin E_1 initially as a continuous infusion and perhaps by stenting the ductus in the catheterization laboratory later if a suitable donor organ is not found. Alteration of flow across the atrial septal defect can be addressed as well by the interventional cardiologist (see Chapter 22). If the balance between systemic and pulmonary blood flow cannot be managed medically, pulmonary artery banding may be necessary to reduce pulmonary over-circulation while waiting for a donor organ.

SURGICAL TECHNIQUE

The original orthotopic technique devised by Lower and Shumway in adults was popular for many years in pediatric cases when the anatomy was straightforward.[260] This technique avoided individual systemic and pulmonary venous anastomoses by leaving a large cuff of right and left atrial recipient tissue behind and anastomosing the donor right and left atria to these cuffs. The resulting atrial chambers were a combination of donor and recipient atria that contracted asynchronously. Because the atrial contribution to CO may be augmented with total cardiac transplantation, most centers have converted to the "bicaval" technique with a modification to use the standard left atrial anastomosis.[261-263] This technique improves sinus node function, causes less tricuspid regurgitation, and improves exercise tolerance.[264,265]

Cardiac transplantation in children with CHD may require surgery of greater complexity involving reconstruction of the great vessels or alterations in venous anastomoses. It is important that the donor-harvesting team understand the recipient's anatomy and the potential harvest needs that may require large portions of aorta, pulmonary arteries, and venae cavae. In children with HLHS who require aortic arch reconstruction, deep hypothermic circulatory arrest may be necessary.[266-268]

The recipient is placed on cardiopulmonary bypass (CPB) after median sternotomy with aortic and bicaval cannulation.

TABLE 31.5	OPTN/UNOS Heart Allocation Policy

Pediatric Status 1A Requirements

1. Continuous mechanical ventilation and admitted to the hospital where the candidate is registered
2. Assistance of an intraaortic balloon pump and admitted to the hospital where the candidate is registered
3. Ductal dependent pulmonary or systemic circulation, with ductal patency maintained by stent or prostaglandin infusion and admitted to the hospital where the candidate is registered
4. Congenital heart disease diagnosis, requiring infusion of multiple intravenous inotropes or a high dose of a single intravenous inotrope, and admitted to the transplant hospital where the candidate is registered
5. Assistance of a mechanical circulatory support device

Pediatric Status 1B Requirements

1. Infusion of one or more inotropic agents but does not qualify for pediatric status 1A
2. Less than 1 year old at the time of the candidate's initial registration and has a diagnosis of hypertrophic or restrictive cardiomyopathy

Cannulation may be modified depending on the cardiac anatomy encountered. The aorta is cross-clamped, and both the aorta and the pulmonary artery are divided at the level of their semilunar valves. The superior and inferior vena cavae are transected, preserving a cuff of atrial tissue on each to facilitate the anastomoses. The interatrial groove is prepared, and an encircling left atriotomy is performed and the recipient heart is removed from the field. The donor organ is prepared and brought to the field. The left atrial anastomosis is completed first, followed by the aortic anastomosis. A vent is placed in the left ventricular cavity for decompression and evacuation of air as the caval anastomoses are completed while the child is rewarming. The cross-clamp is removed, and the donor heart is reperfused while the pulmonary arterial anastomosis is completed. Ventilation is resumed, and the child is separated from CPB after return of cardiac function is documented by TEE. Epicardial pacing wires are placed, mediastinal drainage tubes are positioned, and the chest is closed.

INTRAOPERATIVE PROBLEMS AND MANAGEMENT

Some children listed for cardiac transplantation may be hemodynamically stable and living at home. In these children, preoperative fasting and NPO status may be an issue when a donor organ becomes available. The anesthesiologist must carefully assess the relative risks of a full stomach compared with the potential complications associated with an unexpected difficult airway in a child undergoing a rapid-sequence induction. It is equally likely that the pediatric recipient is hospitalized and requires a host of treatments designed to promote hemodynamic stability while a donor organ is sought. These children have minimal cardiovascular reserve. Anesthetic agents, positive-pressure ventilation, and surgical stress frequently result in hemodynamic instability. Anesthetic preparation should include the immediate availability of a variety of medications for the perioperative manipulation of myocardial function and hemodynamics. Vasoactive drugs and inotropic agents such as epinephrine, phenylephrine, dopamine, dobutamine, isoproterenol, milrinone, nitroprusside, and nitroglycerin should be readily available.[269] For children with underlying CHD, the anesthesiologist needs to understand the child's underlying pathophysiology. The anesthetic management before CPB is similar to that for nontransplant cardiac surgery. For children with end-stage myocardial dysfunction, the sympathetic nervous system is chronically activated with downregulation of the cardiac β_1-receptors and an impaired response to β-agonists.[270] Reduced renal perfusion (reduced filtration) stimulates the renin-angiotensin system, leading to increases in vasoconstriction, venoconstriction, and increased intravascular volume. These compensatory changes further aggravate the congestive heart failure by increasing preload and afterload. A dysfunctional, dilated myocardium is very sensitive to changes in preload, afterload, heart rate, and contractility. Both systolic and diastolic myocardial function are impaired, and a high mean atrial pressure is needed to ensure adequate ventricular filling volume. Increasing heart rate results in a decreased diastolic filling time and, therefore, a diminution in stroke volume because of the poor systolic and diastolic ventricular function, atrial pressure increase, and atrial enlargement. There is a loss of preload reserve, resulting in CO becoming more dependent on the heart rate. Finally, small increases in afterload result in an increased end-systolic volume, decreased stroke output, and a further decrease in CO. Naturally, dysrhythmias are poorly tolerated in these children.

Coordination of the arrival of the child to the operating room with the donor team ensures the briefest possible ischemic time for the donor organ. Premedication is best administered under monitored conditions. If the child was receiving supplemental oxygen, it should be continued during the preinduction period. Before induction, monitoring devices such as ECG, noninvasive blood pressure cuff, and pulse oximeter are applied. Meticulous airway management is critical because hypoxemia and hypercarbia may alter PVR and further depress CO. A wide variety of anesthetic agents have been used depending on the nature of the cardiac disease and the risk of pulmonary aspiration. After induction, invasive monitoring does not differ from that used during routine pediatric cardiac open-heart surgery. Some centers avoid right internal jugular vein cannulation because that vessel may be repeatedly accessed for posttransplant endomyocardial biopsy. TEE is useful to assess graft function, mechanical issues, and pulmonary hypertension. In children, TEE has been shown to be cost-effective and clinically useful.[271] Many experienced centers do not use pulmonary artery catheters routinely because the value of the information gained does not warrant the additional risk. In children who have undergone multiple cardiac operations, the potential risks of reoperation should be addressed and include the need for adequately sized vascular catheters, the availability of blood products and a rapid transfusion device in the operating room, the preparation for alternate cannulation sites, and the use of antifibrinolytics. The use of ultrafiltration during CPB may be beneficial by removing free water, hemoconcentrating the red blood cells and coagulation factors, and modulating the inflammatory response.[272–277]

Anesthesia is generally maintained with opioids, benzodiazepines, isoflurane, and a nondepolarizing neuromuscular blocking drug.[269] In children with CHD, this anesthetic technique preserves CO better than some inhalational agents, provided the heart rate is maintained.[278] In the preparation for termination of CPB, it is critical that the hemodynamics are optimized. A stable cardiac rhythm and acceptable heart rate are desirable. Chronotropic support using IV therapy with β-adrenergic agents such as epinephrine or the use of epicardial pacing may be needed to maintain an appropriate heart rate between 120 and 150 beats/minute. The denervated transplanted heart does not respond in the normal fashion to hypotension. Medications with indirect cardiac effects such as atropine, glycopyrrolate, or ephedrine will likewise be ineffective. Direct-acting medications such as dopamine, dobutamine, epinephrine, or isoproterenol are required if inotropic or chronotropic support is needed (Table 31.6).[279] Some children benefit from vasodilator infusions to improve left ventricular stroke volume and CO.[280] The use of inotropic agents to separate from CPB and provide early postoperative stability is common, and the choices are based largely on the perceived balances between pulmonary and systemic vascular resistance and myocardial dysfunction to blood pressure and CO.[269] Ventilation should be managed to ensure mild respiratory alkalosis and adequate oxygenation. Factors that potentially increase PVR such as hypothermia, acidosis, hypercarbia, hypoxemia, increased adrenergic tone secondary to light anesthesia, and polycythemia should be eliminated. Children with increased PAP before bypass show a greater response to ventilatory changes than those without increased PAP. In addition, children with CHD and associated pulmonary hypertension may develop severe pulmonary hypertension in response to hypoxemia.[281–283] The narrow range of afterload that the donor right ventricle is capable of handling is critical; if success in managing the pulmonary hypertension with conservative methods fails, more aggressive pharmacotherapy is warranted. The use of prostaglandin, prostacyclin, nitroglycerin, high-dose milrinone, calcium channel blockers, sildenafil, and inhaled NO

TABLE 31.6 | Properties of Vasoactive Drugs After Heart Transplantation

Drug	Peripheral Vasoconstriction	Cardiac Contractility	Peripheral Vasodilation	Chronotropic Effect	Arrhythmia Risk
Isoproterenol	0	++++	+++	++++	++++
Dobutamine	0	+++	++	+	+
Dopamine	++	+++	+	+	+
Epinephrine	+++	++++	+	++	+++
Milrinone	0	+++	+	++	++
Norepinephrine	++++	+++	0	+	+
Phenylephrine	++++	0	0	0	0
Vasopressin	++++	0	0	0	0

Modified from Costanzo MR, Dipchand A, Starling R, et al. The International Society of Heart and Lung Transplantation guidelines for the care of heart transplant recipients. *J Heart Lung Transplant*. 2010;29(8):914–956.

(iNO) have all been effective in treating pulmonary hypertension in children (see Chapter 18).[284–296] In extreme cases, mechanical assist devices or ECMO have been used (see Chapter 21).[297,298]

Dysrhythmias may be common in the postbypass period and, depending on the technique of implantation, there may be two independent P waves on the ECG, one from the recipient sinoatrial node and the other from the donor sinoatrial node. It is only the donor sinoatrial node that transmits impulses to the atrioventricular node and thus to the ventricle. The most common dysrhythmias are junctional rhythms, underscoring the utility of direct-acting β-agonists and epicardial atrioventricular sequential pacing. This denervated state results in the loss of the baroreceptor reflex, forcing CO to become primarily dependent on venous return and circulating catecholamines and thus unable to respond acutely to changes in the circulating blood volume and blood pressure.[299,300]

After separation from CPB, hemodynamic stabilization, and control of surgical bleeding, protamine sulfate is administered slowly to reverse anticoagulation. Risk factors for hypotension in children after protamine administration include female sex, larger protamine doses, and smaller heparin doses.[301] Transfusion of blood products should be guided by the balance of the need weighed against the associated risks of administration. Significant acid-base and electrolyte disturbances may be associated with large volume transfusions. These disturbances may be decreased by washing the cells before transfusion.[302–304] Donor blood should be screened for CMV and, ideally, CMV-negative recipients should receive blood screened negative for CMV.[305] Leukocyte reduction by filtration may be associated with a diminished risk of exposure to CMV through transfusion.[306,307] Another concern associated with transfusion in cardiac transplant recipients is the risk of transfusion-associated graft-versus-host disease (TAGVHD). This results from active T lymphocytes in the transfused blood of a recipient who is unable to reject them, such as a neonate, those undergoing chemotherapy, and the otherwise immunocompromised child.[308,309] To limit the risk of TAGVHD in cardiac transplant recipients, some centers routinely gamma-irradiate cellular blood products before administration. At recommended doses, gamma irradiation has an insignificant effect on platelet, red blood cell, or granulocyte function but it may increase the potassium concentrations (see Chapter 12).[310]

Transport of the child from the operating room proceeds as in any other open-heart procedure. In selected recipients with excellent allograft function and hemodynamics, extubation of the trachea is possible in the operating room or within a few hours

of arrival in the ICU. It is important that these children are comfortable but otherwise ventilating adequately to prevent atelectasis, hypoxemia, or hypercarbia that may increase PAP and thus strain the donor right ventricle. Sedative agents such as dexmedetomidine may facilitate early extubation in these children.[311] Other children may require sedation and mechanical ventilation because of hemodynamic instability or delayed sternal closure, particularly if a large donor-to-recipient size mismatch is present.

IMMEDIATE POSTOPERATIVE MANAGEMENT

Early postoperative management consists primarily of maintaining hemodynamic stability. Infusions and volume needs are adjusted to maintain an optimal balance of preload, afterload, CO, and peripheral perfusion. Attention should be directed toward maintaining normal acid-base and electrolyte balance. In some children, pulmonary hypertension remains a serious concern and management of sedation, ventilation, inotrope infusions, and pulmonary vasodilator administration is required to optimize right ventricular function. Ventilation modes may need to be adjusted to reduce the mean intrathoracic (airway) pressure. Additional approaches for management of right ventricular function are illustrated in Fig. 31.7. Renal dysfunction continues to be a major source of morbidity and mortality after cardiac transplantation; the UNOS database showed a 7% incidence of perioperative renal failure after pediatric heart transplants.[312] There was a significant risk for decreased posttransplant survival rates in children with posttransplant renal failure. Risk factors for developing posttransplant renal failure include the use of ECMO and the need for mechanical ventilation and inotropic support at the time of transplant listing. A peritoneal dialysis catheter placed during transplantation can be used to reduce ascites and improve ventilatory mechanics in those with right-sided heart dysfunction and in the treatment of renal insufficiency. Arrhythmias in the postoperative period may herald rejection.

Induction of immunosuppression can begin with corticosteroids, antithymocyte immunoglobulin, or IL-2 receptor antagonists. Induction therapy has increased from 59% of pediatric transplant patients during the years of 2004 to 2009 to 68% from 2009 to June 2014, although there is no evidence to support improved graft survival in primary pediatric heart transplantation with induction.[202] However, transplant recipients with panel reactive antibodies greater than 50% or with CHD were found to benefit from induction immunosuppression through improved survival.[313] Maintenance therapy is guided largely by institutional experience

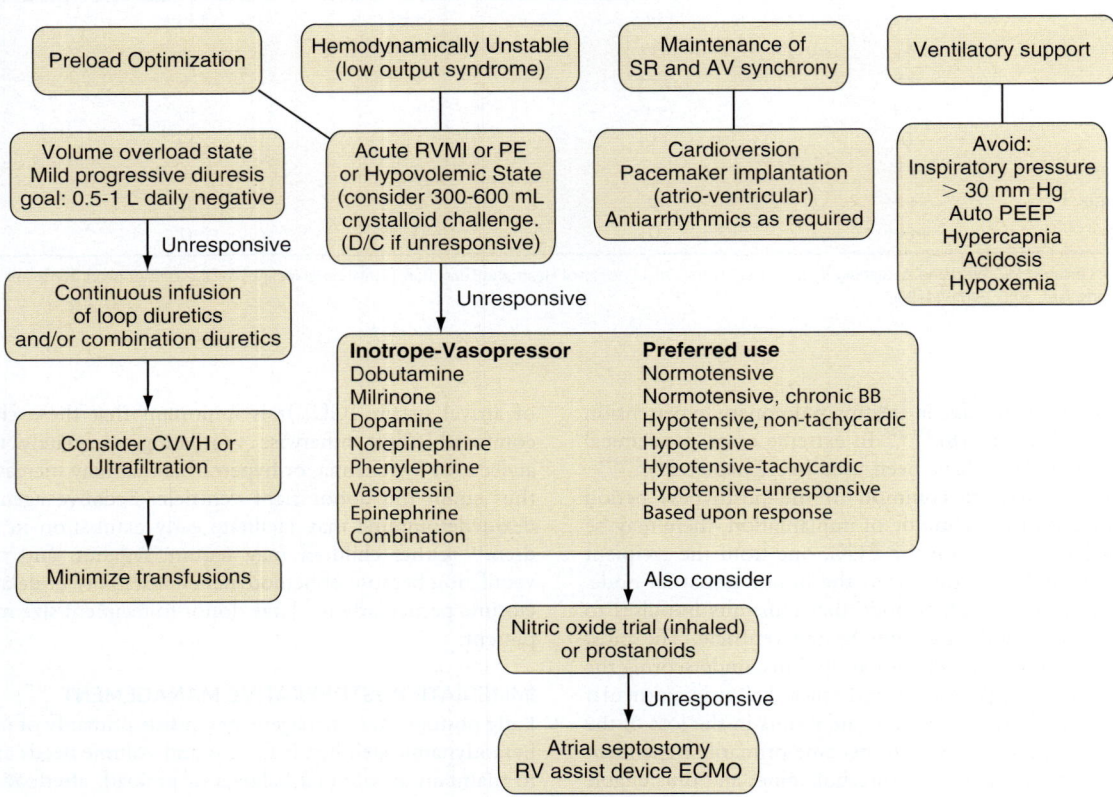

FIGURE 31.7 Management of right ventricular dysfunction. *AV*, atrioventricular; *BB*, beta blocker therapy; *CVVH*, continuous venovenous hemofiltration; *D/C*, discontinue; *ECMO*, extracorporeal membrane oxygenation; *MI*, myocardial infarction; *PE*, pulmonary embolism; *PEEP*, positive end-expiratory pressure; *RV*, right ventricular; *RVMI*, right ventricular myocardial infarction; *SR*, sinus rhythm. (Modified Figure 6 from Haddad F, Hunt SA, Rosenthal DN, Murphy DJ. Right ventricular function in cardiovascular disease, part II: pathophysiology, clinical importance, and management of right ventricular failure. *Circulation* 2008;117:1717–1731.)

and the recipient's clinical profile. The goal of maintenance therapy is to prevent acute and chronic rejection while minimizing the adverse effects of immunosuppression. All maintenance regimens involve a calcineurin phosphatase inhibitor (tacrolimus more commonly than cyclosporine) along with antiproliferative agents such as azathioprine or mycophenolate mofetil (CellCept). Corticosteroids may also be used, although most centers limit or avoid their long-term use. Sirolimus (rapamycin) is a macrolide antibiotic that acts synergistically with the calcineurin phosphatase inhibitors and can be used to reduce the dose of cyclosporine or tacrolimus. Sirolimus may also inhibit the process of coronary arteriopathy.[314]

First-line therapy for acute rejection is high-dose corticosteroids. Other agents, including monoclonal and polyclonal anti–T-lymphocyte antibodies, are reserved for refractory or recurrent severe acute rejection or rejection with severe hemodynamic compromise. Recurrent moderate rejection is usually controlled with modulation of the maintenance therapy dosing.[315]

Graft failure continues to remain the major cause of death after transplantation, with the greatest mortality risk in the first year post transplant (Table 31.7).[202] Fortunately, there has been a decline in early rejection in the more recent era, decreasing from

60% to only 40% in the first year after transplant.[316] Some studies suggest that transplant before 1 year of age offers protection from episodes of acute rejection and significantly greater freedom from rejection and time to first rejection.[317] Monitoring and diagnosis of allograft rejection remain a challenge. The clinical assessment includes nursing and parental accounts of changes in the child's activity and appetite, nausea, emesis, malaise, resting heart rate 15 to 20 beats/minute above normal, and presence of ectopy. Echocardiography plays a very important role in the postoperative follow-up, especially in neonates. These studies are performed frequently, especially in the first months after transplant. Acute changes in left ventricular end-diastolic dimension, posterior wall thickness, and shortening fraction are potential signs of acute rejection.[318] Endomyocardial biopsy remains the gold standard in the diagnosis of acute cardiac allograft rejection. It provides tissue for both precise documentation of the presence or absence of rejection and allows more accurate titration of immunosuppression to avoid the adverse effects of increased use of immunosuppression based on clinical and noninvasive examinations only. Biopsy specimens are also analyzed for signs of humoral and vascular rejection. The biopsy specimen is examined for evidence of lymphocytic accumulations in the graft interstitium and perivascular tissue, and in severe forms of cellular rejection, myocardial necrosis and polymorphonuclear cell infiltrates. Over time, it is also possible to develop chronic rejection, which is primarily a vasculopathy[319] that involves vascular inflammation with binding of IgG and/or IgM and complement. This produces a diffuse and concentric stenosis affecting the mid and distal coronary arteries and is often asymptomatic. Although annual coronary angiography is recommended, accelerated graft arteriosclerosis is underestimated angiographically.

SURVIVAL AND QUALITY OF LIFE

The survival of pediatric heart transplant recipients continues to improve. The overall median survival for pediatric heart transplant recipients is grouped by age at time of transplantation, with a median of 20.6 year for infants, 17.2 years for children with

transplants at 2 to 5 years of age, 13.9 years for children with transplants at 6 to 10 years of age, and 12.4 years for adolescents with transplants at 11 to 17 years of age (Fig. 31.8).[202] Mortality in the first year after the transplant is the greatest, so the median conditional survival after 1 year is even better (Fig. 31.9). The most common causes of death in the first year after transplant include graft failure (28%), multisystem organ failure (16.6%), acute rejection (12.2%), cerebrovascular event (9.1%), and non-CMV infection (8.5%) (see Table 31.7). By 10 years after transplant, graft failure and coronary artery vasculopathy account for the majority of mortality. Patients who had transplants for the diagnosis of CHD have a greater risk for mortality after transplantation compared with those with a diagnosis of cardiomyopathy (Fig. 31.10). Other risk factors for mortality in the first year after transplant include retransplant, pretransplant ECMO support, and pretransplant dialysis.[202]

Pediatric cardiac recipients often return to the operating room for noncardiac procedures. Preoperative evaluation requires an understanding of the unique features associated with the transplanted heart, such as its denervation, risk of vasculopathy (coronary artery disease), and arrhythmias.[269] The interaction of the immunosuppressive regimens with anesthetic agents and their association with hypertension and renal dysfunction are additional considerations. Medication and monitoring choice should be tailored to the individual needs of the child to minimize anesthetic morbidity. Most medically stable cardiac transplant patients can undergo routine noncardiac surgical procedures in a similar fashion to children without transplants (see Chapter 23). It is important to remember that reflex mechanisms are impaired in the denervated heart and changes as a result of light anesthesia, hypovolemia, or contractility will be delayed until circulating catecholamines can influence the cardiac β-receptors directly.[320,321] As cardiac transplant patients live longer, the risks of coronary vasculopathy increase, with coronary ischemia becoming a major concern. Therefore

TABLE 31.7	Risk Factors for 1-Year Mortality: Pediatric Heart Transplants (January 2002–December 2015)	
Cause of Death	**N (493)**	**Percent**
Graft failure	138	28
Multisystem organ failure	82	16.6
Acute rejection	60	12.2
Cerebrovascular event	45	9.1
Infection, non-CMV	42	8.5
Technical	20	8.5

CMV, cytomegalovirus.
Adapted from Dipchand AI, Rossano JW, Edwards LB. The Registry of the International Society for Heart and Lung Transplantation: Eighteenth Official Pediatric Heart Transplantation Report—2015; focus theme: early graft failure. *J Heart Lung Transplant.* 2015;34(10):1233–1243.)

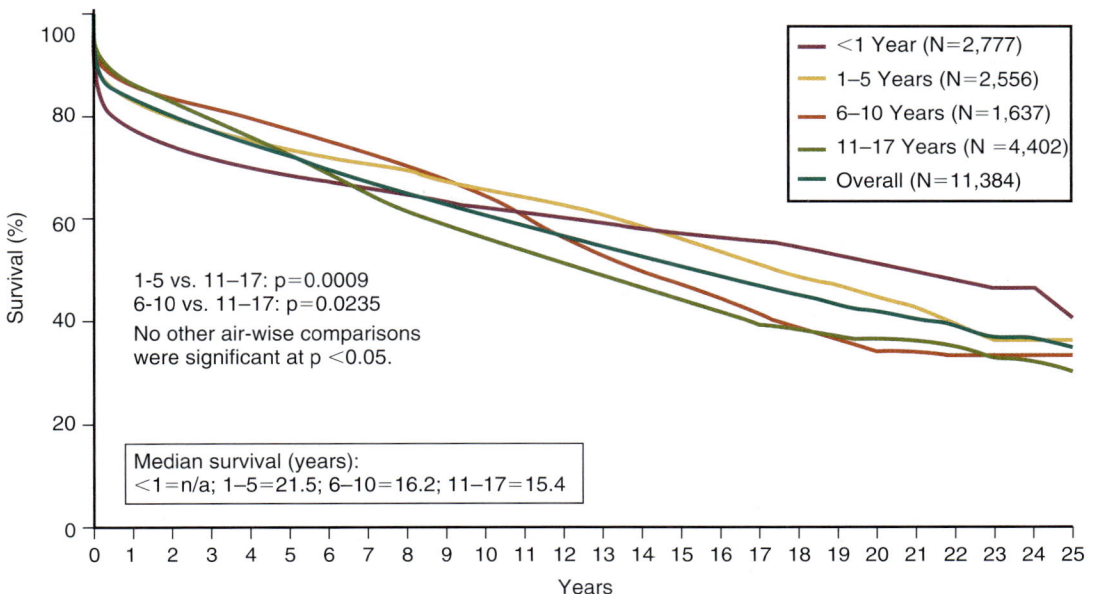

1-5 vs. 11–17: p=0.0009
6-10 vs. 11–17: p=0.0235
No other air-wise comparisons were significant at p <0.05.

Median survival (years):
<1=n/a; 1–5=21.5; 6–10=16.2; 11–17=15.4

Legend:
— <1 Year (N=2,777)
— 1–5 Years (N=2,556)
— 6–10 Years (N=1,637)
— 11–17 Years (N =4,402)
— Overall (N=11,384)

FIGURE 31.8 Survival curve for pediatric heart transplant recipients (Kaplan-Meier). *n/a,* not available. (Figure 9 from Dipchand AI, Rossano JW, Edwards LB. The Registry of the International Society for Heart and Lung Transplantation: Eighteenth Official Pediatric Heart Transplantation Report—2015; focus theme: early graft failure. *J Heart Lung Transplant.* 2015;34[10]:1233–1243.)

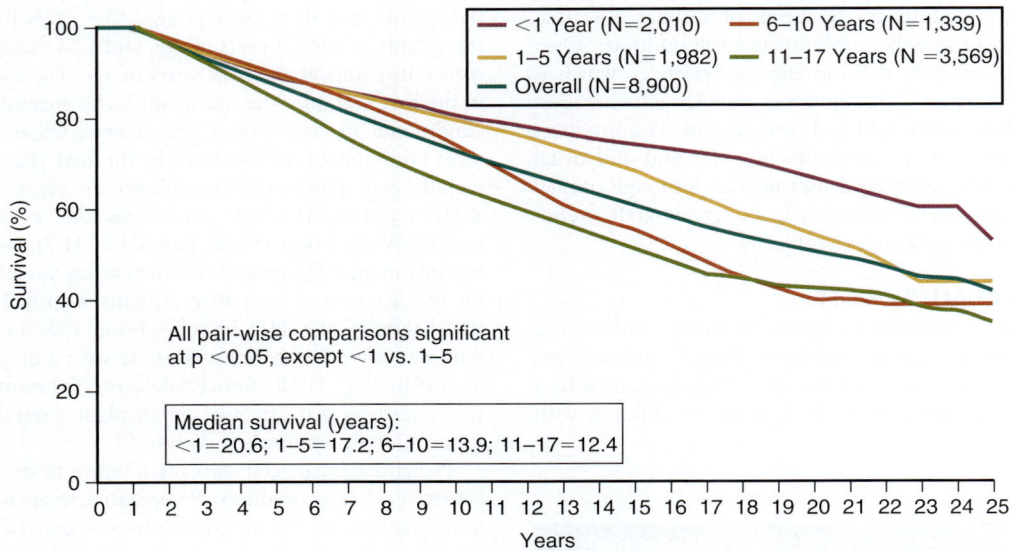

FIGURE 31.9 Conditional survival curve for pediatric heart transplant recipients (Kaplan-Meier). (Modified Figure 11 from Dipchand AI, Rossano JW, Edwards LB. The Registry of the International Society for Heart and Lung Transplantation: Eighteenth Official Pediatric Heart Transplantation Report—2015; focus theme: early graft failure. *J Heart Lung Transplant.* 2015;34[10]:1233–1243.)

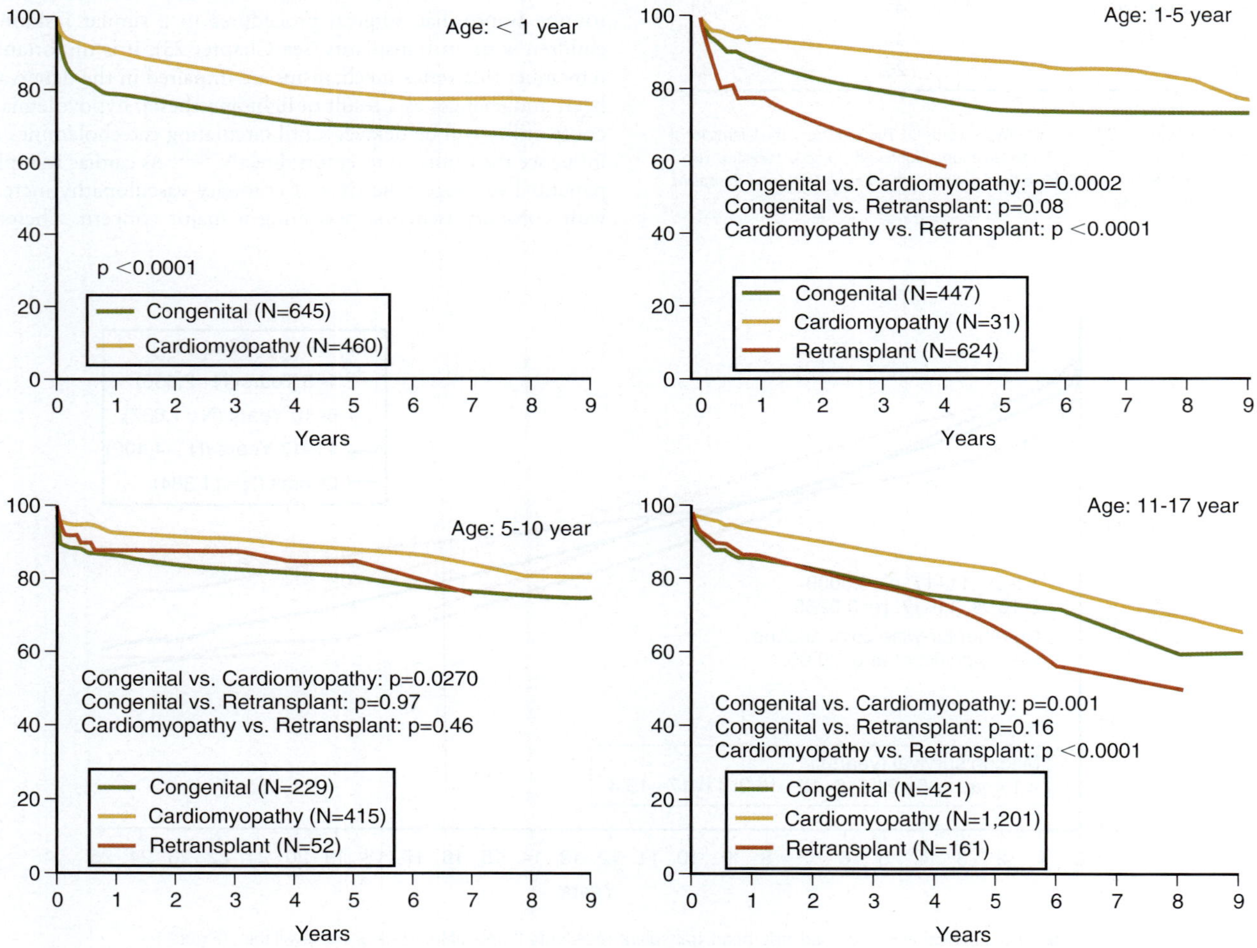

FIGURE 31.10 Survival by diagnosis for pediatric heart transplant recipients (Kaplan-Meier). (Figure 12 from Dipchand AI, Rossano JW, Edwards LB. The Registry of the International Society for Heart and Lung Transplantation: Eighteenth Official Pediatric Heart Transplantation Report—2015; focus theme: early graft failure. *J Heart Lung Transplant.* 2015;34[10]:1233–1243.)

attention to the maintenance of coronary perfusion is paramount. As in all immunocompromised patients, these children are vulnerable to infection, and strict adherence to aseptic and sterile technique is mandatory.

Pediatric Lung and Heart-Lung Transplantation

DEMOGRAPHICS AND EPIDEMIOLOGY

Pediatric lung and heart-lung transplant patients are similar and share many underlying disease management processes. These children, with end-stage pulmonary and cardiopulmonary disease, undergo a variety of pretransplant and posttransplant interventions and require special considerations in all phases of their anesthetic care. While the first adult lung transplant was performed in 1962, it was another two decades before pediatric lung and heart-lung transplantation occurred. Advances in surgical technique and immunosuppressive therapy ushered in the modern era of lung transplantation in the early 1980s. Lung and heart-lung transplantation became a well-accepted treatment for children with end-stage pulmonary and cardiopulmonary disease.[322] The first successful pediatric heart-lung transplant was performed at the Children's Hospital of Pittsburgh in 1985. Since 1988, there have been ~199 heart-lung transplants performed in the United States. Pediatric lung transplantation followed in Toronto in 1986. Since 1988, there have been 1237 lung transplants with over 1800 in adults and children performed in the United States.[323] In 2015, 23 hospitals performed 86 pediatric lung transplants and 5 centers performed 9 heart-lung transplants.[324]

Patients listed on all transplant waiting lists continually exceed donor supply. Donor identification and management are more selective for heart-lung and lung transplant candidates compared with donors for isolated heart transplants. Thoracic capacity of the lung donor should not be greater than that of the recipient because the mismatch increases risk of postoperative atelectasis and infections in the transplanted lungs.[325] While the trend is an increase in organ donations, donor supply remains the largest obstacle in transplantation. As many as one-third of children listed die before receiving lung transplantation. Patients aged 12 to 17 years have the greatest mortality of 19.7 per 100 transplant wait-list years.[326-328] The average waiting time for cadaveric lungs is 20 months for adolescents and 6 to 12 months for children younger than 2 years.

A variety of strategies, including television, radio, and print advertisements, have been used to increase donation. Everyone in the United States may declare themselves a potential donor when obtaining a driver's license. Some states (e.g., Pennsylvania) requires nurses to ask family members of patients whose wishes are not known at their time of death whether they consent for donation. Barriers to donation may fall with education. More often it takes a dramatic event, such as the death of Nicholas Green, a seven-year-old American shot in the head by a random act of violence and subsequently declared brain dead while vacationing in Italy in 1999, to effect change. Nicholas' parents donated his organs, saving seven Italian citizens. In the wake of the publicity of this tragedy and subsequent organ donations, signed organ donation cards in Italy quadrupled and donations tripled. Nicholas' father, as is common among donor families, found solace in helping others: *"There is some consolation with the process. It puts something on the other side of the balance. It will never bring my son back, but it can help somewhat with the grief."*[329]

PATHOPHYSIOLOGY OF THE DISEASE

The indication for lung and heart-lung transplantation is severe end-stage pulmonary disease for which there is no other medical treatment and a life expectancy less than 18 months. The listing criteria for the prospective transplant patient additionally include consideration of the functional status of the patient, the patient's hemodynamic parameters, and the natural history of the underlying disease. Most pediatric lung transplant patients are between 11 and 17 years old, although there is a smaller subset of children younger than 2 years of age.[330] The most common underlying disease in the older pediatric lung transplantation is cystic fibrosis. Cystic fibrosis accounts for nearly half of all pediatric lung transplants. Ninety-five percent of nontransplanted patients with cystic fibrosis will eventually die from pulmonary causes. Factors associated with a less than 50% expected survival for the patient with cystic fibrosis include an FEV_1 less than 30%, PaO_2 less than 55 mm Hg, or a $PaCO_2$ greater than 50 mm Hg.[331] Pulmonary vascular disease accounts for nearly a quarter of the remaining transplants. Infants requiring transplantation most often have a variety of relatively rare diseases, such as surfactant B deficiency, primary alveolar proteinosis, or pulmonary vascular disease (Table 31.8).[332] These infants are often severely ill at the time of their transplants and are frequently intubated and ventilated or on ECMO support.[333,334] Independent risks for mortality after lung transplant include repeat transplant, mechanical ventilation at time of transplant,[332] and CHD.[335,336] Primary contraindications for lung transplantation are (1) active malignant disease within the prior 2 years, (2) significant active infectious processes (including HIV and hepatitis B and C), (3) significant coexisting cardiac disease, (4) hepatic or renal disease (although these patients may be candidates for multiple-organ transplants), (5) collagen vascular disease, (6) major irreversible neurologic injury, and (7) patient or family history of poor medical compliance or severe psychiatric illness that would preclude the patient from effective posttransplant care. Relative contraindications include (1) significant musculoskeletal disease, (2) invasive ventilation, (3) colonization with atypical mycobacterium or fungi, (4) poor nutritional status (body mass index [BMI] at either extreme), and (5) inability to reduce dependency on corticosteroids. A lung allocation score is calculated for each patient on the waiting list who is 12 years or older.[337] The score is based on the individual patient's age, underlying illness, forced vital capacity, functional status, and need for supplemental oxygen.[338] UNOS also includes ABO compatibility and distance between the donor and the recipient in its considerations for organ allocation.

UNOS adopted a new allocation system for children younger than 12 years of age in 2012. There are now two distinct priority levels, with the most ill children given a priority 1 ranking. Priority 1 candidates have respiratory failure requiring continuous mechanical ventilation, a fractional inspired oxygen (FiO_2) greater than 0.5 to maintain arterial oxygen saturation levels of more than 90%, an arterial or capillary PCO_2 of more than 50 mm Hg, or a venous PCO_2 of more than 56 mm Hg and/or significant pulmonary hypertension despite medical therapy. Children not meeting the above conditions are listed as priority 2. Donor lungs are first allocated to the priority 1 candidate longest on the waiting list who matches the donor's blood type and size. If there is no suitable priority 1 candidate, the lungs are then offered to the priority 2 candidate with the most waiting time.

Donor sources include organs from brain dead individuals, non-heart-beating donors (NHBD), and LDs. Donor care is critical. For lung donation, the donor should have been intubated

31

TABLE 31.8	Indications for Pediatric Lung Transplants by Age Group (Transplants January 2000–June 2014)			
Diagnosis	**<1 year** N (%)	**1–5 years** N (%)	**6–10 years** N (%)	**11–17 years** N (%)
Cystic fibrosis	0 (0)	5 (5.7)	99 (50.5)	726 (69.1)
IPAH	7 (13.0)	19 (21.8)	20 (10.2)	83 (7.9)
Obliterative bronchiolitis				
Retransplant	0 (0)	4 (4.6)	6 (3.1)	33 (3.1)
No transplant	0 (0)	8 (9.2)	21 (10.7)	48 (4.6)
Congenital heart disease	8 (14.8)	7 (8.0)	3 (1.5)	8 (0.8)
Pulmonary fibrosis				
Idiopathic	4 (7.4)	11 (12.6)	8 (4.1)	29 (2.8)
Other	7 (13.0)	10 (11.5)	15 (7.7)	28 (2.7)
Retransplant, not obliterative bronchiolitis	0 (0)	4 (4.6)	3 (1.5)	24 (2.3)
Interstitial pneumonitis	0 (0)	2 (2.3)	2 (1.0)	1 (0.1)
Pulmonary vascular disease	2 (3.7)	5 (5.7)	2 (1.0)	1 (0.1)
Eisenmenger syndrome	0 (0)	1 (1.1)	1 (0.5)	4 (0.4)
Surfactant protein B deficiency	11 (20.4)	4 (4.6)	0 (0)	0 (0)
COPD/emphysema	0 (0)	0 (0)	0 (0)	0 (0)
Bronchopulmonary dysplasia	4 (7.4)	2 (2.3)	1 (0.5)	6 (0.6)
Bronchiectasis	0 (0)	0 (0)	0 (0)	14 (1.3)
Other	11 (20.4)	5 (5.7)	12 (6.1)	43 (4.1)

COPD, chronic obstructive pulmonary disease; *IPAH*, idiopathic pulmonary arterial hypertension.

less than 5 days to decrease the risk of lung injury, particularly ventilator-associated pneumonia. The donor should have no active infection and tracheal secretions must be void of infection. The donor should have either a PaO_2 greater than 300 mm Hg at an FIO_2 of 1.0 or greater than 100 mm Hg at an FIO_2 of 0.4 with an inflation pressure less than 30 cm H_2O, a tidal volume of 15 mL/kg, and a PEEP of 4. In anticipation of lung donation and lung protection, the donor is maintained euvolemic to slightly hypovolemic, with CVPs ranging from 8 to 10 mm Hg. Once harvested, the lungs are perfused with a preservative solution and prostaglandins. The lungs are inflated and the trachea stapled closed to maintain an inflated position. The organs are then transported to the recipient at a temperature of 4°C. Ischemic times of less than 8 hours are desired, while less than 3 to 4 hours is ideal.[339]

The NHBD for lung transplant is also another source for organ donations[340]; NHBDs are typically younger than traditional donors. Eleven centers have performed more than 300 adult and pediatric controlled NHBD lung transplants (withdrawal of support from ICU patients). One center has performed 29 adult and pediatric uncontrolled (out of ICU arrest) NHBD lung transplants.[341]

Living-related donation of adult lobes for transplantation into the child offers an additional organ donor source as well as elective transplant scheduling.[342,343] Inherent size mismatch limits use of this technique to children 5 years and older. Typically, the left lower lobe is harvested from one donor with the right lower lobe harvested from another donor. The harvest technique is similar to a lobectomy; however, the harvested lobes require an appropriate length of bronchus as well as adequate vascular pedicles. Donor morbidity is significant.[344]

PREOPERATIVE EVALUATION

Children listed for lung transplantation undergo an extensive workup that includes chest radiographs, pulmonary function tests, arterial blood gas, complete metabolic panel, ECG, and echocardiogram. Those with pulmonary hypertension and/or associated cardiac defects will also require cardiac catheterization to better define the anatomy and hemodynamic profile—specifically, PVR.

SURGICAL TECHNIQUE

Children most commonly receive bilateral lung transplants with the use of CPB[345–347] through a bilateral anterolateral transsternal "clamshell" incision. As much dissection as possible is carried out before instituting CPB. Bilateral bronchial anastomosis has been found to produce better results without the concern for tracheal stenosis. The most popular technique is the telescoping anastomosis in which the larger bronchus is telescoped several centimeters over the smaller bronchus portion with peribronchial tissue wrapped around the anastomosis to ensure blood supply, because bronchial blood supply is not reestablished. If the older end-to-end anastomosis technique is used, an omental wrap is placed around the suture line. The pulmonary artery is reanastomosed after the bronchus is reanastomosed. The pulmonary venous component of the donor lung includes an atrial cuff, which is sutured directly to the left atrium of the recipient. This avoids the complication of pulmonary vein stenosis. While donor lungs are selected for size match, occasionally lungs are too large and cannot be used in total without exposing the recipient to significant areas of atelectasis. In this instance, volume reduction of the donated lung is performed to remove areas prone to atelectasis.[348–351]

Single lung transplants are uncommon in children and are specifically avoided in cystic fibrosis patients to avoid soiling from the remaining diseased lung. If single lung transplantation is performed for a non–cystic fibrosis patient, the most diseased lung is transplanted. Additionally, if emphysematous changes are present, the most emphysematous lung is removed to decrease the risk of compression of the donor lung. Single lung transplants are most often performed without cardiopulmonary bypass. After anesthesia is induced, single lung ventilation is achieved, a thoracotomy is performed, and the bronchus and vessels are exposed. A test occlusion by the surgeon of the pulmonary artery to the proposed explant lung is then performed to evaluate the ability of the patient to hemodynamically tolerate the procedure without CPB. Presuming the patient tolerates the test clamp, the surgery proceeds with the removal of the native diseased lung. The donor lung is anastomosed by first connecting the pulmonary vein atrial flap to the native left atrium followed by reanastomosing the pulmonary artery, and then the smaller of the two bronchial ends is telescoped into the other with an overlap of one cartilage ring. The lung is then gently inflated. Air within the lung vasculature is vented via the pulmonary artery or the atrial cuff with the left atrium partially occluded. Once de-airing is accomplished, ventilation and perfusion of the donor lung are both established.

INTRAOPERATIVE PROBLEMS AND MANAGEMENT

Patients arriving for lung and heart-lung transplant are often critically ill. The anesthesiologist commonly has limited time to collate all data and perform the preoperative evaluation. Although preoperative anxiolysis may be beneficial, it is important to not significantly decrease respiratory drive and worsen hypoxemia, hypercarbia, and right heart failure. Commonly used premedications include midazolam, ketamine, and dexmedetomidine.

Before transplant, patients commonly have a "full stomach" because of the often short interval between their notification of impending transplant and the timing of the transplant itself. In such circumstances, a rapid sequence or modified rapid sequence should be used to facilitate induction of anesthesia. A one-size-fits-all anesthetic technique is not appropriate for heart-lung and lung transplants. The choice of induction agents is broad and must consider comorbid illnesses, such as significant right heart dysfunction, or other congenital anomalies in addition to the end-stage pulmonary disease.

Once standard monitors have been applied, propofol, etomidate, ketamine, or volatile anesthetics may be considered as primary induction agents either alone or in combination with narcotics or benzodiazepines. Ketamine does not appear to significantly alter PVR in infants[352] and may be considered as a first-choice drug.[352–355] Given the desire to rapidly intubate and control the airway, a relatively rapid onset neuromuscular blocking agent, such as high-dose rocuronium, is most commonly used.[67] Much of the peritransplant anesthetic considerations focus on the optimization of PVR, particularly with heart-lung transplant patients, and those with significant pulmonary hypertension and right heart dysfunction. Increases in PVR may cause acute right ventricular failure, resulting in reduced CO. Right-sided pressures may increase such that significant right-to-left shunting occurs through intracardiac defects and results in desaturation.

Initial ventilator settings must consider the underlying disease process. Fibrotic lungs may be better served by smaller tidal volumes with a faster respiratory rate that allows for a decreased peak inspiratory and plateau pressures while preserving minute ventilation. Conversely, severe obstructive disease may be best served by a slower respiratory rate, and a prolonged expiratory time. This can prevent hyperinflation (auto-PEEP). PEEP may be beneficial to improve oxygenation and ventilation and decrease atelectasis. Should hemodynamic collapse occur with the institution of positive-pressure ventilation in a patient with severe obstructive lung disease, dynamic hyperinflation should be immediately considered among the possible etiologies. Both dynamic hyperinflation and PEEP, by increasing intrathoracic pressure, may decrease venous return and cause hemodynamic compromise, particularly in relatively hypovolemic patients. Rapid treatment is provided by just disconnecting the patient from the ventilator circuit and allowing the patient to exhale. When ventilation is reinstituted, care must be taken to allow for adequate expiratory time.

Maintenance anesthesia is most commonly a balanced anesthetic, typically opioid-based and supplemented with volatile anesthesia to ensure amnesia. Volatile anesthetic–based techniques are less common because of their cardiovascular depression and vasodilation. Furthermore, volatile anesthetics blunt hypoxic pulmonary vasoconstriction and may make it more difficult to maintain adequate oxygenation should off-CPB lung transplantation be desired. Regional anesthesia may also be considered for intraoperative and postoperative care. Because of the typical use of CPB and its need for systemic heparinization, epidural thoracic catheters used for postoperative pain control are generally placed postoperatively when the patient's coagulation profile has normalized. Additionally, the anesthesiologist commonly administers preoperative antibiotics and immunosuppressive medications required for transplantation. Many transplant centers include the use of immunosuppressive induction therapy, and more than half of all recipients are now receiving either IL-2 receptor antagonists or cytolytics.

The vast majority of pediatric lung transplants are performed with the assistance of CPB, in contrast to the non-CPB technique most commonly used for adults. There are several reasons for this distinction, particularly when considering the two most common indications for pediatric lung transplantation. Cystic fibrosis patients have a significant risk of cross-contamination of the donor lung during a bilateral sequential lung transplant. This risk of soiling is minimized by the simultaneous removal of both lungs. Pediatric patients with pulmonary hypertension are frequently too unstable to tolerate single lung ventilation. Additionally, many children are too small to accommodate a double-lumen tube and single lung ventilation may be difficult. CPB alleviates these issues and allows the surgeon a quiet field with good exposure and predictable hemodynamics, thus speeding the time for anastomosis and decreasing the overall ischemic time.

Nonetheless, if the patient undergoes either single lung transplant or off-pump sequential bilateral lung transplant, continual vigilance and reassessment of the patient's condition is required. These patients are extremely ill, and undergo dramatic homeostatic perturbations. Single lung ventilation often precipitates hypoxemia and hypercarbia. The combination of increased afterload on the right heart by clamping of the pulmonary artery along with hypercarbia and hypoxemic-induced pulmonary hypertension on the other lung may precipitate right heart failure. Pulmonary vascular dilators and inotropes, such as milrinone, prostaglandins, and NO, along with maintaining adequate right-sided filling pressures may be used to diminish pulmonary hypertension. Nonetheless, continued right heart failure may necessitate CPB. If the patient tolerates pulmonary artery clamping, the gas exchange typically improves as the shunting through the nonventilated lung is stopped and the perfusion-ventilation mismatch is diminished.

Bilateral sequential lung transplants performed on CPB do not offer these problems. Nonetheless, CPB comes with a cost. During CPB the patient is typically cooled to 32°C, which introduces the concerns associated with moderate hypothermia. Gas exchange may worsen because of reperfusion injury, pulmonary edema, and decreased lung compliance. CPB also results in inflammatory mediator release that contributes to the reperfusion injury in the transplanted lungs. The systemic heparinization required for CPB increases the risk for perioperative bleeding and the need for transfusion of blood products. Packed red blood cells, platelets, and clotting factors are typically required. Fibrinolytics may somewhat mitigate bleeding.

When the procedure is performed with CPB, airway management is performed with a single-lumen tracheal tube. Cuffed tracheal tubes are typically chosen for the ability to provide a better tracheal fit and allow for the potential ventilation of the lungs with relatively high pressures. In the rare circumstances that the operation of pediatric lung transplantation is performed without CPB, single lung ventilation will be required. Double-lumen tubes may be used in older patients (see Chapter 15). If a double-lumen tube is used, it is exchanged for a single-lumen tube at the conclusion of the operation unless there is a desire to continue with differential lung ventilation or there is a concern about lung soiling. In small children, either a bronchial blocker or selective intubation of a single bronchus may be considered. These options, however, preclude the ability to suction the nonventilated lung. Once the patient has been intubated, additional invasive monitoring is placed, typically an arterial catheter and a central venous catheter, along with two large-bore IV catheters. Some centers place a pulmonary artery catheter in addition to or in place of the percutaneous CVL. Occasionally, the surgeon will place a right atrial catheter. If a pulmonary artery catheter is placed, it must be withdrawn into the main pulmonary artery before the pneumonectomy. A TEE probe is then placed to assist in evaluation of residual cardiac abnormalities and cardiac performance, particularly right ventricular performance, both with pretransplant and posttransplant cardiac assessment.[356]

Perioperative bleeding is common, both in the operating room after coming off CPB and in the immediate postoperative period. Extensive pulmonary to systemic collaterals, coagulopathies caused by hepatic dysfunction, and adhesions from prior surgeries or cystic fibrosis may make the surgical dissection difficult and precipitate blood loss. Fibrinolytics have been demonstrated to reduce bleeding in patients with prior thoracic surgery.[357]

Those with cystic fibrosis are uniformly colonized with bacteria, so after the native lungs are removed, their tracheal stump is irrigated with antibiotic solution to reduce contamination of the transplanted lungs. Despite best efforts, these patients occasionally develop sepsis or a syndrome similar to septic shock owing to liberation of bacteria and toxic mediators during the removal of the native lungs. These patients require intensive therapy and most often do poorly.

After the first lung has been implanted, a small amount of blood is allowed to eject into the pulmonary artery while the second lung is anastomosed, thereby reducing the ischemic time for the first lung. After the second lung is implanted, the lungs are ventilated to remove areas of atelectasis. Posttransplant ventilation strategy limits tidal volumes to maintain peak inspiratory pressures less than 35 cm H_2O and PEEP in the range of 5 to 10 cm H_2O. It is typical to augment myocardial performance with inotropic support before termination of CPB. Occasionally, a combination of inotropes, dilators, or vasopressors may be required. Some centers routinely use NO and/or prostaglandin E_1 (PGE$_1$) to reduce PVR, while others reserve their use only for those in whom pulmonary hypertension is problematic. Fiberoptic bronchoscopy may be performed to assess the bronchial anastomotic sites in the operating room along with a lung perfusion scan performed within the first 24 hours postoperatively.

In the heart-lung transplant patient, weaning from CPB is analogous to that for cardiac transplantation as described earlier. There remains the need to support the denervated heart with adequate fluids and inotropy. Maintaining adequate fluid status in these patients may require a bit more effort because of increased bleeding compared with heart transplant patients. Bleeding is further exacerbated in these patients owing to extensive collaterals and bronchial circulation, which have often developed. Blood products are uniformly required in these patients.

The onset of acute graft dysfunction may present with persistent hypoxemia after weaning from CPB. While this may be attributable to relatively reversible causes, such as inadequate ventilation, atelectasis, or right ventricular dysfunction with right-to-left shunting, a more ominous problem may be reperfusion injury. Free radicals and inflammatory mediators are readily produced by the lung during both the ischemic time as well as during reperfusion. Reperfusion injury is correlated with longer ischemic times and presents as hypoxemia in the face of adequate ventilation and no other clear etiology of the hypoxemia. Pink frothy secretions noted in the tracheal tube may indicate reperfusion injury. PGE$_1$ may reduce reperfusion injury risk and symptoms. The optimal ventilation strategy aims to maintain oxygenation and ventilation with adequate PEEP and as low a peak inspiratory pressure as possible. FiO$_2$ is targeted to keep the PaO$_2$ less than 120 mm Hg to avoid oxygen toxicity. NO, a potent smooth muscle relaxant, has not been shown to prevent reperfusion injury when administered prophylactically. However, NO in the dose range of 20 to 60 ppm has been demonstrated to be effective in patients with increased pulmonary artery and right heart pressures coupled with hypoxemia.[358-363] Inhaled prostacyclin has also been demonstrated to be safe and effective in the treatment of pulmonary hypertension and reperfusion injury.[364] Occasionally, all these measures are inadequate and ECMO is instituted to allow the donor lungs to recover.[365-368]

IMMEDIATE POSTOPERATIVE MANAGEMENT

Immediate postoperative care is individualized based on the child's age, pretransplant diagnosis, and pretransplant comorbidities. Older patients with cystic fibrosis require mechanical ventilation for several days with their time to discharge from the critical care unit averaging less than 1 week.[369] After extubation, these patients may require supplemental oxygen for exercise therapy. Non–cystic fibrosis infants and children, typically more acutely ill before transplant, require an average of more than 3 weeks of mechanical ventilation and average nearly 2 months of critical care stay.[370] These younger transplant patients are smaller, have an increased incidence of airway complications, and may suffer from associated congenital cardiac defects. Patients with significant pretransplant pulmonary hypertension often manifest significant hemodynamic instability postoperatively. As such, these patients remain intubated, sedated, and frequently paralyzed for the first 2 postoperative days.

The cough reflex is absent and mucociliary transport is disrupted across the bronchial suture line in posttransplant patients, necessitating aggressive chest physiotherapy to avoid lung congestion that could lead to infection and respiratory failure. Frequent tracheal suctioning is mandatory; therapeutic bronchoscopy for pulmonary toilet may also be required. In addition to the risk for infections owing to pulmonary considerations, surgical sites, catheters, and drains add to the risk of infection. Prophylactic antibiotics are given perioperatively, including antivirals and antifungals, particularly if underlying fungal infection or viral infection (such as CMV) are present in either the donor or recipient.[371]

Postoperative pain control with judicious use of opioids is critical to ensure effective pulmonary toilet. Patient-controlled analgesia may be considered in patients capable of using such a

TABLE 31.9 Cumulative Morbidity Rates in Pediatric Lung Transplant Survivors Within 1, 5, and 7 Years After Transplant (Follow-Ups April 1994–June 2014)

Outcome	Total With Known Response (N)	Within 1 Year (%)	Total With Known Response (N)	Within 5 Years (%)	Total With Known Response (N)	Within 7 Years (%)
Hypertension[a]	765	41.4	229	67.7	—	—
Renal dysfunction	795	9.4	247	29.6	138	42.8
Creatinine (≤2.5 mg/dL)		6.5		23.1		32.6
(abnormal) >2.5 mg/dL		1.9		4.0		6.5
Chronic dialysis		0.8		1.6		0.7
Renal transplant		0.3		0.8		2.9
Hyperlipidemia[a]	781	5.1	231	17.7	—	—
Diabetes[a]	797	21.3	250	35.2	—	—
BOS	739	12.2	192	35.9	93	41.9

[a]Data are not available 7 years after transplant.

BOS, bronchiolitis obliterans syndrome.

Goldfarb SB, Benden C, Edwards LB, et al. The Registry of the International Society for Heart and Lung Transplantation: Eighteenth Official Pediatric Lung and Heart-Lung Transplantation Report—2015; Focus Theme: Early Graft Failure. *J Heart Lung Transplant*. 2015;34(1):1255–1263 (Table 4).

device. Regional anesthesia may also be used, but because of the systemic heparinization in CPB, many are reluctant to place a catheter before bypass. If regional anesthesia is desired, a thoracic epidural or paravertebral catheters may be placed postoperatively when the coagulation status of the patient has normalized. Dexmedetomidine may also be used for adjunct pain management by providing arousable sedation with minimal effect on respiratory drive with the additional benefit of opioid sparing.

LONG-TERM CONCERNS

With the large endothelial surface in the lungs and the resulting large number of immunologically active cells that predispose to major histocompatibility class antigens, and an extreme lymphocyte-directed host response, immunosuppressive drugs are used in larger doses in lung transplant and heart-lung transplant patients than in other organ transplants. Induction immunosuppression is used in more than half of the heart-lung and lung transplant centers.[372] Most transplant centers use a continuing multiple-drug immunosuppressive regimen.[373] The International Pediatric Lung Transplant Collaborative has recommended that tacrolimus, mycophenolate mofetil, and prednisone constitute the mainstay of immunosuppressive therapy. The most widely used regimens rely on a calcineurin phosphatase inhibitor coupled with a cell cycle inhibitor and a corticosteroid. The most commonly used calcineurin phosphatase inhibitors are cyclosporine and tacrolimus. Both work similarly, and both have significant side effect profiles. Neither one appears to offer a significant benefit over the other in preventing bronchiolitis obliterans (BO) from occurring. The major adverse effects of tacrolimus include hyperglycemia, alopecia, possibly worsening renal function, and possibly increased risk of PTLD. Cyclosporine's major adverse effects include hypercholesterolemia, hirsutism, gingival hyperplasia, and hypertension. Cyclosporine may prolong the neuromuscular blockade of atracurium and vecuronium.[374] Cyclosporine blood concentrations must be monitored closely, particularly in cystic fibrosis patients who are prone to variable absorption. Increased concentrations of cyclosporine have been implicated in central nervous system adverse effects such as seizures, headaches, and even strokes.[375,376] Steroids are included in nearly all lung transplant programs. Over time, the steroid dose is weaned to prevent complications such as hyperglycemia and osteoporosis, yet at 1 and 5 years after transplant, nearly all lung transplant patients continue to take prednisone. Cell cycle inhibitors are used in addition to the calcineurin phosphatase inhibitors and corticosteroids. Mycophenolate use is increasing, but as yet there has been no clearly demonstrated benefit over azathioprine. Azathioprine may prolong the neuromuscular blockade of succinylcholine.[374] Sirolimus acts by blocking IL-2–induced T-cell proliferation. Its role as a primary medication is limited by its hindrance of wound healing, potentially contributing to a dehiscence. It may be used as rescue therapy in patients with BO with mature suture lines.

A variety of perioperative complications may occur (Table 31.9).[377] More than one-third of patients who receive chronic immunosuppression develop hypertension during the first posttransplant year. By 5 years, that number has reached almost three-quarters of all survivors. Additionally, a number of these children, particularly those receiving tacrolimus, develop chronic renal insufficiency with decreasing creatinine clearance. Chronic kidney disease is a major comorbidity in pediatric lung transplant recipients.[378,379] More than one-third of patients have a degree of renal dysfunction within 7 years of transplantation. Occasionally, renal insufficiency progresses such that the child requires dialysis and renal transplantation.[380] Renal dysfunction is associated with increased mortality.

Posttransplant airway complications may be devastating.[381] While life-threatening bronchial dehiscence is uncommon, bronchial stenosis and tracheomalacia remain problematic.[382,383] Bronchial stenosis may be related to relative ischemia at the anastomotic site, recurrent infections, and possibly high-dose corticosteroids. Initial treatment of stenosis is balloon dilation; however, up to half of the patients with bronchial stenosis will require placement of bronchial stents. In younger patients, dynamic obstruction may be a complication that makes extubation difficult. This dynamic airway obstruction usually is self-limited, improves over time, and does not require intervention. Posttransplant patients are followed closely for signs of rejection, infection, and/or bronchiolitis obliterans. Pulmonary function test results are monitored. The choice of anesthetic for posttransplant patients must be individualized, accounting for comorbidities such as continued right heart dysfunction, decreased ability to handle secretions, and particular caution regarding any potential to cross the bronchial suture line. Flexible fiberoptic bronchoscopies with bronchoalveolar lavage and transbronchial biopsies are the most common indications for anesthesia in posttransplant patients.[384] Bronchoscopies are performed at regular intervals, typically every 3 months, to evaluate even very early pathologic changes. Flexible fiberoptic bronchoscopies are most frequently performed with children under general anesthesia. A laryngeal mask airway is the preferred manner of airway management. The laryngeal mask airway lumen is significantly larger than that of the corresponding tracheal tube and allows the bronchoscopist to use a larger fiberoptic bronchoscope, facilitating improved view, improved suctioning, and easier bronchoalveolar lavage along with enhancing the ability to obtain adequate transbronchial biopsies.[385]

Acute rejection is common in the first several weeks to months after transplant. While acute rejection is often asymptomatic, fever and dyspnea may be present. Radiographic findings may include infiltrates and pleural effusions. Pulmonary function tests may demonstrate a decreased FEV_1 and forced vital capacity. Diagnosis is confirmed by bronchoscopy, bronchoalveolar lavage, and transtracheal biopsy. Acute rejection is graded on a scale of A0 to A4. Grade A2 scores and above are treated with increased immunosuppression. The major manifestation of chronic rejection, BO,[386] occurs in up to 50% of all post–lung transplant patients within 5 years of transplant. BO is the leading cause of death after the first posttransplant year. It presents as progressive deterioration of exercise tolerance and deterioration in airflow. BO is characterized by fibrosis of small airways and thickening of blood vessels. Diagnosis is defined by a decrease in FEV_1 compared with the immediately previous FEV_1.[387] Known risk factors for BO include prolonged ischemic time of the donor lung, more than two rejection episodes, and age greater than 3 years.[332] Unfortunately, there is no consistently reliable treatment for BO. A variety of immunosuppressive medications have been used with variable results. The primary treatment is immunosuppressive prevention of acute rejection and prompt CMV treatment. In severe instances of BO, retransplantation is the only treatment option.

Posttransplant vascular complications are uncommon, but when they do occur are most commonly caused by mechanical obstruction of blood flow secondary to redundant tissue in either the pulmonary artery or at the cuff of the atrial tissue, impeding venous return. Vascular complications may be difficult to distinguish from reperfusion injury, presenting with increased right-sided and PAPs with pink frothy secretions in the tracheal tube. Pulmonary arterial or venous stenosis may be diagnosed in the operating room or at bedside with a TEE; in some cases cardiac catheterization may be required. Depending on the findings, the patient may be treated with a stent placed during cardiac catheterization or reoperation to alleviate the stenosis. Additionally, transplanted lungs do not have lymphatics reanastomosed; this loss of lymphatic drainage increases the risk for pulmonary edema postoperatively. Increased parenchymal water and increased vascular filling further serve to decrease the compliance of the posttransplant lungs.[388]

Transplanted lungs are denervated. While this produces minimal effect on airway reflexes, mucociliary transport, and bronchial reactivity,[389] the larger effect is the loss of stimuli to the respiratory drive center and a loss of coordination of the respiratory accessory muscles. This discoordination may be visually apparent. Additionally, in the early posttransplant period, patients often demonstrate episodes of bradycardia. A late effect is a tendency toward an increased sympathetic tone and an increased heart rate.[390]

Phrenic, recurrent laryngeal, and vagus nerve injuries are common after lung transplant.[391] While phrenic nerve injury is typically transient, the resulting diaphragmatic paralysis may result in prolonged need for mechanical ventilation or even consideration of placement of a diaphragmatic pacer. Recurrent laryngeal nerve injury may occur in up to 1 of every 10 pediatric lung transplant patients. The left recurrent laryngeal nerve–induced vocal cord paralysis is the most common, although most children will recover.[391]

Gastroesophageal reflux disease (GERD) is a considerable post–lung transplant problem, which provides an additional risk factor for BO.[392,393] GERD and gastroparesis may be precipitated by vagal nerve injury. Not only do recurrent aspiration pneumonias contribute to transplanted lung failure, but delayed gastric emptying results in unreliable absorption of the patient's immunosuppressive drugs. A number of patients with GERD require a Nissen fundoplication.[394] Additionally, children with cystic fibrosis have a high incidence (10%) of intestinal obstruction after lung transplantation. These children may require gastrostomy, jejunostomy, or other procedures for ileus.[395]

Postlung transplant graft rejections are common. Older children average 10 times more episodes of rejection than infants.[317,391] The signs and symptoms of rejection are nonspecific.

CMV is one of the most common infections in the posttransplant patient. CMV infections may present with mild symptoms, but they may progress to pneumonitis, gastrointestinal symptoms, or even a sepsis syndrome with multiorgan failure. CMV has been associated with both acute cellular rejection and chronic rejection.[396,397] Antiviral medications have decreased the severity of this infection.[398] Prophylactic treatment is often considered if either the donor or the recipient were CMV positive. Children with cystic fibrosis remain at a greater risk for infection postoperatively with *Pseudomonas aeruginosa* or fungal organisms.

A number of malignancies have been reported in the children with cystic fibrosis after transplantation, at greater rates than their age matched counter parts, and may be attributed to immunosuppressive therapy. PTLD has a greater incidence in lung and heart lung transplant patients than in other solid organ transplant, perhaps owing to the greater level of immunosuppression required. Even in this group of children, the cystic fibrosis subgroup after transplant has an increased incidence of PTLD. PTLD includes a group of tumors, ranging from B-cell hyperplasia to immunoblastic lymphoma. Mortality from PTLD has been reported to be up to 60%; a number of these deaths have been attributed to graft failure as a result of treating the PTLD by decreasing immunosuppressive therapy. As many as 25% of children with cystic fibrosis develop PTLD. PTLD is, in most cases, associated with EBV infection, either as a reactivation of the virus with immunosuppression or with new infection acquired from the donor lung. EBV is uncommon in patients who are seropositive for EBV before transplant. For those who are seronegative before transplant, EBV-associated disease occurs in one in five patients. The diagnosis of PTLD is made by the symptoms, biopsy, and the presence of EBV DNA or RNA in the biopsied tissue. PTLD presents with a variety of nonspecific symptoms including a mononucleosis-type syndrome. The most common symptoms include elevated temperature, lymphadenopathy and gastrointestinal symptoms. Most PTLD occurs in the first year after transplant. EBV infection results in both a humoral and cellular immune reaction. In immunodeficient patients, the normal immune responses are blunted. The natural regulation by T cells and natural killer cells is impaired. Natural killer cells function is impaired for several months after transplant. The immunosuppression required to

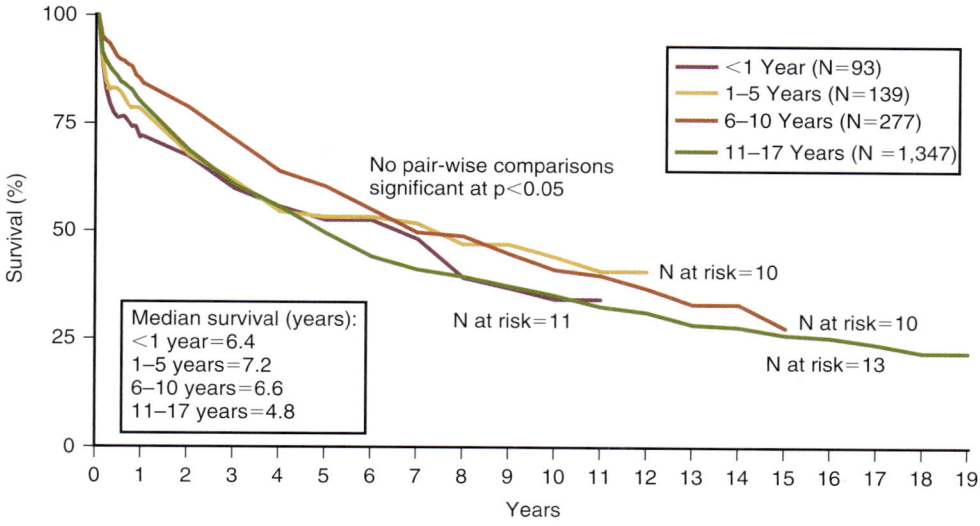

FIGURE 31.11 Pediatric lung transplants. Kaplan-Meier survival by recipient age group (transplants: January 1990–June 2013). (From Figure 10; Goldfarb SB, Benden C, Edwards LB, et al. The registry of the international society for heart and lung transplantation: eighteenth official pediatric lung and heart-lung transplantation report—2015; Focus theme: early graft failure. *J Heart Lung Transplant.* 2015;34(10):1255–1263.)

prevent graft rejection impairs T-cell immunity and allows for unchecked proliferation of EBV-infected B cells.

The treatment of PTLD is reduction or withdrawal of immunosuppressive therapy.[399,400] Unfortunately, reduction or withdrawal of immunosuppressive therapy places these children at risk for graft failure. Additional effective treatments include localized excision of the lesion, antiviral therapy,[401] monoclonal antibodies,[402] interferon,[403,404] immunoglobulin, and cytotoxic T lymphocytes.[405] Chemotherapy does not appear to offer an advantage and may worsen survival.[400]

Dysrhythmias, although possible, are relatively uncommon (<5%) after transplant and typically do not require treatment. Atrial dysrhythmias associated with extensive left atrial suture lines were among the first dysrhythmias to be described.[406,407] However, the types of dysrhythmias after lung transplant surgery includes functional escape rhythm, nonsustained ventricular tachycardia, accelerated junctional rhythm, sinus bradycardia, nonsustained supraventricular tachycardia, ectopic atrial tachycardia, and second-degree heart block; treatment is not generally required.[408] Postoperative lung transplant patients fall behind their contemporaries in height and weight, and their growth curves lie between the 5 and 10 percentiles for age, with the overall growth rate only two-thirds of the predicted value. It appears, based on pulmonary function tests, radiographic studies, and histologic examination, that the growth of the transplanted lung(s) in the recipient is appropriate for the recipient's height and weight. Functional reserve capacity,[409] airway size,[410] and absolute number of alveoli increase as height and weight grow in a manner comparable to their normal counterparts. Furthermore, recipients of mature living-related lobar lungs are also noted to grow. Transplanted mature lung lobes expand and fill the entire chest. In these mature lung lobes, however, while the airways appear to grow in size, the alveoli appear to become distended rather than increasing in absolute number. Pediatric post–lung transplant survival after the first year has remained the same for the past 20 years.[411] The 5-year survival of the transplant patients exceeds 50%. This follows overall 1- and 3-year survival rates of 75% and 66% of the patients, respectively.[372]

Idiopathic pulmonary hypertension patients do slightly better with 1- and 5-year survival rates of 95% and 61%, respectively, but they still have a median survival posttransplant of 5.8 years (Fig. 31.11).[412]

Infants have a substantive early death rate of 25%. Patients with significant pretransplant pulmonary hypertension and those receiving retransplants also have a greater than average death rate. More than one-half of the early (first month) deaths in all ages are due to primary graft failure. The primary causes for later deaths are infections, BO, and malignancies. The leading cause of death from 1 month through 1 year is non-CMV infections. The leading cause of death from 1 to 3 years is BO followed by non CMV infections. After 3 years, BO is the leading cause of death, accounting for nearly half of all deaths. Most malignancies are from PTLD. In those patients who do survive, more than 75% of them have minimal limitation on activity at 1, 3, and 5 years after transplant, respectively.

ANNOTATED REFERENCES

Almond CS, Morales DL, Blackstone EH, et al. Berlin Heart EXCOR pediatric ventricular assist device for bridge to heart transplantation in US children. *Circulation.* 2013;127(16):1702-1711.

The use of ventricular assist devices as a bridge to transplantation has increased significantly over the past decade. The authors describe the overall Berlin Heart EXCOR experience in U.S. children and found that lower patient weight, reduced renal or hepatic function, and use of biventricular device support was associated with death. This paper provides important information in regard to predicting the risk profile when deciding to initiate mechanical support for a patient.

Dharnidharka VR, Fiorina P, Harmon WE. Kidney transplantation in children. *N Engl J Med.* 2014;371(6):549-558.

This review paper summarizes the latest surgical and immunologic advances in pediatric kidney transplantation. The paper includes outcome data of graft and patient survival broken down by patient age and era of time that the transplant was performed.

Henderson HT, Canter CE, Mahle WT, et al. ABO-incompatible heart transplantation: analysis of the Pediatric Heart Transplant Study (PHTS) database. *J Heart Lung Transplant.* 2012;31(2):173-179.

This paper demonstrated equal 1-year survival and rejection outcomes for ABO-incompatible and ABO-compatible heart transplant recipients by analyzing data from the Pediatric Heart Transplant Database. The results from this paper add to the favorable data collected from similar analyses suggesting that UNOS reevaluate the policy of giving priority of ABO-compatible over ABO-incompatible hearts, thus increasing organ availability to children.

Lee J, Yoo YJ, Lee JM, et al. Sevoflurane versus desflurane on the incidence of postreperfusion syndrome during living donor liver transplantation: a randomized controlled trial. *Transplantation.* 2016;100(3): 600-606.

This prospective, randomized, controlled trial investigated postreperfusion syndrome and use of vasoactive agents in 62 adult liver transplant recipients receiving either sevoflurane or desflurane. There was significantly less postreperfusion syndrome (38% vs. 77%) and vasoactive agent (19% vs. 45%) use in adults receiving sevoflurane. There does not appear to be an advantage to using desflurane over sevoflurane during reperfusion.

Sorensen LG, Neighbors K, Martz K, et al. Longitudinal study of cognitive and academic outcomes after pediatric liver transplantation. *J Pediatr.* 2014;165(1):65-72.e2.

This is a prospective multicenter longitudinal study investigating intellect, academic performance, and executive function over time. Pediatric liver transplant recipients 2 or more years after liver transplant were evaluated at 5 to 6 years and 7 to 9 years. A pattern of cognitive and academic deficits were detected in patients that persisted over time. Factors that seemed to predict cognitive deficits included operative complications and intraoperative transfusion volume.

A complete reference list can be found online at ExpertConsult.com.

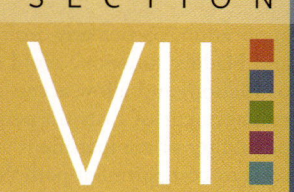

Orthopedic and Spine Surgery 32

NIALL C. WILTON AND BRIAN J. ANDERSON

ANESTHESIA FOR ORTHOPEDIC AND SPINAL SURGERY provides a multitude of challenges. Children often present with concomitant diseases that affect cardiovascular and respiratory function. The ability to maintain a clear airway during anesthesia is not straightforward for some children, such as those with arthrogryposis multiplex congenita.[1] Operating times can be protracted. Significant blood loss can occur that requires strategies for blood product management and transfusion reduction (see Chapter 12). Major trauma causing orthopedic injuries invariably involves other organ systems that may adversely interact with or compromise anesthesia management (see Chapter 39). The risks of pulmonary aspiration of gastric contents and the requisite fasting times, after even minor trauma involving an isolated forearm fracture, continue to be debated. Fat embolus is uncommon in children with long-bone fractures but should be considered in any child with hypoxia and altered consciousness in the perioperative period.[2] Tumor surgery may be complicated by chemotherapy, altered drug disposition, or bone grafting considerations akin to those for plastic and reconstructive surgery (see Chapter 35), and complex postoperative pain management may be required (e.g., phantom pain, reflex sympathetic dystrophy) (see Chapter 45).

Children with chronic illnesses present repeatedly for surgical or diagnostic procedures. A single bad experience can blight attitudes about anesthesia for a long time. Positioning children on the operating table involves care, especially for those with limb deformities and contractures (Video 32.1). Padding, pillows, and special frames are required to protect against damage from inadvertent pressure ischemia while achieving the best posture for surgery. Plaster application, particularly around the hip, should allow for bowel and bladder function, avoid skin breakdown caused by pressure or friction, and allow access to epidural catheters. Postoperative management of casts on peripheral limbs must account for the possibility of compartment syndromes attributable to restrictive casts or compartment pathology. Major plexus blocks may mask pressure effects under plaster casts or compartment syndrome, but epidural blocks using low-dose amide anesthetics do not mask the discomfort of pressure.[3,4] Intraoperative temperature regulation may be affected by tourniquet application or disease (e.g., osteogenesis imperfecta, arthrogryposis multiplex congenita). The use of radiology is common during orthopedic surgery; anesthesiologists should take precautions against excessive radiation exposure.

Regional anesthesia (see Chapter 42) reduces anesthesia requirements intraoperatively and provides analgesia postoperatively. The use of ultrasound techniques to locate neural tissue improves the rate of successful blocks and reduces local anesthetic doses (see Chapter 43).[5,6] This has heralded increasing use of peripheral nerve blockade rather than central blockade for unilateral lower limb surgery. Acetaminophen (paracetamol) and nonsteroidal antiinflammatory drugs (NSAIDs) are the most common analgesics prescribed for moderate pain. Regular administration of acetaminophen and NSAIDs decreases the amount of systemic opioids administered,[7] but NSAIDs decrease osteogenic activity and may increase the incidence of nonunion after spinal fusion.[8,9] Intravenous acetaminophen improves the early effectiveness of this drug before the child is able to tolerate oral intake, but this formulation is not available in all countries.[10] Long-term pain associated with limb-lengthening techniques (e.g., Ilizarov frame) may require oral opioids after hospital discharge.

Scoliosis Surgery

Children presenting for scoliosis surgery represent a spectrum, ranging from uncomplicated adolescents to severely compromised patients with neuromuscular disease, respiratory failure, and cardiac problems. The age range at presentation varies from infancy to young adulthood. Anesthesia techniques for scoliosis surgery vary with individual patient requirements.[11,12] Approaches aimed at minimizing blood loss and transfusion requirements have progressed from extremes of hypotension and hemodilution to a more balanced approach involving moderate degrees of both, use of antifibrinolytic agents, predonation programs, and intraoperative cell salvage. The impact of anesthetic agents on complex physiologic signals has become increasingly important as more sophisticated measurements of neural transmission using somatosensory evoked potentials (SSEPs) and motor evoked potentials (MEPs) have become the standard of care.

TERMINOLOGY, HISTORY, AND SURGICAL DEVELOPMENT

Early Hindu literature (3500 to 1800 BC) describes Lord Krishna curing a woman whose back was "deformed in three places."[13] The terms scoliosis (i.e., crooked), kyphosis (i.e., humpbacked), and lordosis (i.e., bent backward) originated with the Greek physician Galen. *Scoliosis* is a lateral deviation of the normal vertical line of the spine, which is greater than 10 degrees when measured by radiographs. Scoliosis consists of a lateral curvature of the spine with rotation of the vertebrae within the curve. *Lordosis* refers to an anterior angulation of the spine in the sagittal plane, and *kyphosis* refers to a posterior angulation of the spine as evaluated on a side view of the spine. Curves may be simple or complex, flexible or rigid, and structural or nonstructural. Primary curves

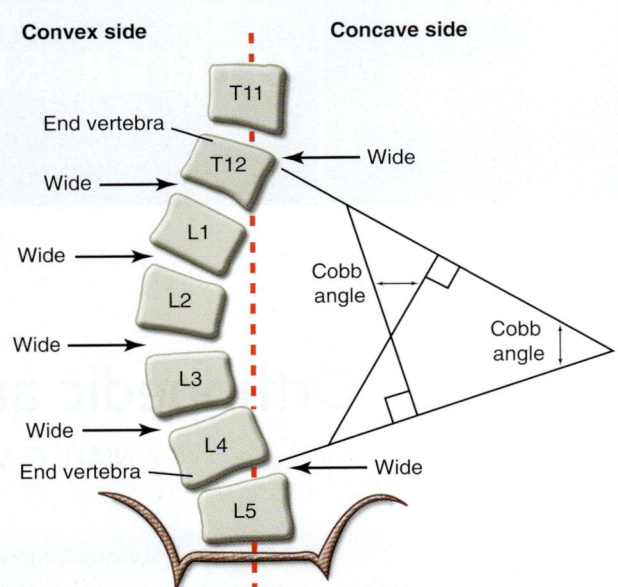

FIGURE 32.1 Diagram of an anteroposterior spinal radiograph shows the Cobb method of scoliosis curve measurement.

are the earliest to appear and occur most frequently in the thoracic and lumbar regions. Secondary (or compensatory) curves can develop above or below the primary curve and evolve to maintain normal body alignment. Various combinations of curve types have different pathophysiologic consequences.

The magnitude of the scoliosis curve is most commonly measured using the Cobb method.[14] Measurement is made from an anteroposterior radiograph and requires accurate identification of the upper and lower end vertebrae involved with the curve. These vertebrae tilt most severely toward the concavity of the curve. The Cobb method of angle measurement is shown in Fig. 32.1.

Hippocrates (circa 400 BC) developed treatments that relied primarily on manipulation and traction, using an elaborate traction table called a *scamnum*.[15] Nonsurgical treatments for spinal deformities persisted until 1839, when a surgical treatment in the form of a subcutaneous tenotomy and myotomy was described by a French surgeon, Jules Guerin.[16]

Posterior spinal fusion was first described by Russell Hibbs for tuberculous spinal deformity in 1911.[17] The original spinal instrumentation system was the Harrington rod system.[18] Modification of this technique that allowed segmental fixation of the rods and early mobilization followed.[19] These systems treated the lateral curve but did not allow for correction of the axial rotation. Subsequent developments allowed both corrections by cantilever maneuvers using Cotrel-Dubousset instrumentation.[20]

Pedicle screws rather than hooks were the next advance. They were initially used as a distal anchor for lumber curves and were found to enhance correction and stabilization, even when used with hooks for the more proximal curves (i.e., hybrid constructs).[21] Pedicle screw instrumentation techniques for total curve correction offer better curve correction than hook techniques[22] and the hybrid pedicle screw and hook technique.[23] Sublaminar polyester bands are often used as part of the hybrid technique in children with dysmorphic or osteoporotic spines because of concerns about pedicle screw placement,[24] although bands may be associated with more neurologic complications.[25]

CLASSIFICATION

Classification of scoliosis deformities is imperfect because the systems used are clinically rather than etiologically based. Most classifications are surgically based and used for surgical decision making. Curves can be described on the basis of age at onset, associated pathology, and anatomic configurations of the curve, such as single, double, or triple curves; amount of pelvic tilt; curve flexibility; and three-dimensional (3D) analysis of the curve.[26] A classification that could indicate the risk of an adverse outcome of anesthesia, particularly respiratory failure, would be of clinical benefit. Children younger than 5 years of age with early-onset scoliosis or with independent cardiac or pulmonary disease appear to be at increased risk for respiratory failure, whereas those with idiopathic scoliosis in whom the curve develops at adolescence appear to have minimal risk.[27] A classification adapted from that proposed by the Scoliosis Research Society in 1973 remains relevant for anesthesiologists (Table 32.1).[28]

TABLE 32.1	Classification of Scoliosis With Associated Key Anesthetic Risk Factors			
Classification	Issues Associated With Scoliosis Surgery	Increased K⁺ With Succinylcholine	Expected High Blood Loss	Respiratory Complications and Ventilatory Support
Idiopathic				
Infantile <3 years	Repeat operations, small size	✓		✓
Juvenile 3–9 years				
Adolescent 9–18 years	Regarded as cosmetic by patient; perfect result expected			
Congenital				
Bony abnormalities	Acute angle deformity; high risk of spinal cord injury, genitourinary malformations			
Neural tube defects Meningomyelocele, spina bifida, syringomyelia	Latex allergy, pressure sores, hydrocephalus, Arnold-Chiari and Chiari malformations (avoid neck extension)			
Neuromuscular *Neuropathic*				
Upper motor neuron Cerebral palsy, cerebral hypoxia	Upper airway obstruction, recurrent pneumonia, postoperative pain management	✓✓		✓✓
Lower motor neuron Poliomyelitis				
Myopathic				
Progressive Duchenne muscular dystrophy	Cardiomyopathy, mitral valve prolapse, conduction abnormalities	✓	✓✓	✓✓
Spinal muscular atrophy	Electrocardiographic abnormalities	✓	✓	✓
Facioscapulohumeral muscular dystrophy	Hypertrophic cardiomyopathy, cardiac failure	✓		
Other Friedrich ataxia		✓		
Neurofibromatosis	Hypertension, other neurofibromas			
Mesenchymal				
Marfan syndrome	Mitral and aortic regurgitation			
Mucopolysaccharidoses (e.g., Morquio syndrome)	Atlantoaxial subluxation, difficult intubation			
Arthrogryposis	Difficult intubation, severe contractures		✓	
Osteogenesis imperfecta	Small size			
Trauma				
Tumor				

✓, anesthetic risk is likely; ✓✓, anesthetic risk is very likely.
Modified from Goldstein LA, Waugh TR. Classification and terminology of scoliosis. *Clin Orthop Relat Res.* 1973;93:10–22.

The Lenke classification system, developed in 2001 for idiopathic scoliosis, provides a means to categorize curves and guide surgical treatment.[29] It is increasingly used by the surgeons as an integral part of their decision making.[30] Major and structural minor curves included in the instrumentation and fusion are used for the classification, and the nonstructural minor curves are excluded. The system has three components: curve type, a lumbar spine modifier, and a sagittal thoracic modifier. The resulting six curve types have specific radiographic characteristics that differentiate structural and nonstructural curves as proximal thoracic, main thoracic, and thoracolumbar/lumbar regions such that the number, curve type, and main structural curves are related as follows:

Type 1, main thoracic: single; main thoracic structural curve

Type 2, double thoracic: double; proximal, and main thoracic structural curves

Type 3, double major: double; main thoracic (major curve) and thoracolumbar/lumbar structural curves

Type 4, triple major: triple; all three structural curves

Type 5, thoracolumbar/lumbar: single; thoracolumbar/lumbar structural curve

Type 6, thoracolumbar/lumbar main thoracic: double; thoracolumbar/lumbar (major curve) and main thoracic structural curves

In types 1 through 4, the main thoracic curve is the major curve, and in types 5 and 6, the thoracolumbar/lumbar curve is the major curve.

PATHOPHYSIOLOGY AND NATURAL HISTORY

Vertebral rotation and rib cage deformity usually accompany any lateral curvature. With progression of the curve, the vertebral bodies in the area of the primary curve rotate the convex aspect of the curve and the spinous process to the concave side. This vertebral rotation can be determined by measurement of the position of the pedicles from the midline (i.e., Moe method).[31] The vertebral bodies and the discs develop a wedge-shaped appearance, with the apex of the wedge toward the concave side. On the convex side of the curve, the ribs are pushed posteriorly, which narrows the thoracic cavity and causes the characteristic hump. On the concave side, the same rotation forces the ribs laterally, with consequent crowding toward their lateral margins (Fig. 32.2). These changes result in an increasingly restrictive lung defect. Exactly when this becomes a problem depends on the child's accompanying pathology. The thoracic and lumbar regions are the most common sites of the primary curve. In children in whom the primary curve is in the lumbar region, the rotation of the vertebral bodies and spinous processes should be taken into consideration when spinal or epidural insertion is attempted because the spinal canal is relatively displaced toward the convex aspect of the curve.

The physical distortion in the thorax results in restriction of lung volumes and function. Ventilation depends on the mobility of the thoracic cage, the volume of each hemithorax, and the muscle power and elastic forces required to move the thorax. Children with idiopathic scoliosis with a mild decrease in vital capacity also have reduced forced expired volume at 1 second (FEV_1), gas transfer factor, and maximal static expiratory airway pressures (PEmax) (see Fig. 13.4 and Table 13.2). The predominant deformity of lateral flexion and vertebral rotation results in the lung on the concave side being able to achieve a near-normal end-expiratory position but not end-inspiratory position, whereas the lung on the convex side achieves a normal end-inspiratory position but cannot reach a normal end-expiratory position. The

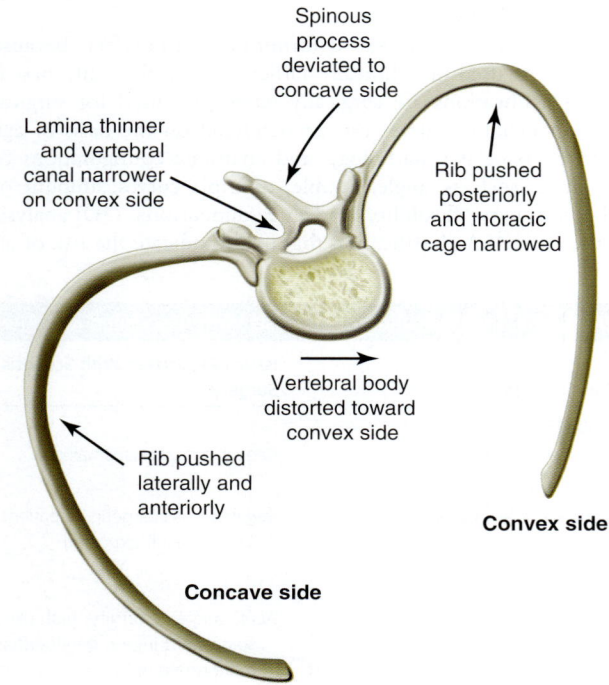

FIGURE 32.2 Characteristic distortion of the vertebra and ribs in thoracic scoliosis. (Modified from Kleim HA. Scoliosis. In: *Ciba Foundation Symposium*. Vol. 1. Summit, NJ: Ciba; 1978:609; Anesthesia for orthopaedic surgery. In: Gregory GA, ed. *Pediatric Anesthesia*. 3rd ed. Edinburgh: Churchill Livingstone; 1994.)

concave side contributes less than normal at total lung capacity, resulting in a decrease in PEmax. Similarly, because the convex side does not reach a normal end-expiratory position, the intercostal muscles and hemidiaphragm will be less efficient, resulting in a reduced maximum static inspiratory airway pressure (PImax), although this reduction may not be quite so marked.[32] The main effect of scoliosis on respiratory function is mechanical, and the anatomic changes in the chest wall cause impaired movement and reduced compliance. Potential long-term respiratory problems when these defects are left untreated include hypoxemia, hypercarbia, recurrent lung infections, and pulmonary hypertension.

Congenital, Infantile, and Juvenile Scoliosis: Early-Onset Scoliosis

Congenital spinal anomalies are caused by failures of formation and segmentation that result in scoliosis and kyphosis. The hemivertebra, caused by failure of formation, is the most common anomaly. Fully segmented hemivertebrae contribute to progressive deformity during periods of rapid spinal growth (e.g., the first 5 years of life). The most severe deformities are seen in the thoracolumbar spine. Congenital spinal anomalies may be associated with malformations of the ribs, chest wall, and hemifacial microsomia.[33] Children with congenital scoliosis have an associated 25% risk of urologic and 10% risk of cardiac abnormalities. Bracing or casting techniques are not effective for this form of scoliosis. These children may have obstructive lung disease in addition to their restrictive impairment, possibly owing to mainstem bronchial compression from spine rotation.[34] Surgical options for these children include fusion in situ, convex hemiepiphysiodesis, hemivertebra excision, growing rods, and vertical expandable prosthetic titanium rib (VEPTR) treatment.[35] Although short-term correction is easily achievable, a short thoracic spine or even thoracic insufficiency syndrome (inability of the thorax to support normal breathing and lung growth) can result.[36] Approximately one-half of the children who have extensive thoracic fusions and those whose fusions involve the proximal thoracic spine develop restrictive pulmonary disease (FEV_1 <50%).[37] Expansion thoraco-plasty and stabilization using a VEPTR may be used.[38]

Infantile and juvenile scoliosis are part of the spectrum of idiopathic scoliosis but are considered here because they manifest and require treatment at an early age. Infantile scoliosis accounts for less than 1% of idiopathic scoliosis and is defined as scoliosis appearing between birth and 3 years of age.[35] It usually occurs in the thoracic spine, and the curve is usually convex to the left. Bracing and serial casting techniques are used for infantile scoliosis; improvement and resolution in some cases have been achieved at 9-year follow-up.[39]

Treatment of infantile scoliosis may begin as early as 4 to 5 months of age or as soon as the diagnosis of scoliosis has been made. Body casting appears useful in selected children, such as those with smaller, flexible spinal curves, but curve progression and the need for secondary treatments affect a significant propor-tion of these children.[40] Bracing is considered when the curve reaches 30 degrees.[35] Success has also been reported for more severe curves (60 degrees) when casting was started before 20 months.[41] After induction of anesthesia, the child is positioned on the frame (first described by Cotrel and Morel[41a]), securing the pelvis to the caudal end of the frame and tethering the head by a chin strap to the rostral end. The spine is mildly distracted, but the main maneuver derotates the spine through the ribs (Fig. 32.3A). General anesthesia with tracheal intubation is required to facilitate positioning the child, stretching the spine, and molding the body cast. Hemoglobin desaturation frequently occurs when the cast is molded to correct the spinal deformity. Hypoxemia or breathlessness may occur following cast application. Peak Inspiratory pressure (PIP) may double if using positive-pressure ventilation intraoperatively; this can be partially improved by cutting a window in the cast.[42]

An oral airway is also needed to prevent compression of the tracheal tube after the chin strap is applied and tightened (Fig. 32.3A). After the cast has hardened, it is cut back and trimmed to maintain the correction to the spine while facilitating breathing, gastrointestinal function, and day-to-day living (see Fig. 32.3B). Halo traction may be used to stretch and improve the curves but infections occur in ~50%.[43]

Juvenile idiopathic scoliosis represents 10% to 15% of idiopathic scoliosis and is defined as scoliosis that is first diagnosed between the ages of 4 and 10 years. Approximately 20% of these children and those with infantile scoliosis with a curve greater than 20% have an underlying spinal condition, most commonly Arnold-Chiari malformation and syringomyelia.[44] Although bracing is used to manage these curves, almost all children in this group with curves greater than 30% require surgical intervention.[45]

Growing rods may be used for congenital, infantile, or juvenile scoliosis to maintain the correction obtained at initial surgery while allowing spinal growth to continue. Several procedures are required before a definitive fusion.[46] All the systems (i.e., growing rods and VEPTR) have a moderate complication rate (i.e., rod breakage and hook displacement).VEPTR systems are being used to correct large-magnitude curves in this group of children when conservative treatment is inadequate.[47]

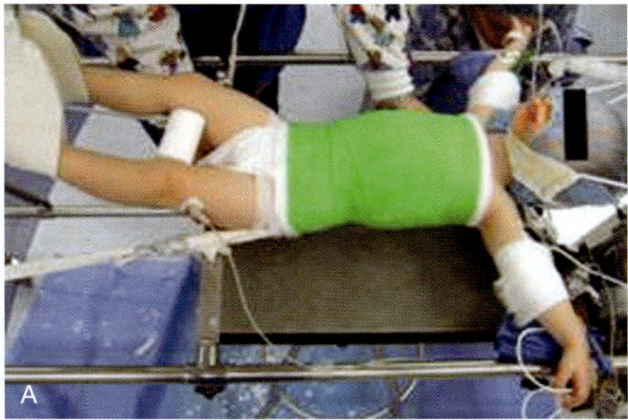

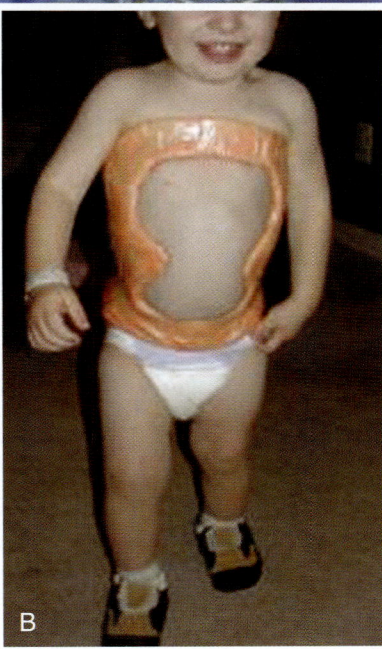

FIGURE 32.3 A, Nonoperative correction of scoliosis in infants and toddlers may be achieved with repeated casting. **B,** Cutting and trimming of the cast allows correction of the spine while facilitating daily living.

Idiopathic Scoliosis

Although adolescent idiopathic scoliosis is relatively common, severe morbidity is seen only in children with early-onset (infantile or juvenile) idiopathic scoliosis.[48] Respiratory deterioration alone is seldom the reason for surgery in those who develop scoliosis after the age of 5 years.[27] This is explained by the fact that the respiratory alveoli are mature by this age.[49,50]

Scoliosis evolves during growth spurts. The earlier the age of onset and the more immature the bone growth at the time the process begins, the more severe the outcome. The relentless progres-sion of infantile-onset idiopathic scoliosis with rapidly deteriorating curves and lung function is often not amenable to surgery. Treatment involving spinal instrumentation and anterior epiphys-iodesis does not prevent the reappearance of the deformity or the decrease in pulmonary function.[51]

Pulmonary impairment correlates directly with the magnitude of the thoracic curve. Severity of the scoliosis is the most accurate predictor of impaired lung function.[52] The morphology of the thoracic curve, the number of vertebrae in the major curve, and the rigidity of the curve also are associated with deteriorating pulmonary function.[53] Conventional wisdom has held that there is minimal impact on the vital capacity until the curve exceeds 60 degrees, with clinically relevant decreases in respiratory function occurring only after the thoracic scoliosis has progressed beyond 100 degrees.[37] However, children with adolescent idiopathic scoliosis may have pulmonary impairment that is disproportionate to the severity of the scoliosis since it occurs before the curve reaches 100 degrees. Forced vital capacity (FVC) may decrease below normal (<80% of predicted) after the magnitude of the thoracic curve exceeds 70 degrees; FEV_1 decreases below normal after the main thoracic curve exceeds 60 degrees.[38] Twenty percent of children with a thoracic curve of 50 to 70 degrees have moderate or severe pulmonary impairment (i.e., <65% of predicted) (Fig. 32.4A).[54] Those with thoracic hypokyphosis are more likely to have moderate

or severe pulmonary impairment; complex curves have a greater prevalence of moderate or severe pulmonary impairment, and the number of vertebrae in the thoracic curve is the most significant predictor of impaired respiratory function (see Fig. 32.4).[55] Children with a structural cephalad thoracic curve, a major thoracic curve spanning eight or more vertebral levels, or thoracic hypokyphosis are at increased risk for moderate to severe pulmonary impairment. Bracing patients with adolescent idiopathic scoliosis (AIS) decreases the progression of high risk curves[56] but is associated with worse pulmonary function test (PFT) results at the time of surgery.[57]

Neuromuscular Scoliosis

Children with neuromuscular scoliosis have the burden of deteriorating muscle function in addition to mechanical distortion. Crowding of the ribs on the concave side of the curve limits chest wall expansion, and the sitting posture restricts diaphragmatic

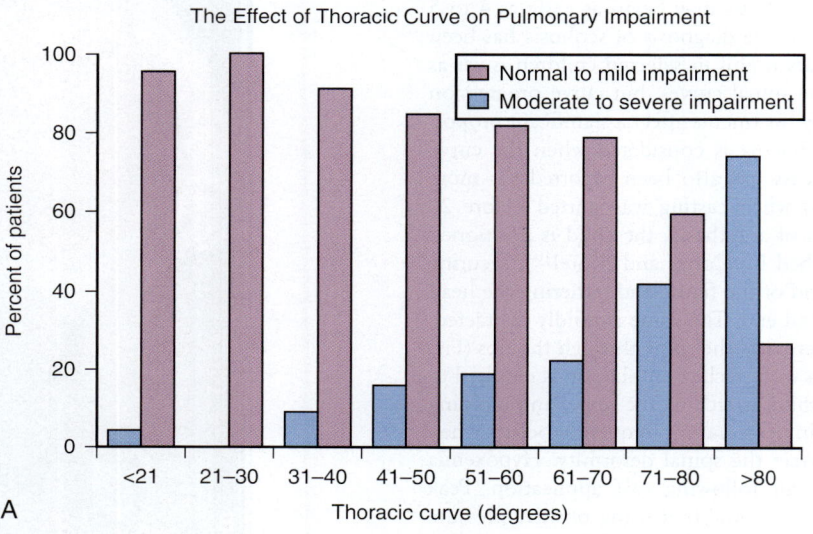

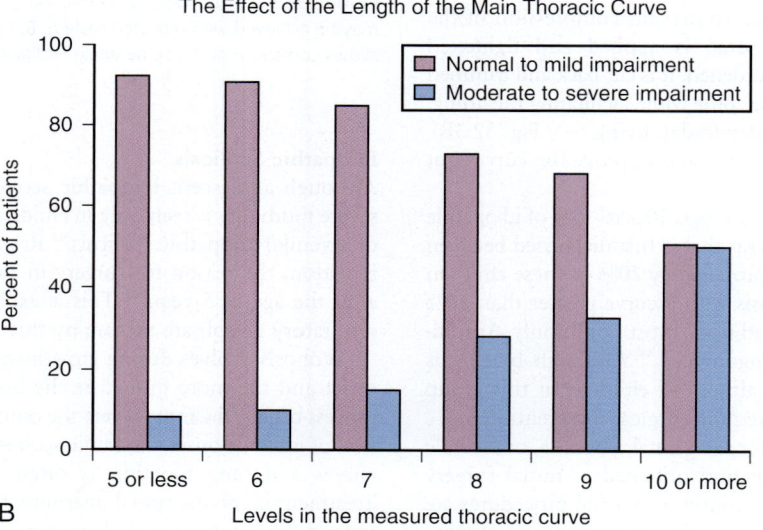

FIGURE 32.4 A, The bar graph demonstrates increasing pulmonary impairment with increasing curve severity as measured by degrees. **B,** Pulmonary impairment increases with increasing length of the thoracic curve. (From Newton PO, Faro FD, Gollogly S, et al. Results of preoperative pulmonary function testing of adolescents with idiopathic scoliosis. A study of six hundred and thirty-one patients. *J Bone Joint Surg Am.* 2005;87:1937–1946.)

excursion. This inevitably leads to more rapid deterioration in the curve and respiratory function. These children also have the potential for rapid and unpredictable deterioration of the curve.[39] It is important to consider the natural history of the specific neuromuscular disease when trying to balance the risks of surgery against conservative management.

Children with Duchenne muscular dystrophy (DMD) suffer from progressive muscular weakness and increasing disability until death occurs, usually by the beginning of the third decade.[58] These children tend to become wheelchair-bound by 8 to 10 years of age because of increasing motor muscle weakness. Scoliosis then progresses with an acute deterioration during the growth spurt between the ages of 13 and 15 years, such that it becomes difficult or impossible to sit unaided. After the lumbar curve exceeds 35 degrees, further progression becomes inevitable.[59] A normal cough requires an inspiratory effort of more than 60% of total lung capacity and effective glottic closure to produce an effective peak flow (more than 160 L/minute in adults). Forced expiratory flows are typically reduced in proportion to the decrease in lung volume. As muscle weakness progresses, patients hypoventilate, initially at night. If nocturnal ventilatory support is not provided at this stage, diurnal hypercapnia will result.[60]

There have been two significant changes in the overall management of children with DMD: the use of steroids and the earlier use of nocturnal noninvasive positive-pressure ventilation (NPPV). Steroid treatment in the early phase of the disease appears to slow disease progression for a few years; treatment with prednisone can stabilize strength and function for 6 months to 2 years.[61,62] This may delay the presentation of children for corrective surgery. Earlier adoption of nocturnal NPPV for nocturnal hypoventilation improves survival and quality of life. Clinically unsuspected nocturnal hypoventilation occurs in about 15% of patients with DMD and can be predicted by moderate impairment according to PFT results (FVC <70% and FEV$_1$ <65% of predicted) and scoliosis. Those with nocturnal hypoventilation have increased gas trapping, decline of muscle strength, and worse perception of health status despite NPPV.[63]

A 2007 multidisciplinary "Consensus Statement on the Respiratory and Related Management of Patients with Duchenne Muscular Dystrophy undergoing Anesthesia or Sedation" provided recommendations to standardize the approach to these patients[64] and others with flaccid neuromuscular diseases undergoing anesthesia. The most important of these recommendations are as follows: an FVC <50% of predicted indicates an increase in postoperative respiratory complications; an FVC <30% suggests a further increase in risk. PFTs should be part of the preoperative evaluation when possible and should include FVC, PImax, PEmax, peak cough flow, oxygen saturation by pulse oximetry (SpO$_2$) on room air, and partial pressure of carbon dioxide (PaCO$_2$) if the SpO$_2$ value is less than 95%. Consider preoperative training and postoperative use of NPPV if FVC is less than 50% of predicted, and strongly consider NPPV if FVC is less than 30%. Consider preoperative training and postoperative use of manual and mechanically assisted cough in those with impaired cough. In older children, this can be predicted by a peak cough flow less than 270 L/minute or maximal expiratory pressure less than 60 cm H$_2$O. Strongly consider planning to extubate the trachea directly to NPPV when the FVC is less than 30%.

Dilated cardiomyopathy occurs in up to 90% of DMD individuals older than 18 years of age; the severity of their physical disability often masks the clinical symptoms of cardiac failure. Cardiomyopathy is responsible for 20% of deaths, but this proportion may increase in the future for individuals in whom NPPV prevents respiratory-related mortality[62] (see also Chapter 23).

Risk Minimization and Improving Outcome From Surgical Intervention

RESPIRATORY FUNCTION AND OTHER COMPLICATIONS IN THE EARLY POSTOPERATIVE PERIOD

Decreases in lung volumes and flow rates similar to thoracic and upper abdominal surgery occur after scoliosis surgery. The FVC and FEV$_1$ decrease with a nadir at 3 days and are about 60% of preoperative values 7 to 10 days after surgery (Fig. 32.5). It is not until 1 to 2 months after surgery that PFTs approach baseline values. The magnitude of this decrease is not affected by the type of surgery performed or whether the scoliosis has an idiopathic or neuromuscular cause.[65] Surveys from the British Scoliosis Society and Scoliosis Research Society report mortality rates of 1.5 to 1.9 per 1000 cases,[66,67] with a smaller rate in children with AIS (0.4 per 1000) and a greater rate in those with neuromuscular disease (3.6 per 1000).[67] Overall, deep infections occurred in 2.8% and permanent neurologic defect in 0.45% of children.[66]

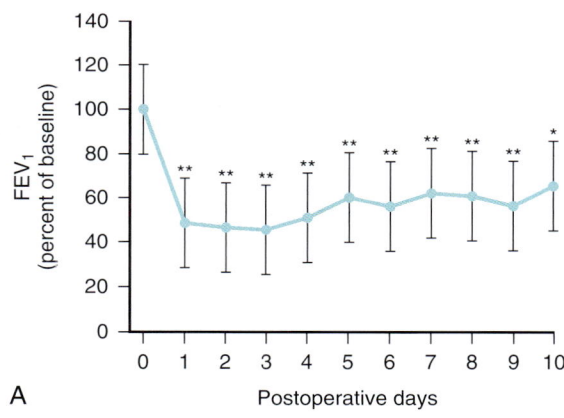

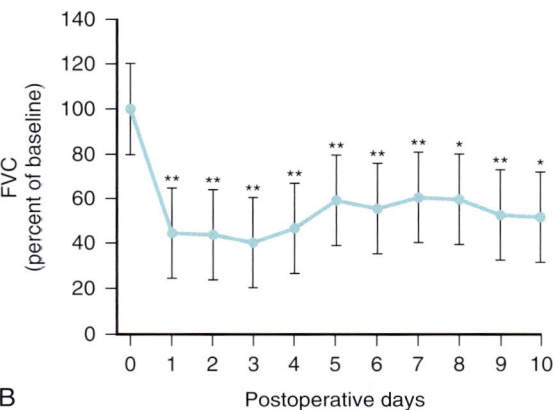

FIGURE 32.5 A, Changes in forced expiratory volume in 1 second (FEV$_1$) during the 10 days after scoliosis surgery. **B,** Changes in forced vital capacity (FVC) during the 10 days after scoliosis surgery. (From Yuan N, Fraire JA, Margetis MM, et al. The effect of scoliosis surgery on lung function in the immediate postoperative period. *Spine* 2005;30:2182–2185.)

Early-Onset Scoliosis

Early-onset scoliosis (EOS) has a dismal prognosis when untreated, and repeated spinal lengthening procedures are associated with a complication rate of 80% and a mortality rate of 18%.[68] Magnetic growing rods, by reducing the number of operative interventions, may be associated with fewer complications and improved pulmonary function.[69]

Idiopathic Scoliosis

Complications in children with AIS are uncommon but an increased body mass index is associated with a threefold increase in postoperative adverse events. Instrumentation of more than 13 segments and operation times longer than 6 hours are associated with an increased length of stay. Any complication during the hospital stay is associated with readmission; the most common cause is surgical site infection (SSI).[70] Scheuermann kyphosis is associated with an 8- to 10-fold increase in major complications, SSI, and reoperations compared with AIS.[71]

Neuromuscular Scoliosis

Children with neuromuscular disease are more likely to require prolonged mechanical ventilation after spinal surgery because of more severe preoperative respiratory impairment.[72] The marked decrease in vital capacity and peak flows is undoubtedly related to the risk of postoperative complications, but determining when it is no longer safe to anesthetize those with a restrictive lung defect remains an imperfect science.

Equipment is available to assist the postoperative management of children with impaired respiratory function. The routine use of NPPV and cough augmentation therapy should be planned if the preoperative FVC is less than 30%. Cough augmentation can be provided manually by hyperinflation and forced expiration, alone or together, and by mechanical insufflation-exsufflation (MIE) therapy.[73] The effectiveness of MIE may be limited in children with a weak or enlarged tongue if it blocks exsufflation flow.

Less extensive surgery with the newer pedicle screw systems decreases the need for pelvic fixation to correct pelvic obliquity. The procedures require less extensive surgery and shorter operating times, which may benefit children with impaired respiratory function.[74–77]

Respiratory complications after surgery for AIS are relatively uncommon; however, these complications are fivefold greater in children with neuromuscular scoliosis.[78,79] Anterior spinal procedures are associated with a greater incidence of complications than posterior spinal fusion; some consider this to be the main risk factor for postoperative respiratory complications.[79] Current pedicle screw systems may decrease the need for anterior procedures, thereby decreasing the complication rate.[80]

Atelectasis, infiltrates, hemothoraces, pneumothoraces, pleural effusions, and prolonged intubation have the greatest incidence, whereas pneumonia, pulmonary edema, and upper airway obstruction occur less frequently. These problems are more common when the scoliosis is associated with developmental delay; the greatest complication rate is in those with cerebral palsy and flaccid neuromuscular scoliosis.[78–81] Respiratory complications increase as the severity of scoliosis and degree of respiratory impairment increase but complication rates vary considerably. Children with neuromuscular scoliosis have a respiratory complication rate of 15% to 30%[81–85] and minimal mortality. One study, which separated three groups according to respiratory impairment (FVC <30%, FVC = 30% to 50%, FVC >50%), reported an overall complication rate of 31% independent of the degree of respiratory impairment,[81] perhaps reflecting improvement with modern management techniques (Table 32.2).

Children with cerebral palsy have additional problems associated with their lack of muscular control (e.g., swallowing incoordination, excessive salivation, gastroesophageal reflux) and sometimes have developmental delay that contributes to a postoperative complication rate of 30%.[82,83,86] Nonambulatory children and those with curves greater than 60 degrees are at increased risk for major complications; nonambulatory patients are almost four times more likely to have a major complication.[86] Gastrointestinal dysmotility in cerebral palsy patients can be exacerbated after scoliosis surgery and cause persistent vomiting and bloating.[87] Pancreatitis may occur in up to 30% of cerebral palsy patients after surgery, with a greater incidence among those with documented gastroesophageal reflux and reactive airway disease.[88]

Surgical Site Infection

SSI results in high morbidity and cost. Rates are much greater after non-idiopathic scoliosis repair, increasing from 2.6% with AIS to 9.2% with neuromuscular scoliosis. The most common pathogens are *Staphylococcus aureus*, coagulase-negative staphylococci, and *Pseudomonas aeruginosa*.[89] Almost half of the infections in children with neuromuscular scoliosis contain at least one gram-negative organism. Despite this, there is little evidence to support the use of intravenous (IV) vancomycin or gentamycin powder to the surgical site or graft.[90] More severe curves, nonambulatory status, and increased length of stay increase the risk of infection.[91]

LONG-TERM CHANGES

Idiopathic Scoliosis

Improvements in pulmonary function are not impressive after correction of idiopathic scoliosis. Early studies suggested that spinal fusion stabilized the respiratory dysfunction that existed preoperatively but failed to offer any improvement.[92] Improvements are possible in certain subgroups of patients with some surgical techniques, but it takes months to years for pulmonary function to improve. Children with a preoperative curve less than 90 degrees undergoing a posterior procedure experienced an increase in vital capacity of slightly greater than 10%, maximum voluntary ventilation, and maximum respiratory mid-flow rate after 2 years; this

TABLE 32.2	Incidence of Pulmonary Complications[81]					
Forced Vital Capacity	Total Number of Patients	Patients With Pulmonary Complications	Pneumonia	Atelectasis	Pneumothorax	Ventilator Care (>3 days)
<30%	18	6	3	0	1	2
30%–50%	18	7	3	1	0	4
>50%	38	10	2	1	0	7

improvement did not occur in those who underwent anterior surgery.[93] Harrington rod instrumentation in children with idiopathic scoliosis resulted in only a small improvement in vital capacity.[94]

The newer instrumentation systems (e.g., Cotrel-Dubousset instrumentation) allow segmental realignment and approximation, resulting in further improvements in pulmonary volumes.[95] Pulmonary function returns to preoperative values within 3 months after the posterior approach using the newer instrumentation systems, with additional improvements occurring and being sustained for 2 years.[96] Pedicle screws provide greater curve correction in AIS, with a trend toward improved pulmonary function after 2 years compared with other instrumentation techniques.[23] Lung volumes measured by 3D computed tomographic scans do not change even with an increase in patient height, suggesting a dynamic improvement from hemithoracic symmetry rather than a static benefit.[97,98] A 10-year follow-up analysis demonstrated an absolute increase in the FVC (3.66 L from 3.25 L) and FEV_1 (3.10 L from 2.77 L) but no changes in percent of predicted values in children who underwent a posterior fusion only. In the same analysis, those with chest wall disruption experienced no change in FVC and FEV_1 over 10 years, but a significant decrease in predicted FVC (79% vs. 85%,) and FEV_1 values (76% vs. 80%).[99]

Chest cage disruption (i.e., thoracoplasty or anterior thoracotomy) is associated with reduced pulmonary function at 3 months and a 10% to 20% decrease in total lung capacity (TLC) and FVC. These values do not return to baseline until 1 to 2 years after surgery. Improvements in lung function with this approach rarely occur.[48,49] Video-assisted thoracoscopic surgery (VATS) for anterior release and instrumentation results in less pulmonary morbidity and a smaller decrease in pulmonary function at 3 months. One year after surgery, values for children treated thoracoscopically return to baseline, but this did not occur for those undergoing open thoracotomy (Fig. 32.6).[100,101] Two- and five-year follow-up evaluations of those undergoing VATS showed no significant changes with regard to the correction of the major Cobb angle (56% ± 11% and 52% ± 14%, respectively) or average predicted TLC (95% ± 14% and 91% ± 10%).[102]

Changing surgical techniques may challenge these findings in the future because some surgeons think that anterior fusions with modern systems offer short-term benefits of reduced blood loss and transfusion and long-term benefits owing to shorter fusions, better maintenance of thoracic kyphosis, and improved spontaneous lumbar curve correction. A 2-year postoperative study concluded that VATS for thoracic curves and open procedures for thoracolumbar curves resulted in minimal to no permanent pulmonary impairment 6 months after the procedure compared with posterior spinal fusion, despite a short-term decrease observed after VATS.[103]

Neuromuscular Scoliosis

Improvements in the scoliosis angle and the degree of pelvic obliquity are achieved after spinal instrumentation in children with neuromuscular disease. Significant improvement in the quality of life perceived by the child or caregiver and in the ability to sit unaided, particularly if children are unable to do so beforehand.[104-108] There is little evidence for any improvement in respiratory function in this group of children, although there may be a period of delay or even stabilization of the inevitable deterioration of respiratory function.[58,105,109] Other investigators have shown no difference in respiratory function after 5 years compared with patients managed conservatively[107,110] or an early loss in vital capacity after surgery with a progressive decrease of 25% over 4 years, with 66% of children requiring mechanical respiratory assistance by that time.[106] A Cochrane review failed to find any data evaluating the effectiveness of scoliosis surgery in patients with DMD, leaving them to suggest: *"Patients should also be informed about the uncertainty of benefits on long-term survival and respiratory function after scoliosis surgery."*[111]

Some retrospective analyses, however, deserve consideration. A review of the long-term survival of children with DMD after spinal surgery and nocturnal ventilation demonstrated that those having spinal surgery and ventilation had a median survival of 30 years, whereas those receiving nocturnal ventilation only survived to 22.2 years. This result occurred despite a decrease in mean vital capacity from 1.4 L to 1.13 L in the first postoperative year.[112] Posterior spinal fusion for scoliosis in DMD was associated with a significant slowing in the rate of decrease in respiratory function; the rate of 4% per year before surgery decreased to 1.75% per year (over 8 years) after surgery.[113] In a study of 14 children with DMD and an FVC of less than 30%, the mean rate of decrease in percent of FVC after surgery was 3.6% per year. Most children and parents thought scoliosis surgery improved their function, sitting balance, and quality of life and gave it high satisfaction scores.[114]

Less outcome information is available for children with cerebral palsy. Surgery is perceived as having a positive impact on patients' quality of life, overall function, and ease of care by parents and other caregivers,[115] despite the high complication rates described earlier. A 3-year follow-up after a pedicle screw construct for scoliosis, which reduced the mean Cobb angle to 31 degrees, demonstrated improved functional ability in 42% of children. Most children had improved sitting balance and nursing care requirements. A 32% complication rate occurred; most were pulmonary in origin but ultimately reversible. One study reported two perioperative deaths and one transient neurologic deficit caused by screw impingement among 56 patients.[80]

Less morbidity has been claimed for the same-day (one-stage) surgery compared with the two-staged approach in children with neuromuscular disease requiring anterior and posterior spinal surgery.[116,117] However, it seems reasonable to avoid anterior thoracotomy in neuromuscular patients in view of the poor respiratory function after chest cage disruption.[96,100] Currently, pedicle screw systems in children with neuromuscular scoliosis produce outcomes similar to those of earlier systems but with shorter operating times and less blood loss.[75]

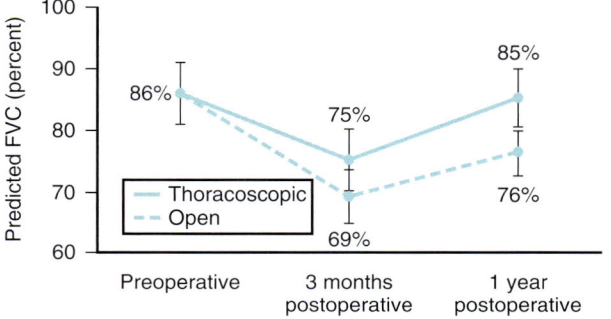

FIGURE 32.6 Changes in percent of forced vital capacity (FVC) for thoracoscopic versus open anterior instrumentation during the first year after surgery. (From Faro FD, Marks MC, Newton PO, Blanke K, Lenke LG. Perioperative changes in pulmonary function after anterior scoliosis instrumentation: thoracoscopic versus open approaches. *Spine* 2005;30:1058–1563.)

Spinal Cord Injury During Surgery

ETIOLOGY

Spinal cord injury can occur by four main mechanisms: direct contusion of the cord during surgical exposure; contusion by hooks, wires, or pedicle screws; distraction by rods or halo traction; and reduction in spinal cord blood flow.[118] Epidural hematoma should be included in the differential diagnosis of deficits occurring postoperatively. The areas of the spinal cord most vulnerable to ischemic injury are the motor pathways, which are supplied by a single anterior spinal artery. This is fed in a segmental manner by the radicular arteries that arise from the vertebral, cervical, intercostals, lumbar, and iliolumbar arteries. The largest radicular artery is the artery of Adamkiewicz, which arises between T8 and L4. A watershed area between T4 and T9 is prone to ischemia because the blood supply in this region of the cord is poorest.[119] Paraplegia is the most feared neurologic complication, but partial spinal cord injury resulting in areas of localized weakness and numbness as well as bladder and bowel disturbances also have been reported.

The increasing use of pedicle screws in spinal surgery raises the possibility of increased risk to individual nerve roots. A systematic review of pedicle screw complications that involved a total of 4570 pedicle screws in 1666 patients reported an overall 4% malposition rate that increased to 16% in studies that systematically examined their patients postoperatively.[120] Eleven patients required revision surgery for the malpositioned screws, and there was one temporary neurologic complication (i.e., epidural hematoma). No vascular injuries were reported, although six cases of aortic abutment were described.

RISK OF SPINAL CORD INJURY AND SPINAL CORD MONITORING

Surveys undertaken by the Scoliosis Research Society investigating idiopathic scoliosis reported in 1975 an incidence of neurologic impairment of 0.72%,[121] which in 2000 had decreased to 0.3%. All of the deficits were partial cord lesions.[118] Patients with curves greater than 100 degrees, congenital scoliosis, kyphosis, and postirradiation deformity appear to be at greatest risk for complications. The use of pedicle screws may have increased the immediate neurologic complication rate. In 2007, 9 neural complications were reported among 1301 patients, for an incidence of 0.69%. Three thecal penetrations occurred, two as a result of pedicle screws, all without sequelae. There were two nerve root injuries and four spinal cord injuries, all of which resolved within 3 months.[122]

A retrospective review of 19,360 cases of pediatric scoliosis showed significantly different overall complication rates among idiopathic (6.3%), congenital (10.6%), and neuromuscular (17.9%) scoliosis. Neurologic deficits had a different distribution, with the greatest rate among congenital cases (2%), and smaller rates with neuromuscular (1.1%) and idiopathic scoliosis (0.8%).[123] Mortality rates of 0.3% were observed for neuromuscular and congenital scoliosis, with an idiopathic scoliosis rate of 0.02%. Rates of new neurologic deficits were greater with anterior screw–only constructs (2%) or wire constructs (1.7%) than with pedicle screw constructs (0.7%). Surgery for high-grade spondylolisthesis appears to be associated with a particularly high risk of neurologic deficit with a rate of 11.5%.[124]

Spinal cord function is monitored to ensure that the complication rate is as small as possible. The Scoliosis Research Society issued a position statement concluding that neurophysiologic monitoring can assist in the early detection of complications and can possibly prevent postoperative morbidity. For any monitoring technique to be effective, it needs to have a sensitivity and specificity that allows true changes to be immediately recognized with very low false-negative and false-positive results to allow the problem to be reversed or prevented. Recognition of the limitation of individual techniques has seen the development of increasingly sophisticated monitoring systems to identify and minimize this risk. Older tests, such as the wake-up test and ankle clonus test, have largely been superseded by monitoring of SSEPs, MEPs, and triggered electromyographic (EMG) techniques The importance of using a multimodal approach is increasingly recognized[125–128]; the capabilities and limitations of the various techniques are summarized in E-Table 32.1.

METHODS OF MONITORING SPINAL CORD FUNCTION

Wake-Up Test

The wake-up test measures gross motor function of the upper and lower extremities.[129] The test requires limiting or reversing muscle relaxation and reducing the depth of anesthesia sufficiently to enable the patient to follow commands during the surgery; failure to move the feet and toes while being able to squeeze a hand suggests a problem with the spinal cord. When the test was initially described, 3 of 124 patients were identified as having no movement and were saved from paraplegia.[129] A major concern is that the test is conducted after maximal spinal correction, which may occur after any neurologic insult has occurred; however, removal or modification of the spinal instrumentation within 3 hours of the onset of the neurologic deficit has been reported to prevent permanent neurologic sequelae.[130] However, the wake-up test is unlikely to detect isolated nerve root injury or sensory changes and is limited to patients with an appropriate developmental age who can follow instructions.

With the clinical application of SSEP and MEP monitoring (Fig. 32.7) well established and in the absence of intraoperative changes, there is no justification to perform the wake-up test.[131] Nonetheless, some surgeons still regard the wake-up test to be the gold standard, and it may be used to confirm changes demonstrated by SSEP or MEP monitoring.[132] Risks associated with the wake-up test include lack of nerve root and sensory information, accidental extubation, dislodgment of the instrumentation, intraoperative recall with subsequent psychological trauma, air embolism, and cardiac ischemia. If a wake-up test is planned, it is prudent to warn the patient at the preoperative visit that they will be awakened during the surgery (but reassure them that they should not feel pain) and the wound will be filled with saline to reduce the risk of an air embolism.

Ankle Clonus Test

The ankle clonus test uses the clonus that occurs just before consciousness is regained during wakening from anesthesia. Rhythmic muscle contractions are thought to result from spinal reflexes returning while the higher neurologic centers remain inhibited by anesthesia, and the oscillations demonstrate an intact spinal cord. Inability to demonstrate clonus suggests spinal cord injury.[133] Like the wake-up test, it is a post hoc test rather than real-time monitoring. However, in a review of more than 1000 patients undergoing spinal procedures in which six postoperative neurologic deficits occurred, this test identified all the deficits but produced three false-positive findings, giving a sensitivity of 100% and a specificity of 99.7%. In comparison, the wake-up test

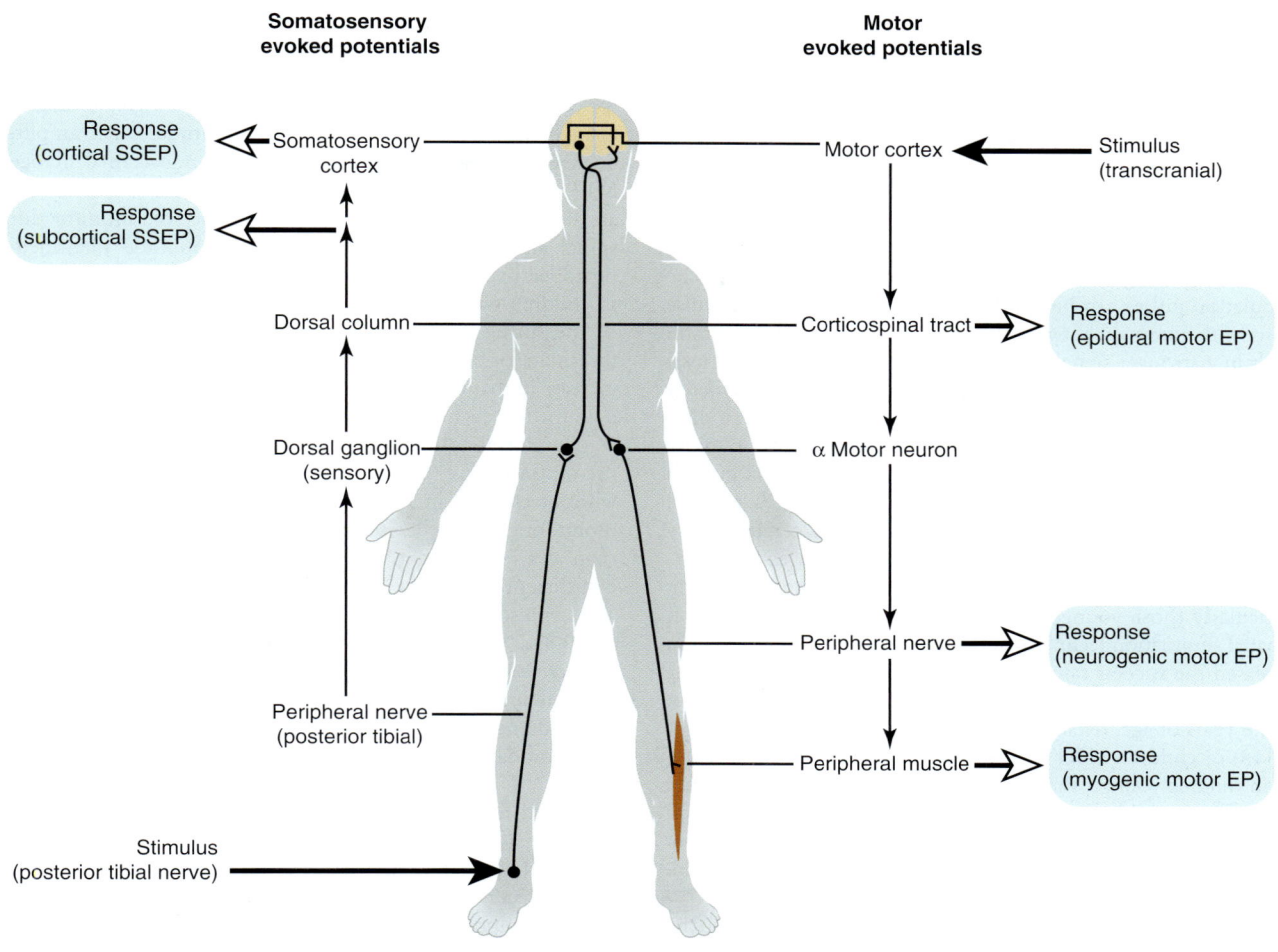

Somatosensory evoked potentials

Response (cortical SSEP) ⇐ Somatosensory cortex

Response (subcortical SSEP) ⇐

Dorsal column

Dorsal ganglion (sensory)

Peripheral nerve (posterior tibial)

Stimulus (posterior tibial nerve)

Motor evoked potentials

Motor cortex ← Stimulus (transcranial)

Corticospinal tract ⇒ Response (epidural motor EP)

α Motor neuron

Peripheral nerve ⇒ Response (neurogenic motor EP)

Peripheral muscle ⇒ Response (myogenic motor EP)

FIGURE 32.7 Comparison of pathways involved in somatosensory evoked potential (SSEP) and motor evoked potential (motor EP) monitoring. (Modified from de Haan P, Kalkman CJ. Spinal cord monitoring: somatosensory- and motor-evoked potentials. *Anesthesiol Clin North Am.* 2001;19:923–945.)

produced false-negative results for four of the five patients who developed deficits.[133]

Somatosensory Evoked Potentials

SSEPs involve stimulating a peripheral nerve and measuring the response to that stimulation using scalp electrodes (i.e., cortical SSEPs).[134,135] Alternatively, the response can be measured subcortically near the spinal cord by electrodes placed in the epidural space, interspinous ligament, or spinous processes of the vertebrae.[136] An intranasally placed pharyngeal electrode can act as a surrogate for these. The advantage of the subcortical evoked potential is that the responses are more stable, reproducible, and resistant to the effects of anesthesic agents.

The signal produced with SSEP monitoring travels from the peripheral nerve through the nerve root and up the ipsilateral dorsal column. The impulses then cross over at the level of the brainstem and progress rostrally through the thalamus to the primary sensory cortex. Up to 30% of patients with AIS may have preoperative abnormal SSEP signals.[137]

The rationale for using SSEP to monitor motor deficits is based on the fact that the sensory tracts are in proximity to the motor

tracts of the spinal cord. Injury to the motor tracts indirectly affects the sensory tracts and causes changes in the SSEP. When spinal cord function is significantly impaired, there is usually an increase in latency and a decrease in amplitude in the SSEP, with eventual loss of signal. A 10% increase in latency of the first cortical peak (P1) or 50% decreases in the peak-to-peak amplitude (P1N1) constitute an indication for intervention.[138,139] Although SSEP signals primarily monitor transmission through the sensory dorsal columns, they are effective,[139] and SSEP monitoring is associated with a 50% decrease in the incidence of neurologic deficits.

It is unusual for motor tract injury to occur when SSEPs remain unchanged, but false-positive and false-negative results have been reported.[139,140] Seventy percent of the postoperative complications were detected by the monitor, but 30% (false negatives) were not detected. Pedicle screw misplacement leading to radiculopathy may not be detected by SSEP monitoring.[141] Several case reports of paraparesis also attest to the limitations of SSEP monitoring. These problems are caused by injury occurring outside the monitored domain of SSEP rather than a failure of this modality. These concerns encouraged development of methods to monitor the motor tracts of the spinal cord. SSEP monitoring is possible in patients with cerebral palsy, whereas MEP monitoring may not be.[142]

Motor Evoked Potentials

The motor pathways can be activated by transcranial stimulation of the motor cortex or by spinal cord stimulation. Transcranial stimulation is achieved using electrical or magnetic stimulation applied to the scalp. Electrical stimulators are most commonly used in spinal surgery and operate by applying high-voltage pulses to the scalp using corkscrew, needle, or surface electrodes. The stimulation pulses can be applied as single stimuli or brief pulse trains with intervals between the pulse trains. Multiple stimuli result in a stronger signal with less variability owing to temporal summation of the excitatory postsynaptic potential.[143] Epilepsy and proconvulsant medicines are considered relative contraindications to MEP monitoring because of concerns about brain injury from prolonged seizure activity caused by the electrical current required for stimulation.[144,145] Not surprisingly, MEPs may be difficult to record and interpret in patients with cerebral palsy and should not be attempted if the child has seizures.

MEP monitoring may be a problem in younger children, particularly those younger than 6 or 7 years of age.[144,146] Use of a spatial summation technique in addition to temporal summation increased the success rate from 78% to 98% over all ages. Using this technique along with ketamine anesthesia in children younger than 6 years of age, reliable MEPs were documented in 98% (111 of 113) of children older than 6 years of age and in 86% (18 of 21) in children younger than 6 years of age.[146] There is also evidence that younger children require a greater stimulating voltage and pulse train frequency for MEP monitoring, probably because of immaturity of the central nervous system, specifically the descending corticospinal tracts.[147]

Spinal cord stimulation is achieved electrically and can be applied using electrodes placed outside or inside the spinal cord rostral to the area of interest. Single stimuli rather than brief pulse trains typically are used for spinal cord stimulation.[148] This approach is not commonly used in scoliosis surgery.

Responses can be recorded anywhere distal to the area of interest. They have included the lower lumbar epidural space (i.e., epidural MEP), peripheral nerve (i.e., neurogenic MEP), and peripheral muscles using compound muscle action potential (CMAP) (see Fig. 32.7).[149] Each recording site has its limitations regarding the accuracy of the information displayed and the susceptibility to anesthetic drug interference. Epidural MEPs are the least affected by neuromuscular blocking drugs (NMBDs), but they monitor only conduction in the corticospinal tract and provide no information about the anterior horn grey matter.[150] They have a much slower response to acute spinal cord ischemia compared with myogenic responses (i.e., CMAPs).[151] Neurogenic MEPs are also resistant to anesthetic interference but appear to not accurately measure motor conduction. Most of the spinally elicited peripheral nerve responses seen with neurogenic MEPs occur through the dorsal columns in a retrograde fashion and are sensory rather than motor.[152] Anterior spinal cord injury has been demonstrated with normal neurogenic MEPs.[153] CMAPs after transcranial stimulation are thought to be exclusively generated by motor tract conduction, and unlike epidural MEPs, they include the ischemia-sensitive anterior horn alpha motor neurons.[149] These responses are very sensitive to anesthetic agents. The responses obtained with CMAPs after spinal cord stimulation also appear to contain signals that include transmission through the dorsal columns and may represent a mixed response.[154]

One outstanding problem with MEP monitoring is deciding when and how much change in the signal is indicative of spinal cord ischemia. Some centers use the same criteria they adopted for SSEP monitoring, whereas others require a greater degree of change, such as a 75% decrease in amplitude.[155] An amplitude decrease of 80% at one of six sites using transcranial myogenic MEP monitoring was demonstrated to have a sensitivity of 1.0 and a specificity of 0.91 when used as the sole monitor during spinal surgery.[156] A 65% decrease in amplitude identified all postoperative motor deficits (SSEP changes identified only 43%) in children with idiopathic scoliosis.[157] An alternative technique of measuring MEP has been described in which a minimum threshold for producing a response is established, and a significant increase in that threshold is used to signal a problem.[158] Supportive data for this technique are lacking.

The dorsal columns may be injured without involvement of the motor tract.[159] Occasionally, adverse changes in SSEPs occur without changes in MEPs.[148,160] Because of these reports, MEP monitoring should be used in addition to SSEP monitoring rather than as a replacement.[125-128,161] Whether SSEP monitoring alone is sufficient to reliably identify neurologic deficits remains debatable, with some institutions reporting sensitivity of 95%, specificity of 99.8%, a positive predictable value of 95%, and a negative predictive value of 99.8% for this monitoring.[162] However, multimodal intraoperative monitoring (combination of SSEP and MEP) demonstrated improved sensitivity when compared with either modality alone.[163]

Triggered Electromyographic Techniques

The increasing use of pedicle screws allows greater curve and rotational correction than earlier techniques but has an additional risk of direct nerve root trauma. Triggered EMGs using a monopolar needle or bipolar handheld stimulator have been described, with a threshold stimulation level of more than 8 mA considered to be normal, 5 to 8 mA to be critical, and less than 5 mA to be pathologic, indicating that there was not enough distance between the screws and the neural tissue.[161] This technique requires monitoring rectus abdominis or intercostal muscles when used for thoracic curves.[164,165]

Preoperative Assessment and Postoperative Planning

RESPIRATORY ASSESSMENT AND PLANNING FOR POSTOPERATIVE VENTILATORY SUPPORT

The preoperative pulmonary assessment should identify patients at increased risk for postoperative respiratory compromise. Since patients with idiopathic scoliosis generally have less compromised pulmonary function, most studies have focused on non-idiopathic patients.[78] The rate of postoperative pulmonary complications correlates broadly with the decrease in vital capacity.[72,166,167] Vital capacity less than 30% to 35% of predicted values indicates marginal respiratory reserve and a level at which complications and a need for postoperative respiratory support are likely. Many patients with these low vital capacities are unable to cough effectively, rendering them prone to postoperative atelectasis, pneumonia, and respiratory failure.

Studies of a mixed population of disorders (but a limited number with neuromuscular disorders) with a vital capacity less than 40% reported that despite the occurrence of short-term and middle-term pulmonary complications, these patients can be successfully discharged home, although some require prolonged postoperative ventilation.[168,169] Modest numbers with a vital capacity less than 25% of the predicted value are included in these studies and do not have greater complication rates than those with greater vital capacities. Anterior or combined approaches increase the likelihood of respiratory complications, particularly owing to pleural effusion.[168,169]

Children with neuromuscular scoliosis are likely to need postoperative ventilation that is often prolonged.[72,167] These patients may also have abnormalities in the central control of breathing and impaired airway defense mechanisms. Impaired coordination of laryngeal and pharyngeal muscles may result in impaired swallowing and inadequate cough with increased risk of aspiration. Initial research suggested that as the vital capacity decreased to less than 35% of predicted, most patients would need a brief period of postoperative ventilation.[101] The earlier use of nocturnal NPPV and use of NPPV in the postoperative period may alter our perception of this risk by decreasing the impact or severity of postoperative respiratory complications while allowing children with increasingly severe respiratory impairment to be considered for surgery. Scoliosis surgery can be successfully undertaken in patients with a vital capacity less than 35% of predicted, often with no more than 24 hours of planned ventilation followed by a period of noninvasive ventilation (e.g., bilevel positive airway pressure [BiPAP]).[72,81,170,171] In one study (n = 30), the overall complication rate was similar whether the FVC was greater than or less than 30%, and the average hospital stay was approximately 3 weeks (see Table 32.2). Tracheostomy was required in two children, and the overall pulmonary complication rate was 30%[171]; similar results are reported by others.[81] It seems reasonable to anticipate using noninvasive ventilator support for several days after spine stabilization surgery in children with a vital capacity less than 25% of predicted values. Children with a mean FVC of 20% of predicted have been successfully managed with a brief period of postoperative ventilation and transition to BiPAP within 48 hours.[172]

Whether a child should be denied surgery requires consideration of individual patient factors. The successful management of children with a vital capacity of 15% to 20% of predicted has been reported, although the sample size was small.[168–171] Although the risk of an unsuccessful outcome can increase at this level of pulmonary dysfunction, individual circumstances may justify the risk. The successful introduction of perioperative NPPV will likely lead to children who were previously considered unsuitable for surgery now being offered surgery, challenging the established limitations.[173]

CARDIOVASCULAR ASSESSMENT

Many children with complex cardiac comorbidities can successfully undergo scoliosis surgery as a result of improvements in understanding, monitoring, anesthesia, and surgical techniques. A greater need for blood transfusion should be expected. A preoperative curve greater than 80 degrees is a risk factor for major complications in children who have had congenital cardiac defects corrected.[174] Children with residual cardiac abnormalities will require prolonged stays in the intensive care unit and hospital. Those with single ventricle or Fontan physiology have increased morbidity and mortality.[175] Increased bleeding is almost always a problem because of high venous pressures; the need for inotropic support and the occurrence of arrhythmias and pleural effusions are common.[175]

Muscle disorders may affect the myocardium and the skeletal system. Children with DMD develop a cardiomyopathy in the second decade that may be difficult to evaluate because the child is wheelchair bound by that age. Sinus tachycardia is an early manifestation. Cardiac function deteriorates during early adolescence[176] as more than 90% of adolescents with DMD have subclinical or clinical cardiac involvement.[177] Echocardiography is an essential aspect of the preoperative evaluation of any wheelchair-bound patient presenting for scoliosis surgery (see also Chapters 17 and 23). Cardiac magnetic resonance imaging may be better than echocardiography for assessment of children with DMD.[178]

POSTOPERATIVE PAIN MANAGEMENT

Scoliosis surgery is associated with severe pain that lasts for at least 3 days.[179] Effective analgesia minimizes postoperative respiratory complications by allowing deep breathing, chest physiotherapy, early ambulation, and rehabilitation. Postoperative pain may be managed with systemic or epidural analgesics. A multimodal approach is likely to be most effective.

Intraoperative Intrathecal and Intravenous Opioids

Intraoperative intrathecal morphine (2–5 µg/kg) has provided potent analgesia during the first 24 hours after spinal fusion in children.[180,181] Intrathecal morphine also decreases the amount of remifentanil required intraoperatively, contributing to less pain when remifentanil is discontinued.[182,183] However, perioperative administration of IV morphine, when using remifentanil as part of the anesthesia technique, does not result in any measurable benefit.[184]

Methadone (0.2 mg/kg) decreases pain scores and opioid requirements for 36 hours in children undergoing surgery, but it seems to have been ignored in modern practice.[185] This drug is used in adult spinal surgery and reports of its use in children are increasing.[186,187] An IV bolus (0.25 mg/kg) followed by an infusion (0.1–0.15 mg/kg per hour) for 4 hours during spinal surgery has been proposed to maintain adequate plasma concentrations for 24 hours.[187]

Nonsteroidal Antiinflammatory Drugs

NSAIDs, but not acetaminophen, impair fracture healing in animal models.[188] Cyclooxygenase-2 (COX-2) activity plays an important role in bone healing, and the use of NSAIDs decreases osteogenic activity that may increase the incidence of nonunion after spinal fusion.[8,9] The effect on osteogenic activity is dose dependent and reversible.[189] Similar effects have not been demonstrated in humans and the use of these drugs after scoliosis surgery varies in different parts of the world.[190] Nonetheless, based on animal evidence, NSAIDs should be used with caution and in consultation with the surgeon during the first 3 to 5 days after scoliosis surgery.[191]

Systemic Analgesics

Morphine remains the mainstay of systemic analgesic regimens. Morphine infusions of 20 to 40 µg/kg per hour are required during the first 48 hours after surgery. Achieving a balance of effective analgesia while avoiding sedation can be difficult in children with neurodevelopmental delay. Regular evaluation of these children is important if complications are to be avoided. Patient-controlled analgesia (PCA) is appropriate for children older than 6 to 7 years of age. It can be used with a typical bolus dose of 20 µg/kg and a lockout interval of 5 to 10 minutes. The use of a background morphine infusion may be effective in some patients, although its inclusion is controversial.[192,193] Our preference is to use a nighttime background infusion at 5 to 10 µg/kg per hour but to use PCA alone during the day (see also Chapter 44). The addition of acetaminophen improves analgesia but does not decrease opioid requirements.[194] Nurse- and parent-controlled analgesia are effective if the child is too young or unable to use PCA.[195] Intrathecal morphine plus PCA appears to offer the optimal combination of effective analgesia and minimal adverse effects in patients with idiopathic scoliosis compared with PCA morphine alone or epidural morphine.[196] The demands/deliveries ratio of PCA is predictive of increased opioid requirements, with a ratio greater than 1.5 associated with greater pain scores, opioid-related adverse effects, and duration of hospitalization; a ratio greater than 2.5 suggests a benefit from switching opioids.[197]

Low-dose ketamine infusion (0.05-0.2 mg/kg per hour) has been used as an adjunct to morphine infusions or PCA, although its role is debated.[198-203] Ketamine may be initiated intraoperatively (initial infusion of 5 µg/kg per minute, decreasing to 2 µg/kg per minute at the end of surgery) as part of the anesthetic technique to minimize the hyperalgesia reported after high-dose remifentanil infusions. A postoperative 72-hour ketamine infusion did not decrease morphine consumption or pain scores.[204] Ketamine added to morphine PCA has produced mixed results, with no clear beneficial effect in orthopedic surgery, despite such evidence being apparent for thoracic surgery.[205] If added to PCA, the optimal combination of morphine/ketamine is a 1:1 ratio.[201] Although scoliosis is a very painful surgery, it is probably best to reserve the use of ketamine for those with significant preoperative pain or morphine-resistant pain.

Gabapentin and pregabalin may provide some benefit with an opioid-sparing effect,[206] although postoperative nausea and vomiting benefits are limited.[207] Gabapentin (15 mg/kg followed by 5 mg/kg three times daily for 3 days) reduced morphine consumption by about 30% during the study period but without any improvement in morphine's adverse effects. Improved pain relief was observed only until the morning after surgery.[208] All the effects of gabapentin for postoperative pain may have been overestimated by statistically significant small study effects.[209]

Epidural Analgesia

Continuous epidural analgesia using single- and double-catheter techniques may provide effective analgesia after spinal surgery.[210] The single-catheter technique using bupivacaine-fentanyl and sited at T6-7 for patients undergoing a mean 12-level scoliosis surgery resulted in analgesia similar to that of PCA but with more postoperative nausea and vomiting and pruritus. Bowel sounds returned earlier in the epidural group, but liquid intake and hospitalization time were similar.[211] Similar results were reported with a bupivacaine-morphine combination in patients undergoing 10-level spinal fusions. Full diet and discharge from hospital were achieved one-half day earlier with the epidural technique than with PCA.[212] A retrospective review of more than 600 patients treated with an epidural or PCA for analgesia after scoliosis surgery that involved an average 8.5 fused segments confirmed the effectiveness of epidural analgesia.[213] In that study, a bupivacaine-hydromorphone epidural combination effectively controlled the pain, although it was associated with more complications. Respiratory depression and transient neurologic changes were the most common complications observed. Thirteen percent of patients with an epidural catheter required discontinuation of the epidural, most commonly for inadequate pain relief.[213] Effective analgesia and a large incidence of postoperative nausea and vomiting and pruritus have been features of studies that combined bupivacaine and morphine.[214,215]

Patient-controlled epidural analgesia (PCEA) has been successfully used in children older than 5 years of age for orthopedic surgery and thoracotomies.[216] In scoliosis surgery, the pain score with PCEA with bupivacaine and hydromorphone was slightly superior to that with PCA, although there was a 37% failure rate with the former.[217] PCEA with a single- or double-catheter technique (as discussed later), depending on the number of spinal segments involved, with a combined bupivacaine-fentanyl-clonidine solution effectively controlled pain with a relatively small incidence of complications.[218]

Improved pain control and bowel function with decreased adverse effects may be possible by using a double-epidural technique using moderate amounts of fentanyl and clonidine with local anesthetics.[219] Double-epidural techniques use an upper catheter positioned in the upper to middle thoracic segments and a lower catheter at the upper to middle lumbar level.[220,221] This technique improved pain control and was associated with fewer gastrointestinal adverse effects when compared with a single epidural catheter and morphine PCA.[210]

Anesthetic and Intraoperative Management

POSITIONING AND RELATED ISSUES

The patient must be positioned so that extreme pressure points are avoided, the limb positions are adjusted to prevent nerve injury, and the abdomen is free to minimize venous congestion. This is usually achieved by the use of the Relton-Hall frame or a variant.[222] The frame consists of four well-padded supports arranged into **V**-shaped pairs, with the upper pads supporting the thoracic cage and the lower pair supporting the anterolateral aspects of the pelvic girdle at the anterior iliac crests. The arms must not be abducted or extended more than 90 degrees from their natural position. The weight of the arms is evenly distributed across the forearm to avoid pressure on the ulnar nerve at the elbow. The range of motion of the shoulders should be assessed preoperatively for optimal positioning during anesthesia. This can present quite a challenge in children with severe deformities, and creative positioning may be required. In some centers, the nipples are covered with Tegaderm (3M, St. Paul, MN) and positioned free of direct pressure. It is also essential that the head is maintained in a neutral position and that pressure is evenly distributed between the forehead and face, avoiding direct pressure on the eyeballs. Care must be taken to avoid any direct pressure on the knees, and the patient's weight should be distributed throughout the lower limb (Fig. 32.8). Reston self-adhering foam (3M, St. Paul, MN) may be used to pad the pelvic brim and knees.

Not all spinal tables and frames affect cardiac function in the same way. There is some evidence that the Jackson spine table (Mizuho OSI, CA, USA) or longitudinal bolsters have fewer effects on cardiac function, whereas Wilson and Andrews frames may negatively impact cardiac function.[223] However, an average decrease in cardiac index of 18.5% (0.5 L, 95% confidence e interval [CI] 0.3–0.7L) was observed after placing patients prone on the Jackson table, without a significant change in blood pressure.[224] The use of two chest pads rather than a single pad with the Jackson frame results in smaller average and maximum chest pressures at the expense of increasing the pelvic pressures.[225]

Postoperative visual loss is an uncommon, unpredictable, and devastating complication associated with spinal surgery in the prone position. It may occur in up to 0.2% of cases, and although most of the reports involve adult patients, older children are not immune.[226,227] The most common cause is ischemic optic neuropathy, but the cause remains obscure. Prolonged operating time (>6 hours) and increased or uncontrolled blood loss are features of most reports.[228–231] The phenomenon is unrelated to pressure on the globe and usually occurs without evidence of any other ischemia-related complications.[231] There are conflicting reports regarding the association with issues such as hypotension, controlled hypotension, anemia, hemodilution, blood loss, rotational positioning of the head, diabetes, and others.[228,231–233]

TEMPERATURE REGULATION

The long preparation time and exposure of undraped patients on a spinal frame render them susceptible to hypothermia. Hypothermia is associated with hemodynamic instability and increased blood loss.[234] A threefold increase in surgical wound infection occurs with a 2°C-decrease in core temperature.[235] Preoperative warming reduces the amount of time that the patient is hypothermic during surgery by almost 2 hours without affecting the temperature at the end of surgery.[236] Efforts should be made to increase the ambient temperature in the operating room while the patient is prepared for surgery. Subsequent hypothermia can be minimized if the room temperature is maintained at 24°C during this period rather than at 18°C to 21°C, as is often encountered during surgery.[237] After the patient has cooled during preparation and positioning, it may take several hours before the core temperature begins to return toward normal. Even with forced-air warming systems, it is often difficult to restore normothermia because only a small amount of the patient's body is exposed to these devices. It may be possible to position a warming blanket underneath the frame so that warming from below and above occurs (see Fig. 32.8 and Video 32.1).

PATIENT MONITORING

Patient monitoring needs to be tailored to the individual case, but at minimum, arterial oxygen saturation, end-tidal carbon dioxide (CO_2), electrocardiographic (ECG) patterns, core temperature, and urine output should be recorded. In most cases, invasive arterial and central venous pressures are monitored because of large blood losses, fluid shifts, and the risk of cardiovascular instability. Externally applied pressure by the surgeon during dissection or curve correction may compromise cardiac function or filling. Central venous pressure is an accurate and valid measurement in the prone position, providing the zero is adjusted for the patient's position on the spinal frame. Patients with a significant

kyphotic component are at increased risk for venous air embolism and should be monitored for this possibility. Depth of anesthesia monitoring should be considered; particularly when MEP monitoring limits the concentrations of anesthetic drugs and total IV anesthesia (TIVA) is used. Care should be taken when positioning the head because pressure on the forehead by the sensor while the patient is in the prone position for many hours may cause erythema, localized swelling, and tissue necrosis; contact dermatitis from the adhesive has been reported.[238] Mixed venous oxygen tension trends may be helpful for children with myocardial compromise. Transesophageal echocardiography can be useful for determining ventricular filling and function when hemodynamic compromise is identified or suspected preoperatively.

MINIMIZING BLOOD LOSS AND DECREASING TRANSFUSION REQUIREMENTS

Scoliosis surgery involves exposure of a large wound over a considerable period. Positioning the patient with the abdomen free to avoid venous compression is important to control and minimize blood loss. Increased intraabdominal pressure attributable to positioning can double intraoperative blood loss.[239]

More blood tends to be lost in posterior spinal fusion procedures than in anterior procedures. This loss probably corresponds to the greater number of vertebral levels fused with the posterior approach. Blood loss increases as the number of vertebrae included in the fusion increases. The estimated blood loss (EBL) is approximately 750 to 1500 mL in patients with idiopathic scoliosis, or 60 to 150 mL per vertebral segment fused. The blood loss of 1300 to 2200 mL (100–190 mL per vertebral segment) is significantly greater in patients with cerebral palsy. Children with DMD experience the largest EBL: 2500 to 4000 mL (200–280 mL per vertebral level).[240]

Children with neuromuscular scoliosis demonstrate a prolonged prothrombin time and a decrease in factor VII activity intraoperatively, suggesting that consumption of clotting factors and dilution of clotting factors enhance the blood loss.[241] It has been postulated that children with DMD lack dystrophin in all muscle types and that the poor vascular smooth muscle vasoconstrictor response may be a factor in the increased blood loss.[242] Hypothermia exacerbates blood loss by decreasing platelet function, decreasing coagulation factor activity, and slowing vasoconstriction.[234]

Adverse reactions to blood appear to be more common in children than adults, with human error as the most common cause.[243] Several techniques have been used to decrease blood loss and minimize exposure to blood products (see also Chapter 12).

Hypotensive Techniques

Controlled hypotension has been used to minimize blood loss during scoliosis surgery since it was first described more than 30 years ago. A greater than 50% decrease in blood loss with a decreased need for blood replacement and a reduced operating time was demonstrated in early studies. Ganglion-blocking agents (i.e., pentolinium and trimethaphan) have been superseded by β-blockers, direct arterial vasodilators, calcium channel blockers, and α_2-agonists. It remains uncertain whether the reduced blood loss results from the reduced blood pressure[244] or reduced cardiac output.[245] A target mean arterial pressure (MAP) of 50 to 65 mm Hg has been recommended. Although this appears to be safe, concerns that the margin of safety for optic, cerebral, and spinal cord ischemia has reduced the use of controlled hypotension, particularly for operations of prolonged duration. Additionally,

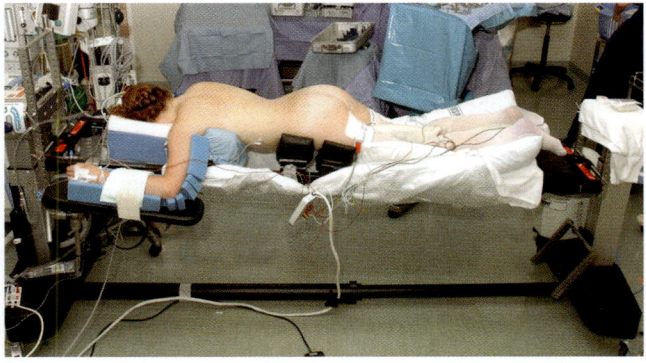

FIGURE 32.8 Positioning on the Orthopedic Systems Incorporated (OSI) Jackson frame (Mizuho OSI, CA, USA), showing protected pressure points and an underframe forced-air warming blanket.

there is the potential that periods of unexpected hypovolemic hypotension may exacerbate and complicate drug-induced (controlled) hypotension.[246,247] The incidence of these feared complications is fortunately very small with or without hypotension. Renal function appears well preserved even when hypotensive anesthesia is used during scoliosis surgery.[248,249] Because of these concerns and the concomitant use of hemodilution, less extreme degrees of hypotension are usually used. Robust data supporting the beneficial effects of controlled hypotension in scoliosis surgery are limited, although clear benefits have been demonstrated for orthognathic and orthopedic surgery.[250,251]

In modern practice, moderate hypotension with good control of the heart rate can often be achieved without the use of specific vasoactive drugs by using a remifentanil infusion titrated to the desired blood pressure.[252] Although not considered a hypotensive agent, intrathecal morphine decreases blood loss and may facilitate blood pressure control, particularly with a remifentanil infusion. At an analgesic dose of 5 µg/kg, a decrease in EBL from 41 to 14 mL/kg has been reported.[181] Using this technique, blood pressure control can frequently be achieved without any additional agents. The use of an anesthetic combination of less than 1 minimum alveolar concentration (MAC) of inhalational agent plus remifentanil with clonidine (2 µg/kg)[253] provides controlled hypotension in most patients without the need for additional agents. Dexmedetomidine may be used as part of a technique for controlling blood pressure.[254,255] Its use resulted in a mean blood pressure of 66 mm Hg (a 20% decrease compared with nonuse), with reduced blood loss (782 vs. 465 mL) and fewer children requiring transfusion.[256]

Short-acting calcium channel blockers have been used to control hypotension in patients undergoing scoliosis surgery, and although these agents are effective, experience is limited. The blood loss during nicardipine for hypotension was less at the same MAP compared with sodium nitroprusside, although blood pressure returned to baseline more slowly (27 vs. 7 minutes) with the former.[257,258] Clevidipine has been used without evidence of clear benefit, but it may be associated with an increase in heart rate.[259] If a hypotensive technique is to be used, invasive arterial monitoring is essential, and central venous pressure catheters are useful for the safe conduct of anesthesia (see also Chapter 12).

Hemodilution

Decreasing the hemoglobin concentration by removing red blood cells and replacing the volume with a combination of crystalloid and colloid means that for a given volume loss, fewer red blood cells are lost (see also Chapter 12). The decreased metabolic rate during anesthesia suggests that oxygen delivery can be maintained with a reduced hemoglobin concentration if normovolemia is maintained.

It has been estimated that more than 2 to 3 units of blood must be removed during hemodilution to significantly reduce transfusion requirements. Hemodilution modeling in adult patients has suggested that as many as 5 units of blood must be removed before there is a decrease in transfusion requirements.[260] Deciding on the degree of hemodilution and establishing a threshold for transfusion may be difficult. In scoliosis surgery, reduction to an initial hematocrit of 30% has been effective for reducing and minimizing transfusion requirements.[261] Some posit that only modest benefits are gained from this technique.[262] Hypotensive anesthesia, hemodilution, and a cell saver used as part of a "bloodless surgery" program with erythropoietin and supplemental iron resulted in an average EBL of 855 mL (blood returned by the

cell saver averaged 341 mL), with an average decrease in hemoglobin after surgery of 3.1 g/dL.[263]

Tachycardia and hemodynamic instability are common at hemoglobin concentrations less than 7 g/dL. Myocardial ischemia becomes a risk at hemoglobin concentrations less than 5 g/dL.[264] At this level of anemia, cyanosis cannot develop because 5 g/dL of desaturated hemoglobin is required for cyanosis to be detected. Extreme hemodilution techniques such as these are reserved for patients who oppose blood transfusion. One report detailed patients who had hemodilution during scoliosis surgery to a hemoglobin concentration of 3 g/dL in the absence of preexisting cardiac disease.[265] Cardiac output increased by more than 30%, with only a modest increase in heart rate and decrease in blood pressure.[265] Although no cerebral sequelae were reported, *this degree of extreme hemodilution is not recommended.*

Autologous Predonation

Preoperative strategies, including predonation of blood and preoperative red cell augmentation, may be used alone or in addition to intraoperative techniques to minimize exposure to blood (see also Chapter 12). In idiopathic scoliosis surgery, pre-autologous blood donation plus intraoperative red cell salvage and controlled hypotension resulted in an average EBL of 1055 mL, avoided transfusion, and decreased the hematocrit by only 10% 35.6% preoperatively to 32.4% at discharge.[266] The advantages of preoperative erythropoietin in addition to preautologous blood donation include a greater preoperative hemoglobin concentration and fewer donated units. Its effect on blood use depends on the total blood loss.[267,268] In children with neuromuscular scoliosis, erythropoietin alone did not affect the amount of blood transfused, although the preoperative and discharge hematocrits were greater in treated patients.[269]

Antifibrinolytic Agents

The use of synthetic antifibrinolytic agents to decrease perioperative blood loss after scoliosis surgery has produced mixed results. To be most effective, an effective plasma concentration of the antifibrinolytics should be established before skin incision (see also Chapter 20). ε-Aminocaproic acid (Amicar) decreases the EBL by 25% during the perioperative period,[270] mainly attributable to decreasing the postoperative suction drainage.[271] In contrast, an initial dose of tranexamic acid (10 mg/kg) followed by an infusion of 1 mg/kg per hour failed to significantly decrease blood loss in a small sample.[272] High-dose tranexamic acid (100 mg/kg loading dose, followed by an infusion of 10 mg/kg per hour), reduced blood loss by 40% but did not affect transfusion requirements. Post hoc analysis in patients with secondary (neuromuscular) scoliosis showed significant reduction in blood loss and transfusion requirements.[273] The correct dose of tranexamic acid remains elusive, but it may be one-half of the high-dose reported previously.[274]

A meta-analysis of aprotinin, tranexamic acid, and ε-aminocaproic acid on blood loss and use of blood products in children undergoing scoliosis surgery showed that all antifibrinolytic drugs decreased the amount of blood transfused and that aprotinin, tranexamic acid, and ε-aminocaproic acid were equally effective.[275] A similar meta-analysis of major pediatric surgery showed that in the scoliosis studies, aprotinin and tranexamic acid reduced blood loss compared with placebo (385 mL, 95% CI 42–727 mL vs. 682 mL, 95% CI 214–1149 mL).[276] In all operations, both drugs also decreased red blood cell transfusion. Demonstration that tranexamic acid is as effective as aprotinin is fortunate, because aprotinin has been withdrawn in many countries after reports of increased morbidity and mortality in adults after cardiac surgery.[277] However, after a review of the evidence, aprotinin has been reintroduced in Canada, citing off-label use of the drug as the cause of complications. Studies are being conducted in the United States. Use of ε-aminocaproic acid reduced mean intraoperative blood loss (1125 mL vs. 2194 mL), total perioperative blood loss (1805 mL vs. 3055 mL), and transfusion requirements (660 mL vs. 1548 mL) compared with placebo.[278] However, a multicenter study involving 37 hospitals across the United States suggested that ε-aminocaproic acid but not tranexamic acid use was associated with a lower odds ratio (0.42) of transfusion in patients with AIS, but neither drug resulted in a decrease in odds for children with neuromuscular scoliosis.[279]

Reduced blood loss has significant cost savings from decreased operating room time and blood product use.[280] Desmopressin is ineffective in decreasing blood loss associated with spinal surgery. Initial beneficial results with desmopressin[281] have not been reproduced in patients with idiopathic scoliosis[282,283] or in those with neuromuscular scoliosis.[284,285]

Intraoperative Salvage of Shed Blood

Decisions concerning the use of intraoperative salvage of shed blood (e.g., cell saver) depend on the anticipated blood loss, size of the child, and use of other methods to minimize blood transfusion, such as predonation and hemodilution (see also Chapter 12). It is important to have some idea of the blood loss associated with idiopathic scoliosis in your institution when deciding to use cell saver techniques. For example, the cell saver was found to be beneficial in less than 5% of adolescents with idiopathic scoliosis involved with an autologous predonation program or modest intraoperative hemodilution in one institution.[261] At another institution, however, allogeneic transfusion rates were reduced from 55% to 18% when the cell saver was used. The allogeneic transfusion relative risk was 2.04 for patients undergoing surgery lasting longer than 6 hours and 5.87 for patients not receiving cell saver blood.[286] Donor transfusion reduction is most effective when intraoperative cell salvage is combined with either preoperative autologous blood donation or postoperative collection and retransfusion.[287]

Pediatric systems are available with small spinning bowls (55 to 75 mL). These systems benefit children with smaller body weights and greater than anticipated blood loss such as patients with neuromuscular scoliosis undergoing extensive spinal fusion.[288,289] Among children undergoing anterior instrumentation for thoracolumbar curves, cell saver use decreased the number requiring allogenic blood transfusion from 39.4% to 6.7% and with similar mean postoperative hemoglobin values (10.2 vs. 9.6 g/dL).[290]

MANAGING BLOOD LOSS

Autologous blood donation before surgery requires an organized schedule of donation with or without the administration of erythropoietin.[291,292] This may be the safest and most effective method of avoiding or minimizing the use of allogenic blood products.[293] A predonation program was effective in minimizing blood exposure in AIS patients undergoing surgical correction for their scoliosis. A mean of 3.7 units of blood was donated by each patient before surgery, and 97% of adolescents avoided the use of allogeneic blood during and after surgery.[291] Similar results have been reported without predonation. Ninety-five percent of patients with AIS avoided transfusion just by using a cell saver with a transfusion trigger of 7 g/dL. The average drop in Hb was 4.1 g/dL with nadir on postoperative day 2.[294]

However, preoperative blood typing for crossmatch is always warranted.

Measurement of blood loss during scoliosis surgery is difficult. Accuracy is lost as measurements embrace blood suctioned from the operative field that includes irrigation fluid, weighing or estimating blood collected on swabs and sponges, approximations of blood on drapes and gowns, and estimations of evaporation from the wound.

The decision about when to administer blood component therapy (i.e., non–red cell blood components) is often based on clinical judgment. Dilutional thrombocytopenia is expected only after several blood volumes have been lost and depends on the preoperative platelet count (see also Chapter 12). Platelet concentrations should be measured after loss of one blood volume and at periodic intervals after this. Dilution of coagulation factors may also lead to surgical bleeding when only packed red blood cells are used to replace blood loss. Prolongation of prothrombin time and activated partial thromboplastin time may occur when the blood loss exceeds one blood volume, and these times should be checked at this time. These coagulation tests are not usually associated with increased bleeding until values are greater than 1.5 times mean control values, at which time increased surgical bleeding can be effectively treated with fresh frozen plasma.[295] Platelet counts after one blood volume loss, whether associated with normal or abnormal clotting, were within the normal range.[295] Blood component therapy should probably be based on abnormal clotting test results, uncontrolled bleeding, or the absence of normal clotting in the surgical field. It is preferable to intervene with blood component therapy before uncontrolled bleeding develops. If pooled blood in a dependent part of the operative field fails to show evidence of clotting, it is time to transfuse with blood components, starting with fresh frozen plasma and administering platelets only if this approach is not effective.[295]

Massive transfusion protocols, in which predefined ratios of red blood cells, plasma factors, and platelets (usually in a 1 : 1 : 1 ratio) are administered early in the resuscitation phase of massive trauma, are being increasingly used in all situations of uncontrolled blood loss (see Chapter 12).[296,297] Evidence that these protocols decrease morbidity and mortality in the trauma setting has resulted in their implementation in surgery, in which significant and uncontrolled bleeding may be expected.[298,299] By adopting these protocols, proportionally greater quantities of factors and platelets are transfused compared with conventional approaches in severe hemorrhage, but it is associated with increased survival.[300] However, there is no evidence that this approach is beneficial in elective surgery.

The thromboelastogram is useful in refining blood product administration if multiple blood volumes are required for resuscitation.[298,300] Scoliosis surgery in patients with neuromuscular scoliosis or cerebral palsy, particularly in those with severe complex curves in whom pelvic stabilization and iliac crest grafts are considered, fulfill these criteria. In this group of patients, early administration of blood and factors using a massive transfusion protocol may be beneficial.[301] Recombinant factor VIIa may be a useful therapy for patients with a dilutional coagulopathy who are unresponsive to blood component replacement therapy. Successful use with doses as small as 20 µg/kg has been described in spinal surgery.[302–305]

EFFECTS OF ANESTHETICS ON SOMATOSENSORY EVOKED AND MOTOR EVOKED POTENTIALS

Anesthetic agents act by directly inhibiting synaptic pathways or by indirectly changing the balance of inhibitory and excitatory influences.[306,307] The greater the number of synapses and the more complex the neuronal pathway being monitored, the greater the potential impact of anesthetic agents on the evoked potentials. Most anesthetic agents depress the amplitude and increase the latency of SSEPs and MEPs. For this reason, cortical SSEPs are more sensitive than spinal cord– or brainstem-measured SSEPs. MEPs are susceptible to anesthetic agents at three sites: the motor cortex, the anterior horn cell, and the neuromuscular junction. Consequently, transcranial stimulation with peripheral muscle detection (using CMAPs) is most susceptible to anesthetic interference. Although inhalational anesthetics and most IV anesthetics markedly depress SSEPs and MEPs, ketamine and etomidate appear to enhance the amplitudes of both, possibly by attenuating inhibition.[307]

Inhalational Anesthetics

Inhalational anesthetics cause a dose-dependent depression of both SSEP and myogenic MEP, although at equipotent concentrations, the MEP is affected to a greater degree than the SSEP. This means that while inhalation agents can be used during SSEP monitoring, they often need to be administered in subanesthetic doses during MEP monitoring. Adequate cortical SSEPs and subcortical SSEPs can be measured with up to 1 MAC of isoflurane, sevoflurane, and desflurane, although some increase in latency and decrease in amplitude may be detected.[308,309] It is important to maintain constant end-tidal concentrations throughout anesthesia after baseline measurements have been established. The concentrations of these inhalational anesthetics that allow adequate monitoring are significantly less than was possible with halothane.[310]

Myogenic MEPs (i.e., CMAPs) are recordable only at low concentrations of inhalational anesthetics. The exact concentration depends on the system being used and is greatly influenced by the number of pulses in the stimulus. Single-pulse transcranial stimuli may be inhibited by end-tidal concentrations as small as 0.2 MAC and abolished by end-tidal concentrations as small as 0.5 MAC.[311–313] This suppression can be partially overcome by using greater intensity stimuli with multipulse stimulation of up to 6 pulses per stimulus. An increasing number of patients lose recordable myogenic MEPs, even when multipulse stimuli are used, as the concentration of inhalational anesthetic exceeds 0.5 MAC. At end-tidal concentrations in excess of 0.75% isoflurane, monitoring conditions become unacceptable.[314–318] Stimulus intensity and pulse train frequency probably are factors in determining successful myogenic MEPs with inhalational anesthetics. Using direct stimulation of the cortex during craniotomy, CMAP was easily recordable at 1 MAC of isoflurane and sevoflurane.[319] Similar results have been demonstrated with sevoflurane using transcranial stimulation.[320] Information regarding desflurane is limited, and although it causes a dose-dependent depression, myogenic MEPs have been successfully recorded at 0.5 MAC.[318,321] Using a multipulse stimulation technique, intraoperative recording of MEPs was equally successful during desflurane or propofol anesthesia.[322] Desflurane anesthesia allowed MEP monitoring when used to provide a depth of anesthesia that maintained the bispectral index (BIS) at 40 to 60 or at a concentration of 0.6 to 0.8 MAC.[323,324] There was no difference in the amplitude or latency of SSEPs compared with propofol (150–300 μg/kg per minute) titrated to a similar BIS.[324] Low-dose desflurane is a viable alternative to propofol infusion and may be associated with a quicker wake-up time.[324]

Nitrous Oxide

Nitrous oxide reduces the amplitude of the cortical SSEP, but comparisons with other inhalational anesthetics are limited. Nitrous oxide (0.5 MAC) depresses SSEPs to a greater extent than isoflurane at a similar MAC.[325] Similarly, 66% nitrous oxide depressed SSEPs to a greater extent than propofol (6 mg/kg per hour; 100 μg/kg per minute).[326] Nitrous oxide depresses myogenic MEPs.[309] The effect relative to other inhalational anesthetics is difficult to determine. Nitrous oxide appears to affect CMAP amplitude to a lesser extent than isoflurane.[327] Multipulse stimulus techniques can partially reverse nitrous oxide–induced depression of amplitude. Compared with a propofol infusion designed to maintain a target concentration of 3 μg/mL, 50% nitrous oxide decreases CMAPs with single or paired stimuli to a lesser extent.[328] When 60% nitrous was added to low-dose propofol infusion at a target concentration of 1 μg/mL, adequate CMAPs were obtained using multipulse transcranial stimulation.[329] Conversely, the addition of nitrous oxide to a variety of different total IV techniques significantly depressed the CMAP such that some were not recordable.[330] With the widespread availability of remifentanil and the variable but mostly negative effects of nitrous oxide on SSEP and MEP signals, the latter is best avoided when monitoring spinal cord potentials.

Propofol

Propofol decreases the amplitude of the cortical SSEP, but adequate signals can be recorded, even in the presence of nitrous oxide, at doses used for anesthesia (6 mg/kg per hour; 100 μg/kg per minute).[331] Propofol better preserves cortical SSEP amplitude and provides a deeper level of hypnosis as measured by processed electroencephalographic values than combinations of low-dose isoflurane and nitrous oxide or low-dose isoflurane or sevoflurane alone.[332–334]

Propofol depresses the amplitude of myogenic MEPs. In addition to its cortical effect, it suppresses activation of the alpha motor neuron at the level of the spinal grey matter.[335,336] Low-dose propofol infusions have become popular as part of the anesthetic technique used with MEP monitoring owing to the rapid improvement of signals when the drug is terminated and because multipulse stimulation techniques can improve the response amplitude.[315,337] Propofol, even in combination with nitrous oxide, depresses multipulse transcranial CMAPs less than isoflurane.[315] Propofol (5 mg/kg per hour; 83 μg/kg per minute) combined with 66% nitrous oxide produced satisfactory CMAP recordings in 75% of patients when a four-pulse stimulation sequence was used. In contrast, no recordings were possible with 1 MAC of isoflurane.[316] The infusion rates or target concentrations that allow acceptable myogenic MEP recordings vary considerably and reflect different adjuvants (e.g., opioids, ketamine, nitrous oxide), degrees of neuromuscular blockade, and transcranial pulse rates. Propofol at a target of 4 μg/mL or at an infusion rate of 6 mg/kg per hour (100 μg/kg per minute) produces acceptable signals with multipulse stimuli.[337–339] Target-controlled infusion models have poor performance characteristics in children undergoing scoliosis repair. Using the Paedfusor model, measured propofol concentration was almost always greater than predicted (see Chapter 8).[340] Because MEPs appear particularly sensitive to depth of anesthesia, it is important that a BIS monitor is used with propofol infusions.

α₂-Adrenoreceptor Agonists: Clonidine and Dexmedetomidine

The cerebral effects of the α₂-agonists appear to act mainly at the locus coeruleus, rather than by the more generalized inhibition of synaptic pathways, as in the case of general anesthetics.[341] Clonidine at IV doses of 2 to 5 μg/kg had minimal effects on cortical SSEPs when added to isoflurane.[342-344] In view of its lack of effect on SSEPs and its anesthetic-sparing properties with inhalational agents and propofol,[344-346] it seems reasonable to consider clonidine at a dose of 2 to 4 μg/kg as part of an anesthetic technique. Dexmedetomidine has similar beneficial properties on SSEPs.[347,348]

There are no published studies on the effects of clonidine on MEPs, but a few publications have examined dexmedetomidine and MEPs with variable results.[349-352] Dexmedetomidine, like other anesthetic agents, produces a dose-dependent depression of MEPs, rendering the ability to interpret these signals dependent on the depth of anesthesia. This suggests that the depth of anesthesia should be monitored when recording MEPs to maintain a plane of anesthesia that is adequate to prevent recall but still ensure meaningful MEP signals. When dexmedetomidine is added to a propofol infusion, it decreases the dose of propofol required to maintain anesthesia at a BIS of 40 to 60 by more than 50%, provides moderate hypotension, decreases blood loss, and allows monitoring of MEPs and SSEPs, but at the expense of slightly prolonged waking.[256] During the loading dose of dexmedetomidine, MEP decreased transiently in some patients in parallel with a decrease in the BIS from 50 to 30. However, the BIS rebounded to greater than 40 once the maintenance infusion was started.

We have observed similar effects with clonidine as an adjunct; a temporary decrease in MEPs sometimes occurs if clonidine is administered too rapidly, but the signals improve if the BIS is maintained in the 50 to 60 range.

Opioids

Alfentanil, fentanyl, sufentanil, and remifentanil minimally depress SSEP and MEP signals.[353,354] Dose-dependent depression of the CMAP occurs at doses of opioids that far exceed those used in clinical anesthesia.[355,356] Comparison of alfentanil, fentanyl, and sufentanil at doses sufficient to suppress noxious stimuli suggested that sufentanil exerted the least effect of the three opioids.[355] A similar study that included remifentanil showed that it depressed the signals the least, with CMAPs measurable at infusion rates of 0.6 μg/kg per minute.[356] It is likely that greater doses can be used if clinically indicated.

Ketamine and Etomidate

Ketamine enhances the cortical SSEP amplitude and has a minimal effect on subcortical and peripheral SSEP responses.[357] It also produces minimal effects on the myogenic MEP responses as a bolus of 0.5 mg/kg[358] or when used in moderate doses (1-4 mg/kg per hour; 17-83 μg/kg per minute) as a supplement to a nitrous oxide–opioid anesthesia.[358,359] Experimental evidence suggests S(+)-ketamine modulates the CMAP by a peripheral mechanism at or distal to the spinal alpha motor neuron.[360] Ketamine (4 μg/kg per minute) has been successfully used with MEP monitoring during propofol-remifentanil anesthesia for scoliosis correction.[146,361]

Although capable of inducing general anesthesia, etomidate behaves more like ketamine in its effect on evoked potentials. It improves the quality of SSEPs and enhances the amplitude of MEPs.[362] It produces minimal changes in MEPs compared with barbiturates or propofol.[335] Etomidate infusions (10-35 μg/kg per minute) produce adequate MEP monitoring signals.[358,363] Concerns regarding adrenocortical depression with etomidate infusions remain and limit its widespread use.[364] Bolus doses of etomidate, however, can transiently depress MEPs.[358] A new etomidate analog is under investigation that will have a half-life of minutes with no associated adrenocortical depression and no active

metabolites[365,366]; when commercially available, this drug may provide an alternative to propofol.

Midazolam

IV midazolam (0.2 mg/kg) decreases the SSEP amplitude by 60%.[367] This does not occur with subcortical SSEPs, for which a slight increase in latency but no change in amplitude has been demonstrated.[368] Although midazolam (0.5 mg/kg) caused marked depression of MEPs in nonhuman primates that persisted during awakening,[369] this finding does not hold true in human studies. MEP amplitude was unaffected by a midazolam-ketamine infusion technique compared with propofol-ketamine or propofol-alfentanil techniques.[330] Midazolam did not suppress myogenic MEPs, even at doses sufficient to produce anesthesia.[356] Effects were similar to those with etomidate.[356]

Neuromuscular Blockade

NMBDs exert little or no effect on the SSEP. They prevent or limit recording of CMAPs during myogenic MEP recording because of their effects on the neuromuscular junction. Partial neuromuscular blockade, however, is commonly used during MEP monitoring because it improves conditions for surgery by providing adequate muscle relaxation when retraction of the tissues is required and limits any patient movement during the stimulus generation. Partial muscle relaxation may also reduce noise caused by spontaneous muscle movement. Constant neuromuscular blockade must be maintained during the procedure. Many centers avoid neuromuscular blockade after intubation, the initial incision, and muscle dissection.

Two methods have been used to assess the degree of neuromuscular blockade for MEP monitoring. One is measurement of the amplitude of the CMAP produced by single supramaximal stimulation (T1) before an NMBD is administered. When T1 is maintained between 20% and 50% of the baseline level, reproducible CMAP responses can be obtained with a degree of muscular blockade that allows surgery.[363,370] The other technique is adjustment of the neuromuscular blockade based on the train-of-four responses. Comparison of the fourth twitch (T4) with that of first twitch (T1) suggests acceptable CMAP monitoring is possible when two of the four twitches remain.[370-372] Neuromuscular blockade should be evaluated in the specific muscle groups that are used for electrophysiologic monitoring because different muscle groups have different sensitivities to the NMBDs. Patients with preoperative neuromuscular dysfunction tend to demonstrate greater effect after partial neuromuscular blockade than those with normal preoperative motor function. It is appropriate to avoid neuromuscular blockade in most of these patients.[363]

CHOOSING ANESTHETIC DRUGS AND TECHNIQUES

The choice of anesthesia depends on the patient's pathology and the type of electrophysiologic monitoring for the operation. A marked increase in the use of MEPs and advances in MEP techniques have occurred worldwide. CMAPs appear to provide the most useful data for minimizing the risk of spinal cord injury.

The key to success is to use a technique that allows a stable concentration of the hypnotic component of anesthesia. There are nominal differences between the inhalational anesthetics (<1 MAC) and propofol (<6 mg/kg per hour; 100 μg/kg per minute). Concentrations of the inhalational anesthetics approaching 1 MAC are now compatible with multipulse MEP monitoring systems that did not appear possible several years ago. Short-acting medications offer greater flexibility if the monitored signals deteriorate.

The use of a remifentanil infusion allows a rapidly titratable analgesic component with minimal effect on spinal cord monitoring. Clonidine or dexmedetomidine may be used to decrease the concentration of hypnotic drugs during SSEP monitoring and MEP monitoring, but the depth of anesthesia should be also be monitored. Although propofol infusions appear to have become a popular anesthetic technique, there is no reason desflurane at equi-anesthetic doses should not be used with the benefit of a quicker wake-up, should neuromonitoring signals rapidly deteriorate.

Ketamine as the main component of anesthesia may improve MEP monitoring because it better preserves the MEP signals and allows reduced doses of other hypnotic agents to be used, but low-dose ketamine used as an adjunct to a conventional anesthetic does not. If processed electroencephalographic monitoring is used to determine anesthetic depth, the addition of ketamine may confound the reading by increasing it.[373,374] This occurs despite a deepening level of hypnosis.[373] An NMBD improves the SSEP monitoring and may be used in conjunction with MEP monitoring within the confines described earlier. However, even in patients with idiopathic scoliosis, adequate operating conditions after the initial muscle dissection can be produced in the absence of neuromuscular blockade. In the absence of muscle relaxation, muscle contractions, including those of the masseter muscles, occur during stimulation. In this situation, it is prudent to insert a bite block to prevent obstructing the tracheal tube or to intubate the patient nasally.

Tourniquets

INDICATIONS AND DESIGN

The tourniquet was used by the Romans to control bleeding during amputation.[375] The arterial tourniquet is used during orthopedic procedures to reduce blood loss and provide good operating conditions, for IV regional blockade and sympathectomy, and for isolated limb perfusion in the management of localized malignancy.[376]

The word *tourniquet* is derived from the French verb *tourner,* meaning "to turn," referring to the twisting or screwing action applied to the constricting bandage to tighten it. In 1873, von Esmarch introduced the use of a flat rubber bandage wrapped repeatedly around a limb.[375] Although this rubber bandage is still used to render a limb bloodless, the pneumatic tourniquet, introduced by Cushing in 1904, has replaced the rubber bandage to maintain ischemia. Compressed nitrogen or air is used for inflation. The target pressure is preset, and compensatory feedback mechanisms maintain that pressure during inflation. Curved and wider tourniquet cuffs, which are designed to fit conical limbs, are associated with lower arterial occlusion pressures than standard cuffs.[377] A soft dressing applied to the limb before tourniquet application helps to prevent wrinkles and blisters that may occur when the skin is pinched.[378] Adequate exsanguination can also be achieved by elevation of the arm at 90 degrees or the leg at 45 degrees for 5 minutes.[379,380]

PHYSIOLOGY

Ischemia

Ischemia leads to tissue hypoxia and acidosis. The severity and consequences of the associated changes (e.g., increased capillary permeability, coagulation alteration, cell membrane sodium pump activity) depend on the tissue type, duration of ischemia, and collateral circulation. Muscle is more susceptible to ischemic damage than nerves. Histologic changes are more pronounced in muscle beneath the tourniquet compared with muscle distal to the tourniquet.

Reperfusion

Reperfusion removes toxic metabolites and restores energy supplies. There is a sudden release of lactic acid, creatinine phosphokinase (i.e., creatine kinase), potassium (peak increase of 0.32 mEq/L), and CO_2 (peak increase of 0.8–18 mm Hg) when the cuff is deflated suddenly. Metabolic changes increase after longer periods of ischemia but return to baseline within 30 minutes. Muscle damage may release myoglobin, which can collect in the collecting tubules of the kidney, precipitating renal failure.

Systemic effects after deflation of the tourniquet include a shift of blood volume back into the limb with a transient decrease in blood pressure that is exacerbated by a postischemic reactive hyperemia in the limb. CO_2 release transiently increases the minute volume. The rapid increase in CO_2 is also associated with a transient (8–10 minutes) increase in cerebral blood volume that may affect patients with raised intracranial pressure.[376]

Increased microvascular permeability of muscle and nerve tissue occurs with tourniquet release after 2 to 4 hours of ischemia. Interstitial and intracellular edema and capillary occlusion owing to endothelial edema and leukocyte aggregation may take months to resolve.

Ischemic Conditioning

Short periods of ischemia followed by reperfusion render muscle more resistant to subsequent ischemia. Ischemic preconditioning improves skeletal muscle force, contractility, and performance and decreases fatigue of skeletal muscle. This preconditioning may enable prolongation of orthopedic and reconstructive procedures.[381]

COMPLICATIONS

Local Complications

Muscle Damage

Histologic changes in the muscle beneath the tourniquet occur after 2 hours of tourniquet time (at 200 mm Hg [26.7 kPa]), but similar changes can occur in the distal ischemic muscle after 4 hours of tourniquet use. Direct pressure and mechanical deformation contribute to increased severity of muscle damage under the cuff.[376] These changes include an increase in the number of inflammatory cells in the perivascular space, focal fiber necrosis, and signs of hyaline degeneration.

The combination of muscle ischemia, edema, and microvascular congestion contributes to posttourniquet syndrome: edema, stiffness, pallor, weakness without paralysis, and subjective numbness of the extremity without objective anesthesia. The common use of postoperative casts may conceal the true incidence of this syndrome. Recovery usually occurs over 7 days.[382]

Nerve Damage

The cause of nerve injuries after tourniquet use probably is direct compression under the cuff rather than ischemia. Sheer forces that are maximal at the upper and lower edges of the tourniquet cause the most damage. These forces are greater with the Esmarch bandage than with the pneumatic tourniquet. The incidence of nerve injuries in the upper limb (1 case per 11,000 patients) is greater than in the lower limb (1 case per 250,000 patients); the radial nerve is the most vulnerable nerve in the upper extremity, and the sciatic nerve is the most vulnerable in the lower extremity.[383]

Vascular Damage

Arterial injury is uncommon in children. It is an injury of adults with atheromatous vessels, and the tourniquet should be avoided in patients with absent distal pulses, poor capillary return, a calcified femoropopliteal system, or a history of vascular surgery on the involved limb.[384]

Skin Safety

Pressure necrosis and friction burns may occur with poorly applied tourniquets, and some form of skin protection should be used routinely.[385] A "limb protection sleeve" may help reduce wrinkling, shearing, and pinching of soft tissues. Chemical burns may result from antiseptic skin preparations that seep beneath the tourniquet and are then retained and compressed against the skin.

Tourniquet Pain

The tourniquet causes a vague, dull ache that becomes intolerable after approximately 30 minutes.[386] This pain is associated with an increase in heart rate and blood pressure that is not ameliorated by general anesthesia and neuraxial blockade.[386] The pain is transmitted by unmyelinated C fibers, which are normally inhibited by fast pain impulses transmitted by myelinated A-delta fibers, but in this case, mechanical compression reduces transmission through the larger A-delta fibers.[387] Narrow silicon ring tourniquets may be associated with less pain than wide tourniquets.[388]

Systemic Complications

Temperature Regulation

The combination of decreased heat loss from the ischemic limb and reduced heat transfer from the central to ischemic peripheral compartment increases core body temperature.[389,390] Bilateral tourniquets increase the temperature more than unilateral tourniquets.[390] Children who require intraoperative tourniquets should not be aggressively warmed during surgery.[390] Redistribution of body heat and the efflux of hypothermic venous blood from the ischemic area into the systemic circulation after deflation of the tourniquet decreases the core body temperature, which may switch off thermoregulatory vasodilation and decrease the skin-surface temperature.[391]

Deep Vein Thrombosis and Emboli

The incidence of emboli after release of the tourniquet in children is unclear. The tourniquet appears to have no influence on deep vein thrombosis, but release of the tourniquet may be associated with an increased risk of embolism in adults. Some clinicians have suggested that heparin be used during total joint arthroplasty in adults to prevent emboli formation,[392] although this practice is not routine in children. Some surgeons use such therapy in adolescents.

Sickle Cell Disease

Hypoxia, acidosis, and circulatory stasis contribute to the sickling of sickle cells in susceptible individuals. However, several institutions routinely use tourniquets in children with sickle cell disease while maintaining acid-base status, hydration, and oxygenation throughout the procedure.[393,394] Each case must be assessed individually for the balance between the advantages of a bloodless field and the risks of precipitating sickling crises (see Chapter 10).

Drug Effects

Antibiotics given after the tourniquet is inflated do not produce effective concentrations in the blood and tissue of the ischemic limb. Inflation of the tourniquet should be delayed at least 5 minutes after administration of the antibiotics.[395,396] Medications administered before inflation of the tourniquet may be sequestered in the ischemic limb and then re-released into the systemic circulation when the tourniquet is deflated. The antibiotic effect depends on the amount of antibiotic sequestered, the tissue binding, and the concentration-response relationship for the antibiotic, although the impact is minimal for most medications used in anesthesia. Volume of distribution may be reduced if the drug is administered after the tourniquet is inflated, but the plasma clearance remains unaffected.

RECOMMENDED CUFF PRESSURES

Most clinicians limit the duration of tourniquet inflation to a maximum of 1.5 to 2 hours. Techniques such as hourly release of the tourniquet for 10 minutes, cooling of the affected limb, and alternating dual cuffs may reduce the risk of injury.[397] Nerve and muscle injuries that occur beneath the tourniquet cuff are related to the pneumatic pressure. Consequently, the minimum pressure that maintains ischemic conditions should be sought. Hypotensive anesthetic techniques have been used in adults to reduce the need for high cuff inflation pressures,[358] but there seems to be little need for this in children. One study recommended that the arterial occlusion pressure in each child should be measured by Doppler and the tourniquet pressure set to 50 mm Hg in excess of this value.[399] Alternatively, the tourniquet pressure may be set to 20 mm Hg in excess of the arterial occlusion pressure for similar results.[400] However, these empiric formulas ignore the typical fluctuations in blood pressure that occur during surgery. The optimal tourniquet pressure may be one that fluctuates with the systemic blood pressure.[401] Maximum mean pressures recommended for the upper and lower extremities are 173.4 ± 11.6 mm Hg (range, 155–190 mm Hg) and 176.7 ± 28.7 mm Hg (range, 140–250 mm Hg), respectively.[399] Wider cuffs exert less force per unit area and reduce the risk of local sequelae. Recommendations for adults suggest that the cuff should exceed the circumference of the extremity by 7 to 15 cm. This is difficult to achieve in infants, in whom the proximal limb length is proportionally shorter than in adults and the wide cuffs impinge on the surgical field. New disposable narrow elastic ring tourniquets may improve access for short-duration adult surgery, but concerns about injury risk limit their use in children.[402]

Acute Bone and Joint Infections

The mainstays of management for osteomyelitis and septic arthritis are antibiotics and surgical drainage. The incidence of these infections is increasing, particularly in immunocompromised children with HIV infection. Tuberculosis remains a scourge in many developing countries. Mortality rates for hospital-acquired staphylococcal disease in compromised children[403] and community-acquired disease in healthy children[404–406] range from 8% to 47% for those presenting with severe sepsis.[407] *Mycobacterium* and *Staphylococcus* species resistant to conventional antibiotics increase morbidity and mortality rates.

PATHOPHYSIOLOGY

Staphylococcus aureus is the most common pathogen. Osteomyelitis develops after bacteremia and occurs mostly in prepubertal children. Normal bone is highly resistant to infection, but *S. aureus* adheres to bone by expressing receptors for components of bone matrix, and the expression of collagen-binding adhesin permits the attachment to cartilage.[408] After the microorganisms adhere to bone, they express phenotypic resistance to antimicrobial treatment.[408]

The metaphyseal region around the growth plate is the predominant area of infection. Sluggish blood flow in the metaphysis predisposes children to bacterial infection, and endothelial gaps in developing vessels allow bacteria to escape into the metaphysis. Subsequent abscesses may decompress into the joint or subperiosteally. Infection may involve adjacent tissue planes, and hematogenous spread causes multiple pathologic processes beyond the primary site of infection.

Septic arthritis is more common in neonates because transphyseal vessels link the metaphysis and epiphysis. Growth plate and epiphyseal destruction may occur in this age group. Articular cartilage damage is attributable to the release of proteolytic enzymes by the pathogen and activated neutrophils.

CLINICAL PRESENTATION

Most children with staphylococcal disease present with musculoskeletal symptoms and fever, but those with disseminated disease may be critically ill (4%–10%) with severe sepsis, lung disease, and extracutaneous foci.[404,405] One report found that one-half of extracutaneous foci of staphylococcal infection were not detected on hospital admission, and one-third of these lesions were observed for the first time at autopsy.[403] There is often a history of trauma.[404,405] An absolute polymorphonuclear cell count of greater than 10,000/mm³ or an absolute band-form count of greater than 500/mm³, or both, correlates with the presence of one or more inadequately treated sites of staphylococcal infection.[403] Tuberculosis is the great mimic and must always be suspected in endemic areas.

Diagnosis is confirmed by blood, bone, or joint aspirate culture. Radiologic procedures (e.g., plain radiographs, computed tomography, magnetic resonance imaging, radionuclide scans) are often required to identify foci, and the anesthesiologist is often requested to provide sedation.[409]

TREATMENT OPTIONS

Antibiotic therapy is the mainstay of treatment. Initial antibiotic choice is dictated by age and by local pathogen and sensitivity profiles. Antibiotic treatment should be extended to cover gram-negative enterococci in neonates and *Streptococcus* in older children. *Haemophilus influenzae* remains a pathogen in unvaccinated regions. Surgical decompression of acute osteomyelitis that is responding poorly to antimicrobial therapy may release intramedullary or subperiosteal pus and lead to clinical improvement. Pus within fascial planes also requires release. Venous thrombosis attributable to pus in soft tissue planes around major joints was associated with a high mortality rate in one series.[404] Determining and eradicating the primary focus improves the mortality and reduces recurrence rates.[410] An aggressive search for foci and surgical drainage of infective foci is required.

Highly active antiretroviral therapy (HAART) has positively altered the mortality rates for HIV-infected children. However, acute bone and joint infections still occur,[411] and these drugs can cause significant morbidity resulting from changes in fat distribution, lipid profiles, glucose concentrations, homeostasis, and bone turnover.[412] Infarction may replace infection as the major cause of morbidity and mortality from HIV.[412] It is uncertain whether HAART should be continued during acute osteomyelitis. Worsening cell-mediated immune function may occur during tuberculosis treatment if HAART is continued.[413] The combination of HIV infection and tuberculosis can be lethal in children; antituberculosis treatment is continued for 12 to 18 months.

ANESTHESIA CONSIDERATIONS

Anesthesiology services are commonly required for sedation during diagnostic investigation, anesthesia for surgical exploration and release of pus or fixation of pathologic fractures, management of pulmonary complications (e.g., intercostal chest drain insertion, pleurodesis), central venous cannulation for long-term antibiotic treatment, and analgesic modalities.

Children with disseminated staphylococcal disease may be critically ill with multisystem disease and require fluid volume augmentation, inotropic support, positive-pressure ventilation, extracorporeal renal support, and coagulation factor replacement. Others may appear clinically stable before induction of anesthesia; the assessment of hypovolemia in children is subject to moderate to poor interrater agreement.[414] IV access and rehydration are required before beginning anesthesia to avoid a precipitous blood pressure drop immediately after induction. Bacteremic showering during manipulation and drainage of pus causes further decompensation. Excessive bleeding owing to altered coagulation status should also be anticipated.

The presence of a septic arthritis in the shoulder or neck may cause cervical ligamentous laxity predisposing to C1–2 subluxation during intubation.[415] Pneumatoceles from staphylococcal pneumonia can rupture during positive-pressure ventilation. A spontaneous breathing mode, however, may be difficult to achieve because of laryngospasm, breath-holding, increased secretions, and bronchospasm. The use of NMBDs and positive-pressure ventilation in these patients with a low threshold for introducing inotropes to support the cardiovascular system is an easier option. Vigilance is required for acute pneumothorax.

Myocarditis, pericarditis, and pericardial effusions compromise myocardial function. A 12% prevalence of infective endocarditis among children with hospital-acquired *S. aureus* bacteremia has been reported.[416] This prevalence of infective endocarditis is frequently associated with congenital heart disease and the necessity for multiple blood cultures.[416] The incidence of infective endocarditis among children with community-acquired disease without preexisting cardiac abnormalities is low,[404] suggesting that echocardiography could be reserved for children with preexisting cardiac disease, those with suspicious clinical findings, those whose temperature fails to stabilize, or those who have prolonged bacteremia without an obvious source of infection.

PAIN MANAGEMENT

Morphine and acetaminophen are the analgesics commonly used for postoperative pain management. The use of tramadol in children is increasing as our understanding of the pharmacokinetics of this medication increases.[417,418] The low incidence of respiratory depression and constipation, fewer controls on use, and similar frequency of nausea and vomiting (10%–40%) compared with opioids make tramadol an attractive alternative.[419–421] NSAIDs are relatively contraindicated in the presence of coagulation disorders, altered renal function, and COX-2–mediated osteogenesis.

The performance of regional blockade in children with acute bone or joint infection is controversial. There are no studies addressing the risk/benefit ratios of regional techniques in this population. It seems reasonable to use these techniques only after 24 hours of appropriate antibiotic therapy in apyrexial children who show no signs of a coagulopathy.

Common Syndromes

Children with some specific conditions present repeatedly for orthopedic procedures. It is worthwhile maintaining a database that details their anesthetic management. There should be 24-hour access to standard texts or electronic information concerning anesthesia and uncommon pediatric diseases.

CEREBRAL PALSY

Clinical Features

Cerebral palsy is an umbrella term that describes a group of nonprogressive, but often changing, motor impairment syndromes caused by lesions or anomalies in the brain that occur during the early stages of its development.[422] It is the leading cause of motor disability during childhood, with a prevalence of approximately 2 per 1000 live births in developed countries.[423]

Disorders include cognitive impairment, sensory loss (i.e., vision and hearing), seizures, and communication and behavioral disturbances. Systemic disorders resulting from cerebral palsy affect the gastrointestinal, respiratory, urinary tract, and orthopedic systems. Cerebral palsy is divided into three broad categories: spastic (70%), dyskinetic (10%), and ataxic (10%). Children with spastic cerebral palsy commonly present for orthopedic procedures because of contractures at major peripheral joints.[424,425] Functional improvement after surgery in children with spastic diplegia and spastic hemiplegia is better than in those suffering spastic quadriplegia.[424]

Orthopedic Considerations

Orthopedic manipulations form only part of the treatments designed to improve performance or improve the ease of care.[426] Management, including orthopedic surgery, physical and occupational therapy, recreational therapy, orthotics, and assistive devices, improves functional outcomes. Medical modalities such as intramuscular injections of botulinum toxin and intrathecal administration of baclofen by means of an implanted pump may also be of benefit.[427] Selective dorsal rhizotomy has been used to control spasticity.[428,429]

The indications for and timing of surgical interventions vary. Gait analysis increases the age of the patient at the first orthopedic surgical procedure, and botulinum toxin type A treatment delays and reduces the frequency of surgical procedures on the lower extremities.[430,431] Bone and soft tissue surgical procedures are designed to lengthen or weaken spastic muscles to give opposing muscles a chance to attain muscle balance.

Anesthetic Considerations

Children with cerebral palsy who present for orthopedic surgery often have previous experience with operating rooms. They should be handled with sensitivity because communication disorders and sensory deficits may mask mildly impaired or normal intellect. They may be accompanied by a parent or caregiver or be premedicated for induction of anesthesia or in the recovery room. If there is a communication problem, the parent or caregiver should be present before and after anesthesia.[424,432] These children have an increased risk of postoperative complications, which correlates with the severity of the child's preoperative condition.[433] Preoperative risk factors associated with increased risk included an American Society of Anesthesiologists physical status score exceeding 2, history of seizures, upper airway hypotonia, general surgery procedures, and adults.[433]

Medical conditions (e.g., seizure control, respiratory function, gastroesophageal reflux) should be optimized preoperatively. Contracture deformities, spinal deformities, decubitus ulceration, and skin infection must be considered when positioning the child for anesthesia and surgery. Poor nutritional status affects postoperative wound healing and the risk of infection. Concurrent medications may influence anesthesia; sodium valproate can cause platelet dysfunction and affect drug metabolism, and anticonvulsant use increases resistance to NMBDs.[434] A history of latex allergy should be sought because of exposure to latex allergens from an early age.[435]

IV access may be difficult. Drooling, a decreased ability to swallow secretions, and gastroesophageal reflux may dissuade some from performing inhalational inductions in these children, although there is no evidence that a rapid-sequence induction is safer. Succinylcholine may be used because it does not cause hyperkalemia in these children, whose muscles have never become denervated. Noncommunicative or nonverbal children with cerebral palsy require less propofol to obtain the same BIS values (i.e., 35–45) than do otherwise healthy children.[436] The MAC of halothane is 20% less in children with cerebral palsy regardless of whether they took anticonvulsant drugs (MAC of 0.62 and 0.71, respectively).[437]

Intraoperative hypothermia is common in children with disordered temperature regulation cause by hypothalamic dysfunction, reduced muscle bulk, and fat deposits. Thermal homeostasis should be managed aggressively from the moment the child enters the operating room.

Extensive plaster casting is an important component of bone and soft tissue surgical procedures. These casts may conceal blood loss, and limb swelling within the cast may contribute to compartment syndromes. Plaster jackets and hip spicas have been associated with mesenteric occlusion and acute gastric dilatation.

Pain and spasm are regular features postoperatively. Epidural analgesia is particularly valuable when major orthopedic procedures are performed. Occasionally, two epidurals at different spinal sites may be required for multilevel surgery. The addition of either fentanyl or clonidine to bupivacaine in an epidural reduced the incidence of muscle spasm, although the incidence of vomiting was greater in the fentanyl group.[438] Systemic benzodiazepines, baclofen, dantrolene, and clonidine have been used to reduce muscle spasms. Selective dorsal rhizotomy is associated with severe pain, muscle spasms, and dysesthesia. Epidural and intrathecal forms of morphine as well as IV morphine and midazolam have been used to control this pain.[439] Oral benzodiazepines may be required to reduce the incidence and severity of muscle spasms but should be used with caution if combined with opioid analgesia.

Pain assessment is difficult in these children, but several scoring systems are available (see also Chapter 44).[440,441] The opinions of parents and caregivers are extremely valuable in the assessment of pain and discrimination from other factors, such as irritability on anesthetic emergence, poor positioning, a full bladder, or nausea.

SPINA BIFIDA

Spina bifida is characterized by developmental abnormalities of the vertebrae and spinal cord that may be associated with changes in the cerebrum, brainstem, and peripheral nerves. The failure of fusion of the vertebral arches is commonly known as *spina bifida*. *Spina bifida occulta* refers to spina bifida that occurs when skin and soft tissues cover the defect. *Spina bifida aperta* is used to describe lesions that communicate with the outside as a meningocele or a myelomeningocele (incidence of 1 per 1000 live births). The myelomeningocele sac contains nerve roots that do not function below the level of the lesion.

Clinical Features

Nerve root dysfunction results in muscle paralysis and a neurogenic bowel and bladder. Eighty percent of children develop hydrocephalus because of aqueductal stenosis (Arnold-Chiari [type II] malformation). Skeletal abnormalities such as clubfoot and congenital dislocation of the hip are common. Scoliosis may result from congenital vertebral abnormalities or, more commonly, abnormal neuromuscular control. Epilepsy and learning disorders can also occur, but most children have normal intelligence.

Orthopedic Considerations

Denervation causes muscle imbalance that results in abnormalities at the hip, knee, and foot. The aims of surgery are to reduce flexor posture at the hip and knee and plantigrade feet. Children with clubfeet, hip subluxation, or scoliosis commonly present for orthopedic correction.

Anesthetic Considerations

The potential for infection of the central nervous system dictates closure of the sac within the first few days of life. Subsequent surgical procedures and urinary catheterizations set the stage for sensitivity to latex.[442] Primary prophylaxis (i.e., avoiding all latex materials and using a latex-free operating room) is recommended for prevention of latex allergy and anaphylaxis.[443]

Preoperative assessment should include motor and sensory deficits, respiratory and renal function, and functioning of a ventriculoperitoneal shunt. Positioning on the operating table may require additional pillows for support of limbs with contractures. As a result of hypesthesia in the lower extremities, IV cannulae can be inserted painlessly. However, venous access is usually poor in the lower extremities because of limited limb use. The risk of endobronchial intubation is increased because of a short trachea (36% of children).[444] Kyphoscoliosis may distort tracheal anatomy. Renal dysfunction may dictate the choice of NMBD as well as the avoidance of NSAIDs. Succinylcholine may be used because it does not cause hyperkalemia in these children.[445] A reduced hypercapnic ventilation response means that these children should be closely observed in the recovery period.

OSTEOGENESIS IMPERFECTA

Osteogenesis imperfecta (OI) is thought to have afflicted Ivar the Boneless (Ivar Ragnarsson), a Viking chieftain who led a successful invasion of the East Anglia region of England in AD 865. Because he "had legs as soft as cartilage," he was unable to walk and had to be carried on a shield. Ivar's name is also associated with an early form of thoracoplasty. When King Ælla of Northumbria was captured, Ivar subjected him to the horrific "Blood Eagle" ordeal. His ribs were torn out and folded back to form the shape of an eagle's wings, and his lungs were removed.

Clinical Features

OI is a genetically determined disorder of connective tissue that is characterized by bone fragility. The disease state encompasses a phenotypically and genotypically heterogeneous group of inherited disorders that result from mutations in the genes that code for type I collagen.[446] The disorder manifests in tissues in which the principal matrix protein is type I collagen—mainly bone, dentin, sclerae, and ligaments. Musculoskeletal manifestations vary in severity along a continuum ranging from perinatal lethal forms with crumpled bones to moderate forms with deformity and propensity for fracture to clinically silent forms with subtle osteopenia and no deformity.[446]

Classification (types I through IV) is based on the timing of fractures or on multiple clinical, genetic, and radiologic features. Type I is the most common (1 case per 30,000 live births), and types I and type IV have autosomal dominant inheritance patterns. These children have the classic triad of blue sclera, multiple fractures, and conductive hearing loss in adolescence. Bowing of the lower limbs, genu valgum, flat feet, and scoliosis develop with age. Type IV is characterized by osteoporosis, leading to bone fragility without many of the other features of type I. Types II and III are more severe forms of OI and have autosomal recessive inheritance patterns. Molecular genetic studies have identified more than 150 mutations of the *COL1A1* and *COL1A2* genes, which encode for type I procollagen.[446]

Orthopedic Considerations

The goals of treatment of OI are to maximize function, minimize deformity and disability, maintain comfort, achieve relative independence in activities of daily living, and enhance social integration. Physiotherapy, rehabilitation, and orthopedic surgery are the mainstays of treatment for moderate and severe forms of OI.[447] Medical treatment with the antiresorptive bisphosphonates (e.g., pamidronate) can decrease pain, lower the fracture incidence, and improve mobility.[448] Initial investigations have demonstrated an acceptable safety profile for pamidronate, although long-term follow-up data are lacking and will be necessary for the development of responsible therapeutic guidelines.[449] Long-term IV bisphosphonate therapy was associated with higher z scores for lumbar spine, bone mineral density, and vertebral reshaping, but long-bone fracture rates were still common and the majority of patients developed scoliosis.[450] Medical therapies other than bisphosphonates, such as growth hormone and parathyroid hormone, have only minor roles; gene-based therapy remains in the early stages of preclinical research.[451,452]

Operative intervention is indicated for recurrent fractures or deformity that impairs function.[446] Fractures in mild to moderately severe cases of OI type I are treated using the same methods as for patients without OI. Deformed bones that are fracturing are realigned, frequently followed by providing external or internal support. In selecting various modes of treatment, it is important to consider the natural history of the particular type of OI and to set realistic goals.[453–457]

Anesthetic Considerations

In common with other children suffering chronic disabilities, children with OI are veterans of the operating room. Chronic pain from frequent fractures complicates handling; deafness may hinder communication. Preoperative assessment centers on the chest wall deformity because it determines the severity of restrictive lung disease and subsequent cardiovascular compromise. Neck mobility, mouth opening, and dentition should also be assessed.

There is a risk of further fractures with positioning, tourniquet application, airway handing, and use of a blood pressure cuff. Invasive pressure monitoring may be less traumatic than a blood pressure cuff for some patients. If noninvasive blood pressure monitoring is used, less frequent monitoring of the blood pressure is recommended if possible. A laryngeal mask airway may avoid pressure from face masks. An individual history may help determine the risk/benefit ratio for each child. Succinylcholine has the potential to cause fasciculation-induced fractures.

Abnormal temperature homeostasis may result in intraoperative hyperthermia that may be severe and accompanied by tachycardia and metabolic acidosis. This response is different from that of malignant hyperthermia in that there is an absence of respiratory acidosis and muscle rigidity.[458] Surface cooling is usually effective in restoring thermal homeostasis.

DUCHENNE MUSCULAR DYSTROPHY
Clinical Features
DMD is the most common of the progressive muscular dystrophies. It is an X-linked recessive disorder with an incidence of 3 per 10,000 births (see also Chapter 24). The *DMD* gene (located at Xp21.2) codes for a large sarcolemmal membrane protein, dystrophin, which is associated muscle cell membrane integrity and signal transduction. Dystrophin is missing or nonfunctional in DMD patients; both sexes can carry the *DMD* mutation, but girls rarely exhibit signs of the disease.

Children usually present before school age with a waddling gait and later develop a lumbar lordosis and difficulty climbing stairs. Children use their arms to assist standing up (i.e., Gowers sign) because of proximal weakness of the hip girdle. Distal muscles, such as the calves, appear hypertrophied. The disease process is progressive, with increasing muscle weakness occurring with age. These boys often become wheelchair-bound by 10 to 11 years of age. Respiratory weakness, often exacerbated by scoliosis and by difficulty swallowing secretions related to pharyngeal involvement, can progress to a terminal pneumonia in the late teenage years.[459] By late adolescence, most children with DMD have cardiac disease, whether it is an abnormal electrocardiogram, arrhythmias, or a cardiomyopathy. Death from cardiorespiratory failure usually occurs before age 30, although respiratory support is extending life expectancy.

DMD is not a static disease but evolves in end-organ implications with age. In early childhood, skeletal muscle is constantly catabolized and becomes unstable. The use of membrane-destabilizing medications such as succinylcholine and potent inhalational anesthetics (halothane in particular) in these young children can result in hyperkalemia, rhabdomyolysis, and cardiac arrest.[460] However, after the children reach adolescence, the bulk of the skeletal muscle catabolism has arrested, and membrane-destabilizing medications are left with no substrate. Succinylcholine and potent inhalational anesthetics may be used in the majority of cases without sequelae in adolescents with DMD who are undergoing scoliosis surgery and instrumentation,[461] although other anesthetic techniques are generally recommended (see also Chapter 24). In contrast to its very limited effect on cardiac and smooth muscles in childhood, in adolescence DMD may cause substantive and life-threatening cardiac complications. The anesthesiologist must appreciate the developmental changes of DMD with age and recognize the varying risks that may be associated with the use of succinylcholine and inhalational anesthetics in children and adolescents with this disease.

DMD can affect cardiac smooth muscle. Right ventricular function may be compromised by nocturnal oxygen desaturation and sleep apnea contributing to pulmonary hypertension. Sinus tachycardia and arrhythmias may occur at an early age, but clinically apparent cardiomyopathy usually does not develop before 10 years of age. One-third of children have some degree of intellectual impairment.

DMD should be suspected in male preschool children with delayed walking ability; measurement of high serum creatinine phosphokinase concentrations provides a screening tool. Steroids are increasingly used for the management of DMD because they appear to increase muscle mass by decreasing protein breakdown.[462]

Becker muscular dystrophy (BMD) is a milder form of DMD with an onset at puberty or later in adolescence. Clinical expression varies, but even adolescents presenting with mild or subclinical weakness can develop cardiomyopathy with age progression. Death from cardiac or respiratory failure does not usually occur until the fourth or fifth decade. Because of improvements in respiratory care, dilated cardiomyopathy has become the major cause of death.[463]

BMD is an autosomal recessive myopathy that also results from mutations of dystrophin caused by a deletion of the exons 11 to 13 in the *DMD* gene (located at Xp21.2).[464] Dystrophin exerts its effect at the voltage-gated chloride channel 1 (CLCN1). Genetic analysis is an essential step in confirming the diagnosis. Additional EMG procedures may be of diagnostic value even when muscle biopsy may reveal no evidence of dystrophy.

Of importance to anesthesiologists, two-thirds of patients with mild or subclinical BMD have evidence of right ventricular dilation, and one-third have evidence of left ventricular dysfunction.[465] A thorough cardiac evaluation (similar to that for DMD) is recommended before scoliosis surgery.[463] Hyperthermia and heart failure, mimicking malignant hyperthermia and hyperkalemia with rhabdomyolysis after inhalational agents, have been reported in patients with BMD.[466,467] Therefore inhalation agents and succinylcholine should be avoided in these patients. Despite these reports, the relationship between BMD and malignant hyperthermia remains unclear.

Orthopedic Considerations
Orthopedic surgery is indicated to improve or maintain ambulation and standing. Early treatment of contractures of the hips and the lower limbs prevents severe contractures and delays the progression of scoliosis.[468] Techniques designed to improve deformities and permit early postoperative mobilization include subcutaneous release of contracted tendons and percutaneous removal of cancellous bone with corrective manipulation of the feet. Maintenance of upright posture extends the ability of patients to attend to the tasks of daily living.[469] Spinal deformities attributable to muscle imbalance or a collapsing spine are corrected to improve or maintain sitting posture. Spinal fusion may also decrease the rate of deterioration of respiratory function, although this has been questioned.[470]

Anesthetic Considerations
Respiratory and cardiovascular compromise dominates preoperative assessment. Deformities and contractures of limb joints hinder vascular access, regional anesthetic techniques, and positioning on the operating table. Hypertrophy of the tongue[471] may cause difficulty during intubation. Gastric motility is delayed, and gastric emptying times are prolonged.[472] Tracheobronchial tree compression has been described in a child positioned prone for spinal instrumentation.[473] These children often have greater blood loss during surgery. The precise cause remains unclear, but it may be because fat and connective tissue have replaced muscle or because of abnormalities in the blood vessels.[242]

Nondepolarizing NMBDs have a slow onset and prolonged duration of action.[474-476] All NMBDs should be monitored with a peripheral nerve stimulator.[477] *Succinylcholine is contraindicated in these children because of the risk of hyperkalemia, muscle rigidity, rhabdomyolysis, myoglobinuria, arrhythmias, and cardiac arrest.* There is no known link between DMD and malignant hyperthermia.[478,479] The predominant candidate gene (*RYR1*) for malignant hyperthermia is located on the long arm of chromosome 19, whereas the *DMD* gene is located on the short arm of the X chromosome.[480] Although inhalational anesthetic agents continue to be used in young children with DMD, rhabdomyolysis and hyperkalemia have been reported in the recovery room after halothane, isoflurane, desflurane, and sevoflurane anesthesia.[481-485] Potent inhalational anesthetics are best avoided in young children with DMD; instead, alternative anesthetics that do not trigger rhabdomyolysis and hyperkalemia, such as propofol, ketamine, opioids, α_2-agonists, and benzodiazepines, are preferred.[486] Ketamine supplemented with dexmedetomidine or propofol has proven useful for brief procedures such as muscle biopsy.[487,488]

Regional techniques such as epidurals may be technically more difficult because of kyphoscoliosis and obesity. The use of ultrasound-guided peripheral nerve blockade can improve the quality and reduce complications of neuronal blockade.[6] Opioids are not contraindicated in the postoperative period but should be used with caution in children with respiratory compromise. Tramadol is an effective alternative. Noninvasive ventilation support using BiPAP or continuous positive airway pressure is sometimes required after major surgery or in those already receiving this treatment overnight.

ARTHROGRYPOSIS MULTIPLEX CONGENITA

Clinical Features

Arthrogryposis multiplex congenita is a spectrum syndrome of multiple, persistent limb contractures often accompanied by associated anomalies, including cleft palate, genitourinary defects, gastroschisis, and cardiac defects.[489] The incidence is 1 case per 3000 births. Joint contractures are present at birth and are a result of immobility in utero, commonly related to a neurogenic abnormality or myopathy.[490] These children have been likened to a "thin, wooden doll," because muscles connected to affected joints are atrophic and replaced by fibrous tissue and fat.[491] The temporomandibular joint may also be involved, causing restricted mouth opening (microstomia) and micrognathia. Scoliosis commonly develops. Restrictive lung disease, rib cage deformities, and pulmonary hypoplasia predispose to recurrent chest infections.

Orthopedic Considerations

The aim of surgery is to improve function. Most operations involve the soft tissues, tendons, and osteotomies of the lower limbs and hips.[492] Upper limb surgery is less common. Extension contracture of the elbow joint makes it impossible to reach the mouth or to perform hygienic necessities. Improvement in passive elbow flexion by capsulotomy or in active flexion by triceps transfer can increase independence and personal hygiene. When both arms are involved, consideration may be given to maintaining one arm in flexion for reaching the head and mouth passively or even actively and one arm in extension for basic hygiene cares.[493]

Anesthetic Considerations

Arthrogryposis multiplex congenita is commonly associated with other syndromes that may complicate anesthesia.[489,494] Venous cannulation is difficult because veins tend to be small and fragile. The concavity of joints is difficult to access. Regional blockade can also be difficult, although use of ultrasound improves success rates for the femoral and sciatic nerve block.[495] Care must be taken in positioning the patient on the operating table and protecting skin overlying bony joints to prevent pathologic fractures.

These children should be evaluated for a difficult airway because of temporomandibular joint limitation and micrognathia.[496-498] Fusion or underdevelopment of the first and second cervical vertebrae may further complicate laryngoscopy and tracheal intubation with a severe reduction in neck mobility. Tracheal intubation may become progressively more difficult with age. During infancy, however, evaluating mouth opening may be difficult; it may be necessary to insert a tongue blade into the mouth to determine whether the mandible can be distracted from the maxilla.

Succinylcholine has been used without incident in these children, although teleologically, the use of a depolarizing muscle relaxant in the presence of anterior horn cell disease is contentious. The response to nondepolarizing NMBDs should be monitored.

Hyperthermia and persistent tachycardia have been reported during general anesthesia.[489,499-501] These signs occur irrespective of the anesthetic agent and are not associated with malignant hyperthermia. In this case, hyperthermia responds to simple cooling techniques.

Pulmonary dysfunction and an increased sensitivity to opioids dictate suitable monitoring postoperatively. Regional techniques may be difficult in the presence of contractures, but if successful, they offer intraoperative and postoperative analgesia.[491] Success can be improved by using ultrasound-guided techniques.

ANNOTATED REFERENCES

Harper CM, Ambler G, Edge G. The prognostic value of preoperative predicted forced vital capacity in corrective spinal surgery for Duchenne's muscular dystrophy. *Anaesthesia*. 2004;59:1160-1162.

Performing scoliosis surgery on children with Duchenne muscular dystrophy who have a forced vital capacity (FVC) of 30% has been questioned because of the high incidence of postoperative pulmonary complications. This clinical paper demonstrated that with careful attention to detail, children with an FVC less than 30% can undergo scoliosis surgery with results similar to those with an FVC greater than 30%. Early extubation followed by the use of noninvasive ventilation was identified as key to reducing respiratory complications.

Holdefer RN, Furman M, Sangare Y, Slimp JC. A comparison of the effects of desflurane versus propofol on transcranial motor-evoked potentials in pediatric patients. *Childs Nerv Syst*. 2014;30:2103-2108.

Mackenzie WG, Matsumoto H, Williams BA, et al. Surgical site infection following spinal instrumentation for scoliosis: a multicenter analysis of rates, risk factors, and pathogens. *J Bone Joint Surg Am*. 2013;95:800-806.

This multicenter retrospective review of surgical site infections from pediatric hospitals in the United States demonstrated rates increasing from 2.6% in those with AIS to 9.2% in those with neuromuscular scoliosis (NMS). Almost all infections involving gram-negative organisms occurred in patients with NMS, and half of the infections in these patients contained at least one gram-negative organism. Whether targeted antimicrobial prophylaxis in these patients will reduce the high infection rate is currently unknown.

Malhotra NR, Shaffrey CI. Intraoperative electrophysiological monitoring in spine surgery. *Spine*. 2010;35:2167-2179.

The authors undertook a pooled data analysis to review intraoperative neuromonitoring changes that occur during the course of spine surgery, and they describe the appropriate application of this monitoring.

Martin DP, Bhalla T, Thung A, et al. A preliminary study of volatile agents or total intravenous anesthesia for neurophysiological monitoring during posterior spinal fusion in adolescents with idiopathic scoliosis. *Spine*. 2014;39:E1318-E1324.

32

These two studies demonstrate that adequate neurophysiologic status using SSEPs and MEPs during scoliosis surgery can be obtained with either a desflurane- or propofol-based anesthetic technique. Current prevailing opinion appears to favor a total IV anesthetic (propofol) technique, but desflurane is an acceptable alternative. Both studies used modest doses of either agent (0.6–0.8 MAC desflurane, propofol 150–300 µg/kg per minute) adjusted to keep the BSI between 40 and 60. Adequate SSEPs and MEPs were obtained in all patients, but a higher stimulating voltage was required in both papers when desflurane was used. A potential benefit of desflurane is a shorter wake-up time, which may be advantageous if signal changes are observed.

McLeod LM, French B, Flynn JM, et al. Antifibrinolytic use and blood transfusions in pediatric scoliosis surgeries performed at US children's hospitals. *J Spinal Disord Tech.* 2015;28:E460-E466.

This cohort of more than 4000 scoliosis surgeries from U.S. children's hospitals challenges the information from randomized clinical trials and systematic reviews suggesting antifibrinolytic use reduces the odds of transfusion.

ε-Aminocaproic acid but not tranexamic acid was associated with lower odds of transfusion in AIS patients, whereas neither drug had benefits in those with NMS.

Yuan N, Fraire JA, Margetis MM, et al. The effect of scoliosis surgery on lung function in the immediate postoperative period. *Spine.* 2005;30:2182-2185.

This study clearly demonstrated the dramatic decrease in pulmonary function in the days after scoliosis surgery, readily explaining why children are at risk for pulmonary complications during this period. Pulmonary function tests (FEV_1, FVC, FEV_1/FVC, and $FEF_{25-75\%}$) were measured daily for 10 days after scoliosis repair. Results of pulmonary function tests decreased by up to 60% after surgery, with a nadir at 3 days. The FEV_1 and FVC values were still only at 60% of the preoperative values on the 10th postoperative day.

A complete reference list can be found online at ExpertConsult.com.

33 Otorhinolaryngologic Procedures

RAAFAT S. HANNALLAH, KAREN A. BROWN, AND SUSAN T. VERGHESE

OTORHINOLARYNGOLOGIC PROCEDURES REPRESENT a large segment of elective surgery in infants and children. Anesthetic management is provided by both pediatric and general anesthesiologists, commonly in ambulatory surgery centers and office practices.[1] Additionally, anesthesiologists are often consulted to help manage potentially life-threatening pediatric otolaryngologic emergencies. These include airway obstruction caused by croup, foreign body aspiration, airway trauma, bacterial tracheitis, and, rarely, acute epiglottitis.[2] In both the elective and emergent scenarios, it is essential to understand the pathophysiology, and to discuss the anesthetic plan in advance with the surgeon who will frequently be sharing the airway with the anesthesiologist. This ensures safe anesthetic management and ideal conditions for both children and surgeons.

Anesthesia for Otologic Procedures

MYRINGOTOMY AND VENTILATING TUBE INSERTION

Chronic serous otitis media is common in young children. If untreated or poorly managed, it can lead to hearing loss and formation of cholesteatoma. When conservative medical management fails, surgical drainage of accumulated middle ear fluid is indicated. Myringotomy creates an opening in the tympanic membrane through which fluid can drain. If only a myringotomy is performed, the drainage path is occluded when the incision heals. Therefore myringotomy is frequently accompanied by placing a small plastic tube (a variation of the grommet or the T-tube) in the incision in the tympanic membrane to serve as a stent for the ostium, facilitating continuous drainage from the middle ear until the tubes are naturally extruded in 6 to 12 months, or surgically removed at an appropriate time.

Children with cleft palate have a high frequency of middle ear disease compared with those without a cleft because of associated abnormalities of the cartilage and muscles surrounding the eustachian tubes. Surgical drainage and ventilation tube insertion is a standard treatment for chronic otitis media in these children; this is usually performed at the time of cleft repair.

Most young children require general anesthesia for tympanotomy tube placement, although occasionally older children tolerate the procedure with only topical anesthesia. This may be accomplished by iontophoresis or instillation of EMLA (eutectic mixture of local anesthetics) cream, which remains in the ear canal for an hour and is then suctioned out before the procedure.

Myringotomy with tube insertion is a very brief operation, usually performed in the ambulatory surgery setting using a potent inhalational agent (e.g., sevoflurane), oxygen, and nitrous oxide administered by face mask with spontaneous respiration. An oropharyngeal airway may assist in maintaining a patent airway when the head is laterally rotated and together with resting the forearm of the anesthesiologist on the table, reduces head movement during respiration (which is amplified through the microscope). Gentle manual assistance of ventilation can also reduce head movement. Occasionally, a laryngeal mask airway (LMA) may be used in children in whom the procedure is expected to be prolonged (e.g., children with narrow ear canals) or those with a difficult airway. Most children can be managed safely without intravenous (IV) access,[3] but it is recommended to have IV equipment set up on standby. Some children with severe underlying medical or surgical conditions will require IV access despite the anticipated brief duration of the minor procedure. Although premedication is often omitted because its duration of effect exceeds that of the procedure, an anxious child may still benefit from a sedative premedication and/or having the parents present during induction of anesthesia.

In some instances, it is desirable to remove a retained tympanotomy tube. This can be easily accomplished in the surgeon's office without anesthesia; however, some stiff-flanged grommet tubes require general anesthesia for removal. If the incision does not heal spontaneously, a paper patch or fat graft may have to be applied over the ostium to stimulate healing of the tympanic membrane. The anesthetic would be the same as that for the tube placement, except that nitrous oxide is best avoided to minimize the chance of graft dislodgment (see later discussion).

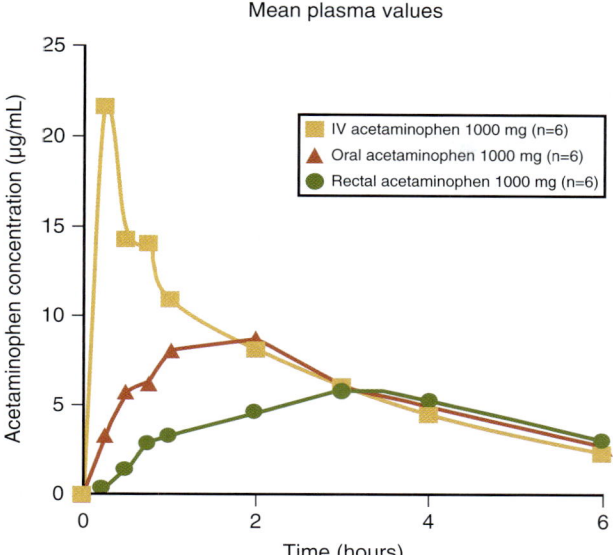

FIGURE 33.1 Plasma time-concentration profile for 1000 mg acetaminophen via three routes: intravenous, oral, and rectal (IV, PO, and PR, respectively). PR acetaminophen reflects standardization of 1300 mg dose to 1000 mg (linear kinetics). (Adapted from: Singla NK, Parulan C, Samson R, et al. Plasma and cerebrospinal fluid pharmacokinetic parameters after single-dose administration of intravenous, oral, or rectal acetaminophen. *Pain Pract.* 2012;12[7]: 523–532.)

Discomfort after myringotomy and tube insertion is usually managed by the administration of nonsteroidal antiinflammatory drugs (NSAIDs) such as acetaminophen, ketorolac, or opioids. The recommended dose of acetaminophen to achieve therapeutic blood concentrations is 10 to 20 mg/kg when administered orally, and 30 to 40 mg/kg when administered rectally.[4-6] Oral acetaminophen is very rapidly absorbed, achieving therapeutic blood concentrations within minutes, whereas rectal acetaminophen is slowly absorbed, with a time to onset of action of 60 to 90 minutes, and a time to peak effect of 1 to 3 hours (Figs. 4.2 and 33.1).[7-10] Consequently, the oral route is preferred for this procedure.

Preschool-aged children who receive sevoflurane without an analgesic for myringotomy and tube insertion may exhibit emergence delirium and postoperative agitation (see Chapter 4). Although pain may be partially responsible for these responses, their etiologies are not completely understood. Because the procedure is so brief and IV access is not usually established, intranasal (IN) fentanyl, 1 to 2 µg/kg, has been shown to provide analgesia and to reduce the frequency of emergence agitation.[11,12] Other analgesics, including IV/intramuscular (IM) ketorolac (0.5–1 mg/kg), or rectal diclofenac or IN butorphanol (25 µg/kg), and IN dexmedetomidine (1–2 µg/kg), reduce the pain after myringotomy and tube insertion.[13-15] However, larger doses of dexmedetomidine (2 µg/kg) significantly prolong the duration of stay in the postanesthesia care unit (PACU). A large retrospective pediatric study of bilateral myringotomy and tube insertion found that the combination of IM fentanyl (1.5–2 µg/kg) and ketorolac (1 mg/kg) was strongly associated with superior PACU analgesia and reduced the need for oxycodone rescue without clinically significant increases in recovery time or the incidence of emesis. This dual therapy appears similarly effective in children of European Caucasian, African ancestry, or those of Hispanic ethnicity.[16] A nerve of Arnold block is also a reasonable alternative (see Chapter 42).[17] Emergence delirium is

often brief (lasting 10–20 minutes) and, provided that analgesia has been addressed, can be managed by maternal or nurse comforts (e.g., cuddling) without pharmacologic intervention. Voluntary rather than forced oral fluid administration reduces the incidence of postoperative nausea and vomiting (PONV).[18]

Children with chronic otitis media frequently have persistent rhinorrhea and suffer recurrent upper respiratory tract infection (URI) (see Chapter 13). Eradication of middle ear congestion and improved fluid drainage often resolves the concomitant symptoms. The frequency of perioperative complications in children with mild URIs is similar to that in children who are asymptomatic. In general, morbidity is not increased in children who present for minor surgery with acute, uncomplicated mild URIs, provided tracheal intubation can be avoided.[19,20] Canceling this surgery because of rhinorrhea or recurrent mild respiratory symptoms is not usually justifiable as the vicious cycle of repeated URIs and chronic ear infections require an intervention (e.g., myringotomy) to break the cycle. It is, however, recommended that children with respiratory symptoms have their oxygen saturation (SpO₂) measured before induction of general anesthesia, and that supplemental oxygen be administered postoperatively to those whose SpO₂ readings are less than 93%.[21]

MIDDLE EAR AND MASTOID SURGERY

Tympanoplasty and mastoidectomy are two of the most common major ear operations performed in children. General anesthesia usually consists of an inhalational anesthetic and IV opioids. Surgical identification and preservation of the facial nerve are necessary because of its proximity to the surgical field. To ensure the facial nerve can be identified using electrical stimulation, neuromuscular blockade is usually avoided. If a neuromuscular blocking drug (NMBD) must be used, a small dose should be given to facilitate tracheal intubation; if an NMBD is used for maintenance, suppression of the twitch response should not exceed 70%.

To gain access to the surgical site, the child's head is placed on a headrest, which may be positioned below the operating table. In addition, extreme degrees of lateral rotation may be required to visualize the middle ear anatomy. The anesthesiologist and surgeon must be especially vigilant to ensure that nerves, muscles, and bony structures are not injured as a result of this unusual positioning; the sternocleidomastoid muscles generally limit the safe degree of lateral head rotation. Left or right tilting (airplaning) of the operating room (OR) table minimizes the need for extreme lateral head rotation, which is an important consideration for children with Down syndrome. The laxity of the ligaments of the cervical spine, as well as immaturity of the odontoid process in children with Down syndrome, predisposes them to C1–C2 subluxation; 15% to 31% of children with Down syndrome or achondroplasia have atlantoaxial instability.[22-25] Anteroposterior positioning requires the utmost care to avoid injury.

Positioning of the OR table to allow access to the respective middle ear and accommodate all the extra surgical equipment can also pose a challenge. Depending on the room configuration, the table may be rotated 90 degrees or even 180 degrees away from the anesthesia machine, necessitating the use of an extra-long breathing circuit (Fig. 33.2). As a result of the limited access to the airway, very careful attention must be paid to securing the tracheal tube. Draping must allow immediate access to the airway should that be required.

Bleeding must be kept to a minimum during surgery on the small structures of the middle ear; relative hypotension (i.e., mean arterial pressure 10%–25% less than baseline) may help to reduce bleeding. Concentrated epinephrine solution (1 : 10,000) is frequently applied to the tympanic membrane to induce vasoconstriction of the blood vessels. Close attention should be paid to the dose of epinephrine used to prevent arrhythmias and wide swings in blood pressure. The maximum dose of topical epinephrine is 10 µg/kg, which may be repeated after 30 minutes. Alternatively, topical oxymetazoline 0.05% may be used to induce vasoconstriction.

The middle ear and sinuses are air-filled, nondistensible cavities; an increase in the volume of gas within these cavities increases the pressure. Nitrous oxide diffuses along a concentration gradient into air-filled middle ear spaces more rapidly than nitrogen moves out because nitrous oxide is 34 times more soluble in blood than nitrogen. The middle ear is vented through the opening of the eustachian tube. Normal passive venting of the eustachian tube occurs at 20 to 30 cm H_2O pressure. Nitrous oxide increases the pressures within the middle ear such that they exceed the ability of the eustachian tube to vent the middle ear within 5 minutes, leading to pressure buildup.[26] If the function of the eustachian tube is compromised during the surgical procedure, then pressure in the middle ear can further increase. Venting the middle ear occurs intermittently, and leads to constant fluctuations in middle ear pressure that cause movement of the tympanic membrane.[27] During procedures in which the tympanic membrane is replaced or a perforation is patched, nitrous oxide should be discontinued before the application of the tympanic membrane graft to reduce the potential for pressure-related displacement.[28] The omission of nitrous oxide does not significantly increase the requirements (minimum alveolar concentration) for the less-soluble inhaled anesthetics (desflurane and sevoflurane) in children.[29] After nitrous oxide is discontinued, it is quickly reabsorbed, creating a void

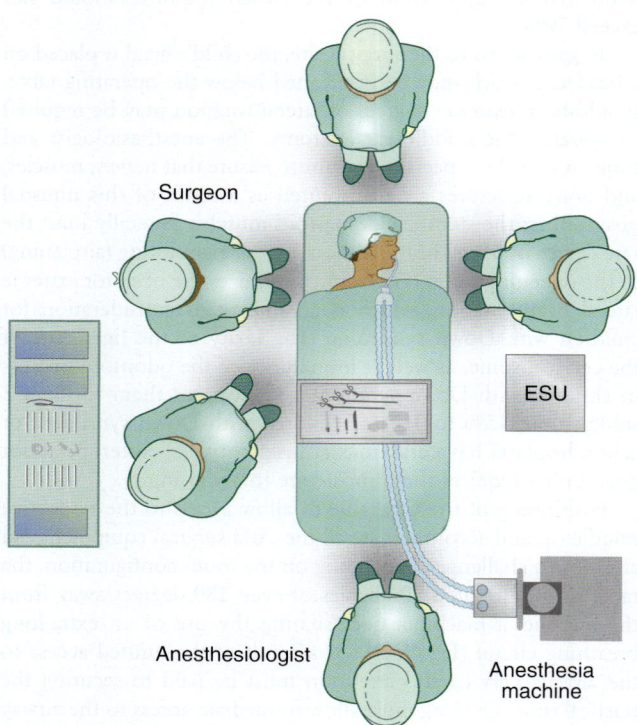

FIGURE 33.2 An operating room table turned 180 degrees may limit access to the child during ear surgery. *ESU* is the electrosurgical unit.

in the middle ear, with resulting negative pressure. This negative pressure may result in serous otitis, disarticulation of the ossicles in the middle ear (especially the stapes), and hearing impairment, which may last up to 6 weeks postoperatively. The use of nitrous oxide may increase the incidence of postoperative nausea and vomiting (PONV), as a direct result of negative middle ear pressure during recovery. The negative pressure created by the reabsorption of nitrous oxide stimulates the vestibular system by producing traction on the round window. Although all children are at risk for PONV, older children and adolescents, in particular, are at the greatest risk.[30] Multimodal prophylactic administration of antiemetics (e.g., dexamethasone and ondansetron) is usually warranted. Local infiltration of the great auricular nerve can provide pain relief equivalent to that of opioids and may reduce the incidence of opioid-induced vomiting (see Chapter 42).[31]

A smooth, quiet emergence is desirable. Deep tracheal extubation can be accomplished if the child breathes spontaneously during the last 15 to 20 minutes of surgery, the concentration of inhalational anesthetic is greater than 1.3 times the minimal alveolar concentration, and opioids are titrated to produce regular slow respirations. Gentle suctioning of the oropharynx and possibly the use of IV lidocaine (1–1.5 mg/kg) in children older than 1 year of age can minimize or even prevent coughing after the tracheal tube is removed. Alternately, total IV anesthesia may be used for middle ear procedures because nitrous oxide is avoided, postoperative vomiting is reduced and the frequency of emergence delirium is minimal (see Chapter 8).

COCHLEAR IMPLANTS

The first multichannel cochlear implant was developed in Australia in 1978. After a series of clinical trials, the US Food and Drug Administration (FDA) approved the use of the Australian cochlear implant in adults in 1985, and subsequently in infants and children as young as 6 months of age.[32] In recent years, the indications for cochlear implants have broadened and continue to evolve. With the application of universal neonatal hearing screening programs, a large pool of hearing-impaired infants has been identified. The benefits of early intervention with cochlear implants are being explored. Younger children with severe to profound hearing loss markedly improve their auditory, speech, and language skills after cochlear implants, and more of these children can be mainstreamed with their age-appropriate hearing peers when they receive an implant early in life. Experience has shown that cochlear implant surgery is safe in infants older than 6 months of age, provided that special attention is paid to the physiologic and anatomic differences present in this age group. The majority of children presenting for surgery have no significant health issues other than deafness. However, in a recent review, 40% had comorbidities that have been categorized into syndromes associated with deafness, problems associated with premature births, neurologic problems, and cardiac abnormalities.[33] For these children, the availability of skilled postoperative nursing and a pediatric intensive care unit (ICU) are essential.[34]

Surgery requires meticulous care with hemostasis, soft tissue dissection, and bone drilling because bleeding from bone can be difficult to control and can complicate the surgical outcome. The surgical procedure itself needs the facial nerve to be identified; thus if an NMBD is used for intubation, spontaneous recovery should be confirmed and communicated to the surgeon. Postoperative fitting of the externally worn speech processor is very important for successful use of the cochlear implant. However, this fitting process can be difficult, particularly in infants and young children, because of limited communication capabilities. Electrically elicited stapedius reflex thresholds (ESRTs) obtained intraoperatively are used to determine the maximum comfort level, which is defined as the loudest sound tolerated without pain. It has been used for postoperative speech processor fitting, although the influence of anesthetics on the threshold values must be taken into account. More reliable threshold values can be obtained by adjusting the dosage of hypnotics to achieve a lighter level of hypnosis during ESRT measurement.[35] In most children, increasing the concentration of inhalational anesthetics increases the stapedius reflex threshold, whereas propofol and nitrous oxide have minimal effects on the ESRT. Consequently, total IV anesthesia (TIVA) is popular in some countries. Dexmedetomidine has been used to decrease inhaled anesthetic requirements, prevent intraoperative hypertension (and bleeding), and ensure a smooth emergence. As always, appropriate communication with the surgeon and audiologist will help ensure a successful outcome.

While cochlear implants are indicated in children with profound sensoneural or nerve deafness, many children with conductive hearing loss who cannot use traditional hearing aids (because of draining ears or chronic infection) can be candidates for bone-anchoring hearing aid devices (BAHA). The BAHA implant is a titanium device placed in the skull behind the ear and vibrates the bone to transmit sound directly to the inner ear. Although most children who are BAHA candidates are older than 5 years of age, some infants can now be fitted. The surgical and anesthetic approach is less challenging than that for cochlear implants.

Anesthesia for Rhinologic Procedures

Chronic sinusitis in children can be caused by antibiotic-resistant bacteria and is usually treated with broad-spectrum antibiotics. In some children with obstructive adenoid pads, adenoidectomy will improve the signs and symptoms of sinusitis. Functional endoscopic sinus surgery (FESS) using sharp biting instruments and/or a microdebrider has become the primary method of surgical therapy for chronic sinusitis.[36] Current techniques aim to leave the mucosa intact to prevent scarring in the frontal recess. Although sometimes controversial, there is no evidence at present that FESS affects facial growth in children. Of interest to the anesthesiologist is that many children who require FESS have coexisting medical problems, such as asthma and cystic fibrosis. These conditions must be optimized before surgery (see Chapter 13).

An alternative to FESS is balloon sinuplasty. This technique uses ballooned catheters to dilate the maxillary, frontal, and sphenoidal natural ostia without bone or soft tissue removal.[37] This should result in less bleeding and reduced anesthetic morbidity.

Anesthetic management usually requires tracheal intubation to secure the airway; the use of an oral preformed tracheal tube (e.g., the Ring-Adair-Elwyn [RAE] tube) allows secure fixation to the mandible and unobstructed access to the maxilla and sinuses. The use of a cuffed tracheal tube is particularly advantageous to eliminate a gas leak that could fog up the endoscopic instruments. A throat pack is frequently inserted to absorb blood in the oropharynx and limit the gas escaping around an uncuffed endotracheal tube (ETT). It is critically important that the pack is removed before tracheal extubation. Occasionally, an LMA may be used to facilitate a quick "second look."

Because bleeding is inevitable with this surgery and can interfere with the surgical exposure, packing the nasal cavity with a vasoconstricting solution before surgery is common. Typically used topical vasoconstrictors include oxymetazoline 0.025% to 0.05%, phenylephrine 0.25% to 1%, and less frequently, cocaine 4% to 10%. It is important for the anesthesiologist to be aware of the type and dose of the vasoconstrictor and to ensure that no more than the maximum effective dose is applied. Application of topical phenylephrine or other potent vasoconstrictors to mucous membranes or open surgical sites can cause severe hypertension, reflex bradycardia, and even cardiac arrest.[38] Hypertension induced by topically applied vasoconstrictors often resolves spontaneously and may not require aggressive treatment. The use of β-adrenergic blockers or calcium-channel blockers to control blood pressure in these circumstances can depress cardiac output, leading to pulmonary edema and cardiac arrest.[38] It is recommended that the initial topical dose of phenylephrine should not exceed 20 µg/kg in children.[38]

Corticosteroids, such as IV dexamethasone (0.25–0.5 mg/kg), are usually administered to reduce swelling and scarring. Frequently, the surgeon will want to leave an absorbable stenting material, such as MeroGel (Medtronic ENT, Jacksonville, FL), at the end of surgery. Unfortunately, this will interfere with nasal breathing and may increase the incidence of emergence delirium. An anesthetic technique that ensures adequate analgesia and rapid return of consciousness at the end of surgery is therefore desirable. One of the authors (RSH) has found that a combination of desflurane, fentanyl, and low-dose propofol works well in this regard. Alternatively, a pure TIVA technique (propofol + remifentanil) or desflurane + remifentanil can be used; the remifentanil dose is adjusted to the desired mean arterial pressure.

A unilateral or bilateral infraorbital nerve block can also be performed via the intraoral or extraoral route to provide analgesia (see Chapter 42).[39] One further concern is the need to avoid NSAIDs in children with asthma and sinusitis secondary to nasal polyps (Samter triad).[40,41]

Adenotonsillectomy

Adenotonsillectomy is one of the oldest pediatric surgical procedures, yet its conduct and practice continue to evolve. In the past decade, notable changes have been introduced. These include the indications for adenotonsillectomy, the criteria for postoperative hospital admission, and recommended postoperative analgesic regimens. Additionally, the American Academy of Otolaryngology-Head and Neck Surgery (AAO-HNS) no longer recommends prophylactic antibiotics during adenotonsillectomy surgery.[42–44]

Adenotonsillectomy is one of the most commonly performed pediatric surgical procedures worldwide; one in eight American children will undergo adenotonsillectomy.[45] Chronic or recurrent tonsillitis and obstructive adenotonsillar hyperplasia are the major indications for surgical removal (Table 33.1). Surgical treatment is required when tonsillitis recurs despite adequate medical therapy, when associated with peritonsillar abscess, or when acute or chronic airway obstruction compromises breathing. Halitosis, persistent pharyngitis, and cervical adenitis may accompany chronic tonsillitis. Tonsillar hyperplasia may lead to chronic airway obstruction, resulting in obstructive sleep apnea (OSA), failure to thrive, swallowing disorders, speech abnormalities, pulmonary hypertension, right-sided heart failure, and eventually cor pulmonale (Fig. 33.3). Certain children with cardiac lesions may be at risk for endocarditis caused by recurrent streptococcal bacteremia secondary to infected tonsils and will require prophylactic antibiotics (see Chapter 16).

Adenoidectomy is usually performed in conjunction with tonsillectomy, although in some situations it is performed as the sole

TABLE 33.1	Indications for Adenotonsillectomy

Infection

Acute tonsillitis or adenoiditis
Recurrent tonsillitis or adenoiditis
Chronic tonsillitis or adenoiditis
Peritonsillar abscess
Halitosis

Obstruction

Nasal airway (adenoids)
Pharyngeal airway (tonsils)
Obstructive sleep apnea/sleep-disordered breathing
Cyanosis
Failure to thrive
Cor pulmonale due to airway obstruction

Mass Lesion

Tonsillar/adenoidal
Benign
Malignant

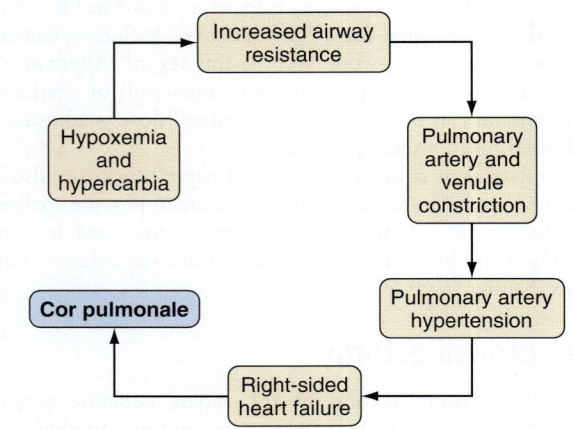

FIGURE 33.3 Children with chronic tonsillar hypertrophy may have long-standing hypoxemia and hypercarbia, which can lead to pulmonary hypertension, right ventricular hypertrophy, and cor pulmonale.

surgical procedure. Indications for adenoidectomy alone include chronic or recurrent purulent adenoiditis, recurrent otitis media with effusion secondary to adenoidal hyperplasia, and chronic sinusitis. Advanced degrees of adenoidal hyperplasia may lead to nasopharyngeal obstruction, obligate mouth breathing, poor feeding resulting in failure to thrive, speech disorders, and sleep-disordered breathing (SDB). Long-standing nasal obstruction can result in orofacial abnormalities with a narrowing of the upper airway and dental abnormalities (so-called adenoid facies or long face syndrome).

Surgical techniques for adenotonsillectomy include guillotine and snare techniques, cold and hot knife dissection, suction, radiofrequency ablation, and unipolar and bipolar electrocautery techniques. Electrocautery dissection offers two advantages over the other techniques with less intraoperative blood loss and a reduced risk of postoperative hemorrhage, although these are offset, in part, by more pain and poor oral intake postoperatively.

A meta-analysis of 23 retrospective studies (N = 13,537 children) reported an overall frequency of postoperative complications after adenotonsillectomy of 19%. Respiratory compromise was

the most frequent complication (9.4%) followed by secondary hemorrhage (5–10 days after surgery) (2.6%).[46] Age has a major influence on these complications. Children older than age of 10 years more commonly have a secondary hemorrhage, whereas younger children more commonly have both poor oral intake and respiratory complications. The majority of children younger than 3 years of age experience airway problems after adenotonsillectomy for obstructive breathing.[47,48]

Surgical complications after adenotonsillectomy are rare but include uvular amputation, uvular edema, velopharyngeal insufficiency, and nasopharyngeal stenosis. Atlantoaxial subluxation manifesting as neck pain and torticollis, mandibular subluxation and condylar fracture, cervical adenitis, and cervical osteomyelitis have also been reported.[49,50] Bleeding, burns, and airway fires account for over one-third of malpractice claims associated with this procedure.[51] The mortality associated with adenotonsillectomy is estimated at 1 per 16,000 to 1 per 41,000 procedures.[49,52,53] Throat pain, otalgia, emesis, poor oral intake, and dehydration are common morbidities.

PREOPERATIVE EVALUATION

The general health of the child and the indications for surgery must be reviewed. URIs are frequent in these children and can interfere with the timing of adenotonsillectomy because the risk of respiratory compromise and hemorrhage is increased.[49,54–56] Obese children often have SDB and they are at increased risk for postoperative hemorrhage.[57–62] A history of bleeding tendencies requires investigation. Medications that interfere with coagulation include aspirin, NSAIDs, and valproic acid. Discontinuation of these drugs preoperatively is sometimes problematic, and preoperative consultation with neurology, cardiology, and hematology specialists may be indicated.

A careful cardiorespiratory history and physical examination is essential. Children with chronic tonsillar hypertrophy may have long-standing hypoxemia and hypercarbia, which can lead to cor pulmonale (see Fig. 33.3). The oropharynx should be evaluated and the tonsillar size classified (Fig. 33.4).[63] In some centers, a complete blood cell count and coagulation profile is required before adenotonsillectomy. There is no evidence that routinely performed preoperative coagulation studies are beneficial unless they are indicated by history or the presence of a disorder of hemostasis.[64,65] The indications for the procedure should be clearly delineated in the surgical plan of care.

Special Considerations for the Child With Obstructive Sleep Apnea Syndrome

SDB describes abnormal breathing patterns during sleep. These abnormal patterns include obstructive breathing, including snoring, paradoxical chest wall motion, and increased respiratory effort, apneas, hypopneas leading to hypercarbia, and desaturation followed by arousals. The spectrum of SDB ranges from primary "benign" snoring to the obstructive sleep apnea syndrome (OSAS). The Childhood Adenotonsillectomy Trial (CHAT), a randomized controlled trial, compared watchful waiting for 7 months with early adenotonsillectomy in more than 400 children with OSAS. The primary outcome, attention and executive function, did not differ between the two groups. However, secondary outcomes for polysomnographic, behavioral, and quality-of-life metrics normalized in 79% of the children after adenotonsillectomy compared with 46% who did not undergo adenostonsillectomy.[45,66]

The single most important task during the preoperative evaluation of the child for adenotonsillectomy is to distinguish the child with the OSAS

A Standardized System for
Evaluation of Tonsillar Size

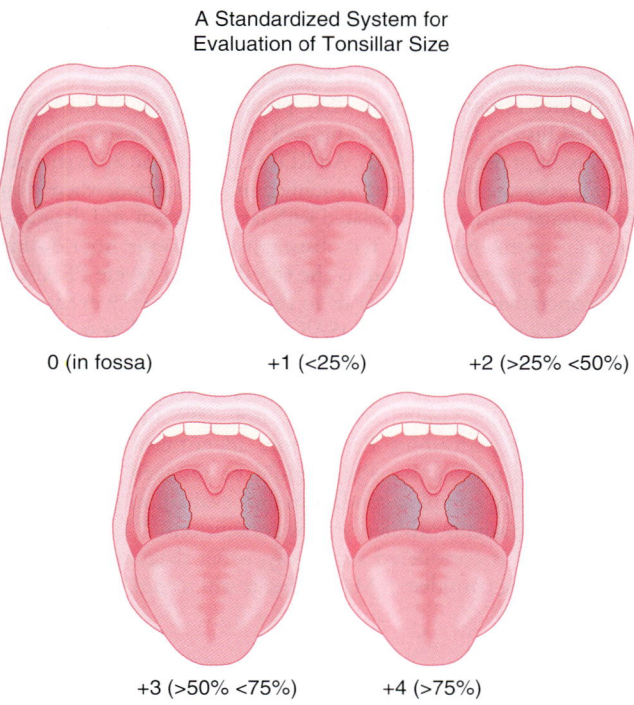

0 (in fossa)   +1 (<25%)   +2 (>25% <50%)

+3 (>50% <75%)   +4 (>75%)

FIGURE 33.4 Classifying tonsil size may be helpful in evaluating the degree of airway obstruction. Children classified as +3 or greater (i.e., having more than 50% of the pharyngeal area occupied by hypertrophied tonsils) are at an increased risk of developing airway obstruction during anesthetic induction. (Modified from Brodsky L. Modern assessment of tonsils and adenoids. *Pediatr Clin North Am.* 1989;36[5]:1551–1569; illustration by Jon S. Krasner.)

TABLE 33.2	Medical Conditions in Children That Predispose to the Development of Obstructive Sleep Apnea

Craniofacial Syndromes

Crouzon syndrome
Apert syndrome
Pfeiffer syndrome
Treacher Collins syndrome
Pierre Robin sequence
Goldenhar syndrome
Larsen syndrome

Disorders of Cranial Base

Arnold-Chiari malformation
Achondroplasia
Syringobulbia

Neuromuscular Disorders

Cerebral palsy

Trisomy 21

Infiltrative Disorders

Mucopolysaccharidoses
Acromegaly
Obesity
Prader-Willi syndrome

Temporomandibular Joint Ankylosis

from the child with isolated obstructive breathing (e.g., primary snoring) and chronic infectious tonsillitis, because the former children are at greater risk for developing severe perioperative respiratory adverse events (PRAEs), possibly including death, after adenotonsillectomy.[67–72] Several recent studies have reported unexpected deaths after adenotonsillectomy from presumed sleep apnea after discharge from a monitored setting, including to home.[59,72,73] A meta-analysis of 3 retrospective studies (N = 371 children) revealed that children with OSAS proven by polysomnography (PSG) criteria have a 5-fold increase in the odds for PRAEs compared with children without OSAS. In contrast, they were less likely to have postoperative hemorrhage (odds ratio 0.4, 95% confidence interval [CI] 0.2–0.7).[46]

The OSAS encompasses a range of severity. At the most extreme, it includes pulmonary and systemic hypertension, cor pulmonale, ventricular hypertrophy, the metabolic syndrome, neurocognitive dysfunction, and life-threatening nocturnal hypoxemia.[74–77] Because adenotonsillectomy is often the initial treatment for OSAS, the majority of these children may present with a spectrum of disease affecting multiple organ systems. Failure to thrive is common. Infections affecting the lower respiratory tract have been linked to chronic aspiration.[78]

A high index of suspicion is required to identify the child with OSAS on clinical criteria. Clinical criteria do not always distinguish primary snoring from OSAS in children.[79] There is a greater incidence of OSAS in Asian and African American populations.[80,81] African American children desaturate more profoundly during sleep-related obstructive airway events than do Caucasian and Hispanic children.[82] Obese children (BMI > 95th percentile)

are at greater risk for OSAS and postoperative hemorrhage.[59,73] Anatomic features may underlie the pathogenesis of OSAS; common medical conditions and syndromes that predispose to the development of OSAS are listed in Table 33.2. Infants who have suffered an acute life-threatening event (ALTE) have a greater incidence of OSAS in childhood and adolescence.[83–85]

Parents should be asked if the child snores loudly, if the snoring can be heard through a closed door, if there are gasps or pauses in respirations, if there is daytime somnolence, night terrors, nocturnal enuresis, attention deficit disorder, or poor school performance.[62,86,87] However clinical features obtained from demography, parental report, and physical findings do not robustly identify OSAS severity[88,89] and parental report of symptoms has a poor positive predictive value.[90–94]

Although it is important to recognize the significance of OSAS in children who are scheduled for adenotonsillectomy, children who do not meet the criteria for OSAS but who have less severe forms of SDB, such as upper airway resistance syndrome (UARS) or obstructive hypopnea, may also be at increased risk for morbidity after surgery. Guidelines for the perioperative management of these children continue to be developed.[71,87,95,96]

The obstructive events that characterize OSAS result in recurrent episodes of hypoxia, hypercarbia, and sleep disruption, a trilogy that has been linked to the development of medical sequelae that accompany severe OSAS. The severity of OSAS is assessed by the frequency and severity of the obstructive respiratory events during sleep; both occur most often during rapid eye movement (REM) sleep. The frequency and severity of obstructive events worsen after midnight.[97–99]

The polysomnogram (PSG) is the gold standard diagnostic test for evaluation of SDB. The PSG simultaneously records the electroencephalogram, electromyogram, electrocardiogram, pulse oximetry, airflow, and thoracic and abdominal movement during sleep (Fig. 33.5). Some cardiorespiratory studies limit the recording devices to pulse oximetry with sensors for thoracic and abdominal movement. A common definition of OSA in children is an obstructive effort that includes more than two obstructive breaths, regardless of the duration of the apnea.[97] An obstructive apnea index of 1 is the cutoff for normality in children.[100] The diagnostic criteria for pediatric OSAS according to the American Academy of Sleep Medicine are: mild OSAS corresponds to an apnea index >1 <5 events per hour; moderate OSAS corresponds to an apnea index >5 <10 events per hour, and severe OSAS corresponds to an apnea index ≥10 events per hour.[71,76] Apneas are classified as central, obstructive, and mixed (see Fig. 33.5). A central apnea occurs when there is no apparent respiratory effort. An obstructive apnea is associated in the presence of apparent, often vigorous, inspiratory efforts that are ineffective because the upper airway is not patent. A mixed obstructive apnea is diagnosed when both central and obstructive components are present without interruption by effective respirations.

Hypopnea is defined as a reduction in airflow of more than 50%.[97] The apnea hypopnea index (AHI) is the summation of the number of obstructive apnea and hypopnea events and is analogous to the respiratory disturbance index (RDI). The PSG study also records oxygen-desaturation indexes.

Metrics obtained during PSG predict the risk of PRAEs; a detailed history from the parents will also help to assess children likely to be at risk (Table 33.3). An RDI of greater than 20 events per hour is associated with breath-holding during induction, whereas an RDI greater than 30 is associated with laryngospasm and desaturation during emergence.[101] Ten obstructive events per hour during a screening polysomnogram is the threshold for severe PRAEs.[68] A preoperative RDI, analogous to the AHI, above 19 events per hour may predict persistent OSAS in long-term follow-up.[79,102,103]

Fewer than 10% of children in North America are assessed with PSG before adenotonsillectomy.[104] Many tertiary care children's hospitals in the United States do not have uniform criteria for routinely performing PSG before adenotonsillectomy (Fig. 33.6).[105] The notion that PSG should be reserved for children with medically complex conditions and evaluation of persistent SDB despite adenotonsillectomy is contentious.[106] If PSG is not available, or is considered too costly, other diagnostic tests for OSAS may be considered. Many parents will record audio and/or

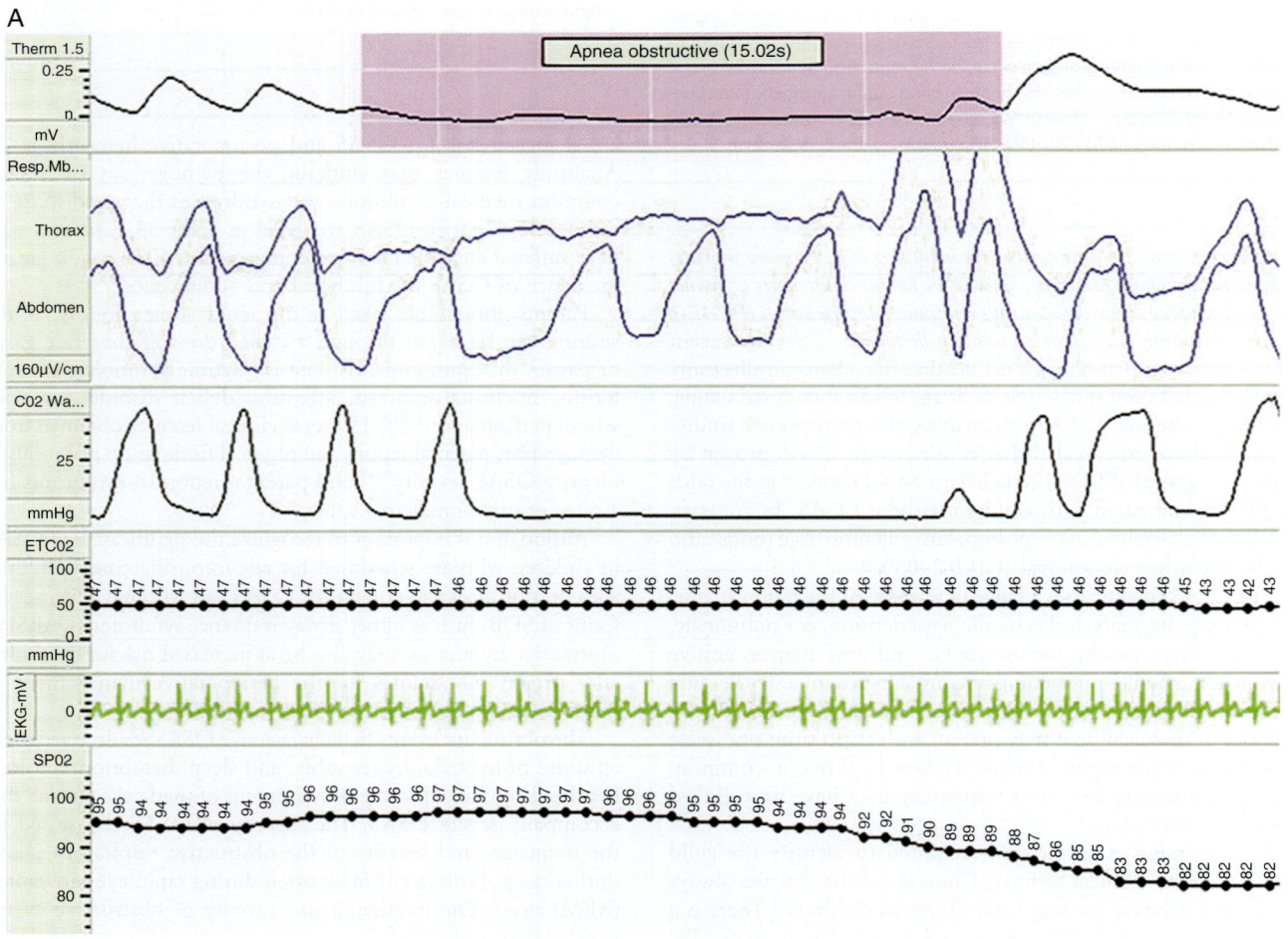

FIGURE 33.5 Typical polysomnographic recordings demonstrating obstructive apnea **(A)**, hypopnea **(B)**, and central apnea **(C)**. (From Schwengel DA, Sterni LM, Tunkel DE, Heitmiller ES. Perioperative management of children with obstructive sleep apnea. *Anesth Analg.* 2009;109[1]:60–75. With permission.)

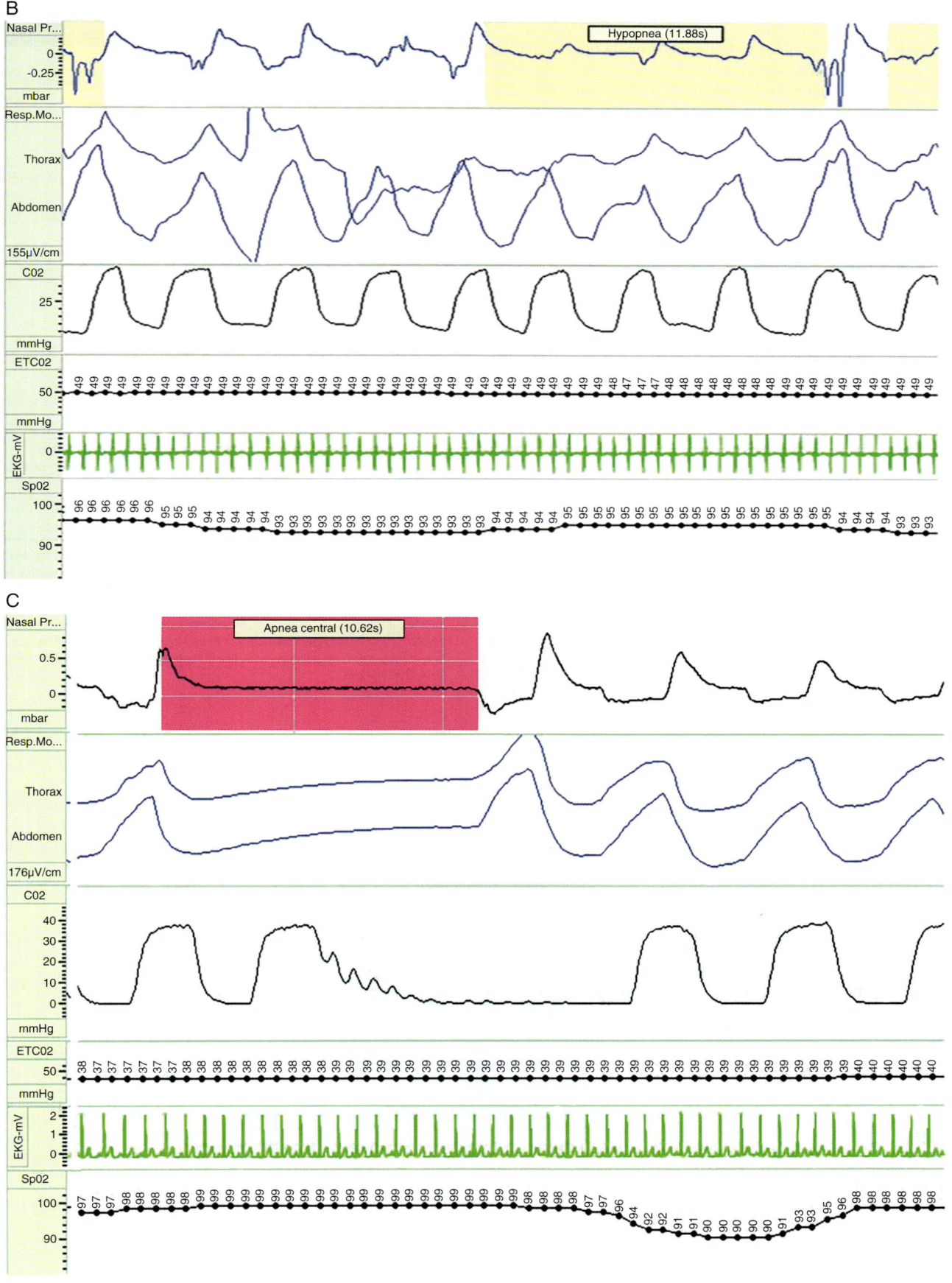

FIGURE 33.5, cont'd

videotapes of their child's breathing pattern during sleep. These have reasonably high positive and negative predictive values.[107,108] Although home sleep apnea tests are increasingly used in adults, there are no published guidelines for their use in children. Nap PSG is an abbreviated study that records sleep and breathing in the laboratory during daytime naps. Because of the limited recording time and the likely absence of REM sleep, they are best regarded as screening tools.[109]

Sleep evaluation with oximetry alone offers a low-cost, easy-to-use alternate test to PSG.[104,110,111] Published normative data in children indicate that the 2.5th percentile for the baseline SpO_2 is 95%. The nadir saturation (nSAT) is the lowest SpO_2 recorded during sleep and correlates inversely with the AHI.[102] An nSAT of 92% is the minimum normal SpO_2 in children[100,104,112]; however, an nSAT of <80% is a robust predictor of the risk for PRAEs and sensitivity to opioids.[67,70,113]

A commonly reported index of desaturation events, the oxygen desaturation index (ODI), is the number of decreases in SpO_2 ≥4% from baseline (ODI_4). In children, the 95th percentile for the ODI_4 is 2.2 episodes per hour. The ODI_4 is a sensitive metric used to evaluate the response to adenotonsillectomy in long-term outcome follow-up.[104] As obstructive respiratory events in children usually occur during REM and stage 2 sleep, the desaturation events tend to cluster at 60- to 90-minute intervals. A cluster of desaturation is defined as 5 or more decreases in SpO_2 (≥4%) within a 10- to 30-minute interval.[46] At least 3 clusters of desaturation with at least 3 SpO_2 decreases to less than 90% during a 6-hour nocturnal oximetry recording is diagnostic of OSA: positive predictive value for an AHI >1 event per hour of 97%; sensitivity 40%. For ≥2 clusters of desaturation along with at least 1 decrease in $Sp_{\geq 2}$ to ≤90% increases the sensitivity of this measurement to predict OSA to 80%.

The McGill Oximetry Scoring (MOS) system further classifies the severity of nocturnal hypoxemia (Fig. 33.7). The MOS correlates

TABLE 33.3	Clinical Diagnostic Criteria for Pediatric Obstructive Sleep Apnea Syndrome

1. Predisposing physical characteristics
   a. Body mass index greater than 95th percentile for age and gender
   b. Craniofacial abnormalities affecting the airway
   c. Anatomic nasal obstruction
   d. Tonsils nearly touching or touching in the midline
2. History of apparent airway obstruction during sleep (two or more of the following)
   a. Loud snoring (loud enough to be heard through a closed door)
   b. Frequent snoring
   c. Observed pauses in breathing during sleep
   d. Frequent arousals from sleep
   e. Intermittent vocalization during sleep
   f. Parental report of restless sleep, difficulty breathing, or struggling respiratory efforts during sleep
   g. Child with night terrors
   h. Child sleeps in unusual positions
   i. New-onset nocturnal enuresis
3. Somnolence (one or more of the following)
   a. Parent or teacher comments that the child appears sleepy during the day, is easily distracted, is overly aggressive, or has difficulty concentrating
   b. Child often is difficult to arouse at the usual awakening time

Note: If signs and symptoms in at least two categories are present, there is a significant probability of moderate obstructive sleep apnea (OSA). If severe abnormalities are present, children should be treated as having severe OSA.
Modified from Table 1 in American Society of Anesthesiologists. Practice guidelines for the perioperative management of patients with obstructive sleep apnea: an updated report by the American Society of Anesthesiologists Task Force on Perioperative Management of Patients with Obstructive Sleep Apnea. *Anesthesiology* 2014;120:268–286.

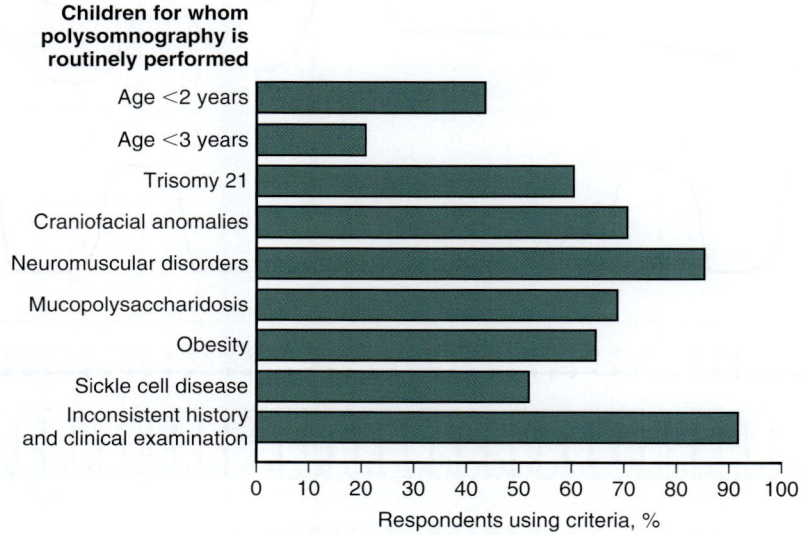

Children for whom polysomnography is routinely performed

FIGURE 33.6 Preoperative polysomnography criteria. Percentage of respondents using criteria shown as indication for polysomnography before adenotonsillectomy. (With permission from Nardone HC, McKee-Cole KM, Friedman NR. Current pediatric tertiary care admission practices following adenotonsillectomy. *JAMA Otolaryngol Head Neck Surg.* 2016;142[5]:452–456. doi:10.1001/jamaoto.2016.0051.)

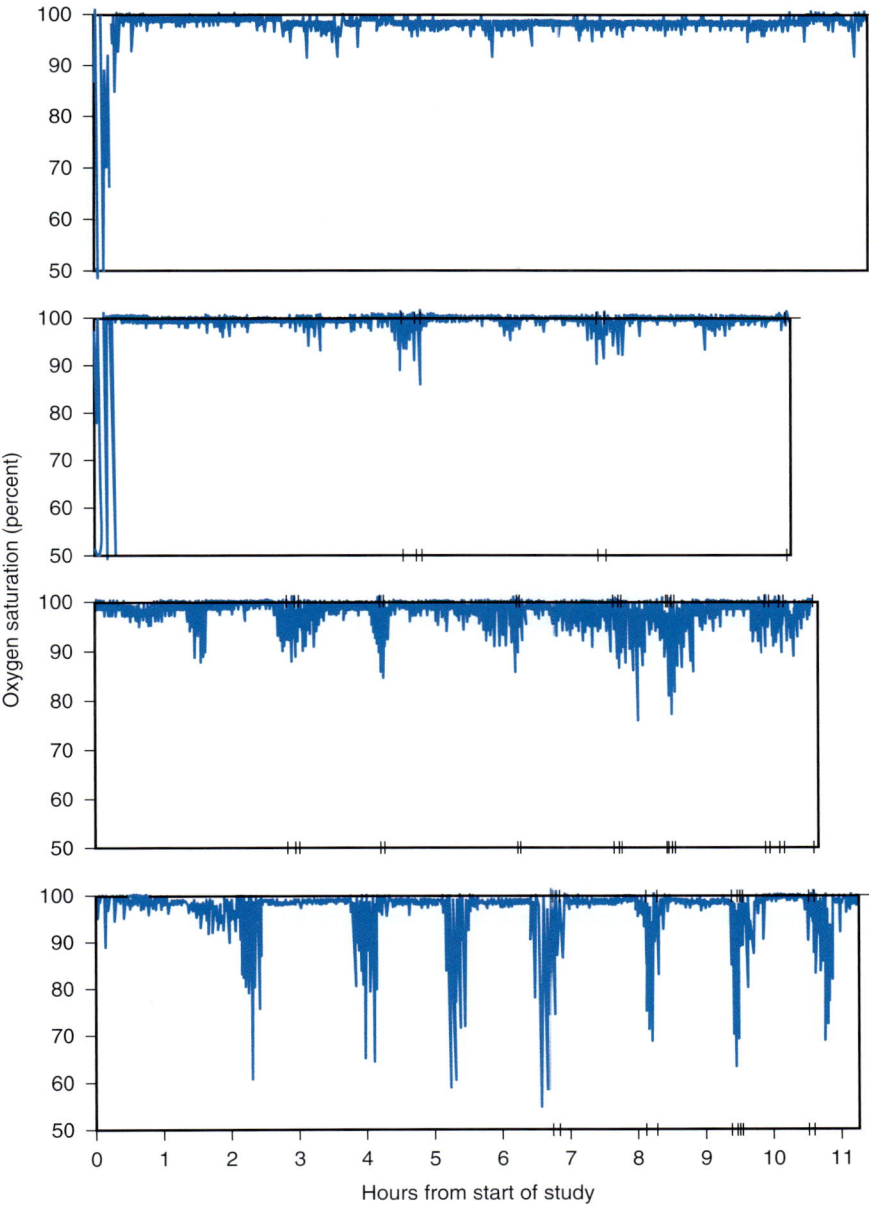

FIGURE 33.7 Representative figures for McGill oximetry scores 1 to 4 (*top to bottom*). McGill oximetry scores 2 to 4 are abnormal in that they all show at least three clusters of desaturation. The severity of the SpO₂ nadir determines the score such that McGill oximetry scores 2, 3, and 4 correspond to SpO₂ nadirs of less than 90%, less than 85%, and less than 80%, respectively. (From Nixon GM, Kermack AS, Davis GM, et al. Planning adenotonsillectomy in children with obstructive sleep apnea: the role of overnight oximetry. *Pediatrics* 2004;113[1 Pt 1]:e19–25.)

with both the AHI and the risk of PRAEs after adenotonsillectomy in children. The MOS4 is defined as >3 decreases in SpO₂ to <80%; corresponding to a mean AHI of 40 events per hour. The risk for major PRAEs, including reintubation, for children with MOS4 managed with a standard opioid regimen was 20% to 24%.[114]

These findings are clinically relevant in at least two respects: the morphine (or morphine equivalent) dose required to achieve a uniform analgesic endpoint in children with OSAS who exhibited a preoperative nSAT <85% was half that required in controls (Fig. 33.8).[115] In updated statements from both the American Academy of Pediatrics (AAP) and the AAO-HNS, the criteria to admit children after adenotonsillectomy is an nSAT <80%.[43,44]

Consultations to plan the perioperative care of children with severe OSAS are important. In contrast to children without OSAS, children with severe OSAS may require additional preoperative testing. A capillary blood gas sample collected in the morning may reveal an increased concentration of bicarbonate, consistent with a chronic respiratory acidosis. A preoperative electrocardiogram or echocardiogram may show evidence of right ventricular hypertrophy and/or pulmonary hypertension. A chest radiograph may demonstrate lower airway disease or cardiomegaly.

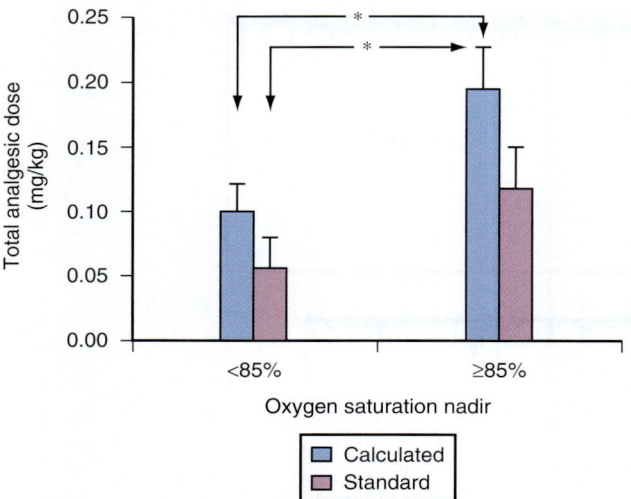

FIGURE 33.8 The total analgesic dose of morphine required to achieve a uniform analgesic endpoint in children with obstructive sleep apnea (OSA). Children were grouped by severity of OSA into those who had a preoperative SpO₂ nadir of <85% or ≥85%. The asterisks indicate post hoc differences between groups, $P < 0.05$. (From Brown KA, Laferrière A, Lakheeram I, Moss IR. Recurrent hypoxemia in children is associated with increased analgesic sensitivity to opiates. *Anesthesiology* 2006;105[4]:665–669.)

In a review of 9023 children with a mean age of 3.8 years evaluated over a 7-year period, 35 (0.4%) required urgent adenotonsillectomy within 48 hours of PSG.[116] Urgent adenotonsillectomy for severe OSAS is associated with significant respiratory morbidity after surgery.[69,116,117] On occasion, adenotonsillar hypertrophy may progress to compromise the upper airway during wakefulness. In some instances, the anesthetic considerations for obstructed and difficult airways may overlap; some may develop postobstructive pulmonary edema after intubation or surgery. Young children with profound oxygen desaturation during sleep, high obstructive indexes, and carbon dioxide (CO_2) retention may require admission to the pediatric ICU for optimization before and/or after adenotonsillectomy.[114,118]

Although adenotonsillar hypertrophy is the primary cause of OSAS in children, those with comorbidities such as obesity, Down syndrome, and craniofacial abnormalities may experience airway obstruction that is unrelated to the tonsils and adenoids.[119] Diagnostic, preoperative evaluation of these airways such as cine magnetic resonance imaging (MRI) and sleep endoscopy may be required before surgery; combinations of sevoflurane, propofol, remifentanil, dexmedetomidine, and ketamine anesthesia have been used.[119] Dexmedetomidine, an α-agonist, mimics non-REM sleep, facilitating the maintenance of airway patency. However, as obstructive events in pediatric OSA occur primarily during REM sleep, dexmedetomidine may not replicate the breathing pattern during natural sleep.

Sleep endoscopy, also known as drug-induced sleep endoscopy (DISE), is a technique that enables the surgeon to evaluate the level of obstruction in an anesthetized child with suspected OSAS.[120] The considerations for DISE are complex, requiring endoscopic evaluation of an obstructive airway in the supine position during spontaneous ventilation. Administration of lidocaine and oxymetazoline to the nasal mucosa may be useful. When DISE is indicated in children whose clinical evaluation is unremarkable or when OSAS persists after adenotonsillectomy, it should be performed by experienced otolaryngologists and anesthesiologists. A retrospective study determined that the frequency of oxygen desaturations to <85% during DISE with dexmedetomidine and ketamine was less than with either propofol alone or a combination of propofol and sevoflurane.[121]

ANESTHETIC MANAGEMENT AND POSTOPERATIVE CONSIDERATIONS

The anesthetic goals for adenotonsillectomy are to (1) provide a smooth, atraumatic induction; (2) provide the surgeon with optimal operating conditions; (3) establish IV access for volume expansion and medications as indicated; and (4) provide rapid emergence so that the child is awake and able to protect the recently instrumented airway. The need for a premedication is determined during the preanesthetic evaluation. *Children with symptoms of SDB who require premedication should be closely observed*, although the desaturation is transient and infrequent (1.5% of cases) after oral midazolam premedication.[122] *In children with severe OSA, premedication with short-acting, reversible drugs is advised and monitoring with pulse oximetry is indicated.*[122]

The anesthetic techniques for adenotonsillectomy are varied and include the choice of an inhalational or TIVA technique, the choice of an ETT or LMA, and the choice of spontaneous or controlled ventilation. Children who are scheduled for adenotonsillectomy have a greater incidence of airway reactivity and laryngospasm than those undergoing non-airway surgery. Of the currently available inhalational agents, sevoflurane provides a smooth induction of anesthesia. Maintenance of anesthesia with desflurane (for those whose airway is secured with an ETT) provides a rapid emergence and recovery.[123,124] An infusion of dexmedetomidine (1 to 2 μg/kg IV over 5 to 10 minutes) combined with an inhalation agent can provide satisfactory intraoperative conditions for adenotonsillectomy without adverse hemodynamic effects. However, clinical experience and a recent study suggest a quicker time frame (0.49 μg/kg over 5 seconds) might be safe.[125] Some authors have reported good results with a single IV dose of clonidine (1 μg/kg).[126]

Cuffed ETTs have become increasingly used in children of all age groups,[127] preventing the air leak and the consequent bubbling of gas in secretions and blood that can interfere with surgery. These tubes also minimize pollution by anesthetic gases and may decrease the risk of an airway fire when electrocautery is used.

Blood, secretions, and/or irrigation fluids may be present in the oropharynx at the conclusion of surgery and should be carefully suctioned by the surgeon or the anesthesiologist before emergence from anesthesia. Emptying the stomach with an orogastric tube, a maneuver frequently performed by surgeons under direct vision after completion of surgery, does not reduce the incidence of PONV.[128]

Many anesthesiologists prefer to wait until the child is fully awake before removing the ETT as the presence of an intact airway and pharyngeal reflexes are of utmost importance in preventing aspiration, laryngospasm, and airway obstruction.[129] However, with current surgical (use of electrocautery) and anesthetic (dexmedetomidine) techniques, a careful deep extubation is frequently chosen. The incidence of major respiratory complications requiring positive airway pressure, administration of drugs, airway manipulation, or instrumentation after deep or awake extubation is similar (~11%).[130] At the time of extubation, a common practice is to position the child in the lateral "recovery" or "tonsil" position with the head slightly down to permit blood and secretions to pool in the dependent cheek and drain out of the mouth rather than accumulate at the laryngeal inlet. The child should remain in the tonsil position postoperatively, while being carefully observed and monitored during transport to the PACU. The lateral position has the additional benefit of increasing both the cross-sectional area of the upper airway and total volume of the upper airway compared with children in the supine position.[131]

The use of the LMA for adenotonsillectomy was described in 1990, but it was not until the availability of a model with a flexible spiral, metallic reinforced shaft that made it practical for use in adenotonsillectomy (E-Fig. 33.1).[132,133] Advantages cited for the LMA over the ETT included a decrease in the incidence of postoperative stridor and laryngospasm[134]; recent evidence disputes these advantages.[135]

Analgesic Management

Children experience significant pain and severe functional limitations for up to 7 days after adenotonsillectomy.[136,137] Recovery from pain and return to normal daytime activities are considerably faster after isolated adenoidectomy.[137] Surgical technique has a major impact on the speed of recovery from pain because electrocautery techniques are generally associated with greater pain, presumably owing to increased thermal injury,[138–140] although this remains controversial.[141] Intracapsular tonsillectomy causes less pain and morbidity than the conventional extracapsular techniques and the outcomes appear comparable[142–144]; this technique may provide an alternative that may reduce the risk for posttonsillectomy apnea because of the reduced pain.

Infiltration of local anesthetics into the tonsillar fossa during tonsillectomy decreases postoperative pain, but the pain relief is brief (E-Fig. 33.2).[145] Life-threatening complications have been reported after local anesthetic infiltration in the tonsillar fossa, including intracranial hemorrhage, bulbar paralysis, deep cervical abscess, cervical osteomyelitis, medullopontine infarct, and cardiac arrest. The risks associated with injection of local anesthesia in the tonsillar fossa may outweigh its potential benefits, particularly in inexperienced hands.[146,147]

Over the past decade, there has been a shift away from opioids as the mainstay of perioperative analgesia to nonopioid regimens, including dexmedetomidine, acetaminophen, NSAIDs, dexamethasone, and ketamine. An infusion of dexmedetomidine (2 µg/kg IV over 5 to 10 minutes followed by 0.7 µg/kg per hour) may reduce postoperative opioid requirements.[148] After larger doses of dexmedetomidine (2 and 4 µg/kg), the opioid-free interval increases and the postoperative opioid requirements decrease; however, duration of stay in the PACU is markedly prolonged.[149]

A single intraoperative dose of dexamethasone reduces postadenotonsillectomy pain and edema when electrocautery has been used. These doses overlap the doses of dexamethasone to mitigate PONV (see later text). Dexamethasone (0.3–1 mg/kg) administration is associated with reduced parental- and physician-rated pain scores after adenotonsillectomy (Table 33.4).[139] The minimum morphine-sparing dose for dexamethasone is reported to be 0.5 mg/kg.[150] The use of dexamethasone in adenotonsillectomy remains routine in most US centers. Single doses of dexamethasone have not been associated with aseptic necrosis of the hip or infections, but have been responsible for precipitating the acute tumor lysis syndrome.[151–153]

In 2008, a report suggested that posttonsillectomy bleeding was increased in children who had received dexamethasone up to 0.5 mg/kg (maximum 20 mg).[158] A retrospective review of 31,934 children investigated whether a single IV dose of either dexamethasone or hydrocortisone administered on the day of surgery resulted in posttonsillectomy hemorrhage that required reoperation.[159] The rate of reoperation for secondary hemorrhage in children who received either steroid, 1.2% (adjusted odds ratio 2.5, 95% CI 1.5–4.2), was significantly greater than that in those who received steroids, 0.5% ($P < 0.001$)[159]; this finding was not present in adults. However, several subsequent studies have refuted these claims.[160–164] The consensus opinion and practice is that a single intraoperative dose of dexamethasone does not cause clinically important hemorrhage. Despite concerns that the routine use of NSAIDs for adenotonsillectomy might increase the risk for postadenotonsillectomy hemorrhage,[165,166] the AAO-HNS now recommends their use for postoperative analgesia. An audit of more than 4800 pediatric tonsillectomies in which the NSAIDs diclofenac and ibuprofen were routinely used, reported a primary hemorrhage rate of 0.9%.[167] Because the effects of ketorolac on platelet function are reversible, the effect depends on the presence of ketorolac within the body.[168] Unlike the effect of aspirin on bleeding, the effects of these NSAIDs is short-lived. However, we recommend avoiding NSAIDs, especially ketorolac, *during* surgery. When used for postoperative analgesia, they should be administered after hemostasis is achieved.[169] The use of ibuprofen in children who have been taking aspirin can result in severe posttonsillectomy bleeding.[170]

A recent editorial suggested that perhaps we need a clean start with a new class of analgesic drugs such as selective cyclooxygenase-2 (COX-2) inhibitors for adenotonsillectomy patients.[171] Although not available in the United States, parecoxib is a selective COX-2 inhibitor drug that reduces the production of inflammation-promoting prostaglandins. It spares platelet aggregation, bronchial tone, and gastric mucosal integrity unlike nonselective NSAIDs, and may reduce the need for rescue morphine and decreased the frequency of vomiting after adenotonsillectomy.[172,173] Celebrex, a COX-2 available in the United States, reduces early postoperative pain and the need for supplemental analgesics.[173a] More evidence is

TABLE 33.4	Effect of Single Intraoperative Dose of Dexamethasone on Postoperative Pain in Pediatric Tonsillectomy or Adenotonsillectomy: a Comparison of Randomized, Double-Blind Studies

Source	No. of Children	Dexamethasone Dose	Electrocautery Technique	Effect on Pain
Catlin and Grimes[154]	25	8 mg/m²	No	No difference
Ohlms et al.[155]	69	0.5 mg/kg	No	No difference
Tom et al.[156]	58	1.0 mg/kg	Yes	Reduced
April et al.[157]	80	1.0 mg/kg	Yes	No difference
Hanasono et al.[139]	219	1.0 mg/kg	Yes	Reduced

Modified from Hanasono MM, Lalakea ML, Mikulec AA, et al. Perioperative steroids in tonsillectomy using electrocautery and sharp dissection techniques. *Arch Otolaryngol Head Neck Surg.* 2004;130(8):917–921.

needed before COX-2 agents can be recommended for children during adenotonsillectomy.

Acetaminophen is commonly used as a component of multimodal analgesic approach in these children.[174] An IV formulation of acetaminophen is available in many countries, offering the theoretical advantage of greater predictability than the oral and rectal routes (see Fig. 33.1). Although the peak blood concentration is greater, the duration of analgesia after 15 mg/kg of IV acetaminophen is less than that after 40 mg/kg given rectally.[175] Reports of 10-fold overdoses of IV acetaminophen with near-catastrophic outcomes in infants should alert clinicians to potentially fatal dosing errors with this medication.[176,177]

Postdischarge pain management strategies vary among practitioners and institutions. Acetaminophen, dexamethasone, and ibuprofen are frequently prescribed in various combinations. Acetaminophen and NSAIDs (e.g., ibuprofen and diclofenac) have additive effects, prolonging the duration of analgesia when combined[178,179]; codeine is no longer indicated (see later text). Oxycodone may be used in older children. Scheduled dosing of any combination of these drugs is more effective than as-needed (pro re nata [PRN]) dosing in reducing pain intensity.[180]

Postoperative Nausea and Vomiting

Emesis and poor oral intake are common comorbid conditions after adenotonsillectomy. Opioids increase the incidence of PONV,

with two-thirds of treated children experiencing PONV.[167,181–184] Propofol,[185,186] ondansetron,[187–189] and dexamethasone[190,191] are widely used to reduce the incidence of emesis after adenotonsillectomy. A single intraoperative dose of dexamethasone reduces the incidence of emesis during the first 24 hours after adenotonsillectomy.[192] The number of children needed to treat was only four, which means that the use of dexamethasone in four children undergoing adenotonsillectomy results in one less child experiencing PONV. In addition, children who received dexamethasone were more likely than those receiving placebo to advance to a soft diet on postoperative day 1, with a number needed to treat of five. Given the antiemetic and possible morphine-sparing advantages of a single dose of dexamethasone, and its low cost and safety profile, the evidence suggests that routine use of dexamethasone reduces morbidity after adenotonsillectomy in children.[139,192] The smallest effective dose remains unclear. One study reported no difference in postoperative vomiting, pain scores, time to first liquid, and time to first analgesics among IV dexamethasone doses between 0.0625 and 1.0 mg/kg (Fig. 33.9).[190]

Postdischarge vomiting continues for days in some children. The use of at-home oral ondansetron disintegrating tablets may prevent emesis during the first 3 days after adenotonsillectomy.[193] Acupuncture, acupressure at the P6 (Nei-Kuwan) point, as well as therapeutic suggestion, have also been used with variable results.[194–196]

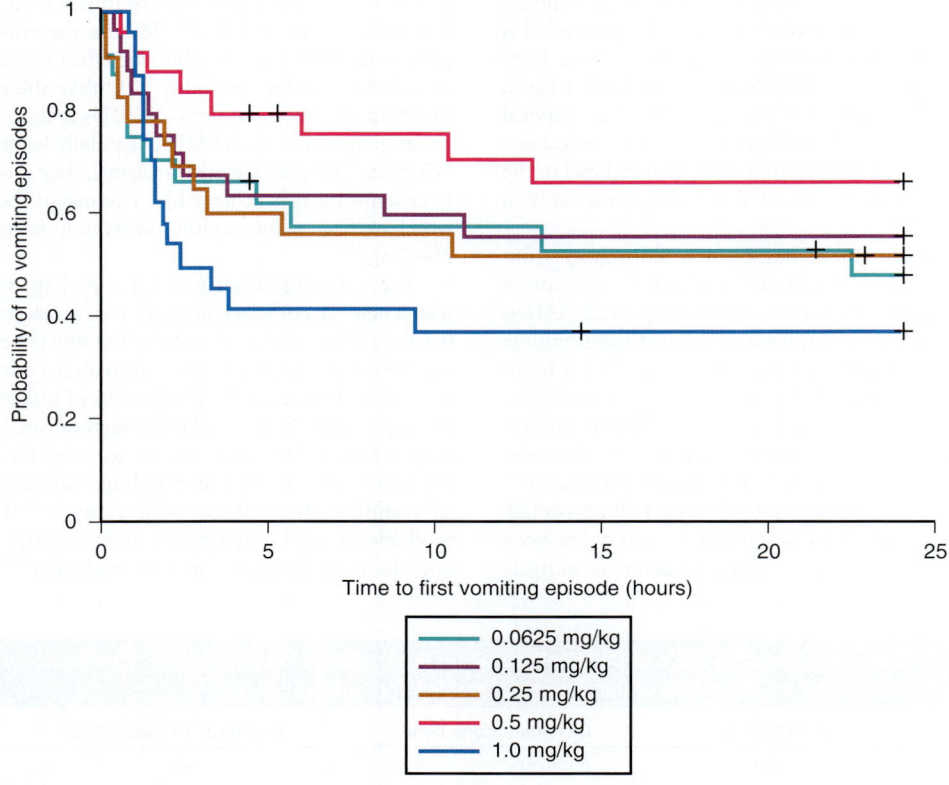

FIGURE 33.9 No dose-escalation response to dexamethasone to prevent vomiting in children undergoing tonsillectomy. Time-to-event analysis for first vomiting episode was performed; tick marks indicate time of censoring for patients who did not have complete follow-up (*N* = 13). No significant difference was found between dose levels, *P* = 0.28 (Cox proportional hazard likelihood ratio test). (Redrawn with permission from Kim MS, Coté CJ, Cristoloveanu C, et al. There is no dose-escalation response to dexamethasone [0.0625–1.0 mg/kg] in pediatric tonsillectomy or adenotonsillectomy patients for preventing vomiting, reducing pain, shortening time to first liquid intake, or the incidence of voice change. *Anesth Analg 2007*. 104[5]:1052–1058.)

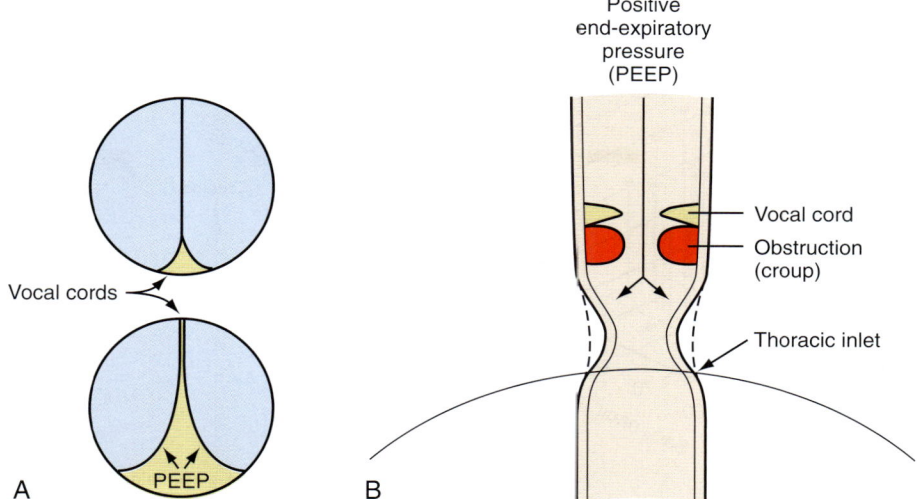

FIGURE 33.10 When a child has upper airway obstruction caused by laryngospasm **(A)** or mechanical obstruction **(B)**, application of approximately 10 cm H$_2$O of positive end-expiratory pressure (PEEP) during spontaneous breathing often relieves obstruction. PEEP helps to hold the vocal cords apart **(A)** and the airway open (*dashed lines* in **B**). (From Coté CJ. Pediatric anesthesia. In Miller RD, ed. *Miller's Anesthesia*. 8th ed. New York: Churchill Livingstone; 2012.)

Special Considerations for Children With OSA

Children with OSA who require premedication should be closely observed because transient oxygen desaturation that did not require any intervention has been reported in 1.5% of children with OSA who received 0.5 mg/kg oral midazolam.[122] This study excluded those with severe OSAS. Accordingly, caution should be exercised when premedicating children with severe OSAS.

Induction of Anesthesia

Compared with children undergoing adenotonsillectomy for chronic tonsillitis, children with OSAS experienced more respiratory complications during anesthetic induction including supraglottic obstruction and desaturation.[46,101] The vulnerability of the upper airway musculature described for halothane in cats[197] has subsequently been reported for most anesthetic agents in humans, resulting in a graded reduction in airway caliber with increasing anesthetic concentrations.[198–202] As airway collapse occurs in the upper two-thirds of the pharyngeal airway[201] during induction, airway obstruction may require a jaw thrust maneuver, insertion of an oral or nasopharyngeal airway, and/or the application of continuous positive airway pressure (CPAP). The application of CPAP acts as a pneumatic splint to increase the caliber of the pharyngeal airway (Fig. 33.10).[203] Of equal importance, CPAP increases longitudinal tension on the pharyngeal airway, thereby decreasing the collapsibility of the upper airway (see Fig. 14.10), and increases lung volumes.[204,205] Small increments in CPAP between 5 and 10 cm H$_2$O increase the dimension of the pharyngeal airway dramatically (Fig. 33.11).[206,207] In children with severe OSA, it is prudent to consider securing IV access before induction of anesthesia to expedite administration of an NMBD or IV agents should pharyngeal obstruction or laryngospasm occur.

Analgesic Management in Children With OSA

Severe OSA is characterized by recurrent episodes of hypoxia and hypercarbia during sleep. In animal models, exposure to

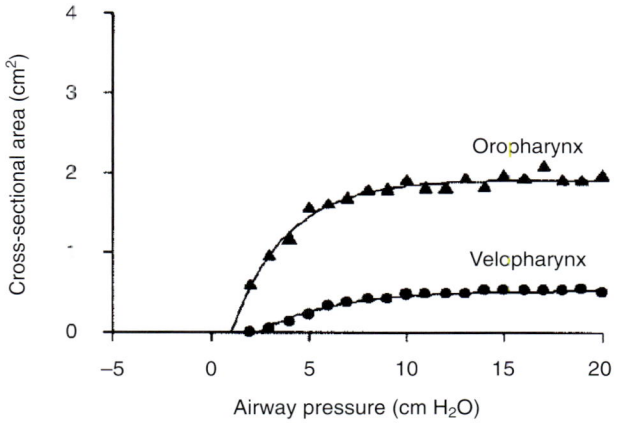

FIGURE 33.11 The relationship between airway pressure and the cross-sectional area of the pharynx. Maximal airway dimension is achieved between 15 and 20 cm H$_2$O. At reduced airway pressures, around 5 cm H$_2$O, small increments in airway pressure make a large difference in airway caliber. (From Isono S, Tanaka A, Nishino T. Dynamic interaction between the tongue and soft palate during obstructive apnea in anesthetized patients with sleep-disordered breathing. *J Appl Physiol*. 2003;95[6]:2257–2264.)

intermittent hypoxia during development is associated with an increase in the density of μ-opioid receptors in the respiratory-related areas of the brainstem. The cellular mechanism whereby this increased density is achieved has yet to be elucidated, but it may represent an adaptive response to the effects of recurrent intermittent hypoxia that allows μ-receptor–mediated opioid respiratory effects to predominate.[208–211]

In young children with severe OSA, the severity of the nocturnal oxygen desaturation correlates with the sensitivity to exogenously administered opioids (Fig. 33.12).[115,212,213] The morphine dose

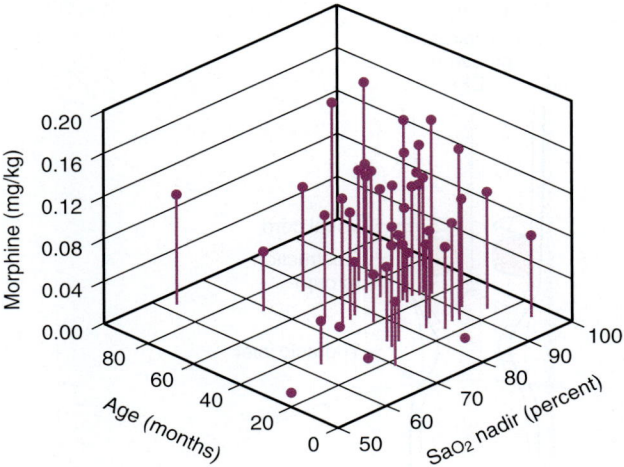

FIGURE 33.12 Relationship between morphine requirement, age, and the preoperative arterial oxygen-saturation nadir in 46 children who were otherwise well. The lengths of the stems supporting the 46 dots are proportional to the morphine dose. The stems in the foreground are shorter than those in the background, indicating a significant correlation between the three variables. SaO_2, arterial oxygen saturation. (From Brown KA, Laferrière A, Moss IR. Recurrent hypoxemia in young children with obstructive sleep apnea is associated with reduced opioid requirements for analgesia. *Anesthesiology* 2004;100[4]:806–810.)

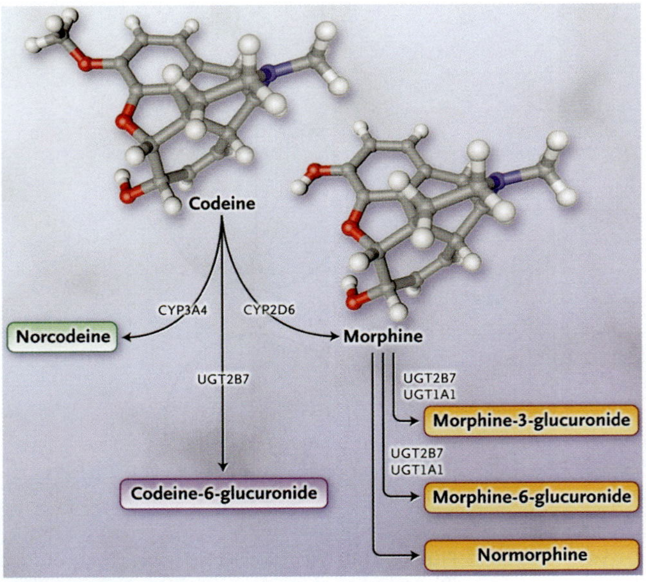

FIGURE 33.13 Codeine metabolic pathways. The CYP-2D6 pathway is responsible for converting the prodrug codeine to the active drug morphine. (From Racoosin JA, Roberson DW, Pacanowski MA, Nielsen DR. New evidence about an old drug—risk with codeine after adenotonsillectomy. *N Engl J Med.* 2013;368[23]:2155–2157 [June 6, 2013] with permission.)

required to achieve a uniform analgesic endpoint in children with OSA who exhibited a low preoperative nSAT (<85%) (see Fig. 33.8) was less than in those whose preoperative nSAT was 85% or more.[115] Children with severe OSAS who exhibit nocturnal hypoxemia require OSA-appropriate opioid regimens. Young age was also associated with an increased sensitivity to opioids. In a retrospective review of 880 children, of whom 116 had PSG-confirmed OSA, a total intraoperative opioid administration of 0.1 mg/kg or more of morphine equivalents increased the risk for intraoperative respiratory complications (adjusted odds ratio of 0.4, 95% CI 0.2–0.8).[130] *An unforeseen risk of perioperative opioid use in children with severe OSA is that age-appropriate doses of opioids may produce exaggerated respiratory depression.* Of children with severe OSAS who were anesthetized with halothane, 46% experienced apnea after a single IV dose of fentanyl (0.05 µg/kg) compared with 4% of controls.[214] This increased sensitivity to the respiratory depressant effects of fentanyl in children with OSAS is supported by the exaggerated respiratory depression to subsequent administration of a uniform dose of fentanyl in rat pups exposed to intermittent hypoxia.[215] Hence, allowing spontaneous respirations during maintenance of anesthesia enables an assessment of the response to small challenges of opioid analgesics.[213,216] In this manner, the anesthesiologist can assess the sensitivity of the child with OSAS to opioids; controlling respirations precludes such an evaluation. Sleep fragmentation blunts the arousal response to acute airway occlusion during sleep.[217,218] In addition, exposure to intermittent hypoxia during development is associated with an increase in the arousal latency to hypoxia.[219–221] Morphine acting at the level of the basal forebrain blunts arousal.[222] If the increased sensitivity to both the analgesic and respiratory effects of exogenously administered opioids reported in children with OSA extends to arousal mechanisms, the use of opioids in children with severe OSA may further impair arousal mechanisms. This heightened

sensitivity may have been a contributing factor in the reports of death from apparent apnea after hospital discharge,[59,72,73,223] prompting the shift to nonopioid and reduced opioid postoperative analgesic regimens.[179,224,225]

Guidelines for the perioperative management of OSAS[112] suggest that the use of codeine, previously thought to be a "low-risk" oral opioid commonly used in the ambulatory setting, is problematic. Codeine is a prodrug that is metabolized by the cytochrome P450 debrisoquine 4-hydroxylase (CYP2D6) to its active analgesic morphine metabolites (Fig. 33.13). The CYP2D6 gene displays polymorphism, including gene duplication that results in ultra-rapid metabolism, which for prodrugs such as codeine, results in a greater fraction of morphine.[226] Respiratory arrest after codeine has been reported in both adults and children who are ultra-rapid metabolizers of codeine.[227–229] Whereas the ultra-rapid metabolizing genotype is present in 3% of Caucasians, it is present in 10% to 30% of Arabian and Northeast African populations. In contrast, almost 10% of children lack CYP2D6, rendering codeine an ineffective analgesic because there is no conversion to morphine. Given the broad variability in codeine metabolism and our lack of knowledge of which polymorphism is carried by each child, the FDA recently required that the manufacturers of all codeine-containing products add a boxed warning to the labeling of their product that describes the risk posed by codeine after a child has undergone tonsillectomy or adenoidectomy and codeine use is restricted in such patients.[230,231] On April 20, 2017, that warning was changed to a *contraindication* in children <18 years of age undergoing tonsillectomy. One approach to manage pain in children at home has been to determine the 2D6 genotyping. In one report of more than 600 children with sickle cell disease who required codeine for painful crises, those who were ultra-rapid or poor metabolizers of 2D6 were treated with analgesics other than codeine and the remainder were treated with codeine; no complications occurred.[232] For children after tonsillectomy, hydrocodone and oxycodone are also affected by polymorphisms in 2D6, thereby rendering them vulnerable to the same risks as those conferred by codeine. The French Society of Otorhinolaryngologists and the Swedish ENT Association for Otorhinolaryngology, Head and Neck Surgery formulated guidelines to manage posttonsillectomy pain in their respective countries.[225,233] With the demise of codeine, the French guidelines based their postoperative treatment on tramadol, whose metabolism by 2D6 is considered less variable in analgesic potency than codeine, whereas the Swedish guidelines adopted a pain management strategy based on oxycodone among other medications. Some have advocated oral morphine to treat these children postoperatively. The pharmacokinetics of oral morphine in children differ substantively from those in adults.[234,235] Initial studies with oral morphine to supplement NSAIDs after tonsillectomy have shown that it does not improve analgesia, but increased side effects such as hemoglobin desaturation.[236,237] Further studies are required before a consensus regarding the optimal pain management strategy for children after tonsillectomy can be recommended.

One very important observation worth emphasis is that children with severe OSA may be exquisitely sensitive to the respiratory depressant effects of opioids such that the usual doses should be reduced by $\frac{1}{2}$ to $\frac{2}{3}$ of the usual starting dose and then titrated to effect. Obese, African American, and Hispanic children are at increased risk. The report of two children who died in the PACU after tonsillectomy, presumably after removal of monitors during emergence, and another who died within a hospital ward emphasizes the insidiousness of this issue and why increased vigilance is needed.[59]

Neural Blockade

Blockade of neural input to the upper airway dilator musculature in children with OSA is also problematic. Serious life-threatening complications, including severe upper airway obstruction (UAO) and pulmonary edema, have been reported after local anesthetics have been infiltrated in the tonsillar fossa to prevent pain after adenotonsillectomy. The pharynx in children with OSA is not only smaller in size,[201,238] but also more collapsible, even during wakefulness.[239–241] Topical anesthesia applied to the mucosa of the pharynx of children with OSA reduces the caliber of the pharynx and may thereby compromise airway patency.[242]

Extubation Strategy and Management of the Postoperative Period in Children With OSA

Full antagonism of neuromuscular blockade is strongly recommended as residual neuromuscular blockade in the PACU will selectively depress the function of the upper airway dilators relative to the diaphragm, promoting collapse of the pharyngeal airway.[243] Antagonism of neuromuscular blockade with atropine and neostigmine after tonsillectomy has been associated with less PONV than antagonism with glycopyrrolate and neostigmine.[244]

The trachea is usually extubated when the child is fully awake. Techniques that involve minimally stimulating the airway have been suggested.[129] Although the incidence of major respiratory complications after deep or awake extubation is similar, a greater proportion of children in the awake extubation group had PSG-proven OSA.[130] Placing a nasopharyngeal or oropharyngeal airway before extubation is sometimes useful.[95]

Several other factors may increase the risk of respiratory difficulties after adenotonsillectomy in children with OSAS. For reasons that are unclear, children with severe OSAS, whose adenotonsillectomy was performed in the morning, were less likely to desaturate

when managed in a PACU setting than those whose surgery was performed in the afternoon.[245] Two drugs, atropine and naloxone, have the potential to augment the function of the upper airway. Atropine administered after induction of anesthesia decreased the risk of postadenotonsillectomy respiratory complications.[69] Of possible relevance is the report that blockade of the muscarinic receptors in the rat hypoglossal nucleus enhances activity of the genioglossus muscle.[246] Agonists of opioid μ-receptors depress activity in the pharyngeal dilator muscles, including the genioglossus muscle.[209,247–249] Given the increased sensitivity to both analgesic and respiratory effects of exogenously administered opioids in children with severe OSAS, a similar sensitivity may also apply to the pharyngeal musculature. Small doses of naloxone may alleviate UAO after adenotonsillectomy if a relative "overdose" of exogenous opioids has been administered.

Children with OSAS continue to demonstrate obstructive apnea and desaturation in the immediate postoperative period. Avoiding opioids, or using both age- and OSAS-appropriate opioid regimens ($\frac{1}{3}$ to $\frac{1}{2}$ the normal starting dose) in both the intraoperative and postoperative periods, decreases the frequency of these events.[96] Measures to support airway patency in the postoperative period include insertion of a nasal airway, administration of noninvasive ventilatory support (e.g., CPAP), reintubation, ventilation, and the administration of bronchodilators, racemic epinephrine, and heliox. Bilevel positive airway pressure and/or CPAP may be useful in children with preexisting neurologic disorders.[250] However, nasal secretions may be copious after adenotonsillectomy, limiting the efficacy of noninvasive ventilatory support. Children with complex medical diseases, who are critically dependent on the function of upper airway musculature, may benefit from delayed extubation. Acute relief of chronic UAO favors the exudation of intravascular fluid into the pulmonary interstitium and noncardiogenic pulmonary edema, which may present preoperatively, intraoperatively, or postoperatively. Supportive measures include the administration of oxygen, tracheal intubation, mechanical ventilation with positive end-expiratory pressure, and administration of furosemide.[251–253]

Despite removal of the hypertrophied tonsils and adenoids, children with OSAS continue to demonstrate obstructive apnea and desaturation during sleep on the first night after adenotonsillectomy, with the frequency of the obstructive events and the severity of desaturation usually greater in those children with severe OSAS (Fig. 33.14).[254,255] This underscores the need to admit these children for continuous overnight monitoring postoperatively. In addition to pulse oximetry, common monitors include photoplethysmography, transthoracic impedance, and capnography. The majority of desaturation events on the first postoperative night are the result of obstructive apnea.[254] Obstructive respiratory efforts act to change thoracic impedance. A limitation of this monitor is that it will falsely detect paradoxical chest wall motion as breathing when in fact the airway is obstructed.[256,257] Nasal capnography is poorly tolerated in postoperative children and nasal secretions may be problematic. Transcutaneous CO_2 monitors may be useful in somnolent children. The AAP and the AAO-HNS now recommend that children with an AHI >24 or an AHI >10 events per hour be admitted to the hospital after adenotonsillectomy.[43,71] Current pediatric tertiary care admission practices after adenotonsillectomy show considerable variability among institutions despite clear guidelines from several societies (Fig. 33.15).[105]

Long-term follow-up studies more than 6 months after tonsillectomy in children with OSAS show that symptoms completely resolve in those with mild OSAS (AHI <10) but are persistent in up

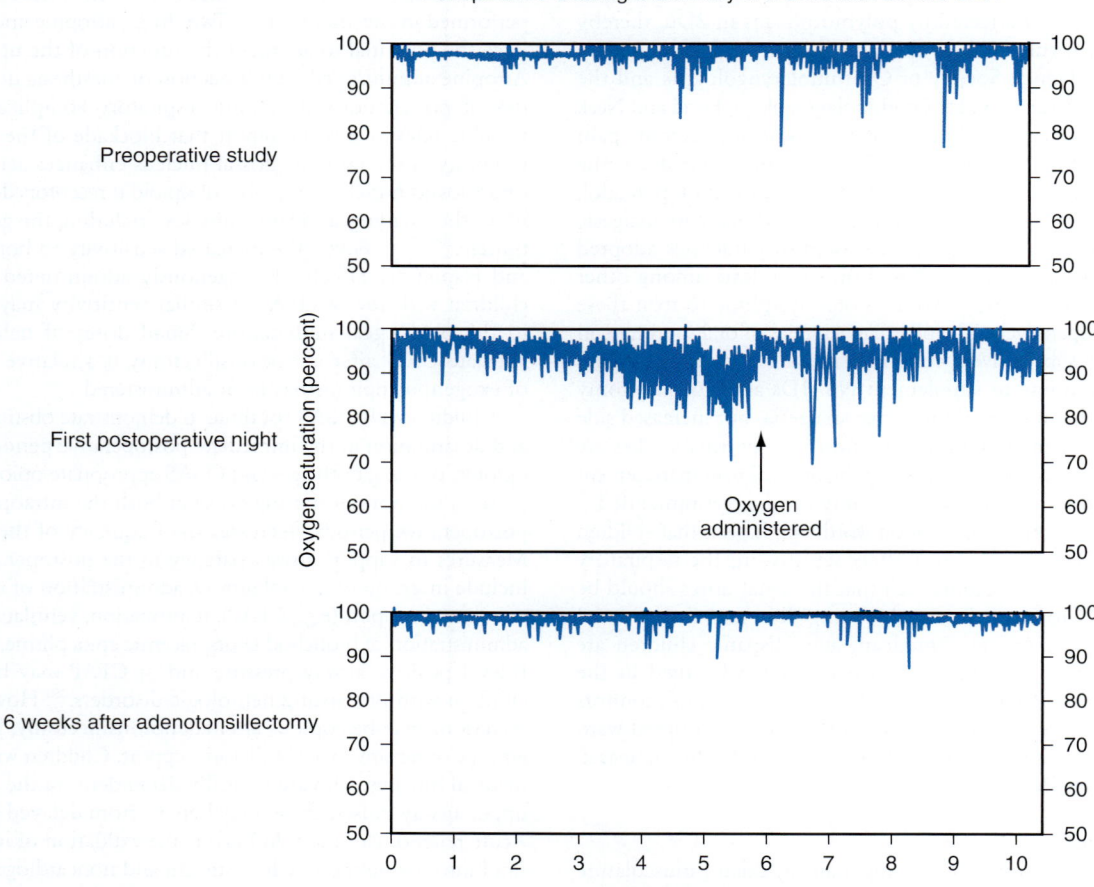

Perioperative Overnight Oximetry in a Child with Severe OSA

FIGURE 33.14 Three oximetry trend records from an otherwise healthy child. The x-axis is time ranging from bedtime on the left to arousal the following morning on the right. The *top* panel is the preoperative record showing clusters of desaturation. The *middle* panel is the record from the first night after adenotonsillectomy. With sleep onset, a decrease in saturation is evident that worsens after midnight. Oxygen therapy is administered after midnight (*arrow*). The *bottom* panel is the recording 6 weeks after adenotonsillectomy, which is within normal limits. (From Nixon GM, Kermack AS, McGregor CD, et al. Sleep and breathing on the first night after adenotonsillectomy for obstructive sleep apnea. *Pediatr Pulmonol.* 2005;39[4]:332–338.)

to 35% of those with severe OSAS (AHI >20).[258–260] Furthermore, recent epidemiologic evidence suggests that residual SDB is more likely to be present after adenotonsillectomy in older children (>7 years of age) and obese children. It has also been suggested that obese children with large tonsils and OSA also show evidence of systemic inflammatory disease that persists after tonsillectomy.[258,261]

DISCHARGE POLICY FOR AMBULATORY ADENOTONSILLECTOMY

Although children undergoing adenotonsillectomy for obstructive breathing without apnea may undergo ambulatory surgery, those with OSAS should not. The AAO-HNS revised the clinical practice guidelines for tonsillectomy in children, including indications for postoperative hospitalization.[42,87]

In otherwise healthy children, conversion from ambulatory to inpatient status was most frequently prompted by respiratory events in children whose indication for surgery was obstructive breathing.[262] In a retrospective review of 6681 cases, implementation of these guidelines decreased the overall rate of unplanned admission to the hospital after adenotonsillectomy from 2.4% to 1.4%,[263] reducing the indications for respiratory complications from 9% to zero and for hemorrhage from 3% to zero.[48,264] A systematic reduction in postoperative morphine use was associated with a reduced rate of hospital admission from 8% to 2.4%.[167] A systematic use of age- and OSAS-appropriate opioid regimens reduced the incidence of PRAEs and the recovery time.[96]

In North America, the indication for adenotonsillectomy in 77% of children is obstructive breathing.[262,265,266] The reality is that fewer than 10% are evaluated with a sleep test before surgery. The challenge is to evaluate the severity of SDB based on clinical criteria alone.[89] Different algorithms are available to guide the disposition of children with OSAS and the indications for postoperative admission (Fig. 33.16).[87,95,257] Because the onset of respiratory complications in children with severe OSAS may be delayed,[68,245,254] practice guidelines from the AAO-NHS, the AAP, and the American Society of Anesthesiologists all recommend that discharge criteria from a monitored setting should include observation with SpO_2 monitoring during sleep. A survey of North

Criteria for admission

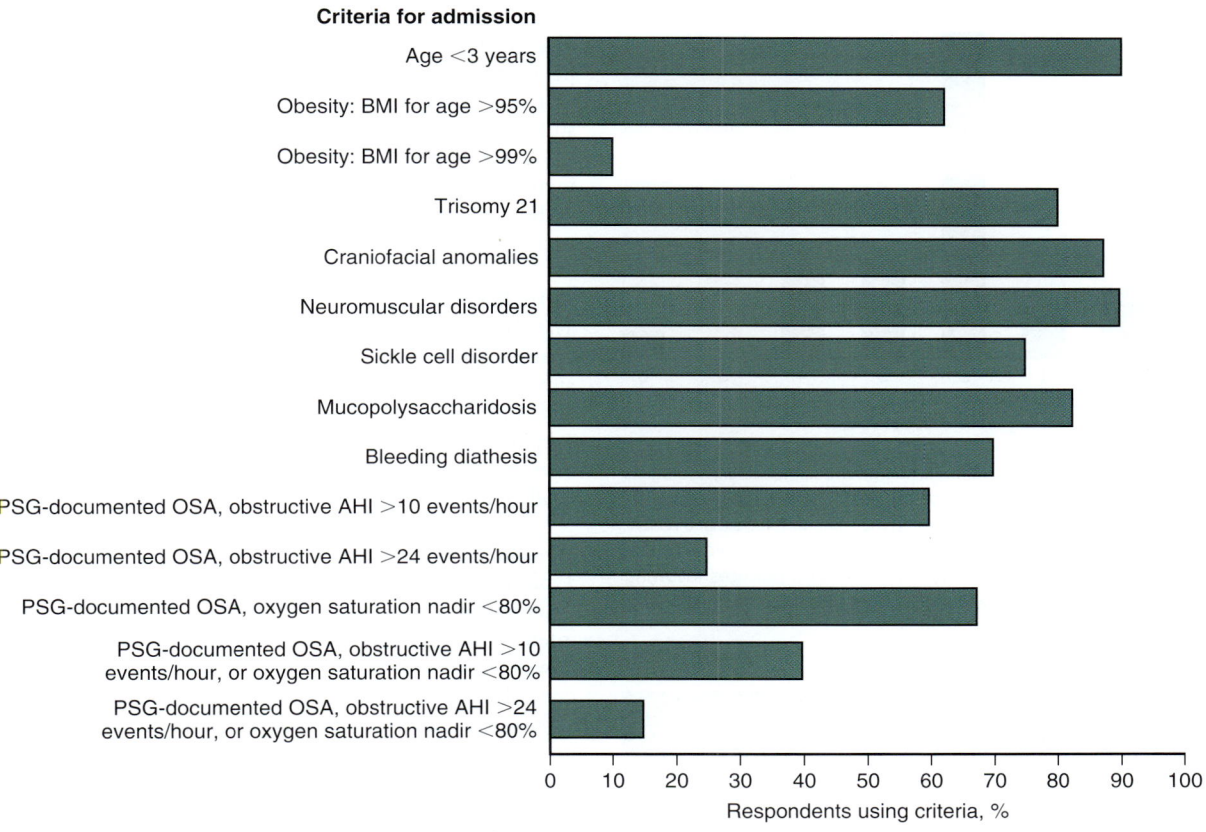

FIGURE 33.15 Admission criteria after adenotonsillectomy. Percentage of respondents from 72 pediatric otolaryngology divisions at tertiary care children's hospitals using the criteria shown as an indication for admission. It is surprising and counterintuitive that the children with documented obstructive sleep apnea (OSA) and the highest apnea hypopnea index (AHI) or desaturation (<80%) criteria had the lowest use by otolaryngologists. *BMI*, body mass index; *PSG*, polysomnography. (From Nardone HC, McKee-Cole KM, Friedman NR. Current pediatric tertiary care admission practices following adenotonsillectomy. *JAMA Otolaryngol Head Neck Surg.* 2016;142[5]:452–456.)

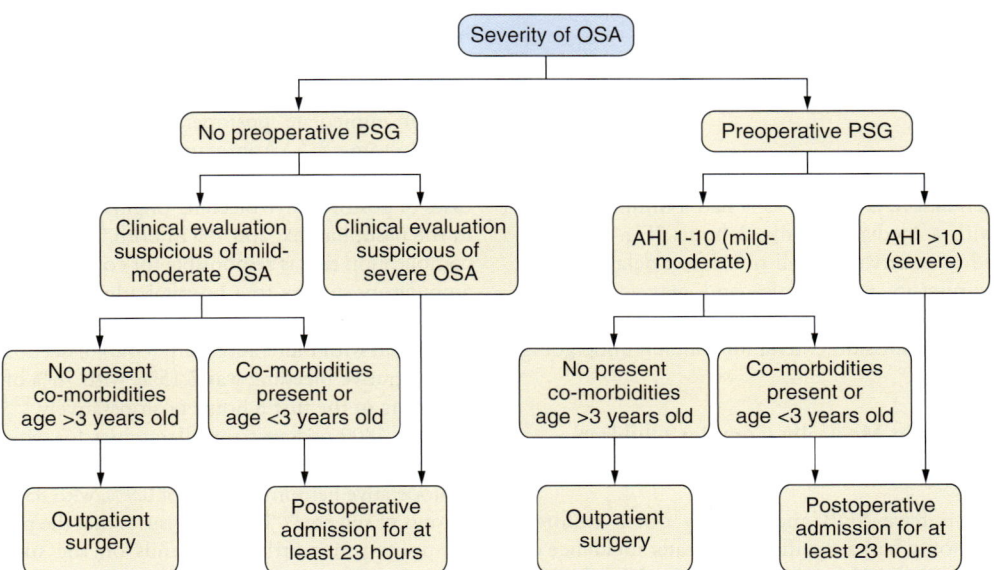

FIGURE 33.16 Pathway showing management pathways for children with obstructive sleep apnea *(OSA)* after adenotonsillectomy. *AHI*, apnea hypopnea index; *PSG*, polysomnography. (From Patino M, Sadhasivam S, Mahmoud M. Obstructive sleep apnoea in children: perioperative considerations. *Br J Anaesth*, 2013;111[Suppl 1]:i83–i95. With permission.)

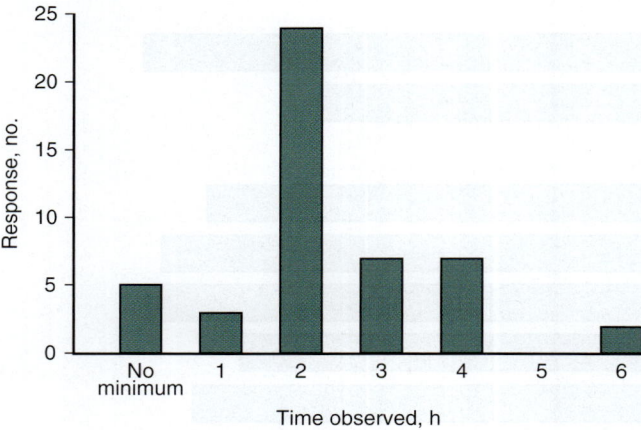

FIGURE 33.17 A survey of observation time from pediatric otolaryngologists from 72 pediatric otolaryngology divisions at tertiary care children's hospitals after outpatient adenotonsillectomy regarding the minimum time that a patient was observed before discharge home. (From Nardone HC, McKee-Cole KM, Friedman NR. Current pediatric tertiary care admission practices following adenotonsillectomy. *JAMA Otolaryngol Head Neck Surg.* 2016;142[5]:452–456. doi:10.1001/jamaoto.2016.0051 March 24, 2016.)

TABLE 33.5	Criteria for Overnight Admission After Tonsillectomy and Adenoidectomy
• Obstructive sleep apnea	
• Sleep disturbance	
• <3 years of age	
• Craniofacial abnormalities (e.g., Down syndrome, Treacher Collins syndrome)	
• Lives >1 hour away	
• Lives in an unstable home environment that precludes adequate supervision	
• Postoperative problems (e.g., fever, failure to take oral fluids, or continued vomiting)	
• Possible or documented coagulopathy	
• Extreme obesity	

From Zalzal G: Personal communications, survey of major pediatric hospitals, 2006.

American pediatric tertiary centers showed that 73% complied with this recommendation, although 93% had a minimum time for observation with a median of only 2 hours (Fig. 33.17).[105] This 2-hour period of observation will not detect delayed onset of sleep-related respiratory compromise and may explain the deaths from apparent apnea after adenotonsillectomy.[72,73] Table 33.5 presents common admission criteria for children undergoing elective tonsillectomy.

Special Considerations in Medically Complex Children With OSAS

Severe Obesity

Obese children often have SDB and severely obese children undergoing tonsillectomy had a significantly greater incidence of comorbid conditions than normal children. Severely obese children (body mass index [BMI] >98th percentile) have an almost 9-fold increase in the odds for perioperative respiratory adverse events (PRAEs), a greater incidence of bleeding,[59,73] and an increase rate of unplanned admission to hospital after adenotonsillectomy.[267]

Down Syndrome

The incidence of OSAS in children with Down syndrome may be as great as 50%.[104] Nocturnal oximetry may be the preferred first test as these children may not be cooperative for a PSG study. An abnormal MOS could help identify children with severe OSA. However, children with Down syndrome may exhibit an increased central apnea index and a reduced obstructive AHI without desaturation events, so that a negative MOS does not exclude severe OSA.

Pierre Robin Sequence

The Pierre Robin sequence (PRS) affects 1 in 3000 to 8000 live births. PRS is an association of micrognathia, glossoptosis, and airway obstruction and feeding difficulties within the first 24 hours after birth. Surgical management includes tongue-lip adhesion, subperiosteal release of the floor of the mouth, and mandibular distraction osteogenesis. Airway management may be a major challenge.[268]

Abnormalities of Ventilatory Control

Typically, oximetry studies in pediatric OSA show clusters of desaturation with an intercluster SpO$_2$ in excess of 90%. A low intercluster SpO$_2$ is reported in children with diseases of the lower airways, such as bronchiolitis, and abnormalities of ventilatory control.[269–271] As young children with undiagnosed disorders of ventilatory control may also have adenotonsillar hypertrophy, a low intercluster SpO$_2$ should prompt further investigation. Late-onset central hypoventilation syndrome, rapid-onset obesity hypoventilation hypothalamic and autonomic dysfunction (ROHHAD) syndrome, and the Prader-Willi syndrome may be associated with adenotonsillar hypertrophy.

POSTTONSILLECTOMY BLEEDING

Posttonsillectomy bleeding is a surgical emergency. It occurs either within the first 24 hours after surgery (primary bleeding) or 5 to 10 days after surgery when the eschar covering the tonsillar bed retracts (secondary bleeding). Primary bleeding is considered a surgical complication as the result of failure to establish surgical hemostasis, whereas secondary bleeding is attributed to nonsurgical complications, including certain medications, a bleeding diathesis, or infection. Obesity and older age are associated with an increased risk of immediate postoperative hemorrhage after outpatient tonsillectomy.[58,59,73] Approximately 75% of postoperative tonsillar bleeding occurs within 6 hours of surgery. Sixty-seven percent of cases of postoperative bleeding originate in the tonsillar fossa, 27% in the nasopharynx, and 7% in both.[272] It is considered a surgical complication that is responsible for converting tonsillectomy from ambulatory surgery to a hospital admission in 1.6% of cases.[262]

In a review of more than 9000 adenotonsillectomies in children performed with blunt and sharp (cold) dissection, the incidence of postoperative bleeding was 2.15%, with 76% of the hemorrhages occurring in the first 6 hours postoperatively.[273] The authors of an audit of 4800 pediatric tonsillectomies for which hemostasis was secured with electrocautery (hot) techniques reported a primary postoperative hemorrhage rate of 0.9%, with 83% presenting within 4 hours of surgery.[167] The consensus is that the period of observation for primary hemorrhage depends on the surgical technique: 6 hours and 4 hours, for cold and hot dissection, respectively,[167,272,273] although abbreviated periods of observation have been advocated by some.[262] IV steroid administration on the day of tonsillectomy in children was reported to be an independent risk factor for severe bleeding requiring reoperation.[159] The impact of revised practice guidelines recommending against the prophylactic antibiotic use on the incidence of bleeding after adenotonsillectomy is still not clear. A retrospective review of 5359 cases reported the incidence of surgery for bleeding increased from 1.4% to 3.5% (95% CI 1.9% to 5.1%) after the change in practice.[274]

The management of anesthesia in this situation can be challenging even in the hands of an experienced pediatric anesthesiologist.[275] It often requires dealing with anxious parents, an upset surgeon, and a frightened anemic, hypovolemic child with a stomach full of blood. A thorough review of the anesthetic record of the original surgery will provide pertinent information about any existing medical condition, use of medications (such as aspirin), difficulty with airway management, and a rough estimate of intraoperative blood loss and fluid replacement, as well as the duration of known bleeding and the volume of blood vomited since the bleeding began. A quick history and examination of the child will provide vital information about the child's current volume status. A history of dizziness and the presence of orthostatic hypotension may suggest a loss of more than 20% of the circulating blood volume and the need for aggressive fluid resuscitation and crossmatch of blood before induction.[276] Even when severe hypotension is not present, the child with the bleeding tonsil may be hypovolemic with a decreased cardiac output secondary to ongoing blood loss. If blood loss is severe, and/or fluid resuscitation is not vigorous, lactic acidosis and shock will develop.

The compensatory response to acute blood loss is an outpouring of catecholamines. This causes peripheral vasoconstriction, which delays the clinical onset of hypotension in the awake child. When anesthesia-induced vasodilation occurs, profound hypotension may develop. Vigorous fluid resuscitation with crystalloids (repeated boluses of 20 mL/kg of balanced salt solution) and/or colloids is therefore the key to improve the cardiac output and achieve hemodynamic stability before induction of anesthesia. Hemoglobin or hematocrit determination should be interpreted in light of the child's volume status and the type of fluid resuscitation administered. If the hemoglobin concentration is reduced after fluid resuscitation, blood may be required; however, blood is rarely the primary solution for volume replacement in these children. If severe hypovolemia is suspected or if there may be a delay in obtaining blood, blood should be crossmatched for two or more units of packed red blood cells before the child reaches the OR. If a child bleeds after the tonsillectomy and a bleeding blood vessel is not identified, it may be necessary to measure the prothrombin time, partial thromboplastin time, platelet count, and a bleeding time to rule out a bleeding diathesis. *It cannot be overemphasized that the child must be adequately volume resuscitated before proceeding to the OR.*

A child who presents with a bleeding tonsil has a full stomach (filled with swallowed blood) and may still be hypovolemic. A child who is spitting bright red blood may quickly exsanguinate, but the bleeding may be temporarily controlled by compression of the carotid artery ipsilateral to the bleeding source. The anesthesiologist may have difficulty visualizing the larynx because of the bleeding tonsillar bed and clots in the pharynx. A stiletted ETT, two sets of well-illuminated laryngoscope blades and handles, and two large-bore Yankauer-type suction tubes must be available before induction of anesthesia (see also Chapter 4 and Fig. 39.5). On arrival in the OR and application of routine monitors, the child who is actively bleeding from the oropharynx should be preoxygenated while positioned in the left lateral position and head down to drain blood out of the mouth (Fig. 33.18). When rapid-sequence induction is performed, cricoid pressure (Sellick

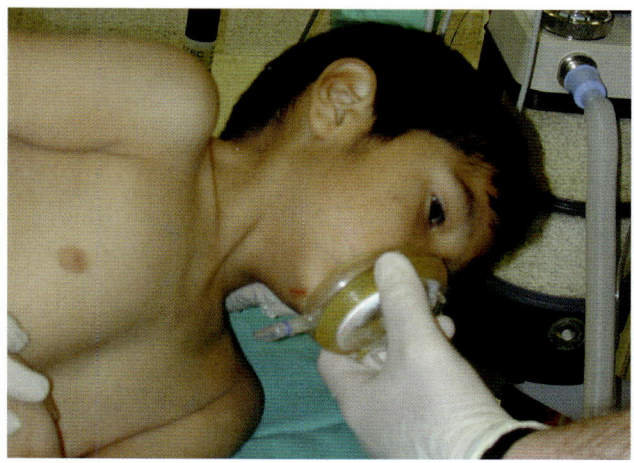

FIGURE 33.18 Preoxygenation with the patient in the lateral position to control posttonsillectomy bleeding before induction of anesthesia.

maneuver) should be applied by an assistant as the child loses consciousness to minimize the risk of aspirating blood into the lungs.[277] The child is then turned supine, and the trachea intubated, although intubation can be performed with the child in the left lateral decubitus position. That a rapid-sequence induction with cricoid pressure decreases the risk of aspiration in children with full stomachs is not evidence-based, although it is commonly practiced. Aspiration of blood into the lungs does not cause the same pathologic changes as acid particulate aspiration unless the volume of blood aspirated compromises pulmonary oxygenation. The use of a full induction dose of propofol in a hypovolemic child could result in significant hypotension. A reduced dose of these induction agents (e.g., propofol, 1–2 mg/kg), or ketamine (1–2 mg/kg) or etomidate (0.2 mg/kg) followed by atropine (0.02 mg/kg) combined with succinylcholine (1.5–2 mg/kg) or rocuronium (1.2 mg/kg) for tracheal intubation should facilitate a rapid control of the airway without hypotension. The change in systolic blood pressure after induction of anesthesia will provide an indication of the volume status of the child. The use of rocuronium instead of succinylcholine is cautiously recommended in these cases, particularly if sugammadex is unavailable; an unexpected difficult intubation combined with arterial bleeding in the oropharynx could rapidly lead to hypoxic brain damage if the airway cannot be secured in a timely manner and the child is paralyzed with a large dose of rocuronium. The surgeon should be scrubbed and immediately available to secure surgical airway if needed.

A cuffed ETT (0.5 mm ID smaller than the usual uncuffed for age or weight) with a stylet should be used to rapidly secure the airway and minimize the chance of aspirating blood. The sevoflurane or desflurane concentration should be titrated with nitrous oxide in oxygen[123] and supplemented with a small dose of opioid, such as fentanyl (1–2 µg/kg); this approach will facilitate a rapid recovery after surgery.[278] Often these surgeries are not excessively painful because surgery is limited to the area of bleeding. Controlling the bleeding vessel in the tonsillar bed can be accomplished rapidly if the blood pressure is maintained in the normal range. Hence, these surgeries are often quite brief and the anesthetic should be planned accordingly. Suctioning the stomach with a large-bore catheter under direct vision after the procedure does not guarantee an empty stomach, because much of the blood may be clotted and the clots are often too large to pass through the catheter lumen. The use of prophylactic antiemetic therapy (e.g., ondansetron 0.1 mg/kg up to 4 mg) is indicated.

The most important postoperative consideration is to extubate these children when they are fully awake and able to control their airway reflexes. Extubating the trachea while the child is in the lateral position may be the safest practice to minimize the risk of aspiration. If there is a medical indication to substitute high-dose rocuronium (1.2 mg/kg) for succinylcholine, then a prolonged period of relaxation may be anticipated. Sugammadex may allow early reversal of residual deep neuromuscular blockade with high-dose rocuronium.[279–281] Postoperatively, a repeat determination of the hemoglobin level may be indicated.

PERITONSILLAR ABSCESS

Peritonsillar abscess (quinsy tonsil) occurs in older children and young adults. It is the most common deep neck-space infection treated by otolaryngologists. Infection originates in the tonsil and spreads to the peritonsillar space between the tonsillar capsule and the superior constrictor muscle, and usually into the soft palate in the region of the superior pole of the tonsil. Commonly cultured organisms include aerobes, such as *Streptococcus pyogenes, S. milleri, S. viridans,* β-hemolytic streptococci, *Haemophilus influenzae,* as well as anaerobes, such as *Fusobacterium* and *Prevotella* species.[282]

Clinically, these children present with fever, pharyngeal swelling, sore throat, dysphagia, odynophagia, and often trismus. Trismus is caused by compression of nerves by the tense peritonsillar mass, spasm of the pterygoid muscles, and inflammation of the muscles of the face and neck. Dehydration can ensue because of fever and the persistent difficulty with swallowing.

Preoperative evaluation includes careful assessment of the airway, with special emphasis on the degree of trismus. Blood specimens should be analyzed for total and differential white blood cell count to ascertain the response to the infection, and for cultures for appropriate antibiotic therapy. Computed tomography of the tonsillar area will identify airway deviation or compromise and the extent of spread of the abscess (Fig. 33.19); transcutaneous ultrasound has been increasingly used to confirm the diagnosis.[283]

While awaiting the results of the cultures, treatment should begin with establishing IV access, hydration, and appropriate antibiotic coverage. The majority of organisms, including anaerobes, are penicillin sensitive. Consequently, penicillin is usually the antibiotic of choice.[282] The three different procedures currently used to drain a peritonsillar abscess are needle aspiration, incision and drainage, and abscess tonsillectomy.[284] Most children undergo general anesthesia for treatment of peritonsillar abscess by incision and drainage, although in some centers, moderate to deep sedation has been successfully used.[285] If the abscess is small and well confined, immediate tonsillectomy is performed.

The anesthetic management of these children can be challenging. Rupture of the abscess and possible aspiration of purulent material during laryngoscopy and intubation should be avoided. Although the airway may appear to be compromised, most peritonsillar abscesses are in a fixed location in the lateral pharynx and do not interfere with mask ventilation. Visualization of the vocal cords is usually not impaired, because the pathology is supraglottic and well above the laryngeal inlet, although a right-sided abscess may interfere with the usual sweeping of the tongue to the left during laryngoscopy. Laryngoscopy must be carefully approached to avoid excessive manipulation of the larynx and surrounding structures. Occasionally, the pharyngeal swelling and the distortion of normal anatomy, along with excessive secretions, may create difficulty for

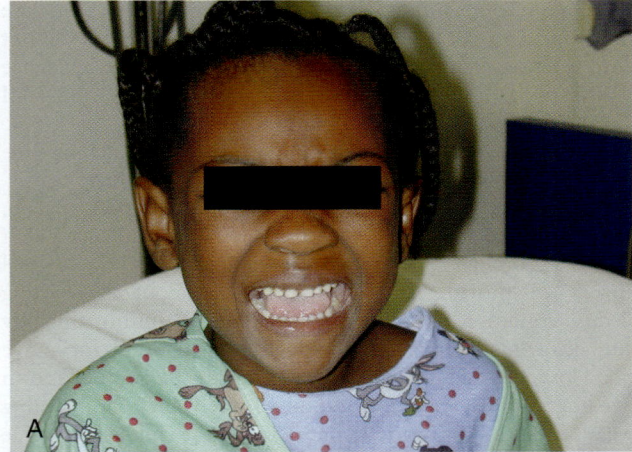

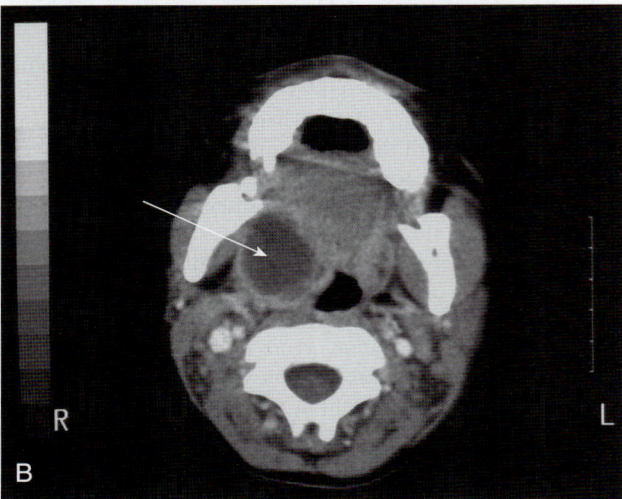

FIGURE 33.19 A, Peritonsillar abscess with trismus. **B,** Axial enhanced computed tomography scan through the oropharynx showing a 3-cm ring-shaped, enhancing, low-density mass (*arrow*) replacing the left tonsil, typical of a tonsillar abscess.

laryngoscopy and intubation. The OR should be prepared as for any difficult airway case, with different sizes of ETTs, stylets, two sets of well-illuminated laryngoscopes, a GlideScope (Verathon, Bothell, WA) or other advanced airway device to facilitate difficult intubation, and a tonsil-tip suction catheter attached to a powerful suction device. The surgeon must be present in the OR during induction of anesthesia should airway obstruction occur. Equipment for cricothyrotomy or tracheotomy must be readily available.

These children are often older and do not require preoperative sedation. If trismus is present, an inhalational induction should be performed, using sevoflurane and oxygen while the anesthesiologist assesses mobility of the temporomandibular joint under anesthesia. An oropharyngeal airway is best avoided, lest the abscess is traumatized. Usually awake trismus resolves once an adequate depth of anesthesia has been achieved. When this is confirmed, or if there was minimal trismus to begin with, then a short-acting NMBD (or propofol) should be given to facilitate tracheal intubation. Alternatively, if there is minimal trismus and the preoperative airway assessment indicates minimal distortion, a rapid-sequence IV induction after adequate preoxygenation may be the best way to avoid trauma to the pharyngeal structures while struggling with a mask induction, needing to insert an oropharyngeal airway, and possibly rupturing the abscess.[2]

To avoid aspiration of purulent material during intubation and drainage, a cuffed ETT is recommended and the child is placed in Trendelenburg position. At the end of surgery, the trachea should be extubated with the child awake, preferably in the lateral decubitus position.[2]

Anesthesia for Endoscopy

Anesthesia for rigid bronchoscopy in young children presents a significant challenge. Not only does the child have a compromised airway, but that airway also must be shared with the surgeon. The importance of constant communication between the endoscopist and the anesthesiologist cannot be overstated. In general, the goals of anesthesia for endoscopy are analgesia, an unconscious child, and a quiet surgical field.[286] Coughing, bucking, or straining during instrumentation with a rigid bronchoscope may cause difficulty for the surgeon and damage the child's airway. At the conclusion of the procedure, children should be returned to consciousness quickly with airway reflexes intact to protect the recently instrumented airway. General principles for the anesthetic management will be outlined first. Disease-specific requirements will be discussed under appropriate subheadings.

For most children, a pulse oximeter, blood pressure cuff, electrocardiographic leads, and precordial stethoscope are applied before induction. Continuous monitoring of ventilation by capnography is not always possible during bronchoscopy, particularly when the Hopkins optical telescope is in place for optimal viewing. Clinical observation of the chest wall movement and the use of a precordial stethoscope are useful. In many cases, intermittent capnography is possible when the bronchoscope is withdrawn by the surgeon. Although greater than normal CO_2 tensions are inevitable with intermittent ventilation, they are generally well tolerated in the presence of sevoflurane or propofol. Hypoxia, on the other hand, is not well tolerated, and the procedure should be stopped while the child is oxygenated.

In many instances, endoscopists prefer that the child breathes spontaneously throughout the procedure; this allows observation of dynamic changes during respiration. Inhalation induction by mask is accomplished with oxygen and an inhalational agent, usually sevoflurane. Nitrous oxide can be used initially, if tolerated, to speed the induction and then discontinued before the examination. Once a sufficient depth of anesthesia has been achieved, IV access is established and the depth of anesthesia is increased. Alternatively, in those children in whom IV access was established before anesthesia, anesthesia may be induced IV with a sleep dose of propofol, followed by mask ventilation with a volatile agent. A hybrid technique that uses an inhalational agent supplemented by small increments of propofol is also common.

An antisialagogue (atropine or glycopyrrolate) may be administered IV to decrease secretions that may impair the view through the bronchoscope. Topically treating the vocal cords and subglottic airway with local anesthetic decreases the incidence of coughing or bucking during instrumentation, and allows the child to tolerate a lighter level of anesthesia. Lidocaine, usually 2%, is the most frequently used topical anesthetic. The dose of lidocaine should be limited to 3 to 4 mg/kg divided between the laryngeal and tracheal surfaces because rapid absorption via the tracheal mucosa occurs. It is important to confirm whether the surgeon intends to observe for movement of the vocal cords or evaluate tracheal or bronchial dynamics so that the anesthetic may be planned accordingly (i.e., spontaneous respirations preserved during light levels of anesthesia versus no respiratory efforts and the use of short-acting muscle relaxants).

DIAGNOSTIC LARYNGOSCOPY AND BRONCHOSCOPY

Although diagnostic laryngoscopy and bronchoscopy procedures are usually of brief duration, the anesthetic management can be challenging in small infants with an already compromised airway. Stridor, or noisy breathing caused by obstructed airflow, is a common indication for a diagnostic laryngoscopy and bronchoscopy in infants and children. Inspiratory stridor results from UAO, expiratory stridor and prolonged expiration result from lower airway obstruction, and biphasic stridor is present with mid-tracheal lesions (see Chapters 13 and 14). Subglottic stenosis may follow prolonged tracheal intubation in an infant who was born preterm.

The evaluation of a child with stridor begins with taking a thorough history. The age at symptom onset helps suggest a cause; for instance, laryngotracheomalacia and vocal cord paralysis are usually present at or shortly after birth, whereas cysts or mass lesions develop later in life (Table 33.6). Information indicating positions that make the stridor better or worse should be obtained, because placing a child in a position that allows gravity to aid in reducing obstruction can be of benefit during induction.

Physical examination reveals the general condition of a child or infant, as well as the degree of the airway compromise. Laboratory examination may include a chest radiograph and barium swallow, which can aid in identifying lesions that may be compressing the trachea. Computed tomography, magnetic resonance imaging, and tomograms may be helpful in isolated instances but are not routinely indicated.

Laryngomalacia is the most common cause of stridor in infants and most often results from a long epiglottis that prolapses

TABLE 33.6	Causes of Stridor
Supraglottic Airway	
Choanal atresia	
Cyst	
Mass	
Large tonsils	
Large adenoids	
Craniofacial abnormalities	
Foreign body	
Larynx	
Laryngomalacia	
Vocal cord paralysis	
Hemangiomas	
Cysts	
Laryngocele	
Laryngeal web	
Infection (tonsillitis, peritonsillar abscess)	
Foreign body	
Subglottic Airway	
Subglottic stenosis	
Tracheomalacia	
Tracheal web	
Vascular ring	
Foreign body	
Infection (croup, epiglottitis)	
Hemangiomas	

posteriorly and prominent arytenoid cartilages with redundant aryepiglottic folds that prolapse into the glottic opening during inspiration.[287] The definitive diagnosis is obtained by direct laryngoscopy and by rigid or flexible bronchoscopy.

Preliminary examination is usually carried out in the surgeon's office. A small flexible fiberoptic bronchoscope is inserted through the nares into the oropharynx. Nasal insertion provides an excellent view of the movement of the vocal cords and pharyngeal structures. Topically treating the nasopharynx with lidocaine facilitates passage of the nasal pharyngoscope or bronchoscope. Alternatively, the examination can be accomplished in the OR in a lightly anesthetized child during spontaneous respirations. Children must be spontaneously breathing so that the vocal cords move freely. After movement of the vocal cords is observed and recorded, the anesthetic level can be increased as appropriate, a rigid bronchoscope (or just the telescope in small infants) is inserted through the vocal cords, and the subglottic area, the lower trachea, and bronchi are evaluated.

The use of premedication in these children should be individualized. Small infants may be brought into the OR unpremedicated; older children may experience respiratory depression and worsening of airway obstruction if heavily premedicated.

Usually an inhalational induction with sevoflurane is performed. Nitrous oxide can be used initially, if tolerated, to speed the induction and then discontinued before the examination. Because sevoflurane is relatively insoluble and is rapidly eliminated, ventilation will be intermittently interrupted during the examination, and the Hopkins optical telescope prevents adequate ventilation through the smallest-diameter bronchoscopes, supplementation with IV agents, such as propofol (1-mg/kg boluses or a 50- to 100-µg/kg per minute infusion), may be necessary to maintain an appropriate depth of anesthesia. If an inhaled technique is used by insufflation, scavenging may be attempted by positioning a suction device near the child's mouth.

A propofol-based TIVA technique has the advantage that it can be given continuously during the procedure, resulting in a more stable level of anesthesia than can be achieved with inhalational agents and intermittent ventilation. Propofol can be supplemented with small (0.5–1.0 mg/kg) doses of ketamine to enhance analgesia. Opioids can also be used but will frequently induce apnea. Dexmedetomidine as a single IV bolus (0.5 µg/kg) or low-dose infusion can also be used to minimize the need for opioids.

The key to a stress-free bronchoscopy is properly applied topical anesthesia. Although topically treating the laryngeal structures with local anesthetic helps the child tolerate the procedure, it may interfere with assessment of normal vocal cord movement. After completion of pharyngoscopy and/or laryngoscopy, the surgeon generally proceeds to rigid bronchoscopy. The size of a rigid bronchoscope refers to the internal diameter (ID). Because the external diameter may be significantly greater than that of an ETT of similar size, care must be taken to select a bronchoscope of proper external diameter to avoid damage to the laryngeal structures (Table 33.7). The rigid bronchoscope can be used for ventilation through the side port attached to the anesthesia circuit with a flexible extension. It is often most useful to paralyze the child with a fixed lesion, which diminishes the risk of vocal cord injury secondary to movement. For nonfixed lesions, such as an aspirated foreign body, and for assessment for bronchomalacia or tracheomalacia, it is preferable to proceed with spontaneous ventilation, a deep level of anesthesia, and good topical anesthesia of the vocal cords and carina. Adequate oxygenation should be maintained in these infants throughout the procedure. Because ventilation may be

TABLE 33.7	External Diameter of Standard Endotracheal Tubes Versus Rigid Bronchoscopes	
Internal Diameter (mm)	**EXTERNAL DIAMETER (MM)**	
	Endotracheal Tube[a]	**Rigid Bronchoscope**[b]
2.0	2.9	
2.5	3.6	4.2
3.0	4.3	5.0
3.5	4.9	5.7
3.7 (bronchoscope)		6.3
4.0	5.6	6.7
5.0	6.9	7.8
6.0	8.2	8.2

[a]Mallinckrodt Medical, Inc., St. Louis, Missouri.
[b]Karl Storz Endoscopy-America, Inc., El Segundo, California.

intermittent and at times suboptimal, it is recommended that 100% oxygen be used as the carrier gas during the bronchoscopic examination. During ventilation of the infant with the optical telescope in place, high resistance may be encountered as a result of partial occlusion of the lumen. This is especially likely when the 2.5-, 3.0-, and 3.5-mm ID scopes are used. Large fresh-gas flow rates, large tidal volumes with high inflation pressures, and large concentrations of inspired inhalational anesthetic (or TIVA) are often necessary to compensate for leaks around the ventilating bronchoscope and the high resistance encountered when the optical telescope is in place. Hand ventilation at greater than normal rates is most effective in achieving adequate ventilation. Sufficient time for exhalation must be provided for passive recoil of the chest. Alternatively the surgeon may remove the optical scope, occlude the bronchoscope with his/her thumb, and allow unimpeded ventilation for several breaths. In small infants, there may be room for only the optical telescopic light source, which does not have a ventilation channel. In these cases, insufflation of oxygen via a small tube placed in the hypopharynx via the nose or mouth will delay the onset of desaturation in a spontaneously breathing child. If (when) desaturation occurs, the surgeon must stop and allow the child to be oxygenated before continuing with the examination.

At the conclusion of bronchoscopy, the surgeon may wish to determine the size of the larynx and determine the degree of airway narrowing. An uncuffed ETT is inserted beyond the narrowest portion of the obstructed airway, and the airway is assessed by applying positive pressure between 10 and 25 cm H_2O to the airway and listening with a stethoscope for an air leak around the ETT at the level of the suprasternal notch. The outer diameter of the appropriate ETT is compared with the inner diameter of the child's larynx and trachea, and the percentage of obstruction is calculated. Grade I obstruction involves up to 50% of the airway, grade II is from 51% to 70%, and grade III is greater than 70% (Fig. 33.20).[288]

An alternative method of ventilation during bronchoscopy is the Sanders jet ventilation technique. The principle of jet ventilation involves intermittent bursts of oxygen delivered at a maximum pressure of 50 psi from a hand-regulated pressure-reducing valve to the lungs, through a 16-gauge catheter attached to a rigid bronchoscope.[289] Current jet ventilators include adjustable pressure-control valves that permit attenuation of the peak pressure; the inflation pressure should begin at 10–15 psi and increase until

Percent Subglottic Stenosis by Endotracheal Tube Size (mm ID)

A

Age	ETT	2	2.5	3	3.5	4	4.5	5	5.5	6
Preterm (<1500 gm)		40								
Preterm (>1500 gm)			30							
0-3 months			48	26		No obstruction				
3-9 months	No detectable lumen	75		41	22					
9 months to 2 years		80			38	20				
2 years		84	74		50	35	19			
4 years		86	78			45	32	17		
6 years		89	81	73			43	30	16	
	Grade IV	Grade III			Grade II		Grade I			

B

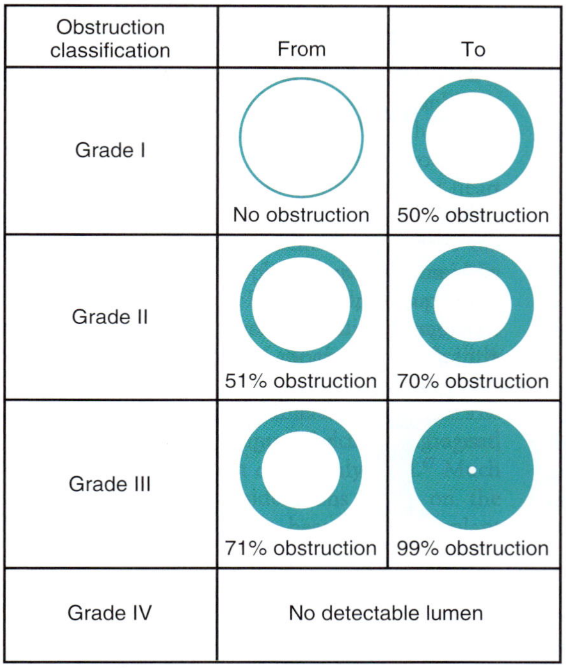

Obstruction classification	From	To
Grade I	No obstruction	50% obstruction
Grade II	51% obstruction	70% obstruction
Grade III	71% obstruction	99% obstruction
Grade IV	No detectable lumen	

FIGURE 33.20 A, Method for estimating the percentage of airway obstruction. After easy passage of an uncuffed endotracheal tube (*ETT*), a manometer is placed at the connection of the elbow of the anesthesia circuit and the ETT. A stethoscope is placed over the larynx and the circuit is slowly pressurized. The pressure at which a leak is auscultated (10–25 cm H$_2$O) is matched with the age of the child and the size of the ETT to estimate the percent of laryngeal narrowing shown in numbers in teal boxes. Clear boxes indicate the usual size ETT for child's age. Grade I, *light teal*; Grade II, *medium teal*; and Grade III, *dark teal*. **B,** Schematic representation of subglottic stenosis classification system. This chart is based on one institution's experience, and the manufacturer of the ETTs was not described, thus the actual external diameter of the ETTs used is unknown. *ID,* internal diameter. (Reproduced and modified with permission from Myer CM III, O'Connor DM, Cotton RT. Proposed grading system for subglottic stenosis based on endotracheal tube sizes. *Ann Otol Rhinol Laryngol.* 1994;103[4]:319–323.)

adequate chest movement is detected visually. Intermittent flow is accomplished by depressing the lever of an on-off valve. A jet of oxygen is released at the tip of the 16-gauge catheter, creating a Venturi effect that entrains room air into the bronchoscope. This jet of oxygen and room air mixture directly inflates the lungs. Exhalation is passive and depends on the recoil of the chest wall. Although this technique is usually effective for both oxygenation and ventilation in experienced hands, a number of potential problems exist. Because of potentially high inflation pressure, pneumothorax, pneumomediastinum, and death have occurred.[290] Blood, infectious, or particulate matter in the airway may be forced distally by high-pressure bursts. There is also the possibility of hypoxemia in some children, because the high-pressure oxygen entrains room air, diluting the oxygen.

High-frequency jet ventilation is also possible for upper airway endoscopy and laryngotracheal surgery. Obstruction to expiratory flow is a major concern and is dependent on good positioning of the rigid laryngoscope. Complications, such as barotrauma, pneumopericardium, CO_2 retention, necrotizing tracheobronchitis, and gastric rupture, dictate a fastidious technique.[291]

Dexamethasone in a dose of 0.3 to 0.5 mg/kg IV (maximum dose, 10–20 mg) is frequently administered during the procedure to decrease postoperative laryngeal swelling and the possibility of croup. At the conclusion of rigid bronchoscopy, an ETT can be placed to control the airway during recovery or, if ventilation is adequate and the anesthetic depth is not excessive, the child can be allowed to emerge breathing 100% oxygen by a face mask.

Children who undergo supraglottoplasty for laryngomalacia pose a special challenge during and after surgery. The most common approach is division of the aryepiglottic folds and/ or trimming of the arytenoid mucosa. This may be performed endoscopically around a small ETT or by surgical excision during suspension laryngoscopy. Because of concerns about postoperative airway edema, aspiration, or decompensation, these children must be watched closely either in an ICU or a monitored bed with continuous pulse oximetry.[292] Some of these children may need to remain intubated overnight if significant swelling is anticipated.

Upper Airway Obstruction

LARYNGOTRACHEOBRONCHITIS (CROUP)

Croup is a symptom complex of inspiratory stridor; suprasternal, intercostal, and substernal retractions; barking cough; and hoarseness that results from swelling of the mucosa in the subglottic area of the larynx.[2] Two common entities account for most cases of croup: spasmodic croup and laryngotracheobronchitis. Spasmodic croup has been diagnosed in about 3% of children with stridor.[293] The child is otherwise healthy and afebrile, presenting with nocturnal episodes of spasmodic cough, which is described as barking and high-pitched. The disease is self-limiting. In addition to viruses, allergic and psychological factors are blamed for this acute phenomenon. It differs from acute laryngotracheitis in that it is considered an allergic reaction to viral antigens rather than a true viral infection.[294] Besides lack of fever, spasmodic croup is usually remarkable for lack of severe laryngeal inflammation, and, in general, supportive therapy on an outpatient basis is all that is required.

Viral laryngotracheitis is by far the most common form of infectious croup. The disease has a gradual onset, usually after a URI in a young child. Low-grade fever is common. Children who have more than two episodes of croup requiring hospitalization should be evaluated for subglottic narrowing from stenosis or cysts. Clinical scoring systems based on objective criteria are helpful in following the progress of the disease and in judging the effectiveness of therapy (Table 33.8).[295]

Anteroposterior radiographs of the neck will confirm the diagnosis of the possibility of a foreign body in the airway (Table 33.9), but a lateral neck x-ray would be required to rule out epiglottitis.[296] The viral infection affects the subglottic region of the larynx, causing edema. The characteristic radiograph of croup, therefore, includes blurring of the tracheal air shadow on

TABLE 33.8	Clinical Croup Score		
	0	1	2
Inspiratory Breath Sounds	Normal	Harsh with rhonchi	Delayed
Stridor	None	Inspiratory	Inspiratory/expiratory
Cough	None	Hoarse cry	Barking
Retractions	None	Flaring and suprasternal retractions	Flaring, suprasternal and intercostal retractions
Cyanosis	None	In air	In 40% O_2

Modified from Downes JJ, Raphaely RC. Pediatric intensive care. *Anesthesiology* 1975;43(22):238–250.

TABLE 33.9	Differential Diagnosis of Croup and Epiglottitis	
	Croup[a]	Epiglottitis
Incidence	More common	Less common
Obstruction	Subglottic	Supraglottic
Age	Younger (<3 years)	Older (3–6 years)
Etiology	Viral	Bacterial
Recurrence	Possible (5%)	Rare
Clinical Features		
Onset	Gradual (days)	Sudden (hours)
Fever	Low grade	High
Dysphagia	None	Marked
Drooling	None	Present
Posture	Recumbent	Sitting
Toxemia	None	Present
Cough	Barking	Usually none
Voice	Hoarse	Clear to muffled
Respiratory rate	Rapid	Normal/slow
Larynx palpation	Not tender	Tender
Leukocytosis	+ (Lymphocytic)	+++ (Polymorphonuclear cells)
Neck radiographs	Anteroposterior: steeple sign	Lateral: thumb-like mass
Clinical course	Longer	Shorter
Treatment		
Primary therapy	Medical and supportive	Secure airway first
O_2 and humidity	Essential	Usually desirable
Hydration	Oral or intravenous	Intravenous
Racemic epinephrine	Usually effective	No value
Corticosteroids	Controversial, commonly used	Not indicated
Antibiotics	Not indicated	Effective
Airway support	Occasionally needed (<3%)	Always indicated (100%)
Preferred airway	Nasotracheal Tracheostomy (rarely)	Nasotracheal
Extubation	4–7 days	1–3 days

[a]Foreign bodies in the airway should also be considered.
From Hannallah R. Epiglottitis. In: Stehling L, ed. *Common Problems in Pediatric Anesthesia.* 2nd ed. St. Louis: Mosby-Year Book; 1992:277–281.

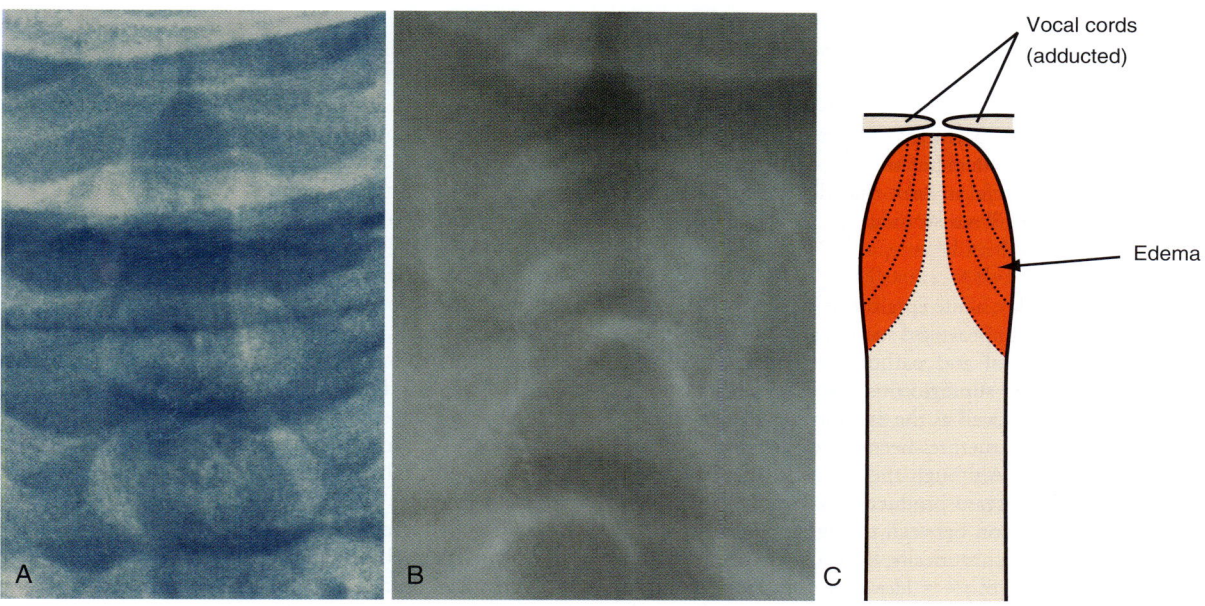

FIGURE 33.21 A, Xerogram radiograph of the normal upper airway (anteroposterior view). Note that the subglottic area is rounded. **B,** Laryngotracheobronchitis (croup) produces swelling (edema and inflammation), which obliterates the normal rounded subglottic area, producing the so-called sharpened pencil or steeple sign. **C,** Schematic representation showing progressive swelling of the subglottic area. For an additional view, see E-Fig. 31.3.

lateral neck films, and symmetric narrowing of the subglottic air shadow, described as a "church steeple" or "sharpened pencil" sign on anteroposterior films (Fig. 33.21 and E-Fig. 33.3). The lateral neck radiographs show normal supraglottic structures and normal epiglottic shadow.

Most cases will resolve quickly with simple conservative measures, such as breathing humidified air or oxygen. Less than 10% of cases require hospitalization because of significant respiratory difficulty, and fewer still require an artificial airway.[287] Humidification of inspired gases is usually effective in improving respiratory distress, and it prevents drying of secretions, although despite the popularity of cool mist therapy, it is not evidence-based practice.[297] Oxygen is obviously essential to prevent or to treat hypoxemia, which may result from ventilation-perfusion mismatching caused by accumulation of secretions. Hydration prevents thickening of tracheal secretions.

Racemic epinephrine is the most effective drug therapy for these children, although L-epinephrine has also been effective.[298] Racemic epinephrine is available as a 2.25% solution, which is diluted in water or saline solution, and administered either by intermittent positive-pressure ventilation via a face mask or nebulization.[299] Nebulized racemic epinephrine is administered in cases of mild-to-moderate obstruction. The solution is prepared by diluting a volume of 2.25% racemic epinephrine in 2 mL of saline solution or sterile water according to the child's weight in kilograms (i.e., 0.25 mL of racemic epinephrine for 0–20 kg, 0.5 mL for 20–40 kg, and 0.75 mL for >40 kg).[300] Because the duration of action of racemic epinephrine is brief, rebound edema may occur. Treatments are required every 1 to 2 hours, and the child should be observed for at least 2 hours after treatment. Racemic epinephrine is no longer available in many countries and L-epinephrine (1/1000) is equally effective; the dose of a 1% solution is 0.5 mL/kg (maximum 5 mL).

If treatment with nebulized epinephrine is unsuccessful, in addition to edema, the underlying problem may be obstruction caused by thick, inspissated secretions possibly related to bacterial superinfection, such as bacterial tracheitis.[301,302] In this situation, or if the child appears exhausted from the increased work of breathing, relief of the obstruction must be obtained through tracheal intubation, followed by pulmonary suctioning. The clinical assessment of "exhaustion" in children with croup may be difficult. An alternative approach is to consider intubating the trachea of children who have an SpO$_2$ <90% when breathing air, despite nebulized epinephrine and steroid treatment. Laryngotracheobronchitis is also a disease of the lower airways. An inability to clear secretions contributes to atelectasis and arterial oxygen desaturation. Tracheal intubation is often required to allow suctioning of the copious yellow secretions.

One large series (512 consecutive admissions in a single year) reported that approximately 6% of children who had sternal and chest retractions on admission and failed to respond to conventional medical therapy required tracheal intubation.[303] Intubation should be performed in the OR under controlled anesthetic conditions, as for a child with severe epiglottitis. The uncuffed tracheal tube selected should be at least one-half size smaller (0.5-mm ID) than would normally be chosen, to avoid aggravating the subglottic edema and possibly causing subglottic stenosis.[304–306] Children whose airways have been intubated are admitted to the ICU, and special care is provided for suctioning of inspissated secretions. The tracheal tube usually remains in place for 2 to 4 days.

Corticosteroid therapy for laryngotracheobronchitis has become the standard of care.[307] Single-dose corticosteroid therapy appears safe and effective,[308] although large studies of the risk of progression of viral infection or the development of secondary bacterial infections in moderate to severe laryngotracheobronchitis are lacking; reports suggest that IV dexamethasone (0.5–1 mg/kg) may be effective.[309] Rapid clinical improvement 12 and 24 hours after steroid treatment significantly reduces the incidence of tracheal intubation.[310-312] Antibiotics are generally not indicated in the treatment of uncomplicated viral croup.

The child is usually ready for extubation within 2 to 4 days. Criteria to consider include abatement of fever, diminished tracheal secretions, change in the character of secretions to a thin and watery type, and an audible air leak that develops around the nasotracheal tube as the edema subsides.

ACUTE EPIGLOTTITIS

Although rarely seen today, acute epiglottitis can be fatal because it can produce seemingly unprovoked sudden and complete airway obstruction. It is a clinical and pathologic entity that should more correctly be termed supraglottitis, because the arytenoids and aryepiglottic folds, as well as the epiglottis itself, are usually affected. All supraglottic structures become swollen and stiffened by inflammatory edema. Although the main focus of infection is the oropharynx, the disease produces a generalized toxemia. Epiglottitis is most common between the ages of 3 and 5 years, but it can occur in any age; historically, the causative organism was typically *H. influenzae* type B.[2,313-315] However, with the widespread use of *H. influenzae* vaccination, the incidence of epiglottitis in children has all but disappeared in medically advantaged countries.[316,317] *Streptococcus*,[318] *Staphylococcus*,[319] *Candida*,[320] and other fungal pathogens[321] have become more frequent causes of this now rare disorder in children,[322] although the incidence in adults has not diminished substantially.[323] It should be noted that vaccine failures may occur or parents may refuse proper immunizations of their child, resulting in susceptibility to *H. influenzae* type B infection.[324,325] Epiglottitis has become more a disease of adults.[326]

The onset is usually abrupt, with a brief history of high fever, severe sore throat, and difficulty in swallowing. Stridor, if present, is usually inspiratory, and because the subglottic structures are usually unaffected, there is little or no hoarseness. An expiratory snore, rather than inspiratory stridor can often be heard. The child appears toxic, and, in an attempt to improve airflow past the swollen epiglottis, assumes the sitting position, leaning forward in the sniffing position (E-Fig. 33.4). The mouth is open, with the tongue protruding. The child frequently drools because of difficulty and pain on swallowing. The mnemonic *SNORED* is often useful for diagnosis: **S**eptic, **NO** cough, **R**apid onset, **E**xpiratory snore, **D**rool.

In addition to high fever, other signs of generalized toxemia may include tachycardia, a flushed face, and prostration. The respiratory pattern is usually slow and quiet to allow more comfortable breathing.

Acute epiglottitis is a clinical diagnosis. It must remain prominent in the differential diagnosis of a child presenting with signs and symptoms of UAO. However, in some early cases, the clinical presentation alone may be inconclusive. If so, a lateral radiograph of the neck will usually demonstrate a swollen epiglottis and aryepiglottic folds (Fig. 33.22 and E-Fig. 33.5). The vallecula may be obliterated, but subglottic structures are usually clear. A physician capable of establishing an airway should always be in the child's attendance (especially if in a remote area of the hospital, such as the Radiology Department), because total airway obstruction can develop during the radiologic examination, especially if the child is forced to lie supine. This is one reason the use of lateral neck radiographs in the differential diagnosis of UAO is avoided. Examination of the pharynx and larynx should only be attempted in an area with adequate equipment and staff prepared to

intervene should UAO develop; ideally, the OR. The safest, most conservative approach to the management of acute epiglottitis is to establish an artificial airway as soon as the diagnosis is made, and then, with the airway secured, to proceed with appropriate antibiotic and supportive therapy. The child should remain in the sitting position at all times and never be forced into the supine position. No attempts to examine the larynx should be made in the emergency room.[2]

These children should not be premedicated. Instead they should be brought to the OR calm and undisturbed. If it takes the presence of a parent to achieve this, then that is what should be done. In the OR, with equipment and personnel who can insert a surgical airway immediately present, a precordial stethoscope, pulse oximeter, and other standard monitors are applied. General anesthesia is induced with oxygen and sevoflurane with the child still sitting up (sometimes a parent may assist sitting on the OR table next to the child). Spontaneous respiration is continued as the child is gently allowed to recline. If the child is moribund, then, after preoxygenation with gentle CPAP, an awake intubation may be considered.

When a surgical stage of anesthesia is achieved, IV access is established and secured. A large fluid bolus of balanced salt solution is infused (20–40 mL/kg) because these children are often dehydrated and will require a deep plane of anesthesia to permit tracheal intubation while spontaneous respirations are preserved. Some anesthesiologists would also administer an antisialagogue to reduce secretions. Epiglottitis is marked by progressive swelling of the lingual surface of the epiglottis with resultant obliteration of the vallecula (see Fig. 33.22). Viewing the glottic opening without traumatizing the epiglottis may usually be accomplished by forcing the tip of the laryngoscope blade along the center of the base of the tongue into the vallecula, where the vallecula has been obliterated by the swollen lingual surface of the epiglottis (see Fig. 33.22C). Lifting the base of the tongue, without directly touching the epiglottis, can then expose the glottis. A stylet within the ETT may be helpful because it provides increased rigidity to facilitate introduction through a partially obstructed glottic aperture. The size of the ETT should be one-half size smaller (0.5-mm ID) than otherwise selected for the same age child. By choosing an ETT with a smaller ID than usual, one also lessens the risks of pressure necrosis on the mucosa. Fig. 33.23 illustrates a case of severe epiglottitis (before [A] and after [B] the airway was secured). A stiletted orotracheal tube is inserted first, and may be replaced by a nasotracheal tube of appropriate size. However, if the glottic opening was difficult to visualize, then no attempt should be made to replace the oral tube with a nasal one. The orotracheal tube may displace supraglottic edema, improving the view of the glottic opening and facilitating placement of the nasotracheal tube. An air leak at 20 to 25 cm of H_2O, when present, confirms the selection of an appropriate size tube. Because the airway obstruction in epiglottitis is supraglottic, not subglottic, the nasotracheal tube size is often the usual size or one-half size smaller for the child's age. A larger tube is not necessary and may contribute to the possible development of serious laryngeal complications, such as subglottic stenosis. The child should be able to breathe around the tube, as well as through it. If the anesthesiologist is unable to intubate the trachea, then a rigid bronchoscope should be used. If both of those maneuvers fail, then a tracheostomy or cricothyrotomy should be performed (see Fig. 14.25).[327,328]

Once the airway is secured, a culture of the pharynx and blood cultures are obtained, and aggressive medical therapy beginning with antibiotics should be commenced. It is recommended that

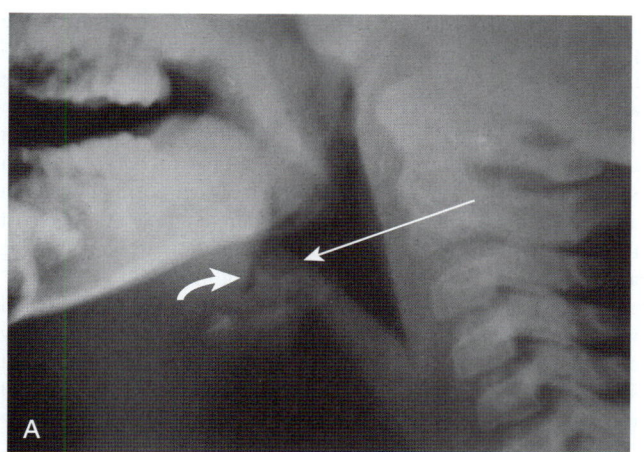

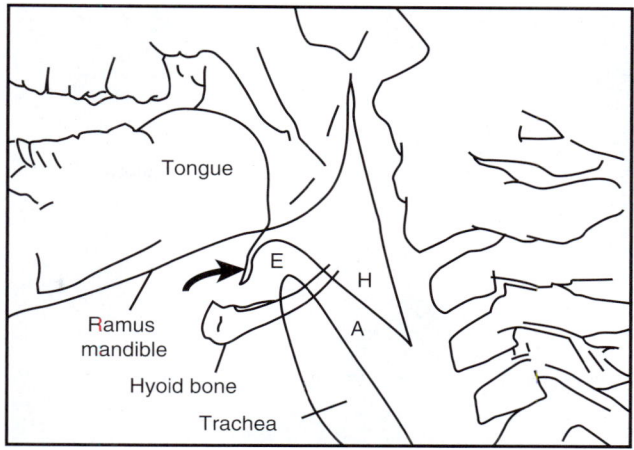

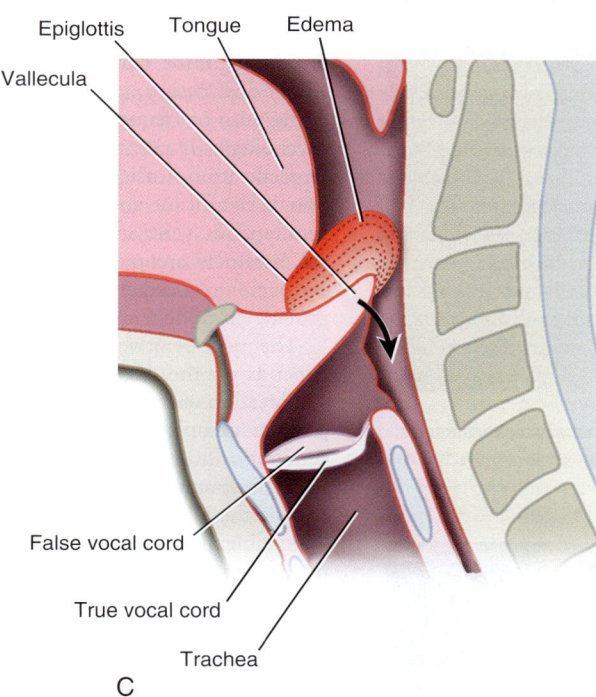

FIGURE 33.22 **A,** Lateral neck radiograph of child with epiglottitis. Note the marked thickening of the aryepiglottic folds (*arrow*). **B,** Schematic representation of **A**. Note the marked thickening of the aryepiglottic folds (*A*), loss ("amputation") of the vallecula (*curved arrow*), swelling of the epiglottis (*E*), and distention of the hypopharynx (*H*). **C,** Schematic representation of epiglottitis demonstrating progressive swelling of the lingual surface of the epiglottis, resulting in "amputation" of the vallecula. Progressive swelling leads to trapdoor-like occlusion of the glottic opening (*curved arrow*). For additional views, see E-Fig. 33.5.

cephalosporins (such as ceftriaxone 50 mg/kg per day)[329–331] be used initially for antibiotic therapy, with the first dose immediately after the diagnosis is made and appropriate cultures taken.[2] The duration of the treatment is controversial, but at least 3 to 5 days of IV antibiotics followed by oral therapy is usually the minimum. Steroids are not indicated. Supportive measures include IV hydration, airway care, sedation as necessary, and acetaminophen for fever. Negative-pressure pulmonary edema can develop after tracheal intubation in children with severe epiglottitis.[251] When the child resumes swallowing and the fever abates, usually 24 to 48 hours after initiation of therapy, the acute supraglottic edema should be resolving and the child may be prepared for tracheal extubation.

OBSTRUCTIVE LARYNGEAL PAPILLOMATOSIS

Recurrent respiratory papillomatosis, also known as juvenile laryngeal papillomatosis, is the most commonly found tumor in the larynx and upper airway in children. Recurrent respiratory papillomatosis is caused by the human papilloma virus (HPV). The incidence is ~1 in 400 births, even though active or latent viral infection is present in 10% to 25% of pregnant women.[332] This disease is caused by HPV 6 and 11; the incidence may markedly

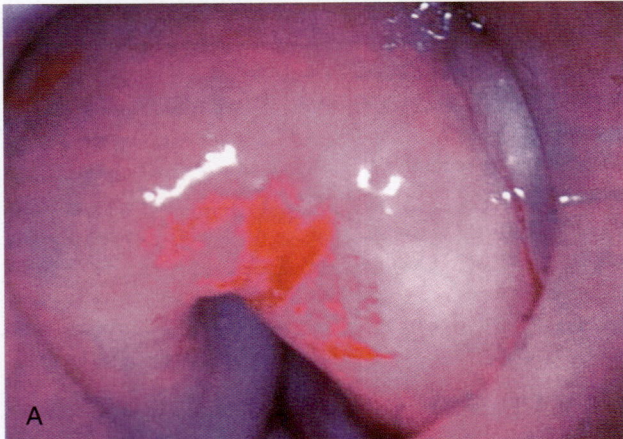

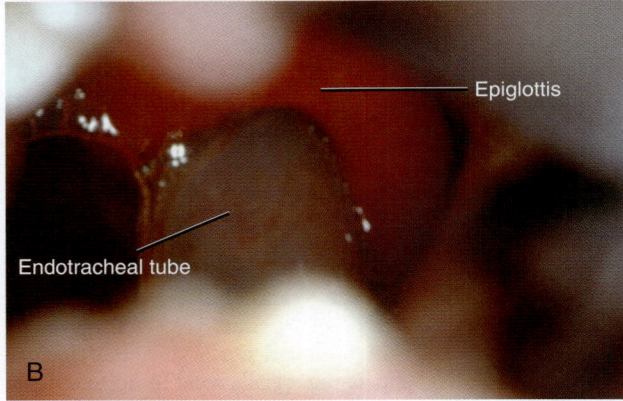

FIGURE 33.23 Acute epiglottitis. **A,** The entire upper airway is inflamed and there is marked swelling of the epiglottis. **B,** Photograph taken after securing the airway with an endotracheal tube.

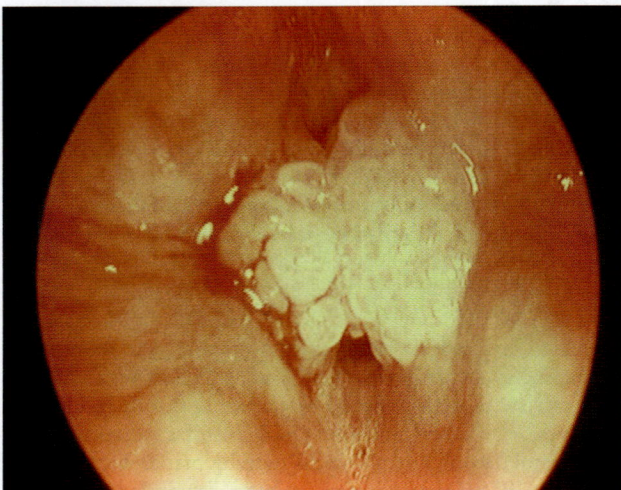

FIGURE 33.24 Large pedunculated papillomas obstructing the laryngeal inlet.

decrease in the future with the introduction of a maternal vaccine to prevent HPV infection for types 6, 11, 16, and 18.[333–336] The papillomas are usually found in the larynx on the vocal cord margins, epiglottis, pharynx, or trachea (Fig. 33.24). If left untreated, symptoms of aphonia, respiratory distress, hoarseness, stridor, right ventricular hypertrophy, and cor pulmonale may occur.

The current treatment is primarily surgical removal of the papillomatous tissue using the CO_2 laser under microscopic visualization. Alternatively, papillomas can be surgically debulked using an ultrasonic microdebrider or cup forceps before laser treatment. Topical application of mitomycin C (usually in combination with debulking procedures) has also been shown to be effective in suppressing these tumors. Nonsurgical treatment using interferon alfa-n1 has been beneficial in some children.[337] The main goal of the treatments is to reduce the bulk of the lesion without scarring and permanent damage to the underlying mucosa.

Because of the recurrent nature of this condition, most children will return frequently for treatment. Many may require monthly scheduled visits to the OR to prevent recurring obstruction. If some of these scheduled sessions are missed, or if the progress of the disease is accelerated, the child will present with an acute exacerbation of obstructive symptoms requiring emergent endoscopic resection. In all cases, it is important to obtain a careful history, including inquiry about changes in voice or increased difficulty breathing during daily activities, that may indicate progressive airway obstruction.

Because of frequent hospitalizations, these children become psychologically sensitized to the perioperative experience. Premedication is usually avoided if the degree of airway obstruction is significant and there are concerns about compromising spontaneous ventilation. In selected cases, when the children are extremely anxious and/or upset, the parents (or a child-life surrogate) may accompany the child to the OR for induction, to provide emotional support.

The perioperative care can be very challenging and often depends on the degree of obstruction to airflow and the type and location of the papillomas.[338–341] Pedunculated papillomas can produce complete ball-valve obstruction of the upper airway in certain positions. It is therefore prudent to avoid paralysis and to maintain spontaneous respirations until the airway is examined and the anesthesiologist is certain that assisted or controlled ventilation is possible. These children must be approached and monitored in the same manner as any child with anticipated severe airway obstruction (e.g., acute epiglottitis). The surgeon must be present in the OR when anesthesia is induced, with equipment immediately available to deal with complete airway obstruction, including rigid bronchoscopes and a tracheostomy-cricothyrotomy set. The problem of sharing the already compromised airway with the surgeon is worsened by the need to use a laser to excise these lesions. A laser (an acronym for **L**ight **A**mplified by **S**timulated **E**mission of **R**adiation) consists of a tube with reflective mirrors at either end with an amplifying medium between them to generate electron activity in the form of light. The CO_2 laser is the most widely used in medical practice, having particular application in the treatment of laryngeal or vocal cord papillomas, laryngeal webs, and resection of subglottic tissue and hemangiomas. A laser is useful for endoscopic procedures because the beam may be directed down open-tube endoscopes and is invisible, thereby affording the surgeon an unobstructed view of the lesion during resection. Laser energy is absorbed by tissue water, rapidly increasing its temperature, denaturing protein, and causing vaporization of the target tissue. The thermal energy produced by the laser beam cauterizes capillaries as it vaporizes tissues; therefore bleeding is minimal and very little postoperative edema occurs.

These properties give the laser a high degree of specificity; however, they also provide the route by which a misdirected laser beam may cause injury to a child or to unprotected OR personnel.[342] Laser radiation increases the temperature of absorbent material; therefore flammable objects, such as surgical drapes, must be kept away from the path of the laser beam. Unprotected surfaces, such as skin, can be burned and must be shielded. Wet towels should be applied to cover the skin of the face and neck when the laser is being used to avoid burns from deflected beams.

The anesthetic management of these children depends on the approach the surgeon will use to remove the lesions. The basic choice is between intubation and nonintubation techniques. For the latter approach, the choice is between intermittent apnea versus jet ventilation.[290] The ETT used during laser surgery can affect the safety of the technique. All standard polyvinylchloride ETTs are flammable and can be ignited and vaporized by a laser beam. Although red rubber ETTs do not vaporize, they deflect the laser beam when wrapped with metallic tape. The metallic tape can only be applied along the stem of the tube down to the cuff; thus the laser may damage the tube below the vocal cords. Alternatively, non-latex ETTs are manufactured specifically for use during laser surgery. Some have a double cuff to protect the airway in the event the outer cuff is damaged by the laser beam. Others have a special matte finish that is effective in deflecting the laser beam along its entire length. Nonreflective flexible metal ETTs and specifically wrapped ETTs are also manufactured for use during laser surgery (Fig. 33.25). The outer diameters of these special tubes are considerably larger than the polyvinylchloride counterpart, especially in the small sizes. Thus they may not be appropriate for use in very small infants or children with a severely narrowed airway. Table 33.10 presents a variety of such specialized tubes compared with standard ETTs. Although these ETTs offer some advantage, they are considerably more expensive than metallic-tape–wrapped red rubber ETTs. A syringe or a bag (500 or 1000 mL) of normal saline solution should be immediately available to douse ignited tissues in the event of an airway fire.

Once the airway is secured, one anesthetic approach is to use intermittent apnea with paralysis, TIVA, and topical lidocaine. An antisialagogue, such as glycopyrrolate, is often given at the beginning of the anesthesia, together with dexamethasone (0.5 mg/kg [maximum dose 10–20 mg]) to reduce mucosal swelling resulting from repeated intubations. However, this dose of dexamethasone is empiric and not evidence-based. Anesthesia is typically induced with oxygen and sevoflurane while the anesthesiologist gradually assists respirations as the depth of anesthesia increases. Once IV access is established, the anesthesia is deepened further and the

larynx is anesthetized with topical lidocaine (3–4 mg/kg). The airway is then evaluated and tracheal intubation performed. The ETT is usually several sizes smaller than what is normally appropriate for the child's age, because most of these children have some degree of laryngeal scarring from repeated resections, and there

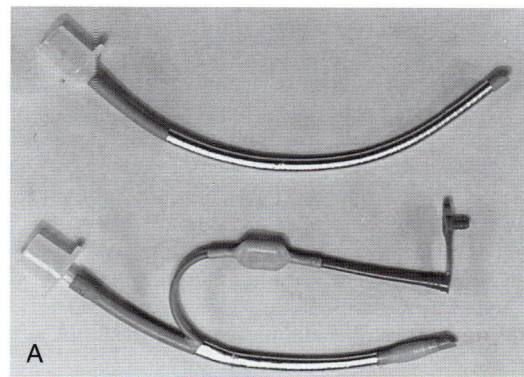

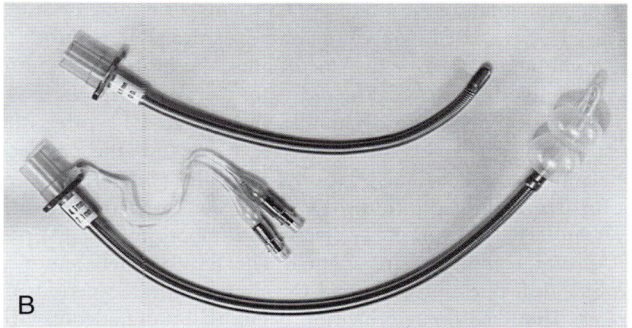

FIGURE 33.25 A, Cuffed and uncuffed red rubber endotracheal tubes may be wrapped with reflective metallic tape for use during laser airway surgery. Note that this metallic tape is not approved by the Food and Drug Administration for this application. Cuffed and uncuffed commercially available foil-wrapped laser tubes are available (Laser-Shield II, Medtronic Xomed, Jacksonville, FL). B, An example of several commercially available stainless steel laser endotracheal tubes (Becton, Dickinson and Company, Franklin Lakes, NJ). Note that the external diameters of these devices are greater than those of standard ETTs.

TABLE 33.10	External Diameter of Standard Plastic Versus Endotracheal Tubes Used for Laser Surgery						
	EXTERNAL DIAMETER (mm)						
ID (mm)	Standard ETT (Uncuffed)[a]	Standard ETT (Cuffed)[a]	Laser-Shield (Cuffed)[b]	Laser-Flex (Uncuffed)[a]	Laser-Flex (Cuffed)[a]	Lasertubus (Double Cuffed)[c]	Red Rubber (Cuffed Without Copper Wrap)
3.0	4.2	4.2		5.2			4.7
3.5	4.9	4.9		5.7			5.3
4.0	5.5	5.5	6.6	6.1		6.0	6.0
4.5	6.2	6.2	7.3		7.0		6.7
5.0	6.8	6.8	8.0		7.5	7.3	7.3
5.5	7.5	7.5	8.6		7.9		8.0
6.0	8.2	8.2	9.0		8.5	8.7	8.7

ETT, endotracheal tube; *ID*, internal diameter.
[a]Mallinckrodt Inc., St. Louis, Missouri.
[b]Medtronic Inc., Minneapolis, Minnesota.
[c]Willy Rüsch GmbH, Kernen, Germany.

is the need to prevent the ETT from obscuring the surgeon's view and interfering with access to the lesions. If the surgeon is planning a non-laser approach, spontaneous ventilation can be maintained by first achieving an adequate depth of anesthesia and then insufflating oxygen in air to reduce the FIO_2 to 30% or less and inhalation agent (usually sevoflurane) via a very small tracheal tube. The use of a double-lumen central venous catheter for this purpose has also been described.[343]

Although the goal is to achieve the desired depth of anesthesia to secure the airway with the child still spontaneously breathing, partial obstruction is frequently encountered before an adequate depth of anesthesia for laryngoscopy is achieved. In these cases, thrusting the jaw forward and applying positive pressure in the anesthetic circuit will maintain an open airway in most situations (see Chapter 14). If complete obstruction is encountered, then a single IV bolus of propofol (2–3 mg/kg) or a short-acting NMBD may be necessary for immediate laryngoscopy and intubation or to allow the surgeon to perform rigid bronchoscopy.

Once the correct position of the ETT is confirmed, an NMBD (e.g., rocuronium) can be administered and the TIVA technique with propofol (200–300 µg/kg per minute) and fentanyl (2–3 µg/kg) or remifentanil infusion (0.1–0.25 µg/kg per minute or more, as needed) is started. Muscle relaxation is desirable to produce an immobile surgical field. A neuromuscular blockade monitor is recommended to assess the degree of relaxation.

An apneic anesthetic technique without an ETT offers the best unobstructed view of the larynx and avoids the presence of flammable material (e.g., the ETT) in the path of the laser beam. The child is positioned for suspension laryngoscopy with eyes protected with moist eye pads, and the otomicroscope and CO_2 laser equipment are aligned. The ETT is then removed and surgical resection is carried out during repeated periods of apnea. The need for reintubation is guided by the adequacy of oxygenation as reflected by the pulse oximeter. Reintubation can be readily performed by the surgeon by introducing the tracheal tube through the suspension laryngoscope under direct vision. After each reintubation, the lungs are ventilated manually to restore both the SpO_2 and end-tidal CO_2 to baseline. When those baselines are reached, the trachea is extubated and surgery can resume. This process is repeated until the surgery is complete.[2]

A modification of the apneic technique that avoids tracheal intubation is the jet ventilator. The operating laryngoscope may be fitted with a catheter through which O_2 flows, entraining ambient air. In this manner, the lungs are intermittently inflated by the pressure delivered by the jet. The advantage of this technique is twofold. The surgical field is extremely quiet because large excursions of the diaphragm are eliminated and ventilation is uninterrupted. However, transtracheal jet ventilation carries a greater risk of pneumothorax in children than the transglottic approach.[290] In the past, tension pneumothorax and pneumomediastinum occurred because of excessive peak inspiratory pressures during jetting. Maximum peak inspiratory jet pressures of approximately 15 mm Hg have reduced this risk dramatically. In morbidly obese children and those with severe disease of the small airways, effective ventilation may be difficult with this technique, and an alternate approach should be used.[344] In addition, jet ventilation may theoretically distribute papilloma virus throughout the tracheobronchial tree, although this technique continues to be used.

When surgery is completed, the ETT is reinserted and secured until the child is completely awakened. Postoperative measures to prevent laryngeal edema, such as racemic epinephrine inhalation and/or the use of dexamethasone, are usually indicated.

ASPIRATED FOREIGN BODIES

Curious young children push small objects into almost every orifice in their body. Objects inserted in the nose or ear are usually benign in nature and simple to remove once the child is anesthetized. Small button-sized battery foreign bodies require urgent removal because of their potential for extensive local damage.[345] Impacted or displaced objects present greater challenges for the anesthesiologist and endoscopist, and the danger of misplacement into the respiratory tract must always be considered.[346]

Tracheobronchial foreign body aspiration is most common in toddlers 1 to 3 years of age. The majority (95%) of foreign bodies lodge in the right main-stem bronchus.[347] A history of choking while eating or playing, persistent cough, or wheezing that does not respond to medical treatment may be the only manifestations. If the foreign body completely obstructs a bronchus or creates a ball-valve phenomenon, distal hyperinflation from air trapping may occur; a hyperinflated lung during the expiratory phase may be the only indication of an aspirated foreign body on chest radiography (Fig. 33.26). The more distal the object is lodged in the airway, the more atelectatic changes are noted.

Foreign bodies lodge in the trachea (<5% of airway foreign bodies) if they are too large to pass the carina.[348] The signs of a tracheal foreign body may include a brassy cough with or without abnormal voice, bidirectional stridor, or complete airway obstruction in the case of laryngeal foreign bodies. Any sharp object, or any object that causes acute UAO with cyanosis and an inability to maintain ventilation, requires emergent removal. Unroasted peanuts (with unsaturated double bonds in the oils) should be removed promptly because the oil can leach out and induce an inflammatory response, that may result in pneumonitis (Fig. 33.27).[349] In contrast, roasted peanuts (with saturated double bonds in the oils) may be present in the lungs for greater periods without inducing as severe an inflammatory response. In addition, peanuts tend to swell, fragment, and crumble over time, making removal "en bloc" extremely difficult. Most children who aspirate foreign bodies do not become cyanotic. However, the child who presents with a history of cyanosis after aspiration of a nut very likely has aspirated material into the trachea or into the lungs bilaterally (as in the case of a broken nut or multiple nuts) and should be assessed emergently. It should be noted that esophageal foreign bodies may compress the trachea as well (Fig. 33.28).

The anesthetic management of these children depends on the level, degree, and duration of obstruction. A child who aspirates a foreign body while eating, or soon thereafter, presents with the additional risk of a full stomach. Waiting for the stomach to empty may not be appropriate or even effective in the acute situation. IV metoclopramide (0.15 mg/kg) may be used to hasten stomach emptying but does not guarantee that the stomach empties.[350] If time permits, the administration of an anticholinergic agent may be useful to reduce secretions. In the debate of how best to anesthetize a child with a full stomach and a compromised airway from an aspirated foreign body, concern for the airway takes precedence over the full stomach and an inhalational induction is recommended.

One of the major controversies in the anesthetic management of foreign body aspiration is whether to control ventilation or allow spontaneous respirations during bronchoscopy.[351,352] Some endoscopists prefer a spontaneously breathing child to allow them to remove the lens from the end of the scope and use a large grabbing forceps to "grab" the foreign body as it is being retrieved out of the airway. Sevoflurane is the preferred inhalational anesthetic

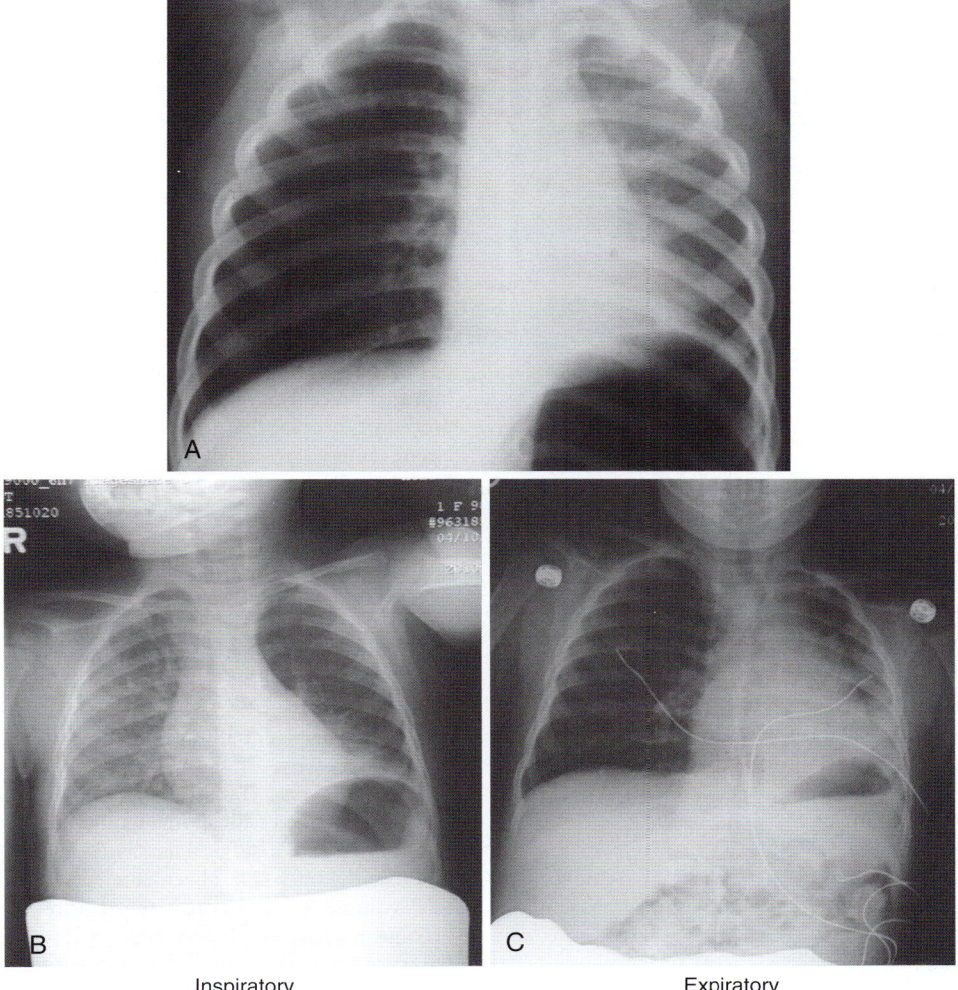

Inspiratory

Expiratory

FIGURE 33.26 A, Expiratory radiograph of the chest demonstrates marked right-sided hyperinflation because of air trapping by the ball-valve effect of the foreign body. The chest radiograph may appear normal during inspiration after foreign body aspiration. **B,** A hyperinflated right lung and **C,** a leftward mediastinal shift during expiration suggest a foreign body in the right main-stem bronchus. (Radiographs courtesy Sjirk J. Westra, MD, Division of Pediatric Radiology, Massachusetts General Hospital.)

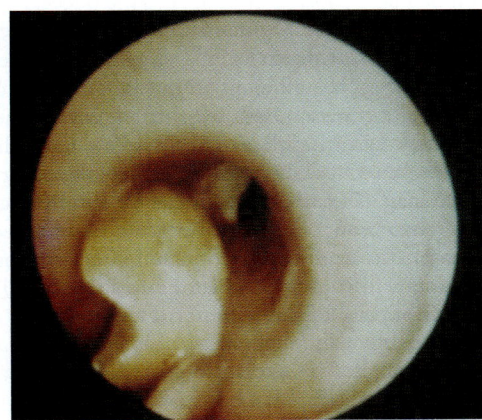

FIGURE 33.27 A classic peanut in the bronchus. Note the irritation caused by the oil of the peanut.

in these children because it maintains spontaneous respirations, does not trigger upper airway reflex responses, and maintains hemodynamic stability.[353] Anesthesia is usually maintained with 100% oxygen and sevoflurane, or a propofol-based TIVA technique.[2] A propofol TIVA technique allows a steady level of anesthesia that is independent of ventilation and does not expose the OR personnel to waste anesthetic agents that inevitably egress from the airway around the bronchoscope. In some cases, a combined approach of sevoflurane in oxygen, as well as IV propofol or dexmedetomidine, may be used. Often these children have very irritable airways because of the presence of the foreign body. The use of topical lidocaine (3–4 mg/kg) divided between the laryngeal structures and tracheal mucosa may be used to suppress airway reflexes and prevent coughing and bronchospasm.

Tracheostomy

Tracheostomy in infants and children is usually performed electively, as a planned procedure after an airway has already been established

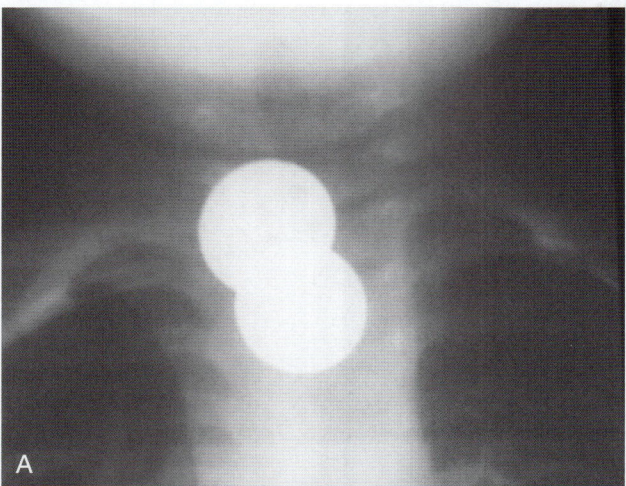

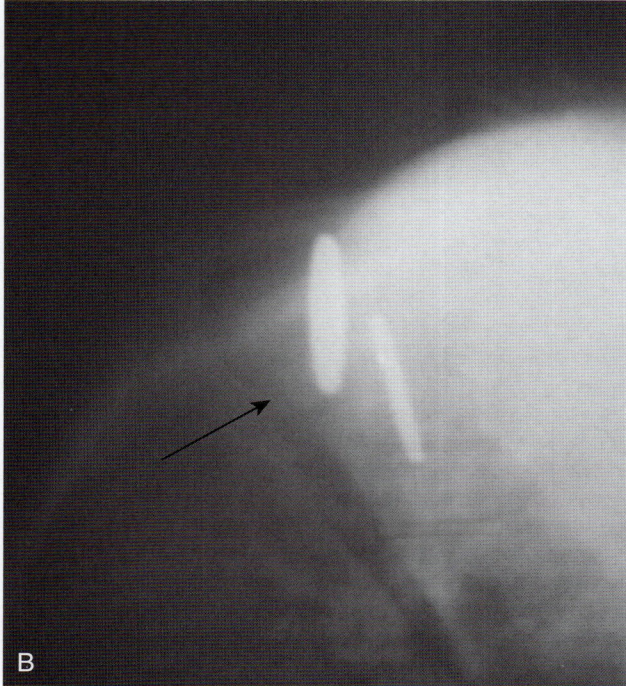

FIGURE 33.28 Anteroposterior **(A)** and lateral **(B)** neck radiographs of a child who swallowed two coins. Note tracheal compression caused by these foreign bodies in the esophagus (*arrow*).

with an ETT. Indications for a planned tracheostomy include need for long-term ventilation or lesions such as congenital or acquired vocal cord paralysis, central hypoventilation syndrome (Ondine curse), craniofacial abnormalities (e.g., Pierre Robin malformation), persistent laryngotracheomalacia, and congenital or acquired subglottic stenosis.[354] Usually these children have had a period of watchful waiting, with the hope of avoiding tracheostomy. However, persistent hypoxemia, hypercarbia, intermittent obstruction that cannot be eliminated with the natural airway, or failed extubation will force the need to secure the airway via a tracheostomy. Children from intensive care sometimes require tracheostomy for long-term ventilation or secretion management. Still other children have acute deteriorations of the airway and require tracheostomy on an emergent basis.

In such cases, the surgeon will frequently want to perform a thorough examination of the airway (i.e., diagnostic laryngoscopy and bronchoscopy) before proceeding with the tracheostomy. This requires that the tracheal tube be removed, the airway examined with a rigid bronchoscope, and then the trachea reintubated for the procedure. After the diagnostic laryngoscopy and bronchoscopy and reintubation, the child is positioned supine, with the head maximally extended over a shoulder roll, and the head taped to the end of the bed. It is a good practice to have a separate clean anesthesia circuit, or an extension, to hand to the surgeon to connect to the freshly inserted tracheostomy cannula.

Anesthesia is maintained with spontaneous respirations of inhalational agents so that, if there is airway compromise at any point, the child may still be able to maintain oxygenation. One hundred percent oxygen should be administered throughout the procedure, because the airway may be lost at any time. If, however, electrocautery is required, then fire prevention precautions should be taken. IV opioids or local anesthetic infiltration, or both, should be used to manage postoperative pain. A thrashing, crying child who is in pain will compromise the integrity of the newly established surgical airway.

Children whose airways cannot be intubated may undergo an "awake" tracheostomy with sedation and local anesthesia. Ketamine is an attractive alternative, but promotes secretions, which may further compromise an already marginal airway; an antisialagogue may reduce the secretions. Children who can be anesthetized with an inhalational agent administered by mask, but who cannot be intubated because of severe subglottic stenosis or inability to visualize the vocal cords by direct laryngoscopy, may have the airway maintained with spontaneous ventilation and a face mask or an LMA until a surgical airway is obtained.

Once the trachea has been entered, a portion of the delivered tidal volume is lost through the incision, and ventilation may become inadequate. This is less of a problem if spontaneous respirations are maintained. It is prudent to leave the ETT within the lumen of the trachea but withdrawn just proximal to the tracheal incision, so that it can be readily advanced should difficulty be encountered with passing the tracheotomy tube. Once the tracheotomy tube is in place and ventilation is confirmed, the ETT is removed, the sterile distal end of the clean anesthesia circuit is attached to the tracheotomy tube (and the proximal end to the anesthesia machine), and the wound is closed. In the event of the tracheostomy tube becoming dislodged or removed, the tracheal incision will close and attempts at reinsertion may cause bleeding, the creation of a false passage, or trauma to the tracheal wall. The tracheal lumen is identified by internal traction sutures, which are placed by the surgeon at the end of the surgical procedure (E-Fig. 33.6). With the surgeon pulling up on the external ends of these sutures, the tracheal incision is identified and the tracheotomy is opened so that an artificial airway can be inserted. The child should not leave the OR without the potentially lifesaving sutures in place and their laterality (right vs. left) properly identified. Flexible fiberoptic bronchoscopy through the new tracheostomy tube is performed to confirm appropriate location of the tip of the tracheostomy tube above the carina with the child in the position for postoperative care.

Laryngotracheal Reconstruction

Glottic and subglottic stenosis, although rare, can be life-threatening and difficult to manage, from both the surgeon's and anesthesiologist's points of view. Congenital laryngeal atresia and congenital laryngeal webs can be incompatible with life unless an emergent tracheostomy is performed at birth. When diagnosed antenatally, such an intervention can be undertaken before placental separation, described as an operation on placental support, or the ex utero intrapartum treatment (EXIT) procedure (see Chapter 38). Unrecognized tracheal webs may result in death shortly after delivery. Treatment depends on the severity of laryngeal obstruction. In some instances, the defects are sufficiently severe to require immediate intubation or tracheostomy (see Fig. 38.13). Others may be discovered as an incidental finding while attempting to intubate the trachea for an unrelated surgical problem.[89,355] Most membranous defects can be broken by passing a bronchoscope through the lumen or incised using a surgical knife or scissors. Thin anterior webs can be managed by microendoscopic incision with a microsurgical knife or CO_2 laser, staging the procedure for each side separately to avoid recurrence. The anesthetic management is similar to that for children undergoing laser excision of laryngeal papillomatosis.

Acquired subglottic stenosis is usually the result of prolonged tracheal intubation for respiratory support of infants born prematurely. In older children, it is often the result of laryngeal trauma. Symptoms usually relate to airway, voice, and feeding and, in the case of a laryngeal insult, often occur 2 to 4 weeks later. Progressive respiratory difficulty with biphasic stridor, dyspnea, air hunger, and retractions are typical. These children usually have a tendency toward prolonged courses of URIs. Soft tissue radiographs of the neck and computed axial tomography will locate the exact site and length of the stenotic segment. Because both gastroesophageal and gastrolaryngopharyngeal reflux disease are thought to contribute to the development and exacerbation of subglottic stenosis, these conditions must be excluded, usually by a 24-hour esophageal pH probe placement. However, direct endoscopic visualization of the larynx is ultimately required to fully evaluate the stenosis. Rigid and flexible endoscopy of the airway and esophagus is performed in the OR. Because of the small diameter of the airway, the rigid rod-lens telescope and/or a flexible bronchoscope are used to visualize the larynx and trachea beyond the obstruction. The trachea is then intubated, and the degree of air leak around the ETT helps establish the degree of stenosis (see Fig. 33.20).

The surgical management of these infants must be individualized according to the degree of obstruction and the general condition of the child.[356] Most cases of moderate or severe subglottic stenosis require a tracheostomy at or below the third tracheal ring to establish a safe airway. The presence of a tracheostomy also helps to facilitate the airway management during subsequent procedures. For less severe cases, endoscopic balloon dilation or CO_2-laser endoscopic scar excision may be sufficient. This approach, however, has limited application in severe cases, and in some cases can be even detrimental by increasing the risk of unplanned urgent intervention compared with laryngotracheoplasty.[357]

The more severe cases of laryngeal stenosis require external reconstruction. Of the many available options, an anterior cricoid split operation and laryngotracheal reconstructions are more frequently used. The cricoid split operation is performed with the use of general endotracheal anesthesia. The largest possible tracheal tube is inserted through the nose. An incision is made through the cricoid, and the cartilage springs open. The ETT will be readily visible in the lumen. Frequently, the incision will be extended to include the proximal two tracheal rings and even the distal third of the thyroid cartilage (Fig. 33.29). Stay sutures are placed on each side of the incised cricoid, and the skin is loosely approximated. The ETT is left in place for about 7 days to act as a splint while the mucosal swelling subsides and the split cricoid heals. Endoscopy is not usually required, but corticosteroids are administered before extubation.

Open reconstructive surgical techniques are done at the youngest age possible to help the development of speech and language skills. They basically combine the use of laryngeal and cricoid splits, cartilage grafts, and stenting.

For laryngotracheal reconstruction procedures, the infant is positioned with a roll under the shoulders and the head is extended. The tracheostomy cannula is replaced with an ETT that is introduced through the stoma to allow easy and secure access to the airway. A sterile, shortened, preformed oral RAE tube is ideal to allow secure fixation. The distal end is cut to an appropriate length to avoid bronchial intubation and then sutured to the skin of the neck. A costal cartilage graft is harvested and fashioned to fit the intended site of transplantation (anterior or posterior splits). Repair of laryngotracheal stenosis in almost all cases, except anterior subglottic stenosis, requires brief stenting to keep the graft in place and lend support to the reconstructed area. Stents will counteract scar contracture and provide a scaffold for epithelium to cover the lumen of the airway. Many types of stents

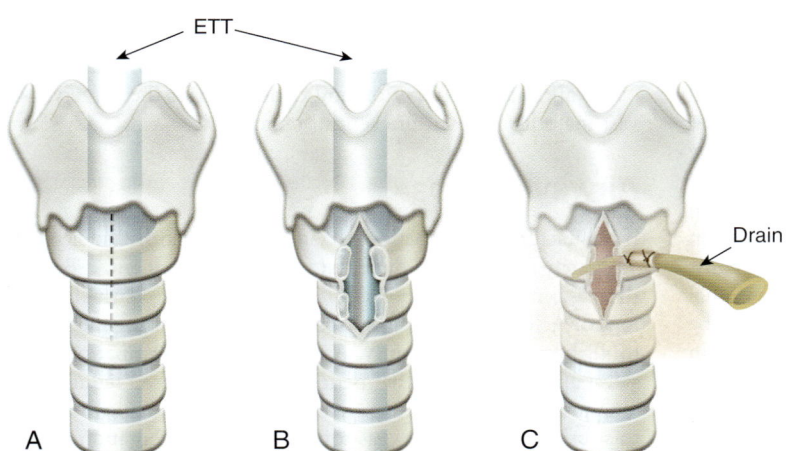

FIGURE 33.29 Anterior cricoid split. After a midline laryngeal incision through cartilage and mucosa **(A)**, the cricoid cartilage is decompressed and the large endotracheal tube (*ETT*) is properly positioned with the tip distal to the incision **(B)**. The skin is loosely closed with a *drain* **(C)**. (From Zalzal GH, Cotton RT. Glottic and subglottic stenosis. In: Cummings CE, ed. *Cummings Otolaryngology Head & Neck Surgery*. 4th ed. St. Louis: Mosby; 2005:2912–2924.)

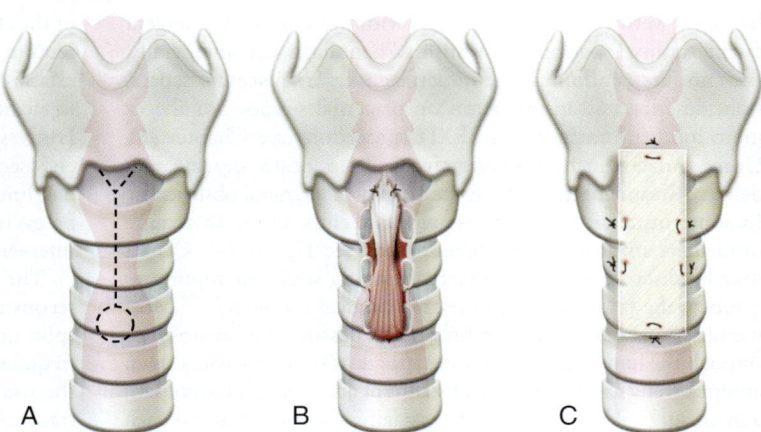

FIGURE 33.30 A, Laryngotracheal resection with anterior cartilage graft. **B,** After a midline incision into the thyroid cartilage, the intraluminal scar and lining mucosa are incised along the length of the stenotic segment **(C)**. A piece of costal cartilage is shaped into a modified "boat" and placed in position with the lining of the perichondrium facing internally. (From Zalzal GH, Cotton RT. Glottic and subglottic stenosis. In: Cummings CE, ed. *Cummings Otolaryngology Head & Neck Surgery*. 4th ed. St. Louis: Mosby; 2005:2912–2924.)

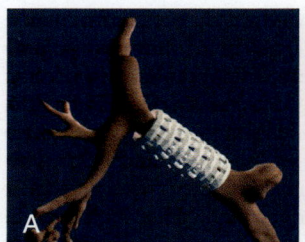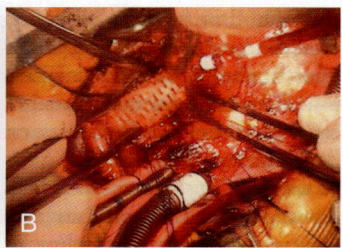

FIGURE 33.31 A, Three-dimensionally printed airway anatomic model clearly defining the airway anatomy with a 3D rendering of airway splint individually designed to fit over the left main-stem bronchus. **B,** Intraoperative photograph of splint being placed on model in vitro and on the patient's left main-stem bronchus in vivo. (From Van Koevering KK, Hollister SJ, Green, GE. Advances in 3-dimensional printing in otolaryngology: a review. *JAMA Otolaryngol Head Neck Surg.* 2017;143[2]:178–183 [with permission].)

have been used. T-tubes are popular in adults, but are associated with more complications and blockage in children. The lower end of the stent is sutured in place during surgery. The stent is eventually removed endoscopically, after cutting the sutures and retrieving the tube.

Single-stage laryngotracheal reconstruction is sometimes used in children without significant obstruction. A full-length nasotracheal tube is used to support the graft for 3 to 7 days, depending on the type of graft. The advantages of immediate decannulation, and possible avoidance of a tracheostomy altogether, make this approach appealing in appropriate candidates (Fig. 33.30). The evolving technology of creating patient-specific three-dimensional (3D) printed models designed with the help of high-resolution imaging (e.g., computed tomography) is likely to revolutionize the approach to these cases through a more precise understanding of the anatomy (Fig. 33.31).[358-362] Additionally, 3D designed external stents will provide a completely new approach to these children (Fig. 33.31). The anesthetic challenges in these cases are many. The general condition of the child may not be perfect. Residual stigmata of prematurity are often present. The airway will be shared with the surgeon, and the tracheal tube that is placed in the stoma will need to be intermittently removed for surgical access and stent placement. A quiet surgical field is essential. The possibility of a pneumothorax during the cartilage graft harvesting should be kept in mind. The need to ensure that the

stent, or the tracheal tube in case of a single-stage laryngotracheal reconstruction, is not dislodged in the ICU cannot be overstated. Accidental extubation cannot be allowed. A combination of sedation techniques and/or pharmacologic relaxation is necessary. The choice is often dictated by the individual policy in each ICU. Dexmedetomidine sedation may offer advantages as an alternative to propofol by providing a relatively rapid recovery from short-term sedation.[363,364]

TRACHEOCUTANEOUS FISTULA

Approximately 12% of children who have had their tracheostomy removed will retain a tracheocutaneous fistula.[365] Surgical repair is generally required to remove the fistula track, followed by a primary closure of the defect.[366-368] In some, this may be accomplished with simple endoscopic cauterization.[369] Usually there is a preliminary endoscopic assessment of the stoma site, removal of residual granuloma, and then a determination of the best approach to closure.[370] A multilayered closure is commonly used to close the fistula,[371,372] whereas others recommend direct primary closure of the defect.[373] The anesthesia approach generally includes maintenance of spontaneous respirations and methods to avoid coughing or straining at the time of extubation. The main concern is the potential for the development of subcutaneous emphysema caused by residual air leak if the child coughs or strains.[369,374-377] This complication may result in life-threatening pneumothorax or pneumomediastinum, which may occur up to 7 days after closure[370]; these complications require emergent removal of sutures, reestablishment of a tracheostomy, and thoracostomy and/or pericardial drainage.[378] Some children may require postoperative ventilation, but most are extubated and admitted for observation after extubation and conclusion of the surgery. The vast majority have an uneventful recovery.

Airway Trauma

Nasal fractures are frequently seen in older children and adolescents. They may result from a direct hit (fight) or an accident.[379] Because the nasal mucosa is very vascular, a lot of blood is usually swallowed. A stomach full of blood is to be assumed for the first 24 to 48 hours after the injury. A rapid-sequence intubation is the safest approach during that period. However, closed reduction of a nasal fracture is often delayed for a few days to allow swelling to subside. At that time, gastroparesis has resolved and an LMA may be considered. These operations can be very brief. Frequently,

33

the surgeon will leave a nasal pack in situ and apply an external splint over the nose. If a throat pack was not inserted, then the pharynx and stomach should be suctioned to remove blood that may have accumulated during the surgery. The tracheal tube or LMA should be removed only when the child is awake, cooperative, and understands the need for mouth breathing; a combative, semi-awake adolescent who is unable to breathe through the nose can hurt himself or herself and others.

Closed or open injuries to the larynx and trachea in children can result from bicycle accidents, falls, direct trauma from sharp objects, and, rarely, a "clothesline" injury. The more cephalad cervical position of the pediatric larynx behind the mandibular arch and the pliability of the cricothyroid structures usually limit the extent of injury and prevent severe fractures.[379] However, the small size of the laryngotracheal airway and the potential for massive soft tissue swelling because of the loose attachment of the submucosal tissue to the perichondrium make early diagnosis and treatment critical. The injury can range from minor laryngeal hematoma to a severe form of laryngotracheal separation. This extreme and often fatal condition can occur after a clothesline mechanism of injury and is often associated with bilateral vocal cord paralysis resulting from recurrent laryngeal nerve damage.[380] Hoarseness, cough, dyspnea, hemoptysis, and voice changes suggest laryngeal damage. Clinical subcutaneous emphysema, pneumothorax, and pneumomediastinum signify definite disruption of the laryngotracheal complex. Computed tomography is the most appropriate imaging modality to identify the extent of laryngeal injury.[381]

Positive-pressure ventilation by mask, excessive coughing, or struggling can worsen the subcutaneous emphysema and cause the airway to further deteriorate. Administration of nitrous oxide, application of cricoid pressure, multiple vigorous attempts at laryngoscopy and intubation, and passage of blind nasotracheal tubes or nasogastric tubes should be avoided to prevent further trauma by creating a false passage through a mucosal tear. A good approach to this type of injury, if the child is stable, is to use the fiberoptic bronchoscope to visualize the airway before tracheal intubation. Ideally, the airway should be secured in the OR after induction of general anesthesia with an inhalational agent, and with the child breathing spontaneously. However, tracheostomy below the level of the injury, under local anesthesia or over a bronchoscope, may be necessary if there is extensive injury to the mouth and larynx that requires major reconstruction.

Postoperatively, these children require management in a monitored setting, usually the ICU. The resolution of other complications, such as subcutaneous emphysema, pneumothorax, or pneumomediastinum, will dictate the duration of the child's stay. Postoperative analgesia must be carefully titrated to balance the need for pain relief with the adequacy of ventilation.

ACKNOWLEDGMENT

The authors wish to acknowledge the prior contributions to this chapter by Lynne R. Ferrari, MD, Susan A. Vassallo, MD, Lucinda L. Everett, Gennadiy Fuzaylov, and I. David Todres.

ANNOTATED REFERENCES

American Society of Anesthesiologists. Practice guidelines for the perioperative management of patients with obstructive sleep apnea: an updated report by the American Society of Anesthesiologists Task Force on Perioperative Management of Patients with Obstructive Sleep Apnea. *Anesthesiology.* 2014;120(2):268-286.

A practice guideline by a panel of experts discussing different levels of evidence for guidelines has been updated with additional guidance for pediatric patients.

Brown KA, Laferrière A, Lakheeram I, Moss IR. Recurrent hypoxemia in children is associated with increased analgesic sensitivity to opiates. *Anesthesiology.* 2006;105(4):665-1283.

This study makes a clear case that younger children with OSA syndrome are at increased risk from opioid-induced respiratory depression; equal analgesia can be achieved with one-third to one-half the usual opioid dose.

Coté CJ, Posner KL, Domino KB. Death or neurologic injury following tonsillectomy in children with a focus on obstructive sleep apnea: Houston, we have a problem! *Anesth Analg.* 2014;118(6):1276-1283.

Results of a survey of members of the Society for Pediatric Anesthesia and the American Society of Anesthesiologists Closed Claims Project revealed at least 16 reports of deaths or neurologic injury after tonsillectomy owing to apparent apnea. Some of the risk factors are presented. The need to develop an improved safety net for these at-risk children is discussed.

Marcus CL, Brooks LJ, Draper KA, et al. Diagnosis and management of childhood obstructive sleep apnea syndrome. *Pediatrics.* 2012;130(3):576-584.

A comprehensive review from the American Academy of Pediatrics regarding assessment and management of children with OSA.

Nixon GM, Kermack AS, Davis GM, et al. Planning adenotonsillectomy in children with obstructive sleep apnea: the role of overnight oximetry. *Pediatrics.* 2004;113(1 Pt 1):e19-e25.

When a full sleep study in a sleep pathology laboratory is not possible, overnight oximetry can be a more practical approach.

Nixon GM, Kermack AS, McGregor CD, et al. Sleep and breathing on the first night after adenotonsillectomy for obstructive sleep apnea. *Pediatr Pulmonol.* 2005;39(4):332-338.

At-risk children become more hypoxemic on the first night after tonsillectomy than they were preoperatively. This study makes a compelling case for in-hospital monitoring postoperatively.

Patino M, Sadhasivam S, Mahmoud M. Obstructive sleep apnoea in children: perioperative considerations. *Br J Anaesth.* 2013;111(suppl 1):i83-i95.

This review focuses on the epidemiology, pathogenesis, and diagnosis of OSA, and the state of-the-art and future directions in the perioperative management of children with OSA.

Schwengel DA, Sterni LM, Tunkel DE. Heitmiller ES. Perioperative management of children with obstructive sleep apnea. *Anesth Analg.* 2009;109(1):60-75.

A review of the pathophysiology, current treatment options, and recognized approaches to perioperative management of pediatric OSA patients.

Tan GX, Tunkel DE. Control of pain after tonsillectomy in children—a review. *JAMA Otolaryngol Head Neck Surg.* 2017;143(9):937-942.

A recent review focusing on the risks of opioids in children with obstructive sleep apnea syndrome (OSAS) and the possible increases in post-tonsillectomy hemorrhage with the use of alternative nonsteroidal antiinflammatory drugs (NSAIDs).

Verghese ST, Hannallah RS. Pediatric otolaryngological emergencies. *Anesthesiol Clin North Am.* 2001;19(2):237-256.

A comprehensive review of pediatric airway emergencies.

A complete reference list can be found online at ExpertConsult.com.

34

Ophthalmology

JOSEPH R. TOBIN AND R. GREY WEAVER, JR.

THE INFANT OR CHILD who presents for elective ophthalmic surgery requires careful preanesthesia assessment. In addition to ophthalmologic issues, the infant or child may have associated or unassociated systemic disorders. In this chapter, we review the essential issues that should be addressed preoperatively and difficulties that may be anticipated in the perioperative period.

Many ophthalmologic diagnoses can be confirmed only by examining a cooperative infant or child. An examination under anesthesia (EUA) is essential for an accurate diagnosis and evaluation of many processes, including trauma, tumors, infiltrative diseases, coloboma, glaucoma and other vascular diseases of the retina, Coats disease, and incontinentia pigmenti. Inpatient preterm infants often require serial EUAs to monitor the development and progress of retinopathy of prematurity (ROP) and the response to previous therapies. These examinations are performed in the neonatal intensive care unit or operating room and may require either sedation or general anesthesia.[1] Inpatient trauma victims may require serial EUAs to monitor the development of glaucoma or retinal injury. Serial EUAs are also necessary to monitor progress during outpatient retinoblastoma radiation treatments. As a result, the anesthesiologist assumes an integral role as a member of the team, providing suitable conditions for the provision of pediatric ophthalmologic diagnostic and therapeutic techniques.

Ophthalmologic procedures that require an immobile child for maximal safety include surgery in which the globe is open (e.g., cataract removal), vitrectomy, laser or cryotherapy for retinopathy, retinal detachment repair, anterior chamber paracentesis, and repair of an open globe injury. Other procedures may require a child to be cooperative only for a nonpainful examination, but because the target organs (orbits) are close to the airway, a strategy must be devised to ensure safe airway management.

The child in need of ophthalmologic surgery typically requires general anesthesia or deep sedation rather than exclusive use of local or regional anesthesia. Many infants and children cannot cooperate for anything beyond a brief eye examination. Although the ophthalmologist may be able to tolerate small movements during an EUA, unnecessary head or eye globe movement during an ophthalmologic procedure should be prevented. Regional blocks (e.g., subtenon, retrobulbar, peribulbar) are infrequently performed for postoperative analgesia before emergence from general anesthesia[2]; all complications associated with these blocks identified in adults may also occur in children.[3,4]

Preoperative Evaluation

The perioperative environment should be welcoming to the child and family.[5,6] All team members should be comfortable with the anesthesia considerations for infants and children for ophthalmologic procedures.[6] Anticipation and prevention of postoperative nausea and vomiting (PONV) and understanding of anesthesia emergence and postoperative analgesia are essential.[7]

Before an elective ophthalmologic procedure, the child undergoes a thorough physical examination, including a review of all systems, and a complete medical history is obtained, including a surgical and anesthesia history, list of current medications, known allergies, and family history.[8] Because many ophthalmologic diagnoses are commonly associated with systemic conditions, all implications of the systemic illness are a concern for the anesthesiologist.

The physical examination should evaluate whether the ophthalmologic condition demands an alteration in airway management or affects the ability to obtain an appropriate mask fit. The airway should be carefully assessed for issues arising from other systemic

TABLE 34.1	Common Ophthalmologic Procedures in Children
Examination under anesthesia	
Strabismus repair	
Retinopathy of prematurity: laser or cryotherapy	
Ptosis repair	
Cataract excision with or without intraocular lens placement	
Corneal transplantation	
Evaluation of penetrating eye injuries	
Dacryocystorhinotomy and dacryocystocele repair	
Enucleation	
Retro-orbital cellulitis decompression	
Vitrectomy	

TABLE 34.2	Ophthalmologic Conditions Associated With Systemic Syndromes and Illnesses
Syndrome or Illness	**Ophthalmologic Conditions**
Fetal alcohol syndrome	Strabismus, optic nerve hypoplasia
Galactosemia	Neonatal cataracts
Mucopolysaccharidoses	Corneal involvement; may require transplantation
Retinitis pigmentosa	Heart block
Sturge-Weber syndrome	Glaucoma
Prematurity	Retinopathy of prematurity, strabismus
Fabry disease	Whorled corneal opacities
Tay-Sachs disease	Cherry-red macular spot
Osteogenesis imperfecta	Blue sclerae
Craniofacial syndromes (e.g., Crouzon, Apert, Pfeiffer)	Proptosis, strabismus, glaucoma

34

conditions. Assessments of cardiorespiratory and neurologic systems are important in formulating the anesthesia plan.

Common Ophthalmologic Diagnoses Requiring Surgery

Common pediatric diagnoses and surgical procedures are listed in Table 34.1. A diagnosis may exist in isolation or be one aspect of a more complex group of diagnoses. Many involve systemic illnesses, and the anesthesiologist should be familiar with the implications of ophthalmologic disease in these settings.

Some procedures and examinations can be performed without insertion of an artificial airway; however, communication with the ophthalmologist about position and possible immobility requirements is essential when planning the anesthetic prescription. Other procedures may be performed very quickly and require only induction of anesthesia (often by mask in children) and then removal of the face mask from the nasal bridge to give the ophthalmologist full access to both orbits, eyelids, and nasolacrimal ducts. With experience and the use of soft, inflatable-cushion face masks, a close fit can be obtained to reduce environmental contamination with anesthetic gases while maintaining a suitable plane of anesthesia. The EUA may be brief or intermediate in length, and as information is generated, surgical correction may be contemplated during the same episode of anesthesia, possibly requiring insertion of an artificial airway.

Communication and flexibility are essential since anesthesia may start with a plan for a brief EUA using an inhalational anesthetic with a face mask and no intravenous (IV) catheter; however, if corrective surgery becomes necessary, then airway control may require placement of a laryngeal mask airway (LMA) or tracheal tube. IV access is usually required to administer medications, including those to prevent or treat the oculocardiac reflex (OCR), postoperative pain, and nausea and vomiting.[9]

For procedures of brief or intermediate duration, the use of an LMA generally allows excellent access to all periorbital structures. Compared with mask anesthesia, the LMA has the advantage of decreasing environmental contamination by inhalational anesthetics. It is relatively easy to insert and remains secure while avoiding the need for the anesthesiologist to hold a face mask near the surgical site. Compared with a tracheal tube, an LMA does not increase the heart rate, blood pressure, and intraocular pressure (IOP) to the same degree.[10]

The more common ophthalmologic presentations and associated systemic illnesses or syndromes are listed in Table 34.2. Some conditions have significant cardiorespiratory and/or central nervous system (CNS) implications for perioperative management and should be fully evaluated before anesthesia (see Chapter 4). Many procedures are performed on preterm infants or formerly preterm infants, and appropriate monitoring for apnea spells after anesthesia is essential.[11,12]

Ophthalmologic Conditions Associated With Systemic Disorders

PREMATURITY

The preterm infant may present for many surgical procedures early in life. ROP, congenital cataracts, and glaucoma may require surgery even when the infant weighs less than 1000 g. The preterm infant may have significant systemic illnesses. Common complications of prematurity include acute and chronic pulmonary disease,[13] respiratory failure and pulmonary hypertension, CHD (unrepaired or with a limited palliative repair), and intraventricular hemorrhage,[14] with or without obstructive hydrocephalus.

Acutely ill preterm infants and those younger than 1 year of age are at greater risk than older children and adults for perioperative complications.[15] Careful attention to airway management, assisted ventilation, and titration of oxygen therapy with specified goals are essential for success.[16] In preterm infants, whose airways are already intubated and whose lungs are ventilated mechanically, the anesthesiologist should confirm the position of the tracheal tube, transport the infant safely to the operating room, and limit the exposure to high concentrations of oxygen. Although institutional goals are not uniform regarding supplemental oxygen therapy,[17] communication with the neonatal team is often helpful in gauging the infant's previous oxygen requirement and current targeted goals (e.g., hemoglobin-oxygen saturation levels of 91%–95%).[18,19] Because most inhalational anesthetics impair hypoxic pulmonary vasoconstriction, a greater fraction of inspired oxygen (FIO_2) may be necessary to maintain the targeted hemoglobin saturation.

Hypercarbia and hypoxia may increase choroidal blood volume and increase IOP. Partial pressures of carbon dioxide (PCO_2) and oxygen (PO_2) should be monitored continuously and controlled. Infants may be at greater risk for the OCR than older children and adults, and IV access should be obtained before the surgical procedure or any examination that may involve traction on the extraocular muscles or pressure on the globe.

Infants of extremely low birth weight require many weeks to grow and develop to a weight of approximately 1800 g and to maintain normothermia without special environmental control. These infants commonly have a history of short-term or intermediate-term assisted ventilation and may or may not require supplemental oxygen before an EUA or planned operative procedure for ROP.[20] Many of these infants undergo ophthalmologic examinations while their lungs are ventilated in the neonatal intensive care unit.[21] During surgical therapy (i.e., laser or cryosurgical stabilization) for ROP, these infants require anesthesia to provide optimal conditions (Fig. 34.1). Perioperative apnea may preclude tracheal extubation or require close postoperative monitoring after anesthesia.[11,12]

Perioperative apnea in the preterm infant is widely described.[11,12,22] Whether the child is still hospitalized or presenting for elective surgery as an outpatient, the preoperative assessment should determine the pattern and frequency of apnea before the planned surgical procedure and anesthesia. The current use of respiratory stimulants (i.e., caffeine or theophylline) and oxygen should be determined. Is an apnea monitor being used, or has it been discontinued? Guidelines have not been developed to manage some of the scenarios, but infants who continue to require supplemental oxygen, who are younger than 60 weeks postconceptional age, or who are monitored for apnea or bradycardia should have continuous cardiorespiratory and oxygen saturation monitoring postoperatively for at least 12 hours or until they are apnea free (see Chapter 4). The risk of apnea after general anesthesia and sedation decreases with advancing gestational age at birth and with advancing

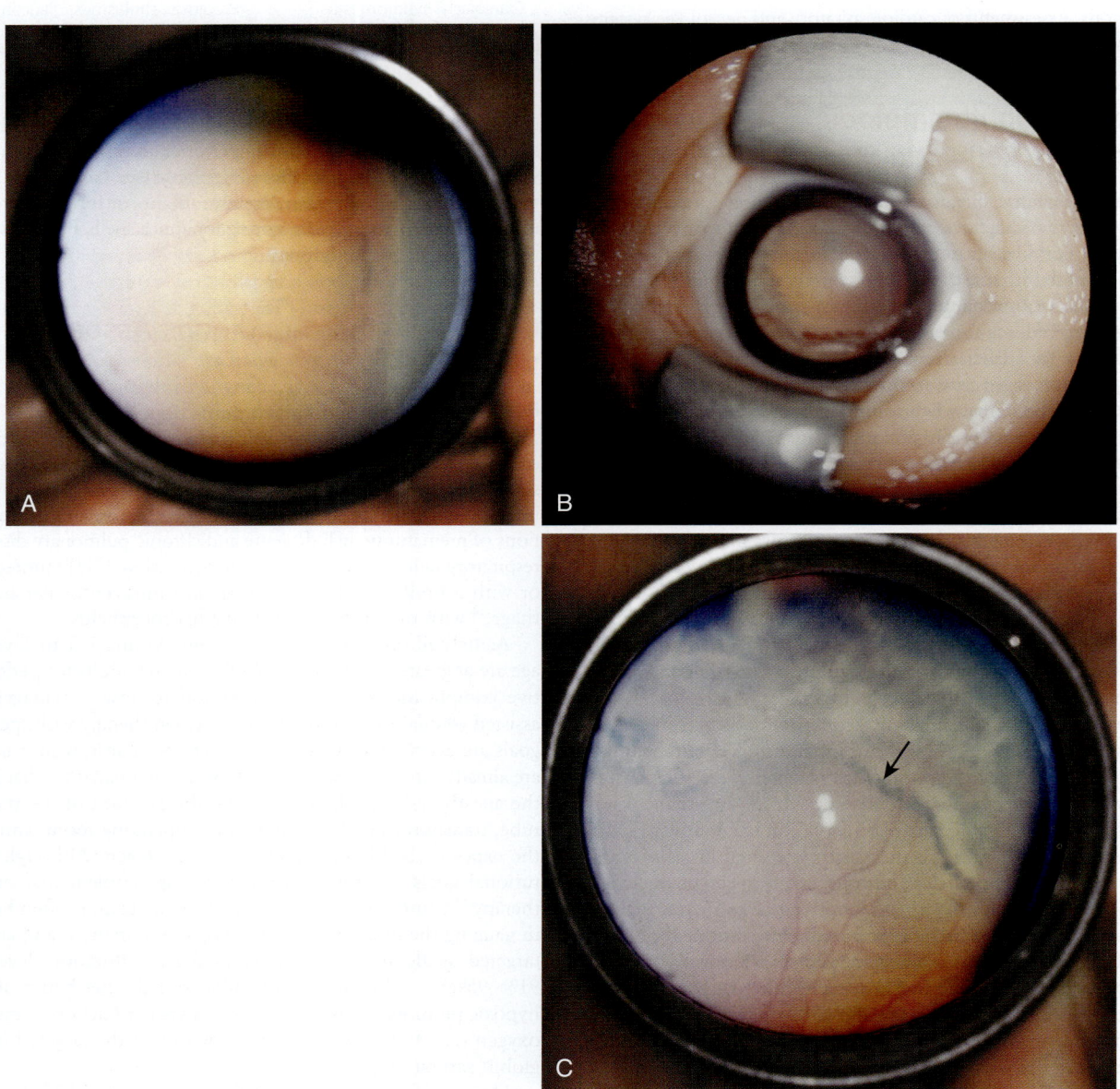

FIGURE 34.1 A, Grade III retinopathy of prematurity with neovascularization of the retina requires surgical therapy to halt the growth of vessels. **B,** Retinal detachment caused by retinopathy of prematurity. This degree of damage results in permanent visual impairment. **C,** Appearance after cryotherapy. Cryotherapy causes a well-demarcated ridge of tissue scarring *(arrow)* that prevents further growth of the neovasculature *(left to right in the middle).*

postnatal-postconceptional age. The risk of apnea is independent of opioid use; its multifactorial origins include the presence of general and neuraxial anesthetics and the immature CNS and respiratory center in the preterm infant. Flexible planning for possible postoperative ventilatory support is essential, and families should be informed of this possibility preoperatively.

The airway of the preterm infant who is younger than 52 to 60 weeks postconceptional age is usually intubated for ophthalmologic surgery (except for a very brief EUA) owing to the immature respiratory drive, unpredictable respiratory response to anesthetic agents, and possible lag before recovery of respiratory drive after completion of the procedure and discontinuation of anesthetic agents. If the infant does not appear to have a stable respiratory drive and strength after anesthesia, postoperative assisted ventilation should be continued as indicated; planning for this contingency is vital. *Ophthalmologic procedures may be brief and have a low risk of blood loss, but the risks of general anesthesia mandate full postoperative support.* Intensive care resources for assisted ventilation in preterm and formerly preterm infants should be available before embarking on anesthesia.

Although chronic lung disease related to prematurity is prevalent, its intensity has been reduced with the routine use of surfactant and advances in ventilator management strategies. Long-lasting respiratory effects from prematurity may include reactive airway disease, subglottic stenosis from prolonged intubation, and alveolar or interstitial disease with an oxygen requirement lasting weeks to years.[13] Because many anesthetics impair hypoxic pulmonary vasoconstriction, an increased oxygen requirement in the perioperative period should be anticipated. Tracheal intubation, a light level of anesthesia, or topical use of β-adrenergic antagonists may exacerbate reactive airway disease, requiring further treatment to reduce air trapping and hypercarbia.

In addition to assessing for airway and alveolar diseases, the anesthesiologist should determine whether pulmonary hypertension or right ventricular dysfunction is or was present.[23] Some infants may be receiving continuing oxygen therapy (and/or surfactant) as treatment for pulmonary hypertension and to reduce intermittent episodes of hypoxemia owing to crying or while sleeping. If pulmonary hypertension was diagnosed previously, an updated evaluation is warranted. Because pulmonary hypertension is exacerbated by hypoxia and hypercarbia, tracheal intubation is indicated to ensure control of ventilation and oxygenation. At emergence, pulmonary hypertension may be exacerbated as hypercapnia develops, causing physiologic or anatomic shunting with systemic hemoglobin-oxygen desaturation. Immediate and continued evaluation of the airway is imperative to rule out an independent respiratory contribution to the systemic hypoxia.

Congenital cardiac disease may be diagnosed in the preterm neonate, infant, or child who presents for ophthalmologic procedures. A patent ductus arteriosus may not close spontaneously or after administration of cyclooxygenase inhibitors. This may lead to persistent congestive failure, reduced pulmonary compliance, and complications of fluid management. Congenital cardiac anomalies require assessment before elective surgery. The various complex congenital cardiac lesions have a wide spectrum of interactions with multiple anesthetic agents.[24] Many cardiac conditions require surgery or palliation (e.g., systemic-to-pulmonary shunts) before elective ophthalmologic procedures. Correction of congenital heart disease (CHD) is limited by the difficulty of using cardiopulmonary bypass in infants weighing less than 2 kg. There may be an urgent need for ophthalmologic evaluation (e.g., congenital tumor, cataract, glaucoma) before repair of the congenital cardiac condition. Preoperative consultation with the infant's pediatric cardiologist can provide useful information on the infant's current ventricular function and the risk of dysrhythmias associated with cardiac defects. Medical management must be optimized before undertaking anesthesia and surgery.

Intraventricular hemorrhage is a major source of morbidity and mortality in preterm infants.[14] Obstructive hydrocephalus may occur and require cerebrospinal fluid diversion procedures to decompress the obstructed ventricular system and treat the associated increased intracranial pressure. Many of these infants require ophthalmologic surgery for repair of strabismus caused by a neurologic insult. If a ventriculoperitoneal shunt is in place, its proper function should be determined by direct evaluation. The anesthesiologist should assess whether there is inappropriate macrocephaly or a bulging or tense fontanelle. Obstructive hydrocephalus may occur after the infant's discharge from hospital, even though a ventriculoperitoneal shunt was not required previously. The preoperative assessment should include the child's developmental and neurologic status at the time of surgery. Because intraventricular hemorrhage is associated with long-term morbidity, any history of seizures should be elicited, and the antiepileptic drugs being used should be documented.

Preterm and small infants rapidly lose heat when anesthetized. Prevention of hypothermia is essential in the perioperative environment. Hypothermia can decrease metabolism of most drugs and depresses respiratory drive in preterm infants (see Chapter 37).

DOWN SYNDROME

Children with Down syndrome (i.e., trisomy 21) frequently present for ophthalmologic surgery because of associated pathologic processes such as neonatal cataracts, significant refractive errors (e.g., hypermetropia, astigmatism), strabismus, glaucoma, keratoconus, nasolacrimal duct obstruction, and nystagmus.[25-27] Infants with trisomy 21 should have an ophthalmologic evaluation in the neonatal period. If this requires an EUA, the anesthesiologist should be prepared for the extensive medical implications associated with trisomy 21.[28,29] Almost half of these infants are born with CHD, including septal defects, complete or partial atrioventricular canal, tetralogy of Fallot, transposition of the great arteries, and valvular insufficiency or stenosis. Any child with a left-to-right shunt may develop pulmonary hypertension, and children with Trisomy 21 develop irreversible pulmonary hypertension at an earlier age. Bradycardia (25%–60%) and hypotension (12%–73%) have been reported during sevoflurane anesthesia in these children.[30,31] The child's cardiac defects should be clearly defined before planning the anesthetic prescription (see Chapters 16 and 18).

Airway abnormalities such as narrowed nasopharyngeal passages, macroglossia, pharyngeal hypotonia, and subglottic stenosis, as well as obstructive sleep apnea, are frequently observed in children with Trisomy 21. These abnormalities may contribute to development of chronic intermittent hypoxia, further exacerbating pulmonary hypertension, and these children should be expected to demonstrate exacerbations of airway obstruction and hypoxia after general anesthesia.[32]

Children with Trisomy 21 have a wide spectrum of developmental delays. Cervical spine instability occurs, and occiput-C1 and C1-2 instabilities have been described.[33,34] Subluxation of the cervical spine has rarely been reported in these children during anesthesia. Nonetheless, the anesthesiologist and the surgeon should avoid extremes of neck flexion and extension and lateral rotation during head positioning for laryngoscopy and surgery. While the child is awake, the range of motion of the neck in flexion and extension should be assessed, along with complaints of numbness or tingling in the hands or feet in a particular position. Previous spine and neck investigations or operations should be reviewed. No consensus exists for the need to radiologically investigate a child with Trisomy 21 who has an asymptomatic cervical spine, although many children are evaluated before 5 years of age.

Children with Trisomy 21 may be born with congenital hypothyroidism or it may develop at any time during their life span. If the child is found to have a goiter on examination or has symptoms consistent with hypothyroidism (i.e., prolonged jaundice, hypothermia, constipation, dry skin, macroglossia, or relative bradycardia), thyroid function studies should be obtained before anesthesia for an elective procedure. They may develop junctional bradycardia during sevoflurane anesthesia.[35] The bradycardia may be associated with or result from occult hypothyroidism.

ALPORT SYNDROME

Alport syndrome (i.e., progressive hereditary nephritis) is a disorder in a group of familial oculorenal syndromes that includes Lowe (oculocerebral) syndrome and familial renal-retinal dystrophy. Alport syndrome involves sensorineural hearing loss, progressive renal disease, and multiple ophthalmologic disorders, including cataracts, retinal detachment, and keratoconus.[36,37] Development of a myopathy and renal failure constitutes the major anesthesia concerns. If the patient has a myopathy, it is prudent to avoid succinylcholine and the risk of a hyperkalemic response and rhabdomyolysis. Renal insufficiency may alter the choice of pharmacologic agents to very–short-acting agents or agents that are not excreted by the kidney.

MARFAN SYNDROME, HOMOCYSTINURIA, AND EHLERS-DANLOS SYNDROME

Marfan syndrome, homocystinuria, and Ehlers-Danlos syndrome are considered together only from the perspective of a general body phenotype. The metabolic and molecular causes of these syndromes are well described.[38,38a] They share problems with connective tissue development, possible joint laxity, and cardiovascular disorders.

Marfan syndrome is caused by a defect in the fibrillin 1 gene (FBN1), which affects elastic and nonelastic connective tissues. These children have an increased risk of retinal detachment, lens dislocation, glaucoma, and cataract formation (E-Fig. 34.1).[39] They may have significant pulmonary (scoliosis) and cardiovascular problems,[40] which may include aortic, mitral, or pulmonic valve insufficiency. Preoperative cardiovascular evaluation is indicated to determine the progression of cardiovascular abnormalities that inevitably occur. Acute and chronic blood pressure control is essential to prevent aortic dissection.

Homocystinuria has at least three forms and different inborn errors. Enzymatic deficiency of the metabolism of sulfur-containing amino acids causes the intermediate metabolite, homocysteine, to accumulate. These children suffer from cataracts, retinal degeneration, optic atrophy, glaucoma, and lens dislocation. The cardiovascular pathology includes coronary artery disease at a young age. Thromboembolic phenomena occur more frequently because they may be hypercoagulable.[41] Nitrous oxide should be avoided because it inhibits methionine synthase, further limiting the conversion of homocysteine to methionine.

At least 10 forms of Ehlers-Danlos syndrome have been described. Not all forms express significant ocular pathology. From the anesthesiologist's perspective, positioning is important to avoid trauma to the skin because these children develop hemorrhages

with minor trauma and experience delayed wound healing. A thorough preoperative assessment should be performed for cardiac lesions. Hypertension should be avoided to reduce the risk of rupturing an aneurysm. The duration of effect of local anesthetics in patients with type III Ehlers-Danlos syndrome may be less than that in normal patients, and contingency plans should be in place to address these possibilities, including retrobulbar block or general anesthesia.[42]

MUCOPOLYSACCHARIDOSES

The mucopolysaccharidoses are a group of disorders with enzyme defects that result in incomplete degradation of glycosaminoglycans. Affected children have various degrees of cognitive dysfunction, macroglossia, airway obstruction, cervical spine instability, and systemic involvement with deposition of mucopolysaccharide material. This leads to cardiac and respiratory dysfunction, airway obstruction, corneal opacities, and glaucoma.

The systemic complications of these disorders are sufficiently severe that even well-planned anesthesia management for ophthalmologic procedures may cause death.[43] Airway management can be extremely difficult with poor mask fit, dynamic airway obstruction with narrowed passages, a floppy epiglottis, and difficulty visualizing the larynx.[44] Infiltrative material may be deposited in the laryngeal inlet and pretracheal tissues; an LMA is particularly useful in maintaining a patent airway. Tracheal intubation may require the use of advanced airway visualization and management techniques, and the anesthesiologist should have several plans for airway management (see Chapter 14). Cardiac evaluation should be considered before an elective procedure to assess ventricular function and arrhythmias. IV access may be difficult due to subcutaneous deposition of mucopolysaccharides.

CRANIOFACIAL SYNDROMES

Craniofacial syndromes may manifest as craniosynostosis or have only middle and lower facial structure involvement.[45] Apert and Crouzon syndromes are both disorders of craniofacial development, but syndactyly occurs only in the former (E-Fig. 34.2). They share the potential for many ocular disorders, including severe proptosis, making mask airway management difficult.[46] Other mutations of the fibroblast growth factor receptor 2 gene (FGFR2) cause Antley-Bixler and Pfeiffer syndromes. These children may develop chronic airway obstruction, and some have complete tracheal rings; tracheal narrowing should be anticipated, and smaller tracheal tube sizes should be used.

Children with asymmetry of facial and mandibular bone growth may present with limited mouth opening. Children with Goldenhar syndrome (i.e., hemifacial microsomia), Treacher Collins syndrome, and Pierre Robin sequence can be expected to present a challenge to airway management (see Chapters 14 and 35).[46a] Children with craniosynostosis have an increased risk of CHD and a cardiac evaluation should be performed before anesthesia.[47] Neurologic morbidity and seizure disorders occur more frequently in this group of patients.

PHAKOMATOSES

The phakomatoses are neurocutaneous syndromes with multiple ocular pathologic processes. These syndromes include neurofibromatosis,[48,49] encephalotrigeminal angiomatosis (i.e., Sturge-Weber syndrome),[50] tuberous sclerosis,[51,52] incontinentia pigmenti, and ataxia telangiectasia. CNS involvement varies with each of these diseases. Patients may have developmental delay, seizures, and significant neurologic morbidity. Preoperative electrolyte and hepatic function studies should be assessed. Anticonvulsant drug history and effectiveness should be reviewed; continue these medications in the perioperative period.

OPHTHALMOLOGIC PHYSIOLOGY

Two major considerations of ophthalmologic physiology are of great interest to the anesthesiologist. The first is the dynamics of aqueous humor production and transport and the effects on IOP. The second is the OCR that may occur during any surgery around the orbit. Anesthetic agents affect the IOP. In a patient with a penetrating eye injury, any increase of IOP may be associated with extravasation of elements of the globe and irretrievable loss of vision.

INTRAOCULAR PRESSURE

IOP is the pressure exerted by the internal components of the globe on the covering (i.e., sclera and conjunctiva). The normal IOP is 12 to 15 mm Hg. An IOP greater than 20 mm Hg is considered abnormal. Aqueous humor is a clear fluid that is secreted by the ciliary body and released into the anterior chamber of the globe. It traverses the anterior chamber and bathes the iris. It flows through the canal of Schlemm into the pores of Fontana and then drains into the episcleral and then systemic veins (Fig. 34.2). The posterior chamber, which is larger than the anterior chamber, is composed of a gelatinous mix known as vitreous humor. The sclera and globe that encase the intraocular constituents are relatively noncompliant and are protected by the bony orbit. However, intraorbital masses may impinge on the globe and increase the relative IOP or alter the flow of aqueous humor, resulting in increased IOP. Any obstruction to the drainage of aqueous humor causes fluid to build up within the anterior chamber and increases IOP.[53] Increased central venous pressure (e.g., Trendelenburg position,

coughing, Valsalva maneuver, straining, increased intrathoracic pressure) attenuates the drainage of aqueous humor from the eye and may further exacerbate the increased IOP. Arterial pressure changes within the normal range do not directly affect the IOP. However, as arterial blood pressure increases beyond the normal range, approximately 30% of the increase in systolic blood pressure is reflected in IOP increases.

Aqueous humor formation is described in the following equation:

$$IOP = K[(OP_{aq} - OP_{pl}) + P_c],$$

where K is the coefficient of outflow, OP_{aq} is the osmotic pressure of aqueous humor, OP_{pl} is the osmotic pressure of plasma, and P_c is the capillary pressure. These variables allow calculation to intervene by increasing the plasma osmolality acutely with mannitol to lower the IOP. This increases the gradient of osmolality and draws water out of the aqueous humor, thereby reducing the IOP.

In the relatively noncompliant globe, any pharmacologic or metabolic process that increases choroidal blood volume (e.g., hypercapnia, coughing, increased central venous pressure) produces choroidal congestion and an increased IOP. Although well tolerated in the healthy eye, this congestion may lead to extrusion of contents if the globe is ruptured. The anesthesiologist should carefully control the child's physiology during the induction and maintenance of anesthesia to minimize increases in IOP, regardless of whether there is a preoperative concern about increased IOP.

Congenital or trauma-induced glaucoma requires therapy to reduce the IOP. If the IOP remains elevated, blood flow in the retina will be impaired, possibly leading to loss of vision. Unfortunately, there are many causes of glaucoma in childhood. Hypercarbia, hypoxia, and drugs known or suspected to increase IOP (e.g., succinylcholine, ketamine) should be avoided or used with care. Reducing a child's apprehension and crying and avoiding increases in central venous pressure are also important considerations.

The effect of succinylcholine on IOP is well documented.[54,55] Succinylcholine increases IOP 6 to 10 mm Hg, an effect that begins within 1 minute after administration and continues for up to 10 minutes, at which time the IOP returns to normal. This effect has been attributed to four possible mechanisms:

- Cycloplegia induced by succinylcholine, which obstructs the outflow of aqueous humor
- Tonic contraction of extraocular muscles
- Increased choroidal blood volume
- Relaxation of orbital muscles, which increases external pressure on the globe

Specific muscles develop a sustained tonic tension after succinylcholine that may in the presence of a ruptured globe cause extrusion of intraocular contents.[56] Extrusion in response to increased IOP depends on the diameter of the orifice; a smaller laceration (<2 mm) is less likely to facilitate extrusion of intraocular contents than a larger laceration (>4 mm). Pretreatment with a nondepolarizing agent (one-tenth the usual intubating dose) and paralysis with succinylcholine are still advocated by some anesthesiologists to minimize the risk of aspiration when dealing with an open globe injury. Alternatively, rocuronium (1.2 mg/kg IV) can provide optimal intubating conditions in 30 seconds for the child with an open globe injury while minimizing the risk for aspiration or succinylcholine-associated increases in IOP. Sugammadex has been used in Europe for some years and is now approved for use in the United States; concerns of prolonged paralysis from

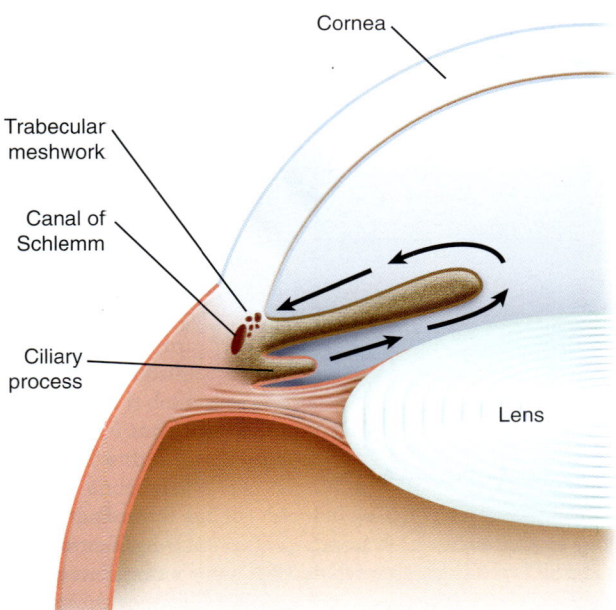

FIGURE 34.2 Aqueous humor is synthesized in the ciliary process and then circulates around the iris, past the lens, and into the anterior chamber. After flowing through the trabecular meshwork, aqueous humor enters the canal of Schlemm (*arrows*), which drains into the episcleral venous system. Pathologic conditions that increase venous pressure, obstruct the canal of Schlemm, or increase aqueous humor production may increase intraocular pressure.

Labels on figure: Cornea, Trabecular meshwork, Canal of Schlemm, Ciliary process, Lens rocuronium or a failed intubation are lessened since even profound neuromuscular blockade can be rapidly reversed.

Most general anesthetics decrease IOP,[57] although ketamine has been shown to increase IOP in some studies and decrease it in others—an effect that may be attributed to ventilation control and consequent Pa_{CO2} rather than the drug.[58-60] When IV access is unavailable or the cardiovascular status of the patient warrants the use of ketamine, the child's overall safety takes precedence over the possible ramifications of ketamine on IOP.

Measurement of IOP is performed by applanation tonometry on the external surface of the globe. Tonometry is often performed along with the EUA during general anesthesia to avoid an overestimation of IOP in struggling, uncooperative infants or children. Borderline measurements must consider the possibility of anesthetic agents temporarily reducing or increasing the IOP.

OCULOCARDIAC REFLEX

First described in 1908, the OCR is triggered during ophthalmologic surgery and other conditions.[53] Traction on the extraocular muscles and levator (eyelid elevator) or external pressure applied to the globe triggers an afferent signal through the trigeminal nerve that activates parasympathetic output through the vagus nerve, resulting in many types of dysrhythmias (Fig. 34.3A), which include sinus or junctional bradycardia, atrioventricular block, ventricular ectopy, and asystole (Fig. 34.3B). Retrobulbar block with local anesthetic may precipitate the trigeminovagal (oculocardiac) reflex as a result of external pressure sensed on the globe, and the local anesthetic may not completely prevent the OCR response to further surgical stimulation or manipulation. For this reason, an anticholinergic medication, such as atropine (20 µg/kg) or glycopyrrolate (10-20 µg/kg), is routinely given IV at induction of anesthesia or early

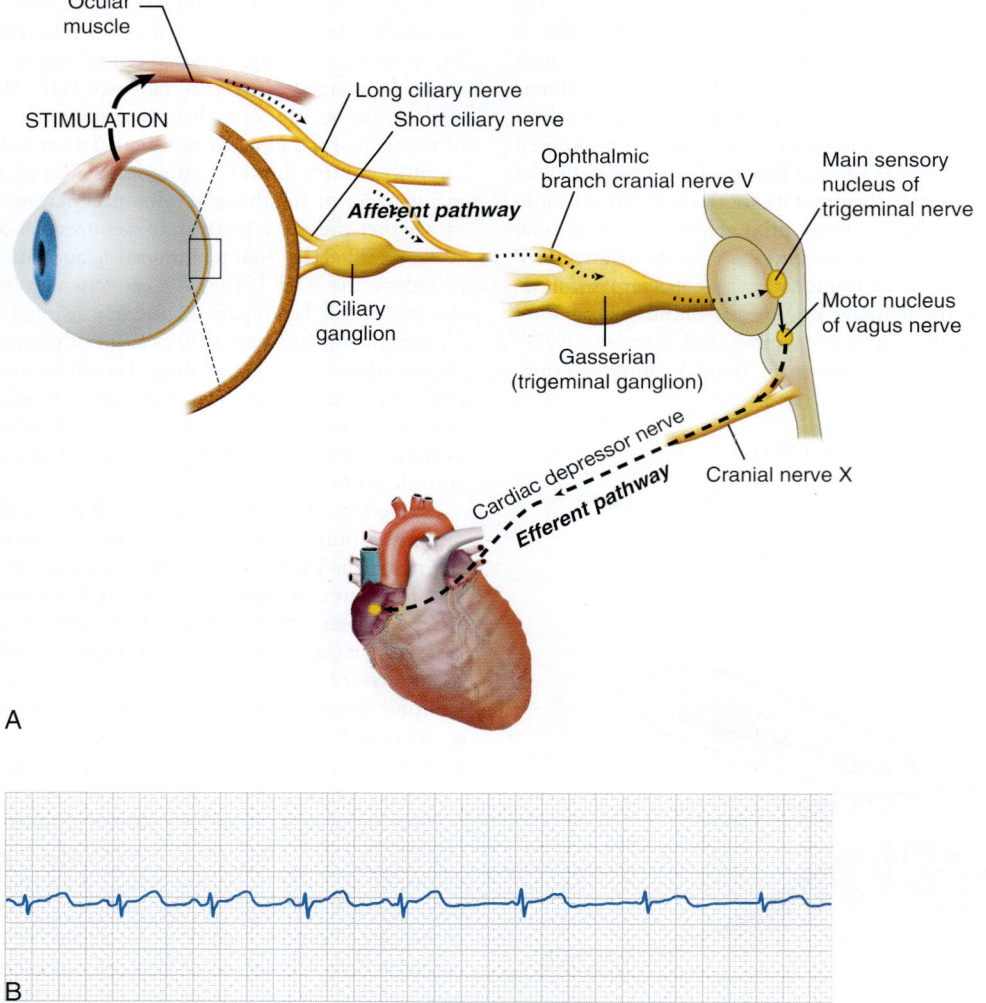

FIGURE 34.3 Traction on the extraocular muscles elicits the oculocardiac reflex. **A,** The afferent limb consists of the long and short ciliary nerves, which synapse in the ciliary ganglion *(dotted arrows)*. The ophthalmic division of the trigeminal nerve (cranial nerve V) carries the impulse to the gasserian ganglion, and the arc continues to the sensory nucleus of cranial nerve V in the brainstem. Fibers in the reticular formation synapse with the nucleus of the vagus nerve (cranial nerve X). Efferent fibers from the vagus nerve terminate in the heart *(dashed arrow)*. The neurotransmitter from the vagus nerve to the sinoatrial node is acetylcholine, and the reflex is blocked by antimuscarinic pharmacologic agents (i.e., atropine and glycopyrrolate). **B,** Electrocardiogram shows conversion from normal sinus rhythm to a nodal rhythm.

thereafter. Although these medications do not preclude the occurrence of bradycardia, both decrease its severity and duration. Because anticholinergics cause pupillary dilatation, they do not present a problem for the ophthalmologist, but they may slightly increase the IOP.

If significant bradycardia occurs, the anesthesia team should ask the surgeon to release the traction on the extraocular muscle or stimulation in the surgical field. An additional IV dose of atropine (5–10 μg/kg) usually interrupts the reflex and restores the heart rate, although the correction may be evanescent and the dysrhythmia may recur. IV epinephrine (1–10 μg/kg) is rarely necessary but should always be available. The anesthesiologist should ensure adequate oxygenation and ventilation because hypercarbia or hypoxia may compound or intensify the reflex activity.

Other strategies to attenuate the OCR include topically applied lidocaine[61] or IV ketamine.[62] In a four-armed study, the incidence of OCR with a ketamine-based anesthetic (10–12 mg/kg per hour) was less compared with the three other anesthetic regimens: propofol/alfentanil, sevoflurane/nitrous oxide, or halothane/nitrous oxide.[63] The prevalence of the OCR during sevoflurane and desflurane anesthesia was similar.[64]

Ophthalmologic Pharmacotherapeutics and Systemic Implications

Topical ophthalmologic medications are usually placed directly on the cornea or in the inferior cul-de-sac. Most of these agents need many minutes to 1 hour for maximal effectiveness and as such are usually administered soon after induction. Medications delivered topically to the eye are absorbed through the conjunctiva and nasal mucosa into the systemic circulation; their pharmacologic mechanisms of action predict the systemic consequences. Therefore some medications are diluted for use in children to reduce the concentration presented and possible systemic toxicity. Anticholinergics, sympathomimetics, and antihistamines can cause pupillary dilation and decrease the movement of aqueous humor, thus increasing the IOP. Table 34.3 lists the more commonly used pediatric topical agents.

Topical mydriatic agents dilate the pupil. The most common mydriatic is phenylephrine (2.5% solution), an α_1-adrenergic agonist that is rapidly absorbed but may cause significant hypertension in small infants. If severe hypertension occurs, reflex bradycardia may ensue.

Topical cycloplegic agents also dilate the pupil, as well as eliminate lens accommodation by paralyzing the ciliary muscle. This aids in retinal evaluation with the indirect ophthalmoscope and scleral depression and in evaluating refractive errors for which the child is using accommodation for compensation. These agents are muscarinic cholinergic antagonists (i.e., antimuscarinic agents). One such agent is cyclopentolate hydrochloride (0.5%), which can cause CNS toxicity with disorientation, seizures, and blurred vision. Atropine (0.5%–2.0%) and scopolamine (0.25%) solutions are also cycloplegics that dilate the pupil. Tropicamide (0.5% and 1.0%) is less commonly used in children. When systemically absorbed, these agents may cause antimuscarinic, anticholinergic toxicity, including tachycardia, dry mouth, pupillary dilation, flushing of the skin, heat intolerance or fever, and disorientation (E-Fig. 34.3).

β-Adrenergic blockers (e.g., timolol, betaxolol) are used to reduce IOP in the treatment of glaucoma. Systemic absorption causes symptoms of sympathetic nervous system blockade. β-Adrenergic antagonists induce bradycardia and cardiovascular collapse and may precipitate bronchospasm. If β-adrenergic intoxication is suspected, direct-acting cardiovascular stimulants (epinephrine) should be used to antagonize the β-adrenergic blockade rather than indirect-acting stimulants such as ephedrine.

Topical local anesthetics are infrequently used in children except for the very cooperative child for tonometry or removal of sutures. Proparacaine and tetracaine (ester local anesthetics) may be used topically, whereas lidocaine and bupivacaine (or levobupivacaine, ropivacaine, which are amide local anesthetics) are used for ophthalmic blocks. Ester local anesthetics confer a small risk for systemic toxicity because they are extensively metabolized by plasma cholinesterases. Ophthalmic amide agents, however, do have the potential to cause systemic toxicity (i.e., cardiac dysrhythmias and seizures), but these agents are not frequently used in children. Topical cocaine is rarely used in pediatric ophthalmology except to test for Horner syndrome and as a vasoconstrictor to reduce nasal bleeding during nasal and nasolacrimal duct surgery.

Nonsteroidal antiinflammatory drugs (NSAIDs) are used for certain inflammatory conditions of the eye, but perioperative use in a child is uncommon. Some NSAIDs (i.e., ketorolac and ibuprofen) pose a concern for ophthalmology because their anticoagulant profiles may increase local perioperative bleeding. However, five NSAIDs are approved for ocular use: diclofenac, bromfenac, flurbiprofen, ketorolac, and nepafenac. Diclofenac, bromfenac, and nepafenac are used postoperatively for their antiinflammatory effects. Ketorolac has been used to treat macular edema after cataract extraction.

Echothiophate (i.e., phospholine iodide) is a cholinesterase inhibitor used to induce miosis in the treatment of glaucoma. When absorbed systemically, it impairs plasma cholinesterase, reducing the metabolism of some drugs (e.g., succinylcholine) and prolonging their duration of action. Decreased metabolism of acetylcholine may result in increased relative cholinergic tone, inducing bradycardia and bronchiolar muscle activity and resulting in bronchospasm. Toxicity from echothiophate may be antagonized by administration of pralidoxime (2-pyridine aldoxime methyl chloride [2-PAM]) (25 mg/kg IV). Otherwise, its action to reduce effective systemic cholinesterases lasts 4 to 6 weeks.

Pilocarpine, a direct-acting cholinergic agonist that is commonly used to treat glaucoma, has replaced echothiophate iodide. Through multiple actions, it improves the flow of aqueous humor; if absorbed, it may acutely cause bradycardia.

Many vitreal substitutes are used in ophthalmologic procedures. They include nonexpansile and expansile gases (e.g., sulfur hexafluoride), perfluorocarbon liquids, and silicone oils. The anesthesia team should be informed when the ophthalmologist plans intraocular use of one of these substances. If a gas pocket is anticipated, nitrous oxide should be discontinued or avoided completely. The patient and parent should be informed of any intraocular gas use, and the patient should wear an alert bracelet for the expected duration of absorption, usually no longer than 6 to 12 weeks, so that inadvertent use of nitrous oxide does not occur during that interval. When a perforated globe is closed, any residual environmental air pocket can be expanded by nitrous oxide; increased ocular pressure and reduced retinal blood flow may result.

A novel agent being studied in the treatment of retinal angiogenic diseases (e.g., ROP, retinoblastoma) is bevacizumab (a recombinant monoclonal antibody), which inhibits the formation

TABLE 34.3	Commonly Used Ophthalmologic Agents	
Drug	**Indication**	**Side Effect Profile**
Cholinergic Agonists		
Carbachol	Induce miosis	Corneal edema, retinal detachment
Pilocarpine	Glaucoma	Corneal edema, retinal detachment
Cholinesterase Inhibitors		
Physostigmine	Glaucoma	Retinal detachment, miosis
Echothiophate	Glaucoma	Retinal detachment, miosis
Muscarinic Antagonists		
Atropine	Cycloplegic retinoscopy	Photosensitivity, blurred vision, increased heart rate, dry mouth
Scopolamine	Cycloplegic retinoscopy	Photosensitivity, blurred vision, increased heart rate, dry mouth
Homatropine	Cycloplegic retinoscopy	Photosensitivity, blurred vision, increased heart rate, dry mouth
Cyclopentolate	Cycloplegic retinoscopy	Photosensitivity, blurred vision, increased heart rate, dry mouth
Tropicamide	Cycloplegic retinoscopy	Photosensitivity, blurred vision, increased heart rate, dry mouth
Sympathomimetic Agents		
Dipivefrin	Glaucoma	Photosensitivity, hypersensitivity
Epinephrine	Glaucoma	Photosensitivity, hypersensitivity
Phenylephrine	Mydriasis	Photosensitivity, hypersensitivity
Apraclonidine	Glaucoma	Photosensitivity, hypersensitivity
Brimonidine	Glaucoma	Photosensitivity, hypersensitivity
Cocaine	Local anesthetic	Anisocoria, corneal injury, photosensitivity, hypersensitivity
Hydroxyamphetamine	Glaucoma	Anisocoria, photosensitivity, hypersensitivity
Naphazoline	Decongestant	Photosensitivity, hypersensitivity
Tetrahydrozoline	Decongestant	Photosensitivity, hypersensitivity
α- and β-Adrenergic Antagonists		
Dapiprazole (α)	Reverse mydriasis	Conjunctival hyperemia
Betaxolol (β_1-selective)	Glaucoma	Bradycardia, hypotension
Carteolol (β)	Glaucoma	Decreased heart rate, blood pressure, bronchospasm
Levobunolol (β)	Glaucoma	Decreased heart rate, blood pressure, bronchospasm
Metipranolol (β)	Glaucoma	Decreased heart rate, blood pressure, bronchospasm
Timolol (β)	Glaucoma	Decreased heart rate, blood pressure, bronchospasm
Recombinant Monoclonal Antibodies		
Bevacizumab	ROP, retinoblastoma, retinal venous thrombosis, diabetic retinopathy	Drug introduced directly into eye and systemic effects minimal

ROP, retinopathy of prematurity.
Modified from Brunton LL, Lazo, JS, Parker KL, eds. *Goodman and Gilman's The Pharmacological Basis of Therapeutics*. 11th ed. New York: McGraw-Hill; 2006.

of new blood vessels.[65–67] In the doses prescribed, it should not raise concerns for anesthesia. The visual outcome of any infant must be monitored for all perioperative care provided.

EMERGENT, URGENT, AND ELECTIVE PROCEDURES

One of the greatest controversies in pediatric anesthesia is defining the optimal technique to induce anesthesia in a child with an open globe injury and a full stomach.[56] The issue of aspiration while securing the airway versus the possible extravasation of intraocular contents caused by an increase in IOP is a difficult risk/benefit assessment. The debate is likely to continue because the risks are real and the incidence of either phenomenon is rare, difficult to study, and probably underreported.

Among adults, aspiration is an uncommon event with a small mortality rate. The incidence of aspiration in children is ~1/10,000 elective cases but is greater in emergent cases; mortality secondary to aspiration is less than 1/200,000 children.[68–71] The use of succinylcholine for rapid-sequence induction in the treatment of a perforated globe has been challenged because of its known propensity to increase IOP. High-dose rocuronium (1.2 mg/kg) has an onset equivalent to that of succinylcholine, provides excellent intubating conditions,[72] and offers the advantage of reducing IOP by blocking the neuromuscular junction of extraocular muscles. However, if the child is not adequately anesthetized and fully paralyzed during instrumentation of the airway, any episode of coughing, retching, or increased systolic blood pressure may increase IOP. Lidocaine (1–2 mg/kg IV) usually attenuates the hemodynamic responses to laryngoscopy and tracheal intubation, but this is not a consistent experience.[73,74] Pretreatment with opioids (0.05–0.15 μg/kg of sufentanil, 0.03 mg/kg of morphine, or 0.1 μg/kg of remifentanil) has been proposed to achieve a similar effect, although they are not consistently recommended. Opioids blunt the IOP response to intubation, but may also induce vomiting, indirectly increasing the IOP transiently.

IV access is essential for a rapid induction of anesthesia. In most instances, children with ruptured globes present with IV access because IV antibiotics must be started as soon as possible (i.e., within 6 hours of the rupture) to prevent endophthalmitis, which if untreated may result in complete loss of vision in the affected eye. In some instances, however, IV access has not been established. In this case, other options may be used to induce anesthesia. Of the approaches in the following list, the one most widely favored is ultrasound guidance:

- Ultrasound-guided IV catheter placement with topical anesthesia
- Intramuscular (IM) ketamine (and succinylcholine or rocuronium)
- Mask induction with sevoflurane or halothane
- Placement of a central line (e.g., femoral vein)
- Placement of an intraosseous needle
- Rectal methohexital or ketamine

The increase in IOP after IM succinylcholine is less than that after IV administration[75]; however, absorption of agents given IM varies widely. Although IM succinylcholine (4–5 mg/kg) will paralyze a child in 2 to 8 minutes depending on the dose, the child may cry from pain, develop hypertension, or vomit during the induction, all of which may increase IOP. Knowing that the airway reflexes are gradually lost after an IM injection in the child with a full stomach is a clinically important risk that must be considered when selecting a method to secure the airway. Placement of a central line may be challenging and potentially risky in a nonsedated or uncooperative child, although ultrasound has been used to secure femoral access.

Some clinicians recommend placement of an intraosseous needle for induction when IV access has not already been established. Even when preceded by local anesthesia infiltrated into the site of insertion of the needle, placement of an intraosseous needle may be poorly tolerated in conscious children, although the pain upon insertion is much less than when fluids are infused rapidly.

Despite the presence of a full stomach, a mask induction with sevoflurane may be used, but a deeper plane of anesthesia is required before inserting an IV line or manipulating the airway because coughing and vomiting may occur with a light plane of anesthesia. IV access should then be established. If this is unsuccessful, an IM dose of a neuromuscular blocking drug may be administered.[76–78] In this circumstance, IOP may increase and regurgitation remains a possibility. Rectal methohexital (30 mg/kg) is used only in infants; if the child evacuates part of the dose, induction is incomplete.[79] Because there is no reliable absorption of neuromuscular relaxant rectally, IM or IV administration is necessary.

A moderate approach to the child who needs emergent or urgent ophthalmologic surgery is to secure IV access as quickly and painlessly as possible (ultrasound with topical analgesia). An attempt is made to preoxygenate the child without causing distress. If a tight mask fit is not easily achieved, forcing the tight fit to the child's face is not desirable because of the likelihood of increasing the IOP as the child resists. Anesthesia may be induced via IV access with lidocaine, propofol, and rocuronium. After 30 to 60 seconds by the clock or with train-of-four monitoring, tracheal intubation is expeditiously performed and gastric contents evacuated. The ophthalmologist should be intimately involved in the induction. He or she can physically protect the injured eye with a metal or plastic shield to prevent further injury and assist the anesthesiologist by holding the tracheal tube and suction apparatus immediately within reach of the field of view of the airway, our preferred team approach.

Other urgent procedures may include treatment of retinopathy or decompression of orbital cellulitis. These procedures may be urgent but still allow several hours of *nil per os* (NPO) status. Concern about aspiration may not be as great. Nonetheless, the surgeon will wish to proceed as expeditiously as is safe. Options for induction and maintenance may or may not include succinylcholine.

Most ophthalmologic procedures are performed on a scheduled basis, allowing routine preoperative evaluation and planning. This includes establishing all relevant medical information about the child, implementing NPO status, and placing an IV catheter if desired.

INDUCTION AND MAINTENANCE OF ANESTHESIA

Infants do not generally require a premedicant for anxiolysis, and the use of premedication after the first year of life is usually discussed between the anesthesiologist and the parents and child. Separation anxiety or struggling during induction usually does not affect most ophthalmologic diagnoses, except for a penetrating eye injury, which may become worse if the child struggles. IV propofol, etomidate, or ketamine produce a smooth induction, as does an inhalational induction with oxygen, nitrous oxide, and sevoflurane or halothane. If laryngospasm develops during induction, an IV bolus of propofol (1–2 mg/kg IV) should be promptly administered. Atropine (20 μg/kg) may be given IV or IM before bradycardia occurs. IM succinylcholine or rocuronium may also break laryngospasm if an IV catheter has not been placed.[70–74,76–78,80–82] For elective tracheal intubation, an IV nondepolarizing muscle relaxant is preferred because succinylcholine may increases the IOP.

Alternative induction methods include IM ketamine (4–10 mg/kg) and, in infants, rectal methohexital (25–30 mg/kg). Ketamine may increase IOP, but it has been successfully used in ophthalmologic procedures in children.[62] Rectal methohexital has a dependable latency to induction of general anesthesia of 7 to 8 minutes, but its elimination can vary widely and its respiratory depressant effects may linger (see Chapter 7). Currently, rectal methohexital is infrequently used.

Tracheal intubation is our preference for most pediatric ophthalmologic procedures, except for a brief EUA or nasolacrimal duct probing. With the tracheal tube secured, the child and operating table may be safely turned 90 or 180 degrees for optimal positioning of the table and child for surgery.

An immobile child may be essential to ensure the optimal surgical outcome. If the surgeon requires immobility, a tracheal tube should be placed and neuromuscular relaxants administered. A cuffed or uncuffed oral Ring-Adair-Elwyn preformed tracheal tube (Mallinckrodt, Inc. St. Louis, MO) or straight tracheal tube may be used. The tracheal tube is secured so that the sterile surgical field is maintained during the procedure. Access to the tracheal tube and anesthesia circuit by the anesthesia care team without trespass of the surgical field is imperative. Extensions to the individual limbs of the anesthetic circle circuit have no bearing on the dead space of the breathing circuit, whereas extensions between the Y connector in the circuit and the patient (i.e., adjacent to the tracheal tube) add dead space that may increase $PaCO_2$.

Anesthesia can be maintained with a variety of techniques. Inhalational sevoflurane, isoflurane, or desflurane provide excellent conditions for maintenance of anesthesia[64] and rapid emergence. Total IV anesthesia is also gaining popularity (see Chapter 8) and reduces PONV. When neuromuscular blockade is necessary to reduce the potential for movement, we routinely use nondepolarizing neuromuscular relaxants and train-of-four monitoring to ensure the adequacy of neuromuscular blockade. Carefully titrated doses of opioids are used as an anesthetic adjunct if postoperative pain is anticipated.

The anesthetic and type of surgery affect the incidence of PONV. Strabismus surgery in children is associated with the greatest incidence (45%–85%) of PONV.[83,84] The type of ventilation does not attenuate the incidence of PONV.[85] Large-volume (30 mL/kg) balanced salt solution replacement significantly decreases the incidence of PONV after strabismus surgery.[86] Avoiding opioids during strabismus surgery may also be effective.[87,88] Nonopioid analgesics such as acetaminophen,[89] diclofenac,[90] and ketorolac[87,88] may be used. If opioids are needed, short-acting medications are preferred: remifentanil, alfentanil, or fentanyl. Some evidence suggests that the more extraocular muscles that require surgery and specific muscles that require more traction (e.g., inferior oblique), the greater the incidence of PONV, although these data have not been firmly established.

A host of medications can significantly affect the risk of PONV.[91] Preoperative use of benzodiazepines,[92] avoidance of nitrous oxide,[93] and superhydration with balanced salt solutions[86]; use of propofol,[93,94] clonidine,[95] 5-HT$_3$ receptor antagonists,[96-100] dimenhydrinate,[101,102] metoclopramide,[100,103] or dexamethasone[104-108]; and delaying oral fluid ingestion after surgery[109] attenuate the incidence of PONV. With clonidine and 5-HT$_3$ receptor blockers, but not dexamethasone, there is a dose-response relationship with PONV.[95,96,104] Older antiemetics such as droperidol that have been very effective in attenuating the incidence of PONV[89,110-113] have fallen into disfavor because of their sedative side effects and concerns associated with prolonged QT intervals,[114] although the latter has not been a common problem in children.[115] Anesthesiologists have adopted a multimodal approach to PONV in the case of strabismus surgery.[115] A commonly used regimen includes premedication with oral midazolam, choice of anesthesia, superhydration with IV fluid, and the combination of 5-HT$_3$ receptor antagonists and dexamethasone. There is no evidence in children undergoing strabismus surgery that dosing of 5-HT$_3$ receptor antagonists at the end of surgery provides better protection against PONV than earlier in the surgery.[116] However, dosing of 5-HT$_3$ receptor antagonists during emergence in children with congenital prolonged QT interval increases the risk of adverse events.[117] There is a dichotomy of practice with respect to maintenance of anesthesia. Some avoid nitrous oxide, maintaining anesthesia by propofol infusion and including the previously mentioned supplementary medications. Others use nitrous oxide and an inhalational anesthetic for maintenance but also include the remainder of the preoperative and intraoperative supplementary medications.

IV fluid replacement can reduce PONV.[118] Children who present for elective surgery may drink clear fluids up to 2 hours before surgery, reducing the fasting period. However, it is important to identify those who have fasted for a prolonged period and to administer sufficient IV fluids to reestablish euvolemia, thus avoiding the activation of antidiuretic hormone and aldosterone that may cause fluid retention. When using balanced salt solutions, children should receive 20 to 30 mL/kg IV to reestablish euvolemia and to avoid activation of the antidiuretic hormone and aldosterone pathways. This should be followed postoperatively by a maintenance IV fluid infusion rate at one-half of the previously considered rate, using 2 mL/kg per hour for the first 10 kg, 1 mL/kg per hour for the next 10 kg, and 0.5 mL/kg per hour for every kilogram greater than 20 kg until the child takes fluids by mouth.[119-121] The incidence of PONV is reduced when large volumes of balanced salt solution (20–30 mL/kg) are administered intraoperatively compared with smaller volumes (10 mL/kg).[86] When the surgical procedure is not likely to involve an increased IOP, we routinely replace almost 100% of the calculated deficit. We have not observed children to experience urinary retention or hypertension from this strategy, most likely because children can redistribute the excess fluid more efficiently than adults.[122] However, if the duration of surgery exceeds 3 hours, we catheterize the bladder to reduce the risk of urinary retention and overdistention of the bladder.

At the completion of surgery, neuromuscular blockade is antagonized, maintenance agents are discontinued, and the child is allowed to awaken. Deep extubation is preferred by some to reduce coughing and increases in IOP at the time of extubation.[123] Others prefer extubating the trachea when the child is fully awake with intact airway reflexes, although coughing and increases in IOP may occur. For most procedures in children, a short interval of increased IOP does not damage a surgical correction, such as strabismus, ptosis, or ROP treatment. Appropriate postoperative analgesics may include local anesthetics, acetaminophen, and opioids. Nonsteroidal agents usually are not given to these children owing to concerns about perioperative bleeding at the surgical site because of their mild anticoagulant profile, but ketorolac has been useful.[87] Lorazepam may also have some utility.[92] Postoperatively, withholding oral fluids until the child expresses a desire to drink reduces the incidence of PONV.[109]

Specific Ophthalmologic Procedures

Strabismus repair is common in children.[99] Corrective surgery realigns the divergent visual axes of the eyes by detaching and reattaching extraocular muscles to the globes (Fig. 34.4). The procedures may be brief if only one or two muscles are involved. In infants, inhalational or IV induction is performed, and neuromuscular blockade is provided with nondepolarizing neuromuscular blocking drugs. Strabismus may be an isolated finding in a child or a manifestation of other systemic diseases or syndromes.[124] The anesthesiologist should carefully review the birth history, history of prematurity, CNS, disorders, syndrome identification, possible coexistent myopathy, and cardiovascular and respiratory history. If OCR is anticipated, prophylactic prevention with IV atropine or glycopyrrolate may be warranted. PONV is common and may be reduced by multiple strategies (Table 34.4).

We usually avoid the routine use of succinylcholine in children; however, in this circumstance, if succinylcholine is used, the surgeon should be informed because it may alter the forced duction testing and affect the planned repair.[125] After induction of anesthesia and tracheal intubation, the operating room table is rotated to permit complete access to the orbits. It is common to use a preformed tube that lies flat against the mandible.[126] The tracheal tube is positioned away from the surgical field. Ventilation may be spontaneous or controlled if the surgery is extraocular. If the surgery is intraocular or medical conditions dictate, controlled ventilation should be considered. Some anesthesiologists are willing to perform strabismus repair using an LMA with spontaneous ventilation.[127] Although regional block is performed in some adults, strabismus surgery in children is routinely performed with general anesthesia.

ANTERIOR CHAMBER PARACENTESIS

An anterior chamber paracentesis may be performed in children for evaluation of uveitis, infection,[128] or leukemia[129] or for removal of fluid to decrease IOP. Because the field needs to be sterile and

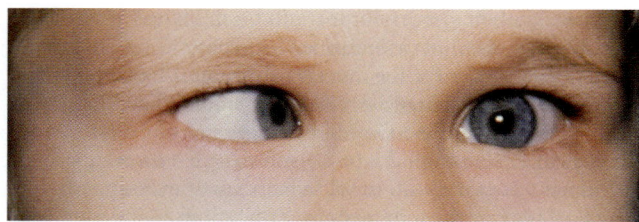

FIGURE 34.4 Strabismus repair is a common pediatric ophthalmologic procedure. The child demonstrates significant right esotropia that requires surgical correction.

TABLE 34.4	Antiemetic Strategies for Prophylaxis and Treatment of Postoperative Nausea and Vomiting
Strategy	**Drug and Dose**
Butyrophenone (dopamine antagonist)	Droperidol (10–70 μg/kg)
Serotonin (5HT$_3$ receptor antagonists)	Ondansetron (0.1 mg/kg) Granisetron (10–40 μg/kg) Dolasetron (0.35 mg/kg)
Propofol-based total IV anesthesia	Propofol (100–175 μg/kg per minute)
Local anesthetic	Lidocaine local-topical and systemic (1–1.5 mg/kg)
Opioid-sparing analgesics or anesthetics	Retrobulbar block with bupivacaine
Other pharmacology	Dexamethasone (10–500 μg/kg); maximum, 8 mg
	Dimenhydrinate (0.5–1 mg/kg)
	Metoclopramide (0.15–0.25 mg/kg)
	Benzodiazepines (e.g., lorazepam, midazolam) (10–100 μg/kg)
	Avoid nitrous oxide (N$_2$O)
	Avoid opioids
	Use ketorolac (Toradol) (0.5 mg/kg PO, IV, IM), acetaminophen (30–40 mg/kg PR or 15 mg/kg IV), or diclofenac (1 mg/kg PR), or short-acting opioids (e.g., remifentanil, alfentanil, fentanyl)
Nonpharmacologic adjuvants	IV hydration
	Gastric decompression

IV, intravenous; *IM,* intramuscular; *PO,* per os (oral); *PR,* per rectum (suppository).

the needle must enter a small target area of the anterior chamber, the child should undergo general anesthesia to make the field immobile for the surgeon.

DACRYOCYSTORHINOSTOMY

Infants may be born with nasolacrimal duct stenosis (i.e., congenital dacryostenosis) (Fig. 34.5 and E-Fig. 34.4). If conservative measures do not improve the drainage of tears, the ophthalmologist may need to dilate the duct or pierce a hole in the intact membrane using a metal probe.[130,131] These infants are induced with general anesthesia, and when the level of anesthesia is sufficient, the ophthalmologist completes the procedure in a few minutes. To confirm that the duct is patent, the ophthalmologist should establish metal-metal contact using one probe within the duct and a second probe within the nostril.[132] Alternatively, the ophthalmologist may inject

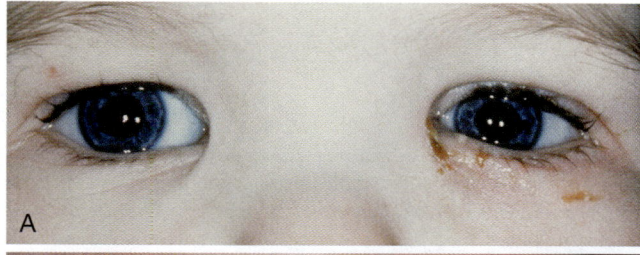
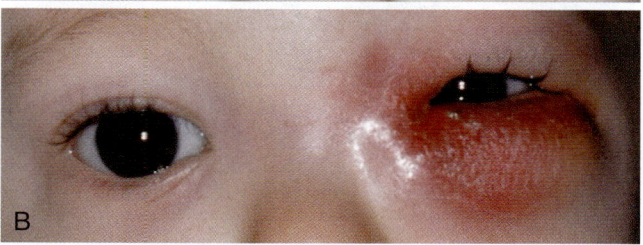

FIGURE 34.5 Nasolacrimal duct obstruction manifests with different degrees of infraorbital inflammation, from mild obstruction with minor infection and mucoid material accumulation **(A)** to severe obstruction with periorbital or preseptal cellulitis **(B)**. Both may require dacryocystorhinostomies.

fluorescein into the nasolacrimal duct and detect the fluorescein on a pipe cleaner in the nasal airway. In both instances, fluorescein or blood may reach the larynx and trigger breath-holding or laryngospasm. To avoid this, it is prudent to tilt the operating table to a 5- to 10-degree Trendelenburg position and place a small roll under the child's shoulders to pool the fluids away from the larynx. These secretions are suctioned out of the oropharynx and nasopharynx before emergence. Anesthesia may be maintained by face mask inhalation or with IV agents. The infant is awakened, and postoperative analgesia may be offered with acetaminophen or opioids, or both, as necessary.

Alternatively, an endonasal endoscopic approach may be used for complicated or recurrent dacryorhinocystotomy.[133,134] Endoscopic-assisted probing significantly increases the duration of the procedure and requires airway control to facilitate the surgeon's approach and to protect the child from aspirating blood during the procedure, but this approach yields results similar to an external approach.[135] In older children with bilateral obstruction, endoscope-assisted probing increased the long-term success rate.[136]

PTOSIS REPAIR

Ptosis (i.e., blepharoptosis) means "drooping of the eyelid." This condition can be congenital or acquired, and it may be associated with amblyopia or astigmatism. If eyelid closure is complete in infancy, occlusion amblyopia will occur, and this may require urgent attention. Otherwise, surgery for ptosis is often performed in later childhood. These children should be investigated for an underlying disease (e.g., muscle diseases such as myasthenia gravis, malignant hyperthermia).[137] The surgical approaches require a quiet surgical field, and the surgeon makes a great effort to produce a symmetric repair.

CATARACT SURGERY

Cataracts are opacifications of the lens of the eye (Fig. 34.6). Cataracts in children may be congenital, posttraumatic, or metabolic in origin.[138] Congenital cataracts require surgery very early in life to permit photostimulation of the retina.[139] Although the surgery can be performed as an outpatient, the formerly premature and young infant may require monitoring for postoperative anesthetic-induced

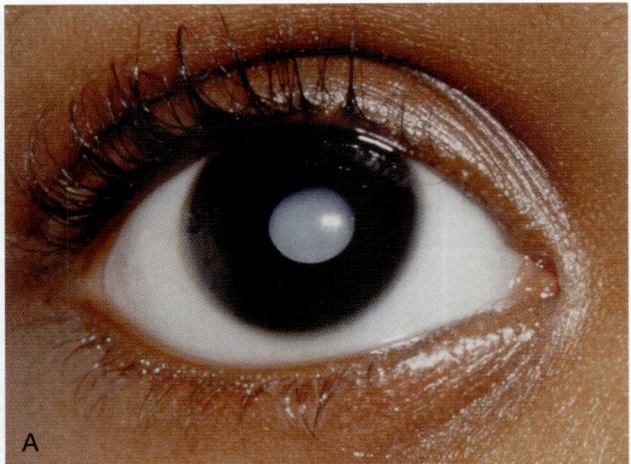

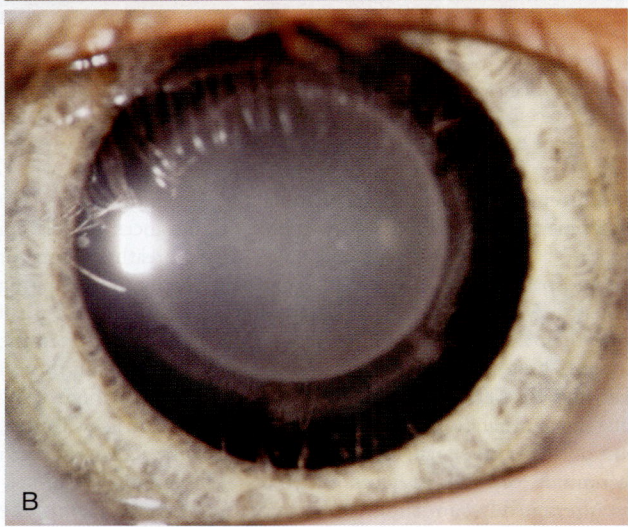

FIGURE 34.6 A, The right red reflex is absent in a child with a cataract that requires removal. **B,** The close-up photograph shows a nuclear cataract, which is associated with many inborn errors of metabolism in childhood. Cataracts that are not central or spherical may be caused by trauma or abuse.

respiratory depression or apnea. Cataracts are associated with some systemic diseases, and intraocular lens implants are often offered to improve the long-term visual prognosis.[140] The child should be examined carefully for dysmorphology, with close attention to issues of airway management and the cardiorespiratory system. One study demonstrated superior postoperative analgesia with a subtenon block compared with IV fentanyl.[141]

RETINOBLASTOMA

Retinoblasoma occurs in about 9000 children yearly.[142,143] Mutations in specific genes are believed to cause these tumors, which are the most common primary malignant tumors in children. The pathognomonic defect is a mutation in the *RB1* gene on chromosome 13. These tumors have a strong familial and hereditary component with sporadic mutations and may be unilateral or bilateral.[144] They are most commonly recognized by a lack of the typical red light reflex in the infant's pupil.[145] Treatment includes chemotherapy,[146] injection of bevacizumab,[147,148] intraarterial chemotherapy, and multiple treatments with proton beam radiation.[149,150] Many children retain useful vision with proton beam

treatments and there does not seem to be an increased incidence of associated secondary malignacy.[151] These children require multiple anesthetics for the initial evaluation, CT planning, and construction of a fiberglass mask for immobilization during treatments. This is then followed by placement of central venous access, which allows all 25 to 30 subsequent treatments to be performed under deep propofol sedation with maintenance of a natural airway with spontaneous respirations. Children with extraocular disease are treated with larger doses of chemotherapy followed by delayed enucleation.[152]

ENUCLEATION

Enucleation of the eye may be necessary when a child has an intraocular tumor (e.g., retinoblastoma) (Fig. 34.7),[153] a ruptured globe or ocular trauma,[154] recurrent or chronic infections, or a blind, painful eye. *Leukocoria* is the term meaning "white pupil." The differential diagnosis is extensive and includes many intraocular tumors. Other disorders causing leukocoria include Coats disease, cataract, coloboma, and *Toxocara canis* infection. When necessary, the entire globe must be removed, and all bleeding points are coagulated. The OCR may occur during this procedure and may be attenuated by infiltration with a local anesthetic. Prophylactic antiemetics are often administered because PONV is common.

VITRECTOMY

Vitrectomy may be necessary for retinal injury or detachment induced in circumstances of nonaccidental trauma or ROP.[155] Any infant or child presenting acutely with a closed head injury from suspected abuse should have an ophthalmologic consultation to completely evaluate all orbital structures.[156] These delicate tissues may demonstrate pathology that requires long-term follow-up or urgent medical or surgical therapy. Glaucoma may occur with hyphema or lens subluxation or dislocation with tearing of the support tissue. Early diagnosis is paramount if surgical intervention is to have the greatest benefit.

RETINOPATHY OF PREMATURITY TREATMENT

Preterm infants may present with multiple ocular pathologic conditions, but none is more common than ROP. It has been extensively studied,[20] and multiple collaborative trials have reported their results and recommendations for medical and surgical interventions, including intravitreal bevacizumab.[157–166] The cause is unknown, but oxygen-related theories have been described for more than 40 years. Because of this concern, oxygen range targeting has become common[167–169] to reduce the oxidative stress[170] on the infant in general and to reduce the effect of oxygen on neovascularization in the eye.

Laser and cryotherapy are common treatments for this condition.[157,158] Because of the delicacy and exacting accuracy required in laser procedures, we routinely intubate the trachea and use neuromuscular relaxants. This facilitates the immobile field necessary for the surgeon and provides better perioperative physiologic stability for the infant.[171] The complications of prematurity determine whether extubation is possible, and many infants require postoperative ventilation, if only for a brief period or overnight.[172] The operative environment should be kept warm to reduce thermal stress on the infant.

ACKNOWLEDGMENT

We wish to acknowledge the prior contributions to this chapter of Susan A. Vassallo, MD, and Lynne R. Ferrari, MD.

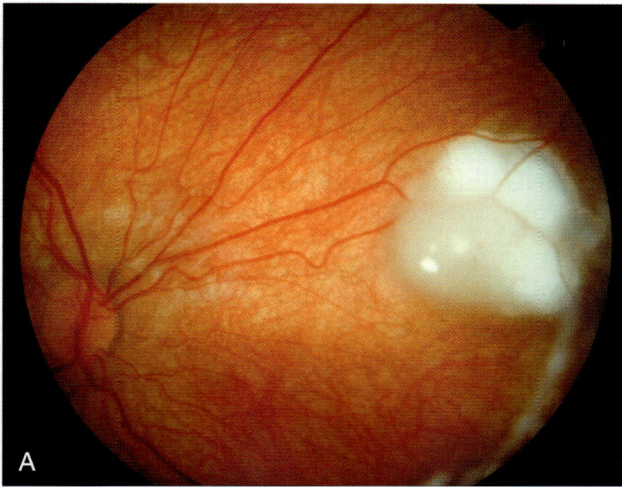
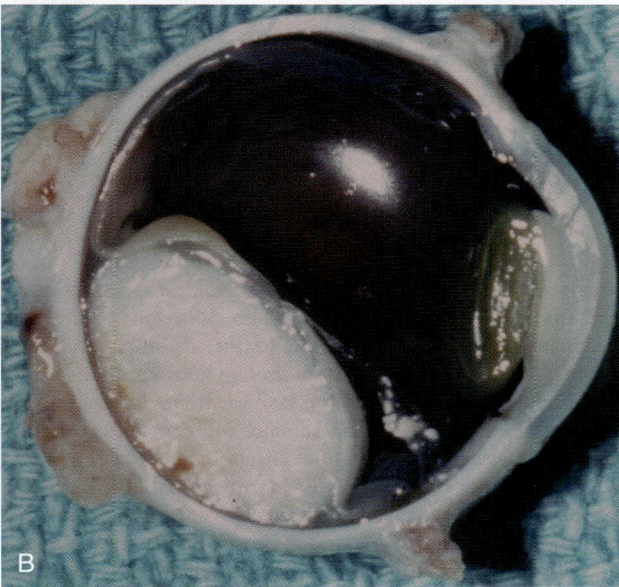

FIGURE 34.7 Retinoblastoma is one of many intraocular tumors that may require enucleation. **A,** Retinoblastoma seen by direct ophthalmoscopy. **B,** Pathologic specimen of a retinoblastoma in the globe after enucleation.

ANNOTATED REFERENCES

Cunningham AJ, Barry P. Intraocular pressure–physiology and implications for anaesthetic management. *Can Anaesth Soc J.* 1986;33:195-208.

This review elegantly details the physiology of intraocular pressure and conditions that may increase it. Structural, physiologic, and pharmacologic considerations are reviewed in detail.

Donahue SP. Clinical practice. Pediatric strabismus. *N Engl J Med.* 2007;356:1040-1047.

Strabismus is a common presenting condition requiring surgical therapy in children. Significant improvements in the detection and treatment of strabismus are reviewed. Surgical approaches and recent advances are presented.

Lewanda AF, Matisoff A, Revenis M, et al. Preoperative evaluation and comprehensive risk assessment for children with Down syndrome. *Pediatr Anesth.* 2016;26:356-362.

Children with Down syndrome have multiple systemic conditions of importance to the anesthesiologist. They are not exclusively of interest owing to CHD. Anesthesia-related complications occur more frequently in children with Down syndrome than other children presenting for noncardiac surgery, and prevention of complications is essential by means of thorough evaluation and planning, particularly appropriate consultation with cardiologists regarding residual or current CHD and the possibility of cervical spine instability.

Saugstad OD, Aune D. In search of the optimal oxygen saturation for extremely low birth weight infants: a systematic review and meta-analysis. *Neonatology.* 2011;100:1-8.

Advances in neonatology continue to reduce morbidity and mortality for these fragile children. Oxygen-saturation targeting is becoming a mainstream technique. This has implications for the management and oxygen support strategies for infants coming to the operating room for ocular and other surgical procedures. Because volatile anesthetics impair hypoxic pulmonary vasoconstriction, a supplemental oxygen requirement should be anticipated, but oxygen-saturation targets should be considered for optimal care.

Shen YD, Chen CY, Wu CH, et al. Dexamethasone, ondansetron, and their combination and postoperative nausea and vomiting in children undergoing strabismus surgery: a meta-analysis of randomized controlled trials. *Paediatr Anaesth.* 2014;24(5):490-498.

This metaanalysis examined 13 randomized controlled trials and found that PONV occurred in 68% of placebo-treated children compared with 34% of dexamethasone-treated children and 37% of ondansetron-treated children. The combination was significantly more effective at reducing PONV than either drug alone.

Stephen E, Dickson J, Kindley AD, et al. Surveillance of vision and ocular disorders in children with Down syndrome. *Dev Med Child Neurol.* 2007;49:513-515.

Children with Down syndrome have many different ocular disorders. In addition to the multiple systemic issues of concern for the anesthesiologist described in the chapter, this reference provides insight into the ocular diseases that may require surgical therapy.

A complete reference list can be found online at ExpertConsult.com.

34

35 Plastic and Reconstructive Surgery

PAUL A. STRICKER, JOHN E. FIADJOE, AND JERROLD LERMAN

PEDIATRIC PLASTIC SURGERY is performed in children of all ages, even in utero.[1] However, the majority of children who undergo plastic surgical and reconstructive procedures are between 2 and 9 years of age, with a median age of 5 years. A wide spectrum of associated craniofacial abnormalities, underlying medical conditions, and surgical procedures characterizes this pediatric population. Consequently, a thorough preoperative assessment, consultation with medical and surgical teams, and anticipation and preparation for potential complications are of paramount importance to ensure a successful perioperative outcome. Many procedures are performed on the head and neck and require thoughtful coordination between the anesthesiologist and surgeon. A thorough understanding of the procedure allows for selection of the optimal anesthetic plan. The incidence of major morbidity and mortality has been reduced over the past 30 years from 16.5% and 1.6% to less than 0.1% and 0.1%, respectively, in children undergoing major craniofacial surgeries.[2]

Cleft Lip and Palate

Cleft lip and palate are among the more common congenital malformations, occurring with an estimated incidence of approximately 1 in 600 births worldwide.[3,4] More common in males than in females and more common in Asians and Latin Americans and least in Africans, this malformation likely results from both environmental and genetic causes. Parental occupation, in particular paternal farming, increases the risk of cleft lip or palate in the offspring, whereas the maternal occupation presents no additional risk.[5] Folate metabolism disturbances and increased maternal homocysteine concentrations also may be contributory.[6] Cleft lip with or without cleft palate has been linked to several loci on chromosomes 1, 2, 4, 6, 14, 17, 19, and 22, suggesting a genetic basis for some of these anomalies.[7–10] Three genes have been associated with syndromic cleft lip and palate: T-box transcription factor-22, poliovirus receptor–like-1, and interferon regulatory factor-6 (IRF6). Gene mutations have been identified in only a small fraction of nonsyndromic cleft lip and palate.

These disorders are associated with more than 400 syndromes; the more common syndromes are presented in Table 35.1. Cleft lip and palate begin as a defect in palatal growth in the first trimester of pregnancy. Fetal magnetic resonance imaging (MRI) provides a greater degree of resolution of defects in the posterior palate and lateral extent of cleft with greater diagnostic accuracy than ultrasound. MRI also enables early detection of potential syndromic conditions by providing a complete study of the fetal head and biometric development of the facial bones.[11]

Primary cleft lip repair is usually undertaken at approximately 2 to 3 months of age, whereas primary cleft palate repair occurs at 6 to 10 months. Surgery for lip or nose revision usually takes place in early childhood, and palatal revision and alveolar bone grafts occur at approximately 10 years of age. Rhinoplasty and maxillary osteotomy to complete the repair may take place at 17 to 20 years of age. Pharyngoplasty may be required for velopharyngeal incompetence secondary to anatomic or neurologic dysfunction to improve speech development and prevent nasal regurgitation during eating.

ANESTHETIC CONSIDERATIONS

Surgical correction of a cleft lip defect is usually performed at 2 to 3 months of age to allow sufficient time for maturation and associated abnormalities to become apparent. Preoperative assessment may reveal abnormalities such as mandibular hypoplasia in Pierre Robin sequence (PRS) (Fig. 35.1 and E-Fig. 35.1) or restricted neck movement as in Klippel-Feil syndrome (E-Fig. 35.2).[3] PRS is defined as the triad of micrognathia, glossoptosis (caudally displaced insertion of the tongue), and respiratory distress in the first 24 to 48 hours after birth. The presence of other anomalies might warrant additional clinical or laboratory investigations. Cleft lip repair usually involves minimal blood loss, so for children with hematocrit values greater than 30%, additional preoperative

TABLE 35.1	Syndromes Commonly Associated With Cleft Lip and Palate
Pierre Robin sequence	
Down syndrome	
Klippel-Feil syndrome	
Treacher Collins syndrome	
Velocardiofacial syndrome	
Fetal alcoho syndrome	
Nager syndrome	
Goldenhar syndrome	

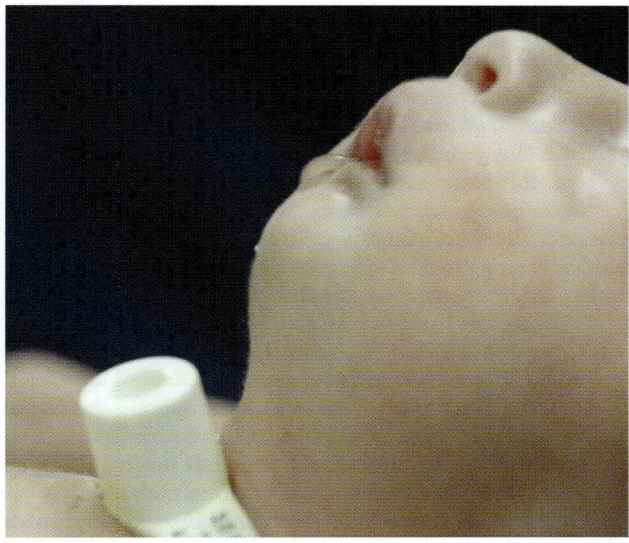

FIGURE 35.1 Child with Pierre Robin sequence who required a tracheostomy because of respiratory distress in the first 24 hours postnatally. The retrognathia is often associated with glossoptosis, which makes visualization of the glottic aperture more difficult.

laboratory testing is unnecessary. A sample for type and screen is usually sufficient for infants with a hematocrit value less than 30%.[12]

The frequency of difficult airways in children with cleft lip and palate varies from 2.9% to 23%.[13–17] The incidence of difficult intubation in children with bilateral cleft is greater than that with unilateral cleft.[15] Furthermore, micrognathia is an independent predictor of a difficult airway. The incidence of difficult direct laryngoscopy is approximately 50% in children with micrognathia but only about 4% in those without. In infants and young children, micrognathia may be subtle and not always easily detected. However, the presence of microtia, which is associated with a 42% incidence of difficult intubation with bilateral compared with 2% with unilateral microtia, should prompt a closer examination of the mandible for hypoplastic growth and raise the possibility of a hemifacial microsomia or Treacher Collins syndrome.[18] Intubation difficulty (by direct laryngoscopy) with isolated micrognathia decreases with increasing age, with the greatest difficulty presenting in infants younger than 6 months. This has been attributed to rapid growth of the mandible, which catches up to the maxilla, thereby aligning the two bones, by 2 years of age in most cases. A careful review of previous anesthetic records may forewarn of a difficult airway. In a second study that reported the frequency of difficult intubations in young infants with cleft lip, cleft palate without PRS, cleft-lip-palate and cleft palate, and

cleft palate with PRS was 0, 2.7%, 10%, and 23%.[17] Difficult airways increased with early airway and feeding problems (P < 0.0001). In the isolated cleft palate, a wider cleft was associated with a significantly more difficult laryngoscopy.

Induction of anesthesia via face mask is usually uncomplicated in infants with cleft lip and palate. Laryngoscopy should be performed using a straight blade via a right paraglossal approach (blade inserted into the pharyngeal gutter with tongue displaced to the left),[19] taking care to avoid dropping the blade into the cleft (see also Fig. 14.28A-C). If the mandible is hypoplastic, external laryngeal manipulation may be required to bring the larynx into view. In some centers, the tongue is sutured to either the mandible or lower lip to preclude airway obstruction in infants with PRS in the postnatal period. In such instances, the tongue cannot be displaced to the left to expose the larynx. To facilitate laryngoscopy in such cases, the tongue is first released from the lower lip using ketamine sedation followed by direct laryngoscopy. Alternatively, selection of a primary airway management strategy other than direct laryngoscopy (e.g., video laryngoscopy, fiberoptic intubation through a supraglottic airway) circumvents this problem and may be a preferable approach with a greater success rate on the first attempt (see Chapter 14).[20]

A variety of tracheal tubes can be used to secure the airway for cleft lip and palate surgery, although the ideal tracheal tube is perhaps the oral Ring-Adair-Elwyn (RAE) tube, which can be fixed centrally to the chin to facilitate optimal surgical access. It should be noted that preformed tracheal tubes vary in length from bend to tip for uncuffed and cuffed tubes.[21] Seven brands of preformed tracheal tubes were compared for the same size inner diameter tubes; the distance from the bend to the tip varied by 0 to 1 cm for oral cuffed tubes but 0 to 4 cm for uncuffed oral tubes. Of greater concern was that the variability for preformed nasal tubes was even greater; cuffed nasal tubes varied by 0 to 5.5 cm and uncuffed varied from 2 to 9 cm (bend to tip). The risk of an endobronchial intubation when a cuffed oral preformed tube replaced an uncuffed tube of the same diameter was 0%–27%, whereas when a cuffed nasal preformed tube replaced an uncuffed tube of the same size, the risk of an endobronchial intubation increased to 50%–100%. Thus the risk for endobronchial intubation varies among manufacturers and is greater with nasal than oral preformed tracheal tubes.

Throat packs usually impinge on the surgical field and are not normally required for cleft palate repair. Ventilation is usually controlled for the duration of the procedure (~1–2 hours). Inhalational or intravenous (IV) anesthetics combined with a short-acting opioid such as fentanyl (1–2 µg/kg) can be used for maintenance of anesthesia. Bilateral infraorbital nerve blocks may be used to provide postoperative analgesia for cleft lip repairs (see Fig. 42.12A-C and Chapter 42 videos). Such blocks reduce the need for opioids and antiemetics, improve the ability to feed,[22,23] and increase parental satisfaction.[24] Additional evidence suggests that the incidence of emergence agitation is reduced with the use of infraorbital nerve blocks.[25] A combination of infraorbital and external nasal nerve blocks for pain control after cleft lip repair is an alternative.[26]

During cleft palate surgery, the pharyngeal space is reduced dramatically; postoperative nasal trumpets may be required (often placed by the surgeon) to maintain airway patency and permit suctioning the airway without damaging the palatal repair (Fig. 35.2 and E-Fig. 35.3A and B). At the end of surgery, the trachea is extubated after the upper airway reflexes have returned and the child is completely awake. These children are at particular risk

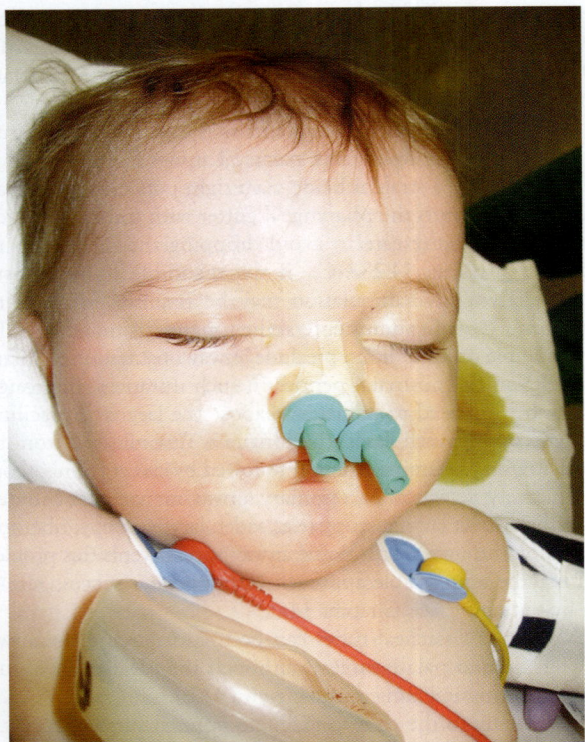

FIGURE 35.2 Nasal airways are often placed at the end of cleft palate or pharyngoplasty surgery to ensure that a patent airway is maintained.

TABLE 35.2	Classification of Craniosynostosis
Nonsyndromic (primary) ~80%: Single suture closed, isolated finding	
Syndromic ~20%: Two or more sutures closed, often with associated clinical findings. More than 150 syndromes have been described; the more common syndromes are as follows:	
Crouzon	
Apert	
Pfeiffer	
Saethre-Chotzen	
Carpenter (acrocephalopolysyndactyly type II)	
Muenke	
Crouzonodermoskeletal	
Shprintzen-Goldberg	
Loeys-Dietz	
Jackson-Weiss	
Beare-Stevenson	
Cole-Carpenter	
Kleeblattschädel	
Fibroblast growth factor receptor mutations 1 and 2	
Metabolic and other causes	
Rickets	
Bone metabolic disorders (hypophosphatasia)	
Achondroplasia	
Prematurity	

for acute upper airway obstruction in the immediate postextubation period as a result of upper airway narrowing, edema, blood, and residual anesthetic effects.[27–32] Accordingly, it is very important to extubate the trachea only when the child is completely awake. Intraoperative dexamethasone (0.5 mg/kg) may be administered to mitigate postoperative airway edema. Late postoperative edema[33] and severe subcutaneous emphysema are additional complications. Upper respiratory tract infections are common in this age group. If airway infections are present, they should weigh heavily in favor of delaying surgery until they are resolved. Antibiotics may reduce the incidence of postoperative respiratory complications.[34] Adverse airway events, including postoperative airway obstruction, oxyhemoglobin desaturation, bronchospasm, laryngospasm, reintubation, and unplanned postoperative intensive care unit (ICU) admission have been identified in as many as 23% of children undergoing cleft palate repair[35]; the presence of a craniofacial syndrome, history of preoperative airway problems, and both surgeon and anesthesiologist inexperience were significantly associated with airway complications.

Arm restraints are used in many centers to prevent suture disruption. These children are monitored for signs of upper airway obstruction during the recovery period for approximately 48 hours.[27] As soon as the child is awake, feeding with clear fluids is allowed. Postoperative pain is managed with a combination of opioids and acetaminophen. Rectal acetaminophen administered before surgery did not reduce postoperative opioid requirements in children undergoing cleft palate repair. In part this may be attributed to local infiltration at the surgical site and the slow and variable absorption of acetaminophen by the rectal route. However, IV acetaminophen has opioid-sparing effects in these children that may be useful in certain scenarios.[36,37] Sphenopalatine

and infraorbital nerve blocks (see Chapter 42, Fig. 42.12) with a long-acting local anesthetic can be placed at the end of the procedure to prevent pain after cleft lip and palate repair.[22] Palatal nerve block (nasopalatine, greater and lesser palatine)[38] or a bilateral suprazygomatic maxillary nerve block reduce postoperative pain and favor early feeding.[39]

Children who are scheduled for elective pharyngoplasty are usually school age, having undergone cleft palate repair at an earlier age. The primary objective of this procedure is to restore velopharyngeal competence for speech development, which can be achieved by a pharyngeal flap, sphincter pharyngoplasty, or palatal lengthening (Furlow double-opposing Z-plasty palatoplasty). The anesthetic goals and management are similar to those discussed for cleft palate repair.

Craniosynostosis

Craniosynostosis, a congenital anomaly in which one or more cranial sutures close prematurely, occurs in approximately 1 in 2000 to 3000 births, affecting males more frequently than females.[40–42] Embryologically, the cranial vault starts to ossify at 8 weeks after conception; fusion of the parietal and frontal bones is usually completed by 7 months after conception. Postnatally, the anterolateral fontanelle closes by 3 months, the posterior fontanelle by 3 to 6 months, the anterior fontanelle by 9 to 18 months, and the posterolateral fontanelle by 2 years. Premature osseous obliteration of a bony suture might result from the absence of osteoinhibitory signals from the suture. Craniosynostosis may be categorized as simple (or nonsyndromic) (60%-80% of cases), involving closure of one suture, or complex (or syndromic) (20%–30%), involving closure of two or more sutures and is often associated with a variety of clinical features and metabolic diseases (Table 35.2).[41,43,44]

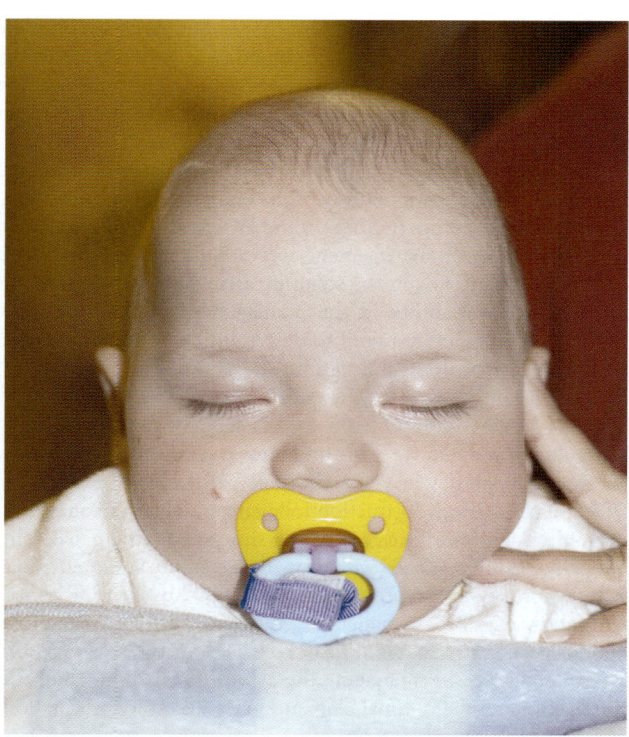

FIGURE 35.3 Infant with classic craniosynostosis. The shape of the child's head may not reflect the severity of the defect. The defect is best appreciated by three-dimensional magnetic resonance imaging reconstruction.

In the child with craniosynostosis, fusion of a cranial suture restricts normal bone growth perpendicular to the affected suture. Compensatory growth and expansion of the cranial vault occurs parallel to the affected suture, and there is a characteristic skull deformity associated with the different sutures involved (Fig. 35.3 and E-Fig. 35.4).[41] The frequency of single suture closures varies with the specific suture: sagittal (50%), coronal (20%), and metopic (10%).[43] The coronal suture (especially bicoronal synostosis) is more commonly associated with syndromic craniosynostosis. Although approximately 80% of premature suture closures are isolated defects, the remaining 20% involve multiple suture closures associated with more than 400 syndromes that present with a myriad of clinical features (see Table 35.2); the more common syndromes that require craniofacial reconstruction are described later.[41,43] Syndromic craniosynostoses are commonly associated with gene defects in the fibroblast growth factor receptor (FGFR), which is involved in bone and cartilage development.

Apert syndrome occurs in less than 1 in 100,000 live births, usually as a sporadic mutation, although autosomal dominant inheritance patterns can occur with the FGFR2 gene on chromosome 10. This syndrome phenotypically manifests as cloverleaf skull (craniosynostosis), hypertelorism, proptosis, midface hypoplasia, and syndactyly (upper or lower extremity). Development is often complicated by increased intracranial pressure (ICP) and obstructive sleep apnea (OSA).[45,46] Whether children with Apert syndrome develop normal intelligence quotients (IQs) is unclear; one study reported that 32% had IQs greater than 70.[47] The timing of cranial surgery may affect the child's IQ; surgery in the first year of life was associated with an IQ greater than 70 in more than 50% of children in one study, whereas surgery after the first year of life was associated with an IQ greater than 70 in only

7%.[47] Two other factors predicted improved IQ indexes: absence of a defect in the septum pellucidum and noninstitutional residence (i.e., family home residence). In contrast, more recent evidence failed to substantiate a salutary effect of early surgery on cognitive development. Indeed, cognitive development was related to the quality of the family environment and parental education and unrelated to brain malformation and the age of surgery.[48]

Crouzon syndrome is phenotypically similar to Apert syndrome but has different ophthalmologic defects, specifically, optic atrophy occurring in up to 20%, and the absence of hand and foot defects (e.g., syndactyly).[41,49] Fifty percent of Crouzon syndrome defects are sporadic mutations, and the remainder are familial with the same gene defect as Apert; FGFR2 on chromosome 10. Pfeiffer syndrome occurs in approximately 1 in 25,000 live births. Most cases are familial with an autosomal dominant inheritance pattern that has its origin in defects in the FGFR1 and FGFR2 genes on chromosome 10, although many remain sporadic. The phenotype of Pfeiffer syndrome is similar to that of Apert syndrome but includes broad thumb, large first toe, polydactyly, and may be associated with a cartilaginous sleeve trachea. Children with Pfeiffer syndrome have normal intelligence. Carpenter syndrome is associated with craniosynostosis, syndactyly, cardiac defects, and obesity.[50] Cognitive impairment is common.[50] Muenke syndrome is more common, occurring in 1 in 30,000 births. It results from a mutation in the FGFR3 gene. Affected patients have midface hypoplasia, ocular hypertelorism, strabismus, developmental delays, and intellectual disabilities.[41] A relatively new but rare syndrome, Shprintzen-Goldberg, is characterized by craniosynostosis and a phenotype that resembles that of Marfan syndrome.

Indications for cranial vault reconstruction include increased ICP, severe exophthalmos, OSA, craniofacial deformity, and psychosocial reasons. If uncorrected, the deformed cranium may cause severe neurologic sequelae, including visual loss and developmental delay.[51-63] Because rapid brain growth during infancy determines skull shape, surgical correction is undertaken within the first months of life to achieve the best cosmetic results.

Cranial vault reconstruction may involve the anterior or posterior aspect of the skull or both (total cranial vault reconstruction).[42] Less invasive approaches to correct craniosynostosis are available and may be associated with reduced morbidity. Surgical correction may use an open approach where the synostotic suture is excised followed by barrel-stave osteotomies to release the adjacent cranium and allow for normalization of skull shape with subsequent brain growth (Fig. 35.4 and E-Fig. 35.5). This technique is used in children younger than 6 months of age and is believed to be less invasive than total cranial vault reconstruction.[64,65] Endoscopic strip craniectomy is increasingly being used in early infancy because of benefits including reduced transfusion requirements and reduced hospital stay, compared with the open procedures. The principal disadvantage of endoscopic techniques is the requirement of 4 to 6 months of wearing a helmet postoperatively to promote normalization of skull shape.[42] Spring-assisted cranioplasty, a technique preferentially used in infants younger than 6 months, involves performing a midline osteotomy along the fused sagittal suture and placing springs across the osteotomy to increase the biparietal dimension.[42] Spring-assisted cranioplasty may be associated with reduced intraoperative blood loss, reduced transfusion requirement, and shorter duration of hospital stay.[66] In a single-center study of 100 children with spring-assisted craniosynostosis repair, no child was transfused and none was admitted to the ICU.[67] The primary disadvantage of this approach is the need for a second surgery to remove the springs. A meta-analysis

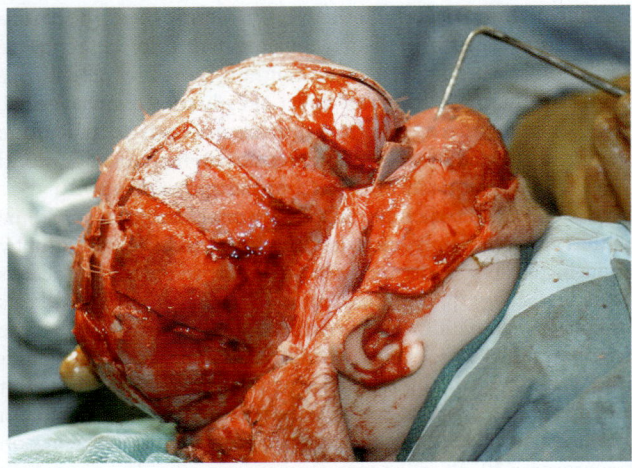

FIGURE 35.4 Child immediately before surgical closure after total cranial vault reshaping using strip craniectomy for sagittal craniosynostosis.

of the outcomes from calvarial remodeling, strip craniectomy, and spring-mediated cranioplasty in nonsyndromic sagittal synostosis demonstrated that the cephalic index (which is the ratio of the width of the outermost tables of the vault to the length of the outermost tables)[68] with calvarial vault was superior to strip craniectomy and that the former approach required more surgical time, involved more blood loss, a greater duration of stay, and greater costs than the other two approaches (P < 0.0001).[69]

The application of cranial vault distractors to achieve distraction osteogenesis is a technique increasingly used in children with syndromic forms of craniosynostosis.[70–72] This procedure involves a craniotomy (usually without reconstruction of the cut bone flap) combined with placement of distractors that are sequentially incrementally lengthened by turning an externalized screw beginning a few days postoperatively and continuing until the targeted cranial vault expansion is achieved. This technique has the advantage of shorter surgery and allows for greater expansion of the cranial vault than what can be achieved with a traditional cranial vault reconstruction. These children also need to return to the operating room for removal of the distraction hardware.

Preoperative assessment of children with craniosynostosis should focus on airway management, eye protection, and ICP. An important consideration in children with syndromic midfacial hypoplasia is its common association with OSA (50%–70% incidence) owing to associated narrowing of the nasopharyngeal space.[46,73,74] Although some recommend preoperative adenotonsillectomy to treat OSA in children with syndromic craniosynostosis, neither airway dimensions nor propensity toward airway collapse are improved. Midfacial advancement may be required to resolve OSA, and even then, residual airway obstruction may persist.[46,73] Preoperative endoscopy has been recommended to assess the severity of midfacial hypoplasia and whether OSA is likely to persist after midface advancement. Careful titration of opioids in the perioperative period is indicated if the child exhibits severe nocturnal desaturation (i.e., if the SaO$_2$ nadir is <85%) (see Chapter 33); children with OSA who have severe nocturnal desaturation require half the dose of opioids that children without nocturnal desaturation require, so a normal dose of opioid is actually a relative overdose in this population.[75] Upper airway obstruction may also occur postoperatively in children who received opioids as a direct effect of opioids on the hypoglossal nucleus.[76]

Preoperative laboratory assessment should include a complete blood cell count and a specimen for blood type, antibody screening, and crossmatching of blood. Many centers also routinely screen for coagulation abnormalities with a preoperative prothrombin time and the activated partial thromboplastin time.

Postoperative pain is generally not severe and is managed effectively with a combination of acetaminophen, nonsteroidal antiinflammatory drugs (NSAIDs), and IV opioids. Opioids remain the mainstay of pain management, but careful titration is indicated if OSA is present. Given the small incidence of craniosynostosis and the large variability in the management of these patients, multicenter trials are required to determine the optimal management strategy for these children.[77]

AIRWAY MANAGEMENT

Meticulous preoperative planning and evaluation of the airway are essential, particularly for children with known or possible OSA.[73] Upper airway obstruction following induction of anesthesia in children with midface hypoplasia should be anticipated. This is usually readily managed with a jaw-thrust/subluxation technique or insertion of an oral airway. Occasionally, however, face mask ventilation may prove challenging owing to difficulty obtaining a good mask seal.[78] External fixator devices on the face may also present challenges in managing the airway (E-Fig. 35.6), and it is essential to craft the optimal plan and make necessary preparations should problems arise (e.g., emergent hardware removal, wire cutting). A laryngeal mask is a valuable rescue tool in these scenarios and should be readily available before anesthetic induction.

In the majority of children with craniosynostosis, the anatomy of the mandible and the temporomandibular joint is normal, as are upper airway dimensions, resulting in an easy direct laryngoscopy and tracheal intubation. Rarely, mandibular hypoplasia may complicate an otherwise straightforward laryngoscopy and tracheal intubation. Abnormal neck mobility also may pose additional challenges for laryngoscopy and tracheal intubation.

BLOOD LOSS, COAGULOPATHY, AND HYPONATREMIA

Crystalloid solutions are commonly administered for minimal to moderate surgical blood loss and fluid shifts during craniosynostosis surgeries. Although lactated Ringer's solution (or Hartmann's solution) is most commonly used in North America, some advocate using normal saline solution because it may be less likely to induce hyponatremia and an acid-base disturbance than lactated Ringer's solution. However, a recent study comparing the two solutions suggests that normal saline solution is more likely to induce (metabolic) acidosis than lactated Ringer's solution in infants undergoing craniosynostosis.[79] Additionally, hyponatremia is usually mild, self-limited, and asymptomatic. The results of large adult cohort studies have demonstrated an association between hyperchloremic metabolic acidosis after normal saline and major complications, morbidity, mortality, and increased resource use.[80,81] Isotonic balanced solutions may be the best choice for crystalloid management.

Surgery for craniosynostosis is associated with the potential for cardiac arrest as a result of sudden massive blood loss or underestimated blood loss.[2,43,82,83] Although these procedures are extradural, significant bleeding from the scalp and cranium can occur, especially following inadvertent tears of dural venous sinuses. The blood loss can be so rapid during the surgery that the expression "trauma in progress" is applicable. The risks of massive blood loss and the need for invasive monitoring are primarily determined by the type of surgery.[83] In children undergoing endoscopic strip craniectomy, weight less than 5 kg, those undergoing sagittal endoscopic craniectomy, those with syndromic craniosynostosis, and earlier date of surgery are associated with blood transfusion.[84] Some centers advocate commencing blood transfusions at the time of skin incision (particularly in infants) to prevent hemodynamic instability and the need for a rapid transfusion, but this must be tempered by whether the surgery is open or endoscopic (see later discussion).

To manage the large volume and rapidity of the blood loss, it is essential to establish large-bore peripheral venous access. Central venous access (see also Figs. 49.3 and 49.4), usually via the internal jugular vein, is most commonly reserved for children in whom obtaining adequate peripheral venous access proves difficult but overall has been used in a minority of cases for rapid transfusion.[85] Strategies that are important to preclude hyperkalemic cardiac arrest include infusing blood stored less than 7 days old (see Wake Up Safe; http://www.wakeupsafe.org/Hyperkalemia_statement.pdf?201501300915; accessed January 7, 2015) and (most importantly) avoiding hypovolemia.[86,87] If only older blood is available, it should be warmed and administered slowly through a peripheral IV line to reduce the risk that hyperkalemia is present when the blood reaches the right atrium.[42] Estimation of ongoing blood loss can be difficult because of the use of large volumes of irrigation fluid and difficulty quantifying blood loss onto surgical drapes and gowns.[88] Invasive arterial blood pressure monitoring and serial blood gas sampling are indicated in this type of surgery (see Fig. 49.11A-D). A urinary catheter should be inserted to monitor urine output.

Several blood conservation strategies have been proposed for this type of surgery, including preoperative recombinant human erythropoietin, acute normovolemic hemodilution, antifibrinolytics, and induced hypotension (see Chapter 12 for a more detailed discussion). Of primary importance is meticulous surgical technique and attention to hemostasis. Bleeding from the scalp incision may be reduced by infiltration with a dilute (1 : 400,000) epinephrine-containing solution. The use of the reverse Trendelenburg position may help to decrease venous pressure and blood loss from osteotomy sites but may increase the risk of venous air embolism (with a reported frequency of 5%–80%; see later discussion). For this reason, the horizontal position is preferred.

Blood-conserving dual therapy with recombinant human erythropoietin (to optimize preoperative hematocrit) and use of a cell saver has reduced transfusion in children undergoing craniosynostosis repair.[89] Administration of preoperative recombinant human erythropoietin, in combination with elemental iron (4 mg/kg per day orally to a maximum of 200 mg/day for 6 weeks) increases the preoperative hematocrit value and may decrease the need for autologous blood transfusion.[90,91] If iron stores are at all compromised, iron therapy combined with oral vitamin C (to increase gastrointestinal absorption) should begin 3 weeks before erythropoietin therapy.[92] Currently this technique is rarely used, likely because of high costs as well as the black box warning applied to synthetic erythropoietin drugs related to increased likelihood of major complications in adult populations receiving these drugs.

Little evidence exists to suggest that autologous blood donation decreases perioperative morbidity in craniosynostosis surgery.[93,94] While infants as young as 3 months have predonated, this technique is of questionable value and should not be pursued in this population. Instead, simpler and more cost-effective techniques should be used such as meticulous surgical attention to hemostasis and administration of antifibrinolytics.[95]

Acute normovolemic hemodilution is a labor-intensive technique in which blood is collected from the child after induction of anesthesia but immediately before surgery and replaced with an appropriate volume of crystalloid or colloid, such as 5% albumin. This technique has been used in combination with other techniques, especially preoperative erythropoietin to reduce transfusion in craniosynostosis surgery.[96,97] The maximum potential blood savings with this technique is modest at best.[98] Despite some reports of efficacy, owing to the labor-intensive nature of the technique and modest blood savings, this technique is rarely used in craniofacial surgery.

The coagulation profile and clotting factors after fresh frozen plasma (FFP) or 5% albumin during craniofacial surgery have been compared in a nonrandomized study in infants younger than 12 months of age.[99] The increases in activated partial thromboplastin time and decreases in the plasma concentration of factors XI and XIII and antithrombin III were less after intraoperative FFP than after 5% albumin. Fibrinogen concentrations remained stable in the FFP-treated group but decreased in the albumin-treated group. A hemostatic resuscitation strategy, similar to that used in massive hemorrhage from trauma, has been applied in pediatric craniofacial surgery. With this approach, blood loss is replaced using red blood cells and FFP in a 1 : 1 ratio. The central tenet of this approach is to prevent dilutional coagulopathy (see also Chapter 12). At one center where blood loss frequently exceeds a blood volume, FFP and packed red blood cells from the same blood donors were used for blood loss replacement; this technique essentially eliminated coagulopathy, resulted in fewer perioperative blood donor exposures,[100] and is most likely to be useful where blood loss is expected to approach or exceed the circulating blood volume. Recombinant factor VIIa has been used successfully for intractable hemorrhage during cranial vault reconstruction in an infant, although this was an extreme circumstance in an isolated case.[101]

Antifibrinolytic therapy may decrease blood loss during craniosynostosis repair in children. Tranexamic acid reduces blood loss and transfusions in pediatric craniofacial surgery[102,103]; the recommended dosing regimen is a loading dose of 10 mg/kg followed by a continuous infusion of 5 mg/kg per hour. The incidence of adverse events, including seizures and thromboembolic events, in children treated with or without antifibrinolytics during craniofacial reconstructive surgery was similar.[104]

Another antifibrinolytic, ε-aminocaproic acid (EACA), is effective in reducing bleeding in cardiac and spinal procedures. In observational studies, EACA has been associated with reduced blood loss and transfusion in craniosynostosis surgery; these findings have yet to be confirmed in a controlled study.[105,106] The dosing for infants undergoing craniofacial surgery is a loading dose of 100 mg/kg followed by 40 mg/kg per hour.[107] A recent single-center prospective study of 120 infants undergoing craniosynostosis repair used thromboelastography and the platelet fibrinogen product to guide the administration of blood products.[108] Using multivariate analysis and receiver operating curves to assess four parameters: K-time $>2 : 1$, MA <55 mm, α-angle <62 degrees, and the platelet-fibrinogen product <343, infants with all four predictors had a 92% probability of a blood loss of 60 mL/kg or more, whereas those with none of these parameters had an approximately 10% probability.

Induced hypotension, defined as a 10% to 20% reduction in the mean arterial blood pressure, may decrease intraoperative surgical blood loss and operating time,[109] although studies demonstrating its effectiveness and safety during craniosynostosis surgery are lacking. The lower limits of safe blood pressure reduction in infants are unknown. A variety of pharmacologic agents have been used to induce hypotension, including inhalational agents, vasodilators, β-blockers, and remifentanil.[109,110] Invasive arterial pressure monitoring is essential whenever hypotensive anesthesia is used. Induced hypotension should be used with great caution in the presence of increased ICP because of the risk of compromising cerebral perfusion pressure (i.e., the difference between mean arterial pressure [MAP] and either ICP or central venous pressure, whichever is greater). The risks of inadequate cerebral and end-organ oxygen delivery during hypotension are magnified by coexistent anemia. It is considered prudent to maintain normovolemia and normocapnia when induced hypotension is used (see Chapter 12). Many practitioners have determined that the potential benefits (reduction of blood loss, shorter surgery) of this technique are outweighed by the risks (cerebral ischemia and irreversible brain injury, blindness, end-organ damage). Rather than an approach of induced hypotension, some use a strategy of deliberate normotension, where the anesthetic is tailored to avoid blood pressures greater than baseline.

Whether used alone or in combination,[97,111,112] the preceding techniques seldom obviate the need for any blood transfusions during craniofacial surgery. In a retrospective review of 60 children who underwent craniofacial surgery at a single institution, half of the children required fewer transfusions and had a reduced length of stay that were attributed to the preoperative use of iron and erythropoietin, the use of a blood-recycling device intraoperatively, and a reduced minimum hemoglobin concentration for transfusion (<7 mg/dL) compared with a placebo group.[113] Given the potential for acute large-volume blood loss IV access with large-bore catheters remains essential and at least 2 units of packed red blood cells (PRBCs) should be crossmatched and available in the operating room at all times. IV fluids should be administered via a fluid warmer to prevent hypothermia. Maintaining normothermia preserves coagulation function and theoretically reduces bleeding and transfusion-related complications.[114] Based on adult data, coagulopathy from dilution of soluble clotting factors on average develops when 142% of the circulating blood volume has been lost and replaced with PRBCs and crystalloid, and with thrombocytopenia developing after an average of 2.3 blood volumes were lost (see also Chapter 12).[115] Estimating the blood loss based on the number of blood volumes of blood products administered, physical estimates of blood loss, and an assessment of hemostasis in the surgical field are useful empiric and clinical indicators for the need for hemostatic blood product administration. Serial determinations of the international normalized ratio prothrombin time (INR), partial thromboplastin time (PTT), platelet count, and fibrinogen concentration and the use of thromboelastography help to identify coagulopathy and guide hemostatic blood product administration.[108,116]

Endoscopic repair of craniosynostosis has become a rapidly growing surgical approach to reduce bleeding and decrease morbidity.[117,118] Independent risk factors for bleeding during endoscopic strip craniectomy include low body weight (<5 kg), sagittal suture surgery (related to proximity to the sagittal venous sinus), syndromic craniosynostosis, and earlier date of surgery.[84]

Hyponatremia and cerebral salt-wasting syndrome are associated with craniosynostosis repair.[119–123] Both intraoperative and postoperative hyponatremia have been described, with the latter occurring in approximately 30% of children. In a retrospective review of a cleft palate and craniofacial database, postoperative hyponatremia was associated with preoperative increased ICP, blood loss, and female gender with normal preoperative ICP.[123] The average reduction

in sodium concentration was more pronounced in children who received hyponatremic (hypotonic) (5% dextrose and 0.2% or 0.5% NaCl) compared with normonatremic (isotonic) postoperative IV fluids.[123] The perioperative use of balanced salt solutions is recommended to prevent hyponatremia (see also Chapter 9).

Increased Intracranial Pressure

Early surgery for craniosynostosis is often indicated to prevent increases in ICP.[44,45] One-third of children with craniofacial dysostosis syndrome and 15% to 20% of children with single-suture craniosynostosis have increased ICP (>15 mm Hg).[124] Approximately 40% to 50% of children with syndromic craniosynostosis have associated hydrocephalus, although differentiation from nonprogressive ventriculomegaly may be difficult.[124–126] Timing of surgery may affect neurocognitive development and intelligence because these are adversely affected by sustained increased ICP. Associated OSA resulting in hypoxemia and hypercapnia may lead to an increase in cerebral blood volume and thereby exacerbate intracranial hypertension.[127] Untreated intracranial hypertension may lead to optic atrophy and visual impairment.[49,128] As a consequence, when increased ICP has been identified either preoperatively or postoperatively, placement of a ventriculoperitoneal shunt should be considered[126]; this occurs more commonly in Crouzon and Pfeiffer syndromes.[126]

For children who present with signs of intracranial hypertension, it is important to follow basic principles of neuroanesthesia to prevent further increases in ICP and decreases in cerebral perfusion pressure (see also Chapter 26). It may be prudent to use protective measures to attenuate the hypertensive response to laryngoscopy and intubation, including the administration of a short-acting opioid, a β-blocker, or topical local anesthesia to the upper airway. Intraoperatively, the anesthesiologist faces numerous challenges to control ICP. Strategies to control ICP include mild to moderate hyperventilation (end-tidal carbon dioxide [ETCO$_2$] of 30 to 35 mm Hg), especially when signs of herniation are evident; avoidance of hypervolemia; and, where indicated, appropriate use of hypertonic (3%) saline solution, mannitol, furosemide, and dexamethasone to reduce ICP, reduce brain volume, and facilitate brain retraction. Although cranial vault reconstruction increases intracranial volume and reduces ICP,[129] children remain at risk of increased ICP after surgery and require close ophthalmologic and clinical follow-up, even after a cosmetically successful cranial expansion.[130,131]

Venous Air Embolism

Venous air embolism (VAE) may occur during any operative procedure in which the operative site is above the level of the heart and noncollapsible veins are exposed to atmospheric pressure.[132–139] The incidence of VAE in children undergoing craniectomy for craniosynostosis repair has been reported to be as great as 83%,[139] although hemodynamically significant VAE is rare. The incidence associated with endoscopic craniectomy may be as small as 2%.[84] Significant hypovolemia resulting from surgical blood loss can lead to a decrease in both systemic and central venous pressures and the development of a pressure gradient between the right atrium and the surgical site. This gradient increases the potential to entrain air via open dural sinuses or bony venous sinusoids.[139,140] If the entrained volume of air is sufficiently large, right ventricular outflow obstruction may ensue, causing acute right-sided heart failure and cardiovascular collapse. Smaller volumes of air may cause a reduction in cardiac output, hypotension, and myocardial or cerebral ischemia.[137] Transesophageal echocardiography (documenting the presence of air in the right ventricular outflow tract), precordial Doppler ultrasonography (continuous windmill murmur), end-tidal carbon dioxide (precipitous decrease in carbon dioxide tension), and nitrogen monitoring (sudden increase in nitrogen concentration in the exhaled breath) have been used to identify VAE with different sensitivities, well before cardiovascular collapse occurs (see Figs. 26.6 and 26.7).[137,141–144] Applying bone wax to the open edges of cut bone, reducing the degree of or avoiding the reverse Trendelenburg position, maintaining positive-pressure ventilation with 5 cm of PEEP, and ensuring normovolemia help to prevent VAE. Fluid resuscitation, vasopressors, and aspiration of air from the right side of the heart may prevent episodes of VAE from progressing to cardiovascular collapse.[133,139,144]

Prolonged Surgery

As with all surgeries that last several hours, preventing the complications associated with prolonged anesthesia is paramount.[145] Nerve palsies, pressure ulcers of the skin, ophthalmic complications, hypothermia, and acidosis may occur. Careful positioning of the extremities, use of an egg-crate–type mattress or foam padding, and avoiding pressure to the eyes, particularly when the surgical procedure requires the prone position, will prevent the majority of these adverse outcomes. In children with proptosis, such as Crouzon syndrome, it may be necessary to suture the eyelids closed after applying lubrication to prevent corneal abrasions. Anterior ischemic optic neuropathy that can cause transient or permanent postoperative blindness is a rare complication that occurs in the absence of external pressure to the eyes.[146,147]

Hypothermia is another major concern and is a largely preventable complication when the appropriate steps are taken. Factors that predispose to hypothermia include the large surface area exposed during surgery and the potential infusion of large volumes of relatively cold IV fluids. Effective measures to prevent hypothermia include warming the operating room, the use of forced-air warmers and radiant warming lamps, insulating the child, and warming devices for blood and IV fluids. Preventing hypothermia and limiting blood loss and transfusion requirements are key factors in preventing the development of perioperative metabolic disturbance[148]; even mild hypothermia has been associated with increased blood loss and transfusion.[149]

Orbital Hypertelorism

The term *orbital hypertelorism* describes abnormally widely separated orbits. This deformity may occur in isolation or in association with other congenital abnormalities, such as facial clefts and Apert syndrome (Fig. 35.5). Surgical repair involves mobilization and repositioning of the orbit through either a subcranial approach, which leaves the roof of the orbit intact, or an intracranial approach via a frontal craniectomy. This procedure is performed in children older than 5 years of age who may have already undergone extensive surgical reconstruction. Surgical manipulation of the globe may elicit the oculocardiac reflex, resulting in bradyarrhythmias or asystole. Oculocardiac reflex may also occur during midface and orthognathic procedures (see also Fig. 34.3A and B).[150] These arrhythmias are usually without significant hemodynamic consequence and extinguish over time. Usually release by the surgeon of any orbital/periorbital pressure/tension being applied will allow the heart rate to return to normal. Hemodynamically significant bradycardia can be treated and further episodes prevented by administering a prophylactic anticholinergic such as atropine (10–20 µg/kg) or glycopyrrolate (5–10 µg/kg).

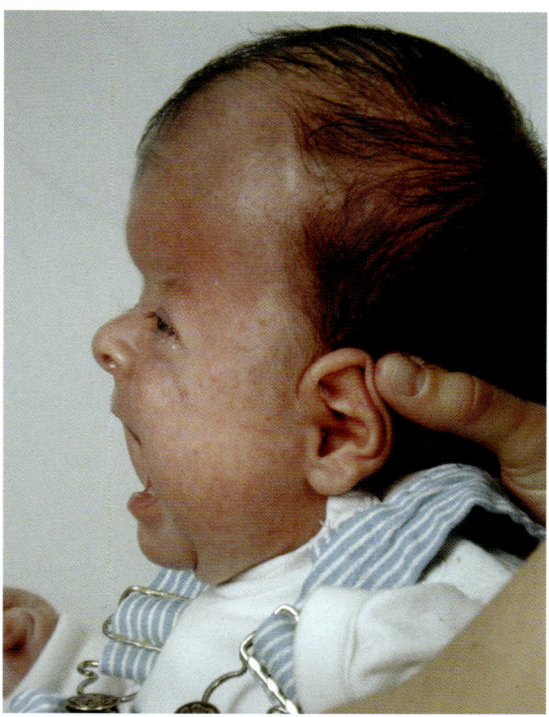

FIGURE 35.5 Child with Apert syndrome. Notable features include proptosis, cloverleaf skull, maxillary hypoplasia, and syndactyly (syndactyly is present in Apert syndrome but not in Crouzon syndrome).

After establishing IV access, the airway should be secured using a preformed orotracheal tube; confirmation of bilateral breath sounds is essential after positioning.[21] Blood loss from multiple osteotomies may be significant, and, as in the case of craniosynostosis surgery, methods to reduce the use of homologous blood should be considered. Intraoperative management follows the principles outlined for craniosynostosis surgery. At the conclusion of surgery, the trachea is extubated and the child is monitored overnight in a high-dependency setting with the capability of managing acute airway obstruction and monitoring of neurologic status.

Midface Procedures

Midface advancement to improve facial appearance is commonly required for children with maxillary hypoplasia, such as those with Crouzon, Apert (see Fig. 35.5), and Pfeiffer syndromes (E-Fig. 35.7).[151–153] This procedure is typically performed in children ages 5 to 7 years, although complications such as proptosis, corneal ulceration, ocular dislocations, and airway obstruction may necessitate earlier intervention.[153–156] A LeFort II procedure is similar to a LeFort III, with the difference that the osteotomy is oriented vertically through the infraorbital rim. Thus the nasal pyramid and the maxilla move forward as a single unit. Le Fort III osteotomy and monobloc procedures (Fig. 35.6) have the potential for significant complications, including massive blood loss, airway difficulties, blindness, cerebrospinal fluid leak, and infection.[145,147,157–159]

Anesthetic concerns are similar to those for orbital hypertelorism and craniosynostosis. Children with Apert and Crouzon syndromes often present with incomplete or complete nasal obstruction that

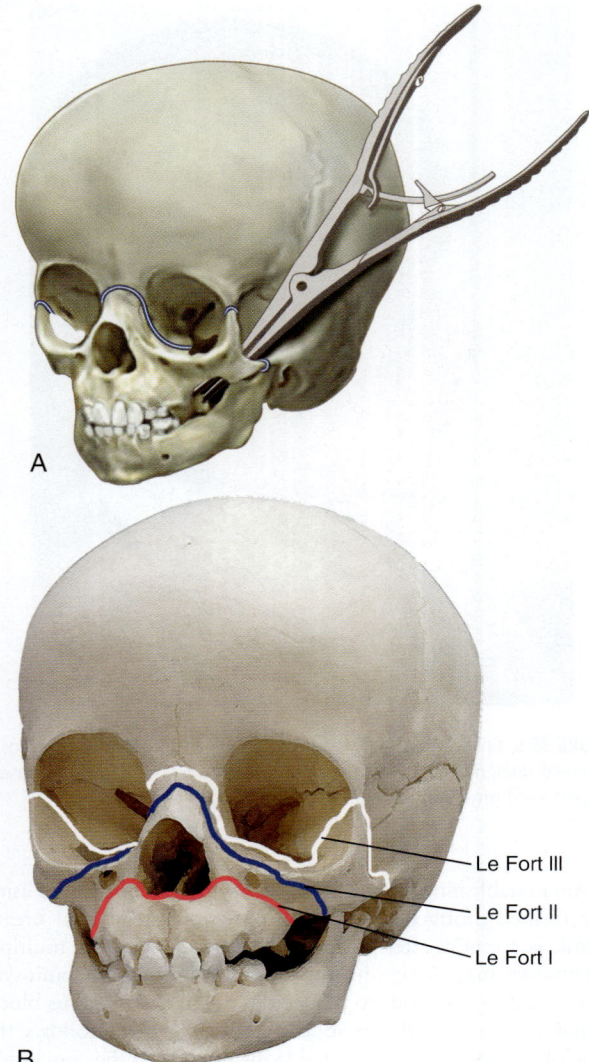

FIGURE 35.6 Le Fort III and monobloc procedures for correction of midface hypoplasia. **A,** The osteotomies in the Le Fort III procedure pass through the nasofrontal junction, across the medial orbital wall and floor, and into the inferior orbital fissure. A cut through the frontozygomatic suture, pterygomaxillary junction, and zygomatic arch allows separation of the midface. **B,** The monobloc procedures are similar, but the nasofrontal junction and frontozygomatic suture are not mobilized. This technique allows simultaneous correction of supraorbital and midface deformities at the expense of an increased incidence of postoperative complications.

results from choanal atresia or midface hypoplasia. As a consequence, mask anesthesia can be difficult, even with an oral airway in situ. However, laryngoscopy and tracheal intubation in these children is usually uncomplicated. The diameter of the tracheal tube requires careful consideration because these children may require prolonged postoperative ventilation until postoperative facial and laryngeal edema has resolved. The decision to intubate the trachea via the oral or nasal route must be discussed with the surgeon before induction of anesthesia. A nasotracheal tube can be used throughout the procedure, or the surgeon may request an intraoperative change from the oral to the nasal tracheal position after completing the midfacial osteotomies.[160] To perform the latter maneuver, the anesthesiologist wears a sterile surgical gown

and gloves and uses sterile equipment, including laryngoscope, Magill forceps, and tube exchange catheter (see E-Fig. 14.3A–H). Visualizing the glottis during surgery may be difficult because of the presence of airway edema and blood in the hypopharynx. A tube exchange catheter is passed through a naris and into the trachea alongside the orotracheal tube. The nasal tube is then passed over the exchange catheter, and its tip is positioned at the glottic opening. The oral tube is then removed, and the nasal tube is advanced (rotating the bevel 90 degrees clockwise or counterclockwise as needed to pass the vocal cords and arytenoids)[161,162] and visualized as it passes through the glottic aperture. Once the tube position is confirmed, the catheter is removed and the nasal tube is sutured securely to the nasal septum after confirmation of bilateral breath sounds.[21] Given the proximity of the tracheal tube to the surgical site, damage to the tracheal tube can occur during surgery.[163,164] Vigilance is required at all times to detect an accidental disconnection or damage to the tracheal tube. The anesthesiologist must be prepared to respond immediately to an unexpected interruption in ventilation and replace the tracheal tube. A nasogastric tube is placed after surgery to prevent gastric distention and reduce the likelihood of postoperative nausea and vomiting. A wire cutter must be available at the bedside at all times if intermaxillary fixation is used to stabilize the facial bones and mandible. In the ICU, the presence of an audible leak around the tracheal tube is an important criterion to determine absence of laryngeal or periglottic edema and therefore readiness for tracheal extubation.[163] Intraoperative blood loss is not typically as great as for craniosynostosis surgery. Hypotensive anesthesia may reduce or prevent the need for blood transfusions during maxillary orthognathic surgery.[165]

Hemifacial Microsomia, Treacher Collins Syndrome, and Goldenhar Syndrome

Hemifacial microsomias, also known as otomandibular dysostosis (Fig. 35.7), result from a malformation of the first and second branchial (or pharyngeal) arches. This is the second most common facial defect after clefts. These disorders are classified according to the classification **O**rbital distortion, **M**andibular hypoplasia, **E**ar anomaly, **N**erve involvement, and **S**oft tissue deficiency (OMENS).[3,166–169] Piezosurgery is a relatively new technique used to perform osteotomies using ultrasonic frequencies during mandibular distraction in children with hemifacial microsomia.[170] Airway difficulty increases with the complexity of the defect from unilateral to bilateral mandibular or temporomandibular involvement. The disorder may include mandibular hypoplasia, temporomandibular joint dysostosis, cleft palate, and auricular, ophthalmologic, and facial nerve defects. Goldenhar syndrome (Fig. 35.8 and E-Fig. 35.8) is the most common form of this disorder. Vertebral anomalies are present in 40% and congenital heart defects occur in 35% of children with this syndrome. Airway management is complicated by midfacial hypoplasia, asymmetry of mouth opening, and mandibular retrognathia. Overall, tracheal intubation in children with unilateral hemifacial microsomia is easy in 70% and very difficult in 9%.[166] In contrast, tracheal intubation in children with bilateral mandibular hypoplasia is evenly distributed among easy, difficult, and very difficult.[166] The airway anomalies associated with this syndrome predispose to OSA.

The craniofacial abnormalities of mandibular hypoplasia, macrostomia, and cleft palate in Treacher Collins syndrome (E-Fig. 35.9) often present difficulties for airway management

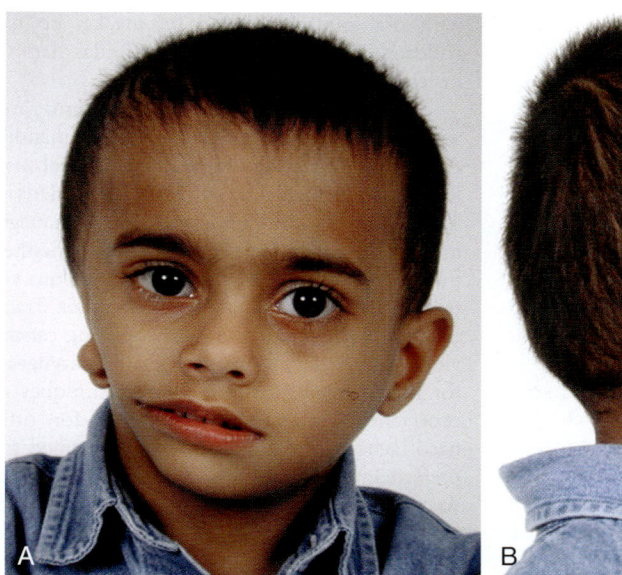
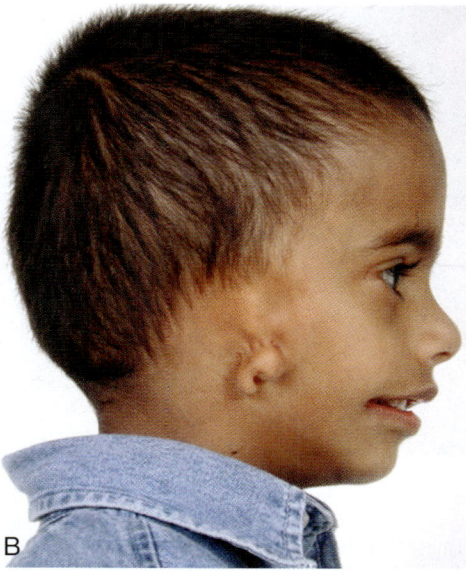

FIGURE 35.7 Frontal (A) and lateral (B) views of unilateral hemifacial microsomia. In the lateral view, microstomia and mandibular and ocular deformities are evident. These children may present with either unilateral or bilateral hemifacial microsomia, a hypoplastic mandible and maxilla, and ear deformities.

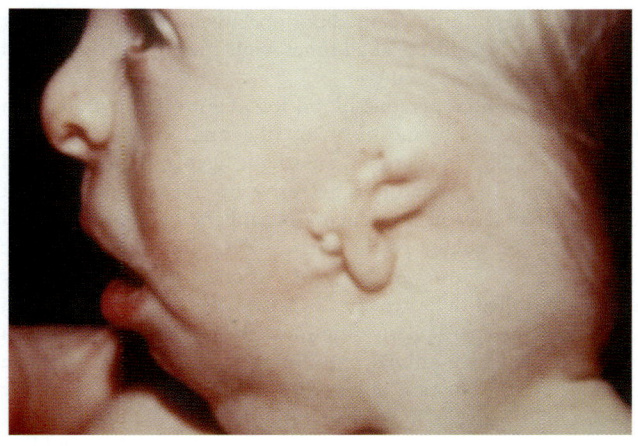

FIGURE 35.8 Goldenhar syndrome in an infant. This is one of the most common forms of hemifacial microsomia. With unilateral hemifacial microsomia, the airway is usually managed and instrumented without difficulty, but with bilateral mandibular hypoplasia, the airway may be very difficult to manage in one third of afflicted children.

that increase with increasing age.[3,166] Other clinical features of the syndrome include hypoplastic zygomatic arches, ophthalmic features (including sloping palpebral fissures, coloboma of the eyes, and notched lower eyelids), microtia, choanal atresia, cardiovascular defects, and renal anomalies. Mandibular distraction osteogenesis is a surgical option considered when upper airway obstruction is due to mandibular deficiency. This avoids tracheostomy or other surgical intervention and allows for future growth of the mandible. Children with hemifacial microsomia have a poor psychosocial outcome.[171]

AIRWAY MANAGEMENT

Airway management of children with hemifacial dysostoses is traditionally known to be difficult. It is essential that all equipment

for management of the difficult airway be present in the operating room before induction of anesthesia (or administration of sedatives/local anesthetic in cases where a sedated/awake approach is used) (see Table 14.10). For infants and children with difficult airways, an inhalational induction is the most commonly used technique. In contrast, in older children and adolescents, either an inhalational induction or IV sedation (using dexmedetomidine or propofol) with topical local anesthesia applied to the upper airway may be used to facilitate tracheal intubation. In all cases, it is essential that primary and backup plans for airway management be in place together with the equipment and personnel required to execute them.

A variety of techniques may be used to control the difficult airway, including a flexible fiberoptic bronchoscope, GlideScope (Verathon Inc., Bothell, WA), the Airtraq (Prodol Meditec S.A., Vizcaya, Spain) disposable optical laryngoscope, Truview Infant laryngoscope (Teleflex Medical, Netanya, Israel), supraglottic airway devices,[172] and others (see Chapter 14). We have used the two-person intubation technique, in which the first anesthesiologist applies external posterior laryngeal pressure while performing laryngoscopy to optimize the view of the glottis, while the second anesthesiologist inserts the tracheal tube into the trachea when the view is adequate (see Fig. 35.9).[173] The second anesthesiologist also may assist with more advanced airway management both in terms of helping to observe the child and assisting with the use of advanced airway devices.

Preformed tracheal tubes are generally used via the oral or nasal route, depending on the site of surgery. When a nasotracheal tube is used, it can be secured by suturing it to the membranous nasal septum or taping it after the skin has been prepared with benzoin. An oral tube may be wired to the mandible or to a non-deciduous tooth. Care must be taken to ensure that the tip of the preformed tube is mid-tracheal as the length of preformed nasotracheal and, to a lesser extent orotracheal tubes, exceeds that of the uncuffed version of the same diameter tube.[21] A laryngeal mask airway can be very effective in maintaining airway patency

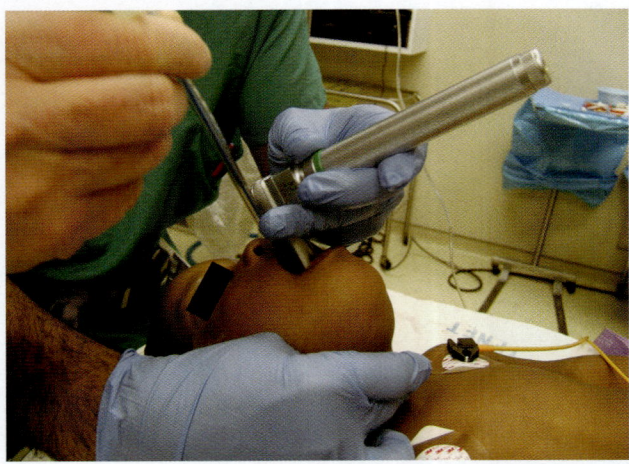

FIGURE 35.9 Two-person intubation technique. The intubator (first person) performs laryngoscopy and manipulates the larynx with external laryngeal manipulation (gloved hands). With the larynx in view, the intubator cocks his or her head to the left while holding position and the assistant (second person, nongloved hand), who is standing on the intubator's right, then passes the tracheal tube through the larynx.[173]

during induction of anesthesia or as a guide to facilitate fiberoptic bronchoscopy.

For children with a history of upper airway obstruction or midfacial hypoplasia who present with a tracheostomy, the tracheostomy tube can be replaced with a cuffed tracheostomy tube or an armored tube that is sutured in place for the duration of the surgery. The use of a cuffed tracheostomy tube allows for separation of the aerodigestive tracts, controlled ventilation, delivery of adequate PEEP, and prevention of atelectasis during long procedures. Changes in the position of the head and neck can cause displacement of the tracheal tube, so care should be taken to confirm tracheal tube position after the child is positioned for surgery.[21,174] This is especially important for cranial vault procedures that involve extremes of neck extension, such as might occur during reconstruction of the supraorbital bar. Airway equipment and additional tracheal tubes must be available in the operating room at all times. It is essential to document an audible leak around the tracheal tube at the time of tracheal intubation (with the cuff on the tracheal tube deflated), because the presence of a leak is often used postoperatively to determine suitability for extubation when significant airway edema has developed. OSA associated with midfacial anomalies may result in upper airway obstruction during induction and emergence.[73,78]

Orthognathic Surgery

Malocclusion secondary to maxillary or mandibular hypoplasia (such as occurs in hemifacial microsomia and Treacher Collins syndrome), tumors, trauma, as well as temporomandibular joint dysfunction are generally accepted indications for orthognathic surgery. LeFort I procedures for maxillary hypoplasia involve a transverse incision through the maxilla to advance the upper teeth into normal occlusion with the mandible. These procedures are usually performed in adolescents because surgery is performed once maxillary and mandibular growth is complete. Because this age group usually exhibits increased perioperative anxiety, preoperative assurance and education as well as premedication

with oral midazolam (0.3–0.5 mg/kg, up to 20 mg for older children and adolescents) or IV midazolam (2–4 mg) are often necessary.

Airway management is a major concern, particularly in children with a hypoplastic mandible or temporomandibular dysfunction.[3] A high index of suspicion for atlantoaxial instability is required if juvenile rheumatoid arthritis is the underlying disease process. The anticipated difficult airway can be managed using fiberoptic intubation, with sedation or topical local anesthesia or an inhalation induction and maintenance of spontaneous ventilation until the trachea is intubated, as discussed earlier. Tracheal intubation in children with adequate mouth opening can be managed with a video/indirect laryngoscope or using a laryngeal mask as a conduit for fiberoptic intubation. These techniques are best suited for orotracheal intubations; frequently for orthognathic surgery nasotracheal intubation (using a preformed tracheal tube) is the preferred method of tracheal intubation. Careful stabilization and fixation of the tube using transseptal suturing to prevent unintended extubation is often used.[21] Excessive pressure on the ala nasi (causing ischemia) can be avoided by fixing the nasal RAE tube to the forehead with the nasal curve positioned away from the ala. LeFort I advancements require close communication between the surgery and anesthesia teams because the nasotracheal tube can be dislodged once the maxilla is fully mobilized. An additional potential intraoperative complication is inadvertent cutting of the tracheal tube when the maxillary osteotomies are performed. If intermaxillary fixation is used postoperatively, wire cutters must be immediately available at all times while the child is monitored in an intensive care setting.

To reduce intraoperative blood loss, controlled hypotension is commonly used by means of any of a range of pharmacologic agents, including inhalational anesthetic agents, β-blockers, and remifentanil. The literature is extensive on the salutary effect of induced hypotension in reducing intraoperative blood loss and improving the quality of the surgical field during orthognathic surgery.[165,175–184] However, many practitioners have moved away from controlled hypotension because of concerns regarding complications, particularly blindness. Regardless of anesthesia technique, invasive arterial monitoring is indicated to facilitate intraoperative evaluation of blood gases and hematocrit. In many cases, a mild degree of hypotension is sufficient for optimal surgical conditions (systolic blood pressure 85–90 mm Hg), thus avoiding a greater degree of hypotension. Dexamethasone (0.5 mg/kg) may reduce postoperative airway edema.[185] After awakening the child and return of protective airway reflexes, the trachea is extubated and the child is monitored overnight in a high-dependency setting with the ability to establish an airway should acute airway obstruction develop. In some cases, at the conclusion of surgery mandibulomaxillary fixation may be used with either metal wires or elastic bands. Emergency wire cutters should be immediately available in the postoperative period in the event of the need for emergency airway management.

Cystic Hygromas and Hemangiomas

Cystic hygroma is a rare congenital malformation of the lymphatic system occurring with an incidence of 1 in 16,000 births, most frequently involving the axilla and neck (Fig. 35.10 and E-Fig. 35.10). The pathology consists of multiple loculated cysts that contain lymph fluid or blood (see Fig. 35.10B). In most cases, cystic hygromas are present at birth, although 80% to 90% are diagnosed within the first 2 years of life. The natural history is

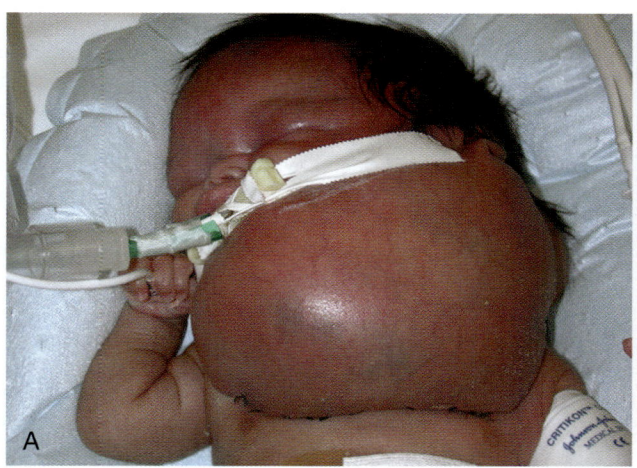
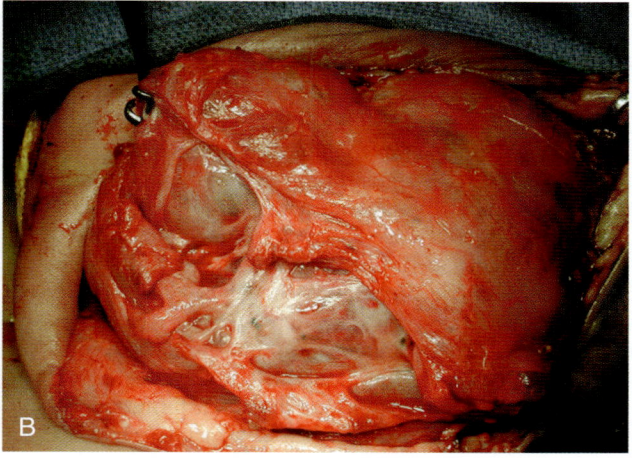

FIGURE 35.10 **A,** Cystic hygroma. Note that the bulk of the tumor is extraoral and extralaryngeal, although extension into the tongue and supraglottic region may complicate direct laryngoscopy. The tumor on the surface of the neck may rapidly expand owing to bleeding into the cysts or accumulation of fluid in the lymphatics. Such large tumors may put the overlying skin under great tension. They may also be situated such that they preclude tracheostomy. **B,** Gross pathologic condition in cystic hygromas consists of a combination of multiloculated cysts that may contain a combination of lymph fluid and blood. Debulking may result in substantial blood loss. Sequential debulking of the hygroma may be required as the residual cysts expand with fluid and blood and reexpand the hygroma.

spontaneous resolution, although most require repeated aspirations, sclerotherapy, or surgical excision to debulk the mass (see E-Fig. 35.10B).[186-188] Cystic hygroma can be associated with other chromosomal abnormalities such as Noonan and Turner syndromes, in which case the anesthetic management is guided by the underlying syndrome. Some children require an urgent tracheostomy at birth or in the first hours of life to relieve an obstructed airway (see Chapter 38). During the preoperative assessment, the airway should be examined and evaluated by radiographs for involvement of supraglottic and infraglottic structures. Acute airway obstruction can occur during induction if cystic lesions are present in the upper airway. Fiberoptic intubation may be required if the larynx is distorted by the lesions, in which case spontaneous ventilation should be maintained until the airway is secured.[189] Postoperative complications of surgical excision include laryngeal edema, airway obstruction, pneumonia, facial palsy, and infection.[186,187,190]

Hemangiomas, also known as juvenile or infantile hemangiomas, are the most common benign tumors in infancy, affecting up to 10% of infants.[191] The majority of hemangiomas are uncomplicated and require no treatment. The natural course begins with a proliferation phase that starts within the first few months of life, followed by an involution phase of variable length. It is estimated that involution occurs at a rate of 10% per year. Hemangiomas can affect all organs, and intervention is required when the lesion affects the function of vital organs such as the eyes, airway, or liver.[192] Hemangiomas that occur in the subglottic region must be considered in the differential diagnosis of a noninfectious cause of croup in infants younger than 3 months of age. When present around the eyes and on the face (Fig. 35.11), hemangiomas are often associated with lesions in the airway.[193,194] They can occur in any part of the airway and can cause airway and feeding difficulties. Airway procedures to resect or remove hemangiomas are generally undertaken between 1 and 11 months of age.[195] Limb hemangiomas generally present with cosmetic concerns and bleeding. Rarely, children with large hemangiomas develop high-output heart failure.

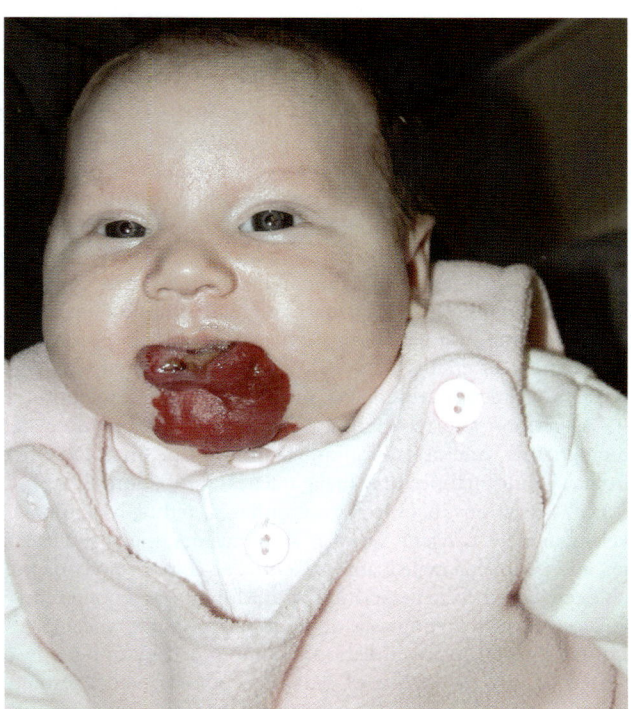

FIGURE 35.11 Facial hemangioma in the cheek of a child. The hemangioma involves the skin overlying the mandible centrally from the lower lip to the tip of the mandible. Hemangiomas vary widely in size but can enlarge precipitously as a result of bleeding into the tumor.

Treatment options for hemangiomas include nonintervention, systemic corticosteroid treatment, corticosteroid injection, surgical excision, and laser ablation. Propranolol is an emerging treatment option for hemangiomas.[196-199] It appears to act on hemangioma stem cells in a variety of ways, including through suppression of cyclic adenosine monophosphate–mediated kinase pathways, promotion of cell death through adipogenesis, and downregulation of vascular endothelial growth factor.[200-202] It may be used in children without contraindications either as an oral monotherapy at a dose of 2 mg/kg per day divided into three doses or in combination with oral prednisone 3 mg/kg per day tapered after 4 to 6 weeks of therapy. Propranolol reduces the need for surgical intervention but requires 6 months to 1 year of therapy.[203] Surgical treatment is reserved for superficial hemangiomas in locations that are surgically accessible.[192] Laser treatment for superficial lesions is commonly performed as an outpatient procedure,[204] and routine anesthetic precautions should be taken. Children with hemangiomas who had airway procedures received more steroids and had increased admissions and mortality compared with those without airway procedures.[195]

Arteriovenous malformations are present at birth but can go unrecognized for years, especially when they are intracranial. Large arteriovenous malformations may cause high-output cardiac failure, necessitating therapeutic intervention. Treatment options may include chemotherapy, corticosteroid therapy, embolization, and surgical excision.[205-207] Children who undergo excision of the hemangiomas often require blood products during surgery, but platelets should be transfused with care because an accumulation within the malformation may increase its size.[208] NSAIDs should be avoided because of their effects on platelet function.

Möbius Syndrome

Möbius sequence is a rare neurologic disorder (2–20 in 1,000,000 births) characterized by congenital palsy of the facial (VII) and abducens (VI) cranial nerves, resulting in unilateral or bilateral facial weakness and defective extraocular eye movement (E-Fig. 35.11), which is now thought to arise from abnormal rhombencephalic development and is therefore primarily a disorder of the caudal brainstem.[209,210] These classic features may be associated with other cranial nerve palsies, ophthalmic abnormalities, developmental delay, and various craniofacial, limb, and musculoskeletal malformations, resulting in a variable pattern of clinical expression.[211-215] Involvement of cranial nerves IX and X is associated with pharyngeal dysfunction, dysphagia, feeding difficulties, retention of oral secretions, and recurrent aspiration pneumonia. Associated micrognathia, microstomia, limited mouth opening, and other orofacial abnormalities may make tracheal intubation difficult.[216] Other associations include gastroesophageal reflux, hypotonia of skeletal muscles, congenital cardiac abnormalities, spinal abnormalities, and peripheral neuropathies. Central alveolar hypoventilation has been described in association with Möbius sequence and may be secondary to hypoplasia of midbrain respiratory centers.[217] Central alveolar hypoventilation, compounded by upper airway hypotonia and the effects of sedatives, opioids, and anesthetic agents, can predispose to postoperative respiratory compromise. The absence of facial expression secondary to paresis of the facial nerve can make it difficult to assess and evaluate postoperative pain.[218] The anesthetic plan for the child with Möbius sequence must be tailored to the individual based on the clinical expression of the syndrome. There is a single, isolated report of fatal malignant hyperthermia in a 7-month-old. The absence of other reported cases renders a connection between malignant hyperthermia and Möbius syndrome exceedingly unlikely.[219]

The most common surgical procedure performed in children with Möbius sequence is segmental gracilis muscle transplantation, in which the muscle is transplanted to the face and revascularized to the facial artery and vein.[220] Motor innervation of the gracilis requires a functioning cranial nerve such as the masseter branch of the trigeminal nerve. The aim of this facial reanimation is to facilitate facial expression and provide lower lip support to reduce drooling and improve speech.[220] Anesthetic considerations include those for prolonged surgery, avoidance of neuromuscular block to facilitate intraoperative nerve stimulation, and avoidance of hypocapnia, hypothermia, and hypotension to ensure graft perfusion. The latter considerations are also applicable to the postoperative period. Other surgical procedures commonly performed in children with Möbius sequence include strabismus surgery and orthopedic procedures to improve limb function.

Congenital Intraoral Fibrous Bands

Congenital intraoral fibrous bands (e.g., pterygium syndrome and syngnathia) can present an almost impossible airway to secure even with advanced pediatric fiberoptic skills (E-Fig. 35.12). Syngnathia reduces mouth opening as a result of fusion of maxilla and mandible and often presents as a part of Van der Woude and popliteal pterygium syndromes.[221] These children often present with airway and feeding difficulties. Depending on the severity of the bands, these children may present formidable anesthetic challenges. IV ketamine anesthesia in the spontaneously breathing neonate may allow division of the adhesions in the first few days of life, precluding the need for a surgical airway or facilitating tracheal intubation if other surgery is required.[221]

Intraoral Tumors

Intraoral tumors are rare in children (E-Fig. 35.13) but, if massive, may present great challenges in securing the airway. Those that present the greatest difficulties preclude visualizing the larynx (E-Fig. 35.14) and present an increased risk of intraoperative bleeding. Preoperative radiographic studies are required to delineate the extent of involvement of the upper airway and whether the supraglottic region or the nasopharynx is clear for passage of a bronchoscope. If the tumors are sufficiently large that laryngoscopy is precluded, fiberoptic nasal intubation must be considered. If the tumor is resectable, a tracheostomy could be a backup plan. The risk of bleeding depends on the vascularity of the tumor and whether the tongue is involved. If the vascular supply of the tumor can be isolated, bleeding should be easily controlled. If, however, the tumor cannot be separated from the tongue, bleeding can be controlled only by clamping the tongue (and lingual arteries) before resecting the tumor. This should prevent excessive blood loss and permit a hemostatic closure of the resected surface. The trachea should remain intubated postoperatively until both airway and lingual edema have abated.

Brachial Plexus Surgery

Brachial plexus injury occurs in 0.5 to 5 infants per 1000 live births as a result of birth trauma.[222,223] Erb palsy involves damage to nerve roots C5, C6, and C7, whereas Klumpke palsy involves roots C8 and T1.[223] Complete plexus palsies are the most devastating injuries, resulting in a flail and insensate arm.[223,224] Although 75% of brachial plexus injuries resolve spontaneously and completely within the first month after birth, 25% result in permanent disability and impairment.[223,225-227] Surgical intervention is indicated if the motor function does not improve after 3 months of age.[225,226] Clinically significant diaphragmatic palsy is associated with 2.4% of neonates with brachial plexus injury. In the very young, diaphragmatic palsy requires aggressive intervention before brachial plexus repair. For brachial plexus surgery to be successful, the nerve root cannot be completely avulsed from the spinal cord. Therefore detailed imaging is required to characterize the nature of the injury: avulsion of the nerve root from the spinal cord, disruption of the nerve within the nerve sheath, or disruption of the nerve and the nerve sheath. Because irreversible loss of the neuromotor end plate may occur, surgery is often undertaken before 12 months of age.[222,225,226,228–230] Microsurgical intervention is performed in infants with global lesions and Horner syndrome by 3 months of age. The aim is to improve function with no expectation of complete recovery; without intervention these children have severe functional deficits. Conversely, if recovery of the biceps occurs by 3 months, treatment is performed without microsurgical intervention.[231] The treatment of choice includes resection of neuromas with interpositional nerve grafting.[232] Nerve grafting is being increasingly performed for treating neonatal brachial plexus injury. Donor nerves include motor branches of C4, intercostal nerves, inferior branches of cranial nerve XI, pectoral nerves, and sural nerves.[233] Synthetic collagen nerve conduits have been approved as nerve guidance channels in microsurgery and may be an option for the future.[234]

Preoperative MRI for assessing bone and joint deformities may require administration of general anesthesia. Repair of the brachial plexus may be challenging because the only extremity for IV access and monitoring (blood pressure and pulse oximetry) is the contralateral upper extremity. Both lower extremities are usually prepped and draped for harvesting the sural nerves or other donor nerves for the repair. Because these infants are usually 9 to 12 months of age, they are chubby, making IV access more difficult. This surgery often takes up to 12 hours, so the considerations for prolonged anesthesia must be invoked, such as protecting pressure points during positioning. Muscle relaxants are avoided to facilitate intraoperative electrophysiologic testing.[235] An indwelling urinary catheter is essential to decompress the bladder. Analgesic requirement is minimal except during brief periods of surgical stimulation. Remifentanil provides excellent intraoperative analgesia and permits rapid adjustment of the depth of anesthesia. Maintenance of normothermia and prevention of fluid overload are important during this prolonged surgery. Blood loss is minimal, and maintenance fluids usually suffice.[222] Prolonged administration of propofol is not recommended because of the risk of propofol infusion syndrome and delayed emergence. In its stead, remifentanil combined with inhalation agent or dexmedetomidine may be a more appropriate regimen. Postoperative analgesia requirements are minimal, and acetaminophen and NSAIDs usually provide adequate pain relief. Shoulder spica casts may be applied to avoid sudden neck movements postoperatively if the lower branches of the accessory nerve are used for reconstruction.[235]

Otoplasty

Protruding ears (commonly known as "bat ears") are common in the Caucasian population, occurring with an incidence of up to 5% (E-Fig. 35.15).[236] Children with protruding ears are generally healthy, with about two-thirds undergoing surgical correction before the age of 8 years or as soon as the child expresses concern about the deformity.[237] Younger children are more likely to require general anesthesia, whereas those older than age 8 years may tolerate the procedure using local anesthetic infiltration or nerve blocks.[238] Laser techniques are now used increasingly to perform cartilage reshaping.[239] The main complication of general anesthesia is postoperative nausea and vomiting, which can last up to 2 days after surgery in approximately 80% of children.[240] However, postoperative nausea and vomiting may be reduced by surgical

and anesthetic techniques, including multimodal techniques with combined pharmacotherapy (ondansetron and dexamethasone), anesthetic maintenance with a propofol infusion, and avoidance of packing of the external auditory meatus and concha.[240,241] To provide optimal surgical access and positioning of the child, a preformed, low-profile tracheal tube, such as the RAE tube, may be required, but flexible laryngeal mask airways provide equally satisfactory conditions in the ventilated or spontaneously breathing child.[242] Infiltration with local anesthetic (usually <10 mL of 1% lidocaine with 1:100,000 epinephrine) attenuates the surgical stimulus and reduces the intraoperative opioid requirements. The use of a long-acting local anesthetic combined with a nerve block, acetaminophen, and NSAIDs provides adequate postoperative analgesia in most children. This multimodal approach may obviate the need for opioids and thereby reduce the incidence of postoperative nausea and vomiting.[243]

Congenital Hand Anomalies

Congenital limb malformations exhibit a wide spectrum of phenotypic manifestations. Syndactyly may occur as an isolated malformation (Fig. 35.12 and E-Fig. 35.16) or part of a syndrome, the most common being Apert syndrome but also with Poland syndrome, in association with skeletal abnormalities and gastrointestinal and cardiac malformations. Limb malformations are more frequent in males than females, and they affect both upper and lower limbs in approximately 50% of children with a deformity. Early separation of digits is favored if the ring and little fingers or index finger and thumb are involved, because the differing longitudinal growth rates will lead to greater deformities.[244] Surgery is usually

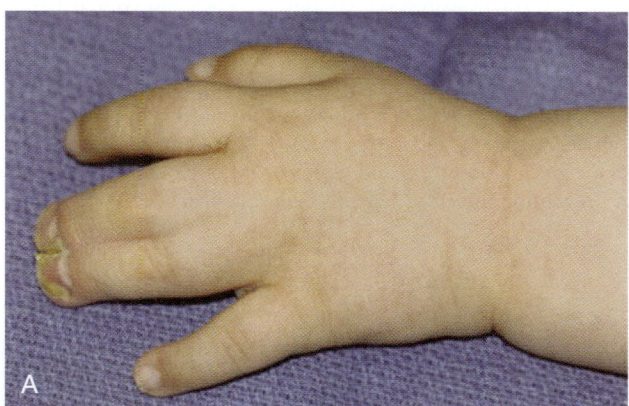

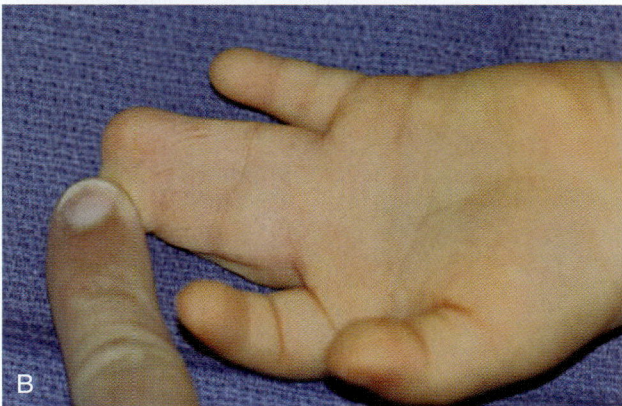

FIGURE 35.12 Syndactyly of the first and second digit of an infant: dorsal aspect **(A)** and volar aspect **(B)**.

performed between 6 and 18 months of age.[245,246] An association has been reported between syndactyly and prolonged QT interval, with life-threatening arrhythmias reported in one child during anesthesia.[247] Timothy syndrome is a multisystem disorder with cardiac, facial, limb, and neurodevelopmental features.[248]

Duplicated thumb can be present as an isolated anomaly and is present in approximately 1 in 3000 births. Hypoplastic thumbs are associated with systemic syndromes such as Holt-Oram syndrome; **V**ertebral, **A**nal, **C**ardiac, **T**racheal, **E**sophageal, **R**enal, **L**imb (VACTERL) anomalies; Fanconi anemia; Nager syndrome; and thrombocytopenia-absent radius.[249] A complete evaluation of the child is generally warranted because abnormalities can occur in the cardiovascular, neurologic, and hematopoietic systems.[249] Genetic testing is not generally needed in isolated thumb duplications.

Tissue Expanders

Tissue expansion has become a major treatment modality in the management of giant congenital hairy pigmented nevi (E-Fig. 35.17), hemangiomas, meningomyelocele, abdominal wall defects, and secondary reconstruction of extensive burn scars.[250–258] Tissue expanders effectively allow removal of the affected area and preserve sensation in a durable flap with minimal donor site morbidity.[259] These devices consist of a silicone shell that stretches to accommodate serial injections of saline solution when placed subcutaneously or, in the case of the scalp, under the galea, through an incision made in normal tissue adjacent to the lesion or defect (Fig. 35.13).[254,260] Osmotic tissue expanders have been used in burn scars, congenital nevi, alopecia, or foot deformities with reduced infection rates and low cost. Tissue expansion requires at least two surgical procedures—one to insert the expander and a second to remove it when expansion is complete; some children may require serial insertions or multiple expanders.[254] Reconstruction of areas of the head and neck constitute a particular challenge because expansion without oral, visual, or airway compromise is required.[261] Complications of tissue expansion include infection, skin erosion, leakage, migration, and flap necrosis.[257,262–265] Perioperative antibiotics are given at insertion and removal, although their effectiveness in preventing infection has not been established.[252,257,259,263,264]

Hairy Pigmented Nevi

Congenital melanocytic nevi characteristically vary in size, shape, surface texture, and hairiness. They are frequently excised because they are disfiguring and have the potential to become malignant. Serial surgical excision is common, but skin grafting and tissue expanders are also used (see E-Fig. 35.17).[259] The position and size determine the frequency of excision and anesthetic technique. If the face, head, or neck is involved, airway management should be discussed with the surgeon to allow optimal surgical access (Fig. 35.14).

In general, these children are healthy. In the cooperative and motivated child, subcutaneous infusion of a very dilute long-acting local anesthetic (e.g., ropivacaine 0.08%) mixed with epinephrine 1:1,000,000 can be used to provide painless tumescent anesthesia.[266] The local anesthetic is infused through a 30-gauge needle at an initial rate of 120 mL/hour. Blanching of skin identifies the area that is anesthetized. This method has been used successfully in children 7 years of age and older.[267] To avoid toxicity, local anesthetic volume and dosing guidelines should be followed (see Chapter 42). Repeated reconstructive procedures are often required, and attention should be paid to providing appropriate premedication where necessary (see Chapter 4).

Cosmetic Procedures

According to the American Society of Plastic Surgeons, the most common cosmetic surgeries performed in adolescents are nose reshaping, male breast reduction, ear surgery, laser hair removal, laser treatment of leg veins, and laser skin resurfacing.[268] Breast implants and liposuction are the most controversial cosmetic procedures performed, although combined they represent only 5% of cosmetic surgery in this age group. In 2011, 73% of male breast reduction and 28% of otoplasty occurred in this age group.[268] The breast augmentation procedures were performed on an outpatient basis.[269] These patients are generally healthy. Routine anesthetic induction with endotracheal intubation with no additional invasive monitoring is generally all that is required.

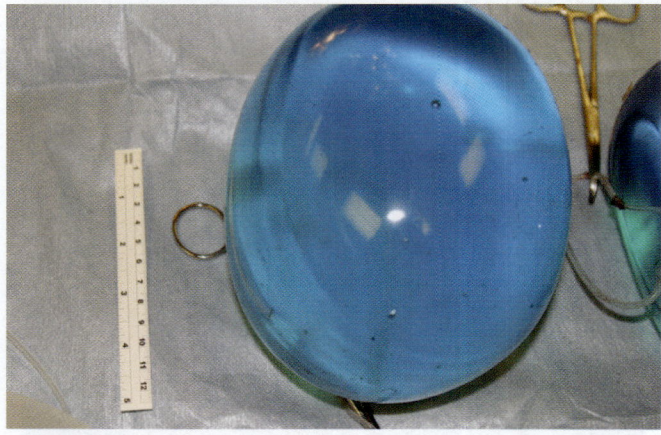

FIGURE 35.13 Tissue expander that is approximately 18 cm long. These expanders are inserted in a partially deflated state and then expanded by sequentially injecting saline solution over a period of weeks.

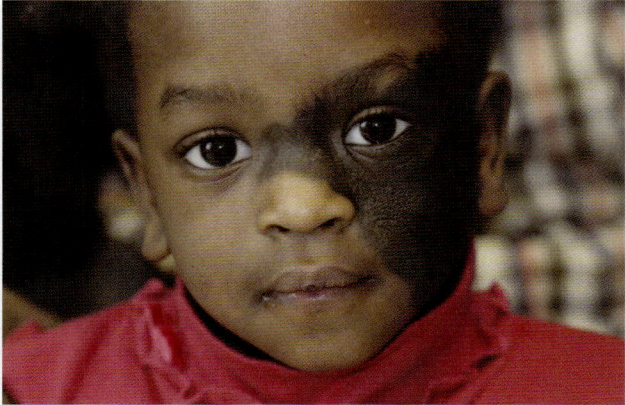

FIGURE 35.14 A heavily pigmented nevus covers the lateral aspect of the face from the eyebrow, over the bridge of the nose, and down to the skin covering the mandible. These large and disfiguring pigmented nevi must be resected in staged events.

This group of patients may be at increased risk of postoperative nausea and vomiting and will benefit from multimodal prophylaxis. Postoperative discomfort is common, requiring administration of systemic opioids or nerve blocks.

Liposuction is usually scheduled as outpatient surgery, although extensive liposuction may require an overnight admission to the hospital. This latter procedure is associated with acute complications, including itching, bruising, and swelling; damage to nerves or vital organs; blood loss; and embolization of fat or blood. Lidocaine toxicity and fluid accumulation at the surgical site are directly proportional to the volume of aspirated fat and number of treated sites.[270] The maximum safe dose of lidocaine is 28 mg/kg without liposuction and 45 mg/kg with liposuction; the difference is likely attributable to the delayed absorption during liposuction.[271] However, surgeons are increasingly using bupivacaine without adequate clinical study to determine the appropriate dose, the maximum dose, and safety recommendations.[272]

Trauma

A considerable proportion of plastic surgical procedures in children are performed for trauma and emergency surgery. Procedures include treatment of simple lacerations, animal bites, tendon, nerve and vascular repair, reimplantation of digits and limbs, and treatment of burns (see Chapter 36). The cooperative and fasted child with minor trauma can often undergo minor surgical procedures using local anesthesia, commonly administered by the plastic surgeon in the emergency department. This can be supplemented with inhalation of a 50:50 mixture of nitrous oxide and oxygen (Entonox),[273] IV administration of small doses of a benzodiazepine and opioid (e.g., midazolam 50 μg/kg, and fentanyl 0.5 μg/kg) or ketamine according to locally established sedation protocols (see Chapter 48). Alternatively, a single-injection digital nerve block is safe and effective for minor surgical procedures.[274]

Surgery for extensive injuries to digits and limbs usually requires general anesthesia because children do not tolerate prolonged application of a tourniquet. The severity and urgency of the injury dictate the timing of the surgery. The general principles of care for the child with trauma should be followed (see Chapter 39), with particular attention directed to identifying more life-threatening injuries. For urgent surgery in the presence of a full stomach, precautions against aspiration of gastric contents should be considered. For postoperative pain control, a combination of regional anesthesia or systemic analgesia is usually adequate. Continuous brachial plexus or other nerve blocks may improve tissue perfusion[275] and facilitate cooperation during postoperative physiotherapy for procedures such as digital reimplantation. Continuous nerve block may attenuate the signs associated with compartment syndrome, and frequent and meticulous attention must be paid to perfusion of the extremity.

ACKNOWLEDGMENTS

The authors acknowledge the prior contribution to this chapter from Thomas Engelhardt, MD, PhD, FRCA; Mark W. Crawford, MBBS, FRCPC; and Rajeev Subramanyam, MBBS, MD, DNB, MNAMS. The authors also thank R. Zuker, MD, FRCS, Professor of Surgery, Division of Plastic Surgery; C. Forrest, MD, FRCS, Associate Professor of Surgery, Head of the Division of Plastic Surgery, The Hospital for Sick Children, University of Toronto, Toronto, Ontario; and J. Girotto, MD, Assistant Professor of Pediatrics, Neurosurgery and Plastic Reconstructive Surgery, Director of the Cleft and Craniofacial Center, Golisano Children's Hospital at Strong Memorial Hospital, University of Rochester, Rochester, NY, for providing photographs to illustrate this chapter.

ANNOTATED REFERENCES

Antony AK, Sloan GM. Airway obstruction following palatoplasty: analysis of 247 consecutive operations. *Cleft Palate Craniofac J.* 2002;39(2):145-148.
Two hundred forty-seven children underwent palatoplasty, yielding a 6% incidence of perioperative airway obstruction. The airway obstruction occurred as late as 48 hours postoperatively. Of the 14 children with severe airway compromise, 12 required continued tracheal intubation, reintubation, and tracheostomy. Of these 14 children (93%), 13 had coexisting craniofacial abnormalities, with 7 having Pierre Robin sequence.

Faberowski LW, Black S, Mickle JP. Incidence of venous air embolism during craniectomy for craniosynostosis repair. *Anesthesiology.* 2000;92(1):20-23.
This case series of 23 children undergoing craniosynostosis reported an 83% incidence of venous air embolism using precordial Doppler monitoring. Although cardiovascular collapse did not occur, 32% developed hypotension. Detection and early intervention are important strategies to prevent cardiovascular collapse associated with this type of surgery.

Goobie SM, Haas T. Bleeding management for pediatric craniotomies and craniofacial surgery. *Paediatr Anaesth.* 2014;24(7):678-689.
This review summarizes patient blood conservation techniques and their application in pediatric craniofacial surgery and in children undergoing craniotomies. The management of massive blood loss and North American and European guidelines for transfusion management are discussed.

Goobie SM, Meier PM, Pereira LM, et al. Efficacy of tranexamic acid in pediatric craniosynostosis surgery: a double-blind, placebo-controlled trial. *Anesthesiology.* 2011;114(4):862-871.
This randomized, placebo-controlled trial examined the effects of tranexamic acid on blood loss during reconstructive craniosynostosis surgery. Both blood loss and blood transfusion requirements were significantly reduced, by almost 50%.

Jackson O, Basta M, Sonnad S, et al. Perioperative risk factors for adverse airway events in patients undergoing cleft palate repair. *Cleft Palate Craniofac J.* 2013;50(3):330-336.
Three hundred children younger than 2 years of age undergoing primary cleft palate repair using the modified Furlow technique were reviewed for the occurrence of perioperative adverse airway events. Adverse airway events occurred in 23% of patients overall. Airway complications were more likely in children with a craniofacial syndrome, preoperative airway problems, and with less experienced providers.

Lavoie J. Blood transfusion risks and alternative strategies in pediatric patients. *Paediatr Anaesth.* 2011;21(1):14-24.
This review summarizes blood conservation modalities such as acute normovolemic hemodilution, hypervolemic hemodilution, deliberate hypotension, antifibrinolytics, intraoperative blood salvage, and autologous blood donation. The transfusion triggers and algorithms and the current literature in blood transfusion alternatives are discussed.

Meier PM, Goobie SM, DiNardo JA, et al. Endoscopic strip craniectomy in early infancy: the initial five years of anesthesia experience. *Anesth Analg.* 2011;112(2):407-414.
This retrospective chart review studied 100 infants ranging from 4 to 34 weeks of age (weight: 3.2-10.1 kg) who underwent single and multiple endoscopic strip craniectomies. Four infants had a craniofacial syndrome; 87 infants underwent single and 13 multiple craniectomy. The risk factors for bleeding are identified, along with an emphasis on venous air embolism, intensive care unit admissions, and reoperation.

Nargozian C. The airway in patients with craniofacial abnormalities. *Paediatr Anaesth.* 2004;14(12):53-59.
This review summarizes the salient features and airway implications of the major craniofacial disorders that affect children, including Pierre Robin sequence, Treacher Collins syndrome, Goldenhar syndrome, and Klippel-Feil syndrome. The anatomic pathology is very well described, and the clinical implications of the pathologic condition are thoroughly discussed.

A complete reference list can be found online at ExpertConsult.com.

36

Burn Injuries

ERIK S. SHANK, CHARLES J. COTÉ, AND J.A. JEEVENDRA MARTYN

Pathophysiology	**Pharmacology**
Cardiac	**Resuscitation and Initial Evaluation**
Pulmonary	Airway and Oxygenation
Renal	Carbon Monoxide and Cyanide Poisoning
Hepatic	Adequacy of Circulation
Central Nervous System	Associated Injury
Hematologic	Circumferential Burns
Gastrointestinal	Electrical Burns
Endocrine	**Guidelines to Anesthetic Management**
Skin	Special Considerations
Metabolic	Pain Management and Postoperative Care
Calcium Homeostasis	**Summary**
Neuropsychiatric	

MILLIONS OF PEOPLE ARE TREATED FOR BURNS every year in the United States: hundreds of thousands of those who are hospitalized have a significant mortality rate.[1-3] The National Burn Repository Report for 2014 reviewed its 10-year experience (2003–2013)[4]; overall mortality from 191,848 records in both males (3.4%–2.7%) and females (4.6%–3.3%) was reduced compared with the previous epoch. Children younger than 5 years of age accounted for 19% of cases (27,379), with most children burned in their homes (~73%). The racial distribution was ~59% Caucasian, ~20% African American, 14% Hispanic, 2.4% Asian, and other ~5% with most pediatric injuries caused by scalds or contact with hot objects. Inhalation injury was reported in 5.4% of cases. Approximately 1861 cases were suspected child abuse. Mortality varied from 0.6% in those with less than 10% body surface area (BSA) burns to ~84% for those with more than 90% BSA burns. It is estimated that approximately 200,000 children with burn injuries are treated in the emergency department each year in the United States; the majority are younger than 6 years.[4,5] Children with burn injuries are well managed only when their care providers thoroughly understand the pathophysiologic and pharmacologic abnormalities associated with burn injury.[6,7] These abnormalities include metabolic derangements, neurohumoral responses, massive fluid shifts, sepsis, and the systemic effects of massive tissue destruction. In this chapter we address the pathophysiology, the initial evaluation and resuscitation, and the anesthetic and pain management of children with burn injuries. Some of the principles presented are the result of more than 40 years of experience in caring for children with burn injuries, and others are derived from experiences with adults and applied to children.

Approximately 486,000 people suffered burn injuries in the United States in 2015, with about 15,000 children hospitalized with burn injuries.[1] The mortality rate from burn injuries has declined steadily over the past decades, owing to the advent of dedicated hospital burn centers,[8,9] improved surgical techniques, and safer anesthetic management. However, almost 1100 children still die each year from fire and burn injuries (http://burninjuryguide.com/burn-statistics/). Safety prevention efforts such as smoke detectors have not reduced pediatric flame injuries because many flame injuries are related to children playing with matches,[10,11] although there has been a small overall decrease in total burn injuries to children.[12]

Pathophysiology

Thermal injury to the skin disrupts the vital barrier responsible for thermal regulation, bacterial defenses, and fluid and electrolyte balance.[13] Even minor, localized burn injuries may be associated with diffuse and dramatic systemic responses that can have an impact on all systems of the body.[6] Mediators released from the burned areas (complement, arachidonic acid metabolites, cytokines, and oxygen radicals) activate local and systemic inflammatory responses.[7,14] Abnormal cytokine values reflect the severity of injury, and these abnormalities may persist for years after injury.[15-19] Endotoxins are frequently detected immediately after the burn, correlate with burn size, and are predictive of multiorgan failure and the subsequent patient demise.[20] The clinical symptoms and pathologic changes are relatively more severe in children, and unfortunately the gravity of the injury is often underestimated because of their greater BSA/weight ratio (Fig. 36.1).[21,22]

Soon after the injury, massive fluid volumes shift from the vascular compartment to burned tissues and nonburned areas of the body resulting in hemoconcentration.[6,23] Despite this massive fluid loss, systemic blood pressure is usually maintained by vasoconstriction through an outpouring of catecholamines and antidiuretic hormone.[24] In the first 4 days after a moderate- or larger (~40% BSA)-sized burn, an amount of albumin equal to

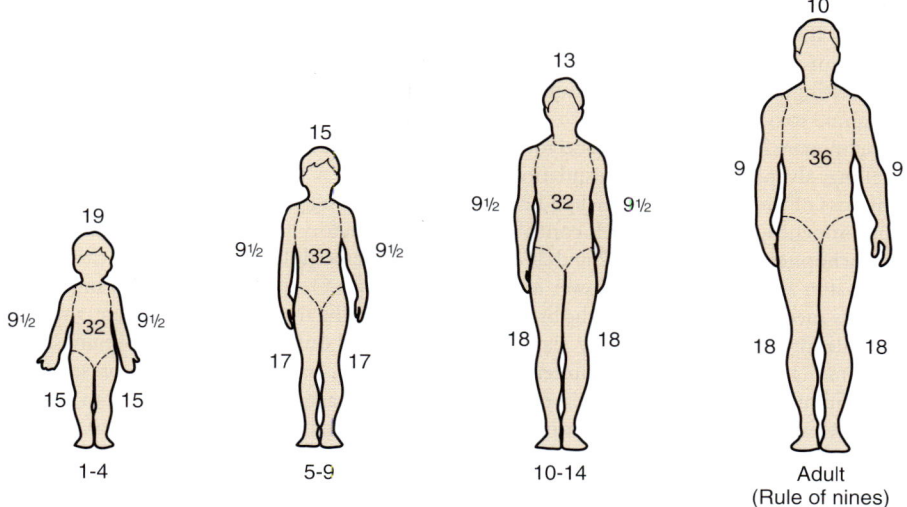

FIGURE 36.1 The different proportions of body surface area are illustrated for the calculation of percentage of burn according to a patient's age. Note the large proportion of body surface area that the head and face account for in an infant. (From Carvajal HF, Goldman AS. Burns. In: Vaughan VC III, McKay RJ, Nelson WE, eds. *Nelson's Textbook of Pediatrics.* Philadelphia: WB Saunders; 1975:281.)

approximately twice the total body plasma content is lost through the wound. In addition to the direct effects of the burn (thrombosis, increased capillary permeability), changes in vascular integrity occur in areas remote from the injury, resulting in widespread edema,[25] including life-threatening pulmonary edema.

A review of 821 pediatric patient outcomes noted a very high mortality rate when three or more organs failed. Respiratory failure occurred primarily in the first 5 days, cardiac and renal failure in the first 3 weeks, and hepatic failure with increasing the duration of hospital stay.[26]

CARDIAC

Immediately after an injury, cardiac output is dramatically reduced.[27,28] This is related to both the rapid reduction in circulating blood volume and the severe compressive effects of circumferential burns on the abdomen and chest that impair venous return.[29] Despite volume replacement and adequate cardiac filling pressures, cardiac output often remains reduced because of direct myocardial depression from circulating myocardial depressant factors such as interleukins, tumor necrosis factors, altered β-adrenergic receptor modulation,[30] or oxygen free radicals in victims with extensive third-degree burns.[31–34] Transesophageal echocardiography may be helpful in guiding supportive care in the early phase.[35] Our experience is that acutely burned children frequently require inotropic support during this acute period of depressed cardiac function; inotropes improve cardiac output while avoiding volume overload. Decreased cardiac output may also be caused by gram-negative sepsis or ongoing hypovolemia.

Children develop a hypermetabolic state 3 to 5 days after a burn injury. This state is associated with a twofold to threefold increase in cardiac output, which persists for weeks to months, depending on the extent of the injury and the time needed for wound closure; heart rate, cardiac output, cardiac index, and rate-pressure product are increased for at least 2 years after burns that involve 40% or more of BSA.[36] Some children develop a reversible cardiomyopathy.[37] Hypertension also occurs during this hypermetabolic period, which may in part, be related to inadequate

pain control. However, mediators such as increased catecholamines, atrial natriuretic factor, renin-angiotensin, endothelin-1, vasopressin, and others can cause intermittent or persistent hypertension.[38–42] Closure of the burn wound usually decreases metabolic demand, resulting in a concomitant reduction in cardiac output.[43,44] Some children may benefit from treatment with propranolol, which reduces cardiac work and decreases the systemic inflammatory response but does not appear to have any impact on mortality.[45–47] Despite the widespread use of propranolol in both adults and children to attenuate this hypermetabolic response, neither randomized studies nor a consensus regarding the dosing have been forthcoming.[48]

PULMONARY

Pulmonary function may be adversely affected from the upper airway to terminal alveoli.[49,50] The upper airway is an excellent heat exchanger; just as it warms cold air, it cools hot air. The air in a closed space (e.g., house or automobile fire) may reach 538°C (1000°F) 2 feet above floor level; cooling of hot inspired air causes a severe thermal injury to laryngeal structures, particularly those above the glottis.[51] These airway burns cause massive edema of all laryngeal and tracheal structures above the carina (see later discussion). The thermal insult also injures or destroys the ciliated epithelium and mucosa in the proximal bronchi. The inhalation of toxic fumes, such as nitrogen dioxide and sulfur dioxide released from burning plastic that combine with water in the tracheobronchial tree to form nitric and sulfuric acids, may damage the distal bronchi and alveoli. These acid gases and phosgene are small aerosolized particles that penetrate deep into the tracheobronchial tree, damaging alveolar membranes and surfactant.[52] Thus upper airway injury is usually a thermal insult, whereas lower airway injury is a chemical or toxic insult. Wool and cotton combustion forms aldehydes, which in concentrations as small as 10 ppm may cause coughing and "respiratory braking" that reduce the rate and depth of breathing and cause pulmonary edema.[53,54] Combustion of synthetic materials (insulation, wall paneling), particularly in enclosed-space fires, releases hydrogen cyanide[55] leading to histotoxic hypoxia and death,[56] while mimicking carbon monoxide (CO) poisoning.[57] Inhalation of hydrogen cyanide is an often unrecognized cause of immediate death.[58,59] The role of hydroxocobalamin in this setting is unclear but is recommended by some centers when cyanide toxicity is suspected.[60-63]

The overall effect of a pulmonary inhalation injury is necrotizing bronchitis, bronchial swelling, alveolar destruction, exudation of protein, loss of surfactant, loss of the protective bronchial lining, loss of cilial function, and bronchospasm, all of which contribute to the development of bronchopneumonia (Figs. 36.2 and 36.3).[49] Inhalation of particulate matter (smoke, soot) and lower airway edema also obstruct the airway mechanically. Edema of the bronchi, combined with loss of integrity of the pulmonary capillary endothelium, decreases pulmonary compliance. Circumferential chest burns may have a tourniquet-like effect that decreases chest wall compliance; escharotomy even in the prehospital setting may be lifesaving.[29,64] All of these injuries lead to ventilation-perfusion abnormalities and right-to-left intrapulmonary shunting, with hypoxemia and hypercarbia. In adults, the PaO_2/FIO_2 ratio and

baseline carboxyhemoglobin (COHb) concentrations are predictive of mortality.[65] One center has reported improved early oxygenation in children with the use of high-frequency oscillation ventilation[66]; the use of extracorporeal membrane oxygenation has had mixed results with no apparent improvement in outcomes.[67]

One pediatric trial of inhaled heparin and acetylcysteine suggested a benefit with decreased airway cast formation and mucus plugging.[68] However, subsequent studies have yielded contradictory results.[69,70] CO inhalation can further compromise both hemoglobin's oxygen (O_2)-carrying capacity and its ability to deliver O_2 to tissues. CO also impairs O_2 usage at the cellular level (cellular respiration). Severe smoke inhalation alone may occur without externally visible injuries.[58,59,71] One clue that smoke inhalation has occurred is the presence of singed nasal hairs or nasal passages. Steam inhalation can also cause supraglottic edema that presents with symptoms similar to epiglottitis related to edema rather than infection.[72]

Reduction in cardiac output also can contribute to hypoxemia. Thus correction of arterial O_2 desaturation requires evaluation of

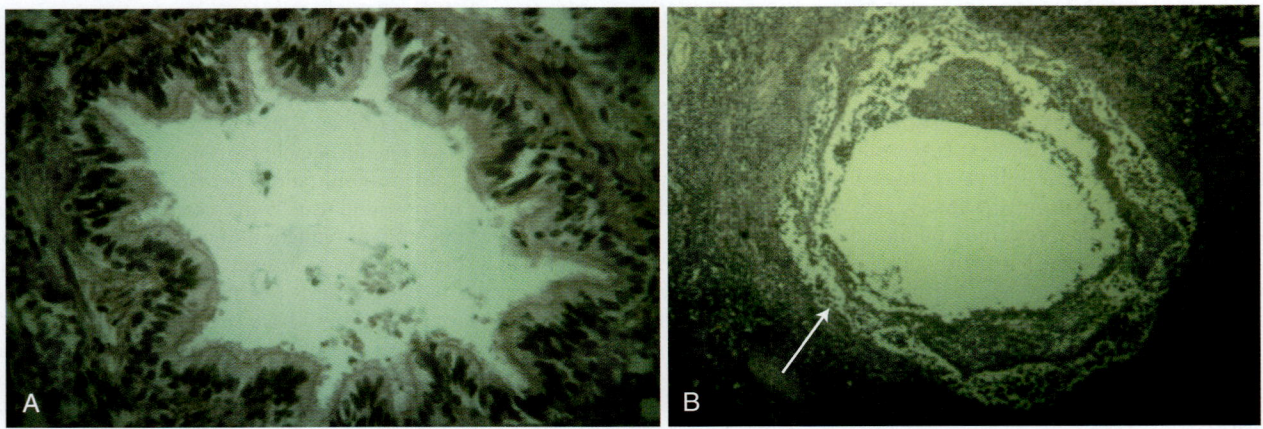

FIGURE 36.2 A, Cross section of a normal bronchiole. Note the ciliated epithelial layer. **B,** Compare with a cross section of a distal bronchiole from a child who died of an inhalation injury. Note the marked thickening of the bronchial wall, the massive inflammatory cell infiltrate, the sloughing of the mucosa *(arrow)*, and the total destruction of the ciliated columnar epithelium.

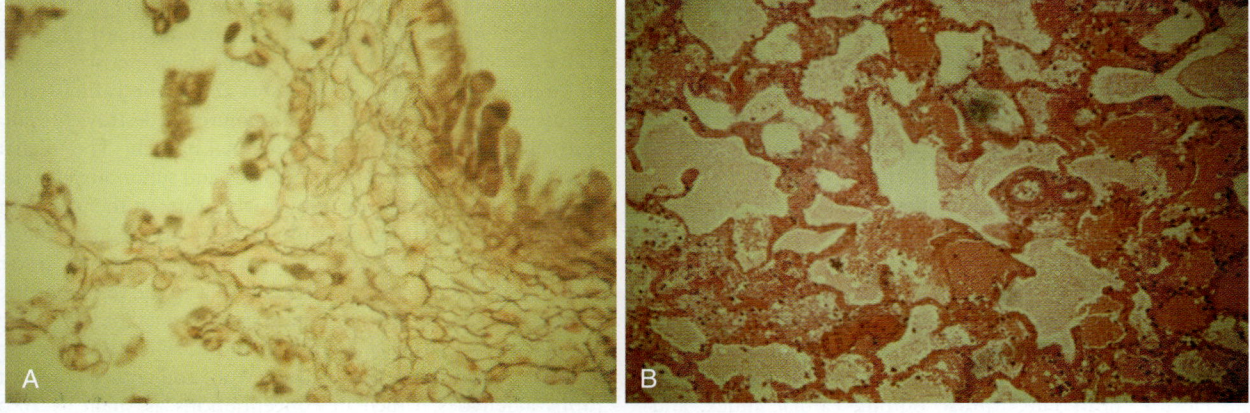

FIGURE 36.3 A, Normal alveoli. **B,** Inhalation alveolar injury is generally related to noxious fumes such as nitrogen dioxide and sulfur dioxide that are carried far down the tracheobronchial tree, combine with exhaled water, and form nitric acid and sulfuric acid, resulting in pulmonary congestion, alveolar injury, and hyaline membrane formation.

both extrapulmonary and intrapulmonary factors,[25,73] including cardiac output, mixed venous O_2 content or saturation, and shunt fraction.[27] In general, the prognosis for survival is diminished by the presence of an inhalation injury that doubles the mortality from cutaneous burns[52]; in children mortality is reported to be approximately 16%.[74]

RENAL

Renal function may be adversely affected soon after the injury, primarily as a result of myoglobinuria and hemoglobinuria but also from hypoxemia, hypotension, or inhaled toxins leading to acute tubular necrosis.[75] Myoglobinemia most commonly occurs after electrical injury,[76,77] whereas hemoglobinemia is common after severe cutaneous burns covering 40% or more of BSA. Catecholamines, angiotensin, and vasopressin production increase; and release of vasoactive peptides such as endothelin-1 cause systemic vasoconstriction, compounding the renal dysfunction.[78–81] Fluid retention is common during the first 3 to 5 days after a burn injury and is followed thereafter by a diuresis. Glomerular filtration rate (GFR) decreases soon after the injury, although 3 to 7 days after the burn injury, it actually increases pari passu with an increased cardiac output and metabolic rate, thus affecting the clearance (increased or decreased) of many antibiotics and other medications that depend on renal excretion.[82–87] Children who sustain a burn affecting 40% or more of BSA demonstrate renal tubular dysfunction with an inability to concentrate urine.[24] Even during hyperosmolar states, antidiuresis is not observed, suggesting an inadequate renal response to antidiuretic hormone and aldosterone. Thus an adequate urine output may be observed even in the presence of hypovolemia.[88] Episodic or persistent hypertension is frequent in children, in part mediated by an increase in renin and catecholamine production[89,90]; in some children treatment with propranolol may be indicated.

HEPATIC

The liver may also be damaged by hypoxemia, hypoperfusion as a result of inhaled or absorbed chemical toxins, hypovolemia, or hypotension during the early postburn phase.[91,92] Reperfusion injury may harm the liver when an adequate circulation is reestablished. Hepatic dysfunction may also result from drug toxicity, sepsis, the hypermetabolic response to burns, or blood transfusions.[19] Studies in adults and animal models have found increased hepatic blood flow, increased protein synthesis and breakdown, and increased hepatic gluconeogenesis during the hypermetabolic phase of burn injury.[93] Sustained increases in hepatic blood flow deliver more drug to the liver; this effect, combined with drug-induced enzyme induction, may increase the clearance of drugs.[94] Although all studies of animals suggest decreased clearance of drugs after burn injury, clinical studies of the capacity of the liver to metabolize drugs are conflicting, even for the same class of drugs.[95–100] The magnitude of the burn, the time after injury, and the effects of coadministered drugs, alone or in combination, as well as alterations in protein binding and volume of distribution, may have contributed to the conflicting reports regarding drug half-lives. With the onset of sepsis, hepatic glucose output and alanine uptake may decrease sharply but hepatic blood flow and O_2 usage can remain increased.[91,101] Fatty infiltration of the liver has also been reported.[102]

CENTRAL NERVOUS SYSTEM

The central nervous system (CNS) may be adversely affected by inhalation of neurotoxic chemicals or by hypoxic encephalopathy; other contributing factors include sepsis, hyponatremia, and hypovolemia.[103] CNS dysfunction includes hallucinations, personality changes, delirium, seizures, abnormal neurologic symptoms, and coma,[104] which may be due to the burn injury or to the drugs necessary for sedation, anxiolysis, and analgesia[105]; these effects usually clear after several weeks. Abnormalities of CNS neurotransmitters have been postulated to mediate the anorexia associated with extensive burn injury.[106] The possibility of cerebral edema and increased intracranial pressure must also be considered during the initial phases of burn injury. Under such circumstances, the usual measures for treating increased intracranial pressure would be instituted (see Chapter 26). Rapid overcorrection of hyponatremia also may be associated with cerebral injury.[107]

HEMATOLOGIC

The hematopoietic system is also adversely affected after burn injury. Blood viscosity may increase with hemoconcentration secondary to fluid shifts and alterations in plasma protein content.[108] Ongoing microangiopathic hemolytic anemia is common.[109] An inhibitor of erythroid stem cells may contribute to the anemia of burns, but burned patients have a normal erythropoietin response to anemia.[110] The half-life of red blood cells is diminished and multiple blood draws further contribute to the development of anemia.[111,112] The possible role of recombinant erythropoietin in the care of children with burns has yet to be defined.[113–116] One study in adults reported no reduction in either mortality or blood transfusion requirements in patients who received recombinant erythropoietin compared with controls.[117] However, evolving evidence suggests that recombinant erythropoietin may promote skin and burn wound healing when administered systemically or locally injected.[118–121]

In the early stage, thrombocytopenia secondary to increased platelet aggregation with a nadir at approximately 3 days and trapping of platelets in the lungs is followed by an increase in platelet count 10 to 14 days after the burn injury. A prolonged period of thrombocytopenia and reduced nadir in platelet count compared with survivors are both associated with sepsis and increased mortality.[122,123] In some patients, thrombocytopenia may persist for several months.[112,122] An increase in fibrin split products (disseminated intravascular coagulopathy), which lasts for 3 to 5 days, may also occur.[85] Factors V, VII, and VIII and fibrinogen are increased several-fold over baseline for the first 3 months after severe injury uncomplicated by sepsis.[124,125] Children with increased platelet counts (thrombocytosis) (>1 million/mm³) who then developed sepsis in our unit experienced a marked decrease in the platelet count; the sudden onset of thrombocytopenia should prompt an evaluation of the child for sepsis.[122,123,126] Likewise, large swings in the fibrinogen concentration can occur (up to 2 g/dL),[127] although these do not appear to herald an increase in the incidence of thrombotic events.

GASTROINTESTINAL

Gastrointestinal function is diminished immediately after thermal injury secondary to the onset of gastric stasis and intestinal ileus.[128] Because of the risk of pulmonary aspiration of gastric contents during this time, the stomach should be adequately vented and appropriate gastric acid ulcer prophylaxis instituted. At 48 to 72 hours after a burn injury, when generalized edema is resolving, gastrointestinal function usually resumes. Enteral feeding should be established at this time to provide calories, to blunt the hypermetabolic response, and to attenuate gluconeogenesis and stress ulceration.[108,129–132] Early enteral feeding has the added advantages of diminishing muscle catabolism, reducing bacterial translocation through the intestinal mucosa, and being associated with reduced mortality.[133-136]

In children who do not tolerate enteral feeding, parenteral nutrition must be initiated.[129,132,137,138] Stress ulcers (Curling ulcers) are associated with any burn injury and may be life-threatening, although the incidence has decreased in critically ill patients because of better management of systemic hypoperfusion, early gut feeding, and improved pharmacologic control of gastric acidity.[139] Prospective studies of pediatric and adult burn patients and patients in intensive care indicate that cimetidine or ranitidine in the usual doses does not adequately protect critically ill patients from increases in gastric acidity.[83,84] The increased requirement for drugs is due to alterations in their pharmacokinetics.[83] Therefore frequent feedings when tolerated and the liberal use of antacids, combined with larger or more frequent doses of H_2-receptor antagonists (or proton pump inhibitors), may be required to prevent stress ulcers.[83,108,128,140]

ENDOCRINE

The endocrinologic response to acute thermal injury involves most organ systems. Stimuli that trigger endocrine responses include the thermal injury itself, type of burn (scald vs. flame) and subsequent fluid shifts, as well as the stress responses associated with critical illness.[141,142] These may include decreased circulating hormone concentrations (e.g., triiodothyronine, dehydroepiandrosterone, and testosterone), as well as increased concentrations of other hormones (antidiuretic hormone, catecholamines, renin, angiotensin II, and cortisol).[143] Replacement therapy with synthetic androgenic steroids (e.g., oxandrolone) reduces acute hospital stay, improves body composition (lean body mass), muscle protein deposition,[144] and hepatic protein synthesis.[145,146] A 5-year follow-up study found that oxandrolone-treated children had improved height percentile, bone mineral content, and improved cardiac function and muscle strength; no adverse effects from long-term administration were noted.[147] Glucose control may be poor, owing to the increased levels of cortisol and insulin resistance; abnormal glucose control may persist for up to 36 months after the burn injury.[148-151] Tight control of hyperglycemia may improve mitochondrial oxidative capacity,[152] reduce protein turnover,[153] decrease the incidence of urinary tract infection, and improve the survival of critically ill burn patients, although the last finding resulted from a single study.[154,155] However, this needs to be balanced with the increased likelihood of hypoglycemic events, which in turn are associated with increased mortality.[153,156] Avoiding hyperglycemia may attenuate the risk of cerebral injury from hypoperfusion states (see Chapters 26 and 39); one group recommends a target blood glucose level of 130 mg/dL.[155] Blocking the renin-angiotensin system may improve the insulin response after burn injury.[45-47,157]

SKIN

Extensive skin destruction, proportional to the number of layers of tissue damaged, results in the inability to regulate body heat, conserve fluids and electrolytes, and protect against bacterial invasion.[158] Because children have a much greater BSA/weight ratio compared with adults, they are more likely to become hypothermic (see Fig. 36.1). Thus it is important to keep children covered as much as possible, to increase the environmental temperature, and to use radiant warmers, plastic wrap around extremities, reflective insulated blankets, artificial "noses" (in-line moisture and heat exchangers), and hot-air heating blankets. Late

complications affecting the skin include progressive scar formation, which results in movement-restricting contractures.[29,159] Topical antibiotic and antibacterial therapy are necessary to prevent burn wound sepsis.[160-165] There is evolving evidence and intensive investigation regarding the role of stem cell therapy that may improve burn would healing and reduce scar formation.[166-174]

METABOLIC

Many metabolic changes follow extensive burn injury.[175] Increased use of glucose, fat, and protein (particularly muscle breakdown)[176] results in greater O_2 demand and increased carbon dioxide (CO_2) production.[a] Mediators that have been implicated in these metabolic changes include interleukin-1, tumor necrosis factor, catecholamines, prostanoids, and other stress hormones.[2,184] Centrally mediated or sepsis-induced hyperthermia also increases O_2 consumption and CO_2 production. Some of these abnormalities may persist even after complete closure of burn wounds, when metabolic demand is already reduced.[b] Intravenous (IV) alimentation, particularly with increased glucose concentrations, may also increase CO_2 production and therefore increase ventilatory requirements.[137] The increase in O_2 demand[186] and CO_2 production must be compensated for during controlled mechanical ventilation; treatment of fever reduces metabolic demand.[187]

CALCIUM HOMEOSTASIS

The ionized calcium concentrations in acutely burned patients are dramatically decreased. Marked abnormalities of calcium and magnesium metabolism, including hypoparathyroidism in both acute and recovery phases, may persist for weeks after injury (E-Fig. 36.1).[188,189] Increased bone resorption with failure of bone calcium uptake, as well as low levels of vitamin D and a markedly reduced conversion in burned skin of dehydrocholesterol to previtamin D, result in bone density loss.[190-192] Treatment with pamidronate, a drug that inhibits bone resorption, conserves bone mass and reduces muscle protein turnover after burn injury in children.[193-195] Hypophosphatemia and hypermagnesemia revert toward normal during the latter phase of recovery from the acute injury. The usual reciprocal relationship between calcium and inorganic phosphate is not evident in those with major burns. Therefore supplemental calcium therapy is extremely important, particularly when rapid intraoperative colloid and fresh frozen plasma (FFP) infusions are required, because ionized hypocalcemia dramatically impairs cardiovascular homeostasis. Frequent small boluses of calcium are safer and more effective than intermittent large boluses (see also Figs. 12.8 and 12.9).[196] Doses of 5 mg/kg calcium chloride or 15 mg/kg calcium gluconate ionize at equivalent rates and produce equivalent increases in serum calcium concentration. During and after recovery from burn injury, high-dose vitamin D supplements are strongly recommended to offset the decreased conversion of 7-dehydrocholesterol to previtamin D_3.[197-199]

NEUROPSYCHIATRIC

It is imperative to recognize that physical trauma is not the only trauma sustained by the pediatric burn patient; psychological trauma and its associated long-term sequelae are also common.[200,201] A large percentage of acutely burned children and their parents present with acute stress or develop posttraumatic stress disorders[200-204];

---

[a]References 2, 91, 108, 137, 161, and 177–183.
[b]References 15, 18, 19, 44, 46, and 185.

risk factors include the size of burn, the degree of pain, the pulse rate, and parental issues.[205] Treatment with fluoxetine or imipramine may ameliorate these stress disorders,[206–208] although one randomized controlled study found no difference from placebo.[209] Another study found risperidone to be of value in reducing stress symptoms.[210] There is an increased incidence of attention-deficit disorders in pediatric burn patients, likely owing to impulsivity.[211,212] Another concern is that sleep efficiency with markedly decreased rapid eye movement time persists for years in children after burn injury, which might necessitate consultation with a sleep specialist.[213] A study of the pharmacokinetics of zolpidem prescribed to reduce sleep fragmentation and insomnia reported an increased frequency or dose may be required for children with large burns.[214] Furthermore, after a burn injury, obese children are at significant risk for obstructive sleep apnea, abnormal respiratory disturbance index, episodes of desaturation, and apneic events.[215] Additionally, a normal psychosocial support network may be impaired in the families of burn patients, even before the burn injury.[216–218]

Pharmacology

Burn injury induces many physiologic changes that affect drug pharmacokinetics and pharmacodynamics. During the hypovolemic period, uptake and clearance of drugs may decrease because of impaired organ perfusion.[2,94–97,219] During the hypermetabolic phase, the activity of organs that clear drugs from the circulation (e.g., the liver and kidneys) are enhanced because of enzyme induction and increased blood flow.[a] Massive edema and loss of drugs through burn wounds increase the volume of drug distribution.[226]

Many drugs are highly bound by plasma proteins, rendering only a small unbound fraction that determines the drug activity. The two major binding proteins, α_1-acid glycoprotein and albumin, increase and decrease, respectively, after a burn injury. These changes exert substantive effects on the free fractions of the drugs they bind.[94,223,227] For example, the clearance of morphine and meperidine is enhanced or impaired, depending on the size of the burn, with a trend to reduced morphine or meperidine clearance after large burns compared with moderate burns. In general, burned children clear drugs more readily than those without burn injuries.[96–98,226,228,229] Similarly, pharmacokinetic studies of lorazepam and diazepam indicate that the clearance of the former is increased, whereas that of the latter is decreased.[99,100] In the case of oral ketamine, the clearance was unaffected in children with small burns, although gastric absorption of the oral formulation was delayed.[230]

Evidence indicates that burn injury, with its complications and hormonal responses, may affect the number of receptors in tissues.[99,106,219,223,231–238] Therefore reports of aberrant responses to drugs acting on adrenergic and cholinergic receptors are not surprising. These include altered sensitivity to succinylcholine at the neuromuscular junction, increased sensitivity to dopamine in the pulmonary circulation, and decreased sensitivity to nondepolarizing neuromuscular blocking drugs (NDBDs).[94,231,233–235,239–241] Other examples of drugs affected by burn-induced kinetic and dynamic changes include aminoglycoside antibiotics, diazepam, and cimetidine. Burn-induced alterations in kinetics and dynamics make the clinical response to any medication unpredictable. Therefore clinical effects should always be closely monitored and

plasma concentrations, protein binding, and clearance evaluated when possible.[83,86,94,242–246] Dexmedetomidine (see later discussion) also may have altered pharmacodynamics in the burned child; because of the known hypotensive effects of the α_{2a}-adrenoceptor agonists, particular attention to limit the dose and to ensure euvolemia may minimize the hemodynamic consequences.[247]

Resuscitation and Initial Evaluation

Resuscitation of children with a burn injury requires a clear and secure airway, as well as maintenance of adequate oxygenation, perfusion, and circulating blood volume. The diagnosis and evaluation of associated injuries also must be considered.

AIRWAY AND OXYGENATION

Every burn patient, especially those with inhalation injuries, must be considered hypoxemic and exposed to CO. Therefore during transport to the hospital and on admission, administration of high inspired concentrations of O_2 is mandatory, pending evaluation of the severity of CO poisoning and pulmonary injury (see later discussion).[246] Direct injury to the airway and alveoli occurs in children with inhalation of smoke, flames, superheated air, noxious gases, or steam.[b] When a child is burned in an enclosed space (house, automobile) or if thermal burns or carbonaceous materials are evident about the mouth and nose, inhalational injury is probable.[258,276] Upper airway obstruction caused by edema of the lips, nose, tongue, pharynx, glottis, and subglottis is very common. The resultant airway obstruction can be compared with the combined effects of acute macroglossia, epiglottitis, macro uvula, and laryngotracheobronchitis. The decreasing patency of the airway resulting from rapidly increasing edema, beginning in the first hours after the injury and lasting several days, makes delayed intubation hazardous if not impossible (Fig. 36.4). Prophylactic intubation should be performed in any case of severe facial burns or when pulmonary burn and upper airway inhalation injury are suspected. Mortality is related to the presence or absence of inhalation injury.[71,74,265–275,277]

Control of the airway in children is usually accomplished with the child under general anesthesia. Our early clinical experience showed that tracheal tubes could be left in place in these children for weeks with fewer risks than the alternative, tracheostomy.[278,279] Tracheostomy in thermally injured children was associated with high mortality rates; in one pediatric series the death rate approached 100%.[280] However, in recent years and with the development of superior antibiotics, there has been a move back to performing tracheostomy for children expected to require long-term ventilation, although one review of burn centers in North America found that the practice of performing a tracheostomy in burned children varied.[281] Some report that an early tracheostomy reduces the risk of subglottic stenosis[282,283]; the duration of tracheostomy is related to BSA burn and not age.[284] When early airway instrumentation is indicated, a cuffed tracheal tube is preferred to reduce the need for changing the tube to deliver high peak inspiratory pressures should they be required.[285] We routinely use cuffed tracheal tubes, appreciating the added flexibility they offer as airway edema recedes, and it is common to allow permissive hypercarbia to reduce barotrauma.[286] Tracheal tubes with a more distal cuff and made of thinner material may reduce the potential for airway injury (see also Figs. 14.15 and

[a]References 32, 83, 86, 91, 94, 100, and 219–225.

[b]References 53, 71, 74, 159, 184, and 248–275.

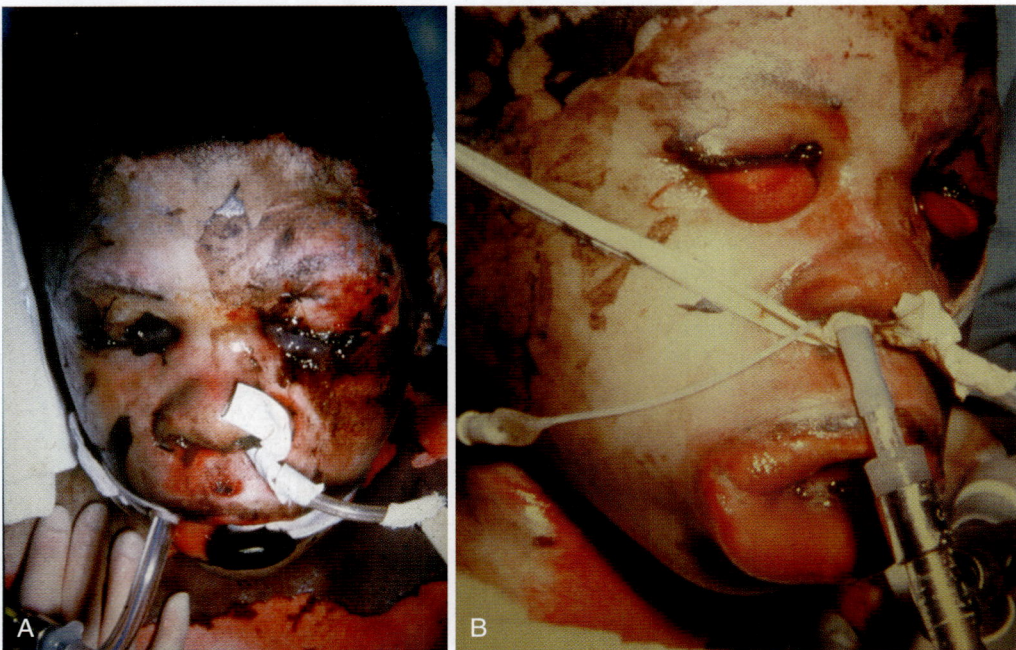

FIGURE 36.4 A, A young child who had just sustained a facial burn in a closed space. Note the early onset of facial edema. **B**, Several hours later there is massive edema that extends into the oropharynx, larynx, and trachea (similar to the combined effects of macroglossia, epiglottitis, and laryngotracheobronchitis). Early prophylactic intubation is mandatory in any facial burn or in any child when there is potential for inhalation injury. Note that the cuffed endotracheal tube was changed from an oral to a nasal position and that it is secured with cloth tape rather than adhesive tape.

14.17), but in the hot environment of a burn unit, they may have a greater tendency toward kinking.[287–293]

CARBON MONOXIDE AND CYANIDE POISONING

Most smoke inhalation victims have CO poisoning; direct measurement of COHb is important to guide treatment. Estimates of COHb concentrations may be derived by measuring (not calculating) O_2 saturation or arterial O_2 content. The half-life of COHb is approximately 5 hours when the patient is breathing room air but decreases to 90 minutes when 100% O_2 is administered.[294,295] Immediate administration of O_2 is essential to achieve the maximum possible PaO_2. Positive-pressure ventilation[296–298] and hyperbaric O_2 may also be indicated (see later discussion).

Standard pulse oximeters cannot accurately monitor oxygen saturation in patients with CO poisoning because COHb produces an overestimation of O_2 saturation; the photodetector is "fooled" into interpreting COHb as oxyhemoglobin.[299–301] An eight-wavelength pulse oximeter is capable of measuring COHb and methemoglobin, but the sensors are quite expensive.[302–305] Concern arose from a study of 1363 patients that compared the Rad-57 device with cooximetry (Masimo Corporation, Irvine, CA), which reported a 9% incidence of false-positive values and an 18% incidence of false-negative values. The authors concluded that pulse oximetry with eight-wavelength sensors yields both greater and lesser values than standard measures of carboxyhemoglobin and that it should not be used for patient management decisions.[306] It is important to be aware that in neonates and young infants, the presence of fetal hemoglobin will result in a false increase in COHb.[307,308]

COHb is produced by the combination of CO with the iron of the heme radical at the O_2-binding site. CO combines more slowly with hemoglobin than O_2 but is bound 200 times more firmly.[309,310] Inhalation of 1% CO for just 2 minutes can result in COHb values of 30% (E-Fig. 36.2).[311] The toxic effects of CO poisoning are due to tissue, organ, and cellular hypoxia from decreased O_2 delivery because CO reduces O_2 binding capacity to the hemoglobin molecule at the tissue level and to cytochromes in the respiratory chain at the cellular level; even in small amounts, COHb shifts the O_2 dissociation curve to the left (E-Fig. 36.3), reducing release of O_2 from hemoglobin.[53,246,296,310–314] For example, if an individual had 40% COHb, this would reduce the O_2-carrying capacity from 20 mL/100 g of hemoglobin to 12 mL/100 g with the leftward shift, further compromising O_2 delivery.

Evidence supporting the use of hyperbaric oxygenation (HBO) therapy as an adjunct therapy for burns remains controversial.[108,315–319] A Cochrane review concluded that insufficient data exist to demonstrate reduced adverse neurologic outcomes with HBO therapy and that additional research is needed to "better define the role, if any, of HBO in the treatment of patients with CO poisoning."[320] The most common indication for hyperbaric therapy in burned children is concomitant CO poisoning.[53,321–325] Children with significant CO exposure are at risk of developing both acute and delayed neurologic sequelae. The pathophysiology of neurologic sequelae is unknown, although imaging studies suggest a potentially reversible demyelinating process.[326,327] The important practical question is whether hyperbaric treatment will decrease the frequency and severity of delayed neurologic sequelae in children with CO poisoning. This is a difficult question because the incidence of delayed sequelae is unknown and determining the severity of the CO poisoning is difficult to pinpoint because there is a poor correlation between serum COHb and degree of CO exposure.[328,329] One study suggests that prolonged loss of consciousness and rescue by ventilation are major indicators for later neurologic sequelae.[330] Another study suggests that increased blood concentrations of lactate at the time of admission may provide additional guidance regarding duration of loss of consciousness.[331] Some clinicians believe that a history of unconsciousness indicates that an exposure has been severe enough to warrant treatment.[330–335] However, the relatively few randomized prospective studies evaluating this have returned conflicting results.[336,337] Hyperbaric O_2 treatment is not without expense, inconvenience, and risk, and the indications for treatment of burned children with concomitant CO poisoning are debated.[325,338] One study described complications during treatment of a heterogeneous group of patients: emesis (6%), seizures (5%), agitation requiring restraints or sedation (2%), cardiac dysrhythmias or cardiac arrests (2%), arterial hypotension (2%), and tension pneumothorax (1%).[325] Complications may be expected more frequently in the critically ill.[339]

The severity of delayed neuropsychological sequela do not seem to be related to the COHb concentration at the time of presentation.[340] Delayed sequelae include headaches, irritability, personality changes, confusion, memory loss, and gross motor deficits; a symptom-free interval of several days is commonly reported. Delayed hyperbaric treatment may relieve symptoms, and spontaneous resolution of delayed sequelae may be expected in up to 75% of patients within 1 year.[332,341–346] Data supporting the use of hyperbaric O_2 to prevent and treat these complications may be weak[336,337,347–352] but cannot be discounted given the seriousness of these sequelae.[317,318,353,354] Hyperbaric O_2 treatment is probably appropriate in burned children with documented or strongly suspected serious CO poisoning who are hemodynamically stable, not requiring ongoing burn resuscitation, and not wheezing or showing evidence of air trapping and in whom such treatment does not require interfacility transport.

Cyanide toxicity is another complication associated with inhalational burn injuries.[355] If cyanide poisoning is confirmed, administration of hydroxycobalamin or sodium thiosulfate, alone or in combination, is warranted (see Chapter 12).[57,356] HBO therapy has been shown to facilitate movement of cyanide out of tissues and into blood, thereby potentially facilitating treatment,[355] although the use of HBO for cyanide poisoning remains investigational.

ADEQUACY OF CIRCULATION

The various formulas for determining fluid replacement are estimates and often need modification, depending on clinical and laboratory findings.[a] The most widely accepted fluid protocols in current use are the Parkland (Baxter) and Brooke formulas. Both formulas provide estimates of the fluid volume required for resuscitation, in addition to the calculated normal maintenance fluid requirement for each day. *These formulas are of great value in guiding the fluid resuscitation of older children; however, serious underestimation of the fluid volume may occur if applied to infants weighing less than 10 kg.* In such infants, it is reasonable to estimate the normal hourly maintenance fluid requirements and then add to this the fluid volume of the Parkland or Brooke formula.[2,369] Alternatively, the crystalloid fluid regimen for resuscitation can

TABLE 36.1   Parkland and Brooke Formulas

Formula	FLUID THERAPY		
	Crystalloid (mL/kg)	Colloid (mL/kg)	
Parkland	4.0	+0	× Percent burn × wt (kg)
Brooke	0.45	+1.5	× Percent burn × wt (kg)

NOTE: Half this volume is administered during the first 8 hours and the remainder during the next 16 hours. **Infants who weigh less than 10 kg may have even greater fluid requirements (see text).**

be increased to 6 mL/kg × the percent surface area burn per 24 hours.[370,371] All formulas and guidelines for fluid therapy require modification according to the individual child's response (Table 36.1)[7]; the most important metric of fluid homeostasis remains a good urine output (0.5 to 1 mL/kg per hour).

Goal-directed fluid therapy, using a noninvasive or a minimally invasive monitor, may be beneficial for tailoring fluid administration.[372] The development of continuous noninvasive cardiac output monitors may soon be routinely used in the fluid and inotropic management of burn victims. These devices include Fick calculation using expired carbon dioxide rebreathing, esophageal Doppler, pulse contour analysis, thoracic impedance, and bioreactance.[373–381] We are currently investigating esophageal Doppler monitors (EDMs) for our pediatric burn patients (Deltex Medical, Chichester, West Sussex, England; see E-Fig. 36.4), which are approved by the U.S. Food and Drug Administration (FDA) for use in children weighing 3 kg or more. The EDM measures blood flow velocity in the descending aorta via a soft Doppler probe placed in the esophagus at approximately the thoracic fifth vertebral level. Based on the flow velocity and diameter of the aorta (estimate based on a normogram of age, weight, and height), a cardiac output is calculated. The advantage of this technology is that it can be used in children with burn injuries of the chest and neck, which precludes the use of other devices that require placement of skin electrodes (bioimpedance and bioreactance require this). One of these latter devices, ICON (Cardiotronic-Osypka, La Jolla, CA), is FDA approved for use even in neonates and could be used in infants and children whose airways are unintubated and who are without injury to the left chest and left neck (E-Fig. 36.4).

The degree of edema depends on the volume and composition of the resuscitation fluid administered. Consequently, colloids or hypertonic saline solution (with or without albumin) are used in some burn centers during early burn wound resuscitation; these modified regimens are purported to be particularly effective in the very young and the elderly, resulting in less tissue edema.[b] A Cochrane review of 15 studies using hypertonic saline solution found that less IV fluid was needed for resuscitation and greater sodium concentrations occurred, although the overall morbidity and mortality was unchanged.[384] Further work is required before advocating hypertonic fluid regimens in burned children routinely.[385]

A growing practice in burn programs has been to begin the fluid resuscitation with colloid, usually 5% albumin, early during resuscitation of seriously burned children[386–388]; however, no consensus has been reached on colloid protocols.[383] In seriously burned children, we begin with 5% albumin at a maintenance

---

[a]References 2, 6, 20, 108, 181, 184, and 357–368.

[b]References 2, 108, 184, 362, 363, 368, 370, 371, 382, and 383.

rate immediately upon admission. We administer an amount equal to that of their calculated crystalloid requirements, tapering the crystalloid first and continuing the albumin infusion for 48 hours.

The syndrome of hyperosmolar hyperglycemic nonketotic coma (severe dehydration, marked hyperglycemia, serum hyperosmolality, and coma in the absence of ketoacidosis) may be associated with burns. Avoiding this syndrome is critically important because it carries a high mortality.[357] Glucose-containing solutions should be restricted at all times, particularly during the initial volume resuscitation. Serum glucose concentrations should be measured frequently during this period; we recommend administering insulin as indicated to maintain a target blood glucose of approximately 130 mg/dL.[155]

The general appearance of the child and his or her sensorium provide important guides to the effectiveness of the resuscitative therapy. In addition, urine output is a useful metric to determine the need for additional fluid administration, recognizing that antidiuretic hormone secretion may be increased and renal tubular dysfunction may be present.[24,220] Every effort must be made to protect kidney function by providing adequate perfusion and fluid replacement.[2,385] Renal failure in the presence of a major burn is usually lethal.[26] However, overly aggressive fluid administration may induce pulmonary and tissue edema. Therefore, when a burned child is volume resuscitated, the fluids we administer to replace the circulating blood volume must be carefully titrated. Commonly used endpoints of satisfactory fluid resuscitation include heart rate, systemic arterial blood pressure, urinary output, central venous pressure (CVP), arterial oxygenation, and pH. Echocardiography may be of great value in critically ill patients but, as described earlier, methods of continuous cardiac output assessment may provide better goal-directed fluid resuscitation than clinical assessments alone regarding the decision to use a vasopressor or provide additional volume loading.

The evaporative fluid losses in a child exceed 4000 mL/m² of burn surface each day, compared with only 2500 mL/m² in an adult.[362] Concomitantly, for each square meter of burn surface, 2500 to 4000 kcal of heat is lost each day. Minimizing caloric expenditure and providing caloric supplementation simultaneously are the only ways to minimize catabolism of body tissues. The tendency for children to be poikilothermic, particularly in the absence of protective skin as a result of the burn injury, causes profound temperature derangements. Efforts to maintain a normal body temperature are essential in both the operating room and the intensive care unit. These measures are especially important during the initial volume resuscitation and in the operating room when dressings are removed for examination and excision (Fig. 36.5).

ASSOCIATED INJURY

Associated injuries such as a tension pneumothorax, a ruptured spleen or liver, long-bone fractures, or head injury may be missed, especially during the initial assessment and early phase of burn wound fluid resuscitation. Taking a detailed history, especially from the emergency medical personnel and family, combined with a careful physical examination, is mandatory during the initial resuscitation because such injuries may compound or be hidden by the need for an increased volume of resuscitation fluids. The type of burn injury (e.g., explosion, electrical) may trigger concerns for associated injuries (e.g., shrapnel wounds).

CIRCUMFERENTIAL BURNS

Adverse cardiovascular and respiratory responses are immediate consequences to circumferential burns of the chest, abdomen,

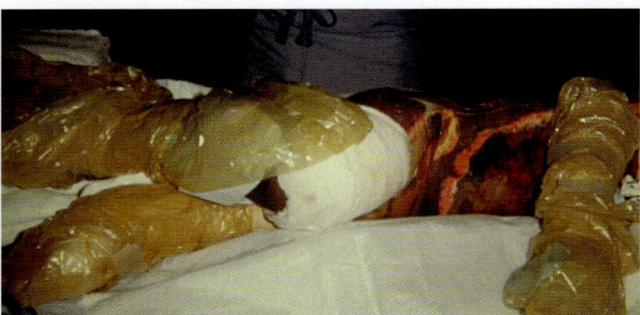

FIGURE 36.5 Children with extensive burn injury can be kept warm by having the extremities wrapped with sterile plastic bags. Covering the head is also an important method of heat preservation.

and extremities.[2,29,159,262] Circumferential burns of the thorax can restrict respiratory effort, resulting in respiratory failure from decreased chest wall compliance; functional residual capacity is reduced with airway closure and atelectasis, resulting in profound hypoxemia.[53,159,249–253,256–263,389] Deep circumferential burns of the chest and abdomen may generate excessive intrathoracic and intraabdominal pressure, which, in addition to restricting movement of the thorax and diaphragm, may further reduce the already decreased cardiac output by impairing venous return (Fig. 36.6).[29,159,262] When this occurs, both extrapulmonary and intrapulmonary factors can contribute to arterial desaturation.[73]

The edema of damaged tissues also can generate severe compressive forces, restricting or occluding the blood flow to burned extremities. The net result may be ischemia of the limb, which if left untreated, may lead to partial or total amputation. Escharotomies of circumferential burns of the chest, abdomen, and extremities must be performed urgently because impaired hemodynamics and respiratory mechanics can cause irreversible damage within hours of the burn injury. Escharotomy is often undertaken without the need for general anesthesia because a full-thickness burn usually destroys skin innervation. Abdominal compartment syndrome may develop in children who require large-volume resuscitation. To detect any evolving compartment syndrome, some burn centers advocate routine monitoring of bladder pressure.[389,390]

ELECTRICAL BURNS

Electrical burns occur with household voltage (electric cords and sockets) and non-household high-voltage current (power line or lightning). Children often disconnect extension cords by stabilizing one end in their mouths and pulling the other end with a hand, resulting in circumoral and lingual burns.[5,76,391,392] High-voltage injuries are often associated with loss of limbs and other injuries that are not immediately obvious.[393–396] The extent of this injury is unpredictable. The surface injury is often small, but the extent of underlying tissue damage and necrosis is massive. Such an injury is a combination of electrical and thermal damage.[396,397] Victims often have concurrent injuries such as fractures of vertebrae or long bones, ruptured organs, myocardial injury, or numerous contusions. Even children with low-voltage injuries may have abnormalities of cardiac conduction.[394] Children with electrical burns may be comatose or have sustained seizures at the time of admission to the hospital. Muscle tissue adjacent to bone is usually more damaged than superficial muscles because bone is a poor conductor of electrical current, and therefore heats up when high currents are passed through it, resulting in damage

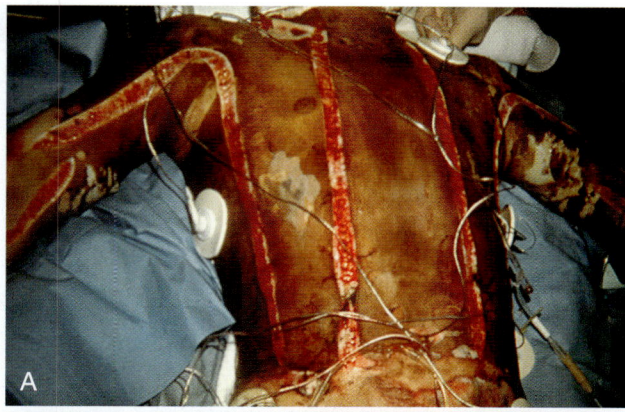

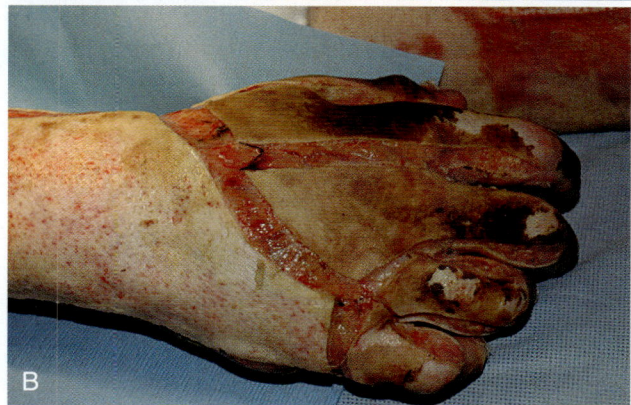

FIGURE 36.6 **A,** Circumferential chest burns result in severe impairment of respirations secondary to the tourniquet effect of the shrinking eschar and subcutaneous edema. The widely separated escharotomy lines indicate the severity of the constriction. **B,** Similar effects occur in circumferentially burned extremities. Early escharotomy may help to preserve blood flow and obviate amputation.

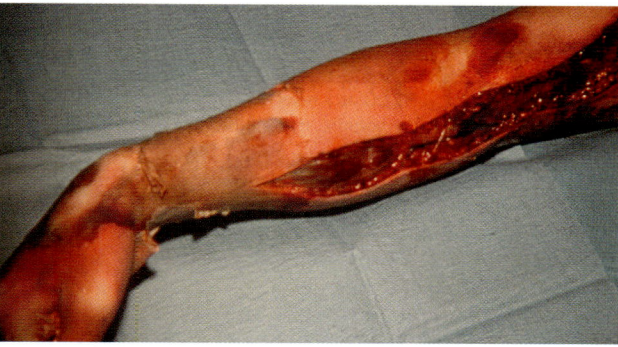

FIGURE 36.7 Electrical injuries tend to follow neurovascular structures and have an entry as well as an exit wound. The skin might appear normal but the underlying structures may have had extensive injury. These children require a fasciotomy rather than just a simple escharotomy to preserve blood flow to the deep structures. In general, this is required on the first day of injury for best results in tissue preservation.

to the surrounding muscles. Early fasciotomy may be needed to preserve the blood flow to extremities (Fig. 36.7). Myonecrosis necessitates general anesthesia during the first day of injury at the time when fluid shifts, hyperkalemia, and myoglobinuria are maximal. Massive myonecrosis and hemolysis may result in hyperkalemia, as well as myoglobinuria and hemoglobinuria. In the presence of hemoglobinuria or myoglobinuria, increased fluids and mannitol will ensure a continuous urine output (>1 mL/kg per hour).[398,399] Alkalization of the urine may prevent these proteins from precipitating in the renal tubules. Follow-up of patients with electrical injuries often reveals unpredictable sequelae, which may manifest months to years later. These injuries may occur in organs or areas that do not appear abnormal during the acute course of illness. These late complications most frequently include neurologic dysfunction, ocular damage, damage to the gastrointestinal tract, circumoral strictures, changes in the electrocardiogram, and delayed hemorrhage from large vessels.[397,399]

Guidelines to Anesthetic Management

Anesthetic management of children with severe thermal injury begins with the initial resuscitation and continues for many years through reconstructive surgery.[400] Knowledge and understanding of the pathophysiology of burn injury enable anesthesiologists

to plan appropriate anesthetic management and recognize and treat complications arising as a result of burn injury or its therapy (Table 36.2).[2,13,23,401]

Children who require surgery for burn wound excision and grafting must be properly prepared physiologically and psychologically, and specific equipment must be available in the operating room. Children who have not had surgical debridement and have had the burn for a week or longer must be considered septic. Such children often demonstrate severe cardiovascular instability during burn wound excision, likely because of acute bacteremia. In such cases, it is advantageous to have infusions of dopamine, epinephrine, or norepinephrine prepared for administration before induction of anesthesia.

Psychological support must be provided by parents, nurses, physicians, and trained psychologists. It is important for anesthesiologists to understand that the families of children who have sustained a severe burn injury feel a great deal of psychological stress and guilt. This stress may be manifested as anger towards the physicians, nurses, and other members of the burn care team. The parents are angry that their child has sustained a devastating injury and occasionally vent their anger and frustration. It is therefore vital that the entire burn care team understand this response, that they spend as much time as possible listening to the parents' concerns, and that they emphasize all that is being done to ensure the very best care for their child. Specific nurses and physicians should be designated to communicate with the family to avoid any misunderstandings and confusion about issues of patient care that result if disparate information comes from multiple sources. The anesthesia care team, while explaining the risks of anesthesia, must emphasize the extensive monitoring and the central role that anesthesiologists have in ensuring the well-being of their child. Special emphasis must be placed on methods for minimizing physical and psychological pain during transport to the operating room, in the operating room, and postoperatively.

Keeping children with severe burn injuries on nothing by mouth (NPO) status for 8 hours or longer before sedation for a dressing change or anesthesia for a surgical procedure severely compromises caloric intake; therefore we advocate the use of continuous orojejunal or nasojejunal alimentation. Generally children can receive calories up to about 4 hours before

TABLE 36.2	Systemic Effects of Burn Injury	
System	**Early Effects**	**Late Effects**
Cardiovascular	↓ CO as a result of decreased circulating blood volume, myocardial depressant factor	↑ CO as a result of sepsis ↑ CO 2 to 3 times > baseline for months (hypermetabolism) Hypertension secondary to vasoactive substances such as renin
Pulmonary	Upper airway obstruction as a result of edema Lower airway obstruction as a result of edema, bronchospasm, particulate matter, sloughing of airway mucosa ↓ FRC ↓ Pulmonary compliance ↓ Chest wall compliance	Bronchopneumonia Tracheal stenosis, vocal cord granuloma ↓ Chest wall compliance
Renal	↓ GFR secondary to ↓ circulating blood volume Myoglobinuria Hemoglobinuria Tubular dysfunction	↑ GFR secondary to ↑ CO Tubular dysfunction
Hepatic	↓ Function as a result of ↓ circulating blood volume, hypoxia, hepatotoxins	Hepatitis ↑ Function as a result of hypermetabolism, enzyme induction, ↑ CO ↓ Function as a result of sepsis, drug interactions
Hematopoietic	↓ Platelets ↑ Fibrin split products, consumptive coagulopathy, anemia	↑ Platelets ↑ Clotting factors
Neurologic	Encephalopathy Seizures ↑ ICP	Encephalopathy Seizures ICU psychosis
Skin	↑ Heat, fluid, electrolyte loss	Contractures, scar formation, difficult IV access, difficult intubation
Metabolic	↓ Ionized calcium	↑ Oxygen consumption ↑ Carbon dioxide production ↓ Ionized calcium
Pharmacokinetics	Altered volume of distribution Altered protein binding Altered pharmacokinetics Altered pharmacodynamics	Tolerance to opioids, sedatives Enzyme induction, altered receptors Drug interaction

↓, decrease in; ↑, increase in; *AIDS*, acquired immunodeficiency syndrome; *CO*, cardiac output; *FRC*, functional residual capacity; *GFR*, glomerular filtration rate; *ICP*, intracranial pressure; *ICU*, intensive care unit.

sedation or induction without fear of significant gastric residual fluid volumes. Some continue these jejunal feeds throughout the perioperative period but insert a nasogastric tube to monitor whether feeds are present in the stomach. If feeds are detected in the stomach, then jejunal feeds are interrupted perioperatively. Feeding can be resumed almost immediately after the procedure. In children with large injuries who will quickly develop a negative nitrogen balance with cessation of enteral feedings, short-term use of parenteral protein-sparing support is justified and safe.[402]

Adequate sedation and pain control are necessary before moving children to the operating room; IV fentanyl and midazolam are particularly helpful to provide analgesia and amnesia. Drug doses should not be based on standard doses used in children without thermal injury because burned children rapidly develop tolerance to most opioids and sedatives, thus requiring increasing doses over time to achieve a satisfactory clinical response.[403,404] The dose of sedative or opioid should be titrated to effect while the child is carefully observed and monitored. It is not unusual for children with burns in excess of 25% of the body surface area to require 1 to 3 mg/kg per hour of both morphine and midazolam to provide adequate analgesia and sedation. However, we believe that opioid-sparing techniques including regional anesthesia and

infusions of dexmedetomidine should be employed before such large doses are used.

Correction of intravascular volume before induction of anesthesia may require fluid boluses during and after sedation and before transport. Establishing adequate IV access preoperatively may be especially difficult in children with large burns. We use both topical anesthetic creams and needle-free subcutaneous local anesthetics to help make this process painless and stress free.

It is critically important to minimize heat loss and maintain normothermia. This is may be difficult to achieve because of the massive evaporative heat loss that occurs through open wounds. Operating room temperatures during extensive excisions are commonly maintained near 98.6°F (37°C).[184] Attention must be paid to minimize heat loss both during transport and in the operating room. Multiple blankets or thermal reflective covers are helpful. Special equipment is used to maintain body temperature, including a warming blanket, radiant warmer, blood warmer, and heat/moisture exchangers and forced hot air warmers. Simply wrapping the extremities in sterile plastic bags and covering the head with plastic or thermal insulation material markedly reduces heat and fluid losses (see Fig. 36.5). Although a hot operating room is uncomfortable for staff, maintaining the child's temperature is essential for maintaining normal blood clotting and reducing loss of valuable calories on thermogenesis. Each calorie saved is one more that can be used for tissue healing.

Adequate monitoring for major blood loss and fluid shifts includes arterial and central venous cannulas, a urinary catheter, an electrocardiograph, a pulse oximeter, a capnograph, and an esophageal stethoscope; continuous noninvasive cardiac output monitoring may be indicated in some children. A secure IV route for volume infusion is essential. If the potential for rapid blood loss exists, multilumen catheters may not be adequate because of their high-flow resistance. Rapid infusion devices may be particularly helpful (see Chapter 52).[405-407] The femoral vein is an alternative cannulation site, in addition to the internal jugular and subclavian veins (see Chapter 49). Sterilized laryngoscope blades, tracheal tubes, airways, and blood pressure cuffs are indicated.

Invasive arterial and CVP monitoring may be established after induction of anesthesia in most children. Propofol, thiopental (if available), or ketamine in incremental doses is usually well tolerated, provided the children are not hypovolemic (onset of effect is noted by lateral nystagmus (see Video 7.1). Studies in children long recovered from acute burn injury found a 40% increase in the thiopental dose needed to ablate the lid reflex, compared with children without burn injury (E-Fig. 36.5).[408] Our experience suggests that the clinical response to propofol appears to be equally shifted to the right; however, clinical studies are lacking. Ketamine may, on occasion, be preferred if the adequacy of intravascular volume is in question or if invasive monitoring lines must be inserted before anesthetic induction; tolerance to ketamine with repeated administration has been reported.[409] High-dose fentanyl or morphine combined with nitrous oxide (N_2O) for those children who will undergo ventilation postoperatively is also an acceptable anesthetic technique. In general, an inhalation agent is titrated to clinical effect to supplement the opioid-based anesthetic. A slow inhalation induction is preferable for children with a compromised airway, bearing in mind the potential for cardiovascular depression[410]; a difficult airway cart with appropriate advanced airway adjuncts should be in the operating room.

Succinylcholine is contraindicated in burned children because of a potentially lethal efflux of potassium from muscle.[231,234,237] However, within the first 24 hours after a burn, succinylcholine can be used without triggering a hyperkalemic response. This abnormal response first appears 24 to 48 hours after the burn and continues for an indeterminate, but prolonged, period. Because the endpoint for succinylcholine-induced hyperkalemia is unknown, we advise avoiding succinylcholine in children with large burns (≥40% BSA) for at least 1½ years. The smallest burn reported to trigger a hyperkalemic response was a 9% BSA burn. This abnormal response occurs because the entire muscle membrane, rather than just the myoneural junction, is occupied by acetylcholine receptors. The muscle tissue of burn victims also demonstrates resistance to nondepolarizing muscle relaxants (NMBD).[234,411] We observed a child who demonstrated marked resistance to NMBDs 463 days after burn injury. This response indirectly suggests that the hyperkalemic response may persist long after the acute injury phase of the burn[412]; nondepolarizing NMBDs are therefore the relaxants of choice in burned children.

Early studies reported that both the total dose of *d*-tubocurarine and the serum concentration necessary to attain a given degree of muscle twitch depression in children with burns in excess of 25% of their BSA are three to five times greater than in children without burn injury.[94,219,222,234,244,245] Although *d*-tubocurarine is no longer used, similar observations have been made with the current NMBDs (Fig. 36.8). If rapid intubation is needed and it is clear that the child's lungs can be ventilated, large doses of rocuronium (1.2–1.5 mg/kg) can be used; because 1.2 mg/kg may not provide adequate conditions for rapid intubation, larger doses may be indicated (Fig. 36.9).[413] Even with these large doses of rocuronium, the onset time is prolonged compared with that in nonburned children.[414] Pharmacologic reversal of neuromuscular blockade, however, poses no special problem in burned children.

Recovery from neuromuscular blockade has been observed at serum concentrations that would cause 100% twitch depression in children without burn injury. Studies with nondepolarizing NMBDs indicate that the hyposensitivity correlates well with the

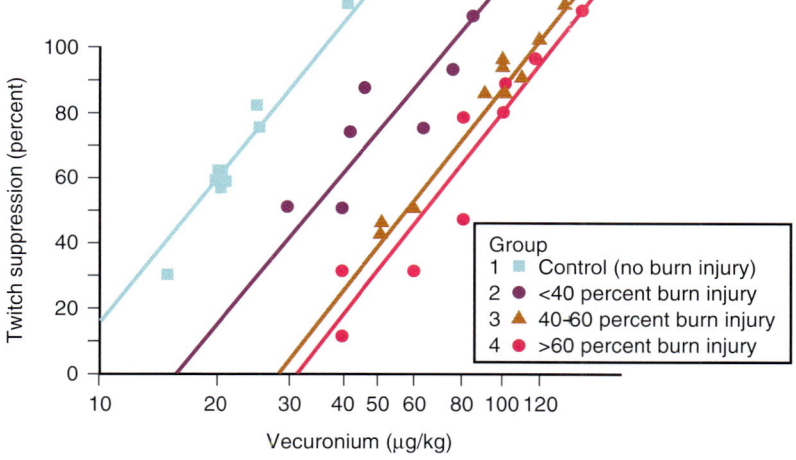

FIGURE 36.8 Logarithm of dose versus twitch suppression for vecuronium in control subjects and burned children. In the presence of acute injury, the vecuronium effective dose values increased with increasing burn size. The slopes of the curves were not different, but the intercepts were significantly different (P < 0.01). *Solid squares,* children without burn injury; *purple circles,* children with less than 40% burn injury; *triangles,* children with 40% to 60% burn injury; *pink circles,* children with greater than 60% burn injury. (From Mills AK, Martyn JA. Neuromuscular blockade with vecuronium in paediatric patients with burn injury. *Br J Clin Pharm.* 1989;28[2]:155–159.)

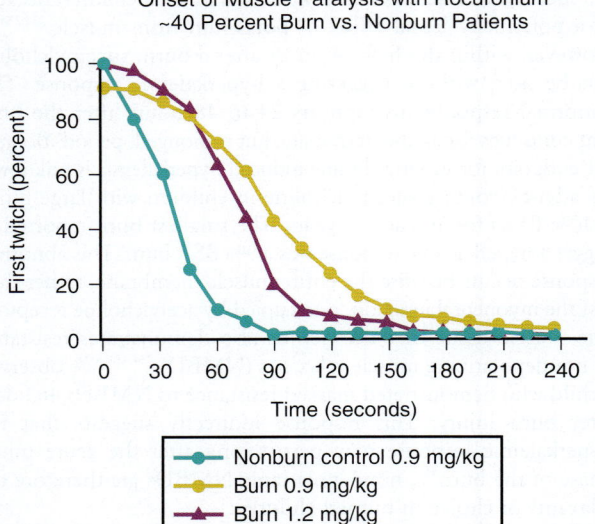

Onset of Muscle Paralysis with Rocuronium
~40 Percent Burn vs. Nonburn Patients

- Nonburn control 0.9 mg/kg
- Burn 0.9 mg/kg
- Burn 1.2 mg/kg

FIGURE 36.9 This dose escalation study of rocuronium in burned adults (approximately 40% BSA) demonstrated severe resistance to the onset of neuromuscular blockade (percent of train-of-four first twitch). The time of onset could be reduced with higher doses; however, a dose of 1.2 mg/kg did not achieve complete paralysis until longer than 2 minutes had elapsed. These data suggest that if a rapid sequence induction were needed in patients with severe burns, an even greater as yet undefined dose would be required to shorten the time to complete relaxation. (Modified from Han TH, Kim HS, Bae JY, et al. Neuromuscular pharmacodynamics of rocuronium in patients with major burns. *Anesth Analg.* 2004;99[2]:386–392.)

magnitude of burn ($r = 0.88$).[245,415–417] Protein binding and pharmacokinetic studies with *d*-tubocurarine indicate that these two factors contribute little to the enhanced requirements.[94,219,222,234] An increase in the number of acetylcholine receptors at junctional and extrajunctional areas and an altered affinity for the NMBD by those receptors have a major role in the elevated demand for nondepolarizing NMBDs.[233,239,411]

Maintenance of anesthesia is usually accomplished with N_2O, O_2, an NMBD, and an opioid or inhalation agent; all potent anesthetic agents can be safely administered to burned children. Sevoflurane offers an advantage of smooth inhalation induction; isoflurane, desflurane, or halothane can be used for maintenance. There is no evidence that repeated halothane anesthetics in burned children cause hepatotoxicity. All anesthetics cause concentration-dependent depression of cardiac output. In very ill children, anesthetic doses, but not NMBD requirements, are drastically reduced. In this injury, high-dose fentanyl-O_2-N_2O/air anesthesia is well tolerated. Ketamine may be the anesthetic agent of choice in specific circumstances, including those in which we wish to avoid airway manipulation after application of fresh facial grafts; for very brief procedures; or for children who are unable to open their mouth for a standard laryngoscopy. Ketamine may also be used along with midazolam for sedation before a trial of extubation. E-Fig. 36.6 illustrates extubation of a child with a severe facial burn with the use of an airway exchange catheter to provide a ready means for possible reintubation should the trial fail. Some burn centers use ketamine as the sole anesthetic and find it quite satisfactory.[418] The postoperative analgesia and somnolence for prolonged periods produced by high-dose ketamine may be considered an advantage in some instances in which postoperative

agitation might dislodge fresh skin grafts.[419] However, prolonged somnolence will delay reinstitution of critical enteral nutrition. Low-dose ketamine may be used postoperatively for its opioid-sparing effects.[420,421] Ketamine, either alone or with propofol, is commonly used for burn dressing changes.[418,422] An emerging experience with dexmedetomidine appears to demonstrate safety and efficacy in reducing otherwise common opioid tolerance and dose escalation.[423]

The inspired O_2 concentration is regulated according to the arterial blood gases and O_2 saturation. A pulse oximeter may not function properly on tissue discolored with silver nitrate; scraping the fingernail and cleaning the skin allow proper transmission and reception of the pulse oximeter light.[424,425] A pulse oximeter probe generally can function even on burned digits; however, if a child's digits are swollen or in the presence of severe vasoconstriction, alternative sites such as the earlobe, nasal septum, or tongue must be sought. We have found the tongue to be particularly valuable[312]; a sealed oximeter probe that prevents electrical current leakage can be easily modified (E-Fig. 36.7).[426,427] Reflectance oximeters may also be valuable in the care of burned children.[428,429]

The combination of increased metabolic rate–induced CO_2 production and inhalation injury often necessitates an increase in alveolar ventilation compared with healthy children. Blood gas analysis must be assessed early and frequently throughout the anesthetic procedure. Constant monitoring of expired CO_2 is vital, but one must be cognizant of the possibility of significant differences between arterial and expired CO_2 values as a result of shunting and dead-space ventilation in children with severe pulmonary injury. *For these reasons, an expired CO_2 monitor may be used for trending and as a disconnect alarm but should not be relied on to adjust and assess ventilation until a correlation with the arterial blood gas value is assessed.* The tracheal tube must be secured with tracheostomy tape because standard adhesive tape does not stick to burned tissue and wet dressings. Electrocardiographic leads also do not adhere and are placed under dependent portions of the body or sutured or stapled onto the skin after the child is anesthetized. The standard measures for protecting the cornea from drying (including ophthalmic ointment and closing the eyelids when possible) and for positioning the limbs to prevent nerve compression must be observed.

The most important consideration of the intraoperative course is monitoring and correcting a child's blood losses. For this reason, invasive intravascular monitoring is essential. Children may lose as much as 1 to 3 blood volumes during each burn excision (this is completely surgeon dependent).[430] It is therefore necessary to be familiar with the surgical approach to burn excision. During a tangential excision (Fig. 36.10 and Videos 36.1 and 36.2), a child might lose 3 to 5 times more blood than during excisions down to fascia (Video 36.3). The liberal use of very dilute concentrations of epinephrine (500 μg/L in normal saline) injected subcutaneously in both donor and excision sites markedly reduces surgical blood loss (Fig. 36.11 and Video 36.4)[431]; our institution uses a 1:2,000,000 epinephrine-containing solution (0.5 μg/mL). Large doses of epinephrine are well tolerated and markedly diminish bleeding. In a series of 25 consecutive children undergoing extensive layered excision, we used a total dose of epinephrine averaging 25 ± 3 μg/kg without complication[431]; as much as 10 μg/kg epinephrine may be injected every 20 minutes.[238] One note of caution is that some centers use electric infusion pumps to inject dilute epinephrine-containing saline solution; such devices have been associated with complications such as acute pulmonary edema and carpal tunnel syndrome, suggesting that hand injection may be safer.[432] Fluid overload may not become evident until several hours after surgery if excessive clysis or tumescent fluid is injected by the surgeons to facilitate harvesting of skin (Video 36.4). We have observed a number of infants (≤10 kg) who later developed pulmonary edema; therefore the amount of fluid injected must be taken into consideration with the amount administered intravenously. Since it is difficult to estimate blood and fluid loss, other indicators of circulating blood volume, such as urine output, CVP, arterial pressure, and shape of the arterial waveform (see Fig. 12.10), must be closely monitored.

Early excision of full-thickness burns has improved survival and shortened hospital stays.[433–435] In the past, we routinely observed that 5% of the blood volume was lost for every 1% BSA excised and grafted.[436,437] This extensive blood loss was a major source of morbidity and expense.[438,439] More recently, effective blood-conserving techniques for excision have drastically reduced intraoperative blood loss. These techniques include (1) clearly planning the excision to be performed before its initiation; (2) performing all extremity excisions under pneumatic tourniquet, exsanguinating the extremity before tourniquet inflation, and

wrapping the extremity in a hemostatic dressing (epinephrine/saline soaked dressings) before tourniquet deflation; (3) conducting all fascial excisions with coagulating electrocautery; (4) performing major layered excisions as soon as possible after injury, before significant wound hyperemia develops; (5) executing all layered torso excisions after subeschar epinephrine clysis; (6) maintaining normothermia, primarily through maintaining a hot operating room (near 98.6°F [37°C]); and (7) subcutaneous injection of saline diluted epinephrine (with and without dilute bupivacaine) in donor areas.[440] Based on preoperative and postoperative hematocrit and known volume of transfusion, the percent of the total blood volume lost per percent of total wound excised generated an average 0.98% ± 0.19% of the blood volume per percent of the body surface excised. This was about one-fifth of our earlier experience with this type of excision.[441,442]

Chronic ionized hypocalcemia is commonly observed with major thermal injury.[188] Prophylactic intermittent administration of calcium chloride or calcium gluconate is strongly recommended during the rapid infusion of citrated blood products.[443–446] Some children experience electromechanical dissociation or cardiac arrest during the rapid administration of FFP. This observation prompted a controlled prospective study in which a highly significant decrease in the serum calcium concentration occurred when FFP was administered at a rate of 1 mL/kg per minute or greater (see Fig. 12.9).[446] Interestingly, there was no correlation between adverse cardiovascular responses, the rate of FFP infusion, and the serum calcium concentration. A careful review of the previous cases of cardiac arrest revealed that all children were anesthetized with halothane, whereas in our prospective study most were anesthetized with "balanced" techniques. Because all inhalation agents depress cardiac function, in part through their calcium channel–blocking activity, a sudden citrate-induced decrease in ionized calcium would be expected to exacerbate the cardiac dysfunction. Studies in our laboratory have, in fact, documented this interaction.[25,446,447] Additional exogenous calcium is administered during rapid infusion of FFP or citrated whole blood, especially in infants (see Chapter 12).[446] It is our clinical impression that the rapid administration of (cold) FFP or citrated whole blood through a central line, without additional exogenous calcium, may be more likely to induce severe hypotension, bradycardia, and electrical mechanical dissociation. Our experience has been that rapid administration of citrated blood products, particularly FFP or whole blood, is safer through peripheral lines; rapid administration of packed red

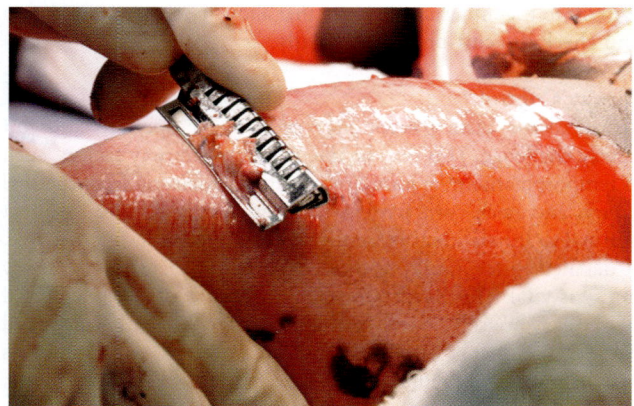

FIGURE 36.10 Tangential skin excision in which multiple thin areas of burn tissue are excised until a viable vascular bed is achieved. This is indicated by brisk bleeding. This type of excision results in less scarring because the majority of fat tissue remains intact. However, this also results in significantly greater blood loss.

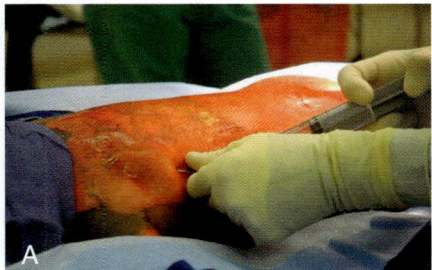
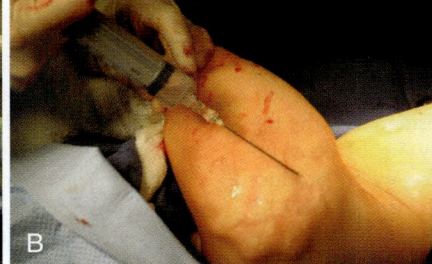
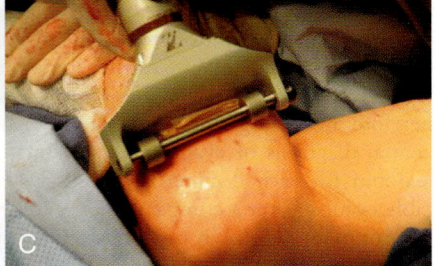

FIGURE 36.11 A, Subcutaneous injection of normal saline with a dilute concentration of epinephrine (0.5 µg/mL) from an area to be excised. **B,** Note the blanching of the donor skin secondary to the epinephrine. This helps to greatly reduce the amount of blood loss from both the donor sites and burn wound excision. It should be noted, however, that in the case of a large quantity administered to a small patient, late absorption can result in fluid overload. **C,** Skin is now harvested with minimal blood loss owing to the vasoconstriction of the tumescence solution.

blood cells does not cause ionized hypocalcemia. However, calcium administered simultaneously in the same IV line with FFP or citrated blood products may precipitate clot formation; we recommend giving exogenous calcium through a separate rapidly running IV line or preferably through a central line.

SPECIAL CONSIDERATIONS

Pharmacologic Responses

As a general rule, children with burn injuries require larger than normal doses of all IV medications, including antibiotics, NMBDs, opioids, and benzodiazepines.[a] Cardiovascular responses to catecholamines may be attenuated because of a reduced affinity of β-adrenergic receptors for ligands and diminished second messenger production,[238] thus the need for greater than standard doses to achieve the desired clinical response. Pharmacokinetic studies in acutely burned children indicate that the increased requirement for antibiotics is due in part to leakage through the burn wound, rapid urinary excretion, and altered volume of distribution.[55] Thermal injuries greater than 30% BSA cause an upregulation of acetylcholine receptors and consequent resistance to NMBDs.[232–234,236–239,448] In addition, there appears to be increased tolerance to sedatives and opioids. In adult burn patients, the free fraction (pharmacologically active component) of diazepam was greater than in nonburned patients, whereas the clearance of free diazepam was reduced. An increased tolerance to diazepam despite a greater fraction of the pharmacologically active compounds combined with a decreased clearance suggests resistance at tissue receptors similar to that observed for NMBDs at the neuromuscular junction.[99] A similar tolerance has been observed with opioids. The persistence of such pharmacodynamic changes for both NMBDs and anesthetic drugs long after recovery from burn injury must be kept in mind and doses titrated according to patient responses.[94,242,408,412] In general, many pharmacokinetic and pharmacodynamic changes are present in this population. Furthermore, these children are frequently taking multiple medications; thus drug interactions, potentiations, and incompatibilities may occur. Of particular importance in this context are the H_2-receptor antagonists, which are commonly used in burned children and are known to inhibit the clearance of many other medications (see Chapter 7).

Methemoglobinemia

A less common, but important, source of intraoperative cyanosis and hypoxemia is the development of methemoglobinemia. When silver nitrate dressings are used on the burn sites, some strains of gram-negative bacteria are capable of reducing nitrates to nitrites, which diffuse into the bloodstream and convert hemoglobin into methemoglobin.[160,161,357] The methemoglobin decreases the available O_2-carrying capacity and increases the affinity of the unaltered hemoglobin for O_2, thereby further impairing O_2 delivery. As a consequence, the O_2-hemoglobin P50 curve is shifted to the left. Therefore methemoglobinemia should be considered in the differential diagnosis of cyanosis. Approximately 5 g of deoxyhemoglobin for each deciliter of blood is necessary to produce visible cyanosis, but a comparable skin color is produced by 1.5 to 2 g of methemoglobin for each deciliter of blood. Blood that contains more than approximately 10% methemoglobin usually appears dark red or even brown, despite a high measured PaO_2, and does not change color even with vigorous agitation in room air. Measured O_2 saturation is low; however, the decrease in saturation provides a falsely increased value.[300,301] Treatment consists of removing the toxic agent and administering methylene blue (2 mg/kg) and high inspired O_2 concentrations. Other possible sources of methemoglobinemia include excessive EMLA (eutectic mixture of local anesthetics) cream or benzocaine cream application for burn wound pruritus.[449,450]

Tracheal Tube Size

Because burned children frequently undergo multiple anesthetic procedures, special considerations must be given to the tracheal tube type and size. As mentioned previously, cuffed tracheal tubes are preferable. The size of the tracheal tube, the volume of air inflated into the cuff, and the pressure at which leakage occurs around the cuff should be recorded on each anesthetic record. It is common to note that the requirement for a smaller diameter tracheal tube as weeks go by suggests the development of a subglottic lesion (stenosis, granuloma, polyps), which should be investigated with bronchoscopy. When N_2O is used, the intraoperative cuff pressure should be checked to avoid excessive pressure on the tracheal mucosa, although Microcuff (Halyard Health, Inc., Alpharetta, GA) tubes provide a greater margin of safety than conventional tracheal tubes (see Chapter 14). We generally inflate the cuff to the minimum pressure that allows controlled ventilation and check the cuff pressure regularly.

Airway Control

The pediatric burn patient may present an especially difficult airway challenge. This may be due to external airway factors, such as temporomandibular joint limitation, macroglossia from thermal injury, and neck contractures.[13,410] It also may be due to direct thermal or inhalational injuries to the glottis and respiratory tree. A detailed history and physical examination focusing on airway injury is vital. History details such as a victim of fire in a closed space (e.g., house or automobile fire [very commonly associated with inhalational injuries]), vocal changes, stridor, and hoarseness may be important predictors of difficulty in establishing an airway.

Fiberoptic intubation is frequently used after induction when we are confident we can maintain a mask airway, as well for "awake" but sedated children who are breathing spontaneously. Recently, we have used dexmedetomidine as our sole sedative while performing fiberoptic intubations on spontaneously breathing children. Dexmedetomidine may provide a relatively stable hemodynamic environment, without respiratory depression, making it an ideal sedative when loss of respiratory drive could be catastrophic.

Fiberoptic intubation is often aided in these children with manual distraction of the tongue (especially if macroglossia is present), a stitch through the tongue, and a jaw lift (Fig. 36.12). If the tongue is difficult to grasp, moderately high suction applied to the tip of the tongue or a gauze wrapped around the tongue and then gently pulling the tongue forward facilitates visualization of glottic structures (Fig. 36.12D; see also Fig. 14.29).[451] Fiberoptic intubation sometimes is more easily performed if the bronchoscope is guided through a laryngeal mask airway (LMA) that has already been seated and used to ventilate the lungs. This can be especially advantageous if there is a great deal of perioral edema from inhalational burn injury.

In addition to direct laryngoscopy, fiberoptic intubations, and LMA-assisted intubations, the GlideScope (Verathon, Bothell, WA) has proven particularly helpful; other techniques including retrograde wires and light-wand intubations may be difficult to use in a child with a severely burned neck and contractures. In

---

[a]References 2, 82–84, 94, 98–100, 222, 223, 226, 228, 229, 234, 242–245, 415–417, and 440.

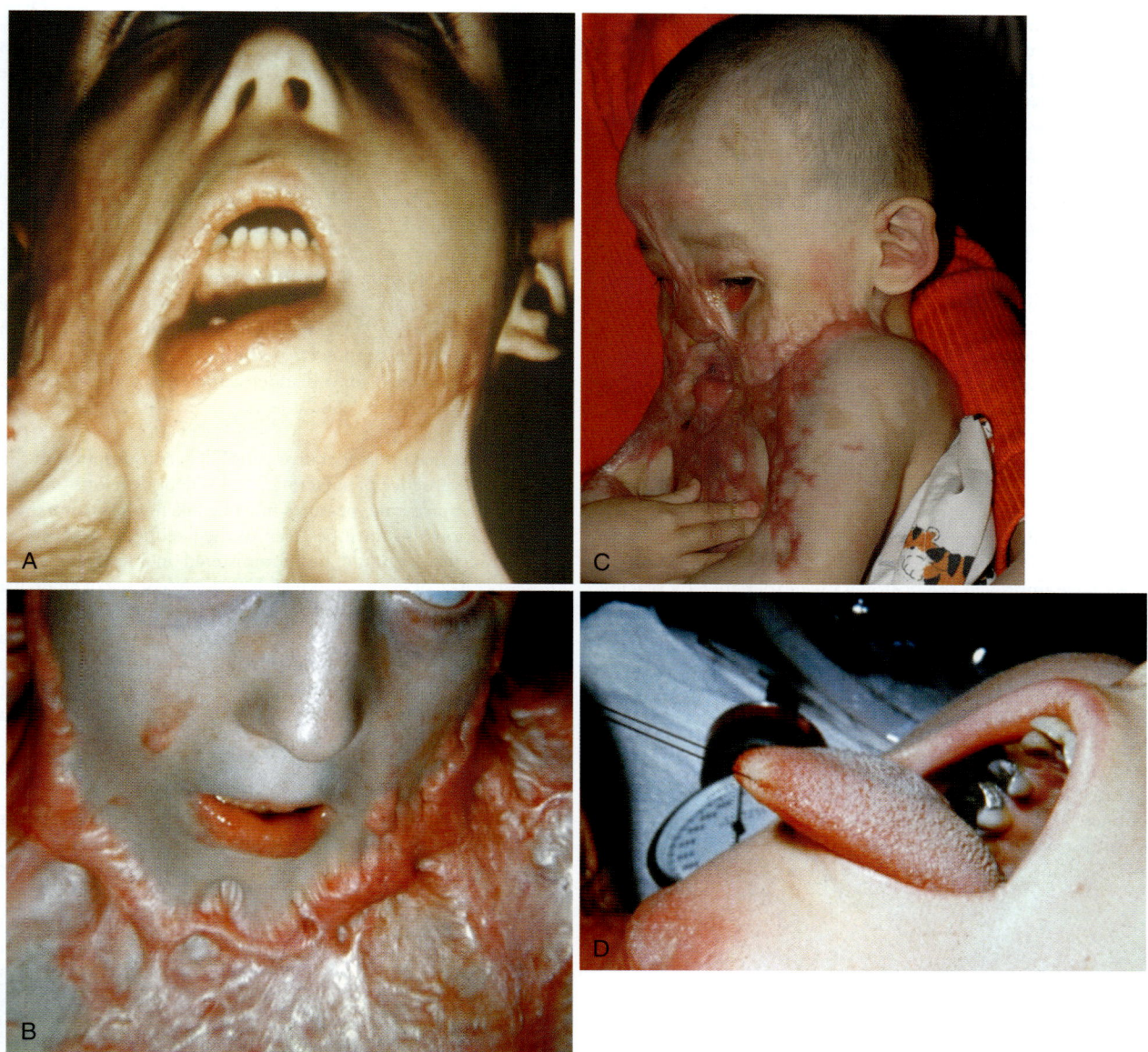

FIGURE 36.12 A, Child with inadequately treated facial burn. Note that skin contracture has resulted in complete distortion of the face with inability to close the right eye. **B**, Child with another example of an inadequately treated neck burn; note that her chin is fused with the sternum, resulting in very difficult airway management. **C**, An acute burn injury with an even more extreme example of inability to access the airway. To manage this child safely for the initial neck release, extracorporeal membrane oxygenation was used. This child is also unable to close her eyes. **D**, Some children with severe neck burns may have their airway visualized only by pulling back on the tongue (0 silk suture, suction applied to the tip of the tongue, or grasping forceps may be used [see also Fig. 14.29]) so as to pull the tongue and larynx cephalad.

these children, the surgeon may release the contracture during ketamine sedation and spontaneous ventilation to facilitate access to the airway (Video 7.1). The airway may then be instrumented either directly or indirectly (see Chapter 14). A useful review of airway management in pediatric head and neck burns that details successful strategies we use for securing the airway is available elsewhere.[452]

Hyperalimentation

Hyperalimentation fluids are frequently administered to burned children.[129,453] These fluids should be continued intraoperatively;

however, we generally reduce the rate of infusion to half to two-thirds of the initial infusion rate because the metabolic rate is usually decreased during anesthesia. These fluids should be administered with a constant-infusion pump to avoid accidental over infusion or under infusion. If the hyperalimentation fluids must be terminated (e.g., to permit blood transfusion), monitoring of blood glucose concentration is recommended. Dangerous rebound hypoglycemia may occur if infusions are abruptly interrupted and no compensation is made with other glucose-containing solutions. Compatibility of hyperalimentation solutions with drugs, blood, and other infusions must be addressed.

Ultrasound-Guided Vascular Access, Regional Analgesia, and Cardiovascular Assessment

High-resolution portable ultrasound is exceedingly helpful in the care of the pediatric burn patient; we commonly use ultrasound as an adjunct for vascular access, regional anesthesia, and cardiopulmonary diagnosis. Placing CVP and arterial catheters in the operating room under carefully controlled conditions is associated with a low rate of acute mechanical complications and deep vein thrombosis (~1%), even in children with multiple prior cannulations, a hypercoagulable state from the burn, and long periods of being bedbound.[454] Ultrasound is useful to rapidly access arteries and veins but also to diagnose clotted vessels, reducing futile attempts at obtaining vascular access.[455] Ultrasound also helps establish the location of cannulae—for example, we use ultrasound to assist in placing peripherally inserted central catheters (PICCs), then place the probe over the internal jugular to verify that the PICC is not traveling cephalad, and then scan the subclavian vein to verify correct placement.

Ultrasound-guided regional anesthesia is also a valuable tool in children undergoing reconstructive surgery. Typically, the complaints children have after reconstructive procedures most often involve the pain of the graft donor site. For the past 10 years we have improved the postoperative experience by placing ultrasound-guided blocks of donor sites, sometimes with catheters for more prolonged postoperative analgesia. These blocks include transversus abdominal plane blocks for truncal analgesia where both single-shot blocks and catheters are used (E-Fig. 36.8). Other specific blocks we have found very useful include the lateral femoral cutaneous nerve and fascia iliaca (Fig. 36.13) to cover the most common donor site: the lateral thigh or lower abdomen. Ultrasound has greatly improved success and reliability over typical blind techniques.[456,457] Our experience is that lateral femoral cutaneous nerve or fascia iliaca blocks provide better pain control for the donor site than infiltrating the donor site with local anesthetics;

more prolonged analgesia is provided by leaving a catheter in place. We usually place fascia iliaca catheters since these are easier to place with a shorter learning curve than for placement of lateral femoral cutaneous nerve catheters.[458,459]

Ultrasound is one of several strategies to rapidly assess intraoperative cardiac function during burn surgery. We have used real-time ultrasound while decompressing a spontaneous pneumothorax in a burn patient as a rapid and reliable indicator of when the lung has reexpanded (as indicated by return of the pleural "sliding" sign).[460–462] Hemodynamic measurements also can be estimated intraoperatively; we use the Bedside Assessment for Trauma/Critical Care (BEAT) examination as a quick assessment of volume status.[463,464] We also use ultrasound as a rapid method of assessing urine output by performing a bladder scan, which may avoid the need for a bladder catheter in some instances.

Awakening

In the immediate postoperative period, O_2 consumption increases even in the absence of shivering.[43] If O_2 debt develops (metabolic acidosis), appropriate measures must be taken to correct it. Special consideration also must be given to the likelihood of severe pain. Analgesic drugs should be administered in increasingly liberal doses because of increased drug tolerance. Adequacy of air exchange and patency of the airway, however, must be given first priority. It is important to assess the leak pressure at the end of the surgical procedure. Airway patency in the burned child is dynamic, and the child whose airway had minimal edema at the beginning of a procedure may have become very edematous at the end and be a poor candidate for extubation.

PAIN MANAGEMENT AND POSTOPERATIVE CARE

Treatment of burn pain, both perioperatively and in the intensive care unit, remains a major challenge. Our experience is that the pain is proportional to the size of the thermal injury. Nearly every

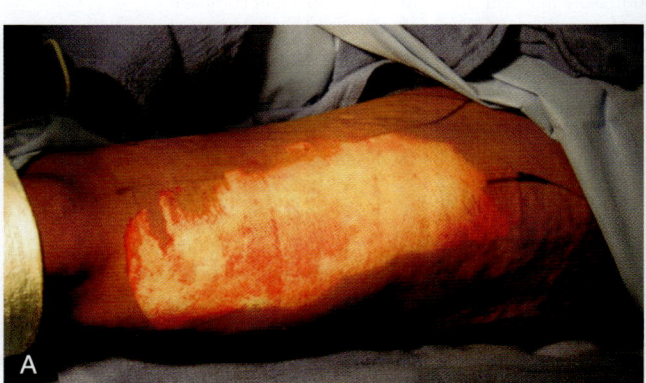
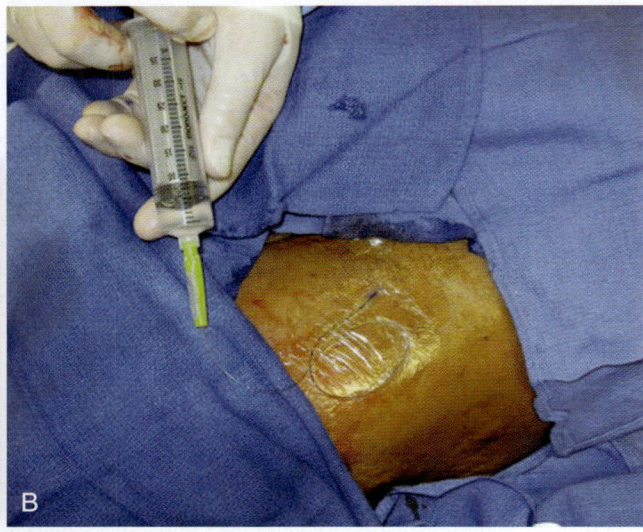

FIGURE 36.13 A, It is common for the thigh to be a donor site. In this case, a single-shot lateral femoral cutaneous nerve block is placed for postoperative analgesia. **B,** The fascia iliaca block will cover the distribution of the lateral femoral cutaneous nerve (lateral thigh) but also covers anterior and medial sensation (femoral and obturator nerves). In this case, the patient's legs are on the left and the lower abdomen to the right. A catheter was placed at the level just above the femoral crease allowing an infusion of low-dose local anesthetic for 2 to 4 days. Note that the catheter is secured with a coil to provide more stable placement.

maneuver involving the care of these children, including dressing changes, excision and grafting, physical therapy, weighing, and line placements, is associated with pain.

Part of the challenge in managing burn pain is due to the overlay of physiologic and psychosocial responses to thermal injury. Besides physical stimulation of nociceptors and other direct pain mechanisms, there is also the very real anticipation, anxiety, and fear associated with these procedures. Evidence suggests that skillful communication and explanations for specific treatments are necessary, despite the pain caused, and decrease analgesic requirements.[403,465-467]

Opioid administration for pain control has been an evolving science; 20 years ago there was significant fear that treatment of pain with opioids would create addictions. However, no reports of children developing opioid addiction after therapeutic uses of opioids have been published and studies in adults revealed a very low addiction rate.[468-472] This has led to liberalization of opioid dosing; it is not unusual for children to receive more than 1 to 3 mg/kg per hour of IV morphine while recovering from burn injuries. Once the thermal wounds are closed, opioid requirements rapidly decrease (Fig. 36.14).

Although the fear of postburn care addiction to opioids has never been realized, there are other reasons this class of drugs may be detrimental to the child with a burn. Animal data suggest that thermal injury itself may lead to a hyperalgesic state with both reduced effectiveness of morphine (presumably from downregulation of spinal μ receptors) and increases in N-methyl-D-aspartate (NMDA) receptors. The increases in NMDA receptors induced by burns provide the rationale for the widespread use of ketamine to treat pain in these children. Opioids may also increase the sensitivity to pain. In a mouse model, morphine downregulates μ-opioid receptors within the spinal cord and causes injury to spinal inhibitory interneurons.[471,472] In the same model, opioids cause postburn immunosuppression.[473] Additionally, opioid tolerance and opioid-induced hyperactive behaviors have, in a rat pup model, been exacerbated when midazolam has been concomitantly administered. This may be important as midazolam is frequently used as a clinical adjunct.[474] These potential opioid disadvantages have led to a search for alternative analgesics. Among these are potentially dexmedetomidine,[475-481] gabapentin,[482] and, until their recent withdrawal from the market, cyclooxygenase-2 inhibitors.[483-485]

Dexmedetomidine is a parenterally administered α2-adrenoceptor agonist with good sedative and anxiolytic properties. In adults, it decreases opioid requirements postoperatively.[476-480,486] In children with burns, it has been used successfully for sedation,[423,475] although larger dexmedetomidine doses may be needed than those required in nonburned adults or nonburned children.[475] Dexmedetomidine does not appear to be a remarkable analgesic for children with burns.[487] In a prospective study of dexmedetomidine in acutely burned children,[488] a bolus dose of dexmedetomidine (1 μg/kg over 10 minutes) was followed by an ascending infusion protocol (0.7 μg/kg per hour to 2.2 μg/kg per hour).[475] We found no instances of heart block, bradycardia, or other arrhythmias, but noted a consistent and significant decrease in mean arterial blood pressure after the bolus dose (approaching 30% change in mean pressure) (Fig. 36.15). This occurred in all ages studied (2–18 years), although the decrease in the mean arterial pressure did not correlate with size of burn, time since the burn, or CVP. Given these observations, we now omit a loading dose of dexmedetomidine, although should a bolus dose be indicated, we recommend 10 mL/kg or more of balanced salt solution or mild pressor support before commencing the dexmedetomidine. Other investigators have retrospectively examined cardiovascular stability of pediatric burn patients sedated

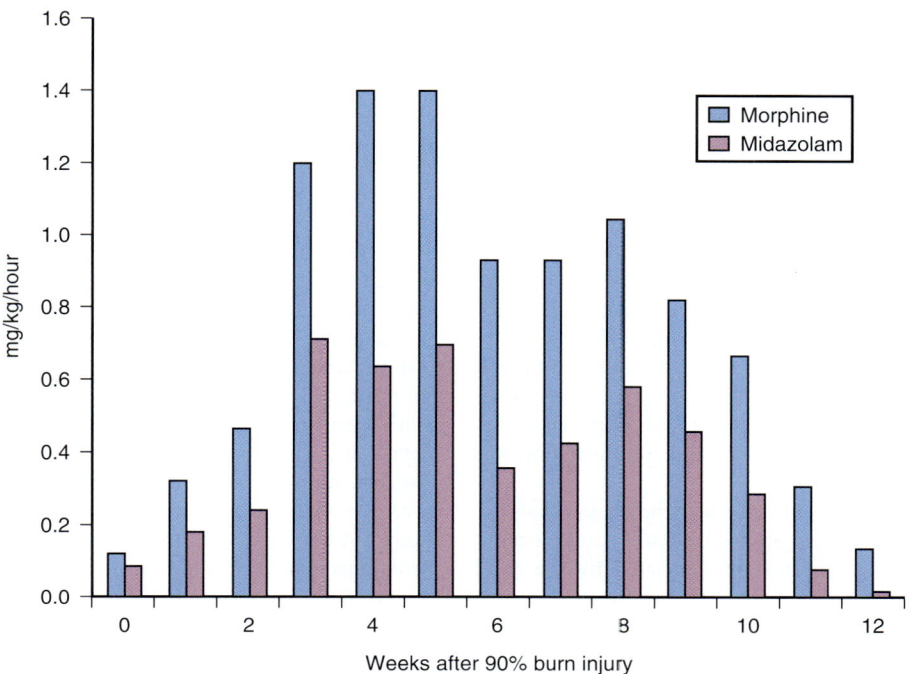

FIGURE 36.14 Morphine and midazolam requirements of a 16-year-old boy who had suffered an approximately 90% BSA burn injury. Note the marked rapid rise in analgesia and sedation requirements during the first 4 to 5 weeks after injury and then the rapid decline in requirements as his wounds were successfully grafted.

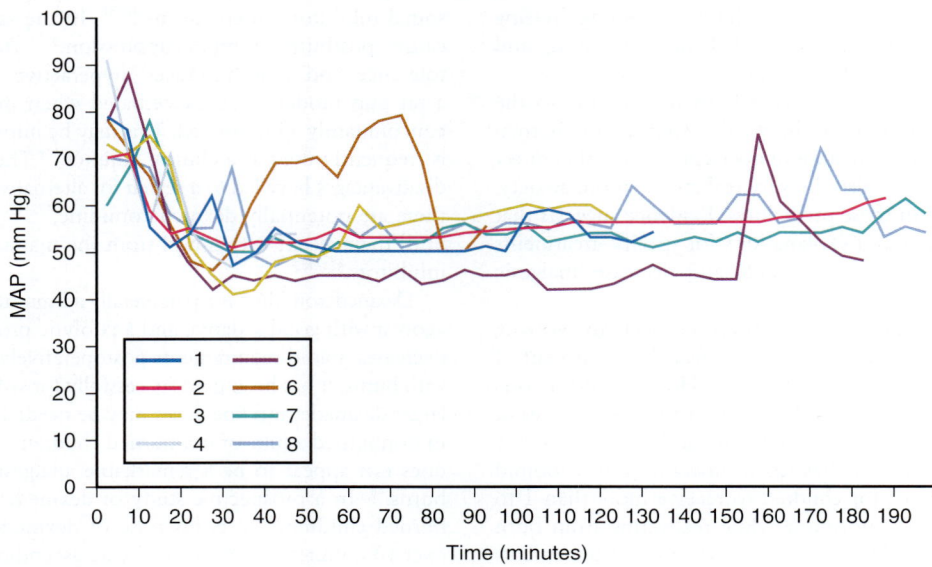

FIGURE 36.15 Change in mean arterial pressure (MAP) after bolus dose of dexmedetomidine in eight consecutive acute pediatric burn patients. *NOTE:* Given these observations, we now avoid a bolus dose; however, should a bolus dose be considered necessary, we suggest that the need for volume resuscitation (≥10 mL/kg of balanced salt solution) or mild pressor support must be anticipated. (From Shank ES, Sheridan RL, Ryan CM, Keaney TJ, Martyn JA. Hemodynamic responses to dexmedetomidine in critically injured intubated pediatric burned patients: a preliminary study. *J Burn Care Res.* 2013;34[3]:311–317.)

with dexmedetomidine and concluded that in the absence of a loading dose, blood pressure was maintained in the dexmedetomidine treatment group.[423] Dexmedetomidine pharmacokinetics in nonburned children appear similar to those in adults, but they have not been reported in pediatric burn patients.[489–491] When dexmedetomidine was compared with midazolam as an adjunct to ketamine in sedation and analgesia for burn dressing changes, the authors determined that both were effective adjuncts but that the dexmedetomidine-ketamine group had better sedation with less hemodynamic instability.[492] Dexmedetomidine has also been used in anxious children with burns as an intranasal premedication.[493] The authors concluded that dexmedetomidine (2 μg/kg) intranasally as a premedication compared with oral midazolam (0.5 mg/kg) induced preoperative sleep faster and was equally effective for induction conditions and rapidity of emergence. In our experience, the majority of our children prefer oral midazolam despite its bitter aftertaste, to intranasal dexmedetomidine. A substantial detractor from dexmedetomidine use is its cost (more than $44 for a 100-μg vial at our institution). One study in adult volunteers compared IV with intranasal dexmedetomidine; pharmacodynamic responses were similar, but the peak blood concentration occurred earlier in the IV group.[494] Bioavailability after nasal administration was 65% (range 35%–93%).

Dressing changes sometimes present one of the greatest analgesic challenges. This is because they are very painful, cause a rapid increase above baseline pain, and are associated by the child with anticipation of impending pain. Strategies to manage this pain include additional opioids and benzodiazepines, ketamine,[418] intranasal fentanyl,[495] remifentanil,[496] immersive virtual reality,[497,498] and music therapy (Video 36.5).[499] Management of the child's pain depends on physiologic and pharmacologic factors, as well as the psychological state of the child. Unfortunately, some children become so tolerant that one author observed that doses of IV fentanyl as

large as 100 μg/kg administered as a bolus to a teenager did not cause respiratory depression nor did it control the pain (CJC).

When poorly controlled, pain and anxiety have adverse psychological[205,500,501] and physiologic effects.[20] Posttraumatic stress disorder occurs in up to 30% of those with serious burns[204,502,503] and may be related to both the accident and the treatment, particularly in the setting of inadequate control of pain and anxiety. An inconsistent approach to pain and anxiety will be associated with inappropriate degrees of child discomfort, nonuniform drug selection with inconsistent dosing of unfamiliar drugs, varying tolerance of child discomfort among staff members, and bedside disagreements over management of the child's distress.

To address this issue, a pain and anxiety guideline should be developed by all facilities that routinely treat burned children.[504–507] We developed one such guideline that we have followed for several years, which is summarized in Table 36.3.[404] The ideal characteristics of such a guideline include (1) safety and efficacy over the broad range of ages and injury acuities seen in the particular unit; (2) explicit recommendations for drug selection, dosing, and escalation of dosing; (3) a limited formulary that generates staff familiarity with agents used; and (4) regular assessment of pain and anxiety levels and guidance for intervention as needed through dose ranging. We have found this structured approach to be very effective over the broad range of injury severity and child ages seen in our unit. Substantial escalation of drug doses, particularly in children with large injuries, is commonly required; doses should be titrated to the child's needs. When the child is being weaned toward extubation, background medications should be tapered to yield a sensorium consistent with airway protection; many tracheas are safely extubated while the children are still receiving opioid and benzodiazepine infusions. Finally, it is essential to emphasize that the most effective of all analgesics and anxiolytics is prompt, definitive wound closure.

TABLE 36.3 | Pain Treatment Plan

Clinical State	Background Anxiety	Background Pain	Procedural Anxiety	Procedural Pain	Transition to Next Clinical State
Mechanically ventilated acute burn	Midazolam infusion	Morphine infusion	Midazolam intravenous titration	Morphine intravenous titration	Wean infusions 10%–20% per day and substitute "nonmechanically ventilated acute burn guideline"
Nonmechanically ventilated acute burn	Scheduled enteral lorazepam	Scheduled enteral morphine	Lorazepam intravenous titration or enteral dose	Morphine enteral or intravenous titration	Wean scheduled drugs 10%–20% per day and substitute "chronic acute burn guideline"
Chronic acute burn	Scheduled enteral lorazepam	Scheduled enteral morphine	Lorazepam enteral dose	Morphine enteral dose	Wean scheduled and bolus drugs 10%–20% per day to outpatient requirements and pruritus medications
Reconstructive surgical patient	Scheduled enteral lorazepam	Scheduled enteral morphine sulfate	Lorazepam enteral dose	Morphine enteral dose	Wean scheduled drugs and bolus drugs to outpatient requirement

Tolerance to opioids occurs over time and must be considered so that adequate analgesia is provided throughout the recovery period. It is common to observe children who receive 1 mg/kg of morphine at the beginning of a 2-hour operative procedure not only to be ready for extubation but also to require additional opioids for continued pain relief postoperatively. Similar trends have been observed for fentanyl.[226] Thus an increased rate of excretion and degradation may attenuate the effects of some opioids. As the child recovers, the painful stimuli diminish and the opioid requirements are gradually reduced. This is generally such a prolonged process that withdrawal is not an issue. Anesthesiologists can have a key role in the treatment of thermal injury pain and, with an understanding of pharmacology, pharmacokinetics, and pharmacodynamics, are a vital resource for the care of these children (see also Chapters 43, 44, and 45).

Summary

The care of burned children involves detailed knowledge of the early and late effects of burn injury on the respiratory, cardiac, renal, central nervous, hepatic, gastrointestinal, hematopoietic, and metabolic systems. An awareness of the pharmacokinetics and pharmacodynamics of anesthetic agents, combined with an understanding of the problems of massive blood transfusion, also contribute to the safe conduct of anesthesia. Finally, the importance of adequate analgesia, sedation, and concern for the psychological well-being of these devastatingly injured children cannot be overemphasized. Knowledge of all of these factors combines to produce a successful outcome.

ACKNOWLEDGMENT
We wish to thank S.K. Szyfelbein for his previous contributions to this chapter.

ANNOTATED REFERENCES

Caruso TJ, Janik LS, Fuzaylov G. Airway management of recovered pediatric patients with severe head and neck burns: a review. *Paediatr Anaesth.* 2012;22(5):462-468.

Pediatric airways in burned children may present some of the greatest airway challenges for the anesthesiologist. This is a useful review of some of these challenges and the techniques used to meet them.

Han T, Kim H, Bae J, et al. Neuromuscular pharmacodynamics of rocuronium in patients with major burns. *Anesth Analg.* 2004;99(2):386-392.

Currently, rocuronium is the fastest-acting nondepolarizing muscle relaxant available. This paper discusses its pharmacodynamics in burn patients and in particular describes both delayed onset and resistance in burned adults with doses as great as 1.2 mg/kg.

Shank ES, Martyn JA, Donelan MB, et al. Ultrasound-guided regional anesthesia for pediatric burn reconstructive surgery: a prospective study. *J Burn Care Res.* 2016;37(3):e213-e237.

This is the first randomized, prospective study in pediatric burn patients demonstrating the efficacy of peripheral regional nerve blocks—especially in patients with continuous indwelling catheters—in the postoperative analgesic management of reconstructive surgery. This study suggests that regional anesthesia should be used for most reconstructive surgeries to minimize narcotics and optimize analgesia.

Song L, Wang S, Zuo Y, et al. Midazolam exacerbates morphine tolerance and morphine-induced hyperactive behaviors in young rats with burn injury. *Brain Res.* 2014;1564:52-61.

This animal study demonstrated that the coadministration of midazolam and morphine did exacerbate morphine tolerance and hyperactive behavior. It appears the morphine tolerance is mediated through a spinal NMDA/protein kinase C mechanism. Since it is very common to sedate pediatric burn-injured patients in the intensive care unit with both midazolam and morphine, this study may have important implications for this population.

A complete reference list can be found online at ExpertConsult.com.

The Extremely Premature Infant (Micropremie) and Common Neonatal Emergencies

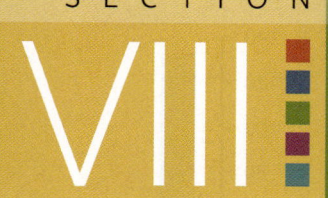

JAMES P. SPAETH AND JENNIFER E. LAM

THE PREMATURE INFANT IS DEFINED as birth before 37 weeks gestation. Premature births can be classified as low-birth-weight (LBW) infants (<2500 g), very low-birth-weight (VLBW) infants (<1500 g), and extremely low-birth-weight (ELBW) infants (<1000 g). Alternatively, they may be classified as moderate to late prematurity (32 to <37 weeks), very premature (28 to <32 weeks), and extremely premature (<28 weeks). A neonate is an infant in the first 28 days after birth. "Premies" are commonly referred to as infants rather than neonates as a group because gestation may be very short (e.g., 24 weeks) and thus even at 37 weeks postmenstrual age (PMA), they are truly infants with a postnatal age of 13 weeks (24 + 13 = 37). These infants should be labeled with both gestational age (i.e., at birth) and postnatal age (i.e., age after birth). The use of current postconception age (PCA) or PMA (approximately 10 days older) helps define maturation of physiologic processes.

Morbidity and mortality in this population has decreased considerably compared with 30 years ago, especially in ELBW infants.[1-3] This decrease is the result of many factors, including the development of specialized maternal fetal medicine and neonatal care units, antenatal corticosteroid administration, surfactant use shortly after birth, increased cesarean deliveries, and implementation of strategies to reduce lung injury, such as decreased delivery room intubations and increased use of continuous positive airway pressure (CPAP).[1,2] Although survival and morbidity-free survival rates continue to increase, the trend over the past 20 years has plateaued. The cost of care is escalating, as are the number of surgical procedures and the need for specialized care these infants require. The first part of this chapter will focus on the VLB and ELBW infant, or "micropremie," and discuss developmental physiology and its impact on anesthetic care.

Physiology of Prematurity Related to Anesthesia

RESPIRATORY SYSTEM

Airway

Anatomic Differences and Work of Breathing

The anatomic differences of the pediatric airway are detailed in Chapter 14; however, there are specific challenges unique to the airway of the premature infant that must be taken into consideration. The small airways predispose the micropremie to obstruction and difficulty with ventilation. Resistance to airflow is inversely proportional to the fifth power of the radius in the upper airway and to the fourth power of the radius beyond the fifth bronchial division (see also Fig. 14.7). As a result, insertion of an endotracheal tube (ETT) increases resistance and work of breathing far greater for the micropremie (2.5- or 3-mm inside diameter [ID]) than for

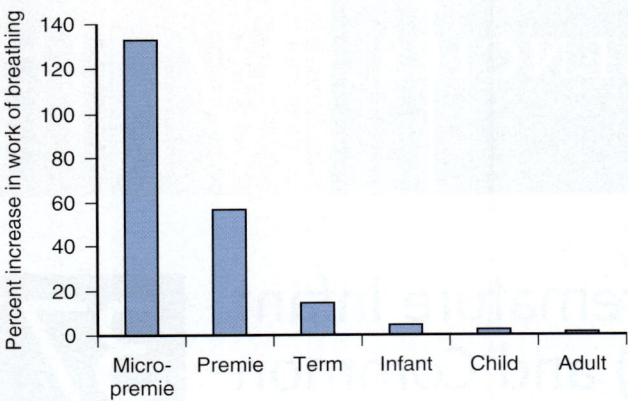

FIGURE 37.1 Change in work of breathing after placement of an appropriately sized endotracheal tube in extremely low-birth-weight infants (<1000 g), premature infants (1500 g), full-term infants, children, and adults (see text for details). (Redrawn with permission from Spaeth JP, O'Hara IB, Kurth CD. Anesthesia for the micropremie. *Semin Perinatol.* 1998;22(5):390–401.)

TABLE 37.1	Lung Function in Infants and Adults		
Variable	Infants	Adults	Infant/Adult Ratio
Oxygen consumption (mL/kg per minute)	5–8	2–3	2
Respiratory rate (breaths/minute)	40–60	12	3–5
Tidal volume (mL/kg per minute)	6–8	7	1.0
Total lung capacity (mL/kg)	53	85	0.6
Airway diameter (mm)			
Trachea	5	14–16	0.3
Bronchus	4	11–14	0.3
Bronchiole	0.1	0.2	0.5

Data from Polgar G, Weng TR. The functional development of the respiratory system: from the period of gestation to adulthood. *Am Rev Respir Dis.* 1979;120(3): 625–695.

a larger infant (4 mm ID), child (5 mm ID), or adult (7 mm ID) (Fig. 37.1). Similarly, partial occlusion of the ETT by secretions, blood, or kinking increases the work of breathing to a much greater extent in the micropremie. Partial occlusion of the natural airway from loss of muscle tone during anesthesia and sedation also increases the work of breathing more in the micropremie. Consequently, general anesthesia often requires placement of an ETT to ensure airway patency and provide assisted ventilation to overcome the increased work of breathing.

Diseases that narrow the airway, such as subglottic stenosis, tracheal stenosis, and tracheobronchomalacia, occur commonly in the micropremie, and the associated reduction in airway diameter further increases both resistance to airflow and work of breathing. Subglottic stenosis necessitates the placement of a smaller ETT than would otherwise be placed, further increasing airflow resistance. Although tracheal stenosis near the carina may not necessitate a smaller ETT, it still increases airway resistance from the stenosis distal to the ETT. With tracheobronchomalacia, the intrathoracic airways collapse during exhalation, again increasing resistance and the work of breathing (see also Figs. 14.10 and 33.10). Positive

end-expiratory pressure (PEEP) or CPAP helps stent open the airway. Mechanical ventilation, rather than spontaneous ventilation during anesthesia, prevents fatigue from increased work of breathing, and maintains ventilation and oxygenation. During anesthesia, the use of smaller inspiratory-to-expiratory ratios prevents air trapping and hyperinflation of lung segments.

The cardiopulmonary system of the neonate is driven by the need to deliver sufficient oxygen (O_2) to maintain a high metabolic rate. The O_2 consumption of an average neonate is 5 to 8 mL/kg per minute, whereas that of an adult is 2 to 3 mL/kg per minute (Table 37.1); the O_2 consumption rate in the premature infant is nearly 3 times that in the adult. It is this enormous O_2 consumption rate that explains the rapid decrease in blood O_2 partial pressures in the neonate during periods of hypoventilation. Although ventilatory gas exchange volume is nearly 10-fold greater in adults than in neonates, the tidal volume relative to body weight for both is approximately equal (6 mL/kg). In neonates, increasing the respiratory rate facilitates the elimination of carbon dioxide (CO_2) generated by their relatively high metabolic processes; alveolar ventilation is approximately 130 mL/kg per minute in the perinatal period, compared with 60 mL/kg per minute in adulthood.

Lungs
Pulmonary Gas Exchange
The structure and function of the immature lung predisposes to alveolar collapse and hypoxia. The premature alveoli are primarily composed of thick-walled, fluid-filled saccular spaces that are surfactant deficient and require greater pressures to initially expand. Production of surfactant by type II alveolar pneumocytes begins between 23 and 24 weeks gestation, although surfactant concentrations often remain inadequate until 36 weeks gestation. These factors lead to the development of respiratory distress syndrome (RDS), which causes reduced lung volumes and lung compliance, increased intrapulmonary shunting, and ventilation-perfusion mismatch. It is clinically characterized by grunting respirations, nasal flaring, and chest retractions that develop shortly after birth. Decreased lung volumes and ventilation-perfusion mismatch may also occur as a consequence of anesthesia. The effects of immature structures, disease, and anesthesia on lung function all increase the risk of hypoxia during surgery and anesthesia.

In neonates, atelectasis might also be caused by anatomic forces that decrease lung volume. For example, the relatively large abdomen in a neonate displaces the diaphragm cephalad, placing the closing capacity within the expiratory reserve volume (see also Fig. 2.5). Moreover, increases in intraabdominal pressure from gastric distention associated with overzealous assisted ventilation with a face mask, replacement of bowel in the abdomen during repair of gastroschisis or omphalocele, or surgical retraction or manipulation of the abdominal contents also might shift the closing capacity to within the infant's expiratory reserve volume. The resulting atelectasis and intrapulmonary shunting may require controlled ventilation with PEEP to recruit closed lung units and improve oxygenation, emptying of the stomach, or changes in surgical maneuvers.

Micropremie lungs are particularly susceptible to volutrauma. Mechanical lung injury is no longer thought to be caused by the use of high peak-inspiratory pressures, but rather related to increased end-inspiratory lung volumes and frequent collapse and reopening of alveoli. A ventilation strategy using small tidal volumes (4–6 mL/kg), greater respiratory rates, PEEP sufficient to avoid alveolar collapse, and permissive hypercapnia reduces lung injury in the premature lung.[4] Permissive hypercapnia

TABLE 37.2	Severity-Based Diagnostic Criteria for Bronchopulmonary Dysplasia (BPD)
Gestational age	<32 weeks
Time point of assessment	36 weeks postmenstrual age or discharge home, whichever comes first
	Therapy with oxygen >21% for at least 28 days
Mild BPD	Breathing room air
Moderate BPD	Need for <30% oxygen
Severe BPD	Need for ≥30% oxygen and/or positive-pressure ventilation or nasal continuous airway pressure

From Ehrenkranz RA, Walsh MC, Vohr BR, et al. Validation of the National Institutes of Health consensus definition of bronchopulmonary dysplasia. *Pediatrics*. 2005;116(6):1353–1360.

(arterial partial pressure of CO_2 [$PaCO_2$] 45–55 mm Hg) results in smaller periods of assisted ventilation and reduced incidence of bronchopulmonary dysplasia (BPD), without an increase in adverse neurodevelopmental outcomes.[5]

Bronchopulmonary Dysplasia

BPD is an important chronic lung disease of prematurity, defined as the need for supplemental oxygen at 28 postnatal days.[6-8] Traditionally, BPD has been associated with premature infants subjected to high levels of O_2 and ventilation therapy that causes a lung injury–induced increase in cytokine activation. Other factors that increase the risk for developing BPD include chorioamnionitis and the persistence of a hemodynamically significant patent ductus arteriosus (PDA).[9]

Alveolarization begins around 36 weeks gestation. Therefore lung injury in the premature infant interrupts pulmonary maturation, resulting in larger but fewer alveoli than normal lungs. Decreased lung development in infants with BPD diminishes the surface area for pulmonary gas exchange, which increases O_2 requirements. Moreover, some infants with BPD have reduced lung compliance and increased airway resistance and hence have prolonged pulmonary time constants. Some infants with severe BPD have abnormal muscularization of the vessels in the periphery of their lungs, leading to pulmonary hypertension and right ventricular hypertrophy.

A number of strategies may be implemented to prevent the development of BPD. Modalities include antenatal corticosteroid administration to the mother and early postnatal administration to the infant, exogenous surfactant therapy, and specific ventilatory strategies, such as early and aggressive use of CPAP instead of intubation with positive-pressure ventilation. Treatment of existing BPD often requires ventilatory and medical therapies.[10] Ventilatory goals should be aimed at the avoidance of intubation if possible, and the use of permissive hypercapnia and smaller tidal volumes in those whose lungs are intubated. Infants with BPD are often treated with diuretics to decrease pulmonary alveolar and interstitial edema. As a result of chronic furosemide treatment, metabolic abnormalities may exist. Hypercalciuria from furosemide may lead to secondary hyperparathyroidism and nephrocalcinosis in some infants. Hydrochlorothiazide and spironolactone produce less severe metabolic abnormalities. Bronchodilators such as aminophylline, albuterol, or ipratropium may be beneficial in reducing airway resistance in some infants with BPD, although

data are conflicting.[7] Finally, large doses of steroids, especially dexamethasone, provide relief for some infants with severe BPD that is refractory to other medical and ventilator therapies.[11,12] However, dexamethasone may cause systemic hypertension, hyperglycemia, hypertrophic cardiomyopathy, and alteration of neurologic and pulmonary development in some children.[13,14]

A severity index for BPD based on the need for supplemental oxygen and/or positive-pressure ventilation or nasal CPAP has been developed and shown to identify a spectrum of risk for adverse pulmonary and neurodevelopmental outcomes in preterm infants (Table 37.2).[15] Although this severity index has not been studied in the context of anesthetic risk, experience suggests that such infants requiring supplemental oxygen, positive pressure, or medications for reactive airways are at greater risk for perioperative pulmonary complications. Anesthetic goals include minimizing the inspired oxygen concentration and tidal volumes while maintaining adequate arterial oxygen saturation (SaO_2 90%–94%) and ventilation ($PaCO_2$ 50–55 mm Hg). The use of smaller tidal volumes decreases the risk of pneumothoraces and interstitial emphysema. Preoperative evaluation of infants with BPD requires a very careful history and physical examination, particularly focused on the pulmonary and cardiovascular systems.

Hyperoxia

Some prematurity-related diseases, such as retinopathy of prematurity (ROP) and BPD, have been associated with neonatal exposure to supplemental oxygen (hyperoxia). Oxygen toxicity from hyperoxia leads to the formation of reactive oxygen intermediaries that impair intracellular macromolecules, leading to cell death. The formation of oxygen free radicals also promotes an extensive inflammatory response, leading to secondary tissue damage and cell death. Oxygen-induced vascular endothelial growth factor (VEGF) signals disturbances associated with abnormal angiogenesis; it may be detected in both ROP and BPD.[8]

Controversy exists over the optimal oxygen saturation to target in the premature infant.[16-20] Two studies, the SUPPORT trial (**S**urfactant, **P**ositive Pressure, and Pulse **O**ximetry **R**andomized **T**rial) from the United States and the BOOST II trial (**B**enefits **O**f **O**xygen **S**aturation **T**argeting) from the United Kingdom, Australia, and New Zealand reported that a reduced oxygen saturation target range of 85% to 89% had a reduced incidence of ROP but an increased mortality compared with a target range of 91% to 95%.[21,22] However, the COT (**C**anadian **O**xygen **T**rial) and BOOST-NZ (BOOST New Zealand) trials found no significant differences in either death or disabilities among the two target ranges.[23,24]

Recent evidence suggests a more graded approach according to gestational age, with increasing oxygen saturation targets with increasing age, rather than a generalized approach that aims to target a single goal.[20] For example, one study suggested that an infant younger than 33 weeks should have an oxygen saturation target between 83% and 89%, whereas an infant between 33 and 36 weeks should have a goal between 90% and 94%.[20] However, the optimal range for the graded approach is controversial, as well. Because of the possible increase in mortality, most practitioners use the 91% to 95% target range of oxygen saturation.

Respiratory Control

Micropremies possess a biphasic ventilatory response to hypoxia. Initially, ventilation increases in response to hypoxia, but after several minutes, ventilation decreases and apnea may ensue.[25] The ventilatory response to CO_2 is decreased in the micropremie, and hypoxia further blunts this response.[26,27] Anesthetic drugs depress

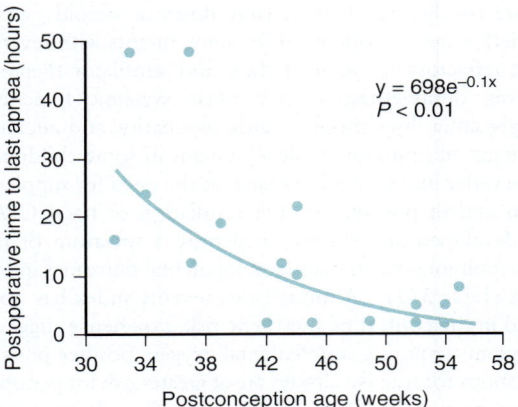

FIGURE 37.2 Time from the end of anesthesia to the last episode of postoperative apnea in prematurely born infants ($r^2 = 0.49$.) (Redrawn with permission from Kurth CD, Spitzer AR, Broennle AM, et al. Postoperative apnea in preterm infants. *Anesthesiology.* 1987;66(4):483–488.)

In the figure: $y = 698e^{-0.1x}$, $P < 0.01$

TABLE 37.3	Primary Categories of Apnea in Infants
Cause	**Treatment**
Central	Increase O_2 delivery
	Increase fraction of inspired O_2
	Increase hematocrit (?)
	Xanthine derivatives:
	Theophylline
	Caffeine
Obstructive	Neck extension
	Prone or lateral position
	Oral airway
	Nasal continuous positive-airway pressure

the ventilatory responses to both hypoxia and hypercapnia. Hypoxia and hypercapnia occur commonly as a result of apnea and hypoventilation during emergence and recovery from anesthesia. Thus the combination of anesthetic effects and an immature respiratory control system (see also Fig. 14.11), as well as immature intercostal and diaphragmatic muscles, increases the risk of hypoxia, hypercapnia, and apnea in the postoperative period (see also Figs. 4.8 and 4.9).[28,29]

Apneic episodes occur commonly in the micropremie but decrease with advancing PCA.[30] PCA is defined as the sum of the conception age and the postnatal age. These apneic episodes usually involve both a failure to breathe (central apnea) and/or a failure to maintain a patent airway (obstructive apnea). Central apnea results from decreased respiratory center output, although it may be precipitated by abrupt changes in oxygenation, pulmonary mechanics, brain hemorrhage, hypothermia, or airway stimulation. Apnea may also occur without a precipitating event (i.e., idiopathic). Preterm infants with apnea do not increase ventilation in response to hypercapnia, compared with those without apnea, thereby delaying resumption of breathing and prolonging the apneic episode.[31] During obstructive apnea, the airway becomes obstructed in the hypopharynx and larynx as a result of pharyngeal muscle incoordination. Anesthetic drugs may further decrease pharyngeal muscle tone, precipitating airway obstruction during recovery from anesthesia. The combination of anesthetic effects and immature respiratory control places the micropremie at risk for central and obstructive apnea for a prolonged period of time during recovery from anesthesia.

Not surprisingly, apnea occurs commonly after anesthesia and surgery in premature infants.[32,33] Like apnea of prematurity, postoperative apnea may be central, obstructive, or mixed in origin.[34] The term *postoperative apnea* usually means prolonged apnea (>15 seconds) or brief apnea accompanied by bradycardia (heart rate ≤80 beats/minute). Postoperative apnea typically occurs as a cluster of episodes over several minutes, with minutes of normal breathing in between the clusters. Bradycardia may occur with apnea, usually beginning at the onset of apnea and is not a response to hypoxia but likely a vagal-mediated response. Arterial oxygen desaturation usually follows the apnea, although many apneic episodes may not have any associated desaturation. Arterial

desaturation is worse with obstructive apnea than with central apnea.[34]

The incidence of postoperative apnea depends on PCA, hematocrit, and the type of surgical procedure (Fig. 37.2; see also Fig. 4.7 and E-Fig. 4.5).[32–35] The most significant risk factor is the PCA; the less the PCA, the greater the risk, with the incidence of postoperative apnea in the micropremie greater than 50%.[32,33] Postoperative apnea can occur in the micropremie even without a history of apnea of prematurity.[32] After the initial decrease in postoperative apneic events in premature infants occurs at approximately 44 weeks PCA, a second significant decrease to near that of full-term infants occurs at 60 weeks PCA.[32] Therefore most centers have adopted a policy where premature infants need to be monitored for 12 continuous hours of apnea-free events after anesthesia when younger than 60 weeks PCA. Many admit these infants for overnight monitoring. Anemia (hematocrit <30%) and younger gestation increase the risk of apnea for a given PCA.[33,35] Postoperative apnea usually begins within an hour of emergence from anesthesia.[32] In the micropremie, it can continue to occur up to 48 hours postoperatively, despite the elimination of anesthetic agents (see Fig. 37.2). In fact, postoperative apnea can occur after surgery with desflurane- or sevoflurane-based anesthetics, or even after surgery for which a regional anesthetic was administered and no general anesthetic drugs were used.[36–39] Although spinal anesthesia may reduce the incidence of apnea within the first 30 minutes in PACU, the incidence of late apnea is the same as that after general anesthesia. Postoperative apnea is more common after major procedures, such as a laparotomy, compared with peripheral surgical procedures, such as inguinal hernia repair. These observations indicate that the neurohormonal response to surgery and postoperative pain may play an important role in the origins of postoperative apnea.

Management of postoperative apnea includes close observation with a cardiorespiratory monitor and pulse oximeter, administration of intravenous (IV) methylxanthines, such as caffeine and theophylline (Table 37.3), and prevention/treatment of anemia or hypovolemia. Caffeine is generally preferred over theophylline as it has a greater half-life and thus needs less frequent dosing (see also E-Fig. 4.6), its enteral absorption is more reliable, has fewer adverse side effects (tachycardia and feeding intolerance), and generally does not require serum drug monitoring. A loading dose of 10 mg/kg (IV or oral [PO]) is followed by a maintenance dose of 2.5 to 5 mg/kg daily.[40] Aminophylline 5–10 mg/kg, a predrug of theophylline, can also be used intravenously. Apnea can be exacerbated by opioids in the premature neonate, so their avoidance, if at all possible, is recommended. Obstructive apnea often responds to

TABLE 37.4	Circulating Blood Volume in Micropremies, Premies, Full-Term Neonates, Infants, and Children			
	Blood Volume (mL/kg)	Weight (kg)	Total Blood Volume (mL)	25-mL Blood Loss Proportion of Total Blood Volume (%)
Micropremie	110	1	110	23
Premie	100	1.75	175	14
Full-term neonate	90	3	270	9
Infant	80	10	800	3
Child	70	20	1400	2

changes in head position, insertion of an oral or nasal airway, or placing the infant in a prone position. Nasal CPAP, high-flow nasal prongs (HFNP), or tracheal intubation and mechanical ventilation may be required for several days postoperatively if these measures fail.[32]

CARDIOVASCULAR SYSTEM

Immature Versus Adult Heart

The micropremie remains at greater risk of cardiovascular collapse during anesthesia and surgery than does the full-term infant for several reasons. The fetal heart differs from the infant heart in that it has more connective tissue, less organized contractile elements, and increased dependence on extracellular calcium concentration. In addition, the less compliant fetal heart has a flatter Frank-Starling curve (see also Figs. 18.3 and 18.4) and is less sensitive to catecholamines because of near-maximal baseline β-adrenergic stimulation (see also Chapter 18).[41,42] Consequently, cardiac output in the micropremie depends more on heart rate than it does in the term neonate. The increased resting heart rate in the micropremie also does not permit cardiac output to increase to the same extent as in an infant or child. Additionally, the vagotonic response caused by succinylcholine or its metabolites (succinylmonocholine) and synthetic opioids may lead to bradycardia. These cardiac reflexes can be offset by the vagolytic effects of pancuronium or atropine.[43,44]

The micropremie has a greater blood volume per kilogram, but it has a smaller absolute blood volume (Table 37.4). Therefore relatively little blood loss during surgery can cause hypovolemia, hypotension, and shock. Because autoregulation is not well developed in the micropremie, the heart rate may not increase with hypovolemia, and blood flow and oxygen delivery to the brain and heart may decrease with relatively little blood loss.[45] Anesthesia blunts baroreceptor reflexes in the micropremie, further limiting the ability to compensate for hypovolemia.[46] The combination of limited ventricular stroke volume reserve, an increased heart rate, small blood volume, and limited autoregulation predispose the micropremie to cardiovascular collapse during major surgery.

Transition From Fetal to Neonatal Circulation

The lungs are not required for gas exchange in utero because the placenta performs this function. The fetal circulatory pattern consists of atria and ventricles working as units in parallel (see Fig. 18.2). As little as 10% of the fetal right ventricular output may circulate through the lungs.[47] Most of the blood returned from the lower extremities and a portion of the umbilical venous

blood supply passes into the pulmonary arteries and subsequently through the ductus arteriosus (DA) into the systemic circulation (see Chapters 16 and 18; Fig. 18.1). The superior vena caval blood supply circulates through the foramen ovale (FO) into the left atria and subsequently into the systemic circulation. With expansion of the lungs and increase in oxygen tension during the first breath, pulmonary vascular resistance decreases and blood flow to the lungs increases, matching perfusion with new ventilation.[47,48] The increased oxygen tension and loss of prostaglandin E_2-based relaxation are thought to result in closure of the DA. Any factor that increases pulmonary vascular resistance (e.g., hypoxia, hypercarbia, acidosis, and hypothermia) may cause the circulation to revert to a fetal circulatory pattern with shunting of deoxygenated blood from the right to the left side of the heart via a patent foramen ovale (PFO) or patent ductus arteriosus (PDA).[49–51] This right-to-left shunting of blood explains in part why some infants remain hypoxemic despite ventilation with 100% O_2 after severe desaturation.

Patent Ductus Arteriosus

In addition to aeration of the lungs, the removal of prostaglandins from the placenta and release of vasoactive substances at birth cause the DA to constrict and functionally close around 12 to 24 hours after birth, with anatomic closure in 2 to 3 weeks. Failure of the DA to close at birth occurs in 1/2000 full-term births, but affects up to 60% of ELBW infants with the incidence increasing with decreasing gestational age.[52,53] It is thought to be due to immaturity and failure of smooth muscle cells within the ductus to constrict, as well as immaturity of the lungs, which are responsible for metabolizing prostaglandins.

With the increase in systemic vascular resistance and decrease in pulmonary vascular resistance at birth, a PDA often results in significant left-to-right shunting of blood, causing excess pulmonary blood flow, congestive heart failure, and respiratory failure. Diastolic runoff of blood into the pulmonary artery leads to a widened pulse pressure (owing to low diastolic blood pressure) and risk of coronary ischemia. In a neonate with RDS or persistent pulmonary hypertension, right-to-left shunting across the PDA may occur, producing cyanosis. Paradoxical embolism is another concern with a PDA, as well as a PFO.[51] Fluid restriction and diuretic therapy, often used to treat congestive heart failure from left-to-right shunting through a PDA, further increase the risk of hypotension during surgery. The use of nonsteroidal antiinflammatory drugs to close the PDA can also cause renal compromise.[54,55]

Persistent Pulmonary Hypertension and Inhaled Nitric Oxide

Persistent pulmonary hypertension (PPHN) and refractory hypoxemia in neonates occurs in approximately 2/1000 live births.[56,57] PPHN is diagnosed when right-to-left shunting of blood occurs through a PDA and/or PFO in the absence of other congenital heart disease. Right-to-left shunting results from the failure of the pulmonary vascular resistance (PVR) to decrease at birth, thus preventing the conversion from fetal to neonatal pulmonary blood flow. The exact etiology of PPHN is not understood, but has been attributed to a variety of factors, including increased muscularization of pulmonary arterial vessels, impaired endothelial release of nitric oxide (NO), increased production of vasoconstrictors (e.g., endothelin-1), and impaired VEGF.[58] It can be associated with circumstances leading to perinatal distress (meconium aspiration, sepsis, asphyxia) or can be idiopathic, and rarely, genetic.[59]

PPHN is suspected in severely hypoxic neonates who do not have a significant increase in postductal O_2 saturation despite mechanical ventilation with an increased fraction of inspired oxygen (FiO_2). A greater preductal versus postductal O_2 saturation supports the diagnosis because it reflects the extrapulmonary right-to-left shunting of deoxygenated blood via the PDA. An echocardiogram excludes the presence of a congenital heart defect as the cause of or a contributing factor in the pulmonary hypertension and/or right to left shunt. It is imperative to diagnose and treat PPHN in a timely fashion as the morbidity, including neurodevelopmental delay, cerebral palsy, deafness, blindness, and mortality are substantive.[60,61] Premature infants tend to have worse outcomes and have more severe PPHN, requiring extracorporeal membrane oxygenation (ECMO) support earlier and more frequently than full-term neonates.[62]

The American Heart Association and American Thoracic Society have published guidelines for the diagnosis and treatment of PPHN. Treatment strategies aim to maintain adequate systemic blood pressure, maximize oxygen delivery, and optimize ventilator management to protect lung volume and function.[62] Normal lung expansion should be the goal of mechanical ventilation. Caution must be taken to avoid overdistending the lung, which can increase PVR. In cases of severe parenchymal lung disease, such as meconium aspiration, in which airway disease can lead to atelectasis and intrapulmonary shunt, PEEP and exogenous surfactant may be used to recruit alveoli. Although inspired O_2 is a potent vasodilator, maximum dilation of the pulmonary vasculature is achieved by relatively low levels of O_2, and hyperoxia can potentiate lung injury. For these reasons, increasing the FiO_2 often does not improve gas exchange in PPHN. Acidosis causes pulmonary vasoconstriction and should be avoided in patients with PPHN. This led to the practice in the past of inducing alkalosis by hyperventilation of the lungs or by infusing sodium bicarbonate. However, there is no evidence of any long-term benefit with this approach, and such management has been shown to worsen pulmonary vascular tone and lead to worse neurodevelopmental outcomes.[62,63] ECMO should be considered in those infants with severe sustained hypoxemia or compromised hemodynamic function.

Inhaled nitric oxide (iNO) is a selective pulmonary vasodilator used to treat PPHN. NO is normally produced by the endothelium and diffuses into subjacent smooth muscle cells, where it increases cyclic guanosine monophosphate (cGMP) levels that play a role in intracellular calcium levels and vasomotor protein function, leading to vascular relaxation (Fig. 37.3). iNO decreases PVR, limiting right-to-left shunting of blood, increases systemic O_2 partial pressures, and reduces the need for ECMO support in neonates with pulmonary hypertension.[62–65] However, not all infants respond to iNO, and studies have failed to demonstrate that iNO reduces mortality, length of stay in the hospital, or risk of neurodevelopmental impairment.[62,63,66] In contrast to full-term neonates, the success of iNO in the micropremie with hypoxic respiratory failure and pulmonary hypertension remains unclear.[62–64] Even among full-term neonates, some conditions such as congenital diaphragmatic hernia (CDH) do not respond well to iNO.[63,67]

When iNO is administered, the optimal initial dose is 20 ppm (Fig. 37.4). There is no advantage in terms of improvement in oxygen requirements to starting iNO at doses greater than 20 ppm. Moreover, doses greater than 20 ppm for extended periods may produce methemoglobinemia and/or nitrogen dioxide. Methemoglobin levels should be monitored if large concentrations of iNO are used. Fig. 37.4 delineates both treatment and weaning algorithms for iNO. Care must be taken to slowly wean the iNO to avoid rebound pulmonary

hypertension. Weaning should cease if the oxygen requirements increase at any stage during the weaning process and resumed once the oxygen requirements stabilize. Some who encounter hypoxemia during weaning may benefit from phosphodiesterase inhibitors such as sildenafil or milrinone. Sildenafil (Revatio) is a phosphodiesterase-5 inhibitor that selectively reduces PVR. It has been recommended for PPHN that is refractory to iNO, although the US Food and Drug Administration (FDA) issued a blackbox warning in 2012 against chronic use of sildenafil in children. It may be administered orally or intravenously. Milrinone may also be added to treat infants with PPHN when left ventricular dysfunction is present. Prostacyclin-I_2 (e.g., epoprostenol IV or treprostinil oral, IV or subcutaenous) has been used to treat PPHN (as well as iNO-resistant PPHN); however, it has a very brief half-life (5 minutes) and requires permanent vascular access for continuous administration.[56,57] Any interruption in therapy will rapidly result in profound rebound pulmonary hypertension with many untoward adverse effects. Inhaled prostaglandin-I_2 analogs (e.g., iloprost) and endothelin receptor antagonists (e.g., bosentan) may also be used in iNO refractory PPHN.

NEUROLOGIC DEVELOPMENT
Immature Brain
The central nervous system (CNS) is incompletely developed at birth. Regions of the CNS develop at different times during gestation; consequently, the impact of premature birth depends on gestational age at birth and the severity of cardiovascular, respiratory, and other postnatal stressors. The area of the brain most susceptible to injury in the micropremie is the periventricular white matter.[65] The white matter consists of preoligodendrocytes, astrocytes, and neuronal axons. Late in the second trimester (24–27 weeks gestation), preoligodendrocytes and astrocytes multiply tremendously and most cortical and subcortical structures begin to develop.[65] The periventricular white matter is perfused by arteries penetrating from the cortical surface and by lenticulostriate arteries from the circle of Willis. During this period, the periventricular white matter is particularly susceptible to neurologic injury as it is a "watershed region," susceptible to poor perfusion and hypoxic-ischemic injury during hypotension, reduced cardiac output, hypoxemia, and hypocarbia.

Neural pathways responsible for the perception of pain develop during the first, second, and third trimesters (see also Chapters 2, 44, and 45).[66] During the first trimester, peripheral sensory receptors and spinal reflex arcs mature, yielding the "withdrawal reflex" to non-noxious stimuli. Neurons that transmit nociception appear in the dorsal root ganglia at 19 weeks gestation, and afferent neurons from the thalamus reach the cortical subplate and cortical plate between 20 and 24 weeks gestation. However, it is not until early in the third trimester (29 weeks) that pathways between the thalamus and somatosensory cortex are functional. Significant controversy exists regarding the exact gestational age at which perception and memory of pain occur.[68,69] The hormonal responses to pain and stress may be exaggerated in neonates, although the clinical significance of this has not been defined.[70,71] Nevertheless, our approach in the micropremie is to administer anesthesia during surgery and provide pain management postoperatively.

Glucose and the Brain
The neonatal brain requires a larger percentage of glucose production because of the greater brain weight in proportion to body weight. Multiple animal models and clinical studies implicate hyperglycemia as detrimental to the adult brain during global

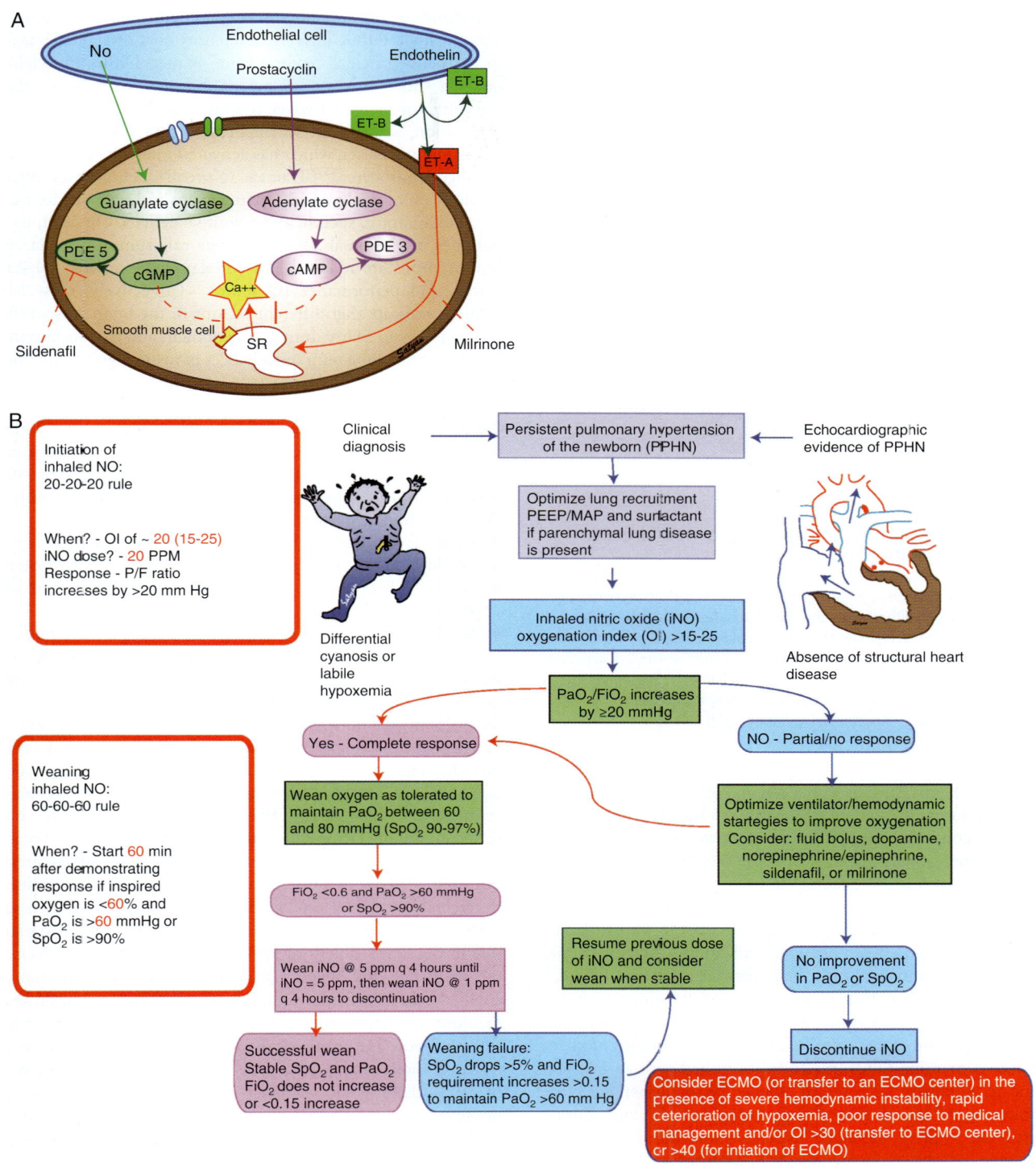

FIGURE 37.3 A, Nitric oxide *(NO)* produced by nitric oxide synthase *(NOS)* in endothelial cells diffuses into subjacent smooth muscle cells, interacts with soluble guanylate cyclase, and increases the concentration of cyclic guanosine monophosphate *(cGMP)* to cause vascular relaxation. The effect of NO is decreased by metabolism of cGMP by specific phosphodiesterases *(PDE).* **B,** Treatment algorithm for PPHN. *ECMO,* extracorporeal membrane oxygenation; *FiO₂,* fraction of inspired oxygen; *L-arg,* L-arginine; *MAP,* mean arterial pressure; *OI,* oxygenation index; *P/F,* Pao₂/ Fraction of inspired oxygen; *Pao₂,* arterial oxygenation; *PEEP,* positive end-expiratory pressure; *Spo₂,* oxygen saturation as measured by pulse oximetry; *SR,* sarcoplasmic reticulum.

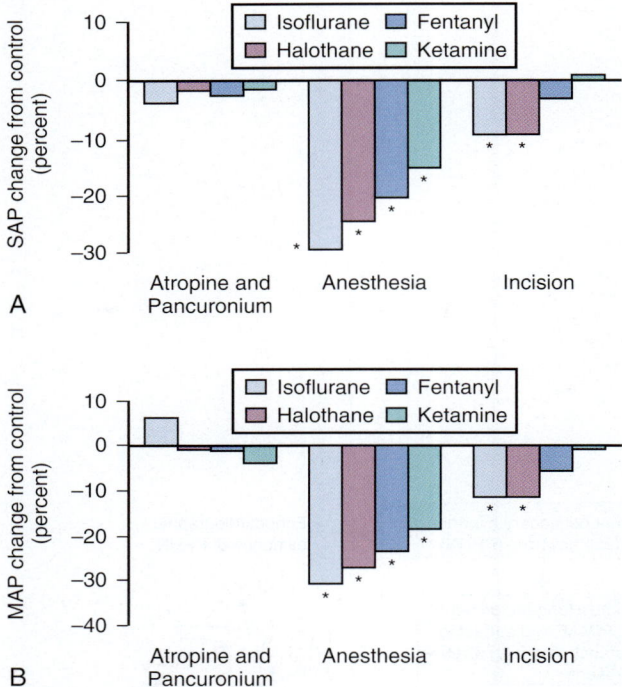

FIGURE 37.4 A, Changes in systolic arterial pressure *(SAP)* in preterm infants after anesthesia with either isoflurane, halothane, fentanyl, or ketamine, and after surgical incision. **B,** Changes in mean arterial pressure *(MAP)* in premature infants after anesthesia with either isoflurane, halothane, fentanyl, or ketamine, and after surgical incision. (Reprinted with permission from Friesen RH, Henry DB. Cardiovascular changes in preterm neonates receiving isoflurane, halothane, fentanyl, and ketamine. *Anesthesiology.* 1986;64(2):238–242.)

and focal ischemia, such as with a cerebral or hypoxemic ischemic event and during cardiac surgery with deep hypothermic cardiac arrest.[72] In contrast, hyperglycemia in neonates appears to protect the brain from ischemic damage or at the very least be less harmful than hypoglycemia.[73,74] Studies in both neonatal rat and pig hypoxia-ischemia models observed less brain damage with greater glucose concentrations. Many mechanisms exist for this strikingly different outcome between neonates and adults.[75] Relatively mild hypoglycemia is known to cause brain damage in preterm infants.[76] Micropremies with critical illness are especially prone to hypoglycemia because they contain limited stores of glucose and consume glucose anaerobically. Thus the administration of dextrose-containing fluids (carefully controlled with an infusion pump to minimize wide serum glucose fluctuations) and close monitoring of blood glucose concentrations are vital during anesthesia. Mild or moderate hyperglycemia during surgery is best managed by reducing the rate of infusion of dextrose-containing solutions and not administering insulin, with its attendant risk of hypoglycemia.

Complications of Prematurity

Despite decreases in mortality in the micropremie, long-term neurologic and developmental disabilities remain common in this group and include cerebral palsy, cognitive deficits, behavioral abnormalities, as well as hearing and visual impairment.[65,77] In a study of ELBW infants, only 25% were classified as "normally developed" at 5 years of age. Twenty percent exhibited major disabilities.[77] Brain magnetic resonance imaging (MRI) has identified

a spectrum of abnormalities in these infants. The most common abnormality is diffuse high signal intensity on T2-weighted imaging in the periventricular cerebral white matter. Diffusion-weighted imaging shows increased apparent diffusion coefficient values, indicative of increased water content and delayed white matter maturation, suggesting ischemia-reperfusion injury in periventricular white matter, which has activated microglia and damaged preoligodendrocytes.[65,78] Damage to preoligodendrocytes impairs myelination of cerebral white matter axons and accounts for many of the fine motor, speech, and cognitive deficits. On MRI, tissue volumes in the basal ganglia, corpus callosum, amygdala, and hippocampus are reduced and correlate with smaller full-scale, verbal, and performance IQ scores.[79] Collectively, these MRI findings indicate that different regions of the brain vary in their susceptibility to injury during development and that such injuries lead to specific long-term disturbances in neurocognitive function.

Intraventricular Hemorrhage

Intraventricular hemorrhage (IVH) occurs in as many as one-third of micropremie infants. Although an association has been noted between the incidence of IVH and fluctuations in blood pressure, it is difficult to confirm any causal relationship. The severity of IVH, as defined by head ultrasound, is graded as follows:

- Grade 1: hemorrhage limited to the germinal matrix
- Grade 2: hemorrhage extending into the ventricular system
- Grade 3: hemorrhage into the ventricular system and with ventricular dilatation
- Grade 4: hemorrhage extending into brain parenchyma.

Although micropremie infants with grade 3 or 4 IVH are more likely to exhibit severe long-term neurocognitive sequelae, even micropremie infants with grade 1 and 2 IVH display poorer neurodevelopmental outcomes compared with those without IVH.[79–81] Early onset of IVH appears during the first day of life. Risk factors include fetal distress, vaginal delivery, reduced Apgar scores, metabolic acidosis, severe hypercapnia, and the need for mechanical ventilation.[82,83] Late onset of IVH appears days to weeks after birth with contributing factors including RDS, seizures, pneumothoraces, hypoxemia, acidosis, severe hypercarbia, and the use of vasopressor infusions.[82,84] Lack of autoregulation leading to rapid fluctuations in cerebral blood flow, cerebral blood volume, and cerebral venous pressure, as well as fragile cerebral blood vessels, appear to play a role in the development of IVH.[45,84,85] Factors that may decrease the incidence and severity of IVH include administration of antenatal glucocorticoids or indomethacin.[86] Indomethacin helps to blunt the hyperemic response to hypoxia, improve cerebral autoregulation, and promote microvessel maturation of the germinal matrix. Although indomethacin decreases the incidence and severity of IVH, there is no evidence that long-term outcomes are improved.[86,87] Corticosteroids produce vasoconstrictive effects on fetal cerebral blood flow, protecting the fetus against IVH at rest and when challenged by conditions causing vasodilatation such as hypercapnia, leading to a significant reduction in IVH.[88]

TEMPERATURE REGULATION

The micropremie is very susceptible to hypothermia. Heat loss occurs by four possible routes: radiation (39%), convection (34%), evaporation (24%), and conduction (3%). In the micropremie, evaporative heat loss and insensible fluid loss are increased because the epidermis has less keratin.[89] Conductive and convective heat losses are also increased because the micropremie has little subcutaneous fat for insulation and a large surface area/mass ratio. Thermal regulation is not well developed in the micropremie.

Even full-term neonates do not have the capability to shiver or sweat, relying instead on nonshivering thermogenesis. Nonshivering thermogenesis, which depends on brown fat stores (which do not develop until 26–30 weeks gestation), is decreased in the micropremie and regulation of skin blood flow is less efficient.[90,91] During anesthesia, measures should be undertaken to minimize radiation and convective heat loss by warming the operating room (OR) to 80°F to 85°F (26.7°C–29.4°C) before the neonate arrives, and minimizing convective heat loss during transport (i.e., use a thermoneutral incubator or a warming mattress). The most effective means to maintain normothermia and to warm the micropremia is a forced-air warmer. Other strategies that may be useful to maintain normothermia include use of a warming pad on the operating table to reduce conductive heat loss, use of overhead heat lamps to reduce radiant heat loss, and keeping the skin dry to reduce evaporative heat loss. Additional strategies to reduce heat loss include using humidified gases in the ventilator circuit, covering the head, and warming IV and irrigation fluids before they are used. Temperature should be carefully monitored as overheating the infant may readily occur.

RENAL AND METABOLIC FUNCTION
Renal Function
The kidneys are not fully developed at birth.[92] Full-term neonates have a glomerular filtration rate (GFR) that is only 30% of normal adult rates owing to fewer nephrons and smaller glomerular size.[93–96] In fact, the GFR does not reach normal adult values until approximately 1 year of age (see Figs. 7.11 and 7.12). Maternal transplacental transfer of creatinine in utero increases the creatinine level in the neonate for the first few days of life.[97] The baseline plasma concentrations of creatinine increase with increasing prematurity and remain increased until approximately 3 weeks of age because of immature renal function and the consequent lower creatinine clearance compared with full-term infants.[98] These factors affect the metabolism of many drugs in the neonate. The renal excretion of medications such as penicillin, gentamicin, and some neuromuscular blocking drugs (NMBDs) such as pancuronium may be prolonged, resulting in increased duration of action or the development of high blood concentrations. This effect is particularly important when administering medications to an extremely premature infant. Thus the use of NMBDs that do not require renal function are most advantageous (e.g., cisatracurium).

Very premature infants easily become hyponatremic because of reduced proximal tubular reabsorption of sodium and water and reduced receptors for hormones that influence tubular sodium transport. As many as one-third of ELBW neonates develop hyponatremia.[95] Frequent assessments of the serum concentration of sodium and free water requirements are important during critical illness. Increased serum concentrations of potassium occur in premature infants during the first few days after birth. The increase results from a shift in potassium from the intracellular to extracellular spaces.[96] These increases are greater as gestational age and birth weight decrease.[99] Reduced cardiac output and urine production may further increase serum concentrations of potassium and predispose to cardiac arrhythmias.[100]

The total body water content in neonates is greater than in infants, children, and adults. In a term infant, 70% of the body weight is water (see also Figs. 7.7 and 7.8).[101] By 6 to 12 months of age, 50% to 60% of the body weight is water. In the premature infant 75% to 85% of the body weight is water. In general, the smaller the PCA of the neonate, the greater the percent of water present. Differences among the total body water, renal maturity, and serum protein concentrations in a neonate affect the volume of distribution of many medications. Because the volume of distribution of drugs confined to the extracellular fluid is increased, the initial doses of some medications (e.g., NMBDs, aminoglycosides) may be greater on a weight basis in neonates than adults to achieve the desired blood concentration. In contrast, because of immaturity of renal function, the interval between doses of these drugs must be increased.

Fluid Management
The basic principles of fluid maintenance in neonates are similar to those in older children and adults. The highly variable body fluid composition, degree of renal maturity, neuroendocrine control of intravascular fluid status, and insensible fluid loss with age make precise estimates of fluid requirements in neonates challenging.[102,103] Urine volume and concentration may be difficult to determine intraoperatively and may not always correlate with volume status. Moreover, blood pressure and heart rate may not correlate with intravascular volume status in premature infants, and anesthetics may mask subtle cardiovascular changes that occur with changes in intravascular volume. Increased insensible fluid loss, which often occurs in the OR environment, requires judicious titration of IV fluids. Congenital abnormalities (e.g., gastroschisis, omphalocele) may markedly increase insensible fluid loss through exposure of large mucosal surfaces. The use of humidified gas mixtures reduces insensible fluid loss through the respiratory tract. However, overzealous intraoperative administration of fluids can result in pulmonary complications and worsened third-spacing of fluids. It is recommended to use volume-controlled devices for fluid management, such as a Buretrol or an IV infusion pump, to ensure accurate fluid administration.

Calcium Homeostasis
During the third trimester, calcium is delivered to the fetus from the mother via placental transfer, resulting in fetal hypercalcemia. At birth serum calcium concentrations decrease with the abrupt loss of maternal calcium and reach a nadir at 2 days. By the third day of life, the combination of parathyroid hormone (PTH) secretion, dietary calcium intake, renal calcium reabsorption, skeletal calcium stores, and vitamin D allow the serum calcium concentrations in the full-term neonate to return to normal.[104]

Infants who are born prematurely do not benefit from the transfer of maternal calcium and are at greater risk for hypocalcemia after birth. In addition, premature infants experience hypocalcemia owing to hypoalbuminemia (reduces serum but not ionized calcium), limited oral intake, impaired secretion and response to PTH, increased calcitonin levels, and increased urinary losses as a result of increased renal excretion of sodium. Hypocalcemia has also been observed in nearly 40% of critically ill neonates.[105–107] Causes of hypocalcemia in the latter population include PTH insufficiency and peripheral resistance to PTH, inadequate calcium supplementation, and altered calcium metabolism caused by transfusion with citrated blood products, bicarbonate administration, or diuretics (e.g., furosemide).

Calcium exists in the serum in three fractions: protein bound, chelated to bicarbonate, phosphate, and citrate, and free or ionized calcium (iCa^{2+}). The ionized fraction is the physiologically active component; however, there is not always a clear relationship between total serum calcium and iCa^{2+}. The correlation is poor with hypoalbuminemia or acid-base disturbances, as seen in premature and critically ill neonates. Hypocalcemia is defined as a total serum calcium concentration less than 8 mg/dL (2 mmol/L) in full-term infants and less than 7 mg/dL (1.75 mmol/L) in premature infants. An iCa^{2+} less than 4 mg/dL (1 mmol/L) defines hypocalcemia in both populations.

Hypocalcemia may be asymptomatic or accompanied by nonspecific symptoms such as neuromuscular irritability (myoclonic jerks, exaggerated startle, or seizures), tachycardia, prolonged QT interval, and decreased cardiac contractility. Diagnosis rests on the determination of total and iCa^{2+} levels. Neonatal hypocalcemia is a feature of DiGeorge syndrome (chromosome 22q11.2 deletion), also known as velocardiofacial syndrome, secondary to underdeveloped or absent parathyroid glands. The syndrome also involves abnormal facial characteristics, cardiac defects, thymic hypoplasia, and cleft palate.

Symptomatic hypocalcemia may be treated with 90 mg/kg calcium gluconate or 30 mg/kg calcium chloride[108] by slow IV infusion over 5 to 10 minutes while monitoring the electrocardiogram, as bradyarrhythmias may develop in response to rapid increases in the serum concentration of calcium.[104] The IV site must also be closely monitored for extravasation of a calcium gluconate infusion, as it may cause tissue necrosis and subcutaneous calcification deposits. Alternatively, if calcium chloride is administered, it should be infused through a central IV line.[104] If using an umbilical venous catheter (UVC), caution must be taken to ensure the tip of the catheter is in the inferior vena cava (IVC) because direct infusion into the portal system can cause hepatic necrosis. Maintenance calcium gluconate dosing is administered at 80 mg/kg per day for the first 48 hours, followed by 40 mg/kg per day for the next 24 hours, and then discontinued. The clinical response and serum iCa^{2+} concentrations should be monitored. Treatment of hypocalcemia is not effective in the presence of hypomagnesemia. In such a situation, parenteral administration of supplemental magnesium and calcium and treatment of the underlying cause of hypocalcemia are necessary.[105] Persistent hypocalcemia necessitates determination of magnesium, phosphorus, PTH, and vitamin D concentrations.

Glucose Homeostasis

Early in gestation, the fetal liver begins to store glycogen while a continuous supply of glucose is delivered by transplacental transfer from the mother. In the third trimester, glycogen stores begin to develop in fetal skeletal and cardiac muscle, as well as in the kidneys, intestines, and brain. At birth neonatal glucose concentrations decrease rapidly to 30 mg/dL within the first 1 to 2 hours, stimulating glycogenolysis and gluconeogenesis.[109,110] The glucose flux usually stabilizes at values greater than 45 mg/dL by 12 hours.[109,110] The premature infant is prone to hypoglycemia owing to immature glucoregulatory mechanisms, reduced levels of glycogen storage, increased energy demands, and limited adipose stores (reduced free fatty acids and ketones available as alternative sources of energy).[109] Full-term infants who have been excessively fasted, small-for-gestational-age (SGA) infants, and infants of diabetic mothers are also prone to develop hypoglycemia.

The definition of hypoglycemia varies in the literature and among institutions. In full-term neonates, hypoglycemia is defined as a glucose concentration less than 40 mg/dL during the first 24 hours after birth and less than 60 mg/dL at 36 hours. In premature infants or those at risk for hypoglycemia, the threshold for hypoglycemia at 24 hours is less than 45 mg/dL and at greater than 24 hours is less than 50 mg/dL.[109,111] Signs and symptoms of hypoglycemia tend to be nonspecific and many are masked under anesthesia.[109,112] Hypoglycemia may manifest as respiratory distress, apnea, cyanosis, seizures, tremors, high-pitched cry, irritability, limpness, lethargy, eye-rolling, poor feeding, temperature instability, and sweating.[112,113]

A bolus of 0.25 to 0.5 g/kg (1–2 mL/kg of $D_{25}W$ or 2.5–5 mL/kg of $D_{10}W$) and an increase in the basal glucose infusion are prudent measures to treat hypoglycemia. Full-term infants require a glucose infusion rate of 5 to 8 mg/kg per minute to prevent hypoglycemia. However, premature and SGA infants have greater glucose requirements, and thus require infusion rates of 8 to 10 mg/kg per minute. It is extremely important to reassess the blood glucose concentration after these treatments to determine the effectiveness of the therapy. A single bolus of glucose without subsequent infusion can stimulate insulin production with consequent return to the hypoglycemic state.

Infants undergoing surgical procedures often require less glucose supplementation.[114] This reduced need may be attributed to hormonal responses that decrease glucose uptake as a result of catecholamine release in excess of insulin activity, as well as a decrease in metabolic demand from the effects of the anesthetic agents.[70,71,115] Nonetheless, it is important to administer glucose-containing solutions using a constant-infusion device to avoid large fluctuations in blood glucose concentrations and to monitor blood glucose concentrations in critically ill neonates. All other fluids (e.g., to replace third-space losses, blood loss, and fluid deficits) should be glucose-free to avoid hyperglycemia.[114] Infants treated with glucose via total parental nutrition (TPN) may develop severe hypoglycemia if the infusion rate is abruptly lowered; thus it is important to continue these infusions (possibly at a slightly reduced rate) during surgery and to check the serum glucose concentrations.

GASTROINTESTINAL AND HEPATIC FUNCTION

The anatomic structures of the fetal gastrointestinal (GI) tract are formed in the second trimester; however, the functional maturation does not occur until later in gestation and continues after birth. For example, compared with adults, gastric emptying in neonates is prolonged and lower esophageal sphincters are incompetent, making reflux of stomach contents common, even in the full-term neonate.

Premature infants, however, are susceptible to a multitude of complications because of the immaturity of the GI system at birth. Intestinal motility significantly increases between 29 and 32 weeks gestation and is stimulated by enteral feeds. A full-term infant usually passes meconium within the first 48 hours; however, less than 50% of micropremies will pass meconium in that time frame, and it may be delayed by days to weeks. Intestinal motility is also important to decrease the time allowed for colonization of harmful bacteria in the GI tract.[116] Increased time for bacterial growth, coupled with decreased bactericidal gastric and pancreatic secretions and immature GI immune defenses, renders the micropremie at risk for infections and the development of necrotizing enterocolitis (NEC). Enteric feeds increase intestinal motility in premature infants. However, controversy exists over the optimal time to start enteral feeds and which type of nutrition is best (mother's milk, donated human milk, or various types of formulas).[117–119] Early feeding of premature infants with hypertonic or trophic feeds (<10–20 mL/kg per day) is well tolerated, although the volume and frequency should be increased very gradually in premature infants to limit the risk of feeding intolerance.[117,120] A recent Cochrane review failed to associate early trophic feeding with the development of NEC or other bowel difficulties in extremely premature infants compared with prolonged enteral fasting.[118,119,121]

Hepatic metabolism is immature in neonates, particularly in premature infants. Drug metabolism may be slow as a result of immaturity of enzymatic processes, reduction of hepatic proteins, and relatively low hepatic perfusion (less drug delivered to the liver). Any factor that further compromises hepatic blood flow (e.g., increased intraabdominal pressure) may have profound adverse effects on drugs with perfusion-limited hepatic clearance.[122] Therefore careful titration of these drugs (e.g., opioids, propofol) is required to optimize therapeutic effects and prevent toxicity. Just as consideration is given to immature renal function, the use of NMBDs that do not require hepatic metabolism is advantageous (e.g., cisatracurium). The use of remifentanil during the procedure followed by a small dose of longer-acting opioid or regional block at the end of the procedure might facilitate early extubation.

In addition, reduced albumin synthesis decreases albumin concentrations compared with term neonates, enhancing the free (unbound) concentration of anesthetic drugs that are highly bound to albumin. Increased concentrations of unbound serum bilirubin introduce the risk of kernicterus, particularly in infants who are premature, hypoxemic, and acidotic and have low serum protein concentrations.[123,124] Highly protein-bound agents such as furosemide, sulfonamides, ceftriaxone, and benzyl alcohol (found as a preservative in many drugs such as diazepam) may displace bilirubin and increase the possibility of kernicterus.[123] The micropremie is also at particular risk for spontaneous liver hemorrhage.[125,126] This occurs most commonly during laparotomy for NEC, is associated with large IV fluid resuscitation, and is difficult to control surgically. One case report described the apparent successful use of recombinant factor VIIa to stop liver hemorrhage when administration of other blood products had failed.[127]

HEMATOLOGIC FUNCTION

Full-term newborns are born with an average hemoglobin (Hgb) concentration of 16.8 g/dL. This increase in Hgb is the results of increased production of fetal Hgb (Hgb-F) during the second and third trimesters, as well as an increase in the production of adult Hgb (Hgb-A) between 34 and 36 weeks gestation. This prepares the infant for the physiologic anemia of the newborn that develops between 8 and 12 weeks of life as the result of the fall in Hgb-F at birth and slow rise in erythropoietin (EPO) levels. The kidneys start transcribing EPO at 17 weeks gestation; however, production is not significant until around 30 weeks. At birth EPO production is initially decreased because of greater oxygen levels, and is subsequently stimulated by the anemia of the neonate. Therefore the premature infant has several reasons for being more susceptible to anemia at birth (average Hgb of 9.4 g/dL), which often occurs earlier and is more pronounced than the full-term neonate (average Hgb of 11.0 g/dL).[128] The leftward shift of the oxygen-Hgb dissociation curve resulting from the decreased affinity of Hgb-F for 2,3-diphosphoglycerate is also more pronounced in the premature infant, further contributing to the anemia.

The ideal hematocrit for the micropremie remains controversial. In the micropremie with reduced oxygen saturations and cardiac output, tissue oxygen delivery is maximized by maintaining the hematocrit between 44% and 48%. In a randomized study of liberal versus restrictive transfusion in neonates weighing between 500 and 1300 g, intraparenchymal brain hemorrhage, periventricular leukomalacia, and episodes of apnea occurred more frequently in the restrictive transfusion group.[129,130] The risks of blood transfusion in the micropremie must be balanced against the benefits of improved oxygen delivery and fewer medical complications.

Thrombocytopenia (platelet count <150,000/mm³) occurs in as many as 70% of micropremies.[131] Although the etiology of thrombocytopenia is often unknown, pathophysiologic processes such as sepsis, disseminated intravascular coagulation, and NEC are common causes. In addition to thrombocytopenia, premature infants are at increased risk for bleeding as the result of increased capillary fragility and decreased concentration of vitamin K–dependent coagulation factors. Preoperative evaluation should include a recent platelet count and coagulation studies and the availability of platelets and fresh frozen plasma and/or cryoprecipitate for major procedures.

Anesthetics and the Neonate/Premature Infant

ANESTHETICS AND THE IMMATURE BRAIN

Research in immature animals indicates that anesthetics are both neuroprotective and neurotoxic. Inhalational anesthetics protect against hypoxic-ischemic injury in neonatal pigs and rats.[132-134] The anesthetic must be administered before and during the ischemic event at a concentration of 1 minimal alveolar concentration (MAC) to be effective. Thus for surgery in which there is a risk of brain ischemia, use of an inhalational anesthetic may afford some advantage over IV agents. Cardiac surgery, ventricular shunt insertion, and vein of Galen embolization represent examples of procedures performed in preterm infants that carry a risk of brain ischemia. The MAC for sevoflurane has not been established in premature infants, and unfortunately many sick preterm infants cannot tolerate even modest concentrations of potent anesthetic agents.

Of particular concern are the reports in immature rats and other animals, including primates, that prolonged exposure to commonly used anesthetics, such as isoflurane, ketamine, and midazolam, induces apoptosis in many regions of the brain (see Chapter 25).[135,136] If this phenomenon applies to humans, the premature infant could potentially be more susceptible to anesthetic neurotoxicity than is the full-term infant.

A confounding factor is that neurodegeneration and apoptosis is a normal developmental phenomenon in the maturing fetal brain. Furthermore, anesthesia-induced neuronal cell death in neonatal animals may not directly translate into long-term neurologic abnormalities. Indeed, evidence suggests that sevoflurane-induced cognitive impairment, in the form of short-term memory deficiency in neonatal rodents, is offset by delayed exercise.[137] Moreover, immature animals that undergo painful procedures without anesthesia experience neuronal degeneration.[138,139] Premature infants who receive anesthesia and sedation for painful procedures experience less morbidity and mortality than those who do not.[140] Curiously, the combination of surgery and anesthesia in neonatal rats produces more apoptosis than either intervention alone, suggesting that in this model, anesthetics are neither neuroprotective themselves nor do they offset the apoptotic effects of surgery.[141] In summary, the neurodegeneration precipitated by inhaled anesthetics, ketamine, and benzodiazepines depends on developmental age, brain region, and duration of exposure. Based on the animal models, the micropremie exposed to several hours of large concentrations of inhaled agents with nitrous oxide (N_2O) and midazolam is potentially at risk, as is the micropremie exposed to surgery with insufficient anesthesia. Thus our approach at the present time for surgery is to use small concentrations of inhaled agent, muscle relaxants, opioids (e.g., remifentanil), and regional anesthesia whenever possible.

Of even greater concern may be the sedatives that are administered for prolonged periods of time in the intensive care unit (ICU), although one study found "no evidence of an association between dose and duration of sedation and/or analgesia drugs given during the preoperative, intraoperative, and postoperative period and major adverse developmental outcomes" in children undergoing repair of congenital heart disease in the first 6 weeks of life.[142]

INHALATIONAL ANESTHETICS

The MAC defines the minimum alveolar concentration for inhaled agents at which 50% of patients respond to a painful skin incision with withdrawal. This measure allows comparison of the effects of inhaled anesthetics at equipotent doses. The MAC of isoflurane in the micropremie (<32 weeks PCA) is approximately 20% less than that in full-term neonates (see also Fig. 7.17), and at equipotent doses of isoflurane (1 MAC), systolic arterial pressure decreased similarly in all age groups, 20% to 30%.[143] Sevoflurane affords a rapid induction and emergence from general anesthesia. Desflurane is contraindicated for induction of anesthesia but is widely used for maintenance of anesthesia administered through an ETT. However, desflurane causes more airway irritability than isoflurane or sevoflurane, and as a result, it is not recommended for infants with severe BPD. Desflurane, sevoflurane, and isoflurane decrease arterial blood pressure in a dose-dependent manner, possibly through decreasing the systemic vascular resistance or by myocardial depression. One possible mechanism to explain the myocardial depression is that the baseline ionized calcium concentrations in premature infants, especially critically ill neonates, are less.[106,107] Premature infants may be more susceptible to the cardiodepressant effects of inhalational anesthetics because inhalational anesthetics block the calcium channels,[144] and the neonatal heart depends on the plasma ionized calcium for contractility to a greater extent than do the hearts of older children[145] (see also Chapter 7).

N_2O is not routinely used in the micropremie for several reasons. First, N_2O must be delivered in inspired concentrations ranging from 50% to 75% to reduce the MAC of other agents; therefore its role in micropremies, a group often requiring supplemental oxygen, is limited. Second, because of its blood gas solubility, N_2O rapidly enters air-filled cavities; therefore it is not recommended for use in infants with bowel obstruction, NEC, pulmonary interstitial emphysema, or pneumothoraces, pathologies that are common disorders in micropremies.[146] Third, in neonatal and young rats, N_2O demonstrates no antinociceptive effects, which contrasts with its antinociceptive effect in adolescent and adult rats.[147] This observation requires validation in humans.

INTRAVENOUS ANESTHETICS

IV agents include opioids, benzodiazepines, barbiturates, propofol, ketamine, and dexmedetomidine. Fentanyl possesses analgesic and sedative properties; however, it does not reliably produce unconsciousness or amnesia and, by itself, is not considered an anesthetic in children or adults. Nonetheless, the use of fentanyl as an anesthetic has been justified in preterm infants because they were deemed to be inherently amnestic by virtue of their age, even though the age at which consciousness and memory occurs is unknown. Premature infants (<1500 g) who receive IV fentanyl (30–50 μg/kg) and pancuronium for ligation of a PDA exhibit remarkable hemodynamic stability, with only a 5% decrease in blood pressure.[148] A dose of 10 to 12.5 μg/kg of fentanyl administered together with an NMBD maintained hemodynamic stability for 75 minutes in neonates undergoing a variety of thoracic and abdominal procedures.[149] Hypertension and tachycardia did not occur with skin incision, suggesting that analgesic concentrations necessary for surgery are achieved with this dose of fentanyl.

The pharmacokinetics of fentanyl (30 μg/kg) in premature infants yielded plasma concentrations that remained constant for up to 120 minutes, indicating a reduced clearance.[150] The elimination half-life of fentanyl ranged from 6 to 32 hours in premature infants, greater than the 2- to 3-hour half-life observed in children and adults.[150] The clearance of fentanyl is 7 mL/minute per kilogram at 25 weeks, 10 mL/minute per kilogram at 30 weeks, and 12 mL/minute per kilogram at 35 weeks PCA.[151] These studies demonstrated that the half-life and volume of distribution of fentanyl are increased, whereas the clearance is reduced in premature infants compared with adults.[122] These changes may be explained by immature CYP450 3A4, the major enzyme responsible for clearance (see also Chapters 6 and 7). In a subset of infants with increased intraabdominal pressure (after repair of a gastroschisis or omphalocele), the elimination half-life of fentanyl is 1.5- to 3-fold greater than that in other infants of the same age.[122] Fentanyl clearance may be impaired consequent to reduced hepatic blood flow as the result of increased intraabdominal pressure, although maldistribution of blood away from regions of concentrated CYP450 3A4 activity and reduced hepatic function may play a greater role.[122,152] The increased volume of distribution decreases the initial plasma concentration of fentanyl compared with that in adults.[122] These pharmacokinetic differences, combined with an increased propensity to apnea, serve to prolong analgesia and respiratory depression, increase the risk of postoperative apnea, and slow recovery of consciousness. In the micropremie, mechanical ventilation may be required for several days after large doses of fentanyl.

Similarly, the elimination half-life of morphine is markedly prolonged in premature infants compared with that in children and adults.[153–156] The elimination half-life of morphine ranges from 6 to 16 hours in the micropremie, compared with 2 to 4 hours in the adult. The clearance (normalized to a 70 kg person) of morphine increased with PMA between 23 and 35 weeks, reaching 50% of the mature clearance by 50 weeks PMA, and mature values by 80 weeks PMA.[154] The active water soluble metabolite, morphine-6-glucuronide, also has reduced elimination because of immature renal function.[157] We prefer fentanyl to large-dose morphine for anesthesia because the former has fewer hemodynamic side effects.[151,156]

Remifentanil is rapidly inactivated by plasma and tissue esterases and, because of its short half-life, is administered by continuous infusion. The half-life of remifentanil in adults is 3 to 4 minutes, independent of the duration of infusion, and similar to that in infants or children.[158] A multicenter study that compared halothane and remifentanil for maintenance of anesthesia in infants undergoing pyloromyotomy showed similar intraoperative hemodynamic stability with the two techniques, but significantly fewer "new-onset apneas" with remifentanil compared with halothane.[159,160] Interestingly, the most rapid clearance of remifentanil was in infants and children younger than 2 years of age, thus allowing an intense opioid effect intraoperatively that rapidly dissipates upon terminating the infusion.[161] Remifentanil has been used to provide anesthesia in infants weighing 400 to 580 g with apparent good hemodynamic stability.[162,163] A study examining cord blood from premature infants found high nonspecific esterase activity, comparable with that of term infants, thus suggesting that preterm infants should be able to rapidly metabolize remifentanil.[164] If a remifentanil infusion is indicated, it is best to use a dilute concentration (5 μg/mL) piggybacked as close to the IV as possible with a continuous carrier to achieve a constant rate of administration.

Ketamine, a phencyclidine derivative, affords several advantages compared with inhaled and other IV agents. It provides analgesia, amnesia, and unconsciousness yet minimally depresses cardiovascular function (Fig. 37.4).[165] However, ketamine anesthesia depresses ventilation and airway reflexes, which predisposes to airway obstruction, apnea, and gastric aspiration. Thus we recommend the use of an ETT when ketamine is used for surgical procedures in the micropremie. In the setting of brief painful procedures, IV ketamine can be used as an anesthetic without an ETT.[166]

Other IV agents include thiopental, propofol, and benzodiazepines. These agents induce loss of consciousness but possess less analgesia than ketamine. Thiopental is a short-acting barbiturate primarily used for the induction of anesthesia. The micropremie requires less thiopental for induction than does the infant (2–3 mg/kg vs. 5–6 mg/kg, respectively), a relationship similar to the MAC of isoflurane.[167] In the past, we used only thiopental for neurosurgical procedures involving increased intracranial pressure in these infants. However, thiopental is no longer available in the United States. Propofol is primarily used to induce anesthesia and has largely replaced thiopental for this purpose. A word of caution is needed regarding the use of propofol for induction of anesthesia in neonates. Several reports highlight episodes in otherwise stable infants of protracted hypotension and low cardiac output that were associated with hypoxia after propofol boluses (1–3 mg/kg IV). The mechanism underlying these responses remains unclear, although systemic vasodilation and acute pulmonary hypertension with reversion to persistent fetal circulation remains a strong possibility.[168,169] In our experience, a propofol infusion (50–200 μg/kg per minute) supplemented with fentanyl as needed for analgesia can anesthetize the micropremie. The use of an infusion pump that accurately allows for delivery of small volumes is vital. The infusion rate of propofol in these small infants must be carefully entered and then double-checked by another provider to avoid a detrimental overdose.[170] Recovery from propofol anesthesia is delayed in micropremies compared with term infants, because micropremies have both less fat and muscle tissue to redistribute the drug, and reduced clearance. In the pediatric ICU, propofol infusions have been implicated in unexpected deaths (propofol infusion syndrome).[171] Until the safety of long-term administration of propofol has been examined in preterm infants, other alternatives for prolonged sedation should be considered.

Benzodiazepines, such as midazolam and diazepam, have been used in the neonatal intensive care unit (NICU) for sedation. As with thiopental and propofol, these drugs do not provide analgesia and are not recommended as the sole anesthetic for surgery. However, the combination of a benzodiazepine and opioid provides complete anesthesia for surgery. Midazolam clearance is markedly decreased in the micropremie compared with the term neonate or infant, and will be further prolonged in the setting of decreased liver function.[172] Midazolam can cause systemic hypotension, depress ventilation, and impair airway reflexes in preterm infants. The hypotension caused by midazolam is greater in the presence of fentanyl; thus both drugs must be titrated in small doses when administered concomitantly.[173] One study noted an 8% to 23% decrease in arterial pressure after a bolus of 0.1 mg/kg of midazolam in premature infants.[174]

REGIONAL ANESTHETICS

Regional anesthesia (see Chapter 42) is possible in premature infants and offers the advantage of the avoidance of sedative, volatile, and opioid medications that may lead to apnea, bradycardia, and hypotension. However, there is conflicting evidence of the superiority and reduction of adverse events of regional anesthesia compared with general anesthesia in this population.[175] In neonates the conus medullaris extends to a lower segment of the spine than adults; however, there does not appear to be a significant difference in location between term and premature neonates (see Fig. 42.3), thus it is generally recommended that lumbar punctures are made at L4-5 or L5-S1 interspaces in this age group.[176] Larger doses of local anesthetics per kilogram are required in infants because of their larger volume of distribution of cerebrospinal fluid (see E-Fig. 42.3), relatively increased surface area of the spinal cord and nerve roots, and increased cardiac output with proportionally greater blood flow to the spinal cord. However, faster drug distribution, uptake, and elimination of local anesthetics from the CSF also abbreviate their duration of action. Adjuncts to local anesthetics, such as clonidine, may increase the duration of the block but also increase the risk of sedation, bradycardia, apnea, and hypotension. The optimal dose, timing and, side effects of these adjuncts in this age group are controversial.[177]

Neonatal Surgical Emergencies

Neonatal emergencies can present at any time, occurring immediately at birth or within weeks after delivery. Thankfully, advances in perinatology have improved the morbidity and mortality of critically ill newborns. Nonetheless, whether acquired or congenital in nature, these emergencies can be truly life-threatening and require the skill and expertise of an anesthesiologist who is knowledgeable about the nuances of neonatal physiology. The goal of this section is to describe common neonatal surgical emergencies and the considerations important to the anesthesiologist caring for this very special population.

PREPARATION FOR SURGERY
The "Urgent" Emergency
In the past, many conditions classified as neonatal emergencies were expeditiously taken to the OR, often within hours of diagnosis. However, with newer technology and medical advances, along with better outcome data, immediate surgical intervention is not always necessary or preferable. In most circumstances, there is time to medically optimize the infants and correct any hemodynamic instability and/or metabolic derangement, although the optimal timing for surgical correction is not always straightforward and must be determined on a case-by-case basis.[178–181]

THE OPERATING ROOM
Environment
Owing to the immature and inefficient measures neonates use to regulate body temperature, precautions must be made to prevent heat loss in the OR. Warming the room to 80°F to 85°F (26.7°C–29.4°C), using radiant warming units, using forced-air heating pads, and adding humidity to the inspired gases in the circuit help maintain the neonate's temperature in the neutral thermal range (see Chapter 52).[182–184] Other methods used to prevent heat loss include using a head cover and warming IV and irrigation fluids before they are used.[185,186] Precautions should also be used during transport, such as the use of an incubator/radiant warmer or a portable heated mattress.

MONITORS

Routine standard monitoring equipment includes an electrocardiograph, chest or esophageal stethoscope, blood pressure monitor, temperature probe, pulse oximeter, and an end-tidal carbon dioxide ($ETCO_2$) and agent analyzer. Cerebral near-infrared spectroscopy (NIRS) is used increasingly in neonates (E-Fig. 42.3) with cardiac pathology, neonatal intensive care, and the OR. Noninvasive continuous cardiac output monitors may become routine in these infants in the future (see Chapter 52).[187,188]

Oxygen Saturation

It is recommended to limit the use of oxygen in neonates to maintain an oxygen saturation as measured by pulse oximetry (SpO_2) of anywhere between 83% and 95% in order to decrease oxidative stress.[16-19] However, an increased inspired fraction of oxygen (FIO_2) may be required during anesthesia and surgery owing to their deleterious effects on oxygenation, such as reduced functional residual capacity (FRC), ventilation-perfusion mismatch, and hypoventilation. Perhaps more importantly, many neonatal emergency surgeries are intrathoracic or intraabdominal in nature, further exacerbating difficulties in oxygenation with limited recruitment maneuvers available. In the event that the ductus arteriosis is still patent, it is recommended to place a preductal pulse oximeter (right hand), as well as a postductal oximeter (left hand or foot) to determine the severity of any extrapulmonary shunting of deoxygenated blood via the PDA. If the patient has a right-sided arch, the pulse oximeter should be placed on the left hand instead of the right for preductal monitoring.

End-Tidal Carbon Dioxide

$ETCO_2$ measurements have been shown to correlate generally well with $PaCO_2$, even in neonates.[187,189-191] However, most of these studies have taken place in ICUs, not in the OR, where the anesthesia circuits tend to carry significantly more dead space (V_D). The increase in V_D, along with a small neonatal tidal volume (T_V) exacerbates the $PaCO_2$-$ETCO_2$ gradient, as evidenced by the Enghoff modification of the Bohr equation:

$$V_D)/V_T = (PaCO_2 - ETCO_2)/PaCO_2$$

In addition, it has been noted that the correlation of $PaCO_2$ to $ETCO_2$ in neonates with severe lung disease who demonstrate an arterial oxygen saturation (PaO_2) to FIO_2 ratio of less than 200 is not as strong.[187] Neonates presenting for emergency surgery may harbor some degree of lung disease, and most will be subject to a large V_D, making it important to recognize that the $ETCO_2$ may significantly underestimate true $PaCO_2$. A more accurate estimate of $ETCO_2$ concentration may be obtained by using a special endotracheal tube with a sample port located at its tip (mainstream monitoring) or by inserting a narrow catheter through the CO_2 sampling port in the elbow and into the lumen of the tracheal tube.[191-193] Measures to limit V_D include eliminating the elbow from the anesthesia circuit and shortening the ventilation circuit as much as possible.

Invasive Monitors

In neonates, changes in blood pressure, heart rate, and the intensity of heart sounds are excellent indicators of cardiac function, intravascular volume status, and depth of anesthesia. Invasive monitors may not be indicated in all cases. They can be difficult to place, lead to adverse events, and contribute to a significant decrease in hematocrit owing to multiple blood draws from a very small circulating volume. However, in cases in which major blood or fluid losses are expected, or the physiology is complicated by the presence of cardiac disease, a central venous catheter is warranted. Likewise, any neonate with significant underlying cardiovascular instability should have an arterial catheter placed for continuous monitoring of blood pressure and to provide means to obtain arterial blood samples for determination of blood pH, serum glucose, and electrolyte concentrations. Some neonates arrive in the OR with umbilical venous (UVC) and/or arterial catheters (UAC) in place. Umbilical catheters can be used during the first 5 to 7 days of life and are rarely used beyond 7 to 10 days. High-lying UACs (above the diaphragm) are associated with fewer complications, such as ischemia, thrombosis, and hypoglycemia, than low-lying catheters (above the aortic bifurcation) (Fig. 49.9).[194] UVCs should lie in the IVC at its junction to the right atrium (Fig. 49.8). A UVC that lies within the portal system or wedged within the liver will not accurately reflect central venous pressure (CVP) and can lead to hepatic necrosis with infusions of hypertonic solutions.[195] Care must be taken to verify where the tips of each of these catheters lie before using them.

Ventilator

As mentioned previously, there is often a large amount of V_D from anesthesia circuits to a neonate who requires a very small T_V. In addition, these infants may have intrinsic lung pathology, which when coupled with intrathoracic or intraabdominal surgery that compresses the lungs, can render it extremely difficult to ventilate with a conventional anesthesia machine. It may be necessary to manually ventilate the lungs in these infants during parts of the surgery, particularly if a primitive ventilator is used. In limited circumstances, it may be beneficial to have the ICU bring one of their ventilators to the OR for use during surgery, but this will preclude the ability to administer volatile agents.

Equipment Setup

Anesthesiologists need to be well prepared for these surgical cases. A sick neonate can have extremely labile hemodynamics even before the induction of anesthesia or surgical incision. Table 37.5 lists basic equipment for conducting emergency anesthesia in a neonate (Figs. 37.5 and 37.6).

Fluids and Medication

Particular attention must be paid to ensuring the accurate delivery of medications and fluids. These infants require only small fractions of the medications in most vials and ampules. As a result, either tuberculin syringes should be used to carefully measure the very small aliquots of medications or the medication in the vial should be diluted so that a measurable and accurate fraction of the content of the vial can be given. Tuberculin syringes present several challenges, including difficulty in removing air bubbles from the syringe, and the very small volume that will be administered. The volume of medication may be so small that it is no larger than the volume of the stem of the clave or stopcock, resulting in less drug than intended being administered to the infant. Diluting medications introduces the risk of a drug dose error that could lead to an overdose or underdose of the medication. In all instances, it is prudent to verify the dose and dilution of the medication with a colleague and carefully label the contents. To ensure the drug is not lost in the V_D of the IV set, each clave or stopcock should be flushed with saline solution after the medication has been given. All medications should be administered into the IV

TABLE 37.5	Suggested Equipment for Emergency Neonatal Anesthesia		
Airway Equipment	**Environment**	**Agents**	**Intravenous Fluids**[a]
Suction catheters	Room temperature (80°–85°F; 26.6°–29.5°C)	Gases Air/O₂/iNO	Lactated Ringer's solution
Oral airways	Forced warm air delivery device	Volatile anesthetics	D₁₀W
Face masks	Underbody warming blanket	Drugs IV anesthetics	Normal saline solution
Breathing circuit	Circuit humidifier	Propofol	5% albumin
Miller 0, 1, blades and handle	IV fluid warmer	Ketamine	PlasmaLyte
Uncuffed endotracheal tubes (ID 2.5, 3.0, 3.5, 4.0 mm)	Infusion pumps for both maintenance fluid and for opioid or vasoactive drugs	Muscle Relaxants Succinylcholine Cisatracurium Vecuronium Pancuronium	
Stylet		Opioids Fentanyl Morphine Remifentanil	
Cuffed endotracheal tubes (ID 3.0, 3.5 mm)		Local Anesthetics Tetracaine 1.0% Bupivacaine 0.25%	
		Emergency Drugs Atropine Epinephrine (1:10,000) Dopamine Calcium Bicarbonate Isoproterenol	

ID, inner diameter; *IV*, intravenous; *NO*, nitric oxide; *O₂*, oxygen.
[a]Some guidelines suggest 1% glucose should be added to an isotonic fluid for maintenance during anesthesia.[301]

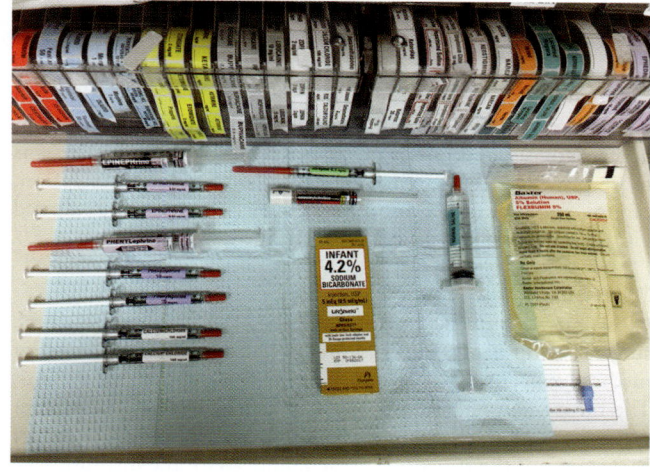

FIGURE 37.5 Example of emergency drug setup on anesthesia cart.

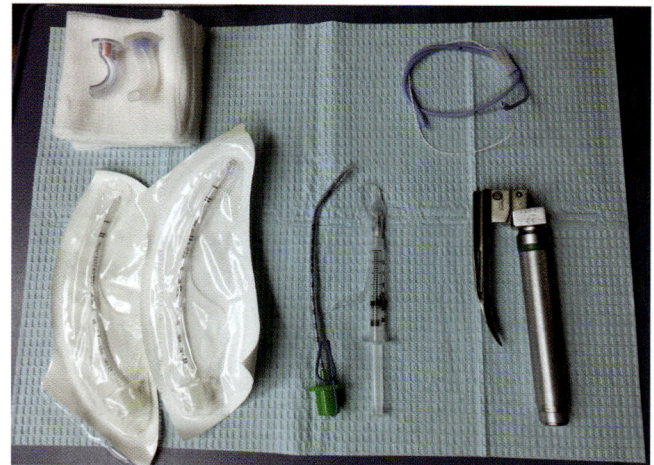

FIGURE 37.6 Example of neonatal airway setup on anesthesia machine.

set as close to the patient as possible to minimize the volume of fluids needed to flush the medication into the child (see Fig. 52.2).

Fluid overload is always a concern in these small infants. To minimize the fluids administered, all IV infusions should be delivered through a pump. Free-flowing IVs are dangerous sources for fluid overload, which may open a DA and cause congestive heart failure. Finally, meticulous care must be taken to remove air bubbles from all IV administration systems, solutions, and medications that are administered. See Chapter 52 for further discussion on infusion pumps and the implications of IV administration VD on drug delivery (see also Figs. 52.2 and 52.3).[196,197]

Intraoperative fluid management in micropremies should begin with continuing the solution that arrives with the infant from the NICU; usually this is a calcium- and/or glucose-containing solution. Alternatively, some infants may arrive with a hyperosmolar glucose or dextrose (10%) parenteral nutrition solution. In both cases, these solutions should not be discontinued, but rather continued at the same rate (by infusion pump) or slightly less throughout the surgery to avoid reactive hypoglycemia from increased circulating insulin concentrations. There is no evidence regarding the

optimal infusion rates for these solutions during anesthesia. If no solution is being infused, a balanced salt solution (e.g., lactated Ringer's solution or PlasmaLyte) could be initiated at 4 mL/kg per hour, supplemented with the same solution for third-space loss (at least 10 mL/kg per hour), and replacement of blood loss. If a glucose solution is not being infused, then a balanced salt solution containing glucose may be administered through a pump. Serum glucose concentrations should be monitored regularly to avoid hypoglycemia. Third-space losses include evaporation and vascular leak and are replaced with a balanced salt solution.

Bedside Procedures in the ICU

Occasionally, neonates may be so critically ill that simply transporting the infant to the OR may be life-threatening. To decrease the risk, many institutions now perform surgical procedures at the infant's bedside or in a specialized surgical suite within the NICU, minimizing the period of transport and providing optimal surgical conditions. Providing surgical and anesthetic care at the bedside has its challenges. There is reduced access to the child, suboptimal lighting, reduced sterility, limited monitors (usually capnography is absent), and an inability to control room temperature, although NICU incubators commonly include a built-in overhead radiant heater.

Adapting to the working environment requires planning and organization in concert with communication with the surgeons, neonatologists, and nurses in the NICU. If bedside anesthesia is to be provided, then appropriate IV equipment for transfusion, pumps, and monitors compatible with electrocautery and expired CO_2 monitoring should be available, just as in the OR.

THE FAMILY

Close interaction between the parents and the anesthesia, medical, surgical, and nursing staff promotes effective communication of medical concerns and continued emotional support for parents. The birth of a premature neonate or illness in a full-term infant often does not allow time for emotional preparation for or acceptance of the situation by the family. With the institution of aggressive medical and surgical interventions, parents sometimes feel excluded from the care of their infant and develop feelings of isolation and lack of control. The development of rapport between the parents of critically ill infants and hospital staff is essential to ensure adequate psychological support during this intensely anxiety-provoking event.

Emergency Surgery

RESPIRATORY PATHOLOGY

Lesions of the respiratory system can be categorized into those that involve the large and small airways and those that involve the lung parenchyma.

ABNORMALITIES OF THE AIRWAY

Airway surgery presents unique operative challenges. The airway must be shared between the anesthesiologist and surgeon, while the OR table is rotated 90 degrees, hindering immediate access to the child's airway. Bronchoscopy with a rigid scope is very stimulating and requires a deep level of anesthesia, which may lead to cardiac and respiratory depression. There is intermittent and often inadequate ventilation because of leakage around the scope or during periods where the insufflation port is removed or just the telescope is used. These factors make it difficult to maintain an adequate level of anesthesia when inhalational agents are used. It may be more prudent to provide anesthesia with IV medications, such as propofol or ketamine, with intermittent boluses or with the use of a constant infusion for longer cases together with opioids (see also Chapters 15 and 33).

Choanal Atresia

Choanal atresia is a developmental failure of the nasal cavity to communicate with the nasopharynx owing to the persistence of the nasobuccal membrane. It occurs in approximately 1/7000 live births with a female predominance.[198] Choanal atresia is often associated with other congenital anomalies, such as CHARGE syndrome (**C**oloboma, **H**eart disease, **A**tresia choanae, **R**etarded growth, **G**enital anomalies, **E**ar anomalies), Treacher-Collins, Pfeiffer, and VATER (**V**ertebral defects, **A**nal atresia, **T**racheoesophageal fistula with **E**sophageal atresia, and **R**adial and renal anomalies).[199,200] Unilateral choanal stenosis is usually diagnosed later in childhood or adulthood and is characterized by unilateral nasal discharge and persistent nasal obstruction. Bilateral stenosis, however, is considered a surgical emergency owing to the obligatory nasal breathing pattern in neonates. They often present within the first days of life with

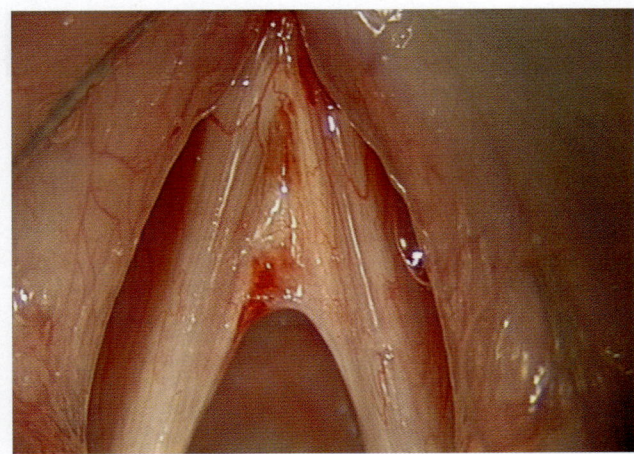

FIGURE 37.7 Laryngeal web in a neonate. (Courtesy Dr. Christopher Hartnick.)

respiratory distress and cyanosis, usually while feeding, which is relieved by crying. Other diagnostic criteria include noisy breathing, difficulty feeding, and the inability to pass a 5/6F catheter into the nasopharynx. Definitive treatment involves perforation of the persistent membrane via an endoscopic transnasal approach (most common) or via a transseptal approach (usually reserved for patients with other significant craniofacial abnormalities).[199,201] Nasal stenting is often performed at the end of the procedure with stents left in place for about 4 weeks. These neonates may develop airway obstruction during anesthetic induction, therefore early placement of an oral airway may aid in airway management.

Laryngeal and Upper Tracheal Obstruction

Because of the narrow diameter of neonatal airways, even a small obstruction can lead to significant resistance to airflow, leading to life-threatening respiratory distress. Therefore timely recognition and treatment of laryngeal and upper tracheal abnormalities, such as webs, congenital subglottic stenosis, and hemangiomas is essential in reducing morbidity/mortality. (Figs. 37.7 and 37.8 and Video 37.1; see also Videos 14.1, 14.5, and 14.18).

As resistance increases inversely with the airway radius to the fifth power, ventilatory assistance is required to overcome this substantial increase in the work of breathing. The greater time constants that result from the increased airway resistance require a greater time for expiration to avoid gas trapping. In the most severe cases of obstruction, tracheal intubation may not be possible or is unable to provide adequate ventilation past the stenosis, and a tracheostomy may have to be placed before treatment.

WEBS. Laryngeal and tracheal webs are fibrous membranes that develop as the result of incomplete recanalization of the larynx during early gestation, resulting in variable degrees of airway obstruction and acute respiratory distress or stridor shortly after birth (see Fig. 37.7).[202,203] Some infants may succumb at birth because of a complete or near-complete tracheal web if this airway defect has not been identified antenatally. If a tracheal web has been identified in utero, an ex utero intrapartum treatment (EXIT) procedure may be a lifesaving maneuver (see Chapter 38). Anterior glottic webs are associated with velocardiofacial syndrome (also known as 22q11.2 deletion or DiGeorge syndrome) in 65% of cases, and many also include concurrent subglottic stenosis.[203] Endoscopic web excision is the preferred treatment via microlaryngoscopy.

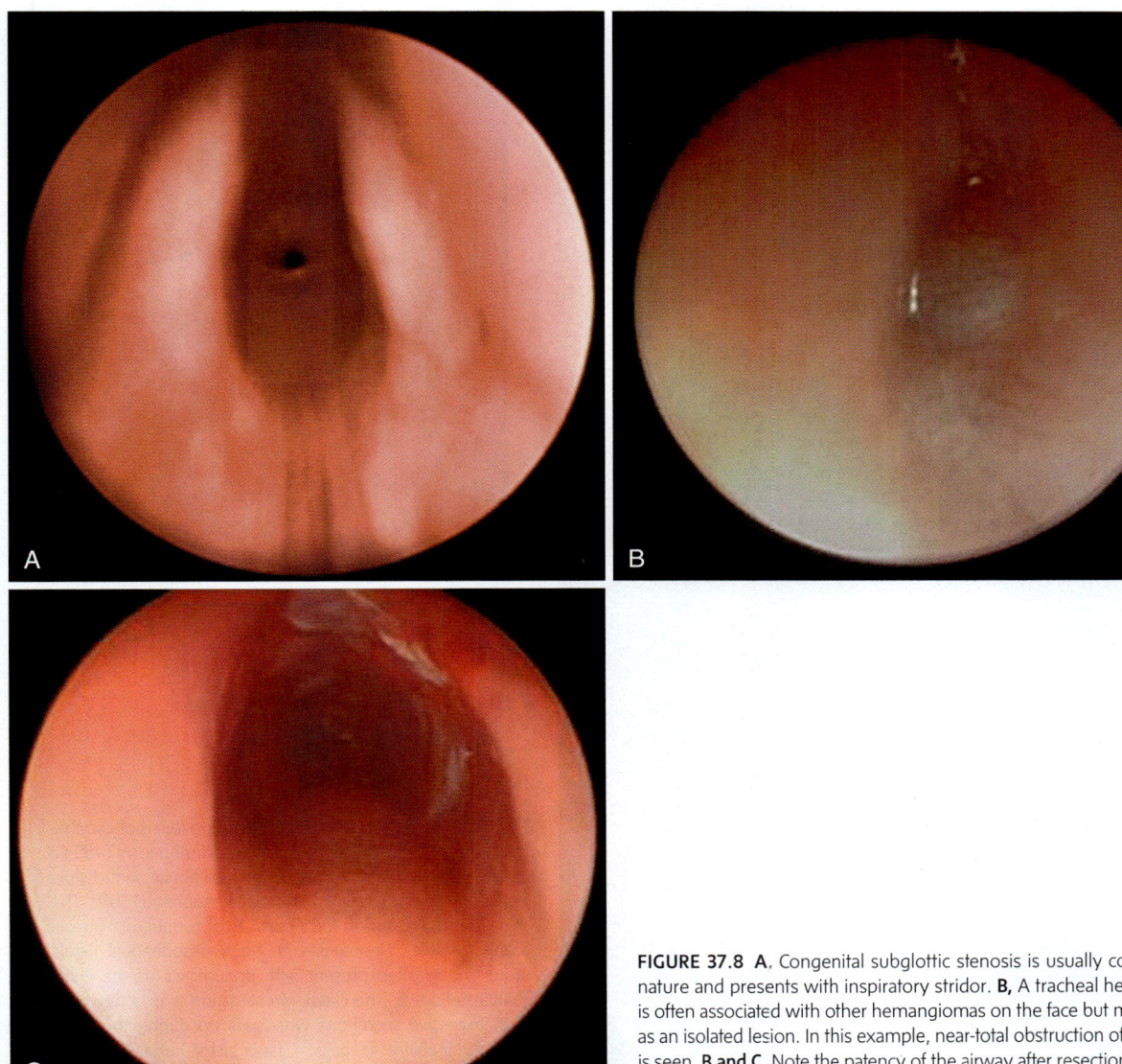

FIGURE 37.8 A. Congenital subglottic stenosis is usually concentric in nature and presents with inspiratory stridor. **B,** A tracheal hemangioma is often associated with other hemangiomas on the face but may present as an isolated lesion. In this example, near-total obstruction of the airway is seen. **B and C,** Note the patency of the airway after resection. (Courtesy Dr. Christopher Hartnick.)

Many surgeons will elect to keep the airway intubated for 24 hours after surgery to allow the raw edges to re-mucosalize.

CONGENITAL SUBGLOTTIC STENOSIS. Subglottic stenosis is the most common indication for neonatal tracheostomy placement.[204] It is thought to be the result of malformed cricoid cartilage in utero, or, in rare cases, owing to severe gastroesophageal reflux, eosinophilic esophagitis, or infection.[203] The degree of symptomatology and treatment options varies with the degree of narrowing. Lower-grade stenoses can be treated with endoscopic interventions such as balloon dilation and steroid injection. However, the more severe stenoses require more extensive surgical repair. In the past, these neonates received long-term tracheostomy placement with the expectation that they would outgrow the stenosis. Currently the surgical options include cricotracheal resection and laryngotracheoplasty, involving an anterior with or without a posterior cricoid split involving the placement of a cartilage graft, usually from the thyroid or costal cartilage, to enlarge the subglottic lumen. This may or may not include the temporary placement of a tracheostomy while the incision heals (see also Chapter 15).[204]

SUBGLOTTIC HEMANGIOMA. Infantile hemangiomas are the most common type of vascular tumor, affecting 4% to 10% of infants, and the most common tumor to involve the pediatric airway (see Fig. 37.8).[205,206] Its cause is not well understood. Any child with a cutaneous hemangioma, especially if in the V3 "beard" distribution on the face, should be evaluated for a concomitant subglottic hemangioma (20%–30% co-incidence), although they can occur anywhere in the airway.[205,207] Airway hemangiomas can also be associated with PHACES syndrome (**P**osterior fossa malformation, **H**emangioma, **A**rterial lesions of the head and neck, **C**ardiac abnormalities, **E**ye abnormalities, **S**ternal cleft or **S**upraumbilical hernia). Symptoms, which include respiratory distress and stridor, are generally absent immediately after birth but can develop quickly as the hemangioma rapidly grows between 6 and 12 weeks of life. This proliferation continues until approximately 12 to 18 months of age, and the hemangioma then gradually begins to shrink. First-line medical therapy includes oral propranolol, followed by systemic and intralesional injection of steroids. Propranolol can cause bradycardia, hypotension,

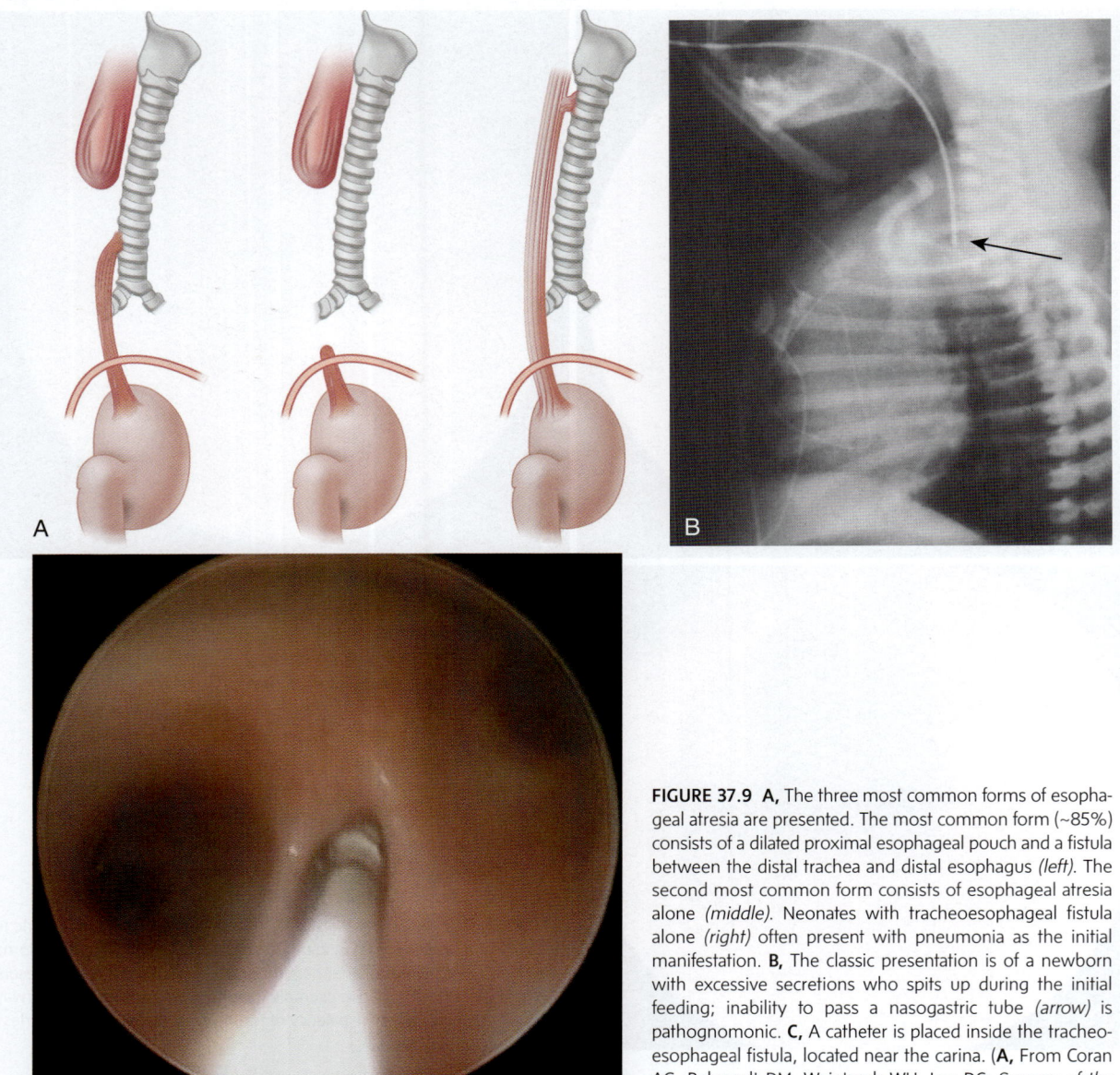

FIGURE 37.9 A, The three most common forms of esophageal atresia are presented. The most common form (~85%) consists of a dilated proximal esophageal pouch and a fistula between the distal trachea and distal esophagus *(left).* The second most common form consists of esophageal atresia alone *(middle).* Neonates with tracheoesophageal fistula alone *(right)* often present with pneumonia as the initial manifestation. **B,** The classic presentation is of a newborn with excessive secretions who spits up during the initial feeding; inability to pass a nasogastric tube *(arrow)* is pathognomonic. **C,** A catheter is placed inside the tracheoesophageal fistula, located near the carina. (**A,** From Coran AG, Behrendt DM, Weintraub WH, Lee DC: *Surgery of the Neonate.* Boston: Little, Brown; 1978:46. **B and C,** Courtesy Dr. Daniel P. Doody.)

hypoglycemia, and hyperkalemia. Surgical options include laser therapy or open excision and are generally offered to those in whom medical therapy with persistent airway obstruction fails. Laser therapy achieves focal tissue ablation with the use of either the yttrium-aluminum-garnet (YAG) laser or a diode laser via an endoscopic approach through direct laryngoscopy. This therapy is reserved for smaller, focal lesions. Open excision is performed via an anterior airway incision around the cricoid cartilage, which may require a rib or thyroid cartilage graft to avoid subglottic stenosis. These children will remain intubated for several days after the procedure.[203,205] Subglottic hemangiomas are easily compressed when a tracheal tube is passed to intubate the airway, although bleeding is always a possibility and should be anticipated. However, when the practitioner is unaware of the presence of a hemangioma, the first recognition of the lesion may be the absence of an air leak around an appropriately sized tracheal tube.

Tracheoesophageal Fistula/Esophageal Atresia

Tracheoesophageal fistulas (TEFs) occur in 1/3000 live births in a mostly sporadic, nonsyndromic manner with no preference for sex or race. They are due to an error in separation of the trachea from the floor of the foregut around the fourth to fifth week of gestation. They are often associated with other congenital anomalies, in particular the VACTERL association (**V**ertebral anomalies, imperforate **A**nus, **C**ongenital heart disease, **T**racheoesophageal fistula, **R**enal abnormalities, **L**imb abnormalities).[208,209] There are two main systems of classifications of TEF (Gross and Vogt) that describe the lesions in terms of whether or not esophageal atresia (EA) is present and where the tracheoesophageal connection occurs in relation to the trachea (Fig. 37.9A) (see also Fig. 15.12). The most common type (Gross classification C) consists of a blind proximal esophageal pouch with a distal TEF just above the carina (80%–90% of cases).

TEF can be diagnosed prenatally with signs of polyhydramnios (fetus cannot swallow), small or absent fetal stomach bubble, and/or blind-ending upper pouch in the fetal neck. Early postnatal signs and symptoms include excessive salivation, choking/coughing/regurgitation at the first feed leading to cyanosis and/or respiratory distress, and a distended abdomen owing to the stomach filling with air every time the baby cries, which can compress the lung and embarrass respiration. Diagnosis of TEF/EA can be confirmed by the inability to pass a nasogastric (NG) tube into the stomach, a dilated proximal esophagus with air in conjunction with air in the distal stomach on x-ray, computed tomography scan, or direct visualization via bronchoscopy/esophagoscopy (Fig. 37.9B and C, E-Fig. 37.1 and Video 37.2) (see also Fig. 15.11).

The Waterston and Okamoto classification systems use weight, congenital anomalies, and comorbidities to determine surgical risk and guide planning. This helps determine whether the child should undergo more immediate surgical correction, should undergo more extensive stabilization before correction, or requires a more drawn-out staged repair. Generally, there is enough time to stabilize and optimize the infant before surgery. This involves establishing IV access, correcting anemia and electrolyte imbalances, typing and crossmatching blood, evaluating for other anomalies (especially cardiac echocardiography), and possible placement of a gastrostomy tube, which can be completed using local anesthesia to vent the stomach.

Surgical repair has traditionally been performed with an open thoracotomy and manual lung retraction. However, in the past two decades, thoracoscopic repair has become increasingly popular.[210] Single-lung ventilation is not required, as low-flow, low pressure intrathoracic CO_2 is used instead to collapse the right lung to improve surgical exposure. The patient is placed in the left lateral decubitus position for a right thoracotomy to avoid the aortic arch. The anesthesiologist will place a nasoesophageal tube to aid the surgeon in identifying the proximal esophageal pouch. The fistula is ligated first to avoid further entrapping air into the stomach, followed by a primary end-to-end anastomosis of the esophagus.

Several approaches may be used to secure the airway in these infants. One option is to keep the infant spontaneously breathing. Avoiding positive-pressure ventilation reduces the amount of gas entering the stomach, which can impede the ability to ventilate. This can be achieved by means of an awake intubation with topicalization and/or sedation, or with an inhalational induction. However, the awake approach can be traumatic and difficult, and a crying infant will only put more air into the stomach. Inhalational inductions in neonates can (but rarely do) cause major cardiovascular instability. An IV induction is quicker (less crying) and may be more stable, allowing for the use of NMBDs to optimize intubating conditions. Positive-pressure ventilation is usually successful because the compliance of the lungs is greater than that of the distended stomach. Gentle mask ventilation with low peak pressure ventilation will decrease the amount of air that enters the stomach. If a gastrostomy has been performed, a Fogarty catheter can be passed retrograde through the gastrostomy to occlude the fistula from below.[211]

Although one-lung ventilation is usually not required, the tip of the ETT must be placed above the carina but distal to the fistula. This can be achieved by purposefully placing the ETT into the right main stem (with the bevel facing anterior to block the aperture of the fistula) and then very slowly withdrawing the ETT while auscultating the left thorax until breath sounds are first heard. A fiberoptic scope can also be used to guide the ETT into position and to confirm correct placement. The ETT must be carefully secured to prevent accidental movement above the fistula. Frequent suctioning of the ETT may be required because of the accumulation of blood and secretions.

After correction of the defect, absorptive atelectasis may require ventilation with long inspiratory times to reexpand alveoli. Early extubation is desirable because it prevents prolonged pressure of the ETT on the suture line. However, many surgeons request that the airway remains intubated postoperatively for several days because the tip of the ETT may perforate the sutured trachea at the level of the fistula during an emergency reintubation or to prevent pneumonia and atelectasis. The ETT provides a means to suction and expand the lungs during the first 24 hours of greatest risk. It is important to maintain the head in a neutral position so as not to pull on the esophageal anastomosis.[212] An epidural catheter threaded from the caudal to the thoracic space may provide a postoperative analgesia and aid in successful extubation (E-Fig. 37.2). An intrapleural catheter is another means of providing analgesia after open surgery, but this may risk local anesthetic toxicity owing to rapid absorption from the pleural cavity.

Abnormalities of the Lung
Congenital Diaphragmatic Hernia
CDH has an incidence of 1 to 2/5000 live births. It occurs around the eighth week of gestation owing to the failure of complete closure of the pleural and peritoneal canal, resulting in herniation of the abdominal organs into the thorax, inhibiting normal lung growth. This affects not only the division of the airways, but also the formation of pulmonary vasculature, leading to a decreased number of bronchi and alveoli (diminished surface area for gas exchange), as well as decreased cross-sectional area and numbers of pulmonary artery branches. This, in turn, increases the PVR and primary pulmonary hypertension. The degree of abnormality depends on the timing of the herniation in utero and the amount of abdominal contents in the thorax. The ipsilateral lung is usually the one affected, but the contralateral lung may be involved as well.

The most common type of CDH occurs at the posterolateral foramen of Bochdalek (90%) and is also the largest and is associated with the greatest degree of pulmonary hypoplasia; CDH occurs five times more frequently on the left rather than right side. Neonates with the Bochdalek hernia are more likely to have other birth defects including a 20% to 40% frequency of congenital heart defects and a 5% to 15% frequency of chromosomal abnormalities.[213] A Morgagni type of defect is reported in about 2% of CDHs with the remaining occurring through the esophageal hiatus. CDH is associated with genitourinary and GI malformations, as well as chromosomal anomalies, including trisomy 13, trisomy 18, tetrasomy, and 12p mosaicism.

Prenatal diagnosis can be made via ultrasound findings of polyhydramnios, an intrathoracic gastric bubble (stomach above the diaphragm), and mediastinal shift away from the herniation site (E-Fig. 37.3) (see also Fig. 15.10).[214] Antenatal predictors of poor outcome rely on the observed/expected lung/head ratio and the presence or absence of a thoracic liver in left-sided lesions. Lung/head ratios of <25% are associated with 25% survival, whereas those with ratios greater than 45% are associated with 100% survival.[214,215] An abdominal chest x-ray displaying intestinal loops and/or abdominal organs in the thorax and ipsilateral lung compression aids in postnatal diagnosis. Signs and symptoms are related to the degree of lung hypoplasia and pulmonary hypertension and associated defects that might be present. Owing to the increase in PVR, right-to-left shunting via the patent foramen ovale and DA may occur with hypoxemia. Infants most often present with respiratory distress, and tachycardia, tachypnea, and cyanosis can be observed shortly after delivery. A scaphoid (concave) abdomen and barrel chest may also occur from displacement of the viscera into the thorax. Bowel sounds in the chest are fairly uncommon.

Emergent surgical closure of the defect used to be the standard of care because of the prevalent belief that reduction of the herniated viscera would facilitate lung growth and a return toward normal lung size and function. However, this was untrue. A thorough understanding of the specific pathophysiology of the defect prompted the application of new medical therapies and changed the timing of open surgical repair.[216] Now the focus is to stabilize these neonates medically, optimize the infant's condition before surgery, and adopt measures to improve pulmonary hypertension and reduce PVR. Respiratory support is given, as needed, which may include tracheal intubation with gentle mechanical ventilation to avoid pneumothorax or barotrauma (especially in the normal [contralateral] lung), as in the use of an oscillator or ECMO. ECMO and/or iNO should be used to bridge ventilation and oxygenation during the early postnatal life if the child is persistently hypoxic and/or acidotic despite conventional ventilation strategies. Care is provided to avoid introducing air into the GI tract via the use of an NG tube and to avoid CPAP and prolonged mask ventilation, which will only further impinge on the lungs. These infants may also need pharmacologic cardiovascular support. Timing of the procedure is uniquely variable but should be based on the individual condition of the infant and institutional experience.[217-220]

Open surgical correction is achieved with a transabdominal approach, and primary closure is usually possible. If the defect is too large, artificial tissue may be used for closure. In most instances, the abdomen is too small to accommodate the bowels when they are returned to the abdominal cavity. The net effect is a dramatic decrease in pulmonary compliance (in the good lung), desaturation, and hypercapnia. Alternately, the viscera are placed in a Silo pouch (Bentec Medical, Woodland, CA) outside the body until growth allows their return to the abdominal cavity. A chest tube may be placed on the contralateral side before surgery in the event of a pneumothorax. In the past two decades, thoracoscopic repair has been used with excellent success in infants who are medically stable.[216,217]

This approach can be performed without single-lung ventilation by use of low-flow, low-pressure CO_2 insufflation, which collapses the lung and gently allows the return of the herniated viscera back into the abdomen. The infant is positioned in the lateral decubitus, with the upper arm supported without interfering with surgical instruments. Both of these techniques can also be performed if the child requires ECMO, but in the latter case these surgeries are usually undertaken in the NICU.[216,217] The surgical timing for neonates who require ECMO remains contentious. Some believe that surgery should be either performed early, before ECMO, whereas others believe that later surgery is preferred. These arguments arise because bleeding during surgery in anticoagulated infants during ECMO can be excessive. In addition, some centers offer advanced treatment options such as fetal-based corrective surgical procedures.[218,221] Temporary fetoscopic tracheal plugging, performed between 25 and 28 weeks gestation, prevents the normal outflow of surfactant-rich fetal lung fluid.[222] The retained volume subsequently enlarges the fetal lungs, accelerates growth, and reduces the mass effect of herniated viscera.

Anesthetic management is aimed at avoiding the harmful effects of volutrauma (by maintaining frequent small TVs and limited peak inspiratory pressures) and those conditions known to increase PVR (hypoxemia, acidosis, hypothermia, hypercarbia). An NG tube should be passed before induction of anesthesia to empty the stomach while the airway is ventilated at low peak inspiratory pressures by face mask before the ETT is placed. N_2O should be avoided because it will expand air-filled cavities (bowel) and limit the inspired oxygen concentration. Postoperatively, the trachea remains intubated. The use of an epidural catheter or intercostal nerve block (thoracoscopic approach) aids in postoperative comfort.

Congenital Lung Malformations

CONGENITAL BRONCHOGENIC AND PULMONARY CYSTS. Congenital bronchogenic and pulmonary cysts result from the abnormal development of the ventral foregut and lung budding during the first trimester.[223] These cysts may be centrally located within the mediastinum and produce obstruction by a mass effect.[224] They may also be located at the carina and cause obstruction or distal gas trapping by a ball-valve effect. Those located in the hilum, in the paratracheal region, or in the lung parenchyma may lead to chronic respiratory illness from infection and abscess formation.[225,226] Congenital cysts are occasionally diagnosed only after rupture of the cyst produces hemorrhage or bronchopulmonary fistula formation.[223,226] Urgent surgical resection via thoracotomy or thoracoscopically is recommended for symptomatic cysts, and at 3 to 6 months of age for asymptomatic cysts to promote lung growth.[227-229]

The anesthetic should be designed to prevent further enlargement of the cyst because a communication may exist with the airway. Awake (sedated) intubation or intubation after an inhalation induction, followed by maintenance of spontaneous ventilation, if possible, until the thorax is opened may reduce the potential risk of a sudden expansion of the cyst. If assisted ventilation is required, low peak inspiratory pressures should be used. Should the cyst be fluid filled or infected, selective bronchial blocking may be helpful to protect the unaffected lung (see Chapter 15).[230,231] N_2O and positive-pressure ventilation without adequate expiratory time should be avoided to decrease the possibility of enlarging the cyst. If these attempts are unsuccessful and the cyst enlarges to the point of occluding the airway or compromising the circulation, needle aspiration may be required to reduce the size of the cyst and facilitate oxygenation and ventilation. If this approach is unsuccessful, emergency thoracostomy may be lifesaving.

CONGENITAL LOBAR EMPHYSEMA. Congenital lobar emphysema, also known as congenital lobar overinflation or infantile lobar emphysema, is the hyperinflation of one or more pulmonary lobes (Fig. 37.10) (see also Fig. 15.9). The incidence is approximately 1/20,000 with a 3 : 1 preference for males. The left upper lobe is most frequently involved (43%), followed by the right middle lobe (32%), and right upper lobe (20%), with bilateral involvement in 20%. In 12% to 14% of cases there is associated congenital heart disease or vascular anomaly.[232] The exact etiology is unknown; however, it is thought to result from a disruption in the development of the bronchial cartilage that causes bronchial collapse.[233,234] This lack of cartilaginous support leads to a ball-valve effect with consequent overinflation. The hyperinflated lung causes an increase in intrathoracic pressure and compression atelectasis on the ipsilateral or contralateral lung, resulting in mediastinal shift and ventilation-perfusion mismatch.[232]

Surgical lobectomy of the affected segments via an open thoracotomy or thoracoscopically is the definitive treatment. Avoiding N_2O and positive-pressure ventilation prevents the expansion of the emphysematous lobe, which could compress

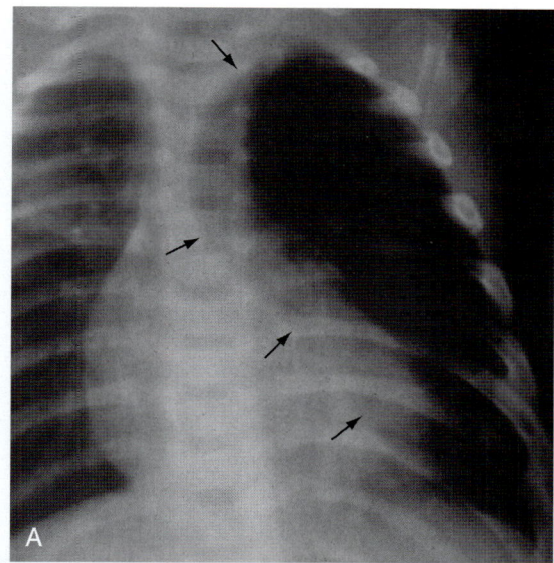

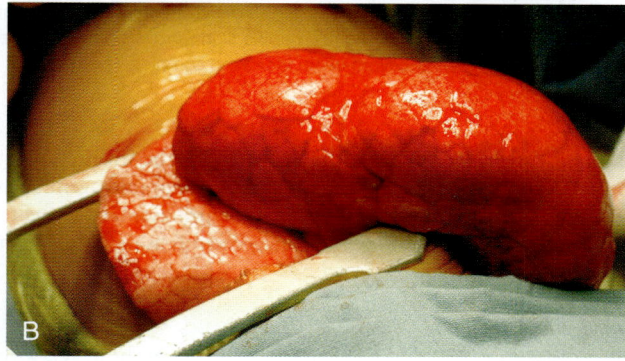

FIGURE 37.10 A, Radiograph from an infant with congenital lobar emphysema demonstrates hyperinflation of the left lung with herniation across the midline *(arrows)* and mediastinal shift. **B,** Intraoperative photograph shows the emphysematous lobe bulging through the thoracotomy incision. (From Coté CJ. The anesthetic management of congenital lobar emphysema. *Anesthesiology.* 1978;49(4):296–298.)

normal lung tissue.[235,236] If positive-pressure is required, low peak pressures and TVs should be used. There have been reports of using single-lung ventilation while the affected lobe is resected. Frequent ETT suctioning is suggested; an epidural catheter threaded from the caudal to the thoracic space may provide pain control.[232,234]

GASTROINTESTINAL PATHOLOGY

Emergency surgical conditions of the GI tract are most frequently due to obstructive lesions, lesions that compromise intestinal blood supply, or both.

Infants with obstructive lesions should be considered to have a full stomach, as the retention of gastric fluid increases the risk of aspiration during induction. A rapid-sequence induction (RSI) should follow suctioning of gastric contents (usually with a vented catheter in supine, right and left positions), and N_2O should be avoided to minimize intestinal distention. Desaturation after a brief period of apnea during an RSI occurs more rapidly in neonates than in older infants,[237] emphasizing the importance of preoxygenation and the rapid establishment of an airway. Some providers advocate the use of a modified RSI technique, with gentle mask

ventilation before tracheal intubation.[238] Unless life-threatening compromise of organ blood flow occurs, these lesions do not require immediate surgical correction, and the priority is to correct any metabolic derangements and establish euvolemia before undergoing corrective surgery.

Infants with lesions that compromise intestinal blood supply and cause ischemia are extremely ill. They may present with hypotension, metabolic abnormalities, particularly hyperkalemia, anemia, and thrombocytopenia. Emergency surgery is required in these circumstances and is directed at removing the necrotic tissue, closing perforations, and reestablishing normal perfusion to the intestine. Blood products and emergency drugs should be readily available. Good IV access is required, and a centrally located catheter may be necessary for the administration of vasoactive drugs, as well as an arterial line for close blood pressure monitoring. Infants with compromised intestinal blood supply are usually considered to have full stomachs and N_2O is avoided, as well.

Obstructed Lesions
Hypertrophic Pyloric Stenosis
Hypertrophic pyloric stenosis is the result of hypertrophy and hyperplasia of the muscularis layer of the pylorus, causing a functional gastric outlet obstruction (Fig. 37.11). It occurs in 1/500 live births and more frequently in first-born males.[239,240] Infants usually present between 2 and 8 weeks of age with protracted nonbilious projectile vomiting, creating a hypokalemic, hypochloremic metabolic alkalosis; severe cases may progress to a metabolic acidosis. The kidneys attempt to maintain a normal blood pH by excreting bicarbonate. To maintain euvolemia and retain sodium cations, the kidneys excrete hydrogen and then potassium cations to maintain charge neutrality. Paradoxical aciduria occurs in the hypovolemic infants (after prolonged vomiting) when the urine appears acidic while the pH in the blood is alkaline. Since this is not a life-threatening emergency, time should be taken to correct the metabolic derangements and ensure proper rehydration; this may take 24 to 48 hours. Before considering an anesthetic in these infants, the skin turgor and the urine output (1–2 mL/kg per hour) should be restored, a serum sodium greater than 130 mEq/L, potassium greater than 3.0 mEq/L, and a chloride concentration greater than 85 mEq/L. Diagnosis is commonly made via ultrasonography or rarely with a barium swallow and radiographic examination.[241,242] Most infants are quickly diagnosed with pyloric stenosis today, rendering a minority who present with severe fluid and electrolyte imbalances compared with the past.[243] Treatment is surgical pyloromyotomy by means of an open periumbilical incision or laparoscopic approach (E-Fig. 37.4 and Video 37.3).[244] The laparoscopic approach speeds time to return to oral feeds, reduces hospital stay, and provides better cosmesis.[245–247] Some assert that the laparoscopic approach may have a greater rate of perforation and incomplete relief of gastric obstruction, although this is not evidence-based.[248,249] A meta-analysis has reported no difference in the rate of incomplete incision, mucosal perforation, and reoperation between open and laparoscopic groups.[250]

Most advocate a modified RSI for induction of anesthesia and tracheal intubation in these infants because of their gastric outlet obstruction, although some have performed inhalational inductions successfully.[251] The duration of surgery whether open or laparoscopic is brief (30 minutes), necessitating the use of a quick-acting inhalational anesthetic (e.g., desflurane) and propofol or a muscle relaxant; the latter is not a requirement in most cases. With postoperative pain of minimal intensity, opioids are generally not

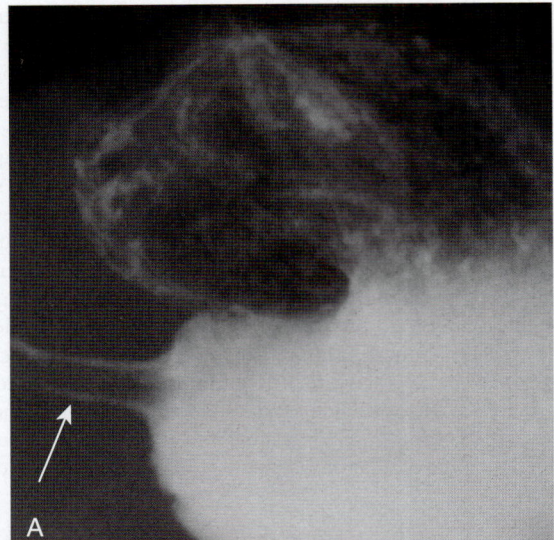

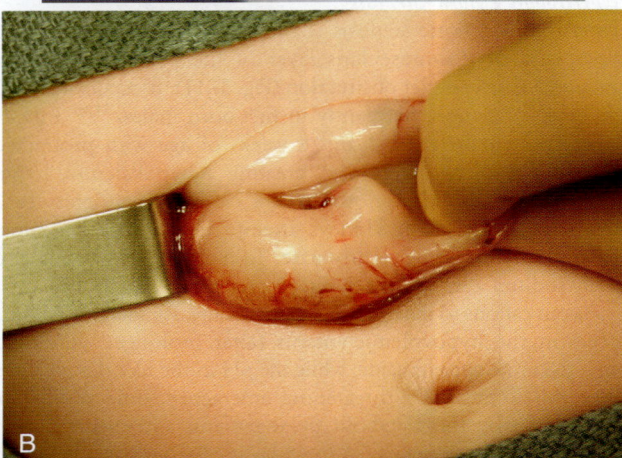

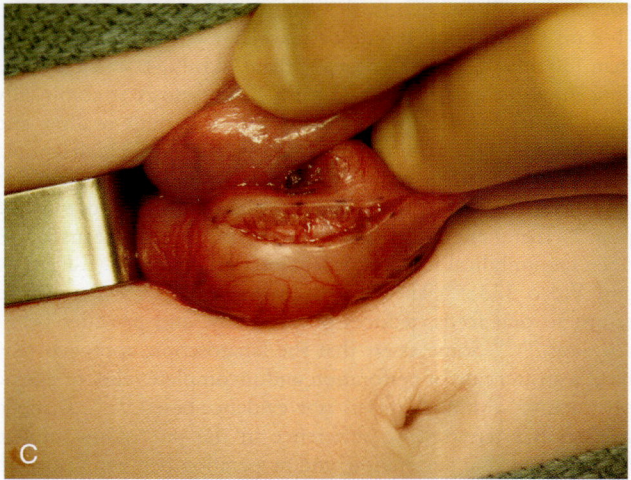

FIGURE 37.11 A, Barium swallow and abdominal radiograph of an infant with pyloric stenosis demonstrates a high degree of obstruction of the gastric outflow tract with a "wisp" of barium escaping through the pylorus *(arrow).* **B,** The hypertrophied pylorus. **C,** Surgical myotomy relieved the obstruction. (Courtesy Dr. Daniel P. Doody.)

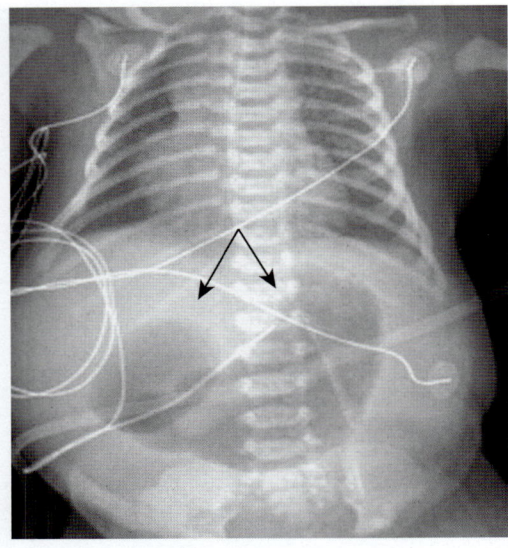

FIGURE 37.12 Abdominal radiograph of a neonate with congenital duodenal atresia demonstrating a classic double-bubble sign *(arrows).* Note that the remainder of the bowel is devoid of air, indicating complete obstruction.

required for this surgery. Pain is managed by the infiltration of local anesthetic into the trochar sites and a nonopioid agent such as acetaminophen or a nonsteroidal antiinflammatory agent. Specific perioperative anesthetic management is as detailed earlier for obstructed lesions.[245,246]

Duodenal Atresia and Meconium Ileus

The exact etiology of duodenal atresia is unknown; however, with its close association with multiple other congenital anomalies (50%–70%), it is believed to occur early in gestation. It is one of the more common causes of intestinal abnormalities, occurring in 1/6000 live births. Approximately 20% to 30% of these neonates also have trisomy 21, and up to 25% of these infants will have a cardiac anomaly. Diagnosis can be made prenatally with ultrasound or postnatally with an abdominal radiograph demonstrating the "double bubble" sign, formed by fluid/air seen in the dilated stomach and proximal duodenum, with the remaining bowel devoid of fluid/air (Fig. 37.12).[252] Neonates born with duodenal atresia usually present with bilious vomiting beginning within the first 24 to 48 hours after birth, leading to dehydration and electrolyte imbalances. After medical stabilization, open or laparoscopic surgical correction is required. A peripherally inserted central catheter (PICC) may be placed in the event of continued obstruction and the need for long-term total parenteral nutrition (TPN).

Meconium ileus is an intestinal obstruction of the newborn caused by inspissated meconium in the terminal ileum. Most cases are associated with cystic fibrosis (10%–15% of neonates with cystic fibrosis will have meconium ileus).[253] Other cases have been reported in premature infants, especially whose with very low birth weight and extremely low birth weight, and is thought to be due to immature intestinal function and dysmotility.[254] Failure to pass meconium within the first 24 hours of birth, abdominal distention, and bilious vomiting support this diagnosis. Abdominal radiographs reveal low small bowel obstruction with numerous air-filled loops of bowel and a soap-bubble effect of gas mixed with meconium in the right lower abdomen. Microcolon is often seen with a barium enema. Conservative management is the initial treatment of choice, consisting of rectal stimulation with *N*-acetylcysteine (NAC) or glycerin, contrast or Gastrografin enemas, or the administration of Gastrografin or NAC via an NG tube.[252,254] Hyperosmolar enemas may result in substantial shifts in intravascular volume, leading to hypovolemia and electrolyte imbalances. If conservative management fails and persistent ileus ensues, the neonate may require surgical evacuation.

Imperforate Anus

The etiology of imperforate anus remains unclear but is thought to occur between 5 and 7 weeks of gestation. The incidence is 1/5000 births and is more prevalent in males. It is a part of the VACTERL association. The diagnosis of imperforate anus is usually made by initial physical examination or by failure to pass meconium within the first 48 hours of life. Milder cases can be treated with a perineal anoplasty, but more complicated cases may require a temporizing colostomy followed by a more definitive repair, such as a colonic pull-through or a posterior sagittal anorectoplasty.

Compromised Intestinal Blood Supply
Inguinal Hernia

Failure of the process vaginalis to close during the last few weeks of gestation can result in the protrusion of abdominal cavity and gonadal structures through the inguinal canal. Most inguinal hernias manifest within the first 6 months of life, affecting 1% to 5% of full-term infants and children, and up to 30% of premature infants. The prevalence is greater in males. In 60% of infants, the hernia occurs on the right, in 30% it occurs on the left, and in 10% there is bilateral involvement. Clinical manifestations include the visualization and/or palpation of a bulge in the inguinal or scrotal region that is more prominent when crying or straining and generally reduces while at rest.

Hernias that do not spontaneously resolve need to be surgically corrected because of the risk of incarceration; however, surgery can be performed on a semi-elective basis as an outpatient. When the contents of the hernia become incarcerated or strangulated, they are at risk for ischemia and necrosis, and emergency surgical correction is indicated. Elective repair can be performed with the infant under either general or regional anesthesia (caudal or spinal block). Premature infants less than 60 weeks PCA should be observed for 24 hours for signs of apnea before discharge. Anesthetic management for incarcerated or strangulated hernias should proceed as mentioned earlier for ischemic lesions.

Necrotizing Enterocolitis

NEC is a multifactorial disease that can lead to bowel necrosis and is a leading cause of neonatal mortality. It affects 5% to 11% of premature and low-birth-weight infants and has a mortality rate of 10% to 50%.[255–257] The pathogenesis is not completely understood, but is thought to be due to unbalanced inflammatory responses of bowel mucosa, alterations in normal intestinal flora by antibiotics and feeds, and lack of a fully developed intestinal mucosal barrier, which leads to the breakdown of the intestinal wall and bowel necrosis.[255,256,258] In addition to prematurity, NEC has also been associated with low systemic cardiac output, hypoxia, PDA, infection, red blood cell transfusion, and enteral feedings (especially formula-fed neonates).[259,260] In fact, human breast milk is now touted as the preferred strategy to prevent NEC in preterm infants.[261]

NEC can be insidious in onset or rapidly progress to multisystem organ failure or death. Early signs tend to be nonspecific and include temperature instability, poor feeding with residual volumes

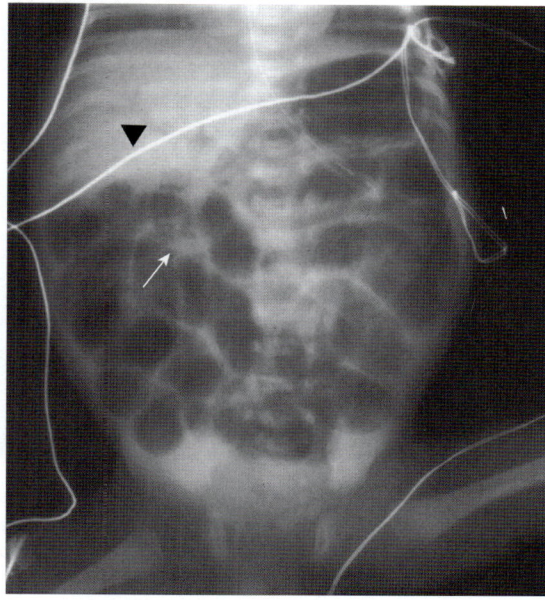

FIGURE 37.13 Abdominal radiograph of a neonate with necrotizing enterocolitis demonstrates generalized bowel distention (ileus), a small amount of pneumatosis intestinalis in the left upper quadrant *(arrow)*, and gas outlining the intrahepatic portal vein *(arrowhead)*. (Courtesy Dr. Sjirk J. Westra.)

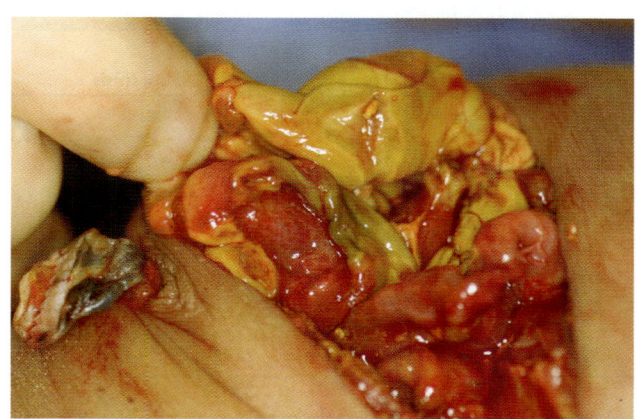

FIGURE 37.14 Early necrotizing enterocolitis with bowel perforation. Note that the perforation was diagnosed early and that there is soiling of the peritoneum but there does not appear to be any dead bowel. This type of perforation is generally associated with a positive outcome.

or vomiting, lethargy, apnea, bradycardia, mild abdominal distention, and bloody stools, although recent evidence points to specific biomarkers to facilitate early diagnosis (fecal calprotectin and S100A12, serum fatty acid–binding protein, and urine biomarkers).[262] Tachycardia, poor perfusion/hypotension, metabolic acidosis, thrombocytopenia, abdominal tenderness, and peritonitis are findings in later, more severe cases.[255,259] An abdominal x-ray may initially suggest an ileus with thickened bowel walls and dilated bowel loops and later demonstrate gas in the intestinal wall (pneumatosis intestinalis) and in the hepatobiliary tract or portal venous system (Fig. 37.13). The finding of free air in the abdominal cavity (pneumoperitoneum) warrants prompt surgical intervention (Fig. 37.14).

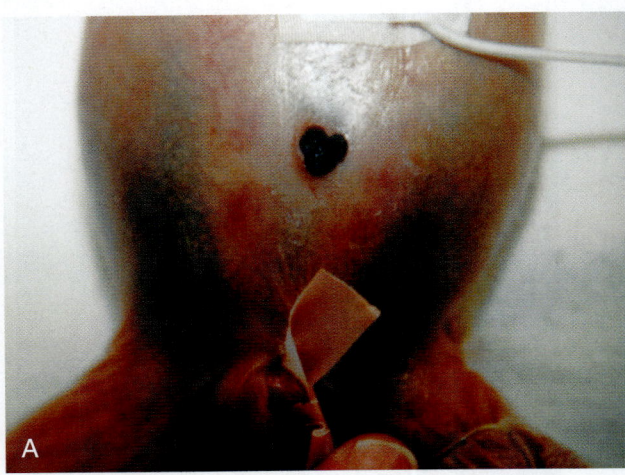
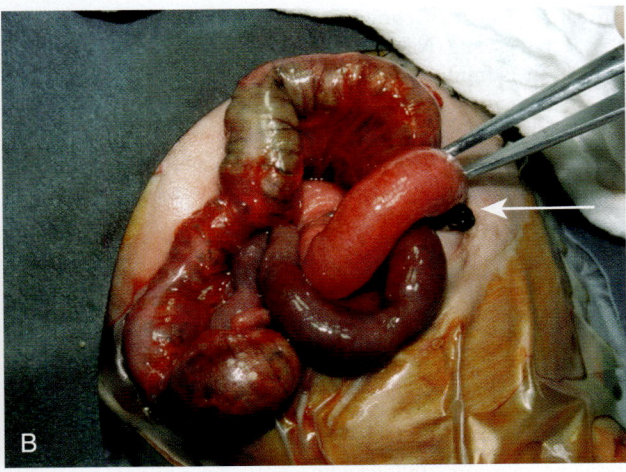

FIGURE 37.15 A preterm neonate with severe necrotizing enterocolitis and intestinal necrosis. **A,** Abdominal discoloration consistent with dead bowel. **B,** Necrotizing enterocolitis with a segment of dead bowel *(top)* and evidence of free stool in the abdomen *(arrow)*. These infants often have bowel perforation and hemorrhage from the bowel or liver. They can have severe hypotension requiring vasopressor support and enormous volume requirements. Moreover, because of hemorrhage and disseminated intravascular coagulopathy, these infants will generally require transfusions of blood, platelets, and fresh frozen plasma. Some practitioners also advocate administration of vitamin K. (Courtesy Dr. Daniel P. Doody.)

TABLE 37.6	Comparison of Omphalocele and Gastroschisis	
Comparison Factors	**Omphalocele**	**Gastroschisis**
Cause	Failure of gut migration from yolk sac into abdomen	Occlusion of omphalomesenteric artery
Location	Within umbilical cord	Periumbilical
Associated lesions	Beckwith-Wiedemann syndrome (macroglossia, gigantism, hypoglycemia, hyperviscosity) Congenital heart disease Exstrophy of bladder	Exposed gut inflammation, edema, dilation, and foreshortened

Initial therapy is conservative and includes making the neonate *nil per os* (NPO), initiating broad-spectrum antibiotics, and decompression of the bowel with low continuous gastric suction. Supportive measures to correct metabolic and hematologic abnormalities, as well as fluid resuscitation, are also involved. If conservative management fails or signs of necrosis or viscus perforation appear, an exploratory laparotomy is indicated for resection of necrotic bowel (Fig. 37.15). These infants are critically ill. Preoperative preparation in a timely fashion is vital. NEC predisposes to hypovolemia, cardiovascular and respiratory failure, capillary leak syndrome, disseminated intravascular coagulation, and hypoglycemia. These infants may be septic and volume depleted with very large fluid requirements as the result of massive third-space losses. Often there is an enormous need for 5% albumin just to maintain intravascular volume (up to 1 blood volume of more) because of third spacing. There is nearly always a need for transfusion of platelets and fresh frozen plasma. Hyperkalemia with renal failure is common, and central venous

access is usually required for inotropic support (dopamine or epinephrine or both).

Omphalocele and Gastroschisis

Defects in the abdominal wall can lead to herniated organs with impaired blood supply, intestinal obstruction, and major intravascular fluid defects in neonates with omphalocele and gastroschisis. The differences between omphalocele and gastroschisis are summarized in Table 37.6.

Omphalocele represents a failure of the gut to migrate from the yolk sac into the abdomen during gestation (Fig. 37.16A).[263,264] It occurs in 1/5000 births.[265] Infants with omphalocele may have associated genetic, cardiac, urologic (exstrophy of the bladder; Fig. 37.16B), and metabolic abnormalities (eg, Beckwith-Wiedemann syndrome with visceromegaly, macroglossia, hypoglycemia, and polycythemia).[266] The herniated viscera emerge from the umbilicus and are covered with a membranous sac. The bowel is morphologically and usually functionally normal.

Gastroschisis develops as a result of occlusion of the omphalomesenteric artery during gestation.[264,267] It occurs in 1/2000 births and is usually not associated with other congenital anomalies.[265] The herniated viscera and intestines are periumbilical, usually on the right, and are exposed to amniotic fluid in utero and to air after delivery, resulting in inflammation, edema, and dilated, foreshortened, functionally abnormal bowel (Fig. 37.16C).[268,269]

Management of these neonates until surgical repair is directed at maintaining perfusion to the herniated viscera and reduction of fluid loss from exposed visceral surfaces by covering the mucosal surfaces with sterile, saline-soaked dressings. A plastic wrap aids in decreasing evaporative volume losses and the tendency to develop hypothermia, which is more pronounced with gastroschisis. These defects represent a wide spectrum of pathology and require individualized assessment of associated anomalies, intravascular volume status, and fluid replacement.[270] If complete reduction is not possible, a staged reduction is carried out.[271,272] The abdominal

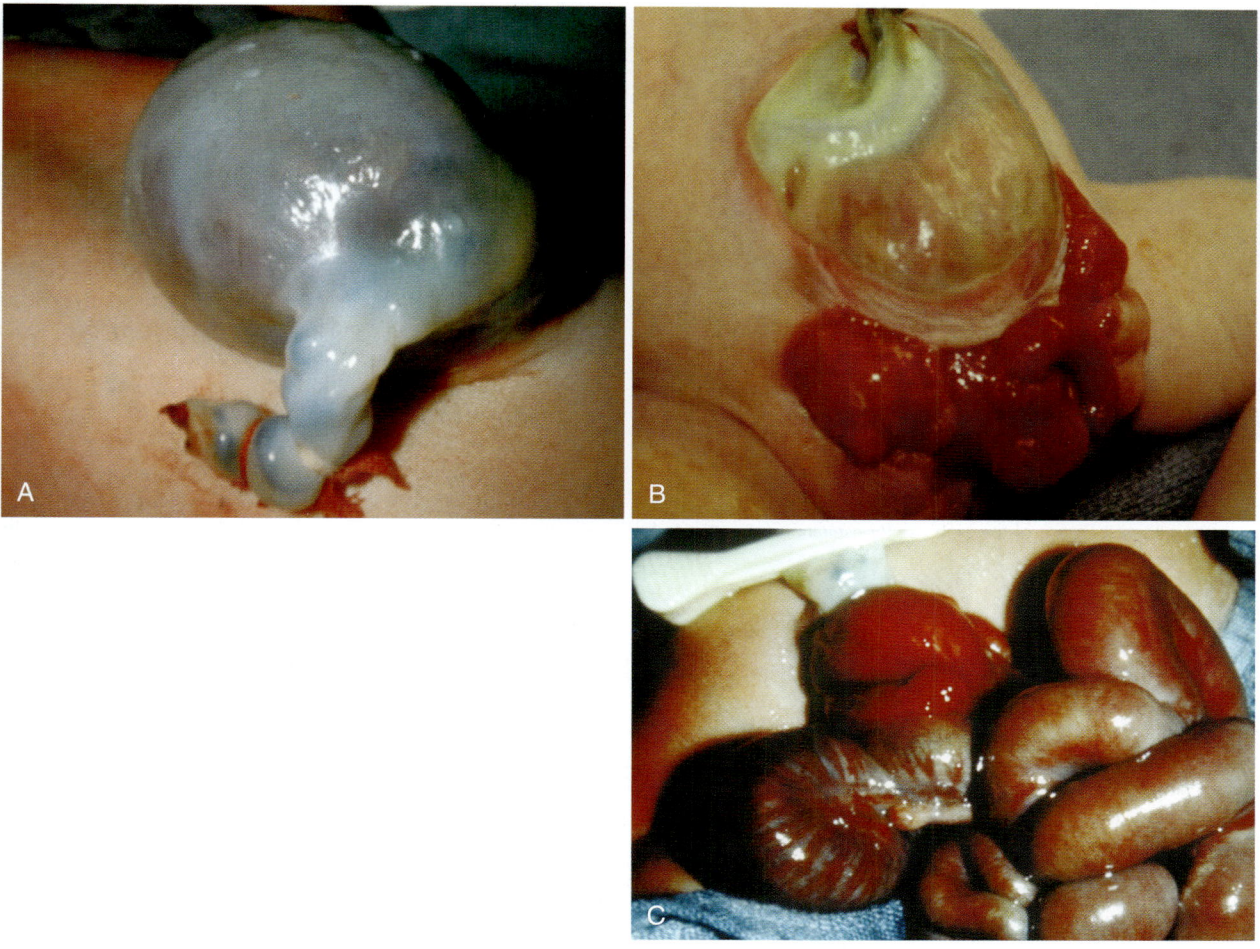

FIGURE 37.16 A, Omphalocele covered with a membranous sac; the defect arises at the umbilicus. **B,** Omphalocele with associated exstrophy of the bladder. **C,** Gastroschisis; note the absence of a membranous sac. In contrast to omphalocele, the gastroschisis anomaly is periumbilical.

contents are covered with a Silastic pouch, and the size of the pouch is subsequently reduced in stages, thus allowing the abdominal cavity gradually to accommodate the increased mass without severely compromising ventilation or organ perfusion.[273,274] Tissue expanders and skin grafting may also be necessary for closure.

Anesthetic management is directed at continued volume resuscitation and measures to prevent hypothermia. Primary abdominal closure may be associated with markedly increased intraabdominal pressure (E-Fig. 37.5). Intraabdominal pressure may be monitored by transducing either a CVP catheter or less invasively, an intragastric tube. A gastric pressure that exceeds 20 mm Hg after primary closure is likely to cause abdominal ischemia and necessitate an urgent reoperation.[275] Increased intraabdominal pressure can decrease organ perfusion and ventilatory reserve, including perfusion of the intestines, kidney, and liver as well as secondarily impaired organ function. This may lead to markedly altered drug metabolism and prolonged drug effects.[122] The bowel may become edematous, and urine output may be reduced as a result of renal congestion. Venous return from the lower body also may be reduced, resulting in lower extremity congestion and cyanosis. Blood pressure and pulse oximetry determinations from a lower extremity may be different from those in the upper extremity. Significantly decreased diaphragmatic function and bilateral lower lobe atelectasis may occur, leading to respiratory failure.[276]

Malrotation and Midgut Volvulus

Malrotation and midgut volvulus result from abnormal migration or incomplete rotation of the intestines from the yolk sac back into the abdomen.[277] It occurs in 1/500 births and 30% to 60% of affected patients have associated congenital anomalies. Rotation of the intestine around the mesentery may produce the abnormal location of the ileocecal valve in the right upper quadrant and kinking or compression of its vascular supply. If the malrotation occurs during development, atretic segments of bowel are formed. If the kinking or compression occurs after the bowel is normally developed, bowel necrosis may result.

These infants present with bilious emesis, a tender and distended abdomen, and increasing abdominal girth. Bloody stools are an ominous sign. They may have hypotension, hypovolemia, and electrolyte abnormalities. Because delay in surgery may result in necrosis of the entire small intestine, fluid and electrolyte resuscitation with stabilization should not delay surgical correction. This is a true neonatal emergency, and surgery should proceed as expeditiously as possible with ongoing perioperative resuscitation.

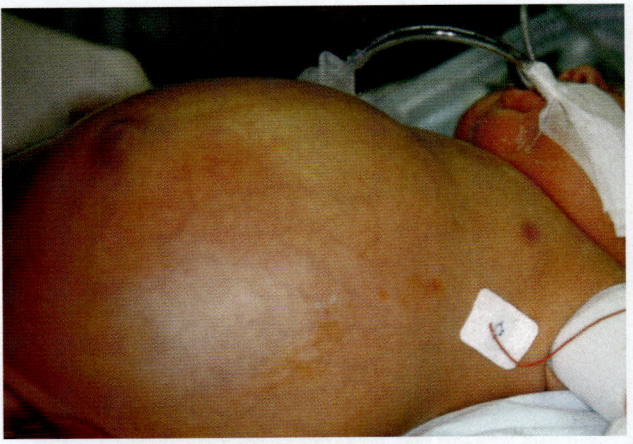

FIGURE 37.17 Toxic megacolon results in massive abdominal distention, fluid requirements, and sepsis. These infants require special consideration in airway management because of the high risk for aspiration and increased abdominal pressure.

Hirschsprung Disease

Hirschsprung disease is the absence of parasympathetic ganglion cells (Auerbach and Meissner plexuses) in the large intestine.[278,279] This deficiency creates a nonperistaltic segment of variable length, a tonically contracted anorectal sphincter, and delayed passage of meconium. Functional obstruction occurs at the level of the affected segment. Its incidence is 1/6000 with a male predominance and is relatively rare in premature infants. Approximately 60% of patients will have an associated anomaly.

Infants with Hirschsprung disease present with symptoms consistent with bowel obstruction, such as bilious vomiting and abdominal distention. However, the bowel may occasionally become distended to the point that its blood supply is compromised, leading to perforation. If left untreated, enteric bacteria may invade the bowel wall and enter the bloodstream, leading to toxic megacolon (Fig. 37.17). These infants are critically ill and may require massive volume replacement and vasopressor support. Surgical repair depends on the extent of intestinal involvement and includes anorectal myomectomy, mucosal resections, diverting colostomies, and transanal pull-throughs.

LIGATION OF PATENT DUCTUS ARTERIOSUS

Controversy exists regarding whether a PDA should be treated at all, the timing of therapy if treated, and merits of medical versus surgical therapy.[280–282] This controversy is the result of several trials that have failed to show early PDA closure leads to significant benefit in premature neonatal outcomes.[282] It is possible that although a PDA is associated with morbidity in the neonate, it is not a causative factor. Medical therapy involves the administration of a cyclooxygenase inhibitor, such as indomethacin or ibuprofen. Indomethacin therapy is less likely to close the PDA in micropremies compared with premature infants, and is more likely to produce complications, including thrombocytopenia, renal failure, hyponatremia, and intestinal perforation.[283] Ibuprofen is equally effective for PDA closure in the micropremie, with a reduced frequency of renal failure.[284] Both the probability of PDA closure and the probability of adverse effects relate to plasma nonsteroidal antiinflammatory drug concentration. The concentration achieved after a standard dose changes with PMA because clearance increases with PMA; failure to account for

a changing clearance with age contributes to confusion in the literature.[285,286] More recently, paracetamol (acetaminophen) has been used with equal effectiveness in those infants in whom cyclooxygenase inhibitor therapy has failed or in whom those drugs are contraindicated, although further efficacy evidence is required.[282,285] Surgical ligation of the PDA has a low incidence of major intraoperative complications when performed by an experienced team.[287] However, as many as one-third of premature infants develop severe cardiovascular instability following PDA ligation, termed postligation cardiac syndrome (PLCS). PLCS is due to an abrupt increase in left ventricular afterload with decreased preload, leading to low cardiac output, hypotension, and myocardial dysfunction.[281,282,288] In addition, some studies show an increased risk of chronic lung disease, ROP, and neurosensory impairment after surgical ligation.[281,289]

Surgical ligation of the PDA can be performed in the OR or in the NICU (usually reserved for micropremies and ELBW neonates). It is achieved via left thoracotomy with manual retraction of the lung. The aorta and pulmonary artery lie in proximity to the PDA; thus severe bleeding may occur abruptly and unexpectedly during the procedure. Blood should be immediately available for transfusion. In addition, it can be difficult to distinguish the PDA from the aorta, as the diameter of the PDA may be the same or even greater than that of the aorta. Monitoring blood pressure and pulse oximetry on the right arm (preductal) and oximetry on the foot (postductal) will assist the surgeon to identify the correct vessel to be ligated. The surgeon will place a temporary clamp on what is believed to be the PDA. A loss in postductal oximetry indicates clamping of the aorta, whereas a decrease in both oximeters and $ETCO_2$ suggests clamping of the pulmonary artery. A successful PDA ligation results in a "step up" in mean arterial pressure owing to an increase in diastolic blood pressure with no decrease in either of the pulse oximeters

Transcatheter occlusion of the PDA can be accomplished using either coils or an occluder device in the catheterization laboratory as an alternative to surgical ligation with similar efficacy (see Chapter 22). Like the surgical option, device occlusion is performed only after failed conservative and medical attempts. In the past, the small vessel size of the extremely premature infant prevented the use of a large enough sheath to implant the device. However, advances over the past 5 to 10 years produced devices capable of transcatheter occlusion in infants weighing less than 1 kg. In some instances, they are even being deployed at the bedside using only echocardiographic guidance. In addition to avoiding the complications of a surgical repair, the transcatheter approach has shown a more rapid recovery of respiratory function. The most common complications include femoral artery thrombosis, left pulmonary artery stenosis, and aortic coarctation.[53,290–293]

RETINOPATHY OF PREMATURITY

ROP can lead to blindness if left uncorrected. The exact cause of ROP is unknown; however, it is associated with prematurity, low birth weight, supplemental oxygen therapy, postnatal hypotension, use of surfactant or inotrope, and need for mechanical ventilation.[294,295] It is thought to be initiated by oxygen-induced retinal vasoconstriction and endothelial cell death, followed by unchecked neovascularization from angiogenic factors, such as VEGF, that do not respond to normal regulation because of immaturity.[296,297] Its incidence increases with decreasing gestational age. ROP may be treated with cryotherapy, laser photocoagulation, scleral buckling surgery, and/or vitrectomy.

37

Cryotherapy involves applying a freezing probe under direct visualization to the avascular retina anterior to the fibrovascular ridge. It requires general anesthesia and is usually performed in the OR. Diode laser photocoagulation is typically performed at the bedside in the NICU. It has been shown to be as effective as cryotherapy for moderate ROP, and is most commonly used because the systemic side effects are significantly less, the ocular tissues are less traumatized, and it has a smaller incidence of late complications than cryotherapy. Laser photocoagulation may be performed using topical anesthesia alone, with IV sedation, or with the patient under general anesthesia. However, the incidence of cardiorespiratory complications is greater with topical anesthesia alone than with topical anesthesia with sedation or general anesthesia.[294] The procedure takes 10 to 30 minutes to perform and often involves a series of treatments every few weeks. Anesthetic goals are to provide optic analgesia and to prevent eye and head movement. Many premature infants younger than 32 weeks PCA are naturally inactive and may remain motionless with topical anesthesia alone.

Scleral buckle surgery and vitrectomy, performed for more severe ROP with retinal detachment, are less frequently used because early detection and treatment with laser photocoagulation prevents ROP progression to severe disease. It is usually performed in older infants between 6 months and 1 year of age and requires general anesthesia in the OR.

The latest form of therapy includes intravitreal injection of bevacizumab, a recombinant humanized monoclonal antibody aimed at reducing VEGF. Results are encouraging; however, more data are needed to establish safety and efficacy.[296,298,299] As discussed previously, the optimal oxygen saturation target is controversial. Hyperoxia should be avoided if at all possible, with a suggested target range of 91% to 95%. It should be noted, however, that ROP has been reported in infants with cyanotic heart disease and infants never exposed to oxygen; thus hyperoxia is but one factor associated with ROP (see also Chapter 34).[298,300]

ANNOTATED REFERENCES

Kamata M, Cartabuke RS, Tobias JD. Perioperative care of infants with pyloric stenosis. *Paediatr Anaesth.* 2015;25(12):1193-1206.

This article reviewed the current techniques in use for the perioperative management of infants with pyloric stenosis. They conclude that the optimal approach to airway management is not known, and several different techniques may be used, such as rapid-sequence induction or modified rapid sequence with gentle mask ventilation.

Sola A, Golombek SG, Montes Bueno MT, et al. Safe oxygen saturation targeting and monitoring in preterm infants: can we avoid hypoxia and hyperoxia? *Acta Paediatr.* 2014;103(10):1009-1018.

This study sought to define a more targeted range of oxygen saturations in premature infants to reduce morbidity and mortality. They concluded that there was an increase in mortality with reduced oxygen saturations, yet a greater morbidity with hyperoxia in the higher ranges, leading them to recommend a broader range of intermediate targets.

Stoll BJ, Hansen NI, Bell E, et al. Trends in care practices, morbidity, and mortality of extremely preterm neonates, 1993–2012. *JAMA.* 2015;314(10):1039-1051.

This prospective study of more than 34,000 premature infants born at the Neonatal Research Network centers looked at maternal and neonatal care, morbidities, and survival. They concluded that over the past 20 years there have been several advances in maternal and neonatal care that have contributed to improved outcomes.

A complete reference list can be found online at ExpertConsult.com.

38

Fetal Intervention and the EXIT Procedure

ROLAND BRUSSEAU

THE ADVENT OF FETAL intervention introduced the concept of surgically correcting or ameliorating known congenital defects in utero. With improvements in prenatal imaging and surgical techniques, fetal interventions have grown to include diagnoses associated with intrauterine demise and significant postnatal morbidity. The goal of fetal intervention is to improve the probability that the fetus will develop normally with minimal postnatal morbidity.[1] Increasingly, advances have changed some procedures from open in utero interventions, which are associated with significant maternal risk, to percutaneous or fetoscopic techniques, thus improving the maternal risk/benefit ratio while diminishing postoperative uterine contractions associated with open procedures.

Fetal surgery often requires the anesthesiologist to care for two or more patients at once, all with distinctive and, at times, conflicting requirements. The first is the mother who can express her level of discomfort, who can be monitored directly, and to whom drugs can be administered easily. The second (and possibly third)

is the fetus. For the latter, detecting pain depends solely on indirect evidence, monitoring is limited at best, administering drugs is more complicated, and there is the possibility of long-term effects from procedures and drugs administered during early development. The anesthesiologist is required to provide both maternal and fetal anesthesia and analgesia while ensuring both maternal and fetal hemodynamic stability; a plan must be prepared to resuscitate the fetus if problems occur during the intervention.

A Range of Anesthetic Options for Mother and Fetus

MOTHER

Fetal interventions have been successfully performed with various anesthetic techniques; both maternal and fetal anesthetic requirements must be considered and may, in fact, be quite different.

With some endoscopic interventions, the site of surgical intervention is not innervated; thus the fetus may not sense a noxious stimulus, and its anesthetic requirements are presumably minimal. Nevertheless, fetal immobility remains essential to procedural safety and success. Other interventions may require that a needle be inserted into the fetus, which may elicit a noxious stimulus and possibly even cause pain. Open procedures can produce significant noxious stimuli. In addition to surgical demands, each mother and fetus exhibit a unique physiologic, pharmacologic, and pathophysiologic profile; the anesthesiologist must evaluate the advantages and disadvantages of each anesthetic technique and select the safest approach.[2]

Local Anesthesia (Field Block)

Local anesthesia is almost exclusively used to insert the trocar for percutaneous procedures. The most obvious advantage is maternal safety because the mother receives no intravenous (IV) medications. The disadvantages of this technique include increased risk of injury to the unanesthetized, nonparalyzed fetus, the absence of analgesia for the fetus, and no uterine relaxation. Patients who receive tocolytic therapy or those with polyhydramnios and uterine contractions may be at even further risk of worsening contractions with this approach.

Monitored Anesthesia Care

IV sedation involves the maternal administration of benzodiazepines, opioids, and occasionally low-dose hypnotic agents. Advantages include possible provision of anesthesia and analgesia to the fetus via transplacental transfer of drugs, as well as decreased maternal anxiety and pain. Depending on the amount and effect of the drugs administered, this sedation may increase the mother's risk of aspiration because of an unprotected airway; this technique is also devoid of uterine relaxation.

Regional Neuraxial Blockade

Neuraxial techniques (spinal, epidural, or combined spinal and epidural anesthesia) have been used with fetoscopic techniques and, rarely, without an adjunct general anesthetic for open techniques. A T4 sensory-level blockade is required for most surgical uterine manipulations. Neuraxial techniques provide neither uterine relaxation nor analgesia or anesthesia for the fetus.

Regional Neuraxial Blockade With Sedation

The addition of IV sedation to regional anesthesia may provide the fetus with analgesia/anesthesia via placental drug transfer. Although IV fentanyl, propofol, and benzodiazepines can be administered to patients receiving regional anesthesia, they may place the mother at increased risk of bradyarrhythmias, respiratory depression, and pulmonary aspiration; the need for a T4 sensory block may produce alterations in respiratory mechanics in addition to those associated with pregnancy. In addition, the level of sympathetic blockade is often two to six levels greater than the sensory level.[3] Hence, a T4 sensory block may completely block cardiac accelerator fibers (T1–T4); severe bradyarrhythmias and cardiac arrest have been reported.[4-6] When IV agents with vagotonic properties are administered in this clinical setting, the risk of significant bradyarrhythmias may be increased.[7]

General Anesthesia

General anesthesia with high-dose inhalational anesthetics (generally desflurane) provides both maternal and fetal anesthesia and dose-dependent uterine relaxation even in patients who have received tocolytic therapy for premature uterine contractions.[8-11] Caution must be exercised as the required depth of maternal anesthesia necessary to provide adequate uterine relaxation may produce maternal hypotension with resultant uteroplacental insufficiency and fetal cardiovascular insufficiency. Particular attention must be paid to maintenance of maternal blood pressure in the normal or perhaps slightly supranormal range.[12]

The adjunctive administration of remifentanil and propofol infusions may reduce the necessary concentration of inhalational anesthetic required without compromising uterine relaxation. With such regimens, maternal hypotension and subsequent fetal depression may be avoided.[13] An additional benefit of this combined approach may be the contribution of remifentanil and propofol to fetal anesthesia, as both readily cross the placenta without known reductions in placental blood flow.[14]

Combined Regional and General Anesthesia

A combined regional and general anesthesia technique is often used for open procedures, as well as for patients with anterior placentas, in whom externalization of the uterus for safe trocar insertion is anticipated. In addition to providing the advantages of both the regional and the general anesthetic techniques listed previously, this method allows for postoperative pain control.[15] The physical window for trocar insertion is often smaller in this patient cohort, necessitating either externalization of the uterus or extreme lateral decubitus position. Externalization of the uterus requires a larger surgical incision than for standard cesarean sections, conferring benefit from epidural anesthesia. However, perceived intraoperative benefits (e.g., reduced requirements for inhalational agents) may be offset by the necessity to provide adequate uterine relaxation.

FETUS

Maternal anesthetic techniques that do not include inhalational anesthetics may not provide adequate analgesia and/or anesthesia for the fetus. However, fetal analgesia and anesthesia may also be accomplished by delivery of anesthetics and analgesics directly to the fetus. Potential methods include transplacental, direct intramuscular, direct intravascular, and intraamniotic administration; each route of administration has advantages and disadvantages that can have a direct impact on overall outcome.

Transplacental Access

Many fetal interventions (open or endoscopic) use transplacental drug administration to provide anesthesia and analgesia for both mother and fetus (Table 38.1). Many, but not all, drugs cross the placenta in accordance with Fick's law of passive diffusion (Fig. 38.1). Lipid solubility, the pH of both maternal and fetal blood, the degree of ionization, protein binding, perfusion, placental area and thickness, and drug concentration are factors that influence the extent of transplacental drug diffusion.[16] The most obvious disadvantage with this approach is that the mother must be exposed to every drug that the fetus is intended to receive, often at large concentrations, to achieve adequate drug concentrations in the fetus. In addition, the uptake of drugs may be impaired if there is reduced placental blood flow. This has implications for successful anesthesia and analgesia both in terms of the delivered fetal dose and the time interval that must be allowed from maternal administration to the start of the fetal intervention. All inhalational anesthetics cross the placental barrier, but uptake in the fetus is slower than in the mother.[16] However, this is offset by the reduced minimum alveolar concentration (MAC) for anesthesia in the

TABLE 38.1	Placental Transfer of Common Anesthetic Drugs[a]
Drugs That DO NOT transfer	**Drugs That DO transfer**
Glycopyrrolate	Atropine
All neuromuscular blocking drugs	Ephedrine
Insulin	Esmolol, labetalol
Heparin	Benzodiazepines
	Propofol
	Ketamine
	Opioids[b]
	Inhalational anesthetics
	Local anesthetics[c]

[a]The major mechanism of transfer is passive diffusion of largely lipid-soluble, nonionized substances with low molecular weight (<500 D). Bulk flow, pinocytosis, and passage through the intervillous spaces are negligible sources of reliable transfer.
[b]Epidural or intrathecal opioids, to a lesser extent, generally produce minimal neonatal effects.
[c]Fetal acidosis produces higher fetal/maternal local anesthetic drug ratios because binding of hydrogen ions to the nonionized form causes trapping of the local anesthetic in the fetal circulation.

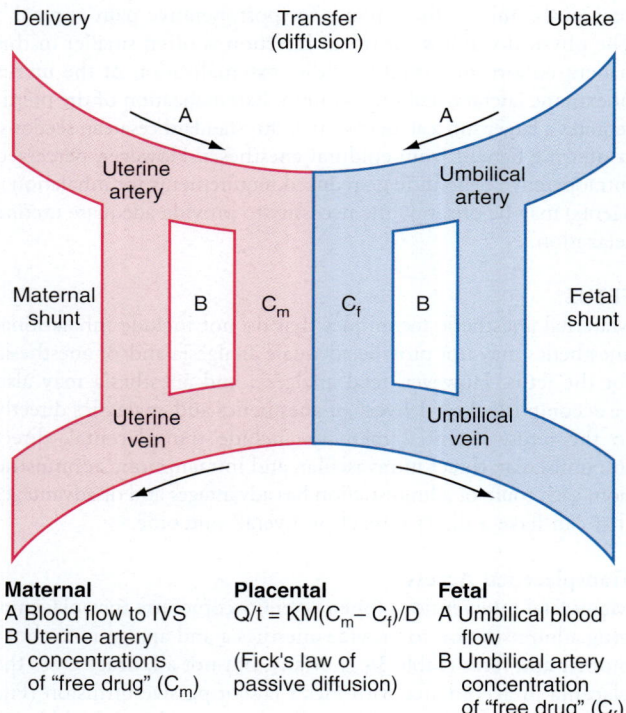

Maternal
A Blood flow to IVS
B Uterine artery concentrations of "free drug" (C_m)

Placental
Q/t = $KM(C_m - C_f)/D$

(Fick's law of passive diffusion)

Fetal
A Umbilical blood flow
B Umbilical artery concentration of "free drug" (C_f)

FIGURE 38.1 Fick's law of passive diffusion described at the intervillous space (*IVS*). *D*, membrane thickness; *K*, diffusion constant of the drug; *M*, membrane surface area; *Q/t*, rate of diffusion.

fetus, resulting in a similar onset of anesthesia as in the mother.[2] Fetal anesthesia is also important to reduce the fetal stress response, which, through catecholamine release, can reduce placental blood flow and exacerbate any asphyxia.[17-20]

Intramuscular Access

Intramuscular (IM) injection involves inserting a needle under ultrasound guidance into a fetal extremity or buttocks. Unlike umbilical cord injection, the noxious stimulus to the fetus by the IM injection stimulates the fetal stress response. Although the bleeding risk from an IM injection is less than that with intravascular injections, there remains a risk of bleeding and injury from the needle itself. Furthermore, if the fetus is already stressed, blood will be diverted away from muscle (the site of drug administration) and toward the fetal heart and brain. In this case, it may be impossible to estimate the time course for the drug to be absorbed from the IM site.

Intravascular Access

Intravascular fetal drug administration ensures immediate fetal drug delivery, and no additional dosing calculations are necessary because placental perfusion does not alter dosing. Intravascular access can be obtained via the umbilical cord (which is not innervated), larger fetal veins (e.g., hepatic vein), or intracardiac, as the specific intervention dictates.[21] One advantage of administering drugs via the umbilical vein is the ability to provide analgesia before the surgical insult. Neuromuscular blocking drugs (NMBDs), analgesics, and vagolytic agents, as well as resuscitation drugs, can be given with assurance of immediate access to the fetal circulation. This method is also useful when alterations in peripheral blood flow occur (i.e., a "central sparing response"), which diminishes the blood distribution to sites of potential IM access.

Establishing intravascular access in the fetus requires inserting a needle in a fetus that is often not sedated from maternally administered agents. The needle may injure the moving fetus, and there is a risk of bleeding from the fetus, umbilical cord, and placenta. Uncontrolled bleeding could impair the surgical view and it places the fetus and mother in jeopardy because an open hysterotomy may be necessary to control the bleeding. Establishing access with the umbilical cord vessels may also produce vascular spasm, potentially compromising fetal perfusion.

Intraamniotic Access

Intraamniotic fentanyl, sufentanil, thyroxine, vasopressin, and digoxin have been safely administered in pregnant large-animal models with only minimal drug detected in the mother.[22,23] If the safety and efficacy of this method of drug delivery hold true in human trials, intraamniotic drug administration may become the preferred method for fetal drug delivery; however, at present, this approach is not currently a part of routine clinical practice.

Fetal Development

PATHOLOGIC LUNG DEVELOPMENT

In the context of fetal interventions, there are two important causes of respiratory morbidity to consider: insufficient amniotic fluid and prematurity. With both, the timing of the insult in terms of the stage of lung development is critical to estimating the degree of likely morbidity. Deficiency of amniotic fluid may result from prelabor premature rupture of the amniotic membranes (PPROM), which may be spontaneous or iatrogenically induced either directly through trauma or by introducing infection into the uterus. Small amniotic fluid volume may also be secondary to reduced fetal urine output, from either poor renal function (e.g., with renal agenesis or urinary tract obstruction) or growth restriction secondary to placental insufficiency. Amniotic fluid deficiency contributes to pulmonary hypoplasia. In general, the likelihood of pulmonary insufficiency is inversely related to gestational age at membrane rupture, a long latency to delivery, and the amount of residual amniotic fluid.[24-26] The risk is relatively small if PPROM occurs after 24 weeks gestation,[27] as demonstrated by one series of fetuses with PPROM before 26 weeks that reported pulmonary hypoplasia in 27% of fetuses.[28] In contrast, in fetuses less than 25 weeks gestation with severe oligohydramnios that persists for more than 2 weeks after PPROM, the predicted neonatal mortality exceeds 90%.[29]

Studies in sheep show that oligohydramnios causes spinal flexion, which compresses the abdominal contents, displacing the diaphragm upward and thus compressing the developing lungs.[30] This increase in the pressure gradient between the lungs and the amniotic cavity causes a net loss of lung fluid through the trachea, preventing lung expansion.[30] Lung fluid produced in the airways is thought to act as a stent for the developing lungs.[31] Normally, it passes out through the trachea and is either swallowed or passes into the amniotic cavity. Ligation of the trachea causes lung hyperplasia[32] or ipsilateral lung hyperplasia if a main bronchus is ligated.[33] Experimental drainage of amniotic fluid in animals has been shown to result in pulmonary hypoplasia.[34] Later restoration of amniotic fluid prevents the onset of pulmonary hypoplasia.[35] There is evidence to support amnioinfusion in humans to maintain fluid volumes around the fetus after PPROM in an effort to improve lung development.[29,36]

Surfactant is a complex of phospholipids secreted by type II alveolar cells that reduces lung surface air tension, thereby preventing the lungs from collapsing at low volumes. Glucocorticoids, thyroid hormone, and β-adrenergic agonists stimulate surfactant synthesis. Surfactant is first detected in the lungs around 23 weeks gestation, but mature levels necessary for unassisted ventilation are not present until about 34 weeks. The degree of lung maturity can be evaluated by amniocentesis using the lecithin/sphingomyelin ratio or, more recently, by the lamellar body count.[37] Acceleration of surfactant synthesis may be achieved with corticosteroids administered to the mother.[38]

FETAL CARDIOVASCULAR DEVELOPMENT

The differences between the fetal and postnatal circulations are complex (Fig. 38.2). In the fetal circulation, oxygenated blood returns from the placenta via the umbilical veins and ductus venosus (bypassing the liver) into the right atrium. At 20 weeks, 30% of the umbilical venous return (40–60 mL/kg per minute) is shunted through the ductus venosus.[39] This flow decreases over the second half of gestation as hepatic blood flow increases so that by term only 20% of umbilical venous return (<20 mL/kg per minute) is shunted through the ductus venosus (see Figs. 18.1 and 18.2).[39] Hypoxia and hemorrhage increase the resistance in the liver, shunting a greater proportion of blood toward the brain and heart through the ductus venosus.[40] The proportion of blood that perfuses the liver, which exits 15% less saturated in oxygen, rejoins the ductus venosus blood in the inferior vena cava. However, this deoxygenated blood has less kinetic energy and flows more slowly into the right atrium toward the right ventricle.[40] The greater-velocity oxygenated blood from the ductus venosus is preferentially directed through the foramen ovale into the left side of the heart and out through the aortic arch to the developing head and upper body. The integrity of the foramen ovale is thus imperative. Blood returning from the placenta along the umbilical vein is 80% to 85% saturated. Despite this streaming within the right atrium, some mixing does occur, resulting in blood that is 65% saturated in the ascending aorta. The blood in the left ventricle, however, is 15% to 20% more saturated than the blood in the right ventricle. Most of the deoxygenated blood in the right ventricle bypasses the high-resistance pulmonary vasculature to enter the ductus arteriosus, and from there the descending aorta

to supply the lower body, or pass through the umbilical arteries for reoxygenation in the placenta. In contrast to extrauterine life, when the two ventricles function in series and thus have equal outputs, before birth they function in parallel. Their outputs, therefore, do not have to be equal and, in fact, are not. In the third trimester, the right side of the heart has a greater output, as determined by Doppler ultrasonography studies, showing a 28% greater stroke volume than the left side.[39,39]

The fetal heart rate (FHR) is maintained above the intrinsic rate of the sinoatrial node by a combination of vagal and sympathetic inputs, as well as circulating catecholamines.[41–43] FHR decreases throughout gestation,[44,45] accompanied by an increase in stroke volume as the heart grows. Hypoxic stress in late gestation produces a reflex bradycardia, with a normal heart rate or tachycardia developing a few minutes later. The chemoreceptor reflex nature of the bradycardia is demonstrated by its abolition after section of the sheep carotid sinus nerves.[46] The later tachycardia is a result of an increase in plasma catecholamines causing β-adrenergic stimulation.[47] Hemorrhage can also produce increases in FHR, probably via a baroreceptor reflex.

Cardiac output in the fetus is determined largely by heart rate.[48] The combined ventricular output of the left and right ventricles in the human fetus is 450 mL/kg per minute.[48] During development, the ability of the fetus to increase stroke volume is limited by a reduced proportion of functioning contractile tissue and a limited ability to increase the heart rate because of a relatively reduced β-adrenergic receptor density and immature sympathetic drive. If the blood volume is reduced by hemorrhage, the heart cannot compensate by increasing stroke volume, or conversely, if volume is increased, the walls are less able to distend and cardiac efficiency is reduced (although this second effect is reduced substantially by the huge, relatively compliant placental circulation). Thus the only mechanism by which the fetus can increase its cardiac output is to increase its heart rate. Despite this homeostatic limitation, the fetus is able to withstand significant hemorrhage. Studies have shown that the fetal lamb can restore arterial blood pressure and heart rate very quickly after acute loss of 20% of its blood volume, without any measurable disturbance in acid-base balance.[49] Even after a 40% reduction in blood volume, the ovine fetal blood pressure recovers to normal within 2 minutes and the heart rate within 35 minutes.[50] Oxygen delivery to the brain and heart is maintained secondary to vascular redistribution (*central sparing effect*) and blood volume replacement from the placenta and extravascular space, with 40% of the hemorrhaged loss being corrected within 30 minutes.[50] The development of acidemia indicates that the fetus is unable to compensate; acidosis shifts the oxygen dissociation curve to the right, thereby decreasing fetal hemoglobin oxygen saturation but improving release of oxygen from hemoglobin. Blood flow during periods of asphyxia increases more than 100% to the brainstem but only 60% to the cerebral hemispheres.[51]

FETAL OXYGENATION

The fetus exists in an environment of low oxygen tension, with arterial oxygen partial pressure (PaO_2) being approximately one-fourth that of the adult. The maximum PaO_2 of umbilical venous blood is approximately 30 mm Hg. The affinity of fetal hemoglobin for oxygen is modulated in utero by two principal factors: fetal hemoglobin and 2,3-diphosphoglycerate (2,3-DPG). The hemoglobin oxygen dissociation curve is shifted to the left because of fetal hemoglobin (hemoglobin F), thereby increasing the affinity for oxygen. In addition, 2,3-DPG is present and might be expected

FETAL CIRCULATION

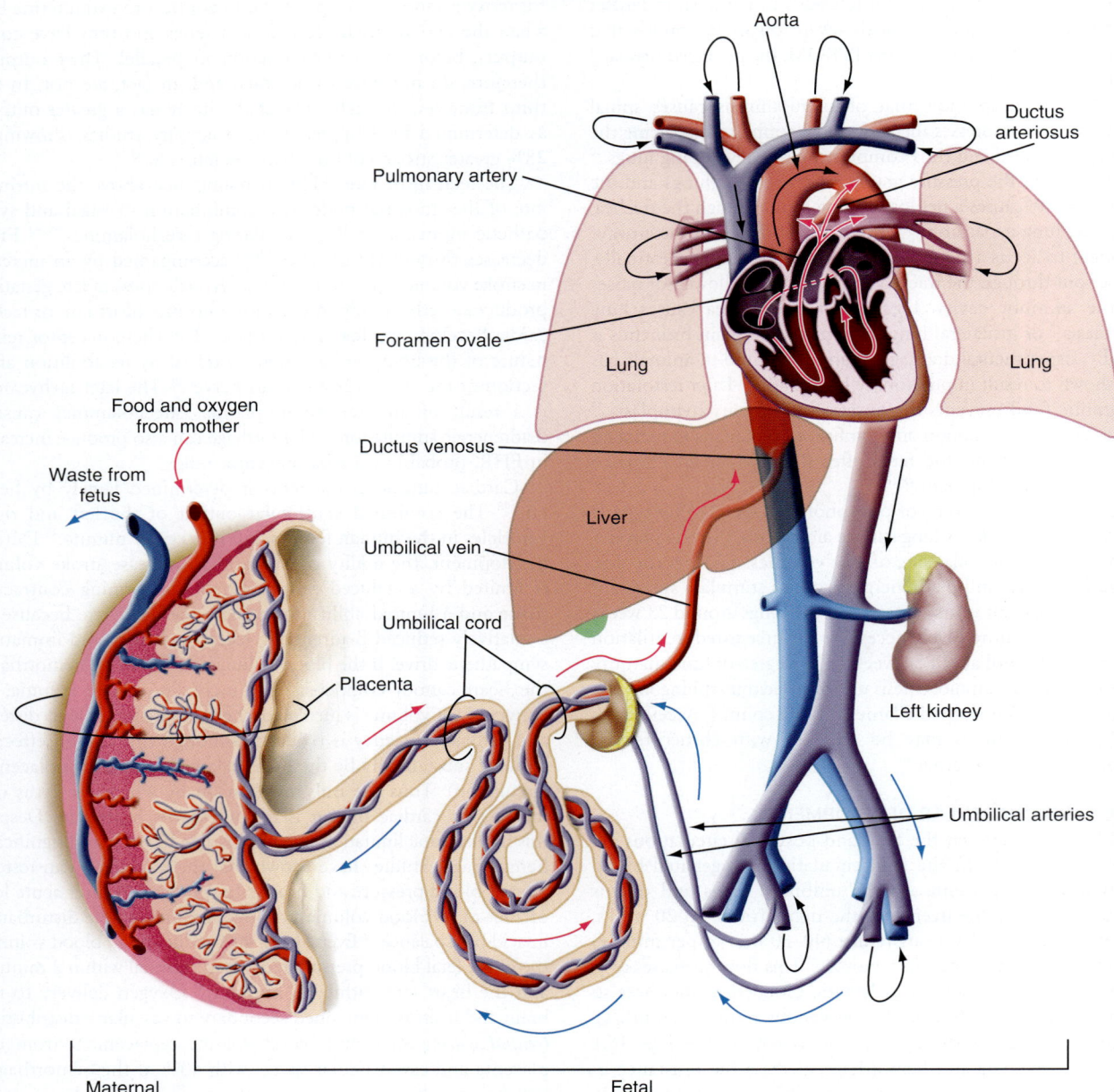

FIGURE 38.2 Fetal circulation. *Red arrows* represent flow of oxygenated blood and *blue arrows* represent flow of deoxygenated blood. *Black arrows* indicate direction of blood flow and represent travel of blood from the central circulation through capillary membranes and return to central circulation. Shading (from red to purple to blue) represents the corresponding relative oxygenation of the blood at that site, from oxygenated to deoxygenated. Note the mixing of blood as the ductus venosus delivers oxygenated blood from the placenta to the central fetal circulation and the progressive desaturation of blood in the fetal aorta secondary to shunts, consumption, and the return of deoxygenated blood from the fetal pulmonary circulation.

to shift the oxyhemoglobin dissociation curve to the right, decreasing the affinity of the fetal hemoglobin for oxygen and favoring oxygen unloading. However, 2,3-DPG appears to only exert approximately 40% of the effect on fetal hemoglobin as it does on adult hemoglobin, thereby preserving a net leftward shift on the oxyhemoglobin dissociation curve. Thus for any given PaO_2, the fetus has a greater affinity for oxygen than does the mother. The P50 (the PaO_2 at which hemoglobin is 50% desaturated)

is approximately 27 mm Hg for the adult and 20 mm Hg for the fetus. The concentration of 2,3-DPG increases with gestation, as does the concentration of hemoglobin A[52]; the greater hemoglobin concentration (18 g/dL) results in a greater total oxygen-carrying capacity.

Oxygen supply to fetal tissues depends on a number of factors (Table 38.2). First, the mother must be adequately oxygenated. Second, there must be adequate flow of well-oxygenated blood

TABLE 38.2	Causes of Impaired Blood Flow and Oxygenation to Fetal Tissues	
Causes of Impaired Uteroplacental Blood Flow/Oxygenation	**Causes of Impaired Umbilical Blood Flow/Fetal Circulatory Redistribution**	
Reduced maternal oxygenation/hemoglobin concentration	Umbilical vessel spasm	
Maternal hemorrhage	Reduced fetal cardiac output	
Aortocaval compression	Fetal hemorrhage/reduced hemoglobin concentration	
Drugs reducing uterine blood flow	Fetal hypothermia	
Uterine trauma	Impaired uteroplacental blood flow/oxygenation	
Uterine contractions	Umbilical cord kinking	
Placental insufficiency (PET, IUGR)		
Polyhydramnios: pressure effect		
Maternal catecholamine production increasing uteroplacental vascular resistance	Fetal catecholamine production increasing fetoplacental vascular resistance	

IUGR, intrauterine growth restriction; *PET,* preeclamptic toxemia.

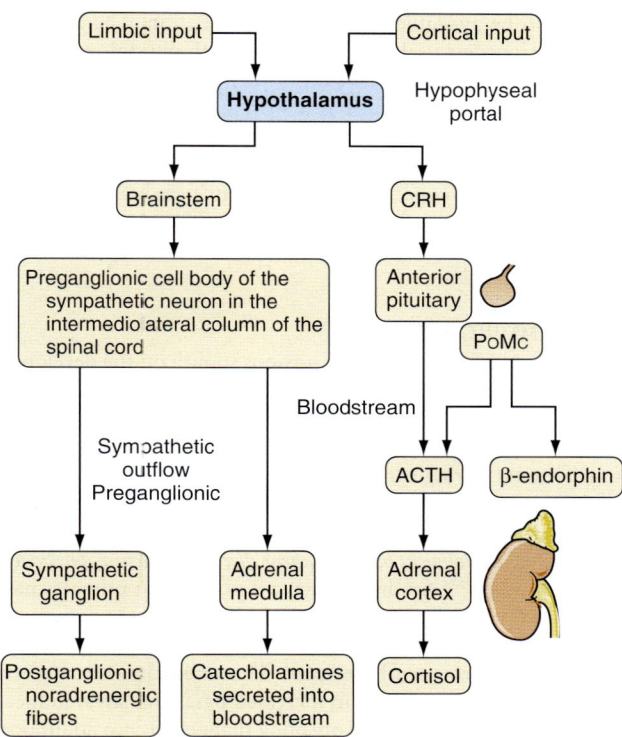

FIGURE 38.3 Human fetal endocrine responses to stress. *ACTH,* adrenocorticotropic hormone; *CRH,* corticotropin-releasing hormone; *PoMc,* proopiomelanocortin.

to the uteroplacental circulation. This blood flow may be reduced from maternal hemorrhage (reduced maternal blood volume) or compression of the inferior vena cava (reduced venous return), which increases uterine venous pressure, thus reducing uterine perfusion. Additionally, aortic compression reduces uterine arterial blood flow.[15] Care must be taken to position the mother in such a way as to prevent aortocaval compression whether by airplaning the table 15 degrees left or by turning the patient to the left decubitus position and then rolling her back to a 15 degrees left tilt.[53,54] The surgical incision of hysterotomy itself reduces uteroplacental blood flow by as much as 73% in sheep, whereas fetoscopic procedures with uterine entry have no effect.[55]

Even if the uterine circulation is adequate, the fetus still depends on uteroplacental blood flow and umbilical venous blood flow for tissue oxygenation. Care must be taken not to interrupt umbilical vessel blood flow by manipulation or kinking the cord, which can cause vasospasm. Umbilical vasoconstriction can also occur as part of a fetal stress reaction resulting from a release of fetal stress hormones (Fig. 38.3). Increases in amniotic fluid volume increase amniotic pressure and impair uteroplacental perfusion.[56,57] Placental vascular resistance may increase, thereby increasing fetal cardiac afterload via a surge in fetal catecholamine production stimulated by surgical stress.[58] Fortunately, animal studies suggest that adverse effects on the arterial blood gas in the fetus do not occur until uteroplacental perfusion has been reduced by 50% or more.[59]

Inhalational anesthetics may cause maternal vasodilatation and thus, in theory, could cause or exacerbate preexisting fetal hypoxia. Studies of anesthetics in hypoxic ovine fetuses have shown that isoflurane exacerbates preexisting acidosis.[60] Isoflurane also attenuates the usual vascular redistribution response to fetal hypoxia, but this is offset by a reduction in cerebral oxygen demand. The net effect is that the balance of cerebral oxygen supply and demand is unaffected. β-Adrenergic blockade, however, renders the fetus less able to cope with asphyxia. Compared with controls, these fetuses have a smaller increase in heart rate, cerebral blood flow, and cardiac output and recover from acidosis more slowly.[61]

CENTRAL AND PERIPHERAL NERVOUS SYSTEM DEVELOPMENT

By the beginning of the second trimester, the spinal cord is largely formed; development of the brain and spinal cord begins as early as postconception week 3. Neural crest cells migrate laterally to form peripheral nerves from about 4 weeks, with the first synapses between them forming a week later.[62] Synapses within the spinal cord develop from about 8 weeks gestation, suggesting the first spinal reflexes may be present at this time. Neuronal development is maximum between 8 and 18 weeks gestation. The first neurons and glial cells develop in the ventricular zone (an epithelial layer) along which the newly formed neurons migrate out in waves to form the neocortex. Synaptogenesis occurs after neural proliferation, first in peripheral structures and, second, more centrally from approximately 20 weeks; this process depends in part on sensory stimulation.[63]

The development of the nociceptive apparatus proceeds in parallel with the development of the basic central nervous system. The first essential requirement for nociception is the presence of sensory receptors, which develop first in the perioral area at around 7 weeks gestation. From here, they develop in the rest of the face and in the palmar surfaces of the hands and soles of the feet from about 11 weeks gestation. By 20 weeks, they are present throughout all of the skin and mucosal surfaces.[64] The nociceptive apparatus is initially involved in local reflex movements at the spinal cord level without higher cortical integration. As these reflex responses become more complex, they in turn involve the brainstem, through which other responses, such as increases in heart rate and blood pressure, are mediated. However, such reflexes to noxious stimuli have not been shown to involve the cortex and, thus, are not thought to be available to conscious perception. The nature of fetal consciousness itself is complicated, both physiologically and philosophically, and a discussion of such is beyond the scope of this chapter. However, there is a working consensus that there must be electrical activity in the cerebral cortex for consciousness to be present.[65] It appears that, far from being "switched on" at any one moment, consciousness evolves in a gradual process that has been likened to a "dimmer switch," making attribution of fetal consciousness to any particular developmental moment a difficult undertaking.

PROGRAMMING EFFECTS

When considering the effects of noxious stimuli on the developing fetus and the rationale for fetal anesthesia and analgesia, we must consider not just the humanitarian need to alleviate the possible distress of pain sensation, but also whether being subjected to surgical stress during early development might cause permanent alterations in physiology. This concept is known as *programming*, defined as *"the process whereby a stimulus or insult at a critical, sensitive period of development has permanent effects on structure, physiology, and metabolism."*[65,66] Studies in rats and nonhuman primates have shown that the numbers of hippocampal and hypothalamic glucocorticoid receptors in the offspring of antenatally stressed animals were permanently reduced. This attenuates the negative feedback response, resulting in increased basal and stress-induced cortisol concentrations in the offspring that persist into adulthood. Behavioral changes, such as poor coping behaviors, have also been observed.[66]

Fetal Monitoring

The goal during any fetal intervention is to optimize fetal well-being by avoiding fetal hypoxia and hypothermia while optimizing stable fetal hemodynamics. It is essential that the physiologic response of the fetus to anesthetic and surgical stresses be understood and addressed to avoid the known detrimental effects of stress on an already compromised fetus. However, access to the fetus is limited at best and the technologies for continuous intraoperative and postoperative fetal vital sign monitoring are still in development.

A hysterotomy is not needed for many surgical interventions; thus the fetus remains within the uterus, often making access for direct monitoring impossible. Even for those fetuses that are partially delivered for an invasive procedure, monitoring is obtainable only intermittently and is frequently unreliable because the fetus must remain within a fluid environment during the procedure. These obstacles make it difficult to directly apply the available monitors. Current methods for assessing fetal well-being include FHR monitoring, direct measurement of fetal blood gases, fetal electrocardiography, fetal pulse oximetry (FPO), fetal echocardiography, and Doppler ultrasonography of fetal cerebral blood flow.

USE OF FETAL HEART RATE MONITORING FOR FETAL INTERVENTIONS

Currently, FHR monitoring with Doppler ultrasonography is the standard for the intrapartum assessment of fetal well-being. FHR monitoring is also used perioperatively during fetal interventions. The FHR is documented before maternal induction of anesthesia to (1) serve as a baseline for comparison and (2) reassure the perinatologist, surgeon, and anesthesiologist that the fetus is stable. The FHR may be continuously monitored intraoperatively by fetal echocardiography and with intermittent palpation of the

umbilical cord in open cases. The most commonly used induction agents for anesthesia (propofol and thiopental) rapidly cross the placenta and thus also rapidly reach the fetus at appropriate doses.[67,68] The inhalational anesthetics also cross the placenta,[69] but their uptake occurs more slowly in the fetus than in the mother.[10,70] These anesthetics decrease FHR and FHR variability. Although it is reassuring if the FHR is within the normal range for the gestational age, fetal bradycardia is a reliable indicator of fetal distress that needs to be immediately addressed.

With the advent of minimally invasive fetal endoscopic surgery, new problems in monitoring have surfaced. The fetus is no longer physically accessible to the surgical team, and the trocars currently used for fetoscopic surgery prevent applying radiotelemetric probes. Currently, fetoscopic or cardiac intervention use direct visualization of the heart with fetal echocardiography, which gives an accurate estimation of the FHR. Although very beneficial, the continuous use of fetal echocardiography requires the presence of a skilled ultrasonographer working in the operative field.

USE OF FETAL BLOOD SAMPLING DURING FETAL INTERVENTIONS

In suspected cases of fetal compromise during an open intervention, fetal blood can be obtained from capillary vessels, a peripheral vein, a central vein, or a puncture of the umbilical vessels. Vascular access is difficult in the fetus because of its small size and friable tissue. Puncture of the umbilical vessels can cause umbilical cord spasm, hematoma, and even fetal death. Hence umbilical cord manipulation should be reserved for circumstances when no other options are available. During an endoscopic intervention, access to the fetal circulation is possible through puncture of the umbilical vessels. With most fetal cardiac interventions, a needle and/or catheter is placed directly through the fetal myocardium, allowing access for blood samples; only a very small sample should be withdrawn because of the small circulating fetal blood volume.

FETAL ELECTROCARDIOGRAPHY

Several groups have used fetal electrocardiography analysis to determine whether changes in time interval (PR and RR interval) and signal morphology (T/QRS ratio) correlate with fetal or neonatal outcome. Studies in animals and humans have shown that under normal conditions, there is a negative correlation between the PR interval and the FHR: as the FHR slows, the PR interval lengthens, and as the FHR increases, the PR interval shortens. *The opposite relationship occurs in acidemic infants.*[71–77] During periods of fetal compromise, it is hypothesized that the sinoatrial node and the atrioventricular node respond differently.[75] Periods of mild hypoxemia induce increases in epinephrine levels, which increase the FHR and shorten the PR interval. However, with periods of prolonged hypoxemia, the oxygen-dependent calcium channels of the sinoatrial node demonstrate reduced sensitivity to epinephrine, thus decreasing the FHR. The fast sodium channels of the atrioventricular node are unaffected by the reduction in the oxygen supply, whereas the increased levels of epinephrine shorten the PR interval. As a result, the relationship between the PR interval and FHR changes from negative to positive.[75,74] Measurements of this relationship have been divided into short-term and long-term measures.[75,76] The short-term measure or the conduction index can be intermittently positive over brief intervals without an adverse outcome. However, a prolonged positive conduction index (>20 minutes) has been associated with an increased risk of fetal acidemia.[77]

FETAL PULSE OXIMETRY

Standard pulse oximeters use the transmission and absorption of light through a vascular bed to a photodetector on the opposite side of the tissue. However, the development of reflectance oximetry allows measurement of oxygen saturation from light-emitting diodes that are positioned next to each other on the same skin surface and absorption is determined from the light that scatters back to the tissue surface[78,79]; any fetal condition that decreases vascular pulsations (e.g., hypotension, vasoconstriction, shock, or strong uterine contractions) can produce inaccurate oximetry readings.[80] Because direct contact of the oximeter must be made with the fetal skin surface, anything that interferes with light transmission or skin adhesion (e.g., fetal or maternal movement, vernix caseosa, caput succedaneum) can influence the signal quality and accuracy of the oximeter.[81–85] Oximetry readings also vary in relation to the site of sensor application; several studies have found reduced baseline oxygen saturation values with the use of the oxygen sensor on the fetal buttock compared with the fetal head.[86–89]

The development of a 735-/890-nm wavelength system (compared with the older 660-/890-nm system) has improved the accuracy in monitoring arterial oxygen saturation ($FSaO_2$) in the fetus.[90] With the normal range of $FSaO_2$ of 30% to 70% in the middle of the oxygen-hemoglobin dissociation curve, small changes in pH or oxygen partial pressure exert large changes in $FSaO_2$.[91] FPO can also identify an acidotic fetus. Increased concentrations of both the hydrogen ion and 2,3-DPG cause a rightward shift of the oxygen dissociation curve (Bohr effect) such that a chronically acidemic or hypoxemic fetus will have a reduced $FSaO_2$ even though the PO_2 is within normal limits.[91]

NEAR-INFRARED SPECTROSCOPY

Near-infrared spectroscopy is a monitoring modality for continuous measurement of mixed-vascular oxygenation of tissues. Using an optical probe to assess light wavelengths in the 650- to 1000-nm range, this tool is able to provide data about tissues several centimeters deep and as such has been particularly useful for assessing cerebral oxygenation as well as detecting changes in fetal tissue oxygenation noninvasively through the maternal abdominal wall in real time in a sheep model.[92] While this monitor has yet to gain widespread clinical use during fetal surgery, in animal models of fetal surgery, near-infrared spectroscopy measurements have been shown to correlate closely with umbilical venous oxygenation.[93]

FETAL ECHOCARDIOGRAPHY

When technically feasible, fetal echocardiography should be available to assess fetal myocardial contractility and function, heart rate, intravascular volume status, and amniotic fluid volume. We have also used echocardiography to correctly identify proper endotracheal tube placement during an EXIT procedure[94] (see later discussion); a sterile sleeve is placed over the ultrasonographic probe, which is then placed over the fetal chest.

DOPPLER ULTRASONOGRAPHY OF FETAL CEREBRAL BLOOD FLOW

Antepartum Doppler ultrasonography studies of the fetal circulation in cases of intrauterine growth restriction with presumed hypoxia have shown a compensatory redistribution, with an increase in peripheral vascular resistance in the fetal body and placenta and a compensatory reduction in peripheral vascular resistance in the fetal brain, producing a brain-sparing effect.[95] Intrapartum Doppler ultrasonography and FPO have verified the brain-sparing response in the presence of intrapartum arterial hypoxemia ($FSaO_2$ <30%

for 5 minutes or more), as reflected by increased mean flow velocity in the fetal middle cerebral artery.[96] Preliminary studies of the middle cerebral artery pulsatility index in minimally invasive procedures, such as fetal blood sampling, transfusion, shunt insertion, tissue biopsy, and ovarian cyst aspiration, have demonstrated significant cerebral hemodynamic responses (decreases in the middle cerebral artery pulsatility index) in fetuses that underwent procedures involving transgression of the fetal body. This response was not noted in the fetuses undergoing procedures at the noninnervated placental cord insertion.[97]

Although not yet advocated for routine intrapartum management, it has been suggested that the combination of reduced arterial oxygen saturation and increased cerebral blood flow may indicate an ominous phase during labor. The redistribution of the fetal circulation is not an unlimited protective mechanism, and with persistent cerebral hypoxia, the active vasodilation of the cerebral vessels may fail, leading to disastrous consequences for the fetus.[98]

Physiologic Consequences of Pregnancy

RESPIRATORY AND AIRWAY CONSIDERATIONS

There is an increase in metabolic demand of both the mother and the fetus, and this, along with anatomic and hormonal influences, accounts for the changes in maternal pulmonary physiology (Table 38.3). Pregnancy results in progressive increases in maternal oxygen consumption and minute ventilation, along with a decreased residual volume and functional residual capacity.[99] The increased metabolic demands and anatomic changes can make adequate oxygenation and perfusion of the parturient and the fetoplacental unit a challenge during maternal general anesthesia. During periods of apnea or hypoventilation, the parturient is prone to rapid development of hypoxia and hypercapnia. Even after adequate preoxygenation, the PaO_2 in an apneic anesthetized parturient decreases about 8 mm Hg more rapidly per minute than in a comparable nonpregnant women.[100] Acidosis rapidly develops from hypoxia during difficult airway situations because of a decreased buffering capacity during pregnancy. The decreased pulmonary oxygen stores and increased oxygen consumption make parturients more susceptible than nonpregnant women to the consequences of airway mismanagement.

Not all physiologic changes of pregnancy are deleterious to the performance of anesthesia. For example, both the induction

TABLE 38.3 Anesthetic Considerations of Respiratory Changes of Pregnancy

Decreased functional residual capacity
  Faster denitrogenation
  Rapidly prone to hypoxia during apnea
  Faster induction and emergence of anesthesia with inhaled agents

Increased oxygen consumption
  Rapidly prone to hypoxia during apnea

Capillary engorgement of the respiratory mucosa
  Predisposes upper airway to trauma, bleeding, and obstruction
  Laryngeal edema increases the frequency of difficult intubation

Decreased $PaCO_2$ and no $PETCO_2$-$PaCO_2$ gradient
  Capnograph reading similar to $PaCO_2$
  Hyperventilation may lead to a reduction in uterine blood flow

$PETCO_2$, end-tidal carbon dioxide pressure.

38

TABLE 38.4	Anesthetic Considerations of Cardiovascular Changes of Pregnancy

Aortocaval compression
Supine position leads to a decline in cardiac output
May lead to supine hypotensive syndrome
Mostly prevented by left or right uterine displacement

Decreased colloid oncotic pressure
Parturient is at greater risk for developing pulmonary edema

Increased maternal blood volume
Parturient tolerates more blood loss than nonparturients
Hypotension and acidosis may develop with significant blood loss

of and emergence from anesthesia with inhalational anesthetics occur faster in parturients than in nonpregnant women because the combination of increased alveolar ventilation and decreased functional residual capacity speeds the rate at which denitrogenation occurs and at which inspired and alveolar concentrations of inhalational anesthetics reach equilibrium[101]; a faster induction, coupled with a decreased MAC, predisposes the parturients to relative anesthetic overdose and severe hypotension.[102]

CARDIOVASCULAR CONSIDERATIONS

Cardiovascular function is appropriately increased during pregnancy to meet the increased metabolic demands and oxygen requirements of the mother (Table 38.4). Cardiac output increases by 35% to 40% by the end of the first trimester and continues to increase steadily throughout the second trimester until it reaches a level 50% greater than that in nonpregnant women.[103] Heart rate increases 15% to 25% and stroke volume increases 25% to 30% compared with prepregnancy values by the end of the second trimester, after which they both remain stable until term.[104,105] Aortocaval compression by the gravid uterus can decrease cardiac output by 30% to 50%; lesser decreases occur in the sitting or semirecumbent positions. Maternal position is a major factor contributing to hypotension and fetal well-being.[106]

Maternal blood flow and pressure are directly linked to fetal perfusion via the placenta, and uterine blood flow represents about 10% of maternal cardiac output. It is imperative to prevent aortocaval compression by left or right uterine displacement. Because large doses of inhalational anesthetics are often necessary to relax the uterus during fetal intervention, prompt treatment of hypotension is vital. A decrease in maternal blood pressure eventually decreases placental blood flow and, therefore, blood flow to the fetus because uteroplacental blood flow is not autoregulated. Ephedrine (5–10 mg IV) or phenylephrine (50–100 μg IV) per dose effectively treats maternal hypotension unless contraindicated.[107]

Careful attention to the volume status of the parturient is imperative; aggressive volume hydration, the normal decrease in colloid oncotic pressure that occurs during pregnancy, and the use of tocolytic agents (e.g., magnesium or β-adrenoceptor agonists) may all predispose the parturient to pulmonary edema.

CENTRAL AND PERIPHERAL NERVOUS SYSTEMS

Pregnancy-mediated analgesia is affected by changes in spinal opioid antinociceptive pathways and peripheral processes, including the effect of ovarian sex steroids (estrogen and progesterone) and uterine afferent neurotransmission. It is thought that pregnancy-mediated analgesia increases the woman's threshold for pain during the latter stages of pregnancy before labor.[108,109] Pregnant women

are more sensitive to the action of many anesthetic agents and require less local anesthetic for spinal and epidural anesthesia and less inhalational anesthetics than their nonpregnant counterparts. The MAC of inhalational anesthetics in pregnancy is approximately 30% less than in nonpregnant females, and yet recent evidence indicated that the hypnotic effects of inhalational anesthetics are similar in pregnant and nonpregnant women.[110] To preclude awareness on the one hand and uterine atony and neonatal depression on the other, the concentration of inhalational anesthetic needs to be carefully titrated.[111]

PHARMACOLOGIC CONSEQUENCES OF PREGNANCY

Physiologic changes of pregnancy alter the pharmacokinetics and pharmacodynamics of many anesthetic drugs. An increase in total body water and adipose tissue, and a decrease in plasma protein concentrations alter the volume of distribution. An increased renal blood flow and glomerular filtration rate can enhance the elimination of renally excreted drugs; hepatic metabolism of some drugs may be inhibited by competition with steroid hormones during pregnancy, whereas others may have a greater clearance associated with the increased basal metabolic rate. Therefore drug administration must consider the pharmacokinetics within the maternal-placental-fetal unit. Most drugs cross the placenta to some extent and the proportion transferred increases with the duration of gestation. The fetus has reduced plasma protein binding, producing relatively greater concentrations of free drug (i.e., unbound and available to cross biologic membranes).[112] Despite detection of oxidation and reduction reactions in the fetal liver from as early as 16 weeks, enzyme concentrations and reaction rates are minimal, exposing the fetus to more prolonged drug effects than occur in the mother.[113] Early in gestation, the primary mode of drug excretion is via blood flow to the placenta, but later, as the fetal kidneys mature, they become a route of drug excretion into the amniotic fluid for water-soluble drugs and metabolites. Amniotic fluid, however, can act as a reservoir for drugs, from which they can be reabsorbed.[112]

Induction

Pregnancy increases the parturient's sensitivity to induction agents.[114] Propofol has been safely used for induction of anesthesia for cesarean delivery in doses of 2 mg/kg, with minimal effects on the neonate.[115] Ketamine has also been used as the sole induction agent for parturients undergoing elective cesarean section; ketamine (1.5 mg/kg) has not been associated with maternal awareness or neonatal depression at delivery and parturients required fewer analgesics in the first 24 hours after delivery.[116] It is speculated that ketamine's analgesic properties may reduce the sensitization of pain pathways and subsequently confer extended benefit into the postoperative period. Induction agents decrease spontaneous uterine contractions of isolated pregnant rat myometrium, but only in concentrations greater than those seen in clinical obstetric practice.[117]

Neuromuscular Blocking Drugs

Although serum cholinesterase activity decreases 30% during pregnancy, recovery from a dose of 1 mg/kg of succinylcholine is not prolonged.[118] Succinylcholine has limited placental transfer, owing to its poor lipid solubility and high degree of ionization.[119] Similarly, *cis*-atracurium has been safely used for cesarean section without routine neostigmine antagonism, despite decreased plasma cholinesterase activity.[120] Pregnant women may be more sensitive to the action of nondepolarizing muscle relaxants, with the administration of vecuronium resulting in a more rapid onset and delayed recovery of neuromuscular blockade compared with nonpregnant control patients. The prolonged action of vecuronium is reported in women 4 days after delivery[121]; the clinical duration of vecuronium in term and postpartum women is twice that of nonpregnant women.[122] However, in a study that compared *cis*-atracurium 0.2 mg/kg for intubation in immediate postpartum women with nonpregnant women, both the mean onset and recovery times in the postpartum women were significantly smaller.[123] Nondepolarizing muscle relaxants have no effect on uterine relaxation and, as quaternary amines, do not cross the placenta.

Inhalational Anesthetics

Pregnant women are more sensitive to the anesthetic action of the inhalational anesthetics (MAC is reduced approximately 30% from nonpregnant females).[124] This may lead to a deeper plane of anesthesia than predicted during fetal surgery and a relative overdose associated with maternal cardiac depression and hypotension. Recent evidence, however, suggests that the hypnotic effects of sevoflurane measured electroencephalographically and with a bispectral index monitor were similar in pregnant and nonpregnant women.[110] The difference in MAC between these two groups may reflect differences in spinal nociceptive responses rather than central hypnotic effects.

All inhalational anesthetics rapidly cross the placenta, but their uptake occurs more slowly in the fetus than in the mother.[125,126] At light (1.0 MAC) isoflurane or halothane anesthesia, neither maternal pulse rate, cardiac output, and acid-base status, nor fetal pulse rate, acid-base status, and oxygen saturation changed significantly.[127] During moderately deep (1.5 MAC) isoflurane or halothane anesthesia, maternal arterial pressure and cardiac output decreased. Uterine vasodilation occurred, but uteroplacental perfusion was maintained; fetal oxygenation and base excess were also maintained. However, at concentrations of inhalational anesthetics that exceeded 2.0 MAC, maternal hypotension decreased uteroplacental perfusion despite uterine vasodilation, leading to fetal hypoxia and acidosis. Inhalational anesthetics produced a dose-related uterine relaxation.[128] At 0.5 MAC of isoflurane, uterine contractility decreases 20%, whereas at 1.5 MAC, contractility decreases 60%.[129] Sevoflurane produces a dose-dependent depression in uterine muscle contractility, with complete abolition of uterine activity at greater than 3.5 MAC.[130] The large concentrations of inhalation anesthetic needed for profound uterine relaxation generally requires tracheal intubation and aggressive use of vasopressors.

Fetal Preoperative Evaluation

Prenatal imaging of all fetal anomalies, including anatomic areas of involvement, the relationship to normal structures, and tracheal location, is needed to plan the most appropriate surgical and anesthetic interventions. The accuracy and quality of preoperative fetal ultrasonography and magnetic resonance imaging (MRI) are of the utmost importance because some lesions, especially pulmonary lesions, may spontaneously regress in utero; an inaccurate diagnosis could lead to suboptimal or inappropriate intervention. In addition, extremely valuable information can be obtained that would aid in the decision-making process for a given treatment—namely, the presence of ascites, hydrops, mediastinal shift, degree of lung hypoplasia and lesion involvement, airway involvement and potential tracheal distortion, or compression from intrathoracic masses. Preoperative imaging can also determine other anticipated

alterations in anatomy that may acutely alter fetal cardiopulmonary physiology (e.g., mediastinal shift and the known associated potential alterations in fetal preload). Serial radiologic examinations can also monitor the growth of certain masses, the development of hydrops, and the response to treatment medications (e.g., transplacental digoxin). Significant fetal ventricular dysfunction or heart failure should alert the anesthesiologist to the possibility of fetal cardiac arrest during a fetal intervention. Other congenital abnormalities may be detected that may render a potential fetal intervention useless.

In addition, a fetal karyotype must be obtained preoperatively to diagnose any genetic disorders that are associated with significant fetal morbidity or mortality and that would preclude further intervention. An estimated fetal weight, obtained by ultrasonography immediately before surgical intervention, allows for preparation of unit doses of fetal medications. Any previous attempts at fetal intervention should be evaluated, including the number of interventions, fetal tolerance of the procedures, transient reversal in fetal symptoms, the presence of fetal cardiac dysfunction, and the reason or reasons for failed intervention. Assuming that fetal hydrops is present, any attempts to treat this condition should also be documented, including the effectiveness of digoxin therapy, total dose administered, method of administration, and response to treatment.

Maternal Evaluation

A complete medical history and physical examination, especially a focused airway evaluation, are of the utmost importance. Details regarding fetal pathophysiology and its effects on secondary maternal morbidity should be addressed. Any patient with significant polyhydramnios and associated preterm contractions is at increased risk for preterm labor and rupture of membranes with uterine manipulation. Patients with polyhydramnios despite multiple amnioreductions require greater amounts of intraoperative tocolysis as well as greater concentrations of inhalational anesthetic to relax the uterus and ensure acceptable surgical conditions.

The presence of fetal hydrops should alert the practitioner to the possibility of maternal mirror syndrome. *Mirror syndrome* refers to characteristic maternal pathophysiologic changes associated with a variety of fetal disorders, including nonimmune hydrops, molar pregnancies, congenital cystic adenomatoid malformation (CCAM) of the lung, and sacrococcygeal teratoma (SCT). Polyhydramnios and placentomegaly are usually present. Although the etiology of this condition is unclear, the end result is a maternal hyperdynamic state with associated hypertension and total body edema.[131] Respiratory insufficiency or pulmonary edema may develop, requiring prompt and aggressive treatment. If preterm uterine contractions develop, treatment options may be limited because tocolytic agents can greatly exacerbate respiratory decompensation. Treatment is aimed at maternal supportive care; even correction of the underlying fetal pathology will not completely resolve the maternal abnormalities. Delivery of the fetus is the only sure method to completely reverse this maternal pathologic process.

The anesthesiologist should specifically investigate for the presence of placentomegaly; increased placental blood flow may alter pharmacologic treatment in both the mother and the fetus because increased drug metabolism may occur. The presence of placentomegaly may also increase the risk for acute massive intraoperative bleeding. Strategies should be in place before incision to permit rapid fluid resuscitation of the mother. Several reports describe inadvertent inclusion of the placental edge during the hysterotomy incision, causing a sudden, massive loss of blood with a completely relaxed uterus.[132,133] Immediate surgical control of the bleeding, resuscitation of the mother with blood products, and liberal use of vasopressors that do not increase placental vascular resistance must be immediately available.

Tocolysis and Tocolytic Agents

The occurrence of contractions and preterm labor is an expectation for the first few postoperative days. Fortunately, in many cases, delivery can be postponed until after 32 weeks, giving the fetus time to heal from the procedure and allowing the lungs to mature. However, for many women, the onset of surgically induced preterm contractions heralds premature labor and delivery that, at best, eliminates the positive results of the procedure, and, at worst, ends in the loss of the pregnancy. Although most women who require fetal surgery can be successfully prevented from delivering immediately after surgery, the current generation of medications used for tocolysis have been ineffective in preventing premature labor and delivery. Preterm labor remains the single most common complication that limits the success of fetal surgery.

HORMONAL RECEPTORS IN LABOR
The adrenergic hormonal system plays a very influential part in the activity of the myometrium; several types of adrenergic receptors are found in the uterus (Fig. 38.4). Stimulation of the α-adrenergic receptor causes an increase in the rate and intensity of uterine contractions, whereas activation of the β₂-adrenergic receptors produce myometrial relaxation.[134] In addition, the term uterus is heavily populated with receptors for endogenously released oxytocin responsible for initiating uterine contractions. Prostaglandins also play a significant role in modulating myometrial tone. In general,

prostaglandins are produced in or near the local environment where they exert their effect; both uterotonic and tocolytic prostaglandins have been identified. The balance of intrauterine and maternal uterotonic prostaglandins is thought to play an essential part in the preparation for both term and preterm labor. Prostaglandins, especially prostaglandin E₂, are an essential component of every aspect of natural labor.[135]

TREATMENT OF ACUTE PRETERM LABOR
Nonsteroidal Antiinflammatory Drugs
Nonsteroidal antiinflammatory drugs (NSAIDs) block the action of cyclooxygenase, preventing the formation of prostaglandins. In vitro studies of indomethacin have found consistent inhibition or complete arrest of overall myometrial activity.

β-Adrenergic–Mimetic Agents
Currently, only β₂-adrenoceptor–selective medications are routinely used for acute preterm labor. Most adverse effects result from their lack of pure specificity—that is, simultaneous stimulation of β₁- and β₂-adrenergic receptors. Adverse effects include fetal tachycardia, maternal tremors, palpitations, tachycardia, a decreased or increased blood pressure, lethargy, sleepiness, ketoacidosis, and pulmonary edema. Pulmonary edema occurs in up to 5% of patients, especially when these medications are used with other tocolytics (e.g., magnesium).[136] Because the β-adrenergic–mimetic agents are nonspecific receptor agonists, in large concentrations these agents can stimulate α-adrenergic receptors, which promotes uterine contractions, leading to treatment failure.

Magnesium
Magnesium competes with calcium for transmembrane channel entry into cells.[137] Because the myometrium depends on stores

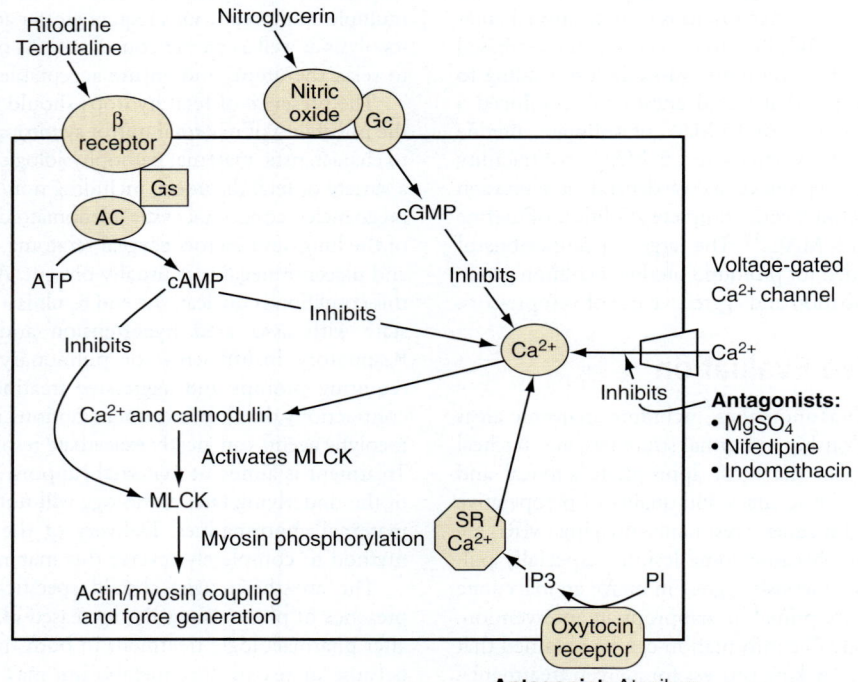

FIGURE 38.4 Biochemistry of uterine contraction and its inhibition. *AC,* adenylate cyclase; *ATP,* adenosine triphosphate; *cAMP,* cyclic adenosine monophosphate; *cGMP,* cyclic guanosine monophosphate; *Gc,* G-protein c; *Gs,* G-protein s; *IP3,* inositol triphosphate; *MLCK,* myosin light-chain kinase; *PI,* phosphatidylinositol; *SR,* sarcoplasmic reticulum.

of calcium for adequate contraction, a decrease in intracellular transport prevents the activation of the actin and myosin complex, resulting in uterine relaxation.

Nitric Oxide Donors

Nitroglycerin is an effective uterine relaxant used in select situations to rapidly relax the uterus (e.g., extraction of a retained placenta and uterine inversion). In pregnant sheep, nitroglycerin causes a decrease in mean maternal arterial pressure and increase in heart rate, without compromising uterine blood flow.[138] During fetal surgery, nitroglycerin has been used to relax the myometrium and arrest breakthrough contractions. Adverse effects include maternal hypotension, tachycardia, headache, development of tachyphylaxis, and a high incidence of maternal pulmonary edema.[139]

Calcium-Channel Blockers

Calcium-channel blockers are better tolerated than β-adrenergic–mimetic agents. Nifedipine may be more effective than β2-adrenergic agonists in postponing delivery, especially in those women with intact membranes.[140] Neonates born to women treated with calcium-channel blockers have a reduced frequency of respiratory distress, necrotizing enterocolitis, and intraventricular hemorrhage.[141] The most serious adverse effect is maternal hypotension; the combination of calcium-channel blockers and magnesium sulfate should generally be avoided.

Pain Control

Pain control after fetal surgery is an essential component of tocolytic therapy, because it is thought that adequate pain control prevents the stress-induced hormonal impetus for preterm labor. Surgical stress elicits the release of adrenocorticotropic hormone that increases production of cortisol; cortisol production, in turn, leads to the deleterious changes in the placenta that increase fetal estrogen and prostaglandin production, promoting increased uterine activity.

Fetal Complications of Tocolytic Therapy

The adverse effects of tocolytics in the fetus present a number of problems, albeit usually less so than in the mother. Sympathomimetics that act through β-adrenoceptors cause fetal tachycardia.[142] Whereas cyclooxygenase inhibitors are more effective than other tocolytics in delaying labor,[143] the adverse effects of fetal oliguria and ductus arteriosus constriction have limited their long-term use.[144] However, after short-term use, these adverse effects are fully reversible within 72 hours from cessation of treatment.[144] Longer-term use of indomethacin has been associated with renal dysfunction and increased rates of necrotizing enterocolitis, intracranial hemorrhage, and patent ductus arteriosus in infants delivered at less than 30 weeks gestation.[145] Magnesium sulfate reduces FHR variability[139] and depresses fetal right ventricular function.[146] Because this drug rapidly crosses the placenta but is excreted more slowly by the fetal kidneys than by the maternal kidneys, there are concerns about fetal toxicity, resulting in respiratory and central nervous system depression.[147] Nitric oxide donors, such as nitroglycerin, appear to have minimal fetal side effects.[11]

POSTOPERATIVE PULMONARY EDEMA

Noncardiogenic pulmonary edema is a known complication of tocolysis. Most often, obstetric pulmonary edema is a result of increased hydrostatic pressures and resolves rapidly with diuretics, cessation of tocolytics, and fluid restriction. One study observed a prevalence of pulmonary edema of 0.5%, but that rate increased to 23% in fetal surgical patients; 93% of those with pulmonary edema required intensive care and 20% required tracheal intubation.[139] It has been hypothesized that extensive uterine manipulation during surgery may result in release of mediators that increase the permeability of lung vasculature. The class of medications most strongly associated with pulmonary edema is β-adrenergic–mimetic agents. An additional important observation is that patients receiving nitroglycerin for tocolysis have demonstrated more pronounced pulmonary edema (more severe hypoxemia, greater time to resolution, worse chest radiograph, and a greater composite lung injury scores) than those who received other tocolytics.[139]

Congenital Cystic Adenomatoid Malformation: the Open Procedure

CCAM serves as a prime example of a fetal condition that requires an open intervention. Fetuses with lung masses that present before extrauterine viability represent a complex group of congenital disorders. Before the advent of preterm fetal intervention, management of fetal lung masses had limited options that included (1) delivery with hydrops once fetal viability was determined based on lung maturity while acknowledging the potential need for emergent postpartum resuscitation, (2) transplacental digoxin therapy in an effort to treat severe forms of cardiac dysfunction,[148,149] and (3) termination of the pregnancy if the fetus was considered nonviable (Fig. 38.5). Fetuses that demonstrate in utero tumor regression documented by serial sonograms are allowed to progress to term gestation. Most infants with smaller lung masses or those with masses demonstrating in utero regression do well with standard delivery and neonatal resection.[145] However, a subset of fetuses experience fetal lung mass growth, ultimately compromising normal lung development. Treatment options for these fetuses have expanded to include cyst aspiration, thoracocentesis, double-J stents for permanent thoracic drainage, and in utero resection of the lung mass.[145,150,151] All treatment options aim to reduce the size of the lung mass to allow the remaining fetal lung to develop.

CONGENITAL CYSTIC ADENOMATOID MALFORMATION OF THE LUNG

CCAM of the lung consists of cystic masses of pulmonary tissue and bronchial structures, neither of which participate in gas exchange,[152,153] that may represent a form of pulmonary hypoplasia.[154] CCAMs can compress surrounding lung tissue and impede normal lung development, resulting in pulmonary hypoplasia.[155] Of all the fetal lung masses, CCAM is the lesion most frequently associated with hydrops fetalis that often indicates a premorbid fetal state. Although the exact mechanisms for the development of hydrops are unclear, it has been suggested that it is secondary to either cardiac compression or vena caval obstruction from the intrathoracic mass.[156,157] This condition is associated with an imbalance of fetal fluid that results in the accumulation of fetal fluid, causing increases in fetal interstitial and total body water, pericardial and pleural effusions, ascites, anasarca, polyhydramnios, or placental thickening.[158,159]

Fetal lung abnormalities themselves may lead to excessive fluid accumulation because the fetal lung is an important organ for amniotic fluid balance. The average fetus produces approximately 300 mL/day or about 4 mL/kg per hour of lung fluid[160] and approximately 700 mL/day of urine output, and swallows approximately

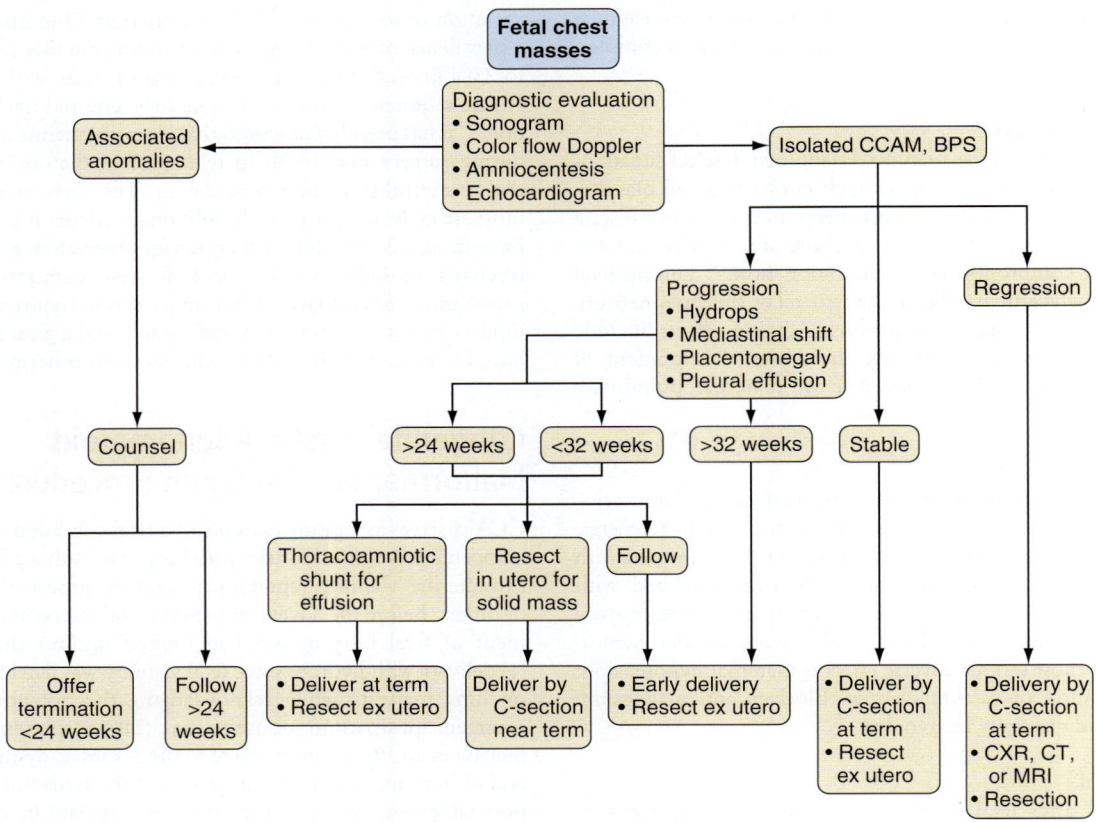

FIGURE 38.5 Algorithm for the management of fetal chest masses. *BPS*, bronchopulmonary syndrome; *CCAM*, congenital cystic adenomatoid malformation; *CT*, computed tomography; *CXR*, chest radiography; *MRI*, magnetic resonance imaging. (Reprinted with permission from Myers LB, Bulich LA, eds. *Anesthesia for Fetal Intervention and Surgery.* Philadelphia: BC Decker; 2005.)

700 mL/day of amniotic fluid. The remaining 300 mL/day is postulated to exit the amnion through the chorioamnionic membrane. CCAMs may impair fetal swallowing via esophageal obstruction and therefore disrupt the normal fluid balance. Fetal swallowing is the major route by which amniotic fluid is returned to the fetal vascular compartment. A second possibility is hypersecretion or transudation of fluid from the CCAM itself.

Management
Experts have formulated guidelines for the fetal surgical management of fetuses diagnosed with CCAM lesions; overall prognosis depends on the size of the lung mass and the presence of secondary physiologic derangements.[145] Special consideration is given to fetuses that exhibit signs of hydrops fetalis, especially those who are less than 32 weeks gestation.[150] Although these conclusions were based primarily on the experience with CCAM infants, it might be appropriate to extend this experience to the management of fetuses with other lung lesions. The primary goal of treatment is to reduce lesion size so that the fetal lung has an improved chance of normal development.

Operating Room Preparation
As with all other types of fetal intervention, ultrasonography should be performed before the induction of anesthesia to assess fetal well-being and to obtain an estimated fetal weight. In addition to the normal preanesthesia preparation checklist, additional

maternal airway equipment, resuscitation drugs, and tocolytic agents should be prepared and immediately available. The availability of type-specific packed red blood cells (PRBCs) for the mother and O-negative irradiated PRBCs, divided into 50-mL aliquots for the fetus must be confirmed. The operating room temperature should be warmed to at least 80°F (26.7°C) to prevent hypothermia of the partially exposed fetus during thoracotomy. Resuscitation drugs for the fetus (atropine 10–20 µg/kg, epinephrine 1–10 µg/kg), as well as an NMBD (e.g., vecuronium 0.2 mg/kg or pancuronium 0.1 mg/kg), and fentanyl (10 µg/kg) are prepared under sterile conditions, thus making them available during the procedure.[51] A rapid infusion system with warmed isotonic saline solution is used to replace amniotic fluid loss during fetal lung resection, and is ready to administer onto the surgical field via a sterile tubing system. A pulse oximeter with a sterile extension cord should be available for application to the upper extremity of the fetus.

Induction
The preferred method of maternal anesthesia for these cases is general anesthesia with tracheal intubation and neuromuscular blockade. IV access is established and sedation is administered as needed before entering the operating room. If the mother has not received indomethacin (50-mg rectal suppository) for tocolysis before arrival, it is administered after induction of general anesthesia. Indomethacin is used in conjunction with magnesium in the postoperative period for tocolysis but does not play a significant

tocolytic role in the intraoperative period. After placement of standard monitors, a lumbar epidural catheter may be inserted for postoperative pain management. With the exception of a test dose, most practitioners avoid local anesthetic administration through the epidural catheter until the fetal intervention is completed. This is done to avoid possible decreases in maternal mean arterial pressure from an epidural-associated sympathectomy. The mother is then positioned in a uterine displacement position, preoxygenated, and a rapid-sequence induction is performed with an induction agent, succinylcholine (and subsequently followed with a short-acting nondepolarizing agent), and a rapid-acting opioid. Anesthesia is maintained with 1 MAC of the inhalational anesthetic of choice (usually sevoflurane or desflurane should a rapid reinstatement of uterine tone be required) in 100% oxygen (with remifentanil and propofol as possible adjuncts), while an ultrasonographic examination maps out surface anatomy with respect to the placenta and fetus, as well as reassuring fetal well-being after anesthetic induction. A second large-bore peripheral IV catheter, radial arterial catheter, urinary catheter, and nasogastric tube are then inserted. Because the maternal anesthesia induction is the same as a standard cesarean section, invasive blood pressure monitoring is not necessary until the inhalational anesthetic (or inhalational plus intravenous equivalent) is increased to 2 to 3 MAC. Fetal hemodynamics (heart rate, right ventricular contractility) are monitored intraoperatively by continuous fetal echocardiography.[51]

Alternatively, if the interval between induction of anesthesia and the hysterotomy is expected to be prolonged, a substitution or combination with an IV anesthetic (typically propofol and remifentanil) may reduce fetal cardiac acidosis that has been reported with greater concentrations of inhalational anesthetics (most notably desflurane).[160] In the past, large concentrations of inhalational anesthetics would be reinstituted before uterine incision to ensure adequate relaxation of the uterus. An alternative approach is to use total IV anesthesia techniques that may include remifentanil, nitrous oxide, midazolam as general anesthetic agents with IV nitroglycerin for uterine relaxation.[12–14,161] Remifentanil, which moves across the placenta freely, has also been described as an agent for fetal immobilization under combined spinal epidural anesthesia.[162]

Maintenance

Historically, the concentration of inhalational anesthetic (typically desflurane) would be increased to 2 MAC before hysterotomy to ensure myometrial relaxation and tocolysis.[51,163] However, as discussed previously,[12–14] a recent trend is to reduce the use of large concentrations of inhalational anesthetics and substitute these with remifentanil and propofol infusions to achieve similar goals. In either case, satisfactory uterine relaxation can be achieved, but these techniques may variably decrease maternal arterial pressure, uteroplacental perfusion, and fetal oxygenation and may require pressor support.[51,164] Although only small increases in fetal PaO$_2$ occur with maternal inspired oxygen concentrations of 100%, this small increase may be advantageous. Furthermore, the increased concentration of inhalational anesthetic needed for uterine relaxation dictates that only medications that augment uterine relaxation be administered.[165] Given that nitrous oxide does not affect the uterine tone to any measurable degree and thus provides no direct surgical benefit, it seems best to omit it and administer 100% oxygen. However, eliminating nitrous oxide from the anesthetic prescription has given rise to an increase in the incidence of perioperative awareness that should be anticipated and prevented.[166] Maternal eucapnia (PaCO$_2$ of 31–33 mm Hg) is the

physiologic goal,[158] because maternal hyperventilation may lead to decreases in fetal PaO$_2$.[167,168] Some have suggested that maternal hypercarbia can, in fact, increase fetal PaO$_2$.[169] At this time, however, extrapolation of these conclusions to fetal intervention cases should be undertaken with caution.

When recovery from the short-acting nondepolarizing agent has been achieved, additional doses of NMBD should be titrated as needed. If preoperative tocolytic agents were administered, combined with the anticipated administration of magnesium sulfate during the abdominal closure, long-acting NMBDs are best avoided to ensure that neuromuscular blockade can be antagonized at the end of the surgery.

Meticulous attention to maternal blood pressure is essential to ensure adequate uterine blood flow and uterine perfusion; maternal systolic pressure is maintained at 110% of mean awake values with IV ephedrine or phenylephrine. Total IV fluids are limited unless blood loss is excessive to minimize the risk of postoperative maternal pulmonary edema.[170]

Once the uterus has been completely exposed, the surgeons assess uterine tone. Because there is no objective method to assess the degree of uterine relaxation, surgical palpation remains the standard. The concentration of inhalational anesthetic is adjusted as needed, with bolus doses of nitroglycerin administered followed by an infusion to diminish uterine tone. Any attempted surgical manipulation before complete uterine relaxation may increase uterine vascular resistance, reduce uterine perfusion, and place the fetus at risk for hypoxia.

After adequate uterine relaxation, the hysterotomy site is prepared by placement of two sutures parallel to the proposed incision site and through the full thickness of the uterine wall. A hemostatic uterine stapling device is inserted. Once the stapler is deployed, the amniotic membranes are secured to the uterine wall, effectively minimizing excessive maternal bleeding. However, if the stapling device misfires or if the placental edge is mistakenly incorporated into the hysterotomy, significant hemorrhage may occur.

Intervention

The fetal hemithorax and upper extremity are delivered through the hysterotomy. Warm fluids are continuously infused into the uterine cavity from a high-volume fluid warmer to replace amniotic fluid losses, provide a thermoneutral environment for the fetus, and prevent umbilical cord kinking or stretching. Limiting the size of the uterine incision helps prevent fetal evaporative fluid loss, uterine hemorrhage, and postoperative uterine contractions. Once the fetal hemithorax and upper extremity have been delivered into the operative field, fentanyl (5–20 µg/kg), atropine (20 µg/kg), and an NMBD (usually vecuronium 0.2 mg/kg or pancuronium 0.1 mg/kg) are given IM as a single injection into the exposed shoulder of the fetus.[51] Fentanyl is administered for intraoperative and postoperative fetal analgesia and to suppress the fetal stress response, atropine ablates the expected bradycardic response with fetal surgical manipulation, and an NMBD will ensure an immobile fetus during surgery. Although the fetus receives anesthesia from transplacental transfer of maternal inhaled anesthetic, these additional IM medications augment fetal anesthesia and ensure fetal analgesia before thoracotomy.

A pulse oximetry probe can be applied to the exposed fetal extremity. Fetal echocardiography provides information about FHR and ventricular filling, which is particularly useful in those procedures in which fetal blood loss is anticipated (Fig. 38.6). Fetal lung lesions, especially if composed of multiple tissue types,

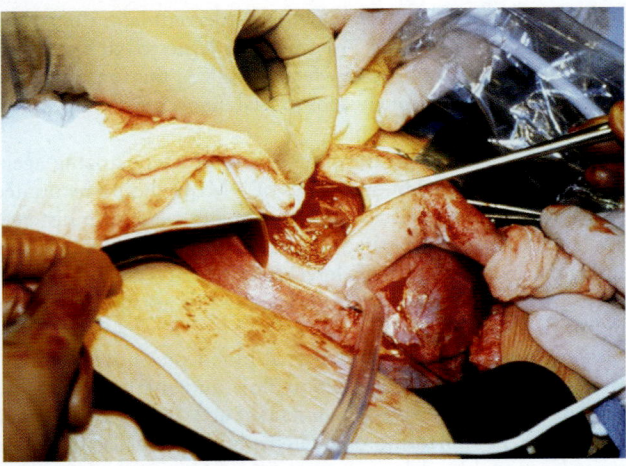

FIGURE 38.6 In utero thoracotomy in a 22-week fetus after excision of congenital cystic adenomatoid malformation. (Courtesy N. Scott Adzick, MD, Children's Hospital of Philadelphia.)

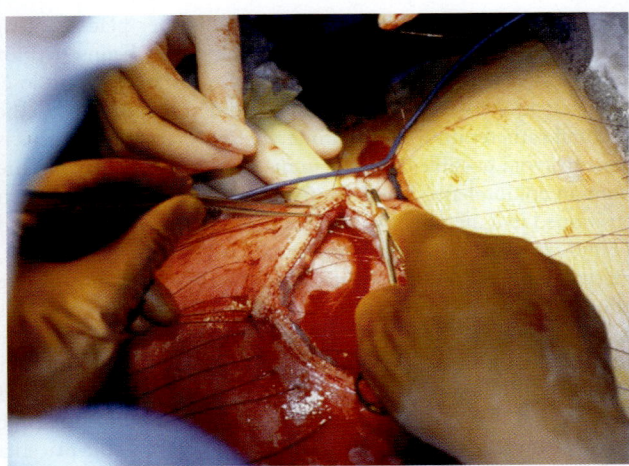

FIGURE 38.7 Hysterotomy closure. (Courtesy N. Scott Adzick, MD, Children's Hospital of Philadelphia.)

may have a very irregular vascular supply, and significant fetal hemorrhage is possible. Direct vascular access in the exposed upper extremity allows immediate resuscitation and blood administration as needed. Even surgical manipulations alone can lead to hemodynamic instability, requiring urgent resuscitation. This may be secondary to mediastinal torsion, resulting in a sudden loss of cardiac preload.

Intraoperative Fetal Resuscitation

Fetal bradycardia (FHR <100 beats/minute) usually results from hypoperfusion with low cardiac output, umbilical cord kinking, or surgical manipulation, but it may also be a result of increased uterine vascular resistance or unrecognized bleeding from the tumor site. Other expected surgery-related complications include blood loss from the tumor, hypothermia, dehydration, and unintended delivery of the fetus. Despite identification and correction of precipitating factors, the fetus may remain severely bradycardic and require resuscitation. Efforts should be made to maximize fetal perfusion and ensure adequate fetal intravascular volume. Maneuvers include confirming maternal FiO_2 of 100%, increasing maternal mean arterial pressure to 15% to 25% above awake values, increasing the concentration of the inhalational anesthetic to minimize the resistance of the uterine vessels, confirming adequate intrauterine volume with warmed replacement Ringer's lactate solution, and identifying the umbilical cord via ultrasonography to verify that twisting or kinking has not occurred are essential to avoiding untoward events. Pharmacologic support may also be needed. In cases with no fetal intravascular access, IM epinephrine (1–2 µg/kg) and atropine (20 µg/kg) can be administered and repeated if necessary. If intravascular access is available, pharmacologic resuscitation should be administered via this route to guarantee immediate effect. In addition, blood transfusions (5–10 mL/kg O-negative irradiated PRBCs) can be administered in cases of severe fetal hypovolemia, by either an upper extremity intravascular route or by percutaneous access to the umbilical vein with ultrasound guidance.

Closure

Once the lung lesion has been resected and fetal well-being is confirmed, the fetus is returned to the intrauterine environment and the hysterotomy incision closed. Closure consists of two separate layers, thus minimizing the risk for postoperative amniotic fluid leak and uterine wall dehiscence (Fig. 38.7). It is important to maintain complete uterine relaxation during closure, because uterine manipulation can alter blood flow and place the fetus at risk of hypoperfusion. Before the last uterine stitches, intraamniotic volume is assessed via ultrasonography and any deficit is replaced with warmed Ringer's lactate solution.

Once the uterine incision is closed, the surgeon begins to close the maternal abdominal wall. At this time, a loading dose of magnesium sulfate (6 g) is administered IV over 20 minutes, followed by an infusion (3 g/hour) that is continued postoperatively. The epidural catheter can be dosed with local anesthetic (15–20 mL of 0.25% bupivacaine) and an opioid (e.g., fentanyl 1–2 µg/kg) as the inhalational anesthetic is decreased or discontinued. Careful attention to the degree of neuromuscular blockade is needed, as magnesium sulfate potentiates the action of the muscle relaxants. Tracheal extubation occurs as soon as the usual criteria for extubation are met.

Postoperative Management

As soon as the procedure is completed, the mother should be monitored by experienced staff with necessary equipment to immediately address any complications that might occur. Ultrasonography is performed in the immediate postoperative setting and frequently over the subsequent week to monitor fetal hemodynamic stability. Tocodynamometers to assess the degree of uterine activity and irritability are used to guide tocolytic therapy.

Serious postoperative complications include premature labor, pulmonary edema, amniotic fluid leak, wound seroma, infection, and fetal demise.[15,51,158,171–173] Virtually all patients experience premature uterine contractions in the immediate postoperative period, thereby necessitating a continuous magnesium sulfate infusion until premature labor risk is significantly diminished. In some instances, additional tocolytic agents may be necessary. Despite maximal tocolytic therapies, continued uterine irritability may result in premature delivery. Amniotic fluid leak can lead to oligohydramnios and significant reductions in amniotic fluid volume that may necessitate replacement. In refractory cases, the mother may need to return to the operating room for reclosure of the hysterotomy incision.

The etiology of fetal demise after open fetal surgery is usually secondary to a primary complication (see earlier discussion). As such, every effort is made to minimize and promptly treat potential postoperative complications to ensure a positive fetal intervention and to provide an environment for a successful term gestation. Surgical stress and pain can lead to release of cortisol and inflammatory cytokines in both the mother and the fetus, which, in turn, may lead to premature uterine maturation and contractions.[174] Maternal pain control can be provided by patient-controlled analgesia and epidural or spinal analgesia. One disadvantage of epidural analgesia is that the systemic opioid concentrations are reduced; therefore less is transferred to the fetus for postoperative analgesia. Maternal IV analgesia improves the likelihood of fetal analgesia. However, IV analgesia does not reliably prevent a maternal stress response. To address this, the optimal choice for epidural analgesia may be a reduced concentration of the local anesthetic with a high concentration of a fat-soluble opioid, such as fentanyl (e.g., bupivacaine [0.05%] and fentanyl [10 µg/mL]).[171]

Other Diseases Eligible for Open Procedures

PULMONARY SEQUESTRATION

Pulmonary sequestration, also known as bronchopulmonary sequestration, accessory lung, or bronchopulmonary foregut malformation, represents 0.5% to 6% of congenital lung disease (0.15% and 1.7% of live births).[33-35] Pulmonary sequestrations consist of nonfunctional lung tissue that does not communicate with the normal tracheobronchial tree and hence does not participate in gas exchange.[34] Pulmonary sequestration may be differentiated from CCAM by investigation of its blood supply. Unlike pulmonary sequestrations, CCAMs derive their blood supply and venous drainage from the pulmonary circulation. A multitude of somatic anomalies have been associated with sequestration, most commonly diaphragmatic hernia. If not treated in utero, these lesions often present as respiratory distress in the neonatal period or as chronic respiratory infections in older children.

BRONCHOGENIC CYSTS AND MIXED OR HYBRID PULMONARY LESIONS

Bronchogenic cysts are embryonic abnormalities considered to be a type of bronchopulmonary foregut malformation.[156] These cysts are thought to result from an abnormal budding of the primitive bronchial tree between weeks 4 and 8 of gestation, thus representing abnormal lung development at an early stage of ontogeny.[175] In most cases, bronchogenic cysts are asymptomatic in the first months of life. A notable exception is a mediastinal cyst that usually manifests as stridor.

Although in utero complications are less likely than with the other fetal lung lesions previously described, the propensity of these lesions to cause life-threatening postnatal complications warrants close attention throughout the prenatal period. Fetal intervention with intermittent or continuous drainage of cysts can prevent the secondary morbidity; definitive fetal surgery with thoracotomy has also been successful.[176]

SACROCOCCYGEAL TERATOMA

SCTs (Fig. 38.8) are one of the most common congenital neonatal tumors (1 per 40,000 live births).[177] A variety of tissues from the three primary germ layers are usually found, and the size of the tumor is quite variable.[178,179] Most SCTs are external, usually protruding from the perineal region. The majority include both solid

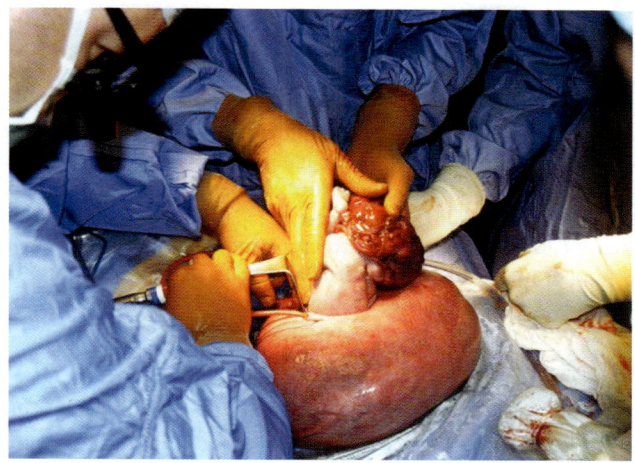

FIGURE 38.8 Fetal sacrococcygeal teratoma before in utero resection in a 22-week fetus. (Courtesy N. Scott Adzick, MD, Children's Hospital of Philadelphia.)

and cystic components, with only 15% being entirely cystic.[180,181] Although usually benign, SCTs can cause significant secondary morbidity in selected cases because of the tumor's mass effect and vast blood supply.[182] With smaller tumors, complete surgical resection usually occurs after delivery under elective, controlled conditions. In extreme cases, the tumor can cause fetal congestive heart failure (usually high output failure), and even fetal demise if no treatment is performed.[131] Death is usually secondary to an enlarged tumor mass and associated polyhydramnios, resulting in preterm labor and delivery, with ultimate survival dependent on fetal lung maturity. Massive hemorrhage into the tumor with fetal exsanguination may occur spontaneously in utero or be precipitated by labor and delivery. Prenatal intervention may be necessary, including intrauterine transfusion or fetal surgery for those fetuses that develop significant secondary morbidity (e.g., hydrops).

Hypoplastic Left Heart Syndrome: Percutaneous and Fetoscopic Procedures

A variety of congenital heart defects (CHDs) may be considered for fetal intervention. To date, the most studied defects include severe aortic stenosis with evolving hypoplastic left heart syndrome (HLHS) and pulmonary valve atresia with an intact ventricular septum with evolving hypoplastic right heart syndrome.[183-187] HLHS and critical aortic stenosis with severely restricted or intact foramen ovale are associated with high neonatal mortality and poor long-term outcome. Prenatal relief of left atrial and pulmonary hypertension may promote normal pulmonary vascular and parenchymal development and improve short- and long-term outcomes. Fetal atrial balloon septostomy, laser perforation, and stenting of the foetal interatrial septum are the current options for fetal therapy.[188]

RATIONALE FOR FETAL CARDIAC INTERVENTION

Most CHDs can be safely repaired in infancy, with excellent surgical survival and long-term prognosis. For these defects, there would be no need for in utero intervention; and for many defects, in utero intervention would not be technically possible (e.g., arterial switch procedure for transposition of the great arteries). For other defects, surgical correction itself may not be possible and the only option is staged surgical palliation, which is often associated with significant surgical morbidity and mortality.[183,189,190] As such, the risk of performing any fetal intervention must be balanced against the potential benefits of improving the anticipated outcome of surgery performed in the neonatal period to correct the specific cardiac defect. It is the intention of prenatal intervention for certain types of CHDs to reverse the pathologic process in an attempt to preserve cardiac structure and function and, thus, it is hoped, prevent serious postnatal disease. A secondary aim of prenatal intervention is to modify the severity of the disease and improve postnatal surgical outcomes.

DEFECTS AMENABLE TO IN-UTERO REPAIR

Certain CHDs cause aberrations in blood flow, which are usually secondary to valvular stenosis or regurgitation. Regardless of the etiology, the end result is often an abnormally developed ventricle.[3] Several case reports have characterized the progression of valvular stenosis to ventricular hypoplasia from reduced flow through the chamber during gestation.[128,191,192] It has been hypothesized that relief of valvular stenosis in utero could reverse the progression toward ventricular hypoplasia. In these cases, there may be a window of opportunity in which ventricular growth can be salvaged. Because most routine prenatal ultrasonographic screening is performed between 16 and 24 weeks gestation, the window of opportunity for prenatal intervention is likely between 20 and 26 weeks gestation.

To date, the defect most amenable to correction is severe aortic stenosis with evolving HLHS.[128,191–193] Without prenatal intervention, severe aortic stenosis can lead to marked left ventricular dysfunction, diminished flow through the left heart, arrest of left ventricular growth, ventricular fibroelastosis, and, consequently, HLHS. Aortic valve dilation may be performed percutaneously with ultrasound guidance. Optimal fetal positioning, placental location, or maternal habitus may require exposure of the uterus through an abdominal incision to obtain ideal access to the fetal thorax. These procedures have been performed with both maternal regional and general anesthesia, although general anesthesia is often preferred to obtain optimal uterine relaxation and an anesthetized fetus. Preliminary results are promising, but larger prospective investigations are warranted to determine long-term outcomes.[48]

TECHNICAL ASPECTS OF FETAL CARDIAC INTERVENTIONS

Open cardiac surgery on the fetus is not presently technically possible.[194–198] In humans, all of the reported procedures to date have been attempted using the transcutaneous or transuterine approach with ultrasound-guided access into the fetal heart.[185–187] Although hysterotomy would provide means for more direct fetal access (e.g., femoral artery, transumbilical or carotid artery access), maternal morbidity would be significantly increased and postoperative premature labor certain. After valvuloplasty, the fetus requires time for the ventricle to recover. Therefore any procedure that substantially increases the likelihood of early delivery would likely be counterproductive.

Although initial percutaneous techniques for fetal cardiac valvuloplasty were performed with only the mother receiving sedation,[185,186] recent advances in surgical techniques have led to the provision of maternal and fetal analgesia and anesthesia.[199] The mother usually receives general anesthesia. After ultrasonographic confirmation of placental location, the maternal abdomen and uterus are punctured with a 22-gauge spinal needle. An IM

injection of fentanyl, atropine, and a NMBD is delivered to the fetus. A 19-gauge needle is subsequently directed into the fetal thorax, and access to the fetal heart is obtained. A small coronary balloon-tipped catheter is threaded over a guidewire through the needle, and passed through the stenotic valve or closed septum. The catheter balloon is then dilated, and blood flow is confirmed using Doppler ultrasonography (Fig. 38.9). The technique has been modified in certain cases, such that a laparotomy to expose the uterus is performed. Using this technique, better ultrasonography and ideal fetal positioning are possible to achieve optimal access to the fetal thorax.

ANESTHETIC MANAGEMENT FOR THE MOTHER

Fetal cardiac interventions are performed using a percutaneous technique or through a laparotomy incision with direct uterine exposure. The surgical approach will vary according to maternal habitus, placental position (anterior vs. posterior), and fetal position. For the less invasive percutaneous approach, the choice of a regional anesthetic accompanied by IV sedation for the mother is preferable for its favorable maternal hemodynamic profile. However, it must be remembered that although the placental transfer of sedative drugs administered to the mother may sedate the fetus, an anesthetized or immobile fetus is not guaranteed and in most cases direct delivery of medications to the fetus will be required. Excessive fetal movement makes most cardiac interventions impossible and even dangerous to both the fetus and mother.

Patients who received an epidural anesthetic technique required significantly more IV fluids but less IV opioid. The administration of large amounts of crystalloid and tocolytics during fetal surgery increases the risk of maternal pulmonary edema.[139,170] Neuraxial techniques (e.g., spinal, epidural, and combined spinal-epidural anesthesia) have been used in other percutaneous and fetoscopic procedures; a T4 sensory-level blockade is required. Neuraxial anesthesia provides no uterine relaxation and no analgesia or anesthesia to the fetus unless supplemented with IV maternal analgesics and sedatives (e.g., fentanyl, benzodiazepines, propofol) or otherwise delivered directly to the fetus. If there is a high suspicion of performing a laparotomy, spinal morphine may be delivered to the mother before the anesthetic induction for postoperative pain relief and resultant suppression of myometrial contractility after laparotomy.[191,192]

ANESTHETIC MANAGEMENT FOR THE FETUS

Anesthesia for percutaneous and fetoscopic interventions, of which fetal cardiac interventions are a significant subset, pose several unique challenges for the anesthesiologist. The combination of immature organ systems and the underlying cardiac anomaly places the fetus at considerable anesthetic risk. Unlike adults and older children, fetal cardiac output depends more on heart rate than on stroke volume. Because fetal myocardial contractility is likely maximally stimulated, the fetus has a limited ability to increase stroke volume. Therefore it is plausible that fetal patients with congenital heart disease and evidence of failure (i.e., hydrops) will exhibit more pronounced physiologic limitations. Notably, anesthetic-induced decreases in contractility, combined with intracardiac catheter manipulation in a structurally compromised heart, can result in fetal hypotension, bradycardia, and eventual cardiac collapse and death. It is generally accepted that neonates manifest a greater degree of hypotension in response to isoflurane and halothane at equipotent anesthetic concentrations compared with older children.[200,201] Because direct exposure of the fetus is not warranted during most cardiac interventions, intraoperative

Normal Heart

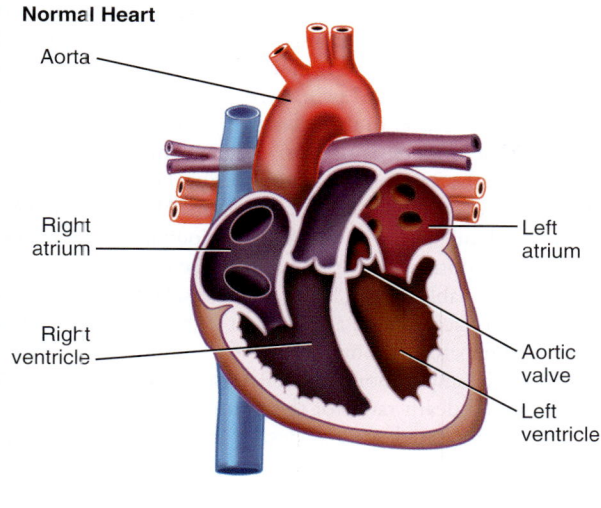

Hypoplastic Left Heart

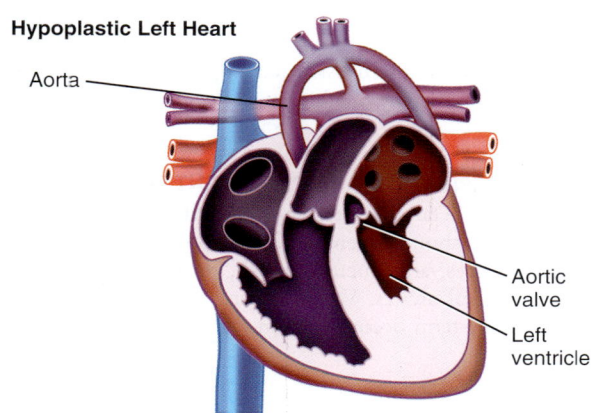

Catheterization Procedure (top view)

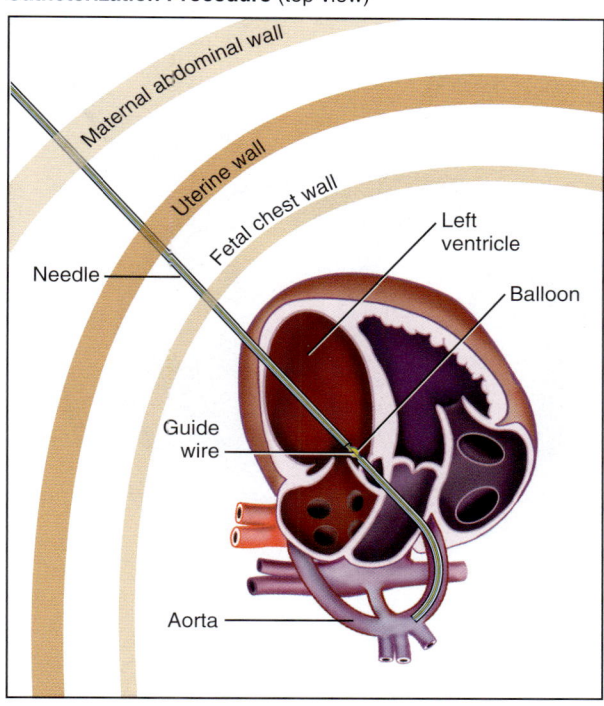

FIGURE 38.9 Technique for balloon dilation of a stenotic aortic valve in a fetus with hypoplastic left heart syndrome. (Reproduced with permission from *Dream Magazine*, Spring/Summer 2002. Boston: Children's Hospital Boston; 2002:20.)

monitoring is limited to echocardiography. An ultrasonographer continually monitors the fetal heart during placement of the intracardiac needle and during catheter balloon inflation. A continuous echocardiogram is also useful for measuring FHR, contractility, and volume status.

INTRAOPERATIVE FETAL RESUSCITATION DURING PERCUTANEOUS INTERVENTIONS

If fetal bradycardia (heart rate <100 beats/minute) or significantly reduced ventricular function develops, resuscitation proceeds immediately. Because direct vascular access to the fetus may not be immediately available, several other treatments can be used. Intracardiac and IM administration of epinephrine (1–2 μg/kg) may be used to treat severe sustained bradycardia. Other maneuvers improve uterine perfusion and hence fetal oxygenation and include increasing maternal mean arterial pressure to 15% to 25% above awake values with volume loading and ephedrine or phenylephrine, and decreasing uterine vascular resistance by ensuring adequate uterine relaxation. Occasionally, pericardial tamponade may impair cardiac function; needle drainage of the effusion may be necessary if the fetus is to survive. If fetal echocardiography indicates a decreased ventricular volume, an intracardiac blood transfusion with O-negative irradiated blood (5–10 mL/kg) may be indicated.

POSTOPERATIVE CONSIDERATIONS

The fetus is monitored postoperatively with intermittent ultrasonographic examinations. The incidence of premature contractions and labor is less after fetoscopic surgery than after open hysterotomy.[37,38] Fetoscopic intervention also appears to have reduced requirements for tocolysis and a reduced rate of premature delivery.[38] (If early delivery should occur, many of these fetuses are considered nonviable owing to their young gestational age [usually <24 weeks gestation] and serious cardiac disease.)

Other Diseases Eligible for Fetoscopic Procedures

TWIN–TWIN TRANSFUSION SYNDROME

Twin–twin transfusion syndrome (TTTS) is a serious complication occurring in 10% to 15% of monozygotic monochorionic twin pregnancies.[202] Although all monochorionic twin pregnancies demonstrate one or more placental vascular anastomoses, TTTS represents a pathologic form of circulatory imbalance between the monochorionic twin fetuses.[203] As a result of this imbalance, a net fetofetal transfusion occurs, from one twin (the donor) to the other (the recipient) (Fig. 38.10). Symptoms develop rapidly and,

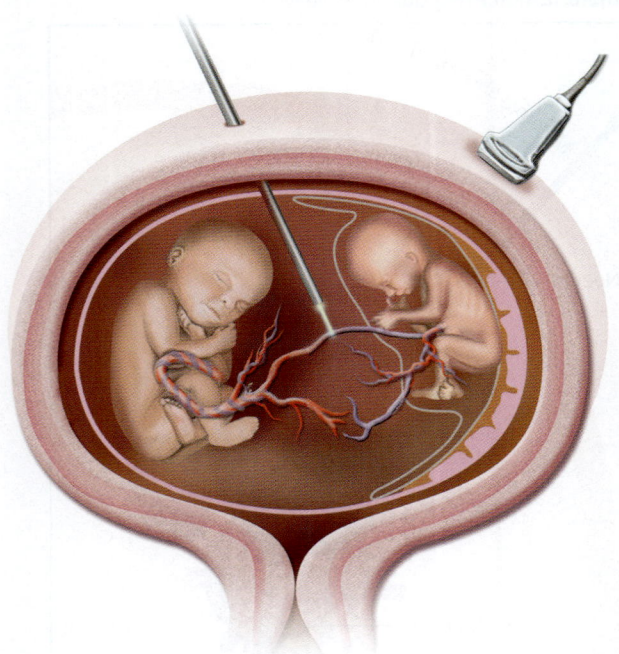

FIGURE 38.10 Schematic representation of umbilical cord ligation in twin reversed arterial perfusion sequence. (Courtesy T.M. Crombleholme, MD.)

in the donor twin, include hypovolemia, oliguria, oligohydramnios, and growth retardation. In turn, the recipient twin develops hypervolemia, polyuria, polyhydramnios, and signs of circulatory volume overload, resulting in congestive heart failure.[202–206] In severe cases, untreated TTTS may result in intrauterine fetal death and miscarriage. Even if twins with TTTS survive, there remains a high incidence of secondary neurologic and pulmonary morbidities.

Fetoscopic laser photocoagulation of the communicating vessels associated with TTTS is based on three fundamental assumptions: (1) the syndrome occurs in the presence of vascular communications between fetuses in a monochorionic gestation, (2) obliteration of these vessels can halt the pathophysiologic process, and (3) both deep and superficial communications can be interrupted at the surface of the placenta.[207] Fetoscopic laser surgical occlusion of superficial communicating vessels is associated with a reported survival rate of 55% to 83% and a reduced neurologic complication rate (5%) among survivors.[202,204]

There are few data on the reported anesthetic techniques used for fetoscopic laser ablation. The procedure has been performed with local, general, epidural, and combined general and epidural anesthesia.[8,208–210] Factors that may influence the anesthetic technique include (1) the planned surgical approach and probability of converting to open fetal surgery; (2) the likelihood of surgical perturbation of innervated fetal tissues; (3) maternal preference; and (4) a history of prior uterine activity. The surgical approach for fetoscopic laser photocoagulation is determined by (1) the location of the placenta (anterior vs. posterior), (2) the position of the fetuses, and (3) the potential window(s) for trocar insertion.[211]

TWIN REVERSED ARTERIAL PERFUSION SEQUENCE

Twin reversed arterial perfusion (TRAP) sequence denotes a common pathophysiology of several different conditions, all of which describe a twin pregnancy in which one twin is normal and the second twin exhibits multisystem malformations, including anencephaly or acardia. The twin with the hemodynamic advantage is denoted as the "pump" twin, perfusing deoxygenated blood in a retrograde direction to the other twin, "the recipient twin." The term *reversed perfusion* is used to describe this scenario because blood enters the acardiac or anencephalic twin through its umbilical artery and exits through the umbilical vein. This eventually places the normal or "pump" twin at a hemodynamic disadvantage because this normal twin provides cardiac output to both itself and the nonviable sibling. This anomaly places the pump twin at risk of cardiac overload and congestive heart failure, often with associated hepatosplenomegaly.

Perinatal complications with TRAP sequence range in severity, with reported death rates for the pump twin ranging from 39% to 59% in untreated pregnancies.[212] Treatment options include observation, medical therapy with digoxin and indomethacin, selective delivery, umbilical cord blockade with a coil, and fetoscopic cord ligation. Although all endoscopic procedures have the primary aim of interrupting umbilical cord blood flow to the nonviable twin, this invasive technique is generally used after failed medical therapy or after signs of cardiac failure in the viable twin.[213,214]

NEEDLE ASPIRATION AND PLACEMENT OF SHUNTS

A variety of fetal disorders may benefit from in utero needle aspiration or shunt placement. These disorders include posterior urethral valves, aqueductal stenosis, fetal hydrothorax, ovarian cyst, and fetal ascites. Various shunts have been attempted to provide long-term decompression, with variable results.[209]

The EXIT Procedure

EX utero **I**ntrapartum **T**reatment, or the EXIT procedure, was initially described as a method for reversal of tracheal occlusion in fetuses with prenatally diagnosed severe congenital diaphragmatic hernia that had undergone in utero tracheal clip application.[215] Although these infants demonstrated no reduced morbidity compared with those who underwent conventional treatment, this novel technique provided a new therapeutic option for fetuses with a variety of potentially fatal diseases. Improvements in prenatal imaging and widespread use of prenatal ultrasonography have increased the identification of potentially lethal fetal structural malformations, which has had a direct impact on perinatal management and outcomes.

Also referred to as the OOPS procedure (**O**peration **O**n **Pl**acental **S**upport),[216] the EXIT procedure allows for a controlled delivery and intrapartum assessment strategy to treat fetuses with certain life-threatening diseases. By maintaining uteroplacental circulation with only partial delivery of the infant, crucial time is provided to perform procedures critical to infant survival. These procedures include direct laryngoscopy, bronchoscopy, intubation, tracheostomy, tumor decompression and resection, and extracorporeal membrane oxygenation (ECMO) cannulation before exteriorizing the entire infant and clamping the umbilical cord (Fig. 38.11). In this way, continuous oxygenation is maintained at all times to the threatened infant, thereby improving the chances of overall survival. The EXIT procedure is now used for infants in whom prenatal imaging suggests a very low probability of survival with conventional treatment methods. This group includes fetuses with known tracheal obstruction and other life-threatening airway abnormalities, as well as those who will likely require

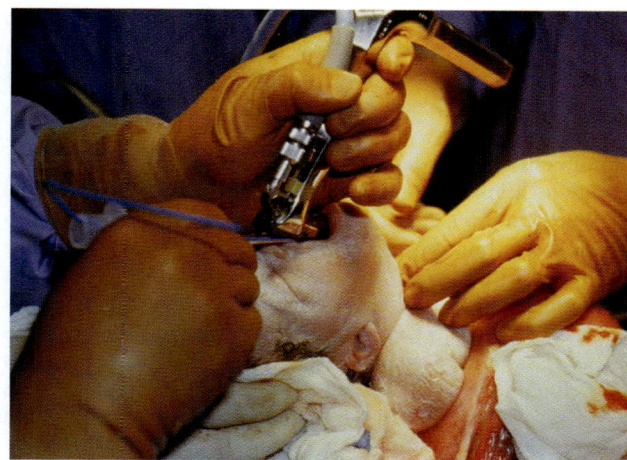

FIGURE 38.11 Fetal rigid bronchoscopy during an ex utero intrapartum treatment procedure. (Courtesy N. Scott Adzick, MD, Children's Hospital of Philadelphia.)

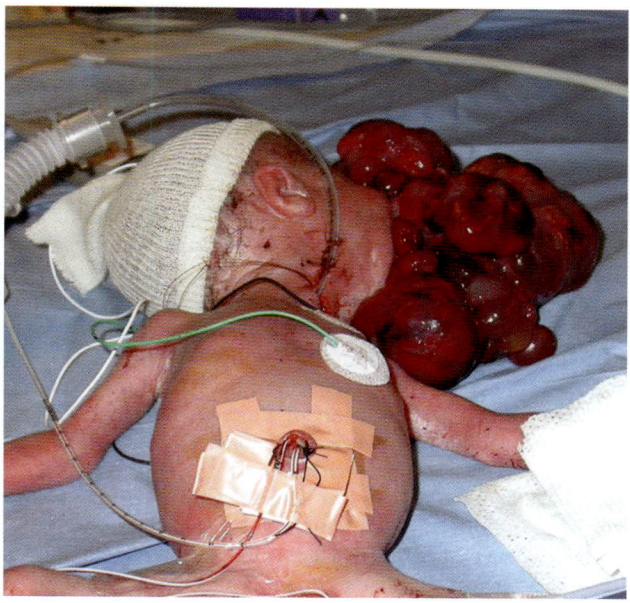

FIGURE 38.12 Newborn with a massive oropharyngeal cervical teratoma immediately after ex utero intrapartum treatment was performed to secure the airway. Immediate resection of the teratoma followed in an adjacent operating room.

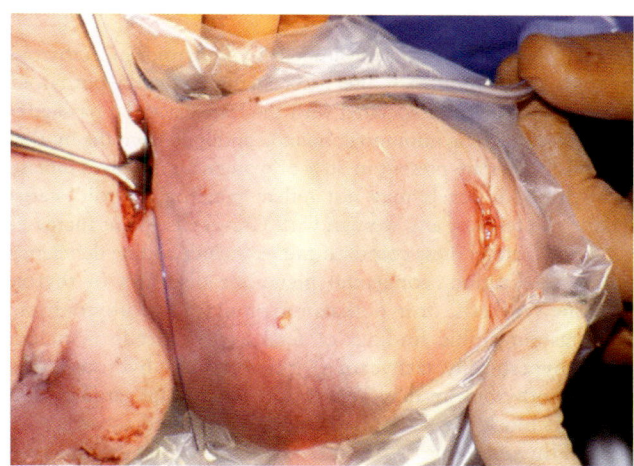

FIGURE 38.13 Fetus (with a cystic hygroma) that underwent ex utero intrapartum treatment to establish a surgical airway before delivery. (Courtesy N. Scott Adzick, MD, Children's Hospital of Philadelphia.)

extracorporeal membrane oxygenation (ECMO) support (i.e., congenital cardiac disease and diaphragmatic hernia).

Unlike many other fetal interventions, however, a planned delivery of the infant is the end result of these interventions. This unique difference creates significant increases in maternal morbidity because these procedures require complete uterine relaxation and serious maternal hemorrhage can occur.[132] An intimate understanding of the EXIT procedure, the fetal pathophysiology involved, and pregnancy-induced alterations directly affecting anesthesia care is required to minimize maternal and fetal morbidity and mortality.

FETAL DISEASES ELIGIBLE FOR THE EXIT PROCEDURE

Cervical Teratoma

Cervical teratomas are rare (1 per 20,000–40,000 live births) and can extend from the mastoid process to the sternal notch inferiorly and to the trapezius muscle posteriorly. They can also invade the oral floor and extend into the anterior mediastinum. Many of the larger teratomas diagnosed prenatally cause maternal polyhydramnios, which is secondary to esophageal compression by the tumor and impaired fetal swallowing. Most of these tumors are benign but are associated with substantial mortality caused by airway compression and difficulty in establishing an adequate airway after delivery (Fig. 38.12).[94] Of neonates with cervical teratomas, 30% die of airway obstruction shortly after delivery[217,214]; for infants whose tumors are not diagnosed prenatally, mortality rates are even greater.[133,159] In addition, some larger tumors may interfere with normal delivery methods and necessitate emergent alterations in maternal care, placing the mother at increased risk.[94,218]

Until recently, treatment options for infants with cervical teratomas who survived the intrauterine period were limited. The standard of care incorporated scheduled cesarean section followed by various airway maneuvers, including the establishment of a surgical airway. Even with skilled help immediately available, dismal outcomes were common.[94,159,217] Despite securing the airway, critical time is needed to perform this task, often at the expense of neonatal oxygenation. With the introduction of the EXIT procedure, precious time is provided to locate the trachea and provide a definitive airway before clamping the umbilical cord,

thereby maintaining continuous fetal oxygenation and decreasing morbidity and mortality.

Cystic Hygroma

Cystic hygromas arise from the failure of the jugular lymph sacs to join the lymphatic system early in fetal development, resulting in the development of endothelium-lined cystic spaces that eventually compress normal surrounding structures. This compression may result in fetal hydrops, including skin edema, ascites, and pleural or pericardial effusions (Fig. 38.13).[133,159] In infants with isolated cervical cystic hygroma and no evidence of hydrops, airway compromise at birth or shortly thereafter is the main therapeutic concern; these infants are candidates for EXIT procedures.

Congenital High Airway Obstruction Syndrome

Congenital High Airway Obstruction Syndrome (CHAOS) is a clinical syndrome consisting of extremely large echogenic lungs, flattened or inverted diaphragms, a dilated tracheobronchial tree, ascites, and evidence of nonimmune hydrops, including fetal ascites, placentomegaly, and pleural or pericardial effusions.[219-221] Airway obstruction may be because of laryngeal atresia, laryngeal cyst, or tracheal atresia. Diagnosis of prenatal CHAOS is confirmed by ultrasonographic evidence of complete or near-complete upper airway obstruction. Most diagnostic findings result from increased intratracheal pressure and distention of the tracheobronchial tree secondary to the accumulation of fluid in the lungs. Cardiac changes include the appearance of an elongated heart, septal shift, and small, compressed heart chambers.[159]

Management guidelines for fetuses with CHAOS are not definitive. In third-trimester fetuses with a diagnosis of CHAOS and no evidence of hydrops, there is most probably incomplete airway obstruction, and management is aimed at establishing an airway before complete delivery. This subset of fetuses would likely benefit from an EXIT procedure.[159,222] Those fetuses with a diagnosis of CHAOS made in the second trimester and those with evidence of complete airway obstruction and/or nonimmune hydrops present a dilemma, because insufficient data exist to determine their best treatment options.

Congenital Goiter

Congenital goiter is associated with fetal hypothyroidism, euthyroidism, or hyperthyroidism. Goiter associated with fetal hypothyroidism is almost always associated with the transplacental passage of a thyroid-stimulating immunoglobulin G antibody from the mother. Such antibodies are present in 90% of women with Graves disease. These antibody levels may not reflect maternal thyroid status, making the fetus of any woman with Graves disease at increased risk for fetal goiter. Less common causes include iodine deficiency, iodine intoxication, congenital metabolic disorders of thyroid hormone synthesis, or hypothalamic-pituitary hypothyroidism.

Ultrasonographic findings of fetal hyperthyroidism include cardiac hypertrophy, tachycardia, or nonimmune hydrops fetalis. Fetal hypothyroidism may be associated with fetal cardiomegaly and heart block. Fetal blood sampling is required to determine the fetal thyroid status.[159,223,224] The possibility of significant airway compression immediately after delivery is similar for all fetuses with goiter. In severe cases, even the presence of experienced personnel in the delivery room may not ensure prompt ability to secure the airway. These infants may benefit from the EXIT procedure; it can provide time to identify and secure the compromised airway.

EXIT TO ECMO

In addition to airway management, the EXIT procedure may be considered for other instances in which separation from uteroplacental support is expected to cause critical cardiac or pulmonary compromise. Fetuses with congenital heart disease who are expected to need emergent ECMO at birth and fetuses with poor-prognosis congenital diaphragmatic hernias may benefit from the "EXIT to ECMO" strategy.[132,225] Neonates undergoing this procedure are partially delivered via the EXIT procedure, and arterial and venous cannulas are inserted while uteroplacental perfusion is maintained. Although congenital diaphragmatic hernia remains

the most common disease entity considered for potential EXIT to ECMO therapy, this technique has been used for neonates with other disease processes associated with almost certain chance of immediate cardiorespiratory collapse after conventional delivery.

Intraoperative Considerations

A multidisciplinary team consisting of an obstetrician, pediatric surgeon, ultrasonographer, anesthesiologist, neonatologist, scrub nurses, and technicians provides the expertise in each respective field to aid in the overall success of the procedure. In cases in which immediate surgical intervention is planned (e.g., resection of a neck mass), a prepared adjacent operating room with separate personnel should be available. A meeting of the entire team is held before the start of the case to clearly identify individual roles and to discuss any concerns or questions. This is also a good opportunity to address any clinical changes, either in radiographic findings or in fetal position, or other factors that may alter the surgical plan.

Uterine Relaxation and Perfusion

To preserve maternal-fetal gas exchange at the placental interface, ensure fetal oxygenation, and avoid life-threatening hypoxemia, it is of primary importance to ensure complete uterine relaxation throughout the duration of fetal uteroplacental support. Factors affecting uterine blood flow include, but are not limited to, anesthetic induction agents, maternal hyperventilation, maternal hypotension, maternal catecholamine release, and other causes of increased noradrenergic activity and uterine tone. Any increase in uterine vascular resistance decreases uterine perfusion, in the same way as uterine contractions do. Of all factors ensuring the overall success of the EXIT procedure, minimal uterine vascular resistance is the most important because decreases in uterine blood flow will cause fetal hypoxia, acidosis, and, potentially, fetal demise.[51]

Surgical Procedure

After the hysterotomy site has been created and hemostasis achieved, the fetal head, neck, and shoulders are delivered. Because many of these procedures involve large neck masses, a generous hysterotomy incision is needed to partially deliver the fetus without injury to the mass or fetus. Furthermore, if a uterine contraction occurs at this time, inadvertent expulsion of the fetus could occur, interrupting the fetoplacental unit and thus critically jeopardizing the viability of the fetus. In some cases, a fetal extremity may be delivered to apply a pulse oximetry probe and to obtain IV access.[174,226] Although the fetus is anesthetized via placental transfer of maternally administered inhalational anesthetics in most cases, additional analgesia and paralytics are administered (e.g., fentanyl, atropine, muscle relaxant). The additional medications may be given as a single IM dose in an upper extremity or can alternatively be delivered under ultrasound guidance before hysterotomy. An advantage to earlier administration is increased time for fetal absorption via the IM route. If peripheral IV access is obtained, additional medications can be given through this route.

ACCESS TO THE FETAL AIRWAY

Most EXIT procedures are currently performed to access a compromised fetal airway before delivery; successful access depends on meticulous preoperative evaluation and careful preparation.[227,228] Portions of the trachea can be completely compressed and distorted such that even successful intubation may result in an inability to achieve adequate ventilation. For this reason, most surgeons perform a direct laryngoscopy and rigid bronchoscopy to examine the status of the fetal airway. In one series, successful tracheal intubation by conventional means was reported in 77% of cases.[132] In those cases in which tracheal intubation is impossible, a surgical tracheostomy can be performed as soon as the trachea is identified. The trachea can be located with the aid of preoperative radiographic studies, often identifying the tracheal location relative to fixed external anatomic landmarks. Gentle surgical palpation may also aid in the identification of cartilaginous tracheal rings. In cases in which the former options have failed, ultrasonography with the sterile probe inserted directly into the surgical incision may help to locate the trachea.[229] When tracheal rings are identified, the trachea may be accessed directly with a tracheal tube by tunneling through the fetal soft tissue, or with the aid of a retrograde wire inserted by the Seldinger technique. The trachea, exposed through a neck incision, may be incised via a temporary tracheotomy to allow passage of a feeding tube or wire from the trachea to the mouth or nose. The guidewire is then attached to the tracheal tube, which is then pulled down into the proper position. After suturing the tracheal tube securely to the mouth, the tracheotomy can then be closed.

Regardless of the method used to secure the trachea, the anesthesiologist must be prepared to control ventilation in the fetus. In some institutions, an anesthesiologist may be scrubbed at the operative field to assume this responsibility. In other institutions, one of the surgeons or neonatologists assumes this role. Adequate ventilation may be difficult to achieve for several reasons. Certain types of tumors—specifically cervical teratomas—may secrete thick mucus into the trachea and this must be aggressively removed before ventilation. As soon as the airway is satisfactorily cleared, surfactant should be administered via the tracheal tube to diminish expected airway resistance. Surfactant is provided for two principal reasons. First, the majority of infants treated for such lesions are delivered at some point before term and their pulmonary development (considered both by gestational age and underlying pathophysiology) cannot be assumed to be normal. Second, the thick mucoid secretions and the aggressive lavage necessary to clear them may interrupt the normal surfactant layering and functionality, suggesting that surfactant therapy may provide a benefit if administered before lung ventilation. These steps should result in increases in fetal oxygen saturation to greater than 90%. If this does not occur, the position of the tracheal tube should be rechecked and the lungs should be auscultated with a sterile stethoscope. Ultrasound examination for the presence of air bronchograms may also be used to confirm tracheal intubation. Ventilation occurs most commonly with the aid of a sterile Jackson-Rees circuit. When adequate ventilation has been established, the fetus can be delivered.

Delivery of the Infant and Maternal Management

Before umbilical cord clamping and delivery, coordination between the surgery and anesthesia teams is crucial to prevent uterine atony and excessive maternal hemorrhage. Because a decrease in the tocolytic agent, whether it is an inhalational or an IV agent, would increase uterine vascular resistance and decrease fetal oxygenation, reversal of the tocolysis must not occur before the umbilical cord is clamped. However, at clamping, a near-total reversal of tocolysis is required to limit uterine bleeding. This is best achieved with an inhalational anesthetic with a low-solubility (e.g., desflurane). As the cord is clamped, the anesthetic is immediately discontinued and oxytocin is administered as a bolus followed by a continuous infusion and titrated to uterine response

(e.g., 40 units oxytocin in 500 mL of normal saline solution over 30 minutes, followed by 20 units over 8 hours). Additional uterotonic medications may be necessary and must be immediately available should uncontrolled maternal hemorrhage occur.[230] These medications include methylergonovine, carboprost, and calcium carbonate. Anticipation of massive and rapid maternal hemorrhage is essential. Appropriate IV access (e.g., rapid infusion catheters, introducer sheaths) with a rapid infusion device in place for blood product administration may be lifesaving, should uncontrolled and persistent bleeding occur. In cases of uncontrolled hemorrhage despite maximal drug therapy, a hysterectomy may be necessary. When maternal hemostasis has been achieved, uterine tone restored, and the placenta delivered, then a low-dose inhalational anesthetic and nitrous oxide can be administered, provided that the mother is hemodynamically stable.

A separate team of neonatologists, anesthesiologists, and nurses should be available for the neonate because additional medications, blood products, and vascular access may be needed. A brief physical examination, confirmation of bilateral breath sounds, and hemodynamic stability must be ensured soon after delivery. In some instances, immediate surgical intervention is planned, necessitating entirely separate anesthetic, surgical, and nursing teams in an adjacent OR as the maternal abdomen is closed.

Postoperative Considerations

Mothers recovering from an EXIT procedure differ from those who undergo standard cesarean deliveries. Potential postoperative complications include wound dehiscence, infection, bleeding, and urinary retention.[132] Although every attempt is made to place the hysterotomy incision in the lower uterine segment during EXIT procedures, those patients with anterior placentas may require incisions in different areas of the uterus. As a result, these patients are at increased risk of uterine rupture in any subsequent pregnancy. Practitioners should also consider the fact that, unlike with a standard cesarean section, the parents cannot immediately interact with or even view their neonates after delivery. Because many of these neonates undergo immediate surgical intervention, the parents' first glimpse of their child will be of an intubated, sedated child with monitors, invasive catheters, and swollen, distorted facies. Continued emotional support, social services, and education will help ease this transition.

Movement Toward Intervention for Non–Life-Threatening Diseases: Myelomeningocele

At present, nearly all human fetal interventions are performed to prevent almost certain fetal demise secondary to a known congenital defect or pathophysiologic process. Myelomeningocele (MMC) is the first nonfatal birth defect to be treated in utero. MMC affects 0.5 to 1 per 1000 live births annually, with variations in both population and geography.[231–233] At least 75% of affected individuals reach early adulthood; most deaths occur during infancy and the preschool years secondary to respiratory and neurologic complications.[234] There is significant risk associated with this early fetal intervention. Many infants with MMC may be delivered prematurely as a direct result of intrauterine intervention, further adding to the risks of an already compromised infant.[233] Some have argued that because MMC is a nonlethal defect, intrauterine intervention for potential reduced secondary morbidity may not justify the significant maternal morbidity or fetal mortality associated with this procedure. However, the severe morbidity associated with MMC combined with the promising results of animal research have led to prenatal intervention for this disorder. Initial human outcomes demonstrated some improvement in secondary morbidity.[233,235,236] The Management of Myelomeningocele Study (or the MOMS trial) demonstrated a reduced need for placement of cerebrospinal fluid shunts and improved motor outcomes (e.g., earlier ambulation) at 30 months in the fetal intervention group, compared with infants whose repairs were deferred until after delivery. Nevertheless, significant maternal and fetal morbidities were reported.[237]

Future Considerations

With the advances in surgical and anesthetic techniques and technologies, significant progress may be made in mid-gestation fetal intervention, and in moving from treatment of only life-threatening fetal pathologic processes toward preemptive management of fetal disorders that are not necessarily life-threatening but have significant, disabling postpartum morbidities. However, these benefits may have to be balanced against the possibility of long-term neurocognitive disorders in anesthetized fetuses, particularly in those fetuses undergoing prenatal repair of anomalies that are not life-threatening, that have been demonstrated in rodents and animals but not in humans.[238–242]

The particular challenges for anesthesiologists are to develop methods to provide selective fetal anesthesia and analgesia, and techniques of targeted uterine relaxation such that safer, specifically tailored anesthesia may be provided to all patients involved in the fetal intervention. Furthermore, techniques and technologies that will enhance tocolysis and retard PPROM and preterm labor will allow increased time for fetuses to heal and mature in utero, while reducing the incidence of postoperative pulmonary edema in mothers. Finally, enhanced fetal monitoring will help the anesthesiologist provide better care for the fetus both in utero and in the postoperative period. With such advances, the provision of fetal anesthesia may become a more routine part of pediatric surgical and anesthetic practice, bringing with it new opportunities for practice and research, and new problems to be solved.

ANNOTATED REFERENCES

Boat A, Mahmoud M, Michelfelder EC, et al. Supplementing desflurane with intravenous anesthesia reduces fetal cardiac dysfunction during open fetal surgery. *Paediatr Anaesth.* 2010;20(5):748-756.
In a retrospective study, Boat and colleagues found that early institution of high concentrations of volatile agents for extended periods before hysterotomy resulted in the development of intraoperative fetal bradycardia, most notably when desflurane was used as the maintenance agent. Based on their findings, they suggest alternative utilization of supplemental IV anesthesia with propofol and remifentanil until just before the hysterotomy incision is made, at which point high volatile-anesthetic concentrations may be used to achieve the desired uterine relaxation.

Fink RJ, Allen TK, Habib AS. Remifentanil for fetal immobilization and analgesia during the ex utero intrapartum treatment procedure under combined spinal-epidural anaesthesia. *Br J Anaesth.* 2011;106(6):851-855.
The authors report three cases of ex utero intrapartum treatment performed under neuraxial anesthesia, with maternal administration of remifentanil used to provide fetal immobilization and analgesia via placental transfer. No clinically significant maternal sedation or respiratory depression were observed. In all cases, the authors argue, remifentanil provided adequate fetal immobilization and obviated the need to administer other analgesics or NMBDs.

Ngamprasertwong P, Michelfelder EC, Arbabi S, et al. Anesthetic techniques for fetal surgery: Effects of maternal anesthesia on intraoperative fetal outcomes in the sheep model. *Anesthesiology.* 2013;118(4):796-808.
Using an instrumented mid-gestational ewe model, the authors compared maternal and fetal hemodynamics, acid-base status, and left ventricular function in the setting of both high-dose desflurane anesthesia and lower-dose desflurane anesthesia with supplemental infusions of propofol and remifentanil. In this crossover design study, high-dose desflurane resulted in more maternal hypotension, reduced uterine blood flow, and greater fetal acidosis when compared with the lower-dose desflurane/intravenous agent technique.

Ngan Kee WD, Khaw KS, Tan PE, et al. Placental transfer and fetal metabolic effects of phenylephrine and ephedrine during spinal anesthesia for cesarean delivery. *Anesthesiology.* 2009;111(3):506-512.
The authors randomly assigned 104 healthy parturients undergoing elective cesarean section under spinal anesthesia to receive infusions of either phenylephrine or ephedrine, titrated to maintain approximate baseline systolic blood pressure. The authors found that, although ephedrine crosses the placenta to a greater extent and undergoes less early metabolism (or redistribution) in the fetus compared with phenylephrine, its associated increased fetal concentrations of lactate, glucose, and catecholamines may favor phenylephrine as the preferred vasopressor for such indications, despite historical evidence suggesting uteroplacental blood flow may be better maintained with ephedrine.

Tran KM, Maxwell LG, Cohen DE, et al. Quantification of serum fentanyl concentrations from umbilical cord blood during ex utero intrapartum therapy. *Anesth Analg.* 2012;114(6):1265-1267.
The authors quantified the concentration of fentanyl in umbilical vein blood drawn following IM injection from 13 human fetal subjects undergoing EXIT procedures. The median dose of fentanyl was 60 μg (range, 45-65 μg) for fetuses with a mean weight at delivery of 3000 g. The median time between IM administration of fentanyl and collection of the sample was 37 minutes (range, 5-86 minutes). Fentanyl was detected in all of the samples, with a median serum concentration of 14.0 ng/mL (range, 4.3-64.0 ng/mL).

A complete reference list can be found online at ExpertConsult.com.

Trauma

39

DAVID A. YOUNG AND DAVID E. WESSON

ANESTHESIOLOGISTS COMMONLY PROVIDE CARE TO CHILDREN who have suffered traumatic injuries of varying complexity. They range from the healthy, older child with an isolated elbow fracture to the infant with a life-threatening epidural hematoma. The anesthesiologist should view the management of children with traumatic injuries as a continuum of care that may originate in the prehospital setting with emergency medical services (EMS), progress to the emergency department, and continue to the operating room, the postanesthesia care unit (PACU), and the intensive care unit (ICU). Anesthesiologists should be integrated into all phases of care of the injured child, with the possible exception of the prehospital setting. The care required to properly manage the injured child may be complex but can be effectively accomplished in a collaborative environment incorporating a standardized process for initial evaluation and management.[1] Anesthesiologists should be familiar with these processes to effectively continue this care into the perioperative setting.

Anesthesiologists provide much needed expertise in the care of injured children. Operative interventions demand the full involvement of the anesthesiologist. In many institutions, anesthesiologists also provide emergency airway and critical care management. In addition, anesthesiologists are highly skilled in airway management, ventilation, hemodynamic resuscitation, metabolic management, and control of pain, all of which can be important in the care of the injured child. Despite major reductions in the overall mortality rate for pediatric trauma within recent years, unintentional injuries remain the leading cause of death and disability in the pediatric population of the United States.[2] Injury has also emerged as the most common public health threat to children around the world.[3]

This chapter reviews the key principles of anesthesia management for children with traumatic injuries. This discussion is intended to augment the principles established in the widely accepted Advanced Trauma Life Support (ATLS) program, which is produced by the American College of Surgeons Committee on Trauma.[4] Additional resources for the management of the pediatric trauma patient include the Advanced Pediatric Life Support (APLS)

course administered by the American Academy of Pediatrics and the American College of Emergency Physicians.[5] Many of the topics discussed in this chapter are currently being investigated to determine the most effective strategy, including fluid resuscitation, evaluation of the cervical spine, and prehospital tracheal intubation.

Epidemiology of Pediatric Trauma

Injuries are the most common cause of death within the United States for children older than 1 year of age[6]; road injuries are the leading cause of death among adolescents globally.[7] Approximately 20,000 children die annually in the United States as a result of trauma. Most traumatic injuries in children result from motor vehicle accidents (the leading cause of death), falls, nonaccidental trauma, drowning, and extremes of temperature. The epidemiology of trauma reflects its continued growth as a significant health risk for children of the world. Table 39.1 lists the death rates for traumatic causes of childhood death within the United States in 2013.[2] Motor vehicle trauma is a major threat to the health of children in the United States. This has spurred research to identify methods to enhance prevention strategies.[8–10] Unintentional injuries consistently rank as the leading causes of death among children older than 1 year of age.[11]

Pediatric and adult injury patterns and their corresponding treatment protocols differ.[12] Head injuries are the leading cause of death among children. One explanation for this is the proportionately larger (and heavier) head of children compared with adults. Thoracic injuries are the second leading cause of death for pediatric trauma patients. Because of increased rib cage pliability from a lack of bony calcification and the presence of a flexible cartilaginous component, severe internal thoracic and upper abdominal injuries can occur in children without obvious external signs such as rib fractures. Blunt abdominal trauma frequently can be treated with close observation, avoiding operative intervention. Penetrating abdominal trauma usually requires surgical exploration. However, diagnostic laparoscopy is being used in lieu of exploratory laparotomy in hemodynamically stable children to evaluate and repair many types of abdominal injuries.[13]

Nonaccidental Trauma

Nonaccidental trauma, also referred to as shaken baby syndrome or child abuse, is an epidemic that continues to grow in virtually every part of the world. Although 3 million reports of nonaccidental trauma are filed every year in the United States, most experts believe that this represents less than one-third of the actual number of cases as many go unreported.[14,15] The youngest children, particularly infants, are the most vulnerable to mistreatment (Fig. 39.1). Every state has stringent laws for reporting nonaccidental trauma. These laws are designed to assist the health care provider who suspects mistreatment and to punish health care providers who do not appropriately report potential abuse and neglect. It is the responsibility of every physician who is involved in a child's care, including the anesthesiologist, to be aware of the potential for nonaccidental trauma in all infants and children and to report all suspicious observations to the appropriate authorities.[16]

Characteristics of nonaccidental trauma include a history inconsistent with the characteristics and extent of the injuries as well as a delay in obtaining medical care.[17,18] Children experiencing nonaccidental trauma have a greater level of injury severity on average when compared with children sustaining injuries from accidental trauma.[19,20] Nonaccidental trauma should be considered when the history appears suspicious. Funduscopic examination may disclose retinal hemorrhages or papilledema, which suggests forceful shaking of the head or increased intracranial pressure (ICP), respectively. Examination of the skin may show bruises, burns, or other injuries in several stages of healing (Fig. 39.2). A skeletal survey may reveal multiple fractures of various ages occurring typically at the metaphysis of long bones. Occasionally, a child who has previously been silent in the company of the parents or caregiver reveals details to operating room or recovery room personnel about the events surrounding his or her injuries. These reports should be carefully documented and conveyed to the appropriate personnel. Mistreated children are often terrified of painful procedures, and the need for sensitivity as well as reassurance in these settings cannot be overemphasized.

The anesthesiologist encountering a potential victim of nonaccidental trauma may be in a position to provide the first impartial assessment of the child's status.[21] Physicians, nurses, and other professionals who provide initial resuscitation may be preoccupied with treating the child's life-threatening injuries. Historical data associated with the event may be inaccurate or fictitious at the time of initial presentation. A careful evaluation by the anesthesiologist in preparation for operative intervention may reveal the first objective evidence of nonaccidental trauma. Indications of mistreatment may be subtle, ranging from lack of parental availability for perioperative evaluation to the irrational refusal of consent for a necessary operative intervention.[22,23]

TABLE 39.1	Death Rates for Traumatic Causes of Childhood Death in the United States (2013)[a]				
	AGE (years)				
Cause of Death	**1–4**	**5–9**	**10–14**	**15–19**	**Overall (1–19)**
Unintentional/ Accidents	8.3	3.6	3.8	17.3	8.3
Assault/homicide	2.1	0.6	0.7	6.6	2.6
Intentional/Self-harm or suicide			1.9	8.3	2.7

[a]The death rate is per 100,000 population within each specified age group. Modified from Osterman MJ, Kochanek KD, MacDorman MF, et al. Annual summary of vital statistics: 2012–2013. *Pediatrics* 2015;135(6):1115–1125.

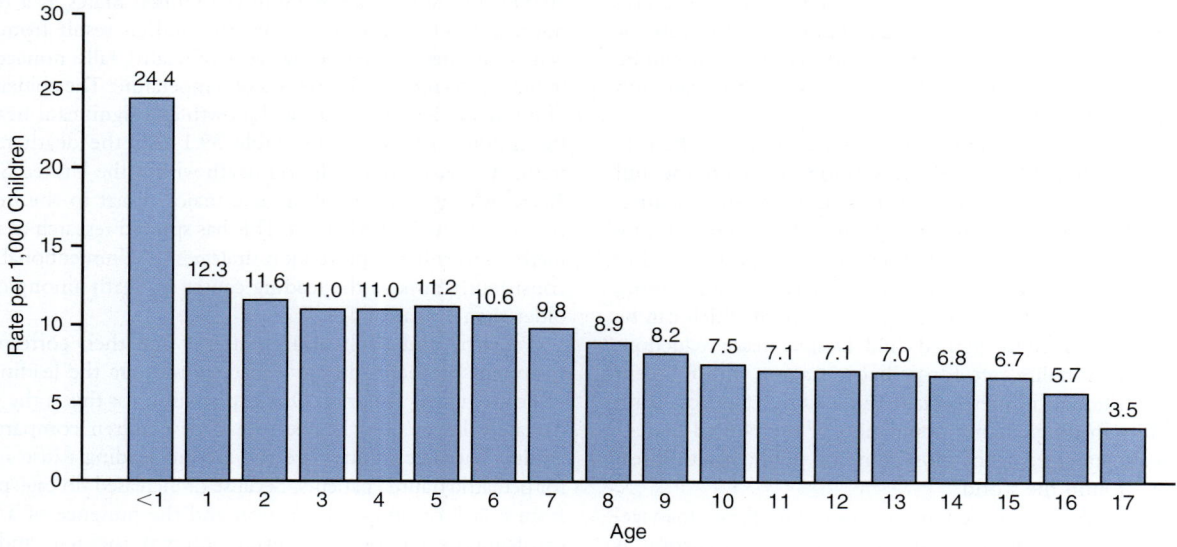

FIGURE 39.1 The rate of maltreatment per 1000 children by age group in years. The youngest children, particularly infants, were the most vulnerable to maltreatment. (Data from the U.S. Department of Health and Human Services, Administration for Children and Families, Administration on Children, Youth, and Families, Children's Bureau; Child Maltreatment 2014. Available at https://www.acf.hhs.gov/sites/default/files/cb/cm2014.pdf#page=65 [accessed June 2017].)

Prehospital Care of the Pediatric Trauma Patient

TRAUMA SYSTEMS

The evolution of pediatric trauma systems has significantly improved outcomes and quality of life for trauma victims.[24,25] Countries such as the United States have a trauma system philosophy more in line with the military approach in which prehospital personnel, such as paramedics, are the first team summoned to make rapid assessments, initiate efforts at stabilization, establish radio contact with the medical facility, and transport the child to the trauma center as rapidly as possible.[26] This philosophy of minimizing the time on the scene and emphasizing prompt transport to the closest trauma center is termed *scoop and run*.

In parts of Canada and several European countries, initial resuscitation of injured children is commonly performed by physicians who are charged with evaluating the child at the scene, securing the airway, initiating resuscitative measures to maintain hemodynamic stability, and transporting the child to an appropriate trauma center. Instituting these management procedures may result in additional time on the scene. This approach has been termed

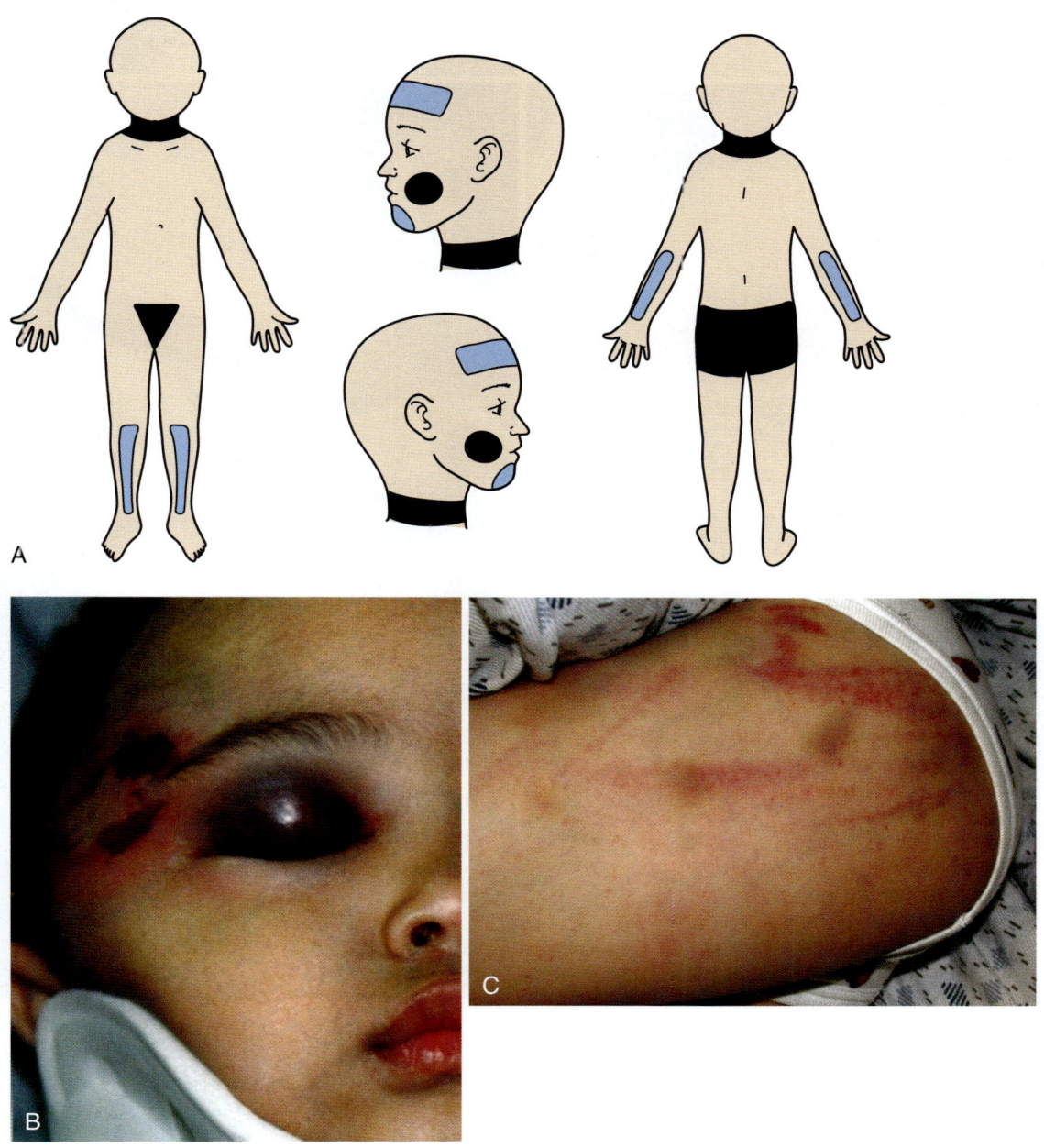

FIGURE 39.2 Common examples of child abuse, also referred to as nonaccidental trauma, are shown. **A**, Typical areas on children where bruising can be detected. The *blue areas* indicate regions where normal bruising may occur. The *black areas* are regions of unusual bruising. Any bruise in the black areas must be considered for possible nonaccidental trauma. **B**, A child with obvious facial trauma. **C**, A whipping injury from a belt plus additional bruises.

Continued

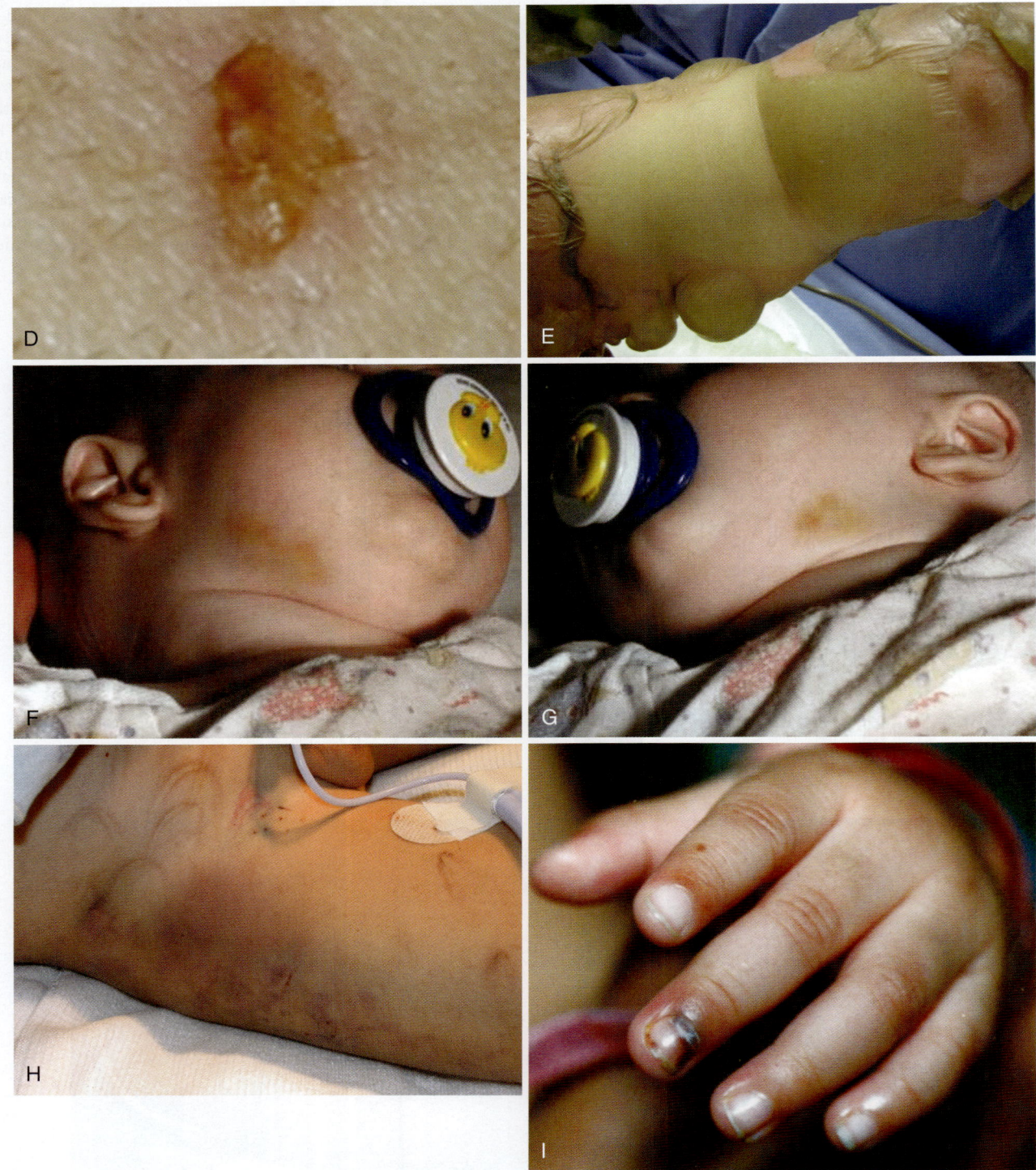

FIGURE 39.2, cont'd D, A cigarette burn. **E**, An immersion burn; notice sparing of the popliteal fossa, which is typical of this type of injury. **F** and **G**, Facial bruises. **H**, Whipping injury from an electrical cord. **I**, Unusual finger injuries in an infant. (Photographs courtesy several child advocates from several institutions who asked to remain anonymous.)

stay and play. Many aspects of this system are being integrated into existing American trauma systems as part of mass casualty disaster management plans.[27,28] The ideal approach is to minimize time on the scene and initiate resuscitation while en route to the hospital.[29]

Developing a systematic approach to the care of the pediatric trauma patient is crucial. This includes acquiring age- and size-appropriate equipment. Broselow and Luten developed a system that provides immediate guidance to identify appropriately sized equipment and drug doses for the trauma victim whose age and

TABLE 39.2 | Modification of the Glasgow Coma Scale for Pediatric Patients

Type of Response	Score[a]	AGE-RELATED RESPONSES		
		>1 Year	<1 Year	
Eye-opening response	4	Spontaneous	Spontaneous	
	3	To verbal command	To shout	
	2	To pain	To pain	
	1	None	None	
		>1 Year	<1 Year	
Motor response	6	Obeys commands	Spontaneous	
	5	Localizes pain	Localizes pain	
	4	Withdraws to pain	Withdraws to pain	
	3	Abnormal flexion to pain (decorticate)	Abnormal flexion to pain (decorticate)	
	2	Abnormal extension to pain (decerebrate)	Abnormal extension to pain (decerebrate)	
	1	None	None	
		>5 Years	2–5 Years	0–2 Years
Verbal response	5	Oriented and converses	Appropriate words, phrases	Babbles, coos appropriately
	4	Confused conversation	Inappropriate words	Cries but is consolable
	3	Inappropriate words	Persistent crying or screaming to pain	Persistent crying or screaming to pain
	2	Incomprehensible sounds	Grunts or moans to pain	Grunts or moans to pain
	1	None	None	None

[a]The total GCS score is determined by adding scores for each of the three sections to predict the extent of neurologic injury: severe, <9; moderate, 9–12; mild, 13–15.
Modified from James HE, Trauner DA. The Glasgow Coma Scale. In: James HE, Anas NG, Perkin RM, eds. *Brain Insults in Infants and Children.* Orlando: Grune & Stratton; 1985;179–182.

weight are unknown (https://www.ebroselow.com/php/static/home.php).[30–33] A folded color-coded tape can be placed next to the child and the height of the child is matched to the color panels on the front and back of the tape (E-Figs. 39.1 and 39.2). The color panel provides weight-based drug doses and other information regarding tracheal tube size and laryngoscope blade size (E-Fig. 39.2). A corresponding color-coded wristband identifies the weight/height category to which the child is assigned. A similarly color-coded crash cart contains appropriately sized airway devices, tracheal tubes, syringes, intravenous (IV) catheter start kits, and other supplies (E-Fig. 39.3). This system is designed to minimize delays, medication errors, and equipment errors.

Dramatic advances in the capability of prehospital providers to initiate resuscitation of pediatric trauma patients have occurred over the past two decades. Part of this progression has been attributed to the development of trauma systems and the commitment of trauma centers to provide more effective medical direction to prehospital providers. Effective management for the continuum of care in trauma patients is optimized if the prehospital personnel communicate the details regarding the child's injuries directly to the responsible hospital-based personnel. This information may include details about the mechanism of injury, traumatic forces involved, time elapsed from the event, loss of consciousness, estimated blood loss, treatment given (e.g., IV access, airway management), and a summary of suspected injuries.

As trauma systems have evolved and emergency departments have become overwhelmed by larger patient volumes, effective triage for the pediatric trauma patient has become increasingly important. Care of traumatically injured children requires the use of personnel and resources from many services, including the operating room and many ancillary services such as diagnostic imaging and transfusion medicine.[34] Inappropriate triage may waste precious time and resources and limit access to patients most in need if every patient with traumatic injuries, regardless of their

severity, is sent to a trauma center. Conversely, failure to recognize a child who needs the resources of a trauma center may increase morbidity and result in preventable deaths.[35–37]

The Glasgow Coma Scale (GCS) and the modified GCS for children (Table 39.2) are the most common scales used to estimate the severity of neurologic injury. The GCS assigns a total score with a range of 3 to 15 that quantifies eye opening, verbal response, and motor function; a GCS score of 8 or less implies severe neurologic injury and the need for placement of an advanced airway. The Pediatric Trauma Score (PTS) was developed to facilitate the initial assessment and triage of injured children by categorizing the overall severity of their injuries (Table 39.3). As trauma systems have matured and prehospital providers have become more experienced with assessment and field management, the GCS and PTS have emerged as effective tools for determination of the need for direct transfer to a trauma center.[38,39]

PREHOSPITAL AIRWAY MANAGEMENT

Providing effective airway management within the prehospital environment has many challenges, including poor access to the child, unavailability of pharmacologic agents, inclement weather, trauma to the face, and demanding environments such as within an ambulance. Several studies of adult patients undergoing tracheal intubation in the prehospital setting have reported an increased incidence of difficult tracheal intubation,[40] the need for multiple attempts,[41] and undiagnosed esophageal intubation. These events have been reported by all levels of providers, including anesthesiologists,[42] although anesthesiologists have more success and fewer complications when performing tracheal intubation compared with other providers.[43–45]

Unsuccessful prehospital airway management in children may be due to a combination of training, experience, equipment, and environmental issues. A significant proportion of the unsuccessful prehospital tracheal intubations results from ineffective operator

TABLE 39.3	The Pediatric Trauma Score			
	SCORE			
Factor	**+2**	**+1**	**−1**	**Totals[a]**
Size (weight)	>20 kg	10–20 kg	<10 kg	
Airway	Patent	Maintainable	Not maintainable	
Systolic blood pressure	>90 mm Hg	50–90 mm Hg	<50 mm Hg	
Central nervous system	Awake	Obtunded or loss of consciousness	Unresponsive	
Open wound	None	Minor	Major or penetrating injury or burns	
Skeletal trauma	None	Closed fracture	Open or multiple fractures	

[a]The Pediatric Trauma Score (PTS) is the sum of all 6 categories. Scoring: minor injury, 12 (maximum); severe injury, <7; uniformly fatal, −6 (minimum).

training and lack of professional experience. Most prehospital providers such as paramedics receive minimal dedicated training in pediatric airway management, insertion of supraglottic airway devices, and tracheal intubation.[46] These providers may not have had an opportunity to either acquire or maintain the necessary skills. Over time, the psychomotor skills required for pediatric tracheal intubation decay, which likely contributes to the increased complication and failure rates associated with tracheal intubation in children.[47]

Guidelines that recommend that instrumentation of the airway be avoided in the prehospital setting may yield similar outcomes to those that recommend intubating the trachea for pediatric trauma patients.[48] For example, the 2015 American Heart Association Pediatric Advanced Life Support (PALS) guidelines state that "*Bag-mask ventilation can be as effective, and may be safer, than endotracheal tube ventilation for short periods during out-of-hospital resuscitation.*"[49] The guideline further states that "*The likelihood of successful endotracheal tube placement with minimal complications is related to the length of training and supervised experience in the operating room and in the field.*"[50] However, if tracheal intubation is performed, it is strongly recommended to utilize carbon dioxide detection devices. The current PALS guidelines state that "*When available, exhaled CO_2 detection (capnography or colorimetry) is recommended as confirmation of tracheal tube position for neonates, infants, and children with a perfusing rhythm in all settings … and during intrahospital or interhospital transport*" (E-Fig. 39.4). Thus many EMS agencies have developed policies based on a scoop-and-run philosophy for pediatric trauma patients that avoid definitive airway management if the transport time is brief and bag-mask ventilation is effective. Several investigators have also questioned whether prehospital tracheal intubation is the best approach in children who require positive-pressure ventilation. The infrequent need for tracheal intubation in pediatric trauma patients has created obstacles for members of the emergency medical teams to maintain their skills. Multiple studies have demonstrated an increased mortality rate or worsening neurologic outcomes for adult patients who received prehospital tracheal intubation compared with those who received standard bag-mask ventilation.[51,52] Several studies focused on children also reported increased complication rates associated with prehospital tracheal intubation,[53–56] particularly in infants.[48]

There is a trend toward using alternative airway devices in the field for adult and pediatric trauma patients. Among the devices that have found support, supraglottic airway devices have proved easy to use with high reliability in the field. Although these devices do not protect the airway from gastric regurgitation and pulmonary aspiration, they may provide adequate oxygenation and ventilation during transport, particularly if traditional bag-mask ventilation is inadequate. One meta-analysis of prehospital alternative airway devices in adults and children indicated that airways (LMAs) were very successful in the hands of anesthesiologists and nonphysician flight crews (success rate 96%) and slightly less successful in the hands of nonphysician clinicians (83%).[57] However, there is no evidence for placement of an LMA in pediatric trauma unless it is used as a rescue device.

Emergency Department Evaluation and Management of the Pediatric Trauma Patient

Anesthesiologists should familiarize themselves with the initial management of pediatric trauma patients in the emergency department because they may be asked to assist in emergency airway management and provide intraoperative care. Rapid establishment of provisional diagnoses and priorities of care is essential in the emergency department management of trauma victims.[58] Most trauma centers use a multilayered assessment system consisting of a primary survey with resuscitation and a secondary survey, followed by definitive management.[1]

Anesthesiologists can provide more effective intraoperative management if they understand the care that pediatric trauma patients commonly receive in the emergency department. During initial resuscitation, a team member should attempt to obtain a history from the parents, the prehospital personnel, and the child if possible. The history should include the usual questions about drug allergies, medications, and past illnesses, as well as inquiries about loss of consciousness, estimated blood loss, and treatment rendered before arrival at the emergency department.

Based on the ATLS program, evaluation of the trauma patient occurs in three progressive steps: primary survey, secondary survey, and definitive care.[4] The initial evaluation of all trauma patients begins with the primary survey. The sequence of the primary survey can be remembered as "ABCDE": **A**irway (A), **B**reathing (B), **C**irculation (C), **D**isability (D), and **E**xposure or environment (E). Many trauma centers have the personnel and resources to concurrently perform several activities and have rooms to accommodate multiple patients simultaneously. In this circumstance, it would be acceptable for the primary and secondary surveys to occur simultaneously—that is, the primary survey (e.g., volume resuscitation) can occur when a part of the secondary survey is being performed (e.g., drawing blood samples).

The primary survey always starts with assessment of the airway. The airway (A) should be evaluated for patency and opened using a jaw-thrust technique if airway obstruction is suspected. Immobilization of the cervical spine should be maintained. The child's breathing (B) and ventilation should be evaluated, and immediate intervention should take place if they are inadequate. Circulation (C) is evaluated by palpation of peripheral or central pulses, blood pressure values, level of sensorium, and degree of skin turgor.

39

TABLE 39.4	The Advanced Trauma Life Support Primary Survey Management Priorities
Priority Level	**Management**
Highest	Airway and cervical spine immobilization
	Breathing and ventilation
	Circulation and hemorrhage control
	Disability and neurologic status
Lowest	Exposure and environmental

Control of external hemorrhage by the application of direct pressure is also part of the circulation phase. Disability (D) is evaluated by examining the child for neurologic injuries and commonly using a neurologic scoring system such as the GCS. A GCS score of 8 or less implies severe neurologic injury (see Table 39.2), and immediate tracheal intubation (with in-line cervical spine immobilization) is strongly recommended (see further). Exposure (E) of the whole child is essential for a complete examination. The environment (E) should consist of a heated treatment area that is ideally prepared in advance of the child's arrival and environmental threats should be determined (i.e., need for chemical decontamination). The ATLS Primary Survey management priorities, listed in order from top (first priority) to bottom, are shown in Table 39.4.

The importance of obtaining an adequate and secure airway cannot be overemphasized. All trauma patients should initially receive 100% supplemental oxygen. The trachea should be intubated in most children with major traumatic injuries using a rapid-sequence induction (RSI) technique with manual in-line stabilization as necessary and appropriate medications or, when it is unclear whether the airway can be secured, while the child remains awake. When increased ICP is suspected, measures to prevent increases in ICP during tracheal intubation should be undertaken. Regardless of the site or mode of tracheal intubation, proper position and patency of the tracheal tube must be confirmed as soon as the child's airway is intubated and again on arrival in the emergency department.[59] Techniques to verify correct tracheal tube position may initially include chest auscultation, direct laryngoscopy, determination of the tracheal tube length from the lips, and the detection of end-tidal carbon dioxide. All children should be monitored with frequent blood pressure measurements as well as continuous electrocardiography and pulse oximetry.

Shock is most commonly the result of hypovolemia in trauma patients. Cardiogenic shock, although rare in children, may also be associated with chest trauma or preexisting cardiovascular disease. Attempts should be made to place two large-bore IV lines that are appropriate for age; if two attempts fail, including femoral access, then intraosseous access is indicated (see also Chapter 49).[60] For the child who is hypotensive, administer a bolus of 20 mL/kg of an isotonic crystalloid solution such as lactated Ringer's solution or normal saline. Fluid administration may be repeated with additional boluses of isotonic crystalloid as required to stabilize the blood pressure within the normal range. Blood products should be considered when the volume of isotonic crystalloid exceeds 40 to 60 mL/kg and the blood pressure remains unstable. Glucose-containing solutions typically are avoided (in the absence of hypoglycemia) because they may lead to hyperglycemia and potentially worsen neurologic outcome.

For traumatic injuries that are primarily located in the abdomen, preference should be made to place vascular access in the upper extremities. Traumatic chest injuries should have vascular access placed in the upper and lower extremities to account for disruption of a major vessel above or below the right atrium.

When the primary survey and initial resuscitation have been completed, a secondary survey is initiated. The secondary survey is a complete head-to-toe examination designed to identify additional injuries not recognized during the primary survey. Frequent reassessment of the vital signs is critical during this phase. If clinical deterioration occurs during the secondary survey, the primary survey and initial resuscitation should be resumed. Head examination should include visual inspection, palpation, assessment of pupillary size and reactivity, and a funduscopic examination. The cervical spine, chest, and abdomen should be evaluated in detail. Chest examination should involve inspection for wounds, palpation for tenderness and crepitus, and auscultation for bilateral breath sounds. The abdomen should also be examined carefully for tenderness, firmness, and external lesions (e.g., gunshot wounds). In children, the physical signs of intraabdominal injuries can be subtle, especially in sedated or neurologically depressed children. The extremities should be inspected for tenderness, bruising, deformities, and vascular insufficiency.

Diagnostic testing is completed during the secondary survey.[61,62] Imaging studies, including computed tomography (CT) scans of the brain, neck, chest, abdomen, and pelvis, may be obtained along with a bedside focused abdominal sonography for trauma (FAST) examination, which is principally used to detect intraperitoneal free fluid but can also be used to identify other life-threatening lesions such as a pneumothorax[63] or pericardial effusion. Standard radiographs of the chest and extremities may also be obtained during the secondary survey. Laboratory studies, including blood cell count, electrolytes, and blood product crossmatching, are completed during this phase. If the child remains unstable despite aggressive resuscitation, the child should be considered for emergent transfer to the operating room for surgical intervention. After the child has been stabilized and all injuries have been identified, plans for definitive care can be made. Disposition options from the emergency department may include admission to the ICU, an acute care bed, an observation unit, discharge home with outpatient follow-up, or transfer to the operating room.

Anesthesia Management of the Pediatric Trauma Patient

Anesthesiologists, surgeons, and other personnel should work as a coordinated team when managing children with traumatic injuries. This collaborative approach can optimize the prompt and reliable identification of suspected injuries so that the anesthesiologist can more effectively anticipate the magnitude of bleeding, physiologic effects, and nature of the surgical procedures. By understanding the appropriate evaluation and initial management of the pediatric trauma patient, the anesthesiologist can recognize injuries that might have been undiagnosed and anticipate the resultant effects intraoperatively.[6]

The approach to diagnosis of and treatment for the pediatric trauma patient is dictated by the degree of urgency. A diagram of the management priorities for pediatric trauma patients appears in Fig. 39.3. For critically ill and hypotensive children who need immediate surgical intervention, resuscitation and the administration of anesthesia may need to be provided simultaneously. The recommended equipment for the management of the pediatric trauma patient is listed in Table 39.5. Basic principles are applied in this circumstance, including establishment and protection of

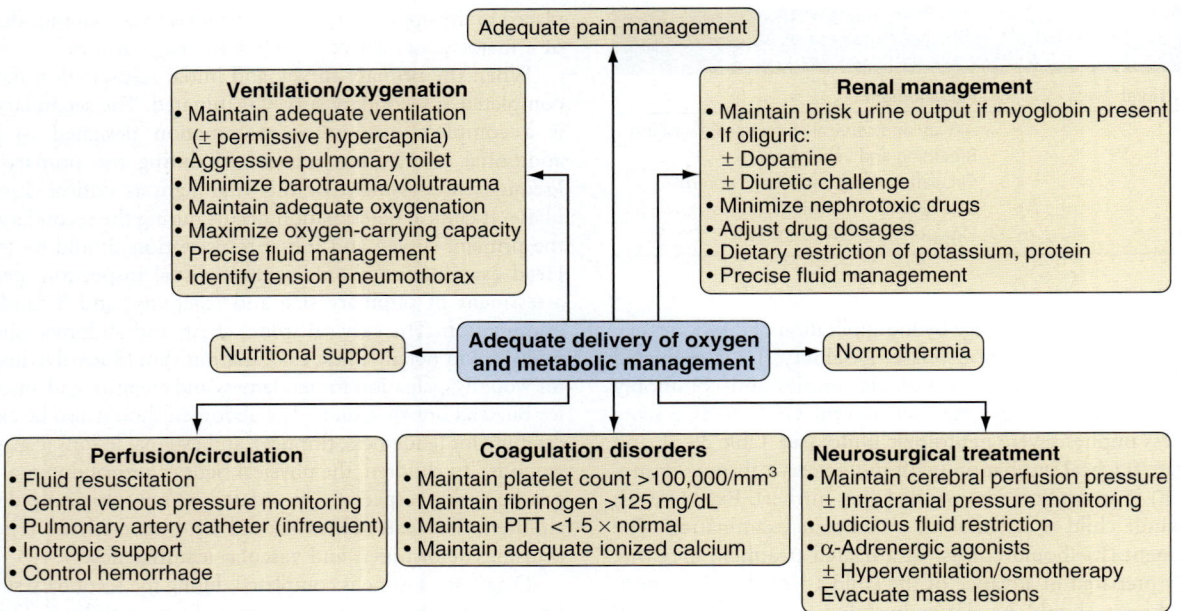

FIGURE 39.3 Diagram of the management priorities for pediatric trauma patients. The primary goals are delivery of oxygen, appropriate ventilation, perfusion to vital organs, maintenance of normothermia to mild hypothermia, stability of renal and neurologic function, correction of coagulopathies, avoidance of overhydration, and meticulous management of metabolic demands. *PPT*, partial thromboplastin time. (Modified from Todres ID, Fugate JH, eds. *Critical Care of Infants and Children.* Boston: Little, Brown; 1996:17.)

the airway, maintenance of adequate ventilation, and support of hemodynamics with fluids, blood products, and vasoactive medications. Establishment of generous vascular access is recommended in the critically injured child; this may necessitate a vascular cutdown or placement of an intraosseous needle (Figs. 49.6 and 49.7) to be used for volume resuscitation. Anesthetic medications should be cautiously administered by carefully titrating the dose to the child's hemodynamic status.

For the child who requires emergent transfer to the operating room, does not have a secure airway in place, and is believed to have a normal airway, induction of anesthesia should begin with preoxygenation followed by IV medications and an RSI technique. If the child is thought to be hypovolemic, a preoperative fluid bolus of an isotonic crystalloid solution (20 mL/kg) should be administered before induction of anesthesia with medications that maintain circulatory homeostasis. If concern exists regarding a possible cervical spine injury, which applies to most trauma patients, the practitioner should also incorporate in-line immobilization of the cervical spine during airway management and all patient transfers (Fig. 39.4).[64] Arterial and central venous line placements should be selected on a case-by-case basis. The anesthesiologist should be vigilant for undiagnosed traumatic injuries that may manifest in the operating room. For a child who is critically ill, surgery should proceed without delay; monitoring may initially include only a blood pressure cuff, pulse oximeter, expired carbon dioxide, and electrocardiogram.

As conditions permit, hemodynamic monitoring with arterial and central venous catheters may be established (see also Chapter 49). Arterial catheters for trauma patients may be helpful in some situations, including concern about the adequacy of ventilation and the need to frequently sample arterial blood gases, the need for frequent and repeated blood sampling (i.e., severe hemorrhage

or metabolic derangements), hemodynamic instability, and the need to alter the blood pressure rapidly. In a setting with significant actual or anticipated blood loss, establishment of large-bore venous access is of much greater priority than obtaining arterial access. Establishment of central venous access may be delayed until hemodynamic stability is established since peripheral venous lines typically can be obtained quickly and can provide effective volume resuscitation. Rotating the neck to place an internal jugular central line in a trauma patient with a possible cervical spine injury should be avoided. Alternative sites should be selected to establish central venous access.

After oxygenation, ventilation, and circulation have been stabilized, the anesthesiologist may need to address additional concerns. If it has not been possible to administer acceptable doses of anesthetic medications, they are administered in stepwise increments after hemodynamic stability has been achieved. Evidence from adult victims of major trauma indicates that recall is more common in these cases. It is reasonable to assume that a similar risk holds true in children.[65-67] IV administration of midazolam is strongly recommended,[68] although a single dose may be insufficient to guarantee amnesia and may contribute to cardiovascular instability. If inhalational anesthetics produce hemodynamic instability, the anesthesiologist may administer a ketamine infusion (titrated to the child's hemodynamic responses), or a total IV anesthetic technique (e.g., high-dose fentanyl and benzodiazepine and vasoactive infusions).

An important principle of trauma anesthesia management is the maintenance of body temperature. Hypothermia occurs commonly in victims of major trauma, especially burn patients, beginning before the child arrives in the emergency department. Hypothermia may potentiate neuromuscular blockade, exacerbate coagulopathy, and contribute to delayed emergence. The evidence

TABLE 39.5	Recommended Equipment for Resuscitation of a Pediatric Trauma Patient

Airway Equipment

Appropriate sizes (neonate to adult) of face masks, endotracheal tubes, stylets, laryngoscopes, oral airways, nasal airways, and supraglottic airway devices

Self-inflating ventilating devices capable of administering >90% oxygen

Anesthesia machine

Difficult airway equipment in appropriate sizes including fiberoptic bronchoscopes, video laryngoscopes, and cricothyrotomy kits

Suction

Monitoring Equipment

Noninvasive blood pressure with appropriately sized cuffs

Pulse oximetry

Electrocardiogram

Capnography

Temperature

Transducers and monitors for direct arterial and central venous pressures

Surgical Instruments

Tracheostomy tray

Thoracotomy, laparotomy, craniotomy trays

Vascular tray

Resuscitation (Code) Cart Immediately Available

Vascular Access Equipment

Intravenous catheters and tubing prepared to administer crystalloids and blood products

Bedside ultrasound device

Intraosseous devices

Medications

Anesthetic drugs

Vasoactive drugs

Other Equipment and Adjuncts

Universal precautions equipment (e.g., gloves, masks, eye protection)

Infusion pumps and pressure bags

External warming devices

Blood-warming devices

Cognitive aids and treatment algorithms

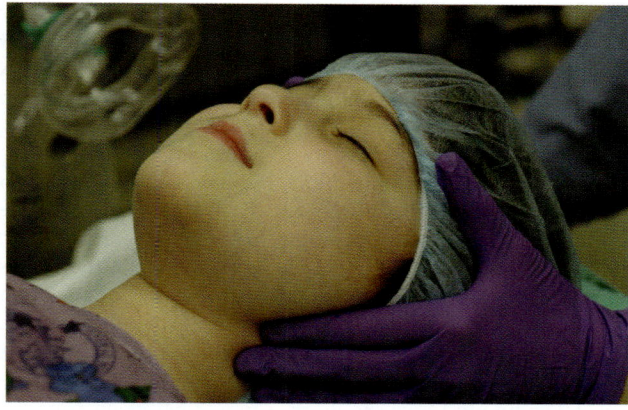

FIGURE 39.4 Cervical spine control must be maintained during tracheal intubation. The child with a known or suspected cervical spine injury requiring a definitive airway should be intubated under controlled circumstances. A dedicated person should immobilize the head and neck during intubation. Oral intubation is the preferred route. Cervical in-line immobilization before attempts at laryngoscopy should occur so that the head is stabilized and prevented from rotating side to side and into flexion or extension.

pneumothorax. Strong consideration should be given to needle decompression or the placement of a chest tube before instituting positive-pressure ventilation in a child with a tension pneumothorax. Chest injuries in children may be overlooked because rib fractures are less common than in adults.[72]

Head injury is the most common cause of traumatic death in children.[73] Although the principles of managing head injuries in polytrauma patients are, for the most part, similar in adults and children, there are some noteworthy differences. In neonates and infants, unlike adults, intracranial bleeding can lead to hypovolemic shock because the head is a significantly larger fraction of the body and the vessel-rich organs receive a substantially greater fraction of the cardiac output in infants and children. The open fontanels in children may provide greater compliance and a potential space for a proportionately larger amount of blood to accumulate. However, the open fontanels may also provide additional protection against initial increases in ICP. A key goal for children with neurosurgical emergencies is maintenance of hemodynamic stability to preserve cerebral perfusion pressure and avoid the development of secondary brain injury. A child with suspected intracranial hemorrhage is at risk for increased ICP. Acute treatment for increased ICP caused by intracranial hemorrhage includes hyperventilation, IV administration of hyperosmolar medications such as hypertonic saline or mannitol, cerebrospinal fluid drainage, raising the head of the bed, and surgical removal of an intracranial hematoma.[74,75]

PREOPERATIVE EVALUATION

Advances in health care have produced an increased patient population with significant preinjury comorbid conditions. For example, children with repaired congenital heart disease may be victims of a traumatic injury. It is common for an acutely injured child to have a preexisting diagnosis of a medical condition such as asthma, developmental delay, seizure disorder, obesity, obstructive sleep apnea, and significant psychosocial issues exacerbated by an unstable home environment. Each of these issues must be carefully considered when planning appropriate anesthesia management and postoperative care.

that moderate hypothermia (34.5°C) might be protective in children with traumatic brain injury[69] is poor.[70,71] Measures to warm the child should be instituted immediately on arrival in the emergency department. These measures include warming all IV fluids and blood products, using forced-air warming devices and heat lamps, wrapping the head and extremities in plastic bags, and increasing the temperature of the operating room. Ideally, the operating room should be warmed in advance of the child's arrival to minimize radiation heat loss.

The features and mechanisms of trauma are different in children than adults. In children, abdominal trauma is more common than thoracic trauma, and blunt traumatic injuries are more common than penetrating traumatic injuries. In thoracic trauma, hemothorax and pneumothorax are common; needle decompression followed by chest tube placement may be lifesaving for a tension

Emergency surgery can be a large source of fear and anxiety for children and their parents.[76] The suddenness of the event provides little time for the child and family to adjust to the crisis and often limits the time the anesthesiologist has to develop rapport with the child and parents. The calm and reassuring anesthesiologist is of great benefit to all parties.

If the child's condition permits, the preoperative evaluation should include a complete assessment. Vital signs should be stable and appropriate for age. Sensorium, urine output, skin turgor, and vital signs can be used to evaluate and estimate the child's preoperative volume status. A comprehensive airway examination should be completed, including assessment of the cervical spine. The past medical and surgical histories, medications, and allergies are recorded when feasible. A list of known injuries and interventions taken up until now should be acquired before entering the operating room. Special attention to fluid management helps to estimate preoperative volume status and assist with intraoperative fluid administration. Assessment should include review of available laboratory reports such as hemoglobin, electrolytes, coagulation studies, and arterial blood gas results. Results from diagnostic imaging studies, including plain radiographs and CT scans, should also be obtained. The suggested items for emphasis during the preoperative evaluation of the pediatric trauma patient are shown in Table 39.6.

Evidence suggests that the gastric residual volume in children undergoing emergency surgery is greater than in those undergoing elective surgery.[77,78] In emergency cases, the size of the gastric residual volume (measured in milliliters per kilograms) depends, in part, on the time interval between the last food ingestion and the injury.[78] There is some reassurance in these numbers, but the anesthesiologist should consider acutely injured children to have full stomachs and take appropriate measures to reduce the risk of pulmonary aspiration of gastric contents.[79–82] The possible value of H_2-blocking agents, metoclopramide, and clear antacids may be considered, although their use in these circumstances is not evidence based.

Premedication for emergency procedures, if indicated, usually is administered by the IV route. Benzodiazepines, such as midazolam, may help to reduce preoperative anxiety. If pain is present, opioids may be beneficial for children who are hemodynamically stable and have no airway compromise. Other than ketamine, anesthetics rarely cause profuse secretions, and the use of antisialagogues before induction should be reserved for specific indications. The administration of premedications to alleviate pain or control anxiety must be balanced against their disadvantages, including the potential for respiratory compromise, increased sedation, or hemodynamic instability.

TABLE 39.6	Items to be Emphasized During the Preoperative Evaluation of the Pediatric Trauma Patient
Vital signs	
Airway/cervical spine evaluation	
Planned surgical procedure(s)	
List of known injuries	
Management since arrival	
Relevant laboratory/imaging results	
Past medical/surgical history/family history	
Allergies/current medications	
Fasting time	

CERVICAL SPINE EVALUATION

Cervical spine injuries occur less often in children than in adults and typically at different spinal levels.[83] Cervical spine injuries in children tend to be located at a more cephalad spinal level than in adults, usually at or above C_3. In contrast to actual injuries, pseudosubluxation of the cervical spine may also be present but is a common and benign finding in children. Pseudosubluxation of the cervical spine usually occurs as the anterior displacement of C_2 on C_3. The physician may need to differentiate benign pseudosubluxation from a true cervical spine injury in the pediatric trauma patient.[84] After consultation with the surgeon, pseudosubluxation can be excluded by placing the child's head in the sniffing position and repeating the radiograph; pseudosubluxation is reduced with this maneuver. In older children, an odontoid or open mouth view can also be considered to evaluate the superior cervical vertebrae. The physician must assume a cervical spine injury exists if the child complains of tenderness in response to palpating the spinous processes of the cervical spine, if the sensorium is decreased, or if neurologic deficits are present. Any of these findings demand a neurosurgical consultation and cervical spine immobilization.

Injury to the cervical spine is less common in children than in adults because the child's spine is more elastic and mobile, and their incompletely calcified vertebrae are less likely to fracture with minor trauma. Nevertheless, the risk of spine injury is increased when the child is subjected to a substantial force from a fall or the considerable forces associated with motor vehicle crashes.[8] Any child with a suspected neck injury should have cervical spine precautions implemented (e.g., placement of a cervical collar). Cervical spine immobilization (see Fig. 39.4) should always be maintained when airway management is attempted. Airway management in a child with a cervical fracture may require up to four individuals: one person to provide in-line immobilization, a second person to perform tracheal intubation, a third person to perform cricoid pressure, hold the tracheal tube, and retract the cheek if needed, and a fourth person to administer the medications (Fig. 39.5).

Challenges in obtaining plain radiographs of the cervical spine include difficulty in obtaining a complete view of the cervical spine below C_6 and the odontoid process. As CT technology has advanced to more rapid and precise imaging, most centers have replaced

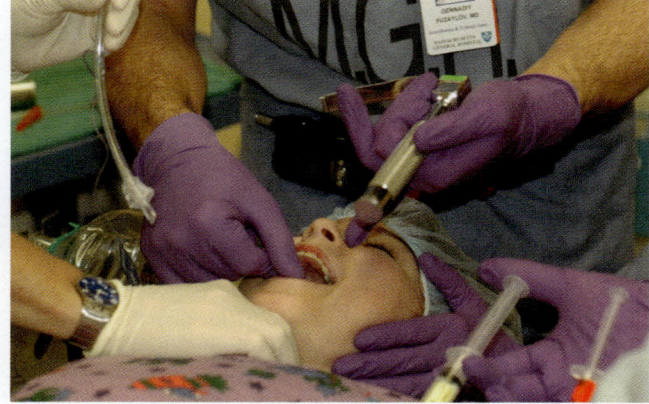

FIGURE 39.5 Intubation of a child with a cervical fracture may require up to four individuals: one person to provide in-line immobilization, a second person to perform tracheal intubation, a third person to perform cricoid pressure, hold the endotracheal tube, and perhaps retract the cheek, and a fourth person to administer the medications.

standard radiographic examinations with CT scans for evaluation of the cervical spine in the trauma patient. The American College of Surgeons updated the ATLS guidelines, stating that a CT scan of the neck can be substituted for a cervical spine radiograph.[4] Replacing plain films with CT scans resulted in a doubling of the rate of cervical spine fractures identified in one study.[85]

It is challenging to rule out spinal cord injuries in children by standard radiography alone because up to 50% of spinal cord injuries may exist without positive radiographic findings. **S**pinal **C**ord **I**njury **W**ithout **R**adiographic **A**bnormality (SCIWORA) has been estimated in as many as 25% to 50% of children with spinal cord injuries.[86,87] These occult cases may reflect ligamentous damage that cannot be detected with standard radiographic examinations or CT scans; however, this ligamentous injury can be visualized using magnetic resonance imaging (MRI), which may require anesthesia care and be performed at a later time because of patient instability.

Imaging must be used in conjunction with the physical examination to evaluate the cervical spine, but the cervical spine cannot be considered cleared of pathology only on the basis of diagnostic imaging studies.[88,89] Appropriate spine immobilization should continue during the intraoperative and postoperative periods if a cervical spine injury cannot be excluded by negative results on an imaging study[90] combined with negative findings on physical examination. The cervical spine cannot be considered cleared if the child is not alert, is nonconversant, has positive neurologic deficits, has midline cervical tenderness, or has a painful, distracting injury. If the cervical spine cannot be clinically cleared in the postoperative period, MRI of the spine should be considered after the child is hemodynamically stable.

AIRWAY MANAGEMENT

Children undergoing emergency surgery are assumed to have full stomachs. They often have considerable gastric contents because of a recent meal,[79] increased acid secretion, delayed gastric emptying caused by pain, trauma, as well as the previous administration of opioids. Many experts recommend using an RSI technique to secure the airway to minimize the risk of pulmonary aspiration of gastric contents. However, evidence-based data supporting this approach are lacking.[91] The anesthesiologist must balance the risks of the RSI technique against the risks of other airway management techniques. RSI may result in the inability to intubate the trachea and rapid oxygen desaturation during periods of apnea.[92] The risks of using this approach must be weighed against the benefit of reducing the risk for pulmonary aspiration. The decision to use an RSI technique assumes that the anesthesiologist has completed an airway evaluation and predicts that the intubation will be uncomplicated and that if mask ventilation is required with cricoid pressure, it will be possible as a backup measure.[93]

In the operating room, induction of anesthesia depends on the child's injuries, condition at the time of presentation, whether the airway has been secured, and anticipated airway difficulty. The most common approach to the initial airway management is to follow a protocol for RSI technique.[94,95] Awake intubation is another approach for airway management but usually is reserved for those with severely depressed consciousness, cardiac arrest, or a suspected difficult airway. The selection of medications depends on individual circumstances (e.g., head injury, hypovolemia, contraindication to succinylcholine) and preferences of the anesthesiologist. Table 39.7 lists the dosages, advantages, and disadvantages of common anesthetic medications used to perform a RSI. Fig. 39.6 presents an algorithm for management of children with multiple traumatic

injuries but without a suspected traumatic brain injury. Specific considerations for children with multiple trauma that includes traumatic brain injury are outlined in Fig. 39.7.

Before RSI is performed, the anesthesiologist must ensure that the proper equipment is present and functioning, including laryngoscope blades and handles, suction, a leak-free anesthesia circuit, an anesthesia machine, monitors, tracheal tubes of appropriate sizes, tracheal tube stylets, and backup equipment such as appropriately sized supraglottic airway devices. If a difficult intubation is suspected, a videolaryngoscope should be present. With the availability of sugammadex (2–16 mg/kg IV), it is reasonable to perform RSI with high-dose rocuronium (1.2 mg/kg) should a cannot intubate/cannot ventilate situation arise.[96] All monitors should be properly functioning, and at a minimum, the pulse oximeter and blood pressure cuff should be applied before induction, even though these monitors may not function properly in a moving, uncooperative child until after induction of anesthesia.

After properly functioning IV access is confirmed, the child's lungs are denitrogenated with 100% oxygen for several breaths (as tolerated). Studies of adult patients demonstrate that oxygen saturation remains greater than 95% for 6 minutes after only four vital capacity breaths of 100% oxygen.[97] Similar studies have not been performed in children, although the rates at which the PaO_2 decreases[98] and the SaO_2 decreases to 95%[99] in infants and younger children after breathing 100% oxygen through a tracheal tube and then performing an apnea maneuver were more rapid than in older children and adults.[100] Even with an uncooperative child, it is possible to increase the PaO_2 by enriching the immediate environment around the child's face with high flows of 100% oxygen. Preoxygenation should not involve forcefully holding the face mask on the awake child; this will likely result in increased anxiety, increased oxygen consumption, and decreased effectiveness of denitrogenation. Premedication (e.g., 0.05–0.1 mg/kg of IV midazolam) in divided doses is one strategy that may alleviate fear and anxiety before induction. All medications intended for use during the RSI should be prepared and labeled along with the doses predetermined for the child's weight and hemodynamic status.

The RSI technique consists of preoxygenation with 100% oxygen and application of cricoid pressure, followed by the bolus administration of an induction agent such as ketamine (2 mg/kg), etomidate (0.2–0.3 mg/kg), or propofol (1–3 mg/kg), as well as atropine (20 μg/kg) if succinylcholine is selected and a neuromuscular blocking agent such as succinylcholine (2 mg/kg) or high-dose rocuronium (1.2 mg/kg). This is followed by laryngoscopy and tracheal intubation. We also recommend the administration of 1 mg/kg of IV lidocaine, before administering the induction agents, to reduce pain from the injection of propofol or etomidate as well as the blunting of hemodynamic responses from airway instrumentation. Positive-pressure ventilation before tracheal intubation is avoided during a "classic" RSI, although many use a "modified" RSI for younger children, which differs from a classic RSI in that it includes manual ventilation at low peak inspiratory pressures before tracheal intubation. Cervical spine immobilization is typically indicated for most trauma patients during RSI (see Fig. 39.4) and requires an assistant dedicated to perform cervical in-line stabilization during laryngoscopy (see Fig. 39.5).

RSI can be a considerable risk for children with cardiovascular problems such as hypovolemia or congenital heart disease. When performing RSI, it may be difficult to select the appropriate anesthetic dose for the child's needs because it may lead to profound hypotension owing to myocardial depression and vasodilation.

TABLE 39.7	Medications, Dosages, Advantages, and Disadvantages of Common Medications Used to Perform a Rapid-Sequence Induction (RSI) in Pediatric Trauma Patients		
Medication	Intravenous Dose (mg/kg)	Advantages	Disadvantages
Atropine	0.01–0.02	Attenuates vagal response	Flushed skin, tachycardia, mild hyperpyrexia; possible sedation/agitation
Glycopyrrolate	0.01	Attenuates vagal response and antisialagogue; lacks sedation/agitation	Longer acting than atropine
Lidocaine	1–1.5	Attenuates hemodynamic and intracranial responses to airway management	Can cause toxicity in large doses (e.g., >5 mg/kg)
Fentanyl	0.001–0.003	Analgesic and attenuates hemodynamic and intracranial responses to airway management	Can cause bradycardia, chest wall and glottic rigidity
Midazolam	0.05–0.2	Sedation, amnesia, anxiolysis, increases seizure threshold, minimal respiratory depression	May cause hypotension when combined with opioids in hypovolemic patients; rarely may cause paradoxical agitation
Ketamine	1–2	Sympathomimetic, used when hypovolemia is suspected, bronchodilation	Increases oral secretions (administer with atropine or glycopyrrolate to reduce secretions), may increase intracranial pressure if $Paco_2$ is uncontrolled, hypotension possible if catecholamine depleted, causes nystagmus
Propofol	1–3	Sedative-hypnotic, some neuroprotective properties, antiemetic, lower intracranial pressure	May cause hypotension especially if hypovolemia present; painful on injection
Etomidate	0.2–0.3	Hemodynamic stability, some neuroprotective properties, used in patients with hypovolemia and cardiac instability	Possible adrenal suppression; painful on injection
Rocuronium	0.6–1.2	Rapid onset/long duration (with high doses), vagolytic properties; is an acceptable substitute for succinylcholine	Intermediate to long duration depending on dose
Succinylcholine	1–2 (precede with atropine or glycopyrrolate)	Rapid onset and ultra-short duration	May cause bradycardia if not preceded by an anticholinergic; may cause hyperkalemia, malignant hyperthermia, and rhabdomyolysis in susceptible children (muscular dystrophy, crush injury, prolonged immobilization, burns, intraabdominal sepsis, and upper and lower motor neuron lesions); may increase intracranial, intraocular, intragastric pressures
Sugammadex	2–16	Dosing to antagonize rocuronium or vecuronium:	Most commonly reported adverse reactions include nausea, vomiting, headache; bradycardia, anaphylaxis, and increases in coagulopathy parameters; not indicated for use in patients with severe renal failure
	2 mg/kg:	At least 2 twitches present with train-of four (TOF)	
	4 mg/kg:	At least 1–2 posttetanic counts but no twitches to TOF	
	16 mg/kg:	No twitches including posttetanic are present; antagonism of neuromuscular blockade quickly, (approximately 3 minutes) after administration of 1.2 mg/kg of rocuronium	

Strategies for dosing IV induction agents in a child with presumed hypovolemia include reduced doses of propofol (e.g., 1 mg/kg) or using agents that are less likely to produce hypotension (e.g., etomidate, ketamine). Conversely, severe hypertension and tachycardia are also possible owing to inadequate dosing during airway management procedures such as prolonged direct laryngoscopy.

Succinylcholine is the neuromuscular blocking agent of choice for an RSI technique because of its rapid onset and short duration of action. A Cochrane review concluded that succinylcholine created superior intubating conditions compared with rocuronium using doses of less than 1.2 mg/kg.[101] However, high-dose rocuronium may also be effectively used as an alternative to succinylcholine for RSI in children.[102] If large doses of rocuronium (e.g., 1.2 mg/kg)

are used in infants and children, the time to achieve a train-of-four recovery to 25% from baseline averages about 45 minutes but can be as long as 75 minutes.[102] It is possible that the duration of action of rocuronium may exceed the planned procedure. Moreover, if the child is unable to be intubated or adequately ventilated, the situation may become life-threatening. The use of high-dose sugammadex (8–16 mg/kg),[103] will reduce the duration of neuromuscular block in these situations, but anesthesiologists should also be aware of several reports of the development of associated hypersensitivity reactions (see Table 39.7).[104] The routine use of succinylcholine for elective tracheal intubation in children has lost popularity among pediatric anesthesiologists because of reports of hyperkalemia-induced cardiac dysrhythmias and cardiac

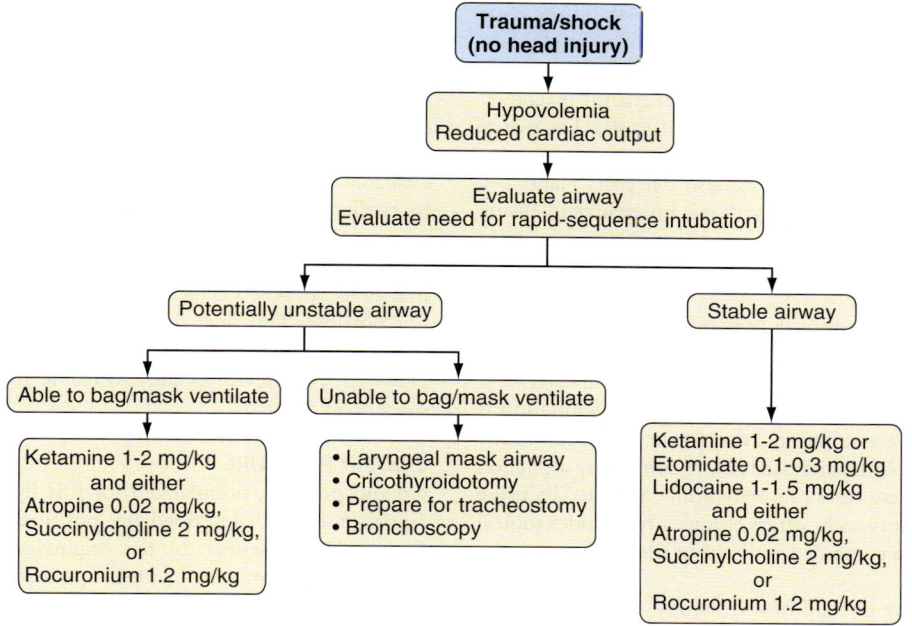

FIGURE 39.6 A proposed algorithm for airway management in children with traumatic injuries but without traumatic brain injury. The selection of medications and airway management techniques should be individualized to each patient. (Modified from Todres ID, Fugate JH, eds. *Critical Care of Infants and Children*. Boston: Little, Brown; 1996:36.)

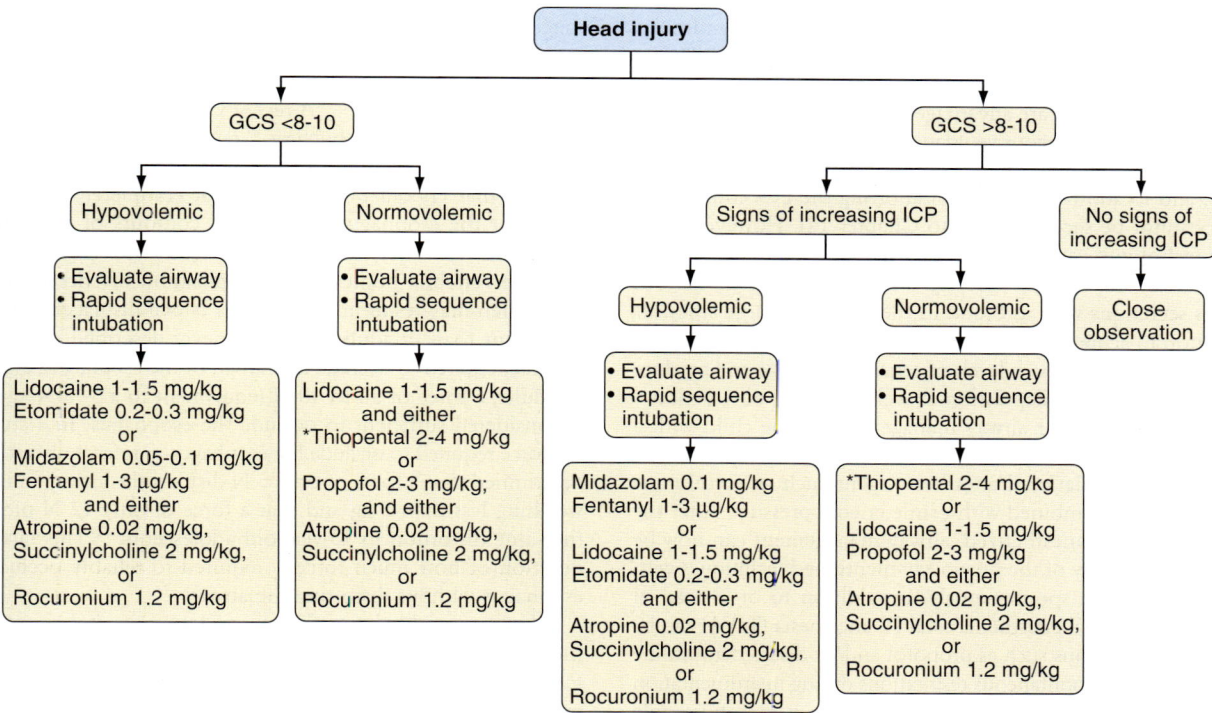

FIGURE 39.7 A proposed algorithm for airway management in children with traumatic injuries including known or suspected traumatic brain injury (TBI). The selection of medications and airway management techniques should be individualized to each patient. *GCS,* Glasgow Coma Scale score; *ICP,* intracranial pressure. *Thiopental is no longer available in the United States. (Modified from Todres ID, Fugate JH, eds. *Critical Care of Infants and Children*. Boston: Little, Brown; 1996:36.)

arrest, which led the U.S. Food and Drug Administration to issue a black box warning about the use of succinylcholine in children undergoing elective surgery.[105] Many of the male children who developed hyperkalemic cardiac arrest were subsequently diagnosed with various forms of muscular dystrophy (mostly Duchenne muscular dystrophy, which may manifest with few clinical signs in boys 8 years of age or younger) (see also Chapters 7 and 24). Whenever succinylcholine is considered, it is imperative to ensure that IV calcium chloride or calcium gluconate is immediately available to antagonize the cardiac manifestations of hyperkalemia should it occur.

Establishing a definitive airway may be required for children with a suspected difficult airway as the result of facial, laryngeal, or thoracic trauma. Alternative approaches for airway management should be considered when difficult intubation or ventilation is anticipated.[106,107] In these situations, the urgency of securing the airway takes priority over the increased risk of pulmonary aspiration of gastric contents. These cases can be typically managed by using an awake intubation approach, which commonly includes topical anesthesia and sedation combined with one of the following airway techniques:

- Direct laryngoscopy or rigid bronchoscopy
- Indirect laryngoscopy using a fiberoptic bronchoscope (FOB) or video laryngoscope
- Supraglottic airway device–assisted tracheal intubation with or without an FOB
- Awake tracheostomy

In the nonemergent situation, the FOB is the gold standard approach to manage a difficult airway. An FOB can be a very effective technique, especially in children with limited mouth opening, restricted neck movement (common in the trauma patient with a cervical collar in place), or associated congenital syndromes that make direct laryngoscopy difficult or impossible.[108,109] Use of a video laryngoscope is also an acceptable alternative. These alternative approaches are advantageous because their main goals are to maintain spontaneous ventilation, to maintain oropharyngeal reflexes to prevent pulmonary aspiration if gastric regurgitation occurs, and to allow the option of aborting the procedure if the airway cannot be secured (see also Chapter 14). However, these airway techniques can be challenging in small children, in those whose airway anatomy is severely distorted, and in those with copious secretions such as blood in the pharynx. Large amounts of sedation to achieve effective patient cooperation during airway interventions may approach levels of general anesthesia and produce significant respiratory depression as well as airway obstruction.

Another strategy for airway management in the child with a suspected difficult airway is to anesthetize the child using a face mask with an inhalational anesthetic agent such as sevoflurane in 100% oxygen combined with gentle cricoid pressure. After the child is effectively anesthetized, airway management can now be performed using any of the previously mentioned techniques with the child breathing spontaneously. In addition to or instead of using an inhalational anesthetic, total IV anesthesia (TIVA) can be used with medications such as propofol and/or dexmedetomidine while maintaining spontaneous respirations during instrumentation of the airway. Alternatively, an infusion of ketamine can provide sedation and analgesia while maintaining spontaneous respirations, although glycopyrrolate may be required to attenuate increased production of oral secretions.

In emergency situations, blind placement of a supraglottic airway device such as an LMA is recommended as part of the American Society of Anesthesiologists' Difficult Airway Algorithm.[110] The LMA does not protect the airway from tracheal aspiration of gastric contents, but it may be used as a conduit to facilitate blind or fiberoptic intubation of the trachea as well as providing reestablishment of adequate oxygenation and ventilation.[111] The development of an LMA ProSeal (Teleflex Medical Inc., Research Triangle Park, NC) with a modified cuff and drainage tube that is available in sizes 1 to 5 may increases the safety of this process by facilitating the evacuation of gastric contents and providing an improved airway seal than earlier LMA devices.[112,113] The Fastrach LMA (Teleflex Medical Inc.) is another type of supraglottic device that is useful when direct visualization of the laryngeal inlet is not possible. This device has been designed to blindly place a tracheal tube into the trachea from within the supraglottic airway.[114] However, this device is only available for children who weigh more than 30 kg.[115]

CRICOID PRESSURE

Cricoid pressure, popularized for RSI by Sellick in his seminal report in 1961,[116] described the position of the head and neck during this maneuver. In the original description, the Sellick maneuver was performed with the patient in the supine position, with the neck fully extended, in a slight head-down tilt, and the nasogastric tube, if present, removed. The concavity of the cervical neck is maintained during cricoid pressure using a firm support placed under the cervical spine. Cricoid pressure is applied by an assistant using the thumb and second finger; the first finger stabilizes the thumb and finger on the cricoid ring. Pressure is applied firmly as consciousness is lost and released only after the tracheal tube cuff has been inflated.

In current practice, the head and neck are often not positioned as described by Sellick. Although Sellick's preliminary evidence suggested that his technique was very effective for occluding the esophagus, no randomized, controlled trials have confirmed its effectiveness or its superiority over other techniques in preventing aspiration during RSI.[117,118] A recent Cochrane review[119] in adults was unable to reach a conclusion regarding the effectiveness of cricoid pressure to prevent regurgitation. Radiologic evidence suggests that cricoid pressure may not completely occlude the lumen of the esophagus because the contours of the vertebral bodies are asymmetric and the esophagus is not aligned directly over the vertebral bodies.[120] The application of cricoid pressure in children may result in even further lateral displacement of the esophagus than in adults.[121] Sellick never described the amount of force required to occlude the lumen of the esophagus, although in adults, a force of 30 to 40 N (equivalent to a 3- to 4-kg mass) is considered sufficient to occlude the esophagus. In a study of the force required to occlude the esophagus in infants, investigators determined that a force of only 5 N distorts the airway in infants weighing less than 5 kg and that a force of only 12 N produces the same distortion in 15-year-old adolescents.[122] This raises the question of how much force is required to reliably occlude the esophagus without distorting the airway.

Many assistants who perform cricoid pressure apply insufficient force,[123] apply force at an incorrect location,[124] or use excessive force that may distort the larynx and make tracheal intubation more difficult. One study found that correctly applied cricoid pressure in children 2 weeks to 8 years of age with or without paralysis resulted in no leak of air into the stomach with up to 40 cm H_2O of peak inflation pressure.[125]

In children, the application of cricoid pressure has been viewed with some skepticism because the force required has been considered excessive in younger children. However, in the current medicolegal climate, many providers have perceived an obligation on their part to perform this technique. In support of this perception, the results of a survey documented that even though 71% do not believe cricoid pressure occludes the esophagus, 90% use it when there is an increased risk for pulmonary aspiration.[126]

VOLUME ADMINISTRATION

Better understanding of the mechanisms of the stress response, and particularly of the factors that contribute to sepsis and ongoing proliferation of proinflammatory cytokines, has helped redefine the immediate and long-term goals of acute resuscitation as well as the definitive management for the unstable trauma patient.[127] The original concept of resuscitation was restoration of adequate circulating volume with appropriate red blood cell mass and adequate oxygenation, but this has evolved to focus on restoration of total body homeostasis. The initial priority is focused on stabilizing the circulation and should progress seamlessly to the aggressive management of metabolic derangements. The anesthesiologist who is involved in immediate resuscitation of the severely injured child should focus on these initial hemodynamic goals.

The preservation of intravascular volume is a primary priority during the initial resuscitation of the severely injured child. When immediate surgical intervention in the operating room is not necessary, it is advisable to replace fluid deficits as much as feasible before induction of anesthesia. Mild to moderate deficits can be replaced with isotonic crystalloid solutions. In severe hypovolemia with ongoing blood loss, colloids such as 5% albumin can be considered for use as an intravascular volume expander along with packed red blood cells. If time permits and if clinically indicated, crossmatched blood products should be administered, starting with an initial dose of 10 mL/kg of packed red blood cells. Type-specific uncrossmatched blood has a very low incidence of transfusion reactions and is typically available before crossmatched blood.[128] In an emergency situation requiring the immediate transfusion of blood products, type O negative packed red blood cells should be administered if the ABO blood type of the child has not been determined. Treatment strategies for managing hemodynamically unstable and actively bleeding adult trauma patients emphasizes rapid transport to definitive care, limits initial surgical interventions and supports the damage control model, uses crystalloid as the initial fluid of choice, and follows an empiric 1:1:1 approach to transfusion with red blood cells, plasma, and platelets.[129] However, the optimal fluid management strategy for trauma resuscitation in pediatric patients has not been established (see also Chapter 12).[130]

Life-threatening exsanguination is most commonly caused by a massive disruption of solid viscera or major vascular structures within the abdomen and chest. External blood loss, typically from the groin, neck, or scalp, can also lead to exsanguination. The most important part of this resuscitation process is restoration of adequate red blood cell mass and circulating volume to promote effective tissue perfusion and oxygenation. Evaluation of 103,434 cases in phases II and III of the National Pediatric Trauma Registry study suggests that massive exsanguination is relatively uncommon.[131] Children who sustain massive exsanguinating injuries typically die at the scene.

There is significant evidence that utilization of massive transfusion protocols (MTPs) improves mortality outcomes and reduces the overall usage of blood products.[132,133] Improvement is likely due to a number of factors relating to human factor behaviors during a crisis,[134] a combination of best evidence practices to reduce the likelihood of coagulopathy,[135] and system organization in reducing delays in blood product delivery.[136,137] Several MTPs have been developed for use in children (see E-Fig. 12.1 and see Chapter 12).

If volume resuscitation is vigorous and large volumes of crystalloid solutions are administered, hemorrhage-induced red blood cell loss may be further exacerbated by dilution. Overzealous fluid resuscitation may worsen bleeding by abruptly increasing the systolic blood pressure that, in turn, disrupts clots from injured vessels. Clinical evidence for this principle has been limited to the assessment of penetrating injuries in adults and elective cardiac surgery, emphasizing the necessity of a proper balance between restoration of adequate peripheral perfusion and avoidance of gross fluid overload.[138,139] Effective circulatory resuscitation of the injured child requires a combination of clinical data, anticipation of future physiologic challenges, and coordination of planned operative interventions by all specialists involved in the child's acute care. Large-volume transfusions without consideration of coagulation status, electrolyte shifts, or critical serum protein depletion may produce coagulopathy. Injudicious or inadequate crystalloid infusions may worsen capillary leak locally within injured organs and remotely in the interstitium of lung and brain. It is postulated that the concentrations of systemic inflammatory mediators increase after traumatic injuries. Increased serum secretory phospholipase A_2 levels have been associated with traumatic injuries.[140] Increased plasma high-mobility group box 1 (HMGB1) levels have also been identified after traumatic injuries, although clear correlations with patient outcomes have not been established.[141]

Injured children tend to be reasonably free of the acquired cardiovascular diseases that complicate the care of injured adults. However, transient myocardial ischemia can quickly undermine contractility of even the healthiest heart. In the presence of cardiovascular collapse from massive or ongoing hemorrhage, this can rapidly lead to cardiac failure and peripheral hypoperfusion. Children who are resuscitated from major hemorrhage and who have been exposed to prolonged low flow states may require inotropic support to maintain adequate perfusion. Since an accurate definition for what was previously referred to as myocardial contusion is not easily quantifiable, a high index of suspicion based on an understanding of the child's mechanism of injury is the best guide to preemptive management, especially if rhythm disturbances or refractory hypotension are observed.[142,143]

Studies are being conducted to determine the ideal products and dosing schedules for fluid resuscitation of injured children; it is possible in the near future that noninvasive continuous cardiac output will provide immediate feedback regarding adequacy of volume resuscitation and/or the need to supplement with inotropic agents[144] (see also Chapter 52 and Fig. 52.9). Several studies have evaluated hypertonic saline for use as a resuscitation solution and for the management of traumatic brain injury[145–147]; recommendations cannot be made at this time since no fluid product has been proven superior.[148–150] However, children with evidence of hypovolemia who are bleeding significantly and receiving isotonic crystalloids probably should be initially resuscitated with lactated Ringer's solution because of its pH of 6.5, compared with a pH of 5.0 for normal saline; solutions such as PlasmaLyte should also be considered since they have a physiologic pH (7.4). The critical objectives during volume resuscitation are immediate control of the sources of hemorrhage, restoration of red blood cell mass to ensure adequate oxygen delivery, and appropriate rheology to enhance tissue microperfusion.

VASCULAR ACCESS

Vascular access can be improperly disregarded as one of the more important priorities in the initial care of injured children. In some circumstances, placement of two large-bore IV lines may be very challenging in the hypovolemic child. In other situations, the child arrives at the emergency department with no vascular access. In the setting of the emergency department or operating room, adequate vascular access can usually be readily obtained by a standard percutaneous approach through a peripheral vein (see Fig. 49.1) or perhaps by direct percutaneous cannulation of the femoral vein (see Fig. 49.5). These two methods are consistently successful in achieving rapid vascular access without resorting to invasive techniques. The success rate for percutaneous femoral catheterizations using a Seldinger technique (see Fig. 49.2) is so high that using a cutdown approach is rarely required. If the child is severely exsanguinated and percutaneous femoral vascular access is unsuccessful, surgical exposure through an incision 1 cm below the inguinal ligament can expose the saphenous vein at the saphenofemoral junction. This provides immediate access to large-caliber venous vessels and also facilitates the placement of a femoral arterial line for ongoing management.

Ultrasound-guided vascular access techniques may also be used to place peripheral and central catheters within the venous and arterial systems.[151,152] Many trauma centers no longer routinely use subclavian or internal jugular veins for vascular access during acute resuscitation. Personnel responsible for airway management usually obstruct access to the neck, as does the cervical collar that should be in place as part of standard prehospital management protocols. In an orchestrated approach, during the primary survey, one individual or group of individuals should concentrate fully on securing adequate access to the vascular system.

Intraosseous infusion devices are being increasingly used in adults and children for whom percutaneous vascular access is unavailable or unsuccessful,[153] particularly within the prehospital setting.[154] In the pediatric population, intraosseous needles are usually placed in the tibial plateau medial to the tibial tuberosity approximately 3 to 5 cm below the knee. These devices can be lifesaving and usually are inserted after several attempts at venous access have failed (see also Chapter 49 and Figs. 49.6 and 49.7). If appropriately placed, they are useful conduits for infusion of all medications, crystalloids, and blood products.[155] Intraosseous needles should be replaced by effective and reliable venous access as soon as possible. One type of intraosseous infusion device, the EZ-IO (Teleflex Medical Inc.) operates like a battery-powered drill and is relatively simple to train providers in its operation and is associated with rare complications (see Fig. 49.7).[156,157]

DAMAGE CONTROL SURGERY

Children with massive anatomic derangements associated with uncontrollable hemorrhage usually require emergent operative intervention. In many trauma centers, these hemodynamically unstable children are initially treated using *damage control surgery*,[158] which is based on the premise that rapid control of abdominal bleeding by placing abdominal packing and immediate coverage of the open abdomen enables more effective resuscitation before exposing the child to a more prolonged definitive repair.

Over the past decade, the use of damage control surgery for the initial stabilization rather than definitive repair has moved the focus of resuscitation away from simple circulatory volume management to a need for immediate correction of whole-body metabolic derangements associated with the stress response.[159] Acute abdominal packing and coverage avoids the development of abdominal compartment syndrome, allows reevaluation of the injured tissue, and provides access for repeated lavage of contaminated spaces. Although there have been concerns that this approach may be used more often than necessary,[160] the risks of leaving an abdomen open are minimal compared with the ventilatory and circulatory consequences that may develop from an abdominal compartment syndrome. Damage control surgery has proved to be a lifesaving technique in isolated circumstances by allowing an unstable child to receive comprehensive resuscitation in a more controlled environment.[161]

PAIN MANAGEMENT

Acute pain that occurs as a result of traumatic injuries is one of the most common adverse sequelae experienced by children.[162] Some practitioners fear that if they treat the pain that follows a traumatic injury, they may mask the symptoms of injury. Historically, adults have received significantly more analgesia after injuries than children.[163] As a result, many physicians withhold significant pain relief, especially opioids, because they fear opioid-related sequelae including respiratory depression or hypotension. All medications used for analgesia and sedation in children can have significant adverse effects; however, careful titration to the desired effect along with appropriate monitoring should ensure their safe administration.

The management of acute pain in the injured child can be accomplished by using nonpharmacologic interventions and pharmacologic therapies. Nonpharmacologic interventions include positive reinforcement, distraction, hypnotherapy, acupuncture, massage and touch relaxation, and guided imagery.[164] Pharmacologic therapies include oral and IV acetaminophen and nonsteroidal antiinflammatory drugs for mild to moderate pain[165] and oral and IV opioids for moderate to severe pain.[166]

Injured children are often in pain at the time of arrival at the emergency department. For unstable children and those with evolving neurologic dysfunction, opioids must be used with caution. In many circumstances, injured children are sufficiently stable to allow judicious administration of opioids. Opioids free of histamine release (e.g., fentanyl) are preferable to those that release histamine (e.g., morphine), especially for children who are potentially hypovolemic. Fentanyl should be titrated in small increments (e.g., 0.5–1.0 µg/kg) to reduce the risk for respiratory depression and side effects such as chest wall or glottic rigidity.

An alternate route to deliver medications, especially when venous or intraosseous access is not initially present, includes the nares. This route can be used until other routes for drug administration are established or in lieu of IV catheters placed solely for minor procedures (i.e., fracture reductions in the emergency department). Nasal diamorphine,[167] sufentanil, ketamine, and fentanyl[168] are commonly used. Improved nasal delivery systems provide accurate dosing and broaden the drug choices (e.g., ketorolac[169]). Drug combinations may show benefits over single-drug therapy. Formulations containing two drugs may improve analgesia by additivity while decreasing adverse effects.[170]

In many cases, regional anesthesia can be used to provide analgesia in the emergency department, as the primary anesthetic in a cooperative or older child to avoid the risks associated with general anesthesia such as pulmonary aspiration, and as a supplement to general anesthesia for postoperative analgesia.[171,172] For example, analgesia for children with midshaft fractures of the femur can be provided by a traditional femoral nerve block or fascia iliaca compartment block, diminishing pain from the femur and quadriceps muscle spasm (see also Chapters 42 and 43). Similarly, an axillary or supraclavicular nerve block may be used in children with forearm fractures.[173] Central neuraxial techniques, such as epidural analgesia, can be useful for children with major thoracoabdominal trauma, including rib fractures, provided no contraindications to regional anesthesia are present.[174] Precise transfer of relevant information with the surgical team is advised so that there are no miscommunications about the ability to perform sensory and motor examinations as well as coordination for the administration of additional analgesic medications.

Future Directions in Pediatric Trauma

As traumatic injuries have become recognized as a significant public health threat, numerous initiatives have emerged to improve prevention of this hazard, management of its victims, and measurement of system performance and outcomes. Exciting areas of investigation continue to emerge in aspects of clinical management, systems development, patient safety, and injury prevention.[175–177]

Prevention and public education are important areas of ongoing research in pediatric trauma. There has been great progress in educating the public that many injuries are avoidable, but there are still many factors that undermine the best intentions to produce a safe and nurturing environment for children. A significant advance in effective prevention and public education has occurred through the Injury Free Coalition for Kids sponsored by the Robert Wood Johnson Foundation.[178–180] This coalition has evolved into a network of more than 30 institutions throughout the country, and each focuses on specific areas of enhanced public education to define opportunities for improvement within the environment of children. Although there is no such thing as a completely risk-free environment, ongoing and effective public awareness campaigns can enhance the likelihood that risks to children throughout the world will diminish.[181,182]

As the transition from fluid resuscitation to metabolic management has evolved, there has been increasing interest in identifying tissue-specific biomarkers that reflect the severity and prognosis of injury.[183,184] The efficacy of resuscitation may be enhanced by the routine assay of biomarkers that accurately reflects the levels of physiologic derangements or effective restoration of homeostasis. Numerous studies are focusing on identification of various components of neuronal tissue markers that reflect the presence and severity of traumatic brain injury.[185]

The combination of hypovolemia, coagulopathy, hypothermia, and acidosis are associated with increased morbidity and mortality. There have been many efforts to control these issues,[186] and most significant has been the evolution of damage control surgery. There is growing laboratory animal evidence that hypothermia, if induced in a rapid and controlled fashion, is cytoprotective.[69,187–189] However, a recent meta-analysis found no benefit from therapeutic hypothermia in children with traumatic brain injury.[190] This is an area that must make the transition from animal observations in the basic science laboratory to well-designed, randomized, controlled trials involving prehospital providers and established trauma programs. Emerging evidence also suggests that premature death in bleeding patients with severe trauma may be attenuated by administering antifibrinolytics, such as tranexamic acid.[191–193] Institution of tranexamic acid within 3 hours of the insult, particularly in countries with low to middle incomes, is likely to have the greatest impact on outcome. However, there is insufficient evidence to recommend antifibrinolytics in patients with traumatic brain injury,[194] although clinical research has demonstrated a reduction in mortality with early use of tranexamic acid in adult trauma patients.[195] Randomized, controlled trials enrolling traumatized children are warranted to identify a possible role for antifibrinolytics to prevent premature death.

Summary

Trauma remains the most common cause of death for children older than 1 year of age. Pediatric patients develop unique traumatic injuries compared with adults, resulting in the need for specific knowledge and specialized anesthesia management. Anesthesiologists may function in several essential roles in the perioperative management of the pediatric trauma patient. They may provide emergent airway management in the emergency department, intraoperative care in the operating room, and anesthesia and pain control in the ICU. The transition from acute resuscitation to definitive care should be a seamless continuum focusing on immediate recognition of threats to life, rapid restoration of homeostasis, definitive treatment of injuries, and effective rehabilitation and convalescence.

Care of the trauma patient is a perfect example of a team-driven approach that requires thoughtful coordination and adherence to established protocols. The investment of time necessary to master this level of multidisciplinary, comprehensive care produces immense returns in diminished mortality and enhanced quality of life for all children.

ACKNOWLEDGMENT
We thank J. Tepas, MD, and H. DeSoto, MD, for their prior contributions to this chapter.

ANNOTATED REFERENCES

Bhalla T, Dewhirst E, Sawardekar A, et al. Perioperative management of the pediatric patient with traumatic brain injury. *Paediatr Anaesth.* 2012;22(7):627-640.
This review presents the current evidence-based medicine regarding the perioperative care of pediatric patients with traumatic brain injury including initial stabilization, airway management, intraoperative mechanical ventilation, hemodynamic support, administration of blood products, and choice of anesthetic technique.

De Ross AL, Vane DW. Early evaluation and resuscitation of the pediatric trauma patient. *Semin Pediatr Surg.* 2004;13:74-79.
This review article focuses on the initial management of the pediatric trauma patient.

Jagannathan N, Ramsey MA, White MC, Sohn L. An update on newer pediatric supraglottic airways with recommendations for clinical use. *Paediatr Anaesth.* 2015;25(4):334-345.
This review presents the current literature on pediatric supraglottic airways and provides recommendations for their use in various clinical scenarios.

Ross AK. Pediatric trauma. Anesthesia management. *Anesthesiol Clin North Am.* 2001;19:309-337.
This article reviews the perioperative implications for managing pediatric trauma patients.

Suresh S, Birmingham PK, Kozlowski RJ. Pediatric pain management. *Anesthesiol Clin.* 2012;30(1):101-117.
This review discusses a comprehensive strategy for the acute pain management in infants, children, and adolescents using regional anesthesia.

A complete reference list can be found online at ExpertConsult.com.

40 Cardiopulmonary Resuscitation

SANDEEP GANGADHARAN, POOJA NAWATHE, AND CHARLES L. SCHLEIEN

THE PEDIATRIC ANESTHESIOLOGIST must be prepared to resuscitate a child who suffers a cardiac arrest in the course of a routine elective anesthetic, during a high-risk surgery, or outside the operating room (OR) during the delivery of an anesthetic or as a vital part of the "code team." The goal of this chapter is to provide pediatric anesthesiologists with an in-depth understanding of cardiopulmonary-cerebral resuscitation physiology and the current recommended resuscitative strategies.

Historical Background

In 1814, a description in poetical form of the Rules of the Humane Society for recovering drowned persons included the following description of mouth-to-mouth resuscitation[1]:

Let one the mouth, and either nostril close
While through the other the bellows gently blows.
Thus the pure air with steady force convey,
To put the flaccid lungs again in play.
Should bellows not be found, or found too late,
Let some kind soul with willing mouth inflate;

Then downward, though but lightly, press the chest.
And let the inflated air be upward prest.

External cardiac massage was successfully performed more than 100 years ago in two children (ages 8 and 13 years) after circulatory arrest precipitated by chloroform anesthesia during a surgical procedure.[2] In 1904, Crile described the effectiveness of external cardiac compressions in maintaining the circulation of dogs.[3]

After multiple reports that attested to the effectiveness of mouth-to-mouth resuscitation,[4–6] in 1958 the National Academy of Sciences National Research Council recommended mouth-to-mouth resuscitation with maximum backward tilt of the head as the preferred technique for all individuals requiring emergency artificial ventilation. In 1960, external cardiac compression was revived as a resuscitation technique when its effectiveness[7] was demonstrated when combined with artificial respirations. Many of the patients had sustained cardiac arrest during anesthesia. Before this study, internal cardiac compression was the accepted technique, with its effectiveness demonstrated by experience in cardiac bypass surgery. In 1947, the first successful internal defibrillation of a human heart was performed,[8] and in 1956, the first successful external defibrillation was performed.[9]

Epidemiology, Prevention, and Outcome of In-Hospital Cardiopulmonary Arrest

A 2009 review of cardiac arrest events submitted to the National Registry of Cardiopulmonary Circulation included 3342 pediatric events, excluding events in a delivery room or neonatal intensive care unit (NICU).[10] Seventy-three percent of the inpatient cardiac arrests had occurred in an ICU, 7% in a general inpatient area, 11% in an emergency department, and 3% in an OR or postanesthesia care unit. Return of spontaneous circulation (ROSC) was achieved in 65%, 24-hour survival occurred in 47%, and 30% of children survived until hospital discharge. Other large series of in-hospital pediatric cardiac arrest reported that between 14% and 44% survived until hospital discharge[11–14] with the 44% survival rate from cardiac arrests that had occurred in a pediatric cardiac ICU. In another multicenter cohort study of in-hospital pediatric cardiac arrest,[15] 48.7% of the 353 children survived until hospital discharge. Survivors had greater body temperatures, greater pH values, and reduced serum lactate concentrations compared with nonsurvivors. Nonsurvivors were more likely to have had a tracheal tube before the arrest and to have received sodium bicarbonate, calcium, and vasopressin during the arrest. In this study, postoperative cardiopulmonary resuscitation (CPR) was associated with decreased mortality. In a retrospective review of more than 29,000 discharges with in-hospital cardiac arrest between 1997 and 2012 revealed a discharge survival of 54% overall, having increased from 49% in 1997 to 60% in 2012.[16] The incidence of in-hospital cardiac arrest was greater for males, neonates and infants, African American children, and children from metropolitan regions and from families with lower median incomes. Survival rates were less for teenagers, African American and Hispanic children, and children from metropolitan regions.

Inpatient quality improvement and patient safety-focused programs have identified interventions and recognized risks that may prevent cardiac arrest events. Rapid response teams and early warning screening scores have become mainstays that reduce the prevalence of cardiac arrest.[17–20] Perioperative physicians have spearheaded the development of risk-stratification instruments for assessing patient's risk of morbidity and mortality such as the American Society of Anesthesiology Classification physical status and airway visualization scoring methods.[21] These screening and stratification instruments identify necessary resources and help to develop plans for high-risk patients.[22–27] In addition, the perioperative physician should identify potential risks to the patient and consult closely with surgical and subspecialty colleagues. The increased survival of children with uncommon chronic morbidities, syndromes, and metabolic illness requires consultation from a host of specialists as the breadth of knowledge and experience required for their safe, effective care is extensive and complex. In complex cases, broad consultation may be necessary before an anesthesia plan is formulated. The operative and anesthesia plan along with potential risks should be conveyed to the patient as well as a management plan for their chronic conditions.

Diagnosis of Cardiac Arrest

For the child who suffers a cardiac arrest in the OR, electronic monitoring usually alerts the anesthesiologist to an actual or impending cardiac arrest. The electrocardiogram (ECG) may indicate nonperfusing rhythms such as ventricular fibrillation (VF), pulseless electrical activity (PEA), and asystole; end-tidal carbon dioxide ($ETCO_2$) may decrease precipitously, reflecting a decrease in cardiac output as a result of a decreased delivery of carbon dioxide (CO_2) to the lungs; and a pulse oximeter may lose its regular waveform in the absence of pulsatile blood flow. Despite the importance of these monitors, the diagnosis of cardiopulmonary arrest still rests on the absence of a pulse in a major artery (e.g., carotid, femoral, or brachial artery) that is determined by palpation in the presence of unconsciousness and apnea.

In the early minutes of CPR, the reason for the cardiac arrest should be sought. A blood gas analysis and serum electrolyte concentrations (ideally as point-of-care testing) may prove helpful in determining the cause of the arrest. In many instances, resuscitation will not be successful without identification and correction of the underlying cause. A focused physical examination should be conducted and a brief history elicited if it is not already known. If not present, a cardiorespiratory monitor should be placed and the ECG examined. In an intraoperative arrest, the surgeon may be able to provide clues to the diagnosis, such as excessive blood loss, compression of major blood vessels, decreasing venous return to the heart, manipulation of anatomic structures (e.g., manipulation of the peritoneum resulting in a severe vagal bradycardia or asystole), or air embolism. Equipment malfunction must always be considered as a potential cause of arrest.

Mechanics of Cardiopulmonary Resuscitation

CPR should follow the airway, breathing, circulation (ABC) algorithm with the exception that the child with VF or pulseless ventricular tachycardia should receive electrical defibrillation without delay. Airway access in children with VF or pulseless ventricular tachycardia should be performed secondarily. CPR should continue without interruption until a shock can be delivered.

AIRWAY

Before tracheal intubation, the child's airway can be managed effectively with bag-valve-mask (BVM) ventilation with proper head positioning and jaw thrust. Although tracheal intubation ensures optimal control of the airway for effective ventilation, multiple attempts at tracheal intubation by an inexperienced operator may seriously compromise the airway and increase the cumulative duration of "no flow" (i.e., no CPR).

In the child without an artificial airway and proper application of the jaw thrust, the use of BVM devices may cause significant gastric inflation that leads to regurgitation and pulmonary aspiration of gastric contents.[28] Abdominal distention (gastric and bowel) can compromise oxygenation; therefore the stomach should be vented when excessive gastric inflation occurs. In one study, the incidence of pulmonary aspiration in a series of failed resuscitations was 28%.[29] For this reason as well as the risk of barotrauma and volutrauma, excessive inflation pressures should be avoided. Visualizing bilateral chest excursions and listening to the quality of the breath sounds rather than setting a preset maximal inflation pressure best judges effective bilateral ventilation. Placement of a supraglottic device such as a laryngeal mask airway (LMA) may serve as a bridge to establishing a more definitive airway in the hands of those inexperienced in airway management.

Tracheal intubation should be performed as soon as appropriate personnel and equipment are available. Some centers advocate placement of an LMA owing to the delay and technical challenge of direct laryngoscopy and endotracheal tube placement. However, this is not a universally reported practice in the care of pediatric cardiac arrest.[30,31] The ETCO$_2$ is a valuable method of confirming correct placement of the tracheal tube. In the absence of capnography, a disposable colorimetric ETCO$_2$ device may be substituted (E-Fig. 39.4). However, it is important to appreciate that ETCO$_2$ measurements are meaningful only in the presence of effective pulmonary circulation, such that a lack of color change may reflect either improper placement of the tube or a lack of pulmonary blood flow resulting from ineffective chest compressions or a massive pulmonary embolism. It is also essential to use the proper size colorimetric device for the child's weight because the adult size may not detect the presence of CO$_2$ and may lead the user to misdiagnose a successful intubation as unsuccessful.

BREATHING

Equipment to artificially ventilate the lungs should be readily available for all inpatients. The anesthesiologist needs to be familiar with the available equipment in different locations within the hospital because equipment for emergency ventilatory support may differ from standard equipment in the OR. Anesthesiologists are skilled providers of ventilatory support, but in the context of a cardiac arrest, must return to the basics and remember that *if there is no chest movement, there is no ventilation.* If no chest movement occurs during BVM ventilation despite an apparently good seal between the mask and the child's face, the underlying cause, be it upper airway obstruction, whether anatomic or caused by the presence of a foreign body, bilateral tension pneumothoraces, or severe bronchospasm, must be considered.

Overventilation is common during CPR, resulting in greater mean intrathoracic pressures than required, which decreases venous return and reduces cardiac output.[32] In cardiopulmonary arrest, less than normal minute ventilation may be appropriate, because cardiac output and delivery of CO$_2$ to the lungs are diminished. If an artificial airway is not in place for single-person rescue, two breaths should be given for each 30 chest compressions. If an artificial airway is not in place for two-person rescue, two breaths should be given after each 15 chest compressions. Once an artificial airway is in place, a ventilator rate of 8 to 10 per minute *without* pausing during rapid chest compressions should be used (Table 40.1).

CIRCULATION

During cardiac arrest, chest compressions provide the sole pump to perfuse a child's vital organs; therefore optimal performance of CPR is critical. Key elements to providing quality chest compressions include (1) ensuring an adequate rate (100 compressions per minute), (2) ensuring adequate chest wall depression (one-third to one-half of the anteroposterior chest diameter), (3) releasing completely between compressions to allow full chest wall recoil, (4) minimizing interruptions in chest compressions, and (5) ensuring that the child is on a sufficiently hard surface to allow effective chest compressions.[33] The strategy for successful CPR is to push hard and push fast, release completely, and do not interrupt compressions unnecessarily. Be mindful that incomplete recoil during CPR is associated with greater intrathoracic pressures and significantly decreased venous return, and coronary and cerebral perfusion.[34]

If the child is younger than 6 months, the person performing chest compressions can comfortably encircle the chest with his or her hands. Chest compressions should be performed using the circumferential technique; with thumbs depressing the sternum and the fingers supporting the infant's back and circumferentially squeezing the thorax (Fig. 40.1). In larger infants, the sternum can be compressed using two fingers; and in the child, either one or two hands can be used, depending on the size of the child and of the rescuer.[34] Whichever method is used, focused attention must remain on delivering effective compressions with *minimal interruptions.*[35] In all cases other than circumferential CPR, a backboard should be used. Properly delivered chest compressions will quickly fatigue the provider. To maintain effective CPR, providers should rotate approximately every 2 minutes to prevent fatigue and deterioration in the quality and rate of chest compressions.[34]

Mechanisms of Blood Flow

External chest compressions generate cardiac output via two mechanisms: the cardiac pump and the thoracic pump. The cardiac pump mechanism generates cardiac output by squeezing blood

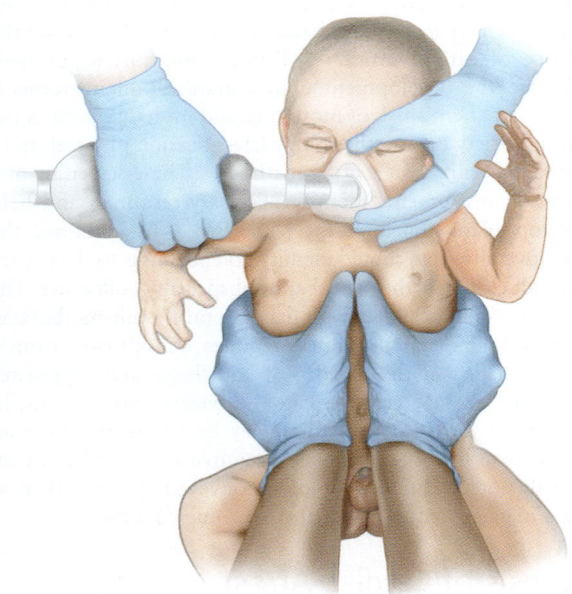

FIGURE 40.1 Chest-encircling method for cardiac compressions in a neonate: thumbs are placed one finger's breadth below the nipple line. (Modified from Todres ID, Rogers MC. Methods of external cardiac massage in the newborn infant. *J Pediatr.* 1975;86:781–782.)

TABLE 40.1	Ventilation and Chest Compressions During Pediatric Cardiopulmonary Pulmonary Resuscitation (all ages)		
	Respirations	Chest Compressions	Notes
Bag-mask ventilation	2 respirations after each 15 chest compressions (if one rescuer only, 2 respirations after each 30 compressions)	100/minute	Aspirate (vent) the stomach if gastric inflation interferes with ventilation.
Endotracheal intubation	8–10/minute	100/minute	Do not pause compressions during ventilation.

Cardiac Pump

Artificial
systole

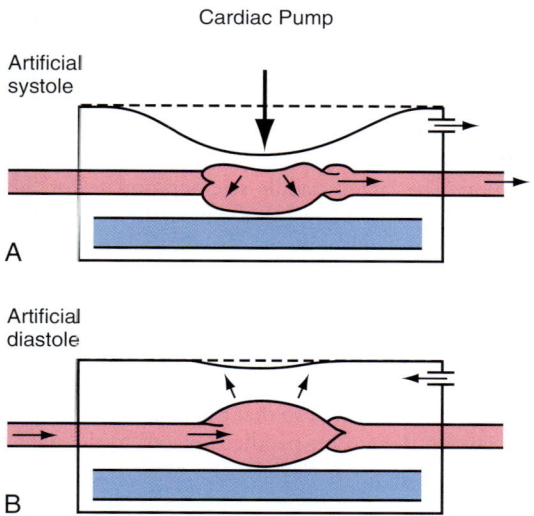

A

Artificial
diastole

B

FIGURE 40.2 A, Cardiac pump mechanism by which the heart is directly squeezed between the sternum and vertebral column, representing artificial systole. **B,** Artificial diastole occurs with relaxation of the compressions. (From Babbs CF. New versus old theories of blood flow during CPR. *Crit Care Med.* 1980;8:191–195; © by Williams & Wilkins.)

Thoracic Pump

Artificial
systole

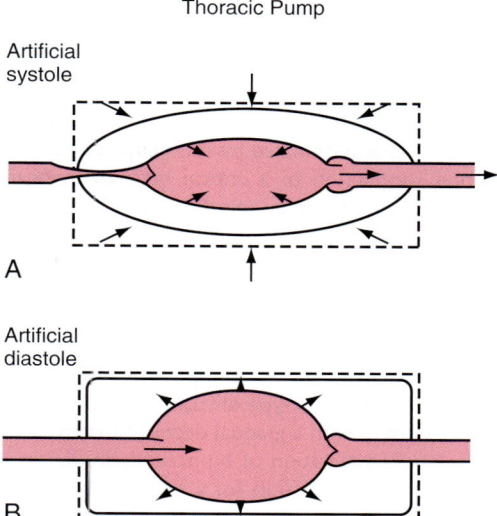

A

Artificial
diastole

B

FIGURE 40.3 A, Thoracic pump mechanism by which blood flow occurs through a general increase in intrathoracic pressure with external compressions (i.e., the heart is a passive conduit). **B,** Artificial diastole occurs with release of external compressions. (From Babbs CF, New versus old theories of blood flow during CPR. *Crit Care Med.* 1980;8:191–195; © by Williams & Wilkins.)

out of the heart when it is compressed between the sternum and the vertebral column. Blood exits the heart in an anterograde direction because the atrioventricular valves close during ventricular compression. Between compressions, ventricular pressure decreases below atrial pressure, allowing the atrioventricular valves to open and fill the ventricles. This sequence of events resembles the normal cardiac cycle. Although the cardiac pump is likely not the dominant mechanism that generates cardiac output during most closed-chest CPR, specific clinical situations have been identified in which the cardiac pump mechanism is more prominent. For example, a smaller, more compliant chest may allow for more direct cardiac compression (Fig. 40.2). Increasing the applied force during chest compressions also increases direct cardiac compression and emptying of the ventricles.

Several observations suggest that the cardiac pump is not the primary mechanism of generating cardiac output during CPR. Angiographic studies show that blood passes from the vena cava through the right heart into the pulmonary artery and from the pulmonary veins through the left heart into the aorta during a single chest compression.[36,37] Echocardiographic studies show that the atrioventricular valves are open during blood ejection.[36,38,39] Without closure of atrioventricular valves during chest compression, the cardiac pump mechanisms cannot account for anterograde movement of blood during CPR.

The thoracic pump mechanism is the second mechanism by which cardiac output is generated during CPR. In 1976, several patients who developed VF during cardiac catheterization were noted to produce enough blood flow to maintain consciousness by repetitive coughing.[40] The increase in thoracic pressure with coughing produced anterograde blood flow without direct cardiac compression. This describes the thoracic pump mechanism, in which the heart acts a passive conduit for blood flow. The intrathoracic pressure is greater than the extrathoracic pressure during the compression phase of CPR, at which time blood flows out of the thorax, with venous valves preventing excessive retrograde blood flow (Fig. 40.3). Experimental and clinical data support both mechanisms of blood flow during CPR in human infants.

Rate and Duty Cycle

The recommended rate of chest compressions for all children is 100 per minute, with great care taken to minimize interruptions in chest compressions and to ensure adequate compression depth.[35] This rate represents a compromise that attempts to maximize contributions from both the thoracic pump and cardiac pump mechanism of blood flow.

Duty cycle is defined as the percent of the compression-relaxation cycle devoted to compression. If blood flow is generated by direct cardiac compression, then the force of compression determines the stroke volume. Prolonging the compression (increasing the duty cycle) beyond the time necessary for full ventricular ejection should not affect the stroke volume. Increasing the rate of compressions should increase cardiac output because a fixed volume of blood is ejected with each cardiac compression. In contrast, if blood flow is produced by the thoracic pump mechanism, the volume of blood that is ejected comes from a large reservoir of blood contained within the capacitance vessels in the chest. With the thoracic pump mechanism, flow is enhanced by increasing either the force of compression or the duty cycle but is not affected by changes in the compression rate over a wide range of rates, given a set duty cycle.[41]

Animal models yield conflicting results as to the optimal compression rate and duty cycle. However, a rate of compressions during conventional CPR of 100 per minute satisfies both those who prefer the faster rates and those who support a longer duty cycle. This is true because it is easier to produce a longer duty cycle when compressions are administered at a faster rate.[42,43]

Defibrillation and Cardioversion

In children with VF or pulseless ventricular tachycardia, the immediate management should be defibrillation, without delay to secure an airway.

ELECTRIC COUNTERSHOCK

Electric countershock, or defibrillation, is the treatment of choice for VF and pulseless ventricular tachycardia. Defibrillation should not be delayed to secure an airway, because the likelihood of restoring an organized rhythm decreases as the duration of fibrillation increases. VF is terminated by simultaneous depolarization and sustained contraction of a critical mass of myocardium,[44] allowing return of spontaneous, coordinated cardiac contractions, assuming the myocardium is well oxygenated and the acid-base status is relatively normal. Drug treatment may be required as an adjunct to defibrillation, but by itself cannot be relied on to terminate VF.

An older generation of defibrillators still present in many hospitals delivers energy in a monophasic damped sinusoidal waveform (Fig. 40.4A). This type of instrument delivers a single, unidirectional current with a gradual decrease to zero current. By contrast, the newer generation of biphasic defibrillators delivers a current in a positive direction for a set period, followed by a reversal in current (Fig. 40.4B). Biphasic defibrillators are more effective than monophasic defibrillators for terminating VF in adults; therefore their use is recommended where possible. Pediatric attenuator pads or a pediatric mode on the automated external defibrillator (AED) should be used in children 1 to 8 years of age if it is available, but if it is not (and a standard defibrillator is similarly unavailable), an unmodified AED can be used.

In the majority of adult cases, energy levels of 100 to 200 J are successful when shocks are delivered with minimal delay.[45,46] The goal of defibrillation is to deliver a minimum amount of electrical energy to a critical mass of ventricular muscle while avoiding excessive current that could further damage the heart.

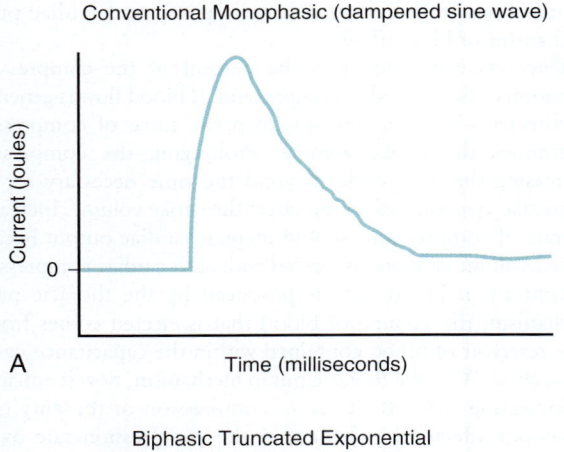

Conventional Monophasic (dampened sine wave)

A — Time (milliseconds) / Current (joules)

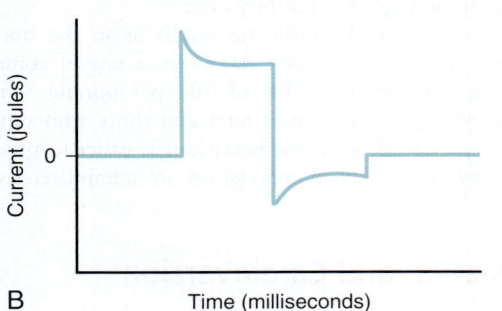

Biphasic Truncated Exponential

B — Time (milliseconds) / Current (joules)

FIGURE 40.4 Energy delivery during conventional monophasic (**A**) and biphasic truncated exponential (**B**) defibrillation.

The most reliable predictor for success of defibrillation is the duration of fibrillation before the first countershock.[47] Acidosis and hypoxemia also decrease the success of defibrillation.[47]

PRACTICAL ASPECTS OF DEFIBRILLATION IN CHILDREN

Correct paddle size and position are critical to the success of defibrillation. The largest paddle size appropriate for the child should be used because a larger size reduces the density of current flow, which in turn reduces myocardial damage. In general, adult paddles should be used in children weighing more than 10 kg and infant paddles should be used in infants weighing less than 10 kg. Paddle force is important as well. If the entire paddle does not rest *firmly* on the chest wall, a current of increased density will be delivered to a small contact point. Paddles should be positioned on the chest wall so that the bulk of myocardium lies directly between them. One paddle is placed to the right of the upper sternum below the clavicle; the other is positioned just caudad and to the left of the left nipple. For children with dextrocardia, the position of the paddles should be a mirror image. An alternative approach is to place one paddle anteriorly over the left precordium and the other paddle posteriorly between the scapulae.

The interface between the paddle and chest wall can be gel pads, electrode cream, or electrode paste. The electrode cream produces less impedance than the paste. *Electric current follows the path of least resistance, so care should be taken that the interface material from one paddle does not touch that of the other paddle. This is especially important in infants, in whom the distance between paddles is small.* If the gel is continuous between paddles, a short circuit is created and an insufficient amount of current will traverse the heart. Use of bare metal paddles increases the risk of arcing and worsens cutaneous burns from defibrillation. The use of self-adhesive pads is preferable when feasible.

In the past, sparking from poorly applied defibrillator paddles has been a fire risk. All sources of free-flowing O_2 were maintained at a distance of at least 1 m from the child. However, the use of pads rather than paddles has reduced the risk of fire, allowing the nasal oxygen or mask oxygen supply to remain in place during defibrillation. It is not necessary to disconnect the ventilator from the child's tracheal tube, but if the ventilator is disconnected, the fresh gas flow should be turned off.

For children with in-hospital VF or pulseless ventricular tachycardia, defibrillation should be attempted as soon as possible, with optimal CPR until the defibrillator is ready to deliver a shock. For the first defibrillation, 2 J/kg of delivered energy should be administered (Fig. 40.5). After delivery of the shock, CPR should resume immediately with chest compressions for five duty cycles (2 minutes). If the first shock fails to restore normal sinus rhythm, the incremental benefit of a second immediate shock is small. Resumption of CPR is likely to confer a greater benefit than a second shock. CPR may restore coronary perfusion, increasing the likelihood of defibrillation with a subsequent shock. It is important to minimize the time interval between chest compressions and delivery of the shock and between delivery of the shock and resumption of post-shock CPR.[35] Approximately 2 minutes of CPR should be delivered before a second shock is delivered at twice the original energy level (4 J/kg).[35]

If VF or pulseless ventricular tachycardia persists beyond the second defibrillation, standard doses of epinephrine should be administered (with subsequent doses every 3 to 5 minutes during persistent cardiac arrest). After 2 minutes of CPR, another defibrillation should be attempted, followed by amiodarone (5 mg/kg)

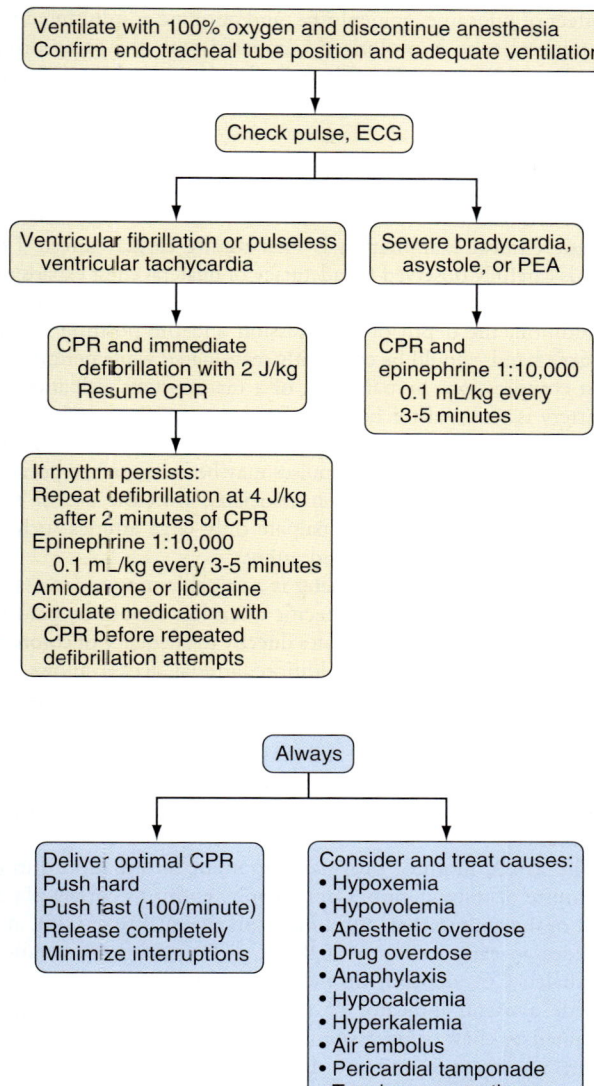

Ventilate with 100% oxygen and discontinue anesthesia
Confirm endotracheal tube position and adequate ventilation

↓

Check pulse, ECG

Ventricular fibrillation or pulseless ventricular tachycardia

Severe bradycardia, asystole, or PEA

CPR and immediate defibrillation with 2 J/kg Resume CPR

CPR and epinephrine 1:10,000 0.1 mL/kg every 3-5 minutes

If rhythm persists:
Repeat defibrillation at 4 J/kg after 2 minutes of CPR
Epinephrine 1:10,000
   0.1 mL/kg every 3-5 minutes
Amiodarone or lidocaine
Circulate medication with
   CPR before repeated
   defibrillation attempts

Always

Deliver optimal CPR
Push hard
Push fast (100/minute)
Release completely
Minimize interruptions

Consider and treat causes:
• Hypoxemia
• Hypovolemia
• Anesthetic overdose
• Drug overdose
• Anaphylaxis
• Hypocalcemia
• Hyperkalemia
• Air embolus
• Pericardial tamponade
• Tension pneumothorax

FIGURE 40.5 Algorithm for diagnosis and treatment of acute cardiac dysfunction in the operating room. *CPR,* cardiopulmonary resuscitation; *ECG,* electrocardiogram; *PEA,* pulseless electrical activity.

or lidocaine (1 mg/kg) intravenously, with subsequent defibrillation attempts. It is not necessary to increase the energy level on each successive shock after the second attempt. However, successful defibrillation has been reported with currents in excess of 4 J/kg, up to a maximum dose not exceeding 10 J/kg or the adult level, whichever is less, without adverse sequelae.[35] This sometimes occurs when a fixed energy level, adult AED is used in a small child.

OPEN-CHEST DEFIBRILLATION

If the chest is already open in the OR or easily opened as in a postoperative cardiac patient, VF should be treated with open-chest defibrillation, using internal paddles applied directly to the heart. These should have a diameter of 6 cm for adults, 4 cm for children, and 2 cm for infants. Handles should be insulated. One electrode is placed behind the left ventricle and the other over the right ventricle on the anterior surface of the heart. The energy level used should begin at 5 J in infants and 20 J in adults.

AUTOMATED EXTERNAL DEFIBRILLATION

The use of AEDs is now standard therapy in out-of-hospital resuscitation of adults.[34,45] AEDs are now deemed appropriate for use in children older than 1 year. If available, pediatric attenuator pads or a pediatric mode on the AED should be used in children 1 to 8 years of age, but if unavailable (and a standard defibrillator is similarly unavailable), an unmodified AED should be used.

TRANSCUTANEOUS CARDIAC PACING

In the absence of in situ pacing wires or an indwelling transvenous or esophageal pacing catheter, transcutaneous cardiac pacing (TCP) is the preferred method for temporary electrical cardiac pacing in children with asystole or severe bradycardia. TCP is indicated for children whose primary problem is impulse formation or conduction, with preserved myocardial function. It is most effective in those with sinus bradycardia or high-grade atrioventricular block, with slow ventricular response but adequate stroke volume. TCP is not indicated for children during prolonged arrest, because in this situation it usually results in electrical but not mechanical cardiac capture and its use may delay or interfere with other resuscitative efforts.

To set up pacing, one electrode is placed anteriorly at the left sternal border and the other posteriorly just below the left scapula. Smaller electrodes are available for infants and children, but adult-sized electrodes can be used in children weighing more than 15 kg. ECG leads should be connected to the pacemaker, the demand or asynchronous mode selected, and an age-appropriate heart rate used. The stimulus output should be set at zero when the pacemaker is turned on and then increased gradually until electrical capture is identified on the monitor. After electrical capture is achieved, whether an effective arterial pulse is generated must be determined. If not, additional resuscitative efforts should be initiated.

The most serious complication of TCP is the induction of a ventricular arrhythmia. Fortunately, this is rare and may be prevented by pacing only in the demand mode. Mild transient erythema beneath the electrodes is common. Skeletal muscle contraction can be minimized by using large electrodes, 40-msec pulse duration, and the smallest stimulus required for capture. If defibrillation or cardioversion is necessary, a distance of 2 to 3 cm must be allowed between the electrode and paddles to prevent arcing of the current.

Vascular Access and Monitoring During Cardiopulmonary Resuscitation

VASCULAR ACCESS AND FLUID ADMINISTRATION

One of the key aspects of successful CPR is the early establishment of a route to administer fluids and medications. If intravenous (IV) access cannot be established rapidly, the intraosseous or endotracheal route should be used (see Chapter 49 and Figs. 49.6 and 49.7).

Intravenous Access

Many children who suffer an in-hospital cardiac arrest will already have established vascular access. For children with impending cardiac arrest and no vascular access, a brief attempt should be made to establish peripheral IV access. If access is not achieved quickly, an intraosseous needle should be placed. For young children in cardiac arrest without vascular access, an intraosseous needle should be placed immediately to avoid any delay from repeated attempts to establish IV access.

Intraosseous Access

The intraosseous route can be used to administer all medications and fluids used during CPR, including whole blood. It may also be used to obtain initial blood samples, although acid-base analysis will be inaccurate after administration of sodium bicarbonate through the intraosseous needle. Intraosseous access should be considered a temporary measure during emergencies when alternate access is not available. Placing an intraosseous needle in an older child (older than 10 years) and adult, although possible, is more difficult because of the thicker bony cortex. Nonetheless, the success rate establishing intraosseous access in these age groups is 50%.[48]

The technique of establishing intraosseous access is straightforward. An intraosseous needle or, if unavailable, a standard 16- or 18-gauge needle, a spinal needle with stylet, or bone marrow needle may be inserted into the anterior surface of the tibia 1 to 2 cm below and 1 cm medial to the tibial tuberosity (avoiding the epiphyseal plate). The needle is directed at 90 degrees to the anteromedial surface of the tibia, just distal to the tuberosity (see Figs. 49.6 and 49.7). When the needle passes through the cortex and into the marrow, a sudden loss of resistance is sensed. If the needle has reached the marrow cavity, it will remain upright without support. If, however, the needle is in the subcutaneous tissue, it cannot remain upright without support. The free flow of infusate without significant subcutaneous infiltration confirms that the tip of the needle is in the bone marrow. Intraosseous access has a small complication rate,[49] although the complications could include osteomyelitis, fat and bone marrow embolism, and compartment syndrome. To avoid these complications, IV access should replace intraosseous access as soon as possible. The onset of action and concentration of most drugs after intraosseous administration are comparable with venous administration.[50] The EZ-IO system (Vidacare, Shavano Park, TX) provides a rapid means to establish intraosseous access (see Fig. 49.7).

ENDOTRACHEAL MEDICATION ADMINISTRATION

In the absence of other vascular access, medications including lidocaine, atropine, naloxone, and epinephrine (mnemonic LANE or LEAN; vasopressin is occasionally used in adults with the mnemonic NAVEL) can be administered through the endotracheal tube.[51,52] Ionized medications such as sodium bicarbonate and calcium chloride should not be administered through the tracheal tube. The peak concentration of epinephrine or lidocaine administered through the endotracheal tube, at similar doses, may be less than that through the IV route.[53] For example, the peak drug concentration of epinephrine after endotracheal administration was only 10% of that after IV administration in anesthetized dogs. The recommended dose for endotracheal epinephrine is 10 times the IV or intraosseous dose or 0.1 mg/kg for bradycardia or pulseless arrest.

The volume and the diluent in which the medications are administered through an endotracheal tube may be important. When large volumes of fluid are used, pulmonary surfactant may be altered or destroyed, resulting in atelectasis. The total volume of fluid delivered into the trachea with each drug administered should not exceed 10 mL in children and 5 mL in infants and neonates.[54] However, administering an adequate volume of a drug is important to reach a large surface area beyond the tip of the endotracheal tube to achieve rapid absorption. Absorption into the systemic circulation may be further enhanced by deep intrapulmonary administration by passing a catheter beyond the tip of the tracheal tube deep into the bronchial tree. The duration

of effect of lidocaine, epinephrine, and atropine administered via the tracheal tube is prolonged compared with the same drugs given by the IV route. This "depot" effect is due to both a slower absorption from the lung and the larger drug doses used via this route.[53]

MONITORING DURING CARDIOPULMONARY RESUSCITATION

A basic clinical examination is vital during cardiac arrest. The chest is carefully observed for adequacy of bilateral chest expansion with artificial ventilation and for equal and normal breath sounds. In addition, the depth of compression and the position of the rescuer's hands should be constantly reevaluated while performing chest compressions by palpation of a major artery. Palpation of an artery is essential for both confirming the absence of a pulse and for assessing the adequacy of blood flow during chest compressions. Palpating the peripheral pulses may be inaccurate, especially during intense vasoconstriction associated with the use of epinephrine, so it is prudent to palpate only large arteries such as the brachial, femoral, or carotid artery.

An indwelling arterial catheter is a valuable monitor to assess the arterial blood pressure. Specific attention should be paid to diastolic blood pressure as it relates directly to adequacy of coronary perfusion during CPR. In addition, arterial access allows for frequent blood sampling, particularly for measurement of arterial pH and blood gases. Pulse oximetry can be used during CPR to determine the O_2 saturation and may be of value in assessing the adequacy of cardiac output, as reflected in the plethysmograph. The ECG can suggest metabolic imbalances and diagnose electrical disturbances.

The $ETCO_2$ monitor provides important information during the course of resuscitation. Capnography confirms correct placement of the endotracheal tube, monitors the quality of CPR, and provides an early indicator of ROSC.[55] Because the generation of exhaled CO_2 depends on pulmonary blood flow, $ETCO_2$ can provide a useful indicator of the adequacy of cardiac output generated by chest compressions. As the cardiac output increases, the $ETCO_2$ increases and the difference between end-tidal and arterial CO_2 becomes smaller.[56] In animal models, $ETCO_2$ during CPR correlates with coronary perfusion pressure and with ROSC.[57,58] A reduced $ETCO_2$ may occur transiently in the presence of adequate chest compressions after administration of epinephrine owing to an increase in intrapulmonary shunting. The International Liaison Committee on Resuscitation (ILCOR) acknowledges that small values of $ETCO_2$ are associated with small probability of survival. The committee believes, however, that there are insufficient data to support or refute a specific cutoff value of $ETCO_2$ as a prognostic indicator of outcome during adult cardiac arrest.[59] $ETCO_2$ monitoring may be considered to evaluate quality of chest compressions, but there is no pediatric evidence that it improves outcomes after cardiac arrest.[60] However, we strongly advocate the use of $ETCO_2$ monitoring as a surrogate to monitor effective chest compressions.

Temperature should be monitored during and after CPR. The resuscitation of the child with hypothermia as the cause of cardiac arrest must be continued until the child's core temperature exceeds 95°F (35°C). A glass bulb thermometer measures the temperature to very low values. Repeated measurements of core body temperature should be made at several sites (rectal, bladder, esophageal, axillary, or tympanic membrane) where possible to avoid misleading temperature readings from a single site, because local body temperature may vary with changes in regional blood flow during

CPR. Hyperthermia should be aggressively treated in the periarrest period, because postarrest hyperthermia is associated with worse outcomes in children.[61] Data suggest a benefit to induced hypothermia after resuscitation from cardiac arrest in adults[62,63] and after perinatal hypoxic or ischemic injury,[64] although recent evidence supports a temperature of 36°C rather than 33°C. The recent Therapeutic Hypothermia After Pediatric Cardiac Arrest (THAPCA) study concluded that therapeutic hypothermia did not confer a significant benefit over therapeutic normothermia for survival with good functional outcome at 1 year.[65]

Medications Used During Cardiopulmonary Resuscitation

α- AND β-ADRENERGIC AGONISTS

In 1963, only 3 years after the original description of closed-chest CPR, early administration of epinephrine in a canine model of cardiac arrest was shown to improve the success rate of CPR.[66] In addition, the administration of α-adrenergic agonists increased the aortic diastolic pressure, which improved the success of resuscitation. The evidence suggested that vasopressors such as epinephrine were valuable during resuscitation because they increased peripheral vascular tone and, hence, coronary perfusion pressure. The relative importance of α- and β-adrenergic agonist actions during resuscitation has been widely investigated. In a canine model of cardiac arrest, only 27% of dogs that received a pure β-adrenergic receptor agonist along with an α-adrenergic antagonist were resuscitated successfully, compared with 100% of dogs that received a pure α-adrenergic agonist and a β-adrenergic antagonist. Others demonstrated that the α-adrenergic effects of epinephrine resulted in intense vasoconstriction of the resistance vessels of all organs of the body, except those supplying the heart and brain.[67] Because of the widespread vasoconstriction in nonvital organs, adequate perfusion pressure and thus blood flow to the heart and brain could be achieved despite the fact that cardiac output was poor during CPR.[67-69]

The increase in aortic diastolic pressure associated with epinephrine administration during CPR is critical for maintaining coronary blood flow and enhancing the success of resuscitation.[70,71] Even though the contractile state of the myocardium is increased in the presence of β-adrenergic agonists in the spontaneously beating heart, β-adrenergic agonists may actually decrease myocardial blood flow by increasing intramyocardial wall pressure and vascular resistance during CPR.[72] By its inotropic and chronotropic effects, β-adrenergic stimulation increases myocardial O_2 demand, which, when superimposed on low coronary blood flow, increases the risk of ischemic injury.

Any medication that causes systemic arterial vasoconstriction can be used to increase aortic diastolic pressure and resuscitate the heart. For example, pure α-adrenergic agonists can be used in place of epinephrine during CPR. Phenylephrine and methoxamine, two α-adrenergic agonists, have been used in animal models of CPR with success equal to that of epinephrine. Their use results in a greater O_2 supply to demand ratio in the ischemic heart and at least a theoretical advantage over the combined α- and β-adrenergic agonist effects of epinephrine. These agonists, as well as other classes of vasopressors such as vasopressin, have been used successfully for resuscitation.

The merits of using a pure α-adrenergic agonist during CPR have been questioned by some investigators. Although the inotropic and chronotropic effects of β-adrenergic agonists may have deleterious hemodynamic effects during CPR for VF, increases in both heart rate and contractility will increase cardiac output when spontaneous coordinated ventricular contractions are achieved.

EPINEPHRINE

Epinephrine (adrenaline) is an endogenous catecholamine with potent α- and β-adrenergic stimulating properties. The β-adrenergic property increases systemic (both systolic and diastolic blood pressures) and pulmonary vascular resistance. The increase in diastolic blood pressure directly increases coronary perfusion pressure, thereby increasing coronary blood flow and increasing the likelihood of ROSC.[70,71] The β-adrenergic effect increases myocardial contractility and heart rate and relaxes smooth muscle in the skeletal muscle vascular bed and bronchi. Epinephrine also increases the vigor and intensity of VF, increasing the likelihood of successful defibrillation.[73]

Larger than necessary doses of epinephrine may be deleterious. Epinephrine may worsen myocardial ischemic injury secondary to increased O_2 demand and may result in postresuscitative tachyarrhythmias, hypertension, and pulmonary edema. Epinephrine causes hypoxemia and an increase in alveolar dead space ventilation by redistributing pulmonary blood flow.[56,74] Prolonged peripheral vasoconstriction by excessive doses of epinephrine may delay or impair reperfusion of systemic organs, particularly the kidneys and gastrointestinal tract.

Routine use of large-dose epinephrine in in-hospital pediatric cardiac arrest should be *avoided*. The use of high-dose epinephrine children with in-hospital cardiac arrest refractory to initial standard-dose epinephrine has not been encouraging. Survival was reduced at 24 hours compared with those given standard-dose epinephrine, with weak evidence of decreased survival to hospital discharge in the children who received large doses of epinephrine.[75] Despite these data, large doses of epinephrine may be considered in special cases (e.g., β-blocker overdose), particularly when diastolic blood pressure remains low despite excellent chest compression and several standard doses of epinephrine.

VASOPRESSIN

Vasopressin is a long-acting endogenous hormone that causes vasoconstriction (V1 receptor) and reabsorption of water in the renal tubule (V2 receptor). In experimental models of cardiac arrest, vasopressin increases blood flow to the heart and brain and improves long-term survival compared with epinephrine.[76,77] In a randomized trial of epinephrine and vasopressin in shock-resistant out-of-hospital VF in adults, vasopressin produced a greater rate of ROSC.[78] In a study of in-hospital adult cardiac arrest, epinephrine and vasopressin produced similar rates of survival to hospital discharge.[79] A recent meta-analysis of vasopressin for cardiac arrest did not demonstrate any overall benefit or harm.[80]

In a pediatric porcine model of prolonged VF, the combination of vasopressin and epinephrine resulted in greater left ventricular blood flow than either drug alone, and both vasopressin alone and vasopressin plus epinephrine increased cerebral blood flow more than epinephrine alone.[81] By contrast, in a pediatric porcine model of *asphyxial* cardiac arrest, ROSC was more likely in piglets treated with epinephrine than in those treated with vasopressin.[82] Pediatric[83-85] case series and reports suggested that vasopressin[83] or its long-acting analog, terlipressin,[84,85] may be effective in refractory cardiac arrest. In the 2009 National Registry of Cardiopulmonary Resuscitation (NRCPR) review, vasopressin was associated with reduced ROSC and weak evidence for reduced 24-hour and discharge survival. There was insufficient evidence to make a recommendation for its routine use during cardiac arrest.[35]

ATROPINE

Atropine, a parasympatholytic agent, blocks cholinergic stimulation of the muscarinic receptors in the heart, increasing the sinus rate and shortening atrioventricular node conduction time. Atropine may activate latent ectopic pacemakers. Atropine has little effect on systemic vascular resistance, myocardial perfusion pressure, or contractility.[86]

Atropine is indicated for the treatment of bradycardia associated with hypotension, second- and third-degree heart block, and slow idioventricular rhythms. Atropine is no longer recommended for asystole or PEA.[87] Atropine is particularly effective in clinical conditions associated with excessive parasympathetic tone. *However, for children with asystole or symptomatic bradycardia associated with severe hypotension, epinephrine is the medication of choice and atropine should be regarded as a second-line drug.*

A dose of 0.02 mg/kg with no minimum dose may be considered when atropine is recommended as a premedication for emergency intubation.[60] Although a minimum dose of 0.1 mg of atropine has been entrenched in the pediatric literature, this dose was not evidence-based.[88,89] There is no minimum dose of atropine in young infants and children.[90] Atropine may be given by any route, including IV, intraosseous, endotracheal, intramuscular, or subcutaneous. After IV administration, its onset of action is within 30 seconds and its peak effect occurs in 1 to 2 minutes. The recommended adult dose is 0.5 mg every 3 to 5 minutes until the desired heart rate is obtained, up to a maximum of 3 mg.

SODIUM BICARBONATE

The routine use of sodium bicarbonate during CPR remains controversial, and it remains American Heart Association Class Indeterminate. Acidosis may depress myocardial function, prolong diastolic depolarization, depress spontaneous cardiac activity, decrease the electrical threshold for VF, and reduce the cardiac response to catecholamines.[91–93] Acidosis also vasodilates systemic vessels and attenuates the vasoconstrictive response of peripheral vessels to catecholamines,[94] which is the opposite of the desired vascular effect during CPR. In children with a reactive pulmonary vascular bed, acidosis causes pulmonary hypertension. Therefore, correction of even mild acidosis may help to resuscitate children with increased pulmonary vascular resistance. In addition, the presence of severe acidosis may increase the threshold for myocardial stimulation in a child with an artificial cardiac pacemaker.[95] Bicarbonate may also be indicated in tricyclic antidepressant overdose, hyperkalemia, hypermagnesemia, and sodium channel blocker poisoning.

Potentially deleterious effects of bicarbonate administration include metabolic alkalosis, hypercapnia, hypernatremia, and hyperosmolality. The use of sodium bicarbonate was associated with increased mortality in a multicenter cohort study of in-hospital pediatric cardiac arrest.[15] Alkalosis causes a leftward shift of the oxyhemoglobin dissociation curve and thus impairs release of O_2 from hemoglobin to tissues at a time when O_2 delivery may already be reduced.[96] Alkalosis also can result in hypokalemia by enhancing potassium influx into cells and in ionic hypocalcemia by increasing protein binding of ionized calcium. The marked hypercapnic acidosis that occurs during CPR in the venous circulation, including the coronary sinus, may be exacerbated by the administration of bicarbonate.[97] Myocardial acidosis during cardiac arrest is associated with decreased myocardial contractility.[93]

Hypernatremia and hyperosmolality may decrease tissue perfusion by increasing interstitial edema in microvascular beds.

Paradoxical intracellular acidosis after bicarbonate administration can occur with the rapid entry of CO_2 into cells with a slow egress of hydrogen ions out of cells; however, in neonatal rabbits recovering from hypoxic acidosis, the administration of bicarbonate increased both arterial pH and intracellular brain pH as measured by nuclear magnetic resonance spectroscopy.[98,99] Likewise, in rats, intracellular brain adenosine triphosphate concentration did not change during severe intracellular acidosis in the brain produced by extreme hypercapnia.[99] In a separate animal study, bicarbonate slowed the rate of decrease of both arterial and cerebral pH during prolonged CPR, suggesting that the blood-brain pH gradient is maintained during CPR.[100] Given the potentially deleterious effects of bicarbonate administration, its use should be *limited to cases in which there is a specific indication*, as discussed earlier.

CALCIUM

Calcium administration during CPR should be restricted to those with a specific indication for calcium (e.g., hypocalcemia, hyperkalemia, hypermagnesemia, and calcium channel blocker overdose). These restrictions are based on the possibility that exogenously administered calcium may worsen ischemia-reperfusion injury. Intracellular calcium overload occurs during cerebral ischemia by the influx of calcium through voltage-dependent and agonist-dependent (e.g., N-methyl-D-aspartate [NMDA]) calcium channels. Calcium plays an important role in the process of cell death in many organs, possibly by activation of intracellular enzymes such as nitric oxide synthase, phospholipase A and C, and others.[101]

The calcium ion is essential in myocardial excitation-contraction coupling, in increasing ventricular contractility, and in enhancing ventricular automaticity during asystole. Ionized hypocalcemia is associated with decreased ventricular performance and the peripheral blunting of the hemodynamic response to catecholamines.[102,103] Severe ionized hypocalcemia has been documented in adults suffering from out-of-hospital cardiac arrest[103] and in animals during prolonged CPR.[104] Children at risk for ionized hypocalcemia should be identified and treated as expeditiously as possible. Both total and ionized hypocalcemia may occur in children with either chronic or acute disease. Ionized hypocalcemia also occurs during massive or rapid transfusion of blood products (particularly whole blood and fresh frozen plasma, see Fig. 12.9) because citrate and other preservatives in stored blood products rapidly bind calcium. Because of this effect, ionized hypocalcemia is a known cause of cardiac arrest in the OR and should be treated immediately with calcium chloride or calcium gluconate (see Chapter 12 and Figs. 12.8 and 12.9). The magnitude of hypocalcemia in this setting depends on the rate and volume of blood products administered and the hepatic and renal function of the child. Administration of fresh frozen plasma at a rate in excess of 1 mL/kg per minute decreases the ionized calcium concentration in anesthetized children.[105]

The pediatric dose of calcium chloride for resuscitation is 20 mg/kg and of calcium gluconate is 60 mg/kg with a maximum dose for both of 2 g. Calcium gluconate is as effective as calcium chloride in increasing the ionized calcium concentration (see Fig. 12.8).[106,107] Calcium should be given slowly through a large-bore, free-flowing IV cannula, or preferably a central venous line. When administered too rapidly, calcium may cause bradycardia, heart block, or ventricular standstill. Severe tissue necrosis occurs when calcium infiltrates into subcutaneous tissue. Calcium administration is not recommended for pediatric cardiopulmonary arrest in the absence of documented hypocalcemia, calcium channel blocker overdose, hypermagnesemia, or hyperkalemia (Class III, level of evidence B). Routine calcium administration in cardiac arrest provides no benefit and may be harmful.[95,108]

GLUCOSE

The administration of glucose during CPR should be restricted to children with documented hypoglycemia because of the possible detrimental effects of hyperglycemia on the brain during or after ischemia. The mechanism by which hyperglycemia exacerbates ischemic neurologic injury may be caused by an increased production of lactic acid in the brain by anaerobic metabolism. During ischemia under normoglycemic conditions, brain lactate concentration reaches a plateau. In a hyperglycemic milieu, however, brain lactate concentration continues to increase for the duration of the ischemic period.[109]

Clinical studies have shown a direct correlation between the initial serum glucose concentration after cardiac arrest and poor neurologic outcome,[110-113] although the greater glucose concentration may be a marker rather than a cause of more severe brain injury.[111] However, given the likelihood of additional ischemic and hypoxic events in the postresuscitation period, it seems prudent to maintain serum glucose concentrations within the normal range. Additional studies are needed to determine if the benefit from tight control of serum glucose after cardiac arrest outweighs the risk of iatrogenic hypoglycemia. Some groups of children, including preterm infants and debilitated children with small endogenous glycogen stores, are more prone to developing hypoglycemia during and after a physiologic stress such as surgery. Bedside monitoring of the serum glucose concentration is critical during and after a cardiac arrest and allows for the opportunity to administer glucose before the critical point of small substrate delivery has been reached. The dose of glucose generally needed to correct hypoglycemia is 0.5 g/kg given as 5 mL/kg of 10% dextrose in infants or 1 mL/kg of 50% dextrose in an older child. The osmolarity of 50% dextrose is approximately 2700 mOsm/L and has been associated with intraventricular hemorrhage in neonates and infants; therefore the more dilute concentration is recommended in infants.

AMIODARONE

Amiodarone was established for the treatment of cardiac arrest after several studies demonstrated that it was more effective than lidocaine in the management of refractory tachyarrhythmias in adults. Compared with lidocaine, amiodarone increases survival to hospital admission of patients with shock-resistant out-of-hospital VF.[114]

Early reports on the use of oral amiodarone in children were favorable.[115-117] Recent data on amiodarone use in children have been limited to case reports and descriptive case series. Nevertheless, it is now used widely for serious pediatric arrhythmias in the nonresuscitation environment. It appears to be effective, with an acceptable short-term safety profile.

The pharmacology of amiodarone is complex and may explain its wide range of usefulness. It is primarily classified as a Vaughn-Williams class III agent that blocks the adenosine triphosphate–sensitive outward potassium channels, causing prolongation of the action potential and refractory period; however, this effect requires intracellular accumulation. After IV loading, the antiarrhythmic effects of amiodarone are primarily due to noncompetitive α- and β-adrenergic receptor blockade, calcium channel blockade, and effects on inward sodium current, causing a decrease in anterograde conduction across the atrioventricular node and an increase in the effective atrioventricular refractory period. The

α-adrenergic blockade leads to vasodilation, which may increase coronary blood flow. It is poorly absorbed orally, requiring IV loading in urgent situations. The full antiarrhythmic impact requires a loading period of up to 1 to 3 weeks to achieve intracellular concentrations and full potassium channel–blocking effects.

Hypotension is commonly reported with IV administration and may limit the rate at which the drug can be given. However, the development of hypotension is less common with the aqueous formulation.[118] The overall hemodynamic impact of IV administration will depend on the balance of its effect on rate control, myocardial performance, and vasodilation. Dosage recommendations for children are based on limited clinical studies. The dose is extrapolated from data on adults; 5 mg/kg intravenously is used for life-threatening arrhythmias. This dose can be repeated if necessary to control the arrhythmia. IV loading doses are followed by a continuous infusion of 10 to 20 mg/kg per day if there is a risk that the arrhythmia will recur. The ideal rate of a bolus administration of amiodarone is unclear; once it has been diluted, it is given as an IV push in adults. Amiodarone is best administered over 20 to 60 minutes to avoid profound vasodilation. We recommend a slow IV push (2 to 3 minutes) for pulseless ventricular tachycardia or VF until the arrhythmia is controlled and then a slower bolus (up to 10 minutes) for the remainder of the dose. An alternative dosing regimen for children is a 1 mg/kg IV push every 5 minutes up to 5 mg/kg. The use of the small aliquot bolus technique may be particularly appropriate for infants younger than 12 months of age.

Amiodarone-induced torsades de pointes has been described.[119] The use of amiodarone should be avoided in combination with other drugs that prolong the QT interval, as well as in the setting of hypomagnesemia and other electrolyte abnormalities that predispose to torsades de pointes. Severe bradycardia and heart block have also been described, especially in the postoperative period, and ventricular pacing wires are recommended in this setting. Both amiodarone and inhalation anesthetic agents prolong the QT interval; however, no specific data exist to evaluate the use of amiodarone for ventricular arrhythmias in children receiving inhalation anesthetics. It would seem prudent to be especially vigilant for this adverse effect in this circumstance.

Noncardiac adverse effects are often seen, especially with chronic dosing.[120] The most serious of these is interstitial pneumonitis seen most commonly in patients with preexisting lung disease.[121] The incidence in children is unknown. Rarely, an acute illness similar to acute respiratory distress syndrome illness has been reported in both infants and adults at the initiation of treatment.[122] The lung disease may remit with early discontinuation of the drug. Hypothyroidism, hepatotoxicity, photosensitivity, and corneal opacities are also common side effects with chronic use.[120]

The 2005 and 2010 Pediatric Advanced Life Support guidelines recommend administering amiodarone in place of lidocaine to manage VF and pulseless ventricular tachycardia. Paradoxically, an observational study demonstrated that the ROSC after lidocaine was superior to that after amiodarone.[123] There was no association between lidocaine or amiodarone use and survival to hospital discharge. Consequently, the 2015 Pediatric Cardiac Arrest Algorithm[60] reflects the change in recommendation that either lidocaine or amiodarone can be used for refractory VF or pulseless VT.

LIDOCAINE

Lidocaine is a class IB antiarrhythmic that decreases automaticity of pacemaker tissue that prevents or terminates ventricular arrhythmias as a result of accelerated ectopic foci. Lidocaine abolishes reentrant ventricular arrhythmias by decreasing the action potential duration and the conduction time of Purkinje fibers and increases the effective refractory period of Purkinje fibers, reducing the nonuniformity of contraction. Lidocaine has no effect on atrioventricular nodal conduction time, so it is ineffective in the treatment of atrial or atrioventricular junctional arrhythmias. In healthy adults, no change in heart rate or blood pressure occurs with lidocaine administration. In patients with cardiac disease there may be a slight decrease in ventricular function when a lidocaine bolus is administered intravenously.

In children with normal cardiac and hepatic function, an initial IV bolus of 1 mg/kg of lidocaine is given, followed by a continuous IV infusion at a rate of 20 to 50 µg/kg per minute. If the arrhythmia recurs, a second IV bolus at the same dose can be given. In children with severely decreased cardiac output, a bolus of no greater than 0.75 mg/kg may be administered followed by an infusion at the rate of 10 to 20 µg/kg per minute. In children with severe hepatic disease and reduced hepatic blood flow, dosages should be decreased by 50%. Children with renal insufficiency have normal lidocaine pharmacokinetics; however, the toxic metabolite (monoethylglycinexylidide) may accumulate in children receiving infusions over a long period and affect sodium channels. In children with hypoproteinemia, the dose of lidocaine also should be reduced because of the increase in free fraction of the drug.

Toxic effects of lidocaine may occur when the serum concentration exceeds 7 to 8 µg/mL. These effects include seizures, psychosis, drowsiness, paresthesias, disorientation, agitation, tinnitus, muscle spasms, and respiratory arrest. The treatment of choice for lidocaine-induced seizures is a benzodiazepine (midazolam or lorazepam) or a barbiturate (e.g., phenobarbital; chronic therapy also increases the hepatic metabolism of lidocaine).[124] Conversion of second-degree heart block to complete heart block has been described,[125] as has severe sinus bradycardia.

Special Cardiac Arrest Situations

PERIOPERATIVE CARDIAC ARREST

The incidence, causes, and risk factors associated with anesthesia- and operative-related cardiac arrest have been evaluated by the Pediatric Perioperative Cardiac Arrest registry.[126,127] Cardiovascular causes of cardiac arrest were the most common (41% of all arrests), with hypovolemia from blood loss and hyperkalemia from transfusion of stored blood the most common identifiable cardiovascular causes. Among respiratory causes of arrest (27%), airway obstruction from laryngospasm was the most common cause. Vascular injury incurred during placement of central venous catheters was the most common equipment-related cause of arrest. The cause of arrest varied by phase of anesthesia care.

Cardiac arrest in the OR should have the greatest potential for a successful outcome, because it is a witnessed arrest with virtually instantaneous availability of skilled personnel, monitoring equipment, resuscitative equipment, and drugs. Whenever a cardiac arrest occurs in the OR, the circumstances causing the arrest should be rapidly determined. The circumstances of the arrest may provide a clue as to the cause, such as hyperkalemia after succinylcholine administration or rapid blood transfusion; hypocalcemia during a rapid infusion of fresh frozen plasma or large blood transfusion; or a sudden fall in ETCO$_2$ indicating air, blood clot, or tumor embolism. The most important causes of bradyarrhythmia are first, hypoxemia, second, an anesthetic overdose (real or relative), and third, a vagal reflex caused by

surgical or airway manipulation. Administering 100% O$_2$ and establishing adequate ventilation should be the first maneuvers to implement, regardless of the cause of the bradycardia. In reflex-induced bradycardia, atropine may be the first drug of choice, but in extreme cases of bradycardia, whatever the mechanism, epinephrine is preferred in place of atropine. Hypotension and a low cardiac output state must be rapidly corrected by administration of IV fluids, vasopressors, and adequate chest compressions to circulate drugs to have the desired clinical effect. Once chest compressions are required, the standard American Heart Association recommendations for CPR apply and these include the frequent administration of epinephrine. Fig. 40.5 presents an algorithm for the differential diagnosis and treatment of the more common causes of acute OR-associated cardiac dysfunction.

HYPERKALEMIA

A child with a hyperkalemic cardiac arrest may be identified by history, by the progression of ECG changes leading up to the arrest (Fig. 9.7), or by initial laboratory results. A high index of suspicion must be maintained for hyperkalemia as a cause of cardiac arrest because it requires specific therapy. Along with the usual resuscitation algorithms, immediate therapy to antagonize the acute effects of the increased serum potassium concentration on the myocardial cells is necessary in order to reestablish sinus rhythm. Calcium gluconate or calcium chloride antagonizes the effects of hyperkalemia on the myocardial cell membrane by increasing the threshold potential so that the gap between the threshold potential and the resting membrane potential is reestablished, curtailing the depolarization of random myocardial cells. Sodium bicarbonate and hyperventilation increase the serum pH and shift potassium from the extracellular to the intracellular compartments. and insulin (with concomitant dextrose) shifts potassium intracellularly (0.1 U/kg of insulin with 0.5 g/kg of dextrose; 2 mL/kg of dextrose 25%). The serum potassium concentration must be monitored frequently during this treatment, preferably by point-of-care testing. Because these therapies simply shift potassium intracellularly, therapy to remove potassium from the body (furosemide, hemodialysis, sodium polystyrene sulfonate) should be instituted (see Chapter 28, Table 28.6).

ANAPHYLAXIS

Anaphylaxis is a rare, but usually reversible, cause of cardiac arrest. Classic anaphylaxis is defined by the triad of dermatologic (usually flushing, pallor, or urticaria), respiratory (airway edema and possible obstruction and bronchospasm), and cardiovascular signs. Anaphylaxis may be particularly severe in situations of decreased endogenous catecholamines, such as in a child taking β-blockers or in children receiving spinal or epidural anesthesia.

Resuscitation of the child with anaphylaxis rests on reversing airway obstruction and restoring intravascular volume and vascular tone. In the child with mild anaphylaxis (as manifested by mild bronchospasm and hypotension), epinephrine 1 to 2 µg/kg IV in repeated doses should be given until signs abate. In the child in cardiac arrest from anaphylaxis, the dose of epinephrine should be 10 µg/kg or 0.01 mL/kg of IV or subcutaneous epinephrine (1:1000 concentration). Children with anaphylactic shock have profound intravascular depletion requiring rapidly administered, large-volume fluid resuscitation (20-mL/kg boluses of balanced salt solutions). In addition to the usual resuscitation medications, treatment should include an antihistamine and corticosteroid, such as diphenhydramine (Benadryl), 1 mg/kg, and methylprednisolone (Solu-Medrol), 2 mg/kg. Inhaled bronchodilators such as albuterol may relieve the bronchospasm. If severe airway obstruction occurs, tracheal intubation or even cricothyroidotomy may become difficult or impossible. Therefore the airway should be secured by a skilled practitioner early in the course of the reaction.

SUPRAVENTRICULAR TACHYCARDIA

Supraventricular tachycardia (SVT), despite being a common arrhythmia in infants and children, is uncommon during the intraoperative period in children without cardiac disease.[128] SVT may be associated with severe circulatory compromise or even cardiac arrest. Therapy for this arrhythmia should be based on the child's hemodynamic status. SVT associated with inadequate circulation should be treated immediately with synchronized cardioversion beginning at a dose of 0.5 J/kg. If IV access is available, adenosine can be administered while cardioversion is being prepared; however, cardioversion should not be delayed to establish IV access.

Adenosine is the medical treatment of choice for SVT. The underlying mechanism in children is usually a reentry circuit involving the atrioventricular node. Adenosine causes a temporary block in the atrioventricular node and interrupts this reentry circuit. The initial dose is 0.1 mg/kg given as a rapid IV bolus. Central venous administration is preferable because the drug is rapidly metabolized by red blood cell adenosine deaminase and therefore has a half-life of only 10 seconds. When the drug is given peripherally, the IV line should be immediately and rapidly flushed with 10 mL of saline. If there is no interruption in the reentry circuit, successive doses of 0.2 and 0.4 mg/kg should be given. In neonates, a smaller initial dose of 0.05 mg/kg is given and increased by 0.05 mg/kg per dose until termination of the arrhythmia up to a maximum dose of 0.3 mg/kg.[129] When SVT appears without any circulatory compromise, conversion of the arrhythmia may first be attempted with a vagal maneuver such as ice to the face. If this is ineffective, then adenosine should be used. Note that the denervated transplanted heart is extremely sensitive to the AV blockade and that half the normal starting dose is recommended.

Other medications used to treat SVT have a greater incidence of adverse effects than adenosine. Digoxin is often ineffective and causes frequent arrhythmias. Verapamil should be avoided in infants because of its association with congestive heart failure and cardiac arrest because of its negative inotropic effects.[130] Flecainide is effective in treating SVT but has many cardiac and noncardiac adverse effects[131]; its role for hemodynamically unstable SVT remains to be established. Other therapies include β-adrenergic blockers, edrophonium, and α-agonists. If SVT persists despite medical therapy and the child progresses to circulatory instability, electrical cardioversion should proceed immediately.

PULSELESS ELECTRICAL ACTIVITY

PEA is defined as organized ECG activity, excluding ventricular tachycardia and fibrillation, without clinical evidence of a palpable pulse or myocardial contractions. It may occur spontaneously after cardiac arrest or as an intervening rhythm associated with treatment for cardiac arrest. The causes of PEA are divided into primary (cardiac) and secondary (noncardiac) causes. Primary PEA, associated with cardiac arrest, is due to depletion of myocardial energy stores and responds poorly to therapy. Drugs used to treat primary PEA include epinephrine, atropine, calcium, and sodium bicarbonate.

The causes of secondary PEA are often remembered using the 4 Hs and 4 Ts mnemonic: **H**ypovolemia, **H**ypoxia, **H**ypothermia, and **H**ypo- or **H**yper-electrolytemia (hyperkalemia, hypocalcemia), **T**ension pneumothorax, pericardial **T**amponade, **T**hromboembolism, and **T**oxins (anesthetic overdose). In secondary PEA, intervention is directed at the underlying disorder and usually results in a successful resuscitation. When the cause of PEA is unknown and the child does not respond to medications, giving a fluid bolus and inserting needles into the pleural space to rule out pneumothorax and into the pericardial space to rule out cardiac tamponade are recommended.

Adjunctive Cardiopulmonary Resuscitation Techniques

OPEN-CHEST CARDIOPULMONARY RESUSCITATION

The use of open-chest cardiac massage, although generally replaced by closed-chest CPR, still has an active role in the OR and ICU, especially during and after thoracic surgery. Compared with closed-chest CPR, open-chest CPR generates greater cardiac output and vital organ blood flow. During open-chest CPR, the intrathoracic, right atrial, and intracranial pressures increase to a lesser extent, resulting in greater coronary and cerebral perfusion pressure and greater myocardial and cerebral blood flow compared with closed-chest CPR.[132,133,134]

Typically, in the OR and ICU, open-chest CPR is preferable to closed-chest CPR in the child who has had a recent sternotomy. Open-chest CPR is also indicated for selected children when closed-chest CPR has failed, although exactly which children should receive this method of resuscitation under this condition is controversial. When initiated early after failure of closed-chest CPR, open-chest CPR may improve outcome.[135-137] When performed after 15 minutes of closed-chest CPR, open-chest CPR significantly improves coronary perfusion pressure and the rate of successful resuscitation.[138]

EXTRACORPOREAL MEMBRANE OXYGENATION

Extracorporeal cardiopulmonary bypass (CPB) may be considered for refractory pediatric cardiac arrest when the condition leading to arrest is reversible and when the period of no flow (cardiac arrest without CPR) was brief. This intervention depends on the institution's ability to rapidly mobilize an extracorporeal circuit. Survival with a good neurologic outcome is possible after more than 50 minutes of CPR in selected children by using extracorporeal CPB.[139,140] Emergency extracorporeal membrane oxygenation (ECMO) in children with in-hospital CPR 10 minutes or longer in duration has been associated with improved survival to hospital discharge and survival with favorable neurologic outcome compared with failed conventional CPR.[141] CPB techniques such as ECMO require major technical support and sophistication but can be rapidly implemented in hospitals set up to do so. However, absence of a formal rapid deployment ECMO team does not preclude resuscitation with ECMO in pediatric cardiac patients with good results.[142]

ACTIVE COMPRESSION-DECOMPRESSION

Active compression-decompression CPR uses a negative-pressure "pull" on the thorax during the release phase of chest compression using a handheld suction device. This technique improves vascular pressures and minute ventilation during CPR in animals and humans.[143-147] The hemodynamic benefit of this technique is attributed to increased venous return by the negative intrathoracic pressure generated during the decompression phase. When this technique was used with a device adding impedance to inspiration, vascular pressures and flow increased further.[148] Its effectiveness in adults shows promise, with increased survival and weak evidence for neurologic improvement in prehospital victims.[149–151] However, larger trials did not demonstrate improved survival in in-hospital or prehospital victims of cardiac arrest, nor did any subgroup demonstrate benefit from active compression-decompression CPR.[152–154] The complication rate, including fatal rib and sternal fractures, may be greater with this technique.[155]

Postresuscitation Stabilization (Post–Cardiac Arrest Care)

The goals of postresuscitation care are to prevent secondary organ injury, preserve neurologic function, diagnose and treat the cause of the illness, and prevent a recurrence of the arrest. Respiratory support should be tailored to minimize the risk of oxidative damage while maintaining adequate O_2 delivery. FiO_2 should be limited to the minimum necessary to maintain an adequate saturation. Ventilation should be closely monitored because both hypercarbia and hypocarbia may confer deleterious effects.

Mitigation of neurologic injury after cardiac arrest has been a goal of many investigator groups. In adult patients with out-of-hospital VF and in asphyxiated newborns,[64] therapeutic hypothermia was believed to offer some benefit. However, the effectiveness of hypothermia therapy was neither supported nor refuted in a retrospective study.[156] A target temperature of 36°C proved better than 33°C in adults.[157] Similar results have been reported in children. Therapeutic hypothermia in children did not confer a significant benefit in survival with a good functional outcome at 1 year.[65]

The 2015 AHA Pediatric Advanced Life Support Guidelines Update[60]

Cardiopulmonary resuscitation of children with a nonnative airway should use ETCO₂ carbon-dioxide monitoring as a surrogate for effective compressions. This is of particular relevance for the perioperative physician as patients should have ETCO₂ monitoring as part of their routine anesthetic care. Attention should focus on an adequate depth and frequency of compressions with sufficient recoil. The compressor should be monitored for fatigue and rapid change of practitioners (every 2 minutes) should be instituted if compressions are judged to be inadequate because of poor technique. Examination of patients for successful ROSC should not occur within the 2-minute epochs of compression as the quality of compressions could be compromised. Compressions should be extended 2 minutes after the confirmation of the ROSC.

ANNOTATED REFERENCES

American Heart Association. American Heart Association guidelines for cardiopulmonary resuscitation and emergency cardiovascular care. *Circulation.* 2015;132(8 suppl 2):S526-S542.[60]
This publication provides comprehensive guidelines for pediatric and adult advanced life support, with comprehensive references.

Nadkarni VM, Larkin GL, Peberdy MA, et al. First documented rhythm and clinical outcome from in-hospital cardiac arrest among children and adults. *JAMA.* 2006;295:50-297.
In this multicenter registry of in-hospital cardiac arrest, the first documented pulseless arrest rhythm was typically asystole or pulseless electrical activity in both children and adults. Because of improved survival after asystole and pulseless electrical activity, children had better outcomes than adults despite fewer cardiac arrests resulting from ventricular fibrillation or pulseless ventricular tachycardia.

Perondi M, Reis A, Paiva E, et al. A comparison of high-dose and standard-dose epinephrine in children with cardiac arrest. *N Engl J Med.* 2004;350:1722-1730.
This blinded, randomized controlled trial compared high-dose and standard-dose epinephrine as rescue therapy in children with in-hospital cardiac arrest. No benefit of high-dose epinephrine was detected. The data suggest that high-dose therapy may be more deleterious than standard-dose therapy.

A complete reference list can be found online at ExpertConsult.com

Malignant Hyperthermia

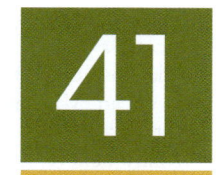

JERROLD LERMAN AND JEROME PARNESS

MALIGNANT HYPERTHERMIA (MH) is a pharmacogenetic disease of skeletal muscle that may precipitate a potentially fatal sequence of metabolic responses in the presence of triggering anesthetics. The primary triggers for MH—inhalational anesthetics and succinylcholine—induce an uncontrollable release of intramyoplasmic calcium (Ca^{2+}) that results in sustained muscle contractures, which produce a hypermetabolic response. The hypermetabolic response manifests with hypercarbia, hyperpnea, tachycardia, and if not treated early, a mixed metabolic and respiratory acidosis. An acute reaction is usually accompanied by muscle rigidity either as isolated muscle rigidity (e.g., masseter muscle tetany in the temporomandibular joint) or total body muscle rigidity (e.g., sustained contraction of major peripheral muscle groups).

MH was first described by Denborough and Lovell in 1960, who reported a 21-year-old man who was hesitant to undergo general anesthesia to repair his leg fracture because family members had died under anesthesia.[1] After 10 minutes of halothane anesthesia, he became hemodynamically unstable with hypotension, tachycardia, and mottled skin that was hot to the touch. The soda lime canister was found to be hot and was changed because it appeared to be exhausted. The anesthetic was discontinued, the patient was packed in ice, and he recovered without sequelae. Postprocedural examination did not reveal any known medical condition. A careful family history disclosed that 10 blood relatives had previously died after ether anesthesia, suggesting an autosomal dominant inheritance pattern. This patient required a subsequent operation and was administered a spinal anesthetic without incident.[2] Subsequent reports from around the world established this disorder as a familial entity that was potentially fatal.[3,4] The term *malignant hyperpyrexia* (later changed to *malignant hyperthermia*) was coined in 1967 at the first international meeting on this disorder in Toronto, Canada.

The incidence of MH based on the frequency of MH reactions has been reported to be 1 case per 50,000 to 100,000 adults and 1 case per 3000 to 15,000 children.[5,6] Regional differences in the prevalence of MH may account for an even greater frequency of reactions (of all levels of severity) in some jurisdictions—for example, 1 case per 16,000 anesthetics in adults in Denmark and 1 case per 4200 adults when an inhaled anesthetic and succinylcholine were combined.[7] A recent review of discharge diagnoses from New York state ambulatory centers reported a prevalence of MH of 1:500,000,[8] a frequency that may reflect the reluctance of these centers to handle patients with MH. A survey in a pediatric hospital in the United States during the halothane era revealed an MH incidence of 1 case per 20,000 to 40,000 children, almost one-half of that reported previously.[9] The incidence of fulminant MH (defined as a rapid increase in temperature accompanied by life-threatening metabolic changes, arrhythmias, and increased serum creatine kinase level) was far less frequent: 1 case per 250,000 general anesthetics in Denmark[7] and 1 case per 200,000 in the United Kingdom.[10] The Danish survey found an incidence of 1 case of masseter muscle spasm per 12,000 anesthetics among children who received succinylcholine, whether in combination with inhalational or intravenous (IV) anesthetics.[7] Clinically, the demographic data suggested that the incidence or suspicion of MH was greater among children than adults and that the incidence was even greater among children in whom succinylcholine was used.

Genetic testing has become sufficiently pervasive to permit estimation of the prevalence of MH based on genetic mutations.[11] On the basis of genetic testing, the prevalence has been estimated between 1:3000 and 1:8500, although some estimates have reached 1:400.[11] The frequency of MH reactions is greatest in childhood (up to 52% of reactions), with a peak age of 3 years, and the youngest confirmed cases in early infancy, 2 months of age.[12] In one case, a known genetic mutation (G2434R) consistent with the diagnosis of MH was identified in the cord blood of a neonate born to an MH-susceptible (MHS) parturient with the same mutation.[13]

Many believe the incidence of MH reactions has decreased in the past 2 decades, although some have challenged this notion.[14] Two reasons for this notion are that (1) families with a genetic predisposition to MH have been identified and patients bring it to the attention of their surgical and anesthetic care providers preoperatively and (2) the routine use of succinylcholine has decreased dramatically as a result of concerns of rare complications, such as hyperkalemic cardiac arrest. The latter has resulted in a black box warning admonishing against the routine use of succinylcholine in children, particularly male children younger than 8 years of age in the United States who may have unrecognized muscular dystrophy or other myopathy.[15,16]

All inhalational anesthetics (except xenon) and succinylcholine trigger MH reactions in susceptible patients[17–23]; no other drugs used for IV or regional anesthesia trigger MH reactions. A comprehensive list of triggering and nontriggering drugs is available from the Malignant Hyperthermia Association of the United States (MHAUS; http://www.mhaus.org/).

The mortality rate from MH has decreased dramatically from more than 80% in the 1960s to 1.4% more recently (Fig. 41.1).[14,24–26] For children, the mortality rate from MH, 0.7%, is 20-fold less than that for adults, 14% based on an inpatient database.[14] The overall decrease in mortality may be attributed to several factors: better identification of MH-susceptible individuals; the routine use of capnography and pulse oximetry, facilitating early identification of the signs and symptoms of an acute MH reaction[27,28]; a better understanding of the pathogenesis of MH; and the widespread availability of dantrolene.[29]

Clinical Presentation

The most common presentation of MH is a hypermetabolic response to the inhalational anesthetics, with or without succinylcholine (Table 41.1). Among the earliest clinical signs is a marked increase in the end-tidal carbon dioxide ($ETCO_2$) that resists control by either mechanical ventilation or an increase in minute ventilation when the patient is breathing spontaneously.[25,30] Other nonspecific early signs include tachycardia and hemodynamic instability with a trend toward hypertension. Severe masseter muscle spasm (i.e., masseter tetany) refers to the inability to insert a laryngoscope blade into the mouth—the so-called jaws of steel—even with no twitches evident on a blockade monitor after administration of succinylcholine. It strongly indicates MH susceptibility (Fig. 41.2). The differential diagnosis of severe masseter spasm should include the possible presence of the ultra-rapid polymorphism of pseudocholinesterase, the C5 (E Cynthiana or Neitlich) variant (see Chapters 6 and 7), which terminates the action of succinylcholine more rapidly than usual.[31] In vitro live muscle biopsy testing revealed a 28% to 50% incidence of MH susceptibility among children with jaws of steel, with an extensive differential diagnosis (Table 41.2).[32–34] Generalized muscle rigidity develops as a result of the excessive accumulation of myoplasmic Ca^{2+} concentrations in MHS skeletal muscle, causing sustained muscle contractures.[30] This occurs even in the presence of neuromuscular blockade with nondepolarizing neuromuscular blocking drugs (NMBDs).

Hyperthermia, often a late sign, results from the greatly increased aerobic and anaerobic metabolic activity of triggered skeletal muscle; the overlying skin soon becomes hot to the touch. In

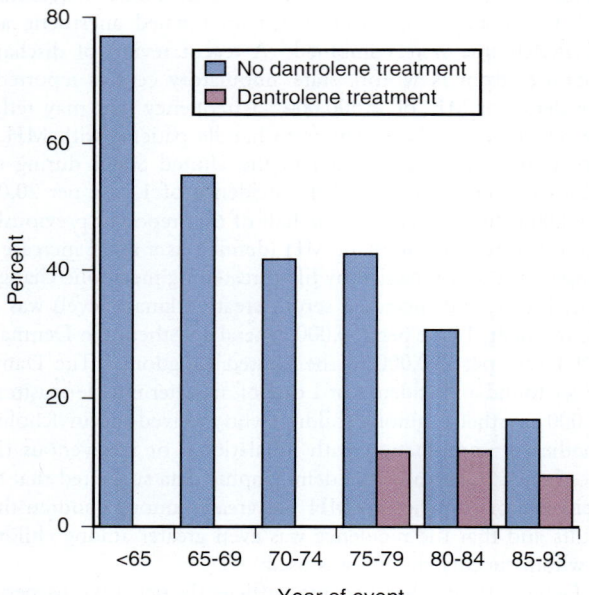

FIGURE 41.1 The trend in fatality rates from malignant hyperthermia is shown over time. The *blue bars* represent data from 361 patients, and the *magenta bars* represent data from 142 patients. Notice the marked decrease in mortality with dantrolene treatment. (Modified from Strazis KP, Fox AW. Malignant hyperthermia: a review of published cases. *Anesth. Analg.* 1993;77[2]:297–304.)

TABLE 41.1	Clinical and Laboratory Findings Associated With Malignant Hyperthermia	
Clinical Findings	**Laboratory Findings**
Tachycardia, tachypnea, and hypertension	
Hypercarbia ($ETCO_2$)	Increased $PaCO_2$
Greatly increased minute ventilation	Acidosis (mixed respiratory and metabolic)
Hemoglobin desaturation	Relative hypoxia, increased alveolar to arterial partial pressure gradient for oxygen
Generalized muscle rigidity (unresponsive to nondepolarizing muscle relaxants)	Hyperkalemia Increased CPK level (usually a late sign) Increased plasma lactate concentration
Skin mottling	
Hyperthermia (late sign)	
Cardiac arrhythmias (hyperkalemia-induced: PVC, VT, VF)	
Cola-colored urine (late sign)	Myoglobinuria, myoglobinemia
Disseminated intravascular coagulation (late)	Abnormal coagulation studies (late sign)

CPK, creatinine phosphokinase; *ETCO₂*, end-tidal carbon dioxide; *PaCO₂*, arterial partial pressure of carbon dioxide; *PVC*, premature ventricular contraction; *VF*, ventricular fibrillation; *VT*, ventricular tachycardia.
Data from Malignant Hyperthermia Association of the United States. Available at http://www.mhaus.org (accessed July 2012).

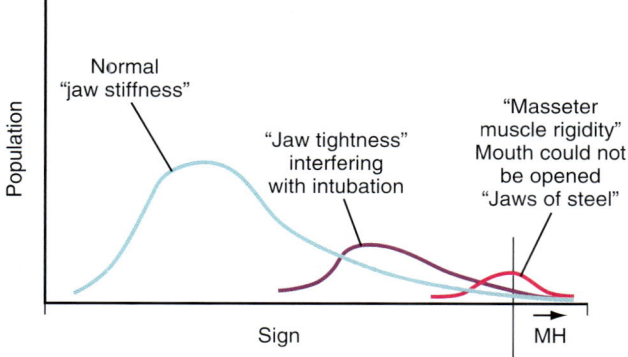

FIGURE 41.2 The spectrum of masseter muscle responses to succinylcholine varies from a slight jaw stiffness that does not interfere with endotracheal intubation to the extreme "jaws of steel," which is masseter muscle tetany that does not allow the mouth to be opened. The latter response is likely highly associated with malignant hyperthermia (MH). Even with the inability to open the mouth, the child's lungs should still be able to be ventilated by bag and mask because all other muscles are relaxed. (From Kaplan RF. Malignant hyperthermia. Annual refresher course lectures. Washington, DC: American Society of Anesthesiologists; 1993.)

TABLE 41.2	Limited Excursion of the Mandible: Differential Diagnosis
Temporomandibular joint dysfunction: congenital, inflammatory/infectious, trauma, neoplasm, collagen vascular disease (rheumatoid arthritis)	
Muscle disease: malignant hyperthermia, Duchenne or Becker muscular cystrophy, myotonia congenita	
Integumentary disease: inflammatory or infectious disease, neoplasm, radiation effects, collagen vascular disease (scleroderma)	
Neurologic injury	
Ultra-rapid metabolizer of succinylcholine (Neitlich or E Cynthiana [C5 enzyme] variant of pseudocholinesterase) (see Chapters 6 and 7)	
Ineffective succinylcholine	

many instances, the large muscle groups such as calf or thigh muscles feel tight or knotted. This is accompanied by exaggerated carbon dioxide (CO_2) production, which usually is the first sign of an evolving MH reaction, and the accumulation of lactate fueled by markedly increased glycogenolysis and glycolysis (i.e., mixed respiratory and metabolic acidosis).[35,36] If an acute MH reaction is diagnosed and treated early in its evolution, before the body becomes unable to maintain this exaggerated aerobic metabolism, arterial blood gases may show an almost pure respiratory acidosis, which can make the diagnosis of MH difficult (Table 41.3). A mixed venous or peripheral venous blood gas analysis can be helpful in establishing the presence of hypermetabolism because it is more likely to demonstrate an increased partial pressure of CO_2, significant oxygen desaturation consistent with increased oxygen consumption ($\dot{V}O_2$ <40 mm Hg, despite administering supplemental oxygen for which the expected $\dot{V}O_2$ is >60 mm Hg), and a possible increased lactate concentration.

In fulminant cases, untreated MH may increase the temperature as rapidly as 1C° every 10 minutes.[30] In one case, the temperature reached 43.8°C (110.8°F) within 18 minutes.[37] In addition to the profound hypercarbia and tachycardia, severe hypoxia, skin mottling, exuberant metabolic acidosis, rhabdomyolysis, coagulopathy, and hyperkalemia may follow unless the reaction is aborted

TABLE 41.3	Arterial Blood Gas Data From a Child in Early Malignant Hyperthermia			
	TIME AT MEASUREMENT			
Data	*08:52*	*08:59*	*09:05*	*09:27*
pH[a]	7.34	7.03	7.29	7.39
PCO_2 (mm Hg)	46.3	109.4	47.9	42.7
PO_2 (mm Hg)	236	159	589	635
Base excess	−1	−2	−3	1
(mmol/L)	25.1	29	23.1	25.6

[a]Notice the pure respiratory acidosis in this patient from Fig. 41.3 and the rapid decrease in $PaCO_2$ after dantrolene administration between 08:59 and 09:05. $PaCO_2$, arterial partial pressure of carbon dioxide; PO_2, partial pressure of oxygen.

following the administration of dantrolene. Unstable hemodynamics and ventricular arrhythmias inevitably follow. Intractable ventricular arrhythmias, pulmonary edema, disseminated intravascular coagulation, cerebral hypoxia or edema, and renal failure as the result of myoglobin deposition in the renal tubules are often associated with fatal outcomes.

In the early years of treating acute MH reactions, before dantrolene was identified as the specific antidote, symptomatic treatment was the mainstay of therapy. This included treatment of the acidosis and hyperkalemia with bicarbonate, and insulin with glucose, respectively; active cooling with iced saline solution gastric lavage; infusion of cold IV saline solution; and infusions of procainamide (a drug that was later shown to be ineffective). These interventions helped to reduce the mortality rate to about 50%, but with the availability of dantrolene, the mortality rate decreased dramatically, to 1.4% to 2.9% based on an MH database and an inpatient pediatric database.[38,39]

The presenting signs of MH vary (see Table 41.1). The syndrome may be fulminant or indolent, not all features of a classic MH reaction may be immediately evident, and it may occur intraoperatively or postoperatively, although the frequency of MH reactions occurring postoperatively is only ~2%.[30,40] The latest that an MH reaction has occurred postoperatively is 11 hours, although a review of reports of postoperative MH from the North American Malignant Hyperthermia Registry failed to find any cases that occurred beyond 40 minutes after the end of the anesthetic.[40,41] The likelihood that an MHS patient will develop MH in the presence of inhalational anesthetics is exasperatingly unpredictable. In one study, 50% of susceptible individuals reported two or more uneventful general anesthetics before an MH reaction was triggered.[25,42] Only 6.5% of probands in a retrospective review reported a family or personal history of MH.[42] A negative personal or family history is insufficient to conclude that a child is not susceptible to MH. Other disease states may be confused with MH (Table 41.4) and must be distinguished from it to provide correct therapy.

Given the variability of the clinical presentation of MH and the dearth of pathognomonic signs for this syndrome, establishing the diagnosis can be difficult. In response to the need for an objective measure to verify a clinical episode of MH, a retrospective, multivariable clinical grading scale was developed.[43] This grading scale was devised to clarify the cutoff value for a positive muscle caffeine halothane contracture test (CHCT) result. It was not intended to be a clinical guide in the operating room. Despite recommendations not to use this scale to guide treatment and to be more conservative in its application, E-Tables 41.1A and 41.1B

TABLE 41.4	Differential Diagnosis of Malignant Hyperthermia
Diagnosis	**Distinguishing Traits**
Hyperthyroidism	Patients often present with similar symptoms and physical findings; blood gas abnormalities gradually evolve; creatine phosphokinase value does not increase substantively. Unresponsive to dantrolene.
Sepsis	Usually, blood gases are normal early, and metabolic acidosis occurs late; creatine phosphokinase remains normal.
Pheochromocytoma	Similar to malignant hyperthermia (MH), except for marked blood pressure swings, hypercarbia, and venous desaturation
Metastatic carcinoid	Flushing, diarrhea, hypotension
Cocaine intoxication	Fever, rigidity, rhabdomyolysis similar to NMS
Heat stroke	Similar to MH, except that the patient is outside the operating room
Masseter muscle rigidity (MMR)	May progress to MH; total body spasm more likely than isolated MMR
Neuroleptic malignant syndrome (NMS)	Similar to MH but evolves over weeks; usually associated with the use of antipsychotics
Serotonergic toxicity	Similar to MH and NMS; associated with the administration of mood-elevating drugs (e.g., selective serotonin reuptake inhibitors)
Nonmalignant hyperthermia syndrome	Reported only once; severe hyperthermia seemingly associated with fentanyl

are provided to help clinicians identify true MH reactions. Although these clinical grading scales are somewhat cumbersome and have not been prospectively validated in clinical settings for use by nonexperts, they do provide a useful guide for the clinician.

Patient Evaluation and Preparation

Optimal treatment begins with prevention and preparation. Obtaining an accurate family history of suspicious or unusual reactions to general anesthesia in blood relatives, unexpected admissions to intensive care after surgery, or unexplained sudden death during or immediately after general anesthesia should signal to the surgeon and anesthesiologist to consider MH or another problem related to anesthesia. These questions assume the patient is part of a classic nuclear family, but with increasing levels of adoption, artificial insemination, surrogate motherhood, and egg donations, standard probing may not elicit clear family histories. The anesthesiologist must be sensitive but decisive in determining the true genetic relationship between the guardians and the child. Despite attempts to obtain an accurate history, misinterpretation of the questions may occur. In one case, an adopted child died of succinylcholine-induced hyperkalemic cardiac arrest, even though the parents denied that anyone in the family had anesthesia problems or muscle disease during the preoperative assessment. Only immediately after the event did the parents reveal that the child had been adopted and that the child's birth uncle had muscular dystrophy.

If the anesthesiologist is informed that the child has a blood relative who had an MH reaction or who has a myopathy with high concordance with MH, the most prudent course of action is to schedule the case for the first of the day to minimize exposing the children to inhalational anesthetics in the operating or recovery room.[44–47] With the abundance of evidence that stress alone can trigger an MH reaction, preoperative anxiolytics such as midazolam are warranted in these children, except for the most minor procedures (e.g., myringotomy and tubes). Prophylactic dantrolene is not warranted in MH patients who receive a trigger-free anesthetic as the frequency of MH reactions is very small.[48–50] The anesthetic prescription must include nontriggering agents such as total IV or regional anesthetics, or both. In the rare circumstance in which triggers must be used (and these are rare), extreme vigilance and anticipation to treat an acute MH reaction are of the utmost importance, although in a recent case of acute epiglottitis, the airway was secured with a total intravenous anesthesia (TIVA) technique rather than an inhalation technique.[48,49,51] When a child with a known susceptibility to MH is scheduled for general anesthesia, the anesthesia machine (i.e., anesthetic workstation [AWS]) must be prepared to preclude the delivery of triggering agents. First, succinylcholine should be removed from the local vicinity to avoid inadvertent administration. Second, all vaporizers should be physically disengaged from the AWS, which is preferable because they can leak trace concentrations of inhalational anesthetics even in the off state, or if they cannot be removed from the AWS, tape should be placed across them in the off position to avoid accidentally turning them on.[52] Third, to accelerate the washout of anesthetics, the CO_2 absorbent should be replaced, a new anesthetic breathing circuit installed, and the ventilator bellows flushed and left operating.[52–54] Fourth, to eliminate inhalational anesthetics from the AWS, many clinicians follow a standardized protocol of flushing the workstation with 10 L/minute of oxygen for 10 to 20 minutes, depending on the AWS manufacturer and age of the machine.[55] However, the assumption that one protocol fits all to reduce the anesthetic concentration to less than 10 ppm, which is assumed to be the threshold below which an MH reaction cannot be triggered,[56] may not hold true for every AWS. This is particularly an issue with the newer AWS, which are more complex in construction and more likely to contain internal working parts made of plastic, which act as sumps for inhalational anesthetics.[57] To address the various types of AWS, the duration of flushing with large fresh gas flows (Table 41.5) and the need to exchange contaminated internal components with clean versions must be determined for each AWS. For some types of AWS, more than 60 minutes may be required to reach anesthetic concentrations less than 10 ppm.[55,57–59] To achieve an anesthetic concentration of 10 ppm or less in the Dräger Primus, Fabius, and Zeus machines (Drägerwerk AG & Co. KGaA, Lübeck, Germany) in a timely manner, the ventilator diaphragm and integrated breathing system should be replaced with autoclaved components and then flushed for 20 minutes at a fresh gas flow of 10 L/minute.[58,59] Table 41.5 lists the published times required to reach an anesthetic concentration of less than 10 ppm without replacing any AWS components.[55,57,59–61] These data support the notion that the previously held protocols to wash out inhalational anesthetics from older AWSs do not hold true for the newer AWSs. The need for a single protocol or intervention that consistently achieves an anesthetic concentration of less than 10 ppm in all AWSs is of even greater importance because none of the available anesthetic agent analyzers is capable of measuring anesthetic concentrations in the 10-ppm range to confirm adequate removal of inhalational anesthetics.

After the AWS has been flushed with 10 L/minute of an air and oxygen mixture, most anesthesiologists reduce the fresh gas flow during anesthesia. However, evidence has shown that

TABLE 41.5	Time to Wash Out Inhalational Anesthetics to Less Than 10 ppm AWSs		
Datex-Ohmeda-GE AWSs	Time (minutes)	Other AWSs	Time (minutes)
Modulus 1[a]	5–15	Narkomed[a] (Dräger)	20
Excel 210	7	Dräger Primus[a,b]	39–70
AS/3[c]	30	Dräger Fabius GS[a]	104
Aestiva (sevoflurane)[d]	22	Dräger Zeus[b,e]	35–85
Aisys (sevoflurane)[d]	25	Kion[f] (Siemens)	>25
Avance[b]	39	Perseus[b] (Dräger)	15
		Felix AInOC[b] (Taema, Air Liquide)	135
		Flow-i[b] (Maquet)	46
		Leon[b] (Heinen + Löwenstein GmBH)	106

AWSs, anesthesia work stations
Data are from the following sources:
[a]Kim TW, Nemergut ME. Preparation of modern anesthesia workstations for malignant hyperthermia-susceptible patients; a review of past and present practice. *Anesthesiology* 2011;114:205–212.
[b]Cottron N, Larcher C, Sommet A, et al. The sevoflurane washout profile of seven recent anesthesia workstations for malignant hyperthermia-susceptible adults and infants: a bench test study. *Anesth Analg.* 2014:119;67–75.
[c]Schonell LHB, Sims C, Bulsara M. Preparing a new generation anaesthetic machine for patients susceptible to malignant hyperthermia. *Anaesth Intens Care.* 2003:31; 58–61.
[d]Sabouri AS, Lerman J, Heard C. Effects of fresh gas flow, tidal volume, and charcoal filters on the washout of sevoflurane from the Datex Ohmeda (GE) Aisys, Aestiva/5 and Excel 210 SE anesthesia workstations. *Can J Anesth.* 2014:61;935–942;
[e]Shanahan H, O'Donoghue R, O'Kelly P, Synnott A, O'Rourke J. Preparation of the Drager Fabius CE and Drager Zeus anaesthetic machines for patients susceptible to malignant hyperthermia. *Eur J Anaesthesiol* 2012;29:229–234.
[f]Petroz GC, Lerman J. Preparation of the Siemens KION anesthetic machine for patients susceptible to malignant hyperthermia. *Anesthesiology.* 2002;96(4): 941–946.

the concentration of inhalational anesthetic surges (≥ 50 ppm) when the fresh gas flow is reduced, and the magnitude of the rebound directly depends on the fresh gas flow rate.[60,62] Those who reduce the fresh gas flow after purging the AWS may be exposing their patients to concentrations of inhalational anesthetics that may trigger an MH reaction, although no MH reactions have been reported in patients in whom a reduced fresh gas flow was used in an AWS that had been purged using a large (>10-L/minute) fresh gas flow. To avoid confusion, a single, consistent, effective, and reliable intervention is required to prevent MH reactions in patients exposed to trace gases from a previously contaminated AWS.

A commercially available charcoal filter (Vapor-Clean, Dynasthetics, LLC, Salt Lake City, UT) fitted to the expiratory and inspiratory limbs of the AWS reduces the concentration of inhalational anesthetics to less than 5 ppm within several minutes.[63] These filters are sold in pairs. The manufacturer recommends that a filter be inserted into both the inspiratory and expiratory limbs of the anesthesia breathing circuit just distal to the valves, which is reasonable during an acute MH reaction. However, when only the machine is contaminated with inhalational anesthetic (e.g., after flushing the AWS for elective MH cases), we apply a single filter in the **inspiratory limb** and keep the second of the pair to replace the first after 60 to 90 minutes, since it may become expended by that time.[63] Another alternate approach is to replace

the breathing circuit and carbon dioxide absorber with new equipment and then insert a filter into the inspiratory limb.

Ambulatory surgery has rapidly expanded to include most pediatric surgery. Consequently, the safety of discharging children with a personal or family history of MH after an uneventful, trigger-free anesthesia on the day of surgery has raised concerns. Several studies demonstrated that the risk of developing an MH reaction after an uneventful, trigger-free anesthesia was exceedingly small.[48–50] Postoperative monitoring for an MH reaction while in the hospital has gradually been reduced from 6 hours to 2 hours or less before discharge.[64–66] For MHS children, parents should be provided with a written description of the signs and symptoms of an MH reaction and the direct phone number to reach the on-call anesthesiologist for further advice and management. Families should contact an anesthesiologist rather than return to the emergency department because the emergency physician may be unfamiliar with MH, particularly in children. Additional advice for the parents should include the use of an oral antipyretic drug (e.g., acetaminophen) to treat a mild fever. If the fever abates after a dose or two of acetaminophen, the fever was not caused by MH. If the fever persists despite acetaminophen and sponge baths and is accompanied by tachycardia and tachypnea, the parents should notify the on-call anesthesiologist and immediately return the child to the hospital.

Monitoring

Capnography and pulse oximetry, key monitors for early signs of an MH reaction, are required for all children who receive general anesthesia, irrespective of the duration of the procedure. Measurement of the body temperature is recommended for all children who undergo general anesthesia when fluctuations may be anticipated, according to the American Society of Anesthesiologists standards for basic anesthesia monitoring, last updated in 2015 (www.asahq.org/quality-and-practice-management/standards-and-guidelines). Monitoring the axillary temperature site (opposite the extremity with the IV line) is recommended rather than a core site for early detection of an MH reaction because the axillary region and the venous drainage thereof may reflect the increased metabolism from sustained contractures of the pectoral shoulder girdle, a large muscle bulk. Although most consider an increasing temperature a late sign of an MH reaction, a retrospective review suggested that an increasing body temperature may occur early in an evolving MH reaction.[42,67] Moreover, data from a retrospective review of MH deaths suggested that the risk of dying during an MH reaction was 14-fold greater if the core temperature was not measured and that the risk of any complication increased 2.9-fold for every 2°C increase in body temperature.[38] Evidence also suggests that crystalline skin temperature tapes may not reliably track temperature changes during MH reactions.[42]

Diagnosis

Because the underlying disorder in MH is a hypermetabolic reaction (i.e., increased CO_2 production and oxygen consumption), massive volumes of CO_2 are released into the circulation, which rapidly increase the partial pressure of CO_2 ($PaCO_2$) and respiratory rate in the unparalyzed child. The cardiovascular response is an increased cardiac output, heart rate, and in some cases, blood pressure (E-Fig. 41.1). The first clinical signs and symptoms of this hypermetabolic reaction in a spontaneously breathing patient are hypercapnia, sinus tachycardia, and tachypnea (see Table 41.1).[42]

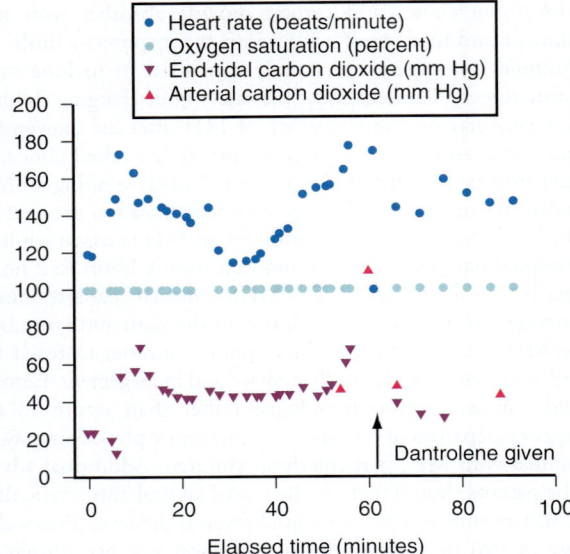

FIGURE 41.3 Response of physiologic parameters to dantrolene during an apparent intraoperative episode of malignant hyperthermia. Notice the rapid decrease in arterial and end-tidal carbon dioxide pressures after dantrolene (2.5 mg/kg) administration (*arrow*). (Courtesy Steven C. Hall, MD.)

In a retrospective review of 264 children in the North American MH Registry, the most common signs of an MH reaction were sinus tachycardia in 73% and hypercarbia in 69%, which were most common in adolescents.[68] Hyperthermia appeared in fewer than half (48%) of the children.[68] Greater temperatures and peak potassium concentrations were present more commonly in adolescents, whereas greater peak lactic acid concentrations and reduced peak creatine kinase concentrations were present in the younger children (<2 years).[68] A steady and relentless increase in the end-tidal CO_2 ($PETCO_2$) is the earliest sign of a reaction and is usually evident regardless of whether respirations are spontaneous or controlled. In some instances, the increase in $PETCO_2$ and heart rate occur contemporaneously, alerting the clinician to consider an evolving MH reaction (Fig. 41.3). Sudden unexpected cardiac arrest is a very rare presentation of MH and suggests a disease process other than MH, such as acute rhabdomyolysis and hyperkalemia after succinylcholine in a (male) child with an undiagnosed myopathy.

The presenting signs of an MH reaction are nonspecific and may suggest several possible disease states or equipment problems. The earliest sign of an MH reaction, an increase in $PETCO_2$, may result from one or more of three factors from the CO_2 mass balance equation:

$$PCO_2 = (\dot{V}CO_2 / \dot{V}A) + FICO_2 \qquad \text{Eq. 41.1}$$

The circulating PCO_2 depends on the production of CO_2 ($\dot{V}CO_2$), the elimination of CO_2 (i.e., alveolar ventilation ([$\dot{V}A$]), and the fraction of inspired concentration of CO_2 ($FICO_2$). The differential diagnosis of an increased PCO_2 can be analyzed by considering the causes for each of these three factors: $\dot{V}CO_2$, $\dot{V}A$, and $FICO_2$. Causes of an increased $\dot{V}CO_2$ include fever, MH, thyroid storm, and sepsis. This may pose a particular challenge to diagnose during laparoscopic surgery.[69,70] Causes of a decreased $\dot{V}A$ include a deep level of anesthesia, endobronchial intubation, bronchospasm, and a kinked tracheal tube or airway breathing circuit. Causes of

increased $FICO_2$ include an incompetent expiratory valve, exogenous source of CO_2, low fresh gas flows with a partial or nonrebreathing circuit, and expired CO_2 absorbent. The initial evaluation should include a rapid assessment of the integrity of the breathing circuit, the presence of bilateral breath sounds and absence of wheezing, and examination of the CO_2 absorbent.

During airway obstruction and hypermetabolic states such as thyrotoxicosis and sepsis, an increased $PETCO_2$ can be readily corrected with mild to moderate hyperventilation. During MH reactions, however, it is very difficult to restore the $PETCO_2$ to the normal range, even with vigorous mechanical hyperventilation.[28] The CO_2 production is sometimes so great that the in-circuit CO_2 absorbent rapidly becomes exhausted in an exothermic reaction, and the absorbent container becomes hot to touch. Thyrotoxicosis can be distinguished from an acute MH reaction by the absence of general muscle rigidity, less severe metabolic acidosis and peak creatine kinase (CK) level, and the absence of an effect by dantrolene on the course of the disease in thyrotoxicosis.

A child's response to surgery during light anesthesia often includes tachycardia and may sometimes include bronchoconstriction. However, a dramatic and unexpected increase in heart rate from 120 to 180 beats/minute in a healthy, 7-year-old child (or an increase from 70 to 120 beats/minute in an adult) strongly suggests a pathologic process, and a differential diagnosis beyond light anesthesia should be seriously considered. Before intervening, it is important to quickly scan all the monitors to determine whether the aggregate indexes point to a specific diagnosis. If tachycardia is associated with an increase in body temperature, a differential diagnosis of fever and tachycardia under anesthesia should be considered. Fever related to sepsis or viral infection usually has a slow onset, whereas fever from an MH reaction typically has a rapid onset. The differential diagnoses include iatrogenic external overheating and an MH reaction (see Table 41.4). A rapid increase in the inspired concentration of desflurane and isoflurane, but not sevoflurane, may cause a sympathetic-based tachycardia that in isolation should not suggest a diagnosis of MH because the $PETCO_2$ remains unchanged.[71,72] Of the inhalational anesthetics, halothane appears to be the most likely to trigger an MH reaction and the best discriminator for the CHCT. Enflurane provides the smallest trigger, sevoflurane and isoflurane are intermediate, and preliminary data suggest that xenon does not trigger MH reactions.[23,56,73–75] If none of these factors appears to be causative and a deeper level of anesthesia (achieved with propofol with or without an opioid) fails to abate the signs, simultaneous venous and arterial blood gases should be analyzed to determine whether the patient has or is developing a hypermetabolic state.

Rhabdomyolysis can occur during an acute MH reaction, but it usually occurs later in the course of an incompletely treated reaction compared with anesthesia-induced rhabdomyolysis (AIR), which is the presenting finding after the administration of succinylcholine with or without an inhaled anesthetic to a young child with an often undiagnosed myopathy (e.g., Duchenne muscular dystrophy).[76] The presenting features of MH and AIR are contrasted in Table 41.6. Note that MH rarely presents with isolated rhabdomyolysis; however, in contrast to AIR, it is responsive to dantrolene.

A moderate but gradual increase in body temperature may occur in children excessively draped, those with forced-air warming devices, those with bilateral limb tourniquets, and those covered with plastic occlusive wrap. However, the sudden onset of a high fever must be more thoroughly investigated because it may result from several potentially fatal causes (see Table 41.4).[77–80]

TABLE 41.6	Differences Between Malignant Hyperthermia and Anesthesia-Induced Rhabdomyolysis		
		Anesthesia-Induced Rhabdomyolysis	**Malignant Hyperthermia**
Early Signs	Clinical		Rigidity Masseter spasm
	ECG	Peaked T waves Bradycardia, dysrhythmia, ± cardiac arrest	Tachycardia
	Oxygen saturation Airway gas monitoring	Normal until arrest	Decreasing ↑ ETCO$_2$ ↑ Oxygen consumption[a]
	Blood results	Marked hyperkalaemia Increased creatine kinase (CK)	Hyperkalaemia
Late Signs		Acidosis ↑ ETCO$_2$ ± ↑ Temperature (rare) Myoglobinemia/urea CK > 1000/μL (may increase to >40,000)	Acidosis ↑ Temperature Myoglobinemia/urea Ventricular arrhythmia Cardiac arrest Bleeding diathesis
Timing (unless succinylcholine has been given)[b]		May occur at any time, particularly later in the anesthetic or in recovery room	Any time
Treatment Priority		CPR Stop halogenated agent Reduce plasma potassium "Clean" source of oxygen	Stop halogenated agent Dantrolene "Clean" source of oxygen

CPR, cardiopulmonary resuscitation; *ECG*, electrocardiogram; *ETCO$_2$*, end-tidal carbon dioxide.
[a]Represented by widening inspired to expired oxygen concentration in the face of unchanged fresh gas flows.
[b]If succinylcholine has been given, malignant hyperthermia or anesthesia-induced rhabdomyolysis may happen precipitously.
Reproduced with permission; from Gray RM. Anesthesia-induced rhabdomyolysis or malignant hyperthermia: is defining the crisis important? *Paediatr Anaesth.* 2017;27(5):490–493.

Management, Susceptibility Screening, and Counseling

TREATMENT

Management of an acute MH reaction is the model for which anesthetic crisis resource management (ACRM) was developed. The decision-making process for every aspect of managing the MH reaction (from differential diagnosis to counseling for MedicAlert bracelets [MedicAlert Foundation, Salida, CA] http://www.medicalert.org) together with excellent communication and human resource management ensure an optimal outcome after the reaction.[81] Given the rarity of these reactions, ACRM can be built into the simulation scenario for MH to teach leadership and decision making in the time of crisis (see Chapter 53).

If the anesthesiologist suspects that a child is experiencing an MH episode, the inhalational anesthetic should be immediately discontinued, 100% oxygen administered at a large fresh gas flow rate (≥10 L/minute), and the surgeon informed; if surgery cannot be aborted, it must be completed expeditiously. Charcoal filters should be inserted into both limbs of a new and previously unused breathing circuit (E-Fig. 41.2). The filters prevent the child from being contaminated by residual anesthetic in the AWS and to prevent the AWS from being contaminated by anesthetic in the patient.[63] The MH cart and additional personnel to assist in dissolving the dantrolene (see later text) should be brought to the operating room immediately (Table 41.7). Minute ventilation should be increased to control the partial pressure of carbon dioxide (PaCO$_2$) and PETCO$_2$.

The anesthesia technique should be converted to total IV anesthesia (TIVA), and if charcoal filters are not available, hyperventilation should be continued using an external self-inflating or anesthesia-type bag with an exogenous source of oxygen that is uncontaminated by inhalational anesthetics. If the airway was not intubated, tracheal intubation should be performed and ventilation controlled mechanically to achieve a normal PETCO$_2$.

Because native dantrolene is quite insoluble in water, several strategies have been developed to speed its solubility. The current formulation (Dantrium, Par Pharmaceutical, Par Sterile Products, Chestnut Ridge, NY) is packaged as a lyophilized yellow powder (E-Fig. 41.3) with constituents that contain mannitol and an alkaline pH to speed the dissolution of dantrolene in water (Table 41.8). Warming the 60 mL of sterile water speeds dissolution.[82] Most of the dantrolene dissolves within 60 seconds of adding the water, turning the solution orange; vigorously shaking the vial quickly dissolves any residual crystals. The solution should be withdrawn immediately and administered intravenously as rapidly as possible. Given the extreme alkaline pH of the dantrolene solution, it should be infused into a large vein to reduce the risk of phlebitis. Extravasation of dantrolene into interstitial tissues may cause tissue necrosis. Prolonged continuous infusions of dantrolene may cause thrombophlebitis or thrombosis of large and small veins.[83–85] Some have recommended continuous infusions of small doses of dantrolene in adults after the initial bolus, although the risk/benefit ratio of this practice is unproved in adults and untested in children.[86] A new formulation of nanocrystalline dantrolene (Ryanodex, Eagle Pharmaceuticals, Woodcliff Lake, NJ) approved in the United States in 2014 rapidly dissolves in a much greater

TABLE 41.7	Contents of a Pediatric Malignant Hyperthermia Emergency Cart		
Fluids			
3 L cold normal saline or Lactated Ringer's solution			
Number of Containers	**Drug**	**Concentration**	**Container**
	Dantrolene IV[a]		
36	Dantrium or Revonto (see Table 41.8)	20 mg in 60 mL of sterile water (0.33 mg/mL)	1 vial
3	Ryanodex	250 mg in 5 mL of sterile water (50 mg/mL)	1 vial
25	Sterile injectable water		100 mL
4	Sodium bicarbonate	1 mEq/mL	50-mL vial
2	50% dextrose	500 mg/mL	50-mL vial
1	Regular insulin	100 units/mL	10-mL vial
2	Calcium gluconate or chloride (10%)		10 mL
3	Lidocaine (2%)[a]	20 mg/mL	5 mL
10	20- and 22-gauge IV catheters		
10	18- and 20-gauge needles		

IV, intravenous; *TB*, tuberculin.
[a]Avoid lidocaine if wide QRS complex is present.
Charcoal filters should be immediately available if they are not on the malignant hyperthermia cart.

TABLE 41.8	Characteristics of Three Formulations of Dantrolene IV		
	Dantrium[a]	**Revonto[b]**	**Ryanodex[c]**
Dose (mg)/vial	20	20	250
Volume of diluent (mL)	60	60	5
Mannitol content (mg)	3000	3000	125
Time to dilute (seconds)	20 or "until solution is clear"[a]	20 or "until solution is clear"[a]	<10
	"Shake the vial to ensure an orange-colored uniform suspension. Visually inspect the vial for particulate matter and discoloration prior to administration."		
pH of reconstituted solution	9.5	9.5	10.3
Number of vials recommended by MHAUS (for a 70 kg patient)	36	36	3 (equivalent to ~720 mg dantrolene)
Shelf-life (years)	3	3	2
Acquisition cost (USD wholesale)	4028	3192	8280

[a]Dantrium (Par Pharmaceutical Companies Inc., Spring Valley, NY).
[b]Revonto (dantrolene sodium; DSM Pharmaceuticals Inc., Greenville, NC); package insert revised November 2016.
[c]Ryanodex (dantrolene sodium; Eagle Pharmaceuticals, Inc., Woodcliff Lake, NJ); package insert revised July 2014.
Data were summarized in part from *Cleveland Clinic Clinical Rx Forum*, 2016:4(5);4–5.

concentration formulation (5 mL of sterile water yielding 250 mg/5 mL) than the previous formulations (http://www.ryanodex.com/wp-content/uploads/2014/09/ryanodex-mh-white-paper.pdf [accessed May 16, 2017]).[87,88] This preparation contains more dantrolene (250 mg) than the standard preparation (20 mg) and less mannitol (125 mg) versus 3 g per vial (see Table 41.8) and requires only 5 mL instead of 60 mL of bacteriostatic water per vial to dissolve the dantrolene.[88] Preliminary evidence suggests that the blood concentration of dantrolene from Ryanodex reaches its maximum concentration (C_{max}) more rapidly (smaller T_{max}) than that from the previous dantrolene formulations.[89] The shelf life of Dantrium is 3 years, whereas that of Ryanodex is only 2 years.[88] Table 41.8 compares and contrasts the characteristics of the three current formulations of dantrolene.

The pharmacokinetics of IV dantrolene have been studied in MHS children 2 to 7 years of age.[90] A loading dose of 2.5 mg/kg produced predictable blood concentrations (≥3 µg/mL) for about 6 hours after the loading dose (Fig. 41.4).[90] Based on these pharmacokinetic data, if half of the loading dose of dantrolene were repeated at 6 hours after the loading dose, therapeutic blood concentrations of dantrolene would be maintained for a total of 15 hours and possibly prevent a recrudescence.[90]

An initial bolus dose of 2.5 mg/kg controls most MH reactions if the dantrolene is administered as soon after the onset of the reaction as possible (see Fig. 41.3).[91] Delay in instituting dantrolene therapy increases the probability of failed therapy and death.[42] For a 70-kg patient, this initial dose requires 8 vials of Dantrium or

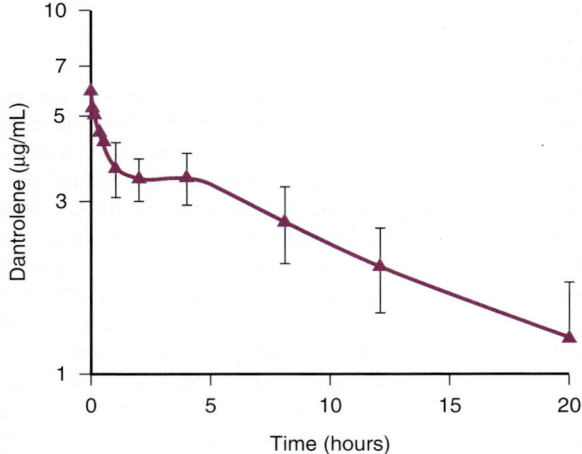

FIGURE 41.4 Pharmacokinetics of dantrolene in children. (From Lerman J, McLeod ME, Strong HA. Pharmacokinetics of intravenous dantrolene in children. *Anesthesiology* 1989;70[4]:625–629.)

1 vial of Ryanodex. Since the likelihood of successfully aborting the MH reaction depends on the speed of administering the dantrolene, we recommend that Ryanodex be used despite its added cost and reduced shelf life. The response to dantrolene should be evident within minutes, with a marked reduction in

$P_{ET}CO_2$, heart rate, and respiratory rate (see Fig. 41.3). If there is no response within 3 to 5 minutes, the initial dose should be repeated until signs that the physiologic variables are abating. The clinical end points include resolution of the hypercapnia, tachypnea, and tachycardia; resolution of muscle rigidity; restoration of clear urine output; return of normal consciousness when sedation is discontinued; self-correction of blood gas abnormalities; and resolution of electrolyte disturbances. If these do not occur or are incomplete, additional doses of dantrolene should be administered until all signs and symptoms of the MH reaction have abated or the diagnosis is reevaluated.[91] There is no upper limit to the amount of dantrolene that can or should be given acutely to stop an MH reaction. In rare instances of persistent MH or recrudescence, a cumulative dose of up to 40 mg/kg has been required.[92] Dantrolene is a fairly potent muscle relaxant, and a child with an unintubated airway (particularly one with respiratory disorders) may become weak and require controlled respirations.

Although dantrolene is effective in terminating acute MH reactions, this effect may wane as the blood concentration of dantrolene decreases and a recrudescence may occur. The prevalence of recrudescence may be as great as 20% and associated with several predictive factors, including muscular body type and a greater time interval between induction of anesthesia and the development of the initial reaction.[93] However, the first episode of recrudescence may occur any time after the initial reaction was successfully treated, up to and as late as 36 hours.[94] The possibility of recrudescence must always be considered during the first 2 to 3 days after an MH reaction has occurred. Because recrudescence cannot be predicted, all children who experience an MH reaction must be admitted to the pediatric intensive care unit or a monitored bed until the reaction resolves and the child's metabolic indices return to and remain normal for 2 to 3 days. MHAUS recommends that 1 mg/kg of dantrolene be administered intravenously every 6 hours for 24 to 48 hours after an MH reaction to prevent recrudescence. This recommendation remains empirical because there are no data to support the effectiveness of dantrolene in preventing recrudescence, although these dosages are consistent with pharmacokinetic data in children.[90] We recommend continued vigilance, frequent physical examinations for muscle tightness (every 30 minutes), repeated laboratory tests (e.g., blood gas analyses), and monitoring of vital signs, particularly heart rate, respiratory rate, and expired CO_2 tension for evidence of a recrudescence during the first 48 hours after an MH episode. If recrudescence does occur, additional IV dantrolene should be administered until the reaction again abates.

There have been no reports of acute dantrolene toxicity, although acute administration of dantrolene may result in side effects that include skeletal muscle weakness (15%), phlebitis (9%) and gastrointestinal upset (4.3%).[84] Respiratory failure was reported in 3.8% of patients who received dantrolene, although distinguishing the cause of the failure to the underlying MH or the dantrolene has proven difficult.[84] Extravasation of dantrolene into subcutaneous tissue may cause necrosis.[88] Not surprisingly, neostigmine is ineffective in reversing the effects of dantrolene because the latter acts intracellularly, not at the neuromuscular junction (see the section on molecular mechanisms of dantrolene). It may be advisable to maintain control of the airway (combined with IV sedation) until there is no further need for dantrolene. Preoperative, orally administered dantrolene, initially recommended in MH-susceptible children 2 decades ago, caused skeletal muscle weakness, dysarthria, sialorrhea, and diplopia and was ineffective in preventing

MH reactions.[48] As a result, this practice was discontinued.[48] Long-term use in the treatment of chronic skeletal muscle spasticity has been reported to cause liver dysfunction and fatal hepatitis in about 1% and 0.1% of patients, respectively.[95] Given the risks of an MH reaction, there seems little downside to treating a child with dantrolene before the diagnosis is certain, provided all the necessary blood work and laboratory tests have been collected, because early treatment reduces mortality and morbidity (see Fig. 41.1).[42] The probability of developing a complication from an MH reaction increases almost threefold for every 2C° increase in body temperature and 1.6-fold for every 30-minute delay in administering IV dantrolene during a reaction.[42] Cardiac arrest and death during an MH reaction correlate with a muscular physique and greater time intervals between induction of anesthesia and the maximal value of $P_{ET}CO_2$.[26] Other possible diagnoses should continue to be considered while the treatment for the suspected MH reaction is organized (see Table 41.4). A positive response to dantrolene is not pathognomonic of an MH reaction, because other conditions may respond with resolution of their signs.

Moderate external cooling measures may be instituted to control a rapidly increasing temperature, although ice should never be applied directly to the skin because it may cause tissue injury and intense cutaneous vasoconstriction. The latter may decrease heat loss further by accelerating acidosis and pyrexia. It is important to avoid overshooting with cooling measures (i.e., stop aggressive cooling at a temperature of about 38.5°C), because hypothermia may ensue, particularly if dantrolene has been administered. A urinary catheter should always be inserted during an MH reaction to identify myoglobinuria and to facilitate bladder emptying because 0.375 g of mannitol/kg body weight is given as part of the initial (2.5 mg/kg) loading dose with the older dantrolene formulations.

Initial laboratory assessments should be obtained before the bolus dose of dantrolene, and in addition to arterial and venous blood gases, determinations should include electrolyte, glucose, blood urea nitrogen, and creatinine levels; a complete blood cell count with platelets; prothrombin and partial thromboplastin times; CK concentrations; and serum and urine myoglobin levels. Because CK concentrations peak 12 to 24 hours after the onset of an MH reaction, it is prudent to obtain a baseline blood sample as soon as an MH reaction is suspected. The provider should be especially aware of the potential for hyperkalemia as the result of muscle breakdown and for acute renal failure as a late complication. Placing an arterial catheter facilitates continuous monitoring of blood pressure and for serial determinations of arterial blood gases, electrolytes, and CK.

The potential for life-threatening acidosis—a pure respiratory acidosis early in the syndrome, followed later by a mixed metabolic/respiratory acidosis—always exists. Metabolic acidosis should be treated with sodium bicarbonate (1–2 mEq/kg IV initially), as would be done for any acutely acidotic child, and continue treatment guided by pH and base deficit, although if hypercapnia persists despite aggressive hyperventilation, administration of sodium bicarbonate should be reconsidered since the severity of the respiratory acidosis may increase. Because an acute MH episode is associated with catecholamine stress, hemodynamic instability, particularly owing to dysrhythmias, may develop and should be treated according to Advanced Cardiac Life Support protocols. Calcium channel blockers must be avoided when treating MH reactions because they may cause cardiovascular collapse or acute hyperkalemia in the presence of dantrolene.[96–98] Acute hyperkalemia is common in patients with MH complicated by rhabdomyolysis and acidosis. Glucose and insulin should be immediately available and combined with the judicious use of exogenous IV calcium for treatment (see also Chapter 9). There is no evidence that the use of calcium in this setting exacerbates an MH reaction but it would be effective in opposing the cardiac effects of hyperkalemia.[99,100]

After the acute crisis has been treated, late complications, including severe rhabdomyolysis, are possible. It is important to follow serial serum concentrations of CK; if they are greater than 10,000 IU or urinary myoglobin concentrations increase, the urine should be alkalinized, and forced diuresis (>2 mL/kg per hour) with mannitol should be induced to prevent myoglobin from precipitating in the renal tubules, causing acute myoglobinuric renal failure. The enormous fluid requirements and edema associated with rhabdomyolysis may produce a compartment syndrome, which requires immediate surgical treatment.

Other organ systems may be affected after an acute episode of MH. It is common for markers of liver function to increase 12 to 36 hours after the crisis; some liver enzymes, including lactate dehydrogenase, aspartate aminotransferase, and alanine aminotransferase, can also originate from muscle. A concomitant increase in CK to more than 10,000 IU strongly suggests a severe and acute muscle disorder. Accompanying increases in γ-glutamyltransferase and bilirubin suggest liver involvement. Disseminated intravascular coagulation as part of multisystem organ failure is an ominous late complication.[101] Coagulation profiles should be followed serially to guide treatment appropriate to the case.

When necessary, the MH treatment algorithm should be accessed, available on the MHAUS website (www.mhaus.org/). We recommend attaching an updated MH treatment algorithm to every MH cart and anesthesia machine and that operating room personnel hold practice drills for the treatment of an MH crisis (see "Emergency Therapy for Malignant Hyperthermia" on the inside back cover of this text and at ExpertConsult.com). If the patient experiences what is believed to be an MH reaction, the care provider should call the MH emergency response line (1-800-644-9737 or 001-1-315-464-7079 if calling from outside the United States) for consultation with experienced anesthesiologists who are available 24 hours every day. We strongly encourage completion of an adverse metabolic reaction to anesthesia (AMRA) report by members of the team who provided anesthesia and postoperative care to the child. These forms can be downloaded (www.mhreg.org), sent by the hotline consultant, or obtained from the MHAUS office through regular mail. The data contained in the completed AMRA forms allow the North American Malignant Hyperthermia Registry (NAMHR) and MHAUS to produce better data regarding the variability of MH crises and the effectiveness of treatment. Because anesthesiologists should take a leading role in managing these patients, the families should be strongly encouraged to register the proband before leaving the hospital for MedicAlert identification (www.medicalert.org) that provides critical health information, such as "malignant hyperthermia susceptible, avoid inhaled anesthetics and succinylcholine."

STRESS-TRIGGERED MALIGNANT HYPERTHERMIA

In 1974, Wingard described an MHS family with a history of exercise- and emotion-induced fevers and sudden death not associated with anesthesia or surgery; he considered the possibility that MH was part of a spectrum of human stress syndromes.[102] Likewise, the porcine model of MH, also known as porcine stress syndrome, was first described as an awake, stress-induced syndrome brought about by tightly packing pigs in a train, car, or truck for shipment.[103] Dantrolene-responsive cases of awake and heat stroke–induced MH have been reported.[104,105] Heat stress–induced MH also seems to be characteristic of susceptible animal models.[106-108] A fatal case of exercise-induced MH in a 12-year-old boy who had previously survived a suspected episode of MH during general anesthesia to set a fractured humerus has been reported.[109] Eight months after surgery, while playing a game of football, the child became hyperthermic, collapsed, and died. Postmortem DNA testing revealed an MH-associated *RYR1* mutation in the child and his surviving father.[109] More cases of stress-induced MH have been reported, substantiated by genetic testing and in vitro contracture testing (IVCT).[110,111]

Screening for MH susceptibility in heat stroke patients and those suffering postexercise cramps or rhabdomyolysis using the in vitro CHCT has led to the laboratory diagnosis of MH susceptibility in some patients.[45,112-115] Although there is laboratory evidence of similarities in skeletal muscle metabolism in exertional heat stroke and MH,[116] and one of the mouse MH knock-in models exhibits environmental heat triggering,[67] there is as yet little evidence that these are anything more than clinically similar presentations.[45] For this reason, dantrolene has rarely been an effective treatment for heat stroke.[117] Nonetheless, it seems reasonable to suggest that subsets of MHS patients may be more sensitive to heat stroke. Therefore it may be helpful to test children with exertional heat illness for MH susceptibility.[118]

MH reactions have been reported infrequently in susceptible patients who received a nontriggering anesthetic.[49,119,120] Of 2214 patients who presented for muscle biopsy for MH susceptibility, 5 (0.46%) of 1082 who had MH-positive biopsy results developed MH reactions in the recovery room. None of the patients with negative biopsy results developed MH reactions. There is a small incidence of MH reactions among susceptible individuals that may occur despite a safe anesthetic regimen. Whether this is caused by stress or trace anesthetic concentrations that were inhaled is unclear. Massive rhabdomyolysis has been reported on rewarming from cardiopulmonary bypass despite the patient having received a nontriggering anesthetic.[119,120] The mechanism of these responses may be stress, but evidence is lacking.

POSTEPISODE COUNSELING

Ideally, after treating a child for MH, the anesthesiologist should arrange for referral of the child and first-degree relatives to an MH diagnostic biopsy center. It is only at such centers that the CHCT can be performed in adults. The CHCT is the only test that can produce a true negative diagnosis (i.e., not MHS),[121] but the sensitivity and specificity of this test are less than 100%. False-negative test results may occur, albeit rarely.[122] When the anesthetic management of a small number of MH biopsy-negative patients was reviewed, more than one-half were given inhalational anesthetics, although the biopsy results for the remainder may not have been known at the time of anesthesia because they were given trigger-free anesthetics.[123]

Because there are no control muscle biopsy data for prepubescent children, contracture testing is not performed in this age group. Instead, children are more often fitted with MedicAlert bracelets, and the parents are counseled regarding their own need for biopsies. The children may be reconsidered for muscle biopsy upon reaching puberty.

Many persons suspected of having MH have normal muscle responses on the CHCT. In the event that an adult who experienced an MH reaction has a normal CHCT result, he or she should be referred to a neurologist with an interest in muscle diseases to determine whether an occult myopathy is responsible for the clinical events. Alternatively, the diagnosis may be incorrect, and other diagnoses should be considered (see Table 41.4). Individuals suspected of being MHS should undergo CHCT; the family should also be evaluated and counseled accordingly.

Patients with strongly positive CHCT results should undergo screening for the ryanodine receptor 1 gene *(RYR1)*, because mutations in this gene have been found in about 60% of family members who had an MH episode (conversely, this means that ~40% test negative genetically but are clinically MH positive). However, if neither an MH reaction nor a positive CHCT result has occurred, DNA testing for *RYR1* gene mutations based on a vague history offers such a poor yield of positive results that it cannot be justified at the present time.[124] If an MH-associated mutation (discussed later) is found in *RYR1*, first-degree relatives have a 50% probability of having a similar defect. Diagnostic testing for *RYR1* is performed on DNA obtained from a blood specimen, obviating the need to travel to an MH diagnostic biopsy center or undergo muscle biopsy for the genetic test. Genetic testing of relatives can be undertaken through the office of the primary care physician or by the anesthesiologist, a process that will simplify evaluation of the family. Failure to identify an MH-causative *RYR1* mutation (E-Fig. 41.4) does not confirm a negative diagnosis (i.e., not MHS) because more than one gene is associated with MH susceptibility, and not all are known.

Genetic testing and counseling can be arranged by the anesthesiologist or primary care physician by scheduling an appointment; one such center is located at the Center for Medical Genetics & Genomics at the University of Pittsburgh. The genetic counselors have extensive experience in counseling patients on the utility of the ryanodine receptor gene test for evaluation of MH susceptibility. The center currently screens 12 exons of genomic *RYR1* that commonly contain MH mutations (exons 6, 9, 11, 14, 17, 39, 40, 44, 45, 46, 101, and 102). A private commercial laboratory that also offers *RYR1* testing is Prevention Genetics (www.preventiongenetics.com), which screens for MH mutations. It has adopted a two-tiered approach: tier 1 involves bidirectional sequencing of exons 2, 6, 8, 9, 11, 12, 14, 15, 17, 39, 40, 41, 44-47, 95, and 100-104. These 22 exons contain most of the conclusively documented MH and central core disease causative mutations in the *RYR1* gene (European Malignant Hypothermia Group, www.emhg.org/genetics/). If the first tier is uninformative, their second-tier screen covers the remaining 84 exons of the 106 making up the human *RYR1* gene. The Prevention Genetics company corresponds only with physicians and does not provide patient or family counseling.

As DNA sequencing has become more automated and the cost has drastically declined, many private companies have arisen that purport to diagnose the entire panoply of human genetic diseases and resultant predispositions, including MH. We have no information about the reliability of their screening or the recommendations based on their findings. If no causative *RYR1* mutations are found, nothing more can be determined from genetic testing about susceptibility, because more than one mutated gene is linked to MH.

Genetics

MH in humans follows an autosomal dominant inheritance pattern with incomplete penetrance and variable expressivity.[30,125,126] In the context of MH, incomplete penetrance means that there are fewer patients with MH susceptibility than would be predicted by simple autosomal dominant inheritance. Variable expressivity means that the presence of a genetic mutation defining susceptibility is documented, but it does not mean that a patient will have an MH reaction when exposed to triggering agents. One patient in the NAMHR received 30 anesthetics before an MH reaction was triggered.[42] Another was discovered to be MHS by IVCT during screening of a proband's family and later was inadvertently anesthetized with succinylcholine and isoflurane, but these drugs did not trigger a reaction.[127] However, it seems that once an MH reaction has been triggered, a reaction will always occur when the patient is exposed to the trigger agents.

The molecular and cellular bases of these phenomena remain unknown. Naturally occurring susceptibility to MH seems to follow autosomal dominant inheritance patterns in dogs[128] and horses[129] but follows a recessive inheritance pattern in pigs.[130] This suggests that other genetic and epigenetic factors may play a role in determining the degree and timing of MH susceptibility.

The first breakthrough in finding a gene that predisposed to MH was the serendipitous finding of a similar syndrome in pigs.[131,132] When anesthetized with halothane and succinylcholine or with halothane alone, the pigs developed full-blown MH reactions (E-Fig. 41.5). The pig model has been a primary pathophysiologic, genetic, and pharmacologic model for the study of MH over the past 5 decades. A second serendipitous event introduced a South African anesthesiologist, G.G. Harrison, to dantrolene, and he successfully tested it in his pig model of MH.[133,134] This observation was quickly followed by the successful treatment of a patient with dantrolene.[135] An interview about Harrison's discovery of dantrolene is available from the Wood Library-Museum of the American Society of Anesthesiologists (www.woodlibrarymuseum.org/library/media).

One of the most surprising findings was that six separate breeds of pigs at different locations worldwide shared this MH susceptibility to inhalational anesthetics and succinylcholine. All reactions were treated successfully with dantrolene, and all were determined to have an autosomal recessive inheritance pattern. It was established that MH was associated with an uncontrolled increase in intramyoplasmic Ca^{2+}, presumably the result of an exaggerated release of Ca^{2+} from the sarcoplasmic reticulum (SR).[136,137] Much effort has been expended in understanding the physiologic basis of excitation–Ca^{2+}-release coupling (ECRC) as part of the general mechanism of skeletal muscle excitation-contraction coupling.

By the mid-1980s, a large channel in the SR membrane, now known as the ryanodine receptor (RyR1), was identified by its ability to bind a plant toxin, ryanodine. It was discovered to have properties consistent with being a Ca^{2+} channel.[138-140] In 1988, this presumed primary Ca^{2+}-release channel of the SR was found to have gap junction–like channel properties.[141] It was hypothesized that the ryanodine receptor might be the site of mutations that caused MH. Within a year, the complementary DNA (cDNA) for the skeletal muscle ryanodine receptor was cloned.[142] In 1990, both porcine and human MH were linked to the same region on chromosome 19q12-13.2 at the glucose phosphate isomerase locus, suggesting that MH in both species was due to mutations in homologous genes.[143] Concurrently, a linkage study in eight families demonstrated that RYR markers cosegregated with MH phenotypes, providing compelling evidence that mutations of *RYR* determine MH susceptibility.[144] Two years after the initial cloning of *RyR1*, the identical single amino acid mutation (Arg615Cys) was discovered in this channel in all six breeds of MH susceptible pigs.[145]

TABLE 41.9	Malignant Hyperthermia Loci	
Designation	**Chromosome Locus**	**Gene**
Ryanodine receptor 1 (skeletal) (formerly malignant hyperthermia susceptibility 1 [MHS1])	19q13.1	*RYR1*
Malignant hyperthermia susceptibility 2	17q11.2-q24	*MHS2*
Malignant hyperthermia susceptibility 4	3q13.2	*MHS4*
Calcium channel, voltage-dependent, L-type, α-1S subunit (formerly malignant hyperthermia susceptibility 5 [MHS5])	1q32	*CACNA1S*
Malignant hyperthermia susceptibility 6	5p	*MHS6*

Detailed genetic evaluations have linked MH susceptibility to chromosome 19q12-13.2, the location of the human *RYR1* gene (19q13.1), in MHS families. This is the locus for malignant hyperthermia susceptibility type 1, symbolized by *RYR1* (formerly designated MHS1) (Table 41.9).[125,146,147] Of the more than 400 variants identified in *RYR1* (ClinVar-National Center for Biotechnology Information; http://www.ncbi.nlm.nih.gov/clinvar/), only about 30 have been shown to cause MH (www.emhg.org provides a comprehensive list of known causative mutations in *RYR1*). *RYR1* mutations account for 50% to 70% of MHS individuals. Not all MHS families have disorders linked to this chromosome (see Table 41.8), indicating that this syndrome is genetically heterogeneous.

The second gene mutation associated with MHS, *MHS5,* codes for the α1 subunit of skeletal muscle dihydropyrimidine receptor L-type calcium channel. This gene, *CACNA1S,* codes for 1% of MHS subjects.

Several additional loci have been mapped to MH susceptibility, although the genes have not been identified. These include *MHS2,* linked to chromosome 17q11.2-q24 in North Americans; *MHS3* locus, located on 3q13; *MHS3* located on 7q21-q22; and *MHS6* located on 5p.[11]

Complicating the potential of genetic testing for MH even further is the phenomenon of gene silencing. This phenomenon mimics a recessive mutation in heterozygous individuals by allowing expression of only the affected allele while silencing the other, normal, allele.[148] Because MH is an autosomal dominant susceptibility, it is conceivable that a mechanism underlying the variability in MH triggering seen in patients with identical, monoallelic *RYR1* mutations results from skeletal muscle–specific silencing of the affected gene. It follows that inhalational anesthetics or succinylcholine, after multiple exposures, may release a gene from the silenced state, allowing triggering to occur. This may be an explanation for discordance among genetics, linkage analysis, and trait expressivity.

Although the inheritance of human MH is described as autosomal dominant, there are a few individuals who are allelically homozygous for an *RYR1* mutation,[149,150] intra-allelically heterozygous for two different *RYR1* mutations, or compound heterozygotes containing one mutation in *RYR1* and a second mutation at another locus for MH susceptibility.[151] Surprisingly, no overt myopathies have been reported in these affected individuals.

Physiology

NORMAL SKELETAL MUSCLE: EXCITATION-CONTRACTION COUPLING

The neurochemical signal that triggers excitation-contraction coupling begins with the release of acetylcholine from the motor nerve terminal at the skeletal muscle nicotinic synapse, resulting in depolarization of the surface membrane, the sarcolemma. Sarcolemmal membrane depolarization is transmitted into the interior of the muscle cell by specialized invaginations of the surface membrane known as transverse tubules (TTs), which occur at regular intervals along the muscle cell (Fig. 41.5). The TT membrane is studded with the skeletal muscle isoform of the voltage-dependent Ca^{2+} channel known as the dihydropyridine receptor (DHPR). In skeletal muscle, this channel does not transmit Ca^{2+} in response to sarcolemmal depolarization, rather, it functions as a sarcolemmal voltage sensor.

In response to depolarization, intrachannel charge movement across the TT membrane results in a conformational change of the DHPR. The TT is surrounded by specialized portions of the cellular organelle (i.e., SR) responsible for maintaining the cellular Ca^{2+} store, and the SR contains a high-capacity Ca^{2+} storage protein called calsequestrin, which regulates the ability of the RyR1 channel to open.[152] The face of the SR junctional membrane apposing the TT contains a packed, regular array of RyR1 proteins in close apposition to the DHPR. Physically, the DHPR and RyR1 receptor proteins overlie each other in a unique arrangement of four DHPRs (tetrad) per one RyR1, with every other RyR1 lacking a tetrad (Fig. 41.6).[153] Physical interaction of the DHPR with RyR1 after depolarization causes the RyR1 channel to open, and SR-stored Ca^{2+} is released into the myoplasm. Orthograde and anterograde communication between the DHPR and RyR1 results in reciprocal regulation of both entities[154,155]

In the myoplasm, the troponin C subunit of the troponin complex is bound to tropomyosin, which in the resting state inhibits myosin interaction with actin and maintains a relaxed muscle. Ca^{2+} binding to troponin C causes a conformational change in troponin and allows the complex to move away from tropomyosin, which rotates along the actin filament in a way that permits myosin head interaction with this fibrous protein. Fiber shortening and muscle contraction then occur in a myosin-ATPase–driven ratcheting reaction. The muscle relaxes when the SR membrane–bound Ca^{2+}-ATPase transports free myoplasmic Ca^{2+} back into the SR against its concentration gradient in an energy-dependent reaction, thereby driving myoplasmic Ca^{2+} concentrations down to resting levels. Troponin I, with its bound Ca^{2+} removed, moves back to block the myosin interaction with actin, thereby preventing muscle contraction and inducing its relaxation. Although a detailed description of the complexity of this process is beyond the scope of this chapter, reviews of excitation-contraction coupling are available.[156,157]

PATHOPHYSIOLOGY OF MALIGNANT HYPERTHERMIA

Advances in the pathophysiology of MH have been reviewed in great detail elsewhere.[158-161] In brief, at the cellular level, MH is characterized by an inhalational anesthetic–induced, uncontrolled increase in intramyoplasmic Ca^{2+} levels,[162,163] which precedes the metabolic and clinical signs of this syndrome[164] (see Fig. 41.6). Increased intramyoplasmic Ca^{2+} has been demonstrated by directly measuring intracellular Ca^{2+} in anesthetic-triggered pigs[162] and by substantiating the sensitivity of stored Ca^{2+} release by isolated SR from MHS pigs.[136,137,165,166] There is also a significant loss in the

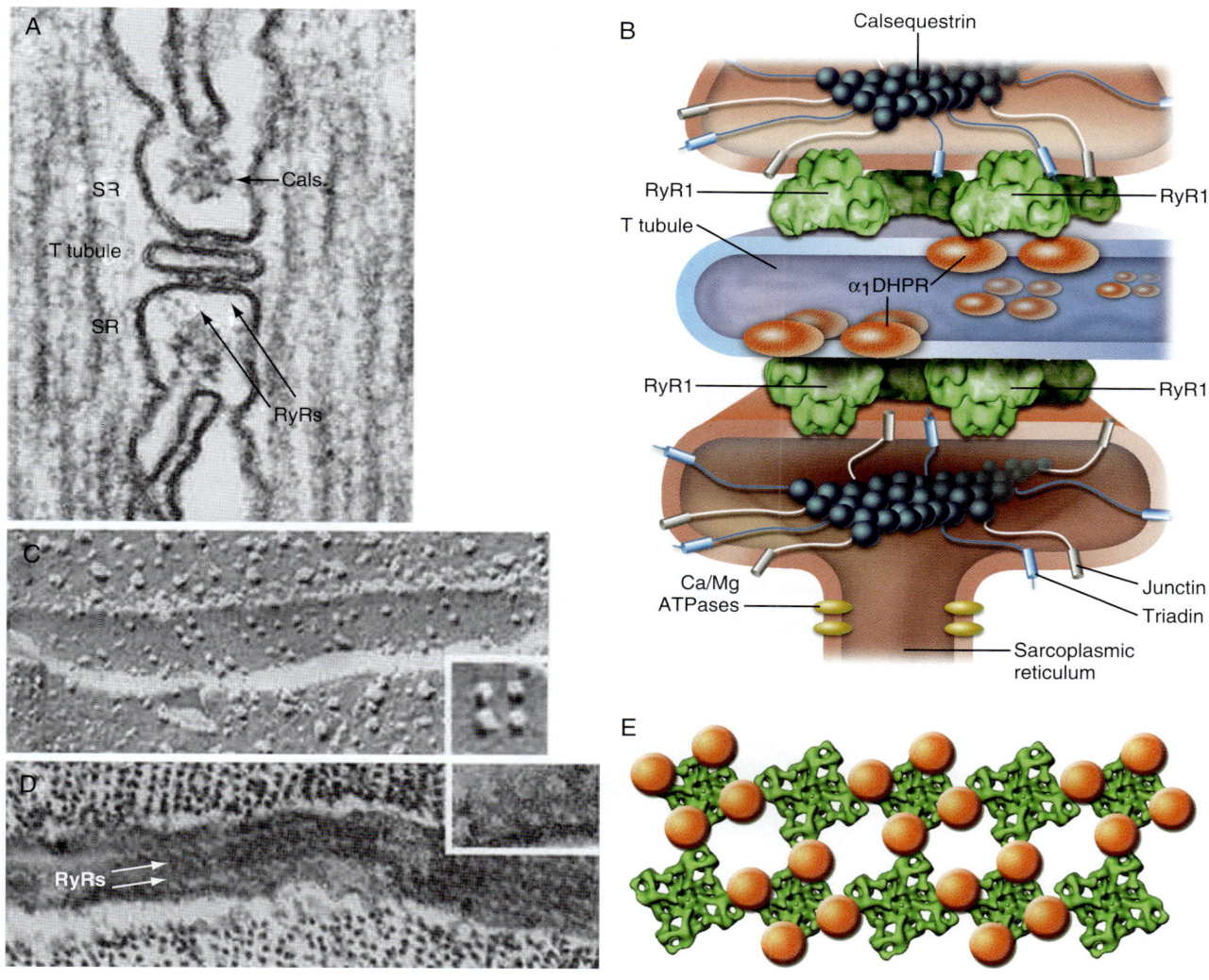

FIGURE 41.5 Structure of calcium release units in adult skeletal muscle fibers. In adult skeletal muscle, junctions are mostly triads: two sarcoplasmic reticulum (*SR*) elements coupled to a central transverse tubule (*T tubule*). **A,** A triad from the toadfish swimbladder muscle in thin-section electron microscopy shows the cytoplasmic domains of the SR Ca^{2+} release channel (*RyR1*), or feet, and calsequestrin (*Cals.*), the SR Ca^{2+} storage protein. **B,** A tridimensional reconstruction of a skeletal muscle triad shows the ultrastructural localization of ryanodine receptors (RyRs), dihydropyridine receptors (*DHPRs*), calsequestrin, triadin, junctin, and Ca^{2+}/Mg^{2+}-ATPases. Notice the localization of DHPRs in the T-tubule membrane; DHPRs are intramembrane proteins that are not visible in thin-section electron microscopy but can be visualized by freeze-fracture replicas of T tubules (in C). **C,** DHPRs in skeletal muscle form tetrads, a group of four receptors (*inset*), that are linked to subunit of alternate RyRs (in **B** and **E**). **D,** In sections parallel to the junctional plane, RyR feet arrays *(white arrows)* are clearly visible in toadfish swimbladder muscle; the feet touch each other close to the corner of the molecule (*inset*). **E,** The model summarizes the findings of **C** and **D**: RyRs (*green*) form two (rarely three) rows, and DHPRs (*orange*) form tetrads that are associated with alternate RyRs. The T tubule is shown in *blue* in **B,** and sandwiched between two portions of the SR in **A**. (**A,** Courtesy Clara Franzini-Armstrong; **B,** courtesy T. Wagenknecht; from Protasi F. Structural interaction between RYRs and DHPRs in calcium release units of cardiac and skeletal muscle cells. *Front Biosci.* 2002;7:d650–d658.)

ability of magnesium (Mg^{2+}), the natural inhibitory divalent cation that competes with Ca^{2+} for binding sites on RyR1, to inhibit Ca^{2+} release in MHS skeletal muscle.[167-169] RyR1 isolated from MHS pigs demonstrate greater open probabilities, greater sensitivity to Ca^{2+} activation, less sensitivity to Ca^{2+} inactivation, and reduced inhibition by Mg^{2+}. As a result, the affected RyR1 channels spend more time in the open state and less time in the closed state than normal channels.[170-174] Although not formally confirmed, this mechanism presumably underlies the sensitivity of RyR1 channels to volatile anesthetics and to the increase in intramyoplasmic Ca^{2+} seen in MHS skeletal muscle.

Similar single-channel studies of the Ca^{2+} responsiveness of human MHS RyR1 channels have yielded more equivocal results,[175] presumably because of the genetic heterogeneity of the human MHS population. Even within a single individual, heterozygosity for an MH mutation permits a given RyR1 channel that is supposed to be made up of four identical subunits to contain any combination of zero to four MHS subunits in combination with wild-type,

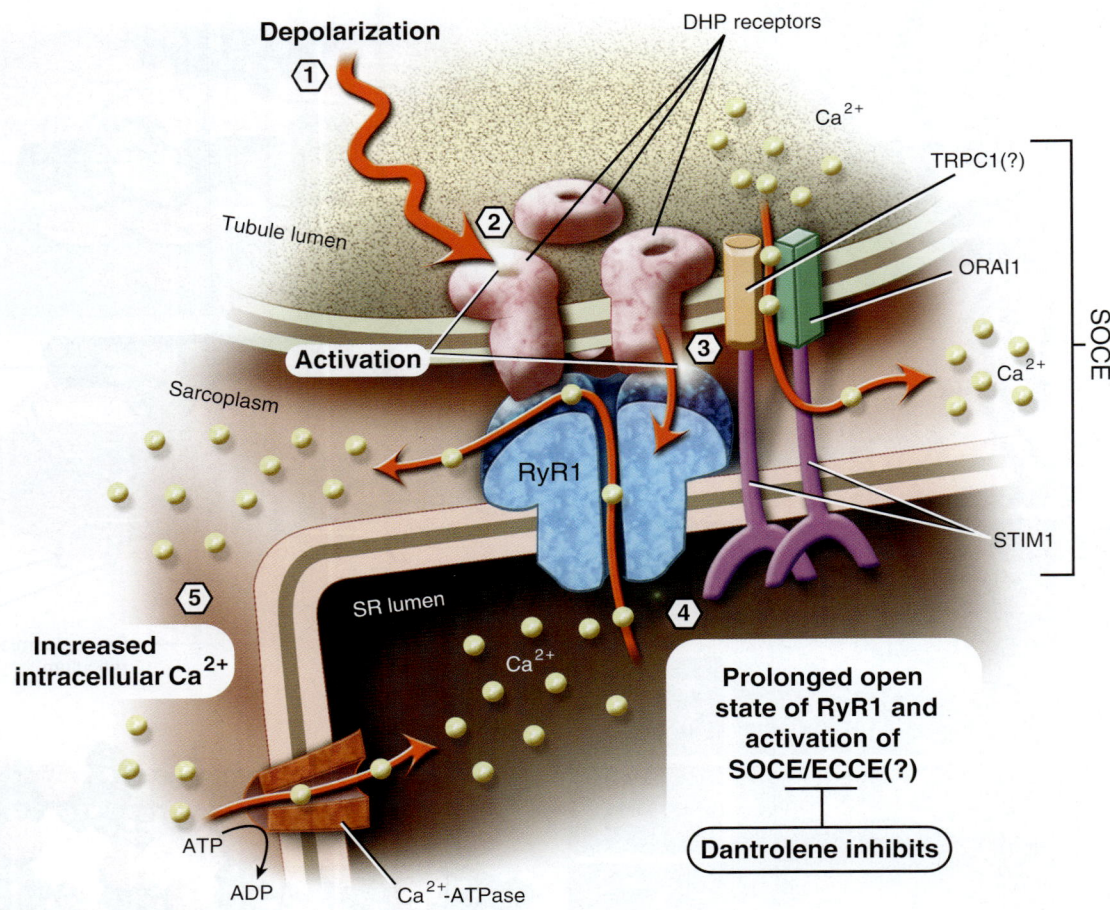

FIGURE 41.6 Schematic of the known pathophysiology of malignant hyperthermia (MH). Exposure of an individual who has a genetic susceptibility because of a ryanodine receptor (*RyR1*) or dihydropyridine (*DHP*) receptor mutation to an anesthetic triggering agent may result in MH. Normally, muscle cell depolarization (**1**) is sensed by the DHP receptor (**2**), which signals RyR1 opening by a direct physical connection (**3**). The conventional view of the genesis of MH is that RyR1 opening is easier and more sustained in the presence of volatile anesthetics (**4**), allowing a sustained rise in the Ca^{2+} concentration in the myoplasm (**5**) that surpasses the sarcoplasmic reticulum Ca^{2+} reuptake activity of the Ca^{2+}/Mg^{2+}-ATPase. This results in unrelenting muscle contraction and uncontrolled anaerobic and aerobic metabolism, which translate into the clinical manifestations of respiratory and metabolic acidosis, muscle rigidity, and hyperthermia. If the process continues unabated, adenosine triphosphate (*ATP*) depletion eventually causes widespread muscle fiber hypoxia with resultant cell death and rhabdomyolysis. Rhabdomyolysis manifests clinically as hyperkalemia and myoglobinuria and an increase in the serum creatine kinase level. Dantrolene sodium binds to RyR1, presumably causing it to favor the closed state and stemming the uninhibited flow of calcium into the myoplasm. The contributions of store-operated Ca^{2+} entry (*SOCE*) to myoplasmic Ca^{2+} fluxes and its inhibition by dantrolene suggest that MH may have a significant component from SOCE or excitation-coupled Ca^{2+} entry (*ECCE*), or both, and dantrolene may inhibit the RyR1-dependent activation of SOCE or ECCE. TRPC1, ORAI1, and STIM1 are proteins involved in calcium transport. *ADP*, adenine diphosphate; *SR*, sarcoplasmic reticulum. (Modified from Litman RS, Rosenberg H. Malignant hyperthermia: update on susceptibility testing. JAMA 2005;293[23]:2918–2924.)

normal RyR1 subunits. When examining single channels from a population of channels isolated from a heterozygous, MHS patient, the clinician can expect a wider range of channel responses than in the homozygous, inbred, porcine population used for MH models.

Several laboratories have reported the creation of knock-in mice containing one of two known MH-related RyR1 mutations: Tyr522Ser and Arg163Cys.[107,108] In contradistinction to the pig model, and like their MHS human counterparts, the knock-in MH mice are heterozygous. Their homozygous littermates die in utero on day 17. These heterozygous mice become rigid, hyperthermic, and hypermetabolic, die after exposure to inhalational anesthetics or heat stress, and respond therapeutically to dantrolene. They display exaggerated responses to the RyR1 agonists caffeine and 4-chloro-*m*-cresol and to potassium depolarization. As with MHS humans and pigs, their muscle is less sensitive to inhibitory

Mg^{2+} and possesses greater resting Ca^{2+} concentrations than wild-type animals. These experimental animals display a physiologic MH phenotype remarkably similar, if not identical, to the human syndrome and should prove extraordinarily useful in working out the details of MH pathophysiology.

Development of MH seems to require some form of neural input to muscle, because epidural anesthesia in the porcine MH model completely inhibits expression of MH.[176] However, complete inhibition of neural input into skeletal muscle in this model by the use of competitive, nondepolarizing, nicotinic cholinergic receptor antagonists such as D-tubocurarine, pancuronium, and vecuronium before a halothane challenge does not inhibit development of MH.[177,178] Together, these results suggest that a neurologically significant contribution to MH arises from the central nervous system by means of sympathetic outflow or the neuroendocrine axis, rather than direct skeletal muscle stimulation. This theory is consistent with the awake or stress-related episodes of MH described earlier.

MOLECULAR MECHANISMS AND PHYSIOLOGIC EFFECTS OF DANTROLENE

Dantrolene (Fig. 41.7) is a hydantoin derivative originally synthesized as part of an effort to examine the muscle relaxant properties of a series of substituted furan derivatives.[179] Thinking that they might have an NMBD, scientists investigated its mechanism of action but found that it differed from the known skeletal muscle relaxants. Dantrolene affected the intrinsic properties of skeletal muscle without affecting the central nervous system, neuromuscular transmission, electrical properties of the sarcolemma or the T tubule, electromyogram, or train-of-four method for testing neuromuscular blockade. Its action was intracellular (Fig. 41.8).[180] Indirect evidence pointed to dantrolene interfering with Ca^{2+} fluxes that were intrinsic to skeletal muscle contraction.[181-183] Direct observations[184,185] demonstrated that dantrolene suppressed the rate and amount of Ca^{2+} released from the SR without completely abolishing it. Subsequently, it was demonstrated that dantrolene inhibited halothane-induced Ca^{2+} release from the isolated SR of MHS pigs,[165,186,187] but was devoid of any effect on calcium reuptake into the SR.[188,189]

After SR Ca^{2+} release was identified as the likely target of dantrolene's activity, several attempts to identify a dantrolene binding partner in the SR proved unsuccessful, primarily because of the difficulties of conducting detailed pharmacologic receptor analyses with a drug as hydrophobic as dantrolene.[190,191] In 1995, an assay for radioactively labeled dantrolene helped to elucidate specific binding sites in porcine skeletal muscle SR.[192] Dantrolene inhibits RyR1-dependent cellular Ca^{2+} fluxes in skeletal muscle,

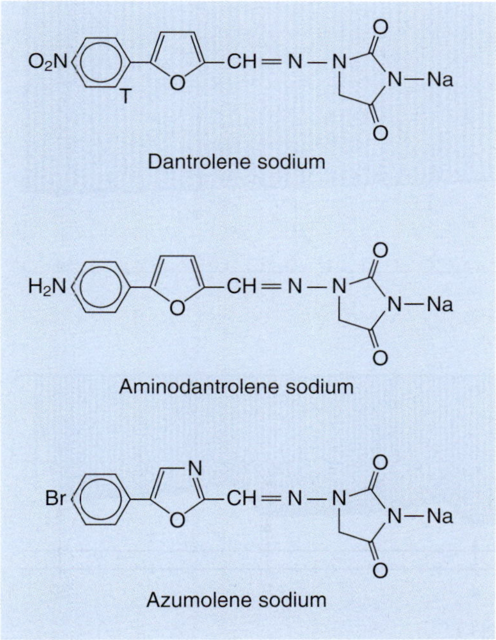

FIGURE 41.7 Dantrolene and its congeners. Dantrolene and azumolene are equipotent drugs, but azumolene is far more water soluble. Only dantrolene is approved by the U.S. Food and Drug Administration for treatment of malignant hyperthermia. Aminodantrolene is a poorly active congener, demonstrating how small changes in drug structure can result in large changes in activity. (Modified from Parness J, Palnitkar SS. Identification of dantrolene binding sites in porcine skeletal muscle sarcoplasmic reticulum. *J Biol Chem.* 1995;270[31]:18465–18472.)

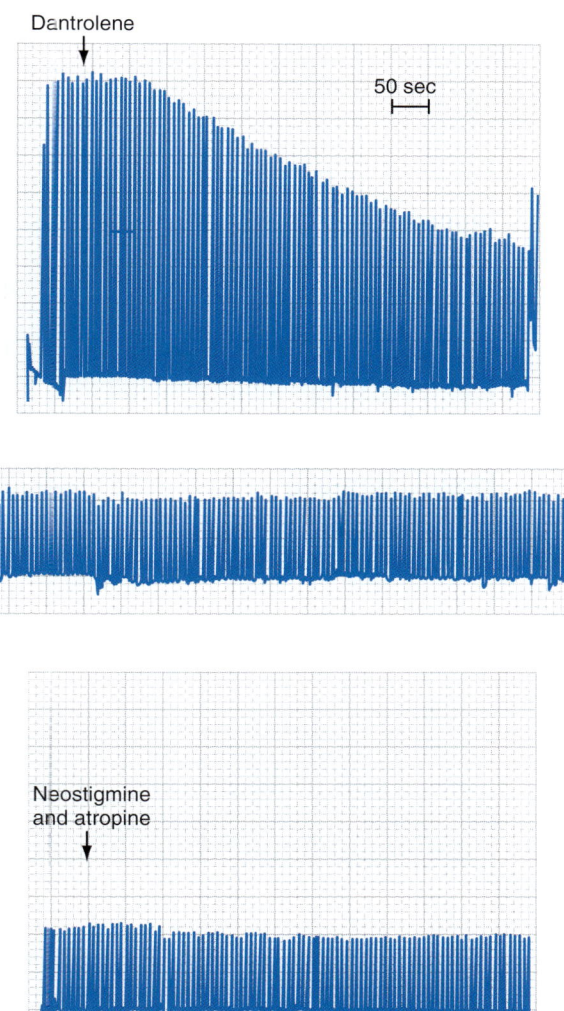

FIGURE 41.8 Intraoperative electromyogram of a child given intravenous dantrolene (2.4 mg/kg). The twitch tension decreased about 75% after dantrolene but was not reversed by administration of neostigmine, demonstrating the lack of involvement of the neuromuscular junction in the action of dantrolene.

albeit incompletely, but it does not seem to affect RyR1 channel activity or its ability to transport Ca^{2+}.[193] Curiously, dantrolene proved to be ineffective in attenuating Ca^{2+} release through single RyRs inserted into lipid bilayers in most in vitro studies.[194] This inconsistency between the in vitro and in vivo studies has been attributed to dantrolene's codependency on adequate concentrations of both calmodulin,[195] which binds to RyR and to Mg^{2+}, which accumulates from the hydrolysis of magnesium adenosine triphosphate (MgATP) during an MH reaction.[196]

A second physiologic process, called store-operated Ca^{2+} entry (SOCE), contributes to the increase in intracellular Ca^{2+} as a result of the RyR1 channel opening in skeletal muscle.[197-199] SOCE is a process by which the SR store of Ca^{2+} is replenished from the extracellular milieu after significant loss of Ca^{2+} from the SR.[200] Experiments with azumolene, a more water-soluble congener of dantrolene, have demonstrated inhibition of skeletal muscle RyR1-dependent SOCE, not SR Ca^{2+} release.[201] These results raise profound questions. Do the induced Ca^{2+} fluxes during excitation-contraction coupling, experimental manipulation, and MH that result in an increase in intracellular Ca^{2+} all result from RyR1-dependent Ca^{2+} release or RyR1-dependent Ca^{2+} entry, or both?

Evidence of a dantrolene-sensitive, excitation-coupled Ca^{2+} entry mechanism of skeletal muscle (ECCE) that is more easily activated in MH skeletal muscle has been described, as well.[202-205] ECCE is different from SOCE in that it does not require depletion of the SR Ca^{2+} store and is activated by high-frequency electrical stimulation of the skeletal muscle membrane. ECCE and SOCE present new physiologic targets of investigation into the pathophysiology of MH that involve Ca^{2+} entry rather than Ca^{2+} release (see Fig. 41.6).

Elucidation of the pathophysiology of MH and the mechanism of action of dantrolene has radically transformed our understanding of muscle physiology and pathophysiology. As our understanding continues to evolve, the future for advances in therapy and testing capabilities hold great promise.

Laboratory Diagnosis

CONTRACTURE TESTING

The standard for testing susceptibility to MH in the human population is an in vitro contracture test that assesses live human muscle fibers from the vastus lateralis in a physiologic bath. With one end of the muscle tissue attached to a strain gauge, the degree of tension developed at baseline and on electrical stimulation is measured as a function of the concentrations of halothane or caffeine. The test is based on the observation that fresh muscle isolated from MHS patients behaved abnormally when exposed to halothane or caffeine in vitro (Fig. 41.9).[206-209] Two variations of this test have been developed and adopted: the CHCT by the North American Malignant Hyperthermia Group (NAMHG) and

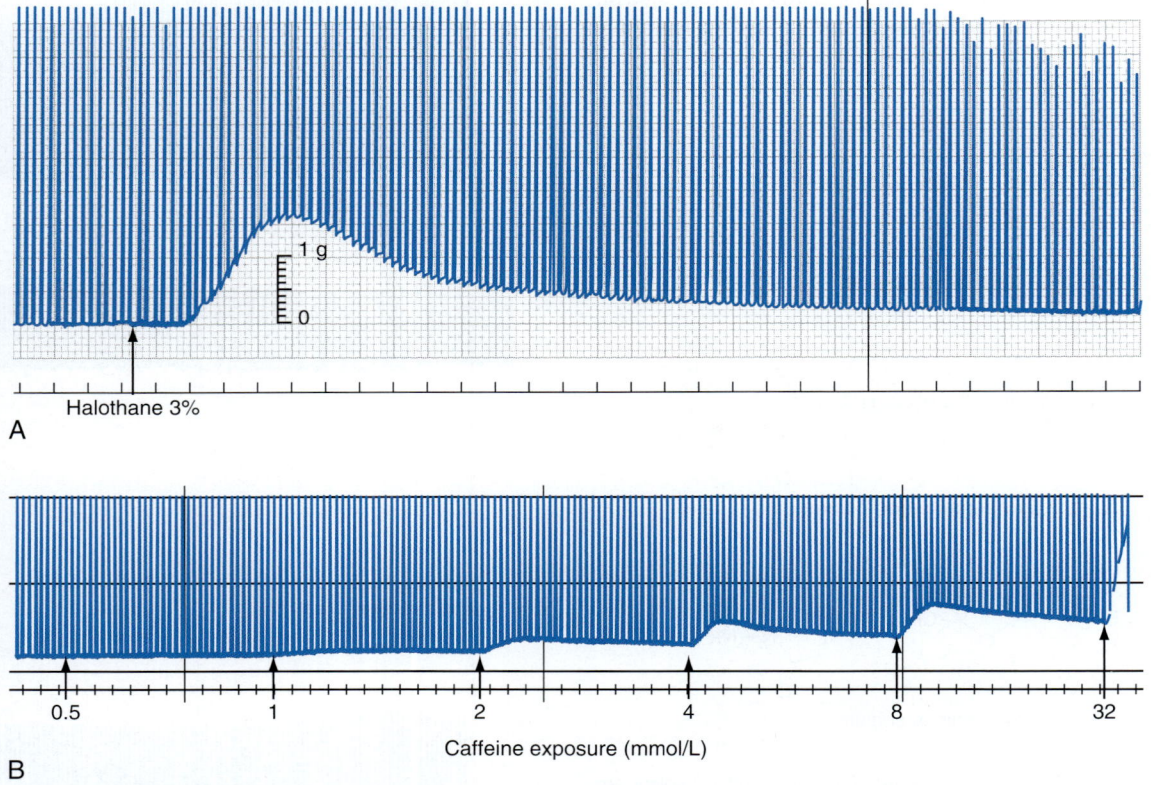

FIGURE 41.9 Caffeine-halothane contracture test. **A,** Abnormal (positive) response to 3% halothane. Each small box represents 0.1 g of tension. The contracture response in this case is 1.6 g. A normal response to 3% halothane is a contracture up to 0.7 g. After exposure to halothane, 32 mmol/L of caffeine is added to the bath to determine maximal response. **B,** Abnormal (positive) response to caffeine. Caffeine exposure is increased to 0.5, 1.0, 2.0, 4.0, 8.0, and 32 mmol/L for 4 minutes. A contracture of greater than 0.3 g to 2 mmol/L of caffeine or less indicates susceptibility. (Modified from Rosenberg H, Antognini JF, Muldoon S. Testing for malignant hyperthermia. *Anesthesiology* 2002;96[1]:232–237.)

the IVCT by the European Malignant Hyperthermia Group (EMHG). The NAMHG test measures the response in separate muscle fascicles to a bolus of 3% halothane or incremental increases in the caffeine concentration,[24,210,211] and it requires a positive response to one of the challenges for a diagnosis of MH susceptibility. Those not responding are considered normal. The EMHG test measures the response to graded increases in the halothane concentration up to 2% and incremental increases in the caffeine concentration in different fascicles. The diagnosis of MH susceptibility by the IVCT requires a positive response to both challenges, whereas a positive response to one of the challenging agents results in equivocal diagnostic categorization (i.e., malignant hyperthermia equivocal).[212–214]

Even though the EMHG protocol may prevent excess false-positive and false-negative results compared with the NAMHG protocol, overall results are comparable.[215] The EMHG reports that the sensitivity and specificity of its protocol are 99% and 94%, respectively,[213] whereas the NAMHG reports that its sensitivity and specificity are 97% and 78%, respectively.[216] Because the North American protocol is less specific and tends to overdiagnose MH susceptibility, it has a very small likelihood of failing to diagnose an MHS individual. The fact that there are some false-positive findings in the contracture testing demonstrates that other myopathic conditions that are not necessarily concordant with MH have muscle tissue that is also capable of giving an abnormal response to halothane and caffeine exposures. Discordance between the results of an IVCT and the presence of MH mutations in *RYR1* can occur in MH families such that 3.1% to 19.4% of family members who do not carry an MH mutation respond positively to an IVCT challenge.[97,213] This presumably indicates that there are other factors (e.g., a second MH susceptibility mutation in *RYR1*, another MH sensitivity locus, a sensitivity to caffeine and halothane that does not reflect MH susceptibility) in these individuals that give a positive IVCT result, but it does not necessarily mean that they are MHS.

GENETIC TESTING

Limited examination of the *RYR1* gene is available for the purpose of diagnosing MH susceptibility at two Clinical Laboratory Improvement Amendments–approved laboratories in North America, as discussed earlier. Any physician can write a prescription for the ryanodine receptor gene test for MH susceptibility or fill out the requisition form and send blood for genetic testing. However, the probability of a positive outcome with genetic testing depends in part on the results of the in vitro CHCT because the clinical signs of MH are nonspecific. Current genetic testing indicates that about 60% of those who have positive CHCT results also have positive genetic results, whereas only 20% of those without a positive CHCT result yield positive genetic results.[97] Thus a negative gene screening test does not eliminate MH susceptibility, but a positive gene screen can be used to trace a family pedigree.

Other Disorders and Malignant Hyperthermia

MYOPATHIC SYNDROMES

An incriminatory association between various myopathies and malignant hyperthermia susceptibility, now known to be far more restricted than originally thought, was described in the 1970s and 1980s with much debate over the biochemical and pathophysiologic

character of the clinical episodes that resulted from exposure to MH-triggering agents.[217,218] Did the clinical episodes represent true MH, did the episodes relate to the instability of myopathic muscle membrane with attendant destruction of muscle cells and release of intracellular proteins, and was there sometimes an associated hyperthermic reaction with these exposures? Although both types of episodes may result in increased CK levels, hyperkalemia, myoglobinemia, and myoglobinuria, one results from exaggerated ramping of cellular energy and heat production, and the other results from cellular destruction that does not involve abnormal cellular metabolism as a primary cause. Of the congenital myopathies, central core disease, the related multi-minicore disease, and the myopathy of King-Denborough syndrome are the only myopathies known to have a definite relationship with true MH (see Chapter 24).[219,220]

MALIGNANT HYPERTHERMIA MIMICS

Malignant Hyperthermia–Like Syndrome in Pediatric Diabetes Mellitus

Diabetes mellitus has two well-characterized, life-threatening childhood presentations: diabetic ketoacidosis (DKA) and hyperglycemic hyperosmotic nonketotic syndrome (HHNS).[221–224] DKA, which is associated with type 1 diabetes, usually manifests as nausea, vomiting, dehydration, and weakness, but shock and coma are uncommon (1%-2%) in the absence of cerebral edema. Fever is rarely a symptom and usually spurs a search for an underlying infection. HHNS is usually associated with type 2 diabetes and classically manifests with symptoms of increasing polyuria, polydipsia, and lethargy that develop over a few days. The estimated mortality rate is between 12% and 46%, somewhat more dramatic than that seen for DKA (2%-10%), presumably because most cases of HHNS occur in adults with many other medical problems. The greatest rates of mortality with HHNS occur in adults older than 75 years of age or those with osmolarity values greater than 350 mOsm/L. The incidence of HHNS among U.S. children has been rapidly increasing and appears to be associated with the increase in childhood obesity. Despite this increase, pediatric HHNS is rare, and the presence of fever, as in DKA, usually prompts the search for an underlying infection.

A novel malignant hyperthermia–like syndrome (MHLS) against the background of pediatric diabetes mellitus was described in six adolescent boys between 14 and 18 years of age; the cases were culled from three tertiary care facilities in the United States.[225] The features of the syndrome included HHNS with coma, fever, rhabdomyolysis, and severe cardiovascular instability. Among the six adolescents with MHLS, five were obese, five had acanthosis nigricans, four were African American, and four died. Two more cases were later described; one patient died 14 hours after admission as a result of too rapid a correction of serum osmolarity and resultant cerebral edema and cardiovascular collapse, and a second patient was treated with dantrolene and completely recovered despite developing compartment syndrome in her left upper extremity as the result of rhabdomyolysis.[226] The survivor was tested for metabolic abnormalities, and a deficiency in short-chain acyl-coenzyme A (acyl-CoA) dehydrogenase was found.

Investigators recommend that anyone presenting with symptoms of HHNS and MHLS should be treated with dantrolene as soon as the syndrome is recognized and that fluid and insulin therapy be used for an appropriate rate of correction of serum osmolarity. A search of the literature reveals a similar case described 10 years earlier as fulminant MH associated with DKA in a patient who survived with the addition of dantrolene to his treatment regimen.[227]

Although it is difficult to ascertain the efficacy of dantrolene in abrogating the deleterious effects on skeletal muscle and in saving critically ill patients with MHLS during HHNS with such a small number of successfully treated patients, it seems prudent to initiate immediate treatment with dantrolene in these cases until the data can inform us about the true efficacy of this drug in MHLS.

Disorders of Fatty Acid Metabolism

Growing numbers of reports have documented cases of rhabdomyolysis in patients with disorders of fatty acid metabolism that in some ways mimic awake MH. These disorders arise from mutations in the enzymes responsible for the metabolism of various fatty acids and for ensuring adequate energy substrate for the mitochondria during periods of reduced glucose availability, such as during stress. Although these disorders have profound effects on energy metabolism, they should not be confused with mitochondrial myopathies, which result from completely different molecular defects and have mutations in the proteins of the mitochondrial respiratory chain (see Chapter 24). In neither case has a real association with MH been established, but there have been case reports of rhabdomyolysis and cardiac arrest in patients with carnitine palmitoyltransferase II deficiency.[228–230]

Various forms of acyl-CoA dehydrogenase deficiencies (i.e., very-long-chain, long-chain, medium-chain, and short-chain forms) lead to different types of myopathy that can have severe clinical consequences, including hypoglycemia and rhabdomyolysis with attendant multiple-organ dysfunction, which in some deficiencies are brought about by stress, particularly heat and severe exercise.[231,232] These diseases can manifest early in childhood or late in adolescence or young adulthood, and they can be a particular problem for individuals in the military or those who participate in intense sports.[232] Patients with the very-long-chain acyl-CoA dehydrogenase deficiency can present with acute hypercapnic respiratory failure.[233] Dantrolene has been used successfully to treat one case of recurrent rhabdomyolysis in a patient with very-long-chain acyl-CoA dehydrogenase deficiency,[234] and it may be useful to treat acute intraoperative rhabdomyolysis in these patients, although there is a dearth of evidence in this regard.

Children may present for surgery without a diagnosis of an inborn error of fatty acid metabolism and develop intraoperative rhabdomyolysis, mimicking aspects of a fulminant MH reaction. This may be the first manifestation of the child's fatty acid metabolism disorder. Preoperative increases in serum CK and uric acid levels, presumably owing to subclinical rhabdomyolysis, suggest an inborn error of metabolism or myopathy,[235] but these tests are not part of the usual preoperative panel of blood tests in normal pediatric anesthesia practice. Perioperative stress that may result from fasting, fear, disease states, and other causes can induce metabolic decompensation and hypoglycemia. As a consequence, an IV glucose-electrolyte solution is recommended for affected children.[236] Because of a few reports of rhabdomyolysis when these children are anesthetized with inhalational anesthetics, there has been some reluctance to use inhalational anesthetics.[236,237] It is, however, likely that the number of patients with inborn errors of fatty acid metabolism who undergo surgery is far greater than the paucity of reports of adverse outcomes with inhalational anesthetics. Because these patients vary considerably in their responses to stress, it is not surprising that most do well with any well-managed anesthetic. The available evidence suggests that the perioperative risk is no greater with any particular anesthetic in these children.

If the clinician elects to avoid inhalational anesthetics, two alternatives remain: regional anesthesia and TIVA. In children, peripheral limb surgery often allows for the use of IV sedation and regional anesthesia that may be suitable depending on the age of the child,[213] but most children do not tolerate this technique. However, a propofol based TIVA (see Chapter 8) is often used in children.[238]

Propofol infusion syndrome, a rare, usually lethal complication of prolonged infusions of propofol, is diagnosed by cardiovascular collapse associated with lipemic plasma, enlarged fatty liver, severe metabolic acidosis, and rhabdomyolysis or myoglobinuria.[239–241] In this syndrome, a large increase in particular fatty acids (i.e., malonylcarnitine and C5-acylcarnitine) that points to impaired entry of long-chain fatty acids into mitochondria and to resultant failure of mitochondrial respiration at complex II has been identified.[242] Others suggest that propofol infusion syndrome may uncover medium-chain acyl-CoA dehydrogenase deficiencies, although this remains unproved.[239] The notion that propofol can impair fatty acid uptake and subsequent oxidation raises the possibility that the acute administration of propofol to a patient with a defect in fatty acid metabolism can precipitate a metabolic crisis, although this has never been reported. It has also been suggested that the lipid load from a propofol infusion in the absence of adequate carbohydrate intake can expose a carnitine deficiency as a model for propofol infusion syndrome.[243] Moreover, propofol itself has been shown to inhibit mitochondrial respiration, possibly compounding the effects of fatty acid oxidation deficiencies.[239] In these children, the use of propofol may be associated with an unclear risk of inducing a metabolic crisis. If their metabolic abnormalities are subclinical, there is no easy, inexpensive preoperative screening tool to establish a diagnosis for a rare abnormality. Even if the child is diagnosed with one of the subsets of fatty acid oxidation deficiencies, it is impossible to predict preoperatively which children will be sensitive to propofol and, if they are, how sensitive they are.

Other TIVA regimens that may be considered include ketamine, dexmedetomidine, benzodiazepines, and opioids. In these instances, the preoperative discussion with the parents, children, and surgeons must address the perioperative risks, including the lack of evidence that any particular anesthetic is more likely to precipitate rhabdomyolysis and an MH-like reaction than another.

NEUROLEPTIC MALIGNANT SYNDROME

Neuroleptic malignant syndrome (NMS) is a rare, potentially lethal reaction to neuroleptics (0.1%-2.5% of patients), which is characterized clinically by the slow onset of fever, muscle rigidity, altered consciousness, and autonomic instability over a protracted period of time.[244] Laboratory findings include increased CK levels, leukocytosis, increased liver enzyme values, and reduced serum iron or potassium concentrations.[244] NMS is similar to MH, and the distinction between the two is often difficult to make, except by medication history; neuroleptics are associated with NMS, and inhalational anesthetics and succinylcholine are associated with MH.

NMS has developed in children taking neuroleptics that block all dopamine D_2 receptors (i.e., high-potency neuroleptics, such as haloperidol; atypical neuroleptics, such as thiothixene; low-potency D_2-receptor antagonists, such as metoclopramide; and tricyclic antidepressants) and in those with the withdrawal of antiparkinsonian medications. Although this syndrome has been attributed to a deficiency of central dopamine, other pathophysiologic mechanisms have also been proposed to explain the many clinical findings that cannot be explained by the lack of dopamine.

Successful therapy for NMS depends on early recognition, cessation of the offending medications, and intensive medical and nursing care geared toward hydration and restoration of electrolyte balance.[244] Specific pharmacologic therapy with dopamine agonists such as bromocriptine or with dantrolene has been advocated, although the use of dantrolene is controversial. Despite the fact that dantrolene is listed in psychiatric textbooks as a first-line pharmacologic treatment for NMS, there is no evidence that it is effective in treating NMS, except for the occasional case report declaring dantrolene to be effective.[244-246]

Children with psychiatric diagnoses who require treatment with neuroleptics make up a significant percentage of these pediatric patients. NMS in this pediatric population continues to be a problem, even with the newest drugs. The perioperative period for the pediatric patient taking neuroleptics is one fraught with potential diagnostic dilemmas. For example, one report described postoperative NMS in a child with severe cerebral palsy and seizure disorder who was not taking any neuroleptics and who was successfully treated three times with dantrolene.[247] Was this NMS or a mild form of MH? The answer remains unclear.

Summary

Many clinical scenarios in pediatric anesthesia can mimic MH and challenge our diagnostic acumen and our ability to deliver anesthesia safely. Not all metabolic syndromes that reveal themselves under inhalational anesthesia are MH, and not all metabolic syndromes that respond to dantrolene are MH. The examples given here underscore the need for expert advice during a case of suspected MH. Providers are urged to make use of the Malignant Hyperthermia Hotline when the need arises.

ANNOTATED REFERENCES

Hopkins PM. Malignant hyperthermia: pharmacology of triggering. *Br J Anaesth*. 2011;107(1):48-56.

Excellent review of the ability of all drugs used in the anesthetic pharmacopaeia and their capacity to trigger MH.

Hopkins PM, Rüffert H, Snoeck MM, et al. European Malignant Hyperthermia Group guidelines for investigation of malignant hyperthermia susceptibility. *Br J Anaesth*. 2015;115(4):531-539.

A European consensus protocol for the laboratory diagnosis of malignant hyperthermia susceptibility. The new guidelines contain a narrative commentary that describes development, changes to previously published protocols and guidelines, and recommendations for patient referral criteria and clinical interpretation of laboratory findings.

Lerman J, McLeod ME, Strong HA. Pharmacokinetics of intravenous dantrolene in children. *Anesthesiology*. 1989;70(4):625-629.

The paper describes the pharmacokinetics of dantrolene in children.

Litman RS, Rosenberg H. Malignant hyperthermia: update on susceptibility testing. *JAMA*. 2005;293(23):2918-2924.

The authors offer an excellent, understandable review of the clinical pathophysiology and testing strategies for malignant hyperthermia.

Robinson R, Carpenter D, Shaw MA, et al. Mutations in RyR1 in malignant hyperthermia and central core disease. *Hum Mutat*. 2006;27(10):977-989.

This comprehensive clinical and genetic review of malignant hyperthermia (MH) and central core disease (CCD) compares data from the United States and the United Kingdom and shows that hot spots of mutations in RyR1 may be population specific. Combined data show that there are many mutations outside of the hot-spot regions. Some mutations are concordant for both MH and CCD, and some are not.

Rosenberg H, Pollock N, Schiemann A, et al. Malignant hyperthermia: a review. *Orphanet J Rare Dis*. 2015;10:93.

This article is a comprehensive review of all aspects of MH, including the clinical diagnosis, management as well as the preparations of dantrolene, genetics and ongoing controversies related to associated medical disorders.

Rossi AE, Dirksen RT. Sarcoplasmic reticulum: the dynamic calcium governor of muscle. *Muscle Nerve*. 2006;33:715-731.

The article reviews the molecular pathophysiology of malignant hyperthermia and central core disease.

A complete reference list can be found online at ExpertConsult.com.

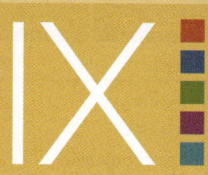

Regional Anesthesia

42

SANTHANAM SURESH, DAVID M. POLANER, AND CHARLES J. COTÉ

THE USE OF REGIONAL anesthesia techniques in children has increased dramatically in the past two decades.[1-9] Regional anesthesia is most commonly used in conjunction with general anesthesia in children, although in certain circumstances regional anesthesia may be the sole technique. In addition to central neuraxial blocks, peripheral nerve blocks are used with increasing frequency; the introduction of high-resolution portable ultrasound imaging has opened up new vistas to ensure that these blocks are safe and effective. Ultrasound-guided visualization of anatomic structures permits both greater precision of needle or catheter placement, confirmation that the drug has been deposited at the site of choice, and may reduce the volume of drug needed to achieve successful blockade while reducing the potential for local anesthetic toxicity (see Chapter 43).[10] Ultrasound guidance has also facilitated the performance of numerous blocks, including truncal blocks, approaches to the brachial plexus (supraclavicular and infraclavicular blocks), and several lower extremity blocks (mid-thigh saphenous and adductor canal blocks) that could not be otherwise performed accurately or safely in children using landmark or nerve stimulation techniques. Evidence from several recent large-scale collaborative studies of regional blockade in children supports the contention that peripheral nerve blockade is assuming greater prominence in pediatric anesthesia, and data from the Pediatric Regional Anesthesia Network (PRAN) suggests that the increased use of ultrasound guidance may, at least in part, be driving this trend.[11,12] Supplementing a general anesthetic with a nerve block can result in a pain-free awakening and postoperative analgesia without the potentially deleterious adverse side effects associated with parenteral opioids (see Chapter 43).[13] This benefit may be of particular importance to neonates, former preterm infants, children with cystic fibrosis and children with other conditions that render them vulnerable to opioid adverse effects.[4] There is also evidence that suggests that regional anesthesia may improve pulmonary function in children who have undergone thoracic or upper abdominal surgery.[14-17] Lastly, the greatly increased number of "same day surgery" cases in recent years has made the advantages of regional anesthesia, such as the rapid awakening, enhanced postoperative analgesia with no sedation or altered sensorium, and lack of opioid-induced nausea or vomiting, even more apparent. The safe and effective use of these techniques in children, however, requires an understanding of both the developmental anatomy of the region in which the block is placed and the developmental pharmacology of local anesthetics. Although there is increasing evidence and consensus that ultrasound guidance affords numerous advantages in safety and precision over landmark techniques for many peripheral nerve blocks,[18,19] this chapter will focus on landmark-guided techniques for those who do not have the advantage of an ultrasound imaging machine. Ultrasound techniques are described in Chapter 43. This chapter will also focus on the general issues of regional anesthetics in children that are applicable to any block technique, and on neuraxial anesthesia.

Pharmacology and Pharmacokinetics of Local Anesthetics

There are two classes of clinically useful local anesthetics, the amino amides (amides) and the amino esters (esters) (Table 42.1). The amides are degraded in the liver by cytochrome P450 enzymes,

TABLE 42.1	Commonly Used Local Anesthetics
Esters	**Amides**
Procaine	Lidocaine
Tetracaine	Mepivacaine
2-Chloroprocaine	Bupivacaine
	Levobupivacaine
	Ropivacaine
	Etidocaine

whereas the esters are hydrolyzed primarily by plasma cholinesterases.[20-24] These degradation pathways account for some of the differences in distribution and metabolism of local anesthetics, particularly in neonates when compared with adults.

AMIDES

Amide local anesthetics commonly used in children include lidocaine, bupivacaine (and its isomer levobupivacaine), and ropivacaine. The choice of agent most often depends on the desired speed of onset and duration of action of the block, but in small infants and children issues related to potential toxicity are also important. Compared with the liver of an adult, the liver of the neonate has limited enzymatic activity to metabolize and biotransform drugs (see also Chapter 7 and Fig. 7.11). The ability to oxidize and to reduce drugs, in particular, is immature.[23-30] Neonates do not metabolize mepivacaine, with most of it excreted unchanged in the urine.[31-37] Conjugation reactions are limited at birth and do not reach adult rates until approximately 6 to 12 months of age.[25-28,33]

The nature of the epidural space in infants differs from that in the adult with increased vascularity, less fat, and a smaller absorptive surface for local anesthetics. Anatomic studies have shown that the epidural fat is spongy and gelatinous in appearance, with distinct spaces between individual fat globules.[38] With increasing age, fat becomes more tightly packed and fibrous. The absorption half-time of epidural levobupivacaine decreases from 0.36 hours at 1 month postnatal age (PNA) to 0.14 hours at 6 months PNA (E-Fig. 42.1). This, combined with reduced clearance (by the cytochrome P450, CYP3A4), decreases the time to maximum plasma concentration (T_{max}) from 2.2 hours at 1 month PNA to 0.75 hours (80% of the mature value) by 6 months PNA.[39]

Older children also differ from adults with respect to the pharmacokinetics of local anesthetics. The steady-state volume of distribution (Vdss) of amides in children is greater than that in adults, whereas their clearances (Cl) are similar.[40-42] Because the elimination half-life ($T_{1/2}$) is related to the volume of distribution and clearance,

$$T_{1/2} = (0.693 \times Vdss)/Cl,$$

a larger Vdss directly prolongs the elimination half-life. However, it is clearance that determines steady-state concentrations with continuous amide infusion; reduced clearance in neonates implies that repeated doses and continuous infusions will lead to an accumulation of local anesthetic (see E-Fig. 42.1).[43-45] Thus infusion rates and local anesthetic concentrations must be reduced in this vulnerable age group when prolonged administration of amides is used for postoperative analgesia.

Further differentiating the pharmacokinetics in adults from children is that pharmacokinetic differences may be amplified by the location and type of block. Children achieve peak plasma concentrations of amide local anesthetics more rapidly than adults after intercostal nerve blocks, but at similar times (~30 minutes with lidocaine and bupivacaine) after caudal epidural administration.[40,46,47] Ilioinguinal nerve blocks in children weighing less than 15 kg may yield plasma concentrations of bupivacaine in the toxic range if more than 1.25 mg/kg is administered.[48]

Bupivacaine

Bupivacaine may still be the most commonly used amide local anesthetic agent for regional blockade in infants and children at some institutions, although ropivacaine (and in Canada and Europe, levobupivacaine) is increasingly used. After a single administration of bupivacaine, analgesia may be expected for up to 4 hours, although its duration of action is somewhat less in small infants. The concentration used depends on the site of injection, the desired density of blockade, consideration of the toxic threshold of the drug, and dose limitations imposed by the concomitant administration of other local anesthetics, such as local infiltration by the surgeon or intravenous (IV) or topical laryngotracheal administration of lidocaine. The most commonly used concentration for peripheral nerve blocks is 0.25%, with reduced concentrations of 0.0625% to 0.1% used for continuous epidural administration. The 0.5% concentration is infrequently used in children, although it may be used for peripheral nerve blocks where subsequent doses and drug accumulation are not of concern and where the volume of administered drug is sufficiently small to permit that concentration to be used without toxicity. Greater concentrations also increase the density of the motor block, an effect that may be desirable depending on the clinical situation.

Bupivacaine is highly bound to plasma proteins, particularly to α_1-acid glycoprotein. It is a racemic mixture of the levorotary and dextrorotary enantiomers; the l-isoform is bioactive with regard to clinical effect, and the d-isoform contributes more to toxicity. Levobupivacaine, the l-enantiomer of bupivacaine, retains the efficacy and duration of blockade as the racemic formulation (demonstrated in both an ovine model and in adult volunteers), yet carries up to a 30% reduced risk of cardiac and central nervous system (CNS) toxicities.[49,50] Although the beneficial toxicity profile of levobupivacaine has resulted in its widespread use, it is currently unavailable in the United States.[51]

Several experimental preparations of local anesthetics have the prospect to prolong analgesia with a reduced potential for toxicity.[52-54] Bioerodible encapsulated microspheres of bupivacaine administered for peripheral neural blockade[55] release local anesthetic over many hours to several days, depending on the formulation of the microsphere, thus producing very prolonged analgesia.[56] The addition of dexamethasone to the microspheres prolongs the block up to 13-fold, and plasma bupivacaine concentrations in animal studies were far below the toxic threshhold.[57] No adverse local reactions were noted. Several different preparations have been developed and studied, including synthetic bioerodible microspheres, protein-lipid-sugar spheres, and liposystems.[58-60] The first such preparation (Exparel, Pacira Pharmaceuticals, Inc., Parsippany, NJ) has been approved for use in patients 18 years of age or older by the U.S. Food and Drug Administration for local site infiltration (i.e., not approved for peripheral nerve blocks); toxicology studies suggest a low risk because of the slow rate of drug release.[52,61-63] In several adult studies (there are no pediatric data), however, the actual duration of analgesia was found to be only marginally prolonged over that produced by bupivacaine with epinephrine.[64] While prolonged action of local anesthetics could be particularly useful for those who require prolonged neural blockade for analgesia but cannot have an indwelling regional anesthetic, it appears that we still await agents with significant clinical efficacy. New drugs with novel mechanisms of action may offer more promise and appear to be on the horizon. Site 1 sodium channel blockers such as neosaxitoxin have low toxicity and high efficacy and are currently undergoing early clinical trials (see Chapter 44).[65-67] Potential applications include intercostal blockade for rib fractures, postoperative analgesia for ambulatory surgery, and children in whom an indwelling epidural catheter poses an excessive risk of infection.

Ropivacaine

Ropivacaine is an amide local anesthetic. Like levobupivacaine, it is an *l*-enantiomer that has reduced risks of cardiac and neurologic toxicities compared with bupivacaine.[68] The lethal dose in 50% of animals (LD_{50}) is greater than that of bupivacaine. Rats of different maturity exhibit a threefold greater tolerance to equipotent doses of ropivacaine than of bupivacaine when administered for a femoral nerve block.[69] Ropivacaine is also reputed to produce a less dense motor block at equianalgesic potency to other local anesthetics, although the data are conflicting in this regard.[70] Some studies report a greater sparing of motor function compared with bupivacaine, whereas others report no difference in motor and sensory block. Ropivacaine produces a denser blockade of the Aδ and C fibers than bupivacaine when low concentrations are used, lending mechanistic credence to the idea of differential blockade.[71] Much of the infant animal data, however, do not support the existence of a greater sensorimotor differential block than that after bupivacaine. The few clinical studies in infants and children currently available do not report a detectable motor-sensory differential, in contrast to the data in adults.[69,72] Several clinical studies in infants and children report a prolonged duration of analgesia with ropivacaine, despite using a solution of reduced potency.[72-74] Although there are still only limited data available in children, the decreased potential for toxicity makes ropivacaine an attractive agent in this age group. Ropivacaine possesses intrinsic vasoconstrictive properties; thus it is not available as an epinephrine-containing solution. Most clinical studies have used a 0.2% solution (2 mg/mL); the volume of drug injected was similar to that of bupivacaine but depended on the type of block and size of the child. We commonly use concentrations of 0.1% for infusions with opioid for continuous neuraxial postoperative analgesia, whereas concentrations up to 0.2% may be used for thoracic epidural infusions and peripheral and plexus blocks.

Lidocaine

Lidocaine has a relatively short duration of action compared with bupivacaine and ropivacaine; it is rarely used for single-injection blocks in pediatric regional anesthesia, where a prolonged effect for postoperative analgesia is usually a priority. However, it can be used effectively in continuous blocks where the drug is continuously infused via a catheter, although here too, ropivacaine, levobupivacaine, and bupivacaine are far more commonly used. In vitro laboratory experiments have suggested that lidocaine might have greater potential for neurotoxicity in the developing nervous system than other local anesthetics, although the clinical implications of these findings remain unclear and unproved.[75]

ESTERS

The pharmacokinetics of the ester local anesthetics are also affected by the quantitative and qualitative difference in plasma proteins. Plasma pseudocholinesterase activity in neonatal umbilical blood is decreased compared with adults;[76] thus the plasma half-life of the ester anesthetics may be prolonged. Despite a prolonged elimination half-life in infants, 2,3-chloroprocaine has been recommended for neonatal regional techniques, particularly for continuous epidural and plexus blockade.[77,78] Limited data suggest that 2,3-chloroprocaine may be safe in this setting and that toxic accumulation does not occur after several hours of use with a 1.5% concentration.

Another enzymatic system with decreased activity in neonates is methemoglobin reductase, which is responsible for maintaining hemoglobin in a reduced valence state where it is capable of binding and transporting oxygen. Hepatic metabolism of prilocaine yields *o*-toluidine, which can produce methemoglobinemia, thereby rendering red blood cells less capable of carrying oxygen.[79] The decreased activity of methemoglobin reductase and the increased susceptibility of fetal hemoglobin to oxidization make prilocaine an unsuitable local anesthetic for use in neonates. Although prilocaine is no longer available for use in the United States as an injected local anesthetic, it is one of the components of EMLA cream (eutectic mixture of local anesthetics, AstraZeneca, Wilmington, DE), a commonly used transdermal local anesthetic. The total dose and surface area for EMLA application must therefore be limited in neonates because methemoglobinemia has been reported (see Chapter 7). Even infants and toddlers are not without increased risk of toxicity, so the dose must be meticulously calculated.[80] Other local anesthetics, particularly topical agents, such as benzocaine, are potentially dangerous in infants because of the risk of methemoglobinemia by this same mechanism.[81] EMLA should only be applied to normal intact skin in appropriate doses[82] (0–3 months or weight <5 kg, 1 g applied to a maximum of approximately 10 cm^2 surface area; 3–12 months and >5 kg, 2 g to a maximum of 20 cm^2; 1–6 years and >10 kg, 10 g applied to a maximum of approximately 100 cm^2 surface area; 7–12 years and >20 kg, 20 g applied to a maximum of approximately 200 cm^2 surface area). The dose must be reduced if EMLA is applied to mucosal surfaces (such as the glans of the penis). The duration of action persists for 1 to 2 hours after the cream is removed. Adverse reactions include skin blanching, erythema, itching, rash, and methemoglobinemia. EMLA should be used with caution and with strict attention to the amount of cream and surface area of application in children younger than 1 month of age. Infants receiving drugs that may induce methemoglobinemia, such as phenytoin, phenobarbital, and sulfonamides, may be at increased risk, and caution is warranted. It is contraindicated in children with congenital or idiopathic methemoglobinemia. Topical amethocaine (Ametop, Smith & Nephew Healthcare, Mississauga, Ontario, Canada) has a more rapid onset of analgesia and increased depth of penetration through the skin and produces minimal vasoconstriction of the skin compared with EMLA.[83] Iontophoresis of lidocaine can also produce excellent transdermal skin analgesia with much faster onset of action (10 minutes) and greater depth of skin penetration than EMLA.[83]

TOXICITY OF LOCAL ANESTHETICS

With the exception of uncommon effects, such as producing methemoglobinemia, the major toxic effects of local anesthetics are on the cardiovascular system and the CNS. Local anesthetics readily cross the blood-brain barrier to cause alterations in CNS function. A consistent sequence of symptoms can be observed as plasma local-anesthetic concentrations progressively increase, although this may not be readily apparent in infants and small children. Because of the smaller threshold for cardiac toxicity with bupivacaine, cardiac and CNS toxicity may occur virtually simultaneously in infants and children, or cardiac toxicity may even precede CNS toxicity. During the intraoperative use of bupivacaine, early recognition of toxicity may be masked by the concomitant use of general anesthetics, which will obscure the signs of CNS toxicity until devastating cardiovascular effects are apparent.[84]

In awake patients, the earliest sign of local-anesthetic toxicity is circumoral paresthesia, which is the result of the high tissue concentrations of local anesthetic rather than CNS effects. The development of circumoral paresthesia is followed by the prodromal CNS symptoms of lightheadedness and dizziness, which progress to both visual and auditory disturbances, such as difficulty in focusing and tinnitus. Objective signs of CNS toxicity during this time are shivering, slurred speech, and muscle twitching. As the plasma concentration of local anesthetic continues to increase, CNS excitation occurs, resulting in generalized seizures. Further increases in the local anesthetic concentration depress the CNS, with respiratory depression leading to a respiratory arrest. In adults, cardiovascular toxicity usually follows CNS toxicity. In this case, the systemic blood pressure decreases (1) because the peripheral vasculature dilates and (2) because of direct myocardial depression, leading to a progressive bradycardia. These effects culminate in a cardiac arrest. In large doses, bupivacaine produces ventricular dysrhythmias, including ventricular tachycardia, peaked T waves, and ST-segment elevation that suggest myocardial ischemia, especially when epinephrine-containing solutions are used. Bupivacaine has a particularly strong affinity for the fast sodium channels, as well as the calcium and slow potassium channels in the myocardium. These effects explain why it is so difficult to resuscitate children from a toxic dose of bupivacaine.[85–87] Stereoselectivity of the sodium channel in the open state, however, has not been demonstrated. There is also evidence that the slow or "flicker" potassium channels may play a significant role in bupivacaine toxicity.[88]

With an intravascular injection of bupivacaine with epinephrine, characteristic changes on the electrocardiogram (ECG) may be observed in the absence of symptoms of CNS toxicity. Fig. 42.1 shows an ECG tracing obtained during an unintended intravenous injection of bupivacaine with and without epinephrine (positive test dose). Even a small IV dose of 1 to 2 µg/kg of epinephrine in a 1:200,000 solution with 0.25% bupivacaine produces peaked

T waves with elevated ST segments, particularly in the lateral chest leads.[89–91] When the ECG effects of bupivacaine, with and without epinephrine, and epinephrine alone were compared in children, the most reliable ECG changes (peaked T waves at 1 minute) and an increase in arterial pressure and heart rate, required the presence of epinephrine.[92] It should be noted, however, that these changes in the T waves depended on age, diminishing in responsiveness beyond 8 years of age. These data suggest that careful observation of the ECG during test dose administration may be a sensitive indicator of unintended intravascular injection of bupivacaine in the child anesthetized with an inhalational anesthetic (see Technique of Administration later).[93]

Plasma protein binding is the most important pharmacologic factor that determines the toxicity of local anesthetics, particularly for amides, because it is the free (unbound) fraction of the drug that produces toxicity. Reduced plasma protein concentrations cause more drug to remain in the unbound active form with greater potential for toxicity (see Chapter 7). Concentrations of α_1-acid glycoprotein in neonates are less than in older infants and children, producing a clinically crucial greater free fraction of amide local anesthetics in neonates. The significantly greater concentrations of free lidocaine and bupivacaine in infants and neonates are attributed to the decreased levels of α_1-acid glycoprotein, the primary binding protein of these drugs, compared with adults.[43,94–98] Current data suggest that the plasma concentration of free drug may be 30% greater in infants younger than 6 months of age and even greater in preterm infants than in adolescents.[99] α_1-Acid glycoprotein is an acute-phase reactant whose concentration increases after surgery. Concentrations of α_1-acid glycoprotein in infants are less in those undergoing elective rather than emergency surgery.[100] It is not known whether these increased α_1-acid glycoprotein concentrations are sufficient to afford any protective effect on the risk of toxicity from bupivacaine accumulation in the perioperative period. Decreased protein binding appears to be especially important in neonates in whom continuous infusions of local anesthetics are used, as reduced clearance contributes to drug accumulation and consequent high concentrations of unbound drug.[101,102]

Plasma concentrations of lidocaine that depress the cardiovascular and respiratory systems in human neonates are about half

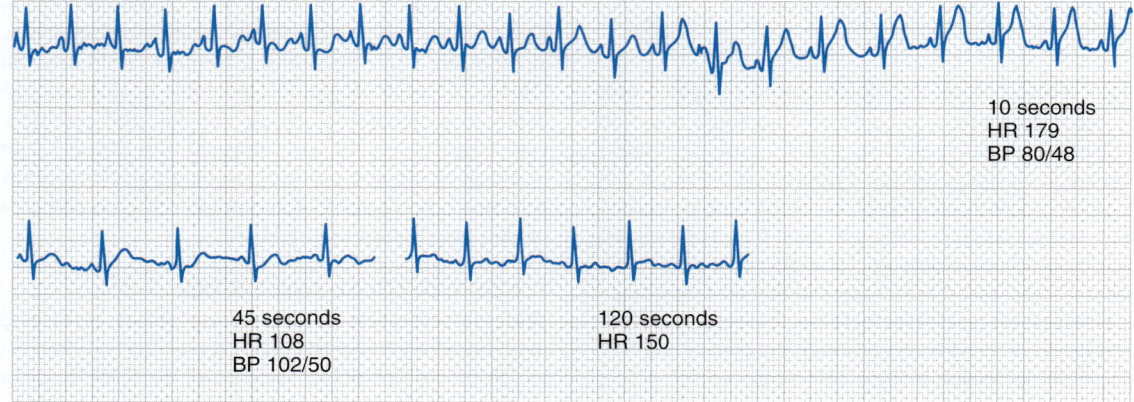

FIGURE 42.1 Electrocardiographic changes associated with the intravenous injection of bupivacaine and epinephrine 1:200,000. Note the marked increase in the height of the T waves at 10 seconds. *BP*, blood pressure; *HR*, heart rate. (From Freid EB, Bailey AG, Valley RD. Electrocardiographic and hemodynamic changes associated with unintentional intravascular injection of bupivacaine with epinephrine in children. *Anesthesiology* 1993;79[2]:394–398.)

those that cause similar toxicity in adults.[103] In contrast, 2-day-old guinea pigs were less susceptible to the toxic effects of bupivacaine than 2-week or 2-month-old guinea pigs, even though the blood concentrations in the 2-day-olds were greater.[84] Data regarding toxicity in infant versus adolescent versus adult rats for both bupivacaine and ropivacaine are similar.[69] Young dogs, however, have a decreased threshold to both seizure and cardiac toxicity caused by excessive doses of bupivacaine.[104] Because species differences are important in toxicity studies, it is difficult to predict which study represents the human neonate.[105] No data exist in humans regarding age-dependent differences in the toxic threshold of bupivacaine at a given blood concentration. Seizures and cardiovascular collapse have been reported in human infants at the same blood concentrations of bupivacaine as in adults. Whereas data from some animal studies suggest that the greater volume of distribution of amides in younger children may protect against bupivacaine toxicity, retrospective analyses of large databases of infants who have received epidural infusions indicate that these findings may not be applicable to the human infant, particularly during continuous infusions or with repeated dosing. Current data on the pharmacokinetic and pharmacodynamic differences associated with early infancy suggest that caution should be exercised when using local anesthetics in infants. Several reports document that infants and children may develop systemic toxicity, including dysrhythmias, seizures, and cardiovascular depression from the accumulation of epidural infusions of bupivacaine.[43,101,106–108] Meticulous attention must be paid to the total dose of local anesthetic administered, the rate of administration, the site of injection, and the use of vasoconstrictors to diminish the rate of uptake of the local anesthetic. This is particularly important when a continuous regional anesthetic technique is used postoperatively or during prolonged surgery when repeated doses of local anesthetic are administered.

We recommend that both the bolus and infusion doses of bupivacaine and lidocaine be reduced by approximately 30% for infants younger than 6 months of age to decrease the risk for toxicity. This would result in a maximal bupivacaine rate of no more than 0.3 mg/kg per hour.[44] Whereas these recommendations are particularly applicable to continuous infusions of bupivacaine for postoperative analgesia, the same caveats apply to large single injections, repeated injections, and continuous infusions of local anesthetics during long surgical procedures.

The *d*-stereoisomer (or enantiomer) of racemic mixtures of local anesthetics may also be a primary factor in the risk for both cardiac and CNS toxicity.[87] As described earlier, both ropivacaine and levobupivacaine, which are *l*-enantiomers, have decreased toxicity compared with bupivacaine, a racemic mixture, as demonstrated in adults and experimental animals.[88] This may be due in part to the reduced affinity of cardiac and CNS tissues for the *l*-enantiomer.[68] The inclusion of levobupivacaine and ropivacaine into the clinical armamentarium may prove beneficial in decreasing local anesthetic toxicity.

PREVENTION OF TOXICITY

Few data have correlated the anesthetic block, blood concentration of local anesthetic, and dose in infants and children. Most dosing guidelines have been extrapolated from studies in adults. Table 42.2 lists the maximum recommended doses of local anesthetics, as well as their approximate durations of action. To avoid overdose and the possibility of toxic effects, it is prudent to remain within these guidelines until studies in children clarify the pharmacokinetics and pharmacodynamics of local anesthetics for specific nerve

TABLE 42.2	Maximum Recommended Doses and Duration of Action of Commonly Used Local Anesthetics	
Local Anesthetic	Maximum Dose (mg/kg)[a]	Duration of Action (minutes)[b]
Procaine	10	60–90
2-Chloroprocaine	20	30–60
Tetracaine	1.5	180–600
Lidocaine	7	90–200
Mepivacaine	7	120–240
Bupivacaine	2.5	180–600
Ropivacaine	3	120–240

[a]These are maximum doses of local anesthetics. Doses of amides should be decreased by 30% in infants younger than 6 months of age. When lidocaine is being administered intravascularly (e.g., during intravenous regional anesthesia), the dose should be decreased to 3 to 5 mg/kg; there is no need to administer long-acting local anesthetic agents for intravenous regional anesthesia, and such a practice is potentially dangerous.

[b]Duration of action depends on the concentration, total dose, site of administration, and the child's age.

blocks. As discussed earlier, all of these doses should be reduced by ~30% in infants younger than 6 months of age.

Toxic reactions from local anesthetics are a function of (1) the total dose administered; (2) the site of administration; (3) the rate of uptake; (4) pharmacologic alterations in toxic threshold; (5) the technique of administration; (6) the rate of degradation, metabolism, and excretion of local anesthetic; and (7) the acid-base status of the child.[109–114] Thus recommendations (including those of the authors) of a specific dose limit for a given drug are both overly simplistic and potentially misleading.[115] Because of the multiplicity of factors that drive the final concentration of unbound local anesthetic, and in the absence of definitive and comprehensive data, conservative dosing remains the most prudent course.

Total Drug Dose

The dose of local anesthetic should be determined by a child's age, physical status, the area to be anesthetized, and *weight according to lean body mass*. A severely ill child who is in congestive heart failure, for example, has a reduced capacity to metabolize amide local anesthetics because of a reduced cardiac output and hepatic blood flow. Similarly, a markedly obese child must not be given a larger dose simply on the basis of increased weight. If a large volume of local anesthetic is required for a particular procedure, a dilute concentration should be used to avoid exceeding the maximum recommended safe dose. Doses are calculated based on the lean body weight of the child (e.g., a 20-kg child could receive up to 50 mg of bupivacaine). An easy approximation for bupivacaine is 1 mL/kg of 0.25% bupivacaine, reduced by approximately one-third for infants younger than 6 months of age.

Site of Injection

Injection of local anesthetics into very vascular areas leads to greater blood concentrations than the same dose injected into less vascular areas. The order of uptake (i.e., maximum blood concentration) of local anesthetics (in order from greatest to least) from regional blocks in adults is (1) intercostal nerve blocks, (2) caudal blocks, (3) epidural blocks, and (4) brachial plexus and femoral-sciatic nerve blocks.[116] An easy way to remember this is by the mnemonic **ICE Block**:

I = intercostal

C = caudal

E = epidural

Block = peripheral nerve blocks

Studies are required to determine whether this order holds true for children. Blood concentrations of bupivacaine twice those measured in older children have been reported in children weighing less than 15 kg after ilioinguinal nerve block for herniorrhaphy using only 1.25 mg/kg of 0.5% bupivacaine without epinephrine, which is half the usual recommended maximal dose.[48] However, the fascia iliaca block in older children produced blood concentrations of bupivacaine that were within the acceptable safe range.[117] Neonates who received a transversus abdominis plane block of 0.125% bupivacaine for a total volume of 1 mL/kg had greatest plasma concentration of 0.38 μg/mL at 30 minutes after the block; one-quarter to one-fifth the toxic threshold, 1.5 to 2.0 μg/L.[118] Local infiltration of the wound in herniorrhaphy has not been associated with increased blood concentrations of local anesthetics,[119] but scalp infiltration during neurosurgery may produce relatively greater blood concentrations.[120] As would be expected, spinal anesthesia results in very small blood concentrations, even in neonates.[98]

Rate of Uptake

The rate of uptake of a local anesthetic depends on the vascularity of the site of injection. Increased perfusion increases uptake, whereas decreased perfusion decreases uptake.[121] The rate of uptake in children is usually more rapid than in adults. In general, the addition of a vasoconstrictor to the local anesthetic reduces the rate of uptake and prolongs the duration of the block. In adults, the dose of epinephrine is usually limited when used in conjunction with potent anesthetic agents because of the risk of inducing cardiac arrhythmias. If epinephrine is combined with the ester anesthetics, there is no increased risk of arrhythmias. For example, in adults anesthetized with halothane, the maximum recommended dose of epinephrine is 1.0 to 1.5 μg/kg. In children, however, larger doses of epinephrine may be safe.[122-124] We have used as much as 10 μg/kg of epinephrine in children, with a maximum dose of 250 μg, during halothane anesthesia without evidence of ventricular irritability, and these doses are likely to be even safer with currently used inhalational anesthetics, which do not sensitize the myocardium to the arrhythmogenic effects of epinephrine. An epinephrine concentration of 1:100,000 should not be exceeded, and 1:200,000 or less is generally used. A quick reference for converting local anesthetic concentrations and the amount of epinephrine in various dilutions is presented in Tables 42.3 and 42.4. *Epinephrine is contraindicated in blocks in which vasoconstriction of an end-artery could lead to tissue necrosis, such as for digital and penile blocks, although this historical practice has recently been challenged, setting the stage for prospective studies.*[125-127]

Alteration in Toxic Threshold

Medications, such as diazepam or midazolam, that increase the seizure threshold (i.e., the threshold for CNS toxicity) can be valuable adjuncts to regional anesthesia. Premedication with diazepam (0.15–0.3 mg/kg) decreases a child's anxiety but also offers some protection from the toxic CNS effects of a local anesthetic overdose.[128] Although diazepam is no longer in common clinical use in children in the perioperative period, evidence in animal models and considerable clinical experience in humans suggests that midazolam is also effective in terminating seizure activity.[129] Animal data, however, suggest that the concomitant use of diazepam and bupivacaine decreases the elimination of bupivacaine from serum and cardiac tissue in mice.[130] This effect is not a result of changes in protein binding.[131] It is not known if this is true for all benzodiazepines or if this is also the case in humans. Although premedication with a benzodiazepine prevents manifestations of CNS toxicity, the threshold for cardiovascular toxicity is unchanged.[132] Thus after premedication with a benzodiazepine, cardiovascular collapse can occur without warning because the symptoms of CNS toxicity may be blunted. Because most regional anesthesia administrations performed in children are placed after induction of general anesthesia (with the exception of some blocks in former preterm infants), this may be a moot point in most circumstances.

Technique of Administration

Whenever regional anesthesia is performed, the operator must be prepared for an adverse reaction and resuscitation supplies, including drugs, suction, and airway equipment, must be immediately available. The needle or catheter must always be inspected for blood as soon as it is positioned, but before injecting the local anesthetic, to determine if the tip is within an artery or a vein. It is preferable to observe the needle or catheter for passive blood flow rather than to actively aspirate for blood because the blood vessels, such as the epidural venous plexus, are thin walled and collapse readily when negative pressure is applied. As a result, the inability to aspirate blood is not absolute proof that the needle or catheter is not in a blood vessel. For this reason, a small volume of local anesthetic with a marker for intravascular injection, such as epinephrine in a concentration of 1:200,000, is administered first, while the ECG is observed for 30 to 60 seconds. Data from awake adults indicate that the heart rate will increase within 1 minute of intravascular administration.[133] When the drugs are administered during general anesthesia, however, the efficacy of the test dose to detect an intravascular injection may be greatly reduced. Heart rate increases in only 73% of children after an IV injection of 0.5 μg/kg of epinephrine during halothane anesthesia, suggesting that this marker of an intravascular injection is not

TABLE 42.3	Epinephrine Dilution and Conversion to μg/mL
Epinephrine Dilution	**μg/mL**
1:100,000	10
1:200,000	5
1:400,000	2.5
1:800,000	1.25

TABLE 42.4	Local Anesthetic Concentration and Its Conversion to mg/mL
Concentration (percent)	**mg/mL**
3	30
2.5	25
2	20
1	10
0.5	5
0.25	2.5
0.125	1.25

completely reliable.[134] Administration of atropine several minutes before the test dose increased the rate of positive responders to 92%, suggesting that vagal tone and the anesthetic's blunting of the sympathetic reflexes are responsible for the reduced sensitivity to the test dose. Test doses during isoflurane anesthesia appear to have the same limitations.[135] With sevoflurane, positive results were obtained in 100% of children if the threshold for a positive response was an increase in heart rate of 10 beats/minute and a dose in excess of 0.5 µg/kg of epinephrine was used; positive results were obtained in 85% if 0.25 µg/kg of epinephrine was used.[136] In all children, a change in the T-wave amplitude was a reliable indicator of intravascular injection with both doses of epinephrine (see Fig. 42.1). All children in that study were pretreated with atropine (10 µg/kg). It is not known if increasing the dose of epinephrine to 1.0 µg/kg or increasing the concentration of epinephrine in the test dose solution to 1:100,000 during general anesthesia would increase the sensitivity of the heart rate response test without atropine. Systolic blood pressure increased by more than 10% within 60 seconds of the test dose injection, suggesting that an increase in blood pressure may be a more sensitive indicator of intravascular injection than heart rate during inhalation anesthesia. ST-segment and T-wave changes also appear to be sensitive indicators of intravascular injection of local anesthetic. Observation of the ECG yields a very sensitive indicator of an intravascular injection of bupivacaine with epinephrine. These ECG changes were present in 97% of infants and children who received an IV dose of bupivacaine and epinephrine.[90] These investigators did not confirm the efficacy of pretreatment with atropine on the heart rate. During total IV anesthesia (TIVA) with propofol and remifentanil, however, quite different results have been reported. A prospective study of children who received an IV injection of bupivacaine with epinephrine as a simulated positive test dose during TIVA found that T-wave alterations were inconsistent and could not be relied on as an indicator of intravascular injection.[115] Only blood pressure (particularly diastolic) was a consistent and reliable marker of intravascular injection, increasing more than 10% in all subjects during TIVA.

Even though no test dose regimen is completely infallible and the difficulty of interpreting a negative test dose has resulted in a European Society of Regional Anaesthesia and Pain Therapy (ESRA)/American Society of Regional Anesthesia and Pain Medicine (ASRA) practice advisory deeming its use as discretionary,[137] it appears most prudent to use an epinephrine-containing test dose before administering the therapeutic dose of local anesthetic, particularly if the block is administered in an anatomic location near a blood vessel.[136] The test dose should be repeated before subsequent bolus injections through a catheter. If the drug injection is visualized in real time using ultrasound, test dosing may be less critical, as the actual drug deposition can be visualized during the injection, although this, too, may not be infallible. If the child is receiving a general inhalation anesthetic, blood pressure and the ST-segment configuration, in addition to the heart rate, should be carefully and frequently observed after injection of the test dose.[93] Pretreatment with atropine (10 µg/kg) may increase the rate of detecting an unintended intravascular injection. In addition, the rate of injection may also be a factor in the development of toxicity. If injection is partially or completely intravascular, a slow injection may not exceed the toxic threshold, whereas a rapid injection could. Thus slow, incremental injection of the therapeutic dose of local anesthetic (over several minutes) may further increase the safety of regional blockade, even though repeated injections within a brief period might also result in toxic reactions.

TREATMENT OF LOCAL ANESTHETIC SYSTEMIC TOXICITY

Treatment of toxic reactions to local anesthetic overdose requires knowledge of the signs and symptoms previously described. The signs of local-anesthetic systemic toxicity (LAST), with the exception of the catastrophic cardiovascular events, are all masked by general anesthesia. Indeed, inhaled anesthetics may actually raise the threshold for seizures and thereby delay the detection of toxicity until cardiovascular collapse occurs. Even in the unanesthetized child, the progression from prodromal signs to cardiovascular collapse may be very rapid and the initial resuscitative therapy in some cases may need to be directed at reestablishing circulation and normal cardiac rhythm, including the timely institution of chest compressions, while definitive treatments are being readied. As always, initial management should consist of establishing and maintaining a patent airway and providing supplemental oxygen. The timely administration of a CNS depressant that alters the seizure threshold may prevent seizures. Administration of midazolam (0.05–0.2 mg/kg IV), thiopental (2–3 mg/kg IV), or propofol (1–3 mg/kg IV) effectively prevents or terminates seizure activity; however, the latter two agents are also potent myocardial depressants and should be used with great caution. If seizure activity is present and the airway is not secured, the use of succinylcholine or other relaxant may facilitate tracheal intubation but does not prevent seizure activity. It should be remembered, however, that the acute morbidity from seizures is the result of airway complications (hypoxia and aspiration) and that securing the airway takes precedence over the actual control of the electrical activity of the seizure. CNS excitability is exacerbated in the presence of hypercarbia; it is, therefore, important to mildly hyperventilate children who have seizures. None of these interventions should in any way supplant or delay the administration of lipid emulsion to directly treat the toxic levels of local anesthetic, and help should be sought to carry out these treatments simultaneously. Indeed, two case reports suggest that lipid emulsion may reverse the CNS symptoms of LAST in the absence of cardiovascular collapse and might be a preferable first-line therapy.[138,139]

Advances in the treatment of LAST have dramatically altered the therapeutic interventions that should be initiated in the event of cardiovascular collapse after a large intravascular injection of an amide local anesthetic. IV lipid emulsion has been shown to be effective for resuscitation of cardiac arrest caused by both bupivacaine and ropivacaine toxicity. In dogs, successful resuscitation after cardiac arrest and 10 minutes of external cardiac massage was demonstrated after lipid administration.[140] Although 100% of the dogs that received an infusion of 20% lipid emulsion were successfully resuscitated, none of the controls that received a saline solution infusion survived. A clear relationship between the tissue concentration and the response has also been established.[141] Lipid emulsion was superior to epinephrine, which fared no better than control in restoring metabolic and hemodynamic indexes in a rat model of bupivacaine toxicity.[142] These animal studies have been corroborated by several anecdotal reports of rescue from cardiac arrest in humans that followed intravascular injections of all of the amide local anesthetics in common use.[143–146] The mechanism of action of lipid emulsions to treat bupivacaine toxicity is not entirely understood, but studies in isolated rat heart preparations suggested that the lipid treatment elutes bupivacaine from the myocardium and accelerates the recovery from bupivacaine-induced asystole.[147] This "lipid sink" hypothesis suggests a novel mechanism of action compared with more conventional antidysrhythmic drugs, and the treatment appears to be more effective as well. An inverse relationship between the concentration of lipid emulsion and the myocardial bupivacaine concentration (greater lipid concentrations were more effective at decreasing the bupivacaine concentration in the myocardium) suggests that this lipid sink hypothesis is correct.[141] Furthermore, a study in infant pigs suggested that administering epinephrine in the initial arrest phase may actually impair resuscitation with lipid emulsion, preventing a sustained response to treatment, and that treatment with lipid alone was superior to both treatment with epinephrine and treatment with lipid plus epinephrine.[148]

The adult and experimental literature suggests that 1 mL/kg of 20% lipid emulsion should be administered over 1 minute and repeated every 3 to 5 minutes, up to a maximum of 3 mL/kg, followed by a maintenance infusion rate of 0.25 mL/kg per minute until the circulation is restored.[149,150] Several pediatric events report success with this intervention, with a range of doses similar to those reported in adults.[144,151,152] However, excess intralipid emulsion has been reported in a child; this reminds us to follow the infusion rate of intralipid carefully in children.[153] Although the dose of lipids in children remains speculative and has not been subject to controlled investigation, the adult guidelines are effective in children as well. There is a consensus that 20% lipid emulsions should be immediately available in any location where regional anesthesia is performed to permit rapid treatment of cardiac toxicity. Although propofol is compounded in a lipid emulsion, it is *not* recommended as a substitute for lipid emulsion to resuscitate patients with LAST because the intralipid in propofol formulation includes propofol, which is a myocardial depressant that may impair recovery.

Because the initial stage of cardiovascular toxicity consists of peripheral vasodilation, supportive treatment should include IV fluid loading (10–20 mL/kg of isotonic crystalloid) and, if necessary, titration of a peripheral vasoconstrictor, such as phenylephrine (initial rate of 0.1 µg/kg per minute), to maintain vascular tone and systemic blood pressure at acceptable limits. As toxicity progresses to cardiovascular collapse, profound decreases in myocardial contractility occur, followed by dysrhythmias. In dogs, echocardiography showed that decreased systolic function always preceded the development of dysrhythmias. Many toxic reactions are self-limited because the local anesthetic redistributes throughout the body and plasma concentrations rapidly decrease. All current data, however, strongly suggest that, in addition to the standard cardiopulmonary resuscitation algorithm, lipid infusion should be immediately administered as the next first line of therapy; see the end pages for a suggested treatment algorithm. To date, there are no reports of treatment failure when lipid emulsion was administered in a timely manner.

HYPERSENSITIVITY TO LOCAL ANESTHETICS

Hypersensitivity reactions to local anesthetics are rare.[154–156] Ester local anesthetics are metabolized to *p*-aminobenzoic acid, which is usually responsible for allergic reactions in this group. However, these agents may cause allergic phenomena in children who are sensitive to sulfonamides, sulfites, or thiazide diuretics.[157,158] Among the amide local anesthetics, only one case of a true allergic reaction has been documented. These drugs may contain the preservative, methylparaben, which can produce allergic reactions in those sensitive to *p*-aminobenzoic acid.[158,159] When in doubt, local anesthetic allergy must be ruled out. Detailed protocols are described elsewhere.[160]

Placement of Blocks in Patients Under General Anesthesia

Although concerns about the risks of neural injury in the unconscious patient have been raised in the adult literature, this is based entirely on individual case reports, and the standard of care in pediatric anesthesia has long been to administer most regional blocks to children who are anesthetized. The safety of this practice has now been confirmed by a large prospective study from the PRAN in an unselected cohort of more than 50,000 regional blocks in children.[161] This is the only prospective investigation of regional anesthesia complications in children under general anesthesia, and researchers detected no serious sequelae in any subject. Block placement in children under general anesthesia was deemed as safe as placement in the awake or sedated child, with postoperative neurologic symptoms occurring at a rate of 0.93/1000 (95% confidence interval [CI] 0.7–1.2) compared with 6.82/1000 (95% CI 4.2–10.5) in sedated and awake patients. The authors concluded that administering regional blocks to children under general anesthesia should be considered safe, remain the standard of care, and that prohibitive recommendations based on anecdotal or case reports were unsupported. These conclusions are further supported in a joint consensus statement by the ASRA and ESRA with level B2 evidence.[137]

Equipment

USE OF ULTRASOUND

Recently there has been great interest in the use of ultrasound-guided peripheral nerve blocks in children.[162] The availability of high-resolution portable ultrasound machines has become increasingly commonplace and has revolutionized the practice of regional anesthesia in children. Many argue that it is already the new standard of care for most peripheral nerve blocks.[19] Emerging evidence suggests ultrasound guidance increased success rates, reduced pain scores, prolonged block duration, and reduced time of block performance and the number of needle passes, particularly in younger children.[19] Although this practice requires sophisticated expensive equipment and the acquisition of new skills, it is likely to have an essential role in pediatric regional blockade because most blocks are performed while the child is anesthetized. The cost-effectiveness of acquiring these devices is justified because they serve a dual purpose for placing invasive central lines, peripheral and arterial catheters. Direct visualization of the nerve may facilitate correct placement of the local anesthetic and may also help reduce the total dose of local anesthetic needed for successful blockade. It is imperative to use an ultrasound machine that is capable of scanning superficially because most of the nerves in children are usually less than a few millimeters from the skin. A more in-depth discussion of ultrasound guidance for peripheral nerve blocks can be found in Chapter 43. Because ultrasound might still not be available to every practitioner, a complete discussion of landmark and nerve stimulator–guided peripheral blockade is included in this chapter.

USE OF A NERVE STIMULATOR

The use of a peripheral nerve stimulator is an alternative safe and effective method to locate the nerve to be blocked. Despite the increasing use of ultrasound to guide the placement of peripheral nerve blocks, some anesthesiologists still use nerve stimulation to verify the position of the tip of the needle when ultrasound is not available, or in combination with ultrasound, particularly when imaging is not available or suboptimal. A nerve stimulator is not a substitute for anatomic knowledge, but it is a useful adjunct that allows the performance of the block in an unconscious or uncooperative heavily sedated child. It avoids the need to seek sensory paresthesias or to rely purely on anatomic landmarks. The tiny amount of current flowing from the uninsulated needle tip stimulates the nerve and produces a motor response when the needle is in close proximity to the nerve. The nerve stimulator is attached to the child as shown in E-Fig. 42.2. The cathode (negative pole) cable is attached to the low-output terminal of the nerve stimulator at one end and to the proximal (uninsulated) shaft of a Teflon-insulated needle via a sterile alligator clip, or to the plug-in lead of a specially designed block needle at the other end (the child). The anode (positive lead) cable is attached to the high-output terminal of the stimulator at the one end and to the child, distant to the block site, via an ECG electrode at the other end.[163 164] The needle is advanced in the appropriate anatomic direction, and when it appears to be in the correct position, the nerve stimulator is adjusted to approximately 0.5 mA with repetitive single-pulse output at 1-second intervals. Local muscle contraction should be minimal at this setting, although direct muscle stimulation can occur and must be distinguished from neural stimulation. The area innervated by the nerves to be blocked is observed for the appropriate muscle contractions. As the uninsulated needle tip approaches the nerve, the muscle contractions will increase in intensity and become weaker as the needle tip moves away from the nerve. One should be able to decrease the current to approximately 0.2 mA with continued elicitation of easily perceptible muscle contraction to ensure that the needle tip is correctly positioned. It should be noted that the injection of even a very small volume of local anesthetic will ablate or dramatically attenuate responses produced by the low current of the nerve stimulator, so the needle position should be optimized before injection (Video 42.1). The responses to stimulation of the radial, median, ulnar, and musculocutaneous nerves are shown in Fig. 42.2.

An insulated epidural catheter may also be advanced cephalad to the abdominal and thorax levels while motor parathesias are stimulated using a low current to determine the dermatomal level of the tip of the catheter.[165,166]

Specific Procedures

CENTRAL NEURAXIAL BLOCKADE
Anatomic and Physiologic Considerations

Several anatomic and physiologic differences between adults and children affect the performance of regional anesthetic techniques. The conus medullaris (the terminus of the spinal cord) in neonates and infants is located at the L3 vertebral level, which is more caudal than in adults.[166a] It does not reach the adult level at L1 until approximately 1 year of age (Fig. 42.3) owing to the difference in the rates of growth between the spinal cord and the bony vertebral column. Thus lumbar puncture for subarachnoid block in neonates and infants should be performed at the L4-5 or L5-S1 interspace to avoid needle injury to the spinal cord. The vertebral laminae are poorly calcified at this age, so a midline approach is preferable to a paramedian one in which the needle is "walked off" the laminae. Another anatomic difference is noted in the sacrum. In neonates, the sacrum is narrower and flatter than in adults (see Fig. 42.3). The approach to the subarachnoid space from the caudal canal is much more direct in neonates than in adults, making dural puncture more likely, so the needle for a caudal block must not be advanced deeply in neonates.[167] The presence of a deep sacral dimple may be associated with spina bifida occulta, greatly increasing the probability of dural puncture. Thus a caudal block may be contraindicated in these children.

The distance from the skin to the subarachnoid space is quite small in neonates (~1.4 cm) and increases progressively with age (Fig. 42.4).[168] The ligamenta flava are much thinner and less dense in infants and children than in adults, which makes the engagement of the epidural needle more difficult to detect and unintended dural puncture during epidural catheter placement

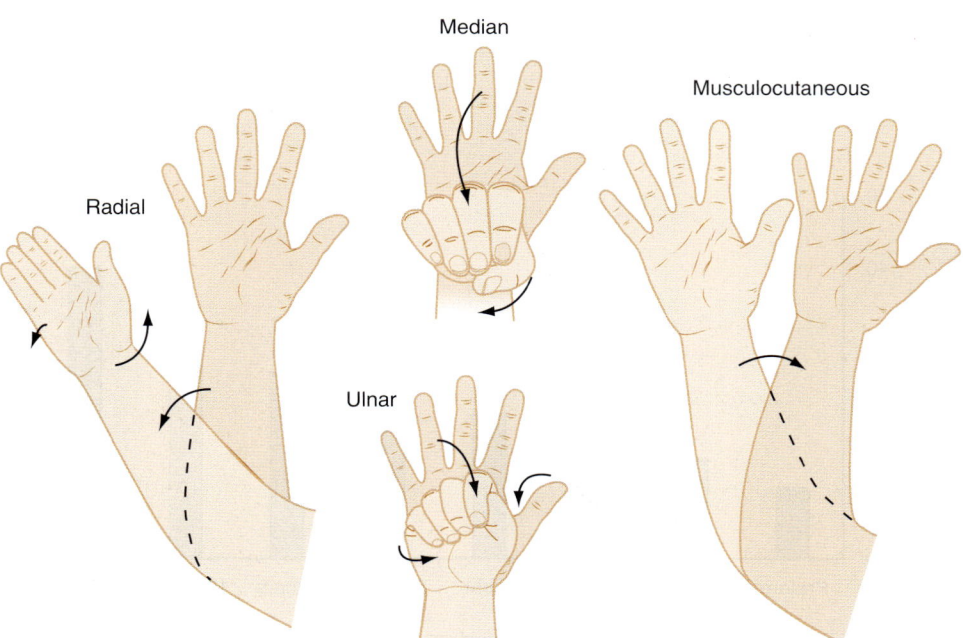

FIGURE 42.2 Characteristic movements of the fingers, wrist, and elbow in response to nerve stimulation of four specific nerves (Modified from Cousins MJ, Bridenbaugh PO, editors. *Neural Blockade in Clinical Anesthesia and Management of Pain.* 2nd ed. Philadelphia: JB Lippincott; 1988:406.)

a greater risk for the infrequent operator. Cerebrospinal fluid (CSF) volume as a percentage of body weight is greater in infants and young children than in adults (E-Fig. 42.3), although these studies are limited.[169-173] This finding may account in part for the comparatively larger doses of local anesthetics required for surgical anesthesia with subarachnoid block in neonates and young infants. The rate of turnover of CSF in infants and children is also greater than that in adults, accounting in part for the much

briefer duration of subarachnoid block with any given agent in the former. These anatomic differences necessitate meticulous attention to detail to achieve successful and uncomplicated spinal or epidural anesthesia.

In contrast to older children and adults, subarachnoid and epidural blockade in infants and small children is characterized by hemodynamic stability, even when the level of the block reaches the upper thoracic dermatomes.[174,175] Although heart rate variability, as determined by spectral analysis, is less, the heart rate is preserved, because the parasympathetic activity modulating the heart rate appears to be attenuated in infants who receive spinal anesthesia.[176] This attenuated vagal tone allows the heart rate to compensate for any changes in peripheral vascular tone, an effect that may be the most important factor in preserving hemodynamic stability compared with any other factor, such as the relatively small venous capacitance in the lower extremities in infants, and the relative lack of resting sympathetic peripheral vascular tone.[177] Very high levels of spinal anesthesia can cause significant bradycardia that may require treatment with vagolytics.[178] Nonetheless, data suggest that alterations in vascular resistance and blood flow to some vascular beds may occur, at least under certain conditions, in infants. In former preterm infants who received isobaric bupivacaine for subarachnoid block, cerebral blood flow decreased concomitant with changes in systemic blood pressure, although the conditions under which the baseline pressures were measured were not clear.[179] In a study in which changes in regional temperature were used as a surrogate sign of sympathetic activity, extremity but not truncal temperature increased during subarachnoid block, together with small insignificant changes in blood pressure.[180] In our clinical experience, and that of others including the University of Vermont neonatal spinal anesthesia database, clinically significant systemic blood pressure changes do not occur in young infants after a subarachnoid block.[178]

Central neuraxial blockade can affect the respiratory mechanics of the chest wall and diaphragm by diminution in intercostal muscle activity. This may be particularly relevant in infants and young children, whose chest walls are very compliant because the ribs are minimally ossified.[181] Infants rely more on excursions of the diaphragm to maintain tidal volume to a greater extent than

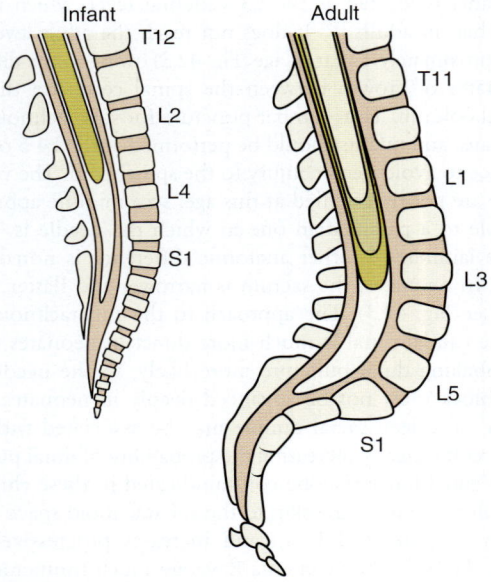

FIGURE 42.3 Anatomic differences between adults and children that affect the performance of spinal and epidural anesthesia; an infant's sacrum (*left*) is flatter and narrower than an adult's (*right*). Note that the tip of the spinal cord in a neonate ends at L3 and does not achieve the normal adult position (L1-2) until approximately 1 year of age. The relative location of the spinal cord with growth to adulthood is illustrated on the *right* as different shades of yellow, the darkest being neonates and the lightest being the final adult configuration.

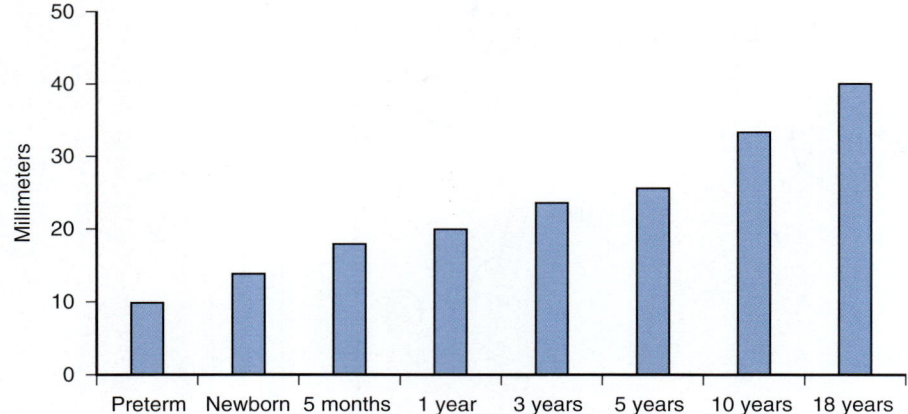

FIGURE 42.4 Distance from the skin to the subarachnoid space as a function of age. (Data from Bonadio WA, Smith DS, Metrou M, et al. Estimating lumbar puncture depth in children. *N Engl J Med.* 1988;319[14]:952–953; Kosaka Y, Sato K, Kawaguchi R. [Distance from the skin to the epidural space in children.] *Masui* 1974;23[9]:874–875 [in Japanese]; Lau HP. [The distance from the skin to the epidural space in a Chinese patient population.] *Ma Tsui Hsueh Tsa Chi* 1989;27:261–264.)

older children and adults. Paradoxical movement of the chest wall—that is, inward displacement of the rostral edge of the rib cage even in the absence of airway obstruction—occurs during inspiration in healthy infants during deep sleep. This paradoxical chest wall motion increases as the force of diaphragmatic excursion increases during rapid eye movement (REM) and deep sleep.[182] In a similar fashion, suppression of intercostal muscle activity leads to decreased rib cage contribution to ventilation in infants during spontaneous respiration under halothane anesthesia.[183] When respiratory inductance plethysmography was used to study rib cage and diaphragmatic contributions to breathing in seven former preterm infants who underwent spinal anesthesia for herniorrhaphy,[181] high thoracic (T2-4) levels of motor blockade were achieved, outward motion of the lower rib cage decreased, and paradoxical motion of the lower rib cage was noted in more than half of the infants. The diaphragmatic contribution to respiration, as estimated by abdominal displacement, was increased in all infants. This suggests a shift of respiratory workload from rib cage to diaphragm in compensation for the loss of the intercostal muscle contribution to breathing. Other factors, such as altered conformation of the diaphragm relative to the chest wall, with concomitant changes in the size of the zone of apposition (the portion of the anterior diaphragm that lies against the lower rib cage), may also contribute. These measurements were compared with each infant's measurements before administration of the spinal anesthetic, but it is not known if these findings would be different if measured in unanesthetized infants during deep sleep. It is likely that these effects are well tolerated and that the ability of the diaphragm to compensate for loss of the contribution of the rib cage to breathing is adequate in the vast majority of infants.

Upper abdominal and thoracic surgery causes changes in respiration in the postoperative period by neurally inhibiting diaphragmatic function.[184-186] The afferent pathways that induce this inhibition are presumed to arise from the chest and abdominal walls and perhaps the diaphragm itself, although they have not been conclusively identified.[187] Contrary to popular belief, pain itself is not a major contributor to postoperative respiratory dysfunction. Numerous studies have demonstrated that opioids administered either parenterally or in the central neuraxis exert limited impact on postoperative respiratory function.[188-190] Regional blockade, on the other hand, has been shown to improve several indexes of postoperative respiratory function.[17,185,191] These data suggest that regional anesthesia has an important role in attenuating diaphragmatic dysfunction postoperatively. Although the mechanism for this improvement has been attributed to blockade of the putative inhibitory neural pathways, other data suggest that alterations in respiratory mechanics, in particular an increase in the resting length of the diaphragm to its control value and a shift in the workload from the rib cage to the diaphragm, may have a greater role in this regard.[16] These data also suggest that the beneficial effects of regional anesthesia on postoperative respiratory function may, in part, be related to the degree of motor blockade. It is not known if the preoperative administration of regional blockade enhances respiratory function compared with postoperative application of the blockade, as has been postulated in "preemptive analgesia."

Spinal Anesthesia

Spinal anesthesia has been successfully performed in children since the first published reports from 1900 to 1910.[192-195] The observation of postanesthetic apnea in former preterm infants led to a resurgence in the use of spinal anesthesia in infants, particularly for herniorrhaphy in the latter 20th century.[196,197] Spinal anesthesia has even been administered for myelomeningocele repair[198] by direct injection of tetracaine into the sac and supplemented as needed by direct application of tetracaine by the surgeon. It has also been used with success for a variety of other surgical procedures performed on infants.[198-201]

It has been recognized since the early 1980s that preterm and former preterm infants are at significant risk for developing perioperative apnea after undergoing general anesthesia.[202-204] The reason for these postanesthetic apneas is not well understood. Spinal anesthesia has been proposed as an alternative to general anesthesia to reduce the incidence of perioperative apnea. However, when the spinal anesthetic was supplemented with ketamine, the incidence of postoperative apnea was even greater than with general anesthesia.[205] In addition to several retrospective reports, some prospective analyses of infants undergoing spinal anesthesia demonstrated fewer or no episodes of postanesthetic apnea compared with those undergoing general anesthesia.[197,205] Although most of these studies were confounded by the absence of preoperative and postoperative pneumograms to control for baseline apnea and bradycardia, a prospective investigation confirmed that neonates who received a subarachnoid block exhibited no changes in heart rate and oxygen saturation when preoperative and postoperative pneumograms were compared.[206] The infants in the general anesthesia group, however, experienced both reduced oxygen saturations and slower heart rates in the postoperative period than those in the spinal anesthesia group, changes that were more severe than those observed preoperatively. These events were not consistently associated with central apnea, defined as a cessation of respirations lasting more than 10 seconds with no demonstrable chest wall movement. These data suggest that the several case reports of apnea after subarachnoid block may have occurred even in the absence of the anesthesia and surgery, but one cannot entirely discount that they may have indeed been caused by the anesthetic or, perhaps, by the stress of surgery itself. Although the data from this study are persuasive, we remain cautious and have not modified the use of routine postoperative monitoring in these infants. The most recent prospective study of spinal versus general anesthesia included apnea as a secondary outcome variable and found that the frequency of early apnea (first 30 minutes after the end of anesthesia) was reduced, but not eliminated, after spinal anesthesia, although the frequency of late apneas (up to 12 hours) was similar in both groups.[207] However, these data should be interpreted with caution as they included infants who were not premature, the data were based on intermittently observed apneas rather than recorded monitored apneas (i.e., without postoperative pneumograms), and reported an overall frequency of apnea that was less than that reported in previous studies. Until studies with greater numbers of infants can distinguish which criteria would define a group with a reduced risk of apnea, all former preterm infants less than approximately 60 weeks postconceptional age should be managed similarly, regardless of the anesthetic technique.[208-211] We believe, however, that the best data available at this time suggest that regional anesthesia is preferred in former preterm infants for whom it would provide adequate operating conditions.

Epidural anesthesia has also been reported for lower extremity and abdominal surgery in former preterm infants. Continuous epidural anesthesia, and even continuous spinal anesthesia, for surgical procedures that outlast the duration of a "single-shot" subarachnoid block have also been reported and are alternative strategies that can achieve the same goals as single-injection subarachnoid block. The risk of LAST with a continuous caudal epidural blockade must be recognized; some have suggested that 2,3-chloroprocaine may be the most prudent agent in this situation.[212] For cardiac surgery, high spinal anesthesia with tetracaine (2.4 mg/kg) has been used for ligation of the patent ductus arteriosus. Because spinal anesthesia in infants is associated with hemodynamic stability, it has been advocated as an ideal anesthetic for cardiac catheterization in infants with congenital heart defects and has been used, in conjunction with a light general anesthetic, for cardiac surgery.[199,213–216] Those infants whose tracheas were not intubated before surgery were successfully extubated immediately after the operation. Hemodynamic stability was maintained without the use of inotropic agents in most children. A series of infants with gastroschisis closures, as well as open pyloromyotomies, have been reported using subarachnoid block.[201,213]

Concerns regarding the potential for adverse neurodevelopmental sequelae of general anesthetics administered to infants has led to additional interest in spinal anesthesia even in term infants. The most recent studies, including one large prospective, randomized controlled trial, show that for procedures lasting an hour or less there is no difference in neurodevelopmental outcome between spinal and general anesthesia (see Chapter 25).[217,218]

When an effective block[38,210,219–222] is achieved, most neonates will fall asleep as a result of *deafferentation*, a reduced level of consciousness because of diminished sensory input to the reticular activating system from the periphery, a mechanism confirmed in an animal model using spectral edge frequency analysis.[223] Sedation levels have been measured using bispectral index and spectral edge frequency analysis in infants undergoing spinal anesthesia without the use of adjunctive agents.[224] The investigators found a decrease in bispectral index, from 97 to 66.5 after 30 minutes, and in spectral edge frequency, from 26.1 to 9.9. These data indicate that sedation with dense regional blockade is a real physiologic phenomenon and can be used to the anesthesiologist's advantage during spinal anesthesia in infants. They also suggest that if sedation is administered to these infants, smaller doses than usual should be considered to avoid oversedation.

Technique

After routine monitors (ECG, blood pressure cuff, pulse oximeter, and precordial stethoscope) are affixed, the child is placed in a sitting or lateral decubitus position. For neonates and infants, care must be taken to avoid excessive flexion of the neck because this position may obstruct the airway (Fig. 42.5A).[225,226] The sitting position may aid in recognizing successful dural puncture increasing CSF hydrostatic pressure, which increases flow through the spinal needle. The skin is infiltrated with a minute quantity of 1% lidocaine (<0.2 mL is sufficient; the authors use a 30-gauge needle on an insulin syringe); alternatively, a small amount of EMLA or other transcutaneous local anesthetic cream is applied to the infant's lumbar area at least 1 hour before spinal placement. The lumbar puncture is performed using a midline approach with a 22-gauge or smaller, 1.5-inch styletted spinal needle (see Fig. 42.5B and C). We do not routinely use a 25-gauge spinal needle because of the time delay between entering the subarachnoid space and the appearance of CSF in the needle hub. This delay may make it difficult to recognize that the subarachnoid space has been entered. Whitacre, Sprotte, Marx, and other "pencil point" needles are available in pediatric sizes.[227,228] Lumbar puncture is performed only at the L4-5 or L5-S1 interspaces, for reasons previously described. The

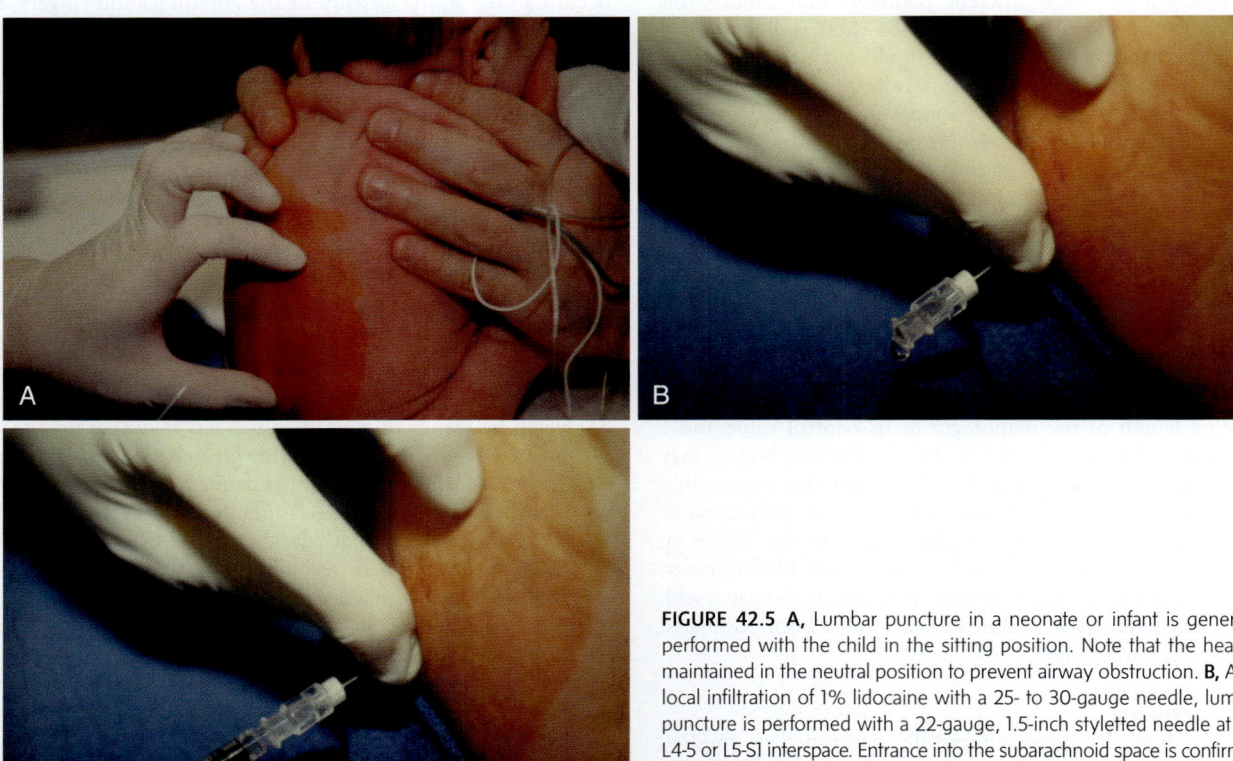

FIGURE 42.5 **A,** Lumbar puncture in a neonate or infant is generally performed with the child in the sitting position. Note that the head is maintained in the neutral position to prevent airway obstruction. **B,** After local infiltration of 1% lidocaine with a 25- to 30-gauge needle, lumbar puncture is performed with a 22-gauge, 1.5-inch styletted needle at the L4-5 or L5-S1 interspace. Entrance into the subarachnoid space is confirmed by free flow of cerebrospinal fluid. **C,** Local anesthetic is injected with a tuberculin syringe. Care must be taken not to inject rapidly or a high level of blockade might result.

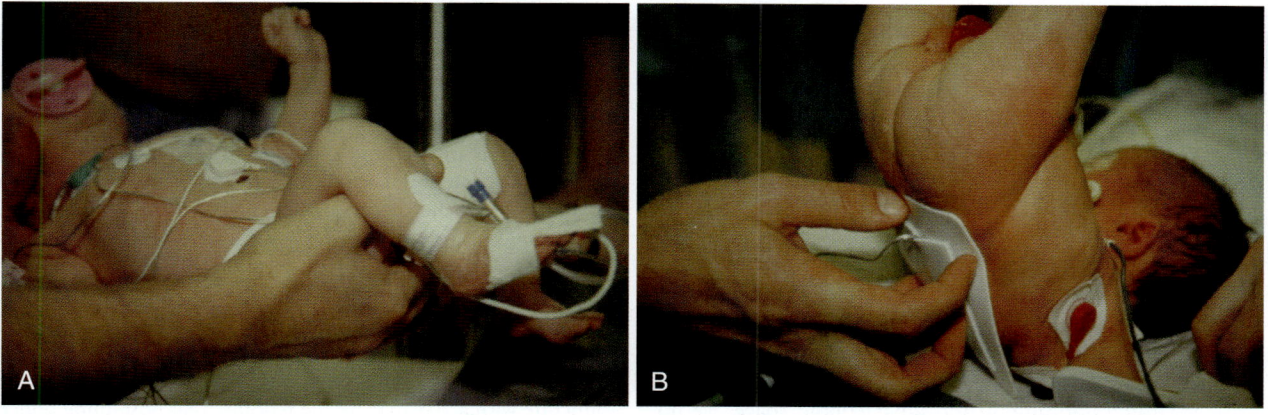

FIGURE 42.6 A, The proper method of applying an electrocautery pad; the infant's entire body is elevated while maintaining the horizontal position or the infant is log-rolled along its long axis to avoid excessively high spread of subarachnoid blockade. **B,** Improper method of applying an electrocautery pad in a neonate after subarachnoid administration of local anesthetic; the legs should never be elevated as this may lead to a high or total spinal block.

subarachnoid space in infants less than 60 weeks postconceptional age is approximately 1.5 cm from the skin (see Fig. 42.4); care must be taken not to pass the needle too deeply, passing beyond the subarachnoid space.[168] When the subarachnoid space is located, the local anesthetic is slowly administered. Immediately thereafter, the child is placed in the supine position. Once the block is in place, the child should remain completely horizontal to preclude cephalad spread of the local anesthetic. If the legs are raised soon after the block is placed, a "total" spinal anesthetic may occur (Fig. 42.6A and B).[229] The grounding pad is best applied by lifting the entire infant while maintaining the body in the horizontal plane or simply log-rolling the infant, or the pad can be affixed to the anterior thigh if sufficient space and muscle mass are available. *The legs should never be raised above the torso once the spinal block is in place as this may produce a high spinal block.*

Because spinal anesthesia maintains remarkable hemodynamic stability in infants, some pediatric anesthesiologists have advocated starting the IV line after the onset of lower extremity analgesia. Although this may be relatively safe in this setting, if a "total spinal" occurred and the airway had to be instrumented or resuscitation drugs had to be administered, having IV access before the spinal block would be important. In addition, should IV access prove difficult, valuable operating time and spinal block time would be lost while searching for a suitable vein. We have found that applying the pulse oximeter to a toe of one leg and the blood pressure cuff to the thigh of the other allows the neonate to remain undisturbed during the surgical procedure (e.g., inguinal herniorrhaphy) (E-Fig. 42.4).

Because the addition of sedatives has been associated with postanesthetic apnea with an incidence at least as great as that of general anesthesia, we try to avoid all sedatives, especially ketamine.[205] Most neonates will fall asleep once the block has set. A pacifier dipped in 50% dextrose will also help the infant to remain quiet and still. Gentle restraint is necessary in many cases, particularly during the most stimulating phase of the operation, when traction is applied to the hernia sac, and the peritoneum. It is particularly important for the infant to be still and not bear down when the hernia sac is dissected to avoid both tearing of the sac and extrusion of abdominal contents through the open hernia. Should the infant become agitated or unsettled at this point, one should administer inhalational anesthesia by mask until the stimulation abates, allowing the operation to proceed without difficulty.

Selection of Drug

NEONATES AND INFANTS. The proportional dose of local anesthetic required for subarachnoid block in neonates is much greater than that required for adults. When calculated on a per-kilogram basis, the drug requirement in neonates is 5- to 10-fold greater than that in adults to achieve a similar dermatomal distribution. In addition, the duration of the relatively larger dose lasts only about one-third to one-half as long as in the adult. This appears to be due in part to the greater volume of CSF per kilogram and to the more rapid turnover of CSF in neonates. The drugs that have commonly been used for spinal anesthesia in neonates and infants include tetracaine, bupivacaine, and lidocaine.[169,230-234] Hyperbaric bupivacaine (0.75 mg/kg of 0.75% bupivacaine in 8.25% dextrose), isobaric bupivacaine (0.5–1.0 mg/kg of a 0.5% solution), or hyperbaric tetracaine (0.75–1.0 mg/kg [equal volumes of tetracaine 1.0% and 10% dextrose]) with 0.01 mL/kg of epinephrine (1 : 100,000) is commonly used to achieve an adequate height and duration of blockade. Isobaric levobupivacaine (1 mg/kg of 0.5% levobupivacaine) has also been reported.[235] Isobaric and hyperbaric bupivacaine have a reported duration similar to that of tetracaine, although the duration of action of the isobaric solution is slightly greater than for the hyperbaric solution.[233,234,236] Epinephrine prolongs the duration of tetracaine blockade by more than 30%[237] but does not prolong bupivacaine blockade.[237] This can be best compounded by drawing a 1 : 1,000 epinephrine solution into a tuberculin or glass syringe and expelling the contents, leaving only a residual amount of epinephrine "wash" in the hub of the needle. These doses usually provide adequate analgesia for inguinal hernia repair with a duration of motor block of 70 to 90 minutes and a dermatome height in the mid to upper thoracic region. For surgeries of limited duration that involve a lower extremity, smaller doses (0.5–0.6 mg/kg) may be used. A dose-ranging study reported that the addition of clonidine (1 µg/kg) prolonged the duration of blockade from a mean of 67 minutes (plain bupivacaine) to 111 minutes.[238] The use of larger doses of clonidine (2 µg/kg), however, caused transient hypotension and apnea, which required treatment with caffeine. Although lidocaine (2 mg/kg) is useful for a block of brief duration,

TABLE 42.5	Local Anesthetics for Spinal Anesthesia in Neonates and Infants	
Anesthetic Drug	**Usual Dose (mg/kg)**	**Range (mg/kg)**
1% Tetracaine in 10% dextrose	0.75	0.75–1
0.5% Bupivacaine (isobaric)	0.8	0.5–1
0.75% Bupivacaine in 8.25% dextrose	0.75	0.5–1

such as for a muscle biopsy of the lower extremity, the duration of useful block is only approximately 30 minutes. In light of concerns regarding lidocaine in the subarachnoid space, we no longer recommend its use in infants.[239-241] A summary of doses for commonly used local anesthetics for subarachnoid block in neonates and infants is provided in Table 42.5.

CHILDREN. There is little information regarding the dose of local anesthetics for spinal anesthesia in children, as subarachnoid block is much less commonly used beyond infancy. When a regional technique is desirable in children, an epidural or caudal block together with a "light" general anesthetic is often preferred. For spinal anesthesia, 0.3 to 0.5 mg/kg of bupivacaine (5 mg/mL concentration) may be used in children 2 months to 12 years of age.[228] Doses of 0.3 to 0.4 mg/kg hyperbaric tetracaine have been used for subarachnoid block in children between 12 weeks and 2 years of age, and 0.2 to 0.3 mg/kg in children older than 2 years of age.[242-244] These limited data suggest that the dose requirement for spinal anesthesia decreases with increasing age. Because there are few data available on drug doses and the height of anesthetic block produced in this age group, it is prudent to use these values as an appropriate reference point and to revise the dose as determined by clinical experience.

Complications

Complications of spinal anesthesia include block failure, total spinal anesthesia, post–dural puncture headache, backache, neurologic sequelae, and the risk of lumbar epidermoid tumors if nonstyletted needles are used for subarachnoid puncture.[227-229,245-250,251]

Block failure is a risk with any regional anesthetic technique, although this is uncommon with spinal anesthesia in infants. The General Anesthesia Compared to Spinal Anesthesia Study (GAS) consortium reported that fewer than 10% of patients in that trial required conversion from spinal to general anesthesia, and just 6.8% required a brief period of sedation. The overall failure rate for spinal anesthesia, however, was approximately 19%.[207,211,235]

Total spinal anesthesia has been reported in neonates. It is most commonly manifested by apnea with no change in systemic blood pressure or heart rate, although should pronounced bradycardia occur, a reduction in cardiac output is likely and should be treated aggressively.[178,229,252] It can occur after a dose of as little as 0.6 mg/kg of tetracaine.[229] Alteration in position, particularly by raising the lower body above the level of the head or thorax, may be the most common cause of a high spinal block. Although the rate of administration of the local anesthetic does not appear to affect the level of spinal anesthesia in adults, similar studies have not been conducted in neonates or infants.[253] It is possible that factors, such as the use of a relatively large-bore needle (22-gauge) and a tuberculin syringe providing the means for injecting with high pressure, along with the small distance between vertebrae, combine to make the rate of injection an important consideration

in neonates and infants by producing unintended barbotage. We have observed this complication with rapid drug administration. Management consists of assisted or controlled ventilation until the return of spontaneous respiratory function.

The incidence of post–dural puncture headache appears to be infrequent in infants and children, although the incidence in preverbal children is unknown. An early study reported an incidence of spinal headache of approximately 2% using 20- to 22-gauge needles in children 2 to 17 years of age.[244] However, no details were provided about the distribution of headache with respect to age. Other studies reported a 5% incidence of headaches in children ranging from 2 months to nearly 10 years of age, but again, no age distribution was cited.[227,228] A prospective study of pediatric oncology patients undergoing diagnostic or therapeutic lumbar puncture with a 20-gauge needle reported that post–dural puncture headache was relatively rare in children younger than 13 years of age.[246] In most instances, the headaches were mild and resolved spontaneously. It is not entirely clear why young children should have a very low incidence of post–dural puncture headache. Several possible reasons include reduced CSF pressure,[247] the increased rate of CSF production, and hormonal changes with age.[246] As more pediatric regional anesthesia equipment becomes readily available, we expect that the use of pencil point (e.g., Whitacre, Marx, or Sprotte) needles will become more commonplace and will further reduce this already low incidence of headache.

Backache is a frequent postoperative complaint after both general and regional anesthesia in adults. It is thought to occur because of flattening of the normal lordotic lumbar curve secondary to muscle and ligament relaxation that occurs with spinal anesthesia. The incidence in children is unknown. Neurologic sequelae after spinal anesthesia are exceedingly rare. There are no reports in the literature of permanent neurologic injury caused by subarachnoid block, but good data in children are lacking. There have been no cases detected in more than 1700 consecutive spinal anesthetics at the University of Vermont Medical Center, in another large series from Schneider Children's Medical Center (Petah Tikva, Israel), or in the PRAN database.[11,126,252]

Epidural Anesthesia

Epidural anesthesia administered by the caudal, lumbar, or thoracic route can be used for the same types of surgical procedures and indications as spinal anesthesia. The most common indication, however, is for augmentation of general anesthesia and for postoperative pain management. The details of postoperative epidural infusions are discussed in Chapter 44.

Caudal Epidural Anesthesia

Caudal epidural anesthesia is the regional technique used with the greatest frequency in children, although this may decline as familiarity with lumbar and thoracic epidural techniques and peripheral nerve blocks increases. Although epidural use was first described in 1933,[254] it was not until the early 1960s that caudal anesthesia gained any degree of popularity.[254-269] Improvements in catheter material, the availability of pediatric-sized needles and catheters, and the growing recognition of the benefits of regional analgesia in general have increased the interest in this technique for children. Caudal anesthesia has a well-deserved reputation for safety in children. In a prospectively collected cohort of more than 18,000 children, the PRAN investigators detected no sequelae after caudal blockade.[270]

TECHNIQUE. The child is placed either in the lateral decubitus or prone position with a small roll beneath the anterior iliac crests.

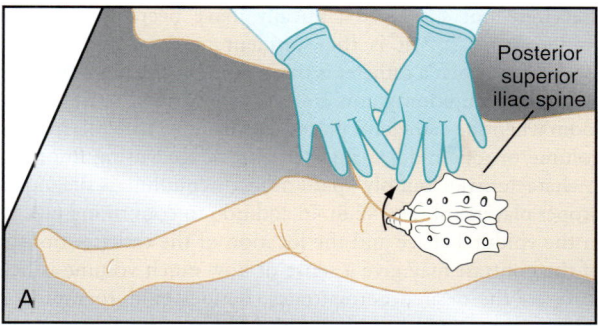

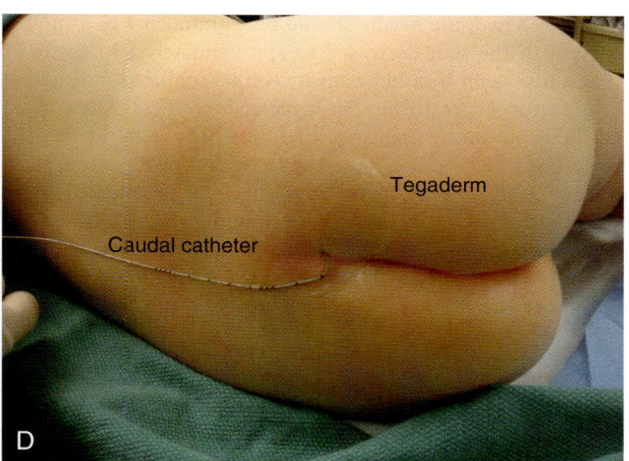

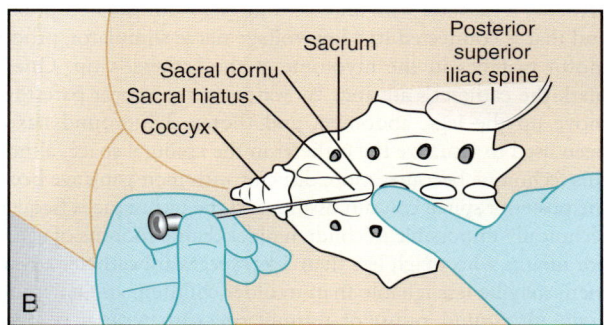

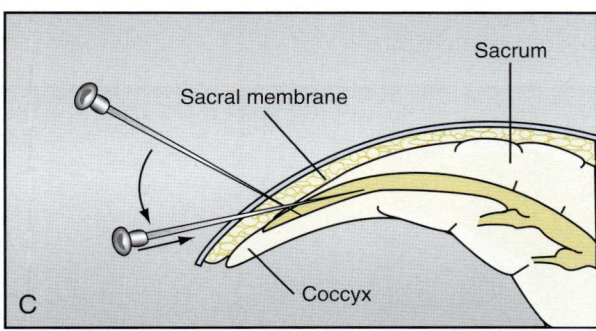

FIGURE 42.7 Performing a caudal block. **A,** The child is placed in a lateral decubitus position. **B,** The posterior superior iliac spines are located and the sacral cornu is palpated; an intravenous needle, an intravenous catheter, or a Crawford needle of appropriate size is advanced at an angle of approximately 45 degrees until a distinct "pop" is felt as the needle pierces the sacrococcygeal ligament. **C,** The angle of the needle with the skin is reduced parallel to the sacrum, and the needle or intravenous catheter is advanced into the caudal canal. **D,** If a continuous technique is used, the caudal catheter is advanced to the mid level of the surgical incision (it usually readily passes in children younger than 5 years of age) and the introducing needle or catheter is withdrawn. The catheter is secured with benzoin and an occlusive dressing.

The cornua of the sacral hiatus are most easily palpated as two bony ridges, about 0.5 to 1.0 cm apart, when the examiner moves his or her finger in a medial to lateral direction (Fig. 42.7A). When the sacral cornua are not prominent or easily appreciated, it may prove easier to locate the space by palpating the L4-5 intervertebral space in the midline and then palpate moving caudally until the sacral hiatus is reached. Because the space between the sacrum and coccyx may be mistaken for the sacral hiatus, the latter technique may make identification of the landmarks easier. The proper location is often, but not always, located just at the beginning of the crease of the buttocks. A short-bevel styletted needle, 22-gauge, should be used because a long-bevel needle may increase the risk of intravascular injection.[271] Some practitioners think that a styletted needle avoids the possibility of introducing a dermal plug into the caudal space, whereas others think that if the skin and subcutaneous

tissues are punctured with an 18-gauge needle, an IV catheter can be inserted without entraining a dermal plug and transferring it to the subarachnoid space. Still others suggest that if an IV catheter is used, it should be inserted with the bevel facing down because once in place, easy advancement of the IV catheter off the needle suggests that the caudal canal has been entered and may reduce the risk of intravascular placement. Although smooth and easy advancement of the cannula off the stylet is not a completely reliable sign that placement is correct, difficulty in doing so, or buckling of the catheter, is virtually always a sign that the needle has penetrated bone or another extraspinal structure. The needle is initially directed cephalad at a 45- to 75-degree angle to the skin until it "pops" through the sacrococcygeal ligament (see Fig. 42.7B) into the caudal canal, which is contiguous with the epidural space. If bone is encountered before the sacrococcygeal ligament is reached, the needle should be withdrawn 1 to 2 mm, the angle with the skin decreased to approximately 30 degrees, and the needle again should be advanced in a cephalad direction until the sacrococcygeal ligament is pierced (see Fig. 42.7C). As the needle is advanced slightly farther, bone (the anterior table of the sacrum) may be encountered. Orientation of the needle should be altered slightly before it is advanced, parallel to the plane of the child's back. The needle should then be advanced into the caudal-epidural space with the needle advanced only a few millimeters. Advancing the needle any farther should not be attempted because the dural sac lies relatively caudad in infants and may be entered a very short distance from the ligament (Video 42.2).[167,272]

Once it is confirmed that neither blood nor CSF has been aspirated, a test dose of local anesthetic is administered. If neither ECG changes during inhalational anesthesia nor blood pressure changes during TIVA are evident after the test dose, the remainder of the dose of local anesthetic should be slowly injected in an incremental fashion over 1 to 2 minutes while observing the ECG for peaked T waves and changes in heart rate and/or blood pressure. We strongly recommend the use of a test dose, even with single-shot caudal anesthesia. In addition to the risk of intravascular injection, it is also possible that the needle could be misplaced in the intramedullary cavity of the sacrum. Intraosseous injection of drugs results in very rapid uptake, similar to direct IV injection. The authors are aware of at least one case of circulatory collapse that occurred from this complication when a test dose was not used.

The block may be placed before the onset of surgery without a significant decrement in duration of postoperative analgesia for short surgical procedures.[273] This has the advantage of reducing the amount of general anesthesia needed, resulting in a more rapid recovery. In addition, there is adequate time for the block to "set up," improving the chances of a pain-free awakening.

Inserting a catheter for a continuous caudal block follows a similar procedure (Video 42.3). First, one should determine the length of catheter that should be inserted into the caudal space by measuring the distance from the sacral hiatus to the desired site where the catheter tip will be positioned. Instead of a small-gauge needle or catheter, an 18-gauge IV catheter[274] or an 18-gauge Crawford needle is used to enter the epidural space (see Fig. 42.7D). Because the internal diameters of different IV cannulae vary, it is advisable to test that the epidural catheter easily passes through the IV cannula before puncturing the sacrococcygeal membrane. Once the epidural space has been accessed, the IV catheter and needle are advanced several millimeters. The catheter is then advanced off the needle several millimeters. Localization of the IV catheter tip in the epidural space is confirmed by lack of resistance to the injection of a small volume of saline solution and the absence of CSF or blood. During injection, the area of the back overlying the IV catheter tip should be palpated; swelling or a fullness on injection of local anesthetic indicates a subcutaneous (SC) rather than an epidural catheter placement. It is also possible to use ultrasound to confirm the injection and cannula in the epidural space.[275] The epidural catheter is advanced through the IV catheter and the IV catheter is withdrawn. After confirming the presence of neither blood nor CSF, a test dose of local anesthetic containing 1:200,000 epinephrine may be administered (see earlier). Test doses should be repeated each time a catheter is reinjected with a bolus dose of local anesthetic.

For those younger than 5 years of age, the catheter can often be advanced to any level desired without exiting a dural sleeve or becoming tangled or knotted, although catheter misplacements

that were not suspected clinically, have been identified using epidurograms.[38,276] It is thus prudent to use some method of localization when a catheter is threaded cephalad more than several centimeters. Epidurograms are easily performed in the operating room when the catheter is placed. A small (0.5 to 2 mL maximum) volume of iopamidol is injected and imaged using fluoroscopy. A characteristic "bubbly" pattern in the midline is diagnostic of proper placement (Fig. 42.8). In addition to confirming placement in the epidural space and the location of the catheter tip, spread of the contrast may give a sense of how much volume is needed to cover the desired dermatomes. Besides epidurography, there are two other useful localizing techniques. The Tsui stimulating catheter, a catheter with an electrode at its uninsulated proximal end that is connected to a low voltage nerve stimulator, produces motor twitches in the myotome at the catheter's tip. One can mark the catheter's advance by watching the motor paresthesias move up the legs, abdomen, and thorax. Ultrasound has also been used to visualize the catheter in the epidural space, although this technique becomes more difficult with increasing age because the posterior spinal column ossifies and the technique is frequently technically impossible in children older than 6 months of age.[277,278] For infants who weigh less than 5 kg, successful catheter advancement may be less reliable than in older children, and an epidurogram, ultrasound, or use of a stimulating catheter may be needed to confirm proper placement of the catheter tip if the catheter is

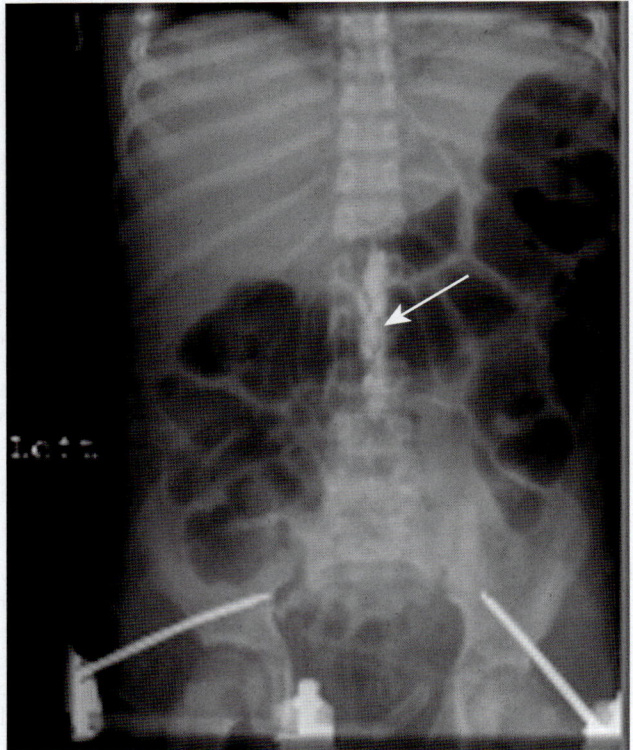

FIGURE 42.8 Epidurogram, performed with 0.5 to 2 mL (maximum) of iopamidol nonionic contrast agent, demonstrating the "bubbly" appearance of contrast in the epidural space (*arrow*). Note the central localization of contrast within the borders bounded by the vertebral bodies. On occasion, contrast may be seen only on one side of the epidural space, with a sharp line of demarcation in the midline. This usually results in unilateral blockade, and is theorized to result from septation or some other impediment to bilateral spread of anesthetic within the epidural space.

not radiopaque.[279] An epidurogram can be useful in any situation in which the catheter is threaded or when there is concern for proper catheter position, although the routine use of an epidurogram is not standard practice. We usually strive to place the catheter tip at a level near or at the midpoint of the dermatomes encompassing the surgical incision. This position allows a more specific site of administration for both intraoperative anesthesia and continuous infusions for postoperative pain management, with the attendant advantage of being able to use reduced doses of medication. If the catheter does not pass easily to the desired level, it should be withdrawn several millimeters and a localizing technique used to ascertain its location. The catheter should never be forced or advanced against resistance. It is thus prudent to use some method of localization when a catheter is threaded cephalad more than several centimeters.

Because caudal catheters are at increased risk of contamination from fecal soiling in children who are not yet continent of stool, meticulous attention to the dressing is necessary. Our practice is to use Mastisol (Ferndale Pharma Group, Ferndale, MI) or tincture of benzoin to secure the catheter with several layers of an adherent clear dressing, such as Tegaderm (3M, St. Paul, MN) or OpSite (Smith & Nephew, Andover, MA), to affix the dressing in the crease of the buttocks (Video 42.4). This transparent dressing permits the observation of the insertion site, which is the most likely source of infection (see later). A piece of single adhesive-edged plastic drape (e.g., Steri-Drape 1010; 3M, St. Paul, MN) can be affixed just caudad to the lower edge of the dressing in a similar manner; this helps prevent direct soiling of the dressing. If there is any question of contamination, the catheter should be promptly removed.

In an observational study of 307 neonates with caudal or epidural catheters, 2.9% of infants had a catheter contamination requiring premature removal, which contributed to an overall complication rate of 13.3% (95% CI 9.8%–17.4%). Catheter malfunction was the primary complication (4.8%).[280]

Lumbar and Thoracic Epidural Anesthesia

It may be preferable to place epidural catheters at a lumbar or thoracic interspace when the area of operation is innervated by higher dermatomes. Advantages include less risk of contamination by stool and urine, closer proximity to the desired tip location, and smaller volume of drug required for a more cephalad dermatomal level (if the caudal catheter is not threaded cephalad). Both lumbar and thoracic epidural catheters may be safely placed in anesthetized infants and children by experienced anesthesiologists.[281]

The technique for both lumbar and thoracic epidural catheter placement is similar to that in adults, with several important differences (see Chapter 43 for ultrasound techniques). The midline approach is most commonly used, for the same reasons cited earlier regarding subarachnoid block. The ligamenta flava are considerably thinner and less dense in infants than in older children and adults. This makes recognition of engagement in a ligament more difficult and requires both extra care and slower, more deliberate passage of the needle to avoid subarachnoid puncture. It takes experience to perceive the more subtle differences in "feel" that are characteristic of the tissue planes in small children. The angle of approach to the epidural space is slightly more perpendicular to the plane of the back than in older children and adults, owing to the orientation of the spinous processes in infants and small children. The loss-of-resistance technique should be used with saline solution, not air. There are several reports of venous air embolism in infants and children when air was used to test

for loss-of-resistance.[282–284] Another method used to identify the epidural space is to attach an IV infusion chamber with a minidrip or other free-flowing fluid delivery device to the epidural needle; commencement of dripping identifies entry into the epidural space.[285–287] We use a short (5-cm) 18-gauge Tuohy needle and a 20- or 21-gauge catheter in infants and children. The shorter length offers much better control than an adult-length (9- to 10-cm) needle. These catheters have fewer problems than the 24-gauge catheters, which in our experience are prone to kinking under the skin, resulting in very high resistance to injecting the solution. Epidural kits specifically for infants and children are available, but aside from the substitution of a shorter needle, they are identical to the adult sets.

SELECTION OF DRUG. The drug dose required for epidural blockade to reach a given dermatomal level depends on the volume (not the concentration) of the local anesthetic and the volume and capacitance of the epidural space, which changes with age. The greater the volume of local anesthetic, the higher the level of block achieved. In two studies, the height of the block achieved when local anesthetic was administered caudal epidurally varied inversely with age using ultrasound to detect the spread; for example, the maximum spinal level of local anesthetic in infants younger than 1 year of age was one to two levels more cephalad than in those older than 1 year.[275,288] This effect of age on the spread of local anesthetic however has been disputed.[288,289] Numerous studies investigated the doses of local anesthetic drugs used for caudal anesthesia in children.[a] The volumes of local anesthetic reported to block from a T4 to a T10 dermatome level span a fivefold range. In our experience, the volume of local anesthetic required is 0.05 mL/kg per dermatome to be blocked.[261]

Thus in a 10-kg child in whom we wish to produce a T10 dermatome level, we would use a volume of (0.05 mL/kg per dermatome) × (10 kg) × (12 dermatomes) = 6 mL.

Another simple method is to administer 1 mL/kg (up to 20 mL) of local anesthetic (usually 0.125% bupivacaine with 1:200,000 epinephrine). This generally provides a sensory block with minimal motor block up to the T4-6 level; this volume limits the potential for toxicity for children older than 6 months of age and is on the border for younger infants. If repeated doses are anticipated, or in infants younger than 6 months of age, it is prudent to reduce the concentration or volume to avoid the risk of accumulation.

A third simple regimen for a caudal block used in the United Kingdom and Australasia is that of Armitage[268]: 0.5 mL/kg for lumbosacral, 1 mL/kg thoracolumbar, and 1.25 mL/kg mid thoracic. If the total volume is less than 20 mL, then use bupivacaine 0.25%. If the volume exceeds 20 mL, then use bupivacaine 0.19%.

Because the level of the block depends on the volume of drug administered, the concentration of the local anesthetic should be based on the desired density of the block (less dense for postoperative analgesia, more dense for intraoperative anesthesia) and on the risk of toxicity.

Continuous Epidural Infusions

Although intermittent doses of local anesthetic are often used to maintain epidural anesthesia during a prolonged surgical procedure, it is also common practice to initiate continuous infusions of local anesthetics during surgery. Continuous infusions maintain the block at a constant level, assuming that the infusion rate is appropriate. This obviates the need for repetitive test dosing.

---

[a]References 254, 256–258, 260, 261, 263–269, 288, and 289.

Theoretically, fewer entries into the epidural catheter may reduce the risk of infection and the risk of accidental administration of the wrong drug. Strict attention to the total drug administered per hour (i.e., the drug concentration and infusion rate) is required to preclude potentially toxic drug doses. We recommend that the same dosing guidelines for postoperative infusion rates be followed intraoperatively: *a maximum of 0.4 mg/kg per hour of bupivacaine after the initial block is established, with this dose reduced by approximately 30% for infants younger than 6 months of age.*[44] The concentration of local anesthetic solution depends on the age of the child, the surgical procedure, and the extent of the area that needs to be blocked. When a denser block is required in a small infant, it may be beneficial to use 2,3-chloroprocaine because its action is terminated by ester hydrolysis and has a minimal risk of accumulation compared with amide local anesthetics. A denser block with a more concentrated solution may then be achieved. The amides ropivacaine and levobupivacaine, because they are levorotary enantiomers and carry reduced risks of toxicity, may also successfully address these issues and allow the administration of more concentrated agents to produce denser blockade with less potential for adverse effects (see Chapters 43 and 44). In a study of children 1 to 9 years of age, infusion rates of up to 0.4 mg/kg per hour of ropivacaine that followed a 2-mg/kg bolus were found to result in stable levels of unbound ropivacaine in plasma, all well below the toxic threshold; clearance did not differ with age.[290]

Epidural Opioids

Epidural opioids can be safely used to augment intraoperative anesthesia in children, as well as to provide postoperative analgesia. Their use is discussed in detail in Chapter 44. If extubation of the trachea is expected at the end of the surgical procedure, one must account for both the systemic and the central neuraxial opioid doses to avoid excessive respiratory depression.

Adjunctive Drugs

Numerous agents have been injected into the epidural space in attempts to prolong analgesia, to improve the quality of analgesia while reducing the dose of opioid and local anesthetic, or to replace the local anesthetic or opioid with a drug that may have fewer adverse effects. It is concerning, however, that several of these agents have neither undergone exhaustive neurotoxicity testing nor are prepared or labeled for neuraxial use.[291] In the United States, the only adjunctive drug accepted for epidural administration is clonidine, an α_2-adrenoceptor agonist. The effect of clonidine to prolong the duration of epidural analgesia remains controversial in the literature. Several studies, including a meta-analysis, reported clonidine prolonged the duration of analgesia by 2 hours, as measured by the time to first supplemental analgesic requirement.[291–295] Other investigators found no significant increase in the duration of analgesia, including one double-blind, randomized trial.[296,297] In neonates, neuraxial clonidine at doses of 2 μg/kg or greater has been associated with apnea. Increased sedation has been reported after epidural clonidine in older infants and children at the same doses. We recommend a dose of 1 μg/kg, especially in ambulatory patients.

Complications

Complications after epidural anesthesia or analgesia include cardiac arrest from an intravascular or intraosseous injection, hematoma, neural injury, and infection. E-Fig. 42.5 illustrates sites of unintended needle placement during the performance of a caudal epidural block. Injection of local anesthetic into an epidural blood vessel or intraosseous injection into the marrow cavity may result in a rapid increase in the blood concentration of the local anesthetic and a toxic reaction as discussed previously. It is also possible to pass the needle through the sacrum and perforate bowel or the pelvic organs, particularly in infants in whom ossification of the sacrum is incomplete.

There are now several large-scale prospective audits that examined both the incidence and the nature of complications in regional anesthetics in children. The prospective audit from the United Kingdom and Ireland is the largest and most carefully described study on complications of epidural anesthesia in pediatrics to date.[298] A total of 10,633 cases were accrued over a period of 5 years, and all complications were reviewed and categorized by severity and type. Only five complications were graded as serious, and of these only one, the result of a drug error, had lasting sequelae. The French-Language Society of Pediatric Anesthesiologists (ADARPEF) published a follow-up prospective study on regional anesthetics in children in which they reported on 10,098 epidural blocks without a single child sustaining permanent sequelae.[75] The PRAN consortium in the United States reported data from their first prospective cohort in which 9073 epidural and caudal blocks were accrued: 6127 single-injection (mostly caudal) and 2946 continuous caudal or epidural anesthesias.[11] In this study there were no complications of any kind that lasted more than 3 months. The most common complication was catheter displacement or malfunction in the postoperative period in continuous blocks. Caudal safety was further supported in a subsequent PRAN analysis of 18,650 single-injection caudal epidurals, which detected an overall incidence of complications of 1.9% (95% CI 1.7%–2.1%) and no instances of temporary or permanent sequelae, calculated as 0.005% (95% CI 0% to 0.03%).[270]

Infection is of grave concern when it occurs in either the subarachnoid or the epidural space.[299] A study of 1620 children over a 6-year period reported a zero frequency of epidural abscess.[300] Catheters remained in situ for a mean of 2 days (maximum 8 days). The adult literature also suggests that infection is an uncommon complication.[301,302] However, both superficial and deep abscesses may rarely occur, particularly in those children with immunodeficiency syndromes or cancer who are receiving long-term infusions.[303] Epidural abscess and meningitis are the most potentially serious complications.[299,304] The development of an epidural abscess is a surgical emergency, because failure to treat it can lead to a permanent neurologic injury. The signs and symptoms (Table 42.6) are the same as those for epidural hematomas, although fever, increased erythrocyte sedimentation rate, and increased leukocyte count with a leftward shift are also often present. Surgical drainage may be necessary. In a British audit, three serious infections (two epidural abscesses and one case of meningitis) were noted. These infections were all related to infections at the insertion site. All cultures grew *Staphylococcus aureus*. Twenty-five local infections were reported, mostly *S. aureus*, and 80% were associated with catheters left in place more than 48 hours. Of note is that some localized infections that developed at the catheter insertion site only became apparent several days after the catheter had been removed (see Fig. 44.9). Similar findings were reported in the PRAN data. In the British study, one case progressed to an epidural abscess. Whether these infections developed while the catheter was in place, leaving bacteria to track through the open site in the skin after the catheter was removed, or by hematologic spread is unknown, although the former etiology is most frequently cited. Infants and toddlers who are in diapers require meticulous management of these catheters and their insertion site. A mild erythema occasionally occurs at the site of catheter insertion when children have indwelling catheters in place for several days, and this must be distinguished from a cellulitis (see Fig. 44.9). In most cases these superficial infections resolve with removal of the catheter and local care. On occasion, these superficial infections may require treatment with a systemic antibiotic. If there is any question that the site is infected, the catheter should be removed. Although no serious systemic infection occurred in a prospective study of 210 children with 170 caudal catheters (age 3 ± 1 years) and 40 lumbar epidural catheters (age 11 ± 3 years) that were in place for 3 ± 1 days, 35% were colonized with bacteria.[305] This rate of colonization was similar with both caudal (25%) and lumbar epidural (23%) approaches. These results suggest that colonization

is not synonymous with infection and that caudal catheters are not necessarily associated with greater infectious risk than lumbar epidural catheters. The factors that transform colonization into infection remain unknown.

It is common to have epidural fluid leak from the insertion site in caudal epidural catheters, especially in the presence of presacral edema. If an indwelling caudal epidural catheter is in place when a child develops a fever of unknown origin, the catheter should be removed because it may be causing the infection or become seeded by the infection (see Chapter 44).

Epidural hematoma is also a rare complication after epidural blockade. Optimal outcome depends on rapid diagnosis and prompt treatment and decompression. Signs and symptoms are presented in Table 42.6. The presence of clinically important coagulopathy or thrombocytopenia is an unacceptable risk for developing an epidural hematoma and is a contraindication to central neuraxial blockade. Guidelines for the conduct of neural blockade in the anticoagulated patient have been published by the ASRA.[306] Of particular note is that there is a difference in the management of the patient who is receiving conventional (unfractionated) heparin and low–molecular-weight heparins, such as enoxaparin. Guidelines for the management of patients who are anticoagulated are shown in Table 42.7.[306]

Postoperatively, *urinary retention* has been associated with the presence of both epidural and spinal anesthesia. In this regard, it is important to distinguish between the effects of local anesthetics and central neuraxial opioids in the blocks. There is no evidence that regional anesthesia with local anesthesia causes urinary retention, and, indeed, there are data to the contrary. In a prospective study of infants and children undergoing inguinal herniorrhaphy or orchiopexy, caudal blockade, ilioinguinal-iliohypogastric nerve block by the surgeon, or a control consisting of caudal injection of 1:200,000 epinephrine (no local anesthetic) yielded similar times to voiding postoperatively.[307] In a retrospective study of 326 children undergoing inguinal herniorrhaphy and urologic surgery, 237 received a caudal block and 66 received local anesthesia by the surgeon. The incidence of urinary retention was similar for the two groups, with the type of surgery being the primary determinant of urinary retention.[308]

TABLE 42.6 Signs and Symptoms of Epidural Hematoma and Abscess

Abscess	Hematoma
Fever	Afebrile
± Increased WBC	WBC normal
± Increased sedimentation rate	Sedimentation rate normal or slightly increased
± Left WBC shift	
Localized back pain	Localized back pain
Radicular pain	Radicular pain
Paraplegia	Paraplegia
Sensory loss	Sensory loss
Urinary and fecal retention	Urinary and fecal retention
Incontinence	Incontinence
Local tenderness	Local tenderness
Defect on myelography	Defect on myelography
Localized lesion on magnetic resonance imaging	Localized lesion on magnetic resonance imaging

WBC, white blood cell count.

TABLE 42.7 Guidelines for the Use of Regional Anesthesia in the Anticoagulated Patient

Drug (Generic)	Common Trade Names	Interval for Catheter Placement After Last Dose	Interval for Catheter Removal After Most Recent Dose	Time Interval to Restart Anticoagulant After Catheter Is Removed
Enoxaparin[a] (therapeutic)	Lovenox (>60 mg daily or 1 mg/kg bid or 1.5 mg/kg daily)	24 hours	Catheter should be removed before first dose. If med given, wait >24 hours	2–4 hours after catheter removed
Enoxaparin[a] (prophylactic)	Lovenox (≤60 mg per day)	12 hours	12 hours	2–4 hours
Heparin SC bid	Heparin	No significant risk at dose of 5000 units bid		
Heparin SC tid	Heparin	Unknown risk at 5000 units tid: suggest check PTT. 10,000 units tid: check PTT		
Heparin IV	Heparin	2–4 hours, PTT < 35 seconds	2–4 hours, PTT < 35 seconds	2 hours
NSAID, ASA	Celebrex, Motrin, Naprosyn, and so on	No significant risk		
Streptokinase	Streptase	10 days	10 days	Uncertain; at least 24 hours
Warfarin	Coumadin	3–5 days, INR ≤ 1.5	If >24 hours, check INR ≤ 1.5	Same day

[a]Note for low–molecular-weight heparin: Prophylactic dosing may be started 6 to 8 hours postoperatively. Therapeutic dosing or bid dosing should be started at least 24 hours postoperatively. Epidural catheters should be removed before initiation of therapy.
ASA, acetylsalicylic acid; *INR*, international normalized ratio; *IV*, intravenous; *NSAID*, nonsteroidal antiinflammatory drug; *PTT*, partial thromboplastin; *SC*, subcutaneous.
Modified from the guidelines of the Massachusetts General Hospital Department of Anesthesia, Critical Care and Pain Medicine, 2011.

The epidural and subarachnoid use of opioids, however, is associated with an increased incidence of urinary retention. Epidural morphine in a dose of 70 µg/kg (a dose that would now be considered excessive) was associated with a 50% incidence of urinary retention[309]; 70% of those with urinary retention required treatment. Another study reported an incidence of urinary retention of 27% after caudally administered morphine, 33 to 100 µg/kg, although most of the children had urinary catheters.[310] Finally, 50 µg/kg diacetylmorphine was associated with an 11% incidence of urinary retention.[311] A dose of 33 µg/kg epidural morphine is the most common recommended in current practice.

Data from the large prospective databases indicate that the incidence of *neural injury* after epidural blockade is very small and that long-term neurologic sequelae of neuraxial blockade is rare. One must slightly temper these conclusions, however, based on the limited follow-up of children in these studies who did not have problems reported within the immediate time frame of the block. A prospective study of more than 2500 infants and children who received epidural blocks demonstrated no evidence of neurologic complications, although a retrospective review of the first ADARPEF data determined that 1 in 5000 infants younger than 3 months of age had neurologic complications with magnetic resonance imaging evidence of spinal cord ischemia.[106,312] In four of the five cases reported in that study, the epidural space was identified using loss-of-resistance to air (in the fifth case, the technique was not specified) and the authors concluded that the etiology of the neurologic injury was an air embolus. Based on these data, the use of air for loss of resistance in infants and children has been strongly discouraged, using saline solution instead. However, this reasoning has been questioned. The use of loss of resistance to saline solution with an air bubble has been advocated by some experts.[137] In the follow-up ADARPEF study there were no cases of neurologic injury.[75] The British epidural audit found 6 cases of neural injury in 10,633 (1 : 1770) children in that prospective study. Of particular note was the delay in recognition of the injury, as no cases were discovered before 2 days had elapsed from the time the block was placed, and some diagnoses were not made for 10 days after the block. All children had complete resolution of their symptoms within 1 year. Two children were referred to a chronic pain service and treated with gabapentin, and one child developed a common peroneal nerve injury that was attributed to malpositioning of the leg during surgery. In our experience, one child who developed symptoms of complex regional pain syndrome after common peroneal nerve injury from positioning in the postoperative period sustained persistent motor block, which emphasizes (1) the importance of early recognition of motor blockade as a potential for injury after surgery and (2) the critical importance of positioning and nursing care in preventing pressure injuries. There were no cases of persistent neurologic injury in the initial PRAN data cohort. In young rabbits, a decrease in blood pressure coincident with epidural anesthesia with lidocaine, decreased spinal cord blood flow was detected using colored microspheres.[313] The addition of epinephrine to the local anesthetic solution did not increase the incidence of ischemia. These studies suggest that it may be particularly important to maintain adequate systemic blood flow during "combined technique" anesthesia in infants and children, and to treat hypotension promptly. Because blood pressure changes caused by neuraxial blockade are uncommon in infants and small children, hypotension in these patients is most likely to be due to other causes and should prompt an assessment of intravascular filling pressures, inotropic state, and the depth of general anesthesia.

PERIPHERAL NERVE BLOCKS

Peripheral nerve blocks are useful adjuvants to general anesthesia. These blocks are also useful as a means for providing postoperative pain relief. Peripheral nerve blocks differ from central neuraxial blocks in several respects:

- A targeted area is anesthetized.
- Side effects, such as weakness of extremities, are minimal.
- The dose of local anesthetic is reduced.
- There is no risk of an unintended spinal anesthetic.
- There is no risk of urinary retention.
- Peripheral blocks can be used in areas where a central neuraxial block is not possible (e.g., face and scalp).

There are many peripheral nerve blocks that can be used in the practice of pediatric anesthesia and each is described in the following text (Table 42.8; see also Chapter 43).

Selection of a Local Anesthetic

Local anesthetics commonly used for peripheral blocks in children include lidocaine, mepivacaine, bupivacaine, and, more recently, levobupivacaine and ropivacaine.[72,74,314] Longer-acting agents have a greater role in peripheral blocks than shorter-acting agents because of the increased duration of postoperative analgesia. Lidocaine can be combined with bupivacaine to provide both a rapid onset and a long duration of action, a practice that we advocate if the child is having the procedure performed with a local block under sedation. If this is done, one must be careful to calculate the doses of the two drugs properly to avoid toxicity. Alternatively, the addition of sodium bicarbonate (1 mEq of bicarbonate/10 mL

TABLE 42.8	Peripheral Nerve Blocks
Head and Neck	
Supraorbital and supratrochlear	
Infraorbital nerve	
Greater occipital nerve	
Great auricular nerve	
Chest Wall	
Intercostal nerve	
Upper Extremity	
Brachial plexus	
Elbow blocks (ulnar, radial, and median nerves)	
Wrist blocks (ulnar, radial, and median nerves)	
Digital	
Abdomen and Genitalia	
Ilioinguinal nerve	
Penile	
Rectus sheath	
Lower extremity	
Femoral nerve	
Lateral femoral cutaneous	
Fascia iliaca	
Sciatic nerve	
Classic approach	
Lateral approach (popliteal fossa)	
Ankle	
Digital	

of local anesthetic [lidocaine]) can speed the onset and reduce the pain of injection of the block by increasing the pH of the solution.[315-318] This alters the pKa of the solution, increasing the active cationic form of the local anesthetic in the solution.[319] Bicarbonate should be added to the local anesthetic solution immediately before administration because precipitation of the local anesthetic and therefore loss of bioavailability increases over time (it should be administered within 10 minutes after alkalinization).[320] This is particularly a problem with mepivacaine, bupivacaine, and ropivacaine in which the addition of 0.1 mL of 8.4% bicarbonate precipitates the anesthetic within 10 minutes.[319,320] The total drug dose administered should not exceed the maximum milligram per kilogram dose permitted for the local anesthetic (see Table 42.2). The addition of epinephrine (1:200,000) may decrease both the vascular absorption and the potential for toxicity; for some local anesthetics the addition of epinephrine will also extend the duration of the block. The exact dose of local anesthetic in terms of volume or concentration needed for most peripheral blocks in children has not been adequately studied. Most blocks performed in children are based on adult experience. Suggested dosing for common peripheral blocks based on volume per kilogram and our experience is presented in Table 42.9.

HEAD AND NECK BLOCKS

Peripheral nerve blocks for postoperative pain relief for the head and neck can be performed with the child under general anesthesia.[321] These blocks can also be used for the provision of pain relief in children with chronic painful problems, such as headaches. Anatomically, two major nerves, the ophthalmic division (V₁) of the trigeminal nerve and the branches of the cervical root C2, supply the sensory innervations of the face and scalp (Fig. 42.9).

Supraorbital and Supratrochlear Nerve Block

ANATOMY. The supraorbital and supratrochlear are the end branches of the ophthalmic division (V₁) of the trigeminal nerve. The supraorbital nerve, the terminal branch of V₁, exits the supraorbital foramen to supply the scalp anterior to the coronal suture. The supratrochlear nerve leaves the orbit between the trochlea and the supraorbital foramen and innervates the lower part of the forehead (Fig. 42.10A). We use this combined block to provide pain relief in children undergoing frontal craniotomies and in children undergoing frontal ventriculoperitoneal shunt revisions. The technique can be used as the sole anesthetic in very sick neonates,[322] and to control postoperative pain in children undergoing excision of scalp lesions.[323] The major advantage is the avoidance of opioids, thereby facilitating an early hospital discharge.

TECHNIQUE. With the child supine and the head in the neutral position, the supraorbital notch is palpated by running a finger from the midline laterally along the eyebrow (the supraorbital

TABLE 42.9	Suggested Dosing for Local Anesthetic Volumes for Common Peripheral Nerve Blocks
Technique	**Dose (mL/kg)**
Head and neck blocks	0.05
Brachial plexus blocks	0.2–0.3
Ilioinguinal nerve block	0.075
Rectus sheath block	0.1
Femoral nerve block	0.2–0.3
Sciatic nerve	0.2–0.3
Digital nerves	0.05

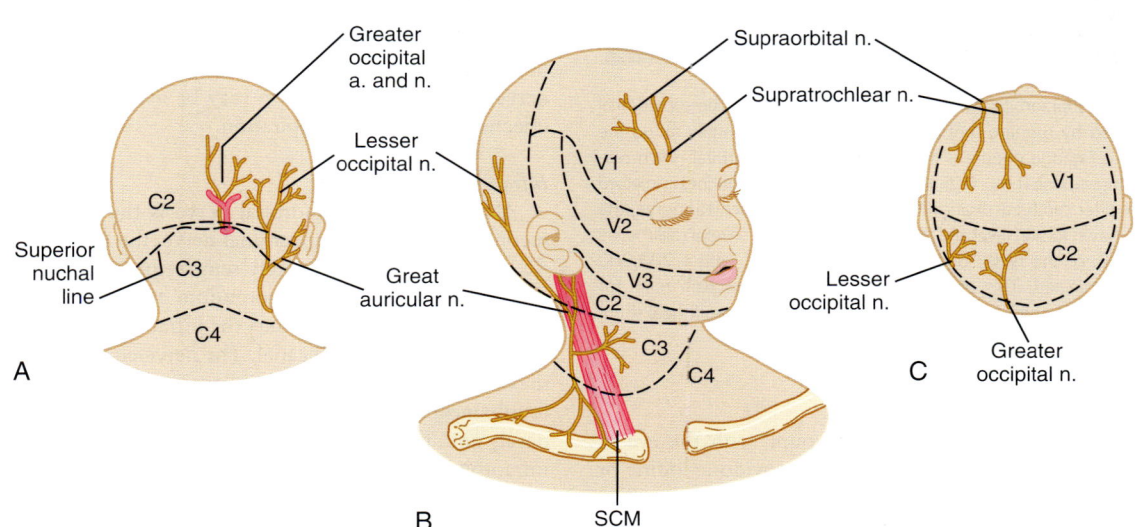

FIGURE 42.9 Dermatomal innervation of head and neck. Sensory and dermatomal innervation of greater and lesser occipital nerves and the innervation of the anterior head by the first division of the trigeminal nerve. Note the sensory innervation anterior to the coronal suture is from the first division of the trigeminal nerve (supraorbital and supratrochlear nerves) and posterior to the coronal suture is from branches of C2 (greater and lesser occipital nerves). These nerves can be blocked individually and in combination to provide postoperative analgesia for a wide variety of procedures; see text for details. **A,** Posterior view. **B,** Anterolateral view. **C,** Axial view. *a,* artery; *C2, C3, C4,* cervical sensory branches of the nerve roots; *n,* nerve; *SCM,* sternocleidomastoid muscle; *V₁, V₂, V₃,* branches of the trigeminal nerve. (Modified from Brown DL, Wong GY. Occipital nerve block. In: Waldman S, Winnie AP, eds. *Interventional Pain Management.* Philadelphia: WB Saunders; 1996:227.)

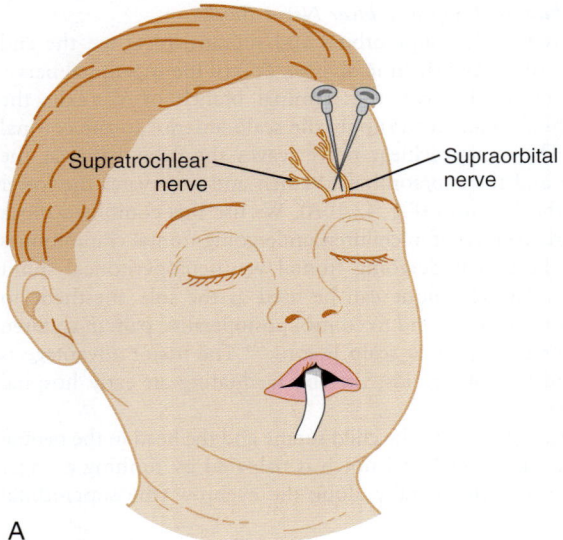

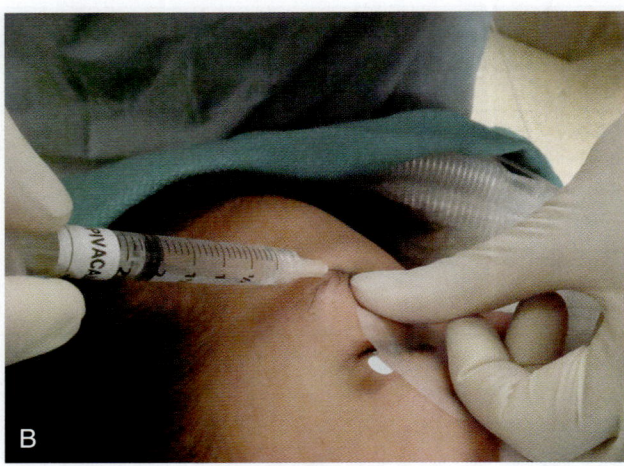

FIGURE 42.10 A, Supraorbital and supratrochlear nerve block. The supraorbital notch is palpated by running a finger from the midline laterally along the eyebrow. **B,** A 27-gauge needle is inserted into the supraorbital notch perpendicularly; bupivacaine (1 mL, 0.25% with 1:200,000 epinephrine) is injected into the space after careful aspiration. To block the supratrochlear nerve, the needle is withdrawn to skin level and then directed medially several millimeters toward the apex of the nose; bupivacaine (1 mL, 0.25% with 1:200,000 epinephrine) is injected. This block provides postoperative pain relief for children undergoing frontal craniotomies or frontal ventriculoperitoneal shunt insertion.

notch is usually located in line with the pupil with the eye in midline position). The skin is prepared with povidone-iodine or chlorhexidine and care is taken to avoid spilling the solution into the eye. A 27-gauge needle is inserted in the proximity of the supraorbital notch; 0.5 to 1.0 mL of bupivacaine (0.25% with epinephrine 1:200,000) is injected into the space after careful aspiration to prevent intravascular placement (see Fig. 42.10B). To block the supratrochlear nerve, the needle is withdrawn to the skin level and then directed and advanced several millimeters medially toward the apex of the nose; 0.5 to 1.0 mL of bupivacaine (0.25% with epinephrine 1:200,000) is injected (Video 42.5).

COMPLICATIONS. Because of the loose adventitious tissue of the eyelid, gentle pressure should be applied to the supraorbital

area; this prevents the dissection of the local anesthetic into the eyelid and supraorbital tissue, and may reduce the potential for ecchymosis and/or hematoma.

Greater Occipital Nerve Block

The greater occipital nerve block is used to diagnose and treat occipital pain. If this technique is used for the diagnosis of occipital neuralgia, a careful history and physical examination is performed to rule out other pathologic causes of headaches, including posterior fossa tumors and Arnold-Chiari malformation.[324] It can also be used to treat postoperative pain in the posterior fossa after posterior fossa surgery, and in children undergoing posterior ventriculoperitoneal shunt revisions.[325]

ANATOMY. The cervical spinal nerves innervate the posterior head and neck. The dorsal rami of C2 end in the greater occipital nerve, which provides the cutaneous innervation to the major portion of the posterior scalp (Fig. 42.11A). The nerve becomes subcutaneous slightly inferior to the superior nuchal line by passing above the aponeurotic sling; here it is in close proximity and medial to the occipital artery.

TECHNIQUE. With the child supine and the head laterally rotated or with the child prone, the occipital artery is palpated at the level of the superior nuchal line. The occipital artery is usually located at approximately one-third of the distance from the external occipital protuberance to the mastoid process on the superior nuchal line (see Fig. 42.11B). A total volume of 2 mL of bupivacaine (0.25% with 1:200,000 epinephrine) is injected SC (Video 42.6). A recent technique using ultrasound guidance has been used in children for performing occipital nerve blocks.[326]

COMPLICATIONS. It is rare to see complications with this block because of the superficial location of the nerve. One has to bear in mind the close proximity to the spinal canal, particularly in children who have had surgery in the area. Thus the needle must remain just beneath the skin during injection of local anesthetic. It is more difficult to perform this block at the C2 nerve root without the aid of either ultrasonography or fluoroscopy and hence it cannot cover the entire distribution of the greater occipital nerve. Intravascular injection may be avoided with incremental injection and frequent aspiration.

Infraorbital Nerve Block

ANATOMY. The infraorbital nerve is the termination of the second division of the trigeminal nerve, the maxillary nerve (Fig. 42.12A). This nerve is entirely sensory in function. It leaves the skull through the foramen rotundum and enters into the pterygopalatine fossa. It then enters the infraorbital groove and passes through the infraorbital canal. The nerve emerges in front of the maxilla through the infraorbital foramen and then divides into four branches: the inferior palpebral, the external nasal, the internal nasal, and the superior labial. The anatomic location of the infraorbital foramen has been studied using CT scans: the average distance from the midline (in millimeters) is 21.3 + 0.5 × age (years).[327,328] The branches of the infraorbital nerve innervate the lower eyelid, the lateral inferior portion of the nose and its vestibule, the upper lip, the mucosa along the upper lip, and the vermilion. This block is effective for surgery of the upper lip and the vermilion after a cleft lip repair,[329] for reconstructive procedures on the nose (including septal reconstruction and rhinoplasty),[330] and for endoscopic sinus surgery.[331] There are two approaches to the infraorbital nerve: intraoral and extraoral.

INTRAORAL APPROACH. This is our preferred method for this block. The infraorbital foramen is located by palpation of the

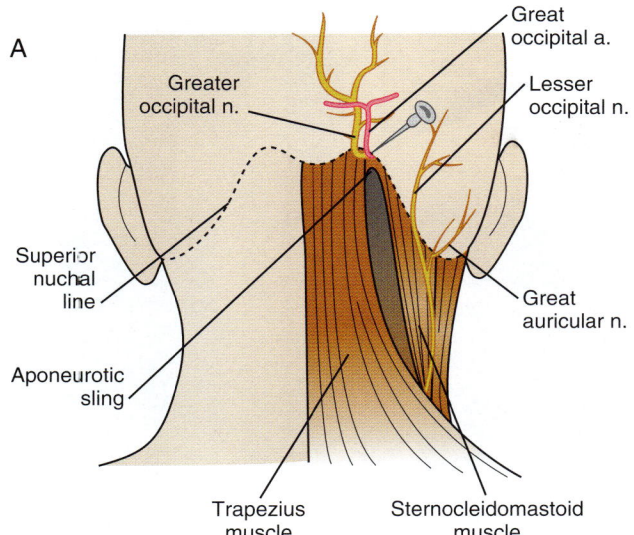

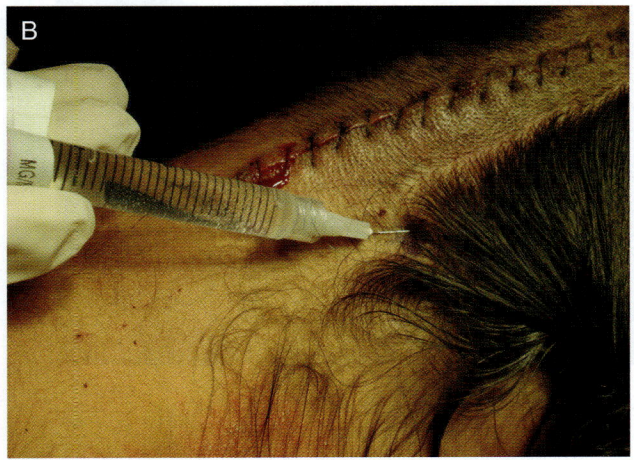

FIGURE 42.11 A, Greater occipital nerve and site of block. **B,** With the patient supine and with the head turned to one side or with the patient prone, the occipital artery is palpated at the level of the superior nuchal line. The occipital artery is located about one-third of the distance from the external occipital protuberance (*dashed line,* part **A**) to the mastoid process on the superior nuchal line. A total volume of 2 mL of bupivacaine (0.25% with 1 : 200,000 epinephrine) is injected subcutaneously to form a skin wheal. Frequent aspiration and incremental injection may avoid intravascular injection. This block is used to diagnose occipital neuralgia and as a means for providing postoperative pain relief for children undergoing posterior fossa tumor resection or posterior ventriculoperitoneal shunt insertion. *a,* artery; *n,* nerve. (Modified from Brown DL, Wong GY. Occipital nerve block. In: Waldman S, Winnie AP, eds. *Interventional Pain Management.* Philadelphia: WB Saunders; 1996:228.)

infraorbital notch. After folding back the upper lip, a 27-gauge needle is inserted through the buccal mucosa approximately parallel to the maxillary second molar and passed SC with the tip of the needle directed toward the infraorbital foramen. It is important to place a finger over the infraorbital foramen so as to palpate the progress of the needle beneath the skin and prevent unintended passage of the needle into the orbit. With the tip of the needle at the level of the infraorbital foramen and after careful aspiration, 0.5 to 1.0 mL of local anesthetic is injected (see Fig. 42.2B and Video 42.7). Bupivacaine (0.25% with epinephrine 1 : 200,000) provides prolonged postoperative analgesia with this block.

EXTRAORAL APPROACH. The infraorbital ridge of the maxillary bone should be identified and the infraorbital foramen palpated. A 27-gauge needle is advanced toward the foramen at a 45-degree angle to the maxilla (see Fig. 42.12C). After careful aspiration, 0.5 to 1.0 mL of bupivacaine (0.25% with epinephrine 1 : 200,000) is injected.

COMPLICATIONS. Because of the loose adventitious tissue, children can develop ecchymosis and swelling. Pressure should be applied to the infraorbital area to retain the solution within the infraorbital foramen, prevent dissection of the local anesthetic into the periorbital area, and reduce the potential for the formation of a hematoma or ecchymosis. Care should be taken to avoid direct injection into the orbit or eye. Intravascular injection may be avoided with incremental injection and frequent aspiration. This block can be achieved with low volumes in infants and toddlers; hence every attempt should be made to decrease the volume of the local anesthetic solution. Using other additives, including clonidine, may be helpful, although there are no randomized controlled trials to demonstrate the improved efficacy of this block using additives.

Great Auricular Nerve Block

The great auricular nerve supplies the sensory innervation to the mastoid area and the external ear. It is a branch of the superficial cervical plexus. Cervical plexus blocks were first performed by Halstead in 1884. This block has been used to provide postoperative analgesia in children undergoing otoplasty repair,[332] as well as in tympanomastoid surgery.[333] We found that the great auricular nerve block decreases the incidence of nausea and vomiting, which is a major morbidity associated with tympanomastoid surgery.[333] It provides surface analgesia but not muscle relaxation and hence can be used for intraoperative analgesia despite the need for facial nerve monitoring in children undergoing tympanomastoid procedures.

ANATOMY. The cervical plexus is formed by the anterior primary division of the anterior and posterior roots of cervical nerves C2-4. The great auricular nerve is derived from C3, which was described by McKinney. The anatomic location of the nerve for blockade has been described as the McKinney point.[334] The great auricular nerve wraps around the belly of the sternocleidomastoid muscle at the level of the cricoid cartilage and emerges to supply the area of the mastoid and external ear (Fig. 42.13A).

TECHNIQUE. With the child under general anesthesia, the cricoid cartilage is identified. A line is drawn from the superior margin of the cricoid cartilage laterally to the posterior border of the sternocleidomastoid muscle (McKinney point). Bupivacaine (2–3 mL, 0.25% with epinephrine 1 : 200,000) is injected superficially at this point (see Fig. 42.13B and Video 42.8).

COMPLICATIONS. Deep rather than superficial injection can result in a deep cervical plexus block and the risk of Horner syndrome, phrenic nerve block, or unintended central neuraxial blockade. A small erythematous area may be seen at the site of the needle injection. Intravascular injection may be avoided by incremental injection of the solution and frequent aspiration.

Nerve of Arnold (Auricular Branch of Vagus)

The auricular branch of the vagus supplies the sensory nerve that supplies the innervation to the auditory canal, as well as the inferior portion of the tympanic membrane. This is useful for providing analgesia to the tympanic membrane after myringotomy and tube placement, as well as for tympanoplasty surgery. In a

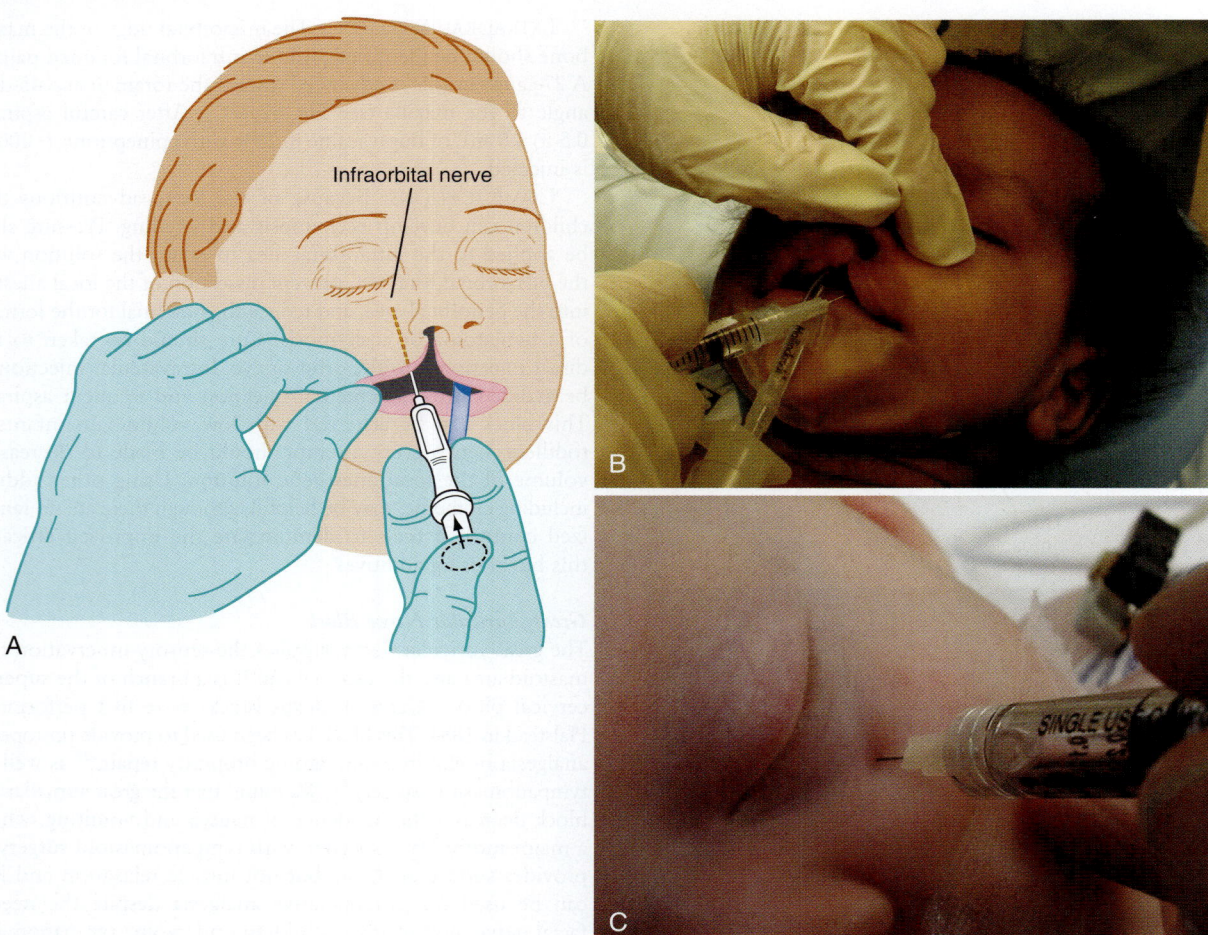

FIGURE 42.12 A, Infraorbital block (intraoral approach): The infraorbital foramen is located by palpation of the infraorbital notch (right-sided block). **B,** The lip is folded back and a 27-gauge needle is inserted through the buccal mucosa approximately parallel to the maxillary second molar. The tip of the needle is directed toward the infraorbital foramen. A finger is placed over the infraorbital foramen to avoid accidental placement of the needle into the orbit. After careful aspiration to avoid intravascular injection, 0.5 to 1.0 mL of bupivacaine (0.25% with 1:200,000 epinephrine) is injected (left-sided block). **C,** For the extraoral approach (left-sided block) the infraorbital ridge of the maxillary bone should be identified and the infraorbital foramen is palpated. A 27-gauge needle is advanced toward the foramen at a 45-degree angle to the maxilla (midpupillary point). After careful aspiration, 0.5 to 1.0 mL of bupivacaine (0.25% with epinephrine 1:200,000) is injected. This block is used to provide postoperative pain relief for children undergoing upper lip or cleft lip repair, reconstructive procedures of the nose (e.g., rhinoplasty), and endoscopic sinus surgery.

randomized controlled trial, intranasal fentanyl and blockade of the auricular branch of the vagus provided equivalent analgesia without adverse effects.[335]

INDICATIONS. This block is used to provide analgesia for myringotomy and tube placement, and for tympanoplasty.

TECHNIQUE. After induction of anesthesia, and with the child turned to one side, the tragus is cleaned and reflected laterally, a 30-gauge needle is inserted into the tragus to pierce the cartilage; after aspiration, 0.2 mL of local anesthetic solution is injected (Video 42.9). Mild pressure is applied to prevent any bleeding following the procedure.

COMPLICATIONS. It is rare to see complications, although occasionally there can be some brisk bleeding from the needle entry site, which can be offset by applying pressure.

TRUNCAL BLOCKS

Truncal blocks are performed in children for a variety of different surgical procedures. The most common blocks include intercostal blocks,[46] ilioinguinal blocks, penile blocks, rectus sheath blocks, and paravertebral blocks.

Intercostal Nerve Block

Intercostal blocks after thoracotomy are useful in reducing opioid requirements, optimizing respiratory mechanics, and encouraging early ambulation.[46,336,337] Their major disadvantage is the limited duration of analgesia. Currently, we more commonly use epidural blockade for this purpose. The development of degradable bupivacaine microspheres and the recent approval of liposomal encapsulated bupivacaine, which produce analgesia of dramatically to 5 mL of 0.25% bupivacaine with epinephrine to block each intercostal nerve, depending on the size of the child and the number of ribs to be blocked. A maximum of 2 mg/kg of bupivacaine is used, although this amount should be reduced by about 30% for infants younger than 6 months of age. The concentration of bupivacaine should be decreased to provide adequate volume for the desired number of intercostal blocks while avoiding the risk of systemic toxicity.

ANATOMY. The intercostal nerves are derived from the ventral rami of the first through the twelfth thoracic nerves. There are four branches. The first is the gray rami communicans, which goes to the sympathetic ganglion. The second branch arises as the posterior cutaneous branch, which supplies the skin in the paravertebral area. The third branch, the lateral cutaneous branch, arises anterior to the midaxillary line and sends subcutaneous branches both anteriorly and posteriorly. The final branch provides cutaneous innervation to the midline of the chest and abdomen. The dura mater and the arachnoid membrane fuse with the epineurium as they exit the vertebral foramen. This could lead to subarachnoid block if the posterior paravertebral approach is used.

TECHNIQUE. The site of injection may be either paravertebral or in the midaxillary line. The lower rib margin is located, and the skin is retracted cephalad (Fig. 42.14A). The needle is inserted perpendicular to the skin over the rib and advanced until the rib is encountered (see Fig. 42.14B). The skin through which the needle is passed is allowed to retract caudally, and the needle is then walked off the lower edge of the rib a distance of 2 to 3 mm (see Fig. 42.14C). This method may reduce the potential for pneumothorax, because the needle strikes the rib and is not advanced more than half of the thickness of the rib. A distinct pop may be felt as the needle enters the neurovascular sheath. After negative aspiration for blood, an appropriate volume of anesthetic is injected. Recently, with the use of ultrasound guidance, we can visualize the pleura, thereby avoiding puncturing the pleura because it can be adequately visualized while performing the block (E-Fig. 42.6; see also Fig. 43.11).

COMPLICATIONS. Pneumothorax has been reported after intercostal blockade, with an incidence of approximately 0.07% in adults.[340] However, the majority of the blocks in that study were performed by residents in training. If a small pneumothorax occurs, reabsorption is facilitated with the use of oxygen. Placement of a chest tube is indicated only if breathing is compromised. A more significant complication is the toxic effect of absorbed local anesthetic drugs. Using smaller volumes of more dilute local anesthetic may reduce the risk of achieving toxic plasma concentrations. The risk of intravascular injection may be reduced with incremental injection and frequent aspiration. A third complication is a high subarachnoid block, usually associated with the posterior paravertebral approach.

Inguinal Block (Ilioinguinal and Iliohypogastric Nerves)

Inguinal block, supplemented by wound infiltration, is sometimes used in adult patients undergoing inguinal hernia repair. However, in children, an inguinal nerve block is used almost exclusively as an adjunct to general anesthesia and to manage postoperative pain. This block is as effective as caudal anesthesia for inguinal repairs.[341,342] Blockade of the ilioinguinal and iliohypogastric nerves is very successful for this purpose and has few associated complications, although injection into the femoral vessels and potential femoral nerve block are possible adverse outcomes.[343,344] The risks of toxicity from excessive drug doses may be greater than previously recognized, as discussed earlier, but ultrasound guidance has

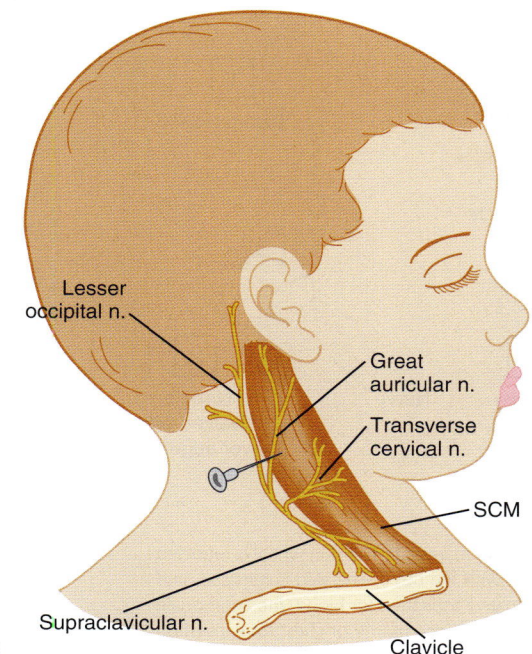

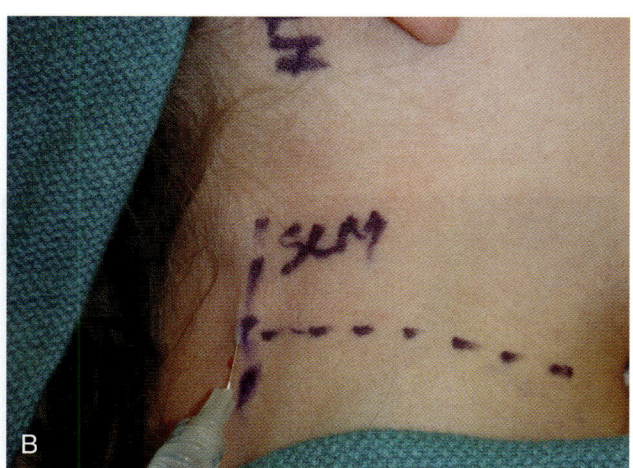

FIGURE 42.13 **A,** Great auricular nerve block. The cricoid cartilage is identified. **B,** A broken line drawn from the superior border of the cricoid cartilage laterally to the posterior border of the sternocleidomastoid (*SCM*) (McKinney point) is identified; bupivacaine (2–3 mL, 0.25% with 1:200,000 epinephrine) is injected subcutaneously at this point. Gentle massage after the injection allows spread of the local anesthetic in the injected site. This block is used to provide postoperative analgesia for children undergoing tympanomastoid surgery or otoplasty. *n,* nerve. (Modified from Brown DL, ed. *Atlas of Regional Anesthesia.* Philadelphia: WB Saunders; 1999:185.)

greater duration, may change this practice in the future.[52,61–63,69,338] There are, however, still situations in which intercostal blocks are useful, particularly in children who cannot have a neuraxial catheter placed.

The uptake of local anesthetic after intercostal blocks is the most rapid of all sites of regional anesthesia, yielding the greatest plasma concentrations of local anesthetics after any other regional block. Furthermore, plasma concentrations in children increase more rapidly than after identical blocks in adults.[339] For this reason, epinephrine (1:200,000) should always be added to reduce the absorption of local anesthetic. We commonly use 1

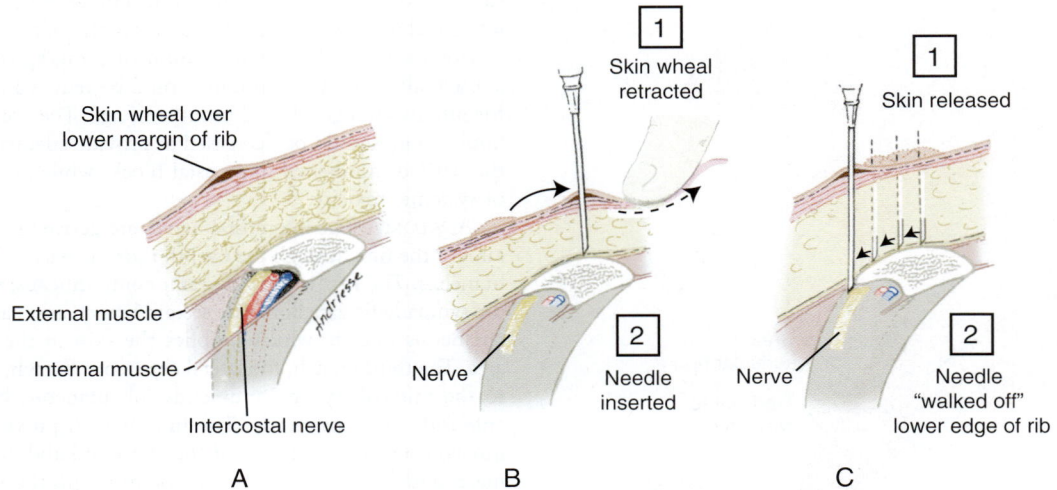

FIGURE 42.14 Intercostal block. **A,** A skin wheal is inserted on the lower rib margin. **B,** The skin wheal is retracted over the body of the rib, and a needle is inserted until contact is made with the rib. **C,** The skin is released, and the needle is carefully "walked" off the edge of the rib margin. After negative aspiration for blood, the appropriate volume of drug is injected. This block is used for postoperative analgesia for thoracotomy or chest tube insertion (see also E-Fig. 42.6).

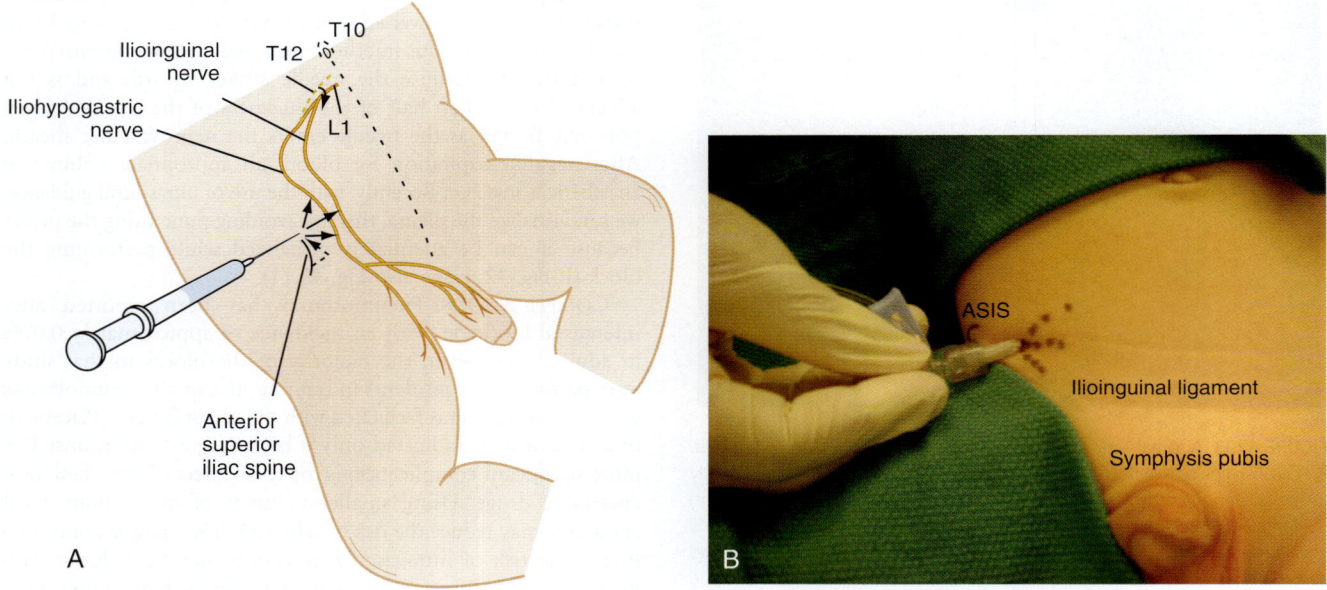

FIGURE 42.15 Ilioinguinal and iliohypogastric nerve blocks. **A** and **B,** The anterior superior iliac spine *(ASIS)* is palpated, and a point 1.0 to 1.5 cm cephalad and toward the midline is located *(dashed line)*. A 22-gauge needle is passed through the external and internal oblique muscles, and 1.0 to 5.0 mL of local anesthetic is deposited in a fan-like fashion cephalad toward the umbilicus, medially, and caudad toward the groin *(solid arrows)*. Just before removal from the skin, another 0.5 to 1.0 mL of local anesthetic is injected subcutaneously to block the iliohypogastric nerve. Blockade of these nerves provides postoperative analgesia for inguinal hernia and orchiopexy procedures (see also E-Fig. 42.7).

demonstrated adequate analgesia with reduced doses of local anesthetic solution because the drug is placed in the optimal location.[345] This block may be (and commonly is) performed in conjunction with infiltration of the wound. The use of ultrasound may also avoid the risk of bowel perforation (see also Chapter 43, and Figs. 43.34 and 43.35).[346]

ANATOMY. The inguinal area is innervated by the subcostal nerve (T12) and the iliohypogastric and ilioinguinal nerves (derived from L1). These nerves lie in close proximity to each other medial and superior to the anterior superior iliac spine (Fig. 42.15A). After piercing the internal oblique 2 to 3 cm medial to the anterior superior iliac spine, the nerve then lies between the internal oblique and the external oblique aponeurosis. Here it accompanies the spermatic cord (in males) to the genital area.

TECHNIQUE. The block may be performed either at the beginning of surgery or before the end of general anesthesia. If bupivacaine is used, a minimum of 15 minutes is usually required from the completion of the block until maximal analgesia is obtained. Thus blocks placed at the beginning of the surgical procedure (our preference) are usually more effective than those performed at the end of surgery. Blocks performed before skin incision may also provide "preemptive analgesia," although the evidence for this is still under debate and somewhat confusing.[347–350] The duration of postoperative analgesia is unaffected by the timing of placing the block at the beginning of the procedure, assuming that the surgical procedure is not of more than 1.5 hours in duration or at the end. A short-bevel 27-gauge needle is inserted at a 45-degree angle at a point one-fourth of the way toward the midline along a line drawn from the anterior superior iliac spine to the umbilicus (1.0–1.5 cm cephalad and toward the midline from the anterior superior iliac spine in a 10- to 15-kg child). As the needle is advanced through the external and internal oblique muscles (see Fig. 42.15B), two pops are elicited and provide useful guides of proper needle placement. Negative aspiration should be confirmed several times during the incremental injection of local anesthetic. A volume of 0.3 mL/kg of local anesthetic solution is injected in a fan-like fashion, cephalad toward the umbilicus, caudad toward the groin, and medially. Before removal of the needle from the skin, an additional 0.5 to 1.0 mL of local anesthetic is injected SC to block the iliohypogastric nerve (Video 42.10). Care must be taken to avoid entering the peritoneum, which has been reported after the blind injection approach.[346] For inguinal herniorrhaphy, orchiopexy, or other inguinal procedures, local anesthetic deposited directly into the wound before it is closed has also proved effective for postoperative analgesia.[342] The volume of drug used by this approach, like the volume of drug used for wound infiltration, must be accounted for when calculating the maximal dose of local anesthetic that can be used. It is important to note that this block will not provide pain relief for scrotal procedures because this is supplied by the genitofemoral nerve and hence it is important to have the surgeon infiltrate the scrotum for complete pain relief after orchiopexy or any other scrotal procedures. As mentioned earlier, an ultrasound-guided technique may be easier to perform and is associated with fewer complications (E-Fig. 42.7).[345]

COMPLICATIONS. Complications are rare. Care should be taken not to enter the peritoneal cavity. Intravascular injection may be avoided by incremental injection with frequent aspiration.

Penile Block

A penile block is used for anesthesia and postoperative analgesia for circumcision, urethral dilatation, and hypospadias repair. Caudal anesthesia is superior for proximal shaft or penoscrotal hypospadias repair because a penile block provides analgesia only for the distal two-thirds of the penis.[265,351,352] The block is easily performed with very good success. Bupivacaine, levobupivacaine, and ropivacaine are the most useful agents because of their prolonged duration of action. *Epinephrine is avoided for this block because the dorsal artery of the penis is an end artery and vasospasm caused by epinephrine could cause necrosis.*

ANATOMY. The nerve supply of the penis is from the pudendal nerve and the pelvic plexus (Fig. 42.16A). Along the dorsal artery to the penis are two dorsal nerves that separate at the level of the symphysis pubis; they supply the sensory innervation to the penis.

TECHNIQUE. There are two commonly used techniques for penile block: (1) a ring block and (2) blockade of the dorsal nerve. One investigation compared the efficacy of these techniques and concluded that the ring block provided analgesia of prolonged duration, although both techniques provided analgesia superior to EMLA cream.[353] The ring block is performed by inserting a 27-gauge needle at the base of the penis and, after negative aspiration, injecting the local anesthetic without epinephrine in a ring-shaped pattern around the base of the penile shaft. The needle may be inserted once in the midline and then redirected to each side (see Fig. 42.16B). The alternate dorsal nerve block is performed with a 27-gauge needle inserted 1 cm above the symphysis pubis, in the midline, at a 30-degree angle and directed caudally (see Fig. 42.16C). The needle is advanced 1 cm after it pierces the penile fascia. After negative aspiration for blood, 1 to 4 mL of local anesthetic *without epinephrine* is injected slowly. There is a small risk of injury to the adjacent neurovascular structures.

COMPLICATIONS. The major complication is compromise of organ blood flow. *Vasoconstrictors, such as epinephrine, must never be used for this block.* Applying pressure after the injection may minimize hematoma formation. Intravascular injection may be avoided with incremental injection and frequent aspiration.

Rectus Sheath Block

Although reported almost 20 years ago,[354] this block has recently become popular for children undergoing repair of an umbilical hernia.[355–357] The rectus sheath contains the thoracic intercostal nerves (T10) that can be blocked at the paraumbilical area using a small volume of local anesthetic solution.

TECHNIQUE. On either side of the umbilicus, about 1 cm from midline a needle is inserted into the rectus sheath (Fig. 42.17). A pop can be felt as the needle advances beyond the anterior rectus sheath, through the rectus abdominis muscle, and then just anterior to the posterior rectus sheath. After aspiration, a volume of 0.1 mL/kg of local anesthetic solution is injected (Video 42.10). This provides excellent analgesia for most umbilical area surgery, including laparoscopic surgery. Use of ultrasound may facilitate performing this block[358] (see Figs. 42.17A and B; see also Chapter 43, and E-Figs. 43.3 and 43.4).

Paravertebral Block

This block is also gaining some popularity for use in children. The main advantage is that deposition of local anesthetics in the paravertebral space will lead to strict unilateral anesthesia of one or more adjacent dermatomes (Fig. 42.18); the main indications for a paravertebral nerve block are unilateral thoracic or abdominal surgical procedures.

ANATOMY. The paravertebral space is a triangular wedge-shaped area situated in the angle between the lateral border of the vertebral body and the anterior surface of the transverse process (Fig. 42.19). The paravertebral space exists only between T1 and T12. Below T12 the space is sealed off by the origin of the psoas muscle from the vertebral body and the transverse process.[359] Cranially the space appears to communicate with fascial planes in the neck, because an upper thoracic paravertebral block may cause Horner syndrome. The communication of different thoracic levels of the paravertebral space is the foundation for spread of local anesthetic to multiple segments (see Fig. 42.18). The medial boundary of the paravertebral space is the lateral part of the vertebral body and disk, the dorsal limitation is the transverse process and costotransverse ligament, and the anterolateral boundary is the

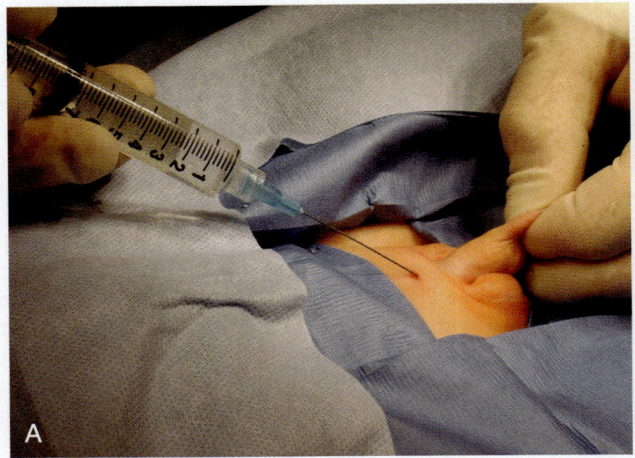
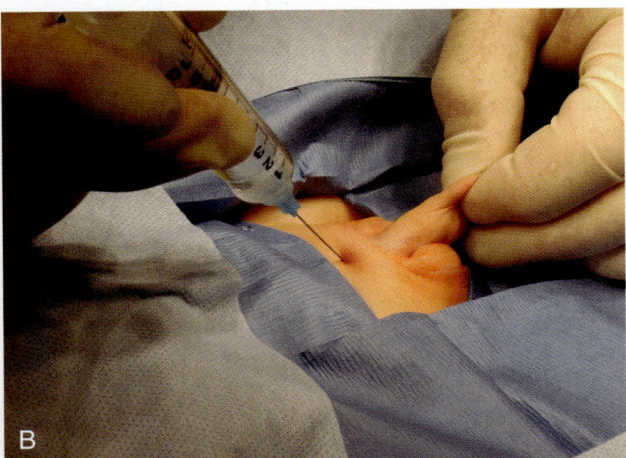

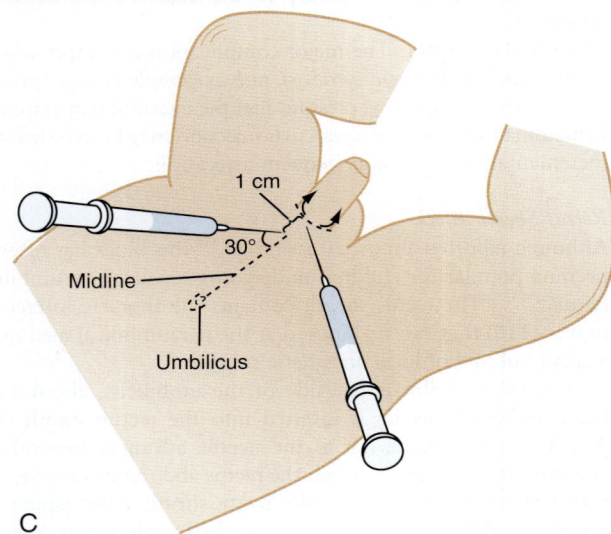

FIGURE 42.16 Penile block. **A,** Dorsal nerve block: a 27- or 25-gauge needle is inserted in the midline, 1 cm above the symphysis pubis at an angle of 30 degrees from the plane of the abdominal wall and directed caudad. **B,** After piercing the penile fascia (0.5–1.0 cm) and negative aspiration for blood, 1.0 to 4.0 mL of local anesthetic without epinephrine is injected. **C,** Ring block: a 25-gauge needle is inserted at the base of the penis at a 45-degree angle, and a ring of local anesthetic is deposited (*curved arrows*). This may be done through a single needle placement by redirecting the needle. This block may be used in children in whom a caudal block is contraindicated.

parietal pleura. Structures that pass through the paravertebral space include the spinal nerve root–intercostal nerve, the sympathetic chain, and the intercostal vessels. The paravertebral space is not like the epidural space, because the pleura are very adhesive to the other structures but should instead be viewed as a "potential space." This accounts for the slight difficulty in introducing a percutaneous catheter into the paravertebral space. In the lumbar region a paravertebral block is still possible but each individual space must be blocked separately because there are no communications between adjacent lumbar levels.

TECHNIQUE. Three approaches to perform a paravertebral block in children have been described:

Loss-of-Resistance Technique[359]: The skin is punctured laterally to the spinous process and the needle is advanced in a perpendicular manner until contact is made with the transverse process. A Tuohy needle (19- to 20-gauge if the child is younger than 1 year of age, 18-gauge if older than 1 year of age) is then "walked" below (underneath) the transverse process and by means of a loss-of-resistance technique the costotransverse ligament is pierced and the paravertebral space located. Alternatively, the needle can be "walked" above (over the top of) the transverse process, but by using this approach there is the risk of striking the neck of the rib before entering the paravertebral space. Occasionally this will redirect the needle, making it virtually impossible to obtain access

to the paravertebral space. The approach from below the transverse process is clearly advantageous.

Once in the paravertebral space, the bolus dose of local anesthetic can be injected after careful aspiration to exclude the presence of blood or air. If a continuous technique is preferred, a catheter can be introduced 1 to 2 cm into the paravertebral space through the Tuohy needle. The insertion of the catheter frequently needs manipulation of the Tuohy needle to be successful, and occasionally one will have to make the injection of the bolus dose to "open up" or "create" a space to allow catheter insertion. One should not insert more than 1 to 2 cm of the catheter into the paravertebral space because further advancement may cause the catheter to migrate into the spinal canal through the intervertebral foramen (causing an epidural distribution of the block) or to go laterally, following the path of the intercostal nerve (giving a dense block of only one dermatome).

An estimate of the distance from the spinous process to the skin puncture site (spinous process to paravertebral space distance) and the distance from the skin to the paravertebral space can be approximated by the following equations[360,361]:

$$\text{Spinous process to paravertebral space distance (mm)} = 0.12 \times \text{kg} + 10.2$$

$$\text{Skin to paravertebral space distance (mm)} = 0.53 \times \text{kg} + 21.2.$$

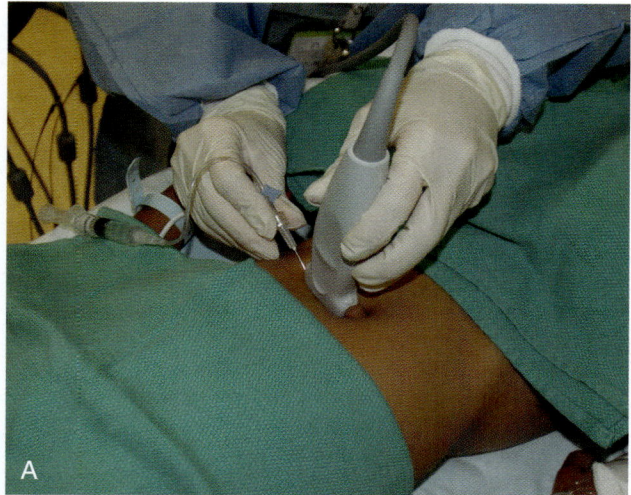

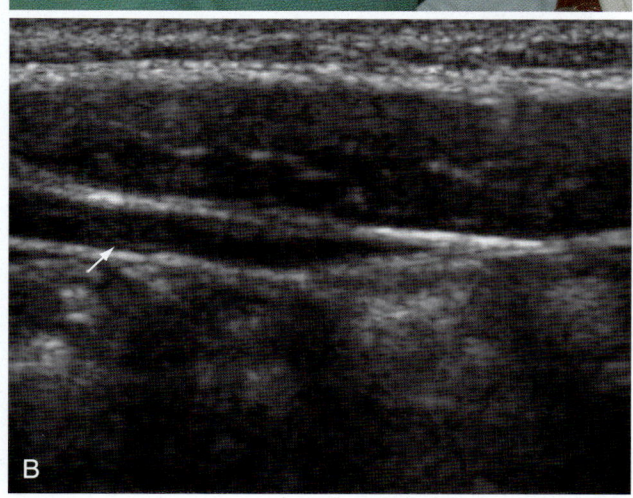

FIGURE 42.17 Rectus sheath block. The rectus sheath is encompassed between the rectus abdominis muscle anteriorly and the posterior rectus sheath. **A,** A linear ultrasound probe is placed lateral to the umbilicus, and the anterior rectus sheath, the rectus abdominis muscle, and the posterior rectus sheath are identified. **B,** With the use of an in-plane approach, a 27-gauge needle is inserted through the rectus abdominis muscle anterior to the posterior rectus sheath and 0.1 mL/kg of local anesthetic solution is injected (*arrow*).

The level of the puncture depends on the surgical intervention, but for a thoracotomy the puncture is best performed at T5-6 and for renal surgery at T9-10.

Nerve-Stimulator–Guided Technique.[362] The intervertebral lines corresponding to the specific dermatomes are determined by manual palpation. The site of injection is marked 1 to 2 cm laterally from the midline on the intervertebral line according to the child's weight. A 21-gauge insulated needle of appropriate length, attached to a nerve stimulator (initial stimulating current: 2.5–5 mA, 1 Hz), is introduced perpendicularly to the skin in all planes. A contraction of the paraspinal muscles is initially observed, and the needle is advanced until the costotransverse ligament is reached. At this point the contraction of the paraspinal muscles will disappear. After piercing the costotransverse ligament, muscle contractions of the corresponding level are sought and the needle tip is manipulated into a position allowing continued muscular contractions while reducing the stimulating current to 0.4 to 0.6 mA; the desired local anesthetic dose and volume is injected.

Manipulation of the needle tip within the paravertebral space is not an "in and out" movement but is rather an angular manipulation and circumferential rotation around the axis of the needle to reach an optimal position of the needle tip with regard to the nerve within the paravertebral space.

Ultrasound-Aided Approach. With the aid of ultrasound the position of the transverse processes and the depth to the paravertebral space can be determined; ultrasound is very helpful regardless of whether a loss-of-resistance or nerve-stimulator–guided technique is used.

SELECTION OF DRUG. After a negative aspiration test and administration of a test dose, 0.5 mL/kg of the local anesthetic (levobupivacaine 0.25% with epinephrine 1:200,000, bupivacaine 0.25% with epinephrine 1:200,000, or lidocaine 1% with epinephrine 1:200,000) is injected in toddlers and older children. This dose will usually spread to cover at least five dermatomes. A typical distribution of the block will be unilateral analgesia of the trunk ranging from T4 to T12 (see Fig. 42.18). In neonates and infants, slightly modified dosage regimens are recommended;[363-365] these dosages have been found to be both effective and associated with acceptable plasma concentrations of bupivacaine.[363]

COMPLICATIONS. The use of a percutaneous loss-of-resistance technique in a mixed adult and pediatric population was found to be associated with an overall failure rate of approximately 10%, and the complications experienced were hypotension (5%; only adults), vascular puncture (4%), pleural puncture (1%), and pneumothorax (0.5%).[366] The risk for block failure is reduced to less than 5% when a nerve-stimulator–guided technique is used, and this technique also appears to be associated with a reduced risk for complications.[362,367] Use of ultrasound may further improve success while reducing complications.

UPPER EXTREMITY BLOCKS

Brachial Plexus Block

Of the four techniques used to block the brachial plexus (axillary, infraclavicular, supraclavicular, and interscalene), the axillary approach is most commonly used in children when using nerve stimulation or landmark approaches.[368] Advantages include ease of insertion, a high rate of success in experienced hands, and low morbidity. The block is also well suited for orthopedic or plastic surgical repairs on the hand or forearm in a child with a full stomach.[369,370] In the latter situation, the child is at greater risk for aspiration of gastric contents with deeper levels of sedation, an intravascular injection, or a drug overdose. Because it is unnecessary to elicit a sensory paresthesia, the block can also be performed in an anesthetized child for postoperative pain management. Toxicity is avoided if the dose of bupivacaine is less than 2.5 mg/kg.

With the use of ultrasound guidance, infraclavicular, supraclavicular and interscalene blocks have largely supplanted the axillary block in children. The infraclavicular block is our preferred technique for the placement of a continuous catheter in the postoperative period. Unintentional block of the phrenic and recurrent laryngeal nerves is much more common in young children because these nerves are close to the site of injection, especially with an interscalene block. Data suggest that some degree of phrenic nerve blockade is present in all children who receive interscalene blocks.[371,372] Phrenic nerve blockade may cause respiratory failure in very young children whose breathing depends almost completely on the diaphragm, whereas blockade of the recurrent laryngeal nerve will paralyze the vocal cords and increase airway resistance. The risk of pneumothorax is greater because the apex of the lung is situated more rostral in infants and small children.

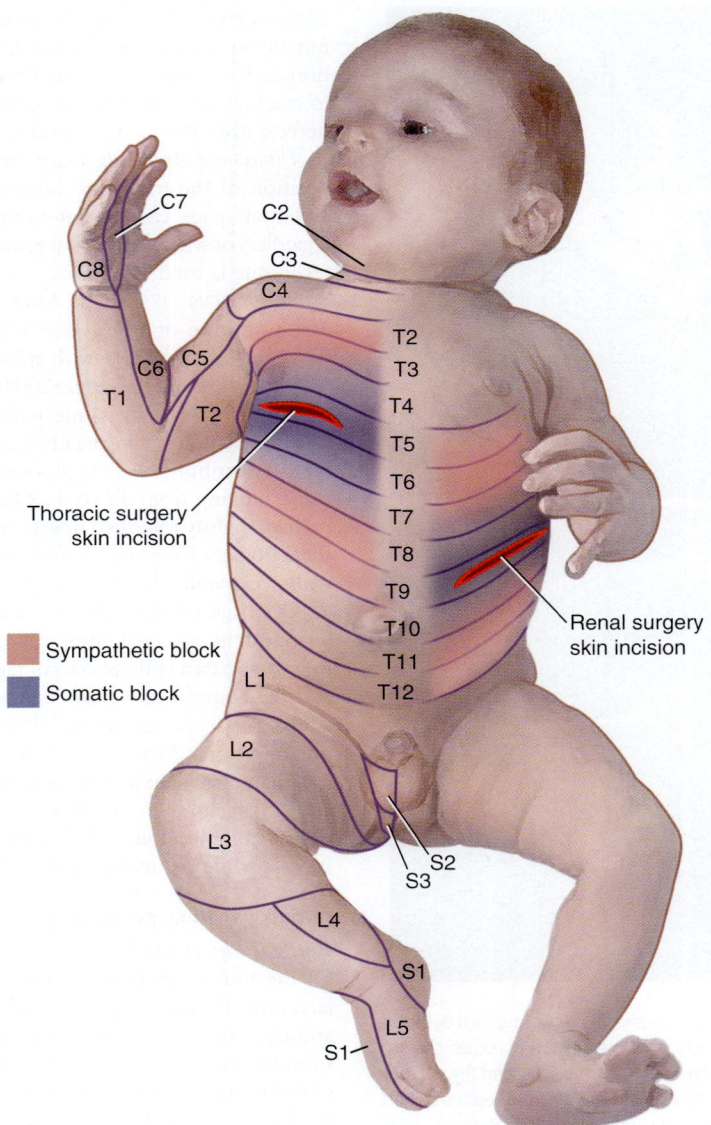

Labels on figure: C7, C2, C8, C3, C4, C5, C6, T1, T2, C5, T2, T3, T4, T5, T6, T7, T8, T9, T10, T11, T12, L1, L2, L3, L4, L5, S1, S2, S3

Thoracic surgery skin incision

Renal surgery skin incision

■ Sympathetic block
■ Somatic block

FIGURE 42.18 Distribution of somatic and sympathetic blockade after thoracic paravertebral blocks. *Blue shading* indicates the approximate spread of somatic blockade and *pink shading* indicates the approximate extent of sympathetic blockade. (See text for details.) (From Lönnqvist PA, Richardson J. Use of paravertebral blockade in children. *Tech Region Anesth Pain Manage.* 1999;3[3]:184–188.)

FIGURE 42.19 Anatomic relationship of the paravertebral block and correct position of Tuohy needle and catheter. (From Lönnqvist PA, Richardson J. Use of paravertebral blockade in children. *Tech Region Anesth Pain Manage.* 1999;3[3]:184–188.)

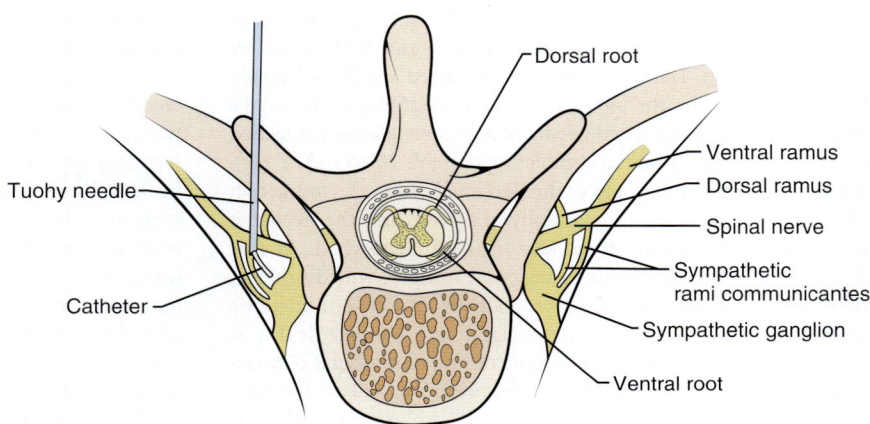

Labels: Dorsal root, Ventral ramus, Dorsal ramus, Spinal nerve, Sympathetic rami communicantes, Sympathetic ganglion, Ventral root, Tuohy needle, Catheter

Total spinal anesthesia is also more likely with the interscalene approach to axillary plexus blockade.[373]

ANATOMY. The brachial plexus arises in the neck from spinal nerves C5, C6, C7, C8, and T1, passes between the clavicle and first rib, and extends into the axilla. At that point, the axillary artery is surrounded by a narrow fascial sheath that contains the median nerve anteriorly, the ulnar nerve posteriorly, and the radial nerve on the posterolateral aspect (Fig. 42.20A). In children, the axillary artery and, at times, the axillary sheath itself may be palpable.

TECHNIQUE. Several techniques can be used to establish that the needle is within the axillary sheath. The first is by eliciting a sensory paresthesia with the needle, but this has little application in pediatric practice, particularly in young children and in those who are anesthetized. The use of a nerve stimulator allows precise placement of the needle in the neurovascular sheath without either the cooperation of the child or the need for painful sensory paresthesias (see Fig. 42.2). In thin children, the sheath can often be palpated as a cord-like structure inferior to the coracobrachialis muscle, allowing the placement of the needle in the sheath by "feel." A transarterial approach can also be used.[374] With all techniques, it is useful to attach a short piece of extension tubing between the needle and syringe to facilitate precise handling during needle placement, aspiration, and drug injection.

The use of a nerve stimulator for the axillary approach to the brachial plexus is best accomplished by abducting the arm to 90 degrees (see E-Fig. 42.2). Care should be taken not to hyperabduct the arm, obscuring the axillary pulse. The artery is palpated in the axilla, and a short beveled needle is advanced toward it (see Fig. 42.20B and C). When using a nerve stimulator, a distal motor response is elicited in the distribution of the radial, ulnar, or median nerves at a threshold of less than 0.2 mA (see E-Fig. 42.2). If one is not using a nerve stimulator, the needle is advanced until a distinct pop is felt as the needle pierces the axillary sheath. The axillary sheath may be divided into fascial compartments for each nerve, and these may limit the spread of local anesthetic within the axillary sheath. Although distinct paresthesias to the distribution of all three nerves may be elicited with the nerve stimulator, and divided doses of anesthetic may be administered to each of those locations, in practice it becomes extremely difficult to find the second and third motor paresthesias after the administration of even a very small amount of local anesthetic with the first injection (Video 42.12). Alternatively, the transarterial technique, which involves direct puncture of the axillary artery, allows deposition of local anesthetic at two sites within the sheath. The needle is aimed directly toward the axillary pulse. As soon as blood is aspirated, the needle is advanced through the posterior wall of the artery. When blood can no longer be aspirated, half of the dose of local anesthetic is deposited posterior to the artery. The needle is withdrawn through the anterior wall of the artery, and the remainder of the dose is deposited anterior to the artery after reconfirming a negative aspiration for blood. Regardless of technique, the local anesthetic is administered in incremental quantities with intermittent aspiration to confirm that the needle is still outside the blood vessel. It is sometimes difficult to block the musculocutaneous nerve, which carries sensory fibers to the radial aspect of the forearm, because it exits the brachial plexus proximal in the axillary fossa. Therefore, some practitioners advocate applying a tourniquet distal to the site where the block is to be performed. Applying a tourniquet promotes proximal spread of local anesthetic and enhances the chances of a successful block of this nerve. Alternatively, the musculocutaneous nerve may be blocked by infiltrating 1 to 3 mL (proportional to the size of the child) of local anesthetic into the body of the coracobrachialis muscle. Regardless of the technique chosen, an additional 1 to 3 mL of local anesthetic is deposited as a subcutaneous cuff to block the intercostobrachial nerve and its communications with the musculocutaneous nerve. These additional quantities of local anesthetic must be accounted for when calculating the total drug dose. An ultrasound may also be used in conjunction with a nerve stimulator to further improve the localization of each nerve bundle (see Figs. 42.20D, 43.16, and 43.21).[370]

SELECTION OF DRUG. Local anesthetics commonly used in our practice include lidocaine and bupivacaine (see Table 42.2). As with other regional techniques that involve larger volumes of local anesthetic, the addition of both levobupivacaine and ropivacaine to the armamentarium is likely to prove beneficial in reducing the risk of toxicity from local anesthetics. Because it is desirable to have a prolonged duration of postoperative analgesia, longer-acting agents are usually used in place of lidocaine. To help ensure block of the musculocutaneous nerve, we use large volumes (0.5 mL/kg), diluting the concentration of local anesthetic with normal saline solution as needed to avoid toxicity. Care must always be taken not to exceed the maximal allowable doses of bupivacaine on a milligram per kilogram basis (2.5 mg/kg).[375] Adding epinephrine (1:200,000) may decrease vascular absorption and the potential for toxicity. Sodium bicarbonate (1 mEq/10 mL of local anesthetic) added to the local anesthetic will speed the onset of blockade by increasing the pH of the solution; this is particularly the case with the premixed anesthetic-epinephrine formulations that have a reduced pH.

COMPLICATIONS. All of the nerves of the brachial plexus occupy a neurovascular bundle and hence are prone to unintended injection into a blood vessel. A hematoma may form at the site of injection. If it is large enough, the hematoma may compress the neurovascular bundle, rendering the limb ischemic. Hence it is important to know the child's coagulation status before attempting the block. Intravascular injection may be avoided with incremental injection and frequent aspiration. Intraneural injection may be minimized by use of a nerve stimulator. Practitioners may feel the importance to check the viability of the radial, median, and ulnar nerves before injecting local anesthetic solution. This block can be carried out in the recovery room after the function of the nerves is determined. A simple rule of thumb is to check the radial nerve (extension of the thumb), median nerve (flexion of the proximal interphalangeal joint of the thumb), and ulnar nerve (scissoring of the fingers) (Video 42.13). This can functionally check the nerves before injection of local anesthetic solution.[376]

INFRACLAVICULAR APPROACH. This approach to the brachial plexus is very helpful, particularly in children who may have fractures making it painful to abduct the arm. A vertical approach to the infraclavicular brachial plexus is performed using the coracoid process as a landmark to access the nerve.[377] We routinely use this technique in children who require continuous infusions of local anesthetic solution in the postoperative period.

TECHNIQUE. With the arm in abduction, the acromial process is palpated. A line drawn 2 cm below and medial to the coracoid process is usually where the needle is introduced (Fig. 42.21A). At this level, the pleura is not usually affected. A sheathed needle with a nerve stimulator is introduced, and the nerve is stimulated at about 1 mA. Any stimulation other than forearm flexion is taken as a positive stimulation of the brachial plexus. Forearm flexion denotes stimulation of the musculocutaneous nerve. The needle should then be directed medial to provide a blockade of the cords of the brachial plexus (see Fig. 42.2B). An ultrasound-guided

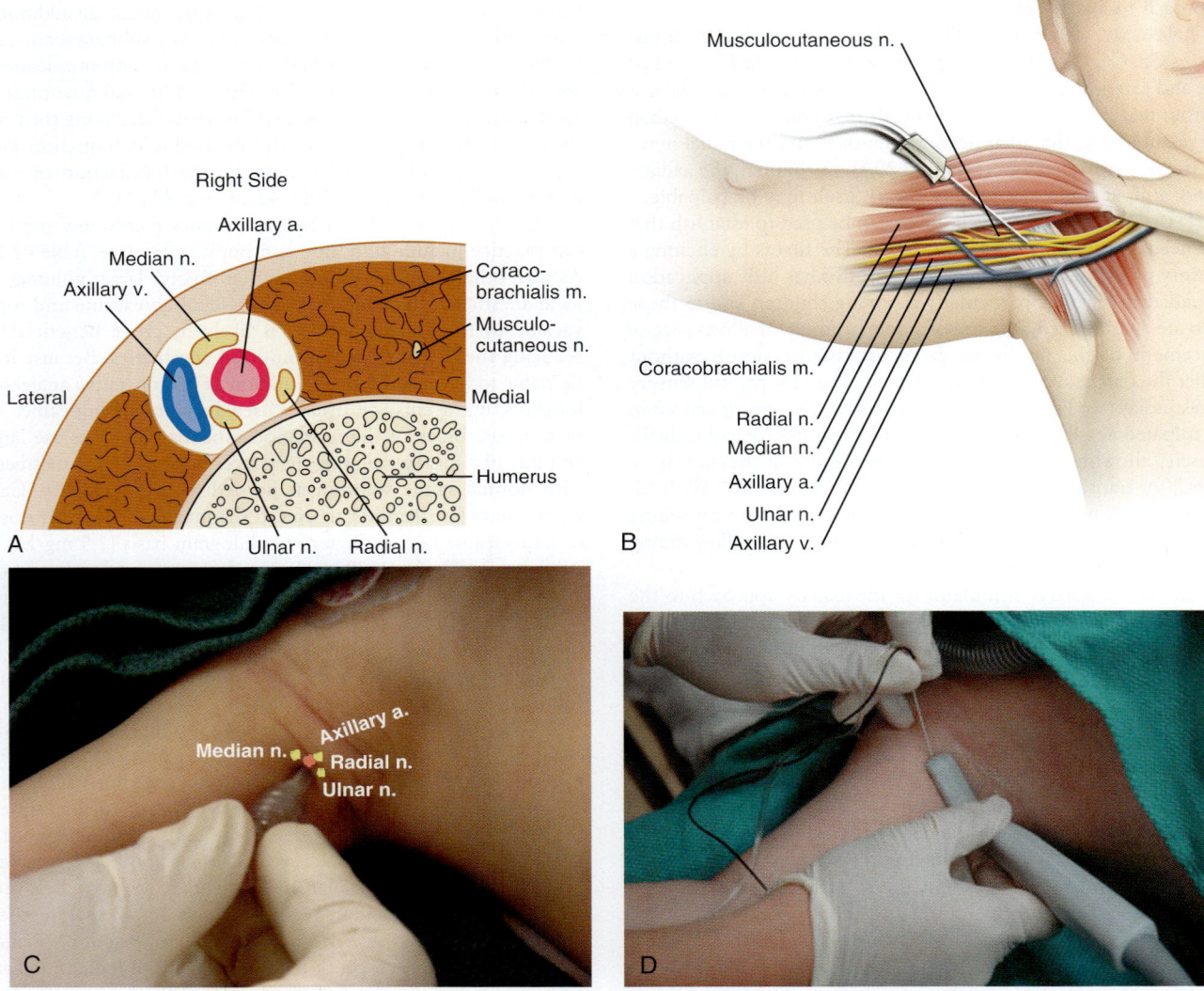

FIGURE 42.20 A and **B,** The anatomic relationships of the brachial plexus are presented. Note that the fascial sheath envelops the nerves and the axillary artery and vein; the musculocutaneous nerve lies within the body of the coracobrachialis muscle. Local anesthetic injected within the sheath (on either side of the axillary artery) produces a satisfactory block. There may be septation within the sheath in some individuals (not pictured). **C,** The axillary artery is palpated with the arm in abduction in the axilla. A needle is introduced superior to the pulsation to block the median nerve. If a nerve stimulator is used, opposition of the thumb can be elicited as the median nerve is stimulated. The needle is then gently positioned below the artery; the ulnar nerve can be blocked in this position. If a nerve stimulator is used, flexion of the fifth finger is elicited. For blocking the radial nerve situated posterior to the artery, it may be necessary to pass the needle posterior to the artery while constantly aspirating to avoid intravascular placement. If the needle does encounter the axillary artery, continue to advance the needle so that the aspirate is negative while the needle is situated posterior to the artery. If a nerve stimulator is used, biceps flexion may be observed. A total volume of 0.1 to 0.15 mL/kg in divided doses between all three nerves will provide an adequate blockade of the nerves. If the axillary artery is encountered while accessing the radial nerve, it is imperative to apply pressure after the block is placed to avoid hematoma formation. **D,** An ultrasound is particularly useful for successful placement of an axillary block. A linear ultrasound probe or a hockey stick probe is placed on the axilla. With the use of an in-plane approach, the median nerve (located anterior to the artery), then the radial nerve (located posterior to the axillary artery), and then the ulnar nerve (located below the artery) are blocked individually. Careful aspiration before injection may prevent intravascular injection. *a,* artery; *m,* muscle; *n,* nerve; *v,* vein.

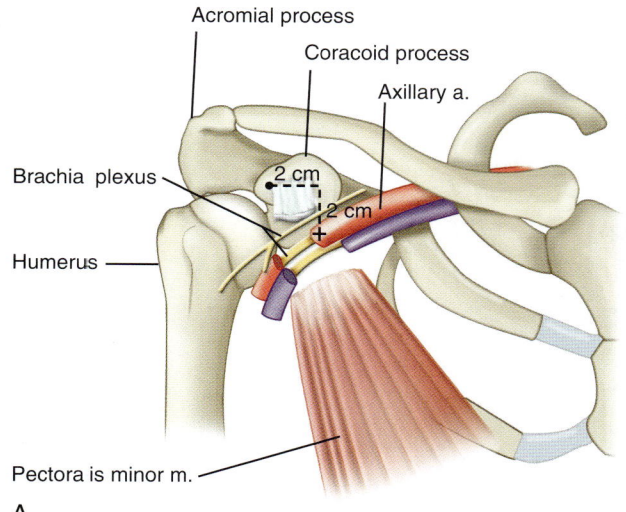

Acromial process
Coracoid process
Axillary a.
Brachia plexus
2 cm
2 cm
Humerus
Pectora is minor m.

A

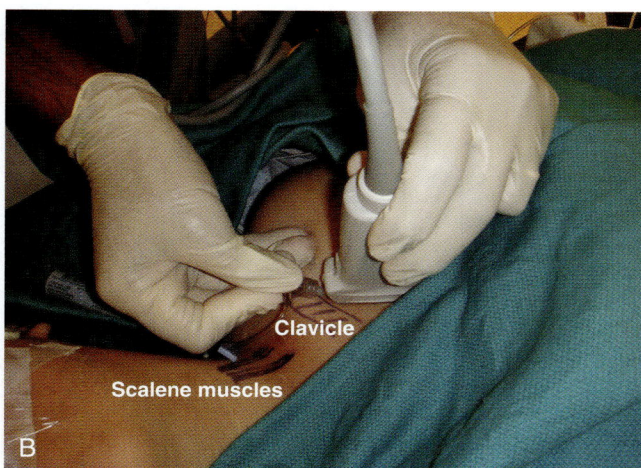

Clavicle

Scalene muscles

B

FIGURE 42.21 A, Anatomic landmarks for the infraclavicular approach to the brachial plexus. Note that the arm is in an abducted position, which may be quite useful for children with fractures. **B,** The coracoid process is palpated. With the arm abducted, a needle is inserted 2 cm medial and inferior to the coracoid process. A nerve stimulator is used and stimulation is initiated at 1 mA and then decreased to 0.4 mA as the nerve is accessed. Elicitation of hand flexion or extension is used as an indicator of being close to the nerve. After asp ration, 0.2 mL/kg of local anesthetic solution is injected. Use of ultrasound may also improve the success of this block. *a*, artery; *m*, muscle. (Modified from Wilson JL, Brown DL, Wong GY, et al. Infraclavicular brachial plexus block: parasagittal anatomy important to the coracoid technique. *Anesth Analg.* 1998;87[4]:870–873.)

technique may also be used and is preferred (see also Chapter 43 and Figs. 43.17 to 43.19).

COMPLICATIONS. There is the potential for intrapleural injection and pneumothorax, especially if the needle is directed medially. Because of the proximity of the plexus to the subclavian vein and artery, it is imperative that the procedure not be attempted on children who have coagulation abnormalities.

SUPRACLAVICULAR APPROACH. This is an easy approach to the brachial plexus in children and can be readily performed, particularly with the aid of ultrasound guidance. The risk with performing this procedure without ultrasound guidance is the potential for injection into the vertebral artery. It can be used for most procedures performed on the upper arm and forearm. The cervical pleura is also located close to the supraclavicular plexus; thus caution should be exercised while performing this block. The entire brachial plexus, including the musculocutaneous and the axillary nerves, is located lateral to the artery. Occasionally, the suprascapular nerve may leave the upper trunk more cranially.

INDICATIONS. This block is used for analgesia or anesthesia for upper arm surgery and can be performed with either a single injection or catheter technique.

TECHNIQUE. The supraclavicular plexus is located above the clavicle and is approximately at the middle of the sternocleidomastoid. A stimulating needle (1 mA) is passed above the clavicle lateral to the arterial pulsation and close to the inferior margin of the anterior scalene. The plexus is located superficially and can be easily stimulated as soon as the skin is pierced. Any movement of the child's fingers or arm is accepted as an adequate stimulation to the plexus. The energy is reduced to 0.4 mA and, if continued response to the stimulation is observed, 0.15 to 0.2 mL/kg of local anesthetic solution is injected in graduated doses after careful aspiration.

The ultrasound-guided technique is now our preferred method for blocking the supraclavicular plexus. We use a linear probe or a hockey stick probe and, using the in-plane technique, pass the needle close to the plexus. If a stimulating needle is used, the needle is advanced until we see movement of the hand. We have been able to decrease the dose of local anesthetic solution to 0.15 to 0.2 mL/kg (Fig. 42.22 and Video 42.14; see also Fig. 43.16).

COMPLICATIONS. Pleural puncture and intravascular injection can occur from misplacement of the needle.

Interscalene Approach

This approach is not commonly used in children. The main indication for this technique is for children undergoing shoulder surgery; this approach is generally reserved for the older teenager or young adult.

ANATOMY. The interscalene groove is formed by the anterior and middle scalene muscles and is located in most children at the lateral border of the sternocleidomastoid muscle (see Fig. 42.22A). The upper three nerve roots are superficial, whereas the lower two roots are in a deeper position. In children the lower nerve roots are close to the pleura, which may increase the potential for a pneumothorax. The phrenic nerve is also close to the nerve roots and may often be unintentionally blocked on the side of the intended nerve block. Therefore this block is clearly avoided in children who may have a compromised pulmonary system. The vertebral artery is located in close proximity to the lower nerve roots (C7) and hence it is important to aspirate and ensure that the needle is not in a vessel.

INDICATIONS. Shoulder and upper arm surgery and ensuing postoperative analgesia can be provided with this block.

Conventional Techniques. Dalens and associates reported a technique of parascalene brachial plexus blockade for pediatric shoulder surgery using an extended head position and placing the puncture between the lower and middle thirds of the line extending from the center of the clavicle to the C6 transverse process (Chassaignac tubercle; see Fig. 42.22A).[378] The rationale for selecting this puncture site was to avoid the vertebral artery and pleura. With the use of a perpendicular needle orientation, the lower roots (C8 and T1) are not blocked at all or require very large amounts of local anesthetic to be successfully blocked. Ultrasound guidance is greatly advantageous in this situation because it paves the way for safe blockade of both roots (C8 and

42

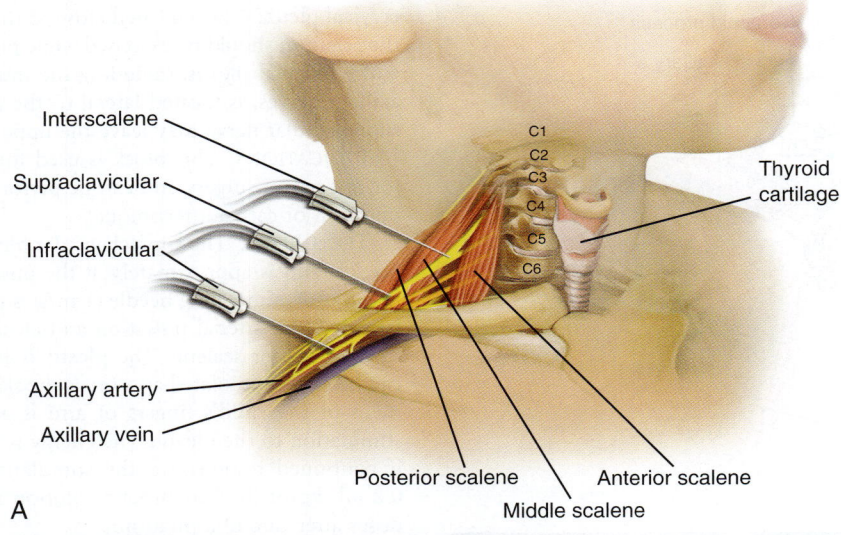

A

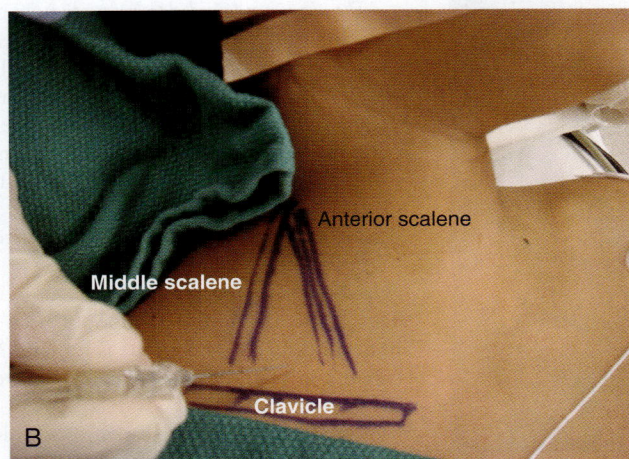

B

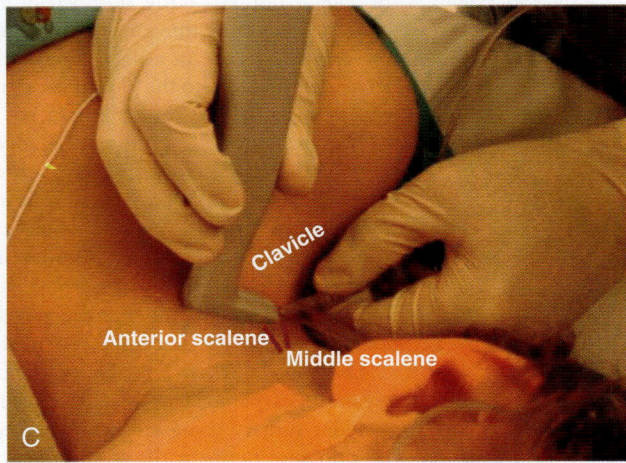

C

FIGURE 42.22 A right-sided supraclavicular block (landmark technique): The supraclavicular block is used frequently in children for most procedures on the hand and elbow. **A,** The divisions and cords are located around the carotid artery cephalad to the clavicle at the inferior margins of the scalene muscles. **B,** A stimulating needle, using 0.5 mA of energy, is introduced at the inferior border of the anterior scalene muscle. Any movement of the patient's fingers (including flexion or extension) suggests adequate positioning of the needle. After aspiration to avoid intravascular injection, 0.15 mL/kg of local anesthetic solution is injected. **C,** Supraclavicular block with ultrasound guidance. A linear ultrasound probe or a hockey stick probe is placed lateral to the suprasternal notch and above the clavicle. The carotid artery is identified. The supraclavicular plexus is located around the carotid artery at this location like a "bunch of grapes." A needle is placed in an in-plane approach (along the axis of the probe), and the plexus is penetrated. Injection of local anesthetic solution will be seen as a hypoechoic spread around the plexus.

T1). With the use of a nerve stimulator, diaphragmatic stimulation may be observed as a result of ventromedial needle position (the phrenic nerve runs ventral to the body of the anterior scalene muscle).

Ultrasound-Guided Technique (see Chapter 43). To visualize the anatomic structures of a child's neck, a high-frequency linear ultrasound probe is used. The process is facilitated by slightly turning the child's head to the contralateral side. The probe should be oriented from the medial to the lateral aspect. Medially, the thyroid gland and the major vessels in the neck area (carotid artery and internal jugular vein) are easily identified. Then the probe is moved along the sternocleidomastoid muscle until its lateral border is reached. At the same time, the transducer is moved in a caudal direction such that the posterior scalene gap and the upper anterior roots (C5-7) of the brachial plexus become visible between the anterior and medial scalene muscles. In very small children, all roots of the brachial plexus (C5-T1) can be simultaneously visualized. The puncture is performed in a tangential direction relative to the neck above the transducer. The C5 nerve root will be encountered superficially, within a few millimeters. As a rule, the needle should be oriented lateral to the C7 root, which will ensure that the neck vessels remain at an adequate distance from the needle insertion site. As soon as the local anesthetic has been injected, it will spread toward the C5 root, which can be visualized in the ultrasound image. Depending on the blockade required, the needle can be advanced to a deeper level for injection after the deep roots (C8 and T1) have been visualized. If the local anesthetic fails to spread adequately in a medial direction, the needle is retracted toward the subcutaneous level and is then repositioned on the medial side of the posterior scalene gap in the area of the C7 root. In the majority of cases, however, the local anesthetic will spread in an adequate manner even when the needle is in a lateral position. The injected volume of local anesthetic should not exceed the amount necessary to fully cover the root surfaces. It is, therefore, inappropriate to recommend a specific volume. In general, however, complete blockade via the interscalene route can be expected with local anesthetic volumes of 0.15 to 0.25 mL/kg.

COMPLICATIONS. Pneumothorax, intravascular injection, and temporary phrenic nerve injury are risks of this block.

Intravenous Regional Anesthesia

IV regional anesthesia was first described in 1908 by August Bier and is frequently referred to as the Bier block.[379] This technique has been advocated for upper extremity procedures lasting 30 to 60 minutes in children because of its rapid onset of anesthesia and its ease of performance.[380-382] *Only dilute lidocaine (0.25% or 0.5%) can be used because of the risk of local-anesthetic toxicity, particularly if the tourniquet is deflated early or inadvertently.* This can be a useful block for upper extremity fracture reduction or suture of a large laceration in children with a full stomach. It is also helpful for chronic painful conditions, including complex regional pain syndrome type 1, in children and adolescents.[383] The exsanguination and manipulation of the limb before administering the local anesthetic may prove to be unduly painful for children with a fracture, and many children may not tolerate the discomfort of the tourniquet without significant sedation. Another disadvantage is the possibility of toxic reactions in the event of tourniquet failure. Strict attention to detail—elevation or exsanguination of the extremity to be blocked, proper application of a double pneumatic cuff, careful attention to anesthetic dose, and care not to deflate the tourniquet until 30 minutes after injection of the local anesthetic—is

important to avoid serious complications and provide a successful block. This block is unsuitable for infants (those younger than 1 year of age) because of the risk of toxic reactions in infants. This technique may also be contraindicated in children in whom the prolonged use of a tourniquet is inadvisable.

TECHNIQUE. A small-gauge IV cannula is inserted in a vein on the dorsum of the hand. Exsanguination of the arm is accomplished either by wrapping the limb with an Esmarch bandage, or by elevating the limb if wrapping is too painful. The proximal compartment of a double tourniquet is inflated to a pressure of 200 to 250 mm Hg, although some have recommended that it be inflated to 150 mm Hg greater than the child's systolic blood pressure. If tourniquet pain develops during the course of the procedure, the distal cuff may be inflated, followed by deflation of the proximal cuff. The tourniquet must remain inflated for a minimum of 30 minutes to prevent a rapid IV infusion of lidocaine and sequelae. It is best to deflate the tourniquet incrementally. Because no residual blockade persists after the tourniquet is released, supplementary analgesia must be considered (e.g., IV opioids, local infiltration with a long-acting local anesthetic).

SELECTION OF DRUG. Use 1 mL/kg of *preservative-free* 0.25 to 0.5% lidocaine without epinephrine for this block because the duration of the block is limited by the tourniquet time and because of the greater potential for cardiac toxicity with longer-acting agents. A very low dose of a nondepolarizing neuromuscular blocking agent, such as rocuronium (0.03 mg/kg), may improve the quality of the motor blockade.[384-386]

COMPLICATIONS. Unintended deflation of the tourniquet results in release of drug into the intravascular compartment; hence, only a short-acting local anesthetic, such as lidocaine, should be used. *Bupivacaine should never be used for this block because of the risk of cardiotoxicity.*

Peripheral Blocks at the Elbow

There is usually no great advantage to blocking the peripheral nerves at the elbow compared with blocking them at the wrist for analgesia or anesthesia of the hand because the forearm is supplied by cutaneous branches that originate in the upper arm. However, on some occasions (e.g., to avoid injections into surgical fields or areas of infection), anesthesia of the hand may be achieved by blocking the appropriate nerves at the elbow because the cutaneous nerve supply to the hand arises at the elbow.

Radial Nerve

ANATOMY. The radial nerve supplies the radial side of the dorsum of the hand and the proximal parts of the radial three-and-a-half digits. Block at the elbow is useful for the provision of anesthesia for an arteriovenous fistula. It is also useful to supplement an inadequate brachial plexus block at the axillary level. The radial nerve passes over the anterior aspect of the lateral epicondyle (Fig. 42.23A).

TECHNIQUE. The intercondylar line is marked. After identification of the biceps tendon, a 27-gauge needle is inserted directly toward the bone of the lateral epicondyle toward the lateral margin; 2.0 to 5.0 mL (depending on the child's weight) of bupivacaine (0.25% with epinephrine 1 : 200,000) is injected into the area (see Fig. 42.23B). Ultrasound guidance can help with determination of the exact location of the nerve in the forearm (see Chapter 43 and Figs. 43.22 and 43.23).

COMPLICATIONS. Intravascular injection and intraneural injections are potential complications. The use of a nerve stimulator or ultrasound can reduce unintended intraneural injection.

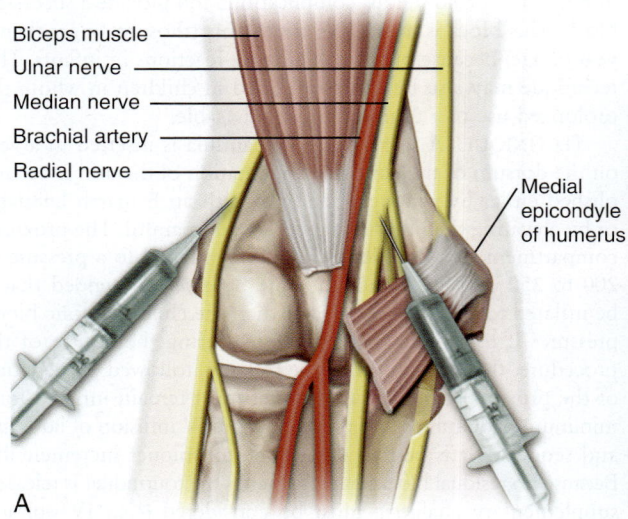

Biceps muscle
Ulnar nerve
Median nerve
Brachial artery
Radial nerve

Medial epicondyle of humerus

A

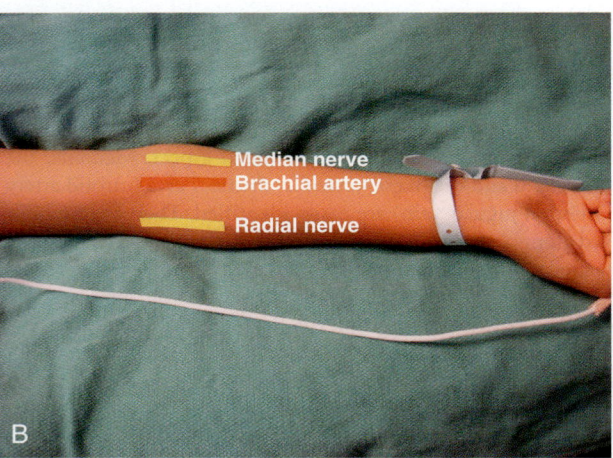

Median nerve
Brachial artery
Radial nerve

B

FIGURE 42.23 A, Anatomic relationship of the nerves around the elbow. **B,** Radial nerve block: the intercondylar line is marked. After identification of the biceps tendon, a 27-gauge needle is inserted directly toward the bone of the lateral epicondyle toward the lateral margin; 2.0 to 5.0 mL (depending on the patient's weight) of bupivacaine (0.25% with epinephrine 1:200,000) is injected into the area. To block the median nerve, the brachial artery is palpated at the elbow crease. The median nerve is located immediately medial to the brachial artery. A nerve stimulator is used, and flexion of the patient's fingers denotes adequate localization of the nerve.

Intravascular injection may be avoided with incremental injection and frequent aspiration.

Median Nerve

ANATOMY. This nerve supplies the radial side of the palm and the three-and-a-half digits of the palmar aspect (see Fig. 42.23A). It accompanies the brachial artery in its course down the arm. It is initially lateral and then crosses the ventral side of the artery and eventually lies medial to the artery at the bend of the elbow. It is deep to the bicipital fascia and superficial to the brachialis muscle.

TECHNIQUE. The arm is abducted and the forearm supinated. After marking the intercondylar line between the medial and the lateral epicondyle of the humerus, the brachial artery is palpated (see Fig. 42.23A). A 27-gauge needle is inserted just medial to the artery and directed perpendicular to the skin; 2.0 to 5.0 mL (depending on the child's weight) of bupivacaine (0.25% with epinephrine 1:200,000) is injected into the site. Caution must be exercised to avoid the artery because it is in close proximity to the nerve. Surface mapping using a nerve stimulator probe generating 5 mA or greater can be used to locate the nerve in the forearm if there is difficulty in palpating the artery (see Fig. 42.23A).[387] An ultrasound-guided technique may also be used for this block (see Chapter 43 and Fig. 43.22).

COMPLICATIONS. Intravascular injection and intraneural injections are potential complications. The use of a nerve stimulator can prevent the unintended intraneural injection. Intravascular injection may be avoided with incremental injection and frequent aspiration.

Ulnar Nerve

ANATOMY. The ulnar nerve is the superficial nerve to the arm and the ulnar side of the forearm and the hand. It is the terminal continuation of the medial cord of the brachial plexus. At the elbow, it pierces the medial intermuscular septum and follows along the medial head of the triceps to the groove between the olecranon and the medial epicondyle of the humerus. It is covered only by skin and fascia and can be easily palpated and blocked at this level (see Figs. 42.13 and 42.24A and B).

TECHNIQUE. With the child supine, the elbow is flexed. The medial epicondyle and the ulnar groove are palpated (see Fig. 42.24). A 27-gauge needle is advanced perpendicular to the skin along the line of the nerve; 1 to 3 mL (depending on the child's weight) of bupivacaine (0.25% with epinephrine 1:200,000) is injected into the area. An ultrasound-guided technique may also be used for this block (see Chapter 43 and Fig. 43.22).

COMPLICATIONS. Intravascular injection and intraneural injections are potential complications. Because this is a very superficial nerve, injection just after the skin is pierced in the area of the ulnar nerve usually produces a good block. Intravascular injection may be avoided with incremental injection and frequent aspiration.

Wrist Blocks

Blocking the median, radial, and ulnar nerves at the wrist can be easily achieved. These blocks provide very good analgesia and, because they are easy to perform, they generally have a predictable successful outcome.

Radial Nerve

The cutaneous branches of the radial nerve supply the radial side of the dorsum of the hand and the proximal parts of the radial three-and-a-half digits.

ANATOMY. The superficial branch of the radial nerve runs along the lateral border of the forearm under the brachioradialis muscle. In the distal third of the forearm it angles dorsally under the tendon of the brachioradialis toward the dorsum of the wrist. It pierces the deep fascia and divides into two branches: (1) the lateral branch supplies the radial side and the tip of the thumb

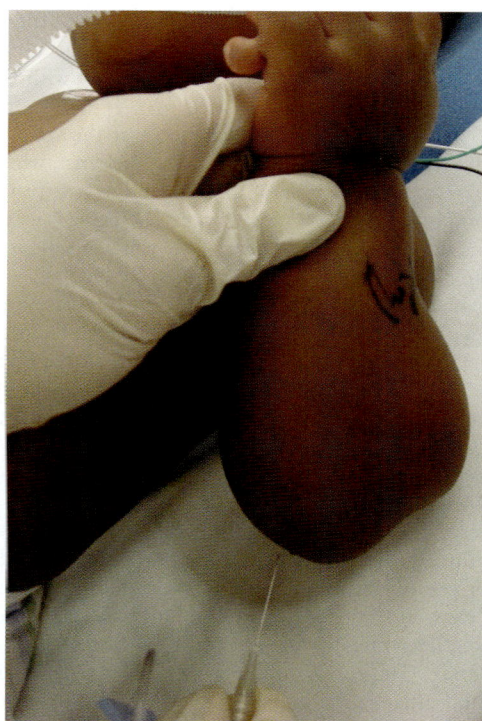

FIGURE 42.24 Ulnar nerve block at the elbow. The olecranon process is palpated. The ulnar nerve is located in the olecranon groove; after aspiration, 1 to 3 mL of local anesthetic solution is injected. It is important not to deposit the local anesthetic deep into the olecranon groove because the nerve is superficial and can be easily blocked by a subcutaneous injection.

and (2) the medial branch communicates with the dorsal branch of the ulnar nerve. This then divides into the four digital nerves that supply the ulnar side of the thumb, the radial side of the index finger, and the space between the index finger and thumb. A communicating branch with the ulnar nerve supplies the adjacent sides of the middle and ring finger (Fig. 42.25A).

TECHNIQUE. This is essentially a field block of the superficial terminal branches. An attempt to make the "anatomic snuffbox" prominent by extension of the thumb before anesthesia is desirable. The extensor pollicis and brevis tendons are marked. A 27-gauge needle is inserted close to the dorsal radial tubercle over the extensor longus tendon, and 2.0 mL of bupivacaine (0.25% with epinephrine 1:200,000) is injected SC. An attempt to fan the local anesthetic in the anatomic snuffbox helps to distribute the local anesthetic over the radial nerve (see Fig. 42.25B).

COMPLICATIONS. Intravascular injection may be avoided with incremental injection and frequent aspiration. Post–nerve block dysesthesia may be occasionally experienced with a radial nerve block and is usually self-limited.

Median Nerve

ANATOMY. In the palm of the hand, the median nerve is very superficial and is covered only by skin and the palmar aponeurosis and rests on the tendons of the flexor muscles. It emerges from under the retinaculum and splits into muscular and digital branches. The muscular division of the median nerve supplies the muscles of the thenar eminence. The palmar digital nerve supplies the thumb, index finger, middle finger, and ring finger. These nerves also supply the lumbricals (Fig. 42.26A).

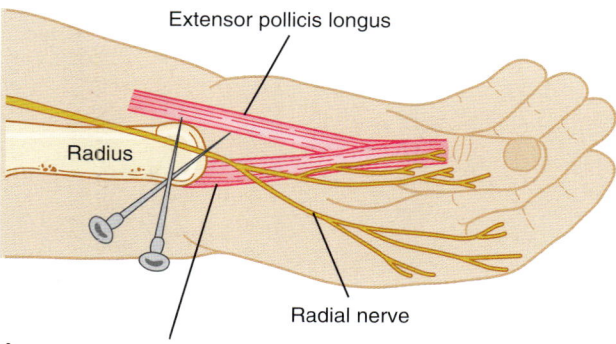

Extensor pollicis longus

Radius

Extensor pollicis brevis

Radial nerve

A

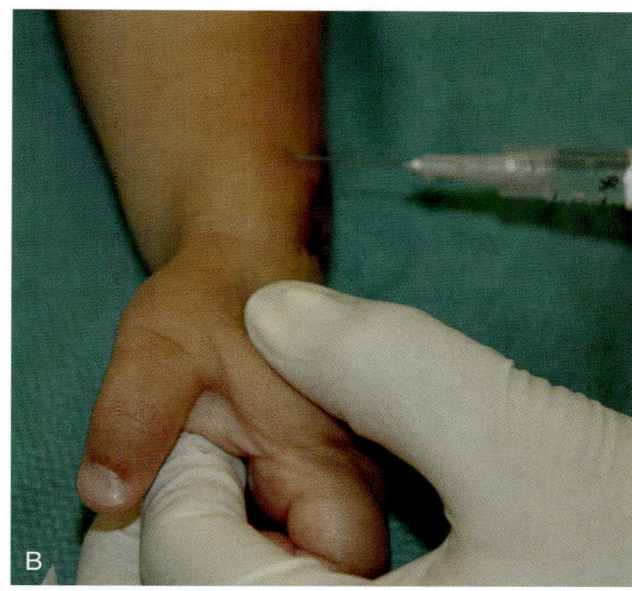

B

FIGURE 42.25 Wrist block: radial nerve. **A,** This is a superficial block of the terminal branches of the radial nerve. An attempt to make the "anatomic snuffbox" prominent by extension of the thumb before anesthesia is desirable. The extensor pollicis and brevis tendons are marked. **B,** A 27-gauge needle is inserted close to the dorsal radial tubercle over the extensor longus tendon; bupivacaine (2 mL, 0.25% with 1:200,000 epinephrine) is injected subcutaneously. Fanning the local anesthetic in the anatomic snuffbox helps to distribute the local anesthetic over the radial nerve. (Modified from Raj P, Pai U. Techniques of nerve block ng. In: Raj P, ed. *Handbook of Regional Anesthesia.* New York: Churchill Livingstone; 1985:185.)

TECHNIQUE. The palmaris tendon is identified. This may be done before general anesthesia by asking the child to flex the wrist against resistance. The radial border of the tendon is identified. Cutaneous landmarks include both distal wrist skin creases. A 27-gauge needle is inserted at the level of the second skin crease (1–1.5 cm proximal to the distal crease in teenagers) perpendicular to the skin. The nerve is at a depth of less than 1 cm in the teenager and less in younger children; 1.0 to 2.0 mL of bupivacaine (0.25% with epinephrine 1:200,000) is injected into the area (see Fig. 42.26B). If the child is awake, it is better to elicit paresthesias because the needle may be anterior to the neurovascular bundle and the nerve could be missed altogether.

COMPLICATIONS. Intravascular placement should be avoided by repeated aspiration before injection.

42

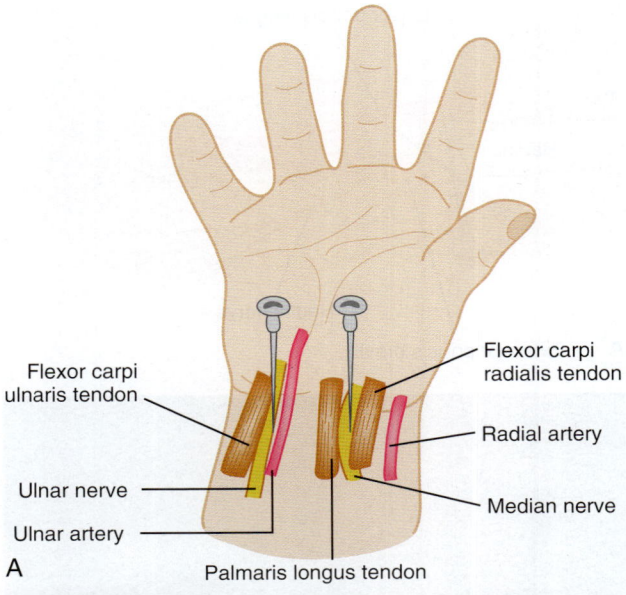

Flexor carpi
ulnaris tendon

Flexor carpi
radialis tendon

Radial artery

Ulnar nerve

Median nerve

Ulnar artery

Palmaris longus tendon

A

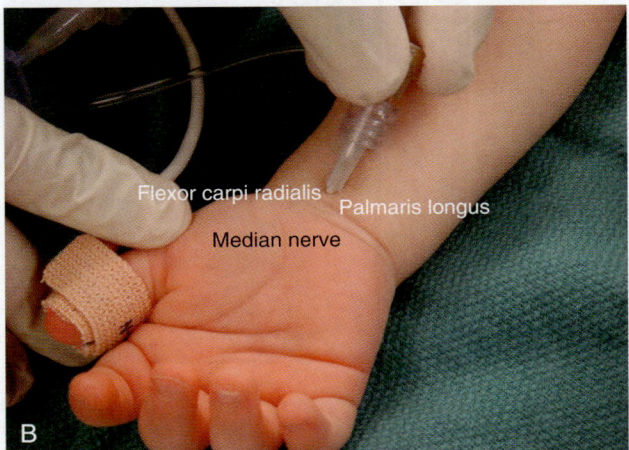

Flexor carpi radialis

Palmaris longus

Median nerve

B

FIGURE 42.26 Wrist block: median and ulnar nerves. **A,** Median nerve: identify the palmaris tendon by asking the child to flex the wrist against resistance. Distal skin creases are identified. **B,** A 27-gauge needle is inserted at the level of the distal skin crease perpendicular to the skin. The nerve is at a depth of less than 1 cm in teenagers and less than that in younger children; 1.0 to 2.0 mL of bupivacaine (0.25% with 1:200.000 epinephrine) is injected in the area. If the child is awake, it is better to elicit paresthesias because the needle may be anterior to the neurovascular bundle, which can be missed altogether. Ulnar nerve: identify the flexor carpi ulnaris tendon, which lies proximal to the pisiform bone. A 27-gauge needle is inserted just proximal to the pisiform bone and directed radially a distance of approximately 0.5 cm. Bupivacaine (2–3 mL, 0.25% with epinephrine 1:200,000) is injected. (Modified from Raj P, Pai U. Techniques of nerve blocking. In: Raj P, ed. *Handbook of Regional Anesthesia.* New York: Churchill Livingstone; 1985:185.)

Ulnar Nerve

ANATOMY. The palmar cutaneous branch of the ulnar nerve arises near the middle of the forearm and accompanies the ulnar artery into the hand (see Fig. 42.26A). It then perforates the flexor retinaculum and ends in the skin of the palm communicating with the palmar branch of the median nerve. There are two dorsal digital nerves and a metacarpal communicating branch. The more medial digital nerve supplies the ulnar side of the little finger and

the digital branch supplies the adjacent sides of the little and ring finger. The palmar or the terminal portion of the ulnar nerve crosses the ulnar border of the wrist in company with the ulnar artery.

TECHNIQUE. Blocking the ulnar nerve at the wrist is easier than at the elbow. The nerve is blocked at the wrist, where it lies under cover of the flexor carpi ulnaris tendon just proximal to the pisiform bone. The best way to access the nerve is to approach it from the ulnar side of the tendon. A 27-gauge needle is inserted just proximal to the pisiform bone and directed radially a distance of approximately 0.5 cm; 2.0 to 3.0 mL of bupivacaine (0.25% with epinephrine 1:200,000) is injected (see Fig. 42.26A).

COMPLICATIONS. The ulnar artery runs in close proximity to the ulnar nerve; every possible effort should be made to avoid intravascular placement. Intravascular injection may be avoided with incremental injection with frequent aspiration.

Digital Nerve Blocks: Hand

Digital nerve blocks are useful for providing pain relief to children who are undergoing procedures to individual fingers. These are useful for postoperative analgesia in procedures, such as trigger finger release, and also for the provision of pain relief in children undergoing laser therapy for warts on their fingers.[388]

ANATOMY. The common digital nerves are derived from the median and ulnar nerves and divide in the palm to volar digital nerves that supply the fingers. All digital nerves are usually accompanied by digital vessels. There are three digital nerves derived from the median nerve. The first common digital nerve divides into three palmar digital nerves that supply the sides of the thumb; the second common digital nerve supplies the web between the index and middle finger; and the third common palmar digital nerve communicates with a branch of the ulnar nerve and supplies the web space between the middle and ring fingers. These common digital nerves then become the proper digital nerves (digital collaterals) that supply the skin of the palmar surface and the dorsal side of the terminal phalanx of their respective digits. All digital nerves ultimately terminate in two branches: one ramifies in the skin of the fingertips and the other ends in the pulp under the nail. Smaller digital nerves are derived from the radial and ulnar nerves and supply the back of the fingers. These tend to lie on the dorsolateral aspect of the finger. There are four dorsal digital nerves: (1) ulnar side of the thumb; (2) radial side of the index finger; (3) adjacent sides of index and middle fingers; and (4) communication to the adjacent sides of middle and ring finger.

TECHNIQUE. There are two techniques for blockade of the digital nerves.

For blockade at the base of the thumb (Fig. 42.27A and B), with the thumb extended, on the palmar surface of the hand, a 27-gauge needle is inserted into the web space between the index finger and thumb. The needle is advanced to the junction of the web space and the palmar skin of the hand, a distance of about 1 cm; 0.5 mL of bupivacaine *without epinephrine* is injected. A second needle is inserted into the thenar eminence on the radial aspect of the thumb; 1.0 mL of bupivacaine *without epinephrine* is injected. Caution has to be exercised if the child has collagen vascular disease, because this may precipitate acute vascular spasm that may not be relieved.

Blockade of the other fingers is accomplished at the bifurcation between the metacarpal heads (see Fig. 42.27B and C). With the fingers extended, a 27-gauge needle is inserted into the web about 3 mm proximal to the junction between the web and the palmar

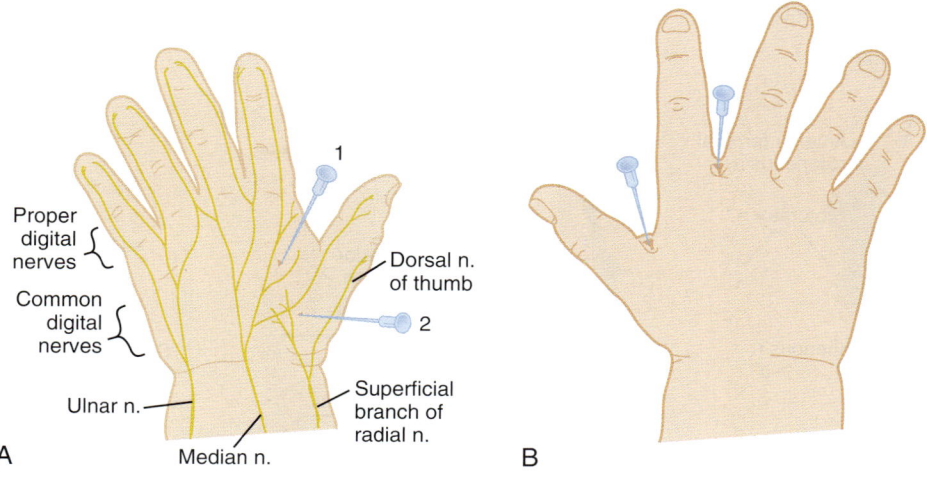

42

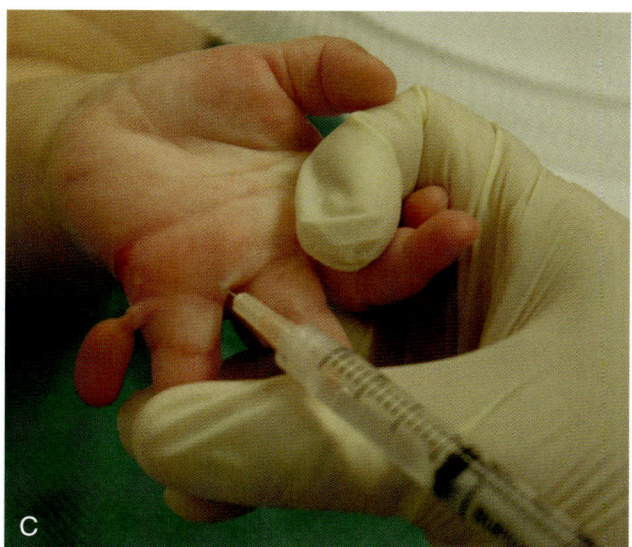

FIGURE 42.27 Digital nerve blocks. **A,** Blockade of the thumb: with the thumb extended, on the palmar surface of the hand, a 27-gauge needle is inserted into the web space between the index finger and thumb (*1*). The needle is advanced to the junction of the web space and the palmar skin of the hand a distance of about 1 cm; bupivacaine (0.5 mL, *without epinephrine*) is injected. A second needle is inserted into the thenar eminence on the radial aspect of the thumb, and 1.0 mL of bupivacaine *without epinephrine* is injected (*2*). Caution has to be exercised if the patient has collagen vascular disease because this may precipitate acute vascular spasm that may not be relieved. **B,** Blockade of other digits: blockade of the other fingers is accomplished at the bifurcation between the metacarpal heads. With the fingers widely extended, a 27-gauge needle is inserted into the web about 3 mm proximal to the junction between the web and the palmar skin; bupivacaine (1.0 to 2.0 mL, *without epinephrine*) is injected. **C,** This can be performed either from a dorsal approach or a volar approach. The web on either side will have to be blocked to provide analgesia for each finger to be anesthetized. *n*, nerve.

skin; 1.0 to 2.0 mL of bupivacaine *without epinephrine* is injected. This can be performed either from a dorsal approach or a volar approach.

Caution: Vasoconstrictors are avoided when blocking digital nerves because these are end vessels and acute vasospasm caused by epinephrine can lead to permanent damage or necrosis of the digits. The use of dilute epinephrine concentrations (1 : 100,000–1 : 200,000) in digital nerve blocks may be undergoing a renaissance as epinephrine with local anesthetics have been in used in almost 3000 digital blocks without sequelae.[389]

COMPLICATIONS. Large volumes of local anesthetic are contraindicated because of the possibility of pressure and vascular

compromise. Vasoconstrictors are generally avoided because they may cause necrosis of the digit. Intravascular injection may be avoided with incremental injection and frequent aspiration.

LOWER EXTREMITY BLOCKS

The major use of nerve blocks of the lower extremity in children is for managing postoperative pain and as an adjunct to general anesthesia. When considering the sensory and cutaneous innervation of the lower extremity (Fig. 42.28), it is not surprising that few surgical procedures can be accomplished under single nerve blocks. However, combinations of sciatic, femoral, and lateral femoral cutaneous blockade can provide both excellent postoperative

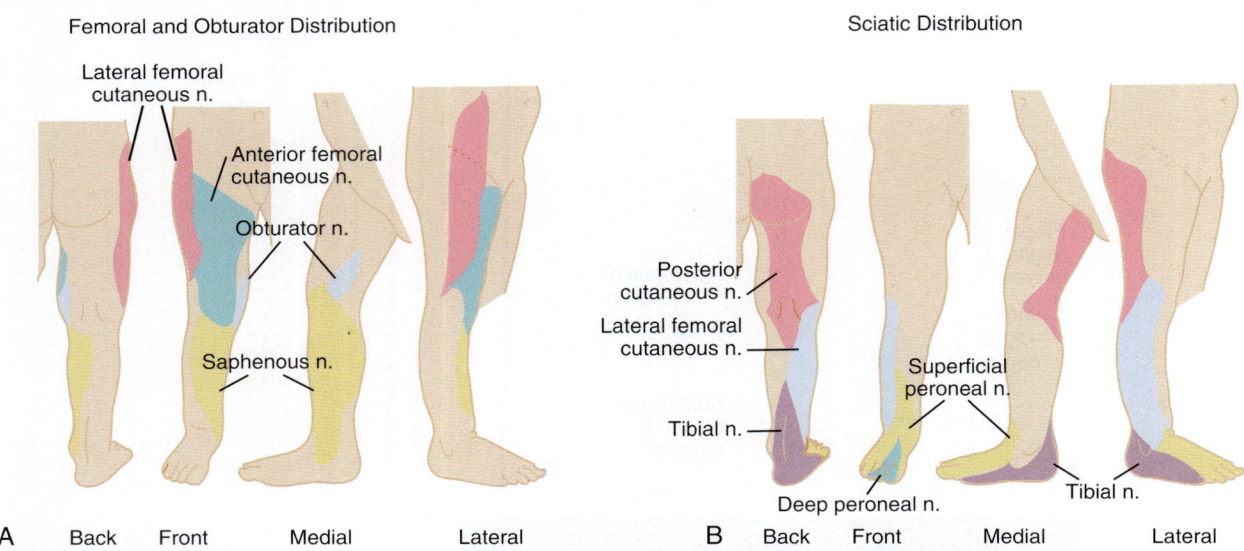

Femoral and Obturator Distribution   Sciatic Distribution

FIGURE 42.28 The sensory innervation of the lower extremity is presented. Note that anesthesia of the lower extremity requires block of the femoral nerve **(A)** (and its branches), as well as the sciatic nerve **(B)**. *n*, nerve.

analgesia and surgical anesthesia for selected operations; the fascia iliaca block produces anesthesia of multiple nerves with a single injection. Continuous peripheral nerve blocks extend the duration of postoperative analgesia with a good safety profile (https://www.asra.com/advisory-guidelines/article/1/anticoagulation-3rd-edition.ia). In a large review of peripheral nerve blocks, with lower extremity blocks accounting for 85% of blocks, the incidence of complications was 12.1% (95% CI 10.7%–13.5%), most commonly catheter malfunction, block failure, superficial infection, and vascular puncture; there were no reports of persistent neurologic problems, catheter malfunctions, or toxicity.[390]

Sciatic Nerve Block

ANATOMY. The sciatic nerve arises from the L4 through S3 roots of the sacral plexus, passes through the pelvis, and becomes superficial at the lower margin of the gluteus maximus muscle. It then descends into the lower extremity in the posterior aspect of the thigh, supplying sensory innervation to the posterior thigh, as well as to the entire leg and foot below the level of the knee, except for the medial aspect, which is supplied by the femoral nerve (see Fig. 42.28A). Although a sciatic nerve block alone is useful for few surgical procedures, it can be combined with a femoral nerve block for operations below the knee and for postoperative pain relief. There are multiple approaches to the sciatic nerve.[391] All blocks in the absence of ultrasound guidance, are performed with the aid of a nerve stimulator to elicit a motor paresthesia in the foot, and, if the block is performed in a lightly sedated trauma victim, the approach that places the child in a greater position of comfort should be chosen. Ultrasound guidance improves the performance of the nerve block (see Chapter 43). A newer approach to the sciatic nerve using a lateral approach to the popliteal fossa has been described. This offers the additional advantage of being able to provide the block in the supine position. An infragluteal-parabiceps approach is another easy method of providing a sciatic nerve block in children.[392]

APPROACH OF LABAT (POSTERIOR APPROACH). The child is placed in the lateral decubitus position lying on the nonoperative leg. The leg to be blocked is flexed and the lower leg is extended (Fig. 42.29A). A line is drawn from the posterior superior iliac spine to the greater trochanter of the femur. Another line is drawn from the greater trochanter to the coccyx. The first line is bisected, and a perpendicular line is drawn from that point to the second line; the point at which it intersects the second line is the site of needle insertion (see Fig. 42.29B). A 22-gauge insulated needle is advanced in the perpendicular plane until it strikes bone. It is possible for the needle to pass through the sciatic notch without either encountering bone or causing a paresthesia. In that case, the needle is redirected in a cephalad direction until bone is encountered. A motor paresthesia is then sought using an organized grid-like approach, fanning medially to laterally.

ANTERIOR APPROACH. As the sciatic nerve emerges from the lower border of the gluteus maximus to extend down the thigh, it passes medial and deep to the lesser trochanter of the femur (Fig. 42.30A; see also Figs. 42.31 and 42.32).

With the child in the supine position, a line is drawn from the anterior superior iliac spine to the pubic tuberosity. The greater trochanter is then located, and another line is drawn parallel to the first line (see Fig. 42.30B); at the medial one-third of the first line, a perpendicular is dropped to the second line. The point of intersection with the line originating at the greater trochanter marks the point of needle entry. The needle is inserted in a perpendicular plane until bone is encountered. It is then partially withdrawn and redirected medially. When the needle is posterior to the medial margin of the femur, ease of injection is determined after negative aspiration for blood. This approach carries a greater risk of unintended puncture of the femoral vessels, and repeated negative aspirations must precede incremental injection. If the needle is in muscle or a fascial bundle, resistance to injection will be felt. In this case, the needle is advanced until minimal resistance to injection is felt. Motor paresthesia is a helpful indicator.

For the previous two techniques, a dose of 0.2 mL/kg of bupivacaine (0.25% with epinephrine 1:200,000) is the dose usually administered for children older than 6 months of age. If the sciatic nerve block is used in conjunction with a femoral nerve block, consideration should be given to diluting the local anesthetic

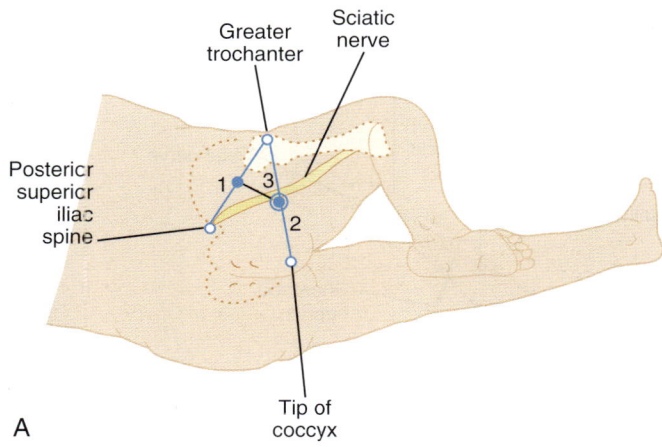

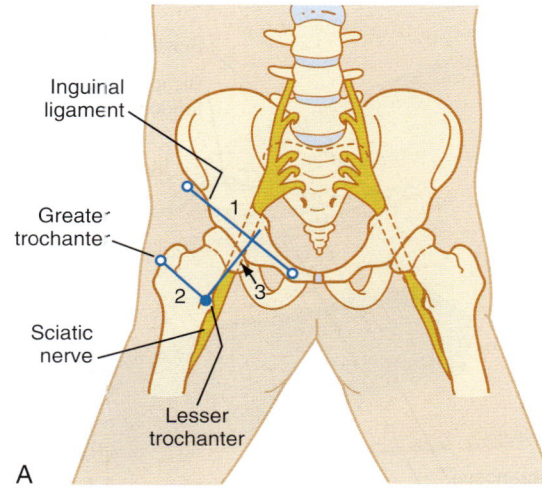

42

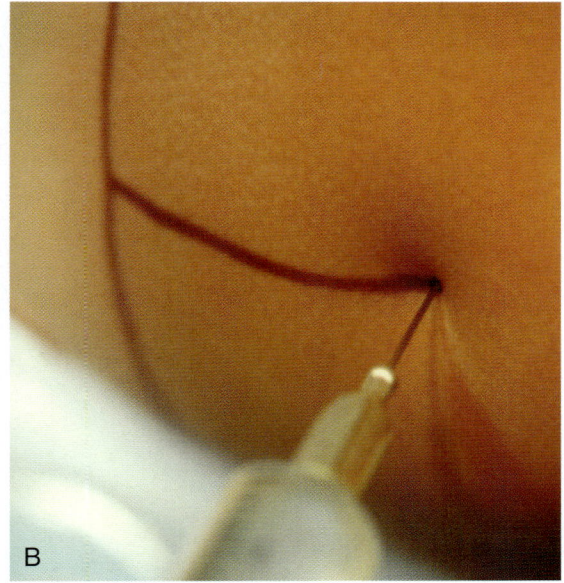

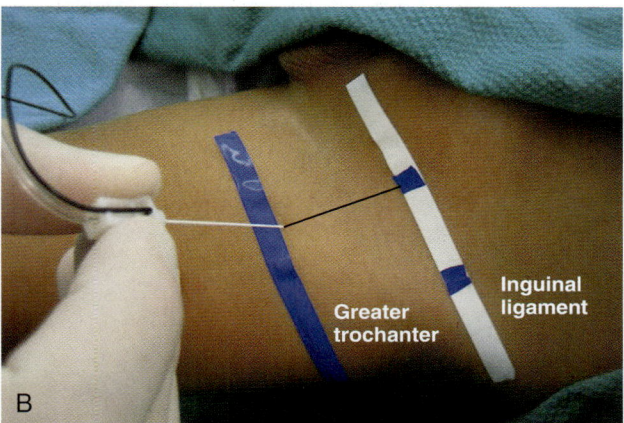

FIGURE 42.30 A, Sciatic nerve block (anterior approach). With the patient supine, a line is drawn from the anterior iliac spine to the pubic tuberosity (*line 1*). The greater trochanter is located, and another line is drawn parallel to the first (*line 2*). A perpendicular line is drawn from line 1 at a point one-third the distance laterally from the pubic tuberosity to the anterior iliac spine (*solid line 3*). **B,** Left sciatic nerve block. A needle is inserted at the intersection of line 2 and the perpendicular line (in **A,** *solid circle*) until bone is encountered. The needle is redirected off the edge of the femur to the approximate posterior margin of the femur and, after negative aspiration for blood, ease of injection is ascertained. Resistance to injection indicates that the needle is within muscle or fascial bundle; the needle should be advanced until there is minimal resistance to injection or until a paresthesia is elicited.

FIGURE 42.29 A, Sciatic nerve block (approach of Labat). The patient is placed in a lateral position with the lower leg extended and the upper leg, the one to be blocked, flexed; a line is drawn from the greater trochanter of the femur to the posterior superior iliac spine (*blue line 1*). A second line is drawn from the greater trochanter to the coccyx (*blue line 2*). Line 1 is bisected, and a perpendicular line is drawn from that point to line 2 (*black line 3*); the point at which the perpendicular broken line intersects line 2 (*encircled dot*) is the point of needle insertion. **B,** A 22-gauge needle is advanced perpendicular to the skin until it strikes bone or, if the child is awake, a paresthesia is elicited. Use of a nerve stimulator will produce either plantar flexion or dorsiflexion of the foot.

concentration further to limit the injected dose to 2.5 mg/kg of bupivacaine.[393]

Lateral Popliteal Sciatic Nerve Block

This approach to the sciatic nerve can be performed with the child in the supine position.[394] This block provides postoperative analgesia in children undergoing surgery to the foot and knee, such as clubfoot repair or triple arthrodesis, and in children having knee surgery, particularly when combined with a femoral nerve

block.[395] It has the advantage of preserving hamstring function and allows early ambulation with crutches.

ANATOMY. The popliteal fossa is a diamond-shaped area located behind the knee. It is bordered by the biceps femoris laterally, medially by the tendons of the semitendinosus and semimembranosus muscles, and inferiorly by the heads of the gastrocnemius muscle. The sciatic nerve, after its formation from L4 through S5, innervates all areas of the leg and foot below the knee except the anteromedial cutaneous areas of the leg and foot, which are supplied by the femoral nerve. The sciatic nerve divides into two branches, the larger tibial nerve located medially and the common peroneal nerve located laterally. The nerves are together at the apex of the popliteal fossa, where they are in close proximity to

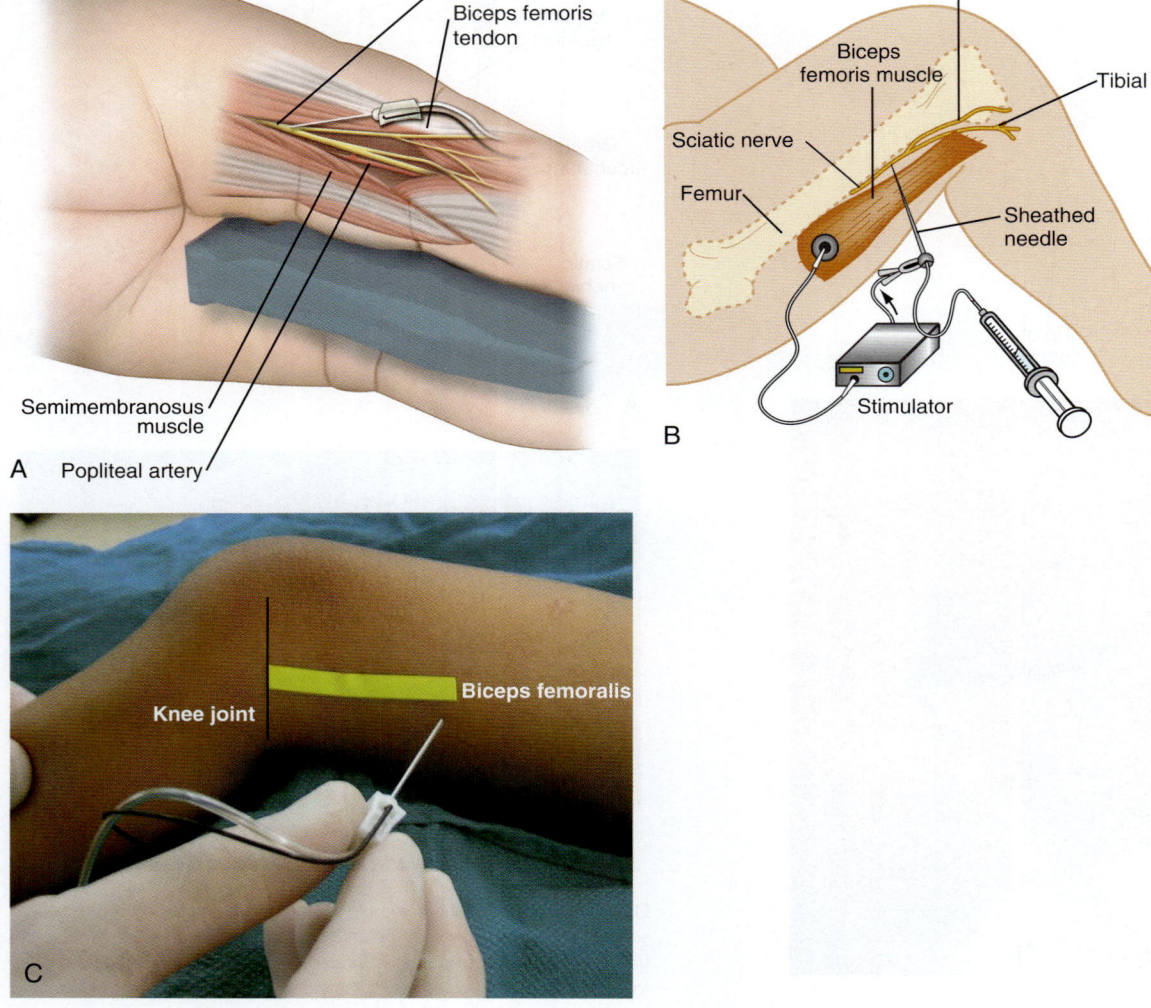

FIGURE 42.31 Lateral popliteal sciatic nerve block. **A,** Anatomy for lateral popliteal approach to the sciatic nerve. The calf is elevated on a pillow and the biceps femoris tendon is palpated. The tendon is traced proximally for 3 to 5 cm. **B,** A 22-gauge insulated needle is inserted anterior to the tendon in a horizontal plane with a cephalad angulation. A nerve stimulator is attached to the needle and with low-voltage stimulation (0.2–0.5 mV), the foot is observed for plantar flexion or dorsiflexion. With injection of the test dose of 1.0 mL of bupivacaine (0.25% with 1:200,000 epinephrine), the twitching is abolished. This confirms the correct placement of the needle. **C,** Then 5 to 10 mL of additional local anesthetic is injected.

each other and are enclosed in a connective tissue sheath for a few more centimeters before dividing into the component nerves (see Fig. 42.31A).

TECHNIQUE. After induction of general anesthesia, the calf is elevated on a pillow. The biceps femoris tendon is palpated. The tendon is then traced upward for 3 to 5 cm. A 22-gauge insulated needle is inserted anterior to the tendon in a horizontal plane with a cephalad angulation (see Fig. 42.31B). A nerve stimulator is attached to the sheathed needle and with low-voltage stimulation (0.2–0.5 mV), the foot is observed for plantar flexion or dorsiflexion. On injection of a test dose of 1 mL bupivacaine (0.25% with epinephrine 1:200,000), the twitching is abolished. This confirms the correct placement of the needle (see Fig. 42.31C); 5 to 10 mL of additional local anesthetic is then injected (see Video 42.1). In adult studies, it has been shown that the sciatic

nerve block is longer lasting than an ankle block or subcutaneous infiltration, and it provides excellent postoperative analgesia.[394] Continuous catheter techniques can be used to provide effective analgesia in children in the postoperative period.[396] An ultrasound-guided technique may also be used (see Chapter 43 and Figs. 42.30 and 43.31).

COMPLICATIONS. Intraneural injection must be avoided. Using a low-voltage nerve stimulator ensures the proper placement of the needle. It is rare to see intravascular placement of the needle with this approach. Intravascular injection may be avoided with incremental injection and frequent aspiration.

Infragluteal-Parabiceps Approach

This approach is a simple way to access the sciatic nerve.[392] It offers an advantage over the popliteal fossa technique because

42

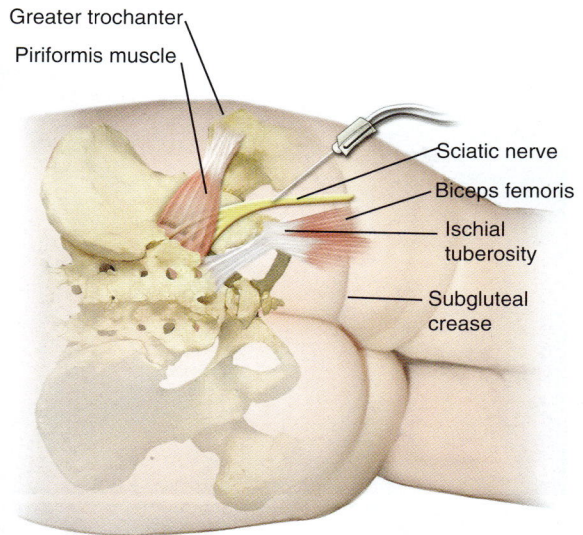

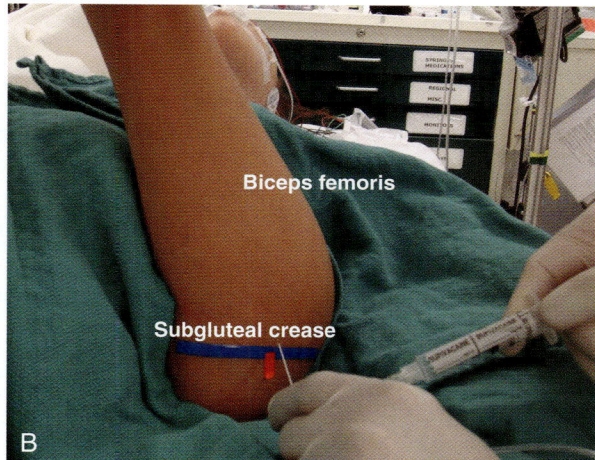

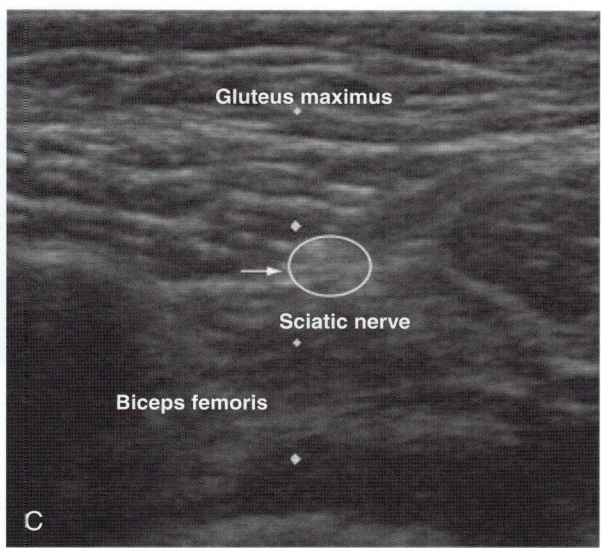

FIGURE 42.32 A, Artist's rendering of infragluteal-parabiceps block. **B, T**he gluteal crease is identified (left leg) in the prone or supine position. The biceps femoris muscle is identified (distal portion not illustrated) and followed cephalad to the gluteal crease. A stimulating needle is inserted at the level of the gluteal crease along the medial border of the biceps femoris muscle *(blue line);* with stimulation at 0.5 mA, plantar flexion or extension or inversion or eversion denotes adequate positioning of the needle. After aspiration to rule out intravascular injection, 0.2 mL/kg of local anesthetic solution is injected to provide an adequate blockade of the sciatic nerve. **C,** An ultrasound technique may also be used. A linear ultrasound probe is placed along the inferior border of the gluteus maximus along the gluteal crease. The biceps femoris muscle and the semitendinosus muscle are identified. The sciatic nerve is seen as a hyperechoic shadow *(arrow).* In this location, the nerve may be isoechoic. This may require mild rotation or movement of the ultrasound probe to recognize the nerve completely. With the use of an in-plane approach, the needle is advanced close to the sciatic nerve. After aspiration, 0.2 mL/kg of local anesthetic solution is injected. A "donut sign" is seen as the nerve is surrounded by the local anesthetic solution.

the posterior cutaneous nerve supplying the posterior portion of the thigh can be blocked with this approach.

TECHNIQUE. The child is placed in the supine position or a lateral position to perform this block. The biceps femoris tendon is palpated and traced cephalad to the distal crease of the buttocks (Fig. 42.32A). A stimulating needle is then inserted perpendicular to the femoral shaft, along the biceps femoris tendon (parabiceps) until a twitch is obtained (see Fig. 42.31B). Either inversion or eversion of the foot is a reasonable response for localization of

the nerve. Next, 0.2 mL/kg of local anesthetic solution is injected into the area (Video 42.15). An ultrasound-guided approach may facilitate this block (see also Chapter 43 and Figs. 42.30 to 42.32).[397]

COMPLICATIONS. Profound motor block can be seen in most children after a subgluteal (infragluteal) parabiceps sciatic nerve block. If the child is discharged home, caution should be exercised because of the motor weakness produced. More recently, we have used continuous catheters in hospitalized children having major lower extremity surgical procedures, with very good results.[398]

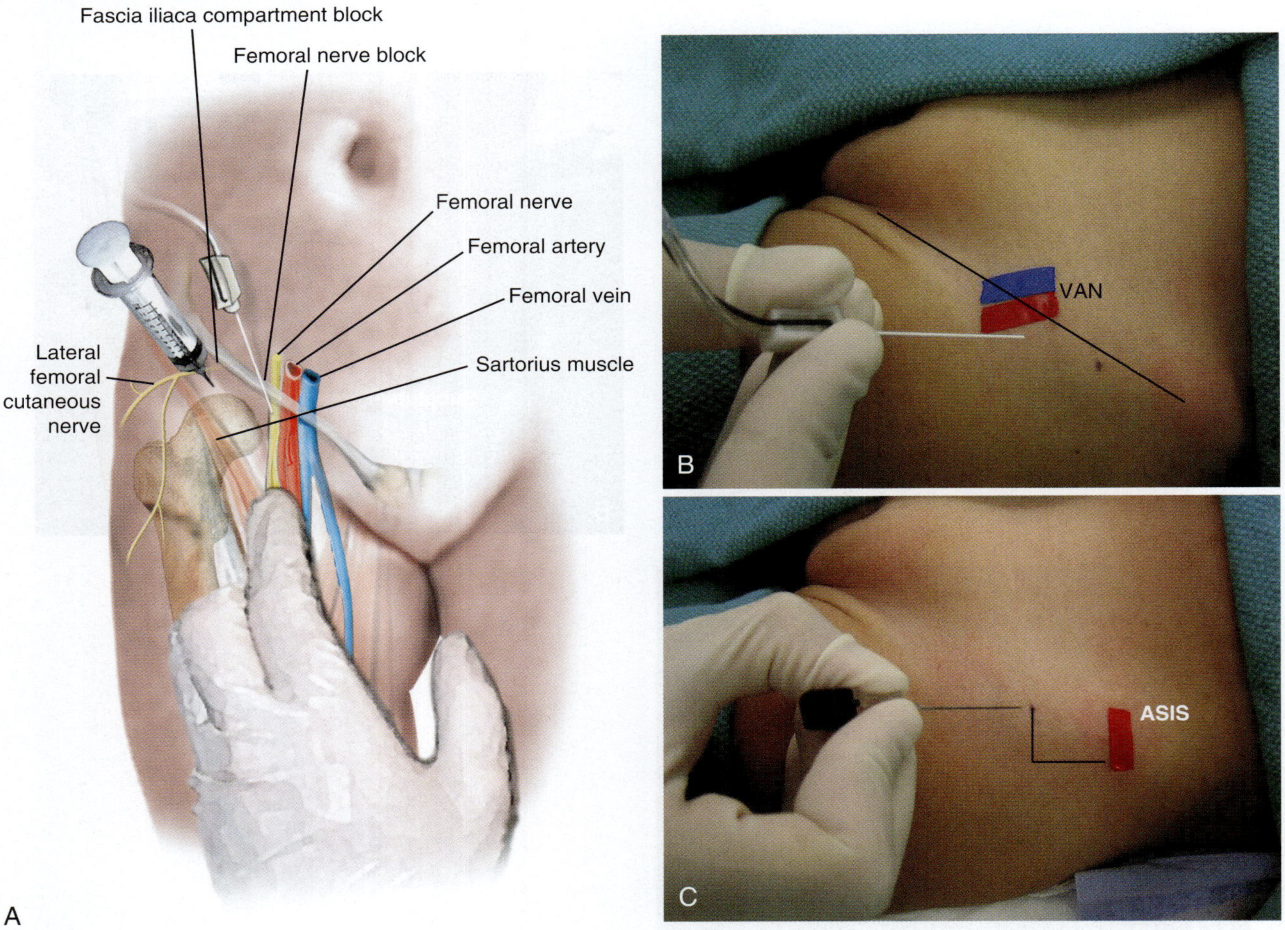

Fascia iliaca compartment block

Femoral nerve block

Femoral nerve

Femoral artery

Femoral vein

Sartorius muscle

Lateral
femoral
cutaneous
nerve

A

B

VAN

C

ASIS

FIGURE 42.33 A, Right femoral nerve block and fascia iliaca compartment block. Note that the femoral nerve lies lateral to the femoral artery. The appropriate dose of local anesthetic is administered while maintaining pressure on the nerve sheath distal to the site of injection just below the inguinal ligament; local anesthetic is thus forced proximally. **B,** For a left femoral nerve block, the point of injection is lateral to the pulse, over the site of the nerve (*V*, vein; *A*, femoral artery; *N*, femoral nerve) (black line indicates inguinal ligament). **C,** The left lateral femoral cutaneous nerve is blocked by injecting 1.0 to 2.0 mL of local anesthetic 1 to 2 cm medial and caudal to the anterior superior iliac crest (*ASIS*). A caudal needle is used so as to better feel the "pop" through tissue planes. For the fascia iliaca block, the point of injection is just lateral to the site depicted for the femoral nerve block, 1 cm inferior to the lateral and middle thirds of the inguinal ligament. An injection at this location will bathe all three nerves in the compartment, resulting in blockade with a single injection.

Femoral Nerve Block

A femoral nerve block is particularly useful in children with a fractured femoral shaft so that transport, radiographic, and other manipulations are not painful.[399–401] This block provides analgesia and relieves muscle spasms around the fracture site.

ANATOMY. The femoral nerve is located immediately lateral to the femoral artery and deep to both the fascia lata and fascia iliaca (Fig. 42.33A).

TECHNIQUE. A 22-gauge blunt B-bevel needle is advanced lateral to the pulsation of the femoral artery. Two fascial planes can be located by the distinct pop that is felt as the needle traverses these fascial tissues. The nerve is blocked by depositing an appropriate volume (5–10 mL) of local anesthetic lateral to the femoral pulse and deep to the fascia iliaca. The needle is advanced in a perpendicular plane (see Fig. 42.33B and Video 42.16). It is not necessary to elicit a motor paresthesia, provided that the two

fascial planes are penetrated. Performance of this block may, on occasion, produce a fascia iliaca block. Repeated aspiration and incremental injection should be used to avoid injection into the femoral artery. With ultrasound guidance, the femoral nerve can be easily visualized and can be blocked (see also Chapter 43 and Fig. 43.26).[397] A catheter can be placed to provide continuous analgesia in the postoperative period.[399]

COMPLICATIONS. It may be preferable to avoid this technique in children who are taking anticoagulants or who may have blood dyscrasias, owing to the close proximity of the nerve to the femoral artery. Intravascular injection may be avoided with incremental injection and frequent aspiration.

Lateral Femoral Cutaneous Nerve

ANATOMY. The lateral femoral cutaneous nerve arises from the L2 and L3 roots of the lumbar plexus. It emerges from the lateral border of the psoas muscle and passes obliquely under the fascia iliaca to enter the thigh 1 to 2 cm medial to the anterior superior iliac crest (see Fig. 42.33A). The nerve innervates the lateral aspect of the thigh. One of its anterior branches forms part of the patellar plexus; thus it must be blocked for regional anesthesia of the knee. Blockade is also indicated for supplementation of femoral and sciatic nerve blocks to provide relief of tourniquet pain. It is also suitable for anesthetizing the lateral aspect of the thigh as a donor site for small skin grafts, fascia iliaca grafts, or muscle biopsy for muscular disorders.[402,403] This block can also be used for both diagnostic and therapeutic purposes in treating meralgia paresthetica, a condition that leads to chronic pain along the lateral aspect of the thigh.[404,405] In most cases, a fascia iliaca block will block this nerve along with the femoral and obturator nerves, thus obviating the need for performing an isolated lateral femoral cutaneous block.

TECHNIQUE. A point approximately 2 cm caudal and 2 cm medial to the anterior superior iliac spine is located (see Fig. 42.33C). A blunt needle is then advanced through the skin and then through the fascia lata. A distinct pop is felt at this point. The fascia lata and fascia iliaca compartments are entered as two distinct pops can be felt as the needle advances into the fascia iliaca compartment. Two to 10 mL of local anesthetic, depending on the size of the child, is deposited in a fan-like fashion (Video 42.17). Recently we have used an ultrasound-guided technique that allows us to visualize the fascia iliaca compartment as it fills up with the local anesthetic solution on injection.

COMPLICATIONS. It is rare to see any complications associated with a lateral femoral cutaneous nerve block. However, care must be taken to avoid an intraneural placement of the local anesthetic solution. Intravascular injection may be avoided with incremental injection and frequent aspiration.

Fascia Iliaca Block

This block is particularly useful in children to provide unilateral anesthesia or analgesia of the lower extremity. The block has been reported to be less reliable in adults than in children.[406] It produces blockade of the femoral, lateral femoral cutaneous, and obturator nerves with a single injection of local anesthetic.

ANATOMY. The compartment is bounded superficially by the fascia iliaca and iliacus muscle, superiorly by the iliac crest, and deeply by the psoas muscle (see Fig. 42.33A). It has the advantage of producing blockade without requiring the needle to be in close proximity to any major nerves or blood vessels. One study reported a greater than 90% success rate and found it far superior in children to the "3 in 1" block described by Winnie.[406]

TECHNIQUE. The injection is made approximately 1 cm inferior to the junction of the outer and middle thirds of the inguinal ligament (see Fig. 42.33A). As the needle is inserted at a perpendicular angle of about 75 degrees to the skin, two characteristic pops are felt as the needle pierces the fascia lata and then the fascia iliaca. Slight pressure on a fluid-filled syringe attached to the needle may aid in placement of the block by producing a subtle loss of resistance when the fascia iliaca compartment is entered. The angle of needle insertion is decreased and directed cephalad, and the local anesthetic is incrementally injected. One should feel little resistance to injection. Digital pressure is exerted distally to the site during the injection and for a short time afterward, and the swelling produced in the groin by the volume of local anesthetic is massaged to promote proximal flow of the drug. A long-acting local anesthetic, such as bupivacaine, ropivacaine, or levobupivacaine, is usually chosen so that postoperative blockade

can provide prolonged analgesia. A volume of 0.3 to 0.5 mL/kg is sufficient in most cases. An ultrasound-guided technique similar to that for the lateral femoral cutaneous block may also be used for this block.

COMPLICATIONS. Because of the larger volume required to provide an adequate block, care has to be taken to not exceed the maximum dosage of the local anesthetic. Intravascular injection may be avoided with incremental injection and frequent aspiration.

Saphenous Nerve Block

The saphenous nerve, the terminal sensory branch of the femoral nerve, provides sensory innervation to the medial aspect of the leg and foot. When blocked in the thigh, as it courses through the adductor canal, it can provide excellent analgesia following operations on the knee while minimizing the weakness of the quadraceps muscle produced by a femoral nerve block (Video 42.18).[406a]

ANATOMY. The nerve lies below the sartorius muscle, and bounded laterally by the vastus medialis and medially by the femoral artery.

An echogenic needle is advanced medially in plane at the mid-thigh level through the sartorius muscle. A pop is felt as the needle exits its investing fascia. The nerve lies lateral to the femoral artery.

COMPLICATIONS. Arterial puncture.

Ankle Block

Block of the nerves of the foot at the ankle is a technique that is valuable to produce both surgical anesthesia and postoperative analgesia for procedures on the foot.

ANATOMY. Three nerves can be blocked from the dorsal aspect of the foot. The deep peroneal nerve (L4, L5, S1, and S2) innervates the web space between the great and second toes. This nerve extends down the anterior aspect of the leg medial to the extensor hallucis longus and lateral to both the anterior tibial muscle and the anterior tibial artery. It is blocked at the level of the ankle crease in the lower part of the leg by inserting a 25-gauge needle through the skin until it contacts the tibia (Fig. 42.34A). Two to three milliliters of local anesthetic are injected, and then an additional amount as the needle is being withdrawn. The superficial peroneal nerve (L4, L5, S1, and S2) innervates the medial and lateral aspects of the dorsum of the foot. Its anatomic course passes through the crural fascia on the anterior aspect of the distal two-thirds of the leg and subcutaneously along the lateral aspect of the foot. It is blocked immediately above the talocrural joint. It can be blocked by subcutaneous infiltration of local anesthetic from the anterior border of the tibia to the lateral malleolus. The last nerve that lies on the dorsal aspect of the foot is the saphenous nerve, which innervates the skin over the medial malleolus. It is blocked by subcutaneous infiltration around the great saphenous vein at the level of the medial malleolus. The tibial and the sural nerves are blocked using a posterior approach. The tibial nerve (L4, L5, S1, S2, and S3) lies posterior to the posterior tibial artery and divides into the medial and lateral plantar branches, which innervate their respective aspects of the sole of the foot. It is blocked at the level of the posterior medial malleolus.

TECHNIQUE. It is not necessary to elicit paresthesias, and an ankle block can be satisfactorily performed in sedated children without the use of a nerve stimulator. Five principal nerves must be blocked to provide analgesia to the entire foot: (1) the deep peroneal, (2) superficial peroneal, (3) saphenous, (4) tibial, and (5) sural nerves (see Fig. 42.34). The technique is the same as in

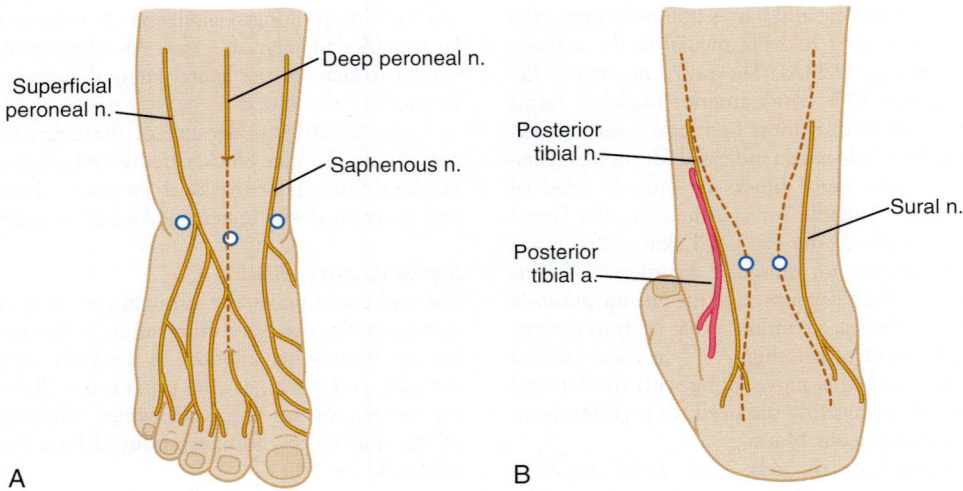

FIGURE 42.34 Ankle block. Block of the ankle generally requires five separate nerves to be blocked. Three nerves can be blocked from the dorsal aspect of the foot **(A)** and two on either side of the Achilles tendon **(B)**. Sites of injection are indicated by the *circles*. *a*, artery; *n*, nerve.

the adult. It should be noted that there might be some variation in the precise distribution of distal innervation from child to child. A 25-gauge needle is inserted at a 90-degree angle to the posterior aspect of the tibia and is directed lateral to the posterior tibial artery until the tibia is contacted. Several milliliters of local anesthetic are deposited at this level and several more are injected as the needle is withdrawn. The sural nerve innervates the heel. It is blocked by subcutaneous infiltration of local anesthetic from the Achilles tendon to the lateral malleolus (see Fig. 42.34B). The deep peroneal nerve is located next to the extensor hallucis longus tendon. Usually it can be located by palpating the dorsalis pedis artery. The needle is inserted lateral to the extensor hallucis longus tendon and is advanced until it meets the periosteum of the metatarsal. It is then withdrawn a few millimeters. After careful aspiration, a volume of 2 to 3 mL of local anesthetic is injected. The superficial peroneal nerve is located under the dorsum of the foot. A superficial injection from the lateral malleolus to the extensor hallucis longus tendon area blocks all the branches of the superficial peroneal nerve.

COMPLICATIONS. It is very rare to see complications from an ankle block. However, the use of vasoconstrictors can theoretically cause necrosis of the toes. Care should be taken to avoid the use of an ankle block in children who may have compromised blood flow to the lower extremity.[407]

Digital Nerve Blocks: Foot

This is an easy block to perform and is useful for surgeries that include trauma to the nails and toes, ingrown toenail surgery, and laser treatment of warts.[388]

ANATOMY. The digital nerves of the foot are derived from the plantar cutaneous branches of the tibial nerve. The proper digital nerve of the great toe pierces the plantar aponeurosis posterior to the tarsal-medial joint and supplies the medial side of the great toe. The three common digital nerves pass between the divisions of the plantar aponeurosis and split into two proper digital nerves each. The first supplies the adjacent areas of the great and second toes; the second supplies the adjacent sides of the second and third toes; the third supplies the adjacent sides of the third and fourth toes. Each proper digital nerve gives off cutaneous

and articular filaments that terminate at the tip of the toe. The superficial peroneal nerve gives off branches that supply the dorsum of the foot. They are derived from two nerves: (1) the dorsal cutaneous divides into two branches, a medial one that supplies the great toe and a lateral one that supplies the adjacent sides of the second and third toes; and (2) the intermediate dorsal cutaneous nerve, which passes along the lateral part of the foot supplying the lateral part of the dorsum of the foot and communicating with the sural nerve. This latter nerve terminates by dividing into two dorsal digital branches, one of which supplies the adjacent sides of the third and fourth toes and another one that supplies the adjacent sides of the fourth and little toes.

TECHNIQUE. Placement of the needle for this block can be initially difficult owing to the thickness of the overlying skin. We prefer using an approach in which we access the nerve from the web space or at the dorsolateral aspect of the toe. Bupivacaine *without epinephrine* is injected (1-2 mL) after aspiration to rule out intravascular placement. These blocks should be avoided in children with already compromised blood flow to the toes.

COMPLICATIONS. Large volumes of local anesthetic are contraindicated because this may cause pressure and vascular compromise. *Vasoconstrictors should be avoided because this may cause necrosis of the digit.*[389] Intravascular injection may be avoided with incremental injection with frequent aspiration.

Summary

Most regional techniques that are suitable for adults can be used in children. Although in most children sedation or general anesthesia is necessary in addition to the regional anesthetic, in certain neonates, regional anesthesia is often used as the sole technique and may reduce the incidence of early but not late postanesthetic apnea in former preterm infants. In addition to the intraoperative benefits, regional anesthesia may improve postoperative analgesia and may offer some improvement to postoperative respiratory function in selected children. Regional anesthesia is particularly useful in outpatient surgery, providing postoperative analgesia with rapid emergence and a low incidence of side effects. It is

42

important to realize, however, that the anatomic, physiologic, and pharmacologic factors unique to children can affect the performance and safety of regional anesthetic techniques. The advent of ultrasound guidance for placement of peripheral, as well as central, neuraxial blockade may increase the use of these blocks. Continuous catheter techniques can also increase the postoperative pain control in these children, with fewer adverse effects related to opioid use.[408] Once these differences are understood, regional anesthesia can be safely and effectively used in children of all ages, either as the sole anesthetic or as a supplement to general anesthesia, to provide a smooth intraoperative course and pain-free awakening.

ACKNOWLEDGMENT

The authors wish to thank Per-Arne Lönnqvist, MD, DEAA, FRCA, PhD, for his generous contribution to the paravertebral block section of this chapter.

ANNOTATED REFERENCES

de Queiroz Siqueira M, Chassard D, Musard H, et al. Resuscitation with lipid, epinephrine, or both in levobupivacaine-induced cardiac toxicity in newborn piglets. *Br J Anaesth*. 2014;112(4):729-734.

A laboratory study documenting both the efficacy of lipid emulsion in treating local anesthetic systemic toxicity in infancy, as well as the risk of adding the usual resuscitation doses of epinephrine in this condition. Lipid is more efficacious than epinephrine.

Polaner DM, Taenzer AH, Walker BJ, et al. Pediatric Regional Anesthesia Network (PRAN): a multi-institutional study of the use and incidence of complications of pediatric regional anesthesia. *Anesth Analg*. 2012;115(6):1353-1364.

The first paper from the Pediatric Regional Anesthetic Network, this is the most comprehensive prospective look at regional anesthesia practice in the United States. The PRAN database now contains 10 times this number of cases and still has documented similarly low numbers of adverse events.

Rosenberg PH, Veering BT, Urmey WF. Maximum recommended doses of local anesthetics: a multifactorial concept. *Reg Anesth Pain Med*. 2004;29(6):564-575, discussion 524.

A scientific and pharmacologic approach to local anesthetic toxicity that describes the important concept that a simple dose per kilogram is insufficient to determine how much drug is safe to administer.

Suresh S, Long J, Birmingham PK, De Oliveira GS Jr. Are caudal blocks for pain control safe in children? An analysis of 18,650 caudal blocks from the Pediatric Regional Anesthesia Network (PRAN) database. *Anesth Analg*. 2015;120(1):151-156.

Caudal block is still the most commonly performed regional anesthetic in children. This analysis demonstrates that it has a high degree of safety, but that one must be careful in choosing the dose.

Taenzer AH, Walker BJ, Bosenberg AT, et al. Asleep versus awake: does it matter? Pediatric regional block complications by patient state: a report from the Pediatric Regional Anesthesia Network. *Reg Anesth Pain Med*. 2014;39(4):279-283.

A landmark study that presents the first prospective data that administering regional blocks in children under general anesthesia does not increase risk. Previous admonitions about the risk of this practice were based on a few case reports. These data show that administering regional anesthesia in anesthetized pediatric patients is at least as safe, and possibly safer, than in awake or sedated children.

Walker BJ, Long JB, De Oliveira GS, et al. Peripheral nerve catheters in children: an analysis of safety and practice patterns from the pediatric regional anesthesia network (PRAN). *Br J Anaesth*. 2015;115(3):457-462.

Peripheral nerve catheters are being increasingly used for ambulatory surgery of the extremities. These catheters can be safely managed at home as long as well-designed follow-up systems are in place. Accidental catheter dislodgment remains the primary problem.

Williams RK, Adams DC, Aladjem EV, et al. The safety and efficacy of spinal anesthesia for surgery in infants: the Vermont Infant Spinal Registry. *Anesth Analg*. 2006;102(1):67-71.

This report from the world's largest database of spinal anesthetics in infants documents a high degree of safety and efficacy, although a minority of patients did require some brief supplementation with general anesthesia or sedation during highly stimulating portions of the operations. The success rate was very high.

A complete reference list can be found online at ExpertConsult.com.

43

Ultrasound-Guided Regional Anesthesia

MANOJ K. KARMAKAR AND WING H. KWOK

PERIPHERAL NERVE BLOCKS ARE frequently performed in children to provide anesthesia or analgesia during the perioperative period.[1-3] Success depends on the ability to accurately place the needle—and thereby the local anesthetic—close to the target nerve without causing injury to the nerve or adjacent structures. Peripheral nerve blocks are not without risk and can pose a serious challenge even to the experienced anesthesiologist because they are usually performed after the child is anesthetized. In the past, clinicians relied on anatomic landmarks,[1-3] fascial clicks,[4] loss of resistance,[5] or nerve stimulation[6] to position the needle in the vicinity of the nerve. Anatomic landmarks provide valuable clues to the position of the nerve, but they are surrogate markers, lack precision,[7] vary among children of different ages, and may be difficult to locate in obese children. Even nerve stimulation, which has been recommended as the gold standard for nerve localization, may not always elicit a motor response[8] and its use does not guarantee success or preclude complications.[9] Moreover, the accuracy of needle placement cannot be predicted with any of these methods, which may lead to multiple attempts to place the needle that may result in pain and possibly an incomplete or failed nerve block.

Various imaging modalities, such as fluoroscopy,[10] computed tomography (CT),[11] and magnetic resonance imaging (MRI),[7]

improve the accuracy of block placement in adults. However, these adjuncts are rarely used in children and are not practical in the operating room. The use of ultrasound (US) to guide peripheral and central neuraxial blocks has improved both accuracy and safety in both adults and children.[12-21] In this chapter, the basic principles of US imaging and US-guided regional anesthesia (USGRA) in children are described. It is assumed that the reader has a basic understanding of common landmark-based nerve block techniques in children (see Chapter 42).

The use of US for regional anesthesia dates back to 1978, when La Grange et al. used a Doppler flow detector to locate the subclavian artery and guide supraclavicular brachial plexus blocks.[22] In 1994, Kapral and colleagues published the first report on direct sonographic visualization in regional anesthesia.[23] They used US to directly visualize the brachial plexus and observe the spread of the local anesthetic in real time during supraclavicular brachial plexus block. Today, US is commonly used to guide regional anesthesia techniques in both adults and children. Improvements in US technology and the availability of portable US machines with high-resolution imaging capabilities allow direct visualization of the peripheral nerves and central neuraxial structures in children; this can be compared to removing a blindfold from

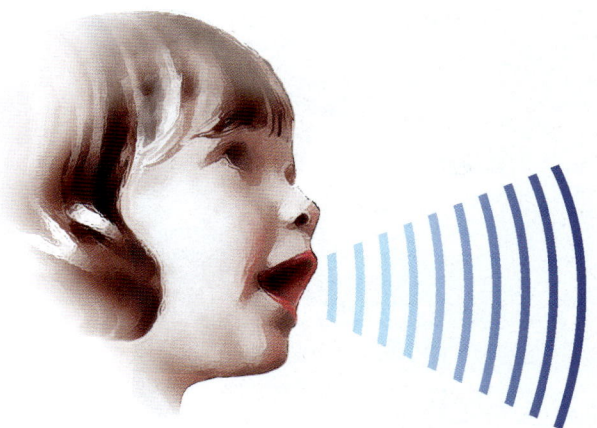

FIGURE 43.1 Sound wave.

TABLE 43.1	Propagation Velocity of Sound in Body Tissues
Tissue	**Propagation Velocity of Sound (m/second)[a]**
Bone	4080
Muscle	1580
Blood	1570
Kidney	1560
Liver	1550
Soft tissue (average)	1540
Water	1480
Fat	1450
Lung	600
Air	330

[a]Medical ultrasound device measurements are based on an assumed average propagation velocity of 1540 m/second.

43

the anesthesiologist performing regional anesthesia. Currently, outcome data that prove US increases the safety and efficacy of regional anesthesia in children are rapidly accumulating.[20,21,24]

Principles of Ultrasound

Sound is a form of mechanical energy that propagates through a medium as a wave of alternating pressure, causing local regions of compression and rarefaction (Fig. 43.1). The frequency (f) of sound is the number of cycles of oscillations per second made by the sound source and the particles in the medium through which it moves. It is expressed in hertz (Hz, cycles per second). Sound waves propagate symmetrically away from the source at a constant velocity (v), which is the speed of sound in the medium. Distance between the wavefronts is the wavelength (λ) of the sound. The speed of sound through a medium can thus be represented as:

$$v = f \times \lambda$$

Amplitude is the strength of a sound wave, and the unit used to describe it is decibels (dB). The velocity of transmission of sound through a medium depends on its acoustic impedance and is determined by factors such as the stiffness, elasticity, and density of the medium. This accounts for the varying velocity of sound transmission through different tissues in the human body (Table 43.1). The average velocity of sound transmission through biologic tissue is 1540 m/second. If the time taken by the US signal to return to the transducer is known, the distance of the target from the transducer (depth) can be computed.

The human ear can detect sound between 20 and 20,000 Hz. US is sound with a frequency beyond 20,000 Hz (20 KHz). For medical imaging, US typically uses a frequency between 1 million and 15 million Hz (megahertz [MHz]) and is produced by a piezoelectric crystal (element) within the transducer. When an electrical field is applied to the surface of an element in a transducer, it undergoes dimensional changes that cause it to vibrate and produce sound. The element is typically driven by a pulsed alternating voltage. This results in the generation of short pulses of US that are emitted into body tissues. Between successive short pulses of US generation, the transducer does not transmit but rather functions as a receiver of the reflected US energy (i.e., the echoes). The percentage of time that a transducer is transmitting is termed the *duty*

factor and is typically less than 1%. The US transducer thus has a dual function—it functions as both a transmitter and a receiver.

The emitted US signal travels through the tissue medium, and when it encounters a tissue interface it is reflected back. The degree of reflection of US from tissues is related to the changes in acoustic impedance (Z) between two tissue interfaces. The reflected echoes are detected by the transducer and converted into electrical energy; they are then processed by the US machine according to their strength and displayed as dots on the monitor. The brightness of each dot corresponds to the strength of the echo signal. Strong echoes produce bright white dots, weak echoes produce gray dots, and anatomic structures that do not reflect US appear as black dots. The position of the dot on the monitor represents the depth from which the echo is received. When all of these dots are combined, they produce a complete image of the area scanned.[25–27]

MODES OF ULTRASOUND
B-Mode (Brightness) or Two-Dimension Mode
B-mode (brightness) or two-dimensional (2D) mode, is the most commonly used US mode. In this mode, the echo is converted to a dot and the brightness of the dot represents the amplitude of the returning signal.[25–27] The position of the dot on the display represents the depth from which the signal is returning and depends on the round-trip time of the US signal. Multiple scan lines across a plane are combined to produce a single 2D gray-scale image. A series of frames are then displayed in rapid succession to give the impression of constant motion, the quality of which depends on the number of images displayed per second, that is, the *frame rate*.

M-Mode (Motion)
Motion, or M-mode, US is directed along a single scan line (sample line), and reflected signals along this scan line are converted to a brightness scale and displayed against a time axis. Because M-mode is produced from US signals along a single scan line, the 2D anatomy of the underlying body tissues should be studied first using the 2D mode. M-mode is of particular interest when time resolution is necessary, such as when examining a target with rapid movement (e.g., the mitral valve during echocardiography).[28]

Doppler Ultrasound
Doppler US (based on the Doppler principle) detects a shift in frequency between the emitted US waves and their echoes. It is

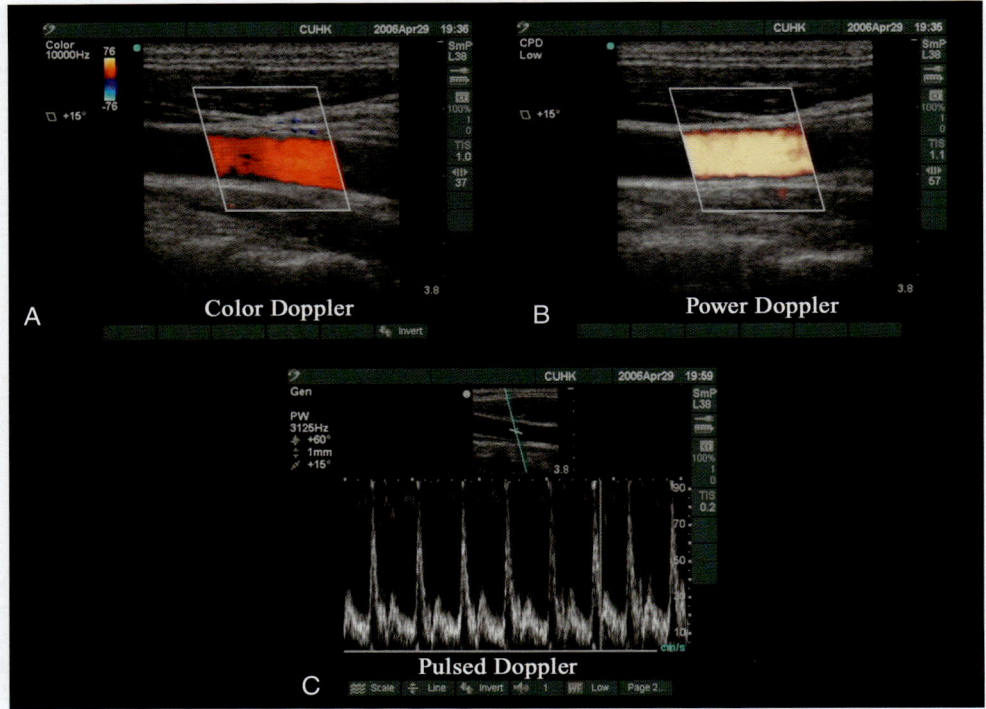

FIGURE 43.2 Doppler ultrasound. **A,** Color Doppler. **B,** Power Doppler. **C,** Pulsed Doppler.

used to detect and measure blood flow, and the major reflector for this purpose are red blood cells.[29-32] Several modes are available:

> *Color Doppler* measures and color codes the direction and magnitude of the mean Doppler frequency shifts that occur in moving red blood cells and superimposes a color depiction of these data on the gray-scale image (Fig. 43.2A).
>
> *Power color Doppler* depicts the amplitude, or power, of the Doppler signals (Fig. 43.2B). This allows better sensitivity for visualization of small vessels, but at the expense of directional information.
>
> *Pulsed Doppler* allows a sampling volume (or gate) to be positioned in a vessel visualized on the gray-scale image and displays a spectrum of the full range of blood velocities within the gate plotted as a function of time (Fig. 43.2C).

THE ULTRASOUND MACHINE

US machines are made up of the following components: a *monitor* (where the clinical images are displayed), the *US unit* (where the signals are processed), the *control panel* (with the knobs and controls), one or more *transducers*, and a *data storage device*.[33-35] For an anesthesiologist's first encounter with a US machine the wide array of knobs and controls available may be confusing. However, several controls are common in most US machines, and a clear understanding of their function—that is, *knobology*—is essential for optimal imaging.

Presets

Most US machines have a number of presets, which are factory set, to allow optimal US imaging of a specific area of the body or type of examination. Some of the categories of presets that are available include small part, vascular, breast, nerve, musculoskeletal, abdominal, and so on. For example, if a small part preset is chosen,

the US machine assumes that the operator is scanning for small, relatively superficial structures and automatically adjusts the depth, power, focus, gain, and time-gain compensation (TGC) to allow optimal imaging of superficial structures. Some US machines also allow customized presets according to clinical requirements. Power output is the amount of energy transmitted from the US transducer. In most machines, the power cannot be adjusted by the operator but is automatically set when a particular preset is chosen.

Frequency

This control is used to select the desired frequency, within certain limits, of a broadband transducer—that is, a transducer that serves a range of frequencies. In some US systems (Edge, SonoSite Inc., Bothell, WA), this is available as an image optimization control. In the "Res" (resolution) setting the highest frequency of the broadband transducer is selected; in the "Pen" (penetration) setting the lowest frequency is selected; and in the "Gen" (general) setting an intermediate frequency is selected.

Gain

The gain control adjusts the amplification of the returning acoustic signals and is used to optimize the US image (Fig. 43.3A). Reduced gain produces a dark image (Fig. 43.3B) and detail is masked. In contrast, too much gain produces a white image and detail is saturated (Fig. 43.3C). Some US machines have separate controls for overall gain and gain for the near and far fields. "Auto-gain," by which the US machine automatically adjusts the gain, is also available in some machines.

Time-Gain Compensation

US energy is progressively attenuated as it travels through tissue. Therefore signals returning from reflectors at a depth are weaker in strength. By selectively amplifying the echoes from greater

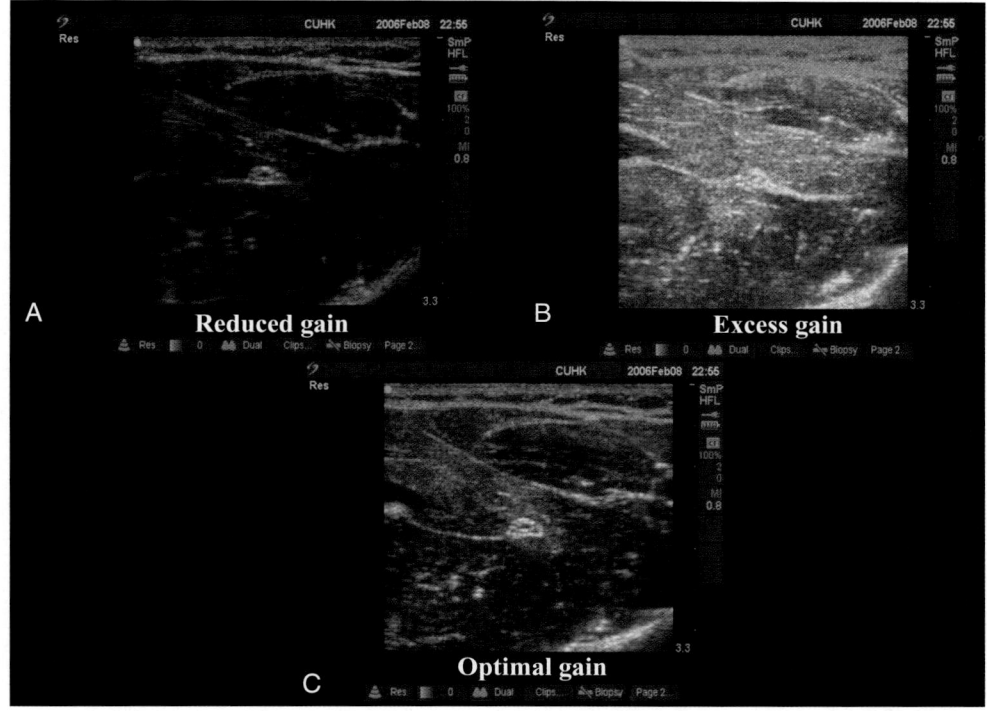

FIGURE 43.3 Transverse sonogram of the forearm demonstrating **A,** reduced gain, **B,** excess gain, and **C,** optimal gain.

depths, using the TGC method or depth-gain compensation (DGC), equal reflectors at unequal depths are displayed as structures of equal brightness on the monitor. TGC is preset to a large degree, and the operator can make fine adjustments if necessary. The TGC control is presented as a series of sliders arranged in a vertical fashion on the control panel. Each of the sliders adjusts the amplification of the returning US signals at a specific image depth.

Depth

Adjustment in the displayed depth may be necessary, depending on the location of the target, the patient's body size, or other anatomic factors. A depth greater than necessary should not be chosen because this reduces the frame rate and resolution of the image.

Focus (Focal Zone)

The focus of the US signal occurs at a point at which the beam is at its narrowest width. It is also the region where lateral resolution is the best. The focus point should therefore be positioned at the depth at which the relevant anatomic structures are located. In some US machines, the operator can select multiple focal zones, but this markedly reduces the frame rate and thus should not be routinely used.

Freeze and Unfreeze

The "freeze" function allows the operator to lock a static image on the monitor. A number of frames (usually 20 or more) are also simultaneously stored in a memory bank. These stored frames can be scrolled back and forth. The selected still image can then be used for annotation, documentation, storage, review, or teaching. Pressing the freeze button once again will unfreeze the image.

Ultrasound Transducers

The transducer functions both as a transmitter and a receiver of the ultrasound signal.[33–35] Three types of transducers are currently used (Fig. 43.4): (1) in a linear-array transducer, the piezoelectric crystals are arranged in a linear fashion and sequentially fired to produce parallel beams of ultrasound in sequence, creating a field of view that is rectangular and as wide as the footprint of the transducer (Fig. 43.4A); (2) a curved linear-array transducer has a curved surface, creating a field of view that is wider than the footprint of the probe (Fig. 43.4B), but at the cost of reduced lateral resolution in the far field as the scan lines diverge; (3) a phased-array transducer has a small footprint, but the ultrasound beam is steered electronically to produce a sufficiently wide far field of view. The ultrasound beam diverges from virtually the same point in the transducer (Fig. 43.4C). Phased-array transducers are routinely used for transthoracic echocardiography.[34] The footprints of these transducers are small enough to fit between the ribs and still produce a wide far field of view to image the heart. US transducers are typically broadband and can serve a range of frequencies. For example, a transducer with the notation HFL38/13-6 indicates that it is a high-frequency broadband (13-6 MHz) linear transducer with a 38-mm footprint. Note that the nomenclature used for transducers varies among manufacturers of US devices.

Ultrasound Transducer Selection

Resolution is the ability to distinguish two objects that are close together. *Axial resolution* is the ability to distinguish two objects that are along the axis of the US beam, and *lateral resolution* is the ability to distinguish two objects that are side by side. High-frequency US (13-6 MHz) has a higher axial and lateral

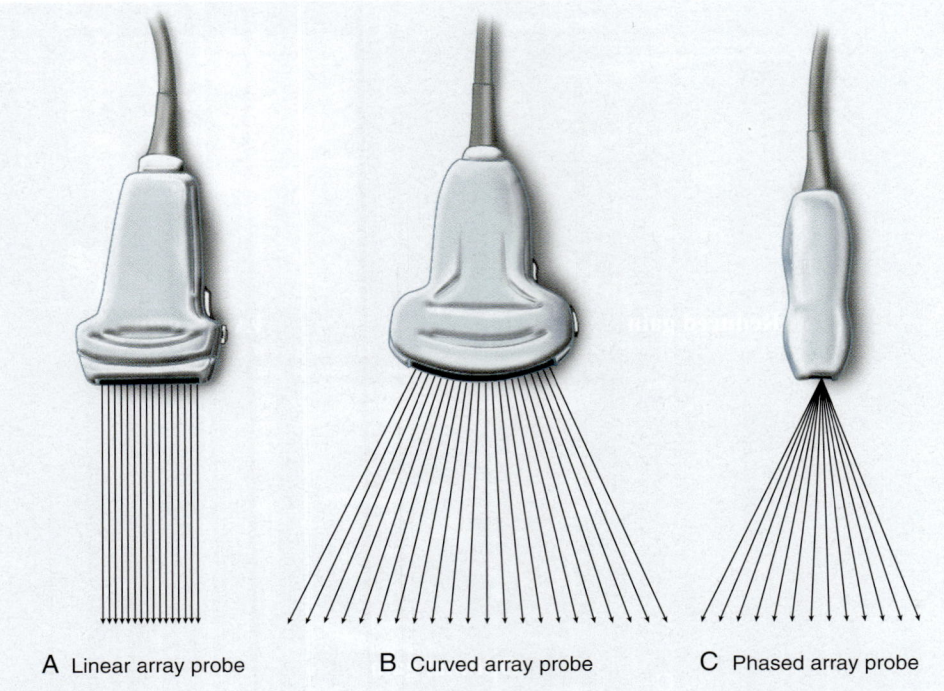

A Linear array probe   **B** Curved array probe   **C** Phased array probe

FIGURE 43.4 Schematic diagram illustrating the different types of ultrasound transducers. Note how the ultrasound beam is emitted from each of these transducers.

resolution compared with low-frequency US but cannot penetrate as deeply into body tissue. Therefore high-frequency US is used to image superficial structures such as the brachial plexus in the interscalene groove or supraclavicular fossa. A lower-frequency US transducer (10-5 MHz) is suited for slightly deeper structures, such as the brachial plexus in the infraclavicular fossa, whereas a low-frequency US transducer (5-2 MHz) is used to image deep structures, such as the lumbar plexus or the sciatic nerve. Broadband transducers allow a single transducer to be used for scanning over a wide range of depths. Because regional blocks are performed at relatively shallow depths in neonates, infants, and young children, high-frequency linear transducers are used for most procedures. High-frequency linear transducers with a small footprint (13-6 MHz, 25 mm), in either a hockey stick or linear configuration, are particularly suited for young children.

Essentials of Musculoskeletal Ultrasound Imaging

AXIS OF SCAN

In diagnostic ultrasonography, scans are performed in the transverse, longitudinal (sagittal), oblique, or coronal axis. During a transverse (axial) scan the transducer is oriented at right angles to the target, producing a cross-sectional display of the structures (Fig. 43.5A). During a longitudinal scan, the transducer is oriented parallel to and along the long axis of the target (e.g., a blood vessel or nerve) (Fig. 43.5 B). During USGRA procedures, US scans are most commonly performed in the transverse axis. In this axis, the nerves, the adjoining structures, and the circumferential spread of the local anesthetic are easily visualized.

PROBE AND IMAGE ORIENTATION

The US image must be properly oriented to accurately identify the anatomic relations of the various structures on the monitor. To facilitate this, all US probes have an orientation marker, which is usually represented by a groove or a ridge on one side of the transducer and corresponds to a green dot (or a logo) on the monitor. By convention, the orientation marker on the transducer is directed cephalad when performing a longitudinal scan and directed toward the right side of the patient when performing a transverse scan. This way the orientation marker on the left upper corner of the monitor always represents the cephalad end during a longitudinal scan or the right side of the patient during a transverse scan. The top of the display monitor therefore represents superficial structures and the bottom of the monitor the deep structures.

ECHOGENICITY

Certain terms are frequently used to describe the sonographic appearance of musculoskeletal structures (Fig. 43.6):

Echogenic: A bright white structure against a dark background
Reflective: Synonymous with an echogenic structure
Isoechoic: A shade of gray that is of the same brightness or echogenicity as the surrounding tissues
Hyperechoic: A shade of gray that is bright white or brighter than the surrounding tissues
Hypoechoic: A shade of gray that is dark or less bright than the surrounding tissues
Anechoic: An absence of echoes, hence blackness

AXIS OF INTERVENTION

The plane of US imaging is approximately 1 mm thick (Fig. 43.7); for a needle to be visible during US imaging it must lie within

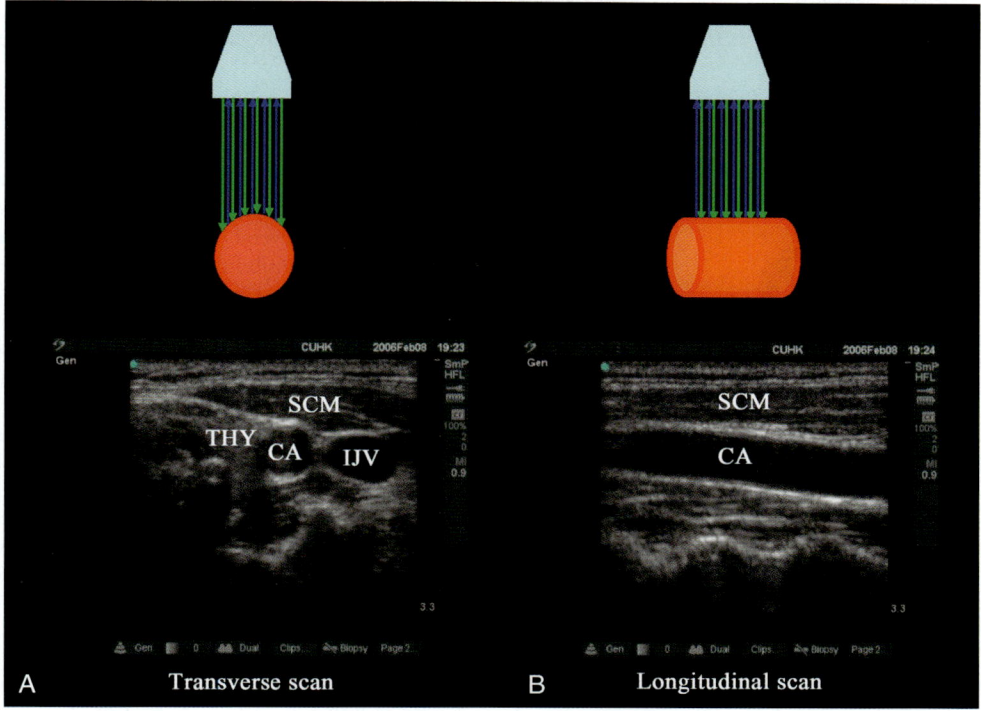

FIGURE 43.5 Axis of scan. **A,** Transverse scan. **B,** Longitudinal scan. *CA,* carotid artery; *IJV,* internal jugular vein; *SCM,* sternocleidomastoid muscle; *THY,* thyroid.

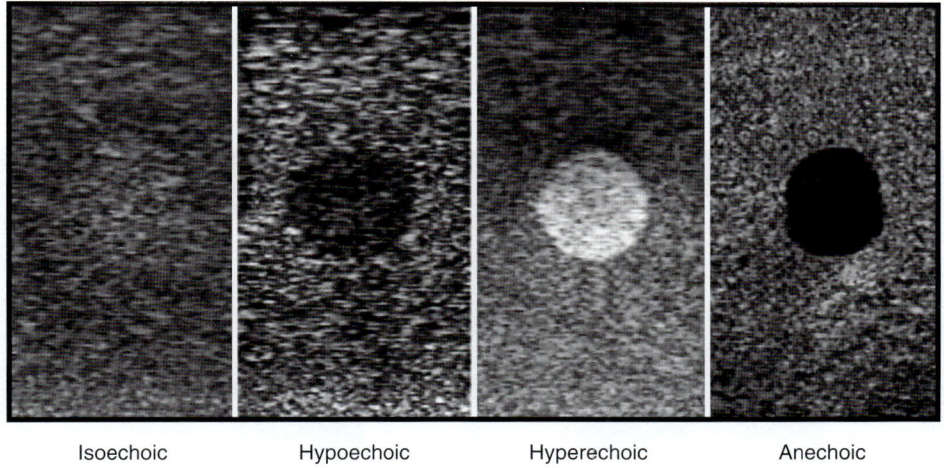

Isoechoic   Hypoechoic   Hyperechoic   Anechoic

FIGURE 43.6 Schematic diagram to demonstrate the relative echogenicity of various tissues.

this narrow plane of imaging. During USGRA procedures, the block needle is inserted either outside of the plane (out-of-plane approach) (Fig. 43.8A) or within the plane of the US beam (in-plane approach) (Fig. 43.8B). In the out-of-plane approach, the needle is inserted in the short axis and is initially outside the plane of imaging and therefore not visible. It becomes visible only when the needle crosses the plane of imaging and is seen as an echogenic dot on the monitor (Fig. 43.8A). It is important to note that this echogenic dot may be just the cross-sectional image of the shaft of the needle as it passes through the plane of the US beam and thus may not represent the tip of the needle. In the in-plane approach, the needle is inserted along the long axis of the transducer

in the plane of imaging and therefore both the shaft and tip of the needle are visible.

Both approaches are commonly used, and no data have shown that one is better than the other. Proponents of the out-of-plane approach[3,14,36] have had great success with this method and claim that it causes less needle-related trauma and pain because the needle is advanced through a shorter distance to the target. However, critics express concerns that the inability to reliably visualize the needle and to use tissue movement as a surrogate marker to locate the needle tip during a procedure can lead to complications. The needle is better visualized in the in-plane approach,[37,38] but this requires good hand–eye coordination.

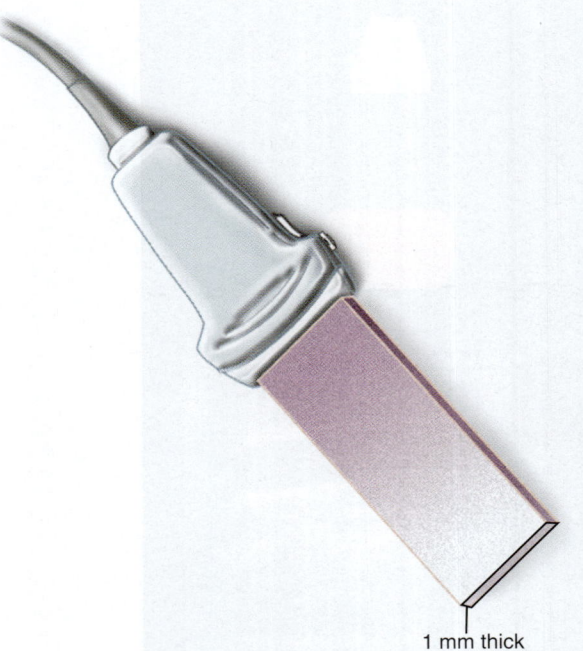

1 mm thick

FIGURE 43.7 The plane of ultrasound imaging. Note that the ultrasound beam is only 1 mm thick and for a needle to be visible during an ultrasound-guided intervention it must lie within this plane of imaging.

Moreover, there are claims that the in-plane approach also causes more discomfort in awake patients because longer needle insertion paths are required.[13,14,36]

NEEDLE VISIBILITY

The ability to visualize the needle during a US (USG) procedure is critical for precision, safety, and success. However, this is often limited by the dispersion of the reflected US signals away from the transducer. Several factors have been identified that can influence needle visibility.[39–41] The shaft of the needle is better visualized in the long axis than in the short axis, and its visibility decreases linearly with steep angles of insertion and smaller needle diameters. The needle tip is better visualized when it is inserted in the long axis for shallow angle of insertion (<30 degrees) and in the short axis when the angle of insertion is steep (>60 degrees). To overcome the effect of angle on needle visibility, some US machines allow the operator to steer the US beam toward the needle ("beam steering") during steep needle insertions.[42] However, this requires experience and decreases in needle visibility can still occur. Manufacturers have incorporated microscopic glass beads or reflectors onto the surfaces of block needles, or have laser-etched the tips of block needles to improve their visibility (echogenic needle).[43–45]

The anesthesiologist's skill in aligning the needle along the plane of imaging is by far the most important factor influencing needle visibility because minor deviations of even a few millimeters from this plane will result in inability to visualize the needle. Even with experience, needle tip visibility is a problem

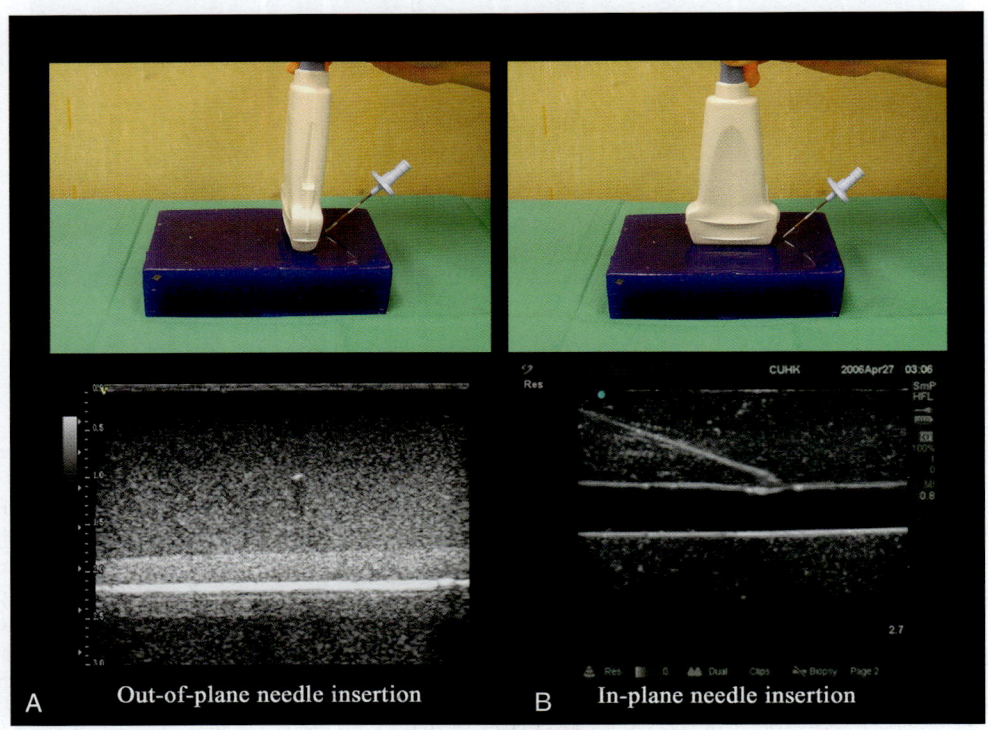

A Out-of-plane needle insertion   **B** In-plane needle insertion

FIGURE 43.8 Axis of intervention. **A,** Out-of-plane and **B,** in-plane techniques.

43

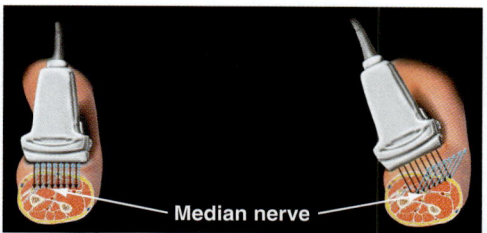

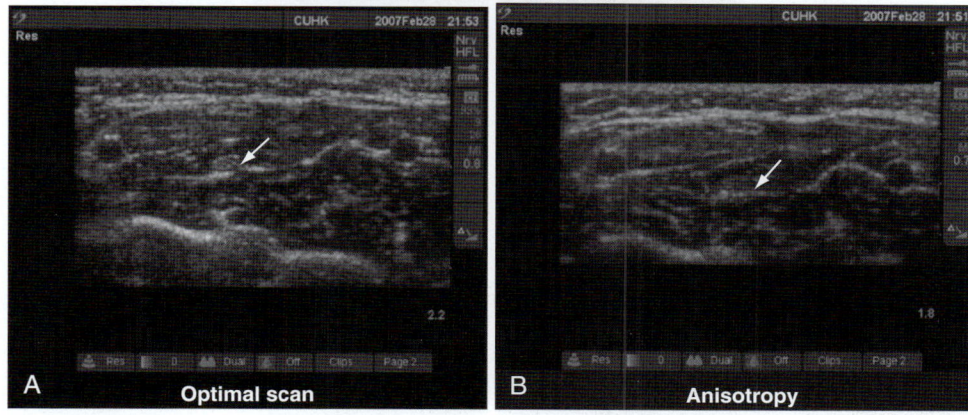

FIGURE 43.9 Anisotropy. Note how a small change in the angle of the ultrasound beam from the neutral position (**A**) has affected the visibility of the median nerve (*white arrow*, **B**) in the forearm.

when performing blocks at a depth in areas that are rich in fatty tissue. Under such circumstances, gently jiggling (rapid in-and-out movement) the needle and observing tissue movement or performing a test injection of saline solution or 5% dextrose (0.5–1 mL) and observing tissue distention can help locate the position of the needle tip. Five percent dextrose is preferred for the latter when nerve stimulation is used because it does not increase the electric current required to elicit a motor response.[46]

ANISOTROPY

Anisotropy, or angular dependence, is a term used to describe the change in echogenicity of a structure with a change in the angle of insonation of the incident US beam (Fig. 43.9).[47] It is frequently observed during scanning of nerves, muscles, and tendons. This occurs because the amplitude of the echoes returning to the transducer varies with the angle of insonation. Nerves are best visualized when the incident beam is at right angles (Fig. 43.9A); small changes in the angle away from the perpendicular can significantly reduce their echogenicity (Fig. 43.9B). Therefore during USGRA procedures, the transducer should be tilted, from side to side, to minimize anisotropy and optimize visualization of the nerve.[48]

Identification of Nerves, Tendons, Muscle, Fat, Bone, Fascia, Blood Vessels, and Pleura

NERVES

On a transverse scan, nerves appear round, oval, triangular, lip-shaped, or even flat.[49] Nerves also assume different shapes along their course, depending on the surrounding structures. The echogenicity of nerves also varies and depends on the nerve and

area scanned. They are generally hyperechoic and stand out in the background of the hypoechoic muscles (Fig. 43.10A), but they can also appear hypoechoic with a hyperechoic rim (Fig. 43.10B). They also have been described to have a fascicular or honeycomb appearance (i.e., echogenic structures with internal punctate, echo-poor spaces) (Fig. 43.10C). On longitudinal scan, the appearance of peripheral nerves has been likened to a "tram track"; that is, parallel hyperechoic lines are seen against a background of echo-poor space (Fig. 43.10D).

TENDONS

Tendons appear to have numerous fine, parallel hyperechoic lines separated by fine hypoechoic lines (fibrillar pattern) on long-axis scans.[50] Compared with nerves, tendons have more hyperechoic lines and move more than adjacent nerves when the corresponding muscle is contracted or passively stretched.

MUSCLE

Muscle fibers are hypoechoic, but the connective tissue structure enveloping the entire muscle (epimysium) is hyperechoic.[51,52] The perimysium that envelops individual muscle fascicles is also hyperechoic. Muscle fibers converge to become tendons or aponeurosis.

FAT

Fat lobules appear as round to oval hypoechoic nodules separated by fine hyperechoic septa. Fat tends to be superficially distributed (subcutaneous fat), slightly compressible, and similar on transverse and longitudinal scans.

BONE

Bone reflects most of the US energy. Therefore it appears bright and has a hyperechoic edge on US imaging, with a large anechoic shadow (acoustic shadow) distal to it (Fig. 43.11).

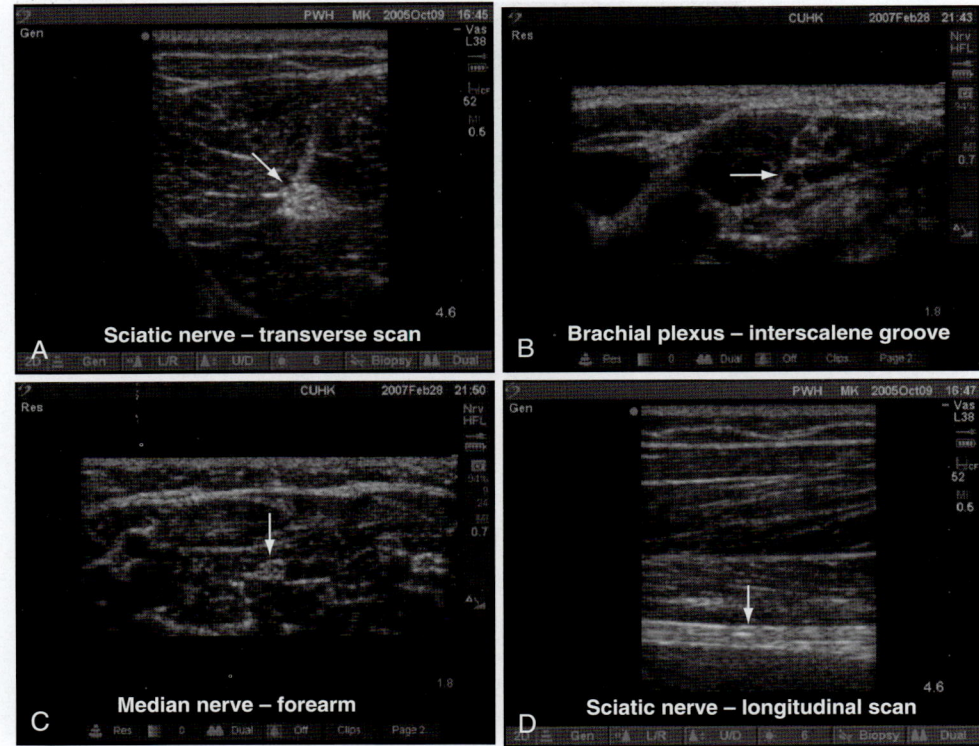

FIGURE 43.10 Ultrasound appearance of peripheral nerves. **A,** Transverse sonogram of the sciatic nerve in the thigh. **B,** Transverse sonogram of the brachial plexus in the interscalene groove. **C,** Transverse sonogram of the median nerve in the forearm. **D,** Longitudinal sonogram of the sciatic nerve in the thigh.

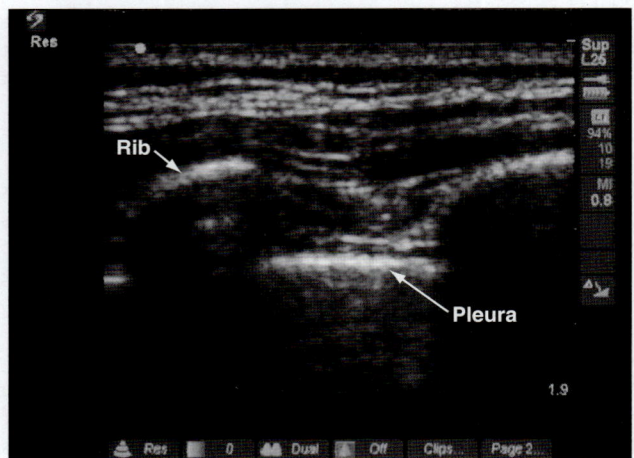

FIGURE 43.11 Longitudinal sonogram of the intercostal space demonstrating the ultrasound appearances of bone and pleura.

FASCIA

Fascia, peritoneum, and aponeurosis appear as thin hyperechoic layers on US imaging.

BLOOD VESSELS

Arteries are identified by their pulsatility, are not easily compressible, and have anechoic lumens. Veins are not pulsatile, are easily compressible, and have anechoic lumens. Color Doppler or power Doppler modes can also be used to demonstrate blood flow pattern and differentiate arteries from veins (see Fig. 43.2).

PLEURA

The pleura appear as a hyperechoic line on US imaging (see Fig. 43.11).[53–55] During scanning of the intercostal space, the pleural line is located slightly below the hyperechoic ribs. "Comet-tail" artifacts may be present as a series of vertical lines arising from the pleura. On real-time imaging, lung sliding movement between the parietal and visceral pleura can be discerned from movement of the comet-tail artifacts ("lung sliding sign").

Special Techniques

TISSUE HARMONIC IMAGING

The term *harmonic* refers to frequencies that are integral multiples of the frequency of the transmitted pulse (which is also called the fundamental frequency or first harmonic). The second harmonic has a frequency of twice the fundamental frequency. Harmonics are generated in the tissues by the nonlinear propagation of sound.[56–58] Tissue harmonic imaging (THI) is a technique in which the harmonic signals reflected from tissue interfaces are selectively displayed. This results in reduced image artifacts, haze, and clutter and improved contrast resolution (Fig. 43.12).

COMPOUND IMAGING

US imaging depends on the reflection of the US from tissue interfaces. Not all tissues are good reflectors, and certain structures

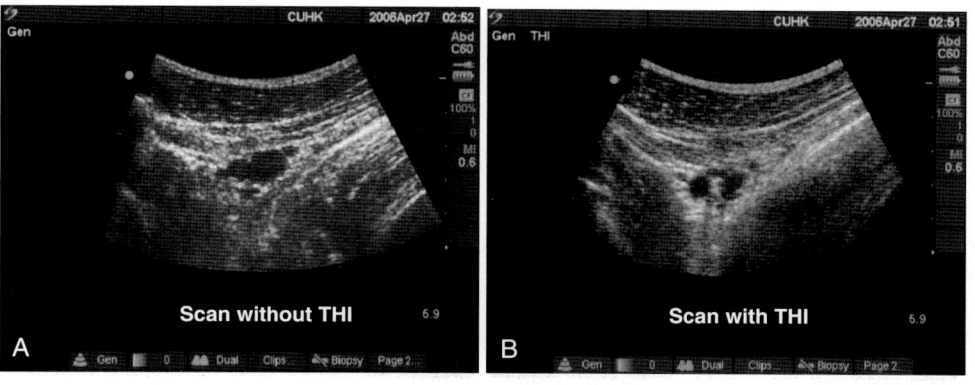

FIGURE 43.12 Tissue harmonic imaging *(THI)*. Sagittal sonogram of the infraclavicular fossa. **A,** Conventional scan. **B,** Conventional scan with THI.

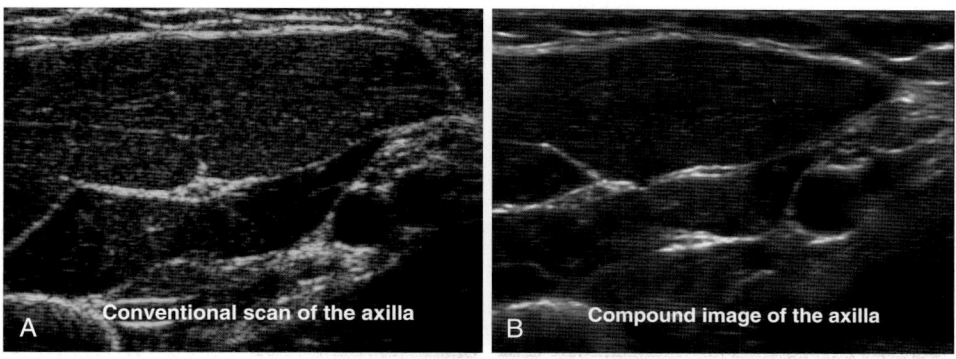

FIGURE 43.13 Compound imaging. Transverse sonogram of the axilla. **A,** Conventional scan. **B,** Conventional scan with compound imaging.

also cause scattering of the US signals. Unlike reflected signals, scattered signals radiate in all directions. As a result, only a small amount of energy is reflected back to the transducer. The scattering of the US signal results in speckle artifacts, also described as noise, which reduces image resolution and makes the US image appear grainy or noisy. Compound imaging is a technique used to improve resolution by reducing the contrast-to-noise ratio.[59] The US beam from the transducer is electronically steered, and the same structure is imaged from several different angles. The returning echoes are then processed with simultaneous filtering of the artifacts in real time, producing a composite image that has reduced noise or speckle and improved definition (Fig. 43.13).

PANORAMIC IMAGING

B-mode (2D) ultrasonography has a limited field of view and allows visualization of only a small portion of any large structure. Panoramic imaging, as the name implies, is a technique used to extend the field of view so that larger structures and their surrounding tissues can be visualized together.[60] During a panoramic scan, the operator slowly slides the US transducer across an area of interest. During this motion, multiple images are acquired from many different transducer positions across the area of interest. The registered image data are accumulated in a large buffer and then combined to form the composite panoramic image (Fig. 43.14). Although useful for annotation, documentation, teaching, and research, it is rarely used in children during USGRA procedures.

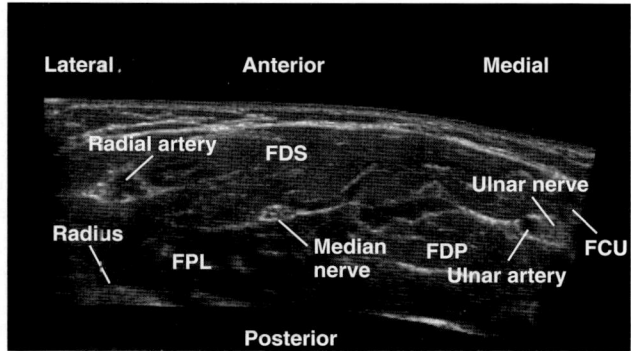

FIGURE 43.14 Panoramic imaging. Transverse panoramic scan of the forearm. *FCU,* flexor carpi ulnaris; *FDP,* flexor digitorum profundus; *FDS,* flexor digitorum superficialis *FPL,* flexor pollicis longus.

ARTIFACTS

US artifacts are structures that are visible in the US image that do not correlate with any anatomic structure.[61] The US machine makes the following assumptions when generating an image:
1. The US beam is considered to travel only in a straight line, with a constant rate of attenuation.
2. The average speed of sound through body tissue is considered to be 1540 m/second.

3. The US beam is assumed to be infinitely thin, with all echoes originating from its central axis.

4. The depth of a reflector is calculated by determining the round-trip time of the US signal.

When a deviation from any of these assumptions occurs, the US machine is unable to determine it. This results in the display of an echo that has no relation with the interface that actually produced the echo; that is, an artifact is produced. Some artifacts are undesirable and interfere with interpretation, whereas others help identify certain structures. It is essential to recognize them to avoid misinterpretation. Therefore when a structure appears abnormal on ultrasonography, it must be examined in two planes to avoid making a wrong interpretation. Real anatomic structures are visible in both planes of imaging, whereas artifacts are visible in only one plane.

Contact Artifact

The contact artifact is the most common artifact produced when loss of acoustic coupling occurs between the skin and the transducer. This could occur because the transducer is not touching the skin, but more frequently it is due to air bubbles that are trapped between the skin and the transducer. Therefore it is prudent to apply liberal amounts of gel to exclude air from the skin and transducer interface.

Reverberation Artifact

Reverberation artifacts, also known as repetitive echoes, occur when repeated reflection of US occurs between two highly reflective surfaces.[62] Some of the US signals returning to the transducer are reflected back, then strike the original interface, and are reflected back toward the transducer a second time. As a result, the first reverberation artifact is twice as far from the skin surface as the original interface. A second or third reverberation artifact also may be seen. Because of attenuation, the intensity of the artifacts decreases with increasing distance from the transducer. Reverberation artifacts are frequently seen during USG axillary brachial plexus block, particularly when the needle is inserted in the long axis.

Mirror Image Artifact

Mirror image artifact is a type of reverberation artifact that occurs at highly reflective interfaces.[63] The first image is displayed in the correct position, and a false image is produced on the other side of the reflector because of its mirrorlike effect.

Propagation Speed Artifact

Propagation speed artifacts occur when the medium through which the US beam passes does not propagate at 1540 m/second, resulting in echoes that appear at incorrect depths on the monitor. An example of propagation speed artifact is the "bayonet artifact," which has been reported during a USG axillary brachial plexus block.[64] The shaft of the needle appeared bent when it accidentally traversed the axillary artery. This happens because of the difference in the velocity of sound between whole blood (1580 m/second) and soft tissue (1540 m/second).

Acoustic Shadowing

Acoustic shadow is an echo-free area behind surfaces that are highly reflective or attenuating, such as bone (see Fig. 43.11) or metallic implants. The implication for regional anesthesia is that tissues in the area of the shadow cannot be imaged.

TABLE 43.2	Scanning Routine
1.	Turn on the ultrasound machine.
2.	Select a scanning mode.
3.	Select an appropriate transducer.
4.	Dim the lights in the room.
5.	Assume a comfortable position.
6.	Apply liberal amount of ultrasound gel.
7.	Perform a scout scan.
8.	Orient the transducer and image.
9.	Select the appropriate ultrasound settings (preset, frequency—for broadband transducers, depth, gain, and focus point).
10.	Mark the position of the transducer on the patient's skin once an optimal image is obtained before the intervention.

SCANNING ROUTINE

Being able to consistently produce high-quality images of the area scanned is vital for safety and success during any USGRA procedure. Without optimal images, it is not possible to accurately identify musculoskeletal structures or perform interventions with precision. We have found that following a "scanning routine," or a set of simple steps that are repeatable, is essential for optimal imaging; the routine that we follow is outlined in Table 43.2. Although the suggested routine may appear complicated at first, with repetition these steps are gradually internalized. Attaching a card with the scanning routine to the US machine facilitates easy recall.

Scout Scan

The aim of the scout scan, or the preintervention scan, as the name implies, is to examine the area of interest before the intervention. This has also been referred to as a "mapping scan." During the scout scan, steps 8 and 9 described in Table 43.2 are performed, the sonoanatomy of the area is visualized, and the image is optimized. Once an optimal view with the target structure is obtained and the best possible site for needle insertion is determined, it is advisable to mark the position of the transducer on the patient's skin so the transducer can be returned to the same position after sterile preparations have been completed. It is common to diagnose anatomic variations during the scout scan.[65] The operator can then decide whether to continue with the block in the same location or to choose an alternative approach or technique that may be safer. This assessment of anatomic variation is one of the major benefits of using US for regional anesthesia.

GENERAL CONSIDERATIONS IN CHILDREN

Preparations for a USG nerve block should begin during the preoperative visit by adequately explaining the technique, its benefits and risks, and, more importantly, the possibility of a failed block to the parents. In the event of failure, a contingency plan to quickly convert to general anesthesia or another form of postoperative analgesia must always be in place. In children, most regional anesthetic procedures are performed while the child is anesthetized. However, in a cooperative child or under special circumstances, such as in a child with difficult airway or a child predisposed to malignant hyperthermia, it is possible to perform the block after light sedation. We find that it is easy to explain the procedure to children who are older than 8 years of age. Some of them may even express a wish to stay awake and observe the US images during the block. Eutectic mixture of local anesthetic

(EMLA) cream applied an hour before the procedure to the skin over the area where the block needle and the intravenous catheter are to be inserted helps reduce needle-related pain. Parental presence during the nerve block may also be helpful. In older children, allowing the child to listen to favorite music through a personal stereo or watch a video are useful distraction techniques that make the whole experience a more pleasant one for the child. We have connected a DVD player to our US machine, and this is used to play movies or cartoons through the monitor during the surgical procedure (E-Fig. 43.1).

Before any USGRA procedure, intravenous access is established, standard monitoring is applied, and equipment and drugs appropriate for the child are prepared. Aseptic precautions are maintained, and the skin over the needle puncture site is prepared with antiseptic solution in the usual fashion. The US probe is placed inside a custom-designed sterile transducer plastic cover.[66]

TIPS AND TRICKS FOR SUCCESS

Certain steps are common to all USG procedures, and, if followed, they may increase success. The lights in the room must be dimmed to avoid any glare or reflection from the US monitor. The operator must assume a comfortable position (Fig. 43.15).[67] For upper extremity blocks, the operator sits at the ipsilateral head end of the child, and the US machine is placed directly in front. For lower extremity blocks, such as femoral nerve block, the operator stands on the ipsilateral side of the child, and the US machine is placed on the opposite side. For lower extremity or central neuraxial blocks in the lateral position, the operator sits behind the child, and the US machine is placed in front, with the monitor in the line of view of the operator. Because of the small muscle bulk in young children the nerves are relatively superficial and can most frequently be easily visualized using high-frequency linear transducers. The exact choice of transducer depends on the area scanned, but a high-frequency linear transducer with a small footprint (13-6 MHz, 25-mm footprint) is particularly suited for young children. The 15-6–MHz broadband linear-array transducer

is also useful for most blocks in young children. In older children, a 10-7–MHz broadband linear-array transducer, which allows greater flexibility with the depth of scan, is adequate for most procedures. Low-frequency (5-2 MHz) curved-array transducers are rarely used in children but are useful for imaging deeper structures such as the lumbar plexus and sciatic nerve in older children.

To improve dexterity, hold the transducer with the nondominant hand and perform interventions with the dominant hand. Holding the transducer steady for even short periods can be quite trying. We have found that gently resting the hand that is holding the transducer on the child during a block helps to keep the transducer steady (see Fig. 43.15). It is important to maintain light contact between the transducer and the skin because excessive pressure will cause the veins to collapse or distort the anatomy of the area of interest. Always apply liberal amounts of US gel to maintain adequate acoustic coupling between the skin and the transducer because even small amounts of air trapped between the two can result in artifacts. We use sterile US gel from single-use sachets for all USG peripheral nerve blocks. At any given time during a USG intervention either the transducer or the needle must be moved. It is impossible to maintain the needle within the plane of imaging if both are moving, a common error by novices. This results in an inability to visualize the needle. If the needle is not visible in the US image, a good strategy is to keep the needle steady and manipulate the transducer (slide, tilt, or rotate) until the needle becomes visible on the monitor. Thereafter the transducer should be held steady and the needle should be gently advanced to the target nerve, maintaining it in the imaging plane. When the angle of insertion of the needle is steep (>60 degrees), it is preferable to introduce the needle in the short axis using the out-of-plane technique. However, if the in-plane approach is used for all USG interventions, as in our case, inserting the needle a few centimeters away from the edge of the transducer may improve needle visibility by decreasing the angle between the needle and the imaging plane.

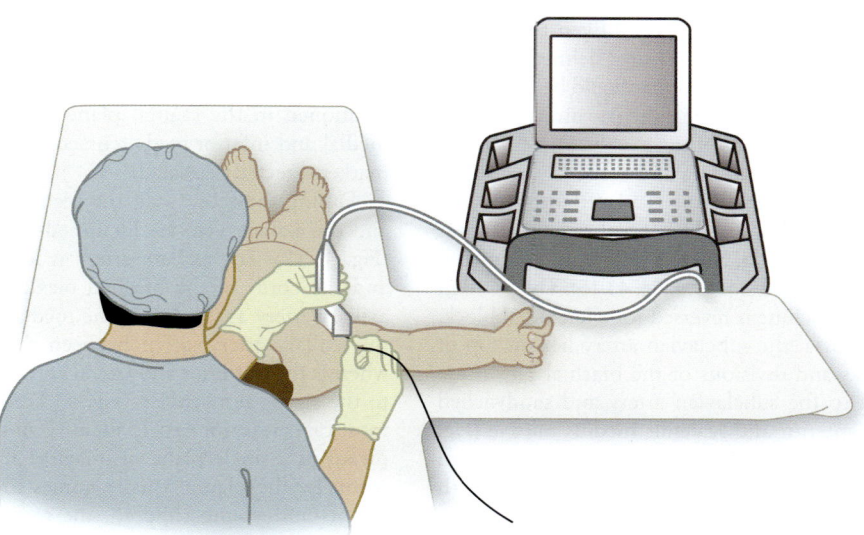

FIGURE 43.15 Position of the child, anesthesiologist, and ultrasound machine during an ultrasound-guided regional anesthesia procedure.

Injecting air into the area of the intervention must be avoided because air bubbles will degrade the image. We routinely purge the block needle with saline solution or local anesthetic to remove air before proceeding with the block. An assistant aids with the injection. When the needle tip is close to the target nerve, the assistant gently aspirates to exclude unintended intravascular placement. The assistant must avoid generating excessive negative pressure because small blood vessels are prone to collapse. A short length of extension tubing attached between the needle and the local anesthetic syringe allows the operator to hold the needle steady while the assistant performs the injection.[68] We routinely perform a test injection with 0.5 to 1 mL of saline solution or 5% dextrose (when nerve stimulation is also used)[46] and visualize the distribution of the injectate in real time before injecting the local anesthetic. Failure to visualize the injectate in the US image indicates that the needle is not in the plane of imaging or it is intravascular until proven otherwise. No further injection should be made until the needle is repositioned and the distribution of the injectate is confirmed.

ANCILLARY EQUIPMENT

Most single-shot peripheral nerve blocks can be performed with a standard short-bevel needle designed for regional anesthesia; an echogenic block needle is preferred because the echogenic coating allows it to be more easily identified. In older children, a 22-gauge block needle is a good choice. Most block needles also allow the use of peripheral nerve stimulation together with US-guidance. Indwelling catheters also can be placed under US guidance. A standard continuous peripheral nerve block kit (stimulating catheter with echogenic introducing needle) of an appropriate size can be used for catheter placement.

Specific Ultrasound-Guided Nerve Blocks

UPPER EXTREMITY BLOCKS

Supraclavicular Brachial Plexus Block

The supraclavicular brachial plexus block in children[69] is rarely used because of fear of pleural puncture and pneumothorax. However, USG supraclavicular brachial plexus block has been performed in children younger than 6 years.[70] Even though the brachial plexus and cervical pleura are clearly delineated using US in the supraclavicular fossa, this technique should be performed by experienced operators because of the close proximity between the cervical pleura and the brachial plexus.

The child's head rests on a head ring and is slightly turned to the contralateral side, and a small roll is placed between the scapula. For a right-sided block, a right-handed operator stands or sits at the head end of the child, and the US machine is placed directly in front on the ipsilateral side (see Fig. 43.15). The position of the operator and US machine is reversed for a left-sided block. In the supraclavicular fossa, the subclavian artery lies on top of the first rib. The trunks and divisions of the brachial plexus are superficial and lateral to the subclavian artery and sandwiched between the scalenus anterior and scalenus medius muscle (Fig. 43.16). A linear-array transducer (13-10 MHz) is used to perform the block; the hockey stick probe or a linear-array transducer with a small footprint (25 mm) is particularly suited for this block.

During the scout scan the transducer is positioned parallel to and against the clavicle and the subclavian artery is identified. The trunks and divisions of the brachial plexus often resemble a bunch of grapes on the superficial and lateral aspect of the subclavian artery (see Fig. 43.16). The cervical pleura and lung are

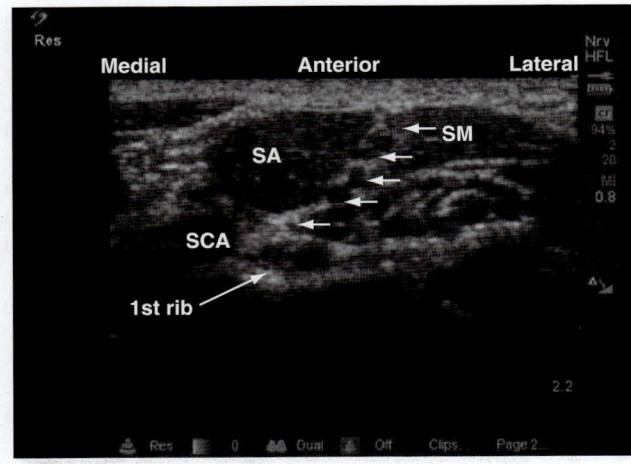

FIGURE 43.16 Sonographic appearance of the brachial plexus *(white arrows)* in the supraclavicular fossa. *SA,* scalenus anterior; *SCA,* subclavian artery; *SM,* scalenus medius.

deep to the first rib. The operator should bear in mind that the acoustic shadow of the first rib can obscure the view of the pleura and lung. The block needle is inserted in the long axis (in-plane) of the transducer in a lateral to medial direction, keeping the pleura in view. A test injection with saline solution is performed to ensure optimal needle position, after which the calculated dose of local anesthetic is injected in aliquots.

Infraclavicular Brachial Plexus Block

USG infraclavicular brachial plexus block is performed with the child in the supine position. The block can be performed with the arms by the side, but it is preferable to abduct the arm (to 90 degrees) whenever possible because it elevates the lateral part of the clavicle, which makes more space available below the clavicle for transducer placement. The operator sits at the ipsilateral head end of the child, and the US machine is positioned directly in front. Because the cords of the brachial plexus are relatively superficial in the infraclavicular fossa in children, a linear-array transducer (13-10 MHz in young children and 10-7 MHz in the older child) is used to perform the block. The transducer is positioned in the sagittal plane over the deltopectoral region, medial and inferior to the coracoid process, with its orientation marker directed cephalad.

During the scout scan the second part of the axillary artery and the axillary vein are identified deep to the pectoral muscles (Fig. 43.17). The axillary artery is located superior to the vein, and the cords of the brachial plexus are closely related to the axillary artery at this level. The medial cord is situated caudal to the axillary artery, often between the axillary artery and vein, whereas the posterior and lateral cords are posterior and cephalad to the artery, respectively (Fig. 43.17A). Despite this relation, in most cases it is not easy to identify all three cords of the brachial plexus in a single plane of imaging. If the transducer is moved medially, the pleura usually comes into view (Fig. 43.17B). In infants and young children, the margin of safety between the cords of the brachial plexus and the pleura is relatively small and pleural puncture is a risk if the block is performed in this medial position. Therefore we recommend that the infraclavicular brachial plexus block be performed laterally where the pleura is not visible in the US image.

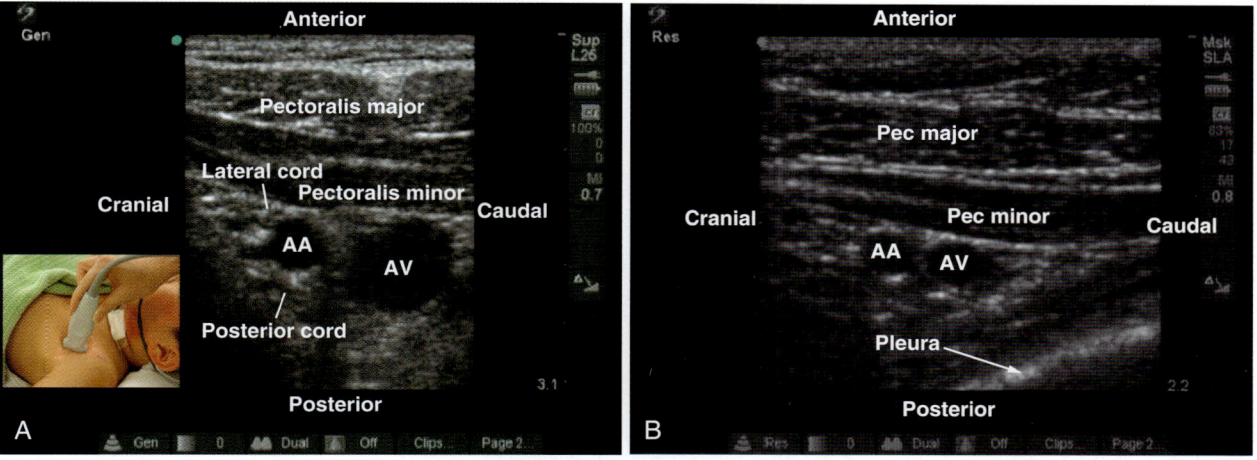

FIGURE 43.17 A, Sagittal sonogram of the left infraclavicular fossa. **B,** Sagittal sonogram of the infraclavicular fossa with the transducer positioned medially. Note the hyperechoic pleura in the lower right corner of the image *(arrow). AA,* axillary artery; *AV,* axillary vein; *Pec,* pectoralis.

We prefer to perform multiple injections targeting the areas where the three cords of the brachial plexus are located. The aim is to produce a circumferential spread of the local anesthetic around the axillary artery, the "doughnut sign" (Fig. 43.18), which correlates well with successful brachial plexus anesthesia. This perivascular injection technique is best visualized by imagining the transverse image of the axillary artery as a clock face with its 12-o'clock position in its anterior aspect and the 6-o'clock position in the posterior aspect of the artery (Fig. 43.19). The block needle is inserted in-plane and from a cranial to caudal direction (see Fig. 43.19), and one-third of the total dose of local anesthetic is injected close to each of the posterior (6-o'clock position), lateral (9-o'clock position), and medial (3-o'clock position) cords.[71-77] Because the angle of needle insertion is fairly steep with this approach, the needle is rarely seen on the US image, and the operator has to gently jiggle the needle to locate the needle tip. A subtle pop may be felt as the needle tip traverses the epimysium of the pectoralis minor muscle. A test injection with 1 mL of saline solution should be performed before the local anesthetic injection to ensure optimal needle position and distribution of the injectate (Video 43.1) (see also Fig. 42.20 for landmark-guided techniques).

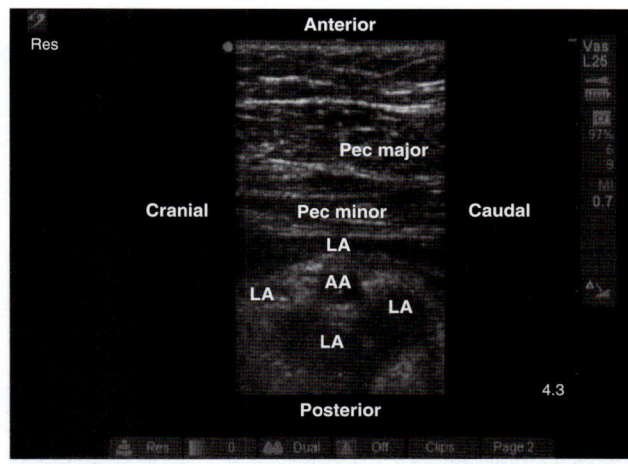

FIGURE 43.18 Infraclavicular brachial plexus block. Sagittal sonogram of the infraclavicular fossa after local anesthetic injection demonstrating the circumferential spread of local anesthetic around the axillary artery—the "doughnut sign." *AA,* axillary artery; *LA,* local anesthetic; *Pec,* pectoralis.

Axillary Brachial Plexus Block

USG axillary brachial plexus block is typically performed with the child in the supine position.[78-80] The arm is abducted (to 90 degrees) and externally rotated so that the palm of the hand is facing up. The operator sits at the ipsilateral head end of the child, and the US machine is positioned directly in front (see Fig. 43.15). Because the nerves of the brachial plexus are relatively superficial in the axilla, a high-frequency linear-array transducer (13-6 MHz) is used. During the scout scan, the transducer is positioned just below the lateral border of the pectoralis major muscle, with its orientation marker directed laterally (Fig. 43.20). The resultant image on the monitor is a transverse scan of the axillary structures. The pulsatile vessel in the image is the axillary artery. The axillary vein is medial to the artery; it is common to see more than one vein (see Fig. 43.20).

At this level, the three major nerves of the brachial plexus (the median, ulnar, and radial nerves) lie very close to the axillary artery. In adults, when the arm is abducted and externally rotated, the median nerve is located on the anterior or anterolateral side of the axillary artery (97.9%), the ulnar nerve is located on the anteromedial side of the artery (91.3%), and the radial nerve is located posterior to the axillary artery (89.9%)[81] (Fig. 43.21). To accurately identify these three nerves it may be necessary to trace the nerve distally along its course. The musculocutaneous nerve frequently courses between the coracobrachialis and the biceps muscle or within the substance of the coracobrachialis muscle (see Fig. 43.21).[82,83] Occasionally, the musculocutaneous nerve also may be located very close to the median nerve, and local anesthetic injected close to the median nerve may affect the musculocutaneous nerve. The shape of the musculocutaneous nerve varies along its course, and it may appear oval, round, elliptical, or even triangular.

We prefer the in-plane approach for needle insertion during axillary brachial plexus block in both sedated and anesthetized

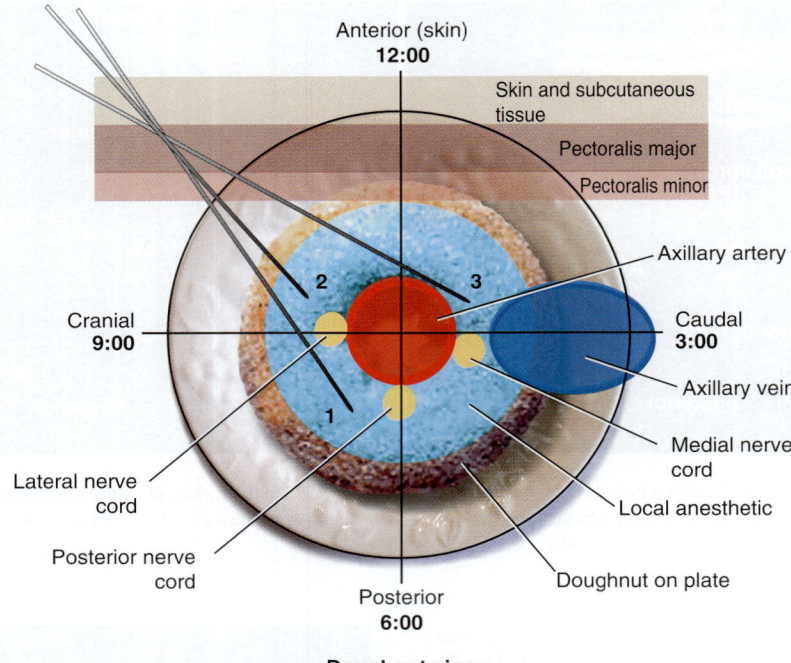

Doughnut sign

FIGURE 43.19 Infraclavicular brachial plexus block (oriented as with a wall clock). Schematic diagram showing the positions of the cords of the brachial plexus and the sites at which the local anesthetic is injected: (**1**) posterior cord, (**2**) lateral cord, and (**3**) medial cord.

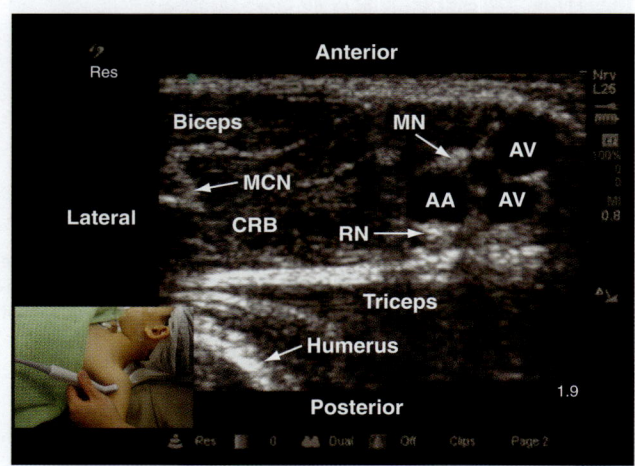

FIGURE 43.20 Transverse sonogram of the left axilla. *AA,* axillary artery; *AV,* axillary vein; *CRB,* coracobrachialis muscle; *MCN,* musculocutaneous nerve; *MN,* median nerve; *Res,* resolution; *RN,* radial nerve.

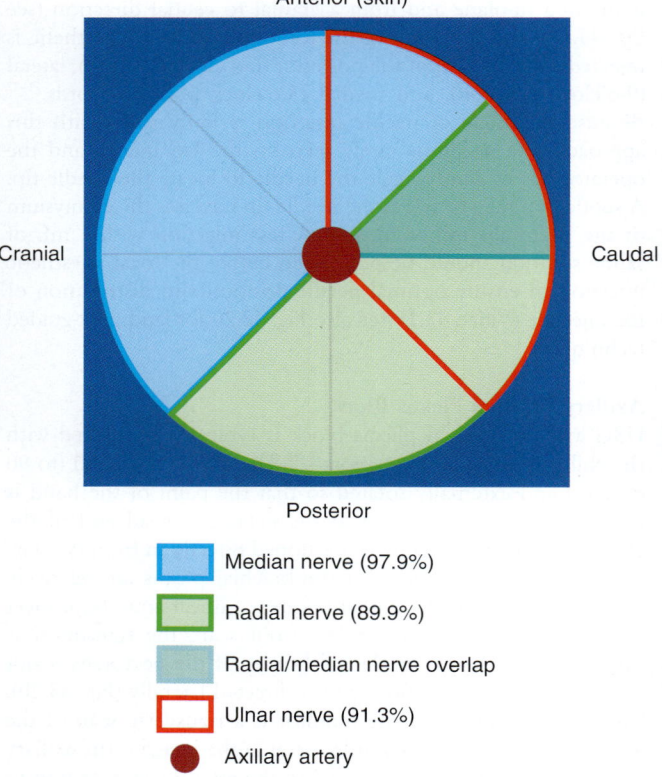

FIGURE 43.21 Schematic diagram showing the positions of the three main nerves (median, radial, and ulnar) of the brachial plexus in relation to the axillary artery, as identified on transverse ultrasonography, at the axilla.

children. The block needle is inserted from the lateral to the medial side of the arm, keeping it within the plane of the US imaging. A subtle pop is often felt when the tip of the needle traverses the epimysium of the biceps muscle and enters the fascial plane containing the neurovascular bundle. Multiple injections are required to block the median, radial, and ulnar nerves. The objective is to produce a circumferential spread of local anesthetic around the artery (i.e., "the doughnut sign" in the US image). To achieve this, local anesthetic is injected close to the anterior (12-o'clock position), posterior (6-o'clock position), and lateral

(9-o'clock position) aspects of the axillary artery. The musculocutaneous nerve is then identified and selectively blocked using a few milliliters of local anesthetic. We have found this approach to be technically simple, safe, and effective in producing brachial plexus blockade in children (Video 43.2) (see also Fig. 42.19 in Chapter 42 for landmark-guided techniques).

SELECTIVE PERIPHERAL NERVE BLOCKS OF THE UPPER EXTREMITY

Selective blockade of the nerves of the upper extremity can be used to rescue incomplete or partial axillary brachial plexus block or provide analgesia or anesthesia over a specific dermatome.[84] It has been successfully used in the emergency department for pain control and interventions involving the hand after trauma.[85] We have also found it to be useful for USG differential nerve blockade in children undergoing ambulatory hand surgery. This technique combines an axillary brachial plexus block with a short-acting local anesthetic agent such as lidocaine and a peripheral nerve block (e.g., a median or ulnar nerve block, depending on the dermatomes involved) in the forearm using a long-acting drug (bupivacaine or ropivacaine). Because of the shorter duration of action of lidocaine compared with bupivacaine or ropivacaine, the child regains protective motor function of the elbow fairly quickly after surgery (2–4 hours) while still enjoying prolonged postoperative analgesia from distal nerve blockade. All of the major nerves of the upper extremity (median, ulnar, and radial) can be identified using high-frequency linear-array transducers (13-10 MHz), and it is possible to selectively block these nerves at various sites along their course with only 1 to 2 mL of local anesthetic. In an adult study, the mean 95% effective dose (ED95) of 1% mepivacaine to block the ulnar nerve at the forearm is only 0.7 mL.[86] We prefer the in-plane needle insertion technique and use a short-beveled nerve block needle.

Median Nerve

The median nerve is closely related to the brachial artery throughout its course in the arm. Proximally it is lateral to the artery; in the middle of the upper arm it crosses to the medial side and then continues on the medial side distal to the elbow. In the antecubital fossa, the median nerve lies medial to the brachial artery, behind the bicipital aponeurosis, and in front of the brachialis muscle (Fig. 43.22A). In the forearm, the median nerve is deep to the flexor digitorum superficialis and on the surface of the flexor digitorum profundus (Fig. 43.22B) and accompanied by the median artery that is a branch of the anterior interosseous artery. Pulsations of the latter can occasionally be observed on the US image. A few centimeters proximal to the wrist, the median nerve becomes superficial and lies between the tendon of the flexor carpi radialis (laterally) and the flexor digitorum superficialis (medially) and may also be overlapped by the tendon of the palmaris longus.

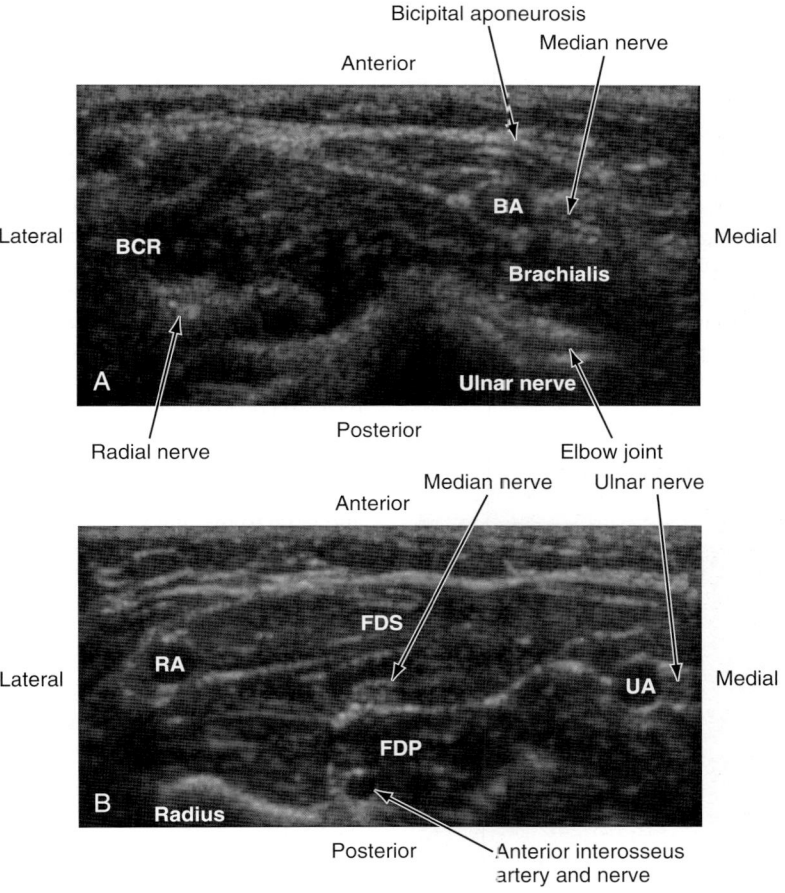

FIGURE 43.22 A, Transverse sonogram of the cubital fossa. **B,** Transverse sonogram of the forearm. *BA,* brachial artery; *BCR,* brachioradialis. *FDP,* Flexor digitorum profundus; *FDS,* flexor digitorum superficialis; *RA,* radial artery; *UA,* ulnar artery.

Because the nerve is superficial at this level and it can be difficult to differentiate the nerve from the tendons, we prefer to perform median nerve block at the midforearm, where it is clearly delineated (Video 43.3) (see also Fig. 42.25 for landmark-guided techniques).

Ulnar Nerve

Proximally, the ulnar nerve runs medial to the brachial artery to about the midhumeral level or the insertion of the coracobrachialis muscle, where it pierces the medial intermuscular septum and enters the posterior compartment of the arm. At the elbow, it passes behind the medial epicondyle to enter the ulnar nerve sulcus. Although the nerve is palpable and superficial at the sulcus, it is often difficult to visualize using US because of bony and contact artifacts. The ulnar nerve then enters the proximal forearm and runs between the flexor digitorum profundus (posterior) and the flexor digitorum superficialis (laterally) muscles, and in the distal forearm it is accompanied by the ulnar artery (lateral) (see Fig. 43.22B). Close to the wrist, the ulnar nerve is lateral to the flexor carpi ulnaris muscle. The ulnar artery may be used as a reference to locate the ulnar nerve. Once the artery is located, the nerve is traced backward and the local anesthetic injected away from the artery (see Video 43.3) (see also Fig. 42.25 for landmark-guided techniques).[87]

Radial Nerve

Proximally the radial nerve is posterior to the brachial artery. It then diverges from the artery to enter the radial (spiral) groove on the back of the arm, where it is accompanied by the profunda brachii artery. In the distal arm the radial nerve pierces the lateral intermuscular septum and enters the anterior compartment. In the antecubital fossa it is lateral to the biceps tendon and lies in an intermuscular gap between the brachialis (medially), the brachioradialis, and the extensor carpi radialis longus (laterally) (Fig. 43.23). At the level of the lateral epicondyle the radial nerve gives off the posterior interosseous nerve (deep branch of the radial nerve), which leaves the fossa by piercing the supinator muscle. In the forearm, the radial nerve (superficial branch of the radial nerve) continues as a pure cutaneous nerve and supplies the radial half of the dorsum of the hand and the proximal parts of the dorsal surfaces of the thumb and index finger. The radial nerve

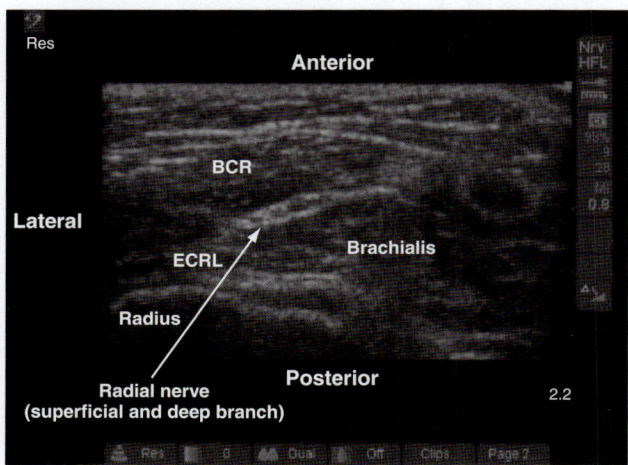

FIGURE 43.23 Transverse sonogram of the arm, just above the elbow, showing the radial nerve. *BCR*, brachioradialis; *ECRL*, extensor carpi radialis longus.

is best blocked before its division in the antecubital fossa (see also Fig. 42.22 for landmark-guided techniques).[84]

LOWER EXTREMITY BLOCKS

Lumbar Plexus Block

The lumbar plexus results from the union of the ventral rami of the first four lumbar spinal nerves within the substance of the psoas major muscle. The plexus may also receive contributions from the 12th thoracic nerve or the 5th lumbar nerve. In adults, the plexus is located between the fleshy anterior part of the psoas major muscle, which arises from the anterolateral part of the vertebral bodies and the intervertebral disk, and the accessory posterior part of the muscle that originates from the anterior surface of the transverse process. Local anesthetic injected into this intramuscular plane, also referred to as the psoas compartment, produces an ipsilateral lumbar plexus block.

A US scan for the lumbar plexus block can be performed in the transverse or sagittal axis at the L3-4 vertebral level. The child is positioned in the lateral position with the side to be blocked uppermost with the hip and knees flexed. A linear-array transducer (10-5 MHz) is adequate for imaging in young children, whereas in the older child (>6 to 8 years) a curved-array transducer (8-5 or 5-2 MHz) is required.

For a transverse scan, the US transducer is positioned approximately 2 to 3 cm lateral to the lumbar spine at the L3-4 vertebral level, with its orientation marker directed laterally. We also prefer to align the transducer slightly medially to produce a paramedian oblique transverse scan (PMOTS) of the lumbar paravertebral region.[88–92] Also during a PMOTS of the lumbar paravertebral region, the US beam can be insonated either at the level of the transverse process (PMOTS-TP, Fig. 43.24A) or through the gap between the two adjacent transverse process (i.e., the intertransverse space [ITS]), producing a PMOTS-ITS scan (Fig. 43.24B). In a typical PMOTS-ITS sonogram of the lumbar paravertebral region, the erector spinae muscle, the vertebral body, the psoas major muscle, the quadratus lumborum muscle, and the anterolateral surface of the vertebral body are clearly visualized (Fig. 43.24B). The inferior vena cava (on the right side) and the aorta (on the left side) are also identified anterior to the vertebral body. The lower pole of the kidney is closely related to the anterior surfaces of the quadratus lumborum and psoas muscle and is seen as an oval structure that moves with respiration in the retroperitoneal space. The lumbar plexus is not sonographically visualized in all patients, but when it is visualized, it appears as an oval hyperechoic structure in the posterior part of the psoas muscle (see Fig. 43.24B) and close to the intervertebral foramen. In contrast, because the acoustic shadow of the transverse process obscures the posterior part of the psoas muscle and the area close to the intervertebral foramen during a PMOTS-TP, the lumbar plexus is rarely visualized in this US scan window (see Fig. 43.24A). Therefore if a transverse scan is performed during a USG lumbar plexus block, it is our recommendation to use the PMOTS-ITS.[91,92]

For a sagittal scan of the lumbar paravertebral region, the US transducer is positioned approximately 2 to 3 cm lateral and parallel to the lumbar spine, with its orientation marker directed cranially. In a typical sagittal sonogram of the lumbar paravertebral region, the L2, L3, and L4 transverse processes with their acoustic shadow produce what we refer to as the "trident sign" (Fig. 43.25) because of its similarity to the trident (Limia tridens or tridentis) that is often associated with Poseidon (the god of the sea in Greek mythology) and the trishula of the Hindu god Shiva.[93] The hypoechoic psoas muscle is seen between the transverse processes,

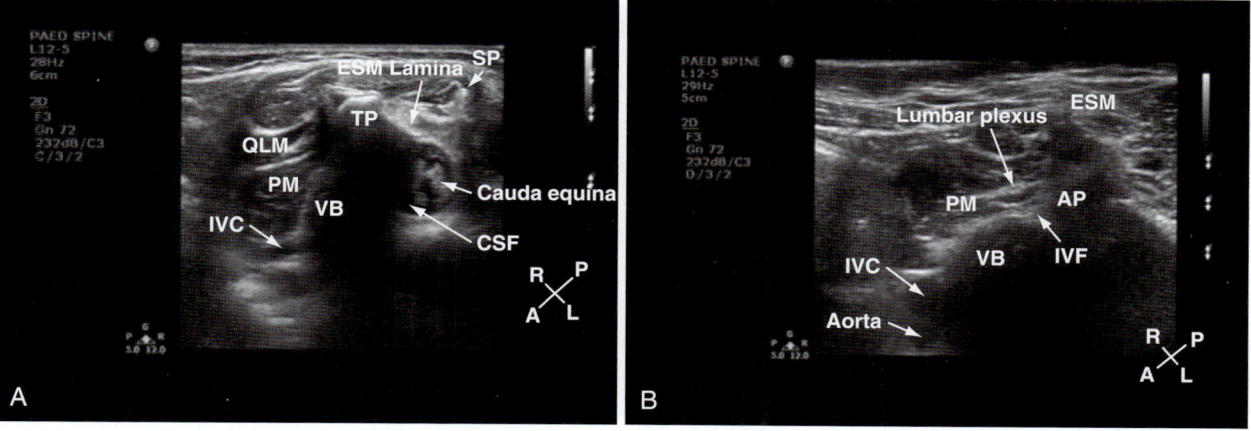

FIGURE 43.24 A, Paramedian oblique transverse scan of the right lumbar paravertebral region at the level of the transverse process (PMOTS-TP) in an 11-month old infant. Note how the acoustic shadow of the transverse process (TP) obscures the posterior part of the psoas muscle (PM) and how parts of the spinal canal and neuraxial structures (dura, intrathecal space, and cauda equina) are seen through the interlaminar space. **B,** Paramedian oblique transverse scan of the right paravertebral region through the gap between two adjacent transverse processes (PMOTS-ITS) in a 14-month old child. Note the intervertebral foramen (IVF), articular process (AP), and the lumbar plexus in the posterior part of the PM. A, anterior; CSF, cerebrospinal fluid; ESM, erector spinae muscle; IVC, inferior vena cava; L, left; P, posterior; PM, psoas muscle; QLM, quadratus lumborum muscle; R, right; SP, spinous process; VB, vertebral body.

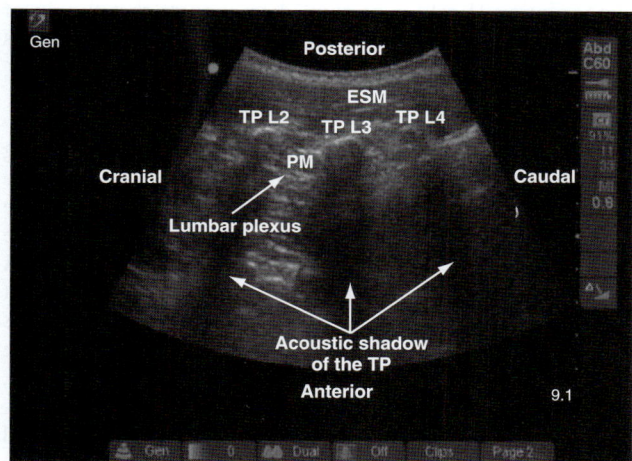

FIGURE 43.25 Longitudinal sonogram of the lumbar paravertebral region showing the lumbar plexus. ESM, erector spinae muscle; PM, psoas muscle; TP, transverse process ("trident sign").

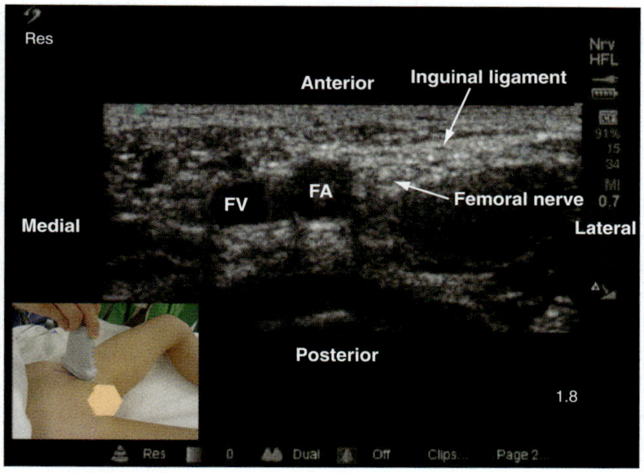

FIGURE 43.26 Transverse sonogram of the inguinal region showing the femoral nerve and its relations. FA, femoral artery; FV, femoral vein.

and the lumbar plexus is identified as hyperechoic longitudinal striations within the posterior aspect of the muscle. A laterally positioned transducer will produce a suboptimal scan without the trident, and the lower pole of the kidney, which can reach the L4-5 level in young children, will come into view.

Once an optimal image of the lumber paravertebral region is obtained, the insulated block needle is inserted in the plane of the US beam. The needle is inserted from the medial side of the transducer when a PMOTS-ITS is used or from the caudal end of the transducer when a sagittal scan is used. The needle is slowly advanced under ultrasound guidance to the posterior part of the psoas muscle, and the correct position of the needle tip close to the lumbar plexus is confirmed by observing ipsilateral quadriceps muscle contraction. After negative aspiration, an appropriate dose

of local anesthetic is injected in aliquots over 2 to 3 minutes and the patient is closely monitored.

Femoral Nerve Block

The femoral nerve is the largest branch of the lumbar plexus and is the major nerve of the anterior (extensor) compartment of the thigh. It is formed by the dorsal division of the anterior primary rami of spinal nerves L2, L3, and L4. It exits the pelvis and enters the femoral triangle in the thigh by passing under the inguinal ligament just lateral to the femoral artery. In the thigh it lies in the groove between the iliacus and the psoas major muscle, outside the femoral sheath, and lateral to the femoral artery. A high-frequency (13-10 MHz) linear-array transducer is used to scan the femoral nerve. On a transverse sonogram the femoral nerve is seen as an oval or triangular hyperechoic structure lateral to the femoral artery (Fig. 43.26). The femoral nerve exhibits marked anisotropy, and it may be necessary to tilt or rotate the transducer during the scan before it can be visualized.[48] In young children one must avoid exerting too much pressure during the scan because it is easy to compress the femoral vein.

A femoral nerve block is used to provide postoperative analgesia after femoral fractures. It is performed with the child in the supine position. The ipsilateral lower limb is slightly abducted and externally rotated, and the knee is also slightly flexed. A right-handed operator stands on the right side of the child, and the US machine is positioned directly in front on the contralateral side. The sides of the operator and the US machine are reversed for a left-handed operator. The scout scan is performed with the transducer positioned parallel and just below the inguinal ligament. This ensures that the femoral nerve is scanned before its division. Once an optimal view of the femoral nerve is obtained, the block needle is inserted in the long axis (in-plane) of the US transducer from the lateral to medial side and directed to the lateral aspect of the femoral nerve.[48,94] A test injection with saline solution is performed before the local anesthetic is injected to confirm that the needle is deep to the fascia iliaca and to observe the distribution of the injectate in relation to the femoral nerve (see also Fig. 42.32 for landmark-guided techniques).

Subsartorial Saphenous Nerve Block
The saphenous nerve is a branch of the anterior division of the femoral nerve and supplies the skin on the medial aspect of the leg and foot up to the ball of the big toe. In the thigh, the saphenous nerve is located in the subsartorial canal, and local anesthetic injected into this intramuscular space produces a saphenous nerve block. The subsartorial canal is also referred to as the adductor canal or Hunter canal and is situated on the medial side of the middle one third of the thigh and extends from the apex of the femoral triangle, above, to the tendinous opening in the adductor magnus muscle, below. The canal is triangular in cross-section, and its anterior wall is formed by the vastus medialis muscle, the posterior wall or floor is formed by the adductor longus, and the medial wall or roof is formed by a strong fibrous membrane that is overlapped by the sartorius muscle (Fig. 43.27). The subsartorial canal contains the following structures: femoral artery and vein, saphenous nerve, nerve to vastus medialis, and the two divisions

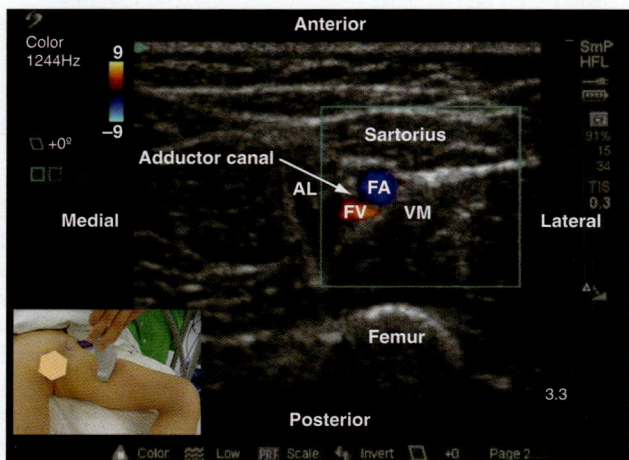

FIGURE 43.27 Transverse sonogram of the thigh showing the adductor canal. *AL*, adductor longus; *FA*, femoral artery; *FV*, femoral vein; *VM*, vastus medialis.

of the obturator nerve. The femoral vein lies posterior to the artery in the upper part and lateral to the artery in the lower part of the canal. The saphenous nerve crosses the femoral artery anteriorly from the lateral to the medial side in the canal.[95–98]

A high-frequency (13-6 MHz) linear-array probe is used to scan the saphenous nerve in the subsartorial canal with the child the supine position. The ipsilateral lower limb is slightly abducted and externally rotated, and the knee is also slightly flexed. For a right-sided block, a right-handed operator stands on the right side of the patient, and the US machine is positioned directly in front on the contralateral side. The transducer is positioned in the transverse axis over the middle one-third of the thigh. The triangular subsartorial canal can be identified between the epimysium of the vastus medialis (closely related to the femur), the adductor longus, and the sartorius muscles. The pulsatile femoral artery lies anterior to the vein in the canal, and the saphenous nerve is seen as a round or oval hyperechoic structure anterior to the artery (12-o'clock position). Because the saphenous nerve is a small nerve, it may not always be visible on US imaging in children. However, owing to the close relation of the saphenous nerve to the femoral artery in the subsartorial canal, a perivascular (arterial) injection in the canal will produce a saphenous nerve block. The block needle is inserted in the long-axis (in-plane) of the US transducer from the medial to lateral side and is directed to the anterior aspect of the femoral artery. A test injection of saline solution (1 mL) is performed to confirm that the tip of the needle is in the canal, after which the local anesthetic is injected.

Sciatic Nerve Block
The sciatic nerve is the largest mixed nerve in the body, arising from the lumbosacral plexus (L4, L5, S1-3). It innervates the posterior aspect of the thigh and the entire lower limb below the knee except for a small patch of skin on the medial aspect of the leg and ankle, which is innervated by the saphenous nerve. A sciatic nerve block is frequently used to provide analgesia for foot (clubfoot) and leg surgery in children. Several different approaches to the sciatic nerve have been described; most rely on surface anatomic landmarks (anterior, transgluteal, infragluteal, lateral, posterior subgluteal, proximal thigh, or at the popliteal fossa). USG sciatic nerve block also has been described[99–110]; a proximal approach is selected when surgery involves the hip (rare in children) or block of the posterior cutaneous nerve of the thigh is warranted. Because a sciatic nerve block is most frequently used for foot (clubfoot) surgery in children, a distal approach to the sciatic nerve at the popliteal fossa is usually preferred (see also Fig. 42.30 for landmark-guided techniques).

Sciatic Nerve Block at the Subgluteal Space
The sciatic nerve exits the pelvis through the greater sciatic foramen, between the piriformis and the superior gemelli muscles, and enters the subgluteal space below the piriformis muscle. It then descends over the dorsum of the ischium, lying on the dorsal surface of the superior gemellus muscle, tendon of obturator internus, inferior gemellus muscle, and quadratus femoris muscle (in a cranial to caudal relation) before it enters the hollow between the greater trochanter and the ischial tuberosity and then goes on to the posterior compartment of the thigh. The anterior surface of the gluteus maximus covers the upper part of the sciatic nerve; immediately distal to its lower border (infragluteal position), the sciatic nerve is fairly superficial. In between the greater trochanter and the ischial tuberosity, the sciatic nerve lies in the subgluteal

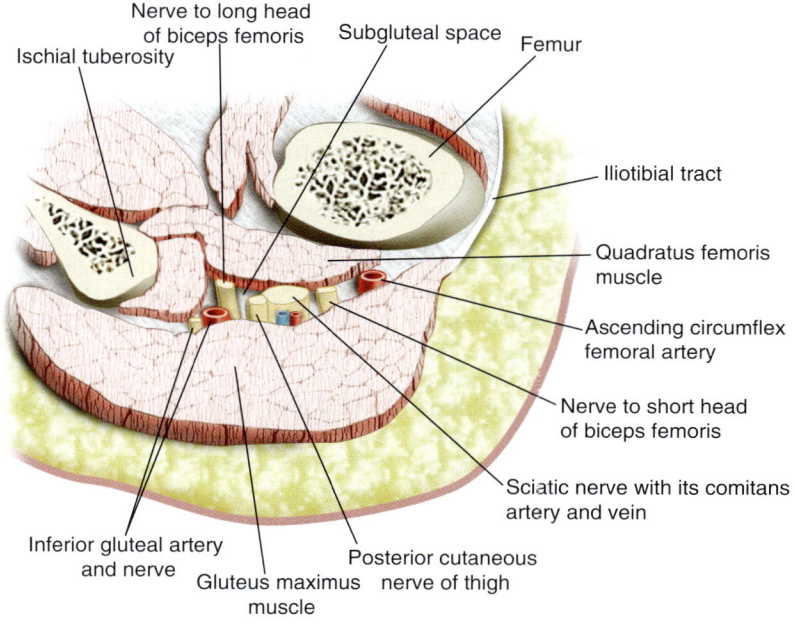

Nerve to long head
of biceps femoris
Ischial tuberosity
Subgluteal space   Femur
Iliotibial tract
Quadratus femoris
muscle
Ascending circumflex
femoral artery
Nerve to short head
of biceps femoris
Sciatic nerve with its comitans
artery and vein
Inferior gluteal artery
and nerve
Gluteus maximus
muscle
Posterior cutaneous
nerve of thigh

FIGURE 43.28 Transverse section through the gluteal region at the level of the quadratus femoris muscle showing the subgluteal space and its contents.

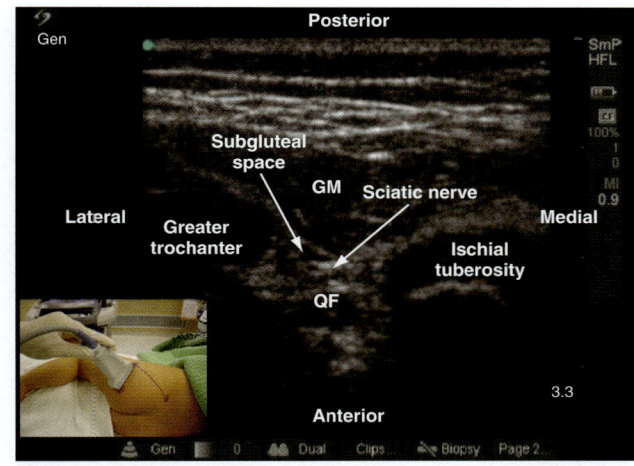

FIGURE 43.29 Transverse sonogram between the greater trochanter and the ischial tuberosity showing the hypoechoic subgluteal space between the hyperechoic perimysium of the gluteus maximus and the quadratus femoris muscle. The sciatic nerve is seen as a hyperechoic structure in the medial aspect of the subgluteal space. *GM*, gluteus maximus; *QF*, quadratus femoris.

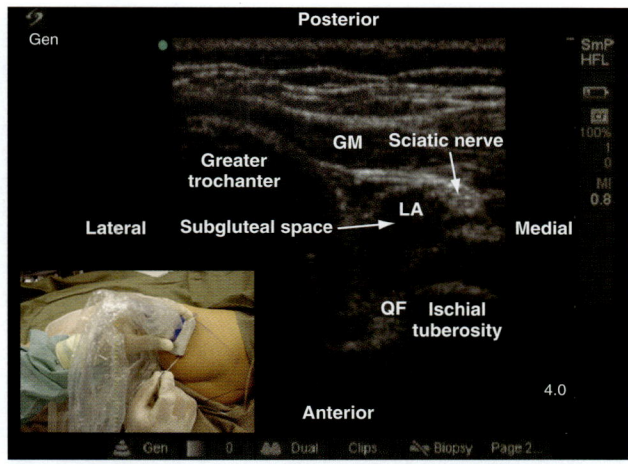

FIGURE 43.30 Transverse sonogram of the sciatic nerve at the subgluteal space after local anesthetic injection. Note the distention of the subgluteal space caused by the local anesthetic and the distribution of local anesthetic around the sciatic nerve. *GM*, gluteus maximus; *LA*, local anesthetic; *QF*, quadratus femoris.

space, which is a well-defined anatomic space between the anterior surface of the gluteus maximus and the posterior surface of the quadratus femoris muscle (Fig. 43.28).[99] Other structures present in the subgluteal space include the posterior cutaneous nerve of the thigh, the inferior gluteal vessels and nerve, the nerve to the short and long head of the biceps femoris, the comitans artery and vein of the sciatic nerve, and the ascending branch of the medial circumflex artery (Fig. 43.29). Local anesthetic injected into the subgluteal space blocks the sciatic nerve and the posterior cutaneous nerve of the thigh, which is useful when anesthesia over the posterior aspect of the thigh is needed.

USG sciatic nerve block at the subgluteal space is performed with the child in the lateral position. The side to be anesthetized is placed uppermost, and the hip and knees are flexed (Fig. 43.30). The operator sits or stands behind the child, and the US machine is positioned directly in front. In young children, a linear-array transducer (10-5 MHz) is adequate for imaging the sciatic nerve; in children older than 6 to 8 years, the sciatic nerve can also be imaged using a curved linear array transducer (8-5 or 5-2 MHz) (preferred) because the increased depth of scan required (as a result of increased muscle bulk) limits the field of vision when a linear transducer is used.

The greater trochanter and the ischial tuberosity are identified, and a line is drawn between these two landmarks. The US transducer is placed parallel to this line, with its orientation marker directed toward the greater trochanter to obtain a transverse scan of the sciatic nerve and the subgluteal space.[99-101] It may be necessary to slide the transducer slightly cephalad or caudad before an optimal image of the sciatic nerve in the subgluteal space can be obtained. On a transverse sonogram, the subgluteal space is seen as a hypoechoic area between the hyperechoic epimysium of the gluteus maximus and quadratus femoris muscle (see Fig. 43.30) extending from the greater trochanter laterally to the ischial tuberosity medially. The subgluteal space is not so well delineated in young children and is better visualized in older children. The sciatic nerve is seen as an oval or triangular hyperechoic structure within the subgluteal space (see Fig. 43.30). The medial limit of the space is obscured by the attachments of the semimembranosus, semitendinosus, and biceps femoris muscles to the ischial tuberosity. Pulsations of the inferior gluteal artery often can be detected medial to the sciatic nerve on the sonogram.

The block needle is inserted using an in-plane technique from the ischial tuberosity side and advanced slowly toward the sciatic nerve.[99,102] Once the block needle is deemed to be in the subgluteal space, the position is confirmed by injecting 1 to 2 mL of saline solution and observing a distention of the subgluteal space (i.e., separation of the epimysium of the gluteus maximus and quadratus femoris muscle) on the US image (Fig. 43.31). However, if the test injection of saline solution spreads posterior to the epimysium of the gluteus maximus muscle, it indicates that the tip of the needle is not in the subgluteal space. The needle should be reoriented and advanced a little farther until the typical distention of the subgluteal space to the saline solution test injection is seen. Occasionally, a subtle pop is felt when the needle tip traverses the epimysium of the gluteus maximus muscle and enters the subgluteal space. Local anesthetic is then injected in aliquots over 2 to 3 minutes while observing for the distention of the subgluteal space and the spread of local anesthetic in relation to the sciatic nerve. It is also easy to pass a catheter into the subgluteal space when a continuous sciatic nerve block is planned. Because the catheter is inserted into an anatomic space, the catheter is also more likely to stay in situ (Video 43.4) (see also Figs. 42.28–42.30. for landmark-guided techniques).

Sciatic Nerve Block at the Popliteal Fossa

The sciatic nerve block at the popliteal fossa is the preferred approach for children undergoing foot surgery. The popliteal fossa is a diamond-shaped space lying behind the knee joint, the lower part of the femur, and the upper part of the tibia. It is bound superolaterally by the biceps femoris tendon, superomedially by the semitendinosus and the semimembranosus tendons, inferolaterally by the lateral head of the gastrocnemius, and inferomedially by the medial head of the gastrocnemius. The sciatic nerve enters the posterior aspect of the thigh at the lower border of the gluteus maximus and runs vertically downward to the apex of the superior triangle of the popliteal fossa, where it terminates by dividing into the tibial and the common peroneal nerve, usually 3 to 7 cm above the popliteal crease in adults.[103-106] The division of the sciatic nerve into its terminal branches may, however, takes place anywhere above this level. This accounts for the occasional sparing of either division of the sciatic nerve after distal sciatic nerve block techniques using a nerve stimulation.

Although the classic teaching is to perform a popliteal sciatic nerve block with the patient in the prone position, it is very commonly performed in children with the child in the supine position with the leg elevated by an assistant (Fig. 43.32). During USG popliteal sciatic nerve block the operator sits on the ipsilateral side facing the head of the patient, and the US machine is positioned directly in front. In young children, a linear-array transducer (10-5 MHz) is adequate for imaging the sciatic nerve in the popliteal fossa; in the adolescent child or children with muscular thighs, a curved-array transducer (8-5 MHz) may be preferable. The transducer is positioned just above the apex of the upper triangle of the popliteal fossa in the transverse axis (see Fig. 43.29). It may be necessary to first scan for the sciatic nerve in the middle of the thigh and then trace it distally to the popliteal fossa, where the sciatic nerve is seen as a round, hyperechoic structure. Division of the sciatic nerve into the tibial and common peroneal nerves varies widely but can be visualized in children.[107] In the popliteal fossa and proximal to the popliteal crease, the tibial and common peroneal nerves are seen as hyperechoic structures superficial and lateral to the popliteal artery.

The block needle is inserted using in-plane technique from the lateral aspect of the thigh with its point of entry being anterior to the tendon of the biceps femoris (if it is palpable). This places

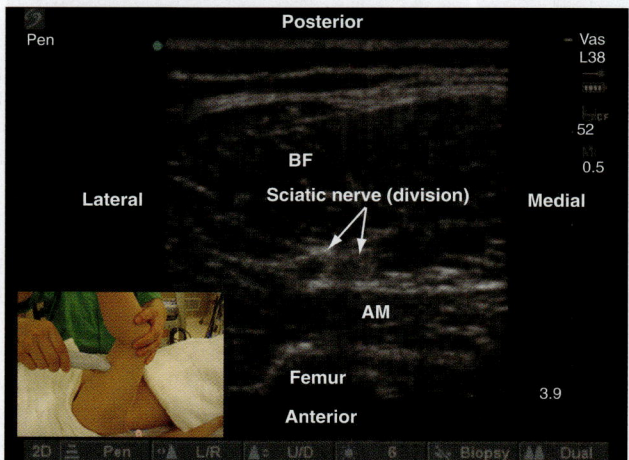

FIGURE 43.31 Popliteal sciatic nerve block. Transverse sonogram of the sciatic nerve at the apex of the popliteal fossa. *AM*, adductor magnus; *BF*, biceps femoris.

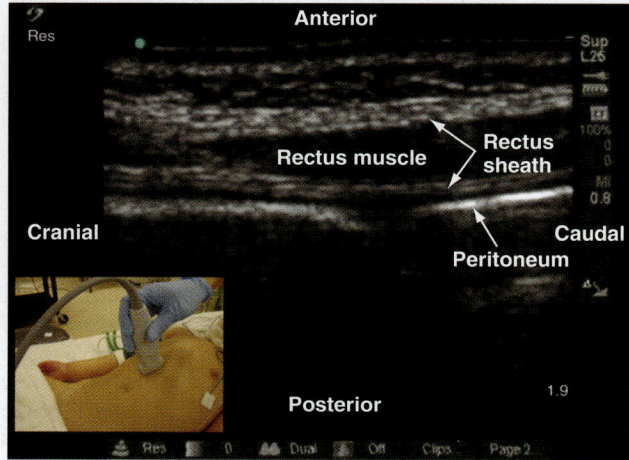

FIGURE 43.32 Longitudinal sonogram of the rectus muscle showing the anterior and posterior rectus sheath.

the needle in the same orientation as for the lateral approach to the sciatic nerve at the popliteal fossa. The exact point of needle entry will depend on where the sciatic nerve is best visualized. The needle is gradually advanced under US guidance, and the tip is positioned just posterior to the sciatic nerve. This is confirmed by injecting 1 to 2 mL of saline solution through the needle, after which half of the calculated dose of local anesthetic is injected. The same process is repeated by repositioning the tip of the needle anterior to the sciatic nerve. This ensures that the local anesthetic spreads optimally around the sciatic nerve (see also Fig. 42.30 for landmark-guided techniques).

TRUNCAL BLOCKS
Rectus Sheath Block

The rectus sheath block is the technique of injecting local anesthetic into the potential space between the rectus muscle and the posterior rectus sheath. This produces anesthesia of the ventral rami of the intercostal nerves as they traverse the rectus muscle to supply the skin of the anterior abdominal wall on either side of the midline. Because the seventh and eighth intercostal nerves also provide motor innervation to the rectus abdominis muscle, a rectus sheath block at this level should also produce relaxation of the muscle. Bilateral rectus sheath blocks are frequently used in children to provide perioperative analgesia during umbilical and paraumbilical hernia repair.[108,109] We have also found it to be useful for analgesia after laparoscopic procedures in children in whom the port insertion sites are close to the midline.

The rectus abdominis muscle arises as two tendinous heads from the lateral part of the pubic crest and the anterior pubic ligament. The fibers run vertically upward and are inserted to the front of the chest wall through the xiphoid process and the fifth, sixth, and seventh costal cartilages. The muscle is enclosed in a fibrous aponeurotic sheath, the rectus sheath, which is formed by the aponeurosis of the external oblique, internal oblique, and transversus abdominis muscles. The anterior rectus sheath is complete and covers the muscle from end to end. However, the posterior rectus sheath is incomplete, being deficient above the costal cartilage and below the arcuate line (or the fold of Douglas), which is located midway between the umbilicus and the pubic symphysis. The rectus sheath on both sides is held together in the midline by a raphe, the linea alba, which is formed by the fusion of the fibers of the three aponeuroses that form the rectus sheath. The ventral rami of the 7th to 12th intercostal nerves pass anteriorly and downward from the intercostal spaces and pierce the posterolateral aspect of the rectus sheath before passing anteriorly through the muscle to supply the skin of the anterior abdominal wall. Three transverse fibrous bands (tendinous insertions)—one at the level of the umbilicus, one at the level of the xiphoid process, and one midway between the two—divide the rectus muscle into three smaller parts. These fibrous bands are adherent to the anterior rectus sheath and traverse only the anterior half of the rectus muscle. Therefore a potential space exists between the rectus muscle and the posterior rectus sheath that communicates from the xiphisternum to the pubic crest. Local anesthetic injected into this space can spread up and down the sheath and is the basis of a rectus sheath block.

A linear-array transducer (13-10 MHz) with a small footprint (25 mm) is used for imaging in children (see Fig. 43.32). The operator stands or sits on one side of the anesthetized child, and the US machine is positioned directly opposite on the contralateral side. The transducer is positioned in the longitudinal axis midway between the umbilicus and the xiphisternum. The rectus muscle

is seen as a hypoechoic structure between the hyperechoic anterior and posterior rectus sheath (see Fig. 43.32). Deep to the posterior rectus sheath the hyperechoic peritoneum can be recognized by its typical peritoneal sliding movement and the comet-tail artifacts produced. The fibrous bands (tendinous insertions) in the rectus sheath can also be recognized in the longitudinal sonogram as hyperechoic areas on the anterior surface of the hypoechoic muscle that do not traverse the whole muscle belly.[110-112] The linea alba can be recognized on a transverse sonogram, and the posterior deficiency of the rectus sheath is also readily recognized below the level of the arcuate line.

The block needle is inserted using the in-plane technique in a caudal to cranial direction (Fig. 43.33A and B). When the tip of the needle is visualized in the potential space between the rectus muscle and the posterior rectus sheath, a test injection of saline solution (1–2 mL) is performed to confirm the longitudinal spread of the injectate between the muscle and the rectus sheath and the widening of the space (Fig. 43.33 C and D). Injection into the muscle will offer resistance to injection and is readily recognized in the sonogram. The needle should be repositioned, and the typical spread of the test injection under the rectus muscle should be confirmed before a calculated dose of the local anesthetic is injected.[113] For umbilical hernia surgery, bilateral rectus sheath blocks are performed just above the umbilicus on either side.

Ilioinguinal and Iliohypogastric Nerve Blocks

Ilioinguinal and iliohypogastric nerve blocks are used to provide analgesia after inguinal hernia repair, orchidopexy, or hydrocele surgery. The analgesia is comparable to caudal epidural analgesia, and it offers the advantage of not affecting micturition after surgery, making it ideal for an outpatient procedure. Currently anatomic landmarks and tactile sensations are relied upon to perform the block, which unfortunately can result in failure in up to 20% to 30% of cases. Moreover, it can also lead to complications such as femoral nerve palsy, pelvic hematoma, and bowel perforation.[114] A USG ilioinguinal iliohypogastric nerve block has been compared with the traditional landmark-based method; USG ilioinguinal iliohypogastric nerve block is more accurate, uses smaller volumes of local anesthetic, and has a greater success rate.[115]

The ilioinguinal and iliohypogastric nerves are branches of the primary ventral ramus of L1, which arises from the lumbar plexus. It also receives contributions from the T12 spinal nerve. Superomedial to the anterior superior iliac spine (ASIS), the two nerves pierce the transversus abdominis muscle to lie between it and the internal oblique muscle. The iliohypogastric nerve is situated superior to the ilioinguinal nerve and continues inferomedially for a short distance, after which their ventral rami transverse the internal oblique muscle to lie between the internal and external oblique muscles before giving off branches that pierce the external oblique muscle to provide cutaneous sensation. The iliohypogastric nerve supplies sensory innervation to the skin over the inguinal region. The ilioinguinal nerve continues anteroinferiorly with the spermatic cord or the round ligament in the inguinal canal and becomes superficial by emerging through the superficial inguinal ring to innervate the skin of the upper medial aspect of the thigh and either the skin of the upper part of the scrotum and the root of the penis or the skin covering the labia majora and mons pubis.

A linear-array transducer (13-10 MHz) is used for imaging the ilioinguinal and iliohypogastric nerves, which are best visualized close to the ASIS.[115-117] The operator stands on the ipsilateral side to be blocked, and the US machine is positioned directly opposite

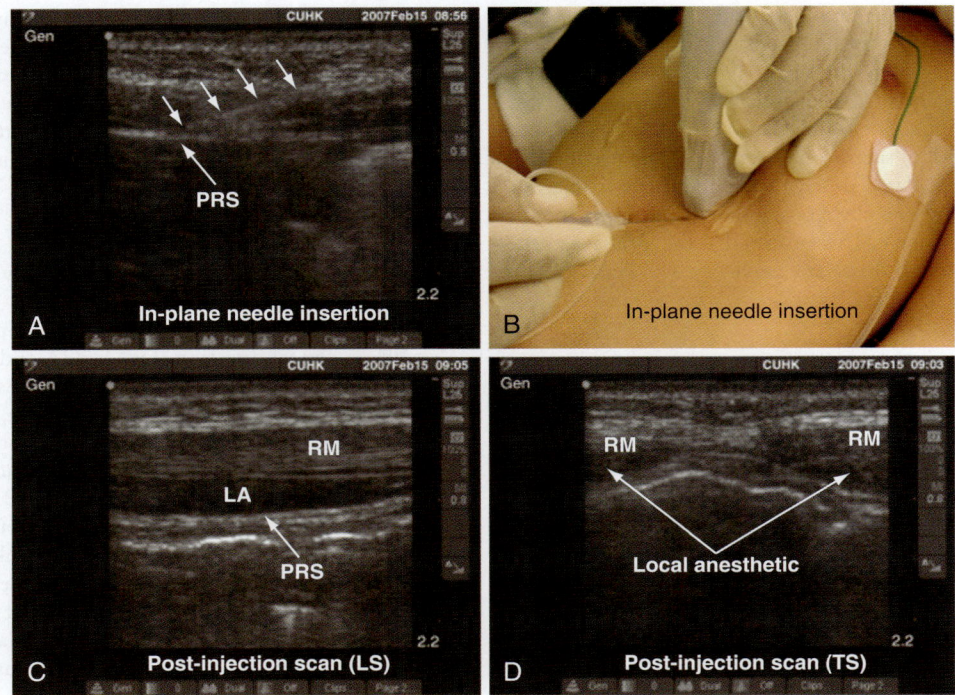

FIGURE 43.33 Rectus sheath block. The in-plane needle insertion technique. *LA*, local anesthetic; *LS*, longitudinal sonogram; *PRS*, posterior rectus sheath; *RM*, rectus muscle; *TS*, transverse sonogram.

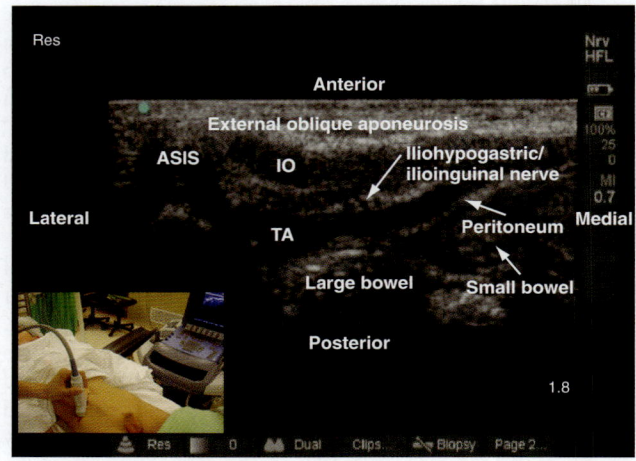

FIGURE 43.34 Transverse sonogram of the inguinal region showing the ilioinguinal and iliohypogastric nerves and its relation to the abdominal musculature. *ASIS*, anterior superior iliac spine; *IO*, internal oblique; *TA*, transverse abdominis.

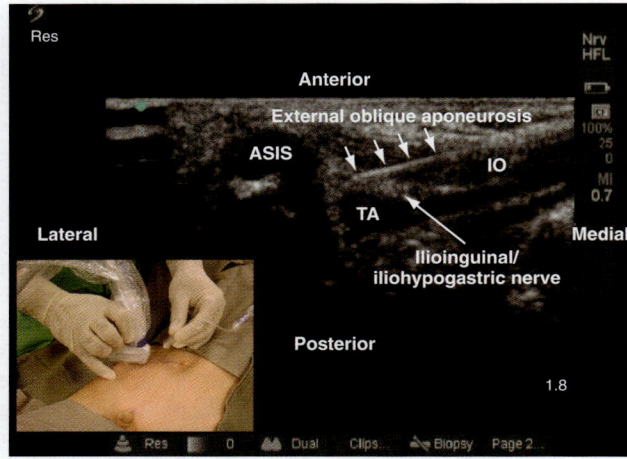

FIGURE 43.35 Ilioinguinal iliohypogastric nerve block. The in-plane needle insertion technique. *ASIS*, anterior superior iliac spine; *IO*, internal oblique; *TA*, transverse abdominis.

on the contralateral side. The transducer is positioned close to the ASIS and parallel to a line joining the ASIS and the umbilicus (Fig. 43.34). The ilioinguinal and iliohypogastric nerves are identified as two small, rounded structures lying side by side between the internal oblique and transversus abdominis muscle (see Fig. 43.34). The external oblique is frequently identified only as a hyperechoic aponeurotic layer at the point of needle insertion. Deep to the transversus abdominis muscle, the peritoneum and the bowel are also visualized (see Fig. 43.34).

The block needle is inserted in the long axis (in-plane) of the US beam in a medial to lateral direction (Fig. 43.35). We prefer this orientation because it facilitates visualization of the needle (in-plane) and, in the event that the needle is inadvertently inserted too deep, further passage is obstructed by the iliac bone, thus reducing the potential for a major complication such as bowel perforation.[114] When the tip of the needle is close to the two nerves, a test injection is performed with 0.5 to 1 mL of normal saline solution. Correct position of the needle tip is confirmed by observing the widening of the tissue plane between the internal oblique and transversus abdominis muscles. A calculated dose of a long-acting local anesthetic (e.g., 0.4 mL/kg) is then injected and the spread of local anesthetic to both nerves visualized (Video 43.5) (see also E-Fig. 42.8B for landmark-guided techniques).

Transversus Abdominis Plane Block

The sensory supply of the abdominal wall is provided by the anterior rami of the T7 to L1 thoracolumbar nerves. T7 to T9 innervate the skin above the umbilicus, T10 innervates the skin around the umbilicus, and T11, T12 (cutaneous branches of the subcostal nerve), and L1 (iliohypogastric and ilioinguinal nerves) innervate the skin below the umbilicus. These nerves pass infero-anteriorly in a plane between the internal oblique and transversus abdominis muscles, also known as the transversus abdominis plane (TAP). The lateral cutaneous branch is given off at the midaxillary line and innervates the abdominal wall up to the lateral edge of the rectus abdominis muscle. The segmental nerve then courses anteriorly and medially toward the midline in the TAP to penetrate the lateral margin of the rectus sheath and emerge anteriorly through the rectus muscle as the anterior cutaneous branch. The lateral and anterior cutaneous branches of the thoracolumbar nerves supply the skin from the midline to the anterior axillary line. The thoracolumbar nerves, as they course through the TAP, also supply muscular branches to the abdominal musculature.

Local anesthetic injected into the TAP plane produces senso-rimotor blockade (segmental) of the abdominal wall. TAP block techniques can be classified according to the site of needle insertion (i.e., the posterior, lateral, and subcostal TAP blocks).[118] The posterior TAP block is discussed together with the quadratus lumborum block (QLB) in the next section. For the lateral TAP block, local anesthetic is injected in the TAP plane between the iliac crest and the costal margin at the midaxillary line; for a subcostal TAP block the local anesthetic is injected into the TAP plane just below the costal margin at the mid-clavicular line.[119] Anesthesia and analgesia produced by a TAP block is unilateral; thus it is useful for surgical procedures (e.g., orchidopexy, herniotomy, appendectomy) in which the incision does not cross the midline. Bilateral TAP blocks are indicated for abdominal surgical procedures in which the surgical incision is in the midline or crosses the midline. It is also the authors' practice to perform bilateral TAP blocks for laparoscopic procedures.[120–122] However, since TAP blocks do not produce visceral analgesia, they should be used as part of a multimodal analgesic regimen for perioperative analgesia. TAP blocks may be useful as an alternative when central neuraxial blocks are contraindicated (e.g., in children with underlying coagulopathy or spinal dysraphism).

For a lateral TAP block, a high-frequency linear array transducer (15-7 MHz) is placed midway between the iliac crest and the costal margin along the midaxillary line (Fig. 43.36A). For infants and young children, a linear transducer with a small footprint (25 mm) is preferred. The operator stands or sits on one side of the child, and the US machine is positioned directly opposite on the contralateral side. The various layers of the abdominal wall are identified on the sonogram (Fig. 43.36B). From superficial to deep, they include a layer of subcutaneous tissue and fat and the three abdominal muscles with their fascial layers (i.e., the external oblique, internal oblique, and the transversus abdominis muscles, respectively). Deep to the transversus abdominis muscle the hypoechoic peritoneum is also visualized (Fig. 43.36B). The block

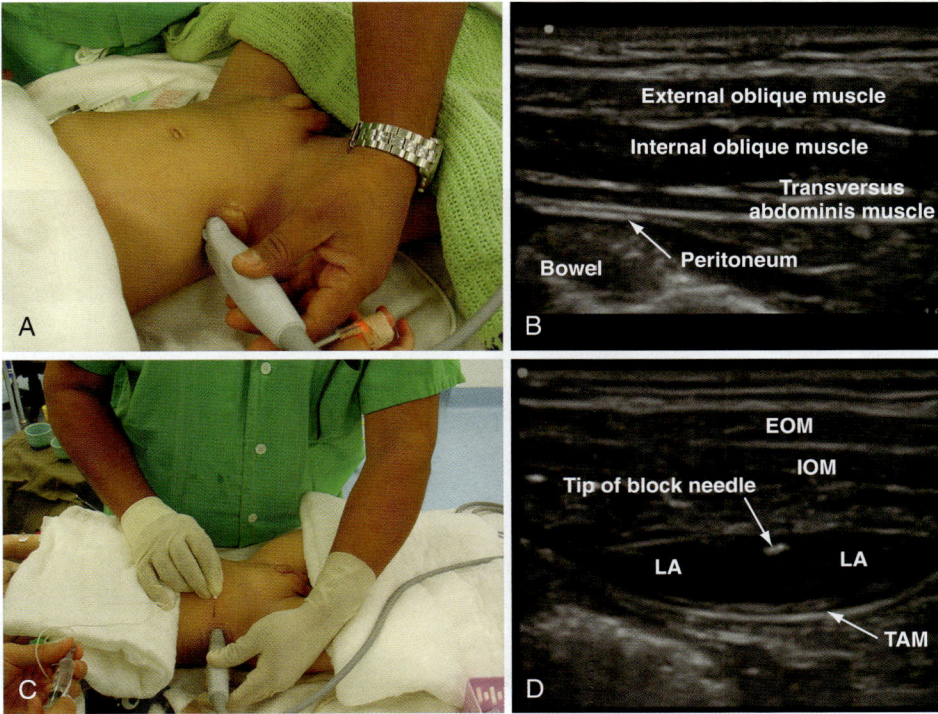

FIGURE 43.36 Posterior transverse abdominis plane (TAP) block. **A,** Note how the ultrasound transducer is positioned between the iliac crest and the costal margin along the mid-axillary line. **B,** The three layers of the abdominal musculature. **C,** In-pane needle insertion during a posterior TAP block. **D,** Distention of the TAP by the injected local anesthetic (*LA*). *EOM,* external oblique muscle; *IOM,* internal oblique muscle; *TAM,* transversus abdomen muscle.

needle (50 mm) is inserted 1 to 2 cm medial to the medial edge of the ultrasound transducer (Fig. 43.36C) in the plane of the US beam. Because the abdominal wall in infants and young children is relatively thin, and to avoid inadvertent deep needle insertion and visceral puncture, it is the authors' practice to initially insert the block needle directed toward the US transducer rather than in an anteroposterior direction. Once the needle tip penetrates the skin and enters the abdominal muscle, it is redirected and slowly advanced under direct vision and penetration of the tip through the external oblique and internal oblique muscles, and finally the TAP is identified between the internal oblique and transversus abdominis muscles. A test injection (1 mL) of saline solution is performed to confirm correct needle placement in the TAP, which is indicated by distention of the TAP by the hypoechoic fluid. A calculated dose of a long-acting local anesthetic is then injected through the needle, while distention of the TAP is visualized in real time (Fig. 43.36D) (Video 43.6).

For a subcostal TAP block, a high-frequency linear-array transducer (15-6 MHz) is placed immediately below the costal margin along the midclavicular line and the block needle (50–80 mm) is inserted in the plane of the US beam and from a medial to lateral direction until the tip is identified to be in the TAP. Saline solution 1 to 2 mL is injected to confirm correct needle placement in the TAP. A calculated dose of local anesthetic is then injected, and as the local anesthetic hydro-dissects the TAP plane, the block needle is advanced posteriorly in the TAP to improve spread of the local anesthetic. Bilateral subcostal TAP blocks are indicated for midline upper abdominal incisions. Currently, published data on the use of subcostal TAP blocks in children are limited, and its role in children is still not defined.

Quadratus Lumborum Block (QLB)

The QLB is a recently introduced abdominal wall field block in which the local anesthetic is injected into a fascial plane located deep to the fascia transversalis (the deep fascia of the abdominal wall) and on the anterolateral aspect of the quadratus lumborum muscle (Fig. 43.37).[123–127] The point of injection is believed to approximate to the landmark-based technique of performing posterior TAP block at the lumbar triangle of Petit.[128,129] Several USG techniques for QLB or their variations have been described in the literature, QLB-I, QLB-II, and transmuscular QLB (Fig. 43.38), but the optimal technique or the best site of injection is still not known.[130–132]

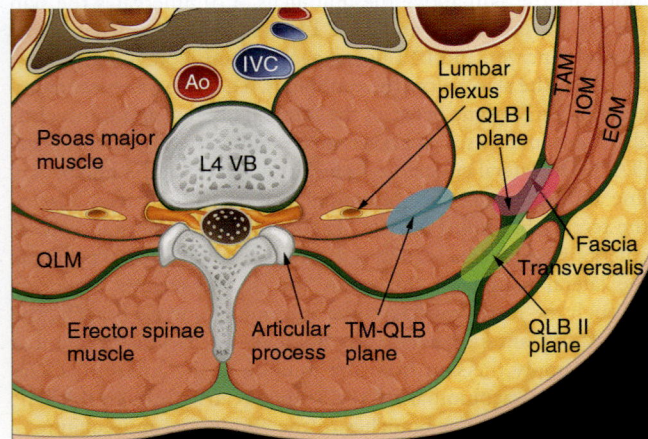

FIGURE 43.37 Cross-sectional anatomy at the L4 level illustrating the anatomy relevant for quadratus lumborum block (QLB). The QLB I block involves injecting the local anesthetic at the anterolateral aspect of the quadrates lumborum muscle (*pink region*). QLB II involves injection posterior to the quadratus lumborum muscle (*green region*). QLB III block, also known as transmuscular QLB (*TM-QLB*), involves advancing the needle through the quadratus lumborum muscle and injecting the local anesthetic between the quadratus lumborum and psoas muscle (*blue region*). *Ao,* aorta; *EOM,* external oblique muscle; *IOM,* internal oblique muscle; *IVC,* inferior vena cava; *QLM,* quadratus lumborum muscle; *TAM,* transversus abdominis muscle; *VB,* vertebral body.

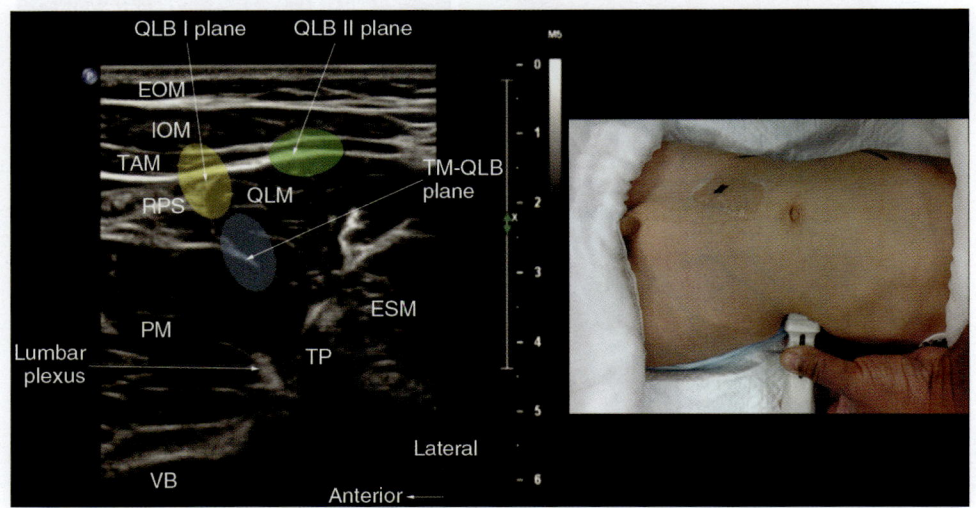

FIGURE 43.38 Quadratus lumborum block in a child. Note how the ultrasound transducer is positioned in the posterior flank immediately above the iliac crest. Transverse sonogram demonstrating the relevant sonoanatomy and the anatomic planes for local anesthetic injection during a quadratus lumborum block. *EOM,* external oblique muscle; *ESM,* erector spinae muscle; *IOM,* internal oblique muscle; *PM,* psoas major; *QLM,* quadratus lumborum muscle; *RPS,* retroperitoneal space; *TAM,* transversus abdominis muscle; *TM-QLB,* transmuscular quadratus lumborum block; *TP,* transverse process; *VB,* vertebral body.

The fascia transversalis of the abdominal wall blends medially with the anterior layer of the quadratus lumborum fascia and the psoas fascia (psoas sheath) (see Fig. 43.37). The subcostal (T12), iliohypogastric (L1), and ilioinguinal (L1) nerves course anterior to and in close contact with the quadratus lumborum muscle and the lateral femoral cutaneous nerve of the thigh (L2, L3) crosses the lateral border of the psoas muscle at the level of the inferior border of the L4 vertebra in this fascial plane.

Currently there are limited data on QLB in children,[124,125,127,133] but studies in adults show that a QLB produces multidermatomal ipsilateral anesthesia of the thoracolumbar nerves. A bilateral single-injection QLB (20 mL of 0.375% ropivacaine on each side) produces loss of sensation to cold from (T7–L1)[134] compared with bilateral lateral TAP blocks (T10–T12).[130–132] Also the duration of analgesia after a bilateral QLB in adults is significantly greater (attributed to paravertebral spread of local anesthetic) than that produced by bilateral lateral TAP blocks.[134] QLB may also produce ipsilateral sympathetic blockade since paravertebral spread of contrast has been demonstrated. Therefore QLB may be effective in relieving sympathetic-mediated visceral pain, which is otherwise not affected by a lateral TAP block. However, since there is a paucity of data on the use of bilateral QLB for major abdominal surgery in children, no recommendations can be made at this time, but QLB holds promise as a technique for perioperative pain management.

A QLB is performed with the child in the lateral or supine position (see Fig. 43.38). The lateral position is preferable for unilateral QLB because the transmuscular approach can be easily performed. For bilateral QLBs the child is placed in the supine position (see Fig. 43.38). The abdomen is exposed between the costal margin and the iliac crest. The operator stands on one side of the subject, and the ultrasound machine is placed directly opposite on the contralateral side. A high-frequency (13-8 MHz) linear-array transducer is used in young children; a curved-array transducer (5-1 MHz), which produces a wider field of view, may be used in older or obese children. The transducer is placed in the transverse orientation in the flank immediately above the iliac crest. The operator then gently slides the transducer posteriorly, aiming to identify the anterolateral surface of the vertebral body and the transverse process in the transverse sonogram. Once the transverse process is located and the relevant anatomy is identified, the operator tilts or slides the transducer slightly caudally to perform the transverse scan through the ITS. The acoustic shadow of the transverse process will now no longer be visible and will be replaced by the hyperechoic articular process. On the transverse sonogram the vertebral body and transverse process of the vertebra appear as hyperechoic structures with a corresponding acoustic shadow (see Fig. 43.38). The psoas major, quadratus lumborum, and erector spinae muscles are easily recognized surrounding the transverse process. Also, depending on the side scanned, the inferior vena cava (on the right) and aorta (on the left) are visualized anterolateral to the vertebral body. The arrangement of the three muscles around the transverse process—that is, the psoas muscle lying anterior, the erector spinae muscle lying posterior, and the quadratus lumborum muscle lying at the apex—produces a sonographic pattern that has been likened to a "shamrock" with the muscles representing the three leaves.[135] Superficial and anterior to these three muscles, the external oblique, internal, and transversus abdominis muscles are identified. In the transverse sonogram through the lumbar ITS, the acoustic shadow of the transverse process is no longer visualized, and the intervertebral foramen and spinal canal may also be visualized in addition to the psoas major, quadratus lumborum, and erector spine muscles (Fig. 43.39).

A 22-G (50- to 80-mm) nerve block needle is inserted in-plane from the anterior to posterior direction, and the needle tip is positioned between the anterior border of QLM and its fascia (QLB-I) (see Fig. 43.37 to Fig. 43.39). Correct needle tip position is confirmed by injection of 1 to 2 mL of normal saline solution and observing the spread of the injectate in relation to the quadratus lumborum muscle (see Fig. 43.39). After negative aspiration, a calculated dose of local anesthetic (e.g., 0.2–0.3 mL/kg per side) is injected. It is prudent to identify the lower pole of the kidney and the limits of the peritoneal cavity during the scout scan to avoid deep needle insertion and visceral injury (Video 43.7).

Thoracic Paravertebral Block

A thoracic paravertebral block (TPVB) is the technique of injecting local anesthetic alongside the thoracic vertebra close to the

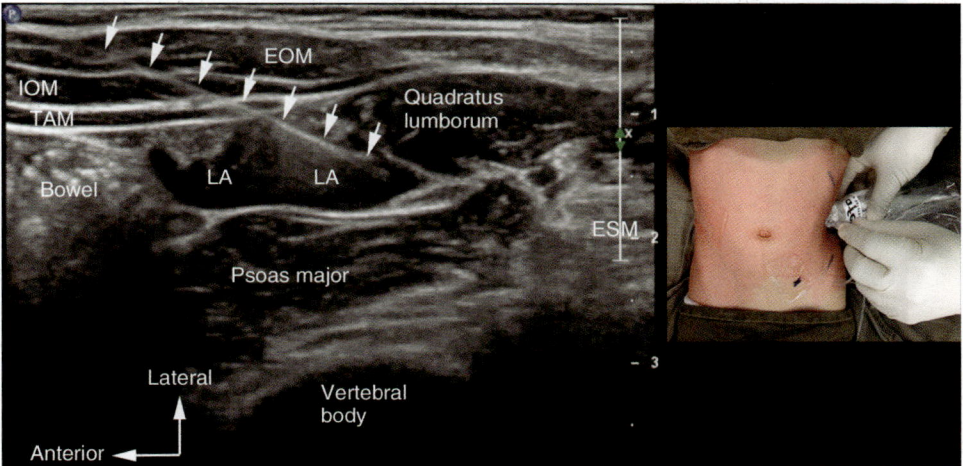

FIGURE 43.39 Quadratus lumborum block II with the patient in the supine position. Note the needle is inserted in-plane and advanced into a fascial plane deep to the fascia transversalis and on the anterolateral aspect of the quadratus lumborum muscle. *EOM,* external oblique muscle; *ESM,* erector spinae muscle; *IOM,* internal oblique muscle; *LA,* local anesthetic; *TAM,* transversus abdominis muscle.

intervertebral foramen. This produces ipsilateral, segmental, somatic, and sympathetic nerve blockade that is effective for relieving postoperative pain of unilateral origin from the chest and abdomen. Traditionally, TPVB is performed using surface anatomic landmarks or a catheter is placed in the thoracic paravertebral space (TPVS) under direct vision during thoracic surgery. Currently, there is a paucity of data on USG TPVB in children.[136,137] The following section describes how the authors perform real-time, in-plane USG TPVB and paravertebral catheter placement in young infants and children.[138–141]

USG TPVB is performed with the child in the lateral position and with the side to be blocked uppermost (Fig. 43.40). The operator sits or stands behind the child, and the US machine is positioned directly in front on the opposite side of the operating table. In most children a 15-6 or 13-8 MHz linear-array transducer is adequate for imaging the paravertebral anatomy. However, a high-frequency linear-array transducer with a small footprint (25 mm) is ideal for USG TPVB in neonates and young infants.

The thoracic paravertebral region can be imaged in the transverse or sagittal axis. We prefer the transverse axis, and the ultrasound scan is performed by sequentially imaging three contiguous sites at the target thoracic level (Fig. 43.41). Each of the three transverse ultrasound scan windows produces a very distinct sonogram, reflecting the different osseous (Fig. 43.42A-C) and musculoskeletal

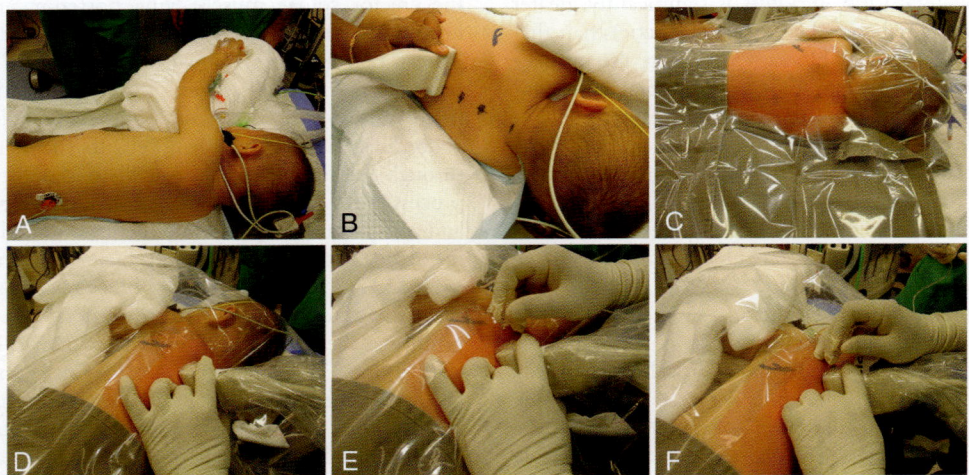

FIGURE 43.40 Ultrasound-guided thoracic paravertebral block in a child. **A,** The child is positioned in the lateral position with the side to be blocked uppermost. **B,** Transverse scan using a 13–8 MHz linear-array transducer. **C,** Aseptic precautions. **D,** The ultrasound transducer is placed inside a sterile cover. **E,** In-plane needle insertion, **F,** Local anesthetic is injected by an assistant.

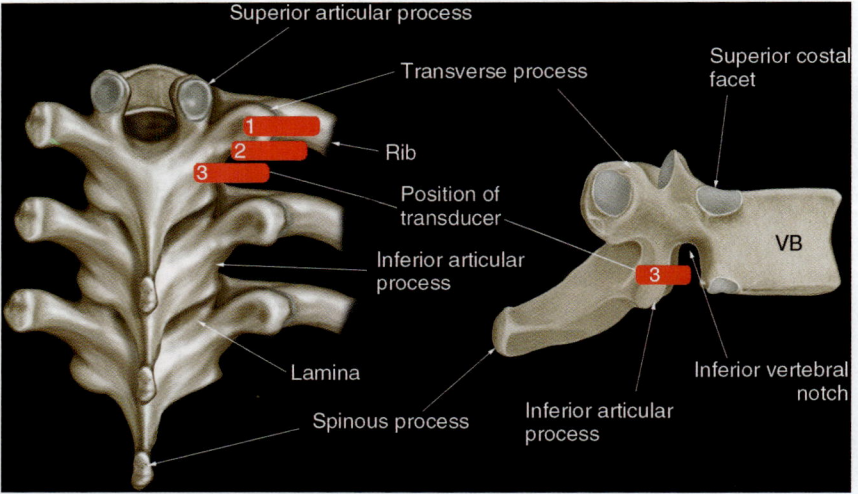

FIGURE 43.41 Schematic diagram showing the positions of the ultrasound transducer at the three contiguous sites over the paravertebral region relevant for thoracic paravertebral block. *Position 1,* The ultrasound transducer is placed over the ipsilateral spinous process, lamina, transverse process, and the rib. *Position 2,* The ultrasound transducer is placed over the ipsilateral lamina and transverse process. *Position 3,* From position 2 the ultrasound transducer is gently slid or tilted caudally until the inferior articular process of the vertebral body is visualized medially.

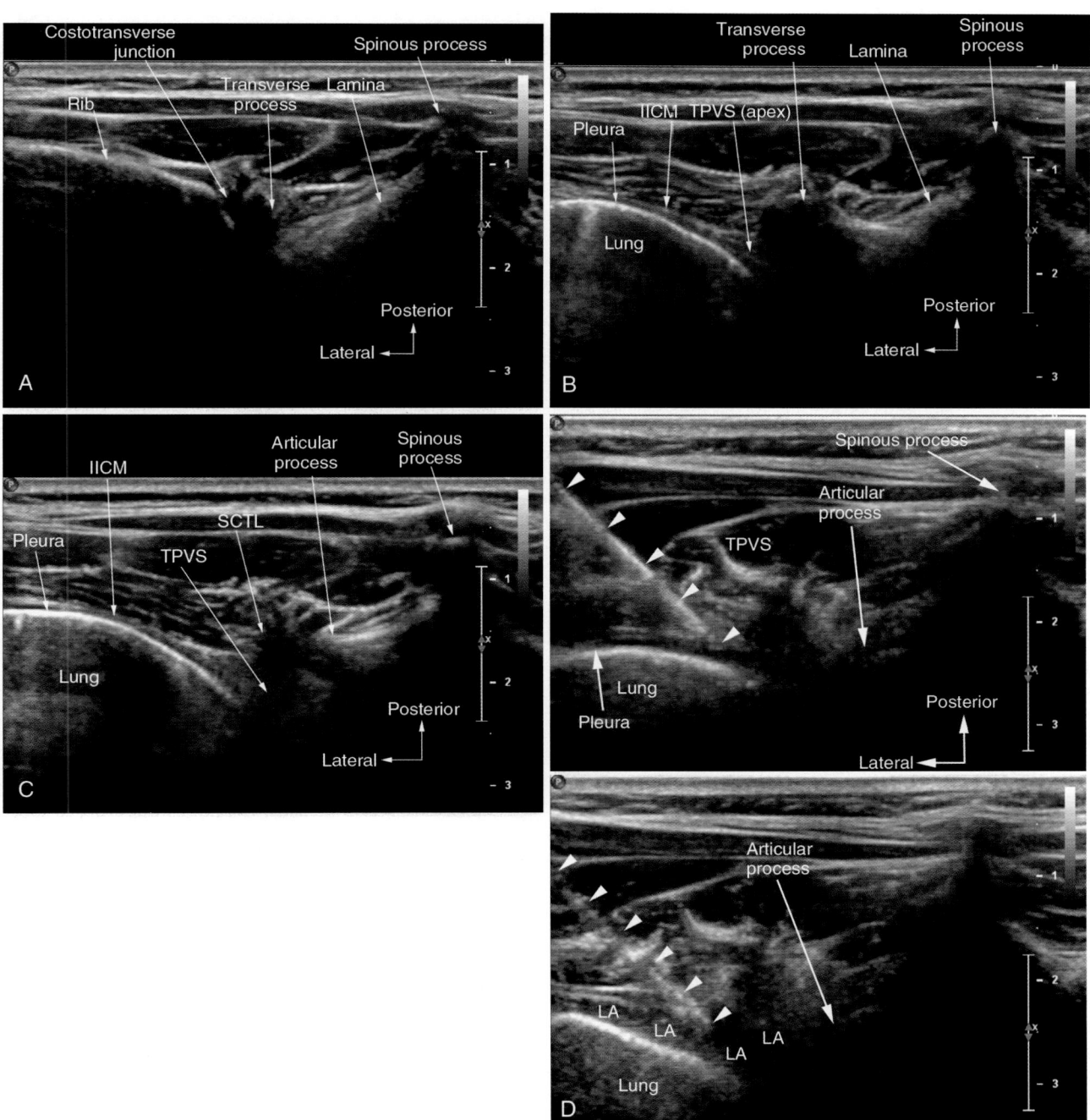

FIGURE 43.42 A, Transverse sonogram of thoracic praravertebral region at the T5 level with the ultrasound transducer placed over position 1 (Fig. 43.41). The hyperechoic outlines of the ipsilateral spinous process, lamina, transverse process, and the rib with their corresponding acoustic shadow anteriorly are clearly delineated from a medial to lateral direction. **B,** Transverse sonogram of thoracic paravertebral block region at the T5 level with the ultrasound transducer placed over position 2 (Fig. 43.41). The hyperechoic outline of transverse process and the lamina with their acoustic shadow are visualized medially. **C,** Transverse sonogram of thoracic paravertebral block region at T5 level with the ultrasound transducer placed over position 3 (Fig. 43.41). Note the acoustic shadow of the transverse process is no longer visualized and the hyperechoic inferior articular process is visualized medially. The outlines of the thoracic paravertebral space are also clearly delineated. **D,** Ultrasound guided thoracic paravertebral block with the block needle being inserted in plane and at the level of the articular process in the transverse sonogram; *arrowheads* indicate the path of the needle. Note the anterior displacement of the parietal pleura and distention of the paravertebral space after the local anesthetic *(LA)* injection. *IICM,* internal intercostal membrane; *SCTL,* superior costotransverse ligament; *TPVS,* thoracic paravertebral space.

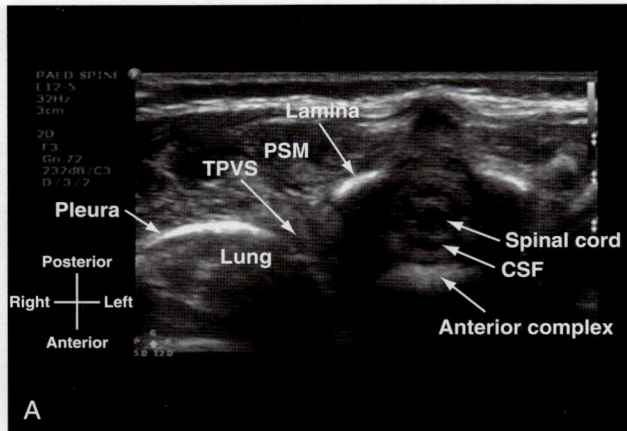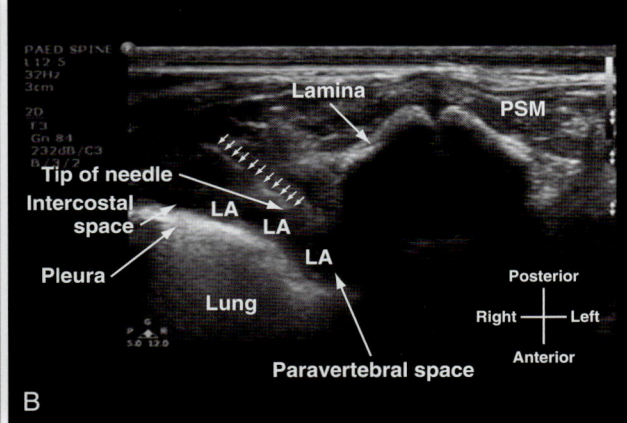

FIGURE 43.43 A, Transverse sonogram demonstrating the sonoanatomy of the right thoracic paravertebral region in a neonate. Note the hyperechoic pleura anteriorly and the hypoechoic apical part of the thoracic paravertebral space *(TPVS)* posterior to the pleura. Also note the large acoustic window resulting from incomplete ossification of the posterior spinal elements that allows visualization of the neuraxial structures within the spinal canal. **B,** Transverse sonogram of the right thoracic paravertebral region in a neonate after an ultrasound-guided thoracic paravertebral block. Note the direction of needle insertion and distention of the right thoracic paravertebral and intercostal spaces, adjacent to the level of injection, with the local anesthetic *(LA)*. *CSF,* cerebrospinal fluid; *PSM,* paraspinal muscles.

structures that are visualized in the sonograms. On a transverse sonogram with the ultrasound beam being insonated over the ipsilateral spinous process, lamina, transverse process, and the rib (position 1, Fig. 43.42A), the hyperechoic outlines of the osseous structures with their corresponding acoustic shadows are clearly delineated from a medial to lateral direction. This ultrasound window does not demonstrate the paravertebral anatomy per se but is the initial ultrasound window that one should acquire after which identification of the transverse sonoanatomy of the paravertebral region becomes relatively simple. From position 1, one can gently slide or tilt the transducer caudally until the acoustic shadow of the rib is no longer visualized (position 2) (see Fig. 43.41), and the hyperechoic outline of the lamina and transverse process with their acoustic shadow are seen (see Fig. 43.42B). Lateral to the transverse process the hyperechoic pleura and lung are visualized anteriorly, the hyperechoic internal intercostal membrane (IICM) posteriorly, and a hypoechoic triangular space that represents the apex of the TPVS is interposed between the two (see Fig. 43.42B). If one now gently slides or tilts the ultrasound transducer slightly more caudally (position 3) (see Fig. 43.41), the acoustic shadow of the transverse process disappears and the hyperechoic inferior articular process is visualized medially (see Fig. 43.42C). The thick superior costotransverse ligament (SCTL), parietal pleura, lung, and the apical part of the paravertebral space are also delineated. Continuation of the SCTL to the IICM laterally can also be delineated in some children (see Fig. 43.42C). However, since the acoustic shadow of the transverse process is no longer visualized, outlines of the entire TPVS can now be seen (see Fig. 43.42C). The location of the intervertebral foramen, which lies anteromedial to the inferior articular process, can also be defined (Video 43.8).

Currently the majority of the published data on USG TPVB in children exclusively use the transverse axis, and the scan is performed at the level of the transverse process (position 2, see Fig. 43.42B).[136,137] There are also no data describing the use of the transverse ultrasound scan window at the level of the articular

process for TPVB. The latter is our preferred ultrasound window for imaging and needle insertion during USG TPVB because it not only delineates the entire TPVS but there is also less bony obstruction during needle insertion. Furthermore, one can also accurately define the location of the intervertebral foramen, "a no-go zone" during TPVB (position 3) (see Fig. 43.42C).

For a USG thoracic paravertebral block, a transverse view of the paravertebral space at the target level and at the articular process level, is obtained (see Fig. 43.42C). The block needle (50 mm) is inserted lateral to the US transducer and advanced toward the apical part of the paravertebral space in the plane of the US beam (Fig. 43.42D). The advancing needle is visualized in real time, and entry into the TPVS is confirmed using a test bolus injection (1 mL) of saline solution. Correct placement of the needle in the paravertebral space is indicated by anterior displacement of the parietal pleura, distention of the paravertebral space, and increased echogenicity of the parietal pleura (see Fig. 43.42D). A calculated dose of local anesthetic (e.g., 0.4 mL/kg) is then injected with the needle in situ before a catheter is inserted through the needle, leaving approximately 2 cm of catheter in situ if a continuous thoracic paravertebral block is planned. The technique described above can also be used for USG TPVB in young infants and neonates (see Fig. 43.43 A and B and Video 43.9) (see also Figs. 42.18 and 42.19 for landmark-guided techniques).

CENTRAL NEURAXIAL BLOCKS

Spinal Sonography

Since the early 1980s, spinal ultrasonography has been used as a diagnostic screening tool in neonates and infants suspected of having a spinal dysraphism and for detecting spinal tumors, vascular malformations, and trauma.[142–147] Today it is considered the first-line screening test for spinal dysraphism, with a diagnostic sensitivity comparable to that of MRI. Spinal ultrasonography is possible in neonates and infants because the incomplete ossification of the predominantly cartilaginous posterior spinal elements creates an acoustic window that allows the transmission of the US beam.

The overall visibility of neuraxial structures decreases with age. Neuraxial structures are best visualized in neonates and infants younger than 3 months of age; progressive ossification of the posterior spinal elements makes detailed sonographic evaluation of the spine difficult beyond 6 months of age unless the child has a persistent posterior spinal defect. Some reports have demonstrated that neuraxial structures can be visualized in older children, although their details are limited. The overall visibility of neuraxial structures also decreases as one progresses up the spine, with the best visibility in the sacral level followed by the lumbar and then at the thoracic level.

In diagnostic radiology, spinal US is most frequently performed with the child in the prone position, whereas in an anesthetized child it is generally performed with the child in the lateral position. Because the neuraxial structures are relatively superficial in children, they are best visualized using high-frequency (10-5 MHz) transducers, which also produce better images than sector transducers. Scans are obtained in both the transverse (axial) and longitudinal (sagittal) axes, and they are performed either through the midline or parallel and lateral (paramedian) to the spinous processes. The paramedian scan is preferable in older children because it avoids the ossified spinous processes that can interfere with US

transmission. In neonates and young infants, the spinal canal can be scanned with the transducer placed directly over the spinous processes (i.e., a median longitudinal scan). Beyond this age group a paramedian longitudinal scan provides the best overall view of neuraxial structures.

On a longitudinal sonogram, the neonatal spinal cord is seen as a hypoechoic tubular structure with hyperechoic anterior and posterior walls. A thin strip of variable intense echo, "the central echo complex" (Fig. 43.44A), extends longitudinally through the center of the spinal cord and represents the area between the myelinated ventral white commissure and the central portion of the anterior median fissure. This produces the "triplet echoes" that are characteristic of the spinal cord at all levels (Fig. 43.44B). The diameter of the spinal cord varies, being largest in the cervical and lumbar regions and smallest at the thoracic region. Anterior and posterior to the spinal cord are two well-defined linear and hyperechoic echoes that represent the arachnoid-dural layer (see Fig. 43.44A). The ligamentum flavum, which is relevant for epidural access, is also readily visualized in young children and appears less echogenic than the dura (see Fig. 43.44B). The dural layers taper distally to close the thecal sac at the S2 level. The epidural space is the hypoechoic area between the dura and the ligamentum

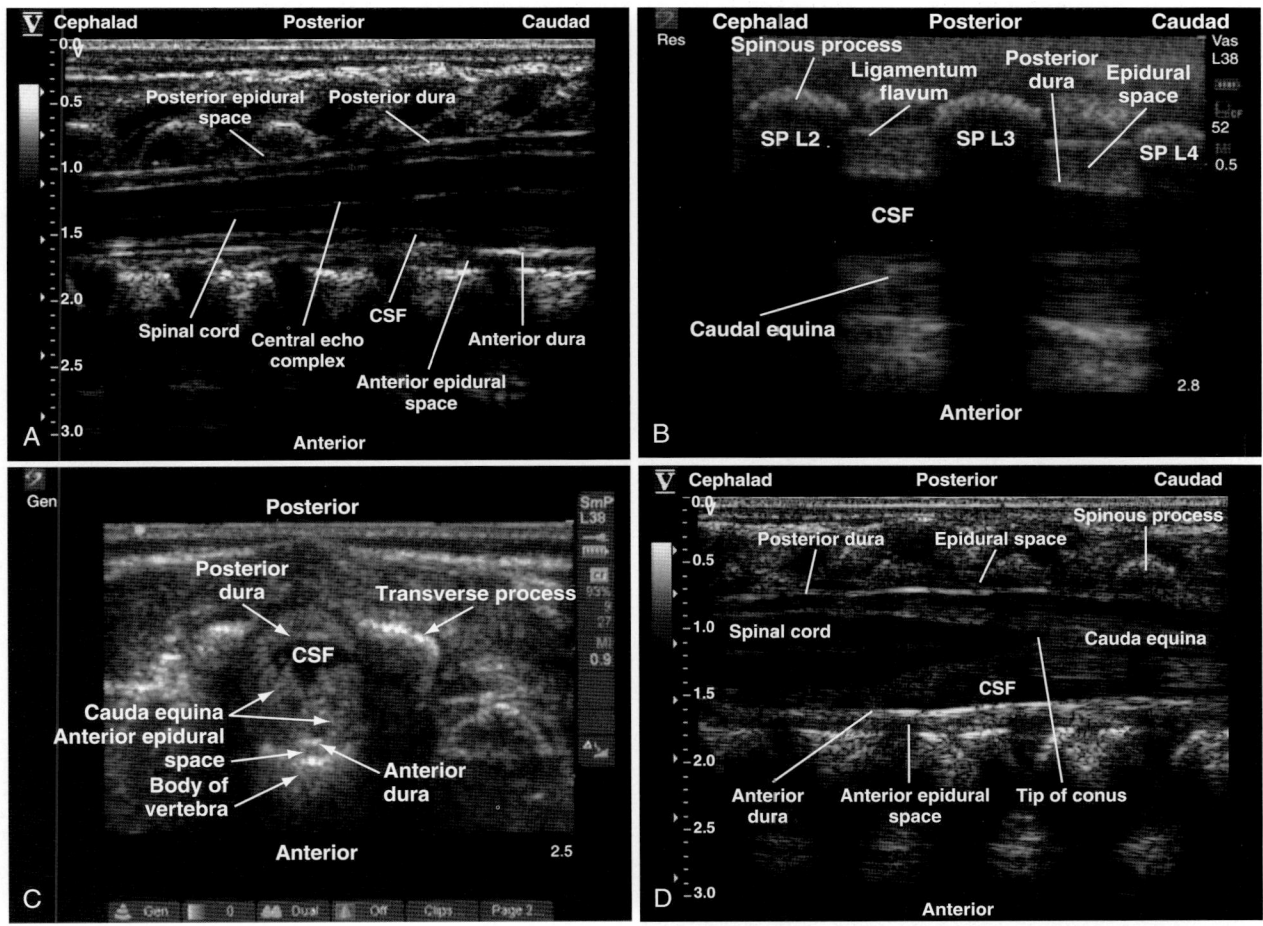

FIGURE 43.44 A, Longitudinal paramedian sonogram of the thoracic spine in a neonate. **B,** Longitudinal midline sonogram of the lumbar spine in a neonate. **C,** Transverse sonogram of the lumbar spine in a neonate showing the cauda equina. **D,** Longitudinal paramedian sonogram of the thoracolumbar spine in a neonate showing the termination of the spinal cord. *CSF,* cerebrospinal fluid; *SP L2,* spinous process of L2; *SP L3,* spinous process of L3; *SP L4,* spinous process of L4.

flavum (see Fig. 43.44B) and arterial pulsations also may be visible on US between these two layers. The cerebrospinal fluid (CSF) surrounds the spinal cord as an anechoic layer between the dura and spinal cord (Fig. 43.44C). The vertebral bodies are seen as echogenic structures anterior to the spinal cord. The spinal cord tapers distally to form the conus medullaris (Fig. 43.44D) at the level of the first and second lumbar vertebral bodies. The conus medullaris is continuous with the filum terminale, which extends into the sacral canal as a hyperechoic structure. It is surrounded by the roots of the cauda equina, which appear as multiple parallel echogenic lines surrounding the filum terminale (Fig. 43.45A). Differentiation of the filum terminale from the roots of the cauda equina can sometimes be difficult. The cauda equina typically lies in the anterior half of the spinal canal when the child is in the prone position, but it moves freely within the CSF with change in position and with crying. Slight anteroposterior movement of the spinal cord, superimposed on the arterial pulsations, is commonly seen during real-time imaging.

On a transverse (axial) sonogram, the spinal cord is seen as a round or oval hypoechoic structure, with its bright central echo complex (see Fig. 43.45B). The spinal cord is fixed laterally by the dentate ligament (see Fig. 43.45B), which represents the transversely oriented, echogenic arachnoid duplications that are seen in parts of the thoracic spinal canal. Paired (ventral and dorsal) echogenic nerve roots are seen below the L2 level. Farther caudally in the lumbar region, a transverse scan shows the filum terminale surrounded by the nerve roots of the cauda equina (see Fig. 43.45C). The arachnoid–dura mater complex is hyperechoic and forms the anterior and posterior border of the subarachnoid space in the lumbar region (see Fig. 43.45C). The vertebral bodies are the hyperechoic structures anterior to the spinal canal. The vertebral arches are also echogenic and cast an acoustic shadow anteriorly (see Fig. 43.45C). The paraspinal muscles appear hypoechoic on US.

Caudal Epidural Anesthesia

Single-shot caudal epidural injection is the most frequently used regional anesthetic technique in children and almost always is used in combination with general anesthesia for surgery involving the lower thoracic, lumbar, and sacral dermatomes.[148-150] Several methods are used to perform a caudal epidural injection.

Detecting the characteristic pop or give as the needle traverses the sacrococcygeal ligament to enter the caudal epidural space is by far the most commonly used method in children. However, even in experienced hands it can result in failure, and the overall failure rate varies between 2.8% and 11%. US has been used to guide caudal epidural injection in children,[151-153] providing correct

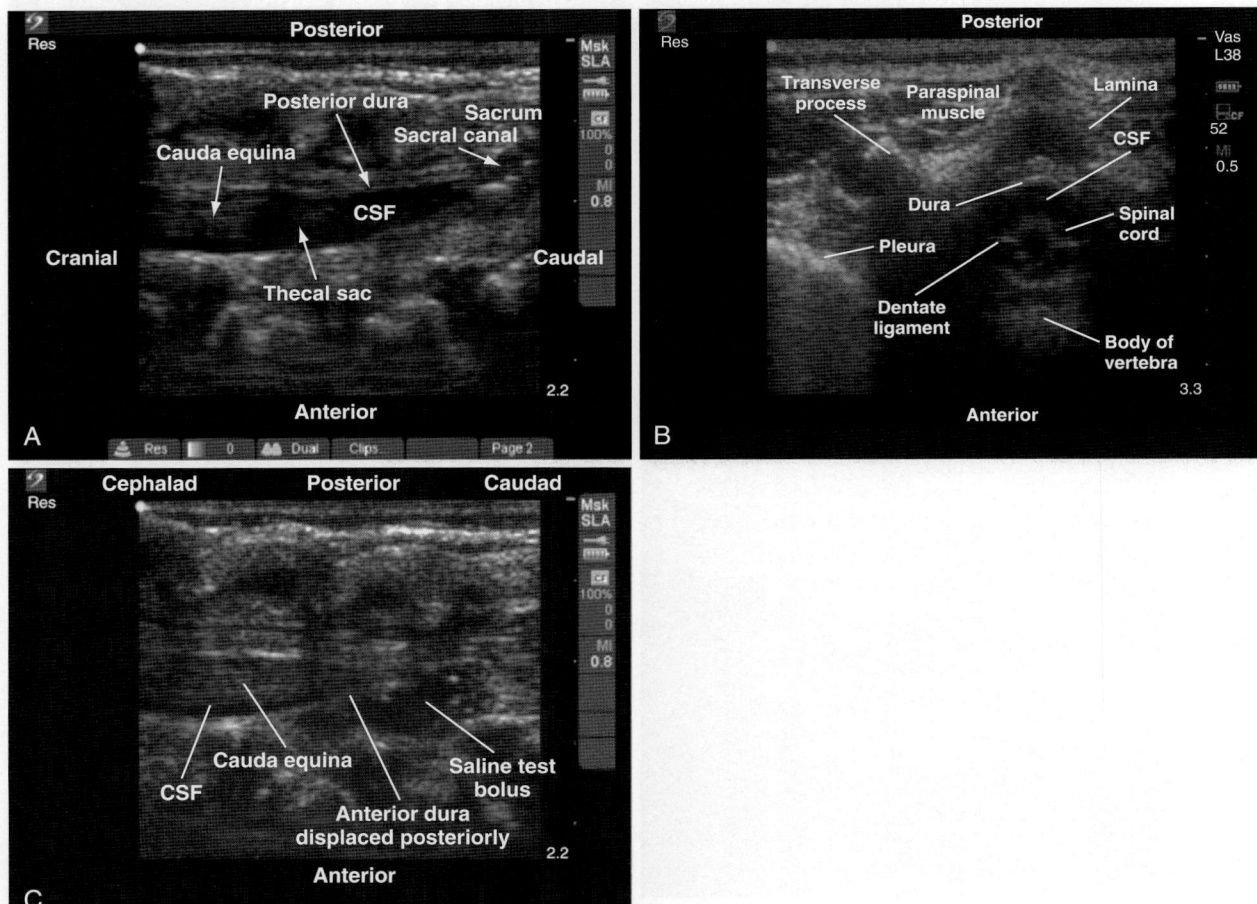

FIGURE 43.45 A, Longitudinal sonogram of the sacrum showing the tapered end of the thecal sac. **B,** Transverse sonogram of the thoracic spine in a neonate. **C,** Longitudinal sonogram of the sacrum after a test bolus injection of saline solution through an indwelling caudal catheter during a single-shot caudal epidural injection. Note the displacement of the dura. *CSF,* cerebrospinal fluid.

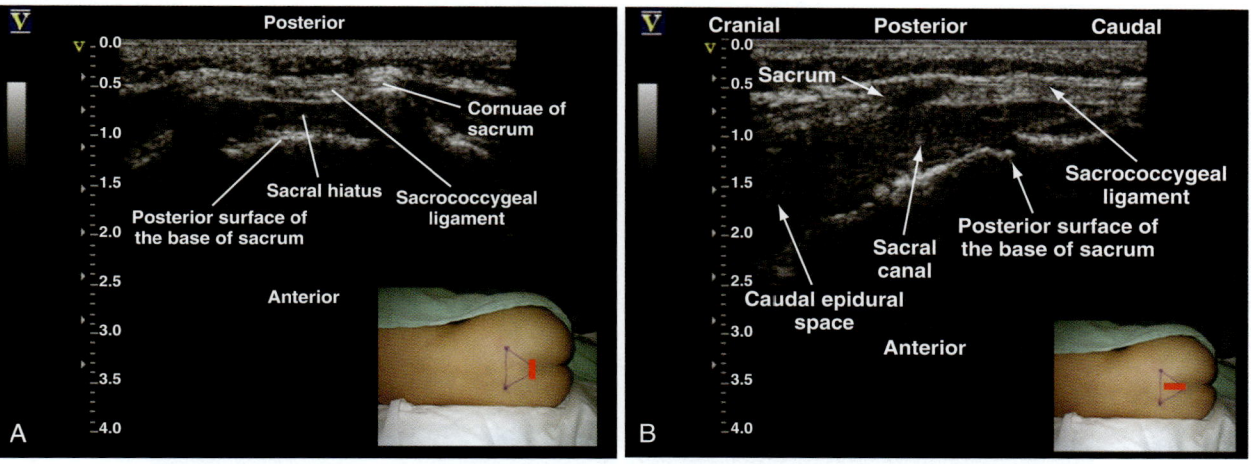

FIGURE 43.46 A, Transverse sonogram of the sacrum ("frog-eye sign"). **B,** Longitudinal sonogram of the sacrum.

needle or catheter positioning in the caudal epidural space confirmed by real-time US visualization in the sacral canal, or by observing dural displacement after a saline solution test bolus (1–10 mL) injection.

The anesthetized child is positioned in the lateral position with the knee and hips flexed. The operator sits or stands behind the child, and the US machine is positioned directly in front. A linear-array transducer (13-10 MHz) is used to image the sacrum. A transducer with a wide footprint is preferable because it allows a greater length of the spine to be examined in a single view. The transducer is initially positioned directly over the sacral cornua in the transverse axis (Fig. 43.46A). On a transverse sonogram at the level of the sacral hiatus, the sacral cornua are seen as two hyperechoic reverse U-shaped structures, one on either side of the midline. Connecting the two sacral cornua and deep to the skin and subcutaneous tissue is a hyperechoic band, the sacrococcygeal ligament (see Fig. 43.46A). Anterior to the sacrococcygeal ligament is another linear hyperechoic structure, which represents the posterior surface of the sacrum. The hypoechoic area between the sacrococcygeal ligament and the bony posterior surface of the sacrum is the sacral hiatus. The two sacral cornua and the posterior surface of the sacrum produce a US image that we refer to as the "frog-eye sign" because of its resemblance to the eyes of a frog. On a longitudinal sonogram of the sacrum, the sacrococcygeal ligament, the base of the sacrum, and the sacral hiatus can be clearly seen (Fig. 43.46B). In neonates and young infants the tapered end of the thecal sac with CSF, the anterior and posterior epidural space filled with fat, and the cauda equina may be visualized in the sacral canal (see Fig. 43.46B) (Video 43.10).

For USG caudal epidural injection, either the in-plane or out-of-plane technique can be used. We prefer the in-plane approach, and the needle is advanced under real-time guidance into the sacral canal through the sacrococcygeal ligament. During insertion, the needle is maintained at an angle (approximately 20 degrees) so that it is parallel to the posterior surface of the sacrum. Correct position of the needle in the caudal epidural space is confirmed objectively by performing a test bolus injection of saline solution and observing in real time the displacement of the dura (Fig. 43.47) (Video 43.11). Anterior displacement of the posterior dura is more frequently seen than posterior displacement of the anterior dura. If dural displacement is not seen in the US image, it implies that the needle or catheter is not in the correct

position, the needle or catheter is not in the plane of US imaging, or the needle is intravascular. The needle should be withdrawn and the procedure repeated until the typical dural displacement is visualized. The calculated dose of local anesthetic is then injected in aliquots. The cephalad spread of the local anesthetic within the epidural space also can be visualized in real time.[154] Depending on the volume of local anesthetic injected, progressive widening of the epidural space and a resultant compression of the thecal sac occur (see Fig. 43.47). These changes are visualized in the sacral canal and at the lumbar and thoracic levels. In some cases the thecal sac is almost completely obliterated in the sacral and lumbar region. Because the compression and obliteration of the thecal sac occurs in a caudal to cranial direction, it indicates that there is a net cranial displacement of CSF (Video 43.12).

US guidance during a caudal epidural injection in children offers several advantages. It is safe, noninvasive, radiation free, simple, and quick to perform; it provides real-time images that are easy to interpret; and, unlike the nerve stimulation technique, is not affected by the use of neuromuscular blocking drugs or epidural local anesthetics. Moreover, US can demonstrate the underlying caudal anatomy, which is useful in children with cutaneous markers of dysraphism when it can be used to screen the underlying spinal anatomy. Thus many children who may have otherwise been excluded from a caudal block can benefit from its effects (see also Fig. 42.6 and E-Fig. 42.6 for landmark-guided techniques).

Epidural Catheterization

Continuous epidural analgesia via an indwelling epidural catheter is a well-established method of providing perioperative analgesia in children. The loss-of-resistance technique is the most frequently used method of identifying the epidural space. Although popular, this technique relies on the operator's tactile sensation and can occasionally result in dural puncture or serious neurologic complication (e.g., a spinal cord injury). Alternative methods for identifying the epidural space in children have been described but have not gained widespread acceptance. Epidural catheters have been successfully placed in young children under US guidance.[155–157] Compared with the traditional loss-of-resistance method, when epidural catheterization is performed using the loss-of-resistance method in conjunction with US guidance, fewer bony contacts occur during the procedure, and the time required for catheter placement is reduced. The spread of local anesthetic in the epidural

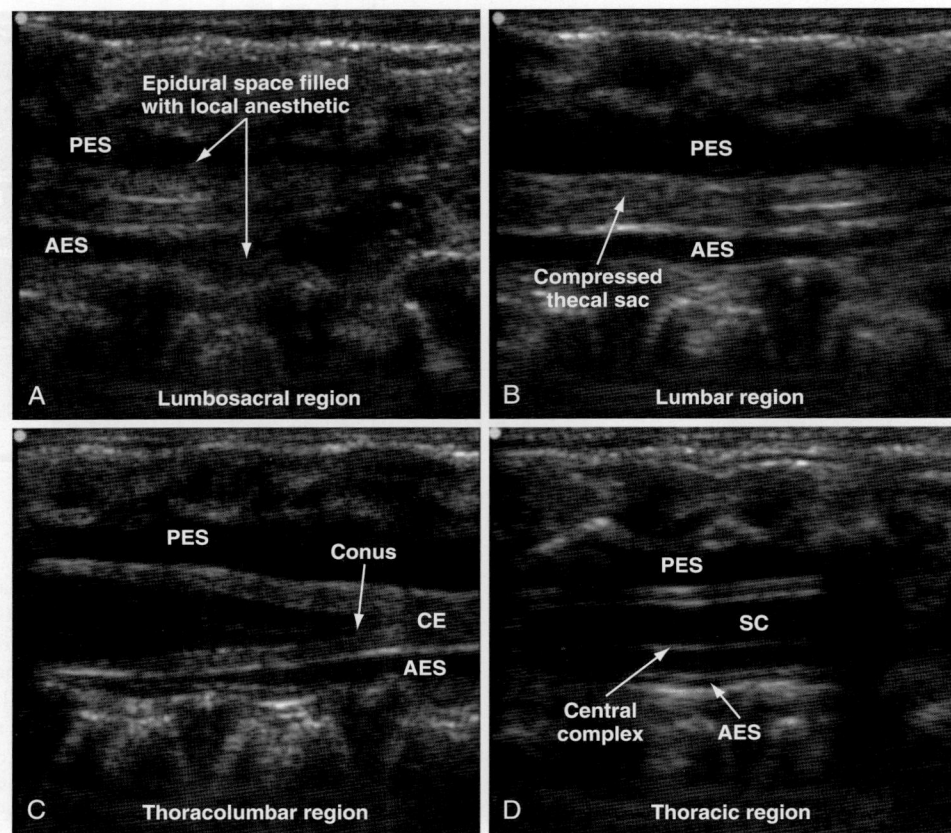

FIGURE 43.47 Longitudinal sonogram of the spine after a single-shot caudal epidural injection at the **A,** lumbosacral, **B,** lumbar, **C,** thoracolumbal, and **D,** thoracic levels. Note the displacement of the anterior and posterior dura, widening of the epidural space, and the compression of the thecal sac at the various levels. *AES,* anterior epidural space; *CE,* cauda equina; *PES,* posterior epidural space; *SC,* spinal cord.

space can also be visualized in real time. In addition, the underlying anatomy and the depth from the skin to the ligamentum flavum, dura, and epidural space can be assessed before needle insertion. However, epidural catheterization under US guidance requires two anesthesiologists who are familiar with epidural anesthesia and spinal sonography in children. The first anesthesiologist performs the scan in the longitudinal paramedian axis and maintains a steady image while the second anesthesiologist performs the needle insertion through the midline. Entry of the needle into the epidural space is confirmed by the loss of resistance to saline solution and observing the local sonographic changes resulting from the saline solution injection (i.e., anterior displacement of the posterior dura, widening of the epidural space, and compression of the thecal sac). USG epidural catheterization in young children is a very demanding procedure and requires a great deal of skill and dexterity; it should be undertaken only by those with adequate training and skill in USG regional anesthesia.

Assessment of Indwelling Epidural Catheters

For optimal epidural anesthesia or analgesia, the epidural catheter tip must be located in the correct dermatomal level. This is often achieved by directly placing the catheter in the desired level via the lumbar or thoracic route. Even with this approach, and in particular when loss of resistance is used to locate the epidural space, it is not possible to determine with any certainty the exact location of the catheter tip. Epidurography can locate the

catheter tip, but this exposes the child to radiation and the risk of anaphylaxis from the contrast medium (see Fig. 42.8).[158,159] An epidural catheter inserted via the caudal route can be advanced to the lumbar or thoracic epidural space. However, this is technically difficult in children older than 1 year of age, and even in children younger than 6 months of age, the catheter can be misplaced in the sacral, lumbar, and even the cervical region. Greater success has been reported with styletted catheters.[160] Even if a catheter is successfully advanced to the thoracic epidural space, a radiographic can confirm the position of the catheter tip.[158,159] Electric nerve stimulation through an indwelling styletted epidural catheter and observation of myotomal contractions have been used to locate the position of the catheter tip.[161] In experienced hands this technique has a success rate of 89%. However, this test cannot be performed if neuromuscular blocking drugs or local anesthetics have been administered. Epidural electrocardiography also can be used to locate the position of a thoracic epidural catheter and is not affected by the use of neuromuscular blocking drugs or local anesthetics in the epidural space.[162] This method relies on matching the evolving electrocardiogram (ECG) recorded from the tip of a specially adapted epidural catheter, as it is advanced, to the surface ECG recorded at the target vertebral level. However, this method is not specific because even a subcutaneous electrocardiographic electrode at the same position relative to the heart will produce a similar electrocardiographic pattern.

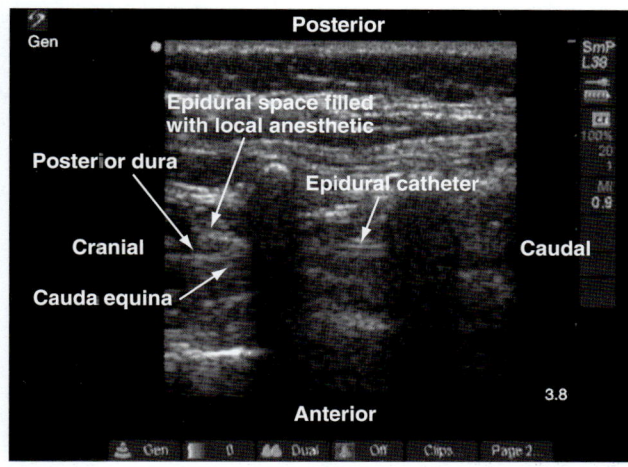

FIGURE 43.48 Longitudinal paramedian sonogram of the lumbar spine demonstrating an indwelling epidural catheter.

US has been used to directly visualize the position of epidural catheters in children (Fig. 43.48).[163,164] US localization noninvasively provides real-time images of the catheter during placement. However, not all epidural catheters or their tips can be identified using US, and it may be limited by the acoustic window available for scanning in children of different ages. Gently jiggling the catheter and observing tissue movement within the epidural space also has been used to facilitate epidural catheter localization. Injecting saline solution with air bubbles may improve catheter localization using US, but the use of air in the injectate can lead to inadvertent air embolism or a patchy block.[165] A small volume of contrast material may be injected under x-ray guidance as well to localize the tip of the catheter. Therefore it is suggested that observing surrogate markers such as the widening of the epidural space, dural displacement, and compression of the thecal sac, subsequent to a saline solution test injection, may be more accurate in locating the position of an epidural catheter in children (Video 43.13).

ADVANTAGES OF ULTRASOUND IMAGING

USG regional anesthetic blocks appear to offer several advantages. US imaging is noninvasive and simple to use and does not involve exposure to radiation. It allows the target nerves and the surrounding structures to be directly visualized during block placement, which is particularly advantageous in children with difficult or variant anatomy, obesity, or amputated limbs in whom the evoked motor responses cannot be visualized. US is also useful in young children because the majority of regional anesthetic procedures in this age group are performed with the child under general anesthesia when the use of a muscle relaxant makes nerve stimulation impractical. US guidance also helps determine the best possible site and maximum safe depth for needle insertion, allows real-time guidance of the needle and needle tip to the target site, avoids unintended vascular or pleural puncture, and allows visualization of the spread of the injected local anesthetic in real time. Together, these should lead to fewer needle insertions, improved comfort during block placement in awake and sedated children, reduced complications, improved quality of block, and greater success rates. Evidence (from adults and children) suggests that US speeds the execution of peripheral nerve and central neuraxial blocks, reduces the discomfort experienced during block placement, reduces the amount of local anesthetic required, speeds the onset of sensory blockade, improves the quality of sensorimotor blockade, and prolongs the duration of sensory blockade.[24,166–168]

Education and Training

Learning USG nerve block techniques takes time and patience. The state of the art of regional anesthesia demands a high degree of manual dexterity and hand–eye coordination and an ability to conceptualize 2D information into a 3D image. In addition, to produce good-quality US images, the anesthesiologist must also possess a sound knowledge of anatomy, the physical principles of US, and musculoskeletal imaging. Therefore individuals who intend to perform USGRA should start by learning the basics of US and USG interventions by attending a course or workshop[169–173] and by working with individuals who already possess these skills. Initial experience of musculoskeletal scanning can also be acquired in volunteer situations, and USG interventions can be practiced using a US phantom. Once the basic skills are acquired, it is best to start by performing superficial peripheral nerve blocks (e.g., axillary brachial plexus block, femoral and sciatic nerve block) under supervision before attempting deeper blocks (e.g., lumbar plexus block), which can be technically demanding even for an experienced operator. Whenever possible, it is advisable to use a peripheral nerve stimulator in conjunction with US during the learning phase of USG nerve blocks. With proficiency, it is possible to perform most techniques without nerve stimulation. Fortunately, the learning curve is steep,[174,175] and most anesthesiologists are able to acquire the required skills very quickly. It is preferable to perfect these techniques in adults or older children before performing them in young children.

Summary

USGRA is a promising alternative to anatomic landmark-guided techniques, and almost all regional anesthetic techniques that are commonly performed in children can be performed using US guidance. US allows the anesthesiologist to visualize the target nerves and surrounding structures in real time during block placement. There is increasing evidence to support the routine use of US for regional anesthesia in children. We believe that anesthesiologists who care for children must acquire the skills necessary to perform USGRA and embrace this technology. US guidance is rapidly becoming the standard of care in pediatric regional anesthesia.[176]

ACKNOWLEDGMENT

Figures, sonograms, and videos in this chapter were reproduced with permission from http://www.aic.cuhk.edu.hk/usgraweb.

ANNOTATED REFERENCES

Guay J, Suresh S, Kopp S. The use of ultrasound guidance for perioperative neuraxial and peripheral nerve blocks in children. *Cochrane Database Syst Rev.* 2016 19;(2):CD011436.

This is the most updated evidence-based review article to support the use of ultrasound guidance in neuraxial and peripheral nerve blocks for children.

Kapral S, Krafft P, Eibenberger K, et al. Ultrasound-guided supraclavicular approach for regional anesthesia of the brachial plexus. *Anesth Analg.* 1994;78(3):507-513.

In 1994, Kapral and colleagues, from Vienna, Austria, published the first randomized controlled study on direct sonographic visualization in regional anesthesia. They

43

used ultrasound to directly visualize the brachial plexus and observe the spread of the local anesthetic in real time during supraclavicular brachial plexus block.

La Grange P, Foster PA, Pretorius LK. Application of the Doppler ultrasound bloodflow detector in supraclavicular brachial plexus block. *Br J Anaesth.* 1978;50(9):965-967.

In 1978, La Grange and associates were the first to describe the use of a Doppler flow detector to locate the subclavian artery and guide supraclavicular brachial plexus block.

Marhofer P, Frickey N. Ultrasonographic guidance in pediatric regional anesthesia Part I: theoretical background. *Pediatr Anesth.* 2006;16(10):1008-1018.

In this review article, Marhofer and Frickey, from Vienna, Austria, discuss the basic principles of ultrasound that are a prerequisite for the safe application of ultrasound for regional anesthesia in children.

A complete reference list can be found online at ExpertConsult.com.

Acute Pain

BENJAMIN J. WALKER, DAVID M. POLANER, AND CHARLES B. BERDE

THE PRACTICE OF PAIN MANAGEMENT in children continues to advance. Since the early 1980s, clinicians have recognized that neonates and infants experience pain and process those learning experiences. Research has demonstrated long-term adverse consequences of unrelieved pain, including harmful neuroendocrine responses, disrupted eating and sleep cycles, and increased pain perception during subsequent painful experiences.[1-3] Adequate pain control is second only to correct diagnosis when parents are surveyed about their priorities and concerns surrounding hospital admission.[4] Disparities in pain treatment led organizations, such as the Agency for Healthcare Research and Quality (AHRQ) and the American Pain Society (APS), to provide guidelines and the Joint Commission (formerly the Joint Commission on Accreditation of Healthcare Organizations) to issue mandates that further enhanced pediatric pain management.[5-7] The availability of reliable and valid pain assessment tools for children and governmental incentives encouraged the inclusion of children in analgesic drug trials. Many children's hospitals have dedicated multidisciplinary teams that manage acute and chronic pain. The increasing use of regional analgesia techniques led to the development of the Pediatric Regional Anesthesia Network (PRAN), a registry of practice patterns and complications of regional anesthetics in children. An enormous expansion of the breadth of techniques for acute pain management in children, the establishment of pediatric pain services, and the investigation and introduction of innovative modalities of therapy all attest to the importance accorded to this aspect of perioperative care.

Developmental Neurobiology of Pain

Nociceptive pathways in the periphery, spinal cord, and brain develop in a series of stages through the second and third trimester in humans. By 26 weeks postconception age, there is sufficient maturation of peripheral and spinal afferent transmission for the late-gestation fetus or preterm neonate to respond to tissue injury or inflammation with withdrawal reflexes, autonomic arousal, and hormonal metabolic stress responses. There are also changes in responsiveness after injury or repetitive stimulation indicative of central sensitization. In general, preterm neonates have reduced thresholds for withdrawal to noxious thermal and mechanical stimuli and immature descending inhibitor pathways that are necessary for modulating the pain response compared with older infants and children. One mechanism that may contribute to these low-threshold responses involves projections of low-threshold peripheral afferents to superficial as well as deep laminae in the spinal dorsal horn; later in development these afferents project only to deeper dorsal horn laminae. Most of the neural pathways that conduct nociception from the periphery through the central nervous system (CNS) are present and functional at 24 weeks gestational age, although the central connections, particularly in the thalamocortical pathways that are involved in the integration and perception of conscious pain, are not as well developed.[8-10] Controversy remains as to the meaning and implications of this neural immaturity. Opioid receptors and responses are present in the spinal cord at the time of birth, although spinal glial inflammatory mechanisms are immature. Because these mechanisms are central to the cyclooxygenase (COX-1 and COX-2) responses, this may imply that there is limited or no analgesic response to nonsteroidal antiinflammatory drugs (NSAIDs) and COX inhibitors in preterm infants or neonates, whereas opioid responses are active. γ-Aminobutyric acid (GABA) receptors and associated pathways, which play an important role in the effects of analgesics and anesthetics, can be either excitatory or inhibitory, depending on the stage of development.[11] The neuroplasticity that is characteristic of these infants may be a double-edged sword. Animal models and some clinical evidence suggest that repeated noxious stimuli may result in heightened sensitivity to nociceptive input and adverse behavioral sequelae.[2,12-16] On the other hand, nerve injury in infant animals may result in less pain than in older animals.[15,16] In humans, the neural injury to the brachial plexus after shoulder dystocia during delivery rarely results in chronic pain. It may be that there are both vulnerable periods and periods of greater resiliency during development, so that the consequences of pain in young children may not be easily predictable.

Investigators have examined indexes suggestive of cortical activation, including near-infrared spectroscopy[17] and electroencephalography,[18] in response to noxious events. Using near-infrared spectroscopy, a unilateral heel stick (performed for clinical purposes) produces signal changes suggestive of contralateral cortical activation.[17-19] Despite these lines of evidence, the nature of pain in neonates, viewed as conscious suffering, remains unknown. Other investigators have looked for long-term consequences of painful events (with or without treatment) in humans and in animal models. Despite attempts by these investigators to correct for confounding factors, in our view, the interpretation of these studies, especially in humans, should be quite cautious. Neonates who undergo painful procedures are commonly those who are more medically ill. It appears difficult to distinguish consequences of pain per se from the consequences of other factors, such as prematurity, critical illness (including episodes of hypoxia or ischemia), deprivation of tactile and social contact, and nutritional deprivation. Many clinicians and investigators have adopted the view that, in the absence of better information about either the nature of suffering experienced by neonates or the potential adverse consequences of pain in terms of long-term development, caregivers should err on the side of providing, rather than withholding, analgesia. Although this is a compelling perspective, it is important to highlight three concerns: (1) in general, available studies have had difficulty showing effects of routine administration of analgesia (e.g., morphine infusions) on immediate behavioral indexes of distress in neonates undergoing intensive care; (2) repeated or prolonged administration of anesthetics and sedatives in animal models have been shown to have deleterious effects on brain development, (the human implications of these animal studies remain unclear at this time [see also Chapters 7 and 25])[12,20-25]; and (3) as detailed later, younger organisms develop tolerance to opioids and benzodiazepines more rapidly than older organisms, so that the management of tolerance and withdrawal has now become a nearly universal consequence of prolonged administration of these medications to critically ill neonates, infants, and children.

Pain Assessment

The International Association for the Study of Pain (IASP) has defined *pain* as an unpleasant sensory and emotional experience associated with actual or potential tissue damage, or *described* in terms of such damage. The IASP and others have acknowledged that the inability to communicate verbally, as in the preverbal, nonverbal, or the cognitively impaired, does not preclude the possibility that an individual is experiencing pain and is in need of appropriate pain management.[26,27] Table 44.1 summarizes various pain assessment tools in terms of appropriate age, target population, ease of use, and practicality; commonly used scales are discussed in more detail later.

Consensus guidelines have been published with recommendations for appropriate tools to use for research studies, many of which are simple to use in routine clinical settings.[28] It should be emphasized that pain intensity is only one of many factors that should be considered when performing a global pain assessment. Other important outcomes include functional recovery, patient satisfaction, adverse effects, emotional recovery, and economic factors. The Revised American Pain Society Patient Outcomes Questionnaire (APS-POQ-R) consists of 12 questions pertaining to multiple pain outcomes.[29] A study is currently under way to validate a modified version in children. Although this tool is likely too cumbersome for daily use, it can be helpful for quality assurance and research studies.

SELF-REPORT METRICS

Self-report metrics in which a patient is asked to quantify the severity of the pain between 0 (no pain) and 10 (maximum pain) most accurately reflect acute pain because pain is a subjective experience. Because many children lack the cognitive skills to use such scales, pain assessment metrics have been developed to include developmentally appropriate self-report tools, behavioral-observational tools, and physiologic-biologic measures (see Table 44.1). Given the multidimensional nature of the individual pain experience, and the complexity and inherent biases associated with self-report, the use of unidimensional numeric scales alone to reflect pain is overly simplistic.[30-33] Therefore, regardless of the metric used, it must be emphasized that a complete pain assessment is more than just a number attempting to quantify the severity of pain. Estimating the impact of pain on the suffering and the quality of the individual's life and recovery process, targeting appropriate therapeutic metrics, and evaluating the efficacy and side effects of such measures are additional key components of a global and ongoing pain assessment and treatment strategy.

For children to use numeric scales, they must understand the concepts of magnitude and ordinal position—that is, they must be able to identify which of different-sized objects is bigger and place them in order from smallest to largest. They must also be able to arrange geometric figures or numbers in a series *(seriation)*. These skills are typically not present until about 7 years of age; thus pain assessment tools that use graphic facial displays representing different degrees of pain expression are used to facilitate self-report of pain in young children.

Faces Pain Scales

Faces pain scales consist of a series of line diagrams of faces with expressions of increasing distress.[34-39] Some versions have a smiling face, whereas others, notably the Faces Pain Scale and Faces Pain Scale-Revised (FPS-R), have a neutral face to represent the "no pain" end of the scale (Fig. 44.1).[39,40] Unlike the numeric scales, the faces scales do not require the concept of magnitude or seriation and can therefore be used by preschool-aged children. The Wong-Baker Faces Pain Scale has been extensively studied and its reliability and validity confirmed in children 3 to 18 years of age. Strong correlations have been reported between the Wong-Baker Scale scores and other faces scales, the Visual Analog Scale (VAS), as well as nurses' ratings based on behavior.[41-44] Data suggest that versions with the smiling face at the no-pain end of the spectrum, such as the Wong-Baker Scale, may overestimate pain because children without pain, but with distress from other sources, may be reluctant to choose the smiling face.[39] The Wong-Baker Scale was preferred by children to the numeric rating scale, the graphic rating scale, and the Color Analog Scale.[34,36,42,45] Overall, the FPS-R is the faces scale with the largest support for its validity.[46] The International Association for the Study of Pain (IASP) has the FPS-R available in dozens of languages on its website (http://www.iasp-pain.org/education).

Numeric Scales
Visual Analog Scale
Several versions of the VAS are available, including horizontal and vertical lines, word anchors representing extremes of pain, and lines with divisions and numeric values (Fig. 44.2). When using the vertical versions of this scale, the severity of the pain

TABLE 44.1	Appropriate Pain Assessment Measures by Age Group: Self-Report, Observational/Behavior, and for the Cognitively Impaired	
Self-Report Tools	**Appropriate Age Groups**	**Comments**
Faces Pain Scale	3–18 years	Simple and quick to use; extensively validated in healthy school children with postoperative and cancer pain
Oucher	3–18 years	Photographic for ≥3-year-olds, numeric 0–10 scale for ≥6-year-olds; less clinical utility and feasibility compared with other faces scales
Manchester Pain Scale	3–18 years	Panda bear faces eliminate gender and ethnic bias; tested in emergency department setting
Computer Face Scale	4–18 years	Offers option for continuous rather than categorical format; good construct validity; preferred by children over the Wong-Baker Faces Scale; further testing needed
Sydney Animated Facial Expression Scale (SAFE)	4–18 years	Animated version of Faces Pain Scale; rated by children as easiest to use; no psychometric advantage compared with other scales
Visual Analog Scale (VAS)	6–18 years	Simple and quick to use; requires the concepts of order, magnitude, and seriation (the ability to place or visualize in series); widely used across settings; preferred to other self-report tools by children ≥8 years old and adolescents
Numeric Rating Scale (NRS)	7–18 years	Simplest and most commonly used in clinical as well as research settings
Observational/Behavioral Measures		
Comfort Scale	0–18 years	Developed for use in intensive care settings; useful in mechanically ventilated children and in the postoperative setting
Face, Legs, Activity, Cry, Consolability (FLACC)	2 months–7 years	Excellent pragmatic and psychometric qualities; widely adopted in clinical and research settings; has been translated into several languages other than English
Children's Hospital of Eastern Ontario Pain Scale (CHEOPS)	1–7 years	Good psychometric properties; lengthy with inconsistent scoring among categories; cumbersome; extensively used both in clinical and research settings
Cognitively Impaired Children		
Revised FLACC	All ages	Allows for scoring individualized pain behaviors; good psychometric properties; highest clinical utility compared with the Non-Communicating Children's Pain Checklist–Postoperative Version (NCCPC-PV) and Nursing Assessment of Pain Intensity (NAPI)
Non-Communicating Children's Pain Checklist (NCCPC)	All ages	Requires 5-minute observation period; comprehensive but cumbersome; used in clinical and research setting
University of Wisconsin Pain Scale	All ages	Inconsistent scoring style compared with other clinical scoring systems; scoring style may permit flexibility but limits precision
The Pain Indicator for Communicatively Impaired Children	All ages	Useful for pain assessment in cognitively impaired children in the home setting.

44

increases as one ascends the ladder. Although moderate to strong correlations have been reported between the VAS, faces pain scales, the Oucher (E-Fig. 44.1), and ethnic versions of the Oucher (E-Fig. 44.2),[47,48] the effect of user age on VAS ratings are conflicting.

Numeric Rating Scale

The Numeric Rating Scale (NRS) is the simplest and most commonly used numeric scale in which the child rates the pain from 0 (no pain) to 10 (worst pain). Its validity has been established with good correlations between NRS and FPS-R scores in children 7 to 17 years of age and NRS and VAS scores in children 9 to 17 years of age.[49] The NRS also correlates well with perceived need for analgesia, pain relief, and patient satisfaction in children.[50] An important caveat when using numeric scales is to verify the denominator that the child is using. For example, a pain score of 9 on a 0 to 100 scale would reflect mild pain and may not require treatment, whereas a score of 9 on a 0 to 10 scale would reflect severe pain that warrants aggressive treatment.

Selection Criteria

Selection of a self-report tool for a child requires careful consideration of the age and cognitive and developmental level. Fig.

44.3 depicts the percentages of children of different ages who can self-report their pain and the tools most appropriate for various age ranges. Children who are unable to use a self-report tool may be able to report their pain intensity using simple words, such as "small," "medium," and "big." However, self-reports of pain are subject to the modulating influences of many factors, including the child's previous pain experience and response to treatment, psychosocial factors, and parental preferences and influences. Consequently, in many cases, it may be necessary to complement self-reported pain scores with behavioral observations, particularly in preschool-aged children. Regardless of the tool selected, assessment of postoperative pain is greatly facilitated by the introduction of the concept of rating pain and of the tool itself during the preoperative preparation of the child.

Novel Self-Report Tools

These self-report tools use a categorical format and the static faces do not allow for "fine-tuning" of the ratings before a final assessment regarding the severity of pain is reached.[51] In recent years, there has been interest in developing computer-based self-report assessment tools that use a continuous rather than categorical format.[52]

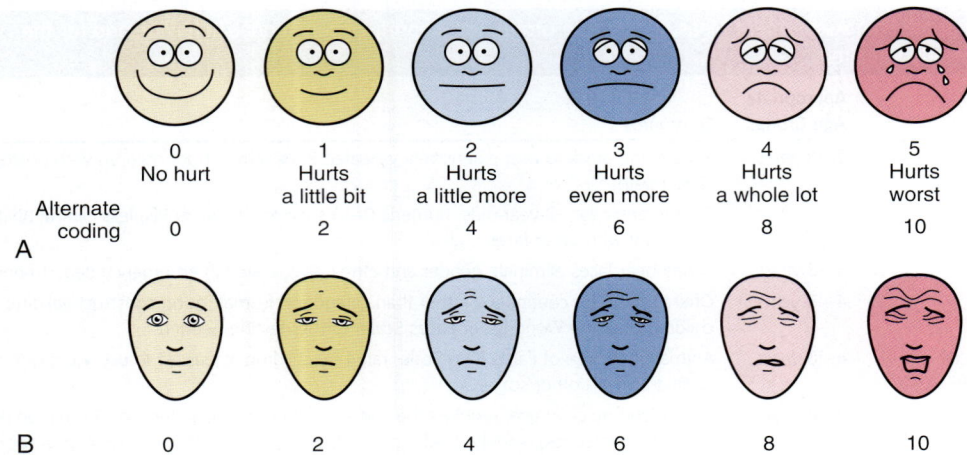

FIGURE 44.1 **A,** The Wong-Baker Faces Pain Scale. **B,** The Bieri Faces Pain Scale. (**B** modified from Bieri D, Reeve RA, Champion GD, et al. The Faces Pain Scale for the self-assessment of the severity of pain experienced by children: development, initial validation, and preliminary investigation for ratio scale properties. *Pain* 1990;41(2):139–150.)

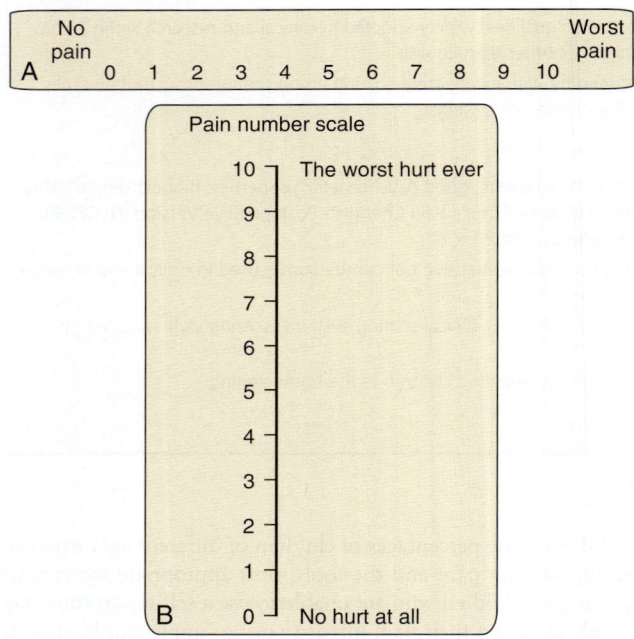

FIGURE 44.2 Numerical self-report scales. **A,** Horizontal Visual Analog Scale. **B,** Vertical Visual Analog Scale.

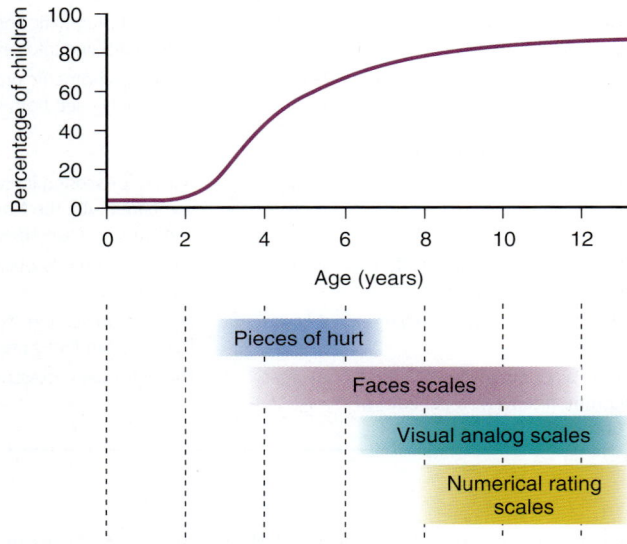

FIGURE 44.3 Self-report tools most appropriate for different age ranges. The percentage of children at different ages who can self report their pain is shown in the upper panel. The lower panel shows suitable pain measure for different ages.

The Computer Face Scale allows the child to adjust the shape of the mouth of a cartoon face from smiling to frowning and simultaneously to adjust the eyes from completely open to completely closed.[51,53] The suggested benefits of this scale include increased sensitivity (given the ability to select from a wide range of faces) and computerized storage of the results, with ready access and data display. Preliminary work with this scale has demonstrated its construct validity, and it was preferred by children over the Wong-Baker Faces Scale.[51]

The Sydney Animated Facial Expression Scale (SAFE) is an animated version of the Faces Pain Scale[54] and consists of a series of 101 faces. To administer this scale, the child pushes the left or right arrow key on a computer, causing the expression of the single face to change until it corresponds with the child's pain intensity (http://www.usask.ca/childpain/research/safe). At this point, a keystroke records a score between 0 and 100. The SAFE scale was rated to be easiest to use by children aged 4 to 16 years compared with other scales, including the Faces Pain Scale, the Color Analog Scale, and Pieces of Hurt,[55] although it offered no psychometric advantage over the other scales. Further research with this tool is needed before its role can be clearly defined.

OBSERVATIONAL-BEHAVIORAL MEASURES

Despite the availability of several age-appropriate methods for self-reporting, assessing pain in children who are unable or unwilling to self-report depends on observations of their behaviors. Five behaviors shown to be reliable, specific, and sensitive when predicting analgesic requirements are facial expression, vocalization or cry, leg posture, body posture, and motor restlessness.[56] Variations in these behaviors have been used in several observational pain tools. Table 44.2 describes the content validity of some commonly used observational tools. Behavior checklists provide a list of pain behaviors that are marked as present or absent, and the extent of pain is estimated on the basis of the number of behaviors present at the time of the assessment.[57,58] Behavior rating scales also incorporate a rating of the intensity or frequency and duration of each behavior.[59] Global rating scales provide a rating of the observer's overall impression of the child's pain.

Children's Hospital of Eastern Ontario Pain Scale

The Children's Hospital of Eastern Ontario Pain Scale (CHEOPS), one of the earliest behavioral rating scales (Table 44.3),[60] incorporates six categories of behavior scored individually from 0 to 2 or 1 to 3 and then sums them to provide a pain score ranging from 4 to 13. Scores of 6 or less indicate no pain. Its validity and reliability for brief painful events and for postoperative pain has been well established, with good to excellent correlations with faces pain scales and the VAS.[48,61] However, the time required to complete the evaluation and inconsistent scoring among categories of the CHEOPS make it cumbersome and impractical to use in a busy clinical setting.

TABLE 44.2	Content Validity of Behavioral Pain Tools: Categories of Behavior in Pain Assessment Tools				
FLACC	**CHEOPS**	**OPS**	**TPPPS**	**Büttner/Finke**
Face	Facial expression		Facial pain expression	Facial expression
Legs	Leg movement	Movement		Leg position
Activity	Torso movement	Agitation	Bodily pain expression	Position of torso
				Motor restlessness
Cry	Cry	Cry	Vocal pain expression	Cry
Consolability	Touching of the wound	Blood pressure		Consolability
	Verbal report of pain	Verbal complaint and body language		

CHEOPS, Children's Hospital of Eastern Ontario Pain Scale; *FLAAC*, Face, Legs, Activity, Cry, Consolability scale; *OPS*, Objective Pain Scale; *TPPPS*, Toddler Preschool Preoperative Pain Scale.

TABLE 44.3	Children's Hospital of Eastern Ontario Pain Scale (CHEOPS)[a]		
Item	**Behavioral**	**Score**	**Definition**
Cry	No cry	1	Child is not crying.
	Moaning	2	Child is moaning or quietly vocalizing silent cry.
	Crying	2	Child is crying, but the cry is gentle or whimpering.
	Scream	3	Child is in a full-lunged cry; sobbing; may be scored with complaint or without complaint.
Facial	Composed	1	Child has neutral facial expression.
	Grimace	2	Score only if definite negative facial expression.
	Smiling	0	Score only if definite positive facial expression.
Child Verbal	None	1	Child is not talking.
	Other complaints	1	Child complains, but not about pain, e.g., "I want to see mommy" or "I am thirsty."
	Pain complaints	2	Child complains about pain.
	Both complaints	2	Child complains about pain and about other things, e.g., "It hurts; I want my mommy."
	Positive	0	Child makes any positive statement or talks about others things without complaint.
Torso	Neutral	1	Body (not limbs) is at rest; torso is inactive.
	Shifting	2	Body is in motion in a shifting or serpentine fashion.
	Tense	2	Body is arched or rigid.
	Shivering	2	Body is shuddering or shaking involuntarily.
	Upright	2	Child is in a vertical or in upright position.
	Restrained	2	Body is restrained.
Touch	Not touching	1	Child is not touching or grabbing at wound.
	Reach	2	Child is reaching for but not touching wound.
	Touch	2	Child is gently touching wound or wound area.
	Grab	2	Child is grabbing vigorously at wound.
	Restrained	2	Child's arms are restrained.
Legs	Neutral	1	Legs may be in any position but are relaxed; includes gentle swimming or discrete movements.
	Squirming/kicking	2	Definitive uneasy or restless movements in the legs and/or striking out with foot or feet.
	Drawn up/tensed	2	Legs tensed and/or pulled up tightly to body and kept there.
	Standing	2	Standing, crouching, or kneeling.
	Restrained	2	Child's legs are being held down.

[a]Recommended for children 1 to 7 years old; a score greater than 6 indicates pain.

Face, Legs, Activity, Cry, Consolability Scale

The Face, Legs, Activity, Cry, Consolability (FLACC) scale was developed in an effort to improve on the pragmatic qualities of the existing behavioral pain tools by providing a simple framework for quantifying pain behaviors in children.[59] This tool includes five categories of behaviors previously found to reliably correlate with pain in young children: facial expression, leg movement, activity, cry, and consolability (Table 44.4).[56] The acronym FLACC facilitates recall of these categories, each of which is scored from 0 to 2 to provide a total pain score ranging from 0 to 10. The FLACC tool has been extensively tested and determined to have good interrater reliability and excellent validity based on changes in pain scores from before to after analgesic administration and excellent correlation with the Objective Pain Scale (OPS), the CHEOPS, the Toddler Preschool Preoperative Pain Scale (TPPPS), and good correlation with self-reported pain scores using faces pain scales.[59,61-63] The FLACC scale has been translated into several languages, including Spanish, Chinese, Swedish, French, Italian, Portuguese, Norwegian, and Thai.

Comfort Scale

The Comfort scale (Table 44.5), developed for use in an intensive care setting, consists of six behavioral and two physiologic measures, each of which has five response categories, thereby allowing detection of subtle changes in the child's distress.[64] Initial evaluation of the Comfort scale found acceptable interrater reliability and good correlations with VAS scores in 37 mechanically ventilated infants.[64] Another study evaluated the reliability and validity of the Comfort scale as a postoperative pain instrument in children after thoracic or abdominal surgery.[65] This study found good to excellent interrater agreement for all categories except respiratory response, for which there was moderate agreement. Additionally,

---

TABLE 44.4 The FLACC Behavioral Pain Scale

Categories	SCORING		
	0	1	2
Face	No particular expression or smile	Occasional grimace or frown, withdrawn, disinterested	Frequent to constant frown, clenched jaw, quivering chin
Legs	Normal position or relaxed	Uneasy, restless, tense	Kicking, or legs drawn up
Activity	Lying quietly, normal position, moves easily	Squirming, shifting back and forth, tense	Arched, rigid, or jerking
Cry	No cry (awake or asleep)	Moans or whimpers, occasional complaint	Crying steadily, screams or sobs, frequent complaints
Consolability	Content, relaxed	Reassured by occasional touching, hugging, or being talked to, distractible	Difficult to console or comfort

Each of the five categories, (F) Face; (L) Legs; (A) Activity; (C) Cry; (C) Consolability, is scored from 0 to 2, which results in a total score between 0 and 10.
©2002, The Regents of the University of Michigan. All rights reserved.

TABLE 44.5 Comfort Scale

	1	2	3	4	5
Alertness	Deeply asleep	Lightly asleep	Drowsy	Fully awake and alert	Hyper-alert
Calmness or Agitation	Calm	Slightly anxious	Anxious	Very anxious	Panicky
Respiratory Response	No coughing and no spontaneous respirations	Spontaneous respiration with little or no response to ventilation	Occasional cough or resistance to ventilator	Actively breathes against ventilator or coughs regularly	Fights ventilator; coughing or choking
Physical Movement	No movement	Occasional, slight movement	Frequent slight movement	Vigorous movement limited to extremities	Vigorous movement including torso and head
Blood Pressure	Less than baseline	Consistently at baseline	Infrequent increases of 15% or more (1–3 episodes during observation period)	Frequent increases of 15% or more (>3 episodes)	Sustained increase >15%
Muscle Tone	Muscles totally relaxed; no muscle tone	Reduced muscle tone	Normal muscle tone	Increased muscle tone and flexion of fingers and toes	Extreme muscle rigidity and flexion of fingers and toes
Facial Tension	Facial muscles totally relaxed	Facial muscle tone normal; no facial muscle tension evident	Tension evident in some facial muscles	Tension evident throughout facial muscles	Facial muscles contorted and grimacing
Heart Rate	Below baseline	Consistently at baseline	Infrequent elevations of 15% or more above baseline	Frequent elevations of 15% or more above baseline	Sustained elevation of 15% or more above baseline

strong correlations between Comfort and VAS pain scores support the use of the Comfort scale as a postoperative pain assessment instrument in children.

After a systematic review of observational pain measures, the FLACC and the CHEOPS[60] scales were recommended for assessment of pain associated with medical procedures, the FLACC for postoperative pain, and the Comfort scale for pain in children in critical care.[30] Despite the extensive science supporting the use of behavioral tools, it may be difficult to separate behaviors caused by pain from those caused by other sources of distress in some children.[66] Accurate pain assessment therefore requires careful consideration of the context of the behaviors. Input from the parents or caregivers may be valuable as proxy measures, although some parents may lose objectivity in such a situation. Similarly, a regular caregiver may best assess older children with significant developmental delay. When in doubt regarding the source of distress, a trial of analgesics is appropriate and may be both diagnostic and therapeutic.

Parents' Postoperative Pain Measure

The Parents' Postoperative Pain Measure (PPPM) is a 15-item yes/no questionnaire that is completed by a parent/caregiver and designed specifically for use at home without involvement of a health professional (E-Table 44.1). A score of 6 or greater correlates with clinically significant pain. This tool has been validated for children 2 to 12 years old[58,67] and is useful for research and quality improvement projects, especially as more operations are done on an outpatient basis.[68]

LIMITATIONS OF PAIN ASSESSMENT

It remains unclear whether integration of routine pain assessment into clinical practice improves patient outcomes. A critical review of the studies that addressed this question determined that in two of six studies, children experienced a reduction in pain intensity when a standardized pain assessment tool was used; in two studies there was no change in pain intensity; and in two studies pain intensity decreased when pain assessment was combined with pain management interventions.[69] Studies that examined sustainability of the benefits over time reported conflicting results, and most studies were identified as having major methodologic problems.[70,71] Additional investigation is required to determine whether routine pain assessment has any effect on pain outcomes.

Despite the large body of evidence supporting the psychometric properties of numerous structured pain assessment tools, there remains considerable variability in the interpretation of the clinical relevance of pain scores.[33] Attempts have been made to define what range of pain scores is associated with a perceived need for medicine or what magnitude of change in pain score is associated with a perception of better or worse pain.[50,72,73] A survey of 6- to 16-year-old hospitalized children found that a median pain score of 3 or a 0-to-6 Faces Pain Scale was associated with the child's perceived need for medicine.[72] Others have reported that a 10-mm change in a 0-to-100-mm VAS score was the minimum difference whereby children in the emergency department perceived their pain to be slightly better or slightly worse.[73] In the postoperative period, children with a median pain score of 6 on a 0-to-10 NRS scale perceived the need for an analgesic, whereas those with a score of 3 felt there was "no need" for treatment.[50] In addition, children felt "a little better" or "worse" if the NRS scale changed by at least 1. Despite these findings, there was large variability and overlap in scores associated with these outcomes.

Evaluations of the effectiveness of pain treatment algorithms based on numerical pain scores have yielded conflicting results. One study reported increased prescription of opioid and nonopioid analgesics, an increased administration of nonopioids, and reduced pain scores in children who received postoperative pain treatment based on a pain score–based algorithm.[74] Children whose pain management was algorithm-based experienced more nausea, but no other adverse effects. In contrast, hospitalized adults whose pain management was based on a numerical pain treatment algorithm experienced a 2-fold increase in episodes of oversedation and a 49% increase in opioid-related adverse drug events.[75] This latter study highlights the potential for harm when numeric pain scores alone are used to guide decisions regarding pain treatment. A comprehensive approach to pain assessment that includes consideration of the child's self-reporting (when available), combined with behavioral observation and the overall clinical context, is required to direct treatment decisions.[76]

It has been suggested that the widespread adoption of a pain score as the fifth vital sign contributes to the overprescribing of analgesics and sedatives.[77] National survey data demonstrate that approximately 276,000 adolescents in the United States abused prescription pain relievers in 2015, second only to marijuana. Unfortunately, even prescription use of opioids in the teenage years has been identified as an independent risk factor for nonmedical use of opioids in early adulthood.[78] Adult data show that many patients use only a fraction of their prescribed opioid after common outpatient procedures.[79] At one author's institution (BW), quality improvement data showed that children used only 10% to 20% of the opioid prescribed to them after tonsillectomy, and data from other institutions demonstrate that significant amounts of opioid are prescribed regardless of patient age or weight.[80] These data highlight the need for procedure-specific opioid prescribing guidelines for children, as well as the importance of patient and family education regarding proper use, storage, and disposal of prescription opioids.

SPECIAL CONSIDERATIONS FOR THE COGNITIVELY IMPAIRED CHILD

Children who are cognitively impaired experience pain more frequently than cognitively intact children because of many inherent conditions, such as spasticity, muscle spasms, the need for assistive devices for positioning and mobility, and the need for invasive surgical procedures. Indeed, as many as 60% of children with cerebral palsy undergo orthopedic surgery by 8 years of age, and many of them require repeated procedures.[81] Yet both children and adults who are cognitively impaired receive fewer analgesics than those who are cognitively intact with similar painful conditions.[82,83] Barriers to effective pain management in the cognitively impaired include the complexity of pain assessment in those who cannot verbalize their pain, outdated beliefs that these children have altered or blunted pain perception, limited evidence for the safety and efficacy of analgesic regimens, and an exaggerated concern regarding opioid adverse effects, particularly respiratory depression. Although there is also evidence of cognitive impairment as an independent risk factor for needing a rescue intervention when patient-controlled analgesia (PCA) by proxy is used,[84] this may reflect challenges in thorough assessment of these patients rather than inherent differences in pain tolerance or opioid metabolism. Difficulties with pain assessment have led to the virtual exclusion of these children from clinical drug trials, leading to deficits in our knowledge of how to effectively manage their pain. A survey of clinicians who treat children who are cognitively

TABLE 44.6 Revised FLACC for Pain Assessment in the Cognitively Impaired[a]

	0	1	2
Face	No particular expression or smile	Occasional grimace/frown; withdrawn or disinterested (Appears sad or worried)	Consistent grimace or frown; frequent/constant quivering chin, clenched jaw (Distressed-looking face; expression of fright or panic)
Legs	Normal position or relaxed	Uneasy, restless, tense (Occasional tremors)	Kicking, or legs drawn up (Marked increase in spasticity, constant tremors or jerking)
Activity	Lying quietly, normal position, moves easily	Squirming, shifting back and forth, tense (Mildly agitated [e.g., head back and forth, aggression]; shallow, splinting respirations, intermittent sighs)	Arched, rigid, or jerking (Severe agitation head banging; shivering [not rigors]; breath-holding, gasping or sharp intake of breath; severe splinting)
Cry	No cry (awake or asleep)	Moans or whimpers, occasional complaint (Occasional verbal outburst or grunt)	Crying steadily, screams, or sobs; frequent complaints (Repeated outbursts, constant grunting)
Consolability	Content, relaxed	Reassured by occasional touching, hugging, or "talking to"; distractible	Difficult to console or comfort (Pushing away caregiver, resisting care or comfort measures)

[a]Revised descriptors for children with disabilities shown in parentheses.

impaired identified inadequate pain assessment tools and inadequate training and knowledge of providers as significant barriers to effective pain management, despite respondents' beliefs that children who are cognitively impaired perceive pain to a similar extent as cognitively intact children.[85]

Revised Face, Legs, Activity, Cry, Consolability (r-FLACC) Observational Tool

Initial evaluation of the FLACC tool in children with cognitive impairment found a good correlation between scores assigned independently by different observers and by parent global ratings of pain.[86] Although measures of exact agreement between observers were acceptable for the face, cry, and consolability categories, measure of agreement for the legs and activity categories were less acceptable, likely because of coexisting motor impairments such as spasticity. The FLACC tool was therefore revised to incorporate additional descriptors of behaviors most consistently associated with pain in children with cognitive impairment (Table 44.6).[87] Interrater reliability for the total FLACC scores, as well as for each of the categories, improved when the evaluation included the revised FLACC (r-FLACC) in 52 cognitively impaired children. Also, good correlation among r-FLACC, parent, and child scores supported its criterion validity. r-FLACC scores were noted to decrease after an opioid was administered, supporting the construct validity of the tool. The pragmatic attributes of the r-FLACC were compared with those of the Nurses' Assessment of Pain Intensity (NAPI) and the Non-Communicating Children's Pain Checklist (NCCPC-PV) (E-Tables 44.2 and 44.3).[88] Clinicians using these tools to score pain rated the complexity as less and the relative advantage and overall clinical utility of the FLACC and the NAPI to be greater compared with the NCCPC-PV, suggesting that these tools may be more readily adopted into clinical practice.

Strategies for Pain Management

Pain is a complex phenomenon that occurs because of the transmission of nociceptive stimuli from the peripheral nervous system through the spinal cord to the cerebral cortex. Pain perception is further influenced by emotions, behavior, and previous pain experiences via multiple synapses in the limbic system, frontal cortex, and thalamus. Given the complexity of the pain mechanism, effective treatment of pain requires the use of multimodal therapies that target multiple sites along the pain pathways, as illustrated in Fig. 44.4. Multimodal treatment includes many nonpharmacologic techniques that are used more commonly for brief procedures (e.g., comfort position, cold/vibration, distraction) in addition to pharmacologic interventions (see further). *The primary goal of this approach is to minimize opioid needs and opioid-related side effects.*

Analgesics with additive or synergistic activity and different adverse effect profiles should be selected so that adequate analgesia can be provided with fewer adverse consequences. Thus pain can be treated at the peripheral level using local anesthetics, peripheral nerve blockade, NSAIDs, antihistamines, or opioids. At the spinal cord level, pain can be treated with local anesthetics, neuraxial opioids, α_2-adrenoceptor agonists, and N-methyl-D-aspartate (NMDA) receptor antagonists. Finally, at the cortical level systemic opioids, α_2-agonists, and voltage-gated calcium channel $\alpha_2\delta$ proteins (targets for anticonvulsants) can be used.[89] Most cases of moderate to severe pain are best treated with a multimodal approach.

The strategy for postoperative pain management is an integral part of the preanesthetic plan, so that informed consent for procedures, such as placement of peripheral or regional blocks, can be obtained (see Chapters 42 and 43). Additionally, appropriate teaching of techniques such as PCA should begin in the preoperative period. An honest discussion with the child that, although some discomfort is inevitable, every effort will be made to minimize pain after surgery, decreases the anxiety related to the perioperative experience. This, together with the use of nonpharmacologic techniques, may even reduce the need for opioids and other analgesics. Selection of an analgesic regimen requires careful consideration of many factors, including scope and requirements of the surgical procedure, age and cognitive abilities of the child, the child's previous pain experience and response to treatment, underlying medical conditions that might alter the response to pain medications, and child and family preferences. The goal should be for the child to emerge from anesthesia in reasonable comfort, because it is generally easier to maintain analgesia in a pain-free child than to achieve analgesia in a child with severe pain. Fig. 44.5 presents a flowchart describing strategies for assessment and management of acute postoperative pain in a child.

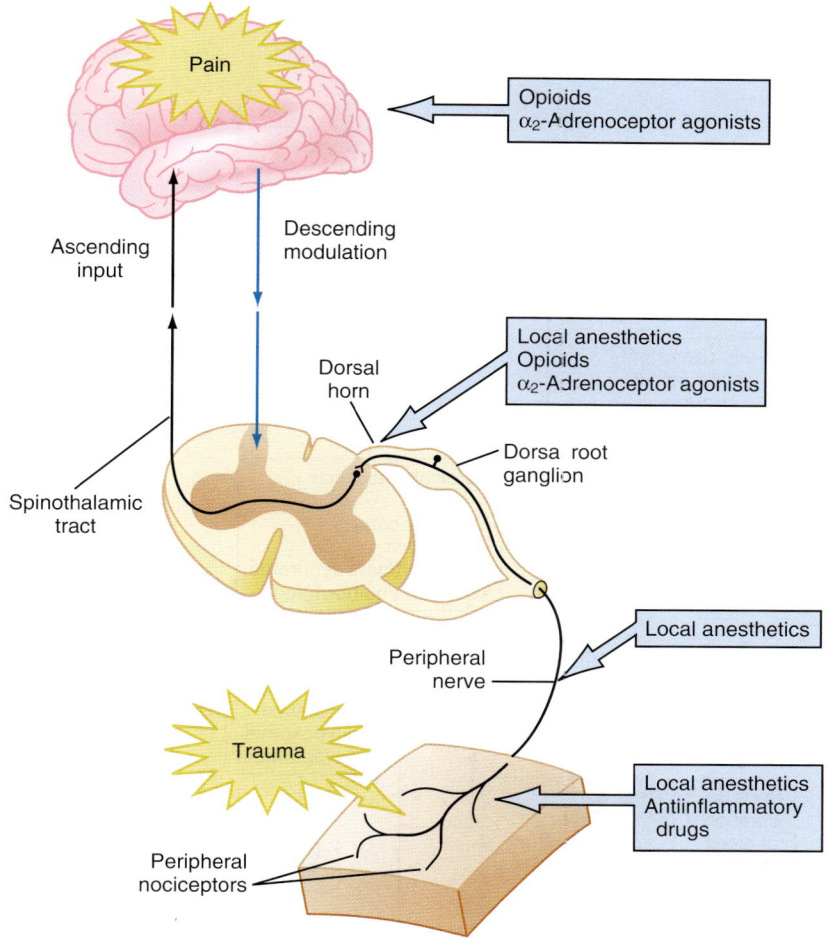

FIGURE 44.4 Schematic diagram of the pain pathways and multimodal measures to provide pain relief. (From Kehlet H, Dahl JB. The value of "multimodal" or "balanced analgesia" in postoperative pain treatment. *Anesth Analg.* 1993;77:1049.)

SURGICAL CONSIDERATIONS

The scope and requirements of the surgical procedure, as well as specific postoperative issues, should be discussed with the surgical team before choosing an analgesic regimen, particularly if a regional technique is planned. For example, the site of placement of an epidural catheter and choice of epidural solution will differ in a child with a vertical midline incision from a child with a transverse suprapubic incision. With certain procedures, an epidural catheter may intrude into the surgical field or access to the catheter site in the postoperative period may be obscured by a cast or dressing. In such cases, the catheter may be tunneled subcutaneously away from the surgical field. Alternatively, one or more epidural catheters may be placed under direct vision by the surgeon at the end of the procedure (e.g., spinal fusion or selective dorsal rhizotomy).[90] Postoperative pain is managed using an infusion of local anesthetic and/or opioid solutions through the catheter.[91] Painful muscle spasms after certain procedures are often ameliorated by continuous regional analgesia.[91-93] This effect is partly related to the density of blockade and may also require supplemental oral or parenteral benzodiazepines if the block alone is inadequate. Refractory spasms of the bladder, which can be quite problematic after some surgeries (e.g., ureteral reimplantation), can also be effectively treated with NSAIDs (e.g., ketorolac) or anticholinergics.[94] Intravesical bupivacaine has also been used to manage bladder spasm, although

close attention must be paid to dosing to avoid toxicity.[95,96] Epidural blockade may favorably alter diaphragmatic mechanics after thoracotomy and upper abdominal surgery. This effect is likely a result of the motor blockade of the intercostal muscles and alteration in the resting length of the diaphragm and is not solely a result of reversal of diaphragmatic inhibition.[97-100] However, it remains uncertain whether analgesia alone, achieved by systemic opioids or central neuraxial blockade, diminishes postoperative diaphragmatic inhibition or significantly improves postoperative pulmonary function.[101,102] Effective analgesia, however, does improve child compliance with measures such as deep breathing and early mobilization, thereby reducing the incidence of postoperative complications.[103]

Child-Related Considerations
Age and Cognitive Abilities
Analgesic techniques, such as infiltration of the wound with local anesthetics, peripheral nerve blocks, or regional blockade that minimize the use of opioids and central respiratory depressants, may be ideal for preterm or very young infants with impaired central respiratory drive.[104,105] Acetaminophen can be a useful adjunct, because when used within its recommended dose range, it has a large therapeutic window with few untoward effects. Although the judicious use of opioids is not contraindicated,

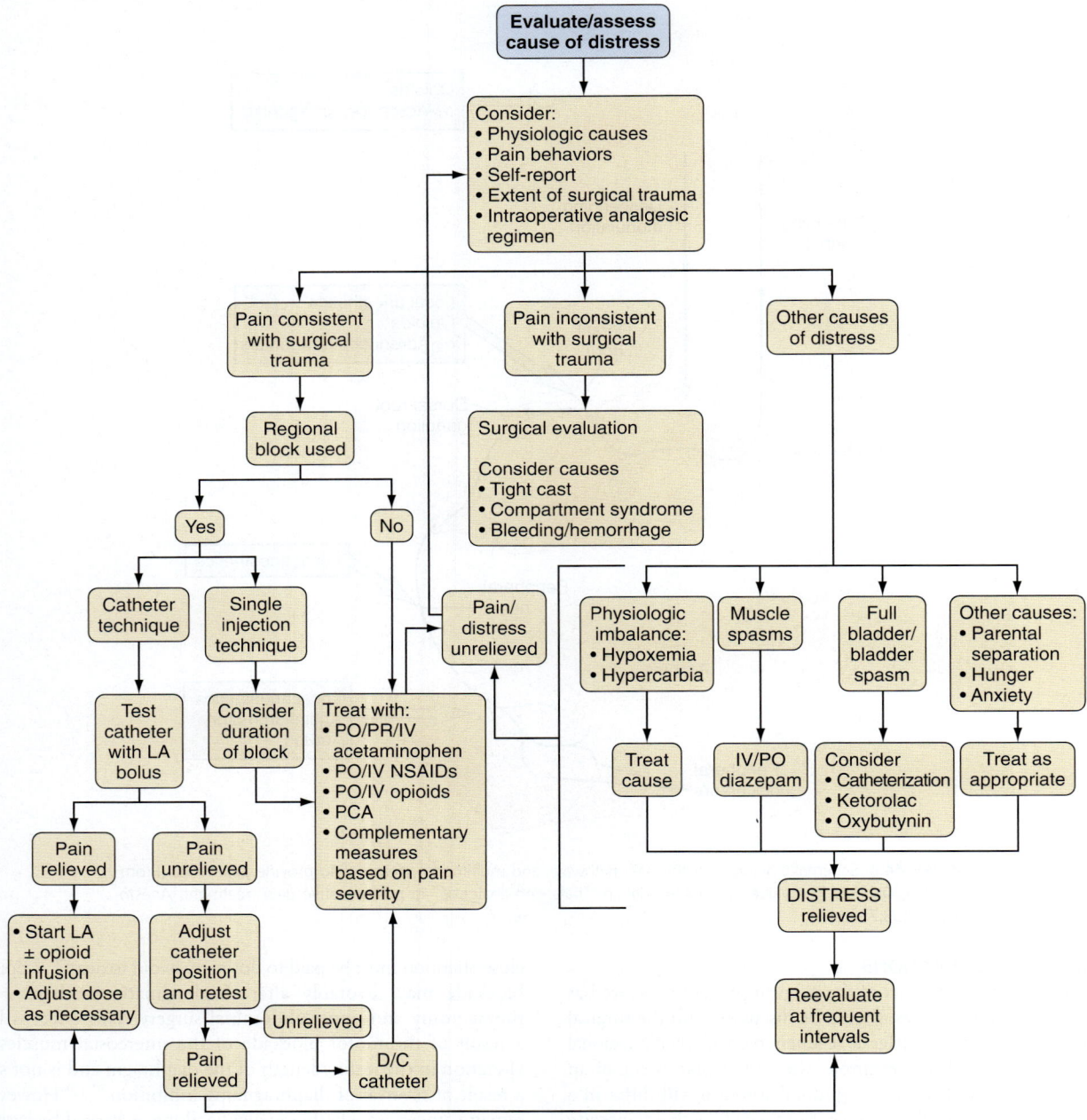

FIGURE 44.5 Flowchart for assessment and management of acute postoperative pain in a child. *D/C*, discontinue; *IV*, intravenous; *LA*, local anesthetic; *NSAIDs*, nonsteroidal antiinflammatory drugs; *PCA*, patient-controlled analgesia; *PO*, orally; *PR*, per rectum.

preterm or term infants younger than 1 month of age who receive these medications require careful observation and monitoring to detect respiratory depression.[106] The use of local anesthetics in infants younger than 6 months of age also requires more careful attention to dose because decreased protein binding of local anesthetics puts them at increased risk for toxicity.[107]

Older infants and toddlers who are expected to experience moderate to severe pain may be adequately treated with oral opioids when oral intake resumes. Alternatively, low-dose continuous opioid infusions, nurse-controlled analgesia (NCA),[108] or regional blockade may be required in those undergoing extensive surgery. Nonpharmacologic techniques that focus on distraction,

such as child-life therapy and the presence of a comforting parent, can augment the analgesic therapy.

Preschool- and school-aged children have greater fears and better understanding of the postoperative experience than do their younger counterparts. Most cognitively intact children 7 years of age or older are able to understand the concept of PCA, which may help to give a sense of control back to the child during a period in which all other aspects of control are removed.[109] Such issues of control and dependency assume even greater importance in adolescents; allowing them to participate in decision making will contribute to the success of any analgesic technique.[109] Regional techniques are excellent for providing analgesia in all age groups and are associated with a reduced incidence of adverse effects compared with systemic opioids (e.g., nausea, vomiting, excessive sedation, dysphoria, and respiratory depression). Children with significant developmental delay require special consideration of their physical disability, as well as cognitive abilities, although in most cases the pharmacologic actions of the drugs are not altered.

Regardless of the child's age, a detailed history regarding the child's previous pain experience, analgesic history, response to treatment, and adverse effects from previous analgesic regimens should be carefully considered when selecting a pain management technique. An opioid-naive child undergoing surgery for the first time requires smaller doses of opioids for a shorter duration compared with a child with chronic pain who has developed opioid tolerance because of long-term or repeated opioid use. Analgesic selection should also be modified based on the effectiveness of analgesics for that particular child in the past. As the use of genomic testing becomes more available and clinically feasible, identification of target polymorphisms, particularly in the cytochrome P450 enzyme system, may be used to tailor drug selection and dosing.

Pharmacologic Treatment of Pain

NONOPIOID ANALGESICS

Nonopioid analgesics are used as sole agents for mild pain and as important adjuncts for multimodal treatment of moderate to severe pain. Although most nonopioid analgesics produce dose-dependent responses, they are limited by a ceiling effect in the analgesia achieved—that is, larger doses of the medication provide no additional analgesia. Hence, more severe pain is resistant to therapy from these medications alone.[110] Ideally, nonopioid medications (Table 44.7) are delivered on a scheduled basis for at least the first few days postoperatively, while opioids are available pro re nata (PRN) for breakthrough pain.

Acetaminophen

Acetaminophen is the most common antipyretic and nonopioid analgesic used in children. Despite years of study, the predominant mechanism of its analgesic action remains unclear. It may exert its analgesic effects by blocking central and peripheral prostaglandin synthesis, reducing substance P–induced hyperalgesia, and modulating the production of hyperalgesic nitric oxide in the spinal cord.[111-113] In addition, acetaminophen might produce analgesia via activation of descending serotonergic pathways.[114-116] One putative site of action may be inhibition of prostaglandin H_2 synthetase at the peroxidase site.[115] Effective analgesia and

antipyresis have been described with plasma concentrations of 5 to 20 µg/mL[117-121]; a target effect-site (similar to cerebrospinal fluid) concentration of 10 µg/mL reduces pain after tonsillectomy by 3.6/10 pain units.[122] The total daily dose of acetaminophen via any route is age- and weight-based, but should not exceed 75 mg/kg for children, 60 mg/kg for neonates 32–44 weeks postconceptual age, and 40 mg/kg for preterm neonates 28–32 weeks.

The recommended dose for oral administration is 10 mg/kg every 4 hours or 15 mg/kg every 6 hours, or a total daily dose of 60 mg/kg per day, which is less than the upper daily limit of 75 mg/kg. Acetaminophen has a wide margin of safety when administered in the recommended therapeutic dose range. However, hepatotoxicity has been reported with doses only slightly above the recommended dose, suggesting that acetaminophen may have a narrow therapeutic index in some children.[123,124] Because of these reports and on the advice of a U.S. Food and Drug Administration panel, the manufacturers have reduced the maximum daily dose to 3 g. Acetaminophen is available in a wide variety of formulations, alone or in combination with decongestants, for oral use in a variety of cold remedies, and with opioids for the treatment of moderate to severe pain. There are currently more than 600 over-the-counter acetaminophen-containing products, increasing the risk of an overdose because children may take more than one formulation that contains the drug. Frequent review of medications and parental education is needed to minimize the risk of overdose. In the past, pediatric liquid formulations of acetaminophen as in infant drops were commonly supplied in larger concentrations than that in elixirs, resulting in dosing errors. As a result, the 80-mg/mL concentration has been removed from the U.S. market by the manufacturer, and liquid formulations have been standardized to 32 mg/mL. This concentration equals approximately 0.5 mL/kg of acetaminophen if given as a 15-mg/kg dose. Since both gastric fluid volume and pH are unchanged after liquid acetaminophen (40 mg/kg of a 50 mg/mL elixir, 0.8 mL/kg) administered orally 90 minutes before induction of anesthesia, it is feasible to use this preoperatively. Whether these results are applicable to acetaminophen that is administered closer to the time of induction is not known.[125]

Intravenous (IV) formulations of paracetamol (acetaminophen) have been used in Europe and Australia for many years and are now available in the United States. IV acetaminophen is available as a 10-mg/mL solution and should be infused over ~15 minutes in a dose of 12.5 mg/kg every 4 hours or 15 mg/kg every 6 hours, with a total daily limit of 75 mg/kg (although at the time of writing, the IV manufacturer continues to recommend a 4 grams per day

TABLE 44.7	Oral Dosing Guidelines for Commonly Used Nonopioid Analgesics				
Medication	Individual Dose for Children <60 kg (mg/kg)	Individual Dose for Children ≥60 kg (mg)	Dosing Interval (hours)	Maximum Daily Dose for Children <60 kg (mg/kg)	Maximum Daily Dose for Children ≥60 kg (mg)
Acetaminophen	10–15	650–1000	4–6	75[a]	3000
Ibuprofen	5–10	400–600	6	40	2400
Naproxen	5–6	250–375	12	10	1000
Diclofenac	1	50	8	3	150
Ketorolac[b]	0.5	30	6–8	2	120
Tramadol	1–2	50	6	8	400

[a]See text for new age-related dosing.
[b]Ketorolac should be administered for a maximum of 5 days or 20 doses up to 15 mg per dose for children <60 kg or 30 mg per dose for children >60 kg.
Modified from Berde CB, Sethna NF. Analgesics for the treatment of pain in children. *N Engl J Med.* 2002;347(14):1094–1103; and World Health Organization. *World Health Organization Guidelines on the Pharmacological Treatment of Persisting Pain in Children with Medical Illnesses.* WHO: Geneva, Switzerland; 2012.

limit, unlike the recommendations for oral acetaminophen). In neonates between 32 and 44 weeks postconception age, a loading dose of 20 mg/kg should be followed by 10 mg/kg every 6 hours (every 12 hours in 28–31 weeks postconception age).[126] Each dose of IV acetaminophen must be documented in a timely manner to avoid overdoses from multiple dosing; several cases of frank overdoses have occurred in young infants who received excessive doses of IV acetaminophen on the ward.[124,127–129] Dosing recommendations for premature and full-term neonates continues to be an active area of research, and one study has shown weight to be a better predictor of individual pharmacokinetics than either postconception or gestational age.[130]

After IV administration of acetaminophen, analgesic onset occurs within 15 minutes and antipyresis within 30 minutes.[131,132] IV acetaminophen rapidly penetrates the blood-brain barrier, yielding detectable concentrations in the cerebrospinal fluid (CSF) within 5 minutes of administration, and peak CSF concentrations within 57 minutes after injection (compared with 2 to 3 hours after rectal or oral administration). This explains the fast onset of its analgesic and antipyretic effects.[133] A large multicenter trial reported that 1 gram of IV paracetamol and 2 grams of IV propacetamol (equivalent to 1 gram acetaminophen) provided superior analgesia with a reduced need for morphine compared with placebo in adults after lower extremity joint replacement.[134] The propacetamol group experienced a greater incidence of local skin reactions and pain on injection compared with the IV paracetamol group. A controlled randomized trial reported that both rectal acetaminophen, 40 mg/kg, and IV acetaminophen, 15 mg/kg, administered after induction of anesthesia in children undergoing adenotonsillectomy provided good analgesia for the first 6 hours after surgery.[135] However, children who received acetaminophen rectally had a greater duration of analgesia and did not require rescue analgesia as early as those in the IV group.[135] This is attributable to the slow absorption of rectal acetaminophen, causing sustained effective concentrations (see also Fig. 4.2).[136] When compared with oral acetaminophen, there was evidence of lower intraoperative opioid requirements (again attributable to differing time to peak effect-site concentration), but no difference in postoperative opioid consumption in young children undergoing cleft palate repair when children received scheduled acetaminophen via the oral or IV route.[137]

Slow and unpredictable absorption of acetaminophen after rectal administration, however, results in variable blood concentrations, with peak concentrations reached between 60 and 180 minutes after administration (Fig. 4.2).[120,138,139] This unpredictability was illustrated in a series of studies from the same group of investigators examining opioid-sparing with rectal and IV acetaminophen in infants undergoing major abdominal and thoracic surgery. In the rectal study, no opioid-sparing effect was detected, and plasma concentrations of acetaminophen varied 50-fold among patients.[140] In a follow-up study in the same population using IV acetaminophen, opioid consumption was reduced by 60% and the frequency of apnea was also reduced.[141] In children undergoing orthopedic surgery, a loading dose of 40 mg/kg rectal acetaminophen followed by 20 mg/kg every 6 hours yielded serum concentrations of 10 to 20 µg/mL in half of the patients, with no evidence of accumulation over a 24-hour period.[138] This dosing scheme is now the one most commonly recommended when the rectal route is used, but it should be noted that scheduled dosing with this scheme would result in a dose of 80 mg/kg per day (or 100 mg/kg on the first day with the loading dose). Contrary to previous assumptions, acetaminophen is relatively evenly distributed in

most suppositories, allowing them to be split to achieve a desired dose, although accuracy of dosing is problematic.[142]

In conclusion, acetaminophen has opioid-sparing potential with very few adverse effects and a low risk of toxicity with appropriate dosing. The oral and IV routes produce equivalent analgesia when differences in onset time are considered. The rectal route should be considered a "last resort" because of unpredictable absorption and limited dosing options. Financial considerations have limited the routine use of IV acetaminophen at many centers in the United States.[143]

Nonsteroidal Antiinflammatory Drugs

NSAIDs provide excellent analgesia for mild to moderate pain resulting from surgery, injury, and disease. Their principal mechanism of action is via inhibition of the enzyme prostaglandin H_2 synthetase at the COX site, causing a reduction in the production of prostaglandins at the site of tissue injury and attenuation of the inflammatory cascade. In addition to their peripheral effects, the NSAIDs have also been shown to exert a direct spinal action by blocking the hyperalgesic response induced by activation of spinal glutamate and substance P receptors.[144] Decreased production of leukotrienes, activation of serotonin pathways, and inhibition of excitatory amino acids, NMDA-mediated hyperalgesia, and central inhibition of prostaglandin biosynthesis have been proposed as additional mechanisms of action.[145,146] The COX-1 enzyme is present in the brain, gastrointestinal tract, kidneys, and platelets and is expressed constitutively. It preserves gastric mucosal integrity and function, platelet aggregation, and renal perfusion. COX-2 expression is induced by inflammation or tissue injury. Selective COX-2 inhibitors reduce inflammation but have less effect on gastric mucosal function and have fewer effects on platelet aggregation, thereby resulting in fewer adverse effects. Their deleterious effects on renal perfusion, however, are no different than the nonselective COX drugs, because COX-2 is constitutively expressed in renal tissues and may be involved in prostaglandin-dependent renal homeostatic processes.[147] The risks of renal toxicity increase in the presence of hypovolemia, cardiac failure, preexisting renal dysfunction, or with the concurrent use of other nephrotoxic drugs. Reports of thrombotic cardiovascular and CNS events after both long-term and short-term use in adults led to withdrawal of two of the COX-2 inhibitors, rofecoxib and valdecoxib, from the market[148,149]; the risk of these agents causing thrombotic complications in children remains unknown. Most pediatric studies have evaluated the use of nonselective COX medications. In adult studies, COX-2 inhibitors have generally, but not always, produced analgesia roughly equivalent to that of traditional NSAIDs.

Ibuprofen, one of the oldest orally administered NSAIDs, has been used extensively for treatment of fever and pain related to surgery, trauma, arthritis, menstrual cramps, and sickle cell disease. A large, controlled, randomized, double-blind study reported a greater decrease in VAS pain scores with ibuprofen than with acetaminophen or codeine in children presenting to the emergency department with acute pain after musculoskeletal trauma.[150] Additionally, more children who received ibuprofen had VAS scores less than 30 on a 0-to-100-mm VAS scale than in the other two groups. The recommended dose of ibuprofen is 5 to 10 mg/kg every 6 hours. Like acetaminophen, ibuprofen is available in a variety of formulations and concentrations, placing children at risk for an overdose. For pediatric use, ibuprofen is available as follows:

- Concentrated drops containing 50 mg ibuprofen in 1.25 mL
- Oral suspension containing 100 mg of ibuprofen in 5 mL

- Junior Strength chewable tablets or caplets containing 100 mg of ibuprofen in each

Diclofenac provides effective analgesia after minor surgical procedures in children. It is available only as an oral tablet in the United States, but it is available as a suppository and in the injectable form in several countries. The pediatric dose of diclofenac is 1 mg/kg every 8 hours orally, 0.5 mg/kg rectally, and 0.3 mg/kg IV.[151] The oral and rectal doses reflect bioavailabilities of 0.36, 0.35, and 0.6 for suspension, dispersible tablets, and suppository forms, respectively. When diclofenac was administered rectally, the relative bioavailability was greater and the peak concentration was reached earlier than after enteric-coated tablets administered orally.[152] Children who received diclofenac experienced analgesia comparable to those who received caudal bupivacaine or IV ketorolac for inguinal hernia repair.[153-155] In children undergoing tonsillectomy and/or adenoidectomy, diclofenac yielded superior analgesia with less supplemental opioid dosing, less nausea and vomiting, and earlier resumption of oral intake compared with acetaminophen.[156,157] Although there are occasional reports of increased bleeding and restlessness in the recovery room in children who received diclofenac compared with those who had received papaveretum during tonsillectomy,[158] a Cochrane review established that NSAIDs did not cause any increase in bleeding that required a return to the operating room (OR) for children. However, when examining the bleeding risk with different types of NSAIDS, ketorolac (but not other NSAIDS) was associated with a statistically significant increase in bleeding after tonsillectomy.[159,160] Overall, there was less nausea and vomiting with NSAIDs compared with alternative analgesics, suggesting their benefits outweigh their negative aspects. A prospective, randomized trial assigned 91 children with sleep-disordered breathing to acetaminophen with ibuprofen or morphine for analgesia after tonsillectomy. There was an almost 4-fold increase in the number of desaturation events (from preoperative levels) during the first postoperative night in the morphine group, and a decrease in the number of desaturation events during the same period in the ibuprofen group. Overall, the pain scores in the morphine group were less, but there was no statistically significant difference. The study was terminated early as a result of preliminary results and an incident of respiratory depression at home, resulting in admission to the pediatric intensive care unit (ICU) in the morphine group.[161]

Ketorolac, indomethacin, and ibuprofen are the only injectable NSAIDs available in the United States. Indomethacin is the most commonly used NSAID used for closure of patent ductus arteriosus in preterm neonates. The IV formulation of ibuprofen is labeled for children and adults in the United States. Ketoprofen, parecoxib, and diclofenac are other injectable NSAIDs that are available outside the United States. A large multicenter study compared the risks of serious adverse events from IV ketorolac, ketoprofen, and diclofenac in more than 11,000 adults undergoing major surgery.[162] The results indicated that 1.4% of adults experienced a serious adverse outcome, including surgical site bleeding (1%), death (0.17%), severe allergic reactions (0.12%), renal failure (0.09%), and gastrointestinal bleeding (0.04%), with no differences in outcomes among the groups. Similar large-scale studies are not available for children, but one placebo-controlled study of 161 children undergoing tonsillectomy who received IV ibuprofen (10 mg/kg IV) (n = 82) demonstrated an opioid-sparing effect without an increase in bleeding,[163] consistent with the findings of larger reviews.[160]

Ketorolac has been shown to provide postoperative analgesia similar to opioids in children of all ages.[164-167] Its benefits include lack of opioid adverse effects (respiratory depression, sedation, nausea, and pruritus), making it an attractive choice for the treatment of postoperative pain. However, in common with all NSAIDs, it carries risks of platelet dysfunction, gastrointestinal bleeding, and renal dysfunction. Ketorolac (1 mg/kg) given to 18 preterm and term neonates undergoing painful procedures in the OR or the neonatal ICU,[165] revealed reduced pain scores (Neonatal Infant Pain Scale) with no incidents of systemic or local bleeding and no hematologic, hepatic, or renal complications (note that this dose is twice the usually recommended dose of 0.5 mg/kg). Similarly, no adverse effects on surgical drain output, renal or hepatic function tests, or oxygen saturation after major surgery were noted in 37 infants and toddlers between 6 and 18 months of age.[168] Children in that study received continuous morphine infusions postoperatively, confounding the evaluation of the analgesic efficacy of ketorolac. In single dose studies, the pharmacokinetics (PK) of ketorolac in infants and small children (2–18 months of age) appear to be homogeneous and show a relatively rapid elimination of the analgesic S enantiomer, with slower clearance of the R enantiomer.[168,169] Finally, ketorolac has been used to supplement opioid analgesia, with no increase in renal or bleeding complications in infants and children after open heart surgery.[170-172] Nevertheless, because ketorolac can reduce renal blood flow, many recommend that its course be limited to 48 to 72 hours, and that renal function be checked if a course of administration greater than 72 hours is required.[168,169]

Another contentious issue regarding NSAIDs relates to their effects on bone healing and their use in children undergoing spinal fusion. Prostaglandins play an integral role in bone metabolism and significantly influence bone resorption and formation; however, their effects on bone formation predominate. NSAIDs inhibit the formation of prostaglandins, thereby raising the concern that they could promote nonunion after spinal fusion. Studies in rabbits and some studies in adults have reported a greater incidence of nonunion or pseudarthrosis, particularly with the use of large doses of ketorolac.[173,174] However, no differences in curve progression, hardware failure, pseudarthrosis, or need for reoperation have been found in children and adolescents who received ketorolac in the immediate postoperative period compared with those who did not.[175-177] Of note, the majority of the pediatric data are from otherwise healthy children with idiopathic scoliosis, making it problematic to extrapolate these data to children with comorbidities or those with neuromuscular scoliosis. There is no unique advantage of the IV route with NSAIDs. There is also no evidence that IV ketorolac is a more potent analgesic than comparable (i.e., equipotent) doses of a number of other NSAIDs administered by oral or rectal routes.[178]

A meta-analysis of the use of NSAIDs for postoperative pain that included 27 studies compared 567 children who received NSAIDs with 418 children who did not.[179] The coadministration of NSAIDs and opioids during the perioperative period decreased opioid requirement in the postanesthesia care unit (PACU) and the first 24 hours after surgery, decreased pain intensity in the PACU, and reduced postoperative nausea and vomiting (PONV) during the first 24 hours postoperatively. Although NSAIDS appear to be more effective than acetaminophen for acute pain,[180] modeling studies show that combination therapy prolongs the duration of analgesia of both drugs.[181] Many studies have also demonstrated the benefits of scheduled combination therapy in children, often performing better than either drug alone.[182,183] Therefore these two medications are part of the World Health Organization global guidelines on treating pain in children[184] and should serve as the foundation of a safe, effective, and opioid-sparing analgesic regimen.

Tramadol

Tramadol is a synthetic analog of codeine that exerts its analgesic properties by two complementary mechanisms. One of its metabolites has a weak affinity for the μ opioid receptor with no affinity for the δ or the κ receptors. In addition to its mild opioid effects, it also inhibits serotonin and norepinephrine uptake. Its main advantages over opioids include reduced incidences of respiratory depression, sedation, nausea, and vomiting. However, tramadol undergoes metabolism via the CYP2D6 pathway, and there are concerns that "ultrametabolizers" could produce excessive amounts of the potent O-desmethyltramadol metabolite, a metabolite with 200-fold greater affinity for μ receptors than tramadol.[185,186] A common formulation of oral tramadol is an elixir in a concentration of 100 mg/mL, a formulation that is easily inadvertently overdosed. This concentrated dose should be administered as "drops," but some have mistakenly administered this concentration in milliliters, resulting in an overdose. To preclude such overdoses, many jurisdictions have limited the concentration of oral tramadol to 5 to 10 mg/mL. Toxicity occurs after administration of 7 to 10 mg/kg of tramadol.[187] Other adverse effects associated with its use include nausea and vomiting (9%–10% of cases), pruritus (7%), and rash (4%).[188] It is reported to cause dizziness, and its use has been associated with seizures. Tramadol is available only in tablet form alone or in combination with acetaminophen in the United States. However, it is available in a liquid formulation (see earlier text), as a suppository, and as an injectable solution in other countries, allowing for greater flexibility of dosing. Therefore it has been used to provide analgesia by many routes, including oral, rectal, IV (including PCA devices), epidural, and by local infiltration.

Tramadol is used for postoperative pain treatment in children undergoing ambulatory surgery and has also been used when transitioning from IV opioids to oral analgesics. Two doses of tramadol (1 mg/kg and 2 mg/kg orally) were compared in children who were being transitioned from morphine PCA. Children who received 2 mg/kg required fewer supplemental analgesics with no difference in adverse effects compared with those who had received 1 mg/kg.[188] Tramadol, 2 mg/kg IV, produced similar analgesia and sedation, with fewer episodes of oxygen desaturation compared with morphine 0.1 mg/kg IV, in children with obstructive sleep apnea undergoing adenotonsillectomy.[189] Tramadol has also been found to produce a similar analgesic effect as that of ilioinguinal and iliohypogastric nerve blocks in children undergoing herniorrhaphy.[190] The tramadol group, however, experienced a greater incidence of nausea and vomiting. The incidence of PONV can be reduced by using a slow-release oral formulation; this reduces early peak concentrations and allows sustained plasma concentrations. Tramadol PCA has also been found to provide adequate analgesia with less sedation, earlier awakening, and earlier extubation in children undergoing atrial or ventricular septal defect repair compared with those who received morphine via PCA.[191]

Tramadol has also been effective when administered via the neuraxial route. Caudal tramadol (2 mg/kg) produced reliable postoperative analgesia comparable with that produced by caudal morphine (30 μg/kg) in children undergoing inguinal hernia repair.[192] No additional pain medications were required in the first 24 hours in more than 90% of children in each group. Rigorous drug-specific neurotoxicity studies, however, are lacking, and

therefore this route of administration is not recommended until such data are available and confirmed. Another study compared the analgesic efficacy of 2 mg/kg tramadol administered IV or by peritonsillar infiltration in children undergoing adenotonsillectomy.[193] Both groups experienced excellent analgesia in the first hour. However, the local infiltration group experienced more prolonged analgesia and required fewer rescue doses of acetaminophen compared with the IV group. Overall, tramadol appears to be an analgesic of medium potency with a low incidence of adverse effects that may be used alone for mild to moderate pain and for its opioid-sparing effect in children with severe pain.

Ketamine

There has been increasing interest in the use of ketamine, an NMDA-receptor antagonist, in the treatment of both chronic and acute pain. Its professed benefits include an opioid-sparing effect, avoidance of opioid tolerance, prevention of central sensitization and wind-up, mitigation of opioid-induced hyperalgesia, and provision of synergistic analgesia in multimodal regimens by virtue of its own antinociceptive properties. Case series in children with intractable pain resulting from advanced stages of cancer have reported reduction in opioid requirement, decreased opioid adverse effects, improvement in pain control and function, and increased ability to interact with their families.[194-196] Ketamine is also very popular as a single agent for both analgesia and sedation for burn care.[197]

Studies evaluating the use of ketamine alone or in combination with opioids for acute postoperative pain in children have yielded equivocal results. In one study, children undergoing tonsillectomy who received IV ketamine 0.5 mg/kg after induction or at the end of surgery experienced reduced pain scores and required fewer rescue analgesics compared with those who received placebo.[198] All children in this study received a standardized analgesic regimen, including rectal diclofenac before the start of surgery and oral acetaminophen at scheduled intervals postoperatively. Another study reported reduced pain scores and reduced requirement for rescue analgesics in children who received ketamine as a bolus dose and by infusion that began before the start of a tonsillectomy, compared with those who received a single bolus dose of ketamine at the end of surgery.[199] Intramuscular (IM) ketamine 0.5 mg/kg has also produced equivalent analgesia in terms of similar pain scores and need for rescue analgesics compared with IM morphine 0.1 mg/kg as sole analgesics for tonsillectomy.[200] Other studies have found no such benefits when ketamine was compared with placebo for tonsillectomy, urologic, and orthopedic surgery.[201-204]

A meta-analysis of 35 randomized controlled trials compared 567 children who received ketamine as an adjuvant analgesic by a variety of routes for a variety of surgical procedures with 418 who did not receive ketamine.[205] Although the use of ketamine was associated with reduced pain intensity in the PACU and there was a reduced need for nonopioids, there was no opioid-sparing effect. A systematic review of 37 studies included 4 in children, 2 of which demonstrated beneficial effects of ketamine administered as an adjuvant analgesic and 2 of which found no benefits.[206] The investigators could draw no conclusions regarding the use of ketamine as an adjuvant analgesic. The use of ketamine in all the previous studies was associated with only a few mild and self-limiting adverse effects. Further investigation is needed to evaluate the benefits of low-dose ketamine for acute postoperative pain before its routine use can be recommended.

Gabapentin

Gabapentin is an anticonvulsant that exhibits an analgesic effect through binding to presynaptic calcium-channels and modulating the release of glutamate and other excitatory neurotransmitters. It is available in 100-, 300-, 600-, and 900-mg tablets as well as a 50-mg/mL oral solution. Although it has been studied most extensively for chronic neuropathic pain, there is substantial evidence in adults for its analgesic effects on acute pain,[207] and it is also useful in preventing PONV.[208] There is comparatively less evidence for its benefit in pediatric acute pain, but a prospective, randomized study of children undergoing posterior spinal fusion demonstrated a significant reduction in morphine consumption in the early postoperative period when given as a preoperative loading dose of 15 mg/kg followed by 5 mg/kg three times daily.[209] Another study using only a single preoperative dose did not show an opioid-sparing effect.[210] Gabapentin does not cause respiratory depression, but sedation is a common adverse effect, which may confound patient assessment when coadministered with opioids

OPIOID ANALGESICS

Opioids are indicated for moderate to severe pain after surgery or trauma, for acute painful crises such as in sickle cell disease, as well as for chronic painful conditions such as cancer. Opioids mimic the effects of endogenous ligands known as endorphins, exerting their effects by binding to specific opioid receptors located at presynaptic and postsynaptic sites in the brain, spinal cord, and peripheral nerve cells. There are four opioid receptors in the CNS: μ, κ, δ, and σ.[211-213] When these receptors are activated, they inhibit neurons by decreasing the release of excitatory neurotransmitters from presynaptic terminals. The μ receptors are further subdivided into μ_1 receptors, responsible for supraspinal analgesia and physical dependence; and μ_2 receptors, responsible for respiratory depression, bradycardia, physical dependence, and gastrointestinal dysmotility.[214] Activation of the κ receptors causes analgesia without significant respiratory depression, whereas activation of the σ receptors causes dysphoria, tachycardia, tachypnea, hypertonia, and mydriasis. The δ receptors modulate the activity of the μ receptors.

Drugs that exert their effects on opioid receptors are classified as agonists, antagonists, partial agonists, and mixed agonist-antagonists. Agonists are neurotransmitters that bind to a receptor and exert their pharmacologic effects. Antagonists, on the other hand, bind to the receptor but do not initiate any effects; yet by occupying the receptor they block the effects of agonists. Partial agonists have reduced intrinsic activity and produce less than a maximal response. They act as antagonists as well because they block the agonists from access to the receptor. The mixed agonist-antagonist drugs act as agonists at certain opioid receptors and antagonists at others. E-Table 44.4 depicts the various opioid receptors, their effects, as well as the drugs that exert activity on each of them. The opioids that are used most commonly in the management of pain are μ-receptor agonists, including morphine, hydromorphone, the fentanyls, methadone, hydrocodone, and oxycodone. Of these, morphine is the opioid that is most commonly used as first-line therapy for moderate to severe pain in children and, consequently, is the agent with which clinicians have the greatest experience. Table 44.8 lists the relative potencies and suggested initial doses of the opioids in common clinical use. Developmental pharmacology, PK, and side effects of opioids are discussed in depth in Chapter 7.

Delivery Techniques

The blood concentration of opioids must be maintained within a therapeutic range to provide effective analgesia and avoid undesirable adverse effects, such as excessive sedation and respiratory depression. Both the dose and the route by which the opioid is delivered determine how well one is able to maintain the blood concentration within this therapeutic window and minimize adverse effects.

TABLE 44.8   Opioid Analgesics: Relative Potency and Initial Dosing Guidelines[a]

Drug	Potency Relative to Morphine	Oral Dose	Intravenous Dose	IV/PO Dose Ratio
Morphine	1	0.3 mg/kg every 3–4 hours Sustained release: 20–35 kg: 10–15 mg every 8–12 hours 35–50 kg: 15–30 mg every 8–12 hours	Bolus: 0.1 mg/kg every 2–4 hours Infusion: 0.01–0.03 mg/kg per hour	1:3
Hydromorphone	5–7	0.04–0.08 mg/kg every 3–4 hours	Bolus: 0.02 mg/kg every 2–4 hours Infusion: 0.002–0.006 mg/kg per hour	1:4
Fentanyl	80–100	NA	Bolus: 0.5–1 µg/kg every 30 minutes to 2 hours Infusion: 0.5–2 µg/kg per hour	NA
Codeine	0.1	0.5–1 mg/kg every 4–6 hours	NR	NA
Oxycodone	1–1.5	0.1–0.2 mg/kg every 4–6 hours	NA	NA
Hydrocodone	1–1.5	0.1–0.2 mg/kg every 4–6 hours	NA	NA
Methadone[b]	1	0.1–0.2 mg/kg every 6–12 hours	0.1 mg/kg every 6–12 hours	1:2
Nalbuphine	0.8–1	NA	50–100 µg/kg every 3–6 hours	1:4–5

IV, intravenous; *NA*, not applicable; *NR*, not recommended; *PO*, oral.
[a]Recommended doses are for infants >6 months of age. For younger infants, reduce initial doses to 25% of these doses and increase as needed.
[b]Methadone has a long half-life and can accumulate, causing delayed sedation or respiratory depression. If sedation or respiratory depression occurs, doses should be withheld until sedation resolves. Then the drug is restarted at a smaller dose and extended dosing interval.
Modified from Berde CB, Sethna NF. Analgesics for the treatment of pain in children. *N Engl J Med.* 2002;347(14):1094–1103.

Oral Administration

Oral opioids are well tolerated and suited for children with mild to moderate pain, for those who undergo outpatient surgery, or as adjuncts to regional anesthetics. For those with regional anesthetics, oral administration of an opioid just before the block is expected to wear off may provide a smooth transition and more stable and satisfactory analgesia. In most cases, oral opioids are better tolerated after resumption of oral intake.

Hydrocodone and oxycodone are two of the most commonly prescribed oral opioids. Both are available in a variety of formulations either alone or in combination with acetaminophen. Both hydrocodone and oxycodone are available in liquid form, making them easy to prescribe for infants and young children. Oxycodone is available in 1-mg/mL and 20-mg/mL strengths. The 1-mg/mL strength is easy to dose and administer to infants, whereas the 20-mg/mL strength is reserved for older children with chronic pain and should rarely be used to treat acute postoperative pain. Although the different formulations allow flexibility in dosing, extreme caution is required in prescribing and dispensing the correct concentration to avoid a potentially lethal overdose.

There are many combination products containing oral opioids and a nonopioid adjuvant, such as acetaminophen. Although the primary advantage of these combinations is to reduce the number of tablets needed, this is outweighed by the disadvantage of a potential overdose of acetaminophen, and also results in suboptimal dosing (i.e., PRN) when scheduled dosing of adjuvant medications results in the greatest amount of opioid sparing. Therefore we discourage the use of combination products and encourage the practice of scheduled dosing of nonopioids complemented by as-needed dosing of opioids for breakthrough pain. *Indeed, this strategy is an important trend in the contemporary use of opioids for acute pain that can ameliorate the problems of opioid adverse effects and overuse. A multimodal analgesic approach, which leverages the synergistic interactions between nonopioid and opioid analgesics, can result in enhanced analgesia with fewer untoward effects and reduced opioid requirements.*[215-217] Although randomized controlled trials are still limited in infants and children, we believe that the preponderance of evidence and clinical experience support a multimodal strategy as logical and clinically beneficial to children and should be used as the principal approach to treating most acute pain.

It should be noted that many oral opioids (oxycodone, hydrocodone, codeine) undergo metabolism via the CYP2D6 pathway (see Chapters 6 and 7). Hydrocodone and oxycodone have intrinsic analgesic properties, but codeine is a prodrug that requires conversion to morphine via demethylation. There are significant genetic polymorphisms that affect the relative production of active metabolites of these drugs (oxymorphone, hydromorphone, and morphine, respectively). These differences result in individuals who are poor-, rapid-, or ultra-metabolizers, depending on the number of functional copies of the CYP2D6 allele present, and they account for significant variability in the response to these drugs. Ineffective conversion of codeine to morphine may be present in up to 7% to 10% of Caucasian children. On the other hand, another polymorphism, present in about 0.5% of children, results in rapid demethylation of codeine to morphine, producing exaggerated conversion to morphine and excessive sedation and respiratory depression when codeine is administered to children with this polymorphism.[186,218] These incidences differ with ethnicity, with a significantly greater incidence of polymorphisms in North African descendants.[219-223] Numerous case reports have described severe and sometimes fatal respiratory depression in ultra-metabolizers who were prescribed codeine, most often in children with obstructive sleep apnea.[186] These reports have prompted the U.S. Food and

Drug Administration to issue a black box warning for codeine and tramadol in children undergoing tonsillectomy (http://www.fda.gov/downloads/Drugs/DrugSafety/UCM339116.pdf) and has further contraindicated use in children <18 years (https://www.fda.gov/Drugs/DrugSafety/ucm549679.htm). To minimize the risk of complications from codeine, one institution identified those children with polymorphisms to CYP2D6 and restricted the codeine use to those without a polymorphism, eliminating complications from codeine.

Therefore, because of both its lack of effect in some children (poor-metabolizers) and an exaggerated effect in others (ultra-metabolizers), we strongly discourage the use of codeine unless their polymorphisms have been characterized. It is also important to note that with active metabolites of codeine excreted in breast milk, there has been a report of an opioid overdose in a neonate who was breastfed by a mother who was an ultra-metabolizer,[224] and mothers taking oxycodone while breastfeeding reported similar rates of infant sedation as those taking codeine.[225] Other oral opioids metabolized by CYP2D6 have also resulted in serious and fatal complications as a result of polymorphisms.[185,226,227] Thus all opioids, including oxycodone, hydrocodone, and tramadol, are at risk for similar complications associated with polymorphisms as codeine. Alternatively, if pain is of moderate or lower intensity, another class of analgesics (e.g., NSAIDs, ketamine, or dexmedetomidine) may be substituted.

Methadone is a synthetic opioid with a very prolonged elimination half-life (mean of 19 hours) in children between 1 and 18 years of age, and a large bioavailability (approximately 80%) after oral administration. Oral or IV methadone has been considered a good alternative to the use of continuous opioid infusions because repeated dosing at intervals of every 6 to 12 hours can achieve relatively stable plasma drug concentrations.[228] Although it is used most frequently to facilitate weaning of opioid-tolerant children, it has also been recommended for postoperative analgesia and for transitioning children from parenteral to oral opioid therapy.[229-231] Methadone is especially useful for children with cancer, burns, or other serious illnesses who require a long-acting oral opioid, because it is available in an elixir formulation. Unlike some sustained-release formulations of other opioids, oral methadone is also relatively inexpensive. Note that crushing tablets of most sustained-release formulations of other opioids renders them into immediate-release, relatively short-acting medications. Methadone should be thought of as virtually a combination analgesic. It is supplied as a racemic mixture. The *l*-isomer acts as a μ opioid, whereas the *d*-isomer acts as an antagonist at the NMDA subclass of excitatory amino acid receptors. Action at NMDA receptors makes methadone uniquely effective in the treatment of neuropathic pain. This NMDA-blocking action, and a differential activation of receptor-mediated endocytosis versus protein kinase activation,[232,233] may lead to a relatively slower rate of development of tolerance for methadone compared with some other opioids. Despite these advantages of methadone, it requires careful titration and repeated reassessment to avoid delayed oversedation. This challenge in methadone dosing is due, in part, to its slow and widely variable clearance, as well as to its effects on NMDA antagonism, generating incomplete cross tolerance on conversion to methadone from other opioids. In opioid-naive subjects, a single dose of IV morphine is roughly equipotent to a single dose of methadone. Although morphine has active metabolites, the slower clearance of methadone compared with morphine translates, in opioid-naive subjects, into daily IV methadone requirements that are roughly one-third those of morphine. *However, in the setting of marked opioid tolerance, such as in the case of children with advanced cancer or in the setting of intensive care, the equipotent daily dose of IV methadone may be as small as one-tenth the preceding daily dose of IV morphine.*[121,228,234–236] A convenient web-based calculation tool (http://www.globalrph.com/narcoticonv.htm) has synthesized the information from these and other studies to aid in opioid conversions in both opioid-naive and opioid-tolerant subjects. In our practice, this calculation tool appears quite useful, although it must be noted that it has not received independent assessment for use in children. Smartphone applications for multiple platforms are also available.

Intravenous Administration

Intermittent IV injections with opioids of short or moderate duration administered on an as-needed basis (PRN) do not achieve stable blood concentrations and predispose to periods of excessive sedation alternating with periods of inadequate analgesia. Yet this technique remains the most common method of treating postoperative pain in many centers. A partial solution to this problem is to prescribe the opioid at closer intervals (such as 2 hourly) and then use a "reverse-PRN" schedule, in which the medication is offered at the prescribed interval but the child can choose to take it or refuse it. Children should be assessed frequently, with the goal of administering the next dose before moderate to severe pain recurs. The use of a long-acting opioid, such as methadone, has been recommended to provide more prolonged and stable periods of analgesia than could be achieved with shorter-acting opioids, approaching the efficacy of continuous infusions.[237] However, careful titration of dosing and frequent assessment of the child are required because of methadone's slow and variable clearance. Alternatively, administration of shorter-acting opioids via continuous infusion or a PCA device should be considered.

Continuous IV opioid infusions are an excellent means of providing analgesia to children with moderate to severe pain who are unable to use PCA, such as infants, young children, and those who are cognitively impaired or physically disabled.[238] Once a therapeutic blood concentration of the opioid is achieved by administering an initial loading dose, an infusion rate can be selected to maintain that concentration without excessive fluctuations. Additionally, rescue doses of IV opioids may be required for breakthrough pain. Opioids, however, cause a dose-dependent respiratory depression by shifting the CO_2 response curve, reducing its slope, and decreasing the hypoxic ventilatory response. Residual and synergistic effects of sedatives and hypnotics in the early postoperative period further increase the risk of opioid-induced respiratory depression. This is particularly true in preterm and term infants because of age-related differences in elimination and clearance of opioids and other sedating medications (see also Chapter 7). This is of particular concern with the use of continuous opioid infusions because inappropriate dosing or prolonged elimination may lead to drug accumulation, placing children at risk for side effects. In a recent prospective audit of 10,726 opioid infusions in the United Kingdom and Ireland, the overall risk of permanent harm was found to be 1 in 10,000 cases, and serious events without permanent harm 1 in 383, with half of the serious events being respiratory depression.[239] Therefore the rate of the infusion should be carefully selected, based on the child's age, comorbidities, and clinical condition. Additionally, children who receive opioid infusions should be monitored and assessed frequently for depth of sedation and respiratory rate. *The onset of sedation and bradypnea is an important clinical index of incipient respiratory depression* and should alert the nursing staff and physicians to decrease the infusion rate and observe the child more closely.

Use of pulse oximetry is widely recommended during continuous opioid infusions, especially in opioid-naive children and other children at increased risk for respiratory depression. Another method of IV opioid delivery is via PCA (see further). With any infusion technique, scrupulous attention must be paid to protocols for checking pump settings to avoid errors. Pump programming errors, none of which caused serious harm, but which had the potential to do so, occurred in 17 instances in the U.K. audit, all from a single center, highlighting the critical importance of system safeguards to prevent patient harm.[239]

Intramuscular and Subcutaneous Routes

Intermittent IM and subcutaneous (SC) injections of opioids are obsolete because they are frightening and unpleasant for children and are often perceived as worse than the pain for which they are administered.[240] Additionally, they have the PK disadvantage of unpredictable and erratic uptake if regional blood flow is impaired, and they produce pronounced wide swings in blood concentrations. The goal of maintaining an even level of analgesia is thus nearly impossible to achieve with these routes of administration. An important exception is the use of indwelling SC catheters for continuous infusions and PCA as in palliative care.

Selection of Opioids for Parenteral Use

Morphine is the opioid most commonly used for postoperative analgesia and has been extensively studied in all pediatric age groups. After major abdominal, thoracic, and orthopedic surgery, children who received continuous morphine infusions had reduced pain scores compared with those who received intermittent IM or IV injections.[241–243] However, other investigators were only able to demonstrate reduced pain scores with continuous morphine infusions compared with intermittent IV injections of morphine in children between 1 and 3 years of age, and not in infants in the first year of life.[244,245] Similarly, evidence of the beneficial effects of opioid analgesia in ameliorating the postoperative response to surgical stress are conflicting. A significant reduction in serum β-endorphin concentrations has been reported in neonates after the initiation of a continuous infusion of postoperative morphine.[246] In neonates whose lungs were mechanically ventilated, both epinephrine and norepinephrine concentrations decreased after the initiation of morphine or fentanyl infusions.[247] However, β-endorphin concentrations decreased only in the children who received fentanyl. When the effects of continuous infusions of morphine were compared with those of intermittent IV injections of morphine on the stress response in children between 1 and 3 years of age, reduced glucose concentrations in the continuous infusion group suggested only a modest ablation of the stress response in this age group.[244]

Several studies have described the PK of morphine administered as a continuous infusion and evaluated the pharmacodynamic effects of morphine on respiratory indexes in neonates, infants, and children after various surgical procedures. In children 14 months to 17 years of age who underwent cardiac surgery,[248] morphine infusions were adjusted between 10 and 50 μg/kg per hour to minimize discomfort and avoid excessive sedation. Supplemental boluses of 100 μg/kg morphine were administered for breakthrough pain. Steady-state morphine concentrations were achieved in 4 hours. Those children who could self-report their pain reported good analgesia with morphine concentrations in excess of 12 ng/mL. Morphine infusions of 10 to 30 μg/kg per hour yielded mean serum concentrations between 10 and 22 ng/mL with less than 2% experiencing evidence of respiratory depression (partial pressure of carbon dioxide [$PaCO_2$] > 50 mm Hg).

Furthermore, children who received morphine infusions of 10 to 30 µg/kg per hour breathed spontaneously after extubation of the trachea, and those who were weaned from assisted to spontaneous ventilation maintained a normal $PaCO_2$. On the other hand, 60% (3 of 5 children) who received a greater infusion rate of morphine, 40 to 50 µg/kg per hour, experienced hypercarbia ($PaCO_2$ 48-66 mm Hg). A subsequent study by the same investigators evaluated the severity of respiratory depression in infants and children aged 2 days to 18 months treated with morphine. Of those whose morphine concentrations exceeded 20 ng/mL, approximately 70% experienced respiratory depression ($PaCO_2 >$ 55 mm Hg and/or a depressed slope of the CO_2 response curve) compared with 15% to 28% of those whose concentrations were less than 20 ng/mL.[249] The investigators suggested a steady-state morphine concentration of 20 ng/mL as a threshold concentration for respiratory depression in this age group.

Previous studies determined that the clearance of morphine is impaired in preterm infants and that clearance increases with postmenstrual age (see Fig. 7.11).[250] Additionally, morphine clearance is impaired in full-term infants up to 1 to 2 months of age, at which time it is comparable with that in older children and adults.[106,251] Preterm and full-term neonates, therefore, have a narrower therapeutic window for morphine analgesia compared with older children. Indeed, these groups have reduced morphine requirements postoperatively, requiring fewer rescue doses of morphine when receiving continuous infusions or intermittent bolus doses.[252] Therefore opioids should be carefully titrated in infants in a monitored environment with significantly reduced continuous infusion rates. Based on PK modeling and morphine clearance predictions, a target morphine concentration of 10 ng/mL can be achieved with morphine infusions ranging from 5 µg/kg per hour in term neonates to 16 µg/kg per hour in 1- to 3-year-old children (see Chapter 7).[253] In addition, reduced clearance in patients with renal insufficiency can result in accumulation of the potent morphine-6-glucuronide metabolite, which can cause delayed respiratory depression, so morphine should be avoided in these patients.[254]

Pharmacodynamic differences between infants and children have been postulated as the mechanism responsible for the greater sensitivity of infants (compared with older children) to the respiratory depressant effects of opioids. However, this may not be the case. Although rodent data suggest that the brain concentrations of opioids in neonates are greater than those in older children at similar serum concentrations,[255] these findings may not be applicable to humans. Neonatal rats have a relatively immature brain and a far more permeable blood-brain barrier than that in human infants. Consequently, the rodent may not be an appropriate model to depict the human condition.[256] It appears that the "increased sensitivity" is related, at least in part, to PK variables, perhaps in some measure as a result of a neonate's decreased conjugating ability.

Regardless of the mechanism, respiratory depression remains the most feared adverse effect of opioids administered by any route. Current monitoring technologies have numerous advantages and disadvantages (see the "Monitoring the Child Using PCA" section). Neonates and infants younger than 6 months of age are at greater risk for opioid-induced respiratory depression because the ventilatory responses to airway obstruction, hypoxemia, and hypercapnia are immature at birth and mature over the first several months of life in preterm as well as full-term infants (see also Figs. 4.8 and 4.9). Indeed, there was a 4.5% incidence of failure to wean from the ventilator and a 13.5% incidence of

apnea (30 seconds or more that required intervention) or severe respiratory depression in spontaneously breathing neonates who received opioids for postoperative pain.[257] Another report of a 3-year surveillance period for adverse drug reactions described 15 children aged 2 days to 17 years who experienced opioid-induced respiratory depression.[258] Respiratory depression in the latter study was defined as apnea, hypoxemia, cyanosis, a marked decrease in respiratory rate, or a need for naloxone. Although this study was unable to define the incidence of respiratory depression because the denominator was unknown, it did identify several predisposing factors, including age younger than 1 year (7 of 15 children), drug errors (including prescription and administration errors; 6 of 15 children), concurrent medical problems (diminished respiratory reserve, hepatic, and/or renal impairment), and concurrent sedative drugs. A prospective U.K. audit found 14 cases of respiratory depression (out of 10,726 total infusions, or 0.13%), 10 with NCA, 2 with continuous infusions, and 2 with PCA.[239] Potentially contributing risk factors in half of the cases included very young age and neurodevelopmental, respiratory, or cardiac disease. In contrast to the earlier studies, no case of respiratory depression was reported in 110 children older than 3 months of age who received opioid infusions postoperatively.[259] Interpretation of this literature is confounded by different monitoring techniques and different definitions of respiratory depression. For instance, in the latter study, a 4.5% incidence of clinically significant hypoxemia was reported but was not included in their definition of respiratory depression. Additionally, children in that study were monitored with hourly documentation of respiratory rate, but oxygen saturation was not monitored after discharge from the PACU, thereby reducing the ability to detect more subtle episodes of respiratory depression. In summary, the results of these studies suggest that children who receive opioids require careful monitoring for respiratory depression, with appropriate age-based reduction of dosage, particularly for neonates and infants younger than 6 months of age.

The most common adverse effect of opioid therapy is nausea and vomiting. One study reported nausea and vomiting in 34 of 80 children (42.5%) who received postoperative morphine infusions. These were well managed with antiemetic therapy in all but two children who required discontinuation of the opioids.[259] In the same study, the incidence of pruritus and urinary retention was 13% for both and that of dysphoria was 7%. Seizures have been reported in two neonates who received bolus doses of morphine followed by infusions of 32 and 40 µg/kg per hour and whose serum morphine concentrations were 61 and 90 ng/mL, respectively.[260] Irregular jerking movements, as well as one case of a generalized seizure, have been reported in children 1 to 15 years of age receiving postoperative morphine infusions.[241] Metoclopramide, 0.10 to 0.15 mg/kg (100–150 µg/kg) given IV, is an effective antiemetic but may also cause sedation and dystonia. The serotonin-receptor antagonist antiemetics, such as ondansetron and dolasetron, have the advantage of virtually eliminating the risk of dystonic or oculogyric reactions that occur with phenothiazines, butyrophenones, and metoclopramide. However, headaches occur in a small number of those who receive serotonin-receptor antagonists. A "microdose" naloxone infusion (0.25–1.0 µg/kg per hour) reverses the incidence of both nausea and pruritus after opioids without affecting the analgesia or opioid consumption.[261,262] A more recent dose-escalation study demonstrated that doses of 1 to 1.65 µg/kg per hour resulted in greater efficacy in reducing adverse effects, particularly pruritus, without degrading analgesia.[262] It is likely that these results may be generalized to other routes of opioid administration.

44

Opioid-induced bowel dysfunction, reported in more than 90% of patients receiving opioid therapy, occurs by blocking propulsive peristalsis, inhibiting secretion and increasing reabsorption of intestinal fluids, and decreasing the activity of excitatory and inhibitory neurons in the myenteric plexus. Bowel dysfunction manifests as abdominal distention and bloating, delayed gastric emptying, and constipation. Aggressive prophylactic measures, including osmotic, lubricant, or stimulant laxatives, should be prescribed early in the course of treatment. A newer selective gastrointestinal peripheral μ-opioid receptor antagonist, methylnaltrexone, was approved for use in adults in 2008. Although adult studies have shown promising results with the use of this agent,[263,264] its pediatric use has been described in only a few case series.[265,266]

Fentanyl may be a useful substitute for morphine in children with hemodynamic instability, in whom a decrease in peripheral vascular tone is undesirable, and in whom histamine release caused by morphine is not well tolerated. Additionally, its rapid onset of analgesia makes it ideal for children with severe escalating pain who require urgent pain relief. Fentanyl is metabolized by the liver into an inactive metabolite, norfentanyl, which is excreted via the kidneys. It is 80 to 100 times more potent than morphine. Although its elimination half-life is significantly less than that for morphine, its context-sensitive half-life during chronic infusion increases exponentially as a result of growing tissue storage (see Chapter 7). Like morphine, the elimination half-life of fentanyl in neonates is nearly twice that in adults, predisposing them to a greater risk for accumulation compared with older infants.[267,268] As with morphine, a reduction in hepatic blood flow in very young infants further decreases fentanyl clearance. For a given bolus of fentanyl, plasma concentrations in infants between 3 months and 1 year of age are less than those in older children and adults.[269] This finding is consistent with the almost 2-fold greater clearance of fentanyl in children compared with neonates. In children 18 days to 14 years of age who were mechanically ventilated, the clearance of fentanyl was age related yet quite variable, with the slowest clearance occurring in infants younger than 6 months of age and the most rapid in those between 6 months and 6 years of age.[270] The clearance of fentanyl is slow in preterm infants, with the clearance correlating with the postnatal age.[271]

Fentanyl is known to cause all the adverse effects reported with opioids, including pruritus, nausea, vomiting, constipation, and sedation. Respiratory depression and chest wall and glottic rigidity, however, are its most feared adverse effects. One study compared the incidence of respiratory depression in full-term and former preterm infants and young infants receiving 2-μg/kg bolus doses of fentanyl every 2 hours or a continuous infusion of 1 μg/kg per hour after abdominal or thoracic surgery.[272] Randomization was terminated prematurely because of a 6-fold greater incidence of apnea that required intervention in the bolus dose group compared with the continuous infusion group (89% vs. 14%). The continuous infusion arm was continued for another 20 children, resulting in a 25% incidence of apnea in this group. In contrast, the incidence of respiratory depression (based on transcutaneous $PaCO_2$ measurements and the incidence of apnea) for a given plasma fentanyl concentration in infants 1 to 12 months of age and children 1 to 5 years of age was less than that in adults undergoing hernia repair or other peripheral surgery.[273] Differences in surgical procedures and the inclusion of preterm infants in the former study may account for the significant difference in the incidence of apnea found in these two studies.

Although chest wall rigidity usually occurs after the rapid bolus administration of high-dose fentanyl, it has also been reported

in an infant after a low-dose continuous infusion of fentanyl. Chest wall rigidity was reported in 9% of preterm and full-term neonates who received an average of 4.9 μg/kg over a 2- to 3-minute period for a procedure or for perioperative analgesia.[274] In every case, naloxone reversed the chest wall rigidity. Additionally, a case of chest wall rigidity has been reported in a preterm neonate after high-dose fentanyl was administered to the parturient before a cesarean section.[275] Although administration of naloxone has been used successfully to treat cases of chest wall rigidity, severe cases associated with rapid oxygen desaturation may require the use of neuromuscular blocking drugs and mechanical ventilation.

The use of continuous fentanyl infusions in infants and children has been associated with a rapid development of tolerance, as indicated by a steady increase in infusion rate to maintain the desired effect[276,277] and a large incidence of opioid withdrawal syndrome after termination of the infusion.[277,278] The incidence of opioid withdrawal is directly related to the total dose administered and the duration of infusion.[277,278] Iatrogenic opioid withdrawal was reported in 21 of 37 neonates (57%) after continuous fentanyl infusions during extracorporeal membrane oxygenation.[277] Both a cumulative fentanyl dose greater than 1.6 mg/kg and extracorporeal membrane oxygenation that lasted more than 5 days were predictors of opioid withdrawal. A similar incidence has been reported in 23 children 1 week to 22 months of age who received continuous fentanyl infusions during mechanical ventilation.[278] This study also found that a cumulative dose of 1.5 mg/kg of fentanyl over 5 days was associated with a greater than 50% incidence of withdrawal symptoms. Furthermore, a cumulative dose of 2.5 mg/kg as a continuous infusion over 9 days was 100% predictive of the occurrence of withdrawal. Finally, movement disorder and irritability have been reported after withdrawal of fentanyl infusion in five infants who were mechanically ventilated.[279] None of the infants who developed the movement disorder had received another opioid after withdrawal of fentanyl, whereas five of eight controls who did not develop withdrawal during the same period had received a substitute opioid. These data suggest that opioid withdrawal occurs earlier and with greater frequency after fentanyl infusions compared with other opioids. Therefore it seems prudent to use fentanyl infusions for pain relief during periods of hemodynamic instability, such as in the early postoperative period, and to transition to another opioid, such as morphine, as soon as the child is stabilized. Children who require fentanyl infusions for 5 days or more should undergo a slow taper (e.g., 10% decrease every 12 hours) or be transitioned to another parenteral or oral opioid regimen.

Hydromorphone has a spectrum of action similar to that of morphine. Adult opioid equipotency data suggest that it is 3.5 to 7 times as potent as morphine.[280-283] A study performed in children with mucositis pain after bone marrow transplant reported that a 7:1 conversion ratio of morphine to hydromorphone underestimated hydromorphone requirements by 27%.[284] These data suggest that a 5:1 conversion ratio may be more appropriate, particularly in children with chronic pain. Despite its widespread use, there are very few studies that evaluated the use of hydromorphone in children. One small pediatric study randomized patients to morphine or hydromorphone PCA (5:1 ratio) and showed no difference in analgesia or side effects.[285] A meta-analysis of adult studies showed very similar analgesia and side effect profiles.[286] Overall, morphine and hydromorphone are very similar for most outcomes. Because side effect profiles for each drug may differ within an individual patient, it remains common practice to prescribe a trial of hydromorphone in children who experience unacceptable adverse effects with morphine (or vice versa). Hydromorphone does have more rapid effect-site equilibration compared with morphine,[286] so there is a theoretical risk of dose stacking and subsequent respiratory depression with morphine compared with hydromorphone, but the requisite large studies needed to examine the clinical significance of this risk have not been done. It should be noted that the analogous hydromorphone-3-glucuronide has been associated with dose-dependent neuroexcitatory effects in hospice patients with renal insufficiency, but no significant cases have been reported in children. Therefore hydromorphone (or fentanyl or methadone) is a preferential choice in patients with kidney disease.[287] Although hydromorphone has an active glucuronide metabolite that is cleared by the kidney, it is considered intermediate in risk, better than morphine, but worse than fentanyl and methadone, for patients with renal failure.

Meperidine, used clinically for many years,[288,289] is approximately one-tenth as potent as morphine. Accumulation of normeperidine, its active metabolite (which has CNS stimulant properties), after repeated doses places children at risk for seizures.[290] Therefore its use has been restricted to the treatment of postoperative shivering[291,292] or rigors after amphotericin. A single dose of dexmedetomidine (0.5 μg/kg) has been used successfully for the treatment of postoperative shivering and may replace meperidine for this indication.[293] Although its short-term use continues by a small number of clinicians for procedural sedation and analgesia, other analgesics are preferable choices. Meperidine is not recommended for PCA or as a continuous infusion and has been removed from the formulary of many children's hospitals.

Patient-Controlled Analgesia

PCA was first studied in adults in 1965. The initial interest with this technique was as a research tool for the study of pain. By the early 1970s, it was identified as an excellent strategy for treating pain in the clinical setting, with studies demonstrating that pain relief was achieved by PCA with relatively smaller doses of opioids and with greater patient satisfaction than with conventional methods.[294] However, it was not until the late 1980s that PCA was studied in children.[295] Since that time, it has become the preferred method for opioid delivery in children older than 6 to 7 years of age (depending on their level of understanding) for acute pain, as well as chronic pain associated with cancer or sickle cell disease.[284,295-298] The primary benefit of PCA is that it allows children to titrate the analgesic to the extent of their pain. The goal is for the child to self-regulate a blood opioid concentration within the therapeutic range. Most children strike a balance between adequate pain relief on the one hand and adverse effects of the drug on the other. This approach, which grants the child some degree of autonomy, is the rationale given since pain is an entirely subjective and individual experience and that opioid metabolism and pain perception varies among individuals. It also reduces the apprehension of older children and adolescents regarding pain relief because they can control it and they can tailor the opioid delivery to the extent of pain they have at a given time—for example, before physical therapy, removal of tubes or drains, dressing changes, or getting out of bed. Additionally, the use of PCA avoids delays in administration of analgesics associated with standard "as-needed" orders of IV opioids and allows smaller doses of opioids to be delivered more frequently without increasing nursing workload. Therefore PCA is thought to provide more consistent pain relief with less total opioid dosing, resulting in fewer adverse effects, such as sedation, nausea, and vomiting. Purportedly, children using PCA report better analgesia and reduced pain scores compared with children who must rely on the nursing staff to administer analgesics when they are in pain. These and other benefits of PCA have been extensively touted in the medical literature,[298-300] as well as in the lay press.[301] Recently, however, risks associated with PCA use have also been highlighted and are discussed later.[302-304] Recognition of these risks has led to recommendations for careful dosing and monitoring of all children who are receiving opioids, particularly those receiving continuous infusions and those with specific risk factors.[305]

Child training is a necessary part of PCA, because successful use of PCA requires that both the child and family understand how it works.[306] The instructions should be clear that the pump should be activated whenever the child feels pain, that children cannot give themselves "too much medication" because of the computer lockout interval, that the child should not wait for severe pain to activate the pump, and that a dose can also be given in anticipation of painful stimuli, such as ambulation or chest physiotherapy. Most importantly, PCA does not mean *parent*-controlled analgesia, and parents should never activate the pump unless specifically authorized to do so by the primary care or pain service physician (see the "Nurse-/Caregiver-Controlled Analgesia" section later in this chapter).[305]

PCA Equipment

PCA devices are microprocessor-driven pumps connected to the child's IV line via Y tubing. For safety reasons, the IV tubing should incorporate a one-way valve to prevent backflow of the PCA drug up the tubing and an unintended delivery of a large bolus of opioid. Alternatively, PCA may be delivered through a separate IV line. These pumps allow programming of the individual dose to be administered, the minimal interval between doses (lockout interval), and the maximal cumulative allowable dose over a 4-hour period. Some pumps allow programming of a maximum number of doses per hour. Most pumps allow delivery of a continuous basal infusion (CBI) in addition to the demand dose. All PCA pumps should have a locking mechanism, so that neither the settings nor the medication cartridge can be changed without using a key, making the device virtually tamper-proof. The child is able to self-administer the preprogrammed doses by pushing a button. A liquid crystal display on the pump displays the programmed settings, the cumulative dosage, the number of doses administered, and the number of times that the button was pushed but no dose was given either because it was during the lockout interval or the 4-hour limit had been reached. This information allows clinicians to track opioid usage and make appropriate changes to the PCA prescription based on the usage pattern. Most children older than 6 to 7 years are able to push the button themselves. In general, a child who can play video games has the cognitive skills required to push a button to achieve a desired response and use PCA effectively.

Choice of Drug and Drug Dosages

Morphine remains the most common opioid administered via PCA, although hydromorphone is a valid first-line option, especially for patients with renal disease or a history of intolerance to morphine. Fentanyl is also used, but the disadvantage is a more rapid development of tolerance. Suggested initial dosages for opioids via PCA for opioid-naive children are presented in Table 44.9. Children with opioid tolerance require adjustments to these settings, considering the previous opioid history and the opioid doses that the child was receiving before the acute painful stimulus. Indeed, one study reported that children with sickle cell disease

TABLE 44.9 | Patient-Controlled Analgesia Dosing Guidelines

Drug	Demand Dose (μg/kg)	Lockout Interval (minutes)	Continuous Basal Infusion (μg/kg per hour)	4-Hour Limit (μg/kg)
Morphine	10–30	8–15	0–20	250–400
Hydromorphone	2–6	8–15	0–4	50–80
Fentanyl	0.5	5–10	0–0.5	7–10

44

self-administered more than double the dose of morphine via PCA, required more nonopioid adjuvant analgesics, reported greater pain scores, and stayed in the hospital for twice the duration compared with non–sickle cell disease–affected children after laparoscopic cholecystectomy.[307]

Fentanyl PCA has been used with success as a first-line and a secondary drug in children with cancer pain, as well as acute postoperative pain.[300,308] Most of the adverse effects, including nausea and pruritus, were mild and easily managed. However, some reported an overall incidence of apnea and hypoxemia of 3.5% in 212 children receiving PCA, of whom 144 had received fentanyl.[300] Finally, children who received tramadol PCA after heart surgery were extubated earlier and had less sedation, comparable pain scores, and a similar incidence of emesis as those who received morphine PCA.[191] The IV formulation of tramadol is not yet available in the United States, but some studies from Europe and China support its use in the postoperative period.[191,309] The benefits that hydromorphone PCA offers over morphine PCA in the chronic and acute pain settings require further investigation.

Pump Settings
Most PCA pumps have five settings to adjust:

- A *loading dose* of opioid ranging from 0.025 to 0.1 mg/kg of morphine divided into incremental doses is usually given to establish adequate analgesia before therapy is turned over to the child, because self-administered doses with this technique are generally small. A sufficient interval between incremental doses must be allowed, so that the morphine achieves its peak effect before the next dose, thereby avoiding an overdose. If PCA is started in the PACU, opioid doses administered during surgery must be considered before prescribing a loading dose. Additionally, it may be desirable to administer the loading dose via the PCA pump so that it is included in the initial 4-hour or hourly limit of the PCA since children who receive IV-PRN doses of opioids in the PACU, followed by initiation of PCA, may be at risk for oversedation and respiratory depression from opioid stacking. Children who have received opioids toward the end of surgery, those who awaken in comfort, or those who receive nerve blocks may not need a loading dose and may start to use the demand doses as needed on awakening.
- A *patient bolus dose*—that is, the dose that will be administered with each child's activation of the pump—must be prescribed. These small boluses are usually in the range of 0.01 to 0.02 mg/kg of morphine in opioid-naive subjects.
- A *lockout interval* of usually 5 to 15 minutes prevents a child from activating the pump until the full effect from the previous bolus is achieved, and it should correspond to the time from IV injection to the peak effect of the drug.
- A *continuous basal infusion* ranging from 0.00 to 0.02 mg/kg per hour of morphine (or more, in opioid-tolerant subjects) may be used in selective cases (see later text).
- A *maximum hourly dose or a 4-hour limit* may be chosen to limit the cumulative amount of drug a child can administer. Once

this limit is reached, the child cannot activate the pump until the 4-hour limit has passed. Four-hour limits allow for increased flexibility in dosing over greater periods of time and pain intensity. Typically, the maximum hourly dose ranges from 0.05 to 0.1 mg/kg and 4-hour limits from 0.25 to 0.4 mg/kg of morphine in opioid-naive subjects. This amount may be chosen based on the average hourly use of morphine during the past 24 hours or, in children started on PCA immediately after surgery, at the reduced range of the dosage scale. Fig. 44.6 presents sample PCA orders, including choice of drugs, dosing, and suggested monitoring.

Continuous Basal Infusions
The use of a CBI of the opioid to supplement child-administered doses remains a subject of controversy. The primary benefit of CBI is improved quality of sleep[310] as near-therapeutic plasma opioid concentrations are maintained, as illustrated in Fig. 44.7A. On the other hand, as depicted in Fig. 44.7B, a child who receives only PCA bolus dosing with no CBI is likely to awaken with unrelieved pain that may require multiple doses to again achieve adequate pain relief. Decreased nocturnal awakenings secondary to pain, improved restfulness or sleep patterns, reduced total opioid consumption, fewer adverse effects, and improved analgesic effectiveness are all potential reasons for using CBI. However, the use of CBI commits the child to receiving a fixed dose of opioid regardless of the level of sedation, and has the theoretical potential for overriding one of the inherent safety features of PCA—that is, an excessively sedated or somnolent child is unlikely to push the button and therefore receives no additional opioid but, with a fixed infusion, drug may accumulate (Fig. 44.7C), with the potential for hypoventilation.[311] Furthermore, it has also been argued that programming errors with CBI can lead to more serious adverse events because the opioid medication is delivered regardless of the child's level of sedation.[309,312]

Some studies in adults have suggested that the use of CBI has limited benefit in terms of efficacy and is associated with a greater incidence of opioid adverse effects, including respiratory depression.[313-315] Studies in children, however, have yielded conflicting results.[297,298,316-320] Children 7 to 19 years of age who received PCA with CBI after orthopedic surgery reported significantly reduced pain scores compared with those who received PCA boluses alone or IM morphine.[298] There were no differences in morphine consumption or in opioid adverse effects among the three groups, with no incidents of respiratory depression. Notably, child satisfaction was greatest in the PCA with CBI group. Similar pain scores with improved sleeping patterns have also been reported with the use of PCA with CBI, compared with those who received PCA alone, on the first two postoperative nights in children after abdominal surgery. No incidents of respiratory depression or excessive sedation were reported in either group.[297] Children who received CBI with PCA or NCA in one study reported slightly reduced pain scores without differences in morphine use or adverse effects after spine fusion surgery compared with those who received

Pediatric Acute Pain Service (APS) Patient Controlled Analgesia (PCA) Initial Orders	BIRTHDATE NAME Reg. No.

| Date: _____ Time: _____

Clerk's Initials: _____ Unit: _____ | |

| No other OPIOIDS or SEDATIVES to be administered while on PCA unless Pain Service has ordered them or been notified.
Please page Pain Service before discontinuing PCA at pager xxxx.

AGE: _____ months/year   WEIGHT: _____ kg | MODE: ☐ PCA ONLY
        ☐ PCA & Continuous
        ☐ Nurse Controlled
        ☐ Continuous
        ☐ Other: _____ |

Select drug to be used	☐ Morphine		☐ Hydromorphone		☐ Fentanyl _____
Drug Concentration	☐ 1 mg/mL	☐ 100 µg/mL (3000 µg/30 mL use for pts ≤10 kg)	☐ 0.5 mg/mL (use only for pts requiring excessive dosing)	☐ 100 µg/mL (3000 µg/30 mL)	20 µg/mL
PCA Dose	_____ mg 0.01-0.03 mg/kg	_____ µg 10-30 µg/kg	_____ mg 0.002-0.006 mg/kg	_____ µg 2-6 µg/kg	_____ µg 0.2-0.5 µg
Lockout Interval	_____ minute 8-15 minutes	_____ minute 8-15 minutes	_____ minute 8-15 minutes	_____ minute 8-15 minutes	_____ minute 8-15 minutes
Continuous Infusion Rate	_____ mg/h 0.01-0.02 mg/kg/h	_____ µg/h 10-20 µg/kg/h	_____ mg/h 0.002-0.004 mg/kg/h	_____ µg/h 2-4 µg/kg/h	_____ /h 0.1-0.5 µg/kg/h
4-Hour Limit	_____ mg 0.25-0.4 mg/kg	_____ µg 250-400 µg/kg	_____ mg 0.05-0.08 mg/kg	_____ µg 50-80 µg/kg	_____ 7-10 µg/kg
Double-check	Double-check pump settings against the order. Document double-check on the PCA/Epidural Flowsheet.				

Emergency Measures	**For sedation score >2 or respiratory rate < _____ :
	   Hold PCA and page Pain Service
	
	**For sedation score = 4 or respiratory rate < _____ :
	   Hold PCA, give Naloxone and STAT page Primary Service **FIRST**, then Pain Service
	   Naloxone Dose:
	   Under 10 kg _____ mg IV STAT (0.01 mg/kg/dose, maximum of 0.1 mg), may repeat every 2 minutes × 2
	   Over 10 kg 0.1 mg IV STAT, may repeat every 2 minutes × 2
	
	   For O₂ Saturation < _____ : (Consider baseline saturation) Stimulate patient and encourage deep breathing
	      Administer O₂ by face mask or nasal cannula and page the Primary Service and Pain Service

Antipruritic	☐ Naloxone (Narcan) 0.25 µg/kg/h. Add 0.25 mg to 100 mL normal saline (0.1 mL/kg/h = 0.25 µg/kg/h) to be infused at 0.1 mL/h × weight (kg) = _____ mL/h or Nalbuphine 0.05 mg/kg = _____ mg IV every 4 hours
Antiemetic	☐ Ondansetron (Zofran) _____ mg IV every 6 hours PRN (0.1 mg/kg/dose up to 4 mg) MAX single dose: 4 mg ☐ Per Primary Service ☐ Other: _____
Other	☐ Other: _____

1. Monitoring:

   Continuous pulse oximetry while on PCA except while patient is out of bed. Record pulse oximetry readings at same frequency as respiratory rate. Respiratory rate and sedation level:

      Initiation of therapy: every 30 minutes × 1 hour and then every 2 hours for the first 24 hours and then every 4 hours
      Transfer to a new unit: every 30 minutes × 1 hour then either every 2 or 4 hours (depends upon start of PCA therapy)
      With loading dose and increases in doses, infusions, limits: every 30 minutes × 2 then every 2 or 4 hours (depends upon start of PCA therapy)
      Regularly scheduled Day/Night changes: every 4 hours if therapy has been initiated longer than 24 hours.

   Pain Scores:
      every 2 hours × 8 hours, then every 4 hours. If pain not controlled after 1 hour, page xxxx or xxxx

2. The Acute Pain Service (APS) nurse may change PCA orders by increasing or decreasing pump settings by 20% and stop the continuous infusion.
3. Any order changes in #2 must be documented on a subsequent PCA order form.

Verbal ☐ Telephone ☐ Print name/title of person giving order	Signature/title of person taking order	Date	Time
Physician Signature	Dr. #	Date	Time

FIGURE 44.6 Sample patient-controlled analgesia orders. *IV*, intravenous; *MAX*, maximum; *PCA*, patient-controlled anesthesia; *PRN*, as needed; *STAT*, immediately. (Modified from the University of Michigan Hospitals & Health Centers.)

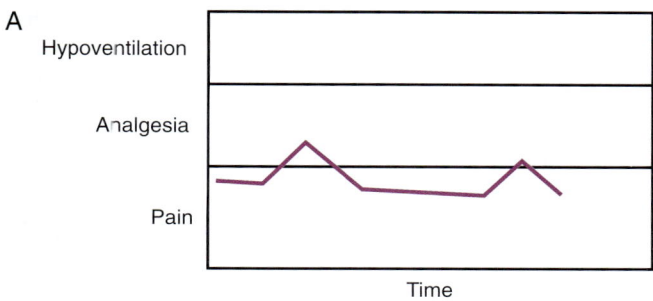

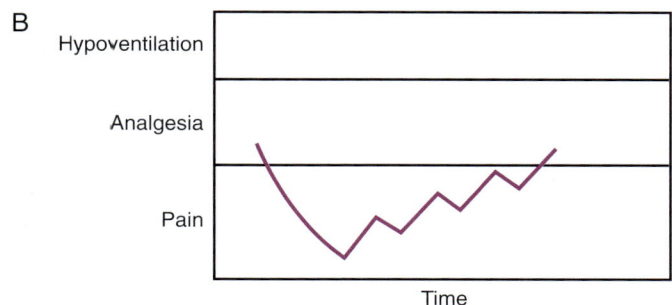

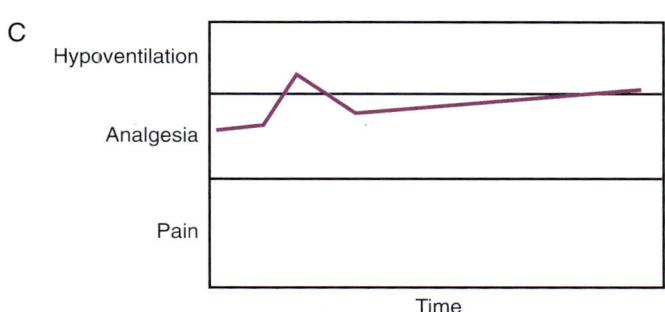

FIGURE 44.7 Patient-controlled analgesia (PCA) with an appropriate dose of continuous basal infusion. **A,** Use of an appropriate dose of continuous basal infusion (CBI) maintains near-therapeutic plasma opioid concentrations during sleep with rapid increase to analgesic concentrations as soon as the child awakens and activates the PCA button. **B,** Chart depicts plasma opioid concentrations in a child who is receiving PCA bolus doses only, with no CBI. Plasma concentrations decrease significantly when the child is asleep, necessitating multiple doses to achieve analgesic concentrations. **C,** An excessive dose of CBI results in opioid accumulation with delayed hypoventilation even when the PCA button is not activated. (Reproduced with permission from Berde CB, Solodiuk J. Multidisciplinary programs for management of acute and chronic pain in children. In: Schecter NL, Berde CB, Yaster M, eds. *Pain in Infants, Children and Adolescents.* 2nd ed. Philadelphia: Lippincott Williams and Wilkins; 2003:476.)

PCA or NCA alone.[320] In contrast, others have reported greater morphine use and a greater incidence of hypoxemia with similar pain scores in children who received PCA plus CBI after surgery compared with those who received PCA alone.[318,319] A subsequent study found that children who received PCA with a CBI of morphine (4 µg/kg per hour) experienced fewer adverse effects and less hypoxia than children who received PCA with 10 to 20 µg/kg per hour) CBI or those who received PCA bolus doses alone, noting similar pain scores in all three groups.[317] Both of the PCA with CBI groups reported better sleep at night than did the PCA alone group.

A meta-analysis of data from the previously mentioned studies found no difference in pain scores or opioid consumption between children who received a CBI and those who received a bolus-only PCA. Improved sleep quality was reported in three of the four studies that examined this outcome. Although there was a 4.6% incidence of excessive sedation (a marker of respiratory depression risk) in the CBI groups as opposed to none in the bolus-only group, this difference was not statistically significant. Overall, the pooled studies had significant heterogeneity and small sample sizes (and thus lower-quality evidence). Therefore the authors concluded that further large-scale randomized trials are necessary.[310]

Based on these studies and our own experience, we hold the view that the use of CBI may benefit some children, although it requires careful selection of dose, based on the surgical severity and the child's comorbid conditions and vigilant monitoring to ensure safety. CBI should be used as a routine for most children with pain resulting from cancer, for most children with mucositis resulting from cancer treatment or bone marrow transplantation, and for a large number of children with sickle cell vasoocclusive episodes. A sensible compromise may be to (1) use CBI at night with the goal of improved sleep quality and (2) allow patients to self-regulate during daytime hours. At our institutions, the standard practice is to use CBI, unless limited by somnolence or hypoventilation, for the first night in most children after selected major painful surgeries, such as scoliosis surgery, pelvic osteotomies, and thoracotomies, unless concomitant regional analgesia techniques are used.

Nurse-/Caregiver-Controlled Analgesia

Activation of the PCA pump by the bedside nurse, a parent, or a caregiver (such as a grandparent) has been used with success in children who are unable to push the button because of young age or because of physical or cognitive impairments.[84,299,300,320,321] In much of the literature, and in some policy statements by the Joint Commission and other organizations, there is, in our view, too little distinction between activation of PCA pumps by nurses and activation by nonclinician surrogates. The term *caregiver* is used variably in this literature; here it is used to mean nonclinician surrogates. In pediatrics, this means primarily parents and other family members. A small study of 12 children who received NCA after spine fusion surgery reported adequate analgesia, parent and nurse satisfaction, and no complications.[320] Children who received NCA received smaller total morphine doses compared with those who could use the PCA device themselves, likely because of the tendency for nurses to underestimate their patients' pain. A larger observational study of 212 children who received parent- or nurse-controlled analgesia with morphine, fentanyl, or hydromorphone reported effective analgesia (pain scores 3/10 or 2/5 or below) in more than 80% of children.[300] Pruritus occurred in 8% and vomiting in 15% of the children on the first day of treatment. Nine children (4.2%) required naloxone for the following: apnea (n = 4), hypoxemia (n = 1), excessive sedation (n = 3), or to facilitate extubation (n = 1). Six of these children had significant comorbid conditions, and five received additional sedatives. These investigators emphasized the importance of close monitoring to minimize risk and permit early intervention when using nurse-/caregiver-controlled analgesia (NCA/CCA). Another study found that the incidence of overall adverse events in opioid-naive children who received NCA was similar to that in children who received PCA after surgery (22% and 24%, respectively).[84] However, children who were able to self-administer PCA required only minor interventions (stimulation, reduction in opioid dosage, or supplemental oxygen), whereas those who received NCA were more likely to require more aggressive interventions, such as opioid reversal, airway management, or escalation of care. They found that cognitive impairment and opioid dose on the first postoperative day independently predicted adverse events. Although the mean time to the occurrence of adverse events was 16 to 27 hours, some events occurred during the third postoperative day, suggesting that monitoring, including continuous pulse oximetry, should be continued as long as the PCA is used. In a study of children with cancer, five respiratory and/or neurologic serious adverse effects were reported, with one child requiring naloxone during the 576 days of treatment with NCA/CCA.[321] In that study, pulse oximetry was used only at the discretion of the provider, perhaps reducing the investigator's ability to recognize hypoxemia in some children. Furthermore, the reduced incidence of adverse events may be explained by the fact that most children in that study were not opioid naive and may have developed some degree of opioid tolerance. A study of 10,000 pediatric patients receiving NCA further confirms the safety and tolerability of this delivery method.[108] For infants younger than 1 year of age, few studies have examined the role of NCA. One study of almost 800 infants, NCA fentanyl, morphine, or hydromorphone all provided similar analgesia, although rapid response team calls (total of 39) were significantly more frequently associated with morphine than with fentanyl use.[322] Only one rapid response call was for apnea.

For safety reasons, however, it is important to distinguish between authorized and unauthorized use of the PCA button by an individual other than the child. Several reports describe serious adverse events, including excessive sedation, severe respiratory depression, respiratory arrest, and death, attributed to unauthorized activation of the PCA device by parents, spouses, other family members, and health care providers.[84,323-326] The practice of PCA by proxy has therefore come under scrutiny and its safety questioned by the Joint Commission and the Institute for Safe Medication Practices (ISMP).[327-329] In 2004, the Joint Commission issued a sentinel event alert based on PCA errors reported to the U.S. Pharmacopeia. Of 460 errors that resulted in death or some level of harm to the patient, 15 resulted from PCA by proxy, including 12 attributed to family members, 2 to a nurse, and 1 to a pharmacist.[327] In interpreting this report and some other reports, it should be emphasized that many do not cite denominator data (total numbers of patients receiving PCA vs. NCA/CCA), so it is difficult to assign numbers for relative or absolute risks of these techniques. Recognition of these risks has led the Joint Commission and ISMP to strongly recommend that specific policies and procedures be developed and implemented related to the use of PCA by individuals other than the child. Such policies must address the following issues:

- Appropriate selection of children. Many pediatric centers restrict parent-controlled analgesia to children with chronic pain, those who require palliative care, and in special circumstances for children who undergo repeated and extensive surgery. In pediatric centers worldwide, NCA is increasingly being used, with appropriate observation, for both opioid-naive and opioid-tolerant children.
- The specific process of identifying suitable caregivers who will be allowed to activate the PCA button.
- Communication among clinicians, including the primary service physician, the pain service team, and the primary bedside nurse, regarding the suitability of CCA.

- An educational plan for health care providers involved in the decision making.
- Education of caregivers, including pain assessment, recognition of opioid adverse effects, and scenarios when not to activate the PCA button (e.g., when the child is asleep or somnolent). The caregiver should be encouraged to call the nursing staff when in doubt.
- Monitoring protocols, including assessment of sedation depth, respiratory status, and pain assessment at regular intervals. It must be emphasized that the primary responsibility for monitoring the safety and effectiveness of analgesia remains with the nursing staff. Electronic monitoring, including pulse oximetry, is widely used in this setting.

With carefully defined policies and procedures, adequate education of clinicians and caregivers, prevention of unauthorized dosing, and vigilant monitoring, it may be possible to reduce the frequency of adverse events from PCA, NCA, and, especially, CCA. However, large outcomes studies are needed after implementation of such policies to confirm the safety and efficacy of practice based on these recommendations. Our view is that NCA is a well-established practice and should be encouraged as a generally safe and effective means for delivering opioids to children who are unable to self-administer.

Risks and Adverse Events With PCA

Despite its numerous benefits, the use of PCA has been associated with a wide range of adverse effects, adverse events, and unfavorable outcomes in adults.[302,303,324,330-333] Although some adverse effects from PCA therapy may be attributed to the opioid drugs themselves or to patient comorbidities, a significant number of harmful effects occur as a result of human error, with incorrect prescribing, dispensing, administration, or equipment failure. E-Table 44.5 describes the causes of PCA medication errors as identified by the ISMP.[328-330,334] Increasing awareness of preventable adverse events from PCA has led to improved pump technology directed at minimizing the likelihood of programming errors, including the development of smart PCA pumps that use bar-coded syringes and an integral bar-code reader to prevent incorrect programming of drug concentration. Potential PCA pump errors have been reduced with "smart pumps."[335] Children are at greater risk for medication-related adverse events resulting from calculation errors in drug doses (because all doses are based on body weight or body surface area) and to developmental differences in PK. However, data for PCA-related adverse events in children are limited.[304,336-338] The reported incidence of respiratory depression in children receiving PCA ranges from 0% to 25%.[84,336,337,339,340] Risk factors for respiratory depression identified by these studies include cumulative opioid dose, use of basal infusions, concomitant administration of sedatives, and comorbid conditions, including renal failure and cognitive impairment. Recognition of the risks from PCA[341,342] has led organizations, such as the ISMP, to emphasize the importance of monitoring children who use PCA and of the need for detailed child and staff education regarding its use.[343]

Monitoring the Child Using PCA

Despite the recommendation from the ISMP that practitioners should identify children at risk for opioid-related respiratory depression and define the appropriate level of monitoring, there remains no consensus regarding the risk/benefit ratio and effectiveness of any specific forms of monitoring for children receiving PCA, NCA, or CCA. No monitor in widespread use today detects respiratory depression in all circumstances, so nursing staff are the frontline personnel for detection. Extensive nursing education and standard monitoring protocols are essential to the safe use of PCA (especially with CBI) in children.

The Anesthesia Patient Safety Foundation (APSF) recommended the use of continuous respiratory monitoring (minimally pulse oximetry and a continuous measure of respiratory rate) for children receiving PCA, neuraxial, or serial doses of parenteral opioids.[344] Additionally, the APSF recommended that reliable alerting methods, such as audible alarms, central stations, or pagers, be implemented to ensure timely and appropriate clinician response to deteriorating respiratory status of those receiving opioid therapy. The impact of implementing such technology on the incidence of PCA-related adverse events requires investigation. *It must be emphasized that pulse oximetry can detect hypoventilation only if the child is breathing room air.*[345] Oximetry is *not* a measure of ventilation but rather of oxygenation. The use of supplemental oxygen interferes with the ability of pulse oximetry to detect respiratory depression by delaying the onset of desaturation.[345,346] Any patient requiring supplemental oxygen while using a PCA should have additional measures in place to detect hypoventilation. Additionally, respiratory monitoring that uses impedance changes across electrocardiogram leads to detect chest wall movement will not detect partial upper airway obstruction and does not ensure that ventilation is adequate.

Sidestream sampling of end-tidal carbon dioxide ($ETCO_2$) via a nasal cannula or noninvasive capnography detects respiratory depression earlier and more frequently than does pulse oximetry or periodic checks of respiratory rate in adults who are receiving opioids via PCA, or for procedural sedation/analgesia.[347,348] Although similar data for children receiving PCA therapy are not available, studies in children undergoing procedural sedation in the emergency department and ICU have reported that capnography detected respiratory events that would have been unrecognized by pulse oximetry, periodic respiratory rate monitoring, and/or clinical examination.[349-352] Additionally, these studies identified instances of respiratory depression that were recognized by abnormal capnography before oxygen desaturation was detected. Thus capnography may provide the earliest warning of impending respiratory compromise and may alert clinicians to carefully evaluate the children under their care and adjust opioid doses accordingly. Conversely, in real-world practice, capnography cannulas can be difficult to maintain in proper position in children on a busy postoperative ward, readings can be influenced by mouth breathing, and this technology also has the potential for false-positive and false-negative conclusions.[353] Acoustic impedance (usually on the neck) is better tolerated than nasal capnography by children,[354] and has the advantage over chest wall impedance of detecting upper airway obstruction. However, it is not 100% sensitive, and episodes of oxygen desaturation are not always correlated to a low respiratory rate.[355]

Newer technology incorporates a fully integrated PCA system with modules for continuous monitoring of oxygen saturation and $ETCO_2$.[356] Some of these pumps also have a feature that shuts off PCA delivery if preset threshold parameters for oxygen saturation and $ETCO_2$ are reached. Studies evaluating the benefits of such technology in reducing PCA-related adverse events in children are needed. Although electronic monitoring has an important role in patient safety, all currently available methods are imperfect. Moreover, they generate frequent false alarms that annoy children and families, disturb the restorative sleep of both children and parents, and contribute to desensitization of nurses' vigilance. Despite these limitations of electronic monitoring, it has been reported that the use of computerized physician order entry and involvement of dedicated pediatric pain teams improved compliance with routine monitoring and increased the likelihood of early identification of adverse events.[357]

REGIONAL BLOCKADE AND ANALGESIA

The use of local anesthetics, both with and without the addition of central neuraxial opioids and other adjuncts, offers many advantages in the postoperative setting. Blockade with long-acting local anesthetic or continuous peripheral nerve blockade with infusion of local anesthetic via catheters and elastomeric infusion pumps can provide postoperative analgesia for outpatient surgery so that a child can be discharged home in comfort. Reducing or eliminating the need for systemic analgesics diminishes the potential for adverse effects associated with their use (see Chapters 42 and 43). Regional blockade affords the ability to provide excellent analgesia to children who might otherwise not tolerate larger doses of opioids. This group includes some neonates, especially preterm and former preterm infants who are at risk for apnea; children with problems of central ventilatory control, respiratory disease, or precarious airways; or those who risk obstruction with sedation (e.g., children with obstructive sleep apnea). Epidural analgesia that covers thoracic dermatomes improves resolution of ileus and return to normal feeding after major abdominal surgery.[358,359]

There are few absolute contraindications to regional blockade. Anatomic anomalies, such as myelodysplasia, sacral dysgenesis, and other abnormalities, either disrupting the epidural space or making access to it impossible, may prevent the performance of a caudal or epidural block. A report of epidural analgesia in children with myelodysplasia, however, suggests that catheters may be used safely in these children when placed at a level above the anatomic neural abnormality.[360] In cases involving these types of anatomic anomalies, we encourage consultation with experts in pediatric regional anesthesia, prior review of imaging studies, and consideration of fluoroscopic guidance. A needle and block should never be placed through infected tissue or near it. Children with burn injuries may be candidates for continuous regional techniques, provided the burned area is distant from the catheter insertion site (see Chapter 36). We do not believe that the benefits of regional analgesia outweigh the potential risks inherent in inserting catheters through burned tissue or close to it.

Sepsis presents a similar problem. In general, it is not advisable to place caudal or epidural catheters in children with sepsis for fear of seeding the epidural space during a period of bacteremia. Peripheral nerve, plexus, or intrapleural catheters may pose less of a problem in this regard, but there are no data to provide guidance regarding this issue. Coagulopathy and thrombocytopenia are relative contraindications to regional anesthesia, with mild abnormalities in hemostasis not necessarily precluding a regional block. When considering the risk of hematoma, it is safer to place a catheter in a site that can be compressed (e.g., femoral) as opposed to a site that cannot (e.g., epidural, paravertebral). In unusual cases, and with proper consideration of risk/benefit issues, fresh frozen plasma or platelets can be infused at the time of a regional procedure to provide temporary correction of coagulopathy. The considerations regarding regional anesthesia, coagulopathy, and anticoagulation are complex and have been reviewed extensively for adults by consensus groups from the American and European Societies of Regional Anesthesia.[539] In the absence of additional pediatric data, we recommend that clinicians review these adult publications as provisional guides for pediatric regional anesthesia as well. When placing a catheter for continuous blockade, consideration of the state of coagulation must include the time of catheter withdrawal as well as placement. If a child is to receive postoperative anticoagulation, for example, a continuous block should not be considered unless anticoagulation therapy can be held temporarily around the time of catheter removal.

When a nerve repair or revision is planned for an extremity, some surgeons may wish to assess motor or sensory function postoperatively. In these cases, consultation with the surgeon should precede a plan for postoperative regional analgesia. If the surgery involves the legs, a caudal or lumbar epidural catheter can be used with opioids or adjunctive drugs such as clonidine without local anesthetics. Very dilute concentrations of local anesthetics (e.g., 0.05%–0.075% bupivacaine or ropivacaine) often can provide additive analgesia if needed without significantly impairing motor function.

There is no consensus on the timing of a regional block (at the beginning or end of the surgical procedure). Placing a single-injection caudal block before incision confers a similar duration of postoperative analgesia, after a surgical procedure of 1 hour or less, as placing it at the end of surgery. For example, the times from recovery until the first request for analgesics after caudal blocks placed before incision or after surgery for inguinal herniorrhaphy were similar.[361] For more prolonged procedures, the block may be renewed with a second caudal injection before emergence or a catheter placed and redosed at appropriate intervals (usually approximately 1.5 hours). A volume of half of the original dose is usually sufficient if less than 2 hours have elapsed. A reduced concentration of local anesthetic is usually effective for postoperative analgesia. Adjunctive additives, such as clonidine, have also been shown in some studies to prolong the action of "single-shot" central neuraxis and some peripheral blocks (see later discussion) permitting a single-injection block placed before the incision to augment both intraoperative and postoperative analgesia for longer operations. In cases of major surgery on the extremities and shoulders, there is a growing trend toward placement of indwelling plexus or peripheral nerve catheters for local anesthetic infusions for several days, both for adults and children, as detailed subsequently in the section on catheter techniques.[362,363]

Evidence suggests that placing a block at the beginning of surgery offers several potential advantages.[364] Although preemptive or preventive analgesia is a reproducible phenomenon in laboratory studies, the results in humans have been conflicting. For example, initial studies in adults demonstrated a dramatic decrease in the incidence of phantom limb pain when an epidural block was administered before an amputation, although subsequent studies did not consistently reaffirm the initial observations.[365-367] Similarly, children who receive intraoperative neural blockade may experience less postoperative pain than those managed with general anesthesia alone, with the duration of analgesia in some cases lasting beyond the pharmacologic action of the block. On the other hand, a blinded study of caudal anesthesia administered either before or after inguinal surgery failed to show a difference in postoperative analgesia.[368]

It is theorized that interruption of nociceptive impulses at the spinal cord level attenuates imprinting of painful stimuli on the sensory cortex or forestalls the development of spinal cord hyperexcitability and "wind-up," thereby reducing the neural input and persistent postoperative pain.[367,369-372] It has also become increasingly evident, however, that if preemptive or preventative analgesia is to have a beneficial effect, other conditions must be met: the block must be of sufficient duration in relation to the nociceptive stimulus, it must extend into the postoperative period, and it must be effective at preventing central transmission of the nociceptive signals.[364] This third requirement suggests that a multimodal analgesic approach may offer the greatest benefit. The presence of poorly controlled preoperative pain may sensitize the CNS, rendering pain difficult to control via intraoperative or postoperative interventions.[373] Additionally, epidural opioids have been shown to reduce the inflammatory response after surgery in adults, as indicated by interleukin-2 concentrations, suggesting that attenuating the stress response to surgery may improve postoperative analgesia.[374]

Further evidence suggests that local anesthetic infiltration of the incision site, especially when performed in conjunction with a regional anesthetic technique, may be an effective means of providing prolonged analgesia after surgery.[375,376] This simple and effective approach can be used before or at the end of virtually any surgical procedure. A major limitation of wound infiltration with currently available local anesthetics is that the duration of analgesia is usually only 4 to 6 hours. Because postoperative pain commonly persists for several days, it would be more useful to administer local anesthetics for 2 to 4 days. To achieve this, the surgeon must place a multi-orifice catheter in the tissue planes of the wound during closure, through which local anesthetics can be infused.[377] Several commercially available kits using these "soaker hoses" have been shown to be effective. A disposable elastomeric pump, filled with local anesthetic that infuses local anesthetic continuously into the surgical tissues, can be placed at the end of surgery and the child sent home with it infusing for several days. Although this is an effective supplemental strategy to achieve postoperative analgesia, practitioners should be aware of complications that have been reported in adults.[378] *A note of caution: the concentration of local anesthetics, such as bupivacaine, and the infusion rate must be carefully prepared to avoid a local anesthetic overdose if such an approach is planned, particularly after chest surgery and in neonates and small infants.*[379]

A suspension of biodegradable polymer microspheres or lipospheres that contain bupivacaine has been used in experimental preparations and a commercially available liposomal foam. After injection, these microspheres release bupivacaine in a controlled manner to provide blockade of peripheral nerves for periods of 2 to 6 days, depending on dose, formulation, and site of injection.[380-383] Despite considerable initial enthusiasm in adults, the clinical utility of this formula has not proven to provide significantly extended analgesia in adults compared with conventional bupivacaine.[384,385] An alternative experimental approach to providing prolonged analgesia is the use of modified neurotoxins. Site 1 sodium channel blockers, such as tetrodotoxin and neosaxitoxin, have very strong affinity for sodium channels in vitro. Tetrodotoxin and neosaxitoxin are nonneurotoxic and do not significantly block sodium channels in the myocardium.[386] In animals, the combination of these toxins with bupivacaine, epinephrine, or clonidine markedly prolongs the nerve block and reduces systemic toxicity. Neosaxitoxin shows no cardiotoxicity in animals[387] and has shown promise for wound infiltration in clinical trials.[388,389]

Peripheral nerve and plexus blocks tend to provide blocks of greater duration than do central neuraxial blocks, the former lasting 8 to 12 hours, and on occasion exceeding 24 hours. Depending on the nature of the surgery, this may permit the child to transition to nonopioid analgesics at the time the block wears off, thereby eliminating or reducing the use of opioids and their potential untoward effects. Children undergoing outpatient surgery may be discharged after a single-injection regional block, but follow-up the next day with the family is necessary to ensure that the block has receded and no complications have developed. This is especially the case after peripheral nerve blocks. Parents must further be cautioned that there may be some degree of motor blockade present, and that the blocked limb must be protected from injury. If a lower extremity is blocked, assistance with ambulation is mandatory. Techniques for regional anesthesia and analgesia are discussed in detail in Chapters 42 and 43.

Choice of Local Anesthetics, Additives, and Dosing

Dilute long-acting local anesthetics, such as bupivacaine 0.125% to 0.25% or ropivacaine 0.1% to 0.2%, are the most commonly used local anesthetics for regional blockade. In Europe and Canada, levobupivacaine is available and has the advantage of smaller risk of toxicity than bupivacaine (see Chapter 42). Ropivacaine and levobupivacaine have the dual advantages when compared with bupivacaine of a relatively prolonged duration of action and decreased motor blockade. Epinephrine (1 : 200,000–1 : 400,000) is often added to bupivacaine to decrease systemic absorption and increase duration of action, although *caution is advised when a digital or penile block is performed, because of the risk of inducing ischemia by direct vasoconstriction.* (Note that the avoidance of epinephrine for digital blocks is based on limited and historical evidence [concentrations of epinephrine of 1 : 80,000 in the past, not 1 : 200,000 as is currently used], and current proponents of the practice have used epinephrine without complications).[390–393] There is probably little advantage to adding epinephrine to the local anesthetic in continuous infusions, since prolonging the block effect is not a consideration.

Initial studies concluded that the optimal concentration of bupivacaine that provides maximum sensory blockade without motor blockade for caudal analgesia was 0.125%,[394] although subsequent studies demonstrated that the optimal concentration was actually 0.175% (7 mL of 0.25% bupivacaine combined with 3 mL of saline solution).[395,396] More concentrated solutions of bupivacaine (0.2%–0.25%) may be used for blocks that do not significantly affect motor function, such as for an ilioinguinal-iliohypogastric nerve block after herniorrhaphy.

Block duration correlates most closely with total local anesthetic dose. The use of a higher concentration such as 0.5%, as is common in adult practice, will produce a block that is 40% longer in duration than an equal volume of 0.25%.[397] This will, of course, increase the incidence of motor blockade. The clinical significance of motor blockade (e.g., site of blockade, need for early ambulation) versus the benefit of prolonged duration (i.e., a block lasting until the following morning instead of wearing off in the middle of the night) must be weighed for each patient. Because most peripheral single-injection blocks can be accomplished with 0.2 to 0.3 mL/kg, it is feasible to stay well under the maximum allowable dose of 2.5 mg/kg (i.e., 0.5 mL/kg of a 0.5% solution). Supraclavicular brachial plexus block using a combination of perineural 0.5% ropivacaine and dexamethasone or IV dexamethasone produces a block with an average duration of 25 hours, ensuring a first postoperative night with an excellent analgesia.[398] Pediatric peripheral nerve blockade can be extended with the addition of α_2-adrenoreceptor agonists (9.75 vs. 3.75 hours).[399] Another example is that thoracic epidural analgesia after Nuss bar placement may be enhanced with a denser blockade. For these blocks, motor block is of less significance because most lung expansion is produced by the diaphragm.[100] For thoracic epidural blocks, we use ropivacaine 0.2% with an opioid and clonidine.

Ropivacaine, an *l*-enantiomer amide local anesthetic, is widely used in children, particularly in neonates and infants.[400–403] In both pediatric and adult studies, the duration of analgesia after ropivacaine is similar to that after bupivacaine, although motor block occurs more frequently with bupivacaine. In a review of 16 pediatric studies of caudal blockade, ropivacaine and bupivacaine were both effective. Ropivacaine caused less motor block than bupivacaine in 6 studies and similar motor block in 8 studies. For caudal block, the duration of motor block with either local anesthetic was short-lived.[404] Ropivacaine is less cardiotoxic than bupivacaine, but it is also less potent in adult studies than bupivacaine,[405] although similar results are obtained with larger doses of ropivacaine.[406] In terms of developing terminal apnea, infant rats tolerate 1.5 times the dose of ropivacaine compared with bupivacaine. The doses for the onset of respiratory distress and seizures are similarly increased with ropivacaine.[402] These differences are more pronounced in infant rats than in adult rats. Animal data suggest that the toxic thresholds for both CNS and cardiovascular toxicity are increased 20% to 30% with this agent in both adults and infants, although seizures can still occur with ropivacaine if the dose exceeds the toxic threshold. Although recommended dose limits are similar for bupivacaine and ropivacaine (2.5 mg/kg bolus, 0.4–0.5 mg/kg per hour infusion), pharmacokinetic modeling suggests that larger doses of ropivacaine are likely safe.[407] Based on these data, some institutions have increased the allowable infusion limits for ropivacaine to 0.6 mg/kg per hour.

The authors recommend using a levorotatory enantiomer (levo-enantiomer), such as ropivacaine, in preference to the racemic mixture, bupivacaine, in infants younger than 6 months of age because of the potential increased margin of safety.[403,408] Another option for continuous infusion is chloroprocaine, which undergoes rapid ester metabolism in the bloodstream, and thus has a low risk of toxicity. Because of chloroprocaine's favorable therapeutic margin in infants, larger volumes can be infused to achieve adequate spread of blockade, an important consideration with epidural analgesia following extensive intraabdominal or intrathoracic operations. Another option with a similar decreased toxicity is levobupivacaine (the levorotatory isomer of bupivacaine). This drug possesses properties similar to bupivacaine with a moderate reduction in the toxicity risks inherent with bupivacaine.[409–411] However, levobupivacaine has become difficult to obtain in the United States, although it is commonly used in place of bupivacaine elsewhere.[412]

Opioids have been injected in the epidural and intrathecal spaces for analgesia in children, both with and without local anesthetics. Central neuraxial opioids have been used for more than two decades to produce effective analgesia in children. However, opioids administered into the central neuraxis have the potential to cause delayed respiratory depression and are generally avoided in the outpatient setting to ensure the safety of children after discharge (see further).[413]

Adjuvant drugs have been added to the local anesthetic administered for caudal blockade to prolong the duration of the sensory block, an obviously desirable attribute for a single-injection block. However, their use is not without controversy. Many drugs have been injected into the epidural space with only limited laboratory evidence for safety and lack of neurotoxicity; therefore some caution is necessary.[414] Clonidine, 0.5 to 2 µg/kg, has been shown to lack evidence of neurotoxicity. It increases the duration of analgesia after bupivacaine in caudal blocks by approximately 3 hours, with insignificant hemodynamic effects, mild sedation, and no delay in recovery times.[415–421] Despite these reported beneficial effects of clonidine, one double-blind investigation found no difference between IV and caudally administered clonidine in a dose of 2 µg/kg as an adjunct to caudal blocks using bupivacaine, and another found no difference in duration or quality of analgesia when compared with caudal bupivacaine alone.[422,423] Conversely, when clonidine was used in conjunction with levobupivacaine, children who received clonidine in the caudal space demonstrated a significant delay in the need for rescue analgesia and reduced pain scores compared with those who received IV clonidine, suggesting that the prolonged analgesia occurs at a spinal cord site of action.[420,421,424] Caudal clonidine produces less nausea, itching, ileus, and urinary retention than opioid additives, although it may increase postoperative somnolence or respiratory depression at doses in excess of 1 µg/kg, particularly in the neonate.[423,425–427] The clearance of clonidine in infants is approximately one-third that of older children.[428] The preponderance of evidence, as shown in a meta-analysis,[429] supports the use of clonidine to prolong the analgesic effect of central neuraxial blocks, but we caution against the use of more than 1 µg/kg for outpatient procedures, especially in younger infants, because of an increased risk of respiratory depression. The use of adjuvant caudal dexmedetomidine 1 µg/kg, another α_2-adrenoreceptor agonist, is increasing. Sensory block duration is reported to increase by 8.21 hour (95% confidence interval 5.02, 11.40 hours).[430]

Dexamethasone has been studied in both perineural and systemic administration with results similar to clonidine. For caudal block, both perineural and IV dexamethasone (0.5 mg/kg) provide improved quality and duration of analgesia.[431,432] Adult data with peripheral blocks show equivalence between perineural and IV dexamethasone as well.[398] There is increased potential for neurotoxicity with any adjuvant compared with local anesthetic alone, so using IV agents to prolong blockade is likely the safest approach.[433]

Preservative-free ketamine has also been used for caudal analgesia, both alone and in combination with bupivacaine. Doses of 0.5 mg/kg appear to provide adequate analgesia, without untoward behavioral effects, such as those reported with IV or oral administration.[434] When combined with bupivacaine, the duration of analgesia approached 24 hours.[206,435,436] In a comparison with IV ketamine, caudal (*S*)-(+)-ketamine significantly prolonged the duration of analgesia, despite similar plasma concentrations.[436] One clinical study suggested a specific spinal site of action. *Only preservative-free ketamine should be used because preservatives have been associated with neurotoxicity.*[437,438] In the United States, preservative-free ketamine is currently unavailable.[417,439]

When performing a regional block, the total safe dose of local anesthetic should be calculated first and the volume and concentration of the solution adjusted if necessary to avoid administering a toxic dose. Most peripheral blocks can be performed with 0.2 to 0.3 mL/kg of local anesthetic, but single-injection caudal blocks require 0.75 to 1.25 mL/kg. Since a larger volume equates to a greater risk of administering a toxic dose, more dilute concentrations should be used. This is particularly important when performing blocks in infants. For example, a 7-kg infant has a maximal allowable dose of 17.5 mg of bupivacaine (or 2.5 mg/kg). If a 0.25% solution (2.5 mg/mL) were administered, the total volume would be limited to 7 mL. The maximum dose should probably be slightly more restrictive in infants younger than 6 months of age. At this age, a cautious approach is to further reduce

the allowable dose by 25% to 30%, particularly if an infusion is to be used following the initial bolus. For example, a 4-kg 2-month-old infant would be permitted to receive 2.7 mL (6.6 mg) of the same solution. A simple rule of thumb for calculating the maximum bolus dose of bupivacaine and ropivacaine in children older than 6 months is 1 mL/kg of 0.25% or 0.5 mL/kg of 0.5% solution. For most circumstances, there is little benefit in using 0.5% concentration. Use of different concentrations increases the odds of a dose calculation error. To prevent this type of error, some hospitals have standardized dosing for infiltration and boluses to a single concentration, namely, 0.2% for ropivacaine or 0.25% for bupivacaine.

Choice of Block and Techniques
Single-Injection Techniques

There are many circumstances in which the simplicity and duration of action of a single-injection block is desirable. Both neuraxial blocks and peripheral plexus and nerve blocks can be effective as single-injection techniques. The caudal block remains the most commonly used technique in pediatric regional anesthesia. It provides analgesia of the lower extremity and lower abdomen, and is easily and quickly performed in most infants and children (see Chapter 42). When an operation is performed on both legs, it is often preferable to bilateral lower extremity blocks.

The use of ultrasound makes the identification of plexuses and peripheral nerves much easier in an anesthetized child. Peripheral nerve stimulation using Teflon-coated needles remains an effective technique, but it is being used less frequently as familiarity with ultrasound and its benefits increases.[440] To precisely position the needle in the target area and avoid piercing adjacent structures, one must develop skill in coordinating its trajectory with the ultrasound image so that the needle tip does not pass out of the plane of view. Although it remains unknown whether ultrasound and more precise needle placement will reduce nerve injury, there is evidence that it reduces the volume of local anesthetic needed to produce an effective block.[441,442] Ultrasound visualization of the local anesthetic surrounding a nerve or plexus provides reliable confirmation that a block will be successful. Nerve blocks of the lower extremity can often be used instead of caudal blockade (see Chapters 42 and 43). The primary disadvantage is that multiple blocks (i.e., femoral and sciatic) are needed to cover the entire extremity. They provide a field of analgesia limited to the operative site, but they have a prolonged duration of analgesia (usually at least twice that of caudal block) and eliminate some of the potential undesirable effects of central neuraxis blockade, such as urinary retention (and need for a urinary catheter) or unintentional unilateral blockade (of the nonoperative leg). Blockade of the femoral nerve, the sciatic nerve, and the nerves of the ankle is easily performed in children by using similar techniques to those in adults (see Chapters 42 and 43). Regional blockade of the upper extremity may involve an interscalene, supraclavicular, infraclavicular, or axillary block, or less commonly, blockade of the individual nerves at the level of the arm or wrist. Unlike the lower extremity, a single block of the brachial plexus can provide anesthesia to the entire extremity. Paravertebral blocks may be used in lieu of an epidural after thoracic or upper abdominal surgery. This block may be considered for procedures of limited scope, such as open-lung biopsy or thoracostomy for drainage, but the duration of blockade is limited to several hours. An emerging approach is ultrasound-guided placement of paravertebral catheters for continuous infusion for thoracic and upper abdominal surgery.[443,444] For open-chest procedures, intercostal blocks by the surgeon pose a low risk and may be indicated, although their effectiveness is limited by their short duration. Epinephrine is commonly included in the local anesthetic for these blocks to limit the rate of uptake. More extensive surgery anticipated to cause postoperative pain of longer duration may be best managed with a catheter (continuous infusion) technique.

An ilioinguinal-iliohypogastric nerve block provides excellent postoperative analgesia for inguinal herniorrhaphy, a common outpatient procedure in children (see Chapters 42 and 43). It appears similar in efficacy to a caudal block, with a duration of analgesia of at least 4 hours when bupivacaine with epinephrine is used. For orchiopexy, ilioinguinal nerve block has been found to be as effective as caudal blockade to the T10 level in a randomized and blinded investigation.[445] In our experience, however, postoperative analgesia for procedures that involve considerable manipulation and traction on the spermatic cord and testis may be better managed with caudal blockade in younger children. Penile block is effective for both circumcision and distal, simple hypospadias repair. More extensive procedures on the penis, especially repair of penile-scrotal hypospadias, require a caudal or pudendal block, rather than a penile block, to produce effective analgesia.[446]

The use of single-injection neuraxial opioids is an additional technique that can provide longer-lasting analgesia, but must be used in inpatients only because of the need for respiratory monitoring. Intrathecal morphine has been administered to infants and children for several decades and provides long-acting analgesia (up to 24 hours) after a single injection.[447,448] It is absolutely essential that only preservative-free preparations of the drug be used because preservative-containing solutions may result in injury to the central neuraxis. Intrathecal doses ranging from 4 to 10 μg/kg are usually chosen. Because of the hydrophilicity of this agent, respiratory monitoring is mandated. Respiratory depression, as well as pruritus, nausea, and urinary retention, are reported after intrathecal morphine. We most commonly use this modality for analgesia after posterior spinal fusion. The drug can be administered by the surgeon under direct vision of the dura, but if administered at the beginning of the case, it has been reported to reduce intraoperative blood loss.[449,450] This route of administration has also been used before cardiac surgery.[451] The effective intrathecal dose of opioid is roughly one-fifth to one-tenth that of the epidural dose, and the duration of action, especially with morphine, is significantly prolonged. Therefore observation in a monitored setting must be continued for 24 hours or until no further evidence of respiratory compromise exists (without the use of naloxone).

Catheter Techniques

A catheter placed in the epidural space or adjacent to a nerve or plexus can be used to provide continuous uninterrupted analgesia for prolonged periods after surgery. These catheters are commonly used for about 3 days but may be used for more prolonged periods in selected situations. However, the risk of infection does increase when catheters are left in place for more than 3 days.[452] If necessary, catheters tunneled under the skin may be left in situ for more than 7 days,[453,454] and they have been left in place for longer periods without infectious complications in palliative care patients.[455] Catheters can also be placed in intrapleural or extrapleural and/or retropleural locations to provide analgesia after thoracic surgery.[456] In our experience, intrapleural analgesia reduces but does not eliminate the need for systemic opioids, especially if thoracostomy drains are present. We rarely use this technique

because toxic concentrations of local anesthetic and seizures have been reported.[457] Continuous extrapleural, intercostal, and paravertebral catheters can be placed either through the operative field or percutaneously. In adult studies, and in a smaller series of pediatric studies, these techniques appear to provide excellent analgesia at rest, but with movement they provide only partial opioid sparing. Some clinicians regard these techniques as providing many of the advantages of thoracic epidural analgesia, with the potential for reducing the risks and adverse effects of thoracic epidural analgesia.

Continuous regional blockade is remarkably effective and safe, although as with any technique, monitoring for untoward effects is necessary to prevent complications. New technology for the delivery of drugs to peripheral nerves and plexuses has made it possible for children to receive the benefits of continuous neural blockade after discharge from the hospital or day surgery unit.[362] Catheters may deliver local anesthetics and other medications via controlled infusion devices that use a pressurized elastomer-bulb reservoir that controls the infusion rate with a flow limiter (ON-Q pump, I-Flow LLC, Lake Forest, CA; Infusor, Baxter Healthcare Corporation, Deerfield, IL; Accufuser, Moog Medical Devices, Salt Lake City, UT; Easypump, B Braun Melsungen AG, Melsungen, Germany; and others) (E-Fig. 44.3). These devices can be used at home after discharge, for infusion of medication into a tissue plane to provide a continuous field blockade or a continuous peripheral nerve block. As the use of peripheral nerve blocks continue to increase, we believe that these techniques may eventually become more common than neuraxial analgesia for suitable indications.

Infusion of local anesthetics in the subcutaneous (SC) tissues at the incision site or into the surgical plane using these devices provides prolonged analgesia in both adults and children. Several types of these infusion systems are available, including ones that have options for fixed, variable, or continuous infusion rates with a bolus option. The latter two must be used with caution in smaller children in whom local anesthetic toxicity from excessive dosage may be a risk; we generally use the fixed-rate devices. When continuous peripheral nerve or plexus blocks are used for outpatients, a carefully designed system must be in place to follow up with these children to avoid complications and achieve early detection of potentially adverse events. Patient and family education to recognize potential complications, along with telephone follow-up, are necessary to ensure safe use of catheters at home. Cases have been reported of possible excessive doses of local anesthetic from a continuous infusion pump used at home, although no catastrophic events have been reported.[458]

CAUDAL AND EPIDURAL CATHETERS. With experience and proper equipment, the lumbar or thoracic routes are feasible at any age, but specific expertise is required for infants and toddlers. Regardless of the level of insertion, the goal should be to place the tip of the catheter as close as possible to the dermatome(s) most affected by the operation. Practitioners who have less experience with direct epidural catheterization in children should consider placing the catheter via the caudal route for children younger than 6 years of age. In infants and children up to about 6 years of age, catheters may be advanced freely from the caudal canal cephalad to thoracic levels with excellent success.[459] This is possible in part because young children have a less developed vascular plexus and more compact and globular fat than do older children and adults.[459,460] However, other authors describe less reliability with caudal-to-thoracic advancement of catheters in children larger than 10 kg.[461] This has been attributed to the more mature composition of the contents of the epidural space and the lumbar lordosis that occurs with walking. With age, the epidural fat appears to lose the spongy gelatinous character noted in infants and the spaces between the fat globules become less distinct.[459,460] Catheters made of nylon or polyamide may be less likely to kink beneath the skin and seem to thread more easily than those made of Teflon or other materials. The catheter should never be advanced if resistance is felt. Similar difficulties in advancing catheters that resulted in catheters looping backward, kinking, or puncturing the dura have been reported in neonates weighing less than 3.5 kg.[462] If a caudal catheter is threaded to higher lumbar or thoracic levels, the position should be confirmed with imaging or other functional assessment.

Epidurography has been used to confirm the position of the catheter tip. In one series of 20 preterm infants, epidurography revealed misplaced catheters in 3 infants or 15%. New data suggest that misplacement of threaded catheters in all ages may be more common than is generally recognized.[463] In this series of 724 epidurograms, unexpected misplacement was detected in 11 or 1.5%, including 3 intravascular catheters, despite negative test doses; 2 intrathecal without cerebrospinal fluid aspiration; 4 that were intraperitoneal; and 1 each in the rectum and psoas compartments. These authors recommended epidurography in all cases, although this is not the current standard of practice and must be weighed against the risks of radiation exposure in young children. If specific dermatomal placement of a catheter is sought, one should consider obtaining an imaging study to confirm the dermatomal level of the tip of the catheter, and the aforementioned data suggest that imaging might be advisable whenever a catheter is advanced to a level substantially more rostral than its insertion level.

As an alternative to epidurography, ultrasound can be used and is especially useful in infants weighing less than 10 kg. It is readily available in most ORs and does not expose the child to radiation. Ultrasound can be used to estimate the skin–ligamentum flavum distance to aid in placement, as well as imaging proper catheter placement. In general, it is more difficult to image the actual catheter but local anesthetic spread can be easily visualized with anterior depression of the dura on injection.[464,465]

Another alternative is a nerve-stimulating catheter, which allows real-time monitoring of the location of the tip of the catheter as it is advanced cephalad.[466,467] If a stimulating catheter is not available, a saline solution–filled catheter can serve in its stead. The technique requires the use of saline loss-of-resistance and avoiding air bubbles in the epidural space or in the catheter-connector-injection system, because air impedes electrical conduction. With either system, neuromuscular blockade must be avoided because it abolishes the motor response. Used in conjunction with a nerve stimulator set to very low milliamperage (approximately 6 mA), the muscles supplied by a nerve root will twitch as the catheter approaches the segments that supply that dermatome, thereby confirming the catheter tip's location. Specifically, twitches in the feet and ankles occur with catheter tips around L5 to S1, hip flexion occurs with catheter tips around T12 to S1, abdominal muscle twitches without hip flexion imply thoracic positioning above T12, and intercostal muscle twitches imply midthoracic tip positioning. Finger twitches would imply advancement to around T1. This technique can also be used to detect catheter malpositioning. Bilateral twitching at a current less than 0.6 mA generally implies subarachnoid positioning. Unilateral twitches in a narrow motor distribution at a current less than 1 mA may suggest advancement out a root foramen. Unilateral twitches at

TABLE 44.10	Estimated Dermatomal Level With Epidural Catheter Advancement	
Amperage (mA)	Estimated Dermatomal Level	Twitch Response Level
6	L5-S1	Feet and ankles
6	T12-S1	Hip flexors
6	Above T12	Abdominal muscle without hip flexion
6	Midthoracic	Intercostal muscles
6	T1	Fingers
<0.6	Subarachnoid malposition	Bilateral motor response
<1	Nerve root	Unilateral
<1	Subdural	Unilateral but broad motor distribution
15	Out of epidural space	No twitches observed

a current less than 1 mA in a very broad motor distribution may indicate subdural positioning. Absence of twitches as the current is increased to about 15 mA (in the absence of air bubbles or neuromuscular blockade) generally indicates that the epidural catheter is not in the epidural space (Table 44.10). Our experience is that the use of one of these confirmatory techniques when catheters are threaded cephalad can help avoid problems with failed or incomplete blocks in the postoperative period.

The choice of drugs for epidural infusions depends on several factors, including site of surgery, site of the epidural catheter tip, and child risk factors. Local anesthetics, lipophilic opioids, and, to some extent, clonidine all have more restricted cephalad distribution of action during infusions compared with hydrophilic opioids, such as hydromorphone or morphine. Consequently, optimal positioning of the catheter tip during insertion can improve the analgesic action postoperatively. Experience in adults suggests that when local anesthetics are used, analgesia is optimized when the tip of the epidural catheter is positioned at or slightly above the dermatomal levels involved in the surgery. This effect may be more pronounced when children are moving than when they are at rest. Positioning at levels slightly above the dermatomal levels involved in surgery is more relevant for surgery in lumbosacral dermatomes compared with upper thoracic dermatomes because of the greater distance between root level and dorsal horn level in these two circumstances.[468]

Placement of catheters at thoracic levels requires consideration of risk/benefit trade-offs. Therefore if a catheter tip is at the lumbar or caudal level and the surgery is in thoracic and upper abdominal dermatomes, continuous infusions containing local anesthetics alone or with lipophilic opioids, such as fentanyl or sufentanil, are likely to be ineffective. Increasing the infusion volume is limited by the maximum allowable systemic local anesthetic concentrations. In this circumstance, a reasonable alternative is to administer hydrophilic opioids (e.g., morphine or hydromorphone) through lumbar or caudal catheters. Such a technique, however, precludes the optimal use of local anesthetics and the considerable benefit that may accrue from a multimodal approach to regional analgesia. Overall, we do not endorse the practice of placing lumbar catheters for thoracic dermatomal coverage.

An epidural catheter can be placed in an awake, sedated, or anesthetized child. A prospective analysis of data from the PRAN database found that the risk of inserting an epidural catheter in

44

an anesthetized child by an experienced clinician is not greater (and may be less) than attempting such placement in an awake adult, nor is it clear that a child can accurately report sensations of paresthesia or differentiate the discomfort of needle passage from more ominous pain.[107,469,470] There is a perception that placing an epidural in the thoracic region is more dangerous than in other spinal levels, but current data do not support this. In the U.K. epidural audit, serious (grade 1) complications were independent of the level of insertion. Overall, there was a greater risk of all types of complications in thoracic epidurals placed in neonates and infants, but half of these complications were the less severe grade 3. Risk is likely more related to the age of the patient rather than level of insertion.[470] In a report of four cases of neurologic complications in children with epidurals, three of four catheters were at T11 or lower.[471] We believe that data and experience support the safety of placement of epidural catheters in anesthetized children by anesthesiologists trained and experienced in this procedure, although the tolerances for error in infants are smaller than in adults and older children.[107,470,472,473]

It is extremely important to secure caudal catheters to the skin with a clear occlusive dressing to avoid contamination or dislodgment and to allow daily inspection of the site. In addition, tincture of benzoin or other adhesive solution reduces the incidence of catheter and dressing displacement. For a caudal catheter, the use of an adhesive-edged plastic drape, covering the area from the gluteal crease over the dressing, also helps prevent fecal soiling of the dressing by children who are in diapers. Another option is to tunnel the caudal catheter in a cephalad-lateral direction, which decreases colonization rates to that seen with epidural catheters.[454] Despite the above precautions, if a dressing becomes detached and the insertion site is contaminated, it is prudent to remove the catheter. The use of lumbar or thoracic catheters removes the insertion site from the diaper area and thereby further reduces the potential for contamination of the catheter and the insertion site.

Successful management of children with an epidural catheter requires carefully coordinated monitoring protocols, nursing management, and medical management of drug selection and dosing. As with PCA or continuous-infusion opioids, the orders should be standardized and written in consultation with the nursing staff, so that misinterpretations are less likely to occur (Fig. 44.8). Because the single most sensitive monitor of children receiving epidural opioids is the nurse, rather than a mechanical or electronic device, education of the nursing staff is of paramount importance to ensure safety. Nursing staff can also assess the adequacy of analgesia and thereby help to titrate the drug dose. Catheter insertion sites should be inspected at least once daily by the pain service, both for the integrity of the dressing and for any evidence of erythema or skin infection (Fig. 44.9). *When continuous infusions are used, the tubing connecting the infusion pump to the catheter should not have any injection ports and it should be clearly labeled as an epidural catheter to preclude unintended epidural administration of drugs intended for IV use.* We use color-coded tubing and a color-coded drug cassette for the continuous administration of regional agents. Although the same pumps are used for IV PCA administration, it is immediately obvious what route the drug is intended for simply by recognizing the tubing and cassette color.

A variation of traditional epidural analgesia and PCA is the technique of patient-controlled epidural analgesia (PCEA).[474] With this variation of traditional PCA, children are generally maintained with an infusion of epidural analgesics (frequently opioid alone or an opioid–local anesthetic mixture) and have the capability of self-administering supplemental doses when needed. When using this technique, the background infusion is used to provide the majority of the analgesia and the child can add to this when needed. It must be emphasized that the time needed for a bolus dose to effect a change with epidural administration is more prolonged than it is with IV agents. Therefore with PCEA lockout intervals are greater (often 15 to 30 minutes) than with PCA.[475,476] The considerations one would use for choosing this technique include the same child-monitoring factors for IV PCA and epidural analgesia, and maximum local anesthetic doses must be carefully calculated to cover the contingency of the greatest possible activation of the PCEA demand doses. Smart pump technology has been demonstrated to improve safety of this technique.[477]

SELECTION OF DRUGS AND DOSES. Local anesthetics, opioids, and adjuvant agents were discussed previously; this section addresses the specifics of drug choices for continuous infusion through indwelling catheters. Many drugs and combinations have been administered via continuous infusion to the epidural space to provide postoperative analgesia.[421] The most common choices involve mixtures of local anesthetics and opioids, such as bupivacaine and fentanyl, although increasingly, clonidine is being added (Table 44.11). Continuous infusions for peripheral nerve and plexus blocks are generally limited to local anesthetics, as evidence for the efficacy of other agents in these blocks is equivocal at best.

The choice of drug is based on several factors: the age and size of the child, the operation, and the underlying medical conditions that may decrease the margin of safety of one of the agents. The volume of solution required to fill the epidural space on a milliliter-per-kilogram basis appears to decrease with age; therefore older children and adolescents may require less volume than infants and young children, based on weight. In children older than 1 year of age, continuous infusions of ropivacaine up to 0.4 mg/kg per hour for up to 72 hours produced stable blood concentrations of unbound ropivacaine without evidence of accumulation or toxicity.[478,479] In very young or preterm infants, however, the risk of accumulation of the amino-amide local anesthetics, and thus the potential for toxicity, is particularly problematic.[480,481] Neonates are at increased risk for potential local anesthetic toxicity because of decreased protein binding (resulting in increased unbound drug) and possibly immature drug metabolism. The manifestations of local anesthetic toxicity in infants and neonates may be more difficult to recognize than in adults. Hence, we recommend a conservative maximum infusion dose for ropivacaine of 0.2 mg/kg per hour for infants younger than 6 months, which produces stable plasma levels for up to 72 hours.[482] Bupivacaine is generally not recommended because of evidence of accumulation in some neonates and small infants, and its lower therapeutic index, especially in this population; however, if ropivacaine is not available, the same reduced maximal dose limits apply (i.e., <0.2 mg/kg per hour).[481,483] Of the five cases of local anesthetic toxicity reported to the PRAN, four were in infants 3 months of age or younger, highlighting the greater risk in this age group.[107] Because safe infusion rates of ropivacaine in the neonate frequently provide insufficient analgesia when wide dermatomal coverage is needed, the amino-ester local anesthetic chloroprocaine may be used in an epidural infusion instead.[484,485] Although the amino-amide local anesthetics are slowly cleared in neonates and young infants, the amino-ester chloroprocaine is cleared extremely rapidly, even in preterm infants, via ester hydrolysis, with an elimination half-life of several minutes.[484] This permits large doses and infusion rates with a reduced risk for

Child's weight: _____ kg

Allergies: _____

Continuous regional analgesia via (check appropriate modality)

☐ Caudal epidural   ☐ Lumbar epidural   ☐ Thoracic epidural   ☐ Plexus or peripheral nerve catheter (specify)

_____

The catheter is _____ cm at the skin.   Loss of resistance (for lumbar and thoracic epidurals) was at _____ cm.

Infusion:

(Choose one only) ☐ Bupivacaine   ☐ Ropivacaine   ☐ Chloroprocaine

(Concentration) ☐ 0.075%   ☐ 0.1%   ☐ 0.2%   ☐ 1% (chloroprocaine only)

Additives (caudal and epidural only):

Opioid (choose one only) ☐ Fentanyl   ☐ Hydromorphone   ☐ Morphine

Concentration (μg/mL): ☐ 1   ☐ 2   ☐ 3   ☐ 5 (hydromorphone and morphine only)   ☐ 7 (morphine only)

☐ 10 (morphine only)

☐ Clonidine   Concentration (μg/mL): ☐ 0.5   ☐ 1

Infusion rate: Start at _____ mL/h. Range: _____ to _____ mL/h. This is a maximum of _____ mg/kg/h of local anesthetic and _____ μg/kg/h of opioid.

Dosing guidelines for regional anesthesia/analgesia solution

	Local anesthetics		Opioids			
	Bupivacaine or ropivacaine	Chloroprocaine	Fentanyl	Hydromorphone	Morphine	Clonidine
Concentration	0.05%-0.1% (0.5-1 mg/mL) May use up to 0.2% for ropivacaine	1%-1.5% (10-15 mg/mL)	1-3 μg/mL	3-7 μg/mL	5-10 μg/mL	0.5-1 μg/mL
Suggested dose	Less than 6 months of age: 0.2 mg/kg/h; Maximum dose: 0.2 mg/kg/h 6 months of age or older: 0.2-0.4 mg/kg/h Maximum dose: 0.4–0.5 mg/kg/h	0.2-0.8 mL/kg/h (neonates)*	0.3-1 μg/kg/h	1-2.5 μg/kg/h	1-5 μg/kg/h	0.1-0.2 μg/kg/h

*Note that the concentration of additives must be proportionally reduced with chloroprocaine if higher infusion rates are administered to avoid overdose.

Treatment of side effects:

Respiratory depression: For RR < _____ BPM, immediately stop epidural infusion and call acute pain service STAT. Administer O₂, ensure clear airway, and assist ventilation if necessary.

☐ Naloxone (Narcan) 1 μg/kg IV = _____ μg, repeat q1min as needed

Nausea and vomiting: ☐ Ondansetron 0.1 mg/kg (4 mg maximum) = _____ mg IV q6h

☐ Metoclopramide 0.1 mg/kg (10 mg maximum) = _____ mg IV q6h

Pruritus: ☐ Nalbuphine 0.05 mg/kg = _____ mg IV q4h

☐ For any of above, begin naloxone infusion at 0.25 μg/kg/h = _____ μg/h

Adjunctive medications: ☐ Acetaminophen 10 mg/kg PO q4h for 24 hours then q4h prn

Inadequate analgesia: ☐ Morphine 0.05-0.1 mg/kg IV = _____ mg q3-4h prn for pain

☐ Ketorolac 0.5 mg/kg IV = _____ mg q6h prn for pain (up to 15 mg ≤ 50 kg; up to 30 mg > 50 kg)

Muscle spasms: ☐ Diazepam 0.05-0.1 mg/kg IV = _____ mg q6h prn

Monitoring and equipment: must choose for patients receiving epidural opioids

☐ Continuous pulse oximetry and respiratory monitoring

☐ O₂ and bag/mask delivery system, suction at the bedside

Nursing orders:

VS: ☐ q4h: temp, HR, RR, BP, pain score

☐ Dermatome level for caudal and epidural

☐ SpO₂ and sedation score (required if opioids are used). Call acute pain service for RR < _____ bpm.

☐ Record Bromage score q8hr; call acute pain service if 4 or less (choose for children receiving local anesthetics).

Call acute pain service for any questions or problems: inadequate analgesia despite intervention, loose or contaminated dressing, catheter disconnect, sedation score >3, increased somnolence, confusion, agitation, dizziness, tinnitus, hypotension, bradycardia, fever >38.2°C; inflammation, tenderness, or swelling at catheter site; Bromage score >0.

Maintain IV access.

For epidural or peripheral nerve block of lower extremity: Ambulate with assistance only with order from primary service and Bromage score of 0. Pad block extremities and elevate heels off of bed.

FIGURE 44.8 Sample Epidural Orders. BP, blood pressure; *BPM,* breaths per minute; *HR,* heart rate; *RR,* respiratory rate; *PO,* orally; *prn,* as needed; *SpO₂,* oxygen saturation measured by pulse oximetry; *STAT,* immediately; *VS,* vital signs. (Modified from the University of Michigan Hospitals & Health Centers.)

44

systemic toxicity. Case reports of chloroprocaine toxicity in infants are rare, generally short-lived (<1 minute), and self-limiting owing to its rapid metabolism.[486,487] Previous concerns regarding neurotoxicity after chloroprocaine involved a succession of formulations with preservatives, including metabisulfite, methylparaben, and ethylenediaminetetraacetic acid, although the current formulation is preservative-free. An epidural solution of 1% to 1.5% chloroprocaine can be infused at rates of 0.2 to 0.8 mL/kg per hour.

When a block is not previously established in the OR, it is useful to dose through catheters with local anesthetic (without opioids) at a volume of 0.05 mL/kg per spinal segment or between 0.5 and 1 mL/kg of local anesthetic, not to exceed 5 mg/kg of lidocaine, or 2.5 mg/kg of bupivacaine or ropivacaine. Some clinicians administer a loading dose of opioid as well, such as 1 to 3 µg/kg of hydromorphone. Bupivacaine infusion rates should not exceed 0.4 mg/kg per hour (e.g., 0.4 mL/kg per hour for 0.1% bupivacaine) for children because toxicity may result.[488] If epidural

local anesthetic infusions are begun without either opioids or clonidine (e.g., 0.0625%–0.125% bupivacaine) and inadequate analgesia occurs at infusion rates of 0.3 to 0.4 mL/kg per hour (a maximum dosage of 0.4 mg/kg per hour), further increases in the local anesthetic infusion rate or concentration should be avoided. Instead, correct placement of the catheter should be confirmed (e.g., with an epidurogram or chloroprocaine/lidocaine test dose) if dermatomal levels cannot be unequivocally determined. If the catheter is properly located, an epidural opioid or clonidine can be added to the local anesthetic infusion. It is imperative to confirm that an epidural catheter is properly functioning immediately after an infant or child arrives in the PACU or if there is any question of its proper location later. If an amino-amide local anesthetic has been given during or after surgery as an initial bolus followed by a continuous infusion, then use of a repeat bolus dose of these amino amides may result in a "stair casing" of plasma concentrations, with a risk for systemic toxicity. Although administration of epidural or systemic opioids may provide analgesia, they may not clarify the site of the epidural catheter. For this reason, confirmation of the catheter location is imperative whenever the clinical picture is not clear. Several means of accomplishing this are described later.

Local anesthetic and opioid combinations (e.g., 0.1% bupivacaine or ropivacaine with fentanyl 2 to 3 µg/mL or hydromorphone 3 to 5 µg/mL at infusion rates of 0.2 to 0.4 mL/kg per hour) via lumbar epidural catheters or caudal catheters advanced to a lumbar position, provide adequate analgesia in most children undergoing lower abdominal or lower extremity surgery. Fentanyl alone (0.3 µg/kg per hour) has been shown to provide 90% effective postoperative analgesia after a levobupivacaine block was established during surgery.[489] However, the blood concentrations achieved with epidural fentanyl are in the therapeutic range, suggesting that much of the therapeutic effect is due to systemic absorption, not entirely surprising with a highly lipophilic agent.[490] We do not recommend the use of epidural fentanyl for this reason. Epidural opioids should be used with great caution, or at considerably reduced doses, in children at risk for apnea or hypoventilation (e.g., former preterm infants, children with chronic respiratory failure or disorders of central control of ventilation, or those with

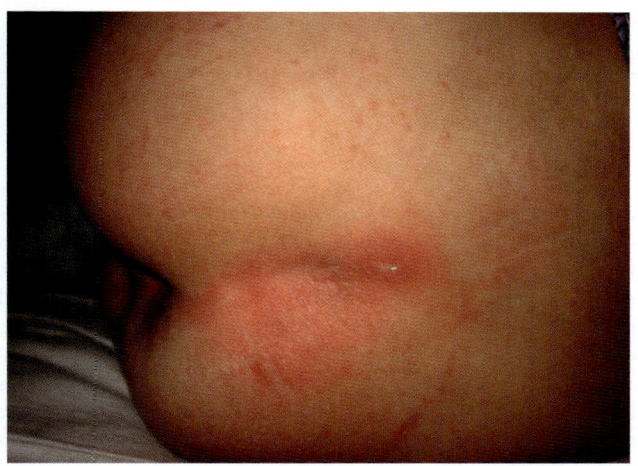

FIGURE 44.9 Superficial skin infection at the site of an epidural catheter insertion. The catheter was withdrawn, and the problem resolved with local skin care only.

TABLE 44.11	Commonly Used Medications for Epidural Administration		
	Dose Range	Untoward Effects	Comments
Local Anesthetics		Motor block	
Bupivacaine	0.2–0.4 mg/kg per hour		Maximum dose 0.2 mg/kg per hour for infants <6 months
Ropivacaine	0.2–0.5 mg/kg per hour		Levo-enantiomer; 20%–30% less toxicity than racemic amino amides. Maximum dose 0.2 mg/kg per hour for infants <6 months.
Levobupivacaine	0.2–0.5 mg/kg per hour		
Chloroprocaine	1%–1.5%; 0.2–0.8 mL/kg per hour (neonates)		
Opioids		Respiratory depression, sedation, pruritus, urinary retention	
Fentanyl	0.3–1 µg/kg per hour		Lipophilic; high rate of systemic absorption
Hydromorphone	1–3 µg/kg per hour	Delayed respiratory depression from rostral spread	Hydrophilic; use when surgery is more extensive. Hydromorphone recommended over morphine due to less rostral spread.
Morphine	1–5 µg/kg per hour		
Adjuncts			
Clonidine	0.1–0.2 µg/kg per hour	Sedation, respiratory depression at greater doses, hypotension (possibly postural) at high doses	Increased risk of apnea with high doses in neonates

TABLE 44.12	Treatment of Untoward Effects of Epidural Opioids	
Adverse Effect	**Treatment**	**Infusion Rate**
Pruritus	Naloxone, 0.5–1 µg/kg IV or infusion at 0.25–1 µg/kg per hour	No change, or decrease opioid concentration, or remove opioid if pruritis persists
	Nalbuphine, 0.025–0.05 mg/kg IV every 6 hours	
Nausea and vomiting	NPO for 24 hours	Decrease opioid concentration or decrease rate by 10%–20% or remove opioid if nausea persists
	Naloxone, 0.5 µg/kg IV or infusion at 0.25–1 µg/kg per hour	
	Ondansetron 0.1 mg/kg (maximum 4 mg) IV every 6 hours	
	Metoclopramide, 0.1–0.15 mg/kg IV every 6–8 hours	
Urinary retention	Bladder catheterization (one time; some institutions keep urinary catheters in these children routinely)	Decrease opioid concentration
	Naloxone, 0.5 µg/kg IV or infusion at 0.25–1 µg/kg per hour	
	Indwelling urinary catheter	
Respiratory depression[a]; child unarousable, hypoxemic, hypercarbic, or apneic	Oxygen by mask; assisted ventilation if needed
Naloxone, 5–10 µg/kg IV
Transfer child to monitored setting until episode is fully resolved.
Consider naloxone infusion (0.25–1 µg/kg per hour)	Discontinue infusion; consider possibility of intrathecal catheter migration (check by aspirating)
	Consider naloxone infusion (0.25–1 µg/kg per hour)	

IV, intravenous; *NPO*, nothing by mouth.
[a]Stop infusion until the child is alert, if using morphine or hydromorphone.

obstructive sleep apnea). In very young infants, epidural infusions of both local anesthetics and opioids and other adjuvants can be used safely, but they require increased surveillance and reduced initial infusion rates. This is because (1) drug clearance may be reduced; (2) protein binding, which is decreased, may increase the free serum drug concentrations; and (3) titration to clinical end points (e.g., pain scoring) is less precise. A double-blind randomized study demonstrated that the combination of 0.1% bupivacaine with 1 µg/mL of fentanyl provided superior analgesia compared with local anesthetic alone, with no increase in adverse effects, when infused through thoracic catheters after thoracotomy in infants younger than 6 months of age.[491] In contrast, another study found no incremental benefits in children after abdominal surgery from the addition of fentanyl to epidural catheters with greater local anesthetic concentrations (e.g., 0.125% bupivacaine at 0.3 mL/kg per hour).[489,492] The use of fentanyl as an adjunct may increase PONV.[492] In some centers, application of epidural infusions, especially with opioids, for children younger than 3 to 6 months of age is restricted to intensive care areas. Acetaminophen or NSAIDs can also be administered if adjunctive analgesia is needed.

If the catheter tip is positioned at the thoracic dermatomes, bupivacaine or ropivacaine with opioid may be used for thoracic and upper abdominal surgery.[93,103,493–496] Infusion rates may need to be decreased for thoracic catheters compared with lumbar catheters because the capacitance or volume of the epidural space appears to be less than in lumbar regions. The authors have noted that some older children and adolescents require greater than expected infusion rates to achieve adequate dermatome levels for analgesia. Using hydromorphone may be of benefit in these instances, as its greater hydrophilicity results in wider spread. We rarely use epidural morphine and prefer a continuous epidural infusion of hydromorphone when greater spread is desired, as its adverse effect profile appears to be preferable. Studies in adults suggest an epidural potency ratio of between 2:1 and 3:1, compared with 5:1 for systemic morphine.[497] When mixed with

a local anesthetic for lumbar epidural infusion, concentrations of 3 to 5 µg/mL of hydromorphone yield a solution that results in an appropriate infusion rate of both drugs. Hydrophilic opioids, especially when administered by infusion, require prolonged careful observation (see later discussion). If somnolence, shallow breathing, or hypopnea occurs, the infusion must be stopped, not simply decreased, until these effects subside and appropriate therapy is instituted (Table 44.12). Common epidural infusions and alternative modalities for pain management of sample cases are provided in Appendix 44.1.

Adjuvant agents, particularly clonidine, can be administered continuously via epidural catheter, most commonly in combination with or in place of local anesthetics and opioids. The primary analgesic effect appears to be via an α-adrenergic mechanism. Although epidural clonidine has been found to be less potent in terms of analgesic efficacy compared with epidural opioids, such as fentanyl, it has occasionally been substituted for neuraxial opioids because it is associated with a smaller incidence of untoward effects, such as respiratory depression, nausea, and pruritus.[498–501] This also suggests that the combination of all three agents, each at smaller concentrations than required individually, might be beneficial at reducing the incidence of adverse effects while optimizing analgesia, but carefully controlled studies have yet to be performed.

Risks and Untoward Effects

Adverse effects associated with regional analgesia can be grouped according to those caused by the technique (e.g., the catheter) and those related to the medications (e.g., local anesthetics, opioids, other adjuvants). Three large prospective studies have confirmed the safety of regional anesthetics in children, detecting very small complication rates.[470,472,502]

Local anesthetics in the dilute concentrations used for postoperative analgesia have a very small incidence of untoward effects. Motor blockade occurs less frequently with dilute concentrations, but can be observed even with small concentrations of bupivacaine,

TABLE 44.13	Bromage Score[a] for Assessment of Motor Function of the Legs	
Full motor function: can flex hip, knee, and ankle		0
Can't flex hip (unable to perform straight-leg lift)		1
Can't flex hip or knee		2
Can't flex hip, knee, or ankle		3

[a]Note that alternative scoring schemes for the Bromage scale exist that range from 1 to 4 (sometimes denoted I–IV) that directly correspond to the 0–3 scale depicted here.

44

such as 0.1%. As discussed earlier, children with neuromuscular disorders causing motor weakness are especially at risk and should be observed carefully for exacerbation of their motor weakness. Motor weakness and blockade can result in several problems. Inability or difficulty in ambulation may impede recovery. The inability of a child to move a limb can result in skin breakdown or peripheral nerve compression injuries, especially if meticulous attention to frequent repositioning does not occur. We are aware of a case of complex regional pain syndrome in the distribution of the peroneal nerve that arose in this manner. Motor blockade should be avoided, and frequent examinations can quantify motor function using the Bromage score (Table 44.13). At our institutions, motor function is assessed every 8 hours along with the other vital signs pertinent to regional blockade. If motor blockade occurs, the clinician should (1) reduce the dose (volume or concentration) of local anesthetic, (2) pay strict attention to padding and to frequent repositioning of the extremity involved, and (3) consider stopping the infusion until motor function returns. *Rapid onset of more profound motor block during epidural infusion should raise immediate concern about erosion of the catheter into the subarachnoid space.* Motor blockade may occur more frequently with peripheral nerve or plexus analgesia than with epidural blocks, and is subject to the same precautions. When children are discharged home with a peripheral nerve catheter, it is particularly important to teach the parents how to deal with motor blockade and to protect the extremity from unintended injury.

The PK of bupivacaine have been studied in infants and children after both single-injection doses[503] and continuous infusions. Reduced protein binding increases the free fraction of circulating bupivacaine, which increases the risk of bupivacaine toxicity.[504] Neonates and infants with immature clearance may be at particular risk for bupivacaine accumulation.[483] Seizures and cardiac arrest have been reported when large doses of bupivacaine have been administered, usually after excessive infusion rates or unintended intravascular injection. Limited information is available regarding extended administration over days, although low concentration solutions (and therefore low total doses) reduce the risk for toxicity. *l*-Enantiomers of amino amides (ropivacaine and levobupivacaine) have toxic thresholds that are greater than that of bupivacaine by as much as 30%, and such drugs should be considered in smaller children and for blocks that require greater infusion rates and for greater durations. A particular "hidden" risk occurs when a block is functioning less than optimally and bolus doses are administered in an attempt to broaden the dermatome level. Even though the infusion rate is kept within the recommended range, the bolus doses can raise the blood concentration above the toxic threshold. *Whenever a local anesthetic is administered by continuous infusion, nursing and medical staff must be aware of the signs and symptoms of local-anesthetic toxicity, be vigilant in monitoring for the early detection*

of those signs, and be familiar with the use of lipid rescue protocols to treat toxicity if it occurs. The use of lipid emulsion for treating local anesthetic toxicity is discussed in detail in Chapter 42.

Tachyphylaxis during prolonged administration of local anesthetics is a theoretic consideration, although no systematic studies have addressed this phenomenon in children. In animal models, tachyphylaxis is accelerated by hyperalgesia and prevented by agents that prevent hyperalgesia at spinal sites. One rationale for coadministration of opioids or clonidine in epidural infusions may be to reduce the incidence or severity of tachyphylaxis. As discussed in Chapter 42, hemodynamic stability is maintained in children younger than 6 years of age during spinal or epidural blockade, even with extensive sympathetic blockade. As children approach school age, however, rapid position changes may produce hemodynamic responses after extensive sympathetic blockade, and this must be considered in children who receive continuous epidural blockade. Orthostatic changes may be exacerbated when epidural clonidine is infused, and extra caution should be taken.

Neuraxial opioids confer several potential adverse effects, including respiratory depression, nausea, urinary retention, and pruritus. Indeed, despite their proven analgesic efficacy, not all practitioners are proponents of their use because of these effects, preferring other adjuvants instead.[505] The most effective means of treating or preventing the adverse effects is the use of opioid antagonists or mixed agonist-antagonists. This approach directly targets the etiology of the signs rather than simply treating their manifestations. Low-dose naloxone infusions, which have been shown to be effective in children receiving parenteral opioids, are also effective for treating the adverse effects of neuraxial opioids, although pediatric data are lacking.[506–510] We have used rates similar to those shown effective in the PCA studies, beginning at 0.25 µg/ kg per hour.[261] This infusion rate can be titrated upward as needed to 1 µg/kg per hour without adversely affecting analgesic efficacy.[262]

The most worrisome and dangerous complication is respiratory depression. The lipophilic agents (fentanyl and sufentanil) have the widest therapeutic indexes. This results from greater receptor binding in the substantia gelatinosa of the spinal cord adjacent to the area of drug administration, thus limiting the rostral spread of the drug, but systemic absorption is considerably greater, resulting in risk of respiratory depression owing to greater blood concentrations. Even though the hydrophilic opioids, hydromorphone and morphine, pose a risk for respiratory depression, the incidence remains small when prudent dosing is followed. Nevertheless, reports in the pediatric literature of respiratory depression after epidural administration of morphine demonstrate that vigilance in monitoring is mandatory.[413,511,512] *The hallmark of impending overdose of central neuraxial opioids is increasing sedation and decreasing DEPTH AND RATE of respiration. It is important to recognize that the depth of respiration must be assessed, not just the rate, because children frequently develop decreased tidal volume before the respiratory rate decreases, leading to alveolar hypoventilation and the potential for hypercarbia and hypoxemia.*[513] Monitoring patients receiving neuraxial opioids entails considerations similar to those with systemic opioids as discussed earlier. As previously noted, pulse oximetry becomes a poorly sensitive monitor for hypoventilation if the child is using supplemental oxygen, and capnographic techniques are plagued by a high rate of false alarms and not well tolerated by children. Again, it is emphasized that no monitor can replace vigilance and frequent clinical assessment.

Oversedation, diminished respiratory depth, and slowing of the respiratory rate are treated by decreasing the rate of opioid administration and, if necessary, administering small incremental doses of naloxone (0.5–1 µg/kg) every few minutes until the adverse effects are reversed (see earlier discussion). A continuous low-dose infusion of naloxone, as described earlier (0.25–1 µg/kg per hour) may need to be started. More profound respiratory depression, including inability to arouse the child and apnea, must be treated more aggressively. *The new development of respiratory depression in a child receiving what appears to be an appropriate opioid dose should always raise the question of catheter migration into the subarachnoid space. Whenever central neuraxial opioids are administered, facilities must be immediately available at the child's bedside for resuscitation, in the unlikely event of respiratory depression.* It is recommended that emergency equipment, including a bag-valve device, appropriate sizes of masks and airways, and suction, be at the child's bedside or in a "code cart" that is accessible within seconds, should the need arise. Naloxone should similarly be immediately available, without the need to obtain the drug from the pharmacy. All children receiving continuous regional analgesia should also have an IV line (a heparin lock is adequate in those children not requiring IV fluids).

Pruritus is a common adverse effect associated with epidural or intrathecal opioid use, occurring in as many as 30% to 70% of children. Antihistamines are less effective antipruritics in this situation, because the primary mechanism is a central opioid, not a histamine effect. Thus opioid antagonists, used in small doses, are most effective. Again, low-dose infusions of naloxone can be administered with good results.[262,506,507,509,510] Some practitioners have found low-dose nalbuphine to be effective to antagonize pruritus (25 to 50 µg/kg every 6 hours PRN).[507,508] In the only pediatric study of nalbuphine, it was no better than placebo. However, the placebo arm in this study had a remarkable efficacy of 58% (nalbuphine 57%).[514]

Nausea and vomiting can also occur in association with opioids (both systemic and neuraxial) and may be more common with morphine than with fentanyl. Children who are fasted during the first 24 hours after surgery do not vomit excessively, even when given caudal morphine.[515] As with all other opioid adverse effects, nausea and vomiting respond to the previously mentioned doses of naloxone or mixed agonist-antagonists, such as nalbuphine. Some antiemetics, such as antihistamines and butyrophenones (e.g., droperidol), may cause sedation and should be used with caution. Serotonin receptor antagonists, such as ondansetron (0.1–0.15 mg/kg, maximum 4 mg) or dolasetron (0.35 mg/kg, maximum 12.5 mg), may be effective and not cause sedation.[516] Metoclopramide in doses of 0.1 to 0.15 mg/kg IV every 6 to 8 hours may provide adequate relief, with less sedation than other drugs of its class. It is sometimes prudent to decrease the infusion rate of the epidural (if the block level permits) or the opioid concentration in the infusate when untoward effects require treatment. Untoward effects of epidural opioids and their treatment are summarized in Table 44.12.

Urinary retention is a relatively common complication of neuraxial opioids. Studies of single-injection caudal blocks have found that this complication does not occur when epidural local anesthetics are used, only when neuraxial opioids are added.[517] Neuraxial opioids depress detrusor contractility in a dose-dependent manner, and this effect may actually outlast the analgesic effect of the drug by hours.[518,519] Different approaches have been used for this problem, including indwelling urinary catheterization and the use of opioid antagonists.[520]

Concerns have been raised that regional analgesia could mask or delay the detection of compartment syndrome of an extremity because of the intensity or quality of analgesia produced by neural blockade.[521] Despite the theoretical worries, this has not been demonstrated in numerous studies, and indeed, the opposite has been observed, that the onset of pain in a patient with previously adequate analgesia from an epidural or nerve block is an early warning sign that may herald the onset of compartment syndrome.[522,523] The concentration of local anesthetics used for postoperative analgesia appears to be inadequate to mask the intensity of ischemic pain caused by compartment syndrome.[524] In addition, epidural blockade is not effective in controlling the discomfort from intense pressure (as demonstrated by the parturient's ability to perceive pressure during labor contractions despite being pain-free). The loss of effective analgesia in a child at risk of compartment syndrome should raise suspicion and prompt urgent investigation before any changes are made to the analgesic regimen (see also Chapter 30).

Catheter-Related Complications

Catheter-related complications are common, with an incidence of around 5% in most studies.[452,502] Although they are generally minor, a nonfunctioning catheter usually results in premature discontinuation of the infusion and a reliance on opioids for analgesia. Inadequate analgesia must prompt an examination of the child and a review of the operative procedure and the analgesic technique. The dermatome level should be determined using differentiation between cold and warm sensation in children who are cognitively and developmentally able to cooperate. Presence of a dermatome level suggests a successful block of inadequate height. No demonstrable blockade suggests a primary malfunction, although low concentrations of local anesthetic may make differentiation of the level difficult in some children. If there were difficulties during catheter placement coupled with a lack of effective analgesia when the child emerges from general anesthesia, the catheter is likely malpositioned. We often use epidurography in this situation to determine whether the catheter is in the epidural space. Misplacement in various locations has been reported, including the subdural space, paravertebral space, tissue planes adjacent to the spine, and even in an epidural blood vessel after a negative test dose.[463,525–527] The catheter's location can be easily visualized on a plain radiograph (or with fluoroscopy in the OR) after the injection of a small volume of nonionic contrast agent. Contrast agent in the epidural space has a characteristic "bubbly" appearance, with the contrast agent centrally located over the spinal column (Fig. 44.10). The existence of a median raphe in the epidural space has been postulated and may be the cause of unilateral multi-dermatome blockade.[528] This has been demonstrated on epidurography when unilateral blockade has occurred (Fig. 44.11). A single unilateral dermatomal band of analgesia or temperature-sensation change may indicate that the catheter has passed through a spinal foramen. In some cases, simply withdrawing the catheter 1 or 2 cm may allow proper repositioning within the epidural space. A functional, rather than anatomic, method of confirming epidural placement is the "chloroprocaine test," which has the advantage of both providing rapid analgesia (with a properly located catheter) and confirming the site of placement. A chloroprocaine test is presented in Fig. 44.12.

On occasion, a collection of fluid may be found at the skin insertion site and pooling under the dressing. Experience suggests that in most cases this is not, as one may fear, cerebrospinal fluid, but rather edema fluid, or occasionally local anesthetic solution, tracking along the catheter's course and leaking through a hole in the skin from the subcutaneous tissues. Local anesthetic solutions

The catheter site should be inspected daily to ensure that the dressing is intact and to assess for the presence of infection. Infections are exceedingly rare, perhaps in part because of the bactericidal properties of the local anesthetics themselves.[530] Although colonization of catheters, usually with *Staphylococcus epidermidis* and other gram-positive organisms, appears common, adult and pediatric studies have shown that this is not associated with neuraxial infection.[531,532] In the U.K. epidural audit, there were three cases of deep tissue infection and 25 local infections reported out of 10,660 epidural catheters, and longitudinal data from a single institution showed similar rates of infection.[470,533] Tunneling a catheter subcutaneously may reduce the risk of bacteriologic contamination and permit the use of a catheter for a greater period of time.[454] A study of the microbiology of the infusion fluids and delivery systems has demonstrated that catheter-related infections of the deep tissues, including epidural abscess, appear to have their origin in local skin infections that track along the catheter's path or via a bacteremia.[534] *Any sign of local infection is cause for immediate catheter removal.* Epidural abscess is a catastrophic complication that can be generally avoided if the catheter is removed early, when only a localized cutaneous infection is present.[535] Clinical signs include fever, malaise, and back pain. Specific neurologic signs, paresthesias, and motor symptoms (e.g., flaccid paralysis as cord compression develops, eventually progressing to spasticity) may occur late in the course if early warning signs are not heeded, but may progress rapidly once established. Children who develop fever or sepsis need to be evaluated on an individual basis. If a clear source for the fever is found, it is acceptable to leave the catheter in place with regular and frequent observation and reassessment, although we remove it if a child is overtly septic or if the situation is unclear.

Plexus Catheters

Catheters may be placed adjacent to upper and lower extremity plexuses. The prolonged duration of analgesia after a single-injection plexus blocks reduces the need for an indwelling catheter in many instances, and duration of action can be further prolonged by the adjunctive use of dexamethasone.[398,536] Specialized kits for peripheral nerve and plexus cannulation are commercially available. These catheters are inserted using the same landmarks and techniques as for placing a single-injection block. After initial dosing, 0.125% bupivacaine or 0.2% ropivacaine at 0.1 to 0.2 mL/kg per hour may be infused. Potential complications of continuous brachial plexus blockade include infection and nerve injury, although these are quite rare, and no persistent neurologic deficits have been reported in major pediatric databases.[452,458]

Infusions can be delivered with conventional infusion pumps or disposable elastomeric controlled infusion devices described earlier. We often use conventional infusion pumps for inpatients owing to reduced cost and to the increased safety that may be inherent in the familiarity of the inpatient nurses with such systems. The disposable devices permit the child to be discharged home and still receive long-lasting analgesia with a regional anesthetic. Most commonly, 0.2% ropivacaine is used at rates of 0.1 to 0.2 mL/kg per hour.[452] An organized system of daily follow-up by telephone or visiting nurses is essential for safety and efficacy of such a service, but both limited published and anecdotal experience suggests that ambulatory analgesia with peripheral neural blockade can be an effective modality in pediatric outpatients.[458] Catheters with multiple side holes can be placed in a fascial plane or wound bed by the surgeon at the time of closure and local anesthetics are infused over several days for postoperative analgesia. There

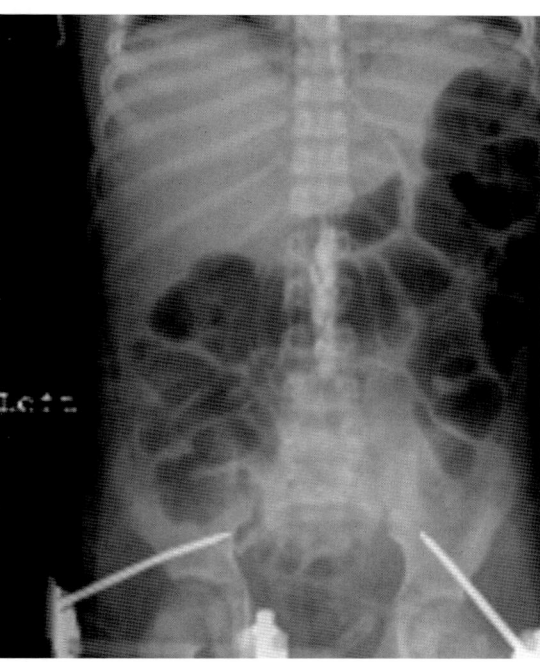

FIGURE 44.10 An epidurogram shows the appearance of the contrast agent centered in the spinal column and also the bubbly appearance of the contrast agent, presumably produced by the epidural fat and plexus.

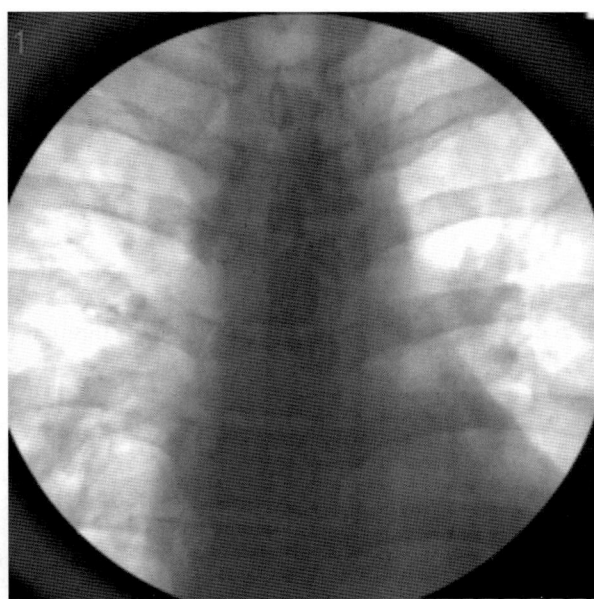

FIGURE 44.11 Epidurogram taken with fluoroscopy demonstrating unilateral spread of contrast agent. The contrast agent appears to have a very sharp edge precisely in the center of the spinal column, demarcating one side of the epidural space from the other.

would test negative for glucose and protein, whereas cerebrospinal fluid and edema fluid would test positive for glucose and protein. It usually requires no special treatment except reinforcing the dressing. It subsides as the edema and third-space fluids are mobilized in the first days after surgery. Application of collodion or cyanoacrylate skin bonding over the insertion site can reduce leakage around the catheter.[529]

PROCEDURE FOR THE CHLOROPROCAINE TEST

An anesthesiologist is present for the procedure with use of standard monitors and supplies for providing respiratory or hemodynamic support.

1. A loading dose of chloroprocaine 3% is divided in five equal increments, each given at 1- to 2-minute intervals (over 5-10 minutes total) according to weight approximately as follows: (doses may be adjusted according to clinical circumstances)

Weight Group	Increment Volume	Total Volume
0-10 kg	0.125 mL/kg	0.6 mL/kg
10-20 kg	0.1 mL/kg	0.5 mL/kg
20-35 kg	2.5 mL (fixed volume)	12.5 mL (fixed volume)
35-60 kg	3 mL (fixed volume)	15 mL (fixed volume)
≥60 kg	3.5 mL (fixed volume)	17.5 mL (fixed volume)

2. Incremental dosing is stopped before giving the full dose if there are clear signs of bilateral lower extremity sensory or motor block, or a very definite reduction in heart rate (e.g., 30 beats/min) and blood pressure (e.g., 25-mm Hg drop in systolic pressure). In most cases, because you are performing this test because of signs of pain, there is some tachycardia and hypertension relative to baseline values at the start of the test. Transient cessation of crying in an infant or toddler is not a sufficiently specific positive response to warrant interruption of the test.

3. A catheter positioned in the **thoracic** epidural space will generally not show lower extremity sensory or motor block with the chloroprocaine test, but should give a very clear drop in heart rate and blood pressure, as well as a clear and persistent reduction in pain reports or pain behaviors.

4. If the chloroprocaine test is positive (i.e., confirms epidural placement), this implies that a stronger or different epidural solution is needed for steady-state pain relief. Because hydromorphone is sufficiently hydrophilic to spread from lumbar to thoracic spinal levels, **switching the solution from bupivacaine-fentanyl to bupivacaine-hydromorphone will provide good steady-state pain relief in >90% of these cases**. A typical loading dose of hydromorphone of 2 µg/kg (0.002 mg/kg) will provide analgesia within 30 minutes in most cases.

If the chloroprocaine test fails to confirm epidural placement, the catheter is repositioned, removed, or replaced according to clinical circumstances.

FIGURE 44.12 Chloroprocaine test to determine regional catheter function as performed at Children's Hospital, Boston. (Personal communication, C. Berde.)

are very limited data in children, but such techniques have been reported to be effective.[377,537,538] There are no studies to date comparing infusion rates; volumes of 2 to 5 mL/hour of 0.2% ropivacaine have most commonly been used, infused via the elastomeric pumps previously described.

Removal of Catheters and Transition to Oral Analgesics

The transition from continuous regional blockade to oral analgesics should ideally be achieved without a significant decrement in the quality of pain relief for the child and should permit the clinician to revert to more aggressive modalities, should the decision prove to be premature. The duration of continuous blockade is, of course, in large part dependent on the type of operation and the underlying medical and/or surgical problems of the child. Some children do well with transition to oral analgesics on the morning after surgery. This is often the case for the child who has undergone an uncomplicated ureteral reimplantation. For more painful procedures, such as Nuss bar placement for pectus excavatum in an adolescent, strong analgesics will be required for a greater duration. The norm in this situation is up to 3 days. We find it most effective to begin the transition from regional analgesia to oral therapy early in the morning. As soon as the regional infusion is discontinued, a dose of oral analgesic, usually an oral opioid

such as oxycodone, is administered. In addition, by this time the child should already be receiving scheduled nonopioid oral adjuvants (i.e., NSAID, acetaminophen). This ensures that the oral agents have provided their full effect before the block recedes. The catheter is not removed until the child has demonstrated that the oral agents provide adequate comfort without any residual analgesia from the block, so that blockade can be reestablished if transition fails.

Children who are anticoagulated require special consideration before removing epidural catheters. Although there are no specific pediatric data, the recommendations of the consensus panel of the American Society of Regional Anesthesia and Pain Medicine, last published in 2010, are generally accepted.[539] The report notes *"the initiation of systemic therapeutic heparin therapy for medical or surgical indications in the presence of a neuraxial catheter potentially increases the risk of hematoma formation during catheter removal"* (https://www.asra.com/advisory-guidelines/article/1/anticoagulation-3rd-edition). Recommendations regarding how long to withhold heparin therapy before removing the catheter and how long to wait before restarting heparin vary based on whether the patient is receiving subcutaneous prophylactic doses (withhold 4–6 hours before removing the catheter, and restart immediately after removing it) or a therapeutic IV infusion (withhold 2–4 hours before removing the catheter, restart the infusion 1 hour after removal). Fractionated or low–molecular-weight heparins pose a risk as well, compounded by several different regimens in common clinical use (once-a-day vs. twice-a-day dosing), differences between different agents, and the inability to assess the degree of anticoagulation with commonly available tests of coagulation (prothrombin time and partial thromboplastin time). The consensus panel recommends that catheters should be removed no sooner than 10 to 12 hours after the last dose of low–molecular-weight heparin with once-a-day administration, and dosing should resume no sooner than 4 hours after the catheter's removal. The use of continuous regional techniques is not recommended when twice-a-day administration is used. Many national societies have also published evidence-based guidelines that can assist in decision making, and the American Society of Regional Anesthesia and Pain Medicine has developed a smartphone app on this subject.

Pain Management in the Cognitively Impaired Child

The goals of pain management in the child with cognitive impairment are to minimize discomfort, maximize function, and improve the quality of life. With these goals in mind, the child's pain management plans should include multimodal pharmacologic and nonpharmacologic strategies tailored to the severity and etiology of pain. The World Health Organization's analgesic guideline[184] provides a framework for decision making related to analgesic use based on severity and persistence of pain.

OPIOID ANALGESICS

The use of opioids in children with cognitive impairment has been limited by concerns regarding potential adverse effects and a perceived reduced margin of safety because of diminished cardiorespiratory reserve and neurologic impairment. Indeed, one study identified that cognitive impairment was an independent predictor of adverse events from PCA/NCA.[84] It is, therefore, necessary to carefully balance the goals of providing adequate analgesia while minimizing adverse events related to analgesic treatments. For moderate to severe pain, scheduled nonopioid analgesics combined with judicious use of opioids titrated to effect is a suitable option. Children with cognitive impairment may lack the cognitive and motor skills to use PCA devices successfully. In these children, NCA or CCA will permit titration of small amounts of opioids to effect, without significantly increasing nursing workload.[540] A study of children whose postoperative pain was managed by parent- or nurse-controlled analgesia reported low pain scores and modest opioid requirements, with the use of basal infusions in addition to bolus dosing, in the majority of children.[541] Adverse effects included nausea and vomiting, and pruritus requiring treatment in 14% and 32% of children, respectively. Supplemental oxygen was required in 79% of the children, and respiratory depression requiring naloxone was noted in 2.8%. The management of two children was remarkable, in that one had received an average morphine dose of 0.045 mg/kg per hour and four concomitant sedatives, including diphenhydramine, diazepam, droperidol, and chloral hydrate, and the second had received only a small dose of morphine and no other sedatives, but the basal infusion of morphine was implicated as the cause of respiratory depression. Both recovered without sequelae. The studies noted previously highlight the importance of frequent and careful assessment of pain, depth of sedation, and respiratory status (using continuous pulse oximetry and/or noninvasive capnography) to ensure the safety and the comfort of children with cognitive impairment receiving opioid therapy

NONOPIOID ANALGESICS

Nonopioid adjuvants, such as acetaminophen, NSAIDs, or tramadol, should be added to provide synergistic analgesia and to reduce opioid requirements. They may be administered orally or via gastrostomy tubes. IV ketorolac provides excellent analgesia in children who have not initiated oral intake after surgery, although the risks of platelet dysfunction must be considered if ongoing bleeding is an issue. The α_2-agonist clonidine has also been used for its synergistic analgesic effects in these patients. However, it has the potential to cause sedation and hypotension.

Muscle spasms and clonus are an ongoing source of pain that may be difficult to differentiate in children who are cognitively impaired, and may be exacerbated after surgical procedures, particularly orthopedic and neurosurgical procedures. Diazepam, baclofen, and tizanidine all effectively treat acute painful muscle spasms after surgery in children with spasticity, but all of these medications have sedative effects, which can confound patient assessment when used with opioids. Benzodiazepines in particular have synergistic respiratory depressant effects when used in conjunction with opioids, so judicious use is essential.

EPIDURAL AND REGIONAL ANALGESIA

Epidural analgesia has been used with success in children who are cognitively impaired who are undergoing lower extremity orthopedic procedures, selective dorsal rhizotomy, and Nissen fundoplication.[91,542] Epidural catheters may be technically difficult to place in some of these children because of contractures and spine deformities. However, when feasible, this technique provides excellent analgesia, reduces muscle spasms, and promotes overall child comfort, with a small incidence of sedation and respiratory depression. Some children will still experience muscle spasms and will require intermittent benzodiazepines. Epidurals have been compared with systemic opioids in children with cerebral palsy undergoing selective dorsal rhizotomy.[91,543] Epidural catheters were placed under direct visualization by the neurosurgeon at the end of surgery. Both studies showed improved analgesia in the epidural groups, and one study demonstrated a lower incidence of desaturation in the epidural group, which allowed patients in this group to go directly to the general ward (instead of the pediatric ICU).[543] In summary, these studies support the attributes and safety of epidural analgesia in children with cognitive impairment.

Children with cerebral palsy who received continuous infusion of local anesthetics via catheters tunneled into the incision site following orthopedic surgery experienced significantly lower pain scores and required less oral analgesics on the first two postoperative days, compared with controls who received oral analgesics alone.[537] Although data related to peripheral and plexus blocks in cognitively impaired children are limited, our experience suggests that these, too, are safe and effective in this population and can contribute to reducing the reliance on systemic analgesics and, thereby, their adverse effects.

Emerging data must be used to guide treatment plans and protocols that incorporate frequent evaluation and careful monitoring of children with cognitive impairment. Involving a multidisciplinary pain team that includes the primary care provider, pain specialist, psychologist, nurse, physical therapist, and occupational therapist is required to provide the level of expertise to care for these children with special needs.

Summary

Postoperative analgesia is an integral and essential component of any pediatric anesthetic plan. Contemporary knowledge of anatomy, physiology, pharmacokinetics, and pharmacodynamics in infancy and childhood permits the anesthesiologist to apply advanced anesthetic and analgesic techniques with excellent efficacy and safety to all children. Analgesic plans should use a balanced approach, including nonopioid analgesics and regional anesthetic techniques, with the goal of minimizing opioid consumption and side effects. Clinical examples of postoperative management strategies are presented in Appendix 44.1. The optimal use of these modalities requires an understanding of the techniques outlined in this chapter, as well as the integration of multiple medical and nursing disciplines in the assessment and care of these children. A well-organized pediatric pain service and an educated nursing staff are the keys to the successful management of acute pain, which, in turn, can be expected to result in improved care for infants and children.[544]

ACKNOWLEDGMENT

We wish to thank Charles J. Coté, Maurice Zwass, and Shobha Malviya for their prior contributions to this chapter.

ANNOTATED REFERENCES

Berde CB, Sethna NF. Analgesics for the treatment of pain in children. *N Engl J Med.* 2002;347(14):1094-1103.

This authoritative reference provides a succinct yet complete review of the pharmacology of effective analgesic regimens in children.

Llewellyn N, Moriarty A. The national pediatric epidural audit. *Paediatr Anaesth.* 2007;17(6):520-533.

The largest prospective study on epidural anesthesia to date followed patients into the postoperative period and highlights the incidence and nature of complications and adverse events, which were rare. This should be read in conjunction with the French study and the PRAN studies.

Lynn AM, Nespeca MK, Opheim KE, Slattery JT. Respiratory effects of intravenous morphine infusions in neonates, infants, and children after cardiac surgery. *Anesth Analg.* 1993;77(4):695-701.

This old but important study identified the threshold serum morphine concentration for respiratory depression in neonates, infants, and children receiving continuous morphine infusions following heart surgery to be 20 ng/mL and, as such, provides a framework to guide appropriate dosing of morphine in these populations. The authors recommended careful observation of all children receiving morphine because of the wide variability in the CO_2 response slope seen in their subjects.

Malviya S, Voepel-Lewis T, Burke C, et al. The revised FLACC observational pain tool: improved reliability and validity for pain assessment in children with cognitive impairment. *Pediatr Anesth.* 2006;16:258-265.

The FLACC tool was revised to incorporate behavioral descriptors consistently associated with pain in cognitively impaired children. This paper describes the development of the Revised Face, Legs, Activity, Cry, Consolability (r-FLACC) scale and demonstrates its reliability and validity in assessing pain in this vulnerable population.

Maxwell LG, Kaufmann SC, Bitzer S, et al. The effects of a small-dose naloxone infusion on opioid-induced side effects and analgesia in children and adolescents treated with intravenous patient-controlled analgesia: a double-blind, prospective, randomized, controlled study. *Anesth Analg.* 2005;100(4):953-958.

This study demonstrated that a low-dose naloxone infusion significantly reduced the incidence and severity of opioid-induced adverse effects, including pruritus and nausea, without affecting opioid-induced analgesia. These data address the important clinical problem of opioid-induced adverse effects that frequently limits the utility of opioids in the treatment of pain.

Michelet D, Andreu-Gallien J, Bensalah T, et al. A meta-analysis of the use of nonsteroidal anti-inflammatory drugs for pediatric postoperative pain. *Anesth Analg.* 2012;114(2):393-406.

This meta-analysis shows that perioperative NSAID administration reduces opioid consumption and PONV during the postoperative period in children. In 27 randomized controlled trials, perioperative administration of NSAIDs reduced opioid requirement in the postanesthesia care unit (PACU) and for the first 24 hours after surgery, decreased pain intensity in the PACU and PONV during the first 24 hours postoperatively. Results from this study suggest that multimodal analgesia should be used in an effort to reduce opioid consumption and adverse effects in children undergoing surgery.

Morton NS, Errera A. APA national audit of pediatric opioid infusions. *Paediatr Anaesth.* 2010;20(2):119-125.

This very large prospective audit of opioid infusions of all types (continuous, PCA, NCA) confirmed the safety of these techniques, but highlights the potential complications and pitfalls that are always present. Respiratory depression and pump programming errors each occurred in about 1 of 766 cases and 1 of 631 cases, respectively, and there was one permanent injury (1 of 10,000 cases).

Polaner DM, Taenzer AH, Walker BJ, et al. Pediatric regional anesthesia network: a multi-institutional study of the use and incidence of complications of pediatric regional anesthesia. *Anesth Analg.* 2012;115(6):1353-1364.

This is the first report from this network in the United States that prospectively examined the incidence of adverse events and complications in nearly 15,000 regional blocks in children. There were no permanent complications detected. PRAN now has over 140,000 cases accrued. These data provided similar results to those reported in the French study.[472]

Voepel-Lewis T, Burke CN, Jeffreys N, et al. Do 0-10 numeric rating scores translate into clinically meaningful pain measures for children? *Anesth Analg.* 2011;112(2):415-421.

This study provides important information regarding the clinical interpretation of NRS pain scores in children. Ten NRS scores were found to be reliably associated with the child's perceived need for medicine, perceived pain relief, and satisfaction with pain treatment. However, a significant overlap in scores associated with these outcomes suggests that the use of specific cutoff scores to guide treatment decisions would be inappropriate in children.

von Baeyer CL, Spagrud LJ. Systematic review of observational (behavioral) measures of pain for children and adolescents aged 3 to 18 years. *Pain.* 2007;127(1-2):140-150.

This is a comprehensive review of the numerous behavioral observational measures of pain for children and identifies the most appropriate tools for assessing pain in various settings, including the postoperative period and in critical care.

A complete reference list can be found online at ExpertConsult.com.

Chronic Pain

ROBERT BAKER, ALEXANDRA SZABOVA, AND KENNETH GOLDSCHNEIDER

THE PRACTICING PEDIATRIC ANESTHESIOLOGIST is involved in chronic pain in one of three main venues: a child who is scheduled for a procedure, in consultation, or during acute pain management rounds. In this chapter, we focus on the essential approaches to children with chronic pain and provide guidelines to help the children and colleagues who request anesthesiology assistance.

Chronic Pain in Children

Chronic pain affects a large number of children.[1] Back pain has been reported in up to 50% of children by the mid-teens,[2] and abdominal pain occurs weekly in up to 17%.[3] Other conditions, such as headaches, complex regional pain syndrome (CRPS), fibromyalgia, limb pain, chest pain, and joint pain, are also common and may substantively affect their quality of life.[4-7]

Several chronic medical conditions are strongly associated with pain and blur the boundaries between acute and chronic pain treatment, including sickle cell disease, cystic fibrosis,[8] epidermolysis bullosa,[9] and cancer. These children require frequent hospitalizations, and their pain can be severe. Because these children present with pain in the hospital, treatment often follows the model for acute pain management based on medication use. However, psychosocial factors heavily influence the child's ability to cope with the pain and have a variable effect on the child's suffering, depending on personal and family factors.[10,11] It is appropriate to include psychology, child-life, and physical therapy consultations as part of the comprehensive team approach to developing a therapeutic plan for these children. The ultimate goal for each of these medical conditions is to stabilize the child's condition and return her or him home. For many, the painful disease and dysfunction are persistent, thus necessitating a long-term plan that is integrated with acute management.

Multidisciplinary Approach

The model of care that appears to work optimally for children with chronic pain is one in which multiple disciplines are involved in developing a coordinated care plan.[4,12] In the outpatient setting, there is a pain physician, a psychologist, nurses, and a physical therapist. Sometimes, a neurologist or physiatrist may be involved. Anesthesiologists managing children with chronic pain should make use of these disciplines when recommending a plan of care. Advocating for the involvement of other therapeutic specialties can advance the child's care beyond suggesting a regional block or medication.

THE PAIN PHYSICIAN

The consulting anesthesiologist in an inpatient setting may be called on to provide care for one of three reasons. First, the child may need a regional nerve block, such as an epidural steroid injection for magnetic resonance imaging–confirmed discogenic pain or epidural catheter placement to assist physical therapy. This consultation is fairly straightforward and is an extension of basic regional anesthesia principles. Second, the child who has been prescribed long-term use of opioids or other medications that interact with anesthetic or postoperative pain drugs may present for consultation. The anesthesiologist must investigate which chronic medications have been prescribed and determine whether drug interactions may exist. Opioid requirements of patients who take opioids chronically may have different requirements during and after surgery that may differ from those who are opioid naïve. This approach is an extension of basic perioperative anesthesia management. Third, a consultation may be requested to assess and diagnose the source of pain. This scenario is the most complex and requires a detailed history and thorough physical examination. These children often require multidisciplinary care beginning with the initial evaluation and extending through treatment.

THE PSYCHOLOGIST

Pain is more than just a physical phenomenon. It can cause and be exacerbated by stress, suffering, family dysfunction, social tension, anxiety, and depression.[7,13] Pain can disrupt almost any aspect of the life of the child and family. Family and school problems can worsen a painful condition and dramatically reduce a child's level of function. The family is invariably involved in the child's suffering and should be included in the process of evaluating the pain.

Families are often wary about seeing a psychologist and are afraid of being stigmatized. It is important to emphasize that pain is what the child says it is, regardless of whether an organic cause can be identified. The child should be treated as a person, not just as the painful body part. Such an approach should be emphasized to the child's family to begin to address the pain.

Psychology-based therapy includes relaxation training, biofeedback, hypnotherapy, coping skills training, and psychotherapy. Together, these therapies are referred to as cognitive behavioral therapy, which is a cornerstone of chronic pain treatment. Therapies aimed at parental and familial aspects of the child's pain include teaching strategies for behavioral interventions (e.g., distraction), activity pacing, consistent discipline, coaching skills training, stress management, and occasionally, family therapy.

THE PHYSICAL THERAPIST

Physical therapy is a crucial component of evaluating and treating chronic pain. The painful condition can cause loss of muscle strength and range of motion, which may affect the biomechanics and daily function of the body. Children can become deconditioned and require a conditioning program to regain lost strength and stamina. These changes affect the original pain site and generate secondary pain problems that need to be addressed.

Physical therapy can benefit many painful conditions (e.g., myofascial pain improves with stretching and range-of-motion exercises) and is the foundation of treatment for others (e.g., CRPS).[14] Emphasizing self-reliance and responsibility for their own care is an important aspect of caring for adolescents. However, young and older children in pain cannot be expected to work aggressively at home without the support of a structured program. Parental involvement is especially important for younger children, but the caretakers must be taught techniques to encourage and support the child, while not making them the child's taskmasters.

Therapies provided by physical therapy include stretching, strengthening, and reconditioning programs. Range-of-motion exercises and endurance training are also important. Aquatic therapy is very useful for children who cannot bear weight on their lower limbs or have limited range of motion or strength. Massage, heat, and cold therapies are also helpful adjuncts to increase function and enhance other physical therapy modalities.

Transcutaneous electrical nerve stimulation (TENS) is an effective,[15] low-risk, analgesic therapy that is usually provided under the guidance of a physical therapist. TENS is excellent for localized pain. The fact that it is portable, can be used discreetly, and has few adverse effects makes it attractive for use at school. Because tolerance to TENS can develop with prolonged use, children need to limit use to no longer than 2 hours at a time. They can take a break for an amount of time equal to the TENS use and then restart it.

THE NURSE

Pain nurses play a major role in hospital-wide education of floor nurses regarding assessment and treatment of pain, including the use of epidural and patient-controlled analgesia (PCA) pumps. When beginning a chronic pain program, the first personnel to recruit should be an advanced practice nurse who can be trained to triage, perform the initial evaluation and intake assessment, and assist with all subsequent pain-related issues that do not require the direct input of a physician.

THE CONSULTANT

Anesthesiologists should be cognizant of their limitations and judiciously use consultants to help diagnose conditions and fashion the optimal treatment plan. Neurologists typically are well versed in headache management and familiar with the medications used for neuropathic pain. Physical medicine and rehabilitation specialists can assist in structuring a treatment plan for a variety of musculoskeletal pains and are accomplished in the treatment of spasticity.

General Approach to Management

Most children with chronic, non-cancer pain are adolescents who require special considerations in terms of their history and physical examination. Because they are between childhood and adulthood, their behavior can fluctuate broadly and frequently. It is important to address them directly but also involve the parents to the extent needed to obtain the relevant and complete history. The clinician should not try to be "cool" with the adolescent patient, because teenagers tend to find that approach condescending and may respond negatively. The examiner should instead find a point of common interest and use it to establish rapport.

Adolescents tend to be image conscious. They may or may not want to discuss body functions such as defecation or menstruation, even when these functions are directly relevant to the problem. If a child appears to be uneasy with the questions being asked, the physician should proceed in a straightforward manner, acknowledge their feelings, and reassure them that the information is needed to ensure that appropriate care is delivered. When discussing these children with their parents, clinicians should refer to them as "children and young adults" rather than just "children" because even 12- and 13-year-olds like to think they are no longer children.

HISTORY

The basic history focuses on the pain: location, duration, quality, intensity, aggravating and alleviating factors, associated symptoms, past therapies, and the tests that have been performed and by whom. Pain intensity is often assessed using a 0 to 10 numeric rating scale for children older than approximately 8 years of age. The child must be asked about the current pain level and about the best and worst pain levels to obtain an idea of the pattern of pain and when it peaks. Quality descriptors include *burning, sharp, aching, throbbing, tingling, numb, weird,* and others; each may give a clue about the type of pain the child is experiencing. Odd descriptors, burning, and tingling suggest neuropathic pain; sharp, tight, and aching may indicate bony or muscular causes; throbbing suggests a vascular component; cramping or pain that comes in waves often suggests spasms of a muscle or hollow viscus.

A vital part of the chronic pain evaluation process is to look for *red flags*, which are signs or symptoms that may indicate a serious illness. Some of the red flag signs and symptoms for major pain

45

TABLE 45.1	Red Flag Signs and Symptoms for Abdominal Pain
Persistent right upper or right lower quadrant pain	
Dysphagia	
Persistent or cyclic vomiting	
Gastrointestinal blood loss	
Family history of inflammatory bowel disease, celiac disease, or peptic ulcer disease	
Pain that awakens the child from sleep	
Arthritis	
Nocturnal diarrhea	
Involuntary weight loss	
Deceleration of linear growth	
Delayed puberty	
Unexplained fever	
Hepatosplenomegaly, masses, or perianal lesions	
Bilious emesis	
Costovertebral angle tenderness	

TABLE 45.2	Red Flag Signs and Symptoms for Secondary Headache
Persistent vomiting	
Focal neurologic signs	
Meningeal signs	
Unexplained fever	
Increased intracranial pressure	
Changes in behavior or mental status	
Sudden onset of severe headache	
Morning headaches	
Headaches that awaken the child from sleep	

TABLE 45.3	Red Flag Signs and Symptoms for Back Pain
Unexplained fever	
Night sweats	
Weight loss	
Night pain	
Constant pain	
Bowel function changes	
Urinary retention	
Neurologic changes in legs: trouble walking, foot drop, weakness, loss of reflexes, sensory changes	

has a "bad back" and is functionally compromised, the child also may complain of back pain. This does not mean the child is faking the complaints but simply patterning the behavioral response to pain after a model that he or she understands. Treatment can include reassurance, cognitive behavioral therapy, and gentle physical therapy to restore the child's functional ability and help him or her with any underlying issues. Family and social histories can be useful in fashioning a treatment plan in conjunction with the general history, physical examination, and relevant testing.

PHYSICAL EXAMINATION

The physical examination should focus on the area of interest, but a brief general examination is also important. A full screening examination, including a neurologic examination, takes only a few minutes and can be combined with the social history. A systemic illness may manifest as a localized complaint—for example, diabetes can manifest as abdominal pain or leukemia as focal bone pain.

When examining a child of the opposite sex, the physician should have a nonfamily observer of the same gender as the child present. Some children are very conscious of their bodies and may consider routine examination maneuvers as invasions of their privacy. The occasional child has a history of being abused and can be further traumatized by even a standard examination. Physicians can demonstrate examination techniques that may make the child feel uneasy. For example, a pinprick examination requires a needle or sharp object (a fractured tongue depressor creates a sharp end to test pinprick, but does not look like a needle); the examiner should touch his or her own skin with the object first to demonstrate that blood is not being drawn. Children are often fascinated by the deep tendon reflexes and usually have fun with that examination. Children with chronic pain often have had many examinations, and doing something a little different or fun can help them accept the current evaluation and enhance rapport.

ANCILLARY DATA

By the time patients with chronic pain have reached a pain clinic, they usually have undergone several investigative tests, and those data should be reviewed. After it becomes clear that there is no life-threatening illness, the focus should shift away from further testing. This is often a hard transition for families and children to accept, especially if no concrete diagnosis has been made to explain the pain. It is a challenge for them to embrace the thought that the pain itself is the disease rather than something that is still undiagnosed. Any study that may help to explain the pain or make a diagnosis that had not been entertained should be recommended. However, pursuing tests and imaging in an unfocused manner wastes resources and causes families to postpone treatment while waiting for a diagnosis. Until the patient wholeheartedly endorses the treatment plan and becomes active in it, the child or adolescent's pain will continue unabated.

Chronic Pain Conditions

Any part of the body can hurt, but in practical terms, several diagnostic clusters represent most pediatric pain conditions. The frequency and intensity of the pain can be striking. One study on the 3-month prevalence, characteristics, consequences, and provoking factors of chronic pain described the experience of 749 children and adolescents in one elementary and two secondary schools[19]: 83% experienced pain during the preceding 3 months. The leading sources of pain were headaches (60.5%, also perceived

types can be found in Tables 45.1, 45.2, and 45.3. For example, a child with back pain who also has weak legs and incontinence may have a tethered spinal cord. Headache that is worse in the morning and associated with vomiting suggests increased intracranial pressure. Back pain with pain running down the posterior leg and loss of ankle jerk suggests compression of the S1 nerve root.

A complete pain evaluation comprises further history regarding medications, allergies, family history, and a thorough review of systems. Certain painful conditions, such as migraine headaches,[16] fibromyalgia,[17] irritable bowel syndrome (IBS),[18] and sickle cell disease, have a genetic basis. Knowing the family history can assist in making the correct diagnosis. The child sometimes may model his or her behavior after a family member. For example, if a parent as most bothersome), abdominal pain (43.3%), extremity pain (33.6%), and back pain (30.2%). Many subjects reported associated sleep problems, restriction in hobbies, and eating problems. School absenteeism reached 48.8% in the population with pain. The use of health care resources by children and adolescents with pain was extensive: 50.9% visited the physician's office, and 51.5% reported use of pain medication.

ABDOMINAL PAIN

Abdominal pain is a major source of distress in children that causes anxiety and invites a large amount of testing. This painful condition, formerly referred to as *recurrent abdominal pain*, is now described as *functional gastrointestinal disorders* (FGIDs).[20] Specific criteria exist for the major categories so that FGIDs are no longer considered diagnoses of exclusion. The pain is thought to be caused by abnormal interactions between the enteric nervous system and central nervous system.[21] Research suggests that peripheral sensitization and abnormal central processing of afferent signals at the level of the central nervous system play roles in the pathophysiology of visceral hyperalgesia—a decreased threshold for pain in response to changes in intraluminal pressure.[22] Mast cells are increased in number in the ileum and colon of adults with IBS, and treatment with mast cell stabilizers can improve visceral hypersensitivity in these patients.[23] The history and physical examination focus on excluding warning signs and symptoms of underlying disease (see Table 45.1).[20,24] The role for testing, endoscopy, and radiographic evaluation is limited.

Multidisciplinary treatment of FGIDs includes medication, psychological interventions, and education, which often need to be ongoing. The most important aspect of the treatment plan is to establish realistic goals, which frequently means return of function rather than complete elimination of pain. Although the literature for treatment is sparse, tricyclic antidepressants (TCAs) such as amitriptyline, nortriptyline, or doxepin have been used effectively for FGID-related pain. Anticonvulsants also are useful because they modify nerve conductivity and transmission. Antacids, antispasmodic agents, smooth muscle relaxants, laxatives, and antidiarrheal agents can be added to address symptoms. Data support the use of peppermint oil capsules in managing IBS, although gastroesophageal reflux can be a limiting adverse effect.[25] Probiotics may also be helpful to control IBS symptoms, including abdominal pain.[26] Children with functional bowel disorders can have abnormal bowel reactions to physiologic stimuli, noxious stressful stimuli, or psychological stimuli (e.g., parental separation, anxiety). Children benefit from cognitive behavioral therapy, coping skill development, biofeedback, hypnosis, and relaxation techniques (Table 45.4).[27,28]

HEADACHE

Headaches can be categorized as primary or secondary. Primary headaches include migraine, tension, cluster, and trigeminal neuralgia headaches. Secondary headaches are those attributable to head and neck traumas; muscle spasms; vascular disorders; nonvascular intracranial disorders; infection; eye, ear, cranium, nose, sinus, and teeth or mouth diseases; homeostatic disturbances; and psychiatric disorders. Headaches represent one of the more poorly tolerated types of chronic pain, with greater medication use than for other types. Of 77 children with long-term headaches who were followed up to 20 years after the initial diagnosis, 27% were headache free, and 66% had improved.[29]

Migraines (especially migraine without aura) and tension-type headaches are the most common types of pediatric headaches.

TABLE 45.4	Care Pathway for Abdominal Pain

Evaluation

Medical examination

Behavioral medicine assessment

Review of records, treatments, history, and physical findings

Consultations with pediatrics, surgery, and gastroenterology specialists as indicated by presence of red flags; assessment may include laboratory testing, ultrasound, computed tomography or magnetic resonance imaging, endoscopy, lactose testing

Treatment of Functional Gastrointestinal Disorders

Medications: tricyclic antidepressants; consider gabapentin; peppermint oil

Behavioral medicine: important and effective to de-medicalize therapy; de-emphasize testing and search for organic diagnoses; redirect focus to treatment and improved function

Physical therapy: not usually involved; trial of transcutaneous electrical nerve stimulation (TENS) if abdominal wall origin found

Other therapy:
  Blocks are rare, except in palliative situation; celiac plexus with local anesthetic and steroid; epidural
  Trigger point injections if abdominal wall trigger points found
  Acupuncture
  Hypnosis
  Meditation
  Dietary management

Prevalence estimates of migraine vary 1% to 3% in children 3 to 7 years of age and 8% to 23% in adolescents.[30] It occurs more frequently in boys than girls between 4 and 7 years of age, and then the prevalence equalizes between 7 and 11 years of age. After 11 years of age, three times as many girls as boys have migraines.[31] Studies are not routinely recommended in the absence of focal neurologic findings. However, the practitioner must be alert to red flag signs and symptoms that warrant imaging and laboratory studies to rule out an underlying condition as a cause of the headaches (see Table 45.2).

There is a genetic component to migraine and chronic tension headaches; 50% to 77% of children with migraines have a positive family history for migraine headaches, especially on the maternal side. The clearest genetic link has been established for familial hemiplegic migraine.[16]

Children with frequent headaches often suffer from medication overuse headaches related to chronic or repeated use of over-the-counter analgesics. Ideally, abortive headache medications should be used no more than two to three times per week to prevent medication overuse headaches from developing. If possible, children should be gradually weaned off analgesics.

Treatments for migraine and tension-type headaches overlap greatly. Pharmacologic interventions can be divided in two types. First, abortive treatment focuses on stopping the acute headache. Second, prophylactic therapy is indicated for those patients with more than two headaches per month, for children with severe attacks, and for those with frequent headaches unresponsive to medication (Table 45.5).[32] The importance of lifestyle modifications when necessary cannot be overstated. These may include improved sleep, increased aerobic exercise, limitation of caffeine intake, stress management, attention to hydration, and avoidance of skipping meals.

Attempts to abort headaches typically begin with nonsteroidal antiinflammatory drugs (NSAIDs). If these are not effective, triptans

TABLE 45.5	Care Pathway for Headaches

Evaluation

Medical examination

Behavioral medicine assessment

Physical therapy if neck or upper back tightness occurs

Review of records, treatments, history, and physical findings

Magnetic resonance imaging and neurology consultations as indicated by red flag signs and symptoms

Treatment

Medications: tricyclic antidepressants, topiramate, trazodone, cyproheptadine

Behavioral medicine: biofeedback, relaxation, coping and pacing skills

Physical therapy: transcutaneous electrical nerve stimulation (TENS) unit on shoulders, posterior neck; stretching

Other therapy:
  Yoga
  Acupuncture
  Meditation
  Occasional neck trigger point injection or occipital nerve block

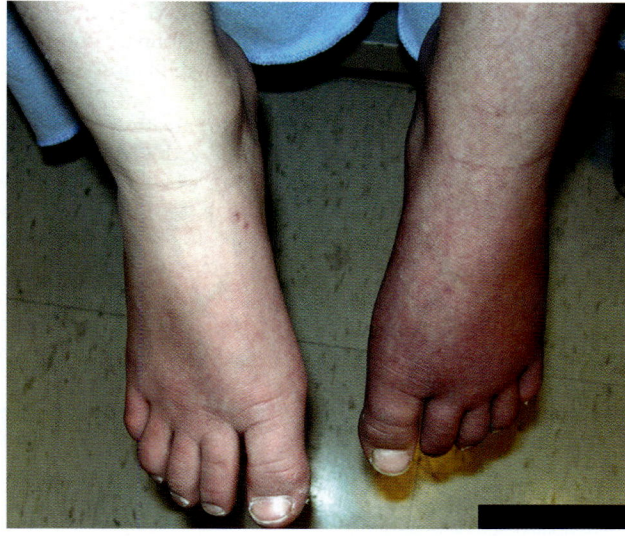

FIGURE 45.1 Complex regional pain syndrome involves the patient's left foot and ankle. Notice the cyanosis and mottling. The affected foot was cool, and allodynia was prominent. Left foot toenails had not been trimmed in 3 months.

may be considered. Only two are approved for use in children by the U.S. Food and Drug Administration (FDA): rizatriptan for children 6 to 17 years old and almotriptan for ages 12 to 17. Opioids are not appropriate in most circumstances. Overall, the lack of randomized, controlled pediatric trials precludes an evidence-based recommendation.[33] However, the anticonvulsant topiramate is a promising medication for the prevention of migraine headaches.[34–36] Tricyclic antidepressants such as amitriptyline may be beneficial, especially when combined with cognitive behavioral therapy.[37]

Coenzyme Q10 is deficient in approximately one-third of children and adolescents who report frequent headaches.[38] A significant number of those experienced both decreased headache frequency and severity after beginning supplementation with coenzyme Q10.

COMPLEX REGIONAL PAIN SYNDROME

Type I and type II CRPS differ only in the presence of a documented nerve injury in type II (formerly called *causalgia*). Pain is an obligatory feature, often occurring alongside allodynia or hyperalgesia. There must be evidence at some time (not necessarily at the time of diagnosis) of edema, changes in skin blood flow, or abnormal sudomotor activity in the region of pain. There are often features of a motor disorder such as tremor, dystonia, and weakness that sometimes lead to a loss of joint mobility. Nail and hair growth can also be affected. In the past, three distinct stages were described. However, it may be that there are phenotypic subtypes instead of stages.[39]

From a clinical standpoint, the typical pediatric CRPS patient is older than 10 years of age, Caucasian, female, and very active or a high achiever from an active family, and the child or adolescent presents with lower extremity pain.[40] A genetic predisposition is suggested by the clinical observation that CRPS is rare in the African American population. The rarity of CRPS in preadolescent children suggests a developmental aspect to its origin.

It is important to obtain a detailed history of the mechanism of trauma and the signs and symptoms. The examiner should specifically look for pain, allodynia, hyperalgesia, and hyperpathia. Edema and color changes do not have to be present at the time of diagnosis, but there should be a history of such changes in the recent past (Fig. 45.1). A complete neurologic examination includes

testing muscle strength, reflexes, sensory responses (e.g., cold, touch, pinprick), capillary refill, temperature, and color differences. The physician should also look for deep tissue hyperalgesia. Occasionally, noninvasive or invasive testing may be helpful, but it is not sensitive or specific. These evaluations may include an electromyogram with nerve conduction velocity (EMG/NCV), quantitative sensory testing (QST), and quantitative sudomotor axon reflex testing (QSART) to detect small fiber dysfunction; thermography; and bone scans. Sympathetic ganglion blocks are not considered necessary for diagnosis, but they can be part of the therapeutic approach.

The therapeutic goal for CRPS is restoration of function. It may seem simple, but in daily practice, this may represent the biggest challenge for the physician and the child. The therapeutic approach to the child with CRPS is multidisciplinary, with a focus on the psychosocial and physical aspects of the disease (Table 45.6). Education is important, and the information available on the Internet is ubiquitous, although it is often discouraging and not applicable to children with CRPS. No isolated treatment technique has been helpful for this condition. Children and physicians should follow an algorithm and adjust the therapeutic strategy every 4 weeks if the child does not respond satisfactorily to chosen measures.

The mainstay of CRPS treatment is physical therapy. However, the pain can be severe and disabling enough to prevent active participation by the child in the physical therapy program. Pharmacologic therapy is often initiated to facilitate physical therapy. Medications prescribed for neuropathic pain such as TCAs and anticonvulsants have been used frequently, although the evidence for this in the pediatric population is limited. It must be emphasized to the patient and family that no medication is curative and that the role of medications is to allow full participation in physical therapy. It is reasonable to use NSAIDs and opioids for a short time until the primary medications take effect. The psychology team must play an active role in the overall treatment program. Psychosocial issues must be aggressively addressed. With physical therapy, psychology, and medications, most children achieve good results and disease resolution. In unusually refractory cases, for which interdisciplinary outpatient programs are insufficient, inpatient pain rehabilitation programs are recommended.

The role of interventional therapy in the treatment of CRPS is to alleviate the pain and provide the child with the opportunity to tolerate and advance in physical therapy. Sympathetic nerve blocks are widely used in adults, although a systematic review revealed a lack of randomized, controlled trials to confirm the effectiveness of this approach in short-term and long-term pain relief.[41] Interventional therapies can be a double-edged sword, representing an easy solution that can demotivate the child from taking an active role in his or her physical therapy. However, pain may be too severe to allow physical therapy and thereby accelerate loss of function.

Several techniques enjoy popularity among pediatric pain specialists. Least invasive is TENS, which is usually provided by a physical therapist. For isolated limb CRPS, intravenous (IV) regional blockade with local anesthetic and adjuncts such as clonidine, ketamine, or ketorolac can be performed, though interventional treatment is not without controversy.[42] General anesthesia or deep sedation is frequently required because placement of IV catheters in the affected limb and inflation of the tourniquet are poorly tolerated. More invasive alternatives include placement of a lumbar sympathetic plexus catheter (Fig. 45.2) and a tunneled epidural catheter at the relevant dermatomal level. The duration of infusion ranges from 3 to 5 days to as long as 4 to 6 weeks, and the procedures require extensive logistical support. An alternative approach is to place a peripheral nerve catheter for a continuous block.[43] Spinal cord stimulation and intrathecal drug delivery are rarely used for pediatric CRPS because of the overall good prognosis with more conservative treatment and the continued growth of the skeleton, which can change the area of paresthesias in the case of spinal cord stimulators. Ketamine infusions are increasingly being used for CRPS, but this treatment is poorly supported by limited quality evidence.[44]

Graded motor imagery (GMI) is an emerging technique that consists of a stepwise approach that includes left-right limb discrimination exercises, limb activity imagery, and mirror therapy[45] that has some early evidence for use in adults.[46]

MUSCULOSKELETAL AND RHEUMATOLOGIC PAIN

Musculoskeletal pain is a recognized problem in children and adolescents, and back pain commonly affects adolescents.[47–50] The most commonly encountered causes of chronic pediatric musculoskeletal pain are diffuse idiopathic musculoskeletal pain (juvenile fibromyalgia), chronic back pain, juvenile idiopathic arthritis, CRPS (discussed previously), and pain secondary to joint hypermobility. Although many factors are blamed for musculoskeletal pain (e.g., heavy backpacks, participation in sports,

TABLE 45.6	Care Pathway for Complex Regional Pain Syndromes

Evaluation

Medical examination

Behavioral medicine assessment

Physical therapy assessment

Review of records, treatments, history, physical findings, and radiographic studies

Treatment

Medications: tricyclic antidepressants, gabapentin, oxcarbazepine

Behavioral medicine: very important, especially in refractory cases

Physical therapy: activate, range of motion, desensitization, strength training. Structured home program extremely important; may use transcutaneous electrical nerve stimulation (TENS) unit

Other therapy:
   Consider intravenous regional block for hand or foot
   Consider lumbar sympathetic block catheter and admission for structured program for lower extremity complex regional pain syndrome (CRPS) that is refractory despite best efforts of patient and family
   Consider high thoracic epidural or continuous brachial plexus catheter for upper extremity CRPS

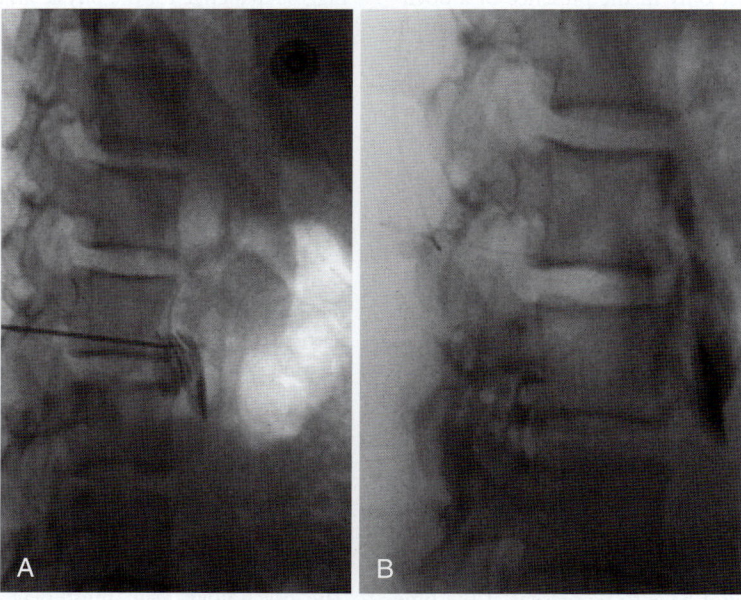

FIGURE 45.2 Lumbar sympathetic block. **A,** In the lateral view, the Tuohy needle is in the proper position. Notice the prepsoas spread of contrast agent. **B,** The dye spreads and clears due to injection of local anesthetic through the catheter. The catheter is tunneled and can be left in place for a week.

| TABLE 45.7 | Care Pathway for Back Pain |

Evaluation

Medical examination

Behavioral medicine assessment

Physical therapy assessment

Review of records, treatments, history, and physical findings

Consultation with specialists in orthopedics; magnetic resonance imaging or computed tomography, as indicated by history and examination findings

Treatment

Medications:
Tricyclic antidepressants
Muscle relaxants (e.g., baclofen, cyclobenzaprine)
Anticonvulsant (if radicular component)
Nonsteroidal antiinflammatory drug of choice
Cyclooxgenase-2 inhibitor for gastrointestinal or bleeding issues
If disk disease with radicular pain is documented, up to three epidural steroid injections may be helpful

Behavioral medicine: biofeedback, coping skills, and relaxation techniques

Physical therapy:
Stretching, postural rehabilitation, general reconditioning, and lifting techniques
Limit bed rest; reactivate
Transcutaneous electrical nerve stimulation (TENS)
Exercise program

Other therapy:
Acupuncture
Yoga
Chiropractic (older patients, lumbar only)
Massage
Trigger-point injections
Additional modalities for specific indications include back bracing, surgery, bisphosphonate therapy

sedentary lifestyle, scoliosis, increased body mass index), only a few have been proven to contribute to musculoskeletal pain. In more than half of cases in one study, the cause could not be identified, and only a minority of children had an underlying disease process (e.g., spondylolysis, infection, tumor, disk problem). Radiologic findings correlated poorly with the pain and failed to distinguish between those with and without pain.[47] Selected red flags for back pain are provided in Table 45.3. A care pathway for the evaluation and treatment of back pain in children and adolescents is presented in Table 45.7.

A special group of children with musculoskeletal pain are those with rheumatologic diseases. Most children referred to the rheumatologist's office report musculoskeletal pain. Only some are diagnosed with a true rheumatologic disease; juvenile idiopathic arthritis is the most common diagnosis. Besides pain, the diseases often manifest as morning stiffness, fatigue, and sleep problems. The process may progress and cause joint deformities and destruction owing to osteoporosis, with resulting growth abnormalities and functional disability. Management combines pharmacologic and nonpharmacologic interventions. The mainstay of therapy includes NSAIDs, acetaminophen, and rarely, opioids for severe breakthrough pain. The rheumatologist may prescribe agents such as methotrexate, cyclophosphamide, or systemic corticosteroids for severe flare-ups. Splints, physical therapy, and psychological interventions such as cognitive-behavioral therapy are often used.[51]

Children with Ehlers-Danlos syndrome (benign joint hypermobility syndrome) and other connective tissue disorders suffer from unstable joints that become very painful from repeated dislocations and mechanical stress. The mainstay of therapy for hypermobility pain is physical therapy that focuses on joint protective strategies. Specific guidelines to assist physical therapists who are unfamiliar with this approach are available.[52] Additionally, low-impact aerobic activity (aquatic physical therapy, elliptical machine, stationary bike) should be encouraged.

Some young women present with fatigue, poor sleep, and pain or unusual tenderness in multiple sites. Fibromyalgia is more common in adolescents than expected, and it can be a significant problem. Although still commonly tested, the presence of tender points is no longer considered diagnostic for fibromyalgia by the American College of Rheumatology. Instead, the newer (2010) criteria focus on the number of body parts that are described as painful, the severity of symptoms, and the chronicity of the pain complaints.[53] Therapy includes education, medications, and general restorative therapy, with a focus on aerobic reconditioning. Traditionally, TCAs and cyclobenzaprine have been prescribed; duloxetine and milnacipran have been shown to be helpful in adults.[54,55] As with many chronic pain conditions, cognitive-behavioral approaches are valuable components of treatment.[56]

Musculoskeletal pain is a particularly difficult problem in children with cerebral palsy.[57] Spasticity itself can be painful, and daily stretching exercises are reported to be painful by many children. Some children with cerebral palsy are nonverbal, making assessment even more difficult. The parents or guardians can provide information about how the child expresses pain and how the pain manifests during daily life. If diaper changes seem to hurt, the practitioner should suspect hip or perineal pain. Pain after eating or a history of hard stools may point to constipation-based abdominal pain. A careful and sometimes staged examination is required. A thoughtful, empirical approach to therapy and judicious use of radiologic and laboratory evaluations can often lead to the diagnosis (Table 45.8).

PAIN IN SICKLE CELL DISEASE, TRAIT, AND VARIANTS

Sickle cell disease is a hereditary disorder characterized by abnormal hemoglobin S (see Chapter 10). About 8% of African Americans carry the sickle cell gene. The homozygous form (sickle cell disease [HbSS]) manifests as a hemolytic anemia with unique vasoocclusive features. The heterozygous form (sickle cell trait [HbAS]) is milder and manifests as a borderline anemia and rarely with vasoocclusive features. Sickle cell/hemoglobin C disease (HbSC) has a clinical presentation similar to that of HbSS, but its vasoocclusive episodes are fewer and usually less intense.

From a pain management perspective, the homozygous HbSS genotype manifests as acute pain attacks (e.g., pain crisis, vasoocclusive episodes, acute chest syndrome) or as underlying chronic pain with acute exacerbations (e.g., avascular necrosis, vertebral collapse, joint involvement). Treatment frequently requires a multidisciplinary approach with close cooperation among the hematologist, psychologist, and pain physician.[58] Most of the episodes can be managed at home with NSAIDs or acetaminophen, supplemented with opioids or with tramadol.[59] In severe cases, children often are hospitalized and treated with IV opioids, although they should be gradually weaned off the opioids as the primary process improves. For episodes of localized, hard-to-control pain or if acute chest syndrome develops, epidural analgesia can provide excellent relief.[60] Rarely, children require opioid maintenance with long-acting preparations of morphine or oxycodone

TABLE 45.8	Care Pathway for Nonverbal Patients

Evaluation

Medical examination
  Often tricky; go slowly
  May need more than one visit to complete the examination
  Try to isolate body part during examination, to avoid generalized effect
  Watch facial or vocal and parent reaction to each examination maneuver

Behavioral medicine assessment: often not possible

Physical therapy assessment: often already engaged in therapy

Review of records, treatments, history, and physical findings

Video documentation: parent may be able to capture pain behaviors for examiner to view

Treatment

Medications: often taking multiple agents at baseline and coordination with other practitioners is important; apply general principles in choosing medications; long-acting opioid is sometimes beneficial for refractory musculoskeletal pain; watch for worsening of constipation.

Behavioral medicine: often not possible if patient's cognitive ability is too low, but the family sometimes can benefit because they carry a large burden when caring for children with multiple medical problems

Physical therapy: often already engaged; if not, engage for musculoskeletal pain or help therapist focus efforts of a particular region of the body

Other therapy:
  Nerve blocks can be used to identify painful areas, if more than one seems active.
  Rarely, a patient must be brought to the operating suite for an infusion of remifentanil to differentiate opioid responsiveness from potentially centralized or behavioral pain phenomena; the latter may respond to anticonvulsant therapy.
  Intrathecal baclofen (and occasionally morphine)
  Surgical therapy for selected conditions

Cautions

Site of pain is often unclear.

Do not forget to look in the ears.

If patient is spastic, strongly consider hip pathology (e.g., subluxation, bursitis, infection).

Constipation, gallbladder pain, and gastroesophageal reflux are possible.

These patients often require more testing than verbal patients.

Be careful with use of nonsteroidal antiinflammatory drugs because gastroesophageal reflux can be a problem and reporting abdominal pain as a signal of gastrointestinal side effects may not be possible.

TABLE 45.9	Care Pathway for Sickle Cell Disease

Evaluation

Medical examination

Behavioral medicine assessment: may be limited to social support in acute setting

Review of records, treatments (need opioid exposure history for dosing), and history

Hematology almost always directly involved, with focused evaluation

Treatment of Vaso-occlusive Episodes

Medications: opioid (often requires basal infusion for several days); nonsteroidal antiinflammatory drug; consider neuropathic medication for hyperalgesia

Behavioral medicine: can be helpful, although learning techniques in the acute setting may be difficult; introducing this modality early in life may be more helpful

Physical therapy: transcutaneous electrical nerve stimulation (TENS) for localized pain

Other therapy:
  Regional anesthesia may be helpful.
  Strongly consider thoracic epidural for acute chest crisis.

Treatment of Chronic Problems

Medications: may involve chronic opioids; otherwise follows treatment of particular pain condition

Behavioral medicine: per particular pain condition; early involvement may reduce need for hospitalizations

Physical therapy: per particular pain condition; may have joint, bone, and deconditioning issues from recurrent vasoocclusive episodes

(Table 45.9). Hyperalgesia over the affected area suggests peripheral or central sensitization, although the role for neuropathic medications is undefined. Fortunately, the use of hydroxyurea by hematologists (to increase hemoglobin F levels and decrease the proportion of HbSS) has had a positive effect on the number and intensity of vasoocclusive episodes.[61]

Pain Pharmacotherapy

Pain treatment has received less study in children than adults; this is also true for much pediatric pharmacologic therapy. In the absence of U.S. FDA–approved indications and experimental data, off-label use of many medications used to treat chronic pain is common. In this situation, the decision to select a particular medication is most often based on extrapolation from adult literature, expert consensus, applied theory, and clinical judgment. Three categories of medications are available for consideration: nonopioid analgesics (i.e., NSAIDs and acetaminophen), opioid analgesics, and a broad spectrum of adjuvant analgesics, including anticonvulsants, antidepressants, muscle relaxants, local anesthetics, N-methyl-D-aspartate (NMDA) receptor antagonists, α_2-agonists, and corticosteroids.

NONSTEROIDAL ANTIINFLAMMATORY DRUGS

NSAIDs are a heterogeneous group of mild analgesics (salicylates, propionic acid derivatives, oxicams, napthylalkanones, and fenamates). Their mechanism of action is to inhibit cyclooxygenases (COXs) at the sites of prostaglandin H_2-synthetase enzymes. There are two subtypes of COXs: COX-1 is constitutive and always present; COX-2 is inducible and produced in the body under proper conditions. NSAIDs have different selectivity for COX-1 or COX-2; selective COX-2 inhibitors have predominant action on inducible COX-2. The benefit of selective blockade is decreased risk of gastrointestinal bleeding. Celecoxib is the only selective COX-2 inhibitor available in the United States. NSAIDs are effective in musculoskeletal pain and as an abortive treatment of migraine headaches.[62,63]

The analgesic and antiinflammatory actions of NSAIDs are dose dependent, reaching a ceiling beyond which there is no additional benefit from increasing the dose. Unlike opioids, NSAIDs do not induce any physical dependence or tolerance.

The choice of NSAID is empirical, based on clinical judgment. If the child provides a history of good response to a particular NSAID, we tend to continue it or to adjust the dose. If the response is inadequate, we select a different medication until we find one that is effective. In children with a history of gastrointestinal side effects, we prescribe combination preparations with protective agents (e.g., misoprostol), add a histamine 2 (H_2)-receptor or proton pump inhibitor, or switch to a selective COX-2 inhibitor. Preexisting renal disease and disorders that reduce actual or effective intravascular volume significantly increase the risk for renal toxicity. In such children, NSAIDs must be used cautiously. Recent research has highlighted an increased risk of cardiovascular events related to use of NSAIDs. We recommend limited, short, intermittent use.[64,65]

OPIOIDS

The current literature does not support the long-term use of opioids for chronic nonmalignant pain. Opioid prescription practices have undergone increased scrutiny by medical, state, and federal authorities as opioid consumption, abuse, and deaths from opioids reached alarming proportions. Regulatory requirements are set by medical or pharmacy boards and vary from state to state. Clinical practice differs among practitioners and institutions. In an attempt to unify the field, several professional societies and governmental organizations have stepped in and published evidence-based guidelines for safe opioid prescribing in nonmalignant pain (e.g., American Pain Society, American Academy of Pain Management [AAPM],[66] and the Centers for Disease Control [CDC][67]). In pediatric pain practice, drug abuse by teens and diversion by proxy are the main concerns. In general, to ensure compliance with regulations and safe opioid prescription practices, several tools have been recommended as parts of clinical routine. Our group uses a controlled substances agreement, which delineates the rules of engagement (e.g., we are the only office prescribing opioids for the patient, lost prescriptions will not be reissued, we will drug screen for compliance, and so on). We obtain informed consent (during which we discuss the risks of long-term opioid use and the potential for drug interactions) and a standard risk of abuse assessment tool.[68] A history of substance abuse (mainly in adolescent and young adult populations) and a family member with substance abuse and a dysfunctional social situation are red flags for opioid prescribing. In these cases, close monitoring (weekly or biweekly visits as opposed to monthly or bimonthly visits) and limited medication quantities are warranted, but not always practical for patients living at a distance. Under those circumstances, we make every effort to collaborate with their local family physician and defer prescribing of medications to them. Additionally, we document side effects, management, and treatment goals in our electronic medical record. These tools are used to provide standardized care for all patients by all providers. State laws vary and providers need to become aware of their particular state's laws. More guidance can be found in the CDC guidelines for safe opioid prescribing,[67] though they are directed at adult practice.

The use of opioids for treatment of pain in children is almost entirely reserved for acute and cancer-related pain. However, there are selected pediatric chronic pain conditions for which opioids can improve the quality of life and the functional capacity without putting patients at significant risk of addiction, tolerance, and toxicity. Opioid agonists are used almost exclusively; agonist-antagonists have less popularity because of a ceiling effect and the potential to precipitate withdrawal when administered alongside a pure agonist. We typically use opioids in two scenarios. The first features opioids as a bridge while titrating other classes of medications to effect or while awaiting physical therapy or an intervention to exert its effect. In the second scenario, we use

TABLE 45.10	Opioid Adverse Effects Associated With Chronic Use
With Development of Tolerance	
Cognitive impairment	
Itching	
Miosis	
Nausea	
Prolonged reaction time	
Respiratory depression	
Sedation	
Urinary retention	
Without Development of Tolerance	
Constipation	
Adverse Effects With Long-Term Use	
Hypogonadism	
Immunosuppression	

opioids as maintenance analgesics in carefully selected children (e.g., chronic musculoskeletal pain in a child with cerebral palsy, severe deformities in patients with neuromuscular disorder, children with juvenile rheumatoid arthritis or Ehlers-Danlos syndrome, epidermolysis bullosa). Medication is titrated in increments toward the main goals of optimal (although rarely complete) pain relief, improved function, and minimal adverse effects. Escalations are usually seen with exacerbations of the primary disease process. Common opioid adverse effects that occur with long-term use can be found in Table 45.10. Morphine, oxycodone, and hydromorphone offer equal flexibility in route of administration (tablets, syrup) and availability of immediate and controlled-release formulations. Active metabolites of morphine (morphine-3-glucuronide and morphine-6-glucuronide) are renally excreted, which is relevant in patients with renal insufficiency. Codeine has been removed from the formularies of many children's hospitals, following the 2013 FDA warning.[69] Codeine is a prodrug of morphine with variable metabolism and efficacy depending on patient's genetic makeup (see Chapters 6 and 7). Without pharmacogenetic screening, drug concentrations can be unpredictable and can range from undetectable to lethal after administration of a single dose. More studies in pharmacogenetics and genomics are becoming available and we are getting closer to personalized analgesia for opioid selection,[59] where effectiveness is maximized and adverse effects are minimized.[70,71]

Alternate Opioids

Several groups of children are at increased risk of developing significant complications related to analgesics. For example, those with inflammatory bowel disease (IBD) face the possibility of toxic megacolon with opioids; children with bleeding disorders and IBD are at increased risk for ulcerations and bleeding with NSAIDs, and those with gastrointestinal dysmotility disorders may develop ileus secondary to opioid agonists. In these situations, tramadol and butorphanol are alternate analgesic treatments. Tramadol provides analgesia for moderate pain without the additional risk of gastrointestinal bleeding or inducing an ileus. Tramadol effects analgesia via several pathways, including a weak μ-receptor opioid agonist action and by blocking monoamine reuptake in the central nervous system (similar to antidepressants). On the basis of its latter action, tramadol is a popular analgesic for neuropathic pain, especially for controlling paresthesias, allodynia, and touch-evoked pain. The likelihood of developing either tolerance or dependence is small, although both have been reported with tramadol. Despite its weak opioid properties, sudden discontinuation of tramadol can cause withdrawal symptoms. The usual dose of tramadol is 1 mg/kg, up to 100 mg every 6 hours (400 mg/d maximum). The dose in children with renal impairment (creatinine clearance <30 mL/minute) should be reduced by 50% and in those with liver impairment by 25%. Pharmacogenetic variability in CYP450 2D6 affects the clearance of tramadol in a manner similar to that of codeine, which has led the FDA to investigate safety issues in children, especially in the post-tonsillectomy population.[72] Common adverse effects include nausea, vomiting, sedation, constipation, diarrhea, dizziness, headache, seizures, and hallucinations. Rare side effects include orthostatic hypotension, syncope, tachyarrhythmia, serotonin syndrome, lowered seizure threshold, and long QT interval.

Butorphanol is a partial opioid agonist-antagonist, approximately 7 to 10 times more potent than morphine. It affects motility to lesser degree than opioid agonists. Butorphanol can be administered via the IV and intranasal routes but may cause dysphoria. Because of its partial agonist nature, its dosing exhibits a ceiling effect. However, butorphanol can be supplemented by opioid agonists if needed for severe breakthrough pain without leading to (theoretical) withdrawal. The advantage of nasal butorphanol is that it bypasses the gastrointestinal system if absorption is a concern. The usual dose is 0.01 mg/kg, up to 1 mg IV, usually 0.5 mg every 3 to 4 hours as needed. The nasal preparation delivers 0.5 mg per spray, which limits its use in smaller children.

Tapentadol is a new μ-opioid receptor agonist and norepinephrine reuptake inhibitor. Tapentadol is 18 times less potent than morphine in binding to human μ-opioid receptor and is 2 to 3 times less potent than analgesics in animal models. Its opioid effect can be reversed using naloxone. Tapentadol has no active metabolites. It has been approved for chronic pain associated with diabetic neuropathy, which makes it a good option treatment for other neuropathic pain states. In children, tapentadol has been used when other opioids failed, although this indication is not evidence-based. Respiratory and gastrointestinal side effects mimic those of standard opioids. In addition, tapentadol decreases the seizure threshold similar to tramadol and may cause a serotonin syndrome if administered in conjunction with other serotonergic drugs. Its use is not recommended in conjunction with monoamine oxidase inhibitors. Dosing is 25 to 50 mg orally q4-6h, maximum 600 mg/day for immediate forms, and 500 mg/day for extended-release forms.

Special consideration should be given to methadone. In addition to being an opioid agonist, methadone is also reasonably effective in controlling neuropathic elements of pain. However, there are a few important caveats for its use. Its prolonged half-life increases the risk of accumulation, sedation, and respiratory depression. The 1:1 methadone/morphine equianalgesic ratio often cited in standard tables is unintentionally misleading. The greater the dose of opioid being converted, the more skewed the conversion ratio; the methadone/morphine ratio ranges from 1:2.5 to 1:14.3 in one study.[73] Because of the prolonged half-life, dose adjustments should be made no more frequently than every 5 days. A unique side effect of methadone is its potential to prolong the QT interval and increase the dispersion of repolarization on the electrocardiogram.[74] Because the dispersion of repolarization is less than 100 msec, it remains unlikely that methadone can trigger torsade de pointes unless used with other medications that prolong the QTc.

Chronic Opioid Exposure and Surgery

When a child receiving long-term opioid therapy presents to the operating room, several simple rules need to be followed to ensure successful perioperative care. We begin with a thorough medication history, including drug dose and frequency. If the patient has not taken a morning dose of opioid, that dose should be replaced by the IV route to avoid withdrawal. It is essential to convert the home medication into morphine equivalents. The daily dose of home opioids should be provided as a baseline, orally or IV (if on non per os status), with all further dosing in addition to the baseline. Because of tolerance to opioids, larger than usual doses may be required. It is advisable to titrate the dose of opioids to achieve an adequate level of analgesia. Opioid consumption during the perioperative period may be more than three times that observed in patients not treated with long-term opioids. Underusing opioids in the perioperative period results in poor pain management and withdrawal phenomena.[75,76]

ADJUVANT DRUGS
Anticonvulsants

Anticonvulsants have been widely used in the pharmacologic treatment of chronic pain since the 1960s. However, pediatric studies are lacking. The clinical practice with anticonvulsants is extrapolated from adult studies and best practice, rather than randomized clinical trials. Often referred to as membrane stabilizers, anticonvulsants exert their effects on neural receptors, ion channels, and nerve conductivity. They modify the level of excitatory and inhibitory neurotransmitters and activation of nerve cells. They are most effective in controlling neuropathic pain. First-generation agents (e.g., carbamazepine) have been largely replaced by second-generation drugs (e.g., oxcarbazepine) with more favorable adverse effect profiles.

Therapeutic effect is achieved with all membrane stabilizers by gradual titrating the dose. The purpose of this approach is twofold: first, to avoid developing adverse effects by allowing the child to develop tolerance (mainly to sedation) and second, to determine the minimal effective dose. The initial treatment course often lasts 3 to 6 months, after which time the child's condition is reassessed. At the completion of the treatment, the child is gradually weaned off the medication in reverse order of its titration. Although weaning is not necessary to prevent seizures, rapid discontinuation may result in pain, sleep, or mood disturbances. Gradual weaning allows rapid re-escalation in case the pain returns, but rarely does it require a full dose. We stop at the minimal effective dose controlling the symptoms and maintain the child on the medication for an additional 3 to 6 months. Although the use of anticonvulsants for pain in children represents an off-label use, this class of agents is a mainstay of therapy for selected pain conditions. The choice of drug is based on thoughtful consideration and expert consensus, as randomized, controlled trials are lacking (even for adults).[77]

Gabapentin and Pregabalin

Gabapentin is an anticonvulsant with a complex mechanism of action. Its name is deceiving; gabapentin does not interact with the γ-aminobutyric (GABA)-ergic system. It binds to the α_2-delta subunit of the voltage-dependent calcium channel and reduces the release of glutamate in the dorsal horn of the spinal cord. This leads to decreased production of substance P, less activation of α-amino-3-hydroxy-5-methylisoxazole-4-propionate (AMPA) receptors on noradrenergic synapses, decreased transmitter release, and decreased neuronal activity. This mechanism is shared by both gabapentin and pregabalin.[76,78]

Gabapentin is usually the drug of choice for neuropathic pain such as CRPS because of its good tolerability, minimal adverse effects, and positive clinical experiences. In addition to causing sedation, its use in children can lead to retention of sodium and water, development of peripheral edema, and weight gain. In adolescents, gabapentin can cause mood swings, irritability, and suicidality. Despite these concerns, gabapentin is used frequently after providing a detailed explanation of its effectiveness and side effects with the child and parents. The target dose is up to 35 mg/kg per day in three divided doses orally, although, doses up to 70 mg/kg per day are possible. The dose of gabapentin does not have to be adjusted in liver failure because it is not metabolized by the liver. However, it is excreted via the kidney, so the dosing interval should be increased in children with renal impairment. Pregabalin is chemically related to gabapentin but has fewer adverse effects and a significantly faster titration schedule. It is approved for postherpetic neuralgia, diabetic neuropathy, and fibromyalgia in adults; experience in children is growing.

Topiramate

Best studied for the treatment of migraine headaches, topiramate can be applied to the full spectrum of neuropathic pain states.[35] It suppresses the appetite as a unique side effect, which makes it a good choice for children with neuropathic pain who are concerned about gaining weight. Topiramate has carbonic anhydrase–inhibiting properties that can cause a metabolic acidosis and renal stones in children with a medical or family history of nephrolithiasis.

Oxcarbazepine

Oxcarbazepine is the second-generation relative of carbamazepine for the treatment of neuropathic pain. Although rare, Stevens-Johnson syndrome can occur with oxcarbazepine and with several other anticonvulsants. Hyponatremia may also occur, as well as adverse effects in common with other anticonvulsants such as sedation, difficulty concentrating, ataxia, and mood instability.

Carbamazepine, Valproic Acid, and Phenytoin

The effectiveness of carbamazepine, valproic acid, and phenytoin for chronic pain has been discussed elsewhere.[79] Carbamazepine has proven effective in the treatment of trigeminal neuralgia, spasticity in multiple sclerosis, and spinal cord injury (compared with tizanidine). Phenytoin has been used alone or in combination with buprenorphine for cancer pain, providing good pain relief in more than 60% of patients. Despite their effectiveness, the use of phenytoin and carbamazepine is limited by liver and renal toxicity (serial laboratory testing is necessary), aplastic anemia, Steven-Johnson syndrome, and syndrome of inappropriate secretion of antidiuretic hormone–like symptoms. Valproate lacks renal side effects but can cause pancreatitis.

Antidepressants

Two major groups of antidepressants are used in the treatment of chronic pain: TCAs (e.g., amitriptyline, nortriptyline, desipramine, doxepin, imipramine) and serotonin reuptake inhibitors. Serotonin reuptake inhibitors are further divided in selective serotonin inhibitors (SSRIs; e.g., fluoxetine, paroxetine) and serotonin-norepinephrine reuptake inhibitors (SNRIs; e.g., venlafaxine, duloxetine, milnacipran).[80] When prescribing antidepressants to adolescents and young adults, we recommend vigilance for the potential increase in suicidal ideation and attempts. Patients and families should be informed in detail about this possibility to ensure that they communicate with the provider should these

occur. It is prudent to refer patients at greater risk for psychiatric comorbidities to a psychologist for evaluation before prescribing this class of medications.

Tricyclic Antidepressants

The efficacy of TCAs in the treatment of neuropathic pain has been confirmed in meta-analyses.[80,81] The doses required to control chronic pain are usually less than those used in the treatment of depression. The adverse effects of TCAs are the major limiting factor in prescribing them. The onset of adverse effects can be reduced by slow dose escalation, as is done with anticonvulsants. The most frequent side effect is sedation, which often benefits patients with disrupted sleep. We prescribe the drug to be taken one hour before bedtime and monitor the child in the morning. If carryover sedation is present, it is reasonable to decrease the dose or encourage the patient to take the medication earlier in the evening. Because of the anticholinergic effects of TCAs, patients may experience a dry mouth, constipation, urinary retention, or weight gain.

TCAs prolong the QT interval, which may lead to lethal arrhythmias. Before initiating therapy, it is prudent to obtain a careful past medical and family history of cardiac symptoms and conduction abnormalities. In addition, a baseline electrocardiogram to rule out congenital long QT syndrome is warranted. Because concomitant use of SSRIs, SNRIs, or tramadol can prolong the QT interval, decrease the seizure threshold in children with a seizure disorder, and cause serotonin syndrome, simultaneous use of these agents should proceed with great caution. Amitriptyline and nortriptyline are the most commonly prescribed TCAs. A starting dose for both drugs is 0.25 mg/kg orally at night, which can be increased as indicated and tolerated to 0.75 to 1 mg/kg over a few weeks. Analgesic effects first appear by 1 to 3 weeks, as with antidepressants effects. Nortriptyline is a metabolite of amitriptyline, with similar utility for pain but less sedation. If top-range dosing is required, periodic electrocardiographic monitoring for QTc changes is recommended.

Selective Serotonin and Norepinephrine Reuptake Inhibitors

The effectiveness of SSRIs and SNRIs in treating neuropathic and nonneuropathic pain such as fibromyalgia and low back pain is poor. SSRIs do not appear to play a role as analgesics.[82] SNRIs have modest support for use in adult fibromyalgia[54,55,83,84] but are not first-line treatments. Minor adverse effects are common, and there is a boxed warning regarding the potential for suicidal ideation in older teens and young adults.[85] Prescribing of both medications in children is best left to those who prescribe them frequently as dosing has not been well established and psychological monitoring is important.

Muscle Relaxants

Muscle relaxants are frequently used as an adjunct to other medications (mostly NSAIDs) in patients with myofascial pain. Data are limited, even in adults, but suggest a role for musculoskeletal conditions and neurologic conditions associated with spasticity,[86] as well as for nonspecific back pain in adults.[87] A caveat for patients with hypermobile joints: muscle relaxants may promote joint subluxations by lowering muscle tone. Therefore they should be used judiciously in this population.

Cyclobenzaprine

Cyclobenzaprine is a centrally acting muscle relaxant. Its major adverse effects are somnolence, dizziness, and asthenia. The usual starting dose is 5 mg orally at night and can be increased to 10 mg after 5 to 7 days, unless the child has difficulties awakening in the morning. The dose can be escalated up to 10 mg three times per day, limited by sedative effects.

Baclofen

Baclofen is one of the most powerful centrally acting muscle relaxants. It interacts with the GABA-B receptor subtype. It is usually indicated in patients with spasticity (cerebral palsy or multiple sclerosis) but can be used for myofascial pain. Patients report fewer sedative effects compared with cyclobenzaprine or tizanidine. The starting daily dose is 10 to 15 mg orally, divided into two or three doses. The dose can be escalated every 3 days by 5 mg. In children 7 years or younger, the maximum daily dose is 40 mg/day and for those older than 8 years, the maximum dose is 60 mg/day. Baclofen is one of a few medications approved for intrathecal administration by implanted pumps, which is usually reserved for children with severe spasticity (e.g., cerebral palsy, spinal cord injury).

Methocarbamol

Methocarbamol is a centrally acting relaxant of skeletal muscle. Its mechanism of action is not fully understood. Methocarbamol gained its popularity because of its minimal sedative adverse effects, which made it a safe adjunct to opioids, enteral or parenteral, in the setting of severe acute postoperative pain after major orthopedic surgeries. Methocarbamol is suitable for daytime administration in patients with chronic musculoskeletal pain and spasms on a short-term scheduled or intermittent basis. The dose of oral and IV forms is 15 mg/kg q6-8h acutely and 10 mg/kg for longer-term use. Methocarbamol should be avoided in patients with renal and liver dysfunction.

Tizanidine

Tizanidine is a centrally acting α_2-adrenergic agonist known to reduce spasticity by presynaptic inhibition of motor neurons. Structurally, tizanidine is similar to clonidine, but only $\frac{1}{10}$ to $\frac{1}{50}$ as potent for lowering blood pressure. Similar to clonidine, tizanidine causes dose-related sedation, more so compared with methocarbamol and baclofen. Predominantly used in patients with spasticity related to multiple sclerosis and spinal cord injury, tizanidine has found its applications in chronic musculoskeletal pain conditions associated with muscle tightness. The usual dosage is 2 to 4 mg orally, usually at night to facilitate sleep.

Local Anesthetics, α_2-Adrenergic Receptor Agonists, Topical Agents, and N-Methyl-D-Aspartate Receptor Antagonists

Many drugs are used in the treatment of pediatric chronic pain,[88] and they have a wide array of mechanisms of action. Oral medications with local anesthetic properties such as mexiletine and clonidine have been used in the treatment of neuropathic pain in patients with CRPS. Mexiletine and others are used orally, as a transdermal patch, or added to local anesthetic solutions in IV regional techniques. The major limiting factor in the use of these drugs is their adverse effect profile, which includes hypotension, sedation, bradycardia, and nausea (particularly mexiletine). The α_2-adrenergic agonist properties are also part of the mechanism of action of the muscle relaxant tizanidine.

The topical agent capsaicin, derived from hot chili peppers, can be helpful in managing neuropathic pain, but its application can cause a burning sensation where it is applied. As a result, it is often poorly tolerated. The topical lidocaine patch has been effective in the controlling symptoms of postherpetic neuralgia and has been used for localized myofascial pain, hyperpathia, and allodynia in other neuropathic conditions.[89] Pharmacokinetic studies in adults have found minimal blood concentrations of lidocaine, suggesting a large margin of safety,[90] although similar studies in children have not been forthcoming.

NMDA receptor antagonists such as ketamine, amantadine, and dextromethorphan have anecdotal evidence supporting their utility in the treatment of neuropathic pain. NMDA receptor antagonists may also exert an opioid-sparing effect. An important limiting factor of the broader use of ketamine in the treatment of chronic pain symptoms is the potential for psychotropic side effects (see reference 88 for a detailed review).

Complementary Therapies

Alternative therapies have appealed to patients for a long time. Because traditional medical therapies have a high failure rate, patients continue to search for better treatments. Many types of therapies have been used to treat chronic pain, including massage, yoga, herbal preparations, tai chi, meditation, chiropractic, and acupuncture. As a consultant, the anesthesiologist should consider suggesting some of these therapies when they seem appropriate. TENS and biofeedback have been discussed earlier. Of note, evidence supporting effectiveness for most of these interventions is minimal,[91] although they have a minimal risk of side effects, except in certain situations.

Acupuncture and its derivative, acupressure, originated in China and constitute an important part of traditional Chinese medicine (Fig. 45.3). In acupuncture, the body energy or qi (pronounced *chi*) circulates in body meridians and collaterals. Meridians and collaterals are pathways that represent body organ systems called the zang-fu organs. In Chinese medicine, pain is caused by alterations in the circulation of qi in these channels owing to multiple causes. Acupuncture has been used in many acute and chronic pain conditions. The data from randomized, controlled trials are insufficient to support or refute the effectiveness of acupuncture.[92]

Summary

The pediatric anesthesiologist may be called on to assist with the care of a child or adolescent with chronic pain.[93,94] The basic tenets of care apply, and a careful history and focused physical

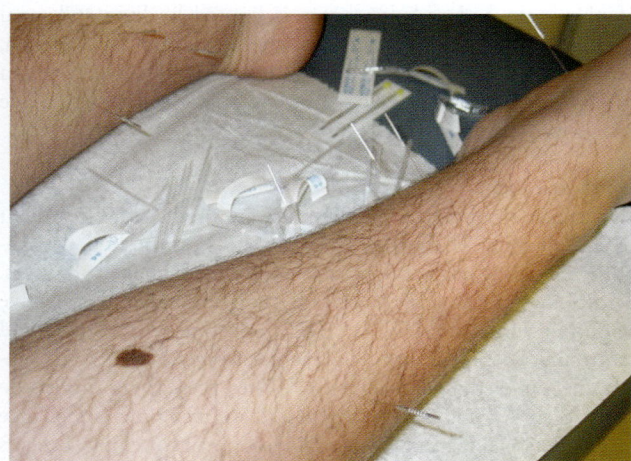

FIGURE 45.3 Acupuncture needles in situ.

examination remain key components of the evaluation. The first step is to ensure that the child is not being physically harmed by the painful condition (i.e., ensuring safety). The second step is to undertake a focused diagnostic evaluation and design of a therapeutic regimen. Treatment for all but the simplest painful conditions uses multiple disciplines in a coordinated attack on the pain. The input of psychologists is a prominent part of chronic pain management, and psychological treatment is not a sign of psychiatric disease or malingering, but a tool that is powerful and effective. Physical therapy and judicious use of medications round out the approach to most chronic pain problems in children. The occasional use of interventional modalities and opioids is warranted, but success will be limited if the problem is viewed in a unidimensional manner. Many patients benefit from alternative approaches to therapy, and these disciplines can be used in a prudent fashion to expand the range of therapies that can be recommended.

ANNOTATED REFERENCES

Brooks MR, Golianu B. Perioperative management of children with chronic pain. *Pediatr Anesth.* 2016;26:794-806.

Geary T, Negus A, Anderson BJ, Zernikow B. Perioperative management of the child taking long-term opioids. *Pediatr Anesth.* 2012;22:189-202.

These two articles outline some of the challenges that children suffering chronic pain present to anesthesiologists when they undergo surgical procedures. Management of these challenges is discussed.

Perquin CW, Hazebroek-Kampschreur AA, Hunfeld JA, et al. Pain in children and adolescents: a common experience. *Pain.* 2000;87:51-58.

This survey article describes the prevalence of chronic pain in children, which is a much more common problem than previously recorded in the general population.

Powers SW, Kashikar-Zuck SM, Allen JR, et al. Cognitive behavioral therapy plus amitriptyline for chronic migraine in children and adolescents: a randomized clinical trial. *JAMA.* 2013;310(24):2622-2630.

This article highlights the importance of the multimodal approach when caring for chronic pain patients; it supports the commonly held notion that medications work best when combined with psychological intervention.

Ripamonti C, Groff L, Brunelli C, et al. Switching from morphine to oral methadone in treating cancer pain: what is the equianalgesic dose ratio? *J Clin Oncol.* 1998;16:3216-3221.

This is an intriguing discussion about the conversion ratio between morphine and methadone. It explodes the commonly held belief (seen in so many opioid conversion tables) that the two opioids are equianalgesic.

Stanton-Hicks M, Baron R, Boas R, et al. Complex regional pain syndromes: guidelines for therapy. *Clin J Pain.* 1998;14:155-166.

The article outlines the multidisciplinary approach to complex regional pain syndromes (CRPS). Multidisciplinary treatment is not just for children with CRPS.

Turk DC. Clinical effectiveness and cost-effectiveness of treatments for patients with chronic pain. *Clin J Pain.* 2002;18:355-365.

The author takes a look at the big picture. Blocks make us money; comprehensive treatment makes patients better.

Wilder RT, Berde CB, Wolohan M, et al. Reflex dystrophy in children: clinical characteristics and follow-up of seventy patients. *J Bone Joint Surg Am.* 1992;74:910-919.

The classic paper describes complex regional pain syndrome in children, its treatment, and patient outcomes. Its observations hold up today.

Wolfe F, Clauw DJ, Fitzcharles MA, et al. The American College of Rheumatology preliminary diagnostic criteria for fibromyalgia and measurement of symptom severity. *Arthritis Care Res.* 2010;62(5):600-610.

Attempts to simplify the diagnosis of fibromyalgia, at the same time attempting to do away with the notoriously unreliable tender point examination-based criteria.

A complete reference list can be found online at ExpertConsult.com

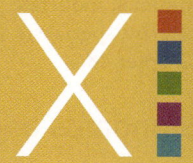

Anesthesia Outside the Operating Room   46

JOSEPH P. CRAVERO AND MARY LANDRIGAN-OSSAR

THE APPROACH TO PROVIDING ANESTHESIA outside the operating room (OR) for children (also known as "non–operating room anesthesia" [NORA] or "Off-site Anesthesia") varies greatly among health care organizations and even from one anesthesia provider to another. Because of its very nature, NORA practice is neither as standardized as anesthesia delivered in the OR nor is it as well studied or reported. As such, it is a difficult topic to review using an evidence-based approach. For instance, although most anesthesiologists would agree on the general approach for delivering anesthesia to a 2-year-old child undergoing an inguinal hernia repair, much more variability (in terms of drugs used, airway management techniques, and general organization of care) exists in providing anesthesia for a magnetic resonance imaging (MRI) scan. This issue is made even more confusing by the fact that NORA procedures that are performed with deep sedation in one institution may be accomplished with general anesthesia and tracheal intubation in another. Furthermore, a procedure that is performed using deep sedation provided by an *anesthesiologist* in one institution may have sedation provided by a specialist *other* than an anesthesiologist at another institution.[1]

The discussion of anesthesia services outside the OR must also include the recognition that the level of sedation/anesthesia for a given child at any moment during a procedure is often a matter of some conjecture. Almost any procedure that involves pain, or absolute movement control in a child, necessitates deep sedation or general anesthesia. The distinction between these two states (defined by the presence or absence of movement in reaction to painful stimuli) is often not completely clear.[2] For anesthesiologists, the difference is more of semantic interest than practical importance. Anesthesia services are often requested outside the OR when deep sedation is what is delivered, and vice versa. Finally, anesthesia is often provided outside the OR for patients with significant comorbidities undergoing routine procedures. Many of these children would be managed with moderate/deep sedation by other specialists were it not for the complexity of the child's underlying illnesses(s). Comorbid conditions that require referral to an anesthesiologist vary among institutions but common (generally accepted) examples include the following[3]:

1. Extremely young age, including healthy children younger than 2 months of age
2. History of prematurity (<32 weeks gestational age at birth) and postmenstrual age less than 60 weeks
3. History of ongoing apnea and bradycardia episodes
4. Craniofacial anomalies or any known difficult functional or anatomic airway problem
5. Cyanotic congenital heart disease or cardiomyopathy
6. Any serious coexisting disease such as sickle cell disease or muscular dystrophy that would qualify a patient as American Society of Anesthesiologists (ASA) status III–IV.
7. Procedures that require elective airway control (intubation) or respiratory control such as breath-holding

With these considerations in mind, this chapter focuses on issues specifically related to the delivery of anesthesia and deep sedation outside the OR *provided by anesthesiologists*. Issues concerning minimal, moderate, and deep sedation, as well as issues involving care by specialists other than anesthesiologists, are covered in Chapter 48.

Standards and Guidelines

Anesthesia outside the OR must meet the same standards as anesthesia given in the OR. Specifically, Medicare's *Conditions for Participation* for hospitals are enforced by The Joint Commission (TJC) regardless of location of care. The *Conditions for Participation* are principles that are articulated to surveyors as instructions in the Interpretive Guidelines published in January 2011, and available at http://www.cms.gov. These guidelines describe appropriate training, credentialing, and oversight of sedation and anesthesia providers and some of the specific requirements for care documentation. The ASA has developed templates for the required policies that help institutions meet the standards of the Interpretive Guidelines. These resources can be downloaded (or links are provided) from the ASA website at http://www.asahq.org. With particular reference to NORA, there are several notable templates, as follows:

1. Preanesthesia Evaluation Policy, Form, and Note

   Within 48 hours immediately before the delivery of the first dose of medication for the purpose of inducing anesthesia, a qualified practitioner must perform a preanesthesia evaluation of the patient that includes, at a minimum: (1) a review of the medical history including anesthesia, drug and allergy history, and (2) an interview if possible, given the patient's condition, and examination of the patient. In addition, the following must be reviewed and updated within 48 hours prior to anesthesia:
   a. Notation of the anesthesia risk.
   b. Identification of potential anesthesia problems.
   c. Additional preanesthesia data or information, if applicable and as required in accordance with standard practice prior to administration of anesthesia (i.e., stress tests).
   d. Development of the plan for the patient's anesthesia care, including the type of medications for induction, maintenance and postoperative care and discussion with the patient (parents) of the risks and benefits of the delivery of anesthesia.
2. Intraoperative record policy. Standard data elements and timing must be included in the intraoperative record—just as in the OR. In other words, the intraoperative electronic record should be accessible from all NORA locations within an institution.
3. Postanesthesia Evaluation Policy, Note, and Form (template). A postanesthesia note must be completed within 48 hours after surgery. The person completing the evaluation does not have to be the person who delivered the anesthetic. The elements of the postanesthesia note include assessment of the following:
   a. Respiratory function
   b. Cardiovascular function
   c. Mental status
   d. Temperature
   e. Pain
   f. Nausea and vomiting
   g. Postoperative hydration

NORA services must be organized in such a way as to meet the *Conditions for Participation* (and thus TJC) standards mentioned earlier, just as they are met in the OR. Depending on how NORA is organized in a particular institution, this can be challenging. The departments that require anesthesia services must appreciate

the need to meet these standards and allow for the infrastructure to meet or exceed them, particularly in preanesthesia assessment and postanesthesia follow-up requirements.

Off-Site Anesthesia: Structure

There is little literature on the organization of pediatric anesthesia services outside the OR. Based on information available from the Pediatric Sedation Research Consortium, we know *some* institutions organize these services through an off-site anesthesia unit that can also be used for general anesthesia or sedation cases.[4] These units have the advantage of providing all anesthesia-related care through one location that contains the personnel and equipment required for anesthesia. Ideally, these units provide a location for preanesthesia assessment, induction, procedure location, and recovery. Children may be transported to remote locations when equipment (such as MRI scanners) cannot be brought to the sedation unit. The advantages of this organizational scheme are many. The uniform environment leads to maximum consistency in the equipment and personnel who interact with children and their families and thus adds to safety, efficiency, parent satisfaction, and effectiveness of care. Specialty teams or microsystems for provision NORA are coordinated groups of professionals who deliver a specific service that achieve the best possible outcomes by developing reliable, efficient, and responsive processes. They are able to meet the individual needs of one child, continually improving care for the next child, and create a user-friendly work environment. The NORA microsystem should be made up of pediatric anesthesiologists, nursing, technical, and administrative personnel who are familiar with the off-site service and dedicated to this care.[5,6] As members gain expertise and comfort with the off-site environment, their care is consistent and reproducible, leading to less confusion with other services. Such systems of care lead to improved effectiveness (decreasing failed anesthesia and sedation cases) and improve patient, family, and staff satisfaction.[7-9]

Another option for NORA organization is the use of standard OR same-day unit admission services and postanesthesia care unit recovery capability while providing induction and procedural anesthesia at the site of the procedure (e.g., endoscopy suite or hematology and oncology unit). This organizational paradigm makes use of existing anesthesia ancillary services but almost always requires patient transport before and after the procedure itself.

Finally, anesthesia services outside the OR may be primarily organized at the site of procedural care (e.g., in radiology departments or gastrointestinal [GI] procedure suites). For this organizational setup, the procedure unit itself may be outfitted for admission and preanesthesia assessment and recovery of children is accomplished in a space contiguous with the procedural location. This kind of organization is most common in children's hospitals, where high volumes of procedures are performed in a given location such as the MRI scanner.[10]

PERSONNEL REQUIREMENTS

Inadequate experience or familiarity with equipment/monitoring devices, poor communications with team members, production pressure, inattention/carelessness, and fatigue have been shown to be critical contributors to anesthesia-related adverse events.[11] The environment and the demands of providing anesthesia outside the OR are unique regardless of the specific organizing strategy. To create a functional and efficient anesthesia microsystem, several common themes lead to optimal safety and effectiveness of care:

1. Anesthesia providers should rotate on this service with a frequency that allows the development of a working relationship among the anesthesiologists, anesthesia extenders, respiratory therapists, registered nurses, patient care technicians, biomedical engineers, and child-life specialists. This familiarity should be based on a common understanding of the routines and protocols for standard procedures and a common agreement on the goals of the service.

2. Effective and efficient communication among personnel is critical to optimize outcomes. Logically, help from all members of the care team, including the supervising anesthesiologist, should be available to provide definitive care for urgent situations within time frames that would allow optimal outcomes for children with critical events—specifically within 3 to 4 minutes. An explicit chain of communication must be established such that in the event of an emergency there is no confusion about how outside resources (additional anesthesia assistance from main OR, hospital code team) will be activated when necessary. The use of cell phones, Internet phones, "stat buttons,"[12] or other devices to optimize communication in NORA locations is often helpful.

3. The ancillary personnel in each location must be familiar with the needs and processes of providing anesthesia to children.

4. Equipment and monitoring standards should mimic that of the OR. Anesthesia carts, machine preparation, and setup should mirror the OR environment as much as possible to maximize the similarity to the most common workspace. It is critical to have a system that allows appropriate restocking and security of anesthesia carts in all off-site locations with the same frequency and organization as the OR. All off-site carts should include a full range of drugs, intravenous (IV) equipment, fluids, and airway equipment such as tracheal tubes, laryngeal mask airways (LMAs), laryngoscopes, oral and nasal airways, masks, and suction equipment in sizes that would fit all possible pediatric age groups.

5. Scheduling off-site anesthesia resources is complex and time-consuming. Timing for some procedures is inexact. In addition, anesthesia time requirements can vary with the child and the associated pathology. Success is enhanced by focusing the task of scheduling NORA procedures with one individual (or a small group) who intimately understands the process involved in anesthesia. This type of organization allows the NORA service to have one focal point for communication between the individuals who perform procedures and the anesthesia service, thus maximizing communication and minimizing incorrect assumptions of staffing or timing for procedures.

6. Successful off-site anesthesia is maximized when arrangements are made for anesthesiologists to be integrated with other sedation/anesthesia providers in a way that allows them to transfer care for those who are *not* successfully sedated—and convert to anesthesia care as needed.[7,13]

SPECIFIC ENVIRONMENTAL REQUIREMENTS

Equipment and monitoring standards must meet those of the main OR environment. The ASA requires that remote locations must have two sources of oxygen (O_2) (preferably a central source of piped O_2 and a backup E cylinder), suction, an anesthesia machine if administering inhalational anesthetics, a scavenging system for waste anesthetic gases, suction, a self-inflating hand resuscitator bag

able to deliver 90% O_2 and positive-pressure ventilation, standard of care monitors and equipment,[10,14] and sufficient electrical outlets, illumination, and space. The ASA Standards for Basic Anesthetic Monitoring include the following:

- Pulse oximetry with audible pulse tone and low-threshold alarm
- Adequate illumination and exposure of the patient to assess color
- Anesthesia machine with O_2 analyzer
- Continuous end-tidal carbon dioxide (ETCO$_2$) analysis with an audible alarm
- Continuous electrocardiogram (ECG)
- Arterial blood pressure and heart rate every 5 minutes or more frequently as indicated
- Temperature monitor, if there is potential for clinically significant changes in body temperature

In addition, it is important to make further adaptations (e.g., duplicates of critical equipment, such as laryngoscope handles and blades). In the MRI unit, it is essential to have MRI-compatible laryngoscope blades and handles, compatible monitoring devices, and MRI-compatible portable oxygen tanks. Each site should be carefully evaluated for important items such as wall-delivered gases (O_2, nitrous oxide [N_2O], and air), the location of suction equipment, and an Ambu bag (Ambu, Copenhagen, Denmark). Every site must have backup gas supplies. If pipeline O_2 is not available, O_2 should be drawn from H cylinders (6600 L) rather than the smaller E tanks (659 L) (oxygen reserves should be checked prior to each use). All equipment for monitoring and resuscitation should be up to date and standardized to that used in the ORs.

Many off-site areas do not have wall suction, especially in the MRI environment. MRI-compatible wall suction is not widely available. An alternative method for providing suction in the MRI suite is to mount a suction canister with 30 feet of suction tubing outside the scanner room.[15] The suction tubing can then be threaded through a hole in the console wall to access for use in the MRI unit.

Scavenging systems should be carefully evaluated in NORA locations. When passive scavenging is not possible, active scavenging may be developed by using the wall-source vacuum or wall suction canisters. A scavenging system dedicated solely to waste gases should be present.[16]

Electrical circuitry in off-site locations must be upgraded to meet OR standards. Specifically, although the outlets tend to be grounded and hospital grade, plug and outlet incompatibility may be a problem. Adapters and conversion plugs must be available. Although off-site locations tend not to have as great a risk of electrical shock or electrocution to the child as in the OR, it is important to remember that these sites do not have line-isolation monitors. In the event of excessive leakage of current, the anesthesiologist would not be warned. Although the National Electrical Code no longer requires line-isolation monitors in nonflammable anesthetizing locations, it is strongly recommended in areas with multiple power sources. To ensure child and health care personnel safety, biomedical engineers must be attentive to the safe maintenance of all electrical equipment.

It is in the nature of NORA that the physical environment and practice patterns are typically that of another medical specialty. It should also be noted that these other specialties practice under standards developed by their own professional organizations that apply to the procedures within their locations reflecting the different procedure goals. The varying specialties involved include (but are not limited to) gastroenterology, dentistry, cardiology, oncology, intensive care, emergency medicine, and radiology.[8] Anesthesia providers who work in these environments are well served by familiarizing themselves with the standards for the given specialty area they are working in, as published on the individual websites for the various professional organizations.

Quality Assurance of Anesthesia Services and Outcome in the Off-Site Areas

It is important to develop a strategy to track all clinically important complications associated with NORA, as we do in the OR. Each department can set its own thresholds for review; however, certain incidents require a full inquiry for example[17]:

- Aspiration events
- Unscheduled admissions to the hospital as a direct result of the sedation (i.e., because of protracted emesis, prolonged sedation, respiratory or cardiac complication)
- Medication errors that lead to patient harm—or that could potentially lead to patient harm
- Failed procedures resulting from inadequate or problematic anesthesia or sedation
- Cardiovascular or respiratory compromise that requires assistance from an outside rescue team or leads to a "call for help"
- Cardiac arrest
- Respiratory arrest or need for airway rescue

Many institutions choose to follow outcomes such as prolonged nausea and vomiting after anesthesia or O_2 desaturation events.[18] Regardless of the data that the quality improvement (QI) committee chooses to review, the process should include anesthesiologists and anesthesia extenders, nurses, and other technical personnel who are routinely involved in anesthesia care and support. It is particularly important to note that in the case of off-site anesthesia, it is critical to include members of the departments (other than anesthesiology) who were involved with the case being reviewed. The timing of QI meetings depends on the number and acuity of the non-OR anesthesia cases provided at a given institution. Review committee meetings should be considered not just an opportunity to evaluate complications but also a forum for exchange of ideas, expertise, and information that can lead to improvements in the systems of patient care.

Anesthesia Versus Sedation for Non–Operating Room Procedures and Tests in Children

Anesthesiologists always have the option to deliver either deep sedation or anesthesia for procedures outside the OR. The choice of whether to deliver general anesthesia with a secured airway (tracheal tube or LMA) using potent inhalational anesthetics versus deep sedation with face mask O_2 and propofol infusion depends on many factors, including the child's comorbid conditions, the procedure, and the experience and comfort level of the anesthesia provider. Several reviews are available on this topic. For MRI scans, propofol deep sedation has been suggested as a safe and effective option in children with airway pathologic conditions or who are premature or very young.[19] For generally healthy children undergoing MRI scans, adverse events were reportedly less common when deep sedation/anesthesia with propofol and a natural airway were used compared with inhaled anesthesia through an LMA.[20] The same report noted that recovery was faster after propofol (alone) compared with inhalational anesthesia. Similarly, multiple

reports have recommended successful outcomes with propofol sedation and general anesthesia with tracheal intubation (GETA) techniques for endoscopies.[21,22] In another study where a direct comparison was made between the techniques for GI procedures, recovery was more rapid and agitation less common after a propofol-based sedation technique rather than an inhaled anesthesia-based anesthetic technique.[23]

No clear evidence exists that one technique is better than another for procedures since both techniques have been reported as effective and safe outside the OR. Recognizing this fact, it is appropriate to carefully evaluate the nature of the sedation/anesthesia provided in the NORA setting and consider all of the possible implications of a given technique for each patient group. For instance, how efficient and effective is the care that is provided? How well does the care provided meet the requirements of the procedure in terms of pain and movement control? How rapid is the emergence from sedation or anesthesia with a given technique? Do the short-term or long-term complications differ? Only after careful analysis can guidelines be established for the optimal technique for a given procedure.[24]

When delivering general anesthesia to children outside the OR, the risk benefit of instrumenting the airway must be carefully evaluated. The LMA has been found to be useful in the MRI or computed tomography (CT) setting because it can be used with spontaneous ventilation, enables the anesthesiologist to monitor $ETCO_2$ continuously, and provides a clear airway for a child who may otherwise have an airway obstruction or who is in a position where the airway is not readily accessible. With the LMA in place, the child can be maintained with a relatively small inspired concentration of anesthesia, allowed to breathe spontaneously, and then rapidly awakened at the conclusion of the scan. After the LMA is placed, anesthesia can be provided with either a continuous infusion of propofol or with a low-dose inhalation agent (e.g., sevoflurane 1.5% in 50% N_2O/O_2). In some circumstances, the LMA may provide a suitable airway in children with bronchopulmonary dysplasia, cystic fibrosis, severe asthma, or active respiratory issues. In children with upper respiratory tract infections, the incidence of mild bronchospasm, laryngospasm, breath-holding, and O_2 desaturation (<90%) in those whose airway was managed with an LMA was reduced compared with those whose airway was managed with a tracheal tube.[25,26] Similarly, the use of LMAs in former preterm infants with bronchopulmonary dysplasia resulted in less coughing and wheezing and greater hemodynamic stability than in those managed with tracheal tubes. In children who underwent a vitrectomy for retinopathy of prematurity, the time to discharge after an LMA was less than that after a tracheal tube.[27] LMAs provide more hemodynamic stability during their removal than during tracheal extubation and may offer a specific advantage in some children.[28]

In healthy children, deep sedation is appropriate (e.g., for an MRI scan); it usually includes a propofol infusion, an optimally positioned upper airway (with a roll under the cervical spine and the neck extended), and noninvasive monitoring (nasal capnometry supplemented with oximetry, an ECG, and noninvasive blood pressure monitoring).[29] The majority of children do not require an airway during deep sedation for medical tests. However, in some (e.g., those with excess secretions or obstructive sleep apnea), the following algorithm of airway intervention may be followed to relieve the obstruction: (1) reposition the head and shoulders, (2) insert an oral or nasal airway,[30,31] (3) if partial obstruction persists, place an LMA, and (4) if the LMA fails to provide adequate gas exchange and oxygenation, place a tracheal tube.

Logistics of Managing Acute Emergencies and Cardiopulmonary Arrest Outside the Operating Room

Although the actual management of a cardiopulmonary arrest should not vary between the OR setting and the non-OR setting, the logistics of performing a resuscitation may be challenged by unanticipated factors, such as personnel who may not be familiar with code situations, an environment that makes performing a resuscitation difficult, or equipment that may be unsafe if used in the particular location (e.g., the MRI environment). It is important that all personnel in the off-site location be familiar with the location and operation of the code cart. The anesthesia cart and the code cart in the off-site location should be stocked in the same precise configuration as all others throughout the hospital and ORs. Standardizing the code carts throughout the hospital ensures that all ancillary personnel can be helpful in locating critical items. If the code cart is kept locked, the key or access code must be readily accessible and in a location that is known to all essential personnel. A hard board on which chest compressions may be performed should be readily available. Each off-site location should have an identified and rehearsed routine for announcing a code situation and summoning aid. Responders to a code must be assured of access to the location to which they are called; in the current age of card-key access, this should be simple but needs to be established in advance of need. The use of patient simulation can be very helpful in testing the team response to critical events. Simulators can be used in place in off-site locations to replicate critical events and evaluate the ability of the care team and backup systems to resuscitate a patient. This methodology has documented significant variation in the ability of rescuers to resuscitate children from sedation or anesthesia critical events in locations outside the OR.[32]

MRI SCANNER

Of all the non-OR environments in which anesthesiologists are asked to provide care, the MRI scanner poses a unique challenge for cardiopulmonary resuscitation. The MRI environment is divided into four zones that correlate with the intensity of the magnetic field and the risk to children and health care providers. These zones are delineated in Table 46.1.

The ASA published a Practice Advisory report in 2009.[33,34] This document advises that in the case of a medical emergency within the scanner, the anesthesia providers should (1) initiate cardiopulmonary resuscitation while immediately removing the patient from zone IV, (2) call for help, and (3) transport the patient to a previously designated safe location in proximity to the MRI suite. This designated location should contain a defibrillator, vital signs monitors, and a code cart with all resuscitation drugs, airway equipment, O_2, and suction. Other acute emergencies that are unique to the MRI environment include a "quench" in the scanner.[33,34] Quenching occurs when the liquid that cools the magnet boils off rapidly and results in helium escaping from the cryogen bath. The magnetic field of the magnet is rapidly decreased because the coils in the magnet cease to be superconducting and become resistive. In addition to performing the institution's protocol in reaction to either of these events, the ASA consultants involved in writing the advisory agree that in the event of a quench (1) the child should be removed from zone IV immediately, (2) O_2 should be administered immediately, and (3) emergency response personnel should be restricted from entering zone IV

TABLE 46.1	Descriptions of the American College of Radiology's Four Zones in the Magnetic Resonance Imaging Suite	
ACR Zones	**Occupants**	**Hazards**
Zone I	General public	Negligible
Zone II	Unscreened MRI patients	Immediately outside area of hazard
Zone III	Screened MRI patients and personnel	Potential biostimulation interference, access to magnet room
Zone IV	Screened MRI patients under constant direct supervision of trained MRI personnel	Biostimulation interference, radiofrequency heating, missile effect, cryogens

ACR, American College of Radiology; *MRI*, magnetic resonance imaging.
From Kanal E, Barkovich AJ, Bell C, et al. ACR guidance document for safe MR practices: 2007. AJR 2007;188:1–27.

because of the powerful magnetic field that can exist even after a quench.

Difficult Airway Management in the Non–Operating Room (Off-Site) Environment

Two potential difficult airway scenarios may occur in non-OR locations: the child with a known difficult airway and the child with an unrecognized difficult airway. There is little peer-reviewed literature that addresses these scenarios, but logic would dictate that children who are identified as having potentially difficult airways should have their airways secured in the controlled environment of the OR. Regardless of an anesthesiologist's comfort level and familiarity with the intended off-site environment, the critical backup personnel and the full array of airway equipment are not generally available in remote locations. It is important to note that a fiberoptic bronchoscope and light source and most video laryngoscopes are not MRI compatible (Tru-MR [Truphatek International Ltd., Netanya, Israel] is an MRI-compatible video laryngoscope). It is easier to secure the airway with these alternative devices in an OR. In this environment, both the nursing and anesthesia support staff (technicians, other anesthesiologists, and otolaryngologists) are readily available and prepared to provide assistance. More recently, the advent of advanced video laryngoscopes has made the requirement for flexible fiberoptic intubations less common.[35] This equipment should be readily available in NORA locations for any child with a proven or suspected difficult laryngoscopy (before and during the procedure). With the trachea intubated, the child may be safely transported to the off-site location for subsequent care. The ASA task force on care in the MRI recommends complex airway management should be performed in a controlled environment outside zone IV.[34]

The more difficult scenario is that of the unrecognized difficult airway[36]; this scenario may best be handled by establishing a local management protocol that can be activated when the situation arises. Each institution has particular equipment, space, and personnel resources. NORA leaders should establish a local protocol for management of the unanticipated difficult airway in an off-site location. In some cases this might involve bringing advanced

46

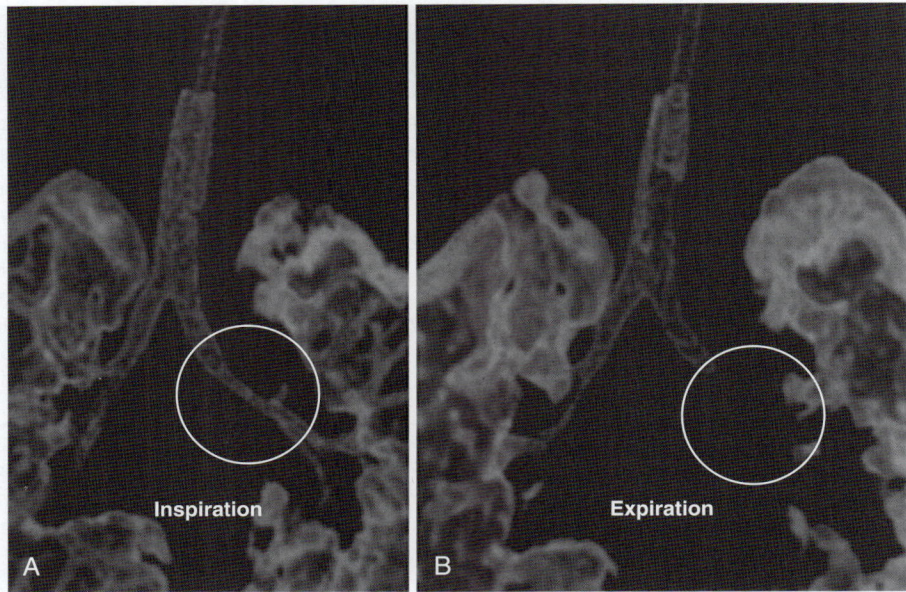

FIGURE 46.1 Three-dimensional dynamic computed tomography scan demonstrating change in caliber of left main-stem bronchus (*circle*) in an intubated child at end-inspiration (pressure held at 15–18 mm Hg) **(A)** versus end-expiration **(B)**.

airway management equipment to the location in a rapid, organized manner. In other cases the best option would include "temporizing" management with alternative airway devices and transporting the child to a location where a definitive airway can be placed in a controlled manner. For this reason, it is important to have alternative airway devices such as LMAs stocked in all anesthesia carts that are designated for off-site locations. In the event that the lungs cannot be ventilated or the trachea intubated, the LMA has a proven track record for providing a lifesaving temporary airway until more definitive action can be taken.[37,38]

Specific Locations for Non–Operating Room Anesthesia

COMPUTED TOMOGRAPHY

CT involves ionizing radiation and can provide a good modality for differentiating between high-density (calcium, iron, bone, contrast-enhanced vascular and cerebrospinal fluid [CSF] spaces) and low-density (O_2, nitrogen, carbon in air, fat, CSF, muscle, white matter, gray matter, and water-containing lesions) structures. Generally, the scan time with the current 64-bit scanners is brief; with actual imaging time ranging from 5 to 50 seconds for image acquisition, many children are able to tolerate CT without sedation or anesthesia. A new generation of high-speed CT scanners obtains images in as little as 0.3 seconds, which should allow even more images to be acquired without sedation and with exposure to less radiation.[39] Children who require anesthesia often have a fragile or unstable respiratory or cardiovascular status. Anesthesia or sedation is often required for children who are unable to cooperate (cognitively impaired children and those younger than 2–3 years of age) or require CT emergently. Emergent indications for CT include head trauma, unstable respiratory status in need of a pulmonary diagnosis, unexplained changes in mental status, neoplasm workup, or radiation therapy planning. Anesthesia

management is also necessary with a potentially unstable airway (peritonsillar abscess, anterior mediastinal mass, craniofacial anomaly, tracheoesophageal fistula, uncontrolled vomiting, or gastroesophageal reflux) or the need for breath-holding during acquisition of images (three-dimensional dynamic airway studies) (Figs. 46.1 and 46.2). Some CT units are particularly concerned about children moving when contrast is injected (because of dose restrictions the contrast injection cannot be repeated) and therefore request anesthesia services for any child they cannot confidently predict will stay motionless for the study.

Children with Down syndrome present a particular risk for atlantoaxial instability and may require a head or neck CT to evaluate cervical and temporomandibular anatomy, recurrent sinusitis, or choanal atresia. The reported incidence of atlantoaxial instability varies from 12% to 32%,[40] although anesthesia-related neck complications are almost nonexistent in children with Down syndrome.[37] These children often require cervical spine radiographs before entering grade school or participating in the Special Olympics. Usually, the parents know the outcome of these tests and can convey the results to the anesthesiologist. These studies alone do *not* indicate to the practitioner whether the child is at risk of dislocation.[37] Rather, it is the presence of neurologic signs or symptoms that would herald a spine that is "at risk": abnormal wide-based gait, incontinence, increased clumsiness, fatigue with ambulation, complaints of numbness, tingling in an extremity, weakness of an extremity, or a new preference for sitting games. In infants, these clinical signs may be difficult to assess. In younger children, developmental milestones (e.g., crawling, sitting up, reaching for objects) should be evaluated. Physical signs may include clonus, hyperreflexia, quadriparesis, neurogenic bladder, hemiparesis, ataxia, and sensory loss. Children with atlantoaxial instability on a radiograph are at less risk for dislocation if they do not exhibit any signs or symptoms of instability. Children who are capable of following commands may be asked to perform full neck flexion and extension maneuvers to determine whether

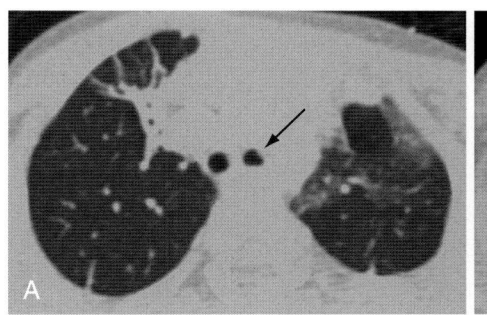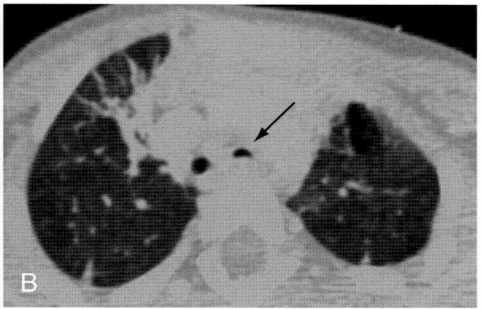

FIGURE 46.2 Three-dimensional CT scan demonstrating change in caliber of left main-stem bronchus *(arrows)* on inspiration **(A)** versus expiration **(B)**.

pain, sensory, or motor manifestations of cord compression develop. When the child is young, unable to cooperate with an examination, or has an uncertain history of atlanto-axial instability, it is wisest to avoid extremes of neck positioning during CT scans and communicate with radiology colleagues about the clinical concerns.

Perhaps the most controversial issue facing anesthesiologists with regard to CT scans is the issue of oral contrast for CT. Because children lack abundant retroperitoneal fat, they do not have the natural contrast needed to elucidate abdominal images. For this reason, children are often required to ingest (orally or via nasogastric tube) diatrizoic acid (Gastrografin) to opacify the stomach and bowel. Oral contrast is useful in the identification of an intraabdominal abscess, mass, fluid collection, bowel injury, pancreatic injury, or other traumatic injury. The oral contrast comes as Gastrografin 3% concentration and may be diluted to a 1:1.5% concentration. Since Gastrografin 3% is hypertonic (2200 mOsm/L) it can cause pulmonary edema, pneumonitis, osmotic effusions, and death if aspirated. Thus the more dilute concentration is recommended for CT, which is thought to be much less dangerous if aspirated. The volume of oral contrast that is administered can be quite large. Neonates typically receive 60 to 90 mL. Infants between 1 month and 1 year of age may receive up to 240 mL. Children between the ages of 1 and 5 years receive between 240 to 360 mL of contrast medium. Risk is introduced when these children require anesthesia within an optimal window after ingestion (usually 30 minutes to 1 hour after receiving the contrast agent) to enhance visualization. By most fasting guidelines (nil per os [NPO]), Gastrografin consumption within 1 to 2 hours of an anesthetic or sedation does not fall within the usual NPO guidelines. On the other hand, the scan must be completed while the Gastrografin is present in the GI tract. Despite the large volume of Gastrografin that may be ingested, there does not appear to be a significant aspiration risk in this population, and many anesthesiologists do not secure the airway with a tracheal tube (Fig. 46.3). A review of the pediatric and adult literature confirms that over the past 35 years (and hundreds of thousands of contrast GI CT scans) only a few case reports have been published of aspiration syndrome attributed to Gastrografin, all in extremely high-risk patients with issues such as bowel obstruction or acute abdomen.[38,41,42]

Several investigators have evaluated the issue of aspiration from different perspectives. In one study, a cohort of 50 children who received oral contrast after blunt abdominal trauma were evaluated for radiologic evidence of aspiration pneumonia or clinical complications of aspiration.[43] Some received general anesthesia and some were neurologically impaired (including several

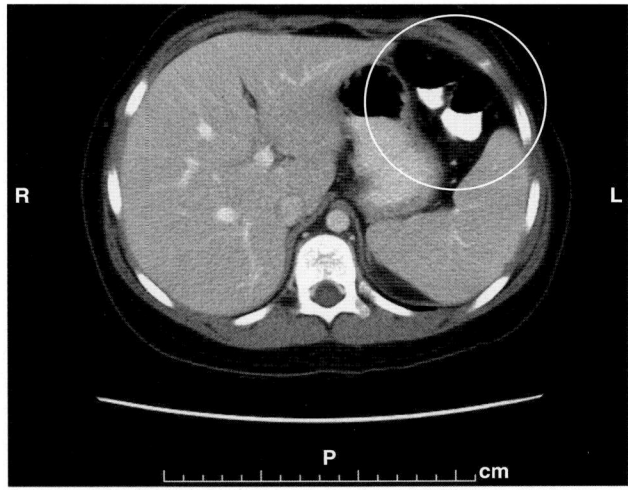

FIGURE 46.3 Four hours after ingestion of Gastrografin, oral contrast is still present in the stomach and small intestine. Although dilute Gastrografin is still frequently present in the stomach at the time of computed tomography, there are as yet no case reports validating an increase in risk of pulmonary aspiration.

with increased intracranial pressure). In this very high-risk group, only one child was thought to have possibly aspirated based on a chest radiograph after the CT scan, although that patient did not develop pulmonary symptoms. Another study evaluated the volume of gastric contents of 365 children undergoing deep sedation or general anesthesia for abdominal CT scans. Omnipaque 3 mL was diluted 50-fold to a volume of 150 mL and given to children younger than 1 year and a volume of 600 mL was given to teenagers—starting 2 hours before the scheduled scan and ending 1 hour before general anesthesia (N = 207) or sedation (N = 158); all were elective scans with standard fasting times. The authors note that gastric contents exceeded 0.4 mL/kg in 49% of those who received gastric contrast[43] (the actual threshold volume for aspiration is likely closer to 0.8 mL/kg as documented in primates[44]). Two cases of vomiting were recorded. None of the children in the study developed clinical evidence of aspiration. When dilute Gastrografin is used, the risks associated with pulmonary aspiration appear to be small, even in children who are moderately to deeply sedated.[45] Despite this evidence, cohort studies with sufficient power to determine the actual incidence of aspiration in this setting have not been performed. Therefore, *no* accepted standard of care for the airway management of these children has been determined. Some anesthesiologists induce anesthesia with an IV or inhalational technique and maintain the anesthetic without securing the airway with a tracheal tube. Others perform rapid-sequence induction and tracheal intubation. The lack of consensus among anesthesiologists and the absence of evidence preclude a clear and consistent recommendation for managing the airway in these children. Common sense would lead one to conclude that a rapid sequence induction with tracheal intubation/general anesthesia would be most appropriate for children with bowel pathology that interfered with gastric emptying.

CT scans that involve imaging the airway are also an area of concern for anesthesiologists.[46] Traditionally, although these scans are brief, they have required breath-holding to allow the capture of images with sufficient clarity to be of diagnostic quality. Appropriate apnea intervals can be obtained under anesthesia with tracheal intubation with or without neuromuscular blockade, or by placing an LMA and providing moderate hyperventilation and a bolus of propofol (which results in apnea when ventilation is discontinued). The current generation of "flash" CT technology with ultra-fast image capture is largely eliminating the need for breath-holding with these studies and may further eliminate the need for sedation or anesthesia for many CT studies in children of any age.[39]

NUCLEAR MEDICINE

Nuclear medicine is one of the oldest functional imaging disciplines; these scans are useful for identification of the extent of disease for many neoplasms.[47] They can also be used to detect epileptic foci in refractory epilepsy, evaluate cerebrovascular disease (e.g., Moyamoya disease) and cognitive and behavior disorders, and detect and delineate renal function and disease, including detection of reflux and acute pyelonephritis.[37] Improvements in the hardware for nuclear imaging have greatly decreased the scan time, although even with the advent of two-level emission and transmission scans and combined CT imaging, some of the scan times can still reach 2 hours or more. The equipment in nuclear medicine imaging emits no ionizing radiation; rather, the radiation is contained within the child and is of very low energy levels. Depending on the nature of the study, the children require IV access for administration of the nuclear tracer well in advance of the scan and therefore usually have IV access for the anesthesia or sedation. Many nuclear scans also require an empty bladder to avoid interference from concentrated tracer in an enlarged bladder. Accordingly, the bladder is often catheterized after anesthesia is induced and the radioactive urine that is collected is disposed of in a radioactive-safe manner.

Two nuclear scans that involve anesthesia and present particular challenges are single-photon emission computed tomography (SPECT) and positron emission tomography (PET) scans. Both of these scans can be combined with a CT scan for optimal imaging. SPECT scans use single-photon gamma-emitting radioisotopes and rotating gamma cameras to produce three-dimensional brain images. SPECT scans involve the use of radiolabeled technetium-99m (half-life of 6 hours), which undergoes extensive first-pass extraction and intracellular trapping in proportion to regional cerebral blood flow. This scan is useful for localizing seizure foci. It appears to be as accurate as invasive direct cortical mapping in this regard.[48] Injection of the radionuclide proximate to the time of a seizure will tag areas of increased cerebral blood flow and localize the seizure foci. The child should be scanned

within 1 to 6 hours of the seizure and injection of the tracer. This technique poses some obvious logistical challenges since there is no way to predict (exactly) when a seizure will occur. The anesthesiology service must be flexible in providing anesthetic services within the window of time allowed to complete the test whenever the next seizure occurs.

PET scans use radionuclide tracers of metabolic activity such as O_2 usage and glucose metabolism. Radionuclide tracers of glucose may be useful when seeking seizure foci or tumor recurrence.[47,49,50] Unlike SPECT scans, PET scans require a seizure-free period of at least 2 hours. Tracer is then injected and the scan is performed after 30 to 45 minutes. Outpatient scans may be scheduled but are canceled if a seizure occurs. In-patient scans required for children who have frequent seizures can be extremely difficult to schedule and must be coordinated between the neurology and anesthesiology services.

Both SPECT and PET scan techniques are noninvasive. There is little noise associated with them, and there are no issues related to electromagnetic field as there is in the MRI scanner. The patients have to hold very still in a specific position, however, and the detector unit is very close to their face/head. This obviates the use of digital movies for distraction, although music can be used and parents can be present if the patient will be awake. Anesthesia/sedation is required for those patients who cannot hold still in a nonthreatening environment for the time periods required for the scans, which can range from 10 minutes for a PET/CT of the head to 2 hours for SPECT scanning of the body.[47]

STEREOTACTIC RADIOSURGERY

Stereotactic radiosurgery (gamma knife) is a major advance in the treatment of selected malignant tumors (ependymoma, glioblastomas), vascular malformations, acoustic neuromas, and pituitary adenomas in children.[51,52] Radiosurgery is indicated, especially for those children with a tumor located deep in the brain or in an area that could put the child at significant surgical risk (e.g., speech, motor, cerebellum, brainstem areas) or for the recurrent brain tumor that has failed prior treatment. Radiosurgery involves the use of a single large fraction of radiation that is directed at a specific target with minimal radiation exposure to the surrounding normal tissues. Optimal results are achieved with small tumor volumes (≤14 cm³).[53]

Stereotactic radiosurgery requires the coordination of the departments of radiology, radiation therapy, and anesthesiology. The procedure averages 9 hours but can take up to 15 hours. The stereotactic portion of the procedure begins in the morning in a CT scanner. A stereotactic head frame is applied after induction of general anesthesia and tracheal intubation. Some older children can tolerate the application of the head frame with local anesthesia alone but then develop anxiety because the pressure sensation produced by the head frame can lead to anxiety, nausea, or vomiting. The vast majority of children require general anesthesia for application of the frame and subsequent imaging and surgery. When the head frame is in place, the key to unlock and remove it should be taped to the frame itself, in the event of a situation necessitating its emergent removal (e.g., vomiting, airway obstruction, or accidental tracheal extubation). For smaller children, nasal intubation may provide better stability during transport from the radiology suite to the OR. After the head frame is in place and the imaging study is completed, the child is transported (trachea intubated, sedated, and appropriately monitored) to the postanesthesia care unit while the radiologists and neurosurgeons review the images and plan radiosurgery. The postanesthesia care unit stay can range from 3 to 5 hours, during which time these children require continuous physiologic monitoring.

After the images are reviewed and the radiosurgery planning is complete, the child is transported to the stereotactic radiosurgery linear accelerator for treatment. The treatment room is equipped with an anesthesia machine and monitors. To minimize radiation exposure to health care personnel, only the child remains in the scanner area during treatment. The child is observed at a distance with video cameras that are focused on both the child and the physiologic monitors. Treatment usually lasts about 1 hour.

After radiosurgery is completed, the child is returned to the postanesthesia care unit where the trachea is extubated under controlled conditions. Risks are inherent with this prolonged anesthesia, which requires multiple transports between sites. Four potentially serious anesthesia-related events were reported in 68 radiosurgery procedures in 65 children.[54] Serious complications in those children who received general anesthesia included obstruction of the tracheal tube while in the head frame and lobar collapse requiring prolonged mechanical ventilation.

RADIATION THERAPY

Radiation therapy for children uses ionizing photons to destroy lymphomas, acute leukemias, Wilms tumor, retinoblastomas, and tumors of the central nervous system. Improved three-dimensional imaging and enhanced computing power have allowed radiation oncologists to conform radiation dose to the shape of the tumor and minimize radiation to the surrounding tissues.[55] The energy absorbed by the tissues is measured in *grays* (Gy), which has replaced the term *rad*. One gray is equivalent to 100 rad. Although most children receive standard x-ray therapy, specific lesions may respond better to bombardment with electron, proton, or neutron beam therapy. The anesthetic considerations are identical regardless of the type of therapy in this respect.[56] A planning session in a simulator is typically scheduled before the initiation of radiation therapy to map the fields that require irradiation while the child is in a fixed position. For proton beam treatments, a planning session is performed in a CT scanner. A fiberglass immobilization mask of the head is made while the child is sedated/anesthetized with propofol and (most often) with a natural airway (Fig. 46.4).

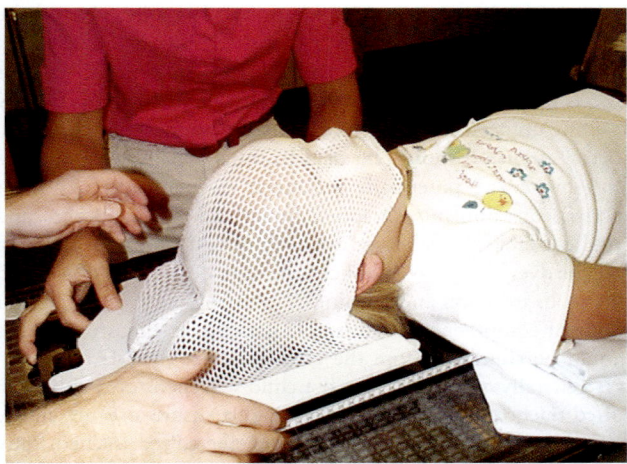

FIGURE 46.4 Child in fiberglass mask for radiation treatment of a cerebral neoplasm.

This cast allows secure positioning to ensure that the child does not move during treatment, but considerable care is required to configure the mask for optimal airway patency while ensuring proper windows for treatments. Once the mask is completed, the use of an oral airway or LMA is not possible as these maneuvers will alter the head position and thus the direction of the radiation beam.

Radiation therapy involves "fractionated" exposure. Repeat sessions are typical. The child must be motionlessness during therapy to precisely target malignant cells. Radiation therapy is typically administered by dividing the total radiation therapy course among daily or twice-daily sessions. In general, most treatment sessions last between 15 and 30 minutes, and the planning simulation session may take as long as 2 hours, depending on the nature and location of the target lesion or area for therapy. For children who require neuraxial treatments for spinal metastases, as many as four fields may be irradiated with the child in both the supine and prone positions. Dividing the total radiation therapy course into discrete daily sessions allows normal tissue repair between sessions while the tumor burden is lessened or destroyed. These children are optimally managed via central venous access that obviates the need for repeated venipunctures. Unless there is a specific airway anomaly, daily anesthetic management typically consists of deep sedation using a propofol infusion (with or without midazolam pretreatment),[57] blow-by oxygen via nasal cannula or face mask, and spontaneous ventilation monitored with $ETCO_2$. Tachyphylaxis does not appear to be an issue even with multiple, frequent treatments.[58] Given all of the challenges, it is somewhat surprising that these treatments have not been associated with an increased adverse event rate. One retrospective review of 177 patients undergoing 3833 radiation treatments documented a 1.3% complication rate.[59] This rate compares favorably with the rate of complications for children undergoing propofol-based anesthesia without cancer.[60]

Dexmedetomidine sedation has been used for radiation therapy, but its use has not become widespread most likely because of the need for a 10-minute loading dose and relatively frequent need for repeated boluses at the doses that have so far been studied.[61] Single-dose IV ketamine 0.5 to 0.8 mg/kg provides effective sedation, albeit with a greater half-life, more movement, and an increased rate of adverse events on emergence (e.g., vomiting) than propofol.[62]

One exceptional case in radiation therapy is retinoblastoma. In this case, the eye must be completely immobile during the treatment. General anesthesia or deep propofol sedation is required to ensure appropriate irradiating conditions; ketamine (in particular), with its side effect of lateral nystagmus, is not appropriate in these cases (see Video 7.1).[62]

The logistics of radiation therapy anesthesia or sedation are complex, even though the treatments themselves are not challenging; only the child remains in the room during treatment. Thus monitoring must be performed using video observation. For this reason, radiation therapy units are equipped with multiple video monitors adjusted to allow viewing of both the child from several views and the physiologic monitors. Children are often moved to allow different angles of access for the radiation treatment; this must be taken into consideration when positioning monitors and power cords. Many cases of spinal irradiation require the child to be prone with the head at a specific angle with respect to the back. Often several adjustments to head position are required to maintain a patent airway with the tight-fitting mask; monitoring expired carbon dioxide is therefore essential.

Most children undergoing radiation therapy are also receiving chemotherapy. As the treatment progresses, nausea, vomiting, and respiratory illness stemming from local radiation effects and chemotherapy can create deteriorating conditions for spontaneous, natural airway ventilation. It is important to work with the child's oncologist to manage symptoms and complete the treatment series as close to the planned treatment regimen as possible, because this is critical to the child's survival and maximizing quality of life.

MAGNETIC RESONANCE IMAGING

MRI, magnetic resonance spectroscopy (MRS), magnetic resonance angiography (MRA), and magnetic resonance venography (MRV) are used for the evaluation of neoplasms, nonhemorrhagic trauma, vascular, cardiac, orthopedic (including joint disorders, osteomyelitis), central nervous system and spinal cord lesions, craniofacial disorders, detecting the origin of developmental delay, behavioral disorders, seizures, failure to thrive, apnea, cyanosis, hypotonia, and in the workup of mitochondrial and metabolic diseases.[63-66] MRA and MRV are especially helpful in evaluating vascular flow and often can replace invasive angiography in follow-up evaluations of vascular malformations, interventional therapy, or radiotherapy.[67,68] All of these imaging modalities are essentially equivalent in terms of the requirements for the provision of anesthesia or sedation and thus can be considered the same as MRI.

Most MRI systems are superconducting magnets set up in a horizontal configuration within the bore so that the magnetic field is directed lengthwise to the child. The magnet is cooled by liquid helium to a temperature of approximately −268°C. The strength of the magnetic field in these scanners is described in tesla (T) units and range from 0.5 to 3.0 T. To put this into perspective, a 1.5-T magnet is the equivalent of 30,000 times the earth's magnetic field.

A variety of safety issues with respect to MRI are important; a review can be found in an American College of Radiology safety paper.[69] All individuals who work in the MR environment should be familiar with the primary recommendations in this paper.

Foremost is the risk of injury from ferromagnetic objects attracted to the magnetic core of the MRI scanner that can cause significant morbidity and mortality (Fig. 46.5). In the presence of an external magnetic field, a ferromagnetic object can develop its own intrinsic magnetic field. The attractive forces created between the intrinsic and extrinsic magnetic fields propel the ferromagnetic object toward the MRI scanner. Numerous injuries including death have been reported from objects accidentally attracted to the MRI magnet, including: an anesthesia cart, a metal fan, pulse oximeter, shrapnel, wheelchair, cigarette lighter, stethoscope, pager, hearing aid, vacuum cleaner, calculator, hair pin, O_2 tank, prosthetic limb, pencil, insulin infusion pump, keys, watches, clipboards, steel-toe or steel-heeled shoes, ferrous jewelry, and even a concealed police revolver.[70,71] Mortality can result from projectile disasters, as when a ferrous O_2 tank was "pulled" from the hands of the respiratory therapist and crushed the skull of the child being scanned.[71a] It is absolutely essential that all portable O_2 tanks are MRI-compatible and that anesthesia carts are not brought into the MRI. Many MRI scanner units now have screening protocols that include a small handheld magnet to test whether objects are ferromagnetic and thus at risk of being pulled into the magnet.

The other major potential morbidity related to MRI scanning results from implanted devices (i.e., cardiac pacemakers, spinal cord stimulators, programmable ventriculoperitoneal shunts) that may malfunction in the powerful magnetic field of the MRI scanner and can cause injury. These injuries are most often caused

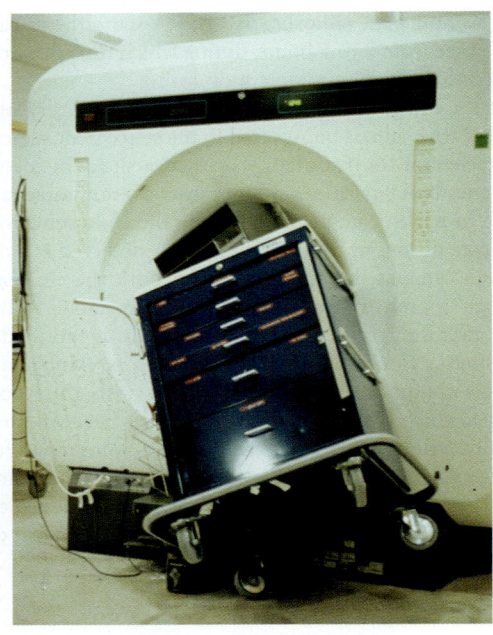

FIGURE 46.5 Magnetic resonance imaging cart that is not compatible inadvertently brought into scanner room. To extricate the cart, the magnet had to be quenched, incurring a cost in excess of $20,000 USD.

by inappropriate patient screening or unfamiliarity with a particular implant's MRI compatibility. The U.S. Food and Drug Administration (FDA) has terminology for designating objects in terms of their safety in the MRI environment. *MRI-safe* is defined as not posing any known hazard in any MR environment. *MRI-conditional* refers to objects that may or may not be safe, depending on the specific conditions that are present. *MRI-unsafe* means the object should never be brought into the MRI environment because it poses a potential or realistic risk or hazard. All objects or medical devices should be referenced and vetted for safety prior to being brought into zone IV. Some devices are compatible with 1.5-T but not with 3.0-T units. Current standards for MRI safety include a magnetic metal detector check of all personnel and patients and/or family each time they enter the scanner.

All implanted objects should be carefully evaluated before a patient or health care provider enters the MRI suite. The website http://www.MRIsafety.com is a useful resource for identifying MRI-safe objects. Note that stainless steel or surgical stainless objects may interact with the external magnetic field, potentially resulting in translational (attractive) and rotational (torque) forces. Special attention should be paid to intracranial aneurysm clips (may move and potentially dislodge), vascular stents, cochlear and stapedial implants, shrapnel, intraorbital metallic bodies, and prosthetic limbs. In fact, some eye make-up and tattoos may contain metallic dyes and are at risk of causing skin, ocular, periorbital, and cutaneous irritation and burning.[72-74] Among the most important pieces of equipment for vulnerable patients, tracheostomy tubes should be checked before the children enter the MRI scanner. It is generally advised to switch a child's tracheostomy tube to a cuffed tracheal tube for MRI scanning to ensure a secure airway during the scan. Currently small-diameter cuffed tracheostomy tubes (Bivona) from Smiths Medical (Minneapolis, MN) are considered MRI-conditional (at www.MRIsafety.com, search for the MRI-compatible object to determine MRI compatibility).

They are acceptable for use, although the pilot balloon must be taped out of the way for use.

Cardiac pacemaker compatibility is a matter of some debate.[75] Historically, the presence of a pacemaker has been considered a contraindication for the MRI environment. Most pacemakers have a reed relay switch that can be activated when exposed to a strong magnetic field and convert the pacemaker to the asynchronous mode. In at least two known cases, patients with pacemakers died from cardiac arrest while in the MRI scanner.[76] Adverse events associated with pacemakers in the MRI scanner include ventricular fibrillation, rapid atrial pacing, asynchronous pacing, inhibition of pacing output, and movement of the device.[77,78]

Since 1996, however, changes in pacemaker electronics have included decreased ferromagnetic content and increased sophistication of the computer capabilities. In 2004, one study reported no changes in pacemaker capabilities or adverse outcomes after 56 patients with pacemakers underwent 62 MRI procedures.[79] Similar results were reported in 68 patients whose pacemakers were reprogrammed to asynchronous or demand mode before undergoing scans in a 1.5-T MRI scanner. Unfortunately, there is a paucity of data on children with pacemakers or implanted defibrillators who underwent MRI scans, particularly with respect to scanners with 3-T field strength. In one large literature review on this topic (mostly adult data) including almost 1500 patient encounters, 82% were found to have no significant changes in pacemaker function after imaging.[80] No deaths or serious adverse events were reported in this study, and the authors echo the sentiments that MRI scans should only be performed after consultation with experts and (even then) only if benefits are thought to outweigh risks.

Auditory considerations exist with respect to MRI. Specifically, a loud banging sound and vibrations are produced as the forces generated within the gradient coils of the MRI scanner cause the gradient coils to vibrate. The noises generated range from 65 to 95 dB in a 1.5-T magnet. Temporary hearing loss after an MRI scan has been reported.[81] This report suggests that earplugs may prevent the temporary hearing loss associated with MRI. Given these data, earplugs or MRI-compatible headphones are routinely used in children undergoing MRI scans.

Temperature regulation for infants and children during sedation or analgesia is a concern. Cool temperatures and humidity are required for proper magnet function, which are a setup for a child's radiant and convective heat loss, particularly since anesthesia limits intrinsic thermoregulation. On the other hand, the MRI generates radiofrequency radiation that is absorbed by the child and may offset heat lost to the environment. The specific absorption rate (SAR), which is measured in watts per kilogram, is used to follow the effects of RF heating. The FDA allows an SAR of 0.4 W/kg averaged over the whole body.[82] Early data suggested that children can increase their core body temperature by 0.5°C during MRI of less than 1-hour duration in a 1.5-T environment.[83,84] The temperature of infants who underwent MRI scans of the brain increased 0.2°C with a 1.5-T scanner and 0.5°C with a 3-T scanner, with minimal efforts to prevent passive heat loss.[85] More recently a study of almost 200 patients undergoing MRI scans found that 52% of children were hypothermic after their MRI scans, whereas none were hyperthermic.[86] Given the cool environment of the MRI scanner, it appears appropriate to pursue simple interventions to preserve warmth in the scanner, such as covering with warm blankets.

Focal heating remains a concern with respect to monitoring equipment in the MRI scanner. For example, the ECG leads

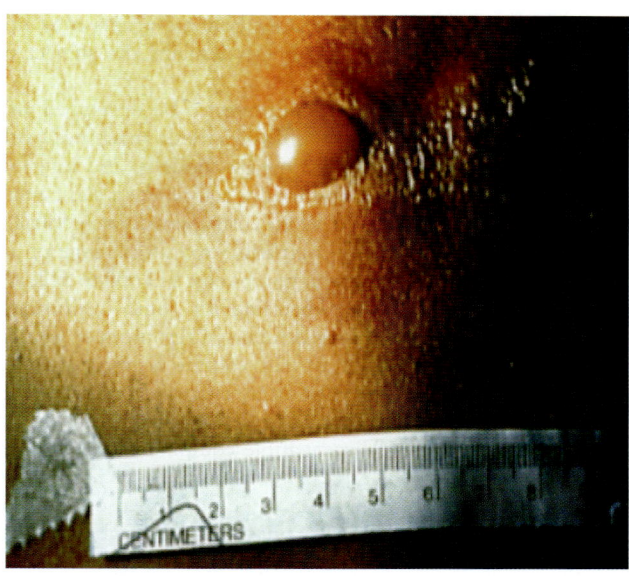

FIGURE 46.6 MRI-induced burn at site of electrocardiogram pad from a frayed lead.

should not have frays or exposed wires; *any coils or loops in a conductor such as ECG wires or a pulse oximeter probe can cause tissue burns* (Fig. 46.6). Cases of first-, second-, and third-degree burns after MRI have been reported.[87] To avoid patient injury, the following precautions should be undertaken: (1) avoid creating a conductive loop between the child and a conductor (ECG monitoring or gating leads, plethysmographic gating wire, and fingertip attachment); (2) do not leave any unconnected imaging coils in the magnet during imaging; and (3) prevent all exposed wires or conductors from touching the child's skin during the scan.

Many MRI scans require contrast administration. Gadolinium (gadopentetate dimeglumine) is an FDA-approved contrast agent that is intravascularly administered for MRI enhancement. Approved for use in 1998, gadolinium provides greater contrast between normal and abnormal tissue throughout the body. Gadolinium forms a complex with chelating agents that facilitates biodistribution to the extracellular compartment and excretion via the kidneys. Unlike iodinated contrast agents, gadolinium complexes do not present a significant osmotic load. Gadolinium agents are considered to be safer than iodine agents with respect to adverse reactions. It is reportedly easily removed with dialysis.[88] On the other hand, recent warnings from the FDA suggest that gadolinium-containing contrast agents may be associated with the development of nephrogenic systemic fibrosis or nephrogenic fibrosing dermopathy in patients with moderate to end-stage kidney disease. The FDA suggests that gadolinium be administered only if necessary in children with advanced kidney failure and that, in those children, prompt dialysis should be considered after gadolinium administration for MRA studies. The incidence of severe anaphylactic or anaphylactoid reactions to gadolinium (0.01%–0.0003%) is less than that of iodine-based contrast media.[89] Another recent concern regarding gadolinium stemmed from evidence that increased uptake and deposition of gadolinium in the dentate nucleus and globus pallidus in normal brain tissue was found at autopsy after repeated scans. Given the lack of long-term follow-up, this has raised safety concerns and prompted some centers to change from using gadolinium to gadoterate meglumine (Dotarem) or other contrast agents. These latter contrast agents may not accumulate in the brain, although this remains the subject of ongoing investigation.[90-92]

MRI-compatible equipment continues to be developed and improved. Multiple MRI-compatible anesthesia machines (with ventilators), monitors (including wireless models), and infusion pumps are now available. The cost for this equipment is substantial: an MRI-compatible anesthesia machine costs approximately $60,000 to $80,000 U.S. dollars; MRI-compatible monitors range up to $140,000 and compatible infusion pumps cost $12,000 to $18,000 each. This cost may be overwhelming for some institutions, especially in facilities with limited financial resources or limited need for MRI anesthetics. If patient volume is insufficient or financial backing to support such an investment is lacking, then special planning may be instituted to deliver anesthesia without a full complement of MRI-compatible equipment. Specifically, a non–MRI-compatible anesthesia machine could be used in the following manner: the machine must be positioned outside the MRI suite, and 30 feet of airway circuit extension may be threaded through the wall of the scanner to the child within. Alternatively, IV sedation or anesthesia can be delivered using MRI-compatible infusion pumps and O_2 can be delivered using a face mask or nasal cannula. If an MRI-compatible ETCO$_2$ monitor is not available, a conventional carbon dioxide (CO_2) monitor may be situated outside the MRI room in a similar fashion.[85] If GETA or LMA is required without an MRI-compatible anesthesia machine, it is safer to anesthetize the child outside the scanner (anesthesia circuit threaded through the console wall and then back out the entrance door to an induction area), secure the airway, and then move the child into the scanner. Similarly, if propofol sedation is intended, the propofol infusion pump can also be situated outside the scanner and equipped with 30 feet of IV infusion tubing. It is important to determine whether the pump is able to infuse accurately through the resistance of the long tubing and that the caliber of the tubing is sufficiently large that the length of tubing required does not trigger the pump's high-pressure alarm. An Ambu bag or Mapleson circuit (Mercury Medical, Clearwater, FL) must always be situated in the MRI suite and connected directly to an O_2 source within the scanner. This is critical, especially when the anesthesia machine is far from the child.

MRI-safe stethoscopes, stylets, laryngoscope, and flashlights should be available. If they are not available, standard equipment can be used with some modification and testing. The only component of the laryngoscope that is usually *not* MRI-safe is the battery. Replacing the standard battery with a lithium battery may be a simple, safe, and less expensive alternative to purchasing a marketed MRI-compatible and safe laryngoscope. Before introducing any equipment into the MRI environment, a rudimentary safety check should be performed by first passing a handheld magnet over the object to confirm that there is no ferrous material within. As a final safety check, an MRI safety expert should carefully introduce the object into the scanner (before bringing in a child) to confirm safety.

Anesthetic management of children in the MRI suite depends to a large extent on the availability of support personnel and equipment, the anesthesiologist's personal anesthetic practice, and the child's medical history. In clinical practice, the choice of anesthetic varies greatly among anesthesiologists. Airway management may include an LMA, a tracheal tube, or a natural airway (with a roll placed under the shoulders). With an LMA or tracheal tube, either inhalational or IV anesthesia may be used to establish a motionless child. With a natural airway, only IV sedation or anesthesia with

propofol or dexmedetomidine is commonly used.[10,93-98] There are few direct comparisons of these two medications in the literature, but investigators have generally found that propofol is more effective and efficient than dexmedetomidine when used alone or in combination with other agents.[29,99] ETCO$_2$ should be monitored; in the case of nasal prongs, a septate design that delivers O_2 (2-4 L/minute) through one nostril while aspirating gas for CO_2 (capnometry) through the other allows for continuous assessment of respirations during spontaneous ventilation. Alternatively, a face mask of oxygen can be used with a sidestream CO_2 monitor placed near the nose or mouth. If respiratory problems occur, immediate access to the airway is not possible while the child is in the bore of the scanner; for this reason, some anesthesiologists may prefer to insert an LMA or tracheal tube in all children. Most LMAs are MRI-compatible, although the pilot balloon should be taped to the circuit tubing when imaging the head or neck because it may create imaging artifacts (Fig. 46.7).

Few studies have directly compared general anesthesia with a controlled airway to IV sedation or anesthesia techniques during MRI. One randomized study of 200 children demonstrated no difference in airway complications between the two groups. However, more pauses occurred during scans (for movement, and so on) with propofol sedation, but much less agitation was experienced on emergence after the scan.[100] To ensure MRI scans without interruption in the majority of children, many begin with infusion rates of propofol 200 to 250 µg/kg per minute in children and either maintain that infusion rate throughout or taper the infusion rate as described previously.[101] For younger children (infants) and children with severe cognitive dysfunction, infusion rates 20% to 50% greater than 250 mg/kg per minute may be required to prevent movement during MRI scans. The addition of remifentanil to propofol using a total intravenous anesthesia technique smooths sedation (see Chapter 8). Other studies documented agitation[102] and prolonged nausea and vomiting[103] after MRI scans performed under general anesthesia with inhalation agents. Some MRI scans (cardiac, thoracic, or abdominal) require breath-holding to obtain adequate images. In such cases, it is necessary to control the airway with an LMA or endotracheal tube and deliver general anesthesia. After reviewing the literature, insufficient evidence exists to recommend a particular anesthetic technique for MRI scans. Anesthesiologists still must consider their own practice environment and expertise, the demands of the scan itself, and the comorbidities of the particular child when selecting an anesthetic technique, particularly for children undergoing a cardiac MRI.

INTERVENTIONAL RADIOLOGY

Interventional radiology (IR) has evolved greatly and the trend is for increased use of IR both as a replacement to and in conjunction with surgical interventions.[104] Many IR procedures are minimally invasive and not particularly painful, although most children require sedation between moderate sedation and general anesthesia to complete their procedure. Procedures vary widely with regard to the level of stimulation, postprocedure pain, and requirements in terms of apnea or positioning. Familiarity with IR procedures and their anesthetic and postoperative requirements are essential for efficient functioning in this area.[105,106] As a large number of cases in IR are scheduled on an urgent or emergent basis, it is vital that anesthesiologists in this area have a well-established habit of mutually respectful communication with the IR team to coordinate patient triage and ensure that cases proceed safely and expeditiously.

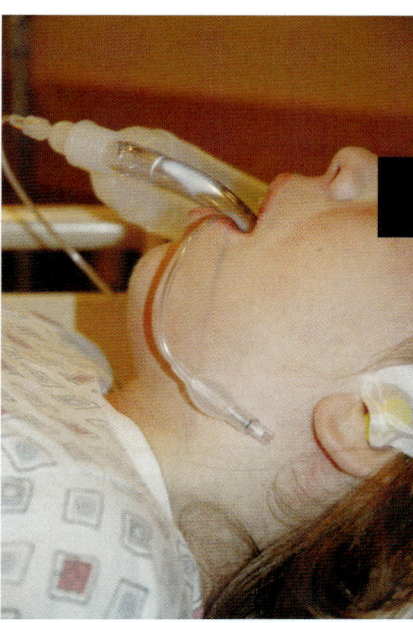
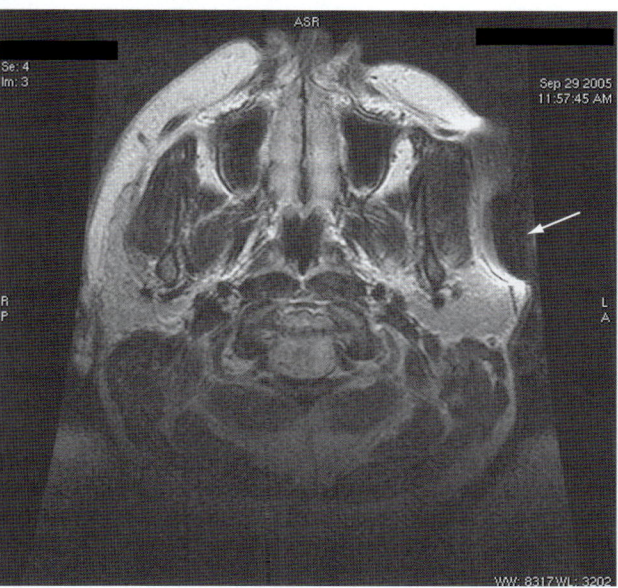

FIGURE 46.7 **A,** Laryngeal mask airway with pilot balloon left adjacent to face; such positioning could cause MRI artifact. We recommend taping to the Y-piece. **B,** MRI scan of the patient in **A** demonstrating artifact *(arrow)* created by ferrous material in pilot balloon.

Safety Radiation and Contrast Reactions

Radiation safety in IR is of paramount concern and tends to be underappreciated by anesthesiologists.[107] In pediatric settings, we are aided by the "Image Gently" campaign to reduce doses for pediatric patients,[108] but it is ultimately our responsibility to reduce our lifelong exposure to ionizing radiation with its attendant long-term health consequences.[109] Appropriate use of portable lead shields, lead aprons (preferably wraparound), thyroid shields, and lead glasses is crucial, as is increasing when possible one's distance from the radiation source and leaving the room when feasible for angiographic "runs." Portable dosimeters should be worn and monitored in compliance with local regulations.

The use of intravascular contrast media is ubiquitous in interventional radiology and cardiac catheterization. It is important that the anesthesiologist be aware of the risks and potential adverse effects of these agents.[110] Reactions to contrast in patients under anesthesia range from rash to bronchospasm to a diffuse anaphylactoid reaction[111] that can be life-threatening. The incidence of acute reactions, both mild and life-threatening, to contrast media has decreased with the advent of low-osmolality nonionic contrast media. Minor reactions are now estimated to occur in approximately 1% to 3% of patients. The risk of a fatal adverse reaction is estimated to occur 1:170,000 times, much improved from the risk in the 1970s of 1:30,000. This reduction is due to the use of newer contrast media and improved recognition and treatment of reactions. Anaphylactic shock is the most worrisome of all contrast reactions and may occur as early as 1 minute and as late as several hours after administration of the contrast material. Although adverse reactions to intravascular contrast media are unpredictable, some risk factors are identifiable. Children who suffer from allergies or an atopic disease; children with asthma, significant cardiovascular disease, or paraproteinemia; and children with prior contrast reactions have an increased incidence of adverse reactions.[112] Children who have been identified as being at increased risk of a contrast reaction should be premedicated with corticosteroids and antihistamines.[112,113] Areas where contrast media is routinely given should have protocols in place for the recognition and treatment of a contrast reaction.

The effect of contrast media on renal function must also be considered. The mechanisms underlying renal injury from contrast media are complex and not fully characterized. Direct renal tubular injury as well as renal hypoperfusion seem to play a role.[114] It is important to note that the trend toward low- and iso-osmolar contrast has been helpful in reducing renal damage from contrast. Nonetheless, in patients at high risk for renal injury, such as those with preexisting renal insufficiency (serum creatine ≥1.5 mg/dL), diabetes mellitus, dehydration, cardiovascular disease, hypertension, and hyperuricemia, good hydration must be maintained, along with careful follow-up of renal function.[115] In some institutions, a protocol of prehydration and posthydration with alkalinized IV fluids is used.

Diagnostic Angiography

Diagnostic angiography of the brain or of the periphery requires absolute control of movement, often with intermittent breath-holding to acquire clear images. For pediatric patients, this implies general anesthesia with a tracheal tube. Mature older children who can cooperate with instructions may be able to tolerate a short diagnostic angiogram with nothing more than minimal sedation, but care should be exercised that they do not become disinhibited or so somnolent that they cannot cooperate with breath-holding. Diagnostic angiography usually takes about 1 hour to complete and requires arterial access (usually of the femoral artery). Once access is obtained, the procedure is not stimulating. During these cases, orogastric and nasogastric tubes, esophageal stethoscopes, and esophageal temperature probes should be used with caution because they may cause artifacts on the angiographic images;

consultation with the IR nurses and technologists is recommended to determine where lines and monitors will be least obtrusive. After any femoral arterial access, patients must lie still for a period of time to reduce the risk of complications at the sheath site.[116]

Cerebral angiography may be indicated in the workup or postoperative follow-up of vascular malformation or tumor resections, stroke, hemorrhagic events, vascular disease, and unexplained mental status changes. Hypercarbia to an ETCO$_2$ of ~50 mm Hg may promote vasodilation to allow better access and visualization of cerebral vasculature (E-Fig. 46.1). Although MRA continues to improve, catheter angiography remains the gold standard for delineating vascular structures in the brain.

Any child who requires a study for the potential or confirmed diagnosis of vasculopathies such as Moyamoya disease should be treated with utmost caution. These children should have an anesthetic that minimizes the risk of transient ischemic attacks and stroke during the procedure.[94] Anesthetic care should begin ideally with the preinduction administration of 10 mL/kg of IV fluid to minimize the risk of hypotension (and potential cerebral ischemia) on induction of anesthesia. Sedating the child before starting the IV line decreases crying and hyperventilation that can lead to cerebral ischemia. Gentle mask induction with close attention to blood pressure has also been used in our institution with success. Blood pressure should be carefully maintained, avoiding hypotension with its potential for cerebral hypoperfusion. Vasoactive drugs are rarely necessary but should be available. Intraarterial blood pressure monitoring for these short procedures is rarely necessary. Hypocarbia should be avoided throughout. In the event of vasospasm or difficult access of small, tortuous vessels, locally administered (through the catheter) vasodilators such as nitroglycerin or calcium channel blockers in small doses may facilitate visualization and access. Although often effective for discretely vasodilating specific areas, these will generally not have a clinically important systemic effect on blood pressure. Specific protocols have been suggested for minimizing perioperative strokes in these children.[95] Close attention to postoperative pain control can similarly improve outcomes (see Chapters 24 and 26).

Peripheral diagnostic angiography is less common but may be useful before complex surgical or orthopedic procedures to delineate arterial anatomy. Angiography of the abdomen and pelvis has unique considerations; N$_2$O can diffuse into the bowel, causing distention and potential distortion of the vasculature of interest; it should be used with caution. In addition, the interventional radiologist may request that the anesthesiologist administer IV glucagon, usually in 0.25-mg increments. Glucagon reduces peristalsis and, as a consequence, reduces motion artifact during image acquisition.[117] However, it may cause nausea, vomiting, hyperglycemia, depression of clotting factors, and electrolyte disturbances[93]; close monitoring is warranted, particularly in neonates and small infants.

Angiography With Embolization

Angiography with interventions can be complex and carry significant risk. Indications for neurointerventional procedures include embolization of intracranial vascular anomalies such as arteriovenous malformations (AVMs), arteriovenous fistulae or aneurysms, targeted injection of intra-arterial chemotherapy for tumors, and presurgical embolization of both AVMs and tumors of the head and neck.[118] These procedures can take up to 10 to 12 hours, and complete immobility is required. Patient padding and positioning must be meticulous for such a long case, as moving the patient once catheters are deployed may be impossible.

Arterial blood pressure monitoring is usually necessary during the treatment of intracranial AVMs. A maximal acceptable blood pressure should be determined with the radiologist owing to the risk of hemorrhage as flow through the AVM is altered by embolization.[119] For the same reason, close blood pressure control immediately after the procedure is essential. Our group has had some success with low-dose dexmedetomidine infusion overnight after extubation in the IR suite. In infants presenting in heart failure from high-flow AVMs such as vein of Galen malformations,[120] immediate improvements in hemodynamics have been described as high-flow AVMs are closed.[121]

Good IV access is necessary for hydration; the chance of significant blood loss is extremely small. Euvolemia to slight hypervolemia is recommended to offset the osmotic diuretic effect of contrast.[122] Note that a continuous infusion of heparinized saline solution is instilled via the femoral sheath to reduce the risk of microemboli.[123] This can result in a considerable volume of fluid delivered to the patient by the neuroradiologist.

Many agents are used for embolization, including various types of glue, metal coils, or polyvinyl alcohol particles.[124] It should be noted that children can become intoxicated if ethanol is used (E-Fig. 46.2). Embolization of brain AVMs carries the risk that perfusion to surrounding normal brain tissue may be compromised with a concomitant loss of function. While there are descriptions of assessment of adult patients' motor, language, or visual function during test injections of agents such as amobarbital before definitive closure of a feeder vessel, this requires an awake cooperative patient and few descriptions of this technique exist in children.[125,126] The goal in treatment of intracranial AVMs in children is to obliterate the lesion; in our institution we favor surgical resection when possible, usually preceded by embolization for better localization and hemostasis.[127,128]

Injection of intraarterial chemotherapy carries some unique challenges for the anesthesiologist. Accessing the ophthalmic artery for injection of chemotherapeutic drug in retinoblastoma has considerable risk of bronchospasm and bradycardia. Agents such as albuterol or anticholinergics are often administered just before chemotherapy instillation.[129] Nausea and vomiting is reported after the procedure, so aggressive antiemetic prophylaxis is encouraged to prevent a child with a femoral puncture from vomiting.

Embolizations of peripheral AVMs have the potential to be of prolonged duration because in many cases the lesion is quite complex. The natural history of AVMs, like all vascular malformations, is to grow over time, with acceleration of growth during puberty[130]; the end stage is tissue destruction and high-output cardiac failure (E-Fig. 46.3). Blood loss is rarely a risk during these minimally invasive procedures, but excellent hydration is necessary both to offset the diuretic effect of the contrast load and to counteract the hemolyzing effect of sclerosing agents (see later discussion). While complete cure is rare, embolization combined with surgical resection in some cases can keep AVMs symptoms manageable.[131]

Embolization for hemorrhage has a long track record of success in cases of trauma, allowing for less insensible fluid loss and not disrupting tamponade.[132] The greatest predictor of success is the volume of blood resuscitation needed before embolization; a larger requirement presages a worse outcome. Anesthetic management for these children is similar to that of any massive transfusion case (see Chapter 12).

Catheter-based embolization of pulmonary vessels for hemoptysis presents several challenges for the anesthesiologist. Embolization is effective for gaining short-term control of hemoptysis, even massive hemoptysis, while not affecting the overall disease course in the case of cystic fibrosis.[133] Massive hemoptysis often necessitates single-lung ventilation and transfusion, coupled with the challenge of securing the airway in the face of ongoing oral blood loss. A grey area exists for more stable patients. Some reports have suggested that positive-pressure ventilation may itself be detrimental in cystic fibrosis patients, and that sedation at most is preferable.[134] This must be weighed against a child's ability to lie flat while in a state of respiratory compromise for a potentially prolonged procedure. With any patient undergoing bronchial embolization, clear communication with the patient and family about goals of care in the event of catastrophe is recommended.

Sclerotherapy of Venous and Lymphatic Malformations

Children may present shortly after birth with vascular malformations that arise from *PIK3CA*-associated overgrowth syndromes such as CLOVES (**C**ongenital, **L**ipomatous, **O**vergrowth, **V**ascular malformations, **E**pidermal nevi, and **S**pinal/skeletal anomalies and/or scoliosis [Fig. 46.8]) or Klippel-Trenaunay,[135] or later in life with isolated lesions that, while present at birth, may have not been recognized. The natural history of venous and lymphatic malformations, which are often discrete and not visible at birth,

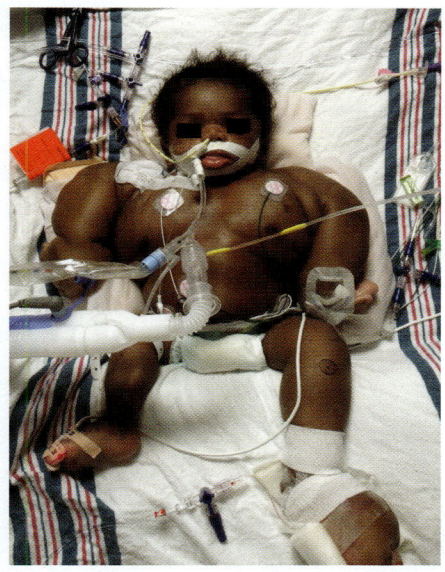

FIGURE 46.8 Neonate with severe CLOVES syndrome, a *PIK3CA*-associated overgrowth syndrome.[33]

is to grow steadily with the child, expanding rapidly and accelerating in size with puberty.[136,137] One review reported that only 18% of patients with lesions presented before 15 years of age.[96] This rapid proliferative phase may occur in response to hormonal changes (pregnancy, puberty), trauma, or other stimuli. Vascular malformations may be classified as high-flow or low-flow lesions, depending on which vessels are involved.[138] High-flow lesions may include arteriovenous fistulas, some large hemangiomas, and AVMs. Low-flow lesions consist of venous, lymphatic, and capillary malformations (see Fig. 46.9). The mainstay of treatment for many high-flow and low-flow vascular anomalies is chemical sclerotherapy, possibly combined with surgical resection; many lesions are inaccessible surgically or have a poor result from primary surgical resection.[139,140]

Sclerotherapy of vascular malformations usually requires a general anesthetic to ensure motionless conditions, especially during complex prolonged procedures that involve injection of potentially painful sclerosants. These procedures require careful planning and discussion between the interventional radiologist and the anesthesiologist for safe airway management, intraprocedural and postprocedural care, and disposition.

The anesthesiologist should be familiar with the mechanism of action and potential risks associated with the various agents used for sclerotherapy (Table 46.2). All sclerosants act by inducing a local tissue reaction that ideally scars closed abnormal vascular channels. Pain and swelling are a result with all sclerosants, to a greater or lesser degree. Ethanol and sodium tetradecyl sulfate produce hemolysis when administered into the vascular bed. They cause hemoglobinuria in a dose-dependent manner, which can result in renal injury necessitating generous hydration and alkalinization of urine to mitigate damage to the kidneys (Fig. 46.10).[141] Hemoglobinuria may not occur until the end of the procedure, sometimes after a large dose of sclerosant has been administered or the tourniquet (if used) has been released. Ethanol in large doses has been associated with serious complications, which has caused its use to fall out of favor as a primary agent in many institutions.[142] The most infrequent but serious risk is cardiovascular collapse, which is generally preceded by hypoxemia and bradycardia. Most reported cases of cardiovascular collapse involved lower extremity malformations,[143] after release of tourniquets in extremities that had been injected with ethanol.

Children with vascular malformations that result in stagnant flow—especially venous malformations—can have preexisting coagulation disturbances that resemble disseminated intravascular coagulation.[144] This is particularly true for patients with *PIK3A*-associated overgrowth syndromes, which have a propensity for huge ectatic veins with slow flow. Children with laboratory indexes

TABLE 46.2	Sclerosants Used for Treatment of Vascular Anomalies[106]			
Agent	**Indications**	**Swelling**	**Pain**	**Complications**
Sodium tetradecyl sulfate	LM, VM	Moderate	Moderate	Hemoglobinuria, skin blistering
Ethanol	LM, VM	Marked	Marked	Nausea, hemoglobinuria, skin blistering, ethanol intoxication, nerve injury, cardiovascular collapse
Doxycycline	LM	Marked	Marked	Minimal
Bleomycin	LM, VM primarily cervicofacial	Moderate	Moderate	Transient fever Concern for pulmonary fibrosis, never described after sclerotherapy
OK-432	LM	Marked	Marked	Not FDA approved for use in the United States

FDA, U.S. Food and Drug Administration; *LM*, lymphatic malformations; *VM*, vascular malformations.

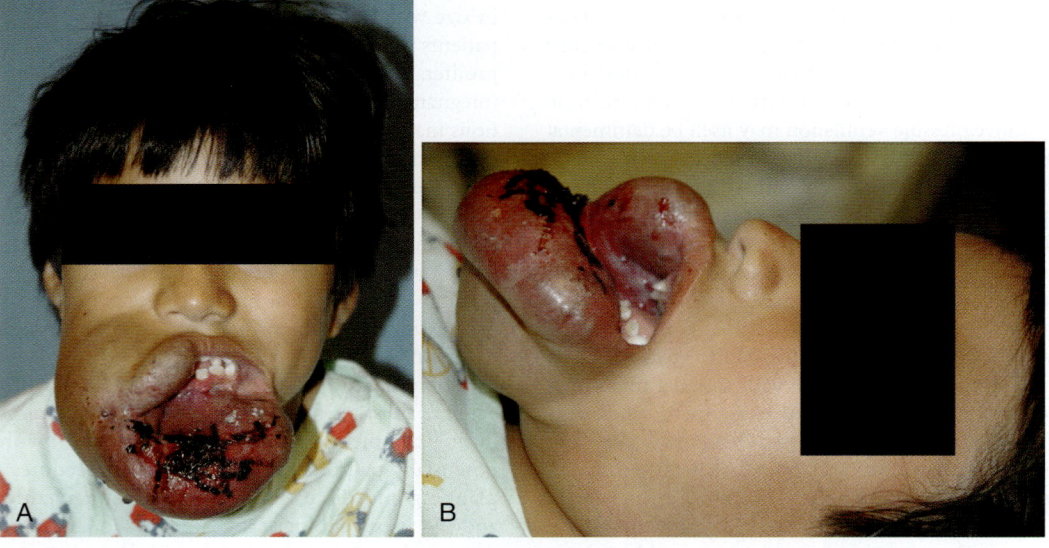

FIGURE 46.9 Venous malformation of the face with patient sitting upright **(A)** and supine **(B)**.

consistent with preexisting consumptive coagulopathy, particularly low fibrinogen, should have a hematology consultation for initiation of anticoagulation before and after the procedure to reduce the chance of a catastrophic periprocedure thromboembolic event.[145]

Vascular malformations that involve the airway are particularly challenging (Fig. 46.9). The anesthesiologist and radiologist should review the imaging studies (preferably MRI) before the procedure. If there is any question of involvement of the oropharynx or nasopharynx, evaluation by a otorhinolaryngologist familiar with vascular anomalies is essential before proceeding with anesthetic induction; nasal fiberoptic endoscopy will provide very useful information and can be performed in the office. Most interventional radiology suites are not situated in the OR. If there is a significant potential for airway compromise, difficulty in attaining a mask airway, or failure to intubate, the airway should be secured in the OR before transport to the radiology suite.

If postsclerotherapy edema and vascular congestion involving the airway structures are anticipated, the child's trachea should be intubated nasally and remain intubated for 48 hours or until the swelling subsides. Nasal intubation is preferred to minimize the risk of dislodging the tracheal tube or premature extubation. The decision to have the child remain intubated after the procedure is usually made after the anesthesiologist and radiologist review the MR images before the procedure. If the trachea remains intubated after the procedure, the trachea is extubated in the intensive care unit after an air leak around the tracheal tube is confirmed or a flexible nasal fiberoptic view of the airway can be performed at the bedside. If there is any doubt about the patency or self-sufficiency of the airway, these children should be transferred to the OR for tracheal extubation in a controlled setting with an otorhinolaryngologist present.

Venous malformations involving the head, neck, or airway structures typically swell with dependency or Valsalva maneuver (e.g., crying). Before extubating the trachea, these children should be positioned head-up to promote venous drainage and reduce swelling. Efforts should be made to minimize coughing before extubation. In the event of respiratory compromise, venous malformations can enlarge when the child coughs, increases

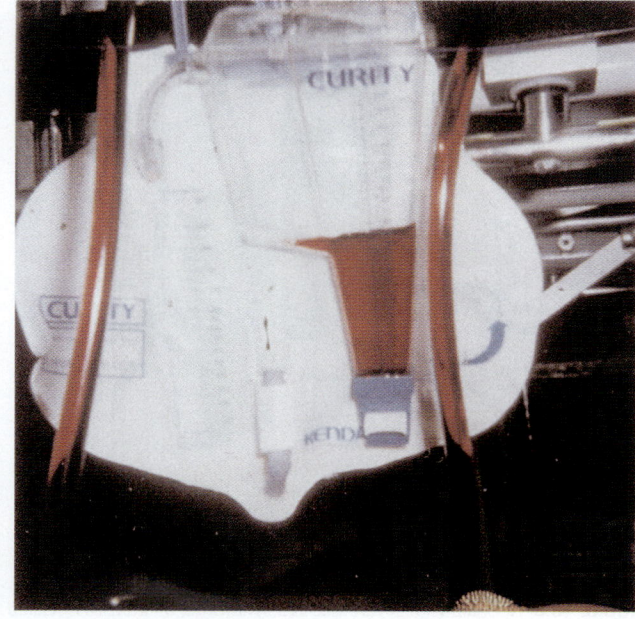

FIGURE 46.10 Hemoglobinuria after ethanol embolization.

intrathoracic pressure, or uses accessory muscles. Attempts at reintubation, cricoid pressure, head extension, and mask ventilation can further enlarge the malformation. Mask ventilation can be challenging, sometimes impossible, if the malformation is swollen and firm. Achieving an occlusive mask seal is particularly difficult when there is swelling of the cheek, tongue, lip, chin, or nares. Venous malformations of the lips and tongue, because of their blue color, can make it difficult to assess the child for hypoxemia in the event of respiratory distress. Reintubation can become impossible in these situations because all of the maneuvers to achieve a mask seal increase venous pressure and swelling. When attempting to reintubate the trachea of a child with intraoral or pharyngeal malformations, special care should be taken to avoid damaging the malformation: even a small nick can create significant bleeding. In the event of oropharyngeal bleeding and inability to mask ventilate and/or intubate, it is critical to have alternative airway devices immediately available. Supraglottic airway (SGA) devices, in particular those with high occluding pressures such as the ProSeal (Teleflex Medical Inc., Research Triangle Park, NC), can be lifesaving. Proper insertion and inflation of the SGA can secure an airway and, more importantly, tamponade bleeding. However, because the SGA rests above the vocal cords, it does not protect the airway from pulmonary aspiration.

ENDOSCOPIC PROCEDURES

GI endoscopy is a common procedure that requires deep sedation or general anesthesia in infants and children. A range of sedation and anesthesia options may be used for both simple[146,147] and more complex procedures, such as foreign body removal, endoscopic retrograde cholangiopancreatography, and percutaneous endoscopic gastrostomy placement.[148] The choice of deep sedation versus general anesthesia (with or without a tracheal tube) depends on the medical condition of the child, the risks associated with the specific procedure, and the anticipated duration. Upper esophagogastroduodenoscopy in infants (<10 kg) generally requires tracheal intubation to prevent airway compression caused by the endoscope pressing the trachealis muscle into the trachea. However, few definitive data exist on this issue (few studies include infants <1 year of age). In some cases, an LMA may be used to secure the airway, deflating the cuff to allow passage of the endoscope, and then reinflating it once the scope has entered the esophagus. It is advised to hold on to either a tracheal tube or an LMA during the procedure to reduce the risk of the endoscopist dislodging it while manipulating the scope.

Many techniques may be used successfully to maintain adequate conditions for upper and lower GI endoscopy. Although all anesthesia-delivery areas must meet ASA standards, scavenging and ventilation in endoscopy suites may not always be up to standard to ensure the safe use of inhalational anesthetics. In these cases, total IV anesthesia can substitute for inhalational anesthetics.[23,149,150] Over the past several years, various combinations of IV agents have been described for the delivery of sedation and anesthesia for GI endoscopy in children. As a general rule, propofol is used either alone,[151] in combination with an opioid (fentanyl or remifentanil),[22,152] or with ketamine.[153] Outcomes after deep sedation or anesthesia with propofol and inhalational anesthesia were similar.[23] However, the time to awakening was more rapid after the inhalational anesthetic, although the incidence of emergence delirium and time to discharge were less after propofol.

Access to the airway is obviously limited once a transoral endoscope is in place. The two most stimulating portions of the esophagogastroduodenoscopy are transoral and transpyloric passage of the endoscope. Once the endoscope has been inserted, the sedation or anesthesia can often be reduced without affecting the procedure conditions. Smooth insertion of the endoscope can be aided by topical spray of local anesthesia to the oropharynx to reduce the discomfort of passing the endoscope and a small bolus of propofol to prevent coughing and gagging. For older children, topicalization of the oropharynx can be accomplished before sedation and the child can position himself or herself for the gastroenterologist (lateral position). Sedation can be subsequently accomplished with the child prepositioned. For cases performed

without tracheal intubation, a CO_2 sampling nasal cannula can be placed in the nares or near the mouth (for those who do not breath through the nose) to supplement O_2 and monitor respiration.

Upper endoscopies have the inherent risk of apnea, laryngospasm, bronchospasm, and airway obstruction. Most problems resolve after withdrawal of the endoscope and positive-pressure ventilation with a face mask.[154] In rare situations, tracheal intubation may be required to complete the procedure or resolve an airway issue. Little published evidence exists on which to base age-related practice in endoscopy sedation and analgesia. Experience led several groups to select all infants up to 6 months of age as the age interval for which general anesthesia with tracheal intubation is required because of a greater frequency of respiratory complications.[146,147] When extubating the tracheas in these infants, be wary that residual air in the stomach can impair effective ventilation and contribute to desaturation or O_2 dependence in the recovery room. It is important to remind the endoscopist to suction all air from the stomach before removing the endoscope.

Few large studies have reported outcomes after pediatric GI endoscopy. The Clinical Outcomes Research Initiative (CORI) is a national registry of endoscopic procedures started in 1995. The PEDS-CORI is the pediatric component started in 1999. A 2007 report collected the complications from pediatric upper endoscopy involving 10,236 encounters from 13 different institutions over 4 years.[155] Overall, there was a 2.3% incidence of complications (of any kind). Of these, 79.9% were cardiopulmonary, 18% were GI, and 5.9% were other complications, including prolonged sedation, drug reactions, or rash. Not surprisingly, children who developed complications were younger and had a greater ASA physical status. General anesthesia was associated with a reduced overall complication rate (1.2%) compared with that in the IV sedation group (3.7%). Although these data were not controlled or randomized, they do shed some insight into the complication rates associated with pediatric sedation outside the OR. Data from closed claims analysis confirm the risk associated with endoscopic procedures in children. Half of NORA closed claims involved the GI unit, 25% involved the diagnostic imaging department, and 25% involved cardiac procedures.[156]

Summary

Technological advancements in many areas such as diagnostic imaging, gastroenterology, and interventional radiology continue to increase the need for pediatric NORA. As the need for anesthesia services for children outside the OR continues to expand, anesthesiologists continue to be requested more and more frequently to provide anesthesia services for these venues. It is in our patients' interests and our own professional interest to accept this responsibility and provide the most effective, efficient, and safe anesthesia and sedation outside the OR. More than in any other aspect of pediatric anesthesia care, communication with other specialists and within anesthesia departments is critical to ensure safe and effective care. The anesthetic configuration and equipment demands are unique at each center. Emergency situations should be simulated so that all personnel are familiar with the location of code equipment and emergency airway equipment. Anesthesia delivery in the areas outside the OR is both rewarding and challenging, and should be approached with a commitment to ensure that children will receive a standard of care equal to the care provided in the OR.

ACKNOWLEDGMENT

We wish to thank Charles J. Coté, Babu V. Koka, and Keira Mason for their prior contributions to this chapter.

ANNOTATED REFERENCES

Coté CJ, Wilson S, American Academy of Pediatrics, American Academy of Pediatric Dentistry. Guidelines for monitoring and management of pediatric patients during and after sedation for diagnostic and therapeutic procedures. *Pediatrics.* 2016;138(1):pii: e20161212.

The most recent American Academy of Pediatrics sedation guideline, this is a landmark paper because it was jointly published by the American Academy of Pediatric Dentistry. Many new recommendations, including the use of capnography and Pediatric Advanced Life Support (PALS) training, have been added to improve the safety net of medical supervision during and after procedural sedation.

Cravero JP, Beach ML, Blike GT, et al. The incidence and nature of adverse events during pediatric sedation/anesthesia with propofol for procedures outside the operating room: a report from the Pediatric Sedation Research Consortium. *Anesth Analg.* 2009;108(3):795-804.

This is the largest study to date that examines the side effects and adverse events associated with the use of propofol for sedation of children during procedures outside the operating room.

Kanal E, Borgstede JP, Barkovich AJ, et al. American College of Radiology White Paper on MR Safety: 2004 update and revisions. *AJR Am J Roentgenol.* 2004;182(5):1111-1114.

Updated paper details the standards and recommendations for providing safe patient care in the MR environment.

Shellock FG, Crues JV. MR procedures: biologic effects, safety, and patient care. *Radiology.* 2004;232(3):635-652.

This detailed article reviews the biologic effects and important safety issues in delivering safe patient care in the MR environment.

A complete reference list can be found online at ExpertConsult.com.

The Postanesthesia Care Unit and Beyond

47

ANDREAS H. TAENZER AND JEANA E. HAVIDICH

EMERGENCE FROM ANESTHESIA IN CHILDREN differs substantially compared with adults. The process is multifaceted, dependent on the nature of the surgery, patient characteristics, and the type of anesthesia administered. In young children, emergence from inhalational agents can be quite rapid as a result of increased minute ventilation, increased blood flow to the vessel-rich group (see Chapter 7), and decreased total body muscle and fat stores, whereas emergence from intravenous (IV) agents may be delayed in infants because of decreased clearance because of immature enzyme systems.

One important aspect to appreciate is the rapidity with which serious complications can develop in the postoperative period. For instance, neonates, infants, and young children have decreased cardiopulmonary reserve compared with adults, resulting in a more rapid physiologic deterioration should airway obstruction or bleeding occur. Vigilant and frequent monitoring by pediatric postanesthesia care nurses and anesthesiologists is essential for appropriate postoperative care as well as to prevent and treat adverse events. Parents or primary caregivers should be considered active partners in the postoperative care of the child. Those who routinely provide comfort and care for the child are essential for the child's sense of well-being. In addition, they should be able to alert medical professionals to changes in the child's status that may require urgent medical attention.

Perioperative Environment

A well-designed, safe perioperative environment is essential for the delivery of high-quality pediatric anesthetic and surgical care. This is evidenced by the fact that several prominent national

organizations have provided recommendations for the perioperative care of children. The American Academy of Pediatrics (AAP) published a policy statement in 2015 delineating the critical elements of the perioperative environment.[1] These recommendations focus on the patient care facility and medical policies, including staff credentialing and necessary supportive services. This document was developed to complement the Society for Pediatric Anesthesia (SPA) statement on the provision of pediatric anesthesia care.[2] Institutions that desire verification by the American College of Surgeons (ACS) Children's Surgery Verification Program must contain a designated postanesthetic care unit (PACU) with appropriately credentialed staff and supportive resources.[3] These guidelines acknowledge that the perioperative environment can be challenging, and health care facilities must understand these challenges and be prepared to manage children and family members through this difficult process. Policies and procedures based on recommendations from national organizations and developed with input from all stakeholders, including physicians, nurses, family members, and child-life specialists, comprise the foundation for a safe, patient- and family-centered perioperative environment.

The ideal perioperative environment is patient- and family-centered, combining aspects of safety, ergonomics, and comfort for patients, family members, and staff. The family and patient experience starts with the admission process and concludes with the discharge to home or the hospital ward. Familiarity with personnel and surroundings reduces stress for patients and families while fostering trust and comfort. Ideally, a child should be under the care of the same team throughout the perioperative period. For example, the child and family benefit if the admitting nurse

TABLE 47.1	Suggested Essential Bedside Equipment

Oxygen supply with regulated flows

Oxygen face masks and face tents for spontaneous ventilation (various sizes)

Oxygen nebulizers for administration of albuterol and racemic epinephrine

Stethoscope

Resuscitation bags, self-inflating (Ambu)

Anesthesia facemasks for positive-pressure ventilation (pediatric sizes: 0, 1, 2, 3; adult sizes: small, medium, large)

Oral airways (sizes 00, 0, 1–5)

Nasal airways (sizes 12F–36F)

Suction and appropriate suction catheters (sizes 6.5F–14F); tonsil-type (Yankauer) attachment

IV supplies: needles, syringes, saline flushes, alcohol wipes, Betadine solution, gauze pads, Tegaderm dressings (3M, Minneapolis, MN), tourniquets, tape

Non-latex gloves (various sizes)

Pulse oximeter and sensors (size appropriate, stick-on type preferred to clip-on type)

Electrocardiograph, monitor, and pads

Manual and automated blood pressure device

All sizes of blood pressure cuffs

TABLE 47.2	Suggested Emergency Supplies for a Crash Cart or Central Location

Cognitive aids for resuscitation (weight-based pediatric advance life support cards) (e.g., Broselow tapes [see E-Figs. 39.1–39.3])

Laryngoscopes with blades: Miller 0, 1, 2, 3; Macintosh 2, 3, 4; extra laryngoscope bulbs and batteries

Endotracheal tubes, sizes 2.0-mm internal diameter (ID) through 8-mm ID; cuffed and uncuffed tubes for all sizes when available

Stylet appropriate for each endotracheal tube size

Syringe for endotracheal cuff inflation

End-tidal carbon dioxide monitor or portable detector

Tape and liquid adhesive for endotracheal tube fixation

Intravenous catheter (14-gauge) with 3-mm ID endotracheal tube adapter for emergency cricothyroidotomy (see Fig. 14.25)

Backup resuscitation bags and masks and oral airways for each bedside

Nasogastric tubes

Intravenous infusion solutions, tubing, drip chambers

Supplies for intravenous cannulation, catheter sizes 24- to 14-gauge

Cutdown tray, tracheostomy, and suture sets

Central venous catheter insertion sets (3F–7F, single- and multiple-lumen)

Tube thoracotomy set and system for suction and underwater seal

Automated electric defibrillator or defibrillator (adult, child paddles)

Electrocardiograph

Pressure transducer system and oscilloscope monitor

Sterile gowns, gloves, masks, towels, drapes

Urinary catheters of appropriate pediatric size

Bed board for cardiopulmonary resuscitation

later cares for the child and the family in the PACU. This may be achieved by creating an integrated perioperative environment, in which children are admitted, prepared, and allowed to recover in the same space, with the same nurses and child-life specialist.

Privacy and shelter from noise are important aspects of the patient and family experience. The ability to spend time with the child without being disturbed is something that many families appreciate, and this helps the child cope with the stress of a strange environment. Most PACUs contain individual patient rooms or cubicles for preoperative and postoperative care, similar to a typical pediatric intensive care unit (PICU).

Equipment (Table 47.1) and available medications (Tables 47.2 and 47.3) should be standardized throughout the unit and be compatible with transport monitors and other devices used in the medical facility (e.g., PICU). Cognitive aids such as preprinted emergency drug cards should be available for every child.[1] This important safety measure may reduce the risk of drug errors in emergency situations. These rapid reference sheets may be attached to each child's bed or chart on admission so that a quick dose recommendation is readily available. Alternatively, the electronic record should have precalculated emergency drug doses for each child.

Nurses, residents, fellows, attending physicians, and other personnel working in the perioperative area must be competent in the provision of neonatal and pediatric advanced life support. Team training in mock codes and enhanced communication have been shown to improve outcomes.[4–6] Continuous medical education in the provision of pediatric care is often required by hospital credentialing committees as well as institutions requesting ACS verification.[3]

TRANSPORT TO THE CARE UNIT

The PACU should be located near the operating room to decrease the amount of time spent in transport of a sedated and/or critically ill patient. If transporting a sedated patient from a remote location, the patient's vital signs and a metric of respiration should be monitored along the route. Appropriate airway equipment and drugs should be immediately available. Transport from the operating room to the PACU should be carried out under the direct supervision of a trained expert. The security and patency of the airway, IV and arterial lines, drains, and urinary catheters should be checked before transport. Children should be covered during transport to maintain normothermia and appear presentable (e.g., remove garments and sheets that contain blood and secretions).

Unless children are awake, with protective airway reflexes intact, or unless there is a specific contraindication, it is appropriate to transport extubated children in the lateral position (i.e., tonsillectomy recovery position) so that the tongue lies away from the larynx and secretions and vomitus leave the mouth rather than enter the larynx, possibly leading to airway obstruction or pulmonary aspiration. To assess ventilation and maintain a patent airway with the child in the decubitus position, we recommend applying the thumb to the forehead to extend the neck and holding the fingers (the finger tips are the most sensitive part of the hand) over the mouth (or nose) to feel for exhalation. A precordial stethoscope may also be used to auscultate respirations. If the child is breathing room air, a pulse oximeter can serve as a crude metric of ventilation because desaturation will occur quickly if hypopnea develops. However, if oxygen is provided to the child, desaturation may not occur for a considerable time in the setting of apnea, and ventilation should be monitored by close observation, a precordial stethoscope, capnography, or ideally, by a combination of these. We recommend that children in a potentially unstable condition be transported with a pulse oximeter, capnogram, an electrocardiographic (ECG) monitor, and a blood pressure cuff or a transduced arterial line. The monitoring lines, IV drips, infusion

TABLE 47.3 | Suggested Recovery Room Medications

Suggested Emergency Medications on Crash Cart[a]

Albuterol (also known as salbutamol outside the United States)
Amiodarone
Atropine
Calcium chloride or gluconate
Dextrose
Diphenhydramine
Dopamine
Epinephrine
Etomidate
Flumazenil
Furosemide
Hydrocortisone, dexamethasone, methylprednisolone
Lidocaine (intravenous and topical)
Naloxone
Neostigmine
Norepinephrine
Physostigmine
Propranolol, atenolol, esmolol, labetalol
Sodium bicarbonate
Sodium nitroprusside
Succinylcholine and rocuronium
Propofol
Verapamil
For inhalation: racemic epinephrine (2.25% at 0.05 mL/kg, common in the United States) *or* epinephrine 1:1000 (0.1%), 0.5 mL/kg, maximum of 5 mL

Medications to Be Kept Under Lock[a]

Diazepam
Fentanyl
Ketamine
Meperidine
Midazolam (intravenous and oral)
Morphine
Potassium chloride

Other Medications for Central Location[a]

Acetaminophen (oral, rectal, and intravenous)
Antibiotics
Antiemetics (e.g., 5-HT$_3$-antagonist, promethazine, metoclopramide)
Dantrolene
Digoxin
Heparin
Insulin
Mannitol
Potassium chloride
Protamine
Ketorolac
Dexmedetomidine
Sugammadex

[a]Alternative or additional medications may be needed.

pumps, and other equipment should be clearly labeled and simplified before transport. A tackle box containing airway equipment and emergency medications is useful, especially when children are transported to or from remote locations.

A child often appears awake after the stimulation of tracheal extubation and transfer to the stretcher but may subsequently become obtunded and obstruct the airway during transit to the PACU or PICU. Just as frequently, a child may become restless during transit. Although restless behavior has many causes, hypoxia should be ruled out first. The guard rails on the stretcher should always be raised when the child is in it and padding with pillows may prevent injury to the child. Most importantly, the anesthesiologist should remain at the head of the stretcher during transport maintaining vigilance of the child and the monitors throughout the transfer.

ARRIVAL IN THE CARE UNIT

The transfer of care from the operating room personnel to the PACU or PICU is a crucial element of quality patient care that deserves considerable focus and the importance of this process cannot be overemphasized. Ideally, it is a stepwise process following an institutional protocol that begins in the operating room with communication to the receiving unit before the end of the procedure that provides pertinent patient information as well as required nonstandard equipment and medication to the receiving care team. On arrival in the PACU, a rapid assessment of the child should be undertaken to ensure that the child has a patent airway and that the vital signs are stable. Once the child has been properly assessed, an admission heart rate, oxygen saturation, respiratory rate, blood pressure, and temperature should be recorded. Supplemental oxygen is administered as indicated, recognizing the limitations of the monitors to detect hypoventilation in such cases. Many children object to having an oxygen mask fixed to their faces; a funnel-type mask or open hose with large flow rates may be less objectionable (although less optimal). In the healthy child, if the child is awake enough to object to a mask with oxygen, the child does not require supplemental oxygen (although the combative, hypoxic child will require not only oxygen but establishment of a patent airway as well).

Numerous patient safety organizations and health care institutions have devoted considerable time and resources to improve patient transfer processes with the primary objective to improve safety, increase the quality of care, and decrease health care costs. Education of health care personnel about the importance of this endeavor is the first step to implementing effective transfers of care; several methods have been suggested.[4,7–12] Standardized handoffs containing validated checklists and protocols are considered essential components of this process. Institutions with effective and organized handoff systems have reported a decrease in the number of medical errors and improved patient outcomes.[6,13–16]

Surgeons, anesthesia providers, and intensive care physicians involved in the care of the child should be present and actively participate during the transfer of care from the operating room to the PACU or PICU. Specific circumstances such as language barriers, developmental delay, or family concerns should be conveyed to members of the team accepting care of the child. Since cultures vary within and among different institutions, we recommend developing a formalized transfer of care process that focuses of critical aspects of patient care, including pertinent patient information and history, surgical procedures, type of anesthesia administered, airway management, medications (especially antibiotics and analgesics), fluids administered, hemodynamics, estimated blood loss, unexpected events, anticipated patient progress, and information that needs to be relayed to parents or hospital staff in the event the patient is being admitted. Any unanticipated or serious events, such as unanticipated difficult airway, hemodynamic instability, or surgical complications, should be clearly communicated. If continuous infusions of local anesthetics are administered (e.g., epidural catheter infusion), the dose, concentration, rate, and maximum infusion rate should be conveyed. Tasks that need to be completed in the near future should be discussed with the team accepting the care of the patient. All stakeholders should have the opportunity to ask questions and confirm the transfer information at the conclusion of the handoff.

The anesthesia team must remain with the child until he or she has stable vital signs and the PACU or PICU team is comfortable and ready to assume responsibility for the child. Physicians who will be in charge of taking care of the child in the PACU or PICU after the anesthesia team leaves must be clearly identified by name, and methods to contact them (e.g., pager number) must be given to surgeons, anesthesiologists, and regional block and pain services. It is important to understand that barriers may exist at several levels and preclude the effective transfer of care. Such circumstances frequently implicated include external distractions, noisy environments, shift changes, and differences in culture and priorities between individuals providing and accepting care of the child.[12,17–20]

Ideally, the nurses taking care of the child postoperatively are already familiar with the child and family from the preoperative setting. The nurse/patient ratio should be 1:1 for sick children and 1:2 or 1:3 for routine cases. It has been reported that staffing ratios, nursing surveillance techniques, and vigilant monitoring of patients in the PACU by pediatric-trained nursing staff improve patient outcomes.[21–23] Available staffing and resources in the PACU or PICU should be in place before transporting the child from the operating room.

All children should be monitored continuously in the PACU. At the very least, this should include continuous pulse oximetry and intermittent noninvasive blood pressure and temperature monitoring. Most PACUs also monitor the electrocardiogram continuously, although some limit this to children with cardiac disease or complex multiple-organ disease. During emergence, many children are so active that it is impossible to maintain the monitoring devices in place. If the child is not hypoxic and is sufficiently awake to remove the monitors, he or she probably does not require the monitors any longer. If the child falls back to sleep, then a pulse oximeter probe should be reapplied, particularly for at-risk children such as those with obstructive sleep apnea (OSA). For a child who is physically or mentally challenged, it may be necessary to apply light restraints until he or she is oriented and awake.

Central Nervous System

PHARMACODYNAMICS OF EMERGENCE
Emergence from anesthesia is a complex process dependent on the dose and types of medications administered, the age, and the physiologic status of the patient. The age of the child exerts a minimal influence on the wash-out of inhalational anesthetic agents and has little impact on the rapidity of emergence, although age may be a factor for infants younger than 1 year.[24] However, the overall clinical implications of age-related differences in emergence are exceedingly difficult to detect.[25] The speed of emergence correlates more closely with the duration of anesthesia. The greater the duration of anesthesia, the more the tissue compartments become filled with anesthetics and the more time it takes to eliminate the anesthetics for recovery. For example, emergence from 30 minutes of sevoflurane anesthesia is significantly faster than emergence from 2 hours of anesthesia, which is more rapid than from 8 hours of anesthesia.[26] This relationship between emergence time and the duration of anesthesia has less relevance as inhalational anesthetics have become less soluble (e.g., desflurane).[27,28]

Emergence from IV agents can vary significantly from that of inhalational agents. Several studies have evaluated the quality and rapidity of emergence after IV anesthetic agents compared with

that after inhalational agents.[29,30] For outpatient surgery, emergence after propofol anesthesia is as rapid as that after sevoflurane but with far less agitation and pain behaviors.[31] The recovery characteristics of propofol with remifentanil (total IV anesthesia [TIVA]; see Chapter 8) have been compared with those after desflurane inhalational anesthesia. Recovery is as rapid as that after desflurane with nitrous oxide, with a similar or reduced incidence of nausea and vomiting but with much less agitation.[32,33]

Although rarely used for maintenance of anesthesia, midazolam is often used as an oral or IV premedication for anxiolysis and amnesia in the preinduction period in children. There is evidence that the addition of midazolam before an inhalational or propofol anesthetic may delay early emergence after brief anesthesia. However, this delay is attenuated as the duration of anesthesia increases and when only late emergence is considered.[34] Midazolam premedication does not affect the incidence of postoperative delirium but has been reported to decrease postoperative nausea and vomiting (PONV).[35–38] IV midazolam at the end of surgery does decrease the incidence of emergence delirium (see later text).

EMERGENCE AGITATION OR DELIRIUM
Emergence agitation refers to an umbrella of signs and symptoms that includes delirium (Videos 47.1 and 47.2), postoperative pain, and behavior disorders. Emergence delirium was first described in a large cohort of postsurgical patients over 50 years ago.[39] From a clinical perspective, it is often impossible to differentiate pure agitation from delirium, although the latter implies a disturbance in attention and represents an acute change from baseline.[40] Despite numerous investigations, differentiating emergence delirium from postoperative pain has proved difficult, although it has been suggested that children who do not make any eye contact or who are unaware of their surroundings are more likely to be experiencing emergence delirium.[41] Emergence delirium typically manifests as thrashing, disorientation, crying, and screaming. The child is unable to recognize parents, familiar objects, or surroundings; is inconsolable; and talks irrationally during early emergence from anesthesia. Emergence delirium occurs more often in children (frequency of 30%–50%) than in adults, particularly in those 2 to 6 years of age.[42,43] The mechanism of emergence delirium in children has not been completely elucidated, but differences in the frontal lobe electroencephalogram[44] and in the locus coeruleus[45] compared with children without delirium may highlight the source of the delirium. Evidence also points to differences in central nervous system (CNS) metabolites in the parietal cortex that may contribute to delirium; lactic acid concentrations and other metabolites after sevoflurane in children correlated with greater Pediatric Anesthesia Emergence Delirium (PAED) scale values than those after propofol.[46]

Several scales have been developed to measure emergence delirium, although only one, the PAED scale, has been validated for this purpose in the postoperative period.[47] Tables 47.4 and 47.5 present two scoring systems that have been used to evaluate emergence behaviors in children. In evaluating emergence delirium with the PAED scale after anesthesia, preliminary evidence suggested that values greater than 10 or possibly greater than 12 were consistent with emergence delirium.[48,49] In the PICU, evidence suggests that a PAED score greater than 8 predicts emergence delirium.[50] The literature regarding postoperative delirium in children is quite confusing in part, because many studies used nonvalidated, unproven scales in children whose pain was not controlled, leaving the cause of the behavior attributable to delirium, pain, or both.

TABLE 47.4 | Pediatric Anesthesia Emergence Delirium Scale

Scored Factor	SCORING				
	0	*1*	*2*	*3*	*4*
Child makes eye contact with caregiver	Extremely	Very much	Quite a bit	Just a little	Not at all
Child's actions are purposeful	Extremely	Very much	Quite a bit	Just a little	Not at all
Child is aware of surroundings	Extremely	Very much	Quite a bit	Just a little	Not at all
Child is restless	Not at all	Just a little	Quite a bit	Very much	Extremely
Child is inconsolable	Not at all	Just a little	Quite a bit	Very much	Extremely
Total score[a]					

[a]Preliminary evidence suggested that a total pediatric anesthesia emergence delirium score greater than 10 defined emergence delirium, but later evidence suggested that a total score greater than 12 might be more specific.

Modified from Sikich N, Lerman J. Development and psychometric evaluation of the pediatric anesthesia emergence delirium scale. *Anesthesiology* 2004;100:1138–1145.

TABLE 47.5 | Postanesthesia Behavior Assessment Scale

Perceptual Disturbances (Maximal Score 3)[a]

0   None evident
1   Feelings of depersonalization (says that situation is not real, comments on "out of body" feelings)
2   Visual illusions or misperceptions (misidentifies objects, such as urinates in trash can)
3   Markedly confused about external reality (misidentifies self or surroundings, such as being at school)

Hallucination Type (Maximal Score 6)[a]

0   None evident
1   Auditory hallucinations only (responds to questions not asked)
2   Visual hallucinations or misperceptions (responds to things only the child can see)
3   Tactile, olfactory (responds to sensations not obvious to others, such as a bug crawling on the leg)

Psychomotor Behavior (Maximal Score 3)[a]

0   No significant agitation
1   Mild restlessness, tremulousness, or anxiety
2   Moderate agitation with pulling at intravenous lines
3   Severe agitation, needs to be restrained, combative

[a]A larger postanesthesia behavior assessment score is associated with a greater degree of postanesthetic distress.

From Przybylo HJ, Martini DR, Mazurek AJ, et al. Assessing behavior in children emerging from anaesthesia: can we apply psychiatric diagnostic techniques? *Pediatr Anesth* 2003;13:609–616.

TABLE 47.6 | Prophylactic Measures to Prevent Emergence Delirium

Prophylactic Measure	Timing
Propofol (IV)	TIVA,[31,67] a brief infusion of 3 mg/kg over 3 minutes after sevoflurane,[68] a single dose at the end of anesthesia (1 mg/kg IV)[61,63,65,69,70]
Thiopental (IV)	After induction, 2–3 mg/kg[71]
Opioid (IV)	Meta-analysis[72] of fentanyl, remifentanil, sufentanil, alfentanil; nalbuphine (0.1 mg/kg)[73]
Midazolam (IV)	0.03–0.05 mg/kg at end of anesthesia[74,75]
(PO)	0.2–0.5 mg/kg[76]; 0.5 mg/kg with parental presence[77]
α₂ Agonist (IV) (caudal)	Clonidine 2 µg/kg at induction[76,78,79]; dexmedetomidine 0.3–1 µg/kg at emergence[60,80–83] Meta-analysis of dexmedetomidine demonstrates effectiveness[60,84] Dexmedetomidine 1 µg/kg followed by 1 µg/kg per hour[85] Clonidine 1 µg/kg[86]
Ketamine (IV)	Ketamine 1 mg/kg followed by 1 mg/kg per hour[85] or 0.25 mg/kg[73]
Melatonin (PO)	0.25 or 0.5 mg/kg premedication[87]
Tropisetron (IV)	0.1 mg/kg at induction[88]
Magnesium sulfate (IV)	30 mg/kg followed by 10 mg/kg per hour[89]
Regional anesthesia	Infraorbital block,[28,90] fascia iliaca block[91]
Acupuncture	Heart 7 site bilaterally during surgery[92]

IV, intravenous; *PO*, oral; *TIVA*; total intravenous anesthesia.

Our understanding of emergence delirium continues to evolve. Delirium occurs after surgical procedures and after procedures that are free from pain, such as magnetic resonance imaging.[41,42,51,52] Factors that have been associated with the development of emergence delirium include age 2 to 6 years, the use of less-soluble inhalational anesthetics (e.g., incidence after sevoflurane, desflurane and isoflurane ≫ TIVA > halothane)[30,32,53,54] and the preoperative mental state.[55] Although some claim that there is a greater incidence of emergence delirium after certain painful surgeries, in most of these instances this cannot be proven as pain was not controlled and a nonvalidated metric of delirium was used.[56] A number of other plausible factors that do not predispose to delirium include a rapid emergence from anesthesia,[57] a greater depth of anesthesia,[58] and preoperative anxiety, although the last factor is contentious. Emergence delirium usually lasts less than 15 to 20 minutes, resolves spontaneously if the children are left undisturbed or they are held by their parents, and does not recur.[42]

Several strategies have been used to prevent emergence delirium (Table 47.6). Effective regional analgesia, dexmedetomidine, opioids, ketamine, melatonin, midazolam, magnesium, and propofol have been used with success.[59–63] Fentanyl (2–2.5 µg/kg intranasally or 1–2 µ/kg IV) decreases the duration and intensity of emergence delirium,[64] even in the absence of painful stimuli, most likely because of its sedating effect.[54] Administration of propofol by continuous infusion or by bolus (1–3 mg/kg) at the end of surgery appears to be preventative, although these findings have not been consistent.[49,65] A dose of propofol at induction of anesthesia does not prevent postoperative emergence delirium.[66] Administration of TIVA has been reported to be superior to inhalational agents in the prevention of emergence delirium.[30,32,53] Some clinicians cannot justify prophylactic treatment to prevent delirium when the local incidence is small.

When emergence delirium does occur, it is important to explain its self-limiting nature to the parents who quickly become frustrated trying to comfort their child. Whether to terminate the delirium pharmacologically or let it take a natural course needs to be discussed with the parents. Many parents prefer to avoid administering additional medications, knowing that the delirium will abate spontaneously after several minutes and that their child will recover to his or her normal disposition soon. Treatment of ongoing delirium has not been widely studied, but current strategies include propofol 1 to 3 mg/kg IV, fentanyl 1 to 2 µg/kg, or dexmedetomidine 0.3 µg/kg. Most use an initial small dose and titrate to effect.

Discharge from the PACU may be delayed while waiting for the delirium to wane or for the effects of the interventional drugs to dissipate. Injury to the child who is delirious, to the site of surgery, or to a parent is a concern, as is pulling out a drain or dressing on a wound or self-extubation. Parental satisfaction decreases when severe emergence delirium occurs. Although the impact of extreme delirium is not fully known, evidence suggests that the incidence of postoperative maladaptive behaviors is greater among children who experience marked emergence delirium.[55]

Respiratory System

CRITERIA FOR EXTUBATION

In most cases, extubation may be safely performed in the operating room. However, a child's condition may necessitate delayed extubation at a more appropriate time in the PACU or PICU. There is widespread agreement that children who have been anesthetized with a full stomach, children at risk for airway obstruction, those with difficult airways, premature infants, and other infants predisposed to apnea should be awake before extubation is attempted. Beyond this, the timing of extubation is a matter of individual judgment. For example, the practice at some institutions is to extubate the trachea when a child is awake and demonstrating eye opening and other purposeful movements, whereas the practice at others is to extubate while the child is deeply anesthetized. Clinicians report only rare problems with either approach.[93,94] Most clinicians agree that either approach is preferable to extubating the trachea during a very light plane of anesthesia (stage 2), when laryngospasm is more likely and vomiting may occur while protective reflexes are impaired.

EXTUBATION IN THE OPERATING ROOM OR POSTANESTHESIA CARE UNIT

Immediately after extubation, oxygen should be administered, and the child should be observed closely to ensure that ventilation, oxygen saturation, and the color of the mucous membranes are adequate and whether airway obstruction, laryngospasm, or vomiting occur. Transport of children out of the anesthetizing location should not begin until the patency of the airway and the adequacy of oxygenation and ventilation have been confirmed.

For children whose tracheas are extubated in the PACU, respiratory insufficiency is the most worrisome and most frequent complication. Respiratory insufficiency represents approximately two-thirds of critical perioperative events when it occurs during emergence from anesthesia.[95] Respiratory insufficiency may manifest in the form of difficulty breathing, or it may present as anxiety, unresponsiveness, tachycardia, bradycardia, hypertension, arrhythmia, or seizures. Cardiac arrest is a late manifestation. When any

of these conditions are present, respiratory insufficiency must be considered as the root cause. Hypoxemia, hypoventilation, and upper airway obstruction are the three most common adverse respiratory events that occur in children in the PACU. This is particularly true for children after tonsillectomy complicated by obesity and possible OSA and for those who have undergone diagnostic bronchoscopy.

HYPOXEMIA

Hypoxemia may result from hypoventilation, upper airway obstruction, bronchospasm, aspiration, pulmonary edema, pneumothorax, atelectasis, or rarely from postobstructive pulmonary edema, cardiac shunting, or pulmonary embolism. Hypoxia occurs more rapidly and may be more profound during emergence from general anesthesia because general anesthesia inhibits the hypoxic and hypercapnic ventilatory drive, reduces functional residual capacity, and alters hypoxic pulmonary vasoconstriction. Shivering may further increase oxygen consumption by a factor of two to five[96,97] and exacerbate hemoglobin desaturation.

Postoperative hemoglobin desaturation is more common in children with or recovering from an active upper respiratory tract infection owing to increased airway reactivity, atelectasis, and increased secretions than in children without a history of upper respiratory tract infection.[98,99] In neonates, hypoxia *increases* ventilation for approximately 1 minute but then *depresses* the respiratory drive (i.e., respiratory rate and tidal volume).[100] The normal ventilatory response to hypoxia is delayed for several months in ex-premature nursery graduates with severe bronchopulmonary dysplasia, placing them at particular risk for desaturation in the perioperative period.[101]

HYPOVENTILATION

Severe hypoventilation causes respiratory acidosis, hypoxemia, carbon dioxide narcosis, and apnea. Hypoventilation may result from a decrease in ventilatory drive, muscle weakness, or mechanical effects. Inhalational anesthetics, opioids, benzodiazepines, and other sedating medications (except α_2-agonists) decrease the ventilatory drive in children in a dose-dependent manner. At particular risk for postoperative hypoventilation are children with underlying disturbances in respiration, such as infants with apnea of prematurity (formerly preterm infants of less than 60 weeks postconception age [PCA]); those with CNS injury such as head injury, strokes, and intracranial surgery; obese children; and those with OSA. These children may require prolonged observation in a setting with continuous monitoring capabilities.

Muscular weakness may contribute to respiratory insufficiency. Preexisting muscular disease (e.g., muscular dystrophy) and inadequate reversal of neuromuscular blockade, electrolyte abnormalities, neurologic disorders, drugs, infection, and endocrine disease may impair the respiratory effort sufficiently to cause hypoventilation and respiratory insufficiency. Inadequate analgesia can lead to splinting and hypoventilation, which may in turn increase ventilation-perfusion mismatch and decrease the oxygen saturation.

AIRWAY OBSTRUCTION

Among the most common and serious problems in the PACU is upper airway obstruction. Airway obstruction is a feature in children with known airway problems resulting from congenital anomalies of the face (particularly those with midfacial hypoplasia as in trisomy 21, achondroplasia, and Crouzon disease) and obese children with a history of OSA. Clinical hallmarks of airway obstruction include hemoglobin desaturation, inspiratory stridor, inspiratory retraction, and paradoxical chest wall motion. Common interventions include stimulating the child, repositioning, suctioning, performing a jaw thrust, insertion of an oral or nasal airway, and application of positive end-expiratory pressure (PEEP) (see Fig. 33.10). If these measures fail, patency of the upper and lower airways should be considered because gas exchange may be compromised by laryngospasm, subglottic narrowing as the result of edema, bronchospasm, atelectasis, or tracheal secretions. Incomplete recovery from general anesthesia or neuromuscular blockade, neck wound hematoma (such as after a thyroidectomy), and vocal cord paralysis may also lead to upper airway obstruction. If the airway is not cleared by any of the previously described maneuvers, oxygen should be administered by mask with continuous positive airway pressure along with the medications necessary to facilitate placement of a tracheal tube.

Postobstructive pulmonary edema is a complication of acute upper airway obstruction and of relief of chronic airway obstruction after tonsillectomy. The mechanism appears to be generation of extreme negative intrathoracic pressure against a closed glottis or obstructed airway and its sudden release, resulting in a dramatic increase in pulmonary blood flow that leads to noncardiogenic or neurogenic pulmonary edema. This complication should be suspected when significant hypoxia, persistent tachypnea, or tachycardia follows a prolonged episode of laryngospasm, airway obstruction, or tonsillectomy and the child has pink, frothy secretions emanating from the airway. Treatment of noncardiogenic pulmonary edema includes tracheal intubation, positive-pressure ventilation with PEEP, 100% oxygen to maintain an adequate oxygen tension, furosemide, and morphine. Furosemide (0.5–1 mg/kg) should be given immediately by IV infusion because it is thought to act by decreasing venous return to the heart by direct venodilatation.[102–105]

Postintubation croup or subglottic edema has been associated with factors such as traumatic intubation, tight-fitting tracheal tubes, multiple intubation attempts, coughing with an in situ tracheal tube, a change in the child's position during surgery, prolonged duration of intubation, surgery of the head and neck, and a history of prematurity (with neonatal intubation), Down syndrome, or croup.[106,107] If the symptoms do not abate, nebulized epinephrine (0.5 mg/kg up to a maximum of 5 mg, or 0.25–0.75 mL of 2.25% racemic epinephrine) should be administered, although its effects are temporary. Repeated use of epinephrine may cause rebound laryngeal edema.[108] If nebulized epinephrine is used, a prolonged period of observation is mandated. Outpatients may require overnight hospital admission or observation in the unit for an extended period. Steroids (e.g., dexamethasone 0.6 mg/kg) are effective for reducing mucosal edema but maximum response is delayed (approximately 6 hours).

RESPIRATORY EFFORT

If the airway is patent, attention turns to the adequacy of ventilatory effort. Residual neuromuscular blockade can be diagnosed by observation (i.e., the patient's ability to lift extremities against gravity or perform a sustained head lift) and quantitatively by assessment with a peripheral nerve stimulator. Depending on the severity and the clinical situation, this condition may be treated with supplemental doses of reversal agents or ventilatory assistance. If the respiratory rate is slow, suggesting opioid-induced respiratory depression, titrated incremental doses of naloxone (0.01–0.1 µg/kg) reverses the respiratory depression without precipitating acute anxiety, pain, or pulmonary edema. If naloxone is effective,

continuous monitoring of respiratory status is advised because naloxone has a short half-life of approximately 20 minutes. The same effective total dose may be given intramuscularly to prevent recrudescence of the opioid-induced respiratory depression. Alternately, nalmefene (Revex), a congener of naltrexone, may be used to reverse opioid-induced respiratory depression with a half-life of 10 hours (see Chapter 48). Residual sedation after benzodiazepines may be antagonized with flumazenil but may require an additional 2 hours of observation to ensure that resedation does not occur after reversal.

Children who have an adequate airway and adequate muscular strength may experience difficulty breathing because of pain, restriction from bandages or casts, abdominal distention, pneumothorax, atelectasis, aspiration pneumonitis, or cardiogenic or postobstructive pulmonary edema. In most cases, the history and physical examination focus the differential diagnosis, and when necessary, investigations that include a chest radiograph, blood gas analysis, and possibly invasive hemodynamic monitoring can identify the underlying cause and guide effective treatment.

DISCHARGE OF PRETERM INFANTS FROM THE POSTANESTHESIA CARE UNIT

Preterm infants (<37 weeks gestation) are at risk for apnea after sedation and general anesthesia; however, the risk decreases as infants age.[109–111] Guidelines for monitoring after the administration of sedation or anesthesia have been suggested, but it should be noted that preterm and former preterm children are considered to be a heterogeneous population with various comorbidities and the decision on the length and extent of monitoring should be individualized for each patient.[112–114] However, it is recommended that formerly preterm infants who are 55 to 60 weeks PCA and who are not anemic and not experiencing apnea be observed for an extended period and, if stable, later discharged. Infants younger than 55 weeks PCA, those who are anemic (hematocrit <30%), and those with ongoing apnea should be admitted for monitoring.[109,114–116] Prophylactic administration of caffeine (10 mg/kg IV or orally) may reduce the risk of apnea after general anesthesia for infants at high risk, although it should not supplant postoperative admission and monitoring.[109,112,117,118] Former preterm infants younger than 55 weeks PCA, those with anemia, or those with major cardiorespiratory or neurologic disorders should be admitted and monitored for at least 12 apnea-free hours after general, regional anesthesia, or sedation (see Chapter 4).[112,115,117]

It has been suggested that preterm infants who undergo surgery with spinal anesthesia are at low risk for the development of adverse events compared with those undergoing general anesthesia; however, it should be noted the infants remain at risk for late apnea whereas those receiving general anesthesia are at risk for early apnea.[119–122] Similarly, caudal anesthesia has been reported as an effective alternative to spinal anesthesia in preterm infants undergoing herniotomy.[123–127] Despite evidence of a reduced risk of apnea after regional anesthesia and no postdischarge complications on the day of surgery in some institutions, there is insufficient evidence to make general recommendations regarding this practice. Our recommendation is to admit and monitor these infants regardless of the type of anesthesia administered.

Full-term neonates typically have a reduced risk of apnea and bradycardia after general anesthesia compared with preterm infants. Opinions vary on the minimum PCA for ambulatory surgery in infants 44 to 50 weeks PCA. Many children's hospitals admit all full-term neonates (<28 days of age) for overnight monitoring after general anesthesia, although this is not evidence-based practice.

All full-term infants with a history of apnea and bradycardia or those who have siblings with sudden infant death syndrome should be observed for an extended period or admitted for overnight monitoring after general anesthesia.

Cardiovascular System

BRADYCARDIA

Bradycardia is the most common dysrhythmia in children and requires immediate attention because of its association with decreased cardiac output. *Until proven otherwise, the most common cause of bradycardia in infants and children is hypoxemia.* Other possible causes for bradycardia include vagal responses (e.g., passage of a nasogastric tube, laryngoscopy), medications (e.g., neostigmine, β-adrenergic blockade, α_2-agonists, opioids such as fentanyl), increased intracranial pressure, and high neuraxial anesthetic block. The definition of bradycardia depends on the age of the child; the incidence decreases with increasing age (see Chapter 2).

Treatment is directed at correcting the underlying cause, including the administration of oxygen and ensuring a patent airway. Bradycardia should be immediately treated with oxygen and, if necessary, with ventilation. If these interventions do not immediately restore the heart rate, atropine (0.02 mg/kg) should be administered; if no response is observed within 30 seconds, administration of epinephrine (2–10 µg/kg) is indicated. For symptomatic bradycardia (e.g., hypotension, decreased level of consciousness), immediate administration of epinephrine is indicated. If there is no response to epinephrine, chest compressions should be instituted and standard cardiopulmonary resuscitation algorithms followed (see Chapter 40).

TACHYCARDIA

Tachycardia is an important postoperative sign that is a marker for one of several disorders, such as inadequate cardiac output or oxygen delivery, a response to pain or a direct drug effect (e.g., epinephrine, atropine). Tachycardia may occur in response to hypoxemia, hypercarbia, hypovolemia, hypervolemia, emergence delirium, anxiety, sepsis, fever, a full bladder, a previously unrecognized cardiac conduction abnormality (see Chapters 16 and 18), or heart failure. The threshold for diagnosing tachycardia varies with the age of the child, and decreases with age.

Treatment is directed at correcting the underlying cause. Occasionally, children present with a sustained tachycardia unrelated to the previously described conditions that is refractory to the usual therapy. A cardiac consultation is required to investigate and identify less common causes, such as an aberrant conduction system or ectopic foci, as a source of supraventricular tachycardia (SVT). SVT, which is defined as more than 220 beats/minute in infants and more than 180 beats/minute in children, may be treated with adenosine when there are no other symptoms. However, SVT with accompanied hypotension or decreased level of consciousness may require cardioversion. Children who have had prior cardiac surgery are particularly at risk.

OTHER ARRHYTHMIAS

With the exception of bradycardia and tachycardia, postoperative arrhythmias are rare in children. Isolated premature ventricular or atrial beats may be observed in the PACU and, unless they progress, are not important. Multifocal premature ventricular beats are uncommon in children. They may occur as a result of inadequately treated pain, cardiac conduction defects, or in rare instances, may be a harbinger of malignant hyperthermia (see

Chapters 16, 18, and 41), acute rhabdomyolysis with hyperkalemia, inadequately treated pain, a congenital conduction defect, or a structural cardiac defect. Electrolyte and arterial blood gas status should be checked. Children with known congenital heart disease should have continuous ECG monitoring in the PACU (see Chapters 16 and 18); all arrhythmias should be recorded and a cardiologist consulted because this may be the first manifestation of a developing ectopic focus.

BLOOD PRESSURE CONTROL

Hypotension

The anesthesiologist should be familiar with the normal blood pressure ranges of infants and children (see Chapter 2). The measurement should be obtained with an appropriately sized blood pressure cuff; the width of the cuff should be two-thirds of the length of the upper arm. An improperly sized cuff produces spurious readings. Small cuffs may overestimate the blood pressure, whereas large cuffs may underestimate it. Proper placement of the cuff is essential to avoid errors in interpretation.

The most common cause of hypotension in children is hypovolemia from inadequate replacement of blood and fluids lost during the surgical procedure or ongoing blood loss. Clinical hallmarks of hypovolemia are hypotension, tachycardia, urine output of less than 0.5 to 1 mL/kg per hour, slow capillary refill (>3 seconds), and narrowing of the pulse pressure. If the hematocrit is adequate, hypovolemia may be treated with an initial bolus of 10 to 20 mL/kg of isotonic crystalloid solution or albumin. This may be repeated until the blood pressure is normalized. If the hematocrit is inadequate, packed red blood cells (PRBCs) or whole blood should be administered. In this case, a rough guide for the volume of blood required is 4 mL/kg of packed cells or 6 mL/kg of whole blood to raise the hemoglobin 1 g/dL in children and adults (see Chapters 10 and 12). To achieve a desired hematocrit more precisely, the volume of PRBCs may be estimated as follows:

$$\frac{(\text{Desired hematocrit} - \text{present hematocrit}) \times \text{estimated blood volume}}{\text{The hematocrit in the PRBCs}}$$

If the child does not respond to volume expansion, other causes for the hypotension need to be considered, such as occult blood loss (e.g., intraabdominal, retroperitoneal, intrathoracic [blocked chest tube], cardiac tamponade), sepsis, or other disorders. Any factor that interferes with venous return can cause hypotension, including positive-pressure ventilation, auto-PEEP, tension pneumothorax, pericardial tamponade, and compression of the inferior vena cava.

Large end-tidal concentrations of inhalational anesthetics, local anesthetics, or opioids and interactions between benzodiazepines and opioids may produce hypotension through vasodilation (i.e., relative hypovolemia) and direct myocardial depression. However, these factors are rarely important in the PACU. Uncommon causes include anaphylaxis (e.g., latex allergy, antibiotics), transfusion reaction, adrenal insufficiency, systemic inflammation, infection, severe liver failure, and administration of antihypertensive, antidysrhythmic, and anticonvulsant medications. Increased body temperature may cause vasodilation and a relative hypovolemia. The increased metabolic demands of fever may compromise an already stressed myocardium. If a child arrives in the PACU requiring vasopressors and subsequently develops hypotension, consider mechanical causes such as a disconnect or kink in the vasopressor infusion, disruption of the IV access, a disconnect from the pump, or pump failure.

Vasodilation caused by sympathetic blockade associated with regional anesthesia occasionally causes hypotension, especially with a high-level blockade and restricted fluid intake. However, this is quite uncommon in children younger than 6 years of age. Because of the developmental changes in the sympathetic nervous system, most children younger than 6 years of age are normally peripherally vasodilated and therefore have little response to further vasodilation with a regional block.[128,129]

Decreased inotropy, dysrhythmia, cardiomyopathy, calcium channel blockers, sepsis, hypothyroidism, negative inotropic agents, and congestive heart failure are uncommon causes of hypotension in children. Treatment is directed at the underlying cause, such as correcting hypovolemia with volume loading, treating the allergic reaction, or treating the sepsis. Decreased cardiac contractility may be treated by diuresis and the administration of inotropic agents that also decrease the afterload (i.e., inodilators).

Hypertension

Postoperative hypertension in children is less common than hypotension and most often reflects incorrect measurement or pain. A blood pressure cuff that is too small may overestimate the blood pressure and should be one of the first considerations in the differential diagnosis, especially if the child has no other symptoms consistent with pain. Causative factors besides pain include hypervolemia, preexisting hypertension (e.g., renal disease), distended bladder, hypercarbia, hypoxemia, agitation and delirium, increased intracranial pressure, and exogenous vasoactive drugs (e.g., epinephrine).

Renal System

Complications related to the renal system are rare in the postoperative period. The most likely cause of low urine output (<0.5–1 mL/kg per hour) is hypovolemia (e.g., postoperative hypotension). Mechanical obstruction downstream from the kidneys may result from direct surgical interference or a misplaced or dysfunctional urinary catheter (i.e., blood clot or kink). If the child has regional (spinal or epidural) anesthesia that includes an opioid and there is no urinary catheter in place, placement of a Foley or straight catheter may be indicated. Renal failure is a rare possibility in children who have had major operations or have systemic inflammatory disease. If screening tests such as blood urea nitrogen, serum creatinine, and urine analysis suggest renal insufficiency, a pediatric nephrologist should be consulted (see also Chapter 28).

Gastrointestinal System

POSTOPERATIVE NAUSEA AND VOMITING

PONV is one of the most bothersome adverse effects of anesthesia and surgery. Unlike adults, most children are unfamiliar with and have never experienced nausea. It is unlikely that they will warn the PACU personnel that they are nauseated. In children, vomiting and complaining about a "sore tummy" are likely the first and only manifestations of gastrointestinal upset. Among children, PONV is inversely related to age.[130] The incidence of PONV is small in very young children, increases throughout childhood, and reaches a zenith in adolescents, for whom the incidence exceeds that for adults.[130,131]

The type of surgery influences the incidence of PONV. The incidence of PONV in children is greatest after tonsillectomy, strabismus repair, hernia repair, orchiopexy, microtia, and middle ear procedures.[130,132] Before puberty, there are no gender-related differences in PONV; after puberty, girls experience much more PONV than boys.[130] The medical complications of PONV include pulmonary aspiration, dehydration, electrolyte imbalance, fatigue, wound disruption, and esophageal tears. PONV can produce psychological effects that may produce anxiety in the children and parents and lead them to avoid further surgery. The cost implications of PONV can be major because of delayed recovery and discharge, increased medical care, and reoperation. Although these problems are seldom life-threatening, the cumulative costs in terms of prolonged PACU stays, unplanned admissions, and patient dissatisfaction are serious.[133]

EVIDENCE-BASED CONSENSUS MANAGEMENT

Management of PONV is complex, and many treatment strategies have been formulated (Fig. 47.1). Most have been shown to be effective in one study or another. However, the superiority of some treatments over others has not been established, in part because of study design flaws such as inadequate dosing, small sample sizes, or various periods of observations and data collection; some studies monitored PONV only during the first few hours after surgery, whereas others monitored the children for 24 to 48 hours after surgery. To make sense of the conflicting data that exist, consensus-based management strategies for the prevention and management of PONV have been suggested.[131,134,135] These guidelines advise to first identify the children at significant risk for developing PONV as outlined earlier and to then administer prophylaxis in that patient population. Studies frequently focus on postoperative vomiting as the primary outcome because nausea may be difficult to identify in children.

The consensus guidelines recognize that the choice of anesthetic can influence the incidence of PONV in children. Propofol-based anesthesia during operations associated with a large incidence of PONV dramatically reduces the incidence of PONV compared with inhalational anesthesia.[32,136,137] Similarly, multimodal therapy that is a combination of PONV treatment strategies is more effective than a single-treatment strategy.[138–140] Although somewhat controversial, avoidance of nitrous oxide is considered to prevent the development of PONV.[33,138,141,142]

Other strategies recommended to decrease the rate of PONV include the use of the smallest dose of opioids that still provides adequate pain control and the use of regional anesthesia if possible. TIVA is associated with reduced PONV (Chapter 8). The use of nonopioids such as acetaminophen, ketamine, and ketorolac should be considered. Adequate parenteral hydration and avoidance of early postoperative fluid ingestion can reduce the incidence of PONV (see Chapter 4).

PROPHYLACTIC THERAPY

Ondansetron has been studied extensively and shown to decrease early and late PONV at doses of 50 to 100 µg/kg.[134,143] Because the 5-HT$_3$-receptor antagonists as a group have greater efficacy in the prevention of vomiting than nausea, they are the drugs of first choice for prophylaxis in children. Dexamethasone also is effective in decreasing PONV.[134,140,142,144] Administration of dexamethasone alone or in combination with other antiemetics can extend the period of effective treatment up to 24 hours. Before the black box warning was added for droperidol, it was also recommended for prophylaxis of PONV in the United States[145]; however, for medicolegal reasons alone, it is no longer a first-tier antiemetic. Droperidol is commonly used in low doses, which limit extrapyramidal and sedation side effects. Adequate fluid

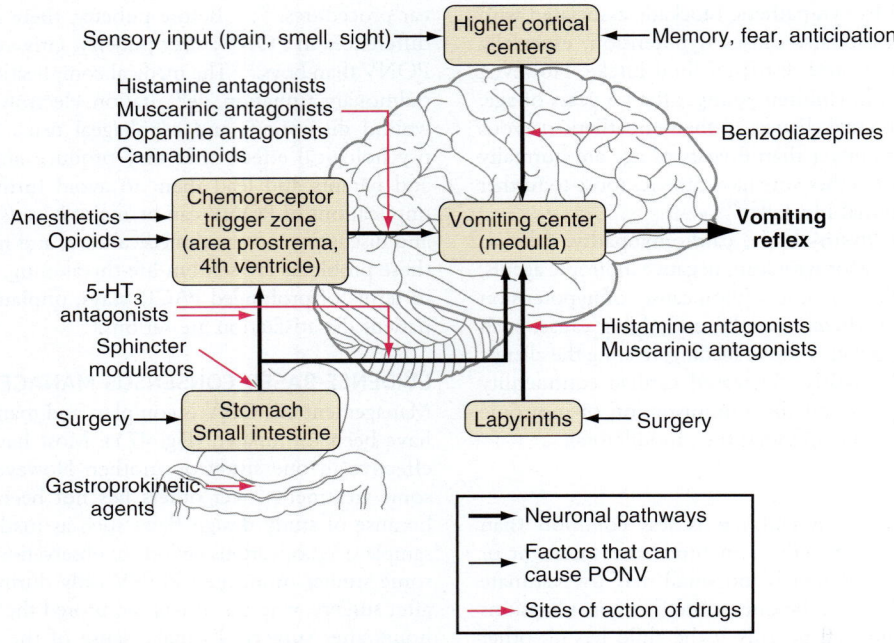

FIGURE 47.1 Treatment strategies for postoperative nausea and vomiting (*PONV*).

resuscitation also plays in important role in PONV prevention. Children given 10 mL/kg of lactated Ringer's solution during strabismus correction had more PONV than those given 30 mL/kg (54% vs. 22%).[138,146]

The most effective prophylaxis strategy in children at moderate or high risk for PONV is to use combination therapy that includes hydration, a 5-HT₃-receptor antagonist, and a second drug such as dexamethasone. Antiemetic rescue therapy should be administered to children who vomit after surgery. An emetic episode more than 6 hours postoperatively can be treated with any of the drugs used for prophylaxis except dexamethasone and transdermal scopolamine.[134,147]

Alternative Treatments

Alternative antiemetic techniques for the prevention and treatment of PONV that have been reported to be successful include acupuncture, electroacupuncture, transcutaneous electrical nerve stimulation, and accupoint stimulation; however, these have not been consistently shown to be effective in children.[148–153]

Postoperative Care and Discharge

PAIN MANAGEMENT IN THE POSTANESTHESIA CARE UNIT

Acute postoperative pain management strategies are discussed in detail in Chapter 44. A child's level of pain (or the perception of pain) changes more rapidly in the PACU than in any other unit of the hospital. Frequent and consistent use of pain scores for children of all ages, including those with developmental disabilities, is essential. Many pain scales have been validated for use in children. More important than the specific scale used, the scale should be used consistently and follow simple principles. For instance, children who are verbal and developmentally appropriate should be encouraged to describe their pain using a self-report scale (e.g., Oucher scale).[154] Young children or those without verbal skills should be assessed using an objective pain behavior scale

(e.g., **F**ace, **L**egs, **A**ctivity, **C**ry, **C**onsolability [FLACC] scale).[155,156] Equally as important is the consistent application of protocols to treat pain; treatment of a given pain level should not vary from shift to shift or from one nurse to another.[157]

As with other areas of pediatric pain control, a multimodal approach to postoperative pain is recommended. A plan for pain management should be discussed among the family, surgical team, and anesthesia team before surgery. Depending on the surgery, the plan may include any or all of the following: acetaminophen, nonsteroidal agents, local anesthesia, nerve blocks, regional anesthesia, α₂-agonists, opioids, patient-controlled analgesia, and patient-controlled epidural analgesia.

Acetaminophen and nonsteroidal drugs act through inhibition of prostaglandins and their metabolites. Most of these drugs are given orally and should be given preoperatively or intraoperatively to be effective in the PACU. Occasionally, they may be indicated in the PACU if they were not administered before arrival. Oral acetaminophen (15 mg/kg) or ibuprofen (10 mg/kg) has been shown to decrease opioid requirements by 20% to 30% after a variety of surgical procedures. IV acetaminophen has become available in the United States for children 2 years of age or older, and it is likely to become a popular analgesic for mild to moderate pain in the PACU and as an opioid-sparing drug.[158] The IV dose of 15 mg/kg every 6 hours is recommended for patients weighing less than 50 kg and should be administered over 15 minutes.[159] Studies on IV formulations of propacetamol and paracetamol have mostly been conducted in the European Union since drug approval in 2002; extreme care regarding dosing must be taken when administering these formulations as the recommended doses vary 2-fold. Studies in neonates have suggested the IV formulation is safe and effective in reducing opioid consumption. However, instances of hepatotoxicity have been reported.[160–164] Several randomized, controlled studies and meta-analyses have demonstrated efficacy of IV administration in adults and children for the treatment of mild to moderate pain or fever.[165,166]

Acetaminophen can also be given rectally in doses of 35 to 45 mg/kg; however, because absorption varies and is delayed (i.e., peak concentration at 60–180 minutes after rectal administration), this route is not recommended for use in the PACU.[167] Because of the pharmacokinetics of the rectal route, a greater interval (6 hours) between doses is recommended, and subsequent doses are reduced (20 mg/kg) so that the total dose per 24 hours does not exceed 100 mg/kg.[168] There are no data to provide guidance for rectal acetaminophen beyond 24 hours. If a child has received rectal acetaminophen, the first oral dose should be delayed until 6 hours after the rectal dose.

The nonsteroidal anti-inflammatory drug (NSAID) ketorolac can decrease opioid requirements by approximately 30%. The recommended dosage is 0.2 to 0.5 mg/kg IV (up to 15 mg for children <50 kg and up to 30 mg for children >50 kg) every 6 hours.[169] Caution is warranted in postoperative children with significant bleeding or a history of renal insufficiency. The use of ketorolac is controversial in the pediatric orthopedic surgical literature since the drug has been linked to adverse outcomes including increased bleeding and nonunion of fractures; however, other researchers have suggested it does not negatively impact patient outcomes.[170-173] Similar considerations also apply to parecoxib, another IV antiinflammatory drug.[174]

Opioids are indicated during the immediate postoperative period for any procedure in which moderate or severe pain is not being managed by other means. Morphine, fentanyl, and hydromorphone have a long history of safe use for infants and children in the PACU when vital signs are monitored appropriately. Meperidine is recommended only to treat shivering for children because of the potential for seizures from epileptogenic metabolites (e.g., normeperidine).[175] Opioid dosing should be initiated according to body weight, physiologic development, underlying medical or surgical conditions, coadministered medications, and severity of pain. The goal should be effective and rapid pain relief. Subsequent dosing of the medications should be titrated based on response to the initial dose. Administration of multiple, small, ineffective doses results in prolongation of pain, stress, and anxiety without improving the safety of care provided. With this caveat in mind, patient-controlled analgesia and patient-controlled epidural analgesia (see Chapters 42 and 44) may be used in the PACU environment, but either intervention should be started only after acute pain has been adequately treated. It is essential to reduce opioid dosing by 33% to 50% in those children at risk for OSA due to their known opioid sensitivity. In this population pulse oximetry must be maintained at all times and deaths in PACU have occurred when monitoring was discontinued due to patient upset treated with sedatives or opioids and monitors not reapplied (see also Chapter 33 and Figs. 33.7 and 33.8).[175a]

Regional analgesia is a common mode of intraoperative pain control in the child that extends into the PACU (see Chapters 42 to 44). The PACU personnel should be competent in assessing the adequacy of the block and familiar with the use and programming of the administration pumps.

Evidence that the regional block is effective should first be detected during surgery since the anesthetic requirements for successful surgical completion are reduced. The addition of hydrophilic opioids or clonidine may extend the level and duration of analgesia to some extent over the course of several hours; however, a block many dermatome segments away from the site of the surgical incision is unlikely to remain adequate for very long. The addition of opioids to an epidural or spinal block increases the risk of pruritus, urinary retention, and emesis. Similarly, visceral pain

such as bladder spasms (which have thoracic innervation) or sore throat after intubation are not attenuated by a lumbar epidural catheter and must be managed by other measures.

The anesthesiologist must verify that the catheter is properly located in the epidural space. Older children can be questioned about their sensation level using ice or other cold sensation to determine the level of sympathectomy. Preverbal or developmentally disabled children require some other objective form of confirmation. Previous reports have focused on electrical stimulation through the epidural catheter at the time of catheter placement to determine the level of insertion.[176,177] Ultrasound methods for detecting epidural catheter placement have been described.[178-180] Perhaps the most practical method may be radiographic confirmation of the dermatome level of the tip of the catheter, often with the use of an appropriate contrast material (i.e., epidurogram) to ensure appropriate placement in the epidural space. A small amount (<1 mL) of contrast (e.g., Omnipaque 180 or 240) can be infused into the catheter while one radiograph is taken to confirm placement (see Fig. 42.7).[181]

TEMPERATURE MANAGEMENT

The literature documents the detrimental effects of hypothermia and suggests optimal outcomes are achieved when children arrive in the PACU with a normal body temperature. Intraoperative normothermia is key to maintaining a normal temperature postoperatively. Hypothermia is associated with discomfort, bleeding, infections, altered metabolism of drugs, delayed return of cognitive functions, and prolonged recovery.[182-185] Because about 90% of heat loss occurs through the skin, only heat exchange through the skin provides an adequate way of warming children. This method of warming is enhanced by the vasodilation properties of most anesthetic agents. Forced-air warming blankets are effective as the sole method for maintaining normothermia in children.[186-188] Given the vasoconstriction that occurs after anesthesia, attempts at warming are less effective postoperatively than intraoperatively, and most of the detrimental physiologic changes have already taken place.

Infants and children may suffer burns from overly aggressive rewarming measures.[189-191] This is particularly true for nonverbal children, children who are somnolent, and children who have decreased sensation owing to disease or use of regional anesthesia techniques.

DISCHARGE CRITERIA

The recovery process and discharge criteria vary from institution to institution. Some institutions require an assessment by a physician before discharge for all patients, but others require an evaluation only if routine discharge criteria are not met. The modified Aldrete scale is the most common system used to assess discharge readiness, but specific criteria depend on the particular situation or environment to which the child will be discharged.[192-194] For example, a child with a slight degree of postextubation croup or stridor may be discharged for monitoring on a pediatric floor or ICU, but the same child is not discharged to parental care and a 2-hour drive home. The criteria for discharge of children to a general inpatient setting are summarized in Table 47.7. For outpatients, these criteria hold, and the additional criteria outlined in Table 47.8 usually must be met before discharge.

Traditionally, children have been allowed to recover in a first-stage recovery unit until the airway was considered stable, consciousness is regained, baseline motor activity is confirmed, vital signs are stable, and oxygen saturation values are stable in room air (or

TABLE 47.7	Discharge Criteria for Inpatients

1. Recovery of airway and respiratory reflexes adequate to support gas exchange and to protect against aspiration of secretions, vomitus, or blood
2. Stability of circulation and control of any surgical bleeding
3. Absence of anticipated instability in criteria 1 and 2
4. Reasonable control of pain and vomiting
5. Appropriate duration of observation after opioid or naloxone flumazenil administration (minimum of 60 minutes after intravenous naloxone and up to 2 hours after flumazenil)
6. Return to baseline level of consciousness unless transfer is to an intensive care unit environment

TABLE 47.8	Discharge Criteria for Outpatients

All Criteria in Table 47.7, Plus the Following:

1. Cardiovascular function and airway patency are satisfactory and stable.
2. The child is easily rousable, and protective reflexes are intact.
3. The child can talk (if age appropriate).
4. The child can sit up unaided (if age appropriate).
5. For a very young or handicapped child, incapable of the usually expected responses, the preanesthetic level of responsiveness or a level as close as possible to the normal level for that child should be achieved unless the child is to be transferred to another monitored location.
6. The state of hydration is adequate.
7. It may be permissible for parents to carry their children without full recovery of gait (parents must be advised that the child is at risk of injury if improperly supervised).
8. Control of pain should be achieved to permit adequate analgesia by the oral route thereafter.
9. Control of nausea and vomiting should be achieved to allow for oral hydration (see "Discharge Criteria" in text).

TABLE 47.9	Discharge Criteria for Fast Tracking	
Criteria		**Score**
Level of Consciousness		
Aware and oriented		2
Arousable with minimal stimulation		1
Responsive only to tactile stimulation		0
Physical Activity		
Able to move all extremities on command		2
Some weakness in movement of extremities		1
Unable to voluntarily move extremities		0
Hemodynamic Stability		
Blood pressure <15% of baseline MAP value		2
Blood pressure 15%–30% of baseline MAP value		1
Blood pressure >30% of baseline MAP value		0
Respiratory Stability		
Able to breathe deeply		2
Tachypneic with good cough		1
Dyspneic with weak cough		0
Oxygen Saturation Status		
Maintains value >95% on room air		2
Requires supplemental oxygen (nasal prongs)		1
Saturation <90% with supplemental oxygen		0
Postoperative Pain Assessment		
None or mild discomfort		2
Moderate to severe pain controlled with intravenous analgesics		1
Persistent, severe pain		0
Postoperative Emetic Symptoms		
None or mild nausea with no active vomiting		2
Transient vomiting or retching		1
Persistent, moderate to severe nausea and vomiting		0
Total[a]		14

[a]Pediatric patients must score 14 to bypass the phase 1 (PACU) recovery unit to be admitted directly to the step-down care unit.
MAP, mean arterial pressure; PACU, postanesthesia care unit.
From White PF, Song D. New criteria for fast-tracking after outpatient anesthesia: a comparison with the modified Aldrete's scoring system. *Anesth Analg.* 1998;88:1069–1072.

at baseline) without respiratory support (unless needed at baseline). Pain should be well controlled. Children then can be transferred to a second-stage recovery unit, where more complete recovery takes place with a reduced nurse/child ratio, until children have met criteria for adequate hydration, minimal emesis, appropriate wound status, stable vital signs, and appropriate ambulation and mental status.

The requirements for children to eat, drink, and void before leaving the secondary recovery area significantly delay discharge. Efforts should be made to reinstate volume homeostasis during surgery, negating any physiologic imperative for oral intake in the immediate postoperative period. Postoperative maintenance fluids should consist of isotonic rather than hypotonic solutions for those expected to remain as inpatients to reduce the risk of hyponatremia (see also Chapter 9).[195–198] Other than children who are at high risk for urinary retention (e.g., history of urinary retention, urethral surgery), there is little evidence that discharge before voiding results in readmission for voiding problems. In fact, this requirement is no longer part of standard discharge criteria.[199] Children who have received a caudal block for surgery are likewise at low risk for urinary retention as long as opioids have not been added to the caudal medication.[194]

Although there are few data on the current status of recovery processes across the country, there appears to be a trend toward one-stage (fast-track) recovery for pediatric outpatients. This process allows selected children to bypass the first-stage recovery and go directly to the second-stage unit based on an appropriate level of consciousness, physical activity, vital signs, respiratory status, and pain control (Table 47.9). This approach has proved successful and quite safe, although appropriate attention to issues such as pain control must be addressed when initiating such a program.

Beyond PACU: Postoperative Monitoring in the General Care Setting

Adult postoperative patients who are taking opioids are a subset of the inpatient population at particular risk for failure to rescue because of respiratory depression[200]; postoperative respiratory failure represents nearly 11% of all inpatient safety events[201] and has the greatest mortality rate per 100 discharges of all classified safety events.[202] A study in adult, noncardiac surgical patients who were continuously monitored with pulse oximetry found that 21% had oxyhemoglobin saturation (SpO_2) of 90% for an average of ≥10 min/h and 8% had average of ≥20 min/h, and 8% had SpO_2 <85% for ≥5 min/h. A further 3% of postsurgical patients had SpO_2 less than 80% for 30 minutes or longer.[203] This increased risk prompted the Anesthesia Patient Safety Foundation to advocate continuous electronic physiologic monitoring for all inpatients receiving postoperative opioids.[204] While equivalent data or recommendations for the pediatric population are missing, there is little reason to assume that these data should be different in children.

Historically, the selective monitoring of children perceived to be at an increased risk for adverse events ("condition monitoring") because of comorbidities, surgical procedures, or opioid use has mostly failed. Recent research in pharmacogenomics as well as error analysis has provided more insight as to why condition monitoring is an inadequate approach to address the problem. Clinicians have been aware of interindividual variation in response to opioids, and advances in pharmacogenetics have provided the scientific background for these variations. The FDA has proscribed the use of codeine in patients after tonsil and adenoidectomies as a result of the single-nucleotide polymorphisms (SNPs) in cytochrome P4502D6, in whom ultrarapid metabolizers experience greater morphine conversion and greater plasma concentrations. The estimated prevalence of ultrarapid metabolizers varies from 1% to 29%, depending on ethnicity (see Chapters 6 and 7).[205] Many of these genetic variations are yet to be discovered but certainly contributed to unanticipated adverse events. According to The Joint Commission's Sentinel Event Database (2004–2011), 47% of respiratory depression events were wrong dosing medication errors, 29% were related to improper monitoring of the patient, and 11% were related to other factors, including excessive dosing, medication interactions, and adverse drug reactions (http://www.jointcommission.org/assets/1/18/SEA_49_opioids_8_2_12_final.pdf, last accessed 04/09/2016).[206] These data provide some insight into why risk stratification and selective, individual monitoring has failed. Future mitigation of drug errors by bar coding medication and their administration as well as medication reconciliation efforts may minimize adverse respiratory events and make selected monitoring a viable option in the future.

There have been some very successful implementations of surveillance systems to dramatically reduce inpatient adverse events by using pulse oximetry–based surveillance reaching back almost a decade. However, the understanding of surveillance monitoring and its approach of applying principles of population health medicine to hospital wards is still in its infancy.[207–209] Using a pulse oximetry surveillance system in an orthopedic inpatient unit, a research group at Dartmouth decreased unanticipated ICU transfers by 50% and activations of the rapid response by 65%. Using a static alarm–based threshold system for heart rate and oxygen saturation, the system redirects attention of nursing staff to these physiologic deteriorations via a paging system, prompting early intervention.[207] Routine surveillance using pulse oximetry for all inpatients on general care units has been institutional policy at Dartmouth since 2009 for adults and since 2012 for children. Because of the physiologic developmental changes in heart rate in children, creating static alarm triggers is more complex in children than in adults. Table 47.10 shows the alarm thresholds used at Children's Hospital at Dartmouth. Strategies to manage alarm fatigue and alerting for actionable events have been described

TABLE 47.10 Patient Surveillance Alarm Thresholds

Age	Heart Rate (beats/minute)	Oxygen Saturation (%)
0–6 months	80–235	80
6–12 months	70–220	80
1–5 years	60–200	80
5–12 years	55–180	80
>12 years	50–140	80

A pulse oximetry-based system used at the Children's Hospital at Dartmouth.

for adults, but they apply equally for children.[207,208] The introduction of pediatric patient surveillance at Dartmouth has decreased the use of the rapid response team because of earlier detection of physiologic deterioration, similar to that in adults.

The role and importance of surveillance monitoring and the needed expertise of pediatric anesthesiologists and intensivists is likely to expand in the future. With the rapid adoption of telemedicine, surveillance monitoring of pediatric patients is likely to exponentially grow not only in the inpatient general care setting, but also is likely to expand to the home setting as length of stay in the hospital will continue to decline.

ACKNOWLEDGMENT
The authors wish to thank A. J. de Armendi, MD, I. D. Todres, MD, and J. P. Cravero, MD, for their prior contributions to this chapter.

ANNOTATED REFERENCES

American Academy of Pediatrics Statement: Critical elements for the pediatric perioperative anesthesia environment. *Pediatrics.* 2015;136(6):1200-1205. doi:10.1542/peds.2015-3595.

Society for Pediatric Anesthesia Policy Statement on Provision of Pediatric Anesthesia Care. http://www.pedsanesthesia.org/about/society-for-pediatric-anesthesia-policy-statement-on-provision-of-pediatric-anesthesia-care/. Accessed April 16, 2016.

American College of Surgeons. Optimal Resources for Children's Surgical Care; 2015. https://www.facs.org/quality-programs/childrens-surgery-verification/standards.

The above citations outline the standards for the perioperative care of children.

Anderson BJ, Woolard GA, Holford NH. Pharmacokinetics of rectal paracetamol after major surgery in children. *Paediatr Anaesth.* 1995;5:237-242.

The authors conducted a pharmacokinetic study in 20 children from 12 months to 17 years of age and demonstrated that paracetamol reached therapeutic plasma concentrations 1 to 2 hours after administration at a dose of 40 mg/kg. Anderson's research group subsequently defined the use of paracetamol in various forms of administration (e.g., oral, rectal, intravenous) in children of all ages.

Boat AC, Spaeth JP. Handoff checklists improve the reliability of patient handoffs in the operating room and postanesthesia care unit. *Paediatr Anaesth.* 2013;23(7):647-654.

The authors demonstrate improvement in effective communication through the implementation of checklists in the postoperative period.

Choong K, Arora S, Cheng J, et al. Hypotonic versus isotonic maintenance fluids after surgery for children: a randomized controlled trial. *Pediatrics.* 2011;128:857-866.

This important paper addresses the issue of postoperative hyponatremia in children. The authors randomly assigned 258 children to two groups receiving isotonic or hypotonic maintenance solutions. Children in the isotonic group had hyponatremia at a rate of 22.7% (vs. 40.8%), with no increased risk for hypernatremia.

Coté CJ, Posner KL, Domino KB. Death or neurologic injury after tonsillectomy in children with a focus on obstructive sleep apnea: Houston, we have a problem! *Anesth Analg.* 2014;118(6):1276-1283.

This paper reported 16 children who died or suffered neurologic injury within 24 hours of their tonsillectomy. Thirteen died at home, one on the ward that evening, but most importantly two died in PACU after monitors were removed; one in his father's lap and the other in bed next to mom. These cases illustrate the insidious nature of OSA and why such children require the utmost attention to opioid dosing and monitoring with a need for postoperative admission and monitoring for those with severe OSA.

Coté CJ, Zaslavsky A, Downes JJ, et al. Postoperative apnea in former preterm infants after inguinal herniorrhaphy. A combined analysis. *Anesthesiology.* 1995;82(4):809-822.

Data presented by the authors are frequently used for admission requirements of formerly preterm neonates.

Cravero JP, Beach M, Thyr B, Whalen K. The effect of small dose fentanyl on the emergence characteristics of pediatric patients after sevoflurane anesthesia without surgery. *Anesth Analg.* 2003;97:364-367.

The authors performed a prospective, randomized, blinded trial in which they studied patients undergoing magnetic resonance imaging with general inhaled sevoflurane anesthesia through a laryngeal mask airway. They concluded that small doses of opioids decrease emergence agitation without increasing unwanted side effects.

Gan TJ, Diemunsch P, Habib AS, et al. Consensus guidelines for the management of postoperative nausea and vomiting. *Anesth Analg.* 2014;118(1):85-113.

The authors review the available literature concerning postoperative nausea and vomiting. They use strength of evidence criteria when possible and expert opinion when data are lacking.

Hicks CW, Rosen M, Hobson DB, et al. Improving safety and quality of care with enhanced teamwork through operating room briefings. *JAMA Surg.* 2014;149(8):863-868.

The authors describe methods to improve operating room communication and provide examples of successful methods.

Kain ZN, Caldwell-Andrews AA, Maranets I, et al. Preoperative anxiety and emergence delirium and postoperative maladaptive behaviors. *Anesth Analg.* 2004;99:1648-1654.

This study is extremely unusual in its ability to correlate perioperative anxiety with the incidence of emergence agitation. Preoperative anxiety is significantly related to the incidence of emergence agitation, and the incidence of agitation is related to the rate of postoperative maladaptive behaviors. This study argues strongly for identifying children at risk for emergence agitation and provides some evidence for why it is worth the effort to prevent or ameliorate this phenomenon.

McNicol ED, Tzortzopoulou A, Cepeda MS, et al. Single-dose intravenous paracetamol or propacetamol for prevention or treatment of postoperative pain: a systemic review and meta-analysis. *Br J Anaesth.* 2011;106:764-775.

The authors performed a meta-analysis of 36 randomized, controlled trials and 3896 patients to study the effect of a single, intravenous dose of acetaminophen. They found that 37% of patients with acute postoperative pain had pain relief for about 4 hours.

Taenzer AH, Pyke JB, McGrath SP. A review of current and emerging approaches to address failure-to-rescue. *Anesthesiology.* 2011;115(2):421-431.

The authors describe and review the current state of failure-to-rescue for inpatients and discuss strategies to mitigate adverse events.

A complete reference list can be found online at ExpertConsult.com.

Sedation for Diagnostic and Therapeutic Procedures Outside the Operating Room

48

JOSEPH P. CRAVERO, RICHARD F. KAPLAN, MARY LANDRIGAN-OSSAR, AND CHARLES J. COTÉ

The Evolution of Pediatric Sedation and the Anesthesiologist's Role

Perhaps more than ever, the care of children in the hospital setting requires the provision of sedation in a timely and effective manner. Many children who require an imaging procedure or invasive test before surgery will not tolerate the procedures without sedation. In addition, children with neurologic, gastroenterologic, or oncologic (medical) illness require repeated tests and procedures for a single course of treatment that may be uncomfortable or invasive. In some, sedation is required because of age, anxiety, or developmental delay. A responsive and accommodating sedation service that helps accomplish these procedures in a safe, efficient, and effective manner is an indispensable component of a functional hospital or health system.

The provision of sedation care for children undergoing tests and procedures outside the operating room continues to evolve. Forty years ago, physical restraint without medications was the preferred method to achieve these objectives in children, but today, that approach is completely eschewed and supplanted with sedation in an atmosphere of respect and safety that is on par with the quality of care provided to children undergoing surgery.[1-4] At the same time, we must recognize that the sheer numbers of children who require sedation exceed the capacity of pediatric anesthesiologists to provide all of this care; partnership with other types of physicians and nurses who are capable and willing to deliver pediatric procedural sedation is required. Furthermore, economic pressures in medicine demand systems that optimize efficiency, throughput, and effectiveness of the care provided. While anesthesiologists may find the practice of sedation only moderately challenging, understanding the environment, guidelines, and organizational issues involving sedation practice for ourselves and our partners is critical if we are to improve the overall delivery of this care to children globally.

Sedation/analgesia for painful procedures performed outside the operating room (OR; e.g., bone marrow aspiration, lumbar puncture, repair of minor surgical wounds, insertion of arterial or venous catheters, burn dressing changes, fracture reduction, bronchoscopy, and endoscopy) requires the same attention to detail as for procedures performed in the OR because the level of sedation needed is usually deep sedation or general anesthesia, particularly for children 6 years of age and younger, as well as for those at any age with developmental delay. Children undergoing diagnostic studies (e.g., computed tomography [CT], magnetic resonance imaging [MRI], positron emission tomography [PET], electroencephalography [EEG], electromyography) and those who require high doses of ionizing radiation require deep levels of sedation or general anesthesia because they must remain absolutely motionless (sometimes with breath-holding).[5] Given these requirements, a coordinated team approach is required to provide safe, optimal conditions for the procedure.

The need for sedation services goes beyond the very young and developmentally challenged patients usually associated with this requirement. Older children and adolescents without developmental delay may also require sedation to undergo a procedure/investigation in a confined space (e.g., MRI scans) because of claustrophobia. Other procedures, such as sexual abuse examinations or urinary catheterization, are more emotionally disturbing than painful, but they still require sedation to control anxiety and fear that can ultimately lead to long-term emotional/psychological harm if they were performed without anxiolytics. Furthermore, a child's emotional state may be worsened by parental anxiety, separation from parents, and the pain (or anticipation of pain) from the procedure (see Chapter 3). Distraction, guided imagery, and the use of videos and music have proven beneficial in this respect, although they may be insufficient to provide the conditions needed to complete all procedures in their entirety.[6-10]

The pharmacologic armamentarium for sedation for diagnostic and therapeutic procedures has greatly expanded over the past 10 years to include potent sedative hypnotics, opioids, and dissociative agents. The determination as to which physicians can use these medications and what qualifications are needed to provide deep sedation/anesthesia has been the subject of some debate.

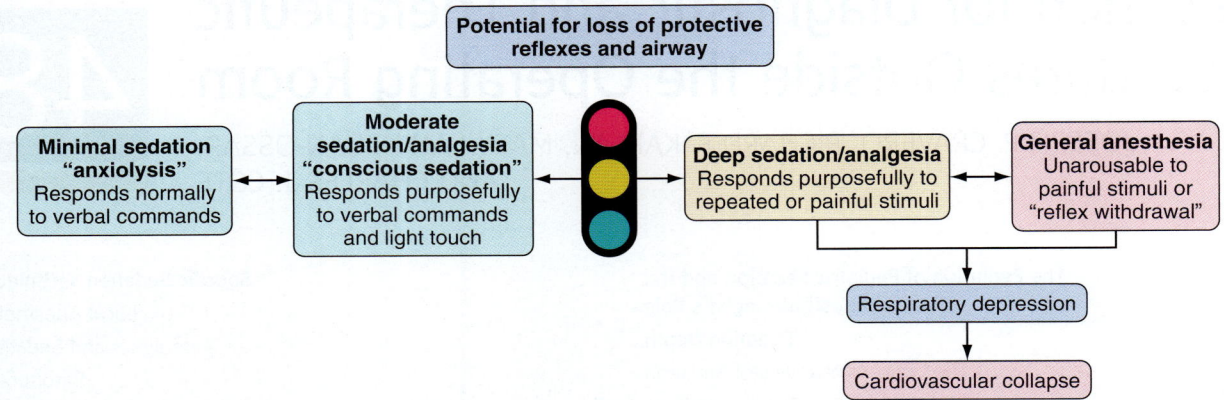

FIGURE 48.1 The sedation continuum. A patient may readily pass from a light level of sedation to deep sedation or general anesthesia. Health care providers must be prepared to increase vigilance and intensity of monitoring consistent with the depth of sedation.

Although the final determination of how this care will be provided remains contentious, the clear trend is toward liberalization of the use of drugs such as propofol, dexmedetomidine, remifentanil, and ketamine.[11] One driving force for this change is the demand for efficient sedation and analgesia outside the OR. Pressure comes from many sources, including hospital administrators, insurance companies, medical specialists, and families, because failures and missed appointments significantly increase hospital costs and frustrate parents.[12] Failed sedations for diagnostic or therapeutic procedures are no longer accepted as part of the sedation process; the use of more potent medications decreases the chance of inadequate sedation. All of these factors have led to the "professionalization" of pediatric sedation with the creation of pediatric sedation services, many of which are led by pediatricians, hospitalists, emergency medicine physicians, intensivists, and dentists. Examples of the changing landscape of sedation abound. A 2005 survey of pediatric sedation practice in 116 children's hospitals in the United States and Canada[13] reported that anesthesiologists exclusively provided the sedation in only 26% of institutions. Similarly, the Pediatric Sedation Research Consortium (PRSC), a collaborative of hospitals heavily committed to improving pediatric sedation, noted that most sedation in the participating institutions (over 100,000 encounters) was delivered by organized sedation services of which anesthesiologists were involved in only 19%.[14] When specifically evaluating the use of propofol in a cohort of 50,000 encounters, the PRSC noted that anesthesiologists were involved only 10% of the time.[15] Despite this changing landscape of sedation, anesthesiologists are still charged by the federal government and the Joint Commission of Hospital Accreditation (JCAHO) in the United States to exercise oversight of sedation practices.[16] To provide effective leadership, anesthesiologists must have a full appreciation of the issues involved in this dynamic area of practice. This chapter focuses on the current definitions of sedation for diagnostic and therapeutic procedures and the goals, risks, and guidelines for creation of safe conditions for children who require sedation for procedures outside the OR.

Sedation Depth

THE CONCEPT OF LEVELS OF SEDATION

Several organizations have defined levels of sedation.[17–20] The definitions of the American Academy of Pediatrics (AAP), the American Society of Anesthesiologists (ASA), JCAHO, and the American Academy of Pediatric Dentistry (AAPD) are the most frequently cited and agreed-upon position statements.[18,19,21-23] These organizations defined sedation and analgesia for procedures as a continuum, including minimal sedation (anxiolysis), moderate sedation, deep sedation, and general anesthesia (Fig. 48.1). All of these definitions are created with the appreciation that a child's depth of sedation may easily pass from one level to another and without easily identifiable signs of any change in condition.[24] The definitions that follow are taken from JCAHO (2010)[25] and are in agreement with the current AAP, AAPD, and ASA definitions[18,19,21]:

- *Minimal sedation (anxiolysis):* A drug-induced state during which patients respond to verbal commands. Although cognitive function and coordination may be impaired, cardiorespiratory functions are unaffected (Video 48.1).
- *Moderate sedation* (previously called "conscious sedation" or sedation/analgesia): A drug-induced depression of consciousness during which patients respond purposefully to verbal commands, either alone or accompanied by light tactile stimulation. No interventions are required to maintain a patent airway, and spontaneous ventilation is adequate. Cardiovascular function is usually maintained (Video 48.2).
- *Deep sedation:* A drug-induced depression of consciousness during which patients cannot be easily aroused but respond purposefully after repeated or painful stimuli. (***Note:* reflex withdrawal from a painful stimulus is not considered a purposeful response.**) The ability to independently maintain respiratory homeostasis may be impaired. Patients may require assistance in maintaining a patent airway and spontaneous ventilation may be inadequate. Cardiovascular function is usually maintained (Video 48.3).
- *General anesthesia:* A drug-induced loss of consciousness during which patients are not arousable, even to painful stimuli. The ability to independently maintain respiratory homeostasis is often impaired. Patients often require assistance in maintaining a patent airway, and positive-pressure ventilation may be required because spontaneous ventilation is depressed or neuromuscular function is compromised. In addition, cardiovascular function may be impaired (Video 48.4).

In clinical practice, procedures that require sedation in children may require deep sedation or general anesthesia for pain control (bone marrow biopsies) or movement control (MRI scans). They

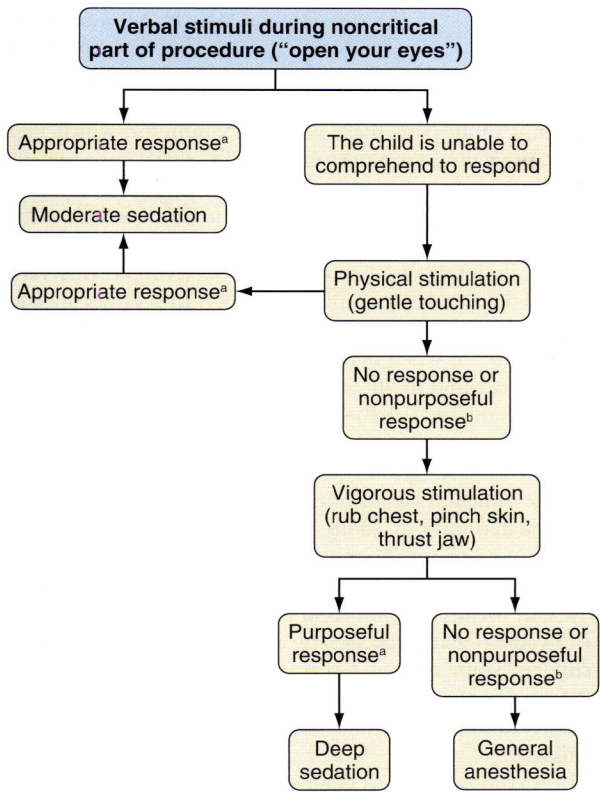

48

TABLE 48.1	Ramsay Scale
Level	**Characteristics**
1	Patient awake, anxious, agitated, or restless
2	Patient awake, cooperative, orientated, and tranquil
3	Patient drowsy, with response to commands
4	Patient asleep, brisk response to glabella tap or loud auditory stimulus
5	Patient asleep, sluggish response to stimulus
6	Patient has no response to firm nail-bed pressure or other noxious stimuli

TABLE 48.2	Modified Ramsay Sedation Scale
Score	**Characteristics**
1	Awake and alert, minimal or no cognitive impairment
2[a]	Awake but tranquil, purposeful responses to verbal commands at conversation level
3[a]	Appears asleep, purposeful responses to verbal commands at conversation level
4[b]	Appears asleep, purposeful responses to verbal commands but at louder than usual conversation level or requiring light glabellar tap
5[b]	Asleep, sluggish purposeful responses only to loud verbal commands or strong glabellar tap
6[c]	Asleep, sluggish purposeful responses only to painful stimuli
7[d]	Asleep, reflex withdrawal to painful stimuli only (no purposeful responses)
8[d]	Unresponsive to external stimuli, including pain

[a]Minimal sedation.
[b]Moderate sedation.
[c]Deep sedation.
[d]General anesthesia.

FIGURE 48.2 Sedated children must be continuously evaluated for depth of sedation and appropriateness of response. As diagrammed here, sedation is a continuum. Note that a purposeful response to voice or light touch is consistent with moderate sedation. A purposeful response to pain is consistent with deep sedation. A nonpurposeful response to pain is consistent with general anesthesia. However, such stimulation often defeats the purpose of the sedation, thus rendering these assessments less helpful unless patient movement is acceptable. None of the current sedation guidelines require such assessments. [a]*Purposeful:* opens eyes, talks back, pushes you out of the way. [b]*Nonpurposeful:* winces, shrugs shoulders, nonspecific withdrawal to pain.

are rarely performed in a child under "moderate sedation." Often moderate sedation is used inappropriately. It is not always easy to accurately describe the depth of sedation based on the child's responses to stimulation (Fig. 48.2). In addition, there are problems with classifying responses when they occur. A child who is under moderate sedation should respond to touch or firm rubbing by an appropriate response, such as saying "ouch," pushing your hand away, or pulling up the covers. *The lack of a purposeful response is a sign that the child has progressed to a deeper sedation level and should lead to an escalation of monitoring and personnel.*[26–29] These differences are seldom appreciated and often lead to inappropriate care. Not surprisingly, an audit in a large pediatric hospital reported that their target level of either moderate or deep sedation was achieved in only 50% to 75% of patients; an awake state was achieved in 12% to 28% of the children, and general anesthesia was reached in 35% of children.[24]

SEDATION SCORING SYSTEMS

There are several validated scoring systems available for assessing sedated patients and grading their level of sedation. The Ramsay scale was described by Ramsay and colleagues[30] in 1974 for the

purpose of monitoring sedation with alphaxalone-alphadolone (Table 48.1). It continues to be the most widely used scale for assessing and monitoring sedation in daily practice, as well as in clinical research. It spans the continuum of sedation but does not clearly separate purposeful from nonpurposeful responses. The Ramsey scale has been modified to more clearly coincide with the AAP and JCAHO guidelines (Table 48.2).[31] A score of 2 to 3 is anxiolysis, 4 to 5 is moderate sedation, 6 is deep sedation, and 7 to 8 is general anesthesia.

The Observer's Assessment of Alertness/Sedation (OAA/S) scale[32] is often cited as a scale for sedation. It is scored as follows: 1, no response to shaking; 2, responds to mild prodding; 3, responds to name called loudly; 4, lethargic response to name; and 5, readily responds to name. Its inability to clearly categorize deep levels of sedation and lack of a clear differentiation between purposeful and nonpurposeful responses limit its usefulness. A more useful clinical scale is the University of Michigan Sedation Scale (UMSS).[33] It is an assessment tool that has been validated against the OAA/S scale and other scales of sedation (Table 48.3). This scale has proven useful in children with significant learning impairment and delays.[34] It separates patients into the sedation categories in line with those defined by the AAP, ASA, and JCAHO.

These responsiveness-based assessment tools require intermittently stimulating the child during the procedure to categorize patients. Unfortunately, poking or prodding the child to determine the depth of sedation defeats the purpose of sedation in many situations (e.g., infants, developmentally delayed children, or procedures requiring immobility). The authors of the guidelines that reference levels of sedation do not require frequent testing of sedation depth. Rather the responsiveness-based definitions are meant to provide a road map for safety that bases the level on the behavior of the patient in response to the procedure itself, with the understanding that a nonresponding child requires an increased level of vigilance.[12] Unfortunately, infrequent testing leaves the sedation provider uncertain about the depth of sedation for significant periods of time during a test or intervention. Concerns regarding these types of assessment tools have led to the suggestion by some experts that there is a need to revise the sedation continuum and to use other monitoring parameters (such as physiologic status) to assess level of sedation.[35] Still others have suggested that the use of an observational scale that simply codifies the "state" of the child at any time during the sedation/procedure is more useful than stimulation (Table 48.4).[36]

For many years, the "holy grail" of sedation has been the non-invasive sedation monitor that would accurately detect and record the depth of sedation without stimulating the child or interfering with a procedure. Over the past 15 years, several monitors have been developed to assess the depth of sedation or anesthesia in a nonstimulating, continuous manner. Examples of the monitors include the BIS (bispectral index) monitor (Medtronic/Covidien, Minneapolis, MN); Narcotrend monitor (Narcotrend-Gruppe, Hannover, Germany); Danmeter AEP monitor/2 (Danmeter DK-5000, Odense C, Denmark); Patient State Monitor (PSA-4000, Pfizer/

Hospira, Lake Forest, IL), the Cerebral State Monitor (Danmeter DK-5000, Odense C, Denmark); and the Entropy module (GE Healthcare/Datex-Ohmeda, Chicago, IL). While each of these has shown some level of utility, the most broadly applied (and thoroughly studied) of these is the BIS monitor, which uses a proprietary method for processing the EEG signal and converting that reading into a number between 0 and 100, which has been correlated with the depth of sedation. The BIS was derived from empirically estimating processed EEG parameters that best predicted OAA/S scale levels in adult volunteers receiving a wide variety of anesthetics, analgesics, and sedatives.[37] BIS values in adults who are awake range from 95 to 100; when lightly to moderately sedated 70 to 95; when deeply sedated with a small probability of explicit recall 60 to 70; and general anesthesia, 40 to 60.[38–40]

Attempts to correlate BIS values with the depth of sedation in children have been met with varying success, particularly when attempting to distinguish moderate from deep sedation.[41–44] In part, these difficulties relate to two factors: (1) the algorithms have been validated only in adults, and (2) many of the anesthetics and drugs used to anesthetize and sedate children have not been adequately studied with the BIS monitor, even in adults. Other issues with the use of the BIS in children include the following:

1. BIS values are not age specific and are relatively inaccurate in children younger than 1 year of age.[45,46]
2. BIS readings may differ from one side of the head to the other.
3. BIS readings are diminished in developmentally delayed children.[47]
4. BIS is completely inaccurate with ketamine sedation because of ketamine-induced central excitation.[48,49]
5. BIS readings are inaccurate during sedation with dexmedetomidine.[50]

Finally, practical problems with the use of BIS-type monitoring include the following:

1. It is not feasible for many procedures, such as MRI scans.
2. BIS is not applicable for procedures involving the mouth and airway (endoscopy, dental, bronchoscopy), because the monitor creates artifacts or is in the way of the proceduralist.
3. Muscular activity around the head creates artifact. Overall, the lack of specificity for levels of sedation, low quality of BIS data, and the lack of information for different age groups or specific drugs preclude recommendation of the BIS for use in procedural sedation in children at this time.[39]

TABLE 48.3	University of Michigan Sedation Scale (UMSS)
Score	Characteristics
0	Awake and alert
1	Minimally sedated: tired/sleepy, appropriate response to verbal conversation and/or sound
2	Moderately sedated: somnolent/sleeping, easily aroused with light tactile stimulation or a simple verbal command
3	Deeply sedated: deep sleep, arousable only with significant physical stimulation
4	Unarousable

TABLE 48.4	The Dartmouth Operative Conditions Scale (DOCS)			
PATIENT STATE			**OBSERVED BEHAVIORS**	
Pain/Stress	(0)	(1)	(2)	
	Eyes closed or calm expression	Grimace or frown	Crying, sobbing, screaming	
Movement	(0)	(1)	(2)	(3)
	Still	Random little movement	Major purposeful movement	Thrashing, kicking, biting
Consciousness	(0)	(–1)	(–2)	
	Eyes open	Ptosis, uncoordinated, "drowsy"	Eyes closed	
Sedation Side Effects	(–1)	(–1)	(–1)	(–1)
	Spo₂ < 92%	Noise with respiration	Respiratory pauses >10 seconds	BP decrease of > 50% from baseline

Patients are scored in four state categories at any one time during sedation for a procedure. The sum of the scores in all four categories is used to determine the DOCS score for any discrete point during a sedation encounter. BP, blood pressure; SpO_2, oxygen saturation as measured by pulse oximetry.

Similar limitations exist for the other monitors of sedation/anesthesia depth. While they may be helpful in specific instances or clinical situations, their general use is not advised.

Sedation Depth Versus Sedation Risk

Sedation scales and sedation depth monitors attempt to quantify the depth of sedation but do not directly measure the "risk" of sedation. While the depth of sedation is defined by response to stimulation, the *important assessment of the child is not the response to stimulation, but the ability to protect and maintain the airway*.[51,52] In fact, each sedative drug or a particular dose of a drug may provide pain relief but may also obstruct the airway or depress ventilation. For example, propofol is a potent, effective sedative that confers no analgesia but has marked effects on the airway tone and respiratory drive.[53] Conversely, dexmedetomidine provides less intense sedation than propofol but modest pain relief with minimal depression of respiration and minimal compromise of airway morphology. In contrast, ketamine produces intense analgesia and decreases the responses to stimulation, but infrequently obstructs the airway or depresses respiratory effort even at very large doses (Table 48.5).[54]

There are also aspects of the *patient* that affect risks for airway-related adverse events as much as sedation depth. For instance, a child with obstructive sleep apnea (OSA) or obesity is much more likely to obstruct his or her airway during deep sedation than one who does not have this comorbidity.[55] A history of prematurity has been shown to increase the risks associated with sedation throughout childhood and adolescence.[56] Furthermore, other comorbidities such as congenital heart disease, airway anomalies, lower respiratory tract disease, and upper respiratory tract infection increase the risk of general anesthesia, and one would expect that they would also increase the risk of sedation, although they have not been studied specifically in this regard. Similarly, the *procedure itself* can increase the risk for a child. A bronchoscopy or upper gastrointestinal endoscopy carries much greater risks of airway-related events than a noninvasive diagnostic test.[57] The environment of the procedure can also increase risk. The MRI scanner (where the observer is remote from the airway during the scan and ferromagnetic objects are forbidden) is a significantly more difficult environment than one where the sedation provider can be situated at the airway and all monitors and rescue equipment are available (as per standard routine). In summary, when assessing the risk of sedation, one must consider the multidimensional aspects of sedation that include the planned level of sedation, existing comorbidities in the child, the procedure to be performed, and the environment in which the procedure will be performed.

The safety of sedation must also focus on appropriate discharge readiness and the subtle differences in recovery from sedation. Adverse events, including deaths, have occurred after premature discharge after procedural sedation.[52] These events were most often associated with sedating medications with a prolonged duration of effect such as chloral hydrate (Fig. 48.3).[51] With this in mind, a simple "maintenance of wakefulness" score (infants had to stay awake for at least 15 to 20 consecutive minutes in a quiet environment before discharge) ensured that more than 90% of children had returned to baseline levels of consciousness, compared with only 55% of children assessed as "street ready" according to usual hospital discharge criteria.[58]

Guidelines

With the definitions of depth of sedation in mind, multiple organizations have produced guidelines for the conduct of sedation in pediatric patients. The first sedation guideline was published in 1985 from the Committee on Hospital Practice and the Section on Anesthesiology of the AAP.[59] The guideline emphasized systems issues pioneered in anesthesiology, such as the need for informed consent, appropriate fasting before sedation, frequent measurement and charting of vital signs, the availability of age- and size-appropriate equipment, the use of continuous physiologic monitoring (pulse oximetry), the need for basic life support skills, as well as proper recovery and discharge procedures. A 2002 amendment of these guidelines[60] eliminated the use of the confusing term *conscious sedation* and replaced it with the term *moderate sedation*. The AAP's guideline was updated again in 2006.[18] It unified the definitions of sedation depth used

TABLE 48.5	Examples of Sedative Drugs That Have Varying Effects on Response to Pain and Airway Protection

Response to Pain Does Not Predict Airway Maintenance
All Drugs Are Different

	Response to Pain	Airway Maintenance
Fentanyl	↓↓	↓
Propofol	±	↓
Ketamine	↓	±
Dexmedetomidine	↓	+

↓↓, large decrease in response to pain or large effect on airway patency; ↓, some decrease in response to pain or some effect on airway patency; ±, minimal to no effect on response to pain or effect on airway patency; +, no effect on airway patency.

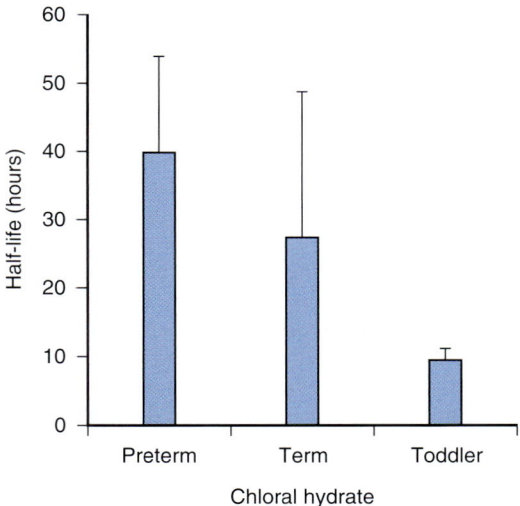

FIGURE 48.3 β-Elimination half-life of the active metabolite of chloral hydrate, trichloroethanol, in preterm infants, term infants, and toddlers. Note the extremely prolonged half-lives and the large standard deviations in all age groups. Although often thought of as a short-acting sedative, chloral hydrate can have profoundly long sedative effects, with a real possibility of resedation after a procedure when the child is left undisturbed. It is for this reason that we recommend a longer period of observation in a step-down area before discharge.

by the ASA and the JCAHO and emphasized further refinements of a systematic approach to sedation that included the following:

- No administration of sedative medications without the safety net of medical supervision (i.e., no sedative medications given at home).
- Careful presedation evaluation to include review of pertinent medical and surgical conditions.
- Careful history for ingestion of nutraceuticals and other medications that may alter drug metabolism and prolong sedation.
- Appropriate fasting guidelines for elective and urgent procedures. There should be a balance between the depth of sedation and the risk for those who are unable to fast because of the urgent nature of the procedure.
- Focused airway examination with particular attention to anatomic airway abnormalities and enlarged tonsils.
- Understanding the pharmacokinetic and pharmacodynamic effects of sedation medications and drug interactions.
- Appropriate training and skills in airway management for sedation providers to allow for rescue. Deep sedation requires training in Pediatric Advanced Life Support (PALS).
- Immediate availability of size- and age-appropriate airway, monitoring, and resuscitation equipment.
- Appropriate emergency medications and reversal agents available for sedation in all cases.
- Sufficient personnel to carry out the procedure *and* monitor the child.
- Appropriate physiologic monitoring during and after the procedure; use of capnography is encouraged.
- A "time-out" should be performed before sedation.
- Recovery personnel, monitoring, and discharge criteria with return to baseline condition before discharge.
- Continuous quality improvement to track common markers of potential safety issues, such as desaturation events, airway obstructions, laryngospasm, unplanned hospital admission, unsatisfactory sedation, and medication errors.
- Use of simulators to practice management of rare adverse events.
- Assume that all children younger than 6 years of age will be deeply sedated for painful procedures or those that are not painful but prolonged.

The most recent version of the AAP guidelines was published in 2016,[61] in which the guidelines for sedation used by pediatric medical and dental practitioners were unified with the same language, the same definitions, and the same goals. The new version added clarifications regarding respiratory monitoring modalities, particularly that continuous capnometry is recommended for moderate sedation and required for deep sedation, provided updated information from the medical and dental literature, and suggested methods for further improvement in safety (incorporating checklists, human simulation training) and documentation. Other important changes included that the responsible practitioner for moderate sedation must have the skills to rescue a child with apnea, laryngospasm, airway obstruction, and perform successful bag-mask ventilation. The practitioner who practices deep sedation must have these same skills and be able to perform tracheal intubation and cardiopulmonary resuscitation. Additionally, the skilled observer for either moderate or deep sedation must be trained in PALS **and be capable to assist with any emergency**. Three decision trees that guide the management of airway obstruction, laryngospasm, and apnea were added.

This recent guideline further emphasized the following:

- *Patient Evaluation.* Clinicians should be familiar with the sedation-related aspects of the patient's medical history. These include (1) abnormalities of major organ systems; (2) previous adverse effects with sedation and general anesthesia; (3) drug allergies, current medications, and drug interactions; (4) time and nature of oral intake; and (5) history of tobacco, alcohol, or substance abuse. A focused physical examination, including vital signs, auscultation of the heart and lungs, and evaluation of the airway, is recommended.
- *Preprocedural Preparation.* Patients should be informed of and agree to sedation, including its risks, benefits, limitations, and alternatives. Sufficient time should elapse before a procedure to allow gastric emptying for elective procedures in healthy children as per the ASA guidelines: minimum fasting intervals of 2 hours after clear liquids, 4 hours after breast milk, 6 hours after infant formula, nonhuman milk, and a light meal (dry toast, tea without milk), and 8 hours after fatty food. If urgent, emergent, or other situations impair gastric emptying, the potential for pulmonary aspiration of gastric contents must be considered when determining the target level of sedation, delay of the procedure/investigation, or the need to secure the airway (e.g., tracheal intubation).
- *Monitoring Level of Consciousness.* Monitoring of verbal commands should be routine during moderate sedation, with the exception of young children and developmentally impaired, uncooperative patients, or when the response would be detrimental. During deep sedation the response to a more profound stimulus should be sought to ensure that the patient has not drifted into general anesthesia.
- *Physiologic Monitoring.* All patients undergoing sedation/analgesia should be monitored by pulse oximetry with appropriate alarms. In addition, respiration should be continuously monitored by observation or auscultation. End-tidal carbon dioxide ($ETCO_2$) is encouraged for moderately sedated children and now required per AAP guideline for all patients receiving deep sedation and for those whose ventilation could not be directly observed during moderate sedation. It should be noted, however, that the ASA standards for basic monitoring were amended in 2012 to include $ETCO_2$ monitoring of those sedated at moderate and deeper levels of sedation.[61,62] In addition, the guidelines recommended that blood pressure should be determined before sedation/analgesia is initiated where possible and at regular intervals during the procedure, unless such monitoring interferes with the procedure (e.g., pediatric MRI, in which stimulation from the blood pressure cuff could arouse an appropriately sedated child). Electrocardiographic (ECG) monitoring should also be used in all children during deep sedation, and during moderate sedation, in those with significant cardiovascular disease, or those who are undergoing procedures in which dysrhythmias are anticipated.
- *Recording of Monitored Parameters.* For both moderate and deep sedation, the child's level of consciousness, respiratory status, and hemodynamic variables should be assessed and recorded at a frequency commensurate with the type and amount of medication administered, the duration of the procedure, and the medical condition of the child. At a minimum, this should be (1) before the beginning of the procedure; (2) after administration of sedative/analgesic agents; (3) at regular intervals during the procedure; (4) during initial recovery; and (5) immediately before discharge. If recording is performed automatically, device alarms should be set to alert the care team to critical changes in patient status.

- *Availability of an Appropriately Trained and Skilled Individual Responsible for Patient Monitoring.* A designated individual, other than the practitioner performing the procedure, should be present to monitor the child throughout procedures performed with sedation/analgesia. During deep sedation, this individual should have no other responsibilities. However, during moderate sedation, this individual may assist with minor, interruptible tasks once the patient's level of sedation/analgesia and vital signs have stabilized, provided that adequate monitoring for the child's level of sedation is maintained.
- *Training of Personnel.* Individuals responsible for children who receive sedation/analgesia should understand the pharmacology of the medications that are administered, as well as the role of pharmacologic antagonists for opioids and benzodiazepines. Individuals who monitor children who receive sedation/analgesia should be able to recognize the associated complications. At least one individual capable of establishing a patent airway and positive-pressure ventilation, as well as a means for summoning additional assistance, should be present whenever sedation/analgesia is administered.
- *Availability of Emergency Equipment.* Pharmacologic antagonists, as well as appropriately sized equipment for establishing a patent airway and providing positive-pressure ventilation with supplemental oxygen, should be present whenever sedation/analgesia is administered. Suction, advanced airway equipment, and resuscitation medications should be immediately available and in good working order. A functional defibrillator should be immediately available whenever deep sedation is administered and when moderate sedation is administered to those with mild or severe cardiovascular disease.
- *Use of Supplemental Oxygen.* Equipment to administer supplemental oxygen should be present when sedation/analgesia is administered. Supplemental oxygen should be considered for moderate sedation and should be administered for deep sedation unless specifically contraindicated for a particular child or procedure. If hypoxemia is anticipated or develops during sedation/analgesia, supplemental oxygen should be administered.
- *Combinations of Sedative/Analgesic Agents.* Combinations of sedative and analgesic agents may be administered as indicated for the procedure being performed and the condition of the child. Ideally, each component should be administered individually to achieve the desired effect (e.g., additional analgesic medication to relieve pain; additional sedative medication to decrease awareness or anxiety). The propensity for combinations of sedative and analgesic agents to cause respiratory depression and airway obstruction emphasizes the need to appropriately reduce the dose of each component, as well as the need to continually monitor respiratory function (Fig. 48.4).
- *Recovery Care.* After sedation for diagnostic and therapeutic procedures, the children should be observed in an appropriately staffed and equipped area until they are near their baseline level of consciousness and are no longer at increased risk for cardiorespiratory depression. Oxygenation should be monitored periodically until they are no longer at risk for hypoxemia. Ventilation and circulation should be monitored at regular intervals until the children are suitable for discharge. Discharge criteria should be designed to minimize the risk of central nervous system (CNS) or cardiorespiratory depression after discharge from observation by trained personnel.
- *Consultation and Availability of an Anesthesiologist.* Whenever possible, appropriate medical specialists should be consulted

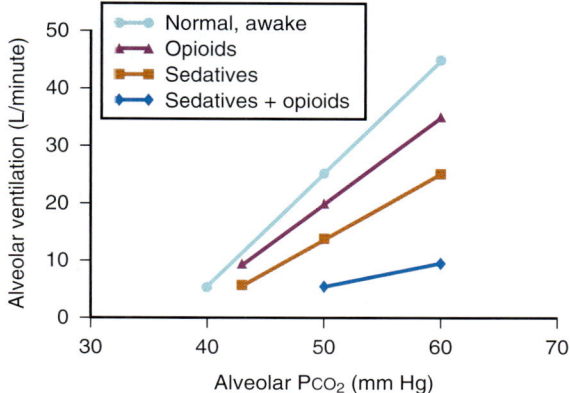

FIGURE 48.4 Relationship between ventilation and carbon dioxide is represented by a family of curves. Each curve has two parameters: an x-intercept and a slope. Sedatives and opioids increase the intercept and decrease the slope. The combination of sedatives and opioids produce the most profound effect. (From Yaster M, Nichols DG, Deshpande JK, Wetzel RC. Midazolam-fentanyl intravenous sedation in children: case report of respiratory arrest. *Pediatrics* 1990;85(3):463–467.)

before sedating children with significant comorbidities. The choice of specialists depends on the nature of the underlying condition and the urgency of the situation. For severely compromised or medically unstable children (e.g., anticipated difficult airway, severe obstructive pulmonary disease, or congestive heart failure), practitioners who are not trained in the administration of general anesthesia should consult an anesthesiologist (Table 48.6).

The ASA also has numerous statements and guidelines for sedation by physicians other than anesthesiologists. The "Practice Guidelines for Sedation and Analgesia by Non-Anesthesiologists" was last updated in 2002 and, in many respects, is in concert with the AAP guidelines.[63] The ASA currently has 10 different statements discussing sedation guidelines available through their website (http://www.asahq.org). Some statements specifically address questions related to the provision of moderate and deep sedation by nonanesthesiologists as well as the use of medications such as propofol by nonanesthesiologist sedationists. Most pertinent of these is the 2010 document "Statement on Granting Privileges for Deep Sedation to Non-Anesthesiologist Sedation Practitioners."[64] The guidelines include the following:

1. Formal training in administration of deep sedation during residency training (within 2 years) or an Accreditation Council for Graduate Medical Education accredited training program
2. Experience and competency in managing sedated patients
3. Clinical experience with more than 35 patients
4. Knowledge of ASA guidelines
5. Advanced cardiac life support training
6. Quality assurance tracking

Separate privileging is required for the care of children. The exact nature of these requirements are not specified, but pediatric sedation training over and above baseline competencies is advised.

Other organizations, notably the American College of Emergency Physicians (ACEP), have published their own sedation guidelines and clinical practice advisories for sedation.[65–69] These guidelines are distinguishable from the AAP and ASA guidelines in several respects, including the definition of the continuum of sedation. The ACEP guideline prefers the term "procedural

TABLE 48.6	Guidelines for the Consultation of an Anesthesiologist

1. **Medical Problems**
   - ASA physical status III or IV
   - Pulmonary: airway obstruction (tonsils/adenoids)—loud snoring, obstructive sleep apnea. Poorly controlled asthma, congenital or acquired anomalies of the airway or face (Trisomy 21, Pierre Robin syndrome, Treacher Collins syndrome, Crouzon disease, tracheomalacia)
   - Morbid obesity (≥2 times ideal body weight, BMI >30 kg/m²)
   - Cardiovascular: cyanosis, repaired or unrepaired congenital heart disease with significant symptoms of cyanosis or congestive heart failure
   - Prematurity: less than 60 weeks postconception age at time of sedation
   - Residual pulmonary, cardiovascular, gastrointestinal, neurologic problems
   - Neurologic: developmental disabilities, poorly controlled seizures, central apnea
   - Gastrointestinal: uncontrolled gastroesophageal reflux
   - Severe liver or renal disease

2. **Procedures requiring deep sedation in patients with a full stomach**
   - Emergency procedures

3. **Management problems**
   - Severe developmental delay
   - Patients who are difficult to control
   - Severe attention-deficit disorder (paradoxically, the child may develop increased agitation during or after the procedure)

4. **History of failed sedation**
   - Oversedation (loss of airway reflexes)
   - Inability to adequately sedate
   - Hyperactive (paradoxical) response to sedatives

ASA, American Society of Anesthesiologists; *BMI,* body mass index.

sedation." It is defined *"as a technique of administering sedatives, analgesics, dissociative agents, alone or in combination to induce a state that allows the child to tolerate unpleasant procedures while maintaining cardiopulmonary function."* It is intended to result in a depressed level of consciousness but one that allows the child to *"independently and continuously"* control his or her own airway. This guideline was updated in 2014 to address several issues with the following recommendations[70]:

1. Do not delay procedural sedation in adults or children in the emergency department based on fasting time. Preprocedural fasting for any duration has not reduced the risk of emesis or aspiration when administering procedural sedation and analgesia.

2. Capnography may be used as an adjunct to pulse oximetry and as a clinical tool to detect hypoventilation and apnea earlier than pulse oximetry and/or clinical assessment alone in children undergoing procedural sedation and analgesia in the ED.

3. During procedural sedation and analgesia, a nurse or other qualified individual should be present to continually observe and monitor the patient, in addition to the provider performing the procedure. Physicians who are working or consulting in the emergency department should coordinate procedures requiring procedural sedation and analgesia with the emergency department staff.

4. Ketamine and etomidate can be safely administered individually to children and propofol can be administered to both children and adults for procedural sedation and analgesia in the emergency department. A combination of propofol and ketamine can be safely administered to children and adults for procedural sedation and analgesia.

The ACEP suggests a very different clinical practice advisory for the fasting interval before sedation based on analysis of reports from the sedation literature and expert consensus. The suggested time frames for fasting start with a 3-hour baseline and vary based on the urgency of the procedure and the planned depth of sedation. In addition, the practitioner can be directing the sedation and performing the procedure, and there is vague language regarding the nurse observer. **The result is a strategy that differs significantly from the standard recommendations from the AAP and ASA.**[71]

It is mandatory that sedation policies used in hospitals conform to JCAHO standards that have been derived from the Department of Health and Human Services (DHHS) Centers for Medicare & Medicaid Services (CMS). These requirements are consistent with the AAP/ASA guidelines but are more explicit in terms of the oversight of sedation services. The standards require documentation (e.g., medical history, physical status, and record-keeping during the procedure and the recovery from the procedure), a fasting protocol, and informed consent procedures that are mandatory for all those undergoing sedation, regardless of the nature, duration, patient's history, and location of the procedure. Similarly, the sedation personnel, monitoring equipment, and recovery facilities must meet uniform standards within an institution. Hospitals risk losing federal funding if they fail to comply. In the most recent CMS regulations published in 2011,[16] the leadership and responsibilities for the delivery of deep sedation are assigned to a "qualified doctor of medicine or osteopathy who leads the department of anesthesia services." This would logically fall under the purview of the Chair of the Department of Anesthesiology in most cases; however, there are many small or unique hospitals where such a position does not exist. In such cases, the hospital administration must designate a physician who will fill this role and meet these qualifications (Fig. 48.5).

Under the CMS directives, deep sedation is placed under anesthesia services and *subject to the anesthesia administration requirements at 42 CFR 482.52(a):* whereas *minimal and moderate sedation* are placed under analgesia/sedation and therefore not subject to anesthesia administrative requirements. To ensure continuity and equanimity of sedation care, CMS states that there should be one anesthesia service that has responsibility for oversight of all anesthesia services. Anesthesia must be administered by a (1) qualified anesthesiologist; (2) certified registered nurse anesthetist (CRNA) or anesthesiologist assistant (AA) with appropriate supervision; (3) doctor of medicine or osteopathy (other than an anesthesiologist); and (4) dentist, oral surgeon, or podiatrist who is qualified to administer anesthesia under state regulations. Credentialing and privileging must be done per hospital policy and is the responsibility of the hospital's director of anesthesia services. The appropriateness and quality of anesthesia, including sedation, must be reviewed and approved by the director of anesthesia services. The standards for sedation require that each hospital develop specific appropriate protocols for patients receiving sedation, but these guidelines offer little detail on the exact content of the protocols (those are left to the individual organizations). These protocols must include delineation of the following:

1. Qualified individuals in sufficient numbers to perform and monitor patients during and after the procedure. A registered nurse must supervise perioperative nursing care.

2. Competency-based education, training, and experience in evaluating patients. These must include the following:
   a. Evaluating patients before the sedation.

48

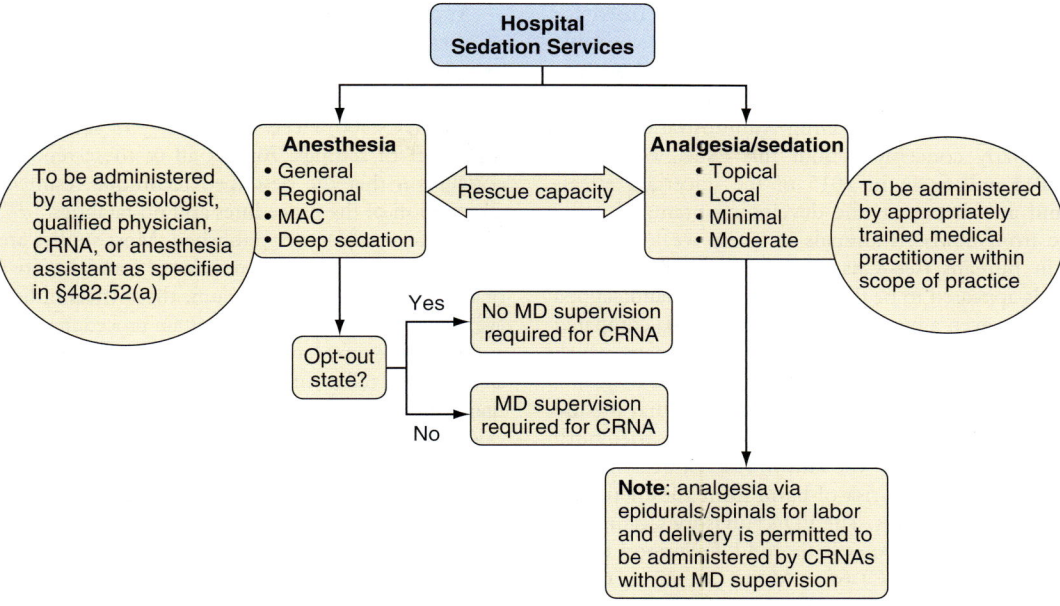

FIGURE 48.5 Centers for Medicare & Medicaid Services organizational chart showing deep sedation under the category of "Anesthesia" and supervised by "Hospital Sedation Services." *CRNA,* certified registered nurse anesthetist; *MAC,* monitored anesthesia care; *MD,* physician.

b. Performing moderate and deep sedation, including rescuing patients who slip into a deeper than desired level of sedation. These include the following:

  i. Moderate sedation—personnel are qualified to rescue patients from deep sedation and are competent to manage a compromised airway and to provide adequate oxygenation and ventilation.

  ii. Deep sedation—personnel are qualified to rescue patients from general anesthesia and are competent to manage an unstable cardiovascular system, as well as a compromised airway and inadequate oxygenation and ventilation.

3. Appropriate equipment for care and resuscitation.

4. The following must occur before moderate or deep sedation:

  a. Appropriate needs of the patient are assessed.

  b. Preprocedural education is provided to the patient according to a plan of care.

  c. A time-out is conducted immediately before starting, as described in universal protocol.

  d. A licensed independent practitioner plans or concurs with the planned procedure.

5. Appropriate monitoring of vital signs during and after the procedure, including, but not limited to, heart rate and oxygenation using pulse oximetry, respiratory frequency and adequacy of pulmonary ventilation, monitoring of blood pressure at regular levels, and cardiac monitoring (by ECG or use of a continuous cardiac monitoring device) in patients with significant cardiovascular disease or when dysrhythmias are anticipated or detected.

6. Documentation of care before, during, and after the procedure.

7. Monitoring of outcomes. In particular, analysis of data is performed on adverse events or patterns of adverse events during moderate or deep sedation.

The guidelines for sedation are actually quite similar among the various organizations and government entities that are responsible for these standards. It is critical that anesthesiologists who oversee and coordinate this care be familiar with the various guidelines and help their colleagues meet or exceed them.

Goals of Sedation

The goals of pediatric sedation are similar to the goals of operative anesthesia[18,29]:

- Guard the child's safety and welfare. This includes ensuring appropriate airway maintenance and cardiovascular stability.
- Minimize physical discomfort and pain.
- Control anxiety and minimize psychological trauma.
- Control movement to allow the safe and efficient completion of the procedure.
- Return the child to a state in which he or she is safe for discharge from medical supervision, as determined by recognized criteria.

It is notable that most of the literature describing various strategies for pediatric sedation focuses on the completion of the procedure rather than the entire spectrum of the goals just outlined. Anesthesia professionals are in a unique position to advocate for a more complete appreciation of the overall goals of sedation that should meet the high standards that have been set in the OR environment. To this end, a useful analysis of issues relating to overall "quality" of sedation is provided by a report from the Society for Pediatric Sedation in which sedation quality is placed in the context defined by the Institute of Medicine[72]: effectiveness, efficiency, family centeredness, timeliness, and equity (in addition to safety) when considering "quality" in the context of sedation.

The Concept of "Safety"

"Safety" in pediatric sedation is multidimensional. Although the adverse events related to the airway hold the greatest risk to cause immediate harm to the child, several additional risks should be considered.

A growing area of concern is the effect of drugs (used for sedation or anesthesia) on the developing brain and the possible association with neuroapoptosis and/or subsequent learning/behavioral deficiencies[73-79] (this topic is covered in detail in Chapter 25). The U.S. Food and Drug Administration (FDA) has been particularly concerned about this issue, warning in editorials in 2011 and again in 2015 of the uncertain effects of sedatives and anesthetics on the developing brain,[80,81] using solid evidence from newborn animals but very weak evidence from studies in humans (see Chapter 25). At face value, the newborn animals appeared to be disproportionately handicapped neurocognitively by even a brief exposure to anesthesia compared with the very mild and inconsistent evidence from humans, which is curious. Specific advisories on the use of anesthesia in young children have been vague and generally recommend that the use of anesthesia for procedures in the first three years after birth should be based on a balance of the known risks of delaying the procedure versus the uncertain risk of harm from anesthetics on the developing brain in humans. The FDA Advisory Committee Background Document to the Anesthetic and Life Support Drugs Advisory Committee (ALSDAC) from March 10, 2011, issued a caveat that exposure to anesthesia drugs should be precluded for purely elective procedures in children younger than 3 years of age.[82]

Practitioners who deliver sedation must balance the risks of inadequate versus excessive sedation. Adverse events related to *inadequate* sedation are more difficult to track than the immediate risk of oversedation; however, this issue should not be discounted—several studies have associated untreated procedural pain with long-term adverse behaviors in animals and children. Specifically, painful experiences in childhood have been linked to excessive pain responses and behaviors later in life.[83-85] In addition, a stressful anesthesia induction has been associated with greater maladaptive behaviors for up to 2 weeks after the experience.[86] The incidence of these behaviors decreases with the use of appropriate preoperative sedation. Similar sequelae have been reported after repeated invasive procedures in pediatric intensive care units (ICUs).[87] Taken together, these data suggest that "less sedation" is not a solution to the various potential adverse effects related to the delivery of sedation in children.

The risks and markers associated with adverse *over*sedation events have been the subject of multiple studies. In 2000, a retrospective review of 95 cases of sedation-related deaths and critical incidents derived from the FDA adverse drug event reporting system, the U.S. Pharmacopeia, and a survey of pediatric specialists[51] revealed that the overwhelming majority of critical events were preventable and caused by operator error or lack of robust rescue systems rather than by specific medications. Drug interactions were the most common causative factor, followed by drug overdose, inadequate monitoring, inadequate cardiopulmonary resuscitation skills, inadequate evaluation before sedation, and premature discharge from medical supervision. The report emphasizes that most sedation complications are related to adverse respiratory events (80%); a majority progressed to cardiac arrest, indicating a lack of rescue skills on the part of the practitioners. A disproportionately large number of severe complications and deaths occurred when sedation was performed in offices outside hospitals (29/60 deaths or neurologic injury occurred during dental procedures), pointing to inadequate rescue planning and training. There was no relationship with class of drug or route of administration, although there was a positive correlation with complications when three or more sedating medications (pointing to drug interactions) were administered.[52]

Another method for analyzing sedation safety is the review of cases performed in a single institution using a particular drug or technique. The literature on pediatric sedation includes a huge number of these studies reporting relatively small numbers of patients (N <200) receiving a variety of sedative medications in a number of settings. Almost all of these reports end with the conclusion that the described technique resulted in successful completion of the procedures and no fatalities.[88-100] Negative trial results are almost never published. Most studies are retrospective and describe different frequencies of transient airway obstruction or oxygen desaturation. In sum, these trials indicate that young age, increased ASA status, and certain procedures such as endoscopy and bronchoscopy have greater rates of adverse events. The sample size of some older studies limits their external validity to evaluate major adverse events or critical incidents, although more recent evidence is more heartening.[101] Accordingly, single-institution trials offer information on sedation techniques but infrequently provide as robust evidence on risk and outcomes as multi-centered, comprehensive studies and databases.[99,102-104]

Simulation may be used to test the abilities of practitioners to diagnose and treat low-frequency adverse effects that occur during pediatric sedation and the ability of systems to rescue patients.[105,106] In one of these studies, a simulated scenario of laryngospasm was programmed so that the physiologic variables either degraded with time after the event if inappropriate interventions were undertaken or improved with time if an effective intervention was performed. The event was videotaped in three different sedation locations. Hypoxia and hypotension lasted less than 90 seconds in the postanesthesia care unit but more than 360 seconds in the emergency department and radiology (CT scanner) settings.[107] Such studies demonstrate that analysis of simulated low-frequency adverse events can identify areas and practitioners within the hospital that need improvement in their rescue systems to improve patient safety.

The advent of the electronic medical record and improved data sharing has allowed the capture of data from the large numbers of pediatric sedation encounters that can lead to an enhanced understanding of the nature and frequency of adverse sedation events. The PRSC consists of a group of more than 30 institutions in North America that shares prospective data on pediatric sedation.[14] Analysis of the first 30,000 records identified demographics, procedures, sedation techniques, outcomes, and adverse events as follows:

1. There were no deaths and only one cardiac arrest was reported.
2. Unanticipated admission occurred infrequently, 1 per 1500 sedations.
3. Vomiting occurred in 1 per 200 sedations, including one aspiration.
4. Stridor, laryngospasm, wheezing, and apnea occurred in 1 per 400 procedures.
5. Airway or ventilatory manipulations were required in 1 per 100 sedations.[107]

Risk factors for adverse events included age younger than 3 months, ASA physical status 3 or greater, and multiple drug combinations for sedation. The PRSC has also reviewed the incidence of adverse events in 49,386 propofol sedation and/or anesthesia encounters for procedures outside of the OR.[15] Propofol was delivered by multiple providers (anesthesiologists, intensivists, emergency medicine physicians, pediatricians, and radiologists). No deaths were recorded. CPR was required in two children and aspiration occurred in four children. The most prominent type of adverse event was related to the airway and occurred in 1 of 65 sedations; 1 in 70 children required airway rescue. Desaturation

(< 90% for more than 30 seconds) occurred 154 times per 10,000 sedations/anesthetics; central apnea or obstruction occurred 575 times per 10,000 sedations, and unexpected admissions occurred 7 times per 10,000 sedations. When all possible adverse events were considered, anesthesiologists reported fewer events than other medical specialists, with an odds ratio of 1.38 (95% confidence interval [CI] 1.21-1.57, P < 0.001).[15] No difference among providers was noted when outcome analysis was limited to major complications. The authors concluded that propofol sedation and/or anesthesia when given in carefully constructed sedation services (i.e., following the AAP sedation guideline with well-trained providers) can result in effective sedation with an acceptable (low) incidence of severe adverse events. They emphasize that the safety of this practice is contingent on the ability to quickly and safely rescue patients from less serious events.

TRAINING AND SYSTEM ISSUES FOR PEDIATRIC PROCEDURAL SEDATION

Education is vital to maintain safety. An institution-wide ongoing educational program on sedation, emphasizing physician (and dentist) responsibility, nursing responsibility, guidelines, and the pharmacology of drugs, should be readily available to all individuals who care for sedated children. Teaching modules, videos, handouts, simulations, and hands-on supervision have been used to supplement such programs.[101] Most institutions have adopted a computerized teaching module that includes a review of hospital policy, equipment, personnel, pharmacology of drugs used, and rescue from deeper levels of sedation. A quiz must be successfully completed at the end of the computerized teaching module. The module is part of the orientation and hospital privileging procedure for each physician and nurse and must be successfully completed before they can administer sedation; the module must be reviewed and successfully completed every 2 years. Staff privileging requirements should include training in PALS or equivalent because this is now a requirement of the 2016 AAP sedation guideline. Further information on the nature of training required for sedation credentialing is sparse. One survey of institutions that provide sedation services for children reported that 51% provided a specific training packet for sedation, whereas 59% depended on sedation training during fellowship, and 49% documented a specific number of procedural sedation encounters.[108]

Specialty organizations are also becoming involved in training of sedation providers. The Society for Pediatric Sedation provides an extensive "primer" on pediatric sedation on its website (http://www.pedsedation.org). This organization also provides a credentialing course for pediatric sedation that uses a test of knowledge based on its written materials (see previous discussion) and the completion of a full-day "Sedation Provider Course," which includes lectures, interactive sessions, and human patient simulation sessions (developed from data relating to pediatric sedation adverse events) to teach and test core competencies. Hands-on simulation-based courses such as this have been shown to improve provider confidence and perceived ability to care for pediatric procedural sedation patients.[109]

Education should also emphasize the limits of sedation and appropriate referral to an anesthesiologist. Of particular concern is upper airway obstruction that would likely become worse with the administration of sedatives (see Table 48.6).[51] Tonsil and adenoid hypertrophy is common in children aged 2 to 12 years and is associated with loud snoring or OSA. OSA occurs in 1% to 3% of all children, in up to 12% of adolescents, is 3-fold more frequent in African American children, and 5-fold more frequent in obese children.[110] Parents often report that their child snores loudly and

then "stops breathing." These children are at increased risk for airway obstruction and should be referred to an airway specialist (anesthesiologist, pediatric intensivist, pediatric emergency medicine specialist) if sedation is required for their procedures. They may also require postsedation overnight admission and monitoring (see also Chapters 4 and 33).[63,111-113] Children with developmental disabilities should raise concern for sedation because they are at increased risk for airway obstruction during sedation and anesthesia.[114] Problems for which consultation with an anesthesiologist or other expert is suggested are listed in Table 48.6.

The importance of nursing in the provision of safe and effective sedation for children cannot be overemphasized. Nurses are the "front line" in sedation safety and frequently are the part of the sedation team that identifies variation in policy compliance. Their support and education is mandatory. In addition, state nursing restrictions on nurses administering certain drugs (such as propofol and ketamine) must be taken into consideration.

Quality improvement is a critical piece of ensuring optimal training and sedation system functioning. Compliance can be monitored by the medical and dental staff office, the department of nursing, as well as a committee charged with the responsibility of continuing quality improvement. Nursing and medical staff offices should monitor compliance with educational certification for appropriate credentialing. It is the responsibility of the department chairperson and nursing supervisors to ensure individual staff compliance. Finally, variance reports should be generated when sedation policy is not followed or when a critical incident occurs. The appropriate institutional committee reviews each incident and informs the sedation committee. The committee should seek system problems and fixes for organizational issues that contribute to care failure. (e.g., inadequate presedation assessment, inadequate monitoring leading to delay in problem recognition, or inadequate recovery procedures). Tracking common problems, such as the need for bag-mask ventilation, apnea, unplanned hospital admissions, or unsatisfactory sedation, can provide direction for developing changes in policy that will prevent more severe but much less frequent events from occurring (Fig. 48.6). This type of critical incident analysis allows recommendations to be made for future adverse event prevention.[115-117]

DOCUMENTATION

A single documentation interface that is used wherever sedation is delivered within an institution will allow for uniformity of care and compliance with sedation policy. The sedation interface should be organized such that the practitioners have a practical guide to the sedation policy. The very act of following and completing the sedation record will ensure compliance with hospital policy (E-Fig. 48.1). The near-universal application of electronic medical records now allows demographic, allergy, and comorbidity data to be gathered from other areas of the electronic medical record and automatically adds vital signs before and during the intervention (Video 48.5). Appropriate electronic record documentation for sedation includes various dropdown menus, which allow the practitioner to access rating scale information and automatically enter vital signs (Video 48.5).

To be in line with standard guidelines on sedation, documentation surrounding sedation should include all of the following:

- *Presedation responsibilities.* During this time, the responsibilities of the registered nurse include evaluation of the child to include learning assessment, NPO (nothing by mouth) status, allergies, current medications, and review of medical problems. The licensed independent practitioner verifies this information with

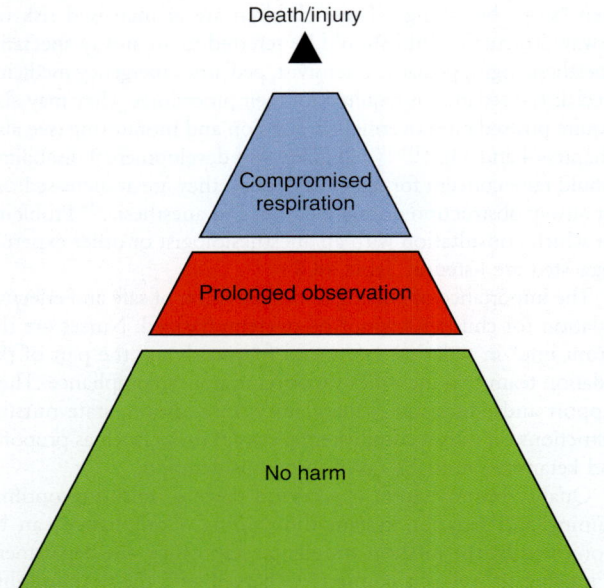

Death/injury

Compromised respiration

Prolonged observation

No harm

FIGURE 48.6 The sedation accident pyramid. The majority of adverse sedation events result in no harm. A smaller number result in no harm but require prolonged observation. An even smaller number result in the need for some intervention, usually related to respiration (repositioning the head, a jaw thrust, bag or mask respirations, or intubation). A very small number result in injury or death because the sentinel event was missed or inadequately treated. The latter cases are the types that occasionally are reported in newspapers, but in general go unreported. The reported cases likely represent just the tip of the pyramid in terms of events that could have indicated a developing problem.

emphasis on assessing the airway. A sedation plan is identified and informed consent is obtained. The licensed independent practitioner assigns an ASA physical status and reassesses the child immediately before the procedure.

- *Presedation pause.* A time out should be performed immediately before sedation medications are given. The time out includes a process of verbal confirmation of the patient and procedure identification, verification of informed consent, as well as ASA physical status and confirmation of the procedure and site of the procedure. No medications are administered without completion of the time out. One advantage of the electronic form is that it forces the licensed independent practitioner to verify time out before it allows further access to the rest of the sedation flow sheet.
- *During sedation.* The time-based flow sheet identifies the type of stimulation needed to elicit a response, as well as which monitors should be used and how frequently the vital signs should be recorded for both moderate and deep sedation. Table 48.7 summarizes monitoring, documentation, personnel, and equipment during sedation.
- *Postsedation.* The criteria for discharge from the sedation area, pain score, and disposition of the child, as well as discharge teaching, are specified. This includes documentation and signature by the licensed independent practitioner and nurse. Space is given for additional documentation and medications given.

Most importantly, both the paper and electronic form have critical parts of the sedation policy for immediate bedside review. This includes pain assessment scales, NPO guideline variations,

reassessment by the licensed independent practitioner before sedation, and the opioid medication order verification. A table that defines the levels of sedation, required monitors, and frequency of monitoring is also present. This, in addition to the online availability of the hospital policy, ensures that sedation practitioners have all information available to be in compliance to safely and successfully sedate children.

Sedation services, however they are configured, may find it helpful to create information sheets on presedation assessment, telephone interviews, and postsedation follow-up. An example of a radiology-nursing database that consists of presedation telephone information, presedation instructions, NPO guidelines, health history, and postexamination telephone call information is shown in E-Figs. 48.2 and 48.3. Samples of presedation and postsedation instruction sheets for pediatric dentistry are shown in E-Figs. 48.4 and 48.5, respectively. These forms are available in Spanish and are explained via interpreters if necessary.

Specific Sedation Techniques

A *sedation treatment plan* that addresses the requirements for analgesics, anxiolytics, or both is necessary for each child, according to the procedure being performed and the anxiety of the child and family. Psychological techniques to allay anxiety and distract children's attention from the procedural environment (computer [e.g., iPad] games/movies, cuddling, parental support, child-life specialists, warm blankets, a gentle reassuring voice, and hypnosis) are extraordinarily useful adjuncts to the sedation plan.[6–10] At times, distraction alone can suffice to produce conditions amenable to accomplishing a simple nonpainful procedure.

Many of the drugs used for sedation and analgesia in children are not approved by the FDA for use in children under certain ages (e.g., fentanyl <2 years; morphine <12 years, bupivacaine <12 years, propofol <2 months, and dexmedetomidine <18 years of age). Although midazolam is approved even in preterm infants, the reversal agent flumazenil is *not* approved in children younger than 1 year of age. The lack of "approval" by the FDA does not imply that a drug can/should not be used; rather, it only means that the manufacturer never carried out the appropriate studies to gain FDA approval.[26,118–121] A number of legislative changes are intended to improve drug research in children and improve drug labeling; however, some of the drugs are no longer under patent protection, and there is no motivation for drug companies to study their use in children.[122–124]

It is important to review the child's presedation medications. It is particularly important to note any chronic opioid or benzodiazepine medications that the child may be taking. Tolerance to either of these medication classes can significantly increase the required dose of sedative medications to achieve the desired depth of sedation. On the other hand, protease inhibitors (e.g., nelfinavir, ritonavir, saquinavir) are potent inhibitors of the cytochrome P450 CYP3A metabolic pathway. This pathway is responsible the metabolism of many sedatives, including midazolam, and may markedly prolong duration of action and may lead to life-threatening respiratory depression. Erythromycin and some calcium channel blockers may also inhibit the cytochrome system and delay metabolism of midazolam.[125–127]

Sedation medications can have significant interactions with other classes of drugs. Dexmedetomidine should not be combined with digoxin (or other atrioventricular node conduction blockers) in infants because severe bradycardia may result.[128] Although not always appreciated as the source of potent interactions, herbal

TABLE 48.7 Recommended Intensity of Monitoring, Documentation, Personnel, and Equipment for Different Levels of Sedation[316]

	Moderate Sedation	Deep Sedation
Monitoring	Pulse oximetry ECG recommended Heart rate Blood pressure Respiration Capnography recommended	Pulse oximetry ECG required Heart rate Blood pressure Respiration Capnography required
Documentation	Name, route, site, time of administration, and dosage of all drugs administered. Continuous oxygen saturation, heart rate, and ventilation (capnography recommended). Parameters recorded q10 minutes	Name, route, site, time of administration, and dosage of all drugs administered. Continuous oxygen saturation, heart rate, and ventilation (capnography required). Parameters recorded at least q5 minutes
Personnel	An observer who will monitor the patient but who may also assist with interruptible tasks—trained in pediatric advanced life support (PALS)	An independent observer whose only responsibility is to continuously monitor the patient—trained in PALS and capable of assisting with any emergency event
Responsible practitioner	Skilled to rescue a child with apnea, laryngospasm, and/or airway obstruction including the ability to open the airway, suction secretions, provide continuous positive airway pressure (CPAP), perform successful bag-valve-mask ventilation. Recommended that at least one practitioner should be skilled in obtaining vascular access in children.	Skilled to rescue a child with apnea, laryngospasm, and/or airway obstruction including the ability to open the airway, suction secretions, provide CPAP, perform successful bag-valve-mask ventilation, tracheal intubation, and cardiopulmonary resuscitation; training in PALS required. At least one practitioner skilled in obtaining vascular access in children immediately available.
Equipment	Pulse oximeter, blood pressure device, stethoscope, capnometer Rescue cart and equipment immediately available properly stocked with rescue drugs and age- and size-appropriate equipment required	Pulse oximeter, blood pressure device, stethoscope, ECG monitor, capnometer Rescue cart and equipment immediately available properly stocked with rescue drugs and age- and size-appropriate equipment required
Other Equipment	Suction equipment Adequate oxygen source/supply	Suction equipment Adequate oxygen source/supply Defibrillator required
Emergency checklists	Recommended	Recommended
Dedicated recovery area: With a rescue cart properly stocked with rescue drugs and age- and size-appropriate equipment with dedicated recovery personnel and adequate oxygen supply	Recommended. Initial recording of vital signs may be needed at least every 10 minutes until the child begins to awaken, then recording intervals may be increased.	Recommended. Initial recording of vital signs may be needed at least 5-minute intervals until the child begins to awaken, then recording intervals may be increased to 10-15 minutes.

medicines can enhance or shorten sedative medication activity.[129-133] Herbal medicines (e.g., St. John's wort or echinacea) may alter drug metabolism through inhibition of the cytochrome P450 system, resulting in prolonged drug effect and altered (increased or decreased) blood drug concentrations. Kava may augment the effects of sedatives, and valerian may itself produce sedation (see also E-Table 4.4).[134]

Several drug classes need to be considered when formulating a plan for procedural sedation. The needs of the procedure and the child will affect the exact choice of drugs in each case. Paramount among the considerations is the issue of whether or not the procedure is accompanied by significant pain. If it is painful (bone marrow biopsy, central line placement), some form of analgesia (with local anesthetics or a systemic drug that offers analgesia) is indicated to achieve all of the goals for the procedural sedation. If the procedure strictly requires sedation and motion control (MRI scans, CT scans), a pure sedative approach is often sufficient and preferable.

LOCAL ANESTHETICS

Local anesthetics play a critical role in analgesia for painful procedures and greatly reduce requirements for systemic opioids. Unlike most drugs used in medicine, local anesthetics must be physically deposited at their site of action to produce their effect. For most blocks and local skin infiltration, epinephrine (1:200,000 [5 µg/mL]) is used as a vasoconstrictor to increase the duration of blockade, decrease bleeding, and reduce systemic toxicity by decreasing vascular uptake. *Historically, the combination of local anesthetics and epinephrine has NOT been advised for digits or the penis. Today the combination is considered safe as long as the concentration of epinephrine is ≤1/200,000.*[135-137] Local anesthetics should be prepared only in labeled syringes immediately before use. No more than the maximum allowable dose (mg/kg) should be prepared in the syringe to minimize the risk of an accidental overdose (see Table 42.2). Local anesthetics can be extremely useful in obtunding airway reflexes when sprayed in the oropharynx or glottis before bronchoscopy or gastrointestinal endoscopy.

Local anesthetics can be administered in the sedated child by subcutaneous (SC) infiltration, field blocks, ultrasound guided nerve blocks, and IV regional anesthesia. A discussion of these topics and treatment of local anesthetic use and toxicity is found in Chapters 42, 43, and 44. Topical administration of local anesthetics is useful for planned sedation patients. EMLA cream is a eutectic mixture of local anesthetics (lidocaine 2.5% and prilocaine 2.5%) (AstraZeneca Pharmaceuticals LP, Wilmington, DE). When placed on the skin for 40 to 60 minutes,[138,139] it is useful for reducing the pain of skin incision, IV cannula insertions, lumbar punctures, and circumcision.[140-142] EMLA must be used with some caution as absorption of excessive amounts of prilocaine can cause methemoglobinemia if applied in inappropriate doses or on mucosal surfaces.[29] That is, for children weighing <10 kg, apply to a maximum of approximately 100 cm² surface area; for those 10–20 kg, apply to a maximum of approximately 600 cm² surface area; and for those >20 kg, apply to a maximum of approximately 2000 cm² surface area. EMLA cream can cause blanching of the skin and local vasoconstriction, which can make IV access difficult.

Other topical anesthetics include ELA-Max and LMX4 (Ferndale Healthcare, Ferndale, MI); these are 4% liposomal lidocaine preparations with onset within 30 minutes. Penetration is slightly deeper than EMLA cream.[143] The S-Caine Patch (ZARS, Inc., Salt Lake City, UT) is a eutectic mixture of 70 mg of lidocaine and 70 mg tetracaine in a bioadhesive layer that contains a heating element. A 20-minute application is effective in lessening pain from venipuncture procedures.[144] Amethocaine (Ametop) is a topical cream of 4% tetracaine (40 mg tetracaine base per gram of gel) that anesthetizes the skin in 20 to 30 minutes without causing vasoconstriction or other sequelae. It is available internationally in the United Kingdom, Canada, Australia, as well as in several other countries (from Smith & Nephew Canada, Mississauga, Ontario). A systematic review of amethocaine versus EMLA cream yielded a weak endorsement of amethocaine over EMLA cream for first-time IV cannulation.[145]

ANXIOLYTICS AND SEDATIVES

Chloral hydrate has historically been a widely used sedative. It is currently not commercially available in the United States but continues to be used internationally and in some U.S. hospitals where it is compounded (Table 48.8).[146-149] Its most common use is as a sedative to facilitate nonpainful diagnostic procedures, such as EEG, CT, or MRI.[148] It is rapidly and completely absorbed when given orally. Rectal administration is erratically absorbed and therefore not recommended. The onset of sedation is 30 to 60 minutes, and the usual clinical duration is 1 hour. Although it has a long history of successful use, it can cause respiratory depression and airway obstruction. Deaths have been associated with its use as a sole sedative agent and when combined with other sedatives; particularly problematic were situations where the drug was administered in an unmonitored setting (such as a car seat).[51,113,150-153] One large series showed a 0.6% incidence of respiratory depression, especially at larger doses (75–100 mg/kg).[154] Chloral hydrate acts primarily through its active metabolite trichloroethanol, which is formed in the liver and erythrocytes.[155] Trichloroethanol has a half-life of 10 hours in toddlers, 18 hours in term infants, and 40 hours in preterm infants (see Fig. 48.3).[156] Agitation and restlessness more than 6 hours in one-third of children sedated with chloral hydrate has been reported, 5% of whom did not return to baseline activity for 2 days after the procedure![58,157]

Benzodiazepines are commonly used in pediatric sedation. They are anxiolytic, amnestic, sedative hypnotics with anticonvulsant activities. Their high lipid solubility at physiologic pH accounts for the rapid CNS effects. As opposed to diazepam, midazolam is delivered in a water-soluble form (pH 3.5), which markedly decreases the incidence of pain on injection and thrombophlebitis.[155] However, the resulting decrease in fat solubility delays transport into the CNS (peak EEG effect 4.8 minutes for midazolam vs. 1.6 minutes for diazepam; Fig. 48.7).[158,159] Benzodiazepines exert their effects by occupying the benzodiazepine receptor that modulates γ-aminobutyric acid (GABA), the major inhibitory neurotransmitter in the brain. The clearance of benzodiazepines is decreased in neonates and also by liver enzyme inhibition that occurs during concomitant use of erythromycin, cimetidine, or protease inhibitors.[126]

When administered at the recommended doses, benzodiazepine-sedated patients become compliant but do not lose consciousness (minimal to moderate sedation). This level of sedation has limited application for achieving ideal procedural conditions for most interventions. Benzodiazepines provide no analgesia; analgesic medications must be added for painful procedures. On the other hand, benzodiazepines have the advantage of providing potent anterograde amnesia that correlates with the onset of slurred speech.[160,161] Midazolam is the preferred drug for pediatric sedation

TABLE 48.8	Sedation Regimens for Children			
Drug Regimen	Dose/Route	Onset (minutes)	Duration (minutes)	Comments
Pentobarbital	4–6 mg/kg IV or PO	IV: 2–5 PO: 20–60	IV: 15–45 PO: 60–240	Long history of safety. Slow onset. Prolonged emergence. May have paradoxical excitement. Half-life increased by valproic acid and MAO inhibitors. Contraindicated in porphyria.
Midazolam	0.25–0.75 mg/kg PO 0.05 mg/kg IV 0.2 mg/kg intranasal 0.1–0.15 mg/kg IM	15–30 1–3 10–15 10–15	60–90 60–90 45–60	Paradoxical response infrequent. Intranasal route very irritating. Increased respiratory depression when used with opioids; reduce midazolam dose by 25%. Prolonged duration with protease inhibitors. Antagonist: flumazenil.
Chloral hydrate	50–100 mg/kg PO (maximum not to exceed 2 g)	30–60	60–120	Very popular for nonpainful radiologic procedures in small children when IV not available. Effects unreliable over 1–2 years of age. Prolonged sedation and paradoxical responses noted. Respiratory depression and obstruction reported with tonsil hypertrophy and anatomic abnormalities. Moderate sedation guidelines required. Markedly prolonged half-life in neonates. Contraindicated in porphyria.

TABLE 48.8	Sedation Regimens for Children—cont'd			
Drug Regimen	Dose/Route	Onset (minutes)	Duration (minutes)	Comments
Etomidate	0.1–0.4 mg/kg IV	<1	5–15	No analgesic effect. Larger doses cause general anesthesia, respiratory depression, and loss of airway. Stable cardiovascular profile. Few data in children. Must be credentialed for deep sedation/anesthesia. No reversal drug. Causes adrenal suppression ~12 hours.
Methohexital	0.25–0.50 mg/kg IV 20–25 mg/kg rectal 10 mg/kg IM	<1 10–15 10–15	10–20 30–60 30–60	Avoid if temporal lobe epilepsy or porphyria. IV doses quickly lead to general anesthesia. Rectal doses cause high frequency of apnea and should be avoided. Deep sedation/anesthesia credentialing. Contraindicated in children <3 months of age, psychosis, stimulation of oropharynx, increased intracranial pressure, head injury, glaucoma.
Dexmedetomidine	IV: 1–2 µg/kg bolus (over 10 minutes) Infusion: 1–2 µg/kg per hour	10	Clinical 30 minutes to 1 hour; half-life 1.5–3 hours	Mimics natural sleep. Rapid bolus may cause hypertension. Minimal respiratory depression. Dose-dependent hypotension and bradycardia. Use with caution with digitalis medications. Glycopyrrolate treatment of bradycardia may induce sustained hypertension of unknown mechanism.
Fentanyl with propofol	Fentanyl 1–2 µg/kg IV with propofol 50–150 mg/kg per minute infusion IV	1–2	30–60	Child may rapidly become anesthetized with loss of airway. Advanced airway management skills required, with appropriate credentialing.
Midazolam with fentanyl	Midazolam 0.02 mg/kg IV with fentanyl 1–2 µg/kg IV	2–3	45–60	Commonly used for painful procedures. Careful titration needed to avoid deep sedation/anesthesia with apnea and hypoxia. Reduce dose of fentanyl when combined with benzodiazepine. Reduce dose with protease inhibitors.
Ketamine	3–4 mg/kg IM 1–2 mg/kg IV 4–6 mg/kg PO	5 1 10–20	30–60 30–60 30–90	Nausea and vomiting common after procedure. Laryngospasm, apnea, agitation, hallucinations reported but uncommon. Midazolam may not prevent emergence delirium. Anticholinergic may be used to control secretions. Larger doses can produce state of general anesthesia. Usually causes tachycardia, hypertension, and bronchodilatation. Paradoxical hypotension in critically ill patients. No antagonist available. Advanced airway management skills required, with appropriate credentialing.
Propofol	Bolus 1–2 mg/kg Infusion 50–250 µg/kg per minute	30 seconds	5–15 minutes after discontinuation	Profound, dose-related respiratory depressant. Assume deep sedation/anesthesia when using in children. Infusions >5 hours may cause propofol infusion syndrome. Caution when used in mitochondrial myopathies. Pain on injection mitigated by IV lidocaine. Advanced airway management skills required, with appropriate credentialing.
Remifentanil	0.1–0.25 µg/kg per minute	1	10–15	Difficulty in titration frequently leads to apnea and general anesthesia. Few studies in children. Exclusively used by anesthesiologists.
Nitrous oxide	50% in 50% oxygen for "minimal sedation"; up to 70% used by some for moderate sedation	<5	On discontinuing	Requires specialized equipment for delivery, monitoring, and scavenging. Use alone (50% in oxygen or less) or with local anesthesia is considered "minimal sedation." Greater doses or addition of other sedatives/analgesics require a minimum of "moderate sedation" guidelines. Contraindications include respiratory failure, altered mental status, otitis media, bowel obstruction, and pneumothorax. No antagonist available.
Opioid antagonist: naloxone	0.01–0.1 mg/kg IV or IM Max 2 mg/dose May repeat every 2 minutes	1–2	IV: 20–40 IM: 60–90	Specifically antagonizes opioid effects. Should not be used for routine reversal of opioid effect. Adverse reactions: nausea, vomiting, tachycardia, hypertension, delirium, pulmonary edema. Reversal after long-term opioid use may lead to acute withdrawal. Children may renarcotize 1 hr after IV dosing.
Benzodiazepine antagonist: flumazenil	IV 0.01–0.02 mg/kg. May repeat every 1 minute to 1 mg	1–2	30–60	Specific benzodiazepine antagonist. Does not antagonize opioids or other sedatives. Resedation may occur in 1 hour. Prolonged observation (2 hours) required. Not for routine sedation reversal. Children using benzodiazepine to control seizures or drug dependency may have exacerbations with flumazenil.

IM, intramuscularly; *IV*, intravenously; *MAO*, monoamine oxidase; *PO*, by mouth.
Data modified from Cravero JP, Burke GT. A review of pediatric sedation. *Anesth Analg*. 2004;99(5):1355–1364; Krauss B, Green SM. Procedural sedation and analgesia in children. *Lancet* 2006;367(9512):766–780; and Coté CJ, Stafford MA. *The Principles of Pediatric Sedation*. Boston: Tufts University School of Medicine; 1998.

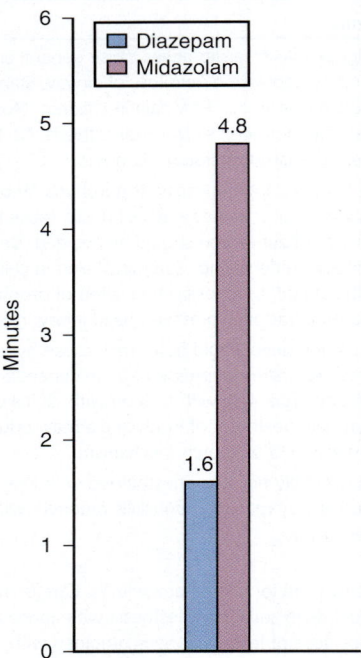

Time to Peak EEG Effect

FIGURE 48.7 Time to peak electroencephalographic (*EEG*) effect of diazepam versus midazolam in adults. Note that it takes nearly three times longer to achieve a peak EEG effect after intravenous (IV) midazolam than after IV diazepam. This is likely caused by the difference in fat solubility; because midazolam is less fat-soluble than diazepam, midazolam does not cross biologic membranes as easily. The clinical importance of this observation is the need to wait 3 to 5 minutes between IV doses of midazolam to avoid stacking of doses and excessive drug effect. (Data from Bührer M, Maitre PO, Crevoisier C, Stanski DR. Electroencephalographic effects of benzodiazepines: II. Pharmacodynamic modeling of the electroencephalographic effects of midazolam and diazepam. *Clin Pharmacol Ther.* 1990;48(5):555–567.)

because of its brief and more consistent half-life compared with diazepam.[162-167] The time to peak effect after IV administration of midazolam is 2 to 4 minutes, with a duration of 45 to 60 minutes. Midazolam can be given IV, intranasally (IN), sublingually, orally, or rectally (see Table 48.8). Nasal administration is well documented and can be very effective; however, it causes nasopharyngeal burning[168]; preadministration of intranasal lidocaine can decrease the irritation.[169] Rectal administration is usually well tolerated in children who have not been toilet trained, but absorption may be irregular owing to many factors, including superior versus inferior hemorrhoidal vein absorption within the rectum.

Benzodiazepines produce mild respiratory depression and upper airway obstruction.[170-172] Small doses of oral midazolam (0.3 mg/kg) that produce minimal sedation were associated with a 6.5% decrease in functional residual capacity and a 7.4% increase in respiratory resistance.[173] Respiratory depression may become marked in children who are neurologically impaired or in children with OSA, although premedication with oral midazolam (0.5 mg/kg) carries an extremely small risk of transient hemoglobin desaturation.[174] The combination of benzodiazepines and opioids can produce a "superadditive effect" on respiratory depression where the total depressant effect from the combination of drugs is much greater than the sum of their anticipated individual effects.[175,176]

Benzodiazepines may have a paradoxical effect in 1% to 15% of children depending on age and personality, rendering the child combative rather than cooperative. A history of this type of paradoxical response should be elicited before administering a benzodiazepine.

Flumazenil is a specific benzodiazepine-receptor antagonist that rapidly reverses the sedative, paradoxical, and respiratory effects of benzodiazepines.[177-181] Children who take benzodiazepines for seizures or drug dependency may experience symptoms rapidly if flumazenil is given.[182] It should also be used with caution in children with increased intracranial pressure and in those taking drugs that decrease the seizure threshold (e.g., cyclosporine, theophylline, and lithium). Because of these concerns, flumazenil should not be administered for the routine reversal of the sedative effects of benzodiazepines but should be reserved for emergency reversal of respiratory depression. The recommended dose of flumazenil is 10 µg/kg up to 200 µg every minute to a maximum cumulative dose of 1 mg IV. Antagonism begins within 1 to 2 minutes after administration and lasts approximately 1 hour. Because resedation after 1 hour may occur, any child who receives flumazenil must be carefully monitored for at least 2 hours. It should be noted that flumazenil does not antagonize respiratory depression induced by opioids.[183]

BARBITURATES

Pentobarbital is an intermediate-acting barbiturate that is now infrequently used. It provides excellent sedation, hypnosis, and amnesia without analgesic. The onset of sedation is 3 to 5 minutes with a peak effect by approximately 10 minutes and duration of action of 1 to 2 (or more) hours. Respiratory obstruction, transient desaturation, and hypotension occur infrequently.[184,185] Barbiturates reduce the threshold for pain in children, so it is best avoided in painful procedures. Recovery after pentobarbital is often protracted, leaving children in a disinhibited state for extended periods. This may lead to a prolonged recovery and, in some cases, the need for restraint (see Table 48.8).[147]

OPIOIDS

Opioid analgesics are rarely effective sedatives in isolation, but their use is essential to manage painful diagnostic and therapeutic procedures. Opioids confer a degree of sedation, but the sedation is usually inadequate to perform procedures in children; thus they are usually combined with sedatives (see Fig. 48.1).[175,186] Combinations require particular caution in infants and children with upper airway obstruction (e.g., tonsil and/or adenoid hypertrophy, Trisomy 21, mucopolysaccharidosis).

Morphine may be used for painful procedures with prolonged duration or when pain is expected after the procedure.[187] Morphine may be given orally (0.2–0.5 mg/kg), IV (0.05–0.1 mg/kg [maximum 0.3 mg/kg]), or intramuscularly (IM) (0.1–0.2 mg/kg), and diamorphine may be given nasally.[188-190] Times to peak effect for oral, IV, and IM administration are 60 minutes, 1 to 2 minutes, and 10 to 30 minutes, respectively.

Fentanyl is the opioid of choice for sedation/analgesia for most procedures in children because of its brief duration of action. It may be given IV, IN or IM.[191-195] IV fentanyl is approximately 50 to 100 times more potent an analgesic than morphine but without amnesic properties. Its high lipid solubility allows for a rapid onset of action (within 30 seconds) and time to peak effect, 2 to 3 minutes. It has a brief clinical duration of 20 to 40 minutes when given in small doses, owing to its rapid redistribution to skeletal muscle, fat, and other inactive sites. Unlike morphine, it has no active metabolites. Fentanyl is frequently used in combination with a short-acting anxiolytic (midazolam). IV doses of fentanyl usually begin at 0.5 to 1 µg/kg. Serial doses may be titrated every 5 to 10 minutes to effect, to a maximum dose not exceeding 5 µg/kg.[196] Fentanyl can also be administered IN at a dose of 1.5 µg/kg, It has been effective at this dose for emergency department procedures.[191,193-195] When carefully titrated and appropriately monitored, fentanyl has few adverse effects. Chest wall rigidity is a centrally mediated idiosyncratic reaction that can interfere with breathing but can be antagonized with either naloxone or muscle relaxants; it is rarely observed in sedation practice.[197-199] Other adverse reactions from fentanyl include bradycardia, dysphoria, delirium, nausea, vomiting, pruritus, urinary retention, hypotension, and smooth muscle spasm. Close postprocedural observation is required because respiratory depression can outlast analgesia (see Table 48.8).

Remifentanil an ultra-short-lived, rapid-acting, potent, lipophilic opioid that is metabolized by plasma and tissue esterases and must be administered as a continuous infusion. It has a half-life of 3 to 6 minutes that is independent of the duration of infusion. Remifentanil has been used for intraoperative and procedural sedation by anesthesiologists and in intubated children in the ICU.[200-205] If postoperative pain is anticipated, another analgesic should be administered before stopping the infusion of remifentanil. Children may develop a degree of opioid tolerance after several hours of infusing remifentanil.[206] Accordingly, provision for pain control after procedures must be anticipated and instituted before emergence from sedation/anesthesia. Remifentanil is also associated with a substantial incidence of apnea, hypoxemia, and chest wall and glottic rigidity, and is not recommended as a sole agent for pediatric sedation (see Table 48.8).[202,204,207] Remifentanil may be administered together with propofol to provide total intravenous anesthesia and sedation (see Chapter 8).

Opioid antagonists reverse the respiratory and analgesic effects of opioids and should be readily available when opioids are used (see Table 48.8). Naloxone (Narcan) is the most commonly used antagonist[208] and may be given IV, IM, or SC.[209] The initial dose for respiratory depression is 10 µg/kg titrated to effect every 2 to 3 minutes. A dose of 10 to 100 µg/kg up to 2 mg may be required for respiratory arrest. Adverse reactions from the rapid reversal of opioid effects include nausea, vomiting, tachycardia, hypertension, delirium, and pulmonary edema.[210-212] Children who have been receiving long-term opioid therapy should be given opioid reversal agents in small doses and with extreme caution because withdrawal seizures, sympathetic overdrive, and delirium may occur. Children given a single dose of IV naloxone may have a recrudescence of the respiratory depression 1 hour later. It is for this reason that the same IV dose is administered IM; otherwise *the child should be observed for a minimum of 2 hours after the IV naloxone.* Nalmefene (Revex), like naltrexone, is a µ-receptor antagonist and weak κ- agonist that boasts a greater half-life (~10 hours) than naloxone.[213] Although experience in children is limited, it accelerates recovery from sedation.[214] Because of its relatively long half-life, it outlasts the effects of fentanyl and may oppose pain treatment for several hours.

α₂-ADRENOCEPTOR AGONIST: DEXMEDETOMIDINE

Dexmedetomidine is highly lipid soluble and quickly crosses the blood-brain barrier. Its mechanism of action in the CNS is via stimulating receptors in the medullary vasomotor center, which decreases sympathetic tone. It also stimulates central parasympathetic outflow and decreases sympathetic outflow from the locus

ceruleus of the brainstem. The decreased outflow from the locus ceruleus increases activity of the inhibitory GABA neurons, which cause sedation and analgesia.[215] Currently, dexmedetomidine is only approved by the FDA for procedural sedation in adults, although it is used off-label to sedate children. In addition to its IV use, it has been administered via the buccal, IN, and IM routes in children.[216-220] When administered in clinical doses, it causes limited effects on ventilation and may mimic natural rapid-eye-movement sleep.[221-223] Because rapid IV boluses can cause transient systemic hypertension, the initial loading dose must be given as a 10-minute infusion and may be followed by a continuous infusion. When given in the recommended fashion, it decreases blood pressure and heart rate in a dose-dependent manner. It should be used with caution in children with preexisting bradycardia, atrioventricular conduction defects, hypotension, and decreased cardiac output.[224-226] It has been associated with severe bradycardia in infants receiving digoxin and β-blockers, and those with preexisting AV nodal conduction delays.[128] Dexmedetomidine has seen a rapid increase in pediatric sedation over the past 10 years largely owing to its lack of respiratory depressant effects.[227-230] To date, dexmedetomidine does not cause neuroapoptosis (unlike all other sedatives). It has been suggested to have neuroprotective properties[231-233] and may therefore hold a unique advantage for sedation in young children when these effects are of greatest concern. Sedation after IV administration has a relatively rapid onset of 10 minutes and a half-life of 1½ to 3 hours. Its minimal effect on respiration has led to its use alone in nonpainful procedures (e.g., EEG, CT, and MRI), in children with Down syndrome and children with OSA. It has also been used in combination with ketamine and propofol for painful procedures (e.g., cardiac catheterizations and complex regional pain syndrome).[234,235] However, caution is advised in children with known congenital heart disease, as it depresses sinus and atrioventricular node function and may pose an increased risk for children prone to bradycardia.[234-238] When analyzed by MRI, the dose-response effects of dexmedetomidine (1–2 µg/kg per hour) on the morphology of the upper airway in children[239,240] revealed minimal changes in the dimensions of the dimensions of the upper airway. Infants and children 5 months to 16 years of age also show minimal effects on respiration.[54] These characteristics make dexmedetomidine a popular choice for children with OSA.[239,240]

Dexmedetomidine has intermediate potency when compared with other sedatives such as etomidate or propofol. The effective dose in children is greater than that in adults. Many studies have investigated the dose of dexmedetomidine needed to successfully complete as close to 100% of the tests and procedures that required sedation. At the top end of the dosing range, a loading dose of 3 µg/kg administered over 10 minutes IV followed by an infusion of 2 µg/kg per hour minimized the need for rescue with pentobarbital (2.4%) for sedation for MRI.[241] At these doses, mean arterial pressure was maintained in all children and oxygen saturation remained greater than 95%; however, 30 of the 747 (4%) experienced bradycardia to less than the 20th percentile for age. No adverse effects were noted, nor were any treatments required. Full recovery may be slow with high doses of dexmedetomidine.[242] Caution should also be used when administering glycopyrrolate to treat the bradycardia from dexmedetomidine because severe and sustained hypertension after traditional doses of 5 µg/kg glycopyrrolate have occurred (e.g., blood pressure 161/113 mm Hg in a 3-year-old).[243] An alternative approach to improving success with dexmedetomidine[244] included a loading dose of 1 µg/kg dexmedetomidine over 10 minutes followed by an infusion of

0.5 μg/kg per hour plus a 0.1-mg/kg bolus of midazolam. With this regimen, a high rate of success with only small changes in ETCO$_2$ and minimal hemodynamic effect has been demonstrated. Combination of propofol with dexmedetomidine has proven highly effective and is associated with few adverse effects.[245] Other investigators reported that a combination of ketamine, propofol, and dexmedetomidine in the cardiac catheterization lab was very effective.[246] Combination regimens offer a preferable mix of successful sedation with few adverse events, although there are insufficient data to recommend a specific regimen to maximize the sedation with dexmedetomidine.

KETAMINE

Ketamine, available since the 1960s, is one of the few sedatives that produces sedation, amnesia, and analgesia. The clinical appearance is that of a child who has open eyes (usually with horizontal nystagmus) but does not respond to pain–the "dissociative" state. Ketamine preserves cardiovascular function and exerts limited effects on respiratory mechanics, allowing spontaneous respirations in most children.[247] Although it is certainly not a new drug, ketamine has experienced a resurgence in popularity for procedural sedation, particularly in the emergency department. Clinical practice guidelines from American College of Emergency Physicians proposed a distinct classification of sedation for ketamine as "Dissociative Sedation"[248,249] because it has unique properties that do not neatly fit into the current definitions of sedation or anesthesia. To date, this reclassification has not been accepted by the AAP, ASA, AAPD, or regulatory agencies.[249-252]

IM and IV ketamine (with and without midazolam) are frequently used for closed fracture reductions and other painful minor procedures in the emergency department (see Table 48.8).[252-254] In a recent systematic review of 41 publications in which ketamine was used for procedural sedation in children (13,876 sedations) in the emergency department, adverse events were infrequent. The most common adverse events were vomiting and agitation, with frequencies of 55 and 18/1000 sedations, respectively.[255] Hypoxia occurred in 1.5% of sedations, apnea in 0.7%, laryngospasm in 2.9/1000 sedations, and 0 cases of aspiration. In a retrospective review of 173 children younger than 2 years of age who were sedated for minor procedures in the emergency department with ketamine/midazolam or morphine/midazolam for the majority of cases, the frequency of complications was 6%, of which all but one were related to ketamine/midazolam. Most were considered minor in severity (3 desaturated, 4 vomited, 1 developed stridor, 2 failed sedation), although one infant (2 months of age) developed bradycardia necessitating tracheal intubation.[256] In a prospective study by the PRSC of more than 22,000 sedations in children (median age 5 years, range <1 month–22 years) with ketamine in radiology and sedation suites, 7.3% experienced adverse events and 1.8% experienced serious adverse events.[257] Two patients with cardiac arrests were successfully resuscitated. Risk factors for adverse events included cardiac and gastrointestinal diseases, lower respiratory tract infections, and coadministration of propofol and anticholinergics.

Ketamine (1–3 mg/kg IV) has also been studied in children undergoing gastroendoscopy procedures, with transient laryngospasm occurring in 8.2%, emesis in 4.1%, emergence agitation in 2.4%, partial airway obstruction in 1.3%, apnea and respiratory depression in 0.5%, and excessive salivation in 0.3%.[95] The analgesic effects of ketamine make it very appealing for use during burn dressing changes. In one study, 4.9% of the ketamine sedations resulted in adverse outcomes, of which 2.9% required an intervention. Eight events were related to the airway.[258] Ketamine sedation/analgesia has a very long history of safety, perhaps offering advantages over other sedation regimens, although these studies indicate that potentially life-threatening events can and do occur even with ketamine sedation. Ketamine is also associated with nonpurposeful motion, which limits its usefulness when immobility is necessary (e.g., use during MRI scans).

Ketamine is contraindicated in a number of clinical scenarios. Human studies support a trend to increase global and regional cerebral blood flow in healthy patients[259] and warrant a relative contraindication for this drug in children with significantly increased intracranial pressure, particularly without controlled respirations. Similarly, ketamine is contraindicated in those with head injury, open globe injury, hypertension, and psychosis. Although it does not directly decrease the ventilatory drive, ketamine decreases the ventilatory response to hypercarbia. Ketamine is associated with a small, but significant rate of laryngospasm and coughing that may require definitive airway management.[260] No antagonist is available. Recovery from ketamine is notable for a greater incidence of emesis and agitation than other sedatives.[255,260,261]

Typical starting doses[262] of ketamine are 3 to 4 mg/kg IM, 0.25 to 1.0 mg/kg IV, and 4 to 6 mg/kg orally.[263-265] The onset after IM injection is 2 to 5 minutes, with a peak at approximately 20 minutes; duration can be 30 to 120 minutes. Onset after IV administration occurs in less than 1 minute, with a peak effect in several minutes and duration of action of approximately 15 minutes. Oral doses of 4 to 6 mg/kg are usually combined with atropine and have an effect in 30 minutes and last up to 120 minutes.[29] In a dose-ranging study of ketamine in the emergency department, doses of 1.5 to 2 mg/kg IV provided similar sedation and satisfaction after the procedures.[266] Although anticholinergics have been recommended when ketamine was used for procedural sedation in the emergency department,[267] recent studies from the emergency department have not only refuted the need for anticholinergics during ketamine sedation but also suggested that the use of anticholinergics may actually increase the odds of adverse events.[257] It is unclear how the use of an anticholinergic could increase the number of adverse events.

Etomidate is a carboxylated imidazole that is primarily used as an induction agent for anesthesia. Its mechanism is thought to be potentiation of GABA inhibitory neurotransmission via alteration of chloride conductance. Loss of consciousness occurs in 15 to 20 seconds. Recovery results from redistribution within 5 to 10 minutes. It is hydrolyzed in the liver to inactive metabolites and excreted (90%) in the urine.[155] Etomidate produces sedation, anxiolysis, and amnesia similar to the barbiturates and propofol. Its major advantage is its lack of adverse cardiovascular effects. It has been used in adults and children for procedural sedation, although the endpoint of sedation is not well described and often is a state of general anesthesia.[91] Etomidate has been compared with pentobarbital for CT sedation. Adverse events were more common with pentobarbital (4.5%) than etomidate (0.9%).[268] Etomidate with fentanyl has been compared with ketamine with midazolam for reduction of limb fractures in children in the emergency department. The combination of etomidate and fentanyl led to a quicker recovery but was less effective in reducing observed patient distress.[269,270] Transient adrenal suppression can occur after etomidate,[271-275] which is why it is infrequently used in acutely ill children.

Propofol is widely used for pediatric sedation and anesthesia with an onset within 30 seconds. It has no analgesic properties, but it does have antiemetic and antipruritic properties. Although small doses of propofol (25–50 μg/kg per minute) can provide moderate sedation in adults, children require larger doses (150–250 μg/kg per minute). It is generally best administered by titration with an infusion pump. Adverse reactions include increased salivary and tracheobronchial secretions, myoclonic movements, anaphylactic reactions, and bacterial contamination. Pain on injection can be lessened by several strategies, although the two most effective strategies are pretreatment with nitrous oxide (N_2O) by inhalation, or a mini-Bier block with 1 mg/kg lidocaine applied for 1 minute.[276,277] Hypotension is mild and usually not clinically significant. Cases of fatal metabolic acidosis, myocardial failure, and lipemic serum have been reported in children who received propofol infusions (propofol infusion syndrome [PRIS]) for more than 48 hours at doses exceeding 5 mg/kg per hour (83 μg/kg per minute), with sporadic cases, which may have been exacerbated by an underlying mitochondrial disorder of the syndrome, appearing after only 5 to 6 hours in some cases.[278-283]

Propofol is also a profound respiratory depressant that may cause apnea. Respiratory complications have been reported in 8% to 30% of children.[284] In a study of propofol sedation (2.5–3 mg/kg IV loading dose with an infusion up to 200 μg/kg per minute) in 105 painful procedures in the pediatric ICU, 21% of the children required airway repositioning, 17% had apnea, 5% had hypotension, and 45% had events that required intervention.[98] In the emergency department, propofol was administered to 113 children in a dose of 4.5 mg/kg in addition to fentanyl 1 to 2 μg/kg[285] that proved to be sufficient to ensure the children were motionless during the reduction of fractures. The net effect was an incidence of desaturation of 21%, laryngospasm in 1%, and a supplemental oxygen requirement in 25%. In a study of sedation by nonanesthesiologists for bone marrow procedures, lumbar punctures, and esophagoscopies titrated propofol to a target of "not arousable"; 21 children from 27 weeks to 18 years of age were studied. Propofol at doses of 520 μg/kg per minute conferred 100% sedation with BIS readings of 45 or less (consistent with general anesthesia).[286] These responses to stimulation, effects on the airway, doses of propofol, and BIS levels are beyond the range of deep sedation and more in keeping with the definition of general anesthesia, with the inherent risk of loss of the airway. More recent studies that reviewed large numbers of sedation encounters involving propofol sedation by a variety of physicians (working in elective sedation services) document that propofol can be used with much fewer severe adverse outcomes (and much smaller doses) than previously reported.[15,104,287,288] In these studies of more than 100,000 total propofol encounters, the rate of significant airway events was less than 2.5%.[100,289]

There has been increasing use of a combination of ketamine (10 mg/mL) with propofol (10 mg/mL), so-called ketofol, for painful procedures in the emergency department and for oncology patients.[290-295] This combination is administered in incremental doses of 0.5 mg/kg of each drug at approximately 1-minute intervals. Other mixture proportions of these two drugs have also been investigated[296] and a better ratio of racemic ketamine to propofol may be 1:3 for brief procedures (5–20 minutes).[296,297] While experience with this combination of drugs is growing, the limited number of prospective studies at this point preclude assessment of safety and efficacy. A literature review found insufficient evidence to recommend routine use of this combination.[294]

Methohexital is a short-acting oxybarburate that is rapidly metabolized and redistributed, and has a rapid recovery (see Table 48.8).[298] Induction of anesthesia occurs with IV doses of 1 to 2 mg/kg. Apnea, hiccups, and methohexital-induced seizures in

children with temporal lobe epilepsy have been reported.[299] IM methohexital has been used in doses of 8 to 10 mg/kg, but the onset of sedation is slow[300] and it is not generally recommended. Rectal methohexital (20–25 mg/kg [from a 100-mg/mL solution]) can induce deep sedation in 7 to 11 minutes[301] with a duration of action of about 30 to 45 minutes.[302] Absorption through the rectal route is erratic.[303] The variability of absorption, tendency to deep sedation, and airway problems have decreased the use of methohexital in favor of newer drugs administered by other routes. This medication should be used only by individuals with advanced airway skills, because upper airway obstruction and apnea may readily occur.[304]

Nitrous oxide (N_2O) is a potent inhalation analgesic with a peak effect in 3 to 5 minutes and very rapid return to baseline when discontinued (see Table 48.8). A premixed tank of no more than 50% N_2O is available (Entonox). Administration of N_2O can be used for "minimal sedation" under the following AAP guidelines:

1. N_2O can be used only in ASA physical status I or II patients.
2. Only 50% N_2O or less is used.
3. Inhalation equipment must have the capacity to deliver 100% oxygen and never less than 25% oxygen.
4. A calibrated oxygen analyzer must be used. The child is able to maintain verbal communication throughout the procedure.

Although 50% N_2O in oxygen usually produces "minimal" sedation, the addition of any sedatives or hypnotic may rapidly produce a deeper level of sedation and require increased monitoring and vigilance.[152,170] N_2O is frequently used by dentists for sedation. The results of a recent questionnaire reported that all dentists performed treatments on patients under sedation during their training and that the majority used N_2O sedation.[305,306] Adverse reactions, drug interactions, and special concerns are listed in Table 48.8.

Summary and Future of Pediatric Sedation

Pediatric sedation has evolved from a clinical "orphan"—with few champions and almost no formal organization—to a well-documented field with clear standards and guidelines for practice. We are in an era where safe, effective, (and efficient) pediatric sedation is demanded by our patients and our professional colleagues. Appropriately, procedural sedation is expected to provide the same level of safety and effectiveness associated with the operating room. At the same time, anesthesiologists must recognize that the literature is replete with reports of *other* pediatric specialists working in sedation systems that provide care with potent medications and excellent outcomes.[227,307-315] Anesthesiologists continue to provide the ultimate "backup" for these services and take on the most challenging sedation cases, while recognizing the capabilities of other professionals. Anesthesiologists must explore ways to collaborate with these other specialists and help them develop optimal sedation monitoring techniques/drug regimens that will result in the best possible sedation results for all patients undergoing sedation for procedures and tests.

ANNOTATED REFERENCES

Coté CJ, Notterman DA, Karl HW, et al. Adverse sedation events in pediatrics: a critical incident analysis of contributory factors. *Pediatrics*. 2000;105(4 Pt 1):805-814.

Landmark study that collated severe adverse outcomes from multiple sources and allowed the identification of sedation practices that led to injury and death. In particular, it highlighted the need for appropriate personnel, monitors, and rescue capability to ensure safety.

Coté CJ, Wilson S, American Academy of Pediatrics, American Academy of Pediatric Dentistry. Guidelines for monitoring and management of pediatric patients before, during, and after sedation for diagnostic and therapeutic procedures: update 2016. *Pediatrics.* 2016;138(1).

These are the most recent American Academy of Pediatrics Sedation Guidelines that now require the use of capnography for all deeply sedated children and encourage its use for moderately sedated children. Important changes are that the responsible practitioner for moderate sedation must have the skills to rescue a child with apnea, laryngospasm, and airway obstruction, and perform successful bag-mask ventilation. The practitioner who practices deep sedation must have these same skills and be able to perform tracheal intubation and cardiopulmonary resuscitation.

Cravero JP, Beach M, Gallagher SM, et al. The incidence and nature of adverse events during pediatric sedation/anesthesia for procedures with propofol outside the operating room: report from the Pediatric Sedation Research Consortium. *Anesth Analg.* 2009;108(3):795-804.

A review of nearly 50,000 sedation encounters using propofol by a variety of sedation providers. The participating providers were highly trained members of organized sedation services with advanced airway education and ongoing quality improvement efforts. Adverse events and requirements for airway interventions are analyzed. The information is useful in understanding the critical competencies necessary for the safe use of this drug.

Cravero JP, Blike GT, Beach M, et al. Incidence and nature of adverse events during pediatric sedation/anesthesia for procedures outside the operating room: report from the Pediatric Sedation Research Consortium. *Pediatrics.* 2006;118(3):1087-1096.

A review of more than 30,000 sedation cases from the Pediatric Sedation Research Consortium. This study is useful as it supplements anecdotal information on sedation complications and aids in understanding the nature and frequency of adverse events in a large group of patients cared for by a variety of sedation providers.

A complete reference list can be found online at ExpertConsult.com.

Procedures for Vascular Access

SAMUEL H. WALD, JULIANNE MENDOZA, FREDERICK G. MIHM, AND CHARLES J. COTÉ

Venous Cannulation	Arterial Cannulation
Peripheral Intravenous Cannulation	Umbilical Artery
Central Venous Pressure Measurement	Radial Artery
Establishing a Large Intravenous Catheter in Small Patients	Axillary Artery
Central Venous Catheterization	Temporal Artery
Intraosseous Infusion	Femoral Artery
Umbilical Vein Catheterization	Dorsalis Pedis and Posterior Tibial Artery

VASCULAR CANNULATION IS AN IMPORTANT PROCEDURE in the anesthetic and perioperative management of children. Its routine use was introduced in the 1950s.[1] The indications are to provide routes to administer fluids, drugs, and blood products, monitor cardiopulmonary function, and access blood for laboratory testing. Although establishing vascular access may be extremely difficult at times, especially in the very young or small child, no child should be denied an indicated procedure because of an operator's inability to access the vascular system; appropriate consultation should be sought as necessary. Regardless of the procedure or the person in whom the procedure is attempted, gloves should be worn to maintain clean or sterile technique and to protect health care professionals from exposure to blood and sharps.[2–6] An update from the Pediatric Perioperative Cardiac Arrest Registry suggests that lack of good vascular access may contribute to an underestimation of the fluid requirement or blood loss and inadequate replacement of fluid or blood in anesthetized children, thus underscoring the importance of appropriate and adequate vascular access and monitoring.[7,8]

Venous Cannulation

PERIPHERAL INTRAVENOUS CANNULATION

Indications
Percutaneous intravenous (IV) access should be present in almost all anesthetized children for the following reasons[9,10]:
- To provide a route for postoperative pain management.
- To administer drugs, fluids and electrolytes, glucose, and blood products, including resuscitation medications.
- To measure central venous pressure; the accuracy of this measurement does not vary according to the location of the catheter[11] but does depend on ensuring direct continuity between the central and peripheral circulation.[9,12] This can be assessed by providing a large, sustained inspiration or occluding the venous return of the extremity, which both cause an increase in the peripheral pressure.[11,13,14] Hypothermia may impair the accuracy of such measurements.[15]

Equipment
- Alcohol pads or chlorhexidine swabs
- Gloves
- Tourniquet
- Gauze
- Clear plastic dressing (Tegaderm, 3M Medical-Surgical Division, St. Paul, MN, or OpSite, Smith & Nephew, Inc., Largo, FL)
- Tape
- Arm board

Consider the possible need for latex-free equipment. In cases of difficult access, the availability of a transillumination light source (Karl Storz, 485 B Type, Tuttlingen, Germany) may improve the success rate of catheter placement.[16] Ultrasonography also may be used to obtain peripheral venous access at the basilic, cephalic, or brachial veins.[17–19] Finally, new near-infrared and infrared technology is available to aid in the identification of peripheral veins (AccuVein, AccuVein, Inc., Huntington, NY; VeinViewer, Christie Digital Systems, Cypress, CA).[20]

Practical Suggestions
1. Awake IV line placement can be facilitated by any combination of good patient rapport, eutectic mixture of local anesthetics (EMLA) cream (lidocaine 2.5% and prilocaine 2.5%), lidocaine and tetracaine patch, lidocaine by iontophoresis, lidocaine by topical cream, topical tetracaine (Ametop), ethyl chloride spray, and/or premedication.[21–30]
2. Prefilling the cannula with saline solution may reduce menisci tension and allow a more rapid blood flashback.
3. A butterfly needle can be inserted for induction, followed by an appropriate-sized catheter after anesthesia.
4. A T-connector (Abbott, Inc., Chicago, IL) may be used to minimize the fluids necessary to flush drugs administered through the IV line; this is particularly important for infants.[31]
5. A calibrated burette should be used to limit the total infusion and provide a means to titrate fluids accurately in infants and young children.
6. A flow-limiting infusion pump may be used for preterm and full-term neonates.
7. Flow rates may be significantly changed by catheter brand, tubing type, and addition of extensions and stopcocks (see also E-Figs. 52.1 and 52.2).[32]
8. One-way valves in the IV tubing to prevent backflow of drugs or infusions.

9. Air filters also may be useful for children at risk for paradoxical gas embolization.

Complications

Hematoma from a failed vascular cannulation is usually of no serious consequence. Infection or thrombosis may be limited by aseptic technique.[33-35] One study of 642 Teflon catheters in 525 patients showed that the risk of catheter complications in children was extremely small and would not be reduced significantly by routine replacement of the catheters.[36] Catheter life span is unrelated to the insertion site, cannula size, or brand in infants younger than 12 months of age.[37,38]

Skin sloughing is usually caused by subcutaneous infiltration of calcium, potassium, or hypertonic solutions; it may be avoided by frequent inspection of the IV line for swelling in the subcutaneous tissues before injecting medications.[39] The risk of subcutaneous infiltration increases with the administration of medications versus no medications and with parenteral nutrition solutions compared with 5% or 10% dextrose solutions, but the risk of infiltration is no different with solutions that contain potassium ($\leq$20 mEq/L vs. >20 mEq/L). In addition, there is no difference between gravity-controlled versus infusion delivery devices.[40] There are insufficient data to support the routine use of heparin to prolong the patency of peripheral IV catheters in neonates and children.[41]

The severity of extravasation injuries depends on many factors, including pH, osmolarity, the diluent, vasoactive properties, and cytotoxic properties. The treatment of extravasation injuries varies with the extent of the injury from simple cessation of the IV solution and removal of the IV catheter while aspirating as much infiltrate as possible, to limb elevation, application of heat or cold packs, saline washout, topical treatments or injections (topical lidocaine, prilocaine, nitroglycerine, antimicrobials, subcutaneous or intradermal hyaluronidase, phentolamine, sodium thiosulfate or dexamethasone), assessment of compartment pressures, escharotomy, and in some cases, skin grafting.[42-46]

CENTRAL VENOUS PRESSURE MEASUREMENT

Some studies in children and adults describe a reasonable correlation between the venous pressure transduced in peripheral IV catheters and central venous catheters, even in critically ill children. Hypothermia (peripheral vasoconstriction) decreases the accuracy of such measurements, but it is useful to understand that transducing the pressure of a peripheral vein may provide valuable information regarding right-sided cardiac filling pressures.[9,10,15,47-49]

ESTABLISHING A LARGE INTRAVENOUS CATHETER IN SMALL PATIENTS

Indications

The following procedure is used for any child in whom there is the potential for massive, rapid hemorrhage:

1. Prepare and drape the appropriate area using standard sterile techniques.
2. Perform a standard IV cannulation of an antecubital, saphenous, or external jugular vein with a small IV catheter (e.g., 22-gauge).
3. Pass a small, flexible guidewire (e.g., 0.018 inch) through the IV catheter, remove the catheter, and with a No. 11 blade, make a small incision at the entry point of the wire at the skin.
4. Pass the next larger size IV catheter over the wire to dilate the vein and leave in place; stiff IV catheters are more effective. An alternative is to use a small dilator from a pulmonary artery catheter introducer and leave the sheath in place. The wire is

removed, and the next larger size wire is inserted (0.025 inch). The catheter (or sheath) is removed, leaving this larger wire within the vein. This process may be repeated with larger catheters and wires until the desired size cannula or sheath is reached. An alternative is to leave progressively larger pulmonary artery introducer sheaths in the vein; both techniques provide a reasonably rapid method of establishing a large-bore IV infusion site.

Rapid Infusion Catheters and Introducer Sheaths

Special rapid volume catheters (6F and larger; Arrow International, Reading, PA) allow venipuncture with a needle or small IV catheter, passage of a guidewire, and then introduction of a dilator and sheath, with fewer steps required.

Intravenous Cutdown
Indications

- Percutaneous cannulation is unsuccessful.
- Percutaneous cannulation is tenuous.
- The catheter in place is inadequate for the planned surgical procedure.

The most common sites for insertion are the saphenous vein at the medial malleolus and the brachiocephalic vein at the antecubital fossa. This procedure may require considerable time to perform and has limited utility for emergent access.[50]

Complications

IV cutdown has a high incidence of infection and therefore should be used only on a short-term basis.

Saphenous Vein Cannulation

The saphenous vein is often a reliable point for IV access in infants and children that may be directly visualized or cannulated with a "blind" technique (Fig. 49.1). It is consistently found lateral to the medial malleolus of the ankle one-half to one finger breadth over the anterior quadrant.

1. Cleanse the area in the standard fashion after a tourniquet is applied to the lower extremity below the knee.
2. The saphenous vein may or may not be palpated, and visualization may not be possible.
3. Enter the skin at a 30-degree angle at the expected site of the saphenous vein at the level of the medial malleolus, with the tip of the needle directed toward the upper two-thirds of the calf. If no evidence of venipuncture is seen on insertion, slowly withdraw the needle because the flash of blood often occurs while exiting the vein.
4. If unsuccessful on the first attempt, fan medially and then laterally from the same insertion point, slowly advancing and withdrawing the catheter until blood return is obtained.
5. Once a flashback is seen, gently advance the entire unit 2 to 3 mm into the lumen before twisting and advancing the catheter off the needle.

Safety Intravenous Catheters

In the United States, federal law requires that retractable or sheathed needles designed to reduce the potential for needlestick injury are available for use by health care personnel (Table 49.1).[51] A study that compared traditional IV catheters with safety devices found that a larger proportion of children younger than 3 years of age required more than one safety catheter to successfully gain IV access. The retractable IV catheter was associated with an almost fourfold greater incidence of splattering and spilling of blood compared with traditional catheters.[52] The excess splatter occurs when the powerful spring-loaded mechanism rapidly retracts the needle into the housing of the safety device; therefore sheathed catheters are regarded as inherently safer because they require no action on the part of the operator to protect the needle tip. Note that U.S. federal legislation requires that these devices be available, but the ultimate decision to use them rests with the physician operator. *Therefore, the type of catheter should not be dictated by the hospital but rather by the individuals who place the catheters.*

CENTRAL VENOUS CATHETERIZATION
Indications
- To provide a secure means to administer fluids and blood when major shifts in intravascular volume are anticipated (e.g., multiple trauma, intestinal obstruction, burns).
- To monitor cardiac filling pressures.

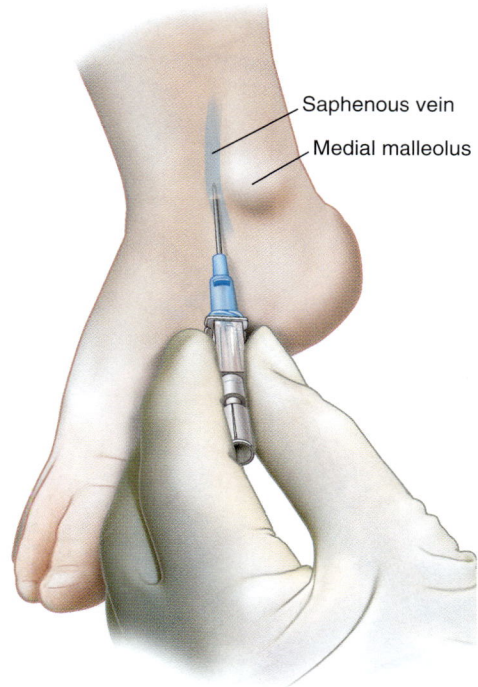

Saphenous vein
Medial malleolus

FIGURE 49.1 Long saphenous vein cannulation.

- To infuse drugs and fluids that are sclerosing to peripheral veins (e.g., antibiotics, vasoactive drugs, or hyperalimentation fluids).
- To access blood for laboratory sampling.
- To measure mixed venous acid-base balance, to estimate cardiac output (Fick principle) or measure cardiac output (dye dilution).
- To aspirate air emboli from the heart.

The common sites for central venous cannulation are the external and internal jugular veins, the subclavian and brachiocephalic veins, the femoral vein in infants and children, and the umbilical vein in neonates. Approaches such as the internal jugular and subclavian veins should be used with extreme caution in the presence of a bleeding diathesis as stopping bleeding may be difficult. The percutaneous approach to central venous cannulation is most successful using a modified Seldinger technique (Fig. 49.2).[53,54] The advantages of this technique are that it avoids the need for a cutdown, only one venipuncture is made with a thin-walled, small-gauge needle, a guidewire directs the catheter within the blood vessel, introducing a large catheter through the small venipuncture site minimizes the chances of significant hematoma formation even after systemic heparinization, and the procedure often can be accomplished when access is required emergently. Whenever a central line is inserted into the heart from above, care must be taken to ensure that the catheter tip is positioned at the junction of the superior vena cava and the right atrium, because other positions have been associated with perforation of large vessels and the myocardium (Fig. 49.3) and with triggering of ventricular arrhythmias.[55]

Ultrasound guidance, pressure waveform analysis, or electrocardiographic guidance may help prevent complications related to central catheter placement.[56,57] Ultrasound-guided access assists successful cannulation of the internal jugular vein,[56] the infraclavicular axillary vein,[57] and the subclavian vein.[58,59] In a meta-analysis of 18 trials with 1646 infants, children, and adults, two-dimensional ultrasound guidance yielded better outcomes than the landmark method.[60] In contrast, a review of 5434 landmark-guided approaches by fully trained anesthesiologists collected over 22 years ($\frac{1}{3}$ < 1 year of age) at 1 institution, 95% of which were internal jugular, reported a 99.5% success rate. Success also depended on experience and the child's age: the success rate was less in junior faculty and smaller children.[61] The greatest benefit with ultrasound was to cannulate the internal jugular vein rather than the subclavian or femoral veins.[60] See Chapter 43 and Videos 49.1 and 49.2 for ultrasound-guided techniques.

TABLE 49.1	Comparison of Intravenous Safety Mechanisms						
Safety Mechanism	Operator Activation Required	Syringe Attachment	Rapid Flash	Bulky	Advantages	Disadvantages	Devices (Manufacturers)
Retractable needle	Yes	No	Yes	Yes	Unobstructed and rapid blood flash; Similarity in use to non-safety devices	Bulky; Requires operator activation; No syringe attachment	Angiocath Autoguard (Becton Dickinson Medical, Franklin Lakes, NJ); Secure IV (Span America Medical Systems, Inc., Greenville, SC)
Blunted needle	No	Yes	No	No	Passive action requiring no operator activation; Syringe attachment possible	Slow blood flash if needle has been partially withdrawn	Introcan Safety IV; Protectiv and Acuvance (Smiths Medical, Kent, UK)

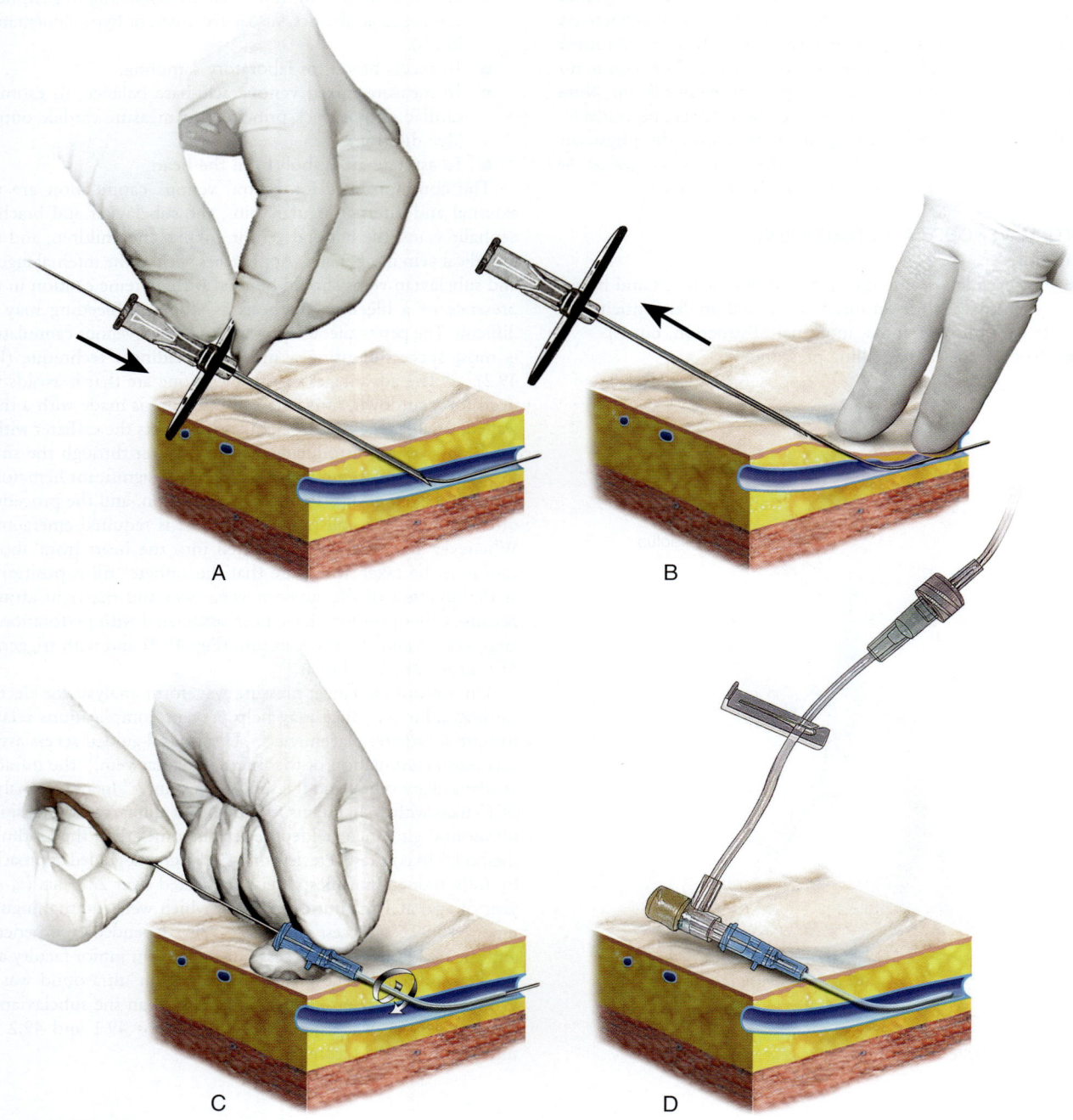

FIGURE 49.2 A, Seldinger technique for catheter placement. The needle is inserted into the target vessel, and the flexible end of the guidewire is passed freely into the vessel. **B,** The needle is then removed, leaving the guidewire in place. **C,** The catheter is advanced with a twisting motion into the vessel. **D,** The wire is removed, and the catheter is connected to an appropriate infusion or monitoring device. (Redrawn with permission from Schwartz AJ, Coté CJ, Jobes DR, et al. Central venous catheterization in pediatrics. Scientific exhibit, American Society of Anesthesiologists, New Orleans, 1977.)

Complications

Pneumothorax, arrhythmia, hematoma, bleeding, infection, thrombosis, inadvertent arterial puncture, cardiac tamponade, air embolus, thoracic duct injury, and malposition are all possible complications associated with central venous cannulation. Data in adults suggest that the smallest catheter and placement from the left subclavian approach may have the least complication rate; similar studies have not been conducted in children.[62] The infection rate reported after 1056 central venous catheters were inserted into 289 children with burn injury varied from 2.0% to 7.3% for catheters in place for less than 11 days, but that rate increased dramatically to 15.8% to 37.5% for catheters left in

49

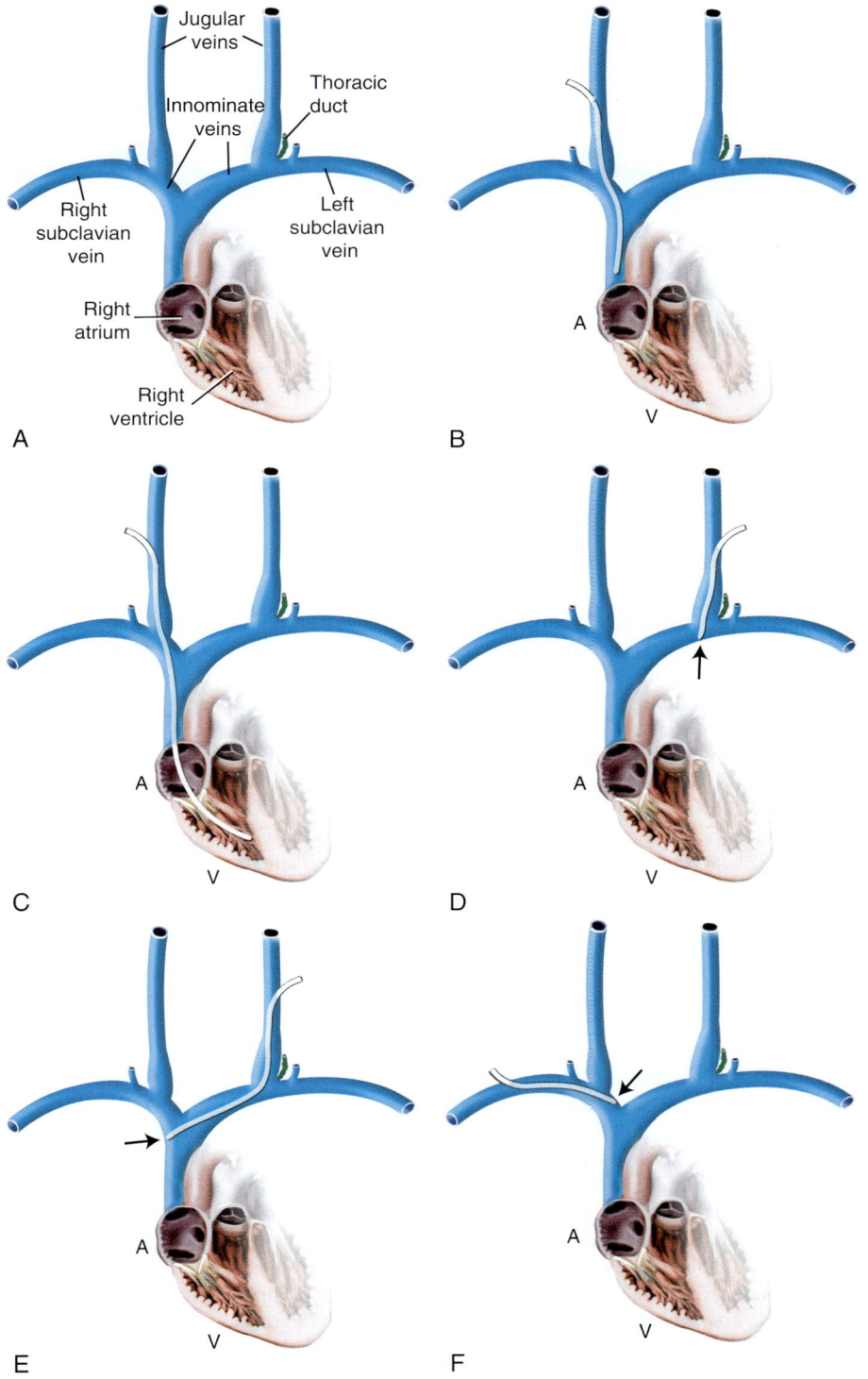

FIGURE 49.3 Proper and improper central venous pressure catheter placement. **A,** Normal vascular anatomy. **B,** Proper location for right internal jugular catheter (i.e., high right atrium or superior vena cava). **C,** Ventricular location of any catheter is dangerous and contraindicated. **D,** A short left-sided internal jugular catheter may erode through the innominate vein (*arrow*). **E,** A left-sided internal jugular catheter striking the lateral wall of the superior vena cava (*arrow*) may erode through it and must be partially withdrawn or advanced. **F,** A short right subclavian catheter may strike the lateral wall of the innominate vein (*arrow*) and erode through it; this catheter should be advanced or withdrawn.   *Continued*

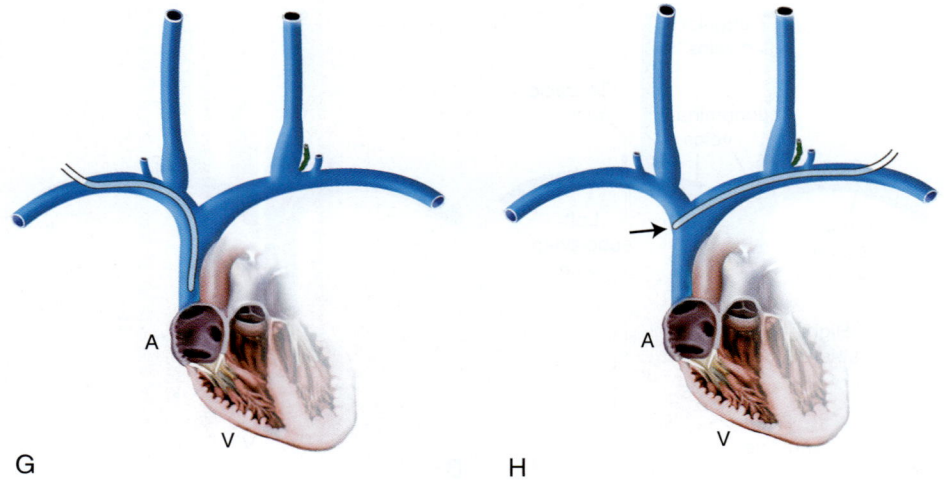

G   H

FIGURE 49.3, cont'd G, Proper location for a right subclavian line. **H,** A short left subclavian line may erode through the superior vena cava (*arrow*); this catheter should be advanced or withdrawn. *A*, atrium; *V*, ventricle.

place for 12 to 14 days.[63] A randomized study that compared the success rate of insertion of the internal jugular versus subclavian approach in 280 pediatric cardiac surgical patients found a similar success rate with the two approaches, although the incidence of positive catheter tip culture results (22% vs. 3.4%) and bloodstream infection (6.9% vs. 0%) were greater with the internal jugular approach.[64] The first attempt success rates were similar with the two approaches (64% vs. 69%). However, the rate of arterial puncture was greater in the internal jugular group (8% vs. 2%) but success rate overall (91% vs. 82%) was greater in the subclavian group. The frequency of catheter malpositions was greater with the subclavian route (17% vs. 1%). In a separate study, catheter-associated bloodborne infections diminished dramatically after initiation of a rigorous hand hygiene program.[65]

Aseptic Technique

Contamination of catheters during insertion may result in catheter colonization or bacterial infection. Evidence suggests that the use of maximum barrier precautions during placement, including the use of sterile gloves, long-sleeved gowns, full-size drapes, and a nonsterile mask and cap, decrease the risk of catheter-related infection.[33,35,66,67] The efficacy of chlorhexidine versus povidone-iodine for preventing bacteremia remains unclear, and the safety of chlorhexidine in infants and children has not been fully established.[68] For older infants and children, chlorhexidine may be safe and effective, but it can cause severe local contact dermatitis in low-birth-weight infants[69,70]; its use in older children has been shown to reduce the incidence of catheter-associated infection compared with povidone-iodine.[71,72] In a case-controlled, prospective, active surveillance study in a pediatric intensive care unit (ICU), independent risk factors for central line–associated bloodstream infection were the duration of central venous catheterization in the ICU, nonoperative cardiovascular disease, gastrostomy tube, parenteral nutrition, central line placement in the ICU, and red blood cell transfusion.[73]

External Jugular Vein Catheterization

1. Place the child in the Trendelenburg position with the head turned 45 degrees away from the side of cannulation.

2. Place a pillow or rolled sheet under the shoulders to extend the head and allow complete access to the neck.
3. Under aseptic conditions, venipuncture and catheter insertion are completed according to the techniques shown in Fig. 49.2. A J-wire is usually more useful to circumvent the plexus of veins at the clavicle.[74,75]
4. Suture or tape appropriately and cover with an occlusive dressing. Many catheters will not pass beyond the clavicle or will pass into the axillary vein; success is generally more often attained on the right side.[76,77] If a shorter catheter is used, infusion and pressure monitoring are very dependent on the position of the head.[78] Continuous free-flowing infusion is best maintained when the head is turned away from the side of catheter insertion. This vein is particularly valuable in children with difficult peripheral venous access and in an emergent situation that suddenly develops intraoperatively that requires establishment of additional IV access.

Internal Jugular Vein Catheterization

Numerous approaches and techniques are used for internal jugular vein cannulation.[79–82] A high approach using the apex of a triangle formed by the two bellies of the sternocleidomastoid muscle and the clavicle may be used as a landmark for insertion (Fig. 49.4). With the use of the Seldinger technique, the success rate, even in neonates, approaches 75% on the first attempt and 90% to 95% on the second attempt.[53] Cannulation of the right side virtually ensures a central location because the internal jugular vein, the superior vena cava, and the right atrium are in a straight line (see Fig. 49.4). Left-sided cannulation risks injury to the thoracic duct and possible pneumothorax because the apex of the lung is more cephalad on the left. In addition, if the catheter inserted on the left is too short, it is not unusual for the tip to rest against the wall of the superior vena cava, be position dependent, and possibly erode through the wall of the vessel. Fig. 49.3 illustrates desirable and less desirable sites for catheter tips that may avoid or result in perforation. The principal advantage of the high approach is that the most common complication (arterial puncture, approximately 10%) is easily recognized and usually treated uneventfully.

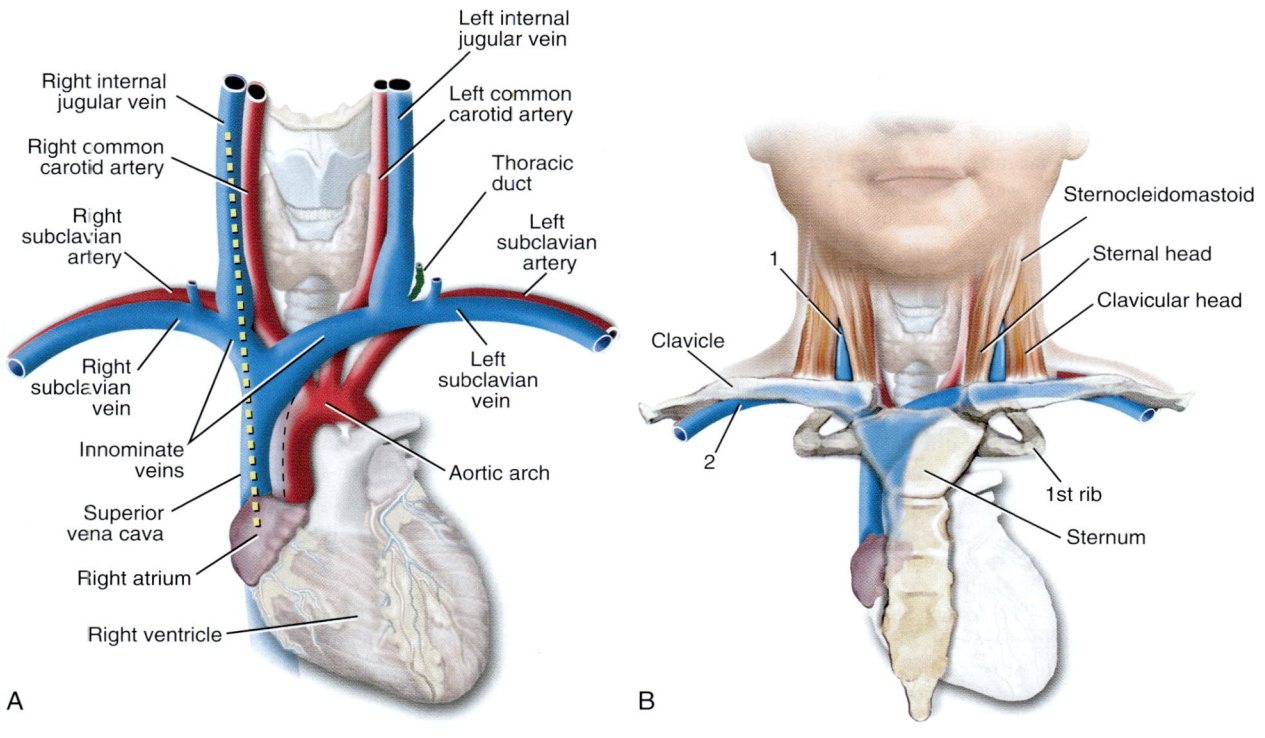

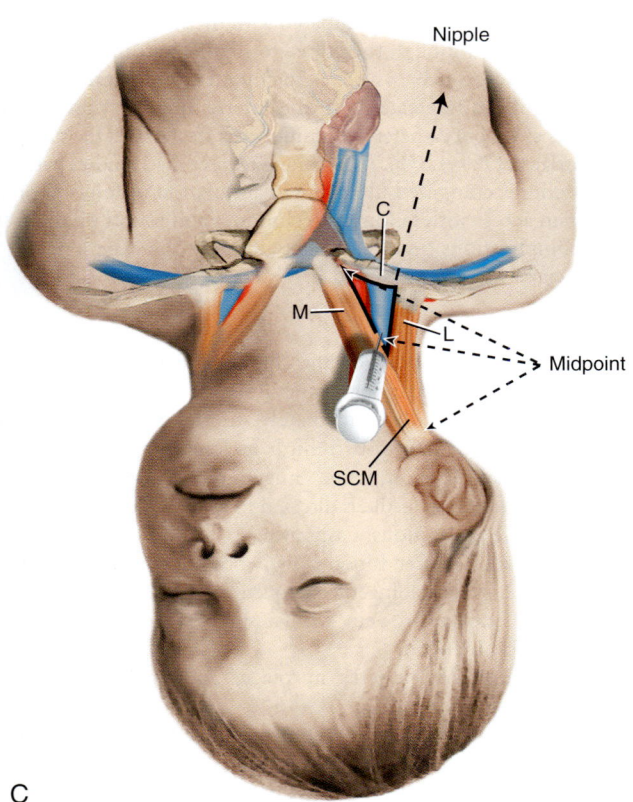

FIGURE 49.4 **A,** The anatomic relationships of major chest and neck structures. Note how the internal jugular vein is in close proximity to the carotid artery. Also, note that a nearly straight line is formed by the internal jugular vein, innominate vein, superior vena cava, and right atrium (*yellow dashed line*); thus it is rare for a right internal jugular catheter to migrate anywhere but to the right atrium. **B,** The relationship of external anatomic landmarks to the anatomy illustrated in **A**. Note the triangle formed by the two bellies of the sternocleidomastoid muscle and the clavicle. *1,* The preferred point of needle insertion at the apex of this triangle for internal jugular vein puncture. *2,* The point of needle insertion for subclavian vein puncture. **C,** The anatomic landmarks as they would appear to an anesthesiologist. The needle is introduced at the apex of the triangle outlined in **C** and is directed at an angle of 30 degrees to the skin toward the ipsilateral nipple. This point of entry is generally half the distance between the mastoid process and the sternal notch. *C,* clavicle; *M* and *L,* medial and lateral bellies of the sternocleidomastoid muscle (*SCM*).

In one study, the effects of a simulated Valsalva maneuver (positive inspiratory pressure of 25 mm Hg for 10 seconds), liver compression, and Trendelenburg position individually or in combination on the cross-sectional area of the right internal jugular vein were studied. The mean increase in cross-sectional area of the right internal jugular vein was maximized at 17.4% ± 16.1% from baseline when all three maneuvers were combined.[83] The magnitude of this maneuver varied with the age of the child: the effect was greatest in children 1 to 6 years of age and clinically negligible in infants younger than 12 months of age. The effect on ease of catheter placement was not investigated, but a larger-sized vessel should improve the success rate.[83] For neonates, a study using skin traction in infants weighing less than 5 kg showed that a technique using tape for skin traction combined with ultrasound guidance increased internal jugular cross-sectional area and decreased the time to place the catheter.[84-86]

Technique

1. Position the child as for external jugular vein cannulation but with a rolled towel under the center of the back to allow the head to be slightly extended (see Fig. 49.3 and Videos 49.1 and 49.2 for positioning and the use of ultrasound to guide insertion). The head is turned slightly away from the side of insertion; *turning the head too far to the side may compress the vein and move the vein in closer proximity to the carotid artery.*

2. Locate the apex of a triangle formed by the two bellies of the sternocleidomastoid muscle. This point is usually where the external jugular vein crosses the sternocleidomastoid muscle or the midpoint between the mastoid process and the sternal notch.

3. Palpate the carotid artery. Introduce the needle just lateral to this artery at an angle of 30 degrees to the skin surface. If the internal jugular vein is superficial, a less acute angle may be indicated. While continuously aspirating, advance the needle toward the ipsilateral nipple a distance of no more than 2.5 cm. If no blood is freely obtained, slowly withdraw the needle while maintaining aspiration. The needle can compress the vessel on entry, and it straightens during withdrawal, allowing free aspiration of blood.

4. Once venipuncture is accomplished, carefully remove the syringe and occlude the end of the needle (to prevent entraining air if the child is breathing spontaneously) until a flexible guidewire is inserted (see Fig. 49.2).[54] The wire should advance easily. However, if the wire cannot be advanced, the needle has passed out of the vessel lumen or its tip rests against the vessel wall. In this situation, the wire and needle should be withdrawn simultaneously to avoid shearing the wire. If the wire passes without difficulty, then cannulation proceeds as demonstrated in Figs. 49.2 and 49.4. The location of the catheter tip should be confirmed with a radiologic study and optimally repositioned as necessary (see Fig. 49.3).

5. Suture the catheter in place, and protect the area with an occlusive dressing.

Contraindications

- A bleeding diathesis (relative contraindication); in life-threatening emergencies, the benefit may outweigh the risk.
- Contralateral pneumothorax.
- Increased intracranial pressure (Trendelenburg position and venous occlusion by the catheter may increase intracranial

pressure); this is a relative contraindication and ultrasound-guided insertion may provide a great advantage because Trendelenburg position may not be required.
- Aberrant vessels (e.g., cervical aortic arch).

Subclavian Vein Catheterization

The subclavian vein is a site frequently used for central vein cannulation.[87,88] Success rates greater than 80% have been reported even in neonates.[89-91] The advantages include fixed landmarks, ease of securing the line to children for long-term management, and patient comfort. Disadvantages include pneumothorax and hemothorax.[92,93] If this site is chosen, we suggest obtaining a chest radiograph after the catheter is inserted and before surgery begins to preclude an unrecognized intraoperative tension pneumothorax. The use of the Seldinger technique (our preference) may reduce the incidence of damage to intrathoracic structures compared with other techniques. As with left-sided internal jugular vein cannulation, if a left subclavian catheter tip rests against the wall of the superior vena cava, it can erode through, resulting in hemothorax or hydrothorax (see Fig. 49.3H). In a comparison of neutral versus lowered shoulder position in 361 adult patients, neutral position significantly reduced the incidence of misplacement of the catheter tip (ipsilateral internal jugular or brachiocephalic vein) with no difference in the rate of arterial puncture or pneumothorax.[94] This maneuver remains to be tested in children. As described earlier, the jugular approach was associated with a greater incidence of positive catheter tip culture results (22% vs. 3.4%) and bloodstream infection (6.9% vs. 0%) compared with the subclavian approach.[64] Importantly, although there was no significant difference in first-attempt success (64% vs. 69%), the frequency of arterial punctures was significantly greater with the internal jugular vein approach (8% vs. 2 %), but catheter malposition was greater with the subclavian approach (17% vs. 1%). A Cochrane review of 13 studies with 2360 procedures compared ultrasound cannulation of femoral or subclavian access with landmark techniques and found no difference in complications or success rate, although the experience of the clinicians was not examined.[95]

Technique

1. Prepare and position the child as previously described for external jugular vein puncture.

2. Insert a needle immediately inferior to the clavicle at a point one-half to two-thirds its length from the sternoclavicular junction; while "hugging" the undersurface of the clavicle, the needle is directed toward the suprasternal notch while continuously aspirating.

3. As soon as free blood flow is obtained, proceed as in Fig. 49.2. If the Seldinger technique is not used, then first locating the subclavian vein with a small-gauge finder needle is recommended.

4. Suture the catheter in place, and apply an occlusive dressing.

If the child's ventilation is controlled, the risk of pneumothorax may be decreased by momentarily ceasing ventilation so that the apex of the lung is away from the needle tip while probing for the subclavian vein. Once successful venipuncture has been achieved, maintaining positive end-expiratory pressure reduces the possibility of air embolism. Optimal depths for right subclavian catheterization have been studied in infants 2 to 5 kg using transesophageal echocardiography and were found to be 40 to 55 mm for catheter tip placement at the junction of the superior vena cava and the right atrium.[96] Contraindications are the same as for internal jugular vein catheterization (see Video 49.1 for illustration of technique).

Brachiocephalic Vein Catheterization

The brachiocephalic vein offers the advantage of being far removed from the intrathoracic structures.[97] The main disadvantage is that a significant number of catheters introduced at this site do not pass centrally—that is, they are caught in the axilla or pass up the jugular vein (internal or external).[98-100] Other disadvantages include significant catheter migration with movement of the arm and possibly an increased incidence of infection. This approach is commonly used by radiologists and pediatric nurses for placement of peripherally inserted central catheters (PICCs), which can be used on a long-term basis.[101-103] These catheters often markedly improve patient care and the quality of life for the child because of the reduced need for peripheral venous access and the reduced number of venipunctures for blood testing. One study examined an ultrasound supraclavicular approach in infants weighing 0.7 to 10 kg; they had a 98.9% success rate with more punctures needed on the right than the left.[104] The routine use of heparin to prevent catheter thrombosis and occlusion is not supported by published studies, but the data are inadequate to reach a conclusion one way or the other.[105]

Technique

1. Prepare and drape the arm with aseptic technique.
2. Cannulate the brachiocephalic vein either by using the modified Seldinger technique (special long catheters and wires for this purpose) or by passing a catheter through a needle (Intracath CVC Catheter, Argon Medical, Plano, Texas). If the catheter cannot be threaded once the vein is entered, initiating rapid IV fluid administration, cephalad positioning of the arm, and anterior displacement of the shoulder may assist advancement. If percutaneous techniques are not possible, direct venous cutdown may be performed.

Femoral Vein Catheterization

The femoral vein may also be used for access to the central circulation.[106] When trainees placed such lines, the ultrasound approach was superior to the palpation/landmark approach,[107] although in more experienced hands, ultrasound did not improve the success rate.[95] The catheter must pass into the thorax to provide accurate measurements of the cardiac filling pressures. Nonetheless, there is a reasonable correlation with central filling pressures even when the catheter tip rests within the abdomen.[108] Occasionally, the catheter is inadvertently advanced into a vertebral vein; this can be confirmed with a lateral radiograph. One advantage of this route is that the vein is large and presents easy access distant from the vital intrathoracic structures (Fig. 49.5). Disadvantages include difficulty in securing the catheter to the child, kinking of the catheter with leg flexion, and problems in maintaining insertion site sterility. Short-term catheterization can provide large-bore venous access for the duration of a procedure with expected large and rapid blood loss if other veins are not accessible. Surprisingly, this site is not associated with a greater incidence of catheter-related sepsis compared with other insertion sites.[63,109] This site is not appropriate if disruption of inferior vena cava blood flow is possible (e.g., Wilms tumor resection with invasion of the inferior vena cava, abdominal trauma). The tip of the catheter should be located either low in the atrium or inferior to the level of the diaphragm but superior to the level of the renal veins to reduce the potential for renal vein thrombosis. Use of this technique also has been reported

to be safe in infants weighing less than 1000 g with the caution of careful catheter advancement to avoid cardiac perforation.[110]

Technique

1. Prepare and drape the groin using an aseptic technique with the legs at 90-degree angles ("frog-leg position") (see Fig. 49.5B). Place a roll under the hips, thereby slightly elevating the hip, to provide optimal conditions
2. Palpate the femoral artery at a point midway between the pubic tubercle and the anterior superior iliac spine (see Fig. 49.5, A).

   Using the Seldinger technique, enter the vein at a point just medial to the femoral artery and 1 to 2 cm below the inguinal ligament. Insert a catheter as in Fig. 49.2. As for the brachiocephalic vein, special long catheters and wires are needed to achieve a central location (see Video 49.2). As with many vascular access methods, ultrasound guidance can be quite useful.[107,111-113]
3. Protect the catheter insertion site as previously described (see discussion of internal jugular vein catheterization). If an alternative technique is used (e.g., catheter through the needle), maintain compression of the cannulation site until hemostasis is ensured. The saphenous vein may be cannulated by direct venous cutdown at its junction with the femoral vein if percutaneous techniques are unsuccessful.

INTRAOSSEOUS INFUSION

The administration of IV fluid into the medullary cavity of long bones is a proven method for volume resuscitation in a hypovolemic child and even in teenagers.[114-121] This method can effectively deliver drugs to the central circulation as quickly as using peripheral IV infusion sites.[122] It is a particularly valuable emergency route of drug administration, even in the hands of emergency medical technicians[123-125] and as part of emergency department resuscitation of pediatric trauma patients.[118,126] Complications such as cellulitis, abscess, fractures, and osteomyelitis have been reported in less than 1% of cases, and this technique does not appear to affect later growth of the tibia with proper insertion technique,[127-129] but the time required for bone healing is unknown.[130] Compartment syndrome may occur if the needle is misplaced. These complications relate in part to duration of infusion, underlying medical conditions, and aseptic technique. The major difficulties with this technique are due to failure to adhere to proper landmarks[131] and bending and clotting of the needle. This technique is used in an emergency situation if several attempts at peripheral or central venous cannulation have failed (suggested "if you cannot achieve reliable access quickly," which generally means after three attempts or 90 seconds).[132,133] Sites for insertion include the upper medial tibia just below the tibial tuberosity, the lower medial tibia just superior to the medial malleolus (to avoid growth plates), the lower femur, and the anterior iliac crest. Intraosseous infusions are discontinued once an alternative IV infusion site has been secured. This technique has been successfully used for resuscitation of burn victims.[134,135] Intraosseous devices should not be used in a fractured leg. For the most recent, complete information, please refer to a review directed to the anesthesiologist caring for pediatric patients.[136]

Technique

1. Palpate the tibial tuberosity.
2. Locate a point on the medial surface of the tibia at least 1 to 2 cm below and medial to the tibial tuberosity for the

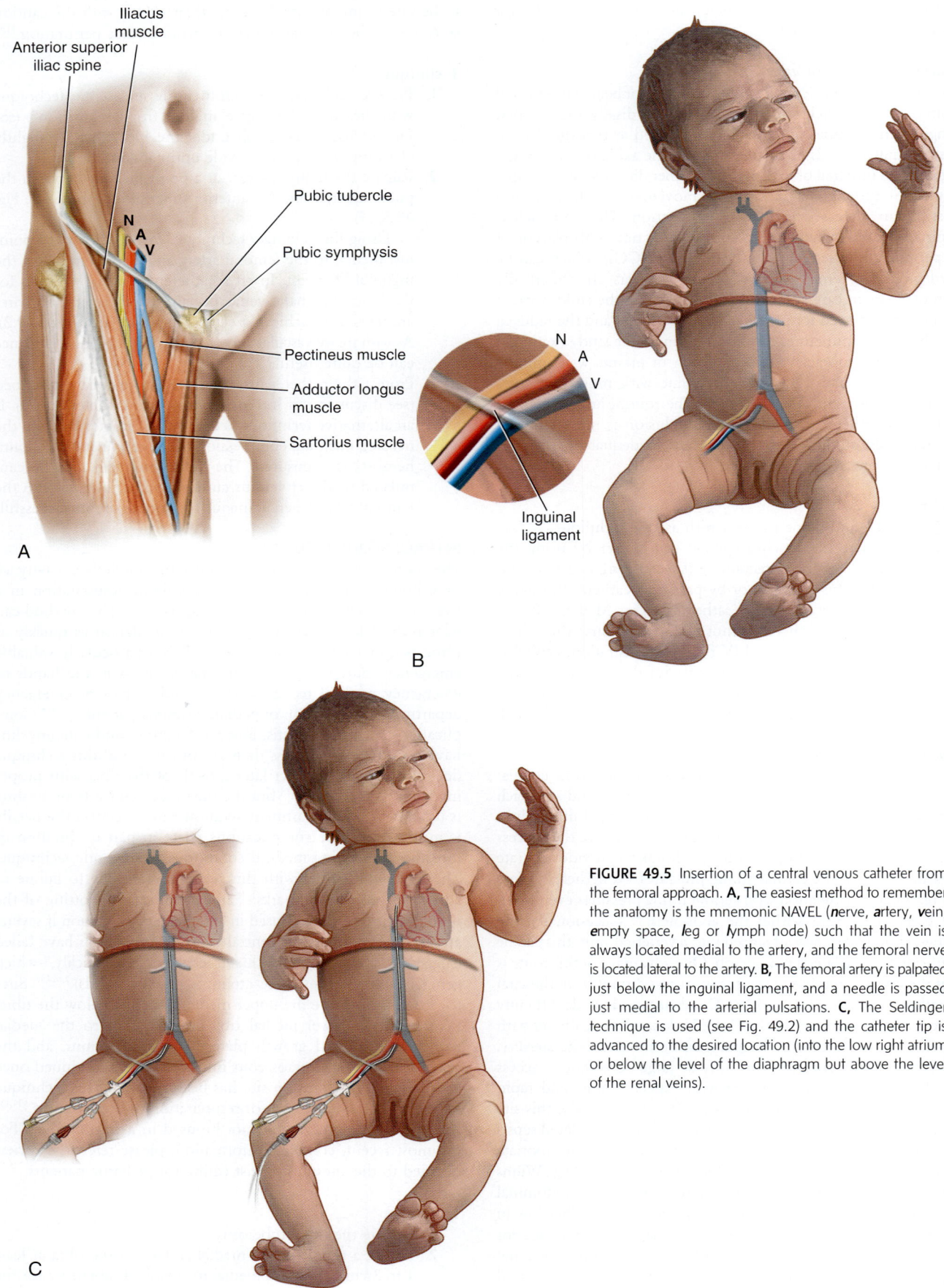

FIGURE 49.5 Insertion of a central venous catheter from the femoral approach. **A,** The easiest method to remember the anatomy is the mnemonic NAVEL (*n*erve, *a*rtery, *v*ein, *e*mpty space, *l*eg or *l*ymph node) such that the vein is always located medial to the artery, and the femoral nerve is located lateral to the artery. **B,** The femoral artery is palpated just below the inguinal ligament, and a needle is passed just medial to the arterial pulsations. **C,** The Seldinger technique is used (see Fig. 49.2) and the catheter tip is advanced to the desired location (into the low right atrium or below the level of the diaphragm but above the level of the renal veins).

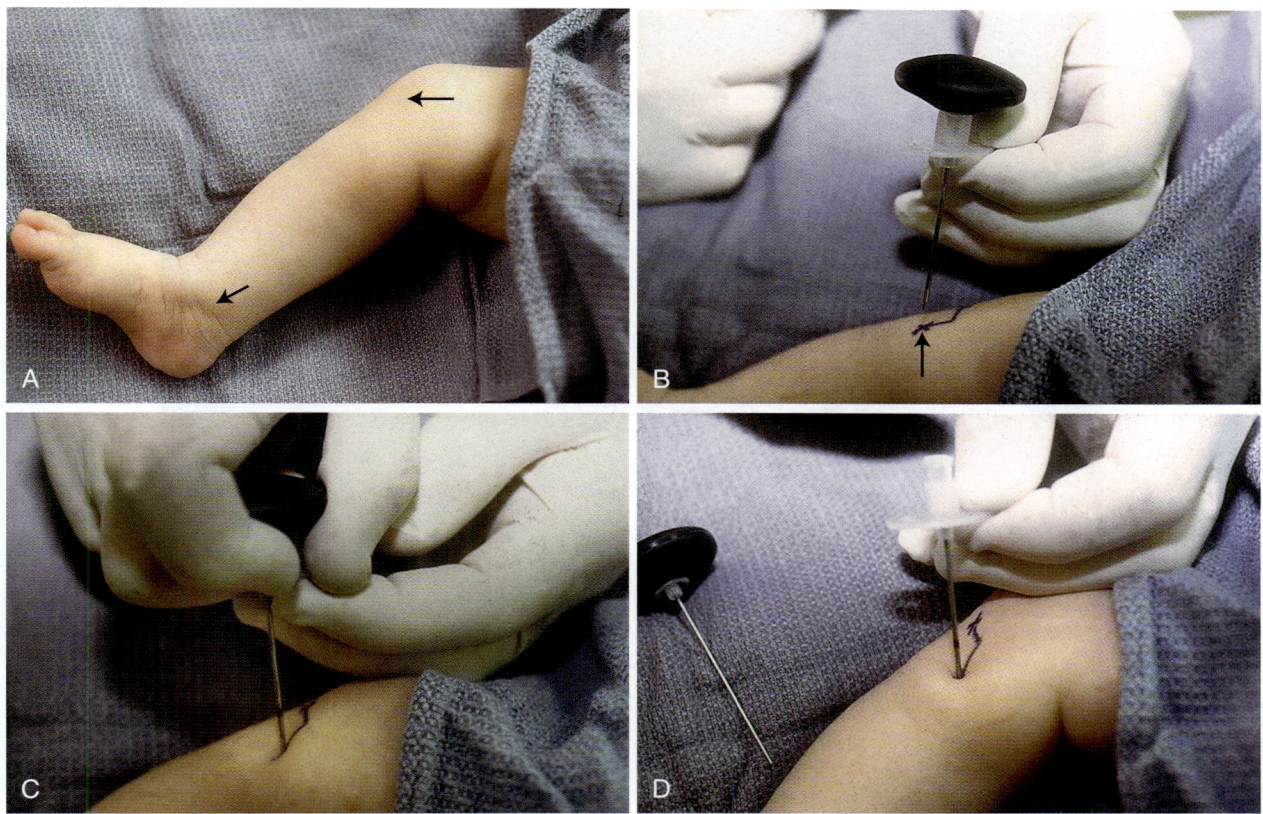

FIGURE 49.6 A, The intraosseous needle may be inserted in either of two locations: at a point 1 to 2 cm below and medial to the tibial tuberosity or at the medial malleolus *(arrows)*. **B** and **C,** The leg is prepared, and the intraosseous needle punctures the skin (note the *X mark (arrow)* connecting the tibial tuberosity with the point of needle insertion); the needle is advanced with a twisting motion in a caudal direction. **D,** The stylet is removed, and the selected solution is infused.

site of needle puncture, because the mantle of the tibia is thin at this location (Fig. 49.6A).

3. Use a special short needle with a stylet to puncture the mantle of the tibia at a 75-degree angle directed toward the feet to avoid the epiphyseal plate (see Fig. 49.6B and C). A styleted spinal needle also may be used.
4. The appropriate position is readily achieved with the loss of resistance; take care to avoid advancing the needle too far (i.e., out the opposite side or against the opposite mantle of the tibia). The needle is usually quite stable if properly positioned.
5. Attach standard IV infusion equipment. Fluid should flow freely without extravasation (see Fig. 49.6D).

A mechanical handheld, battery-powered intraosseous needle insertion device that works much like an electric drill (Fig. 49.7) is the EZ-IO (Teleflex Medical Inc., Research Triangle Park, NC). Several sizes of intraosseous needles (depth of insertion) are available to limit the depth of insertion (determined by patient weight); we recommend that this device be immediately available in all operating rooms[137] and prenatal ICUs because this is the simplest and easiest means for establishing emergent intraosseous access (even in out of hospital venues).[138-143] The specially designed IV fluid low-profile adapter (already primed with IV fluid) is then attached to the sheath, providing clear access for drugs, fluid, or blood administration.

UMBILICAL VEIN CATHETERIZATION
Indications
The umbilical vein provides convenient access to the central circulation of a neonate to restore blood volume and to administer glucose and drugs. This procedure is often carried out blindly with later radiographic confirmation of correct position. A large fraction of catheters are initially malpositioned, which if unrecognized, can lead to life-threatening complications.[144-148] Monitoring changes in the ECG may be helpful (see further). A change in the configuration of the electrocardiogram (ECG) suggests that a small QRS complex reflects catheter position below the diaphragm; a normal-sized QRS complex with a small P wave was associated with location within the inferior vena cava at the thoracic level; and the appearance of a tall P wave indicated positioning within the right atrium.[144] Umbilical vein catheterization also provides a route for the procedure of exchange transfusion and for measuring central venous pressure.

Equipment
- Umbilical artery catheter sizes 3.5F and 5F
- Scalpel and blade
- Fine-curved forceps
- Mosquito hemostats
- Umbilical tape
- Scissors
- Sutures with needle (3-0 silk)

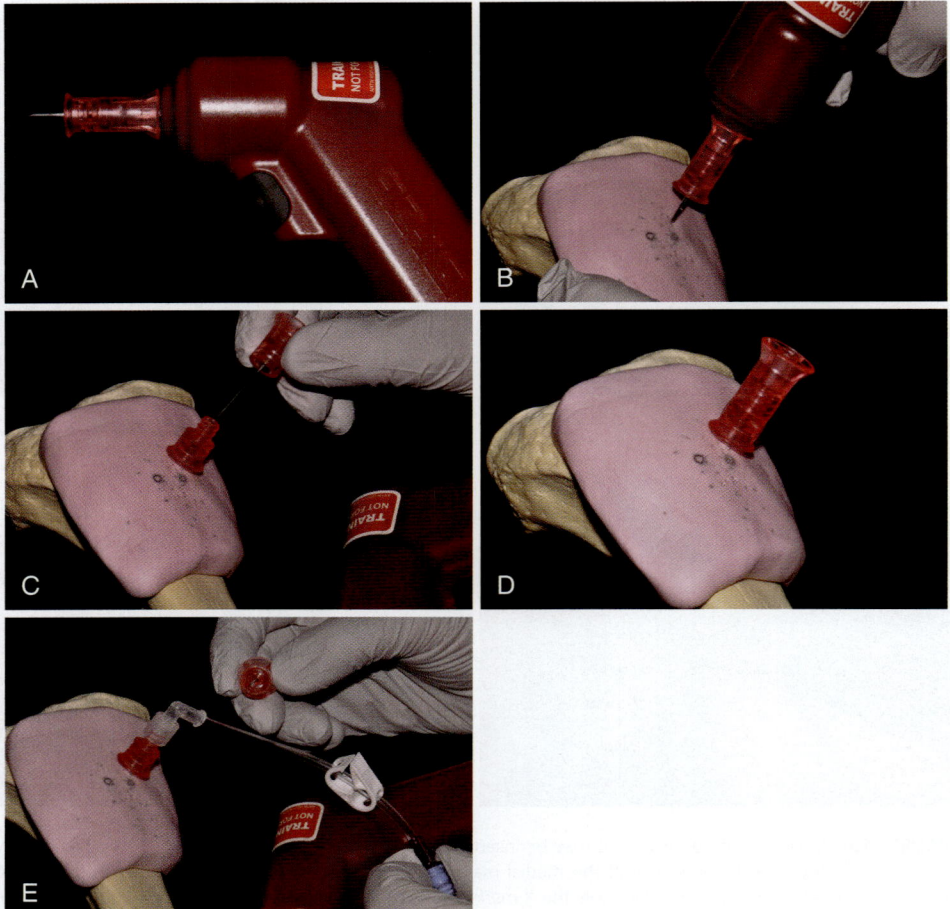

FIGURE 49.7 A, The EZ-IO (Teleflex Medical Inc., Research Triangle Park, NC) is a battery-powered intraosseous needle insertion device that works much like an electric drill. **B,** After appropriate preparation of the skin, at a point 1 to 2 cm below and medial to the tibial tuberosity, the intraosseous needle is directed down and away from the epiphyseal plate. **C,** After successful insertion of the needle and its sheath, the needle is removed, leaving the tip of the metal sheath lodged within the bone marrow cavity. **D,** The intraosseous system is ready for connection and use. **E,** The specially designed intravenous fluid adapter (already primed with intravenous fluid) is then attached to the sheath, providing clear access for drugs, fluid, or blood administration. (Courtesy Charles J. Coté, MD.)

- Antiseptic solutions (e.g., povidone-iodine and alcohol)
- Three-way stopcocks
- 10-mL syringe
- Sterile drapes
- Infusion solution of 10% dextrose in water, with 1 to 2 units of heparin per milliliter at 1 mL/hour
- Calibrated transducer/monitoring system if used for central venous pressure measurement

Technique

1. Prepare and drape the umbilicus with sterile technique; cut the cord approximately 1 cm above the umbilicus. The umbilical vein orifice is more patulous and thin walled than the two umbilical arteries (Fig. 49.8).
2. Holding the catheter filled with heparinized solution 2 cm from the tip, gently introduce it into the vein. In some situations, forceps can aid in directing the catheter. Traction of the umbilical stump *caudad* may help to advance the catheter (see Fig. 49.8). The catheter is passed a distance

that approximates the length between the umbilical stump and the right atrium. Blood should freely aspirate into a syringe. Inability to withdraw blood may occur if the tip of the catheter is resting against a vessel wall or if a clot is present within the catheter lumen. *It is important that the tip of the catheter be placed in the proper position—that is, at the junction of the inferior vena cava and right atrium.* A radiograph confirms proper catheter position. Monitoring changes in the configuration of the ECG during insertion may allow for a more accurate placement within the right atrium but is limited to neonates with a normal tracing.[144] At times, the catheter may fail to traverse the ductus venosus and become wedged in the liver. This position is potentially dangerous because portal necrosis and subsequent cirrhosis may result should hyperosmolar or sclerosing solutions be injected (calcium, sodium bicarbonate, 25%–50% glucose).[148–150] A low position might be acceptable for short-term use if it is not possible to pass the catheter centrally, but the distance of insertion should

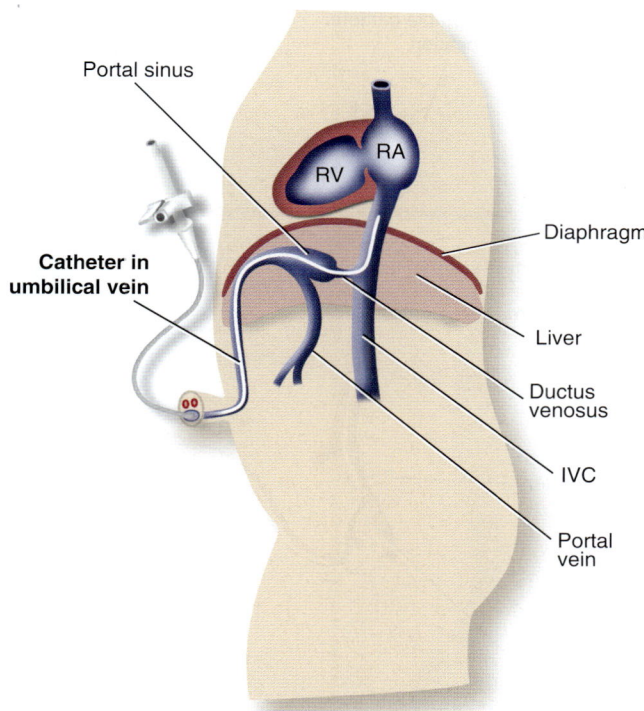

Portal sinus

RA

RV

**Catheter in
umbilical vein**

Diaphragm

Liver

Ductus
venosus

IVC

Portal
vein

FIGURE 49.8 Umbilical vein catheterization. The umbilical vein is thin walled and patulous, whereas umbilical arteries are thicker walled and of smaller diameter. *Caudal* traction on the umbilical stump may facilitate catheter advancement. The catheter should be advanced through the liver into the central circulation within the low right atrium (*RA*) before administration of any medications. *IVC*, Inferior vena cava; *RV*, right ventricle.

be no more than 3 to 4 cm or just until blood is freely aspirated.

3. Suture the catheter in place, cover the insertion site with antibiotic ointment, and tape it to the abdominal wall. The catheter is then connected to a constant-infusion system and should be removed as soon as the indications for its insertion have passed. Complications appear to relate in part to the duration of insertion.[146,148,151]

Complications

- Thrombosis of portal or mesenteric veins[148,152]
- Infection (septicemia)[146]
- Endocarditis
- Pulmonary infarction (misplacement of the catheter into the pulmonary vein through a patent foramen ovale)
- Portal cirrhosis and esophageal varices later in life[153–156]
- Cardiac tamponade[157]
- Liver abscess and subcapsular hematoma[145,158]

Arterial Cannulation

UMBILICAL ARTERY

The umbilical artery in a neonate is a convenient site for monitoring arterial blood pressure, blood gases, and pH. It provides emergency access to an infant's circulation for restoration of blood volume and administration of glucose and drugs.[159–162] Continuous monitoring of arterial O_2 saturation is also possible.[163]

Equipment

The materials used for cannulation are identical to those described for umbilical venous catheterization. Equipment is required for continuous monitoring of blood pressure. *End-hole rather than side-hole catheters may have a smaller incidence of thrombosis or associated ischemic events.*[164]

Technique

1. Prepare and drape the area with sterile technique; cut the umbilical cord approximately 1 cm above the umbilicus. The two umbilical arteries are identified (Fig. 49.9). The cut vessel ends have thicker walls, are smaller than the vein, and are usually in spasm. The artery is entered in the manner described for umbilical vein catheterization, except that *cephalad* traction is applied to the umbilical stump (see Fig. 49.9A) to encourage *caudal* direction of the catheter. The catheter should course through the umbilical artery into the iliohypogastric artery and then into the descending aorta. Proper positioning of the catheter tip is crucial. If the catheter is advanced too far up the aorta, it may pass through the ductus arteriosus and into the pulmonary artery. If this situation is not recognized, blood pressure and blood gas measurements may be misleading. Care should be taken to ensure the placement of the catheter tip in the descending aorta (at T7 to T9). Early reports suggested that a cephalad position, at or above the level of the diaphragm, is easier to maintain but predisposes infants to increased risk of embolization to renal or mesenteric vessels (see Fig. 49.9B).[165–168] However, positioning just above the bifurcation of the descending aorta—that is, at L3 to L5 (see Fig. 49.9A) (below the origin of the renal arteries and visceral branches of the aorta) has not been supported by a Cochrane review; a cephalad position is recommended.[169] The caudad position is difficult to maintain, and the catheter tip may slip into one of the iliac arteries, resulting in tissue ischemia (see Fig. 49.9C).

2. Confirm the position radiographically. Once the catheter is properly positioned, the system is connected to a constant-infusion pump and heparinized fluids (10% dextrose in water or normal saline solution) are infused. Suture and tape the catheter and apply antibiotic ointment as for umbilical vein catheters. A Cochrane review of the use of heparin suggested that low-dose heparinization of the infusate (0.25 unit/mL) reduces the likelihood of catheter occlusion compared with intermittent flushing with heparinized solutions.[170]

Complications

Using the umbilical artery as a source for blood pressure monitoring and blood gas analysis only and reserving alternative sites for glucose and drug administration may minimize complications. Changes in cerebral blood flow are associated with intraventricular hemorrhage and have been documented to occur with umbilical artery blood sampling; fewer changes in cerebral blood flow occur with low-positioned catheters.[171] The incidence of documented intraventricular hemorrhage appears to have a stronger relation with age than with catheter position and is not associated with the use of low-dose heparin.[170,172] The use of an alternate site for monitoring may reduce complications.[173] Other complications are as follows:

- Accidental disconnection of stopcocks and catheters or vessel perforation can lead to potentially dangerous exsanguination.[174]

49

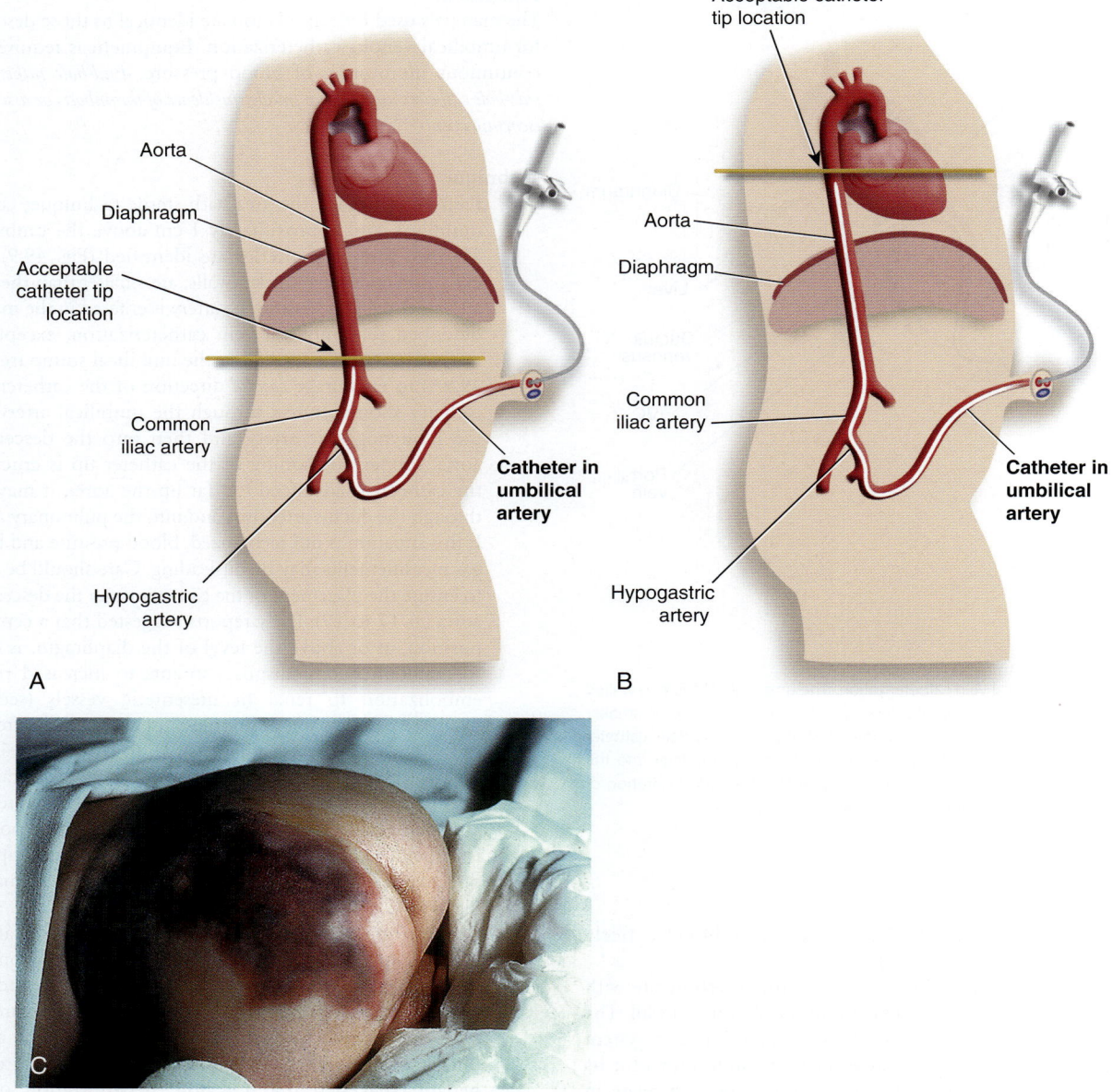

FIGURE 49.9 Umbilical artery catheterization. *Cephalad* traction on the umbilical stump may facilitate catheter advancement. **A,** The catheter tip at L3-4 just above the aortic bifurcation and below the renal arteries is one acceptable location (*arrow to yellow line*). **B,** An alternative acceptable location is in the descending aorta between T7 and T9 (*arrow to yellow line*). **C,** An area of necrosis in the left buttock that resulted from a catheter migrating into the internal iliac vessel, occluding one of its branches.

■ Blood clots may embolize retrograde or, more likely, distally, leading to ischemia or infarction of the infant's gut, kidneys, or lower limbs (see Fig. 49.9C).[175]

■ Vascular spasm is usually transitory and may be resolved by withdrawal of the catheter. Several cases of flaccid paraplegia have been reported resulting from spasm or embolic phenomena.[176]

■ The infant is always at risk for sepsis; therefore clear indications for the insertion of this catheter are mandatory. The catheter should be removed at the earliest possible time. A Cochrane review failed to establish a role for prophylactic antibiotics in reducing catheter-related infections.[177]

■ Hypertension as a result of renal artery emboli may cause ischemia and infarction of the kidney.[168,178]

■ Aortic thrombosis may occur.[179]

RADIAL ARTERY

Radial artery cannulation is a reasonable alternative to umbilical artery cannulation in a neonate and is the primary site of arterial cannulation in infants and children in most pediatric institutions. Percutaneous radial artery cannulation is widely practiced, with minimal morbidity.[146,180–185] The use of ultrasound may improve success rate.[186] Failure to cannulate the artery percutaneously may be followed successfully by direct arterial cutdown. Children with

Down syndrome (trisomy 21) have abnormal radial vessels (both size and location, 16% to 19%), which can make arterial cannulation particularly difficult; some children with Down syndrome have a single median artery.[187,188] The ulnar artery also has been used as an alternative site for arterial catheterization when attempts at insertion in other locations have been unsuccessful; to ensure adequate perfusion of the hand, this site should not be used if previous attempts at cannulation of the ipsilateral radial artery had been attempted.[189]

Indications

Indications for radial artery cannulation include monitoring of arterial blood pressure, arterial blood gases, and pH. The right radial artery is preferred in neonates because it is representative of preductal blood flow.

Technique (Video 49.3)

1. Confirm the adequacy of ulnar artery collateral flow by the modified Allen test (Fig. 49.10A). The color of the hand is noted. The hand is passively clenched, and the radial and ulnar arteries are simultaneously compressed at the wrist (see Fig. 49.10B). The ulnar artery is then released, and flushing (reperfusion) of the blanched hand is noted (see Fig. 49.10C). If the entire hand is well perfused while the radial artery remains occluded, indicating adequate collateral flow, catheterization of the radial artery is performed. Note that the sensitivity of the Allen test is approximately 73%, with a specificity of 97%.[190–192] Many have abandoned the Allen test because of its poor sensitivity as a predictor of ischemia of the hand if the test failed and they simply avoid cannulating the ulnar artery.

2. Secure the hand using an arm board with slight extension of the wrist to avoid excessive median nerve stretching. The fingertips should be left exposed when the hand is taped down so that any peripheral ischemic changes from spasm, clot, or air can be observed.

3. Observe the course of the radial artery in a neonate with the aid of a fiberoptic light source directed toward the lateral side or dorsal aspect of the wrist. Use of a Doppler device or visualization via ultrasound[186] may also be of great value.[193,194]

4. Use a 20-gauge needle to make a small skin puncture over the maximal pulsation of the radial artery, usually at the second proximal wrist crease. This step eases passage of the cannula by reducing resistance offered by the skin and prevents a burr from forming on the catheter tip as it passes through the dermis. A method to avoid accidental puncture of the artery is to pull the overlying skin laterally to make the skin nick.

5. Perform cannulation with a 24- or 22-gauge catheter either on direct entry of the artery at an angle of 15 to 20 degrees or on withdrawing the cannula after transfixion of the artery (Fig. 49.11A to C). A wire (0.018 inch) may be used as an aid to advance 22-gauge and nontapered 24-gauge catheters.

6. Attach the catheter firmly to a T-connector to permit continuous infusion of isotonic saline solution (1 unit/mL) at the rate of 1 to 2 mL/hour via a constant-infusion pump (see Fig. 49.11D). The catheter is securely taped in place. A pressure transducer is connected to allow continuous arterial pressure monitoring. To ensure accurate blood pressure measurement, it is essential that the transducer is calibrated to the neonate's or child's heart level, that all

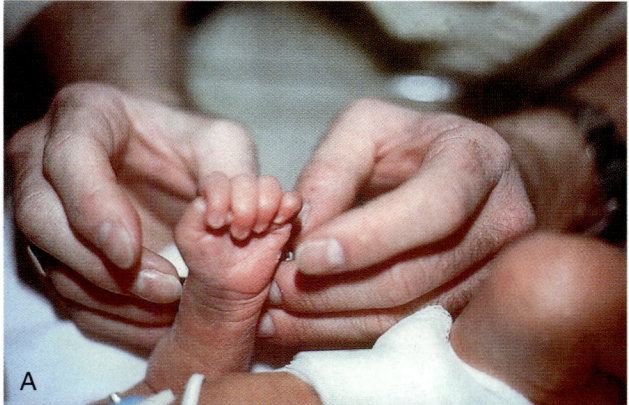

A

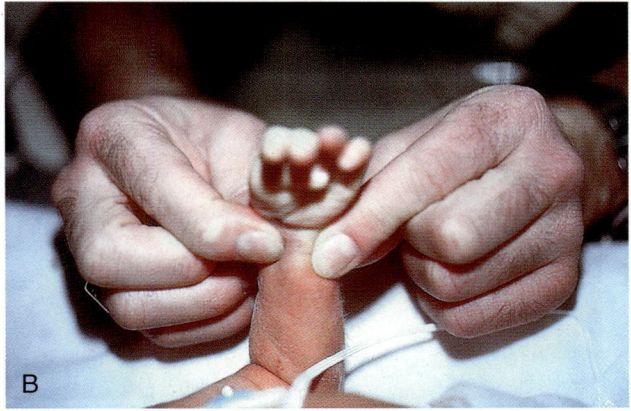

B

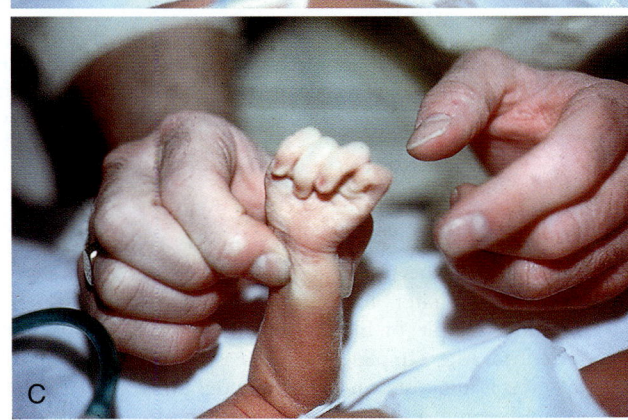

C

FIGURE 49.10 Modified Allen test. **A,** Color and perfusion of the hand are noted. **B,** The hand is first passively clenched, and then both radial and ulnar vessels are occluded. **C,** The ulnar artery is released while the radial artery remains occluded. If flow through the ulnar artery and collateral arch in the hand is adequate, the color and perfusion should rapidly return. If not adequate, then simply do not cannulate the radial artery.

air bubbles are removed from the system, and that no more than 3 feet of tubing is used between the neonate or child and the transducer to minimize artifacts caused by the monitoring tubing.[195]

7. Obtain blood samples by clamping off the distal end of the T-connector, cleaning the injection port of the T-connector with povidone-iodine, introducing a 22-gauge needle, and withdrawing 1 mL of blood. A sample of blood is obtained by heparinized syringe, with minimal blood

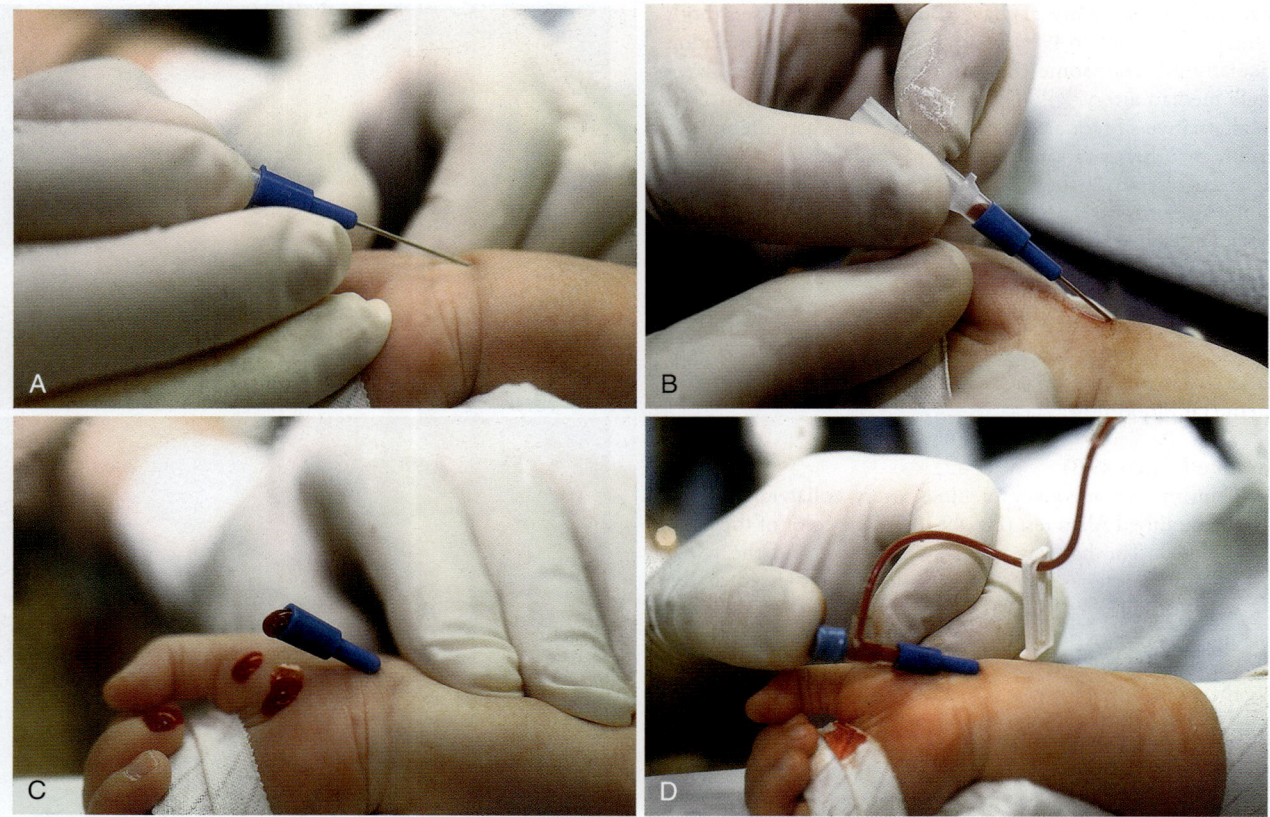

FIGURE 49.11 A, After adequate collateral circulation has been ensured, the radial artery is palpated and the appropriate catheter is advanced into the vessel. **B,** After blood return is noted, the catheter is threaded over the needle and into the artery. **C,** Pulsatile backbleeding confirms intraarterial position. **D,** A T-connector with appropriate flush solution is connected; the catheter is aspirated to clear air bubbles and then gently flushed. Antibiotic ointment and benzoin are applied. The injection port should be clearly marked as "arterial" to minimize accidental drug administration into the artery. A Luer-Lok connection is preferred to prevent accidental disconnection.

loss and minimal manipulation of the system.[180,196] An alternative is the use of a 3-mL syringe on a three-way stopcock: aspirate 2 to 3 mL, clamp the system, and then take the sample of blood from the T-connector as just described. After sampling, the clamp is released, the aspirated blood is readministered, and continuous infusion is resumed or flush is run into the 3-mL syringe and then the system is gently manually flushed intermittently with the syringe but the flush syringe is changed just once per 24 hours. This method of sampling maintains a closed system with reduced potential for sources of infection. Bolus flushes should be very brief or a slow infusion because prolonged flushing in neonates and infants may flush a crystalloid solution retrograde to the brain and cause a stroke. Disastrous results may occur if an air bubble or blood clot should accompany a bolus flush.[197–201] *All arterial lines must be clearly identified (red tape) to avoid accidental infusion of hypertonic solutions and sclerosing medications.*

Complications
- Infection at the site of the catheter insertion, with possible septicemia.
- Arterial thrombus formation. This depends on the size of catheter inserted, the material of which it is constructed, the technique of insertion, and the duration of cannulation.

- Emboli. A blood clot or air may embolize to the digits, resulting in arteriolar spasm or more serious ischemic necrosis.
- Disconnecting the catheter from the infusion system. Blood loss may be life-threatening, especially in an infant.
- Ischemia. The radial artery cannula should be withdrawn if ischemic changes develop.
- Vasospasm. Usually transient but requires careful observation.

The method just described is the traditional percutaneous radial artery cannulation at the ventral aspect of the wrist. The radial artery on the dorsal aspect of the wrist within the anatomic snuff box may be used as an alternative site.[202] Once an attempt at cannulation of the radial artery is made, the ipsilateral ulnar artery should not be instrumented to ensure adequate perfusion of the entire hand. Strict indications for inserting radial artery catheters are necessary, and their removal must be considered at the earliest possible time.[165–168]

AXILLARY ARTERY
Even though axillary arterial cannulation is reported to be used in children as a site when radial or lower extremity access fails, there are few studies specifically related to the risks and benefits of axillary access. In a study of 96 arterial catheters in 56 adult surgical ICU patients, catheter-related infections were increased with prolonged insertion.[203] The infection rate at axillary sites was greater than at the radial and femoral sites. There is only one

publication of axillary arterial monitoring in pediatric patients and it reported no major complications in 16 children.[204] Seven of these patients were neonates with the duration of insertion from 5 to 15 days. There were no differences in systolic blood pressures in either arm after the line was removed or during the time the line was in place. In general, an ultrasound guided technique is highly recommended to minimize damage to surrounding structures (brachial plexus).

TEMPORAL ARTERY

When the radial artery has been previously cannulated or is inaccessible, the temporal artery may be used.[205] Cerebral infarction has been described as a complication of this technique. It appears to be related to retrograde embolization of air or a blood clot.[206] An advantage of this sampling site is that it provides preductal blood gas values. However, in our experience, the tortuous course of the artery and the resultant apposition of the distal tip of the catheter and the arterial wall have caused difficulties in freely drawing blood samples.

FEMORAL ARTERY

Femoral catheterization in infants and children includes a greater risk of vascular injury or thrombosis resulting in ischemia[207] and is not recommended if other peripheral sites are available. In situations in which peripheral arterial cannulation is impossible (e.g., in burned patients, children with poor peripheral perfusion, children with congenital heart disease), the femoral artery should be used rather than not having any invasive arterial monitoring; the remote possibility of a complication must be balanced versus a greater likelihood of life-threatening complications owing to less than ideal monitoring.[208]

Technique

1. Locate the femoral artery by palpation at the groin; this can be confirmed with ultrasonic guidance. Anatomically, it is situated midway between the anterior superior iliac spine and the pubic tubercle (See also Fig. 49.5).
2. After sterile preparation of the skin, insert a catheter of appropriate size into the femoral artery using the Seldinger technique. The artery is entered at the point of maximal pulsation, approximately 1 cm below the line joining the anterior superior iliac spine and the pubic tubercle.
3. After cannulation, connect the catheter to a continuous-flow system and pressure transducer. The catheter is sutured in place, the insertion site is covered, and an occlusive dressing is applied. The possibility of fecal and urinary contamination makes this last step particularly important.

Complications

- Infection
- Emboli of clot and air, leading to ischemic necrosis of the lower limb
- Poor arterial puncture technique, leading to osteoarthritis of the hip joint; severe trauma to the femoral artery has resulted in gangrene of the lower limb, retroperitoneal hemorrhage, and arteriovenous fistula formation.[209–211] Up

to approximately 24% of children will have no resolution of thrombosis and approximately 1% may have partial arrest of bone growth, likely as a result of thrombus formation.[212,213]

- Vasospasm is usually transient but requires careful observation.

DORSALIS PEDIS AND POSTERIOR TIBIAL ARTERY

The dorsalis pedis and posterior tibial arteries are additional sites for arterial cannulation in children when more desirable locations are inaccessible. Collateral circulation should always be checked. Ultrasound guidance may be helpful.[214] If cannulation is attempted or performed in one artery in the foot, the ipsilateral artery should not be instrumented to ensure adequate collateral blood flow.

Technique

The artery is cannulated in the same manner as for the radial artery at a point of maximal pulsation. An understanding of the anatomy of the dorsalis pedis and posterior tibial arteries before attempting this procedure is important. If percutaneous cannulation is impossible, the cutdown technique may be performed. The complications are similar to other arterial line sites of insertion.

ANNOTATED REFERENCES

Camkiran Firat A, Zeyneloglu P, Ozkan M, Pirat A. A randomized controlled comparison of the internal jugular vein and the subclavian vein as access sites for central venous catheterization in pediatric cardiac surgery. *Pediatr Crit Care Med.* 2016;17:e413-e419.

This randomized, prospective study compared the success rate for placement of central venous catheters via the internal jugular route with subclavian routes in 280 children scheduled for cardiac surgery. There was no significant difference in the success rate at first attempt (64% vs. 69%), but the rate of arterial puncture was significantly higher in the internal jugular group (8% vs. 2%) and success rate overall was greater in the subclavian group (91% vs. 82%). However, catheter malposition was greater with the subclavian route (17% vs 1%). Overall, the risk of catheter-associated infection complications was greater with the internal jugular route (22% vs. 3.6%).

Carter JH, Langley JM, Kuhle S, Kirkland S. Risk factors for central venous catheter-associated bloodstream infection in pediatric patients: a cohort study. *Infect Control Hosp Epidemiol.* 2016;37(8):939-945.

This was a within-institution study reviewing their experience from 1995 to 2013 involving 5648 patients that revealed a central line–associated bloodstream infection rate of 3.87/1000 in-hospital line days. Over time there was an 84% reduction in these infections that was primarily related to a vigorous hand hygiene campaign.

Siddik-Sayyid SM, Aouad MT, Ibrahim MH, et al. Femoral arterial cannulation performed by residents: a comparison between ultrasound-guided and palpation technique in infants and children undergoing cardiac surgery. *Paediatr Anaesth.* 2016;26(8):823-830.

This was a randomized prospective study that compared ultrasound-guided with palpation-guided placement of femoral arterial lines in 106 pediatric patients. The number of successful cannulations of first attempt was greater in the ultrasound group (24/5 vs. 13/53), and the time to successful cannulation was also shorter (301 ± 234 seconds ± 420 ± 248 seconds). The ultrasound-guided technique when used by residents was superior to the palpation-guided technique.

A complete reference list can be found online at ExpertConsult.com.

50 Infectious Disease Considerations for the Operating Room

ANDRE L. JAICHENCO AND LUCIANA CAVALCANTI LIMA

THE RABBIT HOLE THAT IS THE PERIOPERATIVE ENVIRONMENT is not well understood by the majority of our general pediatric colleagues. Similarly, the rabbit hole of the primary care clinic or the pediatric inpatient ward is not well understood by the majority of our anesthesiology colleagues. A pediatric patient may repeatedly enter the rabbit hole over the course of a hospital admission, a journey fraught with dangers of airway mishaps, respiratory and/or cardiac arrests, hemorrhage, profound anxiety and stress experienced by the young patient and his or her family, as well as infection risks.[1]

Anesthesiologists have long been patient safety advocates. It is not surprising that anesthesia providers in the 21st century have taken on increasing responsibility for preventing health care–associated infections (HAIs), including surgical site infections (SSIs). Anesthesia providers practice in a nonsterile environment within the operating room (OR) and frequently contact areas of the patient known to have a high rate of contamination such as the axilla, nares, and pharynx. There are two recognized but poorly implemented interventions: preoperative patient skin and other bacterial reservoir decontamination and hand hygiene by anesthesia providers.[2]

Anesthesia providers have an impact on bacterial transmission and infection rates. Specifically, anesthesiologists are known to contaminate their work environment within the OR. Contamination of the work environment includes contamination of intravenous (IV) access ports. Without encouragement, anesthesiologists perform hand hygiene less frequently than once per hour during a case, but with reminders, the rate of hand hygiene is more frequent. Improved hand hygiene reduces contamination of the work area and IV access ports from 32% to 8%, which in turn significantly reduces HAIs.[3,4]

The transmission of infection depends on the presence of three interconnected elements: a causative agent, a source, and a mode of transmission (Fig. 50.1). Understanding the characteristics of each element provides the practicing anesthesiologist with methods to protect susceptible patients and themselves to avoid spreading infection.

There has always been concern about the transmission of infectious agents to the patient from the anesthesiologist and vice versa.[5] In addition, there are many sites within the hospital environment where moist or desiccated organic material with the ability to host potentially pathogenic microbes may survive for extended periods of time (Table 50.1) [6,7]; some may even resist the usual cleaning and disinfection techniques.[8] Their transmission from the source to the host may occur via indirect nonapparent mechanisms (e.g., most commonly through hand contact).

Causative Agent

The infectious vector may be any microorganism capable of causing infection. The pathogenicity is the ability to induce disease, which is characterized by its *virulence* (infection severity, determined by the germ morbidity and mortality rates) and the level of *invasiveness* (capacity to invade tissues). No microorganism is completely avirulent. An organism may have a very low level of virulence, but if the host (i.e., patient or health care provider) is highly susceptible, infection by the organism may cause disease. The risk of infection increases with the *infecting dose* (the number of organisms available to induce disease), the *reservoir* (the site where the organisms reside and multiply), and the *infection source* (the site from where it is transmitted to a susceptible host either directly or indirectly through an intermediary object). The infection source may be a human (e.g., health care providers, children, visitors, housekeeping personnel) with a symptomatic or an asymptomatic infection during the incubation period. The source may also be temporarily or permanently colonized (the most frequently colonized tissues are the skin, digestive, and respiratory tracts).

Host

The presence of a susceptible host is an important element in the chain of infection that paradoxically results from advances in current medical therapies and technology (e.g., children undergoing organ transplantation or chemotherapy, or extremely premature neonates) and the presence of children with diseases that compromise their immune systems (e.g., AIDS, tuberculosis, malnutrition, or burns). The organism may enter the host through the skin, mucous membranes, lungs, gastrointestinal tract, genitourinary tract, or the bloodstream via IV solutions, after laryngoscopy, or from surgical wounds. Organisms may also infect the individual because of work accidents with cutting or piercing devices. The development of

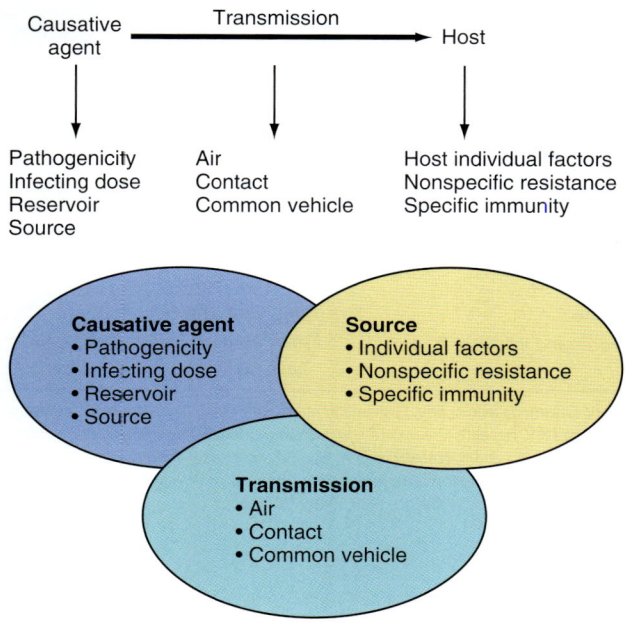

FIGURE 50.1 Elements of the chain of infection.

	TABLE 50.1	Nosocomial Pathogens and Environmental Contamination

Pathogen	Types of Environmental Contamination	Organism Survival Time
Influenza virus	Aerosolization after cleaning; fomites	24–48 hours on nonporous surfaces
Parainfluenza virus	Clothes and nonporous surfaces	10 hours on nonporous surfaces; 6 hours on clothes
Norovirus	Extensive environmental contamination, possible aerosolization	≤14 days on fecal specimens, ≤12 days on carpets
Hepatitis B virus	Environmental contamination with blood	7 days
Coronavirus-SARS	Possible results from emergency department specimens; super-spreading events	24–72 hours on fomites and fecal specimens
Candida	Fomite contamination	3 days for *Candida albicans* and 14 days for *Candida parapsilosis*
Clostridium difficile	Extensive environmental contamination	5 months on hospital floors
Pseudomonas aeruginosa	Drain sink contamination	7 hours on glass slides
Acinetobacter baumannii	Extensive environmental contamination	33 hours on laminated plastic surfaces
MRSA	Extensively contaminated burn units	≤9 weeks after drying; 2 days on laminated plastic surfaces
VRE	Extensive environmental contamination	≤58 days on working surfaces

MRSA, Methicillin-resistant *Staphylococcus aureus; SARS,* severe acute respiratory syndrome; *VRE,* vancomycin-resistant enterococci.
Modified from Hota B. Contamination, disinfection, and cross-colonization: are hospital surfaces reservoirs for nosocomial infection? *Clin Infect Dis.* 2004;39(8):1182–1189.

infection is influenced by the host defense mechanisms that may be classified as either nonspecific or specific:

- *Nonspecific defense mechanisms* include the skin, mucous membranes, secretions, excretions, enzymes, inflammatory responses, genetic factors, hormonal responses, nutritional status, behavior patterns, and the presence of other diseases.
- *Specific defense mechanisms or immunity* may occur because of exposure to an infectious agent (antibody formation) or through placental transfer of antibodies; artificial defenses may be acquired through vaccines, toxoids, or exogenously administered immunoglobulins.

Methods of Transmission

Microorganisms are transmitted in the hospital environment through a number of different routes; the same microorganism may also be transmitted via more than one route. In the OR, the three main routes of transmission are through the air and by direct and indirect contact.

AIR TRANSMISSION

Airborne infections that may infect susceptible hosts are transmitted via two mechanisms: droplets and droplet nuclei.

Droplets

Droplet contamination is considered a direct transmission of organisms because there is a direct transfer of microorganisms from the colonized or infected person to the host. This generally occurs with particles whose diameters are greater than 5 μm that are expelled from an individual's mouth or nose, mainly during sneezing, coughing, talking, or during procedures such as suction, laryngoscopy, and bronchoscopy (Fig. 50.2). Transmission occurs when the microorganism-containing droplets, expelled or shed by the infected person (source), are propelled a short distance (usually not exceeding 60 cm or about 2 feet through the air) and deposited on the host's conjunctivae or oral or nasal mucous membranes. Droplets remain suspended for only a short duration and distance from the source, but this may be affected by temperature, humidity, force of expulsion, and air currents. Larger particle sizes contact the mucosa of the upper airway, whereas aerosols are capable of penetrating into the lower respiratory tract. Infectious agents vary in their affinity for receptors in different regions of the respiratory tract.[9,10] When a person coughs, the exhaled air may reach a speed of up to 965 km/hour (600 mph).[11] However, because the droplets are relatively large, they tend to descend quickly and remain suspended in the air for a very brief period, thus obviating the need for special handling procedures for the OR air. Examples of droplet-borne diseases include influenza, respiratory syncytial virus (RSV), severe acute respiratory syndrome (SARS), diphtheria, *Haemophilus influenzae, Neisseria meningitidis,* mumps, pertussis, rhinovirus, rubella, and Ebola. Droplet precautions include communication of infectious risk

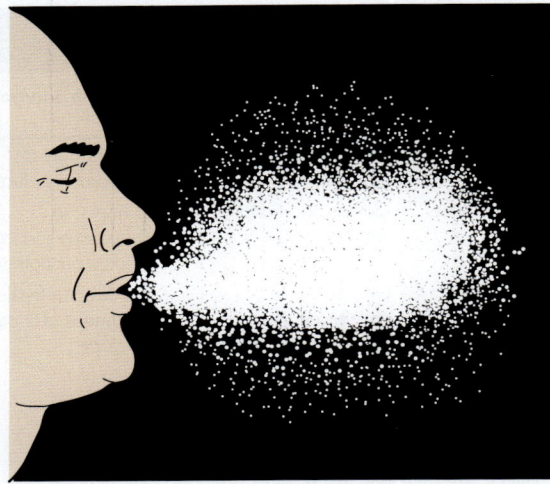

FIGURE 50.2 Droplets expelled during sneezing. (From http://www. vaccineinformation.org/flu/photos.asp.)

TABLE 50.2	Body Fluids and Diseases They May Transmit
Body Fluid	**Disease Transmitted**
Blood	HBV, HIV, HCV, CMV, EBV, NANBH
Seminal fluid	HIV, HBV, CMV
Vaginal discharge	HIV, HBV, CMV
Saliva and sputum	HSV, TB, CMV, respiratory diseases
Cerebrospinal fluid	Encephalopathic organisms (see Table 50.5), HIV
Breast milk	HIV, HBV, CMV
Urine	CMV, EBV, HBV
Feces and intestinal fluid	HAV, gastrointestinal diseases (see Table 50.5)

CMV, Cytomegalovirus; *EBV*, Epstein-Barr virus; *HAV*, hepatitis A virus; *HBV*, hepatitis B virus; *HCV*, hepatitis C virus; *HIV*, human immunodeficiency virus; *HSV*, herpes simplex types I and II; *NANBH*, non-A, non-B hepatitis; *TB*, tuberculosis. Modified with permission from Browne RA, Chernesky MA. Infectious diseases and the anaesthetist. *Can J Anesth*. 1988;35(6):655–665.

between caregivers, single room isolation, gown, glove, mask, and eye protection. Patients undergoing surgery must be brought directly to the OR and recover in isolation. Some medical interventions (intubation, extubation, biphasic airway pressure [BiPAP], continuous positive airway pressure [CPAP], bronchoscopy, sputum induction, open airway suction) are categorized as aerosol-generating procedures. When performing an aerosol-generating procedure on a patient with an infectious disease that can be transmitted through droplets, the recommendation is to maximize protection by using airborne precautions.[10]

Droplet Nuclei

Droplet nuclei result from the evaporation of droplets while suspended in the air. Unlike droplets, the nuclei have an outer layer of desiccated organic material and a very small diameter (1–5 µm) and remain suspended in air indefinitely. The microorganisms contained within these nuclei may be spread by air drafts over great distances, depending on the environmental conditions (dry and cold atmosphere, with limited or no exposure to sunlight favoring the spread).[12] In contrast to droplets, which are deposited on mucous membranes, droplet nuclei may enter the susceptible host by inhalation; examples of droplet nuclei–borne diseases include tuberculosis, varicella, and measles, zoster, smallpox, SARS, and Middle Eastern respiratory syndrome.[10]

CONTACT TRANSMISSION

Direct and indirect contacts are the most significant and frequent methods of hospital infection transmission.

Direct Contact

This type of disease transmission involves direct physical contact between two individuals. The physical transfer of microorganisms from an infected or colonized person to a susceptible host may occur from child to health care provider or from health care provider to child during professional practice (e.g., venous cannulation, laryngoscopy, burn care, or suction of secretions). Health care providers working in the OR may be exposed to skin contamination by body fluids. This is an issue of grave concern because of the potential exposure of health care providers to patients with unrecognized infections, especially hepatitis B virus

(HBV), hepatitis C virus (HCV), and human immunodeficiency virus (HIV). Hepatitis B is a highly infectious virus that requires a small amount of blood (10^{-7}–10^{-9} mL) to transmit the disease. The incidence of skin contamination of anesthesiologists and related personnel by blood and saliva is substantial. One study examined 270 anesthetic procedures during 7 consecutive days. The blood of 35 patients (14%) contaminated the skin of 65 anesthesiologists in 46 incidents. Of these contamination events, 28 (61%) occurred during venous cannulation. Of anesthesiologists who had been contaminated by blood, 5 of 65 (8%) had cuts in the skin of their hands.[13] The importance of this observation is that seroconversion of health care providers has been reported after skin contamination by infected blood from HIV carriers[14] and HBV infection after blood splashing into health care workers' (HCWs') eyes.[15] Scabies, pediculosis, and herpes simplex are among the diseases most frequently transmitted by direct contact.[16–23] Meticulous hand washing before and after every patient contact and routine use of barriers such as gloves and eye protection are essential basic methods for protecting ourselves even during routine procedures such as starting an IV line or performing laryngoscopy.[4]

Indirect Contact

Indirect contact involves the transmission of microorganisms from a source (animate or inanimate) to a susceptible host by means of a vehicle (e.g., an intermediary object) contaminated by body fluids. Tables 50.2 and 50.3 provide examples of diseases associated with bodily fluids to which HCWs may be exposed. The vehicle for transmission may be the hands of a health care provider who is not wearing gloves or a provider who fails to wash his or her hands after providing care to a child.[3,24–26] This type of contact can also come from health care providers who touch (with or without gloves) contaminated monitoring or other patient care devices (e.g., blood pressure cuffs, stethoscopes, electrocardiographic cables, or ventilation systems [respirators, corrugated tubes, Y-pieces, valves]) that are used without proper cleaning or disinfection between each use.[27–29]

Knowledge about the transmission of the spread of bacteria from patients to HCWs' hands and to the hospital environment (Fig. 50.3) has driven many interventions that have reduced patient risks for developing HAIs.[30]

TABLE 50.3	Infectious Agents That May Be Found in the Operating Room
Viral Hepatitis	**Viruses**
Hepatitis A virus	Rhinovirus
Hepatitis B virus	Influenza
Hepatitis C virus	Parainfluenza
Hepatitis delta virus	Adenovirus
Non-A, non-B hepatitis	Respiratory syncytial virus
Human immunodeficiency virus	Measles
Cytomegalovirus	Rubella
Epstein-Barr virus	Cytomegalovirus[a]
Herpes simplex virus	
	Gastrointestinal
Respiratory Bacteria	Viruses: hepatitis A virus,
Streptococcus	rotavirus, adenovirus, enterovirus
Pneumococcus	Bacteria: *Giardia*,[a]
Meningococcus	*Cryptosporidium, Isospora*[a]
Diphtheria	Fungi: *Candida*[a]
Mycobacterium[a]	
Legionella[a]	**Central Nervous System**
	Viruses: Human
Fungi	immunodeficiency virus,[a] herpes
Candida[a]	simplex virus,[a] Epstein-Barr virus[a]
Nocardia[a]	Parasites: *Toxoplasma*[a]
Cryptococcus[a]	Fungi: *Cryptococcus*
Parasites	
Pneumocystis[a]	

[a]Opportunistic infections in immunocompromised patients, especially those with acquired immunodeficiency.
Modified with permission from Browne RA, Chernesky MA. Infectious diseases and the anaesthetist. *Can J Anesth.* 1988;35(6):655–665.

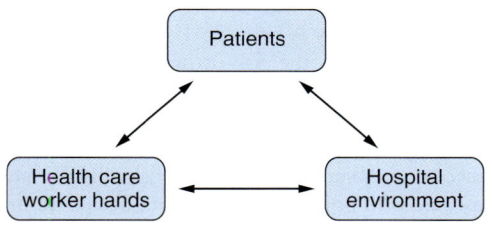

FIGURE 50.3 Epidemiologic links for transmission of multidrug-resistant organisms. (From Munoz-Price LS, Weinstein RA. Fecal patina in the anesthesia work area. *Anesth Analg.* 2015;120(4):703–705.)

Studies on vancomycin-resistant enterococci established the importance of a domino effect of contamination in intensive care units (ICUs) and inpatient wards: spread of vancomycin-resistant enterococci that colonize patients' gastrointestinal tracts ("rectal carriage"), to patients' skin, to the hospital environment, to hands of HCWs, and then to other patients. The skin contamination of patients with enteric organisms inspired the rather graphic description, the patient's "fecal patina."[31] Also referred to as a "stool veneer," this coating with enteric organisms is limited not only to patients' skin but also extends to surfaces in the surrounding environment that are touched, and thereby contaminated, by patients and by HCWs. The environmental contamination spreads out from the patient in a target-like concentric pattern, with the densest contamination closest to the rectum of patients who have rectal carriage of the problem bacteria. This interplay among organisms on patients' body surfaces, hospital environment, and HCWs' hands constitutes the foundation for the development of infection control interventions in the field of hospital epidemiology.[30]

Characterization of the transmission dynamics of frequently encountered gram-negative bacteria in the anesthesia work area environment[32] demonstrates that the spread follows an epidemiologic pattern similar to that seen in ICUs and inpatient wards: from patient, to environment and HCWs' hands, and to other patients (Fig. 50.4). In this report, provider hands were less likely to serve as a transmitter of infection than contaminated environmental or patient skin surfaces. These findings have clinical implications for the risk of colonization and subsequent HCIs—for example, SSIs. This calls attention to the need to develop and enforce strict hand hygiene guidelines for personnel who are providing anesthesia care, but more importantly the need to increase compliance with environmental disinfection of the OR (between cases and terminal cleaning), and to study further the directions of the spread of pathogens in the OR and anesthesia work areas. This study unequivocally underscores our need to improve cleaning procedures in the OR and equipment surfaces to reduce infection risk.

There are also reports of equipment, fomites, and drugs (mainly propofol) that have resulted in hospital-acquired infections.[20,33-51] Propofol is widely used for both inpatient and outpatient anesthesia. This hypnotic agent is a nutrient-rich drug. It is hypothesized that propofol increases bacterial contamination of IV stopcocks and may compromise safety of IV tubing sets when continued to be used after propofol anesthesia. There is a covert incidence of IV stopcock bacterial contamination during anesthesia that is aggravated by the prior presence of propofol. Propofol may increase the risk for postoperative infection because of bacterial growth in IV stopcock dead spaces.[52] Other facets that may also contribute to infection include the following:

- Up to 40% of anesthetic equipment in direct or indirect contact with a child (blood pressure cuffs, cables, oximeters, laryngoscopes, monitors, respirator settings, and horizontal and vertical surfaces) may be contaminated with blood because of inadequate cleansing procedures between uses.[6,7,27,53,54]
- In some institutions, up to 8% of the Bain circuits that were reused without previous sterilization were contaminated.[55]
- Contamination of syringe contents has occurred with glass particles during ampule opening, which in turn may compromise the sterility of the contents, presumably because of the passage of bacteria contained on glass particles into the solution.[56-58]
- IV tubing has both blood contamination as well as contamination by blood from syringes used to inject medications. This can occur with the absence of visible blood reflux in the tubing or syringe. Simply replacing the needle on a syringe that will be reused is ineffective in preventing cross-infection; it is essential to not use the same syringe in multiple patients.[59]
- Refilling both glass and plastic syringes several times has also been shown to result in contamination of the contents; single use is therefore recommended.[59,60]
- Some drug formulations, especially propofol, can sustain bacterial growth under certain conditions. Thus great care should be given to aseptic technique when transferring drugs from the vial to a syringe and to use the contents of the syringe within 4 hours.[61-65] Propofol vials should not be used for multiple patients because of concerns for cross-contamination, particularly since not all countries have added antimicrobials to the propofol emulsion.[66,67]

50

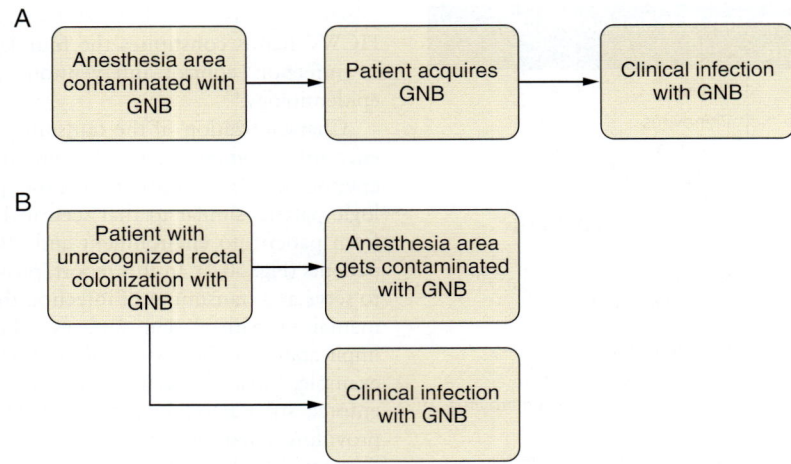

FIGURE 50.4 Possible explanations of subsequent clinical infections caused by the same organism cultured in the anaesthesia work area. **A,** Contaminated environment exposes patient to gram-negative bacilli (GNB) with the subsequent development of a clinical infection. **B,** Patient with unrecognized rectal colonization undergoes surgery, contaminating the anesthesia area with his/her endogenous GNB, and later develops a clinical infection with the same organism. (Data from Loftus RW, Brown JR, Patel HM, et al. Transmission dynamics of gram-negative bacterial pathogens in the anesthesia work area. *Anesth Analg.* 2015;120(4):819–826.)

- Needles that have been used for spinal or epidural anesthesia were contaminated with coagulase-negative staphylococci (15.7%), yeasts (1.5%), enterococci (0.8%), pneumococci (0.8%), and micrococci (0.8%), suggesting that there may be needle contamination despite standard skin preparation and cleansing.[68] It is unclear whether these skin organisms can be transmitted and cause an infection during administration of a neuraxial block.
- Blood and saliva frequently contaminate the skin of anesthetic personnel during routine anesthetic practice.[13]
- Violations of contemporary guidelines for preventing infections (e.g., hand washing, wearing gloves, surgical masks, ocular protection, scrubs, or syringe reuse) by anesthesiologists are frequent.[4] Anesthesia staff are aware that they work in a potentially infectious environment, but they commonly do not adopt appropriate protective measures to reduce infections in both themselves and their patients (11%–99%).[27,69–71]

ACCIDENTS WITH CUTTING OR PIERCING DEVICES

Percutaneous contamination from a cutting or piercing accident is the most effective means to transmit bloodborne pathogens. Evidence suggests that this is the main route of HIV, HBV, and HCV infection,[72–74] especially if the injury is caused by hollow-bore needles that were used to draw blood or establish IV access.[75,76] Over 20 other bloodborne pathogens have been transmitted by this means, including those causing herpes, malaria, and tuberculosis.[77] The risk of exposure to blood and bloodborne pathogens is greater for health care personnel (HCP) than for people who do not work around blood. An exposure to infected blood, tissue, or other potentially infectious body fluids can occur by percutaneous injury or contact with mucous membrane or nonintact skin. The risk of infection after an exposure depends on a number of variables and appears to be greater with exposure to a larger quantity of blood or other infectious fluid; prolonged or extensive exposure of nonintact skin or mucous membrane to blood or other infectious fluid or concentrated virus in a laboratory setting; exposure to

the blood of a patient in an advanced disease stage or with a higher HIV viral load; a deep percutaneous injury; a procedure wherein the sharp was in the vein or artery of an infected source patient; an injury with a hollow-bore, blood-filled needle; and limited or delayed access to postexposure prophylaxis. After exposure, the risk of infection varies for specific bloodborne pathogens. For HBV, if the source patient has active HBV and the HCP do not already have immunity, the risk for infection after percutaneous injury is between 1% and 30%. If the source patient has active HCV, the risk of hepatitis C transmission is approximately 1.8% (range 0%–7%) after a percutaneous injury. If the source patient has HIV infection, the risk of HIV transmission is approximately 0.3% after a percutaneous exposure and 0.09% after a mucous membrane exposure. The risk of HIV transmission for an exposure with nonintact skin has not been determined and is estimated to be less than the risk after a mucous membrane exposure.[78]

Anesthesia staff lacking HBV protective antibodies are at great risk for acquiring the disease.[79,80] These infection rates underscore the need for the use of "safe" needles and the need to advocate the use of "needleless" systems even though they are significantly more expensive.[81,82] This also emphasizes the need for meticulous handling and disposal of needles and other sharp instruments, as well as the use of special "sharps boxes" designed to minimize accidental needlesticks (e.g., "mailbox"-type boxes that do not allow the hand to enter the disposal area).[83–98] The U.S. Centers for Disease Control and Prevention (CDC) has estimated that in the United States there are approximately 385,000 cutting and piercing accidents annually among HCP in hospitals; 25% of these occur in the OR.[77] However, the actual prevalence is thought to be much greater, because many of these events are unreported. The distribution of these accidents among anesthesiologists is shown in Fig. 50.5A; the distribution of the items most frequently associated with cutting and piercing injuries in health care providers is shown in Fig. 50.5B. Should such an accident occur (e.g., needle puncture, exposure to nonintact skin, or mucous membrane

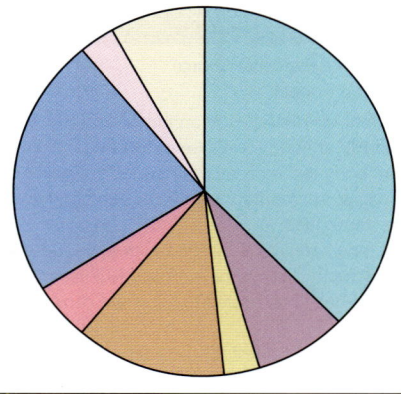

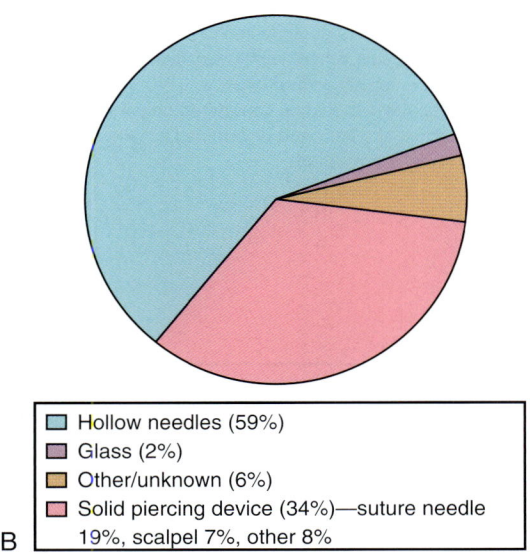

☐ While using the device (38%)
☐ Between steps or during complex procedures (8%)
☐ While removing the needle from the rubber stopper
   or other resistant material (3%)
☐ While capping a used needle (13%)
☐ While setting components apart (5%)
☐ After use, before disposal (23%)
☐ While dumping the device in the waste container (3%)
☐ Other (8%)

A

☐ Hollow needles (59%)
☐ Glass (2%)
☐ Other/unknown (6%)
☐ Solid piercing device (34%)—suture needle
   19%, scalpel 7%, other 8%

B

FIGURE 50.5 A, Percentage distribution of percutaneous injury to anesthesiologists caused by contaminated cutting or piercing devices. **B,** Percentage distribution of items associated with percutaneous injuries in health care work.

exposure), there are now specific recommendations regarding immediate assessment of risk, assessment of the exposure source (chart review, inform the patient that an accident has occurred and ask permission to determine HBV, HCV, and HIV serologic status), and rapid initiation of appropriate antiviral treatment of the HCW.[82] It is advised to obtain as much information regarding the patient as possible—if the patient is known—to (1) obtain a sample of blood from the patient for determination of potential carrier state (Table 50.4) and (2) report to the health service for immediate institution of prophylaxis and follow-up (Table 50.5), especially for HIV exposure (Tables 50.6 and 50.7).

Strategy for Preventing Infection Transmission in Health Care Institutions

Institutional administrative measures aimed at developing, implementing, and monitoring specifically designed accident prevention policies and procedures are important for reducing and preventing transmission of infectious agents in health care centers. To this end, centers should consider the following:[77,99,100]

- Include infection control as a major goal in the organizational mission statement and implement safety programs, both for patients and HCWs.
- Provide sufficient administrative and financial support to carry out this mission.
- Provide sufficient administrative and financial support for the microbiology laboratory and implement an infection surveillance plan, especially for postsurgical infections.
- Establish a multidiscipline cross-functional team (e.g., a team manager, an epidemiologist, a representative from industrial health, and a person trained in quality control) to identify health and safety issues within the institution, analyze trends, assess outcomes, implement interventions, and make recommendations to other members of the organization.
- Provide sufficient administrative and financial support to develop and implement education programs for health care providers, patients, and their families. One positive example of such education is that anesthesiologists who have read the CDC's Universal Precaution Guidelines for the Prevention of Occupational Transmission of HIV and HBV have developed better hygienic practices.[69]
- Provide HCWs with hepatitis A and B vaccine and document that an appropriate immunologic response was achieved. Provide hepatitis A and B immune globulins (HAIG, HBIG) for those exposed who do not have established immunity.[8]
- Provide a health care service for employees for counseling and postexposure prophylaxis should an exposure to HIV occur.[101]
- Provide regular surveillance of HCWs to determine established immunity to infectious diseases such as tuberculosis, measles, mumps, rubella, and chickenpox. Lack of immunity may require immunization; several studies have demonstrated the cost-effectiveness of immunization (for prevention of disease) versus the cost of replacement of HCWs who have become infected.[73,102–107]

Measures for Prevention of Infection Transmission in the Operating Room

PREVENTION OF AIRBORNE PATHOGEN TRANSMISSION

Airborne pathogens may be transmitted through the OR heating, ventilation, and air conditioning systems. It is vital to have in place proper systems to (1) remove contaminated air, (2) facilitate air management requirements to protect susceptible health care providers and children against hospital-related airborne pathogens, and (3) minimize the risk of airborne pathogens being transmitted by children. Many regulatory institutions, such as the National Institute for Occupational Safety and Health; the American Society of Heating, Refrigerating and Air-Conditioning Engineers; the CDC; and the American Institute of Architects (AIA), have developed standards and guidelines for OR ventilation systems. As in any other environment, ventilation in the OR is an important issue to control infection from microbiologic pollutants. Most

50

| TABLE 50.4 | Guide to Postexposure Prophylaxis and Prevention of Infection Transmission |

PEP Step 1: Treat Exposure Site

- Use soap and water to wash areas exposed to potentially infectious fluids as soon as possible after exposure.
- Flush exposed mucous membranes with water.
- Flush exposed eyes with water or saline solution.
- Do NOT apply caustic agents, or inject antiseptics or disinfectants into the wound.

PEP Step 2: Report and Document

- Date and time of exposure.
- Details of the incident: where and how the exposure occurred, exposure site(s) on HCP's body; if related to sharp device, the type and brand of device.
- Details of the exposure: type and amount of fluid or material, severity of exposure.
- Documentation of counseling following exposure and postexposure management plan.
- Details about the exposure source: If the source patient is known or unknown; whether the source material contained HIV, HBV, or HCV; if the source patient is HIV-infected, determine stage of disease, CD4 cell count, HIV viral load, history of antiretroviral therapy, and antiretroviral resistance information as available.
- Details about the exposed HCP: hepatitis B vaccination and vaccine-response status (HBsAb titer); other medical conditions that may influence choice of prophylactic agent(s) if needed; current medications, and drug allergies; pregnancy status or lactation status.

PEP Step 3: Evaluate the Exposure

- The exposure should be evaluated for the potential to transmit HBV, HCV, or HIV based on the type of body substance involved, the route, severity and frequency of exposure.
- Significant exposures to any of the following may pose a risk for bloodborne pathogen transmission and require further evaluation: blood, semen, vaginal secretions, cerebrospinal fluid, synovial fluid, pleural fluid, peritoneal fluid, pericardial fluid, amniotic fluid.
- Body fluids that do NOT pose a risk of bloodborne pathogen transmission unless visibly contaminated with blood include: urine, stool, tears, saliva, gastric secretions or vomitus, sweat, nonpurulent sputum, nasal discharge

PEP Step 4: Evaluate the Exposure Source
When source patient is known:

- Test source patient for HBsAg, HCV antibody, and HIV antibody.
  - Use a rapid HIV antibody test. Use of fourth-generation HIV antigen/antibody testing is recommended if available.
  - HIV viral load assessment for routine screening of source patient is NOT recommended.
  - If the source person is NOT infected with a bloodborne pathogen, further follow-up testing of the exposed HCP is not necessary. Follow state regulations related to informed consent and confidentiality.
- For patients who cannot be tested, consider medical diagnoses, clinical symptoms, and history of risk behaviors.

When source patient is NOT known/unable to be tested immediately:

- Evaluate the likelihood of high-risk exposure:
  - Consider the likelihood of bloodborne pathogen infections among patients in the exposure setting: What is the community infection rate? Does the clinic/hospital unit care for a large number of HIV-, HBV-, or HCV-infected or at-risk patients?
  - Is there a high suspicion for HIV infection and the patient is unable to be tested immediately?
- Do not test discarded needles for bloodborne pathogens; the reliability of these findings is not known.

The "window period":

- To date, there has not been a documented case of occupational HIV transmission from a source patient with a negative HIV antibody test result with risk factors for HIV acquisition.
- Postexposure prophylaxis should be considered only if the source patient has risk factors and has been determined to have symptoms consistent with acute HIV infection.

HBV, hepatitis B virus; HBsAg, hepatitis B surface antigen; HCV, hepatitis C virus; HCP, health care personnel; HIV, human immunodeficiency virus.
From Mountain Plains AIDS Education and Training Center. PEP Steps, A Quick Guide to Postexposure Prophylaxis in the Health Care Setting (April 2006); PEP Steps: A Quick Guide to Postexposure Prophylaxis in the Health Care Setting (March 2014).

wound contamination in the OR is the result of the patient's skin flora and bacteria shed on airborne particles from the OR personnel. Room ventilation affects the distribution of these airborne particles in four ways: total ventilation (dilution), air distribution (directional airflow), room pressurization (filtration barrier), and filtration (contaminant removal). As the air flows of the room increase, the greater the dilutional effect on airborne particles. Balancing this phenomenon is important because while increased flow increases the effectiveness of air exchange, the resultant turbulent flow increases microbial distribution throughout the room. Low-velocity unidirectional flow minimizes the spread of microbes in the room. Directional flow can be inward, from the outside into the OR (negative pressure), or outward, from the OR to the outside (positive pressure). Negative-pressure ventilation is used for highly infective rooms in the hospital (e.g., isolation rooms for tuberculosis patients), and positive-pressure ventilation is used for protective environments (e.g., ORs and

rooms with immunocompromised patients). Most hospital ORs are currently designed with high-efficiency particulate air (HEPA) filtration systems to maximize removal of airborne contaminants. OR ventilation systems should operate at all times, except during maintenance. During unoccupied hours, air exchange can be reduced as long as positive pressure is maintained in each OR. Air is delivered to each OR from the ceiling, with downward movement toward several exhaust or return ducts near the floor. This design helps provide steady movement of clean air through the breathing and working zones.

The AIA has specific guidelines for the location of outside fresh air inlets to minimize contamination from exhaust systems and noxious fumes. A greater air inflow rate and a larger air-inlet area are desirable for contaminant control, but these approaches are detrimental to the thermal comfort of the staff and patient.[108] The AIA recommends an air-change rate in an OR of 20 to 25 air changes per hour (ACH) for ceiling heights between 9 feet

TABLE 50.5	Factors to Consider in Assessing the Need for Follow-Up After Occupational Exposure

Type of Exposure

- Percutaneous injury
- Mucous membrane exposure
- Nonintact skin exposure
- Bites resulting in blood exposure to either person involved

Type and Amount of Fluid/Tissue

- Blood
- Fluids containing blood
- Potentially infectious fluid or tissue
- Direct contact with concentrated virus

Infection Status of Source Patient

- If positive for HBsAg testing for exposed person's vaccination status.
- If positive for HCV antibody, consider measuring HCV viral load.
- If positive for HIV antibody, consider obtaining HIV viral load testing, and evaluating clinical status of patient.

Susceptibility of Exposed HCP

- Hepatitis B vaccine and vaccine response status
- HBV, HCV, and HIV status—baseline testing for HbsAb, anti-HCV, and HIV antibody should be completed as early as possible (preferably within 72 hours)

Accessibility of PEP and Follow-Up

- PEP should be initiated within 2 hours of the exposure.
- The efficacy of PEP initiation is thought to diminish after 24 to 36 hours following an exposure.

Laboratory Tests Used for Evaluation

- If the fourth-generation combination HIV Ag/Ab assay is used to test the source patient, HIV follow-up testing can be completed 4 months after exposure.

HBV, hepatitis B virus; *HBsAb*, hepatitis B surface antigen; *HCV*, hepatitis C virus; *HIV*, human immunodeficiency virus; *PEP*, postexposure prophylaxis.
From Mountain Plains AIDS Education and Training Center. PEP Steps, A Quick Guide to Postexposure Prophylaxis in the Health Care Setting (April 2006); PEP Steps: A Quick Guide to Postexposure Prophylaxis in the Health Care Setting (March 2014).

(2.74 meters) and 12 feet (3.66 meters). Some controversy exists between engineers and clinicians over the need for laminar airflow ventilation in the OR to further minimize airborne infection. Careful mathematical analyses of airflow suggest that laminar airflow is not necessary. Clinical studies are confirmatory. Similarly, the use of ultraviolet light to cleanse the room air is no longer recommended.[109] Table 50.8 shows the 2003 Healthcare Infection Control Practices Advisory Committee and CDC general recommendations for ventilation system specifications for the OR.[12] Children with tuberculosis require special consideration because of the high risk of occupational transmission of *Mycobacterium tuberculosis*,[110,111] especially after the emergence of multidrug-resistant strains (Table 50.9). An easy preventive measure is to screen all children before coming to the OR to determine recent exposure to infectious disease such as measles, mumps, rubella, and chickenpox because these infections can pose a significant risk to HCWs and patients, especially those who are immunocompromised.[73,106] Another potential source for airborne spread of pathogens is through the anesthesia circuit; this may be reduced by the use of circuit filters. However, at present there are no regulatory requirements to use such devices, and performance characteristics vary widely.[28,29,112–116]

STANDARD PRECAUTIONS

Standard precautions[117] assume that any person or patient is potentially infected or colonized by microorganisms that could be transmitted and cause an infectious process. Standard precautions must be implemented with all patients and include the following:

- *Universal precautions—blood and body fluid precautions*, developed to reduce bloodborne pathogen transmission
- *Body substance isolation*, designed to reduce the risk of pathogen transmission by moist body substances

Standard precautions are used to reduce the transmission of all infectious agents from one person to another, thus protecting health care providers and children against exposure to the most common microorganisms. Standard precautions are implemented for any contact with blood and body fluids, secretions, and excretions (except sweat), whether or not they contain visible blood, as well as for any contact with nonintact skin, mucous membranes, and intact skin that is visibly soiled with blood and/or body fluids. *Prevention is primary.* All HCPs should be familiar with standard precautions: wash hands frequently and thoroughly before and after patient care; use personal protective equipment: gloves, gowns, boots, shoe covers, eyewear, masks, and shields, as appropriate for the patient care situation; gloves must be worn when any kind of venous or arterial access is being performed; use sharps with caution: plan ahead (use sharps in a safe environment with a sharps container nearby), dispose of used sharps in puncture-proof receptacles immediately after use, do not recap needles, and use safety devices if available. All HCPs should be vaccinated with the hepatitis B vaccine series and should undergo testing for HBsAb response after completion of the series to document adequate protection. Employees who have not gone through the vaccination series previously should be offered the hepatitis B series through their employer at no cost.[118] Summaries of standard precautions, droplet precautions, airborne precautions, and contact precautions are available on line.[100,119–121]

Hand Washing

Overall hand hygiene compliance across health care providers remains less than 50%, with anesthesia providers identified as a particularly noncompliant group (one study found a compliance rate of only 23%).[122] Bacterial contamination of anesthesia providers has been directly linked to high-risk bacterial transmission events to IV stopcocks and 30-day postoperative infections.[24]

The vast majority of SSIs are caused by *Staphylococcus aureus*. Transmission of specific staphylococcal phenotypes within and between patients is a major contributor to SSIs and HAIs.[3,4,123] The role of anesthesia-provider hand contamination in transmission of *Enterococcus* to the workstation and patient biome is concerning, even though it was not associated with actual infection, because of rising rates of antibiotic-resistant organisms and the observation that *Enterococcus* is becoming a more prevalent pathogen.[3,124] Two approaches are indicated: improved methods of patient reservoir decontamination and more effective and frequent decontamination of provider hands. Hand hygiene is a well-known and effective solution to the problem of bacterial transmission within and across patients. Compliance with the current "5 moments" World Health Organization guidelines could make a major inroad into reducing provider hand and workspace contamination. One study found that only 20% of anesthesia providers demonstrated complete knowledge regarding WHO hand hygiene guidelines.[125] Failure of providers to recognize prior contact with the environment and prior contact with the patient as hand hygiene opportunities contributed to this low percentage. Several cognitive factors were associated

TABLE 50.6 Recommended HIV Postexposure Prophylaxis for Percutaneous Injuries

	INFECTION STATUS OF SOURCE				
Exposure Type	HIV-Positive Class 1[a]	HIV-Positive Class 2[a]	Source of Unknown HIV Status[b]	Unknown Source[c]	HIV-Negative
Less severe[d]	Recommend basic 2-drug PEP	Recommend expanded ≥3-drug PEP	In general, no PEP warranted; however, consider basic 2-drug PEP[e] for source with HIV risk factors[f]	In general, no PEP warranted; however, consider basic 2-drug PEP[e] in settings in which exposure to HIV-infected persons is likely	No PEP warranted
More severe[g]	Recommend expanded 3-drug PEP	Recommend expanded ≥3-drug PEP	In general, no PEP warranted; however, consider basic 2-drug PEP[e] for source with HIV risk factors[f]	In general, no PEP warranted; however, consider basic 2-drug PEP[e] in settings in which exposure to HIV-infected persons is likely	No PEP warranted

HIV, human immunodeficiency virus; PEP, postexposure prophylaxis.

[a]HIV-positive class 1: asymptomatic HIV infection or known low viral load (e.g., <1500 ribonucleic acid copies/mL). HIV-positive class 2: symptomatic HIV infection, AIDS seroconversion, or known high viral load. If drug resistance is a concern, obtain expert consultation. Initiation of PEP should be delayed pending expert consultation, and because expert consultation alone cannot substitute for face-to-face counseling, resources should be available to provide immediate evaluation and follow-up care for all exposures.
[b]For example, deceased source person with no samples available for HIV testing.
[c]For example, a needle from a sharps disposal container.
[d]For example, solid needle or superficial injury.
[e]The recommendation "consider PEP" indicates that PEP is optional; a decision to initiate PEP should be based on a discussion between the exposed person and the treating clinician regarding the risks versus benefits of PEP.
[f]If PEP is offered and administered and the source is later determined to be HIV-negative, PEP should be discontinued.
[g]For example, large-bore hollow needle, deep puncture, visible blood on device, or needle used in patient's artery or vein.
From Centers for Disease Control and Prevention. Updated U.S. Public Health Service guidelines for the management of occupational exposures to HBV, HCV, and HIV and recommendations for postexposure prophylaxis. MMWR Recommendtions and Reports 2001;50(RR11):1–42. Available at http://www.cdc.gov/mmwr/PDF/rr/rr5011.pdf.

TABLE 50.7 Recommended HIV Postexposure Prophylaxis for Mucous Membrane Exposures and Nonintact Skin[a] Exposures

	INFECTION STATUS OF SOURCE				
Exposure Type	HIV-Positive Class 1[b]	HIV-Positive Class 2[c]	Source of Unknown HIV Status[c]	Unknown Source[d]	HIV-Negative
Small volume[e]	Consider basic 2-drug PEP[f]	Recommend basic 2-drug PEP	In general, no PEP warranted[g]	In general, no PEP warranted	No PEP warranted
Large volume[h]	Recommend basic 2-drug PEP	Recommend expanded ≥3-drug PEP	In general, no PEP warranted; however, consider basic 2-drug PEP[f] for source with HIV risk factors[g]	In general, no PEP warranted; however, consider basic 2-drug PEP[f] in settings in which exposure to HIV-infected persons is likely	No PEP warranted

PEP, postexposure prophylaxis.

[a]For skin exposures, follow-up is indicated only if evidence exists of compromised skin integrity (e.g., dermatitis, abrasion, or open wound).
[b]HIV-positive class 1: asymptomatic HIV infection or known low viral load (e.g., <1500 ribonucleic acid copies/mL). HIV-positive class 2: symptomatic HIV infection, acquired immunodeficiency syndrome, acute seroconversion, or known high viral load. If drug resistance is a concern, obtain expert consultation. Initiation of PEP should be delayed pending expert consultation, and because expert consultation alone cannot substitute for face-to-face counseling, resources should be available to provide immediate evaluation and follow-up care for all exposures.
[c]For example, deceased source person with no samples available for HIV testing.
[d]For example, splash from inappropriately disposed blood.
[e]For example, a few drops.
[f]The recommendation "consider PEP" indicates that PEP is optional; a decision to initiate PEP should be based on a discussion between the exposed person and the treating clinician regarding the risks versus benefits of PEP.
[g]If PEP is offered and administered and the source is later determined to be HIV-negative, PEP should be discontinued.
[h]For example, a major blood splash.
From Centers for Disease Control and Prevention. Updated U.S. Public Health Service guidelines for the management of occupational exposures to HBV, HCV, and HIV and recommendations for postexposure prophylaxis. MMWR Recommendtions and Reports 2001;50(RR11):1–42. Available at http://www.cdc.gov/mmwr/PDF/rr/rr5011.pdf.

with a reduced risk of incomplete knowledge, including providers responding positively to washing their hands after contact with the environment, disinfecting their environment during patient care, believing that they can influence their colleagues, and intending to adhere to guidelines. These results suggest that anesthesia providers have knowledge deficits pertaining to opportunity-based hand hygiene in the intraoperative arena[125]—specifically, after interactions with patient skin surfaces and the surrounding environment, the two most important reservoirs of intraoperative bacterial transmission.

Hand washing is considered the most important and cost-effective individual intervention in the prevention of HAIs in children and health care providers.[126] Its importance in medical practice had not been universally accepted, despite the pioneering work by Oliver Wendell Holmes[127] (1843) and Ignaz Semmelweis[128]

TABLE 50.8	Ventilation System Specifications for the Operating Room

- Minimize the circulation of people during surgeries. It has been proved that the level of microbes in the operating room air is directly proportional to the number of people moving inside the room.
- Maintain humidity under 68% and temperature control to prevent environmental conditions that favor the development of germs.
- Maintain positive pressure compared with corridors and surrounding areas to prevent microorganisms from entering the operating room.
- Provide at least 15 air changes per hour in the operating room, 20% of which should be fresh air. Air should be recirculated through a high-efficiency particulate air (HEPA) filter.
- Air should be introduced at ceiling level and disposed of at ground level.

From Centers for Disease Control and Prevention. Guidelines for environmental infection control in health-care facilities: recommendations of CDC and the Healthcare Infection Control Practices Advisory Committee (HICPAC). *MMWR Recommendtions and Reports* 2003;52(RR10):1–42. Available at http://www.cdc.gov/mmwr/preview/mmwrhtml/rr5210a1.htm.

TABLE 50.9	Precautionary Procedures for Patients with Infectious Tuberculosis

Follow Precautionary Procedures for Infectious TB Patients Who Also Require Emergency Surgery. Category IB, IC

1. Use an N95 respirator approved by the National Institute for Occupational Safety and Health without exhalation valves in the operating room. Category IC
2. Intubate the patient in either the AII room or the operating room; if intubating the patient in the operating room, do not allow the doors to open until 99% of the airborne contaminants are removed. Category IB
3. When anesthetizing a patient with confirmed or suspected TB, place a bacterial filter between the anesthesia circuit and the patient's airway to prevent contamination of anesthesia equipment or discharge of tubercle bacilli into the ambient air. Category IB
4. Extubate and allow the patient to recover in an AII room. Category IB
5. If the patient has to be extubated in the operating room, allow adequate time for ACH to clean 99% of airborne particles from the air, because extubation is a cough-producing procedure. Category IB

Use Portable, Industrial-Grade HEPA Filters Temporarily for Supplemental Air Cleaning During Intubation and Extubation for TB Patients Who Require Surgery. Category II

1. Position the units appropriately so that all room air passes through the filter; obtain engineering consultation to determine the appropriate placements. Category II
2. Switch the portable unit off during the surgical procedure. Category II
3. Provide fresh air as per ventilation standards for operating rooms; portable units do not meet the requirements for the number of fresh ACH. Category II

If possible, schedule TB patients as the last surgical cases of the day to maximize the time available for removal of airborne contamination. Category II

No recommendation is offered for performing orthopedic implant operations in rooms supplied with laminar airflow. Unresolved issue

Maintain backup ventilation equipment (e.g., portable units for fans or filters) for emergency ventilation of operating rooms, and take immediate steps to restore the fixed ventilation system. Category IB, IC (AIA: 5.1)

ACH, air changes per hour; *AII*, airborne infection isolation; *HEPA*, high-efficiency particulate air.
Centers for Disease Control and Prevention. Guidelines for environmental infection control in health-care facilities: recommendations of CDC and the Healthcare Infection Control Practices Advisory Committee (HICPAC). 2003. http://apps.who.int/iris/bitstream/10665/44102/1/9789241597906_eng.pdf

(1846), who separately recognized that the contaminated hands of physicians performing autopsies were the vectors responsible for the spread of puerperal fever caused by streptococci. They demonstrated that hand washing before delivering a baby reduced the risk of infectious transmission and maternal mortality by 90%! Unfortunately, the scientific basis for hand washing was not established until the introduction of the germ theory of disease by Louis Pasteur[129] and the discovery of the microorganism that caused anthrax *(Bacillus anthracis)* by Robert Koch[130] in the late 19th century. More than one-and-a-half centuries later, and with strong evidence that health care providers are a leading source of hospital acquired infections,[3,24,131] the average frequency of hand hygiene episodes fluctuates with the method used for monitoring and the setting where the observations are conducted. Hand washing per hour may vary over 30-fold. On the other hand, the average number of opportunities for hand hygiene per HCW varies markedly between hospital wards; nurses in pediatric wards, for example, had an average of eight opportunities for hand hygiene per hour of patient care, compared with an average of 30 for ICU nurses. In some acute clinical situations, the patient is cared for by several HCWs contemporaneously and, on average, as many hand hygiene opportunities per patient per hour of care have been observed per provider as in a postanesthesia care unit (PACU) admission. The number of opportunities for hand hygiene depends largely on the process of care provided[132]: revision of protocols for patient care may reduce unnecessary contacts and, consequently, improve hand hygiene opportunities. In 11 observational studies, the duration of hand cleansing episodes by HCWs ranged, on average, from as little as 6.6 seconds to 30 seconds. In 10 of these studies, the hand hygiene technique monitored was hand washing, while handrubbing was monitored in one study. In addition to washing their hands for very short time periods, HCWs often failed to cover all surfaces of their hands and fingers. Therefore the number of hand hygiene opportunities per hour of care may be very large and, even if the hand hygiene compliance rate is large, the applied cleansing technique may be inadequate. Adherence of HCWs to recommended hand hygiene procedures varies from unacceptably poor (5%) to relatively good (89%) with an overall mean rate of 38.7% in the ICU, OR, and PACU.[133–139] A number of investigators reported improved

adherence after implementing various interventions, but most studies had only short follow-up. Few studies have reported sustained improvement. There are hospital-wide predictors of poor adherence to recommended hand hygiene measures during routine patient care. These include professional category, hospital ward, time of day/week, and type and intensity of patient care, defined as the number of opportunities for hand hygiene per hour of patient care. Nonadherence was the least among nurses and during weekends. Nonadherence was greater in ICUs compared with internal medicine, during procedures that carried a substantial risk of bacterial contamination, and when intensity of patient care was high. In other words, the greater the demand for hand hygiene, the poorer the adherence. The poorest adherence rate (36%) was found in ICUs, where indications for hand hygiene were typically more frequent (on average, 22 opportunities per patient-hour). The greatest adherence rate (59%) was observed in pediatrics, where the average intensity of patient care was smaller than elsewhere (on average, 8 opportunities per patient-hour). The results suggest that full adherence to guidelines is unrealistic and that easy access to hand hygiene at the point of patient care, (i.e., in particular, alcohol-based handrubbing) could help improve adherence to hand hygiene.

Perceived barriers to adherence with hand hygiene practice recommendations include skin irritation caused by hand hygiene agents, inaccessible hand hygiene supplies, interference with HCW–patient relationships, patient needs perceived as a priority over hand hygiene, wearing of gloves, forgetfulness, lack of knowledge of guidelines, insufficient time for hand hygiene, high workload and understaffing, and the lack of scientific information showing a definitive impact of improved hand hygiene on HAI rates. Lack of knowledge of guidelines for hand hygiene, lack of recognition of hand hygiene opportunities during patient care, and lack of awareness of the risk of cross-transmission of pathogens are barriers to good hand hygiene practices. Furthermore, some HCWs believed that they washed their hands when necessary even when observations indicated that they did not. The risk of pathogen transmission via the hands is proportional to the power of the number of times a child is touched.[140] Table 50.10 presents

---

TABLE 50.10   Indications for Hand Hygiene

1. Wash hands with soap and water when visibly dirty or visibly soiled with blood or other body fluids (IB) or after using the toilet (II).

2. If exposure to potential spore-forming pathogens is strongly suspected or proven, including outbreaks of *Clostridium difficile*, hand washing with soap and water is the preferred means (IB).

3. Use an alcohol-based handrub as the preferred means for routine hand antisepsis in all other clinical situations described in terms 4(a) to 4(f) listed below, if hands are not visibly soiled (IA). If alcohol-based handrub is not obtainable, wash hands with soap and water (IB).

4. Perform hand hygiene:
   a. before and after touching the patient (IB);
   b. before handling an invasive device for patient care regardless of whether or not gloves are used (IB);
   c. after contact with body fluids or excretions, mucous membranes, non-intact skin, or wound dressings (IA);
   d. if moving from a contaminated body site to another body site during care of the same patient (IB);
   e. after contact with inanimate surfaces and objects (including medical equipment) in the immediate vicinity of the patient (IB);
   f. after removing sterile (II) or nonsterile gloves (IB).

5. Before handling medication or preparing food, perform hand hygiene using an alcohol-based handrub or wash hands with either plain or antimicrobial soap and water (IB).

6. Soap and alcohol-based handrub should not be used concomitantly (II).

Category IA. Strongly recommended for implementation and strongly supported by well-designed experimental, clinical, or epidemiologic studies.
Category IB. Strongly recommended for implementation and supported by some experimental, clinical, or epidemiologic studies and a strong theoretical rationale.
Category IC. Required for implementation, as mandated by federal and/or state regulation or standard.
Category II. Suggested for implementation and supported by suggestive clinical or epidemiologic studies or a theoretical rationale or a consensus by a panel of experts.
Adapted from *WHO Guidelines on Hand Hygiene in Health Care: First Global Patient Safety Challenge Clean Care Is Safer Care.* Geneva: World Health Organization; 2009.

---

a summary of the indications for and the strength of supporting evidence for hand washing and antisepsis.

Recommendations for surgical hand preparation are as follows: remove rings, wristwatch, and bracelets before beginning surgical hand preparation (II); artificial nails are prohibited (IB); sinks should be designed to reduce the risk of splashes (II); if hands are visibly soiled, wash hands with plain soap before surgical hand preparation (II); remove debris from underneath fingernails using a nail cleaner, preferably under running water (II); brushes are not recommended for surgical hand preparation (IB); surgical hand antisepsis should be performed using either a suitable antimicrobial soap or suitable alcohol-based handrub, preferably with a product ensuring sustained activity, before donning sterile gloves (IB); if the quality of water is not assured in the operating theatre, surgical hand antisepsis using an alcohol-based handrub is recommended before donning sterile gloves when performing surgical procedures (II); when performing surgical hand antisepsis using an antimicrobial soap, scrub hands and forearms for the length of time recommended by the manufacturer, typically 2–5 minutes. Long scrub times (e.g., 10 minutes) are not necessary (IB); when using an alcohol-based surgical handrub product with sustained activity, follow the manufacturer's instructions for application times. Apply the product to dry hands only (IB); do not combine surgical hand scrub and surgical handrub with alcohol-based products sequentially (II); when using an alcohol-based handrub, use sufficient product to keep hands and forearms wet with the handrub throughout the surgical hand preparation procedure (IB); after application of the alcohol-based handrub as recommended, allow hands and forearms to dry thoroughly before donning sterile gloves (IB).

At present, alcohol-based handrubs are the only known means for rapidly and effectively inactivating a wide array of potentially harmful microorganisms on hands. The WHO recommends alcohol-based handrubs based on the following factors: evidence-based, intrinsic advantages of fast-acting and broad-spectrum microbicidal activity with a minimal risk of generating resistance to antimicrobial agents; suitability for use in resource-limited or remote areas with lack of accessibility to sinks or other facilities for hand hygiene (including clean water, towels, and so on); capacity to promote improved compliance with hand hygiene by making the process faster and more convenient; economic benefit by reducing annual costs for hand hygiene, representing approximately 1% of extra costs generated by an HCI; minimization of risks from adverse events because of increased safety associated with better acceptability and tolerance than other products.[118]

After hand washing, it is very important to dry the hands properly with appropriate paper towels, hot air flow, or both, because the level of pathogen transmission from a HCW's hands to a patient is greatly increased if the hands are wet.[141] Sterile cloth towels are most frequently used in ORs to dry wet hands after surgical hand antisepsis. Several methods of drying have been tested without significant differences between techniques.[118]

Transmission may also occur from patients' wet sites, such as groins or armpits, or when a HCW gets his or her hands wet when opening parenteral solutions. It is critical for health institutions to establish written procedures and protocols to support adherence to the recommended hand hygiene practices.

Gloves

Wearing clean or sterile gloves while caring for children is an effective means of reducing HAIs. Gloves remain a supplementary barrier to infection that should not replace proper hand hygiene.

Gloves protect patients by reducing health care provider hand contamination and the subsequent transmission of pathogens to other children, provided the gloves are changed after providing care to each child. Additionally, when the use of gloves is combined with CDC standard precautions, they protect the health care provider against exposure to bloodborne infections or infections transmitted by any other body fluids, such as excretions, secretions (except sweat), mucous membranes, and nonintact skin. Examination gloves are single-use and usually nonsterile. Sterile surgical gloves are required for surgical interventions. Some nonsurgical care procedures, such as central vascular catheter insertion, also require surgical glove use. In addition to their sterile properties, these gloves have characteristics of thickness, elasticity, and strength that differ from other medical gloves.

The use of gloves in situations when their use is not indicated represents a waste of resources without necessarily reducing cross-transmission. The wide-ranging recommendations for glove use have led to very frequent and inappropriate use. Indications for gloving and glove removal are shown in Table 50.11. Situations that require and that do not require glove use are presented in Fig. 50.6.

Ranked consensus recommendations for the use of gloves, categorized according to the CDC/HICPAC system, include the following[118,142,143]:

- Wear gloves in case of contact with blood or any other potentially infecting body fluid, such as excretions, secretions (except sweat), mucous membranes, and nonintact skin (IC).
- Remove the gloves immediately after providing care to a child. Staff should not wear the same pair of gloves to take care of more than one child, nor should they touch the surfaces of any equipment, monitoring devices, or even light switches. Contaminated gloves can pass blood or other body fluids to working surfaces and are vectors for hepatitis transmission (IB).[72]

- Change gloves when taking care of a child if you must move from a contaminated to a clean body site (II).
- Apply hand hygiene measures immediately after removing the gloves because, despite the use of gloves, hands may get contaminated through small (microscopic) holes in the gloves.[131,144,145] Microbial contamination of hands and possible infection transmission have been reported even with the use of gloves.[146]
- Remove the gloves by using an appropriate technique (so as not to contaminate your hands with the contaminated surface of the gloves).

TABLE 50.11	Indications for Gloving and Glove Removal
Indication	
Glove Use	
1. Before a sterile condition	
2. Anticipation of a contact with blood or another body fluid, regardless of the existence of sterile conditions and including contact with non-intact skin and mucous membrane	
3. Contact with a patient (and his/her immediate surroundings) during contact precautions	
Glove Removal	
1. As soon as gloves are damaged (or non-integrity suspected)	
2. When contact with blood, another body fluid, nonintact skin, and mucous membrane has occurred and has ended	
3. When contact with a single patient and his or her surroundings, or a contaminated body site on a patient has ended	
4. When there is an indication for hand hygiene	

From *WHO Guidelines on Hand Hygiene in Health Care. First Global Patient Safety Challenge Clean Care Is Safer Care.* Geneva: World Health Organization; 2009.

STERILE GLOVES INDICATED

Any surgical procedure; vaginal delivery; invasive radiological procedures; performing vascular access and procedures (central lines); preparing total parental nutrition and chemotherapeutic agents.

EXAMINATION GLOVES INDICATED IN CLINICAL SITUATIONS
Potential for touching blood, body fluids, secretions, excertions, and items visibly soiled by body fluids

DIRECT PATIENT EXPOSURE: contact with blood; contact with mucous membrane and with nonintact skin; potential presence of highly infectious and dangerous organism; epidemic; or emergency situations; IV insertion and removal; drawing blood; discontinuation of venous line; pelvic and vaginal examination; suctioning nonclosed systems of endotracheal tubes.

INDIRECT PATIENT EXPOSURE: emptying emesis basins; handling/cleaning instruments; handling waste; cleaning up spills of body fluids.

GLOVES NOT INDICATED (except for CONTACT precautions)
No potential for exposure to blood or body fluids, or contaminated environment

DIRECT PATIENT EXPOSURE: taking blood pressure; temperature and pulse; performing SC and IM injections; bathing and dressing the patient; transporting patient; caring for eyes and ears (without secretions); any vascular line manipulation in absence of blood leakage.

INDIRECT PATIENT EXPOSURE: using the telephone, writing the patient's chart; giving oral medications; distributing or collecting patient dietary trays; removing and replacing linen for patient bed; placing noninvasive ventilation equipment and oxygen cannula; moving patient furniture.

FIGURE 50.6 Situations requiring and not requiring glove use. *IM,* intramuscular; *SC,* subcutaneous. (Adapted from *WHO Guidelines on Hand Hygiene in Health Care: First Global Patient Safety Challenge Clean Care Is Safer Care.* Geneva: World Health Organization; 2009.)

- Alcohol-based handrub dispensers and clean glove boxes (at least two sizes) should be in place near every patient care site (e.g., on top of every anesthesia cart, medication cart, or in the nursing station).
- Disposable gloves should not be washed, resterilized, or disinfected (IB). If gloves are reused, appropriate reprocessing methods should be in place to ensure the physical integrity of the gloves and their full decontamination (II).
- Sterile gloves are much more expensive than clean, disposable gloves and should be used only for certain procedures, such as when hands are in contact with normally sterile body areas or when inserting intravascular or urinary catheters. Clean gloves should be used during any other procedure, including wound dressing.
- Latex-free gloves should be worn when caring for children at risk for latex allergy.

ANTIMICROBIAL PROPHYLAXIS

Surgical antimicrobial prophylaxis is an essential tool to reduce the risk of postoperative infections, and the anesthesia team plays a central role in ensuring the proper timing of drug administration.[147,148] The aim of the perioperative administration of antibiotics is to obtain plasma and tissue drug concentrations exceeding the minimal inhibitory concentration of those organisms most likely to cause an infection. This will reduce the microbial load of the intraoperative contamination; it is not the intent to cover all possible pathogens, because this can lead to the selection of drug-resistant bacteria.

There have been few studies regarding the effectiveness of prophylactic guidelines for prevention of SSIs in children. Currently, prophylactic antibiotic guidelines exist for certain subsets of the pediatric surgical population, but there are no global recommendations, and the guidelines that exist are mostly based on studies from adults or from expert opinion. A retrospective study suggested that the appropriate use of antibiotic prophylaxis was a vital modifiable risk factor and may be the easiest factor to influence. Primary failure to administer the correct dose of antibiotics at the appropriate time resulted in an almost 2-fold increase in the risk of developing an SSI. The importance of correct antibiotic usage and dosing plays a major role in decreasing risk of SSIs in children. Recommendations are provided for adult (age ≥19 years) and pediatric (age 1–18 years) patients. The guidelines do not specifically address newborn (premature and full-term) infants (Table 50.12).[149]

Selection of the Antimicrobial Agent

Although pediatric-specific prophylaxis data are sparse, available data have been evaluated for specific procedures. Selection of antimicrobial prophylactic agents mirrors that in adult guidelines, with the agents of choice being first- and second-generation cephalosporins, reserving the use of vancomycin for patients with documented β-lactam allergies. While the use of a penicillin with a β-lactamase inhibitor in combination with cefazolin or vancomycin and gentamicin has also been studied in pediatric patients, the number of patients included in these evaluations remains small. As with adults, there is little evidence supporting the use of vancomycin, alone or in combination with other antimicrobials, for routine perioperative antimicrobial prophylaxis in institutions that have a high prevalence of methicillin-resistant *S. aureus* (MRSA). Vancomycin may be considered in children known to be colonized with MRSA and decreases MRSA infections.[150] Mupirocin is effective in children colonized with MRSA, but

TABLE 50.12	Antimicrobial Prophylaxis Dosing Recommendations	
Antimicrobial	**Pediatric Recommended Dose**[a]	**Recommended Redosing Interval (From Initiation of Preoperative Dose), hours**[b]
Ampicilin-sulbactam	50 mg/kg of the ampicilin component (up to 3 g)	2
Ampicilin	50 mg/kg (up to 2 g)	2
Azitreonam	30 mg/kg (up to 2 g)	4
Cefazolin	30 mg/kg (up to 2 g, 3 g if >120 kg)	4
Cefuroxime	50 mg/kg (up to 1.5 g)	4
Cefotaxime	50 mg/kg (up to 1 g)	3
Cefoxitin	40 mg/kg (up to 2 g)	2
Cefotetan	40 mg/kg (upto 2 g)	6
Ceftriaxone	50–75 mg/kg (up to 2 g)	N/A
Ciprofloxacin[c]	10 mg/kg (up to 400 mg)	N/A
Clindamycin	10 mg/kg (up to 900 mg)	6
Ertapenem	15 mg/kg (up to 1 g)	N/A
Fluconazole	6 mg/kg (up to 400 mg)	N/A
Gentamicin[d]	2.5 mg/kg based on dosing weight	N/A
Levofloxacin[c]	10 mg/kg (up to 500 mg)	N/A
Metronidazole	15 mg/kg (up to 500 mg) Neonates weighing <1200 g should receive a single 7.5-mg/kg dose	N/A
Moxifloxacin[c]	10 mg/kg (up to 400 mg)	N/A
Piperacilin-tazobactam	Infants 2–9 months: 80 mg/kg of the piperacilin component (up to 3.375 g) Children >9 months and ≤40 kg: 100 mg/kg of the piperacilin component	2
Vancomycin	15 mg/kg	N/A

Oral Antibiotics for Colorectal Surgery Prophylaxis (Used in Conjunction With a Mechanical Bowel Preparation)		
Erythromycin base	20 mg/kg (up to 1 g)	N/A
Metronidazole	15 mg/kg (up to 1 g)	N/A
Neomycin	15 mg/kg (up to 1 g)	N/A

[a]The maximum pediatric dose should not exceed the usual adult dose.

[b]For antimicrobials with a short half-life (e.g., cefazolin, cefoxitin) used before long procedures, redosing in the operating room is recommended at an interval of approximately two times the half-life of the agent in patients with normal renal function. Recommended redosing intervals marked as "not applicable" (N/A) are based on typical case length; for unusually long procedures, redosing may be needed.

[c]While fluoroquinolones have been associated with an increased risk of tendinitis/tendon rupture in all ages, use of these agents for single-dose prophylaxis is generally safe.

[d]In general, gentamicin for surgical antibiotics prophylaxis should be limited to a single dose given preoperatively. Dosing is based on the patient's actual body weight. If the patient's actual weight is more than 20% above ideal body weight (IBW), the dosing weight (DW) can be determined as follows: DW = IBW + 0.4 (actual weight − IBW).

Adapted from Bratzler DW, Dellinger EP, Olsen KM, et al. Clinical practice guidelines for antimicrobial prophylaxis in surgery. *Am J Health Syst Pharm.* 2013;70(3):195–283.

there are limited data supporting its use perioperatively.[151,152] Most recommendations for adults are the same for pediatric patients. Dosing recommendations in pediatric patients are limited and have been extrapolated from adult data; therefore nearly all pediatric recommendations are based on expert opinion. Pediatric efficacy data are few. Fluoroquinolones should not be routinely used for surgical prophylaxis in pediatric patients because of the potential for toxicity in this population. The same principle of preoperative dosing within 60 minutes before incision has been applied to pediatric patients. Additional intraoperative dosing may be needed if the duration of the procedure exceeds two half-lives of the antimicrobial agent or there is excessive blood loss during the procedure. As with adult patients, single-dose prophylaxis is usually sufficient. If antimicrobial prophylaxis is continued postoperatively, the duration should be less than 24 hours, regardless of the presence of intravascular catheters or indwelling drains. There are sufficient pharmacokinetic studies of most agents to recommend pediatric dosages that provide adequate systemic exposure and, presumably, efficacy comparable to that demonstrated in adults. Therefore the pediatric doses recommended in guidelines are based largely on pharmacokinetic data and the extrapolation of adult efficacy data to pediatric patients. Because few clinical trials have been conducted in pediatric surgical patients, strength of evidence criteria have not been applied to these recommendations. With few exceptions (e.g., aminoglycoside dosages), pediatric doses should not exceed the maximum adult recommended dosages. Generally, if a dose is calculated on a milligram-per-kilogram basis for children weighing more than 40 kg, the calculated dosage will likely exceed the maximum recommended dose for adults; adult dosages should therefore be used for larger children.[153]

The Timing of Antibiotic Prophylaxis

The 2013 revised policy paper on prophylactic antibiotics developed jointly by the American Society of Health-System Pharmacists (ASHP), the Infectious Disease Society of America, the Surgical Infection Society, and the Society for Healthcare Epidemiology of America states:

Successful prophylaxis requires the delivery of the antimicrobial to the operative site before contamination occurs. Thus, the antimicrobial agent should be administered at such a time to provide serum and tissue concentrations exceeding the minimum inhibitory concentration (MIC) for the probable organisms associated with the procedure, at the time of incision, and for the duration of the procedure.[154]

Current evidence suggests that for most β-lactams, a bolus dose at 15 to 45 minutes before incision is ideal and provides maximum interstitial fluid concentrations at the time of initial bacterial seeding (see Table 50.12). Because diffusion distances from capillary to pathogen are greater in obese patients, for this patient subset initiating antibiotic infusion 30 minutes or longer before incision is warranted on theoretical grounds.[155] The initial β-lactam bolus dose should be followed by additional doses at every 1 to 2 half-lives per the ASHP guidelines.[154] The use of a SSI prevention bundle in pediatric patients improves compliance with preincision antibiotic administration and decreases the SSI infection rate.[156]

Allergy to β-Lactams

Several studies have shown that the true incidence of allergy to antibiotics is less than that reflected in medical charts.[157] For surgical procedures where cephalosporins are the prophylaxis of choice, alternative antibiotics should be administered to those children at risk of anaphylaxis to β-lactams, based on their history or diagnostic tests (e.g., skin testing). However, the incidence of severe allergic reactions to first-generation cephalosporins in children with reported allergy to penicillin is rare (but not zero)[158,159]; furthermore, skin testing does not reliably predict the likelihood of adverse reactions to cephalosporins in those with reported allergy to penicillin.[160–162] There is no evidence of any risk of cross-reactivity between penicillin and second- and third-generation cephalosporins. For the most part, "allergies" to oral antibiotics that appear on children's charts (rash, vomiting, gastrointestinal disturbances) are reactions to the additives in the antibiotic formulation, including food dyes, fillers, and other compounds, or a manifestation of the underlying infection. IV administration of small test doses of the pure antibiotic in a fully monitored (and anesthetized) child will determine whether the child is at risk for an allergic reaction to the antibiotic. In the case of surgical procedures where antibiotic prophylaxis is mainly directed at gram-positive cocci, children who are truly allergic to β-lactams (cephalosporins) should receive either vancomycin or clindamycin.[163] However, in those children where the history is consistent with either an IgE-mediated penicillin allergy (urticaria, angioedema, anaphylaxis, bronchospasm) or a severe non–IgE-mediated reaction (interstitial nephritis, toxic epidermal necrolysis, hemolytic anemia, or Stevens-Johnson syndrome) it is advisable to switch out the cefazolin. Cross-sensitivity occurs when the R1 side chains of the penicillins and cephalosporins are similar, which perhaps surprisingly is not the case with cefazolin. Cephalosporins with R1 side chains similar to penicillins include cephalexin, cefaclor, and cefadroxil. The risk associated with use of first- or second-generation cephalosporins with dissimilar side chains, or third- or fourth-generation cephalosporins, "*appears to be very low in patients with mild-to-moderate reactions to penicillin G, ampicillin, or amoxicillin. Dismissing cefazolin use when there is a vague history of any penicillin allergy should be reconsidered.*"[155]

Indications for Prophylactic Antibiotics

Surgical wounds are classified into four categories (Table 50.13). The use of antibiotic prophylaxis for postoperative infections is well established for clean-contaminated procedures. Within the clean category, prophylaxis has been traditionally reserved for surgical procedures involving a foreign body implantation or for any surgical procedure where an SSI would be catastrophic (e.g., cardiac surgery or neurosurgical procedures). However, there is evidence that postoperative infections resulting from procedures not involving prosthetic elements are underreported; estimates show that more than 50% of all complications occur after the patient is discharged and are thus unrecognized by the surgical team. Therefore antibiotic prophylaxis is also recommended for certain procedures, such as herniorrhaphy.[164,165] The direct and indirect costs of these complications may not affect the hospital budget; however, they represent a substantial cost for the community at large. In the case of contaminated or dirty procedures, bacterial contamination or infection is established before the procedure begins. Accordingly, the perioperative administration of antibiotics is a therapeutic, not a prophylactic, measure. The use of antibiotics in children has implications not only for the response to the current treatment but also to future treatments. Thus all medical professionals are jointly responsible for the rational use of antibiotics.

Protocols, although effective, require continuous feedback on their acceptance and SSI results.[166] No surgical protocol can replace

TABLE 50.13	Wound Classification System
Wound Category	**Description**
Class I/clean	Uninfected wound with no inflammation, and the respiratory, alimentary, genital, or uninfected urinary tract is not entered. Clean wounds primarily are closed and drained, when necessary, with closed drainage. Operative wounds after blunt trauma may be included in this category if they meet criteria.
Class II/clean contaminated	Operative wound in which the respiratory, alimentary, genital, or urinary tract is entered under controlled conditions and without unusual contamination. Specifically, operations involving the biliary tract, appendix, vagina, and oropharynx are included in the category, provided no evidence of infection or major break in technique is encountered.
Class III/contaminated	Open, fresh, accidental wounds; operations with major breaks in sterile technique (e.g., open cardiac massage) or gross spillage from the gastrointestinal tract; and incisions in which acute, nonpurulent inflammation is encountered
Class IV/dirty-infected	Old traumatic wounds with retained devitalized tissue and those that involve existing clinical infection or perforated viscera, suggesting that the organisms causing postoperative infection were present in the operative field before operation.

From Neville HL, Lally KP. Pediatric surgical wound infections. *Semin Pediatr Infect Dis.* 2001;12:124–129.

the judgment of the medical professional; clinical reasoning must be tailored to the individual circumstances. Finally, children with congenital heart disease and a subgroup of those with repaired congenital heart disease may require bacterial endocarditis prophylaxis (see also Tables 16.2 and 16.3).[167]

ANNOTATED REFERENCES

Fernandez PG, Loftus RW, Dodds TM, et al. Hand hygiene knowledge and perceptions among anesthesia providers. *Anesth Analg.* 2015;120(4):837-843.

Anesthesiologists have long been patient safety advocates. It is not surprising that anesthesia providers have taken on increasing responsibility for preventing health care–associated infections. However, the overall hand hygiene compliance across health care providers remains less than 50%, with anesthesia providers identified as a particularly noncompliant group. In this paper, the authors identified risk factors for knowledge deficits among anesthesia providers and characterized anesthesia provider perceptions, attitudes, awareness of individual group performance, workload and type, and accessibility of hand hygiene agents.

Loftus RW, Brown JR, Koff MD, et al. Multiple reservoirs contribute to intraoperative bacterial transmission. *Anesth Analg.* 2012;114(6):1236-1248.

Bacterial cross-contamination is thought to play an important role in the development of health care–associated infections, but the relative importance of the known hospital bacterial reservoirs (health care providers' hands, patient, and environment, including health care equipment) in this process is unknown. A better understanding of how bacterial cross-contamination occurs can provide the basis for the development of evidence-based preventive measures. This paper examined the relative contributions of anesthesia providers' hands, the patient, and the patient environment to stopcock contamination.

Rizzo M. Striving to eliminate catheter-related bloodstream infections: a literature review of evidence-based strategies. *Semin Anesth Perioper Med Pain.* 2005;24(4):214-225.

This paper reviews and emphasizes the need for preventive measures that could help to avoid or reduce most nosocomial catheter-related infections. The use of evidence-based standardized protocols will result in "best practices" and markedly reduce such infections.

Sagoe-Moses CH, Pearson R, Perry J, Jagger J. Risks to health care workers in developing countries. *N Engl J Med.* 2001;345(7):538-541.

Protecting HCWs in developing countries from exposure to bloodborne pathogens will involve some cost. HCWs are a crucial resource in the health care systems of developing nations. In many countries, including those in sub-Saharan Africa, workers are at increased risk for preventable, life-threatening occupational infections. This paper expands on the need for improved support of HCWs throughout the world with appropriate supplies of gloves, barriers, sharps disposal, and the need for accident education programs.

A complete reference list can be found online at ExpertConsult.com.

Pediatric Anesthesia in Developing Countries

51

ADRIAN T. BÖSENBERG

THE POPULATION IN THE DEVELOPING WORLD CONTINUES TO GROW while world demographics trend toward an aging population in an urbanized, developed world. Children, many orphaned by the ravages of war, human immunodeficiency virus (HIV) infection,[1] and famine, constitute more than one-half of the population in many of these countries.[2] Eighty-five percent will require surgery before their 15th birthday.[3] The burden of surgical disease requires safe anesthesia,[4,5] but provision of safe pediatric anesthesia[6] and intensive care[7-9] in the developing world presents serious challenges.[10-12] Few of these countries have adopted the World Health Organization (WHO) drive for safe surgery.

Poverty, poor educational standards, and limited health resources characterize the developing world.[5,6,13] Debt repayment, housing, education, social services, and health care provision are near-impossible tasks for most governments of these countries. Of the world's poorest countries, 70% are in sub-Saharan Africa, are ravaged by HIV, malaria, Zika virus, and tuberculosis. In addition they are desperately short of health care providers.[4,5]

Pediatric anesthesia in low-income countries has not kept pace with the advances made in developed countries.[4] International standards for the safe practice of anesthesia, adopted by the World Federation of Societies of Anaesthesiologists (WFSA), are seldom met.[14-16] In one survey, only 13% of anesthesiologists were able to provide safe anesthesia for children.[3] Consequently, perioperative mortality and morbidity rates are high by developed world standards,[5,17-21] although local expectations are commensurate with the facilities and quality of the available care.

This chapter outlines some of the many challenges that anesthesiologists face when providing anesthesia for children in a low-income country. Different countries have different problems requiring different solutions. The problems faced in many tropical countries,[8,13] for example, are completely different from those on a tropical island in the South Pacific[22] or West Indies,[23,24] at altitude in Nepal[25] and Afghanistan,[26] or in the humidity of sub-Saharan Africa.[2,3,19,21,27-30] These diverse situations necessitate that generalizations be made. The main differences among these sites are related to the personnel, the spectrum and nature of the disease, the facilities and equipment available, and a tenuous supply of cheap, generic, and perhaps outdated drugs.[10,31]

The Child

Children of the developing world are, for the most part, victims of circumstance: natural disasters, war, refugees, social unrest,[32] and economic crises. For many, medical care or timely access to care can be a remote or nonexistent possibility.[10,25,30,33,34] Fear, poor understanding of medical problems, and poor education often result in delayed presentation. Frequently, prior visits to well-meaning traditional healers expose the child to additional risks caused by potions that may be hepatic or nephrotoxic or enemas that can lead to bowel perforation.[35] Further delays occur when children need to undertake long journeys to the hospital and if the initial diagnosis is incorrect, tertiary referral is often made only when complications occur (Fig. 51.1).[10,30,36,37]

A typical example is acute appendicitis, a relatively uncommon condition in the developing world, where many other causes for a change in bowel habit are initially suspected.[37,38] Most children present for surgery with generalized peritonitis, and perforation is common. In the developing world, the prospect of providing emergent anesthesia for a toxic, acidotic, and dehydrated child is daunting.

Another example is infantile hypertrophic pyloric stenosis, also uncommon in developing countries, where symptoms other than the classic triad of bile-free vomiting, visible peristalsis, and a palpable tumor are more likely. The unsuspecting anesthesiologist, who may have no access to a laboratory[2,13-15] and is limited in the choice of fluid for resuscitation, would be challenged to manage the extreme metabolic derangements in these infants.

Superstition plays a role in compounding the anesthesia risk. For example, rural Vietnamese believe that it is not good to die with an empty stomach. Parents consider surgery to be an enormous risk so they feed their children beforehand. In these circumstances, passage of a nasogastric tube before induction is routine, although it is very unlikely that the stomach can be completely emptied of solids.[24]

Perinatal mortality in some parts of the developing world is 10 times greater than those in developed countries.[5,39-41] The common denominators are early childbearing, poor maternal health, and lack of appropriate and quality medical services.

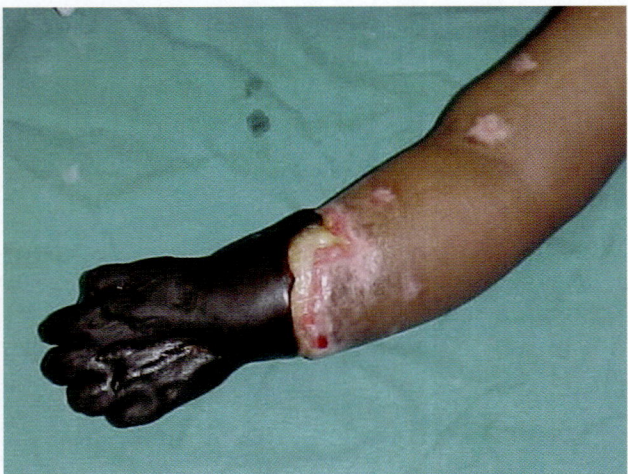

FIGURE 51.1 Peripheral gangrene of the hand. Severe dehydration in this infant was caused by severe gastroenteritis. Dehydration associated with delayed presentation, hypernatremia, herbal medications, and pneumonia are common contributors to this disastrous outcome.

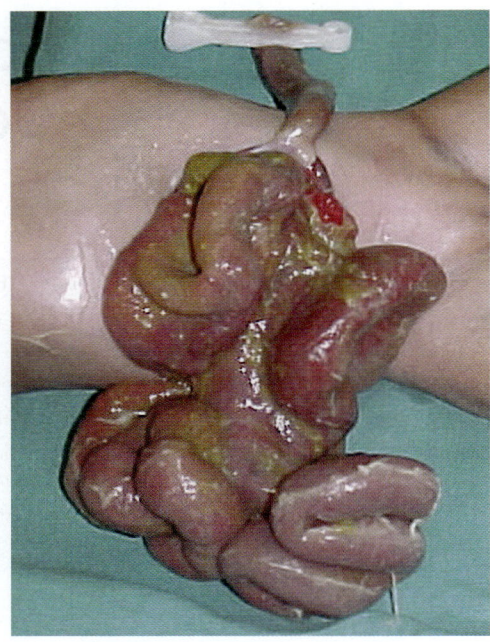

FIGURE 51.2 Gastroschisis is a major problem in the developing world. The outcome is poor because of a paucity of facilities for neonates. This defect was not diagnosed antenatally, and the patient presented late for closure, which proved difficult. Ventilatory support was not available, and a silo was fashioned. Unfortunately, the child died of overwhelming sepsis a week later.

Although lifesaving practices for most infants have been known for decades, one-third of pregnant women still have no access to medical services during pregnancy, and almost 50% do not have access to medical services for childbirth.[30,34,41] Most parturients give birth at home or in rural health centers,[34] where basic neonatal resuscitation equipment is deficient or nonexistent.[30] Those who require surgery may need to be transferred, but specialized transport teams rarely exist.

In some hospitals, neonates are not candidates for surgery because "they always die,"[42] whereas in others, they undergo surgery without anesthesia[23] because "it's safer" and because some still believe that neonates do not feel pain. When neonates undergo surgery, there are additional challenges, particularly in emergency situations.[23] Appropriately sized equipment is lacking,[36] and it may be extremely difficult to maintain normothermia even in relatively warm climates without improvisation. Regional anesthesia can play a significant role in neonatal anesthesia[30,36,43] and in some centers may be the only choice for anesthesia.[34,44] Apart from providing analgesia without respiratory depression, the need for postoperative ventilatory support for conditions such as esophageal atresia,[45] congenital diaphragmatic hernia,[46] and abdominal wall defects can be reduced by continuous epidural analgesia (Fig. 51.2).

Regrettably, even neonates who receive skilled anesthesia and surgery may die because of inadequate postoperative care.[44] Overwhelming infection, sepsis, respiratory insufficiency, and surgical complications are the main causes of morbidity and mortality.[30,34] The development of highly specialized neonatal anesthesia and surgical services,[7,40–42] essential for a good outcome after neonatal surgery,[30,34,36] is a low priority.

Although the burden of disease is dominated by infections and malnutrition,[4,5] pediatric trauma has a low level of advocacy and is given scant attention.[30,36,47] Socioeconomic advances in some countries have introduced a new danger in the form of faster, more powerful vehicles without the necessary maintenance culture or road discipline. Road traffic accidents are inevitable, and effective systems to handle the polytrauma victims that result are hard to find.[36]

Even simple bone fractures may have disastrous outcomes. Inappropriate management by traditional bonesetters frequently results in compartment syndromes or gangrene.[47] Trauma prevention strategies are given low priority despite the acknowledged impact of trauma on the economy of any country. Many developing countries are at war, and this has led to massive trauma and injuries to children who may be either participants in the fighting or innocent bystanders.

CHILDREN AND WAR

Children may be victims of all aspects of violence. They face an intense struggle for survival because of displacement, separation from or loss of parents, poverty, hunger, and disease. They are vulnerable to the abuse of abandonment, abduction, rape, and forced soldiering. An estimated 300,000 children are used as child soldiers in more than 30 countries.[48] Many sustain physical injuries and permanent disabilities, and a large number acquire sexually transmitted disease, including HIV and AIDS. These HIV-positive child soldiers then become vectors in communities where they are deployed.[49]

For many of these children, acts of violence become their form of normality, and former victims become the perpetrators.[32] Survivors are subjected to the total collapse of economic, health, social, and educational infrastructures. Lost and abandoned children sleep on the streets and are forced to beg for food while trying to find their families. Many become child laborers or turn to crime or prostitution for survival.[50]

Children in war-torn areas sustain bullet, machete, or shrapnel injuries, and others are burned. They often sustain mutilating injuries (Figs. 51.3 and 51.4) that are not commonly seen in civilians.[51] Land mines are responsible for killing or maiming an

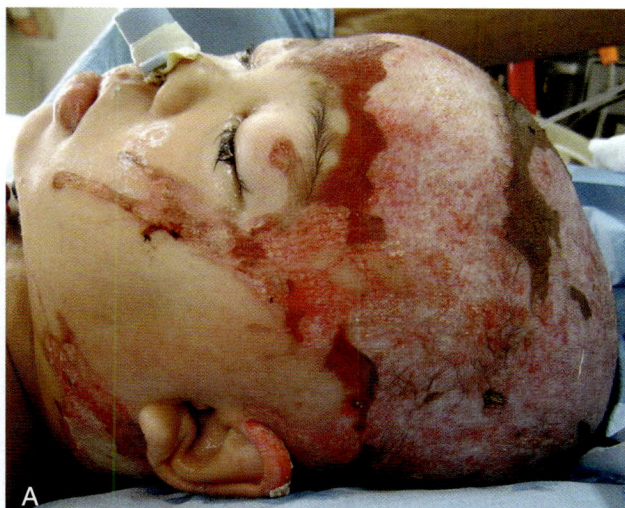

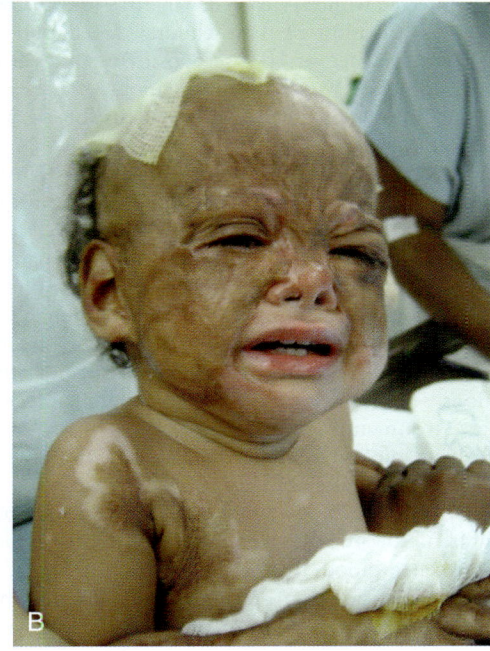

FIGURE 51.3 Facial burn injuries are common in the developing world, and these children may require multiple episodes of anesthesia. **A**, Flame burns of the face are invariably associated with inhalation injuries that may necessitate ventilatory support in intensive care facilities, which are not readily available. **B**, Pain management and pain assessment are challenging. The pained expression on this child's face is one of fear (and possible indignation about having the photograph taken) rather than actual pain.

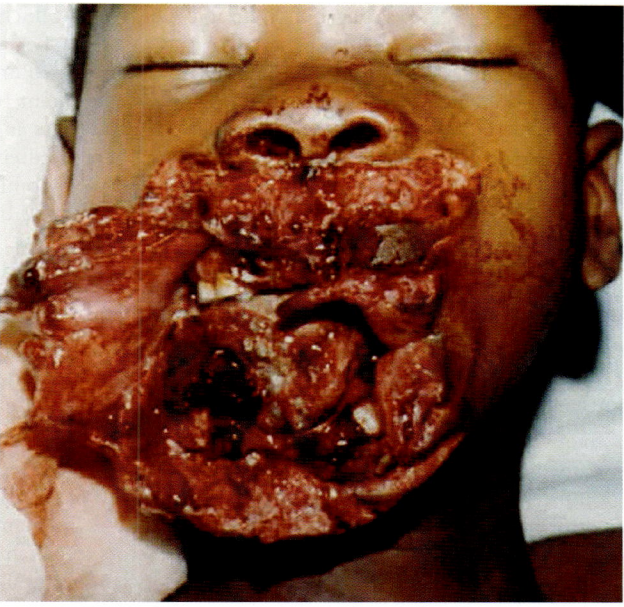

FIGURE 51.4 Children fare poorly in war. This 8-year-boy bit a detonator he found while playing. Endotracheal intubation proved a major challenge without a fiberoptic laryngoscope, which is a luxury in the developing world.

estimated 12,000 civilians per annum. In Angola, a country with the highest rate of amputees in the world, there were an estimated 5.5 land mines for every child. Continuing land mine explosions remain a legacy of this conflict.[51] These blast injuries leave children without feet or lower limbs and with genital injuries, blindness, and deafness—a pattern of injury that has become a post–civil war syndrome encountered by surgeons worldwide.[51] Although the war in Angola is over, the cost of mine removal is beyond the means of local governments. Ironically, artificial limb manufacture has become a developing industry.[51] Tragedies such as these are likely to be repeated in the ongoing conflicts in Afghanistan, Syria, South Sudan, and Somalia.

The terrible psychological effects of war persist even though the armed conflict may be over. Mental and psychiatric disorders with all the ramifications of posttraumatic stress disorder are common among child survivors.

PAIN

Pain management modalities for children in the developed world are vastly different from those available to practitioners working with limited resources.[52] Attempts to apply similar standards are fraught with difficulty. Illiteracy, malnutrition, poor cognitive development, different coping strategies, altitude (e.g., chronic hypoxia),[53] and pharmacogenetic, cultural, and language differences all contribute to the complexity of the problem.[54]

Children of the developing world learn to cope with vastly different problems. Victims of poverty, malnutrition, violence (e.g., war, trauma, abuse), their attitudes toward pain, and pain tolerance are diverse. Children from an impoverished background seem more stoic and indifferent to even severe pain. After cardiac surgery, for example, some appear to need very little pain relief and are easily soothed by lollipops or play therapy.[33] Many can walk from the intensive care unit to the general ward on the first postoperative day.

Pain assessment of children from an impoverished background is difficult[55] (see Fig. 51.3B). Many children in acute pain do not show facial expressions. Is this stoicism or simply a reflection of malnutrition, lack of social stimulation, severity of illness, or even cultural attitude? Language difficulties, cultural barriers, willingness to share information, emotional expressiveness, and outdated attitudes of the caregiver may underpin this quandary. Some cultures convey pain readily, but others teach that expression of pain is inappropriate. Although many pain assessment instruments are available, few have been validated in the developing world.[55–57]

There is an urgent need to develop pain treatment strategies applicable to children of the developing world. Local conditions dictate their use and applicability. Simple pain management strategies may produce the most benefit with the least risk, whereas more complex techniques—offering greater benefit—require minimum standards of monitoring and regular reassessment to titrate analgesia to the needs of the individual. These devices and the necessary personnel are seldom available for these children. The final choice of analgesia is therefore dictated by economic pressures or by the facilities available rather than what would be considered best for the child.

Human Resources

Anesthesia does not enjoy a high profile and lacks the voice to demand access to basic resources in developing countries. The critical shortage of manpower is a barrier to progress.[5,8] Anesthesia is frequently delivered by nonphysicians,[3,6,58] a reality that has remained constant over many decades. Most anesthetics are still administered by nurses or unqualified personnel who have little medical background and are "trained on the job."[3,36] In many African[5,59] and Asian countries,[5,60] the ratio of doctors to patients is often so small that the ideal of employing a physician specifically to provide routine anesthesia is out of the question.[5,61,62] Salaries are insufficient to attract suitably trained and qualified practitioners for more than short periods. Emigration of scarce trained personnel to developed countries in search of better salaries and improved lifestyles exacerbates these human resource shortfalls.[5,10,58,61–64]

Anesthesia is not perceived as an attractive career for many undergraduates,[63] who receive little or no exposure to the specialty.[64] In some countries, surgery is performed without the "luxury" of anesthesia.[65] Few developing countries can afford specialist anesthesiologists, possibly excepting the principal hospitals. Supervision of "nonphysician anesthesiologists" is invariably inadequate,[66] and access to textbooks, journals, or other medical literature is limited. Internet access is invaluable but depends on a reliable electrical supply, telecommunications network, and a computer.[67,68]

Despite these problems, many individuals provide high-quality anesthesia for a limited range of surgical procedures. Few receive formal training in pediatric or neonatal anesthesia. Inadequately trained anesthesiologists tend to shy away from children, particularly neonates and infants, because of the perceived difficulty or fear. This is understandable in view of the lack of supervision, the severity of the child's condition, and equipment that is more suited for adults. Invariably, the "pediatric anesthesiologist" is someone who may simply have a special interest in or affinity for children, or is allocated to pediatric anesthesia for the day because there is no one else. A genuine pediatric trained anesthesiologist is a luxury.

On a more positive note, the WHO has recognized that surgery is a public health issue and has launched the Safe Surgery Saves Lives campaign.[5,16,17,62,69] The WHO has emphasized that safe surgery does not exist without safe anesthesia.[10,11,16,17] Training anesthesiologists in the skills required for pediatric anesthesia is a slow process. Hopefully the WFSA fellowship programs[6,15,69–76] will snowball so that children undergoing surgery in developing countries will reap the benefit.

Pathology

Many pathologic conditions seldom seen in industrialized countries are more prevalent in developing countries because of poor health education, malnutrition, the proximity of livestock to humans, earth-floored homes, poor sanitation, and contaminated water supplies (Fig. 51.5). Some conditions prevalent worldwide and relevant to the anesthesiologist are considered in the following sections.

HUMAN IMMUNODEFICIENCY VIRUS INFECTION AND ACQUIRED IMMUNODEFICIENCY SYNDROME

While the world has committed to ending the AIDS epidemic by 2030, an estimated 36.7 million people are living with HIV, 19 million of whom do not know their HIV status. Only half of those who know their HIV status are accessing antiretroviral therapy. Most cases occur in the developing world (90%), with sub-Saharan Africa (24.7 million) and Southeast Asia (4.8 million) making up two-thirds of the global total. Approximately 8% are children (see Fig. 51.5A).[77] More than 35 million have died of HIV-related diseases since the start of the epidemic in 1981, and as a consequence, there are an estimated 15 million orphans in sub-Saharan Africa alone.[77] Worldwide, more than 500 children were newly infected with HIV each day in 2016 (down from 1000 each day in 2010); most of these children are in sub-Saharan Africa.[78] The prevalence of HIV seropositivity varies from one country to another. In these clinical situations, anesthesiologists and surgeons[79] should assume a positive status for every patient until proven otherwise.[36]

Some success has been achieved in slowing the transmission of HIV in developed countries.[79–85] In sub-Saharan Africa today, 90% of those who know their HIV status have received treatment and 76% have achieved viral suppression. Numerous barriers exist to the treatment of HIV-infected children.[77] Treatment has lagged behind that of adults primarily as a result of poor human resources and infrastructure for administration of antiretroviral treatment,[86] but also because of the expense and the lack of pediatric drug formulations.[82] Only an estimated 25% children infected with HIV receive treatment.[77]

Children are infected by vertical transmission from the mother (>90%) or when sexually abused (≈2%) by an infected adult.[87] Transmission through blood products remains a risk, but with the global trend toward volunteer donors and more sophisticated testing of donated blood, this risk is diminishing.

Vertical transmission can occur in utero, during labor and delivery, or postnatally. Risk factors include maternal viral load and breastfeeding.[78,84] Data indicate that mixed feeding (i.e., breastfeeding with other oral foods and liquids) is associated with the greatest risk of transmission.[88] Perinatal transmission rates are dramatically reduced by universal HIV testing of pregnant women, provision of antiretroviral therapy (when needed for maternal health); or prophylaxis, elective cesarean delivery, and avoidance of breastfeeding.[78,84] Highly active antiretroviral therapy (HAART), the triple antiretroviral therapy, has changed HIV from a fatal illness to a chronic disease with decreased mortality rates and improved quality of life[84]; however, these strategies require resources.

In practical terms, it is difficult to differentiate infants who are infected by vertical transmission from those who are not infected because differentiating between actively or passively acquired antibodies is virtually impossible in low-income countries. All children born to HIV-positive mothers have acquired HIV antibodies for the first 6 to 18 months. Only 30% to 40% of the infants who are infected develop AIDS. The presence of HIV antibody is therefore not a reliable indicator of infection. More sophisticated and expensive tests have been developed but are not widely available. All children born to HIV-positive mothers

Adults and Children Estimated to Be Living with HIV, 2008
Total: 33.4 million (31.1-35.8 million)

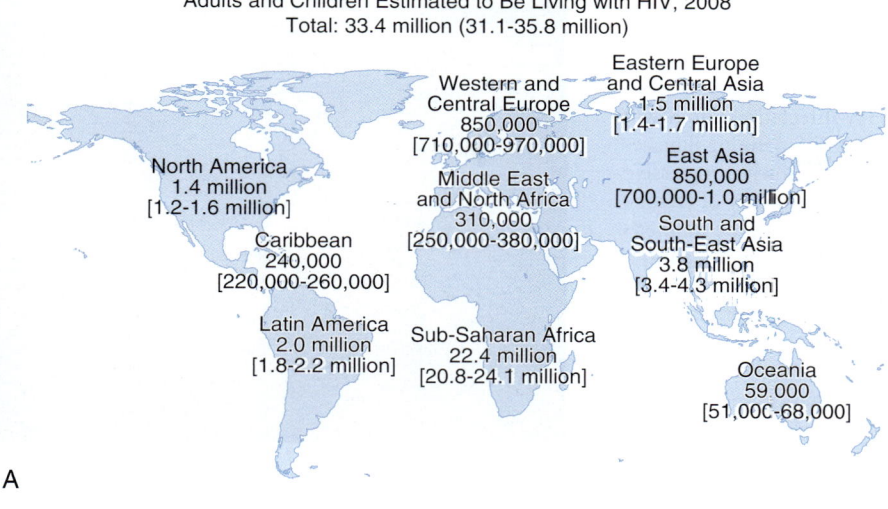

A

Estimated Malaria Incidence, 2005

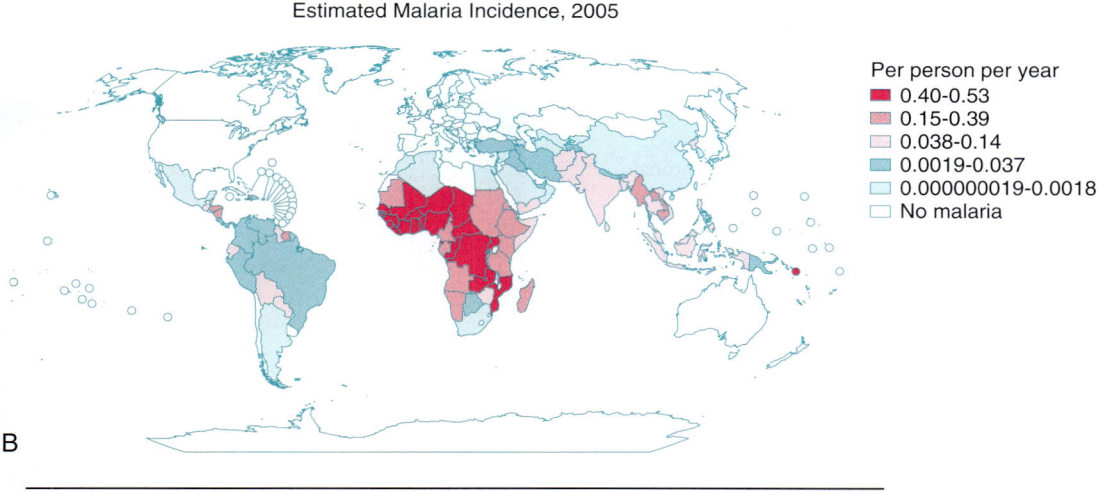

B

Estimated TB Incidence, 2005

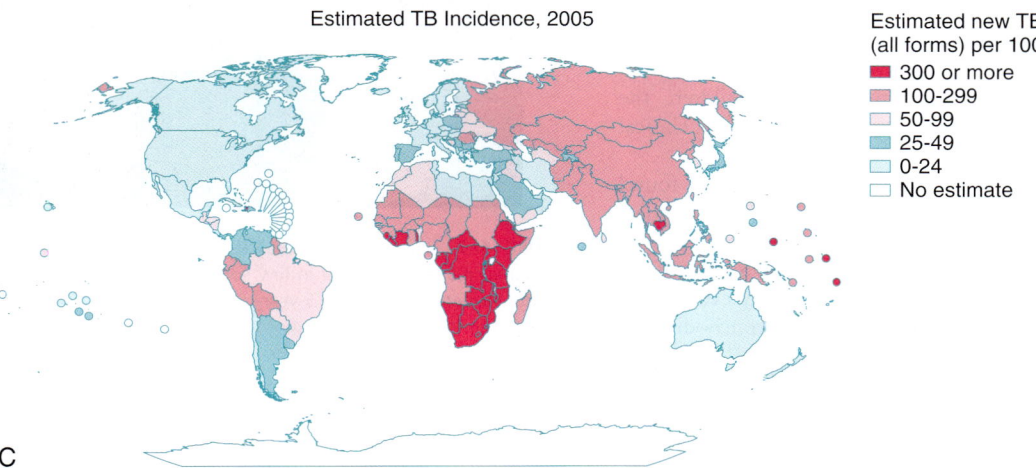

C

FIGURE 51.5 A, Global distribution of human immunodeficiency virus infection and acquired immunodeficiency syndrome (HIV/AIDS). Developing countries, particularly sub-Saharan Africa, carry the greatest health burden with the poor resources. **B,** The global distribution of malaria is remarkably similar to that of HIV/AIDS. Blood products in these regions carry an enormous risk, even if family members act as donors. **C,** Global distribution of tuberculosis (*TB*) in 2005. (**A,** From *AIDS Epidemic Update*, p. 66; available at http://data.unaids.org/pub/EpiReport/2006/2006 _EpiUpdate_en.pdf [accessed September 2017]; **B,** from *World Malaria Report*. Available at http://www.rbm.who. int/wmr2005/html/map3.htm [accessed September 2017]; **C,** from the WHO *World Health Report 2006*. Available at http://www.who.int/whr/2006/en/ [accessed September 2017].)

should be considered infected; if antibody persists beyond 15 months, infection should be assumed.

Progression of the disease depends on the mode of transmission; vertically acquired infection is more aggressive than other forms. Between 20% and 30% of untreated HIV-infected children will develop profound immunodeficiency and AIDS-defining illnesses within a year, whereas two-thirds will have a slowly progressive disease. The course of the disease depends on a variety of factors, including timing of infection in utero, the viral load, the mother's stage of the disease, and whether the mother is receiving antiretroviral therapy. Treatment of children depends on clinical category, CD4 T-cell cell count, viral load, and age at the time of diagnosis. According to the current state of knowledge, after HAART is started, it must be carried on lifelong. This implies great challenges in adherence to avoid development of resistance and to evade long-term adverse effects of HIV therapy. Emerging drug resistance in children in low- and middle-income countries has necessitated new treatment strategies.[82,85]

The clinical manifestation of HIV in infants and children depends on whether they have been managed with antiretrovirals or not.[79,82,85] Most have asymptomatic infections, and the presentation may be subtle, such as failure to thrive, lymphadenopathy, hepatosplenomegaly, interstitial pneumonia, chronic diarrhea, or persistent oral thrush. Some present for the first time with life-threatening disease.

Chronic diarrhea, wasting, and severe malnutrition predominate in Africa, whereas systemic and pulmonary pathologies are more common in the United States and Europe. Recurrent bacterial infections, chronic parotid swelling, lymphocytic interstitial pneumonitis (LIP), and early onset of progressive neurologic deterioration are characteristic of children with AIDS.

Pulmonary disease remains the leading cause of morbidity and mortality.[89-91] Bacterial pneumonia, viral pneumonia, and pulmonary tuberculosis are common, and the course of these infections is more fulminant when associated with HIV infection.[92] As the CD4 T-cell count falls, acute opportunistic infections occur, including *Pneumocystis (carinii) jiroveci* pneumonia (PCP or PJP), cytomegalovirus infection, and the more typical *Haemophilus influenzae, Streptococcus pneumoniae,* and respiratory syncytial virus infections.[89,90,92] The classic presentation of PCP is fever, tachypnea, dyspnea, and marked hypoxemia, but in some children, the presentation is more indolent, with hypoxemia preceding clinical or radiologic changes.[93]

LIP is a slowly progressive, chronic form of lung disease found in older children that can lead to an insidious onset of dyspnea, cough, and chronic hypoxia with normal auscultatory findings but with pulmonary lymphoid hyperplasia in AIDS patients. In contrast to the signs in adults, LIP in children may cause acute respiratory failure that is treated with steroids and bronchodilators. The clinical manifestations affecting otolaryngologists[94] and dental surgeons[95] have been outlined. Management of the upper airway may be difficult in the presence of stomatitis and gingival disease. Intubation may be difficult in the presence of acute (i.e., candidal infection) or chronic epiglottitis (i.e., lymphoid hyperplasia), necrotizing laryngotracheitis, Kaposi sarcoma (Fig. 51.6), or laryngeal papillomas (Fig. 51.7). These comorbid respiratory disorders challenge even the most experienced pediatric anesthesiologist (Fig. 51.8).

Cardiac disease is being diagnosed with increasing frequency in children with HIV. The pathogenesis of cardiomyopathy is multifactorial, including pulmonary insufficiency, anemia, nutritional deficiencies, specific viral infections, and drug therapy. Left

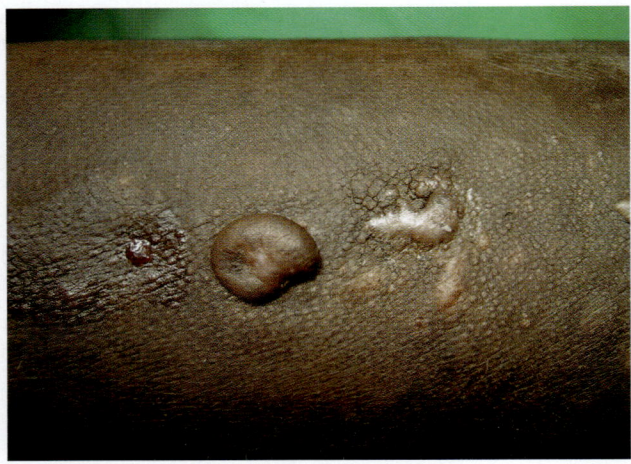

FIGURE 51.6 Human immunodeficiency virus infection and acquired immunodeficiency syndrome (HIV/AIDS) are an increasing problem is developing countries, particularly in sub-Saharan Africa. The skin manifestations in this 8-year-old boy indicate Kaposi sarcoma, an AIDS-defining tumor.

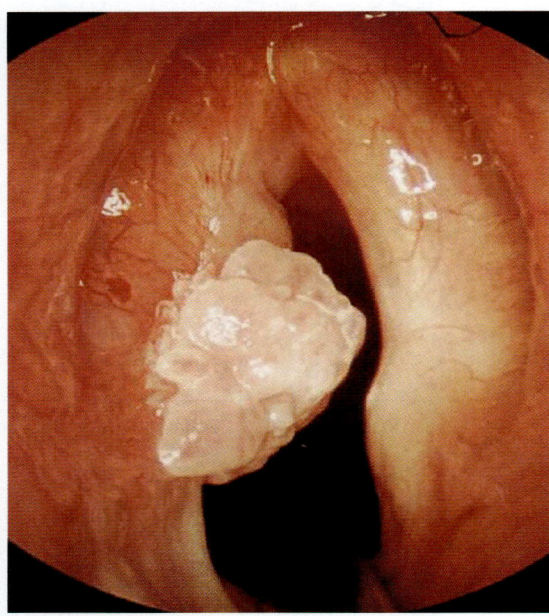

FIGURE 51.7 Laryngeal papilloma. Papillomas, caused by the human papillomavirus, are prevalent in low socioeconomic groups and have the highest incidence in the 2- to 5-year-old age group. This age distribution is changing in the populations exposed to human immunodeficiency virus. Even in well-equipped institutions, anesthesia for these patients can be challenging.

and right ventricular dysfunction, arrhythmias, and pericardial effusions occur, but pulmonary hypertension is rare.[96] HIV may directly infect the myocardium, leading to early electrocardiographic (ECG) changes and abnormal echocardiograms showing hyperdynamic left ventricular dysfunction or evidence of diminished contractility (e.g., dilated cardiomyopathy, myocarditis).

The gastrointestinal tract is commonly involved,[97] particularly in those living in tropical countries. Affected children show evidence of malabsorption (i.e., "slim"), chronic recurrent diarrhea,

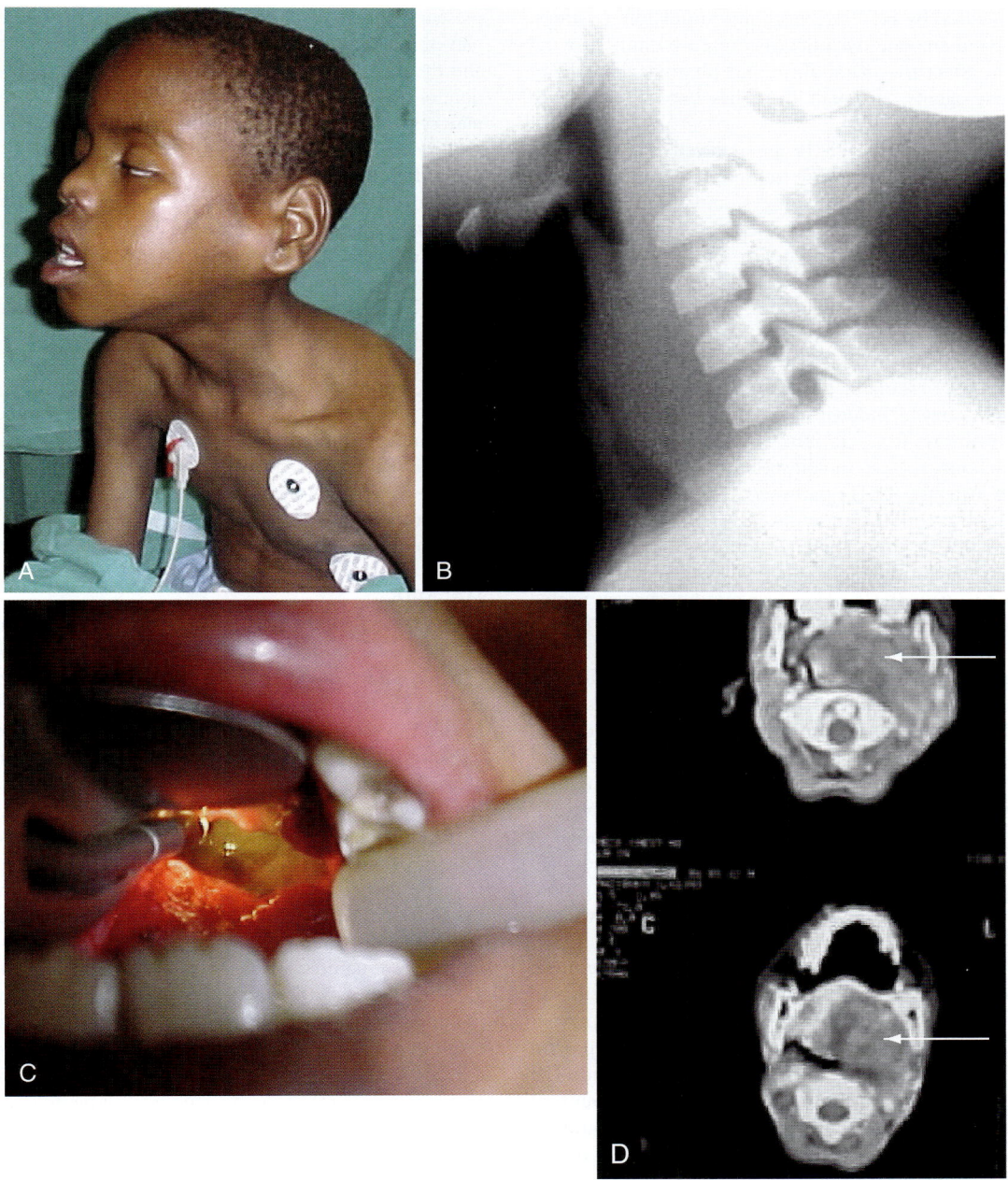

FIGURE 51.8 Kaposi sarcoma is a marker for acquired immunodeficiency syndrome (AIDS). **A,** AIDS was previously considered rare in children, but it may affect the airway at different levels, as shown in this 12-year-old girl. She is clearly fatigued from the respiratory distress caused by Kaposi sarcoma at three levels: base of the tongue, tonsil, and trachea. She also has an underlying pneumonia. Significant supraclavicular recession suggests upper airway obstruction. **B,** The Kaposi sarcoma of the base of the tongue, tonsil, and trachea is shown on a poor-quality, lateral neck radiograph, which illustrates one of the many difficulties faced in remote areas: the lack of high-quality imaging. **C,** Laryngoscopic view of the Kaposi sarcoma at the base of the tongue and the tonsil. **D,** Computed tomography shows a large retropharyngeal Kaposi sarcoma *(arrows)* obstructing the upper airway. The poor quality of the scan reflects inexperienced radiographers using the poor-quality equipment commonly found in developing countries.

dysphagia, failure to thrive, or enteric infection requiring diagnostic endoscopy. From the anesthesiologist's point of view, there is an increased risk of reflux owing to esophagitis caused by infection (e.g., *Candida*, cytomegalovirus) or drugs (e.g., zidovudine). Pseudobulbar palsy, a manifestation of central neurologic involvement, or esophageal strictures may occur.

Nausea and vomiting may have a neurologic, infectious, or drug-related cause. Pancreatitis, lymphomas, or smooth muscle tumors may delay gastric emptying. Hepatomegaly is invariably present, but severe hepatocellular dysfunction is seldom a major problem unless the patient has chronic hepatitis (e.g., hepatitis B or C, cytomegalovirus). Cholestasis and fluctuating transaminase levels may be caused by HIV infection, poor nutrition, or drugs. In theory, hepatic enzyme dysfunction caused by antiretroviral therapy should affect the metabolism and pharmacokinetics of some anesthetic agents, although there has been a paucity of research on this subject.

Medications used to manage HIV are involved in drug interactions on several levels.[98] The reverse transcriptase inhibitors (e.g., zidovudine) are excreted by the kidneys, and drugs that affect renal clearance reduce excretion. Reverse transcriptase inhibitors may induce CYP3A4 (e.g., nevirapine) or inhibit CYP3A4 (e.g., delavirdine) and affect the clearance of other drugs (e.g., midazolam, levobupivacaine, ketamine, methadone). Protease inhibitors are inhibitors of CYP3A enzyme systems and are substrates and inhibitors of P-glycoprotein transporters. Coagulation status with the concomitant use of warfarin, which is metabolized by CYP2C9, may be altered by enzyme induction (e.g., ritonavir) or competition for clearance pathways (e.g., efavirenz, nelfinavir).[99]

Protease inhibitors also can inhibit specific uridine 5′-diphospho-glucuronosyltransferase (UGT) pathways. This accounts for the increase in bilirubin concentration (i.e., UGT1A1 glucuronidates bilirubin) observed in some patients, although UGT1A6 (i.e., acetaminophen glucuronidation) and UGT2B7 (i.e., morphine glucuronidation) are unaffected.[100] Gastric motility changes related to opioids (e.g., methadone) reduce absorption of some reverse transcriptase inhibitors.

HIV, a neurotrophic virus, can have a devastating effect on the immature brain, which can be further compromised by opportunistic infections or neoplasms that occur as a consequence of the associated immunosuppression.[101] Neurologic impairment is observed in most symptomatic HIV-infected children, commonly as a progressive encephalopathy with developmental delay, progressive motor dysfunction, and behavioral changes. Craniofacial dysmorphic features have been described. Hematologic abnormalities can reflect depression of all cell lines. Anemia may be caused by primary marrow failure, malnutrition, or drugs, whereas thrombocytopenia may reflect an autoimmune disorder.

Universal precautions should be strictly applied for all anesthesia procedures. Extra care should be taken when anesthetizing an HIV-infected child. Precautions should be taken to prevent contamination of the anesthetic circuits; disposable equipment, bacterial filters, and disposable circuits are recommended. The prohibitive cost for most institutions in developing countries limits the use of disposables. Reusable equipment should be cleaned, sterilized, and decontaminated according to the manufacturer's instructions as HIV is sensitive to a wide range of disinfectants.[102]

TUBERCULOSIS

Tuberculosis remains an important cause of morbidity and mortality.[36,103–108] The epidemiology of pediatric tuberculosis is shaped by risk factors such as age, race, immigration, poverty, overcrowding, and prevalence of HIV/AIDS (see Fig. 51.5C).[107,108] HIV and tuberculosis form a dangerous synergy that is difficult to manage because of drug interactions between the antituberculosis and antiretroviral agents.[77,104] Even bacillus Calmette–Guérin (BCG) vaccinations can cause significant complications in immuno-compromised HIV patients.[104] The emergence of drug-resistant tuberculosis adds to the burden and is a constant danger to health care workers in general and anesthesiologists in particular.

Primary tuberculosis infection usually does not produce clinical illness in well-nourished, immunized children, whereas reactivated pulmonary tuberculosis is a chronic or subacute disease that may present a variety of challenges for the anesthesiologist, including preventing transmission by contamination of the anesthetic circuits and the risks associated with pleural effusions, pulmonary cavitation, or bronchiectasis.[91,93] Mediastinal and hilar lymphadenopathy may severely compromise the airway.

Primary tuberculosis and its complications are more common in children than in adults. After young children are infected, they are at increased risk for progression to extrapulmonary disease.[107,108] *Mycobacterium tuberculosis* infection can cause symptomatic disease in any organ of the body and is usually a reactivation of a latent site of infection. The most common sites of reactivation are lymph nodes, bones, joints, and the genitourinary tract. Less frequently, the disease may involve the gastrointestinal tract, peritoneum, pericardium, or skin. Tuberculosis meningitis and miliary tuberculosis, both more common in children, carry a high mortality rate.[107] In view of the high prevalence of HIV infection among tuberculous children, HIV testing should be performed in all children with tuberculosis; conversely, tuberculosis should be sought in all HIV-positive children. Tuberculosis is, however, difficult to diagnose in young children, and the search for affordable more sensitive tests continues.[103]

MALARIA

Malaria (see Fig. 51.5B) is a febrile, flu-like illness caused by one of four species of malaria parasites: *Plasmodium falciparum, P. vivax, P. ovale,* and *P. malariae.* Effective and safe prophylaxis against malaria has become increasingly difficult because the species that causes the most severe illness, *P. falciparum,* has become widely resistant to chloroquine and to other antimalarial drugs in some areas.[108] Severe malaria, even when optimally treated, carries a mortality rate of 10% to 25%.[108–110]

Prompt diagnosis and early treatment is an important determinant of outcome. Uncomplicated malaria usually manifests as fever, headache, dizziness, and arthralgia. Gastrointestinal symptoms may predominate and include anorexia, nausea, vomiting, and abdominal discomfort or pain mimicking appendicitis. In children, malaria can manifest with an acute, life-threatening disease or run a chronic course with acute exacerbations. The acute manifestations include three overlapping syndromes: respiratory distress as the result of a severe underlying metabolic acidosis (pH <7.3), usually a lactic acidemia; severe anemia (hemoglobin <5 g/dL) with hypovolemia[111] and thrombocytopenia; or neurologic impairment as a manifestation of cerebral malaria.[109–112] Seizures are an important presenting feature in 60% to 80% of cases. Prolonged seizures refractory to treatment and those that occur on antimalarial treatment are ominous signs and are usually associated with neurologic sequelae or death.[111] Cerebral malaria may also manifest as a prolonged postictal state, status epilepticus, severe metabolic derangement (i.e., hypoglycemia and metabolic acidosis), or a primary neurologic syndrome, ranging from diffuse cortical involvement to brainstem abnormalities.

Children with chronic malaria adjust physiologically to low hemoglobin concentrations but may decompensate rapidly when challenged with a febrile illness or surgery. The characteristic physical findings in children with severe anemia are respiratory distress and a hyperdynamic circulation. Blood transfusion may be administered rapidly in children with metabolic acidosis because most have a depleted intravascular volume.

Although controversial, exchange transfusion has been advocated for severe malaria, particularly for those with cardiorespiratory compromise, hyperparasitemia, or cerebral malaria. The rationale is to remove harmful metabolites, toxins, and cytokines; decrease the parasite load; remove deformed red blood cells; and restore normal red blood cell mass, platelets, and other clotting factors.[111] Unfortunately, many malaria-endemic areas also have a high prevalence of HIV, adding significantly to the risk of blood transfusions.

Chronic recurrent malarial infections may manifest with splenic enlargement. This may cause delayed gastric emptying and pose an aspiration risk on induction of anesthesia. The spleen may enlarge acutely or rupture spontaneously during coughing, vomiting, or defecation. Rupture during external cardiac massage has also been described. Malaria may cause bloody diarrhea with massive fluid loss resembling dysentery in children.

CARDIAC DISEASE

Pediatric cardiac services typically are too expensive for most developing countries, and the increasing economic divide threatens those services that do exist.[113,114] In North America, each cardiac center serves 120,000 people; by contrast, one center serves 16 million people in Asia and 33 million in Africa.[61] Despite the need, few third-world units can treat the required volume of cases. Unless families have the financial means to travel to a developed country, the options for diagnostic or therapeutic cardiac procedures remain poor.[33,113-115] Medical missions may provide immediate help, but their impact on a developing country is short-term and potentially disruptive. These visiting teams ultimately have little effect on the complex socioeconomic and sociopolitical problems that exist.[114]

Rheumatic heart disease is more common than congenital heart disease in many developing countries,[113-115] reflecting the socioeconomic problems of poverty, overcrowding, malnutrition, and lack of antibiotics. Children often present late with life-threatening symptoms as the result of repeated infections and superimposed endocarditis. The acute deterioration precipitated by endocarditis may be the factor that prompts the search for medical attention. Valve replacement can be lifesaving, but long-term follow-up of anticoagulant therapy is often not feasible.

Congenital heart disease is an additional challenge, and it is common to see congenital heart defects in adults in developing countries. Those who have survived without the benefit of palliative or corrective surgery may present with pulmonary hypertension or endocarditis. Total correction of these defects is usually not feasible, and palliative surgery may be the more effective alternative. Excellent palliation with reasonable quality of life can be achieved relatively cheaply.[114]

TETANUS

Tetanus is a disease characterized by painful tonic muscle spasms, hyperreflexia, and autonomic instability.[116] It is caused by the exotoxin of *Clostridium tetani*, an organism that is ever present in the soil and contaminated wounds. Although rarely seen in developed countries, tetanus is prevalent in countries where children are not routinely immunized. Tetanus neonatorum carries a high mortality rate and is still encountered in areas where it is customary to apply feces to the umbilical cord to stop bleeding.

The clinical manifestations of the disease are not the result of invasive tissue injury but are caused by the production of a potent neurotoxin, tetanospasmin, at the site of the injury. The injury may be trivial and may not even be detectable at the time of presentation. The incubation period is inversely proportional to the distance between the site of the injury and the central nervous system. In children, this usually occurs within 14 days of the injury.

Trismus is the presenting sign in most cases, and sustained trismus produces a characteristic sardonic smile (i.e., risus sardonicus). Persistent contraction of the chest and back muscles presents as opisthotonus. Restlessness and irritability may be followed by tetanic seizures, often precipitated by trivial stimuli (e.g., touch, noise). Glottic or laryngeal spasm can cause sudden death. Late deaths may be caused by nosocomial infection, renal failure, sudden cardiac arrest, or cerebral hemorrhage secondary to the autonomic instability.[116]

Treatment consists of surgical debridement of the wound, administration of human tetanus immunoglobulin, antibiotic therapy, and intensive supportive medical care. Ventilatory support is invariably necessary because the frequent spasms impair ventilation already compromised by sedative therapy. Benzodiazepines and opioids are the mainstay of treatment, but numerous protocols have been studied.[116] Magnesium sulfate effectively reduces spasms as well as circulating catecholamines,[117] whereas clonidine does not.[118] Pain management should also be considered, and I have been encouraged by the use of continuous epidural analgesia for these children. Further advantages of epidural analgesia include good control of autonomic instability, earlier weaning from ventilatory support, and possible reduction in the complication rate.[116] From the anesthesiologist's point of view, trismus is overcome by neuromuscular blocking drugs, removing it as an obstacle for tracheal intubation.

Drugs

The supplies of anesthetic gases and drugs for rural medical facilities are erratic and unreliable.[3,8] The cost of many drugs, particularly those used in modern anesthesia, has increased alarmingly above and beyond the reach of most health care budgets. Anesthesiologists in developing countries therefore are forced to use less expensive anesthetics or generic medications.

Halothane and isoflurane are the most widely available inhalational anesthetics, and halothane is still the mainstay of inhalational anesthesia in many countries.[2,3,10,31,119] Halothane has virtually disappeared from the operating rooms in the developed world and has been replaced by sevoflurane and desflurane. As demand for the less expensive agents such as halothane has waned, some manufacturers seeking profitability have threatened its withdrawal. Although this may make commercial business sense, these agents sustain the anesthesia services for millions of patients in the developing world[2] and their loss would be tragic.

Ketamine is probably the most commonly used intravenous (IV) anesthetic.[3,65,119] Ketamine is simple to use, effective, and relatively safe when used as a sole agent for short procedures, used in combination with neuromuscular blocking drugs, or used to supplement general anesthesia for major surgery. It should be used with midazolam to reduce the psychotomimetic effects and nightmares observed after ketamine use. Benzodiazepines, however, are not always available. Morphine and other opioids may not be permitted in some cultures or even available in some institutions. It is sobering to realize that only 6% of the morphine consumption worldwide is used in the low- and middle-income countries that are home to 80% of the world's population.[52]

The choice of neuromuscular blocking drugs is limited. Suxamethonium, gallamine, curare, alcuronium, and pancuronium are the usual options, and the choice is dictated by their availability or the availability of reversal agents. For this reason, neuromuscular blocking drugs are not commonly used.

The cost of nitrous oxide is prohibitive in terms of storage, erratic delivery, and budgetary constraints.[120,121] Closed or semi-closed anesthetic systems are considered dangerous in an environment where the oxygen supply is erratic,[121] agent monitors are seldom available,[25] and the supply of soda lime and compressed gas cylinders is erratic. Consequently, the potential benefits and cost savings of low-flow anesthesia are lost.[121,122]

Regional anesthesia has many benefits in terms of safety, cost savings, and immediate postoperative analgesia.[a] Children in developing countries usually are very accepting of this form of analgesia. However, there seems to be a general reluctance to perform regional anesthesia in children,[29,36] even in some institutions in the developed world. Possible reasons include lack of training or expertise, fear of failure, and the unavailability of drugs, disposables, and other ancillary equipment such as ultrasound.

Improvisation may be the key. In the absence of appropriate equipment, access to the epidural space can be achieved by using a technique first described before the introduction of pediatric epidural needles into clinical practice. A catheter can be threaded through an IV cannula into the epidural space through the sacral hiatus in neonates and small infants.[125] Cheap, uninsulated needles can be used for peripheral nerve blocks when more expensive, insulated needles are not available.[126]

Blood Safety

An estimated 70% of all blood transfusions in Africa are given to children with severe anemia caused by malaria. Blood transfusion services, when they exist, aim to provide a lifesaving service by ensuring an adequate supply of safe blood.[127-129] Patients, particularly children, in developing countries, face the greatest risks from unsafe blood and blood products.[128-131]

Fewer than 30% of developing countries have a nationally coordinated blood transfusion service. Many do not perform the most rudimentary tests for diseases such as HIV or hepatitis B and C because of economic constraints.[131] Even limited testing doubles the basic cost of a unit of blood. It is estimated that about 6 million tests that should be done globally to check for infections are not done annually.[131]

Many countries still rely on paid donors or family members to donate blood before surgery.[131] In Argentina, for example, up to 92% of the blood supply is derived from family members. Although voluntary, unpaid blood donation has increased to 20% in the past 5 years in Pakistan, family donors represented 70% and paid donors 10% of the blood donors in 2004.[129] Public education about the value of blood transfusion is vital to improve supply.[127,128] Through concerted efforts by the WHO to improve blood safety worldwide over the past decade, the number of voluntary, unpaid donors has increased considerably. For example, voluntary blood donation in China increased from 45% of donations in 2000 to 90% in 2004. Similarly, the rate of voluntary, unpaid donations in Bolivia increased from 10% in 2002 to 50% in 2005. Malaysia, China, and India reached 100% screening of donated blood for HIV by the year 2000.[130]

There are risks in any system.[127,128] Family and paid donors may hide aspects of their health and lifestyle that could make the blood unsafe for different reasons. Family members may feel pressured to donate, whereas paid donors are driven by need and

avoid important details about their health status that would negate the transaction. The commercial plasma industry and blood trade can fuel the transmission of HIV. In 1999, for example, 26 million liters of plasma were fractionated for global use,[131] and the major source was paid donors from developing countries. Voluntary, unpaid donors have a greater sense of responsibility to their community and keep themselves healthy to be able to continue giving safe blood. South Africa has had 100% voluntary, unpaid donations since it established a national blood service. With HIV prevalence approaching 30% among the adult population of Africa, only 0.02% of its regular blood donors in South Africa have contracted HIV.

Storage of blood is difficult considering the unreliable and unpredictable electricity supply in many developing countries. To obviate the risk of transmission of malaria, HIV, and other infectious diseases, blood should be transfused only when absolutely necessary. In sophisticated blood transfusion units, the use of predonated autologous blood is an option.[132,133] In poorer countries, this is not practical because malnutrition and chronic anemia are common. There is often a lack of appropriate equipment, and cost is prohibitive. Similarly, intraoperative blood salvage and cell savers appropriate for use in children are not available. Recombinant factor VII, which is being used increasingly to reduce blood use by those who can afford it,[132] is beyond the scope (and cost) of practice in many countries.[133]

Equipment

Electricity is unreliable in many hospitals in the developing world. In some, particularly in rural areas, neither power-line electricity nor a reliable functional backup generator is available.[3,4] Even though recycling disposable equipment such as endotracheal tubes is considered normal practice in many countries, general facilities for infection control, such as running water, disinfectants, or gloves, are also unreliable.[2]

Essential equipment to provide safe anesthesia for children and particularly for neonates is in short supply.[3,25,30,36] Neonatal or pediatric ventilators are virtually nonexistent outside the main centers.[30] Small IV cannulae are a precious commodity, and butterfly needles are still used. Syringe pumps and other control devices are impractical in environments with an erratic electricity supply. Metal or plastic laryngoscopes for children may be available but not well maintained. Batteries may be in short supply and light bulbs unreliable. A full range of pediatric endotracheal tubes is considered a luxury. Laryngeal mask airways in pediatric sizes are usually unavailable. IV fluids are very expensive if not manufactured locally, and many developing countries do not have local production facilities.[10] The choice of IV fluid is therefore limited and in short supply.

Monitoring is very basic: a precordial stethoscope and a finger on the pulse.[2,11] ECG monitoring is used when available but depends on a continuous electricity supply, battery backup, and proper maintenance. Appropriately sized blood pressure cuffs are scarce. Pulse oximetry has been the most useful monitor and should be available in all centers where pediatric surgery is performed.[2,25] Unfortunately, this ideal is far from reality, but it is hoped that the global pulse oximetry project will be rewarded with universal quality improvement.[17]

Anesthetic machines in developing countries fall into two categories: modern, sophisticated machines and simple, low-maintenance equipment. The electronic machines provided by well-meaning donors have a poor track record in austere

---

[a]References 2, 23, 30, 34, 36, 43, and 123-125.

environments. Sophisticated equipment needs to be understood, but operating manuals printed in foreign languages are not helpful. Sophisticated machines require ongoing maintenance, but individuals trained to repair such equipment are seldom available. Service contracts are not considered viable. Unfortunately, these machines are invariably discarded when the first fault occurs, because guarantees are unlikely to be honored and faults are considered too expensive to repair. Poorly maintained equipment becomes hazardous and potentially life-threatening in untrained hands.

Simplicity and safety have long been the keys to anesthetic equipment in developing countries.[2–4,134] Ideally, a suitable anesthetic machine should be inexpensive, versatile, robust, and able to withstand extreme climatic conditions; able to function even if the supply of cylinders or electricity is interrupted; easy to understand and operate by those with limited training; economical to use; and easily maintained by locally available skills.[134–136]

The cheapest, most practical, and most widely used method is inhalational anesthesia administered through an Epstein Macintosh Oxford (EMO) drawover vaporizer (Penlon Ltd., Oxford, UK; Glostavent Penlon Ltd.), or Oxford Miniature Vaporizer (OMV, Penlon Ltd.). Oxygen concentrators supplement oxygen delivery and eliminate the need for expensive oxygen cylinders, whose reducing valves are often faulty or destroyed in these situations. The most appropriate ventilator is the Manley Multivent Ventilator (Penlon Ltd.), which essentially functions like a mechanical version of the Oxford inflating bellows (OIB) and can be used with a drawover system.[136]

A general scheme for inhalational anesthesia, which was first proposed by Ezi-Ashi and colleagues in 1983,[122] for use in developing countries is shown in Fig. 51.9.[134] Applying this scheme, four different modes can be used and modified according to the available supplies and services. The basic mode A is used when there is no

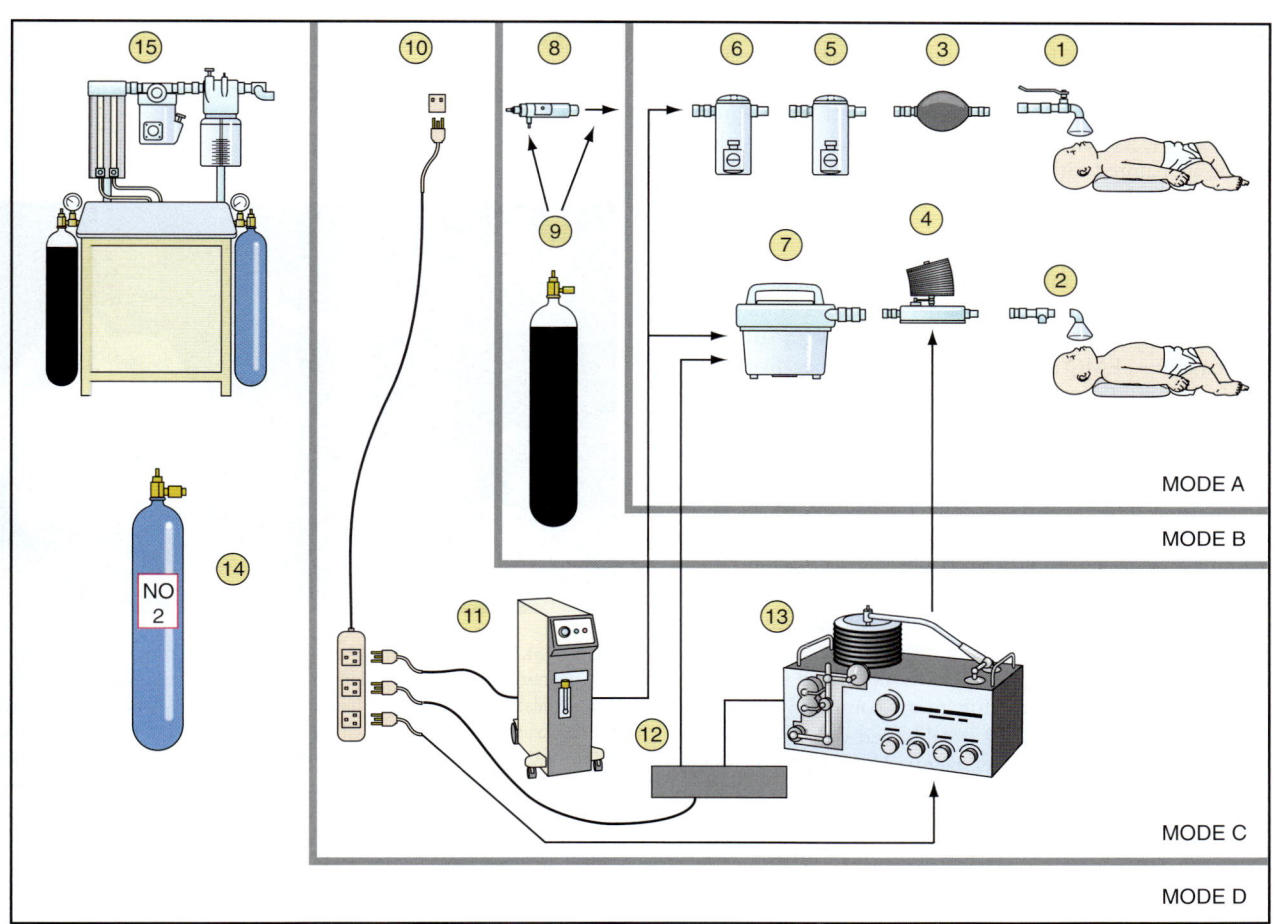

FIGURE 51.9 The schematic diagram shows the use of anesthetic systems, depending on available resources. **Mode A** provides basic inhalational anesthesia with air, spontaneous ventilation, or self-inflating bags. Drawover vaporizers are required. **Mode B** provides oxygen enrichment but requires the availability of oxygen cylinders. Plenum vaporizers can be used. **Mode C** requires electricity to power the oxygen concentrator, air compressor, and ventilator. A mechanical ventilator (e.g., Manley) does not require electrical power. **Mode D** requires a Boyle machine and nitrous oxide cylinders. **1,** T-piece with reservoir tube and face mask. **2,** Ambu Pedi valve. **3,** Self-inflating bag (Ambu). **4,** Oxford Inflating Bellows (OIB). **5,** Oxford Miniature Vaporizer (OMV) with halothane. **6,** OMV with trichloroethylene. **7,** Epstein, Macintosh, Oxford (EMO) vaporizer with ether. These circuits and manual ventilators are interchangeable, and ether, halothane, and trichloroethylene can be used on their own or in series. Farman entrainer **(8)** with an oxygen cylinder **(9)** can be used to supplement oxygen, or an electrical power source **(10)** with an oxygen concentrator **(11)**, air compressor **(12)**, or Manley ventilator **(13)**. Nitrous oxide **(14)** and Boyle apparatus **(15)** allow anesthesia practice equivalent to that of developed countries.

electricity and no supply of compressed gases. The apparatus consists of a low-resistance vaporizer linked by valves to the child to act as a drawover system with room air as the carrier gas. The self-inflating bag or hand bellows makes it possible to provide artificial ventilation while the vaporizer remains as a drawover device. The addition of low-flow oxygen to the inspired gas in mode B depends on the availability of an oxygen cylinder. The addition of a length of reservoir tubing to the circuit enables oxygen to be stored on expiration and to be used on the next inspiration, substantially improving its economy.

When electricity is available, (mode C), operation of the anesthetic apparatus can be extended by permitting the use of an air compressor to provide continuous gas flow (allowing use of a Boyle apparatus and plenum vaporizer), an oxygen concentrator, and ventilators. When nitrous oxide is available (mode D), all types of inhalational anesthesia available in developed countries can be practiced. When services and supplies are interrupted even briefly, it is possible to change from one mode to another without requiring other anesthetic apparatuses.

These techniques may be of little interest to the anesthesiologist working comfortably in the well-maintained, sophisticated environment of developed nations. Their roles, however, are essential in field situations (e.g., war, natural disasters), and all anesthesiologists should be acquainted with their functioning in this unpredictable world (Videos 51.1 and 51.2).

DRAWOVER ANESTHESIA

Drawover anesthesia enables inhalational anesthesia to be administered using atmospheric air as the carrier gas. The essential features of this system consist of a calibrated vaporizer with sufficiently low resistance (i.e., EMO and OMV) to allow the negative pressure created by the child's inspiratory effort to draw room air through the vaporizer during spontaneous ventilation. Positive-pressure ventilation can be provided by means of a self-inflating bag or bellows (OIB), using a valve to prevent the gas mixture from reentering the vaporizer and a unidirectional valve at the child's airway to direct expired gases to the atmosphere, preventing rebreathing (see mode A, Fig. 51.9). In this way, an anesthetic can be administered in the absence of compressed gases. The vaporizer has an inlet for supplementary oxygen that can be attached to the oxygen output tube of an oxygen concentrator or oxygen cylinder when available (see modes B and C, Fig. 51.9).

The EMO and OMV are the more commonly used low-resistance vaporizers. The EMO is calibrated only for ether, but its performance is linear for other agents. The OMV is calibrated for a variety of agents[42,135–137]; despite the lack of temperature compensation, its performance is stable under most conditions. Both vaporizers have been used successfully in pediatric anesthetic practice,[33] but it is recommended that they be converted to form a T-piece for greater safety.

The OMV has been evaluated as a simple drawover system for pediatric anesthesia. Wilson and Bem[42] showed that when a self-inflation bag is used in a drawover mode, more efficient vaporization occurs despite vaporizer cooling. However, the respiratory efforts of neonates or weak infants are insufficient to operate the valve mechanisms of the self-inflating bag (e.g., Ambu bag), necessitating continuous assisted ventilation even in the presence of ether, which stimulates ventilation.

DiaMedica Therapeutics markets a variety of devices specifically designed for use in austere environments where oxygen supply and electricity are unreliable. Examples include a portable anesthesia machine using drawover, which weighs 9.5 kg (Fig. 51.10;

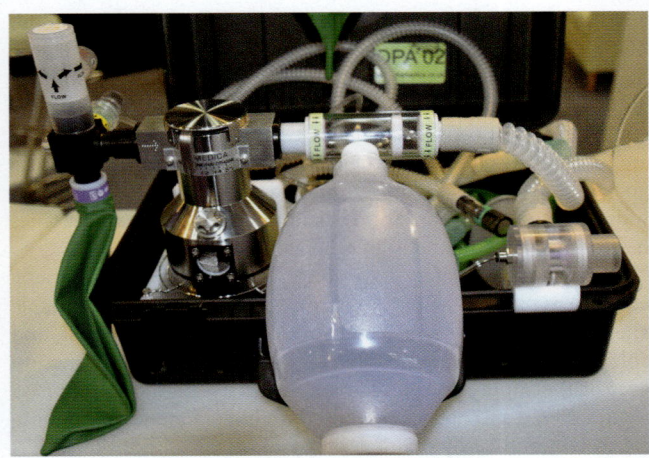

FIGURE 51.10 This portable drawover anesthesia machine weighs 9.5 kg and has a vaporizer capable of delivering halothane, isoflurane, or sevoflurane, packed in a shockproof and waterproof box (47 × 35 × 17 cm). It can work with supplemental oxygen or room air. It may also be used with a portable ventilator for children or adults (see Fig. 51.11). (With permission from DiaMedica Ltd., UK.)

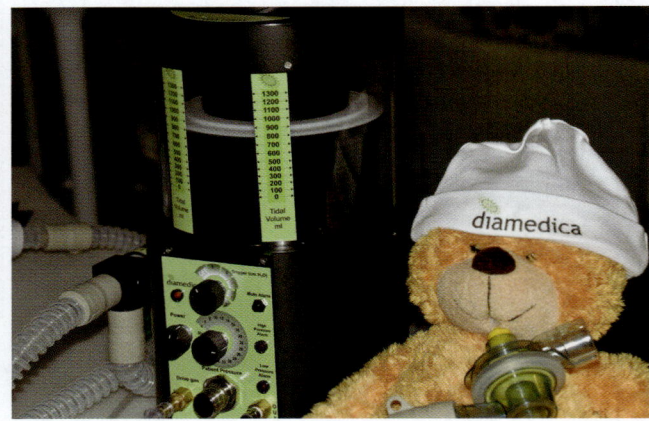

FIGURE 51.11 This is a portable anesthesia ventilator for children or adults. The bellows tidal volume is adjusted by the turn of a screw (see E-Fig. 51.2). The ventilator is equipped with an internal battery, which remains charged for approximately 100 hours without recharge and can be recharged from 100/240-V electrical sources or a 12-V charger. This is a gas-driven ventilator that may be used with an oxygen concentrator, or if no oxygen source is available, a portable battery power pump can run the ventilator using room air. This has a battery life of approximately 20 hours. (See text for further details and video links.) (With permission from DiaMedica Ltd., UK.)

Video 51.3) that may be used with or without oxygen, and the vaporizer may be used with halothane, isoflurane or sevoflurane (E-Fig. 51.1). It allows for both spontaneous and controlled ventilation. A portable ventilator (pediatric or adult) may be used with the portable anesthesia machine (Fig. 51.11); the bellows tidal volume is adjusted by the turn of a screw (E-Fig. 51.2). The ventilator is equipped with an internal battery, which remains charged for approximately 100 hours without recharge and can be recharged from a 100/240-V electrical source or a 12-V charger. This is a gas-driven ventilator (Video 51.4), which may be used with an oxygen concentrator; or if no oxygen source. is available a portable battery power pump can run the ventilator using room air. This has a battery life of approximately 20 hours. The full-size machine (Glostavent Helix; E-Fig. 51.3) with all four components—(1) low-resistance drawover vaporizer, (2) gas-driven ventilator, (3) oxygen concentrator (E-Fig. 51.4), and (4) power supply with battery backup—is shown in E-Fig. 51.5 (Videos 51.5 and 51.6).

OXYGEN CONCENTRATORS

Improved oxygen availability, independent of compressed gas and electrical power supply, can be provided by linking oxygen concentrators[138,139] to a drawover anesthetic apparatus as first described by Fenton.[119] Maintenance requirements are low, and servicing is recommended only after approximately 10,000 hours of usage. The benefits are enormous, but a reliable electricity supply is critical.

The concentrator functions by using a compressor to pump ambient air alternately through one of two canisters containing a molecular sieve of zeolite granules that reversibly absorbs nitrogen from compressed air.[119,134,138] The controls are simple and consists of an on/off switch for the compressor and a flow-control knob to deliver 0 to 5 L/minute. Flow of oxygen continues uninterrupted as the canisters are alternated automatically so that oxygen from one canister is available while the other regenerates. A warning light on a built-in oxygen analyzer illuminates if the oxygen concentration is less than 85%, and the concentrator switches off automatically when the oxygen concentration is less than 70%. This action is heralded by visual and audible alarms. Air is then delivered as the effluent gas. Modern machines are relatively silent.

The oxygen output of the concentrator depends on the size of the unit, the inflow of oxygen, the minute volume, and pattern of ventilation. The addition of dead space (or oxygen economizer tube) at the outlet improves the performance, and predictable concentrations of more than 90% oxygen can be obtained with flows between 1 and 5 L/minute, independent of the pattern of ventilation. Much lower concentrations and less predictability were observed when the dead-space tubing was omitted.[140] An example of a ventilator (mode C, Fig. 51.9) that can use a concentrator for gas supply is shown in E-Fig. 51.6. The possible hazards of oxygen concentrators are few if they are positioned in the operating room so that the in-draw area is free from pollutants. Failure of the power supply or failure of the zeolite canisters results in the delivery of ambient air. A bacterial filter at the outlet combined with the use of dust-free zeolite should prevent contamination of the delivered gas. Dirty internal air filters may produce lower oxygen concentrations and must be checked. An oxygen storage tank and booster pumps afford protection against the vagaries in electrical supply.

Visiting Providers

Personality traits compatible with survival have been suggested as a prerequisite for working in the developing world. These traits include an almost pathologic desire for work, a willingness to merge or at least sympathize with different cultures, patience in relating to and teaching people sometimes far removed educationally, the ability to withstand prolonged periods of cultural isolation, and mostly a never-failing ability to improvise and make the best of a bad situation.[141-145] There is no place for risk-taking "cowboy anesthesiologists."[137,145]

International travel, particularly visits to many parts of the developing world, needs careful preparation and planning, whether the anesthesiologist is part of a volunteer organization[33,143-146] or traveling as an individual.[144] Detailed advice[142-147] is beyond the scope of this chapter, but some generalizations are made based on personal experience and that of colleagues. Changing political climates and international health guidelines dictate visa and vaccination requirements. Expert advice should be sought to tailor the traveler's needs according to the individual's medical and immunization history, the duration of stay, and proposed itinerary.

Physical acclimatization to jet lag, altitude sickness, and heat or sun exposure is necessary, as is adjustment to the local culture and cuisine. Social graces acceptable in a Western culture may be deemed offensive in some other cultures. An interpreter is an important ally. The inability to understand a language or the local dialect places a visiting anesthesiologist at a serious disadvantage, particularly when dealing with children. Children often use subtle ways to describe their feelings that even a skilled interpreter may fail to convey.

The hospital environment may be disconcerting for some. In contrast to the familiar comforts of a clean, child-friendly hospital, the visitor may be struck by the relatively shabby, bland appearance of many hospitals in developing countries. The buildings may not have received a coat of paint since they were built, and broken windowpanes provide the only air conditioning. Children are often cared for in adult wards.

In the operating room, the visitor may be faced with anesthetic equipment barely recognizable from its original manufacture or in a state of disrepair with nonstandard improvisations to make it functional. The choice of drugs may be limited, and the names of locally manufactured generic drugs and the presentation of IV solutions may add to the perplexity. Surgical safety may be the next issue. Informed consent as we know it is unlikely, and identification of the child in the absence of parents may not be obvious to the newcomer. A local or itinerant surgeon may suggest an extensive procedure on a malnourished child without consideration for monitoring, blood transfusion, or availability of intensive care or postoperative analgesia in an unmonitored environment. The anesthesiologist is obligated to consider the risks and benefits carefully in such circumstances.

Summary

The provision of safe anesthesia in a developing country will always be challenging, particularly for those who provide anesthesia for children. The challenges vary, and it is wise to expect the unexpected and have the flexibility to improvise in the face of an ever-changing world racked by famine, violence, natural disasters, and political unrest.

Attracting trained anesthesiologists to work in the developing world is difficult.[5,15,62,70-73,144-148] Temporary sojourns with volunteer medical groups are for the most part stimulating, but volunteers are unlikely to return for longer periods, let alone permanently.

Can anything be done to improve the lot of children who undergo anesthesia in the developing world? The Pediatric Anesthesia Fellowship Program established through the WFSA is commendable, but it produces only a small number of trainees each year.[70,72,73] Audits of morbidity and mortality are the first steps toward improvement if action is taken to address the problems uncovered. Publications reflecting outcomes in developing countries have increased over the past decade.[19-21] Purchasing equipment without ensuring subsequent maintenance is wasteful. Disposables are short-lived items even if they are recycled. Human resources are needed.

Different standards may emerge from different parts of the world. These standards need not necessarily be considered inferior but may open the way for the assimilation of new ideas.[147] The nuances of practice in different communities inevitably vary and may challenge some fondly held beliefs in pediatric anesthesia. A safe anesthetic is not necessarily the most expensive one. It is usually not the agents that we use but the skill with which we use them that determines outcome. It should never be necessary to depart from the dictum *primum non nocere*. Simplicity may be the key, but there is no place for double standards. Guidelines that have evolved over time in the United Kingdom, United States, and Australasia may be untenable in many parts of the world,[145] but every attempt should be made to exercise the same standard of care as expected in developed countries. Our children deserve no less.

ANNOTATED REFERENCES

Chikumbanje S, Bell GT, Kapatuka K, Pollach G. Continuous flow using an entrainer and t-piece vs draw over apparatus for inhalational induction of anesthesia in children. *Paediatr Anaesth*. 2014;24(11):1169-1173.

There are few studies in modern literature that compare circuits that are no longer in use in developed countries. The authors in Malawi compare inhalation induction in children using a Farnham entrainer with the Ayres T-piece (Mapleson F) and a drawover system. There was no difference in oxygen saturation measured by oximetry (SpO₂) recordings, but induction times were slightly (but not clinically significant) longer with the drawover system.

Ekenze SO, Ajuzieogu OV, Nwomeh BC. Challenges of management and outcome of neonatal surgery in Africa: a systematic review. *Pediatr Surg Int*. 2016;32(3):291-299.

This study reviews publications on neonatal surgery from 11 countries in Africa over the past 20 years. Although the overall mortality rate has improved in the past decade, it remains high, around 30%. Although each country has its own problems, delayed presentation, inadequate facilities, a dearth of trained personnel, major neonatal surgery, and an absence of intensive care were the common denominators contributing to this poor outcome.

Hodges SC, Mijumbi C, Okello M, et al. Anaesthesia services in developing countries: defining the problems. *Anaesthesia*. 2007;62(1):4-11.

This paper identifies the difficulties of providing anesthesia in Uganda. The disturbing result was that only 23% of anesthesiologists have the facilities to provide safe anesthesia to adults, 13% for a child, and only 6% for cesarean section.

Walker IA, Merry AF, Wilson IH, et al. Global oximetry: an international anaesthesia quality improvement project. *Anaesthesia*. 2009;64(1):1051-1060.

This paper describes the initial quality assurance program for pulse oximetry in four pilot studies of pulse oximetry in Uganda, Vietnam, India, and the Philippines. The studies determined that formal training in pulse oximetry needed to be a central part of the WHO Safe Surgery Saves Lives project.

Walker IA, Newton M, Bosenberg AT. Improving surgical safety globally: pulse oximetry and the WHO Guidelines for Safe Surgery. *Paediatr Anaesth*. 2011;21(7):825-828.

This paper describes the fact that approximately 78,000 operating rooms worldwide lack pulse oximetry. It discusses the WHO Safe Surgery Saves Lives Program as well as the Global Pulse Oximetry Program.

Zoumenou E, Gbenou S, Assouto P, et al. Pediatric anesthesia in developing countries: experience in the two main university hospitals of Benin in West Africa. *Paediatr Anaesth*. 2010;20(8):741-747.

This article describes anesthesia in Benin. Cardiac arrests occurred at a rate of 156 per 10,000 cases with a mortality rate of approximately 60%, even in two university hospitals. The authors are to be congratulated for studying this issue to gain more financial support from their government for better equipment and monitoring.

A complete reference list can be found online at ExpertConsult.com.

Pediatric Equipment

PATRICK A. ROSS, JERROLD LERMAN, AND CHARLES J. COTÉ

Heating and Cooling Systems

Consider for a moment the design of the surgical gown. It is designed to be a sterile barrier to protect the patient, yet it also must be a barrier to body fluids to protect the wearer. Because it is waterproof, it exchanges air poorly and in turn prevents dissipation of body heat. The surgeon wants to turn down the temperature in the operating room (OR) so the heat is bearable. Consider then the anesthetized infant on the operating table in a cool room. From the moment the infant enters the OR, he or she is partially if not completely uncovered. With a very high surface area to body mass ratio, the infant loses heat through two primary mechanisms: radiation and convection. The OR is unlike an incubator that envelops infants in warm, still air; rather, the cool air of the OR flows continually in a laminar pattern to reduce the risk of infection. Once anesthesia is induced, body heat is redistributed from the central to peripheral compartments through vasodilation. Furthermore, the fluids the child receives, the air that he or she breathes, and the instruments that contact the child's tissues are all colder than the child's body temperature. The neonate and infant in particular are vulnerable to this heat loss, with limited strategies to prevent the decrease in their core temperature.

Several strategies offset heat loss from the child. Before the child enters the OR, the room should be warmed (to >25°C) or as much as tolerable to minimize radiation and convective heat losses. The child should be placed on a forced air warming blanket before the child is unclad. Preferably, inhaled gases and intravenous (IV) fluids should be warmed throughout the surgery.

In some cases, hypothermia is induced deliberately. For example, hypothermia is a necessity for cardiopulmonary bypass[1,2] and continues to be studied for benefit after neonatal asphyxia,[3,4] although the latter has not conferred any benefit after pediatric cardiac arrest or head injury.[5,6] Other than in these specific circumstances, normothermia should be the goal for our patients. Mild to moderate hypothermia may cause apnea in infants, alter the pharmacokinetics of medications, decrease blood clotting and increase surgical site infections,[7] among other complications.[8,9] Conversely, inducing hyperthermia with active warming may increase the metabolic rate and heart rate, introducing concerns of a malignant hyperthermia reaction, thyrotoxicosis, and other metabolic and drug-related disorders. Therefore basic strategies to maintain normothermia and temperature monitoring should be provided for every patient who undergoes general anesthesia, except for those anesthetized for extremely brief procedures.

Infants and children lose heat through four mechanisms: radiation (39%), convection (34%), evaporation (24%), and conduction (3%).[10] Radiation is the transfer of energy through the generation of electromagnetic waves to solid surfaces such as cold walls. Convection is the transfer of energy from the child by the gas or liquid surrounding it. Convection can be passive, as in still air, or active when air flows past the infant. Evaporation is the loss of heat as liquid is converted to gas. This is typically seen through perspiration but can also occur with major open wounds, and evaporation of cleansing preparation solutions. Conduction is the transfer of energy directly from one body to another and can occur in solids, liquids, and gases. Based on their material, objects are conductors (metals) or insulators (gases).

Patient Warming

FORCED AIR WARMERS
Forced air warming devices remain one of the most common and effective strategies to maintain and increase the child's temperature in the OR. These devices consist of a central unit that regulates the air temperature and forces heated air through a hose to a disposable perforated blanket that can be placed underneath or on top of the child or around the child's head. The device must be used in accordance with the manufacturer's instructions to minimize the risk of thermal injury.[11,12] The device very effectively maintains the child's temperature through the combination of active convection and a plastic wrap or blanket that eliminates radiation and evaporative heat losses. Concerns have been raised that these devices develop internal microbial buildup,[13] that they disrupt laminar airflow in the OR,[14,15] and that they cause surgical infections that involve implanted material.[14] However, despite these concerns,[16] forced air warmers continue to be used in children without reports of increased infection rates. Nonetheless, some surgeons prefer that forced air warmers be powered on only after the child has been prepped and draped (e.g., ventriculoperitoneal catheter insertion), a practice that has been applied to many surgical types. Several manufacturers produce forced air warmers and blankets. The devices all operate in a similar manner and may be considered equivalent in effectiveness: 3M (St. Paul, MN), Celsius Medical (Madrid, Spain), Stryker (Kalamazoo, MI), and Medical Solutions, Inc. (Omaha, NE).

WARMING BLANKETS
Warming blankets include circulating water mattresses placed underneath the child and electrical heat-generating conductive blankets that can be placed either underneath or on top of the child. When placed underneath the child, these devices offer complete access to the child without obstruction, transferring heat by conduction, accounting for only 4% of the heat loss. Warming blankets do not have the associated concern of changing airflow in the OR. Typically, these devices are also reusable and require wipe-down disinfection. Since these devices are in direct contact with the child and have a greater thermal density, care must be taken to avoid surface burns at high temperature settings. Circulating water blankets include the Blanketrol by Cincinnati Sub-Zero (Cincinnati, OH), and the Medi-Therm III by Gaymar Industries (Orchard Park, NY).

Manufacturers of non-water–based blankets include Augustine Biomedical (Eden Prairie, MN), Inditherm (Rotherham, United Kingdom), and Novamed USA (Elmsford, NY).

RADIANT WARMERS
Overhead radiant heating units, sometimes referred to as a "french fry light," have become less commonly used in the OR since the introduction of forced air warmers, although they remain in use in the neonatal intensive care unit (NICU) and are built in to many NICU beds. These devices use a temperature sensor on the infant to supply feedback to a servomechanism to adjust the heat output. Without this feedback or if the heating element is placed too close to the neonate, there is a risk of skin burns to the neonate and nearby staff.

PASSIVE HEAT AND MOISTURE EXCHANGERS
Heat and moisture exchangers (HMEs) are reflective filters interposed between the endotracheal tube and the ventilator circuit to preserve the child's temperature and airway humidity. Under the correct circumstances, these devices may maintain body temperature[17] but they cannot increase body temperature. They are less effective at maintaining temperature compared with heated humidifiers in the airway circuit. Even the smallest exchanger can increase the airway dead space and resistance, particularly in neonates,[18] blunting the capnogram until it is almost uninterpretable. These exchangers are effective and useful for preventing the contamination of devices attached to the airway such as pulmonary function testing equipment.

HEATED HUMIDIFIERS
Heated humidifiers or heated breathing circuits are typically a sealed heated wire within one limb of the breathing circuit. Sterile water is introduced into the circuit and the servomechanism controlled heater maintains temperature. These devices are prone to hazards, such as overheating, condensation, changes in the compressible volume of the circuit, leaks in the tubing, and obstruction, if they are not connected correctly. They are superior to any other device for preventing the secretions in the airway from drying out and are universally used with ICU ventilators. However, as the circle breathing circuit supplanted the Mapleson F circuit (Jackson-Rees modification of the Ayre T-piece) in clinical anesthesia care globally, heated humidifiers became anachronistic as it could be difficult to adapt them to the circle circuit. The additional cost and complications of these devices also limit their use except for anesthesia cases of prolonged duration. Manufacturers include Armstrong Medical (Lincolnshire, IL), Carefusion (Becton Dickinson, Franklin Lakes, NJ), Dräger (Telford, PA), Fisher & Paykel (Irvine, CA), Philips Healthcare (Bothell, WA), Teleflex (Morrisville, NC), and Westmed Inc. (Tucson, AZ), among others.

FLUID AND BLOOD WARMERS
When large volumes of IV fluid are infused at a rapid rate, the child's core temperature may decrease precipitously unless a fluid warmer is used. In contrast, when IV fluid is infused at a maintenance flow rate, the effect on the child's temperature is attenuated. One strategy to deliver warmed IV fluid is to warm the IV fluid bags before the fluid is delivered. This can be achieved with blanket warmers already in use in the ORs or with specialized warmers such as the ivNow fluid warmer by Enthermics (Menomonee Falls, WI). The IV fluid bags should be used within a week or two to prevent degradation of the plastic bags. Individuals have warmed IV fluid bags in a standard microwave oven, but

this practice is not recommended because hot spots, overheating, or deterioration of the container might develop.

In general, blood products are stored in refrigerated coolers. When the products are selected for use, they are warmed before administration. Fluid warmers currently marketed are designed to warm crystalloid solutions and blood products. The two main designs for these fluid warmers are a water bath and dry heat. The Level 1 Hotline device (Smiths Medical, Dublin OH) uses a heated water bath and specialized tubing with a sterile inner lumen. Warmed water circulates in the outer lumen, increasing the temperature of the fluid. The Level 1 can deliver warmed fluids with a gravity flow rate up to 83 mL/minute. The dry heat designs use either standard IV tubing or proprietary tubing sets. These are placed in contact with a heat exchanger usually made of metal because of its conductive properties. The device warms the tubing and the fluid as it passes through the tubing. The designs vary in their priming volume, flow rates, portability, and distance they can be placed from the patient. The greater the distance between the device and the patient, the greater the cooling of the fluid before it reaches the patient. Both pressurized and nonpressurized warmers can deliver large fluid flow rates that are commonly necessary for trauma and transplantation surgeries. Nonpressurized warmers that use proprietary tubing sets include the enFlow by Carefusion (Becton Dickinson, Franklin Lakes, NJ) with a 4-mL priming volume and a flow rate up to 200 mL/minute; the Medi-Temp by Stryker (Kalamazoo, MI) with a flow rate up to 500 mL/minute; and the Ranger by 3M (St. Paul, MN) with a flow rate up to 500 mL/minute. Some nonpressurized warmers that adapt to standard IV tubing sets manufactured in Germany include the Nuova/05 by Nuova GmbH (23909 Ratzeburg, Germany) and the Astoflo Plus by Stihler Electronic GmbH (Germany). For massive transfusion of blood, pressurized fluid warmers are used. The Belmont Rapid Infuser RI-2 (Belmont Medical, Billerica, MA) uses electromagnetic induction heating, has an optional blood reservoir, and infuses the warmed fluid with a rapid roller pump. This device can deliver more than 750 mL/minute of warmed blood. The Level 1 h-1200 Fast Flow Fluid Warmer (Smiths Medical, Dublin OH) uses an aluminum heat exchanger, a countercurrent water bath, has two chambers for fluid bags, and uses pressurized air to compress the IV bags and infuse fluids at flows of up to 600 mL/minute, although at the greater rates, the temperature of the IV fluid is not sustained (Fig. 52.1). The flow rate of these devices is limited by the size and length of the inserted venous catheter and, to a lesser extent, by the length of the tubing before the patient (E-Fig. 52.1). These devices have integrated air and pressure detectors that will automatically stop the infusion if a breech is detected. Even with the air detector, it is important to eliminate all air from the bags to avoid the possibility of infusing air into the circulation.

CONTROLLING EXPOSURE

Body temperature can be preserved if the child is covered to reduce radiant and convective heat losses. Plastic wrap used for food is effective, inexpensive, and translucent. Covering the infant's head is an important strategy to prevent heat loss since the infant's head has a large body surface area/volume ratio. Reflective aluminized Mylar blankets are also very effective but more expensive. Using a blanket warmer and uncovering only the necessary small portions of the child during induction and IV placement attenuates heat loss. If the child must be uncovered at any time, warming the air temperature within the OR is effective as it reduces both radiation and convective heat losses. In one study of neonatal

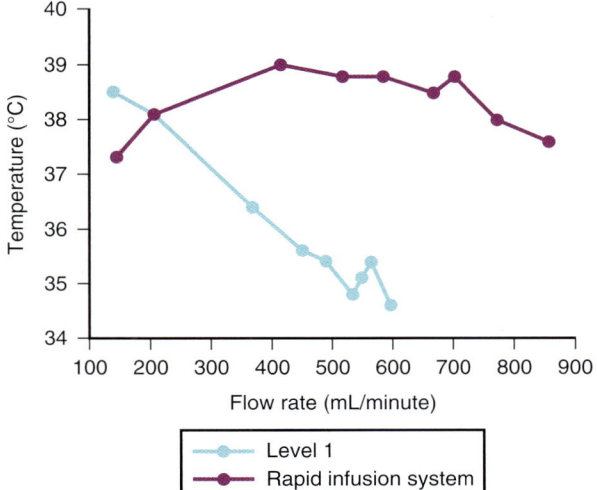

FIGURE 52.1 This figure plots the mean temperature of the fluid at the end of two 2-liter infusions of crystalloid for the Level 1 versus the Rapid Infusion System (RIS). Note that both devices have equivalent warming capacities with flow rates of 200 mL or less per minute, but there is markedly less warming capacity with the Level 1 system at higher flow rates. Note that the RIS was the precursor to the Belmont Rapid Infuser, so the warming characteristics would be similar to those of the RIS. (From Barcelona SL, Vilich F, Coté CJ. A comparison of flow rates and warming capabilities of the Level 1 and Rapid Infusion System with various-size intravenous catheters. *Anesth Analg.* 2003;97[2]:358–363.)

and maternal hypothermia, fewer hypothermic neonates (<36°C) were identified when room temperature was 23°C compared with a room temperature of 20°C (5% vs. 19%).[19] Once the neonate has been covered, the room temperature can be reduced.

Intravenous Therapy

In most children undergoing elective surgery, IV access is secured after induction of anesthesia and before the airway is secured. For emergency surgeries, an IV induction is usually performed and additional IV access is established after the airway is secured.

The basis for determining the adequacy of IV therapy is Poiseuille's law, which is embodied by the equation for laminar flow as follows:

$$Q = \frac{\pi R^4 (P_2 - P_1)}{8\eta L}$$

Here, the volumetric flow rate (Q) of the fluid is directly related to the fourth power of the radius of the catheter lumen (R) and the pressure difference across the tubing ($P_2 - P_1$) and inversely related to the viscosity of the fluid (η) and the length of the tubing (L). Increasing the radius of the catheter has an exponential effect to increase the fluid flow rate by the fourth power. However, for long catheters such as central venous lines or peripherally inserted percutaneous intravenous central catheters (PICC), additional length and fluid viscosity (as in changing from crystalloid to packed red blood cells [PRBCs]) can substantially increase the resistance to flow and thereby dramatically reduce fluid flow rates, even when the fluid bag is pressurized.

The fluid drip rate from a 500-mL solution bag can range from a macrodrip (10–20 drops/mL) to a microdrip (60 drops/mL).

The microdrip set may contain a Buretrol (Baxter International, Deerfield, IL) to finely control the volume of fluid infused and prevent an overdose of IV fluids in neonates and infants. Extension tubing may be small bore in caliber with a small priming volume of 1 to 2 mL or large bore with a larger priming volume of 6 to 10 mL. The latter is recommended as it offers less resistance to flow when fluid resuscitation or blood must be administered. The small-caliber tubing may be "Y'd" into the IV set close to the cannula site to administer drugs to small infants without large volumes of crystalloid. For most neonates and infants, 24-gauge catheters are used, although 22-gauge may be sited in larger veins such as the saphenous. In toddlers and older children undergoing noncomplex surgery, a 22-gauge IV catheter is preferred and for older children to adults 16- to 20-gauge catheters or larger are usually placed. Caution must be used if the caliber of extension tubing is downsized to a small caliber as it may restrict the ability to rapidly transfuse fluids. A three-way stopcock or an access port permits needless injections of medications into the IV tubing.

Fluid can be administered via gravity flow, via mechanical pump, or via an external pressure bag. The addition of a 5-μm bacterial filter increases the resistance and decreases the flow rate. Furthermore, antireflux valves further increase the resistance to flow. However, these valves are essential when infusing fluids or drugs as these may flow retrograde up connected tubing (unnoticed), if an antireflux valve is not in-line. Each medication access point such as the stopcock or needleless hub is a site where air can be introduced; care should be taken to aspirate all air from IV access points (e.g., stopcocks and Luer locks) in all infants and children. The components of the IV set—the tubing, extensions, connectors, and a method of delivery appropriate for the size of the child and the procedure—are determined by individual preferences. There is slight variation among manufacturers, but general flow rates by gravity for IV catheters and central venous lines are listed in Table 52.1; the larger the catheter, the greater the flow rates (E-Fig. 52.2). This information is also printed on the catheter packages.

MAINTENANCE FLUIDS

For neonates and chronically ill infants in whom there is significant risk of hypoglycemia, a dextrose-containing fluid should be used. If the child is receiving 10% dextrose or a similar solution from the NICU, this infusion should be continued at the same rate during anesthesia in the absence of additional data. If the dextrose infusion rate is decreased, the serum dextrose concentration should be measured periodically throughout anesthesia to preclude the development of hypoglycemia. To prevent fluid overload, consider the use of a pump to control the infusion of IV fluids, with a stopcock close to the cannula to infuse medications. Some have recommended in-line filters in IV lines to prevent morbidity and mortality in neonates associated with contamination of the infusions (bacteria, endotoxins, and others). However, a Cochrane review concluded that there was insufficient evidence to recommend in-line filters in neonates to reduce morbidity and mortality.[20] If vasoactive medications and maintenance fluids are infusing and a separate IV catheter is present, the medications should be flushed as close to the patient as possible in the second IV in order to minimize the risk of injecting boluses of vasoactive medications.

RESUSCITATION

If there is an anticipated need for a large volume of fluids for volume resuscitation, the largest IV that can be easily placed should be used, recognizing that attempting to place a catheter that is too

TABLE 52.1	IV Catheter Flow Rate by Gauge and Length[a]	
Gauge	Length (inches)	Flow Rate (mL/minute)
Peripheral IV		
24	0.75	20
22	1.0	37
20	1.0	63
20	1.16	61
20	1.88	54
18	1.16	95
18	1.88	87
16	1.16	193
16	1.77	185
14	2.0	295
Central Venous Line		
4F Double-Lumen		
20		23
22		12
5F Double-Lumen		
20		15
20		20
5F Triple-Lumen		
18		20
23		2
23		2
7F Triple-Lumen		
16		49
18		20
18		20
8F Cordis (4-inch)[b]		133
Percutaneous Intravenous Central Catheters (PICC)		
4F Single-lumen		21.2
5F Single-lumen		20
5F Dual (each lumen)		9.6
6F Dual (each lumen)		12.5

Information regarding central venous catheters was abstracted from Cook Medical "Quick Reference Guide for Spectrum" catheters (https://www.cookmedical.com/data/resources/4%20CC-BM-ABRMQR-EN-201111.pdf). PICC line information is for the PowerPICC Catheter from Bard Access Systems (Salt Lake City, UT).
[a]The standard by which flow rate is measured (by gravity) is that the intravenous bag of crystalloid is suspended 1 meter above the height of measurement.
[b]Cordis (Milpitas, CA).

large may result in failure. It is better to have two working 22-gauge IVs rather than multiple puncture sites from failed attempts with an 18- or 20-gauge IV. Table 52.1 indicates that a shorter catheter delivers a greater flow rate than a longer catheter and that a central venous catheter, which is often a long catheter, is usually limited to infuse low fluid flow rates because of resistance caused by their length. PICC lines cannot be used for resuscitation (and may prevent the rapid administration of a bolus of propofol) because of their narrow caliber and extra length (see Table 52.1).

Large-bore tubing used for blood transfusion or resuscitation has the best flow characteristics. There are multiple strategies to increase the IV flow rate, including using a pressure bag placed around the fluid bag, IV tubing sets with integrated bulb pumps, use of a large (60-mL) syringe[21] and a stopcock to create a pull-push system or large prefilled syringes,[22] and a purpose-built device such as the Level 1 h-1200 Fast Flow Fluid Warmer (Smiths Medical) or Belmont Rapid Infuser RI-2 (Belmont Instrument, Bellerica, MA). If a 20-gauge or larger catheter is already in place, it may be exchanged for an Arrow rapid infusion catheter (Teleflex, Morrisville, NC) that is typically a 7F or 8.5F (internal diameter) 2-inch-long catheter. Fluid resuscitation is limited with the commercially available IV pumps to their maximum flow rates, 999 mL/hour or 16.6 mL/minute. If a pressure infusion bag is used, the IV bag should be de-aired to prevent air from being pumped into the circulation, creating an air embolism, as the bag empties.

The temperature and viscosity of IV fluids greatly affect the infusion rate. Less viscous fluids are infused more rapidly than more viscous fluids (e.g., colloid solutions). Crystalloid solutions are the least viscous fluids followed by colloids, whole blood, and PRBCs. PRBCs may be diluted with normal saline solution to reduce viscosity, improve flow characteristics, and decrease the risk of hemolysis during a rapid infusion.[23]

TOTAL INTRAVENOUS ANESTHESIA AND VASOACTIVE MEDICATIONS

If total IV anesthesia (TIVA) or the use of vasoactive medications is necessary, they are ideally infused through a separate venous access. The speed at which the medication is administered depends on the location of the access point in the infusion line, how much priming volume is present in the tubing, and the speed at which the fluids are infusing (Fig. 52.2). A carrier solution on a pump should be infused at a baseline rate because most vasoactive medications are piggy-backed into the tubing at slow infusion rates. The carrier solution should be adjusted to the child's maintenance infusion rate and the other IV fluids reduced accordingly. Multiple stopcock manifolds allow for the connection of multiple infusions as well as the carrier solution. Fig. 52.3 shows various multiple-drug infusion systems, each of which has slightly different priming volumes, which in turn affect the speed at which medications are infused. Many practitioners prime their medications and then initiate the pumps to run the fluids to the end of the manifold. When connected directly to an IV line, medications should be delivered without delay provided the carrier fluid rate is maintained at the same rate.

Establishing any IV access in infants and toddlers can be difficult, a task that becomes extremely difficult when they are in shock. When peripheral IV access cannot be established quickly and the child is critically ill, placement of an intraosseous catheter should be entertained (see also Chapter 49, Figs. 49.6 and 49.7).

LUER ADAPTERS

Luer-Lok adapters allow for the rapid and secure connection of syringes and IV fluid lines to catheters. This has particular significance in the OR as access to the arterial or venous lines are remote from the caregiver and hidden under the drapes. However, the Luer-Lok adapter is also interchangeable with epidural, spinal and nerve block catheters, feeding tubes, total parenteral nutrition lines, and even sidestream carbon dioxide (CO_2) connectors.[24–26] All of these have the identical six-degree Luer-Lok taper that allows them to be connected interchangeably.[27] This universal connection has led to the accidental injection of drugs not meant for the neuroaxial space into epidural catheters,[28–30] parenteral

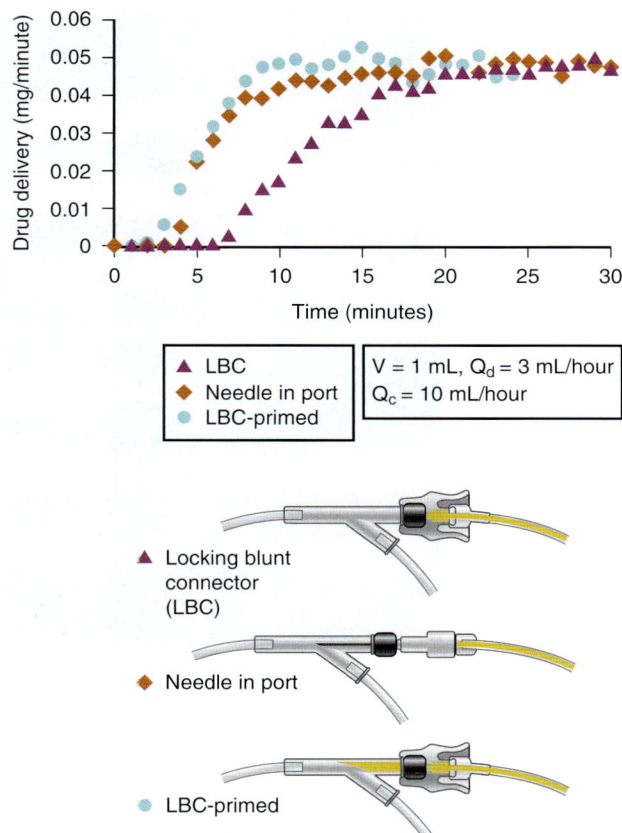

FIGURE 52.2 The time delay in onset of drug delivery to steady-state drug delivery as affected by a needle in an injection port and a locking blunt connector (LBC) or "priming" of the dead space of the injection port are illustrated. Note that the time to initiate drug delivery is delayed by several minutes and the time to achieve a steady-state rate of drug administration may be delayed by 10 minutes or longer when the dead space is not primed or a needle is not used to bypass the dead space of the injection port (in this example, the parameters were: carrier rate [Q_c] 10 mL/hour, drug flow rate [Q_d] 3 mL/hour, dead space volume [V] 1 mL). This concept has important implications regarding drug delivery to all patients, but it is particularly important in infants and neonates in whom small volumes of drug may be administered into a relatively large dead space that must be filled before any drug enters the flow of the intravenous fluid and the hourly rate of the carrier is low. (From Lovich MA, Doles J, Peterfreund RA. The impact of carrier flow rate and infusion set dead-volume on the dynamics of intravenous drug delivery. Anesth Analg. 2005;100[4]:1048–1055.)

chemotherapy (vincristine) given intrathecally (more than 30 times since 1968),[31] local anesthetics (e.g., bupivacaine) injected intravenously.[32,33] a blood pressure (BP) cuff attached to a Hep-Lock IV set (Baxter Healthcare), gastric feeds, and breast milk infused through a central venous catheter,[34] causing significant morbidity and mortality.[35] Labeling of all catheters at the hub, color coding, and vigilance have been effective, in part, to reduce this risk. However, to address this risk formally, an international, multidisciplinary team convened in 2007 to draft a standard by which Luer-Loks will be modified such that a unique Luer-Lok design will be available for each type of Luer-Lok connection (e.g., IV, gastrointestinal, genitourinary, neurologic, anesthesia breathing circuits, and hemodynamic monitoring [BP cuffs]) that will also prevent cross-connection of tubing meant for different uses.[30,36] This meeting resulted in publication of ISO-80369 standard, which

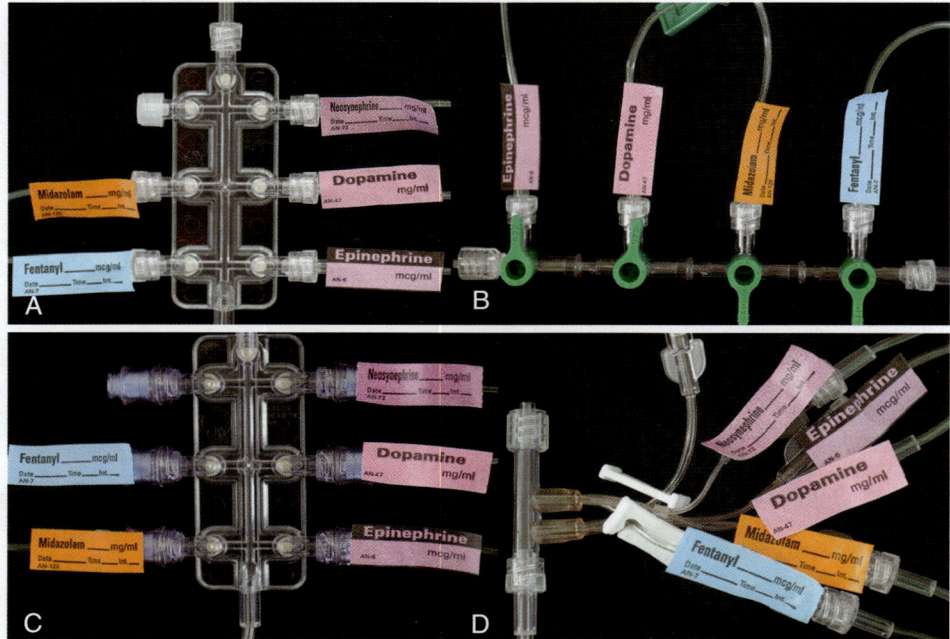

FIGURE 52.3 Several multiple-drug and fluid administration systems are illustrated. Note the wide variation in dead-space volume among the screw-in connectors **(A)**, simple stopcocks **(B)**, screw-in connectors with one-way valves **(C)**, and multiple short tubing connections **(D)**. To avoid variations in rate of drug delivery, it is advised to use a dedicated carrier on a pump. To ensure that the initiation of drug delivery is timely, the following steps are necessary: (1) each dead space port must be flushed and primed with the desired infusion as it is attached to the delivery manifolds; (2) after priming, the stopcock is turned to the off position or the tubing is clamped; (3) the carrier portion of the system is then run through or flushed with the carrier intravenous fluid; and (4) the system is attached to the patient with just the carrier ensuring a constant flow to the patient. When the drug infusion is initiated, the stopcock is turned to the on position or the tubing unclamped and each drug infusion pump turned on at the desired rate. This ensures that no drug is accidentally administered and reduces the time to initial drug delivery by priming the dead space of the system for each drug infusion. It should be borne in mind that this system should be connected as closely as possible to the intravenous catheter to avoid further delay in drug delivery because of the need to fill the dead space between the multiple drug manifolds and the entry into a vein. The use of a pump for the carrier solution also prevents retrograde drug infusion.

after several iterations, is about to be set for implementation.[37] This new standard will modify the six-degree Luer-Lok taper to preclude cross-connection of tubing intended for differences uses by creating non–Luer-Lok connectors for non-IV equipment larger or smaller than the standard Luer-Lok connections.

Airway Apparatus

MASKS

Transparent disposable plastic (latex-free) face masks are available in a wide variety of sizes for children of all ages, to deliver oxygen as well as induce and maintain inhalational anesthesia. These air-filled cushioned masks, which can be inflated to fill the cuff, replaced the old Rendell-Baker/Soucek face masks, which had a very small dead space but often failed to seal completely on the faces of some children. With the wide variability in the morphology of children's facies, especially those who are syndromic, the anesthesiologist should prepare cushioned masks that are smaller and larger than the size chosen for the child. The provider should be able to maintain a tight mask seal on the face with the least amount of dead space. Masks vary according to the manufacturer; however, there are few features that would lead us to recommend one over another. Some masks can be purchased already flavored (with fruit such as strawberry), although most anesthesiologists

prefer to offer flavors (e.g., watermelon or strawberry lip balms) to the child and let him or her choose their favorite and apply the flavor to the mask. Specialized masks with a built-in port for endoscopy or fiberoptic intubation are also available for specific indications (see E-Fig. 14.13).

OROPHARYNGEAL AIRWAYS

Oropharyngeal airways are hard, non-latex plastic that are preformed in different sizes from 40 mm (infant) to 100 mm (large adult). Care should be taken to choose an airway that is the correct size for the child because an airway that is too small displaces the posterior portion of the tongue or epiglottis into the glottic opening, causing upper airway obstruction. Alternatively, if the airway is too large, the airway device may cause damage to laryngeal structures, causing swelling and potential postoperative obstruction (see Fig. 14.13). An oral airway should always be placed midline, without rotating it as it is inserted as is commonly done in adults, since at every age, children have some loose teeth and others that are ready to fall out. Rotating the hard airway may dislodge one or more teeth, leading to a possible pulmonary aspiration. Misplaced oral airways that obstruct venous and/or lymphatic drainage of the tongue can precipitate acute macroglossia.[38] Additional causes of acute macroglossia include retained throat packs,[39] surgical positioning,[40] and the presence of TEE probes.

NASOPHARYNGEAL AIRWAYS

Nasopharyngeal airways are an additional adjunct to reduce or prevent upper airway obstruction.[41,42] Latex-free nasal airways are available in sizes from 12F to 36F. Care should be taken when placing them in the nose as they may injure the mucosa or dissect adenoidal tissue free, causing bleeding. Selecting the correct size of the airway is important because an excessively large nasal airway can apply pressure to the ala of the nose, which can lead to injury and even alar necrosis. If the ala blanches when the airway is seated, it is likely too large for the diameter of the nostril and should be replaced with a smaller-diameter airway. Some nasal airways have a movable flange to prevent them from being inserted too deeply. The flange should be adjusted before it is inserted. The correct nasal airway size approximation is estimated when the airway extends from the nares to the angle of the jaw or the earlobe. In the absence of an appropriately sized nasal airway, one could cut a tracheal tube to the appropriate length. Note that a cut tracheal tube is stiffer than a commercially available nasal airway and has a greater potential for injury. Prewarming the tracheal tube using hot water may soften the tube and reduce the risk of mucosal injury. The lumen of any nasal airway is limited and can be occluded with secretions and/or blood. Therefore they should be removed as quickly as possible if airway obstruction is diagnosed.

LARYNGEAL MASK AIRWAYS

The reusable (Classic) Laryngeal Mask Airway (LMA, Teleflex) is a supraglottic airway device (SGA) developed by Dr. Archibald Brain in the 1980s. Reusable models of the LMA are still available, although most SGAs used today are single-use, disposable airways. Several different types of LMAs are now available, including the LMA Unique (used in emergency setting), LMA Flexible (soft, malleable wired neck), LMA ProSeal (with a second channel to direct gastric contents away from the airway), and the LMA Supreme (the Proseal with a built-in bite block). All of these airways are currently available, although high-quality studies that compared their advantages and disadvantages (with the exception of the Classic and the ProSeal) are lacking in children.[43] The SGA is a lifesaving airway device that should be used to establish ventilation when either ventilation by face mask or tracheal intubation is difficult or impossible. These devices are usually easy to place by inserting them straight into the hypopharynx, although some prefer to rotate the LMAs 90 degrees as they insert them.[44] Occasionally, the LMA will not advance past the posterior pharynx, especially if the bowl has been deflated. This may occur if there is a step-up in the alignment of the mucosa over the vertebral bodies against which the tip of the LMA abuts. Alternately, the tip of the bowl may have flipped backward, toward the nasopharynx, as the LMA is inserted, preventing it from advancing smoothly. To advance the LMA in both circumstances, the tip of the bowl should be lifted using your finger and the LMA then advanced. The bowl should be inflated until there is no air audible leak at ~16 to 20 cm H_2O peak inspiratory pressure. These airways can be used as the sole airway during anesthesia or as a conduit for bronchoscopy or fiberoptic intubation. There are several manufacturers with small to moderate differences among these devices (see also Figs. 14.18 to 14.20). For routine use in children with normal airways these small differences may not matter; some are specifically designed as a conduit for intubation. Supraglottic devices may have either one or two lumens. Dual-lumen SGAs are placed blindly into the oropharynx. They have two separate cuffs that can be inflated to allow isolation of the trachea (see

E-Figs. 14.1 and 14.2). The dual-lumen devices are more typically used for prehospital providers during resuscitation and are not discussed further here. A typical single-lumen SGA is also readily placed blindly into the hypopharynx and makes a nonocclusive seal with the larynx. Single-lumen SGAs have a variety of additional features and design elements, such as nonferrous valves for use in magnetic resonance imaging (MRI); spiral reinforced and flexible, containing a thermoplastic cuff that molds to the airway; drains or sites for drainage of gastric contents; curvature to facilitate fiberoptic intubation; internal bars to prevent the epiglottis from obstructing the lumen; devices specifically designed to facilitate blind endotracheal intubation; and modifications that allow greater airway occlusive pressures during positive-pressure ventilation.

SGAs are available for all age groups from neonates and infants (<5 kg) to children and adolescents (>70 kg). Success rates for inserting the LMA on the first attempt are very high in most age groups, although some report only moderate success rates in neonates and infants (80%).[45] In most infants and children, the epiglottis lies within the bowl of the LMA, without evidence of upper airway obstruction.[46,47] In neonates and infants, it behooves the anesthesiologist to maintain very close vigilance of oxygenation and ventilation as the airway may become compromised quite suddenly and rescue measures must be adopted quickly.

When the LMA was first introduced, most practitioners used it only in children who breathed spontaneously. However, more recently many have adopted the adult practice of using low-pressure volume support and positive end-expiratory pressure (PEEP) with the LMA to minimize the effect of the dead space contributed by the LMA stem and the associated hypercarbia.[48-50] We have had good success with this approach in young children.

ENDOTRACHEAL TUBES

Endotracheal tube (ETT) sizes are polyvinyl chloride in composition, implant tested (based on Z79 standards in rabbits), and non-reusable. ETT sizes range from 2 to 10 mm inner diameter (ID). There may be small differences in wall thickness among manufacturers, although the variability is generally less than that of the anatomy of the upper airway in children of the same age. Additional differences include the bevel angle, tip design, and presence of a Murphy eye. Uncuffed ETTs have been the standard in pediatric anesthesia in infants and children up to 8 years of age for decades, although in the past 10 to 20 years, there has been a shift toward cuffed ETTs, accelerated by the introduction of the Microcuff ETT (Halyard Health, Alpharetta, GA). The reasons behind this shift in practice include the manufacturing of high-volume, low-pressure cuffed ETTs, efforts to reduce OR contamination,[51,52] to decrease anesthetic use with reduced fresh gas flow,[51] to reduce the need to reintubate the airway to prevent a large gas leak,[53] and ICU studies documenting the safety of cuffed ETTs after prolonged tracheal intubation.[54,55] However, Microcuff ETTs completely redesigned the ETT for children, introducing an elliptically shaped cuff that is positioned more distal on the tube, a thinner compliant cuff, and removing the Murphy eye (see Fig. 14.15). The cuff seals at a low pressure (10–12 cm H_2O), is permeable to nitrous oxide (N_2O), and is distal along the shaft of the ETT. Proper positioning is recommended using the markings on the shaft of the tube such that they align with the vocal cords, rather than the number of centimeters at the mandibular gumline.[56]

Several formulas have been developed to predict the ID of the ETT for each age group. The metric most widely used to select the diameter of the ETT is age. In the case of uncuffed

ETTs, Cole originally published his formula in 1957[57] in French catheter gauge, which was subsequently modified by Morgan and Steward in 1982 to:

Uncuffed ETT size (mm ID) = (age (years)/4) + 4 for children 2 years and older.[58]

For infants and children younger than 2 years, most recommend 2.5-mm ID ETT in infants weighing less than 1500 g, 3.0-mm ID for infants 1500 to 3000 g, and 3.5 mm for those who weigh more than 3000 g and full-term.[59]

For cuffed ETTs, Khine published in 1997 that the correct size is:

Cuffed ETT size (mm ID) = (age (years)/ 4) + 3.[52]

Other authors have modified Khine's formula to the size (mm ID) as (age (years)/4 + 3.5) for children older than 1 year.[60]

The outer diameter of cuffed ETTs is 0.5 mm larger than their uncuffed counterparts. One may choose to use the modified Cole formula for the initial ETT size for both cuffed and uncuffed ETTs and subtract 0.5 for the size of the cuffed ETT. Others developed formulas for selecting ETT size based on the child's height.[61,62] Age-based formulas are more accurate than direct comparison with the child's finger width.[63] A number of studies have assessed the accuracy of these formulas,[60,64] but this is a moot point as they should simply be considered a starting point for selecting the correct ETT size. Given the physiologic variability among children, ETT sizes smaller and larger should always be immediately available in the unlikely event that subglottic stenosis is diagnosed or a large trachea is uncovered and the predicted tube size for the child's age is erroneous (see Table 14.2). Some have advocated the use of ultrasound to assess the tracheal dimensions before selecting a tracheal tube to improve the accuracy of the ETT size predicted.[65]

A number of criteria have been proposed to confirm the appropriate fit and placement of the ETT in children. The ETT should pass through the vocal cords and subglottic space without meeting resistance. If resistance is felt, an ETT 0.5-mm ID smaller should be used. Once positioned, many recommend listening for an audible leak between peak inspiratory pressures of 15 and 30 mm H_2O. This pressure range is consistent with the peak inflation pressure for ventilation in most healthy children and maintains mucosal perfusion while avoiding a large gas leak and polluting the OR.[66] The simplest way to test for a leak is to slowly close the adjustable pressure limiting valve until the desired pressure is reached and either listening or placing a stethoscope over the larynx for a leak. However, the leak test is subject to a number of confounding variables, including the head position of the patient and the presence of neuromuscular blockade.[67] Despite these recommendations, several studies have demonstrated that large cuff pressures have not led to subglottic injury and stridor after extubation. If a cuffed ETT is used and there is a substantial leak with the cuff uninflated, then small amounts of air should be injected into the cuff until the leak disappears. If N_2O is used, it can diffuse into the cuff and increase the cuff volume (and pressure). The absence of an initial leak with a cuffed ETT even with the cuff deflated has been associated with postextubation stridor[68] and warrants exchange to the next smaller size ETT. Cuff pressure should be monitored periodically throughout the period of intubation.

A number of specialty ETTs are available, including those for single-lung ventilation, those with preformed curves, for laser surgery near the airway, microlaryngeal tubes for airway surgery, with spiral reinforcement, for neuromonitoring, and with sampling or suction ports (see also Chapters 14, 15, and 33). A preformed oral or nasal Ring, Adair, and Elwyn (RAE) tube allows surgeons to work on the face or in the mouth without the ETT obscuring their view or being at risk for being incised or kinked. They are also useful in head and neck surgery to keep the anesthesia circuit out of the field. It should be noted that the preformed curve has a specific length based on the ETT size predicted from average children. Securing the ETT with the angle of the curve well seated in the mouth or nares may cause the tip of the ETT to be either high or endobronchial, depending on the anatomy of the child. It is essential to pay special attention to the equality of breath sounds after the ETT is taped and the child placed in the position for surgery. Cuffed nasal RAE ETTs begin at 5.0-mm ID, are more difficult to suction through, and more prone to kinking than non-RAE ETTs. Manufacturers of the cuffed oral and nasal RAE ETT aligned the distance from the bend to the tip with an adult-sized ETT of the corresponding diameter rather than pediatric, resulting in longer distances from the bend than corresponds to the distance in the child's airway.[69] This may result in an endobronchial intubation if these ETTs are inserted until the bend is fully inserted into the nares or on the lower lip for the nasal and oral RAE tubes, respectively. As a result of needing to pull back slightly before taping, the bend in these cuffed RAE tubes may sit in the surgical field when the tip of the ETT is properly positioned in the trachea and therefore at risk for kinking (see Chapter 14 for a more in-depth discussion).

For these reasons, smaller versions of these ETTs are not always acceptable for long-term ventilation in the pediatric ICU (PICU); it is worth having this discussion before initiating anesthesia. For children undergoing complex craniofacial reconstructions in which the upper airway may swell postoperatively, their airways should remain intubated for several days and the airway swelling assessed daily for the presence of a leak.

Laser airway surgery places the child at risk for an airway fire. The polyvinylchloride (PVC) of a normal ETT can be damaged by the laser, resulting in mucosal injury or an airway fire. Oxygen and N_2O should both be reduced as much as possible as these are more flammable than air. Designs of specialty ETTs for laser surgery include a flexible stainless steel body, a silicon ETT wrapped in an aluminum material, and rubber tubes with or without metallic wrapping. The use of true natural rubber may put some patients with latex allergies at risk. Previously some institutions have wrapped normal ETTs in metallic tape to reduce the risk of damage to the PVC, but the rough edges of the tape may injure the mucosa. Microlaryngeal ETTs are longer regular ETTs and have a larger cuff providing more space in the airway for surgery; for example, a size 5.0-mm ID microlaryngeal ETT has the length of a 7.0-mm ID ETT. The trade-off is more room for surgical exposure versus a limited increase in airway resistance. Reinforced ETTs have a wire wrapped in a spiral fashion throughout the PVC wall of the ETT. They are often used in circumstances where kinking of the ETT is a risk. A slightly smaller-sized ETT than expected should be selected as reinforced ETTs have a larger outer diameter than the comparable standard ETT of the same size. In addition, a stylet is often needed to manipulate the floppy tube through the larynx. Once in place, a bite block is often used to stabilize the tube and prevent the patient from biting it, which could collapse the lumen.

Another ETT useful in head and neck surgery is the electromyographic ETT that permits neuromonitoring of the recurrent laryngeal nerve during neck dissection or thyroidectomy.[70] This type of specialty ETT is not available in sizes smaller than 6.0-mm

ID. Finally, there are uncuffed ETTs with an extra internal lumen that allows monitoring of airway pressure or exhaled gases (Mallinckrodt Inc., St. Louis, MO).

ETTs have been developed that are designed to reduce ventilator-associated pneumonia in children in the ICU. One such ETT has a suction port that allows continuous aspiration of secretions, whereas another takes advantage of a cone-shaped ETT cuff to prevent microaspiration of airway secretions around the ETT. Evidence for their effectiveness, however, remains weak.[71,72]

Intubation Equipment

LARYNGOSCOPES

A full range of straight (Miller) and curved (Macintosh or Mac) laryngoscope blades for direct laryngoscopy should be available. It is quite possible in a typical pediatric anesthesia practice to use both a Miller 00 and a Mac 4 blade in the same day. Both small and large laryngoscope handles are available to accommodate differences in body habitus among children. The blade and handle combinations should be tested before anesthesia is induced. Backup blades and handles should be immediately available; additional batteries and light bulbs should be in stock. The light source for laryngoscopes has changed over time from a simple light bulb at or near the tip of the blade powered by two D cell batteries to a fiberoptic channel powered by a rechargeable battery that lights a xenon bulb near the tip of the blade. This latter advance has increased the brightness of laryngoscopes and reduced the frequency of bulb changes; however, visual acuity does not appear to improve once illuminance exceeds 700 lux.[73] Disposable laryngoscope handles and blades have also been developed for use on code carts, during transport, and with highly infectious patients. The price of this equipment can be cost-effective if used only occasionally, although in some institutions with large volumes the cost of single-use devices is lower than the need for replacement of lost or stolen handles and blades. MRI-compatible laryngoscopes are also available but are extremely expensive; most use standard laryngoscope handles for use in 2-Tesla magnets but their use is restricted to the side of the magnetic core in zone 4. Laryngoscope blades with a supplemental oxygen channel are available; these delay the time to desaturation[74] in spontaneously breathing infants (see E-Fig. 14.12). This same effect has also been demonstrated with the addition of nasal cannula oxygen during intubation.[75]

A difficult airway cart with all needed equipment should be present in the OR complex (see Table 14.10). These carts should contain fiberoptic bronchoscopes in the three major sizes as well as other airway adjuncts such as LMAs, bougies, and indirect laryngoscopes that use prisms, fiberoptics, or video devices (see also Chapter 14).

Suction Devices

Suction devices include a container for waste and a regulator to control the degree of suction. Although regulators can provide low intermittent suction, systems used in anesthesia are not usually set up this way. Injury can occur to the gastric mucosa if continuous suction is applied to a nasogastric or orogastric tube. Vented tubes (e.g., Salem Sump, Sherwood Medical, St. Louis MO) in a variety of sizes should be available for continuous gastric drainage. If low intermittent suction cannot be provided, we prefer to leave the open end of these tubes sealed in a glove. Suction catheters with a thumb-controlled side port in sizes from 6F to 14 F should be available to suction ETTs. Yankauer tip suction devices are available in small and large sizes and are more effective at clearing material compared with the thumb-controlled catheters. They may be metal or plastic; the latter material is preferable to limit the risk of damaging teeth. Yankauer suction devices should never be inserted into the mouth in the midline (because the child may bite down on it and break or dislodge teeth). Rather, the devices should be inserted between the teeth and the inside of the cheek, reaching the hypopharynx behind the molars or bicuspids. The small size Yankauer works well in infants, limiting damage to the oropharynx. However, if a large amount of material must be cleared, the larger Yankauer is more effective. If a very large volume needs to be suctioned (e.g., gastric bleeding), it is prudent to have two separate suction devices and parallel systems available.

Anesthesia Workstation

An anesthesia machine is a device that allows for mechanical or electronic control of gas titration (O_2 [oxygen], N_2O, and air), titration of anesthetic vapor, and manual or mechanical ventilation. It is also an ergonomically designed workstation that includes storage; a place for computer or hand charting; a work surface for drugs and intubation equipment and patient and machine monitoring; a reservoir bag for hand ventilation with an adjustable pressure limit (APL) valve; a means of scavenging anesthesia and waste gas; and an absorber for CO_2 removal. It is also advisable to have a self-inflating bag readily available should a power failure occur or a patient develop malignant hyperthermia. The anesthesia machine has had a unique role in improving patient safety in the OR. Modern machines cannot deliver a hypoxic gas mixture; they monitor inspired and expired oxygen and anesthesia gases; use an index system to prevent connection of wrong gas lines; and monitor airway pressure and alarms for high pressure, disconnections, high or low minute ventilation, and apnea. The current anesthesia system is a marvel of design that is a very long way from the nonrebreathing open anesthesia systems of the past. The classic example of an open system is the Ayre T-piece, which uses a simple tube as a reservoir for gas (Fig. 52.4). Modifications to this type of system resulted in open breathing circuits that are part of the Mapleson classification (Fig. 52.5);

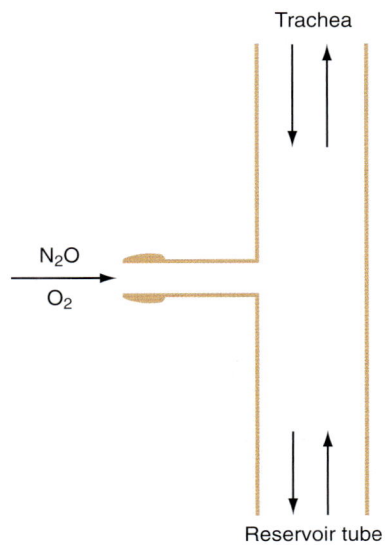

FIGURE 52.4 The T piece as described by Ayre. (From Ayre P. The T-piece technique. *Br J Anaesth*. 1956;28[11]:520–523.)

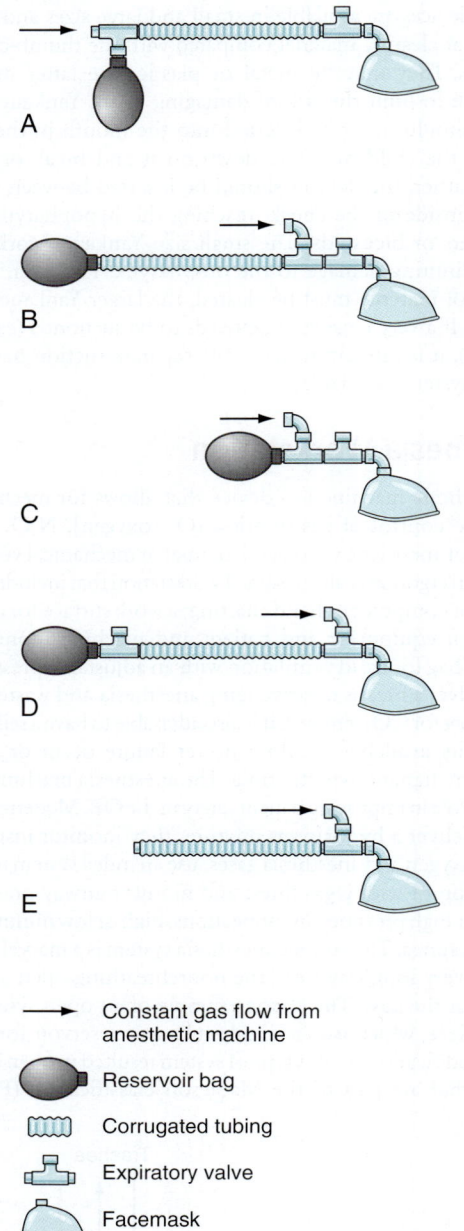

Constant gas flow from anesthetic machine

Reservoir bag

Corrugated tubing

Expiratory valve

Facemask

FIGURE 52.5 The Mapleson categories of breathing circuits. The most commonly used circuit for infants is the Mapleson D configuration. (From Mapleson WW. The elimination of rebreathing in various semi-closed anaesthetic systems. *Br J Anaesth.* 1954;26[5]:323–332.)

advantages and disadvantages of each are described elsewhere.[76] The Mapleson D configuration is frequently used to transport children in the hospital to and from the OR. The Mapleson D circuit is very lightweight and allows for easy adjustment of PEEP while the patient breathes spontaneously and peak inspiratory pressure when ventilation is controlled. The circuit requires three times the minute ventilation to prevent rebreathing of CO_2. The Mapleson D allows the child to breathe spontaneously without additional work to initiate gas flow; this contrasts with a self-inflating (e.g., Ambu bag, Ambu Inc., Columbia, MD) resuscitation bag that must be squeezed to initiate gas flow. However, in the absence of gas flow, a Mapleson D cannot facilitate ventilation as it is not

self-inflating. Therefore for transport of children whose airways are intubated we recommend the Mapleson D but also suggest bringing a self-inflating resuscitation bag (e.g., Ambu bag) should the gas source fail.

Current anesthesia machines are unidirectional semi-closed circuits in which a fixed amount of fresh gas is added to the circle breathing circuit each minute and a means of removing CO_2 is present. These systems contaminate the environment with anesthetic gases less than the open systems, as well as retain the airway gas temperature and humidity better than the open systems. In the following text we describe the key components of the system with specific highlights to pediatrics when applicable including scavenging systems, CO_2 absorption, humidification, and mechanical ventilation.

SCAVENGING SYSTEMS

Scavenger systems are a necessary part of an anesthesia machine to prevent contamination of the OR with waste anesthesia gases. Scavenging systems are either open or closed and movement of waste gas can be either active or passive. An open system uses a reservoir to collect waste gas, which is then actively suctioned from the reservoir. The reservoir in these open systems communicates with the atmosphere, thereby avoiding either positive or negative pressure transmission to the airway. A closed system is not connected to the atmosphere of the OR but waste gas exits the machine and then the OR through a series of valves. In a closed system, scavenging can be either active via means of suction or passive, relying on heavier-than-air anesthesia gases and pressure to move waste gas to evacuation. These systems must have both positive- and negative-pressure relief valves to prevent pressure from being transmitted to the airway. Scavenger systems are necessary and helpful means to reduce the contamination of the OR.[77] In addition, anesthesiologists also contribute substantively to reducing OR contamination; fresh gas flows are not increased until the patient is ready for induction of anesthesia, a tight mask fit is preferred, the leak around the ETT should be minimal, and fresh gas flow rates should be reduced or turned off before disconnecting the anesthesia circuit to move or position the child.

CARBON DIOXIDE ABSORPTION

CO_2 absorption or the removal of CO_2 from the breathing circuit makes a circle system possible. This allows for the rebreathing of exhaled gases and inhalational agents, which reduces waste, pollution of the OR as well as the environment, and retention of heat and humidity within the circuit. All the materials that absorb CO_2 are chemicals that react with CO_2 converting it to stable compounds, hardeners to prevent obstruction of the canister, and dye indicators that identify when the absorption material is expended and should be changed. Soda lime, one typical CO_2 absorbent, contains approximately 80% calcium hydroxide ($Ca(OH)_2$), 15% water (H_2O), 4% sodium hydroxide (NaOH), and 1% potassium hydroxide (KOH). The chemical reactions can be described as a strong alkali with metal hydroxide functioning as a catalyst in the presence of water to convert CO_2 into calcium carbonate. The equations are as follows:

1. $CO_2 + H_2O \rightleftharpoons H_2CO_3$
2. $H_2CO_3 + 2NaOH$ (or KOH) $\rightleftharpoons Na_2CO_3$ (K_2CO_3) $+ 2H_2O +$ Heat
3. Na_2CO_3 (K_2CO_3) $+ Ca(OH)_2 \rightleftharpoons CaCO_3 + 2NaOH$ (KOH)

A number of sequelae occur when potent inhalational anesthetic interact with these absorbents; in the presence of desiccated soda lime, ether anesthetics can degrade to carbon monoxide and in

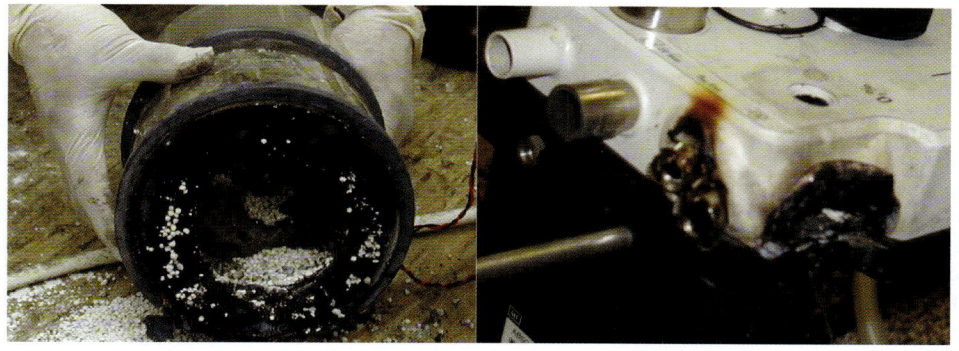

FIGURE 52.6 Sevoflurane/Baralyme interaction produced this fire in an anesthesia machine. (Courtesy Mr. A. Rich.)

the case of sevoflurane, to Compound A,[78-82] a vinyl compound known to cause renal injury in rats.[83,84] In the presence of favorable conditions, carbon monoxide production follows the order desflurane > isoflurane > sevoflurane > halothane.[85] Extreme heat and fire have been associated with the absorbent, Baralyme, which contained barium hydroxide. The reaction of sevoflurane with desiccated Baralyme created such a severe exothermic reaction that it has caused acute respiratory distress syndrome (ARDS),[86] fires[87] and explosions[88,89] in the OR (Fig. 52.6). Both carbon monoxide poisoning and fires typically occurred on a Monday morning after a weekend during which the fresh gas flow had been left running through the anesthesia machine without a reservoir bag, desiccating the absorbent. Baralyme was voluntarily withdrawn from the market in 2004 to prevent additional human injuries; further experiments showed that increased temperatures could occur with desiccated soda lime.[90] These events emphasize that we must remain vigilant and turn off the fresh gas flows between cases, ensure a reservoir bag is in place in the circuit and replace desiccated CO_2 absorbents with fresh absorbent. Concerns about degradation of inhaled anesthetics to carbon monoxide and compound A[91,92] led to the development of a number of CO_2 absorbents that do not contain the strong alkali agents NaOH or KOH and are inert to the ether anesthetics. These include Amsorb Plus (Armstrong Medical Limited, Coleraine, Northern Ireland), Lithely (Allied Healthcare Products, St. Louis, MO), Sodasorb LF (Smiths Medical), and Yabashi Lime-f (Yabashi Holdings Co., Akasaka, Japan). There are also absorbents that contain a reduced amount of NaOH, including Spherasorb (Intersurgical Ltd., Berkshire UK), and Drägersorb 800 Plus (Dräger). In addition, the risk of developing renal injury is related to the dose exposure of compound A and not just to sevoflurane.[93] However, this risk is far less likely than originally thought and now likely eliminated with the newer absorbents.[94-96] However, in a conservative fashion the US Food and Drug Administration in the January 2010 Prescribing Information for Ultane (sevoflurane) recommends: *"To minimize exposure to Compound A, sevoflurane exposure should not exceed 2 MAC·hours at flow rates of 1 to < 2 L/min. Fresh gas flow rates <1 L/min are not recommended"*; in the absence of any ill effects of compound A reported in humans, it is unclear if this recommendation is necessary (see also Chapter 7).

CO_2 absorbents must also include color indicators to identify when the capacity of the absorbent has been exhausted. Ethyl violet is one indicator, which changes from colorless to violet when the pH of the absorbent decreases. Exposure to fluorescent lights can decrease the concentration of functioning ethyl violet.[97] In addition, if consumed absorbent material is left unused for a period of time, it is possible for the color indicator to revert to white or colorless. This can occur when NaOH or KOH regenerates in the absorbent material with a subsequent increase in pH. This does not occur with absorbents that are NaOH- or KOH-free.

HUMIDIFICATION

Oxygen, N_2O, and air from tanks and connecting lines contain no humidity and are room temperature or cold compared with the patient. Warming and humidifying inspired gases help to maintain body temperature and prevent the drying of secretions, improve mucociliary function,[98,99] and reduce the inflammatory response.[100]

A small amount of heat is produced during the exothermic reaction that occurs when CO_2 is removed from the breathing circuit. However, the amount of heat produced is insufficient to maintain a child's temperature. The use of small fresh gas flows increases the humidity relative to high fresh gas flows.[101] However, small fresh gas flows do not increase the humidity sufficiently to preserve mucociliary function. Further, there was no difference in airway temperature between small and large fresh gas flows.[101] Clinicians may choose to use passive humidification with a heat and moisture exchanger (HME). The passive HMEs have a reflective filter or membrane that retains heat and moisture on the patient side of the circuit. HMEs increase the temperature and heat of the inspired gases to the point that they approach physiologic levels.[102] The best results are achieved when an HME is used in conjunction with small fresh gas flows. The downside to using HMEs is that they increase the dead space and can increase the partial pressure of CO_2 (PCO_2) if the minute ventilation is not increased.[103] Humidification of airway gases can also be active with systems that include heated wires within the breathing circuit or reservoirs for sterile water connected to the breathing circuit that can be heated. These systems are very effective at maintaining temperature and humidity but have some drawbacks. Active humidification systems are prone to condensation or "rain out" on the inside of the breathing circuit that can lead to obstruction of the airway, obstruction of the CO_2 gas sampling line, and inaccurate measurement of airway pressure and gas flow. Active humidification systems increase the resistance to gas flow and can alter the compliance and compression volume if they are not in line and warm when the machine check is performed. Finally, if active humidification systems are set incorrectly or malfunction, they can overheat and cause damage to the airway and trachea. The decision to use active or passive systems should be based on factors such as the size of the patient, duration of the case, and difficulty in maintaining an increased minute ventilation.

MECHANICAL VENTILATION

In addition to delivering anesthetic gases and oxygen and eliminating CO_2, one of the primary purposes of the anesthesia workstation is to ventilate the lungs. The complexity of this task is compounded in small infants and children in whom an inaccuracy of 20 mL might double the delivered tidal volume.[104] The determinants of the delivered tidal volume include the compliance of the anesthesia breathing circuit, the fresh gas inflow, the means of delivering the breath, the gas flows, and the dead space of airway circuit.[105] The newest generation of anesthesia machines uses internal electronics to address all of these components except dead space and to compensate for changes in these variables to estimate the minute ventilation.[106]

The electronics of modern anesthesia workstations can compensate for the compliance and compression volume of both the gases delivered and the tubing of the breathing circuit. Breathing circuits are either parallel or coaxial and can be smooth or, more commonly, corrugated. Corrugated breathing circuits come in a variety of sizes to accommodate the patient's size. Larger lumens have reduced resistance to air flow but a greater increase in volume when pressure is applied to the circuit. Compensation calibration can be performed with modern anesthesia workstations to accommodate for the change in volume as the circuit expands under pressure. Recent evidence demonstrated that the compliance of the corrugated circuit tubing is reduced, and therefore the compensation underestimated, if the tubing is not fully expanded before commencing the machine check.[107] The end of the breathing circuit should be occluded and the compensation test performed before use; the workstation increases the volume in the occluded circuit while pressure is being measured. The compliance factor of that breathing circuit is automatically entered into the ventilation system memory and used to compensate for the volume of expansion. This test is specific to the circuit in its current state. If the circuit size is changed or if the corrugated circuit's length is altered, the compliance factor will be inaccurate and therefore the delivered tidal volume will be inaccurate. If either of these changes occur, the compensation test should be repeated to ensure that the displayed respiratory indices are accurate.

One concern with the first generation of anesthesia ventilators was that changing the fresh gas flow could alter the tidal volume delivered to the lungs. The volume of gas set to be delivered entered the bellows mechanism of the ventilator during inspiration, augmenting or diminishing the intended tidal volume with the volume-controlled mode. The most recent generation of anesthesia ventilators does not have this limitation.[106] The mechanism by which this is accomplished varies among manufacturers. One design is to incorporate a valve that shuts off fresh gas flow during the delivery of the inspired breath. Another design is to measure the amount of fresh gas flow and adjust the volume in the bellows, piston, or turbine used to deliver the dialed tidal volume. The ability to measure gas flow very accurately throughout the anesthesia workstation allows for this type of adjustment as well as circuit compensation. Real-time monitoring extends to the ventilation system of the newest generation of anesthesia machines regardless of whether this is accomplished by pneumatics, piston, or turbine.

The latest generation of anesthesia machines also provides multiple modes of mechanical ventilation. These include pressure-controlled ventilation (PCV), volume-controlled ventilation (VCV), and volume-guaranteed ventilation (VGV). These modes can be set as intermittent mechanical ventilation (IMV), or synchronized intermittent mechanical ventilation (SIMV), in which the child's effort to breathe can trigger the ventilator to deliver a breath. Additionally, the ventilator can deliver pressure support (PS) above PEEP. We believe that PCV is the optimal mode for mechanical ventilation of most infants and children in routine practice. This preference may have developed from a time when the measurement of tidal volume with the ventilator was less accurate. At that time, however, pressure could be measured very accurately. For PCV, the clinician sets a positive inspiratory pressure (PIP) level, PEEP level, inspiratory:expiratory (I:E) ratio, and respiratory rate. The adequacy of ventilation is determined by observing the chest rise, auscultating breath sounds, monitoring the end-tidal CO_2 (ETCO2), and intermittent blood gases as indicated. The ventilator delivers a breath with a very fast initial flow, which decreases as the target pressure is achieved. This is known as a decelerating flow pattern. The pressure in the airway is constant throughout the inspiratory breath and forms a square wave. In PCV mode, the tidal volume delivered depends on the compliance of the ventilator circuit and the respiratory system. One disadvantage of this mode of ventilation is that with a decrease in compliance (e.g., surgeon leaning on the infant's chest), the delivered tidal volume decreases. Alternatively, in a VCV mode, the clinician sets a tidal volume to be delivered, PEEP level, rate and I:E ratio. The adequacy of ventilation is determined in the same manner. The inspiratory pressure required to deliver the tidal volume depends on the compliance of the ventilator circuit and respiratory system as well as the time over which the breath is delivered. This inspiratory time is determined by the rate and the I:E ratio. In a VCV mode of ventilation, the rate of air flow is constant throughout the entire inspiratory cycle and forms a square wave. However, the pressure in the airway increases throughout the inspiratory time. Some clinicians argue that the constant air flow throughout the inspiratory breath prevents atelectasis; however, in our view it seems much easier to simply set a level of PEEP and apply an alveolar recruitment maneuver as necessary.

The practical differences between these two modes of ventilation are that if you set the peak pressure, you must monitor the tidal volume and adjust the peak pressure if the compliance changes. If you set the tidal volume, you must monitor pressure and adjust the flow, inspiratory time, and inspiratory waveform or tidal volume when compliance changes. For example, during laparoscopic surgery when the abdomen is inflated with CO_2, the tidal volume decreases and the pressure or rate increases in PCV mode to maintain the same minute ventilation. During the same case in a VCV mode, the ventilator pressure increases and the clinician will need to decide if the increase is tolerable or if the tidal volume needs to be decreased slightly. As a consequence of the differences in the air flow patterns between PCV and VCV modes, a greater pressure is required to achieve the same tidal volume as in the VCV mode. For most children with normally compliant lungs, this difference is negligible. VGV modes of ventilation have different names based on the manufacturer. Some clinicians believe that this mode is the quintessential ventilation strategy of both PCV and VCV. The clinician sets a required tidal volume while the ventilator measures the pressure in the airway over several breaths as it adjusts to deliver the desired tidal volume. Then, in an iterative manner, the ventilator uses pressure to achieve that set volume. The goal is to use the minimum pressure to deliver the prescribed tidal volume. The air flow pattern used is a decelerating waveform and the pressure is constant throughout the inspiratory breath. This would seem like the best of both worlds as this mode can be used for children who are receiving muscle relaxants or are deeply anesthetized. However, when the patient's lung compliance changes rapidly, as in coughing or bucking on the ventilator, it is difficult to maintain the prescribed tidal volume.

The respiratory management of children with acute lung injury or ARDS requires specific barotrauma-sparing ventilator strategies. This newest generation of anesthesia machines ventilators can measure and deliver tidal volumes accurately enough to target 6 to 8 mL/kg. Compared with the overall population of patients, only a small number of children with ARDS come to the OR. Therefore with the current state of the art anesthesia ventilators, there may not be a significant benefit to bringing an ICU ventilator into the OR even for children with poor respiratory compliance. The current anesthesia machines include all the modes of ventilation that are generally used in an ICU setting. In addition, a significant advantage to using an anesthesia machine is the ability to rapidly deepen the depth of anesthesia with inhalational anesthetics. Further, if the APL valve is set to the same value as PEEP, the clinician can switch back and forth between mechanical and hand ventilation without altering PEEP. With an ICU ventilator, the patient is disconnected from the circuit to be hand ventilated; PEEP may be lost, potentially reducing lung recruitment.

Finally, with regard to mode of ventilation, newer anesthesia machines allow clinicians to set PS levels. PS provides additional airway pressure when the patient triggers a breath either by negative pressure on the ventilator circuit or altering the airflow. Sensitivity triggers can be adjusted such that most children are able to initiate PS. If the triggers are set very low, it is possible for "autocycling" to occur. Autocycling occurs when PS breaths are triggered by changes in pressure or flow within the ventilator circuit owing to leaking around an ETT or other non–patient-initiated mechanisms. This can generally be identified by a very rapid ventilator rate with very small tidal volumes.

There are a number of benefits to PS ventilation. For children who are not receiving neuromuscular blocks drugs (NMBDs), PS allows them to set their own ventilator rate. This allows the clinician to use respiratory rate as a measure for depth of anesthesia as well as for titration of opioid pain medications. PS may also provide increased minute ventilation at the end of the procedure compared with spontaneous ventilation, which might decrease the time for emergence. As stated earlier, the conducting portion or shaft of an LMA can substantively increase the mechanical dead space in infants and small children. At times, the patient's tidal volume can be small enough that dead space cannot be overcome. The use of PS and PEEP can assist the child to overcome this dead space and maintain a normal CO_2 level.

The latest generation of anesthesia ventilators can accurately deliver a set PEEP value. They typically have an interruption in fresh gas flow such that tidal volume is neither altered by nor dependent on the fresh gas flow. In earlier anesthesia machines, the constant fresh gas flow would generate small amounts of PEEP. With the current ventilators, it is possible to provide anesthetics with zero PEEP. We can think of very few circumstances (possibly increased intracranial pressure or single-lung ventilation) where even a small amount of PEEP is not beneficial. Even high levels of PEEP do not decrease cardiac output in children who have an adequate intravascular volume.[108,109] Rather than increasing the inspired fraction of oxygen (FiO_2) in response to decreasing saturations, the clinician should perform an alveolar recruitment maneuver followed by the addition of PEEP to keep the alveoli open.[110]

Anesthesia machines have the ability to monitor pressure and flow in the airway. Further, they monitor the inspired and expired concentration of gases from the elbow of the breathing circuit.

These monitors increase patient safety and provide immediate feedback regarding the adequacy of ventilation and the depth of anesthesia. The anesthesia machine can detect increased airway pressure, indicating obstruction of the airway or bronchospasm, airway disconnection, apnea, high and low pressures, as well as minute ventilation, low inspired FiO_2, high anesthesia concentrations, increased inspired CO_2, and increased expired CO_2. Further, continuous CO_2 waveforms and pressure-flow and pressure-volume loops can provide a great deal of information about the respiratory system. The newest-generation anesthesia machines also permit the input of the child's age and weight, thereby enabling specific alarms to be set at initiation of anesthesia based on the child's age, weight, and other variables (see further).

One aspect of monitoring airway gases is that there must be a Luer connection to tightly connect the gas sampling line to the anesthesia machine. Mechanical dead space begins at the Y piece of the anesthesia breathing circuit and extends distally. This includes the elbow itself, HMEs, flexible airway connections or accordion, and the connecting area of the LMA. All of these items can increase the dead space significantly for small children; items with minimum internal volume should be used when possible, particularly in neonates and infants.

It should be noted that anesthesia machines can measure inspiratory and expiratory volumes accurately but have no means to increase the tidal volume to compensate for a leak around the ETT. With large tracheal leaks larger tidal volumes can be used to compensate for leaks. Clinical examination of chest rise, breath sounds, and expired CO_2 values must be used as well as the consideration for intermittent blood gases.

Equipment Cart

It is advantageous to use mobile, lockable, multidrawer carts to stock the wide range and sizes of items necessary to care for the full spectrum of infants and children. The drawers should be organized for ease of use: airway equipment, drugs, IV supplies, monitoring equipment, circuits, and suction catheters, separated into appropriately labeled drawers. To facilitate efficient and safe delivery of anesthesia, it is prudent to design and stock each cart identically. Because pediatric anesthesia is often administered outside the OR suite, these mobile carts simplify the safe practice of anesthesia and guarantee the availability of all necessary equipment in these remote locations for children of all sizes (Table 52.2).

Defibrillator and External Pacemakers

Every OR facility should be equipped with a direct-current defibrillator. It is not necessary to have a unit specifically for use with children provided the energy range may be adjusted to the appropriate levels (e.g., 2 joules/kg) and pediatric paddles are immediately available. Ideally, the design should incorporate all controls in the paddles, facilitating use without leaving the child's side. A sensing circuit that provides the capacity for synchronous defibrillation is desirable. External defibrillators with disposable pads applied to the front and back or right chest and left lateral chest of the child have improved the rapidity of response in some circumstances. These can be placed on high-risk children (e.g., cardiac surgery, cardiomyopathy, atrioventricular conduction defects) before induction of anesthesia.[64,111-115] Similar devices that allow for external cardiac pacing represent a major new advance for high-risk infants and children (see also Chapter 40).[116-118]

TABLE 52.2	Suggested Pediatric Equipment Cart Inventory		

	DRAWER CONTENTS		
Drawer 1	Laryngoscope handles (functioning) (2) Laryngoscope blades (functioning)		
	Miller	Macintosh	Wis-Hipple
	0 (2)	1 (2)	1½ (2)
	1 (2)	2 (2)	
	2 (2)	3 (2)	
	3 (2)		
	Magill forceps: 1 pediatric, 1 adult		
	1-inch tape (4)		
	½-inch waterproof tape (4)		
	Tourniquets of non-latex material:		
	4 each ¾-inch and ¼-inch		
	Scissors		
	Flashlight		
	Extra batteries for laryngoscope handle		
Drawer 2	Masks		
	Neonate (3)		
	Infant (3)		
	Toddler (3)		
	Child (3)		
	Medium adult (3)		
	Large adult (3)		
	Airways		
	3.5 cm (5)		
	5.0 cm (5)		
	6.0 cm (5)		
	7.0 cm (5)		
	8.0 cm (5)		
	9.0 cm (5)		
Drawer 3	Gauze sponges (sterile and nonsterile)		
	Double-stick disks		
	Rubber bands		
	Adhesive bandages		
	Alcohol swabs		
	Antibiotic ointment		
	Water-soluble surgical lubricant		
	Lidocaine ointment 5%		
	Bulldog clips		
	Safety pins		
	Corneal lubricant		
	Pediatric blood tubes (blue, red, purple, and green)		
	Eye patches		
Drawer 4	Adult sodium bicarbonate (2)		
	Pediatric sodium bicarbonate 8.4% (2)		
	Infant sodium bicarbonate 4.2% (2)		
	Cardiac lidocaine 100 mg (2)		
	Dextrose 50% (1)		
	Mannitol 25% (1)		
	Diphenhydramine 50 mg (2)		
	Calcium chloride 10% (4)		

	DRAWER CONTENTS		
Drawer 4—cont'd	Calcium gluconate 10% (4)		
	Sterile water		
	Lidocaine 1% (5)		
	Phenylephrine (5)		
	Neostigmine 1:2000 (10)		
	Ephedrine (5)		
	Atropine (10)		
	Isoproterenol (1)		
	Furosemide (3)		
	Epinephrine 1:1000 (10)		
	Succinylcholine (1)		
	Rocuronium (1)		
	Dexamethasone 4 mg/mL (2)		
	Dopamine (2)		
	Ondansetron (10)		
	Propofol (10)		
Drawer 5	Pediatric uncuffed endotracheal tubes: 2.5 (6); 3.0 (6); 3.5 (6); 4.0 (6); 4.5 (6); 5.0 (6); 6.0 (6)		
	Pediatric cuffed endotracheal tubes: 5.0 (3); 5.5 (3)		
	Adult cuffed endotracheal tubes: 2 each of 6.0; 6.5; 7.0		
	Stylets in various appropriate sizes		
Drawer 6	Pediatric and adult esophageal stethoscopes (6)		
	Adult electrocardiography pads (10)		
	Pediatric electrocardiography pads (10)		
	6.5F suction catheters (6); 10 of each size 8F and 14F		
	Pediatric and adult Yankauer suction devices (10 each)		
Drawer 7	Syringes: 60-mL (2); 20-mL (6); 12-mL (10); 6-mL (10); 3-mL (20); 3-mL (20); 1-mL with 27-gauge needle (20); a variety of needles to facilitate drug withdrawal (18-, 20-, 22-, 25-gauge)		
Drawer 8	Intravenous catheters: 24-gauge; 22-gauge; 20-gauge; 18-gauge; 16-gauge; 14-gauge		
	Pediatric intravenous boards: 2 sizes (4)		
	T-connectors		
	Three-way stopcocks, multiple stopcock manifolds, claves, Luer connectors, small volume (0.5–1 mL) drug administration tubing		
Drawer 9	Pediatric and adult intravenous sets (6)		
	Pediatric Buretrol (2)		
	Intravenous extension sets (2)		
	Lactated Ringer's solution		
	250 mL 0.9 normal saline solution (5)		
	Air trap filters (6)		
	Head strap		
	Blood pressure cuffs (2 each size), 1 adult size with stethoscope		
	Oximeter sensors for infants and children		

NOTE: These are only suggested equipment cart materials. Each hospital should alter the order of drawers and their contents to suit its particular needs and for convenience.

Ultrasound for Regional Anesthesia and Vascular Cannulation

With the availability of ultrasound in the OR, it is reasonable to use ultrasound for certain procedures such as central venous cannulation and regional nerve blocks.[119–122] Improved success and safety have been reported with ultrasound for vascular access (see Chapter 49)[120,123–126] and for regional anesthesia if the practitioner is experienced (see Chapters 42 and 43).[119,127–129]

Most anesthesiologists can use ultrasound to obtain two-dimensional (2D) images but may not be aware of all the features of their ultrasound machines. Newer machines allow the clinician to freeze the image, measure distances, zoom into an area, increase the gain of the image, interrogate a color Doppler signal, print, and possibly transmit images. Color Doppler is the use of a color-coded representation of velocity of the reflecting tissue put on top of the 2D image. Typically blood flow is depicted in red when the flow is directed away from the transducer and in blue when it is directed toward the transducer. The use of color Doppler can improve identification of arterial versus venous vessels, thus improving patient safety. The ability to print or transmit static images to the medical record will likely become important for medicolegal documentation of regional anesthesia in the future.

The physics of ultrasound in some ways favor the pediatric patient. Probes that operate at higher frequencies offer better spatial resolution but with a limited depth of penetration of the image, whereas those that operate at lower frequencies penetrate to identify deeper structures but have decreased resolution. Small children and infants, therefore, have excellent acoustic windows and structures that can easily be identified because the structures are more superficial than in adults (see Chapters 42 and 43). Needles can be difficult to visualize with ultrasound[130] because they do not enter the ultrasound field of view parallel to the transducer. The steeper the angle of the needle, the less reflection and therefore the less the ultrasound waveform. Further, soft tissue is a mix of fluid, fat, connective tissue, and muscle, each with different impedance, which creates difficulty distinguishing the needle from background material. Manufacturers have addressed this issue in two separate ways: by increasing the echogenicity of the needle and by electronically manipulating the ultrasound signal to enhance the needle tissue interface. Manufacturers such as Havel's Incorporated (Cincinnati, OH), Pajunk (Norcross, GA), B. Braun Medical (Bethlehem, PA) and others have insulated the sides of the needle to increase its echogenicity. There are multiple manufacturers of ultrasound equipment for anesthesia. These manufacturers have enhanced software to improve our ability to visualize the needle. BK Ultrasound (Peabody, MA) calls its feature "X-Shine"; GE Healthcare (Little Chalfont, UK) calls its feature LOGIQ-e; Mindray Zonare (Mountain View, CA) calls its feature "iNeedle"; Philips (Foster City, CA) calls its feature "Needle Visualization"; FujiFilm SonoSite (Bothell, WA) calls its feature "Advanced Needle Visualization (AVN)"; and Toshiba Medical Systems (Otawara, Tochigi Prefecture, Japan) calls its feature "Biopsy Enhancement Auto Mode (BEAM)." There are numerous ultrasound workshops each year at various medical society meetings to train practitioners to use ultrasound for vascular access and regional anesthesia.

Monitoring Equipment

THE ANESTHESIA RECORD AND BAR CODE DRUG ADMINISTRATION

Automated anesthesia recording-keeping systems are rapidly becoming ubiquitous in anesthesia practice and likely will replace paper records in all but the smallest anesthetizing sites in the very near future. These systems are also referred to as **A**nesthesia **I**nformation **M**anagement **S**ystems (AIMS). The issue for many practices is not whether to use an AIMS but which system to use and whether to switch to a newer version of the software or vendor. The decision to integrate AIMS into one's practice is beyond the scope of this chapter. These systems are expensive, requiring sizable hardware and software investments along with maintenance contracts that often must integrate efficiently with

hospital-wide electronic health records (EHRs). As a result, hospital administrators usually decide which systems to purchase with advice from their Informatics and Anesthesiology departments.[131-133] An effective AIMS replaces the paper chart and reduces the workload of anesthesiologists, allowing them to focus on patient care. AIMS should ideally integrate information from the anesthesia machine, physiologic monitors, other equipment, and the EHR. Additional functions include automatically calculating cumulative totals for intakes, outputs, and drug infusions, documenting compliance with regulatory requirements such as "time-outs" and administering "antibiotics before surgical incision."[134,135] Whether these functions will reduce perioperative morbidity and mortality remains unclear.[136] The automatic recording of physiologic variables may improve accuracy of data but are not without errors.[137,138] For example, a pulse oximeter signal may be altered by the presence of a tourniquet at the time of IV cannulation, electrocautery may temporarily interfere with both electrocardiographic and temperature readings, and arterial BP readings will be interrupted by blood draws for periodic lab testing. These values can be annotated but most anesthesia providers either miss or disregard these erroneous or absent readings, leaving unusual or missing data in the electronic record. Such errors may have medicolegal implications as well as quality assurance questions.

There are many reasons to use the same manufacturer for AIMS and EHR. However, many of these systems were designed by engineers, not anesthesiologists, with clumsy user interfaces and workflow patterns. The workflow with many of these systems can initially be very taxing and quite different than using paper records. Before these systems are purchased, they should be evaluated under real-world conditions to determine their suitability. With regard to data, the accuracy of the information that one can extract from the AIMS is directly reflected by the accuracy of its input.[137] If data are easy to input and flows directly from the EHR and the OR monitors, the data may be more accurate. Unfortunately, the manufacturers of most AIMS are concerned with replacing a paper record, providing regulatory compliance, and integrating with the EHR and less focused on the need to extract data for research or quality improvement projects. We encourage the adoption of AIMS that record physiologic data such as heart rate, respiratory rate, expired and inspired gases, and CO_2 and oxygen saturation at 10-second intervals for research purposes and for medicolegal defense.

DRUG ERRORS, BAR CODING, AND INTEGRATION

Recent studies in adult patients[139] suggest that medication errors are common in the OR.[140,141] Medication errors are a major concern in pediatric practice and one of the focuses of the Wake Up Safe Quality Improvement campaign.[142] These include wrong drug, wrong dose, wrong route, and wrong patient errors. The process of labeling a medication syringe offers multiple opportunities for medication errors by the person drawing up the wrong drug, mislabeling the syringe, and mislabeling the concentration.[143] Medication errors that result in administration of the wrong drug may be reduced by color-coded labels (e.g., red for NMBDs, blue for opioids, yellow for induction drugs) but advanced technology allows us to consider implementing bar code confirmation of a particular drug. Such systems provide accurate labeling of syringes (date, time, concentration, and initials of provider) and have had great success in reducing medication errors both in and out of the OR.[140,144-148] It does not yet appear that there is significant integration of this technology in pediatric anesthesia. In a 2014 study,[149] none of 34 children's hospital across the United States used bar code technology to identify medications. Bar code labeling can easily be integrated into the AIMS; they can be used to label individual syringes and verify that the correct drug is being administered. We encourage the adoption of this safety feature by all pediatric anesthesiologists, a change we expect will be implemented in the near future.

PRECORDIAL AND ESOPHAGEAL STETHOSCOPES

Precordial and esophageal stethoscopes offer the opportunity for an experienced practitioner to detect cardiac arrhythmias, obstruction of the endotracheal tube, wheezing, airway obstruction, laryngospasm, and decreases in BP compared with baseline (softening of heart tones), among other critical events. Unfortunately, the use of precordial stethoscopes to monitor children in the OR has decreased during the past few decades in a trend that appears to be continuing with each successive generation of anesthesiologists. This problem is underscored by the fact that if clinicians do not use precordial stethoscopes during their training, they are very unlikely to use them upon graduation and thereafter.

The precordial stethoscope is applied to the skin with a double-sided adhesive disk. It can be placed near the apex of the heart to best hear heart sounds, at the suprasternal notch to best hear the combination of heart and breath sounds, or in the left axilla if there is a chance of inadvertent right mainstem intubation (e.g., tetralogy of Fallot repair). Nonferrous versions may be available for use in MRI, but practically speaking, practitioners are more likely to monitor the exhaled CO_2 tension than use a precordial stethoscope.

Disposable esophageal stethoscopes, often combined with a temperature probe, have supplanted precordial stethoscopes as cardiothoracic monitors. The integrated probes are bigger than a simple temperature probe, so they are preferred in children 2 years of age and older. These probes are ideally positioned in a retrocardiac manner by passing the probes down the esophagus until the volume of the auscultated heart sounds is maximized.

Several technologic advances to both the precordial and esophageal stethoscopes have reached the commercial market. A wireless version of these monitors transforms the audio signal into digital data so the "sound" is transmitted wirelessly to a receiver worn by the anesthesiologist. This allows the anesthesiologist to move about in the OR and not be tethered to the short stethoscope tubing. An important advantage of both the precordial and esophageal stethoscopes rests with the fact that they transmit sound waves mechanically and equipment malfunctions are less likely. Even when combined with pulse oximetry and capnography, the stethoscope provides great reassurance that the patient has a BP and cardiac output. *If both the noninvasive blood pressure (NIBP) monitor and the oximeter fail, but the child has strong heart tones, a technical problem likely exists with the former two monitors. However, if the NIBP and pulse oximeter fail and the heart tones are very weak, then cardiac output may be compromised and attention should be immediately focused on resolving that problem rather than troubleshooting the monitors.*

NONINVASIVE BLOOD PRESSURE MONITORING

NIBP monitoring is a mainstay of clinical care. BP cuffs should be available in all age appropriate sizes. The BP cuff should cover approximately two-thirds of the upper arm length. Many practitioners recommend similar-sized BP cuffs on the calf of the lower leg and the upper arm, but there is little evidence to support this recommendation.[150,151] Some individuals may choose to use the thigh to measure BP when the arms are not available, but this is less common. As a result of the propagation of the arterial waveform throughout the body, a BP obtained on the calf may have a slightly greater systolic and lesser diastolic pressures compared with the same values in the upper arm.[150,152] Automatic NIBP units use an oscillatory means to detect the BP. These units are capable of frequent and accurate measurements. To prevent injury to the patient it is important that the NIBP units are set to the correct size (neonate, child, adult). The correct setting will ensure that the range of inflation pressures and deflation time do not cause venous stasis or nerve compression damage. Most devices have two sets of connecting tubing: one for children and adults and one for neonates. Neonatal tubing has different connectors and complementary BP cuffs; they are not interchangeable with adult tubing. Neonatal BP cuffs typically are sized 1 through 5 and fit approximately the same number as the infant's weight in kilograms. It should be noted that the monitor must be set to the correct patient and tubing size for the algorithms to produce accurate information. Backup equipment should be available to obtain BP by auscultation if needed. However, if the NIBP signal is lost, one should immediately attribute the loss of signal to hypotension and treat appropriately (with volume and/or vasopressors) until the equipment is assessed.

ELECTROCARDIOGRAM

The electrocardiogram (ECG) is a mainstay of clinical care. For general pediatric anesthesia, three-lead monitoring of the ECG is usually sufficient to detect arrhythmias and the basic heart rate. A monitor should display a single waveform (usually lead II) and usually does not require ST-segment analyses. The typical placement of leads is white lead to right shoulder, black lead to left shoulder, and red lead to the left flank. Placement of the red lead on the left lower extremity is usually not feasible. Further, lead placement often gets changed slightly based on the surgical field. For pediatric cardiac anesthesia five-lead monitoring of the ECG is used. Five-lead ECG improves the detection of ischemia and three waveforms are usually monitored. Lead placement for a five-lead ECG is the same as three with the addition of a green lead to right flank and a brown lead (V1) to the fourth intercostal space on the right side of the chest. Detection of the QRS is automatic. Signaling of the QRS tone can be set on the monitor to come from either ECG, pulse oximetry, or arterial waveform if present. The choice depends on the surgical type as electrocautery interferes with the ECG signal. Special nonferrous ECG leads and monitors are necessary for use in MRI. Most problems with ECG monitoring occur as a result of poor contact of the leads with the patient. This can sometimes be improved by cleaning the skin first with alcohol and placing new leads. Given the interference during electrocautery and during MRI imaging, the heart rate is best determined from the pulse oximeter.

OXYGEN MONITORS

Sensors that monitor the FiO_2 are built into every modern anesthesia machine. This is in addition to fail-safe devices that detect a decrease in the pressure in the oxygen line. Oxygen monitors with alarms are necessary to prevent the delivery of an hypoxic gas mixture, but they can also be set to alarm for a high FiO_2 as well. Low FiO_2 can be an unintentional consequence of very low flow anesthesia with air-oxygen blends in a closed circle system. However, there are several circumstances when a low FiO_2 is intentional and desirable: (1) a reduced FiO_2 may be necessary in some children with congenital heart disease to reduce the oxygen saturation to balance the pulmonary and systemic blood flows, (2) during airway surgery to reduce the risk of airway fires, and (3) in infants and neonates to reduce the risk of retinopathy of prematurity (see Chapter 34).[153-155] It is not the FiO_2 but the child's arterial partial pressure of oxygen (PaO_2) that is important regarding retinopathy of prematurity. It is common practice to reduce the FiO_2, if otherwise safe for the neonate, to the point where the oxygen saturation measured by pulse oximetry (SpO_2) is between 91% and 95% to minimize the risk of oxygen toxicity without increasing perioperative mortality (see Chapter 37).

TEMPERATURE MONITORS

The child's temperature should be monitored throughout anesthesia to prevent hypothermia or hyperthermia. Hypothermia was a very common problem in pediatric anesthesia, particularly in neonates and infants, that has been resolved to a large extent with the adoption of forced air warmers. Hyperthermia most commonly occurs because of iatrogenic overheating and failure to decrease the temperature of the exogenous heat source in the face of an increasing body temperature. Other causes of hyperthermia include malignant hyperthermia, thyrotoxicosis, sepsis, drug overdose (cocaine, monoamine oxidase inhibitors and meperidine), and in children with arthrogryposis or osteogenesis imperfecta. In a child with malignant hyperthermia, fever is a late sign preceded by other factors, including an increase in end-tidal carbon dioxide tension ($PETCO_2$), tachypnea, and tachycardia. Temperature can be monitored in the axilla, nasopharynx, esophagus, rectum, tympanic membrane, and the skin. Core temperature is most reliably measured on the tympanic membrane or in the esophagus. Rectal temperature is unpredictable as the tip of the probe may be lodged in stool and buffered from the true body temperature. Bladder temperature may be measured via a Foley catheter that has an integrated temperature monitor, but these catheters are sized only for older children. Skin temperature often slowly responds to changes in body temperature and is well known to underestimate the body temperature. The axillary temperature often underestimates the body temperature because the probe tip is not positioned within the axilla. In such a case, the probe measures the ambient temperature, which may be room air or the temperature from a forced air warmer (as great as 43°C). Axillary temperature may detect an increase in temperature that results from malignant hyperthermia because the deltopectoral triangle is the largest muscle group whose venous blood can be sensed with a probe in the axilla.

NONINVASIVE OXYGEN SATURATION MONITORS

Pulse Oximetry

Pulse oximetry is a mainstay of clinical care in pediatric anesthesia, mandated for routine use in every anesthetic in most jurisdictions. Sensors are typically placed on the fingers and toes but can be applied to the ears or other body parts. When pulse oximeters were first introduced, clinicians needed proof that pulse oximetry was better than clinical judgment in detecting oxygen desaturations.[156,157] This notion is now uniformly accepted (E-Figs. 52.3, 52.4, and 52.5). Pulse oximeters determine the arterial oxygen saturation (SaO_2) of hemoglobin by using the absorbance of red (660 nm) and infrared light (930 nm) as it passes through tissue. The presence of two sensors allows the unit to identify blood that is moving (arterial) as opposed to the background oxygen saturation of the tissue. The wavelengths were also chosen to take advantage of the differences in the absorption of light between oxygenated and deoxygenated hemoglobin at these various frequencies. The sensors detect when the volume of the digit increases during systole by making the measurements only when the finger enlarges;

the device can thus separate arterial from venous blood—hence the name "pulse oximeter." The ratio of absorbance of light is converted into an oxygen saturation using an algorithm that is proprietary to each of the manufacturers; that is, their combination of LED lights and detectors produces a certain ratio or signal and it is their own algorithm that produces the saturation value that is displayed. These algorithms are generated by producing various degrees of desaturation in adult volunteers while receiving a hypoxic gas mixture through a face mask. Arterial saturation values from 70% and greater with their paired pulse oximeter ratios are used to calibrate the algorithm. However, the algorithms were created with adult volunteers and then applied to children.

So how accurate are pulse oximeters? The largest study published comparing the SpO_2 values with SaO_2 values measured from arterial samples with co-oximetry in children had 225 subjects and 1980 samples.[158] The bias or the difference between SpO_2 and SaO_2 varied depending on the range of the saturations. SpO_2 values between 90% and 97% exceeded the SaO_2 by only 1%. However, SpO_2 values that were less than 90% exceeded the SaO_2 by 5% (with greater differences as the SpO_2 decreased). In children with some degree of lung injury, the ventilator management should be adjusted to maintain SpO_2 in excess of 90%. However, the accuracy of pulse oximeters in infants and children whose SpO_2 is less than 90% (e.g., in cyanotic heart disease, during laryngospasm) is of greater concern as palliative surgeries or the decision to intervene during an acute event is often based on the pulse oximeter saturation reading much less than 90%. Of the major manufacturers that were studied, no pulse oximeter yielded more accurate measurements than another.

A further technique used by some manufacturers to improve the accuracy of the pulse oximeter signal is to average the measurements over a period of 5 to 10 seconds. This allows the monitor to better characterize the signal produced and minimize the contribution of artifact. The significance of this averaging must be understood by the clinician during episodes of desaturation or hypoxia. For example, with difficult intubations or laryngospasm, the pulse oximeter signal will lag behind the desaturation event. This also means that an improvement in saturation will always take longer than anticipated after an open airway and ventilation have been reestablished. A study of continuous cardiac output in anesthetized children found that stroke index decreased with the severity of desaturation but this was accompanied by a compensatory increase in heart rate with maintained cardiac output; it appears that bradycardia is a relatively late sign of cardiac hypoxemia.[159]

Manufacturers are continually working to improve the algorithms and equipment to eliminate artifact that may be introduced by movement, darker skin color, poor perfusion, hypothermia, or increased ambient light. Improved algorithms and filtering have resulted in significant reductions in movement artifacts. Low perfusion and hypoxemic states provide ongoing challenges for pulse oximeter technology and some manufacturers have generated specific units and sensors to address these issues.

Pulse oximeter manufacturers have moved in two different directions to improve the accuracy of their devices. Masimo Corporation (Masimo Corporation, Irvine, CA) has developed pulse oximeters using multiple wavelength technology: the Masimo Rainbow Pulse Co-oximeters, which can provide much more information beyond oxygen saturation. The presence of additional wavelengths allows the oximeter to provide continuous readings for hemoglobin, carboxyhemoglobin, and methemoglobin. Validation of the hemoglobin measurements in various populations has been studied with varied success.[160-164] Although these devices might not be absolutely accurate, the ability to follow them as a trend monitor during surgery offers promise. There is an additional manufacturer of a pulse oximeter that measures hemoglobin using an occlusion spectroscopy method (OrSense NBM 200 system, OrSense, Raleigh, NC). The accuracy of this device has been studied in adults, mostly for prescreening blood donors.[165-168] Unfortunately, the size of the reusable sensor may limit the use of this device in children. The ability to noninvasively measure carboxyhemoglobin and methemoglobin introduces the possibility of screening large numbers of patients as in an emergency department, bearing in mind some degree of possible inaccuracies. Further validation studies and improved algorithms continue.[163,164,169,170]

Any abnormal value as well as a suspected clinical scenario with a normal result (false negative) should be assessed with a confirmatory test. The presence of abnormal hemoglobin beyond carboxyhemoglobin and methemoglobin can, in theory, affect the accuracy of pulse oximeters,[171] although the most common types of abnormal hemoglobin (fetal and sickle cell) do not have an impact on pulse oximetry.[172-174] It should be further noted that these specialized oximeter probes are quite expensive (three to four times the cost of a normal probe) and thus have a limited role in routine pediatric care. Another advance relates to signal processing, or as Massimo termed it, Signal Extraction Technology (SET). For some manufacturers, the pulse oximeter waveform or plethysmography (commonly referred to as "pleth") is stylized and not an actual reflection of the strength of the arterial waveform. For other manufacturers, the pleth is reflective of the degree of perfusion. During inspiration, there is an increase in the venous return to the heart; during exhalation, there is a decrease in venous return. This periodic variation in venous return with respiration translates to subtle changes in the arterial pulse wave height. This effect (pulsus paradoxus) is more pronounced when there is a decrease in the central venous filling pressure (hypovolemia) or if there is a significant increase in the inspiratory force (upper airway obstruction). The newest generation of pulse oximeters has signal processing technology that can detect these variations. Hypovolemia, vasoconstriction, and decreased cardiac output can also lead to the loss of the pleth signal.[175,176] In addition to providing a visual representation of perfusion, the processing that identifies the pleth can be used to estimate respiratory rate. Taking this a step further with the Masimo SET, the Pleth Variability Index (PVI) is an algorithm used to predict patients whose cardiac output might benefit from fluid boluses. The PVI technology has been investigated and the results show promise in adults and children, although there remains some uncertainty in this regard.[177-179]

Covidien (Boulder, CO) has taken its Nellcor pulse oximeters in a different direction to improve the accuracy of their devices. Rather than producing multiple wavelengths of light, with its OxiMax technology Nellcor has embedded a digital memory chip onto the sensor. This chip contains the calibration and operating characteristics of that sensor that should in turn improve the accuracy. There is some variability in the wavelength of light produced by any light-emitting diode (LED). This chip allows the specific wavelength information to be stored and relayed to the device to use the most accurate algorithm. Nellcor pulse oximeters have respiratory rate monitoring, but they do not appear to yet have an algorithm to assess fluid responsiveness.

In addition, miniaturization and manufacturing of integrated circuits have reduced the size of pulse oximeters to fit on a finger. They have also been integrated into many watches and fitness devices. A number of manufacturers have rushed to market with these devices, although their accuracy has not been tested. Some clinicians are now using these devices for short-distance transports to the recovery room in place of no monitor at all. Whether this will improve clinical outcomes or whether these devices will replace those from the major manufacturers remains to be determined.

REFLECTANCE OXIMETRY

Reflectance oximetry was first created to improve oxygen saturation data in difficult clinical conditions, such as decreased perfusion, movement, and conditions in which optimal sites for standard transmission oximetry probes may not exist (e.g., burns). The technology behind reflectance oximetry involves the emission of multiple wavelengths of red and infrared light that are sensed in two or more photodetectors located a distance away from the diodes on the same probe sensor (Fig. 52.7). These devices measure reflected rather than transmitted light. The technology used to create these oximeter probes permits usage on a flat surface such as the forehead and on the fetal scalp. The forehead devices have had the largest use among pediatric anesthesiologists. Studies of reflectance oximeters in general demonstrate that these devices are more susceptible to erratic measurements when the probe is placed directly over an artery and vein.[180,181] Some potential advantages to using reflectance oximetry on the forehead include better signals during conditions of poor perfusion, lack of motion, and faster response time than conventional peripheral oximeter probes.[182,183] However, possible disadvantages include a high signal dropout rate (no measurable signal) and poor accuracy, often measuring lower than finger transmission oximetry, particularly in cases of venous congestion (e.g., Trendelenburg position or situations that impede venous return). Several studies report good correlation between concurrent measurements of oxygen saturation comparing reflectance oximetry on the forehead[184,185] and around the chest of premature infants[186] compared with extremity pulse oximetry and arterial co-oximetry measurements; these studies also report a clear dropout rate.

The Lifebox Monitoring Initiative

We have long recognized the improvement in patient safety with the use of pulse oximetry technology and its use is ubiquitous in developed nations. Unfortunately, in developing countries the availability of pulse oximetry during general anesthesia cannot be guaranteed (see Chapter 51). In fact, it is estimated that 5 billion people do not have access to safe surgery with approximately 70,000 ORs without basic anesthesia equipment and a shortage of 1 million surgeons, anesthesiologists, and obstetricians worldwide.[187,188] The anesthesia-related death rate is 100 to 1000 times greater than in developed countries.[189] Pulse oximetry is now part of the Safe Surgery Saves Lives project from the World Health Organization.[190,191] The Lifebox Foundation was formed in 2011 as a global patient safety initiative to provide pulse oximeters and education to developing countries.[192] The device has been shown to be accurate in healthy volunteers[193] and it has improved safety under anesthesia for thousands of individuals.[189,194,195] A donation of $250 USD to the Lifebox Foundation will purchase one device for donation, which includes a universal age probe, a pediatric probe for neonates, a multicountry charger, and multilanguage educational DVD; further information is available at www.lifebox.org.

NEAR-INFRARED SPECTROSCOPY

Near-infrared spectroscopy (NIRS) is a noninvasive, optical technology that bears similarities to pulse oximetry in that it uses

52

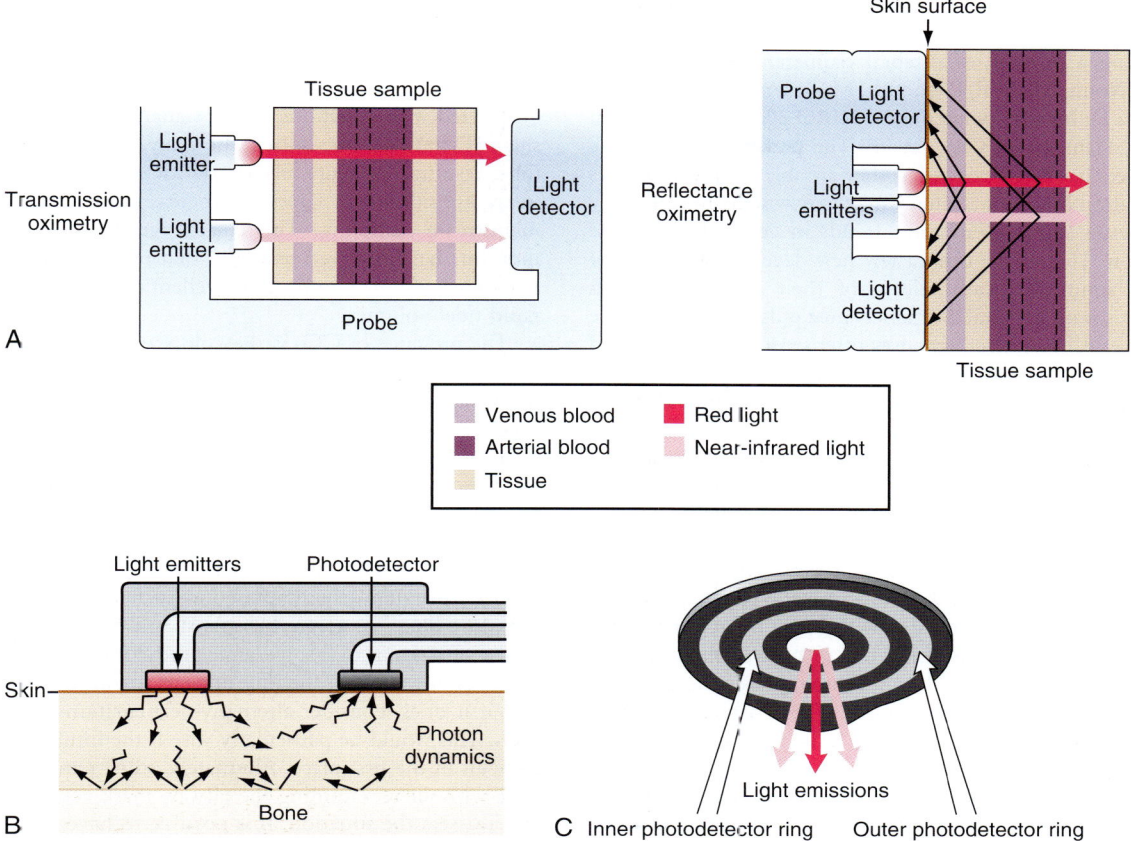

FIGURE 52.7 A, Comparison of conventional transmission pulse oximetry with reflectance oximetry. Note that with conventional oximetry the light detector is located directly opposite on the other side of a digit and detects light transmitted through the digit; with reflectance oximetry the light detector is located next to the light emitters and detects the light reflected back through and from the tissues. **B,** The typical configuration of a reflectance oximeter. **C,** Another configuration, in which several light detectors are located at different distances from the light emitters. In addition, reflectance oximeters may emit light in more than just 2 wavelengths, which is typical of conventional transmission pulse oximeters. (Modified from Kugelman A, Wasserman Y, Mor F, et al. Reflectance pulse oximetry from core body in neonates and infants: comparison to arterial blood oxygen saturation and to transmission pulse oximetry. *J Perinatol.* 2004;24[6]:366–371; and Keogh BF, Kopotic RJ. Recent findings in the use of reflectance oximetry: a critical review. *Curr Opin Anesth.* 2005;18[6]:649–654.)

the relative absorption of near-infrared light, 700 to 900 nm, through biologic tissues to determine tissue oxygenation (E-Fig. 52.6). Oxyhemoglobin and deoxyhemoglobin absorb light at different frequencies, and the use of a probe that emits and detects different frequencies of near-infrared light can be used to estimate tissue oxygenation. In pediatric anesthesia, this device has been widely used to measure "regional" cerebral oxygen saturation (rSO$_2$) for children undergoing and following congenital heart surgery.[196-199] It is also used in this same population to detect renal perfusion[200] and has been shown to predict the development of acute kidney injury.[201,202] NIRS has also been used to detect ischemia in neurosurgery,[203] spine surgery,[204] kidney transplant[205,206] as well as tissue free flaps.[207] NIRS may have applications in an ICU setting,[208] following brain injury[209] and during the use of therapeutic hypothermia.[210] Pulse oximetry requires the measurement of the pulsatile (arterial) component of the total light transmitted by the biologic tissue. Because NIRS does not require the subtraction of the pulsatile component, the signal is more than 100 times stronger and unaffected by poor perfusion compared with pulse oximetry. NIRS is susceptible to motion

artifact and ambient light noise, although software algorithms have significantly decreased these sources of error. A probe placed on the child's forehead (or other tissue beds) measures the concentration of oxyhemoglobin and deoxyhemoglobin in the tissue underlying the probe. The NIRS device functionally measures the oxygenation of blood in the underlying tissues, including blood in the arterioles, capillaries, and venules. The majority (approximately 85%) of the signal originates from the venules; skin and bone and extracranial blood absorb only limited amounts of light, which is subtracted from the signal and does not have a significant impact of the measurement in infants and children. NIRS thus measures the oxygen saturation in venous and arterial blood and represents an average saturation across blood vessels and tissue. In cerebral oximetry, the oxygen saturation of the blood in the tissue (i.e., between the sending and emitting probe) depends on factors that affect oxygen transport, including cerebral blood flow (arterial partial pressure of carbon dioxide [PaCO$_2$]), hemoglobin saturation, hemoglobin–oxygen binding affinity, central venous pressure, and oxygen saturation in the arterial blood. Therapies aimed at improving oxygen delivery or decreasing oxygenation consumption by the brain will potentially increase cerebral oxygenation (rSO_2).[211]

There are a number of cerebral oximeters on the market: Equanox (Nonin Medical, Plymouth, MN); Fore-Sight (Casmed, Branford, CT); Invos (Covidien); and NIRO-200NX (Hamamatsu Photonics, Hamamatsu City, Japan). The performance of these NIRS devices has been reviewed[212]; they are able to detect episodes of desaturation but their accuracy may vary widely. In turn, they may be better suited to monitor trends in cerebral and tissue oxygenation. There have been a few new developments, one of which is Nonin Medical's release of their SenSmart, which incorporates both cerebral and reflectance pulse oximetry in the same device. All manufacturers now offer sensors for infants and children. Normal regional cerebral oxygen saturation (rSv_2) is believed to be between 60% and 80%.[213] The range of rSO_2 has been shown to vary in infants and children with congenital heart disease based on their anatomic lesion as well as their arterial saturations[214,215] and these values can be much less than those in healthy children. In controlled hypoxic-ischemic states in animals, electroencephalogram (EEG) slowing and increased tissue lactic acid levels occur at rSO_2 between 40% and 45%. The EEG becomes flat at rSO_2 between 30% and 35%, and if the cerebral ischemia is protracted, it may be associated with tissue infarction.[216] One other point that requires emphasis is that rSO_2 for cerebral oximetry can be greatly influenced by $PaCO_2$; thus emphasis should be on values during steady-state ventilation. These devices require a period of stabilization at a steady state to be accurate and cannot be considered as beat-to-beat monitors.

NIRS technology has important limitations. These monitors measure only the saturation in tissue below the probes, which reflects focal tissue oxygenation or ischemia. If the probe is placed on the forehead, it will reflect the state of the tissue in the frontal cortex and may not reflect other areas of the brain. The same would be true of renal oxygen saturations. While the kidney is the organ in the flank with the greatest oxygen extraction, all the tissue in that area contributes to the signal. We cannot therefore interpret all decreases in "renal" NIRS as reflecting a global acute kidney injury. One final issue remains with NIRS monitoring. We had hoped that NIRS would provide real-time guidance of regional tissue oxygenation and permit study of the effectiveness of interventions to improve the oxygenation. Research has shown a potential association between reduced saturations and outcomes.[197,198,200–202] However, there is limited information linking any interventions to outcomes. As suggested by recent review articles,[217,218] further research and improvements in NIRS technology are needed to clarify the role of regional tissue oximetry in pediatric patient management.

CARBON DIOXIDE ANALYZERS

Mainstream and Sidestream Analyzers

The most commonly used gas monitor is the infrared CO_2 monitor. This monitor is particularly useful in teaching about ventilation, CO_2 elimination from alveoli, as well as airway and ventilator management. Two configurations of infrared CO_2 monitors are available. They differ only in the location of the CO_2 analysis: (1) the sidestream analyzer, in which expired gas is aspirated from the anesthesia circuit and analyzed remotely; and (2) a mainstream analyzer, in which the gas is analyzed by an optical sensor within a cuvette just proximal to the elbow of the breathing circuit. Sidestream analyzers are lighter and less cumbersome than mainstream analyzers because the former involves no additional pieces to be inserted into the breathing circuit. Sidestream analyzers

aspirate gas through a narrow-gauge flexible tube inserted into the breathing circuit at the elbow. The gas sampling line and water trap can become obstructed with water or secretions, requiring replacement of the parts. Mainstream gas analyzers are less often obstructed with secretions, but the analyzers are heavy, and if a small-ID tracheal tube is used, the analyzer may kink the tracheal tube, resulting in acute airway obstruction. Most OR monitors today use sidestream sampling whereas most ICU monitors use mainstream sampling. The current generation of sidestream monitors has improved precision that reduces the gas sampling rate to just 50 mL/minute and excellent accuracy even with small rapid tidal volumes.

The presence of CO_2 is the gold standard to ensure that the tracheal tube has been inserted within the trachea. In the OR this is generally achieved using capnography but during code situations, this is achieved using litmus color-changing devices (see E-Fig. 39.4). If no expired CO_2 is detected after a presumed tracheal intubation, one must assume that the tracheal tube is in the esophagus, or during a code it is presumed that there is inadequate CO_2 in the exhaled breath because of inadequate chest compressions. One should consider that the lack of CO_2 detected may be due to equipment malfunction such as obstruction of the sampling line[218] or severe bronchospasm. However, the prudent course of action is to first reexamine the glottis with a laryngoscope to determine whether the tube appears to pass through the cords and if it does, consider alternative explanations for the lack of CO_2. This would be particularly wise if the intubation had been difficult in the first place. Alternately, some remove the tracheal tube without reexamining the airway, mask ventilate the lungs, and reassess the situation. It is possible to have CO_2 present on capnography for one or two breaths if the tracheal tube was inserted into the esophagus. This can occur if the stomach had been distended by manual ventilation or crying before tracheal intubation, or if carbonated soft drinks were present in the stomach, CO_2 could be transiently detected immediately after an esophageal intubation.[219,220] This latter event should be very rare with appropriate nil per os (NPO) guidelines. If there is expired CO_2 detected after an esophageal intubation, the CO_2 peak tension will be very low and will decrease rapidly with successive breaths after placing the tracheal tube. Although it is beyond the scope of this chapter, it should be noted that the $ETCO_2$ value can be an indicator of effective cardiopulmonary resuscitation and correlates with outcome (see Chapters 39 and 40).[221–223]

Measurement of expired CO_2 tension is also helpful in detecting other clinical problems. Clinically important air embolism causes a transient but marked reduction in CO_2 excretion because the lungs are ventilated but not perfused; hence dead space is suddenly increased (see Chapter 26, Figs. 26.6 and 26.7). Quantitative measurement allows detection of the change in circuit flows, disconnections, tracheal tube kinking, or accidental extubations.[224] Capnography also signals the earliest clinical sign of an acute malignant hyperthermic reaction and the effectiveness of treatment (see Fig. 41.3).[224–226] The CO_2 waveform may also assist when diagnosing other types of respiratory difficulties (Fig. 52.8).[227] Bronchospasm and its response to treatment may be identified by changes in the CO_2 waveform; bronchospasm causes an increasing slope of the plateau during expiration, and resolution of the bronchospasm restores the plateau to the horizontal (see Fig. 13.9). A slow-speed recorder also allows trending, which we have found particularly useful in diagnosing small circuit leaks, partially kinked tracheal tubes, and rebreathing. In children free from pulmonary shunts, the arterial and alveolar CO_2 values

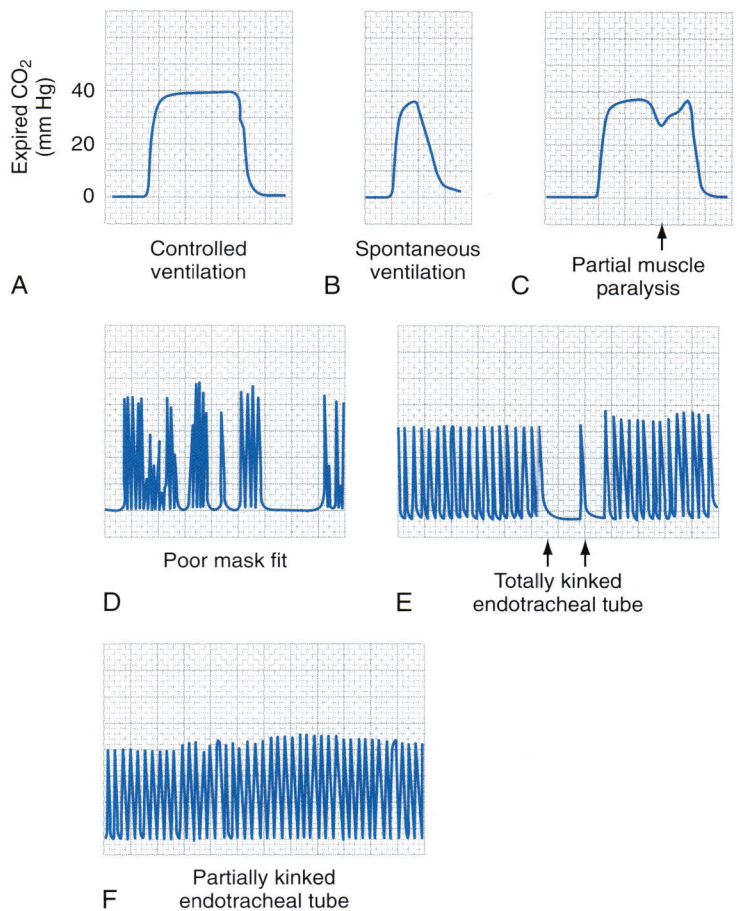

FIGURE 52.8 Expired carbon dioxide (CO_2) tracings (**A, B, C** = rapid recording; **D, E, F** = trend recording). **A,** Normal waveform with a long alveolar plateau indicating good alveolar gas sampling during controlled ventilation. **B,** Spontaneous ventilation with rapid respiratory rate; minimal alveolar plateau. **C,** Patient with partial muscle paralysis; note the change in the CO_2 waveform (*arrow*) during inspiration, which took place during the ventilator expiration. **D,** Poor mask fit with many periods when no CO_2 was detected; this also results in many false alarms. **E,** A totally kinked endotracheal tube was detected by the absence of a CO_2 waveform (*between arrows*); a similar trace could result in a circuit disconnect, esophageal intubation, or a simple pause in respiration. **F,** A partially kinked endotracheal tube may result in a slow change in peak expired CO_2; a similar change could be noted with an unrecognized endobronchial intubation, change in pulmonary compliance, circuit leak, or increase in metabolic rate. The reverse would occur with air embolism, hypothermia (decreased metabolic rate), improved compliance, or, increased fresh gas flow without compensatory change in ventilator settings. (From Coté CJ, Liu LM, Szyfelbein SK, et al. Intraoperative events diagnosed by expired carbon dioxide monitoring in children. *Can Anaesth Soc J.* 1986;33[3 Pt 1]:315–320.)

($PaCO_2$ and $PACO_2$ [as reflected by a true end-expired sample]) should be within 2 to 3 mm Hg. The severity of a shunt or the diagnosis of a shunt may be made if this difference is greater than 5 mm Hg and if the CO_2 sensor is properly calibrated. Children with significant pulmonary problems such as inhalation injury may have larger differences between arterial and expired CO_2 values. In such cases, expired CO_2 monitoring may be used only for trending and as a disconnect alarm.[228] Expired CO_2 will be more accurate in assessing the adequacy of ventilation in children whose trachea is intubated compared with airway management with a facemask. However, even with a facemask the presence of bronchospasm and airway obstruction can be identified. During mechanical ventilation with an LMA the accuracy of $ETCO_2$ monitoring approaches that of an endotracheal tube.[229]

TRANSCUTANEOUS CARBON DIOXIDE MEASUREMENT

Transcutaneous partial pressure of CO_2 ($PtcCO_2$) monitoring has been available for many years for use in preterm and full-term neonates but never achieved widespread acceptance in pediatric anesthesia. The monitor includes a heating element and a variant of the Severinghaus-type CO_2 electrode. Heating the skin increases capillary blood flow as well as the PCO_2 and oxygen. The skin becomes more permeable to diffusion of gas, and the gas tensions are measured by the sensors. CO_2 is calculated using a change in the pH sensed by the electrode. In turn, pH is proportional to the logarithm of the change in CO_2. Previously transcutaneous monitoring was limited because of difficulties preparing and fixing the sensor, preparing the skin, needing to rotate the sensor to prevent burns, calibration time, and concerns for reliability. New transcutaneous monitors have eliminated some of the earlier technical difficulties. These newer versions can limit the temperature so they are less likely to burn children's skin; they remain calibrated for greater intervals, and they appear to be more accurate. One study reported an acceptable correlation with arterial CO_2 among several models[230]: TINA TCM3 (Radiometer, Copenhagen, Denmark); TINA TCM3® (Radiometer, Copenhagen, Denmark), and SenTec (Therwil, Arlesheim, BL, Switzerland). Because the skin must be heated, the CO_2 values are greater than the local arterial values owing to increased local metabolic production; these systems correct for this increase.

The most common use for transcutaneous monitoring has been in intubated premature neonates and small infants because the dead space of a mainstream CO_2 cuvette greatly increases the dead space for these small infants. Another circumstance for which transcutaneous monitors are used is for those who require high-frequency oscillatory ventilation. In this case, it is not possible to monitor $ETCO_2$. There are also some clinical conditions in which $ETCO_2$ monitoring can be inaccurate and a transcutaneous monitor may be helpful. These include uncuffed tracheal tubes with a large gas leak, high respiratory rates, significant cardiopulmonary disease associated with increased dead space and/or right-to-left shunt, and conditions of frequent movement. One clear disadvantage of $PtcCO_2$ is the lack of breath-to-breath monitoring capability for apnea and disordered breathing provided by end-tidal capnography.[231] $PtcCO_2$ monitoring may have a role in anesthetized children with severe pulmonary disease or other pathology that prevents accurate $ETCO_2$ measurement. These devices work less well where there is thickened skin or significant subcutaneous edema. There may be a role for these devices in the monitoring of nonintubated patients who are receiving sedation. However, nasal cannula sidestream CO_2 monitoring will provide more immediate identification of apnea or obstruction.

BLOOD LOSS MONITORS

Close observation of the surgical field is the best single monitor of blood loss. A small-volume trap on the suction line before the major evacuation trap is particularly useful to quantify blood loss in small children. Surgical sponges are often weighed on a dietary scale immediately after they come off the surgical field, assuming that 1 g of weight is equivalent to 1 mL of blood, to assess the blood soaked up by the sponges. This minimizes the evaporative losses from the sponges. Point-of-care testing devices such as the HemoCue (HemoCue America, Brea, CA) and the i-STAT (Abbott Point of Care Inc., Princeton, NJ) rapidly assess hemoglobin values but each may underestimate the hematocrit at lower values. In addition to point-of-care testing, many ORs have blood gas analyzers such as the GEM Premier 3000 (Instrumentation Laboratory, Bedford, MA) that can provide hemoglobin measurements. The accuracy of all of these devices is likely sufficient to follow trends and make decisions about the need to transfuse blood,[232,233] certainly in the face of ongoing blood losses. Noninvasive hemoglobin measurements using multiwavelength pulse oximetry in general may be useful only for trend monitoring.[160-163] Overall, these noninvasive devices underestimate hemoglobin values and may err up to 1 g/dL, thus limiting their value during rapid blood loss where more accurate measurements are essential.

NEUROMUSCULAR TRANSMISSION MONITORS

Measuring the indirectly elicited twitch response is indicated when neuromuscular blocking agents are used (see Chapter 7). Residual or incomplete reversal of neuromuscular blockade is

a common reason that adult patients are delayed in leaving the OR, may have prolonged postanesthesia care unit (PACU) recovery times, and develop respiratory complications in the early postoperative period.[234-236] Evidence confirms that even experienced anesthesiologists cannot assess the decrement in the train-of-four (TOF) accurately without some other monitor. Clinical signs (e.g., sustained head lift) are often difficult to perform in younger children but even if they are, they may fail to uncover significant residual blockade, introducing the potential for respiratory complications.[235,236] In neonates and infants, flexion of the hips is analogous to the clinical signs of recovery of neuromuscular blockade in adults.[237]

Two types of neuromuscular monitoring devices are available for clinical use: mechanomyography and acceleromyography. Mechanomyography models use constant current nerve stimulation. These devices self-calibrate and then deliver a constant stimulus (30-70 mA) to the skin regardless of other influences. Failure to deliver a supramaximal stimulus may result in overestimation of twitch suppression. The power should generally be left off between readings to avoid possible injury secondary to prolonged, repetitious exposure to electric current. Acceleromyography uses a piezoelectric sensor to quantify the acceleration (proportional to force) of the thumb and convert it to an electrical signal. There is considerable disagreement in the published literature as to which of these devices is most accurate.[238-240] Monitors based on acceleromyography are becoming more commonly available and some consider these to be more accurate than mechanomyography-based TOF monitors. However, these monitors are not user-friendly and difficult to use in infants because of the small arc of the displaced thumb. Others regard mechanomyography as more accurate because it is less influenced by external disturbances; that is, it does not go out of calibration.[241] Mechanomyography is currently the simplest and most useful clinical monitor to assess the degree of paralysis when using NMBDs in infants and children (see also E-Figs. 7.14, 7.15, and 7.17). The TOF does not require recording capability or baseline measurement because it compares only the fourth twitch with its own internal standard, the first twitch.[242] The unit may also be used with depolarizing NMBDs, monitoring only the first twitch amplitude. A significant decrement (>50%) between the first and fourth twitch in this context suggests phase II blockade (see E-Fig. 7.15).[243]

Needle electrodes should not be used in children because they may cause bleeding, infection, burns, or nerve injury; current density may be very high owing to the limited contact surface and the resistance of surrounding skin. Self-adhesive electrodes designed specifically for twitch monitors are available, but they are unnecessary, expensive, and tend to be too large for infants and small children. A reasonable alternative is a pair of infant-sized ECG electrodes. The choice of monitoring location depends on the nature of the surgery. It is preferable to select a site where a motor nerve is close to the body surface and its associated muscle group is available for observation. The most common site is the ulnar nerve in the forearm, observing the thumb movement (adductor pollicis brevis); this is the standard site for most research reports. Quantitating the response of other motor nerves is less reliable. Using the facial nerve may result in false-positive responses because the muscles may be directly stimulated, potentially leading to an overdose of NMBDs.

PROCESSED ELECTROENCEPHALOGRAM MONITORS

We anesthetize children daily, often with the use of regional anesthesia as a supplement to general anesthesia. It would be ideal if we were able to monitor the effect of our anesthetic agents on the brain to ensure an adequate depth of anesthesia. Clinically, we have discrete endpoints such as loss of consciousness or limb movement under anesthesia, but we would prefer a monitor that examines awareness and other brain functionality. Therefore as anesthesiologists we may use the processed electroencephalogram (pEEG) in an attempt to provide this information.[244,245] We use a pEEG to reduce the amount of information displayed. A number of different devices are available to gather and present information from an EEG to the clinician. The most commonly used pEEG monitor is the Bispectral Index monitor (BIS Brain Monitoring System, Covidien, Boulder, CO). With the BIS monitor, a sensor is placed on the forehead that detects EEG signals from the frontal lobe of the brain as well as from the frontal motor cortex. The information received is converted into a dimensionless number between 0 and 100. The value of 100 represents a patient who is fully awake and value of 0 represents electroencephalographic silence or complete (isoelectric) suppression.

Like the algorithms for pulse oximeters, the algorithms generating the BIS values are proprietary and based on data from adult subjects, not infants and children. Furthermore, the algorithm was developed during isoflurane and propofol anesthesia, not sevoflurane, the latter having an EEG profile that differs from the former anesthetics. Although there are BIS sensors in pediatric sizes, the EEG changes with both age and development undermine the reliability of BIS values in children, particularly in infants younger than 1 year of age.[246-249] The BIS values in children are affected by several factors. Values are lower in children with developmental delay[250,251]; halothane yields different values from sevoflurane at equipotent MAC concentrations; the pEEG paradoxically increases with values of expired sevoflurane greater than 3%[252-254]; and adjuvant drugs such as opioids and benzodiazepines have variable effects.[255,256] N_2O does not change the BIS value,[257] although it is partially additive to the MAC of insoluble inhalation anesthetics in children; for some devices N_2O actually increases the reported number value. Loss of consciousness with dexmedetomidine as an adjunct to propofol is reported to occur at greater BIS values than propofol alone[258]; ketamine also paradoxically increases the BIS value.[259] Curiously, NMBDs directly interfere with the BIS readings in adults; that is, both succinylcholine and rocuronium decreased BIS readings immediately from values in the mid-90s to mid-80s and 70s and then after about 4 minutes to the 40s and 50s for seconds to longer than 10 minutes.[260] We suspect that the same holds true in children. Accordingly, pEEG signal profiles differ in children according to age and the anesthetics administered, rendering interpretation of the metric confusing and less reliable than it is in adults.

Several other pEEG monitors are clinically available.[261] The SedLine brain function monitor from Masimo refers to its pEEG as the Patient State Index (PSI). The SedLine EEG sensor has four active leads to collect information from both the left and right frontal lobes. The monitor displays a single dimensionless number, a density spectral array, or spectrograms of right and left brain activity and four channels of the bilateral EEG waveforms. The pEEG monitor from Narcotrend (Narcotrend-Gruppe Hannover, Germany) shows the raw EEG, a letter A-E indicating the stage of anesthesia, a dimensionless number, and a cerebrogram. The Response and State Entropy monitor from General Electric (GE Healthcare, Helsinki, Finland) integrates the frontal EEG and electromyography signals to produces its value. Entropy is the measure of irregularity in the EEG and electromyography signals. With anesthesia, the EEG and motor activity decrease and the entropy decreases in parallel.

To recommend the use of pEEG monitoring for most pediatric anesthetic cases, we must be able to demonstrate that such use is reliable, predictable, and associated with a significant benefit or a reduction in adverse events. A number of outcomes have been studied in children and adults. In theory, BIS monitoring might prevent too great of a depth of anesthesia during surgery; the tangible benefits are a reduction in the time to emergence, extubation, and PACU stay. In addition, such monitoring may decrease PONV as well as the amount of anesthetic agent used. Given the age-related differences in anesthetic outcomes, adult studies have also focused on the potential for reduction in delirium and cognitive decline.[262] Alternatively, the use of BIS monitoring would ensure a sufficient depth of anesthesia to prevent the possibility of intraoperative awareness. Thus on the one hand, an adequate depth of anesthesia is achieved, whereas on the other, a more rapid emergence may be established. BIS monitoring has been used to decrease the time to emergence in adults[263] and children,[264] although this has been refuted in another study.[265] In adults, BIS monitoring has decreased PONV[266]; no similar studies have been forthcoming in children. A meta-analysis showed a modest reduction in the consumption of anesthetic, PONV risk, and PACU time for adult ambulatory surgery but the cost savings were not greater than the electrodes and the monitors.[267] One additional issue that affects whether pEEG monitoring shows benefit is the type of anesthetic delivered; the only drug whereby pEEG provided consistent proven relationships with depth of anesthesia was propofol.[268-271] BIS monitoring may have its greatest value as a monitor of depth of anesthesia during TIVA, for which an end-tidal anesthetic concentration for propofol is not currently available, although this may change in the future.[272] It remains unclear if this is true in younger children but certainly it may provide value in teenagers undergoing spinal instrumentation when motor evoked potential monitoring is required.

The use of cerebral monitoring to prevent intraoperative awareness in adults has been studied in several trials. The B-AWARE Trial (2004) showed a decrease in awareness with BIS monitoring.[273] The B-Unaware Trial did not show a decrease in risk of awareness.[274] The BIS or Anesthesia Gas to Reduce Explicit Recall Clinical Trial (BAG-RECALL, 2008) failed to confirm the superiority of the BIS over end-tidal anesthetic concentrations to prevent awareness.[275] The Michigan Awareness Control Study (MACS) (2012) was stopped for futility.[276] The TIVA Trial (2011) was intended to demonstrate the differences between inhaled anesthetics and TIVA, wherein you can monitor depth of anesthesia reasonably well with end-tidal anesthetic gas concentrations. The TIVA Trial (2011) concluded that BIS monitoring prevents awareness during TIVA,[277] but a secondary analysis of the data showed that there was an effect of midazolam on the participants (amnesia of the operating room in the B-Unaware and BAG-RECALL trials).[278] In hospitals where patients receive midazolam in the holding area, the majority do not remember the OR.

A smaller body of literature regards the risk of awareness for children undergoing anesthesia. In 2011, a secondary analysis of five pediatric cohort studies[279] was published investigating awareness.[280-284] The multivariable regression analysis showed that maintenance of anesthesia with N_2O and the use of a tracheal tube were independently associated with awareness, both curious findings since the former confers amnesia and the latter implies use of an inhalational anesthetic (paralysis is infrequently used in pediatric anesthesia). Interestingly, the incidence of awareness in these cohort studies averaged 0.74%, a frequency that exceeded the 0.1% to 0.2% reported in adults by severalfold.[285,286] In contrast to the adults who experienced awareness, none of the children in the earlier cohorts who had awareness reported distress, although 50% reported distress in the 5th National Audit Project (NAP5) recently.[280,287-289] To date, there is no evidence that pEEG devices decrease the frequency of awareness in children as 70% of the events in one report occurred at induction or emergence when the depth of anesthesia may not have stabilized.[289] The adult literature would indicate that there might still be a role for monitoring of pEEG in patients who are at high risk for recall (e.g., trauma patients and obstetric patients who require general anesthesia). A case could be made for their use in pediatrics—for example, for adolescents undergoing posterior spine fusion often with a TIVA anesthetic that the clinician must adjust during the case. In most instances, these patients are unparalyzed and monitored with motor evoked potentials, which requires deep levels of IV anesthesia to prevent movement. By the completion of surgery, recovery may be protracted because of the large amount of propofol infused, unless the dose was adjusted based on a pEEG monitor. Alternately, the anesthetic may need to be adjusted to perform a wake-up test and this too may be protracted if excess anesthesia had been administered. The use of pEEG monitoring or direct feedback from a skilled neurophysiologist who was monitoring the child can provide an indication of the depth of anesthesia. There are other potential cases for which we could consider the use of pEEG monitoring such as neuroanesthesia and otorhinolaryngologic procedures. In certain procedures, placement of the monitors on the forehead could interfere with the surgical site or sterile prep.

Several other issues raised in a recent editorial identified the need for more specific outcomes after pEEG monitoring to clarify potential benefits in children.[290] Currently, it appears that our outcomes focus on the times to removal of a tracheal tube, discharge from the PACU, or the frequency of adverse events. The numbers of patients needed to study or treat to prevent an adverse outcome that is extremely rare are exceedingly large, posing challenges in conducting such studies. Similarly, if we wish to monitor brain function during anesthesia, we may prefer to monitor an index of nociception.[291] The pEEG devices available today are limited to frontal EEG and motor movement and not to detect nociception. New devices under development will be able to monitor the entire brain but they remain experimental at this time.

CONTINUOUS CARDIAC OUTPUT MONITORING

Continuous cardiac output monitoring for anesthesia and critical care has great potential value in some patients. Multiple physiologic, pathophysiologic, and critical events and surgical interventions can affect preload, afterload, cardiac contractility, and heart rate and therefore decrease cardiac contractility and cardiac output (CO). Physicians have few monitors at their disposal to measure cardiac output or systemic vascular resistance non-invasively.[292-294] The next generation of monitors that could greatly advance the care of children may be devices that could accurately continuously assess CO and other indicators of cardiac function such as stroke index, cardiac index, and contractility. The ideal device would be accurate for both individual and trend measurements compared with a gold standard, would be minimally or non-invasive, cheap, portable, and independent of operator technique and experience. Ideally, the accuracy of the device should be unaffected by changes in patient age and size, developmental physiology, position or nature of the procedure (preterm infants to teenagers). Most current

continuous cardiac output monitors do not fulfill all of these criteria.

Multiple different technologies that have been developed to improve CO measurement. These technologies are driven by the needs of the adult anesthesia and critical care market and are subsequently applied to children. In some instances, this has been easily accomplished, whereas in others the physiology and size varies so dramatically in children that they could not be applied. Several techniques may be used to measure CO: indicator dilution, evaluation of the arterial pressure waveform, ultrasound, direct or indirect Fick method, and variations of bioimpedance.[295-299] These devices must be developed with children in mind regarding their size, accuracy of measurements for values in the pediatric range, and integration in the OR for children.

The classic gold standard for the measurement of CO in humans is the direct Fick method. In this method, oxygen consumption ($\dot{V}O_2$) must be measured directly. The oxygen saturations of arterial and venous blood are measured to calculate arterial oxygen content (C_aO_2) and venous oxygen content (C_vO_2), respectively. Cardiac output is calculated using the formula:

$$CO = \dot{V}O_2/(C_aO_2 - C_vO_2)$$

Measurement of oxygen consumption at the bedside is exceedingly difficult. The patient's trachea must be intubated without an air leak around the ETT. A second gold standard for the measurement of CO is the pulmonary artery thermodilution (PAT) catheter. This method requires a catheter placed from a central venous location through the right atrium and ventricle into a pulmonary artery. Successful placement can be technically difficult, is associated with risks (embolism, pneumothorax, hemothorax, chylothorax, cardiac tamponade), and is infrequently used in the PICU. Pediatric use is now confined to limited cardiac surgical populations and during cardiac catheterization. This rare use limits the pediatric population that is available for comparison with data from new CO monitors and the information provided by PAT. Because of the limited use of Fick dilution in children, a number of studies have compared a new method to measure CO with another new technique, which is not a gold standard. Such comparisons limit the validity of the new technique. For devices that may be used for neonates, the accuracy of the CO monitors is usually confirmed in animal studies using ultrasonic flow probes placed around the pulmonary artery. These flow probes are very accurate and produce reproducible assessments. However, the applicability of data from animal models to humans is fraught with pitfalls. With these limitations, pediatric studies of new devices include small sample sizes and are often not tested in children in whom the data would be of greatest value (e.g., those in shock [septic, hypovolemic, cardiogenic]).

Indicator Dilution Method

This technique is based on the Stewart-Hamilton equation, which is the ratio of the amount of dye injected to the area under the concentration-time curve as the dye passes a detector. This is the principle used by PAT CO monitors to estimate CO. Cold saline solution may also be used as the indicator; it is injected into a proximal port of the catheter and then the temperature change is detected using a thermistor at the tip of the catheter. This is an invasive device as the catheter must be placed into the pulmonary artery. Furthermore, 5 to 10 mL of cold saline solution is used for each measurement, which is performed in triplicate. For repeated measurements, the fluid load can be substantial, particularly in neonates, infants, and critically ill patients who require fluid restriction. One means to eliminate or reduce the cold saline solution boluses is by using a thermal filament rather than cold fluid. Edwards Lifescience (Edwards Lifescience, Irvine, CA) has created the Vigilance monitors and continuous CO catheters that have a thermal filament on the catheter. The saline injectate is replaced by thermal energy as an indicator as the filament intermittently heats and cools. The catheter is also able to perform PAT measurements in the usual manner. However, the smallest catheter size is 7.5F, thus limiting this device to adolescents or adults.

Another strategy to reduce the fluid boluses is to use another means of CO measurement between calibrations (that may use cold saline solution) as in both the PiCCO (Pulsion Medical Systems, Munich, Germany) and the LiDCO systems (LiDCO, London, United Kingdom). The PiCCO system uses a combination of central venous and arterial access. Cold saline solution is injected in the central venous line and the dilution curve is measured from the arterial line. This technique is also referred to as transpulmonary thermodilution (TPTD) as the cold injectate traverses the right heart, lungs, and left heart before being measured. The PiCCO devices also measure continuous CO using the arterial pressure-based continuous cardiac output technique (APCCO) (described later). The intermittent injections of cold saline solution are used to calibrate the APCCO measurements. TPTD systems are considered less invasive compared with PAT as they are typically performed with femoral central venous access and peripheral arterial access and do not require a catheter to transverse the heart. Furthermore, the arterial catheter can be used for normal BP monitoring and laboratory testing. However, the arterial catheter required is specific to the device manufacturer, which adds cost to the system. The TPTD technique has been validated in an animal model compared with perivascular flow probes as accurate and capable of tracking CO changes.[300] The TPTD technique using an earlier version of a Pulsion Medical System device (COLD Z-021, Pulsion Medical Systems) has been validated in children compared with the direct Fick method.[301,302] There is some evidence that TPTD can measure CO in subjects with left to right shunting. However, for the moment this appears to have been demonstrated only in animals.[303,304] In 2015, PiCCO catheters were recalled because the devices did not meet company internal standards; there were no patient-related events. However, at the time of this writing, online information regarding PiCCO from the manufacturer "is intended for an audience **outside the United States.**" There have been no updates regarding when these issues will be resolved. More relevant is the fact that this device requires both arterial and central venous access and therefore would be impractical for routine pediatric anesthesia cases.

The LiDCO system uses a bolus of a small amount of lithium chloride as an indicator for the intermittent CO measurements for calibration and also uses an APCCO system for continuous measurement (described later). The LiDCO device uses a peristaltic pump to pull arterial blood through a sensor that detects lithium. However, the measurements will be affected if the patient is already taking lithium for manic depression. In addition, NMBDs with a quaternary ammonia ion will be detected by the sensor. The manufacturer recommends waiting 15 to 30 minutes after a dose of NMBD before performing LiDCO measurements. More importantly, since the measurements are performed in triplicate during various portions of the respiratory cycle to improve accuracy (3 mL of blood per measurement), the volume of blood that may be removed in some infants and children is large (research permits up to 3% of the patient's blood volume). Thus this device is both invasive and requires a large amount of blood sampling. The LiDCO*plus* system is not recommended by the manufacturer for patients who weigh less than 40 kg, and the LiDCO*rapid* system is not approved for use in pediatric patients.

There is an additional CO monitoring device that uses an indicator dilution method but does not also incorporate APCCO. The COstatus monitor from Transonic (Transonic, Ithaca, NY) uses an ultrasound dilution method to measure CO. The system connects the patient's existing arterial and central venous lines with an extracorporeal customized tubing set. During measurement, a pump circulates blood through the arterial to venous tubing loop. Ultrasound measurements are taken of the arterial to venous tubing loop and a bolus of warmed saline solution is given to the patient. The saline solution bolus will dilute the blood in the arterial to venous tubing loop, changing the velocity of the ultrasound signal. The ultrasound velocity of blood is 1560 to 1590 m/second depending on blood protein concentration. The ultrasound velocity of saline solution is 1533 m/second. The difference between the two values creates a conventional indicator dilution curve. The saline solution bolus given is diluted as it transverses the right heart, lungs, and left heart in the same manner as a TPTD measurement. The benefits of this device are the use of a low volume of warmed saline solution, reducing the risk for temperature changes and volume overload. A further advantage is that this system uses normal central venous and arterial catheters that may already be in place. The accuracy of the device has been demonstrated in children.[305–307] This device has been shown to be accurate in the detection of intracardiac shunts as a result of the characteristic changes that occur in the ultrasound dilution curve.[152,304,307] The device is limited to children with central venous and arterial catheters limiting its utility to the PICU or limited children in the OR.

Arterial Pressure-Based Continuous Cardiac Output Monitors

These devices are also referred to as arterial pulse contour-based methods to measure CO. The device is based upon the work and formulas of the renowned physicist Karel H. Wesseling beginning in the mid-1970s.[308] The concept behind the device is that when the heart contracts, the arterial pressure wave of the stroke volume (SV) is transmitted through the arterial tree. It is then possible to use mathematical methods to convert the waveform from the arterial pressure back into a calculated SV. The formulas or equations involved must consider patient factors such as the dispensability and stiffness of the aorta and arteries. The aortic compliance changes not only with age but also with BP. There is also a change in the arterial pressure waveform as it is transmitted from the aorta to the periphery. As the waveform approaches peripheral arteries the systolic pressure increases, the diastolic pressure decreases, and the mean pressure remains about the same as the aorta. Non-patient factors that must be considered include the effect of vasoactive medications, patient temperature, and volume status on vascular tone. From a pediatric standpoint, we must consider that these formulas or algorithms were generated in adults and then applied to children. The specific physiologic changes as a child grows and develops will likely change their accuracy and therefore their validity. The PiCCO™ and LiDCO™ systems mentioned above use APCCO algorithms to calculate continuous cardiac output. For the PiCCO™ system there has been some support that the accuracy of the device is sufficient for use in children,[309,310] although other investigators reported a large inter-individual variability in the measurements obtained.[311] These conflicting results suggest that further studies are needed to validate the accuracy of this device in children. The LiDCO™ system refers to their APCCO method as PulseCO and the majority of validation studies have been in adults; only one pediatric study has demonstrated PulseCO to be accurate compared with pulmonary artery thermodilution (PAT).[312]

Edwards Lifesciences produces a FloTrac system that does not require an additional calibration. The system uses an algorithm that accounts for arterial compliance and vascular resistance based on patient characteristics such as gender, age, weight, and height. There have been multiple studies in adults that addressed the accuracy of this device. One study in children that compared FloTrac™ with PAT concluded that the former was inaccurate in children.[313] However, a second study demonstrated that it was able to identify increased SV variation during normovolemic hemodilution and that this resolved with fluid replacement[314]; the study was further limited by the fact that it was not carried out during surgery but rather at a steady state during hemodilution without surgical stimulation.

An additional method to calculate CO from the arterial pressure curve is referred to as pressure recording analytical method (PRAM). This method samples the pressure wave profile at a very high frequency (1000 Hz) and uses a beat-to-beat analysis of the waveform to calculate cardiac output. The MostCare device (Vytech Health, Padova, Italy), an example of this device, has been shown to be accurate in children.[315-317] The system analyzes the contour of the systolic and diastolic phases, the location of the dicrotic notch, and the area under the entire arterial pressure curve. This might be a promising method of minimally invasive CO monitoring as it only requires an arterial line.

ULTRASOUND DETERMINATION OF CARDIAC OUTPUT

Ultrasound determination of CO includes 2D transthoracic evaluation of the size and flow through the aortic valve to determine SV, transesophageal ultrasound of the descending aorta to determine blood velocity, and transthoracic continuous wave Doppler of the aortic or pulmonary valve determines velocity through the valve to determine SV. Transthoracic 2D echocardiography is frequently obtained for clinical needs. The cross-sectional area of the aortic valve is measured and the velocity of blood through the valve is recorded and then integrated as the velocity time integral (VTI). The area of the valve multiplied by VTI is the SV, and SV multiplied by heart rate is CO. Echocardiography as a technique to estimate CO has been extensively reviewed[318] and deemed to be sufficiently accurate that it is frequently used as the reference standard to compare with other methods of CO determination.[315,319-323] This technique requires considerable expertise and can only be applied intermittently. However, it does provide additional details of the structure and function of the heart, particularly in an ICU setting and cardiac OR.

The velocity of blood moving in the descending aorta can be measured with an ultrasound probe that is positioned in the mid-esophagus. Once in place, the probe is directed to produce the maximum Doppler signal. If the cross-sectional area of the descending aorta is obtained from a nomogram, then the SV of blood flow to the lower half of the body is known. Calculations are made to adjust for the percentage of blood flow to the upper and lower portions of the body and the entire SV and then CO can be measured. Alternatively, without using the cross section of the descending aorta the VTI alone can be used. One system, EDM+ (Deltex Medical, Greenville), has a pediatric probe for use in children who weigh 3 kg or more, are 50 cm or more in height,

and younger than 16 years of age. The measurement of CO in children has been shown to be accurate[318,324,325] and predict fluid responsiveness.[326] Further studies have suggested that measuring the velocity of blood flow in the descending aorta to improve accuracy. It appears that small changes in the angle between the ultrasound probe head and the descending aorta substantively change the VTI, thus requiring frequent adjustments to improve the measurements. The large size of the probe prevents it from being left in small children for a prolonged period of time. In addition, the presence of a nasogastric tube in the esophagus may alter the measurement. When properly used, this technique does seem to be accurate, although it requires frequent repositioning and is limited to intubated children.

Velocity through the aortic or pulmonary valve can also be measured with a continuous-wave Doppler and then VTI calculated from the output. The Ultrasonic Cardiac Output Monitor (USCOM 1A model) (USCOM, Sydney, Australia) is a portable device that uses a small continuous-wave Doppler probe to measure VTI through either the aortic or pulmonary valve. The USCOM software uses the patient's height to determine the area of the aortic or pulmonary valve from a nomogram. The valve area is multiplied by the VTI to SV and SV multiplied by heart rate to give CO. The device was demonstrated to be accurate in animal studies compared with ultrasonic flow probes[327]; it also was inaccurate compared with PAT in children with intracardiac shunting.[326] Our experience differed in that we found that the device is accurate when compared with PAT in children without atrial or ventricular septal defects.[328,329] We found that the measurement technique was easy to learn with good interobserver variability. However, the measurements are intermittent and the clinician must have access to the neck or thorax. Further studies will be needed to demonstrate the response to changes in CO to determine whether the USCOM can be used as a trending device.

Direct and Indirect Fick Measurement of Cardiac Output
CO can be calculated directly using the Fick equation:

$$CO = \text{Oxygen consumption}/(\text{Arterial oxygen content} - \text{Venous oxygen content}).$$

$$\text{Oxygen content} = (\text{Saturation of oxygen} \times \text{Hemoglobin} \times 1.34) + (0.003 \times PaO_2).$$

During cardiac catheterization samples of blood are drawn for arterial and mixed venous saturations and can be used to measure direct Fick CO. However, most catheterization laboratories do not measure oxygen consumption. Rather, they use a nomogram or formula to estimate oxygen consumption.[330,331] Oxygen consumption can be measured with a respiratory mass spectrometer,[332] which can produce extremely precise results. These mass spectrometers are exceedingly expensive and not widely available. Oxygen can also be measured using a photoacoustic infrared gas analyzer such as the Innocor monitor from Innovision (Innovision ApS, Glamsbjerg, Denmark). Oxygen consumption can be calculated breath by breath by measuring the difference between inspired and exhaled oxygen. Further, this same device has a system for inert gas rebreathing as a means of determining CO. If a patient has both arterial and venous access to measure oxygen content, CO can be measured directly. If the patient does not have these catheters, CO can be measured indirectly. During an inert gas rebreathing test the patient breathes from a rebreathing bag for approximately 5 breaths or 15 seconds. In the rebreathing bag is a known, measured, starting concentration of N_2O and sulfur hexafluoride. The N_2O is rapidly taken up by the blood and its rate of decrease in the bag is proportional to the blood flow to the lung. The blood flow to the lung is the effective pulmonary blood flow and in the absence of significant intrapulmonary shunt is equal to CO. The sulfur hexafluoride is not taken up in the blood and the change in its concentration in the bag is measured to determine the lung volume from which the N_2O was taken up. The oxygen consumption technique in the Innocor device yielded excellent correlations with the gold standard of measurement using a Douglas bag method[333] in children weighing more than 15 kg whose airways were intubated.[334] One author (PAR) has used the device and found the measurements of oxygen consumption are not difficult, although learning the inert gas rebreathing technique requires additional skill. Since the concentration of N_2O used is very small, the CO measured in this manner would be in error for any patient who recently received N_2O in the OR. Additionally, the dead space of the equipment is large for infants and small children, which could limit the ability to perform the test. Although it is a noninvasive technique, a further limitation is that the inert gas rebreathing technique is intermittent and it requires an intubated patient.

CO can be measured indirectly by using a modification of the Fick equation. In this case, partial rebreathing of CO_2 is used in place of oxygen consumption. One device that uses partial rebreathing is the Non-Invasive Cardiac Output (NICO) monitoring system, which was produced by Novametrix Medical Systems (Wallingford, CT) beginning in the late 1980s. Novametrix now is a subsidiary of Philips-Respironics and some of the technology has been incorporated into their NM3 device (Respironics NM3 Monitor, Philips Healthcare, Eindhoven, The Netherlands). In brief, the amount of oxygen entering the lungs is directly proportional to the pulmonary blood flow. In the same way, the amount of CO_2 leaving the lungs is proportional to pulmonary blood flow. If there is limited intrapulmonary shunting, then the amount of pulmonary blood flow equals CO. During a measurement with the NICO device the dead space of the breathing circuit is temporarily increased. During that time period, there is a change in the elimination of CO_2 ($\Delta\dot{V}CO_2$) and a rise in the $PETCO_2$. Pulmonary blood flow is calculated from the formula:

$$CO = \Delta\dot{V}CO_2 / \Delta PETCO_2$$

The original NICO monitor used a disposable sensor, which incorporated a CO_2 sensor and a differential pressure flow sensor. The CO_2 elimination rate, $PETCO_2$, and gas flow were closely tracked and the CO calculated. NICO devices are still present in many departments but are no longer commercially available. This is unfortunate as the technique did work for intubated mechanically ventilated older children.[319,335] The NM3 device measures volumetric capnography, which can be used to calculate CO. There are currently no papers describing the accuracy of this technique in children but it does hold scientific promise.

Bioimpedance, Electrical Cardiometry, and Bioreactance

Thoracic electrical bioimpedance (TEB) is a means of using the changes in electrical conductivity of the blood flow in the aortic arch to determine SV and in turn CO. A low-amplitude, high-frequency electrical current is passed through the thorax and the resistance is measured. There are small changes in the volume of the aorta within the thorax during the cardiac cycle, resulting in a change in the electrical resistance. The change in electrical resistance over time is converted through an algorithm into a measure of SV. The theory and technique is several decades old[336]

and had many problems that led to inaccuracies. There have been marked improvements in bioimpedance measurements and are referred to as electrical cardiometry (or as electrical velocimetry). Electrical cardiometry also uses skin sensors to impart high-frequency current into the thorax and measure the change in impedance. This system takes advantage of the difference in thoracic impedance that occurs owing to the arrangement of red blood cells during the cardiac cycle. During diastole, the red blood cells in the heart and aorta are in a random orientation (chaotically oriented) and the electrical resistance is increased. During systole, the red blood cells are in motion and are therefore aligned (parallel oriented) and the electrical resistance is lower. The computer algorithms derive peak acceleration of blood in the aorta, the duration of left ventricular ejection, and then the velocity of blood flow, which then determines the SV. The Osypka Medical Company (Osypka Medical Inc., La Jolla, CA) has two products that measure CO through electrical cardiometry. The Icon model is a handheld, battery-operated, portable monitor. The Aesculon model incorporates the electrical cardiometry measurement but is a complete hemodynamic monitoring system; common settings are to record measurements at ten second intervals that average the prior 20 heart beats. The Aesculon incorporates pulse oximetry, noninvasive BP, and so on and provides data storage for research. In several studies using either the Icon or the Aesculon to measure CO, the latter was shown to be accurate compared with Fick determinations and PAT even in neonates.[320,337-339] In children after a Fontan palliation for congenital heart disease[340,341] and in a general OR setting,[159,342] the Aesculon provided valuable clinical information. The unique value of the device is that it requires application of only four standard ECG electrodes and no other special equipment (Figs. 52.9 and 52.10). This device is approved for use even in neonates.

Bioreactance is another noninvasive technology that measures CO. This device also passes an electrical current through the thorax, although it evaluates the phase shifts that occur as the resistance and reactance of the thorax change during the cardiac cycle. Phase shifts or time delays between the applied current and measured voltage occur as a result of the pulsatile blood flow in the larger arteries of the thorax. The phase shifts are used to estimate SV and therefore CO. Cheetah Medical produces the Nicom monitor (Cheetah Medical, Newton Center, MA). The accuracy of the Nicom model has been demonstrated in adults[343,344] and neonates,[322] but the pediatric trials have limitations. One study[345] showed that the CO measurements were in a range appropriate for the patients being studied, although no reference standard for CO was included. Studies have been conflicting regarding whether Nicom could predict fluid responsiveness.[346,347] This device is not approved for use in children, although studies are ongoing.

BEYOND CARDIAC OUTPUT MEASUREMENTS

Many other physiologic variables can be identified and measured with the previously discussed technology. One of the easiest to identify is the stroke volume variation (SVV). Almost all of the aforementioned technologies can either measure or calculate SV. The change in SV that occurs during the respiratory cycle is a good indicator of intravascular volume or fluid responsiveness. There is strong evidence that SVV is better at predicting fluid responsiveness compared with central venous pressure. In adult studies this has been demonstrated in sepsis,[348] major abdominal surgery,[349] kidney transplantation,[350,351] and major orthopedic surgery,[352] among others. In children, SVV has been shown to predict fluid responsiveness,[346] although, a systematic review

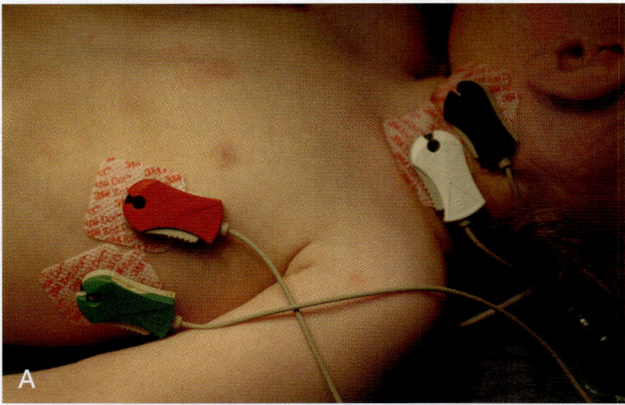

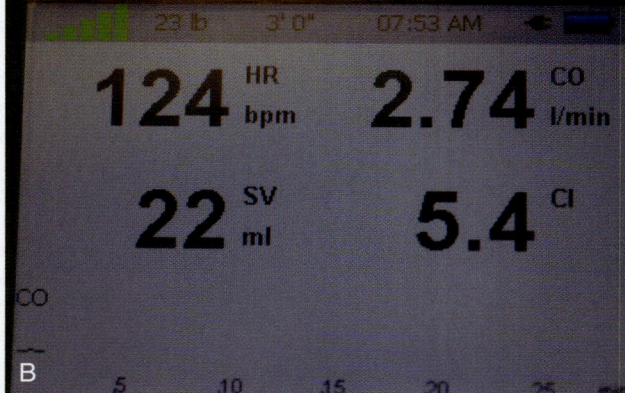

FIGURE 52.9 **A**, Cardiotronic Icon cardiac output device. The only additional equipment is four standard electrocardiogram (ECG) pads placed according to the manufacturer's instructions (Adult: two on left side at the level of xiphoid depression and two on the left neck over the carotid artery; Neonate: one on the left cheek or forehead, one over the left carotid artery, one on the left side at level of xiphoid depression, and the fourth on the left leg). **B**, Electrical cardiometry continuously estimates cardiac output, cardiac index, stroke volume, stroke index, and a variety of other parameters through quantitation of changes in impedance associated with changes in the orientation of red blood cells. During diastole, red blood cells are organized chaotically, but during systole they assume a position parallel to the direction of blood flow. Thus thoracic electrical bioimpedance relates to changes in thoracic aortic blood flow, and by using refined algorithms noninvasive measurement of continuous cardiac output with four ECG pads is achieved.

reported that only the variation in the aortic blood flow peak velocity with respiration predicted fluid responsiveness.[353]

For patients with acute respiratory failure, pulmonary edema can prolong intubation and recovery. Several of the devices that measure CO can be used to compute an extravascular lung water index (EVLWI), which is a measure of pulmonary edema.[354] One study in children[355] found that the increased EVLWI on admission to a PICU predicted both the duration of mechanical ventilation and survival.

Purchasing Anesthesia Equipment

With the increasing sophistication of monitoring and life support equipment, purchasing decisions are no longer intuitive. A complete grounding in the underlying engineering concepts would probably require an advanced degree in engineering, but a reasonable working knowledge of the operating principles, advantages, and special hazards of the various types of apparatus is relatively easy to

obtain. Most hospitals now have a full-time biomedical professional staff, which often have considerable engineering and practical experience to assist in the purchasing, maintenance, and safety of all the equipment and systems used in the hospital setting. The biomedical professionals should be closely integrated into the purchasing, maintenance, and ongoing safety monitoring of all devices. Although vendors are pleased to promote a product, the manufacturer's information literature should be obtained from an unbiased source such as the equipment periodical *Health Devices*, published by ECRI (formerly Emergency Care Research Institute, Plymouth Meeting, PA). The biomedical or hospital safety office of each hospital usually subscribes to this periodical.

Another useful source of information is the specialty pediatric hospital. Whether through inquiry at medical meetings or by direct solicitation, practitioners at these unique resource institutions are often willing to share their special expertise.

The following are useful principles for any equipment purchase:

1. New purchases should interface with equipment that is already present. Considerable cost savings can occur if the same or compatible equipment is used in all the perioperative areas, including the OR, PACU, PICU, and NICU. Another issue to consider is how the equipment will interface with automated record-keeping systems and other hospital information systems if they are present. If an automated recording device is a possible plan for the future, the equipment should be evaluated for how well it will interface with systems that will possibly be purchased. Another compatibility issue to carefully review is the software required to use the equipment. Review the product information carefully to identify the need for software upgrades and compatibility, which can be important for safety and cost-effectiveness.
2. Recognize that the salesperson is inherently biased.
3. Always test proposed equipment in the environment in which it will be used, with the personnel who will be using it. What appears attractive in a display as presented by a salesperson may not function well in practice. It is also important to test the device in unusual circumstances to see how well it performs. The use of simulation is becoming an important modality to test devices under normal and unusual circumstances. Human factors must be considered, such as how easy it is to use the equipment clinically (i.e., the user interface), and equally important, the safety of the equipment or product. Evaluate systems issues that could lead to error or misuse. Software-driven products are harder to test for potential failures when they are connected to existing systems and products in your workstations; always test new equipment in the environment where it will be used.
4. Do not use equipment for any purpose other than that for which it has been designed.
5. Have your hospital biomedical staff be intimately involved with the safety issues of your systems, as described earlier, and periodically check for electrical leakage and other safety issues.
6. Decide explicitly how the product will be maintained. Will the biomedical professionals perform the necessary calibration, testing, and repair of the equipment, or will a member of your department assume this role? Spend the necessary resources to properly maintain the product; this is typically on the order of 10% of the cost of the device per year.

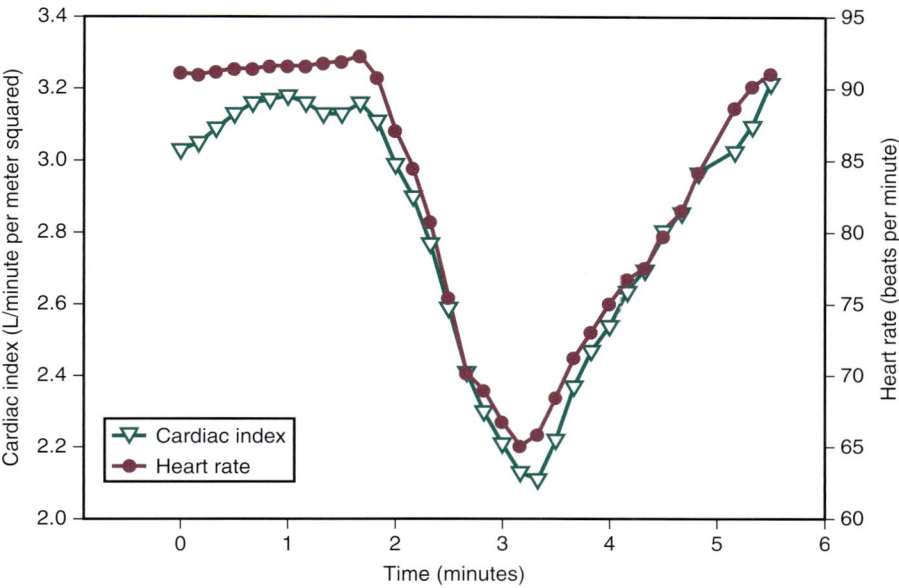

FIGURE 52.10 This graph plots the continuous cardiac index versus heart rate in a 6-year-old child undergoing a posterior fossa procedure. The bradycardia occurred with surgical brainstem irrigation with saline solution that was not adequately warmed. The Icon model averages data from the prior 20 heart beats and records this every 10 seconds. Data plotted here are the average for the six values during each minute of the event. In this case, we asked the surgeon to stop irrigating and administered atropine (0.02 mg/kg). Note how the Icon immediately tracked the improved cardiac index as the atropine took effect.

Consider a maintenance contract, if available. Ask the company to ensure the future availability of parts and the compatibility of subsequent modifications or design evolutions with your equipment.

7. Consider the cost and quality of disposable components of the equipment. This can also have an impact on the safety and cost of the product.

8. If two products are comparable but one has local service facilities, that one may be the better choice.

9. If areas of special needs have been recognized, be as detailed as possible with specifications. For example, if a monitor is to be used strictly in the OR, it may be reasonable to operate it from wall power. Conversely, if the monitor is to serve in the OR and for transport between the OR and the recovery room or ICU, it must have internal battery backup.

The more precisely needs can be defined, the more accurate the comparisons will be between the bids of rival vendors. Note that any given piece of equipment will occasionally be out of service, whether for regular preventive maintenance or for some unanticipated repair. Given this fact, in this era of cost containment it is often difficult to convince the hospital administration of a need for additional spare units.

ANNOTATED REFERENCES

Burn SL, Chilton PJ, Gawande AA, Lilford RJ. Peri-operative pulse oximetry in low-income countries: a cost-effectiveness analysis. *Bull World Health Organ.* 2014;92(12):858-867.

Pulse oximeters are a cost-effective way to reduce the risk of anesthesia-related deaths in developing countries.

Duryea EL, Nelson DB, Wyckoff MH, et al. The impact of ambient operating room temperature on neonatal and maternal hypothermia and associated morbidities: a randomized controlled trial. *Am J Obstet Gynecol.* 2016;214(4):505.e1-505.e7.

An increase of 3°C in the OR temperature (20°C vs. 23°C) during cesarean delivery significantly reduced the number of infants that developed moderate to severe hypothermia. A small change in practice can have a dramatic effect on the temperature of infants during surgery.

Feldman JM. Optimal ventilation of the anesthetized pediatric patient. *Anesth Analg.* 2015;120(1):165-175.

This is an excellent review of the ability to provide mechanical ventilation with an anesthesia workstation.

Moler FW, Silverstein FS, Holubkov R, et al. Therapeutic hypothermia after out-of-hospital cardiac arrest in children. *N Engl J Med.* 2015;372(2):1898-1908.

The largest multicenter randomized pediatric study ever performed. Therapeutic hypothermia following out-of-hospital cardiac arrest did not confer a benefit in survival with a good functional outcome at the time point of 1 year.

Ross PA, Newth CJ, Khemani RG. Accuracy of pulse oximetry in children. *Pediatrics.* 2014;133(1):22-29.

Pulse oximeters are a monitor that we use every day. Many trainees do not know at what point the device becomes inaccurate.

Sutton RM, French B, Meaney PA, et al. Physiologic monitoring of CPR quality during adult cardiac arrest: a propensity-matched cohort study. *Resuscitation.* 2016;106:76-82.

The end-tidal CO_2 value can be an indicator of effective cardiopulmonary resuscitation and correlates with outcome.

A complete reference list can be found online at ExpertConsult.com.

53

Simulation in Pediatric Anesthesia

CHRISTINE L. MAI, DEMIAN SZYLD, AND JEFFREY B. COOPER

THE FIELD OF PEDIATRIC anesthesia has become increasingly subspecialized, with unique challenges that demand high-quality teaching and training. Pediatric anesthesia is focused in detail, diverse in surgical and technical complexity, and tolerates an exceedingly small margin for error.[1] With the advancement of technology in radiology, the rise of procedural sedation and pediatric intensive care unit (ICU) requirements for bedside surgery, there is an increased challenge to provide safe, quality care in remote sites outside the traditional operating theater (see also Chapters 46 and 48). In many countries, tertiary pediatric services are becoming increasingly centralized and working hours of the individual medical professional have been reduced to address concerns of fatigue and burnout. An unintended consequence is a decline in exposure to difficult pediatric scenarios and emergencies for those who are not specialty trained in pediatrics.

There is an inverse correlation between the level of specialization and perioperative morbidity and mortality associated with pediatric anesthesia.[2] With the growth and increased sophistication of pediatric anesthesia, as well as the regionalization of specialty care, anesthesiologists are continually challenged to gain and maintain expertise in the safe and effective delivery of routine and emergency pediatric anesthesia. Early portions of a trainee's learning curve are inconsistent with the demands of safe and efficient patient care, thereby posing challenges for the medical education infrastructure.[3] Simulation education has provided an experiential learning paradigm for training and assessment for the past few decades, offering one solution to many of these challenges.[4–7] These advances provide opportunities to improve medical knowledge, communication, and decision-making skills for common as well as rare events.[8]

Traditionally, medical school education emphasized basic science knowledge and left most of the clinical practice to an apprenticeship model.[9] The focus of medical training had been on individuals gaining knowledge and skills rather than on clinical performance and team dynamics. Unfortunately, once a clinician had completed training, the required level of continued education declined in structure and formality. Within the past decade, there has been rapid progress and growth of simulation in health care training for purposes of improving patient safety and quality of care. Interest in simulation in health care derived from the historical utility of simulation for training purposes in nonmedical industries, such as commercial aviation, nuclear power production, and the military.[10] Similar to health care, these industries are known to be associated with hazards and complexities that benefit from simulation training. Many of the concepts in health care simulation education, including systematic training, rehearsals, performance assessment, situational awareness, and team interactions, have been adopted from the aviation industry and their work with flight simulators. Given that crises in pediatric anesthesia are relatively rare and unpredictable and that anesthesiologists, trainees, and experienced practitioners alike, are expected to be able to successfully manage these situations, simulation technology can fill these important knowledge gaps.[11] In this chapter, we review how simulation is applied in pediatric anesthesiology by describing its uses for learning and practicing basic and advanced skills and by defining key types of technologies and teaching approaches with illustrative videos.

Simulation-Based Training in Anesthesia

In a 1987 review of anesthesia training, gaps were identified in decision making and crisis management and diagnostic decisions were found to be relatively static.[12–14] Today, in the complex, rapidly changing, time-pressured environment of the operating room (OR), anesthesiologists are challenged beyond static decision making, especially when identifying and resolving crises and leading interdisciplinary teams. To reconcile this schism, the *anesthesia crisis resource management* (ACRM) program was developed based on the commercial aviation model: Crew Resource Management.[13,14] These investigators established a framework and curriculum to teach individual and team leadership skills, along with effective communication styles. ACRM provided anesthesia trainees with tools similar to those that made the complex dynamic world of aviation safer through decision making and crisis resource management. The development of anesthesia simulators and OR-simulated settings was critical in the implementation and growth of ACRM as trainees and practitioners needed a safe venue to experience cases that challenged them in diagnostic problem solving, fixation errors, and poor teamwork in order to train and gain ACRM skills.

ACRM was an outgrowth of the patient safety movement that began in anesthesia in the early 1980s in America. In the late 1980s, research funding from the Anesthesia Patient Safety Foundation (APSF) supported the early development of several forms of human patient simulators (HPSs). Further publicity and advocacy from APSF propelled anesthesiology to the forefront of specialties in the application and adoption of simulators, with strong patient safety implications through education (residents attempting new skills for the first time on a mannequin), training (teamwork, critical event management, and situational awareness), and research (human performance).[15] Today, simulation in anesthesiology is global, with emphasis not only on medical knowledge and skills training, but also on ACRM, disaster training, debriefing, and patient safety. To maintain status as board-certified anesthesiologists, the American Board of Anesthesiology (ABA) requires candidates to complete the Maintenance of Certification in Anesthesiology (MOCA) program. One of the approved ways to achieve MOCA credit is to complete a simulation-based course at a simulation center endorsed by the American Society of Anesthesiologists.[5] In some institutions, such training is required as a condition of credentialing for practice and insurance coverage.

What Is Simulation?

Simulation is a *technique* to replace or amplify real experiences with guided experiences that evoke or replicate aspects of the real world. Simulation is enabled by a diverse set of emerging *technologies*.[10] The application of simulation in the health care field is focused on education and training of clinicians. *Education* emphasizes knowledge, skills, and introduction to the actual work. *Training* emphasizes the actual tasks and work to be performed.[10] The term "simulator" is used in the health care field to refer to a device that represents a simulated patient and interacts appropriately in response to the actions of the simulation participant. In aviation, pilots are seated in the cockpit of a flight simulator, whereas in health care, clinicians are in a simulated OR, emergency ward, or patient floor in simulated clinical scenarios, caring for a simulated "patient" experiencing a critical or otherwise challenging event.

Participants in a simulation are "immersed" into a task or setting to the extent necessary to achieve the learning objectives. This may be conducted in a normal classroom or in an environment that extensively replicates the real world. In the latter case, participants and faculty enter into a "fiction contract" such that the instructor prepares an engaging simulation scenario and the participant attempts to care for the "patient" as if he or she were a real person.[15] Most importantly, it is incumbent on those who create and implement the simulation to create sufficient *realism* to enable the learner to feel the reality of the situation and respond accordingly.[16,17]

Participants in a simulation scenario experience *realism* in three distinct domains: *physical, conceptual, and emotional*.[16] Simulations that address all three domains are more likely to instill the intended learning objectives. A high degree of realism appropriate for the specific learning objectives is central to ensure that the learners become mentally and physically engaged. The *physical* properties of the simulator (the patient), such as weight, flexibility, tensile strength, and color, are important for developing kinesthetic awareness and muscle memory. For example, the weight of the

head and force required to effectively perform laryngoscopy are important for teaching tracheal intubation, whereas the rubbery feel of the mannequin skin is not. *Conceptual realism* refers to the causal relationships observed in the scenario, such as a decrease in oxygen saturation during a period of apnea or the resolution of hypotension after an appropriate IV fluid bolus. High conceptual reality enhances clinical reasoning and decision making. Finally, *emotional* and *experiential* fidelity is achieved when participants experience familiar and authentic feelings, such as "emotional activation," anxiety, stress, fear, or excitement. Ultimately, realism in simulation is perceived as "an exciting simulation that captures the imagination, triggering physiologic responses and execution of ingrained clinical algorithms."[16] Although realism is important, it has been said that "when learning is the focus, the flawless recreation of the real world is less important."[17] It is necessary to find circumstances that help participants learn, rather than circumstances that exactly mimic a clinical situation.[17] The degree of realism desired for a successful simulation education program is an amount sufficient to achieve the intended learning outcomes.

Technologies Used in Simulation

PARTIAL TASK TRAINERS

Partial task trainers are mannequins or models (e.g., suturing board, intravenous [IV] arm, airway head) designed to allow participants to practice clinical skills and tasks (Fig. 53.1). They should be reliable, robust, and medically meaningful. Usually they represent a portion of a person rather than the whole. Although many are simple devices designed for learning or practicing a specific procedure (e.g., suturing, IV insertion, arterial line placement, laryngoscopy, cricothyrotomy, or intraosseous access), some are coupled with computers, robotic interphases, and digital graphics to provide sophisticated partial task simulators designed for learning or practicing more involved procedures (e.g., bronchoscopy and endoscopy, endovascular catheterization, or laparoscopic skills). These models are particularly useful for teaching invasive, risky, and rare procedures (e.g., emergency cricothyrotomy, transvenous pacing, or pericardiocentesis), complex psychomotor skills requiring repetitive training (e.g., ultrasound-guided central venous catheterization or awake fiberoptic intubation), or those that are safe but create increased anxiety for either the learner or the patient and his or her family (e.g., neonatal intubation,[18] urethral catheterization, IV insertion, or arterial puncture). The use of partial task trainers in a simulation environment is conducive for coaching and deliberate practice.[19] Curricula that use these types of devices focus on skills training at varying levels of skill-oriented goals, rather than a particular situation. For example, cricothyrotomy training on a partial task simulator aims to teach the procedure, regardless of the indication (e.g., angioedema, burns, obstructing mass, or hemorrhage). Specific partial task trainers used for simulating aspects of pediatric interventions include products to learn or practice lumbar puncture, peripheral IV insertion, intraosseous needle insertion, laryngoscopy and intubation, umbilical vein and artery catheterization, and cardiopulmonary resuscitation (see Video 53.1). In the context of skills training, there is strong evidence that simulation-based mastery learning can improve patient outcomes.[6] Although there are partial task trainers commercially available for many invasive procedures, simulation education faculty and operations specialists frequently design and produce "low-cost" models to teach practice procedures—for example, managing obstetric and neonatal emergencies in Mexico[20] and postpartum hemorrhage in rural Africa.[21]

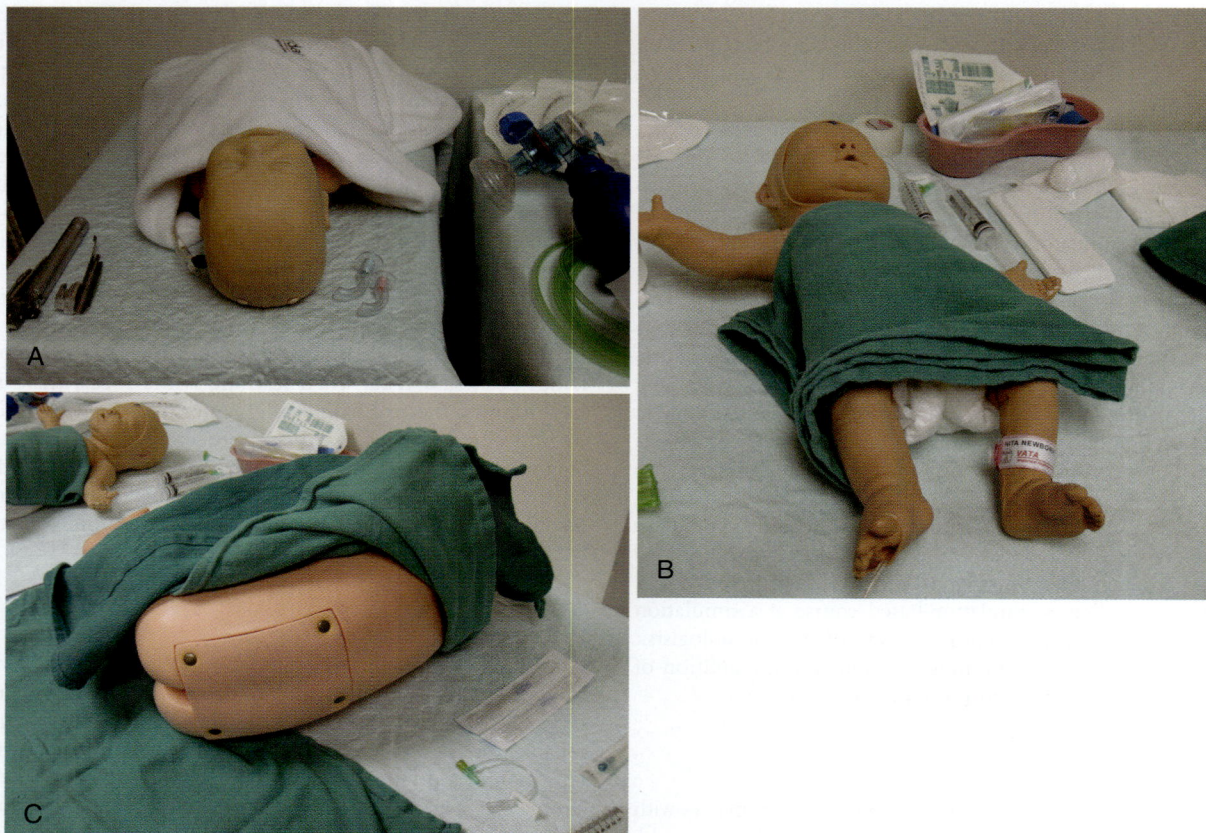

FIGURE 53.1 Examples of partial task trainers to practice **(A)** intubation in neonates (Laerdal SimNewB, Laerdal Medical, Stavanger, Norway); **(B)** peripheral intravenous placement (Nita Newborn Model #1800 Infant Venous Access Simulator, VATA, Canby, OR); and **(C)** central neuraxial techniques (M43C Pediatric Lumbar Puncture Simulator, Kyoto Kagaku, Kyoto, Japan).

HUMAN PATIENT SIMULATORS

An HPS is a representation of the human body constructed on a mannequin, typically made of plastic and metal, without a bony skeletal frame. Although popularized in the 1990s, the first mannequin-based simulator (SimOne) was developed at University of Southern California in the 1960s and was intended to facilitate medical education and training.[22] Adult HPSs became commercially available in the early 1990s; the first high-fidelity pediatric simulator was introduced in 1999. The METI PediaSIM (CAE Healthcare, Sarasota, FL) represented a child between 5 and 7 years of age. Two models of integrated infant HPSs became available in 2005: the METI BabySIM and the Laerdal SimBaby (Laerdal Medical, Stavanger, Norway) (Fig. 53.2). Both models exhibited standard vital signs and variable airway features (e.g., tongue swelling and laryngospasm), breathing patterns and sounds (e.g., retractions to illustrate upper airway obstruction, breath sounds [wheezing], and pneumothorax), cardiovascular features (e.g., heart sounds and peripheral pulses [diminished or absent]), and others (e.g., abdominal sounds and distention, and fontanel bulging). Both infant simulators produce a variety of monitor signals and allow extensive treatment interventions (e.g., intubation, laryngeal mask and nasogastric tube insertion, chest compressions, IV and

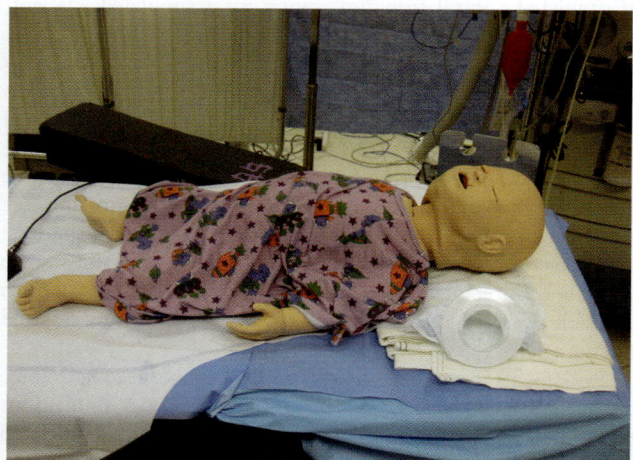

FIGURE 53.2 An infant human patient simulator (Laerdal SimBaby, Laerdal Medical, Stavanger, Norway) exhibits standard vital signs, variable airway features (tongue swelling, laryngospasm), breath sounds (retraction, wheezing), cardiovascular features (palpable pulses, heart sounds), and others (abdominal sounds, bulging fontanel).

intraosseous cannulation, and thoracocentesis) (see Video 53.1).[23] Incorporated into the clinical setting or in a simulation room outfitted with biomedical equipment and teams of health care providers, the HPSs can provide a high degree of clinical authenticity and realism to facilitate participants to fully engage in the care of the simulated patient. Typically, participants in simulation scenarios reflect on their performance during the simulation, for the purpose of sustaining and improving their practice with an instructor, in the process termed *debriefing*[24] (see Video 53.2).

STANDARDIZED PATIENTS

Standardized patients are actors who are trained to represent a patient's condition (e.g., symptoms or social situation) and may also be trained to provide informative feedback. It is common practice to use standardized patients when a simulation session focuses on interviewing, counseling, physical examination of a patient, or a situation that requires high emotional experiences such as giving bad news or de-escalating an upset family member. In pediatrics, actors are more likely to play the role of a parent (e.g., a standardized parent) and team members (e.g., a standardized nurse), although child actors have also been reported, in addition to the use of youthful-appearing actors who role-play adolescents.[25] Going beyond standardized patients, actors can be employed as standardized nurses, surgeons, even residents for the purpose of teaching supervision skills (see Video 53.1). Since 2005, a required portion of the U.S. medical licensing exam (USMLE Step II Clinical Skills) includes a series of standardized patient cases. Exams that use standardized patients and report data based on their ratings are termed objective structured clinical exams (OSCEs). These are common in many undergraduate and graduate medical education programs. OSCEs have also been incorporated into the national board certification exams for anesthesiology in Israel since 2003,[26] in the Royal College of Anaesthetists in the United Kingdom for nearly a decade,[27] and are planned to be introduced into the ABA certification process in the near future.[28]

HYBRID SIMULATION

Hybrid simulation refers to a technique of combining any of the above simulators into a single activity. For instance, in the OR, the simulation scenario may take shape using a combination of three elements: (1) an HPS, to provide the representation of the patient and clinical feedback in the form of the physiologic variables that can be measured and monitored; (2) a partial task simulator deployed to integrate a surgical skill that allows cutting and suturing of tissue; and (3) an actor trained to represent the patient's parent and enact family presence during resuscitation. Hybrids have been used successfully to assess professional, communication, and technical skills.[29]

Hybrid learning (otherwise known as *blended learning*) refers to the combination of web-based instruction incorporated with physical skills practice. As the field of simulation education has matured, it has become clearer that learning with simulation should not be isolated. Integration of simulation into course curricula has given way to hybrid learning techniques. For example, clinicians may complete online pre-course work to strengthen or activate prior knowledge in the days leading up to a simulation session. Subsequently, a simulation session can take place in the simulation-training environment, allowing for integration of new skills and attitudes. This model allows participants to obtain background knowledge to assist them with understanding the planned simulated procedural skills, which can save time and

resources when conducting a training course for a large number of clinicians (e.g., central line maintenance for nursing staff) (see Video 53.1).

SCREEN-BASED SIMULATOR: VIRTUAL PATIENTS AND IMMERSIVE ENVIRONMENTS

Virtual patients are generally two-dimensional avatars on a computer display that serve to help learners maneuver through clinical situations or perform a task, such as the proper technique for taking a patient's medical history. They can also be incorporated into OSCE training when standardized patients are not available. For example, the American Heart Association uses a screen-based simulation to teach and assess knowledge from Advanced Cardiac Life Support (ACLS) and Pediatric Advanced Life Support (PALS) courses.[30]

Immersive environments, such as Second Life (Linden Lab, San Francisco, CA), Advanced Disaster Management Simulator (Environmental Tectonics Corp., Orlando) and multi-user virtual environments, have been used to teach disaster management using interactive virtual simulation systems.[31–33] Other examples include Gas Man (Med Man Simulations, Inc., Boston, MA) for teaching, simulating, and experimenting with the uptake and distribution of inhalational anesthetics,[34] and a virtual reality simulator for training in regional anesthesia.[35] Although virtual reality has been used in ACLS and PALS education,[30] the use of virtual reality simulators in anesthesia is novel and not yet widely incorporated into curricula (see Video 53.1). The American Society of Anesthesiologists recently began a commercial collaboration to develop a screen-based, virtual reality simulator as an adjunct to physical CRM and other skills training.[36]

Sites for Simulation

The number of simulation education centers has increased exponentially from the mid-1990s through the first decade of this century. While there is no exact count, there are at least 1000 centers worldwide incorporated within medical schools and residency training programs in hospital settings,[11] as well as nursing schools and allied health professions colleges.[37] Different settings of simulation education centers include hospital-based or medical school-based simulation centers, freestanding simulation facilities, and in situ simulation located within the actual clinical work environment (Fig. 53.3). Dedicated simulation facilities, either within an existing medical institution or a freestanding center, have been constructed throughout the industrialized world to house high-technology simulator equipment, such as mannequins, laparoscopic surgical equipment, robotics, and audiovisual laboratories. Although simulation education centers are expensive and require significant manpower to operate, they may serve to replace some traditional forms of clinical education for many of the reasons simulation is generally becoming more accepted (e.g., patient safety, clinical production efficiency, and lack of standardized curricula in the apprenticeship model). An in situ simulation location involves setting up the simulator equipment, trainers, and trainees within the actual work environment, such as the OR, emergency room, or ICU. The benefits of an in situ simulation include imitation of the work environment with equipment, personnel, and surroundings that are real and familiar to the trainee. Disadvantages of in situ simulation involve availability of the location, impromptu setup of equipment to operate in different locations, and increased manpower to help with setup and relocation (Table 53.1).

Applications of Simulation in Perioperative Pediatric Education

Perioperative pediatric cardiac arrest is a devastating event. When it occurs, the effects touch the lives of the family and countless health care providers involved. Pediatric cardiac arrest occurs more frequently in neonates than in older children and has a greater mortality.[38,39] The reported incidence of cardiac arrests ranges from 1.4 per 10,000 pediatric anesthetics performed to 3.3 to 4.6 cardiac arrests per 10,000 cases reported by single-institutions.[39–41] In the field of pediatrics, resuscitation skills are taught to pediatric residents using a simulated mock code scenario because perioperative cardiac arrests occur infrequently.[42–45] Furthermore, simulation-based training has been used for anesthesia training to evaluate the ability of anesthesia trainees to manage hyperkalemia after rapid blood transfusion[46] and ventricular fibrillation after hyperkalemia.[47] Newer infant simulators can generate a wide range of pediatric case scenarios and are mobile and wireless for in situ simulation in the OR and ICU. Some examples of simulation-based curricula developed for pediatric critical care medicine include post–congenital heart surgery (using a three-dimensional printed cardiac model),[48] cardiac pulmonary resuscitation skills,[49–52] neonatal resuscitation,[53] as well as specific critical care scenarios including mechanical ventilation of the critically ill patient.[54] Training and managing low-frequency, high-risk cases have been demonstrated in high-fidelity multi-institutional simulation "boot camps" in both pediatric ICU[55] and pediatric anesthesia fellowships.[56] Partial task trainers can be used to teach airway management skills such as difficult airway and neonatal intubation,[18] as well as regional anesthesia techniques.[57–59] High-fidelity simulations have been used in interprofessional health education to improve patient safety, surgical and anesthesia team communication, and patient handovers.[60]

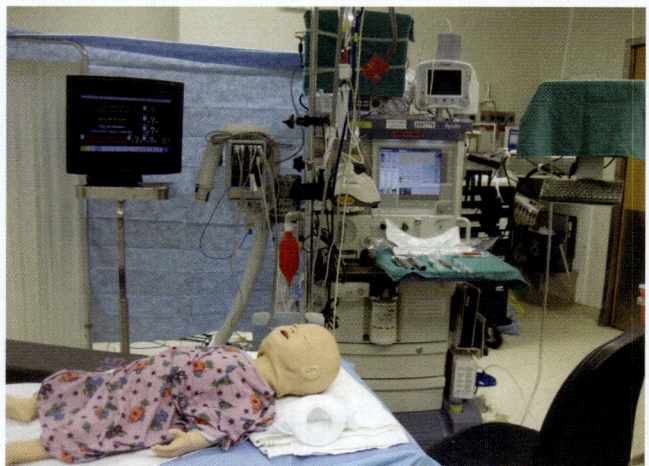

FIGURE 53.3 Simulation in situ setup in an operating room. A human patient simulator (Laerdal SimBaby, Laerdal Medical, Stavanger, Norway) is used in this setting.

TABLE 53.1	Features of Simulation-Based Education by Location			
	Distance	**Features**	**Limitations**	**Operations**
Hospital Simulation Center	*Pro:* Trainees available before, during, and after clinical duties. Other disciplines and professions available. *Con:* Interruptions may occur. Risk of simulation equipment or medication leakage back to clinical environment.	Multimodal education possible (human patient simulators, task trainer, standardized patients, hybrids). Hospital name, numbers, and infrastructure preserved.	Clinical environment may not be accurately represented (outdated equipment, medications not real).	Real estate might be at premium. Equipment and supplies must be ordered separately.
Freestanding Simulation Center	*Pro:* Greatest separation between working and learning environment. Psychological safety and confidentiality are easier to preserve *Con:* Environment and equipment may be significantly different from clinical practice.	Audio and video recording without compromising patient confidentiality. Ability to recreate different clinical environments.	Generic features required to represent multiple-hospital systems may lead to environments that are significantly different from the clinical environment.	Must fund and staff independent organization. May need to pay for transportation. Equipment and supply chain not readily available.
In situ Simulation	*Pro:* Shortest distance to travel. Participants present for work. *Con:* Interruptions are frequent. Family and other practitioners may be disturbed or bothered. Risk of simulation equipment or medication leakage back to clinical environment.	Ability to train in the intended environment enables evaluation of system-level safety features. Findings are readily applicable.	High acuity or census may lead to cancellation of sessions. Emergency equipment may go out of service (MH cart). Equipment may be used for clinical practice during the session (bronchoscope or GlideScope[a]). Difficult to obtain video recording and guarantee patient confidentiality.	Low facility cost (if not charged). Training at work requires no overtime. Disposable material and restocking, including medications, time, and effort to transport equipment to location.

[a]GlideScope (Verathon, Bothell, WA).
MH, malignant hyperthermia.

TABLE 53.2	Five Adult Learning Principles That Apply to the Medical Learner
1.	Adult learners need to know why they are learning.
2.	Adult learners are motivated by the need to solve problems.
3.	The previous experiences of adult learners must be respected and built upon.
4.	The educational approach should match the diversity and background of adult learners.
5.	Adult learners need to be involved actively in the process.

Modified from Okuda Y, Bryson E, DeMaria S Jr, et al. The utility of simulation in medical education: what is the evidence? *Mt Sinai J Med.* 2009;76(4):330–343, and Bryan R, Kreuter M, Brownson R. Integrating adult learning principles into training for public health practice. *Health Promot Pract.* 2009;10(4):557–563.

Comparing Traditional Learning With Simulation-Based Learning

The medical learner at each level of higher education (i.e., undergraduate, graduate, or postgraduate) is an adult learner. An adult learner is one who learns by several methods for different reasons at various stages in his or her education.[61] Adult learning theory teaches that active learning (with simulation) is an effective way to prepare for the dynamic clinical environment.[62] Five adult learning principles that help guide medical learners have been described[61-63] (Table 53.2).

Traditional medical education emphasizes learning and mastering cognitive skills based on textbook readings, lectures, and small group discussions. Evaluation of medical knowledge relies mainly on written or oral examinations. Training models are isolated and sometimes described as being within a "silo," in a static environment where nurses train with nurses, doctors with doctors, pharmacists with pharmacists, and so on. Retention and transfer is weak when passive learning models are employed. According to Kolb's experiential learning theory, simulation-based training allows for active learning, whereby participants are immersed into clinical scenarios and are able to experience how behaviors, interactions, and communication between multi-disciplines affect patient care and, potentially, patient outcomes.[64] The more realistic the case scenario, simulation environment, and actors are, the more those participating are able to become immersed in the task and engaged in the clinical scenario. This engagement with an authentic clinical problem and the need to resolve it as a team serves as the foundation for the debriefing that typically follows a simulation scenario.

Aspects of a High-Fidelity Simulation

High-fidelity simulation requires considerable manpower and preparation. A typical simulation consists of the following: a team leader, actors, high-fidelity mannequin, simulation room, audiovisual equipment, participants and learners, and a debriefer.[65] The team leader may be compared with a director of a film production. He or she is responsible for the smooth execution of the case scenario, from assigning and delegating roles to team members and directing the evolving scenario (usually from a control room), to handling unexpected problems and situations that may arise during the simulation. This position may be the same or different from an "operator," who is responsible for operating the mannequin behind the scenes in the console room. Actors or embedded

simulation participants (ESPs; formerly known as "confederates") are responsible for creating the emotional realism of the case. They may assume roles, such as nurses, physicians, technicians, or administrative staff, to help guide the participants in a way that is clinically familiar. The challenge for actors is to maintain their simulated character and to interact with participants to guide them, but without overt interference with the clinical decisions and management. Communication between actors and the control room personnel using wireless audio devices is helpful in guiding the actors' responses in a manner that maintains conceptual fidelity and smooth flow of the scenario. The clinician caring for the patient or leading a clinical team within a simulated setting is frequently said to be "in the hot seat" because during the scenario the clinician preforms and makes critical decisions that influence the care of the patient. During the debriefing, a debriefer works with the team to aid in transforming a clinical experience into a learning opportunity.

The simulation room is ideally a flexible setting that can be converted into a range of patient care environments, such as the OR, emergency department, obstetric ward, a cafeteria, or other public place—anywhere an anesthesia team might be called to respond. Elaborate scenery, anesthesia, and surgical equipment used in everyday work and moulage (e.g., simulated blood and vomitus) may create very realistic scenarios. The rooms should be equipped with medical air, oxygen, and vacuum suction capabilities to run the high-fidelity mannequins and to provide for their use in the scenario.[65] Audiovisual equipment, such as cameras and microphones, are strategically placed so as to not be obvious to the participants, whose actions are followed in the simulation for debriefing and feedback. The debriefer is responsible for observing the simulation scenario and stimulating learning and discussion in a nonthreatening and organized way at the end of the event. The debriefer identifies elements of the simulation that possess educational value pertinent to the learning objectives of the course and facilitates the discussion of these learning nuggets (e.g., noting where communication broke down or situational awareness was lost) (Video 53.2).

What Is a Debriefing?

A debriefing is a "conversation between two or more people to review a real or simulated event in which participants analyze their actions and interactions, and reflect on the roles of thought processes, psychomotor skills, and emotional states, to improve or sustain performance in the future."[66] Debriefing is considered the most important component of simulation-based education, the time when learning is embedded.[67] As such, it has been exploited through different timing (during or after simulation), conversation facilitation techniques and conversation structure, and different process elements such as scripts, co-debriefers, and the use of video of the simulation session.[68] The debriefing usually follows each simulation, although there is a technique termed "pause-and-discuss," where the instructor interjects during pauses in a scenario.[69] Many simulation centers offer audio and video capture mechanisms, which can be used to review portions of the scenario during a debriefing. Debriefers can show trainees key moments, clarify recall discrepancies, and offer a global view of the room to participants who might have been focused on a task or fixated on a portion of the action. Although many instructors use video during debriefing and students ambivalently appreciate the opportunity to see what they could not appreciate while within the simulation to bridge the gap between experiencing an event and making sense of it, there are limited published data on the specific value of this technique.[70]

There are numerous styles and methods of debriefing in health care simulation. Some of the published debriefing methods are Structured and Supported Debriefing,[71] TeamGAINS,[72] PEARLS,[73] the SAiL Diamond,[74] and Debriefing with Good Judgment.[75]

We describe here the method used at our home institutions: Debriefing with Good Judgment. Like most debriefing methods, we include three phases: *reactions, understanding,* and *summary*.[24,66,76] The *reactions phase* invites participants to share how they felt, allowing the participants to vent and deactivate from the heightened emotional state provoked by participating in a simulation. The debriefer leads the group through a description of the facts of the case to ensure that everyone understands the clinical scenario before tackling the learning objectives. The *understanding phase* is the richest and longest phase, intended to help participants analyze and apply what happened and explore deeper meaning of the interactions. Discussion and teachings are involved in this phase to help simulation participants gain new perspectives and insights into group dynamics and communication. Lessons learned during the simulation can be generalized and applied to the real world, preparing participants to transfer new knowledge into their clinical practice. In the *summary phase*, participants share lessons learned, including individual and group behaviors (both positive and negative), skills, and thinking patterns that they wish to improve, as well as those that were productive and they wish to retain for future performance.[24,66,76]

An effective debriefer requires training and practice to acquire unique skills that are not taught in traditional health care educational programs. Instructors and facilitators are encouraged to learn about the principles of effective debriefing via the literature, formal courses, and mentoring. The Debriefing Assessment for Simulation in Healthcare (DASH) is an example of a testing instrument developed to assess and improve debriefing skills.[77]

Using Simulation for Evaluation

Although patient simulators are well accepted as a core component of CRM and other clinical training, their acceptance and validity as assessment tools for clinical performance have not yet been widely established or validated. In particular, a number of senior professionals are reluctant to be assessed in a simulator environment (e.g., in the process of their recertification). However, some scoring systems for simulator-based performance assessments have been developed, such as the Anaesthetists' Non-Technical Skills (ANTS) system.[23,78] Although validity is not yet rigorous (e.g., based on correlation of training with consistent transfer of skills into clinical use or improvement of patient care), recent studies have shown that simulation-based assessment can be done with sufficient reliability to be used for testing (e.g., reproducible scenarios can be created and implemented, raters can be trained to assign reproducible scores of performance, and critical clinical skills can be simulated).[79] For instance, the Harvard Assessment of Anesthesia Resident Performance Research Group created a validated simulation-based assessment tool to identify critical gaps in safe anesthesia resident performance early in training.[80] Multiscenario, simulation-based assessment has the potential to assess performance of pediatric anesthesia skills in anesthesia residents and pediatric anesthesia fellows; however, further measures of validity, including correlations with direct measures of clinical performance, are needed to establish the true utility and validity of these simulations as assessment tools.[81]

Simulation is widely considered effective in improving clinical skills in a way that is safer than the traditional apprentice model of training. Although there is a dearth of evidence regarding the effectiveness of simulation or the cost relative to its benefit, there is substantial literature that documents its utility. A meta-analysis has established the overall effectiveness of simulation-based training.[4] Furthermore, simulation-based training showed improved outcomes, specifically in survival of children after cardiopulmonary resuscitation.[82]

Challenges Using Simulation

Although simulation centers are increasingly popular worldwide, there are many challenges for establishing and maintaining a simulation program. Trained educators in simulation are few and apprenticeship models require extensive time and effort. Furthermore, availability of faculty members to develop curricula and routinely run simulation case scenarios has been a challenge owing to operational costs and the high demands of clinical practice and patient care.[83] In some institutions where a freestanding simulation center is not feasible, establishing in situ simulations using existing hospital facilities, remodeling old facilities into a simulation room, or having mobile units that contain simulation equipment have been successfully implemented. In the United Kingdom and Canada, the Managing Emergencies in Paediatric Anaesthesia (MEPA) course was developed whereby international centers can share over 60 case scenarios through simulation and telemedicine to train residents.[84] In countries where lack of funding, poor infrastructure, and limited manpower may impede structuring local simulation centers, this "telesimulation" model promotes sharing of knowledge and opportunities for simulation education worldwide[84] (for more details, visit https://mepa.org.uk/about-mepa/mepa-t/).

Future of Simulation

Simulation-based education provides many opportunities for curriculum development in anesthesia residency training, with creative strategies to enhance clinical experiences to practice caring for rare cases and to improve mass-casualty training. Although the apprenticeship model and patient care experience are unlikely to be replaced, incorporation of simulation-based training can help provide solutions to systems-based problems, improve interdisciplinary team training, ease relocation into facilities, and help adapt to new equipment and technology. Since 2004, the Society for Simulation in Healthcare has represented a growing community of educators and researchers who use simulation techniques for education, testing, and research for health care. This consistently growing international society (>3000 members in 2016) is a broad-based, multidisciplinary, multispecialty network that ties together physicians, nurses, and allied health professionals with educators and other social scientists, as well as with industry.[15] Societies such as the Society for Simulation in Healthcare in America and the Society in Europe for Simulation Applied to Medicine, provide technical and political leadership for the simulation community. There are numerous local and profession-specific simulation organizations. The International Pediatric Simulation Society has been meeting for more than eight years (http://ipssglobal.org/).

The long-term impact of simulation on health care still remains to be determined. What is certain is that a large part of anesthesiology and other specialty residency training and maintenance of skills will incorporate simulation-based techniques for education, training, testing, and research. In Israel and the United Kingdom, simulation-based stations are included in the National Anesthesia Board exams and OSCEs in anesthesia, respectively.[26,27] The American Board of Anesthesiology is currently planning to introduce OSCEs into its licensing exam by 2018.[28] Future research must nonetheless focus on addressing questions of how best to use simulation to improve real-life quality of care, patient safety, and long-term outcomes of health care.

ANNOTATED REFERENCES

Andreatta P, Saxton E, Thompson M, Annich G. Simulation-based mock codes significantly correlate with improved pediatric patient cardiopulmonary arrest survival rates. *Pediatr Crit Care Med.* 2011;12(1):33-38.

This is a longitudinal, mixed-method research design to evaluate the viability and effectiveness of a simulation-based mock code program on patient outcomes as well as residents' confidence in performing resuscitations. The study suggests that a simulation-based mock code program may significantly benefit pediatric patient outcome as well as improve learner perceived value and increase learner confidence.

Blum RH, Boulet JR, Cooper JB, et al. Simulation-based assessment to identify critical gaps in safe anesthesia resident performance. *Anesthesiology.* 2014;120(1):129-141.

Valid methods are needed to identify anesthesia residents' performance gaps early in training. However, many assessment tools in medicine have not been properly validated. The authors designed and tested a behaviorally anchored scale used in simulation-based assessment, to identify high- and low-performing residents with regard to domains of concern to expert anesthesiology faculty. The study provides initial evidence to support the validity of a simulation-based performance assessment tool.

Fehr JJ, Boulet JR, Waldrop WB, et al. Simulation-based assessment of pediatric anesthesia skills. *Anesthesiology.* 2011;115(6):1308-1315.

The purpose of this study was to develop a set of relevant simulated pediatric perioperative scenarios and to determine their effectiveness in the assessment of anesthesia residents and fellows. The study showed that the simulation content was relevant and raters could reliably score the scenarios. This study has the potential to contribute to pediatric anesthesia performance assessment, but measures of validity are needed to establish the utility of this approach.

MaGaghie WC, Issenberg SB, Petrusa ER, Scalese RJ. A critical review of simulation-based medical education research: 2003-2009. *Med Educ.* 2010;44(1):50-63.

This review article presents a qualitative synthesis of historical and contemporary research on simulation-based medical education from 2003 to 2009.

Rudolph JW, Simon R, Dufresne RL, Raemer D. There's no such thing as "non-judgmental" debriefing: a theory and method for debriefing with good judgment. *Simul Healthc.* 2009;1:49-55.

The authors describe an approach to debriefing known as "debriefing with good judgment," which emphasizes disclosing instructors' judgment and eliciting trainees' assumptions about the situation and their reasoning for acting as they did. This approach draws on theory and empirical findings from a 35-year research program in the behavioral sciences on how to improve professional effectiveness through "reflective practice."

Weinstock PH, Kappus LJ, Kleinman ME, et al. Toward a new paradigm in hospital-based pediatric education: the development of an onsite simulator program. *Pediatr Crit Care Med.* 2005;6(6):635-641.

This is a descriptive study looking at how an onsite, comprehensive pediatric simulation program in the pediatric intensive care unit can serve as a cost-effective method to enhance the frequency and breadth of critical incident training and education.

A complete reference list can be found online at ExpertConsult.com.

INDEX

Page numbers followed by *f* indicate figures; *t*, tables; *b*, boxes

AAGBI Safety Guideline

Management of Severe Local Anaesthetic Toxicity

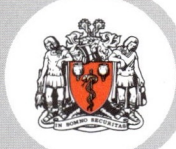

1 **Recognition**	**Signs of severe toxicity:** • Sudden alteration in mental status, severe agitation or loss of consciousness, with or without tonic-clonic convulsions • Cardiovascular collapse: sinus bradycardia, conduction blocks, asystole and ventricular tachyarrhythmias may all occur • Local anaesthetic (LA) toxicity may occur some time after an initial injection
2 **Immediate management**	• Stop injecting the LA • Call for help • Maintain the airway and, if necessary, secure it with a tracheal tube • Give 100% oxygen and ensure adequate lung ventilation (hyperventilation may help by increasing plasma pH in the presence of metabolic acidosis) • Confirm or establish intravenous access • Control seizures: give a benzodiazepine, thiopental or propofol in small incremental doses • Assess cardiovascular status throughout • Consider drawing blood for analysis, but do not delay definitive treatment to do this

3 **Treatment**	**IN CIRCULATORY ARREST** • Start cardiopulmonary resuscitation (CPR) using standard protocols • Manage arrhythmias using the same protocols, recognising that arrhythmias may be very refractory to treatment • Consider the use of cardiopulmonary bypass if available **GIVE INTRAVENOUS LIPID EMULSION** (following the regimen overleaf) • Continue CPR throughout treatment with lipid emulsion • Recovery from LA-induced cardiac arrest may take >1 h • Propofol is not a suitable substitute for lipid emulsion • Lidocaine should not be used as an anti-arrhythmic therapy	**WITHOUT CIRCULATORY ARREST** Use conventional therapies to treat: • hypotension, • bradycardia, • tachyarrhythmia **CONSIDER INTRAVENOUS LIPID EMULSION** (following the regimen overleaf) • Propofol is not a suitable substitute for lipid emulsion • Lidocaine should not be used as an anti-arrhythmic therapy

4
Follow-up
	• Arrange safe transfer to a clinical area with appropriate equipment and suitable staff until sustained recovery is achieved
	• Exclude pancreatitis by regular clinical review, including daily amylase or lipase assays for two days
	• Report cases as follows:
	    in the United Kingdom to the National Patient Safety Agency
	    (via **www.npsa.nhs.uk**)
	    in the Republic of Ireland to the Irish Medicines Board (via **www.imb.ie**)
	If Lipid has been given, please also report its use to the international registry at **www.lipidregistry.org**. Details may also be posted at **www.lipidrescue.org**

Your nearest bag of Lipid Emulsion is kept ....

This guideline is not a standard of medical care. The ultimate judgement with regard to a particular clinical procedure or treatment plan must be made by the clinician in the light of the clinical data presented and the diagnostic and treatment options available.

© The Association of Anaesthetists of Great Britain & Ireland 2010

IMMEDIATELY

Give an initial intravenous bolus injection of 20% lipid emulsion **1.5 ml.kg⁻¹** over 1 min

AND

Start an intravenous infusion of 20% lipid emulsion at **15 ml.kg⁻¹.h⁻¹**

AFTER 5 MIN

Give **a maximum of two** repeat boluses (same dose) if:

- cardiovascular stability has not been restored **or**
- an adequate circulation deteriorates

Leave **5 min** between boluses

A maximum of **three** boluses can be given (including the initial bolus)

AND

Continue infusion at same rate, but:

Double the rate to **30 ml.kg⁻¹.h⁻¹** at any time after 5 min, if:

- cardiovascular stability has not been restored or
- an adequate circulation deteriorates

Continue infusion until stable and adequate circulation restored or maximum dose of lipid emulsion given

Do not exceed a maximum cumulative dose of 12 ml.kg⁻¹

An approximate dose regimen for a 70-kg patient would be as follows:

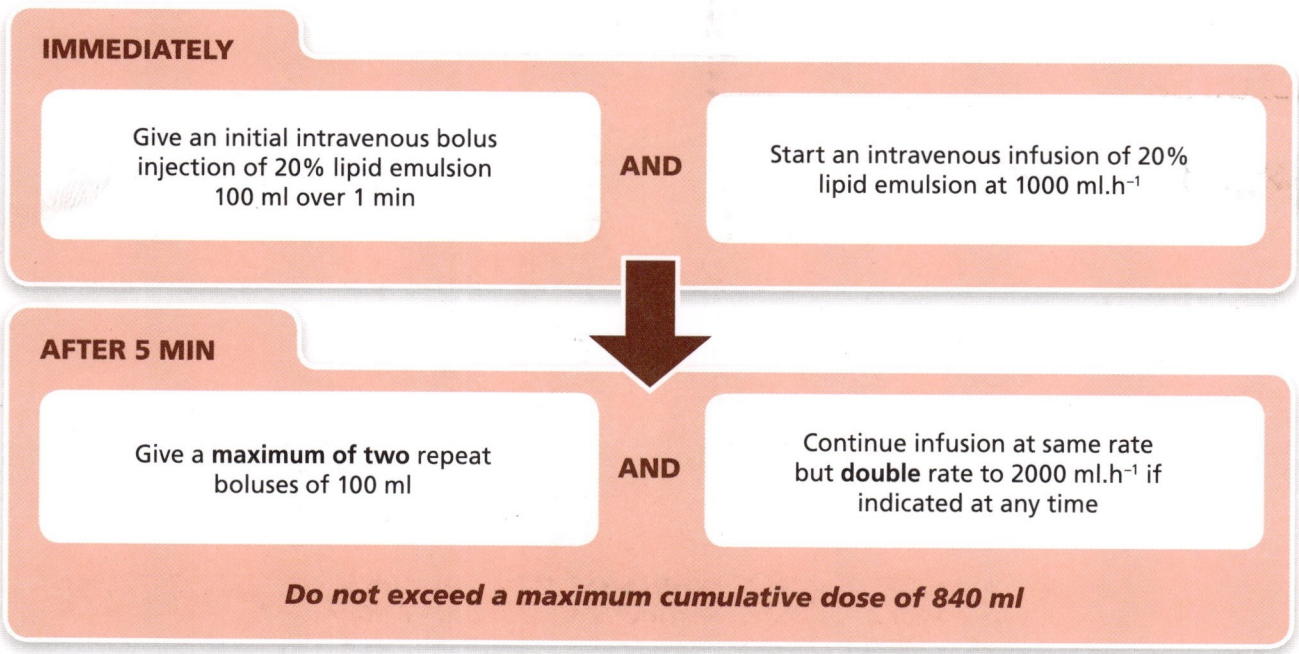

IMMEDIATELY

Give an initial intravenous bolus injection of 20% lipid emulsion 100 ml over 1 min

AND

Start an intravenous infusion of 20% lipid emulsion at 1000 ml.h⁻¹

AFTER 5 MIN

Give a **maximum of two** repeat boluses of 100 ml

AND

Continue infusion at same rate but **double** rate to 2000 ml.h⁻¹ if indicated at any time

Do not exceed a maximum cumulative dose of 840 ml

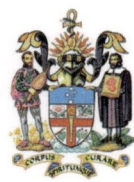

This AAGBI Safety Guideline was produced by a Working Party that comprised:
Grant Cave, Will Harrop-Griffiths (Chair), Martyn Harvey, Tim Meek, John Picard, Tim Short and Guy Weinberg.

This Safety Guideline is endorsed by the Australian and New Zealand College of Anaesthetists (ANZCA).